LEXI-C

Drug Information Handbook *for* Advanced Practice Nursing

Ideal for:

Nurse Practitioners
Nurse Midwives
Clinical Nurse Specialists

4th Edition

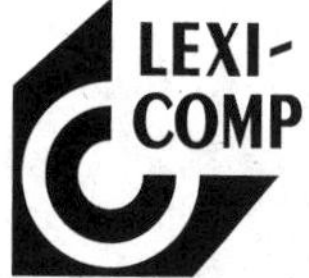

Drug Information Handbook *for* Advanced Practice Nursing

Ideal for

Nurse Practitioners
Nurse Midwives
Clinical Nurse Specialists

4th Edition

Beatrice B. Turkoski, RN, PhD
Assistant Professor
School of Nursing
Kent State University
Kent, Ohio

Brenda R. Lance, RN, MSN
Nurse Coordinator
Ritzman Infusion Services
Akron, Ohio

Mark F. Bonfiglio, BS, PharmD, RPh
Director of Pharmacotherapy Resources
Lexi-Comp, Inc
Hudson, Ohio

Foreword by:
Margaret A. Fitzgerald, MS, RN, CS-FNP

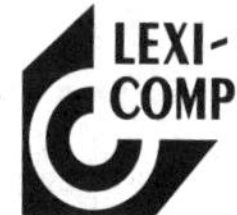

Drug information is constantly evolving because of ongoing research and clinical experience and is often subject to interpretation. While great care has been taken to ensure the accuracy of the information presented, the reader is advised that the authors, editors, reviewers, contributors, and publishers cannot be responsible for the continued currency of the information or for any errors, omissions, or the application of this information, or for any consequences arising therefrom. Therefore, the author(s) and/or the publisher shall have no liability to any person or entity with regard to claims, loss, or damage caused, or alleged to be caused, directly or indirectly, by the use of information contained herein. Because of the dynamic nature of drug information, readers are advised that decisions regarding drug therapy must be based on the independent judgment of the clinician, changing information about a drug (eg, as reflected in the literature and manufacturer's most current product information), and changing medical practices. The authors are not responsible for any inaccuracy of quotation or for any false or misleading implication that may arise due to the text or formulas as used or due to the quotation of revisions no longer official. Further, the *Drug Information Handbook for Advanced Practice Nursing* is not offered as a guide to dosing. The reader, herewith, is advised that information shown under the heading **Dosing** is provided only as an indication of the amount of the drug typically given or taken during therapy. Actual dosing amount for any specific drug should be based on an in-depth evaluation of the individual patient's therapy requirement and strong consideration given to such issues as contraindications, warnings, precautions, adverse reactions, along with the interaction of other drugs. The manufacturers most current product information or other standard recognized references should always be consulted for such detailed information prior to drug use.

The authors and contributors have written this book in their private capacities. No official support or endorsement by any federal agency or pharmaceutical company is intended or inferred.

If you have any suggestions or questions regarding any information presented in this handbook, please contact our drug information pharmacist at 330-650-6506.

This manual was produced using the FormuLex™ Program —
a complete publishing service of Lexi-Comp Inc.

ISBN 1-59195-029-5

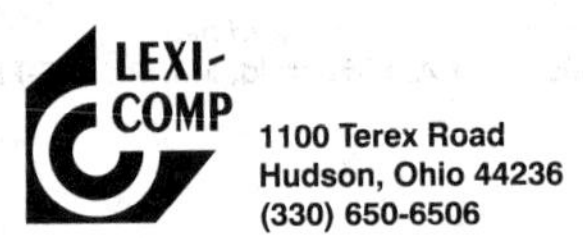

1100 Terex Road
Hudson, Ohio 44236
(330) 650-6506

TABLE OF CONTENTS

FOREWORD

Nationwide, there are now more than 150,000 advanced practice nurses (APNs). As our ranks grow, so do our practice responsibilities. We write thousands of prescriptions daily as we provide care, often to the most vulnerable members of society. As with all busy clinicians, an APN needs references to help guide care, especially in the fast-changing field of pharmacotherapeutics. During the course of APN practice, prescribing questions need to be answered quickly and precisely. When the question is about drug therapy, often the answer is hard to find.

- *Where can you find information on both FDA-approved and unlabeled uses of a drug?*
- *When prescribing a certain agent, are there food, herbal, ethanol, or drug interactions?*
- *How should the drug be started?*
- *How should the dose be adjusted?*
- *How long until a therapeutic dose is reached and therapeutic effect realized?*
- *What is the critical information the prescriber needs to convey to the patient and family in order to ensure safety and facilitate an optimum outcome?*

The *Drug Information Handbook for Advanced Practice Nursing* provides this valuable information and much more, in a clear, concise format. Seldom has so much rich information been found in a single source. A section on pharmacokinetics, pharmacodynamics, and therapeutics sets the stage in this helpful handbook. Each drug monograph features a clear guide to safe prescribing, highlighting important issues, such as information on prescribing for children, adults, the elderly, and during pregnancy/lactation. Details on cytochrome P450 and laboratory value effect, as well as information on monitoring for adverse reactions and required ongoing monitoring, round out each listing. Features of this 4th edition include revised and improved patient education and physical assessment fields critical to each medication, the addition of new products, and updated information on previously approved medications. New to this edition is the highlighting of all generic drug names and cross-references, a helpful feature in an information-intensive text.

The appendix is one of the most valuable portions of this book, providing critical information to informed APN practice. It contains concise summaries of important documents, such as the OBRA Guidelines for use of psychotropic medications in long-term care, in addition to nationally recognized standards of care for common diseases including asthma, diabetes, obesity, community-acquired pneumonia, sexually-transmitted diseases, and hyperlipidemia. Given the current focus on evidenced-based healthcare, a ready-reference for this type of information is critically important.

The publication of the *Drug Information Handbook for Advanced Practice Nursing* comes at an exciting and challenging time. The increasing complexity of clinical care and development of new therapies contribute to the challenges of prescriptive practice. The need for quality references to enhance APN practice continues. In this regard, the *Drug Information Handbook for Advanced Practice Nursing* is a valuable asset.

Margaret A. Fitzgerald, MS, RN, CS-FNP

Ms Fitzgerald is the President and Principal Lecturer with Fitzgerald Health Education Associates, a national provider of NP Board Certification Review and ongoing continuing education for NPs. In addition, she is a family nurse practitioner at the Greater Lawrence Family Health Center in Lawrence, Massachusetts, where her clinical practice focuses on the primary care of multigenerational Latino families and adults with chronic physical and mental health problems. She is also a visiting professor at both Husson College in Bangor, Maine, and Simmons College in Boston, Massachusetts.

PREFACE

The ever-expanding roles of Advanced Practice Nurses require them to be informed and knowledgeable about safe and therapeutic pharmacotherapy. Yet, at the same time, there is an expanding number and complexity of pharmacotherapeutic agents used in both outpatient and institutional settings. In addition, there is an increased availability of over-the-counter (OTC) agents and nonregulated biological and herbal products used by the public, whose information about use and safety may or may not be accurate. The information about current drug therapy is voluminous and the quality of that information varies greatly. Compiling reliable information into a logical guide for therapy when facing the complexities of diverse disease states and the demands of today's changing healthcare environment is difficult. The authors of this book have extensively reviewed the available literature and have developed the *Drug Information Handbook for Advanced Practice Nursing* with the intent to provide pertinent information related to pharmacotherapeutic agents.

In addition to the helpful descriptions of the organization and use of the *Drug Information Handbook for Advanced Practice Nursing*, the introductory section reviews basic pharmacokinetic and pharmacodynamic principles necessary for understanding drug therapy and provides guidelines and approved abbreviations/symbols for safe prescription writing.

The individual drug monographs present information in a concise and consistent manner with cross-referencing to an extensive appendix of helpful information. Each monograph contains pertinent pharmacokinetics, therapeutic purpose, dosing guidelines, and possible adverse effects. Fields highlighted in red contain special issues which may be of particular concern. New to this edition is the introduction of the FDA-proposed "tall-man letters" in generic names to help distinguish those drugs with look-alike names.

The extensive appendix includes sections on antidotes and overdose/toxicology, immunization recommendations and vaccines, ophthalmic and otic agents, over-the-counter medications and common herbal products, maternal and fetal guidelines, OBRA guidelines for long-term care, and selected treatment guidelines for various conditions. Standard laboratory values and conversion information is provided along with updated lists of adverse effects/reactions, and comparison charts of drugs in specific classes. In addition to the updated cytochrome P450 information found in the drug interaction field, the related tables in the appendix have been extensively revised and reformatted to more clearly indicate relevant isoenzyme interactions.

The introductory information, format of drug monographs, and the valuable appendix information in the *Drug Information Handbook for Advanced Practice Nursing* has been designed to provide the Advanced Practice Nurse with information to facilitate safe clinical decision-making.

ABOUT THE AUTHORS

Beatrice B. Turkoski, RN, PhD

Dr Turkoski received her BSN from Alverno College in Wisconsin, an MS in Community Health Nursing from the University of Wisconsin-Milwaukee School of Nursing, and a PhD from the University of Wisconsin. Her extensive professional nursing experience includes several years as a clinician in critical care in Wisconsin and Israel, Director of Nursing, clinician, and researcher in gerontology and chronic adult illness in Wisconsin and Ohio, and clinical nurse specialist in family/community practice in Israel.

In her graduate faculty role at Kent State University School of Nursing, Dr Turkoski developed and teaches the Advanced Pharmacology and Applied Therapeutics courses for students in the Nurse Practitioner and Clinical Nurse Specialist programs. Her expertise in this area is highly regarded by both students and faculty. She also conducts continuing education programs and workshops in geriatric pharmacology for healthcare professionals in hospitals, long-term care, and home care.

Dr Turkoski is an active member and officer in several national and international professional organizations. Her impressive list of professional activities includes presentations in the United States, Europe, China, Korea, Canada, and Israel. In recent publications, Dr Turkoski has addressed the subject of biorhythms and medications, behavioral manifestations of adverse drug reactions, and the impact of age on medication response.

Brenda R. Lance, RN, MSN, DARM

Ms Lance received a diploma in nursing from Methodist Hospital School of Nursing in Lubbock, Texas. She also has earned bachelor's and master's degrees in nursing from Kent State University, Kent, Ohio.

Ms Lance's nursing experiences and expertise are numerous and varied. Her nursing career spans over 30 years, having worked in intensive care, emergency room, ambulatory care clinics, home health, and home infusion. She is currently the Manager of Service Integration for Ritzman Infusion Services, Akron, Ohio.

In addition to many years of direct patient care experience, she is also certified in risk management, has extensive experience in Joint Commission on Accreditation of Healthcare Organizations standards and Medicare regulations for home health, and has been a military nurse for the past 30 years. She retired with the rank of Captain (0-6) from the U.S. Naval Reserve Nurse Corps.

Ms Lance is a member of the Sigma Theta Tau (National Honor Society of Nursing), the Intravenous Nurses Society, and National Association of Vascular Access Networks.

Mark F. Bonfiglio, BS, PharmD, RPh

Dr Bonfiglio received his BA in Biology and BS in Pharmacy from the University of Toledo. He earned his Doctor of Pharmacy degree from Ohio State University and subsequently completed a Residency in Critical Care Pharmacy at the Ohio State University Hospitals. For the next 8 years he was a faculty member of the Ohio Northern University College of Pharmacy, reaching the rank of Associate Clinical Professor. During this time, his appointment was shared by the institutions where he maintained his clinical practice. Initially, he served for 6 years at Akron City Hospital as a Critical Care Pharmacy Specialist, followed by 2 years in practice as a Pharmacotherapy Specialist in Internal Medicine at the Akron General Medical Center. He conducted research activities and authored numerous publications in addition to his activities in practice and education.

Currently, Dr Bonfiglio works at Lexi-Comp Inc as the Director of Pharmacotherapy Resources. He is an invited lecturer to many professional organizations in pharmacy, medical, and nursing and is an author of several courseware modules for the Ohio Council of Colleges of Pharmacy nontraditional PharmD initiative. He has also served as a reviewer for *The Annals of Pharmacotherapy* and *Pharmacotherapy.* Professional memberships include the Society of Critical Care Medicine (SCCM), American College of Clinical Pharmacy (ACCP), and American Society of Health System Pharmacists (ASHP).

EDITORIAL ADVISORY PANEL

ACKNOWLEDGMENTS

This handbook exists in its present form as the result of the concerted efforts of the following individuals: Robert D. Kerscher, publisher and president of Lexi-Comp, Inc; Lynn D. Coppinger, managing editor; Barbara F. Kerscher, production manager; Sheila L. Digman, project manager; David C. Marcus, director of information systems; Matthew C. Kerscher, product manager; and Tracey J. Reinecke, graphic designer.

The authors appreciate the staff's contributions to this handbook and are especially grateful to Joni Stahura, PharmD, and Liz Tomsik, PharmD for their participation in the drafting/review of new monographs and updates to the core pharmacology database. In addition, special acknowledgments to Jeff Lewis, PharmD, for his assistance in the area of drug interactions and Leslie Ruggles for her assistance in managing the core pharmacology database.

Much of the material contained in this book was a result of pharmacy contributors throughout the United States and Canada. Lexi-Comp has assisted many medical institutions to develop hospital-specific formulary manuals that contain clinical drug information as well as dosing. Working with clinical pharmacists, hospital pharmacy and therapeutics committees, and hospital drug information centers, Lexi-Comp has developed an evolutionary drug database that reflects the practice of pharmacy in these major institutions.

The authors wish to sincerely thank Penelope L. Cukr, RN, SNSc, ANP, Director, Adult Nurse Practitioner Program, Kent State University, and Scott Fleming, RN, MSN, cFNP, Instructor, Nurse Practitioner Program, Kent State University for their suggestions and review of this handbook.

The authors also thank their families, friends, and colleagues, who supported them in their efforts to complete this handbook.

DESCRIPTION OF SECTIONS & FIELDS

Introduction

The introductory text includes guidelines for the use of the handbook and sections describing Safe Writing, Pharmacokinetics, Pharmacodynamics, Pharmacotherapeutics, Patient Factors That Influence Drug Therapy, and Patient Education for Management of Common Side Effects.

Individual Drug Monographs

Medications are arranged alphabetically by generic name, which is printed in red. Extensive cross-referencing (with easy visibility marked with a diamond ♦), is provided by U.S. brand names and synonyms. Abbreviated monographs contain unique information, commonly for combination formulations, and a cross-reference to the corresponding individual entity monographs.

Monograph Fields

Generic Name (in red)	U.S. adopted name
Pronunciation Guide	Phonetic pronunciation of generic name
U.S. Brand Names	U.S. trade names (manufacturer specific)
Synonyms	Other names or accepted abbreviations of the generic drug
Restrictions	The controlled substance classification from the Drug Enforcement Agency (DEA); U.S. schedules are I-V; schedules vary by country and sometimes state (ie, Massachusetts uses (I-VI)
Generic Available	Drugs available in generic form
Pharmacologic Category	Systematic classification of medications
Pregnancy Risk Factor	Five categories established by the FDA to indicate the potential of a systemically absorbed drug for causing birth defects
Lactation	Information describing characteristics of using the drug listed in the monograph while breast-feeding (where recommendation of American Academy of Pediatrics differs, notation is made); the following distinctions are made: Does not enter breast milk Enters breast milk/compatible Excretion in breast milk unknown Enters breast milk/use caution Enters breast milk/not recommended Enters breast milk/contraindicated Enters breast milk/consult prescriber No data available
Use	Describes information pertaining to appropriate indications of the drug listed in the monograph; includes FDA approved and non-FDA approved indications
Use - Unlabeled/Investigational	Information pertaining to non-FDA approved and investigational indications of the drug
Mechanism of Action/Effect	A brief description of how the drug works
Contraindications	Information pertaining to inappropriate use of the drug, or disease states and patient populations in which the drug should not be used
Warnings/Precautions	Warnings include hazardous conditions related to use of the drug; precautions include disease states or patient populations in which the drug should be used with caution.
Drug Interactions	
Cytochrome P450 Effect	Drugs which are involved in possible interactions due to their activity with the hepatic cytochrome P450 system are identified and their role as inducers, inhibitors, or substrates for a specific isoenzyme is listed (those in **bold** appear to be of clinical significance).

Decreased Effect	Drug combinations that result in a decreased therapeutic effect between the drug listed in the monograph and other drugs or drug classes
Increased Effect/Toxicity	Drug combinations that result in a increased or toxic therapeutic effect between the drug listed in the monograph and other drugs or drug classes
Nutritional/Ethanol Interactions	Information regarding potential interactions with food, nutritional supplements (including herbal products and vitamins), or ethanol
Effects on Lab Values	A list of assay interferences when taking the drug
Adverse Reactions	Drug-induced side effects are grouped by percentage of incidence (>10%; 1%-10%) and body system. Adverse reactions for <1% incidence are listed as a group. **Side effects of <1% incidence are included only if important or life-threatening.**
Overdose/Toxicology	Comment or considerations with signs/symptoms of excess drug ingestion
Pharmacodynamics/Kinetics	
Absorption	The amount of absorbed drug, including rate and route for the drug listed
Bioavailability	Fraction of administered drug dose that enters systemic circulation
Half-Life Elimination	The reported half-life of elimination for the parent or metabolites of the drug
Time to Peak	Describes the relative time after ingestion when concentration achieves the highest serum concentration
Metabolism	Describes the site of metabolism and may include the percentage of active metabolites.
Onset	The time after drug administration when therapeutic effect is observed; may also include time for peak therapeutic effect
Duration	Length of therapeutic effect
Formulations	A description of the product including strength and formulation (ie, tablet, capsule, injection, syrup, etc)
Dosing	
Adults	The recommended amount of drug to be given to adult patients
Adults and Elderly	This combined field is only used to indicate that no specific adjustments for elderly patients were identified. However, other issues should be considered (ie, renal or hepatic impairment). Also refer to Geriatric Issues for additional information related to the elderly.
Elderly	A suggested amount of drug to be given to elderly patients which may include adjustments from adult dosing; lack of information in the monograph may imply that the drug is not used in the elderly patient or no specific adjustments could be identified
Pediatrics	Suggested dosing for infants and children
Renal Impairment	Suggested dosage adjustments based on compromised renal function, including dosing instructions for patients on dialysis
Hepatic Impairment	Suggested dosage adjustments based on compromised liver function

Administration	
Oral I.M. I.V. Inhalation Topical Other	The administration field contains subfields by route regarding issues relative to appropriately giving a medication; includes suggestions on final drug concentrations and/or rates of infusion for parenteral medications and comments regarding the timing of drug administration relative to meals. Also see Compatibility.
Stability	
Storage	Relates to appropriate storage of the medication prior to opening the manufacturers original packaging; information is only given if recommendations are for storage at other than room temperature; includes storage requirements for reconstituted products
Reconstitution	Includes comments on solution choice with time or conditions for the mixture to maintain full potency before administration
Compatibility	Provides information regarding stability of the drug in solution(s) and lists combinations known to be incompatible when admixed or in syringe
Monitoring Laboratory Tests	Suggested laboratory tests to monitor for safety and efficacy of the drug listed in the monographs
Monitoring and Teaching Issues (printed in red)	
Physical Assessment	Monitoring guidelines
Patient Education	Suggested items to discuss with the patient or caregiver when taking the medication; may include issues regarding contraception, self-monitoring, precautions, and administration
Dietary Issues	Includes information on how the medication should be taken relative to meals or food
Geriatric Considerations	Comments or suggestions of drug use in elderly patients; may include monitoring, dose adjustments, precautions, or comments on appropriateness of use
Breast-feeding Issues	Provides further information relating to taking the drug while nursing
Pregnancy Issues	Comments related to safe drug administration during pregnancy are listed if appropriate.
Other Issues	Any additional pertinent information regarding nursing issues is provided.
Additional Information	Includes dose equivalents, sodium or potassium content, strength equivalents (mg = mEq), or specific brand information
Related Information	Cross-reference with page number to other pertinent drug information found elsewhere in this handbook

Controlled Substance Index

A list of drug names and their corresponding controlled substance classification

Pharmacologic Category Index

Lists all drugs by their unique pharmacologic category and includes cross-references to the drug monographs

Appendix

The last section is an extensive appendix of useful information that includes conversion laboratory information, definitions of specific adverse reactions and a list of drugs associated with specific reactions, comparison charts for selected classes of drugs, maternal and fetal guidelines, OBRA recommendations for long-term care, toxicology information, and treatment guidelines for selected therapy.

FDA NAME DIFFERENTIATION PROJECT: THE USE OF TALL-MAN LETTERS

Confusion between similar drug names is an important cause of medication errors. For years, The Institute For Safe Medication Practices (ISMP), has urged generic manufacturers use a combination of large and small letters as well as bolding (ie, chlorpro**MAZINE** and chlorpro**PAMIDE**) to help distinguish drugs with look-alike names, especially when they share similar strengths. Recently the FDA's Division of Generic Drugs began to issue recommendation letters to manufacturers suggesting this novel way to label their products to help reduce this drug name confusion. Although this project has had marginal success, the method has successfully eliminated problems with products such as diphenhydr**AMINE** and dimenhy**DRINATE**. Hospitals should also follow suit by making similar changes in their own labels, preprinted order forms, computer screens and printouts, and drug storage location labels.

Lexi-Comp Medical Publishing, with this edition of the *Drug Information Handbook for Advanced Practice Nursing*, will begin using these "Tall-Man" letters for the drugs suggested by the FDA.

The following is a list of product names and recommended FDA revisions.

Drug Product	Recommended Revision
acetazolamide	aceta**ZOLAMIDE**
acetohexamide	aceto**HEXAMIDE**
bupropion	bu**PROP**ion
buspirone	bus**PIR**one
chlorpromazine	chlorpro**MAZINE**
chlorpropamide	chlorpro**PAMIDE**
clomiphene	clomi**PHENE**
clomipramine	clomi**PRAMINE**
cycloserine	cyclo**SERINE**
cyclosporine	cyclo**SPORINE**
daunorubicin	**DAUNO**rubicin
dimenhydrinate	dimenhy**DRINATE**
diphenhydramine	diphenhydr**AMINE**
dobutamine	**DOBUT**amine
dopamine	**DOP**amine
doxorubicin	**DOXO**rubicin
glipizide	glipi**ZIDE**
glyburide	gly**BURIDE**
hydralazine	hydr**ALAZINE**
hydroxyzine	hydr**OXY**zine
medroxyprogesterone	medroxy**PROGESTER**one
methylprednisolone	methyl**PREDNIS**olone
methyltestosterone	methyl**TESTOSTER**one
nicardipine	ni**CAR**dipine
nifedipine	**NIFE**dipine
prednisolone	predniso**LONE**
prednisone	predni**SONE**
sulfadiazine	sulfa**DIAZINE**
sulfisoxazole	sulfi**SOXAZOLE**
tolazamide	**TOLAZ**amide
tolbutamide	**TOLBUT**amide
vinblastine	vin**BLAS**tine
vincristine	vin**CRIS**tine

Institute for Safe Medication Practices. "New Tall-Man Lettering Will Reduce Mix-Ups Due to Generic Drug Name Confusion," *ISMP Medication Safety Alert*, September 19, 2001. Available at: http://www.ismp.org.

Institute for Safe Medication Practices. "Prescription Mapping, Can Improve Efficiency While Minimizing Errors With Look-Alike Products," *ISMP Medication Safety Alert*, October 6, 1999. Available at: http://www.ismp.org.

U.S. Pharmacopeia, "USP Quality Review: Use Caution-Avoid Confusion," March 2001, No. 76. Available at: http://www.usp.org.

SYMBOLS & ABBREVIATIONS USED IN THIS HANDBOOK*

°C	degrees Celsius (Centigrade)
<	less than
>	greater than
≤	less than or equal to
≥	greater than or equal to
µg	microgram
µmol	micromole
AAPC	antibiotic associated pseudomembranous colitis
ABG	arterial blood gas
ABMT	autologous bone marrow transplant
ACE	angiotensin-converting enzyme
ACLS	advanced cardiac life support
ADH	antidiuretic hormone
AED	antiepileptic drug
AIDS	acquired immunodeficiency syndrome
ALL	acute lymphoblastic leukemia
ALT	alanine aminotransferase (formerly called SGPT)
AML	acute myeloblastic leukemia
ANA	antinuclear antibodies
ANC	absolute neutrophil count
ANLL	acute nonlymphoblastic leukemia
APTT	activated partial thromboplastin time
ASA (class I-IV)	American Society of Anesthesiology physical status classification of surgical patients according to their baseline health ASA I: Normal healthy patients ASA II: Patients having controlled disease states (eg, controlled hypertension) ASA III: Patients having a disease which compromises their organ function (eg, decompensated CHF, end-stage renal failure) ASA IV: Patients who are extremely critically ill
AST	aspartate aminotransferase (formerly called SGOT)
AUC	area under the curve (area under the serum concentration-time curve)
A-V	atrial-ventricular
BMT	bone marrow transplant
BUN	blood urea nitrogen
cAMP	cyclic adenosine monophosphate
CBC	complete blood count
CHF	congestive heart failure
CI	cardiac index
Cl_{cr}	creatinine clearance
CMV	cytomegalovirus
CNS	central nervous system
COPD	chronic obstructive pulmonary disease
CSF	cerebrospinal fluid
CT	computed tomography
CVA	cerebral vascular accident
CVP	central venous pressure
d	day
D_5W	dextrose 5% in water
D_5/1/2NS	dextrose 5% in sodium chloride 0.45%
$D_{10}W$	dextrose 10% in water
DIC	disseminated intravascular coagulation
DL_{co}	pulmonary diffusion capacity for carbon monoxide
DNA	deoxyribonucleic acid
DVT	deep vein thrombosis
ECHO	echocardiogram
ECMO	extracorporeal membrane oxygenation
EEG	electroencephalogram
EKG	electrocardiogram
ESR	erythrocyte sedimentation rate
E.T.	endotracheal
FEV_1	forced expiratory volume exhaled after 1 second
FSH	follicle-stimulating hormone
FVC	forced vital capacity
g	gram
G6PD	glucose-6-phosphate dehydrogenase
GA	gestational age

GABA	gamma-aminobutyric acid
GE	gastroesophageal
GI	gastrointestinal
GU	genitourinary
h	hour
HIV	human immunodeficiency virus
HPLC	high performance liquid chromatography
IBW	ideal body weight
ICP	intracranial pressure
IgG	immune globulin G
I.M.	intramuscular
INR	international normalized ratio
int. units	international units
I.O.	intraosseous
I & O	input and output
IOP	intraocular pressure
I.T.	intrathecal
I.V.	intravenous
IVH	intraventricular hemorrhage
IVP	intravenous push
JRA	juvenile rheumatoid arthritis
kg	kilogram
L	liter
LDH	lactate dehydrogenase
LE	lupus erythematosus
LH	luteinizing hormone
LP	lumbar puncture
LR	lactated Ringer's
MAC	*Mycobacterium avium* complex
MAO	monoamine oxidase
MAP	mean arterial pressure
mcg	microgram
mg	milligram
MI	myocardial infarction
min	minute
mL	milliliter
mo	month
mOsm	milliosmoles
MRI	magnetic resonance image
MRSA	methicillin-resistant *Staphylococcus aureus*
NCI	National Cancer Institute
ND	nasoduodenal
ng	nanogram
NG	nasogastric
NMDA	n-methyl-d-aspartate
nmol	nanomole
NPO	nothing per os (nothing by mouth)
NSAID	nonsteroidal anti-inflammatory drug
O.R.	operating room
OTC	over-the-counter (nonprescription)
PABA	para-aminobenzoic acid
PALS	pediatric advanced life support
PCA	postconceptional age
PCP	*Pneumocystis carinii* pneumonia
PCWP	pulmonary capillary wedge pressure
PDA	patent ductus arteriosus
PIP	peak inspiratory pressure
PNA	postnatal age
PSVT	paroxysmal supraventricular tachycardia
PT	prothrombin time
PTT	partial thromboplastin time
PUD	peptic ulcer disease
PVC	premature ventricular contraction
PVR	peripheral vascular resistance
qsad	add an amount sufficient to equal
RAP	right arterial pressure
RIA	radioimmunoassay

RNA	ribonucleic acid
S-A	sino-atrial
S.C.	subcutaneous
S_{cr}	serum creatinine
SIADH	syndrome of inappropriate antidiuretic hormone
S.L.	sublingual
SLE	systemic lupus erythematosus
SVR	systemic vascular resistance
SVT	supraventricular tachycardia
SWI	sterile water for injection
T_3	triiodothyronine
T_4	thyroxine
TIBC	total iron binding capacity
TPN	total parenteral nutrition
TSH	thyroid stimulating hormone
TT	thrombin time
UTI	urinary tract infection
V_d	volume of distribution
V_{dss}	volume of distribution at steady-state
VMA	vanillylmandelic acid
w/w	weight for weight
y	year

*Other than drug synonyms

FDA PREGNANCY CATEGORIES

Throughout this book there is a field labeled Pregnancy Risk Factor (PRF) and the letter A, B, C, D, or X immediately following which signifies a category. The FDA has established these five categories to indicate the potential of a systemically absorbed drug for causing birth defects. The key differentiation among the categories rests upon the reliability of documentation and the risk:benefit ratio. Pregnancy Category X is particularly notable in that if any data exists that may implicate a drug as a teratogen and the risk:benefit ratio is clearly negative, the drug is contraindicated during pregnancy.

These categories are summarized as follows:

A — Controlled studies in pregnant women fail to demonstrate a risk to the fetus in the first trimester with no evidence of risk in later trimesters. The possibility of fetal harm appears remote.

B — Either animal-reproduction studies have not demonstrated a fetal risk but there are no controlled studies in pregnant women, or animal-reproduction studies have shown an adverse effect (other than a decrease in fertility) that was not confirmed in controlled studies in women in the first trimester and there is no evidence of a risk in later trimesters.

C — Either studies in animals have revealed adverse effects on the fetus (teratogenic or embryocidal effects or other) and there are no controlled studies in women, or studies in women and animals are not available. Drugs should be given only if the potential benefits justify the potential risk to the fetus.

D — There is positive evidence of human fetal risk, but the benefits from use in pregnant women may be acceptable despite the risk (eg, if the drug is needed in a life-threatening situation or for a serious disease for which safer drugs cannot be used or are ineffective).

X — Studies in animals or human beings have demonstrated fetal abnormalities or there is evidence of fetal risk based on human experience, or both, and the risk of the use of the drug in pregnant women clearly outweighs any possible benefit. The drug is contraindicated in women who are or may become pregnant.

SAFE PRESCRIPTION WRITING

Health professionals and their support personnel frequently produce handwritten copies of information they see in print; therefore, such information is subjected to even greater possibilities for error or misinterpretation on the part of others. Thus, particular care must be given to how drug names and strengths are expressed when creating written healthcare documents.

The following are a few examples of safe writing rules suggested by the Institute for Safe Medication Practices, Inc.*

1. There should be a space between a number and its units, as it is easier to read. There should be no periods after the abbreviations "mg" or "mL" ("2 mg" is correct; "2mg" or "2 mg." is **incorrect**).
2. Never place a decimal and a zero after a whole number ("2 mg" is correct; "2.0 mg" is **incorrect**). If the decimal point is not seen because it falls on a line or because individuals are working from copies where the decimal point is not seen, this causes a tenfold overdose.
3. Just the opposite is true for numbers less than one. Always place a zero before a naked decimal ("0.5 mL" is correct, ".5 mL" is **incorrect**).
4. Never abbreviate the word "unit". The handwritten "U" or "u", looks like a "0" (zero), and may cause a tenfold overdose error to be made.
5. "IU" is not a safe abbreviation for "international units". The handwritten "IU" looks like "IV". Write out "international units" or use "int. units".
6. "Q.D." is not a safe abbreviation for "once daily"; when the "Q" is followed by a sloppy dot, it looks like "QID" which means "four times daily".
7. "O.D." is not a safe abbreviation for "once daily", as it is properly interpreted as meaning "right eye" and has caused liquid medications such as saturated solution of potassium iodide and Lugol's solution to be administered incorrectly. There is **no** safe abbreviation for "once daily". It must be written out **in full**.
8. Do not use chemical names such as "6-mercaptopurine" or "6-thioguanine", as sixfold overdoses have been given when these were not recognized as chemical names. The proper names of these drugs are "mercaptopurine" and "thioguanine".
9. Do not abbreviate drug names (5FC, 6MP, 5-ASA, MTX, HCTZ, CPZ, PBZ, etc), as they are misinterpreted and cause error.
10. Do not use the apothecary system or symbols.
11. Do not abbreviate "microgram" as "µg"; use "mcg", as there is less likelihood of misinterpretation.
12. When writing an outpatient prescription, write a complete prescription. A complete prescription can prevent the prescriber, the pharmacist, and/or the patient from making a mistake and can eliminate the need for further clarification. The legible prescriptions should contain:
    a. patient's full name
    b. for pediatric or geriatric patients: their age (or weight where applicable)
    c. drug name, dosage form and strength; if a drug is new or rarely prescribed, print this information
    d. number or amount to be dispensed
    e. complete instructions for the patient, including the purpose of the medication
    f. when there are recognized contraindications for a prescribed drug, indicate to the pharmacist that you are aware of this fact (ie, when prescribing a potassium salt for a patient receiving an ACE inhibitor, write "K serum level being monitored")

*From "Safe Writing" by Davis NM, PharmD and Cohen MR, MS, Lecturers and Consultants for Safe Medication Practices, 1143 Wright Drive, Huntington Valley, PA 19006. Phone: (215) 947-7566.

ABBREVIATIONS, ACRONYMS, AND SYMBOLS COMMONLY USED IN MEDICAL ORDERS

Abbreviation	Meaning
$\overline{aa}$, aa	of each
AA	Alcoholics Anonymous
ac	before meals or food
ad	to, up to
a.d.	right ear
ADHD	attention-deficit/hyperactivity disorder
ADLs	activities of daily living
ad lib	at pleasure
AIMS	Abnormal Involuntary Movement Scale
a.l.	left ear
AM	morning
amp	ampul
amt	amount
aq	water
aq. dest.	distilled water
ARDS	adult respiratory distress syndrome
a.s.	left ear
ASAP	as soon as possible
a.u.	each ear
AUC	area under the curve
BDI	Beck Depression Inventory
bid	twice daily
bm	bowel movement
bp	blood pressure
BPRS	Brief Psychiatric Rating Scale
BSA	body surface area
c	a gallon
$\bar{c}$	with
cal	calorie
cap	capsule
CBT	cognitive behavioral therapy
cc	cubic centimeter
CGI	Clinical Global Impression
cm	centimeter
CIV	continuous I.V. infusion
comp	compound
cont	continue
CRF	chronic renal failure
CT	computed tomography
d	day
d/c	discontinue
dil	dilute
disp	dispense
div	divide
DSM-IV	Diagnostic and Statistical Manual
DTs	delirium tremens
dtd	give of such a dose
ECT	electroconvulsive therapy
EEG	electroencephalogram
elix, el	elixir
emp	as directed
EPS	extrapyramidal side effects
ESRD	end stage renal disease
et	and
ex aq	in water
f, ft	make, let be made
FDA	Food and Drug Administration
g	gram
GA	Gamblers Anonymous
GAD	generalized anxiety disorder
GAF	Global Assessment of Functioning Scale
GABA	gamma-aminobutyric acid
GERD	gastroesophageal reflux disease

Abbreviation	Meaning
GITS	gastrointestinal therapeutic system
gr	grain
gtt	a drop
GVHD	graft versus host disease
h	hour
HAM-A	Hamilton Anxiety Scale
HAM-D	Hamilton Depression Scale
hs	at bedtime
HSV	herpes simplex virus
I.M.	intramuscular
IU	international unit
I.V.	intravenous
kcal	kilocalorie
kg	kilogram
KIU	kallikrein inhibitor unit
L	liter
LAMM	L-α-acetyl methadol
liq	a liquor, solution
M	mix; Molar
MADRS	Montgomery Asbery Depression Rating Scale
MAOIs	monamine oxidase inhibitors
mcg	microgram
MDEA	3,4-methylene-dioxy amphetamine
m. dict	as directed
MDMA	3,4-methylene-dioxy methamphetamine
mEq	milliequivalent
mg	milligram
mixt	a mixture
mL	milliliter
mm	millimeter
mM	millimolar
MMSE	Mini-Mental State Examination
MPPP	l-methyl-4-proprionoxy-4-phenyl pyridine
MR	mental retardation
MRI	magnetic resonance imaging
NF	National Formulary
NMS	neuroleptic malignant syndrome
no.	number
noc	in the night
non rep	do not repeat, no refills
NPO	nothing by mouth
O, Oct	a pint
OCD	obsessive-compulsive disorder
o.d.	right eye
o.l.	left eye
o.s.	left eye
o.u.	each eye
PANSS	Positive and Negative Symptom Scale
pc, post cib	after meals
PCP	phencyclidine
per	through or by
PM	afternoon or evening
P.O.	by mouth
P.R.	rectally
prn	as needed
PTSD	post-traumatic stress disorder
pulv	a powder
q	every
qad	every other day
qd	every day
qh	every hour
qid	four times a day
qod	every other day
qs	a sufficient quantity
qs ad	a sufficient quantity to make
qty	quantity
qv	as much as you wish
REM	rapid eye movement
Rx	take, a recipe

Abbreviation	Meaning
rep	let it be repeated
$\bar{s}$	without
sa	according to art
sat	saturated
S.C.	subcutaneous
sig	label, or let it be printed
sol	solution
solv	dissolve
$\overline{ss}$	one-half
sos	if there is need
SSRIs	selective serotonin reuptake inhibitors
stat	at once, immediately
STD	sexually transmitted disease
supp	suppository
syr	syrup
tab	tablet
tal	such
TCA	tricyclic antidepressant
TD	tardive dyskinesia
tid	three times a day
tr, tinct	tincture
trit	triturate
tsp	teaspoonful
ULN	upper limits of normal
ung	ointment
USAN	United States Adopted Names
USP	United States Pharmacopeia
u.d., ut dict	as directed
v.o.	verbal order
VZV	varicella zoster virus
w.a.	while awake
x3	3 times
x4	4 times
YBOC	Yale Brown Obsessive-Compulsive Scale
YMRS	Young Mania Rating Scale

BASIC PHARMACOLOGICAL CONCEPTS

There are more pharmacotherapeutic agents (medications/drugs) available today than ever before in history. Many drugs that were formerly legend drugs (available only by prescription) are available over-the-counter (OTC). In addition, the number and variety of drugs available by prescription grows increasingly more complex. Many people use these agents, both over-the-counter and prescription drugs, rather liberally. And, as the population ages, the number of people taking multiple drugs for chronic health problems increases.

Practitioners must be aware that such "routine" use of drugs – the possible interactions or toxic effects – is a major health concern for patients. Understanding both the physiological and psychological changes produced by drugs is a major responsibility of all professional nurses (those advanced practice nurses who may be prescribing medications as well as those nurses who are administering or supervising the administration of drugs prescribed by someone else). Optimal care requires that Advanced Practice Nurses know the name and class of a drug, the type and duration of expected action, the dosage range, contraindications to use of that drug, and the potential adverse or toxic reactions, as well as possible interactions with other drugs the person may be taking. Awareness of how patient traits and lifestyles influence the pharmacodynamics and pharmacokinetics of drugs, and how these same factors influence the therapeutic effects of drugs is vital to safe pharmacotherapeutics. Some very basic concepts related to understanding optimum and safe drug therapy are discussed on the following pages.

1. Pharmacokinetics, Pharmacodynamics, Pharmacotherapeutics
2. Patient Factors That Influence Drug Therapy (pregnancy, age, weight, lifestyle)

PHARMACOKINETICS, PHARMACODYNAMICS, PHARMACOTHERAPEUTICS

PHARMACOKINETICS: ABSORPTION, DISTRIBUTION, AND ELIMINATION (metabolism, excretion)

ABSORPTION

Absorption refers to how a drug progresses from the dosage form to biologically available molecules that can pass through or across membranes and tissues.

Absorption depends on the formulations of the drug, the route of drug administration, and the physiological variables. Drugs administered by the I.V. route require no absorption (they enter the circulatory system immediately). Intramuscularly administered drugs and subcutaneous injections involve some absorption; formulations in oil or microfine crystals (long-acting) have longer absorption times than others. Absorption from the deltoid muscle is faster than absorption from the gluteal muscle because of the increased blood flow in the deltoid muscle.

The oral route of drug administration is the preferred route for most drug therapy because it is more comfortable for the patient and usually safer and easier to use. The oral route, however, has a longer absorption time and is based on the particular drug formulation (compressed tablet, extended release, repeat-action). Anything that reduces systemic blood flow can reduce absorption rates – strenuous exercise decreases splanchnic blood flow because more blood is diverted to the muscles; pain and stress also reduce blood flow in this area. Prolonged intestinal transit time – experienced with high-fat meals, solid food, anticholinergic drugs – may delay absorption rate but increase total drug absorption amount. In addition, some drug-drug interactions or drug-food interactions can reduce overall absorption – highly acidic or basic substances or drugs that significantly alter the gastric pH (eg, H_2-blockers, cimetidine, ranitidine, etc) can, in turn, affect the absorption rates of a drug.

Orally administered drugs must pass through the portal system before they enter the systemic circulation and many drugs undergo metabolic changes in the liver (first-pass effect). The orally administered dose required to achieve a specific therapeutic response may, therefore, be much larger than the dose for a route that bypasses portal circulation such as parenteral or sublingual. [Enterohepatic recycling (reabsorption) is a concern in some cases of drug toxicity. Some drugs (eg, digoxin and levothyroxine) move through the bloodstream after absorption and re-enter the biliary tract to be excreted in bile in their intact form. They are then reabsorbed from the intestine and re-enter the circulatory system. Substances (charcoal, sodium polystyrene sulfonate (Kayexalate®)) which bind the recycled drug in the GI tract may be necessary for rapid reduction of toxic serum levels of a drug.]

Other routes of drug administration (eg, vaginal, rectal, topical, buccal, inhalation) all have positive and negative aspects of absorption. Drugs administered by inhalation are microsized particles that cross thin membranes to reach the target tissues. The type of drugs that can be formulated in the necessary microsized particles is limited and the degree and rate of absorption is less exact than by some other routes, although increasing numbers of drugs are becoming available for inhalation. Rectal absorption for systemic drugs is generally slow, uncomfortable, and sometimes painful. For some drugs and for some patients this is either the only route available or the route of choice. Pharmacists can be remarkably innovative in formulating rectal drugs for extremely debilitated patients (eg, cancer, AIDS, etc). Topical absorption has the advantage of continuous absorption, although onset is generally slow. Drugs for ophthalmic and otic administration are highly specific and designed to take the absorption properties into consideration.

DISTRIBUTION

Distribution of an absorbed drug in the body is dependent on several factors, including blood flow, degree of protein binding, and affinity for lipid or aqueous tissue.

The distribution of a drug affects both the concentration in the body and at the site of action, and thus has direct impact on the therapeutic response to that drug. Many drugs enter the system by one or another means of absorption, circulate through the body via the circulatory system, and are excreted from the body in due course. Those drugs that have a high potential for binding to transport proteins or storage proteins are directly influenced by the amount of albumin available for binding. Only the unbound molecules of the drug remain free in the circulation.

Usually, the degree to which any drug binds to albumin remains constant when albumin levels are normal. However, the degree of binding differs greatly between drugs (eg, gentamicin is <30% bound and warfarin is 97% to 99% bound). When disease states, nutritional status, or other drugs influence the available albumin for binding, toxic serum levels of a drug may occur. Low systemic albumin levels generally mean that a greater than expected amount of an albumin-bound drug will be free in the system, which may be undesirable. Competition between two drugs for albumin-binding sites may also increase the amount of free drug for one of the competitors (eg, aspirin and warfarin may compete for albumin-binding sites; aspirin has a greater affinity for albumin and therefore the free warfarin will be increased).

Distribution is also influenced by physiological barriers (ie, the blood-brain barrier is the network of poreless capillaries in the brain, which are surrounded by a glial sheath that makes them impermeable to water-soluble drugs). Disease states, abscesses, tumors, specific glands, and differences between tissues within a single organ also complicate drug distribution.

ELIMINATION VIA METABOLISM

Elimination via metabolism is the process of biotransformation that occurs when a drug changes from its parent form to a more water-soluble form.

Some drugs are not metabolized and are excreted from the body unchanged (aminoglycosides). However, most drugs are metabolized in the liver, in tissues, in the gastric system, or in the lungs. The metabolites are most often inactive forms of the parent that are more water soluble than the parent drug and can therefore be excreted in the urine. In some instances, metabolism is required to convert a biologically inactive drug (prodrug) to an active form. (Dopamine does not cross the blood-brain barrier; however, levodopa, an inactive precursor of dopamine, does cross the blood-brain barrier where it is metabolized to dopamine.) In other cases, metabolism results in active metabolites (imipramine metabolizes to desipramine).

Hepatic metabolism is a result of enzyme action which can be influenced by other drugs. Some drugs stimulate an increase in specific enzyme activity which increases the metabolism breakdown of other drugs; thereby decreasing the availability of the second drug (eg, phenobarbital induces the enzyme that metabolizes theophylline). Conversely, when a drug inhibits the enzyme activity necessary for metabolism of a second drug, toxic levels of the second drug can result (eg, cimetidine inhibits the enzyme that metabolizes theophylline; theophylline metabolism is inhibited thereby causing an elevated theophylline level). Knowing that a drug is either an enzyme inhibitor or an enzyme inducer should cause a nurse monitoring drug effects to be alert for the effects of any other drugs that may be potentially affected.

Diseases which damage the liver (eg, ethanol abuse, hepatitis) can impact drug metabolism, and genetics may also influence liver metabolism. Patients identified as rapid acetylators may require increased dosage of some medications (eg, hydralazine, procainamide). Smoking, alcohol, diet, disease state, and age also influence enzyme activity (see Patient Factors That Influence Drug Therapy *on page 25*).

ELIMINATION VIA EXCRETION

Elimination via excretion is the process by which a drug or its metabolites is removed from the body.

Drugs can be eliminated through the lungs, kidneys, liver, skin, intestinal tract, or via excretory glands – in sweat, tears, saliva, or breast milk. Peritoneal dialysis or hemodialysis may also be used to remove drugs from the body.

Half-life is the time required for the total amount of a drug to be diminished by one-half (eg, one half-life 50%, second half-life 25%, third half-life 12.5%, etc). With normal functioning excretion, the half-life of a drug will help to determine spacing of dosing schedules. In the presence of decreased kidney function, elimination is slowed or delayed and more of the drug remains in the body than half-life figures would indicate. Elderly persons frequently have decreased kidney function as a part of the aging process – drugs excreted primarily via the kidneys thereby hold the potential for toxic levels for elderly persons when given in "normal" doses.

PHARMACODYNAMICS

Pharmacodynamics is the way drugs bring about biophysical or biochemical changes.

After drugs are absorbed and reach the target site, pharmacological action occurs at the cellular level. The pharmacological action at the cellular level may alter or modify cellular function; it does not cause a new function in a cell or tissue. The action of drug at the cellular level has an effect that can affect body function. The action of the drug is different than the effect or results of that action [eg, insulin facilitates glucose transport across cellular membranes, the expected result is lowered serum glucose; atropine blocks acetylcholine receptors to prevent the action of acetylcholine, the expected result is a decrease in the effects of acetylcholine (anticholinergic response -- see Pharmacologic Category Index *on page 1435*)]. Effects or responses may be beneficial (desired) or nonbeneficial (adverse).

Drug molecules interact with specific receptors on cellular membranes for which they have an affinity in a lock and key type bond. Drugs that stimulate receptor actions are called agonists. Drugs that fit to receptors and prevent or inhibit cellular response to other drugs or endogenous compounds are called antagonists. In some instances, manipulating antagonist action is desirable (eg, naloxone competes with opioids for opioid receptors and may be used to reverse an opioid overdose). In other cases, when two drugs compete for the same receptors the results are to negate the effects of one or both of those drugs (eg, levodopa increases the amount of dopamine that stimulates dopamine receptors and amitriptyline stimulates those same receptors). When given together, one drug negates or reduces the effects of the other.

Some drugs are classified as receptor specific or nonspecific. Some drugs will nonselectively stimulate all of a particular class of receptors [eg, epinephrine will stimulate all beta-adrenergic receptors (stimulating both cardiac tissue and pulmonary smooth muscle tissue), whereas terbutaline is more selective for $beta_2$ adrenergic receptors (acting primarily on the smooth muscle in the lungs)]. Selectivity may be dose-related (ie, at higher doses selectivity may be reduced).

Several factors may also influence the number of specific receptors (up-regulation or down-regulation) and their ability to couple with other drugs or endogenous substances. The changes in number of receptors (increase or decrease) or sensitivity may result in drug tolerance (eg, biogenic amines - antidepressants). The rebound phenomena that follows abrupt withdrawal of some drugs is related to an increase in the availability of receptor sites as the drug is released from the receptor (ie, clonidine). Disease states can influence number and responsiveness of receptors (eg, thyroid hormones can increase the number of beta receptors and their sensitivity to catecholamines in cardiac muscle, which may account for the tachycardia of thyrotoxicosis). Age can decrease responsiveness to insulin. In addition, the concentration of available drug in systemic circulation (bioavailability), metabolism (breakdown), and excretion (elimination) have direct influence on the degree of biophysical or biochemical changes effected by drugs.

Ideally, the dose of a drug should achieve the desired response without the occurrence of adverse effects. Unfortunately, with some drugs, the onset of adverse effects occurs before therapeutic dosage levels can be reached. This precludes the use of this drug. Fortunately, many drugs have a fairly wide window of safety (eg, the relationship between effective dosing levels and adverse effects is wide enough so that adverse or toxic responses can be minimalized). Some drugs, however, have a very narrow therapeutic index (TI); the range between therapeutic effect and toxic response is very small. Drugs with a narrow TI should be monitored (physical assessment and/or serum drug levels) on a regular basis (eg, lithium, digoxin, phenytoin, theophylline, etc).

PHARMACOTHERAPEUTICS

Drug therapy is used for treatment of disease or symptoms of diseases (empiric, supportive, maintenance, or palliative), for prevention (immunization), and for diagnosis (iodine, barium).

Optimal drug therapy should be both effective and safe. It needs to be tailored to the patient (see Patient Factors That Influence Drug Therapy *on page 25*) and the problem. Assessing the problem is the first step – this involves identifying the problem (eg, etiology, laboratory confirmation, subjective and objective symptoms, urgency, severity, and prognosis) and determining what is the goal of therapy. Identifying and assessing the various options require knowledge of what drug therapy is appropriate. These steps lead to clinical decision-making (eg, selecting the drug regimen that is appropriate to meet the goal for this patient).

While professionals responsible for prescribing medications usually select therapy, the implementing of therapy is often a responsibility of nurses, in collaboration with pharmacists. Implementing therapy includes not only the preparation and dispensing of the drug, but also the education of those individual(s) who will administer the drug: nurses, patients, and family members. A major aspect of the education of patients includes how to administer the drug, when to administer the drug, and any dietary or drug-related precautions.

Monitoring the results of that therapy is a major responsibility that involves the prescriber, pharmacist, nurse, patient, and other healthcare providers. A major aspect of monitoring is communicating the subjective and objective responses to the responsible prescriber. Patients, nurses, and other caregivers must know the anticipated results of drug therapy and how to assess and report possible adverse effects.

DRUG INTERACTIONS

Drug interactions are a major concern in drug therapy. Interactions may occur between food and drugs or between different drugs (ie, over-the-counter drugs, herbals, home remedies, and prescription drugs). Careful assessment of **ALL** substances patients are using to treat themselves is imperative for safe drug therapy. Patients may not consider some of the substances they use to treat themselves as drugs and nurses may need to be highly sensitive and very aware when they discuss this subject with the patient.

Drug interactions increase exponentially with the number of drugs a person is taking. Thus, the more illnesses a patient has, the more likely it is he/she will be taking multiple drugs, and the more likely he/she will be to experience drug interactions.

Drugs can interact with other drugs to produce additive effects (when combined they produce more desirable effects with a lesser dose of either drug than they would alone), synergistic effects (the combination produces a greater response than either alone), or antagonistic effect (one drug negates or reverses the effect of the other drug). Such interactions can be a result of altering the pharmacokinetics of the drugs involved; increasing or decreasing either the rate or the quantity in absorption, altering the distribution through competitive receptor binding, changing the metabolism by inducing or reducing actions of liver enzymes, altering blood flow, or excretion by altering renal clearance.

Food, alcohol, and cigarette smoking can interact with drugs. Absorption of some drugs is enhanced with high fat meals (griseofulvin) or by low protein or high carbohydrate meals (theophylline). Whereas, absorption of some drugs is slowed – rather than blocked when the stomach is full and gastric transport is slowed. Other drugs can bind with food to impair or prevent absorption of food byproducts such as carbohydrates or vitamins (eg, cholestyramine, mineral oil). Some drugs, such as isotretinoin, are isomers of vitamins and dietary intake of vitamin A can cause overdose reactions.

Other foods can produce pharmacologic activity on their own and when the patient is also taking a medication that is designed to result in that same pharmacologic activity the result may be life-threatening. For instance, patients using a monamine oxidase (MAO) inhibitor should avoid foods containing tyramines or tryptophan (see Tyramine-Containing Foods *on page 1601*) to prevent excess release of catecholamines resulting in severe potentially life-threatening effects.

Drugs can also impact the results of laboratory tests. This is the basis for instructions from the laboratory to "hold" certain medications prior to some laboratory tests.

ADVERSE DRUG REACTIONS

Adverse reactions to drug therapy can range from mild to debilitating and life-threatening. Mild reactions may either be not severe enough to discontinue the drug or will disappear when the drug is discontinued. Severe or life-threatening reactions may require immediate discontinuance, treatment with other drugs, or dialysis. Adverse reactions may be related to the dosing, they may be inherent in the drug's primary actions, they may be iatrogenic to the drug, or they may be related to individual patient sensitivity or genetics.

Dose-related side effects can be addressed through careful dosage adjustment. Adverse effects associated with inherent properties of the drugs (constipation with opiates or some pain medications) can be addressed through appropriate interventions (ie, increasing fluids, fiber in diets, increased exercise, or stool softeners). Iatrogenic effects (ie, GI irritation and bleeding from aspirin or indomethacin, orthostatic hypotension from antihypertensives) can be reduced by taking a complete patient history, by patient administration and precaution education (eg, safe dose, time, diet, activity, etc), by prescribing another drug to address the anticipated iatrogenic response, or by choosing another drug for treatment. Thorough knowledge of the possible adverse effects, coupled with anticipatory action, will reduce the incidence of adverse side effects.

True allergic responses usually result from previous exposure to one drug or drugs with related chemical composition that sensitizes the patient's immune system. Careful drug histories and assessment of a patient's reported previous adverse responses will help in averting allergic reactions. Idiosyncratic responses are those that are specific to that patient and are generally unpredictable, although many times these are genetically determined.

See Selected Adverse Effects Information *on page 1523*.

PATIENT FACTORS THAT INFLUENCE DRUG THERAPY

Many factors related to an individual patient, or a group of similar patients, can impact the pharmacokinetics of drugs and relate to adverse reactions.

PREGNANCY/LACTATION

The changes that occur during pregnancy may necessitate dosage changes for some drugs. Decreased gastric tract motility, increased blood volume, decreased protein binding sites, and increased glomerular filtration rates may alter the degree of anticipated pharmacotherapeutic response.

Primarily, the concern about drugs during pregnancy is the effect of drugs on the fetus, either teratogenic (causing birth defects) or systemic (causing addiction). Although many drugs cross the placenta, the type of drug, the concentration of that drug, and the gestational age at time of exposure of the fetus are primary determinants of fetal reaction. When prescribing or administering drugs to any childbearing age female, it is vital to ask when her last menstrual period was and, if necessary, to wait for the results of a pregnancy test before starting any drug therapy. Of course, it is best to avoid all drugs during pregnancy, however, in some cases, the physiological context (ie, cardiac output, renal blood flow, etc) may be altered enough to require the use of drugs that are not needed by the same woman when not pregnant.

Most systematically absorbed drugs have been assigned a pregnancy risk factor based on the drugs potential to cause birth defects. This permits an evaluation of the risk:benefit ratio when prescribing or administering drugs becomes necessary. Drugs in the risk factor class "A" are generally considered to be safe for use during pregnancy, class "X" drugs are never safe and are known to be positively teratogenic.

These categories are summarized as follows:

A Controlled studies in pregnant women fail to demonstrate a risk to the fetus in the first trimester with no evidence of risk in later trimesters. The possibility of fetal harm appears remote.

B Either animal-reproduction studies have not demonstrated a fetal risk but there are no controlled studies in pregnant women, or animal-reproduction studies have shown an adverse effect (other than a decrease in fertility) that was not confirmed in controlled studies in women in the first trimester and there is no evidence of a risk in later trimesters.

C Either studies in animals have revealed adverse effects on the fetus (teratogenic or embryocidal effects or other) and there are no controlled studies in women, or studies in women and animals are not available. Drugs should be given only if the potential benefits justify the potential risk to the fetus.

D There is positive evidence of human fetal risk, but the benefits from use in pregnant women may be acceptable despite the risk (eg, if the drug is needed in a life-threatening situation or for a serious disease for which safer drugs cannot be used or are ineffective).

X Studies in animals or human beings have demonstrated fetal abnormalities or there is evidence of fetal risk based on human experience, or both, and the risk of the use of the drug in pregnant women clearly outweighs any possible benefit. The drug is contraindicated in women who are or may become pregnant.

Contraception note: Many drugs will interact with and decrease the effect of oral contraceptives (eg, barbiturates, some antibiotics - minocycline, ampicillin, tetracycline, corticosteroids, and benzodiazepines). When a second drug will decrease the effect of oral contraceptives, the patient needs to be educated about the necessity for using a "barrier" form of contraception. Barrier contraception (alone or in combination with some form of oral contraception) is also often recommended for the patient who must take drugs with pregnancy risk factors "D" (idarubicin) or class "X" (isotretinoin).

Because many drugs and substances used by a mother appear in breast milk, care must be taken to evaluate the drug effects on the lactating woman and the infant. Some drugs are identified as being clearly contraindicated during lactation, others may cross into breast milk but adverse side effects on the fetus have not been identified, and for some drugs the administration times should be distanced from nursing time. Nurses should advise lactating women about the effects that drugs may have on the infant.

AGE

All pharmacokinetics – absorption, distribution, metabolism, and excretion – are different in infants, young adults, and elderly patients. Elderly patients may have mildly decreased or severely decreased blood flow to all organs, gastric motility may be slowed, kidney function may be reduced, decreased nutrition may result in decreased albumin, and sedentary lifestyles may have an impact on drug response. Slower gastric motility means that absorption is slowed, resulting in longer time periods to clinical response. Decreased blood flow means that distribution is altered, resulting in decreased response or longer response time. Decreased available albumin results in higher levels of drug in circulation – more toxic responses with "normal" doses. Excretion may be altered with decreased glomerular filtration rates or slower gastric emptying which can result in increased levels of drug remaining in the system.

The ratio between total body water and total body fat also changes with age; older persons have decreased amounts of total body water and higher body fat. This aspect of aging also influences the blood concentration of some drugs. In a person with increased body fat, fat-soluble drugs are distributed to tissues more than to plasma; resulting in a longer response time as the drug must then be redistributed from tissue to plasma. The idiosyncratic response incidence also increases with an aging population. Responses to drugs may be both more exaggerated or diminished with the "usual" doses of some drugs.

In addition, and of major concern with elderly patients, is the incidence of poly-pharmacy; the increased numbers of drugs the patient may be taking. Older patients may have 2, 3, 4, or 5 (or more) chronic conditions for which they are taking medication. In addition, they may be seeing a different prescriber for each of these conditions. Often, it is a nurse who identifies and coordinates the care of these elderly patients, and the nurse must be aware of the possibility for increased incidence of adverse effects.

BODY WEIGHT/BUILD

Most "recommended" dosages of drugs are based on the average size, young or middle aged adult (usually males). Extremely obese or extremely thin patients may be prone to adverse effects as a result of "nonindividualized" prescribing. Decreased muscle mass can result in reduced creatinine from muscle breakdown which is artificially low or appears normal when dosing is based on "average" or estimated rather than "actual" creatinine clearance.

SMOKING, ALCOHOL, NUTRITION, AND HYDRATION

Smoking has a direct impact on liver enzyme activity, blood flow, and the central nervous system. Excessive alcohol intake impacts liver enzymes, renal function, as well as an additive effect with most antipsychotic, sedative, or anxiolytic medications, as well as altering responses to many other medications. Nutrition and hydration also play an important part in drug responses and possible adverse reactions. Poor hydration may result in reduced blood flow and excretion. Decreased or prolonged gastric motility can result in slowed excretion and/or prolonged absorption. Poor or inadequate nutrition may result in decreased protein available for binding.

It is vital that a patient's current habits are considered when prescribing, administering, or monitoring drug therapy, but in addition, patients must be aware of the need to inform their professional care provider that they have changed their smoking, alcohol, or dietary patterns. When dosage of theophylline is based on the fact that the patient is a smoker, the theophylline dosage must be adjusted to prevent overdose, if the patient quits smoking. When a patient is on warfarin, drastic increases in the amount of vitamin K intake through increased green leafy vegetables can dramatically alter the dose of warfarin.

OTHER PATIENT FACTORS THAT INFLUENCE DRUG RESPONSE

Genetic variations, differences in circadian patterns, psychological temperament, and disease states can also impact the incidence of adverse reactions. Genetic differences in enzymes may influence the incidence of adverse effects (fast acetylators or slow acetylators). Circadian rhythms differ among individuals and have an impact on absorption patterns, hormone secretion, or urinary excretion patterns. Disease states can and do change all aspects of pharmacokinetics: cirrhosis can impair liver enzyme metabolism rate; abnormal thyroid function can influence drug metabolism; diseases which affect blood circulation (eg, hypertension, CHF, Raynaud's phenomena, malignancies, etc) can have an impact on absorption, distribution, and excretion; diabetes impacts response to many drugs; malnutrition commonly associated with disease can drastically reduce albumin levels; and kidney disease will reduce excretion rates for many drugs.

PATIENT EDUCATION FOR MANAGEMENT OF COMMON SIDE EFFECTS

MANAGEMENT OF DRUG-RELATED PROBLEMS

Patients may experience some type of side effect or adverse drug reaction as a result of their drug therapy. The type of effect, the severity, and the frequency of occurrence is dependent on the medication and dose being used, as well as the individual's response to therapy. The following information is presented as helpful tips to assist the patient through these drug-related problems. Pharmacological support may also be required for their management.

Alopecia

- Your hair loss is temporary. Hair usually will begin to grow within 3-6 months of completing drug therapy.
- Your hair may come back with a different texture, color, or thickness.
- Avoid excessive shampooing and hair combing, or harsh hair care products.
- Avoid excessive drying of hair.
- Avoid use of permanents, dyes, or hair sprays.
- Always cover head in cold weather or sunshine.

Anemia

- Observe all bleeding precautions (see Thrombocytopenia).
- Get adequate sleep and rest.
- Be alert for potential for dizziness, fainting, or extreme fatigue.
- Maintain adequate nutrition and hydration.
- Have laboratory tests done as recommended.
- If unusual bleeding occurs, notify prescriber.

Anorexia

- Small frequent meals containing favorite foods may tempt appetite.
- Eat simple foods such as toast, rice, bananas, mashed potatoes, scrambled eggs.
- Eat in a pleasant environment conducive to eating.
- When possible, eat with others.
- Avoid noxious odors when eating.
- Use nutritional supplements high in protein and calories.
- Freezing nutritional supplements sometimes makes them more palatable.
- A small glass of wine (if not contraindicated) may stimulate appetite.
- Mild exercise or short walks may stimulate appetite.
- Request antiemetic medication to reduce nausea or vomiting.

Diarrhea

- Include fiber, high protein foods, and fruits in dietary intake.
- Drink plenty of liquids.
- Buttermilk, yogurt, or boiled milk may be helpful.
- Antidiarrheal agents may be needed. Consult your prescriber.
- Include regular rest periods in your activities.
- Institute skin care regimen to prevent breakdown and promote comfort.

Fluid Retention/Edema

- Elevate legs when sitting.
- Wear support hose.
- Increase physical exercise.
- Maintain adequate hydration; avoiding fluids will not reduce edema.
- Weigh yourself regularly.
- If your prescriber has advised you to limit your salt intake, avoid foods such as ham, bacon, processed meats, and canned foods. Many foods are high in salt content. Read labels carefully.
- Report to prescriber if any of the following occur: sudden weight gain, decrease in urination, swelling of hands or feet, increase in waist size, wet cough, or difficulty breathing.

Headache

- Lie down.
- Use cool cloth on forehead.
- Avoid caffeine.
- Use mild analgesics. Consult prescriber.

Leukopenia/Neutropenia

- Monitor for signs of infections: persistent sore throat, fever, chills, fatigue, headache, flu-like symptoms, vaginal discharge, foul-smelling stools.
- Prevent infection. Maintain strict handwashing at all times. Avoid crowds when possible. Avoid exposure to infected persons.
- Avoid exposure to temperature changes.
- Maintain adequate nutrition and hydration.
- Maintain good personal hygiene.
- Avoid injury or skin breaks.
- Avoid vaccinations (unless recommended by healthcare provider).
- Avoid sunburn.

Nausea and Vomiting

- Eat food served cold or at room temperature. Ice chips are sometimes helpful.
- Drink clear liquids in severe cases of nausea. Avoid carbonated beverages.
- Sip liquids slowly.
- Avoid spicy food. Bland foods are easier to digest.
- Rinse mouth with lemon water. Practice good oral hygiene.
- Avoid sweet, fatty, salty foods and foods with strong odors.
- Eat small frequent meals rather than heavy meals.
- Use relaxation techniques and guided imagery.
- Use distractions such as meals, television, reading, games, etc.
- Sleep during intense periods of nausea.
- Chew gum or suck on hard candy or lozenges.
- Eat in an upright (sitting position), rather than semirecumbant.
- Avoid tight constrictive clothing at meal time.
- Use some mild exercise following light meals rather than lying down.
- Request antiemetic medication to reduce nausea or vomiting.

Postural Hypotension

- Use care and rise slowly from sitting or lying position to standing.
- Use care when climbing stairs.
- Initiate ambulation slowly. Get your bearings before you start walking.
- Do not bend over; always squat slowly if you must pick up something from floor.
- Use caution when showering or bathing (use secure handrails).

Stomatitis

- Perform good oral hygiene frequently, especially before and after meals.
- Avoid use of strong or alcoholic commercial mouthwashes.
- Keep lips well lubricated.
- Avoid tobacco or other products that are irritating to the oral mucosa.
- Avoid hot, spicy, excessively salty foods.
- Eat soft foods and drink adequate fluids.
- Request topical or systemic analgesics for painful ulcerations.
- Be alert for and report signs of oral fungal infections.

Thrombocytopenia

- Avoid aspirin and aspirin-containing products.
- Use electric or safety razor and blunt scissors.
- Use soft toothbrush or cotton swabs for oral care. Avoid use of dental floss.
- Avoid use of enemas, cathartics, and suppositories unless approved by prescriber.
- Avoid valsalva maneuvers such as straining at stool.
- Use stool softeners if necessary to prevent constipation. Consult prescriber.
- Avoid blowing nose forcefully.
- Never go barefoot, wear protective foot covering.
- Use care when trimming nails (if necessary).
- Maintain safe environment; arrange furniture to provide safe passageway.
- Maintain adequate lighting in darkened areas to avoid bumping into objects.
- Avoid handling sharp tools or instruments.
- Avoid contact sports or activities that might result in injury.
- Promptly report signs of bleeding; abdominal pain; blood in stool, urine, or vomitus; unusual fatigue; easy bruising; bleeding around gums; or nosebleeds.
- If injection or bloodsticks are necessary, inform healthcare provider that you may have excess bleeding.

Vertigo

- Observe postural hypotension precautions.
- Use caution when driving or using any machinery.
- Avoid sudden position shifts; do not "rush".
- Utilize appropriate supports (eg, cane, walker) to prevent injury.

ALPHABETICAL LISTING OF DRUGS

A200® Lice [OTC] *see* Permethrin *on page 1061*

Abacavir (a BAK a veer)

U.S. Brand Names Ziagen®

Generic Available No

Pharmacologic Category Antiretroviral Agent, Reverse Transcriptase Inhibitor (Nucleoside)

Pregnancy Risk Factor C

Lactation Excretion in breast milk unknown/contraindicated

Use Treatment of HIV infections in combination with other antiretroviral agents

Mechanism of Action/Effect Nucleoside reverse transcriptase inhibitor which interferes with HIV viral RNA dependent DNA polymerase resulting in inhibition of viral replication

Contraindications Hypersensitivity to abacavir (or carbovir) or any component of the formulation; do not rechallenge patients who have experienced hypersensitivity to abacavir

Warnings/Precautions Should always be used as a component of a multidrug regimen. Fatal hypersensitivity reactions have occurred. **Patients exhibiting symptoms of fever, skin rash, fatigue, respiratory symptoms (eg, pharyngitis, dyspnea, cough) and GI symptoms (eg, abdominal pain, nausea, vomiting) should discontinue therapy immediately and call for medical attention. Abacavir should be permanently discontinued if hypersensitivity cannot be ruled out, even when other diagnoses are possible. Abacavir SHOULD NOT be restarted because more severe symptoms may occur within hours, including LIFE-THREATENING HYPOTENSION AND DEATH. Fatal hypersensitivity reactions have occurred following the reintroduction of abacavir in patients whose therapy was interrupted (interruption in drug supply, temporary discontinuation while treating other conditions). Reactions occurred within hours. In some cases, signs of hypersensitivity may have been previously present, but attributed to other medical conditions (acute onset respiratory diseases, gastroenteritis, reactions to other medications). If abacavir is restarted following an interruption in therapy, evaluate the patient for previously unsuspected symptoms of hypersensitivity. Do not restart if hypersensitivity is suspected or if hypersensitivity cannot be ruled out. To report these events on abacavir hypersensitivity, a registry has been established (1-800-270-0425).** Use with caution in patients with hepatic dysfunction; prior liver disease, prolonged use, and obesity may be risk factors for development of lactic acidosis and severe hepatomegaly with steatosis. Pregnancy factor C.

Drug Interactions

Increased Effect/Toxicity: Ethanol may increase the risk of toxicity. Abacavir increases the blood levels of amprenavir. Abacavir may decrease the serum concentration of methadone in some patients. Concomitant use of ribavirin and nucleoside analogues may increase the risk of developing lactic acidosis (includes adefovir, didanosine, lamivudine, stavudine, zalcitabine, zidovudine).

Adverse Reactions Note: Hypersensitivity reactions, which may be fatal, occur in ~5% of patients (see Warnings/Precautions). Symptoms may include anaphylaxis, fever, rash, fatigue, diarrhea, abdominal pain, respiratory symptoms (eg, pharyngitis, dyspnea, or cough), headache, malaise, lethargy, myalgia, myolysis, arthralgia, edema, paresthesia, nausea and vomiting, mouth ulcerations, conjunctivitis, lymphadenopathy, hepatic failure, and renal failure.

Rates of adverse reactions were defined during combination therapy with lamivudine. Adverse reaction rates attributable to abacavir alone are not available.

Adults:
- Central nervous system: Insomnia (7%)
- Endocrine & metabolic: Hyperglycemia, hypertriglyceridemia (25%)
- Gastrointestinal: Nausea (47%), vomiting (16%), diarrhea (12%), anorexia (11%), pancreatitis
- Neuromuscular & skeletal: Weakness
- Miscellaneous: Transaminases increased, hypersensitivity reaction (5%)

Children:
- Central nervous system: Fever (19%), headache (16%)
- Dermatologic: Rash (11%)
- Gastrointestinal: Nausea (38%), vomiting (38%), diarrhea (16%), anorexia (9%)
- Miscellaneous: Hypersensitivity reaction (5%)

<1% (Limited to important or life-threatening): Anaphylactoid reaction, pulmonary hypertension

Pharmacodynamics/Kinetics

Absorption: Rapid and extensive absorption

Bioavailability: 83%

Half-Life Elimination: 1.5 hours

Time to Peak: 0.7-1.7 hours

Metabolism: Hepatic via alcohol dehydrogenase and glucuronyl transferase to inactive carboxylate and glucuronide metabolites

Formulations

Solution, oral, as sulfate: 20 mg/mL (240 mL) [strawberry-banana flavor]

Tablet, as sulfate: 300 mg

Dosing

Adults & Elderly: HIV treatment: Oral: 600-1200 mg/day in 2-3 divided doses in combination with other antiretroviral agents

Pediatrics: HIV treatment: Oral: 3 months to 16 years: 8 mg/kg body weight twice daily (maximum 300 mg twice daily) in combination with other antiretroviral agents

Monitoring and Teaching Issues

Physical Assessment: Assess for allergy prior to beginning treatment. See Contraindications and Warnings/Precautions for use cautions. Monitor patient response closely on a regular basis throughout therapy (eg, hypersensitivity can be fatal - see Adverse Reactions and Overdose/Toxicology). Teach patient proper use, possible side effects and interventions, and adverse symptoms to report (eg, signs and symptoms of hypersensitivity - see

Patient Education). **Pregnancy risk factor C** - benefits of use should outweigh possible risks. Breast-feeding is contraindicated - CDC recommends that women with HIV not breast-feed in order to prevent transmission of HIV.

Patient Education: Inform prescriber of all prescriptions, OTC medications, or herbal products you are taking, and any allergies you have. Do not take anything new during treatment without consulting prescriber. This drug will not cure HIV; use appropriate precautions to prevent spread to other persons. Take as directed, for full course of therapy; do not discontinue if feeling better. Maintain adequate hydration (2-3 L/day of fluids) unless advised by prescriber to restrict fluids. You may be susceptible to infection (avoid crowds and exposure to known infections and do not have any vaccinations without consulting prescriber). May cause dizziness or weakness (use caution when driving or engaging in tasks requiring alertness until response to drug is known); or nausea or vomiting (small, frequent meals, frequent mouth care, chewing gum, or sucking lozenges may help). Report immediately symptoms of hypersensitivity (eg, fever, skin rash, fatigue, persistent nausea, vomiting, diarrhea, or abdominal pain); respiratory symptoms (eg, pharyngitis, dyspnea, or cough); headache; malaise or lethargy; loss of sensation, pain, tingling, or numbness in toes, feet, muscles or joints; edema, mouth sores, conjunctivitis, swollen glands, alterations in urinary pattern; swelling of extremities or weight gain. If you are instructed to stop the medication, do not take this medication in the future. Do not restart without specific instruction by your prescriber. **Pregnancy/breast-feeding precautions:** Inform prescriber if you are or intend to become pregnant. Do not breast-feed.

Dietary Issues: May be taken with or without food.

Breast-feeding Issues: HIV-infected mothers are discouraged from breast-feeding to decrease potential transmission of HIV.

Pregnancy Issues: It is not known if abacavir crosses the human placenta. Cases of lactic acidosis/hepatic steatosis syndrome have been reported in pregnant women receiving nucleoside analogues. It is not known if pregnancy itself potentiates this known side effect; however, pregnant women may be at increased risk of lactic acidosis and liver damage. Hepatic enzymes and electrolytes should be monitored frequently during the 3rd trimester of pregnancy in women receiving nucleoside analogues. Health professionals are encouraged to contact the antiretroviral pregnancy registry to monitor outcomes of pregnant women exposed to antiretroviral medications (1-800-258-4263).

Additional Information A medication guide is available and should be dispensed with each prescription or refill for abacavir. A warning card is also available and patients should be instructed to carry this card with them.

Abacavir, Lamivudine, and Zidovudine

(a BAK a veer, la MI vyoo deen, & zye DOE vyoo deen)

U.S. Brand Names Trizivir®

Synonyms Azidothymidine, Abacavir, and Lamivudine; AZT, Abacavir, and Lamivudine; Compound S, Abacavir, and Lamivudine; Lamivudine, Abacavir, and Zidovudine; 3TC, Abacavir, and Zidovudine; ZDV, Abacavir, and Lamivudine; Zidovudine, Abacavir, and Lamivudine

Generic Available No

Pharmacologic Category Antiretroviral Agent, Reverse Transcriptase Inhibitor (Nucleoside)

Pregnancy Risk Factor C

Lactation Enters breast milk/not recommended

Use Treatment of HIV infection (either alone or in combination with other antiretroviral agents) in patients whose regimen would otherwise contain the components of Trizivir® (based on analyses of surrogate markers in controlled studies with abacavir of up to 24 weeks; there have been no clinical trials conducted with Trizivir®)

Formulations Tablet: Abacavir 300 mg, lamivudine 150 mg, and zidovudine 300 mg

Dosing

Adults: HIV treatment: Oral: 1 tablet twice daily. **Note:** Not recommended for patients <40 kg.

Elderly: Use with caution.

Pediatrics: HIV treatment: Adolescents: Refer to adult dosing (not recommended for patients <40 kg).

Renal Impairment: Cl_{cr} ≤50 mL/minute: Avoid use.

Monitoring and Teaching Issues

Physical Assessment: See individual components listed in Related Information. **Pregnancy risk factor C** - benefits of use should outweigh possible risks. Breast-feeding is not recommended.

Patient Education: See individual components listed in Related Information. **Pregnancy/breast-feeding precautions:** Inform your prescriber if you are or intend to become pregnant. Breast-feeding is not recommended. HIV-infected mothers are discouraged from breast-feeding to decrease potential transmission of HIV.

Related Information

Abacavir *on page 30*
Lamivudine *on page 768*
Zidovudine *on page 1419*

Abbokinase® *see* Urokinase *on page 1375*

Abbreviations, Acronyms, and Symbols Commonly Used in Medical Orders *see page 18*

ABCD *see* Amphotericin B Cholesteryl Sulfate Complex *on page 92*

Abciximab (ab SIK si mab)

U.S. Brand Names ReoPro®

Synonyms C7E3; 7E3

Generic Available No

Pharmacologic Category Antiplatelet Agent, Glycoprotein IIb/IIIa Inhibitor

Pregnancy Risk Factor C

(Continued)

Abciximab *(Continued)*

Lactation Excretion in breast milk unknown

Use Prevention of acute cardiac ischemic complications in patients at high risk for abrupt closure of the treated coronary vessel and patients at risk of restenosis; an adjunct with heparin to prevent cardiac ischemic complications in patients with unstable angina not responding to conventional therapy when a percutaneous coronary intervention is scheduled within 24 hours

Mechanism of Action/Effect Inhibits fibrinogen binding, platelet aggregation, and prolongs bleeding time.

Contraindications Hypersensitivity to abciximab, to murine proteins, or any component of the formulation; active internal hemorrhage or recent (within 6 weeks) clinically significant GI or GU bleeding; history of cerebrovascular accident within 2 years or cerebrovascular accident with significant neurological deficit; clotting abnormalities or administration of oral anticoagulants within 7 days unless prothrombin time (PT) is ≤1.2 times control PT value; thrombocytopenia (<100,000 cells/μL); recent (within 6 weeks) major surgery or trauma; intracranial tumor, arteriovenous malformation, or aneurysm; severe uncontrolled hypertension; history of vasculitis; use of dextran before PTCA or intent to use dextran during PTCA; concomitant use of another parenteral GP IIb/IIIa inhibitor

Warnings/Precautions Administration of abciximab is associated with increased frequency of major bleeding complications including retroperitoneal bleeding, spontaneous GI or GU bleeding, and bleeding at the arterial access site and in the following: patients weighing <75 kilograms, elderly patients (>65 years), history of previous GI disease, recent thrombolytic therapy.

The risk of major bleeds may increase with concurrent use of thrombolytics. In serious, uncontrolled bleeding, abciximab and heparin should be stopped.

Increased risk of hemorrhage during or following angioplasty is associated with unsuccessful PTCA, PTCA procedure >70 minutes duration, or PTCA performed within 12 hours of symptom onset for acute myocardial infarction.

Safety or efficacy of readministration of abciximab has not been established. Administration of abciximab may result in human antichimeric antibody formation that can cause hypersensitivity reactions (including anaphylaxis), thrombocytopenia, or diminished efficacy. Anticoagulation, such as with heparin, may contribute to the risk of bleeding.

Pregnancy risk C.

Drug Interactions

Increased Effect/Toxicity: The risk of bleeding is increased when abciximab is given with heparin, other anticoagulants, thrombolytics, or antiplatelet drugs. However, aspirin and heparin were used concurrently in the majority of patients in the major clinical studies of abciximab. Allergic reactions may be increased in patients who have received diagnostic or therapeutic monoclonal antibodies due to the presence of HACA antibodies. Concomitant use of other glycoprotein IIb/IIIa antagonists is contraindicated.

Adverse Reactions As with all drugs which may affect hemostasis, bleeding is associated with abciximab. Hemorrhage may occur at virtually any site. Risk is dependent on multiple variables, including the concurrent use of multiple agents which alter hemostasis and patient susceptibility.

>10%:

Cardiovascular: Hypotension (14.4%), chest pain (11.4%)

Gastrointestinal: Nausea (13.6%)

Hematologic: Minor bleeding (4.0% to 16.8%)

Neuromuscular & skeletal: Back pain (17.6%)

1% to 10%:

Cardiovascular: Bradycardia (4.5%), peripheral edema (1.6%)

Central nervous system: Headache (6.45)

Gastrointestinal: Vomiting (7.3%), abdominal pain (3.1%)

Hematologic: Major bleeding (1.1% to 14%), thrombocytopenia: <100,000 cells/mm^3 (2.5% to 5.6%); <50,000 cells/mm^3 (0.4% to 1.7%)

Local: Injection site pain (3.6%)

<1% (Limited to important or life-threatening): Abnormal thinking, allergic reactions/anaphylaxis (possible), AV block, bronchospasm, bullous eruption, coma, confusion, diabetes mellitus, embolism, hyperkalemia, ileus, inflammation, intracranial hemorrhage, myalgia, nodal arrhythmia, pleural effusion, pulmonary embolism, prostatitis, pruritus, stroke, urinary retention, ventricular tachycardia, xerostomia

Overdosage/Toxicology Since abciximab is a platelet antiaggregate, patients who bleed following administration may be best treated with platelet infusions.

Pharmacodynamics/Kinetics

Half-Life Elimination: ~30 minutes

Formulations Injection, solution: 2 mg/mL (5 mL)

Dosing

Adults & Elderly:

Prevention of restenosis (patients at high risk for abrupt closure): I.V.: 0.25 mg/kg bolus administered 10-60 minutes before the start of intervention followed by an infusion of 0.125 mcg/kg/minute (to a maximum of 10 mcg/minute) for 12 hours

Patients with unstable angina not responding to conventional medical therapy and who are planning to undergo percutaneous coronary intervention within 24 hours: I.V.: 0.25 mg/kg intravenous bolus followed by an 18- to 24-hour intravenous infusion of 10 mcg/minute, concluding 1 hour after the percutaneous coronary intervention.

Administration

I.V.: Infuse at a rate of 17 mL/hour (10 mcg/minute) for 12 hours via pump.

Stability

Storage: Vials should be stored at 2°C to 8°C. Do not freeze.

Reconstitution: After admixture, the prepared solution is stable for 12 hours.

Compatibility: Requires separate intravenous line; no incompatibilities have been observed with glass bottles or PVC bags.

Monitoring Laboratory Tests Prothrombin time, activated partial thromboplastin time, hemoglobin, hematocrit, platelet count, fibrinogen, fibrin split products

Monitoring and Teaching Issues

Physical Assessment: Monitor vital signs and laboratory results prior to, during, and after therapy. Assess infusion insertion site and peripheral pulses during and after therapy. Observe and teach patient bleeding precautions (avoid invasive procedures and activities that could result in injury). Monitor closely for signs of excessive bleeding. **Pregnancy risk factor C.** Note breast-feeding caution.

Patient Education: This medication can only be administered I.V. You will have a tendency to bleed easily following this medication; use caution to prevent injury (use electric razor, soft toothbrush, and use caution with knives, needles, or anything sharp). If bleeding occurs, apply pressure to bleeding spot until bleeding stops completely. Report unusual bruising or bleeding; blood in urine, stool, or vomitus; bleeding gums; or vision changes. **Pregnancy/breast-feeding precautions:** Inform prescriber if you are or intend to become pregnant. Consult prescriber if breast-feeding.

Additional Information

Patients at high risk of closure or restenosis:

- Acute evolving myocardial infarction (MI) within 12 hours of onset of symptoms requiring rescue PTCA
- Early postinfarction angina or unstable angina with at least 2 episodes of angina associated with EKG changes during previous 24 hours
- Non-Q-wave myocardial infarction
- Clinical or angiographic characteristic indicating high risk (see "Characteristics of Type A, B, and C Lesions" below)
  - Unfavorable anatomy (ie, 2 or more Type B lesions) **or**
  - One or more Type B lesions with diabetes **or**
  - One or more Type B lesions and a female and over the age of 65 **or**
  - One Type C lesion
- Thrombus score is based upon angiographic evidence

Characteristics of Type A, B, and C Lesions

- Type A lesions (minimally complex)
  - Discrete (length <10 mm)
  - Concentric
  - Readily accessible
  - Nonangulated segment (<45°)
  - Smooth contour
  - Little or no calcification
  - Less than totally occlusive
  - Not ostial in location
  - No major side branch involvement
  - No thrombus
- Type B lesions (moderately complex)
  - Tubular (length 10-20 mm)
  - Eccentric
  - Moderate tortuosity of proximal segment
  - Moderate angulated segment (>45°, <90°)
  - Irregular contour
  - Moderate or heavy calcification
  - Total occlusions <3 months old
  - Ostial in location
  - Bifurcation lesions requiring double lead wires
  - Some thrombus present
- Type C lesions (severely complex)
  - Diffuse (length >20 mm)
  - Excessive tortuosity of proximal segment
  - Extremely angulated segments >90°
  - Total occlusions >3 months old and/or bridging collaterals
  - Inability to protect major side branches
  - Degenerated vein grafts with friable lesions

ABC Pack™ (Avelox®) *see* Moxifloxacin *on page 929*

Abelcet® *see* Amphotericin B (Lipid Complex) *on page 97*

ABLC *see* Amphotericin B (Lipid Complex) *on page 97*

Acarbose (AY car bose)

U.S. Brand Names Precose®

Generic Available No

Pharmacologic Category Antidiabetic Agent, Alpha-Glucosidase Inhibitor

Pregnancy Risk Factor B

Lactation Excretion in breast milk unknown

Use

Monotherapy, as indicated as an adjunct to diet to lower blood glucose in patients with type 2 diabetes mellitus (noninsulin dependent, NIDDM) whose hyperglycemia cannot be managed on diet alone

Combination with a sulfonylurea, metformin, or insulin in patients with type 2 diabetes mellitus (noninsulin dependent, NIDDM) when diet plus acarbose do not result in adequate

(Continued)

Acarbose *(Continued)*

glycemic control. The effect of acarbose to enhance glycemic control is additive to that of other hypoglycemic agents when used in combination.

Mechanism of Action/Effect Delays glucose absorption and lowers postprandial hyperglycemia.

Contraindications Hypersensitivity to acarbose or any component of the formulation; patients with diabetic ketoacidosis or cirrhosis; patients with inflammatory bowel disease, colonic ulceration, partial intestinal obstruction, or in patients predisposed to intestinal obstruction; patients who have chronic intestinal diseases associated with marked disorders of digestion or absorption, and in patients who have conditions that may deteriorate as a result of increased gas formation in the intestine

Warnings/Precautions Patients receiving sulfonylureas: Acarbose given in combination with a sulfonylurea will cause a further lowering of blood glucose and may increase the hypoglycemic potential of the sulfonylurea. If hypoglycemia occurs, appropriate adjustments in the dosage of these agents should be made. Oral glucose (dextrose) should be used in the treatment of mild to moderate hypoglycemia.

Elevated serum transaminase levels: Treatment-emergent elevations of serum transaminases (AST and/or ALT) occurred in 15% of acarbose-treated patients in long-term studies. These serum transaminase elevations appear to be dose related and were asymptomatic, reversible, more common in females, and, in general, were not associated with other evidence of liver dysfunction.

Drug Interactions

Decreased Effect: The effect of acarbose is antagonized/decreased by thiazide and related diuretics, corticosteroids, phenothiazines, thyroid products, estrogens, oral contraceptives, phenytoin, nicotinic acid, sympathomimetics, calcium channel-blocking drugs, isoniazid, intestinal adsorbents (eg, charcoal), and digestive enzyme preparations (eg, amylase, pancreatin).

Increased Effect/Toxicity: Acarbose may increase the risk of hypoglycemia when used with oral hypoglycemics. See Warnings/Precautions.

Nutritional/Ethanol Interactions Ethanol: Limit ethanol.

Adverse Reactions

>10%:

Gastrointestinal: Abdominal pain (21%) and diarrhea (33%) tend to return to pretreatment levels over time, and the frequency and intensity of flatulence (77%) tend to abate with time

Hepatic: Elevated liver transaminases

<1% (Limited to important or life-threatening): Severe gastrointestinal distress

Overdosage/Toxicology An overdose will not result in hypoglycemia. An overdose may result in transient increases in flatulence, diarrhea, and abdominal discomfort which shortly subside.

Pharmacodynamics/Kinetics

Absorption: <2% as active drug

Bioavailability: Low systemic bioavailability of parent compound; acts locally in GI tract

Metabolism: Exclusively via GI tract, principally by intestinal bacteria and digestive enzymes; 13 metabolites identified

Formulations Tablet: 25 mg, 50 mg, 100 mg

Dosing

Adults & Elderly: Type 2 diabetes: Oral:

Initial: 25 mg 3 times/day

Maintenance dose: Should be adjusted at 4- to 8-week intervals based on 1-hour postprandial glucose levels and tolerance until maintenance dose is reached; maintenance dose: 50-100 mg 3 times/day. Dosage must be individualized on the basis of effectiveness and tolerance while not exceeding the maximum recommended dose.

Maximum:

≤60 kg: 50 mg 3 times/day

>60 kg: 100 mg 3 times/day

Patients receiving sulfonylureas: Acarbose given in combination with a sulfonylurea will cause a further lowering of blood glucose and may increase the hypoglycemic potential of the sulfonylurea. If hypoglycemia occurs, appropriate adjustments in the dosage of these agents should be made.

Renal Impairment: Cl_{cr} <25 mL/minute: Peak plasma concentrations were 5 times higher and AUCs were 6 times larger than in volunteers with normal renal function; however, long-term clinical trials in diabetic patients with significant renal dysfunction have not been conducted and treatment of these patients with acarbose is not recommended

Administration

Oral: Drug should be **taken with the first bite of each main meal**.

Stability

Storage: Store at <25°C (77°F) and protect from moisture.

Monitoring Laboratory Tests Postprandial glucose, glycosylated hemoglobin levels, and serum transaminase levels should be checked every 3 months during the first year of treatment and periodically thereafter.

Monitoring and Teaching Issues

Physical Assessment: See Contraindications, Warnings/Precautions, and Dosing for use cautions. Assess potential for interactions with other prescriptions, OTC medications, or herbal products patient may be taking (see Drug Interactions). Assess results of laboratory tests (see above), therapeutic effects, and adverse response (see Adverse Reactions and Overdose/Toxicology) on a regular basis throughout therapy. Teach patient proper use (or refer patient to diabetic educator), possible side effects and appropriate interventions (eg, importance of adequate hydration), and adverse symptoms to report (see Patient Education). Note breast-feeding caution.

Patient Education: Inform prescriber of all prescriptions, OTC medications, or herbal products you are taking, and any allergies you have. Do not take anything new during

treatment unless approved by prescriber. Take this medication exactly as directed, with the first bite of each main meal. Do not change dosage or discontinue without first consulting prescriber. Do not take other medications with or within 2 hours of this medication unless advised by prescriber. Avoid alcohol. It is important to follow dietary and lifestyle recommendations of prescriber. You will be instructed in signs of hypo- or hyperglycemia by prescriber or diabetic educator. If combining acarbose with other diabetic medication (eg, sulfonylureas, insulin), keep source of glucose (sugar) on hand in case hypoglycemia occurs. May cause mild side effects during first weeks of acarbose therapy (eg, bloating, flatulence, diarrhea, abdominal discomfort); these should diminish over time. Report severe or persistent side effects, fever, extended vomiting or flu, or change in color of urine or stool. **Breast-feeding precaution:** Consult prescriber if breast-feeding.

Geriatric Considerations: Monitor change in preprandial blood glucose concentrations to account for potential age-related changes in postprandial glucose.

Pregnancy Issues: Abnormal blood glucose levels are associated with a higher incidence of congenital abnormalities. Insulin is the drug of choice for the control of diabetes mellitus during pregnancy.

Related Information

Antidiabetic Oral Agents Comparison *on page 1556*
Diabetes Mellitus Management *on page 1661*

Accolate® *see* Zafirlukast *on page 1413*

AccuNeb™ *see* Albuterol *on page 52*

Accupril® *see* Quinapril *on page 1160*

Accuretic™ *see* Quinapril and Hydrochlorothiazide *on page 1162*

Accutane® *see* Isotretinoin *on page 751*

ACE *see* Captopril *on page 210*

Acel-Imune® *see page 1498*

Aceon® *see* Perindopril Erbumine *on page 1059*

Acephen® [OTC] *see* Acetaminophen *on page 35*

Acetaminophen (a seet a MIN oh fen)

U.S. Brand Names Acephen® [OTC]; Aspirin Free Anacin® Maximum Strength [OTC]; Cetafen® [OTC]; Cetafen Extra® [OTC]; Feverall® [OTC]; Genapap® [OTC]; Genapap® Children [OTC]; Genapap® Extra Strength [OTC]; Genapap® Infant [OTC]; Genebs® [OTC]; Genebs® Extra Strength [OTC]; Infantaire [OTC]; Liquiprin® for Children [OTC]; Mapap® [OTC]; Mapap® Children's [OTC]; Mapap® Extra Strength [OTC]; Mapap® Infants [OTC]; Redutemp® [OTC]; Silapap® Children's [OTC]; Silapap® Infants [OTC]; Tylenol® [OTC]; Tylenol® Arthritis Pain [OTC]; Tylenol® Children's [OTC]; Tylenol® Extra Strength [OTC]; Tylenol® Infants [OTC]; Tylenol® Junior Strength [OTC]; Tylenol® Sore Throat [OTC]; Valorin [OTC]; Valorin Extra [OTC]

Synonyms APAP; N-Acetyl-P-Aminophenol; Paracetamol

Generic Available Yes

Pharmacologic Category Analgesic, Miscellaneous

Pregnancy Risk Factor B

Lactation Enters breast milk/compatible

Use Treatment of mild to moderate pain and fever; does not have antirheumatic effects (analgesic)

Mechanism of Action/Effect Reduces fever by acting on the hypothalamus to cause vasodilatation and sweating

Contraindications Hypersensitivity to acetaminophen or any component of the formulation; patients with known G6PD deficiency

Warnings/Precautions May cause severe hepatic toxicity on overdose. Use with caution in patients with alcoholic liver disease or who consume large amounts of alcohol. Chronic daily dosing in adults of 5-8 g of acetaminophen over several weeks or 3-4 g/day of acetaminophen for 1 year have resulted in liver damage.

Drug Interactions

Cytochrome P450 Effect: Substrate of CYP1A2, 2A6, 2C8/9, 2D6, 2E1, 3A4

Decreased Effect: Barbiturates, carbamazepine, hydantoins, rifampin, sulfinpyrazone may decrease the analgesic effect of acetaminophen; cholestyramine may decrease acetaminophen absorption (separate dosing by at least 1 hour)

Increased Effect/Toxicity: Barbiturates, carbamazepine, hydantoins, isoniazid, rifampin, sulfinpyrazone may increase the hepatotoxic potential of acetaminophen; chronic ethanol abuse increases risk for acetaminophen toxicity; effect of warfarin may be enhanced

Nutritional/Ethanol Interactions

Ethanol: Excessive intake of ethanol may increase the risk of acetaminophen-induced hepatotoxicity. Avoid ethanol or limit to <3 drinks/day.

Food: May slightly delay absorption of extended-release preparations; rate of absorption may be decreased when given with food high in carbohydrates.

Herb/Nutraceutical: St John's wort may decrease acetaminophen levels.

Effects on Lab Values ↑ chloride, bilirubin, uric acid, glucose, ammonia (B), chloride (S), uric acid (S), alkaline phosphatase (S), chloride (S); ↓ sodium, bicarbonate, calcium (S)

Adverse Reactions <1% (Limited to important or life-threatening): Analgesic nephropathy, anemia, blood dyscrasias (agranulocytosis, thrombocytopenia, neutropenia, pancytopenia, leukopenia), hepatitis, nephrotoxicity with chronic overdose, sterile pyuria

Overdosage/Toxicology Symptoms of overdose include hepatic necrosis, transient azotemia, renal tubular necrosis with acute toxicity, anemia, and GI disturbances with chronic toxicity. Treatment consists of acetylcysteine 140 mg/kg orally (loading) followed by 70 mg/kg every 4 hours for 17 doses; therapy should be initiated based upon laboratory analysis suggesting a high probability of hepatotoxic potential. Activated charcoal is very effective at binding acetaminophen. Intravenous acetylcysteine should be reserved for patients unable to take oral forms.

(Continued)

Acetaminophen *(Continued)*

Pharmacodynamics/Kinetics

Half-Life Elimination: Neonates: 2-5 hours; Adults: 1-3 hours

Time to Peak: Serum: Oral: 10-60 minutes; may be delayed in acute overdoses

Metabolism: At normal therapeutic dosages, hepatic to sulfate and glucuronide metabolites, while a small amount is metabolized by CYP to a highly reactive intermediate (acetylimidoquinone) which is conjugated with glutathione and inactivated; at toxic doses (as little as 4 g daily) glutathione conjugation becomes insufficient to meet the metabolic demand causing an increase in acetylimidoquinone concentration, thought to cause hepatic cell necrosis

Onset: <1 hour

Duration: 4-6 hours

Formulations

Caplet (Genapap® Extra Strength, Genebs® Extra Strength, Tylenol® Extra Strength): 500 mg
Caplet, extended release (Tylenol® Arthritis Pain): 650 mg
Capsule (Mapap® Extra Strength): 500 mg
Elixir: 160 mg/5 mL (5 mL, 10 mL, 20 mL, 120 mL, 240 mL, 500 mL, 3780 mL)
  Genapap® Children: 160 mg/5 mL (120 mL) [cherry and grape flavors]
  Silapap® Children's: 160 mg/5 mL (120 mL, 240 mL, 480 mL)
Gelcap (Genapap® Extra Strength, Tylenol® Extra Strength): 500 mg
Geltab (Tylenol® Extra Strength): 500 mg
Liquid, oral: 160 mg/5 mL (120 mL, 240 mL, 480 mL, 3870 mL); 500 mg/15 mL (240 mL)
  Redutemp®: 500 mg/15 mL (120 mL)
  Tylenol® Sore Throat: 500 mg/15 mL (240 mL) [cherry and honey-lemon flavors]
Solution, oral drops: 100 mg/mL (15 mL, 30 mL) [droppers are marked at 0.4 mL (40 mg) and at 0.8 mL (80 mg)]
  Genapap® Infant: 80 mg/0.8 mL (15 mL)
  Infantaire®, Silapap® Infant's: 80 mg/0.8 mL (15 mL, 30 mL)
  Liquiprin® for Children: 80 mg/0.8 mL (30 mL)
Suppository, rectal: 80 mg, 120 mg, 325 mg, 650 mg
  Acephen®: 120 mg, 325 mg, 650 mg
  Feverall®: 80 mg, 120 mg, 325 mg
  Mapap®: 120 mg, 650 mg
Suspension, oral: 160 mg/5 mL (120 mL)
  Mapap® Children's: 160 mg/5 mL (120 mL) [cherry, grape, and bubblegum flavors]
  Tylenol® Children's: 160 mg/5 mL (120 mL, 240 mL) [cherry, grape, and bubblegum flavors]
Suspension, oral drops: 100 mg/mL (15 mL, 30 mL) [droppers are marked at 0.4 mL (40 mg) and at 0.8 mL (80 mg)]
  Mapap® Infants 80 mg/0.8 mL (15 mL, 30 mL) [cherry flavor]
  Tylenol® Infants: 80 mg/0.8 mL (15 mL, 30 mL) [cherry and grape flavors]
Syrup, oral: 160 mg/5 mL (120 mL)
Tablet: 160 mg, 325 mg, 500 mg
  Aspirin Free Anacin® Maximum Strength, Cetafen® Extra Strength, Genapap® Extra Strength, Genebs® Extra Strength, Mapap® Extra Strength, Redutemp®, Tylenol® Extra Strength, Valorin Extra: 500 mg
  Cetafen®, Genapap®, Genebs®, Mapap®, Tylenol®, Valorin: 325 mg
  Mapap®: 160 mg
Tablet, chewable: 80 mg, 160 mg
  Genapap® Children, Mapap® Children's: 80 mg [contains phenylalanine 3 mg/tablet; fruit and grape flavors]
  Tylenol® Children's: 80 mg [fruit and grape flavors contain phenylalanine 3 mg/tablet; bubblegum flavor contains phenylalanine 6 mg/tablet]
  Tylenol® Junior Strength: 160 mg [contains phenylalanine 6 mg/tablet; fruit and grape flavors]

Dosing

Adults & Elderly: Pain or fever: Oral, rectal: 325-650 mg every 4-6 hours or 1000 mg 3-4 times/day; do **not** exceed 4 g/day. If fever is not controlled with acetaminophen alone, give with full doses of ibuprofen on an every 4- to 6-hour schedule, if not otherwise contraindicated.

Pediatrics: Pain or fever: Oral, rectal (if fever not controlled with acetaminophen alone, administer with full doses of ibuprofen on an every 6- to 8-hour schedule).
Children <12 years: 10-15 mg/kg/dose every 4-6 hours as needed; do **not** exceed 5 doses (2.6 g) in 24 hours; alternatively, the following doses may be used. See table.

Acetaminophen Dosing

Age	Dosage (mg)	Age	Dosage (mg)
0-3 mo	40	4-5 y	240
4-11 mo	80	6-8 y	320
1-2 y	120	9-10 y	400
2-3 y	160	11 y	480

Renal Impairment:
Cl_{cr} 10-50 mL/minute: Administer every 6 hours.
Cl_{cr} <10 mL/minute: Administer every 8 hours (metabolites accumulate).
Moderately dialyzable (20% to 50%)

Hepatic Impairment: Use with caution. Limited, low-dose therapy usually well tolerated in hepatic disease/cirrhosis. However, cases of hepatotoxicity at daily acetaminophen dosages <4 g/day have been reported. Avoid chronic use in hepatic impairment.

Administration

Oral: Shake suspension well before pouring dose.

Stability

Storage: Do not freeze suppositories.

Monitoring Laboratory Tests Serum APAP levels with long-term use in patients with hepatic disease

Monitoring and Teaching Issues

Physical Assessment: **Assess patient for history of liver disease or ethanol abuse** (acetaminophen and excessive ethanol may have adverse liver effects). Assess other medications patient may be taking for additive or adverse interactions (see Drug Interactions). Assess knowledge/teach patient appropriate use. Teach patient to monitor for adverse reactions, adverse reactions to report, and appropriate interventions to reduce side effects.

Patient Education: Take exactly as directed; do not increase dose or frequency. Most adverse effects are related to excessive use. Take with food or milk. While using this medication, avoid or limit alcohol to <3 drinks/day and avoid other prescription or OTC medications that contain acetaminophen. Maintain adequate hydration (2-3 L/day of fluids) unless advised by prescriber to restrict fluids. This medication will not reduce inflammation; consult prescriber for anti-inflammatory, if needed. Report unusual bleeding (stool, mouth, urine) or bruising; unusual fatigue and weakness; change in elimination patterns; or change in color of urine or stool.

Acetaminophen and Codeine (a seet a MIN oh fen & KOE deen)

U.S. Brand Names Capital® and Codeine; Phenaphen® With Codeine; Tylenol® With Codeine

Synonyms Codeine and Acetaminophen

Restrictions C-III; C-V

Generic Available Yes

Pharmacologic Category Analgesic, Narcotic

Pregnancy Risk Factor C

Lactation Enters breast milk/use caution

Use Relief of mild to moderate pain

Formulations

Capsule [C-III]: #3 (Phenaphen® With Codeine): Acetaminophen 325 mg and codeine phosphate 30 mg

Elixir, oral [C-V]: Acetaminophen 120 mg and codeine phosphate 12 mg per 5 mL (5 mL, 10 mL, 12.5 mL, 15 mL, 120 mL, 480 mL, 3840 mL) [contains alcohol 7%]

Tylenol® with Codeine: Acetaminophen 120 mg and codeine phosphate 12 mg per 5 mL (480 mL) [contains alcohol 7%; cherry flavor]

Suspension, oral [C-V] (Capital® and Codeine): Acetaminophen 120 mg and codeine phosphate 12 mg per 5 mL [alcohol free; fruit punch flavor]

Tablet [C-III]:

#2: Acetaminophen 300 mg and codeine phosphate 15 mg

#3 (Tylenol® with Codeine): Acetaminophen 300 mg and codeine phosphate 30 mg [contains sodium metabisulfite]

#4 (Tylenol® with Codeine): Acetaminophen 300 mg and codeine phosphate 60 mg [contains sodium metabisulfite]

Dosing

Adults: Doses should be adjusted according to severity of pain and response of the patient. Adult doses ≥60 mg codeine fail to give commensurate relief of pain but merely prolong analgesia and are associated with an appreciably increased incidence of side effects.

Cough (Antitussive): Oral: Based on codeine (15-30 mg/dose) every 4-6 hours

Pain (Analgesic): Oral: Based on codeine (30-60 mg/dose) every 4-6 hours

1-2 tablets every 4 hours to a maximum of 12 tablets/24 hours

Elderly: Doses should be titrated to appropriate analgesic effect.

1 Tylenol® [#3] or 2 Tylenol® [#2] tablets every 4 hours; do **not** exceed 4 g/day acetaminophen.

Pediatrics: Oral: Analgesic:

Codeine: 0.5-1 mg codeine/kg/dose every 4-6 hours

Acetaminophen: 10-15 mg/kg/dose every 4 hours up to a maximum of 2.6 g/24 hours for children <12 years

3-6 years: 5 mL 3-4 times/day as needed of elixir

7-12 years: 10 mL 3-4 times/day as needed of elixir

>12 years: 15 mL every 4 hours as needed of elixir

Renal Impairment: See individual monographs for Acetaminophen and Codeine.

Hepatic Impairment: Use with caution. Limited, low-dose therapy is usually well tolerated in hepatic disease/cirrhosis; however, cases of hepatotoxicity at daily acetaminophen dosages <4 g/day have been reported. Avoid chronic use in hepatic impairment.

Monitoring and Teaching Issues

Physical Assessment: See individual components listed in Related Information. **Pregnancy risk factor C** - benefits of use should outweigh possible risks. Note breast-feeding caution.

Patient Education: See individual components listed in Related Information. **Pregnancy/breast-feeding precautions:** Inform prescriber if you are or intend to become pregnant. Consult prescriber if breast-feeding.

Related Information

Acetaminophen *on page 35*
Codeine *on page 327*

Acetaminophen and Hydrocodone *see* Hydrocodone and Acetaminophen *on page 667*

Acetaminophen and Oxycodone *see* Oxycodone and Acetaminophen *on page 1022*

Acetaminophen, Butalbital, and Caffeine *see* Butalbital, Acetaminophen, and Caffeine *on page 192*

Acetaminophen, Caffeine, Codeine, and Butalbital *see* Butalbital, Acetaminophen, Caffeine, and Codeine *on page 193*

Acetaminophen, Dichloralphenazone, and Isometheptene *see* Acetaminophen, Isometheptene, and Dichloralphenazone *on page 38*

Acetaminophen, Isometheptene, and Dichloralphenazone

(a seet a MIN oh fen, eye soe me THEP teen, & dye KLOR al FEN a zone)

U.S. Brand Names Midrin®; Migratine®

Synonyms Acetaminophen, Dichloralphenazone, and Isometheptene; Dichloralphenazone, Acetaminophen, and Isometheptene; Dichloralphenazone, Isometheptene, and Acetaminophen; Isometheptene, Acetaminophen, and Dichloralphenazone; Isometheptene, Dichloralphenazone, and Acetaminophen

Restrictions C-IV

Generic Available Yes

Pharmacologic Category Analgesic, Miscellaneous

Pregnancy Risk Factor B

Lactation Excretion in breast milk unknown/use caution

Use Relief of migraine and tension headache

Contraindications Hypersensitivity to acetaminophen, isometheptene, dichloralphenazone, or any component of the formulation; glaucoma; severe renal disease; hypertension; organic heart disease; hepatic disease; MAO inhibitor therapy

Drug Interactions

Cytochrome P450 Effect: Acetaminophen: Substrate of CYP1A2, 2A6, 2C8/9, 2D6, 2E1, 3A4

Nutritional/Ethanol Interactions Ethanol: Excessive intake of ethanol may increase the risk of acetaminophen-induced hepatotoxicity. Avoid ethanol or limit to <3 drinks/day.

Adverse Reactions Frequency not defined.

Central nervous system: Transient dizziness

Dermatological: Rash

Formulations Capsule: Acetaminophen 325 mg, isometheptene mucate 65 mg, dichloralphenazone 100 mg

Dosing

Adults & Elderly:

Migraine headache: Oral: 2 capsules to start, followed by 1 capsule every hour until relief is obtained (maximum: 5 capsules/12 hours)

Tension headache: Oral: 1-2 capsules every 4 hours (maximum: 8 capsules/24 hours)

Hepatic Impairment: Use with caution. Limited, low-dose therapy usually well tolerated in hepatic disease/cirrhosis; however, cases of hepatotoxicity at daily acetaminophen dosages <4 g/day have been reported. Avoid chronic use in hepatic impairment.

Monitoring and Teaching Issues

Physical Assessment: Note breast-feeding caution.

Patient Education: **Breast-feeding precaution:** Consult prescriber if breast-feeding.

Related Information

Acetaminophen *on page 35*

Controlled Substances Comparison *on page 1568*

Acetasol HC® *see page 1519*

AcetaZOLAMIDE (a set a ZOLE a mide)

U.S. Brand Names Diamox®; Diamox Sequels®

Generic Available Yes

Pharmacologic Category Anticonvulsant, Miscellaneous; Carbonic Anhydrase Inhibitor; Diuretic, Carbonic Anhydrase Inhibitor; Ophthalmic Agent, Antiglaucoma

Pregnancy Risk Factor C

Lactation Enters breast milk/compatible

Use Lowers intraocular pressure to treat glaucoma, also as a diuretic, adjunct treatment of refractory seizures and acute altitude sickness; centrencephalic epilepsies (sustained release not recommended for anticonvulsant)

Mechanism of Action/Effect Reversible inhibition of the enzyme carbonic anhydrase resulting in reduction of hydrogen ion secretion at renal tubule and an increased renal excretion of sodium, potassium, bicarbonate, and water. Decreases production of aqueous humor; also inhibits carbonic anhydrase in central nervous system to retard abnormal and excessive discharge from CNS neurons.

Contraindications Hypersensitivity to acetazolamide, to any component of the formulation, or to sulfonamides; patients with hepatic disease or insufficiency; patients with decreased sodium and/or potassium levels; patients with adrenocortical insufficiency, hyperchloremic acidosis, severe renal disease or dysfunction, or severe pulmonary obstruction; long-term use in noncongestive angle-closure glaucoma

Warnings/Precautions Use in impaired hepatic function may result in coma. Use with caution in patients with respiratory acidosis and diabetes mellitus. Impairment of mental alertness and/or physical coordination may occur. I.M. administration is painful. Drug may cause substantial increase in blood glucose in some diabetic patients. Malaise and complaints of tiredness and myalgia are signs of excessive dosing and acidosis in the elderly. Cross-sensitivity between sulfonamide antibiotics and sulfonamide diuretics including various thiazide diuretics. **Sustained release is not recommended for anticonvulsant use.** Pregnancy risk C.

Drug Interactions

Cytochrome P450 Effect: Inhibits CYP3A4

Decreased Effect: Use of acetazolamide may increase lithium excretion and alter excretion of other drugs by alkalinization of urine (eg, amphetamines, quinidine, procainamide, methenamine, phenobarbital, salicylates). Primidone serum concentrations may be decreased.

Increased Effect/Toxicity: Concurrent use with diflunisal may increase the effect of acetazolamide causing a significant decrease in intraocular pressure. Cyclosporine concentrations may be increased by acetazolamide. Salicylate use may result in carbonic anhydrase inhibitor accumulation and toxicity. Acetazolamide-induced hypokalemia may increase the risk of toxicity with digoxin.

Effects on Lab Values May cause false-positive results for urinary protein with Albustix®, Labstix®, Albutest®, Bumintest®.

Adverse Reactions

>10%:

Central nervous system: Malaise, unusual drowsiness or weakness

Gastrointestinal: Anorexia, weight loss, diarrhea, metallic taste, nausea, vomiting

Genitourinary: Polyuria

Neuromuscular & skeletal: Numbness, tingling, or burning in hands, fingers, feet, toes, mouth, tongue, lips, or anus

1% to 10%:

Central nervous system: Mental depression

Renal: Renal calculi

<1% (Limited to important or life-threatening): Blood dyscrasias, bone marrow suppression, cholestatic jaundice, convulsions, hyperchloremic metabolic acidosis, hyperglycemia, hypokalemia

Overdosage/Toxicology Symptoms of overdose include low blood sugar, tingling of lips and tongue, nausea, yawning, confusion, agitation, tachycardia, sweating, convulsions, stupor, and coma. Hypoglycemia should be managed with 50 mL I.V. dextrose 50% followed immediately with a continuous infusion of 10% dextrose in water (administer at a rate sufficient enough to approach a serum glucose level of 100 mg/dL). The use of corticosteroids to treat hypoglycemia is controversial, however, adding 100 mg of hydrocortisone to the dextrose infusion may prove helpful.

Pharmacodynamics/Kinetics

Half-Life Elimination: 2.4-5.8 hours

Onset: Capsule, extended release: 2 hours; I.V.: 2 minutes

Peak effect: Capsule, extended release: 3-6 hours; I.V.: 15 minutes; Tablet: 1-4 hours

Duration: Capsule, extended release: 18-24 hours; I.V.: 4-5 hours; Tablet: 8-12 hours

Formulations

Capsule, sustained release (Diamox Sequels®): 500 mg

Injection, powder for reconstitution: 500 mg

Tablet: 125 mg, 250 mg

Diamox®: 250 mg

Dosing

Adults: Note: I.M. administration is not recommended.

Glaucoma:

Chronic simple (open-angle): Oral: 250 mg 1-4 times/day or 500 mg sustained release capsule twice daily

Secondary, acute (closed-angle): I.M., I.V.: 250-500 mg, may repeat in 2-4 hours to a maximum of 1 g/day

Edema: Oral, I.M., I.V.: 250-375 mg once daily

Epilepsy: Oral: 8-30 mg/kg/day in 1-4 divided doses, not to exceed 1 g/day. **Sustained release capsule is not recommended for treatment of epilepsy.**

Altitude sickness: Oral: 250 mg every 8-12 hours (or 500 mg extended release capsules every 12-24 hours). Therapy should begin 24-48 hours before and continue during ascent and for at least 48 hours after arrival at the high altitude.

Urine alkalinization: Oral: 5 mg/kg/dose repeated 2-3 times over 24 hours

Elderly: Oral: Initial: 250 mg once or twice daily; use lowest effective dose possible.

Pediatrics: Note: I.M. administration is not recommended.

Hydrocephalus: Neonates and Infants: To slow the progression of hydrocephalus in neonates and infants who may not be good candidates for surgery, acetazolamide I.V. or oral doses of 5 mg/kg/dose every 6 hours increased by 25 mg/kg/day to a maximum of 100 mg/kg/day, if tolerated, have been used. Furosemide was used in combination with acetazolamide.

Children:

Glaucoma:

Oral: 8-30 mg/kg/day or 300-900 mg/m^2/day divided every 8 hours

I.M., I.V.: 20-40 mg/kg/24 hours divided every 6 hours, not to exceed 1 g/day

Edema: Oral, I.M., I.V.: 5 mg/kg or 150 mg/m^2 once every day

Epilepsy: Oral: Refer to adult dosing.

Renal Impairment:

Cl_{cr} 10-50 mL/minute: Administer every 12 hours.

Cl_{cr} <10 mL/minute: Avoid use → ineffective.

Moderately dialyzable (20% to 50%)

Administration

I.V.: Recommended rate of administration: 100-500 mg/minute for I.V. push and 4-8 hours for I.V. infusions

Stability

Reconstitution: Reconstituted solution may be refrigerated (2°C to 8°C) for 1 week.

Standard diluent: 500 mg/50 mL D_5W

Minimum volume: 50 mL D_5W

Stability of IVPB solution is 5 days at room temperature (25°C) and 44 days at refrigeration (5°C). Reconstitute with at least 5 mL sterile water to provide a solution containing not more than 100 mg/mL. Further dilution in 50 mL of either D_5W or NS for I.V. infusion administration.

Compatibility: Stable in dextran 6% in D_5W, dextran 6% in NS, D_5LR, D_5NS, $D_5{}^1/_2NS$, $D_5{}^1/_4NS$, D_5W, $D_{10}W$, LR, NS, $^1/_2NS$

Compatibility when admixed: Incompatible with multivitamins

(Continued)

AcetaZOLAMIDE *(Continued)*

Monitoring Laboratory Tests Intraocular pressure, serum electrolytes, periodic CBC with differential

Monitoring and Teaching Issues

Physical Assessment: Assess allergy history prior to beginning therapy. Assess effectiveness and interactions of other medications patient may be taking (see Drug Interactions). See Warnings/Precautions and Contraindications for extensive use cautions. Monitor therapeutic effectiveness, laboratory tests, including serum glucose (see above), and adverse response (see Adverse Reactions and Overdose/Toxicology). Assess knowledge/teach patient appropriate use, possible side effects and appropriate interventions, and adverse symptoms to report (see Patient Education). **Pregnancy risk factor C** - benefits of use should outweigh possible risks.

Patient Education: Take as directed; do not chew or crush long-acting capsule (contents may be sprinkled on soft food). May be administered with food to decrease GI upset. You will need periodic ophthalmic examinations while taking this medication. You may experience drowsiness, dizziness, or weakness (use caution when driving or engaging in tasks that require alertness until response to drug is known); or nausea, loss of appetite, or altered taste (small, frequent meals, frequent mouth care, sucking lozenges, or chewing gum may help). Monitor serum glucose closely (may cause altered blood glucose in some diabetic patients, or unusual response to some forms of glucose testing). You may experience increased sensitivity to sunlight (use sunblock, protective clothing, and avoid exposure to direct sunlight). Report unusual and persistent tiredness; numbness, burning, or tingling of extremities or around mouth, lips, or anus; muscle weakness; black stool; or excessive depression. **Pregnancy precaution:** Inform prescriber if you are or intend to become pregnant.

Dietary Issues: May be taken with food to decrease GI upset. Sodium content of 500 mg injection: 47.2 mg (2.05 mEq).

Geriatric Considerations: Malaise and complaints of tiredness and myalgia are signs of excessive dosing and acidosis in the elderly. Assess blood pressure (orthostatic hypotension can occur).

Related Information

FDA Name Differentiation Project: The Use of Tall-man Letters *on page 12*
Glaucoma Drug Comparison *on page 1575*

Acetic Acid and Hydrocortisone *see page 1519*
Acetic Acid, Propylene Glycol, and Hydrocortisone *see page 1519*
Acetohexamide *see page 1661*
Acetophenazine *see page 1558*
Acetophenazine *see page 1614*
Acetoxymethylprogesterone *see* MedroxyPROGESTERone *on page 842*
Acetylcholine *see page 1509*

Acetylcysteine (a se teel SIS teen)

U.S. Brand Names Mucomyst®; Mucosil™

Synonyms Acetylcysteine Sodium; Mercapturic Acid; NAC; *N*-Acetylcysteine; *N*-Acetyl-L-cysteine

Generic Available Yes

Pharmacologic Category Antidote; Mucolytic Agent

Pregnancy Risk Factor B

Lactation Excretion in breast milk unknown/compatible

Use Adjunctive mucolytic therapy in patients with abnormal or viscid mucous secretions in acute and chronic bronchopulmonary diseases; pulmonary complications of surgery and cystic fibrosis; diagnostic bronchial studies; antidote for acute acetaminophen toxicity

Use - Unlabeled/Investigational Prevention of radiocontrast-induced renal dysfunction

Mechanism of Action/Effect Exerts mucolytic action through its free sulfhydryl group which opens up the disulfide bonds in the mucoproteins thus lowering mucous viscosity. The exact mechanism of action in acetaminophen toxicity is unknown. It is thought to act by providing substrate for conjugation with the toxic metabolite.

Contraindications Hypersensitivity to acetylcysteine or any component of the formulation

Warnings/Precautions Since increased bronchial secretions may develop after inhalation, percussion, postural drainage, and suctioning should follow. If bronchospasm occurs, administer a bronchodilator. Discontinue acetylcysteine if bronchospasm progresses.

Drug Interactions

Decreased Effect: Adsorbed by activated charcoal; clinical significance is minimal, though, once a pure acetaminophen ingestion requiring N-acetylcysteine is established; further charcoal dosing is unnecessary once the appropriate initial charcoal dose is achieved (5-10 g:g acetaminophen)

Adverse Reactions

Inhalation:

>10%:

Stickiness on face after nebulization
Miscellaneous: Unpleasant odor during administration

1% to 10%:

Central nervous system: Drowsiness, chills, fever
Gastrointestinal: Vomiting, nausea, stomatitis
Local: Irritation
Respiratory: Bronchospasm, rhinorrhea, hemoptysis
Miscellaneous: Clamminess

Systemic:

1% to 10%:

Central nervous system: Fever, drowsiness, dizziness (10%; prevention of radiocontrast-induced renal function)

Gastrointestinal: Nausea, vomiting

<1% (Limited to important or life-threatening): Anaphylactoid reaction, bronchospastic allergic reaction, EKG changes (transient)

Overdosage/Toxicology Treatment of acetylcysteine toxicity is usually aimed at reversing anaphylactoid symptoms or controlling nausea and vomiting. The use of epinephrine, antihistamines, and steroids may be beneficial.

Pharmacodynamics/Kinetics

Half-Life Elimination: Reduced acetylcysteine: 2 hours; Total acetylcysteine: 5.5 hours

Time to Peak: Plasma: Oral: 1-2 hours

Onset: Inhalation: 5-10 minutes

Duration: Inhalation: >1 hour

Formulations Solution, as sodium: 10% [100 mg/mL] (4 mL, 10 mL, 30 mL); 20% [200 mg/mL] (4 mL, 10 mL, 30 mL, 100 mL)

Dosing

Adults & Elderly:

Acetaminophen poisoning: Oral: Loading dose: 140 mg/kg; followed by 70 mg/kg every 4 hours (for 17 doses); repeat dose if emesis occurs within 1 hour of administration. Therapy should continue until all doses are administered even though the acetaminophen plasma level has dropped below the toxic range.

Mucolytic:

Inhalation: Acetylcysteine 10% and 20% solution (Mucomyst®) (dilute 20% solution with sodium chloride or sterile water for inhalation); 10% solution may be used undiluted

Nebulization into face-mask, tracheostomy, mouth piece: 1-10 mL of 20% solution or 2-10 mL of 10% solution 3-4 times/day

Closed tent or croupette: Up to 300 mL of 10% or 20% solution treatment

Direct instillation into tracheostomy: 1-2 mL of 10% to 20% solution every 1-4 hours

Percutaneous intratracheal catheter: 1-2 mL of 20% solution or 2-4 mL of 10% solution every 1-4 hours by syringe attached to catheter

Instillation to a particular portion of bronchial tree using small plastic catheter (placed under local anesthesia and with direct visualization): 2-5 mL of 20% solution by syringe attached to catheter

Diagnostic procedures: 2-3 doses of 1-2 mL of 20% solution or 2-4 mL of 10% solution by nebulization or intratracheal instillation before the procedure

Note: Patients should receive an aerosolized bronchodilator 10-15 minutes prior to acetylcysteine.

Prevention of radiocontrast-induced renal dysfunction (unlabeled use): Oral: 600 mg twice daily for 2 days (beginning the day before the procedure); may be given as powder in capsules, some centers use solution (diluted in cola beverage or juice). Hydrate patient with saline concurrently.

Pediatrics:

Mucolytic: Inhalation: Acetylcysteine 10% and 20% solution (Mucomyst®) (dilute 20% solution with sodium chloride or sterile water for inhalation); 10% solution may be used undiluted.

Infants: 1-2 mL of 20% solution or 2-4 mL 10% solution until nebulized given 3-4 times/day

Children: 3-5 mL of 20% solution or 6-10 mL of 10% solution until nebulized given 3-4 times/day

Adolescents: 5-10 mL of 10% to 20% solution until nebulized given 3-4 times/day

Note: Patients should receive an aerosolized bronchodilator 10-15 minutes prior to acetylcysteine.

Meconium ileus equivalent: 100-300 mL of 4% to 10% solution by irrigation or orally

Administration

Oral: For treatment of acetaminophen overdosage, administer orally as a 5% solution. Dilute the 20% solution 1:3 with a cola, orange juice, or other soft drink. Use within 1 hour of preparation. Unpleasant odor becomes less noticeable as treatment progresses.

Inhalation: Acetylcysteine is incompatible with tetracyclines, erythromycin, amphotericin B, iodized oil, chymotrypsin, trypsin, and hydrogen peroxide. Administer separately. Intermittent aerosol treatments are commonly given when patient arises, before meals, and just before retiring at bedtime.

Stability

Storage: Store opened vials in the refrigerator. Use within 96 hours.

Reconstitution: Once diluted for administration, preparation should be used within 1 hour. Light purple color of solution does **not** affect its mucolytic activity.

Monitoring and Teaching Issues

Physical Assessment: Instruct patient on appropriate use, adverse effects to report, and interventions to reduce side effects.

Patient Education: Pulmonary treatment: Prepare solution (may dilute with sterile water to reduce concentrate from impeding nebulizer) and use as directed. Clear airway by coughing deeply before using aerosol. Wash face and face mask after treatment to remove any residual. You may experience drowsiness (use caution when driving), nausea, or vomiting (small, frequent meals may help). Report persistent chills or fever, adverse change in respiratory status, palpitations, or extreme anxiety or nervousness.

Pregnancy Issues: Based on limited reports using acetylcysteine to treat acetaminophen overdose in pregnant women, acetylcysteine has been shown to cross the placenta and may provide protective levels in the fetus.

Acetylcysteine Sodium *see* Acetylcysteine *on page 40*

Acetylsalicylic Acid *see* Aspirin *on page 121*

Achromycin® *see page 1509*

Achromycin [DSC] *see* Tetracycline *on page 1296*

Aciclovir *see* Acyclovir *on page 43*

Aciphex® *see* Rabeprazole *on page 1168*

Aclovate® *see* Topical Corticosteroids *on page 1334*

Acrivastine and Pseudoephedrine (AK ri vas teen & soo doe e FED rin)

U.S. Brand Names Semprex®-D

Synonyms Pseudoephedrine and Acrivastine

Generic Available No

Pharmacologic Category Antihistamine

Pregnancy Risk Factor B

Lactation Enters breast milk/contraindicated

Use Temporary relief of nasal congestion, decongest sinus openings, running nose, itching of nose or throat, and itchy, watery eyes due to hay fever or other upper respiratory allergies

Mechanism of Action/Effect Refer to Pseudoephedrine monograph; acrivastine is a competitive H_1-receptor site blocker.

Contraindications Hypersensitivity to pseudoephedrine, acrivastine (or other alkylamine antihistamines), or any component of the formulation; MAO inhibitor therapy within 14 days of initiating therapy; severe hypertension, severe coronary artery disease; renal impairment (Cl_{cr} ≤48 mL/minute)

Warnings/Precautions Use with caution in patients >60 years of age. Use with caution in patients with high blood pressure, ischemic heart disease, diabetes, increased intraocular pressure, GI or GU obstruction, asthma, thyroid disease, or prostatic hyperplasia. Not recommended for use in children.

Drug Interactions

Decreased Effect: Decreased effect of guanethidine, reserpine, methyldopa, and beta-blockers when given in conjunction with acrivastine and pseudoephedrine.

Increased Effect/Toxicity: Increased risk of hypertensive crisis when acrivastine and pseudoephedrine are given with MAO inhibitors or sympathomimetics. Increased risk of severe CNS depression when given with CNS depressants and ethanol.

Nutritional/Ethanol Interactions Ethanol: Avoid ethanol (may increase sedation)

Adverse Reactions

>10%: Central nervous system: Drowsiness, headache

1% to 10%:

- Cardiovascular: Tachycardia, palpitations
- Central nervous system: Nervousness, dizziness, insomnia, vertigo, lightheadedness, fatigue
- Gastrointestinal: Nausea, vomiting, xerostomia, diarrhea
- Genitourinary: Dysuria
- Neuromuscular & skeletal: Weakness
- Respiratory: Pharyngitis, cough increase
- Miscellaneous: Diaphoresis

Overdosage/Toxicology Symptoms of overdose include trembling, tachycardia, stridor, loss of consciousness, and possible convulsions. There is no specific antidote for pseudoephedrine intoxication, and treatment is primarily supportive.

Pharmacokinetic Note See Pseudoephedrine monograph.

Pharmacodynamics/Kinetics

Time to Peak:

Acrivastine: ~1.1 hours

Metabolism:

Acrivastine: Minimally hepatic

Formulations Capsule: Acrivastine 8 mg and pseudoephedrine hydrochloride 60 mg

Dosing

Adults & Elderly: Rhinitis, nasal congestion, allergic symptoms: Oral: 1 capsule 3-4 times/day

Pediatrics: Refer to adult dosing.

Renal Impairment: Do not use.

Monitoring and Teaching Issues

Physical Assessment: Assess effectiveness and interactions of other medications patient may be taking (see Drug Interactions). See Contraindications and Warnings/Precautions for use cautions. Monitor effectiveness of therapy and adverse reactions (see Adverse Reactions) at beginning of therapy and periodically with long-term use. Assess knowledge/teach patient appropriate use, interventions to reduce side effects, and adverse symptoms to report (see Patient Education). Breast-feeding is contraindicated.

Patient Education: Take as directed; do not exceed recommended dose. Avoid use of other depressants, alcohol, or sleep-inducing medications unless approved by prescriber. You may experience drowsiness or dizziness (use caution when driving or engaging in hazardous activity until response to drug is known); or dry mouth, nausea, or vomiting (small, frequent meals, frequent mouth care, chewing gum, or sucking lozenges may help). Report persistent dizziness, sedation, or agitation; chest pain, rapid heartbeat, or palpitations; difficulty breathing or increased cough; changes in urinary pattern; muscle weakness; or lack of improvement or worsening or condition. **Breast-feeding precaution:** Do not breast-feed.

Related Information

Pseudoephedrine *on page 1150*

ACT *see* Dactinomycin *on page 356*

Acthar® *see page 1461*

ActHIB® *see page 1498*

Acticin® *see* Permethrin *on page 1061*

Actidose® [OTC] *see* Charcoal *on page 266*

Actidose-Aqua® [OTC] *see* Charcoal *on page 266*

Actigall® *see* Ursodiol *on page 1376*

Actimmune® *see* Interferon Gamma-1b *on page 730*

Actinex® *see* Masoprocol *on page 836*

Actinomycin D *see* Dactinomycin *on page 356*

Actiq® *see* Fentanyl *on page 552*

Activase® *see* Alteplase *on page 67*
Activated Carbon *see* Charcoal *on page 266*
Activated Charcoal *see* Charcoal *on page 266*
Activated Ergosterol *see* Ergocalciferol *on page 483*
Activated Protein C, Human, Recombinant *see* Drotrecogin Alfa *on page 455*
Activella™ *see* Estradiol and Norethindrone *on page 499*
Actonel® *see* Risedronate *on page 1192*
Actos® *see* Pioglitazone *on page 1088*
Acular® *see page 1509*
Acular® *see* Ketorolac *on page 761*
Acular® PF *see page 1509*
Acular® PF *see* Ketorolac *on page 761*
ACV *see* Acyclovir *on page 43*
Acycloguanosine *see* Acyclovir *on page 43*

Acyclovir (ay SYE kloe veer)

U.S. Brand Names Zovirax®

Synonyms Aciclovir; ACV; Acycloguanosine

Generic Available Yes

Pharmacologic Category Antiviral Agent

Pregnancy Risk Factor B

Lactation Enters breast milk/compatible

Use Treatment of initial and prophylaxis of recurrent mucosal and cutaneous herpes simplex (HSV-1 and HSV-2) infections; herpes simplex encephalitis; herpes zoster; genital herpes infection; varicella-zoster infections in healthy, nonpregnant persons >13 years of age, children >12 months of age who have a chronic skin or lung disorder or are receiving long-term aspirin therapy, and immunocompromised patients; for herpes zoster, acyclovir should be started within 72 hours of the appearance of the rash to be effective; acyclovir will not prevent postherpetic neuralgias

Mechanism of Action/Effect Inhibits DNA synthesis and viral replication

Contraindications Hypersensitivity to acyclovir, valacyclovir, or any component of the formulation

Warnings/Precautions Use with caution in patients with pre-existing renal disease or in those receiving other nephrotoxic drugs concurrently; maintain adequate urine output during the first 2 hours after I.V. infusion; use with caution in patients with underlying neurologic abnormalities, serious hepatic or electrolyte abnormalities, or substantial hypoxia. Use with caution in immunocompromised patients; thrombocytopenic purpura/hemolytic uremic syndrome (TTP/HUS) has been reported

Drug Interactions

Increased Effect/Toxicity: Increased CNS side effects when taken with zidovudine or probenecid.

Nutritional/Ethanol Interactions Food: Does not appear to affect absorption of acyclovir.

Adverse Reactions

Systemic: Oral:

1% to 10%:
- Central nervous system: Lightheadedness, headache
- Gastrointestinal: Nausea, vomiting, abdominal pain

Systemic: Parenteral:

>10%:
- Central nervous system: Lightheadedness
- Gastrointestinal: Nausea, vomiting, anorexia
- Local: Inflammation at injection site or phlebitis

1% to 10%: Renal: Acute renal failure

Topical:

>10%: Mild pain, burning, or stinging

1% to 10%: Itching

All forms: <1% (Limited to important or life-threatening): Aggression, alopecia, anaphylaxis, anemia, angioedema, ataxia, delirium, encephalopathy, erythema multiforme, hallucinations, hepatitis, hyperbilirubinemia, jaundice, leukocytoclastic vasculitis, leukopenia, local tissue necrosis (following extravasation), mental depression, paresthesia, photosensitization, pruritus, psychosis, renal failure, seizures, somnolence, Stevens-Johnson syndrome, thrombocytopenia, thrombocytopenic purpura/hemolytic uremic syndrome (TTP/HUS), toxic epidermal necrolysis, urticaria

Overdosage/Toxicology Symptoms of overdose include seizures, somnolence, confusion, elevated serum creatinine, and renal failure. In the event of overdose, sufficient urine flow must be maintained to avoid drug precipitation within renal tubules. Hemodialysis has resulted in up to 60% reduction in serum acyclovir levels.

Pharmacodynamics/Kinetics

Absorption: Oral: 15% to 30%

Half-Life Elimination: Terminal: Neonates: 4 hours; Children 1-12 years: 2-3 hours; Adults: 3 hours

Time to Peak: Serum: Oral: Within 1.5-2 hours; I.V.: Within 1 hour

Metabolism: Hepatic (small amounts)

Formulations

Capsule: 200 mg
Injection, powder for reconstitution, as sodium: 500 mg, 1000 mg
Injection, solution, as sodium [preservative free]: 50 mg/mL (10 mL, 20 mL)
Ointment, topical: 5% (3 g, 15 g)
Suspension, oral: 200 mg/5 mL (480 mL) [banana flavor]
Tablet: 400 mg, 800 mg

(Continued)

Acyclovir *(Continued)*

Dosing

Adults & Elderly: Dosing weight should be based on the smaller of lean body weight or total body weight.

Treatment of herpes simplex virus infections:

HSV encephalitis: I.V.: 1500 mg/m^2/day divided every 8 hours or 10 mg/kg/dose for 10 days

Mucocutaneous HSV or severe initial herpes genitalis infection: I.V.: 750 mg/m^2/day divided every 8 hours or 5 mg/kg/dose every 8 hours for 5-10 days

Nonlife-threatening mucocutaneous HSV in immunocompromised patients: Topical: ½" ribbon of ointment for a 4" square surface area every 3 hours (6 times/day) for 7 days

Treatment of genital herpes simplex virus infections:

Oral: 200 mg every 4 hours while awake (5 times/day) for 10 days if initial episode; for 5 days if recurrence (begin at earliest signs of disease)

Topical: ½" ribbon of ointment for a 4" square surface area every 3 hours (6 times/day) for 7 days

Treatment of varicella-zoster virus (chickenpox) infections:

Oral: 600-800 mg/dose every 4 hours while awake (5 times/day) for 7-10 days or 1000 mg every 6 hours for 5 days

I.V.: 1500 mg/m^2/day divided every 8 hours or 10 mg/kg/dose every 8 hours for 7 days

Treatment of herpes zoster (shingles) infections in immunocompromised patients:

Oral: 800 mg every 4 hours (5 times/day) for 7-10 days

I.V.: 10 mg/kg/dose or 500 mg/m^2/dose every 8 hours

Older Adults (immunocompromised): 7.5 mg/kg/dose every 8 hours

If nephrotoxicity occurs: 5 mg/kg/dose every 8 hours

Prophylaxis in immunocompromised patients:

Varicella zoster or herpes zoster in HIV-positive patients: Oral: 400 mg every 4 hours (5 times/day) for 7-10 days

Bone marrow transplant recipients: I.V.:

Allogeneic patients who are HSV seropositive: 150 mg/m^2/dose (5 mg/kg) every 12 hours; with clinical symptoms of herpes simplex: 150 mg/m^2/dose every 8 hours

Allogeneic patients who are CMV seropositive: 500 mg/m^2/dose (10 mg/kg) every 8 hours; for clinically symptomatic CMV infection, consider replacing acyclovir with ganciclovir

Chronic suppressive therapy for recurrent genital herpes simplex virus infections:

Oral: 200 mg 3-4 times/day or 400 mg twice daily for up to 12 months, followed by re-evaluation

Pediatrics: Dosing weight should be based on the smaller of lean body weight or total body weight.

Treatment of herpes simplex virus infections: Children >12 years: I.V.: Refer to adult dosing.

Treatment of varicella-zoster virus (chickenpox) infections:

Oral: Children: 10-20 mg/kg/dose (up to 800 mg) 4 times/day for 5 days; begin treatment within the first 24 hours of rash onset

I.V.: Children: Refer to adult dosing.

Treatment of herpes zoster (shingles) infections:

Oral: Children (immunocompromised): 250-600 mg/m^2/dose 4-5 times/day for 7-10 days

I.V.: Children (immunocompromised): 10 mg/kg/dose or 500 mg/m^2/dose every 8 hours.

If nephrotoxicity occurs: 5 mg/kg/dose every 8 hours

Prophylaxis in immunocompromised patients: Bone marrow transplant recipients: Refer to adult dosing.

Renal Impairment:

Oral: HSV/varicella-zoster:

Cl_{cr} 10-25 mL/minute: Administer dose every 8 hours.

Cl_{cr} <10 mL/minute: Administer dose every 12 hours.

I.V.:

Cl_{cr} 25-50 mL/minute: 5-10 mg/kg/dose: Administer every 12 hours.

Cl_{cr} 10-25 mL/minute: 5-10 mg/kg/dose: Administer every 24 hours.

Cl_{cr} <10 mL/minute: 2.5-5 mg/kg/dose: Administer every 24 hours.

Dialyzable (50% to 100%); administer dose postdialysis.

Peritoneal dialysis effects: Dose as for Cl_{cr} <10 mL/minute.

Continuous arteriovenous or venovenous hemofiltration effects: Dose as for Cl_{cr} <10 mL/minute.

Administration

Oral: May be administered with food.

I.V.: For I.V. infusion only. Avoid rapid infusion. Infuse over 1 hour to prevent renal damage. Maintain adequate hydration of patient. Check for phlebitis and rotate infusion sites.

Stability

Storage: Reconstituted solutions remain stable for 24 hours at room temperature. Do not refrigerate reconstituted solutions as they may precipitate.

Reconstitution: Concentrations >10 mg/mL (usual recommended concentration is <7 mg/mL in D_5W) increase the risk of phlebitis.

Compatibility: Stable in D_5W, D_5NS, D_5¼NS, D_5½NS, LR, NS

Incompatible with blood products and protein-containing solutions

Y-site administration: Incompatible with amifostine, amsacrine, aztreonam, cefepime, dobutamine, dopamine, fludarabine, foscarnet, gemcitabine, idarubicin, levofloxacin, ondansetron, piperacillin/tazobactam, sargramostim, vinorelbine

Compatibility when admixed: Incompatible with dobutamine, dopamine

Monitoring Laboratory Tests

Urinalysis, BUN, serum creatinine, liver enzymes, CBC

Monitoring and Teaching Issues

Physical Assessment: See Warnings/Precautions and Contraindications for use cautions. Assess potential for interactions with other prescriptions, OTC, or herbal medications patient may be taking (see Drug Interactions). **I.V.:** See Reconstitution and Compatibility; monitor closely during infusion. Assess results of laboratory tests (see above), therapeutic effects, and adverse responses (see Adverse Reactions and Overdose/Toxicology). Teach patient appropriate use (if self-administered), possible side effects and appropriate interventions, and adverse symptoms to report (see Patient Education). **Pregnancy risk factor C** - benefits of use should outweigh possible risks.

Patient Education: Inform prescriber of all prescriptions, OTC medications, or herbal products you are taking, and any allergies you have. Do not take anything new during treatment (including creams, lotions, or ointments) unless approved by prescriber. This is not a cure for herpes (recurrences tend to continually reappear every 3-6 months after original infection), nor will this medication reduce the risk of transmission to others when lesions are present; avoid sexual intercourse when visible lesions are present. Take as directed for full course of therapy; do not discontinue even if feeling better. Oral doses may be taken with food. Maintain adequate hydration (2-3 L/day of fluids) unless advised by prescriber to restrict fluids. May cause nausea or vomiting (small, frequent meals, frequent mouth care, sucking lozenges, or chewing gum may help); lightheadedness or dizziness (use caution when driving or engaging in tasks that require alertness until response to drug is known); or headache, fever, muscle pain (consult prescriber for approved analgesic). Report any change in urination (difficulty urinating, dark colored or concentrated urine); persistent lethargy; acute headache; severe nausea or vomiting; confusion or hallucinations; rash; or difficulty breathing. **Pregnancy precaution:** Inform prescriber if you are or intend to become pregnant.

Topical: Apply as directed. Use gloves or finger cot when applying.

Dietary Issues: May be taken with food. Injection formulations have a sodium content of 1 g: 96.6 mg (4.2 mEq).

Geriatric Considerations: Calculate creatinine clearance. Dose adjustment may be necessary depending on renal function.

Adalat® CC *see* NIFEdipine *on page 970*

Adamantanamine Hydrochloride *see* Amantadine *on page 72*

Adapalene (a DAP a leen)

U.S. Brand Names Differin®

Generic Available No

Pharmacologic Category Acne Products

Pregnancy Risk Factor C

Lactation Excretion in breast milk unknown/use caution

Use Treatment of acne vulgaris

Mechanism of Action/Effect Retinoid-like compound which is a modulator of cellular differentiation, keratinization and inflammatory processes, all of which represent important features in the pathology of acne vulgaris

Contraindications Hypersensitivity to adapalene or any component in the vehicle gel

Warnings/Precautions Use with caution in patients with eczema. Avoid excessive exposure to sunlight and sunlamps. Avoid contact with abraded skin, mucous membranes, eyes, mouth, and angles of the nose. Pregnancy risk C.

Adverse Reactions

>10%: Dermatologic: Erythema, scaling, dryness, pruritus, burning, pruritus or burning immediately after application

≤1% (Limited to important or life-threatening): Acne flares, conjunctivitis, contact dermatitis, dermatitis, eczema, eyelid edema, skin discoloration, skin irritation, stinging sunburn, rash (topical cream)

Overdosage/Toxicology Toxic signs of overdose commonly respond to drug discontinuation, with spontaneous resolution in a few days to weeks. When confronted with signs of increased intracranial pressure, treatment with mannitol (0.25 g/kg I.V. up to 1 g/kg/dose repeated every 5 minutes as needed), dexamethasone (1.5 mg/kg I.V. load followed with 0.375 mg/kg every 6 hours for 5 days), and/or hyperventilation should be employed.

Pharmacodynamics/Kinetics

Absorption: Topical: Minimal

Formulations

Cream, topical: 0.1% (15 g, 45 g)

Gel, topical: 0.1% (15 g, 45 g) [alcohol free]

Pledget, topical: 0.1% (60s)

Solution, topical: 0.1% (30 mL)

Dosing

Adults & Elderly: Acne: Topical: Apply once daily before bedtime; results appear after 8-12 weeks of therapy.

Pediatrics: Children >12 years: Refer to adult dosing.

Monitoring and Teaching Issues

Physical Assessment: See Contraindications and Warnings/Precautions for use cautions. Assess knowledge/teach patient appropriate use and adverse symptoms to report (see Patient Education). **Pregnancy risk factor C** - benefits of use should outweigh possible risks. Note breast-feeding caution.

Patient Education: For external use only. Apply with gloves in thin film at night to thoroughly clean/dry skin; avoid area around eyes or mouth. Do not apply occlusive dressing. Results make take 8-12 weeks to appear. You may experience transient burning or stinging immediately after applying. Report worsening of condition or skin redness, dryness, peeling, or burning that persists between applications. **Pregnancy/breast-feeding precautions:** Inform prescriber if you are or intend to become pregnant. Consult prescriber if breast-feeding.

Adderall® *see* Dextroamphetamine and Amphetamine *on page 394*

Adderall XR™ *see* Dextroamphetamine and Amphetamine *on page 394*

Adefovir (a DEF o veer)

U.S. Brand Names Hepsera™

Synonyms Adefovir Dipivoxil

Generic Available No

Pharmacologic Category Antiretroviral Agent, Reverse Transcriptase Inhibitor (Nucleoside)

Pregnancy Risk Factor C

Lactation Excretion in breast milk unknown/not recommended

Use Treatment of chronic hepatitis B with evidence of active viral replication (based on persistent elevation of ALT/AST or histologic evidence), including patients with lamivudine-resistant hepatitis B

Mechanism of Action/Effect Acyclic nucleotide reverse transcriptase inhibitor which interferes with HBV viral DNA polymerase resulting in inhibition of viral replication

Contraindications Hypersensitivity to adefovir or any component of the formulation

Warnings/Precautions Use with caution in patients with renal dysfunction or in patients at risk of renal toxicity (including concurrent nephrotoxic agents or NSAIDs). Chronic administration may result in nephrotoxicity. Dosage adjustment is required in patients with renal dysfunction or in patients who develop renal dysfunction during therapy. May cause the development of resistance in patients with unrecognized or untreated HIV infection. Lactic acidosis and severe hepatomegaly with steatosis (sometimes fatal) have occurred with antiretroviral nucleoside analogues; female gender, obesity, and prolonged treatment may increase the risk of hepatotoxicity. Treatment should be discontinued in patients with lactic acidosis or signs/symptoms of hepatotoxicity (which may occur without marked transaminase elevations). Acute exacerbations of hepatitis may occur (in up to 25% of patients) when antihepatitis therapy is discontinued. Exacerbations typically occur within 12 weeks; monitor patients following discontinuation of therapy. Safety and efficacy in pediatric patients have not been established. Pregnancy risk C.

Drug Interactions

Increased Effect/Toxicity: Ibuprofen increases the bioavailability of adefovir. Concurrent use of nephrotoxic agents (including aminoglycosides, cyclosporine, NSAIDs, tacrolimus, vancomycin) may increase the risk of nephrotoxicity.

Nutritional/Ethanol Interactions

Ethanol: Should be avoided in hepatitis B infection due to potential hepatic toxicity.

Food: Does not have a significant effect on adefovir absorption.

Adverse Reactions

>10%: Renal: Hematuria (11% vs. 10% in placebo-treated)

1% to 10%:

Central nervous system: Fever, headache,

Dermatologic: Rash, pruritus

Gastrointestinal: Dyspepsia (3%), nausea, vomiting, flatulence, diarrhea, abdominal pain

Hepatic: AST/ALT increased, abnormal liver function, hepatic failure

Neuromuscular & skeletal: Weakness

Renal: Serum creatinine increased (4%), renal failure, renal insufficiency

Note: In patients with baseline renal dysfunction, frequency of increased serum creatinine has been observed to be as high as 26% to 37%; the role of adefovir in these changes could not be established.

Respiratory: Cough increased, sinusitis, pharyngitis

Overdosage/Toxicology Limited experience in acute overdose. Chronic overdose may be associated with renal toxicity and gastrointestinal adverse effects. Hemodialysis may be effective in the removal of adefovir (35% of a 10 mg dose removed in 4 hours).

Pharmacodynamics/Kinetics

Bioavailability: 59%

Half-Life Elimination: 7.5 hours; prolonged in renal impairment

Metabolism: Prodrug; rapidly converted to adefovir (active metabolite) in intestine

Formulations Tablet, as dipivoxil: 10 mg

Dosing

Adults & Elderly: Hepatitis B (chronic): Oral: 10 mg once daily

Renal Impairment:

Cl_{cr} 20-49 mL/minute: 10 mg every 48 hours

Cl_{cr} 10-19 mL/minute: 10 mg every 72 hours

Hemodialysis: 10 mg every 7 days (following dialysis)

Hepatic Impairment: Refer to adult dosing. No adjustment required.

Administration

Oral: May be administered without regard to food.

Stability

Storage: Store at 25°C (77 °F); excursions permitted to 15°C to 30°C (59°F to 86°F).

Monitoring Laboratory Tests HIV status (prior to initiation of therapy); serum creatinine (prior to initiation and during therapy)

Monitoring and Teaching Issues

Physical Assessment: See Warnings/Precautions and Dosing for use cautions. Assess potential for interactions with other prescriptions, OTC medications, or herbal products patient may be taking (see Drug Interactions). Assess results of laboratory tests (see above) and patient response on a regular basis throughout therapy (eg, altered hepatic status - see Warnings/Precautions, Adverse Reactions, and Overdose/Toxicology). Teach patient proper use, possible side effects and interventions, and adverse symptoms to report (see Patient Education). **Pregnancy risk factor C** - benefits of use should outweigh possible risks. Breast-feeding is not recommended.

Patient Education: Inform prescriber of all prescriptions, OTC medications, or herbal products you are taking, and any allergies you have. Do not take anything new during treatment without consulting prescriber (some medications may need to be avoided). Use appropriate precautions to prevent spread to other persons. Take as directed. Do not discontinue without consulting prescriber. You will require frequent blood tests; follow recommended schedule. Maintain adequate hydration (2-3 L/day of fluids) unless advised by prescriber to restrict fluids. You may be more susceptible to infection (avoid crowds and exposure to infection and do not have any vaccinations without consulting prescriber). May cause headache or abdominal pain (consult prescriber for approved analgesia); or nausea or vomiting (small, frequent meals, frequent mouth care, sucking lozenges, or chewing gum may help). Report unusual bleeding (blood in urine, tarry stools, or easy bruising); unresolved nausea or vomiting; signs of infection (eg, fever, chills, sore throat, burning urination, flu-like symptoms); persistent fatigue; muscle weakness; changes in urinary pattern; or other persistent adverse effects. **Pregnancy/breast-feeding precautions:** Inform prescriber if you are or intend to become pregnant. Breast-feeding is not recommended.

Dietary Issues: May be taken without regard to food.

Additional Information Adefovir dipivoxil is a prodrug, rapidly converted to the active component (adefovir). It was previously investigated as a treatment for HIV infections (at dosages substantially higher than the approved dose for hepatitis B). The NDA was withdrawn, and no further studies in the treatment of HIV are anticipated (per manufacturer).

Adefovir Dipivoxil *see* Adefovir *on page 46*

Adenine Arabinoside *see* Vidarabine *on page 1399*

Adenocard® *see* Adenosine *on page 47*

Adenoscan® *see* Adenosine *on page 47*

Adenosine (a DEN oh seen)

U.S. Brand Names Adenocard®; Adenoscan®

Synonyms 9-Beta-D-ribofuranosyladenine

Generic Available No

Pharmacologic Category Antiarrhythmic Agent, Class IV; Diagnostic Agent

Pregnancy Risk Factor C

Lactation Excretion in breast milk unknown

Use

Adenocard®: Treatment of paroxysmal supraventricular tachycardia (PSVT) including that associated with accessory bypass tracts (Wolff-Parkinson-White syndrome); when clinically advisable, appropriate vagal maneuvers should be attempted prior to adenosine administration; **not effective in atrial flutter, atrial fibrillation, or ventricular tachycardia**

Adenoscan®: Pharmacologic stress agent used in myocardial perfusion thallium-201 scintigraphy

Mechanism of Action/Effect Slows conduction time through the AV node and restores normal sinus rhythm

Contraindications Hypersensitivity to adenosine or any component of the formulation; second- or third-degree AV block or sick sinus syndrome (except in patients with a functioning artificial pacemaker), atrial flutter, atrial fibrillation, and ventricular tachycardia (this drug is not effective in converting these arrhythmias to sinus rhythm). The manufacturer states that Adenoscan® should be avoided in patients with known or suspected bronchoconstrictive or bronchospastic lung disease.

Warnings/Precautions Patients with pre-existing SA nodal dysfunction may experience prolonged sinus pauses after adenosine. There have been reports of atrial fibrillation/flutter in patients with PSVT associated with accessory conduction pathways after adenosine. Adenosine decreases conduction through the AV node and may produce a short-lasting first-, second-, or third-degree heart block. Because of the very short half-life, the effects are generally self-limiting. Rare, prolonged episodes of asystole have been reported, with fatal outcomes in some cases. At the time of conversion to normal sinus rhythm, a variety of new rhythms may appear on the EKG. A limited number of patients with asthma have received adenosine and have not experienced exacerbation of their asthma. Adenosine may cause bronchoconstriction in patients with asthma, and should be used cautiously in patients with obstructive lung disease not associated with bronchoconstriction (eg, emphysema, bronchitis). Pregnancy risk C.

Drug Interactions

Decreased Effect: Methylxanthines (eg, caffeine, theophylline) antagonize the effect of adenosine.

Increased Effect/Toxicity: Dipyridamole potentiates effects of adenosine. Use with carbamazepine may increase heart block.

Nutritional/Ethanol Interactions Food: Avoid food or drugs with caffeine. Adenosine's therapeutic effect may be decreased if used concurrently with caffeine.

Adverse Reactions

>10%:

Cardiovascular: Facial flushing (18%), palpitations, chest pain, hypotension
Central nervous system: Headache
Respiratory: Dyspnea (12%)
Miscellaneous: Diaphoresis

1% to 10%:

Central nervous system: Dizziness
Gastrointestinal: Nausea (3%)
Neuromuscular & skeletal: Paresthesia, numbness
Respiratory: Chest pressure (7%)

<1% (Limited to important or life-threatening): Dizziness, headache, hyperventilation, hypotension, intracranial pressure, lightheadedness

Overdosage/Toxicology Since adenosine half-life is <10 seconds, adverse effects are rapidly self-limiting. Treatment of prolonged effects requires individualization. Theophylline and other methylxanthines are competitive inhibitors of adenosine and may have a role in reversing its toxic effects.

Pharmacodynamics/Kinetics

Half-Life Elimination: <10 seconds

Metabolism: Blood and tissue to inosine then to adenosine monophosphate (AMP) and hypoxanthine

(Continued)

Adenosine *(Continued)*

Onset: Rapid

Duration: Very brief

Formulations Injection, solution [preservative free]:

Adenocard®: 3 mg/mL (2 mL, 4 mL)

Adenoscan®: 3 mg/mL (20 mL, 30 mL)

Dosing

Adults:

Paroxysmal supraventricular tachycardia (Adenocard®): I.V. (rapid - over 1-2 seconds, via peripheral line): 6 mg; if not effective within 1-2 minutes, 12 mg may be given; may repeat 12 mg bolus if needed; maximum single dose: 12 mg.

Follow each I.V. bolus of adenosine with normal saline flush.

Note: Patients who are receiving concomitant theophylline therapy may be less likely to respond to adenosine therapy. Higher doses may be needed for administration via peripheral versus central vein.

Note: Preliminary results in adults suggest adenosine may be administered via a central line at lower doses (ie, initial adult dose: 3 mg).

Pharmacologic stress agent (Adenoscan®): I.V.: Continuous I.V. infusion via peripheral line: 140 mcg/kg/minute for 6 minutes using syringe or columetric infusion pump; total dose: 0.84 mg/kg. Thallium-201 is injected at midpoint (3 minutes) of infusion.

Elderly: Refer to adult dosing. Elderly may be more sensitive to effects of adenosine.

Pediatrics: Rapid I.V. push (over 1-2 seconds) via peripheral line:

Neonates: Initial dose: 0.05 mg/kg; if not effective within 2 minutes, increase dose by 0.05 mg/kg increments every 2 minutes to a maximum dose of 0.25 mg/kg or until termination of PSVT.

Maximum single dose: 12 mg

Infants and Children: Pediatric advanced life support (PALS): Treatment of SVT: 0.1 mg/kg; if not effective, administer 0.2 mg/kg.

Alternatively: Initial dose: 0.05 mg/kg; if not effective within 2 minutes, increase dose by 0.05 mg/kg increments every 2 minutes to a maximum dose of 0.25 mg/kg or until termination of PSVT; medium dose required: 0.15 mg/kg.

Maximum single dose: 12 mg

Administration

I.V.: For rapid bolus I.V. use only. Administer I.V. push over 1-2 seconds at a peripheral I.V. site as proximal as possible to trunk (ie, not in lower arm, hand, lower leg, or foot).

Stability

Storage: Do **not** refrigerate, precipitation may occur (may dissolve by warming to room temperature).

Compatibility: Stable in D_5LR, D_5W, LR, NS

Monitoring and Teaching Issues

Physical Assessment: Assess other medications patient may be taking for effectiveness and interactions (see Drug Interactions). Requires use of infusion pump and continuous cardiac and hemodynamic monitoring during infusion. Monitor for adverse reactions (see Warnings/Precautions and Adverse Reactions). Note that adenosine could produce bronchoconstriction in patients with asthma (see Warnings/Precautions). **Pregnancy risk factor C.**

Patient Education: Adenosine is administered in emergencies, patient education should be appropriate to the situation.

Geriatric Considerations: Geriatric patients may be more sensitive to the effects of this medication.

Other Issues: Confirm labeling before administration. **Do not use adenosine phosphate (given I.M. for symptomatic relief of varicose veins complications). Have emergency resuscitation and equipment available when using this drug.**

Related Information

Antiarrhythmic Drugs *on page 1551*

ADH *see* Vasopressin *on page 1391*

Adoxa™ *see* Doxycycline *on page 450*

ADR *see* DOXOrubicin *on page 446*

Adrenalin® *see* Epinephrine *on page 470*

Adrenaline *see* Epinephrine *on page 470*

Adriamycin PFS® *see* DOXOrubicin *on page 446*

Adriamycin RDF® *see* DOXOrubicin *on page 446*

Adrucil® *see* Fluorouracil *on page 576*

Adsorbent Charcoal *see* Charcoal *on page 266*

Advair™ Diskus® *see* Fluticasone and Salmeterol *on page 591*

Advil® [OTC] *see* Ibuprofen *on page 688*

Advil® Children's [OTC] *see* Ibuprofen *on page 688*

Advil® Infants' Concentrated Drops [OTC] *see* Ibuprofen *on page 688*

Advil® Junior [OTC] *see* Ibuprofen *on page 688*

Advil® Migraine [OTC] *see* Ibuprofen *on page 688*

AeroBid® *see* Flunisolide *on page 572*

AeroBid®-M *see* Flunisolide *on page 572*

Aerolate III® *see* Theophylline *on page 1300*

Aerolate JR® *see* Theophylline *on page 1300*

Aerolate SR® *see* Theophylline *on page 1300*

Agenerase® *see* Amprenavir *on page 104*

Aggrastat® *see* Tirofiban *on page 1327*

Aggrenox™ *see* Aspirin and Dipyridamole *on page 124*

AHF (Human) *see* Antihemophilic Factor (Human) *on page 109*

Albendazole (al BEN da zole)

U.S. Brand Names Albenza®

Generic Available No

Pharmacologic Category Anthelmintic

Pregnancy Risk Factor C

Lactation Excretion in breast milk unknown/not recommended

Use Treatment of parenchymal neurocysticercosis and cystic hydatid disease of the liver, lung, and peritoneum; albendazole has activity against *Ascaris lumbricoides* (roundworm), *Ancylostoma duodenale* and *Necator americanus* (hookworms), *Enterobius vermicularis* (pinworm), *Hymenolepis nana* and *Taenia* sp (tapeworms), *Opisthorchis sinensis* and *Opisthorchis viverrini* (liver flukes), *Strongyloides stercoralis* and *Trichuris trichiura* (whipworm); activity has also been shown against the liver fluke *Clonorchis sinensis, Giardia lamblia, Cysticercus cellulosae, Echinococcus granulosus, Echinococcus multilocularis*, and *Toxocara* sp.

Mechanism of Action/Effect Active metabolite, albendazole, causes selective degeneration of cytoplasmic microtubules in intestinal and tegmental cells of intestinal helminths and larvae; glycogen is depleted, glucose uptake and cholinesterase secretion are impaired, and desecratory substances accumulate intracellulary. ATP production decreases causing energy depletion, immobilization, and worm death.

Contraindications Hypersensitivity to albendazole or any component of the formulation

Warnings/Precautions Corticosteroids should be administered 1-2 days before albendazole therapy in patients with neurocysticercosis to minimize inflammatory reactions; anticonvulsant therapy should be used concurrently for the first week of therapy to prevent cerebral hypertension. Discontinue therapy if LFT elevations are significant; may restart treatment when decreased to pretreatment values. If retinal lesions exist in patients with neurocysticercosis, weigh risk of further retinal damage due to albendazole-induced changes to the retinal lesion vs benefit of disease treatment. Pregnancy risk C.

Drug Interactions

Cytochrome P450 Effect: Substrate of CYP1A2, 3A4; Inhibits CYP1A2

Decreased Effect: Cimetidine may increase albendazole metabolism.

Increased Effect/Toxicity: Albendazole serum levels are increased when taken with dexamethasone, praziquantel.

Nutritional/Ethanol Interactions Food: Albendazole serum levels may be increased if taken with a fatty meal (increases the oral bioavailability by 4-5 times).

Adverse Reactions N = neurocysticercosis; H = hydatid disease

(Continued)

Albendazole *(Continued)*

Central nervous system: Dizziness, vertigo, fever (≤1%); headache (11% - N; 1% - H); increased intracranial pressure

Dermatologic: Alopecia/rash/urticaria (<1%)

Gastrointestinal: Abdominal pain (6% - H, 0% - N); nausea/vomiting (3% to 6%)

Hematologic: Leukopenia (reversible) (<1%); granulocytopenia/agranulocytopenia/pancytopenia (rare)

Hepatic: Increased LFTs (~15% - H, <1% - N)

Miscellaneous: Allergic reactions (<1%)

Pharmacodynamics/Kinetics

Absorption: <5%; may increase up to 4-5 times when administered with a fatty meal

Half-Life Elimination: 8-12 hours

Time to Peak: Serum: 2-2.4 hours

Metabolism: Hepatic; extensive first-pass effect; pathways include rapid sulfoxidation (major), hydrolysis, and oxidation

Formulations Tablet: 200 mg

Dosing

Adults & Elderly:

Neurocysticercosis: Oral:

<60 kg: 15 mg/kg/day in 2 divided doses (maximum: 800 mg/day) with meals for 8-30 days

≥60 kg: 400 mg twice daily for 8-30 days

Note: Give concurrent anticonvulsant and steroid therapy during first week.

Giardiasis: 400 mg/day for 3 days

Hydatid: Oral:

<60 kg: 15 mg/kg/day in 2 divided doses with meals (maximum: 800 mg/day) for three 28-day cycles with 14-day drug-free interval in-between

≥60 kg: 400 mg twice daily for 3 cycles as above

Strongyloidiasis/tapeworm: Oral: 400 mg/day for 3 days; may repeat in 3 weeks

Hookworm, pinworm, roundworm: Oral: 400 mg as a single dose; may repeat in 3 weeks

Pediatrics:

Neurocysticercosis, Hydatid: Refer to adult dosing.

Strongyloidiasis/tapeworm: Oral: Children >2 years: 400 mg/day for 3 days; may repeat in 3 weeks

Hookworm, pinworm, roundworm: Oral: Children >2 years: 400 mg as a single dose; may repeat in 3 weeks

Monitoring and Teaching Issues

Physical Assessment: See Warnings/Precautions for pretreatment suggestions. Assess potential for interactions with other prescriptions, OTC medications, or herbal products patient may be taking (see Drug Interactions). Assess therapeutic effectiveness and adverse reactions (see Adverse Reactions). Teach patient appropriate use, possible side effects and interventions, and adverse symptoms to report (see Patient Education). **Pregnancy risk factor C** - benefits of use should outweigh possible risks. Breast-feeding is not recommended.

Patient Education: Inform prescriber of all prescriptions, OTC medications, or herbal products you are taking, and any allergies you have. Do not take anything new during treatment unless approved by prescriber. Take as directed, with meals. Follow prescriber's suggestions to prevent reinfection. May cause loss of hair (reversible); nausea or vomiting (small, frequent meals, frequent mouth care, sucking lozenges, or chewing gum may help); or dizziness or headaches (use caution when driving or engaging in tasks that require alertness until response to drug is known). Report unusual fever, persistent or unresolved abdominal pain, vomiting, yellowing of skin or eyes, darkening of urine, or light colored stools. **Pregnancy/breast-feeding precautions:** Inform prescriber if you are or intend to become pregnant. Breast-feeding is not recommended.

Pregnancy Issues: Albendazole has been shown to be teratogenic in laboratory animals and should not be used during pregnancy, if at all possible.

Albenza® *see* Albendazole *on page 49*

Albumarc® *see* Albumin *on page 50*

Albumin (al BYOO min)

U.S. Brand Names Albumarc®; Albuminar®; Albutein®; Buminate®; Plasbumin®

Synonyms Albumin (Human); Normal Human Serum Albumin; Normal Serum Albumin (Human); Salt Poor Albumin; SPA

Generic Available Yes

Pharmacologic Category Blood Product Derivative; Plasma Volume Expander, Colloid

Pregnancy Risk Factor C

Lactation Excretion in breast milk unknown/compatible

Use Plasma volume expansion and maintenance of cardiac output in the treatment of certain types of shock or impending shock; may be useful for burn patients, ARDS, and cardiopulmonary bypass; other uses considered by some investigators (but not proven) are retroperitoneal surgery, peritonitis, and ascites; unless the condition responsible for hypoproteinemia can be corrected, albumin can provide only symptomatic relief or supportive treatment

Use - Unlabeled/Investigational In cirrhotics, administered with diuretics to help facilitate diuresis; large volume paracentesis; volume expansion in dehydrated, mildly-hypotensive cirrhotics

Mechanism of Action/Effect Restores plasma volume

Contraindications Hypersensitivity to albumin or any component of the formulation; patients with severe anemia or cardiac failure

Warnings/Precautions Use with caution in patients with hepatic or renal failure because of added protein load; rapid infusion of albumin solutions may cause vascular overload. All patients should be observed for signs of hypervolemia such as pulmonary edema. Use with caution in those patients for whom sodium restriction is necessary. Avoid 25% concentration in preterm infants due to risk of intraventricular hemorrhage. Nutritional supplementation is not an appropriate indication for albumin. Pregnancy risk C.

Drug Interactions

Increased Effect/Toxicity: ACE inhibitors: May have increased risk of atypical reactions; withhold ACEIs for at least 24 hours prior to plasma exchanges using large volumes of albumin

Adverse Reactions Frequency not defined.

Cardiovascular: CHF precipitation, edema, hypertension, hypervolemia, hypotension, tachycardia

Central nervous system: Chills, fever, headache

Dermatologic: Pruritus, rash, urticaria

Gastrointestinal: Nausea, vomiting

Respiratory: Bronchospasm, pulmonary edema

Miscellaneous: Anaphylaxis

Overdosage/Toxicology Symptoms of overdose include hypervolemia, congestive heart failure, and pulmonary edema.

Formulations Injection, solution, human: 5% [50 mg/mL] (50 mL, 250 mL, 500 mL); 25% [250 mg/mL] (50 mL, 100 mL)

Albumarc®: 5% [50 mg/mL] (250 mL, 500 mL); 25% [250 mg/mL] (50 mL, 100 mL)

Albuminar®: 5% [50 mg/mL] (50 mL, 250 mL, 500 mL, 1000 mL); 25% [250 mg/mL] (20 mL, 50 mL, 100 mL)

Albutein®, Buminate®: 5% [50 mg/mL]: (250 mL, 500 mL); 25% [250 mg/mL] (20 mL, 50 mL, 100 mL)

Plasbumin®: 5% [50 mg/mL] (50 mL, 250 mL, 500 mL); 20% [200 mg/mL] (50 mL); 25% [250 mg/mL] (20 mL, 50 mL, 100 mL)

Dosing

Adults & Elderly:

Note: Use **5%** solution in hypovolemic patients or intravascularly-depleted patients. Use **25%** solution in patients in whom fluid and sodium intake is restricted.

Usual dose (**depends on patient's condition**): 25 g; initial dose may be repeated in 15-30 minutes if response is inadequate; no more than 250 g should be administered within 48 hours.

Hypoproteinemia: I.V.: 0.5-1 g/kg/dose; repeat every 1-2 days as calculated to replace ongoing losses.

Hypovolemia: I.V.: 0.5-1 g/kg/dose; repeat as needed; maximum: 6 g/kg/day.

Pediatrics:

Note: 5% should be used in hypovolemic patients or intravascularly-depleted patients. **25%** should be used in patients in whom fluid and sodium intake must be minimized.

Volume expansion: **Dose depends on condition of patient:** I.V.: Children:

Emergency initial dose: 25 g

Nonemergencies: 25% to 50% of the adult dose

Administration

I.V.: For I.V. administration only. Use within 4 hours after opening vial; discard unused portion. In emergencies, may administer as rapidly as necessary to improve clinical condition. After initial volume replacement:

5%: Do not exceed 2-4 mL/minute in patients with normal plasma volume; 5-10 mL/minute in patients with hypoproteinemia

25%: Do not exceed 1 mL/minute in patients with normal plasma volume; 2-3 mL/minute in patients with hypoproteinemia

Stability

Storage: Store at a temperature ≤30°C (86°F); do not freeze. Do not use solution if it is turbid or contains a deposit; use within 4 hours after opening vial; discard unused portion.

Reconstitution: If 5% human albumin is unavailable, it may be prepared by diluting 25% human albumin with 0.9% sodium chloride or 5% dextrose in water. Do not use sterile water to dilute albumin solutions, as this has been associated with hypotonic-associated hemolysis.

Compatibility: Stable in dextran 6% in D_5W, dextran 6% in NS, D_5LR, D_5NS, $D_5{}^1/_2NS$, $D_5{}^1/_4NS$, D_5W, $D_{10}W$, LR, NS, $^1/_2NS$; **incompatible** with sterile water

Y-site administration: Incompatible with midazolam, vancomycin, verapamil

Compatibility when admixed: Incompatible with verapamil

Monitoring Laboratory Tests Hematocrit

Monitoring and Teaching Issues

Physical Assessment: See Contraindications and Warnings/Precautions for use cautions. See Administration and Reconstitution for appropriate administration. Vital signs, central venous pressure, and fluid balance (intake/output) should be monitored closely during administration with frequent assessment for hypovolemia or fluid overload (see Adverse Reactions and Overdose/Toxicology). If adverse reactions (eg, fever, tachycardia, hypotension, or dyspnea) occur, infusion should be stopped and prescriber notified. **Pregnancy risk factor C** - benefits of use should outweigh possible risks.

Patient Education: Education is provided as appropriate for patient condition. This medication can only be administered intravenously. You will be monitored closely during the infusion. **Pregnancy precaution:** Inform prescriber if you are pregnant.

Additional Information Both 5% and 25% albumin have a sodium concentration of 130-160 mEq/L. There is no risk of hepatitis because albumin is heated to 60°C for 10 hours. Currently, there is no known risk for AIDS.

5% albumin is isotonic; 25% albumin is hypertonic (1500 mOsm/L); dilution of 25% albumin with sterile water can produce hemolysis/renal failure; shelf-life: 3-5 years

Albuminar® *see* Albumin *on page 50*

Albumin (Human) *see* Albumin *on page 50*

Albutein® *see* Albumin *on page 50*

Albuterol (al BYOO ter ole)

U.S. Brand Names AccuNeb™; Proventil®; Proventil® HFA; Proventil® Repetabs®; Ventolin®; Ventolin® HFA; Volmax®

Synonyms Salbutamol

Generic Available Yes

Pharmacologic Category $Beta_2$ Agonist

Pregnancy Risk Factor C

Lactation Excretion in breast milk unknown/use caution

Use Bronchodilator in reversible airway obstruction due to asthma or COPD; prevention of exercise-induced bronchospasm

Mechanism of Action/Effect Relaxes bronchial smooth muscle by action on $beta_2$-receptors with little effect on heart rate

Contraindications Hypersensitivity to albuterol, adrenergic amines, or any component of the formulation

Warnings/Precautions Use with caution in patients with hyperthyroidism, diabetes mellitus, sensitivity to sympathomimetic amines, or with cardiovascular disorders including coronary insufficiency or hypertension. Excessive use may result in tolerance. Pregnancy risk C.

Drug Interactions

Cytochrome P450 Effect: Substrate of **CYP3A4**

Decreased Effect: When used with nonselective beta-adrenergic blockers (eg, propranolol) the effect of albuterol is decreased.

Increased Effect/Toxicity: When used with inhaled ipratropium, an increased duration of bronchodilation may occur. Cardiovascular effects are potentiated in patients also receiving MAO inhibitors, tricyclic antidepressants, and sympathomimetic agents (eg, amphetamine, dopamine, dobutamine). Albuterol may increase the risk of malignant arrhythmias with inhaled anesthetics (eg, enflurane, halothane).

Nutritional/Ethanol Interactions

Food: Avoid or limit caffeine (may cause CNS stimulation).

Herb/Nutraceutical: Avoid ephedra, yohimbe (may cause CNS stimulation).

Effects on Lab Values ↑ renin (S), aldosterone (S)

Adverse Reactions Incidence of adverse effects is dependent upon age of patient, dose, and route of administration.

Cardiovascular: Angina, atrial fibrillation, chest discomfort, extrasystoles, flushing, hypertension, palpitations, tachycardia

Central nervous system: CNS stimulation, dizziness, drowsiness, headache, insomnia, irritability, lightheadedness, migraine, nervousness, nightmares, restlessness, sleeplessness, tremor

Dermatologic: Angioedema, erythema multiforme, rash, Stevens-Johnson syndrome, urticaria

Endocrine & metabolic: Hypokalemia

Gastrointestinal: Diarrhea, dry mouth, gastroenteritis, nausea, unusual taste, vomiting, tooth discoloration

Genitourinary: Micturition difficulty

Neuromuscular & skeletal: Muscle cramps, weakness

Otic: Otitis media, vertigo

Respiratory: Asthma exacerbation, bronchospasm, cough, epistaxis, laryngitis, oropharyngeal drying/irritation, oropharyngeal edema

Miscellaneous: Allergic reaction, lymphadenopathy

Overdosage/Toxicology Symptoms of overdose include hypertension, tachycardia, angina, and hypokalemia. Treatment of hypokalemia and tachyarrhythmias consists of prudent use of a cardioselective beta-adrenergic blocker (eg, atenolol or metoprolol), keeping in mind the potential for induction of bronchoconstriction in an asthmatic individual. Dialysis has not been shown to be of value in the treatment of overdose with albuterol.

Pharmacodynamics/Kinetics

Half-Life Elimination: Inhalation: 3.8 hours; Oral: 3.7-5 hours

Metabolism: Hepatic to an inactive sulfate

Onset: Peak effect: Nebulization/oral inhalation: 0.5-2 hours; Oral: 2-3 hours

Duration: Nebulization/oral inhalation: 3-4 hours; Oral: 4-6 hours

Formulations

Aerosol, oral: 90 mcg/dose (17 g) [200 doses]
- Proventil®: 90 mcg/dose (17 g) [200 doses]
- Ventolin®: 90 mcg/dose (6.8 g) [80 doses] [DSC]; (17 g) [200 doses]

Aerosol, oral, as sulfate [chlorofluorocarbon free]:
- Proventil® HFA: 90 mcg/dose (6.7 g) [200 doses]
- Ventolin® HFA: 90 mcg/dose (18 g) [200 doses]

Solution for oral inhalation, as sulfate: 0.083% (3 mL); 0.5% (20 mL)
- AccuNeb™: 0.63 mg/3 mL (5 vials/pouch); 1.25 mg/3 mL (5 vials/pouch)
- Proventil®: 0.083% (3 mL); 0.5% (20 mL)

Syrup, as sulfate: 2 mg/5 mL (120 mL, 480 mL)
- Ventolin® [DSC]: 2 mg/5 mL (480 mL) [alcohol and sugar free; strawberry flavor]

Tablet, as sulfate: 2 mg, 4 mg

Tablet, extended release, as sulfate:
- Proventil® Repetabs®: 4 mg
- Volmax®: 4 mg, 8 mg

Dosing

Adults:

Bronchospasm (treatment):

Oral: 2-4 mg/dose 3-4 times/day; maximum dose not to exceed 32 mg/day (divided doses)

Extended release: 8 mg every 12 hours; maximum dose not to exceed 32 mg/day (divided doses). A 4 mg dose every 12 hours may be sufficient in some patients, such as adults of low body weight.

Inhalation:
MDI: 90 mcg/spray: 1-2 inhalations every 4-6 hours; maximum: 12 inhalations/day
Capsule: 200-400 mcg every 4-6 hours
Nebulization: 2.5 mg, diluted to a total of 3 mL, 3-4 times/day over 5-15 minutes
Bronchospasm (acute): Asthma exacerbation in intensive care patients: 2.5-5 mg every 20 minutes for 3 doses, then 2.5-10 mg every 1-4 hours as needed, **or** 10-15 mg/hour continuously
Bronchospasm (prophylaxis of exercise-induced): Inhalation:
MDI-CFC aerosol: 2 inhalations 15 minutes before exercising
MDI-HFA aerosol: 2 inhalations 15-30 minutes before exercise
Capsule: 200 mcg 15 minutes before exercise

Elderly:
Inhalation: Refer to adult dosing.
Oral: 2 mg 3-4 times/day; maximum: 8 mg 4 times/day

Pediatrics:
Bronchospasm (treatment):
Oral:
2-6 years: 0.1-0.2 mg/kg/dose 3 times/day; maximum dose not to exceed 12 mg/day (divided doses)
6-12 years: 2 mg/dose 3-4 times/day; maximum dose not to exceed 24 mg/day (divided doses)
Extended release: 4 mg every 12 hours; maximum dose not to exceed 24 mg/day (divided doses)
>12 years: Refer to adult dosing.
Inhalation: ≥4 years:
MDI: 90 mcg/spray: 1-2 inhalations every 4-6 hours; some patients may respond to 1 inhalation every 4 hours
Capsule: 200-400 mcg every 4-6 hours
Nebulization: 0.01-0.05 mL/kg of 0.5% solution every 4-6 hours
2-12 years: AccuNeb™: 0.63 mg or 1.25 mg 3-4 times/day, as needed, delivered over 5-15 minutes
Children >40 kg, patients with more severe asthma, or children 11-12 years: May respond better with a 1.25 mg dose
Bronchospasm (acute): Nebulization: 0.01-0.05 mL/kg of 0.5% solution every 4-6 hours; intensive care patients may require more frequent administration; minimum dose: 0.1 mL; maximum dose: 1 mL diluted in 1-2 mL normal saline; continuous nebulized albuterol at 0.3 mg/kg/hour has been used safely in the treatment of severe status asthmaticus in children; continuous nebulized doses of 3 mg/kg/hour ± 2.2 mg/kg/hour in children whose mean age was 20.7 months resulted in no cardiac toxicity; the optimal dosage for continuous nebulization remains to be determined.
Prophylaxis of exercise-induced bronchospasm: ≥4 years: Inhalation:
MDI-CFC aerosol: 2 inhalations 15 minutes before exercising
MDI-HFA aerosol: 2 inhalations 15-30 minutes before exercise
Capsule: 200 mcg 15 minutes before exercise

Renal Impairment: Not removed by hemodialysis

Administration

Oral: Volmax®: Do not crush or chew.

Inhalation: MDI: Shake well before use; prime prior to first use, and whenever inhaler has not been used for >2 weeks, by releasing 4 test sprays into the air (away from face)

Stability

Storage:
Syrup, nebulization 0.5% solution: Store at 2°C to 30°C (36°F to 86°F)
HFA aerosols: Store at 15°C to 25°C (59°F to 77°F)
Ventolin® HFA: Discard after using 200 actuations or 3 months after removal from protective pouch, whichever comes first. Store with mouthpiece down.
Inhalation solution: AccuNeb™: Store at 2°C to 25°C (36°F to 77°F). Do not use if solution changes color or becomes cloudy. Use within 1 week of opening foil pouch.

Reconstitution: Nebulization 0.5% solution: To prepare a 2.5 mg dose, dilute 0.5 mL of solution to a total of 3 mL with normal saline; also compatible with cromolyn or ipratropium nebulizer solutions.

Monitoring Laboratory Tests Arterial or capillary blood gases (if patients condition warrants)

Monitoring and Teaching Issues

Physical Assessment: Assess effectiveness and interactions of other medications patient may be taking (see Drug Interactions). See Contraindications and Warnings/Precautions for use cautions. Monitor vital signs, effectiveness of therapy, and adverse reactions (see Adverse Reactions) at beginning of therapy and periodically with long-term use. Assess knowledge/teach patient appropriate use, interventions to reduce side effects, and adverse symptoms to report (see Patient Education). **Pregnancy risk factor C** - benefits of use should outweigh possible risks. Note breast-feeding caution.

Patient Education: Use exactly as directed; do not use more often than recommended. Take oral medicine with water 1 hour before or 2 hours after meals. Maintain adequate hydration (2-3 L/day of fluids) unless advised by prescriber to restrict fluids. You may experience nervousness, dizziness, or fatigue (use caution when driving or engaging in hazardous activities until response to drug is known); dry mouth, unpleasant taste, stomach upset (frequent, small meals, frequent mouth care, chewing gum, or sucking lozenges may help); or difficulty urinating (always void before treatment). Report unresolved GI upset, dizziness or fatigue, vision changes, chest pain or palpitations, persistent inability to void, nervousness or insomnia, muscle cramping or tremor, or unusual cough. **Pregnancy/breast-feeding precautions:** Inform prescriber if you are or intend to become pregnant. Consult prescriber if breast-feeding.

Self-administered inhalation: Do not freeze. Shake canister before using. Sit when using medication. Close eyes when administering albuterol to avoid spray getting into eyes.

(Continued)

Albuterol *(Continued)*

Exhale slowly and completely through nose; inhale deeply through mouth while administering aerosol. Hold breath for 5-10 seconds after inhalation. Wait at least 1 full minute between inhalations. Wash mouthpiece between use. If more than one inhalation medication is used, use albuterol first and wait 5 minutes between medications. Prime inhaler prior to first use, and whenever the inhaler has not been used for more than 2 weeks, by releasing 4 test sprays into the air (away from face). Discard inhaler after labeled number of doses are used, even if the canister does not feel empty. **Ventolin® HFA:** Discard canister after 200 actuations or 3 months after removal from foil pouch, whichever comes first. Store with mouthpiece down. Do not allow metal canister to become wet.

Self-administered nebulizer: Wash hands before and after treatment. Wash and dry nebulizer after each treatment. Twist open the top of one unit dose vial and squeeze contents into nebulizer reservoir. Connect nebulizer reservoir to the mouthpiece or face mask. Connect nebulizer to compressor. Sit in comfortable, upright position. Place mouthpiece in your mouth or put on face mask and turn on compressor. If face mask is used, avoid leakage around the mask to avoid mist getting into eyes which may cause vision problems. Breathe calmly and deeply until no more mist is formed in nebulizer (about 5 minutes). At this point treatment is finished.

Volmax®: Tablets should be swallowed whole; do not crush or chew. Outer coating of tablet is not absorbed and may be found eliminated in stool.

Dietary Issues: Oral forms should be administered with water 1 hour before or 2 hours after meals.

Geriatric Considerations: Because of its minimal effect on beta$_1$-receptors and its relatively long duration of action, albuterol is a rational choice in the elderly when a beta agonist is indicated. Elderly patients may find it beneficial to utilize a spacer device when using a metered dose inhaler. The Ventolin Rotahaler® is an alternative for patients who have difficulty using the metered dose inhaler. Oral use should be avoided due to adverse effects.

Related Information

Inhalant (Asthma, Bronchospasm) Agents Comparison *on page 1577*

Albuterol and Ipratropium *see* Ipratropium and Albuterol *on page 735*

Alcaine® *see page 1461*

Alclometasone *see* Topical Corticosteroids *on page 1334*

Alcohol and Hydrocortisone *see page 1519*

Alcohol, Ethyl *see page 1460*

Alconefrin® Nasal [OTC] *see* Phenylephrine *on page 1071*

Aldactazide® *see* Hydrochlorothiazide and Spironolactone *on page 666*

Aldactone® *see* Spironolactone *on page 1244*

Aldara™ *see* Imiquimod *on page 702*

Aldesleukin (al des LOO kin)

U.S. Brand Names Proleukin®

Synonyms Epidermal Thymocyte Activating Factor; ETAF; IL-2; Interleukin-2; Lymphocyte Mitogenic Factor; NSC-373364; T-Cell Growth Factor; TCGF; Thymocyte Stimulating Factor

Generic Available No

Pharmacologic Category Biological Response Modulator

Pregnancy Risk Factor C

Lactation Enters breast milk/contraindicated

Use Treatment of metastatic renal cell cancer, melanoma

Use - Unlabeled/Investigational Investigational: Multiple myeloma, HIV infection, and AIDS; may be used in conjunction with lymphokine-activated killer (LAK) cells, tumor-infiltrating lymphocyte (TIL) cells, interleukin-1, and interferons; colorectal cancer; non-Hodgkin's lymphoma

Mechanism of Action/Effect IL-2 promotes proliferation, differentiation, and recruitment of T and B cells, natural killer (NK) cells, and thymocytes; IL-2 also causes cytolytic activity in a subset of lymphocytes and subsequent interactions between the immune system and malignant cells; IL-2 can stimulate lymphokine-activated killer (LAK) cells and tumor-infiltrating lymphocytes (TIL) cells. LAK cells (which are derived from lymphocytes from a patient and incubated in IL-2) have the ability to lyse cells which are resistant to NK cells; TIL cells (which are derived from cancerous tissue from a patient and incubated in IL-2) have been shown to be 50% more effective than LAK cells.

Contraindications Hypersensitivity to aldesleukin or any component of the formulation; patients with abnormal thallium stress or pulmonary function tests; patients who have had an organ allograft; retreatment in patients who have experienced sustained ventricular tachycardia (≥5 beats), refractory cardiac rhythm disturbances, recurrent chest pain with EKG changes consistent with angina or myocardial infarction, intubation ≥72 hours, pericardial tamponade, renal dialysis for ≥72 hours, coma or toxic psychosis lasting ≥48 hours, repetitive or refractory seizures, bowel ischemia/perforation, GI bleeding requiring surgery

Warnings/Precautions Has been associated with capillary leak syndrome (CLS). CLS results in hypotension and reduced organ perfusion which may be severe and can result in death. Therapy should be restricted to patients with normal cardiac and pulmonary functions as defined by thallium stress and formal pulmonary function testing. Extreme caution should be used in patients with normal thallium stress tests and pulmonary functions tests who have a history of prior cardiac or pulmonary disease.

Intensive aldesleukin treatment is associated with impaired neutrophil function (reduced chemotaxis) and with an increased risk of disseminated infection, including sepsis and bacterial endocarditis, in treated patients. Consequently, pre-existing bacterial infections should be adequately treated prior to initiation of therapy. Additionally, all patients with indwelling central lines should receive antibiotic prophylaxis effective against *S. aureus.*

May exacerbate pre-existing or initial presentation of autoimmune diseases and inflammatory disorders. Patients should be evaluated and treated for CNS metastases and have a negative scan prior to treatment. Mental status changes (irritability, confusion, depression) can occur and may indicate bacteremia, hypoperfusion, CNS malignancy, or CNS toxicity.

Disseminated infections acquired in the course of treatment are a major contributor to treatment morbidity and use of antibiotic prophylaxis, and aggressive treatment of suspected and documented infections may reduce the morbidity of aldesleukin treatment.

Pregnancy risk C.

Drug Interactions

Decreased Effect: Corticosteroids have been shown to decrease toxicity of IL-2, but have not been used since there is concern that they may reduce the efficacy of the lymphokine.

Increased Effect/Toxicity: Aldesleukin may affect central nervous function; therefore, interactions could occur following concomitant administration of psychotropic drugs (eg, narcotics, analgesics, antiemetics, sedatives, tranquilizers).

Concomitant administration of drugs possessing nephrotoxic (eg, aminoglycosides, indomethacin), myelotoxic (eg, cytotoxic chemotherapy), cardiotoxic (eg, doxorubicin), or hepatotoxic (eg, methotrexate, asparaginase) effects with aldesleukin may increase toxicity in these organ systems. The safety and efficacy of aldesleukin in combination with chemotherapies has not been established.

Beta-blockers and other antihypertensives may potentiate the hypotension seen with aldesleukin.

Nutritional/Ethanol Interactions Ethanol: Avoid ethanol (due to CNS adverse effects)

Adverse Reactions

>10%:

Cardiovascular: Sensory dysfunction, sinus tachycardia, arrhythmias, pulmonary congestion; hypotension (dose-limiting toxicity) which may require vasopressor support and hemodynamic changes resembling those seen in septic shock can be seen within 2 hours of administration; chest pain, acute myocardial infarction, SVT with hypotension has been reported, edema

Central nervous system: Dizziness, pain, fever, chills, cognitive changes, fatigue, malaise, disorientation, somnolence, paranoid delusion, and other behavioral changes; reversible and dose related; however, may continue to worsen for several days even after the infusion is stopped

Dermatologic: Pruritus, erythema, rash, dry skin, exfoliative dermatitis, macular erythema

Gastrointestinal: Nausea, vomiting, weight gain, diarrhea, stomatitis, anorexia, GI bleeding

Hematologic: Anemia, thrombocytopenia, leukopenia, eosinophilia, coagulation disorders

Hepatic: Elevated transaminase and alkaline phosphatase, jaundice

Neuromuscular & skeletal: Weakness, rigors which can be decreased or ameliorated with acetaminophen or a nonsteroidal agent and meperidine

Renal: Oliguria, anuria, proteinuria; renal failure (dose-limiting toxicity) manifested as oliguria noted within 24-48 hours of initiation of therapy; marked fluid retention, azotemia, and increased serum creatinine seen, which may return to baseline within 7 days of discontinuation of therapy; hypophosphatemia

Respiratory: Dyspnea, pulmonary edema

1% to 10%: Cardiovascular: Increase in vascular permeability: Capillary-leak syndrome manifested by severe peripheral edema, ascites, pulmonary infiltration, and pleural effusion; occurs in 2% to 4% of patients and is resolved after therapy ends

<1% (Limited to important or life-threatening): Alopecia, coma, CHF, pancreatitis, polyuria, seizure

Overdosage/Toxicology Side effects following the use of aldesleukin are dose related. Administration of more than the recommended dose has been associated with a more rapid onset of expected dose-limiting toxicities. Adverse reactions generally will reverse when the drug is stopped particularly because of its short serum half-life. Provide supportive treatment of any continuing symptoms. Life-threatening toxicities have been ameliorated by the I.V. administration of dexamethasone, but may result in a less than therapeutic effect of aldesleukin.

Pharmacodynamics/Kinetics

Bioavailability: I.M.: 37%

Half-Life Elimination: Initial: 6-13 minutes; Terminal: 80-120 minutes

Formulations Injection, powder for reconstitution: 22 x 10^6 int. units [18 million int. units/mL = 1.1 mg/mL when reconstituted]

Dosing

Adults & Elderly: Refer to individual protocols; all orders must be written in million International units (million int. units).

Renal cell carcinoma: I.V.: 600,000 int. units/kg every 8 hours for a maximum of 14 doses; repeat after 9 days of rest for a total of 28 doses per course. Re-evaluate at 4 weeks. Retreat if needed 7 weeks after hospital discharge from previous course.

Melanoma: I.V.:

Single-agent use: As in renal cell carcinoma

In combination with cytotoxic agents: 24 million int. units/m^2 days 12-16 and 19-23

S.C.:

Single-agent doses: 3-18 million int. units/day for 5 days weekly and repeated weekly up to 6 weeks

In combination with interferon:

5 million int. units/m^2 3 times/week

1.8 million int. units/m^2 twice daily 5 days/week for 6 weeks

Dose modification: In high-dose therapy of RCC, see manufacturer's guidelines for holding and restarting therapy; hold or interrupt a dose - **do not dose reduce**; or refer to specific protocol.

Retreatment: Patients should be evaluated for response approximately 4 weeks after completion of a course of therapy and again immediately prior to the scheduled start of the next treatment course; additional courses of treatment may be given to patients

(Continued)

Aldesleukin *(Continued)*

only if there is some tumor shrinkage or stable disease following the last course and retreatment is not contraindicated. Each treatment course should be separated by a rest period of at least 7 weeks from the date of hospital discharge; tumors have continued to regress up to 12 months following the initiation of therapy

Investigational regimen: S.C.: 11 million int. units (flat dose) daily x 4 days per week for 4 consecutive weeks; repeat every 6 weeks

Administration

I.V.: Infuse over 15 minutes. Administer in D_5W only; incompatible with sodium chloride solutions.

Stability

Storage: Store vials of lyophilized injection in a refrigerator at 2°C to 8°C (36°F to 46°F).

Reconstitution: Reconstituted or diluted solution should be refrigerated. Gently swirl, do not shake.

Concentrations <30 mcg/mL **OR** concentrations between ≥30-70 mcg/mL for infusion via ambulatory infusion pump require addition of albumin (final albumin concentration: 0.1%), see table.

Final Dilution Concentration (mcg/mL)	Final Dilution Concentration (10^6 int. units/mL)	Stability
<30	<0.49	Albumin must be added to bag **prior to addition** of aldesleukin at a final concentration of 0.1% (1 mg/mL) albumin; stable at room temperature or at ≥32°C (89°F) for 6 days*†
≥30 to ≤70	≥0.49 to ≤1.1	Stable at room temperature at 6 days without albumin added or at ≥32°C (89°F) for 6 days only if albumin is added (0.1%)*†
70-100	1.2-1.6	Unstable; avoid use
>100-500	1.7-8.2	Stable at room temperature and at ≥32°C (89°F) for 6 days*†

*These solutions do not contain a preservative; use for more than 24 hours may not be advisable.

†Continuous infusion via ambulatory infusion device raises aldesleukin to this temperature.

Note: As with most biological proteins, solutions containing IL-2 should not be filtered; filtration will result in significant loss of bioactivity.

Compatibility: Stable in D_5W

Y-site administration: Incompatible with ganciclovir, lorazepam, pentamidine, prochlorperazine edisylate, promethazine

Compatibility when admixed: Incompatible with NS

Monitoring Laboratory Tests The following clinical evaluations are recommended for all patients prior to beginning treatment and then daily during drug administration: Standard hematologic tests including CBC, differential, and platelet counts; blood chemistries including electrolytes, renal and hepatic function; chest x-rays.

Monitoring and Teaching Issues

Physical Assessment: See Contraindications, Warnings/Precautions, and Dosing for use cautions. Assess potential for interactions with other prescriptions, OTC medications, or herbal products patient may be taking (see Drug Interactions). See I.V. specifics above. Infusion site should be monitored for extravasation. Vital signs; cardiac, respiratory, and CNS status; fluid balance; and laboratory reports (see above) should be assessed daily prior to beginning infusion and for 2 hours following infusion (see Adverse Reactions and Overdose/Toxicology). Teach patient possible side effects and appropriate interventions and adverse symptoms to report (see Patient Education). **Pregnancy risk factor C** - benefits of use should outweigh possible risks. Breast-feeding is contraindicated.

Patient Education: Inform prescriber of all prescriptions, OTC medications, or herbal products you are taking, and any allergies you have. Do not take anything new during treatment unless approved by prescriber. This drug can only be administered by infusion. Avoid alcohol. Maintain adequate hydration (2-3 L/day of fluids) unless advised by prescriber to restrict fluids. You will be susceptible to infection (avoid crowds and exposure to infection and do not have any vaccinations without consulting prescriber). May cause increased sensitivity to sunlight (use sunblock 15 SPF or greater, wear protective clothing, avoid direct sun exposure); or nausea, vomiting, stomatitis, anorexia (frequent mouth care, small, frequent meals, chewing gum, or sucking lozenges may help). This drug may result in many side effects; you will be monitored and assessed closely during therapy, however, it is important that you report any changes or problems for evaluation. Report any changes in urination, unusual bruising or bleeding, chest pain or palpitations, acute dizziness, difficulty breathing, fever or chills, changes in cognition, rash, feelings of pain or numbness in extremities, severe or persistent GI upset or diarrhea, vaginal discharge or mouth sores, yellowing of eyes or skin, or changes in color of urine or stool. **Pregnancy/breast-feeding precautions:** Inform prescriber if you are pregnant. Do not breast-feed.

Additional Information

1 Cetus unit = 6 int. units

1.1 mg = 18 x 10^6 int. units (or 3 x 10^6 Cetus units)

1 Roche unit (Teceleukin) = 3 int. units

Reimbursement Hotline: 1-800-775-7533

Professional Services: 1-800-244-7668

Aldomet® *see* Methyldopa *on page 879*

Aldoril® *see* Methyldopa and Hydrochlorothiazide *on page 881*

Alendronate (a LEN droe nate)

U.S. Brand Names Fosamax®

Synonyms Alendronate Sodium

Generic Available No

Pharmacologic Category Bisphosphonate Derivative

Pregnancy Risk Factor C

Lactation Excretion in breast milk unknown/use caution

Use Treatment and prevention of osteoporosis in postmenopausal females; treatment of osteoporosis in males; Paget's disease of the bone in patients who are symptomatic, at risk for future complications, or with alkaline phosphatase ≥2 times the upper limit of normal; treatment of glucocorticoid-induced osteoporosis in males and females with low bone mineral density who are receiving a daily dosage ≥7.5 mg of prednisone (or equivalent)

Mechanism of Action/Effect Inhibits bone resorption via actions on osteoclasts or precursors; decreases the rate of bone resorption, leading to an indirect decrease in bone formation. Effects may be enhanced by concurrent estrogen replacement therapy.

Contraindications Hypersensitivity to alendronate, other bisphosphonates, or any component of the formulation; hypocalcemia; abnormalities of the esophagus which delay esophageal emptying such as stricture or achalasia; inability to stand or sit upright for at least 30 minutes

Warnings/Precautions Use caution in patients with renal impairment; hypocalcemia must be corrected before therapy initiation; ensure adequate calcium and vitamin D intake. May cause irritation to upper gastrointestinal mucosa. Esophagitis, esophageal ulcers, esophageal erosions, and esophageal stricture (rare) have been reported; risk increases in patients unable to comply with dosing instructions. Use with caution in patients with dysphagia, esophageal disease, gastritis, duodenitis, or ulcers (may worsen underlying condition). Pregnancy risk C.

Drug Interactions

Decreased Effect: Oral medications (especially those containing multivalent cations, including calcium and antacids): May interfere with alendronate absorption; wait at least 30 minutes after taking alendronate before taking any oral medications

Increased Effect/Toxicity: I.V. ranitidine has been shown to double the bioavailability of alendronate. Estrogen replacement therapy, in combination with alendronate, may enhance the therapeutic effects of both agents on the maintenance of bone mineralization. An increased incidence of adverse GI effects has been noted when >10 mg alendronate is used in patients taking aspirin-containing products.

Nutritional/Ethanol Interactions Food: All food and beverages interfere with absorption. Coadministration with caffeine may reduce alendronate efficacy. Coadministration with dairy products may decrease alendronate absorption. Beverages (especially orange juice and coffee), food, and medications (eg, antacids, calcium, iron, and multivalent cations) may reduce the absorption of alendronate as much as 60%.

Adverse Reactions Note: Incidence of adverse effects increases significantly in patients treated for Paget's disease at 40 mg/day, mostly GI adverse effects.

>10%: Endocrine & metabolic: Hypocalcemia (transient, mild, 18%); hypophosphatemia (transient, mild, 10%)

1% to 10%:

Central nervous system: Headache (0.2% to 3%)

Gastrointestinal: Abdominal pain (1% to 7%), acid reflux (1% to 5%), dyspepsia (1% to 4%), nausea (1% to 4%), flatulence (0.2% to 4%), diarrhea (0.6% to 3%), constipation (0.3% to 3%), esophageal ulcer (0.1% to 2%), abdominal distension (0.2% to 1%), gastritis (0.2% to 1%), vomiting (0.2% to 1%), dysphagia (0.1% to 1%), gastric ulcer (1%), melena (1%)

Neuromuscular & skeletal: Musculoskeletal pain (0.4% to 4%), muscle cramps (0.2% to 1%)

<1% (Limited to important or life-threatening): Angioedema, duodenal ulcer, esophageal erosions, esophageal perforation, esophageal stricture, esophagitis, hypersensitivity reactions, oropharyngeal ulceration, rash, taste perversion, urticaria, uveitis

Overdosage/Toxicology Symptoms of overdose include hypocalcemia, hypophosphatemia, and upper GI adverse affects (eg, upset stomach, heartburn, esophagitis, gastritis, or ulcer). Treat with milk or antacids to bind alendronate. Dialysis would not be beneficial.

Pharmacodynamics/Kinetics

Bioavailability: Fasting: Female: 0.7%; Male: 0.6%; reduced 60% with food or drink

Half-Life Elimination: Exceeds 10 years

Metabolism: None

Formulations Tablet, as sodium: 5 mg, 10 mg, 35 mg, 40 mg, 70 mg

Dosing

Adults & Elderly:

Note: Alendronate must be taken with a full glass (6-8 oz) of plain water first thing in the morning and ≥30 minutes before the first food, beverage, or other medication of the day. Patients should be instructed to stay upright (not to lie down) for at least 30 minutes **and** until after first food of the day (to reduce esophageal irritation). Patients should receive supplemental calcium and vitamin D if dietary intake is inadequate.

Osteoporosis in postmenopausal females: Oral:

Prophylaxis: 5 mg once daily or 35 mg once weekly

Treatment: 10 mg once daily or 70 mg once weekly

Osteoporosis in males: Oral: 10 mg once daily **or** 70 mg once weekly

Paget's disease of bone: Oral: 40 mg once daily for 6 months

Retreatment: Relapses during the 12 months following therapy occurred in 9% of patients who responded to treatment. Specific retreatment data are not available. Retreatment with alendronate may be considered, following a 6-month post-treatment evaluation period, in patients who have relapsed based on increases in serum alkaline phosphatase, which should be measured periodically. Retreatment may also be considered in those who failed to normalize their serum alkaline phosphatase.

Glucocorticoid-induced osteoporosis: Oral: 5 mg once daily; a dose of 10 mg once daily should be used in postmenopausal females who are not receiving estrogen. Patients treated with glucocorticoids should receive adequate amounts of calcium and vitamin D.

Renal Impairment:

Cl_{cr} 35-60 mL/minute: None necessary.

Cl_{cr} <35 mL/minute: Alendronate is not recommended due to lack of experience.

(Continued)

Alendronate *(Continued)*

Hepatic Impairment: No adjustment necessary.

Administration

Oral: Take with a full glass of water (6-8 oz) at least 30 minutes before any food, beverage, or medication. Avoid lying down for at least 30 minutes thereafter.

Stability

Storage: Store at room temperature, 15°C to 30°C (59°F to 86°F). Keep in well-closed container.

Monitoring Laboratory Tests Alkaline phosphatase should be periodically measured; serum calcium and phosphorus; monitor pain and fracture rate; hormonal status (male and female) prior to therapy; bone mineral density (should be done prior to initiation of therapy and after 6-12 months of combined glucocorticoid and alendronate treatment)

Monitoring and Teaching Issues

Physical Assessment: See Contraindications and Warnings/Precautions for use cautions. Assess results of laboratory tests (see above), effectiveness of treatment, and development of adverse reactions (see Adverse Reactions and Overdose/Toxicology). Teach appropriate use and administration of medications (see Administration), lifestyle and dietary changes that will have a beneficial impact on Paget's disease or osteoporosis, possible side effects and interventions, and adverse reactions to report. **Pregnancy risk factor C** - benefits of use should outweigh possible risks. Note breast-feeding caution.

Patient Education: Inform prescriber of all prescriptions, OTC medications, or herbal products you are taking, and any allergies you have. Do not take anything new during treatment unless approved by prescriber. Take as directed, with a full glass of water first thing in the morning and at least 30 minutes before the first food or beverage of the day. Wait at least 30 minutes after taking alendronate before taking anything else. Stay in sitting or standing position for 30 minutes following administration and until after the first food of the day to reduce potential for esophageal irritation. Consult prescriber to determine necessity of lifestyle changes (eg, decreased smoking, decreased alcohol intake, dietary supplements of calcium, or increased dietary vitamin D). May cause GI upset (eg, flatulence, bloating, nausea, acid regurgitation); small, frequent meals may help. Report acute headache or gastric pain, unresolved GI upset, or acid stomach. **Pregnancy/breast-feeding precautions:** Inform prescriber if you are or intend to become pregnant. Consult prescriber if breast-feeding.

Dietary Issues: Ensure adequate calcium and vitamin D intake; however, wait at least 30 minutes after taking alendronate before taking any supplement. Must be taken with plain water first thing in the morning and at least 30 minutes before the first food or beverage of the day.

Geriatric Considerations: Since many elderly patients receive diuretics, evaluation of electrolyte status (calcium, phosphate, magnesium, potassium) may need to be done periodically due to the drug class (bisphosphonate). Should assure immobile patients are at least sitting up for 30 minutes after swallowing tablets. Drink a full glass of water with each dose.

Related Information

Osteoporosis Management *on page 1696*

Alendronate Sodium *see* Alendronate *on page 56*

Aler-Dryl [OTC] *see* DiphenhydrAMINE *on page 422*

Alesse® *see* Ethinyl Estradiol and Levonorgestrel *on page 523*

Aleve® [OTC] *see* Naproxen *on page 948*

Alfentanil *see page 1583*

Alglucerase (al GLOO ser ase)

U.S. Brand Names Ceredase®

Synonyms Glucocerebrosidase

Generic Available No

Pharmacologic Category Enzyme

Pregnancy Risk Factor C

Lactation Excretion in breast milk unknown/use caution

Use Orphan drug: Replacement therapy for Gaucher's disease (type 1)

Mechanism of Action/Effect Replaces the missing enzyme, glucocerebrosidase associated with Gaucher's disease

Contraindications Hypersensitivity to alglucerase or any component of the formulation

Warnings/Precautions Prepared from pooled human placental tissue that may contain the causative agents of some viral diseases. Pregnancy risk C.

Adverse Reactions

>10%: Local: Discomfort, burning, and edema at the site of injection

<1% (Limited to important or life-threatening): Abdominal discomfort, nausea, vomiting

Overdosage/Toxicology No obvious toxicity has been detected after single doses up to 234 units/kg.

Pharmacodynamics/Kinetics

Half-Life Elimination: ~4-20 minutes

Formulations Injection, solution: 10 units/mL (5 mL); 80 units/mL (5 mL)

Dosing

Adults & Elderly: Gaucher's disease: I.V.: Usually administered as a 20-60 units/kg I.V. infusion given with a frequency ranging from 3 times/week to once every 2 weeks. Schedule determined by patient's response to therapy.

Pediatrics: Refer to adult dosing.

Administration

I.V.: Infuse over 1-2 hours.

Stability

Storage: Refrigerate (4°C), do not freeze. Contains no preservatives. Do not store opened vials for future use.

Monitoring Laboratory Tests CBC, platelets, acid phosphatase (AP), plasma glucocerebroside

Monitoring and Teaching Issues

Physical Assessment: See Contraindications and Warnings/Precautions for use cautions. Note infusion specifics above. Assess results of laboratory tests (see above) and therapeutic response (eg, energy level, change in bleeding tendency, reduced joint swelling, or bone pain). Teach patient possible side effects/appropriate interventions and adverse symptoms to report (see Patient Education). **Pregnancy risk factor C** - benefits of use should outweigh possible risks. Note breast-feeding caution.

Patient Education: Inform prescriber of all prescriptions, OTC medications, or herbal products you are taking, and any allergies you have. Do not add anything new during treatment unless approved by prescriber. This medication will not cure Gaucher's disease, but rather, will help control it; treatment is required for life. May cause abdominal discomfort, nausea, or vomiting (small, frequent meals, good mouth care, chewing gum, or sucking lozenges may help); these symptoms should go away with continued use. Inform prescriber if pain, swelling, or redness occurs at injection site or if GI symptoms persist. **Pregnancy/breast-feeding precautions:** Inform prescriber if you are or intend to become pregnant. Consult prescriber if breast-feeding.

Alitretinoin (a li TRET i noyn)

U.S. Brand Names Panretin®

Generic Available No

Pharmacologic Category Antineoplastic Agent, Miscellaneous

Pregnancy Risk Factor D

Lactation Excretion in breast milk unknown/not recommended

Use Orphan drug: Topical treatment of cutaneous lesions in AIDS-related Kaposi's sarcoma; not indicated when systemic therapy for Kaposi's sarcoma is indicated

Mechanism of Action/Effect Binds to retinoid receptors to inhibit growth of Kaposi's sarcoma

Contraindications Hypersensitivity to alitretinoin, other retinoids, or any component of the formulation; pregnancy

Warnings/Precautions Patients with cutaneous T-cell lymphoma have a high incidence of treatment-limiting adverse reactions. Do not use concurrently with topical products containing DEET (a common component of insect repellent products); increased toxicity may result. A common component of insect repellent products. Safety in pediatric patients or geriatric patients has not been established.

Drug Interactions

Increased Effect/Toxicity: Increased toxicity of DEET may occur if products containing this compound are used concurrently with alitretinoin. Due to limited absorption after topical application, interaction with systemic medications is unlikely.

Adverse Reactions

>10%:

- Central nervous system: Pain (0% to 34%)
- Dermatologic: Rash (25% to 77%), pruritus (8% to 11%)
- Neuromuscular & skeletal: Paresthesia (3% to 22%)

5% to 10%:

- Cardiovascular: Edema (3% to 8%)
- Dermatologic: Exfoliative dermatitis (3% to 9%), skin disorder (0% to 8%)

Overdosage/Toxicology There has been no experience with human overdosage of alitretinoin, and overdose is unlikely following topical application. Treatment is symptomatic and supportive.

Pharmacodynamics/Kinetics

Absorption: Not extensive

Formulations Gel: 0.1% (60 g tube)

Dosing

Adults & Elderly: Kaposi's sarcoma: Topical: Apply gel twice daily to cutaneous lesions.

Stability

Storage: Store at room temperature.

Monitoring and Teaching Issues

Physical Assessment: See Contraindications, Warnings/Precautions, and Drug Interactions for use cautions. Assess effectiveness of therapy and adverse reactions at beginning and periodically during therapy. Teach patient appropriate use and adverse symptoms to report (see Patient Education). **Pregnancy risk factor D** - determine that patient is not pregnant before beginning treatment. Teach patients of childbearing age appropriate use of barrier contraceptives. Breast-feeding is not recommended.

Patient Education: For external use only. Use exactly as directed; do not overuse. Avoid use of any product such as insect repellents which contain DEET (check with your pharmacist). Wear protective clothing and/or avoid exposure to direct sun or sunlamps. Wash hands thoroughly before applying. Avoid applying skin products that contain alcohol or harsh chemicals during treatment. Do not apply occlusive dressings. Stop treatment and inform prescriber if rash, skin irritation, redness, scaling, or excessive dryness appears. **Pregnancy/breast-feeding precautions:** Do not get pregnant while taking this medication. Consult prescriber for appropriate contraceptive measures. Breast-feeding is not recommended.

Breast-feeding Issues: Excretion in human breast milk is unknown; women are advised to discontinue breast-feeding prior to using this medication.

Pregnancy Issues: Potentially teratogenic and/or embryotoxic; limb, craniofacial, or skeletal defects have been observed in animal models. If used during pregnancy or if the patient becomes pregnant while using alitretinoin, the woman should be advised of potential harm to the fetus. Women of childbearing potential should avoid becoming pregnant.

Alka-Mints® [OTC] *see* Calcium Supplements *on page 202*

Alkeran® *see* Melphalan *on page 848*

Allegra® *see* Fexofenadine *on page 556*
Allegra-D® *see* Fexofenadine and Pseudoephedrine *on page 557*
Allerest® [OTC] *see page 1509*
Allergan® *see page 1519*
Allergan® Ear Drops *see page 1522*
AllerMax® [OTC] *see* DiphenhydrAMINE *on page 422*

Allopurinol (al oh PURE i nole)

U.S. Brand Names Aloprim™; Zyloprim®

Synonyms Allopurinol Sodium Injection

Generic Available Yes

Pharmacologic Category Xanthine Oxidase Inhibitor

Pregnancy Risk Factor C

Lactation Enters breast milk/compatible

Use

Oral: Prevention of attack of gouty arthritis and nephropathy; treatment of secondary hyperuricemia which may occur during treatment of tumors or leukemia; prevention of recurrent calcium oxalate calculi

Orphan drug: I.V.: Management of patients with leukemia, lymphoma, and solid tumor malignancies who are receiving cancer chemotherapy which causes elevations of serum and urinary uric acid levels and who cannot tolerate oral therapy

Mechanism of Action/Effect Allopurinol inhibits xanthine oxidase, the enzyme responsible for the conversion of hypoxanthine to xanthine to uric acid. Allopurinol is metabolized to oxypurinol which is also an inhibitor of xanthine oxidase; allopurinol acts on purine catabolism, reducing the production of uric acid without disrupting the biosynthesis of vital purines.

Contraindications Hypersensitivity to allopurinol or any component of the formulation

Warnings/Precautions Do not use to treat asymptomatic hyperuricemia. Discontinue at first signs of rash. Reduce dosage in renal insufficiency. Reinstate with caution in patients who have had a previous mild allergic reaction. Monitor liver function and complete blood counts before initiating therapy and periodically during therapy. Use with caution in patients taking diuretics concurrently. Risk of skin rash may be increased in patients receiving amoxicillin or ampicillin. The risk of hypersensitivity may be increased in patients receiving thiazides, and possibly ACE inhibitors. Pregnancy risk C.

Drug Interactions

Decreased Effect: Ethanol decreases effectiveness.

Increased Effect/Toxicity: Allopurinol may increase the effects of azathioprine, chlorpropamide, mercaptopurine, theophylline, and oral anticoagulants. An increased risk of bone marrow suppression may occur when given with myelosuppressive agents (cyclophosphamide, possibly other alkylating agents). Amoxicillin/ampicillin, ACE inhibitors, and thiazide diuretics have been associated with hypersensitivity reactions when combined with allopurinol (rare), and the incidence of rash may be increased with penicillins (ampicillin, amoxicillin). Urinary acidification with large amounts of vitamin C may increase kidney stone formation.

Nutritional/Ethanol Interactions Ethanol: Avoid ethanol (may decrease effectiveness).

Adverse Reactions The most common adverse reaction to allopurinol is a skin rash (usually maculopapular; however, more severe reactions, including Stevens-Johnson syndrome, have also been reported). While some studies cite an incidence of these reactions as high as >10% of cases (often in association with ampicillin or amoxicillin), the product labeling cites a much lower incidence, reflected below. Allopurinol should be discontinued at the first appearance of a rash or other sign of hypersensitivity.

>1%:

Dermatologic: Rash (1.5%)
Gastrointestinal: Nausea (1.3%), vomiting (1.2%)
Renal: Renal failure/impairment (1.2%)

<1% (Limited to important or life-threatening): Acute tubular necrosis, agranulocytosis, angioedema, aplastic anemia, bronchospasm, cataracts, exfoliative dermatitis, granuloma annulare, granulomatous hepatitis, hypersensitivity syndrome, interstitial nephritis, macular retinitis, nephrolithiasis, neuritis, pancreatitis, paresthesia, peripheral neuropathy, Stevens-Johnson syndrome, toxic epidermal necrolysis, toxic pustuloderma, vasculitis

Overdosage/Toxicology If significant amounts of allopurinol have been absorbed, it is theoretically possible that oxypurinol stones could form, but no record of such occurrence exists. Alkalinization of urine and forced diuresis can help prevent potential xanthine stone formation.

Pharmacodynamics/Kinetics

Absorption: Oral: ~80%; Rectal: Poor and erratic

Bioavailability: 49% to 53%

Half-Life Elimination:

Normal renal function: Parent drug: 1-3 hours; Oxypurinol: 18-30 hours
End-stage renal disease: Prolonged

Time to Peak: Plasma: Oral: 30-120 minutes

Metabolism: ~75% to active metabolites, chiefly oxypurinol

Onset: Peak effect: 1-2 weeks

Formulations

Injection, powder for reconstitution, as sodium (Aloprim™): 500 mg
Tablet (Zyloprim®): 100 mg, 300 mg

Dosing

Adults:

Gout: Oral:
Mild: 200-300 mg/day; Severe: 400-600 mg/day

Prevention of hyperuricemia in myeloproliferative neoplastic disorders:
Oral: 600-800 mg/day in 2-3 divided doses for prevention of acute uric acid nephropathy for 2-3 days starting 1-2 days before chemotherapy

I.V.: 200-400 mg/m²/day (maximum: 600 mg/day)

Note: Intravenous daily dose can be given as a single infusion or in equally divided doses at 6-, 8-, or 12-hour intervals. A fluid intake sufficient to yield a daily urinary output of at least 2 L in adults and the maintenance of a neutral or, preferably, slightly alkaline urine are desirable.

Elderly: Oral: Initial: 100 mg/day; increase until desired uric acid level is obtained. Refer to adult dosing.

Pediatrics:

Hyperuricemia in treatment of myeloproliferative neoplastic disorders:

Oral: Children ≤10 years: 10 mg/kg/day in 2-3 divided doses **or** 200-300 mg/m²/day in 2-4 divided doses, maximum: 800 mg/24 hours, for prevention of acute uric acid nephropathy (begin 1-2 days before chemotherapy)

Alternative:

<6 years: 150 mg/day in 3 divided doses

6-10 years: 300 mg/day in 2-3 divided doses

>10 years: Daily doses >300 mg should be administered in divided doses.

I.V.: Starting dose: 200 mg/m²/day

Renal Impairment:

Oral:

Must be adjusted due to accumulation of allopurinol and metabolites; see table.

Adult Maintenance Doses of Allopurinol*

Creatinine Clearance (mL/min)	Maintenance Dose of Allopurinol (mg)
140	400 qd
120	350 qd
100	300 qd
80	250 qd
60	200 qd
40	150 qd
20	100 qd
10	100 q2d
0	100 q3d

*This table is based on a standard maintenance dose of 300 mg of allopurinol per day for a patient with a creatinine clearance of 100 mL/min.

Hemodialysis: Administer dose after hemodialysis or administer 50% supplemental dose.

I.V.:

Cl_{cr} 10-20 mL/minute: Administer 200 mg/day.

Cl_{cr} 3-10 mL/minute: Administer 100 mg/day.

Cl_{cr} <3 mL/minute: Administer 100 mg/day at extended intervals.

Administration

Oral: Should be administered after meals.

I.V.: The rate of infusion depends on the volume of the infusion. Whenever possible, therapy should be initiated at 24-48 hours before the start of chemotherapy known to cause tumor lysis (including adrenocorticosteroids). I.V. daily dose can be administered as a single infusion or in equally divided doses at 6-, 8-, or 12-hour intervals at the recommended final concentration of ≤6 mg/mL.

Stability

Storage: Intravenous solutions should be stored at 20°C to 25°C. Do not refrigerate reconstituted and/or diluted product. Must be administered within 10 hours of solution preparation.

Reconstitution: Allopurinol injection must be reconstituted and diluted. Each 30 mL vial should be reconstituted with 25 mL sterile water for injection, USP. It may then be added to 0.9% sodium chloride injection to 5% dextrose for injection. A final concentration of no greater than 6 mg/mL is recommended.

Compatibility: Stable in D_5W, NS, sterile water for injection

Y-site administration: Incompatible with amikacin, amphotericin B, carmustine, cefotaxime, chlorpromazine, cimetidine, clindamycin, cytarabine, dacarbazine, daunorubicin, diphenhydramine, doxorubicin, doxycycline, droperidol, floxuridine, gentamicin, haloperidol, hydroxyzine, idarubicin, imipenem/cilastatin, mechlorethamine, meperidine, methylprednisolone sodium succinate, metoclopramide, minocycline, nalbuphine, netilmicin, ondansetron, prochlorperazine edisylate, promethazine, sodium bicarbonate, streptozocin, tobramycin, vinorelbine

Monitoring Laboratory Tests CBC, serum uric acid levels, hepatic and renal function, especially at start of therapy

Monitoring and Teaching Issues

Physical Assessment: Assess effectiveness and interactions of other medications patient may be taking (see Contraindications and Drug Interactions). Monitor laboratory values, effectiveness of therapy, and adverse reactions (see Adverse Reactions and Overdose/Toxicology) at beginning of therapy and periodically with long-term use. Assess knowledge/teach patient appropriate use, interventions to reduce side effects, and adverse symptoms to report (see Patient Education). **Pregnancy risk factor C** - benefits of use should outweigh possible risks.

Patient Education: Take as directed. Maintain adequate hydration (2-3 L/day of fluids) unless advised by prescriber to restrict fluids. While using this medication, do not use alcohol, other prescriptions, OTC medications, or vitamins without consulting prescriber. You may experience drowsiness (use caution when driving or engaging in tasks requiring alertness until response to drug is known); nausea, vomiting, or heartburn (small, frequent meals, frequent mouth care, chewing gum, or sucking lozenges may help); or hair loss

(Continued)

Allopurinol *(Continued)*

(reversible). Report skin rash or lesions; painful urination or blood in urine or stool; unresolved nausea or vomiting; numbness of extremities; pain or irritation of the eyes; swelling of lips, mouth, or tongue; unusual fatigue; easy bruising or bleeding; yellowing of skin or eyes; or any change in color of urine or stool. **Pregnancy precaution:** Inform prescriber if you are or intend to become pregnant.

Dietary Issues: Should administer oral forms after meals with plenty of fluid.

Geriatric Considerations: Adjust dose based on renal function.

Allopurinol Sodium Injection *see* Allopurinol *on page 60*

All-*trans*-Retinoic Acid *see* Tretinoin (Oral) *on page 1353*

Almotriptan (al moh TRIP tan)

U.S. Brand Names Axert™

Synonyms Almotriptan Malate

Generic Available No

Pharmacologic Category Serotonin 5-HT_{1D} Receptor Agonist

Pregnancy Risk Factor C

Lactation Excretion in breast milk unknown/use caution

Use Acute treatment of migraine with or without aura

Mechanism of Action/Effect The therapeutic effect for migraine is due to serotonin agonist activity.

Contraindications Hypersensitivity to almotriptan or any component of the formulation; use as prophylactic therapy for migraine; hemiplegic or basilar migraine; cluster headache; known or suspected ischemic heart disease (angina pectoris, MI, documented silent ischemia, coronary artery vasospasm, Prinzmetal's variant angina); peripheral vascular syndromes (including ischemic bowel disease); uncontrolled hypertension; use within 24 hours of another 5-HT_1 agonist; use within 24 hours of ergotamine derivative; concurrent administration or within 2 weeks of discontinuing an MAO inhibitor (specifically MAO type A inhibitors)

Warnings/Precautions Indicated for migraine headaches only. Not for patients with risk factors for coronary artery disease; need cardiac evaluation first. If patient's cardiovascular evaluation is good, healthcare provider should administer the first dose and cardiovascular status should be periodically evaluated. Vasospastic events may occur in the heart, peripheral vascular, or gastrointestinal system. Cerebral/subarachnoid hemorrhage, stroke, and hypertensive crisis have occurred. Use with caution in liver or renal dysfunction. Safety and efficacy in pediatric patients have not been established. Pregnancy risk C.

Drug Interactions

Cytochrome P450 Effect: Substrate of CYP2D6, 3A4

Increased Effect/Toxicity: Ergot-containing drugs prolong vasospastic reactions; ketoconazole and CYP3A4 inhibitors increase almotriptan serum concentration; select serotonin reuptake inhibitors may increase symptoms of hyper-reflexia, weakness, and incoordination; MAO inhibitors may increase toxicity

Adverse Reactions

1% to 10%:

Central nervous system: Headache (>1%), dizziness (>1%), somnolence (>1%)

Gastrointestinal: Nausea (1% to 2%), xerostomia (1%)

Neuromuscular & skeletal: Paresthesia (1%)

<1% (Limited to important or life-threatening): Colitis, coronary artery vasospasm, hypertension, myocardial ischemia, myocardial infarction, neuropathy, rash, syncope, tachycardia, ventricular fibrillation, ventricular tachycardia, vertigo

Overdosage/Toxicology Hypertension or more serious cardiovascular symptoms may occur. Clinical and electrocardiographic monitoring needed for at least 20 hours even if patient asymptomatic. Treatment is symptom-directed and supportive.

Pharmacodynamics/Kinetics

Absorption: Well absorbed

Bioavailability: 70%

Half-Life Elimination: 3-4 hours

Time to Peak: 1-3 hours

Metabolism: MAO type A oxidative deamination (~27% of dose); via CYP3A4 and 2D6 (~12% of dose) to inactive metabolites

Formulations Tablet, as malate: 6.25 mg, 12.5 mg

Dosing

Adults & Elderly: Migraine: Oral: Initial: 6.25-12.5 mg in a single dose; if the headache returns, repeat the dose after 2 hours; no more than 2 doses in 24-hour period

Note: If the first dose is ineffective, diagnosis needs to be re-evaluated. Safety of treating more than 4 migraines/month has not been established.

Renal Impairment: Initial: 6.25 mg in a single dose; maximum daily dose: ≤12.5 mg

Hepatic Impairment: Initial: 6.25 mg in a single dose; maximum daily dose: ≤12.5 mg

Stability

Storage: Store at 15°C to 30°C (59°F to 86°F).

Monitoring and Teaching Issues

Physical Assessment: See Contraindications, Warnings/Precautions (clear diagnosis of migraine), and Dosing for use cautions. Assess potential for interactions with other prescriptions, OTC medications, or herbal products patient may be taking (eg, ergot-containing drugs, MAO inhibitors - see Drug Interactions). Assess effectiveness and adverse response (see Adverse Reactions and Overdose/Toxicology). Teach patient proper use, possible side effects and appropriate interventions, and adverse symptoms to report (see Patient Education). **Pregnancy risk factor C** - benefits of use should outweigh possible risks. Note breast-feeding caution.

Patient Education: Inform prescriber of all prescriptions (including oral contraceptives), OTC medications, or herbal products you are taking, and any allergies you have. This drug is to be used to reduce your migraine, not to prevent or reduce the number of attacks.

Follow exact instructions for use. Do not use more than two doses in 24 hours and do not take within 24 hours of any other migraine medication without consulting prescriber. May cause dizziness, fatigue, or drowsiness (use caution when driving or engaging in tasks requiring alertness until response to drug is known). Report immediately any chest pain, palpitations, or throbbing; feelings of tightness or pressure in jaw or throat; acute headache or dizziness; muscle cramping, pain, or tremors; skin rash; hallucinations, anxiety, panic; or other adverse reactions. **Pregnancy/breast-feeding precautions:** Inform prescriber if you are or intend to become pregnant. Consult prescriber if breast-feeding.

Dietary Issues: May be taken without regard to meals

Almotriptan Malate *see* Almotriptan *on page 62*

Alocril™ *see page 1509*

Alocril™ *see* Nedocromil *on page 953*

Aloe Vesta® 2-n-1 Antifungal [OTC] *see* Miconazole *on page 899*

Alomide® *see page 1509*

Aloprim™ *see* Allopurinol *on page 60*

Alora® *see* Estradiol *on page 494*

Alphagan® [DSC] *see* Ophthalmic Agents, Glaucoma *on page 1002*

Alphagan® P *see* Ophthalmic Agents, Glaucoma *on page 1002*

Alphanate® *see* Antihemophilic Factor (Human) *on page 109*

Alphaquin HP *see* Hydroquinone *on page 679*

Alphatrex® *see* Betamethasone *on page 160*

Alphatrex® *see* Topical Corticosteroids *on page 1334*

Alprazolam (al PRAY zoe lam)

U.S. Brand Names Alprazolam Intensol®; Xanax®

Restrictions C-IV

Generic Available Yes

Pharmacologic Category Benzodiazepine

Pregnancy Risk Factor D

Lactation Enters breast milk/contraindicated (AAP rates "of concern")

Use Treatment of anxiety disorder (GAD); panic disorder, with or without agoraphobia; anxiety associated with depression

Use - Unlabeled/Investigational Anxiety in children

Mechanism of Action/Effect Binds to stereospecific benzodiazepine receptors on the postsynaptic GABA neuron at several sites within the central nervous system, including the limbic system, reticular formation. Enhancement of the inhibitory effect of GABA on neuronal excitability results by increased neuronal membrane permeability to chloride ions. This shift in chloride ions results in hyperpolarization (a less excitable state) and stabilization.

Contraindications Hypersensitivity to alprazolam or any component of the formulation (cross-sensitivity with other benzodiazepines may exist); narrow-angle glaucoma; concurrent use of ketoconazole and itraconazole; pregnancy

Warnings/Precautions Rebound or withdrawal symptoms, including seizures may occur 18 hours to 3 days following abrupt discontinuation or large decreases in dose (more common in patients receiving >4 mg/day or prolonged treatment). Dose reductions or tapering must be approached with extreme caution. Between dose anxiety may also occur. Use with caution in patients receiving concurrent CYP3A4 inhibitors, particularly when these agents are added to therapy. Use with caution in renal impairment or predisposition to urate nephropathy, elderly or debilitated patients, patients with hepatic disease (including alcoholics), renal impairment, respiratory disease, impaired gag reflex, or obese patients.

Causes CNS depression (dose-related) which may impair physical and mental capabilities. Use with caution in patients receiving other CNS depressants or psychoactive agents. Benzodiazepines have been associated with falls and traumatic injury and should be used with extreme caution in patients who are at risk of these events (especially the elderly).

Use caution in patients with depression, particularly if suicidal risk may be present. Episodes of mania or hypomania have occurred in depressed patients treated with alprazolam. May cause physical or psychological dependence - use with caution in patients with a history of drug dependence.

Benzodiazepines have been associated with anterograde amnesia. Paradoxical reactions, including hyperactive or aggressive behavior, have been reported with benzodiazepines, particularly in adolescent/pediatric or psychiatric patients. Does not have analgesic, antidepressant, or antipsychotic properties.

Drug Interactions

Cytochrome P450 Effect: Substrate of **CYP3A4**

Decreased Effect: Carbamazepine, rifampin, rifabutin may enhance the metabolism of alprazolam and decrease its therapeutic effect.

Increased Effect/Toxicity: Alprazolam potentiates the CNS depressant effects of narcotic analgesics, barbiturates, phenothiazines, ethanol, antihistamines, MAO inhibitors, sedative-hypnotics, and cyclic antidepressants. Serum levels and/or effects of alprazolam may be increased by inhibitors of CYP3A4, including amprenavir, cimetidine, ciprofloxacin, clarithromycin, clozapine, diltiazem, disulfiram, digoxin, erythromycin, ethanol, fluconazole, fluoxetine, fluvoxamine, grapefruit juice, isoniazid, itraconazole, ketoconazole, labetalol, levodopa, loxapine, metoprolol, metronidazole, miconazole, nefazodone, nelfinavir, omeprazole, phenytoin, rifabutin, rifampin, ritonavir, troleandomycin, valproic acid, and verapamil.

Nutritional/Ethanol Interactions

Ethanol: Avoid ethanol (may increase CNS depression).

Food: Alprazolam serum concentration is unlikely to be increased by grapefruit juice because of alprazolam's high oral bioavailability.

Herb/Nutraceutical: St John's wort may decrease alprazolam levels. Avoid valerian, St John's wort, kava kava, gotu kola (may increase CNS depression).

(Continued)

Alprazolam *(Continued)*

Effects on Lab Values ↑ with alkaline phosphatase

Adverse Reactions

>10%:

Central nervous system: Drowsiness, fatigue, ataxia, lightheadedness, memory impairment, dysarthria, irritability

Dermatologic: Rash

Endocrine & metabolic: Decreased libido, menstrual disorders

Gastrointestinal: Xerostomia, decreased salivation, increased or decreased appetite, weight gain/loss

Genitourinary: Micturition difficulties

1% to 10%:

Cardiovascular: Hypotension

Central nervous system: Confusion, dizziness, disinhibition, akathisia, increased libido

Dermatologic: Dermatitis

Gastrointestinal: Increased salivation

Genitourinary: Sexual dysfunction, incontinence

Neuromuscular & skeletal: Rigidity, tremor, muscle cramps

Otic: Tinnitus

Respiratory: Nasal congestion

Overdosage/Toxicology Symptoms of overdose include somnolence, confusion, coma, and diminished reflexes. Treatment for benzodiazepine overdose is supportive. Flumazenil has been shown to selectively block the binding of benzodiazepines to CNS receptors, resulting in a reversal of benzodiazepine-induced sedation; however, its use may not reverse respiratory depression.

Pharmacodynamics/Kinetics

Half-Life Elimination: 12-15 hours

Time to Peak: Serum: 1-2 hours

Metabolism: Hepatic; major metabolite inactive

Formulations

Solution, oral (Alprazolam Intensol®): 1 mg/mL (30 mL)

Tablet (Xanax®): 0.25 mg, 0.5 mg, 1 mg, 2 mg

Dosing

Adults:

Anxiety: Oral: Effective doses are 0.5-4 mg/day in divided doses. The manufacturer recommends starting at 0.25-0.5 mg 3 times/day. Titrate dose upward; maximum: 4 mg/day.

Depression: Oral: Average dose required: 2.5-3 mg/day in divided doses

Ethanol withdrawal: Oral: Usual dose: 2-2.5 mg/day in divided doses

Panic disorder: Oral: Many patients obtain relief at 2 mg/day, as much as 10 mg/day may be required.

Note: Treatment >4 months should be re-evaluated to determine the patient's need for the drug.

Elderly: May be more sensitive to the effects of alprazolam including ataxia and oversedation. The elderly may also have impaired renal function leading to decreased clearance. The smallest effective dose should be used.

Pediatrics: Anxiety (unlabeled use): Oral: Initial: 0.005 mg/kg/dose or 0.125 mg/dose 3 times/day; increase in increments of 0.125-0.25 mg, up to a maximum of 0.02 mg/kg/dose or 0.06 mg/kg/day (0.375-3 mg/day)

Hepatic Impairment: Oral: Reduce dose by 50% to 60% or avoid in cirrhosis.

Administration

Oral: Can be administered sublingually with comparable onset and completeness of absorption.

Monitoring and Teaching Issues

Physical Assessment: Assess other medications patient may be taking for effectiveness and interactions (see Drug Interactions). See Contraindications and Warnings/Precautions for use cautions. Assess for history of addiction; long-term use can result in dependence, abuse, or tolerance; periodically evaluate need for continued use. Monitor therapeutic response and adverse reactions at beginning of therapy and periodically with long-term use (see Adverse Reactions and Overdose/Toxicology). Taper dosage slowly when discontinuing. Assess knowledge/teach patient appropriate use, interventions to reduce side effects, and adverse symptoms to report (see Patient Education). **Pregnancy risk factor D** - determine that patient is not pregnant before beginning treatment. Instruct patients of childbearing age about appropriate barrier contraceptive measures. Breast-feeding is contraindicated.

Patient Education: Take exactly as directed; do not increase dose or frequency. Drug may cause physical and/or psychological dependence. Avoid alcohol and do not take other prescription or OTC medications (especially pain medications, sedatives, antihistamines, or hypnotics) without consulting prescriber. Maintain adequate hydration (2-3 L/day of fluids) unless advised by prescriber to restrict fluids. You may experience drowsiness, lightheadedness, impaired coordination, dizziness, or blurred vision (use caution when driving or engaging in hazardous tasks until response to drug is known); nausea, vomiting, or dry mouth (small, frequent meals, frequent mouth care, chewing gum, or sucking lozenges may help); constipation (increased exercise, fluids, fruit, and fiber may help); altered sexual drive or ability (reversible); or photosensitivity (use sunscreen, wear protective clothing and eyewear, and avoid direct sunlight). Report persistent CNS effects (eg, confusion, depression, increased sedation, excitation, headache, agitation, insomnia or nightmares, dizziness, fatigue, impaired coordination, changes in personality, or changes in cognition); changes in urinary pattern; muscle cramping, weakness, tremors, or rigidity; ringing in ears or visual disturbances; chest pain, palpitations, or rapid heartbeat; excessive perspiration; excessive GI symptoms (eg, cramping, constipation, vomiting, anorexia); or worsening of condition. **Pregnancy/breast-feeding precautions:** Do not get pregnant while taking this medication; use appropriate barrier contraceptive measures as recommended by your prescriber. Do not breast-feed.

Geriatric Considerations: Due to short duration of action, it is considered to be a benzodiazepine of choice in the elderly.

Additional Information Not intended for management of anxieties and minor distresses associated with everyday life. Treatment longer than 4 months should be re-evaluated to determine the patient's need for the drug. Patients who become physically dependent on alprazolam tend to have a difficult time discontinuing it; withdrawal symptoms may be severe. To minimize withdrawal symptoms, taper dosage slowly; do not discontinue abruptly. Abrupt discontinuation after sustained use (generally >10 days) may cause withdrawal symptoms.

Related Information

Antiemetics for Chemotherapy-Induced Nausea and Vomiting *on page 1639*
Anxiolytic/Hypnotic Use in Long-Term Care Facilities *on page 1608*
Benzodiazepines *on page 1560*

Alprazolam Intensol® *see* Alprazolam *on page 63*

Alprostadil (al PROS ta dill)

U.S. Brand Names Caverject®; Edex®; Muse® Pellet; Prostin VR Pediatric®

Synonyms PGE_1; Prostaglandin E_1

Generic Available Yes: Injection 5 mcg/mL

Pharmacologic Category Prostaglandin

Pregnancy Risk Factor X

Lactation Not indicated for use in women

Use

Prostin VR Pediatric®: Temporary maintenance of patency of ductus arteriosus in neonates with ductal-dependent congenital heart disease until surgery can be performed. These defects include cyanotic (eg, pulmonary atresia, pulmonary stenosis, tricuspid atresia, Fallot's tetralogy, transposition of the great vessels) and acyanotic (eg, interruption of aortic arch, coarctation of aorta, hypoplastic left ventricle) heart disease;

Caverject®, Edex®, Muse® Pellet: Treatment of erectile dysfunction of vasculogenic, psychogenic, or neurogenic etiology; adjunct in the diagnosis of erectile dysfunction

Use - Unlabeled/Investigational Investigational: Treatment of pulmonary hypertension in infants and children with congenital heart defects with left-to-right shunts

Mechanism of Action/Effect Erectile dysfunction: Causes vasodilation by dilation of cavernosal arteries when injected along the penile shaft, allowing blood flow to, and entrapment in, the lacunar spaces of the penis (ie, corporeal veno-occlusive mechanism)

Contraindications Hypersensitivity to alprostadil or any component of the formulation; hyaline membrane disease or persistent fetal circulation and when a dominant left-to-right shunt is present; respiratory distress syndrome; conditions predisposing patients to priapism (sickle cell anemia, multiple myeloma, leukemia); patients with anatomical deformation of the penis, penile implants; use in men for whom sexual activity is inadvisable or contraindicated; pregnancy

Warnings/Precautions Use cautiously in neonates with bleeding tendencies. Apnea may occur in 10% to 12% of neonates with congenital heart defects, especially in those weighing <2 kg at birth. Apnea usually appears during the first hour of drug infusion.

When used in erectile dysfunction: priapism may occur. Patient must be instructed to report to physician or seek immediate medical assistance if an erection persists for longer than 4 hours. Treat immediately to avoid penile tissue damage and permanent loss of potency; discontinue therapy if signs of penile fibrosis develop (penile angulation, cavernosal fibrosis, or Peyronie's disease). Syncope occurring within 1 hour of administration, has been reported; the potential for drug-drug interactions may occur when prescribed concomitantly with antihypertensives; some lowering of blood pressure may occur without symptoms, and swelling of leg veins, leg pain, perineal pain, and rapid pulse have been reported in <2% of patients during in-clinic titration and home treatment.

Drug Interactions

Increased Effect/Toxicity: Risk of hypotension and syncope may be increased with antihypertensives.

Nutritional/Ethanol Interactions Ethanol: Avoid concurrent use (vasodilating effect).

Adverse Reactions

Intraurethral:

>10%: Genitourinary: Penile pain, urethral burning

2% to 10%:

Central nervous system: Headache, dizziness, pain

Genitourinary: Vaginal itching (female partner), testicular pain, urethral bleeding (minor)

<2% (Limited to important or life-threatening): Tachycardia, perineal pain, leg pain

Intracavernosal injection:

>10%: Genitourinary: Penile pain

1% to 10%:

Cardiovascular: Hypertension

Central nervous system: Headache, dizziness

Genitourinary: Prolonged erection (>4 hours, 4%), penile fibrosis, penis disorder, penile rash, penile edema

Local: Injection site hematoma and/or bruising

<1% (Limited to important or life-threatening): Balanitis, injection site hemorrhage, priapism (0.4%)

Intravenous:

>10%:

Cardiovascular: Flushing

Central nervous system: Fever

Respiratory: Apnea

1% to 10%:

Cardiovascular: Bradycardia, hypotension, hypertension, tachycardia, cardiac arrest, edema

Central nervous system: Seizures, headache, dizziness

(Continued)

Alprostadil *(Continued)*

Endocrine & metabolic: Hypokalemia
Gastrointestinal: Diarrhea
Hematologic: Disseminated intravascular coagulation
Neuromuscular & skeletal: Back pain
Respiratory: Upper respiratory infection, flu syndrome, sinusitis, nasal congestion, cough
Miscellaneous: Sepsis, localized pain in structures other than the injection site

<1% (Limited to important or life-threatening): Anemia, anuria, bleeding, bradypnea, bronchial wheezing, cerebral bleeding, CHF, gastric regurgitation, hematuria, hyperbilirubinemia, hyperemia, hyperextension of neck, hyperirritability, hyperkalemia, hypoglycemia, hypothermia, jitteriness, lethargy, peritonitis, second degree heart block, shock, stiffness, supraventricular tachycardia, thrombocytopenia, ventricular fibrillation

Overdosage/Toxicology Symptoms of overdose when treating patent ductus arteriosus include apnea, bradycardia, hypotension, and flushing. If hypotension or pyrexia occurs, the infusion rate should be reduced until symptoms subside. Apnea or bradycardia requires drug discontinuation. If intracavernous overdose occurs, supervise until systemic effects have resolved or until penile detumescence has occurred.

Pharmacodynamics/Kinetics

Half-Life Elimination: 5-10 minutes

Metabolism: ~75% by oxidation in one pass via lungs

Onset: Rapid

Duration: <1 hour

Formulations

Injection:
- Caverject®: 5 mcg/mL, 10 mcg/mL, 20 mcg/mL
- Edex®: 5 mcg/mL, 10 mcg/mL, 20 mcg/mL, 40 mcg/mL
- Prostin VR Pediatric®: 500 mcg/mL (1 mL)

Pellet, urethral (Muse®): 125 mcg, 250 mcg, 500 mcg, 1000 mcg

Dosing

Adults: Erectile dysfunction:

Penile injection (Caverject®, Edex®): Individualize dose by careful titration; doses >40 mcg (Edex®) or >60 mcg (Caverject®) are not recommended:

Vasculogenic, psychogenic, or mixed etiology: Initiate dosage titration at 2.5 mcg, increasing by 2.5 mcg to a dose of 5 mcg, and then in increments of 5-10 mcg depending on the erectile response until the dose produces an erection suitable for intercourse, not lasting >1 hour. If there is absolutely no response to initial 2.5 mcg dose, the second dose may increased to 7.5 mcg, followed by increments of 5-10 mcg.

Neurogenic etiology (eg, spinal cord injury): Initiate dosage titration at 1.25 mcg, increasing to a dose of 2.5 mcg, and then 5 mcg. Increase further in increments of 5 mcg until the dose is reached that produces an erection suitable for intercourse, not lasting >1 hour.

Note: Patient must stay in the physician's office until complete detumescence occurs. If there is no response, then the next higher dose may be given within 1 hour. If there is still no response, a 1-day interval before giving the next dose is recommended. Increasing the dose or concentration in the treatment of impotence results in increasing pain and discomfort.

Intraurethral (Muse® Pellet): Administer as needed to achieve an erection. Duration of action is about 30-60 minutes; use only two systems per 24-hour period.

Elderly: Elderly patients may have a greater frequency of renal dysfunction; lowest effective dose should be used. In clinical studies with Edex®, higher minimally effective doses and a higher rate of lack of effect were noted.

Pediatrics:

Patent ductus arteriosus (Prostin VR Pediatric®):

I.V. continuous infusion into a large vein, or alternatively through an umbilical artery catheter placed at the ductal opening: 0.05-0.1 mcg/kg/minute with therapeutic response, rate is reduced to lowest effective dosage. With unsatisfactory response, rate is increased gradually; maintenance: 0.01-0.4 mcg/kg/minute.

PGE_1 is usually given at an infusion rate of 0.1 mcg/kg/minute, but it is often possible to reduce the dosage to $^1/_2$ or even $^1/_{10}$ without losing the therapeutic effect. The mixing schedule is shown in the table.

Alprostadil

Add 1 Ampul (500 mcg) to:	Concentration (mcg/mL)	Infusion Rate	
		mL/min/kg Needed to Infuse 0.1 mcg/kg/min	mL/kg/24 h
250 mL	2	0.05	72
100 mL	5	0.02	28.8
50 mL	10	0.01	14.4
25 mL	20	0.005	7.2

Therapeutic response is indicated by increased pH in those with acidosis or by an increase in oxygenation (pO_2) usually evident within 30 minutes.

Administration

Other: Erectile dysfunction: Use a $^1/_2$ inch, 27- to 30-gauge needle. Inject into the dorsolateral aspect of the proximal third of the penis, avoiding visible veins; alternate side of the penis for injections.

Stability

Storage: Refrigerate at 2°C to 8°C until dispensed. After dispensing, stable for up to 3 months at or below 25°C. Do not freeze.

Reconstitution: Use only the supplied diluent for reconstitution (ie, bacteriostatic/sterile water with benzyl alcohol 0.945%).

Monitoring and Teaching Issues

Physical Assessment: After individual dose titration is determined by physician, the Caverject® injection (or Muse®) is generally self-administered by the patient. Assessment and monitoring focus on teaching and evaluating patient knowledge of guidelines for use, appropriate administration and needle disposal, interventions to reduce side effects, and adverse symptoms to report (see Patient Education). **Pregnancy risk factor X** - determine that patient and sexual partner(s) are capable of using barrier contraceptive measures during treatment and for 1 month following discontinuance of therapy.

Patient Education: Use only as directed, no more than 3 times/week, allowing 24 hours between injections. Avoid alcohol. Store in refrigerator and dilute with supplied diluent immediately before use. Use alternate sides of penis with each injection. Dispose of syringes and needle and single dose vials in a safe manner (do not share medication, syringes, or needles). Note that the risk of transmitting blood-borne disease is increased with use of alprostadil injections since a small amount of bleeding at injection site is possible. Stop using and contact prescriber immediately if signs of priapism occur, erections last more than 4 hours, or you experience moderate to severe penile pain. Report penile problems (eg, nodules, new penile pain, rash, bruising, numbness, swelling, signs of infection, abnormal ejaculations); cardiac symptoms (hypo- or hypertension, chest pain, palpitations, irregular heartbeat); flushing, fever, flu-like symptoms; difficulty breathing or wheezing; or other adverse reactions. Refer to prescriber every 3 months to ensure proper technique and for dosage evaluation. **Pregnancy precautions:** This drug will cause severe fetal defects. Consult prescriber for appropriate barrier contraception education for you and your sexual partner(s). Do not give blood while taking this medication and for 1 month following discontinuance.

Geriatric Considerations: Elderly may have concomitant diseases which would contraindicate the use of alprostadil. Other forms of attaining penile tumescence are recommended.

Alrex™ *see page 1509*

Altace® *see* Ramipril *on page 1170*

Alteplase (AL te plase)

U.S. Brand Names Activase®; Cathflo™ Activase®

Synonyms Alteplase, Recombinant; Alteplase, Tissue Plasminogen Activator, Recombinant; tPA

Generic Available No

Pharmacologic Category Thrombolytic Agent

Pregnancy Risk Factor C

Lactation Excretion in breast milk unknown

Use Management of acute myocardial infarction for the lysis of thrombi in coronary arteries; management of acute massive pulmonary embolism (PE) in adults

Acute myocardial infarction (AMI): Chest pain ≥20 minutes, ≤12-24 hours; S-T elevation ≥0.1 mV in at least two EKG leads

Acute pulmonary embolism (APE): Age ≤75 years: As soon as possible within 5 days of thrombotic event. Documented massive pulmonary embolism by pulmonary angiography or echocardiography or high probability lung scan with clinical shock.

Cathflo™ Activase®: Restoration of central venous catheter function

Use - Unlabeled/Investigational Peripheral arterial thrombotic obstruction

Mechanism of Action/Effect Dissolves thrombus (clot)

Contraindications Hypersensitivity to alteplase or any component of the formulation

Treatment of acute MI or PE: Active internal bleeding; history of CVA; recent intracranial or intraspinal surgery or trauma; intracranial neoplasm; arteriovenous malformation or aneurysm; known bleeding diathesis; severe uncontrolled hypertension

Treatment of acute ischemic stroke: Evidence of intracranial hemorrhage or suspicion of subarachnoid hemorrhage on pretreatment evaluation; recent (within 3 months) intracranial or intraspinal surgery; prolonged external cardiac massage; suspected aortic dissection; serious head trauma or previous stroke; history of intracranial hemorrhage; uncontrolled hypertension at time of treatment (eg, >185 mm Hg systolic or >110 mm Hg diastolic); seizure at the onset of stroke; active internal bleeding; intracranial neoplasm; arteriovenous malformation or aneurysm; known bleeding diathesis including but not limited to: current use of anticoagulants or an INR >1.7, administration of heparin within 48 hours preceding the onset of stroke and an elevated aPTT at presentation, platelet count <100,000/mm^3.

Other exclusion criteria (NINDS recombinant tPA study): Stroke or serious head injury within 3 months, major surgery or serious trauma within 2 weeks, GI or urinary tract hemorrhage within 3 weeks, aggressive treatment required to lower blood pressure, glucose level <50 mg/dL or >400 mg/dL, arterial puncture at a noncompressible site or lumbar puncture within 1 week, clinical presentation suggesting post-MI pericarditis, pregnant or lactating women.

Warnings/Precautions Concurrent heparin anticoagulation may contribute to bleeding. Monitor all potential bleeding sites. Doses >150 mg are associated with increased risk of intracranial hemorrhage. Intramuscular injections and nonessential handling of the patient should be avoided. Venipunctures should be performed carefully and only when necessary. If arterial puncture is necessary, use an upper extremity vessel that can be manually compressed. If serious bleeding occurs then the infusion of alteplase and heparin should be stopped.

For the following conditions the risk of bleeding is higher with use of alteplase and should be weighed against the benefits of therapy: recent major surgery (eg, CABG, obstetrical delivery, organ biopsy, previous puncture of noncompressible vessels), cerebrovascular disease, recent gastrointestinal or genitourinary bleeding, recent trauma, hypertension (systolic BP >175 mm Hg and/or diastolic BP >110 mm Hg), high likelihood of left heart thrombus (eg, mitral stenosis with atrial fibrillation), acute pericarditis, subacute bacterial
(Continued)

Alteplase *(Continued)*

endocarditis, hemostatic defects including ones caused by severe renal or hepatic dysfunction, significant hepatic dysfunction, pregnancy, diabetic hemorrhagic retinopathy or other hemorrhagic ophthalmic conditions, septic thrombophlebitis or occluded AV cannula at seriously infected site, advanced age (eg, >75 years), patients receiving oral anticoagulants, any other condition in which bleeding constitutes a significant hazard or would be particularly difficult to manage because of location.

Coronary thrombolysis may result in reperfusion arrhythmias. In treatment of patients with acute ischemic stroke more than 3 hours after symptom onset is not recommended; treatment of patients with minor neurological deficit or with rapidly improving symptoms is not recommended.

Cathflo™ Activase®: When used to restore catheter function, use Cathflo™ cautiously in those patients with known or suspected catheter infections. Evaluate catheter for other causes of dysfunction before use. Avoid excessive pressure when instilling into catheter. Use of Cathflo™ in children <2 years of age (or weighing <10 kg) has not been studied.

Pregnancy risk C.

Drug Interactions

Decreased Effect: Aminocaproic acid (an antifibrinolytic agent) may decrease the effectiveness of thrombolytic therapy. Nitroglycerin may increase the hepatic clearance of alteplase, potentially reducing lytic activity (limited clinical information).

Increased Effect/Toxicity: The potential for hemorrhage with alteplase is increased by oral anticoagulants (warfarin), heparin, low molecular weight heparins, and drugs which affect platelet function (eg, NSAIDs, dipyridamole, ticlopidine, clopidogrel, IIb/IIIa antagonists). Concurrent use with aspirin and heparin may increase the risk of bleeding. However, aspirin and heparin were used concomitantly with alteplase in the majority of patients in clinical studies.

Nutritional/Ethanol Interactions Herb/Nutraceutical: Avoid cat's claw, dong quai, evening primrose, feverfew, red clover, horse chestnut, garlic, green tea, ginseng, ginkgo (all have additional antiplatelet activity).

Effects on Lab Values Altered results of coagulation and fibrinolytic agents

Adverse Reactions As with all drugs which may affect hemostasis, bleeding is the major adverse effect associated with alteplase. Hemorrhage may occur at virtually any site. Risk is dependent on multiple variables, including the dosage administered, concurrent use of multiple agents which alter hemostasis, and patient predisposition. Rapid lysis of coronary artery thrombi by thrombolytic agents may be associated with reperfusion-related atrial and/ or ventricular arrhythmias. **Note:** Lowest rate of bleeding complications expected with dose used to restore catheter function.

1% to 10%:

- Cardiovascular: Hypotension
- Central nervous system: Fever
- Dermatologic: Bruising (1%)
- Gastrointestinal: GI hemorrhage (5%), nausea, vomiting
- Genitourinary: GU hemorrhage (4%)
- Hematologic: Bleeding (0.5% major, 7% minor: GUSTO trial)
- Local: Bleeding at catheter puncture site (15.3%, accelerated administration)

<1% (Limited to important or life-threatening): Allergic reactions: Anaphylaxis, anaphylactoid reactions, laryngeal edema, rash, and urticaria (<0.02%); epistaxis; gingival hemorrhage; intracranial hemorrhage (0.4% to 0.87% when dose is ≤100 mg); pericardial hemorrhage; retroperitoneal hemorrhage

Additional cardiovascular events associated **with use in myocardial infarction:** AV block, cardiogenic shock, heart failure, cardiac arrest, recurrent ischemia/infarction, myocardial rupture, electromechanical dissociation, pericardial effusion, pericarditis, mitral regurgitation, cardiac tamponade, thromboembolism, pulmonary edema, asystole, ventricular tachycardia, bradycardia, ruptured intracranial AV malformation, seizure, hemorrhagic bursitis, cholesterol crystal embolization

Additional events associated **with use in pulmonary embolism:** Pulmonary re-embolization, pulmonary edema, pleural effusion, thromboembolism

Additional events associated **with use in stroke:** Cerebral edema, cerebral herniation, seizure, new ischemic stroke

Overdosage/Toxicology Increased incidence of intracranial bleeding.

Pharmacodynamics/Kinetics

Duration: >50% present in plasma cleared ~5 minutes after infusion terminated, ~80% cleared within 10 minutes

Formulations Injection, powder for reconstitution, recombinant:

Activase®: 50 mg [29 million units]; 100 mg [58 million units]

Cathflo™ Activase®: 2 mg

Dosing

Adults & Elderly:

Coronary artery thrombi: I.V. Front loading dose (weight-based):

Patients >67 kg: Total dose: 100 mg over 1.5 hours; infuse 15 mg (30 mL) over 1-2 minutes. Infuse 50 mg (100 mL) over 30 minutes. See "Note."

Patients ≤67 kg: Total dose: 1.25 mg/kg; infuse 15 mg I.V. bolus over 1-2 minutes, then infuse 0.75 mg/kg (not to exceed 50 mg) over next 30 minutes, followed by 0.5 mg/kg over next 60 minutes (not to exceed 35 mg). See "Note."

Note: Concurrently, begin heparin 60 units/kg bolus (maximum: 4000 units) followed by continuous infusion of 12 units/kg/hour (maximum: 1000 units/hour) and adjust to aPTT target of 1.5-2 times the upper limit of control. Infuse remaining 35 mg (70 mL) of alteplase over the next hour.

Acute pulmonary embolism: I.V.: 100 mg over 2 hours.

Acute ischemic stroke: I.V.: Doses should be given within the first 3 hours of the onset of symptoms; recommended total dose: 0.9 mg/kg (maximum dose should not exceed 90 mg) infused over 60 minutes.

Load with 0.09 mg/kg (10% of the 0.9 mg/kg dose) as an I.V. bolus over 1 minute, followed by 0.81 mg/kg (90% of the 0.9 mg/kg dose) as a continuous infusion over 60 minutes. Heparin should not be started for at least 24 hours after starting alteplase for stroke.

Central venous catheter clearance: Intracatheter: Cathflo™ Activase®:

Patients ≥10 to <30 kg: 110% of the internal lumen volume of the catheter (≤2 mg [1 mg/mL]); retain in catheter for ≤2 hours; may instill a second dose if catheter remains occluded

Patients ≥30 kg: 2 mg (1 mg/mL); retain in catheter for ≤2 hours; may instill a second dose if catheter remains occluded

Peripheral arterial thrombotic obstruction (unlabeled use): 8-10 mg I.V. or injected into the thrombus directly

Pediatrics: Central venous catheter clearance: Intracatheter: ≥10 to <30 kg: 110% of the internal lumen volume of the catheter (≤2 mg [1 mg/mL]); retain in catheter for ≤2 hours; may instill a second dose if catheter remains occluded

Administration

I.V.: Activase®: Acute MI: Accelerated infusion:

Bolus dose may be prepared by one of three methods:

1) removal of 15 mL reconstituted (1 mg/mL) solution from vial
2) removal of 15 mL from a port on the infusion line after priming
3) programming an infusion pump to deliver a 15 mL bolus at the initiation of infusion

Remaining dose may be administered as follows:

50 mg vial: Either PVC bag or glass vial and infusion set

100 mg vial: Insert spike end of the infusion set through the same puncture site created by transfer device and infuse from vial

If further dilution is desired, may be diluted in equal volume of 0.9% sodium chloride or D_5W to yield a final concentration of 0.5 mg/mL AD

Other: Cathflo™ Activase®: Intracatheter: Instill dose into occluded catheter. Do not force solution into catheter. After a 30-minute dwell time, assess catheter function by attempting to aspirate blood. If catheter is functional, aspirate 4-5 mL of blood to remove Cathflo™ Activase® and residual clots. Gently irrigate the catheter with NS. If catheter remains nonfunctional, let Cathflo™ Activase® dwell for another 90 minutes (total dwell time: 120 minutes) and reassess function. If catheter function is not restored, a second dose may be instilled.

Stability

Storage:

Activase®: The lyophilized product may be stored at room temperature (not to exceed 30°C/86°F), or under refrigeration; once reconstituted it must be used within 8 hours

Cathflo™ Activase®: Store lyophilized product in refrigerated; protect from excessive exposure to light when stored for extended periods of time. Once reconstituted, store at 2°C to 30°C (36°F to 86°F).

Reconstitution:

Activase®:

50 mg vial: Use accompanying diluent (50 mL sterile water for injection); do not shake; final concentration: 1 mg/mL

100 mg vial: Use transfer set with accompanying diluent (100 mL vial of sterile water for injection); no vacuum is present in 100 mg vial; final concentration: 1 mg/mL

Cathflo™ Activase®: Add 2.2 mL SWFI to vial; do not shake. Final concentration: 1 mg/mL. Once reconstituted, store at 2°C to 30°C (36°F to 86°F).

Compatibility: Stable in NS, sterile water for injection; **incompatible** with bacteriostatic water

Y-site administration: Incompatible with dobutamine, dopamine, heparin, nitroglycerin

Compatibility when admixed: Incompatible with dobutamine, dopamine, heparin

Monitoring Laboratory Tests CBC, PTT

Monitoring and Teaching Issues

Physical Assessment: See Contraindications, Warnings/Precautions, and Dosing for use cautions. Assess potential for interactions with other prescriptions, OTC medications, or herbal products patient may be taking (especially those medications that may affect coagulation or platelet function - see Drug Interactions). See infusion specifics above. Vital signs, laboratory results (see above), and EKG should be monitored prior to, during, and after therapy. Arrhythmias may occur; antiarrhythmic drugs should be immediately available. Assess infusion site and monitor for hemorrhage every 10 minutes (or according to institutional policy) during therapy and for 1 hour following therapy (see Adverse Reactions and Overdose/Toxicology). Strict bedrest should be maintained and bleeding precautions should be instituted; avoid invasive procedures and activities that could cause trauma. Patient instructions determined by patient condition (see Patient Education). **Pregnancy risk factor C** - benefits of use should outweigh possible risks. Note breast-feeding caution.

Patient Education: Inform prescriber of all prescriptions, OTC medications, or herbal products you are taking, and any allergies you have. This medication can only be administered by infusion; you will be monitored closely during and after treatment. You will have a tendency to bleed easily; use caution to prevent injury (use electric razor, soft toothbrush, and use caution with knives, needles, or anything sharp). Follow instructions for strict bedrest to reduce the risk of injury. If bleeding occurs, report immediately and apply pressure to bleeding spot until bleeding stops completely. Report unusual pain (acute headache, joint pain, chest pain); unusual bruising or bleeding; blood in urine, stool, or vomit; bleeding gums; vision changes; or difficulty breathing. **Pregnancy precaution:** Inform prescriber if you are or intend to become pregnant.

Other Issues: Drug is frequently administered with heparin. Discontinue both if serious bleeding occurs. Avoid invasive procedures.

Alteplase, Recombinant *see* Alteplase *on page 67*

Alteplase, Tissue Plasminogen Activator, Recombinant *see* Alteplase *on page 67*

ALternaGel® [OTC] *see* Aluminum Hydroxide *on page 71*

Altinac™ *see* Tretinoin (Topical) *on page 1355*

Altocor™ *see* Lovastatin *on page 826*

Altretamine (al TRET a meen)

U.S. Brand Names Hexalen®

Synonyms Hexamethylmelamine; HEXM; HMM; HXM; NSC-13875

Generic Available No

Pharmacologic Category Antineoplastic Agent, Miscellaneous

Pregnancy Risk Factor D

Lactation Excretion in breast milk unknown

Use Palliative treatment of persistent or recurrent ovarian cancer following first-line therapy with a cisplatin- or alkylating agent-based combination

Mechanism of Action/Effect Exact mechanism of action that causes cell death is not known. Metabolism in the liver is required for cytotoxicity. Although altretamine clinical antitumor spectrum resembles that of alkylating agents, the drug has demonstrated activity in alkylator-resistant patients; probably requires hepatic microsomal mixed-function oxidase enzyme activation to become cytotoxic. The drug selectively inhibits the incorporation of radioactive thymidine and uridine into DNA and RNA, inhibiting DNA and RNA synthesis. Metabolized to reactive intermediates which covalently bind to microsomal proteins and DNA. These reactive intermediates can spontaneously degrade to demethylated melamines and formaldehyde which are also cytotoxic.

Contraindications Hypersensitivity to altretamine or any component of the formulation; pre-existing severe bone marrow suppression or severe neurologic toxicity; pregnancy

Warnings/Precautions The U.S. Food and Drug Administration (FDA) currently recommends that procedures for proper handling and disposal of antineoplastic agents be considered. Use with caution in patients previously treated with other myelosuppressive drugs or with pre-existing neurotoxicity. Use with caution in patients with renal or hepatic dysfunction. Altretamine may be slightly mutagenic.

Drug Interactions

Decreased Effect: Phenobarbital may increase metabolism of altretamine which may decrease the effect.

Increased Effect/Toxicity: Altretamine may cause severe orthostatic hypotension when administered with MAO inhibitors. Cimetidine may decrease metabolism of altretamine.

Nutritional/Ethanol Interactions Ethanol: Avoid ethanol (due to GI irritation)

Adverse Reactions

>10%:
- Central nervous system: Peripheral sensory neuropathy, neurotoxicity
- Gastrointestinal: Nausea, vomiting
  - Moderate (30% to 60%)
- Hematologic: Anemia, thrombocytopenia, leukopenia

1% to 10%:
- Central nervous system: Seizures
- Gastrointestinal: Anorexia, diarrhea, stomach cramps
- Hepatic: Increased alkaline phosphatase

<1% (Limited to important or life-threatening): Alopecia, hepatotoxicity, myelosuppression, tremor

Overdosage/Toxicology Symptoms of overdose include nausea, vomiting, peripheral neuropathy, severe bone marrow suppression. Treatment is supportive.

Pharmacodynamics/Kinetics

Absorption: Well absorbed (75% to 89%)

Half-Life Elimination: 13 hours

Time to Peak: Plasma: 0.5-3 hours

Metabolism: Hepatic; rapid and extensive demethylation

Formulations Capsule: 50 mg

Dosing

Adults & Elderly: Ovarian cancer (palliative): Oral:

4-12 mg/kg/day in 3-4 divided doses for 21-90 days

Alternatively: 240-320 mg/m²/day in 3-4 divided doses per day for 21 days, repeated every 6 weeks

Alternatively: 260 mg/m²/day in 4 divided doses per day for 14-21 days of a 28-day cycle

Temporarily discontinue for ≥14 days and restart at 200 mg/m²/day if any of the following occurs: GI intolerance unresponsive to symptom measures, WBC <2000/mm³, granulocyte count <1000/mm³, platelet count <75,000/mm³, progressive neurotoxicity.

Administration

Oral: Administer total daily dose as 4 divided oral doses after meals and at bedtime.

Monitoring Laboratory Tests CBC with platelet count and differential should be done routinely before and after drug therapy.

Monitoring and Teaching Issues

Physical Assessment: See Contraindications, Warnings/Precautions, and Dosage for use cautions. Assess potential for interactions with other prescriptions, OTC medications, or herbal products patient may be taking (see Drug Interactions). Assess results of laboratory tests (see above). Assess for therapeutic effectiveness and adverse response (see Adverse Reactions and Overdose Toxicology). Teach patient appropriate use, possible side effects and interventions, and adverse symptoms to report (see Patient Education). **Pregnancy risk factor D** - determine that patient is not pregnant before beginning treatment. Instruct patients of childbearing age about appropriate barrier contraceptive measures. Note breast-feeding caution.

Patient Education: Inform prescriber of all prescriptions, OTC medications, or herbal products you are taking, and any allergies you have. Do not take anything new (including aspirin or any aspirin-containing products) during treatment unless approved by prescriber. Take exactly as directed, preferably after meals. Avoid alcohol. May cause nausea or vomiting during therapy or several weeks after therapy is discontinued (small, frequent meals, good mouth care, chewing gum, or sucking lozenges may help). You will be more susceptible to infection (avoid crowds and exposure to infection). Report any numbness, tingling, or pain in extremities; unrelieved nausea or vomiting; tremors; yellowing of skin or eyes; fever; chills; easy bruising or unusual bleeding; extreme weakness; or increased fatigue. **Pregnancy/breast-feeding precautions:** Do not get pregnant while taking this medication. Consult prescriber for appropriate barrier contraceptive measures. Consult prescriber if breast-feeding.

Dietary Issues: Should be taken after meals.

Alu-Cap® [OTC] *see* Aluminum Hydroxide *on page 71*

Aluminum Acetate and Acetic Acid *see page 1519*

Aluminum Hydroxide (a LOO mi num hye DROKS ide)

U.S. Brand Names ALternaGel® [OTC]; Alu-Cap® [OTC]; Alu-Tab® [OTC]; Amphojel® [OTC]; Dialume® [OTC]

Generic Available Yes

Pharmacologic Category Antacid; Antidote

Pregnancy Risk Factor C

Lactation Excretion in breast milk unknown

Use Treatment of hyperacidity; hyperphosphatemia

Mechanism of Action/Effect Neutralizes or reduces gastric acidity, resulting in increased gastric pH and inhibition of pepsin activity

Contraindications Hypersensitivity to aluminum salts or any component of the formulation

Warnings/Precautions Binds with phosphate ions. Hypophosphatemia may occur with prolonged administration or large doses. Use with caution in patients with CHF, renal failure, edema, cirrhosis, and low sodium diets, and patients who have recently suffered GI hemorrhage. Uremic patients not receiving dialysis may develop aluminum intoxication or osteomalacia and osteoporosis due to phosphate depletion. Pregnancy risk C.

Drug Interactions

Decreased Effect: Aluminum hydroxide decreases the effect of tetracyclines, digoxin, indomethacin, iron salts, isoniazid, allopurinol, benzodiazepines, corticosteroids, penicillamine, phenothiazines, ranitidine, ketoconazole, and itraconazole.

Effects on Lab Values ↓ phosphorus, inorganic (S); may interfere with some gastric imaging techniques or gastric acid secretion tests.

Adverse Reactions

- >10%: Gastrointestinal: Constipation, chalky taste, stomach cramps, fecal impaction
- 1% to 10%: Gastrointestinal: Nausea, vomiting, discoloration of feces (white speckles)
- <1% (Limited to important or life-threatening): Hypomagnesemia, hypophosphatemia

Overdosage/Toxicology Aluminum antacids may cause constipation, phosphate depletion, and bezoar or fecalith formation. In patients with renal failure, aluminum may accumulate to toxic levels. Deferoxamine, traditionally used as an iron chelator, has been shown to increase urinary aluminum output. Deferoxamine chelation of aluminum has resulted in improvement of clinical symptoms and bone histology; however, this remains an experimental treatment for aluminum poisoning and has significant potential for adverse effects.

Formulations

Capsule:
- Alu-Cap®: 400 mg
- Dialume®: 500 mg

Liquid (ALternaGel®): 600 mg/5 mL

Suspension, oral: 320 mg/5 mL, 450 mg/5 mL, 675 mg/5 mL
- Amphojel®: 320 mg/5 mL

Tablet:
- Alu-Tab®: 500 mg
- Amphojel®: 300 mg, 600 mg

Dosing

Adults & Elderly:

Peptic ulcer disease (dosages empirical): Oral: 15-45 mL every 3-6 hours or 1 and 3 hours after meals and at bedtime

Prophylaxis against gastrointestinal bleeding: Oral: 30-60 mL/dose every hour; titrate to maintain the gastric pH >5

Hyperphosphatemia: Oral: 500-1800 mg, 3-6 times/day, between meals and at bedtime; best taken with a meal or within 20 minutes of a meal

Antacid: Oral: 30 mL 1 and 3 hours postprandial and at bedtime
- Amphojel®: 10 mL suspension or two 300 mg tablets 5-6 times/day between meals and at bedtime

Pediatrics:

Peptic ulcer disease (dosages empirical): Oral:
- Children: 5-15 mL/dose every 3-6 hours or 1 and 3 hours after meals and at bedtime

Prophylaxis against gastrointestinal bleeding: Oral:
- Infants: 2-5 mL/dose every 1-2 hours
- Children: 5-15 mL/dose every 1-2 hours
- Titrate to maintain the gastric pH >5

Hyperphosphatemia: Oral:
- Children: 50-150 mg/kg/24 hours in divided doses every 4-6 hours, titrate dosage to maintain serum phosphorus within normal range

Renal Impairment: Aluminum may accumulate in renal impairment.

Administration

Oral: Dose should be followed with water.

Monitoring Laboratory Tests Calcium and phosphate levels periodically when patient is on chronic therapy

Monitoring and Teaching Issues

Physical Assessment: Monitor appropriate laboratory tests and effectiveness of treatment. Assess for constipation and treat accordingly. **Pregnancy risk factor C** - benefits of use should outweigh possible risks. Note breast-feeding caution.

(Continued)

Aluminum Hydroxide *(Continued)*

Patient Education: Take as directed, preferably 1-3 hours after meals (when used as an antacid) or with any other medications. When used to decrease phosphorus, take within 20 minutes of a meal. Dilute liquid dose with water or juice and shake well. Do not increase sodium intake and maintain adequate hydration (2-3 L/day of fluids) unless advised by prescriber to restrict fluids. Chew tablet thoroughly before swallowing with full glass of water. You may experience constipation (increased exercise, fluids, fruit, or fiber may help; if unresolved, contact prescriber). Report unresolved nausea, malaise, muscle weakness, blood in stool or black stool, or abdominal pain. **Pregnancy/breast-feeding precautions:** Inform prescriber if you are or intend to become pregnant. Consult prescriber if breast-feeding.

Dietary Issues: Should be taken 1-3 hours after meals when used as an antacid. When used to decrease phosphorus, should be taken within 20 minutes of a meal.

Geriatric Considerations: Elderly, due to disease and/or drug therapy, may be predisposed to constipation and fecal impaction. This may be managed with a stool softener or laxatives. Careful evaluation of possible drug interactions must be done. Consider renal insufficiency (<30 mL/minute) as predisposition to aluminum toxicity.

Aluminum Sucrose Sulfate, Basic *see* Sucralfate *on page 1254*

Alustra™ *see* Hydroquinone *on page 679*

Alu-Tab® [OTC] *see* Aluminum Hydroxide *on page 71*

Amantadine (a MAN ta deen)

U.S. Brand Names Symmetrel®

Synonyms Adamantanamine Hydrochloride; Amantadine Hydrochloride

Generic Available Yes

Pharmacologic Category Anti-Parkinson's Agent, Dopamine Agonist; Antiviral Agent

Pregnancy Risk Factor C

Lactation Enters breast milk/use caution

Use Prophylaxis and treatment of influenza A viral infection; treatment of parkinsonism; treatment of drug-induced extrapyramidal symptoms

Use - Unlabeled/Investigational Creutzfeldt-Jakob disease

Mechanism of Action/Effect As an antiviral, blocks the uncoating of influenza A virus preventing penetration of virus into host; antiparkinsonian activity may be due to its blocking the reuptake of dopamine into presynaptic neurons or by increasing dopamine release from presynaptic fibers

Contraindications Hypersensitivity to amantadine or any component of the formulation

Warnings/Precautions Use with caution in patients with liver disease, history of recurrent and eczematoid dermatitis, uncontrolled psychosis or severe psychoneurosis, seizures, and in those receiving CNS stimulant drugs. Reduce dose in renal disease. When treating Parkinson's disease, do not discontinue abruptly. In many patients, the therapeutic benefits of amantadine are limited to a few months. Elderly patients may be more susceptible to CNS effects (using 2 divided daily doses may minimize this effect). Has been associated with neuroleptic malignant syndrome (associated with dose reduction or abrupt discontinuation). Has not been shown to prevent bacterial infection or complications when used as prophylaxis or treatment of influenza A. Use with caution in patients with CHF, peripheral edema, or orthostatic hypotension. Avoid in angle closure glaucoma. Pregnancy risk C.

Drug Interactions

Increased Effect/Toxicity: Anticholinergics (benztropine and trihexyphenidyl) may potentiate CNS side effects of amantadine. Hydrochlorothiazide, triamterene, and/or trimethoprim may increase toxicity of amantadine; monitor for altered response.

Nutritional/Ethanol Interactions Ethanol: Avoid ethanol (may increase CNS adverse effects).

Adverse Reactions

1% to 10%:

- Cardiovascular: Orthostatic hypotension, peripheral edema
- Central nervous system: Insomnia, depression, anxiety, irritability, dizziness, hallucinations, ataxia, headache, somnolence, nervousness, dream abnormality, agitation, fatigue, confusion
- Dermatologic: Livedo reticularis
- Gastrointestinal: Nausea, anorexia, constipation, diarrhea, xerostomia
- Respiratory: Dry nose

<1% (Limited to important or life-threatening): Amnesia, CHF, convulsions, decreased libido, dyspnea, eczematoid dermatitis, euphoria, hyperkinesis, hypertension, leukopenia, neutropenia, oculogyric episodes, psychosis, rash, slurred speech, urinary retention, visual disturbances, vomiting, weakness

Overdosage/Toxicology Symptoms of overdose include nausea, vomiting, slurred speech, blurred vision, lethargy, hallucinations, seizures, and myoclonic jerking. Treatment should be directed at reducing CNS stimulation, controlling seizures, and maintaining cardiovascular function.

Pharmacodynamics/Kinetics

Absorption: Well absorbed

Bioavailability: 86% to 90%

Half-Life Elimination: Normal renal function: 16 ± 6 hours (9-31 hours); End-stage renal disease: 7-10 days

Time to Peak: 1-4 hours

Metabolism: Not appreciable; small amounts of an acetyl metabolite identified

Onset: Antidyskinetic: Within 48 hours

Formulations

Capsule, as hydrochloride: 100 mg

Syrup, as hydrochloride (Symmetrel®): 50 mg/5 mL (480 mL) [raspberry flavor]

Tablet, as hydrochloride (Symmetrel®): 100 mg

Dosing

Adults:

Drug-induced extrapyramidal symptoms: Oral: 100 mg twice daily; may increase to 300-400 mg/day, if needed.

Parkinson's disease or Creutzfeldt-Jakob disease (unlabeled use): Oral: 100 mg twice daily as sole therapy; may increase to 400 mg/day if needed with close monitoring; initial dose: 100 mg/day if with other serious illness or with high doses of other anti-Parkinson drugs.

Influenza A viral infection: Oral: 200 mg/day in 1-2 divided doses

Influenza prophylaxis: Oral: Minimum 10-day course of therapy following exposure if the vaccine is concurrently given or for 90 days following exposure if the vaccine is unavailable or contraindicated and re-exposure is possible.

Elderly: Dose is based on renal function. Elderly patients should take the drug in 2 daily doses rather than a single dose to avoid adverse neurologic reactions with improved tolerance.

Pediatrics: Influenza A treatment: Oral: Children:

1-9 years (<45 kg): 5-9 mg/kg/day in 1-2 divided doses to a maximum of 150 mg/day

10-12 years: 100-200 mg/day in 1-2 divided doses

>12 years: Refer to adult dosing.

Note: Prophylaxis: Administer for 10-21 days following exposure if the vaccine is concurrently given or for 90 days following exposure if the vaccine is unavailable or contraindicated and re-exposure is possible.

Renal Impairment:

Cl_{cr} 50-60 mL/minute: Administer 200 mg alternating with 100 mg/day.

Cl_{cr} 30-50 mL/minute: Administer 100 mg/day.

Cl_{cr} 20-30 mL/minute: Administer 200 mg twice weekly.

Cl_{cr} 10-20 mL/minute: Administer 100 mg 3 times/week.

Cl_{cr} <10 mL/minute: Administer 200 mg alternating with 100 mg every 7 days.

Hemodialysis: Slightly hemodialyzable (5% to 20%); no supplemental dose is needed.

Peritoneal dialysis: No supplemental dose is needed.

Continuous arterio-venous or venous-venous hemofiltration: No supplemental dose is needed.

Stability

Storage: Protect from freezing.

Monitoring Laboratory Tests Renal function

Monitoring and Teaching Issues

Physical Assessment: Assess effectiveness and interactions of other medications patient may be taking (see Contraindications and Drug Interactions). Monitor renal function, therapeutic response, and adverse reactions (see Warnings/Precautions, Adverse Reactions, and Overdose/Toxicology) at beginning of therapy and periodically throughout therapy. When treating Parkinson's disease, taper slowly when discontinuing. Assess knowledge/teach patient appropriate use, interventions to reduce side effects, and adverse symptoms to report (see Patient Education). **Pregnancy risk factor C** - benefits of use should outweigh possible risks. Note breast-feeding caution.

Patient Education: Take as directed; do not increase dosage, take more often than prescribed, or discontinue without consulting prescriber. Maintain adequate hydration (2-3 L/day of fluids) unless advised by prescriber to restrict fluids and void before taking medication. Take last dose of day in the afternoon to reduce incidence of insomnia. Avoid alcohol, sedatives, or hypnotics unless consulting prescriber. You may experience decreased mental alertness or coordination (use caution when driving, climbing stairs, or engaging in tasks requiring alertness until response to drug is known); or nausea or dry mouth (small, frequent meals, frequent mouth care, sucking lozenges, or chewing gum may help). Report unusual swelling of extremities, difficulty breathing or shortness of breath, change in gait or increased tremors, or changes in mentation (eg, depression, anxiety, irritability, hallucination, slurred speech). **Pregnancy/breast-feeding precautions:** Inform prescriber if you are pregnant. Consult prescriber if breast-feeding.

Geriatric Considerations: Elderly patients may be more susceptible to the CNS effects of amantadine; using 2 divided daily doses may minimize this effect. The syrup may be used to administer doses <100 mg.

Additional Information Patients with intolerable CNS side effects often do better with rimantadine.

Amantadine Hydrochloride *see* Amantadine *on page 72*

Amaryl® *see* Glimepiride *on page 632*

Ambenonium (am be NOE nee um)

U.S. Brand Names Mytelase®

Synonyms Ambenonium Chloride

Generic Available No

Pharmacologic Category Cholinergic Agonist

Pregnancy Risk Factor C

Lactation Excretion in breast milk unknown/not recommended

Use Treatment of myasthenia gravis

Mechanism of Action/Effect Action increases acetylcholine concentration at transmission sites in parasympathetic neurons and skeletal muscles by inhibiting acetylcholinesterase

Contraindications Routine administration of atropine or other belladonna alkaloids with ambenonium is contraindicated because they may suppress the muscarinic symptoms of excessive gastrointestinal stimulation, leaving only the more serious symptoms of muscle fasciculations and paralysis as signs of overdosage; should not be administered to patients receiving mecamylamine

Warnings/Precautions Prolonged action after cholinergics, drug should be discontinued until the patient is stabilized. Use with caution in patients with asthma, epilepsy, bradycardia, hyperthyroidism, or peptic ulcer. Differentiation of cholinergic/myasthenia crisis is critical, use edrophonium and clinical judgment. Anticholinergic insensitivity may develop for brief or

(Continued)

Ambenonium *(Continued)*

prolonged periods. Reduce or withhold dosages until the patient becomes sensitive again. May require respiratory support. Pregnancy risk C.

Drug Interactions

Decreased Effect: Corticosteroids antagonize effects of anticholinesterases in myasthenia gravis. Procainamide or quinidine may reverse ambenonium cholinergic effects on muscle.

Increased Effect/Toxicity: Succinylcholine neuromuscular blockade may be prolonged.

Effects on Lab Values ↑ aminotransferase [ALT (SGPT)/AST (SGOT)] (S), amylase (S)

Adverse Reactions Frequency not defined.

Cardiovascular: Arrhythmias (especially bradycardia), hypotension, decreased carbon monoxide, tachycardia, AV block, nodal rhythm, nonspecific EKG changes, cardiac arrest, syncope, flushing

Central nervous system: Convulsions, dysarthria, dysphonia, dizziness, loss of consciousness, drowsiness, headache

Dermatologic: Skin rash, thrombophlebitis (I.V.), urticaria

Gastrointestinal: Hyperperistalsis, nausea, vomiting, salivation, diarrhea, stomach cramps, dysphagia, flatulence

Genitourinary: Urinary urgency

Neuromuscular & skeletal: Weakness, fasciculations, muscle cramps, spasms, arthralgias

Ocular: Small pupils, lacrimation

Respiratory: Increased bronchial secretions, laryngospasm, bronchiolar constriction, respiratory muscle paralysis, dyspnea, respiratory depression, respiratory arrest, bronchospasm

Miscellaneous: Diaphoresis (increased), anaphylaxis, allergic reactions

Overdosage/Toxicology Have atropine on hand to reverse cholinergic crisis or hypersensitivity reaction.

Formulations Tablet, as chloride: 10 mg

Dosing

Adults & Elderly: Myasthenia gravis: Oral: 5-25 mg 3-4 times/day

Monitoring and Teaching Issues

Physical Assessment: Assess bladder and sphincter adequacy prior to administering medication. Assess other medications patient may be taking for effectiveness and interactions (see Contraindications and Drug Interactions). Monitor therapeutic effects, and adverse reactions (cholinergic crisis); see Warnings/Precautions, Adverse Reactions, and Overdose/Toxicology. Assess knowledge/teach patient appropriate use, interventions to reduce side effects, and adverse symptoms to report (see Patient Education). **Pregnancy risk factor C** - benefits of use should outweigh possible risks. Breast-feeding is not recommended.

Patient Education: This drug will not cure myasthenia gravis, but it may reduce the symptoms. Use as directed; do not increase dose or discontinue without consulting prescriber. Maintain adequate hydration (2-3 L/day of fluids) unless advised by prescriber to restrict fluids. May cause dizziness, drowsiness, or postural hypotension (rise slowly from sitting or lying position and use caution when driving or climbing stairs); vomiting or loss of appetite (small, frequent meals, frequent mouth care, sucking lozenges, or chewing gum may help); or diarrhea (boiled milk, yogurt, or buttermilk may help). Report persistent abdominal discomfort; significantly increased salivation, sweating, tearing, or urination; flushed skin; chest pain or palpitations; acute headache; unresolved diarrhea; excessive fatigue, insomnia, dizziness, or depression; increased muscle, joint, or body pain; vision changes or blurred vision; or shortness of breath or wheezing. **Pregnancy/breast-feeding precautions:** Inform prescriber if you are or intend to become pregnant. Breast-feeding is not recommended.

Ambenonium Chloride *see* Ambenonium *on page 73*

Ambenyl® Cough Syrup *see page 1522*

Ambien® *see* Zolpidem *on page 1430*

AmBisome® *see* Amphotericin B (Liposomal) *on page 98*

Amcort® *see* Triamcinolone *on page 1356*

Amerge® *see* Naratriptan *on page 950*

Americaine® *see page 1519*

Americaine® [OTC] *see* Benzocaine *on page 156*

Americaine® Anesthetic Lubricant *see* Benzocaine *on page 156*

A-methaPred® *see* MethylPREDNISolone *on page 885*

Amethopterin *see* Methotrexate *on page 874*

Amfepramone *see* Diethylpropion *on page 406*

Amgenal® Cough Syrup *see page 1522*

Amibid LA *see* Guaifenesin *on page 646*

Amifostine (am i FOS teen)

U.S. Brand Names Ethyol®

Synonyms Ethiofos; Gammaphos

Generic Available No

Pharmacologic Category Antidote

Pregnancy Risk Factor C

Lactation Excretion in breast milk unknown/contraindicated

Use Reduce the incidence of moderate to severe xerostomia in patients undergoing postoperative radiation treatment for head and neck cancer, where the radiation port includes a substantial portion of the parotid glands. Reduce the cumulative renal toxicity associated with repeated administration of cisplatin in patients with advanced ovarian cancer or nonsmall cell lung cancer. In these settings, the clinical data does not suggest that the effectiveness of cisplatin-based chemotherapy regimens is altered by amifostine.

Mechanism of Action/Effect Reduces the toxic effects of cisplatin

Contraindications Hypersensitivity to aminothiol compounds or mannitol

Warnings/Precautions Limited data are currently available regarding the preservation of antitumor efficacy when amifostine is administered prior to cisplatin therapy in settings other than advanced ovarian cancer or nonsmall cell lung cancer. Amifostine should therefore not be used in patients receiving chemotherapy for other malignancies in which chemotherapy can produce a significant survival benefit or cure, except in the context of a clinical study.

Patients who are hypotensive or in a state of dehydration should not receive amifostine. Interrupt antihypertensive therapy for 24 hours before amifostine. Patients receiving antihypertensive therapy that cannot be stopped for 24 hours preceding amifostine treatment also should not receive amifostine.

It is recommended that antiemetic medication, including dexamethasone 20 mg I.V. and a serotonin 5-HT_3 receptor antagonist be administered prior to and in conjunction with amifostine. Rare hypersensitivity reactions, including anaphylaxis, have been reported. Discontinue if allergic reaction occurs; do not rechallenge.

Reports of clinically relevant hypocalcemia are rare, but serum calcium levels should be monitored in patients at risk of hypocalcemia, such as those with nephrotic syndrome.

Pregnancy risk C.

Drug Interactions

Increased Effect/Toxicity: Special consideration should be given to patients receiving antihypertensive medications or other drugs that could potentiate hypotension.

Adverse Reactions

>10%:

Cardiovascular: Flushing; hypotension (62%) (see Additional Information)
Central nervous system: Chills, dizziness, somnolence
Gastrointestinal: Nausea/vomiting (may be severe)
Respiratory: Sneezing
Miscellaneous: Feeling of warmth/coldness, hiccups

<1% (Limited to important or life-threatening): Apnea, anaphylactoid reactions, anaphylaxis, arrhythmia, atrial fibrillation, erythema multiforme; hypersensitivity reactions (fever, rash, hypoxia, dyspnea, laryngeal edema); hypocalcemia, mild rashes, myocardial ischemia, rigors, seizure, Stevens-Johnson syndrome, toxic epidermal necrolysis

Overdosage/Toxicology Symptoms of overdose include nausea, vomiting, and hypotension. Treatment includes supportive measures as clinically indicated.

Pharmacodynamics/Kinetics

Half-Life Elimination: 9 minutes

Metabolism: Hepatic dephosphorylation to two metabolites (active-free thiol and disulfide)

Formulations Injection, powder for reconstitution: 500 mg

Dosing

Adults & Elderly:

Prevention of chemotherapy-induced renal toxicity: I.V. (refer to individual protocols): 910 mg/m^2 administered once daily as a 15-minute I.V. infusion, starting 30 minutes prior to chemotherapy. **Note:** A 15-minute infusion is better tolerated than more extended infusions. Further reductions in infusion times have not been systematically investigated. The infusion of amifostine should be interrupted if the systolic blood pressure decreases significantly from the baseline value:

Decrease of 20 if baseline systolic blood pressure <100
Decrease of 25 if baseline systolic blood pressure 100-119
Decrease of 30 if baseline systolic blood pressure 120-139
Decrease of 40 if baseline systolic blood pressure 140-179
Decrease of 50 if baseline systolic blood pressure ≥180

If the blood pressure returns to normal within 5 minutes and the patient is asymptomatic, the infusion may be restarted so that the full dose of amifostine may be administered. If the full dose of amifostine cannot be administered, the dose of amifostine for subsequent cycles should be 740 mg/m^2.

Reduction of xerostomia from head and neck radiation: I.V.: 200 mg/m^2 (as a 3-minute infusion) once daily, starting 15-30 minutes before standard fraction radiation therapy.

Administration

I.V.: Administer over 15 minutes; administration as a longer infusion is associated with a higher incidence of side effects.

Stability

Storage: Store vials of lyophilized powder at refrigeration, 2°C to 8°C.

Reconstitution: Reconstitute with 9.5 mL of sterile 0.9% sodium chloride. The reconstituted solution (500 mg/10 mL) is chemically stable for up to 5 hours at room temperature (25°C) or up to 24 hours under refrigeration 2°C to 8°C. Amifostine should be further diluted in 0.9% sodium chloride to a concentration of 5-40 mg/mL and is chemically stable for up to 5 hours at room temperature (25°C) or up to 24 hours when stored under refrigeration 2°C to 8°C.

Compatibility: Stable in NS

Y-site administration: Incompatible with acyclovir, amphotericin B, cefoperazone, chlorpromazine, cisplatin, ganciclovir, hydroxyzine, minocycline, prochlorperazine edisylate

Monitoring and Teaching Issues

Physical Assessment: Monitor blood pressure closely during infusion (continuously or every 5-7 minutes - see Dosing). Monitor nausea and treat with antiemetic as appropriate. **Pregnancy risk factor C.** Breast-feeding is contraindicated.

Patient Education: This I.V. medication is given to help reduce side effects of your chemotherapy. Report immediately any nausea; you will be given medication. Report chills, severe dizziness, tremors or shaking, or sudden onset of hiccups. **Breast-feeding precaution:** Do not breast-feed.

Additional Information Mean onset of hypotension is 14 minutes into the 15-minute infusion and the mean duration was 6 minutes.

Amigesic® *see* Salsalate *on page 1212*

Amikacin (am i KAY sin)

U.S. Brand Names Amikin®

Synonyms Amikacin Sulfate

Generic Available Yes

Pharmacologic Category Antibiotic, Aminoglycoside

Pregnancy Risk Factor C

Lactation Enters breast milk/compatible

Use Treatment of serious infections due to organisms resistant to gentamicin and tobramycin including *Pseudomonas*, *Proteus*, *Serratia*, and other gram-positive bacilli (bone infections, respiratory tract infections, endocarditis, and septicemia); documented infection of mycobacterial organisms susceptible to amikacin

Mechanism of Action/Effect Inhibits protein synthesis in susceptible bacteria by binding to ribosomal subunits

Contraindications Hypersensitivity to amikacin sulfate or any component of the formulation; cross-sensitivity may exist with other aminoglycosides

Warnings/Precautions Dose and/or frequency of administration must be monitored and modified in patients with renal impairment. Drug should be discontinued if signs of ototoxicity, nephrotoxicity, or hypersensitivity occur. Ototoxicity is proportional to the amount of drug given and the duration of treatment. Tinnitus or vertigo may be indications of vestibular injury and impending bilateral **irreversible** damage. Renal damage is usually reversible. May contain sulfites, use with caution in patients with asthma. Pregnancy risk C.

Drug Interactions

Increased Effect/Toxicity: Amikacin may increase or prolong the effect of neuromuscular blocking agents. Concurrent use of amphotericin (or other nephrotoxic drugs) may increase the risk of amikacin-induced nephrotoxicity. The risk of ototoxicity from amikacin may be increased with other ototoxic drugs.

Effects on Lab Values Penicillin may ↓ aminoglycoside serum concentrations *in vitro*

Adverse Reactions

1% to 10%:

Central nervous system: Neurotoxicity

Otic: Ototoxicity (auditory), ototoxicity (vestibular)

Renal: Nephrotoxicity

<1% (Limited to important or life-threatening): Allergic reaction, dyspnea, eosinophilia

Overdosage/Toxicology Symptoms of overdose include ototoxicity, nephrotoxicity, and neuromuscular toxicity. Treatment of choice following a single acute overdose appears to be maintenance of urine output of at least 3 mL/kg/hour during the acute treatment phase. Dialysis is of questionable value in enhancing aminoglycoside elimination. If required, hemodialysis is preferred over peritoneal dialysis in patients with normal renal function.

Pharmacodynamics/Kinetics

Absorption: I.M.: May be delayed in the bedridden patient

Half-Life Elimination: Renal function and age dependent:

Infants: Low birthweight (1-3 days): 7-9 hours; Full-term >7 days: 4-5 hours

Children: 1.6-2.5 hours

Adults: Normal renal function: 1.4-2.3 hours; Anuria/end-stage renal disease: 28-86 hours

Time to Peak: Serum: I.M.: 45-120 minutes

Formulations Injection, solution, as sulfate: 50 mg/mL (2 mL, 4 mL); 62.5 mg/mL (8 mL); 250 mg/mL (2 mL, 4 mL) [contains metabisulfite]

Dosing

Adults & Elderly: Individualization is critical because of the low therapeutic index

Note: Use of ideal body weight (IBW) for determining the mg/kg/dose appears to be more accurate than dosing on the basis of total body weight (TBW)

In morbid obesity, dosage requirement may best be estimated using a dosing weight of IBW + 0.4 (TBW - IBW)

Susceptible infections: I.M., I.V.: 5-7.5 mg/kg/dose every 8 hours

Adjustment: Initial and periodic peak and trough plasma drug levels should be determined, particularly in critically ill patients with serious infections or in disease states known to significantly alter aminoglycoside pharmacokinetics (eg, cystic fibrosis, burns, or major surgery)

Note: Some clinicians suggest a daily dose of 15-20 mg/kg for all patients with normal renal function. This dose is at least as efficacious with similar, if not less, toxicity than conventional dosing.

Pediatrics: Infants and Children: Refer to adult dosing.

Renal Impairment: Individualization is critical because of the low therapeutic index. Some patients may require larger or more frequent doses if serum levels document the need (ie, cystic fibrosis or febrile granulocytopenic patients).

Cl_{cr} ≥60 mL/minute: Administer every 8 hours.

Cl_{cr} 40-60 mL/minute: Administer every 12 hours.

Cl_{cr} 20-40 mL/minute: Administer every 24 hours.

Cl_{cr} 10-20 mL/minute: Administer every 48 hours.

Cl_{cr} <10 mL/minute: Administer every 72 hours.

Dialyzable (50% to 100%)

Administer dose postdialysis or administer 2/3 normal dose as a supplemental dose postdialysis and follow levels.

Peritoneal dialysis effects: Dose as for Cl_{cr} <10 mL/minute: Follow levels.

Continuous arteriovenous or venovenous hemodiafiltration effects: Dose as for Cl_{cr} 10-40 mL/minute: Follow levels.

Administration

I.M.: Administer I.M. injection in large muscle mass. Administer around-the-clock to promote less variation in peak and trough serum levels. Do not mix with other drugs, administer separately.

I.V.: Infuse over 30-60 minutes.

Stability

Reconstitution: Stable for 24 hours at room temperature and 2 days at refrigeration when mixed in D_5W, $D_5{}^1/_4NS$, $D_5{}^1/_2NS$, NS, LR

Compatibility: Stable in dextran 75 6% in NS, D_5LR, $D_5{}^1/_4NS$, $D_5{}^1/_3NS$, $D_5{}^1/_2NS$, D_5NS, $D_{10}NS$, D_5W, $D_{10}W$, $D_{20}W$, mannitol 20%, $^1/_4NS$, $^1/_2NS$, NS

Y-site administration: Incompatible with allopurinol, amphotericin B cholesteryl sulfate complex, hetastarch, propofol

Compatibility in syringe: Incompatible with heparin

Compatibility when admixed: Incompatible with amphotericin B, ampicillin, cefazolin, chlorothiazide, heparin, phenytoin, thiopental, vitamin B complex with C

Monitoring Laboratory Tests Perform culture and sensitivity testing prior to initiating therapy. Urinalysis, BUN, serum creatinine, appropriately timed peak and trough concentrations. Initial and periodic peak and trough plasma drug levels should be determined, particularly in critically ill patients with serious infections or in disease states known to significantly alter aminoglycoside pharmacokinetics (eg, cystic fibrosis, burns, or major surgery). Aminoglycoside levels measured from blood taken from Silastic® central catheters can sometimes give falsely high readings (draw levels from alternate lumen or peripheral stick, if possible).

Monitoring and Teaching Issues

Physical Assessment: Assess allergy history prior to beginning therapy. See Contraindications and Warnings/Precautions for use cautions. Assess potential for interactions with other prescriptions, OTC medications, or herbal products patient may be taking (see Drug Interactions). Assess results of laboratory tests (see above), therapeutic effectiveness, and adverse response (eg, ototoxicity, nephrotoxicity, neurotoxicity - see Adverse Reactions and Overdose/Toxicology). Hearing and renal status should be assessed before, during, and after therapy. Teach patient possible side effects and interventions and adverse symptoms to report (see Patient Education). **Pregnancy risk factor C** - benefits of use should outweigh possible risks.

Patient Education: Inform prescriber of all prescriptions, OTC medications, or herbal products you are taking, and any allergies you have. Do not take anything new during treatment unless approved by prescriber. This drug can only be administered by I.V. or I.M. injection. It is important to maintain adequate hydration (2-3 L/day of fluids) unless advised by prescriber to restrict fluids. Report immediately any change in hearing acuity, ringing or roaring in ears, alteration in balance, vertigo, feeling of fullness in head; pain, tingling, or numbness of any body part; or change in urinary pattern or decrease in urine. Report signs of opportunistic infection (eg, white plaques in mouth, vaginal discharge, unhealed sores, sore throat, unusual fever, chills); pain, redness, or swelling at injection site; or other adverse reactions. **Pregnancy precaution:** Inform prescriber if you are or intend to become pregnant.

Dietary Issues: Sodium content of 1 g: 29.9 mg (1.3 mEq)

Geriatric Considerations: Adjust dose based on renal function.

Breast-feeding Issues: No specific recommendations. However, aminoglycosides are not systemically available when taken orally. Therefore, the risk to the infant is minimal if ingested with breast milk.

Related Information

Peak and Trough Guidelines *on page 1544*
Tuberculosis *on page 1705*

Amikacin Sulfate *see* Amikacin *on page 76*
Amikin® *see* Amikacin *on page 76*

Amiloride (a MIL oh ride)

U.S. Brand Names Midamor®

Synonyms Amiloride Hydrochloride

Generic Available Yes

Pharmacologic Category Diuretic, Potassium Sparing

Pregnancy Risk Factor B

Lactation Excretion in breast milk unknown/contraindicated

Use Counteracts potassium loss induced by other diuretics in the treatment of hypertension or edematous conditions including CHF, hepatic cirrhosis, and hypoaldosteronism; usually used in conjunction with more potent diuretics such as thiazides or loop diuretics

Use - Unlabeled/Investigational Investigational: Cystic fibrosis; reduction of lithium-induced polyuria

Mechanism of Action/Effect Decreases potassium and calcium excretion in distal tubule, cortical collecting tubule, and collecting direct by inhibiting sodium, potassium, and ATPase; increases sodium, magnesium, and water excretion

Contraindications Hypersensitivity to amiloride or any component of the formulation; presence of elevated serum potassium levels (>5.5 mEq/L); if patient is receiving other potassium-conserving agents (eg, spironolactone, triamterene) or potassium supplementation (medicine, potassium-containing salt substitutes, potassium-rich diet); anuria; acute or chronic renal insufficiency; evidence of diabetic nephropathy. Patients with evidence of renal impairment or diabetes mellitus should not receive this medicine without close, frequent monitoring of serum electrolytes and renal function.

Warnings/Precautions May cause hyperkalemia (patients with renal impairment, diabetes and the elderly are at greatest risk). Should be stopped at least 3 days before glucose tolerance testing. Use caution in severely ill patients in whom respiratory or metabolic acidosis may occur.

Drug Interactions

Decreased Effect: Decreased effect of amiloride with use of NSAIDs. Amoxicillin's absorption may be reduced with concurrent use.

Increased Effect/Toxicity: Increased risk of amiloride-associated hyperkalemia with triamterene, spironolactone, ACE inhibitors, potassium preparations, cyclosporine, tacrolimus, and indomethacin. Amiloride may increase the toxicity of amantadine and

(Continued)

Amiloride *(Continued)*

lithium by reduction of renal excretion. Quinidine and amiloride together may increase risk of malignant arrhythmias.

Nutritional/Ethanol Interactions Food: Hyperkalemia may result if amiloride is taken with potassium-containing foods.

Effects on Lab Values ↑ potassium (S)

Adverse Reactions

1% to 10%:

Central nervous system: Headache, fatigue, dizziness

Endocrine & metabolic: Hyperkalemia, hyperchloremic metabolic acidosis, dehydration, hyponatremia, gynecomastia

Gastrointestinal: Nausea, diarrhea, vomiting, abdominal pain, gas pain, appetite changes, constipation

Genitourinary: Impotence

Neuromuscular & skeletal: Muscle cramps, weakness

Respiratory: Cough, dyspnea

<1% (Limited to important or life-threatening): Alopecia, arrhythmias, bladder spasms, chest pain, dyspnea, dysuria, GI bleeding, increased intraocular pressure, jaundice, orthostatic hypotension, palpitations, polyuria

Overdosage/Toxicology Clinical signs of toxicity are consistent with dehydration and electrolyte disturbance. Large amounts may result in life-threatening hyperkalemia (>6.5 mEq/L). This can be treated with I.V. glucose (dextrose 25% in water), rapid-acting insulin, concurrent I.V. sodium bicarbonate, and (if needed) Kayexalate® oral or rectal solution in sorbitol. Persistent hyperkalemia may require dialysis.

Pharmacodynamics/Kinetics

Absorption: ~15% to 25%

Half-Life Elimination: Normal renal function: 6-9 hours; End-stage renal disease: 8-144 hours

Time to Peak: Serum: 6-10 hours

Metabolism: No active metabolites

Onset: 2 hours

Duration: 24 hours

Formulations Tablet, as hydrochloride: 5 mg

Dosing

Adults: Hypertension, edema (to limit potassium loss): Oral: Initial: 5-10 mg/day (up to 20 mg)

Elderly: Oral: Initial: 5 mg once daily or every other day

Pediatrics: Edema, hypertension: Oral: Although safety and efficacy in children have not been established by the FDA, a dosage of 0.625 mg/kg/day has been used in children weighing 6-20 kg.

Renal Impairment: Oral:

Cl_{cr} 10-50 mL/minute: Administer 50% of normal dose.

Cl_{cr} <10 mL/minute: Avoid use.

Administration

Oral: Administer with food or meals to avoid GI upset.

Monitoring Laboratory Tests Serum electrolytes, renal function

Monitoring and Teaching Issues

Physical Assessment: See Contraindications, Warnings/Precautions, and Dosing for use cautions. Assess potential for interactions with other prescriptions, OTC medications, or herbal products patient may be taking (see Drug Interactions). Assess results of laboratory tests (see above), therapeutic effectiveness, and adverse response (eg, dehydration, hyperkalemia, hyperchloremic metabolic acidosis, hyponatremia - see Adverse Reactions and Overdose/Toxicology). Teach patient proper use, possible side effects and interventions, and adverse symptoms to report (see Patient Education). Breast-feeding is contraindicated.

Patient Education: Inform prescriber of all prescriptions, OTC medications, or herbal products you are taking, and any allergies you have. Do not take anything new during treatment unless approved by prescriber. Take as directed, preferably early in day with food. Do not increase dietary intake of potassium unless instructed by prescriber (too much potassium can be as harmful as too little). May cause dizziness or fatigue (use caution when driving or engaging in tasks that require alertness until response to drug is known); constipation (increased exercise, fluids, fruit, and fiber may help); impotence (reversible); or loss of hair (rare). Report muscle cramping or weakness, unresolved nausea or vomiting, palpitations, or difficulty breathing. **Breast-feeding precaution:** Do not breast-feed.

Dietary Issues: Take with food or meals to avoid GI upset. Do not use salt substitutes or low salt milk without checking with your healthcare provider, too much potassium can be as harmful as too little.

Geriatric Considerations: Use lower initial dose, and adjust dose for renal impairment.

Additional Information Medication should be discontinued if potassium level exceeds 6.5 mEq/L. Combined with hydrochlorothiazide as Moduretic®. Amiloride is considered an alternative to triamterene or spironolactone.

Related Information

Heart Failure *on page 1670*

Amiloride and Hydrochlorothiazide

(a MIL oh ride & hye droe klor oh THYE a zide)

U.S. Brand Names Moduretic®

Synonyms Hydrochlorothiazide and Amiloride

Generic Available Yes

Pharmacologic Category Diuretic, Combination

Pregnancy Risk Factor B

Lactation Excretion in breast milk unknown/contraindicated

Use Potassium-sparing diuretic; antihypertensive

Formulations Tablet: Amiloride hydrochloride 5 mg and hydrochlorothiazide 50 mg

Dosing

Adults: Hypertension, edema: Oral: Initial: 1 tablet/day, then may be increased to 2 tablets/day if needed; usually given in a single dose

Elderly: Oral: Initial: 1/2 to 1 tablet/day

Monitoring and Teaching Issues

Physical Assessment: See individual components listed in Related Information. Breast-feeding is contraindicated.

Patient Education: See individual components listed in Related Information. **Breast-feeding precaution:** Do not breast-feed.

Related Information

Amiloride *on page 77*
Hydrochlorothiazide *on page 664*

Amiloride Hydrochloride *see* Amiloride *on page 77*

2-Amino-6-Mercaptopurine *see* Thioguanine *on page 1305*

2-Amino-6-Trifluoromethoxy-benzothiazole *see* Riluzole *on page 1190*

Aminobenzylpenicillin *see* Ampicillin *on page 101*

Aminoglutethimide (a mee noe gloo TETH i mide)

U.S. Brand Names Cytadren®

Generic Available No

Pharmacologic Category Antineoplastic Agent, Miscellaneous

Pregnancy Risk Factor D

Lactation Excretion in breast milk unknown/contraindicated

Use In postmenopausal patients with breast cancer; third-line salvage agent for metastatic prostate cancer; suppression of adrenal function in selected patients with Cushing's syndrome

Mechanism of Action/Effect Blocks the conversion of cholesterol to delta-5-pregnenolone, thereby reducing the synthesis of adrenal glucocorticoids, mineralocorticoids, estrogens, aldosterone, and androgens. This inhibits growth of tumors that need estrogen to thrive.

Contraindications Hypersensitivity to aminoglutethimide, glutethimide, or any component of the formulation; pregnancy

Warnings/Precautions Monitor blood pressure in all patients at appropriate intervals. Hypothyroidism may occur. **Mineralocorticoid replacement is necessary in up to 50% of patients**. Glucocorticoid replacement is necessary in most patients.

Drug Interactions

Cytochrome P450 Effect: Induces **CYP1A2, 2C19, 3A4**

Decreased Effect: Aminoglutethimide may decrease therapeutic effect of dexamethasone, digitoxin (after 3-8 weeks), theophylline, warfarin, and medroxyprogesterone.

Effects on Lab Values ↑ alkaline phosphatase (S), AST (SGOT), TSH; ↓ plasma cortisol, thyroxine (S), and urinary aldosterone

Adverse Reactions Most adverse effects will diminish in incidence and severity after the first 2-6 weeks

>10%:

- Central nervous system: Headache, dizziness, drowsiness, and lethargy are frequent at the start of therapy, clumsiness
- Dermatologic: Skin rash
- Gastrointestinal: Nausea, vomiting, anorexia
- Hepatic: Cholestatic jaundice
- Neuromuscular & skeletal: Myalgia
- Renal: Nephrotoxicity
- Respiratory: Pulmonary alveolar damage
- Miscellaneous: Systemic lupus erythematosus

1% to 10%:

- Cardiovascular: Hypotension and tachycardia, orthostatic hypotension
- Central nervous system: Headache
- Dermatologic: Hirsutism in females
- Endocrine & metabolic: Adrenocortical insufficiency
- Hematologic: Rare cases of neutropenia, leukopenia, thrombocytopenia, pancytopenia, and agranulocytosis have been reported
- Neuromuscular & skeletal: Myalgia

Overdosage/Toxicology Symptoms of overdose include ataxia, somnolence, lethargy, dizziness, distress, fatigue, coma, hyperventilation, respiratory depression, hypovolemia, and shock. Treatment is supportive.

Pharmacodynamics/Kinetics

Absorption: 90%

Half-Life Elimination: 7-15 hours; shorter following multiple doses

Metabolism: Major metabolite is N-acetylaminoglutethimide; induces its own metabolism

Onset: Adrenal suppression: 3-5 days

Formulations Tablet, scored: 250 mg

Dosing

Adults & Elderly:

Cushing disease: Oral: 250 mg every 6 hours may be increased at 1- to 2-week intervals to a total of 2 g/day

Mineralocorticoid (fludrocortisone) replacement therapy may be necessary in up to 50% of patients. If glucocorticoid replacement therapy is necessary, 20-30 mg hydrocortisone orally in the morning will replace endogenous secretion.

(Continued)

Aminoglutethimide *(Continued)*

Renal Impairment: Dose reduction may be necessary.

Administration

Oral: Give in divided doses, 2-3 times/day to reduce incidence of nausea and vomiting.

Monitoring Laboratory Tests Thyroid function tests, CBC, liver function, electrolytes

Monitoring and Teaching Issues

Physical Assessment: See Contraindications and Warnings/Precautions for use cautions. Assess potential for interactions with other prescriptions, OTC medications, or herbal products patient may be taking (see Drug Interactions). Assess results of laboratory tests (see above), therapeutic response, and adverse reactions (eg, hypothyroidism: slow pulse, lethargy, dry skin, thick tongue; or Cushing syndrome: moon face, hump, hypertension, fragility, hirsutism, mood swings, susceptibility to infection - see Adverse Reactions and Overdose/Toxicology). Teach patient proper use, possible side effects and interventions, and adverse symptoms to report (see Patient Education). **Pregnancy risk factor D** - determine that patient is not pregnant before beginning treatment. Instruct patients of childbearing age about appropriate barrier contraceptive measures. Breast-feeding is contraindicated.

Patient Education: Inform prescriber of all prescriptions, OTC medications, or herbal products you are taking, and any allergies you have. Do not take anything new during treatment unless approved by prescriber. Take exactly as directed; may be taken with food to reduce incidence of nausea. May cause drowsiness or dizziness (avoid driving or engaging in tasks that require alertness until response to drug is known); nausea or vomiting (small, frequent meals, frequent mouth care, chewing gum or sucking lozenges may reduce incidence of nausea or vomiting); or masculinization (reversible when treatment is discontinued). Report rash, unresolved nausea or vomiting, lethargy, yellowing of skin or eyes, easy bruising or bleeding, change in color of urine or stool, increased growth of facial hair, thick tongue, severe mood swings, palpitations, or difficulty breathing. **Pregnancy/breast-feeding precautions:** Do not get pregnant while taking this medication. Consult prescriber for appropriate barrier contraceptive measures. Do not breast-feed.

Aminophylline *see page 1544*

Aminosalicylate Sodium (a MEE noe sa LIS i late SOW dee um)

Synonyms Para-Aminosalicylate Sodium; PAS

Generic Available Yes

Pharmacologic Category Salicylate

Pregnancy Risk Factor C

Lactation Enters breast milk/not recommended

Use Adjunctive treatment of tuberculosis used in combination with other antitubercular agents; has also been used in Crohn's disease

Mechanism of Action/Effect Aminosalicylic acid (PAS) is a highly specific bacteriostatic agent active against *M. tuberculosis*. Most strains of *M. tuberculosis* are sensitive to a concentration of 1 mcg/mL. Structurally related to para-aminobenzoic acid (PABA) and its mechanism of action is thought to be similar to the sulfonamides, a competitive antagonism with PABA. Disrupts plate biosynthesis in sensitive organisms.

Contraindications Hypersensitivity to aminosalicylate sodium or any component of the formulation

Warnings/Precautions Use with caution in patients with hepatic or renal dysfunction, patients with gastric ulcer, patients with CHF, and patients who are sodium restricted. Pregnancy risk C.

Drug Interactions

Decreased Effect: Aminosalicylate sodium may decrease serum levels of digoxin and vitamin B_{12}.

Adverse Reactions

1% to 10%: Gastrointestinal: Nausea, vomiting, diarrhea, abdominal pain

<1% (Limited to important or life-threatening): Agranulocytosis, fever, hemolytic anemia, hepatitis jaundice, leukopenia, thrombocytopenia, vasculitis

Overdosage/Toxicology Acute overdose results in crystalluria and renal failure, nausea, and vomiting. Alkalinization of urine with sodium bicarbonate and forced diuresis can prevent crystalluria and nephrotoxicity.

Pharmacodynamics/Kinetics

Absorption: Readily, >90%

Half-Life Elimination: Reduced with renal impairment

Metabolism: Hepatic (>50%) via acetylation

Formulations Tablet: 500 mg

Dosing

Adults & Elderly: Tuberculosis: Oral: 150 mg/kg/day in 2-3 equally divided doses (usually 12-14 g/day)

Pediatrics: Tuberculosis: Oral: Children: 150 mg/kg/day in 3-4 equally divided doses

Renal Impairment:

Cl_{cr} 10-50 mL/minute: Administer 50% to 75% of dose.

Cl_{cr} <10 mL/minute: Administer 50% of dose.

Administer after hemodialysis: Administer 50% of dose.

Continuous arteriovenous or venovenous hemofiltration: Dose as for Cl_{cr} 10-50 mL/minute.

Hepatic Impairment: Use with caution.

Administration

Oral: Do not use tablets that are discolored (ie, brown or purple).

Monitoring and Teaching Issues

Physical Assessment: Monitor for effectiveness of treatment and indications of adverse effects (see Adverse Reactions). **Pregnancy risk factor C** - benefits of use should outweigh possible risks. Breast-feeding is not recommended.

Patient Education: May be taken with food. Do not take tablets that are discolored (brown or purple); see pharmacist for new prescription. Do not stop taking without consulting prescriber. Report persistent sore throat, fever, unusual bleeding or bruising, persistent nausea or vomiting, or abdominal pain. **Pregnancy/breast-feeding precautions:** Inform prescriber if you are or intend to become pregnant. Breast-feeding is not recommended.

Dietary Issues: May be taken with food.

Geriatric Considerations: See Warnings/Precautions; elderly may require lower recommended dose.

5-Aminosalicylic Acid *see* Mesalamine *on page 858*

Aminoxin® [OTC] *see* Pyridoxine *on page 1156*

Amiodarone (a MEE oh da rone)

U.S. Brand Names Cordarone®; Pacerone®

Synonyms Amiodarone Hydrochloride

Generic Available Yes: Tablet

Pharmacologic Category Antiarrhythmic Agent, Class III

Pregnancy Risk Factor D

Lactation Enters breast milk/contraindicated (AAP rates "of concern")

Use

Oral: Management of life-threatening recurrent ventricular fibrillation (VF) or hemodynamically unstable ventricular tachycardia (VT)

I.V.: Initiation of treatment and prophylaxis of frequency recurring VF and unstable VT in patients refractory to other therapy. Also, used for patients when oral amiodarone is indicated, but who are unable to take oral medication.

Use - Unlabeled/Investigational

Conversion of atrial fibrillation to normal sinus rhythm; maintenance of normal sinus rhythm

Prevention of postoperative atrial fibrillation during cardiothoracic surgery

Paroxysmal supraventricular tachycardia (SVT)

Control of rapid ventricular rate due to accessory pathway conduction in pre-excited atrial arrhythmias [ACLS guidelines]

After defibrillation and epinephrine in cardiac arrest with persistent ventricular tachycardia (VT) or ventricular fibrillation (VF) [ACLS guidelines]

Control of hemodynamically stable VT, polymorphic VT or wide-complex tachycardia of uncertain origin [ACLS guidelines]

Mechanism of Action/Effect Class III antiarrhythmic agent which inhibits adrenergic stimulation, prolongs the action potential and refractory period in myocardial tissue; decreases AV conduction and sinus node function. antiarrhythmic activity may result from both parent compound and active metabolite DEA.

Contraindications Hypersensitivity to amiodarone or any component of the formulation; severe sinus-node dysfunction; second- and third-degree heart block (except in patients with a functioning artificial pacemaker); bradycardia causing syncope (except in patients with a functioning artificial pacemaker); cisapride, ritonavir, sparfloxacin, moxifloxacin, gatifloxacin; pregnancy

Warnings/Precautions Not considered first line therapy due to toxicity profile especially with large doses. Reserve for use in arrhythmias refractory to other therapy. Monitor for pulmonary toxicity, liver toxicity, or exacerbation of the arrhythmia. Use very cautiously and with close monitoring in patients with thyroid or liver disease. Significant heart block or sinus bradycardia can occur. Patients should be hospitalized when amiodarone is initiated. Pre-existing pulmonary disease does not increase risk of developing pulmonary toxicity, but if pulmonary toxicity develops then the prognosis is worse. Due to complex pharmacokinetics, it is difficult to predict when an arrhythmia or interaction with a subsequent treatment will occur following discontinuation of amiodarone. May cause optic neuropathy and/or optic neuritis, usually resulting in visual impairment. Caution in surgical patients; may enhance hemodynamic effect of anesthetics. Corneal microdeposits occur in a majority of patients. Safety and efficacy in pediatric patients have not been established.

Drug Interactions

Cytochrome P450 Effect: Substrate of CYP1A2, **2C8/9**, 2C19, 2D6, 3A4; Inhibits CYP1A2, 2B6, **2C8/9**, 2C19, **2D6, 3A4**

Decreased Effect: Amiodarone blood levels may be decreased by phenytoin and rifampin. Amiodarone may alter thyroid function and response to thyroid supplements; monitor closely.

Increased Effect/Toxicity: Note: Due to the long half-life of amiodarone, drug interactions may take 1 or more weeks to develop. Use of amiodarone with diltiazem, verapamil, digoxin, beta-blockers, and other drugs which delay AV conduction may cause excessive AV block (amiodarone may also decrease the metabolism of some of these agents - see below). Amprenavir, cimetidine, nelfinavir, and ritonavir increase amiodarone levels. Amiodarone may increase the levels of digoxin (reduce dose by 50% on initiation), clonazepam, cyclosporine, flecainide (decrease dose up to 33%), metoprolol, phenothiazines, phenytoin, procainamide (reduce dose), propranolol, quinidine, tricyclic antidepressants, and warfarin. Concurrent use of fentanyl may lead to bradycardia, sinus arrest, and hypotension. The effect of drugs which prolong the QT interval, including amitriptyline, astemizole, bepridil, cisapride, disopyramide, erythromycin, gatifloxacin, haloperidol, imipramine, moxifloxacin, quinidine, pimozide, procainamide, sotalol, sparfloxacin, theophylline, and thioridazine may be increased. Cisapride, gatifloxacin, moxifloxacin, and sparfloxacin are contraindicated. Amiodarone may increase lovastatin-induced myopathy; concurrent use not recommended. Amiodarone may alter thyroid function and response to thyroid supplements. Amiodarone enhances the myocardial depressant and conduction defects of inhalation anesthetics (monitor).

Nutritional/Ethanol Interactions

Food: Increases the rate and extent of absorption of amiodarone.

Herb/Nutraceutical: St John's wort may decrease amiodarone levels or enhance photosensitization. Avoid ephedra (may worsen arrhythmia). Avoid dong quai.

(Continued)

Amiodarone *(Continued)*

Effects on Lab Values Thyroid function tests: Amiodarone partially inhibits the peripheral conversion of thyroxine (T_4) to triiodothyronine (T_3); serum T_4 and reverse triiodothyronine (rT_3) concentrations may be increased and serum T_3 may be decreased. Most patients remain clinically euthyroid, however, clinical hypothyroidism or hyperthyroidism may occur.

Adverse Reactions With large dosages (>400 mg/day), adverse reactions occur in ~75% of patients and require discontinuance in 5% to 20%.

>10%:

- Cardiovascular: Hypotension (I.V., 16%)
- Central nervous system: Between 20% and 40% of patients experience some form of neurologic adverse events (see Central Nervous System and Neuromuscular & Skeletal effects: 1% to 10% category)
- Gastrointestinal: Nausea, vomiting

1% to 10%:

- Cardiovascular: Congestive heart failure, arrhythmias (including atropine-resistant bradycardia, heart block, sinus arrest, ventricular tachycardia), myocardial depression, flushing, edema. Additional effects associated with I.V. administration include asystole, cardiac arrest, electromechanical dissociation, ventricular tachycardia and cardiogenic shock.
- Central nervous system: Fever, fatigue, involuntary movements, incoordination, malaise, sleep disturbances, ataxia, dizziness, headache
- Dermatologic: Photosensitivity (10%)
- Endocrine & metabolic: Hypothyroidism or hyperthyroidism (less common), decreased libido
- Gastrointestinal: Constipation, anorexia, abdominal pain, abnormal salivation, abnormal taste (oral form)
- Genitourinary: noninfectious epididymitis (3% to 11%)
- Hematologic: Coagulation abnormalities
- Hepatic: Abnormal LFTs
- Local: Phlebitis (I.V., with concentrations >3 mg/mL)
- Neuromuscular & skeletal: Paresthesia, tremor, muscular weakness, peripheral neuropathy
- Ocular: Visual disturbances, corneal microdeposits (occur in a majority of patients, and lead to visual disturbance in ~10%); other ocular symptoms are listed under the <1% category
- Respiratory: Pulmonary toxicity has been estimated to occur at a frequency between 2% and 7% of patients (some reports indicate a frequency as high as 17%). Toxicity may present as hypersensitivity pneumonitis, pulmonary fibrosis (cough, fever, malaise), pulmonary inflammation, interstitial pneumonitis, or alveolar pneumonitis; other rare pulmonary toxicities are listed under the <1% category.
- Miscellaneous: Abnormal smell (oral form)

<1% (Limited to important or life-threatening): Acute intracranial hypertension (I.V.), alopecia, anaphylactic shock, angioedema, aplastic anemia, ARDS (postoperative), atrial fibrillation, bone marrow granuloma, brain stem dysfunction, bronchiolitis obliterans organizing pneumonia (BOOP), cholestasis, cirrhosis, delirium, discoloration of skin (slate-blue), dyskinesias, encephalopathy, hypotension (with oral form), impotence, increased QT interval, leukocytoclastic vasculitis, neutropenia, nodal arrhythmia, optic neuritis, optic neuropathy, pancreatitis, pancytopenia, Parkinsonian symptoms, pleuritis, pseudotumor cerebri, pulmonary edema, rash, severe hepatotoxicity (potentially fatal hepatitis), Stevens-Johnson syndrome, thrombocytopenia, toxic epidermal necrolysis, vasculitis, ventricular fibrillation

Overdosage/Toxicology Symptoms include extension of pharmacologic effects, sinus bradycardia and/or heart block, hypotension, and QT prolongation. Patients should be monitored for several days following ingestion. Intoxication with amiodarone necessitates EKG monitoring. Bradycardia may be atropine resistant. Injectable isoproterenol or a temporary pacemaker may be required.

Pharmacodynamics/Kinetics

Bioavailability: ~50%

Half-Life Elimination: 40-55 days (range: 26-107 days); shorter in children than adults

Metabolism: Hepatic, major metabolite active; possible enterohepatic recirculation

Onset: Oral: 3 days to 3 weeks; I.V.: May be more rapid; Peak effect: 1 week to 5 months

Duration: After discontinuing therapy: 7-50 days

Note: Mean onset of effect and duration after discontinuation may be shorter in children than adults

Formulations

Injection, solution, as hydrochloride: 50 mg/mL (3 mL) [contains benzyl alcohol and polysorbate (Tween®) 80]

Tablet, scored, as hydrochloride: 200 mg

- Cordarone®: 200 mg
- Pacerone®: 200 mg, 400 mg

Dosing

Adults:

Ventricular arrhythmias: Oral: 800-1600 mg/day in 1-2 doses for 1-3 weeks, then 600-800 mg/day in 1-2 doses for 1 month; maintenance: 400 mg/day; lower doses are recommended for supraventricular arrhythmias.

Breakthrough VF or VT: I.V.: 150 mg supplemental doses in 100 mL D_5W over 10 minutes

Pulseless VF or VT: I.V. push: Initial: 300 mg in 20-30 mL NS or D_5W; if VF or VT recurs, supplemental dose of 150 mg followed by infusion of 1 mg/minute for 6 hours, then 0.5 mg/minute (maximum daily dose: 2.2 g)

Note: When switching from I.V. to oral therapy, use the following as a guide:

- <1 week I.V. infusion → 800-1600 mg/day
- 1- to 3-week I.V. infusion → 600-800 mg/day
- >3 week I.V. infusion → 400 mg

Recommendations for conversion to intravenous amiodarone after oral administration: During long-term amiodarone therapy (ie, ≥4 months), the mean plasma-elimination half-life of the active metabolite of amiodarone is 61 days. Replacement therapy may not be necessary in such patients if oral therapy is discontinued for a period <2 weeks, since any changes in serum amiodarone concentrations during this period may **not** be clinically significant.

Unlabeled uses:

Prophylaxis of atrial fibrillation following open heart surgery (unlabeled use): **Note:** A variety of regimens have been used in clinical trials, including oral and intravenous regimens:

Oral: 400 mg twice daily (starting in postop recovery) for up to 7 days. An alternative regimen of amiodarone 600 mg/day for 7 days prior to surgery, followed by 200 mg/day until hospital discharge has also been shown to decrease the risk of postoperative atrial fibrillation.

I.V.: 1000 mg infused over 24 hours (starting at postop recovery) for 2 days has been shown to reduce the risk of postoperative atrial fibrillation

Recurrent atrial fibrillation (unlabeled use): No standard regimen defined; examples of regimens include: Oral: Initial: 10 mg/kg/day for 14 days; followed by 300 mg/day for 4 weeks, followed by maintenance dosage of 100-200 mg/day (see Roy D, 2000). Other regimens have been described and are used clinically (ie, 400 mg 3 times/day for 5-7 days, then 400 mg/day for 1 month, then 200 mg/day).

Stable VT or SVT (unlabeled use): First 24 hours: 1000 mg according to following regimen

Step 1: 150 mg (100 mL) over first 10 minutes (mix 3 mL in 100 mL D_5W)

Step 2: 360 mg (200 mL) over next 6 hours (mix 18 mL in 500 mL D_5W): 1 mg/minute

Step 3: 540 mg (300 mL) over next 18 hours: 0.5 mg/minute

Note: After the first 24 hours: 0.5 mg/minute utilizing concentration of 1-6 mg/mL

Elderly: No specific guidelines available. Dose selection should be cautious, at low end of dosage range, and titration should be slower to evaluate response. Refer to adult dosing.

Pediatrics: Arrhythmias:

Oral (calculate doses for children <1 year on body surface area): Loading dose: 10-15 mg/kg/day or 600-800 mg/1.73 m²/day for 4-14 days or until adequate control of arrhythmia or prominent adverse effects occur (this loading dose may be given in 1-2 divided doses/day); dosage should then be reduced to 5 mg/kg/day or 200-400 mg/1.73 m²/day given once daily for several weeks. If arrhythmia does not recur, reduce to lowest effective dosage possible; usual daily minimal dose: 2.5 mg/kg/day; maintenance doses may be given for 5 of 7 days/week.

I.V. (safety and efficacy of amiodarone use in children has not been fully established): sq A multicenter study (Perry, 1996; n=40; mean age 5.4 years with 24 of 40 children <2 years of age) used an I.V. loading dose of 5 mg/kg that was divided into five 1 mg/kg aliquots, with each aliquot given over 5-10 minutes. Additional 1-5 mg/kg doses could be administered 30 minutes later in a similar fashion if needed. The mean loading dose was 6.3 mg/kg. A maintenance dose (continuous infusion of 10-15 mg/kg/day) was administered to 21 of the 40 patients. Further studies are needed. **Note:** I.V. administration at low flow rates (potentially associated with use in pediatrics) may result in leaching of plasticizers (DEHP) from intravenous tubing. DEHP may adversely affect male reproductive tract development. Alternative means of dosing and administration (1 mg/kg aliquots) may need to be considered.

Renal Impairment:

Hemodialysis effects: Not removed by hemodialysis or peritoneal dialysis (0% to 5%); no supplemental doses required.

Hepatic Impairment: Dosage adjustment is probably necessary in substantial hepatic impairment. No specific guidelines available.

Administration

Oral: Administer consistently with regard to meals. Take in divided doses with meals if high daily dose or if GI upset occurs. If GI intolerance occurs with single-dose therapy, use twice daily dosing.

I.V.: Give I.V. therapy using an infusion pump through a central line or a peripheral line at a concentration of <2 mg/mL. Infusions >2 hours must be administered in glass or polyolefin bottles. **Note:** I.V. administration at low flow rates (potentially associated with use in pediatrics) may result in leaching of plasticizers (DEHP) from intravenous tubing. DEHP may adversely affect male reproductive tract development. Alternative means of dosing and administration (1 mg/kg aliquots) may need to be considered.

Stability

Storage: Store at room temperature and protect from light.

Compatibility:

Y-site administration: Incompatible with aminophylline, cefamandole, heparin, sodium bicarbonate

Compatibility in syringe: Incompatible with heparin

Compatibility when admixed: Incompatible with floxacillin

Monitoring Laboratory Tests Thyroid function, pulmonary function

Monitoring and Teaching Issues

Physical Assessment: Assess other medications patient may be taking for effectiveness and interactions (see Drug Interactions). **I.V.:** Requires infusion pump and continuous cardiac/hemodynamic monitoring and observation for adverse reactions (see Warnings and Adverse Reactions). **Oral:** Monitor laboratory tests, therapeutic response, and symptoms of adverse effects (see Warnings/Precautions, Adverse Reactions, and Overdose/Toxicology) at beginning of therapy and regularly during long-term therapy. **Pregnancy risk factor D**. Breast-feeding is contraindicated.

Patient Education: Emergency use: Patient condition will determine amount of patient education.

Oral: May be taken with food to reduce GI disturbance, but be consistent. Always take with food or always take without food. Do not change dosage or discontinue drug without

(Continued)

Amiodarone *(Continued)*

consulting prescriber. Regular blood work, ophthalmic exams, and cardiac assessment will be necessary while taking this medication on a long-term basis. You may experience dizziness, weakness, or insomnia (use caution when driving, climbing stairs, or engaging in tasks requiring alertness until response to drug is known); hypotension (use caution when rising from sitting or lying position); nausea, vomiting, loss of appetite, stomach discomfort, or abnormal taste (small, frequent meals, frequent mouth care, chewing gum, or sucking lozenges may help); photosensitivity (use sunscreen, wear protective clothing and eyewear, and avoid direct sunlight); or decreased libido (reversible). Report persistent dry cough or shortness of breath; chest pain, palpitations, irregular or slow heartbeat; unusual bruising or bleeding; blood in urine, feces (black stool), vomitus; warmth, swelling, pain, in in calves; muscle tremor, weakness, numbness, or changes in gait; skin rash or irritation; or changes in urinary patterns. **Pregnancy/breast-feeding precautions:** Do not get pregnant while taking this medication; use appropriate contraceptive measures. Do not breast-feed.

Dietary Issues: Administer consistently with regard to meals.

Geriatric Considerations: Elderly may be predisposed to toxicity (see Drug Interactions). Half-life may be prolonged due to decreased clearance (see Hepatic/Renal Impairment).

Breast-feeding Issues: Hypothyroidism may occur in nursing infants.

Pregnancy Issues: May cause fetal harm when administered to a pregnant woman, leading to congenital goiter and hypo- or hyperthyroidism.

Related Information

Antiarrhythmic Drugs *on page 1551*

Amiodarone Hydrochloride *see* Amiodarone *on page 81*

Ami-Tex PSE *see* Guaifenesin and Pseudoephedrine *on page 648*

Amitone® [OTC] *see* Calcium Supplements *on page 202*

Amitriptyline (a mee TRIP ti leen)

U.S. Brand Names Elavil®; Vanatrip®

Synonyms Amitriptyline Hydrochloride

Generic Available Yes

Pharmacologic Category Antidepressant, Tricyclic (Tertiary Amine)

Pregnancy Risk Factor D

Lactation Enters breast milk/not recommended (AAP rates "of concern")

Use Relief of symptoms of depression

Use - Unlabeled/Investigational Analgesic for certain chronic and neuropathic pain; prophylaxis against migraine headaches; treatment of depressive disorders in children

Mechanism of Action/Effect Increases the synaptic concentration of serotonin and/or norepinephrine in the central nervous system by inhibition of their reuptake by the presynaptic neuronal membrane

Contraindications Hypersensitivity to amitriptyline or any component of the formulation (cross-sensitivity with other tricyclics may occur); use of MAO inhibitors within past 14 days; acute recovery phase following myocardial infarction; concurrent use of cisapride; pregnancy

Warnings/Precautions May cause drowsiness/sedation, resulting in impaired performance of tasks requiring alertness (ie, operating machinery or driving). Sedative effects may be additive with other CNS depressants and/or ethanol. May worsen psychosis in some patients or precipitate a shift to mania or hypomania in patients with bipolar disease. May cause hyponatremia/SIADH. May increase the risks associated with electroconvulsive therapy. Discontinue, when possible, prior to elective surgery. Therapy should not be abruptly discontinued in patients receiving high doses for prolonged periods.

Use with caution in patients at risk of hypotension (orthostasis) or in patients where transient hypotensive episodes would be poorly tolerated (cardiovascular disease or cerebrovascular disease). Use with caution in elderly patients, patients with diabetes, thyroid disease (or patients receiving thyroid supplements), hepatic dysfunction, renal dysfunction, urinary retention, benign prostatic hyperplasia, narrow-angle glaucoma, xerostomia, visual problems, constipation, or a history of bowel obstruction.

Use caution in patients with depression, particularly if suicidal risk may be present. Use with caution in patients with a history of cardiovascular disease, previous seizure disorder, or condition/drug therapy predisposing to seizures. Not for use in patients <12 years of age.

Drug Interactions

Cytochrome P450 Effect: Substrate of CYP1A2, 2B6, 2C8/9, 2C19, **2D6**, 3A4; Inhibits CYP1A2, 2C8/9, 2C19, 2D6, 2E1

Decreased Effect: Carbamazepine, phenobarbital, and rifampin may increase the metabolism of amitriptyline resulting in a decreased effect of amitriptyline. Amitriptyline inhibits the antihypertensive response to bethanidine, clonidine, debrisoquin, guanadrel, guanethidine, guanabenz, or guanfacine. Cholestyramine and colestipol may bind TCAs and reduce their absorption.

Increased Effect/Toxicity: Amitriptyline increases the effects of amphetamines, anticholinergics, other CNS depressants (sedatives, hypnotics, or ethanol), carbamazepine, tolazamide, chlorpropamide, and warfarin. When used with MAO inhibitors, hyperpyrexia, hypertension, tachycardia, confusion, seizures, and **deaths have been reported** (serotonin syndrome). Serotonin syndrome has also been reported with ritonavir (rare). The SSRIs (to varying degrees), cimetidine, fenfluramine, grapefruit juice, indinavir, methylphenidate, ritonavir, quinidine, diltiazem, valproate, and verapamil inhibit the metabolism of TCAs and clinical toxicity may result. Use of lithium with a TCA may increase the risk for neurotoxicity. Phenothiazines may increase concentration of some TCAs and TCAs may increase the concentration of phenothiazines. Pressor response to I.V. epinephrine, norepinephrine, and phenylephrine may be enhanced in patients receiving TCAs (**Note:** Effect is unlikely with epinephrine or levonordefrin dosages typically administered as infiltration in combination with local anesthetics). Combined use of beta-agonists or drugs which prolong

QT_c (including quinidine, procainamide, disopyramide, cisapride, sparfloxacin, gatifloxacin, moxifloxacin) with TCAs may predispose patients to cardiac arrhythmias.

Nutritional/Ethanol Interactions

Ethanol: Avoid ethanol (may increase CNS depression).

Food: Grapefruit juice may inhibit the metabolism of some TCAs and clinical toxicity may result.

Herb/Nutraceutical: St John's wort may decrease amitriptyline levels. Avoid valerian, St John's wort, kava kava, gotu kola (may increase CNS depression).

Effects on Lab Values Amitriptyline may increase or decrease serum glucose levels, may elevate liver function tests, and may prolong conduction time.

Adverse Reactions Anticholinergic effects may be pronounced; moderate to marked sedation can occur (tolerance to these effects usually occurs).

Frequency not defined.

Cardiovascular: Orthostatic hypotension, tachycardia, nonspecific EKG changes, changes in AV conduction

Central nervous system: Restlessness, dizziness, insomnia, sedation, fatigue, anxiety, impaired cognitive function, seizures, extrapyramidal symptoms

Dermatologic: Allergic rash, urticaria, photosensitivity

Gastrointestinal: Weight gain, xerostomia, constipation

Genitourinary: Urinary retention

Ocular: Blurred vision, mydriasis

Miscellaneous: Diaphoresis

Overdosage/Toxicology Symptoms of overdose include agitation, confusion, hallucinations, urinary retention, hypothermia, hypotension, ventricular tachycardia, and seizures. Treatment is symptomatic and supportive. Alkalinization by sodium bicarbonate and/or hyperventilation may limit cardiac toxicity.

Pharmacodynamics/Kinetics

Half-Life Elimination: Adults: 9-27 hours (average: 15 hours)

Time to Peak: Serum: ~4 hours

Metabolism: Hepatic to nortriptyline (active), hydroxy and conjugated derivatives; may be impaired in the elderly

Onset: Migraine prophylaxis: 6 weeks, higher dosage may be required in heavy smokers because of increased metabolism; Depression: 4-6 weeks, reduce dosage to lowest effective level

Formulations

Injection, as hydrochloride: 10 mg/mL (10 mL)

Tablet, as hydrochloride: 10 mg, 25 mg, 50 mg, 75 mg, 100 mg, 150 mg

Dosing

Adults:

Depression:

Oral: 50-150 mg/day single dose at bedtime or in divided doses; dose may be gradually increased up to 300 mg/day.

I.M.: 20-30 mg 4 times/day

Chronic pain management: Oral: Initial: 25 mg at bedtime; may increase as tolerated to 100 mg/day.

Elderly: Oral: Initial: 10-25 mg at bedtime; dose should be increased in 10-25 mg increments every week if tolerated; dose range: 25-150 mg/day. See Renal/Hepatic Impairment.

Pediatrics:

Chronic pain management (unlabeled use): Oral: Initial: 0.1 mg/kg at bedtime, may advance as tolerated over 2-3 weeks to 0.5-2 mg/kg at bedtime

Depressive disorders (unlabeled use):

Children: Oral: Initial doses of 1 mg/kg/day given in 3 divided doses with increases to 1.5 mg/kg/day have been reported in a small number of children (n=9) 9-12 years of age; clinically, doses up to 3 mg/kg/day (5 mg/kg/day if monitored closely) have been proposed

Adolescents: Initial: 25-50 mg/day; may administer in divided doses; increase gradually to 100 mg/day in divided doses.

Renal Impairment: Nondialyzable

Hepatic Impairment: Use with caution and monitor plasma levels and patient response.

Administration

I.V.: Do **not** administer I.V.

Monitoring and Teaching Issues

Physical Assessment: See Contraindications and Warnings/Precautions for use cautions. Assess other medications patient may be taking for effectiveness and interactions (see Drug Interactions). Assess for suicidal tendencies before beginning therapy. May cause physiological or psychological dependence, tolerance, or abuse; evaluate need for continued use periodically. Caution patients with diabetes; may increase or decrease serum glucose levels. Monitor therapeutic response and adverse reactions at beginning of therapy and periodically with long-term use (see Adverse Reactions and Overdose/Toxicology). Taper dosage slowly when discontinuing. Teach patient appropriate use, interventions to reduce side effects, and adverse symptoms to report (see Patient Education). **Pregnancy risk factor D** - determine that patient is not pregnant before beginning treatment. Teach patients of childbearing age appropriate use of barrier contraceptives. Breast-feeding is not recommended.

Patient Education: Inform prescriber of all prescriptions (including oral contraceptives), OTC medications, or herbal products you are taking, and any allergies you have. Take exactly as directed; do not increase dose or frequency. It may take several weeks to achieve desired results. Restrict use of alcohol or caffeine; avoid grapefruit juice. Maintain adequate hydration (2-3 L/day of fluids) unless advised by prescriber to restrict fluids. If diabetic, monitor glucose levels closely; this medication may alter glucose levels. May turn urine blue-green (normal). May cause drowsiness, lightheadedness, impaired coordination, dizziness, or blurred vision (use caution when driving or engaging in tasks requiring alertness until response to drug is known); constipation (increased exercise, fluids, fruit, or

(Continued)

Amitriptyline *(Continued)*

fiber may help); urinary retention (void before taking medication); postural hypotension (use caution climbing stairs or when changing position from lying or sitting to standing); altered sexual drive or ability (reversible); or photosensitivity (use sunscreen, wear protective clothing and eyewear, and avoid direct sunlight). Report persistent CNS effects (eg, nervousness, restlessness, insomnia, headache, agitation, impaired coordination, changes in cognition); muscle cramping, weakness, tremors, or rigidity; ringing in ears or visual disturbances; chest pain, palpitations, or irregular heartbeat; blurred vision; or worsening of condition. **Pregnancy/breast-feeding precautions:** Do not get pregnant while taking this medication. Consult prescriber for appropriate contraceptive measures. Breast-feeding is not recommended.

Geriatric Considerations: The most anticholinergic and sedating of the antidepressants. Due to pronounced effects on the cardiovascular system (hypotension), many psychiatrists agree it is best to avoid in the elderly.

Breast-feeding Issues: Generally, it is not recommended to breast-feed if taking antidepressants because of the long half-life, active metabolites, and the potential for side effects in the infant.

Related Information

Antidepressant Agents *on page 1553*
Antidepressant Medication Guidelines *on page 1613*
Peak and Trough Guidelines *on page 1544*

Amitriptyline Hydrochloride *see* Amitriptyline *on page 84*

Amlexanox (am LEKS an oks)

U.S. Brand Names Aphthasol™

Generic Available No

Pharmacologic Category Anti-inflammatory, Locally Applied

Pregnancy Risk Factor B

Lactation Excretion in breast milk unknown/use caution

Use Treatment of aphthous ulcers (ie, canker sores)

Use - Unlabeled/Investigational Allergic disorders

Mechanism of Action/Effect As a benzopyrano-bipyridine carboxylic acid derivative, amlexanox has anti-inflammatory and antiallergic properties; it inhibits chemical mediatory release of the slow-reacting substance of anaphylaxis (SRS-A) and may have antagonistic effects on interleukin-3

Contraindications Hypersensitivity to amlexanox or any component of the formulation

Warnings/Precautions Discontinue therapy if rash or contact mucositis develops.

Adverse Reactions

1% to 2%:
- Dermatologic: Allergic contact dermatitis
- Gastrointestinal: Oral irritation

<1% (Limited to important or life-threatening): Contact mucositis

Pharmacodynamics/Kinetics

Absorption: Some from swallowed paste

Half-Life Elimination: 3.5 hours

Time to Peak: Serum: 2 hours

Metabolism: Hydroxylated and conjugated metabolites

Formulations Paste: 5% (5 g)

Dosing

Adults & Elderly: Aphthous ulcers: Topical: Administer (0.5 cm - 1/4") directly on ulcers 4 times/day following oral hygiene, after meals, and at bedtime.

Monitoring and Teaching Issues

Physical Assessment: Assess knowledge/teach patient appropriate application and use, adverse effects to report, and interventions for side-effects. Note breast-feeding caution.

Patient Education: This medication is only for treatment of mouth ulcers; do not apply to ulcers of the eye or any other part of the body. Use as directed. Apply after eating. Wash hands before and after use. Brush teeth and rinse mouth before applying directly to ulcers. Squeeze a small amount of paste on your clean finger tip and dab paste onto each ulcer in the mouth, using gentle pressure. Wash eyes immediately if any paste should come into contact with eyes. Notify prescriber or dentist if rash or irritation occurs, or if condition does not improve after 10 days use. **Breast-feeding precaution:** Consult prescriber if breast-feeding.

Amlodipine (am LOE di peen)

U.S. Brand Names Norvasc®

Generic Available No

Pharmacologic Category Calcium Channel Blocker

Pregnancy Risk Factor C

Lactation Excretion in breast milk unknown/use caution

Use Treatment of hypertension and angina

Mechanism of Action/Effect Inhibits calcium ion from entering the "slow channels" or select voltage-sensitive areas of vascular smooth muscle and myocardium during depolarization

Contraindications Hypersensitivity to amlodipine or any component of the formulation

Warnings/Precautions Increased angina and/or MI has occurred with initiation or dosage titration of calcium channel blockers. Use caution in severe aortic stenosis. Use caution in patients with severe hepatic impairment. Safety and efficacy in children have not been established. Dosage titration should occur after 7-14 days on a given dose. Pregnancy risk C.

Drug Interactions

Cytochrome P450 Effect: Substrate of **CYP3A4**; Inhibits CYP2B6, 2C8/9, 2D6, 3A4

Decreased Effect: Rifampin (and potentially other enzyme inducers) increase the metabolism of amlodipine. Calcium may reduce the calcium channel blocker's hypotensive effects.

Increased Effect/Toxicity: Azole antifungals (itraconazole, ketoconazole, fluconazole), erythromycin, and other inhibitors of cytochrome P450 isoenzyme 3A4 may inhibit amlodipine's metabolism. Grapefruit juice may modestly increase amlodipine levels. Cyclosporine levels may be increased by amlodipine. Blood pressure-lowering effects of sildenafil are additive with amlodipine.

Nutritional/Ethanol Interactions Herb/Nutraceutical: St John's wort may decrease amlodipine levels. Avoid dong quai if using for hypertension (has estrogenic activity). Avoid ephedra, yohimbe, ginseng (may worsen hypertension). Avoid garlic (may have increased antihypertensive effects).

Adverse Reactions

>10%: Cardiovascular: Peripheral edema (1.8% to 14.6% dose-related)

1% to 10%:

Cardiovascular: Flushing (0.7% to 2.6%), palpitations (0.7% to 4.5%)

Central nervous system: Headache (7.3%; similar to placebo)

Dermatologic: Rash (1% to 2%), pruritus (1% to 2%)

Endocrine & metabolic: Male sexual dysfunction (1% to 2%)

Gastrointestinal: Nausea (2.9%), abdominal pain (1% to 2%), dyspepsia (1% to 2%), gingival hyperplasia

Neuromuscular & skeletal: Muscle cramps (1% to 2%), weakness (1% to 2%)

Respiratory: Dyspnea (1% to 2%), pulmonary edema (15% from PRAISE trial, CHF population)

<1% (Limited to important or life-threatening): Abnormal dreams, agitation alopecia, amnesia, anxiety, apathy, arrhythmias, ataxia, bradycardia, cardiac failure, depersonalization, depression, erythema multiforme, exfoliative dermatitis, extrapyramidal symptoms, gastritis, gynecomastia, hypotension, leukocytoclastic vasculitis, migraine, nonthrombocytopenic purpura, paresthesia, peripheral ischemia, photosensitivity, postural hypotension, purpura, rash, skin discoloration, Stevens-Johnson syndrome, syncope, thrombocytopenia, tinnitus, urticaria, vertigo, xerophthalmia

Overdosage/Toxicology Primary cardiac symptoms of calcium channel blocker overdose include hypotension and bradycardia. Noncardiac symptoms include confusion, stupor, nausea, vomiting, metabolic acidosis, and hyperglycemia. Treat other signs and symptoms symptomatically.

Pharmacodynamics/Kinetics

Absorption: Oral: Well absorbed

Bioavailability: 64% to 90%

Half-Life Elimination: 30-50 hours

Metabolism: Hepatic (>90%) to inactive metabolite

Onset: 30-50 minutes; Peak effect: 6-12 hours

Duration: 24 hours

Formulations Tablet: 2.5 mg, 5 mg, 10 mg

Dosing

Adults: Hypertension, angina: Oral: Initial: 2.5-5 mg once daily; usual dose: 5-10 mg once daily; maximum: 10 mg once daily

Elderly: Oral: Initial: 2.5 mg once daily; increase by 2.5 mg increments at 7- to 14-day intervals; maximum recommended dose: 10 mg/day.

Hepatic Impairment: 2.5 mg once daily

Administration

Oral: May be taken without regard to meals.

Stability

Storage: Store at room temperature of 15°C to 30°C (59°F to 86°F).

Monitoring and Teaching Issues

Physical Assessment: See Warnings/Precautions for use cautions. Assess potential for interactions with prescription, OTC medications, or herbal products patient may be taking (eg, nitrates or other drugs that effect blood pressure - see Drug Interactions). Assess therapeutic effects and signs of adverse reactions at beginning of therapy, when changing dose, and periodically during long-term therapy (see Adverse Reactions and Overdose/Toxicology). Teach patient proper use, possible side effects and interventions, and adverse symptoms to report (see Patient Education). **Pregnancy risk factor C** - benefits of use should outweigh possible risks. Note breast-feeding caution.

Patient Education: Inform prescriber of all prescriptions, OTC medications, or herbal products you are taking, and any allergies you have. Do not add anything new during treatment unless approved by prescriber. Take exactly as directed; do not alter dose or discontinue without consulting prescriber. May cause headache (if unrelieved, consult prescriber); nausea or vomiting (small, frequent meals, frequent mouth care, chewing gum or sucking lozenges may help); constipation (increased dietary bulk and fluids may help); or drowsiness (use caution when driving or engaging in tasks that require alertness until response to drug is known). Report unrelieved headache; vomiting, constipation; palpitations; peripheral or facial swelling; weight gain >5 lb/week; or respiratory changes. **Pregnancy/breast-feeding precautions:** Inform prescriber if you are or intend to become pregnant. Consult prescriber if breast-feeding.

Dietary Issues: May be taken without regard to meals.

Geriatric Considerations: Elderly or debilitated persons may experience a greater hypotensive response. Theoretically, constipation may be more of a problem with elderly.

Related Information

Calcium Channel Blockers *on page 1563*

Amlodipine and Benazepril (am LOE di peen & ben AY ze pril)

U.S. Brand Names Lotrel®

Synonyms Benazepril and Amlodipine

Generic Available No

Pharmacologic Category Antihypertensive Agent Combination

Pregnancy Risk Factor C/D (2nd and 3rd trimesters)

(Continued)

Amlodipine and Benazepril *(Continued)*

Lactation

Amlodipine: Excretion in breast milk unknown
Benazepril: Enters breast milk

Use Treatment of hypertension

Formulations

Capsule:
Amlodipine 2.5 mg and benazepril hydrochloride 10 mg
Amlodipine 5 mg and benazepril hydrochloride 10 mg
Amlodipine 5 mg and benazepril hydrochloride 20 mg
Amlodipine 10 mg and benazepril hydrochloride 20 mg

Dosing

Adults & Elderly: Dosage is individualized and adjusted to response:

Hypertension: Oral: 1 capsule/day. May be used as a replacement for separate dosing of components or combination when response to single agent is suboptimal.

Renal Impairment: Cl_{cr} <30 mL/minute: Not recommended since the initial dose of benazepril at this level of renal function is 5 mg. Titration of individual agents is preferred.

Monitoring and Teaching Issues

Physical Assessment: See individual components listed in Related Information. **Pregnancy risk factor C/D** - see see Pregnancy Risk Factor for use cautions. Assess knowledge/instruct patient on need to use appropriate contraceptive measures and the need to avoid pregnancy. Note breast-feeding caution.

Patient Education: See individual components listed in Related Information. **Pregnancy/breast-feeding precautions:** Inform prescriber if you are or intend to become pregnant. Consult prescriber if breast-feeding.

Related Information

Amlodipine *on page 86*
Benazepril *on page 154*

AMO Vitrax® *see page 1509*
AMO Vitrax® *see page 1461*

Amoxicillin (a moks i SIL in)

U.S. Brand Names Amoxicot®; Amoxil®; Moxilin®; Trimox®; Wymox®

Synonyms Amoxicillin Trihydrate; Amoxycillin; *p*-Hydroxyampicillin

Generic Available Yes

Pharmacologic Category Antibiotic, Penicillin

Pregnancy Risk Factor B

Lactation Enters breast milk/compatible

Use Treatment of otitis media, sinusitis, and infections caused by susceptible organisms involving the respiratory tract, skin, and urinary tract; prophylaxis of bacterial endocarditis in patients undergoing surgical or dental procedures; as part of a multidrug regimen for *H. pylori* eradication

Use - Unlabeled/Investigational Postexposure prophylaxis for anthrax exposure with documented susceptible organisms

Mechanism of Action/Effect Interferes with bacterial cell wall synthesis during active multiplication, causing cell wall death and resultant bactericidal activity against susceptible bacteria

Contraindications Hypersensitivity to amoxicillin, penicillin, or any component of the formulation

Warnings/Precautions In patients with renal impairment, doses and/or frequency of administration should be modified in response to the degree of renal impairment. A high percentage of patients with infectious mononucleosis have developed rash during therapy with amoxicillin.

Drug Interactions

Decreased Effect: Decreased effectiveness with tetracyclines and chloramphenicol. Although anecdotal reports suggest oral contraceptive efficacy could be reduced by penicillins, this has been refuted by more rigorous scientific and clinical data.

Increased Effect/Toxicity: Disulfiram and probenecid may increase amoxicillin levels. Amoxicillin may increase the effects of oral anticoagulants (warfarin). Theoretically, allopurinol taken with amoxicillin has an additive potential for amoxicillin rash.

Effects on Lab Values ↑ AST, ALT, protein; altered response to Benedict's reagent in Clinitest®

Adverse Reactions Frequency not defined.

Central nervous system: Hyperactivity, agitation, anxiety, insomnia, confusion, convulsions, behavioral changes, dizziness

Dermatologic: Erythematous maculopapular rashes, erythema multiforme, Stevens-Johnson syndrome, exfoliative dermatitis, toxic epidermal necrolysis, hypersensitivity vasculitis, urticaria

Gastrointestinal: Nausea, vomiting, diarrhea, hemorrhagic colitis, pseudomembranous colitis

Hematologic: Anemia, hemolytic anemia, thrombocytopenia, thrombocytopenia purpura, eosinophilia, leukopenia, agranulocytosis

Hepatic: Elevated AST (SGOT) and ALT (SGPT), cholestatic jaundice, hepatic cholestasis, acute cytolytic hepatitis

Overdosage/Toxicology Symptoms of penicillin overdose include neuromuscular hypersensitivity (eg, agitation, hallucinations, asterixis, encephalopathy, confusion, and seizures). Electrolyte imbalance may occur if the preparation contains potassium or sodium salts, especially in renal failure. Hemodialysis may be helpful to aid in removal of the drug from blood; otherwise, treatment is symptom-directed and supportive.

Pharmacodynamics/Kinetics

Absorption: Oral: Rapid and nearly complete; food does not interfere

Half-Life Elimination:

Neonates, full-term: 3.7 hours

Infants and Children: 1-2 hours
Adults: Normal renal function: 0.7-1.4 hours
Cl_{cr} <10 mL/minute: 7-21 hours

Time to Peak: Capsule: 2 hours; Suspension: 1 hour

Metabolism: Partially hepatic

Formulations

Capsule, as trihydrate: 250 mg, 500 mg
Amoxicot®, Amoxil®, Moxilin®, Trimox®: 250 mg, 500 mg
Wymox®: 250 mg

Powder for oral suspension, as trihydrate: 125 mg/5 mL (5 mL, 80 mL, 100 mL, 150 mL); 250 mg/5 mL (5 mL, 80 mL, 100 mL, 150 mL)
Amoxicot®: 125 mg/5 mL (100 mL, 150 mL); 250 mg/5 mL (100 mL, 150 mL)

Powder for oral suspension [drops], as trihydrate (Amoxil®): 50 mg/mL (15 mL, 30 mL) [strawberry flavor]

Tablet, chewable, as trihydrate: 125 mg, 200 mg, 250 mg, 400 mg
Amoxil® [cherry-banana-peppermint flavor]: 200 mg [contains phenylalanine 1.82 mg/tablet], 400 mg [contains phenylalanine 3.64 mg/tablet]

Tablet, film coated (Amoxil®): 500 mg, 875 mg

Dosing

Adults & Elderly:

Susceptible infections: Oral: 250-500 mg every 8 hours or 500-875 mg twice daily; maximum dose: 2-3 g/day

Endocarditis prophylaxis: 2 g 1 hour before procedure

Helicobacter pylori eradication: Oral: 1000 mg twice daily; requires combination therapy with at least one other antibiotic and an acid-suppressing agent (proton pump inhibitor or H_2 blocker)

Anthrax exposure (unlabeled use): Oral: **Note:** Postexposure prophylaxis only with documented susceptible organisms: 500 mg every 8 hours

Pediatrics:

Susceptible infections: Oral: Children: 20-50 mg/kg/day in divided doses every 8 hours
Acute otitis media due to highly-resistant strains of *S. pneumoniae*: Doses as high as 80-90 mg/kg/day divided every 12 hours have been used
Subacute bacterial endocarditis prophylaxis: Oral: 50 mg/kg 1 hour before procedure
Anthrax exposure (unlabeled use): Oral: **Note:** Postexposure prophylaxis only with documented susceptible organisms:
<40 kg: 15 mg/kg every 8 hours
≥40 kg: 500 mg every 8 hours

Renal Impairment:

Cl_{cr} 10-50 mL/minute: Administer every 12 hours.
Cl_{cr} <10 mL/minute: Administer every 24 hours.
Moderately dialyzable (20% to 50%) by hemodialysis or peritoneal dialysis; approximately 50 mg of amoxicillin per liter of filtrate is removed by continuous arteriovenous or venovenous hemofiltration. Dose as per Cl_{cr} <10 mL/minute guidelines.

Administration

Oral: Administer around-the-clock to promote less variation in peak and trough serum levels.

Stability

Storage: Oral suspension remains stable for 7 days at room temperature or 14 days if refrigerated; unit-dose antibiotic oral syringes are stable for 48 hours

Reconstitution: After reconstitution, the suspension remains stable for 7 days at room temperature or 14 days if refrigerated. Unit-dose antibiotic oral syringes are stable for 48 hours.

Monitoring Laboratory Tests Perform culture and sensitivity testing prior to initiating therapy.

Monitoring and Teaching Issues

Physical Assessment: Assess for allergy history prior to starting therapy. See Contraindications and Warnings/Precautions for use cautions. Assess potential for interactions with other prescriptions, OTC medications, or herbal products patient may be taking (see Drug Interactions). Caution diabetic patients about altered response to Clinitest®. Assess for therapeutic effect and adverse reactions (eg, opportunistic infection: fever, chills, unhealed sores, white plaques in mouth or vagina, purulent vaginal discharge, fatigue - see Adverse Reactions and Overdose/Toxicology). Teach patient proper use, possible side effects and interventions, and adverse symptoms to report (see Patient Education).

Patient Education: Inform prescriber of all prescriptions, OTC medications, or herbal products you are taking, and any allergies you have. Do not add anything new during treatment unless approved by prescriber. Take entire prescription, even if you are feeling better. Take at equal intervals around-the-clock. May be taken with milk, juice, or food. If diabetic, drug may cause false test results with Clinitest® urine glucose monitoring; use of another type of glucose monitoring is preferable. May cause nausea or vomiting (small, frequent meals, frequent mouth care, sucking lozenges, or chewing gum may help). Report rash; unusual diarrhea; vaginal itching, burning, or pain; unresolved vomiting or constipation; fever or chills; abdominal pain; jaundice; unusual bruising or bleeding; or if condition being treated worsens or does not improve by the time prescription is completed.

Dietary Issues: May be taken with food.

Geriatric Considerations: Resistance to amoxicillin has been a problem in patients on frequent antibiotics or in nursing homes. Alternative antibiotics may be necessary in these populations. Consider renal function.

Related Information

Helicobacter pylori Treatment *on page 1676*

Amoxicillin and Clavulanate Potassium

(a moks i SIL in & klav yoo LAN ate poe TASS ee um)

U.S. Brand Names Augmentin®; Augmentin ES-600™; Augmentin XR™

Synonyms Amoxicillin and Clavulanic Acid

(Continued)

Amoxicillin and Clavulanate Potassium *(Continued)*

Generic Available Yes: Excludes extended release

Pharmacologic Category Antibiotic, Penicillin

Pregnancy Risk Factor B

Lactation Enters breast milk/compatible

Use Treatment of otitis media, sinusitis, and infections caused by susceptible organisms involving the lower respiratory tract, skin and skin structure, and urinary tract; spectrum same as amoxicillin with additional coverage of beta-lactamase producing *B. catarrhalis*, *H. influenzae*, *N. gonorrhoeae*, and *S. aureus* (not MRSA). The expanded coverage of this combination makes it a useful alternative when amoxicillin resistance is present and patients cannot tolerate alternative treatments.

Mechanism of Action/Effect Interferes with bacterial cell wall synthesis during active multiplication, causing cell wall death and resultant bactericidal activity against susceptible bacteria. Clavulanic acid binds and inhibits beta-lactamases that inactivate amoxicillin resulting in amoxicillin having an expanded spectrum of activity.

Contraindications Hypersensitivity to amoxicillin, clavulanic acid, penicillin, or any component of the formulation; history of cholestatic jaundice or hepatic dysfunction with amoxicillin/clavulanate potassium therapy

Warnings/Precautions Prolonged use may result in superinfection; in patients with renal impairment, doses and/or frequency of administration should be modified in response to the degree of renal impairment; high percentage of patients with infectious mononucleosis have developed rash during therapy; a low incidence of cross-allergy with cephalosporins exists; incidence of diarrhea is higher than with amoxicillin alone. Use caution in patients with hepatic dysfunction. Hepatic dysfunction, although rare, is more common in elderly and/or males, and occurs more frequently with prolonged treatment, and may occur after therapy is complete. Due to differing content of clavulanic acid, not all formulations are interchangeable. Some products contain phenylalanine.

Drug Interactions

Decreased Effect: Although anecdotal reports suggest oral contraceptive efficacy could be reduced by penicillins, this has been refuted by more rigorous scientific and clinical data.

Increased Effect/Toxicity: Probenecid may increase amoxicillin levels. Increased effect of anticoagulants with amoxicillin. Allopurinol taken with Augmentin® has an additive potential for rash.

Effects on Lab Values Urinary glucose (Benedict's solution, Clinitest®)

Adverse Reactions

>10%: Gastrointestinal: Diarrhea (3% to 34%; incidence varies upon dose and regimen used)

1% to 10%:

- Dermatologic: Diaper rash, skin rash, urticaria
- Gastrointestinal: Abdominal discomfort, loose stools, nausea, vomiting
- Genitourinary: Vaginitis
- Miscellaneous: Moniliasis

<1% (Limited to important or life-threatening): Cholestatic jaundice, flatulence, headache, hepatic dysfunction, prothrombin time increased, thrombocytosis

Additional adverse reactions seen with **ampicillin-class antibiotics:** Agitation, agranulocytosis, ALT elevated, anaphylaxis, anemia, angioedema, anxiety, AST elevated, behavioral changes, black "hairy" tongue, confusion, convulsions, dizziness, enterocolitis, eosinophilia, erythema multiforme, exanthematous pustulosis, exfoliative dermatitis, gastritis, glossitis, hematuria, hemolytic anemia, hemorrhagic colitis, indigestion, insomnia, hyperactivity, interstitial nephritis, leukopenia, mucocutaneous candidiasis, pruritus, pseudomembranous colitis, serum sickness-like reaction, Stevens-Johnson syndrome, stomatitis, thrombocytopenia, thrombocytopenic purpura, tooth discoloration, toxic epidermal necrolysis

Overdosage/Toxicology Symptoms of overdose may include abdominal pain, diarrhea, drowsiness, rash, hyperactivity, stomach pain, and vomiting. Electrolyte imbalance may occur, especially in renal failure. Hemodialysis may be helpful to aid in removal of the drug from blood; otherwise, treatment is supportive or symptom-directed.

Pharmacokinetic Note Amoxicillin pharmacokinetics are not affected by clavulanic acid. See Amoxicillin monograph.

Pharmacodynamics/Kinetics

Metabolism:

Clavulanic acid: Hepatic

Formulations

Powder for oral suspension: 200: Amoxicillin 200 mg and clavulanate potassium 28.5 mg per 5 mL (100 mL) [contains phenylalanine]; 400: Amoxicillin 400 mg and clavulanate potassium 57 mg per 5 mL (100 mL) [contains phenylalanine]

Augmentin®:

- 125: Amoxicillin trihydrate 125 mg and clavulanate potassium 31.25 mg per 5 mL (75 mL, 100 mL, 150 mL) [banana flavor]
- 200: Amoxicillin 200 mg and clavulanate potassium 28.5 mg per 5 mL (50 mL, 75 mL, 100 mL) [contains phenylalanine 7 mg/5 mL; orange-raspberry flavor]
- 250: Amoxicillin trihydrate 250 mg and clavulanate potassium 62.5 mg per 5 mL (75 mL, 100 mL, 150 mL) [orange flavor]
- 400: Amoxicillin 400 mg and clavulanate potassium 57 mg per 5 mL (50 mL, 75 mL, 100 mL) [contains phenylalanine 7 mg/5 mL; orange-raspberry flavor]

Augmentin ES-600™: Amoxicillin 600 mg and clavulanic potassium 42.9 mg per 5 mL (50 mL, 75 mL, 100 mL, 150 mL) [contains phenylalanine 7 mg/5 mL; orange-raspberry flavor]

Tablet: 500: Amoxicillin trihydrate 500 mg and clavulanate potassium 125 mg; 875: Amoxicillin trihydrate 875 mg and clavulanate potassium 125 mg

Augmentin®:

- 250: Amoxicillin trihydrate 250 mg and clavulanate potassium 125 mg
- 500: Amoxicillin trihydrate 500 mg and clavulanate potassium 125 mg
- 875: Amoxicillin trihydrate 875 mg and clavulanate potassium 125 mg

Tablet, chewable: 200: Amoxicillin trihydrate 200 mg and clavulanate potassium 28.5 mg [contains phenylalanine]; 400: Amoxicillin trihydrate 400 mg and clavulanate potassium 57 mg [contains phenylalanine]

Augmentin®:

125: Amoxicillin trihydrate 125 mg and clavulanate potassium 31.25 mg [lemon-lime flavor]

200: Amoxicillin trihydrate 200 mg and clavulanate potassium 28.5 mg [contains phenylalanine 2.1 mg/tablet; cherry-banana flavor]

250: Amoxicillin trihydrate 250 mg and clavulanate potassium 62.5 mg [lemon-lime flavor]

400: Amoxicillin trihydrate 400 mg and clavulanate potassium 57 mg [contains phenylalanine 4.2 mg/tablet; cherry-banana flavor]

Tablet, extended release (Augmentin XR™): Amoxicillin 1000 mg and clavulanic acid 62.5 mg

Dosing

Adults & Elderly: Note: Dose is based on the amoxicillin component; see table.

Augmentin® Product-Specific Considerations

Strength	Form	Consideration
125 mg	CT, S	q8h dosing
	S	For adults having difficulty swallowing tablets, 125 mg/5 mL suspension may be substituted for 500 mg tablet.
200 mg	CT, S	q12h dosing
	CT	Contains phenylalanine
	S	For adults having difficulty swallowing tablets, 200 mg/5 mL suspension may be substituted for 875 mg tablet.
250 mg	CT, S, T	q8h dosing
	CT	Contains phenylalanine
	T	Not for use in patients <40 kg
	CT, T	Tablet and chewable tablet are not interchangeable due to differences in clavulanic acid.
	S	For adults having difficulty swallowing tablets, 250 mg/5 mL suspension may be substituted for 500 mg tablet.
400 mg	CT, S	q12h dosing
	CT	Contains phenylalanine
	S	For adults having difficulty swallowing tablets, 400 mg/5 mL suspension may be substituted for 875 mg tablet.
500 mg	T	q8h or q12h dosing
600 mg	S	q12 h dosing
		Contains phenylalanine
		Not for use in adults or children ≥40 kg
		600 mg/5 mL suspension is not equivalent to or interchangeable with 200 mg/5 mL or 400 mg/5 mL due to differences in clavulanic acid.
875 mg	T	Not for use in Cl_{cr} <30 mL/minute
1000 mg	XR	Not for use in children <16 years of age
		q12h dosing
		Not interchangeable with two 500 mg tablets
		Not for use in Cl_{cr} <30 mL/minute or hemodialysis

Legend: CT = chewable tablet, S = suspension, T = tablet, XR = extended release

Susceptible infections: Oral: Children >40 kg and Adults: 250-500 mg every 8 hours or 875 mg every 12 hours

Acute bacterial sinusitis: Oral: Extended release tablet: Two 1000 mg tablets every 12 hours for 10 days

Community-acquired pneumonia: Oral: Extended release tablet: Two 1000 mg tablets every 12 hours for 7-10 days

Pediatrics: Note: Dose is based on the amoxicillin component; see "Augmentin® Product-Specific Considerations table".

Susceptible infections: Oral: Infants <3 months: 30 mg/kg/day divided every 12 hours using the 125 mg/5 mL suspension

Otitis media: Oral: Children ≥3 months and <40 kg: 90 mg/kg/day divided every 12 hours for 10 days

Lower respiratory tract infections, severe infections, sinusitis: Oral: Children ≥3 months and <40 kg: 45 mg/kg/day divided every 12 hours**or** 40 mg/kg/day divided every 8 hours

Less severe infections: Oral: Children ≥3 months and <40 kg: 25 mg/kg/day divided every 12 hours or 20 mg/kg/day divided every 8 hours

Children >40 kg: Refer to adult dosing.

Renal Impairment:

Cl_{cr} <30 mL/minute: Do not use 875 mg tablet or extended release tablets.

Cl_{cr} 10-30 mL/minute: 250-500 mg every 12 hours

Cl_{cr} <10 mL/minute: 250-500 every 24 hours

Hemodialysis: Moderately dialyzable (20% to 50%)

250-500 mg every 24 hours; administer dose during and after dialysis. Do not use extended release tablets.

Peritoneal dialysis: Moderately dialyzable (20% to 50%)

Amoxicillin: Administer 250 mg every 12 hours

Clavulanic acid: Dose for Cl_{cr} <10 mL/minute

Continuous arteriovenous or venovenous hemofiltration effects:

Amoxicillin: ~50 mg of amoxicillin/L of filtrate is removed

Clavulanic acid: Dose for Cl_{cr} <10 mL/minute

(Continued)

Amoxicillin and Clavulanate Potassium *(Continued)*

Administration

Oral: Administer around-the-clock to promote less variation in peak and trough serum levels. Administer with food to decrease stomach upset; shake suspension well before use. Extended release tablets should be administered with food.

Stability

Storage:

Powder for oral suspension: Store dry powder at room temperature of 25°C (77°F).

Tablet: Store at room temperature of 25°C (77°F).

Reconstitution: Reconstitute powder for oral suspension with appropriate amount of water as specified on the bottle. Shake vigorously until suspended. Reconstituted oral suspension should be kept in refrigerator. Discard unused suspension after 10 days. Unit-dose antibiotic oral syringes are stable for 48 hours.

Monitoring Laboratory Tests Renal, hepatic, and hematologic function periodically with prolonged therapy. Perform culture and sensitivity testing prior to initiating therapy.

Monitoring and Teaching Issues

Physical Assessment: Assess for allergy history prior to starting therapy. See Contraindications and Warnings/Precautions for use cautions. Assess potential for interactions with other prescriptions, OTC medications, or herbal products patient may be taking (see Drug Interactions). Caution diabetic patients about altered response to Clinitest®. Assess results of laboratory tests (see above), therapeutic effectiveness, and adverse reactions (eg, opportunistic infection: fever, chills, unhealed sores, white plaques in mouth or vagina, purulent vaginal discharge, fatigue - see Adverse Reactions and Overdose/Toxicology). Teach patient proper use, possible side effects and interventions, and adverse symptoms to report (see Patient Education).

Patient Education: Inform prescriber of all prescriptions, OTC medications, or herbal products you are taking, and any allergies you have. Do not add anything new during treatment unless approved by prescriber. Take as directed, for as long as directed, even if you are feeling better. (For small children, bottles may contain more suspension than needed, take for number of days prescribed.) Take at equal intervals around-the-clock; may be taken with milk, juice, or food. Extended release tablets should be taken with food. If diabetic, drug may cause false test results with Clinitest® urine glucose monitoring; use of another type of glucose monitoring is preferable. May cause nausea or vomiting (small, frequent meals, frequent mouth care, sucking lozenges, or chewing gum may help). Report rash; unusual diarrhea; vaginal itching, burning, or pain; unresolved vomiting or constipation; fever or chills; abdominal pain; jaundice; unusual bruising or bleeding; or if condition being treated worsens or does not improve by the time prescription is completed. Some products contain phenylalanine. Avoid use in phenylketonurics.

Dietary Issues: May be taken with meals or on an empty stomach; take with meals to increase absorption and decrease GI intolerance; may mix with milk, formula, or juice. Extended release tablets should be taken with food. Some products contain phenylalanine; avoid use in phenylketonurics. All dosage forms contain potassium.

Geriatric Considerations: Resistance to amoxicillin has been a problem in patients on frequent antibiotics or in nursing homes. However, expanded coverage of this combination makes it a useful alternative when amoxicillin resistance is present and patients cannot tolerate alternative treatments. Consider renal function. Considered one of the drugs of choice in the outpatient treatment of community-acquired pneumonia in older adults.

Additional Information Two 250 mg tablets are not equivalent to a 500 mg tablet (both tablet sizes contain equivalent clavulanate). Two 500 mg tablets are not equivalent to a single 1000 mg extended release tablet.

Related Information

Amoxicillin *on page 88*

Amoxicillin and Clavulanic Acid *see* Amoxicillin and Clavulanate Potassium *on page 89*

Amoxicillin, Lansoprazole, and Clarithromycin *see* Lansoprazole, Amoxicillin, and Clarithromycin *on page 774*

Amoxicillin Trihydrate *see* Amoxicillin *on page 88*

Amoxicot® *see* Amoxicillin *on page 88*

Amoxil® *see* Amoxicillin *on page 88*

Amoxycillin *see* Amoxicillin *on page 88*

Amphetamine *see page 1693*

Amphetamine and Dextroamphetamine *see* Dextroamphetamine and Amphetamine *on page 394*

Amphetamine/Methamphetamine *see page 1568*

Amphetamine Variants *see page 1568*

Amphocin® *see* Amphotericin B (Conventional) *on page 94*

Amphojel® [OTC] *see* Aluminum Hydroxide *on page 71*

Amphotec® *see* Amphotericin B Cholesteryl Sulfate Complex *on page 92*

Amphotericin B Cholesteryl Sulfate Complex

(am foe TER i sin bee kole LES te ril SUL fate KOM plecks)

U.S. Brand Names Amphotec®

Synonyms ABCD; Amphotericin B Colloidal Dispersion

Generic Available No

Pharmacologic Category Antifungal Agent, Parenteral

Pregnancy Risk Factor B

Lactation Excretion in breast milk unknown/contraindicated

Use Treatment of invasive aspergillosis in patients who have failed amphotericin B deoxycholate treatment, or who have renal impairment or experience unacceptable toxicity which precludes treatment with amphotericin B deoxycholate in effective doses.

Mechanism of Action/Effect Binds to ergosterol altering cell membrane permeability in susceptible fungi and causing leakage of cell components with subsequent cell death

Contraindications Hypersensitivity to amphotericin B or any component of the formulation

Warnings/Precautions Anaphylaxis has been reported. Facilities for cardiopulmonary resuscitation should be available. Infusion reactions, sometimes severe, usually subside with continued therapy.

Drug Interactions

Decreased Effect: Pharmacologic antagonism may occur with azole antifungals (ketoconazole, miconazole, etc).

Increased Effect/Toxicity: Toxic effect with other nephrotoxic drugs (eg, cyclosporine and aminoglycosides) may be additive. Corticosteroids may increase potassium depletion caused by amphotericin. Amphotericin B may predispose patients receiving digitalis glycosides or neuromuscular blocking agents to toxicity secondary to hypokalemia.

Adverse Reactions

>10%: Central nervous system: Chills, fever

1% to 10%:

Cardiovascular: Hypotension, tachycardia
Central nervous system: Headache
Dermatologic: Rash
Endocrine & metabolic: Hypokalemia, hypomagnesemia
Gastrointestinal: Nausea, diarrhea, abdominal pain
Hematologic: Thrombocytopenia
Hepatic: LFT change
Neuromuscular & skeletal: Rigors
Renal: Elevated creatinine
Respiratory: Dyspnea

Note: Amphotericin B colloidal dispersion has an improved therapeutic index compared to conventional amphotericin B, and has been used safely in patients with amphotericin B-related nephrotoxicity; however, continued decline of renal function has occurred in some patients.

Overdosage/Toxicology Symptoms of overdose include renal dysfunction, anemia, thrombocytopenia, granulocytopenia, fever, nausea, and vomiting. Treatment is supportive.

Pharmacodynamics/Kinetics

Half-Life Elimination: 28-29 hours; prolonged with higher doses

Formulations Injection, suspension: 50 mg (20 mL); 100 mg (50 mL)

Dosing

Adults & Elderly:

Premedication: For patients who experience chills, fever, hypotension, nausea, or other nonanaphylactic infusion-related immediate reactions, premedicate with the following drugs, 30-60 minutes prior to drug administration: a nonsteroidal (eg, ibuprofen, choline magnesium trisalicylate, etc) with or without diphenhydramine; or acetaminophen with diphenhydramine; or hydrocortisone 50-100 mg. If the patient experiences rigors during the infusion, meperidine may be administered.

Susceptible infections: I.V.: Usual range: 3-4 mg/kg/day (infusion of 1 mg/kg/hour); maximum: 7.5 mg/kg/day

A regimen of 6 mg/kg/day has been used for treatment of life-threatening invasive mold infections in immunocompromised patients; maximum: 7.5 mg/kg/day.

Initially infuse at 1 mg/kg/hour. Rate of infusion may be increased with subsequent doses to 3 mg/kg/hour as patient tolerance allows. Treatment should continue as patient tolerance allows, until complete resolution of microbiologic and clinical evidence of fungal disease.

Pediatrics: Refer to adult dosing.

Administration

I.V.: For a patient who experiences chills, fever, hypotension, nausea, or other nonanaphylactic infusion-related reactions, premedication with the following drugs, 30-60 minutes prior to drug administration: A nonsteroidal (ibuprofen, choline magnesium trisalicylate, etc) with or without diphenhydramine; or acetaminophen with diphenhydramine, or hydrocortisone 50-100 mg. If the patient experiences rigors during the infusion, meperidine may be administered. Avoid infusing faster than 1 mg/kg/hour. If severe respiratory distress occurs, the infusion should be immediately discontinued.

Stability

Compatibility: Stable in D_5W; **incompatible** with NS

Y-site administration: Incompatible with alfentanil, amikacin, ampicillin, ampicillin/sulbactam, atenolol, aztreonam, bretylium, buprenorphine, butorphanol, calcium chloride, calcium gluconate, carboplatin, cefazolin, cefepime, cefoperazone, ceftazidime, ceftriaxone, chlorpromazine, cimetidine, cisatracurium, cisplatin, cyclophosphamide, cyclosporine, cytarabine, diazepam, digoxin, diphenhydramine, dobutamine, dopamine, doxorubicin, doxorubicin liposome, droperidol, enalaprilat, esmolol, famotidine, fluconazole, fluorouracil, gatifloxacin, gentamicin, haloperidol, heparin, hydromorphone, hydroxyzine, imipenem/cilastatin, labetalol, leucovorin, lidocaine, magnesium sulfate, meperidine, mesna, metoclopramide, metoprolol, metronidazole, midazolam, mitoxantrone, morphine, nalbuphine, naloxone, ofloxacin, ondansetron, paclitaxel, pentobarbital, phenobarbital, phenytoin, piperacillin, piperacillin/tazobactam, potassium chloride, prochlorperazine, promethazine, propranolol, ranitidine, remifentanil, sodium bicarbonate, ticarcillin, ticarcillin/clavulanate, tobramycin, vancomycin, vecuronium, verapamil, vinorelbine

Monitoring Laboratory Tests Monitor serum electrolytes (especially potassium and magnesium), liver function, and CBC. Perform culture and sensitivity testing prior to initiating therapy.

Monitoring and Teaching Issues

Physical Assessment: See Warnings/Precautions, Contraindications, Dosing, and Administration for use cautions. Assess potential for interactions with other prescription and OTC medications or herbal products patient may be taking (see Drug Interactions). See Administration prior to administering first infusion. Patient should be monitored closely for adverse response (eg, anaphylactoid reaction, hypokalemia, and nephrotoxicity - see

(Continued)

Amphotericin B Cholesteryl Sulfate Complex *(Continued)*

Adverse Reactions and Overdose/Toxicology). Assess results of laboratory tests (see above) and therapeutic effectiveness frequently during therapy. Teach patient possible side effects and appropriate interventions and adverse symptoms to report (see Patient Education). Breast-feeding is contraindicated.

Patient Education: Inform prescriber of all prescriptions, OTC medications, or herbal products you are taking, and any allergies you have. Do not add anything new during treatment unless approved by prescriber. This medication can only be administered by infusion and therapy may last several weeks. Maintain good personal hygiene to reduce spread and recurrence of lesions. Maintain adequate hydration (2-3 L/day of fluids) unless advised by prescriber to restrict fluids. May cause postural hypotension (use caution when changing from lying or sitting position to standing or when climbing stairs); or nausea or vomiting (small, frequent meals, frequent mouth care, sucking lozenges, or chewing gum may help). Report chest pain or palpitations; CNS disturbances; skin rash; chills or fever; persistent nausea, vomiting, or abdominal pain; sore throat; excessive fatigue; swelling of extremities or unusual weight gain; difficulty breathing; pain at infusion site; muscle cramping or weakness; or other adverse reactions. **Breast-feeding precaution:** Do not breast-feed.

Geriatric Considerations: The pharmacokinetics and dosing of amphotericin have not been studied in the elderly. It appears that use is similar to young adults. Caution should be exercised and renal function and desired effect monitored closely.

Breast-feeding Issues: Due to limited data, consider discontinuing nursing during therapy.

Additional Information Controlled trials which compare the original formulation of amphotericin B to the newer liposomal formulations (ie, Amphotec®) are lacking. Thus, comparative data discussing differences among the formulations should be interpreted cautiously. Although the risk of nephrotoxicity and infusion-related adverse effects may be less with Amphotec®, the efficacy profiles of Amphotec® and the original amphotericin formulation are comparable. Consequently, Amphotec® should be restricted to those patients who cannot tolerate or fail a standard amphotericin B formulation.

Related Information

Compatibility of Drugs *on page 1564*

Amphotericin B Colloidal Dispersion *see* Amphotericin B Cholesteryl Sulfate Complex *on page 92*

Amphotericin B (Conventional) (am foe TER i sin bee con VEN sha nal)

U.S. Brand Names Amphocin®; Fungizone®

Synonyms Amphotericin B Desoxycholate

Generic Available Yes: Powder for reconstitution

Pharmacologic Category Antifungal Agent, Parenteral; Antifungal Agent, Topical

Pregnancy Risk Factor B

Lactation Excretion in breast milk unknown/contraindicated

Use Treatment of severe systemic and central nervous system infections caused by susceptible fungi such as *Candida* species, *Histoplasma capsulatum*, *Cryptococcus neoformans*, *Aspergillus* species, *Blastomyces dermatitidis*, *Torulopsis glabrata*, and *Coccidioides immitis*; fungal peritonitis; irrigant for bladder fungal infections; and topically for cutaneous and mucocutaneous candidal infections; used in fungal infection in patients with bone marrow transplantation, amebic meningoencephalitis, ocular aspergillosis (intraocular injection), candidal cystitis (bladder irrigation), chemoprophylaxis (low-dose I.V.), immunocompromised patients at risk of aspergillosis (intranasal/nebulized), refractory meningitis (intrathecal), coccidioidal arthritis (intra-articular/I.M.).

Low-dose amphotericin B 0.1-0.25 mg/kg/day has been administered after bone marrow transplantation to reduce the risk of invasive fungal disease. Alternative routes of administration and extemporaneous preparations have been used when standard antifungal therapy is not available (eg, inhalation, intraocular injection, subconjunctival application, intracavitary administration into various joints and the pleural space).

Mechanism of Action/Effect Binds to ergosterol altering cell membrane permeability in susceptible fungi and causing leakage of cell components with subsequent cell death

Contraindications Hypersensitivity to amphotericin or any component of the formulation

Warnings/Precautions Avoid additive toxicity with other nephrotoxic drugs. Monitor BUN and serum creatinine, potassium, and magnesium levels every 2-4 days, and daily in patients at risk for acute renal dysfunction. I.V. amphotericin is used primarily for the treatment of patients with progressive and potentially fatal fungal infections. Topical preparations may stain clothing. The standard dosage of lipid-based amphotericin B formulations, including amphotericin B cholesteryl sulfate (Amphotec®), amphotericin B lipid complex (Abelcet®), and liposomal amphotericin B (AmBisome®) is manyfold greater than the dosage of conventional amphotericin B. To prevent inadvertent overdose, the product name and dosage must be verified for any amphotericin B dosage exceeding 1.5 mg/kg. Amphotericin B has been administered to pregnant women without obvious deleterious effects to the fetus, but the number of cases reported is small. Use during pregnancy only if absolutely necessary.

Drug Interactions

Decreased Effect: Pharmacologic antagonism may occur with azole antifungal agents (ketoconazole, miconazole).

Increased Effect/Toxicity: Use of amphotericin with other nephrotoxic drugs (eg, cyclosporine and aminoglycosides) may result in additive toxicity. Amphotericin may increase the toxicity of flucytosine. Antineoplastic agents may increase the risk of amphotericin-induced nephrotoxicity, bronchospasms, and hypotension. Corticosteroids may increase potassium depletion caused by amphotericin. Amphotericin B may predispose patients receiving digitalis glycosides or neuromuscular-blocking agents to toxicity secondary to hypokalemia.

Effects on Lab Values ↑ BUN (S), serum creatinine, alkaline phosphate, bilirubin; ↓ magnesium, potassium (S)

Adverse Reactions

Systemic:

>10%:

Cardiovascular: Hypotension, tachypnea

Central nervous system: Fever, chills, headache (less frequent with I.T.), malaise

Endocrine & metabolic: Hypokalemia, hypomagnesemia

Gastrointestinal: Anorexia, nausea (less frequent with I.T.), vomiting (less frequent with I.T.), diarrhea, heartburn, cramping epigastric pain

Hematologic: Normochromic-normocytic anemia

Neuromuscular & skeletal: Generalized pain, including muscle and joint pains (less frequent with I.T.)

Renal: Decreased renal function and renal function abnormalities including: azotemia, renal tubular acidosis, nephrocalcinosis

Local: Pain at injection site with or without phlebitis or thrombophlebitis (incidence may increase with peripheral infusion of admixtures >0.1 mg/mL)

1% to 10%:

Cardiovascular: Hypertension, flushing

Central nervous system: Delirium, arachnoiditis, pain along lumbar nerves (especially I.T. therapy)

Genitourinary: Urinary retention

Hematologic: Leukocytosis

Neuromuscular & skeletal: Paresthesia (especially with I.T. therapy)

<1% (Limited to important or life-threatening): Acute liver failure, agranulocytosis, anuria, bone marrow suppression, cardiac arrest, coagulation defects, convulsions, dyspnea, hearing loss, leukopenia, maculopapular rash, renal failure, renal tubular acidosis, thrombocytopenia, vision changes

Overdosage/Toxicology Symptoms of overdose include renal dysfunction, cardiac arrest, anemia, thrombocytopenia, granulocytopenia, fever, nausea, and vomiting. Treatment is supportive.

Pharmacodynamics/Kinetics

Half-Life Elimination: Biphasic: Initial: 15-48 hours; Terminal: 15 days

Time to Peak: Within 1 hour following a 4- to 6-hour dose

Formulations

Cream: 3% (20 g)

Lotion: 3% (30 mL)

Injection, powder for reconstitution, as desoxycholate: 50 mg

Suspension, oral: 100 mg/mL (24 mL) [with dropper]

Dosing

Adults & Elderly:

Premedication: For patients who experience chills, fever, hypotension, nausea, or other nonanaphylactic infusion-related immediate reactions, premedicate with the following drugs, 30-60 minutes prior to drug administration: a nonsteroidal (eg, ibuprofen, choline magnesium trisalicylate, etc) with or without diphenhydramine; or acetaminophen with diphenhydramine; or hydrocortisone 50-100 mg. If the patient experiences rigors during the infusion, meperidine may be administered.

Test dose: I.V.: 1 mg infused over 20-30 minutes. Many clinicians believe a test dose is unnecessary.

Systemic fungal infections: I.V.: Maintenance dose: Usual: 0.25-1.5 mg/kg/day; 1-1.5 mg/kg over 4-6 hours every other day may be given once therapy is established. Aspergillosis, mucormycosis, rhinocerebral phycomycosis often require 1-1.5 mg/kg/day; do not exceed 1.5 mg/kg/day.

Duration of therapy varies with nature of infection: Usual duration is 4-12 weeks or cumulative dose of 1-4 g.

Meningitis, coccidioidal or cryptococcal: I.T.:

Initial: 25-300 mcg every 48-72 hours; increase to 500 mcg to 1 mg as tolerated; maximum total dose: 15 mg has been suggested.

Oral candidiasis: Oral (suspension): 1 mL (100 mg) 4 times/day

Dermal infection: Topical: Apply to affected areas 2-4 times/day for 1-4 weeks of therapy depending on nature and severity of infection.

Cystitis (Candidal): Bladder irrigation: Irrigate with 50 mcg/mL solution instilled periodically or continuously for 5-10 days or until cultures are clear.

Bone marrow transplantation (prophylaxis): I.V.: Low-dose amphotericin B 0.1-0.25 mg/kg/day has been administered after bone marrow transplantation to reduce the risk of invasive fungal disease.

Note: Alternative routes of administration and extemporaneous preparations have been used when standard antifungal therapy is not available (eg, inhalation, intraocular injection, subconjunctival application, intracavitary administration into various joints and the pleural space).

Pediatrics:

Premedication: For patients who experience chills, fever, hypotension, nausea, or other nonanaphylactic infusion-related immediate reactions, premedicate with the following drugs, 30-60 minutes prior to drug administration: a nonsteroidal (eg, ibuprofen, choline magnesium trisalicylate, etc) with or without diphenhydramine; or acetaminophen with diphenhydramine; or hydrocortisone 50-100 mg. If the patient experiences rigors during the infusion, meperidine may be administered.

Test dose: I.V.: Infants and Children: 0.1 mg/kg/dose to a maximum of 1 mg; infuse over 30-60 minutes. Many clinicians believe a test dose is unnecessary.

Susceptible fungal infections: I.V.: Infants and Children:

Maintenance dose: 0.25-1 mg/kg/day given once daily; infuse over 2-6 hours. Once therapy has been established, amphotericin B can be administered on an every-other-day basis at 1-1.5 mg/kg/dose; cumulative dose: 1.5-2 g over 6-10 week

Duration of therapy varies with nature of infection: Usual duration is 4-12 weeks or cumulative dose of 1-4 g.

(Continued)

Amphotericin B (Conventional) *(Continued)*

Meningitis, coccidioidal or cryptococcal: I.T.:

Children.: 25-100 mcg every 48-72 hours; increase to 500 mcg as tolerated

Renal Impairment:

If renal dysfunction is due to the drug, the daily total can be decreased by 50% or the dose can be given every other day. I.V. therapy may take several months.

Poorly dialyzed; no supplemental dose is necessary when using hemo- or peritoneal dialysis or CAVH/CAVHD.

Administration in dialysate: 1-2 mg/L of peritoneal dialysis fluid either with or without low-dose I.V. amphotericin B (a total dose of 2-10 mg/kg given over 7-14 days).

Administration

I.V.: May be infused over 4-6 hours. For a patient who experiences chills, fever, hypotension, nausea or other nonanaphylactic infusion-related reactions, premedication with the following drugs, 30-60 minutes prior to drug administration: A nonsteroidal (ibuprofen, choline magnesium trisalicylate, etc) with or without diphenhydramine; or acetaminophen with diphenhydramine, or hydrocortisone 50-100 mg. If the patient experiences rigors during the infusion, meperidine may be administered. Bolus infusion of normal saline immediately preceding, or immediately preceding and following amphotericin B may reduce drug-induced nephrotoxicity. Risk of nephrotoxicity increases with amphotericin B doses >1 mg/kg/day. Infusion of admixtures more concentrated than 0.25 mg/mL should be limited to patients absolutely requiring volume contraction.

Topical: Wear gloves to administer. Amphotericin may stain skin and clothing.

Stability

Storage: Amphotericin B does not have a bacteriostatic constituent, subsequently admixture expiration is determined by sterility more than chemical stability.

Reconstitution: Reconstitute only with sterile water without preservatives, not bacteriostatic water. **Benzyl alcohol, sodium chloride, or other electrolyte solutions may cause precipitation.** Short-term exposure (<24 hours) to light during I.V. infusion does **not** appreciably affect potency. Reconstituted solutions with sterile water for injection and kept in the dark remain stable for 24 hours at room temperature and 1 week when refrigerated. Stability of parenteral admixture at room temperature (25°C) is 24 hours; at refrigeration (4°C) is 2 days.

Standard diluent: Dose per 250-500 mL D_5W

Admixture concentration: Standard admixture concentrations are 0.1 mg/mL (peripheral infusion) and 0.25 mg/mL (central administration). Although 0.8 mg/mL in D_5W is physically compatible and chemically stable, the safety of infusing amphotericin B >0.25 mg/mL has not been formally evaluated.

Compatibility:

Solution is **incompatible** with ampicillin, calcium gluconate, carbenicillin, cimetidine, dopamine, gentamicin, lidocaine, potassium chloride, tetracycline, verapamil.

Compatibility when admixed: Some sterile evacuated glass containers have small amounts of ionic liquid buffer that may cause precipitation.

Monitoring Laboratory Tests BUN and serum creatinine levels should be determined every other day when therapy is increased and at least weekly thereafter. Monitor serum electrolytes (especially potassium and magnesium), liver function, and CBC. Perform culture and sensitivity testing prior to initiating therapy.

Monitoring and Teaching Issues

Physical Assessment: See Contraindications, Warnings/Precautions, and Dosing for use cautions. Assess potential for interactions with other prescriptions, OTC medications, or herbal products patient may be taking (see Drug Interactions). See Administration and Compatibility prior to administering first dose. Assess results of laboratory tests (see above), therapeutic effectiveness, and adverse response (eg, anaphylactoid reactions, acute respiratory distress, hypokalemia, and nephrotoxicity - see Adverse Reactions and Overdose/Toxicology) frequently during therapy. Teach patient appropriate use (topical application or oral solution), possible side effects and appropriate interventions, and adverse symptoms to report (see Patient Education). Breast-feeding is contraindicated.

Patient Education: Inform prescriber of all prescriptions, OTC medications, or herbal products you are taking, and any allergies you have. Do not take anything new during treatment unless approved by prescriber. Take entire prescription, even if you are feeling better. Most skin lesions may take 1-3 weeks of therapy; maintain good personal hygiene to reduce spread and recurrence of lesions. Maintain adequate hydration (2-3 L/day of fluids) unless advised by prescriber to restrict fluids. May cause nausea, vomiting, or anorexia (small, frequent meals, frequent mouth care, sucking lozenges, or chewing gum may help); generalized muscle or joint paint (consult prescriber for approved analgesic); or hypotension (use caution when rising from sitting or lying position or when climbing stairs). Report severe muscle cramping or weakness; chest pain or palpitations; CNS disturbances; skin rash; change in urinary patterns or difficulty voiding; black stool; unusual bruising or bleeding; or pain, redness, swelling at infusion site.

Topical: Amphotericin cream may slightly discolor skin and stain clothing; use gloves when applying. Avoid covering topical application with occlusive bandages. Most skin lesions require 1-3 weeks of therapy. Maintain good personal hygiene to reduce the spread and recurrence of lesions.

Breast-feeding precaution: Do not breast-feed.

Geriatric Considerations: Caution should be exercised and renal function and desired effect monitored closely in older adults.

Additional Information Premedication with diphenhydramine and acetaminophen may reduce the severity of acute infusion-related reactions. Meperidine reduces the duration of amphotericin B-induced rigors and chilling. Hydrocortisone may be used in patients with severe or refractory infusion-related reactions. Bolus infusion of normal saline immediately preceding, or immediately preceding and following amphotericin B may reduce drug-induced nephrotoxicity. Risk of nephrotoxicity increases with amphotericin B doses >1 mg/kg/day.

Infusion of admixtures more concentrated than 0.25 mg/mL should be limited to patients absolutely requiring volume contraction. Amphotericin B does not have a bacteriostatic constituent, subsequently admixture expiration is determined by sterility more than chemical stability.

Related Information

Compatibility of Drugs *on page 1564*

Amphotericin B Desoxycholate *see* Amphotericin B (Conventional) *on page 94*

Amphotericin B (Lipid Complex) (am foe TER i sin bee LIP id KOM pleks)

U.S. Brand Names Abelcet®

Synonyms ABLC

Generic Available No

Pharmacologic Category Antifungal Agent, Parenteral

Pregnancy Risk Factor B

Lactation Enters breast milk/contraindicated

Use Treatment of aspergillosis or any type of progressive fungal infection in patients who are refractory to or intolerant of conventional amphotericin B therapy

Mechanism of Action/Effect Mechanism is like amphotericin - includes binding to ergosterol altering cell membrane permeability in susceptible fungi and causing leakage of cell components with subsequent cell death.

Contraindications Hypersensitivity to amphotericin or any component of the formulation

Warnings/Precautions Anaphylaxis has been reported with amphotericin B-containing drugs. If severe respiratory distress occurs, the infusion should be immediately discontinued. During the initial dosing, the drug should be administered under close clinical observation. Acute reactions (including fever and chills) may occur 1-2 hours after starting an intravenous infusion. These reactions are usually more common with the first few doses and generally diminish with subsequent doses.

Drug Interactions

Decreased Effect: Pharmacologic antagonism may occur with azole antifungal agents (ketoconazole, miconazole).

Increased Effect/Toxicity: See Drug Interactions - Increased Effect/Toxicity in Amphotericin B monograph.

Effects on Lab Values ↑ BUN (S), serum creatinine, alkaline phosphate, bilirubin; ↓ magnesium, potassium (S)

Adverse Reactions Nephrotoxicity and infusion-related hyperpyrexia, rigor, and chilling are reduced relative to amphotericin deoxycholate.

>10%:

Central nervous system: Chills, fever
Renal: Increased serum creatinine
Miscellaneous: Multiple organ failure

1% to 10%:

Cardiovascular: Hypotension, cardiac arrest
Central nervous system: Headache, pain
Dermatologic: Rash
Endocrine & metabolic: Bilirubinemia, hypokalemia, acidosis
Gastrointestinal: Nausea, vomiting, diarrhea, gastrointestinal hemorrhage, abdominal pain
Renal: Renal failure
Respiratory: Respiratory failure, dyspnea, pneumonia

Pharmacodynamics/Kinetics

Half-Life Elimination: ~24 hours

Formulations Injection, suspension: 5 mg/mL (10 mL, 20 mL)

Dosing

Adults & Elderly:

Premedication: For patients who experience chills, fever, hypotension, nausea, or other nonanaphylactic infusion-related immediate reactions, premedicate with the following drugs, 30-60 minutes prior to drug administration: a nonsteroidal (eg, ibuprofen, choline magnesium trisalicylate, etc) with or without diphenhydramine; or acetaminophen with diphenhydramine; or hydrocortisone 50-100 mg. If the patient experiences rigors during the infusion, meperidine may be administered.

Susceptible infections: I.V.: 2.5-5 mg/kg/day as a single infusion. Test dose is not recommended.

Pediatrics: Refer to adult dosing.

Renal Impairment: The effects of renal impairment on drug pharmacokinetics or pharmacodynamics are currently unknown. The dose of amphotericin B lipid complex may be adjusted or drug administration may have to be interrupted in patients with acute kidney dysfunction to reduce the magnitude of renal impairment.

Hemodialysis: Supplemental dose is not necessary.
Peritoneal dialysis: Supplemental dose is not necessary.
Continuous arteriovenous or venovenous hemofiltration: Supplemental dose is not necessary.

Administration

I.V.: For a patient who experiences chills, fever, hypotension, nausea, or other nonanaphylactic infusion-related reactions, premedication with the following drugs, 30-60 minutes prior to drug administration: A nonsteroidal (ibuprofen, choline magnesium trisalicylate, etc) with or without diphenhydramine; or acetaminophen with diphenhydramine, or hydrocortisone 50-100 mg. If the patient experiences rigors during the infusion, meperidine may be administered. If infusion time exceeds 2 hours, mix contents by shaking infusion bag every 2 hours.

Stability

Storage: 100 mg vials in 20 mL of suspension in single-use vials (no preservative is present). Intact vials should be stored at 2°C to 8°C (35°F to 46°F) and protected from exposure to light; do not freeze intact vials.

(Continued)

Amphotericin B (Lipid Complex) *(Continued)*

Reconstitution: Shake vial gently to disperse yellow sediment at bottom of container. Withdraw correct volume to prepare dose. Inject into appropriate volume of D_5W through 5-micron filter needle provided by manufacturer. Each filter needle may be used to filter the contents of up to four vials. The final infusion concentration should be 1 mg/mL in D_5W, and is stable for 48 hours at 2°C to 8°C, then an additional 6 hours at room temperature; 2 mg/mL in D_5W may be used for pediatric patients or patients with cardiovascular disease. Infuse 2.5 mg/kg/hour. Do not use an in-line filter during administration. Admixture must be inverted several times before infusion, then every 2 hours, to prevent settling or aggregation of lipid particles. Protect from light.

Compatibility: Do not admix or Y-site with any blood products, intravenous drugs, or intravenous fluids other than D_5W.

Monitoring Laboratory Tests BUN and serum creatinine levels should be determined every other day while therapy is increased and at least weekly thereafter. Monitor serum electrolytes (especially potassium and magnesium), liver function, and CBC. Perform culture and sensitivity testing prior to initiating therapy.

Monitoring and Teaching Issues

Physical Assessment: See Warnings/Precautions, Contraindications, Dosing, and Administration for use cautions. Assess potential for interactions with other prescription and OTC medications or herbal products patient may be taking (see Drug Interactions). See Administration prior to administering first infusion. Patient should be monitored closely for adverse response (eg, anaphylactoid reaction, hypokalemia, and nephrotoxicity - see Adverse Reactions and Overdose/Toxicology). Assess results of laboratory tests (see above) and therapeutic effectiveness frequently during therapy. Teach patient possible side effects and appropriate interventions and adverse symptoms to report (see Patient Education). Breast-feeding is contraindicated.

Patient Education: Inform prescriber of all prescriptions, OTC medications, or herbal products you are taking, and any allergies you have. Do not add anything new during treatment unless approved by prescriber. This medication can only be administered by infusion and therapy may last several weeks. Maintain good personal hygiene to reduce spread and recurrence of lesions. Maintain adequate hydration (2-3 L/day of fluids) unless advised by prescriber to restrict fluids. May cause postural hypotension (use caution when changing from lying or sitting position to standing or when climbing stairs); or nausea or vomiting (small, frequent meals, frequent mouth care, sucking lozenges, or chewing gum may help). Report chest pain or palpitations; CNS disturbances; skin rash; chills or fever; persistent nausea, vomiting, or abdominal pain; sore throat; excessive fatigue; swelling of extremities or unusual weight gain; difficulty breathing; pain at infusion site; muscle cramping or weakness; or other adverse reactions. **Breast-feeding precaution:** Do not breast-feed.

Geriatric Considerations: Caution should be exercised and renal function and desired effect monitored closely in older adults.

Breast-feeding Issues: Due to limited data, consider discontinuing nursing during therapy.

Additional Information As a modification of dimyristoyl phosphatidylcholine:dimyristoyl phosphatidylglycerol 7:3 (DMPC:DMPG) liposome, amphotericin B lipid-complex has a higher drug to lipid ratio and the concentration of amphotericin B is 33 M. ABLC is a ribbon-like structure, not a liposome.

Controlled trials which compare the original formulation of amphotericin B to the newer liposomal formulations (ie, Abelcet®) are lacking. Thus, comparative data discussing differences among the formulations should be interpreted cautiously. Although the risk of nephrotoxicity and infusion-related adverse effects may be less with Abelcet®, the efficacy profiles of Abelcet® and the original amphotericin formulation are comparable. Consequently, Abelcet® should be restricted to those patients who cannot tolerate or fail a standard amphotericin B formulation.

Related Information

Compatibility of Drugs *on page 1564*

Amphotericin B (Liposomal) (am foe TER i sin bee lye po SO mal)

U.S. Brand Names AmBisome®

Synonyms L-AmB

Generic Available No

Pharmacologic Category Antifungal Agent, Parenteral

Pregnancy Risk Factor B

Lactation Excretion in breast milk unknown/contraindicated

Use Empirical therapy for presumed fungal infection in febrile, neutropenic patients. Treatment of patients with *Aspergillus* species, *Candida* species and/or *Cryptococcus* species infections refractory to amphotericin B desoxycholate, or in patients where renal impairment or unacceptable toxicity precludes the use of amphotericin B desoxycholate. Treatment of cryptococcal meningitis in HIV-infected patients. Treatment of visceral leishmaniasis; in immunocompromised patients with visceral leishmaniasis treated with amphotericin B (liposomal), relapse rates were high following initial clearance of parasites.

Mechanism of Action/Effect Amphotericin B, the active ingredient, acts by binding to the sterol component of a cell membrane leading to alterations in cell permeability and cell death. While amphotericin B has a higher affinity for the ergosterol component of the fungal cell membrane, it can also bind to the cholesterol component of the mammalian cell leading to cytotoxicity. AmBisome®, the liposomal preparation of amphotericin B, has been shown to penetrate the cell wall of both extracellular and intracellular forms of susceptible fungi.

Contraindications Hypersensitivity to amphotericin B or any component of the formulation unless, in the opinion of the treating physician, the benefit of therapy outweighs the risk

Warnings/Precautions Anaphylaxis has been reported with amphotericin B desoxycholate and other amphotericin B-containing drugs. Facilities for cardiopulmonary resuscitation should be available during administration. As with any amphotericin B-containing product the drug should be administered by medically trained personnel. During the initial dosing period, patients should be under close clinical observation. AmBisome® has been shown to be significantly less toxic than amphotericin B desoxycholate; however, adverse events may still occur. Acute reactions (including fever and chills) may occur 1-2 hours after starting an intravenous infusion. These reactions are usually more common with the first few doses and generally diminish with subsequent doses.

Drug Interactions

Increased Effect/Toxicity: Drug interactions have not been studied in a controlled manner; however, drugs that interact with conventional amphotericin B may also interact with amphotericin B liposome for injection. See Drug Interactions - Increased Effect/ Toxicity in Amphotericin B (Conventional) monograph.

Adverse Reactions Percentage of adverse reactions is dependent upon population studied and may vary with respect to premedications and underlying illness.

>10%:

Cardiovascular: Peripheral edema (15%), edema (12% to 14%), tachycardia (9% to 18%), hypotension (7% to 14%), hypertension (8% to 20%), chest pain (8% to 12%), hypervolemia (8% to 12%)

Central nervous system: Chills (29% to 48%), insomnia (17% to 22%), headache (9% to 20%), anxiety (7% to 14%), pain (14%), confusion (9% to 13%)

Dermatologic: Rash (5% to 25%), pruritus (11%)

Endocrine & metabolic: Hypokalemia (31% to 51%), hypomagnesemia (15% to 50%), hyperglycemia (8% to 23%), hypocalcemia (5% to 18%), hyponatremia (8% to 12%)

Gastrointestinal: Nausea (16% to 40%), vomiting (10% to 32%), diarrhea (11% to 30%), abdominal pain (7% to 20%), constipation (15%), anorexia (10% to 14%)

Hematologic: Anemia (27% to 48%), blood transfusion reaction (9% to 18%), leukopenia (15% to 17%), thrombocytopenia (6% to 13%)

Hepatic: Increased alkaline phosphatase (7% to 22%), increased BUN (7% to 21%), bilirubinemia (9% to 18%), increased ALT (15%), increased AST (13%), abnormal liver function tests (not specified) (4% to 13%)

Local: Phlebitis (9% to 11%)

Neuromuscular & skeletal: Weakness (6% to 13%), back pain (12%)

Renal: Increased creatinine (18% to 40%), hematuria (14%)

Respiratory: Dyspnea (18% to 23%), lung disorder (14% to 18%), increased cough (2% to 18%), epistaxis (8% to 15%), pleural effusion (12%), rhinitis (11%)

Miscellaneous: Sepsis (7% to 14%), infection (11% to 12%)

2% to 10% (Limited to important or life-threatening):

Cardiovascular: Arrhythmia, atrial fibrillation, bradycardia, cardiac arrest, cardiomegaly, postural hypotension,

Central nervous system: Agitation, coma, convulsion, depression, dizziness (7% to 8%), hallucinations, malaise, somnolence

Dermatologic: Alopecia, rash, petechia, purpura, skin discoloration, urticaria

Endocrine & metabolic: Acidosis, hypernatremia (4%), hyperchloremia, hyperkalemia, hypermagnesemia, hyperphosphatemia, hypophosphatemia

Gastrointestinal: Gastrointestinal hemorrhage (10%), hematemesis, gum/oral hemorrhage, ileus, ulcerative stomatitis

Genitourinary: Vaginal hemorrhage

Hematologic: Coagulation disorder, hemorrhage, decreased prothrombin, thrombocytopenia

Hepatic: Hepatocellular damage, veno-occlusive liver disease

Local: Injection site inflammation

Neuromuscular & skeletal: Arthralgia, bone pain, dystonia, paresthesia, rigors, tremor

Ocular: Conjunctivitis, eye hemorrhage

Renal: Acute kidney failure, toxic nephropathy

Respiratory: Asthma, atelectasis, hemoptysis, pulmonary edema, respiratory alkalosis, respiratory failure, hypoxia (6% to 8%)

Miscellaneous: Allergic reaction, cell-mediated immunological reaction, flu-like syndrome, procedural complication (8% to 10%), diaphoresis (7%)

<1% (Limited to important or life-threatening): Agranulocytosis, angioedema, cyanosis/hypoventilation, erythema, hemorrhagic cystitis, pulmonary edema, urticaria

Overdosage/Toxicology The toxicity due to overdose has not been defined. Repeated daily doses up to 7.5 mg/kg have been administered in clinical trials with no reported dose-related toxicity. If overdosage should occur, cease administration immediately. Symptomatic supportive measures should be instituted. Particular attention should be given to monitoring renal function.

Pharmacodynamics/Kinetics

Half-Life Elimination: Terminal: 174 hours

Formulations Injection, powder for reconstitution: 50 mg

Dosing

Adults & Elderly:

Note: Premedication: For patients who experience chills, fever, hypotension, nausea, or other nonanaphylactic infusion-related immediate reactions, premedicate with the following drugs, 30-60 minutes prior to drug administration: a nonsteroidal (eg, ibuprofen, choline magnesium trisalicylate, etc) with or without diphenhydramine; or acetaminophen with diphenhydramine; or hydrocortisone 50-100 mg. If the patient experiences rigors during the infusion, meperidine may be administered.

Empiric therapy: I.V.: Recommended initial dose: 3 mg/kg/day

Systemic fungal infections (*Aspergillus*, *Candida*, *Cryptococcus*): I.V.: Recommended initial dose of 3-5 mg/kg/day

Cryptococcal meningitis in HIV-infected patients: I.V.: 6 mg/kg/day

Treatment of visceral leishmaniasis: I.V.:

Immunocompetent patients: 3 mg/kg/day on days 1-5, and 3 mg/kg/day on days 14 and 21; a repeat course may be given in patients who do not achieve parasitic clearance

Immunocompromised patients: 4 mg/kg/day on days 1-5, and 4 mg/kg/day on days 10, 17, 24, 31, and 38

(Continued)

Amphotericin B (Liposomal) *(Continued)*

Pediatrics: Refer to adult dosing.

Renal Impairment:

Dosing adjustment in renal impairment: None necessary; effects of renal impairment are not currently known.

Hemodialysis: Supplemental dose is not necessary.

Peritoneal dialysis effects: Supplemental dose is not necessary.

Continuous arteriovenous or venovenous hemofiltration: Supplemental dose is not necessary.

Administration

I.V.: Should be administered by intravenous infusion, using a controlled infusion device, over a period of approximately 2 hours. Infusion time may be reduced to approximately 1 hour in patients in whom the treatment is well-tolerated. If the patient experiences discomfort during infusion, the duration of infusion may be increased. Administer at a rate of 2.5 mg/kg/hour. Discontinue if severe respiratory distress occurs.

For a patient who experiences chills, fever, hypotension, nausea, or other nonanaphylactic infusion-related reactions, premedication with the following drugs, 30-60 minutes prior to drug administration: A nonsteroidal (ibuprofen, choline magnesium trisalicylate, etc) with or without diphenhydramine; or acetaminophen with diphenhydramine, or hydrocortisone 50-100 mg. If the patient experiences rigors during the infusion, meperidine may be administered.

Stability

Reconstitution: Must be reconstituted using sterile water for injection, USP (without a bacteriostatic agent). Vials containing 50 mg of amphotericin B are prepared as follows.

1. Aseptically add 12 mL of sterile water for injection, USP to each vial to yield a preparation containing 4 mg amphotericin B/mL. **Caution:** Do not reconstitute with saline or add saline to the reconstituted concentration, or mix with other drugs. The use of any solution other than those recommended, or the presence of a bacteriostatic agent in the solution, may cause precipitation.

2. Immediately after the addition of water, **shake the vial vigorously** for 30 seconds to completely disperse the powder, it then forms a yellow, translucent suspension. Visually inspect the vial for particulate matter and continue shaking until completely dispersed.

Filtration and Dilution:

3. Calculate the amount of reconstituted (4 mg/mL) to be further diluted.

4. Withdraw this amount of reconstituted powder into a sterile syringe.

5. Attach the 5-micron filter, provided, to the syringe. Inject the syringe contents through the filter, into the appropriate amount of 5% Dextrose Injection. (Use only one filter per vial.)

6. Must be diluted with 5% dextrose injection to a final concentration of 1-2 mg/mL prior to administration. Lower concentrations (0.2-0.5 mg/mL) may be appropriate for infants and small children to provide sufficient volume for infusion. **Discard partially used vials.** Injection should commence within 6 hours of dilution with 5% dextrose injection. An in-line membrane filter may be used for the intravenous infusion; provided, **the mean pore diameter of the filter should not be less than 1 micron.**

Monitoring Laboratory Tests BUN and serum creatinine levels should be determined every other day while therapy is increased and at least weekly thereafter. Serum potassium and magnesium should be monitored closely. Monitor for signs of hypokalemia (muscle weakness, cramping, drowsiness, EKG changes, etc). Monitor electrolytes, liver function, hematocrit, and CBC regularly.

Monitoring and Teaching Issues

Physical Assessment: Assess any history of previous reactions to amphotericin B. See Warnings/Precautions, Contraindications, and Dosing for use cautions. Assess potential for interactions with other prescriptions, OTC medications, or herbal products patient may be taking (see Drug Interactions). See Administration and Compatibility prior to administering first dose. Patient must be monitored closely for adverse reactions (see Adverse Reactions) during and for 2 hours following infusion. Assess results of laboratory tests (see above) during entire course of therapy. Teach patient interventions to reduce side effects, and adverse symptoms to report (see Patient Education). Breast-feeding is contraindicated.

Patient Education: Inform prescriber of all prescriptions, OTC medications, or herbal products you are taking, and any allergies you have. Do not take anything new during treatment unless approved by prescriber. This drug can only be administered I.V. During infusion, report immediately any chills, chest pain, difficulty breathing, tightness in throat, or other adverse reaction. Personal hygiene is very important to help reduce the spread and recurrence of lesions. Most skin lesions require 1-3 weeks of therapy. Maintain adequate hydration (2-3 L/day of fluids) unless advised by prescriber to restrict fluids. May cause hypotension (use caution when changing from lying or sitting position to standing or when climbing stairs); or nausea or vomiting (small, frequent meals, frequent mouth care, sucking lozenges, or chewing gum may help). Report any hearing loss, skin rash, dizziness or weakness, muscle or bone pain, changes in color of urine or stool, persistent GI distress, alteration in voiding or bowel patterns, CNS disturbances, pain at injection site, or other adverse reactions. **Breast-feeding precaution:** Do not breast-feed.

Additional Information Amphotericin B (liposomal) is a true single bilayer liposomal drug delivery system. Liposomes are closed, spherical vesicles created by mixing specific proportions of amphophilic substances such as phospholipids and cholesterol so that they arrange themselves into multiple concentric bilayer membranes when hydrated in aqueous solutions. Single bilayer liposomes are then formed by microemulsification of multilamellar vesicles using a homogenizer. Amphotericin B (liposomal) consists of these unilamellar bilayer liposomes with amphotericin B intercalated within the membrane. Due to the nature and quantity of amphophilic substances used, and the lipophilic moiety in the amphotericin B molecule, the drug is an integral part of the overall structure of the amphotericin B liposomal liposomes. Amphotericin B (liposomal) contains true liposomes that are <100 nm in diameter.

Ampicillin (am pi SIL in)

U.S. Brand Names Marcillin®; Principen®

Synonyms Aminobenzylpenicillin; Ampicillin Sodium; Ampicillin Trihydrate

Generic Available Yes

Pharmacologic Category Antibiotic, Penicillin

Pregnancy Risk Factor B

Lactation Enters breast milk/compatible

Use Treatment of susceptible bacterial infections (nonbeta-lactamase-producing organisms); susceptible bacterial infections caused by streptococci, pneumococci, nonpenicillinase-producing staphylococci, *Listeria*, meningococci; some strains of *H. influenzae*, *Salmonella*, *Shigella*, *E. coli*, *Enterobacter*, and *Klebsiella*

Mechanism of Action/Effect Interferes with bacterial cell wall synthesis during active multiplication, causing cell wall death and resultant bactericidal activity against susceptible bacteria

Contraindications Hypersensitivity to ampicillin, any component of the formulation, or other penicillins

Warnings/Precautions Dosage adjustment may be necessary in patients with renal impairment. A low incidence of cross-allergy with other beta-lactams exists. High percentage of patients with infectious mononucleosis have developed rash during therapy with ampicillin. Appearance of a rash should be carefully evaluated to differentiate a nonallergic ampicillin rash from a hypersensitivity reaction. Ampicillin rash is a generalized dull red, maculopapular rash, generally appearing 3-14 days after the start of therapy. It normally begins on the trunk and spreads over most of the body. It may be most intense at pressure areas, elbows, and knees.

Drug Interactions

Decreased Effect: Although anecdotal reports suggest oral contraceptive efficacy could be reduced by penicillins, this has been refuted by more rigorous scientific and clinical data.

Increased Effect/Toxicity: Ampicillin increases the effect of disulfiram and anticoagulants. Probenecid may increase penicillin levels. Theoretically, allopurinol taken with ampicillin has an additive potential for rash.

Nutritional/Ethanol Interactions Food: Food decreases ampicillin absorption rate; may decrease ampicillin serum concentration.

Effects on Lab Values ↑ protein, positive Coombs' [direct]; alters result of urinary glucose (Benedict's solution, Clinitest®)

Adverse Reactions

>10%: Local: Pain at injection site

1% to 10%:

Dermatologic: Rash (appearance of a rash should be carefully evaluated to differentiate, if possible; nonallergic ampicillin rash from hypersensitivity reaction; incidence is higher in patients with viral infections, *Salmonella* infections, lymphocytic leukemia, or patients that have hyperuricemia)

Gastrointestinal: Diarrhea, vomiting, oral candidiasis, abdominal cramps

Miscellaneous: Allergic reaction (includes serum sickness, urticaria, angioedema, bronchospasm, hypotension, etc)

<1% (Limited to important or life-threatening): Decreased lymphocytes, eosinophilia, granulocytopenia, hemolytic anemia, interstitial nephritis (rare), leukopenia, penicillin encephalopathy, seizures (with large I.V. doses or patients with renal dysfunction), thrombocytopenia, thrombocytopenic purpura

Overdosage/Toxicology Symptoms of penicillin overdose include neuromuscular hypersensitivity (eg, agitation, hallucinations, asterixis, encephalopathy, confusion, and seizures). Electrolyte imbalance may occur if the preparation contains potassium or sodium salts, especially in renal failure. Hemodialysis may be helpful to aid in removal of the drug from blood; otherwise, treatment is supportive or symptom-directed.

Pharmacodynamics/Kinetics

Absorption: Oral: 50%

Half-Life Elimination:

Neonates: 2-7 days: 4 hours; 8-14 days: 2.8 hours; 15-30 days: 1.7 hours

Children and Adults: 1-1.8 hours

Anuria/end-stage renal disease: 7-20 hours

Time to Peak: Oral: Within 1-2 hours

Formulations

Capsule: 250 mg, 500 mg

Marcillin®: 500 mg

Principen®: 250 mg, 500 mg

Injection, powder for reconstitution, as sodium: 125 mg, 250 mg, 500 mg, 1 g, 2 g, 10 g

Powder for oral suspension (Principen®): 125 mg/5 mL (100 mL, 200 mL); 250 mg/5 mL (100 mL, 200 mL)

Dosing

Adults:

Susceptible infections:

Oral: 250-500 mg every 6 hours

I.M.: 500 mg to 1.5 g every 4-6 hours

I.V.: 500 mg to 3 g every 4-6 hours; maximum: 12 g/day

Sepsis/meningitis: 150-250 mg/kg/24 hours divided every 3-4 hours

Elderly: Administer usual adult dose unless renal function is markedly reduced.

Pediatrics:

Susceptible infections:

I.M., I.V.: Infants and Children: 100-400 mg/kg/day in doses divided every 4-6 hours

Oral: Children: 50-100 mg/kg/day in doses divided every 6 hours; maximum dose: 2-3 g/day

(Continued)

Ampicillin *(Continued)*

Meningitis: I.V.: Infants and Children: 200 mg/kg/day in doses divided every 4-6 hours; maximum dose: 12 g/day

Neonatal infections: I.M., I.V.:

Postnatal age ≤7 days:

≤2000 g: Meningitis: 50 mg/kg/dose every 12 hours; other infections: 25 mg/kg/dose every 12 hours

>2000 g: Meningitis: 50 mg/kg/dose every 8 hours; other infections: 25 mg/kg/dose every 8 hours

Postnatal age >7 days:

<1200 g: Meningitis: 50 mg/kg/dose every 12 hours; other infections: 25 mg/kg/dose every 12 hours

1200-2000 g: Meningitis: 50 mg/kg/dose every 8 hours; other infections: 25 mg/kg/dose every 8 hours

>2000 g: Meningitis: 50 mg/kg/dose every 6 hours; other infections: 25 mg/kg/dose every 6 hours

Renal Impairment:

Cl_{cr} 30-50 mL/minute: Administer every 6-8 hours.

Cl_{cr} 10-30 mL/minute: Administer every 8-12 hours.

Cl_{cr} <10 mL/minute: Administer every 12 hours.

Moderately dialyzable (20% to 50%)

Administer dose after dialysis.

Peritoneal dialysis effects: Moderately dialyzable (20% to 50%)

Administer 250 mg every 12 hours.

Continuous arteriovenous or venovenous hemofiltration: Dose as for Cl_{cr} 10-50 mL/minute.

Administration

Oral: Administer around-the-clock to promote less variation in peak and trough serum levels.

I.V.: Administer around-the-clock to promote less variation in peak and trough serum levels. Administer over 3-5 minutes (125-500 mg) or over 10-15 minutes (1-2 g). More rapid infusion may cause seizures.

Stability

Reconstitution:

Oral: Oral suspension is stable for 7 days at room temperature or for 14 days under refrigeration.

I.V.:

Minimum volume: Concentration should not exceed 30 mg/mL due to concentration-dependent stability restrictions. Manufacturer may supply as either the anhydrous or the trihydrate form.

Solutions for I.M. or direct I.V. should be used within 1 hour. Solutions for I.V. infusion will be inactivated by dextrose at room temperature. If dextrose-containing solutions are to be used, the resultant solution will only be stable for 2 hours versus 8 hours in the 0.9% sodium chloride injection. D_5W has limited stability.

Stability of parenteral admixture in NS at room temperature (25°C) is 8 hours.

Stability of parenteral admixture in NS at refrigeration temperature (4°C) is 2 days.

Standard diluent: 500 mg/50 mL NS; 1 g/50 mL NS; 2 g/100 mL NS

Compatibility: Incompatible with D_5W, D_5NS, $D_{10}W$, fat emulsion 10%, hetastarch 6%, LR

Y-site administration: Incompatible with amphotericin B cholesteryl sulfate complex, epinephrine, fluconazole, hydralazine, midazolam, ondansetron, sargramostim, verapamil, vinorelbine

Compatibility in syringe: Incompatible with erythromycin lactobionate, gentamicin, hydromorphone, kanamycin, lincomycin, metoclopramide

Compatibility when admixed: Incompatible with amikacin, chlorpromazine, dopamine, gentamicin, hydralazine, prochlorperazine

Monitoring Laboratory Tests Perform culture and sensitivity testing prior to initiating therapy.

Monitoring and Teaching Issues

Physical Assessment: Assess for allergy history prior to starting therapy. See Contraindications, Warnings/Precautions, and Dosing for use cautions. Assess potential for interactions with other prescriptions, OTC medications, or herbal products patient may be taking (see Drug Interactions). Caution diabetic patients about altered response to Clinitest®. Assess results of laboratory tests (see above), therapeutic effectiveness, and adverse reactions (eg, opportunistic infection: fever, chills, unhealed sores, white plaques in mouth or vagina, purulent vaginal discharge, fatigue - see Adverse Reactions and Overdose/Toxicology). Teach patient proper use, possible side effects and interventions, and adverse symptoms to report (see Patient Education).

Patient Education: Inform prescriber of all prescriptions, OTC medications, or herbal products you are taking, and any allergies you have. Do not add anything new during treatment unless approved by prescriber. Take entire prescription, even if you are feeling better. Take at equal intervals around-the-clock; preferably on an empty stomach with a full glass of water (1 hour before or 2 hours after meals). Maintain adequate hydration (2-3 L/day of fluids) unless advised by prescriber to restrict fluids. If diabetic, drug may cause false test results with Clinitest® urine glucose monitoring; use of another type of glucose monitoring is preferable. May cause nausea or vomiting (small, frequent meals, frequent mouth care, sucking lozenges, or chewing gum may help); or diarrhea (buttermilk, boiled milk, or yogurt may help). Report immediately any rash; swelling of face, tongue, mouth, or throat; or chest tightness. Report if condition being treated worsens or does not improve by the time prescription is completed.

Dietary Issues: Take on an empty stomach 1 hour before or 2 hours after meals.

Sodium content of 5 mL suspension (250 mg/5 mL): 10 mg (0.4 mEq)

Sodium content of 1 g: 66.7 mg (3 mEq)

Geriatric Considerations: See Drug Interactions and Renal Impairment. Adjust dose for renal impairment.

Related Information

Compatibility of Drugs *on page 1564*

Ampicillin and Sulbactam (am pi SIL in & SUL bak tam)

U.S. Brand Names Unasyn®

Synonyms Sulbactam and Ampicillin

Generic Available No

Pharmacologic Category Antibiotic, Penicillin

Pregnancy Risk Factor B

Lactation Enters breast milk/use caution

Use Treatment of susceptible bacterial infections involved with skin and skin structure, intra-abdominal infections, gynecological infections; spectrum is that of ampicillin plus organisms producing beta-lactamases such as *S. aureus*, *H. influenzae*, *E. coli*, *Klebsiella*, *Acinetobacter*, *Enterobacter*, and anaerobes

Mechanism of Action/Effect Interferes with bacterial cell wall synthesis during active multiplication, causing cell wall death and resultant bactericidal activity against susceptible bacteria. The addition of sulbactam, a beta-lactamase inhibitor, to ampicillin extends the spectrum of ampicillin to include beta-lactamase producing organisms.

Contraindications Hypersensitivity to ampicillin, sulbactam, penicillins, or any component of the formulations

Warnings/Precautions Dosage adjustment may be necessary in patients with renal impairment. A low incidence of cross-allergy with other beta-lactams exists. A high percentage of patients with infectious mononucleosis have developed rash during therapy with ampicillin. Appearance of a rash should be carefully evaluated to differentiate a nonallergic ampicillin rash from a hypersensitivity reaction.

Drug Interactions

Decreased Effect: Although anecdotal reports suggest oral contraceptive efficacy could be reduced by penicillins, this has been refuted by more rigorous scientific and clinical data.

Increased Effect/Toxicity: Disulfiram or probenecid can increase ampicillin levels. Theoretically, allopurinol taken with ampicillin has an additive potential for rash.

Effects on Lab Values False-positive urinary glucose levels (Benedict's solution, Clinitest®); may cause temporary decreases in serum estrogens in pregnant women.

Adverse Reactions

>10%: Local: Pain at injection site (I.M.)

1% to 10%:

Dermatologic: Rash

Gastrointestinal: Diarrhea

Local: Pain at injection site (I.V.)

Miscellaneous: Allergic reaction (may include serum sickness, urticaria, bronchospasm, hypotension, etc)

<1% (Limited to important or life-threatening): Interstitial nephritis (rare), leukopenia, neutropenia, penicillin encephalopathy, pseudomembranous colitis, seizures (with large I.V. doses or patients with renal dysfunction), thrombocytopenia, thrombophlebitis

Overdosage/Toxicology Symptoms of penicillin overdose include neuromuscular hypersensitivity (eg, agitation, hallucinations, asterixis, encephalopathy, confusion, and seizures). Electrolyte imbalance may occur if the preparation contains potassium or sodium salts, especially in renal failure. Hemodialysis may be helpful to aid in removal of the drug from blood; otherwise, treatment is supportive or symptom-directed.

Pharmacokinetic Note See Ampicillin monograph.

Pharmacodynamics/Kinetics

Half-Life Elimination:

Sulbactam: Normal renal function: 1-1.3 hours

Formulations Injection, powder for reconstitution:

1.5 g [ampicillin sodium 1 g and sulbactam sodium 0.5 g]

3 g [ampicillin sodium 2 g and sulbactam sodium 1 g]

15 g [ampicillin sodium 10 g and sulbactam sodium 5 g] [bulk package]

Dosing

Adults & Elderly: Note: Recommendations for Unasyn® are based on the ampicillin component

Susceptible infections: I.M., I.V.: 1-2 g ampicillin (1.5-3 g Unasyn®) every 6-8 hours; maximum: 8 g ampicillin/day (12 g Unasyn®)

Pediatrics: Susceptible infections: I.M., I.V.: 3 months to 12 years: 100-200 mg ampicillin/kg/day (150-300 mg Unasyn®) divided every 6 hours; maximum dose: 8 g ampicillin/day (12 g Unasyn®)

Renal Impairment:

Cl_{cr} >50 mL/minute: Administer every 6 hours.

Cl_{cr} 10-50 mL/minute: Administer every 6-12 hours.

Cl_{cr} <10 mL/minute: Administer every 12-24 hours.

Administration

I.V.: Administer around-the-clock to promote less variation in peak and trough serum levels. Administer by slow injection over 10-15 minutes or I.V. over 15-30 minutes.

Stability

Reconstitution: I.M. and direct I.V. administration: Use within 1 hour after preparation. Reconstitute with sterile water for injection or 0.5% or 2% lidocaine hydrochloride injection (I.M.). Sodium chloride 0.9% (NS) is the diluent of choice for I.V. piggyback use. Solutions made in NS are stable up to 72 hours when refrigerated whereas dextrose solutions (same concentration) are stable for only 4 hours.

Compatibility: Stable in NS

Y-site administration: Incompatible with aminoglycosides (eg, gentamicin, tobramycin), amphotericin B cholesteryl sulfate complex, ciprofloxacin, idarubicin, ondansetron, sargramostim

Compatibility when admixed: Incompatible with aminoglycosides

(Continued)

Ampicillin and Sulbactam *(Continued)*

Monitoring Laboratory Tests Hematologic, renal, and hepatic function with prolonged therapy. Perform culture and sensitivity testing prior to initiating therapy.

Monitoring and Teaching Issues

Physical Assessment: Assess for allergy history prior to starting therapy. See Contraindications, Warnings/Precautions, and Dosing for use cautions. Assess potential for interactions with other prescriptions, OTC medications, or herbal products patient may be taking (see Drug Interactions). Caution diabetic patients about altered response to Clinitest®. Assess results of laboratory tests (see above), therapeutic effectiveness, and adverse reactions (eg, opportunistic infection: fever, chills, unhealed sores, white plaques in mouth or vagina, purulent vaginal discharge, fatigue - see Adverse Reactions and Overdose/Toxicology). Teach possible side effects and interventions and adverse symptoms to report (see Patient Education). Note breast-feeding caution.

Patient Education: Inform prescriber of all prescriptions, OTC medications, or herbal products you are taking, and any allergies you have. Do not add anything new during treatment unless approved by prescriber. This medication is administered by infusion/injection. Report immediately pain, redness, swelling, or burning at injection/infusion site or feelings of acute anxiety, chest tightness, or difficulty swallowing. Maintain adequate hydration (2-3 L/day of fluids) unless advised by prescriber to restrict fluids. If diabetic, drug may cause false test results with Clinitest® urine glucose monitoring; use of another type of glucose monitoring is preferable. May cause diarrhea (if persistent, consult prescriber for approved medication). Report rash or persistent, opportunistic infection (eg, fever, chills, unhealed sores, white plaques in mouth or vagina, purulent vaginal discharge, fatigue). **Breast-feeding precaution:** Consult prescriber if breast-feeding caution.

Dietary Issues: Sodium content of 1.5 g injection: 115 mg (5 mEq)

Geriatric Considerations: Adjust dose for renal function.

Related Information

Ampicillin *on page 101*

Ampicillin Sodium *see* Ampicillin *on page 101*

Ampicillin Trihydrate *see* Ampicillin *on page 101*

Amprenavir (am PRE na veer)

U.S. Brand Names Agenerase®

Generic Available No

Pharmacologic Category Antiretroviral Agent, Protease Inhibitor

Pregnancy Risk Factor C

Lactation Excretion in breast milk unknown/contraindicated

Use Treatment of HIV infections in combination with at least two other antiretroviral agents; oral solution should only be used when capsules or other protease inhibitors are not therapeutic options

Mechanism of Action/Effect Binds to the protease activity site and inhibits the activity of the enzyme. HIV protease is required for the cleavage of viral polyprotein precursors into individual functional proteins found in infectious HIV. Inhibition prevents cleavage of these polyproteins, resulting in the formation of immature, noninfectious viral particles.

Contraindications Hypersensitivity to amprenavir or any component of the formulation; concurrent therapy with rifampin, astemizole, bepridil, cisapride, ergot derivatives, midazolam, pimozide, triazolam, lovastatin, simvastatin, and hormonal contraceptives; severe previous allergic reaction to sulfonamides; oral solution is contraindicated in infants or children <4 years of age, pregnant women, patients with renal or hepatic failure, and patients receiving concurrent metronidazole or disulfiram

Warnings/Precautions Because of hepatic metabolism and effect on cytochrome P450 enzymes, amprenavir should be used with caution in combination with other agents metabolized by this system (see Contraindications and Drug Interactions). Avoid concurrent use of St John's wort. Use with caution in patients with diabetes mellitus, sulfonamide allergy, hepatic impairment, or hemophilia. Redistribution of fat may occur (eg, buffalo hump, peripheral wasting, cushingoid appearance). Additional vitamin E supplements should be avoided. Concurrent use of sildenafil should be avoided. Certain ethnic populations (Asians, Eskimos, Native Americans) may be at increased risk of propylene glycol-associated adverse effects; use of the oral solution of amprenavir should be avoided. Use oral solution only when capsules or other protease inhibitors are not options. Pregnancy risk C.

Drug Interactions

Cytochrome P450 Effect: Substrate of CYP2C8/9, **3A4**; Inhibits CYP2C19, **3A4**

Decreased Effect: Enzyme-inducing agents (rifampin, phenobarbital, phenytoin) may decrease serum concentrations/effect of amprenavir; rifampin is contraindicated. The administration of didanosine (buffered formulation) should be separated from amprenavir by 1 hour to limit interaction between formulations. Serum concentrations of estrogen (oral contraceptives) may be decreased, use alternative (nonhormonal) forms of contraception. Dexamethasone may decrease the therapeutic effect of amprenavir. Serum concentrations of delavirdine may be decreased; may lead to loss of virologic response and possible resistance to delavirdine; concomitant use is not recommended. Efavirenz and nevirapine may decrease serum concentrations of amprenavir (dosing for combinations not established). Avoid St John's wort (may lead to subtherapeutic concentrations of amprenavir). Effect of amprenavir may be diminished when administered with methadone (consider alternative antiretroviral); in addition, effect of methadone may be reduced (dosage increase may be required).

Increased Effect/Toxicity: Concurrent use of cisapride, pimozide, quinidine, and rifampin is contraindicated. Serum concentrations/effect of many benzodiazepines may be increased; concurrent use of midazolam or triazolam is contraindicated. Concurrent use of ergot alkaloids (dihydroergotamine, ergotamine, ergonovine, methylergonovine) with amprenavir is also contraindicated (may cause vasospasm and peripheral ischemia).

Concurrent use of oral solution with disulfiram or metronidazole is contraindicated (risk of propylene glycol toxicity). Serum concentrations of amiodarone, lidocaine, quinidine and other antiarrhythmics may be increased, potentially leading to toxicity. HMG-CoA reductase inhibitors serum concentrations may be increased by amprenavir, increasing the risk of myopathy/rhabdomyolysis; lovastatin and simvastatin are contraindicated; fluvastatin and pravastatin may be safer alternatives. Serum concentrations/effect of benzodiazepines, calcium channel blockers, cyclosporine, itraconazole, ketoconazole, rifabutin, tacrolimus, tricyclic antidepressants may be increased. May increase warfarin's effects, monitor INR.

Sildenafil serum concentrations may be increased by amprenavir; when used concurrently, do not exceed a maximum sildenafil dose of 25 mg in a 48-hour period. Concurrent therapy with ritonavir may result in increased serum concentrations: dosage adjustment is recommended. Clarithromycin, indinavir, nelfinavir may increase serum concentrations of amprenavir.

Nutritional/Ethanol Interactions

Ethanol: Avoid ethanol with amprenavir oral solution.

Food: Levels increased sixfold with high-fat meals.

Herb/Nutraceutical: Amprenavir serum concentration may be decreased by St John's wort; avoid concurrent use. Formulations contain vitamin E; avoid additional supplements.

Adverse Reactions Protease inhibitors cause dyslipidemia which includes elevated cholesterol and triglycerides and a redistribution of body fat centrally to cause "protease paunch," buffalo hump, facial atrophy, and breast enlargement. These agents also cause hyperglycemia.

>10%:
- Dermatologic: Rash (28%)
- Endocrine & metabolic: Hyperglycemia (37% to 41%), hypertriglyceridemia (36% to 47%)
- Gastrointestinal: Nausea (38% to 73%), vomiting (20% to 29%), diarrhea (33% to 56%)
- Miscellaneous: Perioral tingling/numbness

1% to 10%:
- Central nervous system: Depression (4% to 15%), headache, paresthesia, fatigue
- Dermatologic: Stevens-Johnson syndrome (1% of total, 4% of patients who develop a rash)
- Endocrine & metabolic: Hypercholesterolemia (4% to 9%)
- Gastrointestinal: Taste disorders (1% to 10%)

Overdosage/Toxicology Monitor for signs and symptoms of propylene glycol toxicity if the oral solution is administered.

Pharmacodynamics/Kinetics

Absorption: 63%

Bioavailability: Not established; increased sixfold with high-fat meal

Half-Life Elimination: 7.1-10.6 hours

Time to Peak: 1-2 hours

Metabolism: Hepatic via CYP (primarily CYP3A4)

Formulations

Capsule: 50 mg, 150 mg

Solution, oral [use only when there are no other options]: 15 mg/mL (240 mL) [contains propylene glycol 550 mg/mL and vitamin E 46 int. units/mL; grape-bubblegum-peppermint flavor]

Dosing

Adults & Elderly: Note: Capsule and oral solution are **not** interchangeable on a mg-per-mg basis.

HIV infection: Oral:
- Capsule:
  - <50 kg: 20 mg/kg twice daily (maximum: 2400 mg/day)
  - ≥50 kg: 1200 mg twice daily
  - **Note:** Dosage adjustments for amprenavir when administered in combination therapy:
    - Efavirenz: Adjustments necessary for both agents:
      - Amprenavir 1200 mg 3 times/day (single protease inhibitor) **or**
      - Amprenavir 1200 mg twice daily plus ritonavir 200 mg twice daily
    - Ritonavir: Adjustments necessary for both agents:
      - Amprenavir 1200 mg plus ritonavir 200 mg once daily **or**
      - Amprenavir 600 mg plus ritonavir 100 mg twice daily
- Solution:
  - <50 kg: 22.5 mg/kg (maximum: 2800 mg/day)
  - ≥50 kg: 1400 mg twice daily

Pediatrics: Note: Capsule and oral solution are **not** interchangeable on a mg-per-mg basis.

HIV infection: Oral:
- Capsule:
  - Children 4-12 years and older (<50 kg): 20 mg/kg twice daily or 15 mg/kg 3 times daily; maximum: 2400 mg/day
  - Children >13 years (>50 kg): 1200 mg twice daily
- Solution:
  - Children 4-12 years or older (up to 16 years weighing <50 kg): 22.5 mg/kg twice daily or 17 mg/kg 3 times daily; maximum: 2800 mg/day
  - Children 13-16 years (weighing at least 50 kg) or >16 years: 1400 mg twice daily

Renal Impairment: Oral solution is contraindicated in renal failure.

Hepatic Impairment:

Child-Pugh score between 5-8:
- Capsule: 450 mg twice daily
- Solution: 513 mg twice daily; contraindicated in hepatic failure.

Child-Pugh score between 9-12:
- Capsule: 300 mg twice daily
- Solution: 342 mg twice daily; contraindicated in hepatic failure.

Monitoring and Teaching Issues

Physical Assessment: See Contraindications, Warnings/Precautions, and Dosing for use cautions. Assess potential for interactions with other prescriptions, OTC medications, or

(Continued)

Amprenavir *(Continued)*

herbal products patient may be taking (see Drug Interactions). Assess patient response (see Adverse Reactions and Overdose/Toxicology) at regular intervals during therapy. Caution patients to monitor glucose levels closely; protease inhibitors may cause hyperglycemia or new-onset diabetes. Teach patient proper use, possible side effects and appropriate interventions, and adverse symptoms to report (see Patient Education). **Pregnancy risk factor C** - benefits of use should outweigh possible risks. Breast-feeding is contraindicated.

Patient Education: Inform prescriber of all prescriptions, OTC medications, or herbal products you are taking, and any allergies you have. Do not take anything new during treatment unless approved by prescriber. This drug is not a cure for HIV, nor has it been found to reduce transmission. Take as directed, at regular intervals around-the-clock. May take with light meal (eg, dry toast, skim milk, corn flakes) to reduce GI upset. Avoid alcohol. Maintain adequate hydration (2-3 L/day of fluids) unless advised by prescriber to restrict fluids. Amprenavir may be prescribed with a combination of other medications; time these medications as directed by prescriber. You may be advised to check your glucose levels (this drug can cause exacerbation or new-onset diabetes). You will be more susceptible to infection (avoid crowds and exposure to infection and do not have any vaccinations unless approved by prescriber). May cause body changes due to redistribution of body fat, facial atrophy, or breast enlargement (normal effects of drug); nausea, vomiting, or flatulence (small, frequent meals, frequent mouth care, chewing gum, or sucking lozenges may help); muscle weakness or flank pain (consult prescriber for approved analgesic); headache or insomnia (consult prescriber for medication); or diarrhea (boiled milk, buttermilk, or yogurt may help). Inform prescriber if you experience muscle numbness or tingling; unresolved persistent vomiting, diarrhea, or abdominal pain; difficulty breathing or chest pain; unusual skin rash; or change in color of stool or urine. **Pregnancy/breast-feeding precautions:** Inform prescriber if you are pregnant and do not get pregnant while taking this medicine. This drug decreases the effect of oral contraceptives; use additional barrier contraceptives. Do not breast-feed.

Dietary Issues: May be taken with or without food; do not take with high-fat meal.

Breast-feeding Issues: HIV-infected mothers are discouraged from breast-feeding to decrease potential transmission of HIV.

Pregnancy Issues: It is not known if amprenavir crosses the human placenta and there are no clinical studies currently underway to evaluate its use in pregnant women. Pregnancy and protease inhibitors are both associated with an increased risk of hyperglycemia. Glucose levels should be closely monitored. Health professionals are encouraged to contact the antiretroviral pregnancy registry to monitor outcomes of pregnant women exposed to antiretroviral medications (1-800-258-4263).

Additional Information Capsules contain 109 int. units of vitamin E per capsule; oral solution contains 46 int. units of vitamin E per mL. Propylene glycol is included in the oral solution; a dose of 22.5 mg/kg twice daily corresponds to an intake of 1650 mg/kg of propylene glycol. Capsule and oral solution are not interchangeable on a mg-per-mg basis.

Related Information

Tuberculosis *on page 1705*

Amvisc® *see page 1509*

Amvisc® *see page 1461*

Amvisc® Plus *see page 1509*

Amvisc® Plus *see page 1461*

Anafranil® *see* ClomiPRAMINE *on page 313*

Ana-Kit® *see page 1460*

Anaprox® *see* Naproxen *on page 948*

Anaprox® DS *see* Naproxen *on page 948*

Anaspaz® *see* Hyoscyamine *on page 685*

Anastrozole (an AS troe zole)

U.S. Brand Names Arimidex®

Generic Available No

Pharmacologic Category Antineoplastic Agent, Miscellaneous

Pregnancy Risk Factor D

Lactation Excretion in breast milk unknown/use caution

Use Treatment of locally-advanced or metastatic breast cancer (ER-positive or hormone receptor unknown) in postmenopausal women; treatment of advanced breast cancer in postmenopausal women with disease progression following tamoxifen therapy; adjuvant treatment of early ER-positive breast cancer in postmenopausal women

Mechanism of Action/Effect Potent and selective nonsteroidal aromatase inhibitor. It significantly lowers serum estradiol concentrations and has no detectable effect on formation of adrenal corticosteroids or aldosterone. In postmenopausal women, the principal source of circulating estrogen is conversion of adrenally generated androstenedione to estrone by aromatase in peripheral tissues.

Contraindications Hypersensitivity to anastrozole or any component of the formulation; pregnancy

Warnings/Precautions Use with caution in patients with hyperlipidemias; total cholesterol and LDL-cholesterol increase in patients receiving anastrozole. Exclude pregnancy before initiating therapy. Tamoxifen should not be used concurrently. Safety and efficacy in pediatric patients have not been established.

Drug Interactions

Cytochrome P450 Effect: Inhibits CYP1A2, 2C8/9, 3A4

Decreased Effect:

Estrogens: Concurrent use may decrease efficacy of anastrozole.

Tamoxifen: Decreased plasma concentration of anastrozole; avoid concurrent use.

Nutritional/Ethanol Interactions Herb/Nutraceutical: Avoid black cohosh, hops, licorice, red clover, thyme, and dong quai.

Effects on Lab Values Lab test abnormalities: GGT, AST, ALT, alkaline phosphatase, total cholesterol and LDL increased; threefold elevations of mean serum GGT levels have been observed among patients with liver metastases. These changes were likely related to the progression of liver metastases in these patients, although other contributing factors could not be ruled out. Mean serum total cholesterol levels increased by 0.5 mmol/L among patients.

Adverse Reactions

>10%:

Cardiovascular: Vasodilatation (25% to 35%)

Central nervous system: Pain (11% to 15%), headache (9% to 13%), depression (5% to 11%)

Endocrine & metabolic: Hot flashes (12% to 35%)

Neuromuscular & skeletal: Weakness (16% to 17%), arthritis (14%), arthralgia (13%), back pain (8% to 12%), bone pain (5% to 11%)

Respiratory: Cough increased (7% to 11%), pharyngitis (6% to 12%)

1% to 10%:

Cardiovascular: Peripheral edema (5% to 10%), hypertension (5% to 9%), chest pain (5% to 7%)

Central nervous system: Insomnia (6% to 9%), dizziness (6%), anxiety (5%), lethargy (1%), fever, malaise, confusion, nervousness, somnolence

Dermatologic: Rash (6% to 10%), alopecia, pruritus

Endocrine & metabolic: Hypercholesteremia (7%)

Gastrointestinal: Vomiting (8% to 9%), constipation (7% to 9%), abdominal pain (7% to 8%), diarrhea (7% to 8%), anorexia (5% to 7%), xerostomia (6%), dyspepsia (5%), weight gain (2% to 8%), weight loss

Genitourinary: Urinary tract infection (6%), vulvovaginitis (6%), vaginal bleeding (5%) leukorrhea (2%), vaginal hemorrhage (2%), vaginal dryness (2%)

Hematologic: Anemia, leukopenia

Hepatic: Liver function tests increased, alkaline phosphatase increased

Local: Deep vein thrombosis, thrombophlebitis

Neuromuscular & skeletal: Osteoporosis (7%), fracture (7%), arthrosis (6%), paresthesia (5% to 6%), hypertonia (3%), myalgia, arthralgia

Ocular: Cataracts (4%)

Respiratory: Dyspnea (6% to 10%), sinusitis, bronchitis, rhinitis

Miscellaneous: Lymph edema (9%), infection (7%), flu-syndrome (5% to 7%), diaphoresis (2% to 4%)

<1% (Limited to important or life-threatening): Angina pectoris, CVA, cerebral ischemia, cerebral infarct, endometrial cancer, erythema multiforme, joint pain, joint stiffness, MI, myocardial ischemia, pulmonary embolus, retinal vein thrombosis, Stevens-Johnson syndrome, thrombophlebitis

Overdosage/Toxicology Symptoms of overdose include severe irritation to the stomach (necrosis, gastritis, ulceration, and hemorrhage). There is no specific antidote; treatment must be symptomatic. Dialysis may be helpful because anastrozole is not highly protein bound.

Pharmacodynamics/Kinetics

Absorption: Well absorbed; not affected by food

Half-Life Elimination: 50 hours

Metabolism: Extensively hepatic (85%) via N-dealkylation, hydroxylation, and glucuronidation; primary metabolite inactive

Onset: Onset of estradiol reduction: 24 hours

Duration: Duration of estradiol reduction: 6 days

Formulations Tablet: 1 mg

Dosing

Adults & Elderly: Breast cancer: Oral (refer to individual protocols): 1 mg once daily

NOTE: In advanced breast cancer, continue until tumor progression. In early breast cancer, optimal duration of therapy unknown.

Renal Impairment: Dosage adjustment is not necessary.

Hepatic Impairment: Plasma concentrations in subjects with stable hepatic cirrhosis were within the range concentrations in normal subjects across all clinical trials; therefore, no dosage adjustment is needed.

Stability

Storage: Store at 20°C to 25°C (68°F to 77°F).

Monitoring Laboratory Tests CBC with differential and platelet count

Monitoring and Teaching Issues

Physical Assessment: See Contraindications and Warnings/Precautions for use cautions. Assess potential for interactions with other prescriptions, OTC medications, or herbal products patient may be taking (see Drug Interactions). Assess results of laboratory results (see above), therapeutic effectiveness, and adverse reactions (see Adverse Reactions and Overdose/Toxicology) periodically during therapy. Teach patient proper use, possible side effects and interventions, and adverse symptoms to report (see Patient Education). **Pregnancy risk factor D** - determine that patient is not pregnant before beginning treatment. Instruct patients of childbearing age about appropriate barrier contraceptive measures. Note breast-feeding caution.

Patient Education: Inform prescriber of all prescriptions, OTC medications, or herbal products you are taking, and any allergies you have. Do not add anything new during treatment unless approved by prescriber. Take exactly as directed. Maintain adequate hydration (2-3 L/day of fluids) unless advised by prescriber to restrict fluids. May cause headache (consult prescriber for approved analgesic); drowsiness, dizziness, anxiety (use caution when driving or engaging in tasks that require alertness until response to drug is known); mild nausea or vomiting (small, frequent meals, frequent mouth care, chewing gum, or sucking lozenges may help); or increased pelvic, bone or tumor pain (may lessen

(Continued)

Anastrozole *(Continued)*

with continued use; if not, consult prescriber for approved analgesic). Report rash; unresolved nausea or vomiting; pain or burning on urination; severe mood swings, confusion, anxiety; palpitations; flu-like symptoms; or difficulty breathing. **Pregnancy/breast-feeding precautions:** Do not get pregnant while taking this medication. Consult prescriber for appropriate contraceptive measures. Consult prescriber if breast-feeding.

Pregnancy Issues: Anastrozole can cause fetal harm when administered to a pregnant woman.

Anatuss LA *see* Guaifenesin and Pseudoephedrine *on page 648*
Anbesol® [OTC] *see* Benzocaine *on page 156*
Anbesol® Baby [OTC] *see* Benzocaine *on page 156*
Anbesol® Maximum Strength [OTC] *see* Benzocaine *on page 156*
Ancef® *see* Cefazolin *on page 234*
Ancobon® *see* Flucytosine *on page 567*
Andehist NR Drops *see* Carbinoxamine and Pseudoephedrine *on page 217*
Androderm® *see* Testosterone *on page 1294*
AndroGel® *see* Testosterone *on page 1294*
Android® *see* MethylTESTOSTERone *on page 887*
Anectine® Chloride *see* Succinylcholine *on page 1252*
Anectine® Chloride Injection *see page 1461*
Anectine® Flo-Pack® *see page 1461*
Anectine® Flo-Pack® *see* Succinylcholine *on page 1252*
Anergan® *see* Promethazine *on page 1133*
Anestacon® *see* Lidocaine *on page 800*
Aneurine Hydrochloride *see* Thiamine *on page 1304*
Anexsia® *see* Hydrocodone and Acetaminophen *on page 667*
Angiotensin Agents *see page 1547*
Animal and Human Bites Guidelines *see page 1626*
Ansaid® *see* Flurbiprofen *on page 585*
Ansamycin *see* Rifabutin *on page 1184*
Antabuse® *see* Disulfiram *on page 427*
Antagon® *see* Ganirelix *on page 620*
Antazoline-V® *see page 1509*
Anthra-Derm® *see* Anthralin *on page 108*

Anthralin (AN thra lin)

U.S. Brand Names Anthra-Derm®; Drithocreme®; Drithocreme® HP 1%; Dritho-Scalp®; Micanol®

Synonyms Dithranol

Generic Available No

Pharmacologic Category Antipsoriatic Agent; Keratolytic Agent

Pregnancy Risk Factor C

Lactation Excretion in breast milk unknown

Use Treatment of psoriasis (quiescent or chronic psoriasis)

Mechanism of Action/Effect Inhibits synthesis of nucleic protein from inhibition of DNA synthesis to affected areas

Contraindications Hypersensitivity to anthralin or any component of the formulation; acute psoriasis (acutely or actively inflamed psoriatic eruptions); use on the face

Warnings/Precautions If redness is observed, reduce frequency of dosage or discontinue application. Avoid eye contact. Should generally not be applied to intertriginous skin areas and high strengths should not be used on these sites. Do not apply to face or genitalia. Use caution in patients with renal disease and in those having extensive and prolonged applications. Perform periodic urine tests for albuminuria. Pregnancy risk C.

Drug Interactions

Increased Effect/Toxicity: Long-term use of topical corticosteroids may destabilize psoriasis and withdrawal may also give rise to a "rebound" phenomenon. Allow an interval of at least 1 week between the discontinuance of topical corticosteroids and the commencement of therapy.

Adverse Reactions 1% to 10%: Dermatologic: Transient primary irritation of uninvolved skin; temporary discoloration of hair and fingernails, may stain skin, hair, or fabrics

Formulations

Cream: 0.1% (50 g); 0.25% (50 g); 0.5% (50 g); 1% (50 g)
Ointment: 0.1% (42.5 g); 0.25% (42.5 g); 0.5% (42.5 g); 1% (42.5 g)

Dosing

Adults & Elderly: Note: Generally, apply once a day or as directed. The irritant potential of anthralin is directly related to the strength being used and each patient's individual tolerance. Always commence treatment for at least 1 week using the lowest strength possible.

Psoriasis: Topical

Skin application: Apply sparingly only to psoriatic lesions and rub gently and carefully into the skin until absorbed. Avoid applying an excessive quantity which may cause unnecessary soiling and staining of the clothing or bed linen.

Scalp application: Comb hair to remove scalar debris and, after suitably parting, rub cream well into the lesions, taking care to prevent the cream from spreading onto the forehead.

Remove by washing or showering; optimal period of contact will vary according to the strength used and the patient's response to treatment. Continue treatment until the skin is entirely clear (ie, when there is nothing to feel with the fingers and the texture is normal).

Monitoring and Teaching Issues

Physical Assessment: See Contraindications and Warnings/Precautions for use cautions. When applied to large areas of skin or for extensive periods of time, monitor for adverse skin or systemic reactions. Assess knowledge/teach patient appropriate application and use and adverse symptoms (see Adverse Reactions) to report. **Pregnancy risk factor C** - systemic absorption may be minimal with appropriate use. Note breast-feeding caution.

Patient Education: For external use only. Use exactly as directed; do not overuse. Before using, wash and dry area gently. Wear gloves to apply a thin film to affected area and rub in gently. Remove by washing; may discolor fabric, skin, or hair. Use a porous dressing if necessary. For lesions on scalp, comb hair to remove scalar debris, part hair, and rub cream into lesions. Do not allow cream to spread to forehead or onto neck. Remove by washing hair. Avoid contact with eyes. Avoid exposing treated areas to direct sunlight; sunburn can occur. Optimal period of contact will vary according to strength used and response to treatment. Report increased swelling, redness, rash, itching, signs of infection, worsening of condition, or lack of healing. **Pregnancy/breast-feeding precautions:** Inform prescriber if you are or intend to become pregnant. Consult prescriber if breast-feeding.

Anthrax Vaccine Adsorbed *see page 1498*

Antiarrhythmic Drugs *see page 1551*

AntibiOtic® Otic *see page 1519*

Anticoagulant Therapy Guidelines *see page 1635*

Antidepressant Agents *see page 1553*

Antidepressant Medication Guidelines *see page 1613*

Antidiabetic Oral Agents Comparison *see page 1556*

Antidigoxin Fab Fragments, Ovine *see* Digoxin Immune Fab *on page 414*

Antidiuretic Hormone *see* Vasopressin *on page 1391*

Antidotes, Antivenins, and Antitoxins *see page 1460*

Antiemetics for Chemotherapy-Induced Nausea and Vomiting *see page 1639*

Antihemophilic Factor (Human) (an tee hee moe FIL ik FAK tor HYU man)

U.S. Brand Names Alphanate®; Hemofil® M; Humate-P®; Koāte®-DVI; Monarc® M; Monoclate-P®

Synonyms AHF (Human); Factor VIII (Human)

Generic Available Yes

Pharmacologic Category Antihemophilic Agent; Blood Product Derivative

Pregnancy Risk Factor C

Lactation Excretion in breast milk unknown/use caution

Use Management of hemophilia A for patients in whom a deficiency in factor VIII has been demonstrated; can be of significant therapeutic value in patients with acquired factor VIII inhibitors not exceeding 10 Bethesda units/mL

Humate-P®: In addition, indicated as treatment of spontaneous bleeding in patients with severe von Willebrand disease and in mild and moderate von Willebrand disease where desmopressin is known or suspected to be inadequate

Orphan status: Alphanate®: Management of von Willebrand disease

Mechanism of Action/Effect Protein (factor VIII) in normal plasma which is necessary for clot formation and maintenance of hemostasis; activates factor X in conjunction with activated factor IX; activated factor X converts prothrombin to thrombin, which converts fibrinogen to fibrin, and with factor XIII forms a stable clot

Contraindications Hypersensitivity to any component of the formulation or to mouse protein (Monoclate-P®, Hemofil® M)

Warnings/Precautions Risk of viral transmission is not totally eradicated. Because antihemophilic factor is prepared from pooled plasma, it may contain the causative agent of viral hepatitis and other viral diseases. Hepatitis B vaccination is recommended for all patients. Hepatitis A vaccination is also recommended for seronegative patients. Antihemophilic factor contains trace amounts of blood groups A and B isohemagglutinins and when large or frequently repeated doses are given to individuals with blood groups A, B, and AB, the patient should be monitored for signs of progressive anemia and the possibility of intravascular hemolysis should be considered. Natural rubber latex is a component of Hemofil® M packaging. Products vary by preparation method; final formulations contain human albumin. Pregnancy risk C.

Adverse Reactions <1% (Limited to important or life-threatening): Acute hemolytic anemia, allergic reactions (rare), anaphylaxis (rare), anemia, blurred vision, chest tightness, chills, edema, fever, headache, hyperfibrinogenemia, increased bleeding tendency, itching, jittery feeling, lethargy, nausea, paresthesias, pruritus, somnolence, stinging at the infusion site, stomach discomfort, tachycardia, tingling, vasomotor reactions with rapid infusion, vomiting

Overdosage/Toxicology Massive doses have been reported to cause acute hemolytic anemia, increased bleeding tendency, or hyperfibrinogenemia. Occurrence is rare.

Pharmacodynamics/Kinetics

Half-Life Elimination: Mean: 12-17 hours with hemophilia A; consult specific product labeling

Formulations Injection, human [single-dose vial]: Labeling on cartons and vials indicates number of int. units

Dosing

Adults: Hemophilia: I.V.: Individualize dosage based on coagulation studies performed prior to treatment and at regular intervals during treatment. 1 AHF unit is the activity present in 1 mL of normal pooled human plasma. Dosage should be adjusted to actual vial size currently stocked in the pharmacy. (General guidelines presented; consult individual product labeling for specific dosing recommendations.)

(Continued)

Antihemophilic Factor (Human) *(Continued)*

Dosage based on desired factor VIII increase (%):

To calculate dosage needed based on desired factor VIII increase (%):

Body weight (kg) x 0.5 int. units/kg x desired factor VIII increase (%) = int. units factor VIII required

For example:

50 kg x 0.5 int. units/kg x 30 (% increase) = 750 int. units factor VIII

Dosage based on expected factor VIII increase (%):

It is also possible to calculate the **expected** % factor VIII increase:

(# int. units administered x 2%/int. units/kg) divided by body weight (kg) = expected % factor VIII increase

For example:

(1400 int. units x 2%/int. units/kg) divided by 70 kg = 40%

General guidelines:

Minor hemorrhage: Required peak postinfusion AHF level: 20% to 40% (10-20 int. units/kg), repeat dose every 12-24 hours for 1-3 days until bleeding is resolved or healing achieved; mild superficial or early hemorrhages may respond to a single dose.

Moderate hemorrhage: Required peak postinfusion AHF level: 30% to 60% (15-30 int. units/kg): Infuse every 12-24 hours for ≥3 days until pain and disability are resolved.

Alternatively, a loading dose to achieve 50% (25 int. units/kg) may be given, followed by 10-15 int. units/kg dose given every 8-12 hours; may be needed for >7 days.

Severe/life-threatening hemorrhage: Required peak postinfusion AHF level: 60% to 100% (30-50 int. units/kg): Infuse every 8-24 hours until threat is resolved.

Alternatively, a loading dose to achieve 80% to 100% (40-50 int. units/kg) may be given, followed by 20-25 int. units/kg dose given every 8-12 hours for ≥14 days.

Minor surgery: Required peak postinfusion AHF level: 30% to 80% (15-40 int. units/kg): Highly dependent upon procedure and specific product recommendations; for some procedures, may be administered as a single infusion plus oral antifibrinolytic therapy within 1 hour. In other procedures, may repeat dose every 12-24 hours as needed.

Major surgery: Required peak pre- and postsurgery AHF level: 80% to 100% (40-50 int. units/kg): Administer every 6-24 hours until healing is complete (10-14 days).

Prophylaxis: May also be given on a regular schedule to prevent bleeding.

If bleeding is not controlled with adequate dose, test for presence of inhibitor. It may not be possible or practical to control bleeding if inhibitor titers >10 Bethesda units/mL; antihemophilic factor (porcine) may be considered as an alternative.

von Willebrand disease:

Treatment of hemorrhage in von Willebrand disease (Humate-P®): 1 int. units of factor VIII per kg of body weight would be expected to raise circulating vWF:RC of approximately 3.5-4 int. units/dL.

Type 1, mild (if desmopressin is not appropriate): Major hemorrhage:

Loading dose: 40-60 int. units/kg

Maintenance dose: 40-50 int. units/kg every 8-12 hours for 3 days, keeping vWF:RC of nadir >50%; follow with 40-50 int. units/kg daily for up to 7 days

Type 1, moderate or severe:

Minor hemorrhage: 40-50 int. units/kg for 1-2 doses

Major hemorrhage:

Loading dose: 50-75 int. units/kg

Maintenance dose: 40-60 int. units/kg daily for up to 7 days

Types 2 and 3:

Minor hemorrhage: 40-50 int. units/kg for 1-2 doses

Major hemorrhage:

Loading dose: 60-80 int. units/kg

Maintenance dose: 40-60 int. units/kg every 8-12 hours for 3 days, keeping vWF:RC of nadir >50%; follow with 40-60 int. units/kg daily for up to 7 days

Elderly: Refer to adult dosing. Dosage should be individualized.

Pediatrics: Refer to adult dosing.

Administration

I.V.: Total dose may be administered over 5-10 minutes (maximum: 10 mL/minute); infuse Monoclate-P® at 2 mL/minute. Adapt based on patient response.

Stability

Storage: Store under refrigeration, 2°C to 8°C (36°F to 46°F); avoid freezing. Use within 3 hours of reconstitution; gently agitate or rotate vial after adding diluent, do not shake vigorously. Do not refrigerate after reconstitution, precipitation may occur.

Alphanate®: May be stored at room temperature for ≤2 months.

Hemofil®M: May be stored at room temperature for ≤12 months.

Humate-P®, Koāte®-DVI; Monoclate-P®: May also be stored at room temperature for ≤6 months.

If refrigerated, the dried concentrate and diluent should be warmed to room temperature before reconstitution.

Monitoring Laboratory Tests In patients with circulating inhibitors, the inhibitor level should be monitored; hematocrit; monitor for signs and symptoms of intravascular hemolysis; bleeding

Monitoring and Teaching Issues

Physical Assessment: See Contraindications, Warnings/Precautions and Dosing for use cautions. Assess potential for interactions with other prescriptions, OTC medications, or herbal products patient may be taking - especially those medications that may affect coagulation or platelet function (see Drug Interactions). See infusion specifics above. During and after therapy patient should be monitored closely (eg, vital signs, cardiac and CNS status) and adverse reactions (eg, acute hypersensitivity reaction - see Adverse Reactions and Overdose/Toxicology). Provide patient education according to patient condition. **Pregnancy risk factor C** - benefits of use should outweigh possible risks. Note breast-feeding caution.

Patient Education: Inform prescriber of all prescriptions, OTC medications, or herbal products you are taking, and any allergies you have. This medication can only be given intravenously. Report immediately any sudden-onset headache, rash, chest or back pain, wheezing or respiratory difficulties, hives, itching, low-grade fever, stomach pain, or nausea/vomiting to prescriber. Wear identification indicating that you have a hemophilic condition. **Pregnancy/breast-feeding precautions:** Inform prescriber if you are or intend to become pregnant. Consult prescriber if breast-feeding.

Antihemophilic Factor (Porcine) (an tee hee moe FIL ik FAK ter POR seen)

U.S. Brand Names Hyate:C®

Synonyms AHF (Porcine); Factor VIII (Porcine)

Generic Available No

Pharmacologic Category Antihemophilic Agent

Pregnancy Risk Factor C

Lactation Excretion in breast milk unknown/use caution

Use Management of hemophilia A in patients with antibodies to human factor VIII (consider use of human factor VIII in patients with antibody titer of <5 Bethesda units/mL); management of previously nonhemophilic patients with spontaneously-acquired inhibitors to human factor VIII, regardless of initial antihuman inhibitor titer

Mechanism of Action/Effect Factor VIII is the coagulation portion of the factor VIII complex in plasma. Factor VIII acts as a cofactor for factor IX to activate factor X in the intrinsic pathway of blood coagulation.

Contraindications Hypersensitivity to porcine or any component of the formulation

Warnings/Precautions Rarely administration has been associated with anaphylaxis. Epinephrine, hydrocortisone, and facilities for cardiopulmonary resuscitation should be available in case such a reaction occurs. Infusion may be followed by a rise in plasma levels of antibody to both human and porcine factor VIII. Inhibitor levels should be monitored both pre- and post-treatment. Pregnancy risk C.

Adverse Reactions Reactions tend to lessen in frequency and severity as further infusions are given; hydrocortisone and/or antihistamines may help to prevent or alleviate side effects and may be prescribed as precautionary measures

1% to 10%:
- Central nervous system: Fever, headache, chills
- Dermatologic: Rashes
- Gastrointestinal: Nausea, vomiting

<1% (Limited to important or life-threatening): Anaphylaxis, thrombocytopenia

Overdosage/Toxicology Massive doses of antihemophilic factor (human) have been reported to cause acute hemolytic anemia, increased bleeding tendency, or hyperfibrinogenemia. Occurrence is rare.

Pharmacodynamics/Kinetics

Half-Life Elimination: 10-11 hours (patients without detectable inhibitors)

Formulations Injection, powder for reconstitution: 400-700 porcine units [to be reconstituted with 20 mL SWFI]

Dosing

Adults & Elderly: Clinical response should be used to assess efficacy.

Factor VIII deficiency: I.V.: Initial dose:

Antibody level to human factor VIII <50 Bethesda units/mL: 100-150 porcine units/kg (body weight) is recommended.

Antibody level to human factor VIII >50 Bethesda units/mL: Activity of the antibody to antihemophilic (porcine) should be determined. **An antiporcine antibody level** >20 Bethesda units/mL indicates that the patient is unlikely to benefit from treatment; for lower titers, a dose of 100-150 porcine units/kg is recommended.

The initial dose may also be calculated using the following method:

1. Determine patient's antibody titer against porcine factor VIII.
2. Calculate average plasma volume:
   (body weight kg) (average blood volume) (1 - hematocrit) = plasma volume
   (body weight kg) (80 mL/kg) (1 - hematocrit) = plasma volume
   Note: A hematocrit of 50% = 0.5 for the equation
3. Neutralizing dose:
   (plasma volume mL) (antibody titer Bethesda units/mL) = neutralizing dose units
   This is the predicted dose required to neutralize the circulating antibodies. An incremental dose must be added to the neutralizing dose in order to increase the plasma factor VIII to the desired level.
4. Incremental dose:
   (desired plasma factor VIII level) (body weight) divided by 1.5 = incremental dose units
5. Total dose = neutralizing dose + incremental dose = total dose units

If a patient has previously been treated with Hyate:C®, this may provide a guide to his likely response and, therefore, assist in estimation of the preliminary dose.

Subsequent doses: Following administration of the initial dose, if the recovery of factor VIII in the patient's plasma is not sufficient, another larger dose should be administered. If recovery after the second dose is still insufficient, a third and larger dose may prove effective. Once appropriate factor VIII levels are achieved, dosing can be repeated every 6-8 hours.

Pediatrics: Refer to adult dosing.

Administration

I.V.: Administer by I.V. route only; infuse slowly, 2-5 mL/minute.

Stability

Storage: Store at -15°C to -20°C (5°F to -4°F); warm to 20°C to 37°C (68°F to 98.6°F) prior to reconstitution; use within 3 hours of mixing.

Monitoring Laboratory Tests Factor VIII levels pre- and postinfusion; inhibitor levels to human and/or porcine factor VIII pre- and postinfusion; bleeding

Antibody levels to human factor VIII >50 Bethesda units/mL: Activity of the antibody to antihemophilic factor (porcine) should be determined.

(Continued)

Antihemophilic Factor (Porcine) *(Continued)*

Antiporcine antibody level >20 Bethesda units/mL: Patient may not benefit from treatment.

Monitoring and Teaching Issues

Physical Assessment: Identify any patient allergies to antihemophilic factor or porcine substances. See Contraindications, Warnings/Precautions, and Dosing for use cautions. Assess potential for interactions with other prescriptions, OTC medications, or herbal products patient may be taking - especially those medications that may affect coagulation or platelet function (see Drug Interactions). Vital signs, cardiac and CNS status should be monitored during and after therapy. Patient should be monitored closely during infusion for adverse reactions. Rarely has administration been associated with anaphylaxis. Epinephrine, hydrocortisone, and facilities for cardiopulmonary resuscitation should be available in case such a reaction occurs (see Adverse Reactions). Provide patient education according to patient condition (see Patient Education). **Pregnancy risk factor C** - benefits of use should outweigh possible risks. Note breast-feeding caution.

Patient Education: Inform prescriber of all prescriptions, OTC medications, or herbal products you are taking, and any allergies you have. This medication can only be given intravenously. Report sudden onset headache, rash, chest or back pain, wheezing or respiratory difficulties, hives, itching, low-grade fever, stomach pain, nausea, or vomiting to prescriber. Wear identification indicating that you have a hemophilic condition. **Pregnancy/ breast-feeding precautions:** Inform prescriber if you are or intend to become pregnant. Consult prescriber if breast-feeding.

Additional Information Sodium ion concentration is not more than 200 mmol/L. The assayed amount of activity is stated on the label, but may vary depending on the type of assay and hemophilic substrate plasma used.

Antihemophilic Factor (Recombinant)

(an tee hee moe FIL ik FAK tor ree KOM be nant)

U.S. Brand Names Helixate® FS; Kogenate® FS; Recombinate™; ReFacto®

Synonyms AHF (Recombinant); Factor VIII (Recombinant); rAHF

Generic Available No

Pharmacologic Category Antihemophilic Agent

Pregnancy Risk Factor C

Lactation Excretion in breast milk unknown/use caution

Use Management of hemophilia A for patients in whom a deficiency in factor VIII has been demonstrated; can be of significant therapeutic value in patients with acquired factor VIII inhibitors not exceeding 10 Bethesda units/mL

Orphan drug: ReFacto®: Control and prevention of hemorrhagic episodes; surgical prophylaxis for hemophilia A (congenital factor VIII deficiency or classic hemophilia)

Mechanism of Action/Effect Protein (factor VIII) in normal plasma which is necessary for clot formation and maintenance of hemostasis; activates factor X in conjunction with activated factor IX; activated factor X converts prothrombin to thrombin, which converts fibrinogen to fibrin, and with factor XIII forms a stable clot

Contraindications Hypersensitivity to mouse or hamster protein (Helixate® FS, Kogenate® FS); hypersensitivity to mouse, hamster, or bovine protein (Recombinate™, ReFacto®); hypersensitivity to any component of the formulation

Warnings/Precautions Monitor for signs of formation of antibodies to factor VIII; may occur at anytime but more common in young children with severe hemophilia. Monitor for allergic hypersensitivity reactions. Products vary by preparation method. Recombinate™ is stabilized using human albumin. Helixate® FS and Kogenate® FS are stabilized with sucrose. Pregnancy risk C.

Adverse Reactions <1% (Limited to important or life-threatening): Allergic reactions, anaphylaxis, angina pectoris, depersonalization, dyspnea, epistaxis, fever, headache, injection site reactions (burning, pruritus, erythema), nausea, rash, somnolence, urticaria, vasodilation, venous catheter access complications, vomiting

Overdosage/Toxicology Massive doses of antihemophilic factor (human) have been reported to cause acute hemolytic anemia, increased bleeding tendency, or hyperfibrinogenemia. Occurrence is rare.

Pharmacodynamics/Kinetics

Half-Life Elimination: Mean: 14-16 hours

Formulations

Injection, powder for reconstitution, recombinant [preservative free]:

Helixate® FS, Kogenate® FS: 250 int. units/vial, 500 int. units/vial, 1000 int. units/vial [contains sucrose 28 mg/vial]

Recombinate™: 250 int. units/vial, 500 units/vial, 1000 int. units/vial [contains human albumin 12.5 mg/mL]

ReFacto®: 250 int. units/vial, 500 units/vial, 1000 int. units/vial, 2000 int. units/vial

Dosing

Adults: Hemophilia: I.V.: Individualize dosage based on coagulation studies. performed prior to treatment and at regular intervals during treatment; 1 AHF unit is the activity present in 1 mL of normal pooled human plasma; dosage should be adjusted to actual vial size currently stocked in the pharmacy. (General guidelines presented; consult individual product labeling for specific dosing recommendations.)

Dosage based on desired factor VIII increase (%):

To calculate dosage needed based on desired factor VIII increase (%):

Body weight (kg) x 0.5 int. units/kg x desired factor VIII increase (%) = int. units factor VIII required

For example:

50 kg x 0.5 int. units/kg x 30 (% increase) = 750 int. units factor VIII

Dosage based on expected factor VIII increase (%):

It is also possible to calculate the **expected** % factor VIII increase:

(# int. units administered x 2%/int. units/kg) divided by body weight (kg) = expected % factor VIII increase

For example:

(1400 int. units x 2%/int. units/kg) divided by 70 kg = 40%

General guidelines:

Minor hemorrhage: Required peak postinfusion AHF level: 20% to 40% (10-20 int. units/kg); mild superficial or early hemorrhages may respond to a single dose; may repeat dose every 12-24 hours for 1-3 days until bleeding is resolved or healing achieved

Moderate hemorrhage/minor surgery: Required peak postinfusion AHF level: 30% to 60% (15-30 int. units/kg); repeat dose at 12-24 hours if needed; some products suggest continuing for ≥3 days until pain and disability are resolved

Severe/life-threatening hemorrhage: Required peak postinfusion AHF level: Initial dose: 80% to 100% (40-50 int. units/kg); maintenance dose: 40% to 50% (20-25 int. units/kg) every 8-12 hours until threat is resolved

Major surgery: Required peak pre- and postsurgery AHF level: ~100% (50 int. units/kg) give first dose prior to surgery and repeat every 6-12 hours until healing complete (10-14 days)

Prophylaxis: May also be given on a regular schedule to prevent bleeding

If bleeding is not controlled with adequate dose, test for presence of inhibitor. It may not be possible or practical to control bleeding if inhibitor titers >10 Bethesda units/mL; antihemophilic factor (porcine) may be considered as an alternative

Elderly: Refer to adult dosing. Dosage should be individualized.

Pediatrics: Refer to adult dosing.

Administration

I.V.: Total dose may be administered over 5-10 minutes (maximum: 10 mL/minute); adapt based on patient response.

Stability

Storage: Store under refrigeration, 2°C to 8°C (36°F to 46°F); avoid freezing. Use within 3 hours of reconstitution; gently agitate or rotate vial after adding diluent, do not shake vigorously. Do not refrigerate after reconstitution, a precipitation may occur.

Kogenate® FS: Avoid prolonged exposure to light during storage.

Recombinate™, ReFacto®: May also be stored at room temperature for up to 3 months; avoid prolonged exposure to light during storage

If refrigerated, the dried concentrate and diluent should be warmed to room temperature before reconstitution.

Monitoring Laboratory Tests In patients with circulating inhibitors, the inhibitor level should be monitored; bleeding

Monitoring and Teaching Issues

Physical Assessment: See Contraindications, Warnings/Precautions, and Dosing for use cautions. Assess potential for interactions with other prescriptions, OTC medications, or herbal products patient may be taking (especially those medications that may affect coagulation or platelet function - see Drug Interactions). See infusion specifics above. During and after therapy, patient should be monitored closely (eg, vital signs, cardiac and CNS status) and observed for adverse reactions (eg, acute hypersensitivity reaction - see Adverse Reactions and Overdose/Toxicology). **Pregnancy risk factor C** - benefits of use should outweigh possible risks. Note breast-feeding caution.

Patient Education: Inform prescriber of all prescriptions, OTC medications, or herbal products you are taking, and any allergies you have. This medication can only be given intravenously. Immediately report any sudden-onset headache, rash, chest or back pain, wheezing or respiratory difficulties, hives, itching, low grade fever, stomach pain, nausea, or vomiting to prescriber. Wear identification indicating that you have a hemophilic condition. **Pregnancy/breast-feeding precautions:** Inform prescriber if you are pregnant. Consult prescriber if breast-feeding.

Anti-inhibitor Coagulant Complex

(an tee-in HI bi tor coe AG yoo lant KOM pleks)

U.S. Brand Names Autoplex® T; Feiba VH Immuno®

Synonyms Coagulant Complex Inhibitor

Generic Available No

Pharmacologic Category Antihemophilic Agent; Blood Product Derivative

Pregnancy Risk Factor C

Lactation Excretion in breast milk unknown/use caution

Use Patients with factor VIII inhibitors who are to undergo surgery or those who are bleeding

Contraindications Disseminated intravascular coagulation; patients with normal coagulation mechanism

Warnings/Precautions Products are prepared from pooled human plasma; such plasma may contain the causative agents of viral diseases. Tests used to control efficacy such as aPTT, WBCT, and TEG do not correlate with clinical efficacy. Dosing to normalize these values may result in DIC. Identification of the clotting deficiency as caused by factor VIII inhibitors is essential prior to starting therapy. Use with extreme caution in patients with impaired hepatic function. Pregnancy risk C.

Effects on Lab Values ↑ ↓ PT, PTT; ↑ fibrin split products; ↓ WBCT, fibrin, platelets

Adverse Reactions <1% (Limited to important or life-threatening): Chills, disseminated intravascular coagulation, fever, headache, hypotension, rash, urticaria

Overdosage/Toxicology Rapid infusion may cause hypotension. Excessive administration can cause DIC.

Formulations

Injection:

Autoplex® T: Each bottle is labeled with correctional units of factor VIII [with heparin 2 units]

Feiba VH Immuno®: Each bottle is labeled with correctional units of factor VIII [heparin free]

Dosing

Adults & Elderly: Bleeding or surgery in patients with factor VIII inhibitors: I.V.: Dosage range: 25-100 factor VIII correctional units per kg depending on the severity of hemorrhage

(Continued)

Anti-inhibitor Coagulant Complex *(Continued)*

Tests used to control efficacy such as APTT, WBCT, and TEG do not correlate with clinical efficacy. Dosing to normalize these values may result in DIC. Identification of the clotting deficiency as caused by factor VIII inhibitors is essential prior to starting therapy.

Pediatrics: Refer to adult dosing.

Hepatic Impairment: Use with extreme caution.

Administration

I.V.: I.V. push (maximum rate: 2 units/kg/minute or 2.5-7.5 mL/minutes).

Stability

Storage: Store at 2°C to 8°C (36°F to 46°F)

Reconstitution: Do **not** shake or refrigerate after reconstitution. Use within 1-3 hours after reconstitution.

Monitoring Laboratory Tests Tests used to control efficacy such as aPTT, WBCT, and TEG do not correlate with clinical efficacy. Dosing to normalize these values may result in DIC.

Monitoring and Teaching Issues

Physical Assessment: See Contraindications, Warnings/Precautions, and Dosing for use cautions. Assess potential for interactions with other prescriptions, OTC medications, or herbal products patient may be taking. **Caution:** See Monitoring Laboratory Tests. Vital signs, cardiac and hemodynamic status should be monitored during and after therapy (see Adverse Reactions and Overdose/Toxicology). If hypotension develops, the rate of infusion should be slowed and prescriber notified. **Pregnancy risk factor C** - benefits of use should outweigh possible risks. Note breast-feeding caution.

Patient Education: Inform prescriber of all prescriptions, OTC medications, or herbal products you are taking, and any allergies you have. This medication can only be given intravenously. Report sudden onset headache, rash, chest or back pain, wheezing or respiratory difficulties, hives, itching, or acute feelings of anxiety. Wear identification indicating that you have a hemophilic condition. **Pregnancy/breast-feeding precautions:** Inform prescriber if you are pregnant. Consult prescriber if breast-feeding.

Antilirium® *see* Physostigmine *on page 1079*

Antimicrobial Drugs of Choice *see page 1628*

Antimigraine Drugs *see page 1557*

Antipsychotic Agents *see page 1558*

Antipsychotic Medication Guidelines *see page 1614*

Antipyrine and Benzocaine *see page 1519*

Antipyrine and Benzocaine *see page 1522*

Antirabies Serum (Equine) *see page 1498*

Antistin-Privin *see page 1509*

Antithymocyte Globulin (Equine) *see* Lymphocyte Immune Globulin *on page 829*

Antithymocyte Immunoglobulin *see* Lymphocyte Immune Globulin *on page 829*

Antivenin *see page 1460*

Antivert® *see* Meclizine *on page 840*

Antizol® *see page 1460*

Antrizine® *see* Meclizine *on page 840*

Anturane® *see* Sulfinpyrazone *on page 1263*

Anucort-HC® *see* Hydrocortisone *on page 673*

Anucort-HC® Suppository *see* Topical Corticosteroids *on page 1334*

Anusol-HC® *see* Hydrocortisone *on page 673*

Anusol® HC-1 [OTC] *see* Hydrocortisone *on page 673*

Anusol® HC-1 [OTC] *see* Topical Corticosteroids *on page 1334*

Anusol® HC-2.5% [OTC] *see* Topical Corticosteroids *on page 1334*

Anusol-HC® Suppository *see* Topical Corticosteroids *on page 1334*

Anxiolytic/Hypnotic Use in Long-Term Care Facilities *see page 1608*

Anzemet® *see* Dolasetron *on page 435*

APAP *see* Acetaminophen *on page 35*

Aphthasol™ *see* Amlexanox *on page 86*

A.P.L.® *see* Chorionic Gonadotropin (Human) *on page 284*

Apothecary/Metric Conversions *see page 1530*

APPG *see* Penicillin G Procaine *on page 1047*

Apraclonidine *see page 1461*

Apraclonidine *see page 1575*

Apraclonidine *see* Ophthalmic Agents, Glaucoma *on page 1002*

Apresazide [DSC] *see* Hydralazine and Hydrochlorothiazide *on page 664*

Apresoline [DSC] *see* HydrALAZINE *on page 662*

Apri® *see* Ethinyl Estradiol and Desogestrel *on page 516*

Aquachloral® Supprettes® *see* Chloral Hydrate *on page 268*

Aqua Gem E® [OTC] *see* Vitamin E *on page 1406*

AquaMEPHYTON® *see* Phytonadione *on page 1080*

Aquanil™ HC [OTC] *see* Hydrocortisone *on page 673*

Aquasol E® [OTC] *see* Vitamin E *on page 1406*

Aquatab® *see* Guaifenesin and Pseudoephedrine *on page 648*

Aquatab® D Dose Pack *see* Guaifenesin and Pseudoephedrine *on page 648*

Aquatab® DM *see* Guaifenesin and Dextromethorphan *on page 647*

Aquazide® H *see* Hydrochlorothiazide *on page 664*

Aqueous Procaine Penicillin G *see* Penicillin G Procaine *on page 1047*

Ara-A *see* Vidarabine *on page 1399*

Arabinofuranosyladenine *see* Vidarabine *on page 1399*

Arabinosylcytosine *see* Cytarabine *on page 348*

Ara-C *see* Cytarabine *on page 348*

Aralen® Phosphate *see* Chloroquine *on page 275*

Aranesp™ *see* Darbepoetin Alfa *on page 365*

Arava™ *see* Leflunomide *on page 774*

Ardeparin *see page 1576*

Aredia® *see* Pamidronate *on page 1027*

Arfonad® Injection *see page 1461*

Argatroban (ar GA troh ban)

Generic Available No

Pharmacologic Category Anticoagulant, Thrombin Inhibitor

Pregnancy Risk Factor B

Lactation Excretion in breast milk unknown/not recommended

Use Prophylaxis or treatment of thrombosis in adults with heparin-induced thrombocytopenia; adjunct to percutaneous coronary intervention (PCI) in patients who have or are at risk of thrombosis associated with heparin-induced thrombocytopenia

Mechanism of Action/Effect A direct, highly selective thrombin inhibitor. Reversibly binds to the active thrombin site of free and clot-associated thrombin. Inhibits fibrin formation; activation of coagulation factors V, VIII, and XIII; protein C; and platelet aggregation.

Contraindications Hypersensitivity to argatroban or any component of the formulation; overt major bleeding

Warnings/Precautions Hemorrhage can occur at any site in the body. Extreme caution should be used when there is an increased danger of hemorrhage, such as severe hypertension, immediately following lumbar puncture, spinal anesthesia, major surgery (including brain, spinal cord, or eye surgery), congenital or acquired bleeding disorders, and gastrointestinal ulcers. Use caution with hepatic dysfunction. Concomitant use with warfarin will cause increased prolongation of the PT and INR greater than that of warfarin alone; alternative guidelines for monitoring therapy should be followed. Safety and efficacy for use with other thrombolytic agents has not been established. Discontinue all parenteral anticoagulants prior to starting therapy. Allow reversal of heparin's effects before initiation. Patients with hepatic dysfunction may require >4 hours to achieve full reversal of argatroban's anticoagulant effect following treatment. Avoid use during PCI in patients with elevations of ALT/AST (>3 x ULN); the use of argatroban in these patients has not been evaluated. Safety and efficacy in children <18 years of age have not been established.

Drug Interactions

Cytochrome P450 Effect: Substrate of CYP3A4

Increased Effect/Toxicity: Drugs which affect platelet function (eg, aspirin, NSAIDs, dipyridamole, ticlopidine, clopidogrel), anticoagulants, or thrombolytics may potentiate the risk of hemorrhage. Sufficient time must pass after heparin therapy is discontinued; allow heparin's effect on the aPTT to decrease

Concomitant use of argatroban with warfarin increases PT and INR greater than that of warfarin alone. Argatroban is commonly continued during the initiation of warfarin therapy to assure anticoagulation and to protect against possible transient hypercoagulability.

Effects on Lab Values Argatroban produces dose-dependent effects on PT, INR, ACT, and TT, however, therapeutic ranges are not established.

Adverse Reactions As with all anticoagulants, bleeding is the major adverse effect of argatroban. Hemorrhage may occur at virtually any site. Risk is dependent on multiple variables, including the intensity of anticoagulation and patient susceptibility.

>10%:

Gastrointestinal: Gastrointestinal bleed (minor, 14%; <1% in PCI)

Genitourinary: Genitourinary bleed and hematuria (minor, 12%)

1% to 10%:

Cardiovascular: Hypotension (7%), cardiac arrest (6%), ventricular tachycardia (5%), atrial fibrillation (3%), cerebrovascular disorder (2%)

Central nervous system: Fever (7%), pain (5%), intracranial bleeding (1%, only observed in patients also receiving streptokinase or tissue plasminogen activator)

Gastrointestinal: Diarrhea (6%), nausea (5%), vomiting (4%), abdominal pain (3%), bleeding (major, 2%)

Genitourinary: Urinary tract infection (5%)

Hematologic: Decreased hemoglobin <2 g/dL and hematocrit (minor, 10%)

Local: Bleeding at the injection site (minor, 2% to 5%)

Renal: Abnormal renal function (3%)

Respiratory: Dyspnea (8% to 10%), coughing (3% to 10%), hemoptysis (minor, 3%), pneumonia (3%)

Miscellaneous: Sepsis (6%), infection (4%)

<1% (Limited to important or life-threatening): Allergic reactions including cough, dyspnea, rash, bullous eruption, and vasodilation (increased to 14% in patients also receiving thrombolytic therapy and/or contrast media); genitourinary bleeding and hematuria (major, 0.9%); hemoglobin and hematocrit decreased (major, 0.7%); limb and below-the-knee stump bleed; multisystem hemorrhage and DIC; retroperitoneal bleeding

Overdosage/Toxicology No specific antidote is available. Treatment should be symptomatic and supportive. Discontinue or decrease infusion to control excessive anticoagulation with or without bleeding. Reversal of anticoagulant effects may be longer than 4 hours in patients with hepatic impairment.

(Continued)

Argatroban *(Continued)*

Pharmacodynamics/Kinetics

Half-Life Elimination: 39-51 minutes; Hepatic impairment: ≤181 minutes

Time to Peak: Steady-state: 1-3 hours

Metabolism: Hepatic via hydroxylation and aromatization. Metabolism via CYP3A4/5 to four known metabolites plays a minor role. Unchanged argatroban is the major plasma component. Plasma concentration of metabolite M1 is 0% to 20% of the parent drug and is three- to fivefold weaker.

Onset: Immediate

Formulations Injection: 100 mg/mL (2.5 mL)

Dosing

Adults & Elderly:

Prophylaxis of thrombosis (heparin-induced thrombocytopenia): I.V.:

Initial dose: 2 mcg/kg/minute

Maintenance dose: Measure aPTT after 2 hours, adjust dose until the steady-state aPTT is 1.5-3.0 times the initial baseline value, not exceeding 100 seconds; dosage should not exceed 10 mcg/kg/minute

Conversion to oral anticoagulant: Because there may be a combined effect on the INR when argatroban is combined with warfarin, loading doses of warfarin should not be used. Warfarin therapy should be started at the expected daily dose.

Patients receiving ≤2 mcg/kg/minute of argatroban: Argatroban therapy can be stopped when the combined INR on warfarin and argatroban is >4; repeat INR measurement in 4-6 hours; if INR is below therapeutic level, argatroban therapy may be restarted. Repeat procedure daily until desired INR on warfarin alone is obtained.

Patients receiving >2 mcg/kg/minute of argatroban: Reduce dose of argatroban to 2 mcg/kg/minute; measure INR for argatroban and warfarin 4-6 hours after dose reduction; argatroban therapy can be stopped when the combined INR on warfarin and argatroban is >4. Repeat INR measurement in 4-6 hours; if INR is below therapeutic level, argatroban therapy may be restarted. Repeat procedure daily until desired INR on warfarin alone is obtained.

Percutaneous coronary intervention (PCI): I.V.:

Initial: Begin infusion of 25 mcg/kg/minute and administer bolus dose of 350 mcg/kg (over 3-5 minutes). ACT should be checked 5-10 minutes after bolus infusion; proceed with procedure if ACT >300 seconds. Following initial bolus:

ACT <300 seconds: Give an additional 150 mcg/kg bolus, and increase infusion rate to 30 mcg/kg/minute (recheck ACT in 5-10 minutes)

ACT >450 seconds: Decrease infusion rate to 15 mcg/kg/minute (recheck ACT in 5-10 minutes)

Once a therapeutic ACT (300-450 seconds) is achieved, infusion should be continued at this dose for the duration of the procedure.

Impending abrupt closure, thrombus formation during PCI, or inability to achieve ACT >300 sec: An additional bolus of 150 mcg/kg, followed by an increase in infusion rate to 40 mcg/kg/minute may be administered.

Renal Impairment: No adjustment is necessary.

Hepatic Impairment: Decreased clearance and increased elimination half-life are seen with hepatic impairment; dose should be reduced. Initial dose for moderate hepatic impairment is 0.5 mcg/kg/minute. **Note:** During PCI, avoid use in patients with elevations of ALT/AST (>3 x ULN); the use of argatroban in these patients has not been evaluated.

Stability

Storage: Store at 25°C (77°F). Protect from light.

Reconstitution: Once mixed, final concentration should be 1 mg/mL. The prepared solution is stable for 24 hours at 25°C (77°F) in ambient indoor light. Do not expose to direct sunlight. Prepared solutions are stable for 48 hours at 2°C to 8°C when stored in the dark.

Compatibility: Stable in 0.9% NS, D_5W, LR; do not expose diluted solution to direct sunlight (light-resistant containers are not necessary with exposure to ambient light)

Y-site administration: Incompatible with other medications

Compatibility when admixed: Incompatible with other medications

Monitoring Laboratory Tests Hemoglobin, hematocrit

Monitoring and Teaching Issues

Physical Assessment: See Warnings/Precautions, Contraindications, and Drug Interactions for use cautions. Monitor therapeutic response (laboratory results) and adverse reactions (see Adverse Reactions) frequently during therapy. Observe bleeding precautions and teach patient interventions to reduce side effects and adverse reactions to report (see Patient Education). Breast-feeding is not recommended.

Patient Education: This medication can only be administered by intravenous infusion and you will be monitored with blood tests during therapy. You may have a tendency to bleed easily; use electric razor, brush teeth with soft brush, floss with waxed floss, avoid all scissors or sharp instruments (knives, needles, etc), and avoid injury or bruising. Report stomach cramping or pain; dark or bloody stools; blood in urine; acute headache or confusion; difficulty breathing; nosebleed; or bleeding from gums. **Pregnancy/breast-feeding precautions:** Inform prescriber if you are or intend to become pregnant. Breast-feeding is not recommended.

Breast-feeding Issues: It is not known if argatroban is excreted in human milk. Because of the serious potential of adverse effects to the nursing infant, a decision to discontinue nursing or discontinue argatroban should be considered.

Additional Information Platelet counts recovered by day 3 in 53% of patients with heparin-induced thrombocytopenia and in 58% of patients with heparin-induced thrombocytopenia with thrombosis syndrome.

Argesic®-SA *see* Salsalate *on page 1212*

8-Arginine Vasopressin *see* Vasopressin *on page 1391*

Aricept® *see* Donepezil *on page 436*

Arimidex® *see* Anastrozole *on page 106*
Aristocort® *see* Topical Corticosteroids *on page 1334*
Aristocort® *see* Triamcinolone *on page 1356*
Aristocort® A *see* Triamcinolone *on page 1356*
Aristocort® Forte *see* Triamcinolone *on page 1356*
Aristocort® Intralesional *see* Triamcinolone *on page 1356*
Aristospan® Intra-Articular *see* Triamcinolone *on page 1356*
Aristospan® Intralesional *see* Triamcinolone *on page 1356*
Arixtra® *see* Fondaparinux *on page 600*
Armour® Thyroid *see* Thyroid *on page 1313*
Aromasin® *see* Exemestane *on page 540*

Arsenic Trioxide (AR se nik tri OKS id)

U.S. Brand Names Trisenox™

Generic Available No

Pharmacologic Category Antineoplastic Agent, Miscellaneous

Pregnancy Risk Factor D

Lactation Excretion in breast milk unknown/contraindicated

Use Induction of remission and consolidation in patients with acute promyelocytic leukemia (APL) which is specifically characterized by t(15;17) translocation or PML/RAR-alpha gene expression. Should be used only in those patients who have relapsed or are refractory to retinoid and anthracycline chemotherapy.

Orphan drug: Treatment of myelodysplastic syndrome; multiple myeloma; chronic myeloid leukemia (CML); acute myelocytic leukemia (AML)

Mechanism of Action/Effect Not fully understood; causes *in vitro* morphological changes and DNA fragmentation to NB4 human promyelocytic leukemia cells; also damages or degrades the fusion protein PML-RAR alpha

Contraindications Hypersensitivity to arsenic or any component of the formulation; pregnancy

Warnings/Precautions The U.S. Food and Drug Administration (FDA) currently recommends that procedures for proper handling and disposal of antineoplastic agents be considered. For use only by physicians experienced with the treatment of acute leukemia. A baseline 12-lead EKG, serum electrolytes (potassium, calcium, magnesium), and creatinine should be obtained. Correct electrolyte abnormalities prior to treatment and monitor potassium and magnesium levels during therapy (potassium should stay >4 mEq/dL and magnesium >1.8 mg/dL). Correct QT_c >500 msec prior to treatment. Discontinue therapy and hospitalize patient if QT_c >500 msec, syncope or irregular heartbeats develop during therapy. May prolong the QT interval. May lead to torsade de pointes or complete AV block. Risk factors for torsade de pointes include CHF, a history of torsade de pointes, pre-existing QT interval prolongation, patients taking potassium-wasting diuretics, and conditions which cause hypokalemia or hypomagnesemia. If possible, discontinue all medications known to prolong the QT interval. May cause retinoic-acid-acute promyelocytic leukemia (RA-APL) syndrome or APL differentiation syndrome (high-dose steroids have been used for treatment). May lead to the development of hyperleukocytosis. Use with caution in renal impairment. Safety and efficacy in children <5 years of age have not been established (limited experience with children 5-16 years of age).

Drug Interactions

Increased Effect/Toxicity: Use caution with medications causing hypokalemia or hypomagnesemia (ampho B, aminoglycosides, diuretics, cyclosporin). Use caution with medications that prolong the QT interval, avoid concurrent use if possible; includes type Ia and type III antiarrhythmic agents, selected quinolones (sparfloxacin, gatifloxacin, moxifloxacin, grepafloxacin), cisapride, thioridazine, and other agents.

Nutritional/Ethanol Interactions

Food: Avoid seafood (due to presence of arsenic as arsenobetaine and arsenocholine).

Herb/Nutraceutical: Avoid homeopathic products (arsenic is present in some homeopathic medications).

Adverse Reactions

>10%:

Cardiovascular: Tachycardia (55%), edema (40%), QT interval >500 msec (38%), chest pain (25%), hypotension (25%)

Central nervous system: Fatigue (63%), fever (63%), headache (60%), insomnia (43%), anxiety (30%), dizziness (23%), depression (20%), pain (15%)

Dermatologic: Dermatitis (43%), pruritus (33%), bruising (20%)

Endocrine & metabolic: Hypokalemia (50%), hyperglycemia (45%), hypomagnesemia (45%), hyperkalemia (18%)

Gastrointestinal: Nausea (75%), abdominal pain (58%), vomiting (58%), diarrhea (53%), sore throat (40%), constipation (28%), anorexia (23%)

Genitourinary: Vaginal hemorrhage (13%)

Hematologic: Leukocytosis (50%), APL differentiation syndrome (23%), thrombocytopenia (19%), anemia (14%), febrile neutropenia (13%)

Hepatic: Elevated ALT (20%), elevated AST (13%)

Local: Injection site: Pain (20%), erythema (13%)

Neuromuscular & skeletal: Rigors (38%), arthralgia (33%), paresthesia (33%), myalgia (25%), bone pain (23%), back pain (18%), tremor (13%)

Respiratory: Cough (65%), dyspnea (53%), epistaxis (25%), hypoxia (23%), pleural effusion (20%), wheezing (13%)

1% to 10% (Limited to important or life-threatening):

Cardiovascular: Hypotension (10%), abnormal EKG (not QT prolongation) (7%)

Central nervous system: Convulsion (8%), somnolence (8%), agitation (5%), coma (5%), confusion (5%)

Dermatologic: Hyperpigmentation (8%), urticaria (8%), local exfoliation (5%)

Endocrine & metabolic: Hypocalcemia (10%), hypoglycemia (8%), acidosis (5%)

(Continued)

Arsenic Trioxide *(Continued)*

Gastrointestinal: Gastrointestinal hemorrhage (8%), hemorrhagic diarrhea (8%), oral blistering (8%)
Genitourinary: Intermenstrual bleeding (8%), incontinence (5%)
Hematologic: Neutropenia (10%), DIC (8%), hemorrhage (8%)
Otic: Tinnitus (5%)
Renal: Renal failure (8%), renal impairment (8%)
Respiratory: Hemoptysis (8%)
Miscellaneous: Hypersensitivity (5%), sepsis (5%)

Overdosage/Toxicology Symptoms of arsenic toxicity include convulsions, muscle weakness, and confusion. Discontinue treatment and begin chelation therapy. One suggested adult protocol: Dimercaprol 3 mg/kg I.M. every 4 hours, continue until life-threatening toxicity has subsided; follow with penicillamine 250 mg orally up to 4 times/day (total daily dose ≤1 g).

Pharmacodynamics/Kinetics

Metabolism: Hepatic; pentavalent arsenic is reduced to trivalent arsenic (active) by arsenate reductase; trivalent arsenic is methylated to monomethylarsinic acid, which is then converted to dimethylarsinic acid via methyltransferases

Formulations Injection: 1 mg/mL (10 mL)

Dosing

Adults:

Induction: I.V.: 0.15 mg/kg/day; administer daily until bone marrow remission; maximum induction: 60 doses

Consolidation: I.V.: 0.15 mg/kg/day starting 3-6 weeks after completion of induction therapy; maximum consolidation: 25 doses over 5 weeks

Elderly: Safety and efficacy have not been established. Clinical trials included patients ≤72 years of age. Use with caution due to the increased risk of renal impairment in the elderly.

Pediatrics: Children >5 years: Refer to adult dosing.

Renal Impairment: Safety and efficacy have not been established; use with caution due to renal elimination.

Hepatic Impairment: Safety and efficacy have not been established.

Administration

I.V.: Dilute in 100-250 mL D_5W or 0.9% sodium chloride. Does not contain a preservative; properly discard unused portion. Do not mix with other medications. Infuse over 1-2 hours. If acute vasomotor reactions occur, may infuse over a maximum of 4 hours. Does not require administration via a central venous catheter.

Stability

Storage: Store at room temperature, 25°C (77°F); do not freeze. Following dilution, stable for 24 hours at room temperature or 48 hours when refrigerated.

Monitoring Laboratory Tests Baseline then weekly 12-lead EKG, baseline then twice weekly serum electrolytes, hematologic and coagulation profiles at least twice weekly; more frequent monitoring may be necessary in unstable patients.

Monitoring and Teaching Issues

Physical Assessment: To be used only by physicians experienced with the treatment of acute leukemia. See Contraindications, Warnings/Precautions, and Dosing for use cautions. Assess potential for interactions with other prescriptions, OTC medications, or herbal products patient may be taking (especially anything that may cause hypokalemia or hypomagnesemia, or antiarrhythmic agents - see Drug Interactions). Assess results of laboratory tests (see above). Assess patient response at beginning and periodically during therapy (especially cardiac and electrolyte status - see Adverse Reactions and Overdose/Toxicology). Teach patient appropriate use and adverse symptoms to report (see Patient Education). **Pregnancy risk factor D** - determine that patient is not pregnant before beginning treatment. Teach patients of childbearing age appropriate use of barrier contraceptives. Breast-feeding is contraindicated.

Patient Education: Inform prescriber of all prescriptions, OTC medications, or herbal products you are taking, and any allergies you have. Do not take anything new during treatment unless approved by prescriber. This medication can only be administered by intravenous infusion. Report immediately any redness, swelling, pain, or burning at infusion site. May cause dizziness, fatigue, blurred vision (use caution when driving or engaging in tasks requiring alertness until response to drug is known); or nausea, vomiting, diarrhea, or decreased appetite (small, frequent meals, frequent mouth care, sucking lozenges, or chewing gum may help). Report immediately unexplained fever; difficulty breathing; chest pain or palpitations; confusion, lightheadedness, or fainting; or other persistent adverse effects. **Pregnancy/breast-feeding precautions:** Inform prescriber if you are pregnant. Do not get pregnant while take this medication. Consult prescriber for appropriate contraceptive methods. Do not breast-feed.

Additional Information Arsenic is stored in liver, kidney, heart, lung, hair, and nails. Arsenic trioxide is a human carcinogen.

Artane® *see* Trihexyphenidyl *on page 1363*
Arthrotec® *see* Diclofenac and Misoprostol *on page 402*
ASA *see* Aspirin *on page 121*
5-ASA *see* Mesalamine *on page 858*
Asacol® *see* Mesalamine *on page 858*
Ascriptin® [OTC] *see* Aspirin *on page 121*
Ascriptin® Arthritis Pain [OTC] *see* Aspirin *on page 121*
Ascriptin® Enteric [OTC] *see* Aspirin *on page 121*
Ascriptin® Extra Strength [OTC] *see* Aspirin *on page 121*

Asparaginase (a SPIR a ji nase)

U.S. Brand Names Elspar®

Synonyms *E. coli* Asparaginase; *Erwinia* Asparaginase; L-asparaginase; NSC-106977 (*Erwinia*); NSC-109229 (*E. coli*)

Generic Available No

Pharmacologic Category Antineoplastic Agent, Miscellaneous

Pregnancy Risk Factor C

Lactation Excretion in breast milk unknown

Use Treatment of acute lymphocytic leukemia, lymphoma; induction therapy

Mechanism of Action/Effect Asparaginase deprives tumor cells of the amino acid for protein synthesis and inhibits cell (malignant) proliferation. There are two purified preparations of the enzyme: one from *Escherichia coli* and one from *Erwinia carotovora*. These two preparations vary slightly in the gene sequencing and have slight differences in enzyme characteristics. Both are highly specific for asparagine and have <10% activity for the D-isomer. The preparation from *E. coli* has had the most use in clinical and research practice.

Contraindications Hypersensitivity to asparaginase or any component of the formulation; history of anaphylaxis to asparaginase; if a reaction occurs to Elspar®, obtain **Erwinia L-asparaginase** and use with caution; pancreatitis (active or any history of)

Warnings/Precautions The U.S. Food and Drug Administration (FDA) currently recommends that procedures for proper handling and disposal of antineoplastic agents be considered. Monitor for severe allergic reactions. May alter hepatic function. Use cautiously in patients with an underlying coagulopathy. Up to 33% of patients who have an allergic reaction to *E. coli* asparaginase will also react to the *Erwinia* form or pegaspargase.

A test dose is often recommended prior to the first dose of asparaginase, or prior to restarting therapy after a hiatus of several days. **False-negative rates of up to 80% to test doses of 2-50 units are reported.** Desensitization should be performed in patients found to be hypersensitive by the intradermal test dose or who have received previous courses of therapy with the drug. See Administration.

Pregnancy risk C.

Drug Interactions

Decreased Effect: Asparaginase terminates methotrexate action.

Increased Effect/Toxicity: Increased toxicity has been noticed when asparaginase is administered with vincristine (neuropathy) and prednisone (hyperglycemia). Decreased metabolism when used with cyclophosphamide. Increased hepatotoxicity when used with mercaptopurine.

Effects on Lab Values ↓ thyroxine and thyroxine-binding globulin

Adverse Reactions Note: Immediate effects: Fever, chills, nausea, and vomiting occur in 50% to 60% of patients.

>10%:

- Central nervous system: Fatigue, somnolence, depression, hallucinations, agitation, disorientation or convulsions (10% to 60%), stupor, confusion, coma (25%)
- Endocrine & metabolic: Fever, chills (50% to 60%), hyperglycemia (10%)
- Gastrointestinal: Nausea, vomiting (50% to 60%), anorexia, abdominal cramps (70%), acute pancreatitis (15%, may be severe in some patients)
- Hematologic: Hypofibrinogenemia and depression of clotting factors V and VIII, variable decreased in factors VII and IX, severe protein C deficiency and decrease in antithrombin III (may be dose-limiting or fatal)
- Hepatic: Transient elevations of transaminases, bilirubin, and alkaline phosphatase
- Hypersensitivity: Acute allergic reactions (fever, rash, urticaria, arthralgia, hypotension, angioedema, bronchospasm, anaphylaxis (15% to 35%); may be dose-limiting in some patients, may be fatal)
- Renal: Azotemia (66%)

1% to 10%:

- Endocrine & metabolic: Hyperuricemia
- Gastrointestinal: Stomatitis

<1% (Limited to important or life-threatening): Acute renal failure, coma (may be due to elevated NH_4 levels), diabetes mellitus (transient), fever, hallucinations, ketoacidosis, laryngeal spasm, Parkinsonian symptoms (tremor), seizures

Inhibition of protein synthesis will cause a decrease in production of albumin, insulin (resulting in hyperglycemia), serum lipoprotein, antithrombin III, and clotting factors II, V, VII, VIII, IX, and X. The loss of the later two proteins may result in either thrombotic or hemorrhagic events. These protein losses occur in 100% of patients.

Myelosuppressive: Myelosuppression is uncommon and usually mild; Onset (days): 7; Nadir (days): 14; Recovery (days): 21

Overdosage/Toxicology Symptoms of overdose include nausea and diarrhea.

Pharmacodynamics/Kinetics

Absorption: I.M.: Produces peak blood levels 50% lower than those from I.V. administration

Half-Life Elimination: 8-30 hours

Metabolism: Systemically degraded

Formulations Injection, powder for reconstitution: 10,000 units

Dosing

Adults & Elderly: Refer to individual protocols; dose must be individualized based upon clinical response and tolerance of the patient.

Single agent induction:

- I.V. infusion:
  - 200 units/kg/day for 28 days **or**
  - 5000-10,000 units/m^2/day for 7 days every 3 weeks **or**
  - 10,000-40,000 units every 2-3 weeks
- I.M.: 6000-12,000 units/m^2; reconstitution to 10,000 units/mL may be necessary. (See pediatric dosage for combination therapy.)

Notes: Some institutions recommended the following precautions for asparaginase administration: Have parenteral epinephrine, diphenhydramine, and hydrocortisone available at the bedside. Have a freely running I.V. in place. Have a physician readily accessible. Monitor the patient closely for 30-60 minutes. Avoid administering the drug at night.

(Continued)

Asparaginase *(Continued)*

A test dose is often recommended prior to the first dose of asparaginase, or prior to restarting therapy after a hiatus of several days. Most commonly, 0.1-0.2 mL of a 20-250 units/mL (2-50 units) is injected intradermally, and the patient observed for 15-30 minutes. False-negative rates of up to 80% to test doses of 2-50 units are reported.

Some practitioners recommend a desensitization regimen for patients who react to a test dose, or are being retreated following a break in therapy. Doses are doubled and given every 10 minutes until the total daily dose for that day has been administered.

One schedule begins with a total of 1 unit given I.V. and doubles the dose every 10 minutes until the total amount given in the planned dose for that day. For example, if a patient was to receive a total dose of 4000 units, he/she would receive injections 1 through 12 during the desensitization. See table.

Asparaginase Desensitization

Injection No.	Elspar Dose (IU)	Accumulated Total Dose
1	1	1
2	2	3
3	4	7
4	8	15
5	16	31
6	32	63
7	64	127
8	128	255
9	256	511
10	512	1023
11	1024	2047
12	2048	4095
13	4096	8191
14	8192	16,383
15	16,384	32,767
16	32,768	65,535
17	65,536	131,071
18	131,072	262,143

Pediatrics: Refer to individual protocols; dose must be individualized based upon clinical response and tolerance of the patient.

Children:

Infusion for induction in combination with vincristine and prednisone: I.V.: 1000 units/kg/day for 10 days

Consolidation: 6000-10,000 units/m^2/day for 14 days

In combination with vincristine and prednisone: I.M.: 6000 units/m^2 on days 4, 7, 10, 13, 16, 19, 22, 25, 28

Refer to information in adult dosing.

Administration

I.M.: Must only be given as a deep intramuscular injection into a large muscle; use two injection sites for I.M. doses >2 mL.

I.V.: The following precautions should be taken when administering. Only administer in a hospital setting. Administer over at least 30 minutes. Give a small test dose first. Note that a negative skin test does not preclude the possibility of an allergic reaction. Desensitization should be performed in patients who have been found to be hypersensitive by the intradermal skin test or who have received previous courses of therapy with the drug. Have epinephrine, diphenhydramine, and hydrocortisone at the bedside. Have a running I.V. in place. A physician should be readily accessible.

Stability

Storage: Intact vials of powder should be refrigerated <8°C; however, the manufacturer states that asparaginase is stable for at least 48 hours at room temperature.

Reconstitution: Lyophilized powder should be reconstituted with 1-5 mL sterile water for I.V. administration or NS for I.M. use, reconstituted solutions are stable 1 week at room temperature. Shake well but not too vigorously. Use of a 5-micron in-line filter is recommended to remove fiber-like particles in the solution (not 0.2 micron filter - has been associated with some loss of potency)

Standard I.M./S.C. dilution: 5000 units/mL: 2 mL/syringe

Standard I.V. dilution: Dose in 50-250 mL NS or D_5W

Stable for 8 hours at room temperature or refrigeration after dilution.

Compatibility: Stable in D_5W, NS

Monitoring Laboratory Tests Intradermal skin test prior to first dose and other doses if more than 1 week between doses; CBC, serum amylase, blood glucose, uric acid, liver function prior to and frequently during therapy

Monitoring and Teaching Issues

Physical Assessment: See Contraindications, Warnings/Precautions, and Dosing for use cautions. Assess potential for interactions with other prescriptions, OTC medications, or herbal products patient may be taking (see Drug Interactions). See Dosing and Administration for premedication recommendations prior to administering first dose. Assess results of pretherapy skin test and regular laboratory tests (see above). With each dose, patient should be monitored closely for adverse reactions (eg, CNS changes and acute hypersensitivity reactions may occur in 10% to 40% of patients; hyperglycemia; nausea or vomiting - see Adverse Reactions and Overdose/Toxicology). In the event of hypersensitivity or hyperglycemia, infusion should be stopped and prescriber notified immediately. Teach patient possible side effects and appropriate interventions and adverse symptoms to report (see Patient Education). **Pregnancy risk factor C** - benefits of use should outweigh possible risks. **Important:** See Pregnancy Issues. Note breast-feeding caution.

Patient Education: Inform prescriber of all prescriptions, OTC medications, or herbal products you are taking, and any allergies you have. Do not take anything new during treatment unless approved by prescriber. This medication can only be given I.M. or I.V. Report immediately any pain or burning at infusion/injection site, rash, chest pain, difficulty breathing or chest tightness, difficulty swallowing, or sharp back pain. It is vital to maintain adequate hydration (2-3 L/day of fluids) unless advised by prescriber to restrict fluids, and good nutritional status (small, frequent meals may help). May cause acute nausea or vomiting (small, frequent meals, frequent mouth care, chewing gum, or sucking lozenges may help - or consult prescriber for approved antiemetic). Report unusual fever or chills; confusion, agitation, depression; yellowing of skin or eyes; unusual bleeding or bruising; unhealed sores; or vaginal discharge. **Pregnancy/breast-feeding precautions:** Inform prescriber if you are or intend to become pregnant. Consult prescriber if breast-feeding.

Pregnancy Issues: Based on limited reports in humans, the use of asparaginase does not seem to pose a major risk to the fetus when used in the 2nd and 3rd trimesters, or when exposure occurs prior to conception in either females or males. Because of the teratogenicity observed in animals and the lack of human data after the 1st trimester exposure, asparaginase should be used cautiously, if at all, during this period.

Additional Information The *E. coli* and the *Erwinia* strains of asparaginase differ slightly in their gene sequencing, and have slight differences in their enzyme characteristics. Both are highly specific for asparagine and have <10% activity for the D-isomer. The *E. coli* form is more commonly used, with the *Erwinia* variety usually being used only in patients who demonstrate allergic reactions to the other form.

Aspercin [OTC] *see* Aspirin *on page 121*

Aspercin Extra [OTC] *see* Aspirin *on page 121*

Aspergum® [OTC] *see* Aspirin *on page 121*

Aspirin (AS pir in)

U.S. Brand Names Ascriptin® [OTC]; Ascriptin® Arthritis Pain [OTC]; Ascriptin® Enteric [OTC]; Ascriptin® Extra Strength [OTC]; Aspercin [OTC]; Aspercin Extra [OTC]; Aspergum® [OTC]; Bayer® Aspirin [OTC]; Bayer® Aspirin Extra Strength [OTC]; Bayer® Aspirin Regimen Adult Low Strength [OTC]; Bayer® Aspirin Regimen Adult Low Strength with Calcium [OTC]; Bayer® Aspirin Regimen Children's [OTC]; Bayer® Aspirin Regimen Regular Strength [OTC]; Bayer® Plus Extra Strength [OTC]; Bufferin® [OTC]; Bufferin® Arthritis Strength [OTC]; Bufferin® Extra Strength [OTC]; Easprin®; Ecotrin® [OTC]; Ecotrin® Low Adult Strength [OTC]; Ecotrin® Maximum Strength [OTC]; Halfprin® [OTC]; St. Joseph® Pain Reliever [OTC]; Sureprin 81™ [OTC]; ZORprin®

Synonyms Acetylsalicylic Acid; ASA

Generic Available Yes

Pharmacologic Category Salicylate

Pregnancy Risk Factor C/D (full-dose aspirin in 3rd trimester - expert analysis)

Lactation Enters breast milk/use caution

Use Treatment of mild to moderate pain, inflammation, and fever; may be used as prophylaxis of myocardial infarction; prophylaxis of stroke and/or transient ischemic episodes; management of rheumatoid arthritis, rheumatic fever, osteoarthritis, and gout (high dose); adjunctive therapy in revascularization procedures (coronary artery bypass graft [CABG], percutaneous transluminal coronary angioplasty [PTCA], carotid endarterectomy)

Use - Unlabeled/Investigational Low doses have been used in the prevention of pre-eclampsia, recurrent spontaneous abortions, prematurity, fetal growth retardation (including complications associated with autoimmune disorders such as lupus or antiphospholipid syndrome)

Mechanism of Action/Effect Inhibits prostaglandin synthesis, acts on the hypothalamus heat-regulating center to reduce fever, blocks prostaglandin synthetase action which prevents formation of the platelet-aggregating substance thromboxane A_2

Contraindications Hypersensitivity to salicylates, other NSAIDs, or any component of the formulation; asthma; rhinitis; nasal polyps; inherited or acquired bleeding disorders (including factor VII and factor IX deficiency); do not use in children (<16 years of age) for viral infections (chickenpox or flu symptoms), with or without fever, due to a potential association with Reye's syndrome; pregnancy (3rd trimester especially)

Warnings/Precautions Use with caution in patients with platelet and bleeding disorders, renal dysfunction, dehydration, erosive gastritis, or peptic ulcer disease. Heavy ethanol use (>3 drinks/day) can increase bleeding risks. Avoid use in severe renal failure or in severe hepatic failure. Discontinue use if tinnitus or impaired hearing occurs. Caution in mild-moderate renal failure (only at high dosages). Patients with sensitivity to tartrazine dyes, nasal polyps and asthma may have an increased risk of salicylate sensitivity. Surgical patients should avoid ASA if possible, for 1-2 weeks prior to surgery, to reduce the risk of excessive bleeding. Pregnancy risk C/D (if full-dose aspirin in 3rd trimester).

Drug Interactions

Cytochrome P450 Effect: Substrate of CYP2C8/9

Decreased Effect: The effects of ACE inhibitors may be blunted by aspirin administration (may be significant only at higher aspirin dosages). Aspirin may decrease the effects of beta-blockers, loop diuretics (furosemide), thiazide diuretics, and probenecid. Aspirin may cause a decrease in NSAIDs serum concentration and decrease the effects of probenecid. Increased serum salicylate levels when taken with with urine acidifiers (ammonium chloride, methionine).

Increased Effect/Toxicity: Aspirin may increase methotrexate serum levels/toxicity and may displace valproic acid from binding sites which can result in toxicity. NSAIDs and aspirin increase GI adverse effects (ulceration). Aspirin with oral anticoagulants (warfarin), thrombolytic agents, heparin, low molecular weight heparins, and antiplatelet agents (ticlopidine, clopidogrel, dipyridamole, NSAIDs, and IIb/IIIa antagonists) may increase risk

(Continued)

Aspirin *(Continued)*

of bleeding. Bleeding times may be additionally prolonged with verapamil. The effects of older sulfonylurea agents (tolazamide, tolbutamide) may be potentiated due to displacement from plasma proteins. This effect does not appear to be clinically significant for newer sulfonylurea agents (glyburide, glipizide, glimepiride).

Nutritional/Ethanol Interactions

Ethanol: Avoid ethanol (may enhance gastric mucosal damage).

Food: Food may decrease the rate but not the extent of oral absorption.

Folic acid: Hyperexcretion of folate; folic acid deficiency may result, leading to macrocytic anemia.

Iron: With chronic aspirin use and at doses of 3-4 g/day, iron-deficiency anemia may result.

Sodium: Hypernatremia resulting from buffered aspirin solutions or sodium salicylate containing high sodium content. Avoid or use with caution in CHF or any condition where hypernatremia would be detrimental.

Benedictine liqueur, prunes, raisins, tea, and gherkins: Potential salicylate accumulation.

Fresh fruits containing vitamin C: Displace drug from binding sites, resulting in increased urinary excretion of aspirin.

Herb/Nutraceutical: Avoid cat's claw, dong quai, evening primrose, feverfew, garlic, ginger, ginkgo, red clover, horse chestnut, green tea, ginseng (all have additional antiplatelet activity). Limit curry powder, paprika, licorice; may cause salicylate accumulation. These foods contain 6 mg salicylate/100 g. An ordinarily American diet contains 10-200 mg/day of salicylate.

Effects on Lab Values False-negative results for glucose oxidase urinary glucose tests (Clinistix®). Interferes with Gerhardt test, VMA determination; 5-HIAA, xylose tolerance test and T_3 and T_4.

Adverse Reactions As with all drugs which may affect hemostasis, bleeding is associated with aspirin. Hemorrhage may occur at virtually any site. Risk is dependent on multiple variables including dosage, concurrent use of multiple agents which alter hemostasis, and patient susceptibility. Many adverse effects of aspirin are dose-related, and are extremely rare at low dosages. Other serious reactions are idiosyncratic, related to allergy or individual sensitivity. Accurate estimation of frequencies is not possible.

Central nervous system: Fatigue, insomnia, nervousness, agitation, confusion, dizziness, headache, lethargy, cerebral edema, hyperthermia, coma

Cardiovascular: Hypotension, tachycardia, dysrhythmias, edema

Dermatologic: Rash, angioedema, urticaria

Endocrine & metabolic: Acidosis, hyperkalemia, dehydration, hypoglycemia (children), hyperglycemia, hypernatremia (buffered forms)

Gastrointestinal: Nausea, vomiting, dyspepsia, epigastric discomfort, heartburn, stomach pains, gastrointestinal ulceration (6% to 31%), gastric erosions, gastric erythema, duodenal ulcers

Hematologic: Anemia, disseminated intravascular coagulation, prolongation of prothrombin times, coagulopathy, thrombocytopenia, hemolytic anemia, bleeding, iron-deficiency anemia

Hepatic: Hepatotoxicity, increased transaminases, hepatitis (reversible)

Neuromuscular & skeletal: Rhabdomyolysis, weakness, acetabular bone destruction (OA)

Otic: Hearing loss, tinnitus

Renal: Interstitial nephritis, papillary necrosis, proteinuria, renal failure (including cases caused by rhabdomyolysis), increased BUN, increased serum creatinine

Respiratory: Asthma, bronchospasm, dyspnea, laryngeal edema, hyperpnea, tachypnea, respiratory alkalosis, noncardiogenic pulmonary edema

Miscellaneous: Anaphylaxis, prolonged pregnancy and labor, stillbirths, low birth weight, peripartum bleeding, Reye's syndrome

Postmarketing and/or case reports: Colonic ulceration, esophageal stricture, esophagitis with esophageal ulcer, esophageal hematoma, oral mucosal ulcers (aspirin-containing chewing gum), coronary artery spasm, conduction defect and atrial fibrillation (toxicity), delirium, ischemic brain infarction, colitis, rectal stenosis (suppository), cholestatic jaundice, periorbital edema, rhinosinusitis

Overdosage/Toxicology Symptoms of overdose include tinnitus, headache, dizziness, confusion, metabolic acidosis, hyperpyrexia, hypoglycemia, and coma. Treatment should be based upon symptomatology.

Pharmacodynamics/Kinetics

Absorption: Rapid

Bioavailability: 50% to 75% reaches systemic circulation

Half-Life Elimination: Parent drug: 15-20 minutes; Salicylates (dose dependent): 3 hours at lower doses (300-600 mg), 5-6 hours (after 1 g), 10 hours with higher doses

Time to Peak: Serum: ~1-2 hours

Metabolism: Hydrolyzed to salicylate (active) by esterases in GI mucosa, red blood cells, synovial fluid, and blood; metabolism of salicylate occurs primarily by hepatic conjugation; metabolic pathways are saturable

Duration: 4-6 hours

Formulations

Caplet, buffered:

Ascriptin® Arthritis Pain: 325 mg [contains aluminum hydroxide, calcium carbonate, and magnesium hydroxide]

Ascriptin® Extra Strength: 500 mg [contains aluminum hydroxide, calcium carbonate, and magnesium hydroxide]

Gelcap:

Bayer® Aspirin: 325 mg

Bayer® Aspirin Extra Strength: 500 mg

Gum (Aspergum®): 227 mg

Suppository, rectal: 60 mg, 120 mg, 125 mg, 200 mg, 300 mg, 325 mg, 600 mg, 650 mg

Tablet: 325 mg, 500 mg

Aspercin: 325 mg

Aspercin Extra, Bayer® Aspirin Extra Strength: 500 mg
Bayer® Aspirin: 325 mg [film coated]
Tablet, buffered:
Ascriptin®: 325 mg [contains aluminum hydroxide, calcium carbonate, and magnesium hydroxide]
Bayer® Plus Extra Strength: 500 mg [contains calcium carbonate]
Bufferin®: 325 mg [contains citric acid]
Bufferin® Arthritis Strength, Bufferin® Extra Strength: 500 mg [contains citric acid]
Tablet, chewable: 81 mg
Bayer® Aspirin Regimen Children's Chewable, St. Joseph® Pain Reliever: 81 mg
Tablet, controlled release (ZORprin®): 800 mg
Tablet, enteric coated: 81 mg, 162 mg, 325 mg, 500 mg, 650 mg, 975 mg
Ascriptin® Enteric, Bayer® Aspirin Regimen Adult Low Strength, Ecotrin® Adult Low Strength, St. Joseph Pain Reliever: 81 mg
Bayer® Aspirin Regimen Adult Low Strength with Calcium: 81 mg [contains calcium carbonate 250 mg]
Bayer® Aspirin Regimen Regular Strength, Ecotrin®: 325 mg
Easprin®: 975 mg
Ecotrin® Maximum Strength: 500 mg
Halfprin: 81 mg, 162 mg
Sureprin 81™: 81 mg

Dosing

Adults:

Analgesic and antipyretic: Oral, rectal: 325-650 mg every 4-6 hours up to 4 g/day
Anti-inflammatory: Oral: Initial: 2.4-3.6 g/day in divided doses; usual maintenance: 3.6-5.4 g/day; monitor serum concentrations
Acute myocardial infarction: 160-325 mg/day
Myocardial infarction prophylaxis: 75-325 mg/day; use of a lower aspirin dosage has been recommended in patients receiving ACE inhibitors
CABG: 325 mg/day starting 6 hours following procedure
PTCA: Initial: 80-325 mg/day starting 2 hours before procedure; longer pretreatment durations (up to 24 hours) should be considered if lower dosages (80-100 mg) are used
Carotid endarterectomy: 81-325 mg/day preoperatively and daily thereafter
Acute stroke: 160-325 mg/day, initiated within 48 hours (in patients who are not candidates for thrombolytics and are not receiving systemic anticoagulation)
Stroke prevention/TIA: 30-325 mg/day (dosages up to 1300 mg/day in 2-4 divided doses have been used in clinical trials)
Pre-eclampsia prevention (unlabeled use): 60-80 mg/day during gestational weeks 13-26 (patient selection criteria not established)

Elderly: Refer to adult dosing; adjust if necessary due to decreased renal function (see Geriatric Considerations).

Pediatrics:

Analgesic and antipyretic: Oral, rectal: Children: 10-15 mg/kg/dose every 4-6 hours, up to a total of 4 g/day
Anti-inflammatory: Oral: Children: Initial: 60-90 mg/kg/day in divided doses; usual maintenance: 80-100 mg/kg/day divided every 6-8 hours; monitor serum concentrations
Antiplatelet effects: Oral: Children: Adequate pediatric studies have not been performed; pediatric dosage is derived from adult studies and clinical experience and is not well established; suggested doses have ranged from 3-5 mg/kg/day to 5-10 mg/kg/day given as a single daily dose. Doses are rounded to a convenient amount (eg, ½ of 80 mg tablet).
Mechanical prosthetic heart valves: Oral: Children: 6-20 mg/kg/day given as a single daily dose (used in combination with an oral anticoagulant in children who have systemic embolism despite adequate oral anticoagulation therapy (INR 2.5-3.5) and used in combination with low-dose anticoagulation (INR 2-3) and dipyridamole when full-dose oral anticoagulation is contraindicated)
Blalock-Taussig shunts: Oral: Children: 3-5 mg/kg/day given as a single daily dose
Kawasaki disease: Oral: Children: 80-100 mg/kg/day divided every 6 hours; monitor serum concentrations; after fever resolves: 3-5 mg/kg/day once daily; in patients without coronary artery abnormalities, give lower dose for at least 6-8 weeks or until ESR and platelet count are normal; in patients with coronary artery abnormalities, low-dose aspirin should be continued indefinitely
Antirheumatic: Oral: Children: 60-100 mg/kg/day in divided doses every 4 hours

Renal Impairment:

Cl_{cr} <10 mL/minute: Avoid use.
Dialyzable (50% to 100%)

Hepatic Impairment: Avoid use in severe liver disease.

Administration

Oral: Do not crush sustained release or enteric coated tablet. Administer with food or a full glass of water to minimize GI distress.

Stability

Storage: Keep suppositories in refrigerator; do not freeze. Hydrolysis of aspirin occurs upon exposure to water or moist air, resulting in salicylate and acetate, which possess a vinegar-like odor. Do not use if a strong odor is present.

Monitoring and Teaching Issues

Physical Assessment: Do not use for persons with allergic reaction to salicylate or other NSAIDs (see Contraindications). Assess other medications patient may be taking for additive or adverse interactions (see Drug Interactions). Monitor therapeutic effectiveness and for signs of adverse reactions or overdose (see Overdose/Toxicology and Adverse Reactions) at beginning of therapy and periodically with long-term therapy. Assess knowledge/teach patient appropriate use. Teach patient to monitor for adverse reactions, adverse reactions to report, and appropriate interventions to reduce side effects. **Pregnancy risk factor C/D** - see Pregnancy Risk Factor for use cautions; benefits of use should outweigh possible risks. Note breast-feeding caution.

(Continued)

Aspirin *(Continued)*

Patient Education: If self-administered, use exactly as directed; do not increase dose or frequency. Adverse reactions can occur with overuse. Take with food or milk. Do not use aspirin with strong vinegar-like odor. Do not crush or chew extended release products. While using this medication, avoid alcohol, excessive amounts of vitamin C, or salicylate-containing foods (eg, curry powder, prunes, raisins, tea, or licorice), other prescription or OTC medications containing aspirin or salicylate, or other NSAIDs without consulting prescriber. Maintain adequate hydration (2-3 L/day of fluids) unless advised by prescriber to restrict fluids. You may experience nausea, vomiting, gastric discomfort (frequent mouth care, small, frequent meals, sucking lozenges, or chewing gum may help); GI bleeding, ulceration, or perforation (can occur with or without pain); or discoloration of stool (pink/red). Stop taking aspirin and report ringing in ears; persistent stomach pain; unresolved nausea or vomiting; difficulty breathing or shortness of breath; unusual bruising or bleeding (mouth, urine, stool); or skin rash. **Pregnancy/breast-feeding precautions:** Inform prescriber if you are or intend to become pregnant. Consult prescriber if breast-feeding.

Dietary Issues: Take with food or large volume of water or milk to minimize GI upset.

Geriatric Considerations: Elderly are at high risk for adverse effects from NSAIDs. Elderly with GI complications can develop peptic ulceration and/or hemorrhage asymptomatically. The concomitant use of H_2 blockers, omeprazole, and sucralfate is not effective as prophylaxis with the exception of NSAID-induced duodenal ulcers which may be prevented by the use of ranitidine. Misoprostol is the only prophylactic agent proven effective. Also, concomitant disease and drug use contribute to the risk for GI adverse effects. Use lowest effective dose for shortest period possible. Consider renal function decline with age. Use of NSAIDs can compromise existing renal function especially when Cl_{cr} is ≤30 mL/minute. Tinnitus may be a difficult and unreliable indication of toxicity due to age-related hearing loss or eighth cranial nerve damage. CNS adverse effects such as confusion, agitation, and hallucination are generally seen in overdose or high-dose situations, but elderly may demonstrate these adverse effects at lower doses than younger adults.

Aspirin and Carisoprodol *see* Carisoprodol and Aspirin *on page 222*

Aspirin and Codeine (AS pir in & KOE deen)

Synonyms Codeine and Aspirin

Restrictions C-III

Generic Available Yes

Pharmacologic Category Analgesic, Narcotic

Pregnancy Risk Factor D

Lactation Enters breast milk/use caution

Use Relief of mild to moderate pain

Formulations Tablet:

#3: Aspirin 325 mg and codeine phosphate 30 mg
#4: Aspirin 325 mg and codeine phosphate 60 mg

Dosing

Adults: Management of pain: Oral: 1-2 tablets (#3 tablet) every 4-6 hours as needed for pain

Elderly: One ASA with codeine 30 mg (#3 tablet), or two ASA with codeine 15 mg (#2 tablet) every 4-6 hours as needed for pain

Renal Impairment:

Cl_{cr} 10-50 mL/minute: Administer 75% of dose.
Cl_{cr} <10 mL/minute: Avoid use.

Hepatic Impairment: Avoid use in severe liver disease.

Monitoring and Teaching Issues

Physical Assessment: See individual components listed in Related Information. **Pregnancy risk factor D** - determine that patient is not pregnant before beginning treatment. Instruct patients of childbearing age about appropriate barrier contraceptive measures. Note breast-feeding caution.

Patient Education: See individual components listed in Related Information. **Pregnancy/breast-feeding precautions:** Inform prescriber if you are or intend to become pregnant. Consult prescriber if breast-feeding.

Related Information

Aspirin *on page 121*
Codeine *on page 327*

Aspirin and Dipyridamole (AS pir in & dye peer ID a mole)

U.S. Brand Names Aggrenox™

Synonyms Aspirin and Extended-Release Dipyridamole; Dipyridamole and Aspirin

Generic Available No

Pharmacologic Category Antiplatelet Agent

Pregnancy Risk Factor B (dipyridamole); D (aspirin)

Lactation Contraindicated

Use Reduction in the risk of stroke in patients who have had transient ischemia of the brain or completed ischemic stroke due to thrombosis

Mechanism of Action/Effect Inhibits generation of thromboxane.

Contraindications Hypersensitivity to dipyridamole, aspirin, or any component of the formulation; allergy to NSAIDs; patients with asthma, rhinitis, and nasal polyps; bleeding disorders (factor VII or IX deficiencies); children <16 years of age with viral infections; pregnancy (especially 3rd trimester)

Warnings/Precautions Cautious use in patients with inherited or acquired bleeding disorders (including those related to liver disease or vitamin K deficiency); ethanol intake >3 drinks per day; hypotension; unstable angina; recent I; hepatic dysfunction. Avoid use in the presence of peptic ulcers, GI bleeding, or renal failure. Discontinue 1-2 weeks prior to elective surgery.

Drug Interactions

Cytochrome P450 Effect: Aspirin: Substrate of CYP2C8/9

Decreased Effect: See individual agents.

Increased Effect/Toxicity: See individual agents.

Nutritional/Ethanol Interactions Ethanol: Avoid ethanol (due to GI irritation).

Adverse Reactions

>10%:

Central nervous system: Headache (38%)

Gastrointestinal: Dyspepsia, abdominal pain (18%), nausea (16%), diarrhea (13%)

1% to 10%:

Cardiovascular: Cardiac failure (2%)

Central nervous system: Pain (6%), seizures (2%), fatigue (6%), malaise (2%), syncope (1%), amnesia (2%), confusion (1%), somnolence (1%)

Dermatologic: Purpura (1%)

Gastrointestinal: Vomiting (8%), bleeding (4%), rectal bleeding (2%), hemorrhoids (1%), hemorrhage (1%), anorexia (1%)

Hematologic: Anemia (2%)

Neuromuscular & skeletal: Back pain (5%), weakness (2%), arthralgia (6%), arthritis (2%), arthrosis (1%), myalgia (1%)

Respiratory: Cough (2%), upper respiratory tract infections (1%), epistaxis (2%)

<1% (Limited to important or life-threatening): Intracranial hemorrhage (0.6%), allergic reaction, coma, paresthesia, cerebral hemorrhage, subarachnoid hemorrhage, ulceration, deafness, arrhythmia, cholelithiasis, jaundice, uterine hemorrhage, bronchospasm, hemoptysis, pulmonary edema, pruritus, urticaria, renal failure, angina pectoris, cerebral edema, pancreatitis, Reye's syndrome, hematemesis, anaphylaxis, hepatitis, hepatic failure, rhabdomyolysis, prolonged PT time, disseminated intravascular coagulation, thrombocytopenia, stillbirths, lower weight infants, antepartum and postpartum bleeding, tachypnea, dyspnea, rash, alopecia, angioedema, Stevens-Johnson syndrome, interstitial nephritis, papillary necrosis, allergic vasculitis, anemia (aplastic), pancytopenia

Overdosage/Toxicology Symptoms of dipyridamole overdose might predominate. Symptoms may include hypotension and peripheral vasodilation.

Pharmacokinetic Note See Aspirin monograph.

Pharmacodynamics/Kinetics

Half-Life Elimination:

Aggrenox™: Salicylic acid: 1.71 hours

Dipyridamole: 13.6 hours

Time to Peak:

Aggrenox™: 0.63 hours

Dipyridamole: 2 hours

Metabolism:

Dipyridamole: Hepatic via conjugation with glucuronic acid

Formulations Capsule: Dipyridamole (extended release) 200 mg and aspirin 25 mg

Dosing

Adults: Stroke prevention: Oral: 1 capsule (200 mg dipyridamole, 25 mg aspirin) twice daily.

Elderly: Plasma concentrations were 40% higher, but specific dosage adjustments have not been recommended.

Renal Impairment: Avoid use in patients with severe renal dysfunction (Cl_{cr} <10 mL/minute).

Hepatic Impairment: Avoid use in patients with severe hepatic impairment.

Administration

Oral: Capsule should be swallowed whole; do not crush or chew. May be given with or without food.

Stability

Storage: Store at 25°C (77°F); excursions permitted to 15°C to 30°C (59°F to 86°F); protect from excessive moisture

Monitoring Laboratory Tests Hemoglobin, hematocrit

Monitoring and Teaching Issues

Physical Assessment: Assess for previous drug allergies before administering first dose. Assess other medications patient may be taking for effectiveness and interactions (see Drug Interactions). See Contraindications and Warnings/Precautions for use cautions. Monitor for signs of stroke or bleeding, laboratory results, therapeutic effect, adverse reactions, and overdose (see Monitoring Laboratory Tests, Adverse Reactions, and Overdose/Toxicology). Assess knowledge/teach patient appropriate use, interventions to reduce side effects, and adverse reactions to report (see Patient Education). **Pregnancy risk factor B/D** - see Pregnancy Risk Factor for use cautions. Instruct patient on need to use appropriate contraceptive measures. Breast-feeding is contraindicated.

Patient Education: See individual agents. **Pregnancy/breast-feeding precautions:** Notify prescriber if you are or intend to become pregnant. Do not breast-feed.

Dietary Issues: May be taken with or without food.

Related Information

Aspirin *on page 121*

Aspirin and Extended-Release Dipyridamole *see* Aspirin and Dipyridamole *on page 124*

Aspirin and Hydrocodone *see* Hydrocodone and Aspirin *on page 669*

Aspirin and Meprobamate (AS pir in & me proe BA mate)

U.S. Brand Names Equagesic®

Synonyms Meprobamate and Aspirin

Restrictions C-IV

Generic Available Yes

Pharmacologic Category Antianxiety Agent, Miscellaneous

Pregnancy Risk Factor D

Lactation Enters breast milk/use caution due to aspirin content

(Continued)

Aspirin and Meprobamate *(Continued)*

Use Adjunct to treatment of skeletal muscular disease in patients exhibiting tension and/or anxiety

Formulations Tablet: Aspirin 325 mg and meprobamate 200 mg

Dosing

Adults: Muscular disorders, anxiety (adjunct): Oral: 1 tablet 3-4 times/day

Elderly: Refer to dosing in individual monographs; use with caution.

Monitoring and Teaching Issues

Physical Assessment: See individual components listed in Related Information. **Pregnancy risk factor D** - determine that patient is not pregnant before beginning treatment. Instruct patients of childbearing age about appropriate barrier contraceptive measures. Note breast-feeding caution.

Patient Education: See individual components listed in Related Information. **Pregnancy/breast-feeding precautions:** Inform prescriber if you are or intend to become pregnant. Consult prescriber if breast-feeding.

Related Information

Aspirin *on page 121*
Meprobamate *on page 853*

Aspirin and Methocarbamol *see* Methocarbamol and Aspirin *on page 874*
Aspirin and Oxycodone *see* Oxycodone and Aspirin *on page 1022*
Aspirin, Caffeine, and Butalbital *see* Butalbital, Aspirin, and Caffeine *on page 194*
Aspirin, Carisoprodol, and Codeine *see* Carisoprodol, Aspirin, and Codeine *on page 223*
Aspirin Free Anacin® Maximum Strength [OTC] *see* Acetaminophen *on page 35*
Aspirin, Orphenadrine, and Caffeine *see* Orphenadrine, Aspirin, and Caffeine *on page 1010*
Asthma *see page 1643*
Astramorph™ PF *see* Morphine Sulfate *on page 926*
Atacand® *see* Candesartan *on page 206*
Atacand HCT™ *see* Candesartan and Hydrochlorothiazide *on page 207*
Atapryl® *see* Selegiline *on page 1221*
Atarax® *see* HydrOXYzine *on page 684*

Atenolol (a TEN oh lole)

U.S. Brand Names Tenormin®

Generic Available Yes: Tablet

Pharmacologic Category Beta Blocker, $Beta_1$ Selective

Pregnancy Risk Factor D

Lactation Enters breast milk/use caution

Use Treatment of hypertension, alone or in combination with other agents; management of angina pectoris, postmyocardial infarction patients

Use - Unlabeled/Investigational Acute ethanol withdrawal, supraventricular and ventricular arrhythmias, and migraine headache prophylaxis

Mechanism of Action/Effect Competitively blocks response to beta-adrenergic stimulation, selectively blocks $beta_1$-receptors with little or no effect on $beta_2$-receptors except at high doses

Contraindications Hypersensitivity to atenolol or any component of the formulation; sinus bradycardia; sinus node dysfunction; heart block greater than first-degree (except in patients with a functioning artificial pacemaker); cardiogenic shock; uncompensated cardiac failure; pulmonary edema; pregnancy

Warnings/Precautions Administer cautiously in compensated heart failure and monitor for a worsening of the condition (efficacy of atenolol in heart failure has not been established). Use caution with concurrent use of beta-blockers and either verapamil or diltiazem; bradycardia or heart block can occur. Avoid concurrent I.V. use of both agents. Beta-blockers should be avoided in patients with bronchospastic disease (asthma) and peripheral vascular disease (may aggravate arterial insufficiency). Atenolol, with B1 selectivity, has been used cautiously in bronchospastic disease with close monitoring. Use cautiously in diabetics - may mask hypoglycemic symptoms. May mask signs of thyrotoxicosis. May cause fetal harm when administered in pregnancy. Use cautiously in the renally impaired (dosage adjustment required). Use care with anesthetic agents which decrease myocardial function. Caution in patients with myasthenia gravis. Beta-blocker therapy should not be withdrawn abruptly (particularly in patients with CAD), but gradually tapered to avoid acute tachycardia, hypertension, and/or ischemia.

Drug Interactions

Decreased Effect: Decreased effect of atenolol with aluminum salts, barbiturates, calcium salts, cholestyramine, colestipol, NSAIDs, penicillins (ampicillin), rifampin, salicylates, and sulfinpyrazone due to decreased bioavailability and plasma levels. Beta-blockers may decrease the effect of sulfonylureas.

Increased Effect/Toxicity: Atenolol may increase the effects of other drugs which slow AV conduction (digoxin, verapamil, diltiazem), alpha-blockers (prazosin, terazosin), and alpha-adrenergic stimulants (epinephrine, phenylephrine). Atenolol may mask the tachycardia from hypoglycemia caused by insulin and oral hypoglycemics. In patients receiving concurrent therapy, the risk of hypertensive crisis is increased when either clonidine or the beta-blocker is withdrawn. Reserpine has been shown to enhance the effect of atenolol. Beta-blockers may increase the action or levels of ethanol, disopyramide, nondepolarizing muscle relaxants, and theophylline although the effects are difficult to predict.

Nutritional/Ethanol Interactions

Food: Atenolol serum concentrations may be decreased if taken with food.

Herb/Nutraceutical: Avoid dong quai if using for hypertension (has estrogenic activity). Avoid ephedra, yohimbe, ginseng (may worsen hypertension). Avoid garlic (may have increased antihypertensive effect).

Effects on Lab Values ↑ glucose; ↓ HDL

Adverse Reactions

1% to 10%:

Cardiovascular: Persistent bradycardia, hypotension, chest pain, edema, heart failure, second- or third-degree AV block, Raynaud's phenomenon

Central nervous system: Dizziness, fatigue, insomnia, lethargy, confusion, mental impairment, depression, headache, nightmares

Gastrointestinal: Constipation, diarrhea, nausea

Genitourinary: Impotence

Miscellaneous: Cold extremities

<1% (Limited to important or life-threatening): Alopecia, dyspnea (especially with large doses), elevated liver enzymes, hallucinations, impotence, lupus syndrome, Peyronie's disease, positive ANA, psoriaform rash, psychosis, thrombocytopenia, wheezing

Overdosage/Toxicology Symptoms of toxicity include lethargy, respiratory drive disorder, wheezing, sinus pause and bradycardia. Additional effects associated with any beta-blocker are congestive heart failure, hypotension, bronchospasm, and hypoglycemia. Treatment includes removal of unabsorbed drug by induced emesis, gastric lavage, or administration of activated charcoal and symptomatic treatment of toxic responses. Atenolol can be removed by hemodialysis.

Pharmacodynamics/Kinetics

Absorption: Incomplete

Half-Life Elimination: Beta:

Neonates: ≤35 hours; Mean: 16 hours

Children: 4.6 hours; children >10 years may have prolonged half-life (>5 hours) compared to children 5-10 years (<5 hours)

Adults: Normal renal function: 6-9 hours, prolonged with renal impairment; End-stage renal disease: 15-35 hours

Metabolism: Limited hepatic

Onset: Peak effect: Oral: 2-4 hours

Duration: Normal renal function: 12-24 hours

Formulations

Injection, solution: 0.5 mg/mL (10 mL)

Tablet: 25 mg, 50 mg, 100 mg

Dosing

Adults & Elderly:

Hypertension:

Oral: 50 mg once daily, may increase to 100 mg/day. Doses >100 mg are unlikely to produce any further benefit.

I.V.: Dosages of 1.25-5 mg every 6-12 hours have been used in short-term management of patients unable to take oral enteral beta-blockers

Angina pectoris: Oral: 50 mg once daily, may increase to 100 mg/day. Some patients may require 200 mg/day.

Postmyocardial infarction: I.V.: Early treatment: 5 mg slow I.V. over 5 minutes; may repeat in 10 minutes. If both doses are tolerated, may start oral atenolol 50 mg every 12 hours or 100 mg/day for 6-9 days postmyocardial infarction.

Postmyocardial infarction: Oral: Follow I.V. dose with 100 mg/day or 50 mg twice daily for 6-9 days postmyocardial infarction.

Pediatrics:

Hypertension: Oral: Children: 0.8-1 mg/kg/dose given daily; range of 0.8-1.5 mg/kg/day; maximum dose: 2 mg/kg/day

Renal Impairment:

Cl_{cr} 15-35 mL/minute: Administer 50 mg/day maximum.

Cl_{cr} <15 mL/minute: Administer 50 mg every other day maximum.

Hemodialysis effects: Moderately dialyzable (20% to 50%) via hemodialysis. Administer dose postdialysis or administer 25-50 mg supplemental dose. Elimination is not enhanced with peritoneal dialysis. Supplemental dose is not necessary.

Administration

I.V.: Administer I.V. at 1 mg/minute. **Intravenous administration requires a cardiac and blood pressure monitor.**

Stability

Compatibility: Stable in D_5W, NS

Y-site administration: Incompatible with amphotericin B cholesteryl sulfate complex

Monitoring and Teaching Issues

Physical Assessment: See Contraindications and Warnings/Precautions for use cautions. Assess potential for interactions with other prescriptions, OTC medications, or herbal products patient may be taking (see Drug Interactions). I.V. administration requires cardiac and hemodynamic monitoring and hypotensive precautions. For oral administration, assess blood pressure and heart rate prior to and following first dose and any change in dosage. Assess therapeutic effectiveness and adverse effects (eg, CHF, edema, new cough, dyspnea, unresolved fatigue - see Adverse Reactions and Overdose/Toxicology). Advise diabetic patients to monitor glucose levels closely (beta-blockers may alter glucose tolerance). Do not discontinue abruptly; taper dose gradually. Teach patient appropriate use, possible side effects/interventions (hypotension precautions), and adverse symptoms to report (see Patient Education).

Pregnancy risk factor D - determine that patient is not pregnant before beginning treatment. Instruct patients of childbearing age about appropriate barrier contraceptive measures. Note breast-feeding caution.

Patient Education: Inform prescriber of all prescriptions, OTC medications, or herbal products you are taking, and any allergies you have. Do not take anything new during treatment unless approved by prescriber. Take exactly as directed; with or without regard to meals; do not take with antacids. Do not adjust dosage or discontinue without consulting prescriber. Take pulse daily (prior to medication) and follow prescriber's instruction about

(Continued)

Atenolol *(Continued)*

holding medication. If diabetic, monitor serum sugar closely (drug may alter glucose tolerance or mask signs of hypoglycemia). May cause fatigue, dizziness, or postural hypotension (use caution when changing position from lying or sitting to standing, when driving, or climbing stairs until response to medication is known). Alteration in sexual performance (reversible); or constipation (increased dietary bulk and fluids and exercise may help). Report unresolved swelling of extremities, difficulty breathing or new cough, unresolved fatigue, unusual weight gain, unresolved constipation, or unusual muscle weakness. **Pregnancy/breast-feeding precautions:** Do not get pregnant or cause a pregnancy (males) while using this medication. Consult prescriber for appropriate contraceptive measures. Consult prescriber if breast-feeding.

Dietary Issues: May be taken without regard to meals.

Geriatric Considerations: Due to alterations in the beta-adrenergic autonomic nervous system, beta-adrenergic blockade may result in less hemodynamic response than seen in younger adults.

Breast-feeding Issues: Symptoms of beta-blockade including cyanosis, hypothermia, and bradycardia have been reported in nursing infants.

Related Information

Beta-Blockers *on page 1561*

Atenolol and Chlorthalidone (a TEN oh lole & klor THAL i done)

U.S. Brand Names Tenoretic®

Synonyms Chlorthalidone and Atenolol

Generic Available Yes

Pharmacologic Category Antihypertensive Agent Combination

Pregnancy Risk Factor D

Lactation Excretion in breast milk unknown

Use Treatment of hypertension with a cardioselective beta-blocker and a diuretic

Formulations Tablet:

50: Atenolol 50 mg and chlorthalidone 25 mg

100: Atenolol 100 mg and chlorthalidone 25 mg

Dosing

Adults & Elderly: Hypertension: Oral: Initial: 1 (50) tablet once daily, then individualize dose until optimal dose is achieved

Renal Impairment:

Cl_{cr} 15-35 mL/minute: Administer 50 mg/day.

Cl_{cr} <15 mL/minute: Administer 50 mg every other day.

Monitoring and Teaching Issues

Physical Assessment: See individual components listed in Related Information. **Pregnancy risk factor D** - determine that patient is not pregnant before beginning treatment. Instruct patients of childbearing age about appropriate barrier contraceptive measures. Note breast-feeding caution.

Patient Education: See individual components listed in Related Information. **Pregnancy/breast-feeding precautions:** Inform prescriber if you are or intend to become pregnant. Consult prescriber if breast-feeding.

Related Information

Atenolol *on page 126*

Chlorthalidone *on page 279*

ATG *see* Lymphocyte Immune Globulin *on page 829*

Atgam® *see* Lymphocyte Immune Globulin *on page 829*

Ativan® *see* Lorazepam *on page 821*

Atolone® *see* Triamcinolone *on page 1356*

Atorvastatin (a TORE va sta tin)

U.S. Brand Names Lipitor®

Generic Available No

Pharmacologic Category Antilipemic Agent, HMG-CoA Reductase Inhibitor

Pregnancy Risk Factor X

Lactation Enters breast milk/contraindicated

Use Adjunct to diet for the reduction of elevated total and LDL-cholesterol, apolipoprotein B, and triglyceride levels in patients with hypercholesterolemia (types IIa, IIb, and IIc); adjunctive therapy to diet for treatment of elevated serum triglyceride levels (type IV); treatment of primary dysbetalipoproteinemia (type III) in patients who do not respond adequately to diet; to increase HDL-cholesterol in patients with primary hypercholesterolemia (heterozygous familial and nonfamilial) and mixed dyslipidemia (Fredrickson types IIa and IIb). Also may be used in hypercholesterolemic patients without clinically evident heart disease to reduce the risk of myocardial infarction, to reduce the risk for revascularization, and reduce the risk of death due to cardiovascular causes

Mechanism of Action/Effect Inhibitor of 3-hydroxy-3-methylglutaryl coenzyme A (HMG-CoA) reductase, the rate limiting enzyme in cholesterol synthesis (reduces the production of mevalonic acid from HMG-CoA); this then results in a compensatory increase in the expression of LDL receptors on hepatocyte membranes and a stimulation of LDL catabolism

Contraindications Hypersensitivity to atorvastatin or any component of the formulation; active liver disease; unexplained persistent elevations of serum transaminases; pregnancy; breast-feeding

Warnings/Precautions Liver function must be monitored by periodic laboratory assessment. Rhabdomyolysis with acute renal failure has occurred. Risk is dose-related and is increased with concurrent use of lipid-lowering agents which may cause rhabdomyolysis (gemfibrozil, fibric acid derivatives, or niacin at doses ≥1 g/day) or during concurrent use with potent CYP3A4 inhibitors (including amiodarone, clarithromycin, cyclosporine, erythromycin, itraconazole, ketoconazole, nefazodone, grapefruit juice in large quantities, verapamil, or protease inhibitors such as indinavir, nelfinavir, or ritonavir). Weigh the risk versus benefit when combining any of these drugs with atorvastatin. Discontinue in any patient experiencing an acute or serious condition predisposing to renal failure secondary to rhabdomyolysis.

Drug Interactions

Cytochrome P450 Effect: Substrate of **CYP3A4**; Inhibits CYP3A4

Decreased Effect: Colestipol, antacids decreased plasma concentrations but effect on LDL-cholesterol was not altered. Cholestyramine may decrease absorption of atorvastatin when administered concurrently.

Increased Effect/Toxicity: Inhibitors of CYP3A4 (amiodarone, amprenavir, clarithromycin, cyclosporine, diltiazem, fluvoxamine, erythromycin, fluconazole, indinavir, itraconazole, ketoconazole, miconazole, nefazodone, nelfinavir, ritonavir, troleandomycin, and verapamil) may increase atorvastatin blood levels and may increase the risk of atorvastatin-induced myopathy and rhabdomyolysis. The risk of myopathy and rhabdomyolysis due to concurrent use of a CYP3A4 inhibitor with atorvastatin is probably less than lovastatin or simvastatin. Cyclosporine, clofibrate, fenofibrate, gemfibrozil, and niacin also may increase the risk of myopathy and rhabdomyolysis. The effect/toxicity of levothyroxine may be increased by atorvastatin. Levels of digoxin and ethinyl estradiol may be increased by atorvastatin.

Nutritional/Ethanol Interactions

Food: Atorvastatin serum concentrations may be increased by grapefruit juice; avoid concurrent intake of large quantities (>1 quart/day).

Herb/Nutraceutical: St John's wort may decrease atorvastatin levels.

Adverse Reactions

>10%: Central nervous system: Headache (3% to 17%)

2% to 10%:

Cardiovascular: Chest pain, peripheral edema

Central nervous system: Weakness (0% to 4%), insomnia, dizziness

Dermatologic: Rash (1% to 4%)

Gastrointestinal: Abdominal pain (0% to 4%), constipation (0% to 3%), diarrhea (0% to 4%), dyspepsia (1% to 3%), flatulence (1% to 3%), nausea

Genitourinary: Urinary tract infection

Neuromuscular & skeletal: Arthralgia (0% to 5%), myalgia (0% to 6%), back pain (0% to 4%), arthritis

Respiratory: Sinusitis (0% to 6%), pharyngitis (0% to 3%), bronchitis, rhinitis

Miscellaneous: Infection (2% to 10%), flu-like syndrome (0% to 3%), allergic reaction (0% to 3%)

<2% (Limited to important or life-threatening): Alopecia, anaphylaxis, angina, angioneurotic edema, arrhythmia, bullous rashes, cholestatic jaundice, deafness, dyspnea, erythema multiforme, esophagitis, facial paralysis, glaucoma gout, hepatitis, hyperkinesias, impotence, migraine, myasthenia, myopathy, myositis, nephritis, pancreatitis, paresthesia, peripheral neuropathy, petechiae, photosensitivity, postural hypotension, pruritus, rectal hemorrhage, rhabdomyolysis, somnolence, Stevens-Johnson syndrome, syncope, tendinous contracture, thrombocytopenia, tinnitus, torticollis, toxic epidermal necrolysis, urticaria, vaginal hemorrhage, vomiting

Overdosage/Toxicology Few symptoms are anticipated. Treatment is supportive.

Pharmacodynamics/Kinetics

Absorption: Rapid

Half-Life Elimination: Parent drug: 14 hours

Time to Peak: Serum: 1-2 hours

Metabolism: To active ortho- and parahydroxylated derivates and an inactive beta-oxidation product; undergoes enterohepatic recirculation

Onset: Initial changes: 3-5 days; Maximal reduction in plasma cholesterol and triglycerides: 2 weeks

Formulations Tablet: 10 mg, 20 mg, 40 mg, 80 mg

Dosing

Adults & Elderly: Dyslipidemia, cardiovascular risk reduction, prevention of MI: Oral: Initial: 10-20 mg once daily; patients requiring >45% reduction in LDL-C may be started at 40 mg once daily; titrate initial dose to achieve goal (maximum dose: 80 mg once daily)

Renal Impairment: No adjustment is necessary.

Hepatic Impairment: Decrease dosage with severe disease (eg, chronic alcoholic liver disease).

Administration

Oral: May take with food if desired; may take without regard to time of day.

Monitoring Laboratory Tests Monitor lipid levels after 2-4 weeks; LFTs prior to initiation and 12 weeks after initiation or first dose or dose elevation, and periodically (semiannually) thereafter; CPK

Monitoring and Teaching Issues

Physical Assessment: See Contraindications and Warnings/Precautions for use cautions. Assess potential for interactions with other prescriptions, OTC medications, or herbal products patient may be taking (see Drug Interactions). Schedule laboratory tests and assess results prior to beginning therapy and at regular periods as recommended above (see Monitoring Laboratory Tests). Assess for therapeutic response and adverse effects (see Adverse Reactions). Teach patient appropriate use, possible side effects and appropriate interventions, and adverse symptoms to report (see Patient Education). **Pregnancy risk factor X** - determine that patient is not pregnant before starting therapy. Do not give to childbearing age females unless capable of complying with effective contraceptive use. Breast-feeding is contraindicated.

Patient Education: Inform prescriber of all prescriptions, OTC medications, or herbal products you are taking, and any allergies you have. Do not take anything new during treatment unless approved by prescriber. May take without regard to food. Maintain adequate hydration (2-3 L/day of fluids) unless advised by prescriber to restrict fluids. You will need laboratory evaluation during therapy. May cause headache (consult prescriber for approved analgesic); diarrhea (buttermilk, boiled milk, or yogurt may help); or euphoria,

(Continued)

Atorvastatin *(Continued)*

giddiness, or confusion (use caution when driving or engaging in tasks that require alertness until response to medication is known). Report unresolved diarrhea, unusual muscle cramping or weakness, changes in mood or memory, yellowing of skin or eyes, easy bruising or bleeding, or unusual fatigue. **Pregnancy/breast-feeding precautions:** Inform prescriber if you are pregnant. Do not get pregnant during therapy. Consult prescriber for instructions on appropriate contraceptive measures. This drug can cause severe fetal defects. Do not donate blood while taking this medication and for same period of time after discontinuing. Do not breast-feed.

Dietary Issues: May take with food if desired; may take without regard to time of day. Before initiation of therapy, patients should be placed on a standard cholesterol-lowering diet for 3-6 months and the diet should be continued during drug therapy.

Geriatric Considerations: A greater degree of LDL lowering may occur (at any dose) in elderly patients as compared to younger adults. The definition of and, therefore, when to treat hyperlipidemia in the elderly is a controversial issue. The National Cholesterol Education Program recommends that all adults 20 years of age and older maintain a plasma cholesterol <200 mg/dL. By this definition, 60% of all elderly would be considered to have a borderline high (200-239 mg/dL) or high (≥240 mg/dL) plasma cholesterol. However, plasma cholesterol has been shown to be a less reliable predictor of coronary heart disease in the elderly. Therefore, it is the authors' belief that pharmacologic treatment be reserved for those who are unable to obtain a desirable plasma cholesterol level by diet alone and for whom the benefits of treatment are believed to outweigh the potential adverse effects, drug interactions, and cost of treatment.

Related Information

Hyperlipidemia Management *on page 1682*
Lipid-Lowering Agents *on page 1582*

Atovaquone (a TOE va kwone)

U.S. Brand Names Mepron®

Generic Available No

Pharmacologic Category Antiprotozoal

Pregnancy Risk Factor C

Lactation Excretion in breast milk unknown/use caution

Use Acute oral treatment of mild to moderate *Pneumocystis carinii* pneumonia (PCP) in patients who are intolerant to co-trimoxazole; prophylaxis of PCP in patients intolerant to co-trimoxazole; treatment/suppression of *Toxoplasma gondii* encephalitis, primary prophylaxis of HIV-infected persons at high risk for developing *Toxoplasma gondii* encephalitis

Mechanism of Action/Effect Has not been fully elucidated; may inhibit electron transport in mitochondria inhibiting metabolic enzymes

Contraindications Life-threatening allergic reaction to the drug or formulation

Warnings/Precautions Has only been used in mild to moderate PCP. Use with caution in elderly patients due to potentially impaired renal, hepatic, and cardiac function. Pregnancy risk C.

Drug Interactions

Decreased Effect: Rifamycins (rifampin) used concurrently decrease the steady-state plasma concentrations of atovaquone.

Increased Effect/Toxicity: Possible increased toxicity with other highly protein-bound drugs.

Nutritional/Ethanol Interactions Food: Ingestion with a fatty meal increases absorption.

Adverse Reactions

>10%:

Central nervous system: Headache, fever, insomnia, anxiety
Dermatologic: Rash
Gastrointestinal: Nausea, diarrhea, vomiting
Respiratory: Cough

1% to 10%:

Central nervous system: Dizziness
Dermatologic: Pruritus
Endocrine & metabolic: Hypoglycemia, hyponatremia
Gastrointestinal: Abdominal pain, constipation, anorexia, heartburn
Hematologic: Anemia, neutropenia, leukopenia
Hepatic: Elevated amylase and liver enzymes
Neuromuscular & skeletal: Weakness
Renal: Elevated BUN/creatinine
Respiratory: Cough
Miscellaneous: Oral *Monilia*

Pharmacodynamics/Kinetics

Absorption: Significantly increased with a high-fat meal

Bioavailability: Tablet: 23%; Suspension: 47%

Half-Life Elimination: 2-3 days

Metabolism: Undergoes enterohepatic recirculation

Formulations Suspension, oral: 750 mg/5 mL (5 mL, 210 mL) [citrus flavor]

Dosing

Adults & Elderly:

Prevention of PCP: Oral: 1500 mg once daily with food
Treatment of mild to moderate PCP: Oral: 750 mg twice daily with food for 21 days

Pediatrics: Adolescents 13-16 years: Refer to adult dosing.

Stability

Storage: Do not freeze.

Monitoring and Teaching Issues

Physical Assessment: Monitor for CNS and respiratory changes, patient knowledge of adverse reactions (see Adverse Reactions). Assess for interactions with other prescription or OTC medications (see Drug Interactions). **Pregnancy risk factor C** - benefits of use should outweigh possible risks. Note breast-feeding caution.

Patient Education: Take as directed. Take with high-fat meals. You may experience dizziness or lightheadedness; use caution when driving or engaging in tasks that require alertness until response to drug is known. Small meals may help reduce nausea. Report unresolved diarrhea, fever, mouth sores (use good mouth care), unresolved headache, or vomiting. **Pregnancy/breast-feeding precautions:** Inform prescriber if you are or intend to become pregnant. Consult prescriber if breast-feeding.

Atovaquone and Proguanil (a TOE va kwone & pro GWA nil)

U.S. Brand Names Malarone™

Synonyms Proguanil and Atovaquone

Generic Available No

Pharmacologic Category Antimalarial Agent

Pregnancy Risk Factor C

Lactation

Atovaquone: Excretion in breast milk unknown

Proguanil: Enters breast milk (small amounts)/use caution

Use Prevention or treatment of acute, uncomplicated *P. falciparum* malaria

Mechanism of Action/Effect

Atovaquone: Selectively inhibits parasite mitochondrial electron transport.

Proguanil: The metabolite cycloguanil inhibits dihydrofolate reductase, disrupting deoxythymidylate synthesis. Together, atovaquone/cycloguanil affect the erythrocytic and exoerythrocytic stages of development.

Contraindications Hypersensitivity to atovaquone, proguanil, or any component of the formulation; prophylactic use in severe renal impairment

Warnings/Precautions Not indicated for severe or complicated malaria. Absorption of atovaquone may be decreased in patients who have diarrhea or vomiting; monitor closely and consider use of an antiemetic. If severe, consider use of an alternative antimalarial. Do not use with other medications containing proguanil. Administer with caution to patients with pre-existing renal disease. Not for use in patients <11 kg. Delayed cases of *P. falciparum* malaria may occur after stopping prophylaxis; travelers returning from endemic areas who develop febrile illnesses should be evaluated for malaria. Recrudescent infections or infections following prophylaxis with this agent should be treated with alternative agent(s). Pregnancy risk C.

Drug Interactions

Cytochrome P450 Effect: Proguanil: Substrate of 1A2, 2C19, 3A4

Decreased Effect: Metoclopramide decreases bioavailability of atovaquone. Rifabutin decreases atovaquone levels by 34%. Rifampin decreases atovaquone levels by 50%. Tetracycline decreases plasma concentrations of atovaquone by 40%.

Nutritional/Ethanol Interactions Food: Atovaquone taken with dietary fat increases the rate and extent of absorption.

Adverse Reactions The following adverse reactions were reported in ≥5% of adults taking atovaquone/proguanil in treatment doses.

>10%: Gastrointestinal: Abdominal pain (17%), nausea (12%), vomiting (12% adults, 10% to 13% children)

1% to 10%:

- Central nervous system: Headache (10%), dizziness (5%)
- Dermatologic: Pruritus (6% children)
- Gastrointestinal: Diarrhea (8%), anorexia (5%)
- Neuromuscular & skeletal: Weakness (8%)

Adverse reactions reported in placebo-controlled clinical trials when used for prophylaxis. In general, reactions were similar to (or lower than) those seen with placebo:

>10%:

- Central nervous system: Headache (22% adults, 19% children)
- Gastrointestinal: Abdominal pain (33% children)
- Neuromuscular & skeletal: Myalgia (12% adults)

1% to 10%:

- Central nervous system: Fever (5% adults, 6% children)
- Gastrointestinal: Abdominal pain (9% adults), diarrhea (6% adults, 2% children), dyspepsia (3% adults), gastritis (3% adults), vomiting (1% adults, 7% children)
- Neuromuscular & skeletal: Back pain (8% adults)
- Respiratory: Upper respiratory tract infection (8% adults), cough (6% adults, 9% children)
- Miscellaneous: Flu-like syndrome (2% adults, 9% children)

In addition, 54% of adults in the placebo-controlled trials reported any adverse event (65% for placebo) and 60% of children reported adverse events (62% for placebo).

Case report: Anaphylaxis

Overdosage/Toxicology

Atovaquone: Overdoses of up to 31,500 mg have been reported. Rash has been reported as well as methemoglobinemia in one patient also taking dapsone. There is no known antidote and it is unknown if it is dialyzable.

Proguanil: Single doses of 1500 mg and 700 mg twice daily for two weeks have been reported without toxicity. Reversible hair loss, scaling of skin, reversible aphthous ulceration, and hematologic side effects have occurred. Epigastric discomfort and vomiting would also be expected. There have been no reported overdoses with the atovaquone/proguanil combination.

Pharmacokinetic Note See Atovaquone monograph.

Pharmacodynamics/Kinetics

Absorption: Proguanil: Extensive

Half-Life Elimination: Proguanil: 12-21 hours

Metabolism: Proguanil: Hepatic to active metabolites, cycloguanil (via CYP2C19) and 4-chlorophenylbiguanide

(Continued)

Atovaquone and Proguanil *(Continued)*

Formulations

Tablet: Atovaquone 250 mg and proguanil hydrochloride 100 mg

Tablet, pediatric: Atovaquone 62.5 mg and proguanil hydrochloride 25 mg

Dosing

Adults: Doses given in mg of atovaquone and proguanil:

Prevention of malaria: Oral: Atovaquone/proguanil 250 mg/100 mg once daily; start 1-2 days prior to entering a malaria-endemic area, continue throughout the stay and for 7 days after returning.

Treatment of acute malaria: Oral: Atovaquone/proguanil 1 g/400 mg as a single dose, once daily for 3 consecutive days

Elderly: Refer to adult dosing. Use with caution due to possible decrease in renal and hepatic function, as well as possible decreases in cardiac function, concomitant diseases, or other drug therapy.

Pediatrics: Doses given in mg of atovaquone and proguanil (dosage based on body weight):

Prevention of malaria: Oral: Children: Start 1-2 days prior to entering a malaria-endemic area, continue throughout the stay and for 7 days after returning. Take as a single dose, once daily.

11-20 kg: Atovaquone/proguanil 62.5 mg/25 mg
21-30 kg: Atovaquone/proguanil 125 mg/50 mg
31-40 kg: Atovaquone/proguanil 187.5 mg/75 mg
>40 kg: Atovaquone/proguanil 250 mg/100 mg

Treatment of acute malaria: Oral: Children: Take as a single dose, once daily for 3 consecutive days.

11-20 kg: Atovaquone/proguanil 250 mg/100 mg
21-30 kg: Atovaquone/proguanil 500 mg/200 mg
31-40 kg: Atovaquone/proguanil 750 mg/300 mg
>40 kg: Atovaquone/proguanil 1 g/400 mg

Renal Impairment: Should not be used as prophylaxis in severe renal impairment (Cl_{cr} <30 mL/minute). No dosage adjustment required in mild to moderate renal impairment.

Hepatic Impairment: No dosage adjustment required in mild to moderate hepatic impairment. No data available for use in severe hepatic impairment.

Administration

Oral: Give with food or a milky drink. If patient vomits within 1 hour of administration, repeat the dose.

Stability

Storage: Store tablets at 25°C (77°F).

Monitoring and Teaching Issues

Physical Assessment: See Contraindications and Warnings/Precautions for safe use. Assess other medications patient may be taking for effectiveness and interactions (see Drug Interactions). Assess therapeutic effectiveness (according to purpose for use), adverse reactions (see Adverse Reactions) to report, and interventions (see Patient Education). **Pregnancy risk factor C** - benefits of use should outweigh possible risks. Note breast-feeding caution.

Patient Education: Complete full course of therapy; do not discontinue or alter dosage without consulting prescriber. Take at the same time each day with full glass of milk or food. If vomiting occurs within 1 hour of taking dose, you may repeat the dose. If GI upset or headache is persistent, contact prescriber. Follow recommended precautions to avoid malaria exposure (use insect repellent, bednets, protective clothing). Notify prescriber if you develop fever after returning from or while visiting a malaria-endemic area. **Pregnancy/breast-feeding precautions:** Inform prescriber if you are or intend to become pregnant. Consult prescriber if breast-feeding.

Dietary Issues: Must be taken with food or a milky drink.

Pregnancy Issues: Because falciparum malaria can cause maternal death and fetal loss, pregnant women traveling to malaria-endemic areas must use personal protection against mosquito bites.

Related Information

Atovaquone *on page 130*

Atracurium (a tra KYOO ree um)

U.S. Brand Names Tracrium®

Synonyms Atracurium Besylate

Generic Available Yes

Pharmacologic Category Neuromuscular Blocker Agent, Nondepolarizing

Pregnancy Risk Factor C

Lactation Excretion in breast milk unknown/use caution

Use Adjunct to general anesthesia to facilitate endotracheal intubation and to relax skeletal muscles during surgery; to facilitate mechanical ventilation in ICU patients; does not relieve pain or produce sedation

Mechanism of Action/Effect Blocks neural transmission at the myoneural junction by binding with cholinergic receptor sites

Contraindications Hypersensitivity to atracurium besylate or any component of the formulation

Warnings/Precautions Reduce initial dosage and inject slowly (over 1-2 minutes) in patients in whom substantial histamine release would be potentially hazardous (eg, patients with clinically important cardiovascular disease); maintenance of an adequate airway and respiratory support is critical; certain clinical conditions may result in potentiation or antagonism of neuromuscular blockade:

Potentiation: Electrolyte abnormalities, severe hyponatremia, severe hypocalcemia, severe hypokalemia, hypermagnesemia, neuromuscular diseases, acidosis, acute intermittent porphyria, renal failure, hepatic failure

Antagonism: Alkalosis, hypercalcemia, demyelinating lesions, peripheral neuropathies, diabetes mellitus

Increased sensitivity in patients with myasthenia gravis, Eaton-Lambert syndrome; resistance in burn patients (>30% of body) for period of 5-70 days postinjury; resistance in patients with muscle trauma, denervation, immobilization, infection, chronic treatment with atracurium. Bradycardia may be more common with atracurium than with other neuromuscular blocking agents since it has no clinically significant effects on heart rate to counteract the bradycardia produced by anesthetics.

Pregnancy risk C.

Drug Interactions

Decreased Effect: Effect of nondepolarizing neuromuscular blockers may be reduced by carbamazepine (chronic use), corticosteroids (also associated with myopathy - see increased effect), phenytoin (chronic use), sympathomimetics, and theophylline.

Increased Effect/Toxicity: Increased effects are possible with aminoglycosides, beta-blockers, clindamycin, calcium channel blockers, halogenated anesthetics, imipenem, ketamine, lidocaine, loop diuretics (furosemide), macrolides (case reports), magnesium sulfate, procainamide, quinidine, quinolones, tetracyclines, and vancomycin. May increase risk of myopathy when used with high- dose corticosteroids for extended periods.

Adverse Reactions

Mild, rare, and generally suggestive of histamine release

1% to 10%: Cardiovascular: Bradycardia, flushing, hypotension, tachycardia

<1%: Bronchial secretions, erythema, itching, urticaria, wheezing

In the ICU setting, reports of prolonged paralysis and generalized myopathy following discontinuation of agent (may be minimized by appropriately monitoring degree of blockade)

Causes of prolonged neuromuscular blockade:

- Excessive drug administration
- Cumulative drug effect, decreased metabolism/excretion (hepatic and/or renal impairment)
- Accumulation of active metabolites
- Electrolyte imbalance (hypokalemia, hypocalcemia, hypermagnesemia, hypernatremia)
- Hypothermia

Overdosage/Toxicology

Symptoms of overdose include respiratory depression and cardiovascular collapse.

Neostigmine 1-3 mg slow I.V. push in adults (0.5 mg in children) antagonizes the neuromuscular blockade, and should be administered with or immediately after atropine 1-1.5 mg I.V. push (adults). This may be especially useful in the presence of bradycardia.

Pharmacodynamics/Kinetics

Half-Life Elimination: Biphasic: Adults: Initial (distribution): 2 minutes; Terminal: 20 minutes

Metabolism: Undergoes ester hydrolysis and Hofmann elimination (nonbiologic process independent of renal, hepatic, or enzymatic function); metabolites have no neuromuscular blocking properties; laudanosine, a product of Hofmann elimination, is a CNS stimulant and can accumulate with prolonged use in ICU patients (no documented evidence of CNS excitation in patients with prolonged administration)

Onset: Dose dependent: 2-3 minutes

Duration: Recovery begins in 20-35 minutes following initial dose of 0.4-0.5 mg/kg under balanced anesthesia; recovery to 95% of control takes 60-70 minutes

Formulations

Injection, as besylate: 10 mg/mL (5 mL, 10 mL)

Injection, as besylate [preservative free]: 10 mg/mL (5 mL)

Dosing

Adults & Elderly: For I.V. administration only (not to be used I.M.): Dose to effect; doses will vary due to interpatient variability; use ideal body weight for obese patients.

Adjunct to surgical anesthesia (neuromuscular blockade):

- I.V. (bolus): 0.4-0.5 mg/kg, then 0.08-0.1 mg/kg 20-45 minutes after initial dose to maintain neuromuscular block, followed by repeat doses of 0.08-0.1 mg/kg at 15- to 25-minute intervals
  - Initial dose after succinylcholine for intubation (balanced anesthesia): Adults: 0.2-0.4 mg/kg
  - Pretreatment/priming: I.V.: 10% of intubating dose given 3-5 minutes before initial dose
- I.V. continuous infusion: Initial: 9-10 mcg/kg/minute at initial signs of recovery from bolus dose; block is usually maintained by a rate of 5-9 mcg/kg/minute under balanced anesthesia.

ICU neuromuscular blockade: I.V.: Initial (bolus) 0.4-0.5 mg/kg, followed by I.V. continuous infusion at an initial rate of 5-10 mcg/kg/min; block is usually maintained by rate of 11-13 mcg/kg/minute (rates for pediatric patients may be higher).

Pediatrics: Adjunct to surgical anesthesia: I.V. (not to be used I.M.): Dose to effect; doses will vary due to interpatient variability; use ideal body weight for obese patients

Children 1 month to 2 years: Initial: 0.3-0.5 mg/kg followed by 0.25 mg/kg maintenance doses as needed to maintain neuromuscular blockade

Children >2 years: Refer to adult dosing.

Renal Impairment: No adjustment is necessary.

Hepatic Impairment: No adjustment is necessary.

Administration

I.M.: Not for I.M. injection due to tissue irritation.

I.V.: May be given undiluted as a bolus injection. Administration via infusion requires the use of an infusion pump. Use infusion solutions within 24 hours of preparation.

Stability

Storage: Refrigerate; unstable in alkaline solutions.

Compatibility: Stable in D_5W, NS, D_5NS; **incompatible** with LR

Y-site administration: Incompatible with diazepam, propofol, thiopental

(Continued)

Atracurium *(Continued)*

Compatibility when admixed: Incompatible with aminophylline, cefazolin, heparin, quinidine gluconate, ranitidine, sodium nitroprusside

Monitoring Laboratory Tests Renal function (serum creatinine, BUN) and liver function when in ICU

Monitoring and Teaching Issues

Physical Assessment: Only clinicians experienced in the use of neuromuscular blocking drugs should administer and/or manage the use of atracurium. Dosage and rate of administration should be individualized and titrated to the desired effect, according to relevant clinical factors, premedication, concomitant medications, age, and general condition of the patient. See Use, Contraindications, and Warnings/Precautions for appropriate use cautions. Ventilatory support must be instituted and maintained until adequate respiratory muscle function and/or airway protection are assured. Assess other medications for effectiveness and safety. Other drugs that affect neuromuscular activity may increase/decrease neuromuscular block induced by atracurium. This drug does not cause anesthesia or analgesia; pain must be treated with appropriate analgesic agents. Continuous monitoring of vital signs, cardiac status, respiratory status, and degree of neuromuscular block (objective assessment with peripheral external nerve stimulator) is mandatory during infusion and until full muscle tone has returned (see Adverse Reactions). Muscle tone returns in a predictable pattern, starting with diaphragm, abdomen, chest, limbs, and finally muscles of the neck, face, and eyes. Safety precautions must be maintained until full muscle tone has returned. **Note:** It may take longer for return of muscle tone in obese or elderly patients or patients with renal or hepatic disease, myasthenia gravis, myopathy, other neuromuscular disease, dehydration, electrolyte imbalance, or severe acid/base imbalance. Provide appropriate patient teaching/support prior to and following administration.

Long-term use: Monitor fluid levels (intake and output) during and following infusion. Reposition patient and provide appropriate skin care, mouth care, and care of patient's eyes every 2-3 hours while sedated. Provide appropriate emotional and sensory support (auditory and environmental).

Pregnancy risk factor C. Note breast-feeding caution.

Patient Education: Patient will usually be unconscious prior to administration. Patient education should be appropriate to individual situation. Reassurance of constant monitoring and emotional support to reduce fear and anxiety should precede and follow administration. Following return of muscle tone, do not attempt to change position or rise from bed without assistance. Report immediately any skin rash or hives, pounding heartbeat, difficulty breathing, or muscle tremors. **Pregnancy/breast-feeding precautions:** Inform prescriber if you are pregnant. Consult prescriber if breast-feeding.

Additional Information Atracurium is classified as an intermediate-duration neuromuscular-blocking agent. It does not appear to have a cumulative effect on the duration of blockade. It does not relieve pain or produce sedation.

Atracurium Besylate *see* Atracurium *on page 132*

Atromid-S® *see* Clofibrate *on page 310*

Atropine (A troe peen)

U.S. Brand Names Atropine-Care®; Atropisol®; Isopto® Atropine; Sal-Tropine™

Synonyms Atropine Sulfate

Generic Available Yes

Pharmacologic Category Anticholinergic Agent; Anticholinergic Agent, Ophthalmic; Antidote; Antispasmodic Agent, Gastrointestinal; Ophthalmic Agent, Mydriatic

Pregnancy Risk Factor C

Lactation Enters breast milk (trace amounts)/use caution (AAP rates "compatible")

Use Preoperative medication to inhibit salivation and secretions; treatment of symptomatic sinus bradycardia; antidote for organophosphate pesticide poisoning; to produce mydriasis and cycloplegia for examination of the retina and optic disc and accurate measurement of refractive errors; uveitis; AV block (nodal level); ventricular asystole; treatment of GI disorders (eg, peptic ulcer disease, irritable bowel syndrome, hypermotility of colon)

Mechanism of Action/Effect Blocks the action of acetylcholine at parasympathetic sites in smooth muscle, secretory glands and the CNS; increases cardiac output, dries secretions, antagonizes histamine and serotonin

Contraindications Hypersensitivity to atropine or any component of the formulation; narrow-angle glaucoma; adhesions between the iris and lens; tachycardia; unstable cardiovascular status in acute hemorrhage; obstructive GI disease; paralytic ileus; intestinal atony of the elderly or debilitated patient; severe ulcerative colitis; toxic megacolon complicating ulcerative colitis; hepatic disease; obstructive uropathy; renal disease; myasthenia gravis; asthma; thyrotoxicosis; Mobitz type II block

Warnings/Precautions Heat prostration can occur in the presence of a high environmental temperature. Rule out intestinal obstruction before treating diarrhea. Psychosis can occur in sensitive individuals. The elderly may be sensitive to side effects. Use caution in patients with myocardial ischemia. Use caution in hyperthyroidism, autonomic neuropathy, BPH, CHF, tachyarrhythmias, hypertension, and hiatal hernia associated with reflux esophagitis. Use with caution in children with spastic paralysis. Pregnancy risk C.

Drug Interactions

Decreased Effect: Effect of some phenothiazines may be antagonized. Levodopa effects may be decreased (limited clinical validation). Drugs with cholinergic mechanisms (metoclopramide, cisapride, bethanechol) decrease anticholinergic effects of atropine.

Increased Effect/Toxicity: Amantadine, antihistamines, phenothiazines, and TCAs may increase anticholinergic effects of atropine when used concurrently. Sympathomimetic amines may cause tachyarrhythmias; avoid concurrent use.

Adverse Reactions

>10%:

Dermatologic: Dry, hot skin

Gastrointestinal: Impaired GI motility, constipation, dry throat, dry mouth
Local: Irritation at injection site
Respiratory: Dry nose
Miscellaneous: Diaphoresis (decreased)

1% to 10%:
Dermatologic: Increased sensitivity to light
Endocrine & metabolic: Decreased flow of breast milk
Gastrointestinal: Dysphagia

<1% (Limited to important or life-threatening): Ataxia, blurred vision, bradycardia (doses <0.5 mg), confusion, delirium, drowsiness, elderly may be at increased risk for confusion and hallucinations, fatigue, headache, increased intraocular pain, loss of memory, mydriasis, orthostatic hypotension, palpitations, restlessness, tachycardia, ventricular fibrillation, ventricular tachycardia

Overdosage/Toxicology Symptoms of overdose include dilated, unreactive pupils; blurred vision; hot, dry flushed skin; dryness of mucous membranes; difficulty swallowing; foul breath; diminished or absent bowel sounds; urinary retention; tachycardia; hyperthermia; hypertension; and increased respiratory rate. For anticholinergic overdose with severe life-threatening symptoms, physostigmine 1-2 mg S.C. or I.V. slowly, may be given to reverse these effects.

Pharmacodynamics/Kinetics

Absorption: Complete

Half-Life Elimination: 2-3 hours

Metabolism: Hepatic

Onset: I.V.: Rapid

Formulations

Injection, solution, as sulfate: 0.1 mg/mL (5 mL, 10 mL); 0.4 mg/mL (1 mL, 20 mL); 0.5 mg/mL (1 mL); 1 mg/mL (1 mL)
Ointment, ophthalmic, as sulfate: 1% (3.5 g)
Solution, ophthalmic, as sulfate: 1% (5 mL, 15 mL)
Atropine-Care®: 1% (2 mL)
Atropisol®: 1% (1 mL)
Isopto® Atropine: 1% (5 mL, 15 mL)
Tablet, as sulfate (Sal-Tropine™): 0.4 mg

Dosing

Adults & Elderly: Doses <0.5 mg have been associated with paradoxical bradycardia.

Asystole: I.V.: 1 mg; may repeat every 3-5 minutes as needed; may give intratracheal in 1 mg/10 mL dilution only, intratracheal dose should be 2-2.5 times the I.V. dose.

Preanesthetic: I.M., I.V., S.C.: 0.4-0.6 mg 30-60 minutes preop and repeat every 4-6 hours as needed.

Bradycardia: I.V.: 0.5-1 mg every 5 minutes, not to exceed a total of 3 mg or 0.04 mg/kg; may give intratracheal in 1 mg/10 mL dilution only, intratracheal dose should be 2-2.5 times the I.V. dose.

Neuromuscular blockade reversal: I.V.: 25-30 mcg/kg 30 seconds before neostigmine or 10 mcg/kg 30 seconds before edrophonium

Organophosphate or carbamate poisoning: I.V.: 1-2 mg/dose every 10-20 minutes until atropine effect (dry flushed skin, tachycardia, mydriasis, fever) is observed, then every 1-4 hours for at least 24 hours; up to 50 mg in first 24 hours and 2 g over several days may be given in cases of severe intoxication.

Mydriasis, cycloplegia: Ophthalmic: Instill 1-2 drops of a 1% solution 1 hour before the procedure.

Uveitis: Ophthalmic:
Solution (1%): Instill 1-2 drops 4 times/day.
Ophthalmic ointment: Apply a small amount in the conjunctival sac up to 3 times/day. Compress the lacrimal sac by digital pressure for 1-3 minutes after instillation.

Pediatrics: Note: Doses <0.1 mg have been associated with paradoxical bradycardia.

Preanesthetic: Oral, I.M., I.V., S.C.: Neonates, Infants, and Children:
<5 kg: 0.02 mg/kg/dose 30-60 minutes preop then every 4-6 hours as needed; use of a minimum dosage of 0.1 mg in neonates <5 kg will result in dosages >0.02 mg/kg. There is no documented minimum dosage in this age group.
>5 kg: 0.01-0.02 mg/kg/dose to a maximum 0.4 mg/dose 30-60 minutes preop; minimum dose: 0.1 mg.

Bradycardia: I.V., intratracheal: Neonates, Infants, and Children:
0.02 mg/kg, minimum dose 0.1 mg, maximum single dose: 0.5 mg in children and 1 mg in adolescents; may repeat in 5-minute intervals to a maximum total dose of 1 mg in children or 2 mg in adolescents. (**Note:** For intratracheal administration, the dosage must be diluted with normal saline to a total volume of 1-2 mL). When treating bradycardia in neonates, reserve use for those patients unresponsive to improved oxygenation and epinephrine.

Mydriasis, cycloplegia (preprocedure): Ophthalmic (0.5% solution): Children: Instill 1-2 drops twice daily for 1-3 days before the procedure.

Uveitis: Ophthalmic (0.5% solution): Children: Instill 1-2 drops up to 3 times/day.

Administration

I.V.: Administer undiluted by rapid I.V. injection; slow injection may result in paradoxical bradycardia

Stability

Storage: Store injection at <40°C; avoid freezing.

Compatibility:

Y-site administration: Incompatible with thiopental

Compatibility in syringe: Incompatible with cimetidine/pentobarbital

Compatibility when admixed: Incompatible with floxacillin, metaraminol, methohexital, norepinephrine

(Continued)

Atropine *(Continued)*

Monitoring and Teaching Issues

Physical Assessment: Assess other medications patient may be taking for effectiveness and interactions (see Warnings/Precautions and Drug Interactions). **Systemic administration:** Monitor therapeutic response, safety measures, and adverse reactions. **Oral, ophthalmic:** Monitor therapeutic response according to purpose for use and adverse response (see Warnings/Precautions, Adverse Reactions, and Overdose/Toxicology). Assess knowledge/teach patient appropriate use, interventions to reduce side effects, and adverse symptoms to report (see Patient Education). **Pregnancy risk factor C** - benefits of use should outweigh possible risks. Note breast-feeding caution. (Systemic effects have been reported following ophthalmic administration.)

Patient Education: Take oral forms exactly as directed, 30 minutes before meals. Maintain adequate hydration (2-3 L/day of fluids) unless advised by prescriber to restrict fluids. Void before taking medication. You may experience dizziness, blurred vision, sensitivity to light (use caution when driving or engaging in tasks requiring alertness until response to drug is known); dry mouth, nausea, or vomiting (small, frequent meals, frequent mouth care, sucking lozenges, or chewing gum may help); orthostatic hypotension (use caution when climbing stairs and when rising from lying or sitting position); constipation (increased exercise, fluids, fruit, or fiber may help; if not effective, consult prescriber); increased sensitivity to heat and decreased perspiration (avoid extremes of heat, reduce exercise in hot weather); or decreased milk if breast-feeding. Report hot, dry, flushed skin; blurred vision or vision changes; difficulty swallowing; chest pain, palpitations, or rapid heartbeat; painful or difficult urination; increased confusion, depression, or loss of memory; rapid or difficult respirations; muscle weakness or tremors; or eye pain.

Ophthalmic: Instill as often as recommended. Wash hands before using. Sit or lie down, open eye, look at ceiling, and instill prescribed amount of solution. Do not blink for 30 seconds, close eye and roll eye in all directions, and apply gentle pressure to inner corner of eye for 1-2 minutes. Do not let tip of applicator touch eye; do not contaminate tip of applicator (may cause eye infection, eye damage, or vision loss). Temporary stinging or blurred vision may occur.

Pregnancy/breast-feeding precautions: Inform prescriber if you are or intend to become pregnant. Consult prescriber if breast-feeding.

Geriatric Considerations: Anticholinergic agents are generally not well tolerated in the elderly and their use should be avoided when possible (see Warnings/Precautions, Adverse Reactions). In the elderly, anticholinergic agents should not be used as prophylaxis against extrapyramidal symptoms.

Additional Information May give intratracheal in 1 mg/10 mL dilution only.

Related Information

Compatibility of Drugs *on page 1564*
Compatibility of Drugs in Syringe *on page 1566*
Ophthalmic Agents *on page 1509*

Atropine and Difenoxin *see* Difenoxin and Atropine *on page 408*
Atropine and Diphenoxylate *see* Diphenoxylate and Atropine *on page 424*
Atropine-Care® *see page 1509*
Atropine-Care® *see* Atropine *on page 134*
Atropine, Hyoscyamine, Scopolamine, and Phenobarbital *see* Hyoscyamine, Atropine, Scopolamine, and Phenobarbital *on page 687*
Atropine Sulfate *see* Atropine *on page 134*
Atropisol® *see page 1509*
Atropisol® *see* Atropine *on page 134*
Atrovent® *see* Ipratropium *on page 733*
A/T/S® *see* Erythromycin (Systemic) *on page 486*
Attenuvax® *see page 1498*
Augmentin® *see* Amoxicillin and Clavulanate Potassium *on page 89*
Augmentin ES-600™ *see* Amoxicillin and Clavulanate Potassium *on page 89*
Augmentin XR™ *see* Amoxicillin and Clavulanate Potassium *on page 89*
Auralgan® *see page 1522*
Auralgan Otic® *see page 1519*
Auro® Ear Drops *see page 1519*
Auroto® *see page 1522*
Auroto Otic® *see page 1519*
Autoplex® T *see* Anti-inhibitor Coagulant Complex *on page 113*
Avage™ *see* Tazarotene *on page 1276*
Avalide® *see* Irbesartan and Hydrochlorothiazide *on page 736*
Avandia® *see* Rosiglitazone *on page 1208*
Avapro® *see* Irbesartan *on page 735*
Avapro® HCT *see* Irbesartan and Hydrochlorothiazide *on page 736*
AVC™ *see* Sulfanilamide *on page 1261*
Avelox® *see* Moxifloxacin *on page 929*
Aventyl® HCl *see* Nortriptyline *on page 986*
Aviane™ *see* Ethinyl Estradiol and Levonorgestrel *on page 523*
Avinza™ *see* Morphine Sulfate *on page 926*
Avita® *see* Tretinoin (Topical) *on page 1355*
Avitene® *see page 1461*
Avonex® *see* Interferon Beta-1a *on page 727*
Axert™ *see* Almotriptan *on page 62*
Axid® *see* Nizatidine *on page 981*
Axid® AR [OTC] *see* Nizatidine *on page 981*

Aygestin® *see* Norethindrone *on page 984*
Azactam® *see* Aztreonam *on page 141*

Azatadine (a ZA ta deen)

U.S. Brand Names Optimine®

Synonyms Azatadine Maleate

Generic Available No

Pharmacologic Category Antihistamine

Pregnancy Risk Factor B

Lactation Excretion in breast milk unknown/not recommended

Use Treatment of perennial and seasonal allergic rhinitis and chronic urticaria

Mechanism of Action/Effect Azatadine has both anticholinergic and antiserotonin activity; has been demonstrated to inhibit mediator release from human mast cells *in vitro*; mechanism of this action is suggested to prevent calcium entry into the mast cell through voltage-dependent calcium channels

Contraindications Hypersensitivity to azatadine, any component of the formulation, or to other related antihistamines including cyproheptadine; patients taking MAO inhibitors should not use azatadine

Warnings/Precautions Use with caution in patients with narrow-angle glaucoma, stenosing peptic ulcer, urinary bladder obstruction, prostatic hyperplasia, asthmatic attacks. Sedation and somnolence are the most commonly reported adverse effects.

Drug Interactions

Cytochrome P450 Effect: Induces CYP3A4

Increased Effect/Toxicity: Potential for increased side effects when used with procarbazine, CNS depressants, tricyclic antidepressants, and alcohol.

Nutritional/Ethanol Interactions Ethanol: Avoid ethanol (may increase CNS depression).

Adverse Reactions

>10%:

Central nervous system: Slight to moderate drowsiness

Respiratory: Thickening of bronchial secretions

1% to 10%:

Central nervous system: Headache, fatigue, nervousness, dizziness

Gastrointestinal: Appetite increase, weight gain, nausea, diarrhea, abdominal pain, dry mouth

Neuromuscular & skeletal: Arthralgia

Respiratory: Pharyngitis

<1% (Limited to important or life-threatening): Hepatitis, bronchospasm, epistaxis

Overdosage/Toxicology Symptoms of overdose include CNS depression or stimulation, dry mouth, flushed skin, fixed and dilated pupils, apnea. There is no specific treatment for antihistamine overdose; however, anticholinesterase inhibitors may be useful.

Pharmacodynamics/Kinetics

Absorption: Rapid and extensive

Half-Life Elimination: ~8.7 hours

Time to Peak: 4 hours

Metabolism: Hepatic

Onset: 1-2 hours

Formulations Tablet, as maleate: 1 mg

Dosing

Adults: Rhinitis, urticaria: Oral: 1-2 mg twice daily

Elderly: 1 mg once or twice daily

Pediatrics: Children >12 years: Refer to adult dosing.

Monitoring and Teaching Issues

Physical Assessment: Assess effectiveness and interactions of other medications patient may be taking (see Drug Interactions). See Contraindications and Warnings/Precautions for use cautions. Monitor effectiveness of therapy and adverse reactions (see Adverse Reactions) at beginning of therapy and periodically with long-term use. Assess knowledge/teach patient appropriate use, interventions to reduce side effects, and adverse symptoms to report (see Patient Education). Breast-feeding is not recommended.

Patient Education: Take as directed; do not exceed recommended dose. Avoid use of other depressants, alcohol, or sleep-inducing medications unless approved by prescriber. You may experience drowsiness or dizziness (use caution when driving or engaging in tasks requiring alertness until response to drug is known); or dry mouth, abdominal pain, or nausea (small, frequent meals, frequent mouth care, chewing gum, or sucking hard candy may help). Report persistent sore throat, difficulty breathing, or expectorating (thick secretions); excessive sedation or mental stimulation; frequent nosebleeds; unusual joint or muscle pain; or lack of improvement or worsening or condition. **Breast-feeding precaution:** Breast-feeding is not recommended.

Geriatric Considerations: Reduce dose in the elderly. Antihistamines are more likely to cause dizziness, excessive sedation, syncope, toxic confusion states, and hypotension in the elderly. See Additional Information and Warnings/Precautions.

Azatadine and Pseudoephedrine (a ZA ta deen & soo doe e FED rin)

U.S. Brand Names Rynatan® Tablet; Trinalin®

Synonyms Pseudoephedrine and Azatadine

Generic Available No

Pharmacologic Category Antihistamine/Decongestant Combination

Pregnancy Risk Factor C

Lactation Excretion in breast milk unknown/not recommended

Use Perennial and seasonal allergic rhinitis and other allergic symptoms including urticaria

Formulations Tablet: Azatadine maleate 1 mg and pseudoephedrine sulfate 120 mg

(Continued)

Azatadine and Pseudoephedrine *(Continued)*

Dosing

Adults: Rhinitis, nasal congestion: Oral: 1 tablet twice daily

Elderly: Refer to dosing in individual monographs.

Monitoring and Teaching Issues

Physical Assessment: See individual components listed in Related Information. **Pregnancy risk factor C** - benefits of use should outweigh possible risks. Breast-feeding is not recommended.

Patient Education: See individual components listed in Related Information. **Pregnancy/breast-feeding precautions:** Inform prescriber if you are or intend to become pregnant. Breast-feeding is not recommended.

Related Information

Azatadine *on page 137*
Pseudoephedrine *on page 1150*

Azatadine Maleate *see* Azatadine *on page 137*

Azathioprine (ay za THYE oh preen)

U.S. Brand Names Imuran®

Synonyms Azathioprine Sodium

Generic Available Yes

Pharmacologic Category Immunosuppressant Agent

Pregnancy Risk Factor D

Lactation Excretion in breast milk unknown/not recommended

Use Adjunct with other agents in prevention of rejection of kidney transplants; also used in severe active rheumatoid arthritis unresponsive to other agents; other autoimmune diseases (ITP, SLE, MS, Crohn's disease)

Use - Unlabeled/Investigational Adjunct in prevention of rejection of solid organ (nonrenal) transplants

Mechanism of Action/Effect Antagonizes purine metabolism and may inhibit synthesis of DNA, RNA, and proteins; may also interfere with cellular metabolism and inhibit mitosis

Contraindications Hypersensitivity to azathioprine or any component of the formulation; pregnancy

Warnings/Precautions Chronic immunosuppression increases the risk of neoplasia. Has mutagenic potential to both men and women and with possible hematologic toxicities. Use with caution in patients with liver disease, renal impairment. Monitor hematologic function closely.

Drug Interactions

Decreased Effect: Azathioprine may result in decreased action of warfarin.

Increased Effect/Toxicity: Allopurinol may increase serum levels of azathioprine's active metabolite (6-MP). Decrease azathioprine dose to $^1/_3$ to $^1/_4$ of normal dose. Azathioprine and ACE inhibitors may induce severe leukopenia. Aminosalicylates (olsalazine, mesalamine, sulfasalazine) may inhibit TPMT, increasing toxicity/myelosuppression of azathioprine.

Nutritional/Ethanol Interactions Herb/Nutraceutical: Avoid cat's claw, echinacea (have immunostimulant properties).

Adverse Reactions Frequency not defined.

Central nervous system: Fever, chills

Dermatologic: Alopecia, erythematous or maculopapular rash

Gastrointestinal: Nausea, vomiting, anorexia, diarrhea, aphthous stomatitis, pancreatitis

Hematologic: Leukopenia, thrombocytopenia, anemia, pancytopenia (bone marrow suppression may be determined, in part, by genetic factors, ie, patients with TPMT deficiency are at higher risk)

Hepatic: Hepatotoxicity, jaundice, hepatic veno-occlusive disease

Neuromuscular & skeletal: Arthralgias

Ocular: Retinopathy

Miscellaneous: Rare hypersensitivity reactions which include myalgias, rigors, dyspnea, hypotension, serum sickness, rash; secondary infections may occur secondary to immunosuppression

Overdosage/Toxicology Symptoms of overdose include nausea, vomiting, diarrhea, and hematologic toxicity. Following initiation of essential overdose management, symptomatic and supportive treatment should be instituted. Dialysis has been reported to remove significant amounts of the drug and its metabolites, and should be considered as a treatment option in those patients who deteriorate despite established forms of therapy.

Pharmacodynamics/Kinetics

Half-Life Elimination: Parent drug: 12 minutes; 6-mercaptopurine: 0.7-3 hours; End-stage renal disease: Slightly prolonged

Metabolism: Extensively hepatic via xanthine oxidase to 6-mercaptopurine (active)

Formulations

Injection, powder for reconstitution, as sodium: 100 mg

Tablet, scored: 50 mg

Dosing

Adults & Elderly: I.V. dose is equivalent to oral dose.

Renal transplantation: Oral, I.V.: 2-5 mg/kg/day to start, then 1-3 mg/kg/day maintenance

Rheumatoid arthritis: Oral: 1 mg/kg/day for 6-8 weeks; increase by 0.5 mg/kg every 4 weeks until response or up to 2.5 mg/kg/day

Pediatrics: Children: Refer to adult dosing.

Renal Impairment:

Cl_{cr} 10-50 mL/minute: Administer 75% of normal dose.

Cl_{cr} <10 mL/minute: Administer 50% of normal dose.

Hemodialysis: Slightly dialyzable (5% to 20%) Administer dose posthemodialysis.

CAPD effects: Unknown; CAVH effects: Unknown

Administration

I.V.: Can be administered IVP over 5 minutes at a concentration not to exceed 10 mg/mL **or** azathioprine can be further diluted with normal saline or D_5W and administered by intermittent infusion over 15-60 minutes.

Stability

Storage: Stability of parenteral admixture at room temperature (25°C) is 24 hours. Stability of parenteral admixture at refrigeration temperature (4°C) is 16 days.

Compatibility: Stable in neutral or acid solutions, but is hydrolyzed to mercaptopurine in alkaline solutions. Stable in D_5W, ½NS, NS.

Monitoring Laboratory Tests CBC, platelet counts, total bilirubin, alkaline phosphatase

Monitoring and Teaching Issues

Physical Assessment: Assess effectiveness and interactions of other medications patient may be taking (see Drug Interactions). Monitor laboratory tests (see above), therapeutic response (according to purpose for use), and adverse reactions at beginning of therapy and periodically throughout therapy, especially opportunistic infection (see Warnings/Precautions, Adverse Reactions, and Overdose/Toxicology). Assess knowledge/teach patient appropriate use, interventions to reduce side effects, and adverse symptoms to report (see Patient Education). **Pregnancy risk factor D** - determine that patient is not pregnant before beginning treatment. Instruct patients of childbearing age about appropriate contraceptive measures. Breast-feeding is not recommended.

Patient Education: Take as prescribed (may take in divided doses or with food if GI upset occurs). You will be susceptible to infection (avoid crowds and exposure to infection and do not have any vaccinations unless approved by prescriber). You may experience nausea, vomiting, loss of appetite (small, frequent meals, frequent mouth care, chewing gum, or sucking lozenges may help). Report abdominal pain and unresolved GI upset (eg, persistent vomiting or diarrhea); unusual fever or chills; bleeding or bruising; sore throat, unhealed sores, or signs of infection; yellowing of skin or eyes; or change in color of urine or stool.

Rheumatoid arthritis: Response may not occur for up to 3 months; do not discontinue without consulting prescriber.

Organ transplant: Azathioprine will usually be prescribed with other antirejection medications.

Pregnancy/breast-feeding precautions: Do not get pregnant while taking this medication; use appropriate contraceptive measures. Breast-feeding is not recommended.

Dietary Issues: May be taken with food.

Geriatric Considerations: Immunosuppressive toxicity is increased in the elderly. Signs or symptoms of infection may differ in the elderly. Lethargy or confusion may be the first signs of infection.

Azathioprine Sodium *see* Azathioprine *on page 138*

Azidothymidine *see* Zidovudine *on page 1419*

Azidothymidine, Abacavir, and Lamivudine *see* Abacavir, Lamivudine, and Zidovudine *on page 31*

Azithromycin (az ith roe MYE sin)

U.S. Brand Names Zithromax®

Synonyms Azithromycin Dihydrate; Zithromax® TRI-PAK™; Zithromax® Z-PAK®

Generic Available No

Pharmacologic Category Antibiotic, Macrolide

Pregnancy Risk Factor B

Lactation Enters breast milk/use caution

Use

Children: Treatment of acute otitis media due to *H. influenzae, M. catarrhalis*, or *S. pneumoniae*; pharyngitis/tonsillitis due to *S. pyogenes*; community-acquired pneumonia due to *C. pneumoniae, H. influenzae, M. pneumoniae*, or *S. pneumoniae*

Adults:

Treatment of mild to moderate upper and lower respiratory tract infections, infections of the skin and skin structure, community-acquired pneumonia, pelvic inflammatory disease (PID), sexually-transmitted diseases (urethritis/cervicitis), pharyngitis/tonsillitis (alternative to first-line therapy), and genital ulcer disease (chancroid) due to susceptible strains of *C. trachomatis, M. catarrhalis, H. influenzae, S. aureus, S. pneumoniae, Mycoplasma pneumoniae*, and *C. psittaci*

Prevention of (or to delay onset of) infection with *Mycobacterium avium* complex (MAC)

Prevention or (or to delay onset of) or treatment of MAC in patients with advanced HIV infection

Prophylaxis of bacterial endocarditis in patients who are allergic to penicillin and undergoing surgical or dental procedures

Acute bacterial exacerbations of chronic obstructive pulmonary disease (COPD) due to *H. influenzae, M. catarrhalis*, or *S. pneumoniae*

Mechanism of Action/Effect Inhibits RNA-dependent protein synthesis at the chain elongation step; binds to the 50S ribosomal subunit resulting in blockage of transpeptidation

Contraindications Hypersensitivity to azithromycin, other macrolide antibiotics, or any component of the formulation

Warnings/Precautions Use with caution in patients with hepatic dysfunction; hepatic impairment with or without jaundice has occurred chiefly in older children and adults; it may be accompanied by malaise, nausea, vomiting, abdominal colic, and fever; discontinue use if these occur; may mask or delay symptoms of incubating gonorrhea or syphilis, so appropriate culture and susceptibility tests should be performed prior to initiating azithromycin; pseudomembranous colitis has been reported with use of macrolide antibiotics; use caution with renal dysfunction; safety and efficacy have not been established in children <6 months of age with acute otitis media or community-acquired pneumonia, or in children <2 years of age with pharyngitis/tonsillitis.

(Continued)

Azithromycin *(Continued)*

Drug Interactions

Cytochrome P450 Effect: Substrate of CYP3A4; Inhibits CYP3A4

Decreased Effect: Decreased azithromycin peak serum concentrations with aluminum- and magnesium-containing antacids (by 24%), however, total absorption is unaffected.

Increased Effect/Toxicity: Concurrent use of pimozide is contraindicated due to potential cardiotoxicity. The manufacturer warns that azithromycin potentially may increase levels of tacrolimus, phenytoin, ergot alkaloids, alfentanil, astemizole, bromocriptine, carbamazepine, cyclosporine, digoxin, disopyramide, and triazolam. However, azithromycin did not affect the response/levels of carbamazepine, terfenadine, theophylline, or warfarin in specific interaction studies; caution is advised when administered together.

Nutritional/Ethanol Interactions Food: Rate and extent of GI absorption may be altered depending upon the formulation. Azithromycin suspension, not tablet form, has significantly increased absorption (46%) with food.

Adverse Reactions

1% to 10%: Gastrointestinal: Diarrhea, nausea, abdominal pain, cramping, vomiting (especially with high single-dose regimens)

<1% (Limited to important or life-threatening): Acute renal failure, allergic reaction, aggressive behavior, anaphylaxis, angioedema, arrhythmias (including ventricular tachycardia), cholestatic jaundice, deafness, enteritis, erythema multiforme (rare), headache (especially with high-dose), hearing loss, hepatic necrosis (rare), hepatitis, hypertrophic pyloric stenosis, hypotension, interstitial nephritis, leukopenia, pancreatitis, paresthesia, pruritus, pseudomembranous colitis, seizures, somnolence, Stevens-Johnson syndrome (rare), syncope, taste abnormality, thrombocytopenia, tinnitus, tongue discoloration (rare), torsade de pointes (case report), urticaria, vertigo

Overdosage/Toxicology Symptoms of overdose include nausea, vomiting, diarrhea, and prostration. Treatment is supportive and symptomatic.

Pharmacodynamics/Kinetics

Absorption: Rapid

Bioavailability: 37%; variable effect with food (increased with oral suspension, unchanged with tablet)

Half-Life Elimination: Terminal: 68 hours

Time to Peak: Serum: 2.3-4 hours

Metabolism: Hepatic

Formulations

Injection, powder for reconstitution, as dihydrate: 500 mg

Powder for oral suspension, as dihydrate: 100 mg/5 mL (15 mL); 200 mg/5 mL (15 mL, 22.5 mL, 30 mL); 1 g [single-dose packet]

Tablet, as dihydrate: 250 mg, 500 mg, 600 mg

Zithromax® TRI-PAK™ [unit-dose pack]: 500 mg (3s)

Zithromax® Z-PAK® [unit-dose pack]: 250 mg (6s)

Dosing

Adults & Elderly:

Mild to moderate respiratory tract, skin, and soft tissue infections: Oral: 500 mg in a single loading dose on day 1 followed by 250 mg/day as a single dose on days 2-5

Alternative regimen for bacterial exacerbation of COPD: 500 mg/day for a total of 3 days

Community-acquired pneumonia: I.V.: 500 mg as a single dose for at least 2 days, follow I.V. therapy by the oral route with a single daily dose of 500 mg to complete a 7- to 10-day course of therapy.

Urethritis/cervicitis:

Due to *C. trachomatis*: Oral: 1 g as a single dose

Due to *N. gonorrhoeae*: Oral: 2 g as a single dose

Chancroid due to *H. ducreyi*: Oral: 1 g as a single dose

Pelvic inflammatory disease (PID): I.V.: 500 mg as a single dose for 1-2 days, follow I.V. therapy by the oral route with a single daily dose of 250 mg to complete a 7-day course of therapy.

Prophylaxis of disseminated *M. avium* complex disease in patient with advanced HIV infection: Oral: 1200 mg once weekly (may be combined with rifabutin)

Prophylaxis for bacterial endocarditis: Oral: 500 mg 1 hour prior to the procedure

Treatment of disseminated *M. avium* complex disease in patient with advanced HIV infection: Oral: 600 mg daily in combination with ethambutol 15 mg/kg

Pediatrics:

Note: Adolescents ≥16 years: Refer to adult dosing.

Community-acquired pneumonia: Oral: Children ≥6 months: 10 mg/kg on day 1 (maximum: 500 mg/day) followed by 5 mg/kg/day once daily on days 2-5 (maximum: 250 mg/day)

Otitis media: Oral: Children ≥6 months:

1-day regimen: 30 mg/kg as a single dose

3-day regimen: 10 mg/kg once daily for 3 days

5-day regimen: 10 mg/kg on day 1 (maximum: 500 mg/day) followed by 5 mg/kg/day once daily on days 2-5 (maximum: 250 mg/day)

Pharyngitis, tonsillitis: Oral: Children ≥2 years: 12 mg/kg/day once daily for 5 days (maximum: 500 mg/day)

M. avium-infected patients with acquired immunodeficiency syndrome: Children (not currently FDA approved for use): 10-20 mg/kg/day once daily (maximum: 40 mg/kg/day) has been used in clinical trials; prophylaxis for first episode of MAC: 5-12 mg/kg/day once daily (maximum: 500 mg/day)

Prophylaxis for bacterial endocarditis: Children: 15 mg/kg 1 hour before procedure

Renal Impairment: Use caution in patients with Cl_{cr} <10 mL/minute

Administration

Oral: Suspension and tablet may be taken without regard to food.

I.V.: Administer over at least 60 minutes. Other medications should not be infused simultaneously through the same I.V. line.

Stability

Storage:

Injection: Store intact vials of injection at room temperature. Reconstituted solution is stable for 24 hours when stored below 30°C/86°F.

Suspension: Store dry powder below 30°C (86°F); following reconstitution, store suspension at 5°C to 30°C (41°F to 86°F).

Tablets: Store between 15°C to 30°C (59°F to 86°F).

Reconstitution: Injection: Prepare initiation solution by adding 4.8 mL of sterile water for injection to the 500 mg vial (resulting concentration: 100 mg/mL). Use of a standard syringe is recommended due to the vacuum in the vial (which may draw additional solution through an automated syringe).

The initial solution should be further diluted to a concentration of 1 mg/mL (500 mL) to 2 mg/mL (250 mL) in 0.9% sodium chloride, 5% dextrose in water, or lactated Ringer's. The diluted solution is stable for 24 hours at or below room temperature (30°C or 86°F) and for 7 days if stored under refrigeration (5°C or 41°F).

Compatibility: Other medications should not be infused simultaneously through the same I.V. line.

Monitoring Laboratory Tests Liver function, CBC with differential. Perform culture and sensitivity testing prior to initiating therapy.

Monitoring and Teaching Issues

Physical Assessment: Assess allergy history prior to beginning therapy. See Contraindications, Warnings/Precautions, and Dosing for use cautions. Assess potential for interactions with other prescriptions, OTC medications, or herbal products patient may be taking (see Drug Interactions). Assess results of laboratory tests (see above), therapeutic effectiveness, and adverse effects (see Adverse Reactions and Overdose/Toxicology). Instruct patients being treated for STDs about preventing transmission. Teach patient appropriate use, possible side effects and interventions, and adverse symptoms to report (see Patient Education). Note breast-feeding caution.

Patient Education: Inform prescriber of all prescriptions, OTC medications, or herbal products you are taking, and any allergies you have. Do not take anything new during treatment unless approved by prescriber. Take as directed. Take all of prescribed medication and do not discontinue until prescription is completed. Suspension may be taken with or without food. Tablet may be taken with meals to decrease GI effects. Maintain adequate hydration (2-3 L/day of fluids) unless advised by prescriber to restrict fluids. If taken to treat sexually-transmitted disease, follow advice of prescriber related to sexual intercourse and preventing transmission. May cause transient abdominal distress, diarrhea, and headache. Report signs of additional infections (eg, sores in mouth or vagina, vaginal discharge, unresolved fever, severe vomiting, or diarrhea). **Breast-feeding precaution:** Consult prescriber if breast-feeding.

Dietary Issues: Oral suspension may be administered with or without food. Tablet may be administered with food to decrease GI effects.

Geriatric Considerations: Dosage adjustment does not appear to be necessary in the elderly. Considered one of the drugs of choice in the treatment of outpatient treatment of community-acquired pneumonia in older adults.

Breast-feeding Issues: Based on one case report, azithromycin has been shown to accumulate in breast milk.

Additional Information Capsules are no longer being produced in the United States.

Azithromycin Dihydrate *see* Azithromycin *on page 139*

Azmacort® *see* Triamcinolone *on page 1356*

Azo-Dine® [OTC] *see* Phenazopyridine *on page 1065*

Azo-Gesic® [OTC] *see* Phenazopyridine *on page 1065*

Azopt™ *see* Ophthalmic Agents, Glaucoma *on page 1002*

Azo-Standard® *see* Phenazopyridine *on page 1065*

AZT *see* Zidovudine *on page 1419*

AZT + 3TC *see* Zidovudine and Lamivudine *on page 1421*

AZT, Abacavir, and Lamivudine *see* Abacavir, Lamivudine, and Zidovudine *on page 31*

Azthreonam *see* Aztreonam *on page 141*

Aztreonam (AZ tree oh nam)

U.S. Brand Names Azactam®

Synonyms Azthreonam

Generic Available No

Pharmacologic Category Antibiotic, Miscellaneous

Pregnancy Risk Factor B

Lactation Enters breast milk/use caution (AAP rates "compatible")

Use Treatment of patients with urinary tract infections, lower respiratory tract infections, septicemia, skin/skin structure infections, intra-abdominal infections, and gynecological infections caused by susceptible gram-negative bacilli; often useful in patients with allergies to penicillins or cephalosporins

Mechanism of Action/Effect Monobactam which is active only against gram-negative bacilli; inhibits bacterial cell wall synthesis during active multiplication, causing cell wall destruction

Contraindications Hypersensitivity to aztreonam or any component of the formulation

Warnings/Precautions Rare cross-allergenicity to penicillins and cephalosporins (rare). Requires dosage reduction in renal impairment.

Drug Interactions

Decreased Effect: Avoid antibiotics that induce beta-lactamase production (cefoxitin, imipenem).

Effects on Lab Values Urine glucose (Clinitest®)

(Continued)

Aztreonam *(Continued)*

Adverse Reactions

1% to 10%:

Dermatologic: Rash

Gastrointestinal: Diarrhea, nausea, vomiting

Local: Thrombophlebitis, pain at injection site

<1% (Limited to important or life-threatening): Anaphylaxis, bronchospasm, *C. difficile*-associated diarrhea, erythema multiforme, exfoliative dermatitis, hepatitis, hypotension, jaundice, leukocytosis, neutropenia, pancytopenia, pruritus, pseudomembranous colitis, purpura, seizures, thrombocytopenia, toxic epidermal necrolysis, urticaria, vaginal candidiasis, vertigo

Overdosage/Toxicology Symptoms of overdose include seizures. Treatment is supportive. If necessary, dialysis can reduce the drug concentration in the blood.

Pharmacodynamics/Kinetics

Absorption: I.M.: Well absorbed; I.M. and I.V. doses produce comparable serum concentrations

Half-Life Elimination:

Neonates: <7 days, ≤2.5 kg: 5.5-9.9 hours; <7 days, >2.5 kg: 2.6 hours; 1 week to 1 month: 2.4 hours

Children 2 months to 12 years: 1.7 hours

Adults: Normal renal function: 1.7-2.9 hours

End-stage renal disease: 6-8 hours

Time to Peak: I.M., I.V. push: Within 60 minutes; I.V. infusion: 1.5 hours

Metabolism: Hepatic (minor %)

Formulations

Injection, powder for reconstitution: 500 mg, 1 g, 2 g

Infusion [premixed]: 1 g (50 mL); 2 g (50 mL)

Dosing

Adults & Elderly:

Urinary tract infection: I.M., I.V.: 500 mg to 1 g every 8-12 hours

Moderately severe systemic infections:

I.M.: 1 g every 8-12 hours

I.V.: 1-2 g I.V. every 8-12 hours

Severe systemic or life-threatening infections (especially caused by *Pseudomonas aeruginosa*): I.V.: 2 g every 6-8 hours; maximum: 8 g/day

Pediatrics:

Susceptible infections: I.M., I.V.: Children >1 month: 90-120 mg/kg/day divided every 6-8 hours

Cystic fibrosis: I.V.: 50 mg/kg/dose every 6-8 hours (ie, up to 200 mg/kg/day); maximum: 6-8 g/day

Renal Impairment:

Cl_{cr} 30-50 mL/minute: Administer every 12 hours.

Cl_{cr} 10-30 mL/minute: Administer every 24 hours.

Cl_{cr} <10 mL/minute: Administer every 48 hours.

Hemodialysis effects: Moderately dialyzable (20% to 50%); administer dose postdialysis or supplemental dose of 500 mg after dialysis.

Peritoneal dialysis: Administer as for Cl_{cr} <10 mL/minute.

Continuous arteriovenous or venovenous hemofiltration: Dose as for Cl_{cr} 10-50 mL/minute.

Administration

I.M.: Inject deep into large muscle mass.

I.V.: I.V. route is preferred for doses ≥1 g or in patients with severe life-threatening infections. Administer by IVP over 3-5 minutes or by intermittent infusion over 20-60 minutes at a final concentration not to exceed 20 mg/mL.

Stability

Reconstitution: Reconstituted solutions are colorless to light yellow straw and may turn pink upon standing without affecting potency. Use reconstituted solutions and I.V. solutions (in NS and D_5W) within 48 hours if kept at room temperature (25°C) or 7 days if kept in refrigerator (4°C).

Compatibility: Stable in D_5LR, D_5¼NS, D_5½NS, D_5NS, D_5W, $D_{10}W$, mannitol 5%, mannitol 10%, LR, NS

Y-site administration: Incompatible with acyclovir, alatrofloxacin, amphotericin B, amphotericin B cholesteryl sulfate complex, amsacrine, chlorpromazine, daunorubicin, ganciclovir, lorazepam, metronidazole, mitomycin, mitoxantrone, prochlorperazine edisylate, streptozocin

Compatibility when admixed: Incompatible with metronidazole, nafcillin

Monitoring Laboratory Tests Obtain specimens for culture and sensitivity before the first dose.

Monitoring and Teaching Issues

Physical Assessment: Assess allergy history before initiating therapy. See Contraindications, Warnings/Precautions, and Dosing for use cautions. See Administration, Reconstitution, and Compatibility above. Assess therapeutic effectiveness and adverse response (see Adverse Reactions and Overdose/Toxicology). Caution diabetic patients about altered response to Clinitest®. Teach patient possible side effects and adverse symptoms to report (see Patient Education). Note breast-feeding caution.

Patient Education: Inform prescriber of all prescriptions, OTC medications, or herbal products you are taking, and any allergies you have. Do not take anything new during treatment unless approved by prescriber. This medication can only be administered by injection or infusion. Report any burning, pain, swelling, or redness at infusion/injection site. May cause nausea or GI distress (frequent mouth care, small, frequent meals, sucking lozenges, or chewing gum may help relieve these symptoms). Report any persistent and unrelieved diarrhea or vomiting, pain at injection site, unresolved fever, unhealed or new sores in mouth or vagina, vaginal discharge, or acute onset of difficulty breathing. **Breast-feeding precaution:** Consult prescriber if breast-feeding.

Geriatric Considerations: Adjust dose relative to renal function.

Additional Information Although marketed as an agent similar to aminoglycosides, aztreonam is a monobactam antimicrobial with almost pure gram-negative aerobic activity. It cannot be used for gram-positive infections. Aminoglycosides are often used for synergy in gram-positive infections.

Azulfidine® *see* Sulfasalazine *on page 1262*

Azulfidine® EN-tabs® *see* Sulfasalazine *on page 1262*

Babee® Teething® [OTC] *see* Benzocaine *on page 156*

Bacid® [OTC] *see Lactobacillus on page 766*

Baciguent® [OTC] *see* Bacitracin *on page 143*

Baci-IM® *see* Bacitracin *on page 143*

Bacitracin (bas i TRAY sin)

U.S. Brand Names AK-Tracin®; Baciguent® [OTC]; Baci-IM®

Generic Available Yes

Pharmacologic Category Antibiotic, Ophthalmic; Antibiotic, Topical; Antibiotic, Miscellaneous

Pregnancy Risk Factor C

Lactation Excretion in breast milk unknown/use caution

Use Treatment of susceptible bacterial infections mainly; has activity against gram-positive bacilli; due to toxicity risks, systemic and irrigant uses of bacitracin should be limited to situations where less toxic alternatives would not be effective; oral administration has been successful in antibiotic-associated colitis and has been used for enteric eradication of vancomycin-resistant enterococci (VRE)

Mechanism of Action/Effect Inhibits bacterial cell wall synthesis by preventing transfer of mucopeptides into the growing cell wall

Contraindications Hypersensitivity to bacitracin or any component of the formulation; I.M. use is contraindicated in patients with renal impairment

Warnings/Precautions Prolonged use may result in overgrowth of nonsusceptible organisms. I.M. use may cause renal failure due to tubular and glomerular necrosis. **Do not administer intravenously** because severe thrombophlebitis occurs. Pregnancy risk C.

Drug Interactions

Increased Effect/Toxicity: Nephrotoxic drugs, neuromuscular blocking agents, and anesthetics (increased neuromuscular blockade).

Adverse Reactions 1% to 10%:

Cardiovascular: Hypotension, edema of the face/lips, tightness of chest
Central nervous system: Pain
Dermatologic: Rash, itching
Gastrointestinal: Anorexia, nausea, vomiting, diarrhea, rectal itching
Hematologic: Blood dyscrasias
Miscellaneous: Diaphoresis

Overdosage/Toxicology Symptoms of overdose include nephrotoxicity (parenteral), nausea, and vomiting (oral). Treatment is symptomatic and supportive.

Pharmacodynamics/Kinetics

Absorption: Poor from mucous membranes and intact or denuded skin; rapidly following I.M. administration; not absorbed by bladder irrigation, but absorption can occur from peritoneal or mediastinal lavage

Time to Peak: Serum: I.M.: 1-2 hours

Duration: 6-8 hours

Formulations

Injection, powder for reconstitution (Baci-IM®): 50,000 units
Ointment, ophthalmic (AK-Tracin®): 500 units/g (3.5 g)
Ointment, topical: 500 units/g (0.9 g, 15 g, 30 g, 120 g, 454 g)
Baciguent®: 500 units/g (15 g, 30 g)

Dosing

Adults & Elderly: Do not administer I.V.:

Antibiotic-associated colitis: Oral: 25,000 units 4 times/day for 7-10 days

Superficial dermal infection: Topical: Apply 1-5 times/day.

Ophthalmic infection: Ophthalmic (ointment): Instill 1/4" to 1/2" ribbon every 3-4 hours into conjunctival sac for acute infections, or 2-3 times/day for mild to moderate infections for 7-10 days.

Local irrigation: Solution: 50-100 units/mL in normal saline, lactated Ringer's, or sterile water for irrigation; soak sponges in solution for topical compresses 1-5 times/day or as needed during surgical procedures.

Pediatrics: Do not administer I.V.

Infants: I.M.:
≤2.5 kg: 900 units/kg/day in 2-3 divided doses
>2.5 kg: 1000 units/kg/day in 2-3 divided doses
Children: I.M.: 800-1200 units/kg/day divided every 8 hours

Administration

Oral: The injection formulation is extemporaneously prepared and flavored to improve palatability.

I.M.: For I.M. administration only. pH of urine should be kept >6 by using sodium bicarbonate. Bacitracin sterile powder should be dissolved in 0.9% sodium chloride injection containing 2% procaine hydrochloride. Do not use diluents containing parabens.

I.V.: Not for I.V. administration.

Stability

Reconstitution: For I.M. use only. Bacitracin sterile powder should be dissolved in 0.9% sodium chloride injection containing 2% procaine hydrochloride. Once reconstituted, bacitracin is stable for 1 week under refrigeration (2°C to 8°C). Sterile powder should be stored in the refrigerator. Do not use diluents containing parabens.

Monitoring Laboratory Tests I.M.: Urinalysis, renal function

(Continued)

Bacitracin *(Continued)*

Monitoring and Teaching Issues

Physical Assessment: Do not administer I.V. Assess effectiveness and interactions of other medications patient may be taking (see Drug Interactions). **Oral, I.M.:** Monitor laboratory results, effectiveness of therapy, and adverse reactions (see Adverse Reactions). **Ophthalmic/topical:** Instruct patient on appropriate application and use, possible adverse reactions, and symptoms to report (see Patient Education). **Pregnancy risk factor C.** Note breast-feeding caution.

Patient Education: Oral/I.M.: Maintain adequate hydration (2-3 L/day of fluids) unless advised by prescriber to restrict fluids. Report rash, redness, or itching; change in urinary pattern; acute dizziness; swelling of face or lips; chest pain or tightness; acute nausea or vomiting; or loss of appetite (small, frequent meals or frequent mouth care may help).

Ophthalmic: Instill as many times per day as directed. Wash hands before using. Gently pull lower eyelid forward, instill prescribed amount of ointment into lower eyelid. Close eye and roll eyeball in all directions. May cause blurred vision; use caution when driving or engaging in tasks that require clear vision. Report any adverse reactions such as rash or itching, swelling of face or lips, burning or pain in eye, worsening of condition, or if condition does not improve.

Topical: Apply a thin film as many times as day as prescribed to the affected area. May cover with porous sterile bandage (avoid occlusive dressings). Do not use longer than 1 week unless advised by prescriber.

Pregnancy/breast-feeding precautions: Inform prescriber if you are or intend to become pregnant. Consult prescriber if breast-feeding.

Additional Information 1 unit is equivalent to 0.026 mg

Related Information

Ophthalmic Agents *on page 1509*

Bacitracin and Polymyxin B (bas i TRAY sin & pol i MIKS in bee)

U.S. Brand Names AK-Poly-Bac®; Betadine® First Aid Antibiotics + Moisturizer [OTC]; Polysporin® Ophthalmic; Polysporin® Topical [OTC]

Synonyms Polymyxin B and Bacitracin

Generic Available Yes

Pharmacologic Category Antibiotic, Ophthalmic; Antibiotic, Topical

Pregnancy Risk Factor C

Lactation Excretion in breast milk unknown/use caution

Use Treatment of superficial infections caused by susceptible organisms

Formulations

Ointment, ophthalmic (AK-Poly-Bac®, Polysporin®): Bacitracin 500 units and polymyxin B sulfate 10,000 units per g (3.5 g)

Ointment, topical [OTC]: Bacitracin 500 units and polymyxin B sulfate 10,000 units per g in white petrolatum (15 g, 30 g)

Betadine® First Aid Antibiotics + Moisturizer: Bacitracin 500 units and polymyxin B sulfate 10,000 units per g (14 g)

Polysporin®: Bacitracin 500 units and polymyxin B sulfate 10,000 units per g (15g, 30 g)

Powder, topical (Polysporin®): Bacitracin 500 units and polymyxin B sulfate 10,000 units per g (10 g)

Dosing

Adults & Elderly:

Ophthalmic infection: Ophthalmic (ointment): Instill ½" ribbon in the affected eye(s) every 3-4 hours for acute infections or 2-3 times/day for mild to moderate infections for 7-10 days.

Superficial dermal infection: Topical ointment/powder: Apply to affected area 1-4 times/day; may cover with sterile bandage if needed.

Pediatrics: Refer to adult dosing.

Monitoring and Teaching Issues

Physical Assessment: See individual components listed in Related Information. **Pregnancy risk factor C** - benefits of use should outweigh possible risks. Note breast-feeding caution.

Patient Education: See individual components listed in Related Information. **Pregnancy/breast-feeding precautions:** Inform prescriber if you are or intend to become pregnant. Consult prescriber if breast-feeding.

Related Information

Bacitracin *on page 143*
Ophthalmic Agents *on page 1509*
Polymyxin B *on page 1100*

Bacitracin, Neomycin, and Polymyxin B

(bas i TRAY sin, nee oh MYE sin, & pol i MIKS in bee)

U.S. Brand Names Mycitracin® [OTC]; Neosporin® Ophthalmic Ointment; Neosporin® Topical [OTC]; Triple Antibiotic®

Synonyms Neomycin, Bacitracin, and Polymyxin B; Polymyxin B, Bacitracin, and Neomycin

Generic Available Yes

Pharmacologic Category Antibiotic, Ophthalmic; Antibiotic, Topical

Pregnancy Risk Factor C

Lactation Excretion in breast milk unknown/use caution

Use Helps prevent infection in minor cuts, scrapes and burns; short-term treatment of superficial external ocular infections caused by susceptible organisms

Formulations

Ointment, ophthalmic (Neosporin®): Bacitracin 400 units, neomycin sulfate 3.5 mg, and polymyxin B sulfate 10,000 units per g (3.5 g)

Ointment, topical (Triple Antibiotic®): Bacitracin 400 units, neomycin sulfate 3.5 mg, and polymyxin B sulfate 5000 units per g (0.9 g, 15 g, 30 g, 454 g)

Mycitracin®: Bacitracin 400 units, neomycin sulfate 3.5 mg, and polymyxin B sulfate 5000 units per g (14 g)

Neosporin®: Bacitracin 400 units, neomycin sulfate 3.5 mg, and polymyxin B sulfate 5000 units per g (0.9 g, 15 g, 30 g)

Dosing

Adults & Elderly:

Ophthalmic infection: Ophthalmic ointment: Instill 1/2" ribbon into the conjunctival sac every 3-4 hours for acute infections or 2-3 times/day for mild to moderate infections for 7-10 days.

Superficial dermal infection: Topical: Apply 1-4 times/day to affected areas and cover with sterile bandage if necessary.

Pediatrics: Refer to adult dosing.

Monitoring and Teaching Issues

Physical Assessment: See individual components listed in Related Information. **Pregnancy risk factor C** - benefits of use should outweigh possible risks. Note breast-feeding caution.

Patient Education: See individual components listed in Related Information. **Pregnancy/breast-feeding precautions:** Inform prescriber if you are or intend to become pregnant. Consult prescriber if breast-feeding.

Related Information

Bacitracin *on page 143*
Neomycin *on page 958*
Ophthalmic Agents *on page 1509*
Polymyxin B *on page 1100*

Bacitracin, Neomycin, Polymyxin B, and Hydrocortisone

(bas i TRAY sin, nee oh MYE sin, pol i MIKS in bee, & hye droe KOR ti sone)

U.S. Brand Names AK-Spore® H.C. [DSC]; Cortisporin® Ointment

Synonyms Hydrocortisone, Bacitracin, Neomycin, and Polymyxin B; Neomycin, Bacitracin, Polymyxin B, and Hydrocortisone; Polymyxin B, Bacitracin, Neomycin, and Hydrocortisone

Generic Available Yes

Pharmacologic Category Antibiotic, Ophthalmic; Antibiotic, Otic; Antibiotic, Topical; Corticosteroid, Ophthalmic; Corticosteroid, Otic; Corticosteroid, Topical

Pregnancy Risk Factor C

Lactation Excretion in breast milk unknown/use caution

Use Prevention and treatment of susceptible superficial topical infections

Formulations

Ointment, ophthalmic (AK-Spore® H.C. [DSC], Cortisporin®): Bacitracin 400 units, neomycin sulfate 3.5 mg, polymyxin B sulfate 10,000 units, and hydrocortisone 10 mg per g (3.5 g)

Ointment, topical (Cortisporin®): Bacitracin 400 units, neomycin sulfate 3.5 mg, polymyxin B sulfate 10,000 units, and hydrocortisone 10 mg per g (15 g)

Dosing

Adults & Elderly:

Ophthalmic infection: Ophthalmic (ointment): Instill 1/2" ribbon to inside of lower lid every 3-4 hours until improvement occurs.

Superficial dermal infection: Topical: Apply sparingly 2-4 times/day.

Pediatrics: Refer to adult dosing.

Monitoring and Teaching Issues

Physical Assessment: See individual components listed in Related Information. **Pregnancy risk factor C** - benefits of use should outweigh possible risks. Note breast-feeding caution.

Patient Education: See individual components listed in Related Information. **Pregnancy/breast-feeding precautions:** Inform prescriber if you are or intend to become pregnant. Consult prescriber if breast-feeding.

Related Information

Bacitracin *on page 143*
Hydrocortisone *on page 673*
Neomycin *on page 958*
Ophthalmic Agents *on page 1509*
Polymyxin B *on page 1100*

Baclofen (BAK loe fen)

U.S. Brand Names Lioresal®

Generic Available Yes: Tablets only

Pharmacologic Category Skeletal Muscle Relaxant

Pregnancy Risk Factor C

Lactation Enters breast milk (small amounts)/compatible

Use Treatment of reversible spasticity associated with multiple sclerosis or spinal cord lesions

Orphan drug: Intrathecal: Treatment of intractable spasticity caused by spinal cord injury, multiple sclerosis, and other spinal disease (spinal ischemia or tumor, transverse myelitis, cervical spondylosis, degenerative myelopathy)

Use - Unlabeled/Investigational Intractable hiccups, intractable pain relief, bladder spasticity, trigeminal neuralgia, cerebral palsy, Huntington's chorea

Mechanism of Action/Effect Inhibits the transmission of both monosynaptic and polysynaptic reflexes at the spinal cord level, possibly by hyperpolarization of primary afferent fiber terminals, with resultant relief of muscle spasticity

Contraindications Hypersensitivity to baclofen or any component of the formulation

Warnings/Precautions Use with caution in patients with seizure disorder or impaired renal function. Avoid abrupt withdrawal of the drug; abrupt withdrawal of intrathecal baclofen has resulted in severe sequelae (hyperpyrexia, obtundation, rebound/exaggerated spasticity, muscle rigidity, and rhabdomyolysis), leading to organ failure and some fatalities. Risk may

(Continued)

Baclofen *(Continued)*

be higher in patients with injuries at T-6 or above, history of baclofen withdrawal, or limited ability to communicate. Elderly are more sensitive to the effects of baclofen and are more likely to experience adverse CNS effects at higher doses. Pregnancy risk C.

Drug Interactions

Increased Effect/Toxicity: Baclofen may decrease the clearance of ibuprofen or other NSAIDs and increase the potential for renal toxicity. Effects may be additive with CNS depressants.

Nutritional/Ethanol Interactions

Ethanol: Avoid ethanol (may increase CNS depression).

Herb/Nutraceutical: Avoid valerian, St John's wort, kava kava, gotu kola.

Effects on Lab Values ↑ alkaline phosphatase, AST, glucose, ammonia (B); ↓ bilirubin (S)

Adverse Reactions

>10%:

Central nervous system: Drowsiness, vertigo, dizziness, psychiatric disturbances, insomnia, slurred speech, ataxia, hypotonia

Neuromuscular & skeletal: Weakness

1% to 10%:

Cardiovascular: Hypotension

Central nervous system: Fatigue, confusion, headache, insomnia

Dermatologic: Rash

Gastrointestinal: Nausea, constipation

Genitourinary: Polyuria

<1% (Limited to important or life-threatening): Chest pain, dyspnea, dysuria, enuresis, hematuria, impotence, inability to ejaculate, nocturia, palpitations, syncope, urinary retention; withdrawal reactions have occurred with abrupt discontinuation (particularly severe with intrathecal use).

Overdosage/Toxicology Symptoms of overdose include vomiting, muscle hypotonia, salivation, drowsiness, coma, seizures, and respiratory depression. Atropine has been used to improve ventilation, heart rate, blood pressure, and core body temperature. Treatment is symptom-directed and supportive.

For toxicity following intrathecal administration: For adults, administer physostigmine 2 mg I.M. or I.V. (not to exceed 1 mg/minute). For pediatric patients, administer physostigmine 0.02 mg/kg I.M. or I.V. (not to exceed 0.5 mg/minute). Consider withdrawal of 30-40 mL of CSF to reduce baclofen concentration. Abrupt withdrawal of intrathecal baclofen has resulted in severe sequelae (hyperpyrexia, obtundation, muscle rigidity, and rhabdomyolysis)

Pharmacodynamics/Kinetics

Absorption: Oral: Rapid; dose dependent

Half-Life Elimination: 3.5 hours

Time to Peak: Serum: Oral: Within 2-3 hours

Metabolism: Hepatic (15% of dose)

Onset: 3-4 days; Peak effect: 5-10 days

Formulations

Injection, solution, intrathecal [preservative free]: 50 mcg/mL (1 mL); 500 mcg/mL (20 mL); 2000 mcg/mL (5 mL)

Tablet: 10 mg, 20 mg

Dosing

Adults:

Spasticity:

Oral: 5 mg 3 times/day, may increase 5 mg/dose every 3 days to a maximum of 80 mg/day

Intrathecal:

Test dose: 50-100 mcg, doses >50 mcg should be given in 25 mcg increments, separated by 24 hours. A screening dose of 25 mcg may be considered in very small patients. Patients not responding to screening dose of 100 mcg should not be considered for chronic infusion/implanted pump.

Maintenance: After positive response to test dose, a maintenance intrathecal infusion can be administered via an implanted intrathecal pump. Initial dose via pump: Infusion at a 24-hourly rate dosed at twice the test dose. Avoid abrupt discontinuation.

Hiccups (unlabeled use): 10-20 mg 2-3 times/day

Elderly: Oral (the lowest effective dose is recommended): Initial: 5 mg 2-3 times/day, increasing gradually as needed; if benefits are not seen withdraw the drug slowly.

Pediatrics: Spasticity:

Oral (avoid abrupt withdrawal of drug): Children:

2-7 years: Initial: 10-15 mg/24 hours divided every 8 hours; titrate dose every 3 days in increments of 5-15 mg/day to a maximum of 40 mg/day.

≥8 years: Maximum: 60 mg/day in 3 divided doses

Intrathecal: Refer to adult dosing.

Renal Impairment: May be necessary to reduce dosage; no specific guidelines have been established

Administration

Other: Intrathecal: For screening dosages, dilute with preservative-free sodium chloride to a final concentration of 50 mcg/mL for bolus injection into the subarachnoid space; for maintenance infusions, concentrations of 500-2000 mcg/mL may be used

Stability

Compatibility: Stable in sterile, preservative free NS

Monitoring and Teaching Issues

Physical Assessment: Assess effectiveness and interactions of other medications patient may be taking (see Drug Interactions). See Contraindications and Warnings/Precautions for use cautions. Monitor effectiveness of therapy and adverse reactions (see Adverse Reactions) at beginning of therapy and periodically with long-term use. Assess knowledge/

teach patient appropriate use, interventions to reduce side effects, and adverse symptoms to report (see Patient Education). **Pregnancy risk factor C** - benefits of use should outweigh possible risks.

Patient Education: Take this drug as prescribed. Do not discontinue without consulting prescriber (abrupt discontinuation may cause hallucinations). Do not take any prescription or OTC sleep-inducing drugs, sedatives, or antispasmodics without consulting prescriber. Avoid alcohol use. You may experience transient drowsiness, lethargy, or dizziness; use caution when driving or engaging in tasks requiring alertness until response to drug is known. Frequent small meals or lozenges may reduce GI upset.

Intrathecal use: Keep scheduled pump refill visits; abrupt interruption can cause serious withdrawal symptoms. Report increased spasticity, itching, numbness, unresolved insomnia, painful urination, change in urinary patterns, constipation, high fever, or persistent confusion.

Pregnancy precaution: Inform prescriber if you are or intend to become pregnant.

Geriatric Considerations: The elderly are more sensitive to the effects of baclofen and are more likely to experience adverse CNS effects at higher doses. Two cases of encephalopathy were reported after inadvertent high doses (50 mg/day and 90 mg/day) were given to elderly patients.

Bactrim™ *see* Sulfamethoxazole and Trimethoprim *on page 1259*

Bactrim™ DS *see* Sulfamethoxazole and Trimethoprim *on page 1259*

Bactroban® *see* Mupirocin *on page 931*

Bactroban® Nasal *see* Mupirocin *on page 931*

Baking Soda *see* Sodium Bicarbonate *on page 1234*

Baldex® *see* Topical Corticosteroids *on page 1334*

BAL in Oil® *see page 1461*

BAL in Oil® *see page 1460*

Bancap HC® *see* Hydrocodone and Acetaminophen *on page 667*

Band-Aid® Hurt-Free™ Antiseptic Wash [OTC] *see* Lidocaine *on page 800*

Banophen® [OTC] *see* DiphenhydrAMINE *on page 422*

Baridium® *see* Phenazopyridine *on page 1065*

Basic Pharmacological Concepts *see page 21*

Basiliximab (ba si LIKS i mab)

U.S. Brand Names Simulect®

Generic Available No

Pharmacologic Category Monoclonal Antibody

Pregnancy Risk Factor B (manufacturer)

Lactation Excretion in breast milk unknown/not recommended

Use Prophylaxis of acute organ rejection in renal transplantation

Mechanism of Action/Effect Mouse-derived monoclonal IgG antibody which blocks the alpha-chain of the interleukin-2 (IL-2) receptor complex; this receptor is expressed on activated T lymphocytes and is a critical pathway for activating cell-mediated allograft rejection

Contraindications Hypersensitivity basiliximab, murine proteins, or any component of the formulation

Warnings/Precautions To be used as a component of immunosuppressive regimen which includes cyclosporine and corticosteroids. Only physicians experienced in transplantation and immunosuppression should prescribe, and patients should receive the drug in a facility with adequate equipment and staff capable of providing the laboratory and medical support required for transplantation.

The incidence of lymphoproliferative disorders and/or opportunistic infections may be increased by immunosuppressive therapy. Severe hypersensitivity reactions, occurring within 24 hours, have been reported. Reactions, including anaphylaxis, have occurred both with the initial exposure and/or following re-exposure after several months. Use caution during re-exposure to a subsequent course of therapy in a patient who has previously received basiliximab. Discontinue the drug permanently if a reaction occurs. Medications for the treatment of hypersensitivity reactions should be available for immediate use. Treatment may result in the development of human antimurine antibodies (HAMA); however, limited evidence suggesting the use of muromonab-CD3 or other murine products is not precluded.

Drug Interactions

Decreased Effect: Basiliximab is an immunoglobulin; specific drug interactions have not been evaluated, but are not anticipated. It is not known if the immune response to vaccines will be impaired during or following basiliximab therapy.

Increased Effect/Toxicity: Basiliximab is an immunoglobulin; specific drug interactions have not been evaluated, but are not anticipated.

Adverse Reactions Administration of basiliximab did not appear to increase the incidence or severity of adverse effects in clinical trials. Adverse events were reported in 96% of both the placebo and basiliximab groups.

>10%:

Cardiovascular: Peripheral edema, hypertension, atrial fibrillation

Central nervous system: Fever, headache, insomnia, pain

Dermatologic: Wound complications, acne

Endocrine & metabolic: Hypokalemia, hyperkalemia, hyperglycemia, hyperuricemia, hypophosphatemia, hypercholesterolemia

Gastrointestinal: Constipation, nausea, diarrhea, abdominal pain, vomiting, dyspepsia

Genitourinary: Urinary tract infection

Hematologic: Anemia

Neuromuscular & skeletal: Tremor

Respiratory: Dyspnea, infection (upper respiratory)

Miscellaneous: Viral infection

(Continued)

Basiliximab *(Continued)*

3% to 10% (Limited to important or life-threatening):

Cardiovascular: Chest pain, cardiac failure, hypotension, arrhythmia, tachycardia, edema, angina pectoris

Central nervous system: Hypoesthesia, neuropathy, agitation, anxiety, depression

Dermatologic: Cyst, hypertrichosis, pruritus, rash

Endocrine & metabolic: Dehydration, diabetes mellitus, fluid overload, hypercalcemia, hyperlipidemia, hypoglycemia, hypomagnesemia, acidosis, hypertriglyceridemia, hypocalcemia, hyponatremia

Gastrointestinal: GI hemorrhage, gingival hyperplasia, melena, esophagitis, ulcerative stomatitis

Genitourinary: Impotence, genital edema, albuminuria, hematuria, renal tubular necrosis, urinary retention

Hematologic: Hematoma, hemorrhage, thrombocytopenia, thrombosis, polycythemia, leukopenia

Neuromuscular & skeletal: Arthralgia, arthropathy, paresthesia

Ocular: Cataract, conjunctivitis, abnormal vision

Respiratory: Bronchospasm, pulmonary edema

Miscellaneous: Sepsis, infection, increased glucocorticoids

Postmarketing and/or case reports: Severe hypersensitivity reactions, including anaphylaxis, have been reported. Symptoms may include hypotension, tachycardia, cardiac failure, dyspnea, bronchospasm, pulmonary edema, urticaria, rash, pruritus, sneezing, capillary leak syndrome, and respiratory failure.

Overdosage/Toxicology There have been no reports of overdose.

Pharmacodynamics/Kinetics

Half-Life Elimination: Children: 9.4 days; Adults: Mean: 7.2 days

Duration: Mean: 36 days (determined by IL-2R alpha saturation)

Formulations Injection, powder for reconstitution: 20 mg

Dosing

Adults & Elderly: Note: Patients previously administered basiliximab should only be re-exposed to a subsequent course of therapy with extreme caution.

Renal transplantation: I.V.: 20 mg within 2 hours prior to transplant surgery, followed by a second 20 mg dose 4 days after transplantation. The second dose should be withheld if complications occur (including severe hypersensitivity reactions or graft loss).

Pediatrics: Note: Patients previously administered basiliximab should only be re-exposed to a subsequent course of therapy with extreme caution.

Children <35 kg: Renal transplantation: I.V.: 10 mg within 2 hours prior to transplant surgery, followed by a second 10 mg dose 4 days after transplantation; the second dose should be withheld if complications occur (including severe hypersensitivity reactions or graft loss)

Children ≥35 kg: Renal transplantation: Refer to adult dosing

Renal Impairment: No specific dosing adjustment is recommended.

Hepatic Impairment: No specific dosing adjustment is recommended.

Administration

I.V.: For central or intravenous administration only. Infuse over 20-30 minutes.

Stability

Storage: Store vials under refrigeration 2°C to 8°C (36°F to 46°F). Reconstituted vials are stable under refrigeration for 24 hours, but only 4 hours at room temperature.

Reconstitution: Reconstitute vials with 5 mL sterile water for injection. Dilute reconstituted contents in 50 mL of normal saline or 5% dextrose.

Monitoring and Teaching Issues

Physical Assessment: See Contraindications and Warnings/Precautions for use cautions. Monitor cardiorespiratory function, renal function, and adverse reactions (see Adverse Reactions) during infusion and periodically following infusion. Assess knowledge/teach patient possible side effects/interventions and adverse symptoms to report as inpatient or following discharge (see Patient Education). Breast-feeding is not recommended (see Pregnancy and Breast-feeding Issues).

Patient Education: This medication, which may help to reduce transplant rejection, can only be given by infusion. You will be monitored and assessed closely during infusion and thereafter, however, it is important that you report any changes or problems for evaluation. You will be susceptible to infection (avoid crowds and exposure to infection). Frequent mouth care and small, frequent meals may help counteract any GI effects you may experience and will help maintain adequate nutrition and fluid intake. Report any changes in urination; unusual bruising or bleeding; chest pain or palpitations; acute dizziness; difficulty breathing; fever or chills; changes in cognition; rash; feelings of pain or numbness in extremities; severe GI upset or diarrhea; unusual back or leg pain or muscle tremors; vision changes; or any sign of infection (eg, chills, fever, sore throat, easy bruising or bleeding, mouth sores, unhealed sores, vaginal discharge). **Breast-feeding precaution:** Breast-feeding is not recommended.

Breast-feeding Issues: It is not known whether basiliximab is excreted in human milk. Because many immunoglobulins are secreted in milk and the potential for serious adverse reactions exists, a decision should be made whether to discontinue nursing or discontinue the drug, taking into account the importance of the drug to the mother.

Pregnancy Issues: IL-2 receptors play an important role in the development of the immune system. Use in pregnant women only when benefit exceeds potential risk to the fetus. Women of childbearing potential should use effective contraceptive measures before beginning treatment and for 2 months after completion of therapy with this agent.

Bayer® Aspirin [OTC] *see* Aspirin *on page 121*

Bayer® Aspirin Extra Strength [OTC] *see* Aspirin *on page 121*

Bayer® Aspirin Regimen Adult Low Strength [OTC] *see* Aspirin *on page 121*

Bayer® Aspirin Regimen Adult Low Strength with Calcium [OTC] *see* Aspirin *on page 121*

Bayer® Aspirin Regimen Children's [OTC] *see* Aspirin *on page 121*

Bayer® Aspirin Regimen Regular Strength [OTC] *see* Aspirin *on page 121*

Bayer® Plus Extra Strength [OTC] *see* Aspirin *on page 121*

BayGam™ *see page 1498*

BayHepB™ *see page 1498*

BayRab™ *see page 1498*

BayRho®-D *see page 1498*

BayRho®-D Mini-Dose *see page 1498*

BayTet™ *see page 1498*

Baza® Antifungal [OTC] *see* Miconazole *on page 899*

BCG Vaccine *see page 1498*

BCNU *see* Carmustine *on page 223*

Beclomethasone (be kloe METH a sone)

U.S. Brand Names Beconase®; Beconase® AQ; QVAR™; Vancenase® AQ 84 mcg; Vancenase® Pockethaler®; Vanceril®

Synonyms Beclomethasone Dipropionate; Beclovent [DSC]

Generic Available No

Pharmacologic Category Corticosteroid, Inhalant (Oral); Corticosteroid, Nasal

Pregnancy Risk Factor C

Lactation Enters breast milk (oral)/use caution

Use

Oral inhalation: Maintenance and prophylactic treatment of asthma; includes those who require corticosteroids and those who may benefit from a dose reduction/elimination of systemically administered corticosteroids. Not for relief of acute bronchospasm

Nasal aerosol: Symptomatic treatment of seasonal or perennial rhinitis and to prevent recurrence of nasal polyps following surgery

Mechanism of Action/Effect Acts at cellular level to prevent or control inflammation

Contraindications Hypersensitivity to beclomethasone or any component of the formulation; status asthmaticus

Warnings/Precautions Not to be used in status asthmaticus or for the relief of acute bronchospasm. May cause suppression of hypothalamic-pituitary-adrenal (HPA) axis, particularly in younger children or in patients receiving high doses for prolonged periods. Fatalities have occurred due to adrenal insufficiency in asthmatic patients during and after transfer from systemic corticosteroids to aerosol steroids; aerosol steroids do **not** provide the systemic steroid needed to treat patients having trauma, surgery, or infections. Withdrawal and discontinuation of the corticosteroid should be done slowly and carefully.

Controlled clinical studies have shown that orally-inhaled and intranasal corticosteroids may cause a reduction in growth velocity in pediatric patients, which appears to be related to dose and duration of exposure.

May suppress the immune system, patients may be more susceptible to infection. Use with caution in patients with systemic infections or ocular herpes simplex. Avoid exposure to chickenpox and measles. Corticosteroids should be used with caution in patients with diabetes, hypertension, osteoporosis, peptic ulcer, glaucoma, cataracts, or tuberculosis. Use caution in hepatic impairment. Beclovent® Oral Inhaler, Beconase® Nasal Inhaler, and Vanceril® Oral Inhaler contain chlorofluorocarbons (CFCs). Safety and efficacy in children <6 years of age have not been established.

Pregnancy risk C.

Drug Interactions

Increased Effect/Toxicity: The addition of salmeterol has been demonstrated to improve response to inhaled corticosteroids (as compared to increasing steroid dosage).

Adverse Reactions Frequency not defined.

Central nervous system: Agitation, depression, dizziness, dysphonia, headache, lightheadedness, mental disturbances

Dermatologic: Acneiform lesions, angioedema, atrophy, bruising, pruritus, purpura, striae, rash, urticaria

Endocrine & metabolic: Cushingoid features, growth velocity reduction in children and adolescents, HPA function suppression

Gastrointestinal: Dry/irritated nose, throat and mouth, hoarseness, localized *Candida* or *Aspergillus* infections, loss of smell, loss of taste, nausea, unpleasant smell, unpleasant taste, vomiting, weight gain

Local: Nasal spray: Burning, epistaxis, localized *Candida* infections, nasal septum perforation (rare), nasal stuffiness, nosebleeds, rhinorrhea, sneezing, transient irritation, ulceration of nasal mucosa (rare)

Ocular: Cataracts, glaucoma, increased intraocular pressure

Respiratory: Cough, paradoxical bronchospasm, pharyngitis, sinusitis, wheezing

Miscellaneous: Anaphylactic/anaphylactoid reactions, death (due to adrenal insufficiency, reported during and after transfer from systemic corticosteroids to aerosol in asthmatic patients), immediate and delayed hypersensitivity reactions

Overdosage/Toxicology Symptoms of overdose include irritation and burning of the nasal mucosa, sneezing, intranasal and pharyngeal *Candida* infections, nasal ulceration, epistaxis, rhinorrhea, nasal stuffiness, and headache. When consumed in high doses over prolonged periods, systemic hypercorticism and adrenal suppression may occur. In those cases, discontinuation of the corticosteroid should be done judiciously.

Pharmacodynamics/Kinetics

Absorption: Readily; quickly hydrolyzed by pulmonary esterases prior to absorption

Bioavailability: Of active metabolite, 44% following nasal inhalation (43% from swallowed portion)

(Continued)

Beclomethasone *(Continued)*

Half-Life Elimination: Initial: 3 hours

Metabolism: Hepatic via CYP3A4 to active metabolites

Onset: Therapeutic effect: 1-4 weeks

Formulations

Aerosol for oral inhalation, as dipropionate:

Beclovent® [DSC], Vanceril®: 42 mcg/inhalation [200 metered doses] (16.8 g)

QVAR™: 40 mcg/inhalation [100 metered doses] (7.3 g); 80 mcg/inhalation [100 metered doses] (7.3 g)

Vanceril® Double Strength: 84 mcg/inhalation [40 metered doses] (5.4 g), 84 mcg/inhalation [120 metered doses] (12.2 g)

Aerosol, intranasal, as dipropionate (Beconase®, Vancenase®): 42 mcg/inhalation: [80 metered doses] (6.7 g); [200 metered doses] (16.8 g)

Suspension, intranasal, aqueous, as dipropionate [spray]:

Beconase® AQ, Vancenase® AQ 0.042%: 42 mcg/inhalation [≥200 metered doses] (25 g)

Vancenase® AQ Double Strength: 84 mcg per inhalation [120 actuations] (19 g)

Dosing

Adults & Elderly: Nasal inhalation and oral inhalation dosage forms are not to be used interchangeably.

Rhinitis:

Intranasal aqueous inhalation:

Vancenase® AQ, Beconase® AQ: 1-2 inhalations each nostril twice daily; total dose 168-336 mcg/day

Vancenase® AQ 84 mcg: 1-2 inhalations in each nostril once daily; total dose 168-336 mcg/day

Intranasal aerosol (Vancenase®, Beconase®): 1 inhalation in each nostril 2-4 times/day or 2 inhalations each nostril twice daily (total dose 168-336 mcg/day); usual maximum maintenance: 1 inhalation in each nostril 3 times/day (252 mcg/day)

Asthma: Oral inhalation (doses should be titrated to the lowest effective dose once asthma is controlled):

Beclovent®, Vanceril®: 2 inhalations 3-4 times/day (alternatively: 4 inhalations twice daily); maximum dose: 20 inhalations/day (840 mcg/day); patients with severe asthma: Initial: 12-16 inhalations/day (divided 3-4 times/day); dose should be adjusted downward according to patient's response

Vanceril® 84 mcg double strength: 2 inhalations twice daily; maximum dose: 10 inhalations/day (840 mcg); patients with severe asthma: Initial: 6-8 inhalations/day (divided twice daily); dose should be adjusted downward according to patient's response

QVAR™: *Patients previously on bronchodilators only:* Initial dose 40-80 mcg twice daily; maximum dose 320 mcg twice day *Patients previously on inhaled corticosteroids:* Initial dose 40-160 mcg twice daily; maximum dose 320 mcg twice daily

NIH Guidelines (NIH, 1997) (give in divided doses):

"Low" dose: 168-504 mcg/day (42 mcg/puff: 4-12 puffs/day or 84 mcg/puff: 2-6 puffs/day)

"Medium" dose: 504-840 mcg/day (42 mcg/puff: 12-20 puffs/day or 84 mcg/puff: 6-10 puffs/day)

"High" dose: >840 mcg/day (42 mcg/puff: >20 puffs/day or 84 mcg/puff: >10 puffs/day)

Pediatrics: Nasal inhalation and oral inhalation dosage forms are not to be used interchangeably.

Rhinitis:

Intranasal aqueous solution:

Vancenase® AQ, Beconase® AQ: Children ≥6 years: 1-2 inhalations each nostril twice daily; total dose 168-336 mcg/day

Vancenase® AQ 84 mcg: Children ≥6 years: 1-2 inhalations in each nostril once daily; total dose 168-336 mcg/day

Intranasal aerosol (Vancenase®, Beconase®): Children 6-12 years: 1 inhalation in each nostril 3 times/day; total dose 252 mcg/day

Children ≥12 years: 1 inhalation in each nostril 2-4 times/day or 2 inhalations each nostril twice daily (total dose 168-336 mcg/day); usual maximum maintenance: 1 inhalation in each nostril 3 times/day (252 mcg/day)

Asthma: Oral inhalation (doses should be titrated to the lowest effective dose once asthma is controlled):

Beclovent®, Vanceril®:

Children 6-12 years: 1-2 inhalations 3-4 times/day (alternatively: 2-4 inhalations twice daily); maximum dose: 10 inhalations/day (420 mcg)

Children ≥12 years: 2 inhalations 3-4 times/day (alternatively: 4 inhalations twice daily); maximum dose: 20 inhalations/day (840 mcg/day); patients with severe asthma: Initial: 12-16 inhalations/day (divided 3-4 times/day); dose should be adjusted downward according to patient's response

Vanceril® 84 mcg double strength:

Children 6-12 years: 2 inhalations twice daily; maximum dose: 5 inhalations/day (420 mcg)

Children ≥12 years: 2 inhalations twice daily; maximum dose: 10 inhalations/day (840 mcg); patients with severe asthma: Initial: 6-8 inhalations/day (divided twice daily); dose should be adjusted downward according to patient's response

QVAR™:

Children 5-11 years: Initial: 40 mcg twice daily; maximum dose: 80 mcg twice daily

Children ≥12 years:

Patients previously on bronchodilators only: Initial dose 40-80 mcg twice daily; maximum dose: 320 mcg twice day

Patients previously on inhaled corticosteroids: Initial dose 40-160 mcg twice daily; maximum dose: 320 mcg twice daily

NIH Guidelines (NIH, 1997) (give in divided doses):

Children:

"Low" dose: 84-336 mcg/day (42 mcg/puff: 2-8 puffs/day or 84 mcg/puff: 1-4 puffs/day)

"Medium" dose: 336-672 mcg/day (42 mcg/puff: 8-16 puffs/day or 84 mcg/puff: 4-8 puffs/day)

"High" dose: >672 mcg/day (42 mcg/puff: >16 puffs/day or 84 mcg/puff >8 puffs/day)

Administration

Inhalation: Shake well before use. Keep oral inhaler clean and unobstructed, wash in warm water and dry thoroughly. Rinse mouth and throat after use to prevent *Candida* infection.

Stability

Storage: Do not store near heat or open flame. Do not puncture canisters. Store at room temperature. Rest QVAR™ on concave end of canister with actuator on top.

Monitoring and Teaching Issues

Physical Assessment: Not to be used to treat status asthmaticus or fungal infections of nasal passages. Monitor therapeutic effects and adverse reactions (see Warnings/Precautions, Adverse Reactions, and Overdose/Toxicology). When changing from systemic steroids to inhalational steroids, taper reduction of systemic medication slowly. Assess knowledge/teach patient appropriate use, interventions to reduce side effects, and adverse symptoms to report (see Patient Education). **Pregnancy risk factor C** - benefits of use should outweigh possible risks. Note breast-feeding caution.

Patient Education: Use as directed; do not increase dosage or discontinue abruptly without consulting prescriber. It may take 1-4 weeks for you to realize full effects of treatment. Review use of inhaler or spray with prescriber or follow package insert for directions. Keep oral inhaler clean and unobstructed. Always rinse mouth and throat after use of inhaler to prevent infection. If you are also using an inhaled bronchodilator, wait 10 minutes before using this steroid aerosol. Report adverse effects such as skin redness, rash, or irritation; pain or burning of nasal mucosa; white plaques in mouth or fuzzy tongue; unresolved headache; or worsening of condition or lack of improvement. Discard after date calculated by prescriber; the amount of medication in canister cannot be guaranteed after using the labeled number of actuations (sprays) even though it may not feel empty. **Pregnancy/breast-feeding precautions:** Inform prescriber if you are or intend to become pregnant. Consult prescriber if breast-feeding.

Inhalation: Sit when using. Take deep breaths for 3-5 minutes, and clear nasal passages before administration (use decongestant as needed). Hold breath for 5-10 seconds after use, and wait 1-3 minutes between inhalations. Follow package insert instructions for use. Do not exceed maximum dosage. If also using inhaled bronchodilator, use before beclomethasone. Rinse mouth and throat after use to reduce aftertaste and prevent candidiasis.

Geriatric Considerations: Older patients may have difficulty with oral metered dose inhalers and may benefit from the use of a spacer or chamber device.

Additional Information Effects of inhaled/intranasal steroids on growth have been observed in the absence of laboratory evidence of HPA axis suppression, suggesting that growth velocity is a more sensitive indicator of systemic corticosteroid exposure in pediatric patients than some commonly used tests of HPA axis function. The long-term effects of this reduction in growth velocity associated with orally-inhaled and intranasal corticosteroids, including the impact on final adult height, are unknown. The potential for "catch up" growth following discontinuation of treatment with inhaled corticosteroids has not been adequately studied.

Related Information

Inhalant (Asthma, Bronchospasm) Agents Comparison *on page 1577*

Beclomethasone Dipropionate *see* Beclomethasone *on page 149*

Beclovent [DSC] *see* Beclomethasone *on page 149*

Beconase® *see* Beclomethasone *on page 149*

Beconase® AQ *see* Beclomethasone *on page 149*

Belladonna and Opium (bel a DON a & OH pee um)

U.S. Brand Names B&O Supprettes®

Synonyms Opium and Belladonna

Restrictions C-II

Generic Available Yes

Pharmacologic Category Analgesic Combination (Narcotic); Antispasmodic Agent, Urinary

Pregnancy Risk Factor C

Lactation Excretion in breast milk unknown/use caution

Use Relief of moderate to severe pain associated with rectal or bladder tenesmus that may occur in postoperative states and neoplastic situations; pain associated with ureteral spasms not responsive to non-narcotic analgesics and to space intervals between injections of opiates

Mechanism of Action/Effect Anticholinergic alkaloids act primarily by competitive inhibition of the muscarinic actions of acetylcholine on structures innervated by postganglionic cholinergic neurons and on smooth muscle; resulting effects include antisecretory activity on exocrine glands and intestinal mucosa and smooth muscle relaxation. Contains many narcotic alkaloids including morphine; its mechanism for gastric motility inhibition is primarily due to this morphine content, resulting in a decrease in digestive secretions, an increase in GI muscle tone, and therefore a reduction in GI propulsion.

Contraindications Glaucoma; severe renal or hepatic disease; bronchial asthma; respiratory depression; convulsive disorders; acute alcoholism; premature labor

Warnings/Precautions Usual precautions of opiate agonist therapy should be observed. Use with caution and generally in reduced doses in the very young or geriatric patients. Pregnancy risk C.

Drug Interactions

Decreased Effect: May decrease effects of drugs with cholinergic mechanisms. Antipsychotic efficacy of phenothiazines may be decreased.

Increased Effect/Toxicity: Additive effects with CNS depressants. May increase effects of digoxin and atenolol. Coadministration with other anticholinergic agents (phenothiazines,

(Continued)

Belladonna and Opium *(Continued)*

tricyclic antidepressants, amantadine, and antihistamines) may increase effects such as dry mouth, constipation, and urinary retention.

Nutritional/Ethanol Interactions Ethanol: Avoid ethanol (may increase sedation).

Effects on Lab Values ↑ aminotransferase [ALT (SGPT)/AST (SGOT)] (S)

Adverse Reactions

>10%:

Dermatologic: Dry skin
Gastrointestinal: Constipation, dry throat, dry mouth
Local: Irritation at injection site
Respiratory: Dry nose
Miscellaneous: Diaphoresis (decreased)

1% to 10%:

Dermatologic: Increased sensitivity to light
Endocrine & metabolic: Decreased flow of breast milk
Gastrointestinal: Dysphagia

<1% (Limited to important or life-threatening): Ataxia, CNS depression, increased intraocular pain, loss of memory, orthostatic hypotension, respiratory depression, tachycardia, ventricular fibrillation

Overdosage/Toxicology Primary attention should be directed to ensuring adequate respiratory exchange. Opiate agonist-induced respiratory depression may be reversed with parenteral naloxone hydrochloride. Anticholinergic toxicity may be caused by strong binding of a belladonna alkaloid to cholinergic receptors. Physostigmine 1-2 mg given slowly S.C. or I.V. may be administered to reverse overdose with life-threatening effects.

Pharmacodynamics/Kinetics

Metabolism:

Opium: Hepatic, with formation of glucuronide metabolites

Onset:

Opium: Within 30 minutes

Formulations Suppository:

#15 A: Belladonna extract 16.2 mg and opium 30 mg
#16 A: Belladonna extract 16.2 mg and opium 60 mg

Dosing

Adults & Elderly: Rectal/bladder tenesmus or ureteral spasm: Rectal: 1 suppository 1-2 times/day, up to 4 doses/day

Administration

Other: Prior to rectal insertion, the finger and suppository should be moistened. Assist with ambulation.

Stability

Storage: Store at 15°C to 30°C; avoid freezing.

Monitoring and Teaching Issues

Physical Assessment: Assess other medications patient may be taking for additive or adverse interactions (see Warnings/Precautions and Drug Interactions). Monitor therapeutic effectiveness, signs of overdose (see Overdose/Toxicology), and adverse effects at beginning of therapy and at regular intervals with long-term use. May cause physical and/or psychological dependence. For inpatients, implement safety measures. Assess knowledge/teach patient appropriate use if self-administered. Teach patient to monitor for adverse reactions (see Adverse Reactions), adverse reactions to report, and appropriate interventions to reduce side effects. **Pregnancy risk factor C** - benefits of use should outweigh possible risks. Note breast-feeding caution.

Patient Education: If self-administered, use exactly as directed; do not increase dose or frequency. Drug may cause physical and/or psychological dependence. While using this medication, do not use alcohol and other prescription or OTC medications (especially sedatives, tranquilizers, antihistamines, or pain medications) without consulting prescriber. Maintain adequate hydration (2-3 L/day of fluids) unless advised by prescriber to restrict fluids. May cause hypotension, dizziness, or drowsiness; use caution when driving, climbing stairs, or changing position (rising from sitting or lying to standing) or when engaging in tasks requiring alertness (until response to drug is known); dry mouth or throat (frequent mouth care, frequent sips of fluids, chewing gum, or sucking lozenges may help); constipation (increased exercise, fluids, fruit, or fiber may help; if unresolved, consult prescriber about use of stool softeners); photosensitivity (use sunscreen, wear protective clothing and eyewear, and avoid direct sunlight); or decreased perspiration (avoid extremes in temperature or excessive activity in hot environments). Report chest pain or palpitations; persistent dizziness; changes in mentation; changes in gait; blurred vision; shortness of breath or difficulty breathing. **Pregnancy/breast-feeding precautions:** Inform prescriber if you are or intend to become pregnant. Consult prescriber if breast-feeding.

Belladonna, Phenobarbital, and Ergotamine

(bel a DON a, fee noe BAR bi tal, & er GOT a meen)

U.S. Brand Names Bellamine S; Bel-Phen-Ergot S®; Bel-Tabs

Synonyms Belladonna, Phenobarbital, and Ergotamine Tartrate; Ergotamine Tartrate, Belladonna, and Phenobarbital; Phenobarbital, Belladonna, and Ergotamine Tartrate

Generic Available Yes

Pharmacologic Category Ergot Derivative

Pregnancy Risk Factor X

Lactation Enters breast milk (ergotamine)/contraindicated

Use Management and treatment of menopausal disorders, GI disorders, and recurrent throbbing headache

Contraindications Hypersensitivity to belladonna alkaloids, phenobarbital, ergotamine, or any component of the formulation; dopamine therapy; hypertension; glaucoma; coronary heart disease and peripheral vascular disease; impaired hepatic or renal function; sepsis; history of manifest or latent porphyria; pregnancy

Warnings/Precautions Total weekly dosage of ergotamine should not exceed 10 mg. May be habit-forming. Use with caution in patients with bronchial asthma or obstructive uropathy. Caution should be used with prolonged use.

Drug Interactions

Cytochrome P450 Effect:

Phenobarbital: Substrate of CYP2C8/9, **2C19**, 2E1; Induces **CYP1A2, 2A6, 2B6, 2C8/9, 3A4**

Ergotamine: Substrate of **CYP3A4**; Inhibits 3A4

Decreased Effect: Phenobarbital may lower plasma levels of dicumarol due to decreased absorption. Possible interaction between ergot alkaloids and beta-blockers.

Increased Effect/Toxicity: Combined administration of phenobarbital and CNS depressants such as ethanol, tricyclic depressants, phenothiazines, and narcotic analgesics may result in potentiation of depressant actions. **Phenobarbital taken with warfarin induces liver enzymes that enhance clearance of warfarin. A reduction in phenobarbital dose in patients receiving warfarin has resulted in fatal bleeding episodes.** Griseofulvin, quinidine, doxycycline, and estrogen have been shown to be metabolized at an increased rate. Belladonna and concomitant administration of tricyclic antidepressants may result in additive anticholinergic effects. Valproic acid appears to decrease barbiturate metabolism (increased barbiturate levels). A similar reaction is possible with phenytoin.

Adverse Reactions

>10%:

Cardiovascular: Peripheral vascular effects (numbness and tingling of fingers and toes)
Central nervous system: Drowsiness, dizziness,
Dermatologic: Dry skin
Gastrointestinal: Constipation, dry mouth and throat, diarrhea, nausea, vomiting
Respiratory: Dry nose
Miscellaneous: Decreased diaphoresis

1% to 10%:

Cardiovascular: Precordial distress and pain, transient tachycardia or bradycardia
Dermatologic: Photosensitivity
Endocrine & metabolic: Decreased flow of breast milk
Gastrointestinal: Difficulty in swallowing
Neuromuscular & skeletal: Muscle pains in the extremities, weakness in the legs

<1% (Limited to important or life-threatening): Drowsiness, increased intraocular pain, loss of memory, orthostatic hypotension, skin rash, tachycardia, ventricular fibrillation

Pharmacokinetic Note See individual agents.

Formulations Tablet: Belladonna alkaloids 0.2 mg, phenobarbital 40 mg, and ergotamine tartrate 0.6 mg

Dosing

Adults: Menopausal disorders, GI disorders, and recurrent throbbing headache: Oral: 1 tablet each morning and evening

Elderly: Refer to dosing in individual monographs.

Monitoring and Teaching Issues

Physical Assessment: See Contraindications and Warnings/Precautions for use cautions. Assess potential for interactions with other prescriptions, OTC medications, or herbal products patient may be taking. This combination drug interacts with many commonly prescribed drugs to potentiate adverse/toxic reactions or to reduce the effectiveness of other drugs (see Drug Interactions). Use caution with prolonged use; may be habit-forming. Monitor for therapeutic effect and adverse reactions (see Adverse Reactions). Teach patient appropriate use, possible side effects and appropriate interventions, and adverse symptoms to report (see Patient Education). **Pregnancy risk factor X** - determine that patient is not pregnant before starting therapy. Do not give to females of childbearing age unless they are capable of complying with barrier contraceptive use. Instruct patient about appropriate barrier contraceptives. Breast-feeding is contraindicated.

Patient Education: Inform prescriber of all prescriptions, OTC medications, or herbal products you are taking, and any allergies you have. Do not take anything new during treatment unless approved by prescriber. Take exactly as directed; do not take more than recommended dose. Maintain adequate nutritional and fluid intake (2-3 L/day) unless advised by prescriber to restrict fluids. May cause drowsiness or dizziness (use caution when driving or engaging in tasks that require alertness until response to drug is known); dry throat or mouth (frequent mouth care or sucking on lozenges may help); dry nose (use humidifier); photosensitivity (use sunscreen, wear protective clothing and eyewear, and avoid direct sunlight); nausea or vomiting (small, frequent meals, frequent mouth care, sucking lozenges, or chewing gum may help); dry skin (mild skin lotion may help); or orthostatic hypotension (use caution when rising from sitting or lying position or climbing stairs). Report any signs of numbness in extremities (fingers and toes); unusual leg pain or cyanosis of extremities; difficulty swallowing; persistent muscle pain or weakness; pain in eye or vision changes; or chest pain, rapid heartbeat, or palpitations. **Pregnancy/breast-feeding precautions:** Inform prescriber if you are pregnant and do not get pregnant during therapy. Consult prescriber for instruction on appropriate contraceptive measures. Do not breast-feed.

Pregnancy Issues: Potential uterotonic effects.

Belladonna, Phenobarbital, and Ergotamine Tartrate *see* Belladonna, Phenobarbital, and Ergotamine *on page 152*

Bellamine S *see* Belladonna, Phenobarbital, and Ergotamine *on page 152*

Bel-Phen-Ergot S® *see* Belladonna, Phenobarbital, and Ergotamine *on page 152*

Bel-Tabs *see* Belladonna, Phenobarbital, and Ergotamine *on page 152*

Benadryl® Allergy [OTC] *see* DiphenhydrAMINE *on page 422*

Benadryl® Dye-Free Allergy [OTC] *see* DiphenhydrAMINE *on page 422*

Benadryl® Gel [OTC] *see* DiphenhydrAMINE *on page 422*

Benadryl® Gel Extra Strength [OTC] *see* DiphenhydrAMINE *on page 422*

Benadryl® Injection *see* DiphenhydrAMINE *on page 422*

Benazepril (ben AY ze pril)

U.S. Brand Names Lotensin®

Synonyms Benazepril Hydrochloride

Generic Available No

Pharmacologic Category Angiotensin-Converting Enzyme (ACE) Inhibitor

Pregnancy Risk Factor C/D (2nd and 3rd trimesters)

Lactation Enters breast milk/compatible

Use Treatment of hypertension, either alone or in combination with other antihypertensive agents; treatment of left ventricular dysfunction after myocardial infarction

Mechanism of Action/Effect Competitive inhibitor of angiotensin-converting enzyme (ACE); prevents conversion of angiotensin I to angiotensin II, a potent vasoconstrictor; results in lower levels of angiotensin II which causes an increase in plasma renin activity and a reduction in aldosterone secretion

Contraindications Hypersensitivity to benazepril or any component of the formulation; angioedema or serious hypersensitivity related to previous treatment with an ACE inhibitor; bilateral renal artery stenosis; primary hyperaldosteronism; patients with idiopathic or hereditary angioedema; pregnancy (2nd and 3rd trimesters)

Warnings/Precautions Anaphylactic reactions can occur. Angioedema can occur at any time during treatment (especially following first dose). Careful blood pressure monitoring with first dose (hypotension can occur especially in volume depleted patients). Dosage adjustment needed in renal impairment. Use with caution in hypovolemia; collagen vascular diseases; valvular stenosis (particularly aortic stenosis); hyperkalemia; or before, during, or immediately after anesthesia. Avoid rapid dosage escalation which may lead to renal insufficiency. Hypersensitivity reactions may be seen during hemodialysis with high-flux dialysis membranes (eg, AN69). Deterioration in renal function can occur with initiation. Use with caution in unilateral renal artery stenosis and pre-existing renal insufficiency. Pregnancy risk C/D (2nd and 3rd trimesters).

Drug Interactions

Decreased Effect: Aspirin (high dose) may reduce the therapeutic effects of ACE inhibitors; at low dosages this does not appear to be significant. Rifampin may decrease the effect of ACE inhibitors. Antacids may decrease the bioavailability of ACE inhibitors (may be more likely to occur with captopril); separate administration times by 1-2 hours. NSAIDs, specifically indomethacin, may reduce the hypotensive effects of ACE inhibitors.

Increased Effect/Toxicity: Potassium supplements, co-trimoxazole (high dose), angiotensin II receptor antagonists (candesartan, losartan, irbesartan, etc), or potassium-sparing diuretics (amiloride, spironolactone, triamterene) may result in elevated serum potassium levels when combined with benazepril. ACE inhibitor effects may be increased by phenothiazines or probenecid (increases levels of captopril). ACE inhibitors may increase serum concentrations/effects of digoxin, lithium, and sulfonlyureas. Diuretics have additive hypotensive effects with ACE inhibitors, and hypovolemia increases the potential for adverse renal effects of ACE inhibitors. In patients with compromised renal function, coadministration with NSAIDs may result in further deterioration of renal function. Allopurinol and ACE inhibitors may cause a higher risk of hypersensitivity reaction when taken concurrently.

Nutritional/Ethanol Interactions Herb/Nutraceutical: Avoid dong quai if using for hypertension (has estrogenic activity). Avoid ephedra, yohimbe, ginseng (may worsen hypertension). Avoid garlic (may have increased antihypertensive effect).

Adverse Reactions

1% to 10%:

Cardiovascular: Postural dizziness (1.5%)

Central nervous system: Headache (6.2%), dizziness (3.6%), fatigue (2.4%), somnolence (1.6%)

Endocrine & metabolic: Hyperkalemia (1%), increased uric acid

Gastrointestinal: Nausea (1.3%)

Renal: Increased serum creatinine (2%), worsening of renal function may occur in patients with bilateral renal artery stenosis or hypovolemia

Respiratory: Cough (1.2% to 10%)

<1% (Limited to important or life-threatening): Alopecia, angina, angioedema, asthma, dermatitis, dyspnea, hemolytic anemia, hypersensitivity, hypotension, impotence, insomnia, pancreatitis, paresthesia, photosensitivity, postural hypotension (0.3%), rash, shock, Stevens-Johnson syndrome, syncope, thrombocytopenia, vomiting

Eosinophilic pneumonitis, neutropenia, anaphylaxis, renal insufficiency and renal failure have been reported with other ACE inhibitors. In addition, a syndrome including fever, myalgia, arthralgia, interstitial nephritis, vasculitis, rash, eosinophilia, and elevated ESR has been reported to be associated with ACE inhibitors.

Overdosage/Toxicology Mild hypotension has been the primary toxic effect seen with acute overdose. Bradycardia may also occur. Hyperkalemia occurs even with therapeutic doses, especially in patients with renal insufficiency and those taking NSAIDs. Treatment is symptom-directed and supportive.

Pharmacodynamics/Kinetics

Absorption: Rapid (37%); food does not alter significantly; metabolite (benazeprilat) itself unsuitable for oral administration due to poor absorption

Half-Life Elimination: Effective: 10-11 hours; Benazeprilat: Terminal: 22 hours

Time to Peak: Parent drug: 1-1.5 hours

Metabolism: Rapidly and extensively hepatic to its active metabolite, benazeprilat, via enzymatic hydrolysis; extensive first-pass effect

Onset:

Reduction in plasma angiotensin-converting enzyme (ACE) activity: Peak effect: 1-2 hours after 2-20 mg dose

Reduction in blood pressure: Peak effect: Single dose: 2-4 hours; Continuous therapy: 2 weeks

Duration: Reduction in plasma angiotensin-converting enzyme (ACE) activity: >90% inhibition for 24 hours after 5-20 mg dose

Formulations Tablet, as hydrochloride: 5 mg, 10 mg, 20 mg, 40 mg

Dosing

Adults: Hypertension or LV dysfunction: Oral: Initial: 10 mg/day in patients not receiving a diuretic; 20-40 mg/day as a single dose or 2 divided doses; base dosage adjustments on peak (2-6 hours after dosing) and trough responses.

Elderly: Patients taking diuretics should have them discontinued 2-3 days prior to starting benazepril. If they cannot be discontinued, then initial dose should be 5 mg; restart after blood pressure is stabilized if needed.

Oral: Initial: 5-10 mg/day in single or divided doses; usual range: 20-40 mg/day; adjust for renal function.

Renal Impairment:

Cl_{cr} <30 mL/minute: Administer 5 mg/day initially; maximum daily dose: 40 mg.

Hemodialysis effects: Moderately dialyzable (20% to 50%); administer dose postdialysis or administer 25% to 35% supplemental dose.

Peritoneal dialysis: Supplemental dose is not necessary.

Monitoring Laboratory Tests CBC, renal function tests, electrolytes

Monitoring and Teaching Issues

Physical Assessment: See Contraindications, Warnings/Precautions, and Dosing for use cautions. Assess potential for interactions with other prescriptions, OTC medications, or herbal products patient may be taking (see Drug Interactions). Assess therapeutic effectiveness, results of laboratory tests (see above), and adverse response on a regular basis during therapy (see Adverse Reactions and Overdose/Toxicology). Teach patient appropriate use, possible side effects and interventions, and adverse symptoms to report (see Patient Education). **Pregnancy risk factor C/D** - see Pregnancy Risk Factor for use cautions. Instruct patient in appropriate use of contraceptives. See Pregnancy Issues.

Patient Education: Inform prescriber of all prescriptions, OTC medications, or herbal products you are taking, and any allergies you have. Do not take anything new without consulting prescriber. Take exactly as directed; do not alter dose or discontinue without consulting prescriber. Take first dose at bedtime. Do not take potassium supplements or salt substitutes containing potassium without consulting prescriber. This drug does not eliminate need for diet or exercise regimen as recommended by prescriber. May cause dizziness, fainting, or lightheadedness (use caution when driving or engaging in tasks that require alertness until response to drug is known); postural hypotension (use caution when rising from lying or sitting position or climbing stairs); nausea, vomiting, abdominal pain, dry mouth, or transient loss of appetite (small, frequent meals, frequent mouth care, sucking lozenges, or chewing gum may help); report if these side effects persist. Report mouth sores; fever or chills; swelling of extremities, face, mouth, or tongue; difficulty breathing or unusual cough; or other persistent adverse reactions. **Pregnancy/breast-feeding precautions:** Inform prescriber if you are or intend to become pregnant. This drug should not be used in the 2nd or 3rd trimester of pregnancy. Consult prescriber for appropriate contraceptive measures if necessary. Consult prescriber if breast-feeding.

Geriatric Considerations: Due to frequent decreases in glomerular filtration (also creatinine clearance) with aging, elderly patients may have exaggerated responses to ACE inhibitors. Differences in clinical response due to hepatic changes are not observed. ACE inhibitors may be preferred agents in elderly patients with congestive heart failure and diabetes mellitus. Diabetic proteinuria is reduced and insulin sensitivity is enhanced. In general, the side effect profile is favorable in elderly and causes little or no CNS confusion. Use lowest dose recommendations initially.

Pregnancy Issues: ACE inhibitors can cause fetal injury or death if taken during the 2nd or 3rd trimester. Discontinue ACE inhibitors as soon as pregnancy is detected.

Related Information

Angiotensin Agents *on page 1547*

Benazepril and Amlodipine *see* Amlodipine and Benazepril *on page 87*

Benazepril and Hydrochlorothiazide

(ben AY ze pril & hye droe klor oh THYE a zide)

U.S. Brand Names Lotensin® HCT

Synonyms Hydrochlorothiazide and Benazepril

Generic Available No

Pharmacologic Category Antihypertensive Agent Combination

Pregnancy Risk Factor C/D (2nd and 3rd trimesters)

Lactation Enters breast milk/compatible

Use Treatment of hypertension

Formulations Tablet:

Benazepril 5 mg and hydrochlorothiazide 6.25 mg

Benazepril 10 mg and hydrochlorothiazide 12.5 mg

Benazepril 20 mg and hydrochlorothiazide 12.5 mg

Benazepril 20 mg and hydrochlorothiazide 25 mg

Dosing

Adults: Hypertension: Oral: Dose is individualized (range: benazepril: 5-20 mg; hydrochlorothiazide: 6.25-25 mg/day)

Elderly: Dose is individualized.

Renal Impairment: Cl_{cr} <30 mL/minute: Not recommended; loop diuretics are preferred.

Monitoring and Teaching Issues

Physical Assessment: See individual components listed in Related Information. **Pregnancy risk factor C/D** - see Pregnancy Risk Factor for use cautions. Assess knowledge/instruct patient on need to use appropriate contraceptive measures and the need to avoid pregnancy.

(Continued)

Benazepril and Hydrochlorothiazide *(Continued)*

Patient Education: See individual components listed in Related Information. **Pregnancy precaution:** Do not get pregnant while taking this medication; use appropriate contraceptive measures.

Related Information

Benazepril *on page 154*
Hydrochlorothiazide *on page 664*

Benazepril Hydrochloride *see* Benazepril *on page 154*

Benemid [DSC] *see* Probenecid *on page 1121*

Benicar™ *see* Olmesartan *on page 997*

Bentiromide *see page 1461*

Benylin® Expectorant [OTC] *see* Guaifenesin and Dextromethorphan *on page 647*

Benzacot® *see* Trimethobenzamide *on page 1365*

Benzamycin® *see* Erythromycin and Benzoyl Peroxide *on page 485*

Benzathine Benzylpenicillin *see* Penicillin G Benzathine *on page 1043*

Benzathine Penicillin G *see* Penicillin G Benzathine *on page 1043*

Benzene Hexachloride *see* Lindane *on page 805*

Benzhexol Hydrochloride *see* Trihexyphenidyl *on page 1363*

Benzmethyzin *see* Procarbazine *on page 1125*

Benzocaine (BEN zoe kane)

U.S. Brand Names Americaine® [OTC]; Americaine® Anesthetic Lubricant; Anbesol® [OTC]; Anbesol® Baby [OTC]; Anbesol® Maximum Strength [OTC]; Babee® Teething® [OTC]; Benzodent® [OTC]; Chiggerex® [OTC]; Chiggertox® [OTC]; Cylex® [OTC]; Detane® [OTC]; Foille® [OTC]; Foille® Medicated First Aid [OTC]; Foille® Plus [OTC]; HDA® Toothache [OTC]; Hurricaine®; Lanacane® [OTC]; Mycinettes® [OTC]; Orabase®-B [OTC]; Orajel® [OTC]; Orajel® Baby [OTC]; Orajel® Baby Nighttime [OTC]; Orajel® Maximum Strength [OTC]; Orasol® [OTC]; Solarcaine® [OTC]; Trocaine® [OTC]; Zilactin®-B [OTC]; Zilactin® Baby [OTC]

Synonyms Ethyl Aminobenzoate

Generic Available Yes

Pharmacologic Category Local Anesthetic

Pregnancy Risk Factor C

Lactation Excretion in breast milk unknown

Use Temporary relief of pain associated with local anesthetic for pruritic dermatosis, pruritus, minor burns, acute congestive and serous otitis media, swimmer's ear, otitis externa, toothache, minor sore throat pain, canker sores, hemorrhoids, rectal fissures, anesthetic lubricant for passage of catheters and endoscopic tubes; nonprescription diet aid

Mechanism of Action/Effect Benzocaine blocks both the initiation and conduction of nerve impulses by decreasing the neuronal membrane's permeability to sodium ions, which results in inhibition of depolarization with resultant blockade of conduction. As a diet aide, the anesthetic effect appears to decrease the ability to detect degrees of sweetness by taste perception.

Contraindications Hypersensitivity to benzocaine, other ester-type local anesthetics, or any component of the formulation; secondary bacterial infection of area; ophthalmic use; see package labeling for specific contraindications

Warnings/Precautions Not intended for use when infections are present. Pregnancy risk C.

Drug Interactions

Decreased Effect: May antagonize actions of sulfonamides.

Adverse Reactions Dose-related and may result in high plasma levels

1% to 10%:

Dermatologic: Angioedema, contact dermatitis

Local: Burning, stinging

<1% (Limited to important or life-threatening): Edema, methemoglobinemia in infants, urethritis, urticaria

Overdosage/Toxicology Methemoglobinemia has been reported with benzocaine in oral overdose. Treatment is primarily symptomatic and supportive; termination of anesthesia by pneumatic tourniquet inflation should be attempted when the agent is administered by infiltration or regional injection. Methemoglobinemia may be treated with methylene blue, 1-2 mg/kg I.V. infused over several minutes. Seizures commonly respond to diazepam, while hypotension responds to I.V. fluids and Trendelenburg positioning. Bradyarrhythmias (when the heart rate is <60) can be treated with I.V., I.M., or S.C. atropine 15 mcg/kg. With the development of metabolic acidosis, I.V. sodium bicarbonate 0.5-2 mEq/kg and ventilatory assistance should be instituted.

Pharmacodynamics/Kinetics

Absorption: Topical: Poor to intact skin; well absorbed from mucous membranes and traumatized skin

Metabolism: Hepatic (to a lesser extent) and plasma via hydrolysis by cholinesterase

Formulations

Aerosol, oral spray (Hurricaine®): 20% (60 mL) [cherry flavor]

Aerosol, topical spray:

Americaine®: 20% (20 mL, 120 mL)

Foille®: 5% (97.5 mL) [contains chloroxylenol 0.63%]

Foille® Plus: 5% (105 mL) [contains chloroxylenol 0.63% and alcohol 57.33%]

Solarcaine®: 20% (90 mL, 120 mL, 135 mL) [contains triclosan, alcohol 0.13%]

Cream, topical: 5% (30 g, 454 g)

Lanacane®: 20% (30g)

Gel, oral:

Anbesol® 6.3% (7.5 g)

Anbesol® Baby, Detane®, Orajel® Baby: 7.5% (7.5 g, 10 g, 15 g)

Anbesol® Maximum Strength, Orajel® Maximum Strength: 20% (6 g, 7.5 g, 10 g)

HDA® Toothache: 6.5% (15 mL) [contains benzyl alcohol]

Hurricaine®: 20% (5 g, 30 g) [mint, pina colada, watermelon, and wild cherry flavors]
Orabase-B®: 20% (7 g)
Orajel®, Orajel® Baby Nighttime, Zilactin®-B, Zilactin® Baby: 10% (6 g, 7.5 g, 10 g)
Gel, topical (Americaine® Anesthetic Lubricant): 20% (2.5 g, 28 g) [contains 0.1% benzethonium chloride
Liquid, oral:
Anbesol®, Orasol®: 6.3% (9 mL, 15 mL, 30 mL)
Anbesol® Maximum Strength: 20% (9 mL, 14 mL)
Hurricaine®: 20% (30 mL) [pina colada and wild cherry flavors]
Orajel®: 10% (13 mL) [contains tartrazine]
Orajel® Baby: 7.5% (13 mL)
Liquid, topical (Chiggertox®): 2% (30 mL)
Lotion, oral (Babee® Teething): 2.5% (15 mL)
Lozenge:
Cylex®, Mycinettes®: 15 mg [Cylex® contains cetylpyridinium chloride 5 mg]
Trocaine®: 10 mg
Ointment, oral (Benzodent®): 20% (30 g)
Ointment, topical:
Chiggerex®: 2% (52 g)
Foille® Medicated First Aid: 5% (3.5 g, 28 g) [contains chloroxylenol 0.1%, benzyl alcohol; corn oil base]
Paste, oral (Orabase®-B): 20% (7 g)

Dosing

Adults & Elderly:

Local anesthetic: Mucous membranes: Dosage varies depending on area to be anesthetized and vascularity of tissues.

Oral mouth/throat preparations: Do not administer for >2 days unless directed by a physician; refer to specific package labeling.

Topical: Apply to affected area as needed.

Pediatrics: Children: Refer to adult dosing.

Administration

Topical: Do not eat for 1 hour after application to oral mucosa. Chemical burns should be neutralized before application of benzocaine. Avoid application to large areas of broken skin, especially in children.

Monitoring and Teaching Issues

Physical Assessment: Monitor for effectiveness of application and adverse reactions (see Adverse Reactions). **Oral:** Use caution to prevent gagging or choking and avoid food or drink for 1 hour. Teach patient adverse reactions to report; use and teach appropriate interventions to promote safety. **Pregnancy risk factor C** - benefits of use should outweigh possible risks. Note breast-feeding caution.

Patient Education: Use as directed; do not overuse. Do not apply when infections are present and do not apply to large areas of broken skin. Do not eat or drink for 1 hour following oral application. Discontinue application and report if swelling of mouth, lips, tongue, or throat occurs; or if skin irritation occurs at application site. **Pregnancy/breast-feeding precautions:** Inform prescriber if you are pregnant. Consult prescriber if breast-feeding.

Dietary Issues: When used as a nonprescription diet aid, take just prior to food consumption.

Related Information

Otic Agents *on page 1519*

Benzocaine, Antipyrine, and Phenylephrine *see page 1519*
Benzodent® [OTC] *see* Benzocaine *on page 156*
Benzodiazepines *see page 1560*

Benzonatate (ben ZOE na tate)

U.S. Brand Names Tessalon®

Generic Available Yes

Pharmacologic Category Antitussive

Pregnancy Risk Factor C

Lactation Excretion in breast milk unknown

Use Symptomatic relief of nonproductive cough

Mechanism of Action/Effect Suppresses cough by topical anesthetic action on the respiratory stretch receptors

Contraindications Hypersensitivity to benzonatate, related compounds (such as tetracaine), or any component of the formulation

Warnings/Precautions Pregnancy risk C.

Adverse Reactions 1% to 10%:

Central nervous system: Sedation, headache, dizziness, mental confusion, visual hallucinations, vague "chilly" sensation
Dermatologic: Rash
Gastrointestinal: Constipation, nausea, vomiting, GI upset
Neuromuscular & skeletal: Numbness in chest
Ocular: Burning sensation in eyes
Respiratory: Nasal congestion

Overdosage/Toxicology Symptoms of overdose include restlessness, tremor, and CNS stimulation. Benzonatate's local anesthetic activity can reduce the patient's gag reflex and, therefore, may contradict the use of ipecac following ingestion. Treatment is supportive and symptomatic.

Pharmacodynamics/Kinetics

Onset: Therapeutic: 15-20 minutes

Duration: 3-8 hours

Formulations Capsule: 100 mg, 200 mg

(Continued)

Benzonatate *(Continued)*

Dosing

Adults & Elderly: Cough: Oral: 100 mg 3 times/day or every 4 hours up to 600 mg/day

Pediatrics: Children >10 years: Refer to adult dosing.

Administration

Oral: Swallow capsule whole (do not break or chew).

Monitoring and Teaching Issues

Physical Assessment: Monitor effectiveness of and adverse reactions (see Adverse Reactions) at beginning of therapy and periodically with long-term use. Assess knowledge/teach patient appropriate use, interventions to reduce side effects, and adverse symptoms to report (see Patient Education). **Pregnancy risk factor C** - benefits of use should outweigh possible risks. Note breast-feeding caution.

Patient Education: Take only as prescribed; do not exceed prescribed dose or frequency. Do not break or chew capsule. Maintain adequate hydration (2-3 L/day of fluids) unless advised by prescriber to restrict fluids. Avoid use of other depressants, or sleep-inducing medications unless approved by prescriber. You may experience drowsiness, impaired coordination, blurred vision, or increased anxiety (use caution when driving or engaging in tasks requiring alertness until response to drug is known); or upset stomach or nausea (small, frequent meals, frequent mouth care, chewing gum, or sucking hard candy may help). Report persistent CNS changes (dizziness, sedation, tremor, or agitation); numbness in chest or feeling of chill; visual changes or burning in eyes; numbness of mouth or difficulty swallowing; or lack of improvement or worsening or condition. **Pregnancy/breast-feeding precautions:** Inform prescriber if you are or intend to become pregnant. Consult prescriber if breast-feeding.

Geriatric Considerations: No specific geriatric information is available about benzonatate. Avoid use in patients with impaired gag reflex or who cannot swallow the capsule whole.

Benzoyl Peroxide and Erythromycin *see* Erythromycin and Benzoyl Peroxide *on page 485*

Benzoyl Peroxide and Hydrocortisone

(BEN zoe il peer OKS ide & hye droe KOR ti sone)

U.S. Brand Names Vanoxide-HC®

Synonyms Hydrocortisone and Benzoyl Peroxide

Generic Available No

Pharmacologic Category Topical Skin Product; Topical Skin Product, Acne

Pregnancy Risk Factor C

Lactation For topical use

Use Treatment of acne vulgaris and oily skin

Formulations Lotion: Benzoyl peroxide 5% and hydrocortisone acetate 0.5% (25 mL)

Dosing

Adults & Elderly: Acne vulgaris: Topical: Apply thin film 1-3 times/day, gently massage into skin.

Pediatrics: Adolescents: Refer to adult dosing.

Monitoring and Teaching Issues

Physical Assessment: See individual components listed in Related Information. **Pregnancy risk factor C** - benefits of use should outweigh possible risks.

Patient Education: Also see Hydrocortisone.

Based on Benzoyl Peroxide component: Shake lotion before using. Cleanse and make sure skin is dry before applying; keep away from eyes, mouth, mucous membranes. If excessive redness or irritation occurs, discontinue use; avoid excessive sunlight, sun lamps, or other topical medication unless directed otherwise by a physician. May bleach color from fabrics; may be worn under make-up.

Pregnancy precaution: Inform prescriber if you are or intend to become pregnant.

Related Information

Hydrocortisone *on page 673*

Benzphetamine *see page 1693*

Benztropine (BENZ troe peen)

U.S. Brand Names Cogentin®

Synonyms Benztropine Mesylate

Generic Available Yes: Tablet

Pharmacologic Category Anticholinergic Agent; Anti-Parkinson's Agent, Anticholinergic

Pregnancy Risk Factor C

Lactation Excretion in breast milk unknown

Use Adjunctive treatment of Parkinson's disease; treatment of drug-induced extrapyramidal symptoms (except tardive dyskinesia)

Mechanism of Action/Effect Possesses both anticholinergic and antihistaminic effects. *In vitro* anticholinergic activity approximates that of atropine; *in vivo* it is only about half as active as atropine. Animal data suggest its antihistaminic activity and duration of action approach that of pyrilamine maleate. May also inhibit the reuptake and storage of dopamine and thereby, prolong the action of dopamine.

Contraindications Hypersensitivity to benztropine or any component of the formulation; pyloric or duodenal obstruction, stenosing peptic ulcers; bladder neck obstructions; achalasia; myasthenia gravis; children <3 years of age

Warnings/Precautions Use with caution in older children (dose has not been established). Use with caution in hot weather or during exercise. May cause anhydrosis and hyperthermia, which may be severe. The risk is increased in hot environments, particularly in the elderly, alcoholics, patients with CNS disease, and those with prolonged outdoor exposure.

Elderly patients frequently develop increased sensitivity and require strict dosage regulation - side effects may be more severe in elderly patients with atherosclerotic changes. Use with caution in patients with tachycardia, cardiac arrhythmias, hypertension, hypotension, prostatic hyperplasia (especially in the elderly), any tendency toward urinary retention, liver or kidney disorders, and obstructive disease of the GI or GU tract. When given in large doses or to susceptible patients, may cause weakness and inability to move particular muscle groups.

May be associated with confusion or hallucinations (generally at higher dosages). Intensification of symptoms or toxic psychosis may occur in patients with mental disorders. Benztropine does not relieve symptoms of tardive dyskinesia.

Pregnancy risk C.

Drug Interactions

Cytochrome P450 Effect: Substrate of CYP2D6

Decreased Effect: May increase gastric degradation of levodopa and decrease the amount of levodopa absorbed by delaying gastric emptying. Therapeutic effects of cholinergic agents (tacrine, donepezil) and neuroleptics may be antagonized.

Increased Effect/Toxicity: Central and/or peripheral anticholinergic syndrome can occur when benztropine is administered with amantadine, rimantadine, narcotic analgesics, phenothiazines and other antipsychotics (especially with high anticholinergic activity), tricyclic antidepressants, quinidine and some other antiarrhythmics, and antihistamines. Benztropine may increase the absorption of digoxin.

Nutritional/Ethanol Interactions Ethanol: Avoid ethanol (may increase CNS depression).

Adverse Reactions Frequency not defined.

Cardiovascular: Tachycardia

Central nervous system: Confusion, disorientation, memory impairment, toxic psychosis, visual hallucinations

Dermatologic: Rash

Endocrine & metabolic: Heat stroke, hyperthermia

Gastrointestinal: Xerostomia, nausea, vomiting, constipation, ileus

Genitourinary: Urinary retention, dysuria

Ocular: Blurred vision, mydriasis

Miscellaneous: Fever

Overdosage/Toxicology Symptoms of overdose include CNS depression, confusion, nervousness, hallucinations, dizziness, blurred vision, nausea, vomiting, and hyperthermia. For anticholinergic overdose with severe life-threatening symptoms, physostigmine 1-2 mg S.C. or I.V. slowly, may be given to reverse these effects.

Pharmacodynamics/Kinetics

Bioavailability: 29%

Metabolism: Hepatic (N-oxidation, N-dealkylation, and ring hydroxylation)

Onset: Oral: Within 1 hour; Parenteral: Within 15 minutes

Duration: 6-48 hours

Formulations

Injection, solution, as mesylate: 1 mg/mL (2 mL)

Tablet, as mesylate: 0.5 mg, 1 mg, 2 mg

Dosing

Adults:

Drug-induced extrapyramidal symptom: Oral, I.M., I.V.: 1-4 mg/dose 1-2 times/day

Acute dystonia: I.M., I.V.: 1-2 mg

Parkinsonism: Oral: 0.5-6 mg/day in 1-2 divided doses; if one dose is greater, give at bedtime. Titrate dose in 0.5 mg increments at 5- to 6-day intervals.

Elderly: Oral: Initial: 0.5 mg once or twice daily; titrate dose in 0.5 mg increments at every 5-6 days; maximum: 4 mg/day.

Pediatrics: Use in children <3 years of age should be reserved for life-threatening emergencies.

Drug-induced extrapyramidal symptom: Oral, I.M., I.V.: Children >3 years: 0.02-0.05 mg/kg/dose 1-2 times/day

Monitoring and Teaching Issues

Physical Assessment: Assess effectiveness and interactions of other medications patient may be taking (see Contraindications and Drug Interactions). Monitor therapeutic response and adverse reactions at beginning of therapy and at regular interval throughout therapy (see Warnings/Precautions, Adverse Reactions, and Overdose/Toxicology). Assess knowledge/teach patient appropriate use, interventions to reduce side effects, and adverse symptoms to report (see Patient Education). **Pregnancy risk factor C** - benefits of use should outweigh possible risks. Note breast-feeding caution.

Patient Education: Take exactly as directed; do not increase, decrease, or discontinue without consulting prescriber. Take at the same time each day. Do not use alcohol and any prescription or OTC sedatives or CNS depressants without consulting prescriber. You may experience drowsiness, dizziness, confusion, and blurred vision (use caution when driving, climbing stairs, or engaging in tasks requiring alertness until response to drug is known); increased susceptibility to heat stroke, decreased perspiration (use caution in hot weather - maintain adequate fluids and reduce exercise activity); or constipation (increased exercise, fluids, fruit, or fiber may help). Report unresolved nausea, vomiting, or gastric disturbances; rapid or pounding heartbeat, chest pain, or palpitation; difficulty breathing; CNS changes (hallucination, loss of memory, nervousness, etc); eye pain; prolonged fever; painful or difficult urination; unresolved constipation; increased muscle spasticity or rigidity; skin rash; or significant worsening of condition. **Pregnancy/breast-feeding precautions:** Inform prescriber if you are or intend to become pregnant. Consult prescriber if breast-feeding.

Geriatric Considerations: Anticholinergic agents are generally not well tolerated in the elderly and their use should be avoided when possible (see Warnings/Precautions and Adverse Reactions). In the elderly, anticholinergic agents should not be used as prophylaxis against extrapyramidal symptoms.

Benztropine Mesylate *see* Benztropine *on page 158*

Benzylpenicillin Benzathine *see* Penicillin G Benzathine *on page 1043*

Benzylpenicillin Potassium *see* Penicillin G (Parenteral/Aqueous) *on page 1045*

Benzylpenicillin Sodium *see* Penicillin G (Parenteral/Aqueous) *on page 1045*

Benzylpenicilloyl-Polylysine *see page 1461*

Beta-Blockers *see page 1561*

Betadine® First Aid Antibiotics + Moisturizer [OTC] *see* Bacitracin and Polymyxin B *on page 144*

9-Beta-D-ribofuranosyladenine *see* Adenosine *on page 47*

Betagan® Liquifilm® *see* Ophthalmic Agents, Glaucoma *on page 1002*

Betamethasone (bay ta METH a sone)

U.S. Brand Names Alphatrex®; Betatrex®; Beta-Val®; Celestone®; Celestone® Phosphate; Celestone® Soluspan®; Diprolene®; Diprolene® AF; Diprosone®; Luxiq™; Maxivate®; Valisone® [DSC]

Synonyms Betamethasone Dipropionate; Betamethasone Dipropionate, Augmented; Betamethasone Sodium Phosphate; Betamethasone Valerate; Flubenisolone

Generic Available Yes

Pharmacologic Category Corticosteroid, Systemic; Corticosteroid, Topical

Pregnancy Risk Factor C

Lactation Excretion in breast milk unknown/use caution

Use Inflammatory dermatoses such as seborrheic or atopic dermatitis, neurodermatitis, anogenital pruritus, psoriasis, inflammatory phase of xerosis

Mechanism of Action/Effect Binds to corticosteroid receptors in cell and acts to prevent or control inflammation

Contraindications Hypersensitivity to betamethasone or any component of the formulation; systemic fungal infections

Warnings/Precautions Not to be used in status asthmaticus or for the relief of acute bronchospasm; topical use in patients ≤12 years of age is not recommended. May cause suppression of hypothalamic-pituitary-adrenal (HPA) axis, particularly in younger children or in patients receiving high doses for prolonged periods. Particular care is required when patients are transferred from systemic corticosteroids to inhaled products due to possible adrenal insufficiency or withdrawal from steroids, including an increase in allergic symptoms. Patients receiving 20 mg per day of prednisone (or equivalent) may be most susceptible. Fatalities have occurred due to adrenal insufficiency in asthmatic patients during and after transfer from systemic corticosteroids to aerosol steroids; aerosol steroids do **not** provide the systemic steroid needed to treat patients having trauma, surgery, or infections. Withdrawal and discontinuation of the corticosteroid should be done slowly and carefully

Controlled clinical studies have shown that orally-inhaled and intranasal corticosteroids may cause a reduction in growth velocity in pediatric patients. (In studies of orally-inhaled corticosteroids, the mean reduction in growth velocity was approximately 1 centimeter per year [range 0.3-1.8 cm per year] and appears to be related to dose and duration of exposure.) The growth of pediatric patients receiving inhaled corticosteroids, should be monitored routinely (eg, via stadiometry). To minimize the systemic effects of orally-inhaled and intranasal corticosteroids, each patient should be titrated to the lowest effective dose.

May suppress the immune system, patients may be more susceptible to infection. Use with caution in patients with systemic infections or ocular herpes simplex. Avoid exposure to chickenpox and measles.

Use with caution in patients with hypothyroidism, cirrhosis, ulcerative colitis; do not use occlusive dressings on weeping or exudative lesions and general caution with occlusive dressings should be observed; discontinue if skin irritation or contact dermatitis should occur; do not use in patients with decreased skin circulation.

Pregnancy risk C.

Drug Interactions

Cytochrome P450 Effect: Inhibits CYP3A4

Decreased Effect: May induce cytochrome P450 enzymes, which may lead to decreased effect of any drug metabolized by P450 (ie, barbiturates, phenytoin, rifampin). Decreased effectiveness of salicylates when taken with betamethasone.

Increased Effect/Toxicity: Inhibitors of CYP3A4 (including erythromycin, diltiazem, itraconazole, ketoconazole, quinidine, and verapamil) may decrease metabolism of betamethasone.

Nutritional/Ethanol Interactions

Ethanol: Avoid ethanol (may enhance gastric mucosal irritation).

Food: Betamethasone interferes with calcium absorption.

Herb/Nutraceutical: Avoid cat's claw, echinacea (have immunostimulant properties).

Adverse Reactions

Systemic:

>10%:

Central nervous system: Insomnia, nervousness

Gastrointestinal: Increased appetite, indigestion

1% to 10%:

Central nervous system: Dizziness or lightheadedness, headache

Dermatologic: Hirsutism, hypopigmentation

Endocrine & metabolic: Diabetes mellitus

Neuromuscular & skeletal: Arthralgia

Ocular: Cataracts, glaucoma

Respiratory: Epistaxis

Miscellaneous: Diaphoresis

<1% (Limited to important or life-threatening): Alkalosis, amenorrhea, Cushing's syndrome, delirium, euphoria, glucose intolerance, growth suppression, hallucinations, hyperglycemia, hypokalemia, pituitary-adrenal (HPA) axis suppression, pseudotumor cerebri, psychoses, seizures, sodium and water retention, vertigo

Topical:

1% to 10%:

Dermatologic: Itching, allergic contact dermatitis, erythema, dryness papular rashes, folliculitis, furunculosis, pustules, pyoderma, vesiculation, hyperesthesia, skin infection (secondary)

Local: Burning, irritation

<1% (Limited to important or life-threatening): Cataracts (posterior subcapsular), Cushing's syndrome, glaucoma, hypokalemic syndrome

Overdosage/Toxicology When consumed in high doses for prolonged periods, systemic hypercorticism and adrenal suppression may occur. In those cases, discontinuation of the corticosteroid should be done judiciously.

Pharmacodynamics/Kinetics

Half-Life Elimination: 6.5 hours

Time to Peak: Serum: I.V.: 10-36 minutes

Metabolism: Hepatic

Formulations

Cream, topical, as dipropionate: 0.05% (15 g, 45 g, 60 g)

Alphatrex®, Diprosone®: 0.05% (15 g, 45 g)

Maxivate®: 0.05% (45 g)

Cream, topical, as dipropionate augmented (Diprolene® AF): 0.05% (15 g, 50 g)

Cream, topical, as valerate: 0.1% (15 g, 45 g)

Betatrex®, Valisone® [DSC]: 0.1% (15 g, 45 g)

Beta-Val®: 0.1% (15 g, 45 g)

Foam, topical, as valerate (Luxiq™): 0.12% (50 g, 100 g) [contains alcohol 60.4%]

Gel, topical, as dipropionate augmented (Diprolene®): 0.05% (15 g, 50 g)

Injection, solution, as sodium phosphate (Celestone® Phosphate): 4 mg/mL (5 mL) [equivalent to 3 mg betamethasone/mL]

Injection, suspension (Celestone® Soluspan®): Betamethasone sodium phosphate 3 mg/mL and betamethasone acetate 3 mg/mL [6 mg/mL] (5 mL)

Lotion, topical, as dipropionate: 0.05% (20 mL, 60 mL)

Alphatrex®, Maxivate®: 0.05% (60 mL)

Diprosone®: 0.05% (20 mL, 60 mL)

Lotion, topical, as dipropionate augmented (Diprolene®): 0.05% (30 mL, 60 mL)

Lotion, topical, as valerate (Beta-Val®, Betatrex®, Valisone® [DSC]): 0.1% (60 mL)

Ointment, topical, as dipropionate: 0.05% (15 g, 45 g)

Alphatrex®, Maxivate®: 0.05% (45 g)

Diprosone®: 0.05% (15 g, 45 g)

Ointment, topical, as dipropionate augmented: 0.05% (15 g, 45 g, 50 g)

Diprolene®: 0.05% (15 g, 50 g)

Ointment, topical, as valerate (Betatrex®, Valisone® [DSC]): 0.1% (15 g, 45 g)

Syrup, as base (Celestone®): 0.6 mg/5 mL (118 mL)

Tablet, as base (Celestone®): 0.6 mg

Dosing

Adults: Base dosage on severity of disease and patient response

Inflammatory conditions:

Oral: 2.4-4.8 mg/day in 2-4 doses; range: 0.6-7.2 mg/day

I.M.: Betamethasone sodium phosphate and betamethasone acetate: 0.6-9 mg/day (generally, 1/3 to 1/2 of oral dose) divided every 12-24 hours

Psoriasis (scalp): Topical (foam): Apply twice daily, once in the morning and once at night to scalp.

Rheumatoid arthritis/osteoarthritis:

Intrabursal, intra-articular, intradermal: 0.25-2 mL

Intralesional:

Very large joints: 1-2 mL

Large joints: 1 mL

Medium joints: 0.5-1 mL

Small joints: 0.25-0.5 mL

Steroid-responsive dermatoses: Topical: Apply thin film 2-4 times/day. Therapy should be discontinued when control is achieved; if no improvement is seen, reassessment of diagnosis may be necessary.

Elderly: Refer to adult dosing. Use the lowest effective dose.

Pediatrics: Base dosage on severity of disease and patient response.

Inflammatory conditions: **Note:** Use lowest dose listed as initial dose for adrenocortical insufficiency (physiologic replacement).

I.M.: 0.0175-0.125 mg base/kg/day divided every 6-12 hours **or** 0.5-7.5 mg base/m^2/day divided every 6-12 hours

Oral: 0.0175-0.25 mg/kg/day divided every 6-8 hours **or** 0.5-7.5 mg/m^2/day divided every 6-8 hours

Topical:

≤12 years: Use is not recommended.

>12 years: Apply a thin film twice daily; use minimal amount for shortest period of time to avoid HPA axis suppression

Administration

Oral: Not for alternate day therapy; once daily doses should be given in the morning.

I.M.: Do **not** give injectable sodium phosphate/acetate suspension I.V.

Topical: Apply topical sparingly to areas. Not for use on broken skin or in areas of infection. Do not apply to wet skin unless directed. Do not apply to face or inguinal area. Do not cover with occlusive dressing.

Monitoring and Teaching Issues

Physical Assessment: See Contraindications, Warnings/Precautions, and Dosing for use cautions. Assess potential for interactions with other prescriptions, OTC medications, or herbal products patient may be taking (see Drug Interactions). Assess therapeutic response, adverse effects according to indications for therapy, dose, route (systemic or topical), and duration of therapy (see Dosing, Warnings/Precautions, Adverse Reactions,

(Continued)

Betamethasone *(Continued)*

and Overdose/Toxicology). When used for long-term therapy (longer than 10-14 days) do not discontinue abruptly; decrease dosage incrementally. With systemic administration, caution patients with diabetes to monitor glucose levels closely (corticosteroids may alter glucose levels). Teach patient proper use (according to formulation), side effects and appropriate interventions, and symptoms to report (see Patient Education). **Pregnancy risk factor C** - benefits of use should outweigh possible risks. Note breast-feeding caution.

Patient Education: Inform prescriber of all prescriptions, OTC medications, or herbal products you are taking, and any allergies you have. Do not take anything new during treatment unless approved by prescriber. Take exactly as directed; do not increase dose or discontinue abruptly, consult prescriber. Take oral medication with or after meals. Avoid alcohol and limit intake of caffeine or stimulants. Prescriber may recommend increased dietary vitamins, minerals, or iron. If diabetic, monitor glucose levels closely (antidiabetic medication may need to be adjusted). Inform prescriber if you are experiencing greater than normal levels of stress (medication may need adjustment). You may be more susceptible to infection (avoid crowds and exposure to infection and do not have any vaccination without consulting prescriber). Some forms of this medication may cause GI upset (small, frequent meals and frequent mouth care may help). Oral medication may be taken with meals to reduce GI upset. Report promptly excessive nervousness or sleep disturbances; signs of infection (eg, sore throat, unhealed injuries); excessive growth of body hair or loss of skin color; vision changes; excessive or sudden weight gain (>3 lb/week); swelling of face or extremities; difficulty breathing; muscle weakness; change in color of stools (tarry) or persistent abdominal pain; or worsening of condition or failure to improve. **Pregnancy/breast-feeding precautions:** Inform prescriber if you are or intend to become pregnant. Consult prescriber if breast-feeding.

Dietary Issues: May be taken with food to decrease GI distress.

Geriatric Considerations: Because of the risk of adverse effects, systemic corticosteroids should be used cautiously in the elderly, in the smallest possible dose, and for the shortest possible time.

Pregnancy Issues: There are no reports linking the use of betamethasone with congenital defects in the literature. Betamethasone is often used in patients with premature labor [26-34 weeks gestation] to stimulate fetal lung maturation.

Related Information

Corticosteroids Comparison, Systemic Equivalencies *on page 1572*

Betamethasone *see* Topical Corticosteroids *on page 1334*

Betamethasone and Clotrimazole (bay ta METH a sone & kloe TRIM a zole)

U.S. Brand Names Lotrisone®

Synonyms Clotrimazole and Betamethasone

Generic Available Yes: Cream

Pharmacologic Category Antifungal Agent, Topical; Corticosteroid, Topical

Pregnancy Risk Factor C

Lactation Excretion in breast milk unknown/use caution

Use Topical treatment of various dermal fungal infections (including tinea pedis, cruris, and corpora in patients ≥17 years of age)

Formulations

Cream: Betamethasone dipropionate 0.05% and clotrimazole 1% (15 g, 45 g)
Lotion: Betamethasone dipropionate 0.05% and clotrimazole 1% (30 mL)

Dosing

Adults:

Tinea corporis, tinea cruris: Topical: Massage into affected area twice daily, morning and evening. Do not use for longer than 2 weeks; re-evaluate after 1 week if no clinical improvement. Do not exceed 45 g cream/week or 45 mL lotion/week.

Tinea pedis: Topical: Massage into affected area twice daily, morning and evening. Do not use for longer than 4 weeks; re-evaluate after 2 weeks if no clinical improvement. Do not exceed 45 g cream/week or 45 mL lotion/week.

Elderly: Use with caution. Skin atrophy and skin ulceration (rare) have been reported in patients with thinning skin. Do not use for diaper dermatitis or under occlusive dressings.

Pediatrics:

Children <17 years: Do not use.
Children ≥17 years: Refer to adult dosing.

Monitoring and Teaching Issues

Physical Assessment: See individual components listed in Related Information. **Pregnancy risk factor C** - benefits of use should outweigh possible risks. Note breast-feeding caution.

Patient Education: See individual components listed in Related Information. **Pregnancy/breast-feeding precautions:** Inform prescriber if you are or intend to become pregnant. Consult prescriber if breast-feeding.

Related Information

Betamethasone *on page 160*
Clotrimazole *on page 322*

Betamethasone Dipropionate *see* Betamethasone *on page 160*
Betamethasone Dipropionate, Augmented *see* Betamethasone *on page 160*
Betamethasone Sodium Phosphate *see* Betamethasone *on page 160*
Betamethasone Valerate *see* Betamethasone *on page 160*
Betapace® *see* Sotalol *on page 1238*
Betapace AF™ *see* Sotalol *on page 1238*
Betaseron® *see* Interferon Beta-1b *on page 729*
Betatrex® *see* Betamethasone *on page 160*
Betatrex® *see* Topical Corticosteroids *on page 1334*

Beta-Val® *see* Betamethasone *on page 160*
Beta-Val® *see* Topical Corticosteroids *on page 1334*

Betaxolol (be TAKS oh lol)

U.S. Brand Names Betoptic® S; Kerlone®

Synonyms Betaxolol Hydrochloride

Generic Available Yes: Solution

Pharmacologic Category Beta Blocker, $Beta_1$ Selective

Pregnancy Risk Factor C (manufacturer); D (2nd and 3rd trimesters - expert analysis)

Lactation Oral: Enters breast milk/use caution

Use Treatment of chronic open-angle glaucoma and ocular hypertension; management of hypertension

Mechanism of Action/Effect Competitively blocks $beta_1$-receptors, with little or no effect on $beta_2$-receptors; ophthalmic reduces intraocular pressure by reducing the production of aqueous humor

Contraindications Hypersensitivity to betaxolol or any component of the formulation; sinus bradycardia; heart block greater than first-degree (except in patients with a functioning artificial pacemaker); cardiogenic shock; uncompensated cardiac failure; pulmonary edema; pregnancy (2nd and 3rd trimester)

Warnings/Precautions Administer cautiously in compensated heart failure and monitor for a worsening of the condition (efficacy has not been demonstrated in heart failure). Use caution with concurrent use of beta-blockers and either verapamil or diltiazem; bradycardia or heart block can occur. Use caution in patients with PVD (can aggravate arterial insufficiency). In general, beta-blockers should be avoided in patients with bronchospastic disease. Betaxolol, with B1 selectivity, has been used cautiously in some patients with bronchospastic disease. Use with caution in patients with diabetes, beta-blockers may mask prominent hypoglycemic symptoms. May mask signs of thyrotoxicosis. Dosage adjustment required in severe renal impairment and those on dialysis. Use care with anesthetic agents which decrease myocardial function. Beta-blocker therapy should not be withdrawn abruptly (particularly in patients with CAD), but gradually tapered to avoid acute tachycardia, hypertension, and/or ischemia. Pregnancy risk C/D (2nd and 3rd trimester).

Drug Interactions

Cytochrome P450 Effect: Substrate of **CYP1A2, 2D6**; Inhibits CYP2D6

Decreased Effect: Decreased effect of betaxolol with aluminum salts, barbiturates, calcium salts, cholestyramine, colestipol, NSAIDs, penicillins (ampicillin), rifampin, salicylates, and sulfinpyrazone due to decreased bioavailability and plasma levels. Beta-blockers may decrease the effect of sulfonylureas.

Increased Effect/Toxicity: The heart rate lowering effects of betaxolol are additive with other drugs which slow AV conduction (digoxin, verapamil, diltiazem). Reserpine increases the effects of betaxolol. Concurrent use of betaxolol may increase the effects of alpha-blockers (prazosin, terazosin), alpha-adrenergic stimulants (epinephrine, phenylephrine), and the vasoconstrictive effects of ergot alkaloids. Betaxolol may mask the tachycardia from hypoglycemia caused by insulin and oral hypoglycemics. In patients receiving concurrent therapy, the risk of hypertensive crisis is increased when either clonidine or the beta-blocker is withdrawn. Beta-blockers may increase the action or levels of ethanol, disopyramide, nondepolarizing muscle relaxants, and theophylline although the effects are difficult to predict.

Nutritional/Ethanol Interactions Herb/Nutraceutical: Avoid dong quai if using for hypertension (has estrogenic activity). Avoid ephedra, yohimbe, ginseng (may worsen hypertension). Avoid garlic (may have increased antihypertensive effect).

Adverse Reactions

Ophthalmic:

>10%: Ocular: Conjunctival hyperemia

1% to 10%:

Ocular: Anisocoria, corneal punctate keratitis, keratitis, corneal staining, decreased corneal sensitivity, eye pain, vision disturbances

Systemic:

>10%:

Central nervous system: Drowsiness, insomnia

Endocrine & metabolic: Decreased sexual ability

1% to 10%:

Cardiovascular: Bradycardia, palpitations, edema, CHF, reduced peripheral circulation

Central nervous system: Mental depression

Gastrointestinal: Diarrhea or constipation, nausea, vomiting, stomach discomfort

Respiratory: Bronchospasm

Miscellaneous: Cold extremities

<1% (Limited to important or life-threatening): Chest pain, thrombocytopenia

Overdosage/Toxicology Symptoms of significant overdose include bradycardia, hypotension, AV block, CHF, bronchospasm, hypoglycemia. Treat initially with fluids. Sympathomimetics (eg, epinephrine or dopamine), glucagon, or a pacemaker can be used to treat toxic bradycardia, asystole, and/or hypotension.

Pharmacodynamics/Kinetics

Absorption: Ophthalmic: Some systemic; Oral: ~100%

Bioavailability: Oral: 89%

Half-Life Elimination: Oral: 12-22 hours

Time to Peak: Ophthalmic: ~2 hours; Oral: 1.5-6 hours

Metabolism: Hepatic to multiple metabolites

Onset: Ophthalmic: 30 minutes; Oral: 1-1.5 hours

Duration: Ophthalmic: ≥12 hours

Formulations

Solution, ophthalmic, as hydrochloride: 0.5% (5 mL, 10 mL, 15 mL) [contains benzalkonium chloride]

(Continued)

Betaxolol *(Continued)*

Suspension, ophthalmic, as hydrochloride (Betoptic® S): 0.25% (2.5 mL, 10 mL, 15 mL) [contains benzalkonium chloride]

Tablet, as hydrochloride (Kerlone®): 10 mg, 20 mg

Dosing

Adults:

Glaucoma: Ophthalmic: Instill 1 drop twice daily.

Hypertension, angina: Oral: 10 mg/day; may increase dose to 20 mg/day after 7-14 days if desired response is not achieved

Elderly:

Ophthalmic: Refer to adult dosing.

Hypertension: Oral: Initial: 5 mg/day

Renal Impairment: Oral: Administer 5 mg/day; can increase every 2 weeks up to a maximum of 20 mg/day.

Cl_{cr} <10 mL/minute: Administer 50% of usual dose.

Administration

Other: Ophthalmic: Shake well before using. Tilt head back and instill in eye. Keep eye open and do not blink for 30 seconds. Apply gentle pressure to lacrimal sac for 1 minute. Wipe away excess from skin. Do not touch applicator to eye and do not contaminate tip of applicator.

Stability

Storage: Avoid freezing.

Monitoring Laboratory Tests Ophthalmic: Intraocular pressure

Monitoring and Teaching Issues

Physical Assessment: See Contraindications, Warnings/Precautions, and Dosing for use cautions. Assess potential for interactions with other prescriptions, OTC medications, or herbal products patient may be taking (especially products that affects cardiac function or blood pressure - see Drug Interactions). Assess results of laboratory tests, therapeutic response, and adverse effects according to indications for therapy, dose, route and duration of therapy (see Adverse Reactions and Overdose/Toxicology). Caution patients with diabetes; beta-blockers may mask prominent hypoglycemic symptoms. Teach patient proper use (according to formulation), side effects and appropriate interventions, and symptoms to report (see Patient Education). **Pregnancy risk factor C/D** - see Pregnancy Risk Factor for use cautions; benefits of use should outweigh possible risks. Note breast-feeding caution. Systemic absorption from ophthalmic instillation is minimal.

Patient Education: Inform prescriber of all prescriptions, OTC medications, or herbal products you are taking, and any allergies you have. Do not take anything new during treatment unless approved by prescriber.

Oral: Take exactly as prescribed and do not discontinue without consulting prescriber. May cause dizziness or blurred vision (use caution when driving engaging in tasks requiring alertness until response to drug is known); or nausea or vomiting (small, frequent meals, frequent mouth care, sucking lozenges, or chewing gum may help). Report chest pain, palpitations or irregular heartbeat; persistent GI upset (eg, nausea, vomiting, diarrhea, or constipation); unusual cough; difficulty breathing; swelling or coolness of extremities; or unusual mental depression.

Ophthalmic: Shake suspension well before using. Tilt head back and instill in eye. Keep eye open; do not blink for 30 seconds. Apply gentle pressure to corner of eye for 1 minute. Wipe away excess from skin. Do not let tip of applicator touch eye; do not contaminate tip of applicator (may cause eye infection, eye damage, or vision loss). Report if condition does not improve or if you experience eye pain, vision changes, or other adverse eye response. **Pregnancy/breast-feeding precautions:** Inform prescriber if you are or intend to become pregnant. Consult prescriber if breast-feeding.

Geriatric Considerations: Oral: Due to alterations in the beta-adrenergic autonomic nervous system, beta-adrenergic blockade may result in less hemodynamic response than seen in younger adults.

Related Information

Beta-Blockers *on page 1561*

Glaucoma Drug Comparison *on page 1575*

Betaxolol *see* Ophthalmic Agents, Glaucoma *on page 1002*

Betaxolol Hydrochloride *see* Betaxolol *on page 163*

Betaxon® *see* Ophthalmic Agents, Glaucoma *on page 1002*

Bethanechol (be THAN e kole)

U.S. Brand Names Urecholine®

Synonyms Bethanechol Chloride

Generic Available No

Pharmacologic Category Cholinergic Agonist

Pregnancy Risk Factor C

Lactation Excretion in breast milk unknown/contraindicated

Use Nonobstructive urinary retention and retention due to neurogenic bladder

Use - Unlabeled/Investigational Treatment and prevention of bladder dysfunction caused by phenothiazines; diagnosis of flaccid or atonic neurogenic bladder; gastroesophageal reflux

Mechanism of Action/Effect Stimulates cholinergic receptors in the smooth muscle of the urinary bladder and GI tract resulting in increased peristalsis, increased GI and pancreatic secretions, bladder muscle contraction, and increased ureteral peristaltic waves

Contraindications Hypersensitivity to bethanechol or any component of the formulation; mechanical obstruction of the GI or GU tract or when the strength or integrity of the GI or bladder wall is in question; hyperthyroidism, peptic ulcer disease, epilepsy, obstructive pulmonary disease, bradycardia, vasomotor instability, atrioventricular conduction defects, hypotension, or parkinsonism

Warnings/Precautions Potential for reflux infection if the sphincter fails to relax as bethanechol contracts the bladder; safety and efficacy in children have not been established; syringe containing atropine should be readily available for treatment of serious side effects. Pregnancy risk C.

Drug Interactions

Decreased Effect: Procainamide, quinidine may decrease the effects of bethanechol. Anticholinergic agents (atropine, antihistamines, TCAs, phenothiazines) may decrease effects.

Increased Effect/Toxicity: Bethanechol and ganglionic blockers may cause a critical fall in blood pressure. Cholinergic drugs or anticholinesterase agents may have additive effects with bethanechol.

Effects on Lab Values ↑ lipase, AST, amylase (S), bilirubin, aminotransferase [ALT (SGPT)/AST (SGOT)] (S)

Adverse Reactions Frequency not defined.

Cardiovascular: Hypotension, tachycardia, flushed skin
Central nervous system: Headache, malaise
Gastrointestinal: Abdominal cramps, diarrhea, nausea, vomiting, salivation, eructation
Genitourinary: Urinary urgency
Ocular: Lacrimation, miosis
Respiratory: Asthmatic attacks, bronchial constriction
Miscellaneous: Diaphoresis

Overdosage/Toxicology Symptoms of overdose include nausea, vomiting, abdominal cramps, diarrhea, involuntary defecation, flushed skin, hypotension, and bronchospasm. Treat symptomatically; atropine for severe muscarinic symptoms, epinephrine to reverse severe cardiovascular or pulmonary sequelae.

Pharmacodynamics/Kinetics

Absorption: Variable

Onset: 30-90 minutes

Duration: Up to 6 hours

Formulations Tablet, as chloride: 5 mg, 10 mg, 25 mg, 50 mg

Dosing

Adults:

Urinary retention, neurogenic bladder, and/or bladder atony:

Oral: Initial: 10-50 mg 2-4 times/day (some patients may require dosages of 50-100 mg 4 times/day). To determine effective dose, may initiate at a dose of 5-10 mg, with additional doses of 5-10 mg hourly until an effective cumulative dose is reached. Cholinergic effects at higher oral dosages may be cumulative.

S.C.: Initial: 2.575 mg, may repeat in 15-30 minutes (maximum cumulative initial dose: 10.3 mg); subsequent doses may be given 3-4 times daily as needed (some patients may require more frequent dosing at 2.5- to 3-hour intervals). Chronic neurogenic atony may require doses of 7.5-10 every 4 hours.

Gastroesophageal reflux (unlabeled): Oral: 25 mg 4 times/day

Elderly: Use the lowest effective dose.

Pediatrics:

Urinary retention (unlabeled use): Oral: 0.6 mg/kg/day divided 3-4 times/day

Gastroesophageal reflux (unlabeled use): Oral: 0.1-0.2 mg/kg/dose given 30 minutes to 1 hour before each meal to a maximum of 4 times/day

Stability

Storage: Store at room temperature of 15°C to 30°C (59°F to 86°F).

Monitoring and Teaching Issues

Physical Assessment: Assess bladder and sphincter adequacy prior to administering medication. Assess other medications patient may be taking for effectiveness and interactions (see Drug Interactions). See Contraindications and Warnings/Precautions for use cautions. Monitor laboratory tests, therapeutic effect, and adverse reactions (see Warnings/Precautions, Adverse Reactions, and Overdose/Toxicology). Assess knowledge/teach patient appropriate use, interventions to reduce side effects, and adverse symptoms to report (see Patient Education). **Pregnancy risk factor C** - benefits of use should outweigh possible risks. Breast-feeding is contraindicated.

Patient Education: Take as directed, on an empty stomach to avoid nausea or vomiting. Do not discontinue without consulting prescriber. Maintain adequate hydration (2-3 L/day of fluids) unless advised by prescriber to restrict fluids. May cause dizziness or hypotension (rise slowly from sitting or lying position and use caution when driving or climbing stairs); or vomiting or loss of appetite (small, frequent meals, frequent mouth care, sucking lozenges, or chewing gum may help). Report persistent abdominal discomfort; significantly increased salivation, sweating, tearing, or urination; flushed skin; chest pain or palpitations; acute headache; unresolved diarrhea; excessive fatigue, insomnia, dizziness, or depression; increased muscle, joint, or body pain; vision changes or blurred vision; or difficulty breathing or wheezing. **Pregnancy/breast-feeding precautions:** Inform prescriber if you are or intend to become pregnant. Do not breast-feed.

Dietary Issues: Should be taken 1 hour before meals or 2 hours after meals.

Geriatric Considerations: Urinary incontinence in an elderly patient should be investigated. Bethanechol may be used for overflow incontinence (dribbling) caused by an atonic or hypotonic bladder, but clinical efficacy is variable (see Contraindications, Warnings/Precautions, and Adverse Reactions).

Bethanechol Chloride *see* Bethanechol *on page 164*
Betimol® *see* Timolol *on page 1322*
Betoptic® S *see* Betaxolol *on page 163*
Betoptic® S *see* Ophthalmic Agents, Glaucoma *on page 1002*

Bexarotene (beks AIR oh teen)

U.S. Brand Names Targretin®

Generic Available No

(Continued)

Bexarotene *(Continued)*

Pharmacologic Category Antineoplastic Agent, Miscellaneous

Pregnancy Risk Factor X

Lactation Excretion in breast milk unknown/contraindicated

Use

Oral: Treatment of cutaneous manifestations of cutaneous T-cell lymphoma in patients who are refractory to at least one prior systemic therapy

Topical: Treatment of cutaneous lesions in patients with cutaneous T-cell lymphoma (stage 1A and 1B) who have refractory or persistent disease after other therapies or who have not tolerated other therapies

Mechanism of Action/Effect Exact mechanism in is unknown. Acts to inhibit the growth of some tumor cell lines of hematopoietic and squamous cell origin.

Contraindications Hypersensitivity to bexarotene or any component of the formulation; pregnancy

Warnings/Precautions Induces major lipid abnormalities in a majority of patients (triglyceride, total cholesterol, and HDL); reversible on discontinuation. Use extreme caution in patients with underlying hypertriglyceridemia. Pancreatitis secondary to hypertriglyceridemia has been reported. Monitor for liver function test abnormalities and discontinue drug if tests are three times the upper limit of normal values for AST (SGOT), ALT (SGPT) or bilirubin. Hypothyroidism occurs in about a third of patients. Monitor for signs and symptoms of infection about 4-8 weeks after initiation (leukopenia may occur). Any new visual abnormalities experienced by the patient should be evaluated by an ophthalmologist (cataracts can form, or worsen, especially in the geriatric population). May cause photosensitization. Safety and efficacy are not established in the pediatric population. Avoid use in hepatically impaired patients. Limit additional vitamin A intake to <15,000 int. units/day. Use caution with diabetic patients: monitor for hypoglycemia.

Drug Interactions

Cytochrome P450 Effect: Substrate of CYP3A4

Decreased Effect: Bexarotene plasma levels may be decreased by rifampin, phenytoin, phenobarbital, or nafcillin.

Increased Effect/Toxicity: Bexarotene plasma concentrations may be increased by azole antifungals, clarithromycin, erythromycin, fluvoxamine, nefazodone, quinine, ritonavir, gemfibrozil, or grapefruit juice.

Nutritional/Ethanol Interactions

Food: Take with a fat-containing meal. Bexarotene serum levels may be increased by grapefruit juice; avoid concurrent use.

Herb/Nutraceutical: Avoid dong quai, St John's wort (may also cause photosensitization). Additional vitamin A supplements may lead to vitamin A toxicity (dry skin, irritation, arthralgias, myalgias, abdominal pain, hepatic changes). St John's wort may decrease bexarotene levels.

Adverse Reactions First percentage is at a dose of 300 mg/m²/day; the second percentage is at a dose >300 mg/m²/day. Grade 3 and grade 4 events that occurred more frequently in patients at both doses were hyperlipidemia, hypertriglyceridemia, pruritus, headache, peripheral edema, leukopenia, rash, and hypercholesterolemia. Frequency of events was dose-related.

>10%:

- Cardiovascular: Peripheral edema (13% to 11%)
- Central nervous system: Headache (30% to 42%), chills (10% to 13%)
- Dermatologic: Rash (17% to 23%), exfoliative dermatitis (10% to 28%)
- Endocrine & metabolic: Hyperlipidemia (about 79% in both dosing ranges), hypercholesteremia (32% to 62%), hypothyroidism (29% to 53%)
- Hematologic: Leukopenia (17% to 47%)
- Neuromuscular & skeletal: Weakness (20% to 45%)
- Miscellaneous: Infection (13% to 23%)

<10% (Limited to important or life-threatening):

- Cardiovascular: Hemorrhage, hypertension, angina pectoris, right heart failure, tachycardia, cerebrovascular accident
- Central nervous system: Fever (5% to 17%), insomnia (5% to 11%), subdural hematoma, syncope, depression, agitation, ataxia
- Dermatologic: Dry skin (about 10% for both dosing ranges), alopecia (4% to 11%), skin ulceration, maculopapular rash, vesicular bullous rash, cheilitis
- Endocrine & metabolic: Hypoproteinemia, hyperglycemia
- Gastrointestinal: Abdominal pain (11% to 4%), nausea (16% to 8%), diarrhea (7% to 42%), vomiting (4% to 13%), anorexia (2% to 23%), colitis, gastroenteritis, gingivitis, melena, pancreatitis
- Genitourinary: Albuminuria, hematuria, dysuria
- Hematologic: Hypochromic anemia (4% to 13%), anemia (6% to 25%), eosinophilia, thrombocythemia, coagulation time increased, lymphocytosis, thrombocytopenia
- Hepatic: LDH increase (7% to 13%), hepatic failure
- Neuromuscular & skeletal: Back pain (2% to 11%), arthralgia, myalgia, myasthenia, neuropathy
- Ocular: Conjunctivitis, blepharitis, corneal lesion, visual field defects, keratitis
- Otic: Ear pain, otitis externa
- Renal: Renal dysfunction
- Respiratory: Pharyngitis, rhinitis, dyspnea, pleural effusion, bronchitis, increased cough, lung edema, hemoptysis, hypoxia
- Miscellaneous: Flu-like syndrome (4% to 13%), infection (1% to 13%)

Topical:

- Cardiovascular: Edema (10%)
- Central nervous system: Headache (14%), weakness (6%), pain (30%)
- Dermatologic: Rash (14% to 72%), pruritus (6% to 40%), contact dermatitis (14%), exfoliative dermatitis (6%)

Hematologic: Leukopenia (6%), lymphadenopathy (6%)
Neuromuscular & skeletal: Paresthesia (6%)
Respiratory: Cough (6%), pharyngitis (6%)
Miscellaneous: Diaphoresis (6%), infection (18%)

Overdosage/Toxicology Doses up to 1000 mg/m^2/day have been used in humans without acute toxic effects. Any overdose should be treated with supportive care focused on the symptoms exhibited.

Pharmacodynamics/Kinetics

Absorption: Significantly improved by a fat-containing meal

Half-Life Elimination: 7 hours

Time to Peak: 2 hours

Metabolism: Hepatic via CYP3A4 isoenzyme; four metabolites identified; further metabolized by glucuronidation

Formulations

Capsule: 75 mg
Gel: 1% (60 g)

Dosing

Adults & Elderly:

Cutaneous T-cell lymphoma (in patients who are refractory to at least one prior systemic therapy):

Oral: 300 mg/m^2/day taken as a single daily dose. If there is no tumor response after 8 weeks and the initial dose was well tolerated, then an increase to 400 mg/m^2/day can be made with careful monitoring. Maintain as long as the patient is deriving benefit. If the initial dose is not tolerated, then it may be adjusted to 200 mg/m^2/day, then to 100 mg/m^2/day or temporarily suspended if necessary to manage toxicity.

Cutaneous lesions of T-cell lymphoma: Topical (gel): Apply to lesions once every other day for first week, then increase on a weekly basis to once daily, 2 times/day, 3 times/day, and finally 4 times/day, according to tolerance.

Renal Impairment: No studies have been conducted; however, renal insufficiency may result in significant protein binding changes and alter pharmacokinetics of bexarotene.

Hepatic Impairment: No studies have been conducted; however, hepatic impairment would be expected to result in decreased clearance of bexarotene due to the extensive hepatic contribution to elimination.

Stability

Storage: Store at 2°C to 25°C (36°F to 77°F). Protect from light.

Monitoring Laboratory Tests If female, pregnancy test 1 week before initiation then monthly while on bexarotene; lipid panel before initiation, then weekly until lipid response established and then at 8-week intervals thereafter; baseline LFTs, repeat at 1, 2, and 4 weeks after initiation then at 8-week intervals thereafter if stable; baseline and periodic thyroid function tests; baseline CBC with periodic monitoring

Monitoring and Teaching Issues

Physical Assessment: See Contraindications, Warnings/Precautions, and Dosing for use cautions. Assess potential for interactions with other prescriptions, OTC medications, or herbal products patient may be taking (see Drug Interactions). Assess results of laboratory tests, therapeutic response (reduction of cutaneous lesions), and adverse reactions (eg, CNS or cardiovascular effects, opportunistic infection, visual abnormalities, hypoglycemia - see Warnings/Precautions, Adverse Reactions, and Overdose/Toxicology). Teach patient proper use (according to formulation), side effects and appropriate interventions, and symptoms to report (see Patient Education). **Pregnancy risk factor X** - determine that patient is not pregnant before beginning treatment (see Monitoring Laboratory Tests). Instruct patients of childbearing age and males who may have intercourse with females of childbearing age about appropriate use of barrier contraceptives 1 month prior to, during, and 1 month following treatment. Breast-feeding is contraindicated.

Patient Education: Inform prescriber of all prescriptions, OTC medications, or herbal products you are taking, and any allergies you have. Do not take anything new during treatment unless approved by prescriber. Maintain hydration (2-3 L/day of fluids) unless advised by prescriber to restrict fluids. You may be more susceptible to infection (avoid crowds and exposure to infection and do not have any vaccinations without consulting prescriber). May cause nausea, vomiting, anorexia, flatulence (frequent, small meals, good mouth care, chewing gum, or sucking lozenges may help); constipation (increased exercise, fluid, fruit, or fiber may help); diarrhea (buttermilk, boiled milk, or yogurt may help); headache, back or muscle pain (consult prescriber for mild analgesic); or photosensitivity (avoid direct sunlight, wear protective clothing and hat, use sunblock, and protective eyewear). Report chest pain, rapid heartbeat; unresolved GI effects; headache, back or muscle pain; skin dryness, skin rash or peeling; mucous membrane lesions; altered urinary patterns; flu syndrome or opportunistic infection (eg, weakness, fatigue, white plaques or sores in mouth, vaginal discharge, chills, fever); CNS disturbances (insomnia, dizziness, agitation, confusion, depression); vision or hearing changes; or any other adverse effects.

Oral: Take exactly as directed, at the same time each day with a fat-containing meal. If you miss a dose, take as soon as possible. If it is almost time for next dose, skip the missed dose and continue on regular schedule. Do not double doses.

Topical: Allow gel to dry before covering. Avoid applying to normal skin or mucous membranes. Do not use occlusive dressings.

Pregnancy/breast-feeding precautions: Pregnancy test is needed 1 week before initiation of therapy and every month during therapy. Consult prescriber for appropriate barrier contraceptives. Effective contraception must be in place 1 month before initiation, during therapy, and for at least 1 month after discontinuation. Male patients with sexual partners who are pregnant, possibly pregnant, or who could become pregnant, must use condoms when having sexual intercourse while using this medication and for 1 month after last dose. Do not breast-feed.

Pregnancy Issues: Bexarotene caused birth defects when administered orally to pregnant rats. It must not be given to a pregnant woman or a woman who intends to become

(Continued)

Bexarotene *(Continued)*

pregnant. If a woman becomes pregnant while taking the drug, it must be stopped immediately and appropriate counseling be given.

Bextra® *see* Valdecoxib *on page 1379*

Biavax® II *see page 1498*

Biaxin® *see* Clarithromycin *on page 304*

Biaxin® XL *see* Clarithromycin *on page 304*

Bicalutamide (bye ka LOO ta mide)

U.S. Brand Names Casodex®

Generic Available No

Pharmacologic Category Antineoplastic Agent, Antiandrogen

Pregnancy Risk Factor X

Lactation Excretion in breast milk unknown

Use In combination therapy with LHRH agonist analogues in treatment of advanced prostatic carcinoma

Mechanism of Action/Effect Nonsteroidal antiandrogen that inhibits androgen uptake or inhibits binding of androgen in target tissues

Contraindications Hypersensitivity to bicalutamide or any component of the formulation; not for use in women, particularly in nonserious or nonlife-threatening conditions; pregnancy

Warnings/Precautions Rare cases of death or hospitalization due to hepatitis have been reported postmarketing. Use with caution in moderate to severe hepatic dysfunction. Hepatotoxicity generally occurs within the first 3-4 months of use. Baseline liver function tests should be obtained and repeated regularly during the first 4 months of treatment, and periodically thereafter. Additionally, patients should be monitored for signs and symptoms of liver dysfunction. Bicalutamide should be discontinued if patients have jaundice or ALT is two times the upper limit of normal. May cause gynecomastia in a high percentage of patients.

Drug Interactions

Increased Effect/Toxicity: Bicalutamide may displace warfarin from protein binding sites which may result in an increased anticoagulant effect, especially when bicalutamide therapy is started after the patient is already on warfarin.

Adverse Reactions

10%:

- Cardiovascular: Flushing (hot flashes), chest pain
- Gastrointestinal: Abdominal pain, constipation, nausea
- Neuromuscular & skeletal: Weakness
- Miscellaneous: Pain (general)

1% to 10%:

- Cardiovascular: Hypertension, chest pain pectoris, CHF, edema, peripheral edema
- Central nervous system: Anxiety, headache, dizziness, depression, confusion, somnolence, nervousness, fever, chills, insomnia
- Dermatologic: Dry skin, pruritus, alopecia, rash
- Endocrine & metabolic: Breast pain, diabetes mellitus (hyperglycemia), decreased libido, dehydration, gout, impotency
- Gastrointestinal: Diarrhea, vomiting, anorexia, heartburn, rectal hemorrhage, dry mouth, melena, weight gain/loss
- Genitourinary: Polyuria, urinary impairment, dysuria, urinary retention, urinary urgency
- Hematologic: Anemia
- Hepatic: Alkaline phosphatase increased
- Neuromuscular & skeletal: Muscle weakness, arthritis, myalgia, leg cramps, pathological fracture, neck pain, hypertonia, neuropathy
- Renal: Creatinine increased
- Respiratory: Cough increased, dyspnea, pharyngitis, bronchitis, pneumonia, rhinitis, lung disorder
- Miscellaneous: Sepsis, neoplasma

Overdosage/Toxicology Symptoms of overdose include hypoactivity, ataxia, anorexia, vomiting, slow respiration, and lacrimation. Management is supportive. Dialysis is of no benefit.

Pharmacodynamics/Kinetics

Absorption: Rapid and complete

Half-Life Elimination: Up to 10 days; active enantiomer 5.8 days

Metabolism: Extensively hepatic; stereospecific metabolism

Formulations Tablet: 50 mg

Dosing

Adults & Elderly: Advanced prostatic carcinoma: Oral: 50 mg once daily (morning or evening), with or without food. It is recommended that bicalutamide be taken at the same time each day; start treatment with bicalutamide at the same time as treatment with an LHRH analog.

Hepatic Impairment: Limited data in subjects with severe hepatic impairment suggest that excretion of bicalutamide may be delayed and could lead to further accumulation. Use with caution in patients with moderate to severe hepatic impairment.

Administration

Oral: Dose should be taken at the same time each day with or without food.

Stability

Storage: Store at room temperature.

Monitoring Laboratory Tests Liver function tests should be obtained at baseline and repeated regularly during the first 4 months of treatment, and periodically thereafter (in addition to monitoring signs/symptoms of liver dysfunction). Discontinue if jaundice is noted or ALT is two or more times the upper limit of normal. Also monitor serum prostate-specific antigen, alkaline phosphatase, acid phosphatase, or prostatic acid phosphatase; prostate gland dimensions; skeletal survey; liver scans; chest x-rays; bone scan every 3-6 months; CBC, EKG, echocardiograms, and serum testosterone and luteinizing hormone (periodically).

Monitoring and Teaching Issues

Physical Assessment: See Contraindications, Warnings/Precautions, and Drug Interactions for use cautions. Assess potential for interactions with other prescriptions, OTC medications, or herbal products patient may be taking (see Drug Interactions). Assess results of laboratory tests (see above), therapeutic effectiveness, and adverse response (see Adverse Reactions and Overdose/Toxicology). Advise diabetics to monitor glucose levels closely (may induce hyperglycemia). Teach patient appropriate use, possible side effects and appropriate interventions, and adverse symptoms to report (see Patient Education). **Pregnancy risk factor X** - instruct patient on absolute need for barrier contraceptives.

Patient Education: Inform prescriber of all prescriptions, OTC medications, or herbal products you are taking, and any allergies you have. Do not take anything new during treatment unless approved by prescriber. Take as directed, at the same time each day with or without food. Do not alter dose or discontinue without consulting prescriber. Void before taking medication. If diabetic, monitor serum glucose closely and notify prescriber of changes (this medication may alter glucose levels). May cause dizziness, confusion, or drowsiness (use caution when driving or engaging in tasks that require alertness until response to drug is known); nausea or vomiting (small, frequent meals, frequent mouth care, sucking lozenges, or chewing gum may help); constipation (increased exercise, fluids, fruit, or fiber may help); hair loss; or impotence. Report easy bruising or bleeding; yellowing of skin or eyes; change in color of urine or stool; unresolved CNS changes (eg, nervousness, chills, insomnia, somnolence); skin rash, redness, or irritation; chest pain or palpitations; difficulty breathing; urinary retention or inability to void; muscle weakness, tremors, or pain; persistent nausea, vomiting, diarrhea, constipation; or other unusual signs or adverse reactions. **Pregnancy/breast-feeding precautions:** This drug will cause fetal abnormalities - consult prescriber for effective contraceptives. Inform prescriber if breast-feeding.

Dietary Issues: May be taken with or without food.

Geriatric Considerations: Renal impairment has no clinically significant changes in elimination of the parent compound or active metabolite; therefore, no dosage adjustment is needed in the elderly. In dosage studies, no difference was found between young adults and elderly with regard to steady-state serum concentrations for bicalutamide and its active R-enantiomer metabolite.

Bicillin® L-A *see* Penicillin G Benzathine *on page 1043*

Bicitra® *see* Sodium Citrate and Citric Acid *on page 1236*

BiCNU® *see* Carmustine *on page 223*

Bimatoprost *see page 1575*

Bimatoprost *see* Ophthalmic Agents, Glaucoma *on page 1002*

Biocef *see* Cephalexin *on page 259*

BioCox® *see page 1461*

Bio-Statin® *see* Nystatin *on page 989*

Bismatrol® [OTC] *see* Bismuth *on page 169*

Bismuth (BIZ muth)

U.S. Brand Names Bismatrol® [OTC]; Colo-Fresh™ [OTC]; Diotame® [OTC]; Pepto-Bismol® [OTC]; Pepto-Bismol® Maximum Strength [OTC]

Synonyms Bismuth Subgallate; Bismuth Subsalicylate; Pink Bismuth

Generic Available Yes

Pharmacologic Category Antidiarrheal

Pregnancy Risk Factor C/D (3rd trimester)

Lactation Excretion in breast milk unknown (salicylates enter breast milk)/use caution

Use Symptomatic treatment of mild, nonspecific diarrhea; indigestion, nausea, control of traveler's diarrhea (enterotoxigenic *Escherichia coli*); as part of a multidrug regimen for *H. pylori* eradication to reduce the risk of duodenal ulcer recurrence; subgallate formulation to control fecal odors in colostomy, ileostomy, or fecal incontinence

Mechanism of Action/Effect Bismuth subsalicylate exhibits both antisecretory and antimicrobial action. This agent may provide some anti-inflammatory action as well. The salicylate moiety provides antisecretory effect and the bismuth exhibits antimicrobial directly against bacterial and viral gastrointestinal pathogens. Bismuth has some antacid properties.

Contraindications Do not use subsalicylate in patients with influenza or chickenpox because of risk of Reye's syndrome; hypersensitivity to salicylates or any component of the formulation; history of severe GI bleeding; history of coagulopathy; pregnancy (3rd trimester)

Warnings/Precautions Subsalicylate should be used with caution if patient is taking aspirin. Use with caution in children, especially those <3 years of age and those with viral illness. May be neurotoxic with very large doses. Pregnancy factor C/D (3rd trimester).

Drug Interactions

Decreased Effect: The effects of tetracyclines and uricosurics may be decreased.

Increased Effect/Toxicity: Toxicity of aspirin, warfarin, and/or hypoglycemics may be increased.

Effects on Lab Values ↑ uric acid, AST; may interfere with radiologic tests since bismuth is radiopaque.

Adverse Reactions

>10%: Gastrointestinal: Discoloration of the tongue (darkening), grayish black stools

<1% (Limited to important or life-threatening): Anxiety, confusion, headache, hearing loss, impaction may occur in infants and debilitated patients, mental depression, muscle spasms, slurred speech, tinnitus, weakness

Overdosage/Toxicology

Symptoms of toxicity:

Subsalicylate: Hyperpnea, nausea, vomiting, tinnitus, hyperpyrexia, metabolic acidoses/respiratory alkalosis, tachycardia, and confusion; seizures in severe overdose,

(Continued)

Bismuth *(Continued)*

pulmonary or cerebral edema, respiratory failure, cardiovascular collapse, coma, and death. **Note:** Each 262.4 mg tablet of bismuth subsalicylate contains an equivalent of 130 mg aspirin (150 mg/kg of aspirin is considered to be toxic; serious life-threatening toxicity occurs with >300mg/kg)

Bismuth: Rare with short-term administrations of bismuth salts; encephalopathy, methemoglobinemia, seizures

Treatment: Gastrointestinal decontamination (activated charcoal for immediate release formulations (10 x dose of ASA in g), whole bowel irrigation for enteric coated tablets or when serially increasing ASA plasma levels indicate the presence of an intestinal bezoar), supportive and symptomatic treatment with emphasis on correcting fluid, electrolyte, blood glucose and acid-base disturbances; elimination is enhanced with urinary alkalinization (sodium bicarbonate infusion with potassium), multiple dose activated charcoal, and hemodialysis. Chelation with dimercaprol in doses of 3 mg/kg or penicillamine 100 mg/kg/day for 5 days can hasten recovery from bismuth-induced encephalopathy; methylene blue 1-2 mg/kg in a 1% sterile aqueous solution I.V. push over 4-6 minutes for methemoglobinemia. This may be repeated within 60 minutes if necessary, up to a total dose of 7 mg/kg. Seizures usually respond to I.V. diazepam.

Pharmacodynamics/Kinetics

Absorption: Minimal (<1%) across GI tract, salt (eg, salicylate) may be readily absorbed (80%); bismuth subsalicylate is rapidly cleaved to bismuth and salicylic acid in the stomach

Half-Life Elimination: Terminal: Bismuth: 21-72 days; Salicylate: 2-5 hours

Metabolism: Bismuth: Oral: Salts undergo chemical dissociation; Salicylate: Extensively hepatic

Formulations

Liquid, as subsalicylate: 262 mg/15 mL (240 mL, 360 mL, 480 mL); 525 mg/15 mL (240 mL, 360 mL)

Bismatrol®: 262 mg/15 mL (240 mL)

Diotame®: 262 mg/15 mL (30 mL)

Pepto-Bismol®: 262 mg/15 mL (120 mL, 240 mL, 360 mL, 480 mL) [wintergreen flavor]

Pepto-Bismol® Maximum Strength: 525 mg/15 mL (120 mL, 240 mL, 360 mL) [wintergreen flavor]

Tablet, as subgallate (Colo-Fresh™): 324 mg

Tablet, chewable, as subsalicylate (Diaotame®, Bismatrol®, Pepto-Bismol®): 262 mg

Dosing

Adults & Elderly:

Nonspecific diarrhea: Subsalicylate: Oral: 2 tablets or 30 mL every 30 minutes to 1 hour as needed up to 8 doses/24 hours

Prevention of traveler's diarrhea: Oral: 2.1 g/day or 2 tablets 4 times/day before meals and at bedtime

Helicobacter pylori eradication: Oral: 524 mg 4 times/day with meals and at bedtime; requires combination therapy

Control of fecal odor in ileostomy or colostomy: Subgallate: Oral: 1-2 tablets 3 times/day with meals (maximum: 5 tablets/day)

Pediatrics:

Nonspecific diarrhea: Subsalicylate:

Children: Up to 8 doses/24 hours:

3-6 years: 1/3 tablet or 5 mL (regular strength) every 30 minutes to 1 hour as needed

6-9 years: 2/3 tablet or 10 mL (regular strength) every 30 minutes to 1 hour as needed

9-12 years: 1 tablet or 15 mL (regular strength) every 30 minutes to 1 hour as needed

Renal Impairment: Should probably be avoided in patients with renal impairment.

Monitoring and Teaching Issues

Physical Assessment: See Contraindications and Warnings/Precautions for use cautions. Assess potential for interactions with other prescriptions, OTC medications, or herbal products patient may be taking (eg, aspirin products - see Drug Interactions). Assess therapeutic effectiveness and adverse response (see Adverse Reactions and Overdose/Toxicology). Teach patient appropriate use, possible side effects and appropriate interventions, and adverse symptoms to report (see Patient Education). **Pregnancy risk factor C/D** - see Pregnancy Risk Factor for use cautions. Instruct patient in appropriate use of contraceptives. Note breast-feeding caution.

Patient Education: Inform prescriber of all prescriptions, OTC medications, or herbal products you are taking, and any allergies you have. Do not take anything new during treatment unless approved by prescriber. Chew tablet well or shake suspension well before using. May darken stools and turn tongue black. If diarrhea persists for more than 2 days, consult healthcare provider. If tinnitus (ringing in the ears) occurs this may indicate toxicity; discontinue use and notify healthcare provider. **Pregnancy/breast-feeding precautions:** Do not get pregnant while taking this medication. Consult prescriber for appropriate contraceptive measures. Consult prescriber if breast-feeding.

Related Information

Helicobacter pylori Treatment *on page 1676*

Bismuth Subgallate *see* Bismuth *on page 169*

Bismuth Subsalicylate *see* Bismuth *on page 169*

Bismuth Subsalicylate, Metronidazole, and Tetracycline

(BIZ muth sub sa LIS i late, me troe NI da zole, & tet ra SYE kleen)

U.S. Brand Names Helidac®

Synonyms Bismuth Subsalicylate, Tetracycline, and Metronidazole; Metronidazole, Bismuth Subsalicylate, and Tetracycline; Metronidazole, Tetracycline, and Bismuth Subsalicylate; Tetracycline, Bismuth Subsalicylate, and Metronidazole; Tetracycline, Metronidazole, and Bismuth Subsalicylate

Generic Available No

Pharmacologic Category Antibiotic, Tetracycline Derivative; Antidiarrheal

Pregnancy Risk Factor D (tetracycline); B (metronidazole)

Lactation Enters breast milk/contraindicated

Use In combination with an H_2 antagonist, as part of a multidrug regimen for *H. pylori* eradication to reduce the risk of duodenal ulcer recurrence

Formulations Each package contains 14 blister cards (2-week supply); each card contains the following:

Capsule: Tetracycline hydrochloride: 500 mg (4)

Tablet:

Bismuth subsalicylate [chewable]: 262.4 mg (8)

Metronidazole: 250 mg (4)

Dosing

Adults & Elderly: Duodenal ulcer associated with *H. pylori* infection: Oral: Chew 2 bismuth subsalicylate 262.4 mg tablets, swallow 1 metronidazole 250 mg tablet, and swallow 1 tetracycline 500 mg capsule plus an H_2 antagonist 4 times/day at meals and bedtime for 14 days; follow with 8 oz of water.

Monitoring and Teaching Issues

Physical Assessment: See individual components listed in Related Information. **Pregnancy risk factor B/D** - see Pregnancy Risk Factor for use cautions. Assess knowledge/instruct patient on need to use appropriate contraceptive measures and the need to avoid pregnancy. Breast-feeding is contraindicated.

Patient Education: See individual components listed in Related Information. **Pregnancy/breast-feeding precautions:** Inform prescriber if you are or intend to become pregnant. Do not breast-feed.

Related Information

Bismuth *on page 169*

Metronidazole *on page 895*

Tetracycline *on page 1296*

Bismuth Subsalicylate, Tetracycline, and Metronidazole *see* Bismuth Subsalicylate, Metronidazole, and Tetracycline *on page 170*

Bisoprolol (bis OH proe lol)

U.S. Brand Names Zebeta®

Synonyms Bisoprolol Fumarate

Generic Available Yes

Pharmacologic Category Beta Blocker, $Beta_1$ Selective

Pregnancy Risk Factor C (manufacturer); D (2nd and 3rd trimesters - expert analysis)

Lactation Enters breast milk/use caution

Use Treatment of hypertension, alone or in combination with other agents

Use - Unlabeled/Investigational Angina pectoris, supraventricular arrhythmias, PVCs

Mechanism of Action/Effect Selective inhibitor of $beta_1$-adrenergic receptors; little or no effect on $beta_2$-receptors at doses <10 mg

Contraindications Hypersensitivity to bisoprolol or any component of the formulation; sinus bradycardia; heart block greater than first-degree (except in patients with a functioning artificial pacemaker); cardiogenic shock; uncompensated cardiac failure; pulmonary edema; pregnancy (2nd and 3rd trimesters)

Warnings/Precautions Administer cautiously in compensated heart failure and monitor for a worsening of the condition. Beta-blocker therapy should not be withdrawn abruptly (particularly in patients with CAD), but gradually tapered to avoid acute tachycardia, hypertension, and/or ischemia. Use caution in patients with PVD (can aggravate arterial insufficiency). Use caution with concurrent use of beta-blockers and either verapamil or diltiazem; bradycardia or heart block can occur. In general, beta-blockers should be avoided in patients with bronchospastic disease. Bisoprolol, with B1 selectivity, has been used cautiously in bronchospastic disease with close monitoring. Use cautiously in diabetics because it can mask prominent hypoglycemic symptoms. Can mask signs of thyrotoxicosis. Can cause fetal harm when administered in pregnancy. Dosage adjustment is required in patients with significant hepatic or renal dysfunction. Use care with anesthetic agents which decrease myocardial function. Pregnancy risk C/D (2nd and 3rd trimesters).

Drug Interactions

Cytochrome P450 Effect: Substrate of CYP2D6, **3A4**

Decreased Effect: Decreased effect of bisoprolol with aluminum salts, barbiturates, calcium salts, cholestyramine, colestipol, NSAIDs, penicillins (ampicillin), rifampin, and salicylates due to decreased bioavailability and plasma levels. The effect of sulfonylureas may be decreased by beta-blockers.

Increased Effect/Toxicity: Bisoprolol may increase the effects of other drugs which slow AV conduction (digoxin, verapamil, diltiazem), alpha-blockers (prazosin, terazosin), and alpha-adrenergic stimulants (epinephrine, phenylephrine). Bisoprolol may mask the tachycardia from hypoglycemia caused by insulin and oral hypoglycemics. In patients receiving concurrent therapy, the risk of hypertensive crisis is increased when either clonidine or the beta-blocker is withdrawn. Reserpine has been shown to enhance the effect of beta-blockers. Beta-blockers may increase the action or levels of ethanol, disopyramide, nondepolarizing muscle relaxants, and theophylline although the effects are difficult to predict.

Nutritional/Ethanol Interactions Herb/Nutraceutical: Avoid dong quai if using for hypertension (has estrogenic activity). Avoid ephedra, yohimbe, ginseng (may worsen hypertension). Avoid garlic (may have increased antihypertensive effect).

Effects on Lab Values ↑ thyroxine (S), cholesterol (S), glucose, triglycerides, uric acid; ↓ HDL; possible false glucose tolerance tests

Adverse Reactions

>10%

Central nervous system: Drowsiness, insomnia

Endocrine & metabolic: Decreased sexual ability

1% to 10%:

Cardiovascular: Bradycardia, palpitations, edema, CHF, reduced peripheral circulation

(Continued)

Bisoprolol *(Continued)*

Central nervous system: Mental depression

Gastrointestinal: Diarrhea or constipation, nausea, vomiting, stomach discomfort

Ocular: Mild ocular stinging and discomfort, tearing, photophobia, decreased corneal sensitivity, keratitis

Respiratory: Bronchospasm

Miscellaneous: Cold extremities

<1% (Limited to important or life-threatening): Arrhythmias, confusion (especially in the elderly), depression, dyspnea, hallucinations, leukopenia, orthostatic hypotension, psoriasiform eruption, thrombocytopenia

Overdosage/Toxicology Symptoms of overdose include severe hypotension, bradycardia, heart failure, bronchospasm, and hypoglycemia. Treat initially with I.V. fluids. Sympathomimetics (eg, epinephrine or dopamine), glucagon, or a pacemaker can be used to treat the toxic bradycardia, asystole, and/or hypotension. Bisoprolol may be removed by hemodialysis. Other treatment is symptomatic and supportive.

Pharmacodynamics/Kinetics

Absorption: Rapid and almost complete

Half-Life Elimination: 9-12 hours

Time to Peak: 1.7-3 hours

Metabolism: Extensively hepatic; significant first-pass effect

Onset: 1-2 hours

Formulations Tablet, as fumarate: 5 mg, 10 mg

Dosing

Adults: Hypertension: Oral: 5 mg once daily, may be increased to 10 mg, and then up to 20 mg once daily, if necessary

Elderly: Oral: Initial: 2.5 mg/day; may be increased by 2.5-5 mg/day; maximum recommended dose: 20 mg/day

Renal Impairment: Oral: Initial: 2.5 mg/day; increase cautiously.

Not dialyzable

Monitoring Laboratory Tests Serum glucose regularly

Monitoring and Teaching Issues

Physical Assessment: See Contraindications and Warnings/Precautions for use cautions. Assess potential for interactions with other prescriptions, OTC medications, or herbal products patient may be taking (see Drug Interactions). Assess blood pressure and heart rate prior to and following first dose and any change in dosage. Assess for therapeutic effectiveness and adverse effects (see Adverse Reactions and Overdose/Toxicology). Instruct diabetic patients to monitor glucose levels closely (beta-blockers may alter glucose tolerance). Teach patient appropriate use, possible side effects and appropriate interventions (hypotension precautions), and adverse symptoms to report (see Patient Education). **Pregnancy risk factor C/D** - see Pregnancy Risk Factor for use cautions; benefits of use should outweigh possible risks. Note breast-feeding caution.

Patient Education: Inform prescriber of all prescriptions, OTC medications, or herbal products you are taking, and any allergies you have. Do not take anything new during treatment unless approved by prescriber. Take exactly as directed, with or without regard to meals. Do not take with antacids. Do not adjust dosage or discontinue without consulting prescriber. Take pulse daily (prior to medication) and follow prescriber's instruction about holding medication. If diabetic, monitor serum sugar closely (drug may alter glucose tolerance or mask signs of hypoglycemia). May cause fatigue, dizziness, or postural hypotension (use caution when changing position from lying or sitting to standing, when driving, or climbing stairs until response to medication is known); alteration in sexual performance (reversible); or constipation (increased dietary bulk and fluids and exercise may help). Report unresolved swelling of extremities, difficulty breathing or new cough, unresolved fatigue, unusual weight gain, unresolved constipation, or unusual muscle weakness. **Pregnancy/breast-feeding precautions:** Inform prescriber if you are or intend to become pregnant. Consult prescriber if breast-feeding.

Dietary Issues: May be taken without regard to meals.

Geriatric Considerations: Due to alterations in the beta-adrenergic autonomic nervous system, beta-adrenergic blockade may result in less hemodynamic response than seen in younger adults.

Related Information

Beta-Blockers *on page 1561*
Heart Failure *on page 1670*

Bisoprolol and Hydrochlorothiazide

(bis OH proe lol & hye droe klor oh THYE a zide)

U.S. Brand Names Ziac®

Synonyms Hydrochlorothiazide and Bisoprolol

Generic Available Yes

Pharmacologic Category Antihypertensive Agent Combination

Pregnancy Risk Factor C/D (2nd and 3rd trimesters)

Lactation Enters breast milk/use caution

Use Treatment of hypertension

Formulations Tablet:

Bisoprolol fumarate 2.5 mg and hydrochlorothiazide 6.25 mg
Bisoprolol fumarate 5 mg and hydrochlorothiazide 6.25 mg
Bisoprolol fumarate 10 mg and hydrochlorothiazide 6.25 mg

Dosing

Adults & Elderly: Hypertension: Oral: Dose is individualized, given once daily.

Hepatic Impairment: Caution should be used in dosing/titrating patients.

Monitoring and Teaching Issues

Physical Assessment: See individual components listed in Related Information. **Pregnancy risk factor C/D** - see Pregnancy Risk Factor for use cautions; benefits of use should outweigh possible risks. Note breast-feeding caution.

Patient Education: See individual components listed in Related Information. **Pregnancy/breast-feeding precautions:** Inform prescriber if you are or intend to become pregnant. Consult prescriber if breast-feeding.

Related Information

Bisoprolol *on page 171*
Hydrochlorothiazide *on page 664*

Bisoprolol Fumarate *see* Bisoprolol *on page 171*

Bitolterol (bye TOLE ter ole)

Synonyms Bitolterol Mesylate; Tornalate [DSC]

Generic Available No

Pharmacologic Category $Beta_2$ Agonist

Pregnancy Risk Factor C

Lactation Excretion in breast milk unknown

Use Prevention and treatment of bronchial asthma and bronchospasm

Mechanism of Action/Effect Selectively stimulates $beta_2$-adrenergic receptors in the lungs producing bronchial smooth muscle relaxation; minor $beta_1$ activity

Contraindications Hypersensitivity to bitolterol or any component of the formulation

Warnings/Precautions Use with caution in patients with unstable vasomotor symptoms, diabetes, hyperthyroidism, prostatic hyperplasia or a history of seizures. Also use caution in the elderly and those patients with cardiovascular disorders such as coronary artery disease, arrhythmias, and hypertension. Excessive use may result in cardiac arrest and death. Do not use concurrently with other sympathomimetic bronchodilators. Safety and efficacy have not been established in children ≤12 years of age. Pregnancy risk C.

Drug Interactions

Decreased Effect: Decreased effect with beta-adrenergic blockers (eg, propranolol).

Increased Effect/Toxicity: Increased toxicity with MAO inhibitors, tricyclic antidepressants, sympathomimetic agents (eg, amphetamine, dopamine, dobutamine), inhaled anesthetics (eg, enflurane). Increased toxicity (cardiotoxicity) with aminophylline, theophylline, or oxtriphylline.

Adverse Reactions

>10%: Neuromuscular & skeletal: Trembling

1% to 10%:

Cardiovascular: Flushing of face, hypertension, pounding heartbeat
Central nervous system: Dizziness, lightheadedness, nervousness, headache
Gastrointestinal: Dry mouth, nausea
Respiratory: Bronchial irritation, coughing

<1% (Limited to important or life-threatening): Arrhythmias, chest pain, paradoxical bronchospasm, tachycardia

Overdosage/Toxicology Symptoms of overdose include tremor, dizziness, nervousness, headache, nausea, coughing. Treatment is symptomatic/supportive. Prudent use of a cardioselective beta-adrenergic blocker (eg, atenolol or metoprolol) should be considered, keeping in mind the potential for induction of bronchoconstriction in an asthmatic individual. Dialysis has not been shown to be of value in the treatment of overdose with bitolterol.

Pharmacodynamics/Kinetics

Half-Life Elimination: 3 hours

Time to Peak: Serum (colterol): Inhalation: ~1 hour

Metabolism: Inhalation: Prodrug, hydrolyzed to colterol (active)

Onset: Rapid

Duration: 4-8 hours

Formulations

Aerosol for oral inhalation, as mesylate: 0.8% [370 mcg/metered spray; 300 inhalations] (15 mL)

Solution for oral inhalation, as mesylate: 0.2% (10 mL, 30 mL, 60 mL)

Dosing

Adults & Elderly:

Bronchospasm: Inhalation: 2 inhalations at an interval of at least 1-3 minutes, followed by a third inhalation if needed

Prevention of bronchospasm: Inhalation: 2 inhalations every 8 hours; do not exceed 3 inhalations every 6 hours or 2 inhalations every 4 hours

Pediatrics: Children >12 years: Refer to adult dosing.

Administration

Inhalation: Administer around-the-clock to promote less variation in peak and trough serum levels.

Monitoring and Teaching Issues

Physical Assessment: Assess effectiveness and interactions of other medications patient may be taking (see Drug Interactions). See Contraindications and Warnings/Precautions for use cautions. Monitor for effectiveness of therapy and adverse reactions (see Adverse Reactions) at beginning of therapy and periodically with long-term use. Assess knowledge/teach patient appropriate use, interventions to reduce side effects, and adverse symptoms to report (see Patient Education). **Pregnancy risk factor C** - benefits of use should outweigh possible risks. Note breast-feeding caution.

Patient Education: Use exactly as directed. Do not use more often than recommended. Maintain adequate hydration (2-3 L/day of fluids) unless advised by prescriber to restrict fluids. You may experience nervousness, dizziness, or fatigue (use caution when driving or

(Continued)

Bitolterol *(Continued)*

engaging in tasks requiring alertness until response to drug is known); or dry mouth, stomach upset (small, frequent meals, frequent mouth care, chewing gum, or sucking hard candy may help). Report unresolved GI upset; dizziness or fatigue; vision changes; chest pain, rapid heartbeat, or palpitations; nervousness or insomnia; muscle cramping or tremor; or unusual cough. **Pregnancy/breast-feeding precautions:** Inform prescriber if you are or intend to become pregnant. Consult prescriber if breast-feeding.

Self-administered inhalation: Store canister upside down; do not freeze. Shake canister before using. Sit when using medication. Close eyes when administering bitolterol to avoid spray getting into eyes. Exhale slowly and completely through nose; inhale deeply through mouth while administering aerosol. Hold breath for 5-10 seconds after inhalation. Wait at least 1 full minute between inhalations. Wash mouthpiece between use. If more than one inhalation medication is used, use bitolterol first and wait 5 minutes between medications.

Self-administered nebulizer: Wash hands before and after treatment. Wash and dry nebulizer after each treatment. Twist open the top of one unit dose vial and squeeze contents into nebulizer reservoir. Connect nebulizer reservoir to the mouthpiece or face mask. Connect nebulizer to compressor. Sit in comfortable, upright position. Place mouthpiece in your mouth or put on face mask and turn on compressor. If face mask is used, avoid leakage around the mask to avoid mist getting into eyes which may cause vision problems. Breathe calmly and deeply until no more mist is formed in nebulizer (about 5 minutes). At this point treatment is finished.

Geriatric Considerations: Elderly patients may find it beneficial to utilize a spacer device when using a metered dose inhaler. Difficulty in using the inhaler often limits its effectiveness (see Adverse Reactions).

Related Information

Inhalant (Asthma, Bronchospasm) Agents Comparison *on page 1577*

Bitolterol Mesylate *see* Bitolterol *on page 173*

Blenoxane® *see* Bleomycin *on page 174*

Bleo *see* Bleomycin *on page 174*

Bleomycin (blee oh MYE sin)

U.S. Brand Names Blenoxane®

Synonyms Bleo; Bleomycin Sulfate; BLM; NSC-125066

Generic Available Yes

Pharmacologic Category Antineoplastic Agent, Antibiotic

Pregnancy Risk Factor D

Lactation Excretion in breast milk unknown/not recommended

Use Treatment of squamous cell carcinomas, melanomas, sarcomas, testicular carcinoma, Hodgkin's lymphoma, and non-Hodgkin's lymphoma

Orphan drug: Sclerosing agent for malignant pleural effusion

Mechanism of Action/Effect Inhibits synthesis of DNA

Contraindications Hypersensitivity to bleomycin sulfate or any component of the formulation; severe pulmonary disease; pregnancy

Warnings/Precautions The U.S. Food and Drug Administration (FDA) currently recommends that procedures for proper handling and disposal of antineoplastic agents be considered. Occurrence of pulmonary fibrosis is higher in elderly patients and in those receiving >400 units total and in smokers and patients with prior radiation therapy. A severe idiosyncratic reaction consisting of hypotension, mental confusion, fever, chills, and wheezing is possible. Check lungs prior to each treatment for fine rales (crackles), which may be the first symptom of pulmonary toxicity.

Drug Interactions

Decreased Effect: Bleomycin and digitalis glycosides may decrease plasma levels of digoxin. Concomitant therapy with phenytoin results in decreased phenytoin levels, possibly due to decreased oral absorption.

Increased Effect/Toxicity: Bleomycin with digoxin may result in elevated serum digoxin levels due to decreased renal clearance. CCNU (lomustine) increases severity of leukopenia. Results in delayed bleomycin elimination due to a decrease in creatinine clearance secondary to cisplatin.

Adverse Reactions

>10%:

- Cardiovascular: Raynaud's phenomenon
- Central nervous system: Mild febrile reaction, fever, chills, patients may become febrile after intracavitary administration
- Dermatologic: Pruritic erythema
  - Integument: ~50% of patients will develop erythema, induration, and hyperkeratosis and peeling of the skin; hyperpigmentation, alopecia, nailbed changes may occur; this appears to be dose-related and is reversible after cessation of therapy
- Gastrointestinal: Mucocutaneous toxicity, stomatitis, nausea, vomiting, anorexia
  - Emetic potential: Moderately low (10% to 30%)
- Local: Phlebitis, pain at tumor site
  - **Irritant chemotherapy**
- Respiratory: Pneumonitis

1% to 10%:

- Dermatologic: Alopecia
- Gastrointestinal: Weight loss
- Respiratory: Pulmonary fibrosis and death
  - Respiratory effects are dose-related when total dose is >400 units or with single doses >30 units; manifested as an acute or chronic interstitial pneumonitis with interstitial fibrosis, hypoxia, and death; symptoms include cough, dyspnea, and bilateral pulmonary infiltrates noted on CXR; it is controversial whether steroids improve symptoms of bleomycin pulmonary toxicity

Miscellaneous: Idiosyncratic: Similar to anaphylaxis and occurs in 1% of lymphoma patients; may include hypotension, confusion, fever, chills, and wheezing. May be immediate or delayed for several hours; symptomatic treatment includes volume expansion, vasopressor agents, antihistamines, and steroids

<1% (Limited to important or life-threatening): Hepatotoxicity, myocardial infarction, myelosuppression (rare), renal toxicity, scleroderma-like skin changes, stroke

Overdosage/Toxicology Symptoms of overdose include chills, fever, pulmonary fibrosis, and hyperpigmentation. Treatment is supportive.

Pharmacodynamics/Kinetics

Absorption: I.M. and intrapleural administration: 30% serum concentrations I.V. administration; intraperitoneal and S.C. routes produce serum concentrations equal to those of I.V.

Half-Life Elimination: Biphasic: Renal function dependent:

Normal renal function: Initial: 1.3 hours; Terminal: 9 hours

End-stage renal disease: Initial: 2 hours; Terminal: 30 hours

Time to Peak: Serum: I.M.: Within 30 minutes

Metabolism: Via several tissues including hepatic, GI tract, skin, pulmonary, renal, and serum

Formulations Injection, powder for reconstitution, as sulfate: 15 units, 30 units [1 unit = 1 mg]

Dosing

Adults & Elderly: Refer to individual protocols; 1 unit = 1 mg; may be administered I.M., I.V., S.C., or intracavitary.

Test dose for lymphoma patient: I.M., I.V., S.C.: 1-5 units of bleomycin before the first dose; monitor vital signs every 15 minutes; wait a minimum of 1 hour before administering remainder of dose.

Single agent therapy:

I.M./I.V./S.C.: Squamous cell carcinoma, lymphosarcoma, reticulum cell sarcoma, testicular carcinoma: 0.25-0.5 units/kg (10-20 units/m^2) 1-2 times/week

Continuous intravenous infusion: 15 units/m^2 over 24 hours/day for 4 days

Combination agent therapy:

I.M./I.V.: 3-4 units/m^2

I.V.: ABVD: 10 units/m^2 on days 1 and 15

Maximum cumulative lifetime dose: 400 units

Pleural sclerosing: Intracavitary: 60-240 units as a single infusion. Dose may be repeated at intervals of several days if fluid continues to accumulate (mix in 50-100 mL of D_5W, NS, or SWFI); may add lidocaine 100-200 mg to reduce local discomfort.

Pediatrics: Refer to adult dosing.

Renal Impairment:

Cl_{cr} 10-50 mL/minute: Administer 75% of normal dose.

Cl_{cr} <10 mL/minute: Administer 50% of normal dose.

Hemodialysis: None

CAPD effects: None

CAVH effects: None

Administration

I.M.: May cause pain at injection site.

I.V.: May be an irritant. I.V. doses should be administered slowly (manufacturer recommends giving over a period of 10 minutes).

Other: S.C.: May cause pain at injection site.

Stability

Storage: Refrigerate intact vials of powder; intact vials are stable for up to one month at 45°C

Reconstitution: Reconstitute powder with 1-5 mL SWI or NS which is stable at room temperature for 28 days or in refrigerator for 14 days. May use bacteriostatic agent if prolonged storage is necessary.

Standard I.V. dilution: Dose/50-1000 mL NS or D_5W

Stable for 96 hours at room temperature and 14 days under refrigeration.

Compatibility: Stable in NS

Compatibility when admixed: Incompatible with aminophylline, ascorbic acid injection, cefazolin, diazepam, hydrocortisone sodium succinate, methotrexate, mitomycin, nafcillin, penicillin G sodium, terbutaline

Monitoring Laboratory Tests Pulmonary function (total lung volume, forced vital capacity, carbon monoxide diffusion), renal function, chest x-ray, CBC with differential and platelet count, liver function

Monitoring and Teaching Issues

Physical Assessment: See Contraindications and Warnings/Precautions for use cautions. Assess potential for interactions with other prescriptions, OTC medications, or herbal products patient may be taking (see Drug Interactions). Respiratory status should be monitored prior to each treatment (special attention to lymphoma patients - see Warnings/Precautions and Adverse Reactions) and prescriber notified of any changes. Test dose may be necessary (see Dosing). Infusion site must be monitored closely to avoid extravasation. Assess results of laboratory tests (see above), therapeutic effectiveness, and adverse effects (see Adverse Reactions and Overdose/Toxicology). Teach patient possible side effects and interventions and adverse symptoms to report (see Patient Education). **Pregnancy risk factor D** - determine that patient is not pregnant before beginning treatment. Instruct patients of childbearing age about appropriate barrier contraceptive measures. Breast-feeding is not recommended.

Patient Education: Inform prescriber of all prescriptions, OTC medications, or herbal products you are taking, and any allergies you have; do not take any new medications during treatment unless approved by prescriber. This medication can only be administered by injection or infusion; report immediately any redness, burning, pain, or swelling at injection/infusion site. May cause loss of appetite, nausea, or vomiting (small, frequent meals, sucking lozenges, or chewing gum may help); mouth sores (frequent mouth care with soft swabs and mouth rinses may help); fever or chills (will usually resolve); redness,

(Continued)

Bleomycin *(Continued)*

peeling, or increased color of skin; or loss of hair (reversible after cessation of therapy). Report any change in respiratory status; difficulty breathing; wheezing; air hunger; increased secretions; difficulty expectorating secretions; confusion; unresolved fever or chills; sores in mouth; vaginal itching, burning, or discharge; sudden onset of dizziness; acute headache; or burning, stinging, redness, or swelling at injection site. **Pregnancy/breast-feeding precautions:** Inform prescriber if you are pregnant. Do not get pregnant during or for 1 month following therapy. Consult prescriber for instruction on appropriate barrier contraceptives. This drug may cause severe fetal defects. Breast-feeding is not recommended

Bleomycin Sulfate *see* Bleomycin *on page 174*

Bleph®-10 *see page 1509*

Bleph®-10 *see* Sulfacetamide *on page 1256*

Blephamide® *see page 1509*

BLM *see* Bleomycin *on page 174*

Blocadren® *see* Timolol *on page 1322*

Body Surface Area of Adults and Children *see page 1531*

Bonine® [OTC] *see* Meclizine *on page 840*

Boric Acid *see page 1519*

B&O Supprettes® *see* Belladonna and Opium *on page 151*

Botox® *see page 1509*

Botulinum Toxin Type A *see page 1509*

Bravelle™ *see* Follitropins *on page 597*

Breonesin® [OTC] [DSC] *see* Guaifenesin *on page 646*

Brethaire [DSC] *see* Terbutaline *on page 1291*

Brethine® *see* Terbutaline *on page 1291*

Bretylium (bre TIL ee um)

Synonyms Bretylium Tosylate

Generic Available Yes

Pharmacologic Category Antiarrhythmic Agent, Class III

Pregnancy Risk Factor C

Lactation Excretion in breast milk unknown

Use Treatment of ventricular tachycardia and fibrillation; treatment of other serious ventricular arrhythmias resistant to lidocaine

Mechanism of Action/Effect Class III antiarrhythmic; after an initial release of norepinephrine at the peripheral adrenergic nerve terminals, bretylium inhibits further release by postganglionic nerve endings in response to sympathetic nerve stimulation

Contraindications Hypersensitivity to bretylium or any component of the formulation; severe aortic stenosis; severe pulmonary hypertension

Warnings/Precautions Use only in areas where there is equipment and staff familiar with management of life-threatening arrhythmias. Use continuous cardiac and blood pressure monitoring. Keep patients supine (postural hypotension common). Initially, may see transient hypertension and increased frequency of arrhythmias. Adjust dose in patients with impaired renal function. Give to a pregnant woman only if clearly needed. Rapid I.V. administration may cause nausea and vomiting, and a higher risk of orthostatic hypotension (particularly in elderly patients). Pregnancy risk C.

Drug Interactions

Increased Effect/Toxicity: Other antiarrhythmic agents may potentiate or antagonize cardiac effects of bretylium. Toxic effects may be additive. The vasopressor effects of catecholamines may be enhanced by bretylium. Toxicity of agents which may prolong QT interval (including cisapride, tricyclic antidepressants, antipsychotics, erythromycin, Class Ia and Class III antiarrhythmics) and specific quinolones (sparfloxacin, gatifloxacin, moxifloxacin) may be increased. Digoxin toxicity may be aggravated by bretylium.

Adverse Reactions

>10%: Cardiovascular: Hypotension (both postural and supine)

1% to 10%: Gastrointestinal: Nausea, vomiting

<1% (Limited to important or life-threatening): Bradycardia, chest pain, dyspnea, flushing, increase in premature ventricular contractions (PVCs), nasal congestion, postural hypotension, renal impairment, respiratory depression, syncope, transient initial hypertension

Overdosage/Toxicology Symptoms of overdose include significant hypertension followed by severe hypotension. Administration of a short-acting hypotensive agent should be used for the hypertensive response. Treatment is symptomatic and supportive. Dialysis is not useful.

Pharmacodynamics/Kinetics

Half-Life Elimination: 7-11 hours; Mean: 4-17 hours; End-stage renal disease: 16-32 hours

Metabolism: None

Onset: I.M.: May require 2 hours; I.V.: 6-20 minutes; Peak effect: 6-9 hours

Duration: 6-24 hours

Formulations

Injection, solution, as tosylate: 50 mg/mL (10 mL)

Injection, solution, as tosylate [premixed in D_5W]: 2 mg/mL (250 mL); 4 mg/mL (250 mL)

Dosing

Adults & Elderly: (**Note:** Patients should undergo defibrillation/cardioversion before and after bretylium doses as necessary.)

Immediate life-threatening ventricular arrhythmias, ventricular fibrillation, unstable ventricular tachycardia: I.V.: Initial: 5 mg/kg (undiluted) over 1 minute; if arrhythmia persists, give 10 mg/kg (undiluted) over 1 minute and repeat as necessary (usually at 15- to 30-minute intervals) up to a total dose of 30-35 mg/kg

Other life-threatening ventricular arrhythmias: I.M., I.V.:

Initial: 5-10 mg/kg, may repeat every 1-2 hours if arrhythmia persist; give I.V. dose (diluted) over 8-10 minutes

Maintenance dose: I.M.: 5-10 mg/kg every 6-8 hours; I.V. (diluted): 5-10 mg/kg every 6 hours; I.V. infusion (diluted): 1-2 mg/minute (little experience with doses >40 mg/kg/day)

Pediatrics: Note: Patients should undergo defibrillation/cardioversion before and after bretylium doses as necessary.

Arrhythmias: **Note:** Not well established, although the following dosing has been suggested:

I.M.: Children: 2-5 mg/kg as a single dose

I.V.: Children: Acute ventricular fibrillation: Initial: 5 mg/kg, then attempt electrical defibrillation; repeat with 10 mg/kg if ventricular fibrillation persists at 15- to 30-minute intervals to maximum total of 30 mg/kg

Maintenance dose: I.M., I.V.: 5 mg/kg every 6 hours

Renal Impairment:

Cl_{cr} 10-50 mL/minute: Administer 25% to 50% of dose.

Cl_{cr} <10 mL/minute: Administer 25% of dose.

Not dialyzable

Administration

I.M.: I.M. injection in adults should not exceed 5 mL volume in any one site.

I.V.: 2 g/250 mL D_5W (infusion pump should be used for I.V. infusion)

Bolus, emergency: Infuse rapidly (1 minute).

Bolus, nonemergency: May be given over 8-10 minutes.

Suggested rate of I.V. infusion: 1-4 mg/minute.

1 mg/minute = 7 mL/hour

2 mg/minute = 15 mL/hour

3 mg/minute = 22 mL/hour

4 mg/minute = 30 mL/hour

Stability

Storage: The premix infusion should be stored at room temperature and protected from freezing.

Reconstitution: Standard diluent: 2 g/250 mL D_5W

Compatibility: Stable in D_5LR, $D_5{}^1/_2NS$, D_5NS, D_5W, mannitol 20%, LR, sodium bicarbonate 5%, NS

Y-site administration: Incompatible with amphotericin B cholesteryl sulfate complex, propofol, warfarin

Compatibility when admixed: Incompatible with phenytoin

Monitoring and Teaching Issues

Physical Assessment: Assess other medications patient may be taking for effectiveness and interactions (see Drug Interactions). **I.V.:** Requires use of infusion pump and continuous cardiac and hemodynamic monitoring. Be alert for adverse cardiovascular reactions (see Warnings/Precautions and Adverse Reactions). Patient education/instruction is according to patient condition (see below). **Pregnancy risk factor C.** Note breast-feeding caution.

Patient Education: Emergency use: Patient education is determined by patient condition. You may experience nausea or vomiting (call for assistance if this occurs, do not try to get out of bed or change position on your own). Report chest pain, acute dizziness, or difficulty breathing immediately. **Breast-feeding precaution:** Consult prescriber if breast-feeding.

Geriatric Considerations: Elderly are particularly at risk of orthostatic hypotension. See Warnings/Precautions and Adverse Reactions.

Related Information

Antiarrhythmic Drugs *on page 1551*

Bretylium Tosylate *see* Bretylium *on page 176*

Brevibloc® *see* Esmolol *on page 491*

Brevicon® *see* Ethinyl Estradiol and Norethindrone *on page 527*

Bricanyl [DSC] *see* Terbutaline *on page 1291*

Brimonidine *see* Ophthalmic Agents, Glaucoma *on page 1002*

Brinzolamide *see page 1575*

Brinzolamide *see* Ophthalmic Agents, Glaucoma *on page 1002*

Brodspec® *see* Tetracycline *on page 1296*

Bromanyl® Cough Syrup *see page 1522*

Bromocriptine (broe moe KRIP teen)

U.S. Brand Names Parlodel®

Synonyms Bromocriptine Mesylate

Generic Available No

Pharmacologic Category Anti-Parkinson's Agent, Dopamine Agonist; Ergot Derivative

Pregnancy Risk Factor B

Lactation Enters breast milk/contraindicated

Use

Amenorrhea with or without galactorrhea; infertility or hypogonadism; prolactin-secreting adenomas; acromegaly; Parkinson's disease

A previous indication for prevention of postpartum lactation was withdrawn voluntarily by Sandoz Pharmaceuticals Corporation

Use - Unlabeled/Investigational Neuroleptic malignant syndrome

Mechanism of Action/Effect Semisynthetic ergot alkaloid derivative and a dopamine receptor agonist which activates postsynaptic dopamine receptors in the tuberoinfundibular and nigrostriatal pathways

Contraindications Hypersensitivity to bromocriptine, ergot alkaloids, or any component of the formulation; uncontrolled hypertension; severe ischemic heart disease or peripheral

(Continued)

Bromocriptine *(Continued)*

vascular disorders; pregnancy (risk to benefit evaluation must be performed in women who become pregnant during treatment for acromegaly, prolactinoma, or Parkinson's disease - hypertension during treatment should generally result in efforts to withdraw)

Warnings/Precautions Use with caution in patients with impaired renal or hepatic function, a history of psychosis, or cardiovascular disease (myocardial infarction, arrhythmia). Patients who receive bromocriptine during and immediately following pregnancy as a continuation of previous therapy (ie, acromegaly) should be closely monitored for cardiovascular effects. Discontinuation of bromocriptine in patients with macroadenomas has been associated with rapid regrowth of tumor and increased prolactin serum levels. Use with caution in patients with a history of peptic ulcer disease, dementia, or concurrent antihypertensive therapy. Safety and effectiveness in patients <15 years of age have not been established.

Drug Interactions

Cytochrome P450 Effect: Substrate of **CYP3A4**; Inhibits **CYP3A4**

Decreased Effect: Antipsychotics may inhibit bromocriptine's ability to lower prolactin.

Increased Effect/Toxicity: Isometheptene and phenylpropanolamine (and other sympathomimetics) should be avoided in patients receiving bromocriptine - may increase risk of hypertension and seizure. Erythromycin, fluvoxamine, and nefazodone may increase bromocriptine concentrations.

Nutritional/Ethanol Interactions

Ethanol: Avoid ethanol (may increase GI side effects or ethanol intolerance).

Herb/Nutraceutical: St John's wort may decrease bromocriptine levels.

Adverse Reactions

>10%:

Central nervous system: Headache, dizziness

Gastrointestinal: Nausea

1% to 10%:

Cardiovascular: Orthostatic hypotension

Central nervous system: Fatigue, lightheadedness, drowsiness

Gastrointestinal: Anorexia, vomiting, abdominal cramps, constipation

Respiratory: Nasal congestion

<1% (Limited to important or life-threatening): Arrhythmias, hair loss, insomnia, paranoia, visual hallucinations

Overdosage/Toxicology Symptoms of overdose include nausea, vomiting, and hypotension. Treatment is symptomatic and supportive.

Pharmacodynamics/Kinetics

Half-Life Elimination: Biphasic: Initial: 6-8 hours; Terminal: 50 hours

Time to Peak: Serum: 1-2 hours

Metabolism: Primarily hepatic

Formulations

Capsule, as mesylate: 5 mg

Tablet, as mesylate: 2.5 mg

Dosing

Adults:

Parkinsonism: Oral: 1.25 mg 2 times/day, increased by 2.5 mg/day in 2- to 4-week intervals (usual dose range is 30-90 mg/day in 3 divided doses), though elderly patients can usually be managed on lower doses.

Neuroleptic malignant syndrome: Oral: 2.5-5 mg 3 times/day

Hyperprolactinemia: Oral: 2.5 mg 2-3 times/day

Acromegaly: Initial: Oral: 1.25-2.5 mg increasing as necessary every 3-7 days; usual dose: 20-30 mg/day

Prolactin-secreting adenomas: Oral: Initial: 1.25-2.5 mg/day; daily range 2.5-10 mg.

Elderly: Refer to adult dosing; however, elderly patients can usually be managed on lower doses.

Pediatrics: Oral: Prolactin-secreting adenoma:

11-15 years (based on limited information): 1.25-2.5 mg daily

16 years to adult: Refer to adult dosing.

Dosage may be increased as tolerated to achieve a therapeutic response (range 2.5-10 mg daily).

Hepatic Impairment: No guidelines are available, however, adjustment may be necessary.

Monitoring and Teaching Issues

Physical Assessment: Assess effectiveness and interactions of other medications patient may be taking (see Contraindications and Drug Interactions). Monitor laboratory tests, therapeutic response (eg, mental status, involuntary movements), and adverse reactions at beginning of therapy and periodically throughout therapy (see Warnings/Precautions, Adverse Reactions, and Overdose/Toxicology). Assess knowledge/teach patient appropriate use, interventions to reduce side effects, and adverse symptoms to report (see Patient Education). Breast-feeding is contraindicated.

Patient Education: Take exactly as directed (may be prescribed in conjunction with levodopa/carbidopa); do not change dosage or discontinue without consulting prescriber. Therapeutic effects may take several weeks or months to achieve and you may need frequent monitoring during first weeks of therapy. Take with meals if GI upset occurs, before meals if dry mouth occurs, after eating if drooling or if nausea occurs. Take at the same time each day. Maintain adequate hydration (2-3 L/day of fluids) unless advised by prescriber to restrict fluids; void before taking medication. Do not use alcohol, prescription or OTC sedatives or CNS depressants without consulting prescriber. Urine or perspiration may appear darker. You may experience drowsiness, dizziness, confusion, or vision changes (use caution when driving, climbing stairs, or engaging in tasks requiring alertness until response to drug is known); orthostatic hypotension (use caution when rising from sitting or lying position); constipation (increased exercise, fluids, fruit, or fiber may help); nasal congestion (consult prescriber for appropriate relief); or nausea, vomiting, loss of appetite, or stomach discomfort (small, frequent meals, frequent mouth care, chewing gum, or sucking lozenges may help). Report unresolved constipation or vomiting; chest pain or irregular heartbeat; acute headache or dizziness; CNS changes (eg, hallucination, loss of memory, seizures, acute headache, nervousness, etc); painful or difficult urination; increased muscle spasticity, rigidity, or involuntary movements; skin rash; or significant worsening of condition. **Breast-feeding precaution:** Do not breast-feed.

Dietary Issues: May be taken with food to decrease GI distress.

Geriatric Considerations: See Adverse Reactions; elderly patients are usually managed on lower doses.

Additional Information Usually used with levodopa or levodopa/carbidopa to treat Parkinson's disease. When adding bromocriptine, the dose of levodopa/carbidopa can usually be decreased.

Bromocriptine Mesylate *see* Bromocriptine *on page 177*

Bromodiphenhydramine and Codeine *see page 1522*

Bromonidine *see page 1575*

Bromotuss® w/Codeine Cough Syrup *see page 1522*

Bronchial® *see* Theophylline and Guaifenesin *on page 1303*

Brontex® *see* Guaifenesin and Codeine *on page 647*

B-type Natriuretic Peptide (Human) *see* Nesiritide *on page 962*

Budesonide (byoo DES oh nide)

U.S. Brand Names Entocort™ EC; Pulmicort Respules™; Pulmicort Turbuhaler®; Rhinocort®; Rhinocort® Aqua™

Generic Available No

Pharmacologic Category Corticosteroid, Inhalant (Oral); Corticosteroid, Nasal; Corticosteroid, Systemic

Pregnancy Risk Factor C/B (Pulmicort Turbuhaler®)

Lactation Excreted in breast milk/use caution

Use

Intranasal: Children ≥6 years of age and Adults: Management of symptoms of seasonal or perennial rhinitis

Nebulization: Children 12 months to 8 years: Maintenance and prophylactic treatment of asthma

Oral capsule: Treatment of active Crohn's disease (mild to moderate) involving the ileum and/or ascending colon

Oral inhalation: Maintenance and prophylactic treatment of asthma; includes patients who require corticosteroids and those who may benefit from systemic dose reduction/elimination

Mechanism of Action/Effect Anti-inflammatory effect on nasal tissues

Contraindications Hypersensitivity to budesonide or any component of the formulation

Inhalation: Contraindicated in primary treatment of status asthmaticus, acute episodes of asthma; not for relief of acute bronchospasm

Warnings/Precautions May cause hypercorticism and/or suppression of hypothalamic-pituitary-adrenal (HPA) axis, particularly in younger children or in patients receiving high doses for prolonged periods. Particular care is required when patients are transferred from systemic corticosteroids to products with lower systemic bioavailability (ie, inhalation). May lead to possible adrenal insufficiency or withdrawal from steroids, including an increase in allergic symptoms. Patients receiving prolonged therapy of ≥20 mg per day of prednisone (or equivalent) may be most susceptible. Aerosol steroids do **not** provide the systemic steroid needed to treat patients having trauma, surgery, or infections.

Controlled clinical studies have shown that orally-inhaled and intranasal corticosteroids may cause a reduction in growth velocity in pediatric patients. (In studies of orally-inhaled corticosteroids, the mean reduction in growth velocity was approximately 1 centimeter per year [range 0.3-1.8 cm per year] and appears to be related to dose and duration of exposure.) To minimize the systemic effects of orally-inhaled and intranasal corticosteroids, each patient should be titrated to the lowest effective dose. Growth should be routinely monitored in pediatric patients.

May suppress the immune system, patients may be more susceptible to infection. Use with caution in patients with systemic infections or ocular herpes simplex. Avoid exposure to chickenpox and measles. Corticosteroids should be used with caution in patients with diabetes, hypertension, osteoporosis, peptic ulcer, glaucoma, cataracts, or tuberculosis. Use caution in hepatic impairment. Enteric-coated capsules should not be crushed or chewed.

Pregnancy risk C.

Drug Interactions

Cytochrome P450 Effect: Substrate of CYP3A4

Decreased Effect: CYP3A4 inducers (including carbamazepine, phenytoin, phenobarbital, rifampin) may decrease budesonide levels and/or effects. Theoretically, proton pump inhibitors (omeprazole, pantoprazole) alter gastric pH may affect the rate of dissolution of enteric-coated capsules. Administration with omeprazole did not alter kinetics of budesonide capsules.

Increased Effect/Toxicity: Cimetidine may decrease the clearance and increase the bioavailability of budesonide, increasing its serum concentrations. In addition, CYP3A4 inhibitors may increase the serum level and/or toxicity of budesonide this effect was shown with ketoconazole, but not erythromycin. Other potential inhibitors include amiodarone, cimetidine, clarithromycin, delavirdine, diltiazem, dirithromycin, disulfiram, fluoxetine, fluvoxamine, grapefruit juice, indinavir, itraconazole, ketoconazole, nefazodone, nevirapine, propoxyphene, quinupristin-dalfopristin, ritonavir, saquinavir, verapamil, zafirlukast, zileuton. The addition of salmeterol has been demonstrated to improve response to inhaled corticosteroids (as compared to increasing steroid dosage).

(Continued)

Budesonide *(Continued)*

Nutritional/Ethanol Interactions

Food: Grapefruit juice may double systemic exposure of orally-administered budesonide. Administration of capsules with a high-fat meal delays peak concentration, but does not alter the extent of absorption.

Herb/Nutraceutical: St John's wort may decrease budesonide levels.

Adverse Reactions Reaction severity varies by dose and duration; not all adverse reactions have been reported with each dosage form.

>10%:

Central nervous system: Oral capsule: Headache (up to 21%)

Gastrointestinal: Oral capsule: Nausea (up to 11%)

Respiratory: Respiratory infection, rhinitis

Miscellaneous: Symptoms of HPA axis suppression and/or hypercorticism (acne, easy bruising, fat redistribution, striae, edema) may occur in >10% of patients following administration of dosage forms which result in higher systemic exposure (ie, oral capsule), but may be less frequent than rates observed with comparator drugs (prednisolone). These symptoms may be rare (<1%) following administration via methods which result in lower exposures (topical).

1% to 10%:

Cardiovascular: Syncope, edema, hypertension

Central nervous system: Chest pain, dysphonia, emotional lability, fatigue, fever, insomnia, migraine, nervousness, pain, dizziness, vertigo

Dermatologic: Bruising, contact dermatitis, eczema, pruritus, pustular rash, rash

Endocrine & metabolic: Hypokalemia, adrenal insufficiency

Gastrointestinal: Abdominal pain, anorexia, diarrhea, dry mouth, dyspepsia, gastroenteritis, oral candidiasis, taste perversion, vomiting, weight gain, flatulence

Hematologic: Cervical lymphadenopathy, purpura, leukocytosis

Neuromuscular & skeletal: Arthralgia, fracture, hyperkinesis, hypertonia, myalgia, neck pain, weakness, paresthesia, back pain

Ocular: Conjunctivitis, eye infection

Otic: Earache, ear infection, external ear infection

Respiratory: Bronchitis, bronchospasm, cough, epistaxis, nasal irritation, pharyngitis, sinusitis, stridor

Miscellaneous: Allergic reaction, flu-like syndrome, herpes simplex, infection, moniliasis, viral infection, voice alteration

<1% (Limited to important or life-threatening): Aggressive reactions, alopecia, angioedema, avascular necrosis of the femoral head, benign intracranial hypertension, depression, dyspnea, growth suppression, hoarseness, hypersensitivity reactions (immediate and delayed; include rash, contact dermatitis, angioedema, bronchospasm), intermenstrual bleeding, irritability, nasal septum perforation, osteoporosis, psychosis, somnolence

Overdosage/Toxicology

Inhaled formulations: Symptoms of overdose include irritation and burning of the nasal mucosa, sneezing, intranasal and pharyngeal *Candida* infections, nasal ulceration, epistaxis, rhinorrhea, nasal stuffiness, headache.

When consumed in excessive quantities, systemic hypercorticism and adrenal suppression may occur, in those cases discontinuation and withdrawal of the corticosteroid should be done judiciously. Treatment should be symptomatic and supportive.

Pharmacodynamics/Kinetics

Absorption: Capsule: Rapid and complete

Bioavailability: Limited by high first-pass effect; Capsule: 9% to 21%; Respules®: 6%; Turbuhaler®: 6% to 13%; Nasal: 34%

Half-Life Elimination: 2-3.6 hours

Time to Peak: Capsule: 30-600 minutes (variable in Crohn's disease); Respules®: 10-30 minutes; Turbuhaler®: 1-2 hours; Nasal: 1 hour

Metabolism: Hepatic via CYP3A4 to two metabolites: 16 alpha-hydroxyprednisolone and 6 beta-hydroxybudesonide; minor activity

Onset: Respules®: 2-8 days; Rhinocort® Aqua™: ~10 hours; Turbuhaler®: 24 hours

Peak effect: Respules®: 4-6 weeks; Rhinocort® Aqua™: ~2 weeks; Turbuhaler®: 1-2 weeks

Formulations

Capsule, enteric coated (Entocort™ EC): 3 mg

Powder for oral inhalation (Pulmicort Turbuhaler®): 200 mcg/inhalation (104 g) [delivers ~160 mcg/inhalation; 200 metered doses]

Suspension for nasal inhalation (Rhinocort®): 50 mcg/inhalation (7 g) [delivers ~32 mcg/inhalation; 200 metered doses]

Suspension, nasal [spray] (Rhinocort® Aqua™): 32 mcg/inhalation (8.6 g) [120 metered doses]

Suspension for oral inhalation (Pulmicort Respules™): 0.25 mg/2 mL (30s), 0.5 mg/2 mL (30s)

Dosing

Adults & Elderly:

Asthma: Inhalation: 1- to 4-inhalations twice daily using Pulmicort Turbuhaler® device; maintenance therapy may be gradually reduced to a single daily inhalation. See table.

Previous Therapy	Recommended Starting Dose	Highest Recommended Dose
Bronchodilators alone	200-400 mcg twice daily	400 mcg twice daily
Inhaled corticosteroids*	200-400 mcg twice daily	800 mcg twice daily
Oral corticosteroids	400-800 mcg twice daily	800 mcg twice daily

*In patients with mild to moderate asthma who are well controlled on inhaled corticosteroids, dosing with Pulmicort® Turbuhaler 200 mcg or 400 mcg once daily may be considered. Pulmicort Turbuhaler® can be administered once daily either in the morning or in the evening.

Crohn's disease: Oral: 9 mg once daily in the morning; safety and efficacy have not been established for therapy duration >8 weeks; recurring episodes may be treated with a repeat 8-week course of treatment

Note: Treatment may be tapered to 6 mg once daily for 2 weeks prior to complete cessation. Patients receiving CYP3A4 inhibitors should be monitored closely for signs and symptoms of hypercorticism; dosage reduction may be required.

Rhinitis: Nasal inhalation:

Rhinocort®: Nasal: Initial: 8 sprays (4 sprays/nostril) per day (256 mcg/day), given as either 2 sprays in each nostril in the morning and evening or as 4 sprays in each nostril in the morning. After symptoms decrease (usually by 3-7 days), reduce dose slowly every 2-4 weeks to the smallest amount needed to control symptoms.

Rhinocort® Aqua™: 64 mcg/day as a single 32 mcg spray in each nostril. Some patients who do not achieve adequate control may benefit from increased dosage. A reduced dosage may be effective after initial control is achieved.

Maximum dose: Children <12 years: 129 mcg/day; Adults: 256 mcg/day

Pediatrics:

Asthma:

Nasal inhalation: ≥6 years: Refer to adult dosing.

Oral inhalation: ≥6 years:

Previous therapy of bronchodilators alone: 200 mcg twice initially which may be increased up to 400 mcg twice daily

Previous therapy of inhaled corticosteroids: 200 mcg twice initially which may be increased up to 400 mcg twice daily

Previous therapy of oral corticosteroids: The highest recommended dose in children is 400 mcg twice daily

NIH Guidelines (NIH, 1997) (give in divided doses twice daily):

"Low" dose: 100-200 mcg/day

"Medium" dose: 200-400 mcg/day (1-2 inhalations/day)

"High" dose: >400 mcg/day (>2 inhalation/day)

Nebulization: Children 12 months to 8 years: Pulmicort Respules™: Titrate to lowest effective dose once patient is stable; start at 0.25 mg/day or use as follows:

Previous therapy of bronchodilators alone: 0.5 mg/day administered as a single dose or divided twice daily (maximum daily dose: 0.5 mg)

Previous therapy of inhaled corticosteroids: 0.5 mg/day administered as a single dose or divided twice daily (maximum daily dose: 1 mg)

Previous therapy of oral corticosteroids: 1 mg/day administered as a single dose or divided twice daily (maximum daily dose: 1 mg)

Hepatic Impairment: Monitor closely for signs and symptoms of hypercorticism; dosage reduction may be required.

Administration

Oral: Oral capsule: Capsule should be swallowed whole; do not crush or chew.

Inhalation:

Inhalation: Inhaler should be shaken well immediately prior to use; while activating inhaler, deep breathe for 3-5 seconds, hold breath for ~10 seconds and allow ≥1 minute between inhalations. Rinse mouth with water after use to reduce aftertaste and incidence of candidiasis.

Nebulization: Shake well before using. Use Pulmicort Respules™ with jet nebulizer connected to an air compressor; administer with mouthpiece or facemask. Do not use ultrasonic nebulizer. Do not mix with other medications in nebulizer. Rinse mouth following treatments to decrease risk of oral candidiasis (wash face if using face mask).

Stability

Storage:

Nebulizer: Store upright at 20°C to 25°C (68°F to 77°F) and protect from light. Do not refrigerate or freeze. Once aluminum package is opened, solution should be used within 2 weeks. Continue to protect from light.

Nasal inhaler: Store with valve up at 15°C to 30°C (59°F to 86°F). Use within 6 months after opening aluminum pouch. Protect from high humidity.

Nasal spray: Store with valve up at 20°C to 25°C (68°F to 77°F) and protect from light. Do not freeze.

Monitoring and Teaching Issues

Physical Assessment: Monitor therapeutic effects and adverse reactions (see Warnings/Precautions, Adverse Reactions, and Overdose/Toxicology). When changing from systemic steroids to inhalational steroids, taper reduction of systemic medication slowly (may take several months). Assess knowledge/teach patient appropriate use, interventions to reduce side effects, and adverse symptoms to report (see Patient Education). **Pregnancy risk factor B/C** - see Pregnancy Risk Factor for use cautions; benefits of use should outweigh possible risks. Note breast-feeding caution.

Patient Education: Use as directed; do not increase dosage or discontinue abruptly without consulting prescriber. May be more susceptible to infection; avoid exposure to chickenpox and measles unless immunity has been established. Report acute nervousness or inability to sleep; severe sneezing or nosebleed; difficulty breathing, sore throat, hoarseness, or bronchitis; difficulty breathing or bronchospasms; disturbed menstrual pattern; vision changes; loss of taste or smell perception; or worsening of condition or lack of improvement. **Pregnancy/breast-feeding precautions:** Inform prescriber if you are or intend to become pregnant. Consult prescriber if breast-feeding.

Oral capsule: Swallow whole; do not crush or chew capsule.

Inhalation/nebulization: This is not a bronchodilator and will not relieve acute asthma attacks. It may take several days for you to realize full effects of treatment. If you are also using an inhaled bronchodilator, wait 10 minutes before using this steroid aerosol. Take

(Continued)

Budesonide *(Continued)*

5-10 deep breaths. Use inhaler on inspiration. Hold breath for 5-10 seconds after inhalation. Allow 1 full minute between inhalations. You may experience dizziness, anxiety, or blurred vision (rise slowly from sitting or lying position and use caution when driving or engaging in tasks requiring alertness until response to drug is known); or taste disturbance or aftertaste (frequent mouth care and mouth rinses may help). Rinse mouth with water following oral treatments to decrease risk of oral candidiasis (wash face if using a face mask).

Dietary Issues: Avoid grapefruit juice when using oral capsules.

Geriatric Considerations: Ensure that patients can correctly use nasal inhaler.

Pregnancy Issues: No adequate or well-controlled studies in pregnant women; use only if potential benefit to the mother outweighs the possible risk to the fetus. Hypoadrenalism has been reported in infants.

Additional Information Effects of inhaled/intranasal steroids on growth have been observed in the absence of laboratory evidence of HPA axis suppression, suggesting that growth velocity is a more sensitive indicator of systemic corticosteroid exposure in pediatric patients than some commonly used tests of HPA axis function. The long-term effects of this reduction in growth velocity associated with orally-inhaled and intranasal corticosteroids, including the impact on final adult height, are unknown. The potential for "catch up" growth following discontinuation of treatment with inhaled corticosteroids has not been adequately studied.

Bufferin® [OTC] *see* Aspirin *on page 121*

Bufferin® Arthritis Strength [OTC] *see* Aspirin *on page 121*

Bufferin® Extra Strength [OTC] *see* Aspirin *on page 121*

Bumetanide (byoo MET a nide)

U.S. Brand Names Bumex®

Generic Available Yes

Pharmacologic Category Diuretic, Loop

Pregnancy Risk Factor C (manufacturer); D (expert analysis)

Lactation Excretion in breast milk unknown/use caution

Use Management of edema secondary to congestive heart failure or hepatic or renal disease including nephrotic syndrome; may be used alone or in combination with antihypertensives in the treatment of hypertension; can be used in furosemide-allergic patients

Mechanism of Action/Effect Inhibits reabsorption of sodium and chloride in the ascending loop of Henle and proximal renal tubule, causing increased excretion of water, sodium, chloride, magnesium, phosphate and calcium

Contraindications Hypersensitivity to bumetanide, any component of the formulation, or sulfonylureas; anuria; patients with hepatic coma or in states of severe electrolyte depletion until the condition improves or is corrected; pregnancy (based on expert analysis)

Warnings/Precautions In cirrhosis, avoid electrolyte and acid/base imbalances that might lead to hepatic encephalopathy. Ototoxicity is associated with I.V. rapid administration, renal impairment, excessive doses, and concurrent use of other ototoxins. Hypersensitivity reactions can rarely occur. Monitor fluid status and renal function in an attempt to prevent oliguria, azotemia, and reversible increases in BUN and creatinine. May cause significant electrolyte disturbances or volume depletion. Coadministration of antihypertensives may increase the risk of hypotension.

Chemical similarities are present among sulfonamides, sulfonylureas, carbonic anhydrase inhibitors, thiazides, and loop diuretics (except ethacrynic acid). Use in patients with sulfonylurea allergy is specifically contraindicated in product labeling, however, a risk of cross-reaction exists in patients with allergy to any of these compounds; avoid use when previous reaction has been severe.

Pregnancy risk C/D.

Drug Interactions

Decreased Effect: Glucose tolerance may be decreased by loop diuretics, requiring adjustment of hypoglycemic agents. Cholestyramine or colestipol may reduce bioavailability of bumetanide. Indomethacin (and other NSAIDs) may reduce natriuretic and hypotensive effects of diuretics. Hypokalemia may reduce the efficacy of some antiarrhythmics.

Increased Effect/Toxicity: Bumetanide-induced hypokalemia may predispose to digoxin toxicity and may increase the risk of arrhythmia with drugs which may prolong QT interval, including type Ia and type III antiarrhythmic agents, cisapride, and some quinolones (sparfloxacin, gatifloxacin, and moxifloxacin). The risk of toxicity from lithium and salicylates (high dose) may be increased by loop diuretics. Hypotensive effects and/or adverse renal effects of ACE inhibitors and NSAIDs are potentiated by bumetanide-induced hypovolemia. The effects of peripheral adrenergic-blocking drugs or ganglionic blockers may be increased by bumetanide.

Bumetanide may increase the risk of ototoxicity with other ototoxic agents (aminoglycosides, cis-platinum), especially in patients with renal dysfunction. Synergistic diuretic effects occur with thiazide-type diuretics. Diuretics tend to be synergistic with other antihypertensive agents, and hypotension may occur.

Nutritional/Ethanol Interactions Herb/Nutraceutical: Avoid ephedra, yohimbe, ginseng (may worsen hypertension). Avoid dong quai if using for hypertension (has estrogenic activity). Avoid garlic (may have increased antihypertensive effect).

Adverse Reactions

>10%:

Endocrine & metabolic: Hyperuricemia (18%), hypochloremia (15%), hypokalemia (15%)

Renal: Azotemia (11%)

1% to 10%:

Central nervous system: Dizziness (1%)

Endocrine & metabolic: Hyponatremia (9%), hyperglycemia (7%), variations in phosphorus (5%), CO_2 content (4%), bicarbonate (3%), and calcium (2%)

Neuromuscular & skeletal: Muscle cramps (1%)

Otic: Ototoxicity (1%)
Renal: Increased serum creatinine (7%)
<1% (Limited to important or life-threatening): Asterixis, dehydration, encephalopathy, hypernatremia, hypotension, impaired hearing, orthostatic hypotension, pruritus, rash, renal failure, vertigo, vomiting

Overdosage/Toxicology Symptoms of overdose include electrolyte depletion and volume depletion. Treatment is symptomatic and supportive.

Pharmacodynamics/Kinetics

Half-Life Elimination: Infants <6 months: Possibly 2.5 hours; Children and Adults: 1-1.5 hours

Metabolism: Partially hepatic

Onset: Oral, I.M.: 0.5-1 hour; I.V.: 2-3 minutes

Duration: 6 hours

Formulations

Injection, solution: 0.25 mg/mL (2 mL, 4 mL, 10 mL)
Tablet: 0.5 mg, 1 mg, 2 mg
Bumex®: 0.5 mg, 1 mg, 2 mg

Dosing

Adults:

Edema:
Oral: 0.5-2 mg/dose (maximum dose: 10 mg/day) 1-2 times/day
I.M., I.V.: 0.5-1 mg/dose; may repeat in 2-3 hours for up to 2 doses if needed (maximum dose: 10 mg/day)
Continuous I.V. infusion: 0.9-1 mg/hour
Hypertension: Oral: 0.5 mg daily (range: 1-4 mg/day, maximum dose: 5 mg/day); for larger doses, divide into 2-3 doses daily

Elderly: Initial: Oral: 0.5 mg once daily, increase as necessary.

Pediatrics: Edema (diuresis); Not FDA-approved for use in children <18 years of age:
<6 months: Dose not established
>6 months:
Oral: Initial: 0.015 mg/kg/dose once daily or every other day; maximum dose: 0.1 mg/kg/day
I.M., I.V.: Dose not established

Administration

I.V.: Administer I.V. slowly, over 1-2 minutes; an alternate-day schedule or a 3-4 daily dosing regimen with rest periods of 1-2 days in between may be the most tolerable and effective regimen for the continued control of edema; reserve I.V. administration for those unable to take oral medications

Stability

Storage: I.V. infusion solutions should be used within 24 hours after preparation. Light sensitive - discoloration may occur when exposed to light.

Compatibility: Stable in D_5W, NS, LR

Y-site administration: Incompatible with midazolam

Compatibility when admixed: Incompatible with dobutamine, milrinone

Monitoring Laboratory Tests Serum electrolytes, renal function

Monitoring and Teaching Issues

Physical Assessment: See Contraindications and Warnings/Precautions for use cautions (especially with I.V. administration). Assess potential for interactions with other prescriptions, OTC medications, or herbal products patient may be taking (see Drug Interactions). Blood pressure, weight, and fluid status should be monitored at beginning of therapy and periodically during therapy. Glucose levels for diabetics should be monitored closely (glucose tolerance may be decreased by loop diuretics, requiring adjustment of hypoglycemic agents). Assess results of laboratory tests (see above), therapeutic effectiveness, and adverse effects (see Adverse Reactions and Overdose/Toxicology). Teach patient proper use, possible side effects and interventions, and adverse symptoms to report (see Patient Education). **Pregnancy risk factor C/D** - see Pregnancy Risk Factor for use cautions; benefits of use should outweigh possible risks. Note breast-feeding caution.

Patient Education: Inform prescriber of all prescriptions, OTC medications, or herbal products you are taking, and any allergies you have. Do not take anything new during treatment unless approved by prescriber. May be taken with food to reduce GI effects. Take single dose early in day (single dose) or last dose early in afternoon (twice daily) to prevent sleep interruptions. Include orange juice or bananas (or other sources of potassium-rich foods) in your daily diet but do not take supplemental potassium without consulting prescriber. If diabetic, monitor glucose levels closely (glucose tolerance may be decreased by loop diuretics). Notify prescriber of noted changes (hypoglycemic agent may need to be adjusted). May cause dizziness, hypotension, lightheadedness, or weakness (use caution when changing position from sitting or lying position, when driving, exercising, climbing stairs, or performing hazardous tasks until response to drug is known). Report palpitations or chest pain; swelling of ankles or feet, weight increase or decrease (>3 lb in any one day), increased fatigue, muscle cramps or trembling, and any changes in hearing. **Pregnancy/breast-feeding precautions:** Inform prescriber if you are or intend to become pregnant; contraceptives may be recommended. Consult prescriber if breast-feeding.

Dietary Issues: May require increased intake of potassium-rich foods.

Geriatric Considerations: See Warnings/Precautions. Severe loss of sodium and/or increases in BUN can cause confusion. For any change in mental status in patients on bumetanide, monitor electrolytes and renal function.

Related Information

Heart Failure *on page 1670*

Bumex® *see* Bumetanide *on page 182*
Buminate® *see* Albumin *on page 50*
Buprenex® *see* Buprenorphine *on page 184*

Buprenorphine (byoo pre NOR feen)

U.S. Brand Names Buprenex®; Subutex®

Synonyms Buprenorphine Hydrochloride

Restrictions Injection: C-V; Tablet: C-III

Prescribing of tablets for opioid dependence is limited to physicians who have met the qualification criteria and have received a DEA number specific to prescribing this product. Tablets will be available through pharmacies and wholesalers which normally provide controlled substances.

Generic Available Yes: Injection

Pharmacologic Category Analgesic, Narcotic

Pregnancy Risk Factor C

Lactation Enters breast milk/not recommended

Use

Injection: Management of moderate to severe pain

Tablet: Treatment of opioid dependence

Use - Unlabeled/Investigational Injection: Heroin and opioid withdrawal

Mechanism of Action/Effect Buprenorphine exerts its analgesic effect via high affinity binding to μ opiate receptors in the CNS; displays both agonist and antagonist activity

Contraindications Hypersensitivity to buprenorphine or any component of the formulation

Warnings/Precautions May cause CNS depression, which may impair physical or mental abilities. Effects with other sedative drugs or ethanol may be potentiated. Elderly may be more sensitive to CNS depressant and constipating effects. May cause respiratory depression - use caution in patients with respiratory disease or pre-existing respiratory depression. Potential for drug dependency exists, abrupt cessation may precipitate withdrawal. Use caution in elderly, debilitated, pediatric patients, depression or suicidal tendencies, or in patients with a history of drug abuse. Tolerance, psychological and physical dependence may occur with prolonged use. Partial antagonist activity may precipitate acute narcotic withdrawal in opioid-dependent individuals.

Use with caution in patients with hepatic, pulmonary, or renal function impairment. Also use caution in patients with head injury or increased ICP, biliary tract dysfunction, pancreatitis, patients with history of ileus or bowel obstruction, glaucoma, hyperthyroidism, adrenal insufficiency, prostatic hyperplasia, urinary stricture, CNS depression, toxic psychosis, alcoholism, delirium tremens, or kyphoscoliosis.

Tablets, which are used for induction treatment of opioid dependence, should not be started until effects of withdrawal are evident.

Pregnancy risk C.

Drug Interactions

Cytochrome P450 Effect: Substrate of **CYP3A4**

Decreased Effect: Enzyme inducers may reduce serum concentrations of buprenorphine, resulting in loss of efficacy (includes barbiturates, carbamazepine, phenytoin rifabutin, and rifampin). Naltrexone may antagonize the effect of narcotic analgesics; concurrent use or use within 7-10 days of injection for pain relief is contraindicated.

Increased Effect/Toxicity: Barbiturate anesthetics and other CNS depressants may produce additive respiratory and CNS depression. Respiratory and CV collapse was reported in a patient who received diazepam and buprenorphine. Effects may be additive with other CNS depressants. CYP3A4 inhibitors may increase serum levels/toxicity of buprenorphine (inhibitors include amiodarone, cimetidine, clarithromycin, erythromycin, delavirdine, diltiazem, dirithromycin, disulfiram, fluoxetine, fluvoxamine, grapefruit juice, indinavir, itraconazole, ketoconazole, nefazodone, nevirapine, propoxyphene, quinupristin-dalfopristin, ritonavir, saquinavir, verapamil, zafirlukast, and zileuton); monitor for altered effects; a decrease in buprenorphine dosage may be required.

Nutritional/Ethanol Interactions

Ethanol: Avoid ethanol (may increase CNS depression).

Herb/Nutraceutical: Avoid valerian, St John's wort, kava kava, gotu kola (may increase CNS depression).

Adverse Reactions

Injection:

>10%: Central nervous system: Sedation

1% to 10%:

Cardiovascular: Hypotension

Central nervous system: Respiratory depression, dizziness, headache

Gastrointestinal: Vomiting, nausea

Ocular: Miosis

Otic: Vertigo

Miscellaneous: Diaphoresis

<1% (Limited to important or life-threatening): Agitation, apnea, appetite decreased, blurred vision, bradycardia, confusion, constipation, convulsion, coma, cyanosis, depersonalization, depression, diplopia, dyspnea, dysphoria, euphoria, fatigue, flatulence, flushing, hallucinations, hypertension, injection site reaction, malaise, nervousness, pallor, paresthesia, pruritus, psychosis, rash, slurred speech, tachycardia, tinnitus, tremor, urinary retention, urticaria, weakness, Wenckebach block, xerostomia

Tablet:

>10:

Central nervous system: Headache (30%), pain (24%), insomnia (21% to 25%), anxiety (12%), depression (11%),

Gastrointestinal: Nausea (10% to 14%), abdominal pain (12%), constipation (8% to 11%)

Neuromuscular & skeletal: Back pain (14%), weakness (14%)

Respiratory: Rhinitis (11%)

Miscellaneous: Withdrawal syndrome (19%; placebo 37%), infection (12% to 20%), diaphoresis (12% to 13%)

1% to 10%:

Central nervous system: Chills (6%), nervousness (6%), somnolence (5%), dizziness (4%), fever (3%)

Gastrointestinal: Vomiting (5% to 8%), diarrhea (5%), dyspepsia (3%)

Ocular: Lacrimation (5%)

Respiratory: Cough (4%), pharyngitis (4%)

Miscellaneous: Flu-like syndrome (6%)

Overdosage/Toxicology Symptoms of overdose include CNS depression, pinpoint pupils, hypotension, and bradycardia. Treatment is supportive. Naloxone may have limited effects in reversing respiratory depression; doxapram has also been used to stimulate respirations.

Pharmacodynamics/Kinetics

Absorption: I.M., S.C.: 30% to 40%

Half-Life Elimination: 2.2-3 hours

Metabolism: Primarily hepatic; extensive first-pass effect

Onset: Analgesic: 10-30 minutes

Duration: 6-8 hours

Formulations

Injection, solution, as hydrochloride (Buprenex®): 0.3 mg/mL (1 mL)

Tablet, sublingual (Subutex®): 2 mg, 8 mg

Dosing

Adults:

Long-term use is not recommended.

Management of moderate to severe pain: I.M., slow I.V.: 0.3-0.6 mg every 6 hours as needed. **Note:** Decrease dose by half in patients with compromised respiratory function or receiving CNS depressants.

Heroin or opiate withdrawal (unlabeled use): I.M., slow I.V.: Variable; 0.1-0.4 mg every 6 hours

Opioid dependence: Sublingual:

Induction: Range: 12-16 mg/day (doses during an induction study used 8 mg on day 1, followed by 16 mg on day 2; induction continued over 3-4 days). Treatment should begin at least 4 hours after last use of heroin or short-acting opioid, preferably when first signs of withdrawal appear. Titrating dose to clinical effectiveness should be done as rapidly as possible to prevent undue withdrawal symptoms and patient drop-out during the induction period.

Maintenance: Target dose: 16 mg/day; range: 4-24 mg/day; patients should be switched to the buprenorphine/naloxone combination product for maintenance and unsupervised therapy

Elderly: Moderate to severe pain: I.M., slow I.V.: 0.15 mg every 6 hours; elderly patients are more likely to suffer from confusion and drowsiness compared to younger patients. **Long-term use is not recommended.**

Pediatrics:

Children 2-12 years: Moderate to severe pain: 2-6 mcg/kg every 4-6 hours

Children ≥13 years: Management of moderate to severe pain: Refer to adult dosing.

Children ≥16 years: Opioid dependence: Refer to adult dosing.

Administration

Oral: Sublingual: Tablet should be placed under the tongue until dissolved; should not be swallowed. If 2 or more tablets are needed per dose, all may be placed under the tongue at once, or 2 at a time; to ensure consistent bioavailability, subsequent doses should always be taken the same way.

I.V.: Administer slowly, over at least 2 minutes.

Stability

Storage:

Injection: Protect from excessive heat of >40°C (>104°F) and light.

Tablet: Store at room temperature of 25°C (77°F).

Compatibility: Injection:

Y-site administration: Compatible: Allopurinol, amifostine, aztreonam, cefepime, cisatracurium, cladribine, docetaxel, etoposide, filgrastim, gatifloxacin, gemcitabine, granisetron, linezolid, melphalan, piperacillin/tazobactam, propofol, remifentanil, teniposide, thiotepa, vinorelbine. **Incompatible:** Amphotericin B cholesteryl sulfate complex, doxorubicin liposome

Compatibility in syringe: Compatible: Midazolam

Compatibility when admixed: Compatible: Atropine, bupivacaine, diphenhydramine, droperidol, glycopyrrolate, haloperidol, hydroxyzine, promethazine, scopolamine. **Incompatible:** Diazepam, floxacillin, furosemide, lorazepam

Monitoring Laboratory Tests LFTs

Monitoring and Teaching Issues

Physical Assessment: Assess other medications patient may be taking for possible additive or adverse interactions (see Drug Interactions). Monitor for effectiveness of pain relief and adverse reactions or overdose (see Adverse Reactions and Overdose/Toxicology) at beginning of therapy and at regular intervals with long-term use. For inpatients, implement safety measures. Assess knowledge/teach patient appropriate use (if self-administered). Teach patient to monitor for adverse reactions (see Adverse Reactions), adverse reactions to report, and appropriate interventions to reduce side effects. **Pregnancy risk factor C** - benefits of use should outweigh possible risks. Breast-feeding is not recommended.

Patient Education: If self-administered, use exactly as directed; do not increase dose or frequency. While using this medication, do not use alcohol and other prescription or OTC medications (especially sedatives, tranquilizers, antihistamines, or pain medications) without consulting prescriber. May cause dizziness, drowsiness, confusion, or blurred vision (use caution when driving, climbing stairs, rising from sitting or lying position, or engaging in tasks requiring alertness until response to drug is known). You may experience nausea or vomiting (frequent mouth care, small, frequent meals, sucking lozenges, or chewing gum may help). Report unresolved nausea or vomiting; difficulty breathing or

(Continued)

Buprenorphine *(Continued)*

shortness of breath; excessive sedation or unusual weakness; or rapid heartbeat or palpitations. **Pregnancy/breast-feeding precautions:** Inform prescriber if you are or intend to become pregnant. Breast-feeding is not recommended.

Additional Information

Buprenorphine injection: 0.4 mg = 10 mg morphine or 75 mg meperidine, has longer duration of action than either agent

Subutex® (buprenorphine) should be limited to supervised use whenever possible; patients should be switched to Suboxone® (buprenorphine/naloxone) for maintenance and unsupervised therapy

Related Information

Narcotic/Opioid Analgesic Comparison *on page 1583*

Buprenorphine and Naloxone (byoo pre NOR feen & nal OKS one)

U.S. Brand Names Suboxone®

Synonyms Buprenorphine Hydrochloride and Naloxone Hydrochloride Dihydrate; Naloxone and Buprenorphine; Naloxone Hydrochloride Dihydrate and Buprenorphine Hydrochloride

Restrictions C-III; Prescribing of tablets for opioid dependence is limited to physicians who have met the qualification criteria and have received a DEA number specific to prescribing this product. Tablets will be available through pharmacies and wholesalers which normally provide controlled substances.

Generic Available No

Pharmacologic Category Analgesic, Narcotic

Pregnancy Risk Factor C

Lactation Buprenorphine: Enters breast milk/not recommended

Use Treatment of opioid dependence

Formulations Tablet, sublingual: Buprenorphine 2 mg and naloxone 0.5 mg; buprenorphine 8 mg and naloxone 2 mg [lemon-lime flavor]

Dosing

Adults: Opioid dependence: Sublingual: **Note:** This combination product is not recommended for use during the induction period; initial treatment should begin using buprenorphine oral tablets. Patients should be switched to the combination product for maintenance and unsupervised therapy.

Maintenance: Target dose (based on buprenorphine content): 16 mg/day; range: 4-24 mg/day

Pediatrics: Children ≥16 years: Opioid dependence: Refer to adult dosing.

Monitoring and Teaching Issues

Patient Education: See individual components listed in Related Information. **Pregnancy/breast-feeding precautions:** Inform prescriber if you are or intend to become pregnant. Consult prescriber if breast-feeding.

Related Information

Buprenorphine *on page 184*

Naloxone *on page 944*

Buprenorphine Hydrochloride *see* Buprenorphine *on page 184*

Buprenorphine Hydrochloride and Naloxone Hydrochloride Dihydrate *see* Buprenorphine and Naloxone *on page 186*

BuPROPion (byoo PROE pee on)

U.S. Brand Names Wellbutrin®; Wellbutrin SR®; Zyban®

Generic Available Yes: Wellbutrin® strength only

Pharmacologic Category Antidepressant, Dopamine-Reuptake Inhibitor; Smoking Cessation Aid

Pregnancy Risk Factor B

Lactation Enters breast milk/not recommended (AAP rates "of concern")

Use Treatment of depression; adjunct in smoking cessation

Use - Unlabeled/Investigational Attention-deficit/hyperactivity disorder (ADHD)

Mechanism of Action/Effect Antidepressant structurally different from all other previously marketed antidepressants; like other antidepressants the mechanism of bupropion's activity is not fully understood; weak inhibitor of the neuronal uptake of serotonin, norepinephrine, and dopamine

Contraindications Hypersensitivity to bupropion or any component of the formulation; seizure disorder; anorexia/bulimia; use of MAO inhibitors within 14 days

Warnings/Precautions Seizure risk is increased at total daily dosage >450 mg, individual dosages >150 mg, or by sudden, large increments in dose. Data for the immediate-release formulation of bupropion revealed a seizure incidence of 0.4% in patients treated at doses in the 300-450 mg/day range. The estimated seizure incidence increases almost tenfold between 450 mg and 600 mg per day. Data for the sustained release dosage form revealed a seizure incidence of 0.1% in patients treated at a dosage range of 100-300 mg/day, and increases to ~0.4% at the maximum recommended dose of 400 mg/day. The risk of seizures is increased in patients with a history of seizures, head trauma, CNS tumor, severe hepatic cirrhosis, abrupt discontinuation of sedative-hypnotics or ethanol, medications which lower seizure threshold, stimulants, or hypoglycemic agents. May cause CNS stimulation (restlessness, anxiety, insomnia) or anorexia. Use with caution in patients where weight loss is not desirable. The incidence of sexual dysfunction with bupropion is generally lower than with SSRIs.

Use caution in patients with cardiovascular disease, history of hypertension, or coronary artery disease; treatment-emergent hypertension (including some severe cases) has been reported, both with bupropion alone and in combination with nicotine transdermal systems.

Use with caution in patients with hepatic or renal dysfunction and in elderly patients. May cause motor or cognitive impairment in some patients. May worsen psychosis in some patients or precipitate a shift to mania or hypomania in patients with bipolar disease. Use caution in patients with depression, particularly if suicidal risk may be present.

Drug Interactions

Cytochrome P450 Effect: Substrate of CYP1A2, 2A6, **2B6**, 2C8/9, 2D6, 2E1, 3A4; Inhibits **CYP2D6**

Decreased Effect: Carbamazepine, phenobarbital, and phenytoin may increase the metabolism (decrease clinical effect) of bupropion. Effect of warfarin may be altered by bupropion.

Increased Effect/Toxicity: Treatment-emergent hypertension may occur in patients treated with bupropion and nicotine patch. Cimetidine may inhibit the metabolism (increase clinical/adverse effects) of bupropion. Toxicity of bupropion is enhanced by levodopa and phenelzine (MAO inhibitors). Risk of seizures may be increased with agents that may lower seizure threshold (antipsychotics, antidepressants, theophylline, abrupt discontinuation of benzodiazepines, systemic steroids). Effect of warfarin may be altered by bupropion.

Nutritional/Ethanol Interactions

Ethanol: Ethanol (may increase CNS depression).

Herb/Nutraceutical : Avoid valerian, St John's wort, SAMe, gotu kola, kava kava (may increase CNS depression).

Effects on Lab Values Decreased prolactin levels

Adverse Reactions Frequency not defined.

Cardiovascular: Arrhythmias, chest pain, flushing, hypertension (may be severe), hypotension, palpitation, syncope, tachycardia

Central nervous system: Agitation, anxiety, confusion, dizziness, euphoria, headache, hostility, insomnia, irritability, memory decreased, migraine, nervousness, sleep disturbance, somnolence

Dermatologic: Pruritus, rash, sweating increased, urticaria

Endocrine & metabolic: Hot flashes, libido decreased, menstrual complaints

Gastrointestinal: Abdominal pain, anorexia, appetite increased, constipation, diarrhea, dyspepsia, dysphagia, nausea, taste perversion, vomiting, xerostomia

Genitourinary: Urinary frequency

Neuromuscular & skeletal: Arthralgia, arthritis, myalgia, neck pain, paresthesia, tremor, twitching

Ocular: Amblyopia, blurred vision

Otic: Auditory disturbance, tinnitus

Respiratory: Cough increased, pharyngitis, sinusitis

Miscellaneous: Allergic reaction, infection

Postmarketing and/or case reports (limited to important or life-threatening): Accommodation abnormality, akinesia, alopecia, amnesia, anemia, angioedema, aphasia, ataxia, atrioventricular block, bronchospasm, bruxism, coordination abnormal, delirium, depersonalization, derealization, diplopia, dry eye, dry skin, dysarthria, dyskinesia, dyspareunia, dysphoria, dystonia, dysuria, edema, EEG abnormality, ejaculation abnormality, emotional lability, enuresis, epistaxis, exfoliative dermatitis, extrapyramidal syndrome, extrasystoles, facial edema, flushing, gastric reflux, glossitis, glycosuria, gynecomastia, hepatitis, hirsutism, hyperglycemia, hyperkinesia, hypertonia, hypesthesia, hypoglycemia, hypokinesia, hypomania, impotence, jaundice, leg cramps, leukocytosis, leukopenia, libido increased, lymphadenopathy, maculopapular rash, manic reaction, mouth ulcers, muscle weakness, musculoskeletal chest pain, mydriasis, myoclonus, neuralgia, neuropathy, nocturia, painful erection, pallor, pancreatitis, pancytopenia, paranoia, peripheral edema, phlebitis, photosensitivity, polyuria, postural hypotension, salivation increased, seizure, SIADH, stomatitis, suicidal ideation, tardive dyskinesia, testicular swelling, thrombocytopenia, tongue edema, urinary incontinence, urinary retention, vaginal irritation, vaginitis, vertigo

Overdosage/Toxicology Symptoms of overdose include labored breathing, salivation, arched back, ataxia, and convulsions. Dialysis may be of limited value after drug absorption because of slow tissue-to-plasma diffusion. Treatment is symptomatic and supportive.

Pharmacodynamics/Kinetics

Absorption: Rapid

Bioavailability: 5% to 20% in animals

Half-Life Elimination: Half-life:

Distribution: 3-4 hours

Elimination: 21 ± 9 hours; Metabolites: Hydroxybupropion: 20 ± 5 hours; Erythrohydrobupropion: 33 ± 10 hours; Threohydrobupropion: 37 ± 13 hours

Time to Peak: Bupropion: ~3 hours; Metabolites: Hydroxybupropion, erythrohydrobupropion, threohydrobupropion: 6 hours

Metabolism: Extensively hepatic to 3 active metabolites: Hydroxybupropion, erythrohydrobupropion, threohydrobupropion

Formulations

Tablet (Wellbutrin®): 75 mg, 100 mg

Tablet, sustained release:

Wellbutrin® SR: 100 mg, 150 mg, 200 mg

Zyban®: 150 mg

Dosing

Adults:

Depression: Oral:

Immediate release: 100 mg 3 times/day; begin at 100 mg twice daily; may increase to a maximum dose of 450 mg/day.

Sustained release: Initial: 150 mg/day in the morning; may increase to 150 mg twice daily by day 4 if tolerated; target dose: 300 mg/day given as 150 mg twice daily; maximum dose: 400 mg/day given as 200 mg twice daily.

Smoking cessation (Zyban®): Oral: Initiate with 150 mg once daily for 3 days; increase to 150 mg twice daily; treatment should continue for 7-12 weeks.

(Continued)

BuPROPion *(Continued)*

Elderly:

Depression: Oral: 50-100 mg/day, increase by 50-100 mg every 3-4 days as tolerated; there is evidence that the elderly respond at 150 mg/day in divided doses, but some may require a higher dose.

Smoking cessation: Refer to adult dosing.

Pediatrics: ADHD (unlabeled use): Oral: Children and Adolescents: 1.4-6 mg/kg/day

Renal Impairment: Effect of renal disease on bupropion's pharmacokinetics has not been studied; elimination of the major metabolites of bupropion may be affected by reduced renal function. Patients with renal failure should receive a reduced dosage initially and be closely monitored.

Hepatic Impairment:

Mild to moderate hepatic impairment: Use with caution and/or reduced dose/frequency

Severe hepatic cirrhosis: Use with extreme caution; maximum dose:

Wellbutrin®: 75 mg/day;

Wellbutrin SR®: 100 mg/day or 150 mg every other day;

Zyban®: 150 mg every other day

Note: The mean AUC increased by ~1.5-fold for hydroxybupropion and ~2.5-fold for erythro/threohydrobupropion; median T_{max} was observed 19 hours later for hydroxybupropion, 31 hours later for erythro/threohydrobupropion; mean half-life for hydroxybupropion increased fivefold, and increased twofold for erythro/threohydrobupropion in patients with severe hepatic cirrhosis compared to healthy volunteers.

Administration

Oral: Sustained release tablet should be swallowed whole; do not crush or chew

Stability

Storage: Store at controlled of 20°C to 25°C (68°F to 77°F).

Monitoring and Teaching Issues

Physical Assessment: Assess other medications patient may be taking for effectiveness and interactions (see Drug Interactions). See Contraindications and Warnings/Precautions for use cautions. Monitor therapeutic response and adverse reactions at beginning of therapy and periodically with long-term use (see Adverse Reactions and Overdose/Toxicology). Taper dosage slowly when discontinuing. Assess knowledge/teach patient appropriate use, interventions to reduce side effects, and adverse symptoms to report (see Patient Education). Breast-feeding is not recommended.

Patient Education: Be aware that bupropion is marketed under different names and should not be taken together; Zyban® is for smoking cessation and Wellbutrin® is for treatment of depression.

Depression: Take as directed, in equally divided doses; do not take in larger dose or more often than recommended. Do not discontinue without consulting prescriber. Do not use alcohol or OTC medications not approved by prescriber. May cause drowsiness, clouded sensorium, restlessness, or agitation (use caution when driving or engaging in tasks requiring alertness until response to drug is known); nausea, vomiting, or dry mouth (small, frequent meals, frequent mouth care, chewing gum, or sucking lozenges may help); constipation (increased exercise, fluids, fruit, or fiber may help); or impotence (reversible). Report persistent CNS effects (eg, agitation, confusion, anxiety, restlessness, insomnia, psychosis, hallucinations, seizures); muscle weakness or tremor; skin rash or irritation; chest pain or palpitations, abdominal pain or blood in stools; yellowing of skin or eyes; or difficulty breathing, bronchitis, or unusual cough.

Smoking cessation: Use as directed; do not take extra doses. Do not combine nicotine patches with use of Zyban® unless approved by prescriber. May cause dry mouth and insomnia (these may resolve with continued use). Report any difficulty breathing, unusual cough, dizziness, or muscle tremors.

Breast-feeding precaution: Breast-feeding is not recommended.

Geriatric Considerations: Limited data is available about the use of bupropion in the elderly. Two studies have found it equally effective when compared to imipramine. Its side effect profile (minimal anticholinergic and blood pressure effects) may make it useful in persons who do not tolerate traditional cyclic antidepressants.

Breast-feeding Issues: Generally, it is not recommended to breast-feed if taking antidepressants because of the long half-life, active metabolites, and the potential for side effects in the infant.

Related Information

Antidepressant Agents *on page 1553*
Antidepressant Medication Guidelines *on page 1613*
FDA Name Differentiation Project: The Use of Tall-man Letters *on page 12*

Burnamycin [OTC] *see* Lidocaine *on page 800*
Burn Jel [OTC] *see* Lidocaine *on page 800*
Burn-O-Jel [OTC] *see* Lidocaine *on page 800*
BuSpar® *see* BusPIRone *on page 188*

BusPIRone (byoo SPYE rone)

U.S. Brand Names BuSpar®

Synonyms Buspirone Hydrochloride

Generic Available Yes

Pharmacologic Category Antianxiety Agent, Miscellaneous

Pregnancy Risk Factor B

Lactation Excretion in breast milk unknown/not recommended

Use Management of generalized anxiety disorder (GAD)

Use - Unlabeled/Investigational Management of aggression in mental retardation and secondary mental disorders; major depression; potential augmenting agent for antidepressants; premenstrual syndrome

Mechanism of Action/Effect The mechanism of action of buspirone is unknown. Buspirone has a high affinity for serotonin 5-HT_{1A} and 5-HT_2 receptors, without affecting benzodiazepine-GABA receptors. Buspirone has moderate affinity for dopamine D_2 receptors.

Contraindications Hypersensitivity to buspirone or any component of the formulation

Warnings/Precautions Safety and efficacy not established in children <18 years of age; use in hepatic or renal impairment is not recommended; does not prevent or treat withdrawal from benzodiazepines; low potential for cognitive or motor impairment. Use with MAO inhibitors may result in hypertensive reactions.

Drug Interactions

Cytochrome P450 Effect: Substrate of CYP2D6, **3A4**

Decreased Effect: Enzyme inducers (phenobarbital, carbamazepine, phenytoin, rifampin) may reduce serum concentrations of buspirone resulting in loss of efficacy.

Increased Effect/Toxicity: Concurrent use of buspirone with SSRIs or trazodone may cause serotonin syndrome. Erythromycin, clarithromycin, diltiazem, itraconazole, ketoconazole, verapamil, and grapefruit juice may result in increases in buspirone concentrations. Buspirone should not be used concurrently with an MAO inhibitor due to reports of increased blood pressure; theoretically, a selective MAO type B inhibitors (selegiline) has a lower risk of this reaction. Concurrent use of buspirone with nefazodone may increase risk of CNS adverse events; limit buspirone initial dose (eg, 2.5 mg/day).

Nutritional/Ethanol Interactions

Ethanol: Ethanol (may increase CNS depression).

Food: Food may decrease the absorption of buspirone, but it may also decrease the first-pass metabolism, thereby increasing the bioavailability of buspirone. Grapefruit juice may cause increased buspirone concentrations; avoid concurrent use.

Herb/Nutraceutical: St John's wort may decrease buspirone levels or increase CNS depression. Avoid valerian, gotu kola, kava kava (may increase CNS depression).

Effects on Lab Values ↑ AST, ALT, growth hormone(s), prolactin (S)

Adverse Reactions

>10%: Central nervous system: Dizziness

1% to 10%:

Central nervous system: Drowsiness, EPS, serotonin syndrome, confusion, nervousness, lightheadedness, excitement, anger, hostility, headache

Dermatologic: Rash

Gastrointestinal: Diarrhea, nausea

Neuromuscular & skeletal: Muscle weakness, numbness, paresthesia, incoordination, tremor

Ocular: Blurred vision, tunnel vision

Miscellaneous: Diaphoresis, allergic reactions

Overdosage/Toxicology Symptoms of overdose include dizziness, drowsiness, pinpoint pupils, nausea, and vomiting. There is no known antidote for buspirone. Treatment is supportive.

Pharmacodynamics/Kinetics

Half-Life Elimination: 2-3 hours

Time to Peak: Serum: Within 0.7-1.5 hours

Metabolism: Hepatic via oxidation; extensive first-pass effect

Formulations Tablet, as hydrochloride: 5 mg, 7.5 mg, 10 mg, 15 mg, 30 mg

BuSpar®: 5 mg, 10 mg, 15 mg, 30 mg

Dosing

Adults: Anxiety disorders (GAD): Oral: 15 mg/day (7.5 mg twice daily); may increase in increments of 5 mg/day every 2-4 days to a maximum of 60 mg/day. Target dose for most people is 30 mg/day (15 mg twice daily).

Elderly: Oral: Initial: 5 mg twice daily, increase by 5 mg/day every 2-3 days as needed up to 20-30 mg/day; maximum daily dose: 60 mg/day (see Geriatric Considerations).

Pediatrics: Children and Adolescents: Generalized anxiety disorder (GAD): Oral: Initial: 5 mg daily; increase in increments of 5 mg/day at weekly intervals as needed, to a maximum dose of 60 mg/day divided into 2-3 doses

Renal Impairment: Use in patients with severe renal impairment cannot be recommended.

Hepatic Impairment: Buspirone is metabolized by the liver and excreted by the kidneys. Patients with impaired hepatic or renal function demonstrated increased plasma levels and a prolonged half-life of buspirone. Therefore, use in patients with severe hepatic or renal impairment cannot be recommended.

Monitoring and Teaching Issues

Physical Assessment: Assess other medications patient may be taking for effectiveness and interactions (see Drug Interactions). See Contraindications and Warnings/Precautions for use cautions. Monitor therapeutic response and adverse reactions (see Adverse Reactions) at beginning of therapy and periodically with long-term use. Assess knowledge/teach patient appropriate use, interventions to reduce side effects, and adverse symptoms to report (see Patient Education). Breast-feeding is not recommended.

Patient Education: Take only as directed; do not increase dose or take more often than prescribed. May take 2-3 weeks to see full effect; do not discontinue without consulting prescriber. Do not use alcohol or other prescription or OTC medications (especially pain medications, sedatives, antihistamines, or hypnotics) without consulting prescriber. Maintain adequate hydration (2-3 L/day of fluids) unless advised by prescriber to restrict fluids. You may experience drowsiness, lightheadedness, impaired coordination, dizziness, or blurred vision (use caution when driving or engaging in tasks requiring alertness until response to drug is known); or upset stomach, nausea (small, frequent meals, frequent mouth care, chewing gum, or sucking lozenges may help). Report persistent vomiting; chest pain or rapid heartbeat; persistent CNS effects (eg, confusion, restlessness, anxiety, insomnia, excitation, headache, dizziness, fatigue, impaired coordination); or worsening of condition. **Breast-feeding precaution:** Breast-feeding is not recommended.

Geriatric Considerations: Because buspirone is less sedating than other anxiolytics, it may be a useful agent in geriatric patients when an anxiolytic is indicated.

(Continued)

BusPIRone *(Continued)*

Additional Information Has shown little potential for abuse; needs continuous use. Because of slow onset, not appropriate for "as needed" (prn) use or for brief, situational anxiety. Ineffective for treatment of benzodiazepine or ethanol withdrawal.

Related Information

FDA Name Differentiation Project: The Use of Tall-man Letters *on page 12*

Buspirone Hydrochloride *see* BusPIRone *on page 188*

Busulfan (byoo SUL fan)

U.S. Brand Names Busulfex®; Myleran®

Generic Available No

Pharmacologic Category Antineoplastic Agent, Alkylating Agent

Pregnancy Risk Factor D

Lactation Contraindicated

Use

Oral: Chronic myelogenous leukemia and bone marrow disorders, such as polycythemia vera and myeloid metaplasia, conditioning regimens for bone marrow transplantation

I.V.: Combination therapy with cyclophosphamide as a conditioning regimen prior to allogeneic hematopoietic progenitor cell transplantation for chronic myelogenous leukemia

Mechanism of Action/Effect Interferes with DNA function; cytotoxic

Contraindications Hypersensitivity to busulfan or any component of the formulation; failure to respond to previous courses; pregnancy

Warnings/Precautions The U.S. Food and Drug Administration (FDA) currently recommends that procedures for proper handling and disposal of antineoplastic agents be considered. May induce severe bone marrow hypoplasia; reduce or discontinue dosage at first sign, as reflected by an abnormal decrease in any of the formed elements of the blood; use with caution in patients recently given other myelosuppressive drugs or radiation treatment. If white blood count is high, hydration and allopurinol should be employed to prevent hyperuricemia. Use caution in patients predisposed to seizures. Discontinue if lung toxicity develops. Busulfan has been causally related to the development of secondary malignancies (tumors and acute leukemias). Busulfan has been associated with ovarian failure (including failure to achieve puberty) in females. Avoid I.M. injections if platelet count falls to <100,000/mm^3.

Drug Interactions

Cytochrome P450 Effect: Substrate of **CYP3A4**

Increased Effect/Toxicity: Itraconazole or other cytotoxic agents may increase risk of pulmonary toxicity.

Nutritional/Ethanol Interactions

Ethanol: Avoid ethanol due to GI irritation.

Food: No clear or firm data on the effect of food on busulfan bioavailability.

Herb/Nutraceutical: St John's wort may decrease busulfan levels.

Adverse Reactions

>10%:

Dermatologic: Skin hyperpigmentation (busulfan tan), urticaria, erythema, alopecia

Endocrine & metabolic: Ovarian suppression, amenorrhea, sterility

Genitourinary: Azoospermia, testicular atrophy; malignant tumors have been reported in patients on busulfan therapy

Hematologic: Severe pancytopenia, leukopenia, thrombocytopenia, anemia, and bone marrow suppression are common and patients should be monitored closely while on therapy; since this is a delayed effect (busulfan affects the stem cells), the drug should be discontinued temporarily at the first sign of a large or rapid fall in any blood element; some patients may develop bone marrow fibrosis or chronic aplasia which is probably due to the busulfan toxicity; in large doses, busulfan is myeloablative and is used for this reason in BMT

Myelosuppressive:

WBC: Moderate

Platelets: Moderate

Onset: 7-10 days

Nadir: 14-21 days

Recovery: 28 days

1% to 10%:

Cardiovascular: Hypotension

Central nervous system: Confusion,

Dermatologic: Hyperpigmentation

Endocrine & metabolic: Amenorrhea, hyperuricemia

Gastrointestinal: Nausea, stomatitis, anorexia, vomiting, diarrhea; drug has little effect on the GI mucosal lining

Emetic potential: Low (<10%)

Hepatic: Elevated LFTs

Neuromuscular & skeletal: Weakness

Ocular: Cataracts

Respiratory: Bronchopulmonary dysplasia

<1% (Limited to important or life-threatening): Adrenal suppression, gynecomastia, isolated cases of hemorrhagic cystitis have been reported, hepatic dysfunction; after long-term or high-dose therapy, a syndrome known as busulfan lung may occur; this syndrome is manifested by a diffuse interstitial pulmonary fibrosis and persistent cough, fever, rales, and dyspnea. May be relieved by corticosteroids.

BMT:

Central nervous system: Generalized or myoclonic seizures and loss of consciousness, abnormal electroencephalographic findings

Gastrointestinal: Mucositis, anorexia, moderately emetogenic

Hepatic: Veno-occulsive disease (VOD), hyperbilirubinemia

Miscellaneous: Transient pain at tumor sites, transient autoimmune disorders

Overdosage/Toxicology Symptoms of overdose include leukopenia and thrombocytopenia. Induction of vomiting or gastric lavage with charcoal is indicated for recent ingestion; the effects of dialysis are unknown.

Pharmacodynamics/Kinetics

Absorption: Rapid and complete

Half-Life Elimination: After first dose: 3.4 hours; After last dose: 2.3 hours

Time to Peak: Serum: Oral: Within 4 hours; I.V.: Within 5 minutes

Metabolism: Extensively hepatic (may increase with multiple dosing)

Duration: 28 days

Formulations

Injection, solution (Busulfex®): 6 mg/mL (10 mL)

Tablet (Myleran®): 2 mg

Dosing

Adults: Refer to individual protocols.

Note: Busulfan should be based on adjusted ideal body weight because actual body weight, ideal body weight, or other factors can produce significant differences in busulfan clearance among lean, normal, and obese patients.

High dose BMT:

Oral:

0.875-1 mg/kg/dose every 6 hours for 16 doses; total dose: 12-16 mg/kg

37.5 mg/m^2 every 6 hours for 16 doses; total dose: 600 mg/m^2

I.V.: 0.8 mg/kg (ideal body weight or actual body weight, whichever is lower) every 6 hours for 4 days (a total of 16 doses)

CML remission: Oral:

Induction: 4-8 mg/day (may be as high as 12 mg/day)

Maintenance doses: Controversial, range from 1-4 mg/day to 2 mg/week; treatment is continued until WBC reaches 10,000-20,000 cells/mm^3 at which time drug is discontinued; when WBC reaches 50,000/mm^3, maintenance dose is resumed.

Unapproved use:

Polycythemia vera: Oral: 2-6 mg/day

Thrombocytosis: Oral: 4-6 mg/day

Elderly: Oral (refer to individual protocols): Start with lowest recommended doses for adults.

Pediatrics: Refer to individual protocols.

Note: Busulfan should be based on adjusted ideal body weight because actual body weight, ideal body weight, or other factors can produce significant differences in busulfan clearance among lean, normal, and obese patients. Refer to individual protocols.

CML remission: Oral: Children: Induction: 0.06-0.12 mg/kg/day **or** 1.8-4.6 mg/m^2/day; titrate dosage to maintain leukocyte count above 40,000/mm^3; reduce dosage by 50% if the leukocyte count reaches 30,000-40,000/mm^3; discontinue drug if counts fall to ≤20,000/mm^3.

BMT marrow-ablative conditioning regimen: Oral: 1 mg/kg/dose (ideal body weight) every 6 hours for 16 doses

Administration

Oral: BMT only: Phenytoin or clonazepam should be administered prophylactically during and for at least 48 hours following completion of busulfan. Risk of seizures is increased in patients with sickle cell disease. Increased risk of VOD when busulfan AUC >3000 µmol(min)/L (mean AUC, 2012 µmol(min)/L). To facilitate ingestion of high doses, insert multiple tablets into clear gel capsules.

I.V.: Intravenous busulfan should be administered via a **central** venous catheter as a 2-hour infusion, every 6 hours for 4 consecutive days for a total of 16 doses. Do not use polycarbonate syringes.

Stability

Storage: Store unopened ampules (injection) under refrigeration (2°C to 8°C). Final solution is stable for up to 8 hours at room temperature (25°C) but the infusion must also be completed within that 8-hour time frame. Dilution of busulfan injection in 0.9% sodium chloride is stable for up to 12 hours at refrigeration (2°C to 8°C) but the infusion must also be completed within that 12-hour time frame. Do not use polycarbonate syringes.

Reconstitution: Dilute busulfan injection in 0.9% sodium chloride injection or dextrose 5% in water. The dilution volume should be ten times the volume of busulfan injection, ensuring that the final concentration of busulfan is ≥0.5 mg/mL.

Monitoring Laboratory Tests CBC with differential and platelet count, liver function

Monitoring and Teaching Issues

Physical Assessment: See Contraindications, Warnings/Precautions, and Administration for use cautions. Assess potential for interactions with other prescriptions, OTC medications, or herbal products patient may be taking (see Drug Interactions). **I.V.:** See Administration and Reconstitution. Assess results of laboratory tests (see above) and therapeutic response and adverse effects (eg, pulmonary or hematologic effects - see Adverse Reactions and Overdose/Toxicology) during therapy and for several months following therapy (pulmonary fibrosis may occur 4-5 months after therapy begins). **Oral:** Teach patient proper use, possible side effects and interventions, and adverse symptoms to report (see Patient Education). **Pregnancy risk factor D** - determine that patient is not pregnant before beginning treatment. Instruct patients of childbearing age about using appropriate barrier contraceptive measures during therapy and for 1 month following therapy. Breast-feeding is contraindicated.

Patient Education: Inform prescriber of all prescriptions, OTC medications, or herbal products you are taking, and any allergies you have. Do not take anything new during treatment unless approved by prescriber. Take oral medication as directed with chilled liquids. Maintain adequate hydration (2-3 L/day of fluids) unless advised by prescriber to restrict fluids. Avoid alcohol, acidic or spicy foods. You will be more susceptible to infection (avoid crowds and exposure to infection and do not have any vaccinations unless approved by prescriber). May cause mouth sores (brush teeth with soft toothbrush or cotton swab); loss of hair or darkening of skin color (reversible when medication is discontinued); nausea, vomiting, or anorexia (small, frequent meals, chewing gum, or sucking hard candy may

(Continued)

Busulfan *(Continued)*

help); constipation (increased exercise, fruit, fluids, or fiber may help); amenorrhea; sterility; or skin rash. Report palpitations or chest pain, excessive dizziness, confusion, difficulty breathing, numbness or tingling of extremities, unusual bruising or bleeding, pain or changes in urination, or other adverse effects. **Pregnancy/breast-feeding precautions:** Inform prescriber if you are pregnant. Do not get pregnant during or for 1 month following therapy. Consult prescriber for instruction on appropriate barrier contraceptive measures. This drug may cause severe fetal defects. Do not breast-feed.

Geriatric Considerations: Toxicity to immunosuppressives is increased in the elderly. Start with lowest recommended adult doses. Signs of infection, such as fever and rise in WBCs, may not occur. Lethargy and confusion may be more prominent signs of infection.

Busulfex® *see* Busulfan *on page 190*

Butalbital, Acetaminophen, and Caffeine

(byoo TAL bi tal, a seet a MIN oh fen, & KAF een)

U.S. Brand Names Esgic®; Esgic-Plus™; Fioricet®; Repan®

Synonyms Acetaminophen, Butalbital, and Caffeine

Generic Available Yes

Pharmacologic Category Barbiturate

Pregnancy Risk Factor D

Lactation Enters breast milk/contraindicated

Use Relief of the symptomatic complex of tension or muscle contraction headache

Contraindications Hypersensitivity to butalbital or any component of the formulation; porphyria; pregnancy

Warnings/Precautions Administer with caution, if at all, to patients who are mentally depressed, have suicidal tendencies, or a history of drug abuse. May be habit-forming.

Drug Interactions

Cytochrome P450 Effect:

Acetaminophen: Substrate of CYP1A2, 2A6, 2C8/9, 2D6, 2E1, 3A4

Caffeine: Substrate of **CYP1A2**, 2C8/9, 2D6, 2E1, 3A4; Inhibits **CYP1A2**

Decreased Effect: Butalbital may diminish effects of uricosuric agents such as probenecid and sulfinpyrazone.

Increased Effect/Toxicity: MAO inhibitors may enhance CNS effects of butalbital. Increased effect (CNS depression) with narcotic analgesics, ethanol, general anesthetics, tranquilizers such as chlordiazepoxide, sedative hypnotics, or other CNS depressants.

Nutritional/Ethanol Interactions Ethanol: Avoid ethanol (may increase CNS depression).

Effects on Lab Values Acetaminophen may produce false-positive test results for urinary 5-hydroxyindoleacetic acid.

Adverse Reactions

>10%:

Central nervous system: Dizziness, lightheadedness, drowsiness

Gastrointestinal: Nausea, heartburn, stomach pains, dyspepsia, epigastric discomfort

1% to 10%:

Central nervous system: Confusion, mental depression, unusual excitement, nervousness, faint feeling, insomnia, nightmares, intoxicated feeling

Dermatologic: Rash

Gastrointestinal: Constipation, GI ulceration

<1% (Limited to important or life-threatening): Agranulocytosis, allergic reaction, bronchospasm, chest pain, epistaxis, exfoliative dermatitis, hallucinations, hepatotoxicity, impaired renal function, iron-deficiency anemia, jitters, leukopenia, megaloblastic anemia, nervousness, occult bleeding, palpitations, prolongation of bleeding time, respiratory depression, Stevens-Johnson syndrome, syncope, tachycardia, thrombocytopenia, thrombophlebitis

Overdosage/Toxicology Symptoms of barbiturate overdose include unsteady gait, slurred speech, confusion, respiratory depression, hypotension, and coma. Treatment is supportive.

Symptoms of acetaminophen overdose include hepatic necrosis, transient azotemia, renal tubular necrosis with acute toxicity, anemia, and GI disturbances with chronic toxicity. Treatment consists of acetylcysteine 140 mg/kg orally (loading) followed by 70 mg/kg every 4 hours for 17 doses; therapy should be initiated based upon laboratory analysis suggesting a high probability of hepatotoxic potential. Activated charcoal is very effective at binding acetaminophen. Intravenous acetylcysteine should be reserved for patients unable to take oral forms.

Formulations

Capsule:

Esgic®: Butalbital 50 mg, caffeine 40 mg, and acetaminophen 325 mg

Esgic-Plus™: Butalbital 50 mg, caffeine 40 mg, and acetaminophen 500 mg

Tablet: Fioricet®, Repan®: Butalbital 50 mg, caffeine 40 mg, and acetaminophen 325 mg

Dosing

Adults: Tension or muscle contraction headache: Oral: 1-2 tablets or capsules every 4 hours; not to exceed 6 tablets or capsules/day

Elderly: Not recommended for use in the elderly.

Renal Impairment: Dosage should be reduced.

Hepatic Impairment: Dosage should be reduced.

Stability

Storage: Store at room temperature below 30°C (86°F). Protect from moisture.

Monitoring and Teaching Issues

Physical Assessment: **Assess patient for history of liver disease or ethanol abuse.** Assess other medications patient may be taking for additive or adverse interactions (see Drug Interactions). Monitor therapeutic effectiveness, signs of overdose, vital signs, and signs of adverse reactions (see Adverse Reactions) at beginning of therapy and at regular intervals with long-term use. Assess knowledge/teach patient appropriate use, adverse reactions to report, and appropriate interventions to reduce side effects. **Pregnancy risk**

factor D - determine that patient is not pregnant before beginning treatment. Instruct patients of childbearing age about appropriate barrier contraceptive measures. Breast-feeding is contraindicated.

Patient Education: If self-administered, use exactly as directed; do not increase dose or frequency. Drug may cause physical and/or psychological dependence. Take with food or milk. While using this medication, do not use alcohol and other prescription or OTC medications (especially sedatives, tranquilizers, antihistamines, or pain medications) without consulting prescriber. Maintain adequate hydration (2-3 L/day of fluids) unless advised by prescriber to restrict fluids. May cause dizziness, lightheadedness, confusion, or drowsiness (use caution when driving, climbing stairs, or changing position - rising from sitting or lying to standing, or when engaging in tasks requiring alertness until response to drug is known); heartburn or epigastric discomfort (frequent mouth care, frequent sips of fluids, chewing gum, or sucking lozenges may help); or constipation (increased exercise, fluids, fruit, or fiber may help). Report chest pain or palpitations; persistent dizziness; confusion, nightmares, excitation, or changes in mentation; shortness of breath or difficulty breathing; skin rash; unusual bleeding or bruising; or unusual fatigue and weakness. **Pregnancy/breast-feeding precautions:** Do not get pregnant while taking this medication; use appropriate barrier contraceptive measures. Do not breast-feed.

Geriatric Considerations: Elderly may react to barbiturates with marked excitement, depression, and confusion.

Butalbital, Acetaminophen, Caffeine, and Codeine

(byoo TAL bi tal, a seet a MIN oh fen, KAF een, & KOE deen)

U.S. Brand Names Fioricet® with Codeine

Synonyms Acetaminophen, Caffeine, Codeine, and Butalbital; Caffeine, Acetaminophen, Butalbital, and Codeine; Codeine, Acetaminophen, Butalbital, and Caffeine

Restrictions C-III

Generic Available Yes

Pharmacologic Category Analgesic Combination (Narcotic); Barbiturate

Pregnancy Risk Factor C (per manufacturer)/D (prolonged use or high doses at term)

Lactation Excreted in breast milk/not recommended

Use Relief of symptoms of complex tension (muscle contraction) headache

Mechanism of Action/Effect Combination product for the treatment of tension headache. Contains codeine (narcotic analgesic), butalbital (barbiturate), caffeine (CNS stimulant), and acetaminophen (nonopiate, nonsalicylate analgesic).

Contraindications Hypersensitivity to butalbital, codeine, caffeine, acetaminophen, or any component of the formulation; porphyria; known G6PD deficiency; pregnancy (prolonged use or high doses at term)

Warnings/Precautions May cause severe hepatic toxicity on overdose; use with caution in patients with alcoholic liver disease; chronic daily dosing in adults of 5-8 g of acetaminophen over several weeks or 3-4 g/day of acetaminophen for 1 year have resulted in liver damage. Use with caution in patients with hypersensitivity reactions to other phenanthrene derivative opioid agonists (eg, morphine, hydrocodone, oxycodone). Use caution with Addison's disease, severe renal or hepatic impairment. Use caution in patients with head injury or other intracranial lesions, acute abdominal conditions, urethral stricture of BPH, or in patients with respiratory diseases. Elderly and/or debilitated patients may be more susceptible to CNS depressants, as well as constipating effects of narcotics. Tolerance or drug dependence may result from extended use. Safety and efficacy in pediatric patients have not been established.

Pregnancy risk C (D in prolonged use or high doses at term).

Drug Interactions

Cytochrome P450 Effect:

Acetaminophen: Substrate of CYP1A2, 2A6, 2C8/9, 2D6, 2E1, 3A4

Caffeine: Substrate of **CYP1A2**, 2C8/9, 2D6, 2E1, 3A4; Inhibits **CYP1A2**

Decreased Effect:

Acetaminophen, caffeine, codeine: See individual agents.

Butalbital: Refer to Phenobarbital monograph.

Increased Effect/Toxicity:

Acetaminophen, caffeine, codeine: See individual agents.

Butalbital: Refer to Phenobarbital monograph.

Nutritional/Ethanol Interactions Ethanol: Avoid ethanol (may increase CNS depression).

Adverse Reactions Frequency not defined.

Cardiovascular: Tachycardia, palpitation, hypotension, edema, syncope

Central nervous system: Drowsiness, fatigue, mental confusion, disorientation, nervousness, hallucination, euphoria, depression, seizure, headache, agitation, fainting, excitement, fever

Dermatologic: Rash, erythema, pruritus, urticaria, erythema multiforme, exfoliative dermatitis, toxic epidermal necrolysis

Gastrointestinal: Nausea, xerostomia, constipation, gastrointestinal spasm, heartburn, flatulence

Genitourinary: Urinary retention, diuresis

Neuromuscular & skeletal: Leg pain, weakness, numbness

Otic: Tinnitus

Miscellaneous: Allergic reaction, anaphylaxis

Note: Potential reactions associated with components of Fioricet® with Codeine include agranulocytosis, irritability, nausea, thrombocytopenia, tremor, vomiting

Overdosage/Toxicology Symptoms of opiate overdose include unsteady gait, slurred speech, confusion, respiratory depression, hypotension, and coma. Opioid symptoms may be reversed by naloxone, 2 mg I.V., with repeated doses as necessary up to a total of 10 mg. Barbiturate treatment is symptomatic and supportive.

Symptoms of acetaminophen overdose include hepatic necrosis, transient azotemia, renal tubular necrosis with acute toxicity, anemia, and GI disturbances with chronic toxicity. Treatment consists of acetylcysteine 140 mg/kg orally (loading) followed by 70 mg/kg every 4 hours for 17 doses; therapy should be initiated based upon laboratory analysis suggesting a

(Continued)

Butalbital, Acetaminophen, Caffeine, and Codeine *(Continued)*

high probability of hepatotoxic potential. Activated charcoal is very effective at binding acetaminophen. Intravenous acetylcysteine should be reserved for patients unable to take oral forms.

Formulations Capsule: Butalbital 50 mg, caffeine 40 mg, acetaminophen 325 mg, and codeine phosphate 30 mg

Dosing

Adults & Elderly: Oral: Adults: 1-2 capsules every 4 hours. Total daily dosage should not exceed 6 capsules.

Hepatic Impairment: Use with caution. Limited, low-dose therapy usually well tolerated in hepatic disease/cirrhosis. However, cases of hepatotoxicity at daily acetaminophen dosages <4 g/day have been reported. Avoid chronic use in hepatic impairment.

Stability

Storage: Store below 30°C (86°F).

Monitoring and Teaching Issues

Physical Assessment: See Contraindications and Warnings/Precautions for use cautions. Assess effectiveness and interactions of other prescription, OTC, or herbal medication patient may be taking (see Drug Interactions). Assess history for allergy to butalbital, codeine, barbiturates, or acetaminophen (see Contraindications). Monitor for effectiveness of pain relief, signs of overdose, and adverse reactions (see Adverse Reactions and Overdose/Toxicology). Discontinue slowly after long-term use. For inpatient use, implement safety precautions. Monitor for effectiveness of therapy and adverse reactions. Assess knowledge/teach patient appropriate use, interventions to reduce side effects, and adverse symptoms to report (see Adverse Reactions and Patient Education). **Pregnancy risk factor C/D (prolonged dose or high doses at term)** - benefits of use should outweigh possible risks. Breast-feeding is not recommended.

Patient Education: Use exactly as directed; do not increase dose or frequency. Drug may cause physical and/or psychological dependence. Take with food or milk. Do not use alcohol, other prescriptions, OTC medications, or herbal products (especially sedatives, tranquilizers, antihistamines, or pain medications) without consulting prescriber. Maintain adequate hydration (2-3 L/day of fluids) unless advised by prescriber to restrict fluids. May cause dizziness, lightheadedness, confusion, or drowsiness (use caution when driving, climbing stairs, or changing position sitting or lying to standing, or when engaging in tasks requiring alertness until response to drug is known); heartburn, nausea (small, frequent meals, frequent mouth care, chewing gum, or sucking lozenges may help); or constipation (increased exercise, fluids, fruit, or fiber may help; if unresolved, contact prescriber). Report chest pain or palpitation; persistent dizziness; confusion; nightmares; excitation or changes in mentation; shortness of breath or difficulty breathing; skin rash or irritation; unusual muscle weakness or leg pain; or ringing in ears. **Pregnancy/breast-feeding precautions:** Inform prescriber if you are or intend to become pregnant. Breast-feeding is not recommended.

Breast-feeding Issues: Codeine, caffeine, barbiturates, and acetaminophen are excreted in breast milk in small amounts. Discontinuation of breast-feeding or discontinuation of the drug should be considered.

Pregnancy Issues: Reproduction studies have not been conducted. Butalbital, codeine, and caffeine cross the placenta and can be found in fetal tissue. Butalbital may cause withdrawal seizures in newborns when taken during pregnancy. Should be administered to a pregnant woman only when clearly indicated, and for as short a period as possible. Use of codeine during labor and delivery may lead to respiratory depression in the neonate.

Butalbital, Aspirin, and Caffeine (byoo TAL bi tal, AS pir in, & KAF een)

U.S. Brand Names Fiorinal®

Synonyms Aspirin, Caffeine, and Butalbital; Butalbital Compound

Restrictions C-III

Generic Available Yes

Pharmacologic Category Barbiturate

Pregnancy Risk Factor C/D (prolonged use or high doses at term)

Lactation Enters breast milk/use caution due to aspirin content

Use Relief of the symptomatic complex of tension or muscle contraction headache

Contraindications Hypersensitivity to butalbital or any component of the formulation; porphyria; pregnancy (prolonged use or high doses at term)

Warnings/Precautions Use with extreme caution in the presence of peptic ulcer or coagulation abnormality - can produce psychological/physical drug dependence. Children and teenagers should not use this product. Pregnancy risk C/D (prolonged use or high doses at term).

Drug Interactions

Cytochrome P450 Effect:

Aspirin: Substrate of CYP2C8/9

Caffeine: Substrate of **CYP1A2**, 2C8/9, 2D6, 2E1, 3A4; Inhibits **CYP1A2**

Decreased Effect: May decrease the effect of uricosuric agents (probenecid and sulfinpyrazone) reducing their effect on gout.

Increased Effect/Toxicity: Enhanced effect/toxicity with oral anticoagulants (warfarin), oral antidiabetic agents, insulin, 6-mercaptopurine, methotrexate, NSAIDs, narcotic analgesics (propoxyphene, meperidine, etc), benzodiazepines, sedative-hypnotics, other CNS depressants. The CNS effects of butalbital may be enhanced by MAO inhibitors.

Nutritional/Ethanol Interactions Ethanol: Avoid ethanol (may increase CNS depression).

Effects on Lab Values Aspirin may interfere with serum amylase, fasting blood glucose, cholesterol, protein, AST (SGOT), uric acid, PT, and bleeding time. Aspirin may interfere with laboratory results in urine of glucose, 5-hydroxyindoleacetic acid, Gerhardt ketone, VMA, uric acid, diacetic acid, and spectrophotometric detection of barbiturates.

Adverse Reactions

>10%:

Central nervous system: Dizziness, drowsiness

Gastrointestinal: Nausea, heartburn, stomach pains, dyspepsia, epigastric discomfort

1% to 10%:

Central nervous system: Lightheadedness

Gastrointestinal: Nausea, vomiting, flatulence

<1% (Limited to important or life-threatening): Bone marrow suppression (one case report), exfoliative dermatitis, Stevens-Johnson syndrome, toxic epidermal necrosis

Formulations Capsule (Fiorinal®): Butalbital 50 mg, caffeine 40 mg, and aspirin 325 mg

Dosing

Adults: Tension or muscle contraction headache: Oral: 1-2 tablets or capsules every 4 hours; not to exceed 6 tablets or capsules/day

Elderly: Not recommended for use in the elderly.

Renal Impairment: Dosage should be reduced.

Hepatic Impairment: Dosage should be reduced.

Stability

Storage: Store below 25°C (77°F).

Monitoring and Teaching Issues

Physical Assessment: Monitor for effectiveness of pain relief. Monitor CNS status, heart rate, blood pressure, fluid balance, and elimination regularly. Combination drug contains aspirin; assess for aspirin sensitivity and see Warnings/Precautions and Drug Interactions. **Pregnancy risk factor C/D** - see Pregnancy Risk Factor for use cautions. Note breast-feeding caution.

Patient Education: Take as directed; do not exceed prescribed amount. Avoid alcohol, aspirin or aspirin-containing medications, or any OTC medications unless approved by prescriber. Maintain adequate hydration to prevent constipation (2-3 L/day) unless advised by prescriber to restrict fluids. You may experience drowsiness, impaired judgment or coordination; use caution when driving or engaging in tasks that require alertness until response to drug is known. Small frequent meals may help reduce GI upset. Report any ringing in ears; abdominal pain; easy bruising or bleeding; blood in urine; severe weakness; acute unresolved dizziness or confusion, nervousness, nightmares, insomnia; or skin rash. **Pregnancy/breast-feeding precautions:** Inform prescriber if you are or intend to become pregnant. Consult prescriber if breast-feeding.

Geriatric Considerations: Elderly may react to barbiturates with marked excitement, depression, and confusion.

Butalbital, Aspirin, Caffeine, and Codeine

(byoo TAL bi tal, AS pir in, KAF een, & KOE deen)

U.S. Brand Names Fiorinal® With Codeine

Synonyms Butalbital Compound and Codeine; Codeine and Butalbital Compound; Codeine, Butalbital, Aspirin, and Caffeine

Restrictions C-III

Generic Available Yes

Pharmacologic Category Analgesic Combination (Narcotic); Barbiturate

Pregnancy Risk Factor C/D (prolonged use or high doses at term)

Lactation Excretion in breast milk unknown/use caution

Use Mild to moderate pain when sedation is needed

Contraindications Hypersensitivity to butalbital, codeine, aspirin, or any component of the formulation; opium derivatives; hemorrhagic diathesis (eg, hemophilia, hypoprothrombinemia, von Willebrand disease, the thrombocytopenias, thrombasthenia, and other ill-defined hereditary platelet dysfunctions, severe vitamin K deficiency, and severe liver damage); peptic ulcer or other serious GI lesions; porphyria; pregnancy (prolonged use or high doses at term)

Warnings/Precautions Habit-forming, potentially abusable; patients on anticoagulant therapy. Pregnancy risk C/D (extended use or high doses near term).

Drug Interactions

Cytochrome P450 Effect:

Aspirin: Substrate of CYP2C8/9

Caffeine: Substrate of **CYP1A2**, 2C8/9, 2D6, 2E1, 3A4; Inhibits **CYP1A2**

Decreased Effect: Aspirin, butalbital, caffeine, and codeine may diminish effects of uricosuric agents such as probenecid and sulfinpyrazone.

Increased Effect/Toxicity: MAO inhibitors may enhance the CNS effects of butalbital. In patients receiving concomitant corticosteroids during the chronic use of ASA, withdrawal of corticosteroids may result in salicylism. Butalbital compound and codeine may enhance effects of oral anticoagulants. Increased effect with oral antidiabetic agents and insulin, 6-mercaptopurine and methotrexate, NSAIDs, other narcotic analgesics, ethanol, general anesthetics, tranquilizers such as chlordiazepoxide, sedative hypnotics, or other CNS depressants.

Nutritional/Ethanol Interactions Ethanol: Avoid ethanol (may increase CNS depression).

Effects on Lab Values

Aspirin: Serum amylase, fasting blood glucose, cholesterol, protein, AST (SGOT), uric acid, PT and bleeding time; urine glucose, 5-hydroxy indoleacetic acid, Gerhardt ketone; vanillylmandelic acid, urine-uric acid, diacetic acid, and spectrophotometric detection of barbiturates

Codeine: Increased serum amylase

Adverse Reactions

>10%:

Central nervous system: Dizziness, lightheadedness, drowsiness

Gastrointestinal: Nausea, heartburn, stomach pains, dyspepsia, epigastric discomfort

1% to 10%:

Central nervous system: Confusion, mental depression, unusual excitement, nervousness, faint feeling, insomnia, nightmares, intoxicated feeling

Dermatologic: Rash

Gastrointestinal: Constipation, GI ulceration

(Continued)

Butalbital, Aspirin, Caffeine, and Codeine *(Continued)*

<1% (Limited to important or life-threatening): Agranulocytosis, allergic reaction bronchospasm, chest pain, epistaxis, exfoliative dermatitis, hallucinations, hepatotoxicity, impaired renal function, iron-deficiency anemia, jitters, leukopenia, megaloblastic anemia, nervousness, occult bleeding, palpitations, prolongation of bleeding time, respiratory depression, Stevens-Johnson syndrome, syncope, tachycardia, thrombocytopenia, thrombophlebitis

Overdosage/Toxicology Symptoms of overdose include unsteady gait, slurred speech, confusion, respiratory depression, hypotension, and coma. Opioid symptoms may be reversed by naloxone, 2 mg I.V., with repeated doses as necessary up to a total of 10 mg. Barbiturate treatment is symptomatic and supportive.

Formulations Capsule: Butalbital 50 mg, caffeine 40 mg, aspirin 325 mg, and codeine phosphate 30 mg

Dosing

Adults: Mild to moderate pain (sedation desired): Oral: 1-2 capsules every 4 hours as needed; up to 6 capsules/day

Elderly: Not recommended for use in the elderly.

Stability

Storage: Store below 25°C (77°F).

Monitoring and Teaching Issues

Physical Assessment: **Do not use for persons with allergic reaction to aspirin, opium, or codeine** (see Contraindications). Assess other medications patient may be taking for additive or adverse interactions (see Drug Interactions). Monitor for effectiveness of pain relief, signs of overdose, and adverse reactions (see Adverse Reactions and Overdose/Toxicology) at beginning of therapy and at regular intervals with long-term use. May cause physical and/or psychological dependence. Discontinue slowly after long-term use. For inpatients, implement safety. Assess knowledge/teach patient appropriate use if self-administered. Teach patient to monitor for adverse reactions, adverse reactions to report, and appropriate interventions to reduce side effects. **Pregnancy risk factor C/D** - see Pregnancy Risk Factor for use cautions; benefits of use should outweigh possible risks. Note breast-feeding caution.

Patient Education: If self-administered, use exactly as directed; do not increase dose or frequency. Drug may cause physical and/or psychological dependence. Take with food or milk. While using this medication, do not use alcohol and other prescription or OTC medications (especially sedatives, tranquilizers, antihistamines, or pain medications) without consulting prescriber. Maintain adequate hydration (2-3 L/day of fluids) unless advised by prescriber to restrict fluids. May cause dizziness, lightheadedness, confusion, or drowsiness (use caution when driving, climbing stairs, or changing position - rising from sitting or lying to standing, or when engaging in tasks requiring alertness until response to drug is known); heartburn or epigastric discomfort (frequent mouth care, frequent sips of fluids, chewing gum, or sucking lozenges may help); or constipation (increased exercise, fluids, fruit, or fiber may help; if unresolved, consult prescriber about use of stool softeners). Report chest pain or palpitations; persistent dizziness; confusion, nightmares, excitation, or changes in mentation; shortness of breath or difficulty breathing; skin rash, unusual bleeding or bruising; or unusual fatigue and weakness. **Pregnancy/breast-feeding precautions:** Inform prescriber if you are or intend to become pregnant. Consult prescriber if breast-feeding.

Other Issues: Abrupt discontinuation after sustained use (generally >10 days) may cause withdrawal symptoms.

Butalbital Compound *see* Butalbital, Aspirin, and Caffeine *on page 194*

Butalbital Compound and Codeine *see* Butalbital, Aspirin, Caffeine, and Codeine *on page 195*

Butorphanol (byoo TOR fa nole)

U.S. Brand Names Stadol®; Stadol® NS

Synonyms Butorphanol Tartrate

Restrictions C-IV

Generic Available Yes: Injection

Pharmacologic Category Analgesic, Narcotic

Pregnancy Risk Factor C/D (prolonged use or high doses at term)

Lactation Enters breast milk/use caution (AAP rates "compatible")

Use

Parenteral: Management of moderate to severe pain; preoperative medication; supplement to balanced anesthesia; management of pain during labor

Nasal spray: Management of moderate to severe pain, including migraine headache pain

Mechanism of Action/Effect Mixed narcotic agonist-antagonist with central analgesic actions; binds to opiate receptors in the CNS, causing inhibition of ascending pain pathways, altering the perception of and response to pain; produces generalized CNS depression

Contraindications Hypersensitivity to butorphanol or any component of the formulation; avoid use in opiate-dependent patients who have not been detoxified, may precipitate opiate withdrawal; pregnancy (prolonged use or high doses at term)

Warnings/Precautions May cause CNS depression, which may impair physical or mental abilities. Effects with other sedative drugs or ethanol may be potentiated. Use with caution in patients with hepatic/renal dysfunction. Tolerance or drug dependence may result from extended use. Concurrent use of sumatriptan nasal spray and butorphanol nasal spray may increase risk of transient high blood pressure. Pregnancy risk C/D (prolonged use or high doses at term).

Drug Interactions

Increased Effect/Toxicity: Increased toxicity with CNS depressants, phenothiazines, barbiturates, skeletal muscle relaxants, alfentanil, guanabenz, and MAO inhibitors.

Nutritional/Ethanol Interactions

Ethanol: Avoid or limit ethanol (may increase CNS depression). Watch for sedation.

Herb/Nutraceutical: Avoid valerian, St John's wort, kava kava, gotu kola (may increase CNS depression).

Adverse Reactions

>10%:

Central nervous system: Drowsiness (43%), dizziness (19%), insomnia (Stadol® NS)
Gastrointestinal: Nausea/vomiting (13%)
Respiratory: Nasal congestion (Stadol® NS)

1% to 10%:

Cardiovascular: Vasodilation, palpitations
Central nervous system: Lightheadedness, headache, lethargy, anxiety, confusion, euphoria, somnolence
Dermatologic: Pruritus
Gastrointestinal: Anorexia, constipation, xerostomia, stomach pain, unpleasant aftertaste
Neuromuscular & skeletal: Tremor, paresthesia, weakness
Ocular: Blurred vision
Otic: Ear pain, tinnitus
Respiratory: Bronchitis, cough, dyspnea, epistaxis, nasal irritation, pharyngitis, rhinitis, sinus congestion, sinusitis, upper respiratory infection
Miscellaneous: Diaphoresis (increased)

<1% (Limited to important or life-threatening): Dependence (with prolonged use), depression, difficulty speaking (transient), dyspnea, hallucinations, hypertension, nightmares, paradoxical CNS stimulation, rash, respiratory depression, syncope, tinnitus, vertigo, withdrawal symptoms

Stadol® NS: Apnea, chest pain, convulsions, delusions, depressions, edema, hypertension, shallow breathing, tachycardia

Overdosage/Toxicology Symptoms of overdose include respiratory depression, cardiac and CNS depression. Treatment is supportive. Naloxone, 2 mg I.V. with repeat administration as necessary up to a total of 10 mg, can also be used to reverse toxic effects of the opiate.

Pharmacodynamics/Kinetics

Absorption: Rapid and well absorbed

Bioavailability: Nasal: 60% to 70%

Half-Life Elimination: 2.5-4 hours

Metabolism: Hepatic

Onset: I.M.: 5-10 minutes; I.V.: <10 minutes; Nasal: Within 15 minutes
Peak effect: I.M.: 0.5-1 hour; I.V.: 4-5 minutes

Duration: I.M., I.V.: 3-4 hours; Nasal: 4-5 hours

Formulations

Injection, solution, as tartrate [preservative free] (Stadol®): 1 mg/mL (1 mL); 2 mg/mL (1 mL, 2 mL)
Injection, solution, as tartrate [with preservative] (Stadol®): 2 mg/mL (10 mL)
Solution, intranasal spray, as tartrate (Stadol® NS): 10 mg/mL (2.5 mL) [14-15 doses]

Dosing

Adults:

Moderate to severe pain:

I.M. Initial: 2 mg, may repeat every 3-4 hours as needed
I.V.: Initial: 1 mg, may repeat every 3-4 hours as needed
Intranasal (spray) (includes use for migraine headache pain): Initial: 1 spray (~1 mg per spray) in 1 nostril; if adequate pain relief is not achieved within 60-90 minutes, an additional 1 spray in 1 nostril may be given; may repeat initial dose sequence in 3-4 hours after the last dose as needed

Note: In some clinical trials, an initial dose of 2 mg (as 2 doses 1 hour apart or 2 mg initially - 1 spray in each nostril) has been used, followed by 1 mg in 1 hour; side effects were greater at these dosages

Migraine: Nasal spray: Refer to "moderate to severe pain" indication
Preoperative medication: I.M.: 2 mg 60-90 minutes before surgery
Supplement to balanced anesthesia: I.V.: 2 mg shortly before induction and/or an incremental dose of 0.5-1 mg (up to 0.06 mg/kg), depending on previously administered sedative, analgesic, and hypnotic medications
Pain during labor (fetus >37 weeks gestation and no signs of fetal distress):

I.M., I.V.: 1-2 mg; may repeat in 4 hours

Note: Alternative analgesia should be used for pain associated with delivery or if delivery is anticipated within 4 hours

Elderly:

I.M., I.V.: Initial dosage should generally be ½ of the recommended dose; repeated dosing must be based on initial response rather than fixed intervals, but generally should be at least 6 hours apart.

Nasal spray: Initial dose should not exceed 1 mg; a second dose may be given after 90-120 minutes.

Administration

Inhalation: See Dosing.

Topical: Intranasal: Consider avoiding simultaneous intranasal migraine sprays; may want to separate by at least 30 minutes

Stability

Storage: Store at room temperature; protect from freezing.

Compatibility:

Y-site administration: Incompatible with amphotericin B cholesteryl sulfate complex, midazolam

Compatibility in syringe: Incompatible with dimenhydrinate, pentobarbital

Monitoring and Teaching Issues

Physical Assessment: Assess other medications patient may be taking for possible additive or adverse interactions (see Warnings/Precautions and Drug Interactions). Monitor for effectiveness of pain relief, signs of overdose, vital signs, and adverse effects at beginning of therapy and at regular intervals with long-term use (see adverse effects and

(Continued)

Butorphanol *(Continued)*

Overdose/Toxicology). For inpatients, implement safety measures. May cause physical and/or psychological dependence. Assess knowledge/teach patient appropriate use (if self-administered), adverse reactions to report, and appropriate interventions to reduce side effects. **Pregnancy risk factor C/D** - see Pregnancy Risk Factor for use cautions. Note breast-feeding caution.

Patient Education: If self-administered, use exactly as directed; do not increase dose or frequency. Drug may cause physical and/or psychological dependence. While using this medication, do not use alcohol and other prescription or OTC medications (especially sedatives, tranquilizers, antihistamines, or pain medications) without consulting prescriber. May cause dizziness, drowsiness, confusion, or blurred vision (use caution when driving, climbing stairs, or changing position - rising from sitting or lying to standing, or when engaging in tasks requiring alertness until response to drug is known); nausea or vomiting, or loss of appetite (frequent mouth care, small, frequent meals, sucking lozenges, or chewing gum may help). Report unresolved nausea or vomiting; difficulty breathing or shortness of breath; restlessness, insomnia, euphoria, or nightmares; excessive sedation or unusual weakness; facial flushing, rapid heartbeat, or palpitations; urinary difficulty; or vision changes.

Nasal administration: Do not use more frequently than prescribed. Blow nose prior to administering. Follow directions on package insert. Insert nozzle of applicator gently into one nostril and exhale. With next breath, squeeze applicator once firmly and quickly once as you breath in. If adequate relief from headache is not achieved within 60-90 minutes, an additional 1 spray may be given. May be repeated in 3-4 hours following last dose, as needed. **Alternately:** Two sprays may be given - one spray in each nostril, if you are able to remain lying down (in the event of drowsiness or dizziness). Additional doses should not be taken for 3-4 hours. Avoid using simultaneously with intranasal migraine sprays. Separate by at least 30 minutes.

Pregnancy/breast-feeding precautions: Inform prescriber if you are or intend to become pregnant. If you are breast-feeding, take dose immediately after breast-feeding or 3-4 hours prior to next feeding.

Geriatric Considerations: Adjust dose for renal function in the elderly.

Related Information

Compatibility of Drugs in Syringe *on page 1566*
Narcotic/Opioid Analgesic Comparison *on page 1583*

Butorphanol Tartrate *see* Butorphanol *on page 196*

BW-430C *see* Lamotrigine *on page 770*

C2B8 *see* Rituximab *on page 1198*

C7E3 *see* Abciximab *on page 31*

311C90 *see* Zolmitriptan *on page 1428*

Caffeine, Acetaminophen, Butalbital, and Codeine *see* Butalbital, Acetaminophen, Caffeine, and Codeine *on page 193*

Caffeine and Sodium Benzoate (KAF een & SOW dee um BEN zoe ate)

Synonyms Sodium Benzoate and Caffeine

Generic Available Yes

Pharmacologic Category Diuretic, Miscellaneous

Pregnancy Risk Factor C

Lactation Caffeine: Enters breast milk/use caution (AAP rates "compatible")

Use Emergency stimulant in acute circulatory failure, diuretic, relief of spinal puncture headache

Drug Interactions

Cytochrome P450 Effect: Caffeine: Substrate of **CYP1A2**, 2C8/9, 2D6, 2E1, 3A4; Inhibits **CYP1A2**

Adverse Reactions Frequency not defined.

Cardiovascular: Tachycardia, extrasystoles, palpitations

Central nervous system: Insomnia, restlessness, nervousness, mild delirium, headache, anxiety

Gastrointestinal: Nausea, vomiting, gastric irritation

Neuromuscular & skeletal: Muscle tension following abrupt cessation of drug after regular consumption of 500-600 mg/day

Renal: Diuresis

Formulations Injection: Caffeine 125 mg and sodium benzoate 125 mg per mL (2 mL)

Dosing

Adults & Elderly:

Stimulant/diuretic: I.M., I.V.: 500 mg, maximum single dose: 1 g

Spinal puncture headaches:

I.V.: 500 mg in 1000 mL NS infused over 1 hour, followed by 1000 mL NS infused over 1 hour; a second course of caffeine can be given for unrelieved headache pain in 4 hours.

Oral: 300 mg

Pediatrics: Children: Stimulant/diuretic: I.M., I.V., S.C.: 8 mg/kg every 4 hours as needed

Monitoring and Teaching Issues

Physical Assessment: See individual components listed in Related Information. **Pregnancy risk factor C** - benefits of use should outweigh possible risks. Note breast-feeding caution.

Patient Education: See individual agents. **Pregnancy/breast-feeding precautions:** Inform prescriber if you are or intend to become pregnant. Consult prescriber if breast-feeding.

Caffeine, Orphenadrine, and Aspirin *see* Orphenadrine, Aspirin, and Caffeine *on page 1010*

Calan® *see* Verapamil *on page 1396*

Calan® SR *see* Verapamil *on page 1396*
Cal Carb-HD® [OTC] *see* Calcium Supplements *on page 202*
Calci-Chew™ [OTC] *see* Calcium Supplements *on page 202*
Calciday-667® [OTC] *see* Calcium Supplements *on page 202*
Calciferol™ *see* Ergocalciferol *on page 483*
Calcijex™ *see* Calcitriol *on page 200*
Calcimar® *see* Calcitonin *on page 199*
Calci-Mix™ [OTC] *see* Calcium Supplements *on page 202*

Calcipotriene (kal si POE try een)

U.S. Brand Names Dovonex®

Generic Available No

Pharmacologic Category Topical Skin Product; Vitamin D Analog

Pregnancy Risk Factor C

Lactation Excretion in breast milk unknown

Use Treatment of moderate plaque psoriasis

Mechanism of Action/Effect Synthetic vitamin D_3 analog which regulates skin cell production and proliferation

Contraindications Hypersensitivity to calcipotriene or any component of the formulation; patients with demonstrated hypercalcemia or evidence of vitamin D toxicity; use on the face

Warnings/Precautions Use may cause irritations of lesions and surrounding uninvolved skin. If irritation develops, discontinue use. Transient, rapidly reversible elevation of serum calcium has occurred during use. If elevation in serum calcium occurs above the normal range, discontinue treatment until calcium levels are normal. For external use only; not for ophthalmic, oral, or intravaginal use. Pregnancy risk C.

Adverse Reactions

>10%: Dermatologic: Burning, itching, skin irritation, erythema, dry skin, peeling, rash, worsening of psoriasis

1% to 10%: Dermatologic: Hyperpigmentation

Formulations

Cream: 0.005% (30 g, 60 g, 100 g)
Ointment: 0.005% (30 g, 60 g, 100 g)
Solution, topical: 0.005% (60 mL)

Dosing

Adults & Elderly: Psoriasis: Topical: Apply in a thin film to the affected skin twice daily and rub in gently and completely.

Administration

Topical: For external use only; apply with gloves.

Monitoring Laboratory Tests Serum calcium

Monitoring and Teaching Issues

Physical Assessment: See Contraindications and Warnings/Precautions for use cautions. When applied to large areas of skin or for extensive periods of time, monitor for adverse skin or systemic reactions. Assess knowledge/teach patient appropriate application and use and adverse symptoms (see Adverse Reactions) to report. **Pregnancy risk factor C** - systemic absorption may be minimal with appropriate use. Note breast-feeding caution.

Patient Education: For external use only. Use exactly as directed; do not overuse. Before using, wash and dry area gently. Wear gloves to apply a thin film to affected area and rub in gently. If dressing is necessary, use a porous dressing. Avoid contact with eyes. Avoid exposing treated area to direct sunlight; sunburn can occur. Report increased swelling, redness, rash, itching, signs of infection, worsening of condition, or lack of healing. **Pregnancy/breast-feeding precautions:** Inform prescriber if you are or intend to become pregnant. Consult prescriber if breast-feeding.

Calcitonin (kal si TOE nin)

U.S. Brand Names Calcimar®; Miacalcin®

Synonyms Calcitonin (Salmon)

Generic Available No

Pharmacologic Category Antidote

Pregnancy Risk Factor C

Lactation Excretion in breast milk unknown

Use Calcitonin (salmon): Treatment of Paget's disease of bone (osteitis deformans); adjunctive therapy for hypercalcemia; used in postmenopausal osteoporosis and osteogenesis imperfecta

Mechanism of Action/Effect Structurally similar to human calcitonin; it directly inhibits osteoclastic bone resorption; promotes the renal excretion of calcium, phosphate, sodium, magnesium and potassium by decreasing tubular reabsorption; increases the jejunal secretion of water, sodium, potassium, and chloride

Contraindications Hypersensitivity to salmon protein or gelatin diluent

Warnings/Precautions A skin test should be performed prior to initiating therapy of calcitonin salmon. Have epinephrine immediately available for a possible hypersensitivity reaction. Use caution with renal insufficiency, pernicious anemia. Pregnancy risk C.

Drug Interactions

Decreased Effect: Calcitonin may be antagonized by calcium and vitamin D in treating hypercalcemia.

Adverse Reactions

>10%:
- Cardiovascular: Facial flushing
- Gastrointestinal: Nausea, diarrhea, anorexia
- Local: Edema at injection site

1% to 10%:
- Genitourinary: Polyuria
- Neuromuscular & skeletal: Back/joint pain

(Continued)

Calcitonin *(Continued)*

Respiratory: Nasal bleeding/crusting (following intranasal administration)

<1% (Limited to important or life-threatening): Dyspnea

Overdosage/Toxicology Symptoms of overdose include nausea, vomiting, hypocalcemia, and hypocalcemic tetany. Treat symptomatically.

Pharmacodynamics/Kinetics

Half-Life Elimination: S.C.: 1.2 hours

Onset: Hypercalcemia: ~2 hours

Duration: Hypercalcemia: 6-8 hours

Formulations

Injection, salmon calcitonin (Calcimar®): 200 units/mL (2 mL)

Solution, intranasal spray, salmon calcitonin (Miacalcin®): 200 units/activation (0.09 mL/dose) [glass bottle with pump] (2 mL)

Dosing

Adults & Elderly:

Paget's disease:

I.M., S.C.: 100 units/day to start, 50 units/day or 50-100 units every 1-3 days maintenance dose

Hypercalcemia: I.M., S.C.: Initial: 4 units/kg every 12 hours; may increase up to 8 units/kg every 12 hours to a maximum of every 6 hours

Osteoporosis prevention (in postmenopausal women):

I.M., S.C.: 100 units/day

Intranasal: 200 units (1 spray)/day

Pediatrics: Osteogenesis imperfecta: I.M., S.C.: 2 units/kg 3 times/week

Administration

I.M.: I.M. route is preferred if volume exceeds 2 mL. Taking medication in the evening may minimize the problems of flushing, nausea, and vomiting.

Other: Skin test should be performed prior to administration of salmon calcitonin

Stability

Storage: Salmon calcitonin:

Injection: Store under refrigeration at 2°C to 6°C (36°F to 43°F); stable for up to 2 weeks at room temperature.

Nasal: Store unopened bottle under refrigeration at 2°C to 8°C. Once the pump has been activated, store at room temperature.

Reconstitution: Salmon calcitonin: Injection: NS has been recommended for the dilution to prepare a skin test.

Monitoring Laboratory Tests Serum electrolytes and calcium, alkaline phosphatase and 24-hour urine collection for hydroxyproline excretion (Paget's disease)

Monitoring and Teaching Issues

Physical Assessment: Monitor skin test after 15 minutes for local inflammatory reaction before initiating therapy (increased erythema or skin wheal indicates positive reaction and allergy - greater with salmon calcitonin). Monitor appropriate laboratory tests as ordered. Monitor for signs or symptoms of adverse or toxic effects as indicated above, especially signs of hypocalcemic tetany, and signs of hypercalcemia. Teach and monitor patient for appropriate administration of subcutaneous or I.M. injections or proper use of nasal spray. If the patient is taking calcitonin for hypercalcemia, give instructions on an appropriate low calcium diet and monitor adherence. **Pregnancy risk factor C** - benefits of use should outweigh possible risks. Note breast-feeding caution.

Patient Education: When this drug is given subcutaneously or I.M. it will be necessary for you or a significant other to learn to prepare and give the injections (keep drug vials in a refrigerator - do not freeze). Report significant nasal irritation if using calcitonin nasal spray. Follow directions exactly. Increased warmth and flushing may be experienced with this drug and should only last about 1 hour after administration (taking drug in the evening may minimize these discomforts). Immediately report twitching, muscle spasm, dark colored urine, hives, significant skin rash, palpitations, or difficulty breathing. **Pregnancy/breast-feeding precautions:** Inform prescriber if you are or intend to become pregnant. Consult prescriber if breast-feeding.

Dietary Issues: Adequate vitamin D and calcium intake is essential for osteoporosis. Patients with Paget's disease and hypercalcemia should follow a low calcium diet as prescribed.

Geriatric Considerations: Calcitonin may be the drug of choice for postmenopausal women unable to take estrogens to increase bone density and reduce fractures. Calcium and vitamin D supplements should also be given. Calcitonin may also be effective in steroid-induced osteoporosis and other states associated with high bone turnover.

Breast-feeding Issues: Has been shown to decrease milk production in animals.

Related Information

Osteoporosis Management *on page 1696*

Calcitonin (Salmon) *see* Calcitonin *on page 199*

Cal-citrate® 250 [OTC] *see* Calcium Supplements *on page 202*

Calcitriol (kal si TRYE ole)

U.S. Brand Names Calcijex™; Rocaltrol®

Synonyms 1,25 Dihydroxycholecalciferol

Generic Available Yes

Pharmacologic Category Vitamin D Analog

Pregnancy Risk Factor C (manufacturer); A/D (dose exceeding RDA recommendation) (expert analysis)

Lactation Enters breast milk/not recommended (per manufacturer)

Use Management of hypocalcemia in patients on chronic renal dialysis; management of secondary hyperparathyroidism in moderate to severe chronic renal failure; management of hypocalcemia in hypoparathyroidism and pseudohypoparathyroidism

Use - Unlabeled/Investigational Decrease severity of psoriatic lesions in psoriatic vulgaris; vitamin D resistant rickets

Mechanism of Action/Effect Promotes absorption of calcium in the intestines and retention at the kidneys thereby increasing calcium levels in the serum; decreases excessive serum phosphatase levels, parathyroid hormone levels, and decreases bone resorption; increases renal tubule phosphate resorption

Contraindications Hypercalcemia; vitamin D toxicity; abnormal sensitivity to the effects of vitamin D; malabsorption syndrome; pregnancy (dose exceeding RDA)

Warnings/Precautions Adequate dietary (supplemental) calcium is necessary for clinical response to vitamin D; maintain adequate fluid intake; calcium-phosphate product (serum calcium times phosphorus) must not exceed 70. Avoid hypercalcemia. Immobilization or excessive dosage may increase risk of hypercalcemia and/or hypercalciuria. Pregnancy factor C (manufacturer).

Drug Interactions

Cytochrome P450 Effect: Induces CYP3A4

Decreased Effect: Cholestyramine and colestipol decrease absorption/effect of calcitriol. Thiazide diuretics, enzyme inducers (phenytoin, phenobarbital), and corticosteroids may reduce the effect of calcitriol.

Increased Effect/Toxicity: Risk of hypercalcemia with thiazide diuretics. Risk of hypermagnesemia with magnesium-containing antacids. Risk of digoxin toxicity may be increased (if hypercalcemia occurs).

Effects on Lab Values ↑ calcium, cholesterol, magnesium, BUN, AST, ALT, calcium (S), cholesterol (S); ↓ alkaline phosphatase

Adverse Reactions

>10%: Endocrine & metabolic: Hypercalcemia (33%)

Frequency not defined:

- Cardiovascular: Cardiac arrhythmias, hypertension, hypotension
- Central nervous system: Headache, irritability, seizures (rare), somnolence, psychosis
- Dermatologic: Pruritus, erythema multiforme
- Endocrine & metabolic: Hypermagnesemia, polydipsia
- Gastrointestinal: Anorexia, constipation, metallic taste, nausea, pancreatitis, vomiting, xerostomia
- Hepatic: Elevated LFTs
- Neuromuscular & skeletal: Bone pain, myalgia, dystrophy, soft tissue calcification
- Ocular: Conjunctivitis, photophobia
- Renal: Polyuria

Overdosage/Toxicology Symptoms of overdose include hypercalcemia and hypercalciuria. Following withdrawal of the drug, treatment consists of bedrest, liberal intake of fluids, reduced calcium intake, and cathartic administration. Severe hypercalcemia requires I.V. hydration and forced diuresis. Urine output should be monitored and maintained at >3 mL/kg/hour during the acute treatment phase. I.V. saline can quickly and significantly increase excretion of calcium into urine. Calcitonin, cholestyramine, prednisone, sodium EDTA, biphosphonates, and mithramycin have all been used successfully to treat the more resistant cases of vitamin D-induced hypercalcemia.

Pharmacodynamics/Kinetics

Absorption: Oral: Rapid

Half-Life Elimination: 3-8 hours

Metabolism: Primarily to 1,24,25-trihydroxycholecalciferol and 1,24,25-trihydroxy ergocalciferol

Onset: ~2-6 hours

Duration: 3-5 days

Formulations

Capsule: 0.25 mcg, 0.5 mcg

Injection: 1 mcg/mL (1 mL); 2 mcg/mL (1 mL)

Solution, oral: 1 mcg/mL

Dosing

Adults: Individualize dosage to maintain calcium levels of 9-10 mg/dL.

Renal failure:

- Oral: 0.25 mcg/day or every other day (may require 0.5-1 mcg/day)
- I.V.: 0.5 mcg (0.01 mcg/kg) 3 times/week; most doses in the range of 0.5-3 mcg (0.01-0.05 mcg/kg) 3 times/week

Hypoparathyroidism/pseudohypoparathyroidism: Oral: 0.5-2 mcg/day

Vitamin D-dependent rickets: Oral: 1 mcg once daily

Vitamin D-resistant rickets (familial hypophosphatemia): Oral: Initial: 0.015-0.02 mcg/kg once daily; maintenance: 0.03-0.06 mcg/kg once daily; maximum dose: 2 mcg once daily

Elderly: Refer to adult dosing. No dosage recommendations, but start at the lower end of the dosage range.

Pediatrics: Individualize dosage to maintain calcium levels of 9-10 mg/dL.

Renal failure:

Children:

- Oral: 0.25-2 mcg/day have been used (with hemodialysis); 0.014-0.041 mcg/kg/day (not receiving hemodialysis); increases should be made at 4- to 8-week intervals.
- I.V.: 0.01-0.05 mcg/kg 3 times/week if undergoing hemodialysis

Hypoparathyroidism/pseudohypoparathyroidism: Oral (evaluate dosage at 2- to 4-week intervals):

Children:

- <1 year: 0.04-0.08 mcg/kg once daily
- 1-5 years: 0.25-0.75 mcg once daily

Children >6 years: 0.5-2 mcg once daily

Vitamin D-dependent rickets: Refer to adult dosing.

Vitamin D-resistant rickets (familial hypophosphatemia): Refer to adult dosing.

(Continued)

Calcitriol *(Continued)*

Administration

Oral: Can be administered without regard to food. Give with meals to reduce GI problems.

Stability

Storage: Store in tight, light-resistant container. Calcitriol degrades upon prolonged exposure to light.

Compatibility: Stable in D_5W, NS, sterile water for injection

Monitoring Laboratory Tests Serum calcium and phosphorus, and renal function. The serum calcium times phosphate product should not be allowed to exceed 70.

Monitoring and Teaching Issues

Physical Assessment: See Contraindications and Warnings/Precautions for use cautions. Assess effectiveness and interactions of other medications patient may be taking (see Drug Interactions). Monitor lab tests, effectiveness of therapy, and adverse effects at beginning of therapy and regularly with long-term use (see Adverse Reactions and Overdose/Toxicology). Assess knowledge/teach patient appropriate use, appropriate nutritional counseling, possible side effects/interventions, and adverse symptoms to report (see Patient Education). **Pregnancy risk factor A/C/D** - see Pregnancy Risk Factor for use cautions. Breast-feeding is not recommended.

Patient Education: Take exact dose as prescribed; do not increase dose. Maintain recommended diet and calcium supplementation. Avoid taking magnesium-containing antacids. You may experience nausea, vomiting, loss of appetite, or metallic taste (small, frequent meals, frequent mouth care, chewing gum, or sucking lozenges may help); or hypotension (use caution when rising from sitting or lying position or when climbing stairs or bending over). Report chest pain or palpitations; acute headache; skin rash; change in vision or eye irritation; CNS changes; unusual weakness or fatigue; persistent nausea, vomiting, cramps, or diarrhea; or muscle or bone pain. **Pregnancy/breast-feeding precautions:** Inform prescriber if you are or intend to become pregnant. Breast-feeding is not recommended.

Dietary Issues: May be taken without regard to food. Give with meals to reduce GI problems.

Geriatric Considerations: Appetite and caloric requirements may decrease with advanced age. Assess diet for adequate nutrient intake with regard to vitamins and minerals. (Daily vitamin supplements are sometimes recommended). Persons >65 years of age have decreased absorption and may have decreased intake of vitamin D. This may require supplement with daily vitamin D intake, especially for those with high risk for osteoporosis.

Calcium Acetate *see* Calcium Supplements *on page 202*

Calcium Carbonate *see* Calcium Supplements *on page 202*

Calcium Channel Blockers *see page 1563*

Calcium Chloride *see* Calcium Supplements *on page 202*

Calcium Citrate *see* Calcium Supplements *on page 202*

Calcium Glubionate *see* Calcium Supplements *on page 202*

Calcium Gluceptate *see* Calcium Supplements *on page 202*

Calcium Gluconate *see* Calcium Supplements *on page 202*

Calcium Lactate *see* Calcium Supplements *on page 202*

Calcium Leucovorin *see* Leucovorin *on page 779*

Calcium Phosphate, Tribasic *see* Calcium Supplements *on page 202*

Calcium Polycarbophil *see page 1581*

Calcium Supplements (KAL see um SUP la ments)

U.S. Brand Names Alka-Mints® [OTC]; Amitone® [OTC]; Cal Carb-HD® [OTC]; Calci-Chew™ [OTC]; Calciday-667® [OTC]; Calci-Mix™ [OTC]; Cal-citrate® 250 [OTC]; Calphron®; Cal-Plus® [OTC]; Caltrate® 600 [OTC]; Caltrate, Jr.® [OTC]; Chooz® [OTC]; Citracal® [OTC]; Dicarbosil® [OTC]; Equilet® [OTC]; Florical® [OTC]; Gencalc® 600 [OTC]; Mallamint® [OTC]; Neo-Calglucon® [OTC]; Nephro-Calci® [OTC]; Os-Cal® 500 [OTC]; Oyst-Cal 500 [OTC]; Oystercal® 500; PhosLo®; Posture® [OTC]; Rolaids® Calcium Rich [OTC]; Tums® [OTC]; Tums® E-X Extra Strength Tablet [OTC]; Tums® Ultra® [OTC]

Synonyms Calcium Acetate; Calcium Carbonate; Calcium Chloride; Calcium Citrate; Calcium Glubionate; Calcium Gluceptate; Calcium Gluconate; Calcium Lactate; Calcium Phosphate, Tribasic

Generic Available Yes

Pharmacologic Category Electrolyte Supplement; Electrolyte Supplement, Parenteral

Pregnancy Risk Factor C

Lactation Excretion in breast milk unknown/use caution

Use Treatment and prevention of calcium depletion; relief of acid indigestion, heartburn; emergency treatment of hypocalcemic tetany; treatment of hypermagnesemia, cardiac disturbances of hyperkalemia, hypocalcemia, or calcium channel blocking agent toxicity; topical treatment of hydrofluoric acid burns; control of hyperphosphatemia in endstage renal failure

Mechanism of Action/Effect Moderates nerve and muscle performance via action potential excitation threshold regulation; neutralizes acidity of stomach (carbonate salt); combines with dietary phosphate to form insoluble calcium phosphate which is excreted in feces and reduces phosphate absorption (acetate and carbonate salts)

Contraindications Hypersensitivity to formulation, hypercalcemia, renal calculi, ventricular fibrillation

Warnings/Precautions Use cautiously in patients with sarcoidosis, respiratory failure, acidosis, renal or cardiac disease. Avoid too rapid I.V. administration. Avoid extravasation. Use with caution in digitalized patients. Avoid or use with caution in phenylketonuria; some products may contain aspartame which is metabolized to phenylalanine and must be avoided in patients with phenylketonuria. Some products may contain tartrazine which may cause allergic reactions in susceptible individuals.

Drug Interactions

Decreased Effect: May antagonize the effects of calcium channel blockers (eg, verapamil); when administered orally, calcium decreases the absorption of tetracycline, atenolol, iron salts, quinolone antibiotics, alendronate, salicylates, sodium fluoride, and zinc; decreases potassium-binding ability of polystyrene sulfonate.

Increased Effect/Toxicity: May potentiate digoxin toxicity; high doses of calcium with thiazide diuretics may result in milk-alkali syndrome and hypercalcemia

Nutritional/Ethanol Interactions Large intakes of dietary fiber may decrease calcium absorption due to a decreased GI transit time and the formation of fiber-calcium complexes. Do not give orally with bran, foods high in oxalates (eg, spinach, rhubarb), or whole grain cereals; may decrease calcium absorption.

Adverse Reactions Frequency not defined.

Cardiovascular: Vasodilation, hypotension, bradycardia, cardiac arrhythmias, ventricular fibrillation, syncope

Central nervous system: Headache, mental confusion, dizziness, lethargy, coma

Dermatologic: Erythema

Endocrine & metabolic: Hypercalcemia, milk-alkali syndrome, hypophosphatemia, hypercalciuria, hypomagnesemia

Gastrointestinal: Constipation, nausea, vomiting, dry mouth, elevated serum amylase

Local: Tissue necrosis (I.V. administration)

Neuromuscular & skeletal: Muscle weakness

Pharmacodynamics/Kinetics

Absorption: Dependent on dose, pH, and vitamin D; in achlorhydric patients and elderly, the citrate salts may be better absorbed

Bioavailability: Generally, 25% to 35% (declines with age); absorption is greatest at individual dose <500 mg

Formulations Elemental calcium listed in brackets:

Calcium acetate:

Capsule (PhosLo®): 333.5 mg [84.5 mg]; 667 mg [169 mg]

Gelcap (PhosLo®): 667 mg [169 mg]

Injection: 0.5 mEq calcium/mL [calcium acetate/mL 39.55 mg] (10 mL, 50 mL, 100 mL)

Calcium carbonate:

Capsule: 1500 mg [600 mg]

Calci-Mix™: 1250 mg [500 mg]

Florical®: 364 mg [145.6 mg] with sodium fluoride 8.3 mg

Powder (Cal Carb-HD®): 6.5 g/packet [2.6 g]

Suspension, oral: 1250 mg/5 mL [500 mg]

Tablet: 650 mg [260 mg], 1500 mg [600 mg]

Calciday-667®: 667 mg [267 mg]

Cal-Plus®, Caltrate® 600, Gencalc® 600, Nephro-Calci®: 1500 mg [600 mg]

Florical®: 364 mg [145.6 mg] with sodium fluoride 8.3 mg

Os-Cal® 500, Oyst-Cal 500, Oystercal® 500: 1250 mg [500 mg]

Tablet, chewable:

Alka-Mints®: 850 mg [340 mg]

Amitone®: 350 mg [140 mg] ®

Caltrate, Jr.®: 750 mg [300 mg]

Chooz®, Dicarbosil®, Equilet®, Tums®: 500 mg [200 mg]

Mallamint®: 420 mg [168 mg]

Rolaids® Calcium Rich: 550 mg [220 mg]

Tums® E-X Extra Strength: 750 mg [300 mg]

Tums® Ultra®: 1000 mg [400 mg]

Calcium chloride:

Injection: 10% = 100 mg/mL [27.2 mg/mL, 1.36 mEq/mL] (10 mL)

Calcium citrate:

Tablet: 950 mg [200 mg]

Cal-Citrate®: 250 mg [100% calcium citrate]

Tablet, effervescent: 2376 mg [500 mg]

Calcium glubionate: Syrup: 1.8 g/5 mL [115 mg/5mL] (480 mL)

Calcium gluceptate: Injection: 220 mg/mL [18 mg/mL, 0.9 mEq/mL] (5 mL)

Calcium gluconate:

Injection: 10% = 100 mg/mL [9 mg/mL] (10 mL, 50 mL, 100 mL, 200 mL)

Tablet: 500 mg [45 mg], 650 mg [58.5 mg], 975 mg [87.75 mg], 1 g [90 mg]

Calcium lactate:

Capsule: 500 mg [90 mg]

Tablet: 325 mg [42.25 mg], 650 mg [84.5 mg]

Calcium phosphate, tribasic: Tablet [sugar free]: 1565.2 mg [600 mg]

Elemental Calcium Content of Calcium Salts

Calcium Salt	Elemental Calcium (mg/1 g of salt form)	mEq Calcium Per Gram	Approximate Equivalent Doses (mg of calcium salt)
Calcium acetate	250	12.7	354
Calcium carbonate	400	20	225
Calcium chloride	270	13.5	330
Calcium citrate	211	10.6	425
Calcium glubionate	64	3.2	1400
Calcium gluceptate	82	4.1	1100
Calcium gluconate	90	4.5	1000
Calcium lactate	130	6.5	700
Calcium phosphate, tribasic	390	19.3	233

(Continued)

Calcium Supplements *(Continued)*

Dosing

Adults: Multiple salt forms of calcium exist; close attention must be paid to the salt form when ordering and administering calcium; incorrect selection or substitution of one salt for another without proper dosage adjustment may result in serious over- or underdosing. For comparison information of calcium salts, see table on previous page.

Oral:

Antacid (calcium carbonate): Adults: 0.5 - 1.5 g as needed

Dosage is in terms of elemental calcium:

Recommended daily allowance (RDA): Adults >24 years: 800 mg/day

Adequate intake (1997 National Academy of Science Recommendations):

19-50 years: 1000 mg/day

>50 years: 1200 mg/day

Prevention of osteoporosis

Oral calcium supplementation: 1000-1500 mg/day (divided in 500 mg increments)

Women >65 years of age receiving estrogen supplements: 1000 mg/day in divided doses

Women >65 years of age who are **not** receiving estrogen supplements or men >55 years of age: 1500 mg/day in divided doses

Hypocalcemia (dose depends on clinical condition and serum calcium level):

Oral:

Dose expressed in mg of **elemental calcium:** 1-2 g or more per day in 3-4 divided doses

Dose expressed in mg of **calcium gluconate:** 10-20 g daily in 3-4 divided doses

Dose expressed in mg of **calcium glubionate:** 6-18 g/day in divided doses

Dose expressed in mg of **calcium lactate:** 1.5-3 g divided every 8 hours

I.V.:

Dosage expressed in mg of **calcium chloride:** 500 mg to 1 g/dose every 6 hours

Dose expressed in mg of **calcium gluceptate:** 500 mg to 1.1 g/dose as needed

Dose expressed in mg of **calcium gluconate:** 2-15 g/day as a continuous infusion or in divided doses

I.V.:

Cardiac arrest in the presence of hyperkalemia or hypocalcemia, magnesium toxicity, or calcium antagonist toxicity:

Dosage expressed in mg of **calcium chloride:** 2-4 mg/kg; may repeat in 10 minutes if necessary

Dose expressed in mg of **calcium gluceptate:** 1.1-1.54 g/dose

Dosage expressed in mg of **calcium gluconate:** 500-800 mg (maximum 3 g/dose)
Note: Calcium chloride is the recommended salt.

Hypocalcemia secondary to citrated blood infusion: Give 0.45 mEq **elemental** calcium for each 100 mL citrated blood infused

Tetany:

Dose expressed in mg of **calcium chloride:** 1 g over 10-30 minutes; may repeat after 6 hours

Dose expressed in mg of **calcium gluconate:** 1-3 g may be administered until therapeutic response occurs

Topical: Hydrofluoric acid (HF) burns (HF concentration <20%): Both calcium gluconate and carbonate have been used at concentrations ranging from 2.5% to 33%: Massage calcium gluconate gel or slurry into exposed area for 15 minutes.

Calcium gluconate gel: Crush 3.5 g calcium gluconate tablets into a fine powder; add to 5 oz tube of water-soluble surgical lubricant (eg, K-Y® Jelly) or add 3.5 g calcium gluconate injection to 5 oz of water-soluble surgical lubricant (calcium carbonate may be substituted; do not use calcium chloride due to potential for irritation)

Calcium carbonate slurry: 32.5% slurry can be prepared by triturating ten 650 mg tablets into a fine powder and adding 20 mL of water-soluble lubricant gel (eg, K-Y® Jelly).

Elderly: Refer to adult dosing and Special Geriatric Considerations.

Pediatrics:

Oral: Dosage is in terms of **elemental calcium:**

Recommended daily allowance (RDA):

<6 months: 400 mg/day

6-12 months: 600 mg/day

1-10 years: 800 mg/day

11-24 years: 1200 mg/day

Adequate intake (1997 National Academy of Science Recommendations):

<6 months: 210 mg/day

6-12 months: 270 mg/day

1-3 years: 500 mg/day

4-8 years: 800 mg/day

9-18 years: 1300 mg/day

Hypocalcemia (dose depends on clinical condition and serum calcium level):

Oral:

Dose expressed in mg of **elemental calcium:**

Neonates: 50-150 mg/kg/day in 4-6 divided doses; not to exceed 1 g/day

Children: 45-65 mg/kg/day in 4 divided doses

Dose expressed in mg of **calcium gluconate:**

Neonates: 500-1500 mg/kg/day in 4-6 divided doses

Infants and Children: 500-725 mg/kg/day in 3-4 divided doses

Dose expressed in mg of **calcium glubionate:**

Neonates: 1200 mg/kg/day in 4-6 divided doses

Infants and Children: 600-2000 mg/kg/day in 4 divided up to a maximum of 9 g/day

Dose expressed in mg of **calcium lactate:**

Neonates and Infants: 400-500 mg/kg/day divided every 4-6 hours

Children: 500 mg/kg/day divided every 6-8 hours; maximum daily dose 9 g

I.V.:

Dosage expressed in mg of **calcium chloride:**

Children (Manufacturer's recommendation): 2.7-5 mg/kg/dose every 4-6 hours

Neonates, Infants, and Children (alternative dosing): 10-20 mg/kg/dose (infants <1 mEq; children 1-7mEq), repeat every 4-6 hours if needed

Dose expressed in mg of **calcium gluceptate:**

Infants and Children: 200-500 mg/kg/day divided every 6 hours

Dose expressed in mg of **calcium gluconate:**

Neonates: 200-800 mg/kg/day as a continuous infusion or in 4 divided doses

Infants and Children: 200-500 mg/kg/day as a continuous infusion or in 4 divided doses

I.V.:

Cardiac arrest in the presence of hyperkalemia or hypocalcemia, magnesium toxicity, or calcium antagonist toxicity:

Dosage expressed in mg of **calcium chloride:**

Neonates, Infants, and Children: 20 mg/kg; may repeat in 10 minutes if necessary

Dose expressed in mg of **calcium gluceptate:** Infants and Children: 110 mg/kg/dose

Dosage expressed in mg of **calcium gluconate:** (Note: Calcium chloride is the recommended salt):

Infants and Children: 60-100 mg/kg/dose (maximum 3 g/dose)

Tetany:

Dose expressed in mg of **calcium chloride:** Neonates, Infants, and Children: 10 mg/kg over 5-10 minutes; may repeat after 6 hours or follow with an infusion with a maximum dose of 200 mg/kg/day

Dose expressed in mg of **calcium gluconate:**

Neonates: 100-200 mg/kg/dose; may follow with 500 mg/kg/day in 3-4 divided doses or as a continuous infusion

Infants and Children: 100-200 mg/kg/dose over 5-10 minutes; may repeat after 6 hours or follow with an infusion of 500 mg/kg/day

Administration

Oral: Administer with plenty of fluids with or following meals. For phosphate binding, administer on an empty stomach before meals to optimize effectiveness.

I.M.: Do not inject calcium salts I.M. or administer S.C. since severe necrosis and sloughing may occur; extravasation of calcium can result in severe necrosis and tissue sloughing. Do not use scalp vein or small hand or foot veins for I.V. administration. Not for endotracheal administration.

I.V.:

For direct I.V. injection, infuse at a maximum rate of 50-100 mg/mL of calcium salt (gluconate, chloride or gluceptate)

I.V. infusion: Dilute to a maximum concentration and infuse over 1 hour or at a maximum rate of infusion as follows:

Salt form (Maximum dilution; Maximum rate of infusion)

Calcium **chloride:** 20 mg/mL; 45-90 mg/kg/hour; 0.6-1.2 mEq/kg/hour

Calcium **gluceptate:** 55 mg/mL: 150-300 mg/kg/hour; 0.6-1.2 mEq/kg/hour

Calcium **gluconate:** 50 mg/mL; 120-240 mg/kg/hour; 0.6-1.2 mEq/kg/hour

Stability

Compatibility: Incompatible with bicarbonates, phosphates, and sulfates

Monitoring Laboratory Tests Serum calcium (ionized calcium preferred if available, see Additional Information), phosphate, magnesium, heart rate, EKG

Monitoring and Teaching Issues

Physical Assessment: Assess other medications patient may be taking for effectiveness and interactions (see Warnings/Precautions and Drug Interactions). Monitor laboratory tests, therapeutic effect, and adverse or toxic effects (see Adverse Reactions and Overdose/Toxicology). Assess knowledge/teach patient appropriate use, interventions to reduce side effects, and adverse symptoms to report (see Patient Education). If administered I.V. monitor EKG, vital signs, and CNS. **Pregnancy risk factor C** - benefits of use should outweigh possible risks. Note breast-feeding caution.

Patient Education: Follow instructions for dosing. Take with a full glass of water or juice, 1-3 hours after meals and other medications and 1-2 hours before any iron supplements. Avoid alcohol, other antacids, caffeine, or other calcium supplements unless approved by prescriber. You may experience constipation (increased exercise, fluids, fiber, or fruits may help) or dry mouth. Report severe, unresolved GI disturbances and unusual emotional lability (mood swings). **Pregnancy/breast-feeding precautions:** Inform prescriber if you are or intend to become pregnant. Consult prescriber if breast-feeding.

Dietary Issues: Avoid foods high in oxalates (eg, spinach, rhubarb).

Geriatric Considerations: Constipation and gas can be significant in the elderly, but are usually mild and may be resolved by switching to another calcium salt form. Achlorhydria is common in the elderly, calcium carbonate may not be the ideal calcium supplement for dietary or treatment use (administration with food will help). Citrate salts may be better absorbed. When using in the elderly, check albumin status and make appropriate decisions concerning reference serum concentrations. Elderly, especially the ill, often have low albumin due to malnutrition.

Additional Information Due to a poor correlation between the serum ionized calcium (free) and total serum calcium, particularly in states of low albumin or acid/base imbalances, direct measurement of ionized calcium is recommended. If ionized calcium is unavailable, in low albumin states, the corrected **total** serum calcium may be estimated by this equation (assuming a normal albumin of 4 g/dL); corrected total calcium = total serum calcium + 0.8 (4 - measured serum albumin).

Related Information

Osteoporosis Management *on page 1696*

Calculations/Conversions/Laboratory Values *see page 1530*

CaldeCORT® [OTC] *see* Hydrocortisone *on page 673*

Calphron® *see* Calcium Supplements *on page 202*
Cal-Plus® [OTC] *see* Calcium Supplements *on page 202*
Caltrate® 600 [OTC] *see* Calcium Supplements *on page 202*
Caltrate, Jr.® [OTC] *see* Calcium Supplements *on page 202*
Camphorated Tincture of Opium *see* Paregoric *on page 1035*
Camptosar® *see* Irinotecan *on page 737*
Camptothecin-11 *see* Irinotecan *on page 737*
Canasa™ *see* Mesalamine *on page 858*
Cancidas® *see* Caspofungin *on page 228*

Candesartan (kan de SAR tan)

U.S. Brand Names Atacand®

Synonyms Candesartan Cilexetil

Generic Available No

Pharmacologic Category Angiotensin II Receptor Blocker

Pregnancy Risk Factor C/D (2nd and 3rd trimesters)

Lactation Enters breast milk/contraindicated

Use Alone or in combination with other antihypertensive agents in treating essential hypertension; may have an advantage over losartan due to minimal metabolism requirements and consequent use in mild to moderate hepatic impairment

Mechanism of Action/Effect Blocks the vasoconstrictor and aldosterone-secreting effects of angiotensin II by binding of angiotensin II at the AT1 receptor in many tissues, such as vascular smooth muscle and the adrenal gland. Independent of pathways for angiotensin II synthesis. Does not affect the response to bradykinin; does not bind to block other hormone receptors or ion channels known to be important in cardiovascular regulation.

Contraindications Hypersensitivity to candesartan or any component of the formulation; hypersensitivity to other A-II receptor antagonists; primary hyperaldosteronism; bilateral renal artery stenosis; pregnancy (2nd and 3rd trimesters)

Warnings/Precautions Avoid use or use a smaller dose in patients who are volume depleted. Deterioration in renal function can occur with initiation. Use with caution in unilateral renal artery stenosis and pre-existing renal insufficiency; significant aortic/mitral stenosis. Pregnancy risk C/D (2nd and 3rd trimesters).

Drug Interactions

Cytochrome P450 Effect: Substrate of CYP2C8/9; Inhibits CYP2C8/9

Increased Effect/Toxicity: The risk of lithium toxicity may be increased by candesartan; monitor lithium levels. Concurrent use with potassium-sparing diuretics (amiloride, spironolactone, triamterene), potassium supplements, or trimethoprim (high-dose) may increase the risk of hyperkalemia.

Nutritional/Ethanol Interactions

Food: Food reduces the time to maximal concentration and increases the C_{max}.

Herb/Nutraceutical: Avoid dong quai if using for hypertension (has estrogenic activity). Avoid ephedra, yohimbe, ginseng (may worsen hypertension). Avoid garlic (may have increased antihypertensive effect).

Adverse Reactions May be associated with worsening of renal function in patients dependent on renin-angiotensin-aldosterone system.

Cardiovascular: Flushing, chest pain, peripheral edema, tachycardia, palpitations, angina, myocardial infarction,

Central nervous system: Dizziness, lightheadedness, drowsiness, fatigue, headache, vertigo, anxiety, depression, somnolence, fever

Dermatologic: Angioedema, rash (>0.5%)

Endocrine & metabolic: Hyperglycemia, hypertriglyceridemia

Gastrointestinal: Nausea, diarrhea, vomiting, dyspepsia, gastroenteritis

Genitourinary: Hyperuricemia, hematuria

Neuromuscular & skeletal: Back pain, arthralgia, paresthesias, increased CPK, myalgia, weakness

Respiratory: Upper respiratory tract infection, pharyngitis, rhinitis, bronchitis, cough, sinusitis, epistaxis, dyspnea

Miscellaneous: Diaphoresis (increased)

<1% (Limited to important or life-threatening): Agranulocytosis, dyspnea, hepatitis, leukopenia, neutropenia, paresthesias, vomiting

Overdosage/Toxicology Symptoms of overdose include hypotension and tachycardia. Treatment is supportive.

Pharmacodynamics/Kinetics

Bioavailability: 15%

Half-Life Elimination: Dose dependent: 5-9 hours

Time to Peak: 3-4 hours

Metabolism: To candesartan by the intestinal wall cells

Onset: 2-3 hours; Peak effect: 6-8 hours

Duration: >24 hours

Formulations Tablet, as cilexetil: 4 mg, 8 mg, 16 mg, 32 mg

Dosing

Adults: Hypertension: Oral: 4-32 mg once daily. Dosage must be individualized. Blood pressure response is dose-related over the range of 2-32 mg. The usual recommended starting dose is 16 mg once daily when it is used as monotherapy in patients who are not volume depleted. It can be administered once or twice daily with total daily doses ranging from 8-32 mg; larger doses do not appear to have a greater effect and there is relatively little experience with such doses.

Elderly: Refer to adult dosing. No initial dosage adjustment is necessary for elderly patients (although higher concentrations (C_{max}) and AUC were observed in these populations), for patients with mildly impaired renal function, or for patients with mildly impaired hepatic function.

Hepatic Impairment: No initial dosage adjustment required in mild hepatic impairment. Consider initiation at lower dosages in moderate hepatic impairment (AUC increased by 145%). No data available concerning dosing in severe hepatic impairment.

Monitoring Laboratory Tests Electrolytes, serum creatinine, BUN, urinalysis

Monitoring and Teaching Issues

Physical Assessment: See Contraindications, Warnings/Precautions, and Dosing for use cautions. Assess potential for interactions with other prescriptions, OTC medications, or herbal products patient may be taking (see Drug Interactions). Assess results of laboratory tests (see above) and patient response at beginning of therapy, when changing dose, and on a regular basis during long-term therapy (see Adverse Reactions and Overdose/Toxicology). Teach patient appropriate use, possible side effects and appropriate interventions, and adverse symptoms to report (see Patient Education). **Pregnancy risk factor C/D** - see Pregnancy Risk Factor for use cautions. Instruct patient of childbearing age about appropriate use of barrier contraceptives (see Pregnancy Issues). Breast-feeding is contraindicated.

Patient Education: Inform prescriber of all prescriptions, OTC medications, or herbal products you are taking, and any allergies you have. Do not take anything new during treatment unless approved by prescriber. Take exactly as directed and do not discontinue without consulting prescriber. Preferable to take on an empty stomach, 1 hour before or 2 hours after meals. This drug does not eliminate need for diet or exercise regimen as recommended by prescriber. May cause dizziness, fainting, or lightheadedness (use caution when driving or engaging in tasks that require alertness until response to drug is known); postural hypotension (use caution when rising from lying or sitting position or climbing stairs); nausea or vomiting (small, frequent meals, frequent mouth care, chewing gum, or sucking lozenges may help); or diarrhea (boiled milk, buttermilk, or yogurt may help). Report chest pain or palpitations; unusual weight gain or swelling of ankles and hands; persistent fatigue; unusual flu or cold symptoms or dry cough; difficulty breathing; swelling of eyes, face, or lips; skin rash; muscle pain or weakness; unusual bleeding (blood in urine or stool, or from gums); or excessive sweating. **Pregnancy/breast-feeding precautions:** Inform prescriber if you are or intend to become pregnant. This drug should not be used in the 2nd or 3rd trimester of pregnancy. Consult prescriber for appropriate contraceptive measures if necessary. Consult prescriber if breast-feeding.

Geriatric Considerations: High concentrations occur in the elderly compared to younger subjects. AUC may be doubled in patients with renal impairment.

Pregnancy Issues: The drug should be discontinued as soon as possible when pregnancy is detected. Drugs which act directly on renin-angiotensin can cause fetal and neonatal morbidity and death.

Related Information

Angiotensin Agents *on page 1547*

Candesartan and Hydrochlorothiazide

(kan de SAR tan & hye droe klor oh THYE a zide)

U.S. Brand Names Atacand HCT™

Synonyms Candesartan Cilexetil and Hydrochlorothiazide

Generic Available No

Pharmacologic Category Angiotensin II Receptor Blocker Combination

Pregnancy Risk Factor C/D (2nd and 3rd trimesters)

Lactation Enters breast milk/contraindicated

Use Treatment of hypertension; combination product should not be used for initial therapy

Formulations Tablet:

Atacand HCT™ 16-12.5: Candesartan 16 mg and hydrochlorothiazide 12.5 mg
Atacand HCT™ 32-12.5: Candesartan 32 mg and hydrochlorothiazide 12.5 mg

Dosing

Adults: Hypertension, replacement therapy: Oral: Combination product can be substituted for individual agents; maximum therapeutic effect would be expected within 4 weeks

Usual dosage range:

Candesartan: 8-32 mg/day, given once daily or twice daily in divided doses
Hydrochlorothiazide: 12.5-50 mg once daily

Elderly: No initial dosage adjustment is recommended in patients with normal renal and hepatic function; some patients may have increased sensitivity.

Renal Impairment: Serum levels of candesartan are increased and the half-life of hydrochlorothiazide is prolonged in patients with renal impairment. Do not use if Cl_{cr} is <30 mL/minute.

Hepatic Impairment: Use with caution.

Monitoring and Teaching Issues

Physical Assessment: See individual components listed in Related Information. **Pregnancy risk factor C/D** - see Pregnancy Risk Factor for use cautions; benefits of use should outweigh possible risks. Breast-feeding is contraindicated.

Patient Education: See individual components listed in Related Information. **Pregnancy/breast-feeding precautions:** Inform prescriber if you are or intend to become pregnant; contraceptives may be recommended. Do not breast-feed.

Related Information

Candesartan *on page 206*
Hydrochlorothiazide *on page 664*

Candesartan Cilexetil *see* Candesartan *on page 206*

Candesartan Cilexetil and Hydrochlorothiazide *see* Candesartan and Hydrochlorothiazide *on page 207*

***Candida albicans* (*Monilia*)** *see page 1461*

Capecitabine (ka pe SITE a been)

U.S. Brand Names Xeloda®

Generic Available No

(Continued)

Capecitabine *(Continued)*

Pharmacologic Category Antineoplastic Agent, Antimetabolite

Pregnancy Risk Factor D

Lactation Excretion in breast milk unknown/not recommended

Use

Treatment of metastatic colorectal cancer.

Treatment of metastatic breast cancer in combination with docetaxel after failure of prior anthracycline therapy.

Monotherapy treatment of metastatic breast cancer resistant to both paclitaxel and an anthracycline-containing chemotherapy regimen or resistant to paclitaxel and for whom further anthracycline therapy is not indicated (eg, patients who have received cumulative doses of 400 mg/m^2 of doxorubicin or doxorubicin equivalents). Resistance is defined as progressive disease while on treatment, with or without an initial response, or relapse within 6 months of completing treatment with an anthracycline-containing adjuvant regimen.

Mechanism of Action/Effect Capecitabine is a prodrug of fluorouracil. It undergoes hydrolysis in the liver and tissues to form fluorouracil. It interferes with DNA (and to a lesser degree RNA) synthesis. Appears to be specific for G_1 and S phases of the cell cycle.

Contraindications Hypersensitivity to capecitabine, fluorouracil, or any component of the formulation; severe renal impairment (Cl_{cr} <30 mL/minute); pregnancy

Warnings/Precautions The U.S. Food and Drug Administration (FDA) currently recommends that procedures for proper handling and disposal of antineoplastic agents be considered. Use with caution in patients with bone marrow suppression, poor nutritional status, on warfarin therapy, ≥80 years of age, or renal or hepatic dysfunction. Dosing adjustment required in moderate renal impairment (Cl_{cr} 30-50 mL/minute). The drug should be discontinued if intractable diarrhea, stomatitis, bone marrow suppression, or myocardial ischemia develop. Use with caution in patients who have received extensive pelvic radiation or alkylating therapy. Use cautiously with warfarin; altered coagulation parameters and bleeding have been reported.

Capecitabine can cause severe diarrhea; median time to first occurrence is 31 days; subsequent doses should be reduced after grade 3 or 4 diarrhea

If grade 2 or 3 hand-and-foot syndrome occurs, interrupt administration of capecitabine until the event resolves or decreases in intensity to grade 1. Following grade 3 hand-and-foot syndrome, decrease subsequent doses of capecitabine.

Use caution in patients with coronary artery disease. Cardiotoxicity has been associated with fluorinated pyrimidine therapy, including myocardial infarction, angina, dysrhythmias, cardiogenic shock, sudden death, and EKG changes (increased risk in CAD).

Drug Interactions

Increased Effect/Toxicity: Taking capecitabine immediately before an aluminum hydroxide/magnesium hydroxide antacid or a meal increases the absorption of capecitabine. The concentration of capecitabine's active metabolite (5-fluorouracil) is increased and its toxicity may be enhanced by leucovorin. Deaths from severe enterocolitis, diarrhea, and dehydration have been reported in elderly patients receiving weekly leucovorin and fluorouracil. Response to warfarin may be increased by capecitabine; changes may occur days to months after starting or stopping capecitabine therapy.

Nutritional/Ethanol Interactions Food: Food reduced the rate and extent of absorption of capecitabine.

Adverse Reactions Frequency listed derived from monotherapy trials.

>10%:

- Cardiovascular: Edema (9% to 15%)
- Central nervous system: Fatigue (~40%), fever (12% to 18%), pain (colorectal cancer: 12%)
- Dermatologic: Palmar-plantar erythrodysesthesia (hand-and-foot syndrome) (~55%, may be dose limiting), dermatitis (27% to 37%)
- Gastrointestinal: Diarrhea (~55%, may be dose limiting), mild to moderate nausea (43% to 53%), vomiting (27% to 37%), stomatitis (~25%), decreased appetite (colorectal cancer: 26%), anorexia (23%), abdominal pain (20% to 35%), constipation (~15%)
- Hematologic: Lymphopenia (94%), anemia (72% to 80%; Grade 3/4: <1% to 3%), neutropenia (13% to 26%; Grade 3/4: 1% to 2%), thrombocytopenia (24%; Grade 3/4: 1% to 3%)
- Hepatic: Increased bilirubin (22% to 48%)
- Neuromuscular & skeletal: Paresthesia (21%)
- Ocular: Eye irritation (~15%)
- Respiratory: Dyspnea (colorectal cancer: 14%)

5% to 10%:

- Cardiovascular: Venous thrombosis (colorectal cancer: 8%), chest pain (colorectal cancer: 6%)
- Central nervous system: Headache (~10%), dizziness (~8%), insomnia (8%), mood alteration (colorectal cancer: 5%), depression (colorectal cancer: 5%)
- Dermatologic: Nail disorders (7%), skin discoloration (colorectal cancer: 7%), alopecia (colorectal cancer: 6%)
- Endocrine & metabolic: Dehydration (7%)
- Gastrointestinal: Motility disorder (colorectal cancer: 10%), oral discomfort (colorectal cancer: 10%), dyspepsia (8%), upper GI inflammatory disorders (colorectal cancer: 8%), hemorrhage (colorectal cancer: 6%), ileus (colorectal cancer: 6%), taste disturbance (colorectal cancer: 6%)
- Neuromuscular & skeletal: Back pain (colorectal cancer: 10%), myalgia (9%), neuropathy (colorectal cancer: 10%), arthralgia (colorectal cancer: 8%), limb pain (colorectal cancer: 6%)
- Respiratory: Cough (7%), sore throat (2%), epistaxis (3%)
- Ocular: Abnormal vision (colorectal cancer: 5%)
- Miscellaneous: Viral infection (colorectal cancer: 5%)

<5% (Limited to important or life-threatening): Angina, asthma, cardiac arrest, cardiac failure, cardiomyopathy, cerebral vascular accident, dysrhythmia, encephalopathy, gastric ulcer, GI hemorrhage, hepatitis, hepatic failure, hepatic fibrosis, hypersensitivity, idiopathic thrombocytopenia purpura, ileus, infections, intestinal obstruction (~1%), myocardial infarction, myocardial ischemia, myocarditis, necrotizing enterocolitis, pericardial effusion, thrombocytopenic purpura, pancytopenia, photosensitivity, pneumonia, pulmonary embolism, radiation recall syndrome, sepsis, toxic dilation of intestine, vertigo

Overdosage/Toxicology Symptoms of overdose include myelosuppression, nausea, vomiting, diarrhea, and alopecia. No specific antidote exists. Monitor hematologically for at least 4 weeks. Treatment is supportive.

Pharmacodynamics/Kinetics

Absorption: Rapid and extensive

Half-Life Elimination: 0.5-1 hour

Time to Peak: 1.5 hours; Fluorouracil: 2 hours

Metabolism: Hepatic: Inactive metabolites: 5′-deoxy-5-fluorocytidine, 5′-deoxy-5-fluorouridine; Tissue: Active metabolite: 5-fluorouracil

Formulations Tablet: 150 mg, 500 mg

Dosing

Adults: Metastatic breast carcinoma, metastatic colorectal cancer: Oral: 2500 mg/m²/day in 2 divided doses (~12 hours apart) at the end of a meal for 2 weeks followed by a 1-week rest period given as 3-week cycles

Capecitabine dose calculation according to BSA table: The following can be used to determine the total daily dose (mg) based on a dosing level of 2500 mg/m²/day. (The number of tablets per dose, given morning and evening, are also listed): See table.

Capecitabine Dose Calculation According to BSA Table

Dose Level 2500 mg/m²/day		# of tablets per dose (morning and evening)	
Surface Area (m²)	**Total Daily Dose (mg)**	**150 mg**	**500 mg**
≤1.25	3000	0	3
1.26-1.37	3300	1	3
1.38-1.51	3600	2	3
1.52-1.65	4000	0	4
1.66-1.77	4300	1	4
1.78-1.91	4600	2	4
1.92-2.05	5000	0	5
2.06-2.17	5300	1	5
≥2.18	5600	2	5

Dosage modification guidelines: Carefully monitor patients for toxicity. Toxicity caused by capecitabine administration may be managed by symptomatic treatment, dose interruptions, and adjustment of dose. Once the dose has been reduced, it should not be increased at a later time.

Dosage reduction for toxicity: The starting dose may be reduced by 25% in patients experiencing significant adverse effects at the full starting dose if symptoms persist, a further reduction (to 50% of the starting dose) may be considered. These recommendations were based on clinical studies reported at the 36th Annual Meeting of the American Society of Clinical Oncology (ASCO). See table.

Recommended Dose Modifications

Toxicity NCI Grades	During a Course of Therapy	Dose Adjustment for Next Cycle (% of starting dose)
Grade 1	Maintain dose level	Maintain dose level
Grade 2		
1st appearance	Interrupt until resolved to grade 0-1	100%
2nd appearance	Interrupt until resolved to grade 0-1	75%
3rd appearance	Interrupt until resolved to grade 0-1	50%
4th appearance	Discontinue treatment permanently	
Grade 3		
1st appearance	Interrupt until resolved to grade 0-1	75%
2nd appearance	Interrupt until resolved to grade 0-1	50%
3rd appearance	Discontinue treatment permanently	
Grade 4		
1st appearance	Discontinue permanently OR If physician deems it to be in the patient's best interest to continue, interrupt until resolved to grade 0-1	50%

Elderly: The elderly may be pharmacodynamically more sensitive to the toxic effects of 5-fluorouracil. Use with caution in monitoring the effects of capecitabine. Insufficient data are available to provide dosage modifications.

Renal Impairment: Baseline calculation of creatinine clearance is required (Cockroft-Gault per manufacturer).

(Continued)

Capecitabine *(Continued)*

Note: In any patient with renal insufficiency, carefully monitor and interrupt therapy if grade 2-, 3-, or 4 toxicity develops.

Cl_{cr} 50-80 mL/minute: No adjustment of initial dose.

Cl_{cr} 30-50 mL/minute: Reduce initial dose to 1900 mg/m^2/day (25% reduction in dose).

Cl_{cr} <30 mL/minute: Do not use.

Hepatic Impairment:

Mild to moderate impairment: No starting dose adjustment is necessary; however, carefully monitor patients.

Severe hepatic impairment: Patients have not been studied.

Administration

Oral: Capecitabine is administered orally, usually in two divided doses taken 12 hours apart. Doses should be taken after meals with water.

Stability

Storage: Tablets are stored at room temperature of 25°C (77°F).

Monitoring Laboratory Tests Renal function should be estimated at baseline to determine initial dose. During therapy, CBC with differential, hepatic function, and renal function should be monitored.

Monitoring and Teaching Issues

Physical Assessment: See Contraindications, Warnings/Precautions, and Dosing for use cautions. Assess potential for interactions with other prescriptions, OTC medications, or herbal products patient may be taking (see Drug Interactions). Assess results of laboratory tests (see above) and patient response at beginning and periodically during therapy (eg, severe diarrhea - see Warnings/Precautions, Adverse Reactions, and Overdose/Toxicology). Teach patient appropriate use, possible side effects and appropriate interventions, and adverse symptoms to report (see Patient Education). **Pregnancy risk factor D** - determine that patient is not pregnant before beginning treatment. Teach patients of childbearing age appropriate use of barrier contraceptives during and for 1 month following therapy. Breast-feeding is not recommended.

Patient Education: Inform prescriber of all prescriptions, OTC medications, or herbal products you are taking, and any allergies you have. Do not take anything new during treatment unless approved by prescriber. Take with food or within 30 minutes after meal. Avoid use of antacids within 2 hours of taking this medication. Do not crush, chew, or dissolve tablets. Maintain adequate hydration (2-3 L/day of fluids) unless advised by prescriber to restrict fluids. You will be more susceptible to infection (avoid crowds and exposure to infection and do not have any vaccinations without consulting prescriber). May cause lethargy, dizziness, visual changes, confusion, anxiety (avoid driving or engaging in tasks requiring alertness until response to drug is known); nausea, vomiting, loss of appetite, or dry mouth (small, frequent meals, frequent mouth care, chewing gum, or sucking lozenges may help); loss of hair (will grow back when treatment is discontinued); photosensitivity (use sunscreen, wear protective clothing and eyewear, and avoid direct sunlight); or dry, itchy, skin, and dry or irritated eyes (avoid contact lenses). Report persistent diarrhea or abdominal pain; skin rash, pain, tenderness, or peeling (especially hands and feet); chills or fever, confusion, persistent or violent vomiting; difficulty breathing; chest pain or palpitations; unusual bleeding or bruising; bone pain; muscle spasms/tremors; or vision changes immediately. **Pregnancy/breast-feeding precautions:** Inform prescriber if you are pregnant. Do not get pregnant while taking this medication. Consult prescriber for appropriate barrier contraceptive measures. Breast-feeding is not recommended.

Dietary Issues: Because current safety and efficacy data are based upon administration with food, it is recommended that capecitabine be administered with food. In all clinical trials, patients were instructed to administer capecitabine within 30 minutes after a meal.

Geriatric Considerations: Patients ≥80 years of age may experience a greater incidence of grade 3 or 4 adverse events (diarrhea, hand-and-foot syndrome, nausea/vomiting).

Breast-feeding Issues: It is not known if the drug is excreted in breast milk. Because of the potential for serious adverse reactions in nursing infants, it is recommended that nursing be discontinued when receiving capecitabine therapy.

Related Information

Antiemetics for Chemotherapy-Induced Nausea and Vomiting *on page 1639*

Capex™ *see* Topical Corticosteroids *on page 1334*

Capital® and Codeine *see* Acetaminophen and Codeine *on page 37*

Capoten® *see* Captopril *on page 210*

Capozide® *see* Captopril and Hydrochlorothiazide *on page 213*

Captopril (KAP toe pril)

U.S. Brand Names Capoten®

Synonyms ACE

Generic Available Yes

Pharmacologic Category Angiotensin-Converting Enzyme (ACE) Inhibitor

Pregnancy Risk Factor C/D (2nd and 3rd trimesters)

Lactation Enters breast milk/compatible

Use Management of hypertension; treatment of congestive heart failure, left ventricular dysfunction after myocardial infarction, diabetic nephropathy

Use - Unlabeled/Investigational Treatment of hypertensive crisis, rheumatoid arthritis; diagnosis of anatomic renal artery stenosis, hypertension secondary to scleroderma renal crisis; diagnosis of aldosteronism, idiopathic edema, Bartter's syndrome, postmyocardial infarction for prevention of ventricular failure; increase circulation in Raynaud's phenomenon, hypertension secondary to Takayasu's disease

Mechanism of Action/Effect Competitive inhibitor of angiotensin-converting enzyme (ACE); prevents conversion of angiotensin I to angiotensin II, a potent vasoconstrictor; results in lower levels of angiotensin II which causes an increase in plasma renin activity and a reduction in aldosterone secretion

Contraindications Hypersensitivity to captopril or any component of the formulation; angioedema related to previous treatment with an ACE inhibitor; primary hyperaldosteronism; idiopathic or hereditary angioedema; bilateral renal artery stenosis; pregnancy (2nd or 3rd trimester)

Warnings/Precautions Angioedema can occur at any time during treatment (especially following first dose). Careful blood pressure monitoring with first dose (hypotension can occur especially in volume depleted patients). Dosage adjustment needed in renal impairment. Use with caution in hypovolemia; collagen vascular diseases; valvular stenosis (particularly aortic stenosis); hyperkalemia; or before, during, or immediately after anesthesia. Avoid rapid dosage escalation which may lead to renal insufficiency. Neutropenia/agranulocytosis with myeloid hyperplasia can rarely occur. Additional hematologic monitoring required in patients with baseline renal impairment. Deterioration in renal function can occur with initiation. Use with caution in unilateral renal artery stenosis and pre-existing renal insufficiency. Pregnancy risk C/D (2nd and 3rd trimesters).

Drug Interactions

Cytochrome P450 Effect: Substrate of **CYP2D6**

Decreased Effect: Aspirin (high dose) may reduce the therapeutic effects of ACE inhibitors; at low dosages this does not appear to be significant. Rifampin may decrease the effect of ACE inhibitors. Antacids may decrease the bioavailability of ACE inhibitors (may be more likely to occur with captopril); separate administration times by 1-2 hours. NSAIDs, specifically indomethacin, may reduce the hypotensive effects of ACE inhibitors. More likely to occur in low renin or volume dependent hypertensive patients.

Increased Effect/Toxicity: Potassium supplements, co-trimoxazole (high dose), angiotensin II receptor antagonists (candesartan, losartan, irbesartan, etc), or potassium-sparing diuretics (amiloride, spironolactone, triamterene) may result in elevated serum potassium levels when combined with captopril. ACE inhibitor effects may be increased by phenothiazines or probenecid (increases levels of captopril). ACE inhibitors may increase serum concentrations/effects of digoxin, lithium, and sulfonlyureas.

Diuretics have additive hypotensive effects with ACE inhibitors, and hypovolemia increases the potential for adverse renal effects of ACE inhibitors. In patients with compromised renal function, coadministration with NSAIDs may result in further deterioration of renal function. Allopurinol and ACE inhibitors may cause a higher risk of hypersensitivity reaction when taken concurrently.

Nutritional/Ethanol Interactions

Food: Captopril serum concentrations may be decreased if taken with food. Long-term use of captopril may result in a zinc deficiency which can result in a decrease in taste perception.

Herb/Nutraceutical: Avoid dong quai if using for hypertension (has estrogenic activity). Avoid ephedra, yohimbe, ginseng (may worsen hypertension). Avoid garlic (may have increased antihypertensive effect).

Effects on Lab Values ↑ BUN, creatinine, potassium, positive Coombs' [direct]; ↓ cholesterol (S); may cause false-positive results in urine acetone determinations using sodium nitroprusside reagent

Adverse Reactions

1% to 10%:

- Cardiovascular: Hypotension (1% to 2.5%), tachycardia (1%), chest pain (1%), palpitation (1%)
- Dermatologic: Rash (maculopapular or urticarial) (4% to 7%), pruritus (2%); in patients with rash, a positive ANA and/or eosinophilia has been noted in 7% to 10%.
- Endocrine & metabolic: Hyperkalemia (1% to 11%)
- Hematologic: Neutropenia may occur in up to 3.7% of patients with renal insufficiency or collagen-vascular disease.
- Renal: Proteinuria (1%), increased serum creatinine, worsening of renal function (may occur in patients with bilateral renal artery stenosis or hypovolemia)
- Respiratory: Cough (0.5% to 2%)
- Miscellaneous: Hypersensitivity reactions (rash, pruritus, fever, arthralgia, and eosinophilia) have occurred in 4% to 7% of patients (depending on dose and renal function); dysgeusia - loss of taste or diminished perception (2% to 4%)

Frequency not defined:

- Cardiovascular: Angioedema, cardiac arrest, cerebrovascular insufficiency, rhythm disturbances, orthostatic hypotension, syncope, flushing, pallor, angina, myocardial infarction, Raynaud's syndrome, CHF
- Central nervous system: Ataxia, confusion, depression, nervousness, somnolence
- Dermatologic: Bullous pemphigus, erythema multiforme, Stevens-Johnson syndrome, exfoliative dermatitis
- Endocrine & metabolic: Increased serum transaminases, increased serum bilirubin, increased alkaline phosphatase, gynecomastia
- Gastrointestinal: Pancreatitis, glossitis, dyspepsia
- Genitourinary: Urinary frequency, impotence
- Hematologic: Anemia, thrombocytopenia, pancytopenia, agranulocytosis, anemia
- Hepatic: Jaundice, hepatitis, hepatic necrosis (rare), cholestasis, hyponatremia (symptomatic)
- Neuromuscular & skeletal: Asthenia, myalgia, myasthenia
- Ocular: Blurred vision
- Renal: Renal insufficiency, renal failure, nephrotic syndrome, polyuria, oliguria
- Respiratory: Bronchospasm, eosinophilic pneumonitis, rhinitis
- Miscellaneous: Anaphylactoid reactions

Postmarketing and/or case reports: Alopecia, aplastic anemia, exacerbations of Huntington's disease, Guillain-Barré syndrome, hemolytic anemia, Kaposi's sarcoma, pericarditis, seizures (in premature infants), systemic lupus erythematosus. A syndrome which may include fever, myalgia, arthralgia, interstitial nephritis, vasculitis, rash, eosinophilia, and elevated ESR has been reported for captopril and other ACE inhibitors.

Overdosage/Toxicology Mild hypotension has been the primary toxic effect seen with acute overdose. Bradycardia may also occur. Hyperkalemia occurs even with therapeutic doses,

(Continued)

Captopril *(Continued)*

especially in patients with renal insufficiency and those taking NSAIDs. Treatment is symptom-directed and supportive.

Pharmacodynamics/Kinetics

Absorption: 60% to 75%; reduced 30% to 40% by food

Half-Life Elimination: Renal and cardiac function dependent: Adults: Healthy volunteers: 1.9 hours; Congestive heart failure: 2.06 hours; Anuria: 20-40 hours

Metabolism: 50%

Onset: Peak effect: Blood pressure reduction: 1-1.5 hours after dose

Duration: Dose related, may require several weeks of therapy before full hypotensive effect

Formulations Tablet: 12.5 mg, 25 mg, 50 mg, 100 mg

Dosing

Adults: Note: Dosage must be titrated according to patient's response

Acute hypertension (urgency/emergency): Oral: 12.5-25 mg, may repeat as needed (may be given sublingually but no therapeutic advantage demonstrated)

Hypertension: Oral:

Initial: 12.5-25 mg 2-3 times/day; may increase by 12.5-25 mg/dose at 1- to 2-week intervals up to 50 mg 3 times/day. Add diuretic before further dosage increases.

Maximum: 150 mg 3 times/day

Congestive heart failure: Oral:

Initial: 6.25-12.5 mg 3 times/day in conjunction with cardiac glycoside and diuretic therapy. Initial dose depends upon patient's fluid/electrolyte status.

Target: 50 mg 3 times/day

Maximum: 100 mg 3 times/day

Prevention of LV dysfunction following MI: Oral: Initial: 6.25 mg; followed by 12.5 mg 3 times/day; increase to 25 mg 3 times/day over the next few days; following by gradual increase to a goal of 50 mg 3 times/day (Some dosage schedules increase the dosage more aggressively to achieve goal dosage within the first few days of initiation).

Diabetic nephropathy: Oral:

25 mg 3 times/day. May be taken with other antihypertensive therapy if required to further lower blood pressure.

Elderly: Note: Dosage must be titrated according to patient's response; use lowest effective dose.

Pediatrics: Note: Dosage must be titrated according to patient's response.

Hypertension: Oral:

Infants: Initial: 0.15-0.3 mg/kg/dose; titrate dose upward to maximum of 6 mg/kg/day in 1-4 divided doses; usual required dose: 2.5-6 mg/kg/day

Children: Initial: 0.5 mg/kg/dose; titrate upward to maximum of 6 mg/kg/day in 2-4 divided doses.

Older Children: Initial: 6.25-12.5 mg/dose every 12-24 hours; titrate upward to maximum of 6 mg/kg/day.

Adolescents: Initial: 12.5-25 mg/dose given every 8-12 hours; increase by 25 mg/dose to maximum of 450 mg/day.

Renal Impairment:

Cl_{cr} 10-50 mL/minute: Administer 75% of normal dose.

Cl_{cr} <10 mL/minute: Administer 50% of normal dose.

Note: Smaller dosages given every 8-12 hours are indicated in patients with renal dysfunction. Renal function and leukocyte count should be carefully monitored during therapy.

Hemodialysis effects: Moderately dialyzable (20% to 50%); administer dose postdialysis or administer 25% to 35% supplemental dose.

Peritoneal dialysis: Supplemental dose is not necessary.

Administration

Oral: Unstable in aqueous solutions; to prepare solution for oral administration, mix prior to administration and use within 10 minutes.

Monitoring Laboratory Tests BUN, serum creatinine, urine dipstick for protein, CBC, electrolytes. If patient has renal impairment then a baseline WBC with differential and serum creatinine should be evaluated and monitored closely during the first 3 months of therapy.

Monitoring and Teaching Issues

Physical Assessment: See Warnings/Precautions, Contraindications, and Dosing for use cautions. Assess potential for interactions with other prescriptions, OTC medications, or herbal products patient may be taking (especially anything that may impact fluid balance or cardiac status - see Drug Interactions). Assess results of laboratory tests (see above), therapeutic effectiveness, and adverse reactions on a regular basis during therapy (eg, hypovolemia, angioedema, postural hypotension - see Adverse Reactions and Overdose/Toxicology). Teach patient appropriate use, possible side effects/ interventions, and adverse symptoms to report (see Patient Education). **Pregnancy risk factor C/D** - see Pregnancy Risk Factor for use cautions. Instruct patient in use of appropriate barrier contraceptives. See Pregnancy Issues.

Patient Education: Inform prescriber of all prescriptions, OTC medications, or herbal products you are taking, and any allergies you have. Do not take anything new during treatment unless approved by prescriber. Do not use potassium supplement or salt substitutes without consulting prescriber. Take exactly as directed; do not discontinue without consulting prescriber. Take first dose at bedtime. Take all doses on an empty stomach, 1 hour before or 2 hours after meals. This drug does not eliminate need for diet or exercise regimen as recommended by prescriber. May cause dizziness, fainting, or lightheadedness (use caution when driving or engaging in tasks that require alertness until response to drug is known); postural hypotension (use caution when rising from lying or sitting position or climbing stairs); or nausea, vomiting, abdominal pain, dry mouth, or transient loss of appetite (small, frequent meals, frequent mouth care, sucking lozenges, or chewing gum may help). Report chest pain or palpitations; mouth sores; fever or chills; swelling of extremities, face, mouth, or tongue; skin rash; numbness, tingling, or pain in muscles; difficulty breathing or unusual cough; and other persistent adverse reactions. **Pregnancy/breast-feeding precautions:** Inform prescriber if you are or intend to become pregnant.

This drug should not be used in the 2nd or 3rd trimester of pregnancy. Consult prescriber for appropriate contraceptive measures if necessary. Consult prescriber if breast-feeding.

Dietary Issues: Should be taken at least 1 hour before or 2 hours after eating.

Geriatric Considerations: Due to frequent decreases in glomerular filtration (also creatinine clearance) with aging, elderly patients may have exaggerated responses to ACE inhibitors. Differences in clinical response due to hepatic changes are not observed.

Breast-feeding Issues: Crosses into breast milk. AAP considers **compatible** with breast-feeding.

Pregnancy Issues: ACE inhibitors can cause fetal injury or death if taken during the 2nd or 3rd trimester. Discontinue ACE inhibitors as soon as pregnancy is detected.

Related Information

Angiotensin Agents *on page 1547*
Heart Failure *on page 1670*

Captopril and Hydrochlorothiazide

(KAP toe pril & hye droe klor oh THYE a zide)

U.S. Brand Names Capozide®

Synonyms Hydrochlorothiazide and Captopril

Generic Available Yes

Pharmacologic Category Antihypertensive Agent Combination

Pregnancy Risk Factor C/D (2nd and 3rd trimesters)

Lactation Enters breast milk/compatible

Use Management of hypertension and treatment of congestive heart failure

Formulations Tablet:

25/15: Captopril 25 mg and hydrochlorothiazide 15 mg
25/25: Captopril 25 mg and hydrochlorothiazide 25 mg
50/15: Captopril 50 mg and hydrochlorothiazide 15 mg
50/25: Captopril 50 mg and hydrochlorothiazide 25 mg

Dosing

Adults:

Hypertension: Oral: Initial: 25 mg 2-3 times/day; may increase at 1- to 2-week intervals up to 150 mg 3 times/day (captopril dosages)

Congestive heart failure: Oral: 6.25-25 mg 3 times/day (maximum: 450 mg/day) (captopril dosages)

Elderly: Refer to dosing in individual monographs.

Renal Impairment: May respond to smaller or less frequent doses.

Monitoring and Teaching Issues

Physical Assessment: See individual components listed in Related Information. **Pregnancy risk factor C/D** - see Pregnancy Risk Factor for use cautions. Assess knowledge/instruct patient on need to use appropriate contraceptive measures and the need to avoid pregnancy.

Patient Education: See individual components listed in Related Information. **Pregnancy precaution:** Inform prescriber if you are or intend to become pregnant.

Related Information

Captopril *on page 210*
Hydrochlorothiazide *on page 664*

Carac™ *see* Fluorouracil *on page 576*

Carafate® *see* Sucralfate *on page 1254*

Carbachol *see page 1575*

Carbachol *see* Ophthalmic Agents, Glaucoma *on page 1002*

Carbamazepine (kar ba MAZ e peen)

U.S. Brand Names Carbatrol®; Epitol®; Tegretol®; Tegretol®-XR

Synonyms CBZ

Generic Available Yes

Pharmacologic Category Anticonvulsant, Miscellaneous

Pregnancy Risk Factor D

Lactation Enters breast milk/compatible

Use Partial seizures with complex symptomatology (psychomotor, temporal lobe), generalized tonic-clonic seizures (grand mal), mixed seizure patterns; pain relief of trigeminal or glossopharyngeal neuralgia

Use - Unlabeled/Investigational Treatment of bipolar disorders and other affective disorders, resistant schizophrenia, ethanol withdrawal, restless leg syndrome, psychotic behavior associated with dementia, post-traumatic stress disorders

Mechanism of Action/Effect In addition to anticonvulsant effects, carbamazepine has anticholinergic, antineuralgic, antidiuretic, muscle relaxant and antiarrhythmic properties; may depress activity in the nucleus ventralis of the thalamus or decrease synaptic transmission or decrease summation of temporal stimulation leading to neural discharge by limiting influx of sodium ions across cell membrane or other unknown mechanisms; stimulates the release of ADH and potentiates its action in promoting reabsorption of water; chemically related to tricyclic antidepressants

Contraindications Hypersensitivity to carbamazepine or any component of the formulation; may have cross-sensitivity with tricyclic antidepressants; marrow depression; MAO inhibitor use; pregnancy (may harm fetus)

Warnings/Precautions MAO inhibitors should be discontinued for a minimum of 14 days before carbamazepine is begun; administer with caution to patients with history of cardiac damage, hepatic, or renal disease; potentially fatal blood cell abnormalities have been reported following treatment; patients with a previous history of adverse hematologic reaction to any drug may be at increased risk; early detection of hematologic change is important; advise patients of early signs and symptoms; carbamazepine is not effective in absence, myoclonic or akinetic seizures; exacerbation of certain seizure types have been seen after initiation of carbamazepine therapy in children with mixed seizure disorders. Elderly may
(Continued)

Carbamazepine *(Continued)*

have increased risk of SIADH-like syndrome. Carbamazepine has mild anticholinergic activity; use with caution in patients with increased intraocular pressure (monitor closely) or sensitivity to anticholinergic effects (constipation, urinary retention). Drug should be discontinued if there are any signs of hypersensitivity.

Drug Interactions

Cytochrome P450 Effect: Substrate of CYP2C8/9, **3A4**; Induces **CYP1A2, 2B6, 2C8/9, 2C19, 3A4**

Decreased Effect: Carbamazepine may decrease the effect of benzodiazepines, citalopram, clozapine, corticosteroids, cyclosporine, doxycycline, ethosuximide, felbamate, felodipine, haloperidol, mebendazole, methadone, oral contraceptives, phenytoin, tacrolimus, theophylline, thyroid hormones, tricyclic antidepressants, valproic acid, and warfarin. Carbamazepine suspension is incompatible with chlorpromazine solution and thioridazine liquid. Schedule carbamazepine suspension at least 1-2 hours apart from other liquid medicinals.

Increased Effect/Toxicity: Carbamazepine levels/toxicity may be increased by amprenavir (and possibly other protease inhibitors), cimetidine, clarithromycin, danazol, diltiazem, erythromycin, felbamate, fluoxetine, fluvoxamine, isoniazid, lamotrigine, metronidazole, propoxyphene, verapamil, fluconazole, itraconazole, and ketoconazole. Carbamazepine may enhance the hepatotoxic potential of acetaminophen. Neurotoxicity may result in patients receiving lithium and carbamazepine concurrently.

Nutritional/Ethanol Interactions

Ethanol: Avoid ethanol (may increase CNS depression).

Food: Carbamazepine serum levels may be increased if taken with food. Carbamazepine serum concentration may be increased if taken with grapefruit juice; avoid concurrent use.

Herb/Nutraceutical: Avoid evening primrose (seizure threshold decreased). Avoid valerian, St John's wort, kava kava, gotu kola (may increase CNS depression).

Effects on Lab Values ↑ BUN, AST, ALT, bilirubin, alkaline phosphatase (S); ↓ calcium, T_3, T_4, sodium (S)

Adverse Reactions Frequency not defined.

Cardiovascular: Edema, CHF, syncope, bradycardia, hypertension or hypotension, AV block, arrhythmias, thrombophlebitis, thromboembolism, lymphadenopathy

Central nervous system: Sedation, dizziness, fatigue, ataxia, confusion, headache, slurred speech, aseptic meningitis (case report)

Dermatologic: Rash, urticaria, toxic epidermal necrolysis, Stevens-Johnson syndrome, photosensitivity reaction, alterations in skin pigmentation, exfoliative dermatitis, erythema multiforme, purpura, alopecia

Endocrine & metabolic: Hyponatremia, SIADH, fever, chills

Gastrointestinal: Nausea, vomiting, gastric distress, abdominal pain, diarrhea, constipation, anorexia, pancreatitis

Genitourinary: Urinary retention, urinary frequency, azotemia, renal failure, impotence

Hematologic: Aplastic anemia, agranulocytosis, eosinophilia, leukopenia, pancytopenia, thrombocytopenia, bone marrow suppression, acute intermittent porphyria, leukocytosis

Hepatic: Hepatitis, abnormal liver function tests, jaundice, hepatic failure

Neuromuscular & skeletal: Peripheral neuritis

Ocular: Blurred vision, nystagmus, lens opacities, conjunctivitis

Otic: Tinnitus, hyperacusis

Miscellaneous: Hypersensitivity (including multiorgan reactions, may include vasculitis, disorders mimicking lymphoma, eosinophilia, hepatosplenomegaly), diaphoresis

Overdosage/Toxicology Symptoms of overdose include dizziness ataxia, drowsiness, nausea, vomiting, tremor, agitation, nystagmus, urinary retention, dysrhythmias, coma, seizures, twitches, respiratory depression, and neuromuscular disturbances. Activated charcoal is effective at binding certain chemicals and this is especially true for carbamazepine. Other treatment is supportive and symptomatic.

Pharmacodynamics/Kinetics

Absorption: Slow

Bioavailability: 85%

Half-Life Elimination: Initial: 18-55 hours; Multiple doses: Children: 8-14 hours; Adults: 12-17 hours

Time to Peak: Serum: Unpredictable, 4-8 hours

Metabolism: Hepatic to active epoxide metabolite; induces hepatic enzymes to increase metabolism

Formulations

Capsule, extended release: 200 mg, 300 mg

Suspension, oral: 100 mg/5 mL (450 mL) [citrus-vanilla flavor]

Tablet: 200 mg

Tablet, chewable: 100 mg

Tablet, extended release: 100 mg, 200 mg, 400 mg

Dosing

Adults:

Epilepsy: Oral (dosage must be adjusted according to patient's response and serum concentrations): 200 mg twice daily to start, increase by 200 mg/day at weekly intervals until therapeutic levels achieved; usual dose: 800-1200 mg/day in 3-4 divided doses; some patients have required up to 1.6-2.4 g/day

Trigeminal or glossopharyngeal neuralgia: Oral: Initial: 100 mg twice daily with food, gradually increasing in increments of 100 mg twice daily as needed usual maintenance: 400-800 mg daily in 2 divided doses; maximum dose: 1200 mg/day

Elderly: Elderly: 100 mg 1-2 times daily, increase in increments of 100 mg/day at weekly intervals until therapeutic level is achieved; usual dose: 400-1000 mg/day

Pediatrics: Epilepsy: Oral (adjust dose according to patient's response and serum concentrations):

<6 years: Initial: 5 mg/kg/day; dosage may be increased every 5-7 days to 10 mg/kg/day; then up to 20 mg/kg/day if necessary; administer in 2-4 divided doses

6-12 years: Initial: 100 mg twice daily or 10 mg/kg/day in 2 divided doses; increase by 100 mg/day at weekly intervals depending upon response; usual maintenance: 20-30 mg/kg/day in 2-4 divided doses; maximum dose: 1000 mg/day

>12 years: 200 mg twice daily to start, increase by 200 mg/day at weekly intervals until therapeutic levels achieved; usual dose: 400-1200 mg/day in 2-4 divided doses; maximum dose: 12-15 years: 1000 mg/day, >15 years: 1200 mg/day; some patients have required up to 1.6-2.4 g/day

Renal Impairment: Cl_{cr} <10 mL/minute: Administer 75% of dose.

Administration

Oral:

Suspension dosage form must be given on a 3-4 times/day schedule versus tablets which can be given 2-4 times/day. When carbamazepine suspension has been combined with chlorpromazine or thioridazine solutions a precipitate forms which may result in loss of effect. Therefore, it is recommended that the carbamazepine suspension dosage form not be administered at the same time with other liquid medicinal agents or diluents. Since a given dose of suspension will produce higher peak levels than the same dose given as the tablet form, patients given the suspension should be started on lower doses and increased slowly to avoid unwanted side effects.

Extended release tablets should be inspected for damage. Damaged extended release tablets (without release portal) should not be administered.

Monitoring Laboratory Tests CBC with platelet count, reticulocytes, serum iron, liver function tests, urinalysis, BUN, serum carbamazepine levels, thyroid function tests, serum sodium; observe patient for excessive sedation, especially when instituting or increasing therapy

Monitoring and Teaching Issues

Physical Assessment: Assess effectiveness and interactions of other medications patient may be taking (see Contraindications, Warnings/Precautions, and Drug Interactions). Monitor therapeutic response, laboratory values, and adverse reactions (see Adverse Reactions) at beginning of therapy and periodically with long-term use. Taper dosage slowly when discontinuing. Observe and teach seizure/safety precautions. Assess knowledge/teach patient appropriate use, interventions to reduce side effects, and adverse symptoms to report (see Patient Education). **Pregnancy risk factor D** (carbamazepine may reduce effects of oral contraceptives) - may cause fetal harm; benefits of use should outweigh possible risks.

Patient Education: Take exactly as directed; do not increase dose or frequency or discontinue without consulting prescriber. Do not use extended release tablets which have been damaged or crushed. While using this medication, do not use alcohol and other prescription or OTC medications (especially pain medications, sedatives, antihistamines, or hypnotics) without consulting prescriber. Maintain adequate hydration (2-3 L/day of fluids) unless advised by prescriber to restrict fluids. You may experience drowsiness, dizziness, or blurred vision (use caution when driving or engaging in tasks requiring alertness until response to drug is known); or nausea, vomiting, loss of appetite, or dry mouth (small, frequent meals, frequent mouth care, chewing gum, or sucking lozenges may help). Wear identification of epileptic status and medications. Report CNS changes, mentation changes, or changes in cognition; muscle cramping, weakness, tremors, sore throat, mouth ulcers, swollen glands, jaundice, changes in gait; persistent GI symptoms (cramping, constipation, vomiting, anorexia); rash or skin irritations; unusual bruising or bleeding (mouth, urine, stool); or worsening of seizure activity, or loss of seizure control. **Pregnancy precaution:** Inform prescriber if you are or intend to become pregnant.

Dietary Issues: Drug may cause GI upset, take with large amount of water or food to decrease GI upset. May need to split doses to avoid GI upset.

Geriatric Considerations: Elderly may have increased risk of SIADH-like syndrome.

Breast-feeding Issues: Crosses into breast milk. AAP considers **compatible** with breast-feeding.

Pregnancy Issues: Crosses the placenta. Dysmorphic facial features, cranial defects, cardiac defects, spina bifida, IUGR, and multiple other malformations have been reported. Epilepsy itself, number of medications, genetic factors, or a combination of these probably influence the teratogenicity of anticonvulsant therapy. Benefit:risk ratio usually favors continued use during pregnancy.

Other Issues:

Timing of serum samples: Absorption is slow, peak levels occur 6-8 hours after ingestion of the first dose. The half-life ranges from 8-60 hours; therefore, steady-state is achieved in 2-5 days.

Therapeutic levels: 6-12 μg/mL (SI: 25-51 μmol/L)

Toxic concentration: >15 μg/mL. Patients who require higher levels of 8-12 μg/mL (SI: 34-51 μmol/L) should be watched closely. Side effects including CNS effects occur commonly at higher dosage levels. If other anticonvulsants are given therapeutic range is 4-8 μg/mL.

Additional Information Investigationally, loading doses of the suspension (10 mg/kg for children <12 years of age and 8 mg/kg for children >12 years of age) were given (via NG or ND tubes followed by 5-10 mL of water to flush through tube) to PICU patients with frequent seizures/status. Five of 6 patients attained mean Cp of 4.3 mcg/mL and 7.3 mcg/mL at 1 and 2 hours postload. Concurrent enteral feeding or ileus may delay absorption.

Related Information

Peak and Trough Guidelines *on page 1544*
Seizure Treatment *on page 1700*

Carbamide Peroxide *see page 1519*

Carbastat® *see* Ophthalmic Agents, Glaucoma *on page 1002*

Carbatrol® *see* Carbamazepine *on page 213*

Carbaxefed RF *see* Carbinoxamine and Pseudoephedrine *on page 217*

Carbenicillin (kar ben i SIL in)

U.S. Brand Names Geocillin®

Synonyms Carbenicillin Indanyl Sodium; Carindacillin

Generic Available No

Pharmacologic Category Antibiotic, Penicillin

Pregnancy Risk Factor B

Lactation Enters breast milk/use caution

Use Treatment of serious urinary tract infections and prostatitis caused by susceptible gram-negative aerobic bacilli

Mechanism of Action/Effect Interferes with bacterial cell wall synthesis during active multiplication

Contraindications Hypersensitivity to carbenicillin, penicillins, or any component of the formulation

Warnings/Precautions Do not use in patients with severe renal impairment (Cl_{cr} <10 mL/minute); dosage modification required in patients with impaired renal and/or hepatic function; oral carbenicillin should be limited to treatment of urinary tract infections. Use with caution in patients with history of hypersensitivity to cephalosporins.

Drug Interactions

Decreased Effect: Decreased effectiveness with tetracyclines. Although anecdotal reports suggest oral contraceptive efficacy could be reduced by penicillins, this has been refuted by more rigorous scientific and clinical data.

Increased Effect/Toxicity: Increased bleeding effects if taken with high doses of heparin or oral anticoagulants. Aminoglycosides may be synergistic against selected organisms. Probenecid and disulfiram may increase levels of penicillins (carbenicillin).

Effects on Lab Values ↑ AST (SGOT), ALT (SGPT)

Adverse Reactions

>10%: Gastrointestinal: Diarrhea

1% to 10%: Gastrointestinal: Nausea, bad taste, vomiting, flatulence, glossitis

<1% (Limited to important or life-threatening): Anemia, elevated LFTs, eosinophilia, epigastric distress, furry tongue, headache, hematuria, hypersensitivity reactions, hyperthermia, hypokalemia, leukopenia, neutropenia, rash, thrombocytopenia, urticaria

Overdosage/Toxicology Symptoms of overdose include neuromuscular hypersensitivity and convulsions. Hemodialysis may be helpful to aid in removal of the drug from blood; otherwise, treatment is supportive or symptom-directed.

Pharmacodynamics/Kinetics

Absorption: 30% to 40%

Half-Life Elimination: Children: 0.8-1.8 hours; Adults: 1-1.5 hours, prolonged to 10-20 hours with renal insufficiency

Time to Peak: Serum: Normal renal function: 0.5-2 hours; concentrations are inadequate for treatment of systemic infections

Formulations Tablet, film coated: 382 mg

Dosing

Adults & Elderly:

Urinary tract infection: Oral: 1-2 tablets every 6 hours

Prostatitis: Oral: 2 tablets every 6 hours for prostatitis

Pediatrics: Susceptible infections: Oral: Children: 30-50 mg/kg/day divided every 6 hours; maximum dose: 2-3 g/day

Renal Impairment:

Cl_{cr} 10-50 mL/minute: Administer every 12-24 hours.

Cl_{cr} <10 mL/minute: Administer every 24-48 hours.

Moderately dialyzable (20% to 50%)

Administration

Oral: Administer around-the-clock to promote less variation in peak and trough serum levels. Give at least 1 hour before aminoglycosides.

Stability

Compatibility: Solution is **incompatible** with aminophylline, amphotericin B, epinephrine, erythromycin, gentamicin, levarterenol, tetracycline, vitamin B and C complex.

Monitoring Laboratory Tests Renal and hepatic function, CBC, serum potassium, bleeding times. Perform culture and sensitivity testing prior to initiating therapy.

Monitoring and Teaching Issues

Physical Assessment: Assess allergy history prior to starting therapy. See Contraindications, Warnings/Precautions, Dosing, and Administration for use cautions. Assess potential for interactions with other prescriptions, OTC medications, or herbal products patient may be taking (see Drug Interactions). Monitor laboratory tests (see above), therapeutic effectiveness, and adverse response (see Adverse Reactions and overdose/Toxicology). Advise diabetics about use of Clinitest®. Teach patient appropriate use, possible side effects and interventions, and adverse symptoms to report (see Patient Education). Note breast-feeding caution.

Patient Education: Inform prescriber of all prescriptions, OTC medications, or herbal products you are taking, and any allergies you have. Do not take anything new during treatment unless approved by prescriber. Take as prescribed, at equal intervals around-the-clock, with a full glass of water, and preferably on an empty stomach, 1 hour before or 2 hours after meals. Do not skip doses and take full course of treatment even if feeling better. If diabetic, drug may cause false test results with Clinitest® urine glucose monitoring; use of another form of glucose monitoring is preferable. May cause diarrhea (boiled milk, buttermilk, or yogurt may help - if diarrhea persists for more than 2 days, contact prescriber for approved antidiarrhea medication); or dry mouth and bitter aftertaste (frequent mouth care may help). Report difficulty breathing; easy bruising or bleeding; rash, itching, hives; or signs of opportunistic infection (eg, sore throat, fever, chills, fatigue, thrush, vaginal discharge, diarrhea). **Breast-feeding precaution:** Consult prescriber if breast-feeding.

Dietary Issues: Should be taken with water on empty stomach. Sodium content of 382 mg tablet: 23 mg (1 mEq).

Geriatric Considerations: Has not been studied in the elderly.

Related Information

Compatibility of Drugs *on page 1564*

Carbenicillin Indanyl Sodium *see* Carbenicillin *on page 216*

Carbidopa and Levodopa *see* Levodopa and Carbidopa *on page 789*

Carbinoxamine and Pseudoephedrine

(kar bi NOKS a meen & soo doe e FED rin)

U.S. Brand Names Andehist NR Drops; Carbaxefed RF; Hydro-Tussin™-CBX; Palgic®-D; Palgic®-DS; Rondec® Drops; Rondec® Tablets; Rondec-TR®

Synonyms Pseudoephedrine and Carbinoxamine

Generic Available No

Pharmacologic Category Adrenergic Agonist Agent; Antihistamine, H_1 Blocker; Decongestant

Pregnancy Risk Factor C

Lactation Enters breast milk/contraindicated

Use Seasonal and perennial allergic rhinitis; vasomotor rhinitis

Mechanism of Action/Effect Carbinoxamine is an antihistamine; pseudoephedrine is a decongestant

Contraindications Hypersensitivity to carbinoxamine, pseudoephedrine, or any component of the formulation; severe hypertension or coronary artery disease; MAO inhibitor therapy; GI or GU obstruction; peptic ulcer disease; narrow-angle glaucoma; avoid use in premature or term infants due to a possible association with SIDS; acute asthma attack

Warnings/Precautions Use caution with hypertension, ischemic heart disease, hyperthyroidism, increased intraocular pressure, diabetes mellitus, BPH, and patients >60 years of age. May cause decreased mental alertness; excitation in younger children; paradoxical reactions (manifested by hyperexcitability) in older children. The elderly may be more sensitive to anticholinergic and antihistamine effects and experience increased adverse effects. Use caution in atopic children. Safety and efficacy in children <1 month of age have not been established. Pregnancy risk C.

Drug Interactions

Decreased Effect: May decrease effects of antihypertensive agents.

Increased Effect/Toxicity: Increased sedation/CNS depression with barbiturates and other CNS depressants; anticholinergic effects may be increased by MAO inhibitors, tricyclic antidepressants

Nutritional/Ethanol Interactions Ethanol: Avoid ethanol (may increase CNS depression).

Adverse Reactions Frequency not defined.

Cardiovascular: Arrhythmias, cardiovascular collapse, hypertension, pallor, tachycardia

Central nervous system: Anxiety, convulsions, CNS stimulation, dizziness, excitability (children; rare), fear, hallucinations, headache, insomnia, nervousness, restlessness, sedation

Gastrointestinal: Anorexia, diarrhea, dyspepsia, nausea, vomiting, xerostomia

Neuromuscular skeletal: Tremors, weakness

Ocular: Diplopia

Renal: Dysuria, polyuria, urinary retention (with BPH)

Respiratory: Respiratory difficulty

Overdosage/Toxicology Symptoms of overdose include dry mouth, flushed skin, dilated pupils, and CNS depression. There is no specific treatment for antihistamine overdose. Clinical toxicity is due to blockade of cholinergic receptors. For anticholinergic overdose with severe life-threatening symptoms, physostigmine 1-2 mg I.V. slowly, may be given to reverse these effects.

Formulations

Solution, oral drops:

Andehist NR: Carbinoxamine maleate 1 mg and pseudoephedrine hydrochloride 15 mg per mL (30 mL) [alcohol and sugar free; raspberry flavor]

Carbaxefed RF, Rondec®: Carbinoxamine maleate 1 mg and pseudoephedrine hydrochloride 15 mg per mL (30 mL) [alcohol free; contains sodium benzoate; cherry flavor]

Syrup (Hydro-Tussin™-CBX, Palgic® DS): Carbinoxamine maleate 4 mg and pseudoephedrine hydrochloride 15 mg per 5 mL (480 mL) [alcohol and sugar free; strawberry/pineapple flavor]

Tablet (Rondec®): Carbinoxamine maleate 4 mg and pseudoephedrine hydrochloride 60 mg

Tablet, sustained release:

Palgic®-D: Carbinoxamine maleate 8 mg and pseudoephedrine hydrochloride 90 mg

Rondec-TR®: Carbinoxamine maleate 8 mg and pseudoephedrine hydrochloride 120 mg

Dosing

Adults & Elderly: Nasal congestion, allergic symptoms: Oral:

Syrup (Hydro-Tussin™-CBX, Palgic®-DS): 10 mL 4 times/day

Tablet (Rondec®): 1 tablet 4 times a day

Tablets, sustained release (Palgic®-D, Rondec-TR®): 1 tablet every 12 hours

Pediatrics: Nasal congestion, allergic symptoms: Oral:

Children:

Drops (Andehist NR, Carbaxefed RF, Rondec®):

1-3 months: 0.25 mL 4 times/day

3-6 months: 0.5 mL 4 times/day

6-12 months: 0.75 mL 4 times/day

12-24 months: 1 mL 4 times/day

Syrup (Hydro-Tussin™-CBX, Palgic®-DS):

1-3 months: 1.25 mL up to 4 times/day

3-6 months: 2.5 mL up to 4 times/day

6-9 months: 3.75 mL up to 4 times/day

9-18 months: 3.75-5 mL up to 4 times/day

18 months to 6 years: 5 mL 3-4 times/day

(Continued)

Carbinoxamine and Pseudoephedrine *(Continued)*

>6 years: Refer to adult dosing.
Tablet (Rondec®): ≥6 years: Refer to adult dosing.
Tablet, sustained release:
6-12 years (Palgic®-D): One-half tablet every 12 hours
≥12 years (Palgic®-D, Rondec-TR®): Refer to adult dosing.

Administration

Oral:
Palgic®-D: Tablets may be broken in half; do not crush or chew
Rondec-TR®: Do not crush or chew

Stability

Storage: Store at room temperature of 15°C to 30°C (59°F to 86°F).

Monitoring and Teaching Issues

Physical Assessment: Assess effectiveness and interactions of other medications patient may be taking (see Drug Interactions). See Contraindications and Warnings/Precautions for use cautions. (especially with patients who have history of bladder problems, ulcers, narrow-angle glaucoma or asthma). Monitor effectiveness of therapy and adverse reactions (see Adverse Reactions) at beginning of therapy and periodically with long-term use. Assess knowledge/teach patient appropriate use, interventions to reduce side effects, and adverse symptoms to report (see Patient Education). **Pregnancy risk factor C** - benefits of use should outweigh possible risks. Breast-feeding is contraindicated.

Patient Education: Take as directed; do not exceed recommended dose. Maintain adequate hydration (2-3 L/day of fluids) unless advised by prescriber to restrict fluids. Avoid use of other depressants, alcohol, or sleep-inducing medications unless approved by prescriber. You may experience drowsiness, impaired coordination, blurred vision, or increased anxiety (use caution when driving or engaging in tasks requiring alertness until response to drug is known); or dry mouth or nausea (small, frequent meals, frequent mouth care, chewing gum, or sucking hard candy may help). Report persistent dizziness, sedation, or agitation; difficulty breathing or increased cough; changes in urinary pattern; muscle weakness; or lack of improvement or worsening or condition. **Pregnancy/breast-feeding precautions:** Inform prescriber if you are or intend to become pregnant. Do not breast-feed.

Geriatric Considerations: Elderly are more predisposed to adverse effects of sympathomimetics since they frequently have cardiovascular diseases and diabetes mellitus as well as multiple drug therapies. It may be advisable to treat with a short-acting/immediate-release formulation before initiating sustained-release/long-acting formulations.

Breast-feeding Issues: Small amounts of antihistamines and pseudoephedrine are excreted in breast milk. Premature infants and newborns have a higher risk of intolerance to antihistamines. Antihistamines may inhibit lactation.

Related Information

Pseudoephedrine *on page 1150*

Carboplatin (KAR boe pla tin)

U.S. Brand Names Paraplatin®

Synonyms CBDCA

Generic Available No

Pharmacologic Category Antineoplastic Agent, Alkylating Agent

Pregnancy Risk Factor D

Lactation Excretion in breast milk unknown/contraindicated

Use Initial treatment of ovarian cancer; secondary treatment of advanced ovarian cancer

Use - Unlabeled/Investigational Lung cancer, head and neck cancer, endometrial cancer, esophageal cancer, bladder cancer, breast cancer, cervical cancer, CNS tumors, germ cell tumors, osteogenic sarcoma, and high-dose therapy with stem cell/bone marrow support

Mechanism of Action/Effect Analogue of cisplatin which covalently binds to DNA; possible cross-linking and interference with the function of DNA

Contraindications History of severe allergic reaction to cisplatin, carboplatin, other platinum-containing formulations, mannitol, or any component of the formulation; pregnancy

Warnings/Precautions The U.S. Food and Drug Administration (FDA) currently recommends that procedures for proper handling and disposal of antineoplastic agents be considered. When carboplatin is dosed using AUC as the endpoint, note that the calculated dose is the dose administered, not the dose based on body surface area. High doses have resulted in severe abnormalities of liver function tests. Bone marrow suppression, which may be severe, and vomiting are dose related; reduce dosage in patients with bone marrow suppression and impaired renal function. Increased risk of allergic reactions in patients previously exposed to platinum therapy. When administered as sequential infusions, taxane derivatives (docetaxel, paclitaxel) should be administered before platinum derivatives (carboplatin, cisplatin) to limit myelosuppression and to enhance efficacy.

Drug Interactions

Increased Effect/Toxicity: Nephrotoxic drugs; aminoglycosides increase risk of ototoxicity. When administered as sequential infusions, observational studies indicate a potential for increased toxicity when platinum derivatives (carboplatin, cisplatin) are administered before taxane derivatives (docetaxel, paclitaxel).

Nutritional/Ethanol Interactions Herb/Nutraceutical: Avoid black cohosh, dong quai in estrogen-dependent tumors.

Adverse Reactions

>10%:
Endocrine & metabolic: Electrolyte abnormalities such as hypocalcemia and hypomagnesemia, hyponatremia, hypokalemia
Gastrointestinal: Nausea, vomiting, stomatitis
Emetic potential: Moderate
Time course for nausea and vomiting: Onset: 2-6 hours; Duration: 1-48 hours
Hematologic: Neutropenia, leukopenia, thrombocytopenia, anemia

Myelosuppressive: Dose-limiting toxicity
WBC: Severe (dose dependent)
Platelets: Severe
Nadir: 21-24 days
Recovery: 28-35 days
Hepatic: Abnormal liver function tests
Local: Pain at injection site
Neuromuscular & skeletal: Weakness
Otic: Hearing loss at high tones (above speech ranges) has been reported in up to 19% in one series; clinically important ototoxicity is not usually seen; routine audiometric testing is not recommended

1% to 10%:
Dermatologic: Alopecia
Gastrointestinal: Diarrhea, anorexia
Hematologic: Hemorrhagic complications
Neuromuscular & skeletal: Peripheral neuropathy (4% to 6%; up to 10% in older and/or previously-treated patients)
Otic: Ototoxicity

<1% (Limited to important or life-threatening): Neurotoxicity has only been noted in patients previously treated with cisplatin; anaphylaxis, hypertension, malaise, nephrotoxicity (uncommon), rash, secondary malignancies, urticaria

BMT:
Dermatologic: Alopecia
Endocrine & metabolic: Hypokalemia, hypomagnesemia
Gastrointestinal: Nausea, vomiting, mucositis
Hepatic: Elevated liver function tests
Renal: Nephrotoxicity

Overdosage/Toxicology Symptoms of overdose include bone marrow suppression and hepatic toxicity. Treatment is symptomatic and supportive.

Pharmacodynamics/Kinetics

Half-Life Elimination: Terminal: 22-40 hours; Cl_{cr} >60 mL/minute: 2.5-5.9 hours

Metabolism: Minimally hepatic to aquated and hydroxylated compounds

Formulations Injection, powder for reconstitution: 50 mg, 150 mg, 450 mg

Dosing

Adults & Elderly: Protocols have utilized IVPB, I.V. infusion, and intraperitoneal administration (refer to individual protocols).

Autologous BMT: I.V.: 1600 mg/m^2 (total dose) divided over 4 days **requires BMT (ie, FATAL without BMT)**

Ovarian cancer: Usual doses range from 360 mg/m^2 I.V. every 3 weeks single agent therapy to 300 mg/m^2 every 4 weeks as combination therapy

In general, however, single intermittent courses of carboplatin should not be repeated until the neutrophil count is at least 2000 and the platelet count is at least 100,000

The following dose adjustments are modified from a controlled trial in previously treated patients with ovarian carcinoma. Blood counts were done weekly, and the recommendations are based on the lowest post-treatment platelet or neutrophil value.

Carboplatin dosage adjustment based on pretreatment platelet counts

- Platelets >100,000 cells/mm^3 and neutrophils >2000 cells/mm^3: Adjust dose 125% from prior course
- Platelets 50-100,000 cells/mm^3 and neutrophils 500-2000 cells/mm^3: No dose adjustment
- Platelets <50,000 cells/mm^3 and neutrophils <500 cells/mm^3: Adjust dose 75% from prior course

Carboplatin dosage adjustment based on the Egorin formula (based on platelet counts):

Previously untreated patients:

$$\text{dosage (mg/m}^2) = (0.091)\ \frac{(\text{Cl}_{cr})}{(\text{BSA})}\ \frac{(\text{Pretreat Plt count - Plt nadir count desired x 100})}{(\text{Pretreatment Plt count})} + 86$$

Previously treated patients with heavily myelosuppressive agents:

$$\text{dosage (mg/m}^2) = (0.091)\ \frac{(\text{Cl}_{cr})}{(\text{BSA})}\ \frac{[(\text{Pretreat Plt count - Plt nadir count desired x 100}) - 17]}{(\text{Pretreatment Plt count})} + 86$$

Pediatrics: Protocols have utilized IVPB, I.V. infusion, intraperitoneal administration (refer to individual protocols).

Solid tumor: I.V.: Children: 300-600 mg/m^2 once every 4 weeks

Brain tumor: I.V.: Children: 175 mg/m^2 once weekly for 4 weeks with a 2-week recovery period between courses; dose is then adjusted on platelet count and neutrophil count values.

Renal Impairment: These dosing recommendations apply to the initial course of treatment. Subsequent dosages should be adjusted according to the patient's tolerance based on the degree of bone marrow suppression.

Cl_{cr} <60 mL/minute: Increased risk of severe bone marrow suppression. In renally impaired patients who received single agent carboplatin therapy, the incidence of severe leukopenia, neutropenia, or thrombocytopenia has been about 25% when the following dosage modifications have been used:

Cl_{cr} 41-59 mL/minute: Recommended dose on day 1 is 250 mg/m^2
Cl_{cr} 16-40 mL/minute: Recommended dose on day 1 is 200 mg/m^2
Cl_{cr} <15 mL/minute: The data available for patients with severely impaired kidney function are too limited to permit a recommendation for treatment

or

Calvert formula:

Total dose (mg) = Target AUC (mg/mL/minute) x (GFR [mL/minute] + 25)

(Continued)

Carboplatin *(Continued)*

Note: The dose of carboplatin calculated is **total mg dose not** mg/m^2. AUC is the area under the concentration versus time curve.

Target AUC value will vary depending upon:

Number of agents in the regimen

Treatment status (ie, previously untreated or treated)

For single agent carboplatin/no prior chemotherapy: Total dose (mg): 6-8 (GFR + 25)

For single agent carboplatin/prior chemotherapy: Total dose (mg): 4-6 (GFR + 25)

For combination chemotherapy/no prior chemotherapy: Total dose (mg): 4.5-6 (GFR + 25)

For combination chemotherapy/prior chemotherapy: A reasonable approach for these patients would be to use a target AUC value <5 for the initial cycle.

Note: The Jelliffe formula (below) substantially underestimates the creatinine clearance in patients with a serum creatinine <1.5 mg/dL. However, the Jelliffe formula is more accurate in estimating creatinine clearance in patients with significant renal impairment than the Cockroft and Gault formula.

Cl_{cr} (mL/minute/1.73 m^2) for males = 98 - [(0.8) (age - 20)]/S_{cr}

Cl_{cr} (mL/minute/1.73 m^2) for females = 98 - [(0.8) (age - 20)]/S_{cr} multiplied by 90%

Intraperitoneal: 200-650 mg/m^2 in 2 L of dialysis fluid have been administered into the peritoneum of ovarian cancer patients.

Hepatic Impairment: There are no published studies available on the dosing of carboplatin in patients with impaired liver function. Human data regarding the biliary elimination of carboplatin are not available; however, pharmacokinetic studies in rabbits and rats reflect a biliary excretion of 0.4% to 0.7% of the dose (ie, 0.05 mL/minute/kg biliary clearance).

Administration

I.V.: Administer as IVPB over 15 minutes up to a continuous intravenous infusion over 24 hours. May also be administered intraperitoneally. When administered as sequential infusions, taxane derivatives (docetaxel, paclitaxel) should be administered before platinum derivatives to limit myelosuppression and to enhance efficacy.

Stability

Storage: Store intact vials at room temperature 15°C to 30°C (59°F to 86°F).

Reconstitution: Reconstitute powder to yield a final concentration of 10 mg/mL which is stable for 5 days at room temperature (25°C). Aluminum needles should not be used for administration due to binding with the platinum ion.

Standard I.V. dilution: Dose/250-1000 mL D_5W or NS

Further dilution to a concentration up to 0.5 mg/mL is stable at room temperature (25°C) for 24 hours in D_5W or NS.

Compatibility: Stable in D_5¼NS, D_5½NS, D_5NS, D_5W, NS

Y-site administration: Incompatible with amphotericin B cholesteryl sulfate complex

Compatibility when admixed: Incompatible with fluorouracil, mesna

Monitoring Laboratory Tests CBC with differential and platelet count, serum electrolytes, urinalysis, creatinine clearance, liver function

Monitoring and Teaching Issues

Physical Assessment: See Contraindications, Warnings/Precautions, and Dosing for use cautions. Assess potential for interactions with other prescriptions, OTC medications, or herbal products patient may be taking (especially anything that is ototoxic or nephrotoxic - see Drug Interactions). Administer antiemetic prior to therapy. See Administration, Reconstitution, and Compatibility for infusion specifics. Observe bleeding precautions. Assess results of laboratory tests (see above), therapeutic effectiveness, and adverse reactions (see Adverse Reactions and Overdose/Toxicology) prior to initiating therapy and on a regular basis throughout therapy. Teach patient (or caregiver) possible side effects and interventions and adverse symptoms to report (see Patient Education). **Pregnancy risk factor D** - determine that patient is not pregnant before beginning treatment. Instruct patients of childbearing age or males who may have intercourse with women of childbearing age about appropriate barrier contraceptive measures during therapy and for 1 month following therapy. Breast-feeding is contraindicated.

Patient Education: Inform prescriber of all prescriptions, OTC medications, or herbal products you are taking, and any allergies you have. Do not take anything new during treatment unless approved by healthcare provider. This medicine can only be administered by I.V. Report immediately any redness, burning, pain, or swelling at infusion site. It is important that you maintain adequate nutrition (small, frequent meals may help) and adequate hydration (2-3 L/day of fluids) unless instructed to restrict fluid intake. You will be susceptible to infection (avoid crowds and exposure to infection and do not have any vaccinations without consulting prescriber). May cause nausea and vomiting (small, frequent meals, frequent mouth care, chewing gum, or sucking lozenges may help - if unresolved, consult prescriber for antiemetic); mouth sores (use soft toothbrush or cotton swabs for mouth care); or loss of hair (reversible). Report chest pain or palpitations; sore throat, fever, chills, unusual fatigue; unusual bruising/bleeding; difficulty breathing; numbness, pain, or tingling in extremities; muscle cramps or twitching; change in hearing acuity; or other persistent adverse effects. **Pregnancy/breast-feeding precautions:** Inform prescriber if you are pregnant. Do not get pregnant during or for 1 month following therapy. Male: Do not cause a female to become pregnant. Male/female: Consult prescriber for instruction on appropriate barrier contraceptive measures. This drug may cause severe fetal defects. Do not breast-feed.

Geriatric Considerations: Peripheral neuropathy is more frequent in patients >65 years of age.

Other Issues: Carboplatin is sometimes confused with cisplatin. Institute measures to prevent mix-ups.

Carboprost *see* Carboprost Tromethamine *on page 221*

Carboprost Tromethamine (KAR boe prost tro METH a meen)

U.S. Brand Names Hemabate™

Synonyms Carboprost

Generic Available No

Pharmacologic Category Abortifacient; Prostaglandin

Pregnancy Risk Factor X

Lactation Excretion in breast milk unknown/opportunity for use is minimal

Use Termination of pregnancy and refractory postpartum uterine bleeding

Use - Unlabeled/Investigational Investigational: Hemorrhagic cystitis

Mechanism of Action/Effect Carboprost tromethamine is a prostaglandin similar to prostaglandin F_2. Carboprost tromethamine stimulates the gravid uterus to contract, which usually results in expulsion of the products of conception. Used to induce abortion between 13-20 weeks of pregnancy.

Contraindications Hypersensitivity to carboprost tromethamine or any component of the formulation; acute pelvic inflammatory disease; pregnancy

Warnings/Precautions Use with caution in patients with history of asthma, hypotension or hypertension, cardiovascular, adrenal, renal or hepatic disease, anemia, jaundice, diabetes, epilepsy, or compromised uterus.

Drug Interactions

Increased Effect/Toxicity: Toxicity may be increased by oxytocic agents.

Adverse Reactions

>10%: Gastrointestinal: Diarrhea, vomiting, nausea

1% to 10%:

Cardiovascular: Flushing

Central nervous system: Dizziness, headache

Gastrointestinal: Stomach cramps

<1% (Limited to important or life-threatening): Abnormal taste, asthma, bladder spasms, blurred vision, bradycardia or tachycardia, breast tenderness, coughing, drowsiness, dry mouth, dystonia, fever, hiccups, hematemesis, hypertension, hypotension, myalgia, nervousness, respiratory distress, septic shock, vasovagal syndrome, vertigo

Formulations Injection: Carboprost 250 mcg and tromethamine 83 mcg per mL (1 mL)

Dosing

Adults & Elderly: I.M.:

Abortion: I.M.: 250 mcg to start, 250 mcg at 1½-hour to 3½-hour intervals depending on uterine response; a 500 mcg dose may be given if uterine response is not adequate after several 250 mcg doses; do not exceed 12 mg total dose.

Refractory postpartum uterine bleeding: I.M.: Initial: 250 mcg; may repeat at 15- to 90-minute intervals to a total dose of 2 mg

Hemorrhagic cystitis: Bladder irrigation (refer to individual protocols): [0.4-1.0 mg/dL as solution] 50 mL instilled into bladder 4 times/day for 1 hour

Administration

I.M.: Give deep I.M.. Rotate site if repeat injections are required.

I.V.: Do not inject I.V.; may result in bronchospasm, hypertension, vomiting, and anaphylaxis.

Stability

Storage: Refrigerate ampuls.

Reconstitution: Bladder irrigation: Dilute immediately prior to administration in NS; stability unknown.

Monitoring and Teaching Issues

Physical Assessment: See Contraindications and Warnings/Precautions for use cautions. Premedication with an antiemetic should be considered. Monitor effectiveness and adverse reactions (see Adverse Reactions). Assess for complete expulsion of uterine contents (fetal tissue). Assess knowledge/instruct patient on adverse symptoms to report (see Patient Education). If used to treat hemorrhagic cystitis (bladder irrigation). If used to treat for bladder irrigation with hemorrhagic cystitis. **Pregnancy risk factor X.**

Patient Education: This medication is used to stimulate expulsion of uterine contents (fetal tissue) or stimulate uterine contractions to reduce uterine bleeding. Report increased blood loss, acute abdominal cramping, persistent elevation of temperature, or foul-smelling vaginal discharge. Increased temperature (elevated temperature) may occur 1-16 hours after therapy and last for several hours. **Pregnancy precaution:** If being treated for hemorrhagic cystitis, inform prescriber if you are pregnant.

Carboptic® *see* Ophthalmic Agents, Glaucoma *on page 1002*

Cardene® *see* NiCARdipine *on page 966*

Cardene® I.V. *see* NiCARdipine *on page 966*

Cardene® SR *see* NiCARdipine *on page 966*

Cardio-Green® *see page 1461*

Cardizem® *see* Diltiazem *on page 418*

Cardizem® CD *see* Diltiazem *on page 418*

Cardizem® SR *see* Diltiazem *on page 418*

Cardura® *see* Doxazosin *on page 441*

Carimune™ *see* Immune Globulin (Intravenous) *on page 703*

Carindacillin *see* Carbenicillin *on page 216*

Carisoprodate *see* Carisoprodol *on page 221*

Carisoprodol (kar i soe PROE dole)

U.S. Brand Names Soma®

Synonyms Carisoprodate; Isobamate

Generic Available Yes

Pharmacologic Category Skeletal Muscle Relaxant

Pregnancy Risk Factor C

Lactation Enters breast milk (high concentrations)/not recommended

(Continued)

Carisoprodol *(Continued)*

Use Skeletal muscle relaxant

Mechanism of Action/Effect Precise mechanism is not yet clear, but many effects have been ascribed to its central depressant actions.

Contraindications Hypersensitivity to carisoprodol, meprobamate or any component of the formulation; acute intermittent porphyria

Warnings/Precautions May cause CNS depression, which may impair physical or mental abilities. Effects with other sedative drugs or ethanol may be potentiated. Use with caution in patients with hepatic/renal dysfunction. Tolerance or drug dependence may result from extended use. Pregnancy risk C.

Drug Interactions

Cytochrome P450 Effect: Substrate of **CYP2C19**

Increased Effect/Toxicity: Ethanol, CNS depressants, psychotropic drugs, and phenothiazines may increase toxicity.

Nutritional/Ethanol Interactions Ethanol: Avoid ethanol (may increase CNS depression).

Adverse Reactions

>10%: Central nervous system: Drowsiness

1% to 10%:

Cardiovascular: Tachycardia, tightness in chest, flushing of face, syncope

Central nervous system: Mental depression, allergic fever, dizziness, lightheadedness, headache, paradoxical CNS stimulation

Dermatologic: Angioedema, dermatitis (allergic)

Gastrointestinal: Nausea, vomiting, stomach cramps

Neuromuscular & skeletal: Trembling

Ocular: Burning eyes

Respiratory: Dyspnea

Miscellaneous: Hiccups

<1% (Limited to important or life-threatening): Aplastic anemia, clumsiness, eosinophilia, erythema multiforme, leukopenia, rash, urticaria

Overdosage/Toxicology Symptoms of overdose include CNS depression, stupor, coma, shock, and respiratory depression. Treatment is supportive.

Pharmacodynamics/Kinetics

Half-Life Elimination: 8 hours

Metabolism: Hepatic

Onset: ~30 minutes

Duration: 4-6 hours

Formulations Tablet: 350 mg

Dosing

Adults: Muscle spasm (including spasm associated with acute temporomandibular joint pain): Oral: 350 mg 3-4 times/day; take last dose at bedtime; compound: 1-2 tablets 4 times/day

Elderly: Not recommended for use in the elderly (see Geriatric Considerations).

Administration

Oral: Give with food to decrease GI upset.

Monitoring and Teaching Issues

Physical Assessment: Assess effectiveness and interactions of other medications patient may be taking (see Drug Interactions). See Contraindications and Warnings/Precautions for use cautions. Monitor effectiveness of therapy (according to rational for therapy) and adverse (see Adverse Reactions) at beginning of therapy and periodically with long-term use. Do not discontinue abruptly; taper dosage slowly (withdrawal symptoms may occur). Assess knowledge/teach patient appropriate use, interventions to reduce side effects, and adverse symptoms to report (see Patient Education). **Pregnancy risk factor C** - benefits of use should outweigh possible risks. Breast-feeding is not recommended.

Patient Education: Take exactly as directed with food. Do not increase dose or discontinue without consulting prescriber. Do not use alcohol, prescriptive or OTC antidepressants, sedatives, and pain medications without consulting prescriber. You may experience drowsiness, dizziness, lightheadedness (avoid driving or engaging in tasks requiring alertness until response to drug is known); nausea, vomiting, or cramping (small, frequent meals, frequent mouth care, or sucking hard candy may help); or postural hypotension (change position slowly when rising from sitting or lying or when climbing stairs). Report excessive drowsiness or mental agitation; palpitations, rapid heartbeat, chest pain; skin rash; muscle cramping or tremors; or difficulty breathing. **Pregnancy/breast-feeding precautions:** Inform prescriber if you are or intend to become pregnant. Breast-feeding is not recommended.

Geriatric Considerations: Because of the risk of orthostatic hypotension and CNS depression, avoid or use with caution in the elderly. Not considered a drug of choice in the elderly.

Carisoprodol and Aspirin (kar i soe PROE dole & AS pir in)

U.S. Brand Names Soma® Compound

Synonyms Aspirin and Carisoprodol

Generic Available Yes

Pharmacologic Category Skeletal Muscle Relaxant

Pregnancy Risk Factor C/D (full-dose aspirin in 3rd trimester)

Lactation Enters breast milk/contraindicated

Use Skeletal muscle relaxant

Formulations Tablet: Carisoprodol 200 mg and aspirin 325 mg

Dosing

Adults: Skeletal muscle relaxant (including TMJ pain/spasm): Oral: 1 or 2 tablets 4 times/day

Elderly: Avoid use in the elderly due to risk of orthostatic hypotension and CNS depression.

Monitoring and Teaching Issues

Physical Assessment: See individual components listed in Related Information. **Pregnancy risk factor C/D** - see Pregnancy Risk Factor for use cautions; benefits of use should outweigh possible risks. Breast-feeding is contraindicated.

Patient Education: See individual components listed in Related Information. **Pregnancy/breast-feeding precautions:** Inform prescriber if you are or intend to become pregnant. Do not breast-feed.

Related Information

Aspirin *on page 121*
Carisoprodol *on page 221*

Carisoprodol, Aspirin, and Codeine

(kar i soe PROE dole, AS pir in, and KOE deen)

U.S. Brand Names Soma® Compound w/Codeine

Synonyms Aspirin, Carisoprodol, and Codeine; Codeine, Aspirin, and Carisoprodol

Restrictions C-III

Generic Available Yes

Pharmacologic Category Skeletal Muscle Relaxant

Pregnancy Risk Factor C/D (full-dose aspirin in 3rd trimester)

Lactation Enters breast milk/contraindicated

Use Skeletal muscle relaxant

Formulations Tablet: Carisoprodol 200 mg, aspirin 325 mg, and codeine phosphate 16 mg

Dosing

Adults: Skeletal muscle relaxant, analgesic: Oral: 1 or 2 tablets 4 times/day

Elderly: Avoid use in the elderly due to the risk of orthostatic hypotension and CNS depression.

Monitoring and Teaching Issues

Physical Assessment: See individual components listed in Related Information. **Pregnancy risk factor C/D** - see Pregnancy Risk Factor for use cautions; benefits of use should outweigh possible risks. Breast-feeding is contraindicated.

Patient Education: See individual components listed in Related Information. **Pregnancy/breast-feeding precautions:** Inform prescriber if you are or intend to become pregnant. Do not breast-feed.

Related Information

Aspirin *on page 121*
Carisoprodol *on page 221*
Codeine *on page 327*

Carmol-HC® Topical *see page 1522*

Carmol® Scalp *see* Sulfacetamide *on page 1256*

Carmustine (kar MUS teen)

U.S. Brand Names BiCNU®; Gliadel®

Synonyms BCNU

Generic Available No

Pharmacologic Category Antineoplastic Agent, Alkylating Agent

Pregnancy Risk Factor D

Lactation Excretion in breast milk unknown/contraindicated

Use Treatment of brain tumors (glioblastoma, brainstem glioma, medulloblastoma, astrocytoma, ependymoma, and metastatic brain tumors), multiple myeloma, Hodgkin's disease, non-Hodgkin's lymphomas, melanoma, lung cancer, colon cancer

Gliadel®: Adjunct to surgery in patients with recurrent glioblastoma multiforme

Mechanism of Action/Effect Interferes with the normal function of DNA by alkylation and cross-linking the strands of DNA, and by possible protein modification

Contraindications Hypersensitivity to carmustine or any component of the formulation; myelosuppression (from previous chemotherapy or other causes); pregnancy

Warnings/Precautions The U.S. Food and Drug Administration (FDA) currently recommends that procedures for proper handling and disposal of antineoplastic agents be considered. Administer with caution to patients with depressed platelet, leukocyte or erythrocyte counts, renal or hepatic impairment. Bone marrow depression, notably thrombocytopenia and leukopenia, may lead to bleeding and overwhelming infections in an already compromised patient. Will last for at least 6 weeks after a dose, do not give courses more frequently than every 6 weeks because the toxicity is cumulative.

Drug Interactions

Increased Effect/Toxicity: Carmustine given in combination with cimetidine is reported to cause bone marrow depression. Carmustine given in combination with etoposide is reported to cause severe hepatic dysfunction with hyperbilirubinemia, ascites, and thrombocytopenia.

Nutritional/Ethanol Interactions Ethanol: Avoid ethanol (due to GI irritation).

Adverse Reactions

>10%:

Cardiovascular: Hypotension is associated with **high-dose** administration secondary to the high content of the diluent

Central nervous system: Dizziness, ataxia; Wafers: Seizures (54%) postoperatively

Dermatologic: Hyperpigmentation of skin

Gastrointestinal: Nausea and vomiting occur within 2-4 hours after drug injection; dose-related

Emetic potential:

<200 mg: Moderately high (60% to 90%)

≥200 mg: High (>90%)

Time course of nausea/vomiting: Onset: 2-6 hours; Duration: 4-6 hours

(Continued)

Carmustine *(Continued)*

Hematologic: Myelosuppressive: Delayed, occurs 4-6 weeks after administration and is dose-related; usually persists for 1-2 weeks; thrombocytopenia is usually more severe than leukopenia. Myelofibrosis and preleukemic syndromes have been reported.
WBC: Moderate
Platelets: Severe
Onset: 14 days
Nadir: 21-35 days
Recovery: 42-50 days
Local: Burning at injection site
Irritant chemotherapy: Pain at injection site
Ocular: Ocular toxicity, and retinal hemorrhages
1% to 10%:
Dermatologic: Facial flushing is probably due to the alcohol used in reconstitution, alopecia
Gastrointestinal: Stomatitis, diarrhea, anorexia
Hematologic: Anemia
<1% (Limited to important or life-threatening): Reversible toxicity; increased LFTs in 20%; fibrosis occurs mostly in patients treated with prolonged total doses >1400 mg/m^2 or with bone marrow transplantation doses; risk factors include a history of lung disease, concomitant bleomycin, or radiation therapy; PFTs should be conducted prior to therapy and monitored; patients with predicted FVC or DLCO <70% are at a higher risk; azotemia; decrease in kidney size; renal failure

BMT:
Cardiovascular: Hypotension (infusion-related), arrhythmias (infusion-related)
Central nervous system: Encephalopathy, ethanol intoxication, seizures, fever
Endocrine & metabolic: Hyperprolactinemia and hypothyroidism in patients with brain tumors treated with radiation
Gastrointestinal: Severe nausea and vomiting
Hepatic Hepatitis, hepatic veno-occlusive disease
Pulmonary: Dyspnea

Overdosage/Toxicology Symptoms of overdose include nausea, vomiting, thrombocytopenia, and leukopenia. Treatment is symptomatic and supportive.

Pharmacodynamics/Kinetics

Half-Life Elimination: Biphasic: Initial: 1.4 minutes; Secondary: 20 minutes (active metabolites: plasma half-life of 67 hours)

Metabolism: Rapidly hepatic

Formulations

Injection, powder for reconstitution: 100 mg/vial [with 3 mL absolute alcohol as diluent]
Wafer (Gliadel®): Carmustine 7.7 mg

Dosing

Adults & Elderly: Refer to individual protocols.

Usual dosage (per manufacturer labeling): 150-200 mg/m^2 every 6-8 weeks as a single dose or divided into daily injections on 2 successive days

Next dose is to be determined based on hematologic response to the previous dose. Repeat dose should not be administered until circulating blood elements have returned to acceptable levels (leukocytes >4000, platelets >100,000), usually 6 weeks

Listed are the suggested carmustine doses, based upon the nadir after the prior dose.

- Leukocytes >4000 mm^3 and platelets >100,000 mm^3: Administer 100% of prior dose.
- Leukocytes 3000-3999 mm^3 and platelets 75,000-99,999 mm^3: Administer 100% of prior dose.
- Leukocytes 2000-2999 mm^3 and platelets 25,000-74,999 mm^3: Administer 70% of prior dose.
- Leukocytes <2000 mm^3 and platelets <25,000 mm^3: Administer 50% of prior dose.

Primary brain cancer: I.V.:
150-200 mg/m^2 every 6-8 weeks as a single dose or divided into daily injections on 2 successive days
20-65 mg/m^2 every 4-6 weeks
0.5-1 mg/kg every 4-6 weeks
40-80 mg/m^2/day for 3 days every 6-8 weeks

Autologous BMT: **ALL OF THE FOLLOWING DOSES ARE FATAL WITHOUT BMT.**
Combination therapy: Up to 300-900 mg/m^2
Single-agent therapy: Up to 1200 mg/m^2 (fatal necrosis is associated with doses >2 g/m^2)

Adjunct to surgery in patients with recurrent glioblastoma multiforme (Gliadel®): Implantation: Up to 8 wafers may be placed in the resection cavity (total dose 62.6 mg); should the size and shape not accommodate 8 wafers, the maximum number of wafers allowed should be placed.

Pediatrics: Refer to individual protocols: Children: I.V.: 200-250 mg/m^2 every 4-6 weeks as a single dose

Hepatic Impairment: Dosage adjustment may be necessary; however, no specific guidelines are available.

Administration

I.V.: Irritant (alcohol-based diluent). Significant absorption to PVC containers - should be administered in either glass or Excel® container. Infusion of drug over 1 hour is recommended.

High-dose carmustine: Maximum rate of infusion ≤3 mg/m^2/minute to avoid excessive flushing, agitation, and hypotension. Infusions should run over at least 2 hours.

Fatal doses if not followed by bone marrow or peripheral stem cell infusions.

Other: Wafers should only be handled by persons wearing surgical gloves (double gloves recommended). Dispose of outer gloves in biohazard waste container after use. A surgical instrument dedicated to the handling of wafers should be used. In the event of removal, wafers should be handled as a potentially cytotoxic agent.

Stability

Storage: Store intact vials under refrigeration; vials are stable for 7 days at room temperature.

Reconstitution: Initially dilute with 3 mL of absolute alcohol diluent. Further dilute with 27 mL SWI to result in a concentration of 3.3 mg/mL with 10% alcohol. Initial solutions are stable for 8 hours at room temperature (25°C) and 24 hours at refrigeration (2°C to 8°C) and protected from light. Further dilution in D_5W or NS is stable for 8 hours at room temperature (25°C) and 48 hours at refrigeration (4°C) in glass or Excel® protected from light.

Standard I.V. dilution: Dose/150-500 mL D_5W or NS

Must use glass or Excel® containers for administration. Protect from light. Stable for 8 hours at room temperature (25°C) and 48 hours under refrigeration (4°C).

Compatibility: Stable in NS

Y-site administration: Incompatible with allopurinol

Compatibility when admixed: Incompatible with sodium bicarbonate

Monitoring Laboratory Tests CBC with differential, platelet count, pulmonary function, liver and renal function

Monitoring and Teaching Issues

Physical Assessment: See Contraindications, Warnings/Precautions, and Dosing for use cautions. Assess potential for interactions with other prescriptions, OTC medications, or herbal products patient may be taking (see Drug Interactions). Administer antiemetic prior to therapy. See Administration, Compatibility, and Reconstitution information. Infusion site should be monitored closely to prevent extravasation (acute cellulitis may occur - see Administration) and bleeding precautions must be observed. Assess results of laboratory tests (see above), therapeutic response, and adverse response (see Adverse Reactions and Overdose/Toxicology) regularly during therapy. Teach patient (or caregiver) possible side effects and interventions and adverse symptoms to report (see Patient Education). **Pregnancy risk factor D** - determine that patient is not pregnant before beginning treatment. Instruct females of childbearing age or males who may have intercourse with females of childbearing age about appropriate barrier contraceptive measures during and for 1 month following therapy. Breast-feeding is contraindicated.

Patient Education: Inform prescriber of all prescriptions, OTC medications, or herbal products you are taking, and any allergies you have. Do not take anything new during treatment unless approved by prescriber. This medication can only be administered by I.V. Report immediately any pain, burning, swelling at infusion site. Limit oral intake for 4-6 hours before therapy to reduce potential for nausea/vomiting. It is important that you maintain adequate nutrition between treatments (small, frequent meals may help) and adequate hydration (2-3 L/day of fluids) unless advised by prescriber to restrict fluids. You will be susceptible to infection (avoid crowds and exposure to infection and do not have any vaccinations without consulting prescriber). May cause nausea, vomiting, or anorexia (small, frequent meals, frequent mouth care, chewing gum, or sucking lozenges may help - if nausea/vomiting are severe, request antiemetic); mouth sores (use soft toothbrush or cotton swabs for mouth care); hyperpigmentation of skin and loss of hair (reversible); or sensitivity to sunlight (use sunblock, wear protective clothing and dark glasses, and avoid direct exposure to sunlight). Report chest pain or palpitations; sore throat, fever, chills, unusual fatigue; unusual bruising/bleeding; change in color of urine or stool; difficulty breathing; change in visual acuity; or pain, redness, or swelling at injection site. **Pregnancy/breast-feeding precautions:** Inform prescriber if you are pregnant. Do not get pregnant or cause a pregnancy (males) during therapy or for 1 month following therapy. Consult prescriber for instruction on appropriate contraceptive measures. This drug may cause severe fetal defects. Do not breast-feed.

Breast-feeding Issues: It is not known if carmustine is excreted in human breast milk. Due to potential harm to infant, breast-feeding is not recommended.

Additional Information Baseline pulmonary function tests are recommended. Delayed onset pulmonary fibrosis occurring up to 17 years after treatment has been reported in children (1-16 years) who received carmustine in cumulative doses ranging from 770-1800 mg/m² combined with cranial radiotherapy for intracranial tumors.

Carnitor® *see* Levocarnitine *on page 787*

Carrington Antifungal [OTC] *see* Miconazole *on page 899*

Carteolol *see* Ophthalmic Agents, Glaucoma *on page 1002*

Cartia XT™ *see* Diltiazem *on page 418*

Carvedilol (KAR ve dil ole)

U.S. Brand Names Coreg®

Generic Available No

Pharmacologic Category Beta Blocker With Alpha-Blocking Activity

Pregnancy Risk Factor C (manufacturer); D (2nd and 3rd trimesters - expert analysis)

Lactation Excretion in breast milk unknown/contraindicated

Use Management of hypertension; can be used alone or in combination with other agents, especially thiazide-type diuretics; mild to severe heart failure of ischemic or cardiomyopathic origin usually in addition to standardized therapy.

Use - Unlabeled/Investigational Angina pectoris

Mechanism of Action/Effect Nonselective beta-adrenoreceptor and alpha-adrenergic blocking agent, lowers heart rate and blood pressure. Has been shown to lower risk of hospitalization and increase survival in patients with mild to severe heart failure.

Contraindications Hypersensitivity to carvedilol or any component of the formulation; patients with decompensated cardiac failure requiring intravenous inotropic therapy; bronchial asthma or related bronchospastic conditions; second- or third-degree AV block, sick sinus syndrome, and severe bradycardia (except in patients with a functioning artificial pacemaker); cardiogenic shock; severe hepatic impairment; pregnancy (2nd and 3rd trimesters)

(Continued)

Carvedilol *(Continued)*

Warnings/Precautions Initiate cautiously and monitor for possible deterioration in CHF. Adjustment of other medications (ACE inhibitors and/or diuretics) may be required. In severe chronic heart failure, trial patients were excluded if they had cardiac-related rales, ascites, or a serum creatinine >2.8 mg/dL. Discontinue therapy if any evidence of liver injury occurs. Use caution in patients with PVD (can aggravate arterial insufficiency). Use caution with concurrent use of beta-blockers and either verapamil or diltiazem; bradycardia or heart block can occur. Patients with bronchospastic disease should not receive beta-blockers. Use cautiously in diabetics because it can mask prominent hypoglycemic symptoms. Can mask signs of thyrotoxicosis. Use care with anesthetic agents that decrease myocardial function. Safety and efficacy in children <18 years of age have not been established.

Pregnancy risk C/D (2nd and 3rd trimesters).

Drug Interactions

Cytochrome P450 Effect: Substrate of CYP1A2, **2C8/9, 2D6**, 2E1, 3A4

Decreased Effect: Rifampin may reduce the plasma concentration of carvedilol by up to 70%. Decreased effect of beta-blockers has also occurred with antacids, barbiturates, calcium channel blockers, cholestyramine, colestipol, NSAIDs, penicillins (ampicillin), and salicylates due to decreased bioavailability and plasma levels. Beta-blockers may decrease the effect of sulfonylureas. Nonselective beta-blockers blunt the effect of beta-2 adrenergic agonists (albuterol).

Increased Effect/Toxicity: Clonidine and cimetidine increase the serum levels and effects of carvedilol. Carvedilol may increase the levels of cyclosporine. Carvedilol may increase the effects of other drugs which slow AV conduction (digoxin, verapamil, diltiazem), alpha-blockers (prazosin, terazosin), and alpha-adrenergic stimulants (epinephrine, phenylephrine). Carvedilol may mask the tachycardia from hypoglycemia caused by insulin and oral hypoglycemics. In patients receiving concurrent therapy, the risk of hypertensive crisis is increased when either clonidine or the beta-blocker is withdrawn. Reserpine has been shown to enhance the effect of beta-blockers. Beta-blockers may increase the action or levels of disopyramide, and theophylline although the effects are difficult to predict.

Nutritional/Ethanol Interactions Herb/Nutraceutical: Avoid dong quai if using for hypertension (has estrogenic activity). Avoid ephedra, yohimbe, ginseng (may worsen hypertension). Avoid garlic (may have increased antihypertensive effect).

Effects on Lab Values ↑ hepatic enzymes, BUN, NPN, alkaline phosphatase; ↓ HDL

Adverse Reactions Note: Frequency ranges include data from hypertension and heart failure trials. Higher rates of adverse reactions have generally been noted in patients with CHF. However, the frequency of adverse effects associated with placebo is also increased in this population. Events occurring at a frequency > placebo in clinical trials.

>10%:
- Central nervous system: Dizziness (6% to 32%), fatigue (4% to 24%)
- Endocrine & metabolic: Hyperglycemia (5% to 12%), weight gain (10% to 12%)
- Gastrointestinal: Diarrhea (2% to 12%)
- Neuromuscular & skeletal: Weakness (11%)
- Respiratory: Upper respiratory tract infection (14% to 18%)

1% to 10%:
- Cardiovascular: Bradycardia (2% to 10%), hypotension (9% to 14%), hypertension (3%), AV block (3%), angina (2% to 6%), postural hypotension (2%), syncope (3% to 8%), dependent edema (4%), palpitations, peripheral edema (1% to 7%), generalized edema (5% to 6%)
- Central nervous system: Pain (9%), headache (5% to 8%), fever (3%), paresthesia (2%), somnolence (2%), insomnia (2%), malaise, hypesthesia, vertigo
- Endocrine & metabolic: Gout (6%), hypercholesterolemia (4%), dehydration (2%), hyperkalemia (3%), hypervolemia (2%), hypertriglyceridemia (1%), hyperuricemia, hypoglycemia, hyponatremia
- Gastrointestinal: Nausea (4% to 9%), vomiting (6%), melena, periodontitis
- Genitourinary: Urinary tract infection (2% to 3%), hematuria (3%), impotence
- Hematologic: Thrombocytopenia (1% to 2%), decreased prothrombin, purpura
- Hepatic: Increased transaminases, increased alkaline phosphatase
- Neuromuscular & skeletal: Back pain (2% to 7%), arthralgia (6%), myalgia (3%), muscle cramps
- Ocular: Blurred vision (3% to 5%)
- Renal: Increased BUN (6%), abnormal renal function, albuminuria, glycosuria, increased creatinine (3%), kidney failure
- Respiratory: Sinusitis (5%), bronchitis (5%), pharyngitis (2% to 3%), rhinitis (2%), increased cough (5%)
- Miscellaneous: Infection (2%), injury (3% to 6%), increased diaphoresis (3%), viral infection (2%), allergy, sudden death

<1% (Limited to important or life-threatening): Aggravated depression, anaphylactoid reaction, anemia, aplastic anemia (rare, all events occurred in patients receiving other medications capable of causing this effect); asthma, AV block (complete), bronchospasm, bundle branch block, convulsion, diabetes mellitus, exfoliative dermatitis, GI hemorrhage, leukopenia, migraine, myocardial ischemia, neuralgia, pancytopenia, peripheral ischemia, pulmonary edema, Stevens-Johnson syndrome

Additional events from clinical trials in heart failure patients occurring at a frequency >2% but equal to or less than the frequency reported in patients receiving placebo: Anemia, arthritis, asthenia, cardiac failure, chest pain, coughing, depression, dyspepsia, flatulence, headache, hyperkalemia, leg cramps, nausea, pain, palpitation, rash, sinusitis, upper respiratory infection

Overdosage/Toxicology Symptoms of intoxication include cardiac disturbances, CNS toxicity, bronchospasm, hypoglycemia, and hyperkalemia. The most common cardiac symptoms include hypotension and bradycardia. Atrioventricular block, intraventricular conduction disturbances, cardiogenic shock, and asystole may occur with severe overdose, especially with membrane-depressant drugs (eg, propranolol). CNS effects include convulsions, coma, and respiratory arrest (commonly seen with propranolol and other membrane-depressant and lipid-soluble drugs). Treatment is symptom-directed and supportive. Carvedilol does not appear to be significantly cleared by hemodialysis.

Pharmacodynamics/Kinetics

Absorption: Rapid; food decreases rate but not extent of absorption; administration with food minimizes risks of orthostatic hypotension

Bioavailability: 25% to 35%

Half-Life Elimination: 7-10 hours

Metabolism: Extensively hepatic, primarily by aromatic ring oxidation and glucuronidation (2% excreted unchanged); three active metabolites (4-hydroxyphenyl metabolite is 13 times more potent than parent drug for beta-blockade); first-pass effect; plasma concentrations in the elderly and those with cirrhotic liver disease are 50% and 4-7 times higher, respectively

Onset: 1-2 hours; Peak antihypertensive effect: ~1-2 hours

Formulations Tablet: 3.125 mg, 6.25 mg, 12.5 mg, 25 mg

Dosing

Adults & Elderly: Reduce dosage if heart rate drops to <55 beats/minute.

Hypertension: Oral: 6.25 mg twice daily; if tolerated, dose should be maintained for 1-2 weeks, then increased to 12.5 mg twice daily. Dosage may be increased to a maximum of 25 mg twice daily after 1-2 weeks. Maximum dose: 50 mg/day

Congestive heart failure: Oral: 3.125 mg twice daily for 2 weeks; if this dose is tolerated, may increase to 6.25 mg twice daily. Double the dose every 2 weeks to the highest dose tolerated by patient. (Prior to initiating therapy, other heart failure medications should be stabilized and fluid retention minimized.)

Maximum recommended dose: Oral:

Mild to moderate heart failure:

<85 kg: 25 mg twice daily

>85 kg: 50 mg twice daily

Severe heart failure: Oral: 25 mg twice daily

Angina pectoris (unlabeled use): Oral: 25-50 mg twice daily

Renal Impairment: None necessary

Hepatic Impairment: Use is contraindicated in liver dysfunction.

Administration

Oral: Administer with food.

Stability

Storage: Store at 30°C (86°F).

Monitoring Laboratory Tests Renal studies, BUN, liver function

Monitoring and Teaching Issues

Physical Assessment: See Contraindications and Warnings/Precautions for use cautions. Assess potential for interactions with other prescriptions, OTC medications, or herbal products patient may be taking (especially anything that will effect blood pressure - see Drug Interactions). Blood pressure and heart rate should be assessed prior to and following first doses and any change in dose. Caution diabetic patients to monitor glucose levels closely (beta-blockers may alter glucose tolerance). Assess results of laboratory tests (see above), therapeutic effectiveness (eg, reduction of hypertension or angina), and adverse response (eg, CHF - see Adverse Reactions and Overdose/Toxicology). Teach patient proper use, possible side effects and interventions, and adverse symptoms to report (see Patient Education). **Pregnancy risk factor C/D** - see Pregnancy Risk Factor for use cautions; benefits of use should outweigh possible risks. Breast-feeding is contraindicated.

Patient Education: Inform prescriber of all prescriptions, OTC medications, or herbal products you are taking, and any allergies you have. Do not take anything new during treatment unless approved by prescriber. Take exactly as directed. Do not alter dose or discontinue without consulting prescriber. Take pulse daily, prior to medication; follow prescriber's instruction about holding medication. If diabetic, monitor serum glucose closely (drug may alter glucose tolerance or mask signs of hypoglycemia). You may experience fatigue, dizziness, or postural hypotension (use caution when changing position from lying or sitting to standing, driving, or climbing stairs until response to medication is known); alteration in sexual performance (reversible); or diarrhea (buttermilk, boiled milk, or yogurt may help). Report unresolved swelling of extremities; difficulty breathing or new cough; unresolved fatigue; unusual weight gain (>5 lbs/week); unresolved constipation or diarrhea; or unusual muscle weakness. **Pregnancy/breast-feeding precautions:** Inform prescriber if you are pregnant. Do not get pregnant while taking this medications. Consult prescriber for appropriate contraceptive use. Do not breast-feed.

Dietary Issues: Should be taken with food to minimize the risk of orthostatic hypotension.

Geriatric Considerations: Due to alterations in the beta-adrenergic autonomic nervous system, beta-adrenergic blockade may result in less hemodynamic response than seen in younger adults.

Additional Information Fluid retention during therapy should be treated with an increase in diuretic dosage.

Related Information

Beta-Blockers *on page 1561*
Heart Failure *on page 1670*

Casanthranol *see page 1581*

Cascara (kas KAR a)

Synonyms Cascara Sagrada

Generic Available Yes

Pharmacologic Category Laxative, Stimulant

Pregnancy Risk Factor C

Lactation Enters breast milk/use caution (AAP rates "compatible")

Use Temporary relief of constipation; sometimes used with milk of magnesia ("black and white" mixture)

(Continued)

Cascara *(Continued)*

Mechanism of Action/Effect Direct chemical irritation of the intestinal mucosa resulting in an increased rate of colonic motility and change in fluid and electrolyte secretion

Contraindications Nausea; vomiting; abdominal pain; fecal impaction; intestinal obstruction; GI bleeding; appendicitis; congestive heart failure

Warnings/Precautions Excessive use can lead to electrolyte imbalance, fluid imbalance, vitamin deficiency, steatorrhea, osteomalacia, cathartic colon, and dependence. Pregnancy risk C.

Drug Interactions

Decreased Effect: Decreased effect of oral anticoagulants.

Effects on Lab Values ↓ calcium (S), potassium (S)

Adverse Reactions 1% to 10%:

Central nervous system: Faintness
Endocrine & metabolic: Electrolyte and fluid imbalance
Gastrointestinal: Abdominal cramps, nausea, diarrhea
Genitourinary: Discoloration of urine (reddish pink or brown)

Pharmacodynamics/Kinetics

Absorption: Oral: Poor, from small intestine
Metabolism: Hepatic
Onset: 6-10 hours

Formulations

Aromatic fluid extract: 120 mL, 473 mL
Tablet: 325 mg

Dosing

Adults & Elderly: Note: Cascara sagrada fluid extract is 5 times more potent than cascara sagrada aromatic fluid extract.

Constipation: Oral (aromatic fluid extract): 5 mL/day (range: 2-6 mL) as needed at bedtime (1 tablet as needed at bedtime)

Pediatrics: Note: Cascara sagrada fluid extract is 5 times more potent than cascara sagrada aromatic fluid extract.

Constipation: Oral (aromatic fluid extract):
Infants: 1.25 mL/day (range: 0.5-1.5 mL) as needed
Children 2-11 years: 2.5 mL/day (range: 1-3 mL) as needed
Children ≥12 years: Refer to adult dosing.

Monitoring and Teaching Issues

Physical Assessment: See Contraindications and Warnings/Precautions for use cautions. Discontinue if patient has abdominal distention, absent bowel sounds, abdominal pain or cramping, rectal pain or bleeding, nausea, vomiting, dehydration, or electrolyte imbalance (eg, muscle cramps, pain, weakness, dizziness, excessive thirst). Assess potential for interactions with other prescriptions, OTC medications, or herbal products patient may be taking (see Drug Interactions). Identify cause of constipation, if possible. Instruct patient in correct use (see Patient Education). **Pregnancy risk factor C** - benefits of use should outweigh possible risks. Note breast-feeding caution.

Patient Education: Inform prescriber of all prescriptions, OTC medications, or herbal products you are taking, and any allergies you have. Take with water on an empty stomach for better absorption. Do not take within 1 hour of antacids, milk, or other medications. Evacuation will usually occur 6-12 hours after taking. Cascara should not be used regularly for more than 1 week. A regular toileting routine, adequate fluids, regular exercise, and a diet that includes roughage and bulk will help to prevent constipation. May discolor urine (black or brown normal). **Pregnancy/breast-feeding precautions:** Inform prescriber if you are or intend to become pregnant. Consult prescriber if breast-feeding.

Dietary Issues: Administer on empty stomach for rapid effect.

Geriatric Considerations: Elderly are often predisposed to constipation due to disease, immobility, drugs, low residue diets, and a decreased "thirst reflex" with age. Avoid stimulant cathartic use on a chronic basis if possible. Use osmotic, lubricant, stool softeners, and bulk agents as prophylaxis. Patients should be instructed for proper dietary fiber and fluid intake as well as regular exercise. Monitor closely for fluid/electrolyte imbalance, CNS signs of fluid/electrolyte loss, and hypotension.

Breast-feeding Issues: Cascara sagrada may have a laxative effect on the infant; use caution.

Related Information

Laxatives: Classification and Properties *on page 1581*

Cascara Sagrada *see* Cascara *on page 227*
Casodex® *see* Bicalutamide *on page 168*

Caspofungin (kas poe FUN jin)

U.S. Brand Names Cancidas®

Synonyms Caspofungin Acetate

Generic Available No

Pharmacologic Category Antifungal Agent, Parenteral

Pregnancy Risk Factor C

Lactation Excretion in breast milk unknown/use caution

Use Treatment of invasive *Aspergillus* infection in patients who do not tolerate or do not respond to other antifungal therapies (including amphotericin B, lipid formulations of amphotericin B, or itraconazole); has not been studied as initial therapy for aspergillosis; treatment of esophageal candidiasis

Mechanism of Action/Effect Blocks synthesis of a vital component of fungal cell wall, limiting its growth. The cell wall component is unique to specific fungi, limiting any potential for toxicity in mammals.

Contraindications Hypersensitivity to caspofungin or any component of the formulation

Warnings/Precautions Has not been studied as initial therapy for *Aspergillus* infection. Avoid concurrent use of cyclosporine, due to a high frequency of hepatic transaminase elevations observed during concurrent use. Limited data are available concerning treatment durations longer than 2 weeks; however, treatment appears to be well tolerated. Use caution in hepatic impairment; dosage reduction required in moderate impairment. An increased daily dosage should be considered in patients receiving enzyme-inducing agents who fail to demonstrate adequate clinical response. Safety and efficacy in pediatric patients have not been established. Pregnancy risk C.

Drug Interactions

Decreased Effect: Caspofungin may decrease blood concentrations of tacrolimus. In limited experience, some enzyme inducers decreased the serum concentrations of caspofungin. Dosage adjustment needed with rifampin and may be needed with other inducers.

Increased Effect/Toxicity: Concurrent administration of cyclosporine may increase caspofungin concentrations. In limited experience, a high frequency of elevated hepatic serum transaminases was observed.

Adverse Reactions Note: Listing includes some reactions/frequencies noted during investigational use for indications other than *Aspergillus*.

>10%:

Central nervous system: Headache (up to 11%), fever (3% to 26%)

Hepatic: Increased serum alkaline phosphatase (3% to 11%), increased transaminases (up to 13%)

Local: Infusion site reactions (2% to 12%), phlebitis (up to 16%)

1% to 10%:

Cardiovascular: Flushing (3%), facial edema (up to 3%)

Central nervous system: Dizziness (2%), chills (up to 3%), pain (1% to 5%), paresthesia (1% to 3%)

Dermatologic: Rash (<1% to 5%), pruritus (2% to 3%), erythema (1% to 2%)

Endocrine & metabolic: Serum potassium decreased (3%)

Gastrointestinal: Nausea (3% to 6%), vomiting (1% to 3%), abdominal pain (2% to 3%), diarrhea (1% to 4%)

Hematologic: Eosinophils increased (3%), hemoglobin decreased (3% to 12%), neutrophils decreased (2% to 3%), WBC increased (5% to 6%), anemia (up to 4%)

Local: Induration (up to 3%)

Neuromuscular & skeletal: Myalgia (up to 3%), paresthesia (1% to 3%)

Renal: Proteinuria (5%), hematuria (2%), serum creatinine increased (<1% to 2%), urinary WBCs increased (up to 8%)

Miscellaneous: Flu-like syndrome (3%)

<1% (Limited to important or life-threatening): Adult respiratory distress syndrome (ARDS), anaphylaxis, dyspnea, dystonia, facial swelling, pruritus, pulmonary edema, rash, stridor

Overdosage/Toxicology No experience with overdosage has been reported. Caspofungin is not dialyzable. Treatment is symptomatic and supportive.

Pharmacodynamics/Kinetics

Half-Life Elimination: Beta (distribution): 9-11 hours; Terminal: 40-50 hours

Metabolism: Slowly, via hydrolysis and *N*-acetylation as well as by spontaneous degradation, with subsequent metabolism to component amino acids

Formulations Injection, powder for reconstitution, as acetate: 50 mg, 70 mg

Dosing

Adults:

Aspergillus infection (invasive): I.V.: Initial dose: 70 mg infused slowly (over 1 hour); subsequent dosing: 50 mg daily (infused over 1 hour)

Esophageal candidiasis: I.V.: 50 mg/day (infused over 1 hour)

Duration of caspofungin treatment should be determined by patient status and clinical response (limited experience beyond 2 weeks of therapy). Efficacy of 70 mg daily dose (in patients not responding to 50 mg/day) has not been adequately studied, although this dose appears to be well tolerated.

Patients receiving rifampin should receive 70 mg caspofungin daily.

Patients receiving carbamazepine, dexamethasone, efavirenz, nelfinavir, nevirapine, phenytoin, and rifampin (and possibly other enzyme inducers) may require an increased daily dose of caspofungin (70 mg/day) if response to 50 mg/day is inadequate.

Elderly: The number of patients >65 years of age in clinical studies was not sufficient to establish whether a difference in response may be anticipated.

Pediatrics: Safety and efficacy in pediatric patients have not been established.

Renal Impairment: No specific dosage adjustment is required; supplemental dose is not required following dialysis.

Hepatic Impairment:

Patients with mild hepatic impairment (Child-Pugh score 5 to 6): No adjustment necessary.

Patients with moderate hepatic insufficiency (Child-Pugh score 7 to 9):

Invasive *Aspergillus* infection: Reduce daily dose to 35 mg (after initial 70 mg dose)

Esophageal candidiasis: 35 mg/day

Administration

I.V.: Infuse slowly, over 1 hour

Stability

Storage: Store vials at 2°C to 8°C (36°F to 46°F). Reconstituted solution may be stored at less than 25°C (77°F) for 1 hour prior to preparation of infusion solution. Infusion solutions may be stored at less than 25°C (77°F) and should be used within 24 hours.

Reconstitution: Reconstitute vial (70 mg loading dose or 50 mg daily dose) with 10.5 mL 0.9% sodium chloride for injection. Transfer 10 mL of the reconstituted solution to 100-250 mL 0.9% sodium chloride. If 70 mg vials are not available for preparation of the loading dose, reconstitute two 50 mg vials and transfer 14 mL to the desired infusion volume. Vials are formulated to provide full-labeled dose when 10 mL is withdrawn from the vial.

Compatibility: Do not mix with dextrose-containing solutions or coadminister with other medications.

(Continued)

Caspofungin *(Continued)*

Monitoring and Teaching Issues

Physical Assessment: See Warnings/Precautions, Contraindications, and Dosing for use cautions. Assess therapeutic response and adverse reactions (see Adverse Reactions). See I.V. Administration. Teach patient possible side and appropriate interventions and adverse symptoms to report (see Patient Education). **Pregnancy risk factor C** - benefits of use should outweigh possible risks. Note breast-feeding caution.

Patient Education: This medication can only be administered by infusion. Report immediately any pain, burning, or swelling at infusion site, or any signs of allergic reaction (eg, difficulty breathing or swallowing, back pain, chest tightness, rash, hives, or swelling of lips or mouth). Report nausea, vomiting, abdominal pain, or diarrhea. **Pregnancy/breast-feeding precautions:** Inform prescriber if you are or intend to become pregnant. Consult prescriber if breast-feeding.

Caspofungin Acetate *see* Caspofungin *on page 228*

Castor Oil *see page 1581*

Cataflam® *see* Diclofenac *on page 400*

Catapres® *see* Clonidine *on page 316*

Catapres-TTS®-1 *see* Clonidine *on page 316*

Catapres-TTS®-2 *see* Clonidine *on page 316*

Catapres-TTS®-3 *see* Clonidine *on page 316*

Cathflo™ Activase® *see* Alteplase *on page 67*

Caverject® *see* Alprostadil *on page 65*

CBDCA *see* Carboplatin *on page 218*

CBZ *see* Carbamazepine *on page 213*

CCNU *see* Lomustine *on page 814*

2-CdA *see* Cladribine *on page 303*

CDDP *see* Cisplatin *on page 298*

Ceclor® *see* Cefaclor *on page 230*

Ceclor® CD *see* Cefaclor *on page 230*

Cedax® *see* Ceftibuten *on page 251*

CeeNU® *see* Lomustine *on page 814*

Cefaclor (SEF a klor)

U.S. Brand Names Ceclor®; Ceclor® CD

Generic Available Yes

Pharmacologic Category Antibiotic, Cephalosporin (Second Generation)

Pregnancy Risk Factor B

Lactation Enters breast milk (small amounts)/use caution

Use Infections caused by susceptible organisms including *Staphylococcus aureus* and *H. influenzae*; treatment of otitis media, sinusitis, and infections involving the respiratory tract, skin and skin structure, bone and joint, and urinary tract

Mechanism of Action/Effect Inhibits bacterial cell wall synthesis by binding to one or more of the penicillin-binding proteins (PBPs)

Contraindications Hypersensitivity to cefaclor, any component of the formulation, or other cephalosporins

Warnings/Precautions Modify dosage in patients with severe renal impairment. Prolonged use may result in superinfection. Cross-sensitivity to penicillins exists (~10%).

Drug Interactions

Increased Effect/Toxicity: Probenecid may decrease cephalosporin elimination. Furosemide, aminoglycosides when taken with cefaclor may result in additive nephrotoxicity. Bleeding may occur when administered with anticoagulants.

Nutritional/Ethanol Interactions Food: Cefaclor serum levels may be decreased slightly if taken with food.

Effects on Lab Values Positive direct Coombs', false-positive urinary glucose test using cupric sulfate (Benedict's solution, Clinitest®, Fehling's solution), false-positive serum or urine creatinine with Jaffé reaction

Adverse Reactions

1% to 10%:

Gastrointestinal: Diarrhea (1.5%)

Hematologic: Eosinophilia (2%)

Hepatic: Elevated transaminases (2.5%)

Dermatologic: Rash (maculopapular, erythematous, or morbilliform) (1% to 1.5%)

<1% (Limited to important or life-threatening): Agitation, anaphylaxis, angioedema, arthralgia, cholestatic jaundice, CNS irritability, confusion, dizziness, hallucinations, hemolytic anemia, hepatitis, hyperactivity, insomnia, interstitial nephritis, nausea, nervousness, neutropenia, prolonged PT, pruritus, pseudomembranous colitis, seizures, serum-sickness, somnolence, Stevens-Johnson syndrome, urticaria, vaginitis, vomiting

Reactions reported with other cephalosporins include abdominal pain, cholestasis, fever, hemorrhage, renal dysfunction, superinfection, toxic nephropathy

Overdosage/Toxicology Symptoms of overdose include neuromuscular hypersensitivity and convulsions. Many beta-lactam containing antibiotics have the potential to cause neuromuscular hyperirritability or convulsive seizures. Hemodialysis may be helpful to aid in removal of the drug from blood; otherwise, treatment is supportive or symptom-directed.

Pharmacodynamics/Kinetics

Absorption: Well absorbed, acid stable

Half-Life Elimination: 0.5-1 hour; prolonged with renal impairment

Time to Peak: Capsule: 60 minutes; Suspension: 45 minutes

Metabolism: Partially hepatic

Formulations

Capsule: 250 mg, 500 mg

Powder for oral suspension: 125 mg/5 mL (75 mL, 150 mL); 187 mg/5 mL (50 mL, 100 mL); 250 mg/5 mL (75 mL, 150 mL); 375 mg/5 mL (50 mL, 100 mL) [strawberry flavor]

Tablet, extended release: 375 mg, 500 mg

Dosing

Adults & Elderly: Susceptible infections: Oral: 250-500 mg every 8 hours or daily dose can be given in 2 divided doses

Pediatrics: Susceptible infections: Oral: Children >1 month: 20-40 mg/kg/day divided every 8-12 hours; maximum dose: 2 g/day (total daily dose may be divided into two doses for treatment of otitis media or pharyngitis)

Renal Impairment:

Cl_{cr} <50 mL/minute: Administer 50% of dose.

Moderately dialyzable (20% to 50%)

Administration

Oral: Administer around-the-clock to promote less variation in peak and trough serum levels. Shake well for oral suspension.

Stability

Reconstitution: Refrigerate suspension after reconstitution. Discard after 14 days. Do not freeze.

Monitoring Laboratory Tests AST (SGOT), ALT (SGPT), CBC, bilirubin, LDH, alkaline phosphatase, Coombs' test monthly if on long-term therapy; perform culture and sensitivity studies prior to initiating drug therapy.

Monitoring and Teaching Issues

Physical Assessment: Assess allergy history prior to therapy. See Contraindications, Warnings/Precautions, and Dosing for use cautions. Assess potential for interactions with other prescriptions, OTC medications, or herbal products patient may be taking (eg, nephrotoxicity - see Drug Interactions). Assess results of laboratory tests (see above), therapeutic response, and adverse reactions (hypersensitivity can occur days after therapy is started - see Adverse Reactions and Overdose/Toxicology). Instruct diabetic patients regarding Clinitest®. Teach patient proper use, possible side effects and interventions, and adverse symptoms to report (eg, nephrotoxicity, opportunistic infection: fever, malaise, rash, diarrhea, itching, fever, chills, or increased cough - see Patient Education). Note breast-feeding caution.

Patient Education: Inform prescriber of all prescriptions, OTC medications, or herbal products you are taking, and any allergies you have. Do not take anything new during treatment unless approved by prescriber. Take as directed, at regular intervals around-the-clock (with or without food). Chilling oral suspension improves flavor (do not freeze). Do not chew or crush extended release tablets. Maintain adequate hydration (2-3 L/day of fluids) unless advised by prescriber to restrict fluids. Complete full course of medication, even if you feel better. May cause false test results with Clinitest®; use of another type of testing is preferable. May cause diarrhea (yogurt, boiled milk, or buttermilk may help). Report rash; difficulty breathing or swallowing; persistent nausea, vomiting, or abdominal pain; changes in urinary pattern or pain on urination; opportunistic infection (eg, vaginal itching or drainage; sores in mouth; blood in stool or urine, vaginal itching or drainage, unusual fever or chills); or CNS changes (eg, irritability, agitation, nervousness, insomnia, hallucinations). **Breast-feeding precaution:** Consult prescriber if breast-feeding.

Dietary Issues: May be taken with or without food.

Breast-feeding Issues: Theoretically, drug absorbed by nursing infant may change bowel flora or affect fever work-up result. **Note:** As a class, cephalosporins are used to treat infections in infants.

Cefadroxil (sef a DROKS il)

U.S. Brand Names Duricef®

Synonyms Cefadroxil Monohydrate

Generic Available Yes

Pharmacologic Category Antibiotic, Cephalosporin (First Generation)

Pregnancy Risk Factor B

Lactation Enters breast milk (small amounts)/use caution (AAP rates "compatible")

Use Treatment of susceptible bacterial infections, including those caused by group A beta-hemolytic *Streptococcus*; prophylaxis against bacterial endocarditis in patients who are allergic to penicillin and undergoing surgical or dental procedures

Mechanism of Action/Effect Inhibits bacterial cell wall synthesis by binding to one or more of the penicillin-binding proteins (PBPs)

Contraindications Hypersensitivity to cefadroxil, other cephalosporins, or any component of the formulation

Warnings/Precautions Modify dosage in patients with severe renal impairment. Prolonged use may result in superinfection. Cross-sensitivity to penicillins exists (~10%).

Drug Interactions

Increased Effect/Toxicity: Bleeding may occur when administered with anticoagulants. Probenecid may decrease cephalosporin elimination.

Nutritional/Ethanol Interactions Food: Concomitant administration with food, infant formula, or cow's milk does **not** significantly affect absorption.

Effects on Lab Values Positive direct Coombs', false-positive urinary glucose test using cupric sulfate (Benedict's solution, Clinitest®, Fehling's solution), false-positive serum or urine creatinine with Jaffé reaction

(Continued)

Cefadroxil *(Continued)*

Adverse Reactions

1% to 10%: Gastrointestinal: Diarrhea

<1% (Limited to important or life-threatening): Abdominal pain, agranulocytosis, anaphylaxis, angioedema, arthralgia, cholestasis, dyspepsia, erythema multiforme, fever, nausea, neutropenia, pruritus, pseudomembranous colitis, rash (maculopapular and erythematous), serum sickness, Stevens-Johnson syndrome, thrombocytopenia, transaminases increased, urticaria, vaginitis, vomiting

Reactions reported with other cephalosporins include abdominal pain, aplastic anemia, BUN increased, creatinine increased, eosinophilia, hemolytic anemia, hemorrhage, pancytopenia, prolonged prothrombin time, renal dysfunction, seizures, superinfection, toxic epidermal necrolysis, toxic nephropathy

Overdosage/Toxicology Symptoms of overdose include neuromuscular hypersensitivity and convulsions. Many beta-lactam containing antibiotics have the potential to cause neuromuscular hyperirritability or convulsive seizures. Hemodialysis may be helpful to aid in removal of the drug from blood; otherwise, treatment is supportive or symptom-directed.

Pharmacodynamics/Kinetics

Absorption: Rapid and well absorbed

Half-Life Elimination: 1-2 hours; Renal failure: 20-24 hours

Time to Peak: Serum: 70-90 minutes

Formulations

Capsule, as monohydrate: 500 mg

Suspension, oral, as monohydrate: 125 mg/5 mL, 250 mg/5 mL, 500 mg/5 mL (50 mL, 100 mL)

Tablet, as monohydrate: 1 g

Dosing

Adults & Elderly:

Susceptible infections: Oral: 1-2 g/day in 2 divided doses

Prophylaxis against bacterial endocarditis: Oral: 2 g 1 hour prior to the procedure

Pediatrics:

Susceptible infections: Oral: Children: 30 mg/kg/day divided twice daily up to a maximum of 2 g/day

Prophylaxis against bacterial endocarditis: Oral: Children: 50 mg/kg 1 hour prior to the procedure

Renal Impairment:

Cl_{cr} 10-25 mL/minute: Administer every 24 hours.

Cl_{cr} <10 mL/minute: Administer every 36 hours.

Administration

Oral: Administer around-the-clock to promote less variation in peak and trough serum levels.

Stability

Reconstitution: Refrigerate suspension after reconstitution. Discard after 14 days.

Monitoring Laboratory Tests AST (SGOT), ALT (SGPT), CBC, bilirubin, LDH, alkaline phosphatase, Coombs' test monthly if on long-term therapy; perform culture and sensitivity studies prior to initiating drug therapy.

Monitoring and Teaching Issues

Physical Assessment: Assess for previous allergy history prior to therapy. See Contraindications and Warnings/Precautions for use cautions. Assess potential for interactions with other prescriptions, OTC medications, or herbal products patient may be taking (eg, nephrotoxicity - see Drug Interactions). Assess results of laboratory tests (see above), therapeutic response, and adverse reactions (eg, hypersensitivity can occur several days after therapy is started - see Adverse Reactions). Instruct diabetic patients regarding Clinitest®. Teach patient proper use, possible side effects and interventions, and adverse symptoms to report (eg, nephrotoxicity, opportunistic infection - see Patient Education). Note breast-feeding caution.

Patient Education: Inform prescriber of all prescriptions, OTC medications, or herbal products you are taking, and any allergies you have. Do not take anything new during treatment unless approved by prescriber. Take as directed, at regular intervals around-the-clock (with or without food). Chilling oral suspension improves flavor (do not freeze). Do not chew or crush extended release tablets. Maintain adequate hydration (2-3 L/day of fluids) unless advised by prescriber to restrict fluids. Complete full course of medication, even if you feel better. May cause false test results with Clinitest®; use of another type of glucose testing is preferable. May cause diarrhea (yogurt, boiled milk, or buttermilk may help). Report changes in urinary pattern or pain on urination; opportunistic infection (eg, vaginal itching or drainage; sores in mouth; blood in urine or stool; unusual fever or chills); or nausea, vomiting, or abdominal pain. **Breast-feeding precaution:** Consult prescriber if breast-feeding.

Geriatric Considerations: Adjust dose for renal function in the elderly.

Breast-feeding Issues: Theoretically, drug absorbed by nursing infant may change bowel flora or affect fever work-up result. **Note:** As a class, cephalosporins are used to treat infections in infants.

Cefadroxil Monohydrate *see* Cefadroxil *on page 231*

Cefadyl® *see* Cephapirin *on page 260*

Cefamandole (sef a MAN dole)

U.S. Brand Names Mandol®

Synonyms Cefamandole Nafate

Generic Available No

Pharmacologic Category Antibiotic, Cephalosporin (Second Generation)

Pregnancy Risk Factor B

Lactation Enters breast milk/use caution

Use Treatment of susceptible bacterial infection; mainly respiratory tract, skin and skin structure, bone and joint, urinary tract and gynecologic, septicemia; surgical prophylaxis. Active against methicillin-sensitive staphylococci, many streptococci, and various gram-negative bacilli including *E. coli*, some *Klebsiella*, *P. mirabilis*, *H. influenzae*, and *Moraxella*.

Mechanism of Action/Effect Inhibits bacterial cell wall synthesis by binding to one or more of the penicillin-binding proteins (PBPs)

Contraindications Hypersensitivity to cefamandole, any component of the formulation, or other cephalosporins

Warnings/Precautions Modify dosage in patients with severe renal impairment. Prolonged use may result in superinfection. Cross-sensitivity to penicillins exists (~10%). Hypoprothrombinemia has been reported rarely which is promptly reversed by vitamin K administration. Episodes more commonly occur in the elderly or medically compromised patients who may have a vitamin K deficiency. Monitor PT in these patients.

Drug Interactions

Increased Effect/Toxicity: Disulfiram-like reaction has been reported when taken within 72 hours of ethanol consumption. Increased cefamandole plasma levels when taken with probenecid. Aminoglycosides, furosemide when taken with cefamandole may increase nephrotoxicity. Increase in hypoprothrombinemic effect with warfarin or heparin and cefamandole.

Nutritional/Ethanol Interactions Ethanol: Avoid ethanol (possible disulfiram reaction).

Effects on Lab Values Positive direct Coombs', false-positive urinary glucose test using cupric sulfate (Benedict's solution, Clinitest®, Fehling's solution), false-positive serum or urine creatinine with Jaffé reaction

Adverse Reactions Contains MTT side chain which may lead to increased risk of hypoprothrombinemia and bleeding.

1% to 10%:

Gastrointestinal: Diarrhea

Local: Thrombophlebitis

<1% (Limited to important or life-threatening): Anaphylaxis, BUN increased, cholestasis, creatinine increased, eosinophilia, fever, nausea, neutropenia, prolonged PT, pseudomembranous colitis, rash (maculopapular and erythematous), thrombocytopenia, transaminases increased, urticaria, vomiting

Reactions reported with other cephalosporins include abdominal pain, aplastic anemia, hemolytic anemia, hemorrhage, pancytopenia, renal dysfunction, seizures, Stevens-Johnson syndrome, superinfection, toxic epidermal necrolysis, nephropathy, vaginitis

Overdosage/Toxicology Symptoms of overdose include neuromuscular hypersensitivity, and convulsions. Many beta-lactam containing antibiotics have the potential to cause neuromuscular hyperirritability or convulsive seizures. Hemodialysis may be helpful to aid in removal of the drug from blood; otherwise, treatment is supportive or symptom-directed.

Pharmacodynamics/Kinetics

Half-Life Elimination: 30-60 minutes

Time to Peak: Serum: I.M.: 1-2 hours

Metabolism: Extensive enterohepatic recirculation

Formulations Injection, powder for reconstitution, as nafate: 1 g (10 mL, 100 mL); 2 g (20 mL, 100 mL); 10 g (100 mL)

Dosing

Adults & Elderly: Susceptible infections: I.M., I.V.: 4-12 g/24 hours divided every 4-6 hours or 500-1000 mg every 4-8 hours; maximum: 2 g/dose

Pediatrics: Susceptible infections: I.M., I.V.: 50-150 mg/kg/day in divided doses every 4-8 hours

Renal Impairment:

Cl_{cr} 50-80 mL/minute: Administer 750-2000 mg every 6 hours.

Cl_{cr} 25-50 mL/minute: Administer 750-2000 mg every 8 hours.

Cl_{cr} 10-25 mL/minute: Administer 500-1250 mg every 8 hours or 1 g every 6 hours.

Cl_{cr} 2-10 mL/minute: Administer 500-1000 mg every 12 hours.

Cl_{cr} <2 mL/minute: Administer 250-750 mg every 12 hours.

Moderately dialyzable (20% to 50%)

Administration

I.M.: Inject deep I.M. into large muscle mass.

I.V.: Inject direct I.V. over 3-5 minutes. Infuse intermittent infusion over 15-30 minutes.

Stability

Reconstitution: After reconstitution, CO_2 gas is liberated which allows solution to be withdrawn without injecting air. Solution is stable for 24 hours at room temperature and 96 hours when refrigerated. For I.V., infusion in NS and D_5W is stable for 24 hours at room temperature, 1 week when refrigerated, or 26 weeks when frozen.

Compatibility: Stable in dextran 40 and dextrose, dextran 40 and NS, dextran 70 and dextrose, dextran 70 and NS, D_5LR, $D_5{}^1/_4NS$, $D_5{}^1/_2NS$, D_5NS, D_5W, $D_{10}W$, fat emulsion, mannitol 10%, mannitol 20%, NS; **incompatible** with LR

Y-site administration: Incompatible with amiodarone, hetastarch

Compatibility in syringe: Incompatible with cimetidine, gentamicin, tobramycin

Compatibility when admixed: Incompatible with calcium gluconate, gentamicin, ranitidine, tobramycin

Monitoring Laboratory Tests Prothrombin times; perform culture and sensitivity studies prior to initiating drug therapy.

Monitoring and Teaching Issues

Physical Assessment: Assess for previous allergy history prior to therapy. See Contraindications and Warnings/Precautions for use cautions. Assess potential for interactions with other prescriptions, OTC medications, or herbal products patient may be taking (eg, nephrotoxicity - see Drug Interactions). Assess results of laboratory tests (eg, hypoprothrombinemia - see above), therapeutic response, and adverse reactions (eg, hypersensitivity can occur several days after therapy is started - see Adverse Reactions and Overdose/Toxicology). Instruct diabetic patients regarding Clinitest®. Teach patient possible side effects and interventions and adverse symptoms to report (eg, nephrotoxicity, opportunistic infection - see Patient Education). Note breast-feeding caution.

(Continued)

Cefamandole *(Continued)*

Patient Education: Inform prescriber of all prescriptions, OTC medications, or herbal products you are taking, and any allergies you have. Do not take anything new during treatment unless approved by prescriber. This medication is administered by infusion or injection. Report immediately any redness, swelling, burning, or pain at injection/infusion site. Maintain adequate hydration (2-3 L/day of fluids) unless advised by prescriber to restrict fluids. Avoid alcohol during therapy and for 72 hours after last dose (may cause severe disulfiram-like reactions). May cause false test results with Clinitest®; use of another type of glucose testing is preferable. May cause diarrhea (yogurt, boiled milk, or buttermilk may help). Immediately report any rash, itching, hives; or difficulty swallowing or difficulty breathing. Report unresolved diarrhea; opportunistic infection (vaginal itching or drainage; sores in mouth; blood, pus, or mucus in stool or urine, unusual fever or chills); or difficulty breathing. **Breast-feeding precaution:** Consult prescriber if breast-feeding.

Geriatric Considerations: The risk of coagulation abnormalities (increased PT) limits the use of cefamandole in the elderly. Adjust dose for renal function in the elderly.

Breast-feeding Issues: Theoretically, drug absorbed by nursing infant may change bowel flora or affect fever work-up result. **Note:** As a class, cephalosporins are used to treat infections in infants.

Cefamandole Nafate *see* Cefamandole *on page 232*

Cefazolin (sef A zoe lin)

U.S. Brand Names Ancef®; Kefzol®

Synonyms Cefazolin Sodium

Generic Available Yes

Pharmacologic Category Antibiotic, Cephalosporin (First Generation)

Pregnancy Risk Factor B

Lactation Enters breast milk (small amounts)/use caution (AAP rates "compatible")

Use Treatment of gram-positive bacilli and cocci (except enterococcus); some gram-negative bacilli including *E. coli*, *Proteus*, and *Klebsiella* may be susceptible

Mechanism of Action/Effect Inhibits bacterial cell wall synthesis by binding to one or more of the penicillin-binding proteins (PBPs)

Contraindications Hypersensitivity to cefazolin sodium, any component of the formulation, or other cephalosporins

Warnings/Precautions Modify dosage in patients with severe renal impairment. Caution in individuals with seizure disorders. Prolonged use may result in superinfection. Cross-sensitivity to penicillins exists (~10%).

Drug Interactions

Increased Effect/Toxicity: High-dose probenecid decreases clearance and increases effect of cefazolin. Aminoglycosides increase nephrotoxic potential when taken with cefazolin.

Effects on Lab Values Positive direct Coombs', false-positive urinary glucose test using cupric sulfate (Benedict's solution, Clinitest®, Fehling's solution), false-positive serum or urine creatinine with Jaffé reaction

Adverse Reactions

1% to 10%:

Gastrointestinal: Diarrhea

Local: Pain at injection site

<1% (Limited to important or life-threatening): Abdominal cramps, anaphylaxis, anorexia, eosinophilia, fever, leukopenia, nausea, neutropenia, oral candidiasis, phlebitis, pruritus, pseudomembranous colitis, rash, seizures, Stevens-Johnson syndrome, thrombocytopenia, thrombocytosis, transaminases increased, vaginitis, vomiting

Reactions reported with other cephalosporins include abdominal pain, aplastic anemia, cholestasis, hemolytic anemia, hemorrhage, pancytopenia, prolonged prothrombin time, renal dysfunction, superinfection, toxic epidermal necrolysis, toxic nephropathy

Overdosage/Toxicology Symptoms of overdose include neuromuscular hypersensitivity and convulsions. Many beta-lactam containing antibiotics have the potential to cause neuromuscular hyperirritability or convulsive seizures. Hemodialysis may be helpful to aid in the removal of drug from blood; otherwise, treatment is supportive or symptom-directed.

Pharmacodynamics/Kinetics

Half-Life Elimination: 90-150 minutes; prolonged with renal impairment

Time to Peak: Serum: I.M.: 0.5-2 hours

Metabolism: Minimally hepatic

Formulations

Infusion, as sodium [premixed in D_5W, frozen] (Ancef®): 500 mg (50 mL); 1 g (50 mL)

Injection, powder for reconstitution, as sodium (Ancef®, Kefzol®): 500 mg, 1 g, 10 g, 20 g

Injection, powder for reconstitution, as sodium [with 50 mL D_5W in DUPLEX™ container]: 500 mg, 1 g

Dosing

Adults & Elderly:

Susceptible infections: I.M., I.V.: 1-2 g every 8 hours, depending on severity of infection; maximum: 12 g/day

Prophylaxis against bacterial endocarditis: 1 g 30 minutes before procedure

Surgical prophylaxis: 1-2 g preoperatively (some procedures require continuation for a limited number of doses)

Pediatrics: Susceptible infections: I.M., I.V.: Children >1 month: 25-100 mg/kg/day divided every 6-8 hours; maximum: 6 g/day

Renal Impairment:

Cl_{cr} 10-30 mL/minute: Administer every 12 hours.

Cl_{cr} <10 mL/minute: Administer every 24 hours.

Moderately dialyzable (20% to 50%); administer dose postdialysis or administer supplemental dose of 0.5-1 g after dialysis.

Peritoneal dialysis: Administer 0.5 g every 12 hours.

Continuous arteriovenous or venovenous hemofiltration: Dose as for Cl_{cr} 10-30 mL/minute. Removes 30 mg of cefazolin per liter of filtrate per day.

Administration

I.M.: Inject deep I.M. into large muscle mass.

I.V.: Inject direct I.V. over 5 minutes. Infuse intermittent infusion over 30-60 minutes.

Stability

Storage:

Store intact vials at room temperature and protect from temperatures exceeding 40°C. Protection from light is recommended for the powder and for the reconstituted solutions.

DUPLEX™: Store at 20°C to 25°C (68°F to 77°F); excursions permitted to 15°C to 30°C (59°F to 86°F) prior to activation

Reconstitution:

Reconstituted solutions of cefazolin are light yellow to yellow. Reconstituted solutions are stable for 24 hours at room temperature and 10 days under refrigeration. Stability of parenteral admixture at room temperature (25°C) is 48 hours. Stability of parenteral admixture at refrigeration temperature (4°C) is 14 days.

Standard diluent: 1 g/50 mL D_5W; 2 g/50 mL D_5W

DUPLEX™: Following activation, stable for 24 hours at room temperature and for 7 days under refrigeration.

Compatibility: Stable in D_5W, D_5LR, D_5¼NS, D_5½NS, D_5NS, $D_{10}W$,LR, NS

Y-site administration: Incompatible with amphotericin B cholesteryl sulfate complex, idarubicin, pentamidine, vinorelbine

Compatibility in syringe: Incompatible with ascorbic acid injection, cimetidine, lidocaine

Compatibility when admixed: Incompatible with amikacin, amobarbital, atracurium, bleomycin, calcium gluconate, clindamycin with gentamicin, colistimethate, kanamycin, pentobarbital, polymyxin B sulfate, ranitidine

Monitoring Laboratory Tests Prothrombin times; perform culture and sensitivity studies prior to initiating drug therapy.

Monitoring and Teaching Issues

Physical Assessment: Assess for previous allergy history prior to therapy. See Contraindications and Warnings/Precautions for use cautions. Assess potential for interactions with other prescriptions, OTC medications, or herbal products patient may be taking (eg, nephrotoxicity - see Drug Interactions). Assess results of laboratory tests (see above), therapeutic response, and adverse reactions (eg, hypersensitivity can occur several days after therapy is started - see Adverse Reactions and Overdose/Toxicology). Instruct diabetic patients regarding Clinitest®. Teach patient possible side effects and interventions and adverse symptoms to report (eg, nephrotoxicity, opportunistic infection - see Patient Education). Note breast-feeding caution.

Patient Education: Inform prescriber of all prescriptions, OTC medications, or herbal products you are taking, and any allergies you have. Do not take anything new during treatment unless approved by prescriber. This medication is administered by injection or infusion. Report immediately any redness, swelling, burning, or pain at injection/infusion site; rash or hives; or difficulty breathing, chest pain, or difficulty swallowing. Maintain adequate hydration (2-3 L/day of fluids) unless advised by prescriber to restrict fluids. If diabetic, drug may cause false test results with Clinitest® urine glucose monitoring; use of another type of glucose monitoring is preferable. May cause diarrhea (yogurt, boiled milk, or buttermilk may help). Report severe, unresolved diarrhea; opportunistic infection (vaginal itching or drainage; sores in mouth; blood in stool or urine; unusual fever or chills); or difficulty breathing. **Breast-feeding precautions:** Consult prescriber if breast-feeding.

Dietary Issues: Sodium content of 1 g: 47 mg (2 mEq)

Geriatric Considerations: Adjust dose for renal function.

Breast-feeding Issues: Theoretically, drug absorbed by nursing infant may change bowel flora or affect fever work-up result. **Note:** As a class, cephalosporins are used to treat infections in infants.

Related Information

Compatibility of Drugs *on page 1564*

Cefazolin Sodium *see* Cefazolin *on page 234*

Cefdinir (SEF di ner)

U.S. Brand Names Omnicef®

Synonyms CFDN

Generic Available No

Pharmacologic Category Antibiotic, Cephalosporin (Third Generation)

Pregnancy Risk Factor B

Lactation Enters breast milk (small amounts)/use caution

Use Treatment of community-acquired pneumonia, acute exacerbations of chronic bronchitis, acute bacterial otitis media, acute maxillary sinusitis, pharyngitis/tonsillitis, and uncomplicated skin and skin structure infections.

Mechanism of Action/Effect Inhibits bacterial cell wall synthesis by binding to one or more of the penicillin-binding proteins (PBPs) which in turn inhibits the final transpeptidation step of peptidoglycan synthesis in bacterial cell walls, thus inhibiting cell wall biosynthesis. Bacteria eventually lyse due to ongoing activity of cell wall autolytic enzymes (autolysins and murein hydrolases) while cell wall assembly is arrested.

Contraindications Hypersensitivity to cefdinir, other cephalosporins, any component of the formulation, or related antibiotics

Warnings/Precautions Administer cautiously to penicillin-sensitive patients. There is evidence of partial cross-allergenicity and cephalosporins cannot be assumed to be an absolutely safe alternative to penicillin in the penicillin-allergic patient. Serum sickness-like reactions have been reported. Signs and symptoms occur after a few days of therapy and resolve a few days after drug discontinuation with no serious sequelae. Pseudomembranous colitis occurs; consider its diagnosis in patients who develop diarrhea with antibiotic use.
(Continued)

Cefdinir *(Continued)*

Drug Interactions

Decreased Effect: Coadministration with iron or antacids reduces the rate and extent of cefdinir absorption.

Increased Effect/Toxicity: Probenecid increases the effects of cephalosporins by decreasing the renal elimination in those which are secreted by tubular secretion. Anticoagulant effects may be increased when administered with cephalosporins.

Adverse Reactions

1% to 10%

Dermatologic: Cutaneous moniliasis (1%)

Gastrointestinal: Diarrhea (8%), rash (3%), vomiting (1%), increased GGT (1%)

<1% (Limited to important or life-threatening): Acute renal failure, anaphylaxis, asthma exacerbation, cardiac failure, chest pain, cholestasis, coagulopathy, DIC, edema, enterocolitis, eosinophilic pneumonia, erythema multiforme, erythema nodosum, exfoliative dermatitis, fever, granulocytopenia, hemolytic anemia, hemorrhagic colitis, hepatic failure, hepatitis, hypertension, idiopathic interstitial pneumonia, ileus, involuntary movements, ITP, jaundice, laryngeal edema, leukopenia, loss of consciousness, myocardial infarction, nausea, nephropathy, pancytopenia, peptic ulcer, pseudomembranous colitis, rash, respiratory failure, rhabdomyolysis, shock, Stevens-Johnson syndrome, thrombocytopenia, toxic epidermal necrolysis, upper gastrointestinal bleeding, vaginal moniliasis, vasculitis

Reactions reported with other cephalosporins include angioedema, aplastic anemia, asterixis, dizziness, encephalopathy, fever, headache, hemorrhage, interstitial nephritis, neuromuscular excitability, prolonged PT, seizures, serum-sickness reactions, superinfection, toxic nephropathy

Overdosage/Toxicology After acute overdose, most agents cause only nausea, vomiting, and diarrhea, although neuromuscular hypersensitivity and seizures are possible, especially in patients with renal insufficiency. Hemodialysis may be helpful to aid in the removal of the drug from the blood but not usually indicated, otherwise most treatment is supportive or symptom-directed following GI decontamination.

Pharmacodynamics/Kinetics

Bioavailability: Capsule: 16% to 21%; Suspension 25%

Half-Life Elimination: 100 minutes

Metabolism: Minimally hepatic

Formulations

Capsule: 300 mg

Suspension, oral: 125 mg/5 mL (60 mL, 100 mL)

Dosing

Adults & Elderly:

Acute maxillary sinusitis: Oral: 300 mg twice daily **or** 600 mg once daily for 10 days

Pharyngitis or chronic bronchitis (exacerbation): Oral: 300 mg twice daily for 5-10 days **or** 600 mg once daily for 10 days

Pneumonia (community-acquired) or skin/skin structure infection (uncomplicated): Oral: 300 mg twice daily for 10 days

Pediatrics:

Children 6 months to 12 years:

Acute maxillary sinusitis: Oral: 7 mg/kg twice daily **or** 14 mg/kg once daily for 10 days

Otitis media or pharyngitis/tonsillitis: Oral: 7 mg/kg twice daily for 5-10 days **or** 14 mg/kg once daily for 10 days

Skin/skin structure infection (uncomplicated): Oral: 7 mg/kg twice daily for 10 days

Children >12 years: Refer to adult dosing.

Renal Impairment: Cl_{cr} <30 mL/minute: 300 mg once daily. Hemodialysis removes cefdinir; recommended initial dose: 300 mg (or 7 mg/kg/dose) every other day. At the conclusion of each hemodialysis session, 300 mg (or 7 mg/kg/dose) should be given. Subsequent doses (300 mg or 7 mg/kg/dose) should be administered every other day.

Stability

Storage: Oral suspension should be mixed with 38 mL water for the 60 mL bottle and 63 mL of water for the 120 mL bottle. After mixing, the suspension can be stored at room temperature (25°C/77°F). The suspension may be used for 10 days. The suspension should be shaken well before each administration.

Monitoring and Teaching Issues

Physical Assessment: Assess for previous allergy history prior to starting therapy. See Contraindications, Warnings/Precautions, and Drug Interactions for use cautions. Assess therapeutic response and adverse reactions (eg, hypersensitivity can occur several days after therapy is started - see Adverse Reactions and Overdose/Toxicology). Teach patient proper use, possible side effects and interventions, and adverse symptoms to report (eg, severe diarrhea, opportunistic infection - see Patient Education). Note breast-feeding caution.

Patient Education: Inform prescriber of all prescriptions, OTC medications, or herbal products you are taking, and any allergies you have. Take as directed, at regular intervals around-the-clock (with or without food). Chilling oral suspension improves flavor (do not freeze). Complete full course of medication, even if you feel better. Maintain adequate hydration (2-3 L/day of fluids) unless advised by prescriber to restrict fluids. May cause false test results with Clinitest®; use of another type of glucose testing is preferable. May cause diarrhea (yogurt, boiled milk, or buttermilk may help); or nausea, vomiting, flatulence (small, frequent meals, frequent mouth care, chewing gum, or sucking lozenges may help). Report severe, unresolved diarrhea; opportunistic infection (vaginal itching or drainage, sores in mouth, blood in stool or urine, unusual fever or chills); skin rash; or difficulty breathing. **Breast-feeding precaution:** Consult prescriber if breast-feeding.

Cefditoren (sef de TOR en)

U.S. Brand Names Spectracef™

Synonyms Cefditoren Pivoxil

Generic Available No

Pharmacologic Category Antibiotic, Cephalosporin

Pregnancy Risk Factor B

Lactation Excretion in breast milk unknown/use caution

Use Treatment of acute bacterial exacerbation of chronic bronchitis or community-acquired pneumonia (due to susceptible organisms including *Haemophilus influenzae, Haemophilus parainfluenzae, Streptococcus pneumoniae*-penicillin susceptible only, *Moraxella catarrhalis*); pharyngitis or tonsillitis (*Streptococcus pyogenes*); and uncomplicated skin and skin-structure infections (*Staphylococcus aureus*-not MRSA, *Streptococcus pyogenes*)

Mechanism of Action/Effect Has bactericidal activity against susceptible gram-positive and gram-negative pathogens. Inhibits bacterial cell wall synthesis by binding to one or more of the penicillin-binding proteins (PBPs)

Contraindications Hypersensitivity to cefditoren, other cephalosporins, milk protein, or any component of the formulation; carnitine deficiency

Warnings/Precautions Use with caution in patients with a history of penicillin allergy, especially IgE-mediated reactions (eg, anaphylaxis, urticaria); may cause antibiotic-associated colitis or colitis secondary to *C. difficile*. Use caution in patients with renal or hepatic impairment. Cefditoren causes renal excretion of carnitine, do not use in patients with carnitine deficiency; not for long-term therapy due to the possible development of carnitine deficiency over time. Cefditoren tablets contain sodium caseinate, which may cause hypersensitivity reactions in patients with milk protein hypersensitivity; this does not affect patients with lactose intolerance. Safety and efficacy have not been established in children <12 years of age.

Drug Interactions

Decreased Effect: Antacids and H_2 receptor antagonists decrease cefditoren levels.

Increased Effect/Toxicity: Increased levels of cefditoren with probenecid.

Nutritional/Ethanol Interactions Food: Moderate- to high-fat meals increase bioavailability and maximum plasma concentration.

Adverse Reactions

>10%: Gastrointestinal: Diarrhea (11% to 15%)

1% to 10%:

- Central nervous system: Headache (2% to 3%)
- Endocrine & metabolic: Glucose increased (1%)
- Gastrointestinal: Nausea (4% to 6%), abdominal pain (2%), dyspepsia (1% to 2%), vomiting (1%)
- Genitourinary: Vaginal moniliasis (3% to 6%)
- Hematologic: Hematocrit decreased (2%)
- Renal: Hematuria (3%), urinary white blood cells increased (2%)

<1% (Limited to important or life-threatening): Allergic reaction, BUN increased, coagulation time increased, positive direct Coombs' test, pseudomembranous colitis, rash, thrombocytopenia

Additional adverse effects seen with cephalosporin antibiotics: Anaphylaxis, aplastic anemia, cholestasis, erythema multiforme, hemorrhage, hemolytic anemia, renal dysfunction, reversible hyperactivity, serum sickness-like reaction, Stevens-Johnson syndrome, toxic epidermal necrolysis, toxic nephropathy

Overdosage/Toxicology Specific information not available. Treatment should be symptom-directed and supportive. Hemodialysis may be helpful (removes ~30% from circulation).

Pharmacodynamics/Kinetics

Bioavailability: ~14% to 16%; increased with moderate to high-fat meal

Half-Life Elimination: 1.6 ± 0.4 hours

Time to Peak: 1.5-3 hours

Metabolism: Cefditoren pivoxil is hydrolyzed to cefditoren (active) and pivalate

Formulations Tablet, as pivoxil: 200 mg [equivalent to cefditoren] [contains sodium caseinate]

Dosing

Adults & Elderly:

- Acute bacterial exacerbation of chronic bronchitis: Oral: 400 mg twice daily for 10 days
- Community-acquired pneumonia: Oral: 400 mg twice daily for 14 days
- Pharyngitis, tonsillitis, uncomplicated skin and skin structure infections: Oral: 200 mg twice daily for 10 days

Pediatrics: Children ≥12 years: Refer to adult dosing.

Renal Impairment:

- Cl_{cr} 30-49 mL/minute: Maximum dose: 200 mg twice daily
- Cl_{cr} <30 mL/minute: Maximum dose: 200 mg once daily
- End-stage renal disease: Appropriate dosing not established

Hepatic Impairment:

- Mild or moderate impairment: Adjustment not required
- Severe impairment (Child-Pugh class C): Specific guidelines not available

Administration

Oral: Should be taken with meals.

Stability

Storage: Store at controlled room temperature of 25°C (77°F). Protect from light and moisture.

Monitoring and Teaching Issues

Physical Assessment: Assess for previous allergy history prior to therapy. See Contraindications, Warnings/Precautions, and Dosing for use cautions. Assess potential for interactions with other prescriptions, OTC medications, and herbal products patient may be taking (see Drug Interactions). Assess therapeutic response and adverse reactions (see Adverse Reactions and Overdose/Toxicology). Teach patient proper use, possible side effects and interventions, and adverse symptoms to report (see Patient Education). Note breast-feeding caution.

Patient Education: Inform prescriber of all prescriptions, OTC medications, or herbal products you are taking, and any allergies you have. Do not take anything new during treatment without consulting prescriber. Take as directed, at regular intervals

(Continued)

Cefditoren *(Continued)*

around-the-clock, with food. Maintain adequate hydration (2-3 L/day of fluids unless instructed to restrict fluid intake). Complete full course of medication, even if you feel better. If diabetic, monitor glucose levels closely; may cause false test results with Clinitest® urine glucose monitoring; use of another type of glucose monitoring is preferable. May cause diarrhea (yogurt, buttermilk, or boiled milk may help); or nausea or vomiting (small, frequent meals, frequent mouth care, sucking lozenges, or chewing gum may help). Report severe, unresolved diarrhea; opportunistic infection (vaginal itching or drainage, sores in mouth, or unusual fever or chills); unusual bleeding or bruising; change in urinary pattern; or rash. **Breast-feeding precaution:** Consult prescriber if breast-feeding.

Dietary Issues: Cefditoren should be taken with meals. Plasma carnitine levels are decreased during therapy (39% with 200 mg dosing, 63% with 400 mg dosing); normal concentrations return within 7-10 days after treatment is discontinued.

Cefditoren Pivoxil *see* Cefditoren *on page 236*

Cefepime (SEF e pim)

U.S. Brand Names Maxipime®

Synonyms Cefepime Hydrochloride

Generic Available No

Pharmacologic Category Antibiotic, Cephalosporin (Fourth Generation)

Pregnancy Risk Factor B

Lactation Enters breast milk/use caution

Use Treatment of uncomplicated and complicated urinary tract infections, including pyelonephritis caused by typical urinary tract pathogens; monotherapy for febrile neutropenia; uncomplicated skin and skin structure infections caused by *Streptococcus pyogenes*; moderate to severe pneumonia caused by pneumococcus, *Pseudomonas aeruginosa*, and other gram-negative organisms; complicated intra-abdominal infections (in combination with metronidazole). Also active against methicillin-susceptible staphylococci, *Enterobacter* sp, and many other gram-negative bacilli.

Children 2 months to 16 years: Empiric therapy of febrile neutropenia patients, uncomplicated skin/soft tissue infections, pneumonia, and uncomplicated/complicated urinary tract infections.

Mechanism of Action/Effect Inhibits bacterial cell wall synthesis by binding to one or more of the penicillin-binding proteins (PBPs)

Contraindications Hypersensitivity to cefepime, any component of the formulation, or other cephalosporins

Warnings/Precautions Modify dosage in patients with severe renal impairment. Prolonged use may result in superinfection. Cross-sensitivity to penicillins exists (~10%). Use in patients less than 2 months of age has not been established.

Drug Interactions

Increased Effect/Toxicity: High-dose probenecid decreases clearance and increases effect of cefepime. Aminoglycosides increase nephrotoxic potential when taken with cefepime.

Effects on Lab Values Positive direct Coombs', false-positive urinary glucose test using cupric sulfate (Benedict's solution, Clinitest®, Fehling's solution), false-positive serum or urine creatinine with Jaffé reaction

Adverse Reactions

>10%: Hematologic: Positive Coombs' test without hemolysis

1% to 10%:

- Dermatologic: Rash, pruritus
- Gastrointestinal: : Diarrhea, nausea, vomiting
- Central nervous system: Fever (1%), headache (1%)
- Local: Pain, erythema at injection site

<1% (Limited to important or life-threatening): Agranulocytosis, anaphylactic shock, anaphylaxis, coma, encephalopathy, hallucinations, leukopenia, myoclonus, neuromuscular excitability, neutropenia, seizures, thrombocytopenia

Other reactions with cephalosporins include aplastic anemia, erythema multiforme, hemolytic anemia, hemorrhage, pancytopenia, prolonged PT, renal dysfunction, Stevens-Johnson syndrome, superinfection, toxic epidermal necrolysis, toxic nephropathy, vaginitis

Overdosage/Toxicology Symptoms of overdose include neuromuscular hypersensitivity and CNS toxicity (including hallucinations, confusion, seizures, and coma). Many beta-lactam containing antibiotics have the potential to cause neuromuscular hyperirritability or convulsive seizures. Hemodialysis may be helpful to aid in removal of the drug from blood; otherwise, treatment is supportive and symptom-directed.

Pharmacodynamics/Kinetics

Absorption: I.M.: Rapid and complete

Half-Life Elimination: 2 hours

Time to Peak: 0.5-1.5 hours

Metabolism: Minimally hepatic

Formulations

Infusion, as hydrochloride (ADD-Vantage®): 1 g, 2 g

Infusion, piggyback, as hydrochloride: 1 g (100 mL); 2 g (100 mL)

Injection, powder for reconstitution, as hydrochloride: 500 mg, 1 g, 2 g

Dosing

Adults:

Most infections: I.V., I.M., 1-2 g every 12 hours for 5-10 days; higher doses or more frequent administration may be required in pseudomonal infections

Urinary tract infections, uncomplicated: I.V., I.M.: 500 mg every 12 hours

Febrile neutropenia: 2 g every 8 hours for 7 days or until neutropenia resolves

Elderly: I.V., I.M.: Should be based on renal function and severity of infection.

Pediatrics:

Febrile neutropenia: I.V.: Children >2 months of age: 50 mg/kg every 8 hours for 7-10 days

Uncomplicated skin/soft tissue infections, pneumonia, and complicated/uncomplicated UTI: I.V.: Children >2 months of age: 50 mg/kg twice daily

Renal Impairment:

Adjustment of recommended maintenance schedule is required:

Normal dosing schedule: 500 mg every 12 hours
- Cl_{cr} 30-60 mL/minute: 500 mg every 24 hours
- Cl_{cr} 11-29 mL/minute: 500 mg every 24 hours
- Cl_{cr} <11 mL/minute: 250 mg every 24 hours

Normal dosing schedule: 1 g every 12 hours
- Cl_{cr} 30-60 mL/minute: 1 g every 24 hours
- Cl_{cr} 11-29 mL/minute: 500 mg every 24 hours
- Cl_{cr} <11 mL/minute: 250 mg every 24 hours

Normal dosing schedule: 2 g every 12 hours
- Cl_{cr} 30-60 mL/minute: 2 g every 24 hours
- Cl_{cr} 11-29 mL/minute: 1 g every 24 hours
- Cl_{cr} <11 mL/minute: 500 mg every 24 hours

Normal dosing schedule: 2 g every 8 hours
- Cl_{cr} 30-60 mL/minute: 2 g every 12 hours
- Cl_{cr} 11-29 mL/minute: 2 g every 24 hours
- Cl_{cr} <11 mL/minute: 1 g every 24 hours

Hemodialysis effects: Removed by dialysis; administer supplemental dose of 250 mg after each dialysis session.

Peritoneal dialysis effects: Removed to a lesser extent than hemodialysis; administer 250 mg every 48 hours.

Continuous arteriovenous hemofiltration: Dose as for Cl_{cr} >30 mL/minute.

Administration

I.M.: Inject deep I.M. into large muscle mass.

I.V.: Inject direct I.V. over 5 minutes. Infuse intermittent infusion over 30-60 minutes.

Stability

Compatibility: Stable in D_5LR, D_5NS, D_5W, $D_{10}W$, NS, bacteriostatic water, sterile water for injection

Y-site administration: Incompatible with acyclovir, amphotericin B, amphotericin B cholesteryl sulfate complex, chlordiazepoxide, chlorpromazine, cimetidine, ciprofloxacin, cisplatin, dacarbazine, daunorubicin, diazepam, diphenhydramine, dobutamine, dopamine, doxorubicin, droperidol, enalaprilat, etoposide, etoposide phosphate, famotidine, filgrastim, floxuridine, ganciclovir, haloperidol, hydroxyzine, idarubicin, ifosfamide, magnesium sulfate, mannitol, mechlorethamine, meperidine, metoclopramide, mitomycin, mitoxantrone, morphine, nalbuphine, ofloxacin, ondansetron, plicamycin, prochlorperazine edisylate, promethazine, streptozocin, vancomycin, vinblastine, vincristine

Compatibility when admixed: Incompatible with aminophylline, gentamicin, netilmicin, tobramycin

Monitoring Laboratory Tests Prothrombin times; perform culture and sensitivity studies prior to initiating drug therapy.

Monitoring and Teaching Issues

Physical Assessment: Assess for previous allergy history prior to therapy. See Contraindications and Warnings/Precautions for use cautions. Assess potential for interactions with other prescriptions, OTC medications, or herbal products patient may be taking (eg, nephrotoxicity - see Drug Interactions). Assess results of laboratory tests (see above), therapeutic response and adverse reactions (eg, hypersensitivity can occur several days after therapy is started - see Adverse Reactions and Overdose/Toxicology). Instruct diabetic patients regarding Clinitest®. Teach patient possible side effects and interventions, and adverse symptoms to report (eg, nephrotoxicity, opportunistic infection - see Patient Education). Note breast-feeding caution.

Patient Education: Inform prescriber of all prescriptions, OTC medications, or herbal products you are taking, and any allergies you have. Do not take anything new during treatment unless approved by prescriber. This medication is administered by infusion or injection. Report immediately any redness, swelling, burning, or pain at injection/infusion site; itching or hives; difficulty swallowing or breathing. Maintain adequate hydration (2-3 L/day of fluids) unless advised by prescriber to restrict fluids. May cause false test results with Clinitest®; use of another type of glucose testing is preferable. May cause diarrhea (yogurt, boiled milk, or buttermilk may help); nausea, and vomiting (small, frequent meals, frequent mouth care, chewing gum, or sucking lozenges may help). Report unresolved diarrhea; opportunistic infection (vaginal itching or drainage; sores in mouth; blood in stool or urine; unusual fever or chills); or difficulty breathing. **Breast-feeding precaution:** Consult prescriber if breast-feeding.

Geriatric Considerations: Adjust dose for changes in renal function.

Breast-feeding Issues: Theoretically, drug absorbed by nursing infant may change bowel flora or affect fever work-up result. **Note:** As a class, cephalosporins are used to treat infections in infants.

Cefepime Hydrochloride *see* Cefepime *on page 238*

Cefixime (sef IKS eem)

U.S. Brand Names Suprax®

Generic Available No

Pharmacologic Category Antibiotic, Cephalosporin (Third Generation)

Pregnancy Risk Factor B

Lactation Excretion in breast milk unknown/use caution

(Continued)

Cefixime *(Continued)*

Use Treatment of urinary tract infections, otitis media, respiratory infections due to susceptible organisms including *S. pneumoniae* and *S. pyogenes*, *H. influenzae* and many Enterobacteriaceae; documented poor compliance with other oral antimicrobials; outpatient therapy of serious soft tissue or skeletal infections due to susceptible organisms; single-dose oral treatment of uncomplicated cervical/urethral gonorrhea due to *N. gonorrhoeae*

Mechanism of Action/Effect Inhibits bacterial cell wall synthesis by binding to one or more of the penicillin-binding proteins (PBPs)

Contraindications Hypersensitivity to cefixime, any component of the formulation, or other cephalosporins

Warnings/Precautions Modify dosage in patients with severe renal impairment. Prolonged use may result in superinfection. Cross-sensitivity to penicillins exists (~10%).

Drug Interactions

Increased Effect/Toxicity: Probenecid increases cefixime concentration. Cefixime may increase carbamazepine.

Nutritional/Ethanol Interactions Food: Delays cefixime absorption.

Effects on Lab Values Positive direct Coombs', false-positive urinary glucose test using cupric sulfate (Benedict's solution, Clinitest®, Fehling's solution), false-positive serum or urine creatinine with Jaffé reaction

Adverse Reactions

>10%: Gastrointestinal: Diarrhea (16%)

1% to 10%: Gastrointestinal: Abdominal pain, nausea, dyspepsia, flatulence

<1% (Limited to important or life-threatening): BUN increased, candidiasis, creatinine increased, dizziness, eosinophilia, erythema multiforme, fever, headache, leukopenia, prolonged PT, pruritus, pseudomembranous colitis, rash, serum sickness-like reaction, Stevens-Johnson syndrome, thrombocytopenia, transaminases increased, urticaria, vaginitis, vomiting

Other reactions with cephalosporins include agranulocytosis, anaphylaxis, aplastic anemia, cholestasis, colitis, hemolytic anemia, hemorrhage, interstitial nephritis, neutropenia, pancytopenia, renal dysfunction, seizures, superinfection, toxic epidermal necrolysis, toxic nephropathy

Overdosage/Toxicology Symptoms of overdose include neuromuscular hypersensitivity and convulsions. Many beta-lactam containing antibiotics have the potential to cause neuromuscular hyperirritability or convulsive seizures. Hemodialysis may be helpful to aid in the removal of drug from blood; otherwise, treatment is supportive or symptom-directed.

Pharmacodynamics/Kinetics

Absorption: 40% to 50%

Half-Life Elimination: Normal renal function: 3-4 hours; Renal failure: Up to 11.5 hours

Time to Peak: Serum: 2-6 hours (15% to 50% higher for oral suspension vs tablets); delayed with food

Formulations

Powder for oral suspension: 100 mg/5 mL (50 mL, 100 mL) [strawberry flavor]

Tablet, film coated: 200 mg, 400 mg

Dosing

Adults & Elderly:

Most susceptible infections: Oral: 400 mg/day divided every 12-24 hours

Uncomplicated cervical/urethral gonorrhea due to *N. gonorrhoeae*: Oral: 400 mg as a single dose

Note: For *S. pyogenes* infections, treat for 10 days; use suspension for otitis media due to increased peak serum levels as compared to tablet form.

Pediatrics: Susceptible infections: Oral:

Children: 8 mg/kg/day divided every 12-24 hours

Adolescents: Refer to adult dosing.

Note: For *S. pyogenes* infections, treat for 10 days; use suspension for otitis media due to increased peak serum levels as compared to tablet form.

Renal Impairment:

Cl_{cr} 21-60 mL/minute: Administer 75% of the standard dose.

Cl_{cr} <20 mL/minute: Administer 50% of the standard dose.

10% removed by hemodialysis

Administration

Oral: Oral: Shake well or oral suspension before use. May be administered with or without food. Administer with food to decrease GI distress.

Stability

Reconstitution: After reconstitution, suspension may be stored for 14 days at room temperature.

Monitoring Laboratory Tests Prothrombin times; perform culture and sensitivity studies prior to initiating drug therapy.

Monitoring and Teaching Issues

Physical Assessment: Assess for previous allergy history prior to therapy. See Contraindications and Warnings/Precautions for use cautions. Assess potential for interactions with other prescriptions, OTC medications, or herbal products patient may be taking (eg, nephrotoxicity - see Drug Interactions). Assess results of laboratory tests (see above), therapeutic response, and adverse reactions (eg, hypersensitivity can occur several days after therapy is started - see Adverse Reactions and Overdose/Toxicology). Instruct diabetic patients regarding Clinitest®. Teach patient proper use, possible side effects and interventions, and adverse symptoms to report (eg, nephrotoxicity, opportunistic infection - see Patient Education). Note breast-feeding caution.

Patient Education: Inform prescriber of all prescriptions, OTC medications, or herbal products you are taking, and any allergies you have. Do not take anything new during treatment unless approved by prescriber. Take as directed, at regular intervals around-the-clock (with or without food). Chilling oral suspension improves flavor (do not freeze). Do not chew or crush extended release tablets. Maintain adequate hydration (2-3

L/day of fluids) unless advised by prescriber to restrict fluids. Complete full course of medication, even if you feel better. May cause false test results with Clinitest®; use of another type of glucose testing is preferable. May cause nausea or vomiting (small, frequent meals, frequent mouth care, sucking lozenges, or chewing gum may help); or diarrhea (yogurt, boiled milk, or buttermilk may help). Report changes in urinary pattern; unresolved diarrhea; opportunistic infection (eg, vaginal itching or drainage, sores in mouth, blood in stool or urine, unusual fever or chills); or difficulty breathing. **Breast-feeding precaution:** Consult prescriber if breast-feeding.

Dietary Issues: May be taken with food.

Geriatric Considerations: Adjust dose for renal function.

Breast-feeding Issues: Theoretically, drug absorbed by nursing infant may change bowel flora or affect fever work-up result. **Note:** As a class, cephalosporins are used to treat infections in infants.

Other Issues: Otitis media should be treated with the suspension since it results in higher peak blood levels than the tablet.

Additional Information Otitis media should be treated with the suspension since it results in higher peak blood levels than the tablet.

Cefizox® *see* Ceftizoxime *on page 252*

Cefobid® *see* Cefoperazone *on page 241*

Cefoperazone (sef oh PER a zone)

U.S. Brand Names Cefobid®

Synonyms Cefoperazone Sodium

Generic Available No

Pharmacologic Category Antibiotic, Cephalosporin (Third Generation)

Pregnancy Risk Factor B

Lactation Enters breast milk (small amounts)/use caution

Use Treatment of susceptible bacterial infection; mainly respiratory tract, skin and skin structure, bone and joint, urinary tract and gynecologic as well as septicemia. Active against a variety of gram-negative bacilli, some gram-positive cocci, and has some activity against *Pseudomonas aeruginosa.*

Mechanism of Action/Effect Inhibits bacterial cell wall synthesis by binding to one or more of the penicillin-binding proteins (PBPs)

Contraindications Hypersensitivity to cefoperazone, any component of the formulation, or other cephalosporins

Warnings/Precautions Cefoperazone may decrease vitamin K synthesis by suppressing GI flora. Monitor prothrombin time and administer vitamin K as needed. Only reported rarely, especially with cefoperazone and cefamandole. Modify dosage in patients with severe renal impairment. Prolonged use may result in superinfection. Cross-sensitivity to penicillins exists (~10%).

Drug Interactions

Increased Effect/Toxicity: Probenecid may decrease cephalosporin elimination resulting in increased levels. Furosemide, aminoglycosides in combination with cefoperazone may result in additive nephrotoxicity.

Nutritional/Ethanol Interactions

Ethanol: Avoid ethanol (may cause a disulfiram-like reaction).

Food: Cefoperazone may decrease vitamin K synthesis by suppressing GI flora; vitamin K deficiency may occur and result in an increased risk of hemorrhage; patients at risk include those with malabsorption states (eg, cystic fibrosis) or poor nutritional status.

Effects on Lab Values Positive direct Coombs', false-positive urinary glucose test using cupric sulfate (Benedict's solution, Clinitest®, Fehling's solution), false-positive serum or urine creatinine with Jaffé reaction

Adverse Reactions Contains MTT side chain which may lead to increased risk of hypoprothrombinemia and bleeding.

1% to 10%:

Dermatologic: Rash (maculopapular or erythematous) (2%)

Gastrointestinal: Diarrhea (3%)

Hematologic: Decreased neutrophils (2%), decreased hemoglobin or hematocrit (5%), eosinophilia (10%)

Hepatic: Increased transaminases (5% to 10%)

<1% (Limited to important or life-threatening): Bleeding, BUN increased, creatinine increased, drug fever, hypoprothrombinemia, induration at injection site, nausea, pain at injection site, phlebitis, pseudomembranous colitis, vomiting

Other reactions with cephalosporins include agranulocytosis, anaphylaxis, aplastic anemia, cholestasis, colitis, hemolytic anemia, pancytopenia, renal dysfunction, seizures, Stevens-Johnson syndrome, superinfection, toxic epidermal necrolysis, toxic nephropathy

Overdosage/Toxicology Symptoms of overdose include neuromuscular hypersensitivity and convulsions. Many beta-lactam containing antibiotics have the potential to cause neuromuscular hyperirritability or convulsive seizures. Hemodialysis may be helpful to aid in removal of the drug from blood; otherwise, treatment is supportive or symptom-directed.

Pharmacodynamics/Kinetics

Half-Life Elimination: 2 hours; prolonged with hepatic disease or biliary obstruction

Time to Peak: Serum: I.M.: 1-2 hours

Formulations

Injection, as sodium [premixed, frozen]: 1 g (50 mL); 2 g (50 mL)

Injection, powder for reconstitution, as sodium: 1 g, 2 g

Dosing

Adults & Elderly: Susceptible infections: I.M., I.V.: 2-4 g/day in divided doses every 12 hours; up to 12 g/day

Pediatrics: Susceptible infections: I.M., I.V.: Children (not approved): 100-150 mg/kg/day divided every 8-12 hours; up to 12 g/day

(Continued)

Cefoperazone *(Continued)*

Renal Impairment: Dosage adjustment is not necessary.

Hepatic Impairment: Reduce dose 50% in patients with advanced liver cirrhosis; maximum daily dose: 4 g.

Administration

I.M.: Inject deep I.M. into large muscle mass.

I.V.: Inject direct I.V. over 3-5 minutes. Infuse intermittent infusion over 30 minutes.

Stability

Reconstitution: Reconstituted solution and I.V. infusion in NS or D_5W solution are stable for 24 hours at room temperature, 5 days when refrigerated or 3 weeks, when frozen. After freezing, thawed solution is stable for 48 hours at room temperature or 10 days when refrigerated.

Compatibility: Stable in bacteriostatic water for injection, D_5LR, $D_5{}^1/_4NS$, D_5NS, D_5W, $D_{10}W$, LR, NS, sterile water for injection

Y-site administration: Incompatible with amifostine, amphotericin B cholesteryl sulfate complex, cisatracurium, doxorubicin liposome, filgrastim, gatifloxacin, gemcitabine, hetastarch, labetalol, meperidine, ondansetron, pentamidine, perphenazine, promethazine, sargramostim, vinorelbine

Compatibility in syringe: Incompatible with doxapram

Compatibility when admixed: Incompatible with aminoglycosides

Monitoring Laboratory Tests Prothrombin times; perform culture and sensitivity studies prior to initiating drug therapy.

Monitoring and Teaching Issues

Physical Assessment: Assess for previous allergy history prior to therapy. See Contraindications and Warnings/Precautions for use cautions. Assess potential for interactions with other prescriptions, OTC medications, or herbal products patient may be taking (eg, nephrotoxicity - see Drug Interactions and Overdose/Toxicology). Assess results of laboratory tests (eg, hypoprothrombinemia - see above), therapeutic response, and adverse reactions (eg, hypersensitivity can occur several days after therapy is started - see Adverse Reactions). Instruct diabetic patients regarding Clinitest®. Teach patient possible side effects and interventions and adverse symptoms to report (eg, nephrotoxicity, opportunistic infection - see Patient Education). Note breast-feeding caution.

Patient Education: Inform prescriber of all prescriptions, OTC medications, or herbal products you are taking, and any allergies you have. Do not take anything new during treatment unless approved by prescriber. This medication is administered by injection or infusion. Report immediately any redness, swelling, pain, or burning at injection/infusion site; itching or hives; difficulty swallowing or breathing. Maintain adequate hydration (2-3 L/day of fluids) unless advised by prescriber to restrict fluids. Avoid alcohol during therapy and for 72 hours after last dose (may cause severe disulfiram-like reactions). May cause false test results with Clinitest®; use of another type of glucose testing is preferable. May cause diarrhea (yogurt, boiled milk, or buttermilk may help); or nausea, vomiting, flatulence (small, frequent meals, frequent mouth care, chewing gum, or sucking lozenges may help). Report severe, unresolved diarrhea; opportunistic infection (eg, vaginal itching or drainage, sores in mouth, blood in stool or urine, unusual fever or chills); rash; or difficulty breathing. **Breast-feeding precaution:** Consult prescriber if breast-feeding.

Dietary Issues: May block activity of vitamin K. Monitor prothrombin time and administer vitamin K as needed. Sodium content of 1 g: 34.5 mg (1.5 mEq).

Geriatric Considerations: No dose adjustment necessary for renal impairment.

Breast-feeding Issues: Theoretically, drug absorbed by nursing infant may change bowel flora or affect fever work-up result. **Note:** As a class, cephalosporins are used to treat infections in infants.

Additional Information Contains the *N*-methylthiotetrazole (NMTT) side chain

Cefoperazone Sodium *see* Cefoperazone *on page 241*

Cefotan® *see* Cefotetan *on page 244*

Cefotaxime (sef oh TAKS eem)

U.S. Brand Names Claforan®

Synonyms Cefotaxime Sodium

Generic Available Yes

Pharmacologic Category Antibiotic, Cephalosporin (Third Generation)

Pregnancy Risk Factor B

Lactation Enters breast milk/use caution (AAP rates "compatible")

Use Treatment of susceptible infection in respiratory tract, skin and skin structure, bone and joint, urinary tract, gynecologic as well as septicemia, and documented or suspected meningitis. Active against most gram-negative bacilli (not *Pseudomonas*) and gram-positive cocci (not enterococcus). Active against many penicillin-resistant pneumococci.

Mechanism of Action/Effect Inhibits bacterial cell wall synthesis by binding to one or more of the penicillin-binding proteins (PBPs)

Contraindications Hypersensitivity to cefotaxime, any component of the formulation, or other cephalosporins

Warnings/Precautions Modify dosage in patients with severe renal impairment; prolonged use may result in superinfection. A potentially life-threatening arrhythmia has been reported in patients who received a rapid bolus injection via central line. Use caution in patients with colitis. Cross-sensitivity to penicillins exists (~10%).

Drug Interactions

Increased Effect/Toxicity: Probenecid may decrease cephalosporin elimination resulting in increased levels. Furosemide, aminoglycosides in combination with cefotaxime may result in additive nephrotoxicity.

Effects on Lab Values Positive direct Coombs', false-positive urinary glucose test using cupric sulfate (Benedict's solution, Clinitest®, Fehling's solution), false-positive serum or urine creatinine with Jaffé reaction

Adverse Reactions

1% to 10%:

Dermatologic: Rash, pruritus

Gastrointestinal: Diarrhea, nausea, vomiting, colitis

Local: Pain at injection site

<1% (Limited to important or life-threatening): Anaphylaxis, arrhythmias (after rapid I.V. injection via central catheter), BUN increased, candidiasis, creatinine increased, eosinophilia, erythema multiforme, fever, headache, interstitial nephritis, neutropenia, phlebitis, pseudomembranous colitis, Stevens-Johnson syndrome, thrombocytopenia, transaminases increased, toxic epidermal necrolysis, urticaria, vaginitis

Reactions reported with other cephalosporins include agranulocytosis, aplastic anemia, cholestasis, hemolytic anemia, hemorrhage, pancytopenia, renal dysfunction, seizures, superinfection, toxic nephropathy.

Overdosage/Toxicology Symptoms of overdose include neuromuscular hypersensitivity and convulsions. Many beta-lactam containing antibiotics have the potential to cause neuromuscular hyperirritability or convulsive seizures. Hemodialysis may be helpful to aid in removal of the drug from blood; otherwise, treatment is supportive or symptom-directed.

Pharmacodynamics/Kinetics

Half-Life Elimination:

Cefotaxime: Premature neonates <1 week: 5-6 hours; Full-term neonates <1 week: 2-3.4 hours; Adults: 1-1.5 hours, prolonged with renal and/or hepatic impairment

Desacetylcefotaxime: 1.5-1.9 hours; prolonged with renal impairment

Time to Peak: Serum: I.M.: Within 30 minutes

Metabolism: Partially hepatic to active metabolite, desacetylcefotaxime

Formulations

Infusion, as sodium [premixed in D_5W, frozen]: 1 g (50 mL); 2 g (50 mL)

Injection, powder for reconstitution, as sodium: 500 mg, 1 g, 2 g, 10 g

Dosing

Adults & Elderly:

Gonorrhea: I.M.: 1 g as a single dose

Uncomplicated infections: I.M., I.V.: 1 g every 12 hours

Moderate/severe infections: I.M., I.V.: 1-2 g every 8 hours

Infections commonly needing higher doses (eg, septicemia): I.V.: 2 g every 6-8 hours

Life-threatening infections: I.V.: 2 g every 4 hours

Preop: I.M., I.V.: 1 g 30-90 minutes before surgery

C-section: 1 g as soon as the umbilical cord is clamped, then 1 g I.M., I.V. at 6- and 12-hours intervals.

Pediatrics:

Most infections: I.M., I.V.: Infants and Children 1 month to 12 years: <50 kg: 50-180 mg/kg/day in divided doses every 4-6 hours

Meningitis: 200 mg/kg/day in divided doses every 6 hours

Children >12 years: Refer to adult dosing.

Renal Impairment:

Cl_{cr} 10-50 mL/minute: Administer every 8-12 hours.

Cl_{cr} <10 mL/minute: Administer every 24 hours.

Moderately dialyzable (20% to 50%)

Continuous arteriovenous hemofiltration: 1 g every 12 hours.

Hepatic Impairment: Moderate dosage reduction is recommended in severe liver disease.

Administration

I.M.: Inject deep I.M. into large muscle mass.

I.V.: Inject direct I.V. over 3-5 minutes. Infuse intermittent infusion over 30 minutes.

Stability

Reconstitution: Reconstituted solution is stable for 12-24 hours at room temperature and 7-10 days when refrigerated and for 13 weeks when frozen; for I.V. infusion in NS or D_5W, solution is stable for 24 hours at room temperature, 5 days when refrigerated, or 13 weeks when frozen in Viaflex® plastic containers; thawed solutions previously of frozen premixed bags are stable for 24 hours at room temperature or 10 days when refrigerated.

Compatibility: Stable in $D_5{}^1/_4NS$, $D_5{}^1/_2NS$, D_5NS, D_5W, $D_{10}W$, LR, NS

Y-site administration: Incompatible with allopurinol, filgrastim, fluconazole, gemcitabine, hetastarch, pentamidine

Compatibility in syringe: Incompatible with doxapram

Compatibility when admixed: Incompatible with aminoglycosides, aminophylline, sodium bicarbonate

Monitoring Laboratory Tests Prothrombin times; perform culture and sensitivity studies prior to initiating drug therapy; CBC with differential (especially with long courses)

Monitoring and Teaching Issues

Physical Assessment: Assess for previous allergy history prior to therapy. See Contraindications and Warnings/Precautions for use cautions (eg, arrhythmia, colitis). Assess potential for interactions with other prescriptions, OTC medications, or herbal products patient may be taking (eg, nephrotoxicity - see Drug Interactions). Assess results of laboratory tests (eg, hypoprothrombinemia - see above and Overdose/Toxicology), therapeutic response, and adverse reactions (eg, hypersensitivity can occur several days after therapy is started - see Adverse Reactions). Instruct diabetic patients regarding Clinitest®. Teach patient possible side effects and interventions and adverse symptoms to report (eg, nephrotoxicity, opportunistic infection - see Patient Education). Note breast-feeding caution.

Patient Education: Inform prescriber of all prescriptions, OTC medications, or herbal products you are taking, and any allergies you have. Do not take anything new during treatment unless approved by prescriber. This medication is administered by injection or infusion. Report immediately any redness, swelling, burning, or pain at injection/infusion site; chest pain, palpitations, difficulty breathing or swallowing; or itching or hives. Maintain adequate hydration (2-3 L/day of fluids) unless advised by prescriber to restrict fluids. May cause false test results with Clinitest®; use of another type of glucose testing is preferable.

(Continued)

Cefotaxime *(Continued)*

May cause diarrhea (yogurt, boiled milk, or buttermilk may help); GI distress or nausea (small, frequent meals, frequent oral care, chewing gum, or sucking lozenges may help). Report unresolved diarrhea; opportunistic infection (vaginal itching or drainage; sores in mouth; blood in stool or urine; easy bleeding or bruising, unusual fever or chills); or difficulty breathing. **Breast-feeding precaution:** Consult prescriber if breast-feeding.

Dietary Issues: Sodium content of 1 g: 50.6 mg (2.2 mEq)

Geriatric Considerations: Adjust dose for renal function.

Breast-feeding Issues: Theoretically, drug absorbed by nursing infant may change bowel flora or affect fever work-up result. **Note:** As a class, cephalosporins are used to treat infections in infants.

Cefotaxime Sodium *see* Cefotaxime *on page 242*

Cefotetan (SEF oh tee tan)

U.S. Brand Names Cefotan®

Synonyms Cefotetan Disodium

Generic Available Yes

Pharmacologic Category Antibiotic, Cephalosporin (Second Generation)

Pregnancy Risk Factor B

Lactation Enters breast milk (small amounts)/use caution

Use Less active against staphylococci and streptococci than first generation cephalosporins, but active against anaerobes including *Bacteroides fragilis*; active against gram-negative enteric bacilli including *E. coli*, *Klebsiella*, and *Proteus*; used predominantly for respiratory tract, skin and skin structure, bone and joint, urinary tract and gynecologic as well as septicemia; surgical prophylaxis; intra-abdominal infections and other mixed infections

Mechanism of Action/Effect Inhibits bacterial cell wall synthesis by binding to one or more of the penicillin-binding proteins (PBPs)

Contraindications Hypersensitivity to cefotetan, any component of the formulation, or other cephalosporins

Warnings/Precautions Modify dosage in patients with severe renal impairment. Prolonged use may result in superinfection. Cross-sensitivity to penicillins exists (~10%).

Drug Interactions

Increased Effect/Toxicity: Probenecid may decrease cephalosporin elimination. Furosemide, aminoglycosides in combination with cefotetan may result in additive nephrotoxicity. May cause disulfiram-like reaction with concomitant ethanol use. Effects of warfarin may be enhanced by cefotetan (due to effects on gastrointestinal flora).

Nutritional/Ethanol Interactions Ethanol: Avoid ethanol (may cause a disulfiram-like reaction).

Effects on Lab Values Positive direct Coombs', false-positive urinary glucose test using cupric sulfate (Benedict's solution, Clinitest®, Fehling's solution), false-positive serum or urine creatinine with Jaffé reaction

Adverse Reactions Contains MTT side chain which may lead to increased risk of hypoprothrombinemia and bleeding.

1% to 10%:
- Gastrointestinal: Diarrhea (1.3%)
- Hepatic: Increased transaminases (1.2%)
- Miscellaneous: Hypersensitivity reactions (1.2%)

<1% (Limited to important or life-threatening): Agranulocytosis, anaphylaxis, bleeding, BUN increased, creatinine increased, eosinophilia, fever, hemolytic anemia, leukopenia, nausea, nephrotoxicity, phlebitis, prolonged PT, pruritus, pseudomembranous colitis, rash, thrombocytopenia, thrombocytosis, urticaria, vomiting

Other reactions with cephalosporins include agranulocytosis, aplastic anemia, cholestasis, colitis, hemolytic anemia, hemorrhage, pancytopenia, renal dysfunction, seizures, Stevens-Johnson syndrome, superinfection, toxic epidermal necrolysis, toxic nephropathy

Overdosage/Toxicology Symptoms of overdose include neuromuscular hypersensitivity and convulsions. Many beta-lactam containing antibiotics have the potential to cause neuromuscular hyperirritability or convulsive seizures. Hemodialysis may be helpful to aid in removal of the drug from blood; otherwise, treatment is supportive or symptom-directed.

Pharmacodynamics/Kinetics

Half-Life Elimination: 3-5 hours

Time to Peak: Serum: I.M.: 1.5-3 hours

Formulations

Infusion, as disodium [premixed, frozen]: 1 g (50 mL); 2 g (50 mL)

Injection, powder for reconstitution, as disodium: 1 g, 2 g, 10 g

Dosing

Adults & Elderly: Susceptible infections: I.M., I.V.: 1-6 g/day in divided doses every 12 hours; 1-2 g may be given every 24 hours for urinary tract infection

Pediatrics: Susceptible infections: I.M., I.V.: Children: 20-40 mg/kg/dose every 12 hours

Renal Impairment: I.M., I.V.:
- Cl_{cr} 10-30 mL/minute: Administer every 24 hours
- Cl_{cr} <10 mL/minute: Administer every 48 hours
- Hemodialysis: Slightly dialyzable (5% to 20%); administer 1/4 the usual dose every 24 hours on days between dialysis; administer 1/2 the usual dose on the day of dialysis.
- Continuous arteriovenous or venovenous hemodiafiltration effects: Administer 750 mg every 12 hours

Administration

I.M.: Inject deep I.M. into large muscle mass.

I.V.: Inject direct I.V. over 3-5 minutes. Infuse intermittent infusion over 30 minutes.

Stability

Reconstitution: Reconstituted solution is stable for 24 hours at room temperature and 96 hours when refrigerated. For I.V. infusion in NS or D_5W solution and after freezing, thawed solution is stable for 24 hours at room temperature or 96 hours when refrigerated. Frozen solution is stable for 12 weeks.

Compatibility: Stable in D_5W, NS

Y-site administration: Incompatible with promethazine, vinorelbine

Compatibility in syringe: Incompatible with doxapram, promethazine

Compatibility when admixed: Incompatible with gentamicin, heparin, tetracyclines

Monitoring Laboratory Tests Prothrombin time; perform culture and sensitivity studies prior to initiating drug therapy.

Monitoring and Teaching Issues

Physical Assessment: Assess for previous allergy history prior to therapy. See Contraindications and Warnings/Precautions for use cautions. Assess potential for interactions with other prescriptions, OTC medications, or herbal products patient may be taking (eg, nephrotoxicity - see Drug Interactions). Assess results of laboratory tests (eg, hypoprothrombinemia - see above), therapeutic response, and adverse reactions (eg, hypersensitivity can occur several days after therapy is started - see Adverse Reactions and Overdose/Toxicology). Instruct diabetic patients regarding Clinitest®. Teach patient possible side effects and interventions and adverse symptoms to report (eg, nephrotoxicity, opportunistic infection - see Patient Education). Note breast-feeding caution.

Patient Education: Inform prescriber of all prescriptions, OTC medications, or herbal products you are taking, and any allergies you have. Do not take anything new during treatment unless approved by prescriber. This medication is administered by injection or infusion. Report immediately any redness, swelling, burning, or pain at injection/infusion site, or immediately report any itching, hives, difficulty swallowing or difficulty breathing. Maintain adequate hydration (2-3 L/day of fluids) unless advised by prescriber to restrict fluids. Avoid alcohol during therapy and for 72 hours after last dose (may cause severe disulfiram-like reactions). May cause false test results with Clinitest®; use of another type of glucose testing is preferable. May cause diarrhea (yogurt, boiled milk, or buttermilk may help). Report severe, unresolved diarrhea; opportunistic infection (vaginal itching or drainage; sores in mouth; blood or mucus in stool or urine; easy bleeding or bruising, unusual fever or chills); rash; difficulty breathing. **Breast-feeding precaution:** Consult prescriber if breast-feeding.

Dietary Issues: Sodium content of 1 g: 34.5 mg (1.5 mEq)

Geriatric Considerations: Cefotetan has not been studied in the elderly. Adjust dose for renal function in the elderly.

Breast-feeding Issues: Theoretically, drug absorbed by nursing infant may change bowel flora or affect fever work-up result. **Note:** As a class, cephalosporins are used to treat infections in infants.

Cefotetan Disodium *see* Cefotetan *on page 244*

Cefoxitin (se FOKS i tin)

U.S. Brand Names Mefoxin®

Synonyms Cefoxitin Sodium

Generic Available No

Pharmacologic Category Antibiotic, Cephalosporin (Second Generation)

Pregnancy Risk Factor B

Lactation Enters breast milk (small amounts)/use caution (AAP rates "compatible")

Use Less active against staphylococci and streptococci than first generation cephalosporins, but active against anaerobes including *Bacteroides fragilis*; active against gram-negative enteric bacilli including *E. coli*, *Klebsiella*, and *Proteus*; used predominantly for respiratory tract, skin and skin structure, bone and joint, urinary tract and gynecologic as well as septicemia; surgical prophylaxis; intra-abdominal infections and other mixed infections; indicated for bacterial *Eikenella corrodens* infections

Mechanism of Action/Effect Inhibits bacterial cell wall synthesis by binding to one or more of the penicillin-binding proteins (PBPs)

Contraindications Hypersensitivity to cefoxitin, any component of the formulation, or other cephalosporins

Warnings/Precautions Use with caution in patients with history of colitis. Cefoxitin may increase resistance of organisms by inducing beta-lactamase. Modify dosage in patients with severe renal impairment. Prolonged use may result in superinfection. Cross-sensitivity to penicillins exists (~10%).

Drug Interactions

Increased Effect/Toxicity: Probenecid may decrease cephalosporin elimination. Furosemide, aminoglycosides in combination with cefoxitin may result in additive nephrotoxicity.

Effects on Lab Values Positive direct Coombs', false-positive urinary glucose test using cupric sulfate (Benedict's solution, Clinitest®, Fehling's solution), false-positive serum or urine creatinine with Jaffé reaction

Adverse Reactions

1% to 10%: Gastrointestinal: Diarrhea

<1% (Limited to important or life-threatening): Anaphylaxis, angioedema, bone marrow suppression, BUN increased, creatinine increased, dyspnea, eosinophilia, exacerbation of myasthenia gravis, exfoliative dermatitis, fever, hemolytic anemia, hypotension, interstitial nephritis, jaundice, leukopenia, nausea, nephrotoxicity (with aminoglycosides), phlebitis, prolonged PT, pruritus, pseudomembranous colitis, rash, thrombocytopenia, thrombophlebitis, toxic epidermal necrolysis, transaminases increased, vomiting

Other reactions with cephalosporins include agranulocytosis, aplastic anemia, cholestasis, colitis, erythema multiforme, hemolytic anemia, hemorrhage, pancytopenia, renal dysfunction, seizures, serum-sickness reactions, Stevens-Johnson syndrome, superinfection, toxic epidermal necrolysis, toxic nephropathy, urticaria, vaginitis

Overdosage/Toxicology Symptoms of overdose include neuromuscular hypersensitivity and convulsions. Many beta-lactam containing antibiotics have the potential to cause neuromuscular hyperirritability or convulsive seizures. Hemodialysis may be helpful to aid in removal of the drug from blood; otherwise, treatment is supportive or symptom-directed.

(Continued)

Cefoxitin *(Continued)*

Pharmacodynamics/Kinetics

Half-Life Elimination: 45-60 minutes; significantly prolonged with renal impairment

Time to Peak: Serum: I.M.: 20-30 minutes

Formulations

Infusion, as sodium [premixed in D_5W, frozen]: 1 g (50 mL); 2 g (50 mL)

Injection, powder for reconstitution, as sodium: 1 g, 2 g, 10 g

Dosing

Adults: Susceptible infections: I.M., I.V.: 1-2 g every 6-8 hours (I.M. injection is painful); up to 12 g/day

Elderly: I.M., I.V.: Usual adult dose adjusted for estimated Cl_{cr}.

Pediatrics: Susceptible infections: I.M., I.V.: Infants >3 months and Children:

Mild to moderate infection: 80-100 mg/kg/day in divided doses every 4-6 hours

Severe infection: 100-160 mg/kg/day in divided doses every 4-6 hours

Maximum dose: 12 g/day

Renal Impairment: I.M., I.V.:

Cl_{cr} 30-50 mL/minute: Administer 1-2 g every 8-12 hours

Cl_{cr} 10-29 mL/minute: Administer 1-2 g every 12-24 hours

Cl_{cr} 5-9 mL/minute: Administer 0.5-1 g every 12-24 hours

Cl_{cr} <5 mL/minute: Administer 0.5-1 g every 24-48 hours

Hemodialysis: Moderately dialyzable (20% to 50%); administer a loading dose of 1-2 g after each hemodialysis; maintenance dose as noted above based on Cl_{cr}

Continuous arteriovenous or venovenous hemodiafiltration effects: Dose as for Cl_{cr} 10-50 mL/minute

Administration

I.M.: Inject deep I.M. into large muscle mass.

I.V.: Inject direct I.V. over 3-5 minutes. Infuse intermittent infusion over 30 minutes.

Stability

Reconstitution: Reconstituted solution is stable for 24 hours at room temperature and 48 hours when refrigerated. I.V. infusion in NS or D_5W, solution is stable for 24 hours at room temperature, 1 week when refrigerated, or 26 weeks when frozen. After freezing, thawed solution is stable for 24 hours at room temperature or 5 days when refrigerated.

Compatibility: Stable in D_5LR, $D_5{}^1/_4NS$, $D_5{}^1/_2NS$, D_5NS, D_5W, $D_{10}W$, LR, NS, mannitol 10%, sodium bicarbonate 5%

Y-site administration: Incompatible with filgrastim, gatifloxacin, hetastarch, pentamidine

Compatibility when admixed: Incompatible with ranitidine

Monitoring Laboratory Tests Prothrombin times; perform culture and sensitivity studies prior to initiating drug therapy.

Monitoring and Teaching Issues

Physical Assessment: Assess for previous allergy history prior to therapy. See Contraindications and Warnings/Precautions for use cautions (eg, colitis). Assess potential for interactions with other prescriptions, OTC medications, or herbal products patient may be taking (eg, nephrotoxicity - see Drug Interactions). Assess results of laboratory tests (eg, hypoprothrombinemia - see above), therapeutic response, and adverse reactions (eg, hypersensitivity can occur several days after therapy is started - see Adverse Reactions and Overdose/Toxicology). Instruct diabetic patients regarding Clinitest®. Teach patient possible side effects and interventions and adverse symptoms to report (eg, nephrotoxicity, opportunistic infection - see Patient Education). Note breast-feeding caution.

Patient Education: Inform prescriber of all prescriptions, OTC medications, herbal products you are taking, and any allergies you have. Do not take anything new during treatment unless approved by prescriber. This medication is administered by injection or infusion. Report immediately any redness, swelling, burning, or pain at injection/infusion site; chest pain, palpitations, difficulty breathing or swallowing; itching or hives. Maintain adequate hydration (2-3 L/day of fluids) unless advised by prescriber to restrict fluids. May cause false test results with Clinitest®; use of another type of glucose testing is preferable. May cause diarrhea (yogurt, boiled milk, or buttermilk may help). Report unresolved diarrhea; opportunistic infection (vaginal itching or drainage, sores in mouth, blood in urine or stool, easy bleeding or bruising, unusual fever or chills); rash; or difficulty breathing. **Breast-feeding precaution:** Consult prescriber if breast-feeding.

Dietary Issues: Sodium content of 1 g: 53 mg (2.3 mEq)

Geriatric Considerations: Adjust dose for renal function in the elderly.

Breast-feeding Issues: Theoretically, drug absorbed by nursing infant may change bowel flora or affect fever work-up result. **Note:** As a class, cephalosporins are used to treat infections in infants.

Cefoxitin Sodium *see* Cefoxitin *on page 245*

Cefpodoxime (sef pode OKS eem)

U.S. Brand Names Vantin®

Synonyms Cefpodoxime Proxetil

Generic Available No

Pharmacologic Category Antibiotic, Cephalosporin (Third Generation)

Pregnancy Risk Factor B

Lactation Enters breast milk (small amounts)/use caution

Use Treatment of susceptible acute, community-acquired pneumonia caused by *S. pneumoniae* or nonbeta-lactamase producing *H. influenzae*; acute uncomplicated gonorrhea caused by *N. gonorrhoeae*; uncomplicated skin and skin structure infections caused by *S. aureus* or *S. pyogenes*; acute otitis media caused by *S. pneumoniae*, *H. influenzae*, or *M. catarrhalis*; pharyngitis or tonsillitis; and uncomplicated urinary tract infections caused by *E. coli*, *Klebsiella*, and *Proteus*

Mechanism of Action/Effect Inhibits bacterial cell wall synthesis by binding to one or more of the penicillin-binding proteins (PBPs)

Contraindications Hypersensitivity to cefpodoxime, any component of the formulation, or other cephalosporins

Warnings/Precautions Modify dosage in patients with severe renal impairment. Prolonged use may result in superinfection. Cross-sensitivity to penicillins exists (~10%).

Drug Interactions

Decreased Effect: Antacids and H_2-receptor antagonists reduce absorption and serum concentration of cefpodoxime.

Increased Effect/Toxicity: Probenecid may decrease cephalosporin elimination. Furosemide, aminoglycosides in combination with cefpodoxime may result in additive nephrotoxicity.

Nutritional/Ethanol Interactions Food: Food delays absorption; cefpodoxime serum levels may be increased if taken with food.

Effects on Lab Values Positive direct Coombs', false-positive urinary glucose test using cupric sulfate (Benedict's solution, Clinitest®, Fehling's solution), false-positive serum or urine creatinine with Jaffé reaction

Adverse Reactions

>10%:
- Dermatologic: Diaper rash (12.1%)
- Gastrointestinal: Diarrhea in infants and toddlers (15.4%)

1% to 10%:
- Central nervous system: Headache (1.1%)
- Dermatologic: Rash (1.4%)
- Gastrointestinal: Diarrhea (7.2%), nausea (3.8%), abdominal pain (1.6%), vomiting (1.1% to 2.1%)
- Genitourinary: Vaginal infections (3.1%)

<1% (Limited to important or life-threatening): Anaphylaxis, anxiety, appetite decreased, chest pain, cough, dizziness, epistaxis, eye itching, fatigue, fever, flatulence, flushing, fungal skin infection, hypotension, insomnia, malaise, nightmares, pruritus, pseudomembranous colitis, purpuric nephritis, salivation decreased, taste alteration, tinnitus, vaginal candidiasis, weakness

Other reactions with cephalosporins include agranulocytosis, aplastic anemia, cholestasis, colitis, erythema multiforme, hemolytic anemia, hemorrhage, interstitial nephritis, toxic nephropathy, pancytopenia, renal dysfunction, seizures, serum-sickness reactions, Stevens-Johnson syndrome, superinfection, toxic epidermal necrolysis, urticaria, vaginitis

Overdosage/Toxicology Symptoms of overdose include neuromuscular hypersensitivity and convulsions. Many beta-lactam containing antibiotics have the potential to cause neuromuscular hyperirritability or convulsive seizures. Hemodialysis may be helpful to aid in removal of the drug from blood; otherwise, treatment is supportive or symptom-directed.

Pharmacodynamics/Kinetics

Absorption: Rapid and well absorbed (50%), acid stable; enhanced in the presence of food or low gastric pH

Half-Life Elimination: 2.2 hours; prolonged with renal impairment

Time to Peak: Within 1 hour

Metabolism: De-esterified in GI tract to active metabolite, cefpodoxime

Formulations

Granules for oral suspension, as proxetil: 50 mg/5 mL (100 mL); 100 mg/5 mL (100 mL) [lemon creme flavor]

Tablet, film coated, as proxetil: 100 mg, 200 mg

Dosing

Adults & Elderly:

Acute community-acquired pneumonia and bacterial exacerbations of chronic bronchitis: Oral: 200 mg every 12 hours for 14 days and 10 days, respectively

Acute maxillary sinusitis: Oral: 200 mg every 12 hours for 10 days

Skin and skin structure: Oral: 400 mg every 12 hours for 7-14 days

Uncomplicated gonorrhea (male and female) and rectal gonococcal infections (female): Oral: 200 mg as a single dose

Pharyngitis/tonsillitis: Oral: 100 mg every 12 hours for 5-10 days

Uncomplicated urinary tract infection: Oral: 100 mg every 12 hours for 7 days

Pediatrics:

Acute otitis media: Oral: Children 2 months to 12 years: 10 mg/kg/day divided every 12 hours (400 mg/day) for 5 days (maximum: 200 mg/dose)

Acute maxillary sinusitis: Oral: Children:
- 2 months to 12 years: 10 mg/kg/day divided every 12 hours for 10 days (maximum: 200 mg/dose)
- ≥12 years: Refer to adult dosing.

Pharyngitis/tonsillitis: Oral: Children:
- 2 months to 12 years: 10 mg/kg/day in 2 divided doses for 5-10 days (maximum: 100 mg/dose)
- ≥12 years: Refer to adult dosing.

Renal Impairment:

Cl_{cr} <30 mL/minute: Administer every 24 hours.

Hemodialysis: Dose 3 times/week following dialysis.

Hepatic Impairment: Dose adjustment is not necessary in patients with cirrhosis.

Administration

Oral: Administer around-the-clock to promote less variation in peak and trough serum levels.

Stability

Reconstitution: After mixing, keep suspension in refrigerator, shake well before using. Discard unused portion after 14 days.

Monitoring Laboratory Tests Prothrombin times; perform culture and sensitivity studies prior to initiating drug therapy.

Monitoring and Teaching Issues

Physical Assessment: Assess for previous allergy history prior to therapy. See Contraindications and Warnings/Precautions for use cautions. Assess potential for interactions with

(Continued)

Cefpodoxime *(Continued)*

other prescriptions, OTC medications, or herbal products patient may be taking (eg, nephrotoxicity - see Drug Interactions). Assess results of laboratory tests (see above), therapeutic response, and adverse reactions (eg, hypersensitivity can occur several days after therapy is started - see Adverse Reactions and Overdose/Toxicology). Instruct diabetic patients regarding Clinitest®. Teach patient proper use, possible side effects and interventions, and adverse symptoms to report (eg, nephrotoxicity, opportunistic infection - see Patient Education). Note breast-feeding caution.

Patient Education: Inform prescriber of all prescriptions, OTC medications, or herbal products you are taking, and any allergies you have. Do not take anything new during treatment unless approved by prescriber. Take as directed, at regular intervals around-the-clock (with or without food). Chilling oral suspension improves flavor (do not freeze). Maintain adequate hydration (2-3 L/day of fluids) unless advised by prescriber to restrict fluids. Complete full course of medication, even if you feel better. May cause false test results with Clinitest®; use of another type of glucose testing is preferable. May cause nausea or vomiting (small, frequent meals, frequent mouth care, sucking lozenges, or chewing gum may help); or diarrhea (yogurt, boiled milk, or buttermilk may help). Report changes in urinary pattern (decreased output); severe, unresolved diarrhea; opportunistic infection (vaginal itching or drainage; sores in mouth; or blood in urine, unusual fever or chills); or rash. **Breast-feeding precaution:** Consult prescriber if breast-feeding.

Dietary Issues: May be taken with food.

Geriatric Considerations: Considered one of the drugs of choice for outpatient treatment of community-acquired pneumonia in older adults. Adjust dosage with renal impairment.

Breast-feeding Issues: Theoretically, drug absorbed by nursing infant may change bowel flora or affect fever work-up result. **Note:** As a class, cephalosporins are used to treat infections in infants.

Cefpodoxime Proxetil *see* Cefpodoxime *on page 246*

Cefprozil (sef PROE zil)

U.S. Brand Names Cefzil®

Generic Available No

Pharmacologic Category Antibiotic, Cephalosporin (Second Generation)

Pregnancy Risk Factor B

Lactation Enters breast milk/use caution (AAP rates "compatible")

Use Treatment of otitis media and infections involving the respiratory tract and skin and skin structure; active against methicillin-sensitive staphylococci, many streptococci, and various gram-negative bacilli including *E. coli*, some *Klebsiella*, *P. mirabilis*, *H. influenzae*, and *Moraxella*.

Mechanism of Action/Effect Inhibits bacterial cell wall synthesis by binding to one or more of the penicillin-binding proteins (PBPs)

Contraindications Hypersensitivity to cefprozil, any component of the formulation, or other cephalosporins

Warnings/Precautions Modify dosage in patients with severe renal impairment. Prolonged use may result in superinfection. Cross-sensitivity to penicillins exists (~10%).

Drug Interactions

Increased Effect/Toxicity: Probenecid may decrease cephalosporin elimination. Furosemide, aminoglycosides in combination with cefprozil may result in additive nephrotoxicity.

Nutritional/Ethanol Interactions Food: Food delays cefprozil absorption.

Effects on Lab Values Positive direct Coombs', false-positive urinary glucose test using cupric sulfate (Benedict's solution, Clinitest®, Fehling's solution), false-positive serum or urine creatinine with Jaffé reaction

Adverse Reactions

1% to 10%:

- Central nervous system: Dizziness (1%)
- Dermatologic: Diaper rash (1.5%)
- Gastrointestinal: Diarrhea (2.9%), nausea (3.5%), vomiting (1%), abdominal pain (1%)
- Genitourinary: Vaginitis, genital pruritus (1.6%)
- Hepatic: Increased transaminases (2%)
- Miscellaneous: Superinfection

<1% (Limited to important or life-threatening): Anaphylaxis, angioedema, arthralgia, BUN increased, cholestatic jaundice, confusion, creatinine increased, eosinophilia, erythema multiforme, fever, headache, hyperactivity, insomnia, leukopenia, pseudomembranous colitis, rash, serum sickness, somnolence, Stevens-Johnson syndrome, thrombocytopenia, urticaria

Other reactions with cephalosporins include agranulocytosis, aplastic anemia, colitis, hemolytic anemia, hemorrhage, interstitial nephritis, pancytopenia, renal dysfunction, seizures, superinfection, toxic epidermal necrolysis, toxic nephropathy, vaginitis

Overdosage/Toxicology Symptoms of overdose include neuromuscular hypersensitivity and convulsions. Many beta-lactam containing antibiotics have the potential to cause neuromuscular hyperirritability or convulsive seizures. Hemodialysis may be helpful to aid in removal of the drug from blood; otherwise, treatment is supportive or symptom-directed.

Pharmacodynamics/Kinetics

Absorption: Well absorbed (94%)

Half-Life Elimination: Normal renal function: 1.3 hours

Time to Peak: Serum: Fasting: 1.5 hours

Formulations

Powder for oral suspension, as anhydrous: 125 mg/5 mL (50 mL, 75 mL, 100 mL); 250 mg/5 mL (50 mL, 75 mL, 100 mL)

Tablet, as anhydrous: 250 mg, 500 mg

Dosing

Adults & Elderly:

Pharyngitis/tonsillitis: Oral: 500 mg every 24 hours for 10 days

Uncomplicated skin and skin structure infections: Oral: 250 mg every 12 hours, or 500 mg every 12-24 hours for 10 days

Secondary bacterial infection of acute bronchitis or acute bacterial exacerbation of chronic bronchitis: Oral: 500 mg every 12 hours for 10 days

Pediatrics:

Otitis media: Oral: Children >6 months to 12 years: 15 mg/kg every 12 hours for 10 days

Pharyngitis/tonsillitis: Oral: Children:

2-12 years: 7.5 -15 mg/kg/day divided every 12 hours for 10 days (administer for >10 days if due to *S. pyogenes*); maximum: 1 g/day

>13 years: Refer to adult dosing.

Uncomplicated skin and skin structure infections: Oral:

2-12 years: 20 mg/kg every 24 hours for 10 days; maximum: 1 g/day

>13 years: Refer to adult dosing.

Renal Impairment:

Cl_{cr} <30 mL/minute: Reduce dose by 50%.

Hemodialysis effects: 55% is removed by hemodialysis.

Administration

Oral: Administer around-the-clock to promote less variation in peak and trough serum levels. Chilling the reconstituted oral suspension improves flavor (do not freeze).

Monitoring Laboratory Tests Prothrombin time; perform culture and sensitivity studies prior to initiating drug therapy.

Monitoring and Teaching Issues

Physical Assessment: Assess for previous allergy history prior to therapy. See Contraindications and Warnings/Precautions for use cautions. Assess potential for interactions with other prescriptions, OTC medications, or herbal products patient may be taking (Drug Interactions). Assess results of laboratory tests (see above), therapeutic response, and adverse reactions (eg, hypersensitivity can occur several days after therapy is started - see Adverse Reactions and Overdose/Toxicology). Instruct diabetic patients regarding Clinitest®. Teach patient proper use, possible side effects and interventions, and adverse symptoms to report (eg, nephrotoxicity, opportunistic infection - see Patient Education). Note breast-feeding caution.

Patient Education: Inform prescriber of all prescriptions, OTC medications, or herbal products you are taking, and any allergies you have. Do not take anything new during treatment unless approved by prescriber. Take as directed, at regular intervals around-the-clock (with or without food). Chilling oral suspension improves flavor (do not freeze). Maintain adequate hydration (2-3 L/day of fluids) unless advised by prescriber to restrict fluids. Complete full course of medication, even if you feel better. May cause false test results with Clinitest®; use of another type of glucose testing is preferable. May cause dizziness (use caution when driving or engaging in potentially hazardous tasks until response to drug is known); nausea or vomiting (small, frequent meals, frequent mouth care, sucking lozenges, or chewing gum may help); or diarrhea (yogurt, boiled milk, or buttermilk may help). Report changes in urinary pattern (decreased output); vaginal burning, itching, or drainage; unresolved diarrhea; or opportunistic infection (vaginal itching or drainage, sores in mouth, blood in urine or stool, unusual fever or chills). **Breast-feeding precaution:** Consult prescriber if breast-feeding.

Dietary Issues: May be taken with food.

Geriatric Considerations: Has not been studied exclusively in the elderly. Adjust dose for estimated renal function.

Breast-feeding Issues: Theoretically, drug absorbed by nursing infant may change bowel flora or affect fever work-up result. **Note:** As a class, cephalosporins are used to treat infections in infants.

Ceftazidime (SEF tay zi deem)

U.S. Brand Names Ceptaz®; Fortaz®; Tazicef®; Tazidime®

Generic Available No

Pharmacologic Category Antibiotic, Cephalosporin (Third Generation)

Pregnancy Risk Factor B

Lactation Enters breast milk (small amounts)/use caution (AAP rates "compatible")

Use Treatment of documented susceptible *Pseudomonas aeruginosa* infection and infections due to other susceptible aerobic gram-negative organisms; empiric therapy of a febrile, granulocytopenic patient

Mechanism of Action/Effect Inhibits bacterial cell wall synthesis by binding to one or more of the penicillin-binding proteins (PBPs)

Contraindications Hypersensitivity to ceftazidime, any component of the formulation, or other cephalosporins

Warnings/Precautions Modify dosage in patients with severe renal impairment. Prolonged use may result in superinfection. Cross-sensitivity to penicillins exists (~10%).

Drug Interactions

Increased Effect/Toxicity: Probenecid may decrease cephalosporin elimination. Aminoglycosides: *in vitro* studies indicate additive or synergistic effect against some strains of Enterobacteriaceae and *Pseudomonas aeruginosa*. Furosemide, aminoglycosides in combination with ceftazidime may result in additive nephrotoxicity.

Effects on Lab Values Positive direct Coombs', false-positive urinary glucose test using cupric sulfate (Benedict's solution, Clinitest®, Fehling's solution), false-positive serum or urine creatinine with Jaffé reaction

Adverse Reactions

1% to 10%:

Gastrointestinal: Diarrhea (1%)

Local: Pain at injection site (1%)

Miscellaneous: Hypersensitivity reactions (2%)

<1% (Limited to important or life-threatening): Anaphylaxis, angioedema, asterixis, BUN increased, candidiasis, creatinine increased, dizziness, encephalopathy, eosinophilia, erythema multiforme, fever, headache, hemolytic anemia, hyperbilirubinemia, jaundice,

(Continued)

Ceftazidime *(Continued)*

leukopenia, myoclonus, nausea, neuromuscular excitability, paresthesia, phlebitis, pruritus, pseudomembranous colitis, rash, Stevens-Johnson syndrome, thrombocytosis, toxic epidermal necrolysis, transaminases increased, vaginitis, vomiting

Other reactions with cephalosporins include agranulocytosis, aplastic anemia, BUN increased, cholestasis, colitis, creatinine increased, hemolytic anemia, hemorrhage, interstitial nephritis, pancytopenia, prolonged PT, renal dysfunction, seizures, serum-sickness reactions, superinfection, toxic nephropathy, urticaria

Overdosage/Toxicology Symptoms of overdose include neuromuscular hypersensitivity and convulsions. Many beta-lactam containing antibiotics have the potential to cause neuromuscular hyperirritability or convulsive seizures. Hemodialysis may be helpful to aid in removal of the drug from blood; otherwise, treatment is supportive or symptom-directed.

Pharmacodynamics/Kinetics

Half-Life Elimination: 1-2 hours, prolonged with renal impairment; Neonates <23 days: 2.2-4.7 hours

Time to Peak: Serum: I.M.: ~1 hour

Formulations

Infusion, as sodium [premixed, frozen] (Fortaz®): 1 g (50 mL); 2 g (50 mL)

Injection, powder for reconstitution:

Ceptaz®: 1 g, 2 g, 10 g [L-arginine formulation]

Fortaz®: 500 mg, 1 g, 2 g, 6 g [contains sodium carbonate]

Tazicef®, Tazidime®: 1 g, 2 g, 6 g [contains sodium carbonate]

Dosing

Adults:

Bone and joint infections: I.V.: 2 g every 12 hours

Cystic fibrosis, lung infection caused by *Pseudomonas* spp: I.V.: 30-50 mg/kg every 8 hours (maximum 6 g/day)

Intra-abdominal or gynecologic infection: I.V.: 2 g every 8 hours

Meningitis: I.V.: 2 g every 8 hours

Pneumonia: I.V.:

Uncomplicated: 500 mg to 1 g every 8 hours

Complicated or severe: 2 g every 8 hours

Skin and soft tissue infections: I.V., I.M.: 500 mg to 1 g every 8 hours

Severe, life-threatening infection (especially in immunocompromised host): I.V.: 2 g every 8 hours

Urinary tract infections: I.V., I.M.:

Uncomplicated: 250 mg every 12 hours

Complicated: 500 mg every 8-12 hours

Elderly: I.M., I.V.: Dosage should be based on renal function with a dosing interval not more frequent then every 12 hours.

Pediatrics: Susceptible infections: I.V.:

Children 1 month to 12 years: 30-50 mg/kg/dose every 8 hours; maximum dose: 6 g/day (higher doses reserved for immunocompromised patients, cystic fibrosis, or meningitis)

Children ≥12 years: Refer to adult dosing.

Renal Impairment:

Cl_{cr} 30-50 mL/minute: Administer every 12 hours

Cl_{cr} 10-30 mL/minute: Administer every 24 hours

Cl_{cr} <10 mL/minute: Administer every 48-72 hours

Hemodialysis: Dialyzable (50% to 100%)

Continuous arteriovenous or venovenous hemodiafiltration effects: Dose as for Cl_{cr} 30-50 mL/minute

Administration

I.M.: Inject deep I.M. into large mass muscle.

I.V.: Ceftazidime can be administered IVP over 3-5 minutes or I.V. intermittent infusion over 15-30 minutes.

Stability

Reconstitution: Reconstituted solution and I.V. infusion in NS or D_5W solution are stable for 24 hours at room temperature, 10 days when refrigerated, or 12 weeks when frozen. After freezing, thawed solution is stable for 24 hours at room temperature or 4 days when refrigerated. After mixing for 96 hours refrigerated.

Compatibility: Stable in D_5NS, D_5W, NS, sterile water for injection

Y-site administration: Incompatible with alatrofloxacin, amphotericin B cholesteryl sulfate complex, amsacrine, doxorubicin liposome, fluconazole, idarubicin, midazolam, pentamidine, warfarin

Compatibility when admixed: Incompatible with aminoglycosides in same bottle/bag, aminophylline, ranitidine

Monitoring Laboratory Tests Prothrombin times; perform culture and sensitivity studies prior to initiating drug therapy.

Monitoring and Teaching Issues

Physical Assessment: Assess for previous allergy history prior to therapy. See Contraindications and Warnings/Precautions for use cautions. Assess potential for interactions with other prescriptions, OTC medications, or herbal products patient may be taking (eg, nephrotoxicity - see Drug Interactions). Assess results of laboratory tests (see above), therapeutic response, and adverse reactions (eg, hypersensitivity can occur several days after therapy is started - see Adverse Reactions and Overdose/Toxicology). Instruct diabetic patients regarding Clinitest®. Teach patient possible side effects and interventions and adverse symptoms to report (eg, opportunistic infection - see Patient Education). Note breast-feeding caution.

Patient Education: Inform prescriber of all prescriptions, OTC medications, or herbal products you are taking, and any allergies you have. Do not take anything new during treatment unless approved by prescriber. This medication is administered by infusion or injection. Report immediately any redness, swelling, burning, or pain at injection/infusion site; itching or hives; or difficulty swallowing or breathing. Maintain adequate hydration (2-3

L/day of fluids) unless advised by prescriber to restrict fluids. May cause false test results with Clinitest®; use of another type of glucose testing is preferable. May cause diarrhea (yogurt, boiled milk, or buttermilk may help). Report unresolved diarrhea; opportunistic infection (vaginal itching or drainage; sores in mouth; blood, pus, or mucus in stool or urine); easy bleeding or bruising; rash; or difficulty breathing. **Breast-feeding precaution:** Consult prescriber if breast-feeding.

Dietary Issues: Sodium content of 1 g: 2.3 mEq

Geriatric Considerations: Changes in renal function associated with aging and corresponding alterations in pharmacokinetics result in every 12-hour dosing being an adequate dosing interval. Adjust dose based on renal function.

Breast-feeding Issues: Theoretically, drug absorbed by nursing infant may change bowel flora or affect fever work-up result. **Note:** As a class, cephalosporins are used to treat infections in infants.

Additional Information With some organisms, resistance may develop during treatment (including *Enterobacter* spp and *Serratia* spp); consider combination therapy or periodic susceptibility testing for organisms with inducible resistance

Ceftibuten (sef TYE byoo ten)

U.S. Brand Names Cedax®

Generic Available No

Pharmacologic Category Antibiotic, Cephalosporin (Third Generation)

Pregnancy Risk Factor B

Lactation Excretion in breast milk unknown/use caution

Use Oral cephalosporin for treatment of bronchitis, otitis media, and pharyngitis/tonsillitis due to *H. influenzae* and *M. catarrhalis*, both beta-lactamase-producing and nonproducing strains, as well as *S. pneumoniae* (weak) and *S. pyogenes*

Mechanism of Action/Effect Inhibits bacterial cell wall synthesis by binding to one or more of the penicillin-binding proteins (PBPs)

Contraindications Hypersensitivity to ceftibuten, any component of the formulation, or other cephalosporins

Warnings/Precautions Modify dosage in patients with severe renal impairment. Prolonged use may result in superinfection. Cross-sensitivity to penicillins exists (~10%).

Drug Interactions

Increased Effect/Toxicity: High-dose probenecid decreases clearance. Aminoglycosides in combination with ceftibuten may increase nephrotoxic potential.

Effects on Lab Values Positive direct Coombs', false-positive urinary glucose test using cupric sulfate (Benedict's solution, Clinitest®, Fehling's solution), false-positive serum or urine creatinine with Jaffé reaction

Adverse Reactions

1% to 10%:

Central nervous system: Headache (3%), dizziness (1%)

Gastrointestinal: Nausea (4%), diarrhea (3%), dyspepsia (2%), vomiting (1%), abdominal pain (1%)

Hematologic: Increased eosinophils (3%), decreased hemoglobin (2%), thrombocytosis

Hepatic: Increased ALT (1%), increased bilirubin (1%)

Renal: Increased BUN (4%)

<1% (Limited to important or life-threatening): Agitation, anorexia, candidiasis, constipation, creatinine increased, diaper rash, dry mouth, dyspnea, dysuria, fatigue, insomnia, irritability, leukopenia, nasal congestion, paresthesia, rash, rigors, transaminases increased, urticaria

Other reactions with cephalosporins include agranulocytosis, anaphylaxis, angioedema, aplastic anemia, asterixis, candidiasis, cholestasis, colitis, encephalopathy, erythema multiforme, fever, hemolytic anemia, hemorrhage, interstitial nephritis, neuromuscular excitability, pancytopenia, paresthesia, prolonged PT, pruritus, pseudomembranous colitis, renal dysfunction, seizures, serum-sickness reactions, Stevens-Johnson syndrome, superinfection, toxic epidermal necrolysis, toxic nephropathy, vaginitis

Overdosage/Toxicology Symptoms of overdose include neuromuscular hypersensitivity and convulsions. Many beta-lactam containing antibiotics have the potential to cause neuromuscular hyperirritability or convulsive seizures. Hemodialysis may be helpful to aid in the removal of drug from blood; otherwise, treatment is supportive or symptom-directed.

Pharmacodynamics/Kinetics

Absorption: Rapid; food decreases peak concentrations, delays T_{max}, and lowers AUC

Half-Life Elimination: 2 hours

Time to Peak: 2-3 hours

Formulations

Capsule: 400 mg

Powder for oral suspension: 90 mg/5 mL (30 mL, 60 mL, 120 mL); 180 mg/5 mL (30 mL, 60 mL, 120 mL) [cherry flavor]

Dosing

Adults & Elderly: Susceptible infections: Oral: 400 mg once daily for 10 days; maximum: 400 mg

Pediatrics: Susceptible infections: Oral:

<12 years: 9 mg/kg/day for 10 days; maximum daily dose: 400 mg

≥12 years: Refer to adult dosing.

Renal Impairment:

Cl_{cr} 30-49 mL//minute: Administer 4.5 mg/kg or 200 mg every 24 hours.

Cl_{cr} 5-29 mL/minute: Administer 2.25 mg/kg or 100 mg every 24 hours.

(Continued)

Ceftibuten *(Continued)*

Administration

Oral: Administer at the same time each day to maintain adequate blood levels.

Stability

Reconstitution: Reconstituted suspension is stable for 14 days in the refrigerator.

Monitoring Laboratory Tests Renal, hepatic, and hematologic function periodically with prolonged therapy; prothrombin time; perform culture and sensitivity studies prior to initiating drug therapy.

Monitoring and Teaching Issues

Physical Assessment: Assess for previous allergy history prior to therapy. See Contraindications and Warnings/Precautions for use cautions. Assess potential for interactions with other prescriptions, OTC medications, or herbal products patient may be taking (see Drug Interactions). Assess results of laboratory tests (see above), therapeutic response, and adverse reactions (eg, hypersensitivity can occur several days after therapy is started - see Adverse Reactions and Overdose/Toxicology). Instruct diabetic patients regarding Clinitest®. Teach patient proper use, possible side effects and interventions, and adverse symptoms to report (eg, nephrotoxicity, opportunistic infection - see Patient Education). Note breast-feeding caution.

Patient Education: Inform prescriber of all prescriptions, OTC medications, or herbal products you are taking, and any allergies you have. Do not take anything new during treatment unless approved by prescriber. Take as directed, at regular intervals around-the-clock (with or without food). Chilling oral suspension improves flavor (do not freeze). Maintain adequate hydration (2-3 L/day of fluids) unless advised by prescriber to restrict fluids. Complete full course of medication, even if you feel better. May cause false test results with Clinitest®; use of another type of testing is preferable. May cause headache or dizziness (use caution when driving or engaging in potentially hazardous tasks until response to drug is known); nausea or vomiting (small, frequent meals, frequent mouth care, sucking lozenges, or chewing gum may help); or diarrhea (yogurt, boiled milk, or buttermilk may help). Report changes in urinary pattern (decreased output); unresolved diarrhea; opportunistic infection (vaginal itching or drainage, sores in mouth; blood in urine or stool); or rash. **Breast-feeding precaution:** Consult prescriber if breast-feeding.

Dietary Issues:

Capsule: Take without regard to food.

Suspension: Take 2 hours before or 1 hour after meals; contains 1 g of sucrose per 5 mL

Geriatric Considerations: Has not been studied specifically in the elderly. Adjust dose for renal function.

Breast-feeding Issues: Theoretically, drug absorbed by nursing infant may change bowel flora or affect fever work-up result. **Note:** As a class, cephalosporins are used to treat infections in infants.

Ceftin® *see* Cefuroxime *on page 255*

Ceftizoxime (sef ti ZOKS eem)

U.S. Brand Names Cefizox®

Synonyms Ceftizoxime Sodium

Generic Available No

Pharmacologic Category Antibiotic, Cephalosporin (Third Generation)

Pregnancy Risk Factor B

Lactation Enters breast milk (small amounts)/use caution

Use Treatment of susceptible bacterial infection, mainly respiratory tract, skin and skin structure, bone and joint, urinary tract and gynecologic, as well as septicemia; active against many gram-negative bacilli (not *Pseudomonas*), some gram-positive cocci (not *Enterococcus*), and some anaerobes

Mechanism of Action/Effect Inhibits bacterial cell wall synthesis by binding to one or more of the penicillin-binding proteins (PBPs)

Contraindications Hypersensitivity to ceftizoxime, any component of the formulation, or other cephalosporins

Warnings/Precautions Modify dosage in patients with severe renal impairment. Prolonged use may result in superinfection. Cross-sensitivity to penicillins exists (~10%).

Drug Interactions

Increased Effect/Toxicity: Probenecid may decrease cephalosporin elimination. Furosemide, aminoglycosides in combination with ceftizoxime may result in additive nephrotoxicity.

Effects on Lab Values Positive direct Coombs', false-positive urinary glucose test using cupric sulfate (Benedict's solution, Clinitest®, Fehling's solution), false-positive serum or urine creatinine with Jaffé reaction

Adverse Reactions

1% to 10%:

Central nervous system: Fever

Dermatologic: Rash, pruritus

Hematologic: Eosinophilia, thrombocytosis

Hepatic: Elevated transaminases, alkaline phosphatase

Local: Pain, burning at injection site

<1% (Limited to important or life-threatening): Anaphylaxis, anemia, bilirubin increased, BUN increased, creatinine increased, diarrhea, injection site reactions, leukopenia, nausea, neutropenia, numbness, paresthesia, phlebitis, thrombocytopenia, vaginitis, vomiting

Other reactions reported with cephalosporins include agranulocytosis, angioedema, aplastic anemia, asterixis, candidiasis, cholestasis, colitis, encephalopathy, erythema multiforme, hemolytic anemia, hemorrhage, interstitial nephritis, neuromuscular excitability, pancytopenia, prolonged PT, pseudomembranous colitis, renal dysfunction, seizures, serum-sickness reactions, Stevens-Johnson syndrome, superinfection, toxic epidermal necrolysis, toxic nephropathy

Overdosage/Toxicology Symptoms of overdose include neuromuscular hypersensitivity and convulsions. Many beta-lactam containing antibiotics have the potential to cause neuromuscular hyperirritability or convulsive seizures. Hemodialysis may be helpful to aid in removal of the drug from blood; otherwise, treatment is supportive or symptom-directed.

Pharmacodynamics/Kinetics

Half-Life Elimination: 1.6 hours; Cl_{cr} <10 mL/minute: 25 hours

Time to Peak: Serum: I.M.: 0.5-1 hour

Formulations

Injection, as sodium [in D_5W, frozen]: 1 g (50 mL); 2 g (50 mL)

Injection, powder for reconstitution, as sodium: 500 mg, 1 g, 2 g, 10 g

Dosing

Adults & Elderly: Susceptible infections: I.M., I.V.: 1-2 g every 8-12 hours, up to 2 g every 4 hours or 4 g every 8 hours for life-threatening infections

Pediatrics: Susceptible infections: I.M., I.V.: Children ≥6 months: 150-200 mg/kg/day divided every 6-8 hours (maximum of 12 g/24 hours)

Renal Impairment:

Cl_{cr} 50-79 mL/minute: Administer 500-1500 mg every 8 hours.

Cl_{cr} 5-49 mL/minute: Administer 250-1000 mg every 12 hours.

Cl_{cr} 0-4 mL/minute: Administer 500-1000 mg every 48 hours or 250-500 mg every 24 hours.

Moderately dialyzable (20% to 50%)

Continuous arteriovenous hemofiltration: Dose as for Cl_{cr} 10-50 mL/minute.

Administration

I.M.: Inject deep I.M. into large muscle mass.

I.V.: Inject direct I.V. over 3-5 minutes. Infuse intermittent infusion over 30 minutes.

Stability

Reconstitution: Reconstituted solution is stable for 24 hours at room temperature and 96 hours when refrigerated. For I.V. infusion in NS or D_5W, solution is stable for 24 hours at room temperature, 96 hours when refrigerated or 12 weeks when frozen. After freezing, thawed solution is stable for 24 hours at room temperature or 10 days when refrigerated.

Compatibility: Stable in $D_5{}^1/_4NS$, $D_5{}^1/_2NS$, D_5NS, D_5W, $D_{10}W$, LR, NS, sodium bicarbonate 5%

Y-site administration: Incompatible with filgrastim

Monitoring Laboratory Tests Prothrombin times; perform culture and sensitivity studies prior to initiating drug therapy.

Monitoring and Teaching Issues

Physical Assessment: Assess for previous allergy history prior to therapy. See Contraindications and Warnings/Precautions for use cautions. Assess potential for interactions with other prescriptions, OTC medications, or herbal products patient may be taking (eg, nephrotoxicity - see Drug Interactions). Assess results of laboratory tests (see above), therapeutic response, and adverse reactions (eg, hypersensitivity can occur several days after therapy is started - see Adverse Reactions and Overdose/Toxicology). Instruct diabetic patients regarding Clinitest®. Teach patient possible side effects and interventions and adverse symptoms to report (see Patient Education). Note breast-feeding caution.

Patient Education: Inform prescriber of all prescriptions, OTC medications, or herbal products you are taking, and any allergies you have. Do not take anything new during treatment unless approved by prescriber. This medication is administered by infusion or injection. Report immediately any redness, swelling, burning, or pain at injection/infusion site; itching or hives; or difficulty swallowing or breathing. Maintain adequate hydration (2-3 L/day of fluids) unless advised by prescriber to restrict fluids. May cause false test results with Clinitest®; use of another type of glucose testing is preferable. Report opportunistic infection (vaginal itching or drainage; sores in mouth; blood, pus, or mucus in stool or urine; or easy bleeding or bruising). **Breast-feeding precaution:** Consult prescriber if breast-feeding.

Dietary Issues: Sodium content of 1 g: 60 mg (2.6 mEq)

Geriatric Considerations: Adjust dose for renal function in the elderly.

Breast-feeding Issues: Theoretically, drug absorbed by nursing infant may change bowel flora or affect fever work-up result. **Note:** As a class, cephalosporins are used to treat infections in infants.

Ceftizoxime Sodium *see* Ceftizoxime *on page 252*

Ceftriaxone (sef trye AKS one)

U.S. Brand Names Rocephin®

Synonyms Ceftriaxone Sodium

Generic Available No

Pharmacologic Category Antibiotic, Cephalosporin (Third Generation)

Pregnancy Risk Factor B

Lactation Enters breast milk/use caution (AAP rates "compatible")

Use Treatment of lower respiratory tract infections, skin and skin structure infections, bone and joint infections, intra-abdominal and urinary tract infections, sepsis and meningitis due to susceptible organisms; documented or suspected infection due to susceptible organisms in home care patients and patients without I.V. line access; treatment of documented or suspected gonococcal infection or chancroid; emergency room management of patients at high risk for bacteremia, periorbital or buccal cellulitis, salmonellosis or shigellosis, and pneumonia of unestablished etiology (<5 years of age); treatment of Lyme disease, depends on the stage of the disease (used in Stage II and Stage III, but not stage I; doxycycline is the drug of choice for Stage I)

Mechanism of Action/Effect Inhibits bacterial cell wall synthesis by binding to one or more of the penicillin-binding proteins (PBPs)

Contraindications Hypersensitivity to ceftriaxone sodium, any component of the formulation, or other cephalosporins; **do not use in hyperbilirubinemic neonates**, particularly those (Continued)

Ceftriaxone *(Continued)*

who are premature since ceftriaxone is reported to displace bilirubin from albumin binding sites

Warnings/Precautions Modify dosage in patients with severe renal impairment. Prolonged use may result in superinfection with yeasts, enterococci, *B. fragilis*, or *P. aeruginosa*. Cross-sensitivity to penicillins exists (~10%).

Drug Interactions

Increased Effect/Toxicity: Aminoglycosides may result in synergistic antibacterial activity. High-dose probenecid decreases clearance. Aminoglycosides increase nephrotoxic potential.

Effects on Lab Values Positive direct Coombs', false-positive urinary glucose test using cupric sulfate (Benedict's solution, Clinitest®, Fehling's solution), false-positive serum or urine creatinine with Jaffé reaction

Adverse Reactions

1% to 10%:

- Dermatologic: Rash (2%)
- Gastrointestinal: Diarrhea (3%)
- Hematologic: Eosinophilia (6%), thrombocytosis (5%), leukopenia (2%)
- Hepatic: Elevated transaminases (3.1% to 3.3%)
- Local: Pain, induration at injection site (I.V. 1%); warmth, tightness, induration (5% to 17%) following I.M. injection
- Renal: Increased BUN (1%)

<1% (Limited to important or life-threatening): Agranulocytosis, anaphylaxis, anemia, basophilia, bronchospasm, candidiasis, chills, diaphoresis, dizziness, dysgeusia, flushing, gallstones, glycosuria, headache, hematuria, hemolytic anemia, jaundice, leukocytosis, lymphocytosis, lymphopenia, monocytosis, nausea, nephrolithiasis, neutropenia, phlebitis, prolonged or decreased PT, pruritus, renal precipitations, renal stones, serum sickness, thrombocytopenia, urinary casts, vaginitis, vomiting; increased alkaline phosphatase, bilirubin, and creatinine

Reactions reported with other cephalosporins include angioedema, aplastic anemia, asterixis, cholestasis, colitis, encephalopathy, erythema multiforme, hemorrhage, interstitial nephritis, neuromuscular excitability, pancytopenia, paresthesia, pseudomembranous colitis, renal dysfunction, seizures, Stevens-Johnson syndrome, superinfection, toxic epidermal necrolysis, toxic nephropathy

Overdosage/Toxicology Symptoms of overdose include neuromuscular hypersensitivity and convulsions. Many beta-lactam containing antibiotics have the potential to cause neuromuscular hyperirritability or convulsive seizures. Hemodialysis may be helpful to aid in removal of the drug from blood; otherwise, treatment is supportive or symptom-directed.

Pharmacodynamics/Kinetics

Absorption: I.M.: Well absorbed

Half-Life Elimination:

- Normal renal and hepatic function: 5-9 hours
- Neonates: Postnatal: 1-4 days old: 16 hours, 9-30 days old: 9 hours

Time to Peak: Serum: I.M.: 1-2 hours

Formulations

Infusion, as sodium [premixed, frozen]: 1 g [in $D_{3.8}W$] (50 mL); 2 g [in $D_{2.4}W$] (50 mL)

Injection, powder for reconstitution, as sodium: 250 mg, 500 mg, 1 g, 2 g, 10 g

Dosing

Adults & Elderly:

- Pneumonia, skin/soft tissue infection, urinary tract infection, septicemia, bone/joint infection, or intra-abdominal infection: I.M., I.V.: 1-2 g every 12-24 hours (depending on the type and severity of infection); maximum: 4 g/day treatment
- Meningitis: I.V.: 2 g every 12 hours
- Uncomplicated gonorrhea: I.M.: 250 mg as a single dose
- Acute epididymitis: I.M.: 250 mg in a single dose

Pediatrics:

- Usual dosage range (nonmeningitis): I.M., I.V.: Infants and Children: 50-75 mg/kg/day divided every 12-24 hours (see below for information on specific infections)
- Chancroid: I.M.: 50 mg/kg as a single dose (maximum dose: 250 mg)
- Chemoprophylaxis for high-risk contacts of patients with invasive meningococcal disease: I.M.:
  - ≤12 years: 125 mg in a single dose
  - >12 years: 250 mg in a single dose
- Epididymitis, acute: I.M.: 250 mg in a single dose
- Gonococcal infections (uncomplicated), sexual assault, and STD prophylaxis: I.M.: 125 mg in a single dose
- Gonococcal infections (complicated): I.M., I.V.:
  - <45 kg:
    - Peritonitis, arthritis, or bacteremia: 50 mg/kg/day once daily for 7 days; maximum dose: 1 g/day
    - Conjunctivitis: 50 mg/kg (maximum dose: 1 g) in a single dose
    - Meningitis or endocarditis: 50 mg/kg/day divided every 12 hours for 10-14 days (meningitis), for 28 days (endocarditis); maximum dose: 2 g/day
  - >45 kg:
    - Disseminated gonococcal infections: 1 g/day once daily for 7 days
    - Meningitis: 1-2 g/dose every 12 hours for 10-14 days
    - Endocarditis: 1-2 g/dose every 12 hours for 28 days
    - Conjunctivitis: I.M.: 1 g in a single dose
- Meningitis: I.M., I.V.: 80-100 mg/kg/day divided every 12-24 hours; loading dose of 75-100 mg/kg may be administered at the start of therapy; maximum dose: 4 g/day
- Otitis media, acute: I.M.: 50 mg/kg as a single dose (maximum dose: 1 g)

Renal Impairment:

No adjustment is necessary.

Not dialyzable (0% to 5%)

Administer dose postdialysis.

Peritoneal dialysis effects: Administer 750 mg every 12 hours.

Continuous arteriovenous or venovenous hemofiltration: Removes 10 mg of ceftriaxone of liter of filtrate per day.

Hepatic Impairment: No adjustment necessary.

Administration

I.M.: Inject deep I.M. into large muscle mass.

I.V.: Infuse intermittent infusion over 15-30 minutes.

Stability

Reconstitution: Reconstituted solution (100 mg/mL) is stable for 3 days at room temperature and 3 days when refrigerated. For I.V. infusion in NS or D_5W, solution is stable for 3 days at room temperature, 10 days when refrigerated, or 26 weeks when frozen. After freezing, thawed solution is stable for 3 days at room temperature or 10 days when refrigerated.

Compatibility: Stable in D_5W with KCl 10 mEq, $D_5{}^1/_4$NS with KCl 20 mEq, $D_5{}^1/_2$ NS, D_5W, $D_{10}W$, NS, mannitol 5%, mannitol 10%, sodium bicarbonate 5%, bacteriostatic water, sterile water for injection

Y-site administration: Incompatible with alatrofloxacin, amphotericin B cholesteryl sulfate complex, amsacrine, filgrastim, fluconazole, labetalol, pentamidine, vinorelbine

Compatibility when admixed: Incompatible with aminophylline, clindamycin, linezolid, theophylline

Monitoring Laboratory Tests Prothrombin times; perform culture and sensitivity studies prior to initiating drug therapy.

Monitoring and Teaching Issues

Physical Assessment: Assess for previous allergy history prior to therapy. See Contraindications and Warnings/Precautions for use cautions. See I.V. specifics above. Assess potential for interactions with other prescriptions, OTC medications, or herbal products patient may be taking (eg, nephrotoxicity - see Drug Interactions). Assess results of laboratory tests (see Monitoring Laboratory Tests and Overdose/Toxicology), therapeutic response and adverse reactions (eg, hypersensitivity can occur several days after therapy is started - see Adverse Reactions). Instruct diabetic patients regarding Clinitest®. Teach patient possible side effects and interventions and adverse symptoms to report (see Patient Education). Note breast-feeding caution.

Patient Education: Inform prescriber of all prescriptions, OTC medications, or herbal products you are taking, and any allergies you have. Do not take anything new during treatment unless approved by prescriber. This medication is administered by infusion or injection. Report immediately any redness, swelling, burning or pain at injection/infusion site; rash, itching, or hives; or difficulty swallowing or breathing. Maintain adequate hydration (2-3 L/day of fluids) unless advised by prescriber to restrict fluids. May cause false test results with Clinitest®; use of another type of glucose testing is preferable. May cause diarrhea (yogurt, boiled milk, or buttermilk may help). Report unresolved diarrhea; opportunistic infection (vaginal itching or drainage; sores in mouth; blood, pus, or mucus in stool or urine); easy bleeding or bruising; unusual fever or chills; rash; or difficulty breathing. **Breast-feeding precaution:** Consult prescriber if breast-feeding.

Dietary Issues: Sodium content of 1 g: 60 mg (2.6 mEq)

Geriatric Considerations: No adjustment for changes in renal function necessary.

Breast-feeding Issues: Theoretically, drug absorbed by nursing infant may change bowel flora or affect fever work-up result. **Note:** As a class, cephalosporins are used to treat infections in infants.

Ceftriaxone Sodium *see* Ceftriaxone *on page 253*

Cefuroxime (se fyoor OKS eem)

U.S. Brand Names Ceftin®; Kefurox®; Zinacef®

Synonyms Cefuroxime Axetil; Cefuroxime Sodium

Generic Available Yes

Pharmacologic Category Antibiotic, Cephalosporin (Second Generation)

Pregnancy Risk Factor B

Lactation Enters breast milk/use caution

Use Treatment of infections caused by staphylococci, group B streptococci, *H. influenzae* (type A and B), *E. coli*, *Enterobacter*, *Salmonella*, and *Klebsiella*; treatment of susceptible infections of the lower respiratory tract, otitis media, urinary tract, skin and soft tissue, bone and joint, sepsis and gonorrhea

Mechanism of Action/Effect Inhibits bacterial cell wall synthesis by binding to one or more of the penicillin-binding proteins (PBPs)

Contraindications Hypersensitivity to cefuroxime, any component of the formulation, or other cephalosporins

Warnings/Precautions Modify dosage in patients with severe renal impairment, prolonged use may result in superinfection; use with caution in patients with a history of penicillin allergy, especially IgE-mediated reactions (eg, anaphylaxis, urticaria); may cause antibiotic-associated colitis or colitis secondary to *C. difficile*; may be associated with increased INR, especially in nutritionally-deficient patients, prolonged treatment, hepatic or renal disease; tablets and oral suspension are not bioequivalent (do not substitute on a mg-per-mg basis)

Drug Interactions

Increased Effect/Toxicity: High-dose probenecid decreases clearance. Aminoglycosides in combination with cefuroxime may result in additive nephrotoxicity.

Nutritional/Ethanol Interactions Food: Bioavailability is increased with food; cefuroxime serum levels may be increased if taken with food or dairy products.

Effects on Lab Values Positive direct Coombs', false-positive urinary glucose test using cupric sulfate (Benedict's solution, Clinitest®, Fehling's solution), false-positive serum or urine creatinine with Jaffé reaction

(Continued)

Cefuroxime *(Continued)*

Adverse Reactions

1% to 10%:

Hematologic: Eosinophilia (7%), decreased hemoglobin and hematocrit (10%)

Hepatic: Increased transaminases (4%), increased alkaline phosphatase (2%)

Local: Thrombophlebitis (1.7%)

<1% (Limited to important or life-threatening): Anaphylaxis, angioedema, BUN increased, cholestasis, colitis, creatinine increased, diarrhea, dizziness, erythema multiforme, fever, GI bleeding, hemolytic anemia, headache, hepatitis, interstitial nephritis, jaundice, leukopenia, nausea, neutropenia, pain at injection site, pancytopenia, prolonged PT/INR, pseudomembranous colitis, rash, seizures, Stevens-Johnson syndrome, stomach cramps, thrombocytopenia, toxic epidermal necrolysis, vaginitis, vomiting

Other reactions with cephalosporins include agranulocytosis, aplastic anemia, asterixis, colitis, encephalopathy, hemorrhage, neuromuscular excitability, serum-sickness reactions, superinfection, toxic nephropathy

Overdosage/Toxicology Symptoms of overdose include neuromuscular hypersensitivity and convulsions. Many beta-lactam containing antibiotics have the potential to cause neuromuscular hyperirritability or convulsive seizures. Hemodialysis may be helpful to aid in removal of the drug from blood; otherwise, treatment is supportive or symptom-directed.

Pharmacodynamics/Kinetics

Absorption: Oral (cefuroxime axetil): Increases with food

Bioavailability: Tablet: Fasting: 37%; Following food: 52%

Half-Life Elimination:

Neonates: ≤3 days old : 5.1-5.8 hours; 6-14 days old: 2-4.2 hours; 3-4 weeks old: 1-1.5 hours

Adults: 1-2 hours; prolonged with renal impairment

Time to Peak: Serum: I.M.: ~15-60 minutes; I.V.: 2-3 minutes

Formulations

Infusion, as sodium [premixed, frozen] (Zinacef®): 750 mg (50 mL); 1.5 g (50 mL)

Injection, powder for reconstitution, as sodium: 750 mg, 1.5 g, 7.5 g

Kefurox®, Zinacef®: 750 mg, 1.5 g, 7.5 g

Powder for oral suspension, as axetil (Ceftin®): 125 mg/5 mL (50 mL, 100 mL, 200 mL); 250 mg/5 mL (50 mL, 100 mL) [tutti-frutti flavor]

Tablet, as axetil (Ceftin®): 250 mg, 500 mg

Dosing

Adults & Elderly: Note: Cefuroxime axetil film-coated tablets and oral suspension are not bioequivalent and are not substitutable on a mg/mg basis.

Acute bacterial maxillary sinusitis: Oral: 250 mg twice daily for 10 days

Bronchitis, acute (and exacerbations of chronic bronchitis):

Oral: 250-500 mg every 12 hours for 10 days

I.V.: 500-750 mg every 8 hours (complete therapy with oral dosing)

Gonococcal infection, uncomplicated:

Oral: 1 g as a single dose

I.M.: 1.5 g as a single dose (administered at two different sites along with 1 g oral probenecid)

Gonococcal infection, disseminated: I.M., I.V.: 750 mg every 8 hours

Lyme disease (early): Oral: 500 mg twice daily for 20 days

Pharyngitis, tonsillitis: Oral: 250 mg twice daily for 10 days

Skin/skin structure infection, uncomplicated:

Oral: 250-500 mg every 12 hours for 10 days

I.M., I.V.: 750 mg every 8 hours

Urinary tract infection, uncomplicated:

Oral: 125-250 mg twice daily for 7-10 days

I.V., I.M.: 750 mg every 8 hours

Pneumonia, uncomplicated: I.M., I.V.: 750 mg every 8 hours

Severe or complicated infections: I.M., I.V.: 1.5 g every 8 hours (up to 1.5 g every 6 hours in life-threatening infections)

Surgical prophylaxis: I.V.: 1.5 g 30 minutes to 1 hour before procedure; 750 mg every 8 hours I.M. when procedure is prolonged

Open heart surgery: I.V.: 1.5 g at the induction of anesthesia and every 12 hours thereafter to a total of 6 g is recommended

Pediatrics: Note: Cefuroxime axetil film-coated tablets and oral suspension are not bioequivalent and are not substitutable on a mg/mg basis.

Children ≥3 months to 12 years:

Pharyngitis, tonsillitis:

Oral:

Suspension: 20 mg/kg/day (maximum: 500 mg/day) in 2 divided doses for 10 days

Tablet: 125 mg every 12 hours for 10 days

I.M., I.V.: 75-150 mg/kg/day divided every 8 hours; maximum dose: 6 g/day

Acute otitis media, impetigo:

Oral:

Suspension: 30 mg/kg/day (maximum: 1 g/day) in 2 divided doses

Tablet: 250 mg every 12 hours

I.M., I.V.: 75-150 mg/kg/day divided every 8 hours; maximum dose: 6 g/day

Meningitis: **Not** recommended (doses of 200-240 mg/kg/day divided every 6-8 hours have been used); maximum dose: 9 g/day

Acute bacterial maxillary sinusitis: Oral:

Suspension: 30 mg/kg/day in 2 divided doses for 10 days; maximum dose: 1 g/day

Tablet: 250 mg twice daily for 10 days

Children ≥13 years: Refer to adult dosing.

Renal Impairment:

Cl_{cr} 10-20 mL/minute: Administer every 12 hours.

Cl_{cr} <10 mL/minute: Administer every 24 hours.

Hemodialysis: Dialyzable (25%)

Note: Cefuroxime axetil film-coated tablets and oral suspension are not bioequivalent and are not substitutable on a mg/mg basis.

Continuous arteriovenous or venovenous hemodiafiltration effects: Dose as for Cl_{cr} 10-20 mL/minute.

Administration

Oral: Administer around-the-clock to promote less variation in peak and trough serum levels. Oral suspension: Administer with food. Shake well before use.

I.M.: Inject deep I.M. into large muscle mass.

I.V.: Inject direct I.V. over 3-5 minutes. Infuse intermittent infusion over 15-30 minutes.

Stability

Reconstitution:

Injectable: Reconstituted solution is stable for 24 hours at room temperature and 48 hours when refrigerated. I.V. infusion in NS or D_5W solution is stable for 24 hours at room temperature, 7 days when refrigerated, or 26 weeks when frozen. After freezing, thawed solution is stable for 24 hours at room temperature or 21 days when refrigerated.

Oral suspension: Store in refrigerator or at room temperature. Discard after 10 days.

Compatibility: Stable in $D_5{}^1/_4NS$, $D_5{}^1/_2NS$, D_5NS, D_5W, $D_{10}W$, LR, NS

Y-site administration: Incompatible with clarithromycin, filgrastim, fluconazole, midazolam, vinorelbine

Compatibility in syringe: Incompatible with doxapram

Compatibility when admixed: Incompatible with aminoglycosides, sodium bicarbonate

Monitoring Laboratory Tests Perform culture and sensitivity studies prior to initiating therapy. Monitor prothrombin time in patients at risk of prolongation during cephalosporin therapy (nutritionally-deficient, prolonged treatment, renal or hepatic disease)

Monitoring and Teaching Issues

Physical Assessment: Assess for previous allergy history prior to therapy. See Contraindications, Warnings/Precautions and Dosing for use cautions. Assess potential for interactions with other prescriptions, OTC medications, or herbal products patient may be taking (see Drug Interactions). Assess results of laboratory tests (see above), therapeutic response, and adverse reactions (eg, hypersensitivity can occur several days after therapy is started - see Adverse Reactions and Overdose/Toxicology). Instruct diabetic patients regarding Clinitest®. Teach patient proper use, possible side effects and interventions, and adverse symptoms to report (see Patient Education). Note breast-feeding caution.

Patient Education: Inform prescriber of all prescriptions, OTC medications, or herbal products you are taking, and any allergies you have. Do not take anything new during treatment unless approved by prescriber.

Oral: Take as directed, at regular intervals around-the-clock (with or without food). Chilling suspension improves flavor (do not freeze). Maintain adequate hydration (2-3 L/day of fluids) unless advised by prescriber to restrict fluids. Complete full course of medication, even if you feel better.

I.V./I.M.: Report immediately any swelling, redness, or pain at injection/infusion site; difficulty breathing or swallowing; chest pain; or rash. May cause false test results with Clinitest®; use of another type of glucose testing is preferable. Report unusual bruising or bleeding; or opportunistic infection (vaginal itching or drainage, sores in mouth, blood in urine or stool).

Breast-feeding precaution: Consult prescriber if breast-feeding.

Dietary Issues: May be taken with food. Sodium content of 1 g: 54.2 mg (2.4 mEq)

Geriatric Considerations: Adjust dose for renal function in the elderly. Considered one of the drugs of choice for outpatient treatment of community-acquired pneumonia in the older adult.

Breast-feeding Issues: Theoretically, drug absorbed by nursing infant may change bowel flora or affect fever work-up result. **Note:** As a class, cephalosporins are used to treat infections in infants.

Cefuroxime Axetil *see* Cefuroxime *on page 255*

Cefuroxime Sodium *see* Cefuroxime *on page 255*

Cefzil® *see* Cefprozil *on page 248*

Celebrex® *see* Celecoxib *on page 257*

Celecoxib (ce le COX ib)

U.S. Brand Names Celebrex®

Generic Available No

Pharmacologic Category Nonsteroidal Anti-inflammatory Drug (NSAID), COX-2 Selective

Pregnancy Risk Factor C/D (3rd trimester)

Lactation Excretion in breast milk unknown/not recommended

Use Relief of the signs and symptoms of osteoarthritis; relief of the signs and symptoms of rheumatoid arthritis in adults; decreasing intestinal polyps in familial adenomatous polyposis (FAP); management of acute pain; treatment of primary dysmenorrhea

Mechanism of Action/Effect Inhibits prostaglandin synthesis by decreasing the activity of the enzyme, cyclooxygenase-2 (COX-2), which results in decreased formation of prostaglandin precursors. Celecoxib does not inhibit cyclooxygenase-1 (COX-1) at therapeutic concentrations.

Contraindications Hypersensitivity to celecoxib, any component of the formulation, sulfonamides, aspirin, or other NSAIDs; pregnancy (3rd trimester)

Warnings/Precautions Gastrointestinal irritation, ulceration, bleeding, and perforation may occur with NSAIDs (it is unclear whether celecoxib is associated with rates of these events which are similar to nonselective NSAIDs). Use with caution in patients with a history of GI disease (bleeding or ulcers), decreased renal function, hepatic disease, CHF, hypertension, or asthma. Anaphylactoid reactions may occur, even with no prior exposure to celecoxib. Use caution in patients with known or suspected deficiency of cytochrome P450 isoenzyme 2C9. (Continued)

Celecoxib *(Continued)*

Safety and efficacy have not been established in patients <18 years of age. Pregnancy risk C/D (3rd trimester).

Drug Interactions

Cytochrome P450 Effect: Substrate of CYP2C8/9, 3A4; Inhibits CYP2D6

Decreased Effect: Efficacy of thiazide diuretics, loop diuretics (furosemide), or ACE-inhibitors may be diminished by celecoxib.

Increased Effect/Toxicity: Fluconazole increases celecoxib concentrations twofold. Other inhibitors of cytochrome P450 isoenzyme 2C9 (ie, amiodarone, fluoxetine, sulfonamides, ritonavir, zafirlukast) theoretically may result in significant increases in celecoxib concentrations. Lithium and methotrexate concentrations may be increased by celecoxib. Celecoxib may be used with low-dose aspirin, however, rates of gastrointestinal bleeding may be increased with coadministration. Celecoxib has been associated with increased prothrombin times and some bleeding episodes (predominantly in elderly patients) during warfarin therapy.

Nutritional/Ethanol Interactions

Ethanol: Avoid ethanol (increased GI irritation).

Food: Peak concentrations are delayed and AUC is increased by 10% to 20% when taken with a high-fat meal.

Adverse Reactions

>10%: Central nervous system: Headache (15.8%)

2% to 10%:

Cardiovascular: Peripheral edema (2.1%)

Central nervous system: Insomnia (2.3%), dizziness (2%)

Dermatologic : Skin rash (2.2%)

Gastrointestinal: Dyspepsia (8.8%), diarrhea (5.6%), abdominal pain (4.1%), nausea (3.5%), flatulence (2.2%)

Neuromuscular & skeletal: Back pain (2.8%)

Respiratory: Upper respiratory tract infection (8.1%), sinusitis (5%), pharyngitis (2.3%), rhinitis (2%)

Miscellaneous: Accidental injury (2.9%)

<2%, postmarketing, and/or case reports (limited to important or life-threatening): Acute renal failure, agranulocytosis, albuminuria, allergic reactions, alopecia, anaphylactoid reactions, angioedema, aplastic anemia, arthralgia, aseptic meningitis, ataxia, bronchospasm, cerebrovascular accident, CHF, colitis, conjunctivitis, cystitis, deafness, diabetes mellitus, dyspnea, dysuria, ecchymosis, erythema multiforme, esophageal perforation, esophagitis, exfoliative dermatitis, flu-like syndrome, gangrene, gastroenteritis, gastroesophageal reflux, gastrointestinal bleeding, glaucoma, hematuria, hepatic failure, hepatitis, hypertension, hypoglycemia, hypokalemia, hyponatremia, interstitial nephritis, intestinal perforation, jaundice, leukopenia, melena, migraine, myalgia, myocardial infarction, neuralgia, neuropathy, pancreatitis, pancytopenia, paresthesia, photosensitivity, prostate disorder, pulmonary embolism, rash, renal calculi, sepsis, Stevens-Johnson syndrome, stomatitis, sudden death, syncope, thrombocytopenia, thrombophlebitis, tinnitus, toxic epidermal necrolysis, urticaria, vaginal bleeding, vaginitis, vasculitis, ventricular fibrillation, vertigo, vomiting

Overdosage/Toxicology Symptoms of overdose may include epigastric pain, drowsiness, lethargy, nausea, and vomiting; gastrointestinal bleeding may occur. Rare manifestations include hypertension, respiratory depression, coma, and acute renal failure. Treatment is symptomatic and supportive. Forced diuresis, hemodialysis and/or urinary alkalinization may not be useful.

Pharmacodynamics/Kinetics

Bioavailability: Absolute bioavailability unknown

Half-Life Elimination: 11 hours

Time to Peak: 3 hours

Metabolism: Hepatic via CYP2C9; forms inactive metabolites

Formulations Capsule: 100 mg, 200 mg, 400 mg

Dosing

Adults:

Osteoarthritis: Oral: 200 mg/day as a single dose or in divided dose twice daily

Rheumatoid arthritis: Oral: 100-200 mg twice daily

Familial adenomatous polyposis (FAP): Oral: 400 mg twice daily

Acute pain or primary dysmenorrhea: Oral: Initial dose: 400 mg, followed by an additional 200 mg if needed on day 1; maintenance dose: 200 mg twice daily as needed

Elderly: Oral: No specific adjustment is recommended; however, the AUC in elderly patients may be increased by 50% as compared to younger subjects. Use the lowest recommended dose in patients weighing <50 kg.

Renal Impairment: No specific dosage adjustment is recommended. Not recommended in patients with advanced renal disease,

Hepatic Impairment: Reduced dosage is recommended (AUC may be increased by 40% to 180%). Decrease dose by 50% in patients with moderate hepatic impairment (Child-Pugh class II).

Stability

Storage: Store at controlled room temperature of 25°C (77°F).

Monitoring and Teaching Issues

Physical Assessment: See Contraindications and Warnings/Precautions for use cautions. Assess effectiveness and interactions of other medications patient may be taking (see Drug Interactions, ie, monitor patients taking lithium closely). Assess allergy history (aspirin, NSAIDs, salicylates). Monitor effectiveness of therapy. Assess knowledge/teach patient appropriate use, possible side effects/interventions, and adverse symptoms to report (see Adverse Reaction, Overdose/Toxicology, and Patient Education). **Pregnancy risk factor C/D** - see Pregnancy Risk Factor for use cautions. Breast-feeding is not recommended.

Patient Education: Do not take more than recommended dose. May be taken with food to reduce GI upset. Do not take with antacids. Avoid alcohol, aspirin, and OTC medication unless approved by prescriber. You may experience dizziness, confusion, or blurred vision (avoid driving or engaging in tasks requiring alertness until response to drug is known); anorexia, nausea, vomiting, taste disturbance, gastric distress (small, frequent meals, frequent mouth care, sucking lozenges, or chewing gum may help). GI bleeding, ulceration, or perforation can occur with or without pain. It is unclear whether celecoxib has rates of these events which are similar to nonselective NSAIDs. Stop taking medication and report immediately stomach pain or cramping; unusual bleeding or bruising (blood in vomitus, stool, or urine). Report persistent insomnia; skin rash; unusual fatigue, muscle pain, tremors, or weakness; sudden weight gain or edema; changes in hearing (ringing in ears) or vision; changes in urination pattern; or difficulty breathing. **Pregnancy/breast-feeding precautions:** Inform your prescriber if you are or intend to become pregnant. This drug should not be used in the 3rd trimester of pregnancy. Breast-feeding is not recommended.

Dietary Issues: Lower doses (200 mg twice daily) may be taken without regard to meals. Larger doses should be taken with food to improve absorption.

Breast-feeding Issues: In animal studies, celecoxib has been found to be excreted in milk; it is not known whether celecoxib is excreted in human milk. Because many drugs are excreted in milk, and the potential for serious adverse reactions exists, a decision should be made whether to discontinue nursing or discontinue the drug, taking into account the importance of the drug to the mother.

Pregnancy Issues: In late pregnancy may cause premature closure of the ductus arteriosus.

Related Information

Nonsalicylate/Nonsteroidal Anti-inflammatory Comparison *on page 1587*

Celestone® *see* Betamethasone *on page 160*

Celestone® Phosphate *see* Betamethasone *on page 160*

Celestone® Soluspan® *see* Betamethasone *on page 160*

Celexa™ *see* Citalopram *on page 301*

CellCept® *see* Mycophenolate *on page 933*

Cellulose, Oxidized *see page 1461*

Cenafed® [OTC] *see* Pseudoephedrine *on page 1150*

Cena-K® *see* Potassium Supplements *on page 1106*

Cenestin® *see* Estrogens (Conjugated A/Synthetic) *on page 502*

Cēpacol® Maximum Strength [OTC] *see* Dyclonine *on page 457*

Cephalexin (sef a LEKS in)

U.S. Brand Names Biocef; Keflex®; Keftab®

Synonyms Cephalexin Hydrochloride; Cephalexin Monohydrate

Generic Available Yes

Pharmacologic Category Antibiotic, Cephalosporin (First Generation)

Pregnancy Risk Factor B

Lactation Enters breast milk (small amounts)/use caution

Use Treatment of susceptible bacterial infections, including those caused by group A beta-hemolytic *Streptococcus, Staphylococcus, Klebsiella pneumoniae, E. coli, Proteus mirabilis*, and *Shigella*; predominantly used for lower respiratory tract, urinary tract, skin and soft tissue, and bone and joint; prophylaxis against bacterial endocarditis in high-risk patients undergoing surgical or dental procedures who are allergic to penicillin

Mechanism of Action/Effect Inhibits bacterial cell wall synthesis by binding to one or more of the penicillin-binding proteins (PBPs)

Contraindications Hypersensitivity to cephalexin, any component of the formulation, or other cephalosporins

Warnings/Precautions Modify dosage in patients with severe renal impairment. Prolonged use may result in superinfection. Cross-sensitivity to penicillins exists (~10%).

Drug Interactions

Increased Effect/Toxicity: High-dose probenecid may decrease clearance of cephalexin. Aminoglycosides in combination with cephalexin may result in additive nephrotoxicity.

Nutritional/Ethanol Interactions Food: Peak antibiotic serum concentration is lowered and delayed, but total drug absorbed is not affected. Cephalexin serum levels may be decreased if taken with food.

Effects on Lab Values Positive direct Coombs', false-positive urinary glucose test using cupric sulfate (Benedict's solution, Clinitest®, Fehling's solution), false-positive serum or urine creatinine with Jaffé reaction

Adverse Reactions

1% to 10%: Gastrointestinal: Diarrhea

<1% (Limited to important or life-threatening): Abdominal pain, agitation, anaphylaxis, anemia, angioedema, arthralgia, cholestasis, confusion, dizziness, dyspepsia, eosinophilia, erythema multiforme, fatigue, gastritis, hallucinations, headache, hepatitis, interstitial nephritis, nausea, neutropenia, pseudomembranous colitis, rash, serum-sickness reaction, Stevens-Johnson syndrome, thrombocytopenia, toxic epidermal necrolysis, transaminases increased, urticaria, vomiting

Other reactions with cephalosporins include agranulocytosis, anaphylaxis, aplastic anemia, asterixis, colitis, encephalopathy, hemolytic anemia, hemorrhage, neuromuscular excitability, pancytopenia, prolonged PT, seizures, superinfection, vomiting

Overdosage/Toxicology Symptoms of overdose include neuromuscular hypersensitivity and convulsions. Many beta-lactam containing antibiotics have the potential to cause neuromuscular hyperirritability or convulsive seizures. Hemodialysis may be helpful to aid in removal of the drug from blood; otherwise, treatment is supportive or symptom-directed.

Pharmacodynamics/Kinetics

Absorption: Delayed in young children; may be decreased up to 50% in neonates

Half-Life Elimination: Neonates: 5 hours old; Children 3-12 months: 2.5 hours; Adults: 0.5-1.2 hours; prolonged with renal impairment

(Continued)

Cephalexin *(Continued)*

Time to Peak: Serum: ~1 hour

Formulations

Capsule, as monohydrate: 250 mg, 500 mg
Tablet, as hydrochloride: 500 mg
Tablet, as monohydrate: 250 mg, 500 mg, 1 g
Powder for oral suspension, as monohydrate: 125 mg/5 mL (5 mL unit dose, 60 mL, 100 mL, 200 mL); 250 mg/5 mL (5 mL unit dose, 100 mL, 200 mL)

Dosing

Adults & Elderly:

Usual dose: Oral: 250-1000 mg every 6 hours; maximum: 4 g/day
Streptococcal pharyngitis, skin/skin structure infections, or uncomplicated cystitis: Oral: 500 mg every 6 hours
Severe infections: Oral: up to 1 g every 6 hours (**Note:** Consider parenteral agents in situations where high doses are needed.)
SBE prophylaxis (dental, oral, respiratory, or esophageal procedures): Oral: 2 g 1 hour before procedure

Pediatrics:

Usual dose: Oral: Children: 25-50 mg/kg/day every 6 hours; severe infections: 50-100 mg/kg/day in divided doses every 6 hours; maximum: 3 g/24 hours
Otitis media: Oral: Children ≥1 year of age: 75-100 mg/kg/day in 4 divided doses
Streptococcal pharyngitis, skin/skin structure infections, or uncomplicated cystitis: Oral:
>1-15 years: Total daily dose may be divided every 12 hours
≥15 years: Refer to adult dosing.
Note: Administer for at least 10 days in the treatment of beta-hemolytic strep.
SBE prophylaxis (dental, oral, respiratory, or esophageal procedures): Oral: 50 mg/kg 1 hour before procedure

Renal Impairment:

Cl_{cr} >50 mL/minute: Administer every 8 hours.
Cl_{cr} 10-50 mL/minute: Administer every 12 hours.
Cl_{cr} <10 mL/minute: Administer every 12-24 hours.
Moderately dialyzable (20% to 50%)

Administration

Oral: Take without regard to food. If GI distress, take with food. Give around-the-clock to promote less variation in peak and trough serum levels.

Stability

Reconstitution: Refrigerate suspension after reconstitution; discard after 14 days.

Monitoring Laboratory Tests Renal, hepatic, and hematologic function periodically with prolonged therapy; perform culture and sensitivity studies prior to initiating drug therapy.

Monitoring and Teaching Issues

Physical Assessment: Assess for previous allergy history prior to therapy. See Contraindications, Warnings/Precautions, and Dosing for use cautions. Assess potential for interactions with other prescriptions, OTC medications, or herbal products patient may be taking (see Drug Interactions). Assess results of laboratory tests (see above), therapeutic response, and adverse reactions (eg, hypersensitivity can occur several days after therapy is started - see Adverse Reactions and Overdose/Toxicology). Instruct diabetic patients regarding Clinitest®. Teach patient proper use, possible side effects and interventions, and adverse symptoms to report (see Patient Education). Note breast-feeding caution.

Patient Education: Inform prescriber of all prescriptions, OTC medications, or herbal products you are taking, and any allergies you have. Do not take anything new during treatment unless approved by prescriber. Take as directed, at regular intervals around-the-clock (with or without food). Chilling oral suspension improves flavor (do not freeze). Maintain adequate hydration (2-3 L/day of fluids) unless advised by prescriber to restrict fluids. Complete full course of medication, even if you feel better. May cause false test results with Clinitest®; use of another type of glucose testing is preferable. May cause diarrhea (buttermilk, boiled milk, or yogurt may help). Report unresolved diarrhea; unusual bruising or bleeding; changes in urinary pattern; or opportunistic infection (vaginal itching or drainage, sores in mouth, blood in urine or stool). **Breast-feeding precaution:** Consult prescriber if breast-feeding.

Dietary Issues: Take without regard to food. If GI distress, take with food.

Geriatric Considerations: Adjust dose for renal function.

Breast-feeding Issues: Theoretically, drug absorbed by nursing infant may change bowel flora or affect fever work-up result. **Note:** As a class, cephalosporins are used to treat infections in infants.

Cephalexin Hydrochloride *see* Cephalexin *on page 259*
Cephalexin Monohydrate *see* Cephalexin *on page 259*

Cephapirin (sef a PYE rin)

U.S. Brand Names Cefadyl®

Synonyms Cephapirin Sodium

Generic Available No

Pharmacologic Category Antibiotic, Cephalosporin (First Generation)

Pregnancy Risk Factor B

Lactation Enters breast milk (small amounts)/use caution

Use Treatment of infections when caused by susceptible strains in respiratory, genitourinary, gastrointestinal, skin and soft tissue, bone and joint infections, septicemia; treatment of susceptible gram-positive bacilli and cocci (never enterococcus); some gram-negative bacilli including *E. coli*, *Proteus*, and *Klebsiella* may be susceptible

Mechanism of Action/Effect Inhibits bacterial cell wall synthesis by binding to one or more of the penicillin-binding proteins (PBPs)

Contraindications Hypersensitivity to cephapirin sodium, any component of the formulation, or other cephalosporins

Warnings/Precautions Modify dosage in patients with severe renal impairment. Prolonged use may result in superinfection. Cross-sensitivity to penicillins exists (~10%).

Drug Interactions

Increased Effect/Toxicity: High-dose probenecid decreases clearance of cephapirin. Aminoglycosides in combination with cephapirin may result in additive nephrotoxicity.

Effects on Lab Values Positive direct Coombs', false-positive urinary glucose test using cupric sulfate (Benedict's solution, Clinitest®, Fehling's solution), false-positive serum or urine creatinine with Jaffé reaction

Adverse Reactions

1% to 10%: Gastrointestinal: Diarrhea

<1% (Limited to important or life-threatening): CNS irritation, fever, leukopenia, rash, seizures, thrombocytopenia, transaminases increased, urticaria

Other reactions with cephalosporins include agranulocytosis, anaphylaxis, angioedema, aplastic anemia, asterixis, cholestasis, dizziness, encephalopathy, erythema multiforme, fever, headache, hemoglobin decreased, hemolytic anemia, hemorrhage, interstitial nephritis, nausea, neuromuscular excitability, pain at injection site, pancytopenia, prolonged PT, pseudomembranous colitis, seizures, serum-sickness reactions, Stevens-Johnson syndrome, superinfection, toxic epidermal necrolysis, toxic nephropathy, vaginitis, vomiting

Overdosage/Toxicology Symptoms of overdose include neuromuscular hypersensitivity and convulsions. Many beta-lactam containing antibiotics have the potential to cause neuromuscular hyperirritability or convulsive seizures. Hemodialysis may be helpful to aid in removal of the drug from blood; otherwise, treatment is supportive or symptom-directed.

Pharmacodynamics/Kinetics

Half-Life Elimination: 36-60 minutes

Time to Peak: Serum: I.M.: ~30 minutes; I.V.: ~5 minutes

Metabolism: Partially hepatic, renal, and in plasma to metabolites (50% active)

Formulations Injection, powder for reconstitution, as sodium: 500 mg, 1 g, 2 g, 4 g

Dosing

Adults & Elderly:

Usual dose: I.M., I.V.: 500 mg to 1 g every 6 hours up to 12 g/day

Perioperative prophylaxis: 1-2 g 30 minutes to 1 hour prior to surgery and every 6 hours as needed for 24 hours following

Pediatrics: Usual dose: I.M., I.V.: Children: 10-20 mg/kg/dose every 6 hours up to 4 g/24 hours

Renal Impairment:

Cl_{cr} 10-50 mL/minute: Administer every 6-8 hours.

Cl_{cr} <10 mL/minute: Administer every 12 hours.

Continuous arteriovenous hemofiltration: Administer 1 g every 8 hours.

Administration

I.M.: Inject deep I.M. into large muscle mass.

I.V.: Inject direct I.V. over 3-5 minutes. Infuse intermittent infusion over 15-30 minutes.

Stability

Reconstitution: Reconstituted solution is stable for 24 hours at room temperature and 10 days when refrigerated. For I.V. infusion in NS or D_5W, solution is stable for 24 hours at room temperature, 10 days when refrigerated or 14 days when frozen. After freezing, thawed solution is stable for 12 hours at room temperature or 10 days when refrigerated.

Compatibility: Discontinue other solutions at the same site to avoid compatibility problems.

Monitoring Laboratory Tests Prothrombin time; perform culture and sensitivity studies prior to initiating drug therapy.

Monitoring and Teaching Issues

Physical Assessment: Assess for previous allergy history prior to therapy. See Contraindications and Warnings/Precautions for use cautions. Assess potential for interactions with other prescriptions, OTC medications, or herbal products patient may be taking (eg, nephrotoxicity - see Drug Interactions). Assess results of laboratory tests (see above), therapeutic response, and adverse reactions (eg, hypersensitivity can occur several days after therapy is started - see Adverse Reactions and Overdose/Toxicology). Instruct diabetic patients regarding Clinitest®. Teach patient possible side effects and interventions and adverse symptoms to report (see Patient Education). Note breast-feeding caution.

Patient Education: Inform prescriber of all prescriptions, OTC medications, or herbal products you are taking, and any allergies you have. Do not take anything new during treatment unless approved by prescriber. This medication is administered by infusion or injection. Report immediately any redness, swelling, burning, or pain at injection/infusion site; itching or hives; or difficulty swallowing or breathing. Maintain adequate hydration (2-3 L/day of fluids) unless advised by prescriber to restrict fluids. May cause false test results with Clinitest®; use of another type of glucose testing is preferable. May cause diarrhea (buttermilk, boiled milk, or yogurt may help). Report unresolved diarrhea; opportunistic infection (vaginal itching or drainage; sores in mouth; blood, pus, or mucus in stool or urine; easy bleeding or bruising); changes in urinary pattern (decreased urine); headache; or CNS changes. **Breast-feeding precaution:** Consult prescriber if breast-feeding.

Dietary Issues: Sodium content of 1 g: 55.2 mg (2.4 mEq)

Geriatric Considerations: Cephapirin has not been studied in the elderly. Adjust dose for renal function.

Breast-feeding Issues: Theoretically, drug absorbed by nursing infant may change bowel flora or affect fever work-up result. **Note:** As a class, cephalosporins are used to treat infections in infants.

Cephapirin Sodium *see* Cephapirin *on page 260*

Cephradine (SEF ra deen)

U.S. Brand Names Velosef®

Generic Available Yes

Pharmacologic Category Antibiotic, Cephalosporin (First Generation)

(Continued)

Cephradine *(Continued)*

Pregnancy Risk Factor B

Lactation Enters breast milk/use caution

Use Treatment of infections when caused by susceptible strains in respiratory, genitourinary, gastrointestinal, skin and soft tissue, bone and joint infections; treatment of susceptible gram-positive bacilli and cocci (never enterococcus); some gram-negative bacilli including *E. coli*, *Proteus*, and *Klebsiella* may be susceptible

Mechanism of Action/Effect Inhibits bacterial cell wall synthesis by binding to one or more of the penicillin-binding proteins (PBPs)

Contraindications Hypersensitivity to cephradine, any component of the formulation, or cephalosporins

Warnings/Precautions Prolonged use may result in superinfection. Use with caution in patients with a history of colitis. Reduce dose in patients with renal dysfunction. Cross-sensitivity to penicillins exists (~10%).

Drug Interactions

Increased Effect/Toxicity: High-dose probenecid decreases clearance of cephradine. Aminoglycosides in combination with cephradine may result in additive nephrotoxicity.

Nutritional/Ethanol Interactions Food: Food delays cephradine absorption but does not decrease extent.

Effects on Lab Values Positive direct Coombs', false-positive urinary glucose test using cupric sulfate (Benedict's solution, Clinitest®, Fehling's solution), false-positive serum or urine creatinine with Jaffé reaction

Adverse Reactions

1% to 10%: Gastrointestinal: Diarrhea

<1% (Limited to important or life-threatening): BUN increased, creatinine increased, nausea, pseudomembranous colitis, rash, vomiting

Other reactions with cephalosporins include agranulocytosis, anaphylaxis, angioedema, aplastic anemia, asterixis, cholestasis, dizziness, encephalopathy, erythema multiforme, fever, headache, hemolytic anemia, hemorrhage, interstitial nephritis, leukopenia, neuromuscular excitability, neutropenia, pancytopenia, prolonged PT, seizures, serum-sickness reactions, Stevens-Johnson syndrome, superinfection, toxic epidermal necrolysis, toxic nephropathy, vaginitis

Overdosage/Toxicology Symptoms of overdose include neuromuscular hypersensitivity and convulsions. Many beta-lactam containing antibiotics have the potential to cause neuromuscular hyperirritability or convulsive seizures. Hemodialysis may be helpful to aid in removal of the drug from blood; otherwise, treatment is supportive or symptom-directed.

Pharmacodynamics/Kinetics

Absorption: Well absorbed

Half-Life Elimination: 1-2 hours; prolonged with renal impairment

Time to Peak: Serum: 1-2 hours

Formulations

Capsule: 250 mg, 500 mg

Powder for oral suspension: 125 mg/5 mL (5 mL, 100 mL, 200 mL); 250 mg/5 mL (5 mL, 100 mL, 200 mL)

Dosing

Adults & Elderly: Susceptible infections, usual dose:

Oral: 250-500 mg every 6-12 hours

Pediatrics: Usual dose: Oral: Children ≥9 months: 25-50 mg/kg/day in divided doses every 6 hours

Renal Impairment:

Cl_{cr} 10-50 mL/minute: Administer 50% of dose.

Cl_{cr} <10 mL/minute: Administer 25% of dose.

Administration

Oral: Administer around-the-clock to promote less variation in peak and trough serum levels. Shake oral suspension well.

Stability

Reconstitution:

Oral suspension: Refrigerated storage maintains potency for 14 days. Room temperature storage maintains potency for 7 days.

Compatibility: Incompatible with LR

Do not mix with other antibiotics.

Monitoring Laboratory Tests Prothrombin time; perform culture and sensitivity studies prior to initiating drug therapy.

Monitoring and Teaching Issues

Physical Assessment: Assess for previous allergy history prior to therapy. See Contraindications and Warnings/Precautions for use cautions. Assess potential for interactions with other prescriptions, OTC medications, or herbal products patient may be taking (see Drug Interactions). Assess results of laboratory tests (see above), therapeutic response, and adverse reactions (eg, hypersensitivity can occur several days after therapy is started - see Adverse Reactions and Overdose/Toxicology). Instruct diabetic patients regarding Clinitest®. Teach patient proper use, possible side effects and interventions, and adverse symptoms to report (see Patient Education). Note breast-feeding caution.

Patient Education: Inform prescriber of all prescriptions, OTC medications, or herbal products you are taking, and any allergies you have. Do not take anything new during treatment with without consulting prescriber. Take as directed, at regular intervals around-the-clock (with or without food). Chilling oral suspension improves flavor (do not freeze). Maintain adequate hydration (2-3 L/day of fluids) unless advised by prescriber to restrict fluids. Complete full course of medication, even if you feel better. May cause false test results with Clinitest®; use of another type of glucose testing is preferable. May cause diarrhea (buttermilk, boiled milk, or yogurt may help). Report unresolved, persistent diarrhea; unusual bruising or bleeding; changes in urinary pattern (decreased output); persistent nausea, vomiting, or abdominal pain; opportunistic infection (vaginal itching or drainage, sores in mouth, blood in urine or stool); or redness, swelling, burning, or pain at injection site. **Breast-feeding precaution:** Consult prescriber if breast-feeding.

Dietary Issues: May administer with food to decrease GI distress.

Geriatric Considerations: Cephradine has not been studied in the elderly. Adjust dose for renal function in the elderly.

Breast-feeding Issues: Theoretically, drug absorbed by nursing infant may change bowel flora or affect fever work-up result. **Note:** As a class, cephalosporins are used to treat infections in infants.

Ceptaz® *see* Ceftazidime *on page 249*

Cerebyx® *see* Fosphenytoin *on page 607*

Ceredase® *see* Alglucerase *on page 58*

Certiva® *see page 1498*

Cerubidine® *see* DAUNOrubicin Hydrochloride *on page 369*

Cerumenex® *see page 1519*

Cervidil® *see* Dinoprostone *on page 421*

C.E.S. *see* Estrogens (Conjugated/Equine) *on page 503*

Cetacort® *see* Hydrocortisone *on page 673*

Cetacort® *see* Topical Corticosteroids *on page 1334*

Cetafen® [OTC] *see* Acetaminophen *on page 35*

Cetafen Extra® [OTC] *see* Acetaminophen *on page 35*

Cetamide® *see page 1509*

Cetamide® *see* Sulfacetamide *on page 1256*

Ceta-Plus® *see* Hydrocodone and Acetaminophen *on page 667*

Cetapred® *see page 1509*

Cetirizine (se TI ra zeen)

U.S. Brand Names Zyrtec®

Synonyms Cetirizine Hydrochloride; P-071; UCB-P071

Generic Available No

Pharmacologic Category Antihistamine

Pregnancy Risk Factor B

Lactation Enters breast milk/not recommended

Use Perennial and seasonal allergic rhinitis and other allergic symptoms including urticaria; chronic idiopathic urticaria

Mechanism of Action/Effect Competes with histamine for H_1-receptor sites on effector cells in the GI tract, blood vessels, and respiratory tract

Contraindications Hypersensitivity to cetirizine, hydroxyzine, or any component of the formulation

Warnings/Precautions Cetirizine should be used cautiously in patients with hepatic or renal dysfunction, or the elderly. Doses >10 mg/day may cause significant drowsiness.

Drug Interactions

Cytochrome P450 Effect: Substrate of CYP3A4

Increased Effect/Toxicity: Increased toxicity with CNS depressants and anticholinergics.

Nutritional/Ethanol Interactions Ethanol: Avoid ethanol (may increase CNS depression).

Adverse Reactions

>10%: Central nervous system: Headache has been reported to occur in 10% to 12% of patients, drowsiness has been reported in as much as 26% of patients on high doses

1% to 10%:

Central nervous system: Somnolence, fatigue, dizziness

Gastrointestinal: Dry mouth

Overdosage/Toxicology Symptoms of overdose include seizures, sedation, and hypotension. There is no specific treatment for antihistamine overdose. Clinical toxicity is due to blockade of cholinergic receptors. For anticholinergic overdose with severe life-threatening symptoms, physostigmine 1-2 mg I.V. slowly, may be given to reverse these effects.

Pharmacodynamics/Kinetics

Absorption: Rapid

Half-Life Elimination: 8-11 hours

Time to Peak: Serum: 30-60 minutes

Metabolism: Limited hepatic

Onset: 15-30 minutes

Formulations

Syrup, as hydrochloride: 5 mg/5 mL (120 mL)

Tablet, as hydrochloride: 5 mg, 10 mg

Dosing

Adults: Allergic rhinitis, urticaria: Oral: 5-10 mg once daily, depending upon symptom severity

Elderly: Oral: Initial: 5 mg once daily; may increase to 10 mg/day; adjust for renal impairment.

Pediatrics: Allergic rhinitis, urticaria: Oral:

Children 2-5 years: Initial dose: 2.5 mg, may be increased to 2.5 mg every 12 hours or up to 5 mg/day

Children ≥6 years: Refer to adult dosing.

Renal Impairment:

Cl_{cr} ≤31 mL/minute: Administer 5 mg once daily.

Hemodialysis: 5 mg once daily

(Continued)

Cetirizine *(Continued)*

Hepatic Impairment: Administer 5 mg once daily.

Administration

Oral: Take without regard to meals.

Monitoring and Teaching Issues

Physical Assessment: Assess effectiveness and interactions of other medications patient may be taking (see Drug Interactions). See Contraindications and Warnings/Precautions for use cautions. Monitor effectiveness of therapy and adverse reactions (see Adverse Reactions) at beginning of therapy and periodically with long-term use. Assess knowledge/teach patient appropriate use, interventions to reduce side effects, and adverse symptoms to report (see Patient Education). Breast-feeding is not recommended.

Patient Education: Take as directed; do not exceed recommended dose. Avoid use of other depressants, alcohol, or sleep-inducing medications unless approved by prescriber. You may experience drowsiness or dizziness (use caution when driving or engaging in tasks requiring alertness until response to drug is known); or dry mouth (small, frequent meals, frequent mouth care, chewing gum, or sucking hard candy may help). Report persistent sedation, confusion, or agitation; persistent nausea or vomiting; changes in urinary pattern; blurred vision; chest pain or palpitations; or lack of improvement or worsening of condition. **Breast-feeding precaution:** Breast-feeding is not recommended.

Geriatric Considerations: Adjust dose for renal function.

Cetirizine Hydrochloride *see* Cetirizine *on page 263*

Cetrorelix (se troh REE liks)

U.S. Brand Names Cetrotide™

Synonyms Cetrorelix Acetate

Generic Available No

Pharmacologic Category Antigonadotropic Agent

Pregnancy Risk Factor X

Lactation Excretion in breast milk unknown/not recommended

Use Inhibits premature luteinizing hormone (LH) surges in women undergoing controlled ovarian stimulation

Mechanism of Action/Effect Competes with naturally occurring GnRH for binding on receptors of the pituitary. This delays luteinizing hormone surge, preventing ovulation until the follicles are of adequate size.

Contraindications Hypersensitivity to cetrorelix or any component of the formulation; extrinsic peptide hormones, mannitol, gonadotropin releasing hormone (GnRH) or GnRH analogs; pregnancy

Warnings/Precautions Should only be prescribed by fertility specialists. Pregnancy should be excluded before treatment is begun.

Drug Interactions

Decreased Effect: No formal studies have been performed.

Increased Effect/Toxicity: No formal studies have been performed.

Adverse Reactions

1% to 10%:

Central nervous system: Headache (1%)

Endocrine & metabolic: Ovarian hyperstimulation syndrome, WHO grade II or III (3%)

Gastrointestinal: Nausea (1%)

Hepatic: Increased ALT, AST, GGT, and alkaline phosphatase (1% to 2%)

Postmarketing and/or case reports: Severe anaphylactic reaction (cough, rash, hypotension) occurred in one patient following several months of treatment in a study not related to fertility. Congenital abnormalities and stillbirths have been reported, however, the relationship to cetrorelix treatment has not been established. Local injection site reactions (bruising, erythema, itching, pruritus, redness, swelling) have also been reported.

Overdosage/Toxicology No cases of overdose have been reported. In nonfertility studies, single doses of up to 120 mg have been well tolerated.

Pharmacodynamics/Kinetics

Absorption: Rapid

Bioavailability: 85%

Half-Life Elimination: 0.25 mg dose: 5 hours; 0.25 mg multiple doses: 20.6 hours; 3 mg dose: 62.8 hours

Time to Peak: 0.25 mg dose: 1 hour; 3 mg dose: 1.5 hours

Metabolism: Transformed by peptidases; cetrorelix and peptides (1-9), (1-7), (1-6), and (1-4) are found in the bile; peptide (1-4) is the predominant metabolite

Onset: 0.25 mg dose: 2 hours; 3 mg dose: 1 hour

Duration: 3 mg dose (single dose): 4 days

Formulations

Injection [prefilled glass syringe; single-dose vial]:

0.25 mg with 1 mL SWFI

3 mg with 3 mL SWFI

Dosing

Adults: Controlled ovarian stimulation in conjunction with gonadotropins (FSH, HMG):

Female: S.C.:

Single-dose regimen: 3 mg given when serum estradiol levels show appropriate stimulation response, usually stimulation day 7 (range days 5-9). If hCG is not administered within 4 days, continue cetrorelix at 0.25 mg/day until hCG is administered

Multiple-dose regimen: 0.25 mg morning or evening of stimulation day 5, or morning of stimulation day 6; continue until hCG is administered.

Elderly: Not intended for use in women ≥65 years of age (Phase 2 and Phase 3 studies included women 19-40 years of age).

Administration

Other: Cetrorelix is administered by S.C. injection following proper aseptic technique procedures. Injections should be to the lower abdomen, preferably around the navel. The injection site should be rotated daily. The needle should be inserted completely into the skin at a 45-degree angle.

Stability

Storage: Store in outer carton. Once mixed, solution should be used immediately.

0.25 mg vials: Store under refrigeration at 2°C to 8°C (36°F to 46°F).

3 mg vials: Store at controlled room temperature at 25°C (77°F).

Monitoring Laboratory Tests Ultrasound to assess follicle size

Monitoring and Teaching Issues

Physical Assessment: This medication should only be prescribed by a fertility specialist. Assess/teach patient use (if medication is to self-administered - demonstrate injection procedures, syringe disposal), interventions to reduce side-effects, and adverse reactions to report (see Adverse Reactions). **Pregnancy risk factor X** - pregnancy must be excluded before starting medication. Breast-feeding is not recommended.

Patient Education: This drug can only be given by injection as demonstrated. An instructional leaflet will be provided if you will be administering this medication to yourself. Instructions will be given on how to administer S.C. injections and proper disposal of syringes and needles. Give at a similar time each day as instructed by prescriber. Do not skip any doses. If you miss an injection, do not double next dose; contact your prescriber. You must keep all scheduled ultrasound appointments. Store in refrigerator in outer carton. Solution should be used immediately after mixing. You may experience headache (use of mild analgesic may help); or nausea (small, frequent meals, good mouth care, chewing gum, or sucking hard candy may help). Report immediately any sudden or acute abdominal pain; shortness of breath; vaginal bleeding; or pain, itching, or signs of infection at injection site. **Pregnancy/breast-feeding precautions:** Do not get pregnant and do not breast-feed while taking this drug.

Pregnancy Issues: Animal studies have shown fetal resorption and implantation losses following administration. Resorption resulting in fetal loss would be expected if used in a pregnant woman.

Cetrorelix Acetate *see* Cetrorelix *on page 264*

Cetrotide™ *see* Cetrorelix *on page 264*

Cevimeline (se vi ME leen)

U.S. Brand Names Evoxac™

Synonyms Cevimeline Hydrochloride

Generic Available No

Pharmacologic Category Cholinergic Agonist

Pregnancy Risk Factor C

Lactation Excretion in breast milk unknown/not recommended

Use Treatment of symptoms of dry mouth in patients with Sjögren's syndrome

Mechanism of Action/Effect Binds to muscarinic (cholinergic) receptors, causing an increase in secretion of exocrine glands (including salivary glands)

Contraindications Hypersensitivity to cevimeline or any component of the formulation; uncontrolled asthma; narrow-angle glaucoma; acute iritis; other conditions where miosis is undesirable

Warnings/Precautions May alter cardiac conduction and/or heart rate; use caution in patients with significant cardiovascular disease, including angina, myocardial infarction, or conduction disturbances. Use with caution in patients with controlled asthma, COPD, or chronic bronchitis. May cause decreased visual acuity (particularly at night and in patients with central lens changes) and impaired depth perception. May cause a variety of parasympathomimetic effects, which may be particularly dangerous in elderly patients; excessive sweating may lead to dehydration in some patients.

Use with caution in patients with a history of biliary stones or nephrolithiasis; cevimeline may precipitate cholangitis, cholecystitis, biliary obstruction, renal colic, or ureteral reflux in susceptible patients. Patients with a known or suspected deficiency of CYP2D6 may be at higher risk of adverse effects. Safety and efficacy have not been established in pediatric patients.

Pregnancy risk C.

Drug Interactions

Cytochrome P450 Effect: Substrate of CYP2D6, CYP3A4

Decreased Effect: Anticholinergic agents (atropine, TCAs, phenothiazines) may antagonize the effects of cevimeline.

Increased Effect/Toxicity: Drugs which inhibit CYP2D6 (including amiodarone, fluoxetine, paroxetine, quinidine, ritonavir) or CYP3A4 (including diltiazem, erythromycin, itraconazole, ketoconazole, verapamil) may increase levels of cevimeline. The effects of other cholinergic agents may be increased during concurrent administration with cevimeline. Concurrent use of cevimeline and beta-blockers may increase the potential for conduction disturbances.

Adverse Reactions

>10%:

Central nervous system: Headache (14%; placebo 20%)

Gastrointestinal: Nausea (14%), diarrhea (10%)

Respiratory: Rhinitis (11%), sinusitis (12%), upper respiratory infection (11%)

Miscellaneous: Increased diaphoresis (19%)

1% to 10%:

Cardiovascular: Peripheral edema, chest pain, edema, palpitation

Central nervous system: Dizziness (4%), fatigue (3%), pain (3%), insomnia (2%), anxiety (1%), fever, depression, migraine, vertigo

Dermatologic: Rash (4%; placebo 6%), pruritus, skin disorder, erythematous rash

Endocrine & metabolic: Hot flashes (2%)

(Continued)

Cevimeline *(Continued)*

Gastrointestinal: Dyspepsia (8%; placebo 9%), abdominal pain (8%), vomiting (5%), excessive salivation (2%), constipation, salivary gland pain, dry mouth, sialoadenitis, ulcerative stomatitis

Genitourinary: Urinary tract infection (6%), vaginitis, cystitis

Hematologic: Anemia

Local: Abscess

Neuromuscular & skeletal: back pain (5%), arthralgia (4%), skeletal pain (3%), rigors (1%), hypertonia, tremor, myalgia

Ocular: Conjunctivitis (4%), abnormal vision, eye pain, eye abnormality, xerophthalmia

Otic: Earache, otitis media

Respiratory: Coughing (6%), bronchitis (4%), pneumonia, epistaxis

Miscellaneous: Flu-like syndrome, infection, fungal infection, allergy, hiccups

<1% (Limited to important or life-threatening): Aggravated multiple sclerosis, aggressive behavior, alopecia, angina, anterior chamber hemorrhage, aphasia, apnea, arrhythmia, arthropathy, avascular necrosis (femoral head), bronchospasm, bullous eruption, bundle branch block, cholelithiasis, coma, deafness, delirium, depersonalization, dyskinesia, eosinophilia, esophageal stricture, esophagitis, fall, gastric ulcer, gastrointestinal hemorrhage, gingival hyperplasia, glaucoma, granulocytopenia, hallucination, hematuria, hypothyroidism, ileus, impotence, intestinal obstruction, leukopenia, lymphocytosis, manic reaction, myocardial infarction, neuropathy, paralysis, paranoia, paresthesia, peptic ulcer, pericarditis, peripheral ischemia, photosensitivity reaction, pleural effusion, pulmonary embolism, pulmonary fibrosis, renal calculus, seizure, sepsis, somnolence, syncope, systemic lupus erythematosus, tenosynovitis, thrombocytopenia, thrombocytopenic purpura, thrombophlebitis, T-wave inversion, urinary retention, vasculitis

Overdosage/Toxicology Symptoms of toxicity may include headache, visual disturbances, lacrimation, sweating, gastrointestinal spasm, nausea, vomiting, diarrhea, AV block, mental confusion, tremor, cardiac depression, bradycardia, tachycardia, or bronchospasm. Atropine may be of value as an antidote, and epinephrine may be required for bronchoconstriction. Additional treatment is supportive. The effect of hemodialysis is unknown.

Pharmacodynamics/Kinetics

Half-Life Elimination: 5 hours

Time to Peak: 1.5-2 hours

Metabolism: Hepatic via CYP2D6 and CYP3A4

Formulations Capsule: 30 mg

Dosing

Adults & Elderly: Xerostomia (in Sjögren's syndrome): Oral: 30 mg 3 times/day

Stability

Storage: Store at 25°C (77°F).

Monitoring and Teaching Issues

Physical Assessment: Assess other medications patient may be taking for effectiveness and interactions (see Drug Interactions). See Contraindications and Warnings/Precautions for use cautions. Monitor for therapeutic effect and adverse reactions (especially with elderly persons) (see Adverse Reactions and Overdose/Toxicology). Assess knowledge/teach patient appropriate use, interventions to reduce side effects, and adverse reactions to report (see Patient Education). **Pregnancy risk factor C** - benefits of use should outweigh possible risks. Breast-feeding is not recommended.

Patient Education: Take exactly as directed; do not alter dosage without consulting prescriber. Take with or without food. You may experience decreased visual acuity (especially at night) (use caution when driving at night or when engaging in other activities in poorly lighted areas until response to medication is known); GI distress or nausea (small, frequent meals, frequent mouth care, sucking lozenges, or chewing gum may help); headache (mild analgesic may help); or diarrhea (boiled milk, yogurt, or buttermilk may help). Report unresolved diarrhea or constipation, abdominal pain, flatulence, anorexia, or excessive salivation; excessive sweating; unresolved respiratory distress, runny nose, cold or flu symptoms; joint, bone, or muscle weakness, pain, tremor, or cramping; chest pain or palpitations, swelling of extremities, weight gain; or other persistent adverse symptoms. **Pregnancy/breast-feeding precautions:** Inform prescriber if you are or intend to become pregnant. Breast-feeding is not recommended.

Dietary Issues: Take with or without food.

Cevimeline Hydrochloride *see* Cevimeline *on page 265*

CFDN *see* Cefdinir *on page 235*

CG *see* Chorionic Gonadotropin (Human) *on page 284*

CGP-42446 *see* Zoledronic Acid *on page 1427*

CGP 57148B *see* Imatinib *on page 695*

CharcoAid® [OTC] *see* Charcoal *on page 266*

Charcoal (CHAR kole)

U.S. Brand Names Actidose® [OTC]; Actidose-Aqua® [OTC]; CharcoAid® [OTC]; Charcocaps® [OTC]; Liqui-Char® [OTC]

Synonyms Activated Carbon; Activated Charcoal; Adsorbent Charcoal; Liquid Antidote; Medicinal Carbon; Medicinal Charcoal

Generic Available Yes

Pharmacologic Category Antidiarrheal; Antidote; Antiflatulent

Pregnancy Risk Factor C

Lactation Does not enter breast milk/compatible

Use Emergency treatment in poisoning by drugs and chemicals; repetitive doses for gastric dialysis in uremia to adsorb various waste products, and repetitive doses have proven useful to enhance the elimination of certain drugs (eg, theophylline, phenobarbital, and aspirin)

Mechanism of Action/Effect Adsorbs toxic substances or irritants, thus inhibiting GI absorption; adsorbs intestinal gas; the addition of sorbitol results in hyperosmotic laxative action causing catharsis

Contraindications Not effective for cyanide, mineral acids, caustic alkalis, organic solvents, iron, ethanol, methanol poisoning, lithium; do not use charcoal with sorbitol in patients with fructose intolerance; charcoal with sorbitol is not recommended in children <1 year.

Warnings/Precautions When using ipecac with charcoal, induce vomiting with ipecac before administering activated charcoal since charcoal adsorbs ipecac syrup. Charcoal may cause vomiting which is hazardous in petroleum distillate and caustic ingestions. If charcoal in sorbitol is administered, doses should be limited to prevent excessive fluid and electrolyte losses. Do not mix charcoal with milk, ice cream, or sherbet. Pregnancy risk C.

Drug Interactions

Decreased Effect: Charcoal decreases the effect of ipecac syrup. Charcoal effect is reduced when taken with milk, ice cream, or sherbet.

Nutritional/Ethanol Interactions Food: Milk, ice cream, sherbet, or marmalade may reduce charcoal's effectiveness.

Adverse Reactions >10%:

Gastrointestinal: Vomiting, diarrhea with sorbitol, constipation
Miscellaneous: Stools will turn black

Formulations

Capsule (Charcocaps®): 260 mg
Granules, activated (CharcoAid®-G): 15 g (120 mL)
Liquid, activated:
- Actidose-Aqua®: 15 g (72 mL); 25 g (120 mL); 50 g (240 mL)
- CharcoAid® 2000: 15 g (72 mL); 50 g (240 mL)
- Liqui-Char®: 15 g (75 mL); 25 g (120 mL); 30 g (120 mL)

Liquid, activated [with propylene glycol]: 12.5 g (60 mL); 25 g (120 mL)
Liquid, activated [with sorbitol]:
- Actidose®: 25 g (120 mL); 50 g (240 mL)
- CharcoAid® 2000: 15 g (72 mL); 50 g (240 mL)
- Liqui-Char®: 25 g (120 mL); 50 g (240 mL)

Powder for suspension, activated: 15 g, 30 g, 40 g, 120 g, 240 g

Dosing

Adults & Elderly:

Acute poisoning: Oral:
- Charcoal with sorbitol: Single-dose: 30-100 g
- Charcoal in water:
  - Single-dose: 30-100 g or 1-2 g/kg
  - Multiple-dose: 20-60 g or 0.5-1 g/kg every 2-6 hours

Gastric dialysis: Oral: 20-50 g every 6 hours for 1-2 days
Intestinal gas, diarrhea, GI distress: Oral: 520-975 mg after meals or at first sign of discomfort; repeat as needed to a maximum dose of 4.16 g/day

Pediatrics: Acute poisoning: Oral:

Charcoal with sorbitol: Single-dose:
- 1-12 years: 1-2 g/kg/dose or 15-30 g or approximately 5-10 times the weight of the ingested poison; 1 g adsorbs 100-1000 mg of poison; the use of repeat oral charcoal with sorbitol doses is not recommended. In young children, sorbitol should be repeated no more than 1-2 times/day.

Charcoal in water:
- Single-dose:
  - <1 year: 1 g/kg
  - 1-12 years: 15-30 g or 1-2 g/kg
- Multiple-dose:
  - <1 year: 0.5 g/kg every 4-6 hours
  - 1-12 years: 20-60 g or 0.5-1 g/kg every 2-6 hours until clinical observations, serum drug concentration have returned to a subtherapeutic range, or charcoal stool apparent.

Administration

Oral: Too concentrated of mixture may clog airway. Flavoring agents (eg, chocolate) and sorbitol can enhance charcoal's palatability. Marmalade, milk, ice cream, and sherbet should be avoided since they can reduce charcoal's effectiveness. If treatment includes ipecac syrup, induce vomiting prior to administration of charcoal.

Stability

Storage: Adsorbs gases from air, store in closed container.

Monitoring and Teaching Issues

Physical Assessment: Monitor for active bowel sounds prior to administration. If antidote treatment includes ipecac syrup, induce vomiting before administering charcoal. May be administered with sorbitol or chocolate to improve palatability; do not administer with milk products. **Pregnancy risk factor C.**

Patient Education: Charcoal will cause your stools to turn black. Do not self-administer as an antidote before calling the poison control center, hospital emergency room, or physician for instructions (charcoal is not the antidote for all poisons). **Pregnancy precaution:** Inform prescriber if you are pregnant.

Charcocaps® [OTC] *see* Charcoal *on page 266*
Chemet® *see page 1460*
Chenix® *see* Chenodiol *on page 267*
Chenodeoxycholic Acid *see* Chenodiol *on page 267*

Chenodiol (kee noe DYE ole)

U.S. Brand Names Chenix®
Synonyms Chenodeoxycholic Acid
Generic Available No
Pharmacologic Category Bile Acid
(Continued)

Chenodiol *(Continued)*

Pregnancy Risk Factor X

Lactation Excretion in breast milk unknown/not recommended

Use Orphan drug: Oral dissolution of cholesterol gallstones in selected patients

Mechanism of Action/Effect Reduces the synthesis of cholesterol and choline acid in the liver; this leads to cholesterol in bile and results in breakdown of cholesterol gallstones

Contraindications Presence of known hepatocyte dysfunction or bile ductal abnormalities; a gallbladder confirmed as nonvisualizing after two consecutive single doses of dye; radiopaque stones; gallstone complications or compelling reasons for gallbladder surgery; inflammatory bowel disease or active gastric or duodenal ulcer; pregnancy

Warnings/Precautions Chenodiol is hepatotoxic in animal models including subhuman Primates. Chenodiol should be discontinued if aminotransferases exceed 3 times the upper normal limit. Chenodiol may contribute to colon cancer in otherwise susceptible individuals.

Drug Interactions

Decreased Effect: Antacids, cholestyramine, colestipol, and oral contraceptives exhibit decreased effectiveness when taken with chenodiol.

Effects on Lab Values ↑ aminotransferases, cholesterol, LDL-cholesterol, bilirubin (I); ↓ triglycerides

Adverse Reactions

>10%: Gastrointestinal: Diarrhea (mild and transient)

<1% (Limited to important or life-threatening): Anorexia, constipation, cramps, diarrhea (severe), frequent urge for bowel movement, hypertransaminasemia (transient), nausea, vomiting

Overdosage/Toxicology Symptoms of overdose include diarrhea. A rise in liver function tests has been observed. There is no specific antidote, institute supportive therapy.

Formulations Tablet, film coated: 250 mg

Dosing

Adults & Elderly: Dissolution of cholesterol gallstones: Oral: 13-16 mg/kg/day in 2 divided doses, starting with 250 mg twice daily the first 2 weeks and increasing by 250 mg/day each week thereafter until the recommended or maximum tolerated dose is achieved

Hepatic Impairment: Contraindicated for use in the presence of known hepatic dysfunction or bile ductal abnormalities.

Monitoring Laboratory Tests Serum aminotransferase, cholesterol

Monitoring and Teaching Issues

Physical Assessment: See Contraindications, Warnings/Precautions and Dosing for use cautions. Assess potential for interactions with other prescriptions, OTC medications, or herbal products patient may be taking (see Drug Interactions). Assess results of laboratory tests (see above), therapeutic response, and adverse reactions (see Adverse Reactions and Overdose/Toxicology) periodically during therapy. Teach patient appropriate use, possible side effects and interventions, and adverse symptoms to report (see Patient Education). **Pregnancy risk factor X** - determine that patient is not pregnant before beginning treatment. Do not give to women of childbearing age unless they are capable of complying with barrier contraceptive use. Instruct patients of childbearing age about appropriate barrier contraceptive measures. Breast-feeding is not recommended.

Patient Education: Inform prescriber of all prescriptions, OTC medications, or herbal products you are taking, and any allergies you have. Do not take anything new during treatment unless approved by prescriber. Take as directed, for entire length of therapy. Do not chew tablets. Medication may need to be taken for several months for effective therapy. Avoid aluminum-based antacids during entire course of therapy. Blood studies and x-rays studies will be necessary during therapy. May cause diarrhea (usually mild and short-term). Report persistent diarrhea; abdominal pain, nausea and vomiting; or yellowing of skin or eyes. **Pregnancy/breast-feeding precautions:** Inform prescriber if you are pregnant. Do not get pregnant during or for 1 month following therapy. Consult prescriber for instruction on appropriate contraceptive measures. This drug may cause severe fetal defects. Do not donate blood during or for 1 month following therapy. Breast-feeding is not recommended.

Cheracol® *see* Guaifenesin and Codeine *on page 647*

Cheracol® D [OTC] *see* Guaifenesin and Dextromethorphan *on page 647*

Cheracol® Plus [OTC] *see* Guaifenesin and Dextromethorphan *on page 647*

Cheratussin DAC *see* Guaifenesin, Pseudoephedrine, and Codeine *on page 649*

Chickenpox Vaccine *see page 1498*

Chiggerex® [OTC] *see* Benzocaine *on page 156*

Chiggertox® [OTC] *see* Benzocaine *on page 156*

Children's Nostril® *see* Phenylephrine *on page 1071*

Children's Silfedrine® [OTC] *see* Pseudoephedrine *on page 1150*

Children's Sudafed® Nasal Decongestant [OTC] *see* Pseudoephedrine *on page 1150*

Chirocaine® *see* Levobupivacaine *on page 786*

Chloral *see* Chloral Hydrate *on page 268*

Chloral Hydrate (KLOR al HYE drate)

U.S. Brand Names Aquachloral® Supprettes®

Synonyms Chloral; Hydrated Chloral; Trichloroacetaldehyde Monohydrate

Restrictions C-IV

Generic Available Yes

Pharmacologic Category Hypnotic, Miscellaneous

Pregnancy Risk Factor C

Lactation Enters breast milk/compatible

Use Short-term sedative and hypnotic (<2 weeks), sedative/hypnotic for diagnostic procedures; sedative prior to EEG evaluations

Mechanism of Action/Effect Central nervous system depressant effects are due to its active metabolite trichloroethanol, mechanism unknown

Contraindications Hypersensitivity to chloral hydrate or any component of the formulation; hepatic or renal impairment; gastritis or ulcers; severe cardiac disease

Warnings/Precautions Use with caution in patients with porphyria. Use with caution in neonates, drug may accumulate with repeated use, prolonged use in neonates associated with hyperbilirubinemia. Tolerance to hypnotic effect develops, therefore, not recommended for use longer than 2 weeks. Taper dosage to avoid withdrawal with prolonged use. Trichloroethanol (TCE), a metabolite of chloral hydrate, is a carcinogen in mice; there is no data in humans. Chloral hydrate is considered a second line hypnotic agent in the elderly. Recent interpretive guidelines from the Health Care Financing Administration (HCFA) discourage the use of chloral hydrate in residents of long-term care facilities. Pregnancy risk C.

Drug Interactions

Increased Effect/Toxicity: Chloral hydrate and ethanol (and other CNS depressants) have additive CNS depressant effects; monitor for CNS depression. Chloral hydrate's metabolite may displace warfarin from its protein binding sites resulting in an increase in the hypoprothrombinemic response to warfarin; warfarin dosages may need to be adjusted. Diaphoresis, flushing, and hypertension have occurred in patients who received I.V. furosemide within 24 hours after administration of chloral hydrate; consider using a benzodiazepine.

Nutritional/Ethanol Interactions

Ethanol: Avoid ethanol (may increase CNS depression).

Herb/Nutraceutical: Avoid valerian, St John's wort, kava kava, gotu kola (may increase CNS depression).

Effects on Lab Values False-positive urine glucose using Clinitest® method; may interfere with fluorometric urine catecholamine and urinary 17-hydroxycorticosteroid tests

Adverse Reactions Frequency not defined.

Central nervous system: Ataxia, disorientation, sedation, excitement (paradoxical), dizziness, fever, headache, confusion, lightheadedness, nightmares, hallucinations, drowsiness, "hangover" effect

Dermatologic: Rash, urticaria

Gastrointestinal: Gastric irritation, nausea, vomiting, diarrhea, flatulence

Hematologic: Leukopenia, eosinophilia, acute intermittent porphyria

Miscellaneous: Physical and psychological dependence may occur with prolonged use of large doses

Overdosage/Toxicology Symptoms of overdose include hypotension, respiratory depression, coma, hypothermia, and cardiac arrhythmias. Treatment is supportive and symptomatic.

Pharmacodynamics/Kinetics

Absorption: Oral, rectal: Well absorbed

Half-Life Elimination: Active metabolite: 8-11 hours

Metabolism: Rapidly hepatic to trichloroethanol (active metabolite); variable amounts hepatically and renally to trichloroacetic acid (inactive)

Onset: Peak effect: 0.5-1 hour

Duration: 4-8 hours

Formulations

Capsule: 500 mg

Suppository, rectal: 324 mg, 500 mg, 648 mg

Syrup: 500 mg/5 mL (5 mL, 10 mL, 480 mL)

Dosing

Adults:

Sedation, anxiety: Oral, rectal: 250 mg 3 times/day

Hypnotic: Oral, rectal: 500-1000 mg at bedtime or 30 minutes prior to procedure, not to exceed 2 g/24 hours

Note: Withdraw gradually over 2 weeks if patient has been maintained on high doses for prolonged period of time. Do not stop drug abruptly.

Elderly: Hypnotic: Initial: Oral: 250 mg at bedtime; adjust for renal impairment. See Geriatric Considerations.

Pediatrics:

Sedation, anxiety: Oral, rectal: 5-15 mg/kg/dose every 8 hours, maximum: 500 mg/dose

Prior to EEG: Oral, rectal: 20-25 mg/kg/dose, 30-60 minutes prior to EEG; may repeat in 30 minutes to maximum of 100 mg/kg or 2 g total

Hypnotic: Oral, rectal: 20-40 mg/kg/dose up to a maximum of 50 mg/kg/24 hours or 1 g/dose or 2 g/24 hours

Conscious sedation: Oral: 50-75 mg/kg/dose 30-60 minutes prior to procedure; may repeat 30 minutes after initial dose if needed, to a total maximum dose of 120 mg/kg or 1 g total

Note: Withdraw gradually over 2 weeks if patient has been maintained on high doses for prolonged period of time. Do not stop drug abruptly.

Renal Impairment:

Cl_{cr} <50 mL/minute: Avoid use.

Hemodialysis effects: Supplemental dose is not necessary; dialyzable (50% to 100%).

Hepatic Impairment: Avoid use in patients with severe hepatic impairment.

Administration

Oral: Chilling the syrup may help to mask unpleasant taste. Do not crush capsule (contains drug in liquid form).

Stability

Storage: Sensitive to light. Exposure to air causes volatilization. Store in light-resistant, airtight container.

Monitoring and Teaching Issues

Physical Assessment: For short-term use. Assess effectiveness and interactions of other medications patient may be taking (see Drug Interactions). See Contraindications and Warnings/Precautions for use cautions. Assess for history of addiction; long-term use can result in dependence, abuse, or tolerance. Evaluate periodically for need for continued use (symptoms of dependence may resemble alcoholism, but usually there is more gastritis). After long-term use, taper dosage slowly when discontinuing. For inpatient use, institute safety measures and monitor effectiveness and adverse reactions. For outpatients, monitor

(Continued)

Chloral Hydrate *(Continued)*

for effectiveness of therapy and adverse reactions (see Adverse Reactions) at beginning of therapy and periodically with long-term use. Assess knowledge/teach patient appropriate use, interventions to reduce side effects, and adverse symptoms to report (see Patient Education). **Pregnancy risk factor C** - benefits of use should outweigh possible risks.

Patient Education: Use exactly as directed; do not increase dose or frequency or discontinue without consulting prescriber. Drug may cause physical and/or psychological dependence. While using this medication, do not use alcohol and other prescription or OTC medications (especially, pain medications, sedatives, antihistamines, or hypnotics) without consulting prescriber. Maintain adequate hydration (2-3 L/day of fluids) unless advised by prescriber to restrict fluids. You may experience drowsiness, dizziness, or blurred vision (use caution when driving or engaging in tasks requiring alertness until response to drug is known); nausea, vomiting, unpleasant taste (small, frequent meals, frequent mouth care, chewing gum, or sucking lozenges may help); or diarrhea (buttermilk, boiled milk, yogurt may help). Report skin rash or irritation, CNS changes (confusion, depression, increased sedation, excitation, headache, insomnia, or nightmares), unresolved GI distress, chest pain or palpitations, or ineffectiveness of medication. **Pregnancy precaution:** Inform prescriber if you are or intend to become pregnant.

Geriatric Considerations: Chloral hydrate is considered a second- or third-line hypnotic agent in the elderly. Interpretive guidelines from the Health Care Financing Administration (HCFA) discourage the use of chloral hydrate in residents of long-term care facilities.

Additional Information Not an analgesic

Related Information

Anxiolytic/Hypnotic Use in Long-Term Care Facilities *on page 1608*

Chlorambucil (klor AM byoo sil)

U.S. Brand Names Leukeran®

Generic Available No

Pharmacologic Category Antineoplastic Agent, Alkylating Agent

Pregnancy Risk Factor D

Lactation Excretion in breast milk unknown

Use Management of chronic lymphocytic leukemia, Hodgkin's and non-Hodgkin's lymphoma; breast and ovarian carcinoma; Waldenström's macroglobulinemia, testicular carcinoma, thrombocythemia, choriocarcinoma

Mechanism of Action/Effect Interferes with DNA replication and RNA transcription by alkylation and cross-linking the strands of DNA

Contraindications Hypersensitivity to chlorambucil or any component of the formulation; pregnancy

Warnings/Precautions The U.S. Food and Drug Administration (FDA) currently recommends that procedures for proper handling and disposal of antineoplastic agents be considered. Use with caution in patients with seizure disorder and bone marrow suppression. Reduce initial dosage if patient has received radiation therapy, myelosuppressive drugs, or has a depressed baseline leukocyte or platelet count within the previous 4 weeks. Can severely suppress bone marrow function; effects human fertility; is carcinogenic in humans and probably mutagenic and teratogenic as well. Chromosomal damage has been documented. Secondary AML may be associated with chronic therapy.

Drug Interactions

Decreased Effect: Patients may experience impaired immune response to vaccines; possible infection after administration of live vaccines in patients receiving immunosuppressants.

Nutritional/Ethanol Interactions

Ethanol: Avoid ethanol (may increase GI irritation).

Food: Avoid acidic foods and hot foods. Avoid spices.

Adverse Reactions

>10%:

Hematologic: Myelosuppressive: Use with caution when receiving radiation; bone marrow suppression frequently occurs and occasionally bone marrow failure has occurred; blood counts should be monitored closely while undergoing treatment; leukopenia, thrombocytopenia, anemia

WBC: Moderate

Platelets: Moderate

Onset (days): 7

Nadir (days): 10-14

Recovery (days): 28

1% to 10%:

Dermatologic: Skin rashes

Endocrine & metabolic: Hyperuricemia, menstrual changes

Gastrointestinal: Nausea, vomiting, diarrhea, oral ulceration are all infrequent

Emetic potential: Low (<10%)

<1% (Limited to important or life-threatening): Agitation, angioneurotic edema, ataxia, confusion, drug fever, epidermal necrolysis, erythema multiforme, fertility impairment (has caused chromosomal damage in men, both reversible and permanent sterility have occurred in both sexes; can produce amenorrhea in females), generalized or focal seizures (rarely), hallucination, hepatic necrosis, hepatotoxicity, increased incidence of AML, muscular twitching, myoclonia, oral ulceration, peripheral neuropathy, pulmonary fibrosis, secondary malignancies, skin hypersensitivity, Stevens-Johnson syndrome, tremors, urticaria, weakness

Overdosage/Toxicology Symptoms of overdose include vomiting, ataxia, coma, seizures, and pancytopenia. There are no known antidotes for chlorambucil intoxication. Treatment is mainly supportive and symptomatic.

Pharmacodynamics/Kinetics

Absorption: 70% to 80% with meals

Bioavailability: Reduced 10% to 20% with food

Half-Life Elimination: 1.5 hours; Phenylacetic acid mustard: 2.5 hours

Metabolism: Hepatic; active metabolite, phenylacetic acid mustard

Formulations Tablet, sugar-coated: 2 mg

Dosing

Adults: Refer to individual protocols.

Usual dose range: Oral: 0.1-0.2 mg/kg/day **or** 3-6 mg/m²/day for 3-6 weeks, then adjust dose on basis of blood counts. Pulse dosing has been used in CLL as intermittent, biweekly, or monthly doses of 0.4 mg/kg and increased by 0.1 mg/kg until the disease is under control or toxicity ensues. An alternate regimen is 14 mg/m²/day for 5 days, repeated every 21-28 days.

Elderly: Oral (refer to individual protocols): Use lowest recommended doses for adults; usual dose for elderly is 2-4 mg/day, particularly for use in treatment of rheumatoid arthritis.

Pediatrics: Refer to individual protocols.

General short courses: Oral: 0.1-0.2 mg/kg/day **or** 4.5 mg/m²/day for 3-6 weeks for remission induction (usual: 4-10 mg/day); maintenance therapy: 0.03-0.1 mg/kg/day (usual: 2-4 mg/day)

Nephrotic syndrome: Oral: 0.1-0.2 mg/kg/day every day for 5-15 weeks with low-dose prednisone

Chronic lymphocytic leukemia (CLL): Oral:

Biweekly regimen: Initial: 0.4 mg/kg/dose every 2 weeks; increase dose by 0.1 mg/kg every 2 weeks until a response occurs and/or myelosuppression occurs

Monthly regimen: Initial: 0.4 mg/kg, increase dose by 0.2 mg/kg every 4 weeks until a response occurs and/or myelosuppression occurs

Malignant lymphomas: Oral:

Non-Hodgkin's lymphoma: 0.1 mg/kg/day

Hodgkin's lymphoma: 0.2 mg/kg/day

Renal Impairment:

Hemodialysis: Supplemental dose is not necessary.

Peritoneal dialysis: Supplemental dose is not necessary.

Administration

Oral: May divide single daily dose if nausea and vomiting occur. Take 1 hour before or 2 hours after meals.

Stability

Storage: Store at room temperature; protect from light.

Monitoring Laboratory Tests Liver function, CBC, platelet count, serum uric acid

Monitoring and Teaching Issues

Physical Assessment: See Contraindications, Warnings/Precautions, and Dosing for use cautions. Assess potential for interactions with other prescriptions, OTC medications, or herbal products patient may be taking (see Drug Interactions). Assess results of laboratory tests (see above), therapeutic effectiveness, and adverse response (eg, hematologic myelosuppression - see Adverse Reactions and Overdose/Toxicology) on a regular basis throughout therapy. Teach patient (or caregiver) proper use, possible side effects and interventions, and adverse symptoms to report (see Patient Education). **Pregnancy risk factor D** - determine that patient is not pregnant before beginning treatment. Instruct patients of childbearing age about appropriate barrier contraceptive measures during therapy and for 1 month following therapy. Note breast-feeding caution.

Patient Education: Inform prescriber of all prescriptions, OTC medications, or herbal products you are taking, and any allergies you have. Do not take anything new during treatment unless approved by prescriber. Take exactly as directed. Maintain adequate hydration (2-3 L/day of fluids) unless advised by prescriber to restrict fluids. Avoid alcohol, acidic, spicy, or hot foods. May cause menstrual irregularities and/or sterility. You will be more susceptible to infection (avoid crowds and exposure to infection and do not have any vaccinations without consulting prescriber). May cause nausea or vomiting (small, frequent meals, good mouth care, chewing gum or sucking lozenges may help); or mouth sores (use soft toothbrush or cotton swab for oral care). Report easy bruising or bleeding; unusual rash; persistent nausea, vomiting, or mouth sores; menstrual irregularities; or difficulty breathing. **Pregnancy/breast-feeding precautions:** Inform prescriber if you are pregnant. Do not get pregnant during or for 1 month following therapy. Consult prescriber for instruction on appropriate contraceptive measures. This drug may cause severe fetal defects. Consult prescriber if breast-feeding.

Geriatric Considerations: Toxicity to immunosuppressives is increased in the elderly. Start with lowest recommended adult doses (Dosage). Signs of infection, such as fever and rise in WBCs, may not occur. Lethargy and confusion may be more prominent signs of infection.

Pregnancy Issues: Carcinogenic and mutagenic in humans.

Chloramphenicol (klor am FEN i kole)

U.S. Brand Names Chloromycetin®; Chloroptic®; Ocu-Chlor®

Generic Available Yes

Pharmacologic Category Antibiotic, Ophthalmic; Antibiotic, Otic; Antibiotic, Miscellaneous

Pregnancy Risk Factor C

Lactation Enters breast milk/not recommended (AAP rates "of concern")

Use Treatment of serious infections due to organisms resistant to other less toxic antibiotics or when its penetrability into the site of infection is clinically superior to other antibiotics to which the organism is sensitive; useful in infections caused by *Bacteroides*, *H. influenzae*, *Neisseria meningitidis*, *Salmonella*, and *Rickettsia*; active against many vancomycin-resistant enterococci

Mechanism of Action/Effect Reversibly binds to 50S ribosomal subunits of susceptible organisms preventing amino acids from being transferred to growing peptide chains thus inhibiting protein synthesis

(Continued)

Chloramphenicol *(Continued)*

Contraindications Hypersensitivity to chloramphenicol or any component of the formulation

Warnings/Precautions Use with caution in patients with impaired renal or hepatic function and in neonates. Reduce dose with impaired liver function. Use with care in patients with glucose 6-phosphate dehydrogenase deficiency. Serious and fatal blood dyscrasias have occurred after both short-term and prolonged therapy. Should not be used when less potentially toxic agents are effective. Prolonged use may result in superinfection. Pregnancy risk C.

Drug Interactions

Cytochrome P450 Effect: Inhibits CYP2C8/9, 3A4

Decreased Effect: Phenobarbital and rifampin may decrease serum concentrations of chloramphenicol.

Increased Effect/Toxicity: Chloramphenicol increases serum concentrations of chlorpropamide, phenytoin, and oral anticoagulants.

Nutritional/Ethanol Interactions Food: May decrease intestinal absorption of vitamin B_{12} may have increased dietary need for riboflavin, pyridoxine, and vitamin B_{12}.

Effects on Lab Values May cause false-positive results in urine glucose tests when using cupric sulfate (Benedict's solution, Clinitest®).

Adverse Reactions

Ophthalmic:

1% to 10%:

Local: Burning or stinging

Ocular: Blurred vision

Miscellaneous: Hypersensitivity reactions

<1% (Limited to important or life-threatening): Blood dyscrasias

Systemic:

1% to 10%:

Gastrointestinal: Diarrhea, nausea, vomiting

Hematologic: Blood dyscrasias

<1% (Limited to important or life-threatening): Aplastic anemia, bone marrow suppression, enterocolitis, gray baby syndrome, headache, nightmares, optic neuritis, peripheral neuropathy, stomatitis

Three major toxicities associated with chloramphenicol include:

Aplastic anemia (idiosyncratic reaction, any route of administration; usually occurs 3 weeks to 12 months after initial exposure to chloramphenicol)

Bone marrow suppression (dose-related; serum concentrations >25 µg/mL)

Gray baby syndrome (circulatory collapse, cyanosis, acidosis, abdominal distention, myocardial depression, coma, and death). Appears to be associated with serum levels ≥50 µg/mL; may result from drug accumulation in patients with impaired hepatic or renal function.

Topical:

>10%: Miscellaneous: Hypersensitivity reactions

<1% (Limited to important or life-threatening): Blood dyscrasias

Overdosage/Toxicology Symptoms of overdose include anemia, metabolic acidosis, hypotension, and hypothermia. Treatment is supportive.

Pharmacodynamics/Kinetics

Half-Life Elimination:

Normal renal function: 1.6-3.3 hours

End-stage renal disease: 3-7 hours

Cirrhosis: 10-12 hours

Neonates: Postnatal: 1-2 days old: 24 hours; 10-16 days old: 10 hours

Time to Peak: Oral: Within 0.5-3 hours

Metabolism: Extensively hepatic (90%) to inactive metabolites, principally by glucuronidation; chloramphenicol palmitate is hydrolyzed by lipases in GI tract to the active base; chloramphenicol sodium succinate is hydrolyzed by esterases to active base

Formulations

Ointment, ophthalmic: 1% [10 mg/g] (3.5 g)

Chloromycetin®, Chloroptic® S.O.P., Ocu-Chlor®: 1% [10 mg/g] (3.5 g)

Injection, powder for reconstitution, as sodium succinate: 1 g

Powder for ophthalmic solution (Chloromycetin®): 25 mg/vial (15 mL)

Solution: 0.5% [5 mg/mL] (7.5 mL, 15 mL)

Solution, ophthalmic (Chloroptic®, Ocu-Chlor®): 0.5% [5 mg/mL] (2.5 mL, 7.5 mL, 15 mL)

Solution, otic (Chloromycetin®): 0.5% (15 mL)

Dosing

Adults & Elderly:

Systemic infections: Oral, I.V.: 50-100 mg/kg/day in divided doses every 6 hours; maximum daily dose: 4 g/day.

Ocular infection: Ophthalmic: Instill 1-2 drops or 1.25 cm (½" of ointment every 3-4 hours); increase interval between applications after 48 hours to 2-3 times/day.

Otitis externa (superficial): Otic solution: Instill 2-3 drops into ear 3 times/day.

Dermal infection: Topical: Gently rub into the affected area 1-4 times/day.

Pediatrics:

Meningitis: I.V.: Infants >30 days and Children: 50-100 mg/kg/day divided every 6 hours

Other infections: I.V.: Infants >30 days and Children: 50-75 mg/kg/day divided every 6 hours; maximum daily dose: 4 g/day

Ophthalmic, Otic, Topical: Refer to adult dosing.

Renal Impairment: Slightly dialyzable (5% to 20%) via hemo- and peritoneal dialysis; no supplemental doses are needed in dialysis or continuous arteriovenous or venovenous hemofiltration.

Hepatic Impairment: Avoid use in severe liver impairment as increased toxicity may occur.

Administration

I.V.: Infuse via direct I.V. over 3-5 minutes; intermittent infusion over 30-60 minutes.

Other: Do not warm ear drops above body temperature. Will decrease its potency.

Stability

Storage: Refrigerate ophthalmic solution.

Reconstitution: Constituted solutions remain stable for 30 days. Use only clear solutions. Frozen solutions remain stable for 6 months.

Compatibility: Stable in dextran 6% in dextrose, dextran 6% in NS, D_5LR, $D_5{}^1/_4NS$, $D_5{}^1/_2NS$, D_5NS, D_5W, $D_{10}W$, fat emulsion 10%, LR, $^1/_2NS$, NS

Y-site administration: Incompatible with fluconazole

Compatibility in syringe: Incompatible with glycopyrrolate, metoclopramide

Compatibility when admixed: Incompatible with chlorpromazine, hydroxyzine, phenytoin, polymyxin B sulfate, prochlorperazine edisylate, prochlorperazine mesylate, promethazine, vancomycin

Monitoring Laboratory Tests CBC with reticulocyte and platelet counts, periodic liver and renal function, serum drug concentration; culture and sensitivity specimen should be taken prior to initiating therapy.

Monitoring and Teaching Issues

Physical Assessment: Assess effectiveness and interactions of other medications patient may be taking (see Drug Interactions). Monitor laboratory tests (see above), therapeutic response, and adverse reactions (see Adverse Reactions). Assess knowledge/teach patient appropriate use appropriate for form prescribed, interventions to reduce side effects, and adverse symptoms to report (see Patient Education). **Pregnancy risk factor C** - benefits of use should outweigh possible risks. Breast-feeding is not recommended.

Patient Education:

I.V.: You may experience a bitter taste during administration, this will pass.

Ophthalmic: Wash hands before instilling. Sit or lie down to instill. Open eye, look at ceiling, and instill prescribed amount of medication. Close eye and apply gentle pressure to inner corner of eye. Do not let tip of applicator touch eye; do not contaminate tip of applicator (may cause eye infection, eye damage, or vision loss). Temporary stinging or burning may occur. Report persistent pain, burning, vision changes, swelling, itching, rash, or worsening of condition.

Otic: Wash hands before instilling. Tilt head with affected ear upward. Gently grasp ear lobe and lift back and upward. Instill prescribed drops into ear canal. Do not push dropper into ear. Remain with head tilted for 2 minutes. Report ringing in ears, discharge, or worsening of condition.

Topical: Wash hands before applying or wear gloves. Apply thin film to affected area. May apply porous dressing. Report persistent burning, swelling, itching, or worsening of condition.

If diabetic, drug may cause false test results with Clinitest® glucose monitoring; use alternative glucose monitoring. This drug may interfere with effectiveness of oral contraceptives. You may experience nausea, vomiting (small, frequent meals, frequent mouth care, sucking lozenges, or chewing gum may help). Report persistent rash, diarrhea; pain, burning, or numbness of extremities; petechiae; sore throat; fatigue; unusual bleeding or bruising; vaginal itching or discharge; mouth sores; yellowing of skin or eyes; dark urine or stool discoloration (blue); CNS disturbances (nightmares acute headache); lack of improvement or worsening of condition.

Pregnancy/breast-feeding precautions: Inform prescriber if you are or intend to become pregnant. Breast-feeding is not recommended.

Dietary Issues: May have increased dietary need for riboflavin, pyridoxine, and vitamin B_{12}. Sodium content of 1 g injection: 51.8 mg (2.25 mEq).

Geriatric Considerations: Chloramphenicol has not been studied in the elderly. It is not necessary to adjust the dose based upon the decrease in renal function associated with age. Chloramphenicol should be reserved for serious infections and the oral form avoided.

Breast-feeding Issues: Excreted in breast milk (even with topical application). Not recommended due to potential bone marrow suppression to the infant.

Related Information

Ophthalmic Agents *on page 1509*

Otic Agents *on page 1519*

Chloramphenicol and Prednisolone *see page 1509*

Chlordiazepoxide (klor dye az e POKS ide)

U.S. Brand Names Librium®

Synonyms Methaminodiazepoxide Hydrochloride

Restrictions C-IV

Generic Available Yes

Pharmacologic Category Benzodiazepine

Pregnancy Risk Factor D

Lactation Enters breast milk/not recommended

Use Management of anxiety disorder or for the short-term relief of symptoms of anxiety; withdrawal symptoms of acute alcoholism; preoperative apprehension and anxiety

Mechanism of Action/Effect Binds to stereospecific benzodiazepine receptors on the postsynaptic GABA neuron at several sites within the central nervous system, including the limbic system, reticular formation. Enhancement of the inhibitory effect of GABA on neuronal excitability results by increased neuronal membrane permeability to chloride ions. This shift in chloride ions results in hyperpolarization (a less excitable state) and stabilization.

Contraindications Hypersensitivity to chlordiazepoxide or any component of the formulation (cross-sensitivity with other benzodiazepines may exist); narrow-angle glaucoma (not in product labeling: however, benzodiazepines are contraindicated); pregnancy

(Continued)

Chlordiazepoxide *(Continued)*

Warnings/Precautions Use with caution in renal impairment or predisposition to urate nephropathy, elderly or debilitated patients, patients with hepatic disease (including alcoholics), renal impairment, respiratory disease, impaired gag reflex, or obese patients. Use with caution in patients receiving concurrent CYP3A4 inhibitors, particularly when these agents are added to therapy. Use with caution in renal impairment or predisposition to urate nephropathy, elderly or debilitated patients, patients with hepatic disease (including alcoholics), renal impairment, respiratory disease, impaired gag reflex, or obese patients.

Parenteral administration should be avoided in comatose patients or shock. Adequate resuscitative equipment/personnel should be available, and appropriate monitoring should be conducted at the time of injection and for several hours following administration. The parenteral formulation should be diluted for I.M. administration with the supplied diluent only. This diluent should not be used when preparing the drug for intravenous administration.

Causes CNS depression (dose-related) which may impair physical and mental capabilities. Use with caution in patients receiving other CNS depressants or psychoactive agents. Benzodiazepines have been associated with falls and traumatic injury and should be used with extreme caution in patients who are at risk of these events (especially the elderly). Active metabolites with extended half-lives may lead to delayed accumulation and adverse effects.

Use caution in patients with depression, particularly if suicidal risk may be present. May cause physical or psychological dependence - use with caution in patients with a history of drug dependence.

Benzodiazepines have been associated with anterograde amnesia. Paradoxical reactions, including hyperactive or aggressive behavior, have been reported with benzodiazepines, particularly in adolescent/pediatric or psychiatric patients. Does not have analgesic, antidepressant, or antipsychotic properties.

Drug Interactions

Cytochrome P450 Effect: Substrate of **CYP3A4**

Decreased Effect: Carbamazepine, rifampin, rifabutin may enhance the metabolism of chlordiazepoxide and decrease its therapeutic effect.

Increased Effect/Toxicity: Chlordiazepoxide potentiates the CNS depressant effects of narcotic analgesics, barbiturates, phenothiazines, ethanol, antihistamines, MAO inhibitors, sedative-hypnotics, and cyclic antidepressants. Serum concentrations/effects of chlordiazepoxide may be increased by inhibitors of CYP3A4, including cimetidine, ciprofloxacin, clarithromycin, clozapine, diltiazem, disulfiram, digoxin, erythromycin, ethanol, fluconazole, fluoxetine, fluvoxamine, grapefruit juice, isoniazid, itraconazole, ketoconazole, labetalol, levodopa, loxapine, metoprolol, metronidazole, miconazole, nefazodone, omeprazole, phenytoin, rifabutin, rifampin, troleandomycin, valproic acid, and verapamil.

Nutritional/Ethanol Interactions

Ethanol: Avoid ethanol (may increase CNS depression).

Food: Serum concentrations/effects may be increased with grapefruit juice, but unlikely because of high oral bioavailability of chlordiazepoxide.

Herb/Nutraceutical: Avoid valerian, St John's wort, kava kava, gotu kola (may increase CNS depression).

Effects on Lab Values ↑ triglycerides (S); ↓ HDL

Adverse Reactions

>10%:

- Central nervous system: Drowsiness, fatigue, ataxia, lightheadedness, memory impairment, dysarthria, irritability
- Dermatologic: Rash
- Endocrine & metabolic: Decreased libido, menstrual disorders
- Gastrointestinal: Xerostomia, decreased salivation, increased or decreased appetite, weight gain/loss
- Genitourinary: Micturition difficulties

1% to 10%:

- Cardiovascular: Hypotension
- Central nervous system: Confusion, dizziness, disinhibition, akathisia, increased libido
- Dermatologic: Dermatitis
- Gastrointestinal: Increased salivation
- Genitourinary: Sexual dysfunction, incontinence
- Neuromuscular & skeletal: Rigidity, tremor, muscle cramps
- Otic: Tinnitus
- Respiratory: Nasal congestion

Overdosage/Toxicology Symptoms of overdose include hypotension, respiratory depression, coma, hypothermia, and cardiac arrhythmias. Treatment for benzodiazepine overdose is supportive. Flumazenil has been shown to selectively block the binding of benzodiazepines to CNS receptors, resulting in a reversal of benzodiazepine-induced CNS depression. Respiratory depression may not be reversed.

Pharmacodynamics/Kinetics

Half-Life Elimination: 6.6-25 hours; End-stage renal disease: 5-30 hours; Cirrhosis: 30-63 hours

Time to Peak: Serum: Oral: Within 2 hours; I.M.: Results in lower peak plasma levels than oral

Metabolism: Extensively hepatic to desmethyldiazepam (active and long-acting)

Formulations

Capsule, as hydrochloride: 5 mg, 10 mg, 25 mg

Injection, powder for reconstitution, as hydrochloride: 100 mg

Dosing

Adults:

Anxiety:

Oral: 15-100 mg divided 3-4 times/day

I.M., I.V.: Initial: 50-100 mg followed by 25-50 mg 3-4 times/day as needed

Preoperative anxiety: I.M.: 50-100 mg prior to surgery

Ethanol withdrawal symptoms: Oral, I.V.: 50-100 mg to start, dose may be repeated in 2-4 hours as necessary to a maximum of 300 mg/24 hours

Note: Up to 300 mg may be given I.M. or I.V. during a 6-hour period, but not more than this in any 24-hour period.

Elderly: Anxiety: Oral: 5 mg 2-4 times/day; adjust for renal impairment. Avoid use if possible. See Geriatric Considerations.

Pediatrics: Anxiety: Oral, I.M.:

<6 years: Not recommended

>6 years: 0.5 mg/kg/24 hours divided every 6-8 hours

Renal Impairment:

Cl_{cr} <10 mL/minute: Administer 50% of dose.

Not dialyzable (0% to 5%)

Hepatic Impairment: Avoid use.

Administration

I.V.: Do not infuse into small veins. Infuse 100 mg or any fraction thereof over a minimum of 1 minute.

Stability

Storage: Refrigerate injection and protect from light.

Reconstitution: Do not use diluent provided with parenteral form for I.V. administration; dissolve with normal saline instead; I.V. form is a powder and should be reconstituted with 5 mL of sterile water or saline prior to administration.

Compatibility: Stable in D_5W; **incompatible** (consult detailed reference) in LR, NS

Y-site administration: Incompatible with cefepime

Monitoring and Teaching Issues

Physical Assessment: Assess other medications patient may be taking for effectiveness and interactions (see Drug Interactions). See Contraindications and Warnings/Precautions for use cautions. Assess for history of addiction; long-term use can result in dependence, abuse, or tolerance; periodically evaluate need for continued use. Monitor therapeutic response and adverse reactions at beginning of therapy and periodically with long-term use (see Adverse Reactions and Overdose/Toxicology). Taper dosage slowly when discontinuing. Assess knowledge/teach patient appropriate use, interventions to reduce side effects, and adverse symptoms to report (see Patient Education). **I.V.:** Monitor vital signs frequently during infusion, observe safety precautions, and maintain bedrest for 2-3 hours following infusion. **Pregnancy risk factor D** - determine that patient is not pregnant before beginning treatment. Instruct patients of childbearing age about appropriate barrier contraceptive measures. Breast-feeding is not recommended.

Patient Education: Oral: Take exactly as directed; do not increase dose or frequency. Drug may cause physical and/or psychological dependence. Do not use alcohol or other prescription or OTC medications (especially pain medications, sedatives, antihistamines, or hypnotics) without consulting prescriber. Maintain adequate hydration (2-3 L/day of fluids) unless advised by prescriber to restrict fluids. You may experience drowsiness, lightheadedness, impaired coordination, dizziness, or blurred vision (use caution when driving or engaging in tasks requiring alertness until response to drug is known); dry mouth (small, frequent meals, frequent mouth care, chewing gum, or sucking lozenges may help); constipation (increased exercise, fluids, fruit, or fiber may help); or altered sexual drive or ability (reversible). Report persistent CNS effects (eg, euphoria, confusion, increased sedation, depression); chest pain, palpitations, or rapid heartbeat; muscle cramping, weakness, tremors, rigidity, or altered gait; or worsening of condition. **Pregnancy/breast-feeding precautions:** Do not get pregnant while taking this medication; use appropriate contraceptive measures. Breast-feeding is not recommended.

Geriatric Considerations: Due to its long-acting metabolite, chlordiazepoxide is not considered a drug of choice in the elderly.

Breast-feeding Issues: There is no significant data for chlordiazepoxide, but a related compound diazepam has been shown to accumulate in nursing infants. It is recommended to discontinue nursing or the drug.

Additional Information Abrupt discontinuation after sustained use (generally >10 days) may cause withdrawal symptoms.

Related Information

Anxiolytic/Hypnotic Use in Long-Term Care Facilities *on page 1608*

Benzodiazepines *on page 1560*

Chlordiazepoxide and Clidinium *see* Clidinium and Chlordiazepoxide *on page 306*

2-Chlorodeoxyadenosine *see* Cladribine *on page 303*

Chloromag® *see* Magnesium Supplements *on page 831*

Chloromycetin® *see page 1519*

Chloromycetin® *see page 1509*

Chloromycetin® *see* Chloramphenicol *on page 271*

Chloroptic® *see page 1509*

Chloroptic® *see* Chloramphenicol *on page 271*

Chloroptic-P® *see page 1509*

Chloroptic® S.O.P. *see page 1509*

Chloroquine (KLOR oh kwin)

U.S. Brand Names Aralen® Phosphate

Synonyms Chloroquine Phosphate

Generic Available Yes

Pharmacologic Category Aminoquinoline (Antimalarial)

Pregnancy Risk Factor C

Lactation Enters breast milk/compatible

Use Suppression or chemoprophylaxis of malaria; treatment of uncomplicated or mild to moderate malaria; extraintestinal amebiasis

(Continued)

Chloroquine *(Continued)*

Use - Unlabeled/Investigational Rheumatoid arthritis; discoid lupus erythematosus, scleroderma, pemphigus

Mechanism of Action/Effect Chloroquine concentrates within parasite acid vesicles and raises internal pH resulting in inhibition of parasite growth

Contraindications Hypersensitivity to chloroquine or any component of the formulation; retinal or visual field changes; patients with psoriasis

Warnings/Precautions Use with caution in patients with liver disease, G6PD deficiency, alcoholism or in conjunction with hepatotoxic drugs, psoriasis, porphyria may be exacerbated. Retinopathy (irreversible) has occurred with long or high-dose therapy. discontinue drug if any abnormality in the visual field or if muscular weakness develops during treatment. Pregnancy risk C.

Drug Interactions

Cytochrome P450 Effect: Substrate of **CYP2D6, 3A4**; Inhibits CYP2D6

Decreased Effect: Decreased absorption if administered concomitantly with kaolin and magnesium trisilicate.

Increased Effect/Toxicity: Chloroquine serum concentrations may be elevated with concomitant cimetidine use.

Nutritional/Ethanol Interactions Ethanol: Avoid ethanol (may increase GI irritation).

Adverse Reactions Frequency not defined.

Cardiovascular: Hypotension (rare), EKG changes (rare)

Central nervous system: Fatigue, personality changes, headache

Dermatologic: Pruritus, hair bleaching, pleomorphic skin eruptions, alopecia, lichen planus eruptions, alopecia, mucosal pigmentary changes (blue-black)

Gastrointestinal: Nausea, diarrhea, vomiting, anorexia, stomatitis

Hematologic: Blood dyscrasias

Ocular: Retinopathy (including irreversible changes in some patients long-term or high dose), blurred vision

Otic: Nerve deafness, tinnitus

Overdosage/Toxicology Symptoms of overdose include headache, visual changes, cardiovascular collapse, seizures, abdominal cramps, vomiting, cyanosis, methemoglobinemia, leukopenia, and respiratory and cardiac arrest. Following initial measures (immediate GI decontamination), treatment is supportive and symptomatic.

Pharmacodynamics/Kinetics

Absorption: Oral: Rapid (~89%)

Half-Life Elimination: 3-5 days

Time to Peak: Serum: 1-2 hours

Metabolism: Partially hepatic

Duration: Small amounts may be present in urine months following discontinuation of therapy

Formulations

Injection, as hydrochloride: 50 mg/mL [equivalent to 40 mg base/mL] (5 mL)

Tablet, as phosphate: 250 mg [equivalent to 150 mg base]; 500 mg [equivalent to 300 mg base]

Dosing

Adults & Elderly: Dosage expressed in terms of mg of base:

Malaria, suppression or prophylaxis: Oral: 300 mg/week (base) on the same day each week; begin 1-2 weeks prior to exposure; continue for 4-6 weeks after leaving endemic area. If suppressive therapy is not begun prior to exposure, double the initial loading dose to 600 mg (base) and give in 2 divided doses 6 hours apart, followed by the usual dosage regimen.

Malaria, acute attack: Oral; 600 mg (base) on day 1, followed by 300 mg (base) 6 hours later, followed by 300 mg (base) on days 2 and 3

Extraintestinal amebiasis: Oral: 600 mg base/day for 2 days followed by 300 mg base/day for at least 2-3 weeks

Pediatrics: Dosage expressed in terms of mg of base:

Malaria, suppression or prophylaxis: Oral: Administer 5 mg base/kg/week on the same day each week (not to exceed 300 mg base/dose). Begin 1-2 weeks prior to exposure; continue for 4-6 weeks after leaving endemic area. If suppressive therapy is not begun prior to exposure, double the initial loading dose to 10 mg base/kg and administer in 2 divided doses 6 hours apart, followed by the usual dosage regimen.

Malaria, acute attack:

Oral: 10 mg/kg on day 1, followed by 5 mg/kg 6 hours later and 5 mg/kg on days 2 and 3

I.M. (as hydrochloride): 5 mg/kg, repeat in 6 hours

Extraintestinal amebiasis: Oral: 10 mg/kg once daily for 2-3 weeks (up to 300 mg base/day)

Renal Impairment:

Cl_{cr} <10 mL/minute: Administer 50% of dose.

Hemodialysis effects: Minimally removed by hemodialysis

Stability

Compatibility: Stable in NS

Compatibility in syringe: Incompatible with promethazine

Monitoring Laboratory Tests Periodic CBC

Monitoring and Teaching Issues

Physical Assessment: See Contraindications, Warnings/Precautions, and Dosing for use cautions. Assess potential for interactions with other prescriptions, OTC medications, or herbal products patient may be taking (see Drug Interactions). Assess results of laboratory tests (see above), therapeutic effectiveness (according to purpose for use), and adverse response (see Adverse Reactions and Overdose/Toxicology) regularly during long-term therapy. Teach patient appropriate use, possible side effects and interventions, and adverse symptoms to report (see Patient Education). **Pregnancy risk factor C** - benefits of use should outweigh possible risks.

Patient Education: Inform prescriber of all prescriptions, OTC medications, or herbal products you are taking, and any allergies you have. Do not take anything new during treatment unless approved by prescriber. It is important to complete full course of therapy, which may take up to 6 months for full effect. May be taken with meals to decrease GI upset and bitter aftertaste. Avoid alcohol. You should have regular ophthalmic exams (every 4-6 months) if using this medication over extended periods. May cause skin discoloration (blue/black), hair bleaching, or skin rash. If you have psoriasis, may cause exacerbation. May turn urine black/brown (normal). May cause headache (if persistent, consult prescriber for analgesic); nausea, vomiting, or loss of appetite (small, frequent meals, frequent mouth care, sucking lozenges, or chewing gum may help); or increased sensitivity to sunlight (wear dark glasses and protective clothing, use sunblock, and avoid direct exposure to sunlight). Report vision changes; rash or itching; persistent diarrhea or GI disturbances; change in hearing acuity or ringing in the ears; chest pain or palpitation; CNS changes; unusual fatigue, easy bruising or bleeding; or any other persistent adverse reactions. **Pregnancy precaution:** Inform prescriber if you are or intend to become pregnant.

Dietary Issues: May be taken with meals to decrease GI upset.

Chloroquine Phosphate *see* Chloroquine *on page 275*

Chlorpheniramine, Phenylephrine, and Methscopolamine *see page 1522*

Chlorpheniramine, Pseudoephedrine, and Codeine *see page 1522*

Chlorpheniramine, Pyrilamine, and Phenylephrine *see page 1522*

ChlorproMAZINE (klor PROE ma zeen)

U.S. Brand Names Thorazine®

Synonyms Chlorpromazine Hydrochloride; CPZ

Generic Available Yes

Pharmacologic Category Antipsychotic Agent, Phenothiazine, Aliphatic

Pregnancy Risk Factor C

Lactation Enters breast milk/not recommended (AAP rates "of concern")

Use Control of mania; treatment of schizophrenia; control of nausea and vomiting; relief of restlessness and apprehension before surgery; acute intermittent porphyria; adjunct in the treatment of tetanus; intractable hiccups; combativeness and/or explosive hyperexcitable behavior in children 1-12 years of age and in short-term treatment of hyperactive children

Use - Unlabeled/Investigational Management of psychotic disorders

Mechanism of Action/Effect Blocks postsynaptic mesolimbic dopaminergic receptors in the brain; exhibits a strong alpha-adrenergic blocking effect and depresses the release of hypothalamic and hypophyseal hormones; believed to depress the reticular activating system, thus affecting basal metabolism, body temperature, wakefulness, vasomotor tone, and emesis

Contraindications Hypersensitivity to chlorpromazine or any component of the formulation (cross-reactivity between phenothiazines may occur); severe CNS depression; coma

Warnings/Precautions Highly sedating, use with caution in disorders where CNS depression is a feature and in patients with Parkinson's disease. Use with caution in patients with hemodynamic instability, bone marrow suppression, predisposition to seizures, subcortical brain damage, severe cardiac, hepatic, renal, or respiratory disease. Esophageal dysmotility and aspiration have been associated with antipsychotic use - use with caution in patients at risk of aspiration pneumonia (ie, Alzheimer's disease). Caution in breast cancer or other prolactin-dependent tumors (may elevate prolactin levels). May alter temperature regulation or mask toxicity of other drugs due to antiemetic effects. May alter cardiac conduction - life-threatening arrhythmias have occurred with therapeutic doses of neuroleptics.

Use with caution in patients at risk of hypotension (orthostasis is common) or those who would tolerate transient hypotensive episodes (cerebrovascular disease, cardiovascular disease, or other medications which may predispose). Significant hypotension may occur, particularly with parenteral administration. Injection contains sulfites and benzyl alcohol.

Use with caution in patients with decreased gastrointestinal motility, urinary retention, BPH, xerostomia, or visual problems (ie, narrow-angle glaucoma - screening is recommended) and myasthenia gravis. Relative to other neuroleptics, chlorpromazine has a moderate potency of cholinergic blockade.

May cause extrapyramidal symptoms, neuroleptic malignant syndrome (NMS) or pigmentary retinopathy.

Pregnancy risk C.

Drug Interactions

Cytochrome P450 Effect: Substrate of CYP1A2, **2D6**, 3A4; Inhibits CYP2D6, 2E1

Decreased Effect: Phenothiazines inhibit the ability of bromocriptine to lower serum prolactin concentrations. Benztropine (and other anticholinergics) may inhibit the therapeutic response to chlorpromazine and excess anticholinergic effects may occur. Cigarette smoking and barbiturates may enhance the hepatic metabolism of chlorpromazine. Antihypertensive effects of guanethidine and guanadrel may be inhibited by chlorpromazine. Chlorpromazine may inhibit the antiparkinsonian effect of levodopa. Chlorpromazine and possibly other low potency antipsychotics may reverse the pressor effects of epinephrine.

Increased Effect/Toxicity: Effects on CNS depression may be additive when chlorpromazine is combined with CNS depressants (narcotic analgesics, ethanol, barbiturates, cyclic antidepressants, antihistamines, or sedative-hypnotics). Chlorpromazine may increase the effects/toxicity of anticholinergics, antihypertensives, lithium (rare neurotoxicity), trazodone, or valproic acid. Concurrent use with TCA may produce increased toxicity or altered therapeutic response. Chloroquine and propranolol may increase chlorpromazine concentrations. Hypotension may occur when chlorpromazine is combined with epinephrine. May increase the risk of arrhythmia when combined with antiarrhythmics, cisapride, pimozide, sparfloxacin, or other drugs which prolong QT interval. Metoclopramide may increase risk of extrapyramidal symptoms (EPS).

(Continued)

ChlorproMAZINE *(Continued)*

Nutritional/Ethanol Interactions

Ethanol: Avoid ethanol (may increase CNS depression).

Herb/Nutraceutical: Avoid St John's wort (may decrease chlorpromazine levels, increase photosensitization, or enhance sedative effect). Avoid dong quai (may enhance photosensitization). Avoid kava kava, gotu kola, valerian (may increase CNS depression).

Effects on Lab Values False-positives for phenylketonuria, amylase, uroporphyrins, urobilinogen. May cause false-positive pregnancy test.

Adverse Reactions Frequency not defined.

Cardiovascular: Postural hypotension, tachycardia, dizziness, nonspecific QT changes

Central nervous system: Drowsiness, dystonias, akathisia, pseudoparkinsonism, tardive dyskinesia, neuroleptic malignant syndrome, seizures

Dermatologic: Photosensitivity, dermatitis, skin pigmentation (slate gray)

Endocrine & metabolic: Lactation, breast engorgement, false-positive pregnancy test, amenorrhea, gynecomastia, hyper- or hypoglycemia

Gastrointestinal: Xerostomia, constipation, nausea

Genitourinary: Urinary retention, ejaculatory disorder, impotence

Hematologic: Agranulocytosis, eosinophilia, leukopenia, hemolytic anemia, aplastic anemia, thrombocytopenic purpura

Hepatic: Jaundice

Ocular: Blurred vision, corneal and lenticular changes, epithelial keratopathy, pigmentary retinopathy

Overdosage/Toxicology Symptoms of overdose include deep sleep, coma, extrapyramidal symptoms, abnormal involuntary muscle movements, and hypotension. Following initiation of essential overdose management, toxic symptom treatment and supportive treatment should be initiated. Neuroleptics often cause extrapyramidal symptoms (eg, dystonic reactions) requiring management with anticholinergic agents such as benztropine mesylate 1-2 mg for adult patients (oral, I.M., I.V.) or diphenhydramine 25-50 mg (oral, I.M., I.V.) may be effective.

Pharmacodynamics/Kinetics

Absorption: Rapid

Bioavailability: 20%

Half-Life Elimination: Biphasic: Initial: 2 hours; Terminal: 30 hours

Metabolism: Extensively hepatic to active and inactive metabolites

Onset: I.M.: 15 minutes; Oral: 30-60 minutes

Formulations

Capsule, sustained action, as hydrochloride: 30 mg, 75 mg, 150 mg, 200 mg, 300 mg

Injection, as hydrochloride: 25 mg/mL (1 mL, 2 mL, 10 mL)

Solution, oral concentrate, as hydrochloride: 30 mg/mL (120 mL); 100 mg/mL (60 mL, 240 mL)

Suppository, rectal, as base: 25 mg, 100 mg

Syrup, as hydrochloride: 10 mg/5 mL (120 mL)

Tablet, as hydrochloride: 10 mg, 25 mg, 50 mg, 100 mg, 200 mg

Dosing

Adults:

Schizophrenia/psychoses:

Oral: Range: 30-800 mg/day in 1-4 divided doses, initiate at lower doses and titrate as needed; usual dose: 200 mg/day; some patients may require 1-2 g/day

I.M., I.V.: Initial: 25 mg, may repeat (25-50 mg) in 1-4 hours, gradually increase to a maximum of 400 mg/dose every 4-6 hours until patient is controlled; usual dose: 300-800 mg/day

Intractable hiccups: Oral, I.M.: 25-50 mg 3-4 times/day

Nausea and vomiting:

Oral: 10-25 mg every 4-6 hours

I.M., I.V.: 25-50 mg every 4-6 hours

Rectal: 50-100 mg every 6-8 hours

Elderly: Behavioral symptoms associated with dementia: Initial: 10-25 mg 1-2 times/day; increase at 4- to 7-day intervals by 10-25 mg/day. Increase dose intervals (bid, tid, etc) as necessary to control behavior response or side effects; maximum daily dose: 800 mg; gradual increases (titration) may prevent some side effects or decrease their severity.

Pediatrics:

Schizophrenia/psychoses: Children ≥6 months:

Oral: 0.5-1 mg/kg/dose every 4-6 hours; older children may require 200 mg/day or higher.

I.M., I.V.: 0.5-1 mg/kg/dose every 6-8 hours; maximum dose for <5 years (22.7 kg): 40 mg/day; maximum for 5-12 years (22.7-45.5 kg): 75 mg/day

Nausea and vomiting: Children ≥6 months:

Oral: 0.5-1 mg/kg/dose every 4-6 hours as needed

I.M., I.V.: 0.5-1 mg/kg/dose every 6-8 hours; maximum dose for <5 years (22.7 kg): 40 mg/day; maximum for 5-12 years (22.7-45.5 kg): 75 mg/day

Rectal: 1 mg/kg/dose every 6-8 hours as needed

Renal Impairment: Not dialyzable (0% to 5%)

Hepatic Impairment: Avoid use in severe hepatic dysfunction.

Administration

Oral: Dilute oral concentrate solution in juice before administration. Chlorpromazine concentrate is not compatible with carbamazepine suspension; schedule dosing at least 1-2 hours apart from each other. **Note:** Avoid skin contact with oral suspension or solution; may cause contact dermatitis.

I.V.: Direct of intermittent infusion: Infuse 1 mg or portion thereof over 1 minute.

Stability

Storage: Protect from light. A slightly yellowed solution does not indicate potency loss, but a markedly discolored solution should be discarded. Diluted injection (1 mg/mL) with NS and stored in 5 mL vials remains stable for 30 days.

Reconstitution: Diluted injection (1 mg/mL) with NS and stored in 5 mL vials remains stable for 30 days.

Compatibility: Stable in dextran 6% in dextrose, dextran 6% in NS, D_5LR, $D_5{}^1/_4NS$, $D_5{}^1/_2NS$, D_5NS, D_5W, $D_{10}W$, LR, $^1/_2NS$, NS

Y-site administration: Incompatible with allopurinol, amifostine, amphotericin B cholesteryl sulfate complex, aztreonam, cefepime, etoposide phosphate, fludarabine, furosemide, linezolid, melphalan, methotrexate, paclitaxel, piperacillin/tazobactam, sargramostim

Compatibility in syringe: Incompatible with cimetidine, dimenhydrinate, heparin, pentobarbital, thiopental

Compatibility when admixed: Incompatible with aminophylline, amphotericin B, ampicillin, chloramphenicol, chlorothiazide, floxacillin, furosemide, methohexital, penicillin G potassium, penicillin G sodium, phenobarbital

Monitoring Laboratory Tests Renal function, CBC, ophthalmic screening

Monitoring and Teaching Issues

Physical Assessment: Assess other medications patient is taking for effectiveness and interactions (see Drug Interactions). See Contraindications and Warnings/Precautions for use cautions. Review ophthalmic exam and monitor laboratory results (see above), therapeutic effects, and adverse reactions at beginning of therapy and periodically with long-term use (see Adverse Reactions and Overdose/Toxicology). **I.V./I.M.:** Significant hypotension may occur. Initiate at lower doses (see Dosing) and taper dosage slowly when discontinuing. Assess knowledge/teach patient appropriate use, interventions to reduce side effects, and adverse symptoms to report (see Patient Education). **Note:** Chlorpromazine may cause false-positive pregnancy test. **Pregnancy risk factor C** - benefits of use should outweigh possible risks. Breast-feeding is not recommended.

Patient Education: Use exactly as directed; do not increase dose or frequency. Do not discontinue without consulting prescriber. Tablets/capsules may be taken with food. Mix oral solution with 2-4 oz of liquid (eg, juice, milk, water). Do not take within 2 hours of any antacid. Store away from light. Avoid alcohol or caffeine and other prescription or OTC medications not approved by prescriber. Maintain adequate hydration (2-3 L/day of fluids) unless advised by prescriber to restrict fluids. May turn urine red-brown (normal). You may experience excess drowsiness, lightheadedness, dizziness, or blurred vision (use caution driving or when engaging in tasks requiring alertness until response to drug is known); dry mouth, upset stomach, nausea, vomiting, anorexia (small, frequent meals, frequent mouth care, sucking lozenges, or chewing gum may help); constipation (increased exercise, fluids, fruit, or fiber may help); postural hypotension (use caution climbing stairs or when changing position from lying or sitting to standing); urinary retention (void before taking medication); ejaculatory dysfunction (reversible); decreased perspiration (avoid strenuous exercise in hot environments); or photosensitivity (use sunscreen, wear protective clothing and eyewear, and avoid direct sunlight). Report persistent CNS effects (trembling fingers, altered gait or balance, excessive sedation, seizures, unusual movements, anxiety, abnormal thoughts, confusion, personality changes); chest pain, palpitations, rapid heartbeat, or severe dizziness; unresolved urinary retention or changes in urinary pattern; altered menstrual pattern, change in libido, swelling or pain in breasts (male or female); vision changes, skin rash, irritation, or changes in color of skin (gray-blue); or worsening of condition. **Pregnancy/breast-feeding precautions:** Inform prescriber if you are or intend to become pregnant. Breast-feeding is not recommended.

Geriatric Considerations: See Warnings/Precautions, Adverse Reactions, and Overdose/Toxicology. Elderly patients have an increased risk of adverse response to side effects or adverse reactions to antipsychotics.

Breast-feeding Issues: Drowsiness and lethargy have been reported in nursing infants; galactorrhea has been reported in mother.

Additional Information Avoid rectal administration in immunocompromised patients.

Related Information

Antiemetics for Chemotherapy-Induced Nausea and Vomiting *on page 1639*
Antipsychotic Agents *on page 1558*
Antipsychotic Medication Guidelines *on page 1614*
Compatibility of Drugs in Syringe *on page 1566*
FDA Name Differentiation Project: The Use of Tall-man Letters *on page 12*

Chlorpromazine Hydrochloride *see* ChlorproMAZINE *on page 277*
Chlorpropamide *see page 1661*
Chlorprothixene *see page 1558*

Chlorthalidone (klor THAL i done)

U.S. Brand Names Thalitone®

Synonyms Hygroton [DSC]

Generic Available Yes

Pharmacologic Category Diuretic, Thiazide

Pregnancy Risk Factor B (manufacturer); D (expert analysis)

Lactation Enters breast milk/use caution (AAP rates "compatible")

Use Management of mild to moderate hypertension when used alone or in combination with other agents; treatment of edema associated with congestive heart failure or nephrotic syndrome. Recent studies have found chlorthalidone effective in the treatment of isolated systolic hypertension in the elderly.

Mechanism of Action/Effect Sulfonamide-derived diuretic that inhibits sodium and chloride reabsorption in the cortical-diluting segment of the ascending loop of Henle

Contraindications Hypersensitivity to chlorthalidone or any component of the formulation; cross-sensitivity with other thiazides or sulfonamides; anuria; renal decompensation; pregnancy

Warnings/Precautions Use with caution in patients with hypokalemia, renal disease, hepatic disease, gout, lupus erythematosus, or diabetes mellitus. Use with caution in severe renal diseases. Correct hypokalemia before initiating therapy. Chemical similarities are present among sulfonamides, sulfonylureas, carbonic anhydrase inhibitors, thiazides, and loop

(Continued)

Chlorthalidone *(Continued)*

diuretics (except ethacrynic acid). Use in patients with thiazide or sulfonamide allergy is specifically contraindicated in product labeling, however, a risk of cross-reaction exists in patients with allergy to any of these compounds; avoid use when previous reaction has been severe.

Drug Interactions

Decreased Effect: Effects of oral hypoglycemics may be decreased. Decreased absorption of chlorthalidone with cholestyramine and colestipol. NSAIDs can decrease the efficacy of chlorthalidone, reducing the diuretic and antihypertensive effects.

Increased Effect/Toxicity: Increased effect of chlorthalidone with furosemide and other loop diuretics. Increased hypotension and/or renal adverse effects of ACE inhibitors may result in aggressively diuresed patients. Beta-blockers increase hyperglycemic effects of thiazides in Type 2 diabetes mellitus. Cyclosporine and thiazides can increase the risk of gout or renal toxicity. Digoxin toxicity can be exacerbated if a thiazide induces hypokalemia or hypomagnesemia. Lithium toxicity can occur with thiazides due to reduced renal excretion of lithium. Thiazides may prolong the duration of action with neuromuscular blocking agents.

Nutritional/Ethanol Interactions Herb/Nutraceutical: Avoid dong quai if using for hypertension (has estrogenic activity). Avoid dong quai, St John's Wort (may also cause photosensitization). Avoid ephedra, yohimbe, ginseng (may worsen hypertension).

Effects on Lab Values ↑ creatine phosphokinase [CPK] (S), ammonia (B), amylase (S), calcium (S), chloride (S), cholesterol (S), glucose, acid (S); ↓ chloride (S), magnesium, potassium (S), sodium (S)

Adverse Reactions

1% to 10%:

Dermatologic: Photosensitivity

Endocrine & metabolic: Hypokalemia

Gastrointestinal: Anorexia, epigastric distress

<1% (Limited to important or life-threatening): Agranulocytosis, aplastic anemia, cholecystitis, cutaneous vasculitis, gout, hypercalcemia, hyperglycemia, hyponatremia, leukopenia, necrotizing angiitis, pancreatitis, paresthesia, purpura, rash, thrombocytopenia, urticaria, vasculitis, vomiting

Overdosage/Toxicology Symptoms of overdose include hypermotility, diuresis, lethargy, confusion, muscle weakness, and coma. Treatment is supportive.

Pharmacodynamics/Kinetics

Absorption: 65%

Half-Life Elimination: 35-55 hours; may be prolonged with renal impairment; Anuria: 81 hours

Metabolism: Hepatic

Onset: Peak effect: 2-6 hours

Formulations

Tablet: 25 mg, 50 mg, 100 mg

Thalitone®: 15 mg

Dosing

Adults: Hypertension, edema: Oral: 25-100 mg/day or 100 mg 3 times/week

Elderly: Oral: Initial: 12.5-25 mg/day or every other day; there is little advantage to using doses >25 mg/day.

Pediatrics: Oral: Children (nonapproved): 2 mg/kg/dose 3 times/week or 1-2 mg/kg/day

Renal Impairment: Cl_{cr} <10 mL/minute: Administer every 48 hours.

Monitoring Laboratory Tests Serum electrolytes, renal function

Monitoring and Teaching Issues

Physical Assessment: Assess allergy history prior to beginning therapy. See Contraindications and Warnings/Precautions for use cautions. Assess potential for interactions with other prescriptions, OTC medications, or herbal products patient may be taking (see Drug Interactions). Assess results of laboratory tests (see above) on a regular basis throughout therapy. Assess therapeutic effectiveness and adverse response (eg, blood pressure, fluid status, and electrolyte balance - see Adverse Reactions and Overdose/Toxicology) regularly during long-term therapy. Caution diabetic patients to monitor glucose levels (may reduce effect of oral hypoglycemics). Teach patient appropriate use, possible side effects and interventions, and adverse symptoms to report (see Patient Education). **Pregnancy risk factor B/D** - see Pregnancy Risk Factor for use cautions; benefits of use should outweigh possible risks. Note breast-feeding caution.

Patient Education: Inform prescriber of all prescriptions, OTC medications, or herbal products you are taking, and any allergies you have. Do not take anything new during treatment unless approved by prescriber. Take once-daily dose in morning or last of daily doses early in the day to avoid night-time disturbances. You may need to make dietary changes; follow dietary suggestions of prescriber (see Dietary Considerations). If using oral hypoglycemics, monitor glucose levels closely (this medication may reduce effect of oral hypoglycemics); contact prescriber with any major changes. May cause sensitivity to sunlight (use sunblock, wear protective clothing, and avoid direct sunlight); or anorexia or GI distress (small, frequent meals, frequent mouth care, chewing gum, or sucking lozenges may help). Report muscle twitching or cramps; nausea or vomiting; confusion; numbness of extremities; loss of appetite or GI distress; severe rash, redness, or itching of skin; chest pain or palpitations; or difficulty breathing. **Pregnancy/breast-feeding precautions:** Do not get pregnant while taking this medication. Consult prescriber for appropriate contraceptive measures. Consult prescriber if breast-feeding.

Dietary Issues: This product may cause a potassium loss; your healthcare provider may prescribe a potassium supplement, another medication to help prevent the potassium loss, or recommend that you eat foods high in potassium, especially citrus fruits; do not change your diet on your own while taking this medication, especially if you are taking potassium supplements or medications to reduce potassium loss; too much potassium can be as harmful as too little.

Geriatric Considerations: Studies have found chlorthalidone effective in the treatment of isolated systolic hypertension in the elderly.

Related Information

Heart Failure *on page 1670*

Chlorthalidone and Atenolol *see* Atenolol and Chlorthalidone *on page 128*

Chlorthalidone and Clonidine *see* Clonidine and Chlorthalidone *on page 319*

Chlorzoxazone (klor ZOKS a zone)

U.S. Brand Names Parafon Forte® DSC

Generic Available Yes

Pharmacologic Category Skeletal Muscle Relaxant

Pregnancy Risk Factor C

Lactation Excretion in breast milk unknown/not recommended

Use Symptomatic treatment of muscle spasm and pain associated with acute musculoskeletal conditions

Mechanism of Action/Effect Acts on the spinal cord and subcortical levels by depressing polysynaptic reflexes

Contraindications Hypersensitivity to chlorzoxazone or any component of the formulation; impaired liver function

Warnings/Precautions Pregnancy risk C.

Drug Interactions

Cytochrome P450 Effect: Substrate of CYP1A2, 2A6, 2D6, **2E1**, 3A4; Inhibits CYP2E1, 3A4

Increased Effect/Toxicity: Increased effect/toxicity when taken with ethanol or CNS depressants.

Nutritional/Ethanol Interactions Ethanol: Avoid ethanol (may increase CNS depression).

Adverse Reactions Frequency not defined.

Central nervous system: Dizziness, drowsiness lightheadedness, paradoxical stimulation, malaise

Dermatologic: Rash, petechiae, ecchymoses (rare), angioneurotic edema

Gastrointestinal: Nausea, vomiting, stomach cramps

Genitourinary: Urine discoloration

Hepatic: Liver dysfunction

Miscellaneous: Anaphylaxis (very rare)

Overdosage/Toxicology Symptoms of overdose include nausea, vomiting, diarrhea, drowsiness, dizziness, headache, absent tendon reflexes, and hypotension. Treatment is supportive following attempts to enhance drug elimination. Dialysis, hemoperfusion, and osmotic diuresis have all been useful in reducing serum drug concentrations. The patient should be observed for possible relapses due to incomplete gastric emptying.

Pharmacodynamics/Kinetics

Absorption: Readily absorbed

Metabolism: Extensively hepatic via glucuronidation

Onset: ~1 hour

Duration: 6-12 hours

Formulations

Caplet (Parafon Forte® DSC): 500 mg

Tablet: 250 mg

Dosing

Adults: Muscle spasm: Oral: 250-500 mg 3-4 times/day up to 750 mg 3-4 times/day

Elderly: Oral: Initial: 250 mg 2-4 times/day; increase as necessary to 750 mg 3-4 times/day.

Pediatrics: Muscle spasm: Oral: 20 mg/kg/day or 600 mg/m^2/day in 3-4 divided doses

Monitoring Laboratory Tests Periodic liver functions

Monitoring and Teaching Issues

Physical Assessment: Monitor results of laboratory tests (see above), effectiveness of therapy (according to rational for therapy), and adverse reactions (see Adverse Reactions) at beginning of therapy and periodically with long-term use. Do not discontinue abruptly; taper dosage slowly. Assess knowledge/teach patient appropriate use, interventions to reduce side effects, and adverse symptoms to report (see Patient Education). **Pregnancy risk factor C** - benefits of use should outweigh possible risks. Breast-feeding is not recommended.

Patient Education: Take exactly as directed with food. Do not increase dose or discontinue without consulting prescriber. Do not use alcohol, prescriptive or OTC antidepressants, sedatives, or pain medications without consulting prescriber. May turn urine orange or red (normal). You may experience drowsiness, dizziness, lightheadedness (avoid driving or engaging in tasks that require alertness until response to drug is known); nausea, vomiting, or cramping (small, frequent meals, frequent mouth care, or sucking hard candy may help); postural hypotension (change position slowly when rising from sitting or lying or when climbing stairs); or constipation (increased exercise, fluids, fruit, or fiber may help). Report excessive drowsiness or mental agitation; palpitations, rapid heartbeat, or chest pain; skin rash or swelling of mouth or face; persistent diarrhea or constipation; or unusual weakness or bleeding. **Pregnancy/breast-feeding precautions:** Inform prescriber if you are or intend to become pregnant. Breast-feeding is not recommended.

Geriatric Considerations: Start dosing low and increase as necessary. The FDA recently approved a stronger warning about hepatotoxicity in the labeling of chlorzoxazone. Because it can cause unpredictable, fatal hepatic toxicity, the use of chlorzoxazone should be avoided.

Cholac® *see* Lactulose *on page 767*

Cholera Vaccine *see page 1498*

Cholestyramine Resin (koe LES tir a meen REZ in)

U.S. Brand Names LoCHOLEST®; LoCHOLEST® Light; Prevalite®; Questran®; Questran® Light

Generic Available Yes

Pharmacologic Category Antilipemic Agent, Bile Acid Sequestrant

Pregnancy Risk Factor C

Lactation Excretion in breast milk unknown/not recommended

Use Adjunct in the management of primary hypercholesterolemia; pruritus associated with elevated levels of bile acids; diarrhea associated with excess fecal bile acids; binding toxicologic agents; pseudomembraneous colitis

Mechanism of Action/Effect Forms a nonabsorbable complex with bile acids in the intestine, releasing chloride ions in the process; inhibits enterohepatic reuptake of intestinal bile salts and thereby increases the fecal loss of bile salt-bound low density lipoprotein cholesterol

Contraindications Hypersensitivity of bile acid sequestering resins or any component of the formulation; complete biliary obstruction; bowel obstruction

Warnings/Precautions Not to be taken simultaneously with many other medicines (decreased absorption). Treat any diseases contributing to hypercholesterolemia first. May interfere with fat-soluble vitamins (A, D, E, K) and folic acid. Chronic use may be associated with bleeding problems (especially in high doses). May produce or exacerbate constipation problems. Fecal impaction may occur. Hemorrhoids may be worsened. Pregnancy risk C.

Drug Interactions

Decreased Effect: Cholestyramine resin may cause decreased absorption of digitalis glycosides (oral), warfarin, thyroid hormones, thiazide diuretics, propranolol, phenobarbital, amiodarone, methotrexate, NSAIDs, and other drugs.

Nutritional/Ethanol Interactions

Food: Cholestyramine (especially high doses or long-term therapy) may decrease the absorption of folic acid, calcium, and iron.

Herb/Nutraceutical: Cholestyramine (especially high doses or long-term therapy) may decrease the absorption of fat-soluble vitamins (vitamins A, D, E, and K).

Effects on Lab Values ↑ prothrombin time (S); ↓ cholesterol (S), iron (B)

Adverse Reactions

>10%: Gastrointestinal: Constipation, heartburn, nausea, vomiting, stomach pain

1% to 10%:

Central nervous system: Headache

Gastrointestinal: Belching, bloating, diarrhea

<1% (Limited to important or life-threatening): Gallstones or pancreatitis, GI bleeding, hyperchloremic acidosis, hypoprothrombinemia (secondary to vitamin K deficiency), peptic ulcer, steatorrhea or malabsorption syndrome

Overdosage/Toxicology Symptoms of overdose include GI obstruction. Treatment is supportive.

Pharmacodynamics/Kinetics

Absorption: None

Onset: Peak effect: 21 days

Formulations

Powder: 4 g of resin/9 g of powder (9 g, 378 g)

Powder for oral suspension:

With aspartame: 4 g of resin/5 g of powder (5 g, 210 g)

With phenylalanine: 4 g of resin/5.5 g of powder (60s)

Dosing

Adults & Elderly: Dyslipidemia: Oral (dosages are expressed in terms of anhydrous resin):

Powder: 4 g 1-2 times/day to a maximum of 16-24 g/day (and a maximum of 6 times/day)

Tablet: Initial: 4 g once or twice daily; maintenance: 8-16 g/day in 2 divided doses

Pediatrics: Dyslipidemia: Oral (dosages are expressed in terms of anhydrous resin): Children:

Powder: 240 mg/kg/day in 3 divided doses; need to titrate dose depending on indication

Renal Impairment: Not removed by hemo- or peritoneal dialysis. Supplemental doses not necessary with dialysis or continuous arteriovenous or venovenous hemofiltration effects.

Administration

Oral: Mix contents of 1 packet or 1 level scoop of powder with 4-6 oz of beverage. Allow to stand 1-2 minutes prior to mixing. May also be mixed with highly fluid soups, cereals, applesauce, etc.

Stability

Storage: Suspension may be used for up to 48 hours after refrigeration.

Monitoring Laboratory Tests Serum cholesterol and triglyceride levels should be obtained before initiating drug treatment and periodically throughout treatment.

Monitoring and Teaching Issues

Physical Assessment: Assess other medications patient may be taking for effectiveness and interactions (see Drug Interactions). Monitor laboratory results, therapeutic response, and adverse reactions (see Adverse Reactions and Overdose/Toxicology) periodically throughout therapy. Assess knowledge/teach patient appropriate use, interventions to reduce side effects, and adverse symptoms to report (see Patient Education). **Pregnancy risk factor C** - benefits of use should outweigh possible risks. Breast-feeding is not recommended.

Patient Education: Take once or twice a day as directed. Do not take the powder in its dry form; mix with fluid, applesauce, pudding, or jello. Chew bars thoroughly. Take other medications 1 hour before or 4-6 hours after cholestyramine. Ongoing medical follow-up and laboratory tests may be required. You may experience GI effects (these should resolve after continued use); nausea and vomiting (small, frequent meals, frequent mouth care, sucking lozenges, or chewing gum may help); or constipation (increased exercise, fluids, fruit, or fiber may help; consult prescriber about use of stool softener or laxative). Report unusual stomach cramping, pain or blood in stool; unresolved nausea, vomiting, or constipation. **Pregnancy/breast-feeding precautions:** Inform prescriber if you are or intend to become pregnant. Breast-feeding is not recommended.

Dietary Issues: Supplementation of vitamins A, D, E, and K, folic acid, and iron may be required with high-dose, long-term therapy.

Geriatric Considerations: The definition of and, therefore, when to treat hyperlipidemia in the elderly is a controversial issue. Treatment is best reserved for those who are unable to obtain a desirable plasma cholesterol level by diet alone and for whom the benefits of treatment are believed to outweigh the potential adverse effects, drug interactions, and cost of treatment.

Related Information

Hyperlipidemia Management *on page 1682*
Lipid-Lowering Agents *on page 1582*

Choline Magnesium Salicylate *see page 1587*

Choline Magnesium Trisalicylate

(KOE leen mag NEE zhum trye sa LIS i late)

U.S. Brand Names Tricosal®; Trilisate®

Generic Available Yes

Pharmacologic Category Salicylate

Pregnancy Risk Factor C/D (3rd trimester)

Lactation Enters breast milk/use caution

Use Management of osteoarthritis, rheumatoid arthritis, and other arthritis; salicylate salts may not inhibit platelet aggregation and, therefore, should not be substituted for aspirin in the prophylaxis of thrombosis; acute painful shoulder

Mechanism of Action/Effect Inhibits prostaglandin synthesis; acts on the hypothalamus heat-regulating center to reduce fever; blocks the generation of pain impulses

Contraindications Hypersensitivity to salicylates, other nonacetylated salicylates, other NSAIDs, or any component of the formulation; tartrazine dye hypersensitivity; bleeding disorders; pregnancy (3rd trimester)

Warnings/Precautions Use with caution in patients with dehydration, impaired renal function, erosive gastritis, or peptic ulcer. Avoid use in patients with suspected varicella or influenza (salicylates have been associated with Reye's syndrome in children <16 years of age when used to treat symptoms of chickenpox or the flu). Tinnitus or impaired hearing may indicate toxicity; discontinue use 1 week prior to surgical procedures.

Elderly are a high-risk population for adverse effects from NSAIDs. As many as 60% of elderly can develop peptic ulceration and/or hemorrhage asymptomatically. Use lowest effective dose for shortest period possible. CNS adverse effects may be observed in the elderly at lower doses than younger adults.

Pregnancy risk C/D (3rd trimester).

Drug Interactions

Decreased Effect: Antacids may decrease choline magnesium trisalicylate absorption/salicylate concentrations.

Increased Effect/Toxicity: Choline magnesium trisalicylate may increase the hypoprothrombinemic effect of warfarin.

Nutritional/Ethanol Interactions

Ethanol: Avoid ethanol (may enhance gastric mucosal irritation).

Food: May decrease the rate but not the extent of oral absorption.

Herb/Nutraceutical: Avoid cat's claw, dong quai, evening primrose, feverfew, garlic, ginger, ginkgo, red clover, horse chestnut, green tea, ginseng (all have additional antiplatelet activity). Limit curry powder, paprika, licorice, Benedictine liqueur, prunes, raisins, tea, and gherkins; may cause salicylate accumulation. These foods contain 6 mg salicylate/100 g.

Effects on Lab Values False-negative results for glucose oxidase urinary glucose tests (Clinistix®); false-positives using the cupric sulfate method (Clinitest®); also, interferes with Gerhardt test (urinary ketone analysis), VMA determination; 5-HIAA, xylose tolerance test, and T_3 and T_4; increased PBI; increased uric acid

Adverse Reactions

<20%:

Gastrointestinal: Nausea, vomiting, diarrhea, heartburn, dyspepsia, epigastric pain, constipation

Ocular: Tinnitus

<2%:

Central nervous system: Headache, lightheadedness, dizziness, drowsiness, lethargy

Ocular: Hearing impairment

<1% (Limited to important or life-threatening): Anorexia, BUN increased, creatinine increased, dysgeusia, edema, epistaxis, gastric ulceration, occult bleeding, pruritus, rash, weight gain

Overdosage/Toxicology Symptoms of overdose include tinnitus, vomiting, acute renal failure, hyperthermia, irritability, seizures, coma, and metabolic acidosis. For acute ingestion, determine serum salicylate levels 6 hours after ingestion. Nomograms, such as the "Done" nomogram, may be helpful for estimating the severity of aspirin poisoning and directing treatment using serum salicylate levels. Treatment is based upon symptomatology.

Pharmacodynamics/Kinetics

Absorption: Stomach and small intestines

Half-Life Elimination: Dose dependent: Low dose: 2-3 hours; High dose: 30 hours

Time to Peak: Serum: ~2 hours

Onset: Peak effect: ~2 hours

Formulations

Liquid: 500 mg/5 mL total salicylate (293 mg/5 mL choline salicylate and 362 mg/5 mL magnesium salicylate)

Tablet:

500 mg total salicylate (293 mg choline salicylate and 362 mg magnesium salicylate)

(Continued)

Choline Magnesium Trisalicylate *(Continued)*

750 mg total salicylate (440 mg choline salicylate and 544 mg magnesium salicylate)
1000 mg total salicylate (587 mg choline salicylate and 725 mg magnesium salicylate)

Dosing

Adults & Elderly: Arthritis, pain: Oral (based on total salicylate content): 500 mg to 1.5 g 2-3 times/day; usual maintenance dose: 1-4.5 g/day

Pediatrics: Children: Oral (based on total salicylate content): <37 kg: 50 mg/kg/day given in 2 divided doses

Renal Impairment: Avoid use in severe renal impairment.

Administration

Oral: Liquid may be mixed with fruit juice just before drinking. Do not administer with antacids. Take with a full glass of water and remain in an upright position for 15-30 minutes after administration.

Monitoring Laboratory Tests Serum magnesium with high-dose therapy or in patients with impaired renal function, serum salicylate levels, renal function

Monitoring and Teaching Issues

Physical Assessment: **Do not use for persons with allergic reaction to salicylates or other NSAIDs** (see Contraindications). Assess other medications patient may be taking for additive or adverse interactions (see Drug Interactions). Monitor for effectiveness of pain relief. Monitor for signs of adverse reactions or overdose (see Overdose/Toxicology and Adverse Reactions) at beginning of therapy and periodically during long-term therapy. Assess knowledge/teach patient appropriate use. Teach patient to monitor for adverse reactions, adverse reactions to report, and appropriate interventions to reduce side effects. **Pregnancy risk factor C/D** - benefits of use should outweigh possible risks. Note breast-feeding caution.

Patient Education: If self-administered, use exactly as directed; do not increase dose or frequency. Adverse reactions can occur with overuse. Take with food or milk. While using this medication, do not use alcohol, excessive amounts of vitamin C, or salicylate-containing foods (curry powder, prunes, raisins, tea, or licorice), other prescription or OTC medications containing aspirin or salicylate, or other NSAIDs without consulting prescriber. Maintain adequate hydration (2-3 L/day of fluids) unless advised by prescriber to restrict fluids. You may experience nausea, vomiting, gastric discomfort (frequent mouth care, small, frequent meals, sucking lozenges, or chewing gum may help). GI bleeding, ulceration, or perforation can occur with or without pain. Stop taking medication and report ringing in ears; persistent stomach pain; unresolved nausea or vomiting; difficulty breathing or shortness of breath; or unusual bruising or bleeding (mouth, urine, stool); or skin rash. **Pregnancy/breast-feeding precautions:** Inform prescriber if you are or intend to become pregnant. Consult prescriber if breast-feeding.

Dietary Issues: Take with food or large volume of water or milk to minimize GI upset. Liquid may be mixed with fruit juice just before drinking.

Magnesium: Hypermagnesemia resulting from magnesium salicylate; avoid or use with caution in renal insufficiency.

Geriatric Considerations: Elderly are at high risk for adverse effects from nonsteroidal anti-inflammatory agents. As much as 60% of elderly can develop peptic ulceration and/or hemorrhage asymptomatically.

Breast-feeding Issues: Excreted in breast milk; peak levels occur 9-12 hours after dose. Use caution if used during breast-feeding.

Additional Information Contains choline salicylate 293 mg and magnesium salicylate 362 mg per tablet or 5 mL of liquid. Salicylate salts do not inhibit platelet aggregation and, therefore, should not be substituted for aspirin in the prophylaxis of thrombosis.

Related Information

Nonsalicylate/Nonsteroidal Anti-inflammatory Comparison *on page 1587*

Chondroitin Sulfate - Sodium Hyaluronate *see page 1509*
Chondroitin Sulfate - Sodium Hyaluronate *see page 1461*
Chooz® [OTC] *see* Calcium Supplements *on page 202*
Chorex® *see* Chorionic Gonadotropin (Human) *on page 284*
Choriogonadotropin Alfa *see* Chorionic Gonadotropin (Recombinant) *on page 285*

Chorionic Gonadotropin (Human)

(kor ee ON ik goe NAD oh troe pin HYU man)

U.S. Brand Names A.P.L.®; Chorex®; Choron®; Gonic®; Novarel™; Pregnyl®; Profasi®

Synonyms CG; hCG

Generic Available Yes

Pharmacologic Category Ovulation Stimulator

Pregnancy Risk Factor C

Lactation Excretion in breast milk unknown/unlikely to be used

Use Induces ovulation and pregnancy in anovulatory, infertile females; treatment of hypogonadotropic hypogonadism, prepubertal cryptorchidism; spermatogenesis induction with follitropin alfa or follitropin beta

Mechanism of Action/Effect Stimulates production of gonadal steroid hormones by causing production of androgen by the testis; as a substitute for luteinizing hormone (LH) to stimulate ovulation

Contraindications Hypersensitivity to chorionic gonadotropin or any component of the formulation; precocious puberty, prostatic carcinoma or similar neoplasms

Warnings/Precautions Use with caution in asthma, seizure disorders, migraine, cardiac or renal disease. **Not** effective in the treatment of obesity. Pregnancy risk C.

Adverse Reactions

1% to 10%:

Central nervous system: Mental depression, fatigue

Endocrine & metabolic: Pelvic pain, ovarian cysts, enlargement of breasts, precocious puberty

Local: Pain at the injection site

Neuromuscular & skeletal: Premature closure of epiphyses

<1% (Limited to important or life-threatening): Gynecomastia, headache, irritability, ovarian hyperstimulation syndrome, peripheral edema, restlessness

Pharmacodynamics/Kinetics

Half-Life Elimination: Biphasic: Initial: 11 hours; Terminal: 23 hours

Formulations Injection, powder for reconstitution, human: 500 units/mL (10 mL); 1000 units/mL (10 mL); 2000 units/mL (10 mL)

Dosing

Adults & Elderly:

Use with menotropins to stimulate spermatogenesis: I.M.: 5000 units 3 times/week for 4-6 months. With the beginning of menotropins therapy, hCG dose is continued at 2000 units 2 times/week.

Induction of ovulation and pregnancy: I.M.: 5000-10,000 units 1 day following last dose of menotropins

Spermatogenesis induction: Male: I.M.: Initial: 1500 int. units twice weekly to normalize serum testosterone levels. If no response in 8 weeks, increase dose to 3000 int. units twice weekly. After normalization of testosterone levels, combine with follitropin beta (Follistim®). Continue hCG at same dose used to normalize testosterone levels. Treatment response was noted at up to 12 months.

Pediatrics:

Prepubertal cryptorchidism: I.M.: Children: 1000-2000 units/m^2/dose 3 times/week for 3 weeks **or** 4000 units 3 times/week for 3 weeks **or** 5000 units every second day for 4 injections **or** 500 units 3 times/week for 4-6 weeks

Hypogonadotropic hypogonadism: I.M.: Children: 500-1000 units 3 times/week for 3 weeks, followed by the same dose twice weekly for 3 weeks **or** 1000-2000 units 3 times/week **or** 4000 units 3 times/week for 6-9 months; reduce dosage to 2000 units 3 times/week for additional 3 months.

Administration

I.M.: I.M. administration only

Stability

Reconstitution: Following reconstitution with the provided diluent, solutions are stable for 30-90 days, depending on the specific preparation, when stored at 2°C to 15°C.

Monitoring and Teaching Issues

Physical Assessment: See Contraindications, Warnings/Precautions, and Dosing for use cautions. Assess therapeutic effectiveness (according to purpose for use) and adverse response (see Adverse Reactions) regularly during long-term therapy. Teach patient appropriate use (if self-administered, include injection technique and needle disposal), possible side effects and interventions, and adverse symptoms to report (see Patient Education). **Pregnancy risk factor C** - benefits of use should outweigh possible risks. Note breast-feeding caution.

Patient Education: This medication can only be administered by injection. If self-administered, follow instruction for reconstitution, injection, and needle disposal as instructed. Follow use directions exactly; do not alter dosage or miss a dose. May cause headache, depression, irritability, or restlessness (use caution when driving or engaging in potentially hazardous tasks until response to drug is known). Contact prescriber if symptoms are severe or do not resolve with use. Contact prescriber if breasts swell; if you experience swelling of legs or feet; or if there is pain, redness, or swelling at injection site. **Pregnancy/breast-feeding precautions:** Inform prescriber if you are or intend to become pregnant. Consult prescriber if breast-feeding.

Chorionic Gonadotropin (Recombinant)

(kor ee ON ik goe NAD oh troe pin ree KOM be nant)

U.S. Brand Names Ovidrel®

Synonyms Choriogonadotropin Alfa; r-hCG

Generic Available No

Pharmacologic Category Gonadotropin; Ovulation Stimulator

Pregnancy Risk Factor X

Lactation Excretion in breast milk unknown/use caution

Use As part of an assisted reproductive technology (ART) program, induces ovulation in infertile females who have been pretreated with follicle stimulating hormones (FSH); induces ovulation and pregnancy in infertile females when the cause of infertility is functional

Contraindications Hypersensitivity to hCG preparations or any component of the formulation; primary ovarian failure; uncontrolled thyroid or adrenal dysfunction; uncontrolled organic intracranial lesion (ie, pituitary tumor); abnormal uterine bleeding, ovarian cyst or enlargement of undetermined origin; sex hormone dependent tumors; pregnancy

Warnings/Precautions For use by infertility specialists; may cause ovarian hyperstimulation syndrome (OHSS); if severe, treatment should be discontinued and patient should be hospitalized. OHSS results in a rapid (<24 hours to 7 days) accumulation of fluid in the peritoneal cavity, thorax, and possibly the pericardium, which may become more severe if pregnancy occurs; monitor for ovarian enlargement; use may lead to multiple births; risk of arterial thromboembolism with hCG products; safety and efficacy in pediatric and geriatric patients have not been established.

Drug Interactions

Increased Effect/Toxicity: Specific drug interaction studies have not been conducted.

Effects on Lab Values May interfere with interpretation of pregnancy tests; may cross-react with radioimmunoassay of luteinizing hormone and other gonadotropins

Adverse Reactions

2% to 10%:

Endocrine & metabolic: Ovarian cyst (3%), ovarian hyperstimulation (<2% to 3%)

Gastrointestinal: Abdominal pain (3% to 4%), nausea (3%), vomiting (3%)

Local: Injection site: Pain (8%), bruising (3% to 5%), reaction (<2% to 3%), inflammation (<2% to 2%)

(Continued)

Chorionic Gonadotropin (Recombinant) *(Continued)*

Miscellaneous: Postoperative pain (5%)

<2% (Limited to important or life-threatening): Abdominal enlargement, albuminuria, back pain, breast pain, cardiac arrhythmia, cervical carcinoma, cervical lesion, cough, diarrhea, dizziness, dysuria, ectopic pregnancy, emotional lability, fever, flatulence, genital herpes, genital moniliasis, headache, heart murmur, hiccups, hot flashes, hyperglycemia, insomnia, intermenstrual bleeding, leukocytosis, leukorrhea, malaise, paresthesias, pharyngitis, pruritus, rash, upper respiratory tract infection, urinary incontinence, urinary tract infection, vaginal hemorrhage, vaginitis

In addition, the following have been reported with menotropin therapy: Adnexal torsion, hemoperitoneum, mild to moderate ovarian enlargement, pulmonary and vascular complications. Ovarian neoplasms have also been reported (rare) with multiple drug regimens used for ovarian induction (relationship not established).

Pharmacodynamics/Kinetics

Bioavailability: 40%

Half-Life Elimination: Initial: 4 hours; Terminal: 29 hours

Time to Peak: 12-24 hours

Formulations Injection [single-dose vial]: 285 mcg r-hCG per vial with 1 mL SWFI [delivers 250 mcg r-hCG following reconstitution]

Dosing

Adults: Assisted reproductive technologies (ART) and ovulation induction in females: S.C.: 250 mcg given 1 day following the last dose of follicle stimulating agent. Use only after adequate follicular development has been determined. Hold treatment when there is an excessive ovarian response.

Elderly: Safety and efficacy have not been established.

Renal Impairment: Safety and efficacy have not been established.

Hepatic Impairment: Safety and efficacy have not been established.

Stability

Storage: Store in original package under refrigeration or at room temperature, 2°C to 25°C (36°F to 77°F). Protect from light.

Monitoring and Teaching Issues

Physical Assessment: For use only under the supervision/direction of an infertility physician. See Use, Contraindications, and Warnings/Precautions for specific use directions and cautions. Monitor for adverse reactions (see Adverse Reactions and Overdose/Toxicology). Assess knowledge/teach patient appropriate use (if self-administered: storage, reconstitution, injection technique, needle/syringe disposal - recommend return demonstration), monitoring requirements, interventions to reduce side effects, and adverse reactions to report (see Patient Education). **Pregnancy risk factor X** - determine that patient is not pregnant before beginning treatment and monitor ovulation closely during treatment (see Monitoring Laboratory Tests). Note breast-feeding caution.

Patient Education: Note that there is a risk of multiple births associated with treatment. This drug must be administered exactly as scheduled (1 day following last dose of follicle stimulating agent); maintain a calendar of treatment days. Follow administration directions exactly (see below). Keep all ultrasound and laboratory appointments as instructed by prescriber. Avoid strenuous exercise, especially those with pelvic involvement. You may experience nausea, vomiting, or GI upset (small, frequent meals, frequent mouth care, sucking lozenges, or chewing gum may help), hot flashes (cool clothes, cool room, adequate rest may help) if persistent consult prescriber. Report immediately any persistent abdominal pain, vomiting, or acute pelvic pain; chest pain or palpitations; shortness of breath; or urinary tract or vaginal infection or urinary incontinence. **Pregnancy/ breast-feeding precautions:** Do not take this medicine if you are pregnant and report to prescriber immediately if you suspect you are pregnant. Consult prescriber if breast-feeding.

Administration: Wash hands and prepare medication in clean environment. Add 1 mL sterile water to vial and gently mix by rotating vial to dissolve powder; do not shake vial. Use only if solution is clear and colorless. Use immediately following reconstitution and inject exactly as directed into stomach area. Do not rub area of injection. Dispose of syringe, needle, and vial in sealed container (do not dispose where others could have access to materials). Wash hands.

Pregnancy Issues: Ectopic pregnancy, premature labor, postpartum fever, and spontaneous abortion have been reported in clinical trials. Congenital abnormalities have also been observed, however, the incidence is similar during natural conception.

Additional Information Clinical studies have shown r-hCG to be clinically and statistically equivalent to urinary-derived hCG products.

Choron® *see* Chorionic Gonadotropin (Human) *on page 284*

Chymex® *see page 1461*

Chymodiactin® *see page 1461*

Chymopapain *see page 1461*

Cidofovir (si DOF o veer)

U.S. Brand Names Vistide®

Generic Available No

Pharmacologic Category Antiviral Agent

Pregnancy Risk Factor C

Lactation Excretion in breast milk unknown/contraindicated

Use Treatment of cytomegalovirus (CMV) retinitis in patients with acquired immunodeficiency syndrome (AIDS). **Note:** Should be administered with probenecid.

Mechanism of Action/Effect Nucleotide analog that selectively inhibits viral DNA polymerase, suppressing viral DNA synthesis

Contraindications Patients with hypersensitivity to cidofovir and in patients with a history of clinically severe hypersensitivity to probenecid or other sulfa-containing medications

Warnings/Precautions Dose-dependent nephrotoxicity requires dose adjustment or discontinuation if changes in renal function occur during therapy (eg, proteinuria, glycosuria, decreased serum phosphate, uric acid or bicarbonate, and elevated creatinine); avoid use in patients with creatinine >1.5 mg/dL; Cl_{cr} <55 mL/minute; use great caution with elderly patients; neutropenia and ocular hypotony have also occurred; safety and efficacy have not been established in children; administration must be accompanied by oral probenecid and intravenous saline prehydration; prepare admixtures in a class two laminar flow hood, wearing protective gear; dispose of cidofovir as directed. Pregnancy risk C.

Drug Interactions

Increased Effect/Toxicity: Drugs with nephrotoxic potential (eg, amphotericin B, aminoglycosides, foscarnet, and I.V. pentamidine) should be avoided during cidofovir therapy.

Adverse Reactions

>10%:

Central nervous system: Infection, chills, fever, headache, amnesia, anxiety, confusion, seizures, insomnia
Dermatologic: Alopecia, rash, acne, skin discoloration
Gastrointestinal: Nausea, vomiting, diarrhea, anorexia, abdominal pain, constipation, heartburn, gastritis
Hematologic: Thrombocytopenia, neutropenia, anemia
Neuromuscular & skeletal: Weakness, paresthesia
Ocular: Amblyopia, conjunctivitis, ocular hypotony
Renal: Tubular damage, proteinuria, Cr elevations
Respiratory: Asthma, bronchitis, coughing, dyspnea, pharyngitis

1% to 10%:

Cardiovascular: Hypotension, pallor, syncope, tachycardia
Central nervous system: Dizziness, hallucinations, depression, somnolence, malaise
Dermatologic: Pruritus, urticaria
Endocrine & metabolic: Hyperglycemia, hyperlipidemia, hypocalcemia, hypokalemia, dehydration
Gastrointestinal: Abnormal taste, stomatitis
Genitourinary: Glycosuria, urinary incontinence, urinary tract infections
Neuromuscular & skeletal: Skeletal pain
Ocular: Retinal detachment, iritis, uveitis, decreased intraocular pressure, abnormal vision
Renal: Hematuria
Respiratory: Pneumonia, rhinitis, sinusitis
Miscellaneous: Diaphoresis, allergic reactions

<1% (Limited to important or life-threatening): Fanconi syndrome, hepatic failure, increased bicarbonate excretion, iritis, metabolic acidosis, pancreatitis, uveitis

Overdosage/Toxicology No reports of acute toxicity have been reported, however, hemodialysis and hydration may reduce drug plasma concentrations. Probenecid may assist in decreasing active tubular secretion.

Pharmacokinetic Note Data is based on a combination of cidofovir administered with probenecid.

Pharmacodynamics/Kinetics

Half-Life Elimination: Plasma: ~2.6 hours

Metabolism: Minimal; phosphorylation occurs intracellularly

Formulations Injection: 75 mg/mL (5 mL)

Dosing

Adults & Elderly: Treatment of cytomegalovirus (CMV) retinitis: I.V.:

Induction treatment: 5 mg/kg once weekly for 2 consecutive weeks
Maintenance treatment: 5 mg/kg administered once every 2 weeks
Note: Probenecid must be administered orally with each dose of cidofovir.
Probenecid dose: 2 g 3 hours prior to cidofovir dose, 1 g 2 hours and 8 hours after completion of the infusion; patients should also receive 1 L of normal saline intravenously prior to each infusion of cidofovir; saline should be infused over 1-2 hours.

Renal Impairment:

Cl_{cr} 41-55 mL/minute:
Induction (weekly x 2 doses): 2 mg/kg
Maintenance (every other week): 2 mg/kg
Cl_{cr} 30-40 mL/minute:
Induction (weekly x 2 doses): 1.5 mg/kg
Maintenance (every other week): 1.5 mg/kg
Cl_{cr} 20-29 mL/minute:
Induction (weekly x 2 doses): 1 mg/kg
Maintenance (every other week): 1 mg/kg
Cl_{cr} <19 mL/minute:
Induction (weekly x 2 doses): 0.5 mg/kg
Maintenance (every other week): 0.5 mg/kg
Patients with clinically significant changes in serum creatinine during therapy: Cidofovir dose should be reduced to 3 mg/kg and discontinued if creatinine rise is >0.5 mg/dL.
Hemodialysis with high-flux filters may reduce serum concentration by as much as 75%.

Administration

I.V.: For I.V. infusion only. Infuse over 1 hour. Hydrate with 1 L of 0.9% NS I.V. prior to cidofovir infusion; a second liter may be administered over a 1- to 3-hour period immediately following infusion, if tolerated

Stability

Storage: Store at controlled room temperature 20°C to 25°C (68°F to 77°F). Store admixtures under refrigeration for ≤24 hours.

Reconstitution: Cidofovir infusion admixture should be administered within 24 hours of preparation at room temperature or refrigerated. Admixtures should be allowed to equilibrate to room temperature prior to use.

Compatibility: Stable in D_5¼NS, D_5W, NS

Monitoring Laboratory Tests Serum creatinine, serum bicarbonate, acid-base status, urine protein, WBC should be monitored with each dose; monitor intraocular pressure frequently.

(Continued)

Cidofovir *(Continued)*

Monitoring and Teaching Issues

Physical Assessment: See Contraindications, Warnings/Precautions, and Dosing for use cautions. Assess potential for interactions with other prescriptions, OTC medications, or herbal products patient may be taking (eg, nephrotoxicity - see Drug Interactions). See Dosing, Administration, and Reconstitution directions. Infusion site should be monitored closely to avoid extravasation. Assess results of laboratory tests with each dose (see above), therapeutic effectiveness, and adverse response (see Adverse Reactions and Overdose/Toxicology) regularly during therapy. For diabetic patients, serum glucose should be monitored closely (may cause hyperglycemia). Teach patient possible side effects and interventions and adverse symptoms to report (see Patient Education). **Pregnancy risk factor C** - determine that patient is not pregnant before beginning treatment. Instruct patients of childbearing age about appropriate barrier contraceptive measures. Breast-feeding is contraindicated.

Patient Education: Inform prescriber of all prescriptions, OTC medications, or herbal products you are taking, and any allergies you have. Do not take anything new during treatment unless approved by prescriber. This drug can only be administered I.V. Report immediately any pain, stinging, swelling at infusion site. You may be more susceptible to infection (avoid crowds and and exposure to infection and do not have any vaccinations without consulting prescriber). May cause hair loss (reversible); headache, anxiety, confusion (use caution when driving or engaging in tasks that require alertness until response to drug is known); diarrhea (buttermilk or yogurt may help); nausea, heartburn, or vomiting (small, frequent meals, frequent mouth care, sucking lozenges, or chewing gum may help); constipation (increased exercise, fluids, fruit, or fiber may help); or postural hypotension (use caution changing from lying to sitting or standing position and when climbing stairs). Report severe unresolved vomiting, constipation, or diarrhea; chills, fever, signs of infection; difficulty breathing or unusual coughing; palpitations, chest pain, or syncope; CNS changes (eg, hallucinations, depression, excessive sedation, amnesia, seizures, insomnia); vision changes; or other severe side effects. **Pregnancy/breast-feeding precautions:** Inform prescriber if you are pregnant and do not get pregnant while taking this medicine. Do not breast-feed.

Geriatric Considerations: Since elderly individuals frequently have reduced kidney function, particular attention should be paid to assessing renal function before and frequently during administration.

Breast-feeding Issues: The CDC recommends **not** to breast-feed if diagnosed with HIV to avoid postnatal transmission of the virus.

Cilostazol (sil OH sta zol)

U.S. Brand Names Pletal®

Synonyms OPC13013

Generic Available No

Pharmacologic Category Antiplatelet Agent; Phosphodiesterase Enzyme Inhibitor

Pregnancy Risk Factor C

Lactation Excretion in breast milk unknown/not recommended

Use Symptomatic management of peripheral vascular disease, primarily intermittent claudication; currently being investigated for the treatment of acute coronary syndromes and for graft patency improvement in percutaneous coronary interventions with or without stenting

Use - Unlabeled/Investigational Investigational: Treatment of acute coronary syndromes and for graft patency improvement in percutaneous coronary interventions with or without stenting

Mechanism of Action/Effect Cilostazol and its metabolites are inhibitors of phosphodiesterase III leading to inhibition of platelet aggregation and vasodilation. Other effects of phosphodiesterase III inhibition include increased cardiac contractility, accelerated AV nodal conduction, increased ventricular automaticity, heart rate, and coronary blood flow.

Contraindications Hypersensitivity to cilostazol or any component of the formulation; heart failure (of any severity)

Warnings/Precautions Use with caution in patients receiving platelet aggregation inhibitors (effects are unknown), hepatic impairment (not studied). Use with caution in patients receiving inhibitors hepatic cytochrome P450 enzymes, particularly CYP3A4 (such as ketoconazole or erythromycin) or inhibitors of CYP2C19 (such as omeprazole). Pregnancy risk C.

Drug Interactions

Cytochrome P450 Effect: Substrate of CYP1A2, 2C19, 2D6, 3A4

Increased Effect/Toxicity: Cilostazol serum concentrations may be increased by erythromycin, diltiazem, and omeprazole. Increased concentrations of cilostazol may be anticipated during concurrent therapy with other inhibitors of CYP3A4 (ie, clarithromycin, ketoconazole, itraconazole, fluconazole, miconazole, fluvoxamine, fluoxetine, nefazodone, and sertraline) or inhibitors of CYP2C19. Aspirin-induced inhibition of platelet aggregation is potentiated by concurrent cilostazol. The effect on platelet aggregation with other antiplatelet drugs is unknown.

Nutritional/Ethanol Interactions Food: Taking cilostazol with a high-fat meal may increase peak concentration by 90%. Avoid concurrent ingestion of grapefruit juice due to the potential to inhibit CYP3A4.

Adverse Reactions

>10%:

Central nervous system: Headache (27% to 34%)

Gastrointestinal: Abnormal stools (12% to 15%), diarrhea (12% to 19%)

Miscellaneous: Infection (10% to 14%)

2% to 10%:

Cardiovascular: Peripheral edema (7% to 9%), palpitation (5% to 10%), tachycardia (4%)

Central nervous system: Dizziness (9% to 10%)

Gastrointestinal: Dyspepsia (6%), nausea (6% to 7%), abdominal pain (4% to 5%), flatulence (2% to 3%)

Neuromuscular & skeletal: Back pain (6% to 7%), myalgia (2% to 3%)

Respiratory: Rhinitis (7% to 12%), pharyngitis (7% to 10%), cough (3% to 4%)

<2% (Limited to important or life-threatening): Arrhythmia, blindness, cardiac arrest, hemorrhage, cerebral infarction/ischemia, cholelithiasis, colitis, CHF, duodenal ulcer, esophageal hemorrhage, esophagitis, gout, hematemesis, hemorrhage, hypotension, melena, myocardial infarction/ischemia, neuralgia, peptic ulcer, postural hypotension, purpura, retinal hemorrhage, retroperitoneal hemorrhage, syncope, urticaria, vaginal hemorrhage

Overdosage/Toxicology Experience with overdosage in humans is limited. Headache, diarrhea, hypotension, tachycardia, and/or cardiac arrhythmias may occur. Treatment is symptomatic and supportive. Hemodialysis is unlikely to be of value. In some animal models, high-dose or long-term administration was associated with a variety of cardiovascular lesions, including endocardial hemorrhage, hemosiderin deposition and left ventricular fibrosis, coronary arteritis, and periarteritis.

Pharmacodynamics/Kinetics

Half-Life Elimination: 11-13 hours

Metabolism: Hepatic via CYP3A4 (primarily), 1A2, 2C19, and 2D6; at least one metabolite has significant activity

Onset: 2-4 weeks; may require up to 12 weeks

Formulations Tablet: 50 mg, 100 mg

Dosing

Adults & Elderly: Peripheral vascular disease: Oral: 100 mg twice daily taken at least 30 minutes before or 2 hours after breakfast and dinner; dosage should be reduced to 50 mg twice daily during concurrent therapy with inhibitors of CYP3A4 or CYP2C19 (see Drug Interactions).

Monitoring and Teaching Issues

Physical Assessment: Assess effectiveness and interactions of other medications patient may be taking (see Drug Interactions, eg, other drugs that inhibit platelet aggregation). See Contraindications and Warnings/Precautions for use cautions. Monitor effectiveness of therapy and adverse reactions at beginning of therapy and periodically with long-term use (see Adverse Reactions). Assess knowledge/teach patient appropriate use, interventions to reduce side effects, and adverse symptoms to report (see Patient Education). **Pregnancy risk factor C** - benefits of use should outweigh possible risks. Breast-feeding is not recommended.

Patient Education: Use exactly as directed; do not discontinue without consulting prescriber. Beneficial effect may take between 2-12 weeks. Take on empty stomach (30 minutes before or 2 hours after meals). Do not take with grapefruit juice. You may experience nervousness, dizziness, or fatigue (use caution when driving or engaging in tasks requiring alertness until response to treatment is known); nausea, vomiting, or flatulence (small, frequent meals, frequent mouth care, chewing gum or sucking hard candy may help); or postural hypotension (change position slowly when rising from sitting or lying position or climbing stairs). Report chest pain, palpitations, unusual heartbeat, or swelling of extremities; unusual bleeding; unresolved GI upset or pain; dizziness, nervousness, sleeplessness, or fatigue; muscle cramping or tremor; unusual cough; or other adverse effects. **Pregnancy/breast-feeding precautions:** Inform prescriber if you are or intend to become pregnant. Breast-feeding is not recommended.

Dietary Issues: It is best to take cilostazol 30 minutes before or 2 hours after meals.

Breast-feeding Issues: It is not known whether cilostazol is excreted in human milk. Because of the potential risk to nursing infants, a decision to discontinue the drug or discontinue nursing should be made.

Pregnancy Issues: In animal studies, abnormalities of the skeletal, renal and cardiovascular system were increased. In addition, the incidence of stillbirth and decreased birth weights were increased.

Ciloxan™ *see page 1509*

Ciloxan® *see* Ciprofloxacin *on page 291*

Cimetidine (sye MET i deen)

U.S. Brand Names Tagamet®; Tagamet® HB [OTC]

Generic Available Yes

Pharmacologic Category Histamine H_2 Antagonist

Pregnancy Risk Factor B

Lactation Enters breast milk/compatible

Use Short-term treatment of active duodenal ulcers and benign gastric ulcers; long-term prophylaxis of duodenal ulcer; gastric hypersecretory states; gastroesophageal reflux; prevention of upper GI bleeding in critically ill patients

Use - Unlabeled/Investigational Part of a multidrug regimen for *H. pylori* eradication to reduce the risk of duodenal ulcer recurrence

Mechanism of Action/Effect Competitive inhibition of histamine at H_2-receptors of the gastric parietal cells resulting in reduced gastric acid secretion, gastric volume and hydrogen ion concentration reduced

Contraindications Hypersensitivity to cimetidine, any component of the formulation, or other H_2 antagonists

Warnings/Precautions Adjust dosages in renal/hepatic impairment or patients receiving drugs metabolized through the cytochrome P450 system.

Drug Interactions

Cytochrome P450 Effect: Inhibits **CYP1A2**, 2C8/9, 2C19, **2D6**, 2E1, **3A4**

Decreased Effect: Ketoconazole, fluconazole, itraconazole (especially capsule) decrease serum concentration; avoid concurrent use with H_2 antagonists. Delavirdine's absorption is decreased; avoid concurrent use with H_2 antagonists.

Increased Effect/Toxicity: Cimetidine increases warfarin's effect in a dose-related manner. Cimetidine may increase serum concentrations of alfentanil, amiodarone, benzodiazepines (except lorazepam, oxazepam, temazepam), beta-blockers (except atenolol, betaxolol, bisoprolol, nadolol, penbutolol), calcium channel blockers, carbamazepine, cisapride (avoid concurrent use), citalopram, flecainide, lidocaine, melphalan, meperidine,

(Continued)

Cimetidine *(Continued)*

metronidazole, moricizine, paroxetine, phenytoin, procainamide, propafenone, quinidine, quinolone antibiotics, tacrine, TCAs, theophylline, and triamterene. Cimetidine increases carmustine's myelotoxicity; avoid concurrent use.

Nutritional/Ethanol Interactions

Ethanol: Avoid ethanol (may enhance gastric mucosal irritation).

Food: Cimetidine may increase serum caffeine levels if taken with caffeine. Cimetidine peak serum levels may be decreased if taken with food.

Herb/Nutraceutical: St John's wort may decrease cimetidine levels.

Effects on Lab Values ↑ creatinine (S), AST, ALT

Adverse Reactions

1% to 10%:

Central nervous system: Headache, dizziness, agitation, drowsiness

Gastrointestinal: Diarrhea, nausea, vomiting

<1% (Limited to important or life-threatening): Agranulocytosis, AST and ALT increased, bradycardia, creatinine increased, hypotension, neutropenia, tachycardia, thrombocytopenia

Overdosage/Toxicology Treatment is symptomatic and supportive. There is no reported experience with intentional overdose. Reported ingestion of 20 g have had transient side effects seen with recommended doses. Animal data has shown respiratory failure, tachycardia, muscle tremor, vomiting, restlessness, hypotension, salivation, emesis, and diarrhea.

Pharmacodynamics/Kinetics

Bioavailability: 60% to 70%

Half-Life Elimination: Neonates: 3.6 hours; Children: 1.4 hours; Adults: Normal renal function: 2 hours

Time to Peak: Serum: Oral: 1-2 hours

Metabolism: Partially hepatic

Onset: 1 hour

Duration: 6 hours

Formulations

Infusion, as hydrochloride, in NS: 300 mg (50 mL)

Injection, as hydrochloride: 150 mg/mL (2 mL, 8 mL)

Liquid, oral, as hydrochloride: 200 mg/20 mL; 300 mg/5 mL [with alcohol 2.8%] (5 mL, 240 mL) [mint-peach flavor]

Tablet: 100 mg, 200 mg, 300 mg, 400 mg, 800 mg

Dosing

Adults & Elderly:

Short-term treatment of active ulcers:

Oral: 300 mg 4 times/day or 800 mg at bedtime or 400 mg twice daily for up to 8 weeks

I.M., I.V.: 300 mg every 6 hours or 37.5 mg/hour by continuous infusion; I.V. dosage should be adjusted to maintain an intragastric pH ≥5

Patients with an active bleed: Give cimetidine as a continuous infusion (see above)

Duodenal ulcer prophylaxis: Oral: 400-800 mg at bedtime

Gastric hypersecretory conditions: Oral, I.M., I.V.: 300-600 mg every 6 hours; dosage not to exceed 2.4 g/day

Helicobacter pylori eradication (unlabeled use): Oral: 400 mg twice daily; requires combination therapy with antibiotics

Pediatrics: Children: Oral, I.M., I.V.: 20-40 mg/kg/day in divided doses every 6 hours

Renal Impairment:

Cl_{cr} 10-50 mL/minute: Administer 50% of normal dose.

Cl_{cr} <10 mL/minute: Administer 25% of normal dose.

Slightly dialyzable (5% to 20%)

Hepatic Impairment: Usual dose is safe in mild liver disease but use with caution and in reduced dosage in severe liver disease. Increased risk of CNS toxicity in cirrhosis suggested by enhanced penetration of CNS.

Administration

Oral: Give with meals so that the drug's peak effect occurs at the proper time (peak inhibition of gastric acid secretion occurs at 1 and 3 hours after dosing in fasting subjects and approximately 2 hours in nonfasting subjects. This correlates well with the time food is no longer in the stomach offering a buffering effect). Stagger doses of antacids with cimetidine.

I.V.: Administer each 300 mg or fraction thereof over a minimum of 5 minutes when giving I.V. push. Give intermittent infusion over 15-30 minutes for each 300 mg dose.

Stability

Storage: Intact vials of cimetidine should be stored at room temperature and protected from light. Cimetidine may precipitate from solution upon exposure to cold but can be redissolved by warming without degradation.

Stability at room temperature for premixed bags: Manufacturer expiration dating and out of overwrap stability: 15 days.

Reconstitution: Stability at room temperature for prepared bags is 7 days. Stable in parenteral nutrition solutions for up to 7 days when protected from light.

Compatibility: Stable in D_5LR, $D_5{}^1/_4NS$, $D_5{}^1/_2NS$, D_5NS, D_5W, $D_{10}W$, $D_{10}NS$, LR, sodium bicarbonate 5%, NS

Y-site administration: Incompatible with allopurinol, amphotericin B cholesteryl sulfate complex, amsacrine, cefepime, indomethacin, warfarin

Compatibility in syringe: Incompatible with atropine/pentobarbital, cefamandole, cefazolin, chlorpromazine, ioxaglate meglumine and ioxaglate sodium, pentobarbital, secobarbital

Compatibility when admixed: Incompatible with amphotericin B, barbiturates

Monitoring Laboratory Tests CBC, gastric pH, occult blood with GI bleeding; monitor renal function to correct dose.

Monitoring and Teaching Issues

Physical Assessment: See Contraindications, Warnings/Precautions, and Dosing for use cautions. Assess potential for interactions with other prescriptions, OTC medications, or herbal products patient may be taking (see extensive list of Drug Interactions). See Dosing, Administration, and Reconstitution directions. Assess results of laboratory tests (see above), therapeutic effectiveness, and adverse effects (eg, changes in CNS, especially in elderly patients - see Adverse Reactions and Overdose/Toxicology) regularly during therapy. Teach patient appropriate use, possible side effects and interventions, and adverse symptoms to report (see Patient Education).

Patient Education: Inform prescriber of all prescriptions, OTC medications, or herbal products you are taking, and any allergies you have. Do not take anything new during treatment unless approved by prescriber. Take with meals. Do not increase dose or frequency without consulting prescriber. Limit xanthine-containing foods and beverages which may decrease iron absorption. To be effective, continue to take for the prescribed time (possibly 4-8 weeks) even though symptoms may have improved. Smoking decreases the effectiveness of cimetidine (stop smoking if possible). Avoid alcohol and caffeine. May cause headache, dizziness, agitation (use caution when driving or engaging in any potentially hazardous tasks until response to drug is known); nausea or vomiting (small, frequent meals, frequent mouth care, chewing gum, or sucking lozenges may help); or diarrhea (buttermilk, boiled milk, or yogurt may help). Report persistent diarrhea; black tarry stools or coffee ground-like emesis; dizziness, confusion, or agitation; rash; unusual bleeding or bruising; sore throat; or fever.

Geriatric Considerations: Patients diagnosed with PUD should be evaluated for *Helicobacter pylori.* When H_2-blockers are indicated, they are the preferred drugs for treating PUD in the elderly due to cost and ease of administration and reduced side effects.

Related Information

Compatibility of Drugs *on page 1564*
Compatibility of Drugs in Syringe *on page 1566*

Cipro® *see* Ciprofloxacin *on page 291*

Ciprofloxacin (sip roe FLOKS a sin)

U.S. Brand Names Ciloxan®; Cipro®

Synonyms Ciprofloxacin Hydrochloride

Generic Available No

Pharmacologic Category Antibiotic, Ophthalmic; Antibiotic, Quinolone

Pregnancy Risk Factor C

Lactation Enters breast milk/contraindicated (AAP rates "compatible")

Use Treatment of documented or suspected infections of the lower respiratory tract, sinuses, skin and skin structure, bone/joints, and urinary tract (including prostatitis) due to susceptible bacterial strains; especially indicated for pseudomonal infections and those due to multidrug-resistant gram-negative organisms, chronic bacterial prostatitis, infectious diarrhea, complicated gram-negative and anaerobic intra-abdominal infections (with metronidazole) due to *E. coli* (enteropathic strains), *B. fragilis*, *P. mirabilis*, *K. pneumoniae*, *P. aeruginosa*, *Campylobacter jejuni* or *Shigella*; approved for acute sinusitis caused by *H. influenzae* or *M. catarrhalis*; also used in treatment of typhoid fever due to *Salmonella typhi* (although eradication of the chronic typhoid carrier state has not been proven), osteomyelitis when parenteral therapy is not feasible, acute uncomplicated cystitis in females, to reduce incidence or progression of disease following exposure to aerolized *Bacillus anthracis*, febrile neutropenia (with piperacillin), and sexually-transmitted diseases such as uncomplicated cervical and urethral gonorrhea due to *Neisseria gonorrhoeae*; used ophthalmologically for superficial ocular infections (corneal ulcers, conjunctivitis) due to susceptible strains

Mechanism of Action/Effect Inhibits DNA-gyrase in susceptible organisms; inhibits relaxation of supercoiled DNA and promotes breakage of double-stranded DNA

Contraindications Hypersensitivity to ciprofloxacin, any component of the formulation, or other quinolones

Warnings/Precautions Not recommended in children <18 years of age (exception - postexposure treatment of inhalational anthrax); has caused transient arthropathy in children. CNS stimulation may occur (tremor, restlessness, confusion, and very rarely hallucinations or seizures). Use with caution in patients with known or suspected CNS disorder. Green discoloration of teeth in newborns has been reported. Prolonged use may result in superinfection; may rarely cause inflamed or ruptured tendons (discontinue use immediately with signs of inflammation or tendon pain). Risk may be increased with concurrent corticosteroids, particularly in the elderly. Quinolones may exacerbate myasthenia gravis.

Severe hypersensitivity reactions, including anaphylaxis, have occurred with quinolone therapy. If an allergic reaction occurs (itching, urticaria, dyspnea, facial edema, loss of consciousness, tingling, cardiovascular collapse), discontinue drug immediately.

Pregnancy risk C.

Drug Interactions

Cytochrome P450 Effect: Inhibits **CYP1A2, 3A4**

Decreased Effect: Enteral feedings may decrease plasma concentrations of ciprofloxacin probably by >30% inhibition of absorption. Aluminum/magnesium products, didanosine, quinapril, and sucralfate may decrease absorption of ciprofloxacin by ≥90% if administered concurrently. (Administer ciprofloxacin at least 4 hours and preferably 6 hours after the dose of these agents.) Calcium, iron, zinc, and multivitamins with minerals products may decrease absorption of ciprofloxacin significantly if administered concurrently. (Administer ciprofloxacin 2 hours before dose or at least 2 hours after the dose of these agents). Antineoplastic agents may decrease quinolone absorption. Intravenous ciprofloxacin may decrease serum phenytoin concentrations.

Increased Effect/Toxicity: Ciprofloxacin increases the levels/effect of cyclosporine, caffeine, theophylline, and warfarin. The CNS-stimulating effect of some quinolones may be enhanced by NSAIDs, and foscarnet has been associated with an increased risk of seizures with some quinolones. Serum levels of some quinolones are increased by loop

(Continued)

Ciprofloxacin *(Continued)*

diuretics, probenecid, and cimetidine (and possibly other H_2-blockers) due to altered renal elimination. This effect may be more important for quinolones with high percentage of renal elimination than with ciprofloxacin. Concurrent use of corticosteroids may increase risk of tendon rupture.

Nutritional/Ethanol Interactions

Food: Food decreases rate, but not extent, of absorption. Ciprofloxacin serum levels may be decreased if taken with dairy products or calcium-fortified juices. Ciprofloxacin may increase serum caffeine levels if taken with caffeine.

Herb/Nutraceutical: Avoid dong quai, St John's wort (may also cause photosensitization).

Adverse Reactions

1% to 10%:

Central nervous system: Headache (1%), restlessness (1%)
Dermatologic: Rash (1%)
Gastrointestinal: Nausea (5%), diarrhea (2%), vomiting (2%), abdominal pain (2%)
Hepatic: Elevated ALT/AST (2%)
Renal: Elevated serum creatinine (1%)

<1% (Limited to important or life-threatening): Acute renal failure, agranulocytosis, allergic reactions, anaphylaxis, angina pectoris, arthralgia, cardiopulmonary arrest, cholestatic jaundice, confusion, delirium, dyspnea, erythema multiforme, gastrointestinal bleeding, hallucinations, hepatic rupture, joint pain, methemoglobinemia, myasthenia gravis (exacerbation), myocardial infarction, nightmares, pancreatitis, photosensitivity, prolongation of PT, pseudomembranous colitis, seizures, Stevens-Johnson syndrome, syncope, tendon rupture, toxic epidermal necrolysis, vasculitis

Overdosage/Toxicology Symptoms of overdose include acute renal failure and seizures. Treatment is supportive. The drug is not removed by peritoneal or hemodialysis.

Pharmacodynamics/Kinetics

Absorption: Oral: Rapid (~50% to 85%)

Half-Life Elimination: Children: 2.5 hours; Adults: Normal renal function: 3-5 hours

Time to Peak: Oral: 0.5-2 hours

Metabolism: Partially hepatic

Formulations

Infusion, as hydrochloride [in D_5W]: 400 mg (200 mL)
Infusion, as hydrochloride [in NS or D_5W]: 200 mg (100 mL) [latex-free PVC]
Injection, as hydrochloride: 200 mg (20 mL); 400 mg (40 mL)
Ointment, ophthalmic, as hydrochloride: 3.33 mg/g [0.3% base] (3.5 g)
Solution, ophthalmic, as hydrochloride: 3.33 mg/g [0.3% base] (2.5 mL, 5 mL. 10 mL)
Suspension, oral: 250 mg/5 mL (100 mL); 500 mg/5 mL (100 mL)
Tablet, as hydrochloride: 100 mg, 250 mg, 500 mg, 750 mg

Dosing

Adults: Usual dosage range:

Oral: 250-750 mg twice daily
I.V.: 200-400 mg every 12 hours
Also refer to the following indication-specific dosing recommendations:

Dermatologic infection:

Skin/skin structure:
Oral: 500-750 mg every 12 hours for 7-14 days
I.V.: 200-400 mg every 12 hours for 7-14 days

Gastrointestinal infection:

Infectious diarrhea: Oral: 500 mg every 12 hours for 5-7 days
Intra-abdominal infection:
Oral (with clindamycin): 500 mg every 12 hours
I.V. (with metronidazole): 400 mg every 12 hours
Typhoid fever: Oral: 500 mg every 12 hours for 10 days

Genitourinary infection:

Chancroid: Oral: 500 mg twice daily for 3 days
Cystitis, uncomplicated (in females): Oral: 100 mg or 250 mg every 12 hours for 3 days
Disseminated gonococcal infection: Oral: 500 mg twice daily to complete 7 days of therapy (initial treatment with ceftriaxone 1 g I.M./I.V. daily for 24-48 hours after improvement begins)
Prostatitis (chronic, bacterial):
Oral: 500 mg every 12 hours for 28 days
I.V.: 400 mg every 12 hours for 28 days
Urethral/cervical gonococcal infections: Oral: 500 mg as a single dose (CDC recommends concomitant doxycycline or azithromycin due to developing resistance; avoid use in Asian or Western Pacific travelers)
Urinary tract infection:
Oral: 250-500 mg every 12 hours for 7-10 days, depending on severity of infection and susceptibility
I.V.:
Mild to moderate: 200 mg every 12 hours for 7-10 days
Severe or complicated: 400 mg every 12 hours for 7-10 days

Ocular infection:

Ophthalmic solution: Instill 1-2 drops in eye(s) every 2 hours while awake for 2 days and 1-2 drops every 4 hours while awake for the next 5 days.
Ophthalmic ointment: Apply a $^1/_2$" ribbon into the conjunctival sac 3 times/day for the first 2 days, followed by a $^1/_2$" ribbon applied twice daily for the next 5 days.

Respiratory infection:

Lower respiratory tract:
Oral: 500-750 mg twice daily for 7-14 days depending on severity and susceptibility
I.V.:
Mild to moderate: 400 mg every 12 hours for 7-14 days
Severe or complicated: 400 mg every 8 hours for 7-14 days

Nosocomial pneumonia (mild to moderate to severe): 400 mg every 8 hours
Sinusitis (mild to moderate):
Oral: 500 mg every 12 hours for 10 days
I.V.: 400 mg every 12 hours for 10 days

Skeletal infection:
Bone/joint infections:
Oral: 500-750 mg twice daily for 4-6 weeks, depending on severity and susceptibility
I.V.:
Mild to moderate: 400 mg every 12 hours for 7-14 days
Severe or complicated: 400 mg every 8 hours for 7-14 days

Miscellaneous infection:
Anthrax:
Inhalational (postexposure prophylaxis):
Oral: 500 mg every 12 hours for 60 days
I.V.: 400 mg every 12 hours
Cutaneous (treatment): Oral: 500 mg every 12 hours for 60 days. **Note:** In the presence of systemic involvement, extensive edema, lesions on head/neck, refer to I.V. dosing for treatment of inhalational/gastrointestinal/oropharyngeal anthrax
Inhalational/gastrointestinal/oropharyngeal (treatment): I.V.: 400 mg every 12 hours. **Note:** Initial treatment should include two or more agents predicted to be effective (per CDC recommendations). Agents suggested for use in conjunction with ciprofloxacin or doxycycline include rifampin, vancomycin, imipenem, penicillin, ampicillin, chloramphenicol, clindamycin, and clarithromycin. May switch to oral antimicrobial therapy when clinically appropriate. Continue combined therapy for 60 days.
Febrile neutropenia (with piperacillin): I.V.: 400 mg every 8 hours for 7-14 days

Elderly: Refer to adult dosing. No adjustment needed in patients with normal renal function.

Pediatrics: Limited use (see Warnings/Precautions). Children:
Usual range:
Oral: 20-30 mg/kg/day in 2 divided doses; maximum: 1.5 g/day
I.V.: 15-20 mg/kg/day divided every 12 hours
Cystic fibrosis:
Oral: 20-40 mg/kg/day divided every 12 hours
I.V.: 15-30 mg/kg/day divided every 8-12 hours
Anthrax:
Inhalational (postexposure prophylaxis): Oral, I.V.: 10-15 mg/kg/dose every 12 hours for 60 days; maximum: 500 mg/dose (oral) or 400 mg/dose (I.V.)
Cutaneous (treatment): Oral: 10-15 mg/kg every 12 hours for 60 days; amoxicillin 80 mg/kg/day divided every 8 hours is an option for completion of treatment after clinical improvement. **Note:** In the presence of systemic involvement, extensive edema, lesions on head/neck, refer to I.V. dosing for treatment of inhalational/gastrointestinal/oropharyngeal anthrax
Inhalational/gastrointestinal/oropharyngeal (treatment): I.V.: Initial: 10-15 mg/kg every 12 hours for 60 days (maximum: 500 mg/dose); switch to oral therapy when clinically appropriate; refer to Adults dosing for notes on combined therapy and duration

Ophthalmic infection: Ophthalmic:
Solution: Children >1 year: Instill 1-2 drops in eye(s) every 2 hours while awake for 2 days and 1-2 drops every 4 hours while awake for the next 5 days.
Ointment: Children >2 years: Apply a ½" ribbon into the conjunctival sac 3 times/day for the first 2 days, followed by a ½" ribbon applied twice daily for the next 5 days.

Renal Impairment:
Cl_{cr} 30-50 mL/minute: Oral: Administer 250-500 mg every 12 hours.
Cl_{cr} 5-29 mL/minute:
Oral: Administer 250-500 mg every 18 hours.
I.V.: Administer 200-400 mg every 18-24 hours.
Dialysis: Only small amounts of ciprofloxacin are removed by hemo- or peritoneal dialysis (<10%); usual dose: 250-500 mg every 24 hours following dialysis.
Continuous arteriovenous or venovenous hemodiafiltration effects: Administer 200-400 mg I.V. every 12 hours.

Hepatic Impairment: Adjustment should be considered in severe hepatic dysfunction.

Administration

Oral: May administer with food to minimize GI upset. Drink plenty of fluids to maintain proper hydration and urine output. Administer at least 2 hours before or 6 hours after antacids or other products containing calcium, iron, or zinc (including dairy products or calcium-fortified juices). Oral suspension should not be administered through feeding tubes (due to its physical characteristics). Patients should avoid chewing on the microcapsules if the suspension is administered orally.

I.V.: Administer by slow I.V. infusion over 60 minutes into a large vein.

Other: Do not administer commercial 5% or 10% oral suspension via enteral feeding tubes (due to physical characteristics of the suspension).

Stability

Storage: Refrigeration and room temperature: Premixed bags: Manufacturer expiration dating; Prepared bags: 14 days; Ophthalmic solution and ointment: 36°F to 77°F (2°C to 25°C), protect from light

Reconstitution: Final concentration for administration should not exceed 2 mg/mL.

Compatibility: Stable in D_5¼NS, D_5½NS, D_5W, $D_{10}W$, LR, NS

Y-site administration: Incompatible with aminophylline, ampicillin/sulbactam, cefepime, dexamethasone sodium phosphate, furosemide, heparin, hydrocortisone sodium succinate, methylprednisolone sodium succinate, phenytoin, propofol, sodium phosphates, warfarin

Compatibility when admixed: Incompatible with aminophylline, clindamycin, floxacillin, heparin

(Continued)

Ciprofloxacin *(Continued)*

Monitoring Laboratory Tests Patients receiving concurrent ciprofloxacin, theophylline, or cyclosporine should have serum theophylline or cyclosporine levels monitored. Culture and sensitivity specimen should be taken prior to initiating therapy.

Monitoring and Teaching Issues

Physical Assessment: See Contraindications, Warnings/Precautions and Dosing for use cautions. Assess potential for interactions with other prescriptions, OTC medications, or herbal products patient may be taking (see extensive list of Drug Interactions). **I.V.:** See Administration, Reconstitution, and Compatibility directions. Assess results of laboratory tests (see above), therapeutic effectiveness, and adverse effects (eg, changes in CNS, especially in elderly patients - see Adverse Reactions and Overdose/Toxicology) regularly during therapy. Teach patient appropriate use, possible side effects and interventions, and adverse symptoms to report (see Patient Education). **Pregnancy risk factor C** - benefits of use should outweigh possible risks. Breast-feeding is contraindicated.

Patient Education: Inform prescriber of all prescriptions, OTC medications, or herbal products you are taking, and any allergies you have. Do not take anything new during treatment unless approved by prescriber. Take exactly as directed, preferably on an empty stomach (2 hours after meals and at least 2 hours before or 6 hours after antacids or other drug products containing calcium, iron, or zinc) to reduce GI upset. Swallow oral suspension; do not chew microcapsules. Shake bottle vigorously with each use. Take entire prescription, even if feeling better. Maintain adequate hydration to avoid concentrated urine and crystal formation (2-3 L/day) unless advised by prescriber to restrict fluids. You may experience nausea, vomiting, or anorexia (small, frequent meals, frequent mouth care, sucking lozenges, or chewing gum may help); or increased sensitivity to sunlight (use sunscreen, wear protective clothing and dark glasses, and avoid direct exposure to sunlight). If signs of inflammation or tendon pain occur, discontinue use immediately and report to prescriber. If signs of allergic reaction (eg, itching urticaria, difficulty breathing, facial edema, difficulty swallowing, loss of consciousness, tingling, chest pain, palpitations) occur, discontinue use immediately and report to prescriber. Report unusual fever or chills, vaginal itching or foul-smelling vaginal discharge, easy bruising or bleeding, or tendon or muscle pain. **Pregnancy/breast-feeding precautions:** Inform prescriber if you are or intend to become pregnant. Do not breast-feed.

Dietary Issues:

Food: Drug may cause GI upset; take without regard to meals (manufacturer prefers that drug is taken 2 hours after meals).

Dairy products, calcium-fortified juices, oral multivitamins, and mineral supplements: Absorption of ciprofloxacin is decreased by divalent and trivalent cations. The manufacturer states that the usual dietary intake of calcium (including meals which include dairy products) has not been shown to interfere with ciprofloxacin absorption. Products may be taken 6 hours before or 2 hours following a dose of ciprofloxacin.

Caffeine: Patients consuming regular large quantities of caffeinated beverages may need to restrict caffeine intake if excessive cardiac or CNS stimulation occurs.

Geriatric Considerations: Ciprofloxacin should not be used as first-line therapy unless the culture and sensitivity findings show resistance to usual therapy. The interactions with caffeine and theophylline can result in serious toxicity in the elderly. Adjust dose for renal function.

Breast-feeding Issues: Not compatible; can resume breast-feeding 48 hours after the last dose. Theoretically, may affect cartilage in weight-bearing joints.

Pregnancy Issues: Reports of arthropathy (observed in immature animals and reported rarely in humans) has limited the use of fluoroquinolones in pregnancy. According to the FDA, the Teratogen Information System concluded that therapeutic doses during pregnancy are unlikely to produce substantial teratogenic risk, but data are insufficient to say that there is no risk. In general, reports of exposure have been limited to short durations of therapy in the first trimester. When considering treatment for life-threatening infection and/or prolonged duration of therapy (such as in anthrax), the potential risk to the fetus must be balanced against the severity of the potential illness.

Related Information

Ophthalmic Agents *on page 1509*
Prophylaxis for Exposure to Common Communicable Diseases *on page 1651*
Tuberculosis *on page 1705*

Ciprofloxacin and Hydrocortisone *see page 1519*
Ciprofloxacin Hydrochloride *see* Ciprofloxacin *on page 291*
Cipro® HC Otic *see page 1519*

Cisapride (SIS a pride)

U.S. Brand Names Propulsid®

Restrictions In U.S., available via limited-access protocol only.

Generic Available No

Pharmacologic Category Gastrointestinal Agent, Prokinetic

Pregnancy Risk Factor C

Lactation Enters breast milk/use caution (AAP rates "compatible")

Use Treatment of nocturnal symptoms of gastroesophageal reflux disease (GERD); has demonstrated effectiveness for gastroparesis, refractory constipation, and nonulcer dyspepsia

Mechanism of Action/Effect Enhances the release of acetylcholine at the myenteric plexus. *In vitro* studies have shown cisapride to have serotonin-4 receptor agonistic properties which may increase GI motility and cardiac rate; increases lower esophageal sphincter pressure and lower esophageal peristalsis; accelerates gastric emptying of both liquids and solids.

Contraindications

Hypersensitivity to cisapride or any component of the formulations; GI hemorrhage, mechanical obstruction, GI perforation, or other situations when GI motility stimulation is dangerous

Serious cardiac arrhythmias including ventricular tachycardia, ventricular fibrillation, torsade de pointes, and QT prolongation have been reported in patients taking cisapride with other drugs that inhibit CYP3A4. Some of these events have been fatal. Concomitant oral or intravenous administration of the following drugs with cisapride may lead to elevated cisapride blood levels and is contraindicated:

Antibiotics: Oral or I.V. erythromycin, clarithromycin, troleandomycin
Antidepressants: Nefazodone
Antifungals: Oral or I.V. fluconazole, itraconazole, miconazole, oral ketoconazole
Protease inhibitors: Indinavir, ritonavir, amprenavir

Cisapride is also contraindicated for patients with a prolonged electrocardiographic QT intervals (QT_c >450 msec), a history of QT_c prolongation, or known family history of congenital long QT syndrome; clinically significant bradycardia, renal failure, history of ventricular arrhythmias, ischemic heart disease, and congestive heart failure; uncorrected electrolyte disorders (hypokalemia, hypomagnesemia); respiratory failure; and concomitant medications known to prolong the QT interval and increase the risk of arrhythmia, such as certain antiarrhythmics, certain antipsychotics, certain antidepressants, astemizole, bepridil, sparfloxacin, and terodiline. The preceding lists of drugs are not comprehensive. Cisapride should not be used in patients with uncorrected hypokalemia or hypomagnesemia or who might experience rapid reduction of plasma potassium such as those administered potassium-wasting diuretics and/or insulin in acute settings.

Warnings/Precautions Safety and effectiveness in children have not been established. Serious cardiac ventricular arrhythmias, including ventricular tachycardia, torsade de pointes, and QT prolongation have been reported in patients taking cisapride with other drugs that inhibit P450 3A4 (eg, clarithromycin, erythromycin, fluconazole, itraconazole, ketoconazole, miconazole injection, troleandomycin). Avoid other medications which may prolong QT. Avoid use when stimulation of GI motility may be dangerous (eg, obstruction, perforation, hemorrhage). Extreme caution with use in the elderly.

A 12-lead EKG should be performed prior to administration of cisapride. Treatment with cisapride should not be initiated if the QT_c value exceeds 450 milliseconds. Serum electrolytes (potassium, calcium, and magnesium) and creatinine should be assessed prior to administration of cisapride and whenever conditions develop that may affect electrolyte balance or renal function.

Pregnancy factor C.

Drug Interactions

Cytochrome P450 Effect: Substrate of 1A2, 2A6, 2B6, 2C8/9, 2C19, **3A4**; Inhibits CYP2D6

Decreased Effect: Cisapride may decrease the effect of atropine and digoxin.

Increased Effect/Toxicity: Cisapride may increase blood levels of warfarin, diazepam, cimetidine, ranitidine, and CNS depressants. The risk of cisapride-induced malignant arrhythmias may be increased by azole antifungals (fluconazole, itraconazole, ketoconazole, miconazole), antiarrhythmics (Class Ia; quinidine, procainamide, and Class III; amiodarone, sotalol), bepridil, cimetidine, maprotiline, macrolide antibiotics (erythromycin, clarithromycin, troleandomycin), molindone, nefazodone, protease inhibitors (amprenavir, indinavir, nelfinavir, ritonavir), phenothiazines (eg, prochlorperazine, promethazine), sertindole, tricyclic antidepressants (eg amitriptyline), and some quinolone antibiotics (sparfloxacin, gatifloxacin, moxifloxacin). Cardiovascular disease or electrolyte imbalances (potentially due to diuretic therapy) increase the risk of malignant arrhythmias.

Nutritional/Ethanol Interactions

Ethanol: Avoid ethanol (may increase CNS depression).

Food: Coadministration of grapefruit juice with cisapride increases the bioavailability of cisapride and concomitant use should be avoided.

Herb/Nutraceutical: St John's wort may decrease cisapride levels.

Adverse Reactions

>10%:

Central nervous system: Headache
Gastrointestinal: Diarrhea (dose dependent)

1% to 10%:

Cardiovascular: Tachycardia
Central nervous system: Extrapyramidal effects, somnolence, fatigue, insomnia, anxiety
Dermatologic: Rash
Gastrointestinal: Abdominal cramping, constipation, nausea
Respiratory: Sinusitis, rhinitis, coughing, upper respiratory tract infection, increased incidence of viral infection

<1% (Limited to important or life-threatening): Apnea, bronchospasm, gynecomastia, hyperprolactinemia, methemoglobinemia, photosensitivity, psychiatric disturbances, seizures (have been reported only in patients with a history of seizures)

Pharmacodynamics/Kinetics

Bioavailability: 35% to 40%

Half-Life Elimination: 6-12 hours

Metabolism: Extensively hepatic to norcisapride

Onset: 0.5-1 hour

Formulations

Suspension, oral: 1 mg/mL (450 mL) [cherry cream flavor]
Tablet, scored: 10 mg, 20 mg

Dosing

Adults & Elderly: GERD or gastrointestinal dysmotility: Oral: Initial: 5-10 mg 4 times/day at least 15 minutes before meals and at bedtime; in some patients the dosage will need to be increased to 20 mg to obtain a satisfactory result.

Pediatrics: Gastrointestinal dysmotility: Oral: Children: 0.15-0.3 mg/kg/dose 3-4 times/day; maximum: 10 mg/dose

Hepatic Impairment: Initiate at 50% usual dose.

Monitoring Laboratory Tests A 12-lead EKG should be performed prior to administration of cisapride. Treatment with cisapride should not be initiated if the QT_c value exceeds

(Continued)

Cisapride *(Continued)*

450 milliseconds. Serum electrolytes (potassium, calcium, and magnesium) and creatinine should be assessed prior to administration of cisapride and whenever conditions develop that may affect electrolyte balance or renal function.

Monitoring and Teaching Issues

Physical Assessment: See Additional Information - **IMPORTANT NOTE**. See Contraindications and Warnings/Precautions for use cautions and limitations. Assess potential for interactions with other prescriptions, OTC medications, or herbal products patient may be taking (see extensive list of Drug Interactions). Assess results of laboratory tests (eg, EKG, electrolyte balance and renal function - see above), therapeutic effectiveness, and adverse response (see Adverse Reactions and Overdose/Toxicology) regularly during therapy. Teach patient appropriate use, possible side effects and interventions, and adverse symptoms to report (see Patient Education). **Pregnancy risk factor C** - benefits of use should outweigh possible risks. Note breast-feeding caution.

Patient Education: It is absolutely vital that you inform prescriber of all prescriptions, OTC medications, or herbal products you are taking, and any allergies you have. Do not take anything new during treatment unless approved by prescriber. Take before meals. Avoid alcohol and grapefruit juice. May cause increased sedation, headache, anxiety (use caution when driving or engaging in hazardous tasks until response to drug is known). Immediately report rapid heartbeat, palpitations, chest pain, or tightness. Report severe abdominal pain, prolonged diarrhea, weight loss, or extreme fatigue. **Pregnancy/breast-feeding precautions:** Inform prescriber if you are or intend to become pregnant. Consult prescriber if breast-feeding.

Geriatric Considerations: Steady-state serum concentrations are higher than those in younger adults; however, the therapeutic dose and pharmacologic effects are the same as those in younger adults and no adjustment in dose recommended for elderly.

Additional Information U.S. - Available Via Limited-Access Protocol Only

IMPORTANT NOTE: On March 24, 2000, the FDA announced that the manufacturer of cisapride would voluntarily withdraw its product from the U.S. market on July 14, 2000. This decision was based on 341 reports of heart rhythm abnormalities including 80 reports of deaths. The company will continue to make the drug available to patients who meet specific clinical eligibility criteria for a limited-access protocol (contact 1-800-JANSSEN).

Cisatracurium (sis a tra KYOO ree um)

U.S. Brand Names Nimbex®

Synonyms Cisatracurium Besylate

Generic Available No

Pharmacologic Category Neuromuscular Blocker Agent, Nondepolarizing

Pregnancy Risk Factor C

Lactation Excretion in breast milk unknown/use caution

Use Adjunct to general anesthesia to facilitate endotracheal intubation and to relax skeletal muscles during surgery; to facilitate mechanical ventilation in ICU patients; does not relieve pain or produce sedation

Mechanism of Action/Effect Blocks neural transmission at the myoneural junction by binding with cholinergic receptor sites

Contraindications Hypersensitivity to cisatracurium besylate or any component of the formulation

Warnings/Precautions Maintenance of an adequate airway and respiratory support is critical; certain clinical conditions may result in potentiation or antagonism of neuromuscular blockade:

Potentiation: Electrolyte abnormalities, severe hyponatremia, severe hypocalcemia, severe hypokalemia, hypermagnesemia, neuromuscular diseases, acidosis, acute intermittent porphyria, renal failure, hepatic failure

Antagonism: Alkalosis, hypercalcemia, demyelinating lesions, peripheral neuropathies, diabetes mellitus

Increased sensitivity in patients with myasthenia gravis, Eaton-Lambert syndrome; resistance in burn patients (>30% of body) for period of 5-70 days postinjury; resistance in patients with muscle trauma, denervation, immobilization, infection, chronic treatment with atracurium. Bradycardia may be more common with cisatracurium than with other neuromuscular blocking agents since it has no clinically significant effects on heart rate to counteract the bradycardia produced by anesthetics.

Pregnancy risk C.

Drug Interactions

Decreased Effect: Effect of nondepolarizing neuromuscular blockers may be reduced by carbamazepine (chronic use), corticosteroids (also associated with myopathy - see increased effect), phenytoin (chronic use), sympathomimetics, and theophylline.

Increased Effect/Toxicity: Increased effects are possible with aminoglycosides, beta-blockers, clindamycin, calcium channel blockers, halogenated anesthetics, imipenem, ketamine, lidocaine, loop diuretics (furosemide), macrolides (case reports), magnesium sulfate, procainamide, quinidine, quinolones, tetracyclines, and vancomycin. May increase risk of myopathy when used with high-dose corticosteroids for extended periods.

Adverse Reactions <1%: Effects are minimal and transient, bradycardia and hypotension, flushing, rash, bronchospasm

Overdosage/Toxicology

Symptoms of overdose include respiratory depression and cardiovascular collapse.

Neostigmine 1-3 mg slow I.V. push in adults (0.5 mg in children) antagonizes the neuromuscular blockade, and should be administered with or immediately after atropine 1-1.5 mg I.V. push (adults). This may be especially useful in the presence of bradycardia.

Pharmacodynamics/Kinetics

Half-Life Elimination: 22 minutes

Metabolism: Undergoes rapid nonenzymatic degradation in the bloodstream, additional metabolism occurs via ester hydrolysis; some active metabolites

Onset: I.V.: 2-3 minutes; Peak effect: 3-5 minutes

Duration: Recovery begins in 20-35 minutes when anesthesia is balanced; recovery is attained in 90% of patients in 25-93 minutes

Formulations Injection, as besylate: 2 mg/mL (5 mL, 10 mL); 10 mg/mL (20 mL)

Dosing

Adults & Elderly: Neuromuscular blockade: I.V. (not to be used I.M.):

Operating room administration:

Intubating doses: 0.15-0.2 mg/kg as components of propofol/nitrous oxide/oxygen induction-intubation technique. (**Note:** May produce generally good or excellent conditions for tracheal intubation in 1.5-2 minutes with clinically effective duration of action during propofol anesthesia of 55-61 minutes.) Initial dose after succinylcholine for intubation: 0.1 mg/kg; maintenance dose: 0.03 mg/kg 40-60 minutes after initial dose, then at ~20-minute intervals based on clinical criteria.

Continuous infusion: After an initial bolus, a diluted solution can be given by continuous infusion for maintenance of neuromuscular blockade during extended surgery; adjust the rate of administration according to the patient's response as determined by peripheral nerve stimulation. An initial infusion rate of 3 mcg/kg/minute may be required to rapidly counteract the spontaneous recovery of neuromuscular function; thereafter, a rate of 1-2 mcg/kg/minute should be adequate to maintain continuous neuromuscular block in the 89% to 99% range in most pediatric and adult patients. Consider reduction of the infusion rate by 30% to 40% when administering during stable isoflurane, enflurane, sevoflurane, or desflurane anesthesia. Spontaneous recovery from neuromuscular blockade following discontinuation of infusion of cisatracurium may be expected to proceed at a rate comparable to that following single bolus administration.

Intensive care unit administration: Follow the principles for infusion in the operating room. At initial signs of recovery from bolus dose, begin the infusion at a dose of 3 mcg/kg/minute and adjust rates accordingly; dosage ranges of 0.5-10 mcg/kg/minute have been reported. If patient is allowed to recover from neuromuscular blockade, readministration of a bolus dose may be necessary to quickly re-establish neuromuscular block prior to reinstituting the infusion. See table.

Cisatracurium Besylate Infusion Chart

Drug Delivery Rate (mcg/kg/min)	Infusion Rate (mL/kg/min) 0.1 mg/mL (10 mg/100 mL)	Infusion Rate (mL/kg/min) 0.4 mg/mL (40 mg/100 mL)
1	0.01	0.0025
1.5	0.015	0.00375
2	0.02	0.005
3	0.03	0.0075
5	0.05	0.0125

Pediatrics: Neuromuscular blockade:

Operating room administration:

Children 2-12 years: I.V. (Not to be used I.M.)

Intubating doses: 0.1 mg over 5-15 seconds during either halothane or opioid anesthesia. (**Note:** When given during stable opioid nitrous oxide/oxygen anesthesia, 0.1 mg/kg produces maximum neuromuscular block in an average of 2.8 minutes and clinically effective block for 28 minutes.)

Continuous infusion: Refer to adult dosing.

Intensive care unit administration: Refer to adult dosing.

Renal Impairment: Because slower times to onset of complete neuromuscular block were observed in renal dysfunction patients, extending the interval between the administration of cisatracurium and intubation attempt may be required to achieve adequate intubation conditions.

Administration

I.M.: Not for I.M. injection, too much tissue irritation.

I.V.: Administer I.V. only. The use of a peripheral nerve stimulator will permit the most advantageous use of cisatracurium, minimize the possibility of overdosage or underdosage and assist in the evaluation of recovery.

Give undiluted as a bolus injection. Continuous administration requires the use of an infusion pump.

Stability

Storage: Refrigerate intact vials at 2°C to 8°C/36°F to 46°F. Use vials within 21 days upon removal from the refrigerator to room temperature (25°C to 77°F). Dilutions of 0.1-0.2 mg/mL in 0.9% sodium chloride or dextrose 5% in water are stable for up to 24 hours at room temperature.

Compatibility: Stable in D_5W, NS, D_5NS

Y-site administration: Incompatible with amphotericin B cholesteryl sulfate complex, cefoperazone

Compatibility when admixed: Incompatible with ketorolac, propofol

Monitoring and Teaching Issues

Physical Assessment: Only clinicians experienced in the use of neuromuscular blocking drugs should administer and/or manage the use of cisatracurium. Dosage and rate of administration should be individualized and titrated to the desired effect, according to relevant clinical factors, premedication, concomitant medications, age, and general condition of the patient. See Use, Contraindications, and Warnings/Precautions for appropriate

(Continued)

Cisatracurium *(Continued)*

use cautions. Ventilatory support must be instituted and maintained until adequate respiratory muscle function and/or airway protection are assured. Assess other medications for effectiveness and safety. Other drugs that affect neuromuscular activity may increase/decrease neuromuscular block induced by cisatracurium. This drug does not cause anesthesia or analgesia; pain must be treated with appropriate analgesic agents. Continuous monitoring of vital signs, cardiac status, respiratory status, and degree of neuromuscular block (objective assessment with peripheral external nerve stimulator) is mandatory during infusion and until full muscle tone has returned (see Adverse Reactions). Muscle tone returns in a predictable pattern, starting with diaphragm, abdomen, chest, limbs, and finally muscles of the neck, face, and eyes. Safety precautions must be maintained until full muscle tone has returned. **Note:** It may take longer for return of muscle tone in obese or elderly patients or patients with renal or hepatic disease, myasthenia gravis, myopathy, other neuromuscular disease, dehydration, electrolyte imbalance, or severe acid/base imbalance. Provide appropriate patient teaching/support prior to and following administration.

Long-term use: Monitor fluid levels (intake and output) during and following infusion. Reposition patient and provide appropriate skin care, mouth care, and care of patient's eyes every 2-3 hours while sedated. Provide appropriate emotional and sensory support (auditory and environmental).

Pregnancy risk factor C. Note breast-feeding caution.

Patient Education: Patient will usually be unconscious prior to administration. Patient education should be appropriate to individual situation. Reassurance of constant monitoring and emotional support to reduce fear and anxiety should precede and follow administration. Following return of muscle tone, do not attempt to change position or rise from bed without assistance. Report immediately any skin rash or hives, pounding heartbeat, difficulty breathing, or muscle tremors. **Pregnancy/breast-feeding precautions:** Inform prescriber if you are pregnant. Consult prescriber if breast-feeding.

Additional Information Cisatracurium is classified as an intermediate-duration neuromuscular-blocking agent. It does not appear to have a cumulative effect on the duration of blockade. Neuromuscular-blocking potency is 3 times that of atracurium; maximum block is up to 2 minutes longer than for equipotent doses of atracurium.

Cisatracurium Besylate *see* Cisatracurium *on page 296*

Cisplatin (SIS pla tin)

U.S. Brand Names Platinol®; Platinol®-AQ

Synonyms CDDP

Generic Available Yes

Pharmacologic Category Antineoplastic Agent, Alkylating Agent

Pregnancy Risk Factor D

Lactation Enters breast milk/contraindicated (AAP rates "compatible")

Use Treatment of head and neck, breast, testicular, and ovarian cancer; Hodgkin's and non-Hodgkin's lymphoma; neuroblastoma; sarcomas, bladder, gastric, lung, esophageal, cervical, and prostate cancer; myeloma, melanoma, mesothelioma, small cell lung cancer, and osteosarcoma

Mechanism of Action/Effect Inhibits DNA synthesis

Contraindications Hypersensitivity to cisplatin, other platinum-containing compounds, or any component of the formulation (anaphylactic-like reactions have been reported); pre-existing renal insufficiency; myelosuppression; hearing impairment; pregnancy

Warnings/Precautions The U.S. Food and Drug Administration (FDA) currently recommends that procedures for proper handling and disposal of antineoplastic agents be considered. All patients should receive adequate hydration prior to and for 24 hours after cisplatin administration, with or without mannitol and/or furosemide, to ensure good urine output and decrease the chance of nephrotoxicity. Reduce dosage in renal impairment. Cumulative renal toxicity may be severe. Dose-related toxicities include myelosuppression, nausea, and vomiting. Ototoxicity, especially pronounced in children, is manifested by tinnitus or loss of high frequency hearing and occasionally, deafness. **Serum magnesium, as well as other electrolytes, should be monitored both before and within 48 hours after cisplatin therapy.** Patients who are magnesium depleted should receive replacement therapy before the cisplatin is administered. If cisplatin contacts the skin, wash and flush thoroughly with water. When administered as sequential infusions, taxane derivatives (docetaxel, paclitaxel) should be administered before platinum derivatives (carboplatin, cisplatin) to limit myelosuppression and to enhance efficacy.

Drug Interactions

Decreased Effect: Sodium thiosulfate theoretically inactivates drug systemically; has been used clinically to reduce systemic toxicity with intraperitoneal administration of cisplatin.

Increased Effect/Toxicity: Cisplatin and ethacrynic acid have resulted in severe ototoxicity in animals. Delayed bleomycin elimination with decreased glomerular filtration rate. When administered as sequential infusions, observational studies indicate a potential for increased toxicity when platinum derivatives (carboplatin, cisplatin) are administered before taxane derivatives (docetaxel, paclitaxel).

Nutritional/Ethanol Interactions Herb/Nutraceutical: Avoid black cohosh, dong quai in estrogen-dependent tumors.

Adverse Reactions

>10%:

Central nervous system: Neurotoxicity: Peripheral neuropathy is dose- and duration-dependent. The mechanism is through axonal degeneration with subsequent damage to the long sensory nerves. Toxicity can first be noted at cumulative doses of 200 mg/m^2, with measurable toxicity at cumulative doses >350 mg/m^2. This process is irreversible and progressive with continued therapy.

Dermatologic: Mild alopecia

Gastrointestinal: Cisplatin is one of the most emetogenic agents used in cancer chemotherapy; nausea and vomiting occur in 76% to 100% of patients and is dose-related. Prophylactic antiemetics should always be prescribed; nausea and vomiting may last up to 1 week after therapy.

Hematologic: Myelosuppressive: Mild with moderate doses, mild to moderate with high-dose therapy

WBC: Mild

Platelets: Mild

Onset: 10 days

Nadir: 14-23 days

Recovery: 21-39 days

Hepatic: Elevation of liver enzymes

Renal: Nephrotoxicity: Related to elimination, protein binding, and uptake of cisplatin. Two types of nephrotoxicity: Acute renal failure and chronic renal insufficiency.

Acute renal failure and azotemia is a dose-dependent process and can be minimized with proper administration and prophylaxis. Damage to the proximal tubules by unbound cisplatin is suspected to cause the toxicity. It is manifested as increased BUN/creatinine, oliguria, protein wasting, and potassium, calcium, and magnesium wasting.

Chronic renal dysfunction can develop in patients receiving multiple courses of cisplatin. Slow release of tissue-bound cisplatin may contribute to chronic nephrotoxicity. Manifestations of this toxicity are varied, and can include sodium and water wasting, nephropathy, hyperuricemia, decreased Cl_{cr}, and magnesium wasting.

Recommendations for minimizing nephrotoxicity include:

Prepare cisplatin in saline-containing vehicles

Infuse dose over 24 hours

Vigorous hydration (125-150 mL/hour) before, during, and after cisplatin administration

Simultaneous administration of either mannitol or furosemide

Pretreatment with amifostine

Avoid other nephrotoxic agents (aminoglycosides, amphotericin, etc)

Otic: Ototoxicity: Ototoxicity occurs in 10% to 30%, and is manifested as high frequency hearing loss. Baseline audiography should be performed. Ototoxicity is especially pronounced in children.

1% to 10%: Local: Extravasation: May cause thrombophlebitis and tissue damage if infiltrated; may use sodium thiosulfate as antidote, but consult hospital policy for guidelines.

Irritant chemotherapy

<1% (Limited to important or life-threatening): Arrhythmias, blurred vision, bradycardia, cerebral blindness, hemolytic anemia, liver enzymes increased, mild alopecia, mouth sores, optic neuritis, papilledema

BMT:

Central nervous system: Peripheral and autonomic neuropathy, ototoxicity

Endocrine & metabolic: Hypokalemia, hypomagnesemia

Gastrointestinal: Highly emetogenic

Hematologic: Myelosuppression

Renal: Acute renal failure, increased serum creatinine, azotemia

Miscellaneous: Transient pain at tumor, transient autoimmune disorders

Overdosage/Toxicology Symptoms of overdose include severe myelosuppression, intractable nausea and vomiting, kidney and liver failure, deafness, ocular toxicity, and neuritis. There is no known antidote. Hemodialysis appears to have little effect. Treatment is supportive.

Pharmacodynamics/Kinetics

Half-Life Elimination: Initial: 20-30 minutes; Beta: 60 minutes; Terminal: ~24 hours; Secondary half-life: 44-73 hours

Metabolism: Nonenzymatic; inactivated (in both cell and bloodstream) by sulfhydryl groups; covalently binds to glutathione and thiosulfate

Formulations

Injection, aqueous: 1 mg/mL (50 mL, 100 mL, 200 mL)

Injection, powder for reconstitution: 10 mg, 50 mg

Dosing

Adults & Elderly: Refer to individual protocols.

Note: An estimated Cl_{cr} should be on all cisplatin chemotherapy orders along with other patient parameters (eg, patient's height, weight, and body surface area). Pharmacy and nursing staff should check the Cl_{cr} on the order and determine the appropriateness of cisplatin dosing.

It is recommended that a 24-hour urine creatinine clearance be checked prior to a patient's first dose of cisplatin and periodically thereafter (ie, after every 2-3 cycles of cisplatin).

Pretreatment hydration with 1-2 L of fluid is recommended prior to cisplatin administration. Adequate hydration and urinary output (>100 mL/hour) should be maintained for 24 hours after administration.

If the dose prescribed is a reduced dose, then this should be indicated on the chemotherapy order.

Advanced bladder cancer: 50-70 mg/m^2 every 3-4 weeks

Head and neck cancer: 100-120 mg/m^2 every 3-4 weeks

Testicular cancer: 10-20 mg/m^2/day for 5 days repeated every 3-4 weeks

Metastatic ovarian cancer: 75-100 mg/m^2 every 3 weeks

Intraperitoneal: cisplatin has been administered intraperitoneal with systemic sodium thiosulfate for ovarian cancer; doses up to 90-270 mg/m^2 have been administered and retained for 4 hours before draining

High dose BMT: Continuous I.V.: 55 mg/m^2/24 hours for 72 hours; total dose: 165 mg/m^2

Pediatrics: Refer to individual protocols.

Intermittent dosing schedule: I.V.: 37-75 mg/m^2 once every 2-3 weeks or 50-100 mg/m^2 over 4-6 hours, once every 21-28 days

Daily dosing schedule: I.V.: 15-20 mg/m^2/day for 5 days every 3-4 weeks

Osteogenic sarcoma or neuroblastoma: I.V.:60-100 mg/m^2 on day 1 every 3-4 weeks

(Continued)

Cisplatin *(Continued)*

Recurrent brain tumors: I.V.: 60 mg/m^2 once daily for 2 consecutive days every 3-4 weeks

Bone marrow/blood cell transplantation: Refer to adult dosing.

Renal Impairment:

Cl_{cr} 10-50 mL/minute: Administer 75% of normal dose.

Cl_{cr} <10 mL/minute: Administer 50% of normal dose.

Hemodialysis: Partially cleared by hemodialysis.

Administer dose posthemodialysis.

CAPD effects: Unknown

CAVH effects: Unknown

Administration

I.V.: Irritant. Perform pretreatment hydration (see Dosage). Aluminum-containing I.V. infusion sets and needles should **not** be used due to binding with the platinum.

I.V.: Rate of administration has varied from a 15- to 120-minute infusion, 1 mg/minute infusion, 6- to 8-hour infusion, 24-hour infusion, or per protocol. Maximum rate of infusion: 1 mg/minute in patients with CHF.

When administered as sequential infusions, taxane derivatives (docetaxel, paclitaxel) should be administered before platinum derivatives to limit myelosuppression and to enhance efficacy.

Stability

Storage: Store intact vials at room temperature 15°C to 25°C (59°F to 77°F) and protect from light. Do not refrigerate solution as a precipitate may form. If inadvertently refrigerated, the precipitate will slowly dissolve within hours to days, when placed at room temperature. The precipitate may be dissolved without loss of potency by warming solution to 37°C (98.6°F).

Multidose (preservative-free) vials: After initial entry into the vial, solution is stable for 28 days protected from light or for at least 7 days under fluorescent room light at room temperature.

Reconstitution: Further dilution stability is dependent on the chloride ion concentration and should be mixed in solutions of NS (at least 0.3% NaCl). Further dilution in NS, D_5/0.45% NaCl or D_5/NS to a concentration of 0.05-2 mg/mL are stable for 72 hours at 4°C to 25°C in combination with mannitol; may administer 12.5-50 g mannitol/L.

Standard I.V. dilution: Dose/250-1000 mL NS, D_5/NS or D_5/0.45% NaCl; stable for 72 hours at 4°C to 25°C (in combination with mannitol).

Compatibility: Stable in D_5¼NS, D_5½NS, D_5NS, ¼NS, ⅓NS, ½NS, NS; **incompatible** with sodium bicarbonate 5%

Y-site administration: Incompatible with amifostine, amphotericin B cholesteryl sulfate complex, cefepime, piperacillin/tazobactam, thiotepa

Compatibility when admixed: Incompatible with fluorouracil, mesna, thiotepa

Monitoring Laboratory Tests Renal function (serum creatinine, BUN, Cl_{cr}), electrolytes (particularly magnesium, calcium, potassium), liver function periodically, CBC with differential and platelet count, urinalysis

Monitoring and Teaching Issues

Physical Assessment: See Contraindications, Warnings/Precautions, and Dosing for extensive use cautions. Assess potential for interactions with other prescriptions, OTC medications, or herbal products patient may be taking (especially anything that is ototoxic or nephrotoxic - see Drug Interactions). Administer antiemetic prior to each treatment and as needed between infusions (see emetic potential). See Administration and Compatibility information. Infusion site must be monitored closely to reduce potential for extravasation (see Administration). Assess results of laboratory tests (see above), auditory evaluation, therapeutic effectiveness, and adverse response (see extensive list of Adverse Reactions and Overdose/Toxicology) prior to each treatment and regularly during therapy. Teach patient (or caregiver) possible side effects and interventions (eg, importance of adequate hydration) and adverse symptoms to report (see Patient Education). **Pregnancy risk factor D** - determine that patient is not pregnant before beginning treatment. Instruct patients of childbearing age about appropriate barrier contraceptive measures. Breast-feeding is contraindicated.

Patient Education: Inform prescriber of all prescriptions, OTC medications, or herbal products you are taking, and any allergies you have. Do not take anything new during treatment unless approved by prescriber. This medication can only be administered by I.V. and numerous side-effects can occur. It is important that you maintain adequate hydration (2-3 L/day of fluids) unless advised by prescriber to restrict fluids, and adequate nutrition (small, frequent meals may help) and. May cause severe nausea or vomiting and can be delayed for up to 48 hours after infusion and last for 1 week (consult prescriber for appropriate antiemetic medication); mouth sores (use soft toothbrush or cotton swabs for mouth care); or loss of hair (reversible). You will be susceptible to infection (avoid crowds and exposure to infection and do not have any vaccinations without consulting prescriber). Report promptly any loss of hearing; rash or hives; difficulty breathing or swallowing; fever or chills; chest pain or palpitations; unusual fatigue; unusual bruising/bleeding; numbness, pain or tingling in extremities; muscle cramps or twitching; pain, redness; swelling at infusion site; or any other unusual symptoms. **Pregnancy/breast-feeding precautions:** Inform prescriber if you are pregnant. Do not get pregnant during or for 1 month following therapy. Consult prescriber for instruction on appropriate contraceptive measures. This drug may cause severe fetal defects. Do not breast-feed.

Dietary Issues: Sodium content: 9 mg/mL (equivalent to 0.9% sodium chloride solution)

Additional Information

Sodium content: 9 mg/mL (equivalent to 0.9% sodium chloride solution)

Osmolality of Platinol®-AQ = 285-286 mOsm

Comments on specific toxicities:

Gastrointestinal: Cisplatin is one of the most emetogenic agents used in cancer chemotherapy; nausea and vomiting occur in 76% to 100% of patients and is dose-related.

Prophylactic antiemetics should always be prescribed; nausea and vomiting may last up to 1 week after therapy.

Nephrotoxicity: Related to elimination, protein binding, and uptake of cisplatin. Two types of nephrotoxicity: Acute renal failure and chronic renal insufficiency.

Acute renal failure and azotemia is a dose-dependent process and can be minimized with proper administration and prophylaxis. Damage to the proximal tubules by unbound cisplatin is suspected to cause the toxicity. It is manifested as increased BUN/creatinine, oliguria, protein wasting, and potassium, calcium, and magnesium wasting.

Chronic renal dysfunction can develop in patients receiving multiple courses of cisplatin. Slow release of tissue-bound cisplatin may contribute to chronic nephrotoxicity. Manifestations of this toxicity are varied, and can include sodium and water wasting, nephropathy, hyperuricemia, decreased Cl_{cr}, and magnesium wasting.

Recommendations for minimizing nephrotoxicity include:

Prepare cisplatin in saline-containing vehicles

Infuse dose over 24 hours

Vigorous hydration (125-150 mL/hour) before, during, and after cisplatin administration

Simultaneous administration of either mannitol or furosemide

Pretreatment with amifostine

Avoid other nephrotoxic agents (aminoglycosides, amphotericin, etc)

Neurotoxicity: Peripheral neuropathy is dose- and duration-dependent. The mechanism is through axonal degeneration with subsequent damage to the long sensory nerves. Toxicity can first be noted at cumulative doses of 200 mg/m^2, with measurable toxicity at cumulative doses >350 mg/m^2. This process is irreversible and progressive with continued therapy.

Ototoxicity: Ototoxicity occurs in 10% to 30%, and is manifested as high frequency hearing loss. Baseline audiography should be performed. Ototoxicity is especially pronounced in children.

Anaphylactic reaction occurs within minutes after intravenous or intraperitoneal administration and can be controlled with epinephrine, antihistamines, and steroids.

13-*cis*-Retinoic Acid *see* Isotretinoin *on page 751*

Citalopram (sye TAL oh pram)

U.S. Brand Names Celexa™

Synonyms Citalopram Hydrobromide; Nitalapram

Generic Available No

Pharmacologic Category Antidepressant, Selective Serotonin Reuptake Inhibitor

Pregnancy Risk Factor C

Lactation Enters breast milk/contraindicated

Use Treatment of depression

Use - Unlabeled/Investigational Investigational: Treatment of dementia, smoking cessation, ethanol abuse, obsessive-compulsive disorder (OCD) in children, diabetic neuropathy

Mechanism of Action/Effect A bicyclic phthalein derivative, citalopram selectively inhibits serotonin reuptake in the presynaptic neurons

Contraindications Hypersensitivity to citalopram or any component of the formulation; hypersensitivity or other adverse sequelae during therapy with other SSRIs; concomitant use with MAO inhibitors or within 2 weeks of discontinuing MAO inhibitors.

Warnings/Precautions Potential for severe reaction when used with MAO inhibitors - serotonin syndrome (hyperthermia, muscular rigidity, mental status changes/agitation, autonomic instability) may occur. May precipitate a shift to mania or hypomania in patients with bipolar disease. May impair cognitive or motor performance (risk relatively low) - caution operating hazardous machinery or driving. Use caution if suicidal risk may be present. Use caution in patients with a previous seizure disorder or condition predisposing to seizures, including concurrent use of drugs lowering seizure threshold. Use with caution in patients with hepatic or renal dysfunction and in elderly patients. May cause hyponatremia/SIADH. May cause or exacerbate sexual dysfunction. Pregnancy risk C.

Drug Interactions

Cytochrome P450 Effect: Substrate of **CYP2C19**, 2D6, **3A4**; Inhibits CYP1A2, 2B6, 2C19, 2D6

Decreased Effect: Cyproheptadine may inhibit the effects of serotonin reuptake inhibitors.

Increased Effect/Toxicity:

MAO inhibitors: Citalopram should not be used with nonselective MAO inhibitors (phenelzine, isocarboxazid) or other drugs with MAO inhibition (linezolid); fatal reactions have been reported. Wait 5 weeks after stopping citalopram before starting a nonselective MAO inhibitor and 2 weeks after stopping an MAO inhibitor before starting citalopram. Concurrent selegiline has been associated with mania, hypertension, or serotonin syndrome (risk may be reduced relative to nonselective MAO inhibitors).

Combined used of SSRIs and amphetamines, buspirone, meperidine, nefazodone, serotonin agonists (such as sumatriptan), sibutramine, other SSRIs, sympathomimetics, ritonavir, tramadol, and venlafaxine may increase the risk of serotonin syndrome. Risk of hyponatremia may increase with concurrent use of loop diuretics (bumetanide, furosemide, torsemide). Citalopram may increase the hypoprothrombinemic response to warfarin. Inhibitors of CYP3A4 or CYP2C19 may increase serum levels/effects of citalopram.

Combined use of sumatriptan (and other serotonin agonists) may result in toxicity; weakness, hyper-reflexia, and incoordination have been observed with sumatriptan and SSRIs. In addition, concurrent use may theoretically increase the risk of serotonin syndrome; includes sumatriptan, naratriptan, rizatriptan, and zolmitriptan.

Nutritional/Ethanol Interactions

Ethanol: Avoid ethanol (may increase CNS depression).

Herb/Nutraceutical: Avoid valerian, St John's wort, SAMe, kava kava, and gotu kola (may increase CNS depression).

(Continued)

Citalopram *(Continued)*

Adverse Reactions

>10%:

Central nervous system: Somnolence, insomnia
Gastrointestinal: Nausea, xerostomia
Miscellaneous: Diaphoresis

<10%:

Central nervous system: Anxiety, anorexia, agitation, yawning
Dermatologic: Rash, pruritus
Endocrine & metabolic: Sexual dysfunction
Gastrointestinal: Diarrhea, dyspepsia, vomiting, abdominal pain, weight gain
Neuromuscular & skeletal: Tremor, arthralgia, myalgia
Respiratory: Cough, rhinitis, sinusitis

Overdosage/Toxicology Symptoms of overdose include dizziness, nausea, vomiting, sweating, tremor, somnolence, and sinus tachycardia. Rare symptoms have included amnesia, confusion, coma, seizures, hyperventilation, and EKG changes (including QT_c prolongation, ventricular arrhythmia, and torsade de pointes). Management is supportive and symptomatic.

Pharmacodynamics/Kinetics

Bioavailability: 80%

Half-Life Elimination: 24-48 hours (average: 35 hours); doubled with hepatic impairment

Time to Peak: Serum: 1-6 hours, average within 4 hours

Metabolism: Extensively hepatic, including CYP, to N-demethylated, N-oxide, and deaminated metabolites

Formulations

Solution, oral: 10 mg/5 mL [alcohol free; peppermint flavor; sugar free]
Tablet, as hydrobromide: 10 mg, 20 mg, 40 mg

Dosing

Adults: Depression: Oral: Initial: 20 mg/day, generally with an increase to 40 mg/day; doses of more than 40 mg are not usually necessary. Should a dose increase be necessary, it should occur in 20 mg increments at intervals of no less than 1 week. Maximum dose: 60 mg/day.

Elderly: Reduce dosage in elderly.

Pediatrics: Children and Adolescents: OCD (unlabeled use): Oral: 10-40 mg/day

Renal Impairment: None necessary in mild-moderate renal impairment; best avoided in severely impaired renal function (Cl_{cr} <20 mL/minute).

Hepatic Impairment: Reduce dosage in those with hepatic impairment.

Stability

Storage: Store below 25°C.

Monitoring Laboratory Tests Liver function tests and CBC with continued therapy

Monitoring and Teaching Issues

Physical Assessment: Assess other medications patient may be taking for possible interaction (especially MAO inhibitors, P450 inhibitors, and other CNS active agents - see Drug Interactions). Note Contraindications and Warnings/Precautions for use cautions (assess patient history carefully). Monitor for effectiveness of therapy and adverse reactions (see Adverse Reactions and Overdose/Toxicology). Assess knowledge/teach patient appropriate use, interventions to reduce side effects (eg, hypotensive precautions), and adverse symptoms to report (see Patient Education). **Pregnancy risk factor C** - benefits of use should outweigh possible risks. Breast-feeding is contraindicated.

Patient Education: The effects of this medication may take up to 3 weeks. Take as directed; do not alter dose or frequency without consulting prescriber. May be taken with or without food. Avoid alcohol, caffeine, and CNS stimulants. You may experience sexual dysfunction (reversible). May cause dizziness, anxiety, or blurred vision (rise slowly from sitting or lying position and use caution when driving or engaging in tasks requiring alertness until response to drug is known); or nausea or dry mouth (small, frequent meals, frequent mouth care, chewing gum, or sucking lozenges may help). Report confusion or impaired concentration, severe headache, palpitations, rash, insomnia or nightmares, changes in personality, muscle weakness or tremors, altered gait pattern, signs and symptoms of respiratory infection, or excessive perspiration. **Pregnancy/breast-feeding precautions:** Inform prescriber if you are or intend to become pregnant. Do not breast-feed.

Dietary Issues: May be taken without regard to food.

Geriatric Considerations: Clearance was decreased, while AUC and half-life were significantly increased in elderly patients and in patients with hepatic impairment. Mild to moderate renal impairment may reduce clearance of citalopram (17% reduction noted in trials). No pharmacokinetic information is available concerning patients with severe renal impairment.

Breast-feeding Issues: Citalopram is excreted in human milk; a decision should be made whether to continue or discontinue nursing or discontinue the drug.

Pregnancy Issues: Animal reproductive studies have revealed adverse effects on fetal and postnatal development (at doses higher than human therapeutic doses). Should be used in pregnancy only if potential benefit justifies potential risk.

Related Information

Antidepressant Agents *on page 1553*
Antidepressant Medication Guidelines *on page 1613*

Citalopram Hydrobromide *see* Citalopram *on page 301*

Citracal® [OTC] *see* Calcium Supplements *on page 202*

Citrate of Magnesia (Magnesium Citrate) *see* Magnesium Supplements *on page 831*

Citric Acid and Potassium Citrate *see* Potassium Citrate and Citric Acid *on page 1104*

Citrovorum Factor *see* Leucovorin *on page 779*

CI-719 *see* Gemfibrozil *on page 625*

CL184116 *see* Porfimer *on page 1101*
Cla *see* Clarithromycin *on page 304*

Cladribine (KLA dri been)

U.S. Brand Names Leustatin™

Synonyms 2-CdA; 2-Chlorodeoxyadenosine

Generic Available Yes

Pharmacologic Category Antineoplastic Agent, Antimetabolite

Pregnancy Risk Factor D

Lactation Enters breast milk/contraindicated

Use Treatment of hairy cell leukemia, chronic lymphocytic leukemia, non-Hodgkin's lymphomas, progressive multiple sclerosis

Mechanism of Action/Effect Incorporates into susceptible cells and into DNA breakage of DNA strand and shutdown of DNA synthesis Cladribine is able to kill resting as well as dividing cells, unlike most other cytotoxic drugs.

Contraindications Hypersensitivity to cladribine or any component of the formulation; pregnancy

Warnings/Precautions The U.S. Food and Drug Administration (FDA) currently recommends that procedures for proper handling and disposal of antineoplastic agents be considered. Because of its myelosuppressive properties, cladribine should be used with caution in patients with pre-existing hematologic or immunologic abnormalities. Prophylactic administration of allopurinol should be considered in patients receiving cladribine because of the potential for hyperuricemia secondary to tumor lysis. Appropriate antibiotic therapy should be administered promptly in patients exhibiting signs or symptoms of neutropenia and infection. If cladribine contacts the skin, wash and flush thoroughly with water. Patients should be considered immunosuppressed for up to 1 year after cladribine therapy.

Nutritional/Ethanol Interactions Ethanol: Avoid ethanol (due to GI irritation).

Adverse Reactions

>10%:

- Central nervous system: Fatigue, headache, fever (temperature ≥101°F has been associated with the use of cladribine in approximately 66% of patients in the first month of therapy. Although 69% of patients developed fevers, <33% of febrile events were associated with documented infection)
- Dermatologic: Rash
- Gastrointestinal: Nausea and vomiting
  - Emetic potential: Mild (10% to 30%)
- Hematologic: Anemia (severe); thrombocytopenia; neutropenia; bone marrow suppression
  - Nadir: 5-10 days
  - Recovery 4-8 weeks
  - **Note:** CD4 counts nadir at 4-6 months after treatments. Patients should be considered immunosuppressed for up to 1 year after cladribine therapy.

1% to 10%:

- Cardiovascular: Edema, tachycardia, phlebitis
- Central nervous system: Dizziness, insomnia, pain, chills, malaise
- Dermatologic: Pruritus, erythema
- Gastrointestinal: Constipation, diarrhea, abdominal pain
- Local: Injection site reactions
- Neuromuscular & skeletal: Myalgia, arthralgia, weakness
- Respiratory: Coughing, dyspnea
- Miscellaneous: Diaphoresis, trunk pain

Pharmacodynamics/Kinetics

Half-Life Elimination: Biphasic: Alpha: 25 minutes; Beta: 6.7 hours; Terminal, mean: Normal renal function: 5.4 hours

Formulations Injection [preservative free]: 1 mg/mL (10 mL)

Dosing

Adults & Elderly: Refer to individual protocols.

- Hairy cell leukemia: I.V. Continuous infusion:
  - 0.09-0.1 mg/kg/day days 1-7; may be repeated every 28-35 days **or**
  - 3.4 mg/m²/day S.C. days 1-7
- Chronic lymphocytic leukemia: I.V. Continuous infusion:
  - 0.1 mg/kg/day days 1-7 **or**
  - 0.028-0.14 mg/kg/day as a 2-hour infusion days 1-5
- Chronic myelogenous leukemia: I.V. 15 mg/m²/day as a 1-hour infusion days 1-5; if no response increase second course to 20 mg/m²/day.

Pediatrics: Refer to individual protocols.

- Acute leukemias: Optimum dose not determined; 6.2-7.5 mg/m²/day continuous infusion for days 1-5; maximum tolerated dose was 8.9 mg/m²/day.

Administration

I.V.:

- Single daily infusion: Administer diluted in an infusion bag containing 500 mL of 0.9% sodium chloride and repeated for a total of 7 consecutive days.
- 7-day infusion: Administer via ambulatory infusion pump into central line; use 0.22 micron filter to infuse.

Stability

Storage: Store intact vials under refrigeration (2°C to 8°C).

Reconstitution: 7-day infusion: Prepare with bacteriostatic 0.9% sodium chloride. Both cladribine and diluent should be passed through a sterile 0.22 micron hydrophilic filter as it is being introduced into the infusion reservoir. The calculated dose of cladribine (7 days x 0.09 mg/kg) should first be added to the infusion reservoir through a filter then the bacteriostatic 0.9% sodium chloride should be added to the reservoir to obtain a total volume of 100 mL.

Further dilution in 100-1000 mL NS is stable for 72 hours. Stable in PVC containers for 24 hours at room temperature and 7 days in Pharmacia Deltec® medication cassettes at room

(Continued)

Cladribine *(Continued)*

temperature. For 7-day infusion, dilute with bacteriostatic NS and filter through 0.22 micron filter prior to addition into infusion reservoir.

Standard I.V. 24-hour infusion dilution: 24-hour dose/500 mL NS
24-hour infusion solution is stable for 24 hours at room temperature.

Standard I.V. 7-day infusion dilution: 7-day dose/qs to 100 mL with bacteriostatic NS
7-day infusion solution is stable for 7 days at room temperature.

Compatibility: Stable in NS; **incompatible** with D_5W

Monitoring Laboratory Tests Liver and renal function tests, CBC with differential, platelets, uric acid

Monitoring and Teaching Issues

Physical Assessment: See Contraindications, Warnings/Precautions, and Dosing for extensive use cautions. See Administration, Compatibility, and Reconstitution information. Assess results of laboratory tests (see above), therapeutic effectiveness, and adverse response (see Adverse Reactions) prior to therapy, regularly during therapy, and following therapy (patients should be considered immunosuppressed for up to 1 year after cladribine therapy). Teach patient (or caregiver) possible side effects and interventions and adverse symptoms to report (see Patient Education). **Pregnancy risk factor D** - determine that patient is not pregnant before beginning treatment. Instruct patients of childbearing age about appropriate barrier contraceptive measures. Breast-feeding is contraindicated.

Patient Education: Inform prescriber of all prescriptions, OTC medications, or herbal products you are taking, and any allergies you have. Do not take anything new during treatment unless approved by prescriber. This drug can only be administered by infusion. It is important to maintain adequate hydration (2-3 L/day of fluids) unless advised by prescriber to restrict fluids, and nutrition during therapy (small, frequent meals may help). You will be more susceptible to infection during therapy and for up to 1 year following therapy (avoid crowds and exposure to infection and do not have any vaccinations without consulting prescriber). May cause nausea or vomiting (small, frequent meals, frequent mouth care, sucking lozenges, or chewing gum may help); muscle weakness or pain (consult prescriber for mild analgesics); or mouth sores (use frequent mouth care with soft toothbrush or cotton swabs and frequent mouth rinses). Report immediately rash, unusual excessive fatigue, and/or signs of infection. Report rapid heartbeat or palpitations; unusual bruising or bleeding; persistent GI disturbances; diarrhea or constipation; yellowing of eyes or skin; change in color of urine or stool; swelling, warmth, or pain in extremities; or difficult respirations. **Pregnancy/breast-feeding precautions:** Do not get pregnant while taking this medication. Consult prescriber for appropriate contraceptive measures. Do not breast-feed until prescriber advises it is safe.

Claforan® *see* Cefotaxime *on page 242*
Clarinex® *see* Desloratadine *on page 379*
Claripel™ *see* Hydroquinone *on page 679*

Clarithromycin (kla RITH roe mye sin)

U.S. Brand Names Biaxin®; Biaxin® XL

Synonyms Cla

Generic Available No

Pharmacologic Category Antibiotic, Macrolide

Pregnancy Risk Factor C

Lactation Excretion in breast milk unknown/use caution

Use

Children:
- Pharyngitis/tonsillitis, acute maxillary sinusitis, uncomplicated skin/skin structure infections, and mycobacterial infections due to the above organisms
- Acute otitis media (*H. influenzae*, *M. catarrhalis*, or *S. pneumoniae*)
- Prevention of disseminated mycobacterial infections due to MAC disease in patients with advanced HIV infection

Adults:
- Pharyngitis/tonsillitis due to susceptible *S. pyogenes*
- Acute maxillary sinusitis and acute exacerbation of chronic bronchitis due to susceptible *H. influenzae*, *M. catarrhalis*, or *S. pneumoniae*
- Pneumonia due to susceptible *H. influenzae*, *Mycoplasma pneumoniae*, *S. pneumoniae*, or *Chlamydia pneumoniae* (TWAR);
- Uncomplicated skin/skin structure infections due to susceptible *S. aureus*, *S. pyogenes*
- Disseminated mycobacterial infections due to *M. avium* or *M. intracellulare*
- Prevention of disseminated mycobacterial infections due to *M. avium* complex (MAC) disease (eg, patients with advanced HIV infection)
- Duodenal ulcer disease due to *H. pylori* in regimens with other drugs including amoxicillin and lansoprazole or omeprazole, ranitidine bismuth citrate, bismuth subsalicylate, tetracycline, and/or an H_2 antagonist
- Alternate antibiotic for prophylaxis of bacterial endocarditis in patients who are allergic to penicillin and undergoing surgical or dental procedures

Mechanism of Action/Effect Exerts its antibacterial action by binding to 50S ribosomal subunit resulting in inhibition of protein synthesis. The 14-OH metabolite of clarithromycin is twice as active as the parent compound against some organisms.

Contraindications Hypersensitivity to clarithromycin, erythromycin, or any macrolide antibiotic; use with ergot derivatives, pimozide, astemizole, cisapride; combination with ranitidine bismuth citrate should not be used in patients with history of acute porphyria or Cl_{cr} <25 mL/minute

Warnings/Precautions Dosage adjustment required with severe renal impairment, decreased dosage or prolonged dosing interval may be appropriate; antibiotic-associated colitis has been reported with use of clarithromycin. Macrolides (including clarithromycin) have been associated with rare QT prolongation and ventricular arrhythmias, including torsade de pointes. Safety and efficacy in children <6 months of age have not been established. Pregnancy risk C.

Drug Interactions

Cytochrome P450 Effect: Substrate of **CYP3A4**; Inhibits CYP1A2, **3A4**

Decreased Effect: Clarithromycin may decrease the serum concentrations of zafirlukast. Clarithromycin may antagonize the therapeutic effects of clindamycin and lincomycin. Peak levels (but not AUC) of zidovudine may be increased; other studies suggest levels may be decreased.

Increased Effect/Toxicity: Avoid concomitant use of the following with clarithromycin due to increased risk of malignant arrhythmias: Astemizole, cisapride, gatifloxacin, moxifloxacin, pimozide, sparfloxacin, thioridazine. Other agents that prolong the QT_c interval, including type Ia (eg, quinidine) and type III antiarrhythmic agents, and selected antipsychotic agents (eg, mesoridazine, thioridazine) should be used with extreme caution.

Clarithromycin may increase the serum concentrations (and possibly the toxicity) of the following agents: Alfentanil (and possibly other narcotic analgesics), benzodiazepines (alprazolam, diazepam, midazolam, triazolam), buspirone, calcium channel blockers, dihydropyridine (felodipine), carbamazepine, cilostazol, clozapine, colchicine, cyclosporine, digoxin, disopyramide, ergot alkaloids (eg, bromocriptine), HMG-CoA reductase inhibitors (except fluvastatin, pravastatin), loratadine, methylprednisolone, rifabutin, tacrolimus, theophylline, sildenafil, valproate, vinblastine, vincristine, zopiclone.

The effects of neuromuscular-blocking agents and warfarin have been potentiated by clarithromycin. Clarithromycin serum concentrations may be increased by amprenavir (and possibly other protease inhibitors). Digoxin serum levels may be increased by clarithromycin; digoxin toxicity and potentially fatal arrhythmias have been reported; monitor digoxin levels. Fluconazole increases clarithromycin levels and AUC by ~25%. Peak levels (but not AUC) of zidovudine may be increased; other studies suggest levels may be decreased.

Nutritional/Ethanol Interactions

Food: Delays absorption; total absorption remains unchanged.

Herb/Nutraceutical: St John's wort may decrease clarithromycin levels.

Adverse Reactions

1% to 10%:

Central nervous system: Headache (adults and children 2%)

Dermatologic: Rash (children 3%)

Gastrointestinal: Diarrhea (adults 6%, children 6%); vomiting (children 6%); nausea (adults 3%); abnormal taste (adults 7%); heartburn (adults 2%); abdominal pain (adults 2%, children 3%)

Hepatic: Elevated prothrombin time (1%)

Renal: Elevated BUN (4%)

<1% (Limited to important or life-threatening): Anaphylaxis, *Clostridium difficile* colitis, dyspnea, hallucinations, hepatitis, hypoglycemia, jaundice, leukopenia, manic behavior, neuromuscular blockade (case reports), neutropenia, pancreatitis, psychosis, QT prolongation, seizures, Stevens-Johnson syndrome, thrombocytopenia, torsade de pointes, toxic epidermal necrolysis, tremor, ventricular tachycardia, vertigo

Overdosage/Toxicology Symptoms of overdose include nausea, vomiting, diarrhea, prostration, reversible pancreatitis, hearing loss with or without tinnitus, or vertigo. Treatment includes symptomatic and supportive care.

Pharmacodynamics/Kinetics

Absorption: Highly stable in presence of gastric acid (unlike erythromycin); food delays but does not affect extent of absorption

Bioavailability: 50%

Half-Life Elimination: 5-7 hours

Time to Peak: 2-4 hours

Metabolism: Partially hepatic; converted to 14-OH clarithromycin (active metabolite)

Formulations

Granules for oral suspension: 125 mg/5 mL (50 mL, 100 mL); 187.5 mg/5 mL (100 mL); 250 mg/5 mL (50 mL, 100 mL)

Tablet, film coated: 250 mg, 500 mg

Tablet, film coated, extended release: 500 mg

Dosing

Adults:

Usual dose: Oral: 250-500 mg every 12 hours **or** 1000 mg (two 500 mg extended release tablets) once daily for for 7-14 days

Upper respiratory tract: Oral: 250-500 mg every 12 hours for 10-14 days

Pharyngitis/tonsillitis: 250 mg every 12 hours for 10 days

Acute maxillary sinusitis: 500 mg every 12 hours **or** 1000 mg (two 500 mg extended release tablets) once daily for 14 days

Lower respiratory tract: Oral: 250-500 mg every 12 hours for 7-14 days

Acute exacerbation of chronic bronchitis due to:

M. catarrhalis and *S. pneumoniae*: 250 mg every 12 hours **or** 1000 mg (two 500 mg extended release tablets) once daily for 7-14 days

H. influenzae: 500 mg every 12 hours for 7-14 days

Pneumonia due to:

C. pneumoniae, *M. pneumoniae*, and *S. pneumoniae*: 250 mg every 12 hours for 7-14 days **or** 1000 mg (two 500 mg extended release tablets) once daily for 7-14

H. influenzae: 250 mg every 12 hours for 7 days **or** 1000 mg (two 500 mg extended release tablets) once daily for 7 days

Mycobacterial infection (prevention and treatment): Oral: 500 mg twice daily (use with other antimycobacterial drugs, eg, ethambutol, clofazimine, or rifampin)

Prophylaxis of bacterial endocarditis: Oral: 500 mg 1 hour prior to procedure

Uncomplicated skin and skin structure: Oral: 250 mg every 12 hours for 7-14 days

(Continued)

Clarithromycin *(Continued)*

Peptic ulcer disease due to *Helicobacter pylori*: Oral (Combination regimen with bismuth subsalicylate, tetracycline, clarithromycin, and an H_2-receptor antagonist; or combination of omeprazole and clarithromycin): 250 mg twice daily to 500 mg 3 times/day

Elderly: Refer to adult dosing. Monitor and adjust dose if necessary.

Pediatrics: Oral:

Children ≥6 months: 15 mg/kg/day divided every 12 hours for 10 days

Mycobacterial infection (prevention and treatment): 7.5 mg/kg twice daily, up to 500 mg twice daily

Prophylaxis of bacterial endocarditis: 15 mg/kg 1 hour before procedure (maximum dose: 500 mg)

Renal Impairment:

Cl_{cr} <30 mL/minute: Half the normal dose or double the dosing interval.

In combination with ritonavir:

Cl_{cr} 30-60 mL/minute: Reduce dose by 50%.

Cl_{cr} <30 mL/minute: Reduce dose by 75%.

Hepatic Impairment: No dosing adjustment is needed as long as renal function is normal.

Administration

Oral: Clarithromycin may be given with or without meals. Give every 12 hours rather than twice daily to avoid peak and trough variation.

Biaxin® XL: Should be given with food. Do not crush or chew extended release tablet.

Stability

Storage: Store tablets and granules for oral suspension at controlled room temperature.

Reconstitution: Reconstituted oral suspension should not be refrigerated because it might gel. Microencapsulated particles of clarithromycin in suspension is stable for 14 days when stored at room temperature.

Monitoring Laboratory Tests Perform culture and sensitivity studies prior to initiating drug therapy.

Monitoring and Teaching Issues

Physical Assessment: Assess for previous allergy history prior to therapy. See Contraindications and Warnings/Precautions for use cautions (eg, renal, cardiac, and GI concerns). Assess potential for interactions with other prescriptions, OTC medications, or herbal products patient may be taking (see Drug Interactions). Assess results of laboratory tests, therapeutic response, and adverse reactions (see Adverse Reactions and Overdose/Toxicology). Teach patient proper use, possible side effects and interventions, and adverse symptoms to report (see Patient Education). **Pregnancy risk factor C** - benefits of use should outweigh possible risks. Note breast-feeding caution.

Patient Education: Inform prescriber of all prescriptions, OTC medications, or herbal products you are taking, and any allergies you have. Do not take anything new during treatment unless approved by prescriber. Take full course of therapy; do not discontinue without consulting prescriber. Tablets or suspension may be taken with or without food or milk. Extended release tablets should be taken with food. Do not crush or chew extended release tablets. Do not refrigerate oral suspension (more palatable at room temperature). Maintain adequate hydration (2-3 L/day of fluids) unless advised by prescriber to restrict fluids. May cause nausea, heartburn, or abnormal taste (small, frequent meals, frequent mouth care, chewing gum or sucking lozenges may help); diarrhea (buttermilk, boiled milk, or yogurt may help); or headache or abdominal cramps (consult prescriber for analgesic). Report rapid heartbeat or palpitations, persistent fever or chills, easy bruising or bleeding, joint pain, severe persistent diarrhea, skin rash, sores in mouth, foul-smelling urine, or difficulty breathing. **Pregnancy/breast-feeding precautions:** Inform prescriber if you are or intend to become pregnant. Consult prescriber if breast-feeding.

Dietary Issues: May be taken with or without meals; may be taken with milk. Biaxin® XL should be taken with food.

Geriatric Considerations: Considered one of the drugs of choice in the outpatient treatment of community-acquired pneumonia in older adults. After doses of 500 mg every 12 hours for 5 days, 12 healthy elderly had significantly increased C_{max} and C_{min}, elimination half-lives of clarithromycin and 14-OH clarithromycin compared to 12 healthy young subjects. These changes were attributed to a significant decrease in renal clearance. At a dose of 1000 mg twice daily, 100% of 13 older adults experienced an adverse event compared to only 10% taking 500 mg twice daily.

Breast-feeding Issues: Erythromycins may be taken while breast-feeding. Use caution.

Related Information

Helicobacter pylori Treatment *on page 1676*

Clarithromycin, Lansoprazole, and Amoxicillin *see* Lansoprazole, Amoxicillin, and Clarithromycin *on page 774*

Claritin® *see* Loratadine *on page 820*

Claritin-D® 12-Hour *see* Loratadine and Pseudoephedrine *on page 821*

Claritin-D® 24-Hour *see* Loratadine and Pseudoephedrine *on page 821*

Clear Eyes® [OTC] *see page 1509*

Cleocin® *see* Clindamycin *on page 307*

Cleocin HCl® *see* Clindamycin *on page 307*

Cleocin Pediatric® *see* Clindamycin *on page 307*

Cleocin Phosphate® *see* Clindamycin *on page 307*

Cleocin T® *see* Clindamycin *on page 307*

Clidinium and Chlordiazepoxide (kli DI nee um & klor dye az e POKS ide)

U.S. Brand Names Librax®

Synonyms Chlordiazepoxide and Clidinium

Generic Available Yes

Pharmacologic Category Antispasmodic Agent, Gastrointestinal; Benzodiazepine

Pregnancy Risk Factor D

Lactation Enters breast milk/contraindicated

Use Adjunct treatment of peptic ulcer; treatment of irritable bowel syndrome

Contraindications Hypersensitivity to clidinium, chlordiazepoxide, or any component of the formulation; glaucoma; prostatic hyperplasia; benign bladder neck obstruction; pregnancy

Warnings/Precautions Use with caution with ethanol or other CNS depressants because of possible combined effects. Do not abruptly discontinue this medication after prolonged use; taper dose gradually.

Drug Interactions

Cytochrome P450 Effect: Chlordiazepoxide: Substrate of **CYP3A4**

Increased Effect/Toxicity: Additive effects may result from concomitant benzodiazepine and/or anticholinergic therapy.

Nutritional/Ethanol Interactions Ethanol: Avoid ethanol (may increase CNS depression).

Adverse Reactions

1% to 10%:

Central nervous system: Drowsiness ataxia, confusion, anticholinergic side effects

Gastrointestinal: Dry mouth, constipation, nausea

<1% (Limited to important or life-threatening): Agranulocytosis, blood dyscrasias, extrapyramidal symptoms, hepatic dysfunction, jaundice, syncope

Formulations Capsule: Clidinium bromide 2.5 mg and chlordiazepoxide hydrochloride 5 mg

Dosing

Adults: Adjunct treatment of peptic ulcer; treatment of IBS: Oral: 1-2 capsules 3-4 times/day, before meals or food and at bedtime. **Caution:** Do not abruptly discontinue after prolonged use; taper dose gradually.

Elderly: Limit dosage to smallest effective amount to preclude the development of ataxia, oversedation, or confusion (not more than 2 capsules/day initially to be increased gradually as needed and tolerated).

Administration

Oral: Caution: Do not abruptly discontinue after prolonged use; taper dose gradually.

Monitoring Laboratory Tests CBC, liver function

Monitoring and Teaching Issues

Physical Assessment: Assess effectiveness and interactions of other medications patient may be taking (see Drug Interactions). See Warnings/Precautions and Contraindications for use cautions. Monitor therapeutic effectiveness, laboratory tests, and adverse response (see Adverse Reactions and Overdose/Toxicology). Assess knowledge/teach patient appropriate use, possible side effects and appropriate interventions, and adverse symptoms to report (see Patient Education). **Pregnancy risk factor D** - determine that patient is not pregnant before beginning treatment. Instruct patients of childbearing age about appropriate barrier contraceptive measure. Breast-feeding is contraindicated.

Patient Education: Take as directed before meals; do not increase dose and do not discontinue without consulting prescriber first. Avoid alcohol and other CNS depressant medications (antihistamines, sleeping aids, antidepressants) unless approved by prescriber. Void before taking medication. This drug may impair mental alertness (use caution when driving or engaging in tasks that require alertness until response to drug is known). Report excessive and persistent anticholinergic effects (blurred vision, headache, flushing, tachycardia, nervousness, constipation, dizziness, insomnia, mental confusion or excitement, dry mouth, altered taste perception, dysphagia, palpitations, bradycardia, urinary hesitancy or retention, impotence, decreased sweating), or change in color of urine or stools. **Pregnancy/breast-feeding precautions:** Do not get pregnant while taking this medication; use appropriate contraceptive measures. Do not breast-feed.

Dietary Issues: Should be taken before meals.

Pregnancy Issues: An increased risk of congenital malformations has been associated with the use of minor tranquilizers during the 1st trimester. Because use of these drugs is rarely a matter of urgency, their use should be avoided during this period.

Other Issues: After extended therapy, abrupt discontinuation should be avoided and a gradual dose tapering schedule followed.

Related Information

Chlordiazepoxide *on page 273*

Climara® *see* Estradiol *on page 494*

Clindagel™ *see* Clindamycin *on page 307*

Clindamycin (klin da MYE sin)

U.S. Brand Names Cleocin®; Cleocin HCl®; Cleocin Pediatric®; Cleocin Phosphate®; Cleocin T®; Clindagel™; Clindets®

Synonyms Clindamycin Hydrochloride; Clindamycin Phosphate

Generic Available Yes

Pharmacologic Category Antibiotic, Miscellaneous

Pregnancy Risk Factor B

Lactation Enters breast milk/compatible

Use Treatment against aerobic and anaerobic streptococci (except enterococci), most staphylococci, *Bacteroides* sp and *Actinomyces*; bacterial vaginosis; prophylaxis in the prevention of bacterial endocarditis in high-risk patients undergoing surgical or dental procedures in patients allergic to penicillin; may be useful in PCP; used topically in treatment of severe acne; vaginally for *Gardnerella vaginalis* or alternate treatment for toxoplasmosis

Mechanism of Action/Effect Reversibly binds to 50S ribosomal subunits preventing peptide bond formation thus inhibiting bacterial protein synthesis; bacteriostatic or bactericidal depending on drug concentration, infection site, and organism

Contraindications Hypersensitivity to clindamycin or any component of the formulation; previous pseudomembranous colitis; hepatic impairment

Warnings/Precautions Dosage adjustment may be necessary in patients with severe hepatic dysfunction. No change necessary with renal insufficiency. Can cause severe and possibly fatal colitis. Use with caution in patients with a history of pseudomembranous colitis.
(Continued)

Clindamycin *(Continued)*

Discontinue drug if significant diarrhea, abdominal cramps, or passage of blood and mucus occurs. Avoid in neonates (contains benzyl alcohol).

Drug Interactions

Increased Effect/Toxicity: Increased duration of neuromuscular blockade when given in conjunction with tubocurarine and pancuronium.

Nutritional/Ethanol Interactions

Food: Peak concentrations may be delayed with food.

Herb/Nutraceutical: St John's wort may decrease clindamycin levels.

Adverse Reactions

Systemic:

>10%: Gastrointestinal: Diarrhea, abdominal pain

1% to 10%:

Cardiovascular: Hypotension

Dermatologic: Urticaria, rashes, Stevens-Johnson syndrome

Gastrointestinal: Pseudomembranous colitis, nausea, vomiting

Local: Thrombophlebitis, sterile abscess at I.M. injection site

Miscellaneous: Fungal overgrowth, hypersensitivity

<1% (Limited to important or life-threatening): Granulocytopenia, neutropenia, polyarthritis, renal dysfunction (rare), thrombocytopenia

Topical:

>10%: Dermatologic: Dryness, burning, itching, scaliness, erythema, or peeling of skin (lotion, solution); oiliness (gel, lotion)

<1% (Limited to important or life-threatening): Pseudomembranous colitis, nausea, vomiting, diarrhea (severe), abdominal pain, folliculitis, hypersensitivity reactions

Vaginal:

>10%: Genitourinary: Vaginitis or vulvovaginal pruritus (from *Candida albicans*), painful intercourse

1% to 10%:

Central nervous system: Dizziness, headache

Gastrointestinal: Diarrhea, nausea, vomiting, stomach cramps

Overdosage/Toxicology Symptoms of overdose include diarrhea, nausea, and vomiting. Treatment is supportive.

Pharmacodynamics/Kinetics

Absorption: Topical: ~10%; Oral: Rapid (90%)

Bioavailability: Topical: <1%

Half-Life Elimination: Neonates: Premature: 8.7 hours; Full-term: 3.6 hours; Adults: 1.6-5.3 hours (average: 2-3 hours)

Time to Peak: Serum: Oral: Within 60 minutes; I.M.: 1-3 hours

Metabolism: Hepatic

Formulations

Capsule, as hydrochloride (Cleocin HCl®): 75 mg [contains tartrazine], 150 mg [contains tartrazine], 300 mg

Cream, vaginal, as phosphate (Cleocin®): 2% (40 g) [packaged with 7 disposable applicators]

Gel, topical, as phosphate: 1% [10 mg/g] (30 g, 60 g)

Cleocin T®: 1% [10 mg/g] (30 g, 60 g)

Clindagel™: 1% [10 mg/g] (42 g, 77 g)

Granules for oral solution, as palmitate (Cleocin Pediatric®): 75 mg/5 mL (100 mL) [cherry flavor]

Infusion, as phosphate [premixed in D_5W] (Cleocin Phosphate®): 300 mg (50 mL); 600 mg (50 mL); 900 mg (50 mL)

Injection, solution, as phosphate (Cleocin Phosphate®): 150 mg/mL (2 mL, 4 mL, 6 mL, 60 mL) [contains benzyl alcohol]

Lotion, as phosphate (Cleocin T®): 1% [10 mg/mL] (60 mL)

Pledgets, topical: 1% (60s)

Clindets®: 1% (69s)

Cleocin T®: 1% (60s)

Solution, topical, as phosphate (Cleocin T®): 1% [10 mg/mL] (30 mL, 60 mL)

Suppository, vaginal, as phosphate (Cleocin®): 100 mg (3s)

Dosing

Adults & Elderly:

Usual dose:

Oral: 150-450 mg/dose every 6-8 hours; maximum dose: 1.8 g/day

I.M., I.V.: 1.2-1.8 g/day in 2-4 divided doses; maximum dose: 4.8 g/day

Pelvic inflammatory disease: I.V.: 900 mg every 8 hours with gentamicin 2 mg/kg, then 1.5 mg/kg every 8 hours; continue after discharge with doxycycline 100 mg twice daily to complete 14 days of total therapy

Pneumocystis carinii pneumonia:

Oral: 300-450 mg 4 times/day with primaquine

I.M., I.V.: 1200-2400 mg/day with pyrimethamine

I.V.: 600 mg 4 times/day with primaquine

Acne: Topical: Apply a thin film twice daily

Bacterial vaginosis:

Oral: 300 mg twice daily for 7 days

Intravaginal:

Suppositories: Insert one ovule (100 mg clindamycin) daily into vagina at bedtime for 3 days

Cream: One full applicator inserted intravaginally once daily before bedtime for 3 or 7 consecutive days

Prevention of bacterial endocarditis in patients unable to take amoxicillin: Oral: 600 mg 1 hour before procedure with no follow-up dose needed; for patients allergic to penicillin and unable to take oral medications: 600 mg I.V. within 30 minutes before procedure

Orofacial infections: 150-450 mg every 6 hours for at least 7 days; maximum dose: 1.8 g/day

Patients with prosthesis allergic to penicillin: Oral: 600 mg 1 hour before procedure; for patients with prosthesis allergic to penicillin and unable to take oral medication: I.V.: 600 mg 1 hour before procedure

Pediatrics: Avoid in neonates (contains benzyl alcohol)

Usual dose:

Oral: Infants and Children: 8-20 mg/kg/day as hydrochloride; 8-25 mg/kg/day as palmitate in 3-4 divided doses; minimum dose of palmitate: 37.5 mg 3 times/day

I.M., I.V.:

<1 month: 15-20 mg/kg/day

>1 month: 20-40 mg/kg/day in 3-4 divided doses

Prevention of bacterial endocarditis: Oral: Children: 20 mg/kg 1 hour before procedure with no follow-up dose needed; for patients allergic to penicillin and unable to take oral medications: 20 mg/kg I.V. within 30 minutes before procedure

Orofacial infections: 8-25 mg/kg in 3-4 equally divided doses

Acne: Topical: Children ≥12 years: Refer to adult dosing.

Babesiosis: Oral: 20-40 mg/kg divided every 8 hours for 7 days plus quinine

Hepatic Impairment: Systemic use: Adjustment is recommended in patients with severe hepatic disease.

Administration

Oral: Administer oral dosage form with a full glass of water to minimize esophageal ulceration. Give around-the-clock to promote less variation in peak and trough serum levels.

I.M.: Deep I.M. sites, rotate sites. Do not exceed 600 mg in a single injection.

I.V.: Never give as bolus. Do not exceed 1200 mg/hour.

Stability

Reconstitution: Oral: Do **not** refrigerate reconstituted oral solution because it will thicken. Oral solution is stable for 2 weeks at room temperature following reconstitution. I.V. infusion solution in NS or D_5W solution is stable for 16 days at room temperature.

Compatibility: Stable in D_5LR, $D_5{}^1\!/_2NS$, D_5NS, D_5W, $D_{10}W$, LR, NS

Y-site administration: Incompatible with allopurinol, filgrastim, fluconazole, idarubicin

Compatibility in syringe: Incompatible with tobramycin

Compatibility when admixed: Incompatible with aminophylline, barbiturates, calcium gluconate, ceftriaxone, ciprofloxacin, gentamicin with cefazolin, magnesium sulfate, phenytoin

Monitoring Laboratory Tests CBC, liver and renal function periodically with prolonged therapy

Monitoring and Teaching Issues

Physical Assessment: Assess previous allergy history prior to beginning therapy. See Contraindications, Warnings/Precautions, and Drug Interactions for use cautions. **I.V.:** Monitor cardiac status and blood pressure. Keep patient recumbent after infusion until blood pressure is stabilized. Assess results of laboratory tests (see above) and patient response according to dose, route of administration, and purpose of therapy (see Adverse Reactions and Overdose/Toxicology). Teach patient proper use, possible side effects and interventions, and adverse symptoms to report (eg, severe diarrhea, opportunistic infection - see Patient Education).

Patient Education: Oral: Take each dose with a full glass of water. Complete full prescription, even if feeling better. You may experience nausea or vomiting (small, frequent meals, frequent mouth care, chewing gum, or sucking lozenges may help). Report dizziness; persistent GI effects (pain, diarrhea, vomiting); skin redness, rash, or burning; fever; chills; unusual bruising or bleeding; signs of infection; excessive fatigue; yellowing of eyes or skin; change in color of urine or blackened stool; swelling, warmth, or pain in extremities; difficult respirations; bloody or fatty stool (do not take antidiarrheal without consulting prescriber); or lack or improvement or worsening of condition.

Topical: Wash hands before applying or wear gloves. Apply thin film of gel, lotion, or solution to affected area. May apply porous dressing. Report persistent burning, swelling, itching, or worsening of condition.

Vaginal: Wash hands before using. At bedtime, gently insert full applicator into vagina and expel cream. Wash applicator with soap and water following use. Remain lying down for 30 minutes following administration. Avoid intercourse during 7 days of therapy. Report adverse reactions (dizziness, nausea, vomiting, stomach cramps, or headache) or lack of improvement or worsening of condition.

Dietary Issues: May be taken with food.

Geriatric Considerations: Elderly patients are often at a higher risk for developing serious colitis and require close monitoring.

Related Information

Compatibility of Drugs *on page 1564*

Clindamycin Hydrochloride *see* Clindamycin *on page 307*

Clindamycin Phosphate *see* Clindamycin *on page 307*

Clindets® *see* Clindamycin *on page 307*

Clinoril® *see* Sulindac *on page 1266*

Clobetasol *see* Topical Corticosteroids *on page 1334*

Clocort™ *see* Hydrocortisone *on page 673*

Clocort® Maximum Strength *see* Topical Corticosteroids *on page 1334*

Clocortolone *see* Topical Corticosteroids *on page 1334*

Cloderm® *see* Topical Corticosteroids *on page 1334*

Clofazimine (kloe FA zi meen)

U.S. Brand Names Lamprene®

Synonyms Clofazimine Palmitate

Generic Available No

(Continued)

Clofazimine *(Continued)*

Pharmacologic Category Leprostatic Agent

Pregnancy Risk Factor C

Lactation Enters breast milk/contraindicated (AAP rates "of concern")

Use Orphan drug: Treatment of dapsone-resistant leprosy; multibacillary dapsone-sensitive leprosy; erythema nodosum leprosum; *Mycobacterium avium-intracellulare* (MAI) infections

Mechanism of Action/Effect Binds preferentially to mycobacterial DNA to inhibit mycobacterial growth; also has some anti-inflammatory activity through an unknown mechanism

Contraindications Hypersensitivity to clofazimine or any component of the formulation

Warnings/Precautions Use with caution in patients with GI problems. Dosages >100 mg/day should be used for as short a duration as possible. Skin discoloration resulting from clofazimine treatment may lead to depression. Pregnancy risk C.

Drug Interactions

Cytochrome P450 Effect: Inhibits CYP3A4

Decreased Effect: Combined use may decrease effect with dapsone (unconfirmed).

Nutritional/Ethanol Interactions

Food: The presence of food increases the extent of absorption.

Effects on Lab Values ↑ ESR, glucose (S), albumin, bilirubin, AST

Adverse Reactions

>10%:

Dermatologic: Dry skin

Gastrointestinal: Abdominal pain, nausea, vomiting, diarrhea

Miscellaneous: Pink to brownish-black discoloration of the skin and conjunctiva

1% to 10%:

Dermatologic: Rash, pruritus

Endocrine & metabolic: Elevated blood sugar

Gastrointestinal: Fecal discoloration

Genitourinary: Discoloration of urine

Ocular: Irritation of the eyes

Miscellaneous: Discoloration of sputum, sweat

<1% (Limited to important or life-threatening): Acneiform eruptions, bowel obstruction, diminished vision, eosinophilia, eosinophilic enteritis, erythroderma, GI bleeding, giddiness, hepatitis, hypokalemia, jaundice, monilial cheilosis, neuralgia, phototoxicity

Overdosage/Toxicology Treatment is supportive.

Pharmacodynamics/Kinetics

Absorption: Slowly (45% to 70%)

Half-Life Elimination: Terminal: 8 days; Tissue: 70 days

Time to Peak: Serum: Chronic therapy: 1-6 hours

Metabolism: Partially hepatic to two metabolites

Formulations Capsule, as palmitate: 50 mg

Dosing

Adults & Elderly:

Dapsone-resistant leprosy: Oral: 100 mg/day in combination with one or more antileprosy drugs for 3 years; then alone 100 mg/day

Dapsone-sensitive multibacillary leprosy: Oral: 100 mg/day in combination with two or more antileprosy drugs for at least 2 years and continue until negative skin smears are obtained, then institute single drug therapy with appropriate agent.

Erythema nodosum leprosum: Oral: 100-200 mg/day for up to 3 months or longer then taper dose to 100 mg/day when possible

Pyoderma gangrenosum: Oral: 300-400 mg/day for up to 12 months

Pediatrics: Leprosy: Oral: Children: 1 mg/kg/day every 24 hours in combination with dapsone and rifampin

Hepatic Impairment: Should be considered in severe hepatic dysfunction.

Monitoring and Teaching Issues

Physical Assessment: See Contraindications, Warnings/Precautions, Drug Interactions, and Dosing for use cautions. Assess therapeutic effectiveness and adverse reactions (eg, type 2 reaction state - onset of tender skin nodules with joint and lymph gland swelling or visual disturbances - see Adverse Reactions and Overdose/Toxicology). Teach patient proper use, possible side effects and interventions, and adverse symptoms to report (see Patient Education). **Pregnancy risk factor C** - benefits of use should outweigh possible risks. Breast-feeding is contraindicated.

Patient Education: Take as directed. May be taken with meals. Drug may cause a pink to brownish-black discoloration of the skin, conjunctiva, tears, sweat, urine, feces, and nasal secretions. Although reversible, it may take months to years for skin discoloration to disappear after therapy is complete. Report promptly bone or joint pain, GI disturbance, or vision changes. **Pregnancy/breast-feeding precautions:** Inform prescriber if you are or intend to become pregnant. Do not breast-feed.

Dietary Issues: May be taken with meals.

Geriatric Considerations: No specific studies in the elderly. Use with caution in diabetics.

Breast-feeding Issues: Increased skin pigmentation may occur in nursing infants.

Related Information

Tuberculosis *on page 1705*

Clofazimine Palmitate *see* Clofazimine *on page 309*

Clofibrate (kloe FYE brate)

U.S. Brand Names Atromid-S®

Generic Available Yes

Pharmacologic Category Antilipemic Agent, Fibric Acid

Pregnancy Risk Factor C

Lactation Excretion in breast milk unknown/contraindicated

Use Adjunct to dietary therapy in the management of hyperlipidemias associated with high triglyceride levels (types III, IV, V); primarily lowers triglycerides and very low density lipoprotein

Mechanism of Action/Effect Increases breakdown of VLDL to LDL. Decreases liver synthesis of VLDL. Inhibits cholesterol formation, lowering serum lipid levels. Has antiplatelet effect.

Contraindications Hypersensitivity to clofibrate or any component of the formulation; significant hepatic or renal dysfunction; primary biliary cirrhosis

Warnings/Precautions Possible increased risk of malignancy and cholelithiasis. No evidence of cardiovascular mortality benefit. Anemia and leukopenia have been reported. Elevations in serum transaminases can be seen. Discontinue if lipid response is not seen. Use with caution in peptic ulcer disease. Flu-like symptoms may occur. Be careful in patient selection; this is not a first- or second-line choice. Other agents may be more suitable. Pregnancy risk C.

Drug Interactions

Cytochrome P450 Effect: Substrate of CYP3A4; Inhibits CYP2A6; Induces CYP2B6, 2E1, 3A4

Decreased Effect: Rifampin (and potentially other inducers of CYP3A4) may reduce blood levels of clofibrate.

Increased Effect/Toxicity: Clofibrate may increase effects of warfarin, insulin, and sulfonylureas. Clofibrate's levels may be increased with probenecid. HMG-CoA reductase inhibitors (atorvastatin, cerivastatin, fluvastatin, lovastatin, pravastatin, simvastatin) may increase the risk of myopathy and rhabdomyolysis. The manufacturer warns against the concomitant use. However, combination therapy with statins has been used in some patients with resistant hyperlipidemias (with great caution).

Effects on Lab Values ↑ creatine phosphokinase [CPK] (S); ↓ alkaline phosphatase (S), cholesterol (S), glucose, uric acid (S)

Adverse Reactions Frequency not defined.

Common: Gastrointestinal: Nausea, diarrhea

Less common:

Central nervous system: Headache, dizziness, fatigue

Gastrointestinal: Vomiting, loose stools, heartburn, flatulence, abdominal distress, epigastric pain

Neuromuscular & skeletal: Muscle cramping, aching, weakness, myalgia

Frequency not defined:

Central nervous system: Fever

Cardiovascular: Chest pain, cardiac arrhythmias

Dermatologic: Rash, urticaria, pruritus, alopecia, dry,brittle hair, toxic epidermal necrolysis, erythema multiforme, Stevens-Johnson syndrome

Endocrine & metabolic: Polyphagia, gynecomastia, hyperkalemia

Gastrointestinal: Stomatitis, gallstones, pancreatitis, gastritis, peptic ulcer, weight gain

Genitourinary: Impotence, decreased libido

Hematologic: Leukopenia, anemia, eosinophilia, agranulocytosis, thrombocytopenic purpura

Hepatic: Increased liver function test, hepatomegaly, jaundice

Local: Thrombophlebitis

Neuromuscular & skeletal: Myalgia, myopathy, myositis, arthralgia, rhabdomyolysis, increased creatinine phosphokinase (CPK), rheumatoid arthritis, tremor

Ocular: Photophobic

Renal: Dysuria, hematuria, proteinuria, renal toxicity (allergic), rhabdomyolysis-induced renal failure

Miscellaneous: Flu-like syndrome, increased diaphoresis, systemic lupus erythematosus

Overdosage/Toxicology Symptoms of overdose include nausea, vomiting, diarrhea, and GI distress. Treatment is supportive.

Pharmacodynamics/Kinetics

Absorption: Complete

Half-Life Elimination: 6-24 hours; significantly prolonged with renal impairment; Anuria: 110 hours

Time to Peak: Serum: 3-6 hours

Metabolism: Hepatic to an inactive glucuronide ester; intestinal transformation required to activate drug

Formulations Capsule: 500 mg

Dosing

Adults & Elderly: Dyslipidemia: Oral: 500 mg 4 times/day; some patients may respond to lower doses.

Renal Impairment:

Cl_{cr} >50 mL/minute: Administer every 6-12 hours.

Cl_{cr} 10-50 mL/minute: Administer every 12-18 hours.

Cl_{cr} <10 mL/minute: Avoid use.

Administration

Oral: Administer with meals or milk if GI upset occurs.

Monitoring Laboratory Tests Periodic lipid panels

Monitoring and Teaching Issues

Physical Assessment: See Contraindications and Warnings/Precautions for use cautions. Assess potential for interactions with other prescriptions, OTC medications, or herbal products patient may be taking (see Drug Interactions). Assess results of laboratory tests, therapeutic effectiveness (eg, lipid levels), and adverse reactions (see Adverse Reactions and Overdose/Toxicology). Teach patient proper use, possible side effects and interventions, and adverse symptoms to report (see Patient Education). **Pregnancy risk factor C** - benefits of use should outweigh possible risks. Breast-feeding is contraindicated.

Patient Education: Inform prescriber of all prescriptions, OTC medications, or herbal products you are taking, and any allergies you have. Do not take anything new during treatment unless approved by prescriber. Take as directed. May take with food or milk to

(Continued)

Clofibrate *(Continued)*

reduce stomach upset. This drug may have to be taken long-term; ongoing follow-up is essential. May cause nausea, vomiting, or stomach upset (small, frequent meals, frequent mouth care, chewing gum, or sucking lozenges may help); headache, dizziness, fatigue (use care when driving or engaging in potentially hazardous tasks until response to drug is known); or muscle cramping or pain (if persistent consult prescriber for analgesic). Report chest pain, shortness of breath, irregular heartbeat, palpitations, severe stomach pain with persistent nausea and vomiting, persistent fever, sore throat, or unusual bleeding or bruising. **Pregnancy/breast-feeding precautions:** Inform prescriber if you are or intend to become pregnant. Do not breast-feed.

Geriatric Considerations: The definition of, and therefore, when to treat hyperlipidemia in the elderly is a controversial issue. Therefore, treatment may be better reserved for those who are unable to obtain a desirable plasma cholesterol level by diet alone and for whom the benefits of treatment are believed to outweigh the potential adverse effects, drug interactions, and cost of treatment. Adjust dose for renal function.

Related Information

Lipid-Lowering Agents *on page 1582*

Clomid® *see* ClomiPHENE *on page 312*

ClomiPHENE (KLOE mi feen)

U.S. Brand Names Clomid®; Milophene®; Serophene®

Synonyms Clomiphene Citrate

Generic Available Yes

Pharmacologic Category Ovulation Stimulator

Pregnancy Risk Factor X

Lactation Excretion in breast milk unknown/contraindicated

Use Treatment of ovulatory failure in patients desiring pregnancy

Use - Unlabeled/Investigational Male infertility

Mechanism of Action/Effect Induces ovulation by stimulating the release of pituitary gonadotropins

Contraindications Hypersensitivity to clomiphene citrate or any of its components; liver disease; abnormal uterine bleeding; enlargement or development of ovarian cyst; uncontrolled thyroid or adrenal dysfunction in the presence of an organic intracranial lesion such as pituitary tumor; pregnancy

Warnings/Precautions Use with caution in patients sensitive to pituitary gonadotropins (eg, polycystic ovary disease). Clomiphene may induce multiple pregnancies, ovarian enlargement, ovarian hyperstimulation syndrome, or abdominal pain, blurring or other visual symptoms.

Drug Interactions

Decreased Effect: Decreased response when used with danazol. Decreased estradiol response when used with clomiphene.

Effects on Lab Values Clomiphene may increase levels of serum thyroxine and thyroxine-binding globulin (TBG)

Adverse Reactions

>10%: Endocrine & metabolic: Hot flashes, ovarian enlargement

1% to 10%:

Cardiovascular: Thromboembolism

Central nervous system: Mental depression, headache

Endocrine & metabolic: Breast enlargement (males), breast discomfort (females), abnormal menstrual flow, ovarian cyst formation, ovarian enlargement, premenstrual syndrome, uterine fibroid enlargement

Gastrointestinal: Distention, bloating, nausea, vomiting

Hepatic: Hepatotoxicity

Ocular: Blurring of vision, diplopia, floaters, after-images, phosphenes, photophobia, scotoma

<1% (Limited to important or life-threatening): Alopecia (reversible), polyuria

Pharmacodynamics/Kinetics

Half-Life Elimination: 5-7 days

Metabolism: Undergoes enterohepatic recirculation

Formulations Tablet, as citrate: 50 mg

Dosing

Adults & Elderly:

Male (infertility): Oral: 25 mg/day for 25 days with 5 days rest, or 100 mg every Monday, Wednesday, Friday

Female (ovulatory failure): Oral: 50 mg/day for 5 days (first course); start the regimen on or about the fifth day of cycle. The dose should be increased only in those patients who do not ovulate in response to cyclic 50 mg Clomid®. A low dosage or duration of treatment course is particularly recommended if unusual sensitivity to pituitary gonadotropin is suspected, such as in patients with polycystic ovary syndrome.

If ovulation does not appear to occur after the first course of therapy, a second course of 100 mg/day (two 50 mg tablets given as a single daily dose) for 5 days should be given. This course may be started as early as 30 days after the previous one after precautions are taken to exclude the presence of pregnancy. Increasing the dosage or duration of therapy beyond 100 mg/day for 5 days is not recommended. The majority of patients who are going to ovulate will do so after the first course of therapy. If ovulation does not occur after 3 courses of therapy, further treatment is not recommended and the patient should be re-evaluated. If 3 ovulatory responses occur, but pregnancy has not been achieved, further treatment is not recommended. If menses does not occur after an ovulatory response, the patient should be re-evaluated. Long-term cyclic therapy is not recommended beyond a total of about 6 cycles.

Stability

Storage: Protect from light.

Monitoring Laboratory Tests Urine estrogens and estriol levels; normal levels indicate appropriateness for clomiphene therapy.

Monitoring and Teaching Issues

Physical Assessment: See Contraindications, Warnings/Precautions, Drug Interactions, and Dosing for use cautions. Assess results of laboratory tests (see above), therapeutic effectiveness (according to purpose for use), and adverse response (see Adverse Reactions) regularly during therapy. Teach patient appropriate use (eg, measuring basal body temperature and timing intercourse), possible side effects and interventions, and adverse symptoms to report (see Patient Education). **Pregnancy risk factor X** - determine that patient is not pregnant before beginning treatment. Breast-feeding is contraindicated.

Patient Education: Inform prescriber of all prescriptions, OTC medications, or herbal products you are taking, and any allergies you have. Do not take anything new during treatment unless approved by prescriber. Follow recommended schedule of dosing exactly. May cause hot flashes (cool clothes and cool environment may help). Report acute sudden headache; difficulty breathing; warmth, swelling, pain, or redness in calves; breast enlargement (male) or breast discomfort (female); abnormal menstrual bleeding; vision changes (blurring, diplopia, photophobia, floaters); acute abdominal discomfort; or fever. **Breast-feeding precaution:** Do not breast-feed.

Related Information

FDA Name Differentiation Project: The Use of Tall-man Letters *on page 12*

Clomiphene Citrate *see* ClomiPHENE *on page 312*

ClomiPRAMINE (kloe MI pra meen)

U.S. Brand Names Anafranil®

Synonyms Clomipramine Hydrochloride

Generic Available Yes

Pharmacologic Category Antidepressant, Tricyclic (Tertiary Amine)

Pregnancy Risk Factor C

Lactation Enters breast milk/contraindicated (AAP rates "of concern")

Use Treatment of obsessive-compulsive disorder (OCD)

Use - Unlabeled/Investigational Depression, panic attacks, chronic pain

Mechanism of Action/Effect Clomipramine appears to affect serotonin uptake while its active metabolite, desmethylclomipramine, affects norepinephrine uptake

Contraindications Hypersensitivity to clomipramine, other tricyclic agents, or any component of the formulation; use of MAO inhibitors within 14 days; use in a patient during the acute recovery phase of MI

Warnings/Precautions May cause seizures (relationship to dose and/or duration of therapy) - do not exceed maximum doses. Use caution in patients with a previous seizure disorder or condition predisposing to seizures, including concurrent therapy with other drugs which lower the seizure threshold. Has been associated with a high incidence of sexual dysfunction. Weight gain may occur. May cause sedation, resulting in impaired performance of tasks requiring alertness (ie, operating machinery or driving). Sedative effects may be additive with other CNS depressants and/or ethanol. May worsen psychosis in some patients or precipitate a shift to mania or hypomania in patients with bipolar disease. May increase the risks associated with electroconvulsive therapy. Discontinue, when possible, prior to elective surgery. Therapy should not be abruptly discontinued in patients receiving high doses for prolonged periods.

Use with caution in patients at risk of hypotension (orthostasis) or in patients where transient hypotensive episodes would be poorly tolerated (cardiovascular disease or cerebrovascular disease). Use caution in patients with thyroid disease, hepatic or renal dysfunction, elderly patients, urinary retention, benign prostatic hyperplasia, narrow-angle glaucoma, xerostomia, visual problems, constipation, history of bowel obstruction, MI, stroke, or dysrhythmia. Use caution in patients with depression, particularly if suicidal risk may be present. Safety and efficacy in pediatric patients <10 years of age have not been established.

Pregnancy risk C.

Drug Interactions

Cytochrome P450 Effect: Substrate of **CYP1A2, 2C19, 2D6**, 3A4; Inhibits **CYP2D6**

Decreased Effect: Clomipramine serum concentrations/effect may be decreased by carbamazepine, cholestyramine, colestipol, phenobarbital, and rifampin. Clomipramine inhibits the antihypertensive response to bethanidine, clonidine, debrisoquin, guanadrel, guanethidine, guanabenz, and guanfacine.

Increased Effect/Toxicity: Clomipramine increases the effects of amphetamines, anticholinergics, lithium, other CNS depressants (sedatives, hypnotics, ethanol), chlorpropamide, tolazamide, phenothiazines, and warfarin. When used with MAO inhibitors or other serotonergic drugs, serotonin syndrome may occur. Serotonin syndrome has also been reported with ritonavir (rare). Clomipramine serum concentrations/toxicity may be increased by SSRIs (to varying degrees), cimetidine, grapefruit juice, indinavir, methylphenidate, ritonavir, quinidine, diltiazem, phenothiazines, and verapamil. Pressor response to I.V. epinephrine, norepinephrine, and phenylephrine may be enhanced in patients receiving TCAs (**Note:** Effect is unlikely with epinephrine or levonordefrin dosages typically administered as infiltration in combination with local anesthetics). Combined use of beta-agonists or drugs which prolong QT_c (including quinidine, procainamide, disopyramide, cisapride, sparfloxacin, gatifloxacin, moxifloxacin) with TCAs may predispose patients to cardiac arrhythmias.

Nutritional/Ethanol Interactions

Ethanol: Avoid ethanol (may increase CNS depression).

Food: Serum concentrations/toxicity may be increased by grapefruit juice.

Herb/Nutraceutical: Avoid valerian, St John's wort, SAMe, kava kava.

Effects on Lab Values ↑ glucose

(Continued)

ClomiPRAMINE *(Continued)*

Adverse Reactions

>10%:

Central nervous system: Dizziness, drowsiness, headache, insomnia, nervousness
Endocrine & metabolic: Libido changes
Gastrointestinal: Xerostomia, constipation, increased appetite, nausea, weight gain, dyspepsia, anorexia, abdominal pain
Neuromuscular & skeletal: Fatigue, tremor, myoclonus
Miscellaneous: Increased diaphoresis

1% to 10%:

Cardiovascular: Hypotension, palpitations, tachycardia
Central nervous system: Confusion, hypertonia, sleep disorder, yawning, speech disorder, abnormal dreaming, paresthesia, memory impairment, anxiety, twitching, impaired coordination, agitation, migraine, depersonalization, emotional lability, flushing, fever
Dermatologic: Rash, pruritus, dermatitis
Gastrointestinal: Diarrhea, vomiting
Genitourinary: Difficult urination
Ocular: Blurred vision, eye pain

<1% (Limited to important or life-threatening): Alopecia, galactorrhea, hyperacusis, marrow depression, photosensitivity, reflux, seizures, SIADH

Overdosage/Toxicology Symptoms of overdose include agitation, confusion, hallucinations, urinary retention, hypothermia, hypotension, tachycardia, ventricular tachycardia, seizures, and coma. Following initiation of essential overdose management, toxic symptoms should be treated.

Pharmacodynamics/Kinetics

Absorption: Rapid

Half-Life Elimination: 20-30 hours

Metabolism: Hepatic to desmethylclomipramine (active); extensive first-pass effect

Formulations Capsule, as hydrochloride: 25 mg, 50 mg, 75 mg

Dosing

Adults & Elderly: Treatment of OCD: Oral: Initial: 25 mg/day and gradually increase, as tolerated, to 100 mg/day the first 2 weeks, may then be increased to a total of 250 mg/day maximum

Pediatrics: Treatment of OCD: Oral: Children >10 years: Initial: 25 mg/day and gradually increase, as tolerated, to a maximum of 3 mg/kg/day or 200 mg/day, whichever is smaller. **Note:** The safety and efficacy of clomipramine in pediatric patients <10 years of age have not been established and, therefore, dosing recommendations cannot be made.

Monitoring Laboratory Tests Monitor EKG/cardiac status in older adults and patients with cardiac disease

Monitoring and Teaching Issues

Physical Assessment: Assess other medications patient may be taking for effectiveness and interactions (see Drug Interactions). See Contraindications and Warnings/Precautions for use cautions. Monitor therapeutic response, and adverse reactions at beginning of therapy and periodically with long-term use (see Adverse Reactions and Overdose/Toxicology). Taper dosage slowly when discontinuing. Assess knowledge/teach patient appropriate use, interventions to reduce side effects, and adverse symptoms to report (see Patient Education). **Pregnancy risk factor C** - benefits of use should outweigh possible risks. Breast-feeding is contraindicated.

Patient Education: Take multiple dose medication with meals to reduce side effects. Take single daily dose at bedtime to reduce daytime sedation. The effect of this drug may take several weeks to appear. Do not use alcohol, caffeine, and other prescriptive or OTC medications without consulting prescriber. May cause dizziness, drowsiness, headache, or seizures (use caution when driving or engaging in tasks that require alertness until response to drug is known); dry mouth or unpleasant aftertaste (sucking lozenges and frequent mouth care may help); constipation (increased exercise, fluids, fruit, or fiber may help); or orthostatic hypotension (use caution when rising from lying or sitting to standing position or when climbing stairs). Report unresolved constipation or GI upset, unusual muscle weakness, palpitations, or persistent CNS disturbances (hallucinations, delirium, insomnia, or impaired gait). **Pregnancy/breast-feeding precautions:** Inform prescriber if you are or intend to become pregnant. Do not breast-feed.

Geriatric Considerations: Not approved as an antidepressant, clomipramine's anticholinergic and hypotensive effects limit its use versus other preferred antidepressants. Elderly patients were found to have higher dose-normalized plasma concentrations as a result of decreased demethylation (decreased 50%) and hydroxylation (25%).

Breast-feeding Issues: Generally, it is not recommended to breast-feed if taking antidepressants because of the long half-life, active metabolites, and the potential for side effects in the infant.

Pregnancy Issues: There are no adequate studies in pregnant women. Withdrawal symptoms (including dizziness, nausea, vomiting, headache, malaise, sleep disturbance, hyperthermia, and/or irritability) have been observed in neonates whose mothers took clomipramine up to delivery. Use in pregnancy only if the benefits to the mother outweigh the potential risks to the fetus.

Related Information

Antidepressant Agents *on page 1553*
Antidepressant Medication Guidelines *on page 1613*
FDA Name Differentiation Project: The Use of Tall-man Letters *on page 12*

Clomipramine Hydrochloride *see* ClomiPRAMINE *on page 313*

Clonazepam (kloe NA ze pam)

U.S. Brand Names Klonopin™

Restrictions C-IV

Generic Available Yes

Pharmacologic Category Benzodiazepine

Pregnancy Risk Factor D

Lactation Enters breast milk/not recommended

Use Alone or as an adjunct in the treatment of petit mal variant (Lennox-Gastaut), akinetic, and myoclonic seizures; petit mal (absence) seizures unresponsive to succimides; panic disorder with or without agoraphobia

Use - Unlabeled/Investigational Restless legs syndrome; neuralgia; multifocal tic disorder; parkinsonian dysarthria; bipolar disorder; adjunct therapy for schizophrenia

Mechanism of Action/Effect The exact mechanism is unknown, but believed to be related to its ability to enhance the activity of GABA; suppresses the spike-and-wave discharge in absence seizures by depressing nerve transmission in the motor cortex

Contraindications Hypersensitivity to clonazepam or any component of the formulation (cross-sensitivity with other benzodiazepines may exist); significant liver disease; narrow-angle glaucoma; pregnancy

Warnings/Precautions Use with caution in elderly or debilitated patients, patients with hepatic disease (including alcoholics), or renal impairment. Use with caution in patients with respiratory disease or impaired gag reflex or ability to protect the airway from secretions (salivation may be increased). Worsening of seizures may occur when added to patients with multiple seizure types. Concurrent use with valproic acid may result in absence status. Monitoring of CBC and liver function tests has been recommended during prolonged therapy.

Causes CNS depression (dose-related) resulting in sedation, dizziness, confusion, or ataxia which may impair physical and mental capabilities. Use with caution in patients receiving other CNS depressants or ethanol. Benzodiazepines have been associated with falls and traumatic injury and should be used with extreme caution in patients who are at risk of these events (especially the elderly).

Use caution in patients with depression, particularly if suicidal risk may be present. Use with caution in patients with a history of drug dependence. Benzodiazepines have been associated with dependence and acute withdrawal symptoms, including seizures, on discontinuation or reduction in dose.

Benzodiazepines have been associated with anterograde amnesia. Paradoxical reactions, including hyperactive or aggressive behavior, have been reported with benzodiazepines, particularly in adolescent/pediatric or psychiatric patients. Does not have analgesic, antidepressant, or antipsychotic properties.

Drug Interactions

Cytochrome P450 Effect: Substrate of **CYP3A4**

Decreased Effect: The combined use of clonazepam and valproic acid has been associated with absence seizures. Carbamazepine, rifampin, rifabutin may enhance the metabolism of clonazepam and decrease its therapeutic effect.

Increased Effect/Toxicity: Combined use of clonazepam and valproic acid has been associated with absence seizures. Clonazepam potentiates the CNS depressant effects of narcotic analgesics, barbiturates, phenothiazines, ethanol, antihistamines, MAO inhibitors, sedative-hypnotics, and cyclic antidepressants. Serum levels and/or toxicity of clonazepam may be increased by inhibitors of CYP3A4, including cimetidine, ciprofloxacin, clarithromycin, clozapine, delavirdine, diltiazem, disulfiram, digoxin, erythromycin, ethanol, fluconazole, fluoxetine, fluvoxamine, grapefruit juice, indinavir, isoniazid, itraconazole, ketoconazole, loxapine, metoprolol, metronidazole, miconazole, nefazodone, nevirapine, quinupristin/dalfopristin, omeprazole, phenytoin, rifabutin, rifampin, ritonavir, saquinavir, troleandomycin, verapamil, zafirlukast, and zileuton.

Nutritional/Ethanol Interactions

Ethanol: Avoid ethanol (may increase CNS depression).

Food: Clonazepam serum concentration is unlikely to be increased by grapefruit juice because of clonazepam's high oral bioavailability.

Herb/Nutraceutical: St John's wort may decrease clonazepam levels. Avoid valerian, St John's wort, kava kava, gotu kola (may increase CNS depression).

Adverse Reactions

>10%: Central nervous system: Drowsiness

1% to 10%:

- Central nervous system: Dizziness, abnormal coordination, ataxia, dysarthria, depression, memory disturbance, fatigue
- Dermatologic: Dermatitis, allergic reactions
- Endocrine & metabolic: Decreased libido
- Gastrointestinal: Anorexia, constipation, diarrhea, xerostomia
- Respiratory: Upper respiratory tract infection, sinusitis, rhinitis, coughing

<1% (Limited to important or life-threatening): Blood dyscrasias, menstrual irregularities

Overdosage/Toxicology May produce somnolence, confusion, ataxia, diminished reflexes, or coma. Treatment for benzodiazepine overdose is supportive. Flumazenil has been shown to selectively block the binding of benzodiazepines to CNS receptors, resulting in a reversal of benzodiazepine-induced CNS depression, but not respiratory depression.

Pharmacodynamics/Kinetics

Absorption: Well absorbed

Half-Life Elimination: Children: 22-33 hours; Adults: 19-50 hours

Time to Peak: Serum: 1-3 hours; Steady-state: 5-7 days

Metabolism: Extensively hepatic via glucuronide and sulfate conjugation

Onset: 20-60 minutes

Duration: Infants and young children: 6-8 hours; Adults: ≤12 hours

Formulations Tablet: 0.5 mg, 1 mg, 2 mg

Dosing

Adults: Seizure disorders: Oral:

Initial daily dose not to exceed 1.5 mg given in 3 divided doses; may increase by 0.5-1 mg every third day until seizures are controlled or adverse effects seen (maximum: 20 mg/day)

Usual maintenance dose: 0.05-0.2 mg/kg; do not exceed 20 mg/day

(Continued)

Clonazepam *(Continued)*

Elderly: Refer to adult dosing. Initiate with low doses and observe closely.

Pediatrics: Seizure disorders (see Use): Oral:

Children <10 years or 30 kg:

Initial daily dose: 0.01-0.03 mg/kg/day (maximum: 0.05 mg/kg/day) given in 2-3 divided doses; increase by no more than 0.5 mg every third day until seizures are controlled or adverse effects seen.

Usual maintenance dose: 0.1-0.2 mg/kg/day divided 3 times/day; not to exceed 0.2 mg/kg/day.

Children >10 years or 30 kg: Refer to adult dosing.

Renal Impairment: Hemodialysis: Supplemental dose is not necessary.

Monitoring Laboratory Tests Renal function

Monitoring and Teaching Issues

Physical Assessment: Assess effectiveness and interactions of other medications patient may be taking (see Contraindications, Warnings/Precautions, and Drug Interactions). Assess for history of addiction - long-term use can result in dependence, abuse, or tolerance; periodically evaluate need for continued use. For inpatients, observe safety/seizure precautions. Monitor therapeutic response, laboratory values, and adverse reactions (see Adverse Reactions) at beginning of therapy and periodically with long-term use. Taper dosage slowly when discontinuing. Assess knowledge/teach patient seizure precautions (if administered for seizures), appropriate use, interventions to reduce side effects, and adverse symptoms to report (see Patient Education). **Pregnancy risk factor D** - benefits of use should outweigh possible risks. Breast-feeding is not recommended.

Patient Education: Take exactly as directed; do not increase dose or frequency. Drug may cause physical and/or psychological dependence. While using this medication, do not use alcohol and other prescription or OTC medications (especially pain medications, sedatives, antihistamines, or hypnotics) without consulting prescriber. Maintain adequate hydration (2-3 L/day of fluids) unless advised by prescriber to restrict fluids. You may experience drowsiness, dizziness, or blurred vision (use caution when driving or engaging in tasks requiring alertness until response to drug is known); nausea, vomiting, loss of appetite, or dry mouth (small, frequent meals, frequent mouth care, chewing gum, or sucking lozenges may help); or constipation (increased exercise, fluids, fruit, or fiber may help). If medication is used to control seizures, wear identification that you are taking an antiepileptic medication. Report excessive drowsiness, dizziness, fatigue, or impaired coordination; CNS changes (confusion, depression, increased sedation, excitation, headache, agitation, insomnia, or nightmares) or changes in cognition; difficulty breathing or shortness of breath; changes in urinary pattern, changes in sexual activity; muscle cramping, weakness, tremors, or rigidity; ringing in ears or visual disturbances, excessive perspiration, or excessive GI symptoms (cramping, constipation, vomiting, anorexia); worsening of seizure activity, or loss of seizure control. **Pregnancy/breast-feeding precautions:** Inform prescriber if you are or intend to become pregnant. Breast-feeding is not recommended.

Geriatric Considerations: Hepatic clearance may be decreased allowing accumulation of active drug. Observe for signs of CNS and pulmonary toxicity.

Breast-feeding Issues: Clonazepam enters breast milk; clinical effects on the infant include CNS depression, respiratory depression reported (no recommendation from the AAP).

Pregnancy Issues: Two reports of cardiac defects; respiratory depression, lethargy, hypotonia may be observed in newborns exposed near time of delivery. Epilepsy itself, number of medications, genetic factors, or a combination of these probably influence the teratogenicity of anticonvulsant therapy. Benefit:risk ratio usually favors continued use during pregnancy.

Additional Information Ethosuximide or valproic acid may be preferred for treatment of absence (petit mal) seizures. Clonazepam-induced behavioral disturbances may be more frequent in mentally handicapped patients. Abrupt discontinuation after sustained use (generally >10 days) may cause withdrawal symptoms. Flumazenil, a competitive benzodiazepine antagonist at the CNS receptor site, reverses benzodiazepine-induced CNS depression.

Related Information

Anxiolytic/Hypnotic Use in Long-Term Care Facilities *on page 1608*
Benzodiazepines *on page 1560*

Clonidine (KLOE ni deen)

U.S. Brand Names Catapres®; Catapres-TTS®-1; Catapres-TTS®-2; Catapres-TTS®-3; Duraclon™

Synonyms Clonidine Hydrochloride

Generic Available Yes: Tablet

Pharmacologic Category Alpha$_2$-Adrenergic Agonist

Pregnancy Risk Factor C

Lactation Enters breast milk/not recommended

Use Management of mild to moderate hypertension; either used alone or in combination with other antihypertensives

Orphan drug: Duraclon™: For continuous epidural administration as adjunctive therapy with intraspinal opiates for treatment of cancer pain in patients tolerant to or unresponsive to intraspinal opiates

Use - Unlabeled/Investigational Heroin or nicotine withdrawal; severe pain; dysmenorrhea; vasomotor symptoms associated with menopause; ethanol dependence; prophylaxis of migraines; glaucoma; diabetes-associated diarrhea; impulse control disorder, attention-deficit/hyperactivity disorder (ADHD), clozapine-induced sialorrhea

Mechanism of Action/Effect Stimulates alpha$_2$-adrenoceptors in the brain stem, thus activating an inhibitory neuron, resulting in reduced sympathetic outflow from the CNS, producing a decrease in peripheral resistance, renal vascular resistance, heart rate, and blood pressure; epidural clonidine may produce pain relief at spinal presynaptic and postjunctional alpha$_2$-adrenoceptors by preventing pain signal transmission; pain relief occurs only for the body regions innervated by the spinal segments where analgesic concentrations of clonidine exist

Contraindications Hypersensitivity to clonidine hydrochloride or any component of the formulation

Warnings/Precautions Gradual withdrawal is needed (over 1 week for oral, 2-4 days with epidural) if drug needs to be stopped. Patients should be instructed about abrupt discontinuation (causes rapid increase in BP and symptoms of sympathetic overactivity). In patients on both a beta-blocker and clonidine where withdrawal of clonidine is necessary, withdraw the beta-blocker first and several days before clonidine. Then slowly decrease clonidine.

Use with caution in patients with severe coronary insufficiency; conduction disturbances; recent MI, CVA, or chronic renal insufficiency. Caution in sinus node dysfunction. Discontinue within 4 hours of surgery then restart as soon as possible after. Clonidine injection should be administered via a continuous epidural infusion device. Epidural clonidine is not recommended for perioperative, obstetrical, or postpartum pain. It is not recommended for use in patients with severe cardiovascular disease or hemodynamic instability. In all cases, the epidural may lead to cardiovascular instability (hypotension, bradycardia). May cause significant CNS depression and xerostomia. Caution in patients with pre-existing CNS disease or depression. Elderly may be at greater risk for CNS depressive effects, favoring other agents in this population.

Pregnancy risk C.

Drug Interactions

Decreased Effect: Tricyclic antidepressants (TCAs) antagonize the hypotensive effects of clonidine.

Increased Effect/Toxicity: Concurrent use with antipsychotics (especially low potency), narcotic analgesics, or nitroprusside may produce additive hypotensive effects. Clonidine may decrease the symptoms of hypoglycemia with oral hypoglycemic agents or insulin. Alcohol, barbiturates, and other CNS depressants may have additive CNS effects when combined with clonidine. Epidural clonidine may prolong the sensory and motor blockade of local anesthetics. Clonidine may increase cyclosporine (and perhaps tacrolimus) serum concentrations. Beta-blockers may potentiate bradycardia in patients receiving clonidine and may increase the rebound hypertension of withdrawal. Tricyclic antidepressants may also enhance the hypertensive response associated with abrupt clonidine withdrawal.

Nutritional/Ethanol Interactions

Ethanol: Avoid ethanol (may increase CNS depression).

Herb/Nutraceutical: Avoid dong quai if using for hypertension (has estrogenic activity). Avoid ephedra, yohimbe, ginseng (may worsen hypertension). Avoid valerian, St John's wort, kava kava, gotu kola (may increase CNS depression).

Effects on Lab Values ↑ sodium (S), transient serum glucose; ↓ catecholamines (U); positive Coombs'

Adverse Reactions Incidence of adverse events is not always reported.

>10%:

Central nervous system: Drowsiness (35% oral, 12% transdermal), dizziness (16% oral, 2% transdermal)

Dermatologic: Transient localized skin reactions characterized by pruritus, and erythema (15% to 50% transdermal)

Gastrointestinal: Dry mouth (40% oral, 25% transdermal)

1% to 10%:

Cardiovascular: Orthostatic hypotension (3% oral)

Central nervous system: Headache (1% oral, 5% transdermal), sedation (3% transdermal), fatigue (6% transdermal), lethargy (3% transdermal), insomnia (2% transdermal), nervousness (3% oral, 1% transdermal), mental depression (1% oral)

Dermatologic: Rash (1% oral), allergic contact sensitivity (5% transdermal), localized vesiculation (7%), hyperpigmentation (5% at application site), edema (3%), excoriation (3%), burning (3%), throbbing, blanching (1%), papules (1%), and generalized macular rash (1%) has occurred in patients receiving transdermal clonidine.

Endocrine & metabolic: Sodium and water retention, sexual dysfunction (3% oral, 2% transdermal), impotence (3% oral, 2% transdermal), weakness (10% transdermal)

Gastrointestinal: Nausea (5% oral, 1% transdermal), vomiting (5% oral), anorexia and malaise (1% oral), constipation (10% oral, 1% transdermal), dry throat (2% transdermal), taste disturbance (1% transdermal), weight gain (1% oral)

Genitourinary: Nocturia (1% oral)

Hepatic: Liver function test (mild abnormalities, 1% oral)

Miscellaneous: Withdrawal syndrome (1% oral)

<1% (Limited to important or life-threatening): Abdominal pain, agitation, alopecia, angioedema, AV block, behavioral changes, blurred vision, bradycardia, chest pain, CHF, contact dermatitis (transdermal), CVA, delirium, depression, dryness of the eyes, EKG abnormalities, gynecomastia, hallucinations, hepatitis, increased sensitivity to ethanol, localized hypo- or hyperpigmentation (transdermal), nightmares, orthostatic symptoms, pseudo-obstruction rash, Raynaud's phenomenon, syncope, tachycardia, thrombocytopenia, urinary retention, urticaria, vomiting, withdrawal syndrome

Overdosage/Toxicology Symptoms of overdose include bradycardia, CNS depression, hypothermia, diarrhea, respiratory depression, and apnea. Treatment is supportive and symptomatic. Naloxone may be utilized in treating CNS depression and/or apnea and should be given I.V., 0.4-2 mg, with repeated doses as needed up to a total of 10 mg, or as an infusion.

Pharmacodynamics/Kinetics

Bioavailability: 75% to 95%

Half-Life Elimination: Adults: Normal renal function: 6-20 hours; Renal impairment: 18-41 hours

Time to Peak: 2-4 hours

Metabolism: Extensively hepatic to inactive metabolites; undergoes enterohepatic recirculation

(Continued)

Clonidine *(Continued)*

Onset: Oral: 0.5-1 hour

Duration: 6-10 hours

Formulations

Injection, as hydrochloride [preservative free]: 100 mcg/mL (10 mL); 500 mcg/mL (10 mL)

Patch, transdermal, as hydrochloride [7-day duration]:

- Catapres-TTS®-1: 0.1 mg/day (4s)
- Catapres-TTS®-2: 0.2 mg/day (4s)
- Catapres-TTS®-3: 0.3 mg/day (4s)

Tablet, as hydrochloride: 0.1 mg, 0.2 mg, 0.3 mg

Dosing

Adults:

Acute hypertension (urgency): Oral: Initial 0.1-0.2 mg; may be followed by additional doses of 0.1 mg every hour, if necessary, to a maximum total dose of 0.6 mg

Hypertension:

Oral: Initial dose: 0.1 mg twice daily, usual maintenance dose: 0.2-1.2 mg/day in 2-4 divided doses; maximum recommended dose: 2.4 mg/day

Transdermal: Apply once every 7 days; for initial therapy start with 0.1 mg and increase by 0.1 mg at 1- to 2-week intervals; dosages >0.6 mg do not improve efficacy

Conversion from oral to transdermal:

Day 1: Place Catapres-TTS® 1; administer 100% of oral dose.

Day 2: Administer 50% of oral dose.

Day 3: Administer 25% of oral dose.

Day 4: Patch remains, no further oral supplement necessary.

Nicotine withdrawal symptoms: 0.1 mg twice daily to maximum of 0.4 mg/day for 3-4 weeks

Epidural infusion: Pain management: Starting dose: 30 mcg/hour; titrate as required for relief of pain or presence of side effects; minimal experience with doses >40 mcg/hour; should be considered an adjunct to intraspinal opiate therapy

Elderly: Oral: Initial: 0.1 mg once daily at bedtime, increase gradually as needed.

Pediatrics:

Hypertension: Oral: Initial: 5-10 mcg/kg/day in divided doses every 8-12 hours; increase gradually at 5- to 7-day intervals to 25 mcg/kg/day in divided doses every 6 hours; maximum: 0.9 mg/day.

Clonidine tolerance test (test of growth hormone release from pituitary): Oral: 0.15 mg/m^2 or 4 mcg/kg as single dose

ADHD (unlabeled use): Oral: Initial: 0.05 mg/day, increase every 3-7 days by 0.05 mg/day to 3-5 mcg/kg/day given in divided doses 3-4 times/day; maximum dose: 0.3-0.4 mg/day

Pain management: Epidural infusion: Reserved for patients with severe intractable pain, unresponsive to other analgesics or epidural or spinal opiates: Initial: 0.5 mcg/kg/hour; adjust with caution, based on clinical effect

Renal Impairment:

Cl_{cr} <10 mL/minute: Administer 50% to 75% of normal dose initially.

Not dialyzable (0% to 5%) via hemo- or peritoneal dialysis; supplemental dose is not necessary.

Administration

Oral: Do not discontinue clonidine abruptly. if needed, gradually reduce dose over 2-4 days to avoid rebound hypertension.

Topical: Transdermal patches should be applied weekly at bedtime to a clean, hairless area of the upper outer arm or chest. Rotate patch sites weekly. Redness under patch may be reduced if a topical corticosteroid spray is applied to the area before placement of the patch.

Monitoring Laboratory Tests Liver function tests

Monitoring and Teaching Issues

Physical Assessment: See Contraindications, Warnings/Precautions, and Dosing for use cautions (eg, pre-existing cardiovascular disease, hemodynamic instability, and CNS status). Assess potential for interactions with other prescriptions, OTC medications, or herbal products patient may be taking (see Drug Interactions). See Administration information. Assess results of laboratory tests (see above), therapeutic effectiveness (according to purpose for use), and adverse response (see Adverse Reactions and Overdose/Toxicology) regularly during therapy. When discontinuing, monitor blood pressure and taper dose slowly over 1 week or more. Teach patient appropriate use, possible side effects and interventions, and adverse symptoms to report (see Patient Education). **Pregnancy risk factor C** - benefits of use should outweigh possible risks. Breast-feeding is not recommended.

Patient Education: Inform prescriber of all prescriptions, OTC medications, or herbal products you are taking, and any allergies you have. Do not take anything new (especially cough or cold remedies and sleep or stay-awake medications that might affect blood pressure) during treatment unless approved by prescriber. Take as directed, at bedtime. If using patch, check daily for correct placement. Avoid alcohol. Do not skip doses or discontinue without consulting prescriber (this drug must be discontinued on specific schedule to prevent serious adverse effects). This medication may cause drowsiness, dizziness, or impaired judgment (use caution when driving or engaging in tasks that require alertness until response is known); decreased libido or sexual function (will resolve when drug is discontinued); postural hypotension (use caution when rising from sitting or lying position or when climbing stairs); constipation (increase roughage, bulk in diet); or dry mouth or nausea (frequent mouth care or sucking lozenges may help). Report difficulty, pain, or burning on urination; increased nervousness or depression; sudden weight gain (weigh yourself in the same clothes at the same time of day once a week); unusual or persistent swelling of ankles, feet, or extremities; wet cough or difficulty breathing; chest pain or palpitations; muscle weakness, fatigue, or pain; or other persistent side effects. **Pregnancy/breast-feeding precautions:** Inform prescriber if you are or intend to become pregnant. Breast-feeding is not recommended.

Dietary Issues: Hypertensive patients may need to decrease sodium and calories in diet.

Geriatric Considerations: Because of its potential CNS adverse effects, clonidine may not be considered a drug of choice in the elderly. If the decision is to use clonidine, adjust dose based on response and adverse reactions.

Breast-feeding Issues: Enters breast milk; AAP has NO RECOMMENDATION.

Additional Information Transdermal clonidine should only be used in patients unable to take oral medication. The transdermal product is much more expensive than oral clonidine and produces no better therapeutic effects.

Clonidine and Chlorthalidone (KLOE ni deen & klor THAL i done)

U.S. Brand Names Combipres®

Synonyms Chlorthalidone and Clonidine

Generic Available Yes

Pharmacologic Category Antihypertensive Agent Combination

Pregnancy Risk Factor C

Lactation

Clonidine: Enters breast milk/not recommended

Chlorthalidone: Enters breast milk/compatible

Use Management of mild to moderate hypertension

Formulations

Tablet:

0.1: Clonidine 0.1 mg and chlorthalidone 15 mg

0.2: Clonidine 0.2 mg and chlorthalidone 15 mg

0.3: Clonidine 0.3 mg and chlorthalidone 15 mg

Dosing

Adults: Hypertension: Oral: 1 tablet 1-2 times/day

Elderly: May benefit from lower initial dose; see individual agents.

Monitoring and Teaching Issues

Physical Assessment: See individual components listed in Related Information. **Pregnancy risk factor C** - benefits of use should outweigh possible risks. Breast-feeding is not recommended.

Patient Education: See individual components listed in Related Information. **Pregnancy/breast-feeding precautions:** Inform prescriber if you are or intend to become pregnant. Breast-feeding is not recommended.

Related Information

Chlorthalidone *on page 279*

Clonidine *on page 316*

Clonidine Hydrochloride *see* Clonidine *on page 316*

Clopidogrel (kloh PID oh grel)

U.S. Brand Names Plavix®

Synonyms Clopidogrel Bisulfate

Generic Available No

Pharmacologic Category Antiplatelet Agent

Pregnancy Risk Factor B

Lactation Excretion in breast milk unknown/not recommended

Use Reduce atherosclerotic events (myocardial infarction, stroke, vascular deaths) in patients with atherosclerosis documented by recent myocardial infarction (MI), recent stroke, or established peripheral arterial disease; prevention of thrombotic complications after coronary stenting; acute coronary syndrome (unstable angina or non-Q-wave MI)

Use - Unlabeled/Investigational In aspirin-allergic patients, prevention of coronary artery bypass graft closure (saphenous vein)

Mechanism of Action/Effect Blocks the ADP receptors, which prevent fibrinogen binding at that site and thereby reduce the possibility of platelet adhesion and aggregation.

Contraindications Hypersensitivity to clopidogrel or any component of the formulation; active pathological bleeding such as PUD or intracranial hemorrhage; coagulation disorders

Warnings/Precautions Use with caution in patients who may be at risk of increased bleeding, including patients with peptic ulcer disease, trauma, or surgery. Consider discontinuing 5 days before elective surgery. Use caution in mixing with other antiplatelet drugs. Use with caution in patients with severe liver disease (experience is limited). Cases of thrombotic thrombocytopenic purpura (usually occurring within the first 2 weeks of therapy) have been reported.

Drug Interactions

Cytochrome P450 Effect: Substrate of CYP1A2, 3A4; Inhibits CYP2C8/9

Increased Effect/Toxicity: At high concentrations, clopidogrel may interfere with the metabolism of amiodarone, cisapride, cyclosporine, diltiazem, fluvastatin, irbesartan, losartan, oral hypoglycemics, paclitaxel, phenytoin, quinidine, sildenafil, tamoxifen, torsemide, verapamil, and some NSAIDs which may result in toxicity. Clopidogrel and naproxen resulted in an increase of GI occult blood loss. Anticoagulants (warfarin, thrombolytics, drotrecogin alfa) or other antiplatelet agents may increase the risk of bleeding.

Nutritional/Ethanol Interactions Herb/Nutraceutical: Avoid cat's claw, dong quai, evening primrose, feverfew, garlic, ginger, ginkgo, red clover, horse chestnut, green tea, ginseng (all have additional antiplatelet activity).

Adverse Reactions As with all drugs which may affect hemostasis, bleeding is associated with clopidogrel. Hemorrhage may occur at virtually any site. Risk is dependent on multiple variables, including the concurrent use of multiple agents which alter hemostasis and patient susceptibility.

>10%: Gastrointestinal: The overall incidence of gastrointestinal events (including abdominal pain, vomiting, dyspepsia, gastritis and constipation) has been documented to be 27% compared to 30% in patients receiving aspirin.

(Continued)

Clopidogrel *(Continued)*

3% to 10%:

Cardiovascular: Chest pain (8%), edema (4%), hypertension (4%)

Central nervous system: Headache (3% to 8%), dizziness (2% to 6%), depression (4%), fatigue (3%), general pain (6%)

Dermatologic: Rash (4%), pruritus (3%)

Endocrine & metabolic: Hypercholesterolemia (4%)

Gastrointestinal: Abdominal pain (2% to 6%), dyspepsia (2% to 5%), diarrhea (2% to 5%), nausea (3%)

Genitourinary: Urinary tract infection (3%)

Hematologic: Purpura (5%), epistaxis (3%)

Hepatic: Liver function test abnormalities (<3%; discontinued in 0.11%)

Neuromuscular & skeletal: Arthralgia (6%), back pain (6%)

Respiratory: Dyspnea (5%), rhinitis (4%), bronchitis (4%), coughing (3%), upper respiratory infections (9%)

Miscellaneous: Flu-like syndrome (8%)

<1% (Limited to important or life-threatening): Agranulocytosis, allergic reaction, anaphylactoid reaction, angioedema, aplastic anemia, bilirubinemia, bronchospasm, bullous eruption, fatty liver, fever, granulocytopenia, hematuria, hemoptysis, hemothorax, hepatitis, hypochromic anemia, intracranial hemorrhage (0.4%), ischemic necrosis, leukopenia, maculopapular rash, menorrhagia, neutropenia (0.05%), ocular hemorrhage, pulmonary hemorrhage, purpura, retroperitoneal bleeding, thrombocytopenia, thrombotic thrombocytopenic purpura, urticaria

Overdosage/Toxicology

Symptoms of acute toxicity include vomiting, prostration, difficulty breathing, and gastrointestinal hemorrhage. Only one case of overdose with clopidogrel has been reported to date, no symptoms were reported with this case and no specific treatments were required.

Based on its pharmacology, platelet transfusions may be an appropriate treatment when attempting to reverse the effects of clopidogrel. After decontamination, treatment is symptomatic and supportive.

Pharmacodynamics/Kinetics

Absorption: Well absorbed

Half-Life Elimination: ~8 hours

Time to Peak: Serum: ~1 hour

Metabolism: Extensively hepatic via hydrolysis; biotransformation to carboxyl acid derivative (active metabolite that inhibits platelet aggregation)

Onset: Inhibition of platelet aggregation detected: 2 hours after 300 mg administered; after second day of treatment with 50-100 mg/day

Peak effect: 50-100 mg/day: Bleeding time: 5-6 days; Platelet function: 3-7 days

Formulations Tablet, as bisulfate: 75 mg

Dosing

Adults & Elderly:

Recent MI, recent stroke, or established arterial disease: Oral: 75 mg once daily

Acute coronary syndrome: Oral: Initial: 300 mg loading dose, followed by 75 mg once daily (in combination with aspirin 75-325 mg once daily)

Prevention of coronary artery bypass graft closure (saphenous vein): Aspirin-allergic patients (unlabeled use): Oral: Loading dose: 300 mg 6 hours following procedure; maintenance: 50-100 mg/day

Renal Impairment: No adjustment is necessary.

Hepatic Impairment: Dose adjustment may be necessary for patients with moderate to severe hepatic disease.

Stability

Storage: Store at 25°C (77°F); excursions permitted to 15°C to 3°C (59°F to 86°F).

Monitoring Laboratory Tests Hemoglobin and hematocrit periodically

Monitoring and Teaching Issues

Physical Assessment: Assess effectiveness or interactions of other medications patient may be taking. Clopidogrel is a P450 enzyme inhibitor (see Drug Interactions). Monitor therapeutic effectiveness and instruct patient what symptoms to report (see Patient Education). Breast-feeding is not recommended.

Patient Education: Take as directed. May cause headache or dizziness; use caution when driving or engaging in tasks that require alertness until response to drug is known. It may take longer than usual to stop bleeding. Small frequent meals, frequent mouth care, sucking lozenges, or chewing gum may reduce nausea or vomiting. Mild analgesics may reduce arthralgia or back pain. Inform physicians and dentists that you are taking this medication prior to scheduling any surgery or dental procedure. Report immediately unusual or acute chest pain or respiratory difficulties; skin rash; unresolved bleeding, diarrhea, or GI distress; nosebleed; or acute headache. **Breast-feeding precaution:** Breast-feeding is not recommended.

Dietary Issues: May be taken without regard to meals.

Geriatric Considerations: Plasma levels of the primary clopidogrel metabolite were significantly higher in the elderly (≥75 years). This was not associated with changes in bleeding time or platelet aggregation. No dosage adjustment is recommended.

Clopidogrel Bisulfate *see* Clopidogrel *on page 319*

Clorazepate (klor AZ e pate)

U.S. Brand Names Tranxene®

Synonyms Clorazepate Dipotassium

Restrictions C-IV

Generic Available Yes

Pharmacologic Category Benzodiazepine

Pregnancy Risk Factor D

Lactation Excretion in breast milk unknown/not recommended

Use Treatment of generalized anxiety disorder; management of ethanol withdrawal; adjunct anticonvulsant in management of partial seizures

Mechanism of Action/Effect Binds to stereospecific benzodiazepine receptors on the postsynaptic GABA neuron at several sites within the central nervous system, including the limbic system, reticular formation. Enhancement of the inhibitory effect of GABA on neuronal excitability results by increased neuronal membrane permeability to chloride ions. This shift in chloride ions results in hyperpolarization (a less excitable state) and stabilization.

Contraindications Hypersensitivity to clorazepate or any component of the formulation (cross-sensitivity with other benzodiazepines may exist); narrow-angle glaucoma; pregnancy

Warnings/Precautions

Causes CNS depression (dose-related) which may impair physical and mental capabilities. Use with caution in patients receiving other CNS depressants or psychoactive agents. Benzodiazepines have been associated with falls and traumatic injury and should be used with extreme caution in patients who are at risk of these events (especially the elderly). May cause physical or psychological dependence - use with caution in patients with a history of drug dependence.

Active metabolites with extended half-lives may lead to delayed accumulation and adverse effects. Use is not recommended in patients with depressive disorders or psychoses. Avoid use in patients with sleep apnea. Use with caution in patients receiving concurrent CYP3A4 inhibitors, particularly when these agents are added to therapy. Use with caution in elderly or debilitated patients, patients with hepatic disease (including alcoholics), renal impairment, respiratory disease, impaired gag reflex, or obese patients.

Benzodiazepines have been associated with anterograde amnesia. Paradoxical reactions, including hyperactive or aggressive behavior, have been reported with benzodiazepines, particularly in adolescent/pediatric or psychiatric patients. Does not have analgesic, antidepressant, or antipsychotic properties. Not recommended for use in patients <9 years of age.

Drug Interactions

Cytochrome P450 Effect: Substrate of **CYP3A4**

Decreased Effect: Carbamazepine, rifampin, rifabutin may enhance the metabolism of clorazepate and decrease its therapeutic effect.

Increased Effect/Toxicity: Clorazepate potentiates the CNS depressant effects of narcotic analgesics, barbiturates, phenothiazines, ethanol, antihistamines, MAO inhibitors, sedative-hypnotics, and cyclic antidepressants. Serum concentrations/toxicity of clorazepate may be increased by inhibitors of CYP3A4, including amprenavir, cimetidine, ciprofloxacin, clarithromycin, clozapine, diltiazem, disulfiram, digoxin, erythromycin, ethanol, fluconazole, fluoxetine, fluvoxamine, grapefruit juice, isoniazid, itraconazole, ketoconazole, labetalol, levodopa, loxapine, metoprolol, metronidazole, miconazole, nefazodone, nelfinavir, omeprazole, phenytoin, rifabutin, rifampin, ritonavir, troleandomycin, valproic acid, and verapamil.

Nutritional/Ethanol Interactions

Ethanol: Avoid ethanol (may increase CNS depression).

Food: Serum concentrations/toxicity may be increased by grapefruit juice.

Herb/Nutraceutical: Avoid valerian, St John's wort, kava kava, gotu kola (may increase CNS depression).

Effects on Lab Values ↓ hematocrit; abnormal liver and renal function tests

Adverse Reactions Frequency not defined.

Cardiovascular: Hypotension

Central nervous system: Drowsiness, fatigue, ataxia, lightheadedness, memory impairment, insomnia, anxiety, headache, depression, slurred speech, confusion, nervousness, dizziness, irritability

Dermatologic: Rash

Endocrine & metabolic: Decreased libido

Gastrointestinal: Xerostomia, constipation, diarrhea, decreased salivation, nausea, vomiting, increased or decreased appetite

Neuromuscular & skeletal: Dysarthria, tremor

Ocular: Blurred vision, diplopia

Overdosage/Toxicology May produce somnolence, confusion, ataxia, diminished reflexes, and coma. Treatment for benzodiazepine overdose is supportive. Rarely is mechanical ventilation required. Flumazenil has been shown to selectively block the binding of benzodiazepines to CNS receptors, resulting in a reversal of benzodiazepine-induced CNS depression, but not respiratory depression.

Pharmacodynamics/Kinetics

Half-Life Elimination: Adults: Desmethyldiazepam: 48-96 hours; Oxazepam: 6-8 hours

Time to Peak: Serum: ~1 hour

Metabolism: Rapidly decarboxylated to desmethyldiazepam (active) in acidic stomach prior to absorption; hepatically to oxazepam (active)

Onset: 1-2 hours

Duration: Variable, 8-24 hours

Formulations Tablet, as dipotassium:

Tranxene®-SD™: 22.5 mg [once daily]

Tranxene®-SD™ Half Strength: 11.25 mg [once daily]

Tranxene® T-Tab®: 3.75 mg, 7.5 mg, 15 mg

Dosing

Adults:

Anxiety:

Regular release tablets (Tranxene® T-Tab®): 7.5-15 mg 2-4 times/day

Sustained release (Tranxene®-SD): 11.25 or 22.5 mg once daily at bedtime

Anxiety: Oral: 7.5-15 mg 2-4 times/day, or given as single dose of 11.25 or 22.5 mg at bedtime

Ethanol withdrawal: Oral: Initial: 30 mg, then 15 mg 2-4 times/day on first day; maximum daily dose: 90 mg; gradually decrease dose over subsequent days.

Seizures (anticonvulsant): Oral: Initial: Up to 7.5 mg/dose 2-3 times/day; increase dose by 7.5 mg at weekly intervals; not to exceed 90 mg/day

(Continued)

Clorazepate *(Continued)*

Elderly: Oral: Anxiety: 7.5 mg 1-2 times/day; use is not recommended in the elderly.

Pediatrics:

Seizures (anticonvulsant): Oral:

Children 9-12 years: Initial: 3.75-7.5 mg/dose twice daily; increase dose by 3.75 mg at weekly intervals, not to exceed 60 mg/day in 2-3 divided doses.

Children >12 years: Refer to adult dosing.

Stability

Compatibility: Incompatible with water

Monitoring and Teaching Issues

Physical Assessment: Assess other medications patient may be taking for effectiveness and interactions (see Drug Interactions). See Contraindications and Warnings/Precautions for use cautions. Assess for history of addiction; long-term use can result in dependence, abuse, or tolerance; periodically evaluate need for continued use. Monitor therapeutic response (eg, mood, affect, anxiety level, sleep pattern) and adverse reactions at beginning of therapy and periodically with long-term use (see Adverse Reactions and Overdose/Toxicology). Taper dosage slowly when discontinuing. Assess knowledge/teach patient appropriate use, interventions to reduce side effects, and adverse symptoms to report (see Patient Education). **Pregnancy risk factor D** - determine that patient is not pregnant before beginning treatment. Instruct patients of childbearing age about appropriate barrier contraceptive measures. Breast-feeding is not recommended.

Patient Education: Take exactly as directed; do not increase dose or frequency. Drug may cause physical and/or psychological dependence. Do not use alcohol and other prescription or OTC medications (especially pain medications, sedatives, antihistamines, or hypnotics) without consulting prescriber. Maintain adequate hydration (2-3 L/day of fluids) unless advised by prescriber to restrict fluids. You may experience drowsiness, lightheadedness, impaired coordination, dizziness, or blurred vision (use caution when driving or engaging in tasks requiring alertness until response to drug is known); nausea, vomiting, or dry mouth (small, frequent meals, frequent mouth care, chewing gum, or sucking lozenges may help); constipation (increased exercise, fluids, fruit, or fiber may help); altered sexual drive or ability (reversible); or photosensitivity (use sunscreen, wear protective clothing and eyewear, and avoid direct sunlight). Report persistent CNS effects (eg, confusion, depression, increased sedation, excitation, headache, agitation, insomnia or nightmares, dizziness, fatigue, impaired coordination, changes in personality, or changes in cognition); changes in urinary pattern; muscle cramping, weakness, tremors, or rigidity; ringing in ears or visual disturbances; chest pain, palpitations, or rapid heartbeat; excessive perspiration; excessive GI symptoms (cramping, constipation, vomiting, anorexia); or worsening of condition. **Pregnancy/breast-feeding precautions:** Do not get pregnant while using this medication; use appropriate contraceptive measures. Breast-feeding is not recommended.

Geriatric Considerations: Clorazepate is not considered a drug of choice in the elderly. Long-acting benzodiazepines have been associated with falls in the elderly.

Breast-feeding Issues: No specific data for clorazepate; however, other benzodiazepines have been shown to be excreted in breast milk. Therefore, it is recommended not to nurse while taking clorazepate.

Additional Information Abrupt discontinuation after sustained use (generally >10 days) may cause withdrawal symptoms.

Related Information

Anxiolytic/Hypnotic Use in Long-Term Care Facilities *on page 1608*
Benzodiazepines *on page 1560*

Clorazepate Dipotassium *see* Clorazepate *on page 320*

Clotrimazole (kloe TRIM a zole)

U.S. Brand Names Cruex® [OTC]; Gyne-Lotrimin® [OTC]; Gyne-Lotrimin® 3 [OTC]; Gynix® [OTC]; Lotrimin®; Lotrimin® AF [OTC]; Mycelex®; Mycelex®-3; Mycelex®-7 [OTC]; Mycelex® Twin Pack [OTC]; Trivagizole 3™

Generic Available Yes

Pharmacologic Category Antifungal Agent, Oral Nonabsorbed; Antifungal Agent, Topical; Antifungal Agent, Vaginal

Pregnancy Risk Factor B (topical); C (troches)

Lactation Excretion in breast milk unknown

Use Treatment of susceptible fungal infections, including oropharyngeal candidiasis, dermatophytoses, superficial mycoses, and cutaneous candidiasis, as well as vulvovaginal candidiasis; limited data suggest that clotrimazole troches may be effective for prophylaxis against oropharyngeal candidiasis in neutropenic patients

Mechanism of Action/Effect Binds to phospholipids in the fungal cell membrane altering cell wall permeability resulting in loss of essential intracellular elements

Contraindications Hypersensitivity to clotrimazole or any component of the formulation

Warnings/Precautions Clotrimazole should not be used for treatment of ocular or systemic fungal infection. Use with caution with hepatic impairment. Safety and effectiveness of clotrimazole lozenges (troches) in children <3 years of age have not been established. When using topical formulation, avoid contact with eyes. Pregnancy risk C (troches).

Drug Interactions

Cytochrome P450 Effect: Inhibits CYP2A6, 2C8/9, 2E1, 3A4

Adverse Reactions

Oral:

>10%: Hepatic: Abnormal liver function tests

1% to 10%:

Gastrointestinal: Nausea and vomiting may occur in patients on clotrimazole troches

Local: Mild burning, irritation, stinging to skin or vaginal area

Vaginal:

1% to 10%: Genitourinary: Vulvar/vaginal burning

<1% (Limited to important or life-threatening): Burning or itching of penis of sexual partner; polyuria; vulvar itching, soreness, edema, or discharge

Pharmacodynamics/Kinetics

Absorption: Topical: Negligible through intact skin

Time to Peak: Serum:

Oral topical: Salivary levels occur within 3 hours following 30 minutes of dissolution time

Vaginal cream: High vaginal levels: 8-24 hours

Vaginal tablet: High vaginal levels: 1-2 days

Formulations

Combination pack:

Gyne-Lotrimin®, Mycelex®-7: Vaginal tablet 100 mg (7s) and vaginal cream 1% (7 g)

Gyne-Lotrimin® 3: Vaginal tablet 200 mg (3s) and vaginal cream 1%

Mycelex® Twin Pack: Vaginal tablet 500 mg (1s) and vaginal cream 1% (7 g)

Cream, topical (Lotrimin®, Lotrimin® AF, Mycelex®, Mycelex® OTC): 1% (15 g, 30 g, 45 g, 90 g)

Cream, vaginal:

Gyne-Lotrimin®, Mycelex®-7: 1% (45 g, 90 g)

Gyne-Lotrimin® 3, Mycelex®-3, Trivagizole 3™: 2% (25 g)

Lotion (Lotrimin®): 1% (30 mL)

Solution, topical (Lotrimin®, Lotrimin® AF, Mycelex®, Mycelex® OTC): 1% (10 mL, 30 mL)

Tablet, vaginal:

Gyne-Lotrimin®, Mycelex®-7: 100 mg (7s)

Troche (Mycelex®): 10 mg

Dosing

Adults & Elderly:

Oropharyngeal candidiasis: Oral:

Prophylaxis: 10 mg troche dissolved 3 times/day for the duration of chemotherapy or until steroids are reduced to maintenance levels

Treatment: 10 mg troche dissolved slowly 5 times/day for 14 consecutive days

Dermatophytosis, cutaneous candidiasis: Topical (cream, lotion, solution): Apply twice daily; if no improvement occurs after 4 weeks of therapy, re-evaluate diagnosis.

Vulvovaginal candidiasis:

Intravaginal:

Cream (1%): Insert 1 applicatorful of 1% vaginal cream daily (preferably at bedtime) for 7 consecutive days.

Cream (2%): Insert 1 applicatorful of 2% vaginal cream daily (preferably at bedtime) for 3 consecutive days.

Tablet: Insert 100 mg/day for 7 days or 500 mg single dose.

Dermatologic infection (superficial): Topical (cream, lotion, solution): Apply to affected area twice daily (morning and evening) for 7 consecutive days.

Pediatrics:

Oropharyngeal candidiasis: Children >3 years: Refer to adult dosing.

Vaginal, Topical infections: Children >12 years: Refer to adult dosing.

Administration

Oral: Allow to dissolve slowly over 15-30 minutes.

Topical: For external use only. Apply sparingly. Protect hands with latex gloves. Do not use occlusive dressings.

Other: Avoid contact with eyes.

Monitoring Laboratory Tests Periodic liver function during oral therapy with clotrimazole lozenges

Monitoring and Teaching Issues

Physical Assessment: See Contraindications and Warnings/Precautions for use cautions. Monitor laboratory values (see above), effectiveness of treatment, and adverse reactions (See Adverse Reactions). Assess knowledge/teach patient appropriate use, interventions to reduce side effects, and adverse symptoms to report (see Patient Education). **Pregnancy risk factor B/C** - see Pregnancy Risk Factor for use cautions. Assess for opportunistic infection. Note breast-feeding caution.

Patient Education: Oral: Do not swallow oral medication whole; allow to dissolve slowly in mouth. You may experience nausea or vomiting (small, frequent meals, frequent mouth care, chewing gum, or sucking lozenges may help). Report signs of opportunistic infection (eg, white plaques in mouth, fever, chills, perianal itching, vaginal itching or discharge, fatigue, unhealed wounds or sores).

Topical: Avoid contact with eyes. Wash hands before applying or wear gloves. Apply thin film of gel, lotion, or solution to affected area. May apply porous dressing. Report persistent burning, swelling, itching, worsening of condition, or lack of response to therapy.

Vaginal: Wash hands before using. Insert full applicator into vagina gently and expel cream, or insert tablet into vagina, at bedtime. Wash applicator with soap and water following use. Remain lying down for 30 minutes following administration. Avoid intercourse during therapy (sexual partner may experience penile burning or itching). Report adverse reactions (eg, vulvar itching, frequent urination), worsening of condition, or lack of response to therapy. Contact prescriber if symptoms do not improve within 3 days or you do not feel well within 7 days. Do not use tampons until therapy is complete. Contact prescriber immediately if you experience abdominal pain, fever, or foul-smelling discharge.

Pregnancy/breast-feeding precautions: Inform prescriber if you are pregnant. Consult prescriber if breast-feeding.

Geriatric Considerations: Localized fungal infections frequently follow broad spectrum antimicrobial therapy. Specifically, oral and vaginal infections due to *Candida*.

Clotrimazole and Betamethasone *see* Betamethasone and Clotrimazole *on page 162*

Clozapine (KLOE za peen)

U.S. Brand Names Clozaril®

Generic Available Yes

(Continued)

Clozapine *(Continued)*

Pharmacologic Category Antipsychotic Agent, Dibenzodiazepine

Pregnancy Risk Factor B

Lactation Enters breast milk/contraindicated (AAP rates "of concern")

Use Treatment of refractory schizophrenia

Use - Unlabeled/Investigational Schizoaffective disorder, bipolar disorder, childhood psychosis

Mechanism of Action/Effect Clozapine is a weak dopamine$_1$ and dopamine$_2$ receptor blocker, but blocks D_1-D_5 receptors; in addition, it blocks the serotonin$_2$, alpha-adrenergic, histamine H_1, and cholinergic receptors

Contraindications Hypersensitivity to clozapine or any component of the formulation; history of agranulocytosis or granulocytopenia with clozapine; uncontrolled epilepsy; severe central nervous system depression or comatose state; myeloproliferative disorders or use with other agents which have a well-known risk of agranulocytosis or bone marrow suppression

In patients with WBC $\leq$3500 cells/mm^3 before therapy; if WBC falls to <3000 cells/mm^3 during therapy the drug should be withheld until signs and symptoms of infection disappear and WBC rises to >3000 cells/mm^3

Warnings/Precautions Medication should not be stopped abruptly; taper off over 1-2 weeks. If conditions warrant abrupt discontinuation (leukopenia, myocarditis, cardiomyopathy), monitor patient for psychosis and cholinergic rebound (headache, nausea, vomiting, diarrhea). Elderly patients are more susceptible to adverse effects (including cardiovascular, anticholinergic, and tardive dyskinesia).

Significant risk of agranulocytosis, potentially life-threatening. WBC testing should occur weekly for the first 6 months of therapy; thereafter, if acceptable WBC counts are maintained (WBC $\geq$3000/mm^3, ANC $\geq$1500/mm^3) then WBC counts can be monitored every other week. WBCs must be monitored weekly for the first 4 weeks after therapy discontinuation. Use with caution in patients receiving other marrow suppressive agents. Eosinophilia has been reported to occur with clozapine and may require temporary or permanent interruption of therapy.

Cognitive and/or motor impairment (sedation) is common with clozapine, resulting in impaired performance of tasks requiring alertness (ie, operating machinery or driving). Use with caution in patients at risk of seizures, including those with a history of seizures, head trauma, brain damage, alcoholism, or concurrent therapy with medications which may lower seizure threshold. Has been associated with benign, self-limiting fever (<100.4°F, usually within first 3 weeks). However, clozapine may also be associated with severe febrile reactions, including neuroleptic malignant syndrome (NMS). Clozapine's potential for extrapyramidal symptoms appears to be extremely low.

May cause anticholinergic effects; use with caution in patients with urinary retention, benign prostatic hyperplasia, narrow-angle glaucoma, xerostomia, visual problems, constipation, or history of bowel obstruction. May cause hyperglycemia; use with caution in patients with diabetes or other disorders of glucose regulation. Use with caution in patients with hepatic disease or impairment; hepatitis has been reported as a consequence of therapy.

May cause orthostatic hypotension and tachycardia; use with caution in patients at risk of hypotension or in patients where transient hypotensive episodes would be poorly tolerated (cardiovascular disease or cerebrovascular disease). Concurrent use of psychotropics and benzodiazepines may increase the risk of severe cardiopulmonary reactions.

Myocarditis, pericarditis, pericardial effusion, cardiomyopathy, and CHF have also been associated with clozapine. Fatalities due to myocarditis have been reported; highest risk in the first month of therapy, however, later cases also reported. Myocarditis or cardiomyopathy should be considered in patients who present with signs/symptoms of heart failure (dyspnea, fatigue, orthopnea, paroxysmal nocturnal dyspnea, peripheral edema), chest pain, palpitations, new electrocardiographic abnormalities (arrhythmias, ST-T wave abnormalities), or unexplained fever. Patients with tachycardia during the first month of therapy should be closely monitored for other signs of myocarditis. Discontinue clozapine if myocarditis is suspected; do not rechallenge in patients with clozapine-related myocarditis. The reported rate of cardiomyopathy in clozapine-treated patients is similar to that in the general population. The majority of patients were over 50 years of age and were taking clozapine for >6 months. Clozapine should be discontinued in patients with confirmed cardiomyopathy unless benefit clearly outweighs risk. Rare cases of thromboembolism, including pulmonary embolism and stroke resulting in fatalities, have been associated with clozapine.

Drug Interactions

Cytochrome P450 Effect: Substrate of **CYP1A2**, 2A6, 2C8/9, 2C19, 2D6, 3A4; Inhibits CYP2C8/9, 2D6, 3A4

Decreased Effect: Carbamazepine, phenytoin, primidone, and valproic acid may increase the hepatic metabolism (decrease serum levels) of clozapine. Cigarette smoking (nicotine) may enhance the metabolism of clozapine. Clozapine may reverse the pressor effect of epinephrine (avoid in treatment of drug-induced hypotension).

Increased Effect/Toxicity: May potentiate anticholinergic and hypotensive effects of other drugs. Benzodiazepines in combination with clozapine may produce respiratory depression and hypotension, especially during the first few weeks of therapy. May potentiate effect/toxicity of risperidone. Clozapine serum concentrations may be increased by inhibitors of CYP1A2, CYP2D6, and CYP3A4. The list of inhibitors is extensive, but includes amiodarone, cimetidine, ciprofloxacin, clarithromycin, delavirdine, diltiazem, erythromycin, fluoxetine, fluvoxamine, indinavir, isoniazid, itraconazole, ketoconazole, nefazodone, paroxetine, quinidine, ritonavir, saquinavir, sertraline, verapamil, zafirlukast, and zileuton. Metoclopramide may increase risk of extrapyramidal symptoms (EPS).

Nutritional/Ethanol Interactions

Ethanol: Avoid ethanol (may increase CNS depression).

Herb/Nutraceutical: St John's wort may decrease clozapine levels. Avoid kava kava, gotu kola, valerian, St John's wort (may increase CNS depression).

Adverse Reactions

>10%:

Cardiovascular: Tachycardia, orthostasis (up to 25%)
Central nervous system: Drowsiness, dizziness
Gastrointestinal: Constipation, weight gain, diarrhea, sialorrhea
Genitourinary: Urinary incontinence

1% to 10%:

Cardiovascular: EKG changes, hypertension, hypotension, syncope
Central nervous system: Akathisia, seizures, headache, nightmares, akinesia, confusion, insomnia, fatigue, myoclonic jerks
Dermatologic: Rash
Gastrointestinal: Abdominal discomfort, heartburn, xerostomia, nausea, vomiting
Hematologic: Eosinophilia, leukopenia
Neuromuscular & skeletal: Tremor
Miscellaneous: Diaphoresis (increased), fever

<1% (Limited to important or life-threatening): Agranulocytosis, arrhythmias, cardiomyopathy (usually dilated), CHF, diabetes mellitus, granulocytopenia, hyperglycemia, impotence, myocardial infarction, myocarditis, narrow-angle glaucoma, neuroleptic malignant syndrome, pericardial effusion, pericarditis, pulmonary embolism, rigidity, stroke, tardive dyskinesia, thrombocytopenia, thromboembolism

Overdosage/Toxicology Symptoms of overdose include altered states of consciousness, tachycardia, hypotension, hypersalivation, and respiratory depression. Following initiation of essential overdose management, toxic symptom treatment and supportive treatment should be initiated.

Pharmacodynamics/Kinetics

Half-Life Elimination: 12 hours (range: 4-66 hours)

Time to Peak: 2.5 hours

Metabolism: Extensively hepatic

Formulations Tablet: 25 mg, 100 mg

Dosing

Adults: Schizophrenia (refractory): Oral: 25 mg once or twice daily initially, and increased as tolerated to a target dose of 300-450 mg/day after 2 weeks, but may require doses as high as 600-900 mg/day

Note: In the event of planned termination of clozapine, gradual reduction in dose over a 1- to 2-week period is recommended. If conditions warrant abrupt discontinuation (leukopenia), monitor patient for psychosis and cholinergic rebound (headache, nausea, vomiting, diarrhea).

Elderly: Oral: Experience in the elderly is limited; initial dose should be 25 mg/day; increase as tolerated by 25 mg/day to desired response. Maximum daily dose in the elderly should probably be 450 mg. Dose titration to 300-450 mg/day may be attained in 2 weeks if tolerated; however, elderly may require slower titration and daily increases may not be tolerated.

Pediatrics: Children and Adolescents: Childhood psychosis (unlabeled use): Oral: Initial: 25 mg/day; increase to a target dose of 25-400 mg/day

Stability

Storage: Dispensed in "clozapine patient system" packaging.

Monitoring Laboratory Tests Complete blood count weekly for 6 months then every other week thereafter, if clozapine is discontinued, continue monitoring for 1 month. WBC testing should occur weekly for the first 6 months of therapy; thereafter, if acceptable WBC counts are maintained (WBC ≥3000/mm^3, ANC ≥1500/mm^3), then WBC counts can be monitored every other week. WBCs must be monitored weekly for the first 4 weeks after therapy discontinuation. EKG, liver function tests should also be monitored.

Monitoring and Teaching Issues

Physical Assessment: Assess other medications patient is taking for effectiveness and interactions (see Drug Interactions). See Contraindications and Warnings/Precautions for use cautions. Initiate at lower doses and taper dosage slowly when discontinuing. Instruct diabetics to monitor blood glucose levels frequently; can cause hyperglycemia. Review ophthalmic exam and monitor laboratory results weekly (see Dosing and Monitoring Laboratory Tests), therapeutic response, and adverse reactions at beginning of therapy and periodically with long-term use (see Adverse Reactions and Overdose/Toxicology). Assess knowledge/teach patient appropriate use, interventions to reduce side effects, and adverse symptoms to report (see Patient Education). Breast-feeding is contraindicated.

Patient Education: Use exactly as directed; do not increase dose or frequency. Do not discontinue without consulting prescriber. Avoid alcohol or caffeine and other prescription or OTC medications not approved by prescriber. Maintain adequate hydration (2-3 L/day of fluids) unless advised by prescriber to restrict fluids. If you are diabetic, monitor blood glucose levels frequently. You may experience headache, excess drowsiness, dizziness, or blurred vision (use caution driving or when engaging in tasks requiring alertness until response to drug is known); dry mouth, constipation, diarrhea; nausea, vomiting (small, frequent meals, frequent mouth care, sucking lozenges, or chewing gum may help); or postural hypotension (use caution climbing stairs or when changing position from lying or sitting to standing). Report persistent CNS effects (insomnia, depression, altered consciousness); palpitations, rapid heartbeat, severe dizziness; vision changes; hypersalivation, tearing, sweating; difficulty breathing; or worsening of condition. Report flu-like symptoms, chest pain, shortness of breath, or excessive fatigue. **Breast-feeding precaution:** Do not breast-feed.

Dietary Issues: May be taken without regard to food.

Geriatric Considerations: Not recommended for use in nonpsychotic patients.

Related Information

Antipsychotic Agents *on page 1558*
Antipsychotic Medication Guidelines *on page 1614*

Clozaril® *see* Clozapine *on page 323*

CMV-IGIV *see* Cytomegalovirus Immune Globulin (Intravenous/Human) *on page 352*

Coagulant Complex Inhibitor *see* Anti-inhibitor Coagulant Complex *on page 113*
Coagulation Factor VIIa *see* Factor VIIa (Recombinant) *on page 541*

Cocaine (koe KANE)

Synonyms Cocaine Hydrochloride

Restrictions C-II

Generic Available Yes

Pharmacologic Category Local Anesthetic

Pregnancy Risk Factor C/X (nonmedicinal use)

Lactation Enters breast milk/contraindicated

Use Topical anesthesia for mucous membranes

Mechanism of Action/Effect Blocks both the initiation and conduction of nerve impulses

Contraindications Hypersensitivity to cocaine or any component of the topical solution; ophthalmologic anesthesia (causing sloughing of the corneal epithelium); pregnancy (nonmedicinal use)

Warnings/Precautions For topical use only. Limit to office and surgical procedures only. Resuscitative equipment and drugs should be immediately available when any local anesthetic is used. Debilitated, elderly patients, acutely ill patients, and children should be given reduced doses consistent with their age and physical status. Use caution in patients with severely traumatized mucosa and sepsis in the region of the proposed application. Use with caution in patients with cardiovascular disease or a history of cocaine abuse. In patients being treated for cardiovascular complication of cocaine abuse, avoid beta-blockers for treatment. Pregnancy risk C/X (nonmedicinal use).

Drug Interactions

Cytochrome P450 Effect: Substrate of **CYP3A4**; Inhibits **CYP2D6**, 3A4

Increased Effect/Toxicity: Increased toxicity with MAO inhibitors. Use with epinephrine may cause extreme hypertension and/or cardiac arrhythmias.

Adverse Reactions

>10%:

- Central nervous system: CNS stimulation
- Gastrointestinal: Loss of taste perception
- Respiratory: Rhinitis, nasal congestion
- Miscellaneous: Loss of smell

1% to 10%:

- Cardiovascular: Heart rate (decreased) with low doses, tachycardia with moderate doses, hypertension, cardiomyopathy, cardiac arrhythmias, myocarditis, QRS prolongation, Raynaud's phenomenon, cerebral vasculitis, thrombosis, fibrillation (atrial), flutter (atrial), sinus bradycardia, CHF, pulmonary hypertension, sinus tachycardia, tachycardia (supraventricular), arrhythmias (ventricular), vasoconstriction
- Central nervous system: Fever, nervousness, restlessness, euphoria, excitation, headache, psychosis, hallucinations, agitation, seizures, slurred speech, hyperthermia, dystonic reactions, cerebral vascular accident, vasculitis, clonic-tonic reactions, paranoia, sympathetic storm
- Dermatologic: Skin infarction, pruritus, madarosis
- Gastrointestinal: Nausea, anorexia, colonic ischemia, spontaneous bowel perforation
- Genitourinary: Priapism, uterine rupture
- Hematologic: Thrombocytopenia
- Neuromuscular & skeletal: Chorea (extrapyramidal), paresthesia, tremors, fasciculations
- Ocular: Mydriasis (peak effect at 45 minutes; may last up to 12 hours), sloughing of the corneal epithelium, ulceration of the cornea, iritis, mydriasis, chemosis
- Renal: Myoglobinuria, necrotizing vasculitis
- Respiratory: Tachypnea, nasal mucosa damage (when snorting), hyposmia, bronchiolitis obliterans organizing pneumonia
- Miscellaneous: "Washed-out" syndrome

Overdosage/Toxicology Symptoms of overdose include anxiety, excitement, confusion, nausea, vomiting, headache, rapid pulse, irregular respiration, delirium, fever, seizures, respiratory arrest, hallucinations, dilated pupils, muscle spasms, sensory aberrations, and cardiac arrhythmias.

Fatal dose: Oral: 500 mg to 1.2 g; severe toxic effects have occurred with doses as low as 20 mg.

Since no specific antidote for cocaine exists, serious toxic effects are treated symptomatically.

Pharmacokinetic Note Data is based on topical administration to mucosa.

Pharmacodynamics/Kinetics

Absorption: Well absorbed through mucous membranes; limited by drug-induced vasoconstriction; enhanced by inflammation

Half-Life Elimination: 75 minutes

Metabolism: Hepatic; major metabolites are ecgonine methyl ester and benzoyl ecgonine

Onset: ~1 minute; Peak effect: ~5 minutes

Duration: Dose dependent: ≥30 minutes; cocaine metabolites may appear in urine of neonates up to 5 days after birth due to maternal cocaine use shortly before birth

Formulations

Powder, as hydrochloride: 5 g, 25 g

Solution, topical, as hydrochloride: 4% [40 mg/mL] (4 mL, 10 mL); 10% [100 mg/mL] (4 mL, 10 mL)

Solution, viscous, topical, as hydrochloride: 4% [40 mg/mL] (4 mL, 10 mL); 10% [100 mg/mL] (4 mL, 10 mL)

Dosing

Adults: Dosage depends on the area to be anesthetized, tissue vascularity, technique of anesthesia, and individual patient tolerance. The lowest dose necessary to produce adequate anesthesia should be used, not to exceed 1 mg/kg.

Local anesthetic: Topical application (ear, nose, throat, bronchoscopy): Concentrations of 1% to 4% are used. Concentrations >4% are not recommended because of potential for increased incidence and severity of systemic toxic reactions.

Elderly: Refer to adult dosing; use with caution.

Administration

Topical: Use only on mucous membranes of the oral, laryngeal, and nasal cavities. Do not use on extensive areas of broken skin.

Stability

Storage: Store in well-closed, light-resistant containers.

Monitoring and Teaching Issues

Physical Assessment: Assess other medications patient may be taking for interactions (see Drug Interactions). See Contraindications and Warnings/Precautions for use cautions. Monitor adverse effects and teach patient adverse symptoms to report (see Adverse Reactions, Overdose/Toxicology, and Patient Education). **Pregnancy risk factor C/X (if nonmedicinal use).** Breast-feeding is contraindicated.

Patient Education: When used orally, do not take anything by mouth until full sensation returns. **Ocular:** Use caution when driving or engaging in tasks that require alert vision (mydriasis may last for several hours). At time of use or immediately thereafter, report any unusual cardiovascular, CNS, or respiratory symptoms. Following use, report skin irritation or eruption; alterations in vision, eye pain, or irritation; persistent GI effects; muscle or skeletal tremors, numbness, or rigidity; urinary or genital problems; or persistent fatigue. **Pregnancy/breast-feeding precautions:** Inform prescriber if you are pregnant. Do not breast-feed.

Breast-feeding Issues: Irritability, vomiting, diarrhea, tremors, and seizures have been reported in nursing infants.

Additional Information Cocaine intoxication of infants who are receiving breast milk from their mothers abusing cocaine has been reported.

Related Information

Controlled Substances Comparison *on page 1568*

Cocaine Hydrochloride *see* Cocaine *on page 326*

Coccidioidin Skin Test *see page 1461*

Codafed® Expectorant *see* Guaifenesin, Pseudoephedrine, and Codeine *on page 649*

Codafed® Pediatric Expectorant *see* Guaifenesin, Pseudoephedrine, and Codeine *on page 649*

Codehist® DH Liquid *see page 1522*

Codeine (KOE deen)

Synonyms Codeine Phosphate; Codeine Sulfate; Methylmorphine

Restrictions C-II

Generic Available Yes

Pharmacologic Category Analgesic, Narcotic; Antitussive

Pregnancy Risk Factor C/D (prolonged use or high doses at term)

Lactation Enters breast milk/use caution (AAP rates "compatible")

Use Treatment of mild to moderate pain; antitussive in lower doses; dextromethorphan has equivalent antitussive activity but has much lower toxicity in accidental overdose

Mechanism of Action/Effect Inhibits perception of and response to pain; causes cough supression; produces generalized CNS depression

Contraindications Hypersensitivity to codeine or any component of the formulation; pregnancy (prolonged use or high doses at term)

Warnings/Precautions Use with caution in patients with hypersensitivity reactions to other phenanthrene derivative opioid agonists (morphine, hydrocodone, hydromorphone, levorphanol, oxycodone, oxymorphone); respiratory diseases including asthma, emphysema, COPD, or severe liver or renal insufficiency; some preparations contain sulfites which may cause allergic reactions; tolerance or drug dependence may result from extended use

Not recommended for use for cough control in patients with a productive cough; not recommended as an antitussive for children <2 years of age; the elderly may be particularly susceptible to the CNS depressant and confusion as well as constipating effects of narcotics

Not approved for I.V. administration (although this route has been used clinically). If given intravenously, must be given slowly and the patient should be lying down. Rapid intravenous administration of narcotics may increase the incidence of serious adverse effects, in part due to limited opportunity to assess response prior to administration of the full dose. Access to respiratory support should be immediately available

Pregnancy risk C/D (prolonged use or high doses at term)

Drug Interactions

Cytochrome P450 Effect: Substrate of **CYP2D6**, 3A4; Inhibits CYP2D6

Decreased Effect: Decreased effect with cigarette smoking.

Increased Effect/Toxicity: May cause severely increased toxicity of codeine when taken with CNS depressants, phenothiazines, tricyclic antidepressants, other narcotic analgesics, guanabenz, MAO inhibitors, and neuromuscular blockers.

Nutritional/Ethanol Interactions

Ethanol: Avoid or limit ethanol (may increase CNS depression). Watch for sedation.

Herb/Nutraceutical: St John's wort may decrease codeine levels. Avoid valerian, St John's wort, kava kava, gotu kola (may increase CNS depression).

Effects on Lab Values ↑ aminotransferase [ALT (SGPT)/AST (SGOT)] (S)

Adverse Reactions

>10%:

Central nervous system: Drowsiness

Gastrointestinal: Constipation

1% to 10%:

Cardiovascular: Tachycardia or bradycardia, hypotension

(Continued)

Codeine *(Continued)*

Central nervous system: Dizziness, lightheadedness, false feeling of well being, malaise, headache, restlessness, paradoxical CNS stimulation, confusion
Dermatologic: Rash, urticaria
Gastrointestinal: Dry mouth, anorexia, nausea, vomiting
Hepatic: Increased transaminases
Genitourinary: Decreased urination, ureteral spasm
Local: Burning at injection site
Neuromuscular & skeletal: Weakness
Ocular: Blurred vision
Respiratory: Dyspnea
Miscellaneous: Physical and psychological dependence, histamine release

<1% (Limited to important or life-threatening): Convulsions, hallucinations, insomnia, mental depression, nightmares

Overdosage/Toxicology Symptoms of overdose include CNS and respiratory depression, GI cramping, and constipation. Naloxone, 2 mg I.V. with repeat administration as necessary up to a total of 10 mg, can also be used to reverse toxic effects of the opiate.

Pharmacodynamics/Kinetics

Absorption: Oral: Adequate

Half-Life Elimination: 2.5-3.5 hours

Metabolism: Hepatic to morphine (active)

Onset: Oral: 0.5-1 hour; I.M.: 10-30 minutes; Peak effect: Oral: 1-1.5 hours; I.M.: 0.5-1 hour

Duration: 4-6 hours

Formulations

Injection, as phosphate: 30 mg (1 mL, 2 mL); 60 mg (1 mL, 2 mL)
Solution, oral, as phosphate: 15 mg/5 mL
Tablet, as sulfate: 15 mg, 30 mg, 60 mg
Tablet, soluble, as phosphate: 30 mg, 60 mg
Tablet, soluble, as sulfate: 15 mg, 30 mg, 60 mg

Dosing

Adults & Elderly: Doses should be titrated to appropriate analgesic effect. When changing routes of administration, note that oral dose is $^2/_3$ as effective as parenteral dose.

Pain (Analgesic): Oral, I.M., I.V., S.C.: 30 mg/dose; range: 15-60 mg every 4-6 hours as needed; maximum: 360 mg/24 hours

Cough (Antitussive): Oral (for nonproductive cough): 10-20 mg/dose every 4-6 hours as needed; maximum: 120 mg/day

Pediatrics: Doses should be titrated to appropriate analgesic effect; when changing routes of administration, note that oral dose is $^2/_3$ as effective as parenteral dose.

Analgesic: Oral, I.M., S.C.: Children: 0.5-1 mg/kg/dose every 4-6 hours as needed; maximum: 60 mg/dose

Antitussive: Oral (for nonproductive cough): Children: 1-1.5 mg/kg/day in divided doses every 4-6 hours as needed: Alternative dose according to age:
2-6 years: 2.5-5 mg every 4-6 hours as needed; maximum: 30 mg/day
6-12 years: 5-10 mg every 4-6 hours as needed; maximum: 60 mg/day

Renal Impairment:

Cl_{cr} 10-50 mL/minute: Administer 75% of dose.
Cl_{cr} <10 mL/minute: Administer 50% of dose.

Hepatic Impairment: Dosing adjustment is probably necessary in hepatic insufficiency.

Stability

Storage: Store injection between 15°C to 30°C, avoid freezing. Do not use if injection is discolored or contains a precipitate. Protect injection from light.

Monitoring and Teaching Issues

Physical Assessment: Assess other medications patient may be taking for possible additive or adverse interactions (see Warnings/Precautions and Drug Interactions). See Contraindications and Warnings/Precautions for use cautions. Monitor for effectiveness of pain relief, for signs of overdose (see Overdose/Toxicology), vital signs and CNS status, and adverse reactions (see Adverse Reactions) at beginning of therapy and at regular intervals with long-term use. May cause physical and/or psychological dependence. For inpatients, implement safety measures. Assess knowledge/teach patient appropriate use (if self-administered). Teach patient to monitor for adverse reactions, adverse reactions to report, and appropriate interventions to reduce side effects. **Pregnancy risk factor C/D** - see Pregnancy Risk Factor for use cautions. Assess knowledge/teach patient use of barrier contraceptives if appropriate. Note breast-feeding caution.

Patient Education: If self-administered, use exactly as directed; do not increase dose or frequency. Drug may cause physical and/or psychological dependence. While using this medication, do not use alcohol and other prescription or OTC medications (especially sedatives, tranquilizers, antihistamines, or pain medications) without consulting prescriber. Maintain adequate hydration (2-3 L/day of fluids) unless advised by prescriber to restrict fluids. May cause dizziness, drowsiness, confusion, agitation, impaired coordination, or blurred vision (use caution when driving, climbing stairs, or changing position - rising from sitting or lying to standing, or when engaging in tasks requiring alertness until response to drug is known); nausea or vomiting, or loss of appetite (frequent mouth care, small, frequent meals, sucking lozenges, or chewing gum may help); or constipation (increased exercise, fluids, fruit, or fiber may help; if unresolved, consult prescriber about use of stool softeners). Report confusion, insomnia, excessive nervousness, excessive sedation or drowsiness, or shakiness; acute GI upset; difficulty breathing or shortness of breath; facial flushing, rapid heartbeat, or palpitations; urinary difficulty; unusual muscle weakness; or vision changes. **Pregnancy/breast-feeding precautions:** Inform prescriber if you are or intend to become pregnant. If you are breast-feeding, take medication immediately after breast-feeding or 3-4 hours prior to next feeding.

Geriatric Considerations: The elderly may be particularly susceptible to CNS depression and confusion as well as the constipating effects of narcotics.

Related Information

Controlled Substances Comparison *on page 1568*
Narcotic/Opioid Analgesic Comparison *on page 1583*

Codeine, Acetaminophen, Butalbital, and Caffeine *see* Butalbital, Acetaminophen, Caffeine, and Codeine *on page 193*

Codeine and Acetaminophen *see* Acetaminophen and Codeine *on page 37*

Codeine and Aspirin *see* Aspirin and Codeine *on page 124*

Codeine and Butalbital Compound *see* Butalbital, Aspirin, Caffeine, and Codeine *on page 195*

Codeine and Guaifenesin *see* Guaifenesin and Codeine *on page 647*

Codeine and Promethazine *see* Promethazine and Codeine *on page 1135*

Codeine, Aspirin, and Carisoprodol *see* Carisoprodol, Aspirin, and Codeine *on page 223*

Codeine, Butalbital, Aspirin, and Caffeine *see* Butalbital, Aspirin, Caffeine, and Codeine *on page 195*

Codeine, Guaifenesin, and Pseudoephedrine *see* Guaifenesin, Pseudoephedrine, and Codeine *on page 649*

Codeine Phosphate *see* Codeine *on page 327*

Codeine, Promethazine, and Phenylephrine *see* Promethazine, Phenylephrine, and Codeine *on page 1136*

Codeine Sulfate *see* Codeine *on page 327*

Cogentin® *see* Benztropine *on page 158*

Co-Gesic® *see* Hydrocodone and Acetaminophen *on page 667*

Cognex® *see* Tacrine *on page 1270*

Colace® [OTC] *see* Docusate *on page 432*

ColBenemid [DSC] *see* Colchicine and Probenecid *on page 330*

Colchicine (KOL chi seen)

Generic Available Yes

Pharmacologic Category Colchicine

Pregnancy Risk Factor C (oral); D (parenteral)

Lactation Enters breast milk/use caution (AAP rates "compatible")

Use Treatment of acute gouty arthritis attacks and prevention of recurrences of such attacks; management of familial Mediterranean fever

Use - Unlabeled/Investigational Primary biliary cirrhosis

Mechanism of Action/Effect Reduces the deposition of urate crystals that perpetuates the inflammatory response

Contraindications Hypersensitivity to colchicine or any component of the formulation; serious renal, gastrointestinal, hepatic, or cardiac disorders; blood dyscrasias; pregnancy (parenteral)

Warnings/Precautions Severe local irritation can occur following S.C. or I.M. administration. Use with caution in debilitated patients or elderly patients or patients with severe GI, renal, or liver disease. Pregnancy risk C (oral)/D (parenteral).

Drug Interactions

Cytochrome P450 Effect: Substrate of **CYP3A4**; Induces CYP2C8/9, 2E1, 3A4

Decreased Effect: Vitamin B_{12} absorption may be decreased with colchicine. Acidifying agents inhibit action of colchicine.

Increased Effect/Toxicity: Increased toxicity may be seen when taken with sympathomimetic agents or CNS depressant (effects are enhanced). Alkalizing agents potentiate effects of colchicine.

Nutritional/Ethanol Interactions

Ethanol: Avoid ethanol.

Food: Cyanocobalamin (vitamin B_{12}): Malabsorption of the substrate. May result in macrocytic anemia or neurologic dysfunction.

Effects on Lab Values May cause false-positive results in urine tests for erythrocytes or hemoglobin

Adverse Reactions

>10%: Gastrointestinal: Nausea, vomiting, diarrhea, abdominal pain

1% to 10%:

- Dermatologic: Alopecia
- Gastrointestinal: Anorexia

<1% (Limited to important or life-threatening): Agranulocytosis, aplastic anemia, arrhythmias (with intravenous administration), bone marrow suppression, hepatotoxicity

Overdosage/Toxicology Symptoms of overdose include acute nausea, vomiting, abdominal pain, shock, kidney damage, muscle weakness, burning in throat, watery to bloody diarrhea, hypotension, anuria, cardiovascular collapse, delirium, convulsions, and respiratory paralysis. Treatment includes gastric lavage and measures to prevent shock, hemodialysis or peritoneal dialysis. Atropine and morphine may relieve abdominal pain.

Pharmacodynamics/Kinetics

Half-Life Elimination: 12-30 minutes; End-stage renal disease: 45 minutes

Time to Peak: Serum: Oral: 0.5-2 hours, declining for the next 2 hours before increasing again due to enterohepatic recycling

Metabolism: Partially hepatic via deacetylation

Onset: Oral: Pain relief: ~12 hours if adequately dosed

Formulations

Injection: 0.5 mg/mL (2 mL)

Tablet: 0.5 mg, 0.6 mg

Dosing

Adults & Elderly:

Prophylaxis of familial Mediterranean fever: Oral: 1-2 mg/day in 2-3 divided doses

(Continued)

Colchicine *(Continued)*

Gouty arthritis, acute attacks:

Oral: Initial: 0.5-1.2 mg, then 0.5-0.6 mg every 1-2 hours or 1-1.2 mg every 2 hours until relief or GI side effects (nausea, vomiting, or diarrhea) occur to a maximum total dose of 8 mg; wait 3 days before initiating another course of therapy.

I.V.: Initial: 1-3 mg, then 0.5 mg every 6 hours until response, not to exceed a total dose of 4 mg. If pain recurs, it may be necessary to administer additional daily doses; the amount of colchicine administered intravenously in an acute treatment period (generally ~1 week) should not exceed a total dose of 4 mg. Do not administer more colchicine by any route for at least 7 days after a full course of I.V. therapy (4 mg); transfer to oral colchicine in a dose similar to that being given I.V.

Gouty arthritis, prophylaxis of recurrent attacks: Oral: 0.5-0.6 mg/day or every other day

Pediatrics: Prophylaxis of familial Mediterranean fever: Oral:

Children ≤5 years: 0.5 mg/day

Children >5 years: 1-1.5 mg/day in 2-3 divided doses

Renal Impairment:

Cl_{cr} <50 mL/minute: Avoid chronic use or administration.

Cl_{cr} <10 mL/minute: Decrease dose by 50% for treatment of acute attacks.

Hemodialysis effects: Not dialyzable (0% to 5%)

Supplemental dose is not necessary.

Administration

I.V.: Injection should be made over 2-5 minutes into tubing of free-flowing I.V. with compatible fluid. Do not give I.M. or S.C.

Stability

Storage: Protect tablets from light.

Compatibility: I.V. colchicine is **incompatible** with dextrose or I.V. solutions with preservatives.

Monitoring Laboratory Tests CBC and renal function on a regular basis

Monitoring and Teaching Issues

Physical Assessment: Assess effectiveness and interactions of other medications patient may be taking (see Contraindications and Drug Interactions). **I.V.** (see Dosing and Administration): Monitor therapeutic response, laboratory values, and adverse reactions (see Adverse Reactions and Overdose/Toxicology) at beginning of therapy and periodically with long-term use. Assess knowledge/teach patient appropriate use, interventions to reduce side effects, and adverse symptoms to report (see Patient Education). **Pregnancy risk factor C/D** - see Pregnancy Risk Factor for use cautions. Assess knowledge/teach patient on the need to use appropriate contraceptive measures and the need to avoid pregnancy. Note breast-feeding caution.

Patient Education: Take as directed; do not exceed recommended dosage. Consult prescriber about a low-purine diet. Maintain adequate hydration (2-3 L/day of fluids) unless advised by prescriber to restrict fluids. Do not use alcohol or aspirin-containing medication without consulting prescriber. You may experience nausea, vomiting, or anorexia (small, frequent meals, frequent mouth care, chewing gum, or sucking lozenges may help); hair loss (reversible). Stop medication and report to prescriber if severe vomiting, watery or bloody diarrhea, or abdominal pain occurs. Report muscle tremors or weakness; fatigue; easy bruising or bleeding; yellowing of eyes or skin; or pale stool or dark urine. **Pregnancy/breast-feeding precautions:** Inform prescriber if you are or intend to become pregnant. Consult prescriber if breast-feeding.

Dietary Issues: May need to supplement with vitamin B_{12}.

Geriatric Considerations: Colchicine appears to be more toxic in the elderly, particularly in the presence of renal, gastrointestinal, or cardiac disease. The most predictable oral side effects are (gastrointestinal) vomiting, abdominal pain, and nausea. If colchicine is stopped at this point, other more severe adverse effects may be avoided, such as bone marrow suppression, peripheral neuritis, etc.

Colchicine and Probenecid (KOL chi seen & proe BEN e sid)

Synonyms ColBenemid [DSC]; Probenecid and Colchicine

Generic Available Yes

Pharmacologic Category Antigout Agent; Anti-inflammatory Agent; Uricosuric Agent

Pregnancy Risk Factor C

Lactation

Colchicine: Compatible

Probenecid: Excretion in breast milk unknown

Use Treatment of chronic gouty arthritis when complicated by frequent, recurrent acute attacks of gout

Formulations Tablet: Colchicine 0.5 mg and probenecid 0.5 g

Dosing

Adults: Gout: Oral: 1 tablet/day for 1 week, then 1 tablet twice daily thereafter

Elderly: Refer to dosing in individual monographs; adjust for renal impairment.

Renal Impairment: Probenecid may not be effective in patients with chronic renal insufficiency particularly when Cl_{cr} is ≤30 mL/minute.

Monitoring and Teaching Issues

Physical Assessment: See individual components listed in Related Information. **Pregnancy risk factor C** - assess knowledge/instruct patient on need to use appropriate contraceptive measures and the need to avoid pregnancy. Note breast-feeding caution.

Patient Education: See individual components listed in Related Information. **Pregnancy/breast-feeding precautions:** Inform prescriber if you are or intend to become pregnant. Consult prescriber if breast-feeding.

Related Information

Colchicine *on page 329*

Probenecid *on page 1121*

Cold-eze® [OTC] *see* Zinc Supplements *on page 1423*

Colesevelam (koh le SEV a lam)

U.S. Brand Names WelChol™

Generic Available No

Pharmacologic Category Antilipemic Agent, Bile Acid Sequestrant

Pregnancy Risk Factor B

Lactation Excretion in breast milk unknown

Use Adjunctive therapy to diet and exercise in the management of elevated LDL in primary hypercholesterolemia (Fredrickson type IIa) when used alone or in combination with an HMG-CoA reductase inhibitor

Mechanism of Action/Effect Colesevelam binds bile acids including glycocholic acid in the intestine, impeding their reabsorption. Increases the fecal loss of bile salt-bound LDL-C.

Contraindications Hypersensitivity to colesevelam or any component of the formulation; bowel obstruction

Warnings/Precautions Use caution in treating patients with triglyceride levels >300 mg/dL (excluded from trials). Safety and efficacy not established in pediatric patients. Use caution in dysphagia, swallowing disorders, severe GI motility disorders, major GI tract surgery, or in patients susceptible to fat soluble vitamin deficiencies. Minimal effects are seen on HDL-C and triglyceride levels. Secondary causes of hypercholesterolemia should be excluded before initiation.

Drug Interactions

Decreased Effect: Sustained-release verapamil AUC and C_{max} were reduced. Clinical significance unknown.

Digoxin, lovastatin, metoprolol, quinidine, valproic acid, or warfarin absorption was not significantly affected with concurrent administration.

Clinical effects of atorvastatin, lovastatin, and simvastatin were not changed by concurrent administration.

Increased Effect/Toxicity: Refer to Decreased Effect.

Adverse Reactions

>10%: Gastrointestinal: Constipation (11%)

2% to 10%:

Gastrointestinal: Dyspepsia (8%)

Neuromuscular & skeletal: Weakness (4%), myalgia (2%)

Respiratory: Pharyngitis (3%)

Overdosage/Toxicology Systemic toxicity low since it is not absorbed.

Pharmacodynamics/Kinetics

Absorption: Insignificant

Half-Life Elimination: 0.05% was excreted in the urine after 1 month of chronic dosing

Onset: Peak effect: Therapeutic: ~2 weeks

Formulations Tablet: 625 mg

Dosing

Adults & Elderly: Dyslipidemia: Oral:

Monotherapy: 3 tablets twice daily with meals or 6 tablets once daily with a meal; maximum dose: 7 tablets/day

Combination therapy with an HMG-CoA reductase inhibitor: 4-6 tablets daily; maximum dose: 6 tablets/day

Administration

Oral: Give with meal(s). Make sure patient understands dietary guidelines.

Stability

Storage: Store at room temperature. Protect from moisture.

Monitoring Laboratory Tests Serum cholesterol, LDL, and triglyceride levels should be obtained before initiating treatment and periodically thereafter (in accordance with NCEP guidelines).

Monitoring and Teaching Issues

Physical Assessment: Assess other medications patient may be taking for effectiveness and interactions (see Drug Interactions). Note Warnings/Precautions and Contraindications Precautions for safe use. Laboratory tests and results should be monitored prior to and on a regular basis during therapy. Assess knowledge/teach patient appropriate use, possible adverse reactions and interventions, and symptoms to report (see Patient Education). Note breast-feeding caution.

Patient Education: Take medication exactly as directed; do not alter dosage without consulting prescriber. Other medications should be taken 1 hour before or 2 hours after colesevelam. You may experience constipation (increased exercise, increased exercise, fluids, fruit, fiber, or stool softener may help). Report persistent GI upset, skeletal or muscle pain or weakness, or respiratory difficulties. **Breast-feeding precaution:** Inform prescriber if breast-feeding.

Dietary Issues: Take with meal(s). Follow dietary guidelines.

Related Information

Lipid-Lowering Agents *on page 1582*

Colestid® *see* Colestipol *on page 331*

Colestipol (koe LES ti pole)

U.S. Brand Names Colestid®

Synonyms Colestipol Hydrochloride

Generic Available No

Pharmacologic Category Antilipemic Agent, Bile Acid Sequestrant

Pregnancy Risk Factor C

Lactation Not recommended

Use Adjunct in management of primary hypercholesterolemia; regression of arteriolosclerosis; relief of pruritus associated with elevated levels of bile acids; possibly used to decrease plasma half-life of digoxin in toxicity

Mechanism of Action/Effect Increases fecal loss of low density lipoprotein cholesterol

(Continued)

Colestipol *(Continued)*

Contraindications Hypersensitivity to bile acid sequestering resins or any component of the formulation; bowel obstruction

Warnings/Precautions Not to be taken simultaneously with many other medicines (decreased absorption). May interfere with fat soluble vitamins (A, D, E, K) and folic acid. Chronic use may be associated with bleeding problems. May produce or exacerbate constipation problems; fecal impaction may occur, hemorrhoids may be worsened. Pregnancy risk C.

Drug Interactions

Decreased Effect: Colestipol can reduce the absorption of numerous medications when used concurrently. Give other medications 1 hour before or 4 hours after giving colestipol. Medications which may be affected include HMG-CoA reductase inhibitors, thiazide diuretics, propranolol (and potentially other beta-blockers), corticosteroids, thyroid hormones, digoxin, valproic acid, NSAIDs, loop diuretics, sulfonylureas, troglitazone (and potentially other agents in this class - pioglitazone and rosiglitazone).

Warfarin and other oral anticoagulants: Absorption is reduced by cholestyramine and may also be reduced by colestipol. Separate administration times (as detailed above).

Effects on Lab Values ↑ prothrombin time (S); ↓ cholesterol (S)

Adverse Reactions

>10%: Gastrointestinal: Constipation

1% to 10%:

Central nervous system: Headache, dizziness, anxiety, vertigo, drowsiness, fatigue

Gastrointestinal: Abdominal pain and distention, belching, flatulence, nausea, vomiting, diarrhea

<1% (Limited to important or life-threatening): Cholecystitis, cholelithiasis, dyspnea breath, gallstones, GI bleeding, malabsorption syndrome, peptic ulceration

Overdosage/Toxicology Symptoms of overdose include GI obstruction, nausea, and GI distress. Treatment is supportive.

Pharmacodynamics/Kinetics

Absorption: None

Formulations

Granules, as hydrochloride: 5 g packet, 300 g, 500 g

Tablet, as hydrochloride: 1 g

Dosing

Adults & Elderly: Dyslipidemia: Oral: 5-30 g/day in divided doses 2-4 times/day

Administration

Oral: Dry powder should be added to at least 90 mL of liquid and stirred until completely mixed. Other drugs should be administered at least 1 hour before or 4 hours after colestipol.

Monitoring and Teaching Issues

Physical Assessment: Assess other medications the patient may be taking for effectiveness and interactions (see Drug Interactions). Monitor knowledge/teach patient appropriate preparation and use, possible adverse reactions, and symptoms to report (see Patient Education). **Pregnancy risk factor C** - benefits of use should outweigh possible risks. Breast-feeding is not recommended.

Patient Education: Take with 3-4 oz of water or fruit juice. Rinse glass with small amount of water to ensure full dose is taken. Other medications should be taken 2 hours before or 2 hours after colestipol. You may experience constipation (increased exercise, fluids, fruit, fiber, or stool softener may help); or drowsiness or dizziness (use caution when driving or engaging in tasks that require alertness until response to drug is known). Report acute gastric pain, tarry stools, or difficulty breathing. **Pregnancy/breast-feeding precautions:** Inform prescriber if you are or intend to become pregnant. Breast-feeding is not recommended.

Geriatric Considerations: Pharmacologic treatment should be reserved for those who are unable to obtain a desirable plasma cholesterol level by diet alone and for whom the benefits of treatment are believed to outweigh the potential adverse effects, drug interactions, and cost of treatment.

Related Information

Hyperlipidemia Management *on page 1682*
Lipid-Lowering Agents *on page 1582*

Colestipol Hydrochloride *see* Colestipol *on page 331*

Colistin, Neomycin, and Hydrocortisone *see page 1519*

Collagenase (KOL la je nase)

U.S. Brand Names Santyl®

Generic Available No

Pharmacologic Category Enzyme, Topical Debridement

Pregnancy Risk Factor C

Lactation Excretion in breast milk unknown

Use Promotes debridement of necrotic tissue in dermal ulcers and severe burns

Orphan drug: Injection: Treatment of Peyronie's disease; treatment of Dupytren's disease

Mechanism of Action/Effect Digests collagen in injured tissue. Collagenase will not attack collagen in healthy tissue or newly formed granulation tissue. In addition, it does not act on fat, fibrin, keratin, or muscle.

Contraindications Hypersensitivity to collagenase

Warnings/Precautions For external use only. Avoid contact with eyes. Monitor debilitated patients for systemic bacterial infections because debriding enzymes may increase the risk of bacteremia. Pregnancy risk C.

Drug Interactions

Decreased Effect: Enzymatic activity is inhibited by detergents, benzalkonium chloride, hexachlorophene, nitrofurazone, tincture of iodine, and heavy metal ions (silver and mercury).

Adverse Reactions Frequency not defined.

Local: Irritation, Pain and burning may occur at site of application

Postmarketing and/or case reports: Hypersensitivity reaction

Overdosage/Toxicology Action of enzyme may be stopped by applying Burow's solution.

Formulations Ointment (Santyl®): 250 units/g (15 g)

Dosing

Adults & Elderly: Dermal ulcers, burns: Topical: Apply once daily.

Pediatrics: Refer to adult dosing.

Administration

Topical: For external use only. Clean target area of all interfering agents listed above. If infection is persistent, apply powdered antibiotic first. Do not introduce into major body cavities. Monitor debilitated patients for systemic bacterial infections.

Monitoring and Teaching Issues

Physical Assessment: See Contraindications and Warnings/Precautions for use cautions. See application directions above. When applied to large areas or for extensive periods of time, monitor for adverse reactions. Assess knowledge/teach patient appropriate application and use and adverse symptoms to report (see Patient Education). **Pregnancy risk factor C.** Note breast-feeding caution.

Patient Education: Use exactly as directed; do not overuse. Wear gloves to apply a thin film to affected area. If dressing is necessary, use a porous dressing. Avoid contact with eyes. Report increased swelling, redness, rash, itching, signs of infection, worsening of condition, or lack of healing. **Pregnancy/breast-feeding precautions:** Inform prescriber if you are or intend to become pregnant. Consult prescriber if breast-feeding.

Geriatric Considerations: Preventive skin care should be instituted in all older patients at high risk for pressure ulcers. Collagenase is indicated in stage 3 and 4 pressure ulcers.

Collyrium Fresh® *see page 1509*

Colo-Fresh™ [OTC] *see* Bismuth *on page 169*

Coly-Mycin® S Otic Drops *see page 1519*

Colyte® *see* Polyethylene Glycol-Electrolyte Solution *on page 1098*

CombiPatch® *see* Estradiol and Norethindrone *on page 499*

Combipres® *see* Clonidine and Chlorthalidone *on page 319*

Combivent® *see* Ipratropium and Albuterol *on page 735*

Combivir® *see* Zidovudine and Lamivudine *on page 1421*

Comfort® [OTC] *see page 1509*

Community-Acquired Pneumonia in Adults *see page 1653*

Compatibility of Drugs *see page 1564*

Compatibility of Drugs in Syringe *see page 1566*

Compazine® *see* Prochlorperazine *on page 1127*

Compound F *see* Hydrocortisone *on page 673*

Compound S *see* Zidovudine *on page 1419*

Compound S, Abacavir, and Lamivudine *see* Abacavir, Lamivudine, and Zidovudine *on page 31*

Compoz® Nighttime Sleep Aid [OTC] *see* DiphenhydrAMINE *on page 422*

Compro™ *see* Prochlorperazine *on page 1127*

Comtan® *see* Entacapone *on page 469*

Concerta™ *see* Methylphenidate *on page 882*

Congestac® *see* Guaifenesin and Pseudoephedrine *on page 648*

Constilac® *see* Lactulose *on page 767*

Constulose® *see* Lactulose *on page 767*

Controlled Substances Comparison *see page 1568*

Cooper AR *see page 1509*

Copaxone® *see* Glatiramer Acetate *on page 631*

Copolymer-1 *see* Glatiramer Acetate *on page 631*

Cordarone® *see* Amiodarone *on page 81*

Cordran® *see* Topical Corticosteroids *on page 1334*

Cordran® SP *see* Topical Corticosteroids *on page 1334*

Coreg® *see* Carvedilol *on page 225*

Corgard® *see* Nadolol *on page 938*

Cormax® *see* Topical Corticosteroids *on page 1334*

CortaGel® Maximum Strength [OTC] *see* Hydrocortisone *on page 673*

Cortaid® Intensive Therapy [OTC] *see* Hydrocortisone *on page 673*

Cortaid® Maximum Strength [OTC] *see* Hydrocortisone *on page 673*

Cortaid® Maximum Strength [OTC] *see* Topical Corticosteroids *on page 1334*

Cortaid® Sensitive Skin With Aloe [OTC] *see* Hydrocortisone *on page 673*

Cortaid® With Aloe [OTC] *see* Topical Corticosteroids *on page 1334*

Cortatrigen® Otic *see page 1519*

Cort-Dome® *see* Topical Corticosteroids *on page 1334*

Cortef® *see* Hydrocortisone *on page 673*

Cortef® Feminine Itch *see* Topical Corticosteroids *on page 1334*

Cortenema® *see* Topical Corticosteroids *on page 1334*

Corticaine® *see* Topical Corticosteroids *on page 1334*

Corticool® [OTC] *see* Hydrocortisone *on page 673*

Corticosteroids *see page 1572*

Corticosteroids Comparison, Systemic Equivalencies *see page 1572*
Corticosteroids, Topical *see* Topical Corticosteroids *on page 1334*
Corticotropin *see page 1461*
Cortifoam® *see* Hydrocortisone *on page 673*
Cortifoam® *see* Topical Corticosteroids *on page 1334*
Cortisol *see* Hydrocortisone *on page 673*
Cortisporin® Ointment *see* Bacitracin, Neomycin, Polymyxin B, and Hydrocortisone *on page 145*
Cortisporin® Ophthalmic Ointment *see page 1509*
Cortisporin® Ophthalmic Solution *see page 1509*
Cortisporin® Otic *see page 1519*
Cortisporin-TC® Otic *see page 1519*
Cortizone®-5 [OTC] *see* Hydrocortisone *on page 673*
Cortizone®-5 [OTC] *see* Topical Corticosteroids *on page 1334*
Cortizone®-10 [OTC] *see* Topical Corticosteroids *on page 1334*
Cortizone®-10 Maximum Strength [OTC] *see* Hydrocortisone *on page 673*
Cortizone®-10 Plus Maximum Strength [OTC] *see* Hydrocortisone *on page 673*
Cortizone® 10 Quick Shot [OTC] *see* Hydrocortisone *on page 673*
Cortizone® for Kids [OTC] *see* Hydrocortisone *on page 673*
Cortrosyn® Injection *see page 1461*
Corvert® *see* Ibutilide *on page 690*
Cosmegen® *see* Dactinomycin *on page 356*
Cosyntropin *see page 1461*
Co-Trimoxazole *see* Sulfamethoxazole and Trimethoprim *on page 1259*
Coumadin® *see* Warfarin *on page 1410*
Covera-HS® *see* Verapamil *on page 1396*
Cozaar® *see* Losartan *on page 824*
CP-99,219-27 *see* Trovafloxacin *on page 1372*
CPM *see* Cyclophosphamide *on page 339*
CPT-11 *see* Irinotecan *on page 737*
CPZ *see* ChlorproMAZINE *on page 277*
Creatinine Clearance Estimating Methods in Patients With Stable Renal Function *see page 1532*
Creon® *see* Pancrelipase *on page 1029*
Cresyl Acetate *see page 1519*
Cresylate® *see page 1519*
Crinone® *see* Progesterone *on page 1130*
Crixivan® *see* Indinavir *on page 708*
Crolom™ *see page 1509*
Crolom® *see* Cromolyn Sodium *on page 334*
Cromoglycic Acid *see* Cromolyn Sodium *on page 334*

Cromolyn Sodium (KROE moe lin SOW dee um)

U.S. Brand Names Crolom®; Gastrocrom®; Intal®; Nasalcrom® [OTC]; Opticrom®
Synonyms Cromoglycic Acid; Disodium Cromoglycate; DSCG
Generic Available Yes: Solution for inhalation, ophthalmic drops
Pharmacologic Category Mast Cell Stabilizer
Pregnancy Risk Factor B
Lactation Excretion in breast milk unknown/use caution
Use
Inhalation: May be used as an adjunct in the prophylaxis of allergic disorders, including rhinitis, asthma; prevention of exercise-induced bronchospasm
Oral: Systemic mastocytosis
Ophthalmic: Treatment of vernal keratoconjunctivitis, vernal conjunctivitis, and vernal keratitis
Use - Unlabeled/Investigational Oral: Food allergy, treatment of inflammatory bowel disease
Mechanism of Action/Effect Prevents the mast cell release of histamine, leukotrienes and slow-reacting substance of anaphylaxis
Contraindications Hypersensitivity to cromolyn or any component of the formulation; acute asthma attacks
Warnings/Precautions Severe anaphylactic reactions may occur rarely; cromolyn is a prophylactic drug with no benefit for acute situations; caution should be used when withdrawing the drug or tapering the dose as symptoms may reoccur; use with caution in patients with a history of cardiac arrhythmias. Transient burning or stinging may occur with ophthalmic use. Dosage of oral product should be decreased with hepatic or renal dysfunction.
Adverse Reactions
Inhalation: >10%: Gastrointestinal: Unpleasant taste in mouth
Nasal:
>10%: Respiratory: Increase in sneezing, burning, stinging, or irritation inside of nose
1% to 10%:
Central nervous system: Headache
Gastrointestinal: Unpleasant taste
Respiratory: Hoarseness, coughing, postnasal drip
<1% (Limited to important or life-threatening): Anaphylactic reactions, epistaxis
Ophthalmic: Frequency not defined:
Ocular: Conjunctival injection, dryness around the eye, edema, eye irritation, immediate hypersensitivity reactions, itchy eyes, puffy eyes, styes, rash, watery eyes
Respiratory: Dyspnea

Systemic: Frequency not defined:
- Cardiovascular: Angioedema, chest pain, edema, flushing, palpitations, premature ventricular contractions, tachycardia
- Central nervous system: Anxiety, behavior changes, convulsions, depression, dizziness, fatigue, hallucinations, headache, irritability, insomnia, lethargy, migraine, nervousness, hypoesthesia, postprandial lightheadedness, psychosis
- Dermatologic: Erythema, photosensitivity, pruritus, purpura, rash, urticaria
- Gastrointestinal: Abdominal pain, constipation, diarrhea, dyspepsia, dysphagia, esophagospasm, flatulence, glossitis, nausea, stomatitis, unpleasant taste, vomiting
- Genitourinary: Dysuria, urinary frequency
- Hematologic: Neutropenia, pancytopenia, polycythemia
- Hepatic: Liver function test abnormal
- Local: Burning
- Neuromuscular & skeletal: Arthralgia, leg stiffness, leg weakness, myalgia, paresthesia
- Otic: Tinnitus
- Respiratory: Dyspnea, pharyngitis
- Miscellaneous: Lupus erythematosus

Overdosage/Toxicology Symptoms of overdose include bronchospasm, laryngeal edema, and dysuria. Treat symptomatically.

Pharmacodynamics/Kinetics

Absorption:
- Inhalation: ~8% reaches lungs upon inhalation; well absorbed
- Oral: <1% of dose absorbed

Half-Life Elimination: 80-90 minutes

Time to Peak: Serum: Inhalation: ~15 minutes

Onset: Onset: Response to treatment:
- Nasal spray: May occur at 1-2 weeks
- Ophthalmic: May be seen within a few days; treatment for up to 6 weeks is often required
- Oral: May occur within 2-6 weeks

Formulations
- Solution, oral spray, as sodium (Intal®): 800 mcg/inhalation (8.1 g) [112 metered inhalations; 56 doses], (14.2 g) [200 metered inhalations; 100 doses]
- Solution for nebulization, as sodium (Intal®): 20 mg/2 mL (60s, 120s)
- Solution, intranasal spray, as sodium (Nasalcrom®): 40 mg/mL (13 mL, 26 mL) [5.2 mg/inhalation]
- Solution, ophthalmic, as sodium (Crolom®, Opticrom®): 4% (2.5 mL, 10 mL) [contains benzalkonium chloride]
- Solution, oral, as sodium (Gastrocrom®): 100 mg/5 mL (96s)

Dosing

Adults & Elderly:
- Allergic rhinitis (treatment and prophylaxis): Nasal: Instill 1 spray in each nostril 3-4 times/day
- Asthma:
  - **Note:** Not effective for immediate relief of symptoms in acute asthmatic attacks; must be used at regular intervals for 2-4 weeks to be effective.
  - Inhalation: Metered spray: 2 inhalations 4 times/day
  - Nebulization solution: Inhalation: Single dose of 20 mg
- Prophylaxis of bronchospasm (allergen- or exercise-induced):
  - **Note:** Administer 10-15 minutes prior to exercise or allergen exposure but no longer than 1 hour before:
  - Nebulization solution: Single dose of 20 mg
  - Metered spray: Single dose of 2 inhalations
- Conjunctivitis and keratitis: Ophthalmic: 1-2 drops in each eye 4-6 times/day
- Mastocytosis: Oral: 200 mg 4 times/day; given 1/2 hour prior to meals and at bedtime. If control of symptoms is not seen within 2-3 weeks, dose may be increased to a maximum 40 mg/kg/day
- Food allergy and inflammatory bowel disease (unlabeled use): Oral: Initial dose: 200 mg 4 times/day; may double the dose if effect is not satisfactory within 2-3 weeks; up to 400 mg 4 times/day

Pediatrics:
- Allergic rhinitis (treatment and prophylaxis): Nasal: Children ≥2 years: Refer to adult dosing.
- Asthma: Inhalation:
  - For chronic control of asthma, taper frequency to the lowest effective dose (ie, 4 times/day to 3 times/day to twice daily):
  - Nebulization solution: Children >2 years: Initial: 20 mg 4 times/day; usual dose: 20 mg 3-4 times/day
  - Metered spray:
    - Children 5-12 years: Initial: 2 inhalations 4 times/day; usual dose: 1-2 inhalations 3-4 times/day
    - Children ≥12 years: Refer to adult dosing.
- Prevention of allergen- or exercise-induced bronchospasm: Administer 10-15 minutes prior to exercise or allergen exposure but no longer than 1 hour before:
  - Nebulization solution: Children >2 years: Refer to adult dosing.
  - Metered spray: Children >5 years: Single dose of 2 inhalations
- Systemic mastocytosis: Oral:
  - Children 2-12 years: 100 mg 4 times/day; not to exceed 40 mg/kg/day; given 1/2 hour prior to meals and at bedtime
  - Children >12 years: Refer to adult dosing.
- Food allergy and inflammatory bowel disease (unlabeled use): Oral:
  - Children <2 years: Not recommended
  - Children 2-12 years: Initial dose: 100 mg 4 times/day; may double the dose if effect is not satisfactory within 2-3 weeks; not to exceed 40 mg/kg/day
  - Children >12 years: Refer to adult dosing.

(Continued)

Cromolyn Sodium *(Continued)*

Note: Once desired effect is achieved, dose may be tapered to lowest effective dose

Renal Impairment: Specific guidelines not available; consider lower dose of oral product.

Hepatic Impairment: Specific guidelines not available; consider lower dose of oral product.

Administration

Oral: Oral concentrate: Open ampul and squeeze contents into glass of water; stir well. Administer at least 30 minutes before meals and at bedtime.

Inhalation: Oral inhalation: Shake canister gently before use; do not immerse canister in water.

Other: Nasal inhalation: Clear nasal passages by blowing nose prior to use.

Stability

Storage: Store at room temperature of 15°C to 30°C (59°F to 86°F); protect from light. Do not use oral concentrate if solution becomes discolored or forms a precipitate.

Compatibility: Nebulizer solution is **compatible** with metaproterenol sulfate, isoproterenol hydrochloride, 0.25% isoetharine hydrochloride, epinephrine hydrochloride, terbutaline sulfate, and 20% acetylcysteine solution for at least 1 hour after their admixture.

Monitoring Laboratory Tests Periodic pulmonary function

Monitoring and Teaching Issues

Physical Assessment: This is prophylactic therapy, not to be used for acute situations (see Contraindications and Warnings/Precautions). Monitor laboratory tests (long-term use) and adverse reactions (see Warnings/Precautions, Adverse Reactions, and Overdose/Toxicology). Assess knowledge/teach patient appropriate use, interventions to reduce side effects, and adverse symptoms to report (see Patient Education). Note breast-feeding caution.

Patient Education: Oral: Use as directed; do not increase dosage or discontinue abruptly without consulting prescriber. Take at least 30 minutes before meals. You may experience dizziness or nervousness (use caution when driving or engaging in tasks requiring alertness until response to drug is known); diarrhea (boiled milk, yogurt, or buttermilk may help); or headache or muscle pain (mild analgesic may offer relief). Report persistent insomnia; skin rash or irritation; abdominal pain or difficulty swallowing; unusual cough, bronchospasm, or difficulty breathing; decreased urination; or if condition worsens or fails to improve. **Breast-feeding precaution:** Consult prescriber if breast-feeding.

Nebulizer: Store nebulizer solution away from light. Prepare nebulizer according to package instructions. Clear as much mucus as possible before use. Rinse mouth following each use to prevent opportunistic infection and reduce unpleasant aftertaste. Report if symptoms worsen or condition fails to improve.

Nasal: Instill 1 spray into each nostril 3-4 times a day. You may experience unpleasant taste (rinsing mouth and frequent oral care may help); or headache (mild analgesic may help). Report increased sneezing, burning, stinging, or irritation inside of nose; sore throat, hoarseness, nosebleed; anaphylactic reaction (skin rash, fever, chills, backache, difficulty breathing, chest pain); or worsening of condition or lack of improvement.

Ophthalmic: For ophthalmic use only. Wash hands before using. Tilt head back and look upward. Put drops of suspension inside lower eyelid. Close eye and roll eyeball in all directions. Do not blink for ½ minute. Apply gentle pressure to inner corner of eye for 30 seconds. Do not let tip of applicator touch eye; do not contaminate tip of applicator (may cause eye infection, eye damage, or vision loss). Do not share medication with anyone else. Temporary stinging or blurred vision may occur. Inform prescriber if condition worsens or fails to improve or if you experience eye pain, redness, burning, watering, dryness, double vision, puffiness around eye, vision changes, or other adverse eye response; or worsening of condition or lack of improvement. Do not wear contact lenses during treatment.

Dietary Issues: Oral: Should be taken at least 30 minutes before meals.

Geriatric Considerations: Assess the patient's ability to empty capsules via the Spinhaler®. Older persons often have difficulty with inhaled and ophthalmic dosage forms.

Breast-feeding Issues: No data available on whether cromolyn enters into breast milk or clinical effects on the infant.

Related Information

Inhalant (Asthma, Bronchospasm) Agents Comparison *on page 1577*
Ophthalmic Agents *on page 1509*

Crotalidae Polyvalent *see page 1460*

Crotamiton (kroe TAM i tonn)

U.S. Brand Names Eurax® Topical

Generic Available No

Pharmacologic Category Scabicidal Agent

Pregnancy Risk Factor C

Lactation Excretion in breast milk unknown

Use Treatment of scabies (*Sarcoptes scabiei*) and symptomatic treatment of pruritus

Mechanism of Action/Effect Mechanism of action unknown

Contraindications Hypersensitivity to crotamiton or any component of the formulation; patients who manifest a primary irritation response to topical medications

Warnings/Precautions Avoid contact with face, eyes, mucous membranes, and urethral meatus. Do not apply to acutely inflamed or raw skin. For external use only. Pregnancy risk C.

Adverse Reactions <1% (Limited to important or life-threatening): Contact dermatitis, irritation, pruritus, warm sensation

Overdosage/Toxicology Symptoms of ingestion include burning sensation in mouth, irritation of the buccal, esophageal and gastric mucosa, nausea, vomiting, and abdominal pain. There is no specific antidote. General measures to eliminate the drug and reduce its absorption, combined with symptomatic treatment, are recommended.

Formulations

Cream: 10% (60 g)

Lotion: 10% (60 mL, 454 mL)

Dosing

Adults & Elderly:

Scabies: Topical: Wash thoroughly and scrub away loose scales, then towel dry; apply a thin layer and massage drug onto skin of the entire body from the neck to the toes (with special attention to skin folds, creases, and interdigital spaces). Repeat application in 24 hours. Take a cleansing bath 48 hours after the final application. Treatment may be repeated after 7-10 days if live mites are still present.

Pruritus: Topical: Massage into affected areas until medication is completely absorbed; repeat as necessary

Pediatrics: Refer to adult dosing.

Administration

Topical: For external use only. Shake lotion well before using. Avoid contact with face, eyes, mucous membranes, and urethral meatus.

Monitoring and Teaching Issues

Physical Assessment: Assess knowledge/teach patient appropriate application and use and adverse symptoms to report (see Patient Education). **Pregnancy risk factor C.** Note breast-feeding caution.

Patient Education: For topical use only. Apply lotion to whole body from the chin down being sure to cover all skin folds and creases. Apply a second application 24 hours later. Avoid eyes. Take a bath 48 hours after application. All contaminated clothing and bed linen should be washed to avoid reinfestation. If cure is not achieved after 2 doses, use alternative therapy. **Pregnancy/breast-feeding precautions:** Inform prescriber if you are or intend to become pregnant. Consult prescriber if breast-feeding.

Cruex® [OTC] *see* Clotrimazole *on page 322*

Crystalline Penicillin *see* Penicillin G (Parenteral/Aqueous) *on page 1045*

Crystamine® *see* Cyanocobalamin *on page 337*

Crysti 1000® *see* Cyanocobalamin *on page 337*

CSA *see* CycloSPORINE *on page 343*

CTX *see* Cyclophosphamide *on page 339*

Cutivate® *see* Fluticasone *on page 588*

Cutivate™ *see* Topical Corticosteroids *on page 1334*

CyA *see* CycloSPORINE *on page 343*

Cyanide Antidote Kit *see page 1460*

Cyanocobalamin (sye an oh koe BAL a min)

U.S. Brand Names Crystamine®; Crysti 1000®; Cyanoject®; Cyomin®; Ener-B®; Nascobal®

Synonyms Vitamin B_{12}

Generic Available Yes

Pharmacologic Category Vitamin, Water Soluble

Pregnancy Risk Factor A/C (dose exceeding RDA recommendation); C (nasal gel)

Lactation Enters breast milk/compatible

Use Treatment of pernicious anemia; vitamin B_{12} deficiency; increased B_{12} requirements due to pregnancy, thyrotoxicosis, hemorrhage, malignancy, liver or kidney disease

Mechanism of Action/Effect Coenzyme for various metabolic functions, including fat and carbohydrate metabolism and protein synthesis, used in cell replication and hematopoiesis

Contraindications Hypersensitivity to cyanocobalamin or any component of the formulation, cobalt; patients with hereditary optic nerve atrophy, Leber's disease

Warnings/Precautions I.M. route used to treat pernicious anemia; vitamin B_{12} deficiency for >3 months results in irreversible degenerative CNS lesions; treatment of vitamin B_{12} megaloblastic anemia may result in severe hypokalemia, sometimes, fatal, when anemia corrects due to cellular potassium requirements. B_{12} deficiency masks signs of polycythemia vera; vegetarian diets may result in B_{12} deficiency; pernicious anemia occurs more often in gastric carcinoma than in general population. Patients with Leber's disease may suffer rapid optic atrophy when treated with vitamin B_{12}. Pregnancy risk C (dose exceeding RDA/nasal gel).

Drug Interactions

Decreased Effect: Ethanol decreases B_{12} absorption. Chloramphenicol, cholestyramine, cimetidine, colchicine, neomycin, PAS, and potassium may reduce absorption and/or effect of cyanocobalamin.

Effects on Lab Values Methotrexate, pyrimethamine, and most antibiotics invalidate folic acid and vitamin B_{12} diagnostic microbiological blood assays

Adverse Reactions

1% to 10%:

Central nervous system: Headache (2% to 11%), anxiety, dizziness, pain, nervousness, hypoesthesia

Dermatologic: Itching

Gastrointestinal: Sore throat, nausea and vomiting, dyspepsia, diarrhea

Neuromuscular & skeletal: Weakness (1% to 4%), back pain, arthritis, myalgia, paresthesia, abnormal gait

Respiratory: Dyspnea, rhinitis

<1% (Limited to important or life-threatening): Anaphylaxis, CHF, peripheral vascular thrombosis, pulmonary edema, urticaria

Pharmacodynamics/Kinetics

Absorption: From the terminal ileum in presence of calcium; gastric "intrinsic factor" must be present to transfer the compound across the intestinal mucosa

Metabolism: Converted in tissues to active coenzymes, methylcobalamin and deoxyadenosylcobalamin

Formulations

Gel, intranasal (Nascobal®): 500 mcg/0.1 mL (5 mL)

(Continued)

Cyanocobalamin *(Continued)*

Injection: 100 mcg/mL (1 mL, 10 mL, 30 mL); 1000 mcg/mL (1 mL, 10 mL, 30 mL)
Tablet [OTC]: 50 mcg, 100 mcg, 250 mcg, 500 mcg, 1000 mcg

Dosing

Adults & Elderly:

Recommended daily allowance (RDA):
Adults: 2.4 mcg
Pregnant women: 2.6 mcg
Lactating women: 2.8 mcg

Nutritional deficiency:
Intranasal gel: 500 mcg once weekly
Oral: 25-250 mcg/day

Pernicious anemia: **Note:** Oral is not generally recommended due to poor absorption and I.V. is not recommended due to more rapid elimination:
Neurologic involvement: I.M. or deep S.C.: 100 mcg/day for 6-7 days; if improvement, administer same dose on alternate days for 7 doses; then every 3-4 days for 2-3 weeks; once hematologic values have returned to normal, maintenance dosage: 100 mcg/month.
Hematologic remission (without evidence of nervous system involvement): Intranasal gel: 500 mcg once weekly

Vitamin B_{12} deficiency: Initial: 30 mcg/day for 5-10 days; maintenance: 100-200 mcg/month
Schilling test: I.M.: 1000 mcg
Familial selective B_{12} malabsorption: I.M.: 1 mg weekly for 3 weeks, followed by a maintenance dose of 250 mcg monthly
Methylmalonic aciduria: I.M.: 1000 mcg daily

Pediatrics:

Recommended daily allowance (RDA): Children: 0.3-2 mcg
Nutritional deficiency: Oral: 25-250 mcg/day
Anemias: I.M. or deep S.C. (oral is not generally recommended due to poor absorption and I.V. is not recommended due to more rapid elimination):
Pernicious anemia, congenital (if evidence of neurologic involvement): 1000 mcg/day for at least 2 weeks; maintenance: 50-100 mcg/month or 100 mcg for 6-7 days; if there is clinical improvement, give 100 mcg every other day for 7 doses, then every 3-4 days for 2-3 weeks; follow with 100 mcg/month for life. Administer with folic acid if needed.
Children: 30-50 mcg/day for 2 or more weeks (to a total dose of 1000-5000 mcg), then follow with 100 mcg/month as maintenance dosage

Vitamin B_{12} deficiency: Children: I.M. or deep S.C.:
Neurologic signs: 100 mcg/day for 10-15 days (total dose of 1-1.5 mg), then once or twice weekly for several months; may taper to 60 mcg every month
Hematologic signs: 10-50 mcg/day for 5-10 days, followed by 100-250 mcg/dose every 2-4 weeks

Administration

Oral: Not recommended
I.M.: I.M. or deep S.C. are preferred routes of administration.
I.V.: Not recommended

Stability

Storage: Clear pink to red solutions are stable at room temperature. Protect from light.
Compatibility: Stable in dextran 6% in dextrose, dextran 6% in NS, D_5LR, $D_5{}^1/_4NS$, $D_5{}^1/_2NS$, D_5NS, D_5W, $D_{10}W$, $D_{10}NS$, LR, $^1/_2NS$, NS
Compatibility when admixed: Incompatible with chlorpromazine, phytonadione, prochlorperazine edisylate, warfarin

Monitoring Laboratory Tests Erythrocyte and reticulocyte count, hemoglobin, hematocrit; monitor potassium concentrations during early therapy.

Monitoring and Teaching Issues

Physical Assessment: See Contraindications and Warnings/Precautions for use cautions. Assess effectiveness and interactions of other medications patient may be taking (see Drug Interactions). Monitor laboratory tests at beginning of therapy and periodically with long-term therapy (see above). Assess knowledge/teach patient appropriate administration (injection technique and needle disposal), appropriate nutritional counseling, and adverse symptoms to report (see Patient Education). **Pregnancy risk factor A/C** - see Pregnancy Risk Factor for use cautions.

Patient Education: Use exactly as directed. Pernicious anemia may require monthly injections for life. Report skin rash; swelling, pain, or redness of extremities; or acute persistent diarrhea. **Pregnancy precaution:** Inform prescriber if you are pregnant.

Geriatric Considerations: There exists evidence that people, particularly elderly whose serum cobalamin concentrations <500 pg/mL, should receive replacement parenteral therapy.

Cyanoject® *see* Cyanocobalamin *on page 337*
Cyclessa® *see* Ethinyl Estradiol and Desogestrel *on page 516*

Cyclobenzaprine (sye kloe BEN za preen)

U.S. Brand Names Flexeril®
Synonyms Cyclobenzaprine Hydrochloride
Generic Available Yes
Pharmacologic Category Skeletal Muscle Relaxant
Pregnancy Risk Factor B
Lactation Excretion in breast milk unknown/not recommended
Use Treatment of muscle spasm associated with acute painful musculoskeletal conditions; supportive therapy in tetanus
Mechanism of Action/Effect Centrally acting skeletal muscle relaxant pharmacologically related to tricyclic antidepressants; reduces tonic somatic motor activity influencing both alpha and gamma motor neurons

Contraindications Hypersensitivity to cyclobenzaprine or any component of the formulation; do not use concomitantly or within 14 days of MAO inhibitors; hyperthyroidism; congestive heart failure; arrhythmias

Warnings/Precautions Cyclobenzaprine shares the toxic potentials of the tricyclic antidepressants and the usual precautions of tricyclic antidepressant therapy and cholinergic blockage should be observed. Use with caution in patients with urinary hesitancy or angle-closure glaucoma. Do not use concomitantly or within 14 days after MAO inhibitors; combination may cause hypertensive crisis, severe convulsions.

Drug Interactions

Cytochrome P450 Effect: Substrate of **CYP1A2**, 2D6, 3A4

Decreased Effect: Cyclobenzaprine may block effect of guanethidine.

Increased Effect/Toxicity: Because of cyclobenzaprine's similarities to the tricyclic antidepressants, there may be additive toxicities and side effects similar to tricyclic antidepressants. Cyclobenzaprine's toxicity may also be additive with other agents with anticholinergic properties. Cyclobenzaprine may enhance effects of alcohol, barbiturates, and other CNS depressants. See Warnings/Precautions for MAO inhibitor precautions.

Nutritional/Ethanol Interactions

Ethanol: Avoid ethanol (may increase CNS depression).

Herb/Nutraceutical: St John's wort may decrease cyclobenzaprine levels. Avoid valerian, St John's wort, kava kava, gotu kola (may increase CNS depression).

Adverse Reactions

>10%:

Central nervous system: Drowsiness, dizziness, lightheadedness
Gastrointestinal: Dry mouth

1% to 10%:

Cardiovascular: Edema of the face/lips, syncope
Gastrointestinal: Bloated feeling
Genitourinary: Problems in urinating, polyuria
Neuromuscular & skeletal: Problems in speaking, muscle weakness
Ocular: Blurred vision
Otic: Tinnitus

<1% (Limited to important or life-threatening): Angioedema, dermatitis, dysuria, hepatitis, rash, syncope

Overdosage/Toxicology Symptoms of overdose include troubled breathing, drowsiness, syncope, seizures, tachycardia, hallucinations, and vomiting. Following initiation of essential overdose management, treatment is supportive and symptomatic.

Pharmacodynamics/Kinetics

Absorption: Complete

Half-Life Elimination: 1-3 days

Time to Peak: Serum: 3-8 hours

Metabolism: Hepatic; may undergo enterohepatic recirculation

Onset: ~1 hour

Duration: 8 to >24 hours

Formulations Tablet, as hydrochloride: 10 mg

Dosing

Adults: Muscle spasm (including spasms associated with acute temporomandibular joint pain), supportive therapy in tetanus: Oral: 20-40 mg/day in 2-4 divided doses; maximum: 60 mg/day. Do not use longer than 2-3 weeks.

Elderly: See Geriatric Considerations.

Pediatrics: Muscle spasm: Oral: Children: Dosage has not been established.

Monitoring and Teaching Issues

Physical Assessment: Assess effectiveness and interactions of other medications patient may be taking (see Drug Interactions). See Contraindications and Warnings/Precautions for use cautions. Monitor effectiveness of therapy (according to rational for therapy) and adverse reactions (see Adverse Reactions) at beginning and periodically during therapy. Assess knowledge/teach patient appropriate use, interventions to reduce side effects (postural hypotension precautions), and adverse symptoms to report (see Patient Education). Breast-feeding is not recommended.

Patient Education: Take exactly as directed. Do not increase dose or discontinue without consulting prescriber. Do not use alcohol, prescriptive or OTC antidepressants, sedatives, or pain medications without consulting prescriber. You may experience drowsiness, dizziness, lightheadedness (avoid driving or engaging in tasks that require alertness until response to drug is known); or urinary retention (void before taking medication). Report excessive drowsiness or mental agitation, chest pain, skin rash, swelling of mouth/face, difficulty speaking, ringing in ears, or blurred vision. **Breast-feeding precaution:** Breast-feeding is not recommended.

Geriatric Considerations: High doses in the elderly caused drowsiness and dizziness; therefore, use the lowest dose possible. Because cyclobenzaprine causes anticholinergic effects, it may not be the skeletal muscle relaxant of choice in the elderly.

Cyclobenzaprine Hydrochloride *see* Cyclobenzaprine *on page 338*

Cyclogyl® *see page 1509*

Cyclogyl® *see page 1461*

Cyclomydril® Ophthalmic *see page 1461*

Cyclopentolate *see page 1509*

Cyclopentolate *see page 1461*

Cyclopentolate and Phenylephrine *see page 1461*

Cyclophosphamide (sye kloe FOS fa mide)

U.S. Brand Names Cytoxan®; Neosar®

Synonyms CPM; CTX; CYT; NSC-26271

Generic Available Yes

Pharmacologic Category Antineoplastic Agent, Alkylating Agent

(Continued)

Cyclophosphamide *(Continued)*

Pregnancy Risk Factor D

Lactation Enters breast milk/contraindicated

Use

Oncologic: Treatment of Hodgkin's and non-Hodgkin's lymphoma, Burkitt's lymphoma, chronic lymphocytic leukemia (CLL), chronic myelocytic leukemia (CML), acute myelocytic leukemia (AML), acute lymphocytic leukemia (ALL), mycosis fungoides, multiple myeloma, neuroblastoma, retinoblastoma, rhabdomyosarcoma, Ewing's sarcoma; breast, testicular, endometrial, ovarian, and lung cancers, and in conditioning regimens for bone marrow transplantation

Nononcologic: Prophylaxis of rejection for kidney, heart, liver, and bone marrow transplants, severe rheumatoid disorders, nephrotic syndrome, Wegener's granulomatosis, idiopathic pulmonary hemosideroses, myasthenia gravis, multiple sclerosis, systemic lupus erythematosus, lupus nephritis, autoimmune hemolytic anemia, idiopathic thrombocytic purpura (ITP), macroglobulinemia, and antibody-induced pure red cell aplasia

Mechanism of Action/Effect Interferes with the normal function of DNA by alkylation and cross-linking the strands of DNA, and by possible protein modification; cyclophosphamide also possesses potent immunosuppressive activity; note that cyclophosphamide must be metabolized to its active form in the liver

Contraindications Hypersensitivity to cyclophosphamide or any component of the formulation; pregnancy

Warnings/Precautions The U.S. Food and Drug Administration (FDA) currently recommends that procedures for proper handling and disposal of antineoplastic agents be considered. Dosage adjustment needed for renal or hepatic failure. Use with caution in patients with bone marrow depression. If cyclophosphamide contacts the skin, wash and flush thoroughly with water.

Drug Interactions

Cytochrome P450 Effect: Substrate of CYP2A6, **2B6**, 2C8/9, **2C19**, 3A4; Induces CYP2B6, 2C8/9

Decreased Effect: Cyclophosphamide may decrease digoxin serum levels.

Increased Effect/Toxicity: Allopurinol may cause an increase in bone marrow depression and may result in significant elevations of cyclophosphamide cytotoxic metabolites.

Anesthetic agents: Cyclophosphamide reduces serum pseudocholinesterase concentrations and may prolong the neuromuscular blocking activity of succinylcholine. Use with caution with halothane, nitrous oxide, and succinylcholine.

Chloramphenicol causes prolonged cyclophosphamide half-life and increased toxicity.

Cimetidine inhibits hepatic metabolism of drugs and may decrease the activation of cyclophosphamide.

Doxorubicin: Cyclophosphamide may enhance cardiac toxicity of anthracyclines.

Phenobarbital and phenytoin induce hepatic enzymes and cause a more rapid production of cyclophosphamide metabolites with a concurrent decrease in the serum half-life of the parent compound.

Tetrahydrocannabinol results in enhanced immunosuppression in animal studies.

Thiazide diuretics: Leukopenia may be prolonged.

Nutritional/Ethanol Interactions Herb/Nutraceutical: St John's wort may decrease cyclobenzaprine levels. Avoid black cohosh, dong quai in estrogen-dependent tumors.

Effects on Lab Values ↑ uric acid in serum and urine; false-positive Pap test; suppression of some skin tests

Adverse Reactions

>10%:

- Dermatologic: Alopecia (40% to 60%) but hair will usually regrow although it may be a different color and/or texture. Hair loss usually begins 3-6 weeks after the start of therapy.
- Endocrine & metabolic: Fertility: May cause sterility; interferes with oogenesis and spermatogenesis; may be irreversible in some patients; gonadal suppression (amenorrhea)
- Gastrointestinal: Nausea and vomiting occur more frequently with larger doses, usually beginning 6-10 hours after administration; anorexia, diarrhea, mucositis, and stomatitis are also seen
- Genitourinary: Severe, potentially fatal acute hemorrhagic cystitis, believed to be a result of chemical irritation of the bladder by acrolein, a cyclophosphamide metabolite, occurs in 7% to 12% of patients and has been reported in up to 40% of patients in some series. Patients should be encouraged to drink plenty of fluids during therapy (most adults will require at least 2 L/day), void frequently, and avoid taking the drug at night. With large I.V. doses, I.V. hydration is usually recommended. The use of mesna and/or continuous bladder irrigation is rarely needed for doses <2 g/m^2.
- Hematologic: Thrombocytopenia and anemia are less common than leukopenia
  - Onset: 7 days
  - Nadir: 10-14 days
  - Recovery: 21 days

1% to 10%:

- Central nervous system: Headache
- Dermatologic: Skin rash, facial flushing
- Renal: SIADH may occur, usually with doses >50 mg/kg (or 1 g/m^2); renal tubular necrosis, which usually resolves with discontinuation of the drug, is also reported
- Respiratory: Nasal congestion occurs when I.V. doses are administered too rapidly (large doses via 30-60 minute infusion); patients experience runny eyes, rhinorrhea, sinus congestion, and sneezing during or immediately after the infusion. If needed, a decongestant or decongestant/antihistamine (eg, pseudoephedrine or pseudoephedrine/triprolidine) can be used to prevent or relieve these symptoms.

<1% (Limited to important or life-threatening): High-dose therapy may cause cardiac dysfunction manifested as CHF; cardiac necrosis or hemorrhagic myocarditis has occurred rarely, but may be fatal. Cyclophosphamide may also potentiate the cardiac toxicity of anthracyclines. Other adverse reactions include anaphylactic reactions, darkening of skin/fingernails, dizziness, hemorrhagic colitis, hemorrhagic ureteritis, hepatotoxicity, hyperglycemia, hyperuricemia, hypokalemia, jaundice, renal tubular necrosis, secondary malignancy, Stevens-Johnson syndrome, toxic epidermal necrolysis; interstitial pneumonitis and pulmonary fibrosis are occasionally seen with high doses

BMT:

Cardiovascular: Heart failure, cardiac necrosis, pericardial tamponade
Endocrine & metabolic: Hyponatremia
Gastrointestinal: Severe nausea and vomiting
Miscellaneous: Hemorrhagic cystitis, secondary malignancy

Overdosage/Toxicology Symptoms of overdose include myelosuppression, alopecia, nausea, and vomiting. Treatment is supportive.

Pharmacodynamics/Kinetics

Absorption: Oral: Well absorbed

Bioavailability: >75%

Half-Life Elimination: 4-8 hours

Time to Peak: Serum: Oral: ~1 hour

Metabolism: Hepatic into its active components: Acrolein, 4-aldophosphamide, 4-hydroperoxycyclophosphamide, and nor-nitrogen mustard

Formulations

Injection, powder for reconstitution: 100 mg, 200 mg, 500 mg, 1 g, 2 g
Tablet: 25 mg, 50 mg

Dosing

Adults: Refer to individual protocols. Patients with compromised bone marrow function may require a 33% to 50% reduction in initial loading dose.

Usual dose:

Oral: 50-100 mg/m^2/day as continuous therapy or 400-1000 mg/m^2 in divided doses over 4-5 days as intermittent therapy

I.V.:

Single doses: 400-1800 mg/m^2 (30-50 mg/kg) per treatment course (1-5 days) which can be repeated at 2- to 4-week intervals
Maximum single dose without BMT is 7 g/m^2 (190 mg/kg) single agent therapy
Continuous daily doses: 60-120 mg/m^2 (1-2.5 mg/kg) per day

High dose BMT:

I.V.:

60 mg/kg/day for 2 days (total dose: 120 mg/kg)
50 mg/kg/day for 4 days (total dose: 200 mg/kg)
1.8 g/m^2/day for 4 days (total dose: 7.2 g/m^2)

Continuous I.V.:

1.5 g/m^2/24 hours for 96 hours (total dose: 6 g/m^2)
1875 mg/m^2/24 hours for 72 hours (total dose: 5625 mg/m^2)
Duration of infusion is 1-24 hours; generally combined with other high-dose chemotherapeutic drugs, lymphocyte immune globulin, or total body irradiation (TBI).

Nephrotic syndrome: Oral: 2-3 mg/kg/day every day for up to 12 weeks when corticosteroids are unsuccessful

Elderly: Refer to individual protocols: Initial and maintenance for induction: 1-2 mg/kg/day; adjust for renal clearance.

Pediatrics: Refer to individual protocols. Patients with compromised bone marrow function may require a 33% to 50% reduction in initial loading dose. Children:

Chemotherapy: Refer to adult dosing.
SLE: I.V.: 500-750 mg/m^2 every month; maximum dose: 1 g/m^2
JRA/vasculitis: I.V.: 10 mg/kg every 2 weeks
Nephrotic syndrome: Refer to adult dosing.

Renal Impairment: A large fraction of cyclophosphamide is eliminated by hepatic metabolism; some authors recommend no dose adjustment unless severe renal insufficiency (Cl_{cr} <20 mL/minute).

Cl_{cr} >10 mL/minute: Administer 100% of normal dose.
Cl_{cr} <10 mL/minute: Administer 75% of normal dose.
Hemodialysis effects: Moderately dialyzable (20% to 50%)
Administer dose posthemodialysis or administer supplemental 50% dose.
CAPD effects: Unknown
CAVH effects: Unknown

Hepatic Impairment: Some authors recommend dosage reductions (of up to 30%); however, the pharmacokinetics of cyclophosphamide are not significantly altered in the presence of hepatic insufficiency.

Administration

Oral: Tablets are not scored and should not be cut or crushed; should be administered during or after meals.

I.V.: May be administered I.M., I.P., intrapleurally, IVPB, or continuous intravenous infusion. I.V. infusions may be administered over 1-2 hours. Doses >500 mg to approximately 1 g may be administered over 20-30 minutes.

To minimize bladder toxicity, increase normal fluid intake during and for 1-2 days after cyclophosphamide dose. Most adult patients will require a fluid intake of at least 2 L/day. High-dose regimens should be accompanied by vigorous hydration with or without mesna therapy.

Stability

Storage: Store intact vials of powder at room temperature (25°C to 35°C).

Reconstitution: Reconstitute vials with SWI to a concentration of 20 mg/mL as follows below; reconstituted solutions are stable for 24 hours at room temperature (25°C) and 6 days at refrigeration (5°C).

(Continued)

Cyclophosphamide *(Continued)*

100 mg vial = 5 mL
200 mg vial = 10 mL
500 mg vial = 25 mL
1 g vial = 50 mL
2 g vial = 100 mL

Further dilutions in D_5W or NS are stable for 24 hours at room temperature (25°C) and 6 days at refrigeration (5°C).

Maximum concentration of cyclophosphamide is limited to 20 mg/mL due to solubility of cyclophosphamide.

Standard I.V. push dilution: Dose up to 500 mg/30 mL syringe

Maximum syringe size for IVP is a 30 mL syringe. Syringe should be ≤75% full.

Standard IVPB dilution: May further dilute in D_5W or NS after initial reconstitution with SWI

Doses up to 2 g/250 mL volume
Doses up to 4 g/500 mL volume

Compatibility: Stable in D_5LR, D_5NS, D_5W, LR, ½NS, NS

Y-site administration: Incompatible with amphotericin B cholesteryl sulfate complex

Monitoring Laboratory Tests CBC with differential, platelet count, ESR, BUN, UA, serum electrolytes, serum creatinine

Monitoring and Teaching Issues

Physical Assessment: See Warnings/Precautions, Contraindications, and Dosing for extensive use cautions. Assess potential for interactions with other prescriptions, OTC medications, or herbal products patient may be taking (eg, increased nephrotoxicity - see Drug Interactions). **I.V.:** See Administration and Compatibility. Monitor infusion site to prevent extravasation. Assess results of laboratory tests (see above), therapeutic effectiveness (according to purpose for use), and adverse response (see extensive list of Adverse Reactions and Overdose/Toxicology) prior to each infusion and regularly during therapy. Teach patient (or caregiver) proper use (oral), possible side effects and interventions (eg, importance of adequate hydration), and adverse symptoms to report (see Patient Education). **Pregnancy risk factor D** - determine that patient is not pregnant before beginning treatment. Instruct patients of childbearing age about appropriate barrier contraceptive measures during therapy and for 1 month following therapy. Breast-feeding is contraindicated.

Patient Education: Inform prescriber of all prescriptions, OTC medications, or herbal products you are taking, and any allergies you have. Do not take anything new during treatment unless approved by prescriber. Take exactly as directed, during or after meals; do not take at night. Maintain adequate hydration (2-3 L/day of fluids) unless advised by prescriber to restrict fluids and void frequently to reduce incidence of bladder irritation. You will be more susceptible to infection (avoid crowds and exposure to infection and do not have any vaccinations without consulting prescriber). May cause loss of hair (reversible, although regrowth hair may be different color or texture); fertility or amenorrhea; nausea or vomiting (small, frequent meals, good mouth care, chewing gum, or sucking lozenges may help - if persistent consult prescriber for antiemetic); headache (consult prescriber for analgesic); nasal congestion or cold symptoms (consult prescriber for decongestant); or mouth sores (use soft toothbrush or cotton swab for oral care). Report any difficulty or pain with urination; chest pain, rapid heartbeat, or palpitations; easy bruising or bleeding; unusual rash; persistent nausea or vomiting; menstrual irregularities; swelling of extremities; difficulty breathing; or unusual fatigue. **Pregnancy/breast-feeding precautions:** Inform prescriber if you are pregnant. Do not get pregnant during therapy or for 1 month following therapy. Consult prescriber for instruction on appropriate contraceptive measures. This drug may cause severe fetal defects. Do not breast-feed.

Dietary Issues: Tablets should be administered during or after meals.

Geriatric Considerations: Toxicity to immunosuppressives is increased in the elderly. Start with lowest recommended adult doses. Signs of infection, such as fever and WBC rise, may not occur. Lethargy and confusion may be more prominent signs of infection; adjust dose for renal function in the elderly.

Additional Information May be used in combination with mesna to prevent hemorrhagic cystitis. Rarely required for doses <1.5-2 g/m^2.

CycloSERINE (sye kloe SER een)

U.S. Brand Names Seromycin® Pulvules®

Generic Available No

Pharmacologic Category Antibiotic, Miscellaneous; Antitubercular Agent

Pregnancy Risk Factor C

Lactation Enters breast milk/compatible

Use Adjunctive treatment in pulmonary or extrapulmonary tuberculosis; has been studied for use in Gaucher's disease

Mechanism of Action/Effect Inhibits bacterial cell wall synthesis by competing with amino acid (D-alanine) for incorporation into the bacterial cell wall; bacteriostatic or bactericidal

Contraindications Hypersensitivity to cycloserine or any component of the formulation

Warnings/Precautions Epilepsy, depression, severe anxiety, psychosis, severe renal insufficiency, chronic alcoholism. Pregnancy risk C.

Drug Interactions

Increased Effect/Toxicity: Alcohol, isoniazid, and ethionamide increase toxicity of cycloserine. Cycloserine inhibits the hepatic metabolism of phenytoin and may increase risk of epileptic seizures.

Nutritional/Ethanol Interactions

Ethanol: Avoid ethanol (may increase CNS depression).

Food: May increase vitamin B_{12} and folic acid dietary requirements.

Adverse Reactions Frequency not defined.

Cardiovascular: Cardiac arrhythmias

Central nervous system: Drowsiness, headache, dizziness, vertigo, seizures, confusion, psychosis, paresis, coma
Dermatologic: Rash
Endocrine & metabolic: Vitamin B_{12} deficiency
Hematologic: Folate deficiency
Hepatic: Liver enzymes increased
Neuromuscular & skeletal: Tremor

Overdosage/Toxicology Symptoms of overdose include confusion, CNS depression, psychosis, coma, and seizures. Decontaminate with activated charcoal. Can be hemodialyzed. Management is supportive. Administer 100-300 mg/day of pyridoxine to reduce neurotoxic effects. Acute toxicity can occur with ingestion >1 g.

Pharmacodynamics/Kinetics

Absorption: ~70% to 90%

Half-Life Elimination: Normal renal function: 10 hours

Time to Peak: Serum: 3-4 hours

Metabolism: Hepatic

Formulations Capsule: 250 mg

Dosing

Adults & Elderly: Some of the neurotoxic effects may be relieved or prevented by the concomitant administration of pyridoxine.

Tuberculosis: Oral: Initial: 250 mg every 12 hours for 14 days, then give 500 mg to 1 g/day in 2 divided doses for 18-24 months (maximum daily dose: 1 g)

Pediatrics: Some of the neurotoxic effects may be relieved or prevented by the concomitant administration of pyridoxine.

Tuberculosis: Oral: Children: 10-20 mg/kg/day in 2 divided doses up to 1000 mg/day for 18-24 months

Renal Impairment:

Cl_{cr} 10-50 mL/minute: Administer every 12-24 hours.
Cl_{cr} <10 mL/minute: Administer every 24 hours.

Monitoring Laboratory Tests Periodic renal, hepatic, hematological tests, plasma cycloserine concentrations

Monitoring and Teaching Issues

Physical Assessment: See Warnings/Precautions, Contraindications, and Drug Interactions for use cautions. Assess results of laboratory tests (see above), therapeutic effectiveness, and adverse response (see extensive list of Adverse Reactions and Overdose/Toxicology) regularly during therapy. Teach patient proper use, possible side effects and interventions (eg, importance of adequate hydration), and adverse symptoms to report (see Patient Education). **Pregnancy risk factor C** - benefits of use should outweigh possible risks.

Patient Education: Take as prescribed; do not discontinue without consulting prescriber. Avoid alcohol. Maintain recommended diet and adequate hydration (2-3 L/day of fluids) unless advised by prescriber to restrict fluids. May cause drowsiness or restlessness (use caution when driving or engaging in tasks that require alertness until response to drug is known). Report skin rash, acute headache, tremors or changes in mentation (confusion, nightmares, depression, or suicide ideation), or fluid retention (difficulty breathing, swelling of extremities, unusual weight gain). **Pregnancy precaution:** Inform prescriber if you are or intend to become pregnant.

Dietary Issues: May be taken with food; may increase vitamin B_{12} and folic acid dietary requirements.

Geriatric Considerations: Adjust dose for renal function.

Related Information

FDA Name Differentiation Project: The Use of Tall-man Letters *on page 12*
Tuberculosis *on page 1705*

Cyclosporin A *see* CycloSPORINE *on page 343*

CycloSPORINE (SYE kloe spor een)

U.S. Brand Names Gengraf™; Neoral®; Sandimmune®

Synonyms CSA; CyA; Cyclosporin A

Generic Available Yes

Pharmacologic Category Immunosuppressant Agent

Pregnancy Risk Factor C

Lactation Enters breast milk/contraindicated

Use Prophylaxis of organ rejection in kidney, liver, and heart transplants, has been used with azathioprine and/or corticosteroids; severe, active rheumatoid arthritis (RA) not responsive to methotrexate alone; severe, recalcitrant plaque psoriasis in nonimmunocompromised adults unresponsive to or unable to tolerate other systemic therapy

Use - Unlabeled/Investigational Short-term, high-dose cyclosporine as a modulator of multidrug resistance in cancer treatment; allogenic bone marrow transplants for prevention and treatment of graft-versus-host disease; also used in some cases of severe autoimmune disease (ie, SLE, myasthenia gravis) that are resistant to corticosteroids and other therapy; focal segmental glomerulosclerosis

Mechanism of Action/Effect Inhibits T-lymphocytes and lymphokine production and release in a reversible manner.

Contraindications Hypersensitivity to cyclosporine or any component of the formulation. Rheumatoid arthritis and psoriasis: Abnormal renal function, uncontrolled hypertension, malignancies. Concomitant treatment with PUVA or UVB therapy, methotrexate, other immunosuppressive agents, coal tar, or radiation therapy are also contraindications for use in patients with psoriasis.

Warnings/Precautions Dose-related risk of nephrotoxicity and hepatotoxicity; monitor. Use caution with other potentially nephrotoxic drugs. Increased risk of lymphomas and other malignancies. Increased risk of infection. May cause hypertension. Use caution when changing dosage forms. Monitor cyclosporine concentrations closely following the addition,
(Continued)

CycloSPORINE *(Continued)*

modification, or deletion of other medications; live, attenuated vaccines may be less effective; use should be avoided.

Transplant patients: May cause significant hyperkalemia and hyperuricemia, seizures (particularly if used with high dose corticosteroids), and encephalopathy. To avoid toxicity or possible organ rejection, make dose adjustments based on cyclosporine blood concentrations. Anaphylaxis has been reported with I.V. use; reserve for patients who cannot take oral form.

Psoriasis: Patients should avoid excessive sun exposure. Safety and efficacy in children <18 have not been established.

Rheumatoid arthritis: Safety and efficacy for use in juvenile rheumatoid arthritis have not been established.

Products may contain corn oil, castor oil, ethanol, or propylene glycol; injection also contains Cremophor® EL (polyoxyethylated castor oil).

Pregnancy risk C.

Drug Interactions

Cytochrome P450 Effect: Substrate of **CYP3A4**; Inhibits CYP2C8/9, 3A4

Decreased Effect:

Drugs that decrease cyclosporine concentrations: Carbamazepine, nafcillin, phenobarbital, phenytoin, rifampin, isoniazid, ticlopidine

Cyclosporine decreases effect of: Live vaccines

Orlistat may decrease absorption of cyclosporine; avoid concomitant use.

Increased Effect/Toxicity: Increased toxicity:

Drugs that increase cyclosporine concentrations include allopurinol, metoclopramide, nicardipine, octreotide

In addition, serum level and/or toxicity of cyclosporine may be increased by CYP3A4 inhibitors. Inhibitors include amiodarone, bromocriptine, cimetidine, clarithromycin, danazol, erythromycin, delavirdine, diltiazem, disulfiram, fluconazole, fluoxetine, fluvoxamine, grapefruit juice, indinavir, itraconazole, ketoconazole, nefazodone, nevirapine, propoxyphene, quinupristin-dalfopristin, ritonavir, saquinavir, verapamil, zafirlukast, zileuton. Voriconazole may increase cyclosporine serum concentrations; decrease cyclosporine dosage by 50% when initiating voriconazole.

Drugs that enhance nephrotoxicity of cyclosporine: Aminoglycosides, amphotericin B, acyclovir, cimetidine, ketoconazole, lovastatin, melphalan, NSAIDs, ranitidine, trimethoprim and sulfamethoxazole, tacrolimus

Cyclosporine increases toxicity of: Digoxin, diuretics, methotrexate, nifedipine

Nutritional/Ethanol Interactions

Food: Grapefruit juice increases absorption; unsupervised use should be avoided.

Herb/Nutraceutical: Avoid St John's wort; as an enzyme inducer, it may increase the metabolism of and decrease plasma levels of cyclosporine. Avoid cat's claw, echinacea (have immunostimulant properties).

Effects on Lab Values Specific whole blood, HPLC assay for cyclosporine may be falsely elevated if sample is drawn from the same line through which dose was administered (even if flush has been administered and/or dose was given hours before).

Adverse Reactions Note: Adverse reactions reported generally reflect dosages used in transplantation, range is approximate/may overlap. [Reactions reported for rheumatoid arthritis (RA) are based on cyclosporine (modified) 2.5 mg/kg/day versus placebo.]

>10%:

Cardiovascular: Hypertension (13% to 53%; RA 8%; psoriasis 25% to 27%)

Central nervous system: Headache (2% to 15%; RA 17%, psoriasis 14% to 16%)

Dermatologic: Hirsutism (21% to 45%), hypertrichosis (5% to 19%)

Endocrine & metabolic: Increased triglycerides (psoriasis 15%), female reproductive disorder (psoriasis 8% to 11%)

Gastrointestinal: Nausea (RA 23%), diarrhea (RA 12%), gum hyperplasia (4% to 16%), abdominal discomfort (RA 15%), dyspepsia (RA 12%)

Neuromuscular & skeletal: Tremor (12% to 55%)

Renal: Renal dysfunction/nephropathy (25% to 38%; RA 10%, psoriasis 21%), creatinine elevation ≥50% (RA 24%), increased creatinine (psoriasis 16% to 20%)

Respiratory: Upper respiratory infection (psoriasis 8% to 11%)

Miscellaneous: Infection (psoriasis 24% to 25%)

1% to 10% (All indications, frequency range approximate):

Cardiovascular: Hypertension, edema, chest pain, arrhythmia, cardiac failure, myocardial infarction

Central nervous system: Dizziness, seizures (up to 5%), psychiatric events (up to 5%), pain, insomnia, depression, migraine, anxiety, vertigo

Dermatologic: Purpura, pruritus, acne, skin disorder, urticaria

Endocrine & metabolic: Menstrual disorder, diabetes mellitus, goiter, hyperkalemia, hyperuricemia, hypoglycemia, hyperglycemia, gynecomastia

Gastrointestinal: Vomiting, nausea, diarrhea, flatulence, gingivitis, gum hyperplasia, constipation, dry mouth, gastritis, gingival bleeding, taste perversion,

Genitourinary: Leukorrhea, urinary incontinence

Hematologic: Anemia, leukopenia, thrombocytopenia

Hepatic: Bilirubinemia, hepatotoxicity (<1% to 7%)

Neuromuscular & skeletal: Paresthesia, tremor, leg cramps/muscle contractions

Renal: Increased BUN, hematuria, renal abscess

Respiratory: Cough, dyspnea, bronchospasm, sinusitis

Miscellaneous: Infection, allergy, lymphoma, flu-like syndrome

<1% (Limited to important or life-threatening): Allergic reaction, bleeding disorder, deafness, death (due to renal deterioration), encephalopathy, gout, hyperbilirubinemia, hyperkalemia,

impaired consciousness, increased cholesterol, increased uric acid, mild hypomagnesemia, neurotoxicity, upper GI bleeding, vestibular disorder

Overdosage/Toxicology Symptoms of overdose include hepatotoxicity, nephrotoxicity, nausea, vomiting, tremor. CNS secondary to direct action of the drug may not be reflected in serum concentrations, may be more predictable by renal magnesium loss. Forced emesis may be beneficial if done within 2 hours of ingestion of cyclosporine capsules (modified). Treatment is symptomatic and supportive. Cyclosporine is not dialyzable.

Pharmacodynamics/Kinetics

Absorption: Oral:

Cyclosporine (non-modified): Erratic and incomplete; dependent on presence of food, bile acids, and GI motility; larger oral doses are needed in pediatrics due to shorter bowel length and limited intestinal absorption

Cyclosporine (modified): Erratic and incomplete; increased absorption, up to 30% when compared to cyclosporine (non-modified); less dependent on food, bile acids, or GI motility when compared to cyclosporine (non-modified)

Bioavailability: Oral:

Cyclosporine (non-modified): Dependent on patient population and transplant type (<10% in adult liver transplant patients and as high as 89% in renal transplant patients); bioavailability of Sandimmune® capsules and oral solution are equivalent; bioavailability of oral solution is ~30% of the I.V. solution

Children: 28% (range: 17% to 42%); gut dysfunction common in BMT patients and oral bioavailability is further reduced

Cyclosporine (modified): Bioavailability of Neoral® capsules and oral solution are equivalent:

Children: 43% (range: 30% to 68%)

Adults: 23% greater than with cyclosporine (non-modified) in renal transplant patients; 50% greater in liver transplant patients

Half-Life Elimination: Oral: May be prolonged with hepatic impairment and shorter in pediatric patients due to the higher metabolism rate

Cyclosporine (non-modified): Biphasic: Alpha: 1.4 hours; Terminal: 19 hours (range: 10-27 hours)

Cyclosporine (modified): Biphasic: Terminal: 8.4 hours (range: 5-18 hours)

Time to Peak: Serum: Oral:

Cyclosporine (non-modified): 2-6 hours; some patients have a second peak at 5-6 hours

Cyclosporine (modified): Renal transplant: 1.5-2 hours

Metabolism: Extensively hepatic via CYP; forms at least 25 metabolites; extensive first-pass effect following oral administration

Formulations

Capsule, soft gel, modified: 25 mg, 100 mg [contains castor oil, ethanol]

Gengraf™: 25 mg, 100 mg [contains ethanol, castor oil, propylene glycol]

Neoral®: 25 mg, 100 mg [contains dehydrated ethanol, corn oil, castor oil, propylene glycol]

Capsule, soft gel, non-modified (Sandimmune®): 25 mg, 100 mg [contains dehydrated ethanol, corn oil]

Injection, solution, non-modified (Sandimmune®): 50 mg/mL (5 mL) [contains Cremophor® EL (polyoxyethylated castor oil), ethanol]

Solution, oral, modified (Neoral®): 100 mg/mL (50 mL) [contains dehydrated ethanol, corn oil, castor oil, propylene glycol]

Solution, oral, non-modified (Sandimmune®): 100 mg/mL (50 mL) [contains olive oil, ethanol]

Dosing

Adults: Note: Neoral® and Sandimmune® are not bioequivalent and cannot be used interchangeably

Newly-transplanted patients: Adjunct therapy with corticosteroids is recommended. Initial dose should be given 4-12 hours prior to transplant or may be given postoperatively; adjust initial dose to achieve desired plasma concentration.

Oral: Dose is dependent upon type of transplant and formulation:

Cyclosporine (modified):

Renal: 9 ± 3 mg/kg/day, divided twice daily

Liver: 8 ± 4 mg/kg/day, divided twice daily

Heart: 7 ± 3 mg/kg/day, divided twice daily

Cyclosporine (non-modified): Initial dose: 15 mg/kg/day as a single dose (range 14-18 mg/kg); lower doses of 10-14 mg/kg/day have been used for renal transplants. Continue initial dose daily for 1-2 weeks; taper by 5% per week to a maintenance dose of 5-10 mg/kg/day; some renal transplant patients may be dosed as low as 3 mg/kg/day

When using the non-modified formulation, cyclosporine levels may increase in liver transplant patients when the T-tube is closed; dose may need decreased

I.V.: Cyclosporine (non-modified): Initial dose: 5-6 mg/kg/day as a single dose (1/3 the oral dose), infused over 2-6 hours; use should be limited to patients unable to take capsules or oral solution; patients should be switched to an oral dosage form as soon as possible

Conversion to cyclosporine (modified) from cyclosporine (non-modified): Start with daily dose previously used and adjust to obtain preconversion cyclosporine trough concentration. Plasma concentrations should be monitored every 4-7 days and dose adjusted as necessary, until desired trough level is obtained. When transferring patients with previously poor absorption of cyclosporine (non-modified), monitor trough levels at least twice weekly (especially if initial dose exceeds 10 mg/kg/day); high plasma levels are likely to occur.

Rheumatoid arthritis: Oral: Cyclosporine (modified): Initial dose: 2.5 mg/kg/day, divided twice daily; salicylates, NSAIDs, and oral glucocorticoids may be continued (refer to Drug Interactions); dose may be increased by 0.5-0.75 mg/kg/day if insufficient response is seen after 8 weeks of treatment; additional dosage increases may be made again at 12 weeks (maximum dose: 4 mg/kg/day). Discontinue if no benefit is seen by 16 weeks of therapy.

(Continued)

CycloSPORINE *(Continued)*

Note: Increase the frequency of blood pressure monitoring after each alteration in dosage of cyclosporine. Cyclosporine dosage should be decreased by 25% to 50% in patients with no history of hypertension who develop sustained hypertension during therapy and, if hypertension persists, treatment with cyclosporine should be discontinued.

Psoriasis: Oral: Cyclosporine (modified): Initial dose: 2.5 mg/kg/day, divided twice daily; dose may be increased by 0.5 mg/kg/day if insufficient response is seen after 4 weeks of treatment; additional dosage increases may be made every 2 weeks if needed (maximum dose: 4 mg/kg/day). Discontinue if no benefit is seen by 6 weeks of therapy. Once patients are adequately controlled, the dose should be decreased to the lowest effective dose. Doses <2.5 mg/kg/day may be effective. Treatment longer than 1 year is not recommended.

Note: Increase the frequency of blood pressure monitoring after each alteration in dosage of cyclosporine. Cyclosporine dosage should be decreased by 25% to 50% in patients with no history of hypertension who develop sustained hypertension during therapy and, if hypertension persists, treatment with cyclosporine should be discontinued.

Focal segmental glomerulosclerosis: Initial: 3 mg/kg/day divided every 12 hours

Autoimmune diseases: 1-3 mg/kg/day

Elderly: Refer to adult dosing (**Note:** Sandimmune® and Neoral® are not bioequivalent and cannot be used interchangeably without physician supervision).

Pediatrics: Transplant: Refer to adult dosing; children may require, and are able to tolerate, larger doses than adults.

Renal Impairment: For severe psoriasis:

Serum creatinine levels ≥25% above pretreatment levels: Take another sample within 2 weeks; if the level remains ≥25% above pretreatment levels, decrease dosage of cyclosporine (modified) by 25% to 50%. If two dosage adjustments do not reverse the increase in serum creatinine levels, treatment should be discontinued.

Serum creatinine levels ≥50% above pretreatment levels: Decrease cyclosporine dosage by 25% to 50%. If two dosage adjustments do not reverse the increase in serum creatinine levels, treatment should be discontinued.

Hemodialysis: Supplemental dose is not necessary.

Peritoneal dialysis: Supplemental dose is not necessary.

Hepatic Impairment: Dosage adjustment is probably necessary; monitor levels closely

Administration

Oral: Oral solution: May dilute Neoral® oral solution with orange juice or apple juice. May dilute Sandimmune® oral solution with milk, chocolate milk, or orange juice. Avoid changing diluents frequently. Mix thoroughly and drink at once. Use syringe provided to measure dose. Mix in a glass container and rinse container with more diluent to ensure total dose is taken. Do not rinse syringe before or after use (may cause dose variation).

I.V.: Following dilution, intravenous admixture should be administered over 2-6 hours. Patients should be under continuous observation for at least the first 30 minutes of the infusion, and should be monitored frequently thereafter.

Stability

Storage:

Capsule: Store at controlled room temperature

Injection: Store at controlled room temperature; do not refrigerate. Ampuls should be protected from light.

Oral solution: Store at controlled room temperature; do not refrigerate. Use within 2 months after opening; should be mixed in glass containers

Reconstitution:

Sandimmune® injection: Injection should be further diluted [1 mL (50 mg) of concentrate in 20-100 mL of D_5W or NS] for administration by intravenous infusion. Light protection is not required for intravenous admixtures of cyclosporine.

Stability of injection of parenteral admixture at room temperature (25°C) is 6 hours in PVC; 24 hours in Excel®, PAB® containers, or glass.

Polyoxyethylated castor oil (Cremophor® EL) surfactant in cyclosporine injection may leach phthalate from PVC containers such as bags and tubing. The actual amount of diethylhexyl phthalate (DEHP) plasticizer leached from PVC containers and administration sets may vary in clinical situations, depending on surfactant concentration, bag size, and contact time.

Compatibility: Stable in D_5W, fat emulsion 10%, fat emulsion 20%, NS

Y-site administration: Incompatible with amphotericin B cholesteryl sulfate complex

Compatibility when admixed: Incompatible with magnesium sulfate

Monitoring Laboratory Tests Cyclosporine levels, serum electrolytes, renal function, hepatic function

Monitoring and Teaching Issues

Physical Assessment: Assess effectiveness and interactions of other medications patient may be taking (see Drug Interactions). See Contraindications and Warnings/Precautions for use cautions. Monitor laboratory tests (see above), therapeutic response, and adverse reactions at beginning of therapy and periodically throughout therapy (see Warnings/Precautions, Adverse Reactions, and Overdose/Toxicology). **I.V.:** Monitor closely for first 30-60 minutes of infusion and frequently thereafter to assess for adverse reactions. **Oral:** Teach patient appropriate administration, possible side effects, and symptoms to report (see Patient Education). **Pregnancy risk factor C** - benefits of use should outweigh possible risks. Breast-feeding is contraindicated.

Patient Education: Diluting oral solution improves flavor. May dilute Neoral® oral solution with orange juice or apple juice. May dilute Sandimmune® oral solution with milk, chocolate milk, or orange juice. Avoid changing what you mix with your cyclosporine. Mix thoroughly and drink at once. Use syringe provided to measure dose. Mix in a glass container (do not use plastic or styrofoam) and rinse container with more juice/milk to ensure total dose is taken. Do not rinse syringe before or after use (may cause dose variation). Take dose at the same time each day. You will be susceptible to infection (avoid crowds and exposure to infection and do not have any vaccinations without consulting prescriber). Practice good oral hygiene to reduce gum inflammation; see a dentist regularly during treatment. Report severe headache; unusual hair growth or deepening of voice; mouth sores or swollen gums; persistent nausea, vomiting, or abdominal pain; muscle pain or cramping; unusual swelling of extremities, weight gain, or change in urination; or chest pain or rapid heartbeat. Increase in blood pressure or damage to the kidney is possible. Your prescriber will need to monitor closely. Do not change one brand of cyclosporine for another; any changes must be done by your prescriber. If you are taking this medication for psoriasis, your risk of cancer may be increased when taking additional medications. **Pregnancy/breast-feeding precautions:** Inform prescriber if you are or intend to become pregnant. Do not breast-feed.

Dietary Issues: Administer this medication consistently with relation to time of day and meals.

Pregnancy Issues: Cyclosporine crosses the placenta. Based on clinical use, premature births and low birth weight were consistently observed. Use only if the benefit to the mother outweighs the possible risks to the fetus.

Additional Information Cyclosporine (modified): Refers to the capsule dosage formulation of cyclosporine in an aqueous dispersion (previously referred to as "microemulsion"). Cyclosporine (modified) has increased bioavailability as compared to cyclosporine (non-modified) and cannot be used interchangeably without close monitoring.

In July, 2000, SangCya® (cyclosporine, modified) was voluntarily recalled due to lack of bioequivalency with Neoral® oral solution when mixed in apple juice. The product was allowed to remain in pharmacies to provide a transition time for changing patients to another cyclosporine product. Patients who were previously stabilized on this product should be instructed not to change how they mix their medication until they can be switched to another product. (SangCya® was previously marketed as a generic Neoral® oral solution.)

Related Information

FDA Name Differentiation Project: The Use of Tall-man Letters *on page 12*
Peak and Trough Guidelines *on page 1544*

Cylert® *see* Pemoline *on page 1042*

Cylex® [OTC] *see* Benzocaine *on page 156*

Cyomin® *see* Cyanocobalamin *on page 337*

Cyproheptadine (si proe HEP ta deen)

U.S. Brand Names Periactin®

Synonyms Cyproheptadine Hydrochloride

Generic Available Yes

Pharmacologic Category Antihistamine

Pregnancy Risk Factor B

Lactation Excretion in breast milk unknown/contraindicated

Use Perennial and seasonal allergic rhinitis and other allergic symptoms including urticaria

Use - Unlabeled/Investigational Appetite stimulation, blepharospasm, cluster headaches, migraine headaches, Nelson's syndrome, pruritus, schizophrenia, spinal cord damage associated spasticity, and tardive dyskinesia

Mechanism of Action/Effect A potent antihistamine and serotonin antagonist

Contraindications Hypersensitivity to cyproheptadine or any component of the formulation; narrow-angle glaucoma; bladder neck obstruction; acute asthmatic attack; stenosing peptic ulcer; GI tract obstruction; concurrent use of MAO inhibitors; avoid use in premature and term newborns due to potential association with SIDS

Warnings/Precautions Do not use in the presence of symptomatic prostate hypertrophy. Antihistamines are more likely to cause dizziness, excessive sedation, syncope, toxic confusion states, and hypotension in the elderly. In case reports, cyproheptadine has promoted weight gain in anorexic adults, though it has not been specifically studied in the elderly. All cases of weight loss or decreased appetite should be adequately assessed.

Drug Interactions

Increased Effect/Toxicity: Cyproheptadine may potentiate the effect of CNS depressants. MAO inhibitors may cause hallucinations when taken with cyproheptadine.

Nutritional/Ethanol Interactions Ethanol: Avoid ethanol (may increase CNS sedation).

Effects on Lab Values Diagnostic antigen skin tests; ↑ amylases (S); ↓ fasting glucose (S)

Adverse Reactions

>10%:
- Central nervous system: Slight to moderate drowsiness
- Respiratory: Thickening of bronchial secretions

1% to 10%:
- Central nervous system: Headache, fatigue, nervousness, dizziness
- Gastrointestinal: Appetite stimulation, nausea, diarrhea, abdominal pain, dry mouth
- Neuromuscular & skeletal: Arthralgia
- Respiratory: Pharyngitis

<1% (Limited to important or life-threatening): Bronchospasm, CNS stimulation, depression, epistaxis, hemolytic anemia, hepatitis, leukopenia, sedation, seizures, thrombocytopenia

Overdosage/Toxicology Symptoms of overdose include CNS depression or stimulation, dry mouth, flushed skin, fixed and dilated pupils, and apnea. There is no specific treatment for antihistamine overdose. Clinical toxicity is due to blockade of cholinergic receptors. For anticholinergic overdose with severe life-threatening symptoms, physostigmine 1-2 mg I.V. slowly, may be given to reverse these effects.

Pharmacodynamics/Kinetics

Absorption: Completely

Metabolism: Almost completely hepatic

Formulations

Syrup, as hydrochloride: 2 mg/5 mL [with alcohol 5%] (473 mL)
Tablet, as hydrochloride: 4 mg

(Continued)

Cyproheptadine *(Continued)*

Dosing

Adults:

Appetite stimulation (including anorexia nervosa): Oral: 2 mg 4 times/day; may be increased gradually over a 3-week period to 8 mg 4 times/day

Allergic conditions: Oral: 4-20 mg/day divided every 8 hours (not to exceed 0.5)

Cluster headaches: Oral: 4 mg 4 times/day

Migraine headaches: Oral: 4-8 mg 3 times/day

Spasticity associated with spinal cord damage: Oral: 4 mg at bedtime; increase by a 4 mg dose every 3-4 days; average daily dose: 16 mg in divided doses; not to exceed 36 mg/day

Elderly: Oral: Initial: 4 mg twice daily

Pediatrics:

Allergic conditions: Oral: Children: 0.25 mg/kg/day or 8 mg/m^2/day in 2-3 divided doses **or**

2-6 years: 2 mg every 8-12 hours (not to exceed 12 mg/day)

7-14 years: 4 mg every 8-12 hours (not to exceed 16 mg/day)

Migraine headaches: 4 mg 2-3 times/day

Spasticity associated with spinal cord damage: Oral: Children ≥12 years: Refer to adult dosing.

Appetite stimulation (Including anorexia nervosa): Children >13 years: Refer to adult dosing.

Hepatic Impairment: Dosage should be reduced in patients with significant hepatic dysfunction.

Monitoring and Teaching Issues

Physical Assessment: Assess effectiveness and interactions of other medications patient may be taking (see Drug Interactions). See Contraindications for use cautions. Monitor effectiveness of therapy and adverse reactions (eg, excess anticholinergic effects - see Adverse Reactions) at beginning of therapy and periodically with long-term use. Assess knowledge/teach patient appropriate use, interventions to reduce side effects, and adverse symptoms to report (see Patient Education). Breast-feeding is contraindicated.

Patient Education: Take as directed; do not exceed recommended dose. Avoid use of other depressants, alcohol, or sleep-inducing medications unless approved by prescriber. You may experience drowsiness or dizziness (use caution when driving or engaging in tasks requiring alertness until response to drug is known); or dry mouth, nausea, or abdominal pain (small, frequent meals, frequent mouth care, chewing gum, or sucking hard candy may help). Report persistent sedation, confusion, or agitation; changes in urinary pattern; blurred vision; chest pain or palpitations; sore throat difficulty breathing or expectorating (thick secretions); or lack of improvement or worsening or condition. **Breast-feeding precaution:** Do not breast-feed.

Geriatric Considerations: Elderly may not tolerate anticholinergic effects.

Additional Information May stimulate appetite; in case reports, cyproheptadine has promoted weight gain in anorexic adults.

Cyproheptadine Hydrochloride *see* Cyproheptadine *on page 347*

Cystospaz® *see* Hyoscyamine *on page 685*

Cystospaz-M® *see* Hyoscyamine *on page 685*

CYT *see* Cyclophosphamide *on page 339*

Cytadren® *see* Aminoglutethimide *on page 79*

Cytarabine (sye TARE a been)

U.S. Brand Names Cytosar-U®

Synonyms Arabinosylcytosine; Ara-C; Cytarabine Hydrochloride; Cytosine Arabinosine Hydrochloride

Generic Available Yes

Pharmacologic Category Antineoplastic Agent, Antimetabolite

Pregnancy Risk Factor D

Lactation Excretion in breast milk unknown/not recommended

Use Ara-C is one of the most active agents in leukemia; also active against lymphoma, meningeal leukemia, and meningeal lymphoma; has little use in the treatment of solid tumors

Mechanism of Action/Effect Inhibition of DNA synthesis in S Phase of cell division; degree of its cytotoxicity correlates linearly with its incorporation into DNA, therefore, incorporation into the DNA is responsible for drug activity and toxicity

Contraindications Hypersensitivity to cytarabine or any component of the formulation; pregnancy

Warnings/Precautions Use with caution in patients with impaired hepatic function. The U.S. Food and Drug Administration (FDA) currently recommends that procedures for proper handling and disposal of antineoplastic agents be considered. Must monitor drug tolerance, protect and maintain a patient compromised by drug toxicity that includes bone marrow depression with leukopenia, thrombocytopenia and anemia along with nausea, vomiting, diarrhea, abdominal pain, oral ulceration, and hepatic impairment. Marked bone marrow depression necessitates dosage reduction in the number of days of administration. If cytarabine contacts the skin, wash and flush thoroughly with water.

Drug Interactions

Decreased Effect: Decreased effect of gentamicin, flucytosine. Decreased digoxin oral tablet absorption.

Increased Effect/Toxicity: Alkylating agents and radiation, purine analogs, and methotrexate when coadministered with cytarabine result in increased toxic effects.

Adverse Reactions

>10%:

High-dose therapy toxicities: Cerebellar toxicity, conjunctivitis (make sure the patient is on steroid eye drops during therapy), corneal keratitis, hyperbilirubinemia, pulmonary edema, pericarditis, and tamponade

Central nervous system: Seizures (when given I.T.), cerebellar toxicity (ataxia, dysarthria, and dysdiadochokinesia; dose-related)
Dermatologic: Oral/anal ulceration, rash
Gastrointestinal: Nausea, vomiting, anorexia, stomatitis, mucositis
Emetic potential:
<500 mg: Moderately low (10% to 30%)
500 mg to 1500 mg: Moderately high (60% to 90%)
>1-1.5 g: High (>90%)
Time course of nausea/vomiting: Onset: 1-3 hours; Duration: 3-8 hours
Hematologic: Bleeding, leukopenia, thrombocytopenia
Myelosuppressive: Occurs within the first week of treatment and lasts for 10-14 days; primarily manifested as granulocytopenia, but anemia can also occur
WBC: Severe
Platelets: Severe
Onset (days): 4-7
Nadir (days): 14-18
Recovery (days): 21-28
Hepatic: Hepatic dysfunction, mild jaundice, increased transaminases
1% to 10%:
Cardiovascular: Cardiomegaly
Central nervous system: Dizziness, headache, somnolence, confusion, neuritis, malaise
Dermatologic: Skin freckling, itching, alopecia, cellulitis at injection site
Endocrine & metabolic: Hyperuricemia or uric acid nephropathy
Gastrointestinal: Esophagitis, diarrhea
Genitourinary: Urinary retention
Hematologic: Megaloblastic anemia
Hepatic: Hepatotoxicity
Local: Thrombophlebitis
Neuromuscular & skeletal: Myalgia, bone pain, peripheral neuropathy
Respiratory: Syndrome of sudden respiratory distress progressing to pulmonary edema, pneumonia
Miscellaneous: Sepsis
<1% (Limited to important or life-threatening): Pancreatitis

BMT:
Dermatologic: Rash, desquamation may occur following cytarabine and TBI
Gastrointestinal: Severe nausea and vomiting, mucositis, diarrhea
Neurologic:
Cerebellar toxicity: Nystagmus, dysarthria, dysdiadochokinesia, slurred speech
Cerebral toxicity: Somnolence, confusion
Ocular: Photophobia, excessive tearing, blurred vision, local discomfort, chemical conjunctivitis
Respiratory: Noncardiogenic pulmonary edema (onset 22-27 days following completion of therapy)

Overdosage/Toxicology Symptoms of overdose include myelosuppression, megaloblastosis, nausea, vomiting, respiratory distress, and pulmonary edema. A syndrome of sudden respiratory distress progressing to pulmonary edema and cardiomegaly has been reported following high doses. Treatment is symptomatic and supportive.

Pharmacodynamics/Kinetics

Half-Life Elimination: Initial: 7-20 minutes; Terminal: 0.5-2.6 hours

Metabolism: Primarily hepatic; aracytidine triphosphate is the active moiety; about 86% to 96% of dose is metabolized to inactive uracil arabinoside

Formulations

Injection, powder for reconstitution: 100 mg, 500 mg, 1 g, 2 g
Cytosar-U®: 100 mg, 500 mg, 1 g, 2 g

Dosing

Adults & Elderly: I.V. bolus, IVPB, and continuous intravenous infusion doses of cytarabine are very different. Bolus doses are relatively well tolerated since the drug is rapidly metabolized. Continuous infusion uniformly results in myelosuppression. Refer to individual protocols.

Induction remission:
I.V.: 200 mg/m^2/day for 5 days at 2-week intervals
100-200 mg/m^2/day for 5- to 10-day therapy course or every day until remission
I.T.: 5-75 mg/m^2 every 2-7 days until CNS findings normalize
Maintenance remission:
I.V.: 70-200 mg/m^2/day for 2-5 days at monthly intervals
I.M., S.C.: 1-1.5 mg/kg single dose for maintenance at 1- to 4-week intervals
High-dose therapies:
Doses as high as 1-3 g/m^2 have been used for refractory or secondary leukemias or refractory non-Hodgkin's lymphoma.
Doses of 3 g/m^2 every 12 hours for up to 12 doses have been used
Bone marrow transplant: 1.5 g/m^2 continuous infusion over 48 hours

Pediatrics: I.V. bolus, IVPB, and CIV doses of cytarabine are very different. Bolus doses are relatively well tolerated since the drug is rapidly metabolized; bolus doses are associated with greater gastrointestinal and neurotoxicity; continuous infusion uniformly results in myelosuppression. Refer to individual protocols.

Children:
Induction remission:
I.V.: 200 mg/m^2/day for 5 days at 2-week intervals
100-200 mg/m^2/day for 5- to 10-day therapy course or every day until remission
I.T.: 5-75 mg/m^2 every 4 days until CNS findings normalize
or
<1 year: 20 mg
1-2 years: 30 mg
2-3 years: 50 mg

(Continued)

Cytarabine *(Continued)*

>3 years: 70 mg

Maintenance remission: Refer to adult dosing.

Renal Impairment: In one study, 76% of patients with a Cl_{cr} <60 mL/minute experienced neurotoxicity. Dosage adjustment of high-dose therapy should be considered in patients with renal insufficiency.

Hepatic Impairment: Dose may need to be adjusted in patients with liver failure since cytarabine is partially detoxified in the liver.

Administration

I.V.: Can be administered I.M., IVP, I.V. infusion, or S.C. at a concentration not to exceed 100 mg/mL. I.V. may be administered either as a bolus, IVPB (high doses >500 mg/m^2) or continuous intravenous infusion (doses of 100-200 mg/m^2). Administer IVP at a rate of each 100 mg over 1-3 minutes. Administer IVPB over 30 minutes.

Other: Can be administered intrathecally.

Stability

Storage: Store intact vials of powder at room temperature 15°C to 30°C (59°F to 86°F).

Reconstitution: Warning: Bacteriostatic diluent should **not** be used for the preparation of either high doses or intrathecal doses of cytarabine. Reconstitute with SWI, D_5W or NS. Dilute to a concentration of 100 mg/mL as follows. Reconstituted solutions are stable for 48 hours at 15°C to 30°C.

100 mg vial = 1 mL
500 mg vial = 5 mL
1 g vial = 10 mL
2 g vial = 20 mL

Further dilution in D_5W or NS is stable for 8 days at room temperature (25°C)

Standard I.V. dilution:

I.V. push: Dose/syringe (concentration: 100 mg/mL)

Maximum syringe size for IVP is 30 mL syringe and syringe should be ≤75% full

IVPB: Dose/100 mL D_5W or NS

Continuous intravenous infusion: Dose/250-1000 mL D_5W or NS

Standard intrathecal dilutions:

Dose/3-5 mL lactated Ringer's ± methotrexate (12 mg) ± hydrocortisone (15-50 mg)

Intrathecal solutions in 3-20 mL lactated Ringer's are stable for 7 days at room temperature (30°C); however, should be used within 24 hours due to sterility concerns.

Compatibility: Stable in D_5LR, $D_5{}^1/_4NS$, D_5NS, $D_{10}NS$, D_5W, LR, NS

Y-site administration: Incompatible with allopurinol, amphotericin B cholesteryl sulfate complex, ganciclovir

Compatibility when admixed: Incompatible with fluorouracil, gentamicin, heparin, insulin (regular), nafcillin, oxacillin, penicillin G sodium

Monitoring Laboratory Tests Liver function, CBC with differential and platelet count, serum creatinine, BUN, serum uric acid

Monitoring and Teaching Issues

Physical Assessment: See Contraindications,Warnings/Precautions, and Dosing for use cautions (eg, antiemetic, steroid eye drops). Assess potential for interactions with other prescriptions, OTC medications, or herbal products patient may be taking (see Drug Interactions). See Administration, Dosing, Reconstitution, and Compatibility for administration specifics. Premedicate with antiemetic; especially with larger doses. Assess results of laboratory tests (see above) and monitor adverse response (see extensive list of Adverse Reactions and Overdose/Toxicology) prior to therapy and on a regular basis throughout therapy. Teach patient possible side effects and interventions (eg, importance of adequate hydration) and adverse symptoms to report (see Patient Education). **Pregnancy risk factor D** - determine that patient is not pregnant before beginning treatment. Instruct patients of childbearing age about appropriate barrier contraceptive measures. Breast-feeding is not recommended.

Patient Education: Inform prescriber of all prescriptions, OTC medications, or herbal products you are taking, and any allergies you have. Do not take anything new during treatment unless approved by prescriber. This drug can only be given by infusion or injection. Report immediately any redness, swelling, burning, or pain at injection/infusion site. Maintain adequate hydration (2-3 L/day of fluids) unless advised by prescriber to restrict fluids. You will be more susceptible to infection (avoid crowds and exposure to infection and do not have any vaccinations without consulting prescriber). May cause nausea, vomiting or loss of appetite (small, frequent meals, frequent mouth care, sucking lozenges, or chewing gum may help - if ineffective, consult prescriber for antiemetic medication); diarrhea (buttermilk, boiled milk, or yogurt may help - if persistent, consult with prescriber); mouth sores (use soft toothbrush or cotton swabs for oral care); or dizziness, headache, or confusion (use caution when driving or engaging in potentially hazardous tasks until response to drug is known). Report immediately any signs of CNS changes, change in gait, respiratory distress or difficulty breathing, easy bruising or bleeding, persistent GI upset, yellowing of eyes or skin, change in color of urine or blackened stool, or any other persistent adverse effects. **Pregnancy/breast-feeding precautions:** Inform prescriber if you are pregnant. Do not get pregnant during or for 1 month following therapy. Consult prescriber for instruction on appropriate contraceptive measures. This drug may cause severe fetal defects. Do not breast-feed.

Additional Information

Supplied with diluent containing benzyl alcohol, which should not be used when preparing either high-dose or I.T. doses.

Latex-free products: 100 mg, 500 mg, 1 g, 2 g vials (Cytosar-U®) by Pharmacia-Upjohn

Cytarabine Hydrochloride *see* Cytarabine *on page 348*

Cytarabine (Liposomal) (sye TARE a been lip po SOE mal)

U.S. Brand Names DepoCyt™

Generic Available No

Pharmacologic Category Antineoplastic Agent, Antimetabolite

Pregnancy Risk Factor D

Lactation Excretion in breast milk unknown/not recommended

Use Treatment of neoplastic (lymphomatous) meningitis

Mechanism of Action/Effect This is a sustained-release formulation of the active ingredient cytarabine. Acts to inhibit DNA polymerase which decreases DNA synthesis and repair.

Contraindications Hypersensitivity to cytarabine or any component of the formulation; active meningeal infection; pregnancy

Warnings/Precautions The U.S. Food and Drug Administration (FDA) currently recommends that procedures for proper handling and disposal of antineoplastic agents be considered. The incidence and severity of chemical arachnoiditis is reduced by coadministration with dexamethasone. May cause neurotoxicity. Blockage to CSF flow may increase the risk of neurotoxicity.

Drug Interactions

Decreased Effect: No formal studies of interactions with other medications have been conducted. The limited systemic exposure minimizes the potential for interaction between liposomal cytarabine and other medications.

Increased Effect/Toxicity: No formal studies of interactions with other medications have been conducted. The limited systemic exposure minimizes the potential for interaction between liposomal cytarabine and other medications.

Effects on Lab Values Since cytarabine liposomes are similar in appearance to WBCs, care must be taken in interpreting CSF examinations in patients receiving liposomal cytarabine

Adverse Reactions Chemical arachnoiditis is commonly observed, and may include neck pain, neck rigidity, headache, fever, nausea, vomiting, and back pain. It may occur in up to 100% of cycles without dexamethasone prophylaxis. The incidence is reduced to 33% when dexamethasone is used concurrently.

>10%:
- Central nervous system: Headache (28%), confusion (14%), somnolence (12%), fever (11%), pain (11%)
- Gastrointestinal: Vomiting (12%), nausea (11%)

1% to 10%:
- Cardiovascular: Peripheral edema (7%)
- Gastrointestinal: Constipation (7%)
- Genitourinary: Incontinence (3%)
- Hematologic: Neutropenia (9%), thrombocytopenia (8%), anemia (1%)
- Neuromuscular & skeletal: Back pain (7%), weakness (19%), abnormal gait (4%)

<1% (Limited to important or life-threatening): Anaphylaxis, neck pain

Overdosage/Toxicology No overdosage with liposomal cytarabine has been reported. See Cytarabine monograph for toxicology related to systemic administration.

Pharmacodynamics/Kinetics

Absorption: Systemic exposure following intrathecal administration is negligible since transfer rate from CSF to plasma is slow

Half-Life Elimination: CSF: 100-263 hours

Time to Peak: CSF: Intrathecal: ~5 hours

Metabolism: In plasma to ara-U (inactive)

Formulations Injection: 10 mg/mL (5 mL)

Dosing

Adults & Elderly:

Lymphomatous meningitis: I.T.:
- Induction: 50 mg intrathecally every 14 days for a total of 2 doses (weeks 1 and 3)
- Consolidation: 50 mg intrathecally every 14 days for 3 doses (weeks 5, 7, and 9), followed by an additional dose at week 13
- Maintenance: 50 mg intrathecally every 28 days for 4 doses (weeks 17, 21, 25, and 29)

If drug-related neurotoxicity develops, dose should be reduced to 25 mg. If toxicity persists, treatment with liposomal cytarabine should be discontinued.

Note: Patients should be started on dexamethasone 4 mg twice daily (oral or I.V.) for 5 days, beginning on the day of liposomal cytarabine injection.

Administration

Other: For intrathecal use only. Dose should be removed from vial immediately before administration (must be administered within 4 hours of removal). An in-line filter should **not** be used. Vials are intended for a single use and contain no preservative. Administer directly into the CSF via an intraventricular reservoir or by direct injection into the lumbar sac. Injection should be made slowly (over 1-5 minutes). Patients should lie flat for 1 hour after lumbar puncture. Patients should be monitored closely for immediate toxic reactions.

Stability

Storage: Store under refrigeration (2°C to 8°C); protect from freezing and avoid aggressive agitation. Solutions should be used within 4 hours of withdrawal from the vial. Particles may settle in diluent over time, and may be resuspended by gentle agitation or inversion of the vial.

Monitoring Laboratory Tests Since cytarabine liposomes are similar in appearance to WBCs, care must be taken in interpreting CSF examinations in patients receiving liposomal cytarabine.

Monitoring and Teaching Issues

Physical Assessment: This medication if only for intrathecal administration. See Contraindications and Warnings/Precautions for use cautions. Patient must be monitored closely for adverse reactions, which may be immediate The incidence and severity of chemical arachnoiditis is reduced by coadministration with dexamethasone (see Adverse Reactions and Overdose/Toxicology). Provide patient teaching according to patient condition (see Patient Education). **Pregnancy risk factor D**. Breast-feeding is not recommended.

Patient Education: Patient instruction will be according to mental status. This medication can only be given I.V. into the spinal cord. You will be monitored closely during and after each infusion. Report immediately any neck pain or rigidity, headache, fever, nausea, or vomiting. Report any swelling of extremities, acute weakness, unusual gait pattern, or other

(Continued)

Cytarabine (Liposomal) *(Continued)*

adverse effects. **Pregnancy/breast-feeding precautions:** Inform prescriber if you are pregnant. Breast-feeding is not recommended.

Cytochrome P450 Enzymes: Substrates, Inhibitors, and Inducers *see page 1588*

CytoGam® *see* Cytomegalovirus Immune Globulin (Intravenous/Human) *on page 352*

Cytomegalovirus Immune Globulin (Intravenous/Human)

(sye toe meg a low VYE rus i MYUN GLOB yoo lin in tra VEE nus HYU man)

U.S. Brand Names CytoGam®

Synonyms CMV-IGIV

Generic Available No

Pharmacologic Category Immune Globulin

Pregnancy Risk Factor C

Lactation Excretion in breast milk unknown

Use Prophylaxis of cytomegalovirus (CMV) disease associated with kidney, lung, liver, pancreas, and heart transplants; concomitant use with ganciclovir should be considered in organ transplants (other than kidney) from CMV seropositive donors to CMV seronegative recipients; has been used as adjunct therapy in the treatment of CMV disease in immunocompromised patients

Mechanism of Action/Effect CMV-IGIV is a preparation of immunoglobulin G (as well as trace amounts of IgA and IgM) derived from pooled healthy blood donors with a high titer of CMV antibodies; administration provides a passive source of antibodies against cytomegalovirus

Contraindications Hypersensitivity to CMV-IGIV, other immunoglobulins, or any component of the formulation; immunoglobulin A deficiency

Warnings/Precautions Monitor for anaphylactic reactions during infusion. May theoretically transmit blood-borne viruses. Use with caution in patients with renal insufficiency, diabetes mellitus, patients >65 years of age, volume depletion, sepsis, paraproteinemia, or patients on concomitant nephrotoxic drugs. Stabilized with sucrose and albumin, contains no preservative. Pregnancy risk C.

Drug Interactions

Decreased Effect: Decreased effect of live vaccines may be seen if given within 3 months of IGIV administration. Defer vaccination or revaccinate.

Adverse Reactions

<6%:

Cardiovascular: Flushing

Central nervous system: Fever, chills

Gastrointestinal: Nausea, vomiting

Neuromuscular & skeletal: Arthralgia, back pain, muscle cramps

Respiratory: Wheezing

<1%: Blood pressure decreased

Postmarketing and/or case reports: Acute renal failure, acute tubular necrosis, AMS, anaphylactic shock, angioneurotic edema, anuria, BUN increase, serum creatinine increase, oliguria, osmotic nephrosis, proximal tubular nephropathy

Overdosage/Toxicology Symptoms related to volume overload would be expected to occur with overdose; treatment is symptom-directed and supportive.

Formulations Injection, powder for reconstitution, detergent-treated: 2500 mg ± 500 mg (50 mL); 1000 mg ± 200 mg (20 mL)

Dosing

Adults:

Kidney transplant: I.V.:

Initial dose (within 72 hours of transplant): 150 mg/kg/dose

2-, 4-, 6-, and 8 weeks after transplant: 100 mg/kg/dose

12 and 16 weeks after transplant: 50 mg/kg/dose

Liver, lung, pancreas, or heart transplant: I.V.:

Initial dose (within 72 hours of transplant): 150 mg/kg/dose

2-, 4-, 6-, and 8 weeks after transplant: 150 mg/kg/dose

12 and 16 weeks after transplant: 100 mg/kg/dose

Severe CMV pneumonia: I.V.: Various regimens have been used, including 400 mg/kg CMV-IGIV in combination with ganciclovir on days 1, 2, 7, or 8, followed by 200 mg/kg CMV-IGIV on days 14 and 21

Elderly: Use with caution in patients >65 years of age; elderly may be at increased risk of renal insufficiency.

Renal Impairment: Use with caution; specific dosing adjustments are not available. Infusion rate should be the minimum practical; do not exceed 180 mg/kg/hour.

Administration

I.V.: For I.V. use only. Administer as separate infusion. Infuse beginning at 15 mg/kg/hour, then increase to 30 mg/kg/hour after 30 minutes if no untoward reactions. May titrate up to 60 mg/kg/hour. Do not administer faster than 75 mL/hour. Begin infusion within 6 hours of entering vial, complete infusion within 12 hours.

Stability

Storage: Store between 2°C and 8°C (35.6°F and 46.4°F)

Reconstitution: Dilution is not recommended. Do not shake vials. Do not use if turbid.

Compatibility: Infusion with other products is not recommended. If unavoidable, may be piggybacked into an I.V. line of sodium chloride, 2.D_5W, D_5W, $D_{10}W$, or $D_{20}W$; do not dilute more than 1:2

Monitoring and Teaching Issues

Physical Assessment: Assess for history of previous allergic reactions (see Contraindications). See Administration for safe infusion. Monitor vital signs during infusion and observe for adverse or allergic reactions (see Adverse Reactions). Teach patient adverse symptoms to report (see Patient Education). **Pregnancy risk factor C** - benefits of use should outweigh possible risks. Note breast-feeding caution.

Patient Education: This medication can only be administered by infusion. You will be monitored closely during the infusion. If you experience nausea ask for assistance, do not get up alone. Do not have any vaccinations for the next 3 months without consulting prescriber. Immediately report chills, muscle cramping, low back pain, chest pain or tightness, or difficulty breathing. **Pregnancy/breast-feeding precautions:** Inform prescriber if you are or intend to become pregnant. Consult prescriber if breast-feeding.

Cytosar-U® *see* Cytarabine *on page 348*

Cytosine Arabinosine Hydrochloride *see* Cytarabine *on page 348*

Cytotec® *see* Misoprostol *on page 912*

Cytovene® *see* Ganciclovir *on page 618*

Cytoxan® *see* Cyclophosphamide *on page 339*

d4T *see* Stavudine *on page 1245*

Dacarbazine (da KAR ba zeen)

U.S. Brand Names DTIC-Dome®

Synonyms DIC; Dimethyl Triazeno Imidazol Carboxamide; DTIC; Imidazole Carboxamide

Generic Available Yes

Pharmacologic Category Antineoplastic Agent, Alkylating Agent

Pregnancy Risk Factor C

Lactation Excretion in breast milk unknown/not recommended

Use Treatment of malignant melanoma, Hodgkin's disease, soft-tissue sarcomas, fibrosarcomas, rhabdomyosarcoma, islet cell carcinoma, medullary carcinoma of the thyroid, and neuroblastoma

Mechanism of Action/Effect Inhibits DNA/RNA and protein synthesis; cytotoxic

Contraindications Hypersensitivity to dacarbazine or any component

Warnings/Precautions The U.S. Food and Drug Administration (FDA) currently recommends that procedures for proper handling and disposal of antineoplastic agents be considered. Use with caution in patients with bone marrow depression. In patients with renal and/or hepatic impairment, dosage reduction may be necessary. Avoid extravasation of the drug.

Dacarbazine preparation should be performed in a Class II laminar flow biologic safety cabinet. Personnel should be wearing surgical gloves and a closed front surgical gown with knit cuffs. Appropriate safety equipment is recommended for preparation, administration, and disposal of antineoplastics. If dacarbazine contacts the skin, wash and flush thoroughly with water.

Pregnancy risk C.

Drug Interactions

Cytochrome P450 Effect: Substrate of **CYP1A2, 2E1**

Decreased Effect: Metabolism may be increased by drugs that induce hepatic enzymes (carbamazepine, phenytoin, phenobarbital, and rifampin), potentially leading to decreased efficacy. Patients may experience impaired immune response to vaccines; possible infection after administration of live vaccines in patients receiving immunosuppressants.

Nutritional/Ethanol Interactions

Ethanol: Avoid ethanol (due to GI irritation).

Herb/Nutraceutical: Avoid dong quai, St John's wort (may also cause photosensitization).

Adverse Reactions

>10%:

Local: Pain and burning at infusion site

Irritant chemotherapy

Gastrointestinal: Anorexia; moderate to severe nausea and vomiting in 90% of patients and lasting up to 12 hours after administration; nausea and vomiting are dose-related and occur more frequently when given as a one-time dose, as opposed to a less intensive 5-day course; diarrhea may also occur

Hematologic: Anemia, leukopenia, thrombocytopenia

Emetic potential:

<500 mg: Moderately high (60% to 90%)

≥500 mg: High (>90%)

Time course of nausea/vomiting: Onset: 1-2 hours; Duration: 2-4 hours

1% to 10%:

Cardiovascular: Facial flushing

Central nervous system: Headache

Dermatologic: Alopecia, rash

Flu-like effects: Fever, malaise, headache, myalgia, and sinus congestion may last up to several days after administration

Gastrointestinal: Anorexia, metallic taste

Hematologic: Myelosuppressive: Mild to moderate is common and dose-related dose-limiting toxicity

WBC: Mild (primarily leukocytes)

Platelets: Mild

Onset (days): 7

Nadir (days): 21-25

Recovery (days): 21-28

Neuromuscular & skeletal: Paresthesias

Respiratory: Sinus congestion

<1% (Limited to important or life-threatening): Alopecia, elevated LFTs, headache, hepatic vein thrombosis, hepatocellular necrosis, orthostatic hypotension, photosensitivity reactions, polyneuropathy, seizures

BMT:

Cardiovascular: Hypotension (infusion-related)

Gastrointestinal: Severe nausea and vomiting

Overdosage/Toxicology Symptoms of overdose include myelosuppression and diarrhea. There are no known antidotes and treatment is symptomatic and supportive.

(Continued)

Dacarbazine *(Continued)*

Pharmacodynamics/Kinetics

Half-Life Elimination: Biphasic: Initial: 20-40 minutes; Terminal: 5 hours

Metabolism: Extensively hepatic; hepatobiliary excretion is probably of some importance; metabolites may also have an antineoplastic effect

Onset: I.V.: 18-24 days

Formulations Injection, powder for reconstitution: 200 mg, 500 mg

DTIC-Dome®: 100 mg, 200 mg

Dosing

Adults & Elderly: Refer to individual protocols. Some dosage regimens include:

Intra-arterial: 50-400 mg/m^2 for 5-10 days

ABVD for Hodgkin's disease: I.V.: 375 mg/m^2 days 1 and 15 every 4 weeks

Metastatic melanoma (alone or in combination with other agents): I.V.: 150-250 mg/m^2 days 1-5 every 3-4 weeks

Metastatic melanoma: I.V.: 850 mg/m^2 every 3 weeks

High dose: Bone marrow/blood cell transplantation: I.V.: 1-3 g/m^2; maximum dose as a single agent: 3.38 g/m^2; generally combined with other high-dose chemotherapeutic drugs

Pediatrics: Refer to individual protocols.

Pediatric solid tumors: I.V.: 200-470 mg/m^2/day over 5 days every 21-28 days

Pediatric neuroblastoma: I.V.: 800-900 mg/m^2 as a single dose on day 1 of therapy every 3-4 weeks in combination therapy

Hodgkin's disease: I.V.: 375 mg/m^2 on days 1 and 15 of treatment course, repeat every 28 days

Renal Impairment: Adjustment is warranted.

Hepatic Impairment: Monitor closely for signs of toxicity.

Administration

I.V.: Irritant. Infuse over 30-60 minutes.

Stability

Storage: Store intact vials under refrigeration (2°C to 8°C) and protect from light. Vials are stable for 4 weeks at room temperature.

Reconstitution: Reconstitute with a minimum of 2 mL (100 mg vial) or 4 mL (200 mg vial) of SWI, D_5W, or NS. Dilute to a concentration of 10 mg/mL as follows. Reconstituted solution is stable for 24 hours at room temperature (20°C) and 96 hours under refrigeration (4°C):

100 mg vial = 9.9 mL
200 mg vial = 19.7 mL
500 mg vial = 49.5 mL

Further dilution in 200-500 mL of D_5W or NS is stable for 24 hours at room temperature and protected from light. Decomposed drug turns pink.

Standard I.V. dilution: Dose/250-500 mL D_5W or NS

Stable for 24 hours at room temperature and refrigeration (4°C) when protected from light.

Compatibility: Stable in NS, sterile water for injection

Y-site administration: Incompatible with allopurinol, cefepime, piperacillin/tazobactam

Compatibility when admixed: Incompatible with hydrocortisone sodium succinate

Monitoring Laboratory Tests CBC with differential, platelet count, liver function

Monitoring and Teaching Issues

Physical Assessment: See Contraindications, Warnings/Precautions, and Dosing for use cautions. Assess potential for interactions with other prescriptions, OTC medications, or herbal products patient may be taking (see Drug Interactions). See Administration, Dosing, Reconstitution, and Compatibility for administration specifics. Premedicate with antiemetic (emetic potential is moderately high). Infusion site must be closely monitored; extravasation can cause severe cellulitis or tissue necrosis (see Administration). Assess results of laboratory tests (see above), therapeutic effectiveness, and adverse response (see Adverse Reactions and Overdose/Toxicology) prior to each treatment and on a regular basis throughout therapy. Teach patient possible side effects and interventions and adverse symptoms to report (see Patient Education). **Pregnancy risk factor C** - benefits of use should outweigh possible risks. Breast-feeding is not recommended.

Patient Education: Inform prescriber of all prescriptions, OTC medications, or herbal products you are taking, and any allergies you have. Do not take anything new during treatment unless approved by prescriber. This drug can only be given by infusion. Report immediately any pain, burning, or swelling at infusion site. Limit oral intake for 4-6 hours before infusion. Maintain adequate hydration (2-3 L/day of fluids) unless advised by prescriber to restrict fluids, and nutrition (small, frequent meals). You will be more susceptible to infection (avoid crowds and exposure to infection and do not have any vaccinations without consulting prescriber). May cause nausea, vomiting, loss of appetite, or diarrhea (consult prescriber for medication); hair loss (reversible); or headache, fever, sinus congestion, or muscles aches (consult prescriber for analgesic). Report immediately any numbness in extremities or change in gait, respiratory distress or difficulty breathing; rash; easy bruising or bleeding; yellowing of eyes or skin, change in color of urine or blackened stool; or any other persistent adverse effects. **Pregnancy/breast-feeding precautions:** Inform prescriber if you are pregnant. Breast-feeding is not recommended.

Daclizumab (dac KLYE zue mab)

U.S. Brand Names Zenapax®

Generic Available No

Pharmacologic Category Immunosuppressant Agent

Pregnancy Risk Factor C

Lactation Excretion in breast milk unknown/use caution

Use Part of an immunosuppressive regimen (including cyclosporine and corticosteroids) for the prophylaxis of acute organ rejection in patients receiving renal transplant

Use - Unlabeled/Investigational Graft-versus-host disease

Contraindications Hypersensitivity to daclizumab or any component of the formulation

Warnings/Precautions Patients on immunosuppressive therapy are at increased risk for infectious complications and secondary malignancies. Long-term effects of daclizumab on immune function are unknown. Severe hypersensitivity reactions have been rarely reported; anaphylaxis is a potential side effect of protein infusion; medications for the management of severe allergic reaction should be available for immediate use. Readministration of daclizumab after an initial course of therapy has not been studied. Anti-idiotype antibodies have been measured in patients that have received daclizumab (adults 14%; children 34%); detection of antibodies may be influenced by multiple factors and may therefore be misleading. Pregnancy risk C.

Adverse Reactions Although reported adverse events are frequent, when daclizumab is compared with placebo the incidence of adverse effects is similar between the two groups. Many of the adverse effects reported during clinical trial use of daclizumab may be related to the patient population, transplant procedure, and concurrent transplant medications. Diarrhea, fever, postoperative pain, pruritus, respiratory tract infections, urinary tract infections, and vomiting occurred more often in children than adults.

≥5%:

- Cardiovascular: Chest pain, edema, hypertension, hypotension, tachycardia, thrombosis
- Central nervous system: Dizziness, fatigue, fever, headache, insomnia, pain, post-traumatic pain, tremor
- Dermatologic: Acne, cellulitis, wound healing impaired
- Gastrointestinal: Abdominal distention, abdominal pain, constipation, diarrhea, dyspepsia, epigastric pain, nausea, pyrosis, vomiting
- Genitourinary: Dysuria
- Hematologic: Bleeding
- Neuromuscular & skeletal: Back pain, musculoskeletal pain
- Renal: Oliguria, renal tubular necrosis
- Respiratory: Cough, dyspnea, pulmonary edema,
- Miscellaneous: Lymphocele, wound infection

≥2% to < 5%:

- Central nervous system: Anxiety, depression, shivering,
- Dermatologic: Hirsutism, pruritus, rash, diaphoresis
- Endocrine & metabolic: Dehydration, diabetes mellitus, fluid overload
- Gastrointestinal: Flatulence, gastritis, hemorrhoids
- Genitourinary: Urinary retention, urinary tract bleeding
- Local: Application site reaction
- Neuromuscular & skeletal: Arthralgia, leg cramps, myalgia, weakness
- Ocular: Vision blurred
- Renal: Hydronephrosis, renal damage, renal insufficiency
- Respiratory: Atelectasis, congestion, hypoxia, pharyngitis, pleural effusion, rales, rhinitis
- Miscellaneous: Night sweats, prickly sensation

<1% (Limited to important or life-threatening): Severe hypersensitivity reactions (rare)

Overdosage/Toxicology Overdose has not been reported.

Pharmacodynamics/Kinetics

Half-Life Elimination: Estimated: Adults: Terminal: 20 days; Children: 13 days

Formulations Injection, solution [preservative free]: 5 mg/mL (5 mL)

Dosing

Adults:

Note: Daclizumab is used adjunctively with other immunosuppressants (eg, cyclosporine, corticosteroids, mycophenolate mofetil, and azathioprine).

Immunoprophylaxis against acute renal allograft rejection: I.V.: 1 mg/kg infused over 15 minutes within 24 hours before transplantation (day 0), then every 14 days for 4 additional doses

Treatment of graft-versus-host disease (unlabeled use, limited data): I.V.: 0.5-1.5 mg/kg, repeat same dosage for transient response. Repeat doses have been administered 11-48 days following the initial dose.

Elderly: Refer to adult dosing. Use with caution.

Pediatrics: Refer to adult dosing.

Renal Impairment: No dosage adjustment needed.

Hepatic Impairment: No data available for patients with severe impairment.

Administration

I.V.: For I.V. administration following dilution. Daclizumab solution should be administered within 4 hours of preparation if stored at room temperature; infuse over a 15-minute period via a peripheral or central vein.

Stability

Storage: Refrigerate vials at 2°C to 8°C (36°F to 46°F). Do not shake or freeze; protect undiluted solution against direct sunlight.

Reconstitution: Dose should be further diluted in 50 mL 0.9% sodium chloride solution. When mixing, gently invert bag to avoid foaming; do not shake. Do not use if solution is discolored. Diluted solution is stable for 24 hours at 4°C or for 4 hours at room temperature.

Compatibility: Do not mix with other medications or infuse other medications through same I.V. line.

Monitoring and Teaching Issues

Physical Assessment: See Contraindications, Warnings/Precautions, and Dosing for use cautions. Assess potential for interactions with other prescriptions, OTC medications, or herbal products patient may be taking. See administration specifics above. Assess cardiorespiratory and renal function (fluid overload) and adverse reactions (see Adverse Reactions) during infusion and periodically between infusions. **Note:** Hypersensitivity reactions can occur; medications for immediate treatment of severe allergic reactions should be available for immediate use. Teach patient possible side effects and appropriate interventions and adverse symptoms to report (see Patient Education). **Pregnancy risk factor C** - benefits of use should outweigh possible risks. Note breast-feeding caution.

(Continued)

Daclizumab *(Continued)*

Patient Education: This medication, which may help transplant rejection, can only be administered by infusion. You will be monitored closely during infusion. Report immediately any difficulty breathing or swallowing; tightness in jaw or throat; chest pain; or rash, pain, burning, redness, or swelling at infusion site. You will be more susceptible to infection (avoid crowds and exposure to infection and do not have any vaccinations without consulting prescriber). Maintain adequate hydration (2-3 L/day of fluids unless instructed to restrict fluid intake) and nutrition (small, frequent meals may be advisable). May cause headache, dizziness, fatigue (use caution when driving or engaged in tasks that require alertness until response to drug is known): back pain, leg cramps, or musculoskeletal pain (consult prescriber for approved analgesic); or nausea, vomiting, dyspepsia, or abdominal discomfort (good mouth care, small, frequent meals, chewing gum, or sucking lozenges may help). Report changes in urinary pattern; unusual bleeding or bruising; chest pain or palpitations; persistent dizziness, tremors, or headache; difficulty breathing or unusual cough; rash; opportunistic infection (vaginal itching or drainage, sores in mouth, unusual fever or chills); or other persistent adverse effects. **Pregnancy/breast-feeding precautions:** Inform prescriber if you are or intend to become pregnant. Consult prescriber if breast-feeding.

Dactinomycin (dak ti noe MYE sin)

U.S. Brand Names Cosmegen®

Synonyms ACT; Actinomycin D

Generic Available No

Pharmacologic Category Antineoplastic Agent, Antibiotic

Pregnancy Risk Factor C

Lactation Excretion in breast milk unknown/contraindicated

Use Treatment of testicular tumors, melanoma, choriocarcinoma, Wilms' tumor, neuroblastoma, retinoblastoma, rhabdomyosarcoma, uterine sarcomas, Ewing's sarcoma, Kaposi's sarcoma, sarcoma botryoides, and soft tissue sarcoma

Mechanism of Action/Effect Causes cell death by inhibiting messenger RNA

Contraindications Hypersensitivity to dactinomycin or any component of the formulation; patients with concurrent or recent chickenpox or herpes zoster; avoid in infants <6 months of age

Warnings/Precautions The U.S. Food and Drug Administration (FDA) currently recommends that procedures for proper handling and disposal of antineoplastic agents be considered. Drug is extremely irritating to tissues and must be administered I.V. If extravasation occurs during I.V. use, severe damage to soft tissues will occur. Use with caution in patients who have received radiation therapy or in the presence of hepatobiliary dysfunction. Reduce dosage in patients who are receiving radiation therapy simultaneously. Pregnancy risk C.

Drug Interactions

Increased Effect/Toxicity: Dactinomycin potentiates the effects of radiation therapy. Radiation may cause skin erythema which may become severe. Also associated with GI toxicity.

Nutritional/Ethanol Interactions Ethanol: Avoid ethanol (due to GI irritation).

Effects on Lab Values May interfere with bioassays of antibacterial drug levels

Adverse Reactions

>10%:

Central nervous system: Unusual fatigue, malaise, fever

Dermatologic: Alopecia (reversible), skin eruptions, acne, increased pigmentation of previously irradiated skin, cheilitis

Endocrine & metabolic: Hypocalcemia

Gastrointestinal: **Highly emetogenic**

Severe nausea and vomiting occurs in most patients and persists for up to 24 hours; stomatitis, anorexia, abdominal pain, esophagitis, diarrhea, dysphagia, GI ulceration, pharyngitis

Time course of nausea/vomiting: Onset: 2-5 hours; Duration: 4-24 hours

Hematologic: Myelosuppressive: Dose-limiting toxicity; anemia, aplastic anemia, agranulocytosis, pancytopenia, leukopenia, thrombocytopenia, reticulopenia

WBC: Moderate

Platelets: Moderate

Onset: 7 days

Nadir: 14-21 days

Recovery: 21-28 days

Hepatic: Liver toxicity, ascites, hepatomegaly, hepatitis

Local: Extravasation: An irritant and should be administered through a rapidly running I.V. line; extravasation can lead to tissue necrosis, pain, and ulceration

Vesicant chemotherapy

1% to 10%: Gastrointestinal: Mucositis

<1% (Limited to important or life-threatening): Anaphylactoid reaction, hepatitis, hyperuricemia, LFT abnormalities

Overdosage/Toxicology Symptoms of overdose include myelosuppression, nausea, vomiting, glossitis, and oral ulceration. There are no known antidotes and treatment is symptomatic and supportive.

Pharmacodynamics/Kinetics

Half-Life Elimination: 36 hours

Time to Peak: Serum: I.V.: 2-5 minutes

Metabolism: Minimally hepatic

Formulations Injection, powder for reconstitution: 0.5 mg [contains mannitol 20 mg]

Dosing

Adults & Elderly: Refer to individual protocols.

Dactinomycin doses are almost ALWAYS expressed in MICROGRAMS rather than milligrams. Some practitioners recommend calculation of the dosage for obese or edematous patients on the basis of body surface area in an effort to relate dosage to lean body mass.

Usual dose: I.V.: 500 mcg daily for a maximum of 5 days; dosage should not exceed 15 mcg/kg/day or 400-600 mcg/m^2/day for 5 days; a second course may be given after at least 3 weeks have elapsed, provided all signs of toxicity have disappeared

Other regimens have included:

0.75-2 mg/m^2 as a single dose given at intervals of 1-4 weeks

400-600 mcg/m^2/day for 5 days, repeated every 3-6 weeks

Pediatrics: Refer to individual protocols.

Dactinomycin doses are almost ALWAYS expressed in MICROGRAMS rather than milligrams. Some practitioners recommend calculation of the dosage for obese or edematous patients on the basis of body surface area in an effort to relate dosage to lean body mass.

Usual dose: I.V.: Children >6 months: 15 mcg/kg/day for 5 days **or** 2.5 mg/m^2 given over 1-week period; a second course may be given after at least 3 weeks have elapsed, provided all signs of toxicity have disappeared

Other regimens have included:

0.75-2 mg/m^2 as a single dose given at intervals of 1-4 weeks

400-600 mcg/m^2/day for 5 days, repeated every 3-6 weeks

Renal Impairment: No adjustment is necessary.

Administration

I.V.: Vesicant. Infuse over 10-15 minutes.

Stability

Storage: Store intact vials at room temperature (30°C) and protect from light. Storage at high temperatures (up to 50°C) for up to 2 weeks is permissible.

Reconstitution: Dilute with 1.1 mL of preservative-free SWI to yield a final concentration of 500 mcg/mL. Do not use preservative diluent as precipitation may occur. Solution is chemically stable for 24 hours at room temperature (25°C). Significant binding of the drug occurs with micrometer nitrocellulose filter materials.

Standard I.V. dilution:

I.V. push: Dose/syringe (500 mcg/mL)

IVPB: Dose/50 mL D_5W or NS

Stable for 24 hours at room temperature.

Compatibility: Stable in D_5W, NS, sterile water for injection

Y-site administration: Incompatible with filgrastim

Monitoring Laboratory Tests CBC with differential and platelet count, liver and renal function

Monitoring and Teaching Issues

Physical Assessment: See Contraindications, Warnings/Precautions, and Dosing for use cautions. Assess potential for interactions with other prescriptions, OTC medications, or herbal products patient may be taking (see Drug Interactions). See Administration, Dosing, Reconstitution, and Compatibility for administration specifics. Premedicate with antiemetic (highly emetic). Infusion site must be closely monitored; extravasation can cause severe cellulitis or tissue necrosis (see Administration). Assess results of laboratory tests (see above), therapeutic response, and adverse response (see Adverse Reactions and Overdose/Toxicology) prior to each treatment and on a regular basis throughout therapy. Teach patient possible side effects and interventions and adverse symptoms to report (see Patient Education). **Pregnancy risk factor C** - benefits of use should outweigh possible risks. Breast-feeding is contraindicated.

Patient Education: Inform prescriber of all prescriptions, OTC medications, or herbal products you are taking, and any allergies you have. Do not take anything new during treatment unless approved by prescriber. This drug can only be given by infusion; report immediately any pain, burning, or swelling at infusion site. Limit oral intake for 4-6 hours before infusion. During therapy, maintain adequate hydration (2-3 L/day of fluids) unless advised by prescriber to restrict fluids, and nutrition (small, frequent meals). Avoid alcohol. You will be more susceptible to infection (avoid crowds and exposure to infection and do not have any vaccinations without consulting prescriber). May cause fatigue or malaise (use caution when driving or engaging in potentially hazardous tasks until response to drug is known); nausea, vomiting, loss of appetite, or diarrhea (consult prescriber for medication); or hair loss (reversible). Report unresolved nausea, vomiting, diarrhea, abdominal pain, or difficulty swallowing; sudden respiratory distress or difficulty breathing; rash; or any other persistent adverse effects. **Pregnancy/breast-feeding precautions:** Inform prescriber if you are or intend to become pregnant. Do not breast-feed.

Breast-feeding Issues: It is not known if dactinomycin is excreted in human breast milk. Due to the potential for serious reactions in the infant, breast-feeding is not recommended.

Pregnancy Issues: Malformations reported in animal studies. No controlled studies in pregnant women. Use only when potential benefit justifies potential risk to the fetus.

D.A.II™ Tablet *see page 1522*

Dalalone® *see* Topical Corticosteroids *on page 1334*

Dalalone L.A.® *see* Topical Corticosteroids *on page 1334*

Dallergy® *see page 1522*

Dalmane® *see* Flurazepam *on page 583*

***d*-Alpha Tocopherol** *see* Vitamin E *on page 1406*

Dalteparin (dal TE pa rin)

U.S. Brand Names Fragmin®

Generic Available No

Pharmacologic Category Low Molecular Weight Heparin

Pregnancy Risk Factor B

Lactation Excretion in breast milk unknown/use caution

Use Prevention of deep vein thrombosis which may lead to pulmonary embolism, in patients requiring abdominal surgery who are at risk for thromboembolism complications (ie, patients

(Continued)

Dalteparin *(Continued)*

>40 years of age, obesity, patients with malignancy, history of deep vein thrombosis or pulmonary embolism, and surgical procedures requiring general anesthesia and lasting longer than 30 minutes); prevention of DVT in patients undergoing hip surgery; acute treatment of unstable angina or non-Q-wave myocardial infarction; prevention of ischemic complications in patients on concurrent aspirin therapy

Use - Unlabeled/Investigational Active treatment of deep vein thrombosis

Mechanism of Action/Effect Low molecular weight heparin analog; the commercial product contains 3% to 15% heparin; has been shown to inhibit both factor Xa and factor IIa (thrombin), however, the antithrombotic effect of dalteparin is characterized by a higher ratio of antifactor Xa to antifactor IIa activity (ratio = 4)

Contraindications Hypersensitivity to dalteparin or any component of the formulation; thrombocytopenia associated with a positive *in vitro* test for antiplatelet antibodies in the presence of dalteparin; hypersensitivity to pork products; patient with active major bleeding; not for I.M. or I.V. use

Warnings/Precautions

Patients with recent or anticipated neuraxial anesthesia (epidural or spinal anesthesia) are at risk of spinal or epidural hematoma and subsequent paralysis. Consider risk versus benefit prior to neuraxial anesthesia. Risk is increased by concomitant agents which may alter hemostasis, as well as traumatic or repeated epidural or spinal puncture. Patient should be observed closely for bleeding if dalteparin is administered during or immediately following diagnostic lumbar puncture, epidural anesthesia, or spinal anesthesia.

Not to be used interchangeably (unit for unit) with heparin or any other low molecular weight heparins. Use caution in patients with known hypersensitivity to methylparaben or propylparaben, renal failure, or a history of heparin-induced thrombocytopenia. Monitor patient closely for signs or symptoms of bleeding. Certain patients are at increased risk of bleeding. Risk factors include bacterial endocarditis; congenital or acquired bleeding disorders; active ulcerative or angiodysplastic GI diseases; severe uncontrolled hypertension, hemorrhagic stroke; or use shortly after brain, spinal, or ophthalmology surgery; in patient treated concomitantly with platelet inhibitors; recent GI bleeding; thrombocytopenia or platelet defects; severe liver disease; hypertensive or diabetic retinopathy; or in patients undergoing invasive procedures. Rare cases of thrombocytopenia with thrombosis have occurred. Multidose vials contain benzyl alcohol and should not be used in pregnant women. Heparin can cause hyperkalemia by affecting aldosterone. Similar reactions could occur with LMWHs. Monitor for hyperkalemia. Discontinue therapy if platelets are <100,000/mm^3. Safety and efficacy in pediatric patients have not been established.

Drug Interactions

Increased Effect/Toxicity: The risk of bleeding with dalteparin may be increased by drugs which affect platelet function (eg, aspirin, NSAIDs, dipyridamole, ticlopidine, clopidogrel), oral anticoagulants, and thrombolytic agents. Although the risk of bleeding may be increased during concurrent warfarin therapy, dalteparin is commonly continued during the initiation of warfarin therapy to assure anticoagulation and to protect against possible transient hypercoagulability.

Nutritional/Ethanol Interactions Herb/Nutraceutical: Avoid cat's claw, dong quai, evening primrose, garlic, ginseng (all have additional antiplatelet activity).

Effects on Lab Values ↑ AST, ALT levels

Adverse Reactions

1% to 10%

Hematologic: Bleeding (3% to 5 %), wound hematoma (0.1% to 3%)

Local: Pain at injection site (up to 12%), injection site hematoma (0.2% to 7%)

<1% (Limited to important or life-threatening): Allergic reaction (fever, pruritus, rash, injection site reaction, bullous eruption), anaphylactoid reaction, gastrointestinal bleeding, injection site hematoma, operative site bleeding, skin necrosis, thrombocytopenia (including heparin-induced thrombocytopenia). Spinal or epidural hematomas can occur following neuraxial anesthesia or spinal puncture, resulting in paralysis. Risk is increased in patients with indwelling epidural catheters or concomitant use of other drugs affecting hemostasis, osteoporosis (3-6 month use).

Pharmacodynamics/Kinetics

Half-Life Elimination: Route dependent: 2-5 hours

Time to Peak: Serum: 4 hours

Onset: 1-2 hours

Duration: >12 hours

Formulations

Injection, solution [multidose vial]: Antifactor Xa 10,000 int. units per 1 mL (9.5 mL) [contains benzyl alcohol]

Injection, solution [preservative free; prefilled syringe]: Antifactor Xa 2500 int. units per 0.2 mL (0.2 mL); antifactor Xa 5000 int. units per 0.2 mL (0.2 mL); antifactor Xa 7500 int. units per 0.3 mL (0.3 mL); antifactor Xa 10,000 int. units per 1 mL (1 mL)

Dosing

Adults & Elderly:

Low-moderate risk patients undergoing abdominal surgery: S.C.: 2500 int. units 1-2 hours prior to surgery, then once daily for 5-10 days postoperatively

High-risk patients undergoing abdominal surgery: S.C.: 5000 int. units 1-2 hours prior to surgery and then once daily for 5-10 days postoperatively

Patients undergoing total hip surgery: S.C.: **Note:** Three treatment options are currently available. Dose is given for 5-10 days, although up to 14 days of treatment have been tolerated in clinical trials:

Postoperative start:

Initial: 2500 int. units 4-8 hours* after surgery

Maintenance: 5000 int. units once daily; start at least 6 hours after postsurgical dose

Preoperative (starting day of surgery):

Initial: 2500 int. units within 2 hours before surgery

Adjustment: 2500 int. units 4-8 hours* after surgery

Maintenance: 5000 int. units once daily; start at least 6 hours after postsurgical dose

Preoperative (starting evening prior to surgery):

Initial: 5000 int. units 10-14 hours before surgery

Adjustment: 5000 int. units 4-8 hours* after surgery

Maintenance: 5000 int. units once daily, allowing 24 hours between doses.

***Dose may be delayed if hemostasis is not yet achieved.**

Patients with unstable angina or non-Q-wave myocardial infarction: S.C.: 120 int. units/kg body weight (maximum dose: 10,000 int. units) every 12 hours for 5-8 days with concurrent aspirin therapy. Discontinue dalteparin once patient is clinically stable.

Administration

I.M.: Do not give I.M.

Other: Administer deep S.C. only, alternate injection site R → L anterolateral/posterolateral abdominal wall. Do not give I.M. Apply pressure to injection site. Do not massage.

Stability

Storage: Store at temperatures 20°C to 25°C (68°F to 77°F).

Monitoring Laboratory Tests Periodic CBC including platelet count, stool occult blood; monitoring of PT and PTT is not necessary.

Monitoring and Teaching Issues

Physical Assessment: See Contraindications, Warnings/Precautions, and Dosing for use cautions. Assess potential for interactions with other prescription and OTC medications or herbal products patient may be taking (especially anything that will impact coagulation or platelet aggregation - see Drug Interactions). Assess laboratory tests (see above), therapeutic effectiveness, and adverse response (eg, thrombolytic reactions - see Adverse Reactions and Overdose/Toxicology). Teach patient possible side effects and interventions and adverse symptoms to report (see Patient Education). Note breast-feeding caution.

Patient Education: Inform prescriber of all prescriptions, OTC medications, or herbal products you are taking, and any allergies you have. Do not take anything new during treatment unless approved by prescriber. This drug can only be administered by injection. You may have a tendency to bleed easily while taking this drug (brush teeth with soft brush, use waxed dental floss, use electric razor, avoid scissors or sharp knives and potentially harmful activities). Report unusual fever; unusual bleeding or bruising (bleeding gums, nosebleed, blood in urine, dark stool); pain in joints or back; severe head pain; skin rash; or redness, swelling, or pain at injection site. **Breast-feeding precaution:** Consult prescriber if breast-feeding.

Pregnancy Issues: Multiple-dose vials contain benzyl alcohol (avoid in pregnant women due to association with fetal syndrome in premature infants).

Additional Information Multidose vial contains 14 mg/mL benzyl alcohol.

Related Information

Heparins *on page 1576*

Damason-P® *see* Hydrocodone and Aspirin *on page 669*

Danaparoid (da NAP a roid)

U.S. Brand Names Orgaran® [DSC]

Synonyms Danaparoid Sodium

Generic Available No

Pharmacologic Category Anticoagulant

Pregnancy Risk Factor B

Lactation Excretion in breast milk unknown/compatible

Use Prevention of postoperative deep vein thrombosis following elective hip replacement surgery

Use - Unlabeled/Investigational Systemic anticoagulation for patients with heparin-induced thrombocytopenia: factor Xa inhibition is used to monitor degree of anticoagulation if necessary

Mechanism of Action/Effect Prevents fibrin formation in coagulation pathway via thrombin generation inhibition by anti-Xa and anti-IIa effects.

Contraindications Hypersensitivity to danaparoid or thrombocytopenia associated with a positive *in vitro* test for antiplatelet antibodies in the presence of danaparoid; hypersensitivity to pork products or to sulfites (contains metabisulfite); patients with active major bleeding; severe hemorrhagic diathesis (hemophilia, idiopathic thrombocytopenic purpura); not for I.M. or I.V. use

Warnings/Precautions

Patients with recent or anticipated neuraxial anesthesia (epidural or spinal anesthesia) are at risk of spinal or epidural hematoma and subsequent paralysis. Consider risk versus benefit prior to neuraxial anesthesia; Risk is increased by concomitant agents which may alter hemostasis, as well as traumatic or repeated epidural or spinal puncture. Patient should be observed closely for bleeding if danaparoid is administered during or immediately following diagnostic lumbar puncture, epidural anesthesia, or spinal anesthesia.

Not to be used interchangeably (unit for unit) with heparin or any other low molecular weight heparins. Use caution in patients with a known hypersensitivity to methylparaben or propylparaben, renal impairment, or a history of heparin-induced thrombocytopenia. Monitor patient closely for signs or symptoms of bleeding. Certain patients are at increased risk of bleeding. Risk factors include bacterial endocarditis; congenital or acquired bleeding disorders; active ulcerative or angiodysplastic GI diseases; severe uncontrolled hypertension; hemorrhagic stroke; use shortly after brain, spinal, or ophthalmology surgery; patient treated concomitantly with platelet inhibitors; recent GI bleeding; thrombocytopenia or platelet defects; severe liver disease; hypertensive or diabetic retinopathy; or patients undergoing invasive procedures. Safety and efficacy in pediatric patients have not been established. Heparin can cause hyperkalemia by affecting aldosterone. A similar reaction could occur with danaparoid. Monitor for hyperkalemia. Discontinue therapy if platelets are $<100,000/mm^3$. Safety and efficacy in pediatric patients have not been established.

(Continued)

Danaparoid *(Continued)*

Drug Interactions

Increased Effect/Toxicity: The risk of hemorrhage associated with danaparoid may be increased with thrombolytic agents, oral anticoagulants (warfarin) and drugs which affect platelet function (eg, aspirin, NSAIDs, dipyridamole, ticlopidine, clopidogrel).

Nutritional/Ethanol Interactions Herb/Nutraceutical: Avoid cat's claw, dong quai, evening primrose, feverfew, garlic, ginger, ginkgo, red clover, horse chestnut, green tea, and ginseng (all have additional antiplatelet activity).

Adverse Reactions As with all anticoagulants, bleeding is the major adverse effect of danaparoid. Hemorrhage may occur at virtually any site. Risk is dependent on multiple variables.

>10%:
- Central nervous system: Fever (22.2%)
- Gastrointestinal: Nausea (4.1% to 14.3%), constipation (3.5% to 11.3%)

1% to 10%:
- Cardiovascular: Peripheral edema (3.3%), edema (2.6%)
- Central nervous system: Insomnia (3.1%), headache (2.6%), asthenia (2.3%), dizziness (2.3%), pain (8.7%)
- Dermatologic: Rash (2.1% to 4.8%), pruritus (3.9%)
- Gastrointestinal: Vomiting (2.9%)
- Genitourinary: Urinary tract infection (2.6% to 4.0%), urinary retention (2.0%)
- Hematologic: Anemia (2.2%)
- Local: Injection site pain (7.6% to 13.7%), injection site hematoma (5%)
- Neuromuscular & skeletal: Joint disorder (2.6%)
- Miscellaneous: Infection (2.1%)

<1% (Limited to important or life-threatening): Spinal or epidural hematomas can occur following neuraxial anesthesia or spinal puncture, resulting in paralysis. Risk is increased in patients with indwelling epidural catheters or concomitant use of other drugs affecting hemostasis, thrombocytopenia, hyperkalemia, wound infection, skin rash, allergic reaction.

Overdosage/Toxicology Symptoms of overdose include hemorrhage. Protamine zinc has been used to reverse effects, but the effects of danaparoid are not effectively antagonized.

Pharmacodynamics/Kinetics

Half-Life Elimination: Plasma: Mean: Terminal: ~24 hours

Onset: Peak effect: S.C.: Maximum antifactor Xa and antithrombin (antifactor IIa) activities occur in 2-5 hours

Formulations Injection, solution, as sodium [prefilled syringe or ampul]: 750 anti-Xa units/0.6 mL (0.6 mL) [contains sodium sulfite]

Dosing

Adults:

Prevention of DVT following hip replacement: S.C.: 750 anti-Xa units twice daily; beginning 1-4 hours before surgery and then not sooner than 2 hours after surgery and every 12 hours until the risk of DVT has diminished, the average duration of therapy is 7-10 days

Treatment (unlabeled uses): See table.

Adult Danaparoid Treatment Dosing Regimens (Not FDA Approved)

	Body Weight (kg)	I.V. Bolus aFXaU	Long–Term Infusion aFXaU	Level of aFXaU/mL	Monitoring
Deep Vein Thrombosis OR Acute Pulmonary Embolism	<55 55-90 >90	1250 2500 3750	400 units/h over 4 h then 300 units/h over 4 h, then 150-200 units/h maintenance dose	0.5-0.8	Days 1-3 daily, then every alternate day
Deep Vein Thrombosis OR Pulmonary Embolism >5 d old	<90 >90	1250 1250	S.C.: 3 x 750/d S.C.: 3 x 1250/d	<0.5	Not necessary
Embolectomy	<90 >90 and high risk	2500 preoperatively 2500 preoperatively	S.C.: 2 x 1250/d postoperatively 150-200 units/hour I.V.; perioperative arterial irrigation, if necessary: 750 units/20 mL NaCl	<0.4 0.5-0.8	Not necessary Days 1-3 daily, then every alternate day
Peripheral Arterial Bypass		2500 preoperatively	150-200 units/h	0.5-0.8	Days 1-3 daily, then every alternate day
Cardiac Catheter	<90 >90	2500 preoperatively 3750 preoperatively			
Surgery (excluding vascular)			S.C.: 750, 1-4 h preoperatively S.C.: 750, 2-5 h postoperatively, then 2 x 750/d	<0.35	Not necessary

S.C.: 750 anti-Xa units twice daily; beginning 1-4 hours before surgery and then not sooner than 2 hours after surgery and every 12 hours until the risk of DVT has diminished; the average duration of therapy is 7-10 days.

Elderly: Dose adjustment may be necessary in elderly patients with severe renal impairment.

Pediatrics: S.C.: Children: Safety and effectiveness have not been established.

Renal Impairment: Adjustment may be necessary in patients with severe renal impairment. Patients with serum creatinine levels ≥2.0 mg/dL should be carefully monitored. S.C.: Hemodialysis: See table.

Hemodialysis With Danaparoid Sodium

Dialysis on alternate days	**Dosage prior to dialysis in aFXaU (dosage for body wt <55 kg)**	
First dialysis	3750 (<55 kg 2500)	
Second dialysis	3750 (<55 kg 2000)	
Further dialysis:		
aFXa level before dialysis (eg, day 5)	**Bolus before next dialysis, aFXaU (eg, day 7)**	**aFXa level during dialysis**
<0.3	3000 (<55 kg 2000)	0.5-0.8
0.3-0.35	2500 (<55 kg 2000)	
0.35-0.4	2000 (<55 kg 1500)	
>0.4	No bolus; if fibrin strands occur, 1500 aFXaU I.V.	
Monitoring: 30 minutes before dialysis and after 4 hours of dialysis		
Daily Dialysis		
First dialysis	3750 (<55 kg 2500)	
Second dialysis	2500 (<55 kg 2000)	
Further dialyses	See above	
As with "dialysis on alternate days", always take the aFXa activity preceding the previous dialysis as a basis for the current dosage.		

Administration

I.M.: Do not administer I.M.

Other: Administer by subcutaneous injection, **not** I.M. Have patient lie down and administer by deep S.C. injection using a fine needle (25- to 26-gauge). Rotate sites of injection.

Stability

Storage: Store intact vials or ampuls under refrigeration

Monitoring Laboratory Tests Platelets, occult blood, anti-Xa activity, if available; the monitoring of PT and/or PTT is not necessary.

Monitoring and Teaching Issues

Physical Assessment: See Contraindications, Warnings/Precautions, and Dosing for use cautions. Assess potential for interactions with other prescription and OTC medications or herbal products patient may be taking (especially anything that will impact coagulation or platelet aggregation - see Drug Interactions). Assess results of laboratory tests (see above), therapeutic effectiveness, and adverse response (eg, thrombolytic reactions - see Adverse Reactions and Overdose/Toxicology). Teach patient appropriate use if self-administered (injection technique and needle disposal), possible side effects and interventions (eg, bleeding precautions), and adverse symptoms to report (see Patient Education).

Patient Education: Inform prescriber of all prescriptions, OTC medications, or herbal products you are taking, and any allergies you have. Do not take anything new during treatment unless approved by prescriber. This drug can only be administered by injection. You may have a tendency to bleed easily while taking this drug (brush teeth with soft brush, floss with waxed floss, use electric razor, avoid scissors or sharp knives and potentially harmful activities). Report unusual fever; unusual bleeding or bruising (bleeding gums, nosebleed, blood in urine, dark stool); pain in joints or back; severe head pain; skin rash; or redness, swelling, or pain at injection site.

Geriatric Considerations: Evaluation of elderly's creatinine serum concentrations is important before initiating therapy.

Additional Information A 750 anti-Xa unit dose of danaparoid is approximately equivalent to 55 mg of danaparoid.

Related Information

Heparins *on page 1576*

Danaparoid Sodium *see* Danaparoid *on page 359*

Danazol (DA na zole)

U.S. Brand Names Danocrine®

Generic Available Yes

Pharmacologic Category Androgen

Pregnancy Risk Factor X

Lactation Enters breast milk/contraindicated

Use Treatment of endometriosis, fibrocystic breast disease, and hereditary angioedema

Mechanism of Action/Effect Suppresses pituitary output of follicle-stimulating hormone and luteinizing hormone that causes regression and atrophy of normal and ectopic endometrial tissue; decreases rate of growth of abnormal breast tissue; reduces attacks associated with hereditary angioedema by increasing levels of C4 component of complement

Contraindications Hypersensitivity to danazol or any component of the formulation; undiagnosed genital bleeding; pregnancy; breast-feeding; porphyria; markedly impaired hepatic, renal, or cardiac function

(Continued)

Danazol *(Continued)*

Warnings/Precautions Use with caution in patients with seizure disorders, migraine, or conditions influenced by edema. Thromboembolism, thrombotic, and thrombophlebitic events have been reported (including life-threatening or fatal strokes). Peliosis hepatis and benign hepatic adenoma have been reported with long-term use. May cause benign intracranial hypertension. Breast cancer should be ruled out prior to treatment for fibrocystic breast disease. May increase risk of atherosclerosis and coronary artery disease. May cause nonreversible androgenic effects. Pregnancy must be ruled out prior to treatment. Safety and efficacy in pediatric patients have not been established.

Drug Interactions

Cytochrome P450 Effect: Inhibits CYP3A4

Decreased Effect: Danazol may decrease effectiveness of hormonal contraceptives. Nonhormonal birth control methods are recommended.

Increased Effect/Toxicity: Danazol may increase serum levels of carbamazepine, cyclosporine, tacrolimus, and warfarin leading to toxicity; dosage adjustment may be needed; monitor. Concomitant use of danazol and HMG-CoA reductase inhibitors may lead to severe myopathy or rhabdomyolysis. Danazol may enhance the glucose-lowering effect of hypoglycemic agents.

Nutritional/Ethanol Interactions Food: Delays time to peak; high-fat meal increases plasma concentration

Adverse Reactions Frequency not defined.

Cardiovascular: Benign intracranial hypertension (rare), edema, flushing, hypertension, diaphoresis

Central nervous system: Anxiety (rare), chills (rare), convulsions (rare), depression, dizziness, emotional lability, fainting, fever (rare), Guillain-Barré syndrome, headache, nervousness, sleep disorders, tremor

Dermatologic: Acne, hair loss, mild hirsutism, maculopapular rash, papular rash, petechial rash, pruritus, purpuric rash, seborrhea, Stevens-Johnson syndrome (rare), photosensitivity (rare), urticaria, vesicular rash

Endocrine & metabolic: Amenorrhea (which may continue post therapy), breast size reduction, clitoris hypertrophy, glucose intolerance, HDL decreased, LDL increased, libido changes, nipple discharge, menstrual disturbances (spotting, altered timing of cycle), semen abnormalities (changes in volume, viscosity, sperm count/motility), spermatogenesis reduction

Gastrointestinal: Appetite changes (rare), bleeding gums (rare), constipation, gastroenteritis, nausea, pancreatitis (rare), vomiting, weight gain

Genitourinary: Vaginal dryness, vaginal irritation, pelvic pain

Hematologic: Eosinophilia, erythrocytosis (reversible), leukocytosis, leukopenia, platelet count increased, polycythemia, RBC increased, thrombocytopenia

Hepatic: Cholestatic jaundice, hepatic adenoma, jaundice, liver enzymes (elevated), malignant tumors (after prolonged use), peliosis hepatis

Neuromuscular & skeletal: Back pain, carpal tunnel syndrome (rare), CPK abnormalities, extremity pain, joint lockup, joint pain, joint swelling, muscle cramps, neck pain, paresthesias, spasms, weakness

Ocular: Cataracts (rare), visual disturbances

Renal: Hematuria

Respiratory: Nasal congestion (rare)

Miscellaneous: Voice change (hoarseness, sore throat, instability, deepening of pitch)

Pharmacodynamics/Kinetics

Half-Life Elimination: Variable: 4.5 hours

Time to Peak: Serum: Within 2 hours

Metabolism: Extensively hepatic, primarily to 2-hydroxymethylethisterone

Onset: Therapeutic: ~4 weeks

Formulations Capsule: 50 mg, 100 mg, 200 mg

Dosing

Adults & Elderly:

Endometriosis: Oral: Initial: 200-400 mg/day in 2 divided doses for mild disease; individualize dosage. Usual maintenance dose: 800 mg/day in 2 divided doses to achieve amenorrhea and rapid response to painful symptoms. Continue therapy uninterrupted for 3-6 months (up to 9 months).

Fibrocystic breast disease (female): Oral: Range: 100-400 mg/day in 2 divided doses

Hereditary angioedema (Male/Female): Oral: Initial: 200 mg 2-3 times/day; after favorable response, decrease the dosage by 50% or less at intervals of 1-3 months or longer if the frequency of attacks dictates. If an attack occurs, increase the dosage by up to 200 mg/day.

Stability

Storage: Store at controlled room temperature of 15°C to 30°C (59°F to 86°F).

Monitoring Laboratory Tests Liver and renal function

Monitoring and Teaching Issues

Physical Assessment: See Contraindications and Warnings/Precautions for use cautions. Assess potential for interactions of other prescriptions, OTC medications, or herbal products patient may be taking (eg, anticoagulants and hypoglycemic agents - see Drug Interactions). Assess results of laboratory tests, therapeutic effectiveness (according to purpose for use), and adverse response (see Adverse Reactions and Overdose/Toxicology). Caution diabetic patients to monitor glucose levels closely (may enhance the glucose-lowering effect of hypoglycemic agents). Teach patient proper use, possible side effects and interventions (eg, good self-breast-exam technique), and adverse symptoms to report (see Patient Education). **Pregnancy risk factor X** - determine that patient is not pregnant before starting therapy. Do not give to female patients of childbearing age unless capable of complying with barrier contraceptive use. Instruct patient in appropriate barrier contraceptive measures. Breast-feeding is contraindicated.

Patient Education: Inform prescriber of all prescriptions, OTC medications, or herbal products you are taking, and any allergies you have. Do not take anything new during

treatment unless approved by prescriber. Take as directed; do not discontinue without consulting prescriber. Therapy may take up to several months depending on purpose for therapy. If diabetic, monitor serum glucose closely and notify prescriber of changes; this medication can alter hypoglycemic requirements. Consult prescriber for appropriate self-breast-exam technique. May cause headache, sleeplessness, anxiety (use caution when driving or engaging in potentially hazardous tasks until response to drug is known); acne, growth of body hair, deepening of voice, loss of libido, impotence, or menstrual irregularity (usually reversible). Report changes in menstrual pattern; deepening of voice or unusual growth of body hair; persistent penile erections; fluid retention (eg, swelling of ankles, feet, or hands, difficulty breathing, or sudden weight gain); change in color of urine or stool; yellowing of eyes or skin; unusual bruising or bleeding; or other adverse reactions.

Pregnancy/breast-feeding precautions: Inform prescriber if you are pregnant. Do not get pregnant during therapy or for 1 month following therapy. Consult prescriber for appropriate contraceptive measures. This drug may cause severe fetal defects. Do not donate blood during or for 1 month following therapy. Do not breast-feed.

Pregnancy Issues: Pregnancy should be ruled out prior to treatment using a sensitive test (beta subunit test, if available). Nonhormonal contraception should be used during therapy. May cause androgenic effects to the female fetus; clitoral hypertrophy, labial fusion, urogenital sinus defect, vaginal atresia, and ambiguous genitalia have been reported.

Danocrine® *see* Danazol *on page 361*

Dantrium® *see* Dantrolene *on page 363*

Dantrolene (DAN troe leen)

U.S. Brand Names Dantrium®

Synonyms Dantrolene Sodium

Generic Available No

Pharmacologic Category Skeletal Muscle Relaxant

Pregnancy Risk Factor C

Lactation Excretion in breast milk unknown/not recommended

Use Treatment of spasticity associated with spinal cord injury, stroke, cerebral palsy, or multiple sclerosis; treatment of malignant hyperthermia

Use - Unlabeled/Investigational Neuroleptic malignant syndrome (NMS)

Mechanism of Action/Effect Acts directly on skeletal muscle by interfering with release of calcium ion from the sarcoplasmic reticulum; prevents or reduces the increase in myoplasmic calcium ion concentration that activates the acute catabolic processes associated with malignant hyperthermia

Contraindications Active hepatic disease; should not be used where spasticity is used to maintain posture or balance

Warnings/Precautions Use with caution in patients with impaired cardiac function or impaired pulmonary function. Has potential for hepatotoxicity. Overt hepatitis has been most frequently observed between the third and twelfth month of therapy. Hepatic injury appears to be greater in females and in patients >35 years of age. Pregnancy risk C.

Drug Interactions

Cytochrome P450 Effect: Substrate of **CYP3A4**

Increased Effect/Toxicity: Increased toxicity with estrogens (hepatotoxicity), CNS depressants (sedation), MAO inhibitors, phenothiazines, clindamycin (increased neuromuscular blockade), verapamil (hyperkalemia and cardiac depression), warfarin, clofibrate, and tolbutamide.

Nutritional/Ethanol Interactions

Ethanol: Avoid ethanol (may increase CNS depression).

Herb/Nutraceutical: Avoid valerian, St John's wort, kava kava, gotu kola (may increase CNS depression).

Effects on Lab Values ↑ aminotransferase [ALT (SGPT)/AST (SGOT)] (S), alkaline phosphatase, LDH, BUN, and total serum bilirubin

Adverse Reactions

>10%:

- Central nervous system: Drowsiness, dizziness, lightheadedness, fatigue
- Dermatologic: Rash
- Gastrointestinal: Diarrhea (mild), vomiting
- Neuromuscular & skeletal: Muscle weakness

1% to 10%:

- Cardiovascular: Pleural effusion with pericarditis
- Central nervous system: Chills, fever, headache, insomnia, nervousness, mental depression
- Gastrointestinal: Diarrhea (severe), constipation, anorexia, stomach cramps
- Ocular: Blurred vision
- Respiratory: Respiratory depression

<1% (Limited to important or life-threatening): Confusion, hepatic necrosis, hepatitis, seizures

Overdosage/Toxicology Symptoms of overdose include CNS depression, hypotension, nausea, and vomiting. For decontamination, lavage with activated charcoal and administer a cathartic. Do not use ipecac. Other treatment is supportive and symptomatic.

Pharmacodynamics/Kinetics

Absorption: Oral: Slow and incomplete

Half-Life Elimination: 8.7 hours

Metabolism: Hepatic

Formulations

Capsule, as sodium: 25 mg, 50 mg, 100 mg

Injection, powder for reconstitution, as sodium: 20 mg [contains mannitol 3 g]

Dosing

Adults & Elderly:

Spasticity: Oral: 25 mg/day to start, increase frequency to 2-4 times/day, then increase dose by 25 mg every 4-7 days to a maximum of 100 mg 2-4 times/day or 400 mg/day

(Continued)

Dantrolene *(Continued)*

Malignant hyperthermia:

Preoperative prophylaxis:

Oral: 4-8 mg/kg/day in 4 divided doses, begin 1-2 days prior to surgery with last dose 3-4 hours prior to surgery

I.V.: 2.5 mg/kg ~1¼ hours prior to anesthesia and infused over 1 hour with additional doses as needed and individualized

Crisis: I.V.: 2.5 mg/kg; may repeat dose up to cumulative dose of 10 mg/kg; if physiologic and metabolic abnormalities reappear, repeat regimen

Postcrisis follow-up: Oral: 4-8 mg/kg/day in 4 divided doses for 1-3 days; I.V. dantrolene may be used when oral therapy is not practical; individualize dosage beginning with 1 mg/kg or more as the clinical situation dictates

Neuroleptic malignant syndrome (unlabeled use): I.V.: 1 mg/kg; may repeat dose up to maximum cumulative dose of 10 mg/kg, then switch to oral dosage

Pediatrics:

Spasticity: Oral: Children: Initial: 0.5 mg/kg/dose twice daily, increase frequency to 3-4 times/day at 4- to 7-day intervals, then increase dose by 0.5 mg/kg to a maximum of 3 mg/kg/dose 2-4 times/day up to 400 mg/day

Malignant hyperthermia: Children: Refer to adult dosing.

Administration

I.V.: Therapeutic or emergency dose can be administered with rapid continuous I.V. push. Follow-up doses should be administered over 2-3 minutes.

Stability

Reconstitution: Reconstitute vial by adding 60 mL of sterile water for injection USP (**not bacteriostatic water for injection**). Protect from light. Use within 6 hours. Avoid glass bottles for I.V. infusion.

Monitoring Laboratory Tests Liver function for potential hepatotoxicity

Monitoring and Teaching Issues

Physical Assessment: Assess effectiveness and interactions of other medications patient may be taking (see Drug Interactions). See Contraindications and Warnings/Precautions for use cautions. **I.V.:** Monitor vital signs, cardiac function, respiratory status and I.V. site (extravasation very irritating to tissues). Monitor effectiveness of therapy and adverse reactions (see Adverse Reactions) at beginning and periodically during therapy. Assess knowledge/teach patient appropriate use, interventions to reduce side effects, and adverse symptoms to report (see Patient Education). **Pregnancy risk factor C** - benefits of use should outweigh possible risks. Breast-feeding is not recommended.

Patient Education: Take exactly as directed. Do not increase dose or discontinue without consulting prescriber. Do not use alcohol, prescriptive or OTC antidepressants, sedatives, or pain medications without consulting prescriber. You may experience drowsiness, dizziness, lightheadedness (avoid driving or engaging in tasks that require alertness until response to drug is known); nausea or vomiting (small, frequent meals, frequent mouth care, or sucking hard candy may help); or diarrhea (buttermilk, boiled milk, or yogurt may help). Report excessive confusion; drowsiness or mental agitation; chest pain, palpitations, or difficulty breathing; skin rash; or vision changes. **Pregnancy/breast-feeding precautions:** Inform prescriber if you are or intend to become pregnant. Breast-feeding is not recommended.

Dantrolene Sodium *see* Dantrolene *on page 363*

Dapiprazole *see page 1461*

Dapsone (DAP sone)

Synonyms Diaminodiphenylsulfone

Generic Available Yes

Pharmacologic Category Antibiotic, Miscellaneous

Pregnancy Risk Factor C

Lactation Enters breast milk/not recommended (AAP rates "compatible")

Use Treatment of leprosy and dermatitis herpetiformis (infections caused by *Mycobacterium leprae*); prophylaxis of toxoplasmosis in severely immunocompromised patients; alternative agent for *Pneumocystis carinii* pneumonia prophylaxis (given alone) and treatment (given with trimethoprim); may be useful in relapsing polychondritis, prophylaxis of malaria, inflammatory bowel disorders, leishmaniasis, rheumatic/connective tissue disorders, brown recluse spider bites

Mechanism of Action/Effect Dapsone is a sulfone antimicrobial that prevents normal bacterial utilization of PABA for the synthesis of folic acid.

Contraindications Hypersensitivity to dapsone or any component of the formulation

Warnings/Precautions Use with caution in patients with severe anemia, G6PD deficiency, hypersensitivity to other sulfonamides, or restricted hepatic function. Pregnancy risk C.

Drug Interactions

Cytochrome P450 Effect: Substrate of CYP2C8/9, 2C19, 2E1, **3A4**

Decreased Effect: Para-aminobenzoic acid and rifampin levels are decreased when given with dapsone.

Increased Effect/Toxicity: Folic acid antagonists (methotrexate) may increase the risk of hematologic reactions of dapsone; probenecid decreases dapsone excretion; trimethoprim with dapsone may increase toxic effects of both drugs Dapsone levels may be increased by protease inhibitors (amprenavir, nelfinavir, ritonavir).

Nutritional/Ethanol Interactions Herb/Nutraceutical: St John's wort may decrease dapsone levels.

Adverse Reactions

>10%:

Hematologic: Hemolytic anemia, methemoglobinemia with cyanosis

Dermatologic: Skin rash

1% to 10%:

Central nervous system: Reactional states

Hematologic: Dose-related hemolysis,

<1% (Limited to important or life-threatening): Agranulocytosis, cholestatic jaundice, exfoliative dermatitis, hepatitis, leukopenia, peripheral neuropathy

Overdosage/Toxicology Symptoms of overdose include nausea, vomiting, hyperexcitability, methemoglobin-induced depression, seizures, cyanosis, and hemolysis. Following decontamination, methylene blue 1-2 mg/kg I.V. is the treatment of choice.

Pharmacodynamics/Kinetics

Absorption: Well absorbed

Half-Life Elimination: 30 hours (range: 10-50 hours)

Metabolism: Hepatic

Formulations Tablet: 25 mg, 100 mg

Dosing

Adults & Elderly:

Leprosy: Oral: 50-100 mg/day for 3-10 years

Dermatitis herpetiformis: Oral: Initial: 50 mg/day, increase to 300. mg/day, or higher to achieve full control. Reduce dosage to minimum level as soon as possible.

Treatment/Prophylaxis: *Pneumocystis carinii* pneumonia: Oral: 100 mg/day in combination with trimethoprim (15-20 mg/kg/day) for 21 days

Pediatrics:

Leprosy: Oral: Children: 1-2 mg/kg/24 hours, up to a maximum of 100 mg/day

Prophylaxis of *Pneumocystis carinii* pneumonia: Oral: Children >1 month: 2 mg/kg/day once daily (maximum dose: 100 mg/day) or 4 mg/kg/dose once weekly (maximum dose: 200 mg)

Renal Impairment: No guidelines are available.

Administration

Oral: May give with meals if GI upset occurs.

Stability

Storage: Protect from light.

Monitoring Laboratory Tests Liver function, CBC

Monitoring and Teaching Issues

Physical Assessment: See Contraindications and Warnings/Precautions for use cautions. Assess potential for interactions of other prescription, OTC medications, or herbal products patient may be taking (see Drug Interactions). Assess results of laboratory tests (see above), therapeutic effectiveness (according to purpose for use), and adverse response (see Adverse Reactions and Overdose/Toxicology). Teach patient appropriate use, possible side effects and interventions, and adverse symptoms to report (see Patient Education). **Pregnancy risk factor C** - benefits of use should outweigh possible risks. Breast-feeding is not recommended.

Patient Education: Inform prescriber of all prescriptions, OTC medications, or herbal products you are taking, and any allergies you have. Do not take anything new during treatment unless approved by prescriber. Take as directed; do not discontinue without consulting prescriber. Do not take with antacids, alkaline foods, or other medication. Therapy may take 3-10 years for leprosy. Frequent blood tests may be required. If rash develops, discontinue and notify prescriber. Report persistent sore throat, fever, chills; constant fatigue; yellowing of skin or eyes; or easy bruising or bleeding. **Pregnancy/ breast-feeding precautions:** Inform prescriber if you are or intend to become pregnant. Breast-feeding is not recommended.

Dietary Issues: Do not administer with antacids, alkaline foods, or drugs.

Daraprim® *see* Pyrimethamine *on page 1157*

Darbepoetin Alfa (dar be POE e tin AL fa)

U.S. Brand Names Aranesp™

Synonyms Erythropoiesis Stimulating Protein

Generic Available No

Pharmacologic Category Colony Stimulating Factor; Growth Factor; Recombinant Human Erythropoietin

Pregnancy Risk Factor C

Lactation Excretion in breast milk unknown/use caution

Use Treatment of anemia associated with chronic renal failure (CRF), including patients on dialysis (ESRD) and patients not on dialysis; anemia associated with chemotherapy for non-myeloid malignancies

Mechanism of Action/Effect Stimulates production of red blood cells within the bone marrow. There is a dose response relationship with this effect. This results in an increase in red blood cell counts followed by a rise in hematocrit and hemoglobin levels. When administered S.C. or I.V., darbepoetin's half-life is ~3 times that of epoetin alfa.

Contraindications Hypersensitivity to darbepoetin or any component of the formulation (including polysorbate 80 and/or albumin); uncontrolled hypertension

Warnings/Precautions Erythropoietic therapies may be associated with an increased risk of cardiovascular and/or neurologic events in chronic renal failure. Darbepoetin alfa should be managed carefully; avoid hemoglobin increases >1 g/dL in any 2-week period, and do not exceed a target level of 12 g/dL. Prior to and during therapy, iron stores must be evaluated. Supplemental iron is recommended if serum ferritin <100 mcg/mL or serum transferrin saturation <20%.

Use with caution in patients with hypertension or with a history of seizures. If hypertension is difficult to control, reduce or hold darbepoetin alpha. **Not** recommended for acute correction of severe anemia or as a substitute for transfusion. Consider discontinuing in patients who receive a renal transplant.

Prior to treatment, correct or exclude deficiencies of vitamin B_{12} and/or folate, as well as other factors which may impair erythropoiesis (aluminum toxicity, inflammatory conditions, infections). Poor response should prompt evaluation of these potential factors, as well as possible malignant processes, occult blood loss, hemolysis, and/or bone marrow fibrosis. Pure red cell aplasia (PRCA) with associated neutralizing antibodies to erythropoietin has been reported, (Continued)

Darbepoetin Alfa *(Continued)*

predominantly in patients with CRF. Patients with loss of response to darbepoetin alfa should be evaluated. Discontinue treatment in patients with PRCA secondary to neutralizing antibodies to erythropoietin.

Due to the delayed onset of erythropoiesis, darbepoetin is of no value in the acute treatment of anemia. Safety and efficacy in patients with underlying hematologic diseases have not been established, including porphyria, thalassemia, hemolytic anemia, and sickle cell disease. Risk of thrombosis, including pulmonary embolism, increased in cancer patients. Safety and efficacy in pediatric patients have not been established.

Pregnancy risk C.

Nutritional/Ethanol Interactions Ethanol: Should be avoided due to adverse effects on erythropoiesis.

Adverse Reactions Note: Frequency of adverse events cited in patients with CRF or cancer and may be, in part, a reflection of population in which the drug is used and/or associated with dialysis procedures.

>10%:

- Cardiovascular: Hypertension (4% to 23%), hypotension (22%), edema (21%), peripheral edema (11%), arrhythmia (10%)
- Central nervous system: Fatigue (9% to 33%), fever (9% to 19%), headache (12% to 16%), dizziness (8% to 14%)
- Gastrointestinal: Diarrhea (16% to 22%), constipation (5% to 18%) vomiting (15%), nausea (14%), abdominal pain (12%)
- Neuromuscular & skeletal: Myalgia (21%), arthralgia (11% to 13%), limb pain (10%)
- Respiratory: Upper respiratory infection (14%), dyspnea (12%), cough (10%)
- Miscellaneous: Infection (27%)

1% to 10%:

- Cardiovascular: Angina/chest pain (6% to 8%), fluid overload (6%), CHF (6%), thrombosis (6%), MI (2%)
- Central nervous system: Seizure (<1% to 1%), stroke (1%), TIA (1%)
- Dermatologic: Pruritus (8%), rash (7%)
- Endocrine & metabolic: Dehydration (5%)
- Local: Injection site pain (7%)
- Neuromuscular & skeletal: Back pain (8%), weakness (5%)
- Respiratory: Bronchitis (6%), pulmonary embolism (1%)
- Miscellaneous: Vascular access thrombosis (8%, annualized rate 0.22 events per patient year), vascular access infection (6%), influenza-like symptoms (6%), vascular access hemorrhage (6%)

Overdosage/Toxicology The maximum amount of darbepoetin which may be safely administered has not been determined. However, cardiovascular and neurologic adverse events have been correlated to excessive and/or rapid rise in hemoglobin. Phlebotomy may be performed if clinically indicated.

Pharmacodynamics/Kinetics

Absorption: S.C.: Slow

Bioavailability: CRF: S.C.: ~37% (range: 30% to 50%)

Half-Life Elimination: CRF: Terminal: I.V.: 21 hours, S.C.: 49 hours; **Note:** Half-life is ~3 times as long as epoetin alfa

Time to Peak: S.C.: CRF: 34 hours (range: 24-72 hours); Cancer: 90 hours (range: 71-123 hours)

Onset: Increased hemoglobin levels not generally observed until 2-6 weeks after initiating treatment

Formulations Injection, solution, with human albumin 2.5 mg/mL [preservative free, single-dose vial]: 25 mcg/mL (1 mL); 40 mcg/mL (1 mL); 60 mcg/mL (1 mL); 100 mcg/mL (1 mL); 150 mcg/0.75 mL (0.75 mL); 200 mcg/mL (1 mL); 300 mcg/mL (1 mL); 500 mcg/mL (1 mL)

Dosing

Adults & Elderly:

Correction of anemia associated with CRF: I.V., S.C.:

- Initial: 0.45 mcg/kg once weekly; dosage should be titrated to limit increases in hemoglobin to <1 g/dL over any 2-week interval, with a target concentration of <12 g/dL.
- Maintenance: Titrated to hematologic response. Some patients may require doses <0.45 mcg/kg once weekly. Selected patients may be managed by administering S.C. doses every 2 weeks.
- Conversion from epoetin alfa to darbepoetin alfa: Initial: Estimate dosage based on weekly epoetin alfa dosage; see table:

Conversion From Epoetin Alfa to Darbepoetin Alfa

Previous Dosage of Epoetin Alfa (units/week)	Darbepoetin Alfa Dosage (mcg/week)
<2500	6.25
2500-4999	12.5
5000-10,999	25
11,000-17,999	40
18,000-33,999	60
34,000-89,999	100
≥90,000	200

Note: In patients receiving epoetin alfa 2-3 times per week, darbepoetin alfa is administered once weekly. In patients receiving epoetin alfa once weekly, darbepoetin alfa is administered once every 2 weeks.

Dosage adjustment: Goal: Dose should be adjusted to achieve and maintain a target hemoglobin not to exceed 12 g/dL.

Inadequate response: Hemoglobin increases <1 g/dL over 4 weeks and iron stores are adequate: Increase by ~25% of the previous dose; increases should not be made more frequently than once monthly.

Excessive response:

Hemoglobin increases >1 g/dL in any 2-week period: Decrease dose

Hemoglobin increases and approaches the target value of 12 g/dL: Decrease weekly dosage by ~25%. If hemoglobin continues to increase, hold dose temporarily until hemoglobin begins to decrease, then restart at a dose 25% below the previous dose.

S.C.: Correction of anemia associated with cancer patients receiving chemotherapy: Initial: 2.25 mcg/kg once weekly; adjust dose as follows to achieve and maintain a target hemoglobin:

Inadequate response: Hemoglobin increases <1 g/dL after 6 weeks of therapy: Increase dose to 4.5 mcg/kg

Excessive responses:

Hemoglobin increases >1 g/dL in a 2-week period **OR** if hemoglobin exceeds 12 g/dL: Reduce dose by 25%

Hemoglobin >13 g/dL: Withhold dose until hemoglobin falls to 12 g/dL, then reinitiate at 25% less than previous dose.

Renal Impairment: Dosage requirements for patients with chronic renal failure who do not require dialysis may be lower than in dialysis patients. Monitor patients closely during the time period in which a dialysis regimen is initiated, dosage requirement may increase.

Administration

I.V.: May be administered by S.C. or I.V. injection. Do not shake; vigorous shaking may denature darbepoetin alfa, rendering it biologically inactive. Do not dilute or administer in conjunction with other drug solutions. Discard any unused portion of the vial; do not pool unused portions. Discontinue immediately if signs/symptoms of anaphylaxis occur.

Stability

Storage: Store at 2°C to 8°C (36°F to 46°F). Do not freeze or shake. Protect from light.

Compatibility: Do not dilute or administer with other solutions.

Monitoring Laboratory Tests Hemoglobin (weekly); prior to and during therapy, iron stores must be evaluated (supplemental iron is recommended in any patient with a serum ferritin <100 mcg/mL or serum transferrin saturation <20%)

Monitoring and Teaching Issues

Physical Assessment: See Contraindications, Warnings/Precautions (eg, pretreatment deficiencies), and Dosing for use cautions. Assess potential for interactions with other prescriptions, OTC medications, or herbal products patient may be taking (eg, nutritional or supplemental iron). See Administration directions. Assess results of laboratory tests prior to and during therapy (see above). Assess therapeutic effectiveness and adverse response (see Adverse Reactions and Overdose/Toxicology) on a regular basis during therapy. Teach patient appropriate injection technique and needle disposal if self-administered, possible side effects and appropriate interventions, and adverse symptoms to report (see Patient Education). **Pregnancy risk factor C** - benefits of use should outweigh possible risks. Note breast-feeding caution.

Patient Education: Inform prescriber of all prescriptions, OTC medications, herbal products, vitamins, or dietary supplements you are taking, and any allergies you have. Do not take anything new during treatment without consulting prescriber. This medication can only be administered by infusion or injection (if self-administered, follow exact directions for injection and needle disposal). You will need frequent blood tests to determine appropriate dosage. Avoid alcohol and do not make significant changes in your dietary iron without consulting prescriber. Check your blood pressure as frequently as recommended and report any significant changes. May cause nausea or vomiting (small, frequent meals, frequent mouth care, sucking lozenges, or chewing gum may help); diarrhea (boiled milk, buttermilk, or yogurt may help); constipation (increased dietary fruit, fiber, fluids, and increased exercise may help); or dizziness, fatigue, or headache (use caution when driving or engaging in tasks that require alertness until response to drug is known). Report signs of edema (swollen extremities, difficulty breathing); sudden onset of acute headache, back pain, or chest pain; muscle tremors or weakness; cough or signs of respiratory infection; or other adverse effects. **Pregnancy/breast-feeding precautions:** Inform prescriber if you are or intend to become pregnant. Consult prescriber if breast-feeding.

Dietary Issues: Supplemental iron intake may be required in patients with low iron stores.

Darvocet-N® 50 *see* Propoxyphene and Acetaminophen *on page 1142*

Darvocet-N® 100 *see* Propoxyphene and Acetaminophen *on page 1142*

Darvon® *see* Propoxyphene *on page 1141*

Darvon® Compound-65 Pulvules® *see* Propoxyphene and Aspirin *on page 1142*

Darvon-N® *see* Propoxyphene *on page 1141*

Daunomycin *see* DAUNOrubicin Hydrochloride *on page 369*

DAUNOrubicin Citrate (Liposomal)

(daw noe ROO bi sin SI trate lip po SOE mal)

U.S. Brand Names DaunoXome®

Generic Available No

Pharmacologic Category Antineoplastic Agent, Anthracycline

Pregnancy Risk Factor D

Lactation Excretion in breast milk unknown/not recommended

Use First-line cytotoxic therapy for advanced HIV-associated Kaposi's sarcoma

Mechanism of Action/Effect Binds to DNA and inhibits DNA synthesis causing cell death

Contraindications Hypersensitivity to daunorubicin or any component of the formulation; pregnancy

(Continued)

DAUNOrubicin Citrate (Liposomal) *(Continued)*

Warnings/Precautions The U.S. Food and Drug Administration (FDA) currently recommends that procedures for proper handling and disposal of antineoplastic agents be considered.

The primary toxicity is myelosuppression. May cause cardiac toxicity, particularly in patients who have received prior anthracyclines or who have pre-existing cardiac disease. Refer to Daunorubicin monograph.

No instances of local tissue necrosis were observed with extravasation. However, refer to Daunorubicin monograph and avoid extravasation.

Reduce dosage in patients with impaired hepatic function. Administer allopurinol prior to initiating antileukemic therapy. Use with caution in patients with systemic infection and cardiac disease. If daunorubicin (liposomal) contacts the skin, wash and flush thoroughly with water.

Drug Interactions

Decreased Effect: Patients may experience impaired immune response to vaccines; possible infection after administration of live vaccines in patients receiving immunosuppressants.

Nutritional/Ethanol Interactions Ethanol: Avoid ethanol (due to GI irritation).

Adverse Reactions

>10%:

- Dermatologic: Alopecia (reversible)
- Gastrointestinal: Mild nausea or vomiting occurs in 50% of patients within the first 24 hours; esophagitis or stomatitis may occur 3-7 days after administration, but is not as severe as that caused by doxorubicin
  - Time course for nausea/vomiting: Onset: 1-3 hours; Duration: 4-24 hours
- Genitourinary: Discoloration of urine (red)

1% to 10%:

- Cardiovascular: Congestive heart failure; maximum lifetime dose: Refer to Warnings/Precautions
- Dermatologic: Darkening or redness of skin
- Endocrine & metabolic: Hyperuricemia
- Gastrointestinal: GI ulceration, diarrhea
- Hematologic: Myelosuppressive: Dose-limiting toxicity; occurs in all patients; leukopenia is more significant than thrombocytopenia
  - WBC: Severe
  - Platelets: Severe
  - Onset (days): 7
  - Nadir (days): 14
  - Recovery (days): 21-28
- Local: **Vesicant chemotherapy**

<1% (Limited to important or life-threatening): Elevation in serum bilirubin, AST, and alkaline phosphatase; myocarditis; pericarditis

Overdosage/Toxicology Symptoms of acute overdose are increased severity of the observed dose-limiting toxicities of therapeutic doses, myelosuppression (especially granulocytopenia), fatigue, nausea, and vomiting. Treatment is symptomatic.

Pharmacodynamics/Kinetics

Half-Life Elimination: Distribution: 4.4 hours; Terminal: 3-5 hours

Metabolism: Similar to daunorubicin, but metabolite plasma levels are low

Formulations Injection, solution: 2 mg/mL (25 mL) [equivalent to 50 mg daunorubicin base]

Dosing

Adults & Elderly: Refer to individual protocols.

Advanced HIV-associated Kaposi's sarcoma: I.V.:

- 20-40 mg/m^2 every 2 weeks
- 100 mg/m^2 every 3 weeks

Renal Impairment:

- S_{cr} 1.2-3 mg/dL: Reduce dose to 75% of normal.
- S_{cr} >3 mg/dL: Reduce dose to 50% of normal.

Hepatic Impairment:

- Serum bilirubin 1.2-3 mg/dL: Reduce to 75% of normal dose.
- Serum bilirubin >3 mg/dL: Reduce to 50% of normal dose.

Administration

I.V.: Vesicant. Infuse over 1 hour; do not mix with other drugs.

Stability

Storage: Store in refrigerator 2°C to 8°C (37°F to 45°F); do not freeze. Protect from light.

Reconstitution: Only fluid which may be mixed with DaunoXome® is D_5W. Must not be mixed with saline, bacteriostatic agents such as benzyl alcohol, or any other solution.

Compatibility: Incompatible with sodium bicarbonate and 5-FU, heparin, dexamethasone

Monitoring Laboratory Tests Cardiac function, CBC with differential and platelet count, liver and renal function prior to each course of treatment; repeat blood counts prior to each dose and withhold if the absolute granulocyte count is <750 cells/mm^3. Monitor serum uric acid levels.

Monitoring and Teaching Issues

Physical Assessment: See contraindications, Warnings/Precautions, and Dosing for use cautions. Assess potential for interactions with other prescriptions, OTC medications, or herbal products patient may be taking (see Drug Interactions). See Administration, Dosing, Reconstitution, and Compatibility for administration specifics. Infusion site must be closely monitored to prevent extravasation (see Administration). Assess results of laboratory tests (see above), therapeutic response, and adverse response (especially cardiac toxicity - see Adverse Reactions and Overdose/Toxicology) prior to each infusion and on a regular basis throughout therapy. Teach patient possible side effects and interventions and adverse symptoms to report (see Patient Education). **Pregnancy risk factor D** - determine that patient is not pregnant before beginning treatment. Instruct patients of childbearing on appropriate barrier contraceptive measures. Breast-feeding is not recommended.

Patient Education: Inform prescriber of all prescriptions, OTC medications, or herbal products you are taking, and any allergies you have. Do not take anything new during treatment unless approved by prescriber. This medication can only be administered I.V. Report immediately any swelling, pain, burning, or redness at infusion site. Avoid alcohol. It is important to maintain adequate hydration (2-3 L/day of fluids) unless advised by prescriber to restrict fluids, and nutrition (small, frequent meals may help). You will be more susceptible to infection (avoid crowds and exposure to infection and do not have any vaccinations without consulting prescriber). May cause nausea or vomiting (small, frequent meals, frequent mouth care, sucking lozenges, or chewing gum may help); diarrhea (buttermilk, boiled milk, or yogurt may help); loss of hair (reversible); or red-pink urine (normal). Report immediately chest pain, swelling of extremities, difficulty breathing, palpitations, or rapid heartbeat. Report unresolved nausea, vomiting, or diarrhea; alterations in urinary pattern (increased or decreased); opportunistic infection (eg, fever, chills, unusual bruising or bleeding fatigue; purulent vaginal discharge; unhealed mouth sores); abdominal pain or blood in stools; excessive fatigue; or yellowing of eyes or skin. **Pregnancy/breast-feeding precautions:** Inform prescriber if you are pregnant. Do not get pregnant or while taking this medication. Consult prescriber for appropriate contraceptive measures to use during and for 1 month following therapy. Breast-feeding is not recommended.

Related Information

FDA Name Differentiation Project: The Use of Tall-man Letters *on page 12*

DAUNOrubicin Hydrochloride (daw noe ROO bi sin hye droe KLOR ide)

U.S. Brand Names Cerubidine®

Synonyms Daunomycin; DNR; Rubidomycin Hydrochloride

Generic Available Yes

Pharmacologic Category Antineoplastic Agent, Anthracycline

Pregnancy Risk Factor D

Lactation Excretion in breast milk unknown/not recommended

Use Treatment of acute lymphocytic (ALL) and nonlymphocytic (ANLL) leukemias

Mechanism of Action/Effect Inhibition of DNA and RNA synthesis; is not cell cycle-specific for the S Phase of cell division; daunomycin is preferred over doxorubicin for the treatment of ANLL because of its dose-limiting toxicity (myelosuppression) is not of concern in the therapy of this disease; has less mucositis associated with its use

Contraindications Hypersensitivity to daunorubicin or any component of the formulation; congestive heart failure or arrhythmias; previous therapy with high cumulative doses of daunorubicin and/or doxorubicin; pre-existing bone marrow suppression; pregnancy

Warnings/Precautions The U.S. Food and Drug Administration (FDA) currently recommends that procedures for proper handling and disposal of antineoplastic agents be considered. I.V. use only, severe local tissue necrosis will result if extravasation occurs. Reduce dose in patients with impaired hepatic, renal, or biliary function. Severe myelosuppression is possible when used in therapeutic doses. Total cumulative dose should take into account previous or concomitant treatment with cardiotoxic agents or irradiation of chest.

Irreversible myocardial toxicity may occur as total dosage approaches:

- 550 mg/m^2 in adults
- 400 mg/m^2 in patients receiving chest radiation
- 300 mg/m^2 in children >2 years of age or
- 10 mg/kg in children <2 years; this may occur during therapy or several months after therapy.

If daunorubicin contacts the skin, wash and flush thoroughly with water.

Drug Interactions

Decreased Effect: Patients may experience impaired immune response to vaccines; possible infection after administration of live vaccines in patients receiving immunosuppressants.

Nutritional/Ethanol Interactions Ethanol: Avoid ethanol (due to GI irritation).

Effects on Lab Values ↑ potassium (S)

Adverse Reactions

>10%:

Dermatologic: Alopecia (reversible)

Gastrointestinal: Mild nausea or vomiting occurs in 50% of patients within the first 24 hours; esophagitis or stomatitis may occur 3-7 days after administration, but is not as severe as that caused by doxorubicin

Time course for nausea/vomiting: Onset: 1-3 hours; Duration: 4-24 hours

Genitourinary: Discoloration of urine (red)

1% to 10%:

Cardiovascular: Congestive heart failure; maximum lifetime dose: Refer to Warnings/Precautions

Dermatologic: Darkening or redness of skin

Endocrine & metabolic: Hyperuricemia

Gastrointestinal: GI ulceration, diarrhea

Hematologic: Myelosuppressive: Dose-limiting toxicity; occurs in all patients; leukopenia is more significant than thrombocytopenia

WBC: Severe

Platelets: Severe

Onset (days): 7

Nadir (days): 14

Recovery (days): 21-28

Local: **Vesicant chemotherapy**

<1% (Limited to important or life-threatening): Elevation in serum bilirubin, AST, and alkaline phosphatase; myocarditis; pericarditis

(Continued)

DAUNOrubicin Hydrochloride *(Continued)*

Overdosage/Toxicology Symptoms of overdose include myelosuppression, nausea, vomiting, and stomatitis. There are no known antidotes. Treatment is symptomatic and supportive.

Pharmacodynamics/Kinetics

Half-Life Elimination: Distribution: 2 minutes; Elimination: 14-20 hours; Terminal: 18.5 hours; Daunorubicinol plasma half-life: 24-48 hours

Metabolism: Primarily hepatic to daunorubicinol (active)

Formulations

Injection, powder for reconstitution, as hydrochloride: 20 mg

Injection, solution, as hydrochloride: 5 mg/mL (4 mL, 10 mL)

Dosing

Adults & Elderly: Refer to individual protocols.

Range: I.V.: 30-60 mg/m^2/day for 3-5 days, repeat dose in 3-4 weeks

AML: I.V.:

Single agent induction: 60 mg/m^2/day for 3 days; repeat every 3-4 weeks

Combination therapy induction: 45 mg/m^2/day for 3 days of the first course of induction therapy; subsequent courses: Every day for 2 days

ALL combination therapy: I.V.: 45 mg/m^2/day for 3 days

Cumulative dose should not exceed 400-600 mg/m^2

Pediatrics: Refer to individual protocols.

ALL combination therapy: I.V.: Children: Remission induction: 25-45 mg/m^2 on day 1 every week for 4 cycles **or** 30-45 mg/m^2/day for 3 days

AML combination therapy: I.V.: Children: Induction (continuous infusion): 30-60 mg/m^2/day on days 1-3 of cycle

Note: In children <2 years or <0.5 m^2, daunorubicin should be based on weight - mg/kg: 1 mg/kg per protocol with frequency dependent on regimen employed

Cumulative dose should not exceed 300 mg/m^2 in children >2 years or 10 mg/kg in children <2 years

Renal Impairment:

Cl_{cr} <10 mL/minute: Administer 75% of normal dose.

S_{cr} >3 mg/dL: Administer 50% of normal dose.

Hepatic Impairment:

Serum bilirubin 1.2-3 mg/dL or AST 60-180 int. units: Reduce dose to 75%.

Serum bilirubin 3.1-5 mg/dL or AST >180 int. units: Reduce dose to 50%.

Serum bilirubin >5 mg/dL: Omit use.

Administration

I.V.: Vesicant. **Never** administer I.M. or S.C. Administer IVP over 1-5 minutes.

Stability

Storage: Store intact vials at room temperature and protect from light.

Reconstitution: Dilute vials with 4 mL SWI for a final concentration of 5 mg/mL. Reconstituted solution is stable for 4 days at 15°C to 25°C. Protect from direct sunlight or fluorescent light to decrease photo-inactivation after storage in solution for several days. Decomposed drug turns purple. For I.V. push administration, desired dose is withdrawn into a syringe containing 10-15 mL NS. Further dilution in D_5W, LR, or NS is stable for 24 hours at room temperature (25°C) and up to 4 weeks if protected from light.

Standard I.V. dilution:

I.V. push: Dose/syringe (initial concentration is 5 mg/mL; however, qs to 10-15 mL with NS)

Maximum syringe size for IVP is a 30 mL syringe and syringe should be <75% full.

IVPB: Dose/50-100 mL NS or D_5W

Stable for 24 hours at room temperature (25°C).

Compatibility: Stable in D_5W, LR, NS, sterile water for injection

Incompatible with heparin, sodium bicarbonate, 5-FU, and dexamethasone

Y-site administration: Incompatible with allopurinol, aztreonam, cefepime, fludarabine, piperacillin/tazobactam

Compatibility when admixed: Incompatible with dexamethasone sodium phosphate, heparin

Monitoring Laboratory Tests CBC with differential, platelet count, liver function, EKG, ventricular ejection fraction, renal function

Monitoring and Teaching Issues

Physical Assessment: See Contraindications, Warnings/Precautions, and Dosing for use cautions. Assess potential for interactions with other prescriptions, OTC medications, or herbal products patient may be taking (see Drug Interactions). See Administration, Dosing, Reconstitution, and Compatibility for administration specifics. Infusion site must be closely monitored; extravasation can cause severe cellulitis or tissue necrosis (see Administration). Assess results of laboratory tests (see above), therapeutic response, and adverse response (especially cardiac toxicity - see Adverse Reactions and Overdose/Toxicology) prior to each infusion and on a regular basis throughout therapy. Teach patient possible side effects and interventions and adverse symptoms to report (see Patient Education). **Pregnancy risk factor D** - determine that patient is not pregnant before beginning treatment. Instruct patients of childbearing age on appropriate barrier contraceptive measures. Breast-feeding is not recommended.

Patient Education: Inform prescriber of all prescriptions, OTC medications, or herbal products you are taking, and any allergies you have. Do not take anything new during treatment unless approved by prescriber. This medication can only be administered I.V. Report immediately any swelling, pain, burning, or redness at infusion site. Avoid alcohol. It is important to maintain adequate hydration (2-3 L/day of fluids) unless advised by prescriber to restrict fluids, and nutrition (small, frequent meals may help). You will be more susceptible to infection (avoid crowds and exposure to infection and do not have any vaccinations without consulting prescriber). May cause nausea or vomiting (small, frequent meals, frequent mouth care, sucking lozenges, or chewing gum may help); diarrhea (buttermilk, boiled milk, or yogurt may help); loss of hair (reversible); or red-pink urine (normal). Report immediately chest pain, swelling of extremities, difficulty breathing, palpitations, or rapid heartbeat. Report unresolved nausea, vomiting, or diarrhea; alterations in urinary pattern (increased or decreased); opportunistic infection (eg, fever, chills, unusual bruising or bleeding fatigue, purulent vaginal discharge, unhealed mouth sores); abdominal pain or blood in stools; excessive fatigue; or yellowing of eyes or skin. **Pregnancy/breast-feeding precautions:** Do not get pregnant or cause a pregnancy (males) while taking this medication. Consult prescriber for appropriate contraceptive measures to use during and for 1 month following therapy. Breast-feeding is not recommended.

Pregnancy Issues: May cause fetal harm when administered to a pregnant woman. Animal studies have shown an increased incidence of fetal abnormalities.

Related Information

FDA Name Differentiation Project: The Use of Tall-man Letters *on page 12*

DaunoXome® *see* DAUNOrubicin Citrate (Liposomal) *on page 367*

1-Day™ [OTC] *see* Tioconazole *on page 1326*

Daypro® *see* Oxaprozin *on page 1013*

DCF *see* Pentostatin *on page 1056*

DDAVP® *see* Desmopressin *on page 380*

ddC *see* Zalcitabine *on page 1415*

ddI *see* Didanosine *on page 403*

1-Deamino-8-D-Arginine Vasopressin *see* Desmopressin *on page 380*

Debrisan® [OTC] *see* Dextranomer *on page 391*

Debrox® Otic *see page 1519*

Decadron® *see* Dexamethasone *on page 382*

Decadron® Phosphate *see* Dexamethasone *on page 382*

Deca-Durabolin® [DSC] *see* Nandrolone *on page 947*

Decaspray® *see* Topical Corticosteroids *on page 1334*

Declomycin® *see* Demeclocycline *on page 374*

Decofed® [OTC] *see* Pseudoephedrine *on page 1150*

Decohistine® DH Liquid *see page 1522*

Deconsal® II *see* Guaifenesin and Pseudoephedrine *on page 648*

Defen-LA® *see* Guaifenesin and Pseudoephedrine *on page 648*

Deferoxamine (de fer OKS a meen)

U.S. Brand Names Desferal®

Synonyms Deferoxamine Mesylate

Generic Available No

Pharmacologic Category Antidote

Pregnancy Risk Factor C

Lactation Excretion in breast milk unknown/contraindicated

Use Acute iron intoxication when serum iron is >450-500 µg/dL or when clinical signs of significant iron toxicity exist; chronic iron overload secondary to multiple transfusions; diagnostic test for iron overload; iron overload secondary to congenital anemias; hemochromatosis; removal of corneal rust rings following surgical removal of foreign bodies

Use - Unlabeled/Investigational Investigational: Treatment of aluminum accumulation in renal failure; treatment of aluminum-induced bone disease

Mechanism of Action/Effect Complexes with trivalent ions (ferric ions) to form ferrioxamine, which are removed by the kidneys

Contraindications Hypersensitivity to deferoxamine or any component of the formulation; patients with anuria, primary hemochromatosis

Warnings/Precautions Use with caution in patients with severe renal disease, pyelonephritis. May increase susceptibility to *Yersinia enterocolitica.* Ocular and auditory disturbances, as well as growth retardation (children only), have been reported following prolonged administration. Has been associated with adult respiratory distress syndrome (ARDS) following excessively high-dose treatment of acute intoxication. Pregnancy risk C.

Drug Interactions

Increased Effect/Toxicity: May cause loss of consciousness when administered with prochlorperazine. Concomitant treatment with vitamin C (>500 mg/day) has been associated with cardiac impairment.

Adverse Reactions Frequency not defined.

Cardiovascular: Flushing, hypotension, tachycardia, shock, edema

Central nervous system: Convulsions, fever, dizziness, neuropathy, paresthesia, seizures, exacerbation of aluminum-related encephalopathy (dialysis), coma, aphasia, agitation

Dermatologic: Erythema, urticaria, pruritus, rash, cutaneous wheal formation

Endocrine & metabolic: Hypocalcemia

Gastrointestinal: Abdominal discomfort, diarrhea

Genitourinary: Dysuria

Hematologic: Thrombocytopenia, leukopenia

Local: Pain and induration at injection site

Neuromuscular & skeletal: Leg cramps

Ocular: Blurred vision, visual loss, scotoma, visual field defects, impaired vision, optic neuritis, cataracts, retinal pigmentary abnormalities

Otic: Hearing loss, tinnitus

Renal: Renal impairment, acute renal failure

Respiratory: Acute respiratory distress syndrome (with dyspnea, cyanosis)

Miscellaneous: Anaphylaxis

Overdosage/Toxicology Symptoms of overdose include hypotension, blurring of vision, diarrhea, leg cramps, and tachycardia. Treatment is symptomatic and supportive.

(Continued)

Deferoxamine *(Continued)*

Pharmacodynamics/Kinetics

Absorption: Oral: <15%

Half-Life Elimination: Parent drug: 6.1 hours; Ferrioxamine: 5.8 hours

Metabolism: Hepatic to ferrioxamine

Formulations Injection, powder for reconstitution, as mesylate: 500 mg, 2 g

Dosing

Adults & Elderly:

Acute iron toxicity:

I.V.: For the first 1000 mg, in fuse at 15 mg/kg/hour (although rates up to 40-50 mg/kg/hour have been given in patients with massive iron intoxication); may be followed by 500 mg every 4 hours for up to 2 doses; subsequent doses of 500 mg have been administered every 4-12 hours

Maximum recommended dose: 6 g/day (however, doses as high as 16-37 g have been administered)

Note: I.V. route is used when severe toxicity is evidenced by systemic symptoms (coma, shock, metabolic acidosis, or severe gastrointestinal bleeding) or potentially severe intoxications (serum iron level >500 μg/dL). When severe symptoms are not present, the I.M. route may be preferred; however, the use of deferoxamine in situations where the serum iron concentration is <500 μg/dL or when severe toxicity is not evident is a subject of some clinical debate.

Chronic iron overload:

I.M.: 500-1000 mg daily; in addition, 2000 mg should be given with each unit of blood transfused (administer separately from blood)

I.V.: 2 g after each unit of blood infusion at 15 mg/kg/hour

S.C.: 1-2 g every day over 8-24 hours

Diagnostic aid, aluminum-associated osteodystrophy: I.V.: Has been used investigationally as a single 40 mg/kg I.V. dose over 2 hours, to promote mobilization of aluminum from tissue stores

Pediatrics:

Acute iron toxicity: Children: Refer to adult dosing.

Chronic iron overload: S.C.: 20-40 mg/kg/day over 8-12 hours (via a portable, controlled infusion device)

Aluminum-induced bone disease (Investigational): 20-40 mg/kg every hemodialysis treatment; frequency dependent on clinical status of the patient.

Renal Impairment: Cl_{cr} <10 mL/minute: Administer 50% of dose.

Administration

I.M.: I.M. administration is preferred in patients not in shock. Add 2 mL sterile water to 500 mg vial. For I.M. or S.C. administration, no further dilution is required.

I.V.: Urticaria, hypotension, and shock have occurred following rapid I.V. administration; give I.M., slow S.C., or I.V. infusion.

The manufacturer states that the I.M. route is preferred; however, the I.V. route is generally preferred in patients with severe toxicity (ie, patients in shock). Maximum I.V. rate: 15 mg/kg/hour.

Stability

Storage: Protect from light.

Reconstitution: Reconstituted solutions (sterile water) may be stored at room temperature for 7 days.

Compatibility: Stable in D_5W, LR, NS, sterile water for injection

Monitoring Laboratory Tests Serum iron, total iron-binding capacity, ophthalmologic exam (fundoscopy, slit-lamp exam) and audiometry with chronic therapy

Monitoring and Teaching Issues

Physical Assessment: See Monitoring Laboratory Tests. **I.V.:** Infuse slowly (see Administration) and monitor infusion site. Monitor for acute reactions; urticaria, hypotension and shock can occur following rapid I.V. administration. Monitor for adverse reactions (eg, cardiac, respiratory, or CNS symptoms - see Adverse Reactions) and teach patient importance of reporting adverse symptoms (see Patient Education). **Pregnancy risk factor C** - benefits of use should outweigh possible risks. Breast-feeding is contraindicated.

Patient Education: I.V.: Instructions depend on patient condition. You will be monitored closely for effects of this medication and frequent blood or urine tests may be necessary. Report chest pain, rapid heartbeat, headache, pain, swelling, or irritation at infusion site; skin rash; changes or loss of hearing or vision; or acute abdominal or leg cramps. **Pregnancy/breast-feeding precautions:** Inform prescriber if you are or intend to become pregnant. Do not breast-feed.

Deferoxamine Mesylate *see* Deferoxamine *on page 371*

Degest® 2[OTC] *see page 1509*

Delatestryl® *see* Testosterone *on page 1294*

Delavirdine (de la VIR deen)

U.S. Brand Names Rescriptor®

Synonyms U-90152S

Generic Available No

Pharmacologic Category Antiretroviral Agent, Reverse Transcriptase Inhibitor (Non-nucleoside)

Pregnancy Risk Factor C

Lactation Excretion in breast milk unknown/contraindicated

Use Treatment of HIV-1 infection in combination with at least two additional antiretroviral agents

Mechanism of Action/Effect Delavirdine binds directly to reverse transcriptase, blocking RNA-dependent and DNA-dependent DNA polymerase activities

Contraindications Hypersensitivity to delavirdine or any component of the formulation; concurrent use of alprazolam, astemizole, cisapride, ergot alkaloids, midazolam, pimozide, or triazolam

Warnings/Precautions Avoid use with benzodiazepines, cisapride, clarithromycin, dapsone, enzyme-inducing anticonvulsants (carbamazepine, phenytoin, phenobarbital, rifampin, rifabutin, or St John's wort); may lead to loss of efficacy or development of resistance. Concurrent use of lovastatin or simvastatin should be avoided (use caution with other statins). Use caution with amphetamines, antacids, antiarrhythmics, benzodiazepines (alprazolam, midazolam, and triazolam are contraindicated), clarithromycin, dihydropyridine, calcium channel blockers, dapsone, immunosuppressants, methadone, oral contraceptives, or sildenafil.

Use with caution in patients with hepatic or renal dysfunction; due to rapid emergence of resistance, delavirdine should not be used as monotherapy; cross-resistance may be conferred to other non-nucleoside reverse transcriptase inhibitors, although potential for cross-resistance with protease inhibitors is low. Long-term effects of delavirdine are not known. Safety and efficacy have not been established in children. Rash, which occurs frequently, may require discontinuation of therapy; usually occurs within 1-3 weeks and lasts <2 weeks. Most patients may resume therapy following a treatment interruption.

Pregnancy risk C.

Drug Interactions

Cytochrome P450 Effect: Substrate of CYP2D6, **3A4**; Inhibits CYP1A2, 2C8/9, 2C19, 2D6, 3A4

Decreased Effect: Decreased plasma concentrations of delavirdine with amprenavir, carbamazepine, dexamethasone, phenobarbital, phenytoin, rifabutin, rifampin, didanosine, and saquinavir. Decreased absorption of delavirdine with antacids, histamine-2 receptor antagonists, proton pump inhibitors (omeprazole, lansoprazole), and didanosine. Delavirdine decreases plasma concentrations of didanosine.

Increased Effect/Toxicity: Delavirdine concentrations may be increased by clarithromycin, ketoconazole, and fluoxetine. Delavirdine increases plasma concentrations of alprazolam, amiodarone, amphetamines, amprenavir, astemizole, bepridil, calcium channel blockers (dihydropyridine-type), cisapride, clarithromycin, dapsone, dexamethasone, ergot alkaloids, flecainide, HMG-CoA reductase inhibitors, indinavir, methadone, midazolam, pimozide, propafenone, quinidine, rifabutin, saquinavir, sildenafil, triazolam, and warfarin.

Nutritional/Ethanol Interactions Herb/Nutraceutical: Delavirdine serum concentration may be decreased by St John's wort; avoid concurrent use.

Adverse Reactions

>10%: Dermatologic: Rash (3.2% required discontinuation)

1% to 10%:

Central nervous system: Headache, fatigue

Dermatologic: Pruritus

Gastrointestinal: Nausea, diarrhea, vomiting

Metabolic: Increased ALT (SGPT), increased AST (SGOT)

<1% (Limited to important or life-threatening): Acute renal failure, allergic reaction, alopecia, angioedema, ataxia, chest pain, confusion, dermal leukocytoblastic vasculitis, desquamation, dyspnea, eosinophilia, epistaxis, erythema multiforme, ethanol intolerance, granulocytosis, hallucination, hematuria, hemolytic anemia, hepatic failure, hepatitis (nonspecific), neuropathy, neutropenia, nystagmus, pancytopenia, paralysis, paranoid symptoms, postural hypotension, proteinuria, renal calculi, rhabdomyolysis, Stevens-Johnson syndrome, syncope, thrombocytopenia, vertigo, vesiculobullous rash

Overdosage/Toxicology Reports of human overdose with delavirdine are not available. GI decontamination and supportive measures are recommended. Dialysis is unlikely to be of benefit in removing this drug since it is extensively metabolized by the liver and is highly protein bound.

Pharmacodynamics/Kinetics

Absorption: Rapid

Bioavailability: 85%

Half-Life Elimination: 2-11 hours

Time to Peak: Plasma: 1 hour

Metabolism: Hepatic via CYP3A4 and 2D6 (**Note:** May reduce CYP3A activity and inhibit its own metabolism.)

Formulations Tablet, as mesylate: 100 mg, 200 mg

Dosing

Adults & Elderly: HIV-1 infection (part of combination): Oral: 400 mg 3 times/day

Administration

Oral: Patients with achlorhydria should take the drug with an acidic beverage. Antacids and delavirdine should be separated by 1 hour. A dispersion of delavirdine may be prepared by adding 4 tablets to at least 3 oz of water. Allow to stand for a few minutes and stir until uniform dispersion. Drink immediately. Rinse glass and mouth following ingestion to ensure total dose administered.

Monitoring Laboratory Tests Liver function tests if administered with saquinavir

Monitoring and Teaching Issues

Physical Assessment: See Contraindications, Warnings/Precautions, and Dosing for use cautions. Assess potential for interactions with other prescriptions, OTC medications, or herbal products patient may be taking (see Drug Interactions). Assess results of laboratory tests (see above), therapeutic response, and adverse reactions (see Adverse Reactions and Overdose/Toxicology) on a regular basis throughout therapy. Teach patient proper use (see Administration), possible side effects and interventions, and adverse symptoms to report (see Patient Education). **Pregnancy Risk Factor C** - benefits of use should outweigh possible risks. Breast-feeding is contraindicated - delavirdine is only used to treat patients with HIV and the CDC recommends that women with HIV not breast-feed in order to prevent transmission of HIV.

(Continued)

Delavirdine *(Continued)*

Patient Education: Inform prescriber of all prescriptions, OTC medications, or herbal products you are taking, and any allergies you have. Do not take anything new during treatment unless approved by prescriber. This drug is not a cure for HIV, nor has it been found to reduce transmission of HIV. Take as directed, with or without food. Do not take antacids within 1 hour of delavirdine. Mix 4 tablets in 3-5 oz of water, allow to stand a few minutes, and stir; drink immediately. May cause nausea or vomiting (small, frequent meals, frequent mouth care, sucking lozenges, or chewing gum may help - consult prescriber if nausea or vomiting persists). Report mouth sores; skin rash or irritation; muscle weakness or tremors; easy bruising or bleeding, fever or chills; CNS changes (eg, hallucinations, confusion, dizziness, altered coordination); swelling of face, lips, or tongue; yellowing of eyes or skin; or dark urine or pale stools. **Pregnancy/breast-feeding precautions:** Inform prescriber if you are or intend to become pregnant. Do not breast-feed.

Dietary Issues: May be taken without regard to food.

Breast-feeding Issues: HIV-infected mothers are discouraged from breast-feeding to decrease potential transmission of HIV.

Pregnancy Issues: It is not known if delavirdine crosses the human placenta. Health professionals are encouraged to contact the antiretroviral pregnancy registry to monitor outcomes of pregnant women exposed to antiretroviral medications (1-800-258-4263).

Additional Information Potential compliance problems, frequency of administration, and adverse effects should be discussed with patients before initiating therapy to help prevent the emergence of resistance.

Related Information

Tuberculosis *on page 1705*

Delcort® *see* Topical Corticosteroids *on page 1334*

Delestrogen® *see* Estradiol *on page 494*

Deltacortisone *see* PredniSONE *on page 1115*

Deltadehydrocortisone *see* PredniSONE *on page 1115*

Deltahydrocortisone *see* PrednisoLONE *on page 1113*

Deltasone® *see* PredniSONE *on page 1115*

Delta-Tritex® *see* Topical Corticosteroids *on page 1334*

Delta-Tritex® *see* Triamcinolone *on page 1356*

Demadex® *see* Torsemide *on page 1342*

Demecarium *see page 1575*

Demecarium *see* Ophthalmic Agents, Glaucoma *on page 1002*

Demeclocycline (dem e kloe SYE kleen)

U.S. Brand Names Declomycin®

Synonyms Demeclocycline Hydrochloride; Demethylchlortetracycline

Generic Available No

Pharmacologic Category Antibiotic, Tetracycline Derivative

Pregnancy Risk Factor D

Lactation Enters breast milk/use caution

Use Treatment of susceptible bacterial infections (acne, gonorrhea, pertussis and urinary tract infections) caused by both gram-negative and gram-positive organisms; used when penicillin is contraindicated (other agents are preferred)

Use - Unlabeled/Investigational Treatment of chronic syndrome of inappropriate secretion of antidiuretic hormone (SIADH)

Mechanism of Action/Effect Inhibits protein synthesis by binding with the 30S and possibly the 50S ribosomal subunit(s) of susceptible bacteria; may also cause alterations in the cytoplasmic membrane; inhibits actions of ADH in patients with SIADH

Contraindications Hypersensitivity to demeclocycline, tetracyclines, or any component of the formulation; pregnancy

Warnings/Precautions Do not administer to children <8 years of age. Photosensitivity reactions occur frequently with this drug, avoid prolonged exposure to sunlight, do not use tanning equipment.

Drug Interactions

Decreased Effect: Decreased effect with antacids (aluminum, calcium, zinc, or magnesium), bismuth salts, sodium bicarbonate, barbiturates, carbamazepine, and hydantoins. Decreased effect of penicillins. Although anecdotal reports suggest oral contraceptive efficacy could be reduced by tetracyclines, this has been refuted by more rigorous scientific and clinical data.

Increased Effect/Toxicity: Increased effect of warfarin, digoxin when taken with demeclocycline.

Nutritional/Ethanol Interactions

Food: Demeclocycline serum levels may be decreased if taken with food.

Herb/Nutraceutical: Avoid dong quai, St John's wort (may also cause photosensitization).

Effects on Lab Values May interfere with tests for urinary glucose (false-negative urine glucose using Clinistix®).

Adverse Reactions

1% to 10%:

Dermatologic: Photosensitivity

Gastrointestinal: Nausea, diarrhea

<1%: Pericarditis, increased intracranial pressure, bulging fontanels in infants, dermatologic effects, pruritus, exfoliative dermatitis, diabetes insipidus syndrome, vomiting, esophagitis, anorexia, abdominal cramps, paresthesia, acute renal failure, azotemia, superinfections, anaphylaxis, pigmentation of nails

Overdosage/Toxicology Symptoms of overdose include diabetes insipidus, nausea, anorexia, and diarrhea. Treatment is supportive.

Pharmacodynamics/Kinetics

Absorption: ~50% to 80%; reduced by food and dairy products

Half-Life Elimination: Reduced renal function: 10-17 hours

Time to Peak: Serum: 3-6 hours

Metabolism: Hepatic (small amounts) to inactive metabolites; undergoes enterohepatic recirculation

Onset: SIADH: Several days

Formulations Tablet, as hydrochloride: 150 mg, 300 mg

Dosing

Adults & Elderly: Oral: 150 mg 4 times/day or 300 mg twice daily

Uncomplicated gonorrhea (penicillin sensitive): 600 mg stat, 300 mg every 12 hours for 4 days (3 g total)

SIADH: 900-1200 mg/day or 13-15 mg/kg/day divided every 6-8 hours initially, then decrease to 600-900 mg/day

Pediatrics: Susceptible infections: Oral: ≥8 years: 8-12 mg/kg/day divided every 6-12 hours

Renal Impairment: Should be avoided in patients with renal dysfunction.

Hepatic Impairment: Should be avoided in patients with hepatic dysfunction.

Administration

Oral: Administer 1 hour before or 2 hours after food or milk with plenty of fluid.

Monitoring Laboratory Tests CBC, renal and hepatic function; perform culture and sensitivity studies prior to initiating therapy to determine the causative organism and its susceptibility to demeclocycline.

Monitoring and Teaching Issues

Physical Assessment: Assess allergy history prior to beginning therapy. See Contraindications and Warnings/Precautions for use cautions. Assess potential for interactions with other prescriptions, OTC medications, or herbal products patient may be taking (see Drug Interactions). Assess results of laboratory tests (see above), therapeutic response, and adverse reactions (see Adverse Reactions and Overdose/Toxicology) on a regular basis throughout therapy. Caution diabetic patients about altered response to Clinitest®. Teach patient proper use, possible side effects and interventions, and adverse symptoms to report (see Patient Education). **Pregnancy risk factor D** - determine that patient is not pregnant before beginning treatment. Instruct patients in appropriate use barrier contraceptive measures. Note breast-feeding caution.

Patient Education: Inform prescriber of all prescriptions, OTC medications, or herbal products you are taking, and any allergies you have. Do not take anything new during treatment unless approved by prescriber. Take on an empty stomach (1 hour before or 2 hours after meals with plenty of fluid). Take at regularly scheduled intervals around-the-clock. Avoid antacids, iron, dairy products, and other medications within 2 hours of taking demeclocycline. May cause photosensitivity (use sunscreen, wear protective clothing and eyewear, and avoid direct sunlight); dizziness or lightheadedness (use caution when driving or engaging in tasks that require alertness until response to drug is known); nausea or vomiting (frequent, small meals, frequent mouth care, sucking lozenges, or chewing gum may help); or diarrhea (buttermilk, yogurt, or boiled milk may help). Report rash or intense itching, yellowing of skin or eyes, change in color of urine or stools, fever or chills, dark urine or pale stools, vaginal itching or discharge, foul-smelling stools, excessive thirst or urination, acute headache, unresolved diarrhea, or difficulty breathing. **Pregnancy/breast-feeding precautions:** Inform prescriber if you are pregnant. Do not get pregnant while taking this medication. Consult prescriber if breast-feeding.

Dietary Issues: Should be taken 1 hour before or 2 hours after food or milk with plenty of fluid.

Geriatric Considerations: Has not been studied exclusively in the elderly.

Demeclocycline Hydrochloride *see* Demeclocycline *on page 374*

Demerol® *see* Meperidine *on page 851*

4-demethoxydaunorubicin *see* Idarubicin *on page 692*

Demethylchlortetracycline *see* Demeclocycline *on page 374*

Demulen® *see* Ethinyl Estradiol and Ethynodiol Diacetate *on page 521*

Denavir™ *see* Penciclovir *on page 1043*

Denileukin Diftitox (de ne LU kin DEFT e tox)

U.S. Brand Names ONTAK®

Generic Available No

Pharmacologic Category Antineoplastic Agent, Miscellaneous

Pregnancy Risk Factor C

Lactation Excretion in breast milk unknown/contraindicated

Use Treatment of patients with persistent or recurrent cutaneous T-cell lymphoma whose malignant cells express the CD25 component of the IL-2 receptor

Mechanism of Action/Effect Interacts with receptors on surface of malignant cells to inhibit intracellular protein synthesis rapidly leading to cell death.

Contraindications Hypersensitivity to denileukin diftitox, diphtheria toxin, interleukin-2, or any component of the formulation

Warnings/Precautions Acute hypersensitivity reactions, including anaphylaxis, may occur; most events occur during or within 24 hours of the first dose of a treatment cycle. Has been associated with a delayed-onset vascular leak syndrome, which may be severe. Denileukin diftitox may impair immune function. Use with caution in patients with pre-existing cardiovascular disease and in patients >65 years of age. Pregnancy risk C.

Adverse Reactions The occurrence of adverse events diminishes after the first two treatment courses. Infusion-related hypersensitivity reactions have been reported in 69% of patients.

Has been associated with vascular leak syndrome (27%), characterized by hypotension, edema, or hypoalbuminemia, usually developing within the first 2 weeks of infusion. Six percent of patients who developed this syndrome required hospitalization. The symptoms may persist or even worsen despite cessation of denileukin diftitox.

(Continued)

Denileukin Diftitox *(Continued)*

>10%:

Cardiovascular: Edema (47%), hypotension (36%), chest pain (24%), vasodilation (22%), tachycardia (12%)

Central nervous system: Fever/chills (81%), headache (26%), pain (48%), dizziness (22%), nervousness (11%)

Dermatologic: Rash (34%), pruritus (20%)

Endocrine & metabolic: Hypoalbuminemia (83%), hypocalcemia (17%)

Gastrointestinal: Nausea/vomiting (64%), anorexia (36%), diarrhea (29%), weight loss (14%)

Hematologic: Decreased lymphocyte count (34%), anemia (18%)

Hepatic: Increased transaminases (61%)

Neuromuscular & skeletal: Asthenia (66%), myalgia (17%)

Respiratory: Dyspnea (29%), increased cough (26%), pharyngitis (17%), rhinitis (13%)

Miscellaneous: Hypersensitivity (69%), infection (48%), vascular leak syndrome (27%), increased diaphoresis (10%), paresthesia (13%)

1% to 10%:

Cardiovascular: Hypertension (6%), arrhythmias (6%), myocardial infarction (1%)

Central nervous system: Insomnia (9%), confusion (8%)

Endocrine & metabolic: Dehydration (9%), hypokalemia (6%), hyperthyroidism (<5%), hypothyroidism (<5%)

Gastrointestinal: Constipation (9%), dyspepsia (7%), dysphagia (6%), pancreatitis (<5%)

Genitourinary: Hematuria (10%), albuminuria (10%), pyuria (10%)

Hematologic: Thrombotic events (7%), thrombocytopenia (8%), leukopenia (6%)

Local: Injection site reaction (8%)

Miscellaneous: Anaphylaxis (1%)

Neuromuscular & skeletal: Arthralgia (8%)

Renal: Increased creatinine (7%), acute renal insufficiency (<5%)

Overdosage/Toxicology Although there is no human experience in overdose, dose-limiting toxicities include nausea, vomiting, fever, chills and persistent asthenia. Treatment is supportive and symptom-directed. Fluid balance, as well as hepatic and renal function, should be closely monitored.

Pharmacodynamics/Kinetics

Half-Life Elimination: Distribution: 2-5 minutes; Terminal: 70-80 minutes

Metabolism: Hepatic via proteolytic degradation (animal studies)

Formulations Injection, solution [frozen]: 150 mcg/mL (2 mL)

Dosing

Adults & Elderly: Persistent or recurrent cutaneous T-cell lymphoma: I.V.: A treatment cycle consists of 9 or 18 mcg/kg/day for 5 consecutive days administered every 21 days. The optimal duration of therapy has not been determined. Only 2% of patients who failed to demonstrate a response (at least a 25% decrease in tumor burden) prior to the fourth cycle responded to subsequent treatment.

Administration

I.V.: For I.V. use only. Should be infused over at least 15 minutes. Should not be given as an I.V. bolus. Patients should be closely observed during the infusion for symptoms of hypersensitivity. If a patient experiences a reaction, the severity of the reaction should be evaluated, and a decision should be made to either reduce the rate or discontinue the infusion. Resuscitation equipment must be readily available. Delay therapy if serum albumin is <3 g/dL.

Stability

Storage: Store frozen at or -10°C; cannot be refrozen.

Reconstitution: Must be brought to room temperature (25°C or 77°F) before preparing the dose. Do **not** heat vials. Thaw in refrigerator for not more than 24 hours or at room temperature for 1-2 hours. Avoid vigorous agitation. Solution may be mixed by gentle swirling.

Compatibility: Do **not** use glass syringes or containers.

Monitoring Laboratory Tests Prior to administration, malignant cells should be tested for expression of CD25. The patient should have a CBC, blood chemistry panel, renal and hepatic function tests as well as a serum albumin level. These tests should be repeated at weekly intervals during therapy.

Monitoring and Teaching Issues

Physical Assessment: See Contraindications, Warnings/Precautions, and Dosing for use cautions. Assess results of laboratory tests (see above) prior to therapy and weekly during therapy. Patient must be monitored closely for acute hypersensitivity reaction during and for 24 hours following first infusion (see Adverse Reactions and Administration). Following infusion, patient should be monitored or taught to monitor for delayed vascular leak syndrome (eg, hypotension, edema, or hypoalbuminemia) and other adverse reactions (see Adverse Reactions). Teach patient appropriate interventions to reduce side effects and adverse reactions to report (see Patient Education). **Pregnancy risk factor C** - benefits of use should outweigh possible risks. Breast-feeding is contraindicated.

Patient Education: This drug can only be administered I.V. During infusion, report immediately any chills; chest pain, difficulty breathing, or tightness in throat; or redness, swelling, pain, or burning at infusion site. Maintaining adequate nutrition and hydration is important (2-3 L/day) unless advised by prescriber to restrict fluids. You may be more susceptible to infection (avoid crowds and exposure to infection and do not have any vaccinations without consulting prescriber). May cause nausea, vomiting, anorexia, flatulence (small, frequent meals, good mouth care, chewing gum, or sucking lozenges may help); constipation (increased exercise, fluids, fruit, or fiber may help); diarrhea (buttermilk, boiled milk, or yogurt may help); headache, back or muscle pain (consult prescriber for mild analgesic); dizziness, weakness, or confusion (use caution when driving, engaging in hazardous activities, or climbing stairs until effect of medication is known). Report unresolved GI effects; headache, back or muscle pain; skin dryness, rash, or sores; altered urinary patterns; flu syndrome or infection (eg, weakness, fatigue, white plaques or sores in mouth, vaginal discharge, chills, fever); CNS disturbances (insomnia, dizziness, agitation, confusion, depression); unusual bleeding or bruising, blood in urine or stool; swelling of extremities; or any other adverse effects. **Pregnancy/breast-feeding precautions:** Inform prescriber if you are or intend to become pregnant. Do not breast-feed.

Breast-feeding Issues: The excretion of denileukin diftitox in breast milk is unknown, however, it is recommended that a breast-feeding woman who is treated with denileukin diftitox should discontinue nursing.

Additional Information Formulation includes EDTA and polysorbate 20, and has a pH of 6.9-7.2.

Deoxycoformycin *see* Pentostatin *on page 1056*

2′-deoxycoformycin *see* Pentostatin *on page 1056*

Depacon® *see* Valproic Acid and Derivatives *on page 1382*

Depakene® *see* Valproic Acid and Derivatives *on page 1382*

Depakote® Delayed Release *see* Valproic Acid and Derivatives *on page 1382*

Depakote® ER *see* Valproic Acid and Derivatives *on page 1382*

Depakote® Sprinkle® *see* Valproic Acid and Derivatives *on page 1382*

depMedalone® *see* MethylPREDNISolone *on page 885*

DepoCyt™ *see* Cytarabine (Liposomal) *on page 350*

Depo®-Estradiol *see* Estradiol *on page 494*

Depoject® *see* MethylPREDNISolone *on page 885*

Depo-Medrol® *see* MethylPREDNISolone *on page 885*

Deponit® [DSC] *see* Nitroglycerin *on page 977*

Depopred® *see* MethylPREDNISolone *on page 885*

Depo-Provera® *see* MedroxyPROGESTERone *on page 842*

Depo®-Testosterone *see* Testosterone *on page 1294*

Deprenyl *see* Selegiline *on page 1221*

Depression *see page 1659*

Dermacort® *see* Topical Corticosteroids *on page 1334*

Dermarest Dricort® [OTC] *see* Hydrocortisone *on page 673*

Derma-Smoothe/FS® *see* Topical Corticosteroids *on page 1334*

Dermatop® *see* Topical Corticosteroids *on page 1334*

Dermatophytin® Injection *see page 1461*

Dermatophytin-O *see page 1461*

Dermazene® *see* Iodoquinol and Hydrocortisone *on page 732*

DermiCort® *see* Topical Corticosteroids *on page 1334*

Dermolate® [OTC] *see* Topical Corticosteroids *on page 1334*

Dermtex® HC [OTC] *see* Hydrocortisone *on page 673*

Dermtex® HC With Aloe *see* Topical Corticosteroids *on page 1334*

DES *see* Diethylstilbestrol *on page 407*

Desferal® *see* Deferoxamine *on page 371*

Desiccated Thyroid *see* Thyroid *on page 1313*

Desipramine (des IP ra meen)

U.S. Brand Names Norpramin®

Synonyms Desipramine Hydrochloride; Desmethylimipramine Hydrochloride

Generic Available Yes

Pharmacologic Category Antidepressant, Tricyclic (Secondary Amine)

Pregnancy Risk Factor C

Lactation Enters breast milk/not recommended (AAP rates "of concern")

Use Treatment of depression

Use - Unlabeled/Investigational Analgesic adjunct in chronic pain; peripheral neuropathies; substance-related disorders; attention-deficit/hyperactivity disorder (ADHD)

Mechanism of Action/Effect Traditionally believed to increase the synaptic concentration of norepinephrine (and to a lesser extent, serotonin) in the central nervous system by inhibition of its reuptake by the presynaptic neuronal membrane. However, additional receptor effects have been found including desensitization of adenyl cyclase, down regulation of beta-adrenergic receptors, and down regulation of serotonin receptors.

Contraindications Hypersensitivity to desipramine, drugs of similar chemical class, or any component of the formulation; use of MAO inhibitors within 14 days; use in a patient during the acute recovery phase of MI

Warnings/Precautions May cause drowsiness/sedation, resulting in impaired performance of tasks requiring alertness (ie, operating machinery or driving). Sedative effects may be additive with other CNS depressants and/or ethanol. May worsen psychosis in some patients or precipitate a shift to mania or hypomania in patients with bipolar disease. May cause hyponatremia/SIADH. May increase the risks associated with electroconvulsive therapy. Discontinue, when possible, prior to elective surgery. Therapy should not be abruptly discontinued in patients receiving high doses for prolonged periods.

Use with caution in patients at risk of hypotension (orthostasis) or in patients where transient hypotensive episodes would be poorly tolerated (cardiovascular disease or cerebrovascular disease). Use with caution in elderly patients, patients with diabetes, thyroid disease (or patients receiving thyroid supplements), hepatic dysfunction, renal dysfunction, urinary retention, benign prostatic hyperplasia, narrow-angle glaucoma, xerostomia, visual problems, constipation, or a history of bowel obstruction.

Use caution in patients with depression, particularly if suicidal risk may be present. Use with caution in patients with a history of cardiovascular disease (including previous MI, stroke, tachycardia, or conduction abnormalities). Use caution in patients with a previous seizure disorder or condition predisposing to seizures such as brain damage, alcoholism, or concurrent therapy with other drugs which lower the seizure threshold.

(Continued)

Desipramine *(Continued)*

Pregnancy risk C.

Drug Interactions

Cytochrome P450 Effect: Substrate of CYP1A2, **2D6**; Inhibits CYP2D6, 2E1

Decreased Effect: Desipramine's serum levels/effect may be decreased by carbamazepine, cholestyramine, colestipol, phenobarbital, and rifampin. Desipramine inhibits the antihypertensive effect of to bethanidine, clonidine, debrisoquin, guanadrel, guanethidine, guanabenz, or guanfacine.

Increased Effect/Toxicity: Desipramine increases the effects of amphetamines, anticholinergics, other CNS depressants (sedatives, hypnotics, or ethanol), chlorpropamide, tolazamide, and warfarin. When used with MAO inhibitors, serotonin syndrome may occur. Serotonin syndrome has also been reported with ritonavir (rare). The SSRIs (to varying degrees), cimetidine, grapefruit juice, indinavir, methylphenidate, ritonavir (and other protease inhibitors), quinidine, diltiazem, and verapamil inhibit the metabolism of TCAs and clinical toxicity may result. Use of lithium with a TCA may increase the risk for neurotoxicity. Phenothiazines may increase concentration of some TCAs and TCAs may increase concentration of phenothiazines. Pressor response to I.V. epinephrine, norepinephrine, and phenylephrine may be enhanced in patients receiving TCAs (**Note:** Effect is unlikely with epinephrine or levonordefrin dosages typically administered as infiltration in combination with local anesthetics). Combined use of beta-agonists or drugs which prolong QT_c (including quinidine, procainamide, disopyramide, cisapride, sparfloxacin, gatifloxacin, moxifloxacin) with TCAs may predispose patients to cardiac arrhythmias.

Nutritional/Ethanol Interactions

Ethanol: Avoid ethanol (may increase CNS depression).

Food: Grapefruit juice may inhibit the metabolism of some TCAs and clinical toxicity may result.

Herb/Nutraceutical: Avoid valerian, St John's wort, SAMe, kava kava (may increase risk of serotonin syndrome and/or excessive sedation).

Effects on Lab Values ↑ glucose; ↓ glucose has also been reported

Adverse Reactions Frequency not defined.

Cardiovascular: Arrhythmias, hypotension, hypertension, palpitations, heart block, tachycardia

Central nervous system: Dizziness, drowsiness, headache, confusion, delirium, hallucinations, nervousness, restlessness, parkinsonian syndrome, insomnia, disorientation, anxiety, agitation, hypomania, exacerbation of psychosis, incoordination, seizures, extrapyramidal symptoms

Dermatologic: Alopecia, photosensitivity, skin rash, urticaria

Endocrine & metabolic: Breast enlargement, galactorrhea, SIADH

Gastrointestinal: Xerostomia, decreased lower esophageal sphincter tone may cause GE reflux, constipation, nausea, unpleasant taste, weight gain/loss, anorexia, abdominal cramps, diarrhea, heartburn

Genitourinary: Difficult urination, sexual dysfunction, testicular edema

Hematologic: Agranulocytosis, eosinophilia, purpura, thrombocytopenia

Hepatic: Cholestatic jaundice, increased liver enzyme

Neuromuscular & skeletal: Fine muscle tremors, weakness, numbness, tingling, paresthesia of extremities, ataxia

Ocular: Blurred vision, disturbances of accommodation, mydriasis, increased intraocular pressure

Miscellaneous: Diaphoresis (excessive), allergic reactions

Overdosage/Toxicology Symptoms of overdose include agitation, confusion, hallucinations, hyperthermia, urinary retention, CNS depression, cyanosis, dry mucous membranes, cardiac arrhythmias, and seizures. Treatment is supportive. Ventricular arrhythmias and EKG changes (eg, QRS widening) often respond with concurrent systemic alkalinization (sodium bicarbonate 0.5-2 mEq/kg I.V. or hyperventilation). Arrhythmias unresponsive to phenytoin 15-20 mg/kg (adults) may respond to lidocaine. Physostigmine (1-2 mg I.V. slowly for adults) may be indicated for reversing life-threatening cardiac arrhythmias.

Pharmacodynamics/Kinetics

Absorption: Well absorbed

Half-Life Elimination: Adults: 7-60 hours

Time to Peak: Plasma: 4-6 hours

Metabolism: Hepatic

Onset: 1-3 weeks; Maximum antidepressant effect: >2 weeks

Formulations Tablet, as hydrochloride: 10 mg, 25 mg, 50 mg, 75 mg, 100 mg, 150 mg

Dosing

Adults: Depression: Oral: Initial: 75 mg/day in divided doses; increase gradually to 150-200 mg/day in divided or single dose; maximum: 300 mg/day

Elderly: Oral: Initial: 10-25 mg/day; increase by 10-25 mg every 3 days for inpatients and every week for outpatients if tolerated; usual maintenance dose: 75-100 mg/day, but doses up to 150 mg/day may be necessary.

Pediatrics: Depression: Oral:

Children 6-12 years: 10-30 mg/day or 1-5 mg/kg/day in divided doses; do not exceed 5 mg/kg/day

Adolescents: Initial: 25-50 mg/day; gradually increase to 100 mg/day in single or divided doses; maximum: 150 mg/day

Renal Impairment: Hemodialysis/peritoneal dialysis effects: Supplemental dose is not necessary.

Monitoring and Teaching Issues

Physical Assessment: See Contraindications, Warnings/Precautions, and Dosing for use cautions. Assess potential for interactions with other prescriptions, OTC medications, or herbal products patient may be taking (see extensive list of Drug Interactions). Assess for suicidal tendencies before beginning therapy. May cause physiological or psychological dependence, tolerance, or abuse; periodically evaluate need for continued use. Caution patients with diabetes to monitor glucose levels closely; may increase or decrease serum glucose levels. Monitor therapeutic response and adverse reactions at beginning of therapy and periodically with long-term use (see Adverse Reactions and Overdose/Toxicology). Taper dose slowly when discontinuing. Teach patient appropriate use, interventions to reduce side effects, and adverse symptoms to report (see Patient Education). **Pregnancy risk factor C** - benefits of use should outweigh possible risks. Breast-feeding is not recommended.

Patient Education: Inform prescriber of all prescriptions, OTC medications, or herbal products you are taking, and any allergies you have. Do not take anything new during treatment unless approved by prescriber. Take exactly as directed; do not increase dose or frequency. It may take 2-3 weeks to achieve desired results. This medicine may cause physical and/or psychological dependence. Avoid alcohol and grapefruit juice. Maintain adequate hydration (2-3 L/day of fluids) unless advised by prescriber to restrict fluids. May cause drowsiness, lightheadedness, impaired coordination, dizziness, or blurred vision (use caution when driving or engaging in tasks requiring alertness until response to drug is known); loss of appetite or disturbed taste (small, frequent meals, good mouth care, chewing gum, or sucking lozenges may help); constipation (increased exercise, fluids, fruit, or fiber may help); urinary retention (void before taking medication); postural hypotension (use caution climbing stairs or when changing position from lying or sitting to standing); altered sexual drive or ability (reversible); or photosensitivity (use sunscreen, wear protective clothing and eyewear, and avoid direct sunlight). Report chest pain, palpitations, or rapid heartbeat; persistent CNS effects (eg, nervousness, restlessness, insomnia, anxiety, excitation, headache, agitation, impaired coordination, changes in cognition); muscle cramping, weakness, tremors, or rigidity; blurred vision or eye pain; breast enlargement or swelling; yellowing of skin or eyes; or worsening of condition. **Pregnancy/breast-feeding precautions:** Inform prescriber if you are or intend to become pregnant. Breast-feeding is not recommended.

Geriatric Considerations: Preferred agent because of its milder side effect profile; patients may experience excitation or stimulation, in such cases, give as a single morning dose or divided dose.

Breast-feeding Issues: Generally, it is not recommended to breast-feed if taking antidepressants because of the long half-life, active metabolites, and the potential for side effects in the infant.

Additional Information Less sedation and anticholinergic effects than with amitriptyline or imipramine

Related Information

Antidepressant Agents *on page 1553*
Antidepressant Medication Guidelines *on page 1613*
Peak and Trough Guidelines *on page 1544*
Pharmacotherapy of Urinary Incontinence *on page 1699*

Desipramine Hydrochloride *see* Desipramine *on page 377*

Desloratadine (des lor AT a deen)

U.S. Brand Names Clarinex®

Generic Available No

Pharmacologic Category Antihistamine, Nonsedating

Pregnancy Risk Factor C

Lactation Enters breast milk/not recommended

Use Relief of nasal and non-nasal symptoms of seasonal allergic rhinitis (SAR) and perennial allergic rhinitis (PAR); treatment of chronic idiopathic urticaria (CIU)

Mechanism of Action/Effect Desloratadine is a long-acting antihistamine with selective H_1 receptor antagonistic activity.

Contraindications Hypersensitivity to desloratadine, loratadine, or any component of the formulation

Warnings/Precautions Dose should be adjusted in patients with liver or renal impairment. Use with caution in patients known to be slow metabolizers of desloratadine (incidence of side effects may be increased). RediTabs® contain phenylalanine. Safety and efficacy have not been established for children <12 years of age. Pregnancy risk C.

Drug Interactions

Increased Effect/Toxicity: With concurrent use of desloratadine and erythromycin or ketoconazole, the C_{max} and AUC of desloratadine and its metabolite are increased; however, no clinically-significant changes in the safety profile of desloratadine were observed in clinical studies.

Nutritional/Ethanol Interactions Food: Does not affect bioavailability.

Adverse Reactions

>10%: Central nervous system: Headache (14%)

1% to 10%:

Central nervous system: Fatigue (2% to 5%), somnolence (2%), dizziness (4%)
Endocrine & metabolic: Dysmenorrhea (2%)
Gastrointestinal: Xerostomia (3%), nausea (5%), dyspepsia (3%)
Neuromuscular & skeletal: Myalgia (3%)
Respiratory: Pharyngitis (3% to 4%)

Postmarketing and/or case reports: Anaphylaxis, bilirubin increased, dyspnea, edema, hypersensitivity reactions, liver enzymes increased, pruritus, rash, tachycardia, urticaria

Overdosage/Toxicology Information is limited to doses studied during clinical trials (up to 45 mg/day). Symptoms included somnolence, and small increases in heart rate and QT_c interval (not clinically significant). In the event of an overdose, treatment should be symptom-directed and supportive. Desloratadine and its metabolite are not removed by hemodialysis.

Pharmacodynamics/Kinetics

Half-Life Elimination: 27 hours

Time to Peak: 3 hours

Metabolism: Hepatic to active metabolite, 3-hydroxydesloratadine (specific enzymes not identified); undergoes glucuronidation. Decreased in slow metabolizers of desloratadine.

(Continued)

Desloratadine *(Continued)*

Not expected to affect or be affected by medications metabolized by CYP with normal doses.

Formulations

Tablet (Clarinex®): 5 mg

Tablet, orally-disintegrating (Clarinex® RediTabs®): 5 mg [contains phenylalanine 1.75 mg/tablet; tutti-frutti flavor]

Dosing

Adults & Elderly: Seasonal or perennial allergic rhinitis, chronic idiopathic urticaria: Oral: 5 mg once daily

Pediatrics: Children ≥12 years: Seasonal or perennial allergic rhinitis, chronic idiopathic urticaria: Oral: Refer to adult dosing.

Renal Impairment: 5 mg every other day

Hepatic Impairment: 5 mg every other day

Administration

Oral: May be taken with or without food.

RediTabs® should be placed on the tongue; tablet will disintegrate immediately. May be taken with or without water.

Stability

Storage:

Tablet: Store between 2°C to 25°C (36°F to 77°F). Protect from moisture and excessive heat (temperatures ≥30°C/86°F).

Orally-disintegrating tablet: Store between 15°C to 30°C (59°F to 86°F). Use immediately after opening blister package.

Monitoring and Teaching Issues

Physical Assessment: Assess effectiveness and interactions of other medications patient may be taking (see Drug Interactions). See Warning/Precautions for use cautions. Monitor effectiveness of therapy and adverse reactions (see Adverse Reactions) at beginning of therapy and periodically with long-term use. Assess knowledge/teach patient appropriate use, interventions to reduce side effects, and adverse symptoms to report (see Patient Education). **Pregnancy risk factor C** - benefits of use should outweigh possible risks. Breast-feeding is not recommended.

Patient Education: Take as directed; do not exceed recommended dose. Avoid use of other depressants, alcohol, or sleep-inducing medications unless approved by prescriber. You may experience drowsiness or dizziness (use caution when driving or engaging in tasks that require alertness until response to drug is known); or dry mouth, dry throat, or nausea (small, frequent meals, frequent mouth care, chewing gum, or sucking hard candy may help). Report rapid heartbeat, shortness of breath, skin rash, persistent flu-like symptoms, or muscle aches. **Pregnancy/breast-feeding precautions**: Inform prescriber if you are or intend to become pregnant. Breast-feeding is not recommended.

Dietary Issues: May be taken with or without food. Orally-disintegrating tablets contain phenylalanine 1.75 mg/tablet.

Desmethylimipramine Hydrochloride *see* Desipramine *on page 377*

Desmopressin (des moe PRES in)

U.S. Brand Names DDAVP®; Stimate™

Synonyms 1-Deamino-8-D-Arginine Vasopressin; Desmopressin Acetate

Generic Available Yes: Injection only

Pharmacologic Category Vasopressin Analog, Synthetic

Pregnancy Risk Factor B

Lactation Excretion in breast milk unknown/use caution

Use Treatment of diabetes insipidus; control of bleeding in hemophilia A, and mild-to-moderate classic von Willebrand disease (type I); primary nocturnal enuresis

Mechanism of Action/Effect Enhances reabsorption of water in the kidneys by increasing cellular permeability of the collecting ducts; possibly causes smooth muscle constriction with resultant vasoconstriction; raises plasma levels of von Willebrand factor and factor VIII

Contraindications Hypersensitivity to desmopressin or any component of the formulation; hemophilia B, severe classic von Willebrand disease (type IIB); patients with ≤5% factor VIII activity level; factor VIII antibodies

Warnings/Precautions Fluid intake should be adjusted downward in the elderly and very young patients to decrease the possibility of water intoxication and hyponatremia. Avoid overhydration especially when drug is used for its hemostatic effect. Use caution with cystic fibrosis or other conditions associated with fluid and electrolyte imbalance due to potential hyponatremia. Use caution with coronary artery insufficiency or hypertensive cardiovascular disease; may increase or decrease blood pressure leading to changes in heart rate. Consider switching from nasal to intravenous solution if changes in the nasal mucosa (scarring, edema) occur leading to unreliable absorption. Use caution in patients predisposed to thrombus formation; thrombotic events (acute cerebrovascular thrombosis, acute myocardial infarction) have occurred (rare). Use may rarely lead to extreme decreases in plasma osmolality, resulting in seizures and coma.

Drug Interactions

Decreased Effect: Demeclocycline and lithium may decrease ADH response.

Increased Effect/Toxicity: Chlorpropamide, fludrocortisone may increase ADH response.

Nutritional/Ethanol Interactions Ethanol: Avoid ethanol (may decrease antidiuretic effect).

Adverse Reactions Frequency not defined (may be dose or route related).

Cardiovascular: Acute cerebrovascular thrombosis, acute MI, blood pressure increased/decreased, chest pain, edema, facial flushing, palpitations

Central nervous system: Agitation, chills, coma, dizziness, headache, insomnia, somnolence

Endocrine & metabolic: Hyponatremia, water intoxication

Gastrointestinal: Abdominal cramps, dyspepsia, nausea, sore throat, vomiting

Genitourinary: Balanitis, vulval pain

Local: Injection: Burning pain, erythema, and swelling at the injection site

Respiratory: Cough, nasal congestion, epistaxis
Miscellaneous: Allergic reactions (rare), anaphylaxis (rare)

Overdosage/Toxicology Symptoms of overdose include drowsiness, headache, confusion, anuria, and water intoxication. In case of overdose, decrease or discontinue desmopressin.

Pharmacodynamics/Kinetics

Bioavailability: Tablet: 5% compared to intranasal; 0.16% compared to I.V.

Half-Life Elimination:
I.V. infusion: Terminal: 75 minutes
Tablet: 1.5-2.5 hours

Metabolism: Unknown

Onset:
Intranasal administration: Onset of increased factor VIII activity: 30 minutes (dose related); peak effect 1.5 hours
I.V. infusion: Onset of increased factor VIII activity: 30 minutes (dose related); peak effect: 1.5-2 hours
Oral tablets: Onset of action: ADH: ~1 hour; peak effect: 4-7 hours

Formulations
Injection, solution, as acetate (DDAVP®): 4 mcg/mL (1 mL, 10 mL)
Solution, intranasal, as acetate (DDAVP®): 100 mcg/mL (2.5 mL) [with rhinal tube]
Solution, intranasal spray, as acetate:
DDAVP®: 100 mcg/mL (5 mL) [delivers 10 mcg/spray]
Stimate™: 1.5 mg/mL (2.5 mL)
Tablet, as acetate (DDAVP®): 0.1 mg, 0.2 mg

Dosing

Adults & Elderly:
Diabetes insipidus:
I.V., S.C.: 2-4 mcg/day (0.5-1 mL) in 2 divided doses or 1/10 of the maintenance intranasal dose
Intranasal (100 mcg/mL nasal solution): 10-40 mcg/day (0.1-0.4 mL) divided 1-3 times/day; adjust morning and evening doses separately for an adequate diurnal rhythm of water turnover. **Note:** The nasal spray pump can only deliver doses of 10 mcg (0.1 mL) or multiples of 10 mcg (0.1 mL); if doses other than this are needed, the rhinal tube delivery system is preferred.
Oral: Initial: 0.05 mg twice daily; total daily dose should be increased or decreased as needed to obtain adequate antidiuresis (range: 0.1-1.2 mg divided 2-3 times/day)
Nocturnal enuresis:
Intranasal (using 100 mcg/mL nasal solution): Initial: 20 mcg (0.2 mL) at bedtime; range: 10-40 mcg; it is recommended that ½ of the dose be given in each nostril. **Note:** The nasal spray pump can only deliver doses of 10 mcg (0.1 mL) or multiples of 10 mcg (0.1 mL); if doses other than this are needed, the rhinal tube delivery system is preferred.
Oral: 0.2 mg at bedtime; dose may be titrated up to 0.6 mg to achieve desired response. Patients previously on intranasal therapy can begin oral tablets 24 hours after the last intranasal dose.
Hemophilia A and mild-to-moderate von Willebrand disease (type I):
I.V.: 0.3 mcg/kg by slow infusion, begin 30 minutes before procedure
Nasal spray: Using high concentration spray (1.5 mg/mL): <50 kg: 150 mcg (1 spray); >50 kg: 300 mcg (1 spray each nostril); repeat use is determined by the patient's clinical condition and laboratory work. If using preoperatively, administer 2 hours before surgery.

Pediatrics:
Diabetes insipidus:
Intranasal (using 100 mcg/mL nasal solution):
Children 3 months to 12 years: Initial: 5 mcg/day (0.05 mL/day) divided 1-2 times/day; range: 5-30 mcg/day (0.05-0.3 mL/day) divided 1-2 times/day; adjust morning and evening doses separately for an adequate diurnal rhythm of water turnover; doses <10 mcg should be administered using the rhinal tube system
Children >12 years: Refer to adult dosing.
Oral: Children ≥4 years: Initial: 0.05 mg twice daily; total daily dose should be increased or decreased as needed to obtain adequate antidiuresis (range: 0.1-1.2 mg divided 2-3 times/day)
Hemophilia A and von Willebrand disease (type I):
I.V.: >3 months: 0.3 mcg/kg by slow infusion; may repeat dose if needed; begin 30 minutes before procedure
Intranasal: ≥11 months: Refer to adult dosing.
Nocturnal enuresis:
Children ≥6 years:
Intranasal (using 100 mcg/mL nasal solution): Initial: 20 mcg (0.2 mL) at bedtime; range: 10-40 mcg; it is recommended that ½ of the dose be given in each nostril. **Note:** The nasal spray pump can only deliver doses of 10 mcg (0.1 mL) or multiples of 10 mcg (0.1 mL); if doses other than this are needed, the rhinal tube delivery system is preferred.
Oral: 0.2 mg at bedtime. Dose may be titrated up to 0.6 mg to achieve desired response. Patients previously on intranasal therapy can begin oral tablets 24 hours after the last intranasal dose.
Children >12 years: Refer to adult dosing.

Administration

I.V.: Dilute in 0.9% sodium chloride and infuse over 15-30 minutes; dose should be diluted in 10 mL NS for children ≤10 kg; 50 mL NS for adults and children >10 kg

Other: DDAVP®: Nasal pump spray delivers 0.1 mL (10 mcg); for other doses which are not multiples, use rhinal tube. DDAVP® Nasal spray delivers fifty 10 mcg doses. Any solution remaining after 50 doses should be discarded. Pump must be primed prior to first use.

(Continued)

Desmopressin *(Continued)*

Stability

Storage:

DDAVP®:

Tablet, nasal spray: Store at controlled room temperature of 20°C to 25°C (68°F to 77°F). Keep nasal spray in upright position.

Rhinal tube: Store refrigerated at 2°C to 8°C (36°F to 46°F). May store at room temperature for up to 3 weeks.

Injection: Store refrigerated at 2°C to 8°C (36°F to 46°F).

Stimate™: Store refrigerated at 2°C to 8°C (36°F to 46°F). May store at room temperature for up to 3 weeks.

Monitoring Laboratory Tests

Diabetes insipidus: Urine volume, specific gravity, plasma and urine osmolality, serum electrolytes

Hemophilia: Factor VIII antigen levels, APTT, bleeding time (for von Willebrand disease and thrombocytopathies)

Monitoring and Teaching Issues

Physical Assessment: See Contraindications, Warnings/Precautions, Drug Interactions, and Dosing for use cautions. Assess results of laboratory tests according to purpose for use (see above), therapeutic effectiveness, and adverse reactions (see Adverse Reactions and Overdose/Toxicology) on a regular basis throughout therapy. Teach patient proper use (if self-administered), possible side effects and interventions, and adverse symptoms to report (see Patient Education). Note breast-feeding caution.

Patient Education: Inform prescriber of all prescriptions, OTC medications, or herbal products you are taking, and any allergies you have. Do not take anything new during treatment unless approved by prescriber. Use specific product as directed. Avoid alcohol.

Diabetes insipidus: Avoid overhydration. Weigh yourself daily at the same time in the same clothes. Report increased weight or swelling of extremities. If using intranasal product, inspect nasal membranes regularly. Report swelling or increased nasal congestion.

All uses: Report unresolved headache, difficulty breathing, acute heartburn or nausea, abdominal cramping, or vulval pain. **Breast-feeding precaution:** Consult prescriber if breast-feeding.

Geriatric Considerations: Elderly patients should be cautioned not to increase their fluid intake beyond that sufficient to satisfy their thirst in order to avoid water intoxication and hyponatremia.

Additional Information 10 mcg of desmopressin acetate is equivalent to 40 int. units

Desmopressin Acetate *see* Desmopressin *on page 380*

Desogen® *see* Ethinyl Estradiol and Desogestrel *on page 516*

Desogestrel and Ethinyl Estradiol *see* Ethinyl Estradiol and Desogestrel *on page 516*

Desonide *see* Topical Corticosteroids *on page 1334*

DesOwen® *see* Topical Corticosteroids *on page 1334*

Desoximetasone *see* Topical Corticosteroids *on page 1334*

Desoxyphenobarbital *see* Primidone *on page 1119*

Desoxyribonuclease and Fibrinolysin *see* Fibrinolysin and Desoxyribonuclease *on page 558*

Desyrel® *see* Trazodone *on page 1351*

Detane® [OTC] *see* Benzocaine *on page 156*

Detrol™ *see* Tolterodine *on page 1333*

Detrol® LA *see* Tolterodine *on page 1333*

Dexacidin® *see page 1509*

Dexamethasone (deks a METH a sone)

U.S. Brand Names Decadron®; Decadron® Phosphate; Dexamethasone Intensol®; Dexasone®; Dexasone® L.A.; DexPak® TaperPak®; Maxidex®; Solurex®; Solurex L.A.®

Synonyms Dexamethasone Acetate; Dexamethasone Sodium Phosphate

Generic Available Yes

Pharmacologic Category Corticosteroid, Nasal; Corticosteroid, Ophthalmic; Corticosteroid, Systemic; Corticosteroid, Topical

Pregnancy Risk Factor C

Lactation Excretion in breast milk unknown

Use Systemically and locally for chronic swelling; allergic, hematologic, neoplastic, and autoimmune diseases; may be used in management of cerebral edema, septic shock, as a diagnostic agent, antiemetic

Use - Unlabeled/Investigational General indicator consistent with depression; diagnosis of Cushing's syndrome

Mechanism of Action/Effect Decreases inflammation by suppression of migration of polymorphonuclear leukocytes and reversal of increased capillary permeability; suppresses normal immune response

Contraindications Hypersensitivity to dexamethasone or any component of the formulation; active untreated infections; ophthalmic use in viral, fungal, or tuberculosis diseases of the eye

Warnings/Precautions Dexamethasone has a low degree of mineralocorticoid activity, which limits potential for fluid retention or hyperkalemia. Use caution in patients with hypothyroidism, cirrhosis, hypertension, CHF, ulcerative colitis, or thromboembolic disorders. Corticosteroids should be used with caution in patients with diabetes, osteoporosis, peptic ulcer, glaucoma, cataracts, or tuberculosis. Use caution in hepatic impairment. May cause suppression of hypothalamic-pituitary-adrenal (HPA) axis, particularly in younger children or in patients receiving high doses for prolonged periods. Fatalities have occurred due to adrenal insufficiency in asthmatic patients during and after transfer from systemic corticosteroids to aerosol steroids; aerosol steroids do **not** provide the systemic steroid needed to treat patients having trauma, surgery, or infections. Withdrawal and discontinuation of the corticosteroid should be done slowly and carefully

Controlled clinical studies have shown that orally-inhaled and intranasal corticosteroids may cause a reduction in growth velocity in pediatric patients, which appears to be related to dose and duration of exposure.

May suppress the immune system, patients may be more susceptible to infection. Use with caution in patients with systemic infections or ocular herpes simplex. Avoid exposure to chickenpox and measles.

Pregnancy risk C.

Drug Interactions

Cytochrome P450 Effect: Substrate of CYP3A4; Induces CYP2A6, 2B6, 2C8/9, 3A4

Decreased Effect: Barbiturates, phenytoin, and rifampin may cause decreased dexamethasone effects. Dexamethasone decreases effect of salicylates, vaccines, and toxoids.

Nutritional/Ethanol Interactions

Ethanol: Avoid ethanol (may enhance gastric mucosal irritation).
Food: Dexamethasone interferes with calcium absorption. Limit caffeine.
Herb/Nutraceutical: Avoid cat's claw, echinacea (have immunostimulant properties).

Adverse Reactions

Systemic:

>10%:
- Central nervous system: Insomnia, nervousness
- Gastrointestinal: Increased appetite, indigestion

1% to 10%:
- Dermatologic: Hirsutism
- Endocrine & metabolic: Diabetes mellitus
- Neuromuscular & skeletal: Arthralgia
- Ocular: Cataracts
- Respiratory: Epistaxis

<1% (Limited to important or life-threatening): Abdominal distention, acne, amenorrhea, bone growth suppression, bruising, Cushing's syndrome, delirium, euphoria, hallucinations, headache, hyperglycemia, hyperpigmentation, hypersensitivity reactions, mood swings, muscle wasting, pancreatitis, seizures, skin atrophy, sodium and water retention, ulcerative esophagitis

Topical: <1% (Limited to important or life-threatening): Acneiform eruptions, allergic contact dermatitis, burning, dryness, folliculitis, hypertrichosis, hypopigmentation, irritation, itching, miliaria, perioral dermatitis, secondary infection, skin atrophy, skin maceration, striae

Overdosage/Toxicology When consumed in high doses over prolonged periods, systemic hypercorticism and adrenal suppression may occur. In these cases, discontinuation of the corticosteroid should be done judiciously.

Pharmacodynamics/Kinetics

Half-Life Elimination: Normal renal function: 1.8-3.5 hours; Biological half-life: 36-54 hours

Time to Peak: Serum: Oral: 1-2 hours; I.M.: ~8 hours

Metabolism: Hepatic

Onset: Acetate: Prompt

Duration: Metabolic effect: 72 hours; acetate is a long-acting repository preparation

Formulations

Elixir, as base: 0.5 mg/5 mL (100 mL, 240 mL) [contains alcohol 5%; raspberry flavor]
Injection, suspension, as acetate: (Dexasone® LA, Solurex LA®): 8 mg/mL (5 mL)
Injection, solution, as sodium phosphate: 4 mg/mL (1 mL, 5 mL, 10 mL, 25 mL, 30 mL); 10 mg/mL (1 mL, 10 mL)
- Decadron® Phosphate: 4 mg/mL (5 mL, 25 mL); 24 mg/mL (5 mL) [contains sodium bisulfite]
- Dexasone: 4 mg/mL (5 mL)
- Solurex: 4 mg/mL (5 mL, 10 mL, 30 mL)

Ointment, ophthalmic, as sodium phosphate: 0.05% (3.5 g)
Solution, oral: 0.5 mg/5 mL (5 mL, 500 mL) [cherry flavor]
Solution, oral concentrate (Dexamethasone Intensol®): 1 mg/mL (30 mL) [contains alcohol 30%]
Suspension, ophthalmic (Maxidex®): 0.1% (5 mL, 15 mL)
Tablet: 0.25 mg, 0.5 mg, 0.75 mg, 1 mg, 1.5 mg, 2 mg, 4 mg, 6 mg [some 0.5 mg tablets may contain tartrazine]
- Decadron®: 0.5 mg, 0.75 mg, 4 mg
- DexPak® TaperPak®: 1.5 mg [51 tablets on taper dose card]

Dosing

Adults:

Antiemetic:
- Prophylaxis: Oral, I.V.: 10-20 mg 15-30 minutes before treatment on each treatment day
  - Continuous infusion regimen: Oral or I.V.: 10 mg every 12 hours on each treatment day
  - Mildly emetogenic therapy: Oral, I.M., I.V.: 4 mg every 4-6 hours
- Delayed nausea/vomiting: Oral:
  - 8 mg every 12 hours for 2 days; then
  - 4 mg every 12 hours for 2 days **or**
  - 20 mg 1 hour before chemotherapy; then
  - 10 mg 12 hours after chemotherapy; then
  - 8 mg every 12 hours for 4 doses; then
  - 4 mg every 12 hours for 4 doses

Anti-inflammatory:
- Oral, I.M., I.V. (injections should be given as sodium phosphate): 0.75-9 mg/day in divided doses every 6-12 hours
- I.M. (as acetate): 8-16 mg; may repeat in 1-3 weeks

(Continued)

Dexamethasone *(Continued)*

Intralesional (as acetate): 0.8-1.6 mg
Intra-articular/soft tissue (as acetate): 4-16 mg; may repeat in 1-3 weeks
Intra-articular, intralesional, or soft tissue (as sodium phosphate): 0.4-6 mg/day

Dexamethasone suppression test (depression indicator) or diagnosis for Cushing's syndrome (unlabeled uses): Oral: 1 mg at 11 PM, draw blood at 8 AM the following day for plasma cortisol determination

Ophthalmic:

Ointment: Apply thin coating into conjunctival sac 3-4 times/day; gradually taper dose to discontinue.

Suspension: Instill 2 drops into conjunctival sac every hour during the day and every other hour during the night; gradually reduce dose to every 3-4 hours, then to 3-4 times/day.

Topical: Apply 1-4 times/day.

Elderly: Refer to adult dosing. Use cautiously in the elderly in the smallest possible dose.

Pediatrics:

Antiemetic (prior to chemotherapy): I.V. (should be given as sodium phosphate): 10 mg/m^2/dose (maximum: 20 mg) for first dose then 5 mg/m^2/dose every 6 hours as needed

Anti-inflammatory immunosuppressant: Oral, I.M., I.V. (injections should be given as sodium phosphate): 0.08-0.3 mg/kg/day **or** 2.5-10 mg/m^2/day in divided doses every 6-12 hours

Extubation or airway edema: Oral, I.M., I.V. (injections should be given as sodium phosphate): 0.5-2 mg/kg/day in divided doses every 6 hours beginning 24 hours prior to extubation and continuing for 4-6 doses afterwards

Cerebral edema: I.V. (should be given as sodium phosphate): Loading dose: 1-2 mg/kg/dose as a single dose; maintenance: 1-1.5 mg/kg/day (maximum: 16 mg/day) in divided doses every 4-6 hours for 5 days then taper for 5 days, then discontinue

Bacterial meningitis in infants and children >2 months: I.V. (should be given as sodium phosphate): 0.6 mg/kg/day in 4 divided doses every 6 hours for the first 4 days of antibiotic treatment; start dexamethasone at the time of the first dose of antibiotic

Physiologic replacement: Oral, I.M., I.V.: 0.03-0.15 mg/kg/day or 0.6-0.75 mg/m^2/day in divided doses every 6-12 hours

Ophthalmic: Refer to adult dosing.

Renal Impairment: Hemodialysis or peritoneal dialysis: Supplemental dose is not necessary.

Administration

Oral: Administer oral formulation with meals to decrease GI upset.

I.M.: Acetate injection is **not** for I.V. use.

Topical: Topical formation is for external use. Do not use on open wounds. Apply sparingly to occlusive dressings. Should not be used in the presence of open or weeping lesions.

Stability

Storage: Dexamethasone 4 mg/mL injection solution is clear and colorless. Dexamethasone 24 mg/mL injection solution is clear and colorless to light yellow. Injection solution should be protected from light and freezing.

Reconstitution: Stability of injection of parenteral admixture at room temperature (25°C) is 24 hours. Stability of injection of parenteral admixture at refrigeration temperature (4°C) is 2 days. Protect from light and freezing. Standard diluent: 4 mg/50 mL D_5W; 10 mg/50 mL D_5W. Minimum volume: 50 mL D_5W.

Compatibility: Stable in D_5W, NS

Y-site administration: Incompatible with ciprofloxacin, idarubicin, midazolam, topotecan

Compatibility in syringe: Incompatible with doxapram, glycopyrrolate

Compatibility when admixed: Incompatible with daunorubicin, diphenhydramine with lorazepam and metoclopramide, metaraminol, vancomycin

Monitoring Laboratory Tests Hemoglobin, occult blood loss, serum potassium, glucose

Dexamethasone suppression test, overnight: 8 AM cortisol <6 mg/100 mL (dexamethasone 1 mg). Plasma cortisol determination should be made on the day after giving dose.

Monitoring and Teaching Issues

Physical Assessment: Assess other medications patient may be taking for effectiveness and interactions (see Drug Interactions). Note Contraindications and Warnings/Precautions for use cautions. Monitor laboratory tests, therapeutic response, and adverse effects according to indications for therapy, dose, route (systemic or topical), and duration of therapy (see Dosing, Warnings/Precautions, Adverse Reactions). With systemic administration, diabetics should monitor glucose levels closely (corticosteroids may alter glucose levels). Instruct patient on appropriate application of particular form of dexamethasone. Advise about appropriate interventions for side effects and instruct about symptoms to report (see Patient Education). When used for long-term therapy (longer than 10-14 days) do not discontinue abruptly; decrease dosage incrementally. **Pregnancy risk factor C** - benefits of use should outweigh possible risks. Note breast-feeding caution.

Patient Education: Take exactly as directed; do not increase dose or discontinue abruptly without consulting prescriber. Take oral medication with or after meals. Avoid alcohol. Limit intake of caffeine or stimulants. Prescriber may recommend increased dietary vitamins, minerals, or iron. If diabetic, monitor glucose levels closely (antidiabetic medication may need to be adjusted). Inform prescriber if you are experiencing greater than normal levels of stress (medication may need adjustment). Some forms of this medication may cause GI upset (oral medication may be taken with meals to reduce GI upset; small, frequent meals and frequent mouth care may reduce GI upset) or increased appetite. You may be more susceptible to infection (avoid crowds and and exposure to infection). Report promptly excessive nervousness or sleep disturbances; any signs of infection (sore throat, unhealed injuries); excessive growth of body hair or loss of skin color; vision changes; excessive or sudden weight gain (>3 lb/week); swelling of face or extremities; difficulty breathing; muscle weakness; change in color of stools (tarry) or persistent abdominal pain; or worsening of condition or failure to improve. **Pregnancy/breast-feeding precautions:** Inform prescriber if you are or intend to become pregnant. Consult prescriber if breast-feeding.

Ophthalmic: For ophthalmic use only. Wash hands before using. Tilt head back and look upward. Put drops of suspension or apply thin ribbon of ointment inside lower eyelid. Close eye and roll eyeball in all directions. Do not blink for 1/2 minute. Apply gentle pressure to inner corner of eye for 30 seconds. Do not use any other eye preparation for at least 10 minutes. Do not let tip of applicator touch eye; do not contaminate tip of applicator (may cause eye infection, eye damage, or vision loss). Do not share medication with anyone else. Wear sunglasses when in sunlight; you may be more sensitive to bright light. Inform prescriber if condition worsens or fails to improve or if you experience eye pain, disturbances of vision, or other adverse eye response.

Topical: For external use only. Not for eyes or mucous membranes or open wounds. Apply in very thin layer to occlusive dressing. Apply dressing to area being treated. Avoid prolonged or excessive use around sensitive tissues, genital, or rectal areas. Inform prescriber if condition worsens (swelling, redness, irritation, pain, open sores) or fails to improve.

Dietary Issues: May be taken with meals to decrease GI upset. May need diet with increased potassium, pyridoxine, vitamin C, vitamin D, folate, calcium, and phosphorus.

Geriatric Considerations: Because of the risk of adverse effects, systemic corticosteroids should be used cautiously in the elderly in the smallest possible dose, and for the shortest possible time.

Pregnancy Issues: Dexamethasone has been used in patients with premature labor (26-34 weeks gestation) to stimulate fetal lung maturation. Effects on the fetus: Crosses the placenta; transient leukocytosis has been reported. Available evidence suggests safe use during pregnancy.

Additional Information Not suitable for every-other-day dosing due to long duration of effect. Effects of inhaled/intranasal steroids on growth have been observed in the absence of laboratory evidence of HPA axis suppression, suggesting that growth velocity is a more sensitive indicator of systemic corticosteroid exposure in pediatric patients than some commonly used tests of HPA axis function. The long-term effects of this reduction in growth velocity associated with orally-inhaled and intranasal corticosteroids, including the impact on final adult height, are unknown. The potential for "catch up" growth following discontinuation of treatment with inhaled corticosteroids has not been adequately studied.

Related Information

Antiemetics for Chemotherapy-Induced Nausea and Vomiting *on page 1639*
Corticosteroids Comparison, Systemic Equivalencies *on page 1572*
Inhalant (Asthma, Bronchospasm) Agents Comparison *on page 1577*

Dexamethasone *see* Topical Corticosteroids *on page 1334*

Dexamethasone Acetate *see* Dexamethasone *on page 382*

Dexamethasone and Neomycin *see* Neomycin and Dexamethasone *on page 959*

Dexamethasone Intensol® *see* Dexamethasone *on page 382*

Dexamethasone Sodium Phosphate *see* Dexamethasone *on page 382*

Dexasone® *see* Dexamethasone *on page 382*

Dexasone® *see* Topical Corticosteroids *on page 1334*

Dexasone® L.A. *see* Dexamethasone *on page 382*

Dexasone® L.A. *see* Topical Corticosteroids *on page 1334*

Dexasporin® *see page 1509*

Dexchlorpheniramine (deks klor fen EER a meen)

U.S. Brand Names Polaramine® [DSC]

Synonyms Dexchlorpheniramine Maleate

Generic Available Yes: Sustained action tablet, syrup

Pharmacologic Category Antihistamine

Pregnancy Risk Factor B

Lactation Excretion in breast milk unknown/not recommended

Use Perennial and seasonal allergic rhinitis and other allergic symptoms including urticaria

Mechanism of Action/Effect Competes with histamine for H_1-receptor sites on effector cells in the GI tract, blood vessels, and respiratory tract

Contraindications Hypersensitivity to dexchlorpheniramine or any component of the formulation; narrow-angle glaucoma

Warnings/Precautions Causes sedation, caution must be used in performing tasks which require alertness (ie, operating machinery or driving). Sedative effects of CNS depressants or ethanol are potentiated. Use with caution in patients with angle-closure glaucoma, pyloroduodenal obstruction (including stenotic peptic ulcer), urinary tract obstruction (including bladder neck obstruction and symptomatic prostatic hyperplasia), hyperthyroidism, increased intraocular pressure, and cardiovascular disease (including hypertension and tachycardia). High sedative and anticholinergic properties, therefore may not be considered the antihistamine of choice for prolonged use in the elderly. May cause paradoxical excitation in pediatric patients, and can result in hallucinations, coma, and death in overdose.

Drug Interactions

Decreased Effect: May increase gastric degradation of levodopa and decrease the amount of levodopa absorbed by delaying gastric emptying. Therapeutic effects of cholinergic agents (tacrine, donepezil) and neuroleptics may be antagonized.

Increased Effect/Toxicity: CNS depressants may increase the degree of sedation and respiratory depression with antihistamines. May increase the absorption of digoxin. Central and/or peripheral anticholinergic syndrome can occur when administered with amantadine, rimantadine, narcotic analgesics, phenothiazines and other antipsychotics (especially with high anticholinergic activity), tricyclic antidepressants, quinidine, disopyramide, procainamide, and antihistamines.

Nutritional/Ethanol Interactions Ethanol: Avoid ethanol (may increase CNS depression).

Effects on Lab Values May interfere with a methacholine bronchial challenge.

(Continued)

Dexchlorpheniramine *(Continued)*

Adverse Reactions

>10%:

Central nervous system: Slight to moderate drowsiness

Respiratory: Thickening of bronchial secretions

1% to 10%:

Central nervous system: Headache, fatigue, nervousness, dizziness

Gastrointestinal: Appetite increase, weight gain, nausea, diarrhea, abdominal pain, dry mouth

Neuromuscular & skeletal: Arthralgia

Respiratory: Pharyngitis

<1% (Limited to important or life-threatening): Bronchospasm, epistaxis, hepatitis, palpitations

Overdosage/Toxicology Symptoms of overdose include dry mouth, flushed skin, dilated pupils, CNS depression. There is no specific treatment for antihistamine overdose. Clinical toxicity is due to blockade of cholinergic receptors. For anticholinergic overdose with severe life-threatening symptoms, physostigmine 1-2 mg I.V. slowly, may be given to reverse these effects.

Pharmacodynamics/Kinetics

Absorption: Well absorbed

Metabolism: Hepatic

Onset: ~1 hour

Duration: 3-6 hours

Formulations

Syrup, as maleate: 2 mg/5 mL (480 mL, 3840 mL) [contains alcohol 6%; orange flavor]

Tablet, as maleate (Polaramine®): 2 mg [DSC]

Tablet, sustained action, as maleate: 4 mg, 6 mg

Dosing

Adults & Elderly: Allergy symptoms: Oral: 2 mg every 4-6 hours or 4-6 mg timed release at bedtime or every 8-10 hours

Pediatrics: Allergy symptoms: Oral:

2-5 years: 0.5 mg every 4-6 hours (do not use timed release)

6-11 years: 1 mg every 4-6 hours or 4 mg timed release at bedtime

Monitoring and Teaching Issues

Physical Assessment: Assess effectiveness and interactions of other medications patient may be taking (see Drug Interactions). See Contraindications and Warnings/Precautions for use cautions. Monitor effectiveness of therapy and adverse reactions (see Adverse Reactions) at beginning of therapy and periodically with long-term use. Assess knowledge/teach patient appropriate use, interventions to reduce side effects, and adverse symptoms to report (see Patient Education). Breast-feeding is not recommended.

Patient Education: Take as directed; do not exceed recommended dose. Do not chew or crush sustained release tablet. Take with food or water. Avoid use of other depressants, alcohol, or sleep-inducing medications unless approved by prescriber. You may experience drowsiness or dizziness (use caution when driving or engaging in tasks requiring alertness until response to drug is known); or dry mouth, nausea, or abdominal pain (small, frequent meals, frequent mouth care, chewing gum, or sucking hard candy may help). Report persistent sedation, confusion, or agitation; changes in urinary pattern; blurred vision; sore throat, difficulty breathing or expectorating (thick secretions); or lack of improvement or worsening or condition. **Breast-feeding precaution:** Breast-feeding is not recommended.

Dietary Issues: May be taken with food or water.

Geriatric Considerations: Anticholinergic action may cause significant confusional symptoms, constipation, or problems voiding urine.

Dexchlorpheniramine Maleate *see* Dexchlorpheniramine *on page 385*

Dexedrine® *see* Dextroamphetamine *on page 392*

Dexferrum® *see* Iron Dextran Complex *on page 741*

Dexmedetomidine (deks MED e toe mi deen)

U.S. Brand Names Precedex™

Synonyms Dexmedetomidine Hydrochloride

Generic Available No

Pharmacologic Category Alpha$_2$-Adrenergic Agonist; Sedative

Pregnancy Risk Factor C

Lactation Excretion in breast milk unknown/use caution

Use Sedation of initially intubated and mechanically ventilated patients during treatment in an intensive care setting; duration of infusion should not exceed 24 hours

Use - Unlabeled/Investigational Unlabeled uses include premedication prior to anesthesia induction with thiopental; relief of pain and reduction of opioid dose following laparoscopic tubal ligation; as an adjunct anesthetic in ophthalmic surgery; treatment of shivering; premedication to attenuate the cardiostimulatory and postanesthetic delirium of ketamine

Mechanism of Action/Effect Selective alpha$_2$-adrenoceptor agonist with sedative properties; alpha$_1$ activity was observed at high doses or after rapid infusions

Contraindications Hypersensitivity to dexmedetomidine or any component of the formulation; use outside of an intensive care setting

Warnings/Precautions Should be administered only by persons skilled in management of patients in intensive care setting. Patients should be continuously monitored. Episodes of bradycardia, hypotension, and sinus arrest have been associated with dexmedetomidine. Use caution in patients with heart block, severe ventricular dysfunction, hypovolemia, diabetes, chronic hypertension, and in the elderly. Use with caution in patients receiving vasodilators or drugs which decrease heart rate. Transient hypertension has been primarily observed during the dose in association with the initial peripheral vasoconstrictive effects of dexmedetomidine. Treatment of this is not generally necessary; however, reduction of infusion rate may be desirable. Pregnancy risk C.

Drug Interactions

Cytochrome P450 Effect: Substrate of **CYP2A6**; Inhibits CYP1A2, 2C8/9, **2D6**, 3A4

Increased Effect/Toxicity:

Possible enhanced effects and pharmacodynamic interaction with sedatives, hypnotics, opioids, and anesthetics; monitor and decrease the dose as necessary of each agent and/or dexmedetomidine. Enhanced effects may occur with sevoflurane, isoflurane, propofol, alfentanil, and midazolam.

Hypotension and/or bradycardia may be increased by vasodilators and heart rate-lowering agents.

Adverse Reactions

>10%:

Cardiovascular: Hypotension (30%)
Gastrointestinal: Nausea (11%)

1% to 10%:

Cardiovascular: Bradycardia (8%), atrial fibrillation (7%)
Central nervous system: Pain (3%)
Hematologic: Anemia (3%), leukocytosis (2%)
Renal: Oliguria (2%)
Respiratory: Hypoxia (6%), pulmonary edema (2%), pleural effusion (3%)
Miscellaneous: Infection (2%), thirst (2%)

Overdosage/Toxicology In reports of overdosages where the blood concentration was 13 times the upper boundary of the therapeutic range, first-degree AV block and second degree heart block occurred. No hemodynamic compromise was noted with the AV block and the heart block resolved spontaneously within one minute. Two patients who received a 2 mcg/kg loading dose over 10 minutes experienced bradycardia and/or hypotension. One patient who received a loading dose of undiluted dexmedetomidine (19.4 mcg/kg) had cardiac arrest and was successfully resuscitated.

Pharmacodynamics/Kinetics

Half-Life Elimination: 6 minutes; Terminal: 2 hours

Metabolism: Hepatic via glucuronidation and CYP2A6

Onset: Rapid

Formulations Injection, solution: 100 mcg/mL (2 mL)

Dosing

Adults:

ICU sedation: I.V.: Initial: Loading infusion of 1 mcg/kg over 10 minutes, followed by a maintenance infusion of 0.2-0.7 mcg/kg/hour (individualized and titrated to desired clinical effect); not indicated for infusions lasting >24 hours

Note: Solution must be diluted prior to administration.

Elderly: Refer to adult dosing. Dosage reduction may need to be considered. No specific guidelines available. Dose selections should be cautious, at the low end of dosage range; titration should be slower, allowing adequate time to evaluate response.

Renal Impairment: Dosage reduction may need to be considered.

Hepatic Impairment: Dosage reduction may need to be considered. No specific guidelines available.

Administration

I.V.: Administer using a controlled infusion device. Must be diluted in 0.9% sodium chloride solution to achieve the required concentration prior to administration. Advisable to use administration components made with synthetic or coated natural rubber gaskets. Parenteral products should be inspected visually for particulate matter and discoloration prior to administration.

Stability

Compatibility: Stable in D_5W, LR, 0.9% NS, 20% mannitol, plasma substitute

May adsorb to certain types of natural rubber; use components made with synthetic or coated natural rubber gaskets whenever possible.

Monitoring and Teaching Issues

Physical Assessment: Administration should be managed by professionals experienced in anesthesia. Dosage and rate of administration should be individualized and titrated to the desired effect, according to relevant clinical factors, premedication, concomitant medications, age, and general condition of patient. Assess other medications for effectiveness and safety. Other drugs that cause CNS depression may increase CNS depression induced by dexmedetomidine (monitor and adjust dosage as necessary). Continuous monitoring of vital signs, cardiac and respiratory status, and level of sedation is mandatory during infusion and until full consciousness is regained (see Adverse Reactions). Safety precautions must be maintained until patient is fully alert. Dexmedetomidine is an anesthetic; pain must be treated with appropriate analgesic agents. Do not discontinue abruptly (may result in rapid awakening associated with anxiety, agitation, and resistance to mechanical ventilation). Titrate infusion rate so patient awakes slowly. Monitor fluid levels (intake and output) during and following infusion. Reposition patient and provide appropriate skin, mouth, and eye care every 2-3 hours, while sedated. Provide appropriate emotional and sensory support (auditory and environmental). **Pregnancy risk factor C.** Note breast-feeding caution.

Patient Education: This is an anesthetic. Patient education should be appropriate to individual situation. Following return of consciousness, do not attempt to change position or rise from bed without assistance. Report immediately any pounding or unusual heartbeat, difficulty breathing, or acute dizziness. **Pregnancy/breast-feeding precautions:** Inform prescriber if you are pregnant. Consult prescriber if breast-feeding.

Dexmedetomidine Hydrochloride *see* Dexmedetomidine *on page 386*

Dexmethylphenidate (dex meth il FEN i date)

U.S. Brand Names Focalin™

Synonyms Dexmethylphenidate Hydrochloride

(Continued)

Dexmethylphenidate *(Continued)*

Restrictions C-II

Generic Available No

Pharmacologic Category Central Nervous System Stimulant

Pregnancy Risk Factor C

Lactation Excretion in breast milk unknown/use caution

Use Treatment of attention-deficit/hyperactivity disorder (ADHD)

Mechanism of Action/Effect CNS stimulant

Contraindications Hypersensitivity to dexmethylphenidate, methylphenidate, or any component of the formulation; marked anxiety, tension, and agitation; glaucoma, motor tics, family history or diagnosis of Tourette's syndrome; use during or within 14 days following MAO inhibitor therapy

Warnings/Precautions Recommended to be used as part of a comprehensive treatment program for ADHD. Use with caution in patients with bipolar disorder, diabetes mellitus, cardiovascular disease, hyperthyroidism, seizure disorders, insomnia, porphyria, or hypertension. Use caution in patients with history of ethanol or drug abuse. May exacerbate symptoms of behavior and thought disorder in psychotic patients. Do not use to treat severe depression or fatigue states. Potential for drug dependency exists - avoid abrupt discontinuation in patients who have received for prolonged periods. Visual disturbances have been reported with methylphenidate (rare). Stimulant use has been associated with growth suppression. Stimulants may unmask tics in individuals with coexisting Tourette's syndrome. Safety and efficacy in children <6 years of age not established. Pregnancy risk C.

Drug Interactions

Decreased Effect: Effectiveness of antihypertensive agents may be decreased. Carbamazepine may decrease the effect of methylphenidate.

Increased Effect/Toxicity: Methylphenidate may cause hypertensive effects when used in combination with MAO inhibitors or drugs with MAO-inhibiting activity (linezolid). Risk may be less with selegiline (MAO type B selective at low doses); it is best to avoid this combination. NMS has been reported in a patient receiving methylphenidate and venlafaxine. Methylphenidate may increase levels of phenytoin, phenobarbital, TCAs, and warfarin. Increased toxicity with clonidine and sibutramine.

Nutritional/Ethanol Interactions

Ethanol: Avoid ethanol (may cause CNS depression).

Food: High-fat meal may increase time to peak concentration.

Herb/Nutraceutical: Avoid ephedra (may cause hypertension or arrhythmias) and yohimbe (also has CNS stimulatory activity).

Adverse Reactions

>10%: Gastrointestinal: Abdominal pain (15%)

1% to 10%:

- Central nervous system: Fever (5%)
- Gastrointestinal: Nausea (9%), anorexia (6%)

Adverse effects seen with **methylphenidate** (frequency not defined):

- Cardiovascular: Angina, cardiac arrhythmias, cerebral arteritis, cerebral occlusion, hypertension, hypotension, palpitations, pulse increase/decrease, tachycardia
- Central nervous system: Depression, dizziness, drowsiness, fever, headache, insomnia, nervousness, neuroleptic malignant syndrome (NMS), Tourette's syndrome, toxic psychosis
- Dermatologic: Erythema multiforme, exfoliative dermatitis, hair loss, rash, urticaria
- Endocrine & metabolic: Growth retardation
- Gastrointestinal: Abdominal pain, anorexia, nausea, vomiting, weight loss
- Hematologic: Anemia, leukopenia, thrombocytopenic purpura
- Hepatic: Abnormal liver function tests, hepatic coma, transaminase elevation
- Neuromuscular & skeletal: Arthralgia, dyskinesia
- Ocular: Blurred vision
- Renal: Necrotizing vasculitis
- Respiratory: Cough increased, pharyngitis, sinusitis, upper respiratory tract infection
- Miscellaneous: Hypersensitivity reactions

Overdosage/Toxicology Signs and symptoms of overdose may include agitation, cardiac arrhythmias, coma, confusion, convulsions, delirium, dry mucous membranes, euphoria, flushing, hallucinations, headache, hyper-reflexia, hyperpyrexia, hypertension, muscle twitching, mydriasis, palpitations, sweating, tachycardia, tremors and vomiting. Treatment is symptom-directed and supportive.

Pharmacodynamics/Kinetics

Absorption: Rapid

Half-Life Elimination: 2.2 hours

Time to Peak: Fasting: 1-1.5 hours

Metabolism: Via de-esterification to inactive metabolite, *d*-α-phenyl-piperidine acetate (*d*-ritalinic acid)

Formulations Tablet, as hydrochloride: 2.5 mg, 5 mg, 10 mg

Dosing

Adults: Treatment of ADHD: Oral: Initial: 2.5 mg twice daily in patients not currently taking methylphenidate; dosage may be adjusted in 2.5-5 mg increments at weekly intervals (maximum dose: 20 mg/day); doses should be taken at least 4 hours apart

When switching from methylphenidate to dexmethylphenidate, the starting dose of dexmethylphenidate should be half that of methylphenidate (maximum dose: 20 mg/day)

Safety and efficacy for long-term use of dexmethylphenidate have not yet been established. Patients should be re-evaluated at appropriate intervals to assess continued need of the medication.

Dose reductions and discontinuation: Reduce dose or discontinue in patients with paradoxical aggravation. Discontinue if no improvement is seen after one month of treatment.

Pediatrics: Children ≥6 years: Treatment of ADHD: Oral: Refer to adult dose.

Administration

Oral: Doses should be taken at least 4 hours apart. May be taken with or without food.

Stability

Storage: Store at 25°C (77°F). Protect from light and moisture.

Monitoring and Teaching Issues

Physical Assessment: This drug should be used as part of a comprehensive treatment program for ADHD. Monitor closely any other medication patient may be taking for effectiveness and possible interactions prior to beginning therapy (see Drug Interactions). See Warnings/Precautions for multiple use cautions. Monitor laboratory results (see Monitoring Laboratory Tests) for effectiveness of therapy, and adverse reactions at beginning of therapy and periodically with long-term use. Assess knowledge/teach patient appropriate use, interventions to reduce side effects, and importance of reporting adverse symptoms promptly (see Patient Education). **Pregnancy risk factor C** - benefits of use should outweigh possible risks. Note breast-feeding caution.

Patient Education: Take exactly as directed; do not change dosage or discontinue without consulting prescriber. Response may take some time. Avoid alcohol, caffeine, or other stimulants. Maintain adequate hydration (2-3 L/day of fluids) unless advised by prescriber to restrict fluids. You may experience decreased appetite or weight loss (small, frequent meals may help maintain adequate nutrition); or restlessness, impaired judgment, or dizziness (use caution when driving or engaging in tasks requiring alertness until response to drug is known). Report unresolved rapid heartbeat; excessive agitation, nervousness, insomnia, tremors, or dizziness; blackened stool; skin rash or irritation; or altered gait or movement. **Pregnancy/breast-feeding precautions:** Inform prescriber if you are or intend to become pregnant. Consult prescriber if breast-feeding.

Dietary Issues: May be taken with or without food.

Dexmethylphenidate Hydrochloride *see* Dexmethylphenidate *on page 387*

Dexone® *see* Topical Corticosteroids *on page 1334*

Dexone® LA *see* Topical Corticosteroids *on page 1334*

DexPak® TaperPak® *see* Dexamethasone *on page 382*

Dexrazoxane (deks ray ZOKS ane)

U.S. Brand Names Zinecard®

Synonyms ICRF-187

Generic Available No

Pharmacologic Category Cardioprotectant

Pregnancy Risk Factor C

Lactation Excretion in breast milk unknown/not recommended

Use Reduction of the incidence and severity of cardiomyopathy associated with doxorubicin administration in women with metastatic breast cancer who have received a cumulative doxorubicin dose of 300 mg/m^2 and who would benefit from continuing therapy with doxorubicin. It is not recommended for use with the initiation of doxorubicin therapy.

Mechanism of Action/Effect Derivative of EDTA and potent intracellular chelating agent. The mechanism of cardioprotectant activity is not fully understood. Appears to be converted intracellularly to a ring-opened chelating agent that interferes with iron-mediated free radical generation thought to be responsible, in part, for anthracycline-induced cardiomyopathy.

Contraindications Do not use with chemotherapy regimens that do not contain an anthracycline

Warnings/Precautions Dexrazoxane may add to the myelosuppression caused by chemotherapeutic agents. There is some evidence that the use of dexrazoxane concurrently with the initiation of fluorouracil, doxorubicin, and cyclophosphamide (FAC) therapy interferes with the antitumor efficacy of the regimen, and this use is not recommended. Dexrazoxane should only be used in those patients who have received a cumulative doxorubicin dose of 300 mg/m^2 and are continuing with doxorubicin therapy. Dexrazoxane does not eliminate the potential for anthracycline-induced cardiac toxicity. Carefully monitor cardiac function. Pregnancy risk C.

Drug Interactions

Decreased Effect: The use of dexrazoxane concurrently with the initiation of FAC therapy may interfere with the antitumor efficacy of the regimen, and this use is not recommended.

Adverse Reactions Adverse experiences are likely attributable to the FAC regimen, with the exception of pain on injection that was observed mainly with dexrazoxane. Patients receiving FAC with dexrazoxane experienced more severe leukopenia, granulocytopenia, and thrombocytopenia at nadir than patients receiving FAC without dexrazoxane; but recovery counts were similar for the two groups.

1% to 10%: Dermatologic: Urticaria, recall skin reaction, extravasation

Overdosage/Toxicology Management includes supportive care until resolution of myelosuppression and related conditions is complete. Retention of a significant dose fraction of unchanged drug in the plasma pool, minimal tissue partitioning or binding, and availability of >90% of systemic drug levels in the unbound form suggest that dexrazoxane could be removed using conventional peritoneal or hemodialysis.

Pharmacodynamics/Kinetics

Half-Life Elimination: 2.1-2.5 hours

Formulations Injection, powder for reconstitution: 250 mg, 500 mg [10 mg/mL when reconstituted]

Dosing

Adults & Elderly: Prevention of doxorubicin cardiomyopathy: I.V.: The recommended dosage ratio of dexrazoxane:doxorubicin is 10:1 (eg, 500 mg/m^2 dexrazoxane:50 mg/m^2 doxorubicin).

Administration

I.V.: Doxorubicin should not be given prior to the I.V. injection of dexrazoxane. Give dexrazoxane by slow I.V. push or rapid drip I.V. infusion from a bag. Give doxorubicin within 30 minutes after beginning the infusion with dexrazoxane.

(Continued)

Dexrazoxane *(Continued)*

Stability

Storage: Store intact vials at controlled room temperature (15°C to 30°C/59°F to 86°F).

Reconstitution: Caution should be exercised in the handling and preparation of the reconstituted solution; the use of gloves is recommended. If dexrazoxane powder or solutions contact the skin or mucosae, immediately wash with soap and water.

Reconstituted and diluted solutions are stable for 6 hours at controlled room temperature or under refrigeration (2°C to 8°C/36°F to 46°F). Must be reconstituted with 0.167 Molar (M/6) sodium lactate injection to a concentration of 10 mg dexrazoxane/mL sodium lactate. Reconstituted dexrazoxane solution may be diluted with either 0.9% sodium chloride injection or 5% dextrose injection to a concentration of 1.3-5 mg/mL in intravenous infusion bags.

Monitoring Laboratory Tests Since dexrazoxane will always be used with cytotoxic drugs, and since it may add to the myelosuppressive effects of cytotoxic drugs, frequent complete blood counts are recommended. Monitor LFTs.

Monitoring and Teaching Issues

Physical Assessment: Assess effectiveness and interactions of other medications patient may be taking (see Drug Interactions). See Contraindications and Warnings/Precautions for use cautions. See Stability/Reconstitution for handling precautions. Monitor for effectiveness of therapy and adverse effects. **Pregnancy risk factor C** - benefits of use should outweigh possible risks. Note breast-feeding caution.

Patient Education: This I.V. medication is given to reduce incidence of cardiac complications with doxorubicin. Report promptly any pain at infusion site. **Pregnancy/breast-feeding precautions:** Inform prescriber if you are pregnant. Consult prescriber if breast-feeding.

Breast-feeding Issues: Discontinue nursing during dexrazoxane therapy.

Other Issues: Follow guidelines for handling cytotoxic agents. If drug comes in contact with skin or mucosa, wash immediately with soap and water.

Additional Information Reimbursement Guarantee Program: 1-800-808-9111

Dextran (DEKS tran)

U.S. Brand Names Gentran®; LMD®

Synonyms Dextran 40; Dextran 70; Dextran, High Molecular Weight; Dextran, Low Molecular Weight

Generic Available Yes

Pharmacologic Category Plasma Volume Expander

Pregnancy Risk Factor C

Lactation Excretion in breast milk unknown

Use Blood volume expander used in treatment of shock or impending shock when blood or blood products are not available; dextran 40 is also used as a priming fluid in cardiopulmonary bypass and for prophylaxis of venous thrombosis and pulmonary embolism in surgical procedures associated with a high risk of thromboembolic complications

Mechanism of Action/Effect Produces plasma volume expansion by virtue of its highly colloidal starch structure, similar to albumin

Contraindications Hypersensitivity to dextran or any component of the formulation; marked hemostatic defects (thrombocytopenia, hypofibrinogenemia) of all types including those caused by drugs; marked cardiac decompensation; renal disease with severe oliguria or anuria

Warnings/Precautions Hypersensitivity reactions have been reported (dextran 40 rarely causes a reaction), usually early in the infusion. Monitor closely during infusion initiation for signs or symptoms of a hypersensitivity reaction. Dextran 1 is indicated for prophylaxis of serious anaphylactic reactions to dextran infusions. Administration can cause fluid or solute overload. Use caution in patients with fluid overload. Use with caution in patients with active hemorrhage. Use caution in patients receiving corticosteroids. Renal failure has been reported. Fluid status including urine output should be monitored closely. Exercise care to prevent a depression of hematocrit <30% (can cause hemodilution). Observe for signs of bleeding. Pregnancy risk C.

Adverse Reactions <1% (Limited to important or life-threatening): Mild hypotension, tightness of chest, wheezing

Overdosage/Toxicology Symptoms of overdose include fluid overload, pulmonary edema, increased bleeding time, and decreased platelet function. Treatment is supportive. Blood products containing clotting factors may be necessary.

Pharmacodynamics/Kinetics

Onset: Minutes to 1 hour (depending upon the molecular weight polysaccharide administered)

Formulations

Injection, solution, high molecular weight:
- Gentran®: 6% dextran 70 [in sodium chloride 0.9%] (500 mL)

Injection, solution, low molecular weight (Gentran®, LMD®):
- 10% dextran 40 [in dextrose 5%] (500 mL)
- 10% dextran 40 [in sodium chloride 0.9%] (500 mL)

Dosing

Adults:

Volume expansion/shock:

Children: Total dose should not exceed 20 mL/kg during first 24 hours

Adults: 500-1000 mL at a rate of 20-40 mL/minute; maximum daily dose: 20 mL/kg for first 24 hours; 10 mL/kg/day thereafter; therapy should not be continued beyond 5 days

Pump prime (Dextran 40): Varies with the volume of the pump oxygenator; generally, the 10% solution is added in a dose of 1-2 g/kg

Prophylaxis of venous thrombosis/pulmonary embolism (Dextran 40): Begin during surgical procedure and give 50-100 g on the day of surgery; an additional 50 g (500 mL)

should be administered every 2-3 days during the period of risk (up to 2 weeks postoperatively); usual maximum infusion rate for nonemergency use: 4 mL/minute

Elderly: Use with extreme caution in patients with renal or hepatic impairment.

Pediatrics: Treatment of shock or impending shock (when blood or blood products are not available): I.V. (requires an infusion pump): Children: Total dose should not be >20 mL/kg during first 24 hours

Renal Impairment: Use with extreme caution.

Hepatic Impairment: Use with extreme caution.

Administration

I.V.: For I.V. infusion only (use an infusion pump). Infuse initial 500 mL at a rate of 20-40 mL/minute if hypervolemic. Reduce rate for additional infusion to 4 mL/minute. **Observe patients closely for anaphylactic reaction.**

Stability

Storage: Store at room temperature. Discard partially used containers. If crystals have formed, can heat in a water bath at 100°C or autoclave at 110°C for 15 minutes.

Compatibility: Dextran 40 is stable in D_5W, NS

Solution **incompatible** with other drugs

To prevent coagulation of blood, flush tubing well or change I.V. tubing before infusing blood after dextran.

Compatibility when admixed: Incompatible with amoxicillin

Monitoring Laboratory Tests Hemoglobin and hematocrit, electrolytes, serum protein

Monitoring and Teaching Issues

Physical Assessment: See Contraindications, Warnings/Precautions, Drug Interactions, and Dosing for use cautions. See Administration and Compatibility. Fluid status, vital signs, and CVP should be monitored during first minute of infusion, every 5-15 minutes for first hour, and periodically thereafter (see Adverse Reactions and Overdose/Toxicology). Patient teaching should be appropriate to patient condition (see Patient Education). **Pregnancy risk factor C**. Note breast-feeding caution.

Patient Education: Since this medication is generally used in emergency situations, patient education should be appropriate to patient condition.

Additional Information Dextran 40 is known as low molecular weight dextran (LMD®) and has an average molecular weight of 40,000; dextran 75 has an average molecular weight of 75,000. Dextran 70 has an average molecular weight of 70,000; sodium content of 500 mL is 77 mEq, with pH ranging from 3.0-7.0.

Dextran 1 (DEKS tran won)

U.S. Brand Names Promit®

Generic Available No

Pharmacologic Category Plasma Volume Expander

Pregnancy Risk Factor C

Lactation Excretion in breast milk unknown

Use Prophylaxis of serious anaphylactic reactions to I.V. infusion of dextran

Mechanism of Action/Effect Binds to dextran-reactive immunoglobulin without bridge formation and no formation of large immune complexes

Contraindications Hypersensitivity to dextrans or any component of the formulation; **dextran** contraindicated

Warnings/Precautions Severe hypotension and bradycardia can occur. If any reaction occurs, do not administer dextran. Mild dextran-induced anaphylactic reactions are not prevented. Pregnancy risk C.

Adverse Reactions <1% (Limited to important or life-threatening): Mild hypotension, tightness of chest, wheezing

Formulations Injection, solution: 150 mg/mL (20 mL)

Dosing

Adults & Elderly: Prophylaxis of severe reactions to dextran infusions: I.V.: 20 mL 1-2 minutes before infusion of dextran. Administer 1 dose only prior to dextran. Give 1-2 minutes before I.V. infusion of dextran. Time between dextran 1 and dextran solution should not exceed 15 minutes.

Pediatrics: Prophylaxis of severe adverse reactions to dextran: I.V. (time between dextran 1 and dextran solution should not exceed 15 minutes): Children: 0.3 mL/kg 1-2 minutes before I.V. infusion of dextran

Administration

I.V.: Infuse over 1 minute.

Stability

Storage: Protect from freezing.

Compatibility: Do not dilute or admix with dextrans.

Monitoring and Teaching Issues

Physical Assessment: See Contraindications, Warnings/Precautions, Drug Interactions, and Dosing for use cautions. Assess therapeutic response and adverse response (see Adverse Reactions and Overdose/Toxicology) during and after dextran infusion (see Dextran monograph). Patient teaching should be appropriate to patient condition (see Patient Education). **Pregnancy risk factor C** - note breast-feeding caution.

Patient Education: Since this medication is generally administered in emergency situations, patient education should be supportive and appropriate to patient condition.

Dextran 40 *see* Dextran *on page 390*

Dextran 70 *see* Dextran *on page 390*

Dextran, High Molecular Weight *see* Dextran *on page 390*

Dextran, Low Molecular Weight *see* Dextran *on page 390*

Dextranomer (deks TRAN oh mer)

U.S. Brand Names Debrisan® [OTC]

Generic Available No

(Continued)

Dextranomer *(Continued)*

Pharmacologic Category Topical Skin Product

Pregnancy Risk Factor C

Lactation For external use

Use Clean exudative ulcers and wounds such as venous stasis ulcers, decubitus ulcers, and infected traumatic and surgical wounds; no controlled studies have found dextranomer to be more effective than conventional therapy

Mechanism of Action/Effect Dextranomer is a network of dextran-sucrose beads possessing a great many exposed hydroxy groups. When this network is applied to an exudative wound surface, the exudate is drawn by capillary forces generated by the swelling of the beads, with vacuum forces producing an upward flow of exudate into the network.

Contraindications Hypersensitivity to dextranomer or any component of the formulation; deep fistulas or sinus tracts

Warnings/Precautions Do not use in deep fistulas or any area where complete removal is not assured. Do not use on dry wounds (ineffective). Avoid contact with eyes. Pregnancy risk C.

Adverse Reactions 1% to 10%:

Local: Transitory pain, blistering

Dermatologic: Maceration may occur, erythema

Hematologic: Bleeding

Formulations

Beads, topical: 4 g, 25 g, 60 g, 120 g

Paste, topical [foil pack]: 10 g

Dosing

Adults & Elderly: Wound/ulcer cleansing: Topical: Apply to affected area every 12 hours or more frequent as needed. Removal should be done by irrigation.

Administration

Topical: For external use only. Debride and clean wound before application. Sprinkle beads into ulcer (or apply paste) to 1/4" thickness. Change dressings 1-4 times/day depending on drainage. Change dressing before it is completely dry to facilitate removal.

Monitoring and Teaching Issues

Physical Assessment: See Contraindications and Warnings/Precautions for use cautions. See application directions above. When applied to large areas or for extensive periods of time, monitor for adverse reactions. Assess knowledge/teach patient appropriate application and use and adverse symptoms to report (see Patient Education). **Pregnancy risk factor C.**

Patient Education: Use exactly as directed; do not overuse. Clean wound as directed. Sprinkle beads into or apply paste to 1/4" thickness. Change dressing 1-4 times/day before dressing is completely dry to facilitate removal. Wash hands carefully following application. Avoid contact with eyes or other nonulcerous tissue. Report increased swelling, redness, rash, itching, signs of infection, worsening of condition, or lack of healing. **Pregnancy precaution:** Inform prescriber if you are or intend to become pregnant.

Geriatric Considerations: Debrisan® is indicated in stage 3 and 4 decubitus ulcers.

Dextroamphetamine (deks troe am FET a meen)

U.S. Brand Names Dexedrine®; Dextrostat®

Synonyms Dextroamphetamine Sulfate

Restrictions C-II

Generic Available Yes

Pharmacologic Category Stimulant

Pregnancy Risk Factor C

Lactation Enters breast milk/contraindicated

Use Narcolepsy; attention-deficit/hyperactivity disorder (ADHD)

Use - Unlabeled/Investigational Exogenous obesity; depression; abnormal behavioral syndrome in children (minimal brain dysfunction)

Mechanism of Action/Effect Blocks reuptake of dopamine and norepinephrine from the synapse, thus increases the amount of circulating dopamine and norepinephrine in cerebral cortex to reticular activating system; inhibits the action of monoamine oxidase and causes catecholamines to be released. Peripheral actions include elevated blood pressure, weak bronchodilator, and respiratory stimulant action.

Contraindications Hypersensitivity or idiosyncrasy to dextroamphetamine or other sympathomimetic amines. Patients with advanced arteriosclerosis, symptomatic cardiovascular disease, moderate to severe hypertension (stage II or III), hyperthyroidism, glaucoma, diabetes mellitus, agitated states, patients with a history of drug abuse, and during or within 14 days following MAO inhibitor therapy. Stimulant medications are contraindicated for use in children with attention-deficit/hyperactivity disorders and concomitant Tourette's syndrome or tics.

Warnings/Precautions Use with caution in patients with bipolar disorder, cardiovascular disease, seizure disorders, insomnia, porphyria, mild hypertension (stage I), or history of substance abuse. May exacerbate symptoms of behavior and thought disorder in psychotic patients. Potential for drug dependency exists - avoid abrupt discontinuation in patients who have received for prolonged periods. Use in weight reduction programs only when alternative therapy has been ineffective. Products may contain tartrazine - use with caution in potentially sensitive individuals. Stimulant use in children has been associated with growth suppression. Pregnancy risk C.

Drug Interactions

Cytochrome P450 Effect: Substrate of **CYP2D6**

Decreased Effect: Amphetamines inhibit the antihypertensive response to guanethidine and guanadrel. Urinary acidifiers decrease the half-life and duration of action of amphetamines.

Increased Effect/Toxicity: Dextroamphetamine may precipitate hypertensive crisis or serotonin syndrome in patients receiving MAO inhibitors (selegiline >10 mg/day, isocarboxazid, phenelzine, tranylcypromine, furazolidone). Serotonin syndrome has also been associated with combinations of amphetamines and SSRIs; these combinations should be avoided. TCAs may enhance the effects of amphetamines. Large doses of antacids or urinary alkalinizers increase the half-life and duration of action of amphetamines. May precipitate arrhythmias in patients receiving general anesthetics.

Nutritional/Ethanol Interactions

Ethanol: Avoid ethanol (may increase CNS depression).

Food: Dextroamphetamine serum levels may be altered if taken with acidic food, juices, or vitamin C.

Herb/Nutraceutical: Avoid ephedra (may cause hypertension or arrhythmias).

Adverse Reactions Frequency not defined.

Cardiovascular: Palpitations, tachycardia, hypertension, cardiomyopathy

Central nervous system: Overstimulation, euphoria, dyskinesia, dysphoria, exacerbation of motor and phonic tics, restlessness, insomnia, dizziness, headache, psychosis, Tourette's syndrome

Dermatologic: Rash, urticaria

Endocrine & metabolic: Changes in libido

Gastrointestinal: Diarrhea, constipation, anorexia, weight loss, xerostomia, unpleasant taste

Genitourinary: Impotence

Neuromuscular & skeletal: Tremor

Overdosage/Toxicology Symptoms of overdose include restlessness, tremor, confusion, hallucinations, panic, dysrhythmias, nausea, and vomiting. There is no specific antidote for dextroamphetamine intoxication and treatment is primarily supportive. Hyperactivity and agitation usually respond to reduced sensory input; however, with extreme agitation, haloperidol (2-5 mg I.M. for adults) may be required.

Pharmacodynamics/Kinetics

Half-Life Elimination: Adults: 10-13 hours

Time to Peak: Serum: T_{max}: Immediate release: 3 hours; sustained release: 8 hours

Metabolism: Hepatic via CYP monooxygenase and glucuronidation

Onset: 1-1.5 hours

Formulations

Capsule, sustained release, as sulfate: 5 mg, 10 mg, 15 mg

Dexedrine® Spansule®: 5 mg, 10 mg, 15 mg

Tablet, as sulfate: 5 mg, 10 mg

Dexedrine®: 5 mg [contains tartrazine], 10 mg

Dextrostat®: 5 mg, 10 mg [contains tartrazine]

Dosing

Adults:

Narcolepsy: Oral: Initial: 10 mg/day, may increase at 10 mg increments in weekly intervals until side effects appear; maximum: 60 mg/day

Exogenous obesity (short-term adjunct): Oral: 5-30 mg/day in divided doses of 5-10 mg 30-60 minutes before meals

Elderly: Refer to adult dosing; start at lowest dose. Use with caution.

Pediatrics:

Narcolepsy: Oral: Children 6-12 years: Initial: 5 mg/day, may increase at 5 mg increments in weekly intervals until side effects appear; maximum dose: 60 mg/day

Attention-deficit/hyperactivity disorder (ADHD): Oral:

3-5 years: Initial: 2.5 mg/day given every morning; increase by 2.5 mg/day in weekly intervals until optimal response is obtained, usual range: 0.1-0.5 mg/kg/dose every morning with maximum of 40 mg/day

≥6 years: 5 mg once or twice daily; increase in increments of 5 mg/day at weekly intervals until optimal response is reached, usual range: 0.1-0.5 mg/kg/dose every morning (5-20 mg/day) with maximum of 40 mg/day

Administration

Oral: Do not crush sustained release drug product. Administer as single dose in morning or as divided doses with breakfast and lunch. Should be administered 30 minutes before meals and at least 6 hours before bedtime.

Stability

Storage: Protect from light.

Monitoring and Teaching Issues

Physical Assessment: Assess effectiveness and interactions of other medications patient may be taking (see Contraindications and Drug Interactions). Assess for history of psychopathology, homicidal or suicidal tendencies, or addiction; long-term use can result in dependence, abuse, or tolerance (see Warnings/Precautions). Periodically evaluate the need for continued use. Monitor therapeutic response, vital signs, and adverse reactions at start of therapy, when changing dosage, and at regular intervals during therapy (see Adverse Reactions). Monitor serum glucose closely with diabetic patients (amphetamines may alter antidiabetic requirements). Taper dosage slowly when discontinuing. Assess knowledge/teach patient appropriate use, possible side effects, and symptoms to report (see Patient Education). **Pregnancy risk factor C** - contraceptive education may be appropriate - benefits of use should outweigh possible risks. Breast-feeding is contraindicated.

Patient Education: Take exactly as directed; do not increase dose or frequency without consulting prescriber. Drug may cause physical and/or psychological dependence. Take early in day to avoid sleep disturbance, 30 minutes before meals. Avoid alcohol, caffeine, or OTC medications that act as stimulants. You may experience restlessness, false sense of euphoria, or impaired judgment (use caution when driving or engaging in tasks requiring alertness until response to drug is known); dry mouth (frequent mouth care, sucking lozenges, or chewing gum may help); nausea or vomiting (small, frequent meals, frequent mouth care may help); constipation (increased exercise, fluids, fruit, or fiber may help); diarrhea (buttermilk, boiled milk, or yogurt may help); or altered libido (reversible). Diabetics need to monitor serum glucose closely (may alter antidiabetic medication

(Continued)

Dextroamphetamine *(Continued)*

requirements). Report chest pain, palpitations, or irregular heartbeat; extreme fatigue or depression; CNS changes (aggressiveness, restlessness, euphoria, sleep disturbances); severe unremitting abdominal distress or cramping; blackened stool; changes in sexual activity; or blurred vision. **Pregnancy/breast-feeding precautions:** Inform prescriber if you are or intend to become pregnant. Do not breast-feed.

Dietary Issues: Should be taken 30 minutes before meals and at least 6 hours before bedtime.

Dextroamphetamine and Amphetamine

(deks troe am FET a meen & am FET a meen)

U.S. Brand Names Adderall®; Adderall XR™

Synonyms Amphetamine and Dextroamphetamine

Restrictions C-II

Generic Available Yes: Tablet

Pharmacologic Category Stimulant

Pregnancy Risk Factor C

Lactation Enters breast milk/contraindicated

Use Attention-deficit/hyperactivity disorder (ADHD); narcolepsy

Mechanism of Action/Effect Blocks reuptake of dopamine and norepinephrine from the synapse, thus increases the amount of circulating dopamine and norepinephrine in cerebral cortex to reticular activating system; inhibits the action of monoamine oxidase and causes catecholamines to be released. Peripheral actions include elevated blood pressure, weak bronchodilator, and respiratory stimulant action.

Contraindications Hypersensitivity to dextroamphetamine, amphetamine, or any component of the formulation; advanced arteriosclerosis; symptomatic cardiovascular disease; moderate to severe hypertension; hyperthyroidism; hypersensitivity or idiosyncrasy to the sympathomimetic amines; glaucoma; agitated states; patients with a history of drug abuse; during or within 14 days following MAO inhibitor (hypertensive crisis)

Warnings/Precautions Use caution in mildly hypertensive patients; amphetamines may impair the ability to engage in potentially hazardous activities. In psychotic children, amphetamines may exacerbate symptoms of behavior disturbance and thought disorder. Stimulants may unmask tics in individuals with coexisting Tourette's syndrome. Not recommended for children <3 years of age. Avoid abrupt discontinuation. Pregnancy risk C.

Drug Interactions

Cytochrome P450 Effect:

Dextroamphetamine: Substrate of **CYP2D6**

Amphetamine: Substrate of **CYP2D6**; Inhibits CYP2D6

Decreased Effect: Amphetamines inhibit the antihypertensive response to guanethidine and guanadrel. Urinary acidifiers decrease the half-life and duration of action of amphetamines. Enzyme inducers (barbiturates, carbamazepine, phenytoin, and rifampin) may decrease serum concentrations of amphetamines.

Increased Effect/Toxicity: Dextroamphetamine and amphetamine may precipitate hypertensive crisis or serotonin syndrome in patients receiving MAO inhibitors (selegiline >10 mg/day, isocarboxazid, phenelzine, tranylcypromine, furazolidone). Serotonin syndrome has also been associated with combinations of amphetamines and SSRIs; these combinations should be avoided. TCAs may enhance the effects of amphetamines, potentially leading to hypertensive crisis. Large doses of antacids or urinary alkalinizers increase the half-life and duration of action of amphetamines. May precipitate arrhythmias in patients receiving general anesthetics. Inhibitors of CYP2D6 may increase the effects of amphetamines (includes amiodarone, cimetidine, delavirdine, fluoxetine, paroxetine, propafenone, quinidine, and ritonavir).

Nutritional/Ethanol Interactions

Ethanol: Avoid ethanol (may increase CNS depression).

Food: Dextroamphetamine serum levels may be altered if taken with acidic food, juices, or vitamin C. Avoid caffeine.

Herb/Nutraceutical: Avoid ephedra (may cause hypertension or arrhythmias).

Effects on Lab Values Increased corticosteroid levels (greatest in evening); may interfere with urinary steroid testing

Adverse Reactions

As reported with Adderall XR™:

>10%:

Central nervous system: Insomnia (1% to 17%)

Gastrointestinal: Appetite decreased (22%), abdominal pain (14%)

1% to 10%:

Central nervous system: Emotional lability (1% to 9%), nervousness (6%), fever (4%), dizziness (2%), weakness (2%)

Gastrointestinal: Vomiting (7%), nausea (5%), anorexia (3%), diarrhea (2%), dyspepsia (2%), weight loss (1%)

Miscellaneous: Infection (2% to 4%)

<1% (Limited to important or life-threatening): Depression

In addition, the following have been reported with amphetamine use: Frequency not defined:

Cardiovascular: Palpitations, tachycardia, hypertension, cardiomyopathy

Central nervous system: Overstimulation, euphoria, dyskinesia, dysphoria, exacerbation of motor and phonic tics, restlessness, insomnia, headache, psychosis, exacerbation of Tourette's syndrome

Dermatologic: Rash, urticaria

Endocrine & metabolic: Changes in libido

Gastrointestinal: Constipation, xerostomia, unpleasant taste

Genitourinary: Impotence

Neuromuscular & skeletal: Tremor

Overdosage/Toxicology Manifestations of overdose vary widely. Symptoms of central stimulation are usually followed by fatigue and depression. Cardiovascular and gastrointestinal symptoms are also reported. Treatment is symptomatic and supportive. Chlorpromazine may be used to antagonize CNS effects.

Pharmacokinetic Note See Dextroamphetamine monograph.

Pharmacodynamics/Kinetics

Absorption: Well-absorbed

Half-Life Elimination:

Children: D-amphetamine: 9 hours; L-amphetamine: 11 hours

Adults: D-amphetamine: 10 hours; L-amphetamine: 13 hours

Time to Peak: T_{max}: Adderall®: 3 hours; Adderall XR™: 7 hours

Metabolism: Hepatic via cytochrome P450 monooxygenase and glucuronidation

Onset: 30-60 minutes

Duration: 4-6 hours

Formulations

Capsule (Adderall XR™):

5 mg [dextroamphetamine sulfate 1.25 mg, dextroamphetamine saccharate 1.25 mg, amphetamine aspartate monohydrate 1.25 mg, amphetamine sulfate 1.25 mg] (equivalent to amphetamine base 3.1 mg)

10 mg [dextroamphetamine sulfate 2.5 mg, dextroamphetamine saccharate 2.5 mg, amphetamine aspartate monohydrate 2.5 mg, amphetamine sulfate 2.5 mg] (equivalent to amphetamine base 6.3 mg)

15 mg [dextroamphetamine sulfate 3.75 mg, dextroamphetamine saccharate 3.75 mg, amphetamine aspartate monohydrate 3.75 mg, amphetamine sulfate 3.75 mg] (equivalent to amphetamine base 9.4 mg)

20 mg [dextroamphetamine sulfate 5 mg, dextroamphetamine saccharate 5 mg, amphetamine aspartate monohydrate 5 mg, amphetamine sulfate 5 mg] (equivalent to amphetamine base 12.5 mg)

25 mg [dextroamphetamine sulfate 6.25 mg, dextroamphetamine saccharate 6.25 mg, amphetamine aspartate monohydrate 6.25 mg, amphetamine sulfate 6.25 mg] (equivalent to amphetamine base 15.6 mg)

30 mg [dextroamphetamine sulfate 7.5 mg, dextroamphetamine saccharate 7.5 mg, amphetamine aspartate monohydrate 7.5 mg, amphetamine sulfate 7.5 mg] (equivalent to amphetamine base 18.8 mg)

Tablet: 5 mg [dextroamphetamine sulfate 1.25 mg, dextroamphetamine saccharate 1.25 mg, amphetamine aspartate 1.25 mg, amphetamine sulfate 1.25 mg] (equivalent to amphetamine base 3.13 mg); 10 mg [dextroamphetamine sulfate 2.5 mg, dextroamphetamine saccharate 2.5 mg, amphetamine aspartate 2.5 mg, amphetamine sulfate 2.5 mg] (equivalent to amphetamine base 6.3 mg); 20 mg [dextroamphetamine sulfate 5 mg, dextroamphetamine saccharate 5 mg, amphetamine aspartate 5 mg, amphetamine sulfate 5 mg] (equivalent to amphetamine base 12.6 mg)

Adderall®:

5 mg [dextroamphetamine sulfate 1.25 mg, dextroamphetamine saccharate 1.25 mg, amphetamine aspartate 1.25 mg, amphetamine sulfate 1.25 mg] (equivalent to amphetamine base 3.13 mg)

7.5 mg [dextroamphetamine 1.875 mg, dextroamphetamine saccharate 1.875 mg, amphetamine aspartate 1.875 mg, amphetamine sulfate 1.875 mg] (equivalent to amphetamine base 4.7 mg)

10 mg [dextroamphetamine sulfate 2.5 mg, dextroamphetamine saccharate 2.5 mg, amphetamine aspartate 2.5 mg, amphetamine sulfate 2.5 mg] (equivalent to amphetamine base 6.3 mg)

12.5 mg [dextroamphetamine sulfate 3.125 mg, dextroamphetamine saccharate 3.125 mg, amphetamine aspartate 3.125 mg, amphetamine sulfate 3.125 mg] (equivalent to amphetamine base 7.8 mg)

15 mg [dextroamphetamine sulfate 3.75 mg, dextroamphetamine saccharate 3.75 mg, amphetamine aspartate 3.75 mg, amphetamine sulfate 3.75 mg] (equivalent to amphetamine base 9.4 mg)

20 mg [dextroamphetamine sulfate 5 mg, dextroamphetamine saccharate 5 mg, amphetamine aspartate 5 mg, amphetamine sulfate 5 mg] (equivalent to amphetamine base 12.6 mg)

30 mg [dextroamphetamine sulfate 7.5 mg, dextroamphetamine saccharate 7.5 mg, amphetamine aspartate 7.5 mg, amphetamine sulfate 7.5 mg] (equivalent to amphetamine base 18.8 mg)

Dosing

Adults & Elderly: Oral: **Note:** Use lowest effective individualized dose; administer first dose as soon as awake; use intervals of 4-6 hours between additional doses.

ADHD: Oral: Initial: 5 mg once or twice daily; increase daily dose in 5 mg increments at weekly intervals until optimal response is obtained; usual maximum dose: 40 mg/day given in 1-3 divided doses per day.

Narcolepsy: Adderall®: Oral: Initial: 10 mg/day; increase daily dose in 10 mg increments at weekly intervals until optimal response is obtained; maximum dose: 60 mg/day given in 1-3 divided doses per day.

Pediatrics:

Note: Use lowest effective individualized dose; administer first dose as soon as awake

ADHD: Oral:

Children: <3 years: Not recommended.

Children: 3-5 years (Adderall®): Initial 2.5 mg/day given every morning; increase daily dose in 2.5 mg increments at weekly intervals until optimal response is obtained; maximum dose: 40 mg/day given in 1-3 divided doses per day. Use intervals of 4-6 hours between additional doses.

Children: ≥6 years:

Adderall®: Initial: 5 mg once or twice daily; increase daily dose in 5 mg increments at weekly intervals until optimal response is obtained; usual maximum dose: 40 mg/

(Continued)

Dextroamphetamine and Amphetamine *(Continued)*

day given in 1-3 divided doses per day. Use intervals of 4-6 hours between additional doses.

Adderall XR™: 5-10 mg once daily in the morning; if needed, may increase daily dose in 5-10 mg increments at weekly intervals (maximum dose: 30 mg/day)

Narcolepsy: Adderall®: Oral:

Children: 6-12 years: Initial: 5 mg/day; increase daily dose in 5 mg increments at weekly intervals until optimal response is obtained; maximum dose: 60 mg/day given in 1-3 divided doses per day.

Children >12 years: Refer to adult dosing.

Administration

Oral:

Adderal®: To avoid insomnia, last daily dose should be administered no less than 6 hours before retiring.

Adderall XR™: Should be given by noon. Capsule may be swallowed whole or it may be opened and the contents sprinkled on applesauce. Applesauce should be consumed immediately without chewing. Do not divide the contents of the capsule.

Stability

Storage: Store at controlled room temperature of 15°C to 30°C (59°F to 86°F)

Monitoring Laboratory Tests CNS activity

Monitoring and Teaching Issues

Physical Assessment: Assess effectiveness and interactions of other medications patient may be taking (see Contraindications and Drug Interactions). Assess for history of psychopathology, homicidal or suicidal tendencies, or addiction; long-term use can result in dependence, abuse, or tolerance (see Warnings/Precautions). Periodically evaluate the need for continued use. Monitor therapeutic response, blood pressure, vital signs, and adverse reactions at start of therapy, when changing dosage, and at regular intervals during therapy (see Adverse Reactions). Monitor serum glucose closely with diabetic patients (amphetamines may alter antidiabetic requirements). Taper dosage slowly when discontinuing. Assess knowledge/teach patient appropriate use, possible side effects, and symptoms to report (see Patient Education). **Pregnancy risk factor C** - contraceptive education may be required - benefits of use should outweigh possible risks. Breast-feeding is contraindicated.

Patient Education: Take exactly as directed; do not increase dose or frequency without consulting prescriber. Drug may cause physical and/or psychological dependence. Take early in the day to avoid sleep disturbance. If you miss a dose, take it as soon as you can. If it is almost time for your next dose, do not take double dose. Avoid alcohol, caffeine, or OTC medications that act as stimulants. You may experience restlessness, false sense of euphoria, or impaired judgment (use caution when driving or engaging in tasks requiring alertness until response to drug is known); dry mouth (frequent mouth care, sucking lozenges, or chewing gum may help); nausea or vomiting (small, frequent meals, frequent mouth care may help); constipation (increased exercise, fluids, fruit, or fiber may help); diarrhea (buttermilk, boiled milk, or yogurt may help); altered libido (reversible); or altered acuity of taste or smell. Diabetics need to monitor serum glucose closely (may alter antidiabetic medication requirements). Report chest pain, palpitations, or irregular heartbeat; extreme fatigue or depression; CNS changes (aggressiveness, restlessness, euphoria, sleep disturbances); severe unremitting abdominal distress or cramping; blackened stool; changes in sexual activity; or blurred vision. **Pregnancy/breast-feeding precautions:** Inform prescriber if you are pregnant. Do not breast-feed.

Pregnancy Issues: Use during pregnancy may lead to increased risk of premature delivery and low birth weight. Infants may experience symptoms of withdrawal. Teratogenic effects were reported when taken during the 1st trimester.

Additional Information Treatment of ADHD may include "drug holidays" or periodic discontinuation of medication in order to assess the patient's requirments, decrease tolerance, and limit suppression of linear growth and weight; the combination of equal parts of *d*, *l*-amphetamine aspartate, *d*, *l*-amphetamine sulfate, dextroamphetamine saccharate and dextroamphetamine sulfate results in a 75:25 ratio of the dextro- and levo isomers of amphetamine.

The duration of action of Adderall® is longer than methylphenidate; behavioral effects of a single morning dose of Adderall® may last throughout the school day; a single morning dose of Adderall® has been shown in several studies to be as effective as twice daily dosing of methylphenidate for the treatment of ADHD (see Pelham et al, *Pediatrics*, 1999, 104(6):1300-11; Manos 1999, Pliszka 2000).

Related Information

Dextroamphetamine *on page 392*

Diabetic Tussin® DM Maximum Strength [OTC] *see* Guaifenesin and Dextromethorphan *on page 647*
Diabetic Tussin® EX [OTC] *see* Guaifenesin *on page 646*
Diagnostics and Surgical Aids *see page 1461*
Dialume® [OTC] *see* Aluminum Hydroxide *on page 71*
Diaminocyclohexane Oxalatoplatinum *see* Oxaliplatin *on page 1012*
Diaminodiphenylsulfone *see* Dapsone *on page 364*
Diamox® *see* AcetaZOLAMIDE *on page 38*
Diamox Sequels® *see* AcetaZOLAMIDE *on page 38*
Diastat® Rectal Delivery System *see* Diazepam *on page 397*

Diazepam (dye AZ e pam)

U.S. Brand Names Diastat® Rectal Delivery System; Diazepam Intensol®; Valium®

Restrictions C-IV

Generic Available Yes: Injection, tablet, solution only

Pharmacologic Category Benzodiazepine

Pregnancy Risk Factor D

Lactation Enters breast milk/contraindicated (AAP rates "of concern")

Use Management of anxiety disorders, ethanol withdrawal symptoms; skeletal muscle relaxant; treatment of convulsive disorders

Orphan drug: Viscous solution for rectal administration: Management of selected, refractory epilepsy patients on stable regimens of antiepileptic drugs (AEDs) requiring intermittent use of diazepam to control episodes of increased seizure activity

Use - Unlabeled/Investigational Panic disorders; preoperative sedation, light anesthesia, amnesia

Mechanism of Action/Effect Binds to stereospecific benzodiazepine receptors on the postsynaptic GABA neuron at several sites within the central nervous system, including the limbic system, reticular formation. Enhancement of the inhibitory effect of GABA on neuronal excitability results by increased neuronal membrane permeability to chloride ions. This shift in chloride ions results in hyperpolarization (a less excitable state) and stabilization.

Contraindications Hypersensitivity to diazepam or any component of the formulation (cross-sensitivity with other benzodiazepines may exist); narrow-angle glaucoma; not for use in children <6 months of age (oral) or <30 days of age (parenteral); pregnancy

Warnings/Precautions Diazepam has been associated with increasing the frequency of grand mal seizures. Withdrawal has also been associated with an increase in the seizure frequency. Use with caution with drugs which may decrease diazepam metabolism. Use with caution in elderly or debilitated patients, patients with hepatic disease (including alcoholics), respiratory disease, impaired gag reflex, or renal impairment. Active metabolites with extended half-lives may lead to delayed accumulation and adverse effects.

Acute hypotension, muscle weakness, apnea, and cardiac arrest have occurred with parenteral administration. Acute effects may be more prevalent in patients receiving concurrent barbiturates, narcotics, or ethanol. Appropriate resuscitative equipment and qualified personnel should be available during administration and monitoring. Avoid use of the injection in patients with shock, coma, or acute ethanol intoxication. Intra-arterial injection or extravasation of the parenteral formulation should be avoided. Parenteral formulation contains propylene glycol, which has been associated with toxicity when administered in high dosages.

Causes CNS depression (dose-related) resulting in sedation, dizziness, confusion, or ataxia which may impair physical and mental capabilities. Use with caution in patients receiving other CNS depressants or psychoactive agents. Effects with other sedative drugs or ethanol may be potentiated. The dosage of narcotics should be reduced by approximately $^1/_3$ when diazepam is added. Benzodiazepines have been associated with falls and traumatic injury and should be used with extreme caution in patients who are at risk of these events (especially the elderly).

Use caution in patients with depression, particularly if suicidal risk may be present, or in patients with a history of drug dependence. Benzodiazepines have been associated with dependence and acute withdrawal symptoms on discontinuation or reduction in dose. Acute withdrawal, including seizures, may be precipitated in patients after administration of flumazenil to patients receiving long-term benzodiazepine therapy.

Diazepam has been associated with anterograde amnesia. Paradoxical reactions, including hyperactive or aggressive behavior, have been reported with benzodiazepines, particularly in adolescent/pediatric or psychiatric patients. Does not have analgesic, antidepressant, or antipsychotic properties.

Drug Interactions

Cytochrome P450 Effect: Substrate of CYP1A2, 2B6, 2C8/9, **2C19, 3A4**; Inhibits CYP2C19, 3A4

Decreased Effect: Carbamazepine, rifampin, and rifabutin may enhance the metabolism of diazepam and decrease its therapeutic effect.

Increased Effect/Toxicity: Diazepam potentiates the CNS depressant effects of narcotic analgesics, barbiturates, phenothiazines, ethanol, antihistamines, MAO inhibitors, sedative-hypnotics, and cyclic antidepressants. Diazepam effect/toxicity may be increased by inhibitors of CYP3A4, including amprenavir, cimetidine, ciprofloxacin, clarithromycin, clozapine, diltiazem, disulfiram, digoxin, erythromycin, ethanol, fluconazole, fluoxetine, fluvoxamine, grapefruit juice, isoniazid, itraconazole, ketoconazole, labetalol, levodopa, loxapine, metoprolol, metronidazole, miconazole, nefazodone, nelfinavir, omeprazole, phenytoin, rifabutin, rifampin, ritonavir, troleandomycin, valproic acid, and verapamil.

Nutritional/Ethanol Interactions

Ethanol: Avoid ethanol (may increase CNS depression).

Food: Diazepam serum levels may be increased if taken with food. Diazepam effect/toxicity may be increased by grapefruit juice; avoid concurrent use.

(Continued)

Diazepam *(Continued)*

Herb/Nutraceutical: St John's wort may decrease diazepam levels. Avoid valerian, St John's wort, kava kava, gotu kola (may increase CNS depression).

Effects on Lab Values False-negative urinary glucose determinations when using Clinistix® or Diastix®

Adverse Reactions Frequency not defined.

Cardiovascular: Hypotension

Central nervous system: Drowsiness, ataxia, amnesia, slurred speech, paradoxical excitement or rage, fatigue, insomnia, memory impairment, headache, anxiety, depression, vertigo, confusion

Dermatologic: Rash

Endocrine & metabolic: Changes in libido

Gastrointestinal: Changes in salivation, constipation, nausea

Genitourinary: Incontinence, urinary retention

Hepatic: Jaundice

Local: Phlebitis, pain with injection

Neuromuscular & skeletal: Dysarthria, tremor

Ocular: Blurred vision, diplopia

Respiratory: Decrease in respiratory rate, apnea

Overdosage/Toxicology Symptoms of overdose include somnolence, confusion, coma, hypoactive reflexes, dyspnea, hypotension, slurred speech, or impaired coordination. Treatment for benzodiazepine overdose is supportive. Flumazenil has been shown to selectively block the binding of benzodiazepines to CNS receptors, resulting in a reversal of benzodiazepine-induced CNS depression, but not respiratory depression.

Pharmacodynamics/Kinetics

Absorption: Oral: 85% to 100%, more reliable than I.M.

Half-Life Elimination: Parent drug: Adults: 20-50 hours; increased half-life in neonates, elderly, and those with severe hepatic disorders; Active major metabolite (desmethyldiazepam): 50-100 hours; may be prolonged in neonates

Metabolism: Hepatic

Onset: I.V.: Status epilepticus: Almost immediate

Duration: I.V.: Status epilepticus: 20-30 minutes

Formulations

Gel, rectal delivery system (Diastat®):

- Adult rectal tip [6 cm]: 5 mg/mL (15 mg, 20 mg) [contains ethyl alcohol, sodium benzoate, benzyl alcohol; twin pack]
- Pediatric rectal tip [4.4 cm]: 5 mg/mL (2.5 mg, 5 mg) [contains ethyl alcohol, sodium benzoate, benzyl alcohol; twin pack]
- Universal rectal tip [for pediatric and adult use; 4.4 cm]: 5 mg/mL (10 mg) [contains ethyl alcohol, sodium benzoate, benzyl alcohol; twin pack]

Injection, solution: 5 mg/mL (2 mL, 10 mL) [may contain benzyl alcohol, sodium benzoate, benzoic acid]

Solution, oral: 5 mg/5 mL (5 mL, 10 mL, 500 mL) [wintergreen-spice flavor]

Solution, oral concentrate (Diazepam Intensol®): 5 mg/mL (30 mL)

Tablet (Valium®): 2 mg, 5 mg, 10 mg

Dosing

Adults: Oral absorption is more reliable than I.M.

Anxiety/sedation/skeletal muscle relaxation:

- Oral: 2-10 mg 2-4 times/day
- I.M., I.V.: 2-10 mg, may repeat in 3-4 hours if needed

Status epilepticus: I.V.: 5-10 mg every 10-20 minutes, up to 30 mg in an 8-hour period; may repeat in 2-4 hours if necessary

Rapid tranquilization of agitated patient (administer every 30-60 minutes): Oral: 5-10 mg; average total dose for tranquilization: 20-60 mg

Elderly: Oral absorption is more reliable than I.M..

Oral: Initial:

- Anxiety: 1-2 mg 1-2 times/day; increase gradually as needed, rarely need to use >10 mg/day.
- Skeletal muscle relaxant: 2-5 mg 2-4 times/day

Pediatrics:

Conscious sedation for procedures:

- Oral:
  - Children: 0.2-0.3 mg/kg (maximum dose: 10 mg) 45-60 minutes prior to procedure
  - Adolescents: 10 mg
- I.V.:
  - Adolescents: 5 mg; may repeat with 2.5 mg if needed

Febrile seizure prophylaxis: Oral: Children: 1 mg/kg/day divided every 8 hours; initiate therapy at first sign of fever and continue for 24 hours after fever is gone

Sedation or muscle relaxation or anxiety:

- Oral: Children: 0.12-0.8 mg/kg/day in divided doses every 6-8 hours
- I.M., I.V.: Children: 0.04-0.3 mg/kg/dose every 2-4 hours to a maximum of 0.6 mg/kg within an 8-hour period if needed

Status epilepticus:

- I.V.:
  - Neonates (not recommended as a first-line agent; conventional injection contains sodium benzoate and benzoic acid; see Precautions): 0.1-0.3 mg/kg/dose given over 3-5 minutes, every 15-30 minutes to a maximum total dose of 2 mg
  - Infants >30 days and Children <5 years: 0.05-0.3 mg/kg/dose given over 3-5 minutes, every 15-30 minutes to a maximum total dose of 5 mg **or** 0.2-0.5 mg/dose every 2-5 minutes to a maximum total dose of 5 mg; repeat in 2-4 hours as needed
  - Children ≥5 years: 0.05-0.3 mg/kg/dose given over 3-5 minutes, every 15-30 minutes to a maximum total dose of 10 mg **or** 1 mg/dose every 2-5 minutes to a maximum of 10 mg; repeat in 2-4 hours as needed

Rectal: 0.5 mg/kg/dose then 0.25 mg/kg/dose in 10 minutes if needed

Anticonvulsant (acute treatment): Rectal gel formulation:

Infants <6 months: Not recommended

Children <2 years: Safety and efficacy have not been studied

Children 2-5 years: 0.5 mg/kg

Children 6-11 years: 0.3 mg/kg

Children ≥12 years and Adults: 0.2 mg/kg

Note: Dosage should be rounded upward to the next available dose, 2.5, 5, 10, 15, and 20 mg/dose; dose may be repeated in 4-12 hours if needed; do not use more than 5 times per month or more than once every 5 days

Muscle spasm associated with tetanus: I.V., I.M.:

Infants >30 days: 1-2 mg/dose every 3-4 hours as needed

Children ≥5 years: 5-10 mg/dose every 3-4 hours as needed

Renal Impairment: Hemodialysis effects: Not dialyzable (0% to 5%); supplemental dose is **not** necessary.

Hepatic Impairment: Reduce dose by 50% in cirrhosis and avoid in severe/acute liver disease.

Administration

I.V.: Continuous infusion is not recommended because of precipitation in I.V. fluids and absorption of drug into infusion bags and tubing. In children, do not exceed 1-2 mg/minute IVP; in adults 5 mg/minute.

Stability

Storage:

Protect parenteral dosage form from light; potency is retained for up to 3 months when kept at room temperature.

Rectal gel: Store at 25°C (77°F); excursion permitted to 15°C to 30°C (59°F to 86°F).

Reconstitution: Most stable at pH 4-8, hydrolysis occurs at pH <3.

Compatibility: Do not mix I.V. product with other medications.

Y-site administration: Incompatible with amphotericin B cholesteryl sulfate complex, atracurium, cefepime, diltiazem, fluconazole, foscarnet, gatifloxacin, heparin, heparin with hydrocortisone sodium succinate, hydromorphone, linezolid, meropenem, pancuronium, potassium chloride, propofol, vecuronium, vitamin B complex with C

Compatibility in syringe: Incompatible with doxapram, glycopyrrolate, heparin, hydromorphone, nalbuphine, sufentanil

Compatibility when admixed: Incompatible with bleomycin, buprenorphine, dobutamine, doxorubicin, floxacillin, fluorouracil, furosemide

Monitoring and Teaching Issues

Physical Assessment: Assess effectiveness and interactions of other medications patient may be taking (see Contraindications, Warnings/Precautions, and Drug Interactions). See Warnings/Precautions for use cautions. Assess for history of addiction - long-term use can result in dependence, abuse, or tolerance; periodically evaluate need for continued use. Monitor therapeutic response, laboratory values, and adverse reactions (see Adverse Reactions) at beginning of therapy and periodically with long-term use. Taper dosage slowly when discontinuing. Assess knowledge/teach patient seizure precautions (if administered for seizures), appropriate use, interventions to reduce side effects, and adverse symptoms to report (see Patient Education). **Pregnancy risk factor D** - determine that patient is not pregnant before beginning treatment. Instruct patients of childbearing age about appropriate barrier contraceptive measures. Breast-feeding is contraindicated.

Patient Education: Take exactly as directed; do not increase dose or frequency. Drug may cause physical and/or psychological dependence. While using this medication, do not use alcohol and other prescription or OTC medications (especially pain medications, sedatives, antihistamines, or hypnotics) without consulting prescriber. Maintain adequate hydration (2-3 L/day of fluids) unless advised by prescriber to restrict fluids. You may experience drowsiness, dizziness, or blurred vision (use caution when driving or engaging in tasks requiring alertness until response to drug is known); nausea, vomiting, loss of appetite, or dry mouth (small, frequent meals, frequent mouth care, chewing gum, or sucking lozenges may help); constipation (increased exercise, fluids, fruit, or fiber may help). If medication is used to control seizures, wear identification that you are taking an antiepileptic medication. Report CNS changes (confusion, depression, increased sedation, excitation, headache, agitation, insomnia or nightmares, dizziness, fatigue, or impaired coordination) or changes in cognition; difficulty breathing or shortness of breath; changes in urinary pattern; changes in sexual activity; muscle cramping, weakness, tremors, or rigidity; ringing in ears or visual disturbances; excessive perspiration; excessive GI symptoms (cramping, constipation, vomiting, anorexia); or worsening of seizure activity or loss of seizure control. **Pregnancy/ breast-feeding precautions:** Do not get pregnant while taking this medication; use appropriate contraceptive measures. Do not breast-feed.

Geriatric Considerations: Due to its long-acting metabolite, diazepam is not considered a drug of choice in the elderly. Long-acting benzodiazepines have been associated with falls in the elderly. Interpretive guidelines from the Health Care Financing Administration (HCFA) discourage the use of this agent in residents of long-term care facilities.

Breast-feeding Issues: Clinical effects on the infant include sedation; AAP reports that USE MAY BE OF CONCERN.

Pregnancy Issues: Crosses the placenta. Oral clefts reported, however, more recent data does not support an association between drug and oral clefts; inguinal hernia, cardiac defects, spina bifida, dysmorphic facial features, skeletal defects, multiple other malformations reported. Hypotonia and withdrawal symptoms reported following use near time of delivery.

Additional Information Intensol® should be diluted before use; diazepam does not have any analgesic effects.

Related Information

Anxiolytic/Hypnotic Use in Long-Term Care Facilities *on page 1608*

Benzodiazepines *on page 1560*

Compatibility of Drugs *on page 1564*

Diazepam Intensol® *see* Diazepam *on page 397*

DIC *see* Dacarbazine *on page 353*

Dicarbosil® [OTC] *see* Calcium Supplements *on page 202*

Dichloralphenazone, Acetaminophen, and Isometheptene *see* Acetaminophen, Isometheptene, and Dichloralphenazone *on page 38*

Dichloralphenazone, Isometheptene, and Acetaminophen *see* Acetaminophen, Isometheptene, and Dichloralphenazone *on page 38*

Diclofenac (dye KLOE fen ak)

U.S. Brand Names Cataflam®; Solaraze™; Voltaren®; Voltaren Ophthalmic®; Voltaren®-XR

Synonyms Diclofenac Potassium; Diclofenac Sodium

Generic Available Yes

Pharmacologic Category Nonsteroidal Anti-inflammatory Drug (NSAID)

Pregnancy Risk Factor B/D (3rd trimester)

Lactation Enters breast milk/use caution

Use

Immediate-release tablets: Acute treatment of mild to moderate pain; ankylosing spondylitis; primary dysmenorrhea; acute and chronic treatment of rheumatoid arthritis, osteoarthritis

Delayed-release tablets: Acute and chronic treatment of rheumatoid arthritis, osteoarthritis, ankylosing spondylitis

Extended-release tablets: Chronic treatment of osteoarthritis, rheumatoid arthritis

Ophthalmic solution: Postoperative inflammation following cataract extraction; temporary relief of pain and photophobia in patients undergoing corneal refractive surgery

Topical gel: Actinic keratosis (AK) in conjunction with sun avoidance

Use - Unlabeled/Investigational Juvenile rheumatoid arthritis

Mechanism of Action/Effect Inhibits prostaglandin synthesis by decreasing activity of the enzyme, cyclooxygenase, which results in decreased formation of prostaglandin precursors

Contraindications Hypersensitivity to diclofenac, any component of the formulation, aspirin or other NSAIDs, including patients who experience bronchospasm, asthma, rhinitis, or urticaria following NSAID or aspirin; porphyria; pregnancy (3rd trimester)

Warnings/Precautions Use with caution in patients with CHF, dehydration, hypertension, decreased renal or hepatic function, history of GI disease, active gastrointestinal ulceration or bleeding, or those receiving anticoagulants. Anaphylactoid reactions have been reported with NSAID use, even without prior exposure; may be more common in patients with the aspirin triad. Use with caution in patients with pre-existing asthma. Rare cases of severe hepatic reactions (including necrosis, jaundice, fulminant hepatitis) have been reported. Vision changes (including changes in color) have been rarely reported with oral diclofenac. Topical gel should not be applied to the eyes, open wounds, infected areas, or to exfoliative dermatitis. Monitor patients for 1 year following application of ophthalmic drops for corneal refractive procedures. Patients using ophthalmic drops should not wear soft contact lenses. Ophthalmic drops may slow/delay healing or prolong bleeding time following surgery. Elderly are at a high risk for adverse effects from NSAIDs. As many as 60% of elderly can develop peptic ulceration and/or hemorrhage asymptomatically.

Use lowest effective dose for shortest period possible. Use of NSAIDs can compromise existing renal function especially when Cl_{cr} is <30 mL/minute. CNS adverse effects such as confusion, agitation, and hallucination are generally seen in overdose or high-dose situations; however, elderly may demonstrate these adverse effects at lower doses than younger adults. Withhold for at least 4-6 half-lives prior to surgical or dental procedures.

Drug Interactions

Cytochrome P450 Effect: Substrate of CYP1A2, 2B6, 2C8/9, 2C19, 2D6, 3A4; Inhibits CYP2C8/9, 2E1

Decreased Effect: Decreased effect of diclofenac with aspirin. Decreased effect of thiazides, furosemide.

Increased Effect/Toxicity: Increased toxicity of digoxin, methotrexate, cyclosporine, lithium, insulin, sulfonylureas, potassium-sparing diuretics, warfarin, and aspirin.

Nutritional/Ethanol Interactions

Ethanol: Avoid ethanol (may enhance gastric mucosal irritation).

Herb/Nutraceutical: Avoid cat's claw, dong quai, evening primrose, feverfew, garlic, ginger, ginkgo, red clover, horse chestnut, green tea, ginseng (all have additional antiplatelet activity).

Adverse Reactions

>10%:

Local: Application site reactions (gel): Pruritus (31% to 52%), rash (35% to 46%), contact dermatitis (19% to 33%), dry skin (25% to 27%), pain (15% to 26%), exfoliation (6% to 24%), paresthesia (8% to 20%)

Ocular: Ophthalmic drops (incidence may be dependent upon indication): Lacrimation (30%), keratitis (28%), elevated IOP (15%), transient burning/stinging (15%)

1% to 10%:

Central nervous system: Headache (7%), dizziness (3%)

Dermatologic: Pruritus (1% to 3%), rash (1% to 3%)

Endocrine & metabolic: Fluid retention (1% to 3%)

Gastrointestinal: Abdominal cramps (3% to 9%), abdominal pain (3% to 9%), constipation (3% to 9%), diarrhea (3% to 9%), flatulence (3% to 9%), indigestion (3% to 9%), nausea (3% to 9%), abdominal distention (1% to 3%), peptic ulcer/GI bleed (0.6% to 2%)

Hepatic: Increased ALT/AST (2%)

Local: Application site reactions (gel): Edema (4%)

Ocular: Ophthalmic drops: Abnormal vision, acute elevated IOP, blurred vision, conjunctivitis, corneal deposits, corneal edema, corneal opacity, corneal lesions, discharge, eyelid swelling, injection, iritis, irritation, itching, lacrimation disorder, ocular allergy

Otic: Tinnitus (1% to 3%)

<1% (Limited to important or life-threatening): Oral dosage forms: Acute renal failure, agranulocytosis, allergic purpura, alopecia, anaphylactoid reactions, anaphylaxis, angioedema, aplastic anemia, aseptic meningitis, asthma, bullous eruption, cirrhosis, CHF, eosinophilia,

erythema multiforme major, GI hemorrhage, hearing loss, hemolytic anemia, hepatic necrosis, hepatitis, hepatorenal syndrome, interstitial nephritis, jaundice, laryngeal edema, leukopenia, nephrotic syndrome, pancreatitis, papillary necrosis, photosensitivity, purpura, Stevens-Johnson syndrome, swelling of lips and tongue, thrombocytopenia, urticaria, visual changes, vomiting

Overdosage/Toxicology Symptoms of overdose include acute renal failure, vomiting, drowsiness, and leukocytosis. Management of NSAID intoxication is supportive and symptomatic.

Pharmacodynamics/Kinetics

Absorption: Topical gel: 10%

Half-Life Elimination: 2 hours

Time to Peak: Serum: Cataflam®: ~1 hour; Voltaren®: ~2 hours

Metabolism: Hepatic to several metabolites

Onset: Cataflam® is more rapid than sodium salt (Voltaren®) because it dissolves in the stomach instead of the duodenum

Formulations

Gel, as sodium (Solaraze™): 30 mg/g (50 g)
Solution, ophthalmic, as sodium (Voltaren Ophthalmic®): 0.1% (2.5 mL, 5 mL)
Tablet, as potassium (Cataflam®): 50 mg
Tablet, delayed release, enteric coated, as sodium (Voltaren®): 25 mg, 50 mg, 75 mg
Tablet, extended release, as sodium (Voltaren®-XR): 100 mg

Dosing

Adults:

Analgesia/primary dysmenorrhea: Oral: Starting dose: 50 mg 3 times/day; maximum dose: 150 mg/day

Rheumatoid arthritis: Oral: 150-200 mg/day in 2-4 divided doses (100 mg/day of sustained release product)

Osteoarthritis: Oral: 100-150 mg/day in 2-3 divided doses (100-200 mg/day of sustained release product)

Ankylosing spondylitis: Oral: 100-125 mg/day in 4-5 divided doses

Cataract surgery: Ophthalmic: Instill 1 drop into affected eye 4 times/day beginning 24 hours after cataract surgery and continuing for 2 weeks

Corneal refractive surgery: Ophthalmic: Instill 1-2 drops into affected eye within the hour prior to surgery, within 15 minutes following surgery, and then continue for 4 times/day, up to 3 days

Actinic keratosis (AK): Topical (gel): Apply gel to lesion area twice daily for 60-90 days

Elderly: Refer to adult dosing. No specific dosing recommendations; elderly may demonstrate adverse effects at lower doses than younger adults, and >60% may develop asymptomatic peptic ulceration with or without hemorrhage. Monitor renal function.

Renal Impairment: Monitor closely in patients with significant renal impairment.

Hepatic Impairment: No adjustment necessary.

Administration

Oral: Do not crush tablets. Administer with food or milk to avoid gastric distress. Take with full glass of water to enhance absorption.

Other: Ophthalmic: Wait at least 5 minutes before administering other types of eye drops.

Stability

Storage: Store above 30°C (86°F); protect from moisture, store in tight container.

Monitoring Laboratory Tests CBC, liver enzymes, urine output and BUN/serum creatinine in patients receiving diuretics, occult blood loss

Monitoring and Teaching Issues

Physical Assessment: Assess other medications patient may be taking for effectiveness and interactions (see Drug Interactions). See Contraindications and Warnings/Precautions for use cautions. Monitor laboratory tests, therapeutic response, and adverse reactions (systemic or ophthalmic) at beginning of therapy and periodically throughout therapy (see Adverse Reactions and Overdose/Toxicology). Schedule ophthalmic evaluations for patients who develop eye complaints during long-term NSAID therapy. Assess knowledge/teach patient appropriate use (oral, ophthalmic, gel), interventions to reduce side effects, and adverse symptoms to report (see Patient Education). **Pregnancy risk factor B/D.** Note breast-feeding caution.

Patient Education: Oral: Take this medication exactly as directed; do not increase dose without consulting prescriber. Do not crush or chew tablets. Take with 8 oz of water, along with food or milk products to reduce GI distress. Maintain adequate hydration (2-3 L/day of fluids) unless advised by prescriber to restrict fluids. Avoid alcohol, aspirin and aspirin-containing medication, or any other anti-inflammatory medications unless consulting prescriber. You may experience dizziness, nervousness, or headache (use caution when driving or engaging in tasks requiring alertness until response to drug is known); nausea, vomiting, dry mouth, or heartburn (small, frequent meals, frequent mouth care, sucking lozenges, or chewing gum may help); or constipation (increased exercise, fluids, fruit, or fiber may help). GI bleeding, ulceration, or perforation can occur with or without pain; discontinue medication and contact prescriber if persistent abdominal pain or cramping, or blood in stool occurs. Report chest pain or palpitations; breathlessness or difficulty breathing; unusual bruising/bleeding or blood in urine, stool, mouth, or vomitus; unusual fatigue; skin rash or itching; jaundice, unusual weight gain, or swelling of extremities; change in urinary pattern; change in vision or hearing (ringing in ears). **Pregnancy/breast-feeding precautions:** Consult prescriber if you are pregnant. This drug should not be used in the 3rd trimester of pregnancy. Consult prescriber if you are breast-feeding.

Ophthalmic: For ophthalmic use only. Apply prescribed amount as often as directed. Wash hands before using. Tilt head back and look upward. Gently pull down lower lid and put drop(s) in inner corner of eye. Do not let tip of applicator touch eye; do not contaminate tip of applicator (may cause eye infection, eye damage, or vision loss). Close eye and roll eyeball in all directions. Do not blink for 1/2 minute. Apply gentle pressure to inner corner of eye for 30 seconds. Wipe away excess from skin around eye. Do not use any other eye preparation for at least 10 minutes. Do not share medication with anyone else. May cause

(Continued)

Diclofenac *(Continued)*

sensitivity to bright light (dark glasses may help); temporary stinging or blurred vision may occur. Inform prescriber if you experience eye pain, redness, burning, watering, dryness, double vision, puffiness around eye, vision changes, other adverse eye response, worsening of condition, or lack of improvement.

Gel: This preparation is for topical use only. Treatment may take up to 3 months. Do not use more often than recommended; use at regular intervals. Wash hands before and after use. Follow directions on prescription label. Gently apply enough of the gel to cover the lesion. Advise prescriber if you are using any other skin preparations. Avoid direct sunlight and sunlamps while using this medication. You may experience dry skin, itching, peeling, swelling, or tingling at site of application. If severe skin reaction develops, stop applications and notify your prescriber at once.

Dietary Issues: May be taken with food to decrease GI distress.

Diclofenac potassium = Cataflam®; potassium content: 5.8 mg (0.15 mEq) per 50 mg tablet

Geriatric Considerations: Elderly are at high risk for adverse effects from NSAIDs.

Pregnancy Issues: Safety and efficacy in pregnant women have not been established. Exposure late in pregnancy may lead to premature closure of the ductus arteriosus and may inhibit uterine contractions.

Related Information

Nonsalicylate/Nonsteroidal Anti-inflammatory Comparison *on page 1587*
Ophthalmic Agents *on page 1509*

Diclofenac and Misoprostol (dye KLOE fen ak & mye soe PROST ole)

U.S. Brand Names Arthrotec®

Synonyms Misoprostol and Diclofenac

Generic Available No

Pharmacologic Category Nonsteroidal Anti-inflammatory Drug (NSAID); Prostaglandin

Pregnancy Risk Factor X

Lactation Enters breast milk/contraindicated

Use The diclofenac component is indicated for the treatment of osteoarthritis and rheumatoid arthritis; the misoprostol component is indicated for the prophylaxis of NSAID-induced gastric and duodenal ulceration

Formulations Tablet: Diclofenac 50 mg and misoprostol 200 mcg; diclofenac 75 mg and misoprostol 200 mcg

Dosing

Adults & Elderly:

Osteoarthritis: Oral: Arthrotec® 50: 1 tablet 2-3 times/day

Rheumatoid arthritis: Oral: Arthrotec® 50: 1 tablet 3-4 times/day

For both regimens, if not tolerated by patient, the dose may be reduced to 1 tablet twice daily.

Note: Arthrotec® 75 may be used in patients who cannot tolerate full daily Arthrotec® 50 regimens. Dose: 1 tablet twice daily. However, the use of these tablets may not be as effective at preventing GI ulceration.

Renal Impairment: In renal insufficiency, diclofenac should be used with caution due to potential detrimental effects on renal function, and misoprostol dosage reduction may be required if adverse effects occur (misoprostol is renally eliminated).

Monitoring and Teaching Issues

Physical Assessment: See individual components listed in Related Information. **Pregnancy risk factor X** - determine that patient is not pregnant before beginning treatment and do not give to women of childbearing age or to males who may have intercourse with women of childbearing age unless both male and female are capable of complying with barrier contraceptive measures during therapy and for 1 month following therapy. Breast-feeding is contraindicated.

Patient Education: See individual components listed in Related Information. Consult your prescriber before use if you have hypertension or heart failure. **Pregnancy/breast-feeding precautions:** Inform prescriber if you are pregnant. Do not get pregnant during or for 1 month following therapy. Male: Do not cause a female to become pregnant. Male/female: Consult prescriber for instruction on appropriate contraceptive measures. The misoprostol ingredient in this drug may cause severe fetal defects, miscarriage, or abortion; do not share medication with others. Do not breast-feed.

Related Information

Diclofenac *on page 400*
Misoprostol *on page 912*

Diclofenac Potassium *see* Diclofenac *on page 400*

Diclofenac Sodium *see* Diclofenac *on page 400*

Dicloxacillin (dye kloks a SIL in)

Synonyms Dicloxacillin Sodium

Generic Available Yes

Pharmacologic Category Antibiotic, Penicillin

Pregnancy Risk Factor B

Lactation Excretion in breast milk unknown (probably similar to penicillin G)

Use Treatment of systemic infections such as pneumonia, skin and soft tissue infections, and osteomyelitis caused by penicillinase-producing staphylococci

Mechanism of Action/Effect Interferes with bacterial cell wall synthesis; causes cell wall death

Contraindications Hypersensitivity to dicloxacillin, penicillin, or any component of the formulation

Warnings/Precautions Monitor PT if patient concurrently on warfarin. Use with caution in patients allergic to cephalosporins.

Drug Interactions

Cytochrome P450 Effect: Induces CYP3A4

Decreased Effect: Although anecdotal reports suggest oral contraceptive efficacy could be reduced by penicillins, this has been refuted by more rigorous scientific and clinical data.

Increased Effect/Toxicity: Disulfiram, probenecid may increase penicillin levels. Increased effect of (warfarin) anticoagulants.

Nutritional/Ethanol Interactions Food: Decreases drug absorption rate; decreases drug serum concentration.

Effects on Lab Values Positive Coombs' test [direct]

Adverse Reactions

1% to 10%: Gastrointestinal: Nausea, diarrhea, abdominal pain

<1% (Limited to important or life-threatening): Agranulocytosis, eosinophilia, hemolytic anemia, hepatotoxicity, hypersensitivity, interstitial nephritis, leukopenia, neutropenia, prolonged PT, pseudomembranous colitis, rash (maculopapular to exfoliative), seizures with extremely high doses and/or renal failure, serum sickness-like reactions, thrombocytopenia, vaginitis, vomiting

Overdosage/Toxicology Symptoms of penicillin overdose include neuromuscular hypersensitivity (eg, agitation, hallucinations, asterixis, encephalopathy, confusion, and seizures). Electrolyte imbalance may occur if the preparation contains potassium or sodium salts, especially in renal failure. Hemodialysis may be helpful to aid in removal of the drug from blood; otherwise, treatment is supportive or symptom-directed.

Pharmacodynamics/Kinetics

Absorption: 35% to 76%; rate and extent reduced by food

Half-Life Elimination: 0.6-0.8 hour; slightly prolonged with renal impairment

Time to Peak: Serum: 0.5-2 hours

Formulations Capsule, as sodium: 250 mg, 500 mg

Dosing

Adults & Elderly: Susceptible infections: Oral: 125-500 mg every 6 hours

Pediatrics: Use in newborns is not recommended.

Susceptible infections: Oral:

Children <40 kg: 12.5-25 mg/kg/day divided every 6 hours; doses of 50-100 mg/kg/day in divided doses every 6 hours have been used for therapy of osteomyelitis

Children >40 kg: 125-250 mg every 6 hours

Renal Impairment:

Dosage adjustment is not necessary.

Not dialyzable (0% to 5%); supplemental dose is not necessary.

Peritoneal dialysis effects: Supplemental dose is not necessary.

Continuous arteriovenous or venovenous hemofiltration: Supplemental dose is not necessary.

Administration

Oral: Administer 1 hour before or 2 hours after meals. Administer around-the-clock to promote less variation in peak and trough serum levels.

Monitoring Laboratory Tests Perform culture and sensitivity studies prior to initiating therapy.

Monitoring and Teaching Issues

Physical Assessment: Assess allergy history prior to beginning therapy. See Contraindications and Warnings/Precautions for use cautions. Assess potential for interactions with other prescriptions, OTC medications, or herbal products patient may be taking (see Drug Interactions). Assess results of laboratory tests (see above), therapeutic response, and adverse reactions (see Adverse Reactions and Overdose/Toxicology) on a regular basis throughout therapy. Teach patient proper use, possible side effects and interventions, and adverse symptoms to report (see Patient Education). Note breast-feeding caution.

Patient Education: Inform prescriber of all prescriptions, OTC medications, or herbal products you are taking, and any allergies you have. Do not take anything new during treatment unless approved by prescriber. Take medication as directed, with a large glass of water 1 hour before or 2 hours after meals. Take at regular intervals around-the-clock and take for length of time prescribed. If diabetic, drug may cause false test results with Clinitest® urine glucose monitoring; use of another type of glucose monitoring is preferable. May cause some gastric distress (small, frequent meals may help) and diarrhea (if this persists, consult prescriber). Report fever, vaginal itching, sores in the mouth, loose foul-smelling stools, yellowing of skin or eyes, or change in color of urine or stool. **Breast-feeding precaution:** Consult prescriber if breast-feeding.

Dietary Issues: Administer on an empty stomach 1 hour before or 2 hours after meals. Sodium content of 250 mg capsule: 13 mg (0.6 mEq)

Breast-feeding Issues: No data reported; however, other penicillins may be taken while breast-feeding.

Dicloxacillin Sodium *see* Dicloxacillin *on page 402*

Didanosine (dye DAN oh seen)

U.S. Brand Names Videx®; Videx® EC

Synonyms ddI; Dideoxyinosine

Generic Available No

Pharmacologic Category Antiretroviral Agent, Reverse Transcriptase Inhibitor (Nucleoside)

Pregnancy Risk Factor B

Lactation Excretion in breast milk unknown/contraindicated

Use Treatment of HIV infection; always to be used in combination with at least two other antiretroviral agents

Mechanism of Action/Effect Didanosine, a purine nucleoside analogue and the deamination product of dideoxyadenosine (ddA), inhibits HIV replication *in vitro* in both T cells and monocytes. Didanosine is converted within the cell to the mono-, di-, and triphosphates of ddA. These ddA triphosphates act as substrate and inhibitor of HIV reverse transcriptase

(Continued)

Didanosine *(Continued)*

substrate and inhibitor of HIV reverse transcriptase thereby blocking viral DNA synthesis and suppressing HIV replication.

Contraindications Hypersensitivity to didanosine or any component of the formulation

Warnings/Precautions Pancreatitis (sometimes fatal) has been reported, incidence is dose related. Risk factors for developing pancreatitis include a previous history of the condition, concurrent cytomegalovirus or *Mycobacterium avium-intracellulare* infection, and concomitant use of stavudine, pentamidine, or co-trimoxazole. Discontinue didanosine if clinical signs of pancreatitis occur. Lactic acidosis, symptomatic hyperlactatemia, and severe hepatomegaly with steatosis (sometimes fatal) have occurred with antiretroviral nucleoside analogues, including didanosine. Hepatotoxicity may occur even in the absence of marked transaminase elevations; suspend therapy in any patient developing clinical/laboratory findings which suggest hepatotoxicity. Pregnant women may be at increased risk of lactic acidosis and liver damage.

Peripheral neuropathy occurs in ~20% of patients receiving the drug. Retinal changes (including retinal depigmentation) and optic neuritis have been reported in adults and children using didanosine. Patients should undergo retinal examination every 6-12 months. Use with caution in patients with decreased renal or hepatic function, phenylketonuria, sodium-restricted diets, or with edema, CHF, or hyperuricemia. Twice-daily dosing is the preferred dosing frequency for didanosine tablets. Didanosine sustained release capsules are indicated for once-daily use.

Drug Interactions

Decreased Effect: Didanosine buffered tablets and buffered pediatric solution may decrease absorption of quinolones or tetracyclines (administer 2 hours prior to didanosine buffered formulations). Didanosine should be held during PCP treatment with pentamidine. Didanosine may decrease levels of indinavir. Drugs whose absorption depends on the level of acidity in the stomach such as ketoconazole, itraconazole, and dapsone should be administered at least 2 hours prior to the buffered formulations of didanosine (not affected by sustained release capsules). Methadone may decrease didanosine concentrations.

Increased Effect/Toxicity: Concomitant administration of other drugs which have the potential to cause peripheral neuropathy or pancreatitis may increase the risk of these toxicities Allopurinol may increase didanosine concentration; avoid concurrent use. Concomitant use of antacids with buffered tablet or pediatric didanosine solution may potentiate adverse effects of aluminum- or magnesium-containing antacids. Ganciclovir may increase didanosine concentration; monitor. Hydroxyurea may precipitate didanosine-induced pancreatitis if added to therapy; concomitant use is not recommended. Coadministration with ribavirin or tenofovir may increase exposure to didanosine and/or its active metabolite increasing the risk or severity of didanosine toxicities, including pancreatitis, lactic acidosis, and peripheral neuropathy; monitor closely and suspend therapy if signs or symptoms of toxicity are noted.

Nutritional/Ethanol Interactions

Ethanol: Avoid ethanol (increases risk of pancreatitis).

Food: Decreases AUC and C_{max}. Didanosine serum levels may be decreased by 55% if taken with food.

Adverse Reactions As reported in monotherapy studies; risk of toxicity may increase when combined with other agent.

>10%:

Gastrointestinal: Increased amylase (15% to 17%), abdominal pain (7% to 13%), diarrhea (19% to 28%)

Neuromuscular & skeletal: Peripheral neuropathy (17% to 20%)

1% to 10%:

Dermatologic: Rash, pruritus

Endocrine & metabolic: Increased uric acid

Gastrointestinal: Pancreatitis; patients >65 years of age had a higher frequency of pancreatitis than younger patients

Hepatic: Increased SGOT, increased SGPT, increased alkaline phosphatase

Postmarketing and/or case reports: Alopecia, anaphylactoid reaction, anemia, anorexia, arthralgia, diabetes mellitus, granulocytopenia, hepatitis, hyperlactatemia (symptomatic), hypersensitivity, lactic acidosis/hepatomegaly, leukopenia, liver failure, myalgia, myopathy, neuritis, optic renal impairment, pain, retinal depigmentation, rhabdomyolysis, seizures, thrombocytopenia, weakness

Overdosage/Toxicology Chronic overdose may cause pancreatitis, peripheral neuropathy, diarrhea, hyperuricemia, and hepatic impairment. There is no known antidote for didanosine overdose. Treatment is symptomatic.

Pharmacodynamics/Kinetics

Absorption: Subject to degradation by acidic pH of stomach; some formulations are buffered to resist acidic pH; ≤50% reduction in peak plasma concentration is observed in presence of food. Sustained release capsules contain enteric-coated beadlets which dissolve in the small intestine.

Bioavailability: 42%

Half-Life Elimination:

Children and Adolescents: 0.8 hour

Adults: Normal renal function: 1.5 hours; however, active metabolite, ddATP, has an intracellular half-life >12 hours *in vitro*; Renal impairment: 2.5-5 hours

Time to Peak: Buffered tablets: 0.67 hours; Sustained release capsules: 2 hours

Metabolism: Has not been evaluated in humans; studies conducted in dogs, show extensive metabolism with allantoin, hypoxanthine, xanthine, and uric acid being the major metabolites found in urine

Formulations

Capsule, sustained release (Videx® EC): 125 mg, 200 mg, 250 mg, 400 mg

Powder for oral solution, buffered [single-dose packet] (Videx®): 100 mg, 167 mg, 250 mg [contains sodium 1380 mg/packet] [DSC]

Powder for oral solution, pediatric (Videx®): 2 g, 4 g [makes 10 mg/mL solution after final mixing]

Tablet, buffered, chewable/dispersible (Videx®): 25 mg, 50 mg, 100 mg, 150 mg, 200 mg [all strengths contain phenylalanine 36.5 mg/tablet; orange flavor]

Dosing

Adults: Treatment of HIV infection: Oral (administer on an empty stomach):

Note: Preferred dosing frequency is twice daily for didanosine tablets

Tablets:

<60 kg: 125 mg twice daily or 250 mg once daily

≥60 kg: 200 mg twice daily or 400 mg once daily

Note: Adults should receive 2-4 tablets per dose for adequate buffering and absorption; tablets should be chewed or dispersed; didanosine has also been used as 300 mg once daily

Buffered Powder:

<60 kg: 167 mg twice daily

≥60 kg; 250 mg twice daily

Sustained release capsule:

<60 kg: 250 mg once daily

≥60 kg; 400 mg once daily

Elderly: Refer to adult dosing. Elderly patients have a higher frequency of pancreatitis (10% versus 5% in younger patients); monitor renal function and dose accordingly.

Pediatrics: Treatment of HIV infection: Oral (administer on an empty stomach):

Children:

2 weeks to 8 months: 100 mg/m^2 twice daily

>8 months: 120 mg/m^2 twice daily

Children <1 year should receive 1 tablet per dose and children >1 year should receive 2-4 tablets per dose for adequate buffering and absorption; tablets should be chewed or dispersed.

Renal Impairment: See table.

Recommended Dose (mg) of Didanosine by Body Weight

Creatinine Clearance (mL/min)	≥60 kg			<60 kg		
	Tablet* (mg)	Buffered Powder† (mg)	Sustained Release Capsule (mg)	Tablet* (mg)	Buffered Powder† (mg)	Sustained Release Capsule (mg)
≥60	400 qd or 200 bid	250 bid	400 qd	250 qd or 125 bid	167 bid	250 qd
30-59	200 qd or 100 bid	100 bid	200 qd	150 qd or 75 bid	100 bid	125 qd
10-29	150 qd	167 qd	125 qd	100 qd	100 qd	125 qd
<10	100 qd	100 qd	125 qd	75 qd	100 qd	‡

*Chewable/dispersible buffered tablet; 2 tablets must be taken with each dose; different strengths of tablets may be combined to yield the recommended dose.

†Buffered powder for oral solution

‡Not suitable for use in patients <60 kg with Cl_{cr} <10 mL/minute; use alternate formulation

Hepatic Impairment: Should be considered; monitor for toxicity.

Administration

Oral:

Chewable/dispersible buffered tablets: At least 2 tablets, but no more than 4 tablets, should be taken together to allow adequate buffering. Tablets may be chewed or dispersed prior to consumption. To disperse, dissolve in 1 oz water, stir until uniform dispersion is formed, and drink immediately. May also add 1 oz of clear apple juice to initial dispersion if additional flavor is needed. The apple juice dilution is stable for 1 hour at room temperature.

Buffered powder for oral solution: Pour contents of packet into 4 ounces of water. Mix until dissolved and drink immediately. Do not mix with fruit juice.

Pediatric powder for oral solution: Prior to dispensing, the powder should be mixed with purified water USP to an initial concentration of 20 mg/mL and then further diluted with an appropriate antacid suspension to a final mixture of 10 mg/mL. Stable for 30 days under refrigeration. Shake well prior to use.

Stability

Storage: Tablets and sustained release capsules should be stored in tightly closed bottles at 15°C to 30°C.

Reconstitution: Undergoes rapid degradation when exposed to an acidic environment. Tablets dispersed in water are stable for 1 hour at room temperature. Reconstituted buffered solution is stable for 4 hours at room temperature. Reconstituted pediatric solution is stable for 30 days if refrigerated. Unbuffered powder for oral solution must be reconstituted and mixed with an equal volume of antacid at time of preparation.

Monitoring Laboratory Tests Serum potassium, uric acid, creatinine, hemoglobin, CBC with neutrophil, platelet count, CD4 cells, liver function, amylase

Monitoring and Teaching Issues

Physical Assessment: See Contraindications, Warnings/Precautions, and Dosing for use cautions. Assess potential for interactions with other prescriptions, OTC medications, or herbal products patient may be taking (see Drug Interactions). Assess results of laboratory tests (see above), therapeutic response, and adverse reactions (eg, peripheral neuropathy, CNS changes, pancreatitis, opportunistic infection - see Adverse Reactions and Overdose/Toxicology) on a regular basis throughout therapy. Teach patient proper use (see Administration, Storage, and Reconstitution), possible side effects and interventions, and adverse symptoms to report (see Patient Education). Breast-feeding is contraindicated.

Patient Education: Inform prescriber of all prescriptions, OTC medications, or herbal products you are taking, and any allergies you have. Do not take anything new during treatment unless approved by prescriber. This drug will not cure HIV; use appropriate

(Continued)

Didanosine *(Continued)*

precautions to prevent spread of HIV to other persons. Take as directed, 1 hour before or 2 hours after meals. Avoid alcohol. Chew tablets thoroughly. Pour powder into 4 oz of water, stir, and drink immediately (do not mix with fruit juice or other acid-containing liquids). Maintain adequate hydration (2-3 L/day of fluids) unless advised by prescriber to restrict fluids. A dilated retinal eye exam is recommended every 6-12 months while on this therapy. You may be susceptible to infection (avoid crowds and exposure to infection and do not have any vaccinations without consulting prescriber). May cause dizziness or weakness (use caution when driving or engaging in tasks requiring alertness until response to drug is known); nausea or vomiting (small, frequent meals, frequent mouth care, chewing gum, or sucking lozenges may help); diarrhea (boiled milk, yogurt, or buttermilk may help); or headache, back or joint pain (mild analgesics may offer relief). Report immediately any loss of sensation, numbness, or tingling in fingers, toes, or feet; persistent unresolved abdominal distress (nausea, vomiting, diarrhea); or signs of infection (burning on urination, perineal itching, white plaques in mouth, unhealed sores, persistent sore throat or cough). **Breast-feeding precaution:** Do not breast-feed.

Dietary Issues:

Videx® EC: Take on an empty stomach; administer at least 1 hour before or 2 hours after eating

Buffered powder: Do not mix with fruit juice. Each single-dose powder packet (for oral solution) contains 1380 mg sodium.

Chewable/dispersible tablet: Chew well or mix in water; if mixed in water, may add 2 tablespoons (1 oz) apple juice for flavor. Do not use other juices. Each chewable tablet contains 36.5 mg phenylalanine and 8.6 mEq magnesium. Sodium content of buffered tablets: 264.5 mg (11.5 mEq).

Geriatric Considerations: Since the elderly often have a creatinine clearance <60 mL/minute, monitor closely for adverse reactions and adjust dose accordingly to maintain efficacy (CD4 counts).

Breast-feeding Issues: HIV-infected mothers are discouraged from breast-feeding to decrease potential transmission of HIV.

Pregnancy Issues: Cases of fatal and nonfatal lactic acidosis, with or without pancreatitis, have been reported in pregnant women. It is not known if pregnancy itself potentiates this known side effect; however, pregnant women may be at increased risk of lactic acidosis and liver damage. Hepatic enzymes and electrolytes should be monitored frequently during the 3rd trimester of pregnancy. Use during pregnancy only if the potential benefit to the mother outweighs the potential risk of this complication. Phase I/II studies have shown limited placental transfer. Health professionals are encouraged to contact the antiretroviral pregnancy registry to monitor outcomes of pregnant women exposed to antiretroviral medications (1-800-258-4263).

Dideoxycytidine *see* Zalcitabine *on page 1415*

Dideoxyinosine *see* Didanosine *on page 403*

Diethylpropion (dye eth il PROE pee on)

U.S. Brand Names Tenuate®; Tenuate® Dospan®

Synonyms Amfepramone; Diethylpropion Hydrochloride

Restrictions C-IV

Generic Available Yes

Pharmacologic Category Anorexiant

Pregnancy Risk Factor B

Lactation Enters breast milk/not recommended

Use Short-term adjunct in a regimen of weight reduction based on exercise, behavioral modification, and caloric reduction in the management of exogenous obesity for patients with an initial body mass index $\geq$30 kg/m^2 or $\geq$27 kg/m^2 in the presence of other risk factors (diabetes, hypertension)

Use - Unlabeled/Investigational Migraine

Mechanism of Action/Effect Diethylpropion is used as an anorexiant possessing pharmacological and chemical properties similar to those of amphetamines. The mechanism of action of diethylpropion in reducing appetite appears to be secondary to CNS effects, specifically stimulation of the hypothalamus to release catecholamines into the central nervous system. Anorexiant effects are mediated via norepinephrine and dopamine metabolism. An increase in physical activity and metabolic effects (inhibition of lipogenesis and enhancement of lipolysis) may also contribute to weight loss.

Contraindications Hypersensitivity or idiosyncrasy to sympathomimetic amines. Patients with advanced arteriosclerosis, symptomatic cardiovascular disease, moderate to severe hypertension (stage II or III), hyperthyroidism, glaucoma, agitated states, patients with a history of drug abuse, and during or within 14 days following MAO inhibitor therapy. Concurrent use with other anorectic agents; stimulant medications are contraindicated for use in children with attention-deficit/hyperactivity disorders and concomitant Tourette's syndrome or tics.

Warnings/Precautions Use with caution in patients with bipolar disorder, diabetes mellitus, cardiovascular disease, seizure disorders, insomnia, porphyria, or mild hypertension (stage I). May exacerbate symptoms of behavior and thought disorder in psychotic patients. Potential for drug dependency exists - avoid abrupt discontinuation in patients who have received for prolonged periods. Stimulant use in children has been associated with growth suppression. Not recommended for use in patients <12 years of age.

Serious, potentially life-threatening toxicities may occur when thyroid hormones (at dosages above usual daily hormonal requirements) are used in combination with sympathomimetic amines to induce weight loss. Treatment of obesity is not an approved use for thyroid hormone.

Drug Interactions

Decreased Effect: Diethylpropion may displace guanethidine from the neuron and antagonize its antihypertensive effects; discontinue diethylpropion or use alternative antihypertensive.

Increased Effect/Toxicity: Concurrent use or use within 14 days following the administration of a MAO inhibitor is contraindicated (hypertensive crisis). Concurrent use of sibutramine and diethylpropion is contraindicated (severe hypertension, tachycardia). Concurrent use with TCAs may result in enhanced toxicity. Concurrent use with other anorectic agents may cause serious cardiac problems and is contraindicated.

Nutritional/Ethanol Interactions Ethanol: Avoid ethanol (may increase CNS depression).

Adverse Reactions Frequency not defined.

Cardiovascular: Hypertension, palpitations, tachycardia, chest pain, T-wave changes, arrhythmias, pulmonary hypertension, valvulopathy

Central nervous system: Euphoria, nervousness, insomnia, restlessness, dizziness, anxiety, headache, agitation, confusion, mental depression, psychosis, CVA, seizure

Dermatologic: Alopecia, urticaria, skin rash, ecchymosis, erythema

Endocrine & metabolic: Changes in libido, gynecomastia, menstrual irregularities, porphyria

Gastrointestinal: Nausea, vomiting, abdominal cramps, constipation, xerostomia, metallic taste

Genitourinary: Impotence

Hematologic: Bone marrow depression, agranulocytosis, leukopenia

Neuromuscular & skeletal: Tremor

Ocular: Blurred vision, mydriasis

Overdosage/Toxicology There is no specific antidote for amphetamine intoxication and treatment is primarily supportive. Hyperactivity and agitation usually respond to reduced sensory input; however, with extreme agitation, haloperidol (2-5 mg I.M. for adults) may be required.

Pharmacodynamics/Kinetics

Onset: 1 hour

Duration: 12-24 hours

Formulations

Tablet, as hydrochloride (Tenuate®): 25 mg

Tablet, controlled release, as hydrochloride (Tenuate® Dospan®): 75 mg

Dosing

Adults & Elderly: Obesity (short-term adjunct): Oral:

Tablet: 25 mg 3 times/day before meals or food

Tablet, controlled release: 75 mg at midmorning

Administration

Oral: Do not crush 75 mg controlled release tablets. Dose should not be given in evening or at bedtime. Take tablets 1 hour before meals. Take controlled-release tablet at midmorning.

Monitoring and Teaching Issues

Physical Assessment: Assess effectiveness and interactions of other medications patient may be taking (see Drug Interactions). Assess for history of psychopathology, homicidal or suicidal tendencies, or addiction; long-term use can result in dependence, abuse, or tolerance. Periodically evaluate the need for continued use. Monitor therapeutic response, vital signs, and adverse reactions at start of therapy, when changing dosage, and at regular intervals during therapy (see Adverse Reactions). Monitor serum glucose closely with diabetic patients (amphetamines may alter antidiabetic requirements). Taper dosage slowly when discontinuing. Assess knowledge/teach patient appropriate use, possible side effects, and symptoms to report (see Patient Education). Breast-feeding is not recommended.

Patient Education: Take exactly as directed; do not increase dose or frequency without consulting prescriber. Drug may cause physical and/or psychological dependence. Do not crush or chew extended release tablets. Take early in day to avoid sleep disturbance, 1 hour before meals. Avoid alcohol, caffeine, or OTC medications that act as stimulants. You may experience restlessness, false sense of euphoria, or impaired judgment (use caution when driving or engaging in tasks requiring alertness until response to drug is known); dry mouth (frequent mouth care, sucking lozenges, or chewing gum may help); nausea or vomiting (small, frequent meals, frequent mouth care may help); constipation (increased exercise, fluids, fruit, or fiber may help); or diarrhea (buttermilk, boiled milk, or yogurt may help); or altered libido (reversible). Diabetics need to monitor serum glucose closely (may alter antidiabetic medication requirements). Report chest pain, palpitations, or irregular heartbeat; muscle weakness or tremors; extreme fatigue or depression; CNS changes (aggressiveness, restlessness, euphoria, sleep disturbances); severe unremitting abdominal distress or cramping; changes in sexual activity; changes in urinary pattern; or blurred vision. **Breast-feeding precaution:** Breast-feeding is not recommended.

Related Information

Obesity Treatment Guidelines for Adults *on page 1693*

Diethylpropion Hydrochloride *see* Diethylpropion *on page 406*

Diethylstilbestrol (dye eth il stil BES trole)

U.S. Brand Names Stilphostrol®

Synonyms DES; Diethylstilbestrol Diphosphate Sodium; Stilbestrol

Generic Available No

Pharmacologic Category Estrogen Derivative

Pregnancy Risk Factor X

Lactation Excretion in breast milk unknown/contraindicated

Use Palliative treatment of inoperable metastatic prostatic carcinoma and postmenopausal inoperable, progressing breast cancer

Mechanism of Action/Effect Competes with estrogenic and androgenic compounds for binding onto tumor cells and thereby inhibits their effects on tumor growth

(Continued)

Diethylstilbestrol *(Continued)*

Contraindications Undiagnosed vaginal bleeding; breast cancer except in select patients with metastatic disease; pregnancy

Warnings/Precautions Use with caution in patients with a history of thromboembolism, stroke, myocardial infarction (especially >40 of age who smoke), liver tumor, hypertension, cardiac, renal or hepatic insufficiency, hypercalcemia, epilepsy, migraine, and metabolic bone disease. Estrogens have been reported to increase the risk of endometrial carcinoma.

Drug Interactions

Decreased Effect: Barbiturates, phenytoin, and rifampin may decrease steroids.

Effects on Lab Values ↑ prothrombin and factors VII, VIII, IX, X; ↑ platelet aggregability; ↑ thyroid-binding globulin; ↑ total thyroid hormone (T_4); ↑ serum triglycerides/phospholipids; ↓ antithrombin III; ↓ serum folate concentration

Adverse Reactions

>10%:

Cardiovascular: Peripheral edema

Endocrine & metabolic: Enlargement of breasts (female and male), breast tenderness

Gastrointestinal: Nausea, anorexia, bloating

1% to 10%:

Central nervous system: Headache, migraine headache

Endocrine & metabolic: Increased libido (female), decreased libido (male)

Gastrointestinal: Vomiting, diarrhea

<1% (Limited to important or life-threatening): Alterations in frequency and flow of menses, amenorrhea, anxiety, breast tumors, decreased glucose tolerance, depression, dizziness, edema, gallbladder obstruction, GI distress, hepatitis, hypertension, increased susceptibility to *Candida* infection, increased triglycerides and LDL, intolerance to contact lenses, myocardial infarction, nausea, stroke, thromboembolism

Overdosage/Toxicology Nausea

Pharmacodynamics/Kinetics

Metabolism: Hepatic

Formulations

Injection, as diphosphate sodium: 0.25 g (5 mL)

Tablet: 50 mg

Dosing

Adults & Elderly:

Prostate carcinoma (inoperable, progressing):

Oral: Diphosphate: 50 mg 3 times/day; increase up to 200 mg or more 3 times/day; maximum daily dose: 1 g

I.V.: Administer 0.5 g, dissolved in 250 mL of saline or D_5W, administer slowly the first 10-15 minutes then adjust rate so that the entire amount is given in 1 hour; repeat for ≥5 days depending on patient response, then repeat 0.25-0.5 g 1-2 times for one week or change to oral therapy

Postmenopausal (inoperable, progressing) breast carcinoma (in females): Oral: 15 mg/day

Stability

Storage: Intravenous solution should be stored at room temperature and away from direct light. Solution is stable for 3 days as long as cloudiness or precipitation has not occurred.

Reconstitution: NS or D_5W

Monitoring and Teaching Issues

Physical Assessment: See Contraindications, Warnings/Precautions, and Drug Interactions for use cautions. Assess therapeutic response and adverse effects (see Adverse Effects). Teach patient use, side effects and appropriate interventions, and symptoms to report (see Patient Education). **Pregnancy risk factor X** - determine that patient is not pregnant before starting therapy. Do not give to childbearing age women unless capable of complying with barrier contraceptive use. Breast-feeding is contraindicated during therapy and for 1 month following therapy.

Patient Education: Inform prescriber of all prescriptions, OTC medications, or herbal products you are taking, and any allergies you have. Do not take anything new during treatment unless approved by prescriber. Use as directed. Take with or after meals. If you are diabetic, monitor serum glucose closely; antidiabetic agent may need to be adjusted. May cause breast tenderness or enlargement (consult prescriber); sensitivity to sunlight (use sunblock, wear protective clothing and dark glasses, and avoid direct exposure to sunlight). Discontinue use and report promptly any warmth, swelling, pain, or redness in calves; sudden onset difficulty breathing; headache; loss of vision; difficulty speaking; sharp or sudden chest pain; severe abdominal pain; or unusual bleeding or speech. **Pregnancy/breast-feeding precautions:** Inform prescriber if you are pregnant. Do not get pregnant while taking this drug and for 1 month following therapy. Consult prescriber for instruction on appropriate contraceptive measures. This drug may cause severe fetal defects. Do not donate blood during or for 1 month following therapy. Do not breast-feed.

Dietary Issues: Should be taken with food to decrease GI distress.

Geriatric Considerations: The benefits of postmenopausal estrogen therapy may be substantial for some women. Diethylstilbestrol is not the drug of choice for vasomotor symptoms, to prevent bone loss, or to treat vaginal atrophy or urinary incontinence secondary to estrogen deficiency. Diethylstilbestrol does have a role in the treatment of inoperable, progressive prostatic carcinoma and inoperable, progressive breast cancer in select men and women.

Diethylstilbestrol Diphosphate Sodium *see* Diethylstilbestrol *on page 407*

Difenoxin and Atropine (dye fen OKS in & A troe peen)

U.S. Brand Names Motofen®

Synonyms Atropine and Difenoxin

Restrictions C-IV

Generic Available No

Pharmacologic Category Antidiarrheal

Pregnancy Risk Factor C

Lactation Enters breast milk/contraindicated

Use Treatment of diarrhea

Mechanism of Action/Effect Slows intestinal motility

Contraindications Hypersensitivity to difenoxin, atropine, or any component of the formulation; severe liver disease; jaundice; dehydrated patient; angle-closure glaucoma; children <2 years of age; diarrhea associated with organisms that penetrate the intestinal mucosa (toxigenic *E. coli*, *Salmonella* sp, *Shigella*), and pseudomembranous colitis associated with broad spectrum antibiotics

Warnings/Precautions Dosage recommendations should be strictly adhered to. If severe dehydration or electrolyte imbalance is manifested, withhold until appropriate corrective therapy has been initiated. Patients with acute ulcerative colitis should be carefully observed. Use with caution in patients with advanced hepatorenal disease. Pregnancy risk C.

Drug Interactions

Increased Effect/Toxicity: Concurrent use with MAO inhibitors may precipitate hypertensive crisis. May potentiate action of barbiturates, tranquilizers, narcotics, and alcohol. Difenoxin has the potential to prolong biological half-life of drugs for which the rate of elimination is dependent on the microsomal drug metabolizing enzyme system.

Nutritional/Ethanol Interactions Ethanol: Avoid ethanol (may increase CNS depression).

Adverse Reactions

1% to 10%:

Central nervous system: Dizziness, drowsiness, lightheadedness, headache

Gastrointestinal: Nausea, vomiting, dry mouth, epigastric distress

<1% (Limited to important or life-threatening): Anaphylaxis, blurred vision, confusion, constipation, tachycardia

Pharmacodynamics/Kinetics

Absorption: Rapid and well absorbed

Time to Peak: Plasma: Within 40-60 minutes

Metabolism: To inactive hydroxylated metabolite

Formulations Tablet: Difenoxin hydrochloride 1 mg and atropine sulfate 0.025 mg

Dosing

Adults: Diarrhea: Oral: Initial: 2 tablets, then 1 tablet after each loose stool; 1 tablet every 3-4 hours, up to 8 tablets in a 24-hour period; if no improvement after 48 hours, continued administration is not indicated

Elderly: Refer to adult dosing; use with caution.

Stability

Storage: Store at room temperature 15°C to 30°C (59°C to 86°C).

Monitoring and Teaching Issues

Physical Assessment: Assess effects and interactions of other prescription and OTC medications or herbal products patient may be taking (see Drug Interactions). Assess therapeutic effectiveness and adverse response (see Adverse Reactions and Overdose/Toxicology). Teach patient proper use, possible side effects and interventions, and adverse effects to report (see Patient Education). **Pregnancy risk factor C** - benefits of use should outweigh possible risks. Breast-feeding is contraindicated.

Patient Education: Inform prescriber of all prescriptions, OTC medications, or herbal products you are taking, and any allergies you have. Do not take anything new during treatment unless approved by prescriber. Take as directed; do not exceed recommended dose. If no relief in 48 hours, contact prescriber. Avoid alcohol. Keep out of reach of children; can cause severe and fatal respiratory depression if accidentally ingested. May cause lightheadedness, depression, dizziness, or weakness (use caution when driving or engaging in tasks that require alertness until response to drug is known). Report acute dizziness, headache, or GI symptoms. **Pregnancy/breast-feeding precautions:** Inform prescriber if you are or intend to become pregnant. Do not breast-feed.

Breast-feeding Issues: Potential for serious adverse reactions in nursing infants.

Related Information

Atropine *on page 134*

Differin® *see* Adapalene *on page 45*

Diflorasone *see* Topical Corticosteroids *on page 1334*

Diflucan® *see* Fluconazole *on page 565*

Diflunisal (dye FLOO ni sal)

U.S. Brand Names Dolobid®

Generic Available Yes

Pharmacologic Category Nonsteroidal Anti-inflammatory Drug (NSAID)

Pregnancy Risk Factor C (1st and 2nd trimesters); D (3rd trimester)

Lactation Enters breast milk/use caution

Use Management of inflammatory disorders usually including rheumatoid arthritis and osteoarthritis; can be used as an analgesic for treatment of mild to moderate pain

Mechanism of Action/Effect Inhibits prostaglandin synthesis by decreasing the activity of the enzyme, cyclooxygenase, which results in decreased formation of prostaglandin precursors

Contraindications Hypersensitivity to diflunisal or any component of the formulation; may be a cross-sensitivity with other NSAIDs including aspirin; should not be used in patients with active GI bleeding; pregnancy (3rd trimester)

Warnings/Precautions Peptic ulceration and GI bleeding have been reported; platelet function and bleeding time are inhibited; ophthalmologic effects; impaired renal function, use lower dosage; dehydration; peripheral edema; possibility of Reye's syndrome; elevation in liver tests. Withhold for at least 4-6 half-lives prior to surgical or dental procedures. Pregnancy risk C (1st and 2nd trimester), D (3rd trimester).

(Continued)

Diflunisal *(Continued)*

Drug Interactions

Decreased Effect: Decreased effect with antacids, aspirin.

Increased Effect/Toxicity: May cause increased toxicity of cyclosporine, digoxin, methotrexate, anticoagulants, phenytoin, sulfonylureas, sulfonamides, lithium, indomethacin, hydrochlorothiazide, and acetaminophen (levels) when coadministered with diflunisal.

Nutritional/Ethanol Interactions

Ethanol: Avoid ethanol (may enhance gastric mucosal irritation).

Herb/Nutraceutical: Avoid cat's claw, dong quai, evening primrose, feverfew, garlic, ginger, ginkgo, red clover, horse chestnut, green tea, ginseng (all have additional antiplatelet activity).

Effects on Lab Values ↑ prothrombin time (S), liver tests; ↓ uric acid (S)

Adverse Reactions

1% to 10%:

Cardiovascular: Chest pain, arrhythmias

Central nervous system: Dizziness, headache

Dermatologic: Rash

Endocrine & metabolic: Fluid retention

Gastrointestinal: Abdominal cramps, bloated feeling, constipation, diarrhea, indigestion, nausea, vomiting, mouth soreness

Genitourinary: Vaginal bleeding

Otic: Tinnitus

<1% (Limited to important or life-threatening): Agranulocytosis, angioedema, chest pain, dyspnea, edema, erythema multiforme, exfoliative dermatitis, hallucinations, hearing loss, hemolytic anemia, hepatitis, interstitial nephritis, itching, mental depression, nephrotic syndrome, renal impairment, seizures, Stevens-Johnson syndrome, thrombocytopenia, toxic epidermal necrolysis, urticaria, vasculitis, wheezing

Overdosage/Toxicology Symptoms of overdose include drowsiness, nausea, vomiting, hyperventilation, tachycardia, tinnitus, stupor, coma, renal failure, and leukocytosis. Management of NSAID intoxication is supportive and symptomatic.

Pharmacodynamics/Kinetics

Absorption: Well absorbed

Half-Life Elimination: 8-12 hours; prolonged with renal impairment

Time to Peak: Serum: 2-3 hours

Metabolism: Extensively hepatic

Onset: Analgesic: ~1 hour

Duration: 8-12 hours

Formulations Tablet: 250 mg, 500 mg

Dosing

Adults & Elderly:

Pain: Oral: Initial: 500-1000 mg followed by 250-500 mg every 8-12 hours; maximum daily dose: 1.5 g

Inflammatory condition: Oral: 500-1000 mg/day in 2 divided doses; maximum daily dose: 1.5 g

Renal Impairment: Cl_{cr} <50 mL/minute: Administer 50% of normal dose.

Monitoring and Teaching Issues

Physical Assessment: **Assess patient for allergic reaction to salicylates or other NSAIDs** (see Contraindications). Assess other medications patient may be taking for additive or adverse interactions (see Drug Interactions). See Warnings/Precautions for use cautions. Monitor therapeutic effectiveness and signs of adverse reactions or overdose (see Overdose/Toxicology Adverse Reactions) at beginning of therapy and periodically during long-term therapy. Schedule ophthalmic evaluations for patients who develop eye complaints during long-term NSAID therapy. Assess knowledge/teach patient appropriate use, appropriate interventions to reduce side effects, and adverse reactions to report (see Patient Education). **Pregnancy risk factor C/D** - see Pregnancy Risk Factor for use cautions; benefits of use should outweigh possible risks. Note breast-feeding caution.

Patient Education: If self-administered, use exactly as directed; do not increase dose or frequency. Adverse reactions can occur with overuse. Consult your prescriber before use if you have hypertension or heart failure. Do not take longer than 3 days for fever, or 10 days for pain without consulting medical advisor. Take with food or milk. While using this medication, do not use alcohol, excessive amounts of vitamin C, or salicylate-containing foods (curry powder, prunes, raisins, tea, or licorice), other prescription or OTC medications containing aspirin or salicylate, or other NSAIDs without consulting prescriber. Maintain adequate hydration (2-3 L/day of fluids) unless advised by prescriber to restrict fluids. You may experience nausea, vomiting, gastric discomfort (frequent mouth care, small, frequent meals, chewing gum, or sucking lozenges may help). GI bleeding, ulceration, or perforation can occur with or without pain. Stop taking medication and report ringing in ears; persistent stomach pain; unresolved nausea or vomiting; difficulty breathing or shortness of breath; unusual bruising or bleeding (mouth, urine, stool); skin rash; unusual swelling of extremities; chest pain; or palpitations. **Pregnancy/breast-feeding precautions:** Inform prescriber if you are or intend to become pregnant. This drug should not be used in the 3rd trimester of pregnancy. Consult prescriber if breast-feeding.

Dietary Issues: Should be taken with food to decrease GI distress.

Geriatric Considerations: Elderly are at high risk for adverse effects from NSAIDs.

Additional Information Diflunisal is a salicylic acid derivative which is chemically different than aspirin and is not metabolized to salicylic acid. It is not considered a salicylate. Diflunisal 500 mg is equal in analgesic efficacy to aspirin 650 mg, acetaminophen 650 mg, and acetaminophen 650 mg/propoxyphene napsylate 100 mg, but has a longer duration of effect (8-12 hours). Not recommended as an antipyretic. Not found to be clinically useful to treat fever; at doses ≥2 g/day, platelets are reversibly inhibited in function. Diflunisal is uricosuric at 500-750 mg/day; causes less GI and renal toxicity than aspirin and other NSAIDs; fecal blood loss is ½ that of aspirin at 2.6 g/day.

Related Information

Nonsalicylate/Nonsteroidal Anti-inflammatory Comparison *on page 1587*

Digibind® *see* Digoxin Immune Fab *on page 414*

DigiFab™ *see* Digoxin Immune Fab *on page 414*

Digitek® *see* Digoxin *on page 411*

Digoxin (di JOKS in)

U.S. Brand Names Digitek®; Lanoxicaps®; Lanoxin®

Generic Available Yes: Excludes capsule

Pharmacologic Category Antiarrhythmic Agent, Class IV; Cardiac Glycoside

Pregnancy Risk Factor C

Lactation Enters breast milk (small amounts)/compatible

Use Treatment of congestive heart failure and to slow the ventricular rate in tachyarrhythmias such as atrial fibrillation, atrial flutter, and supraventricular tachycardia (paroxysmal atrial tachycardia); cardiogenic shock

Mechanism of Action/Effect

Congestive heart failure: Inhibition of the sodium/potassium ATPase pump which acts to increase the intracellular sodium-calcium exchange to increase intracellular calcium leading to increased contractility

Supraventricular arrhythmias: Direct suppression of the AV node conduction to increase effective refractory period and decrease conduction velocity - positive inotropic effect, enhanced vagal tone, and decreased ventricular rate to fast atrial arrhythmias. Atrial fibrillation may decrease sensitivity and increase tolerance to higher serum digoxin concentrations.

Contraindications Hypersensitivity to digoxin or any component of the formulation; hypersensitivity to cardiac glycosides (another may be tried); history of toxicity; ventricular tachycardia or fibrillation; idiopathic hypertrophic subaortic stenosis; constrictive pericarditis; amyloid disease; second- or third-degree heart block (except in patients with a functioning artificial pacemaker); Wolff-Parkinson-White syndrome and atrial fibrillation concurrently

Warnings/Precautions Withdrawal in CHF patients may lead to recurrence of CHF symptoms. Some arrhythmias that digoxin is used to treat may be exacerbated in digoxin toxicity. Sinus nodal disease may be worsened. Adjust doses in renal impairment and when verapamil, quinidine or amiodarone are added to a patient on digoxin. Correct hypokalemia and hypomagnesemia before initiating therapy. Calcium, especially when administered rapidly I.V., can produce serious arrhythmias. When used for rate control in atrial fibrillation, response may be better in a sedentary patients than in active/hypermetabolic patients. Use with caution in acute MI (within 6 months). Reduce or hold dose 1-2 days before elective electrical cardioversion. Pregnancy risk C.

Drug Interactions

Cytochrome P450 Effect: Substrate of CYP3A4

Decreased Effect: Amiloride and spironolactone may reduce the inotropic response to digoxin. Cholestyramine, colestipol, kaolin-pectin, and metoclopramide may reduce digoxin absorption. Levothyroxine (and other thyroid supplements) may decrease digoxin blood levels. Penicillamine has been associated with reductions in digoxin blood levels The following reported interactions appear to be of limited clinical significance: Aminoglutethimide, aminosalicylic acid, aluminum-containing antacids, sucralfate, sulfasalazine, neomycin, ticlopidine.

Increased Effect/Toxicity: Beta-blocking agents (propranolol), verapamil, and diltiazem may have additive effects on heart rate. Carvedilol has additive effects on heart rate and inhibits the metabolism of digoxin. Digoxin levels may be increased by amiodarone (reduce digoxin dose 50%), bepridil, cyclosporine, diltiazem, indomethacin, itraconazole, some macrolides (erythromycin, clarithromycin), methimazole, nitrendipine, propafenone, propylthiouracil, quinidine (reduce digoxin dose 33% to 50% on initiation), tetracyclines, and verapamil. Moricizine may increase the toxicity of digoxin (mechanism undefined). Spironolactone may interfere with some digoxin assays, but may also increase blood levels directly. Succinylcholine administration to patients on digoxin has been associated with an increased risk of arrhythmias. Rare cases of acute digoxin toxicity have been associated with parenteral calcium (bolus) administration. The following medications have been associated with increased digoxin blood levels which appear to be of limited clinical significance: Famciclovir, flecainide, ibuprofen, fluoxetine, nefazodone, cimetidine, famotidine, ranitidine, omeprazole, trimethoprim.

Nutritional/Ethanol Interactions

Food: Digoxin peak serum levels may be decreased if taken with food. Meals containing increased fiber (bran) or foods high in pectin may decrease oral absorption of digoxin.

Herb/Nutraceutical: Avoid ephedra (risk of cardiac stimulation). Avoid natural licorice (causes sodium and water retention and increases potassium loss).

Adverse Reactions Incidence of reactions are not always reported.

Cardiovascular: Heart block; first-, second- (Wenckebach), or third-degree heart block; asystole; atrial tachycardia with block; AV dissociation; accelerated junctional rhythm; ventricular tachycardia or ventricular fibrillation; PR prolongation; ST segment depression

Central nervous system: Visual disturbances (blurred or yellow vision), headache (3.2%), weakness, dizziness (4.9%), apathy, confusion, mental disturbances (4.1%), anxiety, depression, delirium, hallucinations, fever

Dermatologic: Maculopapular rash (1.6%), erythematous, scarlatiniform, papular, vesicular or bullous rashes, urticaria, pruritus, facial, angioneurotic or laryngeal edema, shedding of fingernails or toenails, alopecia

Gastrointestinal: Nausea (3.2%), vomiting (1.6%), diarrhea (3.2%), abdominal pain

<1% (Limited to important or life-threatening): Abdominal pain, anorexia, eosinophilia, gynecomastia, hemorrhagic necrosis of the intestines, increased plasma estrogen and decreased serum luteinizing hormone in men and postmenopausal women and decreased plasma testosterone in men, intestinal ischemia, palpitations, sexual dysfunction, thrombocytopenia, unifocal or multiform ventricular premature contractions (especially bigeminy or trigeminy), vaginal cornification

(Continued)

Digoxin *(Continued)*

Any arrhythmia seen in a child on digoxin should be considered as digoxin toxicity. The gastrointestinal and central nervous system symptoms are not frequently seen in children.

Overdosage/Toxicology Manifested by a wide variety of signs and symptoms difficult to distinguish from effects associated with cardiac disease. Nausea and vomiting are common early signs of toxicity and may precede or follow evidence of cardiotoxicity. Other symptoms include anorexia, diarrhea, abdominal discomfort, headache, weakness, drowsiness, visual disturbances, mental depression, confusion, restlessness, disorientation, seizures, and hallucinations. Cardiac abnormalities include ventricular tachycardia, unifocal or multifocal PVCs (bigeminal, trigeminal), paroxysmal nodal rhythms, AV dissociation, excessive slowing of the pulse, AV block of varying degree, P-R prolongation, S-T depression, and occasional atrial fibrillation. Ventricular fibrillation is a common cause of death (alterations in cardiac rate and rhythm can result in any type of known arrhythmia).

Antidote: Life-threatening digoxin toxicity is treated with Digibind®. Administer potassium except in cases of complete heart block or renal failure. Digitalis-induced arrhythmias not responsive to potassium may be treated with phenytoin or lidocaine. Cholestyramine and colestipol may decrease absorption. Other agents to consider, based on EKG and clinical assessment, include atropine, quinidine, procainamide, and propranolol. **Note:** Other antiarrhythmics appear more dangerous to use in toxicity.

Pharmacodynamics/Kinetics

Absorption: By passive nonsaturable diffusion in the upper small intestine; food may delay, but does not affect extent of absorption

Bioavailability: Oral (formulation dependent): Elixir: 75% to 85%; Tablet: 70% to 80%

Half-Life Elimination:

Age, renal and cardiac function dependent:

Neonates: Premature: 61-170 hours; Full-term: 35-45 hours
Infants: 18-25 hours
Children: 35 hours
Adults: 38-48 hours
Adults, anephric: 4-6 days

Parent drug: 38 hours; Metabolites: Digoxigenin: 4 hours; Monodigitoxoside: 3-12 hours

Time to Peak: Serum: Oral: ~1 hour

Metabolism: Via sequential sugar hydrolysis in the stomach or by reduction of lactone ring by intestinal bacteria (in ~10% of population, gut bacteria may metabolize up to 40% of digoxin dose); metabolites may contribute to therapeutic and toxic effects of digoxin; metabolism is reduced with CHF

Onset: Oral: 1-2 hours; I.V.: 5-30 minutes; Peak effect: Oral: 2-8 hours; I.V.: 1-4 hours

Duration: Adults: 3-4 days both forms

Formulations

Capsule (Lanoxicaps®): 50 mcg, 100 mcg, 200 mcg [contains ethyl alcohol]
Elixir: 50 mcg/mL (2.5 mL, 5 mL, 60 mL) [contains alcohol 10%; lime flavor]
Lanoxin® (pediatric): 50 mcg/mL (60 mL) [contains alcohol 10%; lime flavor]
Injection: 250 mcg/mL (1 mL, 2 mL) [contains alcohol 10%]
Lanoxin®: 250 mcg/mL (2 mL) [contains alcohol 10%]
Injection, pediatric: 100 mcg/mL (1 mL) [contains alcohol 10%]
Tablet: 125 mcg, 250 mcg, 500 mcg
Digitek®, Lanoxin®: 125 mcg, 250 mcg

Dosing

Adults:

Note: When changing from oral (tablets or liquid) or I.M. to I.V. therapy, dosage should be reduced by 20% to 25%.

Atrial dysrhythmias (rate control), CHF: Initial: Total digitalizing dose: Give ½ of the total digitalizing dose (TDD) in the initial dose, then give ¼ of the TDD in each of two subsequent doses at 9- to 12-hour intervals. Obtain EKG 6 hours after each dose to assess potential toxicity.

Oral: 0.75-1.5 mg
I.V. or I.M.: 0.5-1 mg

Daily maintenance dose: Give once daily to children >10 years of age and adults.

Oral: 0.125-0.5 mg
I.V. or I.M.: 0.1-0.4 mg

Elderly: Elderly dose is based on lean body weight and normal renal function for age. Decrease dose in patients with decreased renal function (see Renal Impairment).

Dosage Recommendations for Digoxin

Age	Total Digitalizing Dose† (mcg/kg*)		Daily Maintenance Dose‡ (mcg/kg*)	
	P.O.	I.V. or I.M.	P.O.	I.V. or I.M.
Preterm infant*	20-30	15-25	5-7.5	4-6
Full-term infant*	25-35	20-30	6-10	5-8
1 mo - 2 y*	35-60	30-50	10-15	7.5-12
2-5 y*	30-40	25-35	7.5-10	6-9
5-10 y*	20-35	15-30	5-10	4-8
>10 y*	10-15	8-12	2.5-5	2-3

*Based on lean body weight and normal renal function for age. Decrease dose in patients with ↓ renal function; digitalizing dose often not recommended in infants and children.

†Give one-half of the total digitalizing dose (TDD) in the initial dose, then give one-quarter of the TDD in each of two subsequent doses at 8- to 12-hour intervals. Obtain EKG 6 hours after each dose to assess potential toxicity.

‡Divided every 12 hours in infants and children <10 years of age. Given once daily to children >10 years of age and adults.

Pediatrics: Atrial dysrhythmias (rate control), CHF: When changing from oral (tablets or liquid) or I.M. to I.V. therapy, dosage should be reduced by 20% to 25%. See table.

Renal Impairment:

Cl_{cr} 10-50 mL/minute: Administer 25% to 75% of dose or every 36 hours.

Cl_{cr} <10 mL/minute: Administer 10% to 25% of dose or every 48 hours.

Reduce loading dose by 50% in ESRD.

Not dialyzable (0% to 5%)

Administration

I.M.: Inject no more than 2 mL per injection site. May cause intense pain.

I.V.: Inject slowly 1-5 minutes for undiluted form. May dilute up to fourfold with, SWI, D_5W, or NS.

Stability

Storage: Protect elixir and injection from light.

Compatibility: Stable in $D_5{}^1/_2NS$ with KCl 20 mEq, D_5W, $D_{10}W$, LR, $^1/_2NS$, NS, and sterile water for injection (when diluted fourfold or greater)

Y-site administration: Incompatible with amphotericin B cholesteryl sulfate complex, fluconazole, foscarnet, propofol

Compatibility in syringe: Incompatible with doxapram

Compatibility when admixed: Incompatible with dobutamine

Monitoring Laboratory Tests

When to draw serum digoxin concentrations: Digoxin serum concentrations are monitored because digoxin possesses a narrow therapeutic serum range; the therapeutic endpoint is difficult to quantify and digoxin toxicity may be life threatening. Digoxin serum levels should be drawn **at least 4 hours after an intravenous dose** and **at least 6 hours after an oral dose (optimally 12-24 hours after a dose).**

Initiation of therapy:

If a loading dose is given: Digoxin serum concentration may be drawn within 12-24 hours after the initial loading dose administration. Levels drawn this early may confirm the relationship of digoxin plasma levels and response but are of little value in determining maintenance doses.

If a loading dose is not given: Digoxin serum concentration should be obtained after 3-5 days of therapy.

Maintenance monitoring:

Trough concentrations should be followed just prior to the next dose or at a minimum of 4 hours after an I.V. dose and at least 6 hours after an oral dose.

Digoxin serum concentrations should be obtained within 5-7 days (approximate time to steady-state) after any dosage changes. Continue to obtain digoxin serum concentrations 7-14 days after any change in maintenance dose. **Note:** In patients with end-stage renal disease, it may take 15-20 days to reach steady-state.

Patients who are receiving potassium-depleting medications such as diuretics, should be monitored for potassium, magnesium, and calcium levels.

Digoxin serum concentrations should be obtained whenever any of the following conditions occur:

Questionable patient compliance or to evaluate clinical deterioration following an initial good response

Changing renal function

Suspected digoxin toxicity

Initiation or discontinuation of therapy with drugs (amiodarone, quinidine, verapamil) which potentially interact with digoxin; if quinidine therapy is started; digoxin levels should be drawn within the first 24 hours after starting quinidine therapy, then 7-14 days later or empirically skip one day's digoxin dose and decrease the daily dose by 50%.

Any disease changes (hypothyroidism)

Monitoring and Teaching Issues

Physical Assessment: Closely assess effects and interactions with other prescription and OTC medications patient may be taking (see Drug Interactions). See Contraindications and Warnings/Precautions for use cautions. Monitor laboratory tests (when beginning or changing dosage, especially with I.V. administration and when patients are receiving diuretics or amphotericin) (see Monitoring Laboratory Tests). Monitor therapeutic response and adverse reactions at beginning of therapy, periodically throughout therapy, or when changing dosage (see Adverse Reactions and Overdose/Toxicology). **I.V.:** Monitor EKG continuously. **Oral:** Monitor apical pulse before administering any dose. Assess knowledge/teach patient appropriate use, adverse reactions to report, and appropriate interventions to reduce side effects. **Pregnancy risk factor C** - benefits of use should outweigh possible risks.

Patient Education: Take as directed; do not discontinue without consulting prescriber. Maintain adequate dietary intake of potassium (do not increase without consulting prescriber). Adequate dietary potassium will reduce risk of digoxin toxicity. Take pulse at the same time each day; follow prescriber instructions for holding medication if pulse is below 50. Notify prescriber of acute changes in pulse. Report loss of appetite, nausea, vomiting, persistent diarrhea, swelling of extremities, palpitations, "yellowing" or blurred vision, mental confusion or depression, or unusual fatigue. **Pregnancy precaution:** Inform prescriber if you are or intend to become pregnant.

Dietary Issues: Maintain adequate amounts of potassium in diet to decrease risk of hypokalemia (hypokalemia may increase risk of digoxin toxicity).

Geriatric Considerations: Elderly may develop exaggerated serum/tissue concentrations due to age-related alterations in clearance and pharmacodynamic differences. Elderly are at risk for toxicity due to age-related changes.

Related Information

Antiarrhythmic Drugs *on page 1551*
Heart Failure *on page 1670*
Peak and Trough Guidelines *on page 1544*

Digoxin Immune Fab (di JOKS in i MYUN fab)

U.S. Brand Names Digibind®; DigiFab™

Synonyms Antidigoxin Fab Fragments, Ovine

Generic Available No

Pharmacologic Category Antidote

Pregnancy Risk Factor C

Lactation Excretion in breast milk unknown/use caution

Use Treatment of life-threatening or potentially life-threatening digoxin intoxication, including:
- acute digoxin ingestion (ie, >10 mg in adults or >4 mg in children)
- chronic ingestions leading to steady-state digoxin concentrations > 6 ng/mL in adults or >4 ng/mL in children
- manifestations of digoxin toxicity due to overdose (life-threatening ventricular arrhythmias, progressive bradycardia, second- or third-degree heart block not responsive to atropine, serum potassium >5 mEq/L in adults or >6 mEq in children)

Mechanism of Action/Effect Binds with molecules of digoxin or digitoxin and then is excreted by the kidneys and removed from the body

Contraindications Hypersensitivity to sheep products or any component of the formulation

Warnings/Precautions Suicidal attempts often involve multiple drugs. Consider other drug toxicities as well. Hypersensitivity reactions can occur. Epinephrine should be immediately available. Serum potassium levels should be monitored, especially during the first few hours after administration. Total serum digoxin concentrations will rise precipitously following administration of this drug (has no clinical meaning - avoid monitoring serum concentrations). If digoxin was being used to treat CHF then may see exacerbation of symptoms as digoxin level is reduced. Use with caution in renal failure (experience limited) - the complex will be removed from the body more slowly. Monitor for reoccurrence of digoxin toxicity. Has reversed thrombocytopenia induced by digoxin. Failure of response to adequate treatment may call diagnosis of digitalis toxicity into question. Digoxin immune Fab is processed with papain and may cause hypersensitivity reactions in patients allergic to papaya, other papaya extracts, papain, chymopapain, or the pineapple enzyme bromelain. There may also be cross allergy with dust mite and latex allergens. Pregnancy risk C.

Drug Interactions

Increased Effect/Toxicity: Digoxin: Following administration of digoxin immune Fab, serum digoxin levels are markedly increased due to bound complexes (may be clinically misleading, since bound complex cannot interact with receptors).

Effects on Lab Values Digibind® will interfere with digitalis immunoassay measurements - this will result in clinically misleading serum digoxin concentrations fragment is eliminated from the body (several days to >1 week after Digibind® administration).

Adverse Reactions Frequency not defined.

Cardiovascular: Effects (due to withdrawal of digitalis) include exacerbation of low cardiac output states and CHF, rapid ventricular response in patients with atrial fibrillation; postural hypotension

Endocrine & metabolic: Hypokalemia

Local: Phlebitis

Miscellaneous: Allergic reactions, serum sickness

Overdosage/Toxicology Symptoms of overdose include delayed serum sickness. Treatment of serum sickness includes acetaminophen, histamine$_1$ and possibly histamine$_2$ blockers, and corticosteroids.

Pharmacodynamics/Kinetics

Half-Life Elimination: 15-20 hours; prolonged with renal impairment

Onset: I.V.: Improvement in 2-30 minutes for toxicity

Formulations Injection, powder for reconstitution:

Digibind®: 38 mg

DigiFab™: 40 mg

Dosing

Adults & Elderly: Each vial of Digibind® 38 mg or DigiFab™ 40 mg will bind ~0.5 mg of digoxin or digitoxin.

Estimation of the dose is based on the body burden of digitalis. This may be calculated if the amount ingested is known or the postdistribution serum drug level is known (round dose to the nearest whole vial). See table.

Digoxin Immune Fab

Tablets Ingested (0.25 mg)	Fab Dose (vials)
5	2
10	4
25	10
50	20
75	30
100	40
150	60
200	80

Fab dose based on serum drug level postdistribution:

Digoxin: No. of vials = level (ng/mL) x body weight (kg) divided by 100

Digitoxin: No. of vials = digitoxin (ng/mL) x body weight (kg) divided by 1000

If neither amount ingested nor drug level are known, dose empirically as follows:

For acute toxicity: 20 vials, administered in 2 divided doses to decrease the possibility of a febrile reaction, and to avoid fluid overload in small children.

For chronic toxicity: 6 vials; for infants and small children (≤20kg), a single vial may be sufficient.

Pediatrics:

Acute toxicity: I.V.: Refer to adult dosing.

Chronic toxicity: I.V.: If amount ingested and blood level are unknown: Children ≤ 20 kg: 1 vial may be sufficient. If amount ingested or blood level is known, refer to adult dosing.

Children >20 kg: Refer to adult dosing.

Renal Impairment: Renal elimination of complexed digoxin may be decreased in renal failure. Potential "rebound" may occur when immune fragments are hepatically metabolized, leaving unbound digoxin.

Administration

I.V.: Continuous I.V. infusion over ≥30 minutes is preferred. Small doses (infants/small children) may be administered using tuberculin syringe.

Stability

Storage: Should be refrigerated at 2°C to 8°C.

Reconstitution: Digoxin immune Fab is reconstituted by adding 4 mL sterile water, resulting in 10 mg/mL for I.V. infusion. The reconstituted solution may be further diluted with NS to a convenient volume (eg, 1 mg/mL). Reconstituted solutions should be used within 4 hours if refrigerated.

For very small doses, vial can be reconstituted by adding an additional 36 mL of sterile isotonic saline, to achieve a final concentration of 1 mg/mL.

Monitoring Laboratory Tests Serum potassium, serum digoxin concentration prior to first dose of digoxin immune Fab, subsequent to start of Digibind® therapy; **digoxin levels will greatly increase and are not an accurate determination of body stores.**

Monitoring and Teaching Issues

Physical Assessment: Note Warnings/Precautions. Monitor lab values (see Effects on Lab Values and Monitoring Laboratory Tests), cardiac status, vital signs, blood pressure, and adverse reactions during and following infusion (see Adverse Reactions). **Pregnancy risk factor C.** Note breast-feeding caution.

Patient Education: Patient education and instruction will be determined by patient condition and ability to understand. Immediately report dizziness, palpitations, cramping, difficulty breathing, rash, or itching. **Pregnancy/breast-feeding precautions:** Inform prescriber if you are pregnant. Consult prescriber if breast-feeding.

Dihematoporphyrin Ether *see* Porfimer *on page 1101*

Dihistine® DH Liquid *see page 1522*

Dihistine® Expectorant *see* Guaifenesin, Pseudoephedrine, and Codeine *on page 649*

Dihydrocodeine Compound (dye hye droe KOE deen KOM pound)

U.S. Brand Names Synalgos®-DC

Restrictions C-III

Generic Available Yes

Pharmacologic Category Analgesic, Narcotic

Pregnancy Risk Factor B/D (prolonged use or high doses at term)

Lactation Excretion in breast milk unknown/use caution

Use Management of mild to moderate pain that requires relaxation

Mechanism of Action/Effect Binds to opiate receptors in the CNS, causing inhibition of ascending pain pathways, altering the perception of and response to pain; causes cough suppression by direct central action in the medulla; produces generalized CNS depression

Contraindications Hypersensitivity to dihydrocodeine or any component of the formulation; pregnancy (prolonged use or high doses at term)

Warnings/Precautions Use with caution in patients with hypersensitivity reactions to other phenanthrene derivative opioid agonists (morphine, hydrocodone, hydromorphone, levorphanol, oxycodone, oxymorphone); respiratory diseases including asthma, emphysema, COPD; or severe liver or renal insufficiency. Some preparations contain sulfites which may cause allergic reactions. May be habit-forming. Dextromethorphan has equivalent antitussive activity but has much lower toxicity in accidental overdose.

Drug Interactions

Cytochrome P450 Effect: Substrate of **CYP2D6**

Increased Effect/Toxicity: MAO inhibitors may increase adverse symptoms.

Nutritional/Ethanol Interactions Ethanol: Avoid ethanol (may increase CNS depression).

Adverse Reactions

>10%:

Central nervous system: Lightheadedness, dizziness, drowsiness, sedation

Dermatologic: Pruritus, skin reactions

Gastrointestinal: Nausea, vomiting, constipation

1% to 10%:

Cardiovascular: Hypotension, palpitations, bradycardia, peripheral vasodilation

Central nervous system: Increased intracranial pressure

Endocrine & metabolic: Antidiuretic hormone release

Gastrointestinal: Biliary tract spasm

Genitourinary: Urinary tract spasm

Ocular: Miosis

Respiratory: Respiratory depression

Miscellaneous: Histamine release, physical and psychological dependence with prolonged use

Overdosage/Toxicology Symptoms of overdose include CNS depression, pinpoint pupils, hypotension, and bradycardia. Treatment is supportive. Naloxone, 2 mg I.V. with repeat administration as necessary up to a total of 10 mg, can also be used to reverse toxic effects of the opiate.

(Continued)

Dihydrocodeine Compound *(Continued)*

Pharmacodynamics/Kinetics

Half-Life Elimination: Serum: 3.8 hours

Time to Peak: Serum: 30-60 minutes

Metabolism: Hepatic

Onset: 10-30 minutes

Duration: 4-6 hours

Formulations Capsule: Synalgos®-DC: Dihydrocodeine bitartrate 16 mg, aspirin 356.4 mg, and caffeine 30 mg

Dosing

Adults: Pain: Oral: 1-2 capsules every 4-6 hours as needed

Elderly: Initial dosing should be cautious (low end of adult dosing range).

Monitoring and Teaching Issues

Physical Assessment: Assess for history of allergies (see Warnings/Precautions) and other medications patient may be taking for additive or adverse interactions. Monitor therapeutic effectiveness and adverse reactions (see Adverse Reactions and Overdose/Toxicology) at beginning of therapy and at regular intervals with long-term use. May cause physical and/or psychological dependence. Assess knowledge/teach patient appropriate use (if self-administered), appropriate interventions to reduce side effects, and adverse reactions to report (see Patient Education). **Pregnancy risk factor B/D** - see Pregnancy Risk Factor for use cautions. Note breast-feeding caution.

Patient Education: If self-administered, use exactly as directed; do not increase dose or frequency. Drug may cause physical and/or psychological dependence. While using this medication, do not use alcohol and other prescription or OTC medications (especially sedatives, tranquilizers, antihistamines, or pain medications) without consulting prescriber. Maintain adequate hydration (2-3 L/day of fluids) unless advised by prescriber to restrict fluids. May cause dizziness, drowsiness, impaired coordination, or blurred vision (use caution when driving, climbing stairs, or changing position - rising from sitting or lying to standing or when engaging in tasks requiring alertness until response to drug is known); nausea or vomiting (frequent mouth care, small, frequent meals, chewing gum, or sucking lozenges may help); or constipation (increased exercise, fluids, fruit, or fiber may help; if unresolved, consult prescriber about use of stool softeners). Report chest pain or rapid heartbeat; acute headache; swelling of extremities or unusual weight gain; changes in urinary elimination; acute headache; back or flank pain or spasms; or other adverse reactions. **Pregnancy/breast-feeding precautions:** Inform prescriber if you are or intend to become pregnant. Consult prescriber if breast-feeding.

Breast-feeding Issues:

Acetaminophen: May be taken while breast-feeding.

Aspirin: Use cautiously due to potential adverse effects in nursing infants.

Dihydrocodeine: No data reported.

Related Information

Aspirin *on page 121*

Dihydroergotamine (dye hye droe er GOT a meen)

U.S. Brand Names D.H.E. 45®; Migranal®

Synonyms DHE; Dihydroergotamine Mesylate

Generic Available No

Pharmacologic Category Ergot Derivative

Pregnancy Risk Factor X

Lactation May be excreted in breast milk/contraindicated

Use Treatment of migraine headache with or without aura; injection also indicated for treatment of cluster headaches

Use - Unlabeled/Investigational Adjunct for DVT prophylaxis for hip surgery, for orthostatic hypotension, xerostomia secondary to antidepressant use, and pelvic congestion with pain

Mechanism of Action/Effect Ergot alkaloid alpha-adrenergic blocker directly stimulates vascular smooth muscle to vasoconstrict peripheral and cerebral vessels; also has effects on serotonin receptors

Contraindications Hypersensitivity to dihydroergotamine or any component of the formulation; high-dose aspirin therapy; uncontrolled hypertension, ischemic heart disease, angina pectoris, history of MI, silent ischemia, or coronary artery vasospasm including Prinzmetal's angina; hemiplegic or basilar migraine; peripheral vascular disease; sepsis; severe hepatic or renal dysfunction; following vascular surgery; avoid use within 24 hours of sumatriptan, zolmitriptan, other serotonin agonists, or ergot-like agents; avoid during or within 2 weeks of discontinuing MAO inhibitors; concurrent use with potent CYP3A4 inhibitors (clarithromycin, erythromycin, itraconazole, ketoconazole, protease inhibitors, troleandomycin); pregnancy

Warnings/Precautions Do not give to patients with risk factors for CAD until a cardiovascular evaluation has been performed; if evaluation is satisfactory, the healthcare provider should administer the first dose and cardiovascular status should be periodically evaluated. May cause vasospastic reactions; persistent vasospasm may lead to gangrene or death in patients with compromised circulation. Discontinue if signs of vasoconstriction develop. Rare reports of increased blood pressure in patients without history of hypertension. Rare reports of adverse cardiac events (acute MI, life-threatening arrhythmias, death) have been reported following use of the injection. Cerebral hemorrhage, subarachnoid hemorrhage, and stroke have also occurred following use of the injection. Not for prolonged use. Pleural and peritoneal fibrosis have been reported with prolonged daily use. Cardiac valvular fibrosis has also been associated with ergot alkaloids. Safety and efficacy in pediatric patients have not been established.

Drug Interactions

Cytochrome P450 Effect: Substrate of **CYP3A4**; Inhibits CYP3A4

Increased Effect/Toxicity: CYP3A4 inhibitors (potent) may increase vasoconstrictive effect (concurrent use is contraindicated). Concurrent use of protease inhibitors (amprenavir, indinavir, nelfinavir, and ritonavir) may increase toxicity of dihydroergotamine (use is contraindicated). Increased effect of heparin. Increased toxicity with erythromycin, clarithromycin, nitroglycerin, propranolol, and troleandomycin. Potential for serotonin syndrome if combined with other serotonergic drugs.

Adverse Reactions

>10%: Nasal spray: Respiratory: Rhinitis (26%)

1% to 10%: Nasal spray:

Central nervous system: Dizziness (4%), somnolence (3%)

Endocrine & metabolic: Hot flashes (1%)

Gastrointestinal: Nausea (10%), taste disturbance (8%), vomiting (4%), diarrhea (2%)

Local: Application site reaction (6%)

Neuromuscular & skeletal: Weakness (1%), stiffness (1%)

Respiratory: Pharyngitis (3%)

<1% (Limited to important or life-threatening): Injection and nasal spray: Cerebral hemorrhage, coronary artery vasospasm, hypertension, myocardial infarction, paresthesia, peripheral cyanosis, peripheral ischemia, rash, stroke, subarachnoid hemorrhage, ventricular fibrillation, ventricular tachycardia. Pleural and retroperitoneal fibrosis have been reported following prolonged use of the injection; cardiac valvular fibrosis has been associated with ergot alkaloids.

Overdosage/Toxicology Symptoms of overdose include peripheral ischemia, paresthesia, headache, nausea, and vomiting. Treatment is supportive. Activated charcoal is effective at binding ergot alkaloids.

Pharmacodynamics/Kinetics

Half-Life Elimination: 1.3-3.9 hours

Time to Peak: Serum: I.M.: 15-30 minutes

Metabolism: Extensively hepatic

Onset: 15-30 minutes

Duration: 3-4 hours

Formulations

Injection, solution, as mesylate (D.H.E. 45®): 1 mg/mL (1 mL) [contains ethanol 94%]

Solution, intranasal spray, as mesylate (Migranal®): 4 mg/mL [0.5 mg/spray] (1 mL) [contains caffeine 10 mg/mL]

Dosing

Adults:

Migraine, cluster headache:

I.M., S.C.: 1 mg at first sign of headache; repeat hourly to a maximum dose of 3 mg total; maximum dose: 6 mg/week

I.V.: 1 mg at first sign of headache; repeat hourly up to a maximum dose of 2 mg total; maximum dose: 6 mg/week

Intranasal: 1 spray (0.5 mg) of nasal spray should be administered into each nostril; if needed, repeat after 15 minutes, up to a total of 4 sprays. **Note:** Do not exceed 3 mg (6 sprays) in a 24-hour period and no more than 8 sprays in a week.

Elderly: Refer to adult dosing. Patients >65 years of age were not included in controlled clinical studies.

Renal Impairment: Contraindicated in severe renal impairment

Hepatic Impairment: Dosage reductions are probably necessary but specific guidelines are not available.

Administration

Other: Prior to administration of nasal spray, the nasal spray applicator must be primed (pumped 4 times); in order to let the drug be absorbed through the skin in the nose, patients should not inhale deeply through the nose while spraying or immediately after spraying; for best results, treatment should be initiated at the first symptom or sign of an attack; however, nasal spray can be used at any stage of a migraine attack

Stability

Storage:

Injection: Store below 25°C (77°F), do not refrigerate or freeze; protect from heat and light

Nasal spray: Prior to use, store below 25°C (77°F), do not refrigerate or freeze; once spray applicator has been prepared, use within 8 hours; discard any unused solution

Monitoring and Teaching Issues

Physical Assessment: See Contraindications, Warnings/Precautions, and Dosing for use cautions. Assess potential for interactions with other prescriptions, OTC medications, or herbal products patient may be taking (see Drug Interactions). Assess therapeutic response and adverse reactions (see Adverse Reactions and Overdose/Toxicology) on a regular basis. Teach patient proper use if self-administered (eg, injection technique and needle disposal), possible side effects and interventions, and adverse symptoms to report (see Patient Education). **Pregnancy risk factor X** - determine that patient is not pregnant before starting therapy. Do not give to women of childbearing are patient is unless capable of complying with barrier contraceptive use. Breast-feeding is contraindicated.

Patient Education: Take this drug as rapidly as possible when first symptoms occur. May cause rare feelings of numbness or tingling of fingers, toes, or face (use caution and avoid injury) or drowsiness (use caution when driving or engaging in potentially hazardous tasks until response to drug is known). Report heart palpitations, severe nausea or vomiting, and severe numbness of fingers or toes.

Nasal spray: Follow directions for use on package insert. Prime inhaler before use. Wait 15 minutes between inhalations. Use no more than 4 inhalations (2 mg) for a single administration; do not use >3 mg (6 sprays) in a 24-hour period and no more than 8 sprays in a week.

I.M.: Follow directions for injections and needle disposal.

Pregnancy/breast-feeding precautions: Inform prescriber if you are pregnant. Do not get pregnant during or for 1 month following therapy. Consult prescriber for instruction on appropriate contraceptive measures. This drug may cause severe fetal defects. Do not breast-feed.

(Continued)

Dihydroergotamine *(Continued)*

Geriatric Considerations: Monitor cardiac and peripheral effects closely in the elderly since they often have cardiovascular disease and peripheral vascular impairment (ie, diabetes mellitus, PVD) that will complicate therapy and monitoring for adverse effects.

Breast-feeding Issues: Ergot derivatives inhibit prolactin and it is known that ergotamine is excreted in breast milk (vomiting, diarrhea, weak pulse, and unstable blood pressure have been reported in nursing infants). It is not known if dihydroergotamine would also cause these effects, however, it is likely that it is excreted in human breast milk. Do not use in nursing women.

Pregnancy Issues: Dihydroergotamine is oxytocic and should not be used during pregnancy.

Dihydroergotamine Mesylate *see* Dihydroergotamine *on page 416*

Dihydrohydroxycodeinone *see* Oxycodone *on page 1020*

Dihydromorphinone *see* Hydromorphone *on page 677*

1,25 Dihydroxycholecalciferol *see* Calcitriol *on page 200*

Diiodohydroxyquin *see* Iodoquinol *on page 731*

Dilacor® XR *see* Diltiazem *on page 418*

Dilantin® *see* Phenytoin *on page 1073*

Dilatrate®-SR *see* Isosorbide Dinitrate *on page 749*

Dilaudid® *see* Hydromorphone *on page 677*

Dilaudid-HP® *see* Hydromorphone *on page 677*

Diltia® XT *see* Diltiazem *on page 418*

Diltiazem (dil TYE a zem)

U.S. Brand Names Cardizem®; Cardizem® CD; Cardizem® SR; Cartia XT™; Dilacor® XR; Diltia® XT; Tiazac®

Synonyms Diltiazem Hydrochloride

Generic Available Yes

Pharmacologic Category Calcium Channel Blocker

Pregnancy Risk Factor C

Lactation Enters breast milk/compatible

Use

Capsule: Essential hypertension (sustained release only, alone or in combination); chronic stable angina or angina from coronary artery spasm

Injection: Atrial fibrillation or atrial flutter; paroxysmal supraventricular tachycardia (PSVT)

Use - Unlabeled/Investigational Investigational: Therapy of Duchenne muscular dystrophy

Mechanism of Action/Effect Inhibits calcium ion from entering the "slow channels" or select voltage-sensitive areas of vascular smooth muscle and myocardium during depolarization, producing a relaxation of coronary vascular smooth muscle and coronary vasodilation; increases myocardial oxygen delivery in patients with vasospastic angina

Contraindications Hypersensitivity to diltiazem or any component of the formulation; sick sinus syndrome; second- or third-degree AV block (except in patients with a functioning artificial pacemaker); hypotension (systolic <90 mm Hg); acute MI and pulmonary congestion by x-ray

Warnings/Precautions Concomitant use with beta-blockers or digoxin can result in conduction disturbances. Avoid concurrent I.V. use of diltiazem and a beta-blocker - monitor closely when I.V. diltiazem is used. Use caution in left ventricular dysfunction and CHF (can exacerbate condition). Symptomatic hypotension can occur. Use with caution in hepatic or renal dysfunction. Pregnancy risk C.

Drug Interactions

Cytochrome P450 Effect: Substrate of CYP2C8/9, 2D6, **3A4**; Inhibits CYP2C8/9, 2D6, **3A4**

Decreased Effect: Rifampin markedly reduces diltiazem serum levels resulting in decreased diltiazem effect. Coadministration with other cytochrome P450 enzyme inducers should be avoided (includes phenytoin, barbiturates, and carbamazepine).

Increased Effect/Toxicity: Diltiazem effects may be additive with amiodarone, beta-blockers, or digoxin, which may lead to bradycardia, other conduction delays, and decreased cardiac output. Serum concentrations/toxicity of diltiazem may be increased by inhibitors of CYP3A4, including amprenavir, cimetidine, ciprofloxacin, clarithromycin, clozapine, diltiazem, disulfiram, digoxin, erythromycin, ethanol, fluconazole, fluoxetine, fluvoxamine, isoniazid, itraconazole, ketoconazole, labetalol, levodopa, loxapine, metoprolol, metronidazole, miconazole, nefazodone, nelfinavir, omeprazole, phenytoin, rifabutin, rifampin, ritonavir, troleandomycin, valproic acid, and verapamil. Diltiazem may increase serum levels/toxicity of alfentanil (possibly fentanyl and sufentanil), some benzodiazepines (specifically midazolam and triazolam), carbamazepine, cisapride (QT prolongation, arrhythmia), cyclosporine, digoxin, HMG-CoA reductase inhibitors (atorvastatin, lovastatin, simvastatin), lithium (neurotoxicity), midazolam, moricizine, and tacrolimus.

Nutritional/Ethanol Interactions

Ethanol: Avoid ethanol (may increase risk of hypotension or vasodilation).

Food: Diltiazem serum levels may be elevated if taken with food. Serum concentrations were not altered by grapefruit juice in small clinical trials.

Herb/Nutraceutical: St John's wort may decrease diltiazem levels. Avoid dong quai if using for hypertension (has estrogenic activity). Avoid ephedra (may worsen arrhythmia or hypertension). Avoid yohimbe, ginseng (may worsen hypertension). Avoid garlic (may have increased antihypertensive effect).

Adverse Reactions

>10%: Gastrointestinal: Gingival hyperplasia (21%)

1% to 10%:

Cardiovascular: Sinus bradycardia (2% to 6%), first-degree AV block (2% to 8%), EKG abnormality (4%), peripheral edema (dose-related 5% to 8%), flushing (2% to 3%), hypotension (1%), palpitations (1%)

Central nervous system: Dizziness (3% to 7%), headache (5% to 12%), somnolence (1%), insomnia (1%)
Gastrointestinal: Nausea (1% to 2%), constipation (2%), dyspepsia (1%)
Neuromuscular & skeletal: Weakness (3% to 5%)
Dermatological: Rash (1% to 2%)
Renal: Polyuria (1%)

<1% (Limited to important or life-threatening): Agranulocytosis, akathisia, amnesia, angina, arrhythmia, AV block, bundle branch block, CHF, depression, dysgeusia, dyspnea, erythema multiforme, exfoliative dermatitis, gait abnormalities, hallucinations, hyperglycemia, impotence, leukocytopenia (overdose), mania, myoclonus, nocturia, osteoarticular pain, paresthesia, Parkinsonian-like syndrome, personality change, photosensitivity, pruritus, psychosis, sexual dysfunction, Stevens-Johnson syndrome, syncope, thrombocytopenia, tinnitus, toxic epidermal necrolysis (TEN), tremor, urticaria, vomiting

Overdosage/Toxicology Primary cardiac symptoms of calcium blocker overdose include hypotension and bradycardia. Noncardiac symptoms include confusion, stupor, nausea, vomiting, metabolic acidosis, and hyperglycemia.

Following initial gastric decontamination, if possible, repeated calcium administration may promptly reverse depressed cardiac contractility (but not sinus node depression or peripheral vasodilation). Glucagon, epinephrine, and amrinone may treat refractory hypotension. Glucagon and epinephrine also increase heart rate (outside the U.S., 4-aminopyridine may be available as an antidote). Dialysis and hemoperfusion are not effective in enhancing elimination although repeat-dose activated charcoal may serve as an adjunct with sustained-release preparations.

Pharmacodynamics/Kinetics

Absorption: 80% to 90%

Bioavailability: ~40% to 60%

Half-Life Elimination: 4-6 hours, may be prolonged with renal impairment; Sustained release: 5-7 hours

Time to Peak: Serum: Short-acting tablet: 2-3 hours; Sustained release: 6-11 hours

Metabolism: Hepatic; extensive first-pass effect; following single I.V. injection, plasma concentrations of N-monodesmethyldiltiazem and desacetyldiltiazem are typically undetectable; however, these metabolites accumulate to detectable concentrations following 24-hour constant rate infusion. N-monodesmethyldiltiazem appears to have 20% of the potency of diltiazem; desacetyldiltiazem is about 50% as potent as the parent compound.

Onset: Oral: Short-acting tablets: 30-60 minutes

Formulations

Capsule, extended release, as hydrochloride [once-daily dosing]: 120 mg, 180 mg, 240 mg, 300 mg
Cardizem® CD: 120 mg, 180 mg, 240 mg, 300 mg, 360 mg
Cartia XT™: 120 mg, 180 mg, 240 mg, 300 mg
Dilacor® XR, Diltia XT®: 120 mg, 180 mg, 240 mg
Tiazac®: 120 mg, 180 mg, 240 mg, 300 mg, 360 mg, 420 mg

Capsule, sustained release, as hydrochloride [twice-daily dosing] (Cardizem® SR): 60 mg, 90 mg, 120 mg

Injection, solution, as hydrochloride: 5 mg/mL (5 mL, 10 mL, 25 mL)
Cardizem®: 5 mg/mL (5 mL, 10 mL)

Injection, powder for reconstitution, as hydrochloride (Cardizem®): 25 mg, 100 mg

Tablet, as hydrochloride (Cardizem®): 30 mg, 60 mg, 90 mg, 120 mg

Dosing

Adults & Elderly:

Angina: Oral: Usual starting dose: 30 mg 4 times/day; sustained release: 120-180 mg once daily; dosage should be increased gradually at 1- to 2-day intervals until optimum response is obtained. Doses up to 360 mg/day have been effectively used. Also see product-specific dosing (below) for sustained release products.

Hypertension: Oral: Hypertension is controllable with single daily doses of sustained release products, or divided daily doses of regular release products, in the range of 240-360 mg/day. Also see product-specific dosing (below) for sustained release products.

Product-specific dosing; Sustained-release capsules:

Cardizem® SR: Initial: 60-120 mg twice daily; adjust to maximum antihypertensive effect (usually within 14 days); usual range: 240-360 mg/day

Cardizem® CD, Tiazac®: Hypertension: Total daily dose of short-acting administered once daily or initially 180 or 240 mg once daily; adjust to maximum effect (usually within 14 days); maximum: 480 mg/day; usual range: 240-360 mg/day

Cardizem® CD: Angina: Initial: 120-180 mg once daily; maximum: 480 mg once/day

Dilacor® XR:

Hypertension: 180-240 mg once daily; maximum: 540 mg/day; usual range: 180-480 mg/day; use lower dose in elderly

Angina: Initial: 120 mg/day; titrate slowly over 7-14 days up to 480 mg/day, as needed

Atrial dysrhythmia: I.V. (requires an infusion pump):

- Initial bolus dose: 0.25 mg/kg actual body weight over 2 minutes (average adult dose: 20 mg)
- Repeat bolus dose (may be administered after 15 minutes if the response is inadequate.): 0.35 mg/kg actual body weight over 2 minutes (average adult dose: 25 mg)
- Continuous infusion (infusions >24 hours or infusion rates >15 mg/hour are not recommended.): Initial infusion rate of 10 mg/hour; rate may be increased in 5 mg/hour increments up to 15 mg/hour as needed; some patients may respond to an initial rate of 5 mg/hour.

If Cardizem® injectable is administered by continuous infusion for >24 hours, the possibility of decreased diltiazem clearance, prolonged elimination half-life, and increased diltiazem and/or diltiazem metabolite plasma concentrations should be considered.

Conversion from I.V. diltiazem to oral diltiazem: Start oral approximately 3 hours after bolus dose.

Oral dose (mg/day) is approximately equal to [rate (mg/hour) x 3 + 3] x 10.

(Continued)

Diltiazem *(Continued)*

3 mg/hour = 120 mg/day
5 mg/hour = 180 mg/day
7 mg/hour = 240 mg/day
11 mg/hour = 360 mg/day

Pediatrics:

Children: Minimal information available; some centers use the following:

Hypertension: Oral: Initial: 1.5-2 mg/kg/day in 3-4 divided doses; maximum dose: 3.5 mg/kg/day

Note: Doses up to 8 mg/kg/day given in 4 divided doses have been used for investigational therapy of Duchenne muscular dystrophy

Adolescents: Refer to adult dosing.

Renal Impairment: Use with caution as diltiazem is extensively metabolized by the liver and excreted in the kidneys and bile. Not removed by hemo- or peritoneal dialysis; supplemental dose is not necessary.

Hepatic Impairment: Use with caution as diltiazem is extensively metabolized by the liver and excreted in the kidneys and bile.

Administration

Oral: Do not crush sustained release capsules.

I.V.: Bolus doses given over 2 minutes with continuous EKG and blood pressure monitoring. Continuous infusion should be via infusion pump.

Stability

Compatibility: Stable in $D_5{}^1/_2NS$, D_5W, NS

Y-site administration: Incompatible with diazepam, furosemide, phenytoin, rifampin, thiopental

Monitoring Laboratory Tests Liver function tests

Monitoring and Teaching Issues

Physical Assessment: See Contraindications, Warnings/Precautions, and Dosing for use cautions. Assess potential for interactions with other prescriptions, OTC medications, or herbal products patient may be taking (see Drug Interactions). I.V. requires use of infusion pump and continuous cardiac and hemodynamic monitoring. Assess results of laboratory tests, therapeutic response, and adverse reactions (see Warnings/Precautions, Adverse Reactions, and Overdose/Toxicology) when beginning therapy, when changing dose, and periodically during long-term therapy. Teach patient appropriate use (oral), interventions to reduce side effects, and adverse symptoms to report (see Patient Education). **Pregnancy risk factor C** - benefits of use should outweigh possible risks.

Patient Education: Inform prescriber of all prescriptions, OTC medications, or herbal products you are taking, and any allergies you have. Do not take anything new during treatment unless approved by prescriber. Oral: Take as directed; do not alter dosage or discontinue therapy without consulting prescriber. Do not crush or chew extended release form. Avoid (or limit) alcohol and caffeine. May cause dizziness or lightheadedness (use caution when driving or engaging in tasks requiring alertness until response to drug is known); nausea or vomiting (small, frequent meals, frequent mouth care, chewing gum, or sucking lozenges may help); constipation (increased exercise, fluids, fruit, or fiber may help); or diarrhea (buttermilk, boiled milk, or yogurt may help). Report chest pain, palpitations, irregular heartbeat; unusual cough, difficulty breathing; swelling of extremities; muscle tremors or weakness; confusion or acute lethargy; skin rash; or other adverse reactions. **Pregnancy precaution:** Inform prescriber if you are or intend to become pregnant.

Geriatric Considerations: Elderly may experience a greater hypotensive response.

Breast-feeding Issues: Freely diffuses into breast milk; however, the AAP considers diltiazem to be **compatible** with breast-feeding. Available evidence suggest safe use during breast-feeding.

Pregnancy Issues: Teratogenic and embryotoxic effects have been demonstrated in small animals given doses 5-10 times the adult dose (mg/kg).

Related Information

Antiarrhythmic Drugs *on page 1551*
Calcium Channel Blockers *on page 1563*

Diltiazem Hydrochloride *see* Diltiazem *on page 418*

Dimercaprol *see page 1461*

Dimercaprol *see page 1460*

Dimetapp® Decongestant Liqui-Gels® [OTC] *see* Pseudoephedrine *on page 1150*

Dimethyl Sulfoxide (dye meth il sul FOKS ide)

U.S. Brand Names Rimso®-50

Synonyms DMSO

Generic Available No

Pharmacologic Category Urinary Tract Product

Pregnancy Risk Factor C

Lactation Excretion in breast milk unknown

Use Symptomatic relief of interstitial cystitis

Drug Interactions

Cytochrome P450 Effect: Inhibits CYP2C8/9, 2C19

Adverse Reactions

>10%: Gastrointestinal: Garlic-like breath

1% to 10%:

Central nervous system: Headache, sedation
Gastrointestinal: Nausea, vomiting
Local: Local dermatitis
Ocular: Burning eyes

Formulations Solution, intravesical: 50% [500 mg/mL] (50 mL)

Dosing

Adults & Elderly: Interstitial cystitis: Not for I.M. or I.V. administration; only for bladder instillation. Instill 50 mL of solution directly into bladder and allow to remain for 15 minutes. Repeat in 2 weeks or until symptoms are relieved, then increase intervals between treatments.

Monitoring and Teaching Issues

Physical Assessment: For bladder instillation only (see Dosing). Assess knowledge/teach patient interventions to reduce side effects and adverse symptoms to report (see Patient Education). **Pregnancy risk factor C** - benefits of use should outweigh possible risks. Note breast-feeding caution.

Patient Education: This medication is only for use as a bladder instillation. Maintain adequate hydration (2-3 L/day of fluids) unless advised by prescriber to restrict fluids. Report adverse reactions. **Pregnancy/breast-feeding precautions:** Inform prescriber if you are or intend to become pregnant. Note breast-feeding caution.

Dimethyl Triazeno Imidazol Carboxamide *see* Dacarbazine *on page 353*

Dinoprost *see page 1461*

Dinoprostone (dye noe PROST one)

U.S. Brand Names Cervidil®; Prepidil®; Prostin E_2®

Synonyms PGE_2; Prostaglandin E_2

Generic Available No

Pharmacologic Category Abortifacient; Prostaglandin

Pregnancy Risk Factor C

Lactation Excretion in breast milk unknown/opportunity for use is minimal

Use

Gel: Promote cervical ripening prior to labor induction; usage for gel include any patient undergoing induction of labor with an unripe cervix, most commonly for pre-eclampsia, eclampsia, postdates, diabetes, intrauterine growth retardation, and chronic hypertension

Suppositories: Terminate pregnancy from 12th through 28th week of gestation; evacuate uterus in cases of missed abortion or intrauterine fetal death; manage benign hydatidiform mole

Vaginal insert: Initiation and/or cervical ripening in patients at or near term in whom there is a medical or obstetrical indication for the induction of labor

Mechanism of Action/Effect A synthetic prostaglandin E_2 abortifacient that stimulates uterine contractions similar to those seen during natural labor

Contraindications

Vaginal insert: Hypersensitivity to prostaglandins; fetal distress (suspicion or clinical evidence unless delivery is imminent); unexplained vaginal bleeding during this pregnancy; strong suspicion of marked cephalopelvic disproportion; patients in whom oxytoxic drugs are contraindicated or when prolonged contraction of the uterus may be detrimental to fetal safety or uterine integrity (including previous cesarean section or major uterine surgery); greater than 6 previous term pregnancies; patients already receiving oxytoxic drugs

Gel: Hypersensitivity to prostaglandins or any constituents of the cervical gel, history of asthma, contracted pelvis, malpresentation of the fetus

Gel: The following are "relative" contraindications and should only be considered by the physician under these circumstances: Patients in whom vaginal delivery is not indicated (ie, herpes genitalia with a lesion at the time of delivery), prior uterine surgery, breech presentation, multiple gestation, polyhydramnios, premature rupture of membranes

Suppository: Hypersensitivity to dinoprostone, acute pelvic inflammatory disease, uterine fibroids, cervical stenosis

Warnings/Precautions Dinoprostone should be used only by medically trained personnel in a hospital; caution in patients with cervicitis, infected endocervical lesions, acute vaginitis, compromised (scarred) uterus or history of asthma, hypertension or hypotension, epilepsy, diabetes mellitus, anemia, jaundice, or cardiovascular, renal, or hepatic disease. Oxytocin should not be used simultaneously with Prepidil® (>6 hours of the last dose of Prepidil®). Pregnancy risk C.

Drug Interactions

Increased Effect/Toxicity: Increased effect of oxytocics.

Adverse Reactions

>10%:

Central nervous system: Headache

Gastrointestinal: Vomiting, diarrhea, nausea

1% to 10%:

Cardiovascular: Bradycardia

Central nervous system: Fever

Neuromuscular & skeletal: Back pain

<1% (Limited to important or life-threatening): Bronchospasm, cardiac arrhythmias, chills, coughing, dizziness, dyspnea, flushing, hot flashes, hypotension, pain, shivering, syncope, tightness of the chest, vasomotor and vasovagal reactions, wheezing

Overdosage/Toxicology Symptoms of overdose include vomiting, bronchospasm, hypotension, chest pain, abdominal cramps, and uterine contractions. Treatment is symptomatic.

Pharmacodynamics/Kinetics

Absorption: Vaginal: Slow

Metabolism: In many tissues including the renal, pulmonary, and splenic systems

Onset: Uterine contractions: Within 10 minutes

Duration: Up to 2-3 hours

Formulations

Gel, endocervical (Prepidil®): 0.5 mg/3 g syringes [each package contains a 10 mm and 20 mm shielded catheter]

Insert, vaginal (Cervidil®): 10 mg [releases 0.3 mg/hour]

Suppository, vaginal (Prostin E_2®): 20 mg

(Continued)

Dinoprostone *(Continued)*

Dosing

Adults & Elderly:

Abortifacient: Insert 1 suppository high in vagina, repeat at 3- to 5-hour intervals until abortion occurs up to 240 mg (maximum); continued administration for longer than 2 days is not advisable.

Cervical ripening:

Gel:

Intracervical: 0.25-1 mg

Intravaginal: 2.5 mg

Suppositories, intracervical: 2-3 mg

Vaginal insert (Cervidil®): Intracervical: 10 mg; remove upon onset of active labor or after 12 hours.

Administration

Other: Intracervically: Bring suppository to room temperature just prior to use. Patient should remain recumbent for 2 hours following insertion.

Stability

Storage: Suppositories must be kept frozen, store in freezer not above -4°C (-20°F). Bring to room temperature just prior to use. Cervical gel should be stored under refrigeration 2°C to 8°C (36°F to 46°F).

Monitoring and Teaching Issues

Physical Assessment: See Contraindications and Warning/Precautions for use cautions. Monitor temperature, uterine tone, and vaginal discharge closely throughout procedure and postprocedure. Monitor abortion for completeness (other measures may be necessary if incomplete). Assess knowledge/teach patient interventions to reduce side effects and adverse symptoms to report (see Patient Education).

Patient Education: Nausea and vomiting, cramping or uterine pain, or fever may occur. Report acute pain, difficulty breathing, or skin rash. Closely monitor for vaginal discharge for several days. Report vaginal bleeding, itching, malodorous or bloody discharge, or severe cramping.

Diocto® [OTC] *see* Docusate *on page 432*

Dioctyl Calcium Sulfosuccinate *see* Docusate *on page 432*

Dioctyl Sodium Sulfosuccinate *see* Docusate *on page 432*

Diotame® [OTC] *see* Bismuth *on page 169*

Diovan® *see* Valsartan *on page 1386*

Diovan HCT® *see* Valsartan and Hydrochlorothiazide *on page 1388*

Dipentum® *see* Olsalazine *on page 998*

Diphen® [OTC] *see* DiphenhydrAMINE *on page 422*

Diphen® AF [OTC] *see* DiphenhydrAMINE *on page 422*

Diphen® Cough [OTC] *see* DiphenhydrAMINE *on page 422*

Diphenhist [OTC] *see* DiphenhydrAMINE *on page 422*

DiphenhydrAMINE (dye fen HYE dra meen)

U.S. Brand Names Aler-Dryl [OTC]; AllerMax® [OTC]; Banophen® [OTC]; Benadryl® Allergy [OTC]; Benadryl® Dye-Free Allergy [OTC]; Benadryl® Gel [OTC]; Benadryl® Gel Extra Strength [OTC]; Benadryl® Injection; Compoz® Nighttime Sleep Aid [OTC]; Diphen® [OTC]; Diphen® AF [OTC]; Diphen® Cough [OTC]; Diphenhist [OTC]; Genahist® [OTC]; Hydramine® [OTC]; Hydramine® Cough [OTC]; Hyrexin-50®; Nytol® [OTC]; Nytol® Maximum Strength [OTC]; Siladryl® Allergy [OTC]; Silphen® [OTC]; Sleepinal® [OTC]; Sominex® [OTC]; Sominex® Maximum Strength [OTC]; Tusstat®; Twilite® [OTC]; Unisom® Maximum Strength SleepGels® [OTC]

Synonyms Diphenhydramine Hydrochloride

Generic Available Yes

Pharmacologic Category Antihistamine

Pregnancy Risk Factor B

Lactation Enters breast milk/contraindicated

Use Symptomatic relief of allergic symptoms caused by histamine release which include nasal allergies and allergic dermatosis; can be used for mild nighttime sedation; prevention of motion sickness and as an antitussive; has antinauseant and topical anesthetic properties; treatment of antipsychotic-induced extrapyramidal symptoms

Mechanism of Action/Effect Competes with histamine for H_1-receptor sites on effector cells in the gastrointestinal tract, blood vessels, and respiratory tract; anticholinergic and sedative effects are also seen

Contraindications Hypersensitivity to diphenhydramine or any component of the formulation; acute asthma; not for use in neonates

Warnings/Precautions Causes sedation, caution must be used in performing tasks which require alertness (ie, operating machinery or driving). Sedative effects of CNS depressants or ethanol are potentiated. Use with caution in patients with angle-closure glaucoma, pyloroduodenal obstruction (including stenotic peptic ulcer), urinary tract obstruction (including bladder neck obstruction and symptomatic prostatic hyperplasia), hyperthyroidism, increased intraocular pressure, and cardiovascular disease (including hypertension and tachycardia). Diphenhydramine has high sedative and anticholinergic properties, so it may not be considered the antihistamine of choice for prolonged use in the elderly. May cause paradoxical excitation in pediatric patients, and can result in hallucinations, coma, and death in overdose. Some preparations contain sodium bisulfite; syrup formulations may contain alcohol.

Drug Interactions

Cytochrome P450 Effect: Inhibits CYP2D6

Decreased Effect: May increase gastric degradation of levodopa and decrease the amount of levodopa absorbed by delaying gastric emptying. Therapeutic effects of cholinergic agents (tacrine, donepezil) and neuroleptics may be antagonized.

Increased Effect/Toxicity: CNS depressants may increase the degree of sedation and respiratory depression with diphenhydramine. May increase the absorption of digoxin. Central and/or peripheral anticholinergic syndrome can occur when administered with amantadine, rimantadine, narcotic analgesics, phenothiazines and other antipsychotics (especially with high anticholinergic activity), tricyclic antidepressants, quinidine, disopyramide, procainamide, and antihistamines. Syrup should not be given to patients taking drugs that can cause disulfiram reactions (ie, metronidazole, chlorpropamide) due to high alcohol content.

Nutritional/Ethanol Interactions

Ethanol: Avoid ethanol (may increase CNS depression).

Herb/Nutraceutical: Avoid valerian, St John's wort, kava kava, gotu kola (may increase CNS depression).

Effects on Lab Values May suppress the wheal and flare reactions to skin test antigens.

Adverse Reactions Frequency not defined.

Cardiovascular: Hypotension, palpitations, tachycardia

Central nervous system: Sedation, sleepiness, dizziness, disturbed coordination, headache, fatigue, nervousness, paradoxical excitement, insomnia, euphoria, confusion

Dermatologic: Photosensitivity, rash, angioedema, urticaria

Gastrointestinal: Nausea, vomiting, diarrhea, abdominal pain, xerostomia, appetite increase, weight gain, dry mucous membranes, anorexia

Genitourinary: Urinary retention, urinary frequency, difficult urination

Hematologic: Hemolytic anemia, thrombocytopenia, agranulocytosis

Neuromuscular & skeletal: Tremor, paresthesia

Ocular: blurred vision

Respiratory: Thickening of bronchial secretions

Overdosage/Toxicology Symptoms of overdose include CNS stimulation or depression; overdose may result in death in infants and children. There is no specific treatment for antihistamine overdose. Clinical toxicity is due to blockade of cholinergic receptors. For anticholinergic overdose with life-threatening symptoms, physostigmine 1-2 mg S.C. or I.V. slowly may be given to reverse these effects.

Pharmacodynamics/Kinetics

Bioavailability: Oral: 40% to 60%

Half-Life Elimination: 2-8 hours; Elderly: 13.5 hours

Time to Peak: Serum: 2-4 hours

Metabolism: Extensively hepatic; smaller degrees in pulmonary and renal systems; significant first-pass effect

Onset: Maximum sedative effect: 1-3 hours

Duration: 4-7 hours

Formulations

Capsule, as hydrochloride: 25 mg, 50 mg
- Banophen®, Diphen®, Diphenhist®, Genahist®: 25 mg
- Nytol® Maximum Strength, Sleepinal®: 50 mg

Elixir, as hydrochloride: 12.5 mg/5 mL (5 mL, 10 mL, 20 mL, 120 mL, 480 mL, 3780 mL)
- Banophen®: 12.5 mg/5 mL (120 mL, 480 mL, 3840 mL)
- Diphen AF: 12.5 mg/5 mL (120 mL, 240 mL, 480 mL, 3840 mL) [alcohol free; cherry flavor]
- Genahist®: 12.5 mg/5 mL (120 mL)
- Hydramine®: 12.5 mg/5 mL (120 mL) [alcohol free; cherry flavor]

Gel, topical, as hydrochloride:
- Benadryl®: 1% (120 mL)
- Benadryl® Extra Strength: 2% (120 mL)

Injection, solution, as hydrochloride: 10 mg/mL (30 mL); 50 mg/mL (1 mL, 10 mL)
- Benadryl®: 50 mg/mL (1 mL, 10 mL)
- Hyrexin®: 50 mg/mL (10 mL)

Liquid, as hydrochloride:
- Benadryl® Allergy: 12.5 mg/5 mL (120 mL, 240 mL) [alcohol free; cherry flavor]
- Benadryl® Dye-Free Allergy: 12.5 mg/5 mL (120 mL) [alcohol free, dye free, sugar free; bubble-gum flavor]

Softgel, as hydrochloride
- Benadryl® Dye-Free Allergy: 25 mg [dye-free]
- Unisom® Maximum Strength SleepGels®: 50 mg

Solution, oral, as hydrochloride
- AllerMax®: 12.5 mg/5 mL (120 mL)
- Diphenhist®: 12.5 mg/5 mL (120 mL, 480 mL)

Solution, topical, as hydrochloride [spray]: 1% (60 mL); 2%

Syrup, as hydrochloride: 12.5 mg/5 mL (120 mL, 240 mL, 480 mL)
- Diphen® Cough: 12.5 mg/5 mL (120 mL, 240 mL, 480 mL) [contains alcohol 5.1%; raspberry flavor]
- Diphenhist®: 12.5 mg/5 mL (120 mL)
- Hydramine® Cough: 12.5 mg/5 mL (120 mL, 480 mL) [contains alcohol 5%; fruit flavor]
- Siladryl® Allergy, Silphen® Cough: 12.5 mg/5 mL (120 mL, 240 mL, 480 mL)
- Tusstat:® 12.5 mg/5 mL (120 mL, 240 mL, 3840 mL)

Tablet, as hydrochloride: 25 mg, 50 mg
- Aler-Dryl, AllerMax®, Compoz® Nighttime Sleep Aid, Sominex® Maximum Strength, Twilite®: 50 mg
- Banophen®, Benadryl® Allergy, Diphenhist®, Genahist®, Nytol®, Sominex®: 25 mg

Tablet, chewable, as hydrochloride (Benadryl® Allergy): 12.5 mg [contains phenylalanine 4.2 mg/tablet; grape flavor]

Dosing

Adults:

Minor allergic rhinitis or motion sickness: Oral: 25-50 mg every 4-6 hours; maximum: 300 mg/day

Moderate to severe allergic reactions:
- Oral: 25-50 mg every 4 hours, not to exceed 400 mg/day
- I.M., I.V.: 10-50 mg in a single dose every 2-4 hours, not to exceed 400 mg/day

(Continued)

DiphenhydrAMINE *(Continued)*

Night-time sleep aid: Oral: 50 mg at bedtime
Dystonic reaction: I.M., I.V.: 50 mg in a single dose; may repeat in 20-30 minutes if necessary
Allergic dermatosis: Topical: For external application, not longer than 7 days

Elderly: Initial: 25 mg 2-3 times/day increasing as needed

Pediatrics:

Treatment of dystonic reactions and moderate to severe allergic reactions: Oral, I.M., I.V.: 5 mg/kg/day or 150 mg/m²/day in divided doses every 6-8 hours, not to exceed 300 mg/day

Minor allergic rhinitis or motion sickness: Oral, I.M., I.V.:
- 2 to <6 years: 6.25 mg every 4-6 hours; maximum: 37.5 mg/day
- 6 to <12 years: 12.5-25 mg every 4-6 hours; maximum: 150 mg/day
- ≥12 years: 25-50 mg every 4-6 hours; maximum: 300 mg/day

Night-time sleep aid: 30 minutes before bedtime: Oral, I.M., I.V.:
- 2 to <12 years: 1 mg/kg/dose; maximum: 50 mg/dose
- ≥12 years: 50 mg

Oral: Antitussive: Oral, I.M., I.V.:
- 2 to <6 years: 6.25 mg every 4 hours; maximum 37.5 mg/day
- 6 to <12 years: 12.5 mg every 4 hours; maximum 75 mg/day
- ≥12 years: 25 mg every 4 hours; maximum 150 mg/day

Administration

Oral: Swallow whole, do not crush or chew sustained release product.

Stability

Storage: Injection: Protect from light.

Compatibility: Stable in dextran 6% in dextrose, dextran 6% in NS, D_5LR, $D_5\frac{1}{4}NS$, $D_5\frac{1}{2}NS$, D_5NS, D_5W, $D_{10}W$, fat emulsion 10%, LR, ½NS, NS

Y-site administration: Incompatible with allopurinol, amphotericin B cholesteryl sulfate complex, cefepime, foscarnet

Compatibility in syringe: Incompatible with diatrizoate meglumine 52% and diatrizoate sodium 8%, diatrizoate sodium 60%, haloperidol, iodipamide meglumine, iodipamide meglumine 52%, ioxaglate meglumine 39.3% and ioxaglate sodium 19.6%, pentobarbital, thiopental

Compatibility when admixed: Incompatible with amobarbital, amphotericin B, dexamethasone sodium phosphate with lorazepam and metoclopramide, iodipamide meglumine, phenytoin, phenobarbital, thiopental

Monitoring and Teaching Issues

Physical Assessment: Assess effectiveness and interactions of other medications patient may be taking (see Drug Interactions). See Contraindications and Warnings/Precautions for use cautions. Monitor effectiveness of therapy and adverse reactions (see Adverse Reactions) at beginning of therapy and periodically with long-term use. Assess knowledge/teach patient appropriate use, interventions to reduce side effects, and adverse symptoms to report (see Patient Education). Breast-feeding is contraindicated.

Patient Education: Take as directed; do not exceed recommended dose. Avoid use of other depressants, alcohol, or sleep-inducing medications unless approved by prescriber. You may experience drowsiness or dizziness (use caution when driving or engaging in tasks requiring alertness until response to drug is known); or dry mouth, nausea, or vomiting (small, frequent meals, frequent mouth care, chewing gum, or sucking hard candy may help). Report persistent sedation, confusion, or agitation; changes in urinary pattern; blurred vision; sore throat, difficulty breathing, or expectorating (thick secretions); or lack of improvement or worsening or condition. **Breast-feeding precaution:** Do not breast-feed.

Geriatric Considerations: Diphenhydramine has high sedative and anticholinergic properties, so it may not be considered the antihistamine of choice for prolonged use in the elderly. Its use as a sleep aid is discouraged due to its anticholinergic effects.

Breast-feeding Issues: Infants may be more sensitive to the effects of antihistamines.

Additional Information Its use as a sleep aid is discouraged due to its anticholinergic effects.

Related Information

Antiemetics for Chemotherapy-Induced Nausea and Vomiting *on page 1639*
Anxiolytic/Hypnotic Use in Long-Term Care Facilities *on page 1608*
Compatibility of Drugs in Syringe *on page 1566*
FDA Name Differentiation Project: The Use of Tall-man Letters *on page 12*

Diphenhydramine Hydrochloride *see* DiphenhydrAMINE *on page 422*

Diphenoxylate and Atropine (dye fen OKS i late & A troe peen)

U.S. Brand Names Lomocot®; Lomotil®; Lonox®

Synonyms Atropine and Diphenoxylate

Restrictions C-V

Generic Available Yes

Pharmacologic Category Antidiarrheal

Pregnancy Risk Factor C

Lactation Use caution

Use Treatment of diarrhea

Mechanism of Action/Effect Diphenoxylate inhibits excessive GI motility and GI propulsion; commercial preparations contain a subtherapeutic amount of atropine to discourage abuse

Contraindications Hypersensitivity to diphenoxylate, atropine, or any component of the formulation; severe liver disease; jaundice; dehydration; narrow-angle glaucoma; not for use in children <2 years of age

Warnings/Precautions High doses may cause physical and psychological dependence with prolonged use. Use with caution in patients with ulcerative colitis, dehydration, and hepatic dysfunction. Reduction of intestinal motility may be deleterious in diarrhea resulting from *Shigella*, *Salmonella*, toxigenic strains of *E. coli*, and from pseudomembranous enterocolitis associated with broad spectrum antibiotics. If there is no response within 48 hours, the drug is unlikely to be effective and should be discontinued. If chronic diarrhea is not improved symptomatically within 10 days at maximum dosage of 20 mg/day, control is unlikely with further use. Pregnancy risk C.

Drug Interactions

Increased Effect/Toxicity: MAO inhibitors (hypertensive crisis), CNS depressants when taken with diphenoxylate may result in increased adverse effects, antimuscarinics (paralytic ileus). May prolong half-life of drugs metabolized in liver.

Nutritional/Ethanol Interactions Ethanol: Avoid ethanol (may increase CNS depression).

Adverse Reactions

1% to 10%:

Central nervous system: Nervousness, restlessness, dizziness, drowsiness, headache, mental depression

Gastrointestinal: Paralytic ileus, dry mouth, megacolon

Genitourinary: Urinary retention and difficult urination

Ocular: Blurred vision

Respiratory: Respiratory depression

<1% (Limited to important or life-threatening): Abdominal discomfort, nausea, pancreatitis, stomach cramps, tachycardia, vomiting

Overdosage/Toxicology Symptoms of overdose include drowsiness, hypotension, blurred vision, flushing, dry mouth, and miosis. Administration of activated charcoal will reduce bioavailability of diphenoxylate. Naloxone, 2 mg I.V. with repeat administration as necessary up to a total of 10 mg, can also be used to reverse toxic effects of the opiate. For anticholinergic overdose with severe life-threatening symptoms, physostigmine 1-2 mg S.C. or I.V. slowly, may be given to reverse these effects.

Pharmacokinetic Note See Atropine monograph.

Pharmacodynamics/Kinetics

Absorption:

Diphenoxylate: Well absorbed

Half-Life Elimination:

Diphenoxylate: 2.5 hours

Time to Peak:

Diphenoxylate: Serum: 2 hours

Metabolism:

Diphenoxylate: Extensively hepatic to diphenoxylic acid (active)

Onset:

Diphenoxylate: Antidiarrheal: 45-60 minutes; Peak antidiarrheal effect: ~2 hours

Duration:

Diphenoxylate: Antidiarrheal: 3-4 hours

Formulations

Solution, oral: Diphenoxylate hydrochloride 2.5 mg and atropine sulfate 0.025 mg per 5 mL (5 mL, 10 mL, 60 mL)

Lomotil®: Diphenoxylate hydrochloride 2.5 mg and atropine sulfate 0.025 mg per 5 mL (60 mL) [contains alcohol 15%; cherry flavor]

Tablet (Lomocot®, Lomotil®, Lonox®): Diphenoxylate hydrochloride 2.5 mg and atropine sulfate 0.025 mg

Dosing

Adults & Elderly: Diarrhea: Oral: 15-20 mg/day of diphenoxylate in 3-4 divided doses; maintenance: 5-15 mg/day in 2-3 divided doses

Pediatrics: Diarrhea: Oral: Use with caution in young children due to variable responses:

Liquid: 0.3-0.4 mg of diphenoxylate/kg/day in 2-4 divided doses **or**

<2 years: Not recommended

2-5 years: 2 mg of diphenoxylate 3 times/day

5-8 years: 2 mg of diphenoxylate 4 times/day

8-12 years: 2 mg of diphenoxylate 5 times/day

Stability

Storage: Protect from light.

Monitoring and Teaching Issues

Physical Assessment: Ascertain etiology of diarrhea before beginning treatment if possible. Assess effects and interactions of other prescription and OTC medications or herbal products patient may be taking (see Drug Interactions). Assess therapeutic effectiveness and response (see Adverse Reactions and Overdose/Toxicology). **Note:** There is potential for physical and psychological dependence with prolonged use. Teach patient proper use, possible side effects and interventions, and adverse effects to report (see Patient Education). **Pregnancy risk factor C** - benefits of use should outweigh possible risks. Note breast-feeding caution.

Patient Education: Inform prescriber of all prescriptions, OTC medications, or herbal products you are taking, and any allergies you have. Do not take anything new during treatment unless approved by prescriber. Take as directed; do not exceed recommended dosage. If no response within 48 hours, notify prescriber. Avoid alcohol or other prescriptive or OTC sedatives or depressants. May cause drowsiness, blurred vision, impaired coordination (use caution when driving or engaging in tasks that require alertness until response to drug is known); dry mouth (sucking on lozenges or chewing gum may help). Report difficulty urinating, persistent unrelieved diarrhea, respiratory difficulties, fever, or palpitations. **Pregnancy/breast-feeding precautions:** Inform prescriber if you are or intend to become pregnant. Consult prescriber if breast-feeding.

Geriatric Considerations: Elderly are particularly sensitive to fluid and electrolyte loss. Maintaining hydration and electrolyte balance is vital.

Related Information

Atropine *on page 134*

Diphenylhydantoin *see* Phenytoin *on page 1073*

Diphtheria and Tetanus Toxoid *see page 1498*

Diphtheria Antitoxin *see page 1460*
Diphtheria CRM$_{197}$ Protein *see page 1498*
Diphtheria, Tetanus Toxoids, and Acellular Pertussis Vaccine *see page 1498*
Diphtheria, Tetanus Toxoids, and Whole-Cell Pertussis Vaccine *see page 1498*
Diphtheria, Tetanus Toxoids, Whole-Cell Pertussis Vaccine, and *Haemophilus* B Conjugate Vaccine *see page 1498*
Dipivefrin *see page 1575*
Dipivefrin *see* Ophthalmic Agents, Glaucoma *on page 1002*
Diprivan® *see* Propofol *on page 1138*
Diprolene® *see* Betamethasone *on page 160*
Diprolene® *see* Topical Corticosteroids *on page 1334*
Diprolene® AF *see* Betamethasone *on page 160*
Diprolene® AF *see* Topical Corticosteroids *on page 1334*
Dipropylacetic Acid *see* Valproic Acid and Derivatives *on page 1382*
Diprosone® *see* Betamethasone *on page 160*
Diprosone® *see* Topical Corticosteroids *on page 1334*

Dipyridamole (dye peer ID a mole)

U.S. Brand Names Persantine®

Generic Available Yes

Pharmacologic Category Antiplatelet Agent; Vasodilator

Pregnancy Risk Factor B

Lactation Enters breast milk (low concentrations)/use caution

Use Maintains patency after surgical grafting procedures including coronary artery bypass; used with warfarin to decrease thrombosis in patients after artificial heart valve replacement; used with aspirin to prevent coronary artery thrombosis; in combination with aspirin or warfarin to prevent other thromboembolic disorders. Dipyridamole may also be given 2 days prior to open heart surgery to prevent platelet activation by extracorporeal bypass pump and as a diagnostic agent in CAD.

Use - Unlabeled/Investigational Treatment of proteinuria in pediatric renal disease

Mechanism of Action/Effect Inhibits platelet aggregation and may cause vasodilation. May also stimulate release of prostacyclin or PGD_2 resulting in coronary vasodilation.

Contraindications Hypersensitivity to dipyridamole or any component of the formulation

Warnings/Precautions Use caution in patients with hypotension. Use caution in patients on other antiplatelet agents or anticoagulation. Severe adverse reactions have occurred with I.V. administration (rarely); use the I.V. form with caution in patients with bronchospastic disease or unstable angina. Aminophylline should be available in case of urgency or emergency with I.V. use.

Drug Interactions

Decreased Effect: Decreased vasodilation from I.V. dipyridamole when given to patients taking theophylline. Theophylline may reduce the pharmacologic effects of dipyridamole (hold theophylline preparations for 36-48 hours before dipyridamole facilitated stress test).

Increased Effect/Toxicity: Dipyridamole enhances the risk of bleeding with aspirin (and other antiplatelet agents), heparin, low-molecular weight heparins, and warfarin. Adenosine blood levels and pharmacologic effects are increased with dipyridamole; consider reduced doses of adenosine.

Nutritional/Ethanol Interactions Herb/Nutraceutical: Avoid cat's claw, dong quai, evening primrose, feverfew, garlic, ginger, ginkgo, red clover, horse chestnut, green tea, ginseng (all have additional antiplatelet activity).

Adverse Reactions

>10%:

Cardiovascular: Exacerbation of angina pectoris (20% I.V.)

Central nervous system: Dizziness (14% oral), headache (12% I.V.)

1% to 10%:

Cardiovascular: Hypotension (5%), hypertension (2%), blood pressure lability (2%), EKG abnormalities (ST-T changes, extrasystoles), chest pain, tachycardia (3% I.V.)

Central nervous system: Headache (2% I.V.), flushing (3% I.V.), fatigue (1% I.V.)

Dermatologic: Rash (2% oral)

Gastrointestinal: Abdominal distress (6% oral), nausea (5% I.V.)

Neuromuscular & skeletal: Paresthesia (1% I.V.)

Respiratory: Dyspnea (3% I.V.)

<1% (Limited to important or life-threatening):

I.V.: Arrhythmias (ventricular tachycardia, bradycardia, AV block, SVT, atrial fibrillation, asystole), bronchospasm, depersonalization, intermittent claudication, myocardial infarction, orthostatic hypotension, syncope, vertigo

Oral: Angina pectoris, liver dysfunction.

Postmarketing and/or case reports: Epistaxis, esophageal hematoma, gallstones, pharyngeal bleeding, rapidly progressive glomerulonephritis, respiratory arrest (I.V.), thrombotic thrombocytopenic purpura

Overdosage/Toxicology Symptoms of overdose include hypotension and peripheral vasodilation. Dialysis is not effective. Treatment is symptomatic and supportive.

Pharmacodynamics/Kinetics

Absorption: Readily, but variable

Half-Life Elimination: Terminal: 10-12 hours

Time to Peak: Serum: 2-2.5 hours

Metabolism: Hepatic

Formulations

Injection, solution: 5 mg/mL (2 mL, 10 mL)

Tablet: 25 mg, 50 mg, 75 mg

Dosing

Adults & Elderly:

Prevention of thrombosis: Oral: 75-400 mg/day in 3-4 divided doses

Evaluation of coronary artery disease: I.V.: 0.14 mg/kg/minute for 4 minutes; maximum dose: 60 mg

Pediatrics:

Prevention of thrombosis: Oral: 3-6 mg/kg/day in 3 divided doses

Proteinuria: **Note:** Doses of 4-10 mg/kg/day have been used investigationally to treat proteinuria in pediatric renal disease.

Mechanical prosthetic heart valves: Oral: 2-5 mg/kg/day (used in combination with an oral anticoagulant in children who have systemic embolism despite adequate oral anticoagulant therapy, and used in combination with low-dose oral anticoagulation (INR 2-3) plus aspirin in children in whom full-dose oral anticoagulation is contraindicated).

Renal Impairment: Hemodialysis: Significant drug removal is unlikely based on physiochemical characteristics

Stability

Storage: I.V.: Do not freeze, protect from light.

Monitoring and Teaching Issues

Physical Assessment: See Warnings/Precautions, Contraindications, and Drug Interactions for use cautions. Monitor therapeutic response (dependent on purpose for use) and adverse reactions (see Adverse Reactions and Overdose/Toxicology). Observe bleeding precautions. **I.V.:** Continuous EKG and blood pressure monitoring during infusion. Assess knowledge/teach patient appropriate use, interventions to reduce side effects, and adverse symptoms to report (see Patient Education). **Oral:** Monitor blood pressure on a regular basis. Note breast-feeding caution.

Patient Education: Oral: Take exactly as directed, with water 1 hour before meals. You may experience mild headache, transient diarrhea, or temporary dizziness (sit or lie down when taking medication). You may have a tendency to bleed easy; use caution with sharps, needles, or razors. Report chest pain, redness around mouth, acute abdominal cramping or severe diarrhea, acute and persistent headache or dizziness, rash, difficulty breathing, or swelling of extremities. **Breast-feeding precaution:** Consult prescriber if breast-feeding.

Dietary Issues: Should be taken with water 1 hour before meals.

Geriatric Considerations: Since evidence suggests that clinically used doses are ineffective for prevention of platelet aggregation, consideration for low-dose aspirin (81-325 mg/day) alone may be necessary. This will decrease cost as well as inconvenience.

Dipyridamole and Aspirin *see* Aspirin and Dipyridamole *on page 124*

Disalcid® *see* Salsalate *on page 1212*

Disalicylic Acid *see* Salsalate *on page 1212*

Discoloration of Feces Due to Drugs *see page 1526*

Discoloration of Urine Due to Drugs *see page 1526*

Disodium Cromoglycate *see* Cromolyn Sodium *on page 334*

***d*-Isoephedrine Hydrochloride** *see* Pseudoephedrine *on page 1150*

Disulfiram (dye SUL fi ram)

U.S. Brand Names Antabuse®

Generic Available No

Pharmacologic Category Aldehyde Dehydrogenase Inhibitor

Pregnancy Risk Factor C

Lactation Excretion in breast milk unknown

Use Management of chronic alcoholism

Mechanism of Action/Effect Disulfiram is a thiuram derivative which interferes with aldehyde dehydrogenase. When taken concomitantly with alcohol, there is an increase in serum acetaldehyde levels. High acetaldehyde causes uncomfortable symptoms including flushing, nausea, thirst, palpitations, chest pain, vertigo, and hypotension. This reaction is the basis for disulfiram use in postwithdrawal long-term care of alcoholism.

Contraindications Hypersensitivity to disulfiram and related compounds or any component of the formulation; patients receiving or using ethanol, metronidazole, paraldehyde, or ethanol-containing preparations like cough syrup or tonics; psychosis; severe myocardial disease and coronary occlusion

Warnings/Precautions Use with caution in patients with diabetes, hypothyroidism, seizure disorders, nephritis (acute or chronic), hepatic cirrhosis or insufficiency. Should never be administered to a patient when he/she is in a state of ethanol intoxication, or without his/her knowledge. Patient must receive appropriate counseling, including information on "disguised" forms of alcohol (tonics, mouthwashes, etc) and the duration of the drug's activity (up to 14 days). Pregnancy risk C.

Drug Interactions

Cytochrome P450 Effect: Substrate of CYP1A2, 2A6, 2B6, 2D6, 2E1, 3A4; Inhibits CYP1A2, 2A6, 2B6, 2C8/9, 2D6, **2E1**, 3A4

Increased Effect/Toxicity: Disulfiram may increase serum concentrations of benzodiazepines that undergo oxidative metabolism (all but oxazepam, lorazepam, temazepam). Disulfiram increases phenytoin and theophylline serum concentrations; toxicity may occur. Disulfiram inhibits the metabolism of warfarin resulting in an increased hypoprothrombinemic response. Disulfiram results in severe ethanol intolerance (disulfiram reaction) secondary to disulfiram's ability to inhibit aldehyde dehydrogenase; this combination should be avoided. Combined use with isoniazid, metronidazole, or MAO inhibitors may result in adverse CNS effects; this combination should be avoided. Some pharmaceutic dosage forms include ethanol, including elixirs and intravenous trimethoprim-sulfamethoxazole (contains 10% ethanol as a solubilizing agent); these may inadvertently provoke a disulfiram reaction.

Nutritional/Ethanol Interactions Ethanol: Disulfiram inhibits ethanol's usual metabolism. Avoid all ethanol. Patients can have a disulfiram reaction (headache, nausea, vomiting,

(Continued)

Disulfiram *(Continued)*

chest, or abdominal pain) if they drink ethanol concurrently. Avoid cough syrups and elixirs containing ethanol. Avoid vinegars, cider, extracts, and foods containing ethanol.

Adverse Reactions Frequency not defined.

Central nervous system: Drowsiness, headache, fatigue, psychosis
Dermatologic: Rash, acneiform eruptions, allergic dermatitis
Gastrointestinal: Metallic or garlic-like aftertaste
Genitourinary: Impotence
Hepatic: Hepatitis
Neuromuscular & skeletal: Peripheral neuritis, polyneuritis, peripheral neuropathy
Ocular: Optic neuritis

Overdosage/Toxicology Management of disulfiram reaction: Institute support measures to restore blood pressure (vasopressors and fluids). Monitor for hypokalemia.

Pharmacodynamics/Kinetics

Absorption: Rapid
Metabolism: To diethylthiocarbamate
Onset: Full effect: 12 hours
Duration: ~1-2 weeks after last dose

Formulations Tablet: 250 mg

Dosing

Adults & Elderly: Note: Do not administer until the patient has abstained from ethanol for at least 12 hours.

Alcoholism: Oral: Initial: 500 mg/day as a single dose for 1-2 weeks; maximum daily dose is 500 mg. Average maintenance dose: 250 mg/day; range: 125-500 mg; duration of therapy is to continue until the patient is fully recovered socially and a basis for permanent self control has been established. Maintenance therapy may be required for months or even years.

Administration

Oral: Administration of any medications containing alcohol, including topicals, is contraindicated. Do not administer disulfiram if ethanol has been consumed within the prior 12 hours.

Monitoring Laboratory Tests Monitor liver function before, 10-14 days after beginning therapy, and every 6 months during therapy.

Monitoring and Teaching Issues

Physical Assessment: See Contraindications and Warnings/Precautions for use cautions. Assess for adverse drug interactions with other prescription or OTC drugs (see Drug Interactions). Do not administer until the patient has abstained from ethanol for 12 hours. Monitor laboratory tests (see above) and for CNS changes at beginning of therapy and periodically with long-term therapy (see Adverse Reactions). Advise patient about disulfiram reaction if alcohol is ingested. Assess knowledge/teach patient appropriate use, interventions to reduce side effects, and adverse symptoms to report (see Patient Education). **Pregnancy risk factor C** - benefits of use should outweigh possible risks. Note breast-feeding caution.

Patient Education: Tablets can be crushed or mixed with water or juice. Metallic aftertaste may occur; this will go away. Do not drink any alcohol, including products containing alcohol (such as cough and cold syrups or some mouthwashes), or use alcohol-containing skin products for at least 3 days and preferably 14 days after stopping this medication or while taking this medication. Drowsiness, tiredness, or visual changes may occur. Use care when driving or engaging in tasks requiring alertness until response to drug is known. Notify prescriber of any difficulty breathing, weakness, nausea, vomiting, decreased appetite, yellowing of skin or eyes, or dark-colored urine. **Pregnancy/breast-feeding precautions:** Inform prescriber if you are or intend to become pregnant. Consult prescriber if breast-feeding.

Dithranol *see* Anthralin *on page 108*
Ditropan® *see* Oxybutynin *on page 1019*
Ditropan® XL *see* Oxybutynin *on page 1019*
Divalproex Sodium *see* Valproic Acid and Derivatives *on page 1382*
Dizmiss® [OTC] *see* Meclizine *on page 840*
***dl*-Alpha Tocopherol** *see* Vitamin E *on page 1406*
***D*-Mannitol** *see* Mannitol *on page 835*
4-dmdr *see* Idarubicin *on page 692*
DMSO *see* Dimethyl Sulfoxide *on page 420*
DNase *see* Dornase Alfa *on page 439*
DNR *see* DAUNOrubicin Hydrochloride *on page 369*

DOBUTamine (doe BYOO ta meen)

U.S. Brand Names Dobutrex®

Synonyms Dobutamine Hydrochloride

Generic Available Yes

Pharmacologic Category Adrenergic Agonist Agent

Pregnancy Risk Factor B

Lactation Excretion in breast milk unknown

Use Short-term management of patients with cardiac decompensation

Use - Unlabeled/Investigational Postive inotropic agent for use in myocardial dysfunction of sepsis

Mechanism of Action/Effect Stimulates $beta_1$-adrenergic receptors, causing increased contractility and heart rate, with little effect on $beta_2$- or alpha-receptors

Contraindications Hypersensitivity to dobutamine or sulfites (some contain sodium metabisulfate), or any component of the formulation; idiopathic hypertrophic subaortic stenosis (IHSS)

Warnings/Precautions Can see an increase in heart rate. Patients with atrial fibrillation may experience an increase in ventricular response. An increase in blood pressure is more common, but occasionally a patient may become hypotensive. May exacerbate ventricular ectopy. If needed, correct hypovolemia first to optimize hemodynamics. Ineffective in the presence of mechanical obstruction such as severe aortic stenosis. Use caution post-MI (can increase myocardial oxygen demand). Use cautiously in the elderly starting at lower end of the dosage range.

Drug Interactions

Decreased Effect: Beta-adrenergic blockers may decrease effect of dobutamine and increase risk of severe hypotension.

Increased Effect/Toxicity: General anesthetics (eg, halothane or cyclopropane) and usual doses of dobutamine have resulted in ventricular arrhythmias in animals. Bretylium and may potentiate dobutamine's effects. Beta-blockers (nonselective ones) may increase hypertensive effect; avoid concurrent use. Cocaine may cause malignant arrhythmias. Guanethidine, MAO inhibitors, methyldopa, reserpine, and tricyclic antidepressants can increase the pressor response to sympathomimetics.

Effects on Lab Values May affect serum assay of chloramphenicol.

Adverse Reactions Incidence of adverse events is not always reported.

Cardiovascular: Increased heart rate, increased blood pressure, increased ventricular ectopic activity, hypotension, premature ventricular beats (5%, dose-related), anginal pain (1% to 3%), nonspecific chest pain (1% to 3%), palpitations (1% to 3%)

Central nervous system: Fever (1% to 3%), headache (1% to 3%), paresthesia

Endocrine & metabolic: Slight decrease in serum potassium

Gastrointestinal: Nausea (1% to 3%)

Hematologic: Thrombocytopenia (isolated cases)

Local: Phlebitis, local inflammatory changes and pain from infiltration, cutaneous necrosis (isolated cases)

Neuromuscular & skeletal: Mild leg cramps

Respiratory: Dyspnea (1% to 3%)

Overdosage/Toxicology Symptoms of overdose include fatigue, nervousness, tachycardia, hypertension, and arrhythmias. Reduce rate of administration or discontinue infusion until condition stabilizes.

Pharmacodynamics/Kinetics

Half-Life Elimination: 2 minutes

Metabolism: In tissues and hepatically to inactive metabolites

Onset: I.V.: 1-10 minutes; Peak effect: 10-20 minutes

Formulations

Infusion, as hydrochloride [premixed in dextrose]: 1 mg/mL (250 mL, 500 mL); 2 mg/mL (250 mL), 4 mg/mL (250 mL)

Injection, solution, as hydrochloride: 12.5 mg/mL (20 mL, 40 mL, 100 mL) [contains sodium bisulfite]

Dosing

Adults & Elderly: Cardiac decompensation: I.V. infusion: 2.5-20 mcg/kg/minute; maximum: 40 mcg/kg/minute, titrate to desired response; see table.

Infusion Rates of Various Dilutions of Dobutamine

Desired Delivery Rate (mcg/kg/min)	Infusion Rate (mL/kg/min)	
	500 mcg/mL*	1000 mcg/mL†
2.5	0.005	0.0025
5.0	0.01	0.005
7.5	0.015	0.0075
10.0	0.02	0.01
12.5	0.025	0.0125
15.0	0.03	0.015

* 500 mg per liter or 250 mg per 500 mL of diluent.

†1000 mg per liter or 250 mg per 250 mL of diluent.

Pediatrics: Cardiac decompensation: I.V. infusion: See table.

Neonates: 2-15 mcg/kg/minute, titrate to desired response

Children: Refer to adult dosing.

Administration

I.V.: Always administer via infusion device; administer into large vein.

Stability

Reconstitution: Remix solution every 24 hours. Store reconstituted solution under refrigeration for 48 hours or 6 hours at room temperature. Pink discoloration of solution indicates slight oxidation but **no** significant loss of potency. Stability of parenteral admixture at room temperature (25°C) is 48 hours; at refrigeration (4°C) stability is 7 days.

Standard adult diluent: 250 mg/500 mL D_5W; 500 mg/500 mL D_5W

Compatibility: Do not give through same I.V. line as heparin, hydrocortisone sodium succinate, cefazolin, or penicillin. **Incompatible** with heparin, cefazolin, penicillin, and in alkaline solutions (sodium bicarbonate).

Stable in D_5LR, $D_5\frac{1}{2}NS$, D_5NS, D_5W, $D_{10}W$, LR, ½NS, NS, mannitol 20%; **incompatible** with sodium bicarbonate 5%

Y-site administration: Incompatible with acyclovir, alatrofloxacin, alteplase, aminophylline, amphotericin B cholesteryl sulfate complex, cefepime, foscarnet, indomethacin, phytonadione, piperacillin/tazobactam, thiopental, warfarin

Compatibility in syringe: Incompatible with doxapram

Compatibility when admixed: Incompatible with acyclovir, alteplase, aminophylline, bumetanide, calcium gluconate, diazepam, digoxin, floxacillin, furosemide, insulin (regular), magnesium sulfate, phenytoin, potassium phosphates, sodium bicarbonate

(Continued)

DOBUTamine *(Continued)*

Monitoring Laboratory Tests Serum glucose, renal function

Monitoring and Teaching Issues

Physical Assessment: Assess other medications patient may be taking for effectiveness and interactions (see Drug Interactions). See Warnings/Precautions and Contraindications for use cautions. Infusion pump and continuous cardiac and hemodynamic monitoring are required. Monitor therapeutic response and adverse reactions (see Warnings/Precautions and Adverse Reactions). Instruct patient on adverse symptoms to report (see Patient Education). Note breast-feeding caution.

Patient Education: When administered in emergencies, patient education should be appropriate to the situation. If patient is aware, instruct to promptly report chest pain, palpitations, rapid heartbeat, headache, nervousness, or restlessness, nausea or vomiting, or difficulty breathing. **Breast-feeding precaution:** Consult prescriber if breast-feeding.

Geriatric Considerations: Beneficial hemodynamic effects have been demonstrated in in elderly patients; however, significant hypotension may occur more frequently in elderly patients; monitor closely.

Pregnancy Issues: Since dobutamine has not been given to pregnant women, benefits of use should outweigh the risks.

Additional Information Dobutamine lowers central venous pressure and wedge pressure but has little effect on pulmonary vascular resistance.

Dobutamine therapy should be avoided in patients with stable heart failure due to an increase in mortality. In patients with intractable heart failure, dobutamine may be used as a short-term infusion to provide symptomatic benefit. It is not known whether short-term dobutamine therapy in end-stage heart failure has any outcome benefit.

Dobutamine infusion during echocardiography is used as a cardiovascular stress. Wall motion abnormalities developing with increasing doses of dobutamine may help to identify ischemic and/or hibernating myocardium.

Related Information

FDA Name Differentiation Project: The Use of Tall-man Letters *on page 12*
Inotropic and Vasoconstrictor Comparison *on page 1580*

Dobutamine Hydrochloride *see* DOBUTamine *on page 428*

Dobutrex® *see* DOBUTamine *on page 428*

Docetaxel (doe se TAKS el)

U.S. Brand Names Taxotere®

Generic Available No

Pharmacologic Category Antineoplastic Agent, Natural Source (Plant) Derivative

Pregnancy Risk Factor D

Lactation Excretion in breast milk unknown/contraindicated

Use Treatment of patients with locally advanced or metastatic breast cancer who have progressed during anthracycline-based therapy or have relapsed during anthracycline-based adjuvant therapy; treatment of patients with locally advanced or metastatic nonsmall cell lung cancer after failure of prior platinum-based chemotherapy

Use - Unlabeled/Investigational Investigational: Treatment of gastric, pancreatic, head and neck, ovarian, soft tissue sarcoma, and melanoma

Mechanism of Action/Effect Inhibits cancer cell division by acting on the microtubules

Contraindications Hypersensitivity to docetaxel, Polysorbate 80®, or any component of the formulation; pre-existing bone marrow suppression (neutrophils <1500 cells/mm^3); pregnancy

Warnings/Precautions Hypersensitivity, including severe reactions, may occur (incidence up to 25% in patients who did not receive premedication).

Fluid retention syndrome (pleural effusions, ascites, edema, and 2-15 kg weight gain) may occur. It has not been associated with cardiac, pulmonary, renal, hepatic, or endocrine dysfunction. The incidence and severity of the syndrome increase sharply at cumulative doses ≥400 mg/m^2.

Neutropenia was the dose-limiting toxicity. Patients with an absolute neutrophil count <1500 cells/mm^3 should not receive docetaxel. Hepatic dysfunction increases risk of neutropenia and severe infections. Should generally not be given to patients with bilirubin greater than the upper limit of normal or to patients with AST (SGOT) and/or ALT (SGPT) greater than 1.5x the upper limit of normal concomitantly with alkaline phosphatase greater than 2.5x the upper limit of normal. Obtain baseline levels prior to administration.

If docetaxel contacts the skin, wash and flush thoroughly with water.

When administered as sequential infusions, taxane derivatives (docetaxel, paclitaxel) should be administered before platinum derivatives (carboplatin, cisplatin) to limit myelosuppression and to enhance efficacy.

Drug Interactions

Cytochrome P450 Effect: Substrate of **CYP3A4**

Increased Effect/Toxicity: Increased toxicity with cytochrome P450 substrate agents. Possibility of an inhibition of metabolism of docetaxel in patients treated with ketoconazole, erythromycin, astemizole, or cyclosporine. When administered as sequential infusions, observational studies indicate a potential for increased toxicity when platinum derivatives (carboplatin, cisplatin) are administered before taxane derivatives (docetaxel, paclitaxel).

Nutritional/Ethanol Interactions

Ethanol: Avoid ethanol (due to GI irritation).

Herb/Nutraceutical: St John's wort (may docetaxel decrease levels).

Adverse Reactions Note: Frequencies cited for nonsmall cell lung cancer and breast cancer treatment. Exact frequency may vary based on tumor type, prior treatment, premedication, and dosage of docetaxel.

>10%:

Cardiovascular: Fluid retention, including peripheral edema, pleural effusions, and ascites (33% to 47%); may be more common at cumulative doses ≥400 mg/m². Up to 64% in breast cancer patients with dexamethasone premedication.

Dermatologic: Alopecia (56% to 76%); nail disorder (11% to 31%, banding, onycholysis, hypo- or hyperpigmentation)

Gastrointestinal: Mucositis/stomatitis (26% to 42%, severe in 6% to 7%), may be dose-limiting (premedication may reduce frequency and severity); nausea and vomiting (40% to 80%, severe in 1% to 5%); diarrhea (33% to 43%)

Hematologic: Myelosuppression, neutropenia (75% to 85%), thrombocytopenia, anemia
- Onset: 4-7 days
- Nadir: 5-9 days
- Recovery: 21 days

Hepatic: Transaminase levels increased (18%)

Neuromuscular & skeletal: Neurosensory changes (paresthesia, dysesthesia, pain) noted in 23% to 49% (severe in up to 6%). Motor neuropathy (including weakness) noted in as many as 16% of lung cancer patients (severe in up to 5%). Neuropathy may be more common at higher cumulative docetaxel dosages or with prior cisplatin therapy.

Miscellaneous: Hypersensitivity reactions (6% to 13%; angioedema, rash, flushing, fever, hypotension); frequency substantially reduced by premedication with dexamethasone starting one day prior to docetaxel administration.

1% to 10%:

Cardiovascular: Hypotension (3%)

Dermatologic: Rash and skin eruptions (6%)

Gastrointestinal: Taste perversion (6%)

Hepatic: Bilirubin increased (9%)

Neuromuscular & skeletal: Myalgia (6% to 91%), arthralgia (3% to 9%)

Miscellaneous: Infusion site reactions (up to 4%)

<1% (Limited to important or life-threatening): Atrial fibrillation, acute respiratory distress syndrome (ARDS), dehydration, erythema multiforme, gastrointestinal hemorrhage, gastrointestinal obstruction, gastrointestinal perforation, hepatitis, ileus, interstitial pneumonia, ischemic colitis, lacrimal duct obstruction, MI, neutropenic enterocolitis, radiation recall, seizures, Stevens-Johnson syndrome

Pharmacokinetic Note Administered by I.V. infusion and exhibits linear pharmacokinetics at the recommended dosage range.

Pharmacodynamics/Kinetics

Half-Life Elimination: Alpha, beta, gamma: 4 minutes, 36 minutes, and 11.1 hours, respectively

Metabolism: Hepatic; oxidation via CYP3A4 to metabolites

Formulations Injection, solution [concentrate]: 20 mg/0.5 mL (0.5 mL, 2 mL) [diluent contains ethanol 13%]

Dosing

Adults & Elderly: Corticosteroids (oral dexamethasone 8 mg twice daily for 3 days or 5 days starting 1 day prior to docetaxel administration) are necessary to reduce the potential for hypersensitivity and severe fluid retention.

Refer to individual protocols:

Breast cancer (locally advanced or metastatic): I.V.: 60-100 mg/m² over 1 hour every 3 weeks; patients initially started at 60 mg/m² who do not develop toxicity may tolerate higher doses

Nonsmall-cell lung cancer: I.V.: 75 mg/m² over 1 hour every 3 weeks

Dosing adjustment for toxicity: I.V.:

Note: Toxicity includes febrile neutropenia, neutrophils ≤500/mm³ for >1 week, severe or cumulative cutaneous reactions; in nonsmall cell lung cancer, this may also include other grade 3/4 nonhematologic toxicities.

Breast cancer: Patients dosed initially at 100 mg/m²; reduce dose to 75 mg/m²; **Note:** If the patient continues to experience these adverse reactions, the dosage should be reduced to 55 mg/m² or therapy should be discontinued

Nonsmall cell lung cancer: Patients dosed initially at 75 mg/m² should have dose held until toxicity is resolved, then resume at 55 mg/m²; discontinue patients who develop ≥ grade 3 peripheral neuropathy.

Hepatic Impairment: Total bilirubin ≥ the upper limit of normal (ULN), or AST (SGOT)/ALT (SGPT) >1.5 times the ULN concomitant with alkaline phosphatase >2.5 times the ULN: Docetaxel **should not be administered** secondary to increased incidence of treatment-related mortality.

Administration

I.V.: Irritant. Anaphylactoid-like reactions have been reported: Premedication with dexamethasone (8 mg orally twice daily for 3 or 5 days starting 1 prior to administration of docetaxel). Administer I.V. infusion over 1-hour. When administered as sequential infusions, taxane derivatives should be administered before platinum derivatives (cisplatin, carboplatin) to limit myelosuppression and to enhance efficacy.

Stability

Storage: Docetaxel is available in 20 mg and 80 mg vials prepackaged with a special diluent and formulated in polysorbate 80. Docetaxel is diluted with 13% (w/w) ethanol in water giving a final concentration of 10 mg/mL. Docetaxel is slightly more water soluble than paclitaxel. Intact vials should stored at 2°C to 25°C (36°F to 77°F) and protected from light. Initial diluted solution is stable for 8 hours at room temperature or under refrigeration. Vials should be stored at room temperature for approximately 5 minutes before using. Freezing does not adversely affect the product.

Reconstitution: Intact vials of solution should be further diluted with 13% (w/w) ethanol/water to a final concentration of 10 mg/mL. Docetaxel dose should be further diluted with 0.9% sodium chloride or 5% dextrose in water to a final concentration of 0.3-0.9 mg/mL and must be prepared in a glass bottle, polypropylene, or polyolefin plastic bag to prevent leaching of plasticizers. Non-PVC tubing **must** be used. Diluted solutions are stable for up to 4 weeks at room temperature 15°C to 25°C (59°F to 77°F) in polyolefin containers.

(Continued)

Docetaxel *(Continued)*

(Thiesen J and Kramer I, *Pharm World Sci*, 1999, 21(3):137-41.) The manufacturer recommends using within 4 hours.

Compatibility: Stable in D_5W, NS

Y-site administration: Incompatible with amphotericin B, doxorubicin liposome, methylprednisolone sodium succinate, nalbuphine

Monitoring Laboratory Tests CBC with differential and platelet count; liver function especially bilirubin, AST, ALT, and alkaline phosphatase

Monitoring and Teaching Issues

Physical Assessment: See Contraindications, Warnings/Precautions, and Dosing for use cautions. Assess potential for interactions with other prescriptions, OTC medications, or herbal products patient may be taking (see Drug Interactions). **Caution:** Anaphylactoid-like reactions have been reported; premedication with dexamethasone may be advisable (see Dosing and Administration). See Administration, Storage, and Reconstitution. Assess results of laboratory tests (see above), therapeutic response, and adverse reactions (see Adverse Reactions and Overdose/Toxicology, eg, severe fluid retention, pleural effusion, opportunistic infection) on a regular basis. Teach patient possible side effects and interventions and adverse symptoms to report (see Patient Education). **Pregnancy risk factor D** - determine that patient is not pregnant before beginning treatment. Instruct patients of childbearing age on appropriate barrier contraceptive measures. Breast-feeding is contraindicated.

Patient Education: Inform prescriber of all prescriptions, OTC medications, or herbal products you are taking, and any allergies you have. Do not take anything new during treatment unless approved by prescriber. This medication can only be administered I.V. Report immediately any pain, burning, swelling, or redness at infusion site. It is important to maintain adequate hydration (2-3 L/day of fluids) unless advised by prescriber to restrict fluids, and adequate nutrition (small, frequent meals may help). You will be more susceptible to infection (avoid crowds and exposure to infection and do not have any vaccinations without consulting prescriber). Urine may turn red-brown (normal). May cause nausea or vomiting (small, frequent meals, frequent mouth care, sucking lozenges, or chewing gum may help); loss of hair (reversible); or diarrhea (buttermilk, boiled milk, or yogurt may help - if unresolved, contact prescriber for medication relief). Report immediately swelling of extremities, difficulty breathing, unusual weight gain, abdominal distention, chest pain or palpitations, fever, chills, unusual bruising or bleeding, signs of infection, excessive fatigue, or rash. **Pregnancy/breast-feeding precautions:** Inform prescriber if you are pregnant. Do not get pregnant while taking this drug. Consult prescriber for appropriate barrier contraceptives. Do not breast-feed.

Docusate (DOK yoo sate)

U.S. Brand Names Colace® [OTC]; Diocto® [OTC]; Docusoft-S™ [OTC]; DOS® [OTC]; D-S-S® [OTC]; Ex-Lax® Stool Softener [OTC]; Fleet® Sof-Lax® [OTC]; Genasoft® [OTC]; Phillips'® Stool Softener Laxative [OTC]; Surfak® [OTC]

Synonyms Dioctyl Calcium Sulfosuccinate; Dioctyl Sodium Sulfosuccinate; Docusate Calcium; Docusate Potassium; Docusate Sodium; DOSS; DSS

Generic Available Yes

Pharmacologic Category Stool Softener

Pregnancy Risk Factor C

Lactation Excretion in breast milk unknown/compatible

Use Stool softener in patients who should avoid straining during defecation and constipation associated with hard, dry stools; prophylaxis for straining (Valsalva) following myocardial infarction. A safe agent to be used in elderly; some evidence that doses <200 mg are ineffective; stool softeners are unnecessary if stool is well hydrated or "mushy" and soft; shown to be ineffective used long-term.

Use - Unlabeled/Investigational Ceruminolytic

Mechanism of Action/Effect Reduces surface tension of the oil-water interface of the stool resulting in enhanced incorporation of water and fat allowing for stool softening

Contraindications Hypersensitivity to docusate or any component of the formulation; concomitant use of mineral oil; intestinal obstruction, acute abdominal pain, nausea, or vomiting

Warnings/Precautions Prolonged, frequent, or excessive use may result in dependence or electrolyte imbalance. Pregnancy risk C.

Drug Interactions

Decreased Effect: Decreased effect of warfarin with high doses of docusate.

Increased Effect/Toxicity: Increased toxicity with mineral oil, phenolphthalein.

Effects on Lab Values ↓ potassium (S), chloride (S)

Adverse Reactions 1% to 10%:

Gastrointestinal: Intestinal obstruction, diarrhea, abdominal cramping

Miscellaneous: Throat irritation

Overdosage/Toxicology Symptoms of overdose include abdominal cramps, diarrhea, fluid loss, and hypokalemia. Treatment is symptomatic.

Pharmacodynamics/Kinetics

Onset: 12-72 hours

Formulations

Capsule, as calcium (Surfak®): 240 mg

Capsule, as sodium: 100 mg, 250 mg

Colace®: 50 mg, 100 mg

Docusoft-S™, Fleet® Sof-Lax®,Genasoft®, Phillips'® Stool Softener Laxative: 100 mg

DOS®, D-S-S®: 100 mg, 250 mg

Liquid, as sodium: 150 mg/15 mL (480 mL)

Colace®: 150 mg/15 mL (30 mL)

Diocto®: 150 mg/15 mL (480 mL) [vanilla flavor]

Syrup, as sodium: 50 mg/15 mL (30 mL); 60 mg/15 mL (480 mL)

Colace®, Diocto®: 60 mg/15 mL (480 mL) [contains alcohol]
Tablet, as sodium (Ex-Lax® Stool Softener): 100 mg

Dosing

Adults & Elderly: Note: Docusate salts are interchangeable; the amount of sodium, calcium, or potassium per dosage unit is clinically insignificant.

Stool softener:
Oral: 50-500 mg/day in 1-4 divided doses
Rectal: Add 50-100 mg of docusate liquid to enema fluid (saline or water); give as retention or flushing enema

Pediatrics: Note: Docusate salts are interchangeable; the amount of sodium, calcium, or potassium per dosage unit is clinically insignificant.

Stool softener: Oral:
Infants and Children <3 years: 10-40 mg/day in 1-4 divided doses
Children:
3-6 years: 20-60 mg/day in 1-4 divided doses
6-12 years: 40-150 mg/day in 1-4 divided doses
Adolescents: Refer to adult dosing.
Rectal: Older Children: Refer to adult dosing.

Administration

Oral: Docusate liquid should be given with milk, or fruit juice, to mask the bitter taste. Capsules should be administered with a full glass of water, milk, or fruit juice.

Monitoring and Teaching Issues

Physical Assessment: See Contraindications, Warnings/Precautions, and Drug Interactions for use cautions. Monitor for effectiveness and instruct patient in proper use, side effects and interventions, and adverse effects to report. **Pregnancy risk factor C** - benefits of use should outweigh possible risks.

Patient Education: Docusate should be taken with a full glass of water, milk, or fruit juice. Do not use if abdominal pain, nausea, or vomiting are present. Laxative use should be used for a short period of time (<1 week). Prolonged use may result in abuse, dependence, as well as fluid and electrolyte loss. Report bleeding or if constipation occurs. **Pregnancy precaution:** Inform prescriber if you are or intend to become pregnant.

Dietary Issues: Should be taken with a full glass of water, milk, or fruit juice.

Geriatric Considerations: A safe agent to be used in the elderly. Some evidence that doses <200 mg are ineffective.

Related Information

Laxatives: Classification and Properties *on page 1581*

Docusate Calcium *see* Docusate *on page 432*
Docusate/Casanthranol *see page 1581*
Docusate Potassium *see* Docusate *on page 432*
Docusate Sodium *see* Docusate *on page 432*
Docusoft-S™ [OTC] *see* Docusate *on page 432*

Dofetilide (doe FET il ide)

U.S. Brand Names Tikosyn™

Generic Available No

Pharmacologic Category Antiarrhythmic Agent, Class III

Pregnancy Risk Factor C

Lactation Excretion in breast milk unknown/not recommended

Use Maintenance of normal sinus rhythm in patients with chronic atrial fibrillation/atrial flutter of longer than 1-week duration who have been converted to normal sinus rhythm; conversion of atrial fibrillation and atrial flutter to normal sinus rhythm

Mechanism of Action/Effect Blocks cardiac potassium ion channels and increases action potential duration due to delayed repolarization

Contraindications Hypersensitivity to dofetilide or any component of the formulation; patients with paroxysmal atrial fibrillation; patients with congenital or acquired long QT syndromes, do not use if a baseline QT interval or QT_c is >440 msec (500 msec in patients with ventricular conduction abnormalities); severe renal impairment (estimated Cl_{cr} <20 mL/minute); concurrent use with verapamil, cimetidine, trimethoprim (alone or in combination with sulfamethoxazole), ketoconazole, prochlorperazine, or megestrol; baseline heart rate <50 beats/minute; other drugs that prolong QT intervals (phenothiazines, cisapride, bepridil, tricyclic antidepressants, certain oral macrolides: sparfloxacin, gatifloxacin, moxifloxacin); hypokalemia or hypomagnesemia; concurrent amiodarone

Warnings/Precautions Note: Must be initiated (or reinitiated) by a cardiologist in a setting with continuous monitoring and staff familiar with the recognition and treatment of life-threatening arrhythmias. Patients must be monitored with continuous EKG for a minimum of 3 days, or for a minimum of 12 hours after electrical or pharmacological cardioversion to normal sinus rhythm, whichever is greater. Patients should be readmitted for continuous monitoring if dosage is later increased.

Reserve for patients who are highly symptomatic with atrial fibrillation/atrial flutter. Torsade de pointes significantly increases with doses >500 mcg twice daily. Hold class I or class III antiarrhythmics for at least three half-lives prior to starting dofetilide. Use in patients on amiodarone therapy only if serum amiodarone level is <0.3 mg/L or if amiodarone was stopped for >3 months previously. Correct hypokalemia or hypomagnesemia before starting dofetilide and maintained within normal limits during treatment.

Patients with sick sinus syndrome or with second or third degree heart block should not receive dofetilide unless a functional pacemaker is in place. Defibrillation threshold is reduced in patients with ventricular tachycardia or ventricular fibrillation undergoing implantation of a cardioverter-defibrillator device. Safety/efficacy in children (<18 years of age) have not been established. Use with caution in renal impairment; not recommended in patients receiving drugs which may compete for renal secretion via cationic transport. Use with caution in patients with severe hepatic impairment.
(Continued)

Dofetilide *(Continued)*

Pregnancy risk C.

Drug Interactions

Cytochrome P450 Effect: Substrate of CYP3A4

Increased Effect/Toxicity: Dofetilide concentrations are increased by cimetidine, verapamil, ketoconazole, and trimethoprim (concurrent use of these agents is contraindicated). Dofetilide levels may also be increased by renal cationic transport inhibitors (including triamterene, metformin, amiloride, and megestrol) or inhibitors of cytochrome P450 isoenzyme 3A4 (including amiodarone, azole antifungal agents, clarithromycin, cannabinoids, diltiazem, erythromycin, nefazodone, norfloxacin, protease inhibitors, quinidine, serotonin reuptake inhibitors. verapamil, and zafirlukast). Diuretics and other drugs which may deplete potassium and/or magnesium (aminoglycoside antibiotics, amphotericin, cyclosporine) may increase dofetilide's toxicity (torsade de pointes).

Nutritional/Ethanol Interactions Herb/Nutraceutical: St John's wort may decrease dofetilide levels. Avoid ephedra (may worsen arrhythmia).

Adverse Reactions

Supraventricular arrhythmia patients (incidence > placebo)

>10%: Central nervous system: Headache (11%)

2% to 10%:

- Central nervous system: Dizziness (8%), insomnia (4%)
- Cardiovascular: Ventricular tachycardia (2.6% to 3.7%), chest pain (10%), torsade de pointes (3.3% in CHF patients and 0.9% in patients with a recent MI; up to 10.5% in patients receiving doses in excess of those recommended). Torsade de pointes occurs most frequently within the first 3 days of therapy.
- Dermatologic: Rash (3%)
- Gastrointestinal: Nausea (5%), diarrhea (3%), abdominal pain (3%)
- Neuromuscular & skeletal: Back pain (3%)
- Respiratory: Dyspnea (6%), respiratory tract infection (7%)
- Miscellaneous: Flu syndrome (4%)

<2% (Limited to important or life-threatening): Angioedema, AV block (0.4% to 1.5%), bundle branch block, cardiac arrest, facial paralysis, flaccid paralysis, heart block, hepatotoxicity, myocardial infarction, paralysis, paresthesia, stroke, syncope, ventricular fibrillation (0% to 0.4%)

Overdosage/Toxicology The major dose-related toxicity is torsade de pointes. Treatment should be symptomatic and supportive. Watch for excessive prolongation of the QT interval in overdose situations. Continuous cardiac monitoring is necessary. A charcoal slurry is helpful when given early (15 minutes) after the overdose.

Pharmacodynamics/Kinetics

Absorption: >90%

Bioavailability: >90%

Half-Life Elimination: 10 hours

Time to Peak: Fasting: 2-3 hours

Metabolism: Hepatic via CYP3A4, but low affinity for it; metabolites formed by N-dealkylation and N-oxidation

Formulations Capsule: 125 mcg, 250 mcg, 500 mcg

Dosing

Adults: Antiarrhythmic: Oral:

Note: QT_c must be determined prior to first dose (see Contraindications and Warnings/Precautions).

Initial: 500 mcg orally twice daily. Initial dosage must be adjusted in patients with estimated Cl_{cr} <60 mL/minute. Dofetilide may be initiated at lower doses than recommended based on physician discretion.

Modification of dosage in response to initial dose:

QT_c interval should be measured 2-3 hours after the initial dose. If the QT_c >15% of baseline, or if the QT_c is >500 msec (550 msec in patients with ventricular conduction abnormalities), dofetilide should be adjusted. If the starting dose is 500 mcg twice daily, then adjust to 250 mcg twice daily. If the starting dose was 250 mcg twice daily, then adjust to 125 mcg twice daily. If the starting dose was 125 mcg twice daily, then adjust to 125 mcg every day.

Continued monitoring for doses 2-5:

QT_c interval must be determined 2-3 hours after each subsequent dose of dofetilide for in-hospital doses 2-5. If the measured QT_c is >500 msec (550 msec in patients with ventricular conduction abnormalities) dofetilide should be stopped.

Elderly: No specific dosage adjustments are recommended based on age; however, careful assessment of renal function is particularly important in this population.

Renal Impairment:

- Cl_{cr} >60 mL/minute: Administer 500 mcg twice daily.
- Cl_{cr} 40-60 mL/minute: Administer 250 mcg twice daily.
- Cl_{cr} 20-39 mL/minute: Administer 125 mcg twice daily.
- Cl_{cr} <20 mL/minute: Contraindicated in this group

Hepatic Impairment: No dosage adjustments required in Child-Pugh class A and B; patients with severe hepatic impairment were not studied.

Administration

Oral: Do not open capsules.

Monitoring Laboratory Tests EKG monitoring with attention to QT_c and occurrence of ventricular arrhythmias, baseline serum creatinine, and changes in serum creatinine. Check serum potassium and magnesium levels if on medications where these electrolyte disturbances can occur, or if patient has a history of hypokalemia or hypomagnesemia.

Monitoring and Teaching Issues

Physical Assessment: Assess other medications patient may be taking for effectiveness and interactions (see Drug Interactions). See Contraindications and Warnings/Precautions for use cautions. Must be initiated or reinitiated by a cardiologist in a setting with continuous EKG monitoring for a period of time at beginning or adjustment of therapy (see

Warnings/Precautions). Monitor laboratory results (see Monitoring Lab Tests), therapeutic response, and adverse reactions (see Adverse Reactions and Overdose/Toxicology) at beginning of therapy and on a regular basis with long-term therapy. Assess knowledge/ teach patient appropriate use, interventions to reduce side effects, and adverse reactions to report (see Patient Education). **Pregnancy risk factor C** - benefits of use should outweigh possible risks. Breast-feeding is not recommended.

Patient Education: Take exactly as directed; do not take additional doses or discontinue without consulting prescriber. Do not open capsules. If you miss a dose, take your normal amount at the next scheduled time. You will need regular cardiac checkups and blood tests when taking this medication. You may experience headache, dizziness, or difficulty sleeping (use caution when driving or engaging in tasks requiring alertness until response to drug is known); or abdominal pain, diarrhea, or nausea (small, frequent meals and increased dietary bulk may help). Inform prescriber immediately if you experience fainting; severe GI discomfort or diarrhea; chest palpitations, irregular heartbeat, or chest pain; increased thirst; difficulty breathing; skin rash; back pain; or alteration in muscle strength or gait. **Pregnancy/breast-feeding precautions:** Inform your prescriber if you are or intend to become pregnant. Breast-feeding is not recommended.

Pregnancy Issues: Dofetilide has been shown to adversely affect *in utero* growth, organogenesis, and survival of rats and mice. There are no adequate and well controlled studies in pregnant women. Dofetilide should be used with extreme caution in pregnant women and in women of childbearing age only when the benefit to the patient unequivocally justifies the potential risk to the fetus.

Related Information

Antiarrhythmic Drugs *on page 1551*

Dolasetron (dol A se tron)

U.S. Brand Names Anzemet®

Synonyms Dolasetron Mesylate

Generic Available No

Pharmacologic Category Selective 5-HT_3 Receptor Antagonist

Pregnancy Risk Factor B

Lactation Excretion in breast milk unknown

Use Prevention of nausea and vomiting associated with emetogenic cancer chemotherapy, including initial and repeat courses; prevention of postoperative nausea and vomiting and treatment of postoperative nausea and vomiting (injectable form only)

Mechanism of Action/Effect Selective 5-HT_3 receptor antagonist, blocking serotonin, both peripherally on vagal nerve terminals and centrally in the chemoreceptor trigger zone

Contraindications Hypersensitivity to dolasetron or any component of the formulation

Warnings/Precautions Administer with caution in patients who have or may develop prolongation of cardiac conduction intervals, particularly QT_c intervals. These include patients with hypokalemia, hypomagnesemia, patients taking diuretics which may cause electrolyte disturbances, patients with congenital QT syndrome, patients taking antiarrhythmic drugs or drug which prolong QT interval, and cumulative high-dose anthracycline therapy.

Drug Interactions

Cytochrome P450 Effect: Substrate of CYP2C8/9, 3A4; Inhibits CYP2D6

Decreased Effect: Blood levels of active metabolite are decreased during coadministration of rifampin.

Increased Effect/Toxicity: Increased blood levels of active metabolite may occur during concurrent administration of cimetidine and atenolol. Inhibitors of this isoenzyme may increase blood levels of active metabolite. Due to the potential to potentiate QT_c prolongation, drugs which may prolong QT interval directly (eg, antiarrhythmics) or by causing alterations in electrolytes (eg, diuretics) should be used with caution.

Nutritional/Ethanol Interactions Herb/Nutraceutical: St John's wort may decrease dolasetron levels.

Adverse Reactions Dolasetron may cause EKG changes which are directly related to the concentration of hydrodolasetron, its active metabolite. Other adverse effects include:

Cancer patients:
- >10%
  - Central nervous system: Headache (24%)
  - Gastrointestinal: Diarrhea (15%)
- 1% to 10% (occurring >2% and > placebo):
  - Central nervous system: Fever (4.3%), fatigue (3.6%), pain (2.4%), dizziness (2.2%), chills (2.0%)
  - Gastrointestinal: Increased transaminase levels (3.6%), abdominal pain (3.2%)
  - Cardiovascular: Hypertension (2.9%)

Postoperative patients:
- 1% to 10% (occurring >2% and > placebo):
  - Central nervous system: Headache (9.4%), dizziness (5.5%), drowsiness (2.4%), pain (2.4%)
  - Genitourinary: Urinary retention (2.4%)

<1% (Limited to important or life-threatening):
- Patients in clinical trials involving either cancer patients or surgery: Anaphylaxis, arrhythmias, bronchospasm, hypotension

Overdosage/Toxicology Prolongation of QT, AV block, severe hypotension, and dizziness have been reported. Treatment is supportive, and continuous EKG monitoring (telemetry) is recommended.

Pharmacodynamics/Kinetics

Half-Life Elimination: Dolasetron: 10 minutes; MDL 74,156: 8 hours

Metabolism: Hepatic to a reduced alcohol (active metabolite MDL 74,156)

Formulations

Injection, solution, as mesylate: 20 mg/mL (0.625 mL, 5 mL)

Tablet, as mesylate: 50 mg, 100 mg

(Continued)

Dolasetron *(Continued)*

Dosing

Adults & Elderly:

Nausea and vomiting associated with cancer chemotherapy:

Oral: 100 mg within 1 hour before chemotherapy (doses of 200 mg have been used)

I.V.: 1.8 mg/kg ~30 minutes before chemotherapy (maximum 100 mg)

Postoperative nausea and vomiting;

Prevention:

Oral: 100 mg within 2 hours before surgery (doses of 25-200 mg have been used)

I.V.: 12.5 mg ~15 minutes before stopping anesthesia

Treatment: I.V. (only): 12.5 mg as soon as needed

Pediatrics:

Note: Not recommended in children <2 years

Nausea and vomiting associated with chemotherapy, including initial and repeat courses (Children 2-16 years):

Oral: 1.8 mg/kg within 1 hour before chemotherapy; maximum: 100 mg/dose

I.V.: 1.8 mg/kg ~30 minutes before chemotherapy; maximum: 100 mg/dose

Postoperative nausea and vomiting (Children 2-16 years):

Prevention:

Oral: 1.2 mg/kg within 2 hours before surgery; maximum: 100 mg/dose

I.V.: 0.35 mg/kg (maximum: 12.5 mg) ~15 minutes before stopping anesthesia

Treatment: I.V. (only): 0.35 mg/kg as soon as needed

Administration

Oral: May be diluted in apple or apple-grape juice.

I.V.: May be given either undiluted IVP over 30 seconds or diluted to 50 mL and administered as an IVPB over 15 minutes.

Stability

Reconstitution: After dilution, stable at room temperature for 24 hours or under refrigeration for 48 hours.

Compatibility: Stable in 0.9% NS, D_5W, D_5W and 0.45% NS, D_5W and LR, LR, and 10% mannitol injection

Monitoring and Teaching Issues

Physical Assessment: See Contraindications and Warnings/Precautions for use cautions. Assess potential for interactions with other prescriptions, OTC medications, or herbal products patient may be taking (see Drug Interactions). Assess therapeutic effectiveness and adverse reactions (see Adverse Reactions and Overdose/Toxicology, eg, cardiac abnormalities) on a regular basis. Teach patient possible side effects and interventions and adverse symptoms to report (see Patient Education). Note breast-feeding caution.

Patient Education: This drug is given to reduce the incidence of nausea and vomiting. May cause headache, drowsiness, or dizziness (request assistance when getting up or changing position and do not perform activities requiring alertness). Report immediately any chest pain, rapid heartbeat, or palpitations; unusual pain, chills, or fever; severe headache or diarrhea; chest pain, palpitations, or tightness; swelling of throat or feeling of tightness in throat; or difficulty urinating. **Breast-feeding precaution:** Consult prescriber if breast-feeding.

Additional Information Efficacy of dolasetron, for chemotherapy treatment, is enhanced with concomitant administration of dexamethasone 20 mg (increases complete response from 50% to 76%). Oral administration of the intravenous solution is equivalent to tablets. A single I.V. dose of dolasetron mesylate (1.8 or 2.4 mg/kg) has comparable safety and efficacy to a single 32 mg I.V. dose of ondansetron in patients receiving cisplatin chemotherapy.

Related Information

Antiemetics for Chemotherapy-Induced Nausea and Vomiting *on page 1639*

Dolasetron Mesylate *see* Dolasetron *on page 435*

Dolobid® *see* Diflunisal *on page 409*

Dolophine® *see* Methadone *on page 868*

Donepezil (don EH pa zil)

U.S. Brand Names Aricept®

Synonyms E2020

Generic Available No

Pharmacologic Category Acetylcholinesterase Inhibitor (Central)

Pregnancy Risk Factor C

Lactation Excretion in breast milk unknown/not recommended

Use Treatment of mild to moderate dementia of the Alzheimer's type

Use - Unlabeled/Investigational Attention-deficit/hyperactivity disorder (ADHD)

Mechanism of Action/Effect Alzheimer's disease is characterized by cholinergic deficiency in the cortex and basal forebrain, which contributes to cognitive deficits. Donepezil reversibly and noncompetitively inhibits centrally-active acetylcholinesterase, the enzyme responsible for hydrolysis of acetylcholine. This appears to result in increased concentrations of acetylcholine available for synaptic transmission in the central nervous system.

Contraindications Hypersensitivity to donepezil, piperidine derivatives, or any component of the formulation

Warnings/Precautions May cause bradycardia and/or heart block with or without a history of cardiac disease; syncopal episodes have been associated with donepezil. Use with caution in patients with sick sinus syndrome or other supraventricular cardiac conduction abnormalities, in patients with seizures, COPD, or asthma; avoid use in nursing mothers. Use with caution in patients at risk of ulcer disease (ie, previous history or NSAID use), or in patients with bladder outlet obstruction. May cause diarrhea, nausea, and/or vomiting, which may be dose-related. Pregnancy risk C.

Drug Interactions

Cytochrome P450 Effect: Substrate of CYP2D6, 3A4

Decreased Effect: Donepezil levels may be decreased by enzyme inducers (phenytoin, carbamazepine, dexamethasone, rifampin, and phenobarbital). Anticholinergic agents (benztropine) may inhibit the effects of donepezil.

Increased Effect/Toxicity: Ketoconazole and quinidine inhibit donepezil's metabolism *in vitro* and may increase toxicity. A synergistic effect may be seen with concurrent administration of succinylcholine or cholinergic agonists (bethanechol).

Nutritional/Ethanol Interactions Herb/Nutraceutical: St John's wort may decrease donepezil levels.

Adverse Reactions

>10%:

Central nervous system: Headache

Gastrointestinal: Nausea, diarrhea

1% to 10%:

Cardiovascular: Syncope, chest pain, hypertension, atrial fibrillation, hypotension, hot flashes

Central nervous system: Fatigue, insomnia, dizziness, depression, abnormal dreams, somnolence

Dermatologic: Bruising

Gastrointestinal: Anorexia, vomiting, weight loss, fecal incontinence, GI bleeding, bloating, epigastric pain

Genitourinary: Frequent urination

Neuromuscular & skeletal: Muscle cramps, arthritis, body pain

<1% (Limited to significant or life-threatening): Cholecystitis, CHF, delusions, dysarthria, dysphasia, dyspnea, eosinophilia, hallucinations, heart block, hemolytic anemia, hyponatremia, intracranial hemorrhage, neuroleptic malignant syndrome, pancreatitis, paresthesia, rash, seizures, thrombocytopenia

Overdosage/Toxicology Implement general supportive measures. Donepezil can cause a cholinergic crisis characterized by severe nausea, vomiting, salivation, sweating, bradycardia, hypotension, collapse, and convulsions. Increased muscle weakness is a possibility and may result in death if respiratory muscles are involved.

Tertiary anticholinergics, such as atropine, may be used as an antidote for overdose. I.V. atropine sulfate titrated to effect is recommended with an initial dose of 1-2 mg I.V., with subsequent doses based upon clinical response. Atypical increases in blood pressure and heart rate have been reported with other cholinomimetics when coadministered with quaternary anticholinergics such as glycopyrrolate.

Pharmacodynamics/Kinetics

Absorption: Well absorbed

Bioavailability: 100%

Half-Life Elimination: 70 hours; time to steady-state: 15 days

Time to Peak: Plasma: 3-4 hours

Metabolism: Extensively to four major metabolites (two are active) via CYP2D6 and 3A4; undergoes glucuronidation

Formulations Tablet: 5 mg, 10 mg

Dosing

Adults & Elderly: Alzheimer's disease: Oral: Initial: 5 mg/day at bedtime; may increase to 10 mg/day at bedtime after 4-6 weeks.

Pediatrics: ADHD (unlabeled use): Oral: 5 mg/day

Monitoring and Teaching Issues

Physical Assessment: Assess bladder adequacy prior to administering medication. Assess other medications patient may be taking for effectiveness and interactions (see Drug Interactions). Monitor laboratory tests, therapeutic effect, and adverse reactions (eg, cholinergic crisis - see Warnings/Precautions, Adverse Reactions, and Overdose/Toxicology). Assess knowledge/teach patient appropriate use, interventions to reduce side effects, and adverse symptoms to report (see Patient Education). **Pregnancy risk factor C** - benefits of use should outweigh possible risks. Breast-feeding is not recommended.

Patient Education: This medication will not cure the disease, but may help reduce symptoms. Use as directed; do not increase dose or discontinue without consulting prescriber. Maintain adequate hydration (2-3 L/day of fluids) unless advised by prescriber to restrict fluids. May cause dizziness, sedation, or hypotension (rise slowly from sitting or lying position and use caution when driving or climbing stairs); vomiting or loss of appetite (small, frequent meals, frequent mouth care, chewing gum, or sucking lozenges may help); or diarrhea (boiled milk, yogurt, or buttermilk may help). Report persistent abdominal discomfort; significantly increased salivation, sweating, tearing, or urination; flushed skin; chest pain or palpitations; acute headache; unresolved diarrhea; excessive fatigue, insomnia, dizziness, or depression; increased muscle, joint, or body pain; vision changes or blurred vision; or shortness of breath or wheezing. **Pregnancy/breast-feeding precautions:** Inform prescriber if you are or intend to become pregnant. Breast-feeding is not recommended.

Geriatric Considerations: Donepezil is a new anticholinesterase for the treatment of Alzheimer's disease. It has been shown to cause an improvement in the ADAS-cog scores. As compared to tacrine, donepezil does **not** cause elevations in liver function tests and does not require routine laboratory monitoring. In addition, it is dosed once a day versus tacrine's four doses per day. For these reasons, donepezil may be preferred over tacrine in the treatment of mild to moderate dementia of the Alzheimer's type.

Additional Information Donepezil does not significantly elevate liver enzymes.

Donnatal® [DSC] *see* Hyoscyamine, Atropine, Scopolamine, and Phenobarbital *on page 687*

DOPamine (DOE pa meen)

Synonyms Dopamine Hydrochloride

Generic Available Yes

(Continued)

DOPamine *(Continued)*

Pharmacologic Category Adrenergic Agonist Agent

Pregnancy Risk Factor C

Lactation Excretion in breast milk unknown

Use Adjunct in the treatment of shock (eg, MI, open heart surgery, renal failure, cardiac decompensation, etc) which persists after adequate fluid volume replacement

Use - Unlabeled/Investigational Symptomatic bradycardia or heart block unresponsive to atropine or pacing

Mechanism of Action/Effect Stimulates both adrenergic and dopaminergic receptors, lower doses are mainly dopaminergic stimulating and produce renal and mesenteric vasodilation, higher doses also are both dopaminergic and $beta_1$-adrenergic stimulating and produce cardiac stimulation and renal vasodilation; large doses stimulate alpha-adrenergic receptors

Contraindications Hypersensitivity to sulfites (commercial preparation contains sodium bisulfite); pheochromocytoma; ventricular fibrillation

Warnings/Precautions Use with caution in patients with cardiovascular disease or cardiac arrhythmias or patients with occlusive vascular disease. Correct hypovolemia and electrolytes when used in hemodynamic support. May cause increases in HR and arrhythmia. Avoid infiltration - may cause severe tissue necrosis. Use with caution in post-MI patients. Avoid sudden discontinuation. Pregnancy risk C.

Drug Interactions

Decreased Effect: Tricyclic antidepressants may have a decreased effect when coadministered with dopamine. Guanethidine's hypotensive effects may only be partially reversed; may need to use a direct-acting sympathomimetic.

Increased Effect/Toxicity: Dopamine's effects are prolonged and intensified by MAO inhibitors, alpha- and beta-adrenergic blockers, cocaine, general anesthetics, methyldopa, phenytoin, reserpine, and TCAs.

Adverse Reactions Frequency not defined.

Most frequent:

- Cardiovascular: Ectopic beats, tachycardia, anginal pain, palpitations, hypotension, vasoconstriction
- Central nervous system: Headache
- Gastrointestinal: Nausea and vomiting
- Respiratory: Dyspnea

Infrequent:

- Cardiovascular: Aberrant conduction, bradycardia, widened QRS complex, ventricular arrhythmias (high dose), gangrene (high dose), hypertension
- Central nervous system: Anxiety
- Endocrine & metabolic: Piloerection, serum glucose increased (usually not above normal limits)
- Local: Extravasation of dopamine can cause tissue necrosis and sloughing of surrounding tissues
- Ocular: Intraocular pressure increased, dilated pupils
- Renal: Azotemia, polyuria

Overdosage/Toxicology Symptoms of overdose include severe hypertension, cardiac arrhythmias, acute renal failure. Treat symptomatically.

Important: Antidote for peripheral ischemia: To prevent sloughing and necrosis in ischemic areas, the area should be infiltrated as soon as possible with 10-15 mL of saline solution containing 5-10 mg of Regitine® (brand of phentolamine), an adrenergic blocking agent. A syringe with a fine hypodermic needle should be used, and the solution liberally infiltrated throughout the ischemic area. Sympathetic blockade with phentolamine causes immediate and conspicuous local hyperemic changes if the area is infiltrated within 12 hours. Therefore, phentolamine should be given as soon as possible after extravasation is noted.

Pharmacokinetic Note Dopamine has exhibited nonlinear kinetics in children; with medication changes, may not achieve steady-state for ~1 hour rather than 20 minutes.

Pharmacodynamics/Kinetics

Half-Life Elimination: 2 minutes

Metabolism: Renal, hepatic, plasma; 75% to inactive metabolites by monoamine oxidase and 25% to norepinephrine

Onset: Adults: 5 minutes

Duration: Adults: <10 minutes

Formulations

Infusion, as hydrochloride [premixed in D_5W]: 0.8 mg/mL (250 mL, 500 mL); 1.6 mg/mL (250 mL, 500 mL); 3.2 mg/mL (250 mL)

Injection, solution, as hydrochloride: 40 mg/mL (5 mL, 10 mL); 80 mg/mL (5 mL); 160 mg/mL (5 mL)

Dosing

Adults: Hemodynamic support: I.V. infusion:

1-5 mcg/kg/minute up to 50 mcg/kg/minute, titrate to desired response; infusion may be increased by 1-4 mcg/kg/minute at 10- to 30-minute intervals until optimal response is obtained

If dosages >20-30 mcg/kg/minute are needed, a more direct-acting vasopressor may be more beneficial (ie, epinephrine, norepinephrine).

Hemodynamic effects of dopamine are dose dependent:

- Low-dose: 1-5 mcg/kg/minute, increased renal blood flow and urine output
- Intermediate-dose: 5-15 mcg/kg/minute, increased renal blood flow, heart rate, cardiac contractility, and cardiac output
- High-dose: >15 mcg/kg/minute, alpha-adrenergic effects begin to predominate, vasoconstriction, increased blood pressure

Elderly: Refer to adult dosing. Monitor closely, especially due to increase in cardiovascular disease with age.

Pediatrics: Hemodynamic support: I.V. infusion:

Children: 1-20 mcg/kg/minute, maximum: 50 mcg/kg/minute continuous infusion, titrate to desired response.

Administration

I.V.: Vesicant. **Must be diluted prior to use**. Do not discontinue suddenly - sudden discontinuation may lead to marked hypotension.

Stability

Storage: Protect from light. Solutions that are darker than slightly yellow should not be used.

Compatibility: Stable in D_5LR, $D_5{}^1/_2NS$, D_5NS, D_5W, $D_{10}W$, LR, mannitol 20%, NS; **incompatible** with sodium bicarbonate 5%, and alkaline solutions or iron salts.

Y-site administration: Incompatible with acyclovir, alteplase, amphotericin B cholesteryl sulfate complex, cefepime, indomethacin, insulin (regular), thiopental

Compatibility when admixed: Incompatible with acyclovir, alteplase, amphotericin B, ampicillin, metronidazole with sodium bicarbonate, penicillin G potassium

Monitoring Laboratory Tests Continuous hemodynamic monitoring; serum glucose, renal function

Monitoring and Teaching Issues

Physical Assessment: Assess other medications patient may be taking for effectiveness and interactions (see Drug Interactions). See Warnings/Precautions and Contraindications for use cautions. Infusion pump, continuous cardiac and hemodynamic monitoring, and frequent assessment of I.V. site is required for inpatient therapy (see Administration for extravasation antidote instructions). Low-dose home infusion therapy requires frequent monitoring of cardiac and renal status and adverse reactions. Monitor therapeutic response and adverse reactions (see Warnings/Precautions, Adverse Reactions, Administration, and Patient Education). Instruct patient on adverse symptoms to report. Note breast-feeding caution.

Patient Education: When administered in emergencies, patient education should be appropriate to the situation. If patient is aware, instruct to promptly report chest pain, palpitations, rapid heartbeat, headache, nervousness or restlessness, nausea or vomiting, or difficulty breathing.

Geriatric Considerations: Has not been specifically studied in the elderly.

Additional Information Dopamine is most frequently used for treatment of hypotension because of its peripheral vasoconstrictor action. In this regard, dopamine is often used together with dobutamine and minimizes hypotension secondary to dobutamine-induced vasodilation. Thus, pressure is maintained by increased cardiac output (from dobutamine) and vasoconstriction (by dopamine). It is critical neither dopamine nor dobutamine be used in patients in the absence of correcting any hypovolemia as a cause of hypotension.

Low-dose dopamine is often used in the intensive care setting for presumed beneficial effects on renal function. However, there is no clear evidence that low-dose dopamine confers any renal or other benefit. Indeed, dopamine may act on dopamine receptors in the carotid bodies causing chemoreflex suppression. In patients with heart failure, dopamine may inhibit breathing and cause pulmonary shunting. Both these mechanisms would act to decrease minute ventilation and oxygen saturation. This could potentially be deleterious in patients with respiratory compromise and patients being weaned from ventilators.

Related Information

Compatibility of Drugs *on page 1564*
FDA Name Differentiation Project: The Use of Tall-man Letters *on page 12*
Inotropic and Vasoconstrictor Comparison *on page 1580*

Dopamine Hydrochloride *see* DOPamine *on page 437*

Dornase Alfa (DOOR nase AL fa)

U.S. Brand Names Pulmozyme®

Synonyms DNase; Recombinant Human Deoxyribonuclease

Generic Available No

Pharmacologic Category Enzyme

Pregnancy Risk Factor B

Lactation Excretion in breast milk unknown

Use Management of cystic fibrosis patients to reduce the frequency of respiratory infections that require parenteral antibiotics, and to improve pulmonary function

Use - Unlabeled/Investigational Treatment of chronic bronchitis

Mechanism of Action/Effect The hallmark of cystic fibrosis lung disease is the presence of abundant, purulent airway secretions composed primarily of highly polymerized DNA. Dornase selectively cleaves DNA, thus reducing mucous viscosity and as a result, airflow in the lung is improved and the risk of bacterial infection may be decreased.

Contraindications Hypersensitivity to dornase alfa, Chinese hamster ovary cell products (eg, epoetin alfa), or any component of the formulation

Warnings/Precautions No clinical trials have been conducted to demonstrate safety and effectiveness of dornase in children <5 years of age, in patients with pulmonary function <40% of normal, or in patients for longer treatment periods >12 months.

Adverse Reactions

>10%:

Cardiovascular: Chest pain
Respiratory: Pharyngitis
Miscellaneous: Voice alteration

1% to 10%:

Dermatologic: Rash
Ocular: Conjunctivitis
Respiratory: Laryngitis, cough, dyspnea, hemoptysis, rhinitis, hoarse throat, wheezing

Pharmacodynamics/Kinetics

Onset: Nebulization: Enzyme levels are measured in sputum in ~15 minutes

Duration: Rapidly declines

Formulations Solution for nebulization: 1 mg/mL (2.5 mL)

(Continued)

Dornase Alfa *(Continued)*

Dosing

Adults & Elderly: Mucolytic: Inhalation: 2.5 mg once daily through selected nebulizers

Pediatrics: Mucolytic (CF): Inhalation:

Children >3 months to Adults: 2.5 mg once daily through selected nebulizers; experience in children <5 years is limited

Patients unable to inhale or exhale orally throughout the entire treatment period may use Pari-Baby™ nebulizer. Some patients may benefit from twice daily administration.

Stability

Storage: Must be stored in the refrigerator at 2°C to 8°C (36°F to 46°F) and protected from strong light. Should not be exposed to room temperature for a total of 24 hours.

Compatibility: Should not be diluted or mixed with any other drugs in the nebulizer, this may inactivate the dornase alfa.

Monitoring and Teaching Issues

Physical Assessment: See Contraindications and Warnings/Precautions for use cautions. Assess effectiveness of therapy and adverse reactions (see Adverse Reactions) at beginning of therapy and periodically with long-term use. Teach patient or caregiver appropriate use of nebulizer, interventions to reduce side effects, and adverse symptoms to report (see Patient Education). Note breast-feeding caution.

Patient Education: Use exactly as directed by prescriber (see following administration information). Report any signs of adverse response, skin rash, sore throat, respiratory wheezing, cough, or difficulty breathing. **Breast-feeding precaution:** Consult prescriber if breast-feeding.

Self-administered nebulizer: Store in refrigerator, away from light. Do not combine with any other medications in the nebulizer. Wash hands before and after treatment. Wash and dry nebulizer after each treatment. Twist open the top of one unit dose vial and squeeze contents into nebulizer reservoir. Connect nebulizer reservoir to the mouthpiece or face mask. Connect nebulizer to compressor. Sit in comfortable, upright position. Put on face mask and turn on compressor. Avoid leakage around the mask to avoid mist getting into eyes. Breathe calmly and deeply until no more mist is formed in nebulizer (about 5 minutes). At this point treatment is finished.

Doryx® *see* Doxycycline *on page 450*

Dorzolamide *see page 1575*

Dorzolamide *see* Ophthalmic Agents, Glaucoma *on page 1002*

DOS® [OTC] *see* Docusate *on page 432*

DOSS *see* Docusate *on page 432*

Dovonex® *see* Calcipotriene *on page 199*

Doxacurium (doks a KYOO ri um)

U.S. Brand Names Nuromax®

Synonyms Doxacurium Chloride

Generic Available No

Pharmacologic Category Neuromuscular Blocker Agent, Nondepolarizing

Pregnancy Risk Factor C

Use Adjunct to general anesthesia to facilitate endotracheal intubation and to relax skeletal muscles during surgery; to facilitate mechanical ventilation in ICU patients; does not relieve pain or produce sedation; the characteristics of this agent make it especially useful in procedures requiring careful maintenance of hemodynamic stability for prolonged periods

Mechanism of Action/Effect Prevents depolarization of muscle membrane and subsequent muscle contraction by acting as a competitive antagonist to acetylcholine at the alpha subunits of the nicotinic cholinergic receptors on the motor endplates in skeletal muscle, also interferes with the mobilization of acetylcholine presynaptically; the neuromuscular blockade can be pharmacologically reversed with an anticholinesterase agent (neostigmine, edrophonium, pyridostigmine)

Contraindications Hypersensitivity to doxacurium or any component of the formulation

Warnings/Precautions Use with caution in the elderly, effects and duration are more variable; product contains benzyl alcohol, use with caution in newborns; use with caution in patients with renal or hepatic impairment; certain clinical conditions may result in potentiation or antagonism of neuromuscular blockade

Increased sensitivity in patients with myasthenia gravis, Eaton-Lambert syndrome; resistance in burn patients (>30% of body) for period of 5-70 days postinjury; resistance in patients with muscle trauma, denervation, immobilization, infection; does not counteract bradycardia produced by anesthetics/vagal stimulation.

Pregnancy risk C.

Drug Interactions

Decreased Effect: Effect of nondepolarizing neuromuscular blockers may be reduced by carbamazepine (chronic use), corticosteroids (also associated with myopathy - see increased effect), phenytoin (chronic use), sympathomimetics, and theophylline.

Increased Effect/Toxicity: Increased effects are possible with aminoglycosides, beta-blockers, clindamycin, calcium channel blockers, halogenated anesthetics, imipenem, ketamine, lidocaine, loop diuretics (furosemide), macrolides (case reports), magnesium sulfate, procainamide, quinidine, quinolones, tetracyclines, and vancomycin. May increase risk of myopathy when used with high- dose corticosteroids for extended periods.

Adverse Reactions <1% (Limited to important or life-threatening): Diplopia, fever, hypotension, **produces little, if any, histamine release**, respiratory insufficiency and apnea, skeletal muscle weakness, urticaria, wheezing

In the ICU setting, reports of prolonged paralysis and generalized myopathy following discontinuation of agent (may be minimized by appropriately monitoring degree of blockade)

Overdosage/Toxicology

Overdosage is manifested by prolonged neuromuscular blockage.

Treatment is supportive; reverse blockade with neostigmine, pyridostigmine, or edrophonium.

Pharmacodynamics/Kinetics

Onset: 5-11 minutes

Duration: 30 minutes (range: 12-54 minutes)

Formulations Injection, solution, as chloride: 1 mg/mL (5 mL)

Dosing

Adults & Elderly: Administer I.V.; dose to effect; doses will vary due to interpatient variability; use ideal body weight for obese patients.

Surgery: I.V.: 0.05-0.08 mg/kg with thiopental/narcotic or 0.025 mg/kg after initial dose of succinylcholine for intubation; initial maintenance dose of 0.005-0.01 mg/kg after 100-160 minutes followed by repeat doses every 30-45 minutes

Pretreatment/priming: I.V.: 10% of intubating dose given 3-5 minutes before initial dose

ICU: I.V.: 0.05 mg/kg bolus followed by 0.025 mg/kg every 2-3 hours or 0.25-0.75 mcg/kg/minute once initial recovery from bolus dose observed

Pediatrics: Administer I.V.; dose to effect; doses will vary due to interpatient variability; use ideal body weight for obese patients

Surgery (Children >2 years): I.V.: Initial: 0.03-0.05 mg/kg followed by maintenance doses of 0.005-0.01 mg/kg after 30-45 minutes

Renal Impairment: Reduce initial dose and titrate carefully as duration may be prolonged.

Administration

I.V.: May be given rapid I.V. injection undiluted or via a continuous infusion using an infusion pump. Use infusion solutions within 24 hours of preparation.

Stability

Storage: Stable for 24 hours at room temperature when diluted, up to 0.1 mg/mL in dextrose 5% or normal saline.

Compatibility: Stable in D_5LR, D_5NS, D_5W, LR, NS

Monitoring Laboratory Tests Blockade is monitored with a peripheral nerve stimulator.

Monitoring and Teaching Issues

Physical Assessment: Only clinicians experienced in the use of neuromuscular blocking drugs should administer and/or manage the use of doxacurium. Dosage and rate of administration should be individualized and titrated to the desired effect, according to relevant clinical factors, premedication, concomitant medications, age, and general condition of the patient. See Use, Contraindications, and Warnings/Precautions for appropriate use cautions. Ventilatory support must be instituted and maintained until adequate respiratory muscle function and/or airway protection are assured. Assess other medications for effectiveness and safety. Other drugs that affect neuromuscular activity may increase/decrease neuromuscular block induced by doxacurium. This drug does not cause anesthesia or analgesia; pain must be treated with appropriate analgesic agents. Continuous monitoring of vital signs, cardiac status, respiratory status, and degree of neuromuscular block (objective assessment with peripheral external nerve stimulator) is mandatory during infusion and until full muscle tone has returned (see Adverse Reactions). Muscle tone returns in a predictable pattern, starting with diaphragm, abdomen, chest, limbs, and finally muscles of the neck, face, and eyes. Safety precautions must be maintained until full muscle tone has returned. **Note:** It may take longer for return of muscle tone in obese or elderly patients or patients with renal or hepatic disease, myasthenia gravis, myopathy, other neuromuscular disease, dehydration, electrolyte imbalance, or severe acid/base imbalance. Provide appropriate patient teaching/support prior to and following administration.

Long-term use: Monitor fluid levels (intake and output) during and following infusion. Reposition patient and provide appropriate skin care, mouth care, and care of patient's eyes every 2-3 hours while sedated. Provide appropriate emotional and sensory support (auditory and environmental).

Pregnancy risk factor C.

Patient Education: Patient will usually be unconscious prior to administration. Patient education should be appropriate to individual situation. Reassurance of constant monitoring and emotional support to reduce fear and anxiety should precede and follow administration. Following return of muscle tone, do not attempt to change position or rise from bed without assistance. Report immediately any skin rash or hives, pounding heartbeat, difficulty breathing, or muscle tremors. **Pregnancy precaution:** Inform prescriber if you are pregnant.

Additional Information Doxacurium is a long-acting nondepolarizing neuromuscular blocker with virtually no cardiovascular side effects. Characteristics of this agent make it especially useful in procedures requiring careful maintenance of hemodynamic stability for prolonged periods; reduce dosage in renal or hepatic impairment. It does not relieve pain or produce sedation. It does not appear to have a cumulative effect on duration of blockade.

Doxacurium Chloride *see* Doxacurium *on page 440*

Doxazosin (doks AYE zoe sin)

U.S. Brand Names Cardura®

Generic Available Yes

Pharmacologic Category Alpha$_1$ Blocker

Pregnancy Risk Factor C

Lactation Excretion in breast milk unknown

Use Treatment of hypertension alone or in conjunction with diuretics, cardiac glycosides, ACE inhibitors, or calcium antagonists (particularly appropriate for those with hypertension and other cardiovascular risk factors such as hypercholesterolemia and diabetes mellitus); treatment of urinary outflow obstruction and/or obstructive and irritative symptoms associated with benign prostatic hyperplasia (BPH), particularly useful in patients with troublesome symptoms who are unable or unwilling to undergo invasive procedures, but who require rapid symptomatic relief

(Continued)

Doxazosin *(Continued)*

Mechanism of Action/Effect Competitively inhibits postsynaptic alpha-adrenergic receptors which results in vasodilation of veins and arterioles and a decrease in total peripheral resistance and blood pressure; approximately 50% as potent on a weight by weight basis as prazosin

Contraindications Hypersensitivity to quinazolines (prazosin, terazosin), doxazosin, or any component of the formulation

Warnings/Precautions Can cause significant orthostatic hypotension and syncope, especially with first dose. Prostate cancer should be ruled out before starting for BPH. May need dosage adjustment in severe hepatic dysfunction. Anticipate a similar effect if therapy is interrupted for a few days, if dosage is rapidly increased, or if another antihypertensive drug is introduced. Pregnancy risk C.

Drug Interactions

Decreased Effect: Decreased hypotensive effect with NSAIDs.

Increased Effect/Toxicity: Increased hypotensive effect with beta-blockers, diuretics, ACE inhibitors, calcium channel blockers, and other antihypertensive medications.

Nutritional/Ethanol Interactions Herb/Nutraceutical: Avoid dong quai if using for hypertension (has estrogenic activity). Avoid ephedra, yohimbe, ginseng (may worsen hypertension). Avoid saw palmetto when used for BPH (due to limited experience with this combination). Avoid garlic (may have increased antihypertensive effect).

Effects on Lab Values Increased urinary VMA 17%, norepinephrine metabolite 42%

Adverse Reactions

>10%: Central nervous system: Dizziness (16% to 19%), headache (10% to 14%)

1% to 10%:

Cardiovascular: Orthostatic hypotension (dose-related; 0.3% up to 10%), edema (3% to 4%), hypotension (2%), palpitation (1% to 2%), chest pain (1% to 2%), arrhythmia (1%), syncope (2%), flushing (1%)

Central nervous system: Fatigue (8% to 12%), somnolence (3% to 5%), nervousness (2%), pain (2%), vertigo (2%), insomnia (1%), anxiety (1%), paresthesia (1%), movement disorder (1%), ataxia (1%), hypertonia (1%), depression (1%), weakness (1%)

Dermatologic: Rash (1%), pruritus (1%)

Endocrine & metabolic: Sexual dysfunction (2%)

Gastrointestinal: Abdominal pain (2%), diarrhea (2%), dyspepsia (1% to 2%), nausea (2% to 3%), xerostomia (1% to 2%), constipation (1%), flatulence (1%)

Genitourinary: Urinary tract infection (1%), impotence (1%), polyuria (2%), incontinence (1%)

Neuromuscular & skeletal: Back pain (2%), arthritis (1%), muscle weakness (1%), myalgia (1%), muscle cramps (1%)

Ocular: Abnormal vision (1% to 2%), conjunctivitis (1%)

Otic: Tinnitus (1%)

Respiratory: Rhinitis (3%), dyspnea (1% to 3%), respiratory disorder (1%), epistaxis (1%)

Miscellaneous: Flu-like syndrome (1%), increased diaphoresis (1%)

<1% (Limited to important or life-threatening): Agitation, alopecia, amnesia, angina, bronchospasm, cataplexy, depersonalization, eczema, emotional lability, enuresis, fecal incontinence, fever, gout, hot flashes, impaired concentration, infection, leukopenia, myocardial infarction, paranoia, paresis, peripheral ischemia, photophobia, purpura, renal calculus, rigors, stroke, syncope, systemic lupus erythematosus, urticaria

Overdosage/Toxicology Symptoms of overdose include severe hypotension, drowsiness, and tachycardia. Treatment is supportive and symptomatic.

Pharmacokinetic Note Not significantly affected by increased age.

Pharmacodynamics/Kinetics

Half-Life Elimination: 22 hours

Time to Peak: Serum: 2-3 hours

Metabolism: Extensively hepatic

Duration: >24 hours

Formulations Tablet: 1 mg, 2 mg, 4 mg, 8 mg

Dosing

Adults: Hypertension or urinary outflow obstruction: Oral: 1 mg once daily in morning or evening; may be increased to 2 mg once daily; thereafter titrate upwards, if needed, over several weeks, balancing therapeutic benefit with doxazosin-induced postural hypotension; maximum dose for **hypertension**: 16 mg/day, for **BPH**: 8 mg/day.

Elderly: Oral: Initial: 0.5 mg once daily

Administration

Oral: Syncope may occur usually within 90 minutes of the initial dose.

Monitoring Laboratory Tests White blood count

Monitoring and Teaching Issues

Physical Assessment: See Contraindications and Warnings/Precautions for use cautions. Assess potential for interactions with other prescriptions, OTC medications, or herbal products patient may be taking (see Drug Interactions). Assess results of laboratory tests (see above), therapeutic effectiveness, and adverse reactions (see Adverse Reactions and Overdose/Toxicology) at beginning of therapy and on a regular basis with long-term therapy. When discontinuing, monitor blood pressure and taper dose slowly over 1 week or more. Teach patient proper use, possible side effects and interventions, and adverse symptoms to report (see Patient Education). **Pregnancy risk factor C** - benefits of use should outweigh possible risks. Note breast-feeding caution.

Patient Education: Inform prescriber of all prescriptions, OTC medications, or herbal products you are taking, and any allergies you have. Do not take anything new during treatment unless approved by prescriber. Take as directed, at bedtime. Do not skip dose or discontinue without consulting prescriber. Follow recommended diet and exercise program. May cause drowsiness, dizziness, or impaired judgment (use caution when driving or engaging in tasks that require alertness until response to drug is known); postural hypotension (use caution when rising from sitting or lying position or when climbing stairs); or dry mouth or nausea (frequent mouth care or sucking lozenges may help). Report increased nervousness or depression; sudden weight gain (weigh yourself in the same clothes at the same time of day once a week); unusual or persistent swelling of ankles, feet, or extremities; palpitations or rapid heartbeat; muscle weakness, fatigue, or pain; or other persistent side effects. **Pregnancy/breast-feeding precautions:** Inform prescriber if you are or intend to become pregnant. Consult prescriber if breast-feeding.

Geriatric Considerations: Adverse reactions such as dry mouth and urinary problems can be particularly bothersome in the elderly.

Additional Information First-dose hypotension occurs less frequently with doxazosin as compared to prazosin; this may be due to its slower onset of action.

Related Information

Pharmacotherapy of Urinary Incontinence *on page 1699*

Doxepin (DOKS e pin)

U.S. Brand Names Prudoxin™; Sinequan®; Zonalon®

Synonyms Doxepin Hydrochloride

Generic Available Yes: Capsule, solution

Pharmacologic Category Antidepressant, Tricyclic (Tertiary Amine); Topical Skin Product

Pregnancy Risk Factor C

Lactation Enters breast milk/not recommended (AAP rates "of concern")

Use

Oral: Depression

Topical: Short-term (<8 days) management of moderate pruritus in adults with atopic dermatitis or lichen simplex chronicus

Use - Unlabeled/Investigational Analgesic for certain chronic and neuropathic pain; anxiety

Mechanism of Action/Effect Increases the synaptic concentration of serotonin and norepinephrine in the central nervous system by inhibition of their reuptake by the presynaptic neuronal membrane

Contraindications Hypersensitivity to doxepin, drugs from similar chemical class, or any component of the formulation; narrow-angle glaucoma; urinary retention; use of MAO inhibitors within 14 days; use in a patient during acute recovery phase of MI

Warnings/Precautions May cause drowsiness/sedation, resulting in impaired performance of tasks requiring alertness (ie, operating machinery or driving). Sedative effects may be additive with other CNS depressants and/or ethanol. May worsen psychosis in some patients or precipitate a shift to mania or hypomania in patients with bipolar disease. May cause hyponatremia/SIADH. May increase the risks associated with electroconvulsive therapy. Discontinue, when possible, prior to elective surgery. Therapy should not be abruptly discontinued in patients receiving high doses for prolonged periods.

Use with caution in patients at risk of hypotension (orthostasis) or in patients where transient hypotensive episodes would be poorly tolerated (cardiovascular disease or cerebrovascular disease). Use with caution in elderly patients, patients with diabetes, thyroid disease (or patients receiving thyroid supplements), hepatic dysfunction, renal dysfunction, urinary retention, benign prostatic hyperplasia, narrow-angle glaucoma, xerostomia, visual problems, constipation, or a history of bowel obstruction.

Use caution in patients with depression, particularly if suicidal risk may be present. Use with caution in patients with a history of cardiovascular disease (including previous MI, stroke, tachycardia, or conduction abnormalities). Use caution in patients with a previous seizure disorder or condition predisposing to seizures such as brain damage, alcoholism, or concurrent therapy with other drugs which lower the seizure threshold. Not for use in patients <12 years of age.

Pregnancy risk C.

Drug Interactions

Cytochrome P450 Effect: Substrate of **CYP1A2, 2D6, 3A4**

Decreased Effect: Carbamazepine, phenobarbital, and rifampin may increase the metabolism of doxepin resulting in decreased effect of doxepin. Doxepin inhibits the antihypertensive response to bethanidine, clonidine, debrisoquin, guanadrel, guanethidine, guanabenz, and guanfacine. Cholestyramine and colestipol may bind TCAs and reduce their absorption.

Increased Effect/Toxicity: Doxepin increases the effects of amphetamines, anticholinergics, other CNS depressants (sedatives, hypnotics, or ethanol), chlorpropamide, tolazamide, and warfarin. When used with MAO inhibitors, hyperpyrexia, hypertension, tachycardia, confusion, seizures, and **deaths have been reported** (serotonin syndrome). Serotonin syndrome has also been reported with ritonavir (rare). The SSRIs (to varying degrees), cimetidine, grapefruit juice, indinavir, methylphenidate, ritonavir, quinidine, diltiazem, and verapamil inhibit the metabolism of TCAs and clinical toxicity may result. Use of lithium with a TCA may increase the risk for neurotoxicity. Phenothiazines may increase concentration of some TCAs and TCAs may increase concentration of phenothiazines. Pressor response to I.V. epinephrine, norepinephrine, and phenylephrine may be enhanced in patients receiving TCAs (**Note:** Effect is unlikely with epinephrine or levonordefrin dosages typically administered as infiltration in combination with local anesthetics). Combined use of beta-agonists or drugs which prolong QT_c (including quinidine, procainamide, disopyramide, cisapride, sparfloxacin, gatifloxacin, moxifloxacin) with TCAs may predispose patients to cardiac arrhythmias.

Nutritional/Ethanol Interactions

Ethanol: Avoid ethanol (may increase CNS depression).

Food: Grapefruit juice may inhibit the metabolism of some TCAs and clinical toxicity may result.

Herb/Nutraceutical: Avoid valerian, St John's wort, SAMe, kava kava (may increase risk of serotonin syndrome and/or excessive sedation).

Effects on Lab Values ↑ glucose

Adverse Reactions Frequency not defined.

Cardiovascular: Hypotension, hypertension, tachycardia

(Continued)

Doxepin *(Continued)*

Central nervous system: Drowsiness, dizziness, headache, disorientation, ataxia, confusion, seizure
Dermatologic: Alopecia, photosensitivity, rash, pruritus
Endocrine & metabolic: Breast enlargement, galactorrhea, SIADH, increase or decrease in blood sugar, increased or decreased libido
Gastrointestinal: Xerostomia, constipation, vomiting, indigestion, anorexia, aphthous stomatitis, nausea, unpleasant taste, weight gain, diarrhea, trouble with gums, decreased lower esophageal sphincter tone may cause GE reflux
Genitourinary: Urinary retention, testicular edema
Hematologic: Agranulocytosis, leukopenia, eosinophilia, thrombocytopenia, purpura
Neuromuscular & skeletal: Weakness, tremors, numbness, paresthesia, extrapyramidal symptoms, tardive dyskinesia
Ocular: Blurred vision
Otic: Tinnitus
Miscellaneous: Diaphoresis (excessive), allergic reactions

Overdosage/Toxicology Symptoms of overdose include confusion, hallucinations, seizures, urinary retention, hypothermia, hypotension, tachycardia, and cyanosis. Following initiation of essential overdose management, toxic symptoms should be treated symptomatically.

Pharmacodynamics/Kinetics

Half-Life Elimination: Adults: 6-8 hours

Metabolism: Hepatic; metabolites include desmethyldoxepin (active)

Onset: Peak effect: Antidepressant: Usually >2 weeks; Anxiolytic: May occur sooner

Formulations

Capsule, as hydrochloride (Sinequan®): 10 mg, 25 mg, 50 mg, 75 mg, 100 mg, 150 mg
Solution, oral concentrate, as hydrochloride (Sinequan®): 10 mg/mL (120 mL)
Cream:
Prudoxin™: 5% (45 g)
Zonalon®: 5% (30 g, 45 g) [contains benzyl alcohol]

Dosing

Adults:

Depression and/or anxiety (unlabeled use): Oral: Initial: 30-150 mg/day at bedtime or in 2-3 divided doses; may gradually increase up to 300 mg/day; single dose should not exceed 150 mg; select patients may respond to 25-50 mg/day.

Pruritus: Topical: Apply a thin film 4 times/day with at least 3- to 4-hour interval between applications. (Oral administration of doxepin 25-50 mg has also been used, but systemic adverse effects are increased.)

Elderly: Oral: Initial: 10-25 mg at bedtime; increase by 10-25 mg every 3 days for inpatients and weekly for outpatients if tolerated. Rarely does the maximum dose required exceed 75 mg/day; a single bedtime dose is recommended.

Pediatrics: Depression and/or anxiety (unlabeled use): Oral:
Children: 1-3 mg/kg/day in single or divided doses
Adolescents: Initial: 25-50 mg/day in single or divided doses; gradually increase to 100 mg/day

Hepatic Impairment: Use a lower dose and adjust gradually.

Administration

Oral: Do not mix oral concentrate with carbonated beverages (physically incompatible).

Stability

Storage: Protect from light.

Monitoring and Teaching Issues

Physical Assessment: Assess other medications patient may be taking for effectiveness and interactions (see Drug Interactions). See Contraindications and Warnings/Precautions for use cautions. Monitor laboratory tests, therapeutic response, and adverse reactions at beginning of therapy and periodically with long-term use (see Adverse Reactions and Overdose/Toxicology). Taper dosage slowly when discontinuing. Assess knowledge/teach patient appropriate use, interventions to reduce side effects, and adverse symptoms to report (see Patient Education). **Pregnancy risk factor C** - benefits of use should outweigh possible risks. Breast-feeding is not recommended.

Patient Education: Oral: Take exactly as directed; do not increase dose or frequency. It may take several weeks to achieve desired results. Avoid alcohol, caffeine, and other prescription or OTC medications not approved by prescriber. Maintain adequate hydration (2-3 L/day of fluids) unless advised by prescriber to restrict fluids. You may experience drowsiness, lightheadedness, impaired coordination, dizziness, or blurred vision (use caution when driving or engaging in tasks requiring alertness until response to drug is known); constipation (increased exercise, fluids, fruit, or fiber may help); urinary retention (void before taking medication); postural hypotension (use caution climbing stairs or when changing position from lying or sitting to standing); altered sexual drive or ability (reversible); or photosensitivity (use sunscreen, wear protective clothing and eyewear, and avoid direct sunlight). Report persistent CNS effects (eg, nervousness, restlessness, insomnia, anxiety, excitation, headache, agitation, impaired coordination, changes in cognition); muscle cramping, weakness, tremors, or rigidity; chest pain, palpitations, or irregular heartbeat; blurred vision or eye pain; yellowing of skin or eyes; or worsening of condition. **Pregnancy/breast-feeding precautions:** Inform prescriber if you are or intend to become pregnant. Breast-feeding is not recommended.

Topical: Use as directed. Apply in thin layer; do not overuse. Report increased skin irritation, worsening of condition or lack of improvement.

Geriatric Considerations: Preferred agent when sedation is a desired property. Less potential for anticholinergic effects than amitriptyline and less orthostatic hypotension than imipramine.

Breast-feeding Issues: Generally, it is not recommended to breast-feed if taking antidepressants because of the long half-life, active metabolites, and the potential for side effects in the infant.

Related Information

Antidepressant Agents *on page 1553*

Antidepressant Medication Guidelines *on page 1613*

Doxepin Hydrochloride *see* Doxepin *on page 443*

Doxercalciferol (dox er kal si fe FEER ole)

U.S. Brand Names Hectorol®

Generic Available No

Pharmacologic Category Vitamin D Analog

Pregnancy Risk Factor B

Lactation Excretion in breast milk unknown/compatible

Use Reduction of elevated intact parathyroid hormone (iPTH) in the management of secondary hyperparathyroidism in patients on chronic hemodialysis

Mechanism of Action/Effect Doxercalciferol is metabolized to the active form of vitamin D.

Contraindications History of hypercalcemia or evidence of vitamin D toxicity; hyperphosphatemia should be corrected before initiating therapy

Warnings/Precautions Other forms of vitamin D should be discontinued when doxercalciferol is started. Hyperphosphatemia should be corrected before initiating therapy; hyperphosphatemia diminishes response. Use with caution in patients with hepatic impairment. Safety and efficacy have not been established in pediatrics.

Drug Interactions

Decreased Effect: Absorption of doxercalciferol is reduced with mineral oil and cholestyramine.

Increased Effect/Toxicity: Doxercalciferol toxicity may be increased by concurrent use of other vitamin D supplements or magnesium-containing antacids and supplements.

Effects on Lab Values Serum calcium times phosphorus product should be <70

Adverse Reactions

>10%:

Cardiovascular: Edema (34.4%)

Central nervous system: Headache (28%), malaise (28%), dizziness (11.5%)

Gastrointestinal: Nausea/vomiting (34%)

Respiratory: Dyspnea (11.5%)

1% to 10%:

Cardiovascular: Bradycardia (6.6%)

Central nervous system: Sleep disorder (3.3%)

Dermatologic: Pruritus (8.2%)

Gastrointestinal: Anorexia (4.9%), constipation (3.3%), dyspepsia (4.9%)

Neuromuscular & skeletal: Arthralgia (4.9%)

Miscellaneous: Abscess (3.3%)

Overdosage/Toxicology Doxercalciferol, in excess, can cause hypercalcemia, hypercalciuria, hyperphosphatemia and oversuppression of PTH secretion. Some of the signs and symptoms of hypercalcemia include anorexia, nausea, vomiting, constipation, polyuria, weakness, fatigue, confusion, stupor, and coma. Following withdrawal of the drug and calcium supplements, hypercalcemia treatment consists of a low calcium diet and monitoring.

Pharmacodynamics/Kinetics

Half-Life Elimination: Active metabolite: 32-37 hours; up to 96 hours

Metabolism: Hepatic via CYP27

Formulations

Capsule: 2.5 mcg [contains coconut oil]

Injection, solution: 2 mcg/mL (1 mL, 2 mL)

Dosing

Adults & Elderly: Secondary hyperparathyroidism:

Oral:

If the iPTH >400 pg/mL, then the initial dose is 10 mcg 3 times/week at dialysis. The dose is adjusted at 8-week intervals based upon the iPTH levels.

If the iPTH level is decreased by 50% and >300 pg/mL, then the dose can be increased to 12.5 mcg 3 times/week for 8 more weeks. This titration process can continue at 8-week intervals up to a maximum dose of 20 mcg 3 times/week. Each increase should be by 2.5 mcg/dose.

If the iPTH is between 150-300 pg/mL, maintain the current dose.

If the iPTH is <100 pg/mL, then suspend the drug for 1 week; resume doxercalciferol at a reduced dose. Decrease each dose (not weekly dose) by at least 2.5 mcg.

I.V.:

If the iPTH >400 pg/mL, then the initial dose is 4 mcg 3 times/week after dialysis, administered as a bolus dose

If the iPTH level is decreased by 50% and >300 pg/mL, then the dose can be increased by 1-2 mcg at 8-week intervals as necessary

If the iPTH is between 150-300 pg/mL, maintain the current dose.

If the iPTH is <100 pg/mL, then suspend the drug for 1 week; resume doxercalciferol at a reduced dose (at least 1 mcg lower)

Renal Impairment: No adjustment is required.

Hepatic Impairment: Use caution in these patients; no guidelines for dosage adjustment.

Stability

Storage: Store at controlled room temperature (15°C to 30°C/59°F to 86°F).

Monitoring Laboratory Tests Before initiating, check iPTH, serum calcium, and phosphorus. Check weekly thereafter until stable. Serum iPTH, calcium, phosphorus, and alkaline phosphatase should be monitored.

Monitoring and Teaching Issues

Physical Assessment: Monitor therapeutic response (laboratory results), adverse reactions (see Adverse Reactions and Overdose/Toxicology). Assess knowledge/teach patient appropriate use, interventions to reduce side effects, and adverse reactions to report (see Patient Education).

(Continued)

Doxercalciferol *(Continued)*

Patient Education: Be clear on dose and directions for taking. Stop other vitamin D products. Do not miss doses. Avoid magnesium-containing antacids and supplements. Report headache, dizziness, weakness, sleepiness, severe nausea, vomiting, and difficulty thinking or concentrating to your prescriber. Do not take over-the-counter medicines or supplements without first consulting your prescriber. Follow diet and calcium supplements as directed by your prescriber.

Breast-feeding Issues: Excretion in breast milk is unknown. Other vitamin D derivatives are excreted in breast milk; there is a potential for adverse effects. Therefore, breast-feeding should be discontinued or doxercalciferol discontinued, depending upon importance of the drug to the mother.

Doxil® *see* DOXOrubicin (Liposomal) *on page 448*

DOXOrubicin (doks oh ROO bi sin)

U.S. Brand Names Adriamycin PFS®; Adriamycin RDF®; Rubex®

Synonyms ADR; Doxorubicin Hydrochloride; Hydroxydaunomycin Hydrochloride

Generic Available Yes

Pharmacologic Category Antineoplastic Agent, Anthracycline

Pregnancy Risk Factor D

Lactation Enters breast milk/contraindicated

Use Treatment of leukemias, lymphomas, multiple myeloma, osseous and nonosseous sarcomas, mesotheliomas, germ cell tumors of the ovary or testis, and carcinomas of the head and neck, thyroid, lung, breast, stomach, pancreas, liver, ovary, bladder, prostate, uterus, and neuroblastoma

Mechanism of Action/Effect Inhibits DNA and RNA synthesis of susceptible bacteria, active throughout cell cycle, results in cell death.

Contraindications Hypersensitivity to doxorubicin or any component of the formulation; congestive heart failure or arrhythmias; previous therapy with high cumulative doses of doxorubicin and/or daunorubicin; pre-existing bone marrow suppression; pregnancy

Warnings/Precautions The U.S. Food and Drug Administration (FDA) currently recommends that procedures for proper handling and disposal of antineoplastic agents be considered. Total dose should not exceed 550 mg/m^2 or 400 mg/m^2 in patients with previous or concomitant treatment with daunorubicin, cyclophosphamide, or irradiation of the cardiac region. Irreversible myocardial toxicity may occur as total dosage approaches 550 mg/m^2. I.V. use only, severe local tissue necrosis will result if extravasation occurs. Elderly and pediatric patients are at higher risk of cardiotoxicity (delayed). Reduce dose in patients with impaired hepatic function. Severe myelosuppression is also possible. Administration of live vaccines to immunosuppressed patients may be hazardous. Heart failure may occur during therapy or months to years after therapy. Treatment may increase the risk of other neoplasms. Secondary acute myelogenous leukemia may occur following treatment.

If doxorubicin contacts the skin, wash and flush thoroughly with water.

Drug Interactions

Cytochrome P450 Effect: Substrate of **CYP2D6, 3A4**; Inhibits CYP2D6, 3A4

Decreased Effect: Doxorubicin may decrease plasma levels and effectiveness of digoxin and phenytoin. Phenobarbital increases elimination (decreases effect) of doxorubicin. Doxorubicin may decrease the antiviral activity of zidovudine.

Increased Effect/Toxicity: Allopurinol may enhance the antitumor activity of doxorubicin (animal data only). Cyclosporine may increase doxorubicin levels, enhancing hematologic toxicity or may induce coma or seizures. Cyclophosphamide enhances the cardiac toxicity of doxorubicin by producing additional myocardial cell damage. Mercaptopurine increases doxorubicin toxicities. Streptozocin greatly enhances leukopenia and thrombocytopenia. Verapamil alters the cellular distribution of doxorubicin and may result in increased cell toxicity by inhibition of the P-glycoprotein pump. Paclitaxel reduces doxorubicin clearance and increases toxicity if administered prior to doxorubicin. High doses of progesterone enhance toxicity (neutropenia and thrombocytopenia). Based on mouse studies, cardiotoxicity may be enhanced by verapamil. Concurrent therapy with actinomycin-D may result in recall pneumonitis following radiation.

Nutritional/Ethanol Interactions

Ethanol: Avoid ethanol (due to GI irritation).

Herb/Nutraceutical: St John's wort may decrease doxorubicin levels. Avoid black cohosh, dong quai in estrogen-dependent tumors.

Adverse Reactions

>10%:

Dermatologic: Alopecia

Gastrointestinal: Acute nausea and vomiting may be seen in 21% to 55% of patients; mucositis, ulceration, and necrosis of the colon, anorexia, and diarrhea, stomatitis, esophagitis

Emetic potential:

≤20 mg: Moderately low (10% to 30%)

>20 mg or <60 mg: Moderate (30% to 60%)

≥60 mg: Moderately high (60% to 90%)

Time course for nausea/vomiting: Onset: 1-3 hours; Duration 4-24 hours

Genitourinary: Discoloration of urine (red)

Hematologic: Myelosuppressive: 60% to 80% of patients will have leukopenia; dose-limiting toxicity

WBC: Moderate

Platelets: Moderate

Onset (days): 7

Nadir (days): 10-14

Recovery (days): 21-28

Local: **Vesicant chemotherapy**

1% to 10%:

Cardiovascular: Acute: Arrhythmias, heart block, pericarditis-myocarditis, facial flushing; Delayed: Congestive heart failure (related to cumulative dose; usually a maximum total lifetime dose of 450-550 mg/m^2; possibly higher if given by continuous infusion in breast cancer),

Dermatologic: Hyperpigmentation of nail beds, erythematous streaking along the vein if administered rapidly

Endocrine & metabolic: Hyperuricemia

<1% (Limited to important or life-threatening):

Pediatric patients may be at increased risk of later neoplastic disease, particularly acute myeloid leukemia (pediatric patients). Prepubertal growth failure may result from intensive chemotherapy regimens.

Radiation recall: Noticed in patients who have had prior irradiation; reactions include redness, warmth, erythema, and dermatitis in the radiation port. Can progress to severe desquamation and ulceration. Occurs 5-7 days after doxorubicin administration; local therapy with topical corticosteroids and cooling have given the best relief.

Overdosage/Toxicology Symptoms of overdose include myelosuppression, nausea, vomiting, and myocardial toxicity. Treatment of acute overdose consists of treatment of the severely myelosuppressed patient with hospitalization, antibiotics, platelet and granulocyte transfusions, and symptomatic treatment of mucositis.

Pharmacodynamics/Kinetics

Absorption: Oral: Poor (<50%)

Half-Life Elimination:

Distribution: 10 minutes

Elimination: Doxorubicin: 1-3 hours; Metabolites: 3-3.5 hours

Terminal: 17-30 hours

Male: 54 hours; Female: 35 hours

Metabolism: Primarily hepatic to doxorubicinol (active), then to inactive aglycones, conjugated sulfates, and glucuronides

Formulations

Injection, powder for reconstitution, as hydrochloride: 10 mg, 20 mg, 50 mg [contains lactose]

Adriamycin RDF®: 10 mg, 20 mg, 50 mg, 150 mg [contains lactose; rapid dissolution formula]

Rubex®: 50 mg, 100 mg [contains lactose]

Injection, solution, as hydrochloride [preservative free]: 2 mg/mL (5 mL, 10 mL, 25 mL, 100 mL)

Adriamycin PFS® [preservative free]: 2 mg/mL (5 mL, 10 mL, 25 mL, 37.5 mL, 100 mL)

Dosing

Adults & Elderly: Refer to individual protocols (patient's ideal weight should be used to calculate body surface area).

Usual or typical dose: 60-75 mg/m^2 as a single dose, repeat every 21 days **or** other dosage regimens like 20-30 mg/m^2/day for 2-3 days, repeat in 4 weeks **or** 20 mg/m^2 once weekly.

The lower dose regimen should be given to patients with decreased bone marrow reserve, prior therapy or marrow infiltration with malignant cells.

Currently, the maximum cumulative dose is 550 mg/m^2 or 450 mg/m^2 in patients who have received RT to the mediastinal areas. A baseline MUGA should be performed prior to initiating treatment. If the LVEF is <30% to 40%, therapy should not be instituted; LVEF should be monitored during therapy.

Doxorubicin has also been administered intraperitoneal (phase I in refractory ovarian cancer patients) and intra-arterially.

Pediatrics: Refer to individual protocols.

Usual/typical dosages: I.V.:

Children:

35-75 mg/m^2 as a single dose, repeat every 21 days **or**

20-30 mg/m^2 once weekly **or**

60-90 mg/m^2 given as a continuous infusion over 96 hours every 3-4 weeks

Renal Impairment:

Adjustments are not required.

Hemodialysis effects: Supplemental dose is not necessary.

Hepatic Impairment:

Bilirubin 1.5-3 mg/dL: Administer 50% of dose.

Bilirubin 3.1-5 mg/dL: Administer 25% of dose.

Administration

I.V.: Vesicant. Administer I.V. push over 1-2 minutes or IVPB. Infusion via central venous line recommended.

Stability

Storage: Store intact vials of solution under refrigeration at 2°C to 8°C and protected from light. Store intact vials of lyophilized powder at room temperature (15°C to 30°C).

Reconstitution: Reconstitute lyophilized powder with SWI or NS to a final concentration of 2 mg/mL as follows. Reconstituted solution is stable for 7 days at room temperature (25°C) and 15 days under refrigeration (5°C) when protected from light.

10 mg vial = 5 mL

20 mg vial = 10 mL

50 mg vial = 25 mL

Further dilution in D_5W or NS is stable for 48 hours at room temperature (25°C) when protected from light.

Unstable in solutions with a pH <3 or >7. Avoid aluminum needles and bacteriostatic diluents as precipitation occurs. Decomposing drug turns purple. Protect from direct sunlight.

Standard I.V. dilution:

I.V. push: Dose/syringe (concentration: 2 mg/mL)

Maximum syringe size for IVP is a 30 mL syringe and syringe should be ≤75% full.

(Continued)

DOXOrubicin *(Continued)*

Syringes are stable for 7 days at room temperature (25°C) and 15 days under refrigeration (5°C) when protected from light.

IVPB: Dose/50-100 mL D_5W or NS

IVPB solutions are stable for 48 hours at room temperature (25°C) when protected from light.

Compatibility: Stable in D_5W, LR, NS

Y-site administration: Incompatible with allopurinol, amphotericin B cholesteryl sulfate complex, cefepime, ganciclovir, piperacillin/tazobactam, propofol

Compatibility in syringe: Incompatible with furosemide, heparin

Compatibility when admixed: Incompatible with aminophylline, diazepam, fluorouracil

Monitoring Laboratory Tests CBC with differential, platelet count, echocardiogram, liver function

Monitoring and Teaching Issues

Physical Assessment: See Contraindications, Warnings/Precautions, and Dosing for use cautions. Assess potential for interactions with other prescriptions, OTC medications, or herbal products patient may be taking (see Drug Interactions). See Administration, Dosing, Reconstitution, and Compatibility for administration specifics. Premedication with antiemetic is recommended (especially with larger doses). Infusion site must be closely monitored; extravasation can cause sloughing or tissue necrosis (see Administration). Assess results of laboratory tests (see above), therapeutic effectiveness, and adverse response (see Adverse Reactions and Overdose/Toxicology) prior to each treatment and on a regular basis throughout therapy. Teach patient possible side effects and interventions (eg, importance of adequate hydration) and adverse symptoms to report (see Patient Education). **Pregnancy risk factor D** - determine that patient is not pregnant before beginning treatment. Instruct patients of childbearing age on appropriate barrier contraceptive measures. Breast-feeding is contraindicated.

Patient Education: Inform prescriber of all prescriptions, OTC medications, or herbal products you are taking, and any allergies you have. Do not take anything new during treatment unless approved by prescriber. This medication can only be administered by infusion. Report immediately any swelling, pain, burning, or redness at infusion site. Avoid alcohol. It is important to maintain adequate hydration (2-3 L/day of fluids) unless advised by prescriber to restrict fluids, and adequate nutrition (small, frequent meals may help). You will be more susceptible to infection (avoid crowds and exposure to infection and do not have any vaccinations without consulting prescriber). May cause nausea or vomiting (small, frequent meals, frequent mouth care, sucking lozenges, or chewing gum may help); diarrhea (buttermilk, boiled milk, or yogurt may help); loss of hair (reversible); or red-pink urine (normal). Report immediately chest pain, swelling of extremities, difficulty breathing, palpitations, or rapid heartbeat. Report unresolved nausea, vomiting, or diarrhea; alterations in urinary pattern (increased or decreased); opportunistic infection (fever, chills, unusual bruising or bleeding fatigue, purulent vaginal discharge, unhealed mouth sores); abdominal pain or blood in stools; excessive fatigue; or yellowing of eyes or skin. **Pregnancy/breast-feeding precautions:** Inform prescriber if you are pregnant. Do not get pregnant while taking this medication and for 1 month following therapy; consult prescriber for appropriate barrier contraceptives. Do not breast-feed.

Related Information

FDA Name Differentiation Project: The Use of Tall-man Letters *on page 12*

Doxorubicin Hydrochloride *see* DOXOrubicin *on page 446*

Doxorubicin Hydrochloride (Liposomal) *see* DOXOrubicin (Liposomal) *on page 448*

DOXOrubicin (Liposomal) (doks oh ROO bi sin lip pah SOW mal)

U.S. Brand Names Doxil®

Synonyms Doxorubicin Hydrochloride (Liposomal)

Generic Available No

Pharmacologic Category Antineoplastic Agent, Anthracycline

Pregnancy Risk Factor D

Lactation Enters breast milk/contraindicated

Use Treatment of AIDS-related Kaposi's sarcoma, breast cancer, ovarian cancer, solid tumors

Mechanism of Action/Effect Inhibits DNA and RNA synthesis of susceptible bacteria, active throughout cell cycle, results in cell death

Contraindications Hypersensitivity to doxorubicin, other anthracyclines, or any component of the formulation; pre-existing bone marrow suppression; pregnancy

Warnings/Precautions The U.S. Food and Drug Administration (FDA) currently recommends that procedures for proper handling and disposal of antineoplastic agents be considered. Total dose should not exceed 550 mg/m^2 or 400 mg/m^2 in patients with previous or concomitant treatment (with daunorubicin, cyclophosphamide, or irradiation of the cardiac region); irreversible myocardial toxicity may occur as total dosage approaches 550 mg/m^2. I.V. use only, severe local tissue necrosis will result if extravasation occurs. Reduce dose in patients with impaired hepatic function. Severe myelosuppression is also possible. Acute infusion reactions may occur, some may be serious/life-threatening. Administer at an initial rate of 1 mg/minute to minimize risk.

If doxorubicin (liposomal) contacts the skin, wash and flush thoroughly with water.

Drug Interactions

Cytochrome P450 Effect: Substrate of **CYP2D6, 3A4**; Inhibits CYP2D6, 3A4

Decreased Effect: Doxorubicin may decrease plasma levels and effectiveness of digoxin and phenytoin. Phenobarbital increases elimination (decreases effect) of doxorubicin. Doxorubicin may decrease the antiviral activity of zidovudine.

Increased Effect/Toxicity: Allopurinol may enhance the antitumor activity of doxorubicin (animal data only). Cyclosporine may induce coma or seizures. Cyclophosphamide enhances the cardiac toxicity of doxorubicin by producing additional myocardial cell damage. Mercaptopurine increases toxicities. Streptozocin greatly enhances leukopenia and thrombocytopenia. Verapamil alters the cellular distribution of doxorubicin and may result in increased cell toxicity by inhibition of the P-glycoprotein pump.

Nutritional/Ethanol Interactions

Ethanol: Avoid ethanol (due to GI irritation).

Herb/Nutraceutical: St John's wort may decrease doxorubicin levels. Avoid black cohosh, dong quai in estrogen-dependent tumors.

Adverse Reactions Information on adverse events is based on the experience reported in 753 patients with AIDS-related Kaposi's sarcoma enrolled in four studies.

>10%:

Gastrointestinal: Nausea; emetic potential:

≤20 mg: Moderately low (10% to 30%)

>20 mg or <75 mg: Moderate (30% to 60%)

≥75 mg: Moderately high (49%)

Hematologic: Myelosuppressive: 60% to 80% of patients will have leukopenia; dose-limiting toxicity

WBC: Moderate

Platelets: Moderate

Onset (days): 7

Nadir (days): 10-14

Recovery (days): 21-28

Local: **Irritant chemotherapy**

1% to 10%:

Cardiovascular: Cardiac toxicity (9.7%): Cardiomyopathy, CHF, arrhythmia, pericardial effusion, tachycardia, facial flushing

Dermatologic: Hyperpigmentation of nail beds, erythematous streaking along the vein if administered rapidly

Endocrine & metabolic: Hyperuricemia

Overdosage/Toxicology Symptoms of overdose include increases in mucositis, leukopenia, and thrombocytopenia. For acute overdose, treatment of the severely myelosuppressed patient consists of hospitalization, antibiotics, platelet and granulocyte transfusion, and symptomatic treatment of mucositis.

Pharmacodynamics/Kinetics

Metabolism: Hepatic and in plasma to both active and inactive metabolites

Formulations Injection, solution, as hydrochloride: 2 mg/mL (10 mL, 25 mL)

Dosing

Adults & Elderly: Refer to individual protocols.

AIDS-KS: I.V. (patient's ideal weight should be used to calculate body surface area): 20 mg/m^2 over 30 minutes, once every 3 weeks, for as long as patients respond satisfactorily and tolerate treatment.

Breast cancer: I.V.: 20-80 mg/m^2/dose has been studied in a limited number of phase I/II trials.

Ovarian cancer: I.V.: 50 mg/m^2/dose repeated every 4 weeks (minimum of 4 courses is recommended).

Solid tumors: I.V.: 50-60 mg/m^2/dose repeated every 3-4 weeks has been studied in a limited number of phase I/II trials.

Hepatic Impairment:

Bilirubin 1.2-3 mg/dL: Administer 50% of dose.

Bilirubin >3 mg/dL: Administer 25% of dose.

Administration

I.V.: Irritant. Administer IVPB over 30 minutes; administer at initial rate of 1 mg/minute to minimize risk of infusion reactions; further dilute in D_5W. Do not administer as a bolus injection or undiluted solution. **Do not administer intramuscular or subcutaneous.**

Stability

Storage: Store intact vials of solution under refrigeration at 2°C to 8°C and avoid freezing. Prolonged freezing may adversely affect liposomal drug products, however, short-term freezing (<1 month) does not appear to have a deleterious effect.

Reconstitution: The appropriate dose (up to a maximum of 90 mg) must be diluted in 250 mL of dextrose 5% in water prior to administration. Diluted doxorubicin hydrochloride liposome injection is stable when refrigerated at 2°C to 8°C for 48 hours. When stored at room temperature, remains stable for 24 hours. **Do not use with in-line filters.**

Compatibility: Stable in D_5W

Y-site administration: Incompatible with amphotericin B, amphotericin B cholesteryl sulfate complex, buprenorphine, cefoperazone, ceftazidime, docetaxel, fluorouracil, furosemide, heparin, hydroxyzine, mannitol, meperidine, metoclopramide, mitoxantrone, morphine, ofloxacin, paclitaxel, piperacillin/tazobactam, promethazine, sodium bicarbonate

Monitoring Laboratory Tests CBC with differential, platelet count, echocardiogram, liver function

Monitoring and Teaching Issues

Physical Assessment: See Contraindications, Warnings/Precautions, and Dosing for use cautions. Assess potential for interactions with other prescriptions, OTC medications, or herbal products patient may be taking (see Drug Interactions). See Administration, Dosing, Reconstitution, and Compatibility for administration specifics. Premedication with antiemetic is recommended - especially with larger doses. Infusion site must be closely monitored; extravasation can cause sloughing or tissue necrosis (see Administration). Assess therapeutic response, results of laboratory tests (see above) and adverse reactions (see Adverse Reactions and Overdose/Toxicology) prior to each treatment and on a regular basis throughout therapy. Teach patient possible side effects and interventions (eg, importance of adequate hydration) and adverse symptoms to report (see Patient Education). **Pregnancy risk factor D** - determine that patient is not pregnant before beginning treatment. Instruct patients of childbearing age on appropriate barrier contraceptive measures. Breast-feeding is contraindicated.

(Continued)

DOXOrubicin (Liposomal) *(Continued)*

Patient Education: Inform prescriber of all prescriptions, OTC medications, or herbal products you are taking, and any allergies you have. Do not take anything new during treatment unless approved by prescriber. This medication can only be administered by infusion. Report immediately any swelling, pain, burning, or redness at infusion site. Avoid alcohol. It is important to maintain adequate hydration (2-3 L/day of fluids) unless advised by prescriber to restrict fluids, and adequate nutrition (small, frequent meals may help). You will be more susceptible to infection (avoid crowds and exposure to infection and do not have any vaccinations without consulting prescriber). May cause nausea or vomiting (small, frequent meals, frequent mouth care, sucking lozenges, or chewing gum may help); diarrhea (buttermilk, boiled milk, or yogurt may help); loss of hair (reversible); or red-pink urine (normal). Report immediately chest pain, swelling of extremities, difficulty breathing, palpitations, or rapid heartbeat. Report unresolved nausea, vomiting, or diarrhea; alterations in urinary pattern (increased or decreased); opportunistic infection (fever, chills, unusual bruising or bleedlng fatigue, purulent vaginal discharge, unhealed mouth sores); abdominal pain or blood in stools; excessive fatigue; or yellowing of eyes or skin. **Pregnancy/breast-feeding precautions:** Do not get pregnant while taking this medication and for 1 month following therapy; consult prescriber for appropriate barrier contraceptives. Do not breast-feed.

Doxy-100® *see* Doxycycline *on page 450*

Doxycycline (doks i SYE kleen)

U.S. Brand Names Adoxa™; Doryx®; Doxy-100®; Monodox®; Periostat®; Vibramycin®; Vibra-Tabs®

Synonyms Doxycycline Calcium; Doxycycline Hyclate; Doxycycline Monohydrate

Generic Available Yes

Pharmacologic Category Antibiotic, Tetracycline Derivative

Pregnancy Risk Factor D

Lactation Enters breast milk/not recommended

Use Principally in the treatment of infections caused by susceptible *Rickettsia*, *Chlamydia*, and *Mycoplasma* along with uncommon susceptible gram-negative and gram-positive organisms; alternative to mefloquine for malaria prophylaxis; treatment for syphilis in penicillin-allergic patients; often active against vancomycin-resistant enterococci; used for community-acquired pneumonia and other common infections due to susceptible organisms; anthrax due to *Bacillus anthracis,* including inhalational anthrax (postexposure), to reduce the incidence or progression of disease following exposure to aerolized *Bacillus anthracis*

Use - Unlabeled/Investigational Sclerosing agent for pleural effusion injection

Mechanism of Action/Effect Inhibits protein synthesis by binding with the 30S and possibly the 50S ribosomal subunit(s) of susceptible bacteria; may also cause alterations in the cytoplasmic membrane

Doxycycline inhibits collagenase *in vitro* and has been shown to inhibit collagenase in the gingival crevicular fluid in adults with periodontitis

Contraindications Hypersensitivity to doxycycline, tetracycline or any component of the formulation; children <8 years of age, except in treatment of anthrax (including inhalational anthrax postexposure prophylaxis); severe hepatic dysfunction; pregnancy

Warnings/Precautions Do not use during pregnancy - use of tetracyclines during tooth development may cause permanent discoloration of the teeth and enamel hypoplasia. Prolonged use may result in superinfection, including oral or vaginal candidiasis. Photosensitivity reaction may occur with this drug; avoid prolonged exposure to sunlight or tanning equipment.

Drug Interactions

Cytochrome P450 Effect: Substrate of **CYP3A4**; Inhibits CYP3A4

Decreased Effect: Decreased levels of doxycycline may occur when taken with antacids containing aluminum, calcium, or magnesium. Decreased levels when taken with iron, bismuth subsalicylate, barbiturates, phenytoin, sucralfate, didanosine, quinapril, and carbamazepine. Concurrent use of tetracycline and Penthrane® has been reported to result in fatal renal toxicity. Although anecdotal reports suggest oral contraceptive efficacy could be reduced by tetracyclines, this has been refuted by more rigorous scientific and clinical data.

Increased Effect/Toxicity: Increased digoxin toxicity when taken with digoxin. Increased prothrombin time with warfarin.

Nutritional/Ethanol Interactions

Ethanol: Chronic ethanol ingestion may reduce the serum concentration of doxycycline.

Food: Doxycycline serum levels may be slightly decreased if taken with food or milk. Administration with iron or calcium may decrease doxycycline absorption. May decrease absorption of calcium, iron, magnesium, zinc, and amino acids.

Herb/Nutraceutical: St John's wort may decrease doxycycline levels. Avoid dong quai, St John's wort (may also cause photosensitization).

Effects on Lab Values False-negative urine glucose using Clinistix®

Adverse Reactions Frequency not defined.

Cardiovascular: Intracranial hypertension, pericarditis

Dermatologic: Angioneurotic edema, exfoliative dermatitis (rare), photosensitivity, rash, urticaria

Endocrine & metabolic: Brown/black discoloration of thyroid gland (no dysfunction reported)

Gastrointestinal: Anorexia, diarrhea, dysphagia, enterocolitis, esophagitis (rare), esophageal ulcerations (rare), glossitis, inflammatory lesions in anogenital region, tooth discoloration (children)

Hematologic: Eosinophilia, hemolytic anemia, neutropenia, thrombocytopenia

Renal: Increased BUN

Miscellaneous: Anaphylactoid purpura, anaphylaxis, bulging fontanels (infants), SLE exacerbation

Note: Adverse effects in clinical trials with Periostat® occurring at a frequency more than 1% greater than placebo included nausea, dyspepsia, joint pain, diarrhea, menstrual cramp, and pain.

Overdosage/Toxicology Symptoms of overdose include nausea, anorexia, and diarrhea. Treatment is supportive.

Pharmacodynamics/Kinetics

Absorption: Oral: Almost complete; reduced by food or milk by 20%

Half-Life Elimination: 12-15 hours (usually increases to 22-24 hours with multiple doses); End-stage renal disease: 18-25 hours

Time to Peak: Serum: 1.5-4 hours

Metabolism: Not hepatic; partially inactivated in GI tract by chelate formation

Formulations

Capsule, as hyclate (Vibramycin®): 50 mg, 100 mg
Capsule, as monohydrate (Monodox®): 50 mg, 100 mg
Capsule, coated pellets, as hyclate (Doryx®): 100 mg
Injection, powder for reconstitution, as hyclate (Doxy-100®): 100 mg
Powder for oral suspension, as monohydrate (Vibramycin®): 25 mg/5 mL (60 mL) [raspberry flavor]
Syrup, as calcium (Vibramycin®): 50 mg/5 mL (480 mL) [contains sodium metabisulfite; raspberry-apple flavor]
Tablet, as hyclate: 100 mg
Periostat®: 20 mg
Vibra-Tabs®: 100 mg
Tablet, as monohydrate (Adoxa™): 50 mg, 100 mg

Dosing

Adults & Elderly:

Acute gonococcal infection: Oral, I.V.: 200 mg immediately, then 100 mg at bedtime on the first day followed by 100 mg twice daily for 3 days **or** 300 mg immediately followed by 300 mg in 1 hour

Anthrax:

Inhalational (postexposure prophylaxis): Oral, I.V. (use oral route when possible): 100 mg every 12 hours for 60 days (*MMWR*, 2001, 50:889-93); **Note:** Preliminary recommendation, FDA review and update is anticipated.

Cutaneous (treatment): Oral: 100 mg every 12 hours for 60 days. **Note:** In the presence of systemic involvement, extensive edema, lesions on head/neck, refer to I.V. dosing for treatment of inhalational/gastrointestinal/oropharyngeal anthrax

Inhalational/gastrointestinal/oropharyngeal (treatment): I.V.: Initial: 100 mg every 12 hours; switch to oral therapy when clinically appropriate; some recommend initial loading dose of 200 mg, followed by 100 mg every 8-12 hours (*JAMA*, 1997, 278:399-411).

Note: Initial treatment should include two or more agents predicted to be effective (per CDC recommendations). Agents suggested for use in conjunction with doxycycline or ciprofloxacin include rifampin, vancomycin, imipenem, penicillin, ampicillin, chloramphenicol, clindamycin, and clarithromycin. May switch to oral antimicrobial therapy when clinically appropriate. Continue combined therapy for 60 days

Community-acquired pneumonia, bronchitis: Oral, I.V.: 100 mg twice daily

Syphilis:

Early syphilis: 200 mg/day in divided doses for 14 days
Late syphilis: 200 mg/day in divided doses for 28 days

Uncomplicated chlamydial infections: Oral, I.V.: 100 mg twice daily for ≥7 days

Endometritis, salpingitis, parametritis, or peritonitis: 100 mg I.V. twice daily with cefoxitin 2 g every 6 hours for 4 days and for ≥48 hours after patient improves; then continue with oral therapy 100 mg twice daily to complete a 10- to 14-day course of therapy

Lyme disease: Oral: 100 mg twice daily for 14-21 days

Sclerosing agent for pleural effusion injection (unlabeled use): Intrapleural: 500 mg as a single dose in 30-50 mL of NS or SWI

Dental: Oral (Periostat®): As adjunctive treatment for periodontitis: 20 mg twice daily at least 1 hour before morning and evening meals for up to 9 months (no antimicrobial activity at this dosage)

Pediatrics:

Anthrax:

Inhalational (postexposure prophylaxis) (*MMWR*, 2001, 50:889-893): Oral, I.V. (use oral route when possible):
≤8 years: 2.2 mg/kg every 12 hours for 60 days
>8 years and ≤45 kg: 2.2 mg/kg every 12 hours for 60 days
>8 years and >45 kg: 100 mg every 12 hours for 60 days

Cutaneous (treatment): Oral: See dosing for "Inhalational (postexposure prophylaxis)"

Note: In the presence of systemic involvement, extensive edema, and/or lesions on head/neck, doxycycline should initially be administered I.V.

Inhalational/gastrointestinal/oropharyngeal (treatment): I.V.: Refer to dosing for inhalational anthrax (postexposure prophylaxis); switch to oral therapy when clinically appropriate.

Note: Initial treatment should include two or more agents predicted to be effective (per CDC recommendations). Agents suggested for use in conjunction with doxycycline or ciprofloxacin include rifampin, vancomycin, imipenem, penicillin, ampicillin, chloramphenicol, clindamycin, and clarithromycin. May switch to oral antimicrobial therapy when clinically appropriate. Continue combined therapy for 60 days

Susceptible infections:

Children ≥8 years (<45 kg): Oral, I.V.: 2-5 mg/kg/day in 1-2 divided doses, not to exceed 200 mg/day
Children >8 years (>45 kg): Oral, I.V.: Refer to adult dosing.

Renal Impairment: No adjustment necessary.

Not dialyzable; 0% to 5% by hemo- and peritoneal methods or by continuous arteriovenous or venovenous hemofiltration; supplemental dose is not necessary.

(Continued)

Doxycycline *(Continued)*

Administration

Oral: Administer with adequate fluid to reduce risk of esophageal irritation and ulceration. May give with meals to decrease GI upset.

I.V.: Infuse slowly, usually over 1-4 hours.

Stability

Storage: Capsules/tablets: Store at controlled room temperature; protect from light

Reconstitution: I.V. infusion: Following reconstitution with sterile water for injection, dilute to a final concentration of 0.1-1 mg/mL using a compatible solution. Protect from light. Stability varies based on solution.

Compatibility: Stable in NS, D_5W, LR, D_5LR

Y-site administration: Incompatible with allopurinol, heparin, piperacillin/tazobactam

Monitoring Laboratory Tests Perform culture and sensitivity testing prior to initiating therapy.

Monitoring and Teaching Issues

Physical Assessment: Assess allergy history before beginning therapy. See Contraindications, Warnings/Precautions, and Dosing for use cautions. Assess potential for interactions with other prescriptions, OTC medications, or herbal products patient may be taking (see Drug Interactions). See Administration, Dosing, Reconstitution, and Compatibility for administration specifics. Infusion site must be closely monitored; extravasation can be very irritating to veins (see Administration). Assess therapeutic response, laboratory tests (see above), and adverse reactions (see Adverse Reactions and Overdose/Toxicology) on a regular basis throughout therapy. Caution diabetic patients about altered response to Clinitest®. Teach patient possible side effects and interventions (eg, importance of adequate hydration) and adverse symptoms to report (see Patient Education). **Pregnancy risk factor D** - determine that patient is not pregnant before beginning treatment. Instruct patients of childbearing age on appropriate barrier contraceptive measures. Breast-feeding is not recommended.

Patient Education: Inform prescriber of all prescriptions, OTC medications, or herbal products you are taking, and any allergies you have. Do not take anything new during treatment unless approved by prescriber. Take entire prescription as directed, even if you are feeling better. Take each oral dose with food or a full glass of water to reduce stomach upset. Avoid alcohol and maintain adequate hydration (2-3 L/day of fluids) unless advised by prescriber to restrict fluids. You may be very sensitive to sunlight (use sunblock, wear protective clothing and eyewear, or avoid exposure to direct sunlight). May cause lightheadedness, dizziness, or drowsiness (use caution when driving or engaging in tasks that require alertness until response to drug is known); nausea or vomiting (small, frequent meals, frequent mouth care, sucking lozenges, or chewing gum may help); or diarrhea (buttermilk, boiled milk, or yogurt may help). Report skin rash or itching; easy bruising or bleeding; yellowing of skin or eyes; pale stool or dark urine; unhealed mouth sores; vaginal itching or discharge; fever, chills, or unusual cough. **Pregnancy/breast-feeding precautions:** Inform prescriber if you are pregnant. Do not get pregnant while taking this medication. Breast-feeding is not recommended.

Dietary Issues: Take with food if gastric irritation occurs. While administration with food may decrease GI absorption of doxycycline by up to 20%, administration on an empty stomach is not recommended due to GI intolerance. Of currently available tetracyclines, doxycycline has the least affinity for calcium.

Pregnancy Issues: Exposure during the last half or pregnancy causes permanent yellow-gray-brown discoloration of the teeth. Tetracyclines also form a complex in bone-forming tissue, leading to a decreased fibula growth rate when given to premature infants. According to the FDA, the Teratogen Information System concluded that therapeutic doses during pregnancy are unlikely to produce substantial teratogenic risk, but data are insufficient to say that there is no risk. In general, reports of exposure have been limited to short durations of therapy in the first trimester. When considering treatment for life-threatening infection and/or prolonged duration of therapy (such as in anthrax), the potential risk to the fetus must be balanced against the severity of the potential illness.

Related Information

Prophylaxis for Exposure to Common Communicable Diseases *on page 1651*

Doxycycline Calcium *see* Doxycycline *on page 450*

Doxycycline Hyclate *see* Doxycycline *on page 450*

Doxycycline Monohydrate *see* Doxycycline *on page 450*

DPA *see* Valproic Acid and Derivatives *on page 1382*

DPH *see* Phenytoin *on page 1073*

DPT *see page 1498*

Dramamine® II [OTC] *see* Meclizine *on page 840*

Dri/Ear® *see page 1519*

Drisdol® *see* Ergocalciferol *on page 483*

Drithocreme® *see* Anthralin *on page 108*

Drithocreme® HP 1% *see* Anthralin *on page 108*

Dritho-Scalp® *see* Anthralin *on page 108*

Dronabinol (droe NAB i nol)

U.S. Brand Names Marinol®

Synonyms Tetrahydrocannabinol; THC

Restrictions C-III

Generic Available No

Pharmacologic Category Antiemetic

Pregnancy Risk Factor C

Lactation Enters breast milk/contraindicated

Use When conventional antiemetics fail to relieve the nausea and vomiting associated with cancer chemotherapy, AIDS-related anorexia

Mechanism of Action/Effect Not well defined, probably inhibits the vomiting center in the medulla oblongata

Contraindications Hypersensitivity to dronabinol or any component of the formulation, or marijuana; should be avoided in patients with a history of schizophrenia

Warnings/Precautions Use with caution in patients with heart disease, hepatic disease, or seizure disorders. Reduce dosage in patients with severe hepatic impairment. May have potential for abuse; drug is psychoactive substance in marijuana. Monitor for possible psychotic reaction with first dose. Pregnancy risk C.

Drug Interactions

Increased Effect/Toxicity: Increased toxicity (drowsiness) with alcohol, barbiturates, and benzodiazepines.

Nutritional/Ethanol Interactions

Ethanol: Avoid ethanol (may increase CNS depression).

Herb/Nutraceutical: St John's wort may decrease dronabinol levels.

Effects on Lab Values ↓ FSH, LH, growth hormone, testosterone

Adverse Reactions

>10%:

Central nervous system: Drowsiness (48%), sedation (53%), confusion (30%), dizziness (21%), detachment, anxiety, difficulty concentrating, mood change

Gastrointestinal: Increased appetite (may be troublesome when used as an antiemetic), xerostomia (38% to 50%)

1% to 10%:

Cardiovascular: Orthostatic hypotension, tachycardia

Central nervous system: Ataxia (4%), depression (7%), headache, vertigo, hallucinations (5%), memory lapse (4%)

Neuromuscular & skeletal: Paresthesia, weakness

<1% (Limited to important or life-threatening): Diaphoresis, diarrhea, myalgia, nightmares, syncope, tinnitus

Overdosage/Toxicology Symptoms of overdose include tachycardia, hyper- and hypotension. Treatment is symptomatic.

Pharmacodynamics/Kinetics

Absorption: Oral: 90% to 95%; ~10% to 20% of dose gets into systemic circulation

Half-Life Elimination: THC: 19-24 hours; THC metabolites: 49-53 hours

Time to Peak: Serum: 2-3 hours

Metabolism: Hepatic to at least 50 metabolites, some of which are active; 11-hydroxytetrahydrocannabinol (11-OH-THC) is the major metabolite; extensive first-pass effect

Onset: Within 1 hour

Formulations Capsule, gelatin: 2.5 mg, 5 mg, 10 mg

Dosing

Adults & Elderly:

Antiemetic: Oral: 5 mg/m^2 1-3 hours before chemotherapy, then give 5 mg/m^2/dose every 2-4 hours after chemotherapy for a total of 4-6 doses/day; dose may be increased up to a maximum of 15 mg/m^2/dose if needed (dosage may be increased by 2.5 mg/m^2 increments).

Appetite stimulant (AIDS-related): Oral: Initial: 2.5 mg twice daily (before lunch and dinner); titrate up to a maximum of 20 mg/day.

Pediatrics: Antiemetic: Oral: NCI protocol recommends 5 mg/m^2 starting 6-8 hours before chemotherapy and every 4-6 hours after to be continued for 12 hours after chemotherapy is discontinued.

Hepatic Impairment: Usual dose should be reduced in patients with severe liver failure.

Stability

Storage: Store in a cool place.

Monitoring and Teaching Issues

Physical Assessment: See Contraindications, Warnings/Precautions, and Dosing for use cautions. Assess potential for interactions with other prescriptions, OTC medications, or herbal products patient may be taking (see Drug Interactions). Assess effectiveness of therapy and adverse response (eg, severe psychotic reactions). This drug is the psychoactive substance in marijuana (see Adverse Reactions and Overdose/Toxicology). Teach patient appropriate use, possible side effects and interventions, and adverse symptoms to report (see Patient Education). **Pregnancy risk factor C** - benefits of use should outweigh possible risks. Breast-feeding is contraindicated.

Patient Education: Inform prescriber of all prescriptions, OTC medications, or herbal products you are taking, and any allergies you have. Do not take anything new during treatment unless approved by prescriber (especially barbiturates, and benzodiazepines). Take exactly as directed; do not increase dose or take more often than prescribed. Avoid alcohol. May cause psychotic reaction, impaired coordination or judgment, faintness, dizziness, or drowsiness (do not drive or engage in activities that require alertness and coordination until response to drug is known); or clumsiness, unsteadiness, or muscular weakness (change position slowly and use caution when climbing stairs). Report excessive or persistent CNS changes (euphoria, anxiety, depression, memory lapse, bizarre though patterns, excitability, inability to control thoughts or behavior, fainting); respiratory difficulties; rapid heartbeat; or other adverse reactions. **Pregnancy/breast-feeding precautions:** Inform prescriber if you are or intend to become pregnant. Do not breast-feed.

Related Information

Antiemetics for Chemotherapy-Induced Nausea and Vomiting *on page 1639*

Droperidol (droe PER i dole)

U.S. Brand Names Inapsine®

Generic Available Yes

Pharmacologic Category Antiemetic; Antipsychotic Agent, Butyrophenone

Pregnancy Risk Factor C

Lactation Excretion in breast milk unknown

(Continued)

Droperidol *(Continued)*

Use Antiemetic in surgical and diagnostic procedures; preoperative medication in patients when other treatments are ineffective or inappropriate

Mechanism of Action/Effect Butyrophenone derivative that produces tranquilization, sedation, and an antiemetic effect.

Contraindications Hypersensitivity to droperidol or any component of the formulation; known or suspected QT prolongation, including congenital long QT syndrome (prolonged QT_c is defined as >440 msec in males or >450 msec in females)

Warnings/Precautions Droperidol should be reserved for patients who fail to respond or do not tolerate other treatments. May alter cardiac conduction. Cases of QT prolongation and torsade de pointes have been reported, including some fatal cases, in patients treated within or even below normal dosage range. A 12-lead EKG is recommended prior to initiation; continued monitoring is recommended for 2-3 hours. Use extreme caution in patients with bradycardia (<50 bpm), cardiac disease, concurrent MAOI therapy, Class I and Class III antiarrhythmics or other drugs known to prolong QT interval, and electrolyte disturbances (hypokalemia or hypomagnesemia), including concomitant drugs which may alter electrolytes (diuretics).

Use with caution in patients with seizures, bone marrow suppression, or severe liver disease. May be sedating, use with caution in disorders where CNS depression is a feature. Caution in patients with hemodynamic instability, predisposition to seizures, subcortical brain damage, renal or respiratory disease. Esophageal dysmotility and aspiration have been associated with antipsychotic use. Caution in breast cancer or other prolactin-dependent tumors. May cause orthostatic hypotension - use with caution in patients at risk of this effect. Significant hypotension may occur; injection contains benzyl alcohol; injection also contains sulfites which may cause allergic reaction.

Relative to other neuroleptics, droperidol has a low potency of cholinergic blockade. Use with caution in patients with decreased gastrointestinal motility, urinary retention, BPH, xerostomia, or visual problems. May worsen myasthenia gravis.

May cause extrapyramidal symptoms, including tardive dyskinesia. May be associated with neuroleptic malignant syndrome (NMS) or pigmentary retinopathy. Safety in children <6 months of age has not been established.

Pregnancy risk C.

Drug Interactions

Increased Effect/Toxicity: Droperidol in combination with certain forms of conduction anesthesia may produce peripheral vasodilitation and hypotension. Droperidol and CNS depressants will likely have additive CNS effects. Droperidol and cyclobenzaprine may have an additive effect on prolonging the QT interval. Use caution with other agents known to prolong QT interval (Class I or Class III antiarrhythmics, some quinolone antibiotics, cisapride, some phenothiazines, pimozide, tricyclic antidepressants). Potassium- or magnesium-depleting agents (diuretics, aminoglycosides, amphotericin B, cyclosporine) may increase risk of arrhythmias. Metoclopramide may increase risk of extrapyramidal symptoms (EPS).

Adverse Reactions EKG changes, retinal pigmentation are more common than with chlorpromazine. Relative to other neuroleptics, droperidol has a low potency of cholinergic blockade.

>10%:
- Cardiovascular: QT_c prolongation (dose dependent)
- Central nervous system: Restlessness, anxiety, extrapyramidal reactions, dystonic reactions, pseudoparkinsonian signs and symptoms, tardive dyskinesia, neuroleptic malignant syndrome (NMS), seizures, altered central temperature regulation, akathisia
- Endocrine & metabolic: Swelling of breasts
- Gastrointestinal: Weight gain, constipation

1% to 10%:
- Cardiovascular: Hypotension (especially orthostatic), tachycardia, abnormal T waves with prolonged ventricular repolarization
- Central nervous system: Hallucinations, sedation, drowsiness, persistent tardive dyskinesia
- Gastrointestinal: Nausea, vomiting
- Genitourinary: Dysuria

<1% (Limited to important or life-threatening): Adynamic ileus, agranulocytosis, alopecia, arrhythmia, cholestatic jaundice, decreased visual acuity (may be irreversible), heat stroke, hyperpigmentation, laryngospasm, leukopenia, neuroleptic malignant syndrome (NMS), obstructive jaundice, photosensitivity (rare), priapism, rash, respiratory depression, retinal pigmentation, tardive dystonia, torsade de pointes, urinary retention, ventricular tachycardia

Overdosage/Toxicology Symptoms of overdose include hypotension, tachycardia, hallucinations, and extrapyramidal symptoms. Following initiation of essential overdose management, toxic symptom treatment and supportive treatment should be initiated. Prolonged QT interval, seizures, and arrhythmias have been reported.

Pharmacodynamics/Kinetics

Half-Life Elimination: Adults: 2.3 hours

Metabolism: Hepatic

Onset: Peak effect: Parenteral: Within 30 minutes

Duration: Parenteral: 2-4 hours, may extend to 12 hours

Formulations Injection, solution: 2.5 mg/mL (1 mL, 2 mL)

Dosing

Adults: Titrate carefully to desired effect: Nausea and vomiting: I.M., I.V.: Initial: 2.5 mg; additional doses of 1.25 mg may be administered to achieve desired effect; administer additional doses with caution

Elderly: Elderly patients should be started on lowest dose recommendations for adults; titrate carefully to desired effect.

Pediatrics: Titrate carefully to desired effect: Children 2-12 years: Nausea and vomiting: I.M., I.V.: 0.05-0.06 mg/kg (maximum initial dose: 0.1 mg/kg); additional doses may be repeated to achieve effect; administer additional doses with caution

Administration

I.V.: I.V. should be administered slow IVP (over 2-5 minutes) or IVPB. EKG monitoring for 2-3 hours after administration is recommended.

Stability

Storage: Droperidol ampuls/vials should be stored at room temperature and protected from light.

Reconstitution:

Standard diluent: 2.5 mg/50 mL D_5W

Stability of parenteral admixture at room temperature (25°C): 7 days

Compatibility: Stable in D_5W, LR, NS

Y-site administration: Incompatible with allopurinol, amphotericin B cholesteryl sulfate complex, cefepime, fluorouracil, foscarnet, furosemide, leucovorin, nafcillin, piperacillin/tazobactam

Compatibility in syringe: Incompatible with fluorouracil, furosemide, heparin, leucovorin, methotrexate, ondansetron, pentobarbital

Monitoring Laboratory Tests To identify QT prolongation, a 12-lead EKG prior to use is recommended (use is contraindicated); continued EKG monitoring for 2-3 hours following administration is recommended.

Monitoring and Teaching Issues

Physical Assessment: Assess other medications the patient may be taking for effectiveness and interactions (see Drug Interactions). See Contraindications and Warnings/Precautions for use cautions. Monitor vital signs and respiratory status on a frequent basis immediately following administration and for several hours afterward. Monitor for extrapyramidal symptoms for 24-48 hours after therapy (see Adverse Reactions and Overdose/Toxicology). Teach and use safety precautions until the patient is stable. Teach adverse reactions to report. **Pregnancy risk factor C** - benefits of use should outweigh possible risks. Note breast-feeding caution.

Patient Education: This drug may cause you to feel very sleepy; do not attempt to get up without assistance. Immediately report any difficulty breathing, confusion, loss of thought processes, or palpitations. **Pregnancy/breast-feeding precautions:** Inform prescriber if you are pregnant. Consult prescriber if breast-feeding.

Geriatric Considerations: Use of droperidol in the elderly may result in severe and often irreversible undesirable effects. Before initiating antipsychotic therapy, the clinician should investigate possible reversible causes.

Additional Information Does not possess analgesic effects; has little or no amnesic properties.

Related Information

Antiemetics for Chemotherapy-Induced Nausea and Vomiting *on page 1639*

Drospirenone and Ethinyl Estradiol *see* Ethinyl Estradiol and Drospirenone *on page 519*

Drotrecogin Alfa (dro TRE coe jin AL fa)

U.S. Brand Names Xigris®

Synonyms Activated Protein C, Human, Recombinant; Drotrecogin Alfa, Activated; Protein C (Activated), Human, Recombinant

Generic Available No

Pharmacologic Category Protein C (Activated)

Pregnancy Risk Factor C

Lactation Excretion in breast milk unknown/not recommended

Use Reduction of mortality from severe sepsis (associated with organ dysfunction) in adults at high risk of death (eg, APACHE II score ≥25)

Mechanism of Action/Effect Decreases mortality from severe sepsis by blocking thrombotic activity. Blocks factor Va and VIIIa. In addition, may have other anti-inflammatory effects.

Contraindications Hypersensitivity to drotrecogin alfa or any component of the formulation; active internal bleeding; recent hemorrhagic stroke (within 3 months); severe head trauma (within 2 months); recent intracranial or intraspinal surgery (within 2 months); intracranial neoplasm or mass lesion; evidence of cerebral herniation; presence of an epidural catheter; trauma with an increased risk of life-threatening bleeding

Warnings/Precautions Increases risk of bleeding; careful evaluation of risks and benefit is required prior to initiation (see Contraindications). Bleeding risk is increased in patients receiving concurrent therapeutic heparin, oral anticoagulants, glycoprotein IIb/IIIa antagonists, platelet aggregation inhibitors, or aspirin at a dosage of >650 mg/day (within 7 days). In addition, an increased bleeding risk is associated with prolonged INR (>3.0), gastrointestinal bleeding (within 6 weeks), decreased platelet count (<30,000/mm^3), thrombolytic therapy (within 3 days), recent ischemic stroke (within 3 months), intracranial AV malformation or aneurysm, known bleeding diathesis, severe hepatic disease (chronic), or other condition where bleeding is a significant hazard or difficult to manage due to its location. Discontinue if significant bleeding occurs (may consider continued use after stabilization). Treatment interruption required for invasive procedures. APTT cannot be used to assess coagulopathy during treatment (PT/INR not affected).

Efficacy not established in adult patients at a low risk of death. Patients with pre-existing nonsepsis-related medical conditions with a poor prognosis (anticipated survival <28 days), patients with acute pancreatitis (no established source of infection), HIV-infected patients with a CD4 count ≤50 cells/mm^3, chronic dialysis patients, pre-existing hypercoagulable conditions, and patients who had received bone marrow, liver, lung, pancreas, or small bowel transplants were excluded from the clinical trial which established benefit. In addition, patients with a high body weight (>135 kg) were not evaluated. Safety and efficacy have not been established in pediatric patients.

Pregnancy risk C.

(Continued)

Drotrecogin Alfa *(Continued)*

Drug Interactions

Increased Effect/Toxicity: Concurrent use of antiplatelet agents, including aspirin (>650 mg/day, recent use within 7 days), cilostazol, clopidogrel, dipyridamole, ticlopidine, NSAIDs, or glycoprotein IIb/IIIa antagonists (recent use within 7 days) may increase risk of bleeding. Concurrent use of low molecular weight heparins or heparin at therapeutic rates of infusion may increase the risk of bleeding. However, the use of low-dose prophylactic heparin does not appear to affect safety. Recent use of thrombolytic agents (within 3 days) may increase the risk of bleeding. Recent use of warfarin (within 7 days or elevation of INR ≥3) may increase the risk of bleeding. Other drugs which interfere with coagulation may increase risk of bleeding (including antithrombin III, danaparoid, direct thrombin inhibitors)

Nutritional/Ethanol Interactions Herb/Nutraceutical: Recent use/intake of herbs with anticoagulant or antiplatelet activity (including cat's claw, feverfew, garlic, ginkgo, ginseng, and horse chestnut seed) may increase the risk of bleeding.

Adverse Reactions As with all drugs which may affect hemostasis, bleeding is the major adverse effect associated with drotrecogin alfa. Hemorrhage may occur at virtually any site. Risk is dependent on multiple variables, including the dosage administered, concurrent use of multiple agents which alter hemostasis, and patient predisposition.

>10%

Dermatologic: Bruising

Gastrointestinal: Gastrointestinal bleeding

1% to 10%: Hematologic: Bleeding (serious 2.4% during infusion vs 3.5% during 28-day study period; individual events listed as <1%)

<1% (Limited to important or life-threatening): Gastrointestinal hemorrhage, genitourinary bleeding, immune reaction (antibody production), intracranial hemorrhage (0.2%; frequencies up to 2% noted in a previous trial without placebo control), intrathoracic hemorrhage, retroperitoneal bleeding, skin/soft tissue bleeding

Overdosage/Toxicology No reported experience with overdose. Hemorrhagic complications are likely consequence of overdose. Treatment is supportive, including immediate interruption of the infusion and monitoring for hemorrhagic complications. No known antidote.

Pharmacodynamics/Kinetics

Half-Life Elimination: 1.6 hours

Metabolism: Inactivated by endogenous plasma protease inhibitors; mean clearance: 40 L/hour; increased with severe sepsis (~50%)

Duration: Plasma nondetectable within 2 hours of discontinuation

Formulations Injection, powder for reconstitution [preservative free]: 5 mg, 20 mg

Dosing

Adults: Severe sepsis: I.V.: 24 mcg/kg/hour for a total of 96 hours; stop infusion **immediately** if clinically-important bleeding is identified.

Renal Impairment: No specific adjustment recommended.

Administration

I.V.: Administer via infusion pump or syringe pump. Administration must be completed within 12 hours of solution preparation. Suspend administration for 2 hours prior to invasive procedures or other procedure with significant bleeding risk; may continue treatment immediately following uncomplicated, minimally-invasive procedures, but delay for 12 hours after major invasive procedures/surgery.

Stability

Storage: Store vials under refrigeration at 2°C to 8°C (36°F to 46°F). Protect from light. Do not freeze.

Reconstitution: Reconstitute 5 mg vials with 2.5 mL and 20 mg vials with 10 mL sterile water for injection (resultant solution ~2 mg/mL). Must be further diluted (within 3 hours of reconstitution) in 0.9% sodium chloride, typically to a concentration between 100 mcg/mL and 200 mcg/mL when using infusion pump and between 100 mcg/mL and 1000 mcg/mL when infused via syringe pump. Although product information states administration must be completed within 12 hours of preparation, additional studies (data on file, Lilly Research Laboratories) show that the final solution is stable for 14 hours at 15°C to 30°C (59°F to 86°F). If not used immediately, a prepared solution may be stored in the refrigerator for up to 12 hours. The total expiration time (refrigeration and administration) should be ≤24 hours from time of preparation.

Compatibility: Stable in NS; only NS, dextrose, LR, or dextrose/saline mixtures may be infused through the same line.

Monitoring Laboratory Tests Monitor for signs and symptoms of bleeding, hemoglobin/hematocrit, PT/INR, platelet count

Monitoring and Teaching Issues

Physical Assessment: See Contraindications, Warnings/Precautions, and Dosing for use cautions. Assess potential for interactions with other prescriptions, OTC medications, or herbal products patient may be taking (especially drugs affecting coagulation or platelet activity - see Drug Interactions). See specific Administration, Reconstitution, and Compatibility directions. Assess results of laboratory tests (see Monitoring Laboratory Tests) prior to, during, and following therapy. Patient must be monitored very closely for bleeding during and following infusion (hemorrhage may occur at virtually any site - see Adverse Reactions and Overdose/Toxicology). If significant bleeding occurs, infusion should be stopped and prescriber notified immediately. Bleeding precautions must be observed. Patient instruction should be according to patient condition (see Patient Education). **Pregnancy risk factor C** - benefits of use should outweigh possible risks. Breast-feeding is not recommended.

Patient Education: Inform prescriber of all prescriptions, OTC medications, or herbal products you are taking, and any allergies you have. This medication can only be administered by infusion. You will be monitored closely. Report immediately any unusual or acute abdominal pain or headache, or difficulty breathing. You will be more susceptible to bleeding and bruising; remain in bed and ring for assistance to avoid falling or injuring yourself. Avoid sharps of any kind (knives, scissors, needles, nail clippers, etc; shave with a safety razor). **Pregnancy/breast-feeding precautions:** Inform prescriber if you are pregnant. Breast-feeding is not recommended.

Additional Information Prepared by recombinant DNA technology in human cell line

Drotrecogin Alfa, Activated *see* Drotrecogin Alfa *on page 455*

Droxia™ *see* Hydroxyurea *on page 682*

DSCG *see* Cromolyn Sodium *on page 334*

D-S-S® [OTC] *see* Docusate *on page 432*

DTIC *see* Dacarbazine *on page 353*

DTIC-Dome® *see* Dacarbazine *on page 353*

DTO *see* Opium Tincture *on page 1006*

DuoNeb™ *see* Ipratropium and Albuterol *on page 735*

DuP 753 *see* Losartan *on page 824*

Duraclon™ *see* Clonidine *on page 316*

Duragesic® *see* Fentanyl *on page 552*

Duralone® *see* MethylPREDNISolone *on page 885*

Duramorph® *see* Morphine Sulfate *on page 926*

Duratuss™ *see* Guaifenesin and Pseudoephedrine *on page 648*

Duratuss® DM *see* Guaifenesin and Dextromethorphan *on page 647*

Duratuss-G® *see* Guaifenesin *on page 646*

Duratuss™ GP *see* Guaifenesin and Pseudoephedrine *on page 648*

Dura-Vent®/DA *see page 1522*

Duricef® *see* Cefadroxil *on page 231*

D-Xylose *see page 1461*

Dyazide® *see* Hydrochlorothiazide and Triamterene *on page 667*

Dyclonine (DYE kloe neen)

U.S. Brand Names Cēpacol® Maximum Strength [OTC]; Sucrets® [OTC]

Synonyms Dyclonine Hydrochloride

Generic Available No

Pharmacologic Category Local Anesthetic; Local Anesthetic, Oral

Pregnancy Risk Factor C

Lactation Excretion in breast milk unknown

Use Local anesthetic prior to laryngoscopy, bronchoscopy, or endotracheal intubation; use topically for temporary relief of pain associated with oral mucosa or anogenital lesions

Mechanism of Action/Effect Blocks impulses at peripheral nerve endings in skin and mucous membranes by altering cell membrane permeability to ionic transfer

Contraindications Contraindicated in patients allergic to chlorobutanol (preservative used in dyclonine) or dyclonine

Warnings/Precautions Use with caution in patients with sepsis or traumatized mucosa in the area of application to avoid rapid systemic absorption. May impair swallowing and enhance the danger of aspiration. Use with caution in patients with shock or heart block. Resuscitative equipment, oxygen, and resuscitative drugs should be immediately available when dyclonine topical solution is administered to mucous membranes. **Not for injection or ophthalmic use**. Pregnancy risk C.

Adverse Reactions <1% (Limited to important or life-threatening): Allergic reactions, blurred vision, bradycardia, cardiac arrest, hypotension, respiratory arrest, seizures

Overdosage/Toxicology Symptoms of overdose are CNS (seizures, excitation) and cardiovascular (hypotension, myocardial depression). Treatment is supportive and symptomatic.

Pharmacodynamics/Kinetics

Onset: Local anesthetic: 2-10 minutes

Duration: 30-60 minutes

Formulations

Lozenge, as hydrochloride (Sucrets®): 1.2 mg, 2 mg, 3 mg [cherry, lemon, wintergreen, and assorted flavors]

Spray, oral, as hydrochloride (Cēpacol® Maximum Strength): 0.1% (120 mL) [cherry and menthol flavors]

Dosing

Adults & Elderly: Note: Administered as topical solution, use lowest dose needed to provide effective anesthesia:

Mouth sores: Topical: 5-10 mL of 0.5% or 1% to oral mucosa (swab or swish and then spit) 3-4 times/day as needed; maximum single dose: 200 mg (40 mL of 0.5% solution or 20 mL of 1% solution)

Bronchoscopy: Topical: Use 2 mL of the 1% solution or 4 mL of the 0.5% solution sprayed onto the larynx and trachea every 5 minutes until the reflex has been abolished.

Pediatrics: Refer to adult dosing.

Stability

Storage: Store in tight, light-resistant containers.

Monitoring and Teaching Issues

Physical Assessment: See Warnings/Precautions for use cautions. Monitor for effectiveness of anesthesia and for adverse or toxic reactions. Monitor for return of sensation. Teach patient adverse reactions to report; use and teach appropriate interventions to promote safety. **Pregnancy risk factor C** - benefits of use should outweigh possible risks. Note breast-feeding caution.

Patient Education: This medication is given to reduce sensation in the injected area. When used in mouth or throat; do not eat or drink anything for at least 1 hour following treatment. Take small sips of water at first to ensure that you can swallow without difficulty. Your tongue and mouth may be numb - use caution to avoid biting yourself. Immediately report swelling of face, lips, tongue; chest pain or palpitations; increased restlessness,

(Continued)

Dyclonine *(Continued)*

confusion, anxiety, or dizziness. **Pregnancy/breast-feeding precautions:** Inform prescriber if you are or intend to become pregnant. Consult prescriber if breast-feeding.

Dietary Issues: Food should not be ingested for 60 minutes following application in the mouth or throat area.

Dyclonine Hydrochloride *see* Dyclonine *on page 457*

Dynacin® *see* Minocycline *on page 909*

DynaCirc® *see* Isradipine *on page 754*

DynaCirc® CR *see* Isradipine *on page 754*

E_2C and MPA *see* Estradiol and Medroxyprogesterone *on page 497*

7E3 *see* Abciximab *on page 31*

E2020 *see* Donepezil *on page 436*

Ear-Sol® H.C. *see page 1519*

EarSol® HC *see* Hydrocortisone *on page 673*

Easprin® *see* Aspirin *on page 121*

Echothiophate *see page 1575*

Echothiophate *see* Ophthalmic Agents, Glaucoma *on page 1002*

EC-Naprosyn® *see* Naproxen *on page 948*

***E. coli* Asparaginase** *see* Asparaginase *on page 118*

Econopred® *see* PrednisoLONE *on page 1113*

Econopred® Plus *see* PrednisoLONE *on page 1113*

Ecotrin® [OTC] *see* Aspirin *on page 121*

Ecotrin® Low Adult Strength [OTC] *see* Aspirin *on page 121*

Ecotrin® Maximum Strength [OTC] *see* Aspirin *on page 121*

Edecrin® [DSC] *see* Ethacrynic Acid *on page 511*

Edex® *see* Alprostadil *on page 65*

Edrophonium (ed roe FOE nee um)

U.S. Brand Names Enlon®; Reversol®

Synonyms Edrophonium Chloride

Generic Available Yes

Pharmacologic Category Antidote; Cholinergic Agonist; Diagnostic Agent

Pregnancy Risk Factor C

Lactation Excretion in breast milk unknown

Use Diagnosis of myasthenia gravis; differentiation of cholinergic crises from myasthenia crises; reversal of nondepolarizing neuromuscular blockers; adjunct treatment of respiratory depression caused by curare overdose

Mechanism of Action/Effect Inhibits destruction of acetylcholine by acetylcholinesterase. This facilitates transmission of impulses across myoneural junction and results in increased cholinergic responses such as miosis, increased tonus of intestinal and skeletal muscles, bronchial and ureteral constriction, bradycardia, and increased salivary and sweat gland secretions.

Contraindications Hypersensitivity to edrophonium, sulfites, or any component of the formulation; GI or GU obstruction

Warnings/Precautions Use with caution in patients with bronchial asthma and those receiving a cardiac glycoside. Atropine sulfate should always be readily available as an antagonist. Overdosage can cause cholinergic crisis which may be fatal (DUMBELS - **d**iarrhea, **u**rination, **m**iosis, **b**ronchospasm/**b**radycardia, **e**xcitability, **l**acrimation, **s**alivation/excessive **s**weating), and acute muscle weakness. I.V. atropine should be readily available for treatment of cholinergic reactions. Pregnancy risk C.

Drug Interactions

Decreased Effect: Atropine, nondepolarizing muscle relaxants, procainamide, and quinidine may antagonize the effects of edrophonium.

Increased Effect/Toxicity: Digoxin may enhance bradycardia potential of edrophonium. Effects of succinylcholine, decamethonium, nondepolarizing muscle relaxants (eg, pancuronium, vecuronium) are prolonged by edrophonium. I.V. acetazolamide, neostigmine, physostigmine, and acute muscle weakness may increase the effects of edrophonium.

Effects on Lab Values ↑ aminotransferase [ALT (SGPT)/AST (SGOT)] (S), amylase (S)

Adverse Reactions Frequency not defined.

Cardiovascular: Arrhythmias (especially bradycardia), hypotension, decreased carbon monoxide, tachycardia, AV block, nodal rhythm, nonspecific EKG changes, cardiac arrest, syncope, flushing

Central nervous system: Convulsions, dysarthria, dysphonia, dizziness, loss of consciousness, drowsiness, headache

Dermatologic: Skin rash, thrombophlebitis (I.V.), urticaria

Gastrointestinal: Hyperperistalsis, nausea, vomiting, salivation, diarrhea, stomach cramps, dysphagia, flatulence

Genitourinary: Urinary urgency

Neuromuscular & skeletal: Weakness, fasciculations, muscle cramps, spasms, arthralgias

Ocular: Small pupils, lacrimation

Respiratory: Increased bronchial secretions, laryngospasm, bronchiolar constriction, respiratory muscle paralysis, dyspnea, respiratory depression, respiratory arrest, bronchospasm

Miscellaneous: Diaphoresis (increased), anaphylaxis, allergic reactions

Overdosage/Toxicology Symptoms of overdose include muscle weakness, nausea, vomiting, miosis, bronchospasm, and respiratory paralysis. Maintain an adequate airway. For muscarinic symptoms, the antidote is atropine 0.4-0.5 mg I.V. repeated every 3-10 minutes (initial doses as high as 1.2 mg have been administered). Skeletal muscle effects of edrophonium are not alleviated by atropine.

Pharmacodynamics/Kinetics

Half-Life Elimination: 1.8 hours

Onset: I.M.: 2-10 minutes; I.V.: 30-60 seconds

Duration: I.M.: 5-30 minutes: I.V.: 10 minutes

Formulations Injection, solution, as chloride: 10 mg/mL (15 mL)

Enlon®: 10 mg/mL (15 mL) [contains sodium sulfite]

Reversol®: 10 mg/mL (10 mL) [contains sodium sulfite]

Dosing

Adults & Elderly: Usually administered I.V., however, if not possible, I.M. or S.C. may be used.

Diagnosis:

I.V.: 2 mg test dose administered over 15-30 seconds; 8 mg given 45 seconds later if no response is seen. Test dose may be repeated after 30 minutes.

I.M.: Initial: 10 mg; if no cholinergic reaction occurs, give 2 mg 30 minutes later to rule out false-negative reaction.

Titration of oral anticholinesterase therapy: 1-2 mg given 1 hour after oral dose of anticholinesterase; if strength improves, an increase in neostigmine or pyridostigmine dose is indicated.

Reversal of nondepolarizing neuromuscular blocking agents (neostigmine with atropine usually preferred): I.V.: 10 mg over 30-45 seconds; may repeat every 5-10 minutes up to 40 mg.

Termination of paroxysmal atrial tachycardia: I.V. rapid injection: 5-10 mg

Differentiation of cholinergic from myasthenic crisis: I.V.: 1 mg; may repeat after 1 minute. **Note:** Intubation and controlled ventilation may be required if patient has cholinergic crisis.

Pediatrics: Usually administered I.V., however, if not possible, I.M. or S.C. may be used:

Infants:

I.M.: 0.5-1 mg

I.V.: Initial: 0.1 mg, followed by 0.4 mg if no response; total dose = 0.5 mg

Children:

Diagnosis: Initial: 0.04 mg/kg over 1 minute followed by 0.16 mg/kg if no response, to a maximum total dose of 5 mg for children <34 kg, or 10 mg for children >34 kg

I.M.:

<34 kg: 1 mg

>34 kg: 5 mg

Titration of oral anticholinesterase therapy: 0.04 mg/kg once given 1 hour after oral intake of the drug being used in treatment. If strength improves, an increase in neostigmine or pyridostigmine dose is indicated.

Renal Impairment: Dose may need to be reduced in patients with chronic renal failure.

Monitoring and Teaching Issues

Physical Assessment: Administration of edrophonium for MG diagnosis is supervised by a neurologist and use as a neuromuscular blocking agent is supervised by an anesthesiologist. Patient must be monitored closely during and following procedure, especially for cholinergic crisis; keep atropine at hand for antidote. Patients receiving the medication for MG testing will have been advised by their neurologist about drug effects. Those patients receiving medication for neuromuscular block will be unaware of drug effects. Patient should never be left alone until all drug effects and the possibility of cholinergic crisis have passed. **Pregnancy risk factor C** - benefits of use should outweigh possible risks. Note breast-feeding caution.

Patient Education: **Pregnancy/breast-feeding precautions:** Inform prescriber if you are or intend to become pregnant. Consult prescriber if breast-feeding.

Geriatric Considerations: Many elderly will have diseases which may influence the use of edrophonium. Also, many elderly will need doses reduced 50% due to creatinine clearances in the 10-50 mL/minute range (common in the aged). Side effects or concomitant disease may warrant use of pyridostigmine.

Additional Information Atropine should be administered along with edrophonium when reversing the effects of nondepolarizing agents to antagonize the cholinergic effects at the muscarinic receptors, especially bradycardia. It is important to recognize the difference in dose for diagnosis of myasthenia gravis versus reversal of muscle relaxant, a much larger dose is needed for desired effect of reversal of muscle paralysis.

Edrophonium Chloride *see* Edrophonium *on page 458*

E.E.S.® *see* Erythromycin (Systemic) *on page 486*

Efavirenz (e FAV e renz)

U.S. Brand Names Sustiva®

Generic Available No

Pharmacologic Category Antiretroviral Agent, Reverse Transcriptase Inhibitor (Non-nucleoside)

Pregnancy Risk Factor C

Lactation Excretion is breast milk unknown/contraindicated

Use Treatment of HIV-1 infections in combination with at least two other antiretroviral agents. Also has some activity against hepatitis B virus and herpes viruses.

Mechanism of Action/Effect As a non-nucleoside reverse transcriptase inhibitor, efavirenz has activity against HIV-1 by binding to reverse transcriptase. It consequently blocks the RNA-dependent and DNA-dependent DNA polymerase activities including HIV-1 replication. It does not require intracellular phosphorylation for antiviral activity.

Contraindications Clinically significant hypersensitivity efavirenz or any component of the formulation

Warnings/Precautions Do not use as single-agent therapy. Do not administer with other agents metabolized by cytochrome P450 isoenzyme 3A4 including cisapride, midazolam, triazolam, or ergot alkaloids (potential for life-threatening adverse effects). History of mental illness/drug abuse (predisposition to psychological reactions). Serious psychiatric side effects

(Continued)

Efavirenz *(Continued)*

have been associated with efavirenz, including severe depression, suicide, paranoia, and mania. Discontinue if severe rash (involving blistering, desquamation, mucosal involvement, or fever) develops. Use caution in patients with known or suspected hepatitis B or C infection (monitoring of liver function is recommended); hepatic impairment. Persistent elevations of serum transaminases greater than five times the upper limit of normal should prompt evaluation - benefit of continued therapy should be weighed against possible risk of hepatotoxicity. Children are more susceptible to development of rash; prophylactic antihistamines may be used. Women of childbearing potential should undergo pregnancy testing prior to initiation of therapy. Pregnancy risk C.

Drug Interactions

Cytochrome P450 Effect: Substrate of **CYP2B6, 3A4**; Inhibits CYP2C8/9, 2C19, 3A4; Induces CYP2B6, 3A4

Decreased Effect: Other inducers of this enzyme (including phenobarbital, rifampin, rifabutin, and St John's wort) may decrease serum concentrations of efavirenz. Concentrations of indinavir may be reduced; dosage increase to 1000 mg 3 times/day is recommended. Concentrations of saquinavir may be decreased (use as sole protease inhibitor is not recommended). The AUC of amprenavir may be decreased (36%). Plasma concentrations of clarithromycin are decreased (clinical significance unknown). Serum concentrations of methadone are decreased; monitor for withdrawal. May decrease (or increase) effect of warfarin.

Increased Effect/Toxicity: Coadministration with medications metabolized by these enzymes may lead to increased concentration-related effects. Cisapride, midazolam, triazolam, and ergot alkaloids may result in life-threatening toxicities; concurrent use is contraindicated. The AUC of nelfinavir is increased (20%); AUC of both ritonavir and efavirenz are increased by 20% during concurrent therapy. The AUC of ethinyl estradiol is increased 37% by efavirenz (clinical significance unknown). May increase (or decrease) effect of warfarin.

Nutritional/Ethanol Interactions

Ethanol: Avoid ethanol (hepatic and CNS adverse effects).

Food: Avoid high-fat meals (increase the absorption of efavirenz).

Herb/Nutraceutical: St John's wort may decrease efavirenz serum levels. Avoid concurrent use.

Effects on Lab Values False-positive test for cannabinoids have been reported when the CEDIA DAU Multilevel THC assay is used. False-positive results with other assays for cannabinoids have not been observed.

Adverse Reactions

>10%:

- Central nervous system: Dizziness* (2% to 28%), depression (1% to 16%), insomnia (6% to 16%), anxiety (1% to 11%), pain* (1% to 13%)
- Dermatologic: Rash* (NCI grade 1: 9% to 11%; NCI grade 2: 15% to 32%)
- Endocrine & metabolic: HDL increased (25% to 35%), total cholesterol increased (20% to 40%)
- Gastrointestinal: Diarrhea* (3% to 14%), nausea* (2% to 12%)

1% to 10%

- Central nervous system: Impaired concentration (2% to 8%), headache* (2% to 7%), somnolence (2% to 7%), fatigue (2% to 7%), abnormal dreams (1% to 6%), nervousness (2% to 6%), severe depression (2%), hallucinations (1%)
- Dermatologic: Pruritus (1% to 9%), diaphoresis increased (1% to 2%)
- Gastrointestinal: Vomiting* (6% to 7%), dyspepsia (3%), abdominal pain (1% to 3%), anorexia (1% to 2%)

*Adverse effect reported in ≥10% of patients 3-16 years of age

<1% (Limited to important or life-threatening): Aggressive reaction, agitation, allergic reaction, body fat accumulation/redistribution, convulsions, liver failure, manic reaction, neuropathy, paranoid reaction, Stevens-Johnson syndrome, suicide, visual abnormality

Overdosage/Toxicology Increased central nervous system symptoms and involuntary muscle contractions have been reported in accidental overdose. Treatment is supportive. Activated charcoal may enhance elimination; dialysis is unlikely to remove the drug.

Pharmacodynamics/Kinetics

Absorption: Increased 50% by fatty meals

Half-Life Elimination: Single dose: 52-76 hours; Multiple doses: 40-55 hours

Time to Peak: 3-8 hours

Metabolism: Hepatic

Formulations

Capsule: 50 mg, 100 mg, 200 mg

Tablet: 600 mg

Dosing

Adults & Elderly: Dosing at bedtime is recommended to limit central nervous system effects; should not be used as single-agent therapy.

HIV infection (as part of combination): Oral: 600 mg once daily

Pediatrics: Dosing at bedtime is recommended to limit central nervous system effects; should not be used as single-agent therapy. Dosage is based on body weight.

HIV infection (as part of combination): Oral:

- 10 kg to <15 kg: 200 mg once daily
- 15 kg to <20 kg: 250 mg once daily
- 20 kg to <25 kg: 300 mg once daily
- 25 kg to <32.5 kg: 350 mg once daily
- 32.5 kg to <40 kg: 400 mg once daily
- ≥40 kg: 600 mg once daily

Renal Impairment: No adjustment is necessary.

Hepatic Impairment: Limited clinical experience - use with caution.

Administration

Oral: Administer on an empty stomach.

Stability

Storage: Store below 25°C (77°F).

Monitoring Laboratory Tests False-positive test for cannabinoids have been reported when the CEDIA DAU Multi-Level THC assay is used. False-positive results with other assays for cannabinoids have not been observed. Monitor serum transaminases (discontinuation of treatment should be considered for persistent elevations greater than five times the upper limit of normal), cholesterol, and triglycerides.

Monitoring and Teaching Issues

Physical Assessment: See Contraindications, Warnings/Precautions, and Dosing for use cautions. Assess potential for interactions with other prescriptions, OTC medications, or herbal products patient may be taking (see Drug Interactions). Assess results of laboratory tests (see above), therapeutic response, and adverse reactions (see Adverse Reactions and Overdose/Toxicology) on a regular basis throughout therapy. Teach patient proper use, possible side effects and interventions, and adverse symptoms to report (see Patient Education). **Pregnancy risk factor C** - benefits of use should outweigh possible risks. Women of childbearing potential should undergo pregnancy testing prior to initiation of therapy. Breast-feeding is contraindicated.

Patient Education: Inform prescriber of all prescriptions, OTC medications, or herbal products you are taking, and any allergies you have. Do not take anything new during treatment unless approved by prescriber. This drug is not a cure for HIV nor has it been found to reduce transmission of HIV. Take as directed, with or without food. This drug is usually used in combination with other medications; maintain recommended schedule of all medications. Maintain adequate hydration (2-3 L/day of fluids) unless advised by prescriber to restrict fluids. Avoid alcohol (may cause undesirable reactions). May cause dizziness, anxiety, tremor, impaired coordination, inability to concentrate (use caution when driving or engaging in tasks requiring alertness until response to drug is known); nausea or vomiting (small, frequent meals, good mouth care, chewing gum, or sucking lozenges may help - consult prescriber if nausea or vomiting persists); or diarrhea (buttermilk, boiled milk, or yogurt may help). Report CNS changes (acute headache, abnormal dreams, sleepiness or fatigue, seizures, hallucinations, amnesia, emotional lability, confusion); muscle pain, weakness, tremors, numbness; rash; or other unusual effects. **Pregnancy/breast-feeding precautions:** Inform prescriber if you are or intend to become pregnant. Do not breast-feed.

Dietary Issues: Should be taken on an empty stomach.

Breast-feeding Issues: HIV-infected mothers are discouraged from breast-feeding to decrease potential transmission of HIV.

Pregnancy Issues: Teratogenic effects have been observed in Primates receiving efavirenz; no studies in pregnant humans are currently planned. Pregnancy should be avoided. Women of childbearing potential should undergo pregnancy testing prior to initiation of efavirenz. Barrier contraception should be used in combination with other (hormonal) methods of contraception. Health professionals are encouraged to contact the antiretroviral pregnancy registry to monitor outcomes of pregnant women exposed to antiretroviral medications (1-800-258-4263).

Additional Information Evafirenz oral solution is available only through an expanded access (compassionate use) program. Enrollment information may be obtained by calling 1-877-372-7097.

Related Information

Tuberculosis *on page 1705*

Effer-K™ *see* Potassium Supplements *on page 1106*

Effexor® *see* Venlafaxine *on page 1394*

Effexor® XR *see* Venlafaxine *on page 1394*

Efidac/24® [OTC] *see* Pseudoephedrine *on page 1150*

Eflone® *see* Fluorometholone *on page 575*

Eflornithine (ee FLOR ni theen)

U.S. Brand Names Vaniqa™

Synonyms DFMO; Eflornithine Hydrochloride

Generic Available No

Pharmacologic Category Antiprotozoal; Topical Skin Product

Pregnancy Risk Factor C

Lactation Excretion in breast milk unknown/use caution

Use Cream: Females ≥12 years: Reduce unwanted hair from face and adjacent areas under the chin

Orphan status: Injection: Treatment of meningoencephalitic stage of *Trypanosoma brucei gambiense* infection (sleeping sickness)

Mechanism of Action/Effect Eflornithine exerts antitumor and antiprotozoal effects through specific, irreversible ("suicide") inhibition of the enzyme ornithine decarboxylase (ODC). ODC is the rate-limiting enzyme in the biosynthesis of putrescine, spermine, and spermidine, the major polyamines in nucleated cells. Polyamines are necessary for the synthesis of DNA, RNA, and proteins and are, therefore, necessary for cell growth and differentiation. Although many microorganisms and higher plants are able to produce polyamines from alternate biochemical pathways, all mammalian cells depend on ornithine decarboxylase to produce polyamines. Eflornithine inhibits ODC and rapidly depletes animal cells of putrescine and spermidine; the concentration of spermine remains the same or may even increase. Rapidly dividing cells appear to be most susceptible to the effects of eflornithine. Topically, the inhibition of ODC in the skin leads to a decreased rate of hair growth.

Contraindications Hypersensitivity to eflornithine or any component of the formulation

(Continued)

Eflornithine *(Continued)*

Warnings/Precautions

Injection: Must be diluted before use. Frequent monitoring for myelosuppression should be done. Use with caution in patients with a history of seizures and in patients with renal impairment. Serial audiograms should be obtained. Due to the potential for relapse, patients should be followed up for at least 24 months.

Cream: For topical use by females only. Discontinue if hypersensitivity occurs. Safety and efficacy in children <12 years has not been studied.

Pregnancy risk C.

Drug Interactions

Decreased Effect: Cream: Possible interactions with other topical products have not been studied.

Increased Effect/Toxicity: Cream: Possible interactions with other topical products have not been studied.

Adverse Reactions

Injection:

>10%: Hematologic (reversible): Anemia (55%), leukopenia (37%), thrombocytopenia (14%)

1% to 10%:

Central nervous system: Seizures (may be due to the disease) (8%), dizziness
Dermatologic: Alopecia
Gastrointestinal: Vomiting, diarrhea
Hematologic: Eosinophilia
Otic: Hearing impairment

<1% (Limited to important or life-threatening): Abdominal pain, anorexia, facial edema, headache, weakness

Topical:

>10%: Dermatologic: Acne (11% to 21%), pseudofolliculitis barbae (5% to 15%)

1% to 10%:

Central nervous system: Headache (4% to 5%), dizziness (1%), vertigo (0.3% to 1%)
Dermatologic: Pruritus (3% to 4%), burning skin (2% to 4%), tingling skin (1% to 4%), dry skin (2% to 3%), rash (1% to 3%), facial edema (0.3% to 3%), alopecia (1% to 2%), skin irritation (1% to 2%), erythema (up to 2%), ingrown hair (0.3% to 2%), folliculitis (up to 1%)
Gastrointestinal: Dyspepsia (2%), anorexia (0.7% to 2%)

<1% (Limited to important or life-threatening): Bleeding skin, cheilitis, contact dermatitis, herpes simplex, lip swelling, nausea, numbness, rosacea, weakness

Overdosage/Toxicology No known antidote; treatment is supportive. In mice and rats, CNS depression, seizures, death have occurred. Overdose with topical product is not expected due to low percutaneous penetration.

Pharmacodynamics/Kinetics

Absorption: Topical: <1%

Half-Life Elimination: I.V.: 3-3.5 hours; Topical: 8 hours

Formulations

Cream, topical, as hydrochloride: 13.9% (30 g)
Injection, solution, as hydrochloride: 200 mg/mL (100 mL) [orphan drug status]

Dosing

Adults & Elderly:

Unwanted facial hair (females): Topical: Apply thin layer of cream to affected areas of face and adjacent chin twice daily, at least 8 hours apart.

Trypanosoma infections: I.V. infusion (orphan drug): 100 mg/kg/dose given every 6 hours (over at least 45 minutes) for 14 days.

Pediatrics: Unwanted facial hair (females): Children ≥12 years: Refer to adult dosing.

Renal Impairment: Injection: Dose should be adjusted although no specific guidelines are available.

Stability

Storage:

Injection: Must be diluted before use and used within 24 hours of preparation.
Cream: Store at controlled room temperature 25°C (77°F); do not freeze.

Monitoring Laboratory Tests CBC with platelet counts

Monitoring and Teaching Issues

Physical Assessment: See Warnings/Precautions and Contraindications for safe use. Laboratory tests and results should be monitored on regular basis during therapy. Monitor effectiveness according to purpose for use. Patient should be monitored for adverse reactions - especially with infusion administration (see Adverse Reactions). Assess knowledge/teach patient appropriate use, adverse reactions and possible interventions, and adverse reactions to report (see Patient Education). **Pregnancy risk factor C** - benefits of use should outweigh possible risks. Note breast-feeding caution.

Patient Education: I.V.: This medication can only be administered I.V.; you will be closely monitored during therapy. Report immediately any sings of acute GI upset, seizures, altered hearing. You may lose your hair, however, it will grow back when therapy is discontinued.

Cream: This medication is for external use only. It will not prevent hair growth, but may decrease rate of growth. You will still need to use hair removal techniques while using eflornithine cream. Use only as directed; do not use more often or discontinue without consulting prescriber. Wait at least 5 minutes after removing hair to apply cream. Wash hands thoroughly prior to using cream. Apply thin lay of cream to affected areas of face and chin twice daily (at least 8 hours apart). Rub in thoroughly. Wash hands thoroughly after rubbing cream in. Do not wash area for 8 hours following application. Once cream has dried you may apply make-up over the affected area. Improvement may be seen in 4-8 weeks. Following discontinuation of therapy you may see hair growth return in about 8 weeks. You may be required to have blood tests if used for extended period of time. Report any skin irritation, rash, tingling, or skin eruptions; persistent headache, dizziness; or GI disturbances.

Pregnancy/breast-feeding precautions: Inform prescriber if you are or intend to become pregnant. Consult prescriber if breast-feeding.

Eflornithine Hydrochloride *see* Eflornithine *on page 461*

Efudex® *see* Fluorouracil *on page 576*

E-Gems® [OTC] *see* Vitamin E *on page 1406*

ELA-Max® [OTC] *see* Lidocaine *on page 800*

ELA-Max® 5 [OTC] *see* Lidocaine *on page 800*

Elase® *see* Fibrinolysin and Desoxyribonuclease *on page 558*

Elase-Chloromycetin® *see* Fibrinolysin and Desoxyribonuclease *on page 558*

Elavil® *see* Amitriptyline *on page 84*

Eldecort® *see* Topical Corticosteroids *on page 1334*

Eldepryl® *see* Selegiline *on page 1221*

Eldopaque® [OTC] *see* Hydroquinone *on page 679*

Eldopaque Forte® *see* Hydroquinone *on page 679*

Eldoquin® [OTC] *see* Hydroquinone *on page 679*

Eldoquin Forte® *see* Hydroquinone *on page 679*

Electrolyte Lavage Solution *see* Polyethylene Glycol-Electrolyte Solution *on page 1098*

Elidel® *see* Pimecrolimus *on page 1084*

Eligard™ *see* Leuprolide *on page 781*

Elimite® *see* Permethrin *on page 1061*

Elitek™ *see* Rasburicase *on page 1174*

Elixophyllin® *see* Theophylline *on page 1300*

Ellence® *see* Epirubicin *on page 473*

Elocon® *see* Topical Corticosteroids *on page 1334*

Eloxatin™ *see* Oxaliplatin *on page 1012*

Elspar® *see* Asparaginase *on page 118*

Emcyt® *see* Estramustine *on page 500*

Emgel® *see* Erythromycin (Systemic) *on page 486*

EMLA® *see* Lidocaine and Prilocaine *on page 803*

EmTet® *see* Tetracycline *on page 1296*

ENA 713 *see* Rivastigmine *on page 1200*

Enalapril (e NAL a pril)

U.S. Brand Names Vasotec®; Vasotec® I.V.

Synonyms Enalaprilat; Enalapril Maleate

Generic Available Yes

Pharmacologic Category Angiotensin-Converting Enzyme (ACE) Inhibitor

Pregnancy Risk Factor C/D (2nd and 3rd trimesters)

Lactation Enters breast milk/compatible

Use Management of mild to severe hypertension; treatment of congestive heart failure, left ventricular dysfunction after myocardial infarction

Use - Unlabeled/Investigational

Unlabeled: Hypertensive crisis, diabetic nephropathy, rheumatoid arthritis, diagnosis of anatomic renal artery stenosis, hypertension secondary to scleroderma renal crisis, diagnosis of aldosteronism, idiopathic edema, Bartter's syndrome, postmyocardial infarction for prevention of ventricular failure

Investigational: Severe congestive heart failure in infants, neonatal hypertension, acute pulmonary edema

Mechanism of Action/Effect Competitive inhibitor of angiotensin-converting enzyme (ACE); prevents conversion of angiotensin I to angiotensin II, a potent vasoconstrictor; results in lower levels of angiotensin II which causes an increase in plasma renin activity and a reduction in aldosterone secretion

Contraindications Hypersensitivity to enalapril or enalaprilat; angioedema related to previous treatment with an ACE inhibitor; patients with idiopathic or hereditary angioedema; bilateral renal artery stenosis; primary hyperaldosteronism; pregnancy (2nd and 3rd trimesters)

Warnings/Precautions Anaphylactic reactions can occur. Angioedema can occur at any time during treatment (especially following first dose). Careful blood pressure monitoring with first dose (hypotension can occur especially in volume depleted patients). Dosage adjustment needed in renal impairment. Use with caution in hypovolemia; collagen vascular diseases; valvular stenosis (particularly aortic stenosis); hyperkalemia; or before, during, or immediately after anesthesia. Avoid rapid dosage escalation which may lead to renal insufficiency. Hypersensitivity reactions may be seen during hemodialysis with high-flux dialysis membranes (eg, AN69). Hyperkalemia may rarely occur. Neutropenia/agranulocytosis with myeloid hyperplasia can rarely occur. Use with caution in unilateral renal artery stenosis and pre-existing renal insufficiency. Pregnancy risk C/D (2nd and 3rd trimesters).

Drug Interactions

Cytochrome P450 Effect: Substrate of **CYP3A4**

Decreased Effect: Aspirin (high dose) may reduce the therapeutic effects of ACE inhibitors; at low dosages this does not appear to be significant. Rifampin may decrease the effect of ACE inhibitors. Antacids may decrease the bioavailability of ACE inhibitors (may be more likely to occur with captopril); separate administration times by 1-2 hours. NSAIDs may reduce the hypotensive effects of ACE inhibitors. More likely to occur in low renin or volume dependent hypertensive patients.

Increased Effect/Toxicity: Potassium supplements, co-trimoxazole (high dose), angiotensin II receptor antagonists (candesartan, losartan, irbesartan, etc), or potassium-sparing diuretics (amiloride, spironolactone, triamterene) may result in elevated serum potassium

(Continued)

Enalapril *(Continued)*

levels when combined with enalapril. ACE inhibitor effects may be increased by phenothiazines or probenecid (increases levels of captopril). ACE inhibitors may increase serum concentrations/effects of digoxin, lithium, and sulfonlyureas.

Diuretics have additive hypotensive effects with ACE inhibitors, and hypovolemia increases the potential for adverse renal effects of ACE inhibitors. In patients with compromised renal function, coadministration with NSAIDs may result in further deterioration of renal function. Allopurinol and ACE inhibitors may cause a higher risk of hypersensitivity reaction when taken concurrently.

Nutritional/Ethanol Interactions Herb/Nutraceutical: St John's wort may decrease enalapril levels. Avoid dong quai if using for hypertension (has estrogenic activity). Avoid ephedra, yohimbe, ginseng (may worsen hypertension). Avoid natural licorice (causes sodium and water retention and increases potassium loss). Avoid garlic (may have increased antihypertensive effect).

Effects on Lab Values Positive Coombs' [direct]; may cause false-positive results in urine acetone determinations using sodium nitroprusside reagent

Adverse Reactions Note: Frequency ranges include data from hypertension and heart failure trials. Higher rates of adverse reactions have generally been noted in patients with CHF. However, the frequency of adverse effects associated with placebo is also increased in this population.

1% to 10%:

Cardiovascular: Hypotension (0.9% to 6.7%), chest pain (2%), syncope (0.5% to 2%), orthostasis (2%), orthostatic hypotension (2%)

Central nervous system: Headache (2% to 5%), dizziness (4% to 8%), fatigue (2% to 3%), weakness (2%)

Dermatologic: Rash (1.5%)

Gastrointestinal: Abnormal taste, abdominal pain, vomiting, nausea, diarrhea, anorexia, constipation

Neuromuscular & skeletal: Weakness

Renal: Increased serum creatinine (0.2% to 20%), worsening of renal function (in patients with bilateral renal artery stenosis or hypovolemia)

Respiratory (1% to 2%): Bronchitis, cough, dyspnea

<1% (Limited to important or life-threatening): Agranulocytosis, alopecia, angina pectoris, angioedema, ataxia, bronchospasm, cardiac arrest, cerebral vascular accident, depression, erythema multiforme, exfoliative dermatitis, giant cell arteritis, gynecomastia, hallucinations, hemolysis with G6PD, Henoch-Schönlein purpura, hepatitis, ileus, impotence, jaundice, lichen-form reaction, myocardial infarction, neutropenia, ototoxicity, pancreatitis, paresthesia, pemphigus, pemphigus foliaceus, photosensitivity, psychosis, pulmonary edema, sicca syndrome, Stevens-Johnson syndrome, systemic lupus erythematosus, toxic epidermal necrolysis, toxic pustuloderma, vertigo. Worsening of renal function may occur in patients with bilateral renal artery stenosis or in hypovolemic patients. A syndrome which may include fever, myalgia, arthralgia, interstitial nephritis, vasculitis, rash, eosinophilia and positive ANA, and elevated ESR has been reported for enalapril and other ACE inhibitors.

Overdosage/Toxicology Mild hypotension has been the primary toxic effect seen with acute overdose. Bradycardia may also occur. Hyperkalemia occurs even with therapeutic doses, especially in patients with renal insufficiency and those taking NSAIDs. Following initiation of essential overdose management, toxic symptom treatment and supportive treatment should be initiated.

Pharmacodynamics/Kinetics

Absorption: Oral: 55% to 75%

Half-Life Elimination:

Enalapril: Adults: Healthy: 2 hours; Congestive heart failure: 3.4-5.8 hours

Enalaprilat: Infants 6 weeks to 8 months old: 6-10 hours; Adults: 35-38 hours

Time to Peak: Serum: Oral: Enalapril: 0.5-1.5 hours; Enalaprilat (active): 3-4.5 hours

Metabolism: Prodrug, undergoes hepatic biotransformation to enalaprilat

Onset: Oral: ~1 hour

Duration: Oral: 12-24 hours

Formulations

Injection, solution, as enalaprilat (Vasotec® I.V.): 1.25 mg/mL (1 mL, 2 mL) [contains benzyl alcohol]

Tablet, as maleate (Vasotec®): 2.5 mg, 5 mg, 10 mg, 20 mg

Dosing

Adults & Elderly: Use lower listed initial dose in patients with hyponatremia, hypovolemia, severe congestive heart failure, decreased renal function, or in those receiving diuretics.

Asymptomatic left ventricular dysfunction: Oral: 2.5 mg twice daily, titrated as tolerated to 20 mg/day

Hypertension:

Oral: 2.5-5 mg/day then increase as required, usual therapeutic dose for hypertension: 10-40 mg/day in 1-2 divided doses; usual therapeutic dose for heart failure: 5-20 mg/day. **Note:** Initiate with 2.5 mg if patient is taking a diuretic which cannot be discontinued. May add a diuretic if blood pressure cannot be controlled with enalapril alone.

I.V. (Enalaprilat): 1.25 mg/dose, given over 5 minutes every 6 hours; doses as high as 5 mg/dose every 6 hours have been tolerated for up to 36 hours. **Note:** If patients are concomitantly receiving diuretic therapy, begin with 0.625 mg I.V. over 5 minutes; if the effect is not adequate after 1 hour, repeat the dose and administer 1.25 mg at 6-hour intervals thereafter; if adequate, administer 0.625 mg I.V. every 6 hours.

Heart failure: Oral: As adjunct with diuretics and digitalis, initiate with 2.5 mg once or twice daily (usual range: 5-20 mg/day in 2 divided doses; maximum: 40 mg)

I.V.: Avoid I.V. administration in patients with unstable heart failure or those suffering acute myocardial infarction.

Conversion from I.V. to oral therapy if not concurrently on diuretics: 5 mg once daily; subsequent titration as needed; if concurrently receiving diuretics and responding to 0.625 mg I.V. every 6 hours, initiate with 2.5 mg/day.

Pediatrics:

Hypertension: Oral: Children 1 month to 16 years: Initial: 0.08 mg/kg (up to 5 mg) once daily; adjust dosage based on patient response; doses >0.58 mg/kg (40 mg) have not been evaluated in pediatric patients

Heart failure (non-FDA approved): Infants and Children:

Oral (Enalapril): Initial: 0.1 mg/kg/day in 1-2 divided doses; increase as required over 2 weeks to maximum of 0.5 mg/kg/day; mean dose required for CHF improvement in 39 children (9 days to 17 years) was 0.36 mg/kg/day; investigationally, select individuals have been treated with doses up to 0.94 mg/kg/day

I.V. (Enalaprilat): 5-10 mcg/kg/dose administered every 8-24 hours (as determined by blood pressure readings); monitor patients carefully; select patients may require higher doses

Adolescents: Refer to adult dosing.

Renal Impairment:

Oral: Enalapril: Hypertension:

Cl_{cr} 30-80 mL/minute: Administer 5 mg/day titrated upwards to maximum of 40 mg.

Cl_{cr} <30 mL/minute: Administer 2.5 mg day titrated upward until blood pressure is controlled up to a maximum of 40 mg.

For heart failure patients with sodium <130 mEq/L or serum creatinine >1.6 mg/dL, initiate dosage with 2.5 mg/day, increasing to twice daily as needed; increase further in increments of 2.5 mg/dose at >4-day intervals to a maximum daily dose of 40 mg.

I.V.: Enalaprilat:

Cl_{cr} >30 mL/minute: Initiate with 1.25 mg every 6 hours and increase dose based on response.

Cl_{cr} <30 mL/minute: Initiate with 0.625 mg every 6 hours and increase dose based on response.

Moderately dialyzable (20% to 50%)

Administer dose postdialysis (eg, 0.625 mg I.V. every 6 hours) or administer 20% to 25% supplemental dose following dialysis; Clearance: 62 mL/minute

Peritoneal dialysis effects: Supplemental dose is not necessary, although some removal of drug occurs.

Hepatic Impairment: Hydrolysis of enalapril to enalaprilat may be delayed and/or impaired in patients with severe hepatic impairment, but the pharmacodynamic effects of the drug do not appear to be significantly altered. No dosage adjustment is necessary.

Administration

I.V.: Give direct IVP over at least 5 minutes or dilute up to 50 mL and infuse.

Stability

Storage: Enalaprilat: Clear, colorless solution which should be stored at <30°C.

Reconstitution: Enalaprilat: I.V. is stable for 24 hours at room temperature in D_5W or NS.

Compatibility: Stable in dextran 40 10% in dextrose, D_5LR, D_5NS, D_5W, hetastarch 6%, NS

Y-site administration: Incompatible with amphotericin B, amphotericin B cholesteryl sulfate complex, cefepime, phenytoin

Monitoring Laboratory Tests CBC, renal function tests, electrolytes. If patient has renal impairment then a baseline WBC with differential and serum creatinine should be evaluated and monitored closely during the first 3 months of therapy.

Monitoring and Teaching Issues

Physical Assessment: See Contraindications, Warnings/Precautions, and Dosing for use cautions. Assess potential for interactions with other prescriptions, OTC medications, or herbal products patient may be taking (especially anything that may impact fluid balance or cardiac status - see Drug Interactions). **Infusion:** See Administration details. Assess results of laboratory tests (see above), therapeutic effectiveness, and adverse response on a regular basis during therapy (eg, hypovolemia, angioedema, postural hypotension - see Adverse Reactions and Overdose/Toxicology). Teach patient appropriate use, possible side effects and appropriate interventions, and adverse symptoms to report (see Patient Education). **Pregnancy risk factor C/D** - see Pregnancy Risk Factor for use cautions. Instruct patient in appropriate use of barrier contraceptives. Danger of use during pregnancy must outweigh risk to fetus - see Pregnancy Issues.

Patient Education: Inform prescriber of all prescriptions, OTC medications, or herbal products you are taking, and any allergies you have. Do not take anything new during treatment unless approved by prescriber. Do not use potassium supplement or salt substitutes without consulting prescriber. Take exactly as directed; do not discontinue without consulting prescriber. Take first dose at bedtime. Take all doses on an empty stomach, 1 hour before or 2 hours after meals. This drug does not eliminate need for diet or exercise regimen as recommended by prescriber. May cause dizziness, fainting, or lightheadedness (use caution when driving or engaging in tasks that require alertness until response to drug is known); postural hypotension (use caution when rising from lying or sitting position or climbing stairs); or nausea, vomiting, abdominal pain, dry mouth, or transient loss of appetite (small, frequent meals, frequent mouth care, sucking lozenges, or chewing gum may help). Report persistent nausea and vomiting; chest pain or palpitations; mouth sores; fever or chills; swelling of extremities, face, mouth, or tongue; skin rash; numbness, tingling, or pain in muscles; difficulty breathing or unusual cough; or other persistent adverse reactions. **Pregnancy/breast-feeding precautions:** Inform prescriber if you are or intend to become pregnant. This drug should not be used in the 2nd or 3rd trimester of pregnancy. Consult prescriber for appropriate contraceptive measures if necessary. Consult prescriber if breast-feeding.

Dietary Issues: Limit salt substitutes or potassium-rich diet.

Geriatric Considerations: Due to frequent decreases in glomerular filtration (also creatinine clearance) with aging, elderly patients may have exaggerated responses to ACE inhibitors.

Breast-feeding Issues: Crosses into breast milk. Detectable levels but appears clinically insignificant. AAP considers **compatible** with breast-feeding.

(Continued)

Enalapril *(Continued)*

Pregnancy Issues: ACE inhibitors can cause fetal injury or death if taken during the 2nd or 3rd trimester. Discontinue ACE inhibitors as soon as pregnancy is detected.

Related Information

Angiotensin Agents *on page 1547*
Heart Failure *on page 1670*

Enalapril and Felodipine (e NAL a pril & fe LOE di peen)

U.S. Brand Names Lexxel®

Synonyms Felodipine and Enalapril

Generic Available No

Pharmacologic Category Antihypertensive Agent Combination

Pregnancy Risk Factor C/D (2nd and 3rd trimesters)

Lactation Enters breast milk/use caution

Use Treatment of hypertension, however, not indicated for initial treatment of hypertension; replacement therapy in patients receiving separate dosage forms (for patient convenience); when monotherapy with one component fails to achieve desired antihypertensive effect, or when dose-limiting adverse effects limit upward titration of monotherapy

Formulations Tablet, extended release:

Enalapril maleate 5 mg and felodipine 2.5 mg
Enalapril maleate 5 mg and felodipine 5 mg

Dosing

Adults: Hypertension: Oral: 1 tablet/day, individualize dose to achieve optimal effect. In some patients, the effect of enalapril may diminish toward the end of the dosing interval. Twice daily dosing may be considered.

Elderly: Recommended initial dose of felodipine is 2.5 mg daily. Titration of individual components is preferred.

Renal Impairment: Cl_{cr} <30 mL/minute: Recommended initial dose of enalapril is 2.5 mg/day. Titration of individual components is preferred.

Hepatic Impairment: Recommended initial dose of felodipine is 2.5 mg daily. Titration of individual components is preferred.

Monitoring and Teaching Issues

Physical Assessment: See individual components listed in Related Information. **Pregnancy risk factor C/D** - see Pregnancy Risk Factor for use cautions. Assess knowledge/instruct patient on need to use appropriate contraceptive measures and the need to avoid pregnancy. Note breast-feeding caution.

Patient Education: See individual components listed in Related Information. **Pregnancy/breast-feeding precautions:** Inform prescriber if you are or intend to become pregnant. Consult prescriber if breast-feeding.

Related Information

Enalapril *on page 463*
Felodipine *on page 548*

Enalapril and Hydrochlorothiazide

(e NAL a pril & hye droe klor oh THYE a zide)

U.S. Brand Names Vaseretic®

Synonyms Hydrochlorothiazide and Enalapril

Generic Available No

Pharmacologic Category Antihypertensive Agent Combination

Pregnancy Risk Factor C/D (2nd and 3rd trimesters)

Lactation Enters breast milk (both ingredients)/compatible

Use Treatment of hypertension

Formulations Tablet:

5-12.5: Enalapril maleate 5 mg and hydrochlorothiazide 12.5 mg
10-25: Enalapril maleate 10 mg and hydrochlorothiazide 25 mg

Dosing

Adults: Hypertension: Dose is individualized based on components

Elderly: Refer to dosing in individual monographs; adjust for renal impairment.

Renal Impairment:

Cl_{cr} >30 mL/minute: Administer usual dose.
Severe renal failure: Avoid; loop diuretics are recommended.

Monitoring and Teaching Issues

Physical Assessment: See individual components listed in Related Information. **Pregnancy risk factor C/D** - see Pregnancy Risk Factor for use cautions. Assess knowledge/instruct patient on need to use appropriate contraceptive measures and the need to avoid pregnancy.

Patient Education: See individual components listed in Related Information. **Pregnancy precaution:** Inform prescriber if you are or intend to become pregnant.

Related Information

Enalapril *on page 463*
Hydrochlorothiazide *on page 664*

Enalaprilat *see* Enalapril *on page 463*

Enalapril Maleate *see* Enalapril *on page 463*

Enbrel® *see* Etanercept *on page 510*

Endocet® *see* Oxycodone and Acetaminophen *on page 1022*

Endodan® *see* Oxycodone and Aspirin *on page 1022*

Ener-B® *see* Cyanocobalamin *on page 337*

Engerix-B® *see page 1498*

Enlon® *see* Edrophonium *on page 458*

Enoxaparin (e noks ah PA in)

U.S. Brand Names Lovenox®

Synonyms Enoxaparin Sodium

Generic Available No

Pharmacologic Category Low Molecular Weight Heparin

Pregnancy Risk Factor B

Lactation Excretion in breast milk unknown/use caution

Use

Prevention of deep vein thrombosis following hip or knee replacement surgery or abdominal surgery in patients at risk for thromboembolic complications (high-risk patients include those with one or more of the following risk factors: >40 years of age, obese, general anesthesia lasting >30 minutes, malignancy, history of deep vein thrombosis or pulmonary embolism)

Prevention of deep vein thrombosis in medical patients at risk for thromboembolic complications due to severely restricted mobility during acute illness

Inpatient treatment of acute deep vein thrombosis with and without pulmonary embolism when administered in conjunction with warfarin sodium

Outpatient treatment of acute deep vein thrombosis without pulmonary embolism when administered in conjunction with warfarin sodium

Prevention of ischemic complications of unstable angina and non-Q wave myocardial infarction (when administered with aspirin)

Mechanism of Action/Effect Low molecular weight heparin that blocks factor Xa and IIa to prevent thrombus and clot formation

Contraindications Hypersensitivity to enoxaparin or any component of the formulation; thrombocytopenia associated with a positive *in vitro* test for antiplatelet antibodies in the presence of enoxaparin; hypersensitivity to pork products; active major bleeding; not for I.M. or I.V. use

Warnings/Precautions Patients with recent or anticipated neuraxial anesthesia (epidural or spinal anesthesia) are at risk of spinal or epidural hematoma and subsequent paralysis. Consider risk versus benefit prior to neuraxial anesthesia; risk is increased by concomitant agents which may alter hemostasis, as well as traumatic or repeated epidural or spinal puncture. Patient should be observed closely for bleeding if enoxaparin is administered during or immediately following diagnostic lumbar puncture, epidural anesthesia, or spinal anesthesia.

Not recommended for thromboprophylaxis in patients with prosthetic heart valves (especially pregnant women). Not to be used interchangeably (unit for unit) with heparin or any other low molecular weight heparins. Use caution in patients with history of heparin-induced thrombocytopenia, renal dysfunction, and elderly patients. Monitor patient closely for signs or symptoms of bleeding. Certain patients are at increased risk of bleeding. Risk factors include bacterial endocarditis; congenital or acquired bleeding disorders; active ulcerative or angiodysplastic GI diseases; severe uncontrolled hypertension; hemorrhagic stroke; use shortly after brain, spinal, or ophthalmology surgery; patients treated concomitantly with platelet inhibitors; recent GI bleeding; thrombocytopenia or platelet defects; severe liver disease; hypertensive or diabetic retinopathy; or in patients undergoing invasive procedures. Safety and efficacy in pediatric patients have not been established. Heparin can cause hyperkalemia by affecting aldosterone. Similar reactions could occur with LMWHs. Monitor for hyperkalemia. Discontinue therapy if platelets are <100,000/mm^3.

Drug Interactions

Increased Effect/Toxicity: Risk of bleeding with enoxaparin may be increased with thrombolytic agents, oral anticoagulants (warfarin), drugs which affect platelet function (eg, aspirin, NSAIDs, dipyridamole, ticlopidine, clopidogrel, and IIb/IIIa antagonists). Although the risk of bleeding may be increased during concurrent therapy with warfarin, enoxaparin is commonly continued during the initiation of warfarin therapy to assure anticoagulation and to protect against possible transient hypercoagulability. Some cephalosporins and penicillins may block platelet aggregation, theoretically increasing the risk of bleeding.

Nutritional/Ethanol Interactions Herb/Nutraceutical: Avoid cat's claw, dong quai, evening primrose, feverfew, garlic, ginger, ginkgo, red clover, horse chestnut, green tea, ginseng (all have additional antiplatelet activity).

Effects on Lab Values ↑ AST, ALT levels

Adverse Reactions As with all anticoagulants, bleeding is the major adverse effect of enoxaparin. Hemorrhage may occur at virtually any site. Risk is dependent on multiple variables. At the recommended doses, single injections of enoxaparin do not significantly influence platelet aggregation or affect global clotting time (ie, PT or APTT).

1% to 10%:

- Central nervous system: Fever (5% to 8%), confusion, pain
- Dermatologic: Erythema, bruising
- Gastrointestinal: Nausea (3%), diarrhea
- Hematologic: Hemorrhage (5% to 13%), thrombocytopenia (2%), hypochromic anemia (2%)
- Hepatic: Increased ALT/AST
- Local: Injection site hematoma (9%), local reactions (irritation, pain, ecchymosis, erythema)

<1% (Limited to important or life-threatening): Allergic reaction, anaphylactoid reaction, eczematous plaques, hyperlipidemia, hypertriglyceridemia, itchy erythematous patches, pruritus, purpura, skin necrosis, thrombocytosis, urticaria, vesicobullous rash. Retroperitoneal or intracranial bleed (some fatal). Spinal or epidural hematomas can occur following neuraxial anesthesia or spinal puncture, resulting in paralysis. Risk is increased in patients with indwelling epidural catheters or concomitant use of other drugs affecting hemostasis. Cases of heparin-induced thrombocytopenia with thrombosis (some complicated by organ infarction, limb ischemia, or death) have been reported. Prosthetic valve thrombosis, including fatal cases, has been reported in pregnant women receiving enoxaparin as thromboprophylaxis.

(Continued)

Enoxaparin *(Continued)*

Overdosage/Toxicology Symptoms of overdose include hemorrhage. Protamine zinc has been used to reverse effects.

Pharmacodynamics/Kinetics

Half-Life Elimination: Plasma: 2-4 times longer than standard heparin, independent of dose

Onset: Peak effect: S.C.: Antifactor Xa and antithrombin (antifactor IIa): 3-5 hours

Duration: 40 mg dose: Antifactor Xa activity: ~12 hours

Formulations

Injection, solution, as sodium [ampul; preservative free]: 30 mg/0.3 mL (0.3 mL)

Injection, solution, as sodium [graduated prefilled syringe; preservative free]: 60 mg/0.6 mL (0.6 mL); 80 mg/0.8 mL (0.8 mL); 100 mg/mL (1 mL); 120 mg/0.8 mL (0.8 mL); 150 mg/mL (1 mL)

Injection, solution, as sodium [prefilled syringe; preservative free]: 30 mg/0.3 mL (0.3 mL); 40 mg/0.4 mL (0.4 mL)

Dosing

Adults:

DVT prophylaxis (surgical): S.C.:

Hip replacement:

30 mg twice daily: First dose within 12-24 hours after surgery and every 12 hours until risk of deep vein thrombosis has diminished or the patient is adequately anticoagulated on warfarin. Average duration of therapy: 7-10 days.

40 mg once daily: First dose within 9-15 hours before surgery and daily until risk of deep vein thrombosis has diminished or the patient is adequately anticoagulated on warfarin. Average duration of therapy: 7-10 days unless warfarin is not given concurrently, then 40 mg S.C. once daily should be continued for 3 more weeks (4 weeks total).

Knee replacement: 30 mg twice daily: First dose within 12-24 hours after surgery and every 12 hours until risk of deep vein thrombosis has diminished. Average duration of therapy: 7-10 days; maximum course: 14 days.

Abdominal surgery (high-risk patients): 40 mg once daily, with initial dose given 2 hours prior to surgery; usual duration: 7-10 days and up to 12 days has been tolerated in clinical trials.

DVT prophylaxis in medical patients with severely restricted mobility during acute illness: S.C.: 40 mg once daily; usual duration: 6-11 days; up to 14 days was used in clinical trial

DVT Treatment (acute proximal DVT):

Note: Start warfarin within 72 hours and continue enoxaparin until INR is between 2.0 and 3.0 (usually 7 days).

Inpatient treatment of DVT with or without pulmonary embolism: S.C.: 1 mg/kg/dose every 12 hours or 1.5 mg/kg once daily.

Outpatient treatment of DVT without pulmonary embolism: S.C.: 1 mg/kg/dose every 12 hours.

Unstable angina or non-Q-wave myocardial infarction (prevention of ischemic complications): S.C.: 1 mg/kg twice daily in conjunction with oral aspirin therapy (100-325 mg once daily); treatment should be continued for a minimum of 2 days and continued until clinical stabilization (usually 2-8 days).

Elderly: S.C.: Increased incidence of bleeding with doses of 1.5 mg/kg/day or 1 mg/kg every 12 hours. Injection-associated bleeding and serious adverse reactions are also increased in the elderly. Careful attention should be paid to elderly patients <45 kg.

Pediatrics:

Prophylaxis of DVT following abdominal, hip replacement or knee replacement surgery: S.C.: Safety and effectiveness have not been established. Few studies have been conducted; the Fifth American College of Chest Physicians Consensus Conference on Antithrombotic Therapy (Michelson, 1998) recommends low molecular weight heparin as an alternative to heparin therapy in children ≥2 months with DVT or pulmonary embolism; the following initial doses and titration schedule, based on therapeutic antifactor Xa levels of 0.5-1 unit/mL, are recommended. **Note:** For treatment of DVT or pulmonary embolism in children ≥2 months of age, enoxaparin should be continued for 5-10 days and oral anticoagulation should be overlapped for 4-5 days (Michelson, 1998).

Infants >2 months and Children ≤18 years: Prophylaxis: Initial: 0.5 mg/kg every 12 hours; treatment: Initial: 1 mg/kg every 12 hours

Dosage titration:

Antifactor Xa <0.35 units/mL: Increase dose by 25%; repeat antifactor Xa level 4 hour after next dose

Antifactor Xa 0.35-0.49 units/mL: Increase dose by 10%; repeat antifactor Xa level 4 hour after next dose

Antifactor Xa 0.5-1 unit/mL: Keep same dosage; repeat antifactor Xa level next day, then 1 week later (4 hour after dose)

Antifactor Xa 1.1-1.5 units/mL: Decrease dose by 20%; repeat antifactor Xa level before next dose

Antifactor Xa 1.6-2 units/mL: Hold dose for 3 hour and decrease dose by 30%; repeat antifactor Xa level before next dose, then 4 hour after next dose

Antifactor Xa >2 units/mL: Hold all doses until antifactor Xa is 0.5 units/mL, then decrease dose by 40%; repeat antifactor Xa level before next dose and every 12 hour until antifactor Xa <0.5 units/mL

Renal Impairment: Total clearance is lower and elimination is delayed in patients with renal failure; adjustment may be necessary in elderly and patients with severe renal impairment.

Hemodialysis: Supplemental dose is not necessary.

Peritoneal dialysis: Significant drug removal is unlikely based on physiochemical characteristics.

Administration

Other: Should be administered by deep S.C. injection to the left or right anterolateral and left or right posterolateral abdominal wall. To avoid loss of drug from the 30 mg and 40 mg syringes, do not expel the air bubble from the syringe prior to injection. In order to minimize bruising, do not rub injection site. An automatic injector (Lovenox EasyInjector™) is available with the 30 mg and 40 mg syringes to aid the patient with self-injections. **Note:** Enoxaparin is available in 100 mg/mL and 150 mg/mL concentrations.

Stability

Storage: Store at 15°C to 25°C (59°F to 77°F). Do not freeze. Do not mix with other injections or infusions.

Compatibility: Stable in NS

Monitoring Laboratory Tests Platelets, occult blood, anti-Xa activity, if available; the monitoring of PT and/or PTT is not necessary.

Monitoring and Teaching Issues

Physical Assessment: See Contraindications, Warnings/Precautions, and Dosing for use cautions. Assess potential for interactions with other prescriptions, OTC medications, or herbal products patient may be taking (especially anything that may impact fluid balance or cardiac status - see Drug Interactions). See Administration specifics. Assess results of laboratory tests (see above), therapeutic effectiveness, and adverse response on a regular basis during therapy (eg, hypovolemia, angioedema, postural hypotension - see Adverse Reactions and Overdose/Toxicology). Teach patient appropriate use (injection technique and needle disposal), possible side effects and appropriate interventions, and adverse symptoms to report (see Patient Education). Note breast-feeding caution.

Patient Education: Inform prescriber of all prescriptions, OTC medications, or herbal products you are taking, and any allergies you have. Do not take anything new without consulting prescriber. This drug can only be administered by injection. If self-administered, follow exact directions for injection and needle disposal. You may have a tendency to bleed easily while taking this drug (brush teeth with soft brush, use waxed dental floss, use electric razor, avoid scissors or sharp knives, and potentially harmful activities). Report chest pain; persistent constipation; persistent erection; unusual bleeding or bruising (bleeding gums, nosebleed, blood in urine, dark stool); pain in joints or back; or redness, swelling, burning, or pain at injection site. **Breast-feeding precaution:** Consult prescriber if breast-feeding.

Geriatric Considerations: No specific recommendations.

Breast-feeding Issues: This drug has a high molecular weight that would minimize excretion in breast milk and is inactivated by the GI tract which further reduces the risk to the infant.

Pregnancy Issues: There are no adequate and well-controlled studies using enoxaparin in pregnant women. Animal studies have not shown teratogenic or fetotoxic effects. Postmarketing reports include congenital abnormalities (cause and effect not established) and also fetal death when used in pregnant women. In addition, prosthetic valve thrombosis, including fatal cases, has been reported in pregnant women receiving enoxaparin as thromboprophylaxis.

Related Information

Heparins *on page 1576*

Enoxaparin Sodium *see* Enoxaparin *on page 467*

Enpresse™ *see* Ethinyl Estradiol and Levonorgestrel *on page 523*

Entacapone (en TA ka pone)

U.S. Brand Names Comtan®

Generic Available No

Pharmacologic Category Anti-Parkinson's Agent, COMT Inhibitor

Pregnancy Risk Factor C

Lactation Excretion in breast milk unknown/use caution

Use Adjunct to levodopa/carbidopa therapy in patients with idiopathic Parkinson's disease who experience "wearing-off" symptoms at the end of a dosing interval

Mechanism of Action/Effect Entacapone inhibits COMT peripherally and alters the pharmacokinetics of levodopa so serum levels of levodopa become more sustained when used with levodopa/carbidopa combinations.

Contraindications Hypersensitivity to entacapone or any of component of the formulation

Warnings/Precautions May increase risk of orthostatic hypotension and syncope. May cause diarrhea, hallucinations; may cause or exacerbate dyskinesia. This drug should be slowly withdrawn if discontinuation is needed. Use caution in patients with hepatic impairment and renal impairment. Other drugs metabolized by COMT (see drug interactions) may cause increases in heart rate, arrhythmias, and changes in blood pressure when used concurrently. Pregnancy risk C.

Drug Interactions

Cytochrome P450 Effect: Inhibits CYP1A2, 2A6, 2C8/9, 2C19, 2D6, 2E1, 3A4

Decreased Effect: Entacapone is an iron chelator and an iron supplement should not be administered concurrently with this medicine.

Increased Effect/Toxicity: Cardiac effects with drugs metabolized by COMT (eg, epinephrine, isoproterenol, dopamine, apomorphine, bitolterol, dobutamine, methyldopa) increased other CNS depressants; nonselective MAO inhibitors are not recommended; chelates iron. Caution with drugs that interfere with glucuronidation, intestinal, biliary excretion, intestinal beta-glucuronidase (eg, probenecid, cholestyramine, erythromycin, chloramphenicol, rifampicin, ampicillin).

Nutritional/Ethanol Interactions Ethanol: Avoid ethanol (may increase CNS adverse effects).

Adverse Reactions

>10%:

Gastrointestinal: Nausea (14%)

Neuromuscular & skeletal: Dyskinesia (25%), placebo (15%)

(Continued)

Entacapone *(Continued)*

1% to 10%:

Cardiovascular: Orthostatic hypotension (4.3%), syncope (1.2%)

Central nervous system: Dizziness (8%), fatigue (6%), hallucinations (4%), anxiety (2%), somnolence (2%), agitation (1%)

Dermatologic: Purpura (2%)

Gastrointestinal: Diarrhea (10%), abdominal pain (8%), constipation (6%), vomiting (4%), dry mouth (3%), dyspepsia (2%), flatulence (2%), gastritis (1%), taste perversion (1%)

Genitourinary: Brown-orange urine discoloration (10%)

Neuromuscular & skeletal: Hyperkinesia (10%), hypokinesia (9%), back pain (4%), weakness (2%)

Respiratory: Dyspnea (3%)

Miscellaneous: Increased diaphoresis (2%), bacterial infection (1%)

<1% (Limited to important or life-threatening): Hyperpyrexia and confusion (resembling neuroleptic malignant syndrome), pulmonary fibrosis, retroperitoneal fibrosis, rhabdomyolysis

Overdosage/Toxicology There have been no reported cases of overdose with this drug.

Pharmacodynamics/Kinetics

Absorption: Rapid

Bioavailability: 35%

Half-Life Elimination: B phase: 0.4-0.7 hours; Y phase: 2.4 hours

Time to Peak: Serum: 1 hour

Metabolism: Isomerization to the *cis*-isomer, followed by direct glucuronidation of the parent and *cis*-isomer

Onset: Rapid; Peak effect: 1 hour

Formulations Tablet: 200 mg

Dosing

Adults & Elderly: Parkinson's disease: Oral: 200 mg dose, up to a maximum of 8 times/day; maximum daily dose: 1600 mg/day. Always administer with levodopa/carbidopa. To optimize therapy the levodopa/carbidopa dosage must be reduced, usually by 25%. This reduction is usually necessary when the patient is taking more than 800 mg of levodopa daily.

Renal Impairment: No adjustment is required; dialysis patients were not studied.

Hepatic Impairment: Dosage adjustment in chronic therapy with standard treatment has not been studied.

Monitoring and Teaching Issues

Physical Assessment: Assess other medications patient may be taking for effectiveness and interactions (see Drug Interactions). See Contraindications and Warnings/Precautions for use cautions. Monitor therapeutic response and adverse reactions (see Adverse Reactions). Assess knowledge/teach patient appropriate use, interventions to reduce side effects, and adverse reactions to report (see Patient Education). **Pregnancy risk factor C** - benefits of use should outweigh possible risks. Note breast-feeding caution.

Patient Education: Take exactly as directed; do not alter dosage or discontinue without consulting prescriber. May be taken with food. Notify prescriber if any other prescription medications you are taking. Avoid all alcohol or OTC medications unless approved by your prescriber. Orange-brown urine is normal with this medication. You may experience dizziness, fatigue, or sleepiness (use caution when driving or engaging in tasks requiring alertness until response to drug is known); postural hypotension (rise slowly when getting up from chair or bed, when climbing stairs); or unusual taste, nausea, vomiting, flatulence, or upset stomach (small, frequent meals, good mouth care, chewing gum, or sucking hard candy may help). Report any increased or abnormal skeletal movements or pain; unresolved sedation, nausea, diarrhea, constipation, or GI distress; signs of infection; persistent dizziness or sleepiness; or other unusual responses. **Pregnancy/breast-feeding precautions:** Inform prescriber if you are or intend to become pregnant. Consult prescriber if breast-feeding.

Dietary Issues: May be taken with or without food.

Entex® PSE *see* Guaifenesin and Pseudoephedrine *on page 648*

Entocort™ EC *see* Budesonide *on page 179*

Enulose® *see* Lactulose *on page 767*

Epidermal Thymocyte Activating Factor *see* Aldesleukin *on page 54*

Epifrin® *see* Epinephrine *on page 470*

Epifrin®, Glaucon® *see* Ophthalmic Agents, Glaucoma *on page 1002*

E-Pilo-x® *see* Pilocarpine and Epinephrine *on page 1083*

Epinal® *see* Ophthalmic Agents, Glaucoma *on page 1002*

Epinephrine (ep i NEF rin)

U.S. Brand Names Adrenalin®; Epifrin®; EpiPen®; EpiPen® Jr; Primatene® Mist [OTC]

Synonyms Adrenaline; Epinephrine Bitartrate; Epinephrine Hydrochloride

Generic Available Yes

Pharmacologic Category Alpha/Beta Agonist; Antidote; Ophthalmic Agent, Antiglaucoma

Pregnancy Risk Factor C

Lactation Excretion in breast milk unknown

Use Treatment of bronchospasms, anaphylactic reactions, cardiac arrest, management of open-angle (chronic simple) glaucoma; added to local anesthetics to decrease systemic absorption, increase duration of action, and decrease toxicity of the local anesthetic

Use - Unlabeled/Investigational ACLS guidelines: Ventricular fibrillation (VF) or pulseless ventricular tachycardia (VT) unresponsive to initial defibrillatory shocks; pulseless electrical activity, asystole, hypotension unresponsive to volume resuscitation; symptomatic bradycardia or heart block unresponsive to atropine or pacing

Mechanism of Action/Effect Stimulates alpha-, beta$_1$-, and beta$_2$-adrenergic receptors resulting in relaxation of smooth muscle of the bronchial tree, cardiac stimulation, and dilation of skeletal muscle vasculature; small doses can cause vasodilation via $beta_2$-vascular receptors; large doses may produce constriction of skeletal and vascular smooth muscle; decreases production of aqueous humor and increases aqueous outflow; dilates the pupil by contracting the dilator muscle

Contraindications Hypersensitivity to epinephrine or any component of the formulation; cardiac arrhythmias; angle-closure glaucoma

Warnings/Precautions Use with caution in elderly patients, patients with diabetes mellitus, cardiovascular diseases (angina, tachycardia, prostatic hyperplasia, history of seizures, renal dysfunction, myocardial infarction), thyroid disease, cerebral arteriosclerosis, or Parkinson's. Some products contain sulfites as preservatives. Rapid I.V. infusion may cause death from cerebrovascular hemorrhage or cardiac arrhythmias. Oral inhalation of epinephrine is **not** the preferred route of administration. Pregnancy risk C.

Drug Interactions

Decreased Effect: Decreased bronchodilation with β-blockers. Decreases antihypertensive effects of methyldopa or guanethidine.

Increased Effect/Toxicity: Increased cardiac irritability if administered concurrently with halogenated inhalation anesthetics, beta-blocking agents, or alpha-blocking agents.

Nutritional/Ethanol Interactions Herb/Nutraceutical: Avoid ephedra, yohimbe (may cause CNS stimulation).

Effects on Lab Values ↑ bilirubin (S), catecholamines (U), glucose, uric acid (S)

Adverse Reactions Frequency not defined.

Cardiovascular: Tachycardia (parenteral), pounding heartbeat, flushing, hypertension, pallor, chest pain, increased myocardial oxygen consumption, cardiac arrhythmias, sudden death, angina, vasoconstriction

Central nervous system: Nervousness, anxiety, restlessness, headache, dizziness, lightheadedness, insomnia

Gastrointestinal: Nausea, vomiting, xerostomia,dry throat

Genitourinary: Acute urinary retention in patients with bladder outflow obstruction

Neuromuscular & skeletal: Weakness, trembling

Ocular: Precipitation or or exacerbation of narrow-angle glaucoma, transient stinging, burning, eye pain, allergic lid reaction, ocular irritation

Renal: Decreased renal and splanchnic blood flow

Respiratory: Wheezing, dyspnea

Miscellaneous: Diaphoresis (increased)

Overdosage/Toxicology Symptoms of overdose include hypertension, which may result in subarachnoid hemorrhage and hemiplegia; arrhythmias; unusually large pupils; pulmonary edema; renal failure; and metabolic acidosis. There is no specific antidote for epinephrine intoxication and treatment is primarily supportive.

Pharmacodynamics/Kinetics

Metabolism: Taken up into the adrenergic neuron and metabolized by monoamine oxidase and catechol-o-methyltransferase; circulating drug hepatically metabolized

Onset: Bronchodilation: S.C.: ~5-10 minutes; Inhalation: ~1 minute; Conjunctival instillation: IOP declines ~1 hour

Peak effect: Conjunctival instillation: 4-8 hours

Duration: Conjunctival instillation: Ocular effect: 12-24 hours

Formulations

Aerosol for oral inhalation (Primatene® Mist): 0.22 mg/inhalation (15 mL, 22.5 mL)

Injection, solution [prefilled auto injector]:

EpiPen®: 0.3 mg/0.3 mL [1:1000] (2 mL) [contains sodium metabisulfite; available as single unit or in double-unit pack with training unit]

EpiPen® Jr: 0.15 mg/0.3 mL [1:2000] (2 mL) [contains sodium metabisulfite; available as single unit or in double-unit pack with training unit]

Injection, solution, as hydrochloride: 0.1 mg/mL [1:10,000] (10 mL); 1 mg/mL [1:1000] (1 mL)

Adrenalin®: 1 mg/mL [1:1000] (1 mL, 30 mL)

Solution for oral inhalation, as hydrochloride: Adrenalin®: 1% [10 mg/mL, 1:100] (7.5 mL) [contains sodium bisulfite]

Solution, ophthalmic, as hydrochloride (Epifrin®): 0.5% (15 mL); 1% (15 mL); 2% (15 mL) [contains benzalkonium chloride and sodium metabisulfite]

Dosing

Adults & Elderly:

Asystole:

I.V.: 1 mg every 3-5 minutes; if this approach fails, alternative regimens include: Intermediate: 2-5 mg every 3-5 minutes; Escalating: 1 mg, 3 mg, 5 mg at 3-minute intervals; High: 0.1 mg/kg every 3-5 minutes.

Intratracheal: Although optimal dose is unknown, doses of 2-2.5 times the I.V. dose may be needed

Bronchospasm:

I.M., S.C. (1:1000): 0.1-0.5 mg every 10-15 minutes to 4 hours

Suspension (1:200) S.C.: 0.1-0.3 mL (0.5-1.5 mg)

I.V.: 0.1-0.25 mg (single dose maximum: 1 mg)

Nebulization: Instill 8-15 drops into nebulizer reservoirs; administer 1-3 inhalations 4-6 times/day.

Hypotension (refractory to dopamine/dobutamine): Continuous I.V. infusion: Initial: 1 mcg/minute (range: 1-10 mcg/minute); titrate to desired effect; severe cardiac dysfunction may require doses >10 mcg/minute (up to 0.1 mcg/kg/minute)

Hypersensitivity reaction: I.M., S.C.: 0.2-0.5 mg every 20 minutes to 4 hours (single dose maximum: 1 mg)

Glaucoma: Ophthalmic: Instill 1-2 drops in eye(s) once or twice daily.

Nasal congestion: Intranasal: Apply locally as drops or spray or with sterile swab.

Pediatrics:

Bronchodilator:

S.C.: Infants and Children: 10 mcg/kg (0.01 mL/kg of **1:1000**) (single doses not to exceed 0.5 mg) **or** suspension (1:200): 0.005 mL/kg/dose (0.025 mg/kg/dose) to a maximum of 0.15 mL (0.75 mg for single dose) every 8-12 hours

(Continued)

Epinephrine *(Continued)*

Nebulization: Infants and Children: 0.25-0.5 mL of 2.25% **racemic epinephrine** solution diluted in 3 mL normal saline, or L-epinephrine at an equivalent dose; racemic epinephrine 10 mg = 5 mg L-epinephrine; use lower end of dosing range for younger infants.

Bradycardia:

I.V.: 0.01 mg/kg (0.1 mL/kg of **1:10,000** solution) every 3-5 minutes as needed (maximum: 1 mg/10 mL)

Intratracheal: 0.1 mg/kg (0.1 mL/kg of **1:1000** solution every 3-5 minutes); doses as high as 0.2 mg/kg may be effective

Asystole or pulseless arrest:

I.V. or intraosseous: **First dose**: 0.01 mg/kg (0.1 mL/kg of a **1:10,000** solution); **subsequent doses**: 0.1 mg/kg (0.1 mL/kg of a **1:1000** solution); doses as high as 0.2 mg/kg may be effective; repeat every 3-5 minutes.

Intratracheal: 0.1 mg/kg (0.1 mL/kg of a **1:1000** solution); doses as high as 0.2 mg/kg may be effective.

Hypersensitivity reaction: S.C.: 0.01 mg/kg every 15 minutes for 2 doses then every 4 hours as needed (single doses not to exceed 0.5 mg)

Refractory hypotension (refractory to dopamine/dobutamine): Continuous I.V. infusions of 0.1-1 mcg/kg/minute; titrate dosage to desired effect.

Nasal congestion: Intranasal: Children ≥6 years: Apply locally as drops or spray or with sterile swab.

Administration

I.M.: I.M. administration into the buttocks should be avoided.

I.V.: Central line administration only. I.V. infusions require an infusion pump.

Endotracheal: Doses (2-2.5 times the I.V. dose) should be diluted to 10 mL with NS or distilled water prior to administration.

Epinephrine can be administered S.C., I.M. (Sus-Phrine®), I.V.

Stability

Storage: Epinephrine is sensitive to light and air. Protection from light is recommended. Oxidation turns drug pink, then a brown color. **Solutions should not be used if they are discolored or contain a precipitate.**

Reconstitution:

Standard diluent: 1 mg/250 mL NS

Preparation of adult I.V. infusion: Dilute 1 mg in 250 mL of D_5W or NS (4 mcg/mL). Administer at an initial rate of 1 mcg/minute and increase to desired effects. At 20 mcg/minute pure alpha effects occur.

1 mcg/minute: 15 mL/hour
2 mcg/minute: 30 mL/hour
3 mcg/minute: 45 mL/hour, etc

Stability of injection of parenteral admixture at room temperature (25°C) or refrigeration (4°C) is 24 hours.

Compatibility: Stable in dextran 6% in dextrose, dextran 6% in NS, D_5LR, $D_5{}^1/_4NS$, $D_5{}^1/_2NS$, D_5NS, D_5W, $D_{10}W$, $D_{10}NS$, LR, NS; **incompatible** with sodium bicarbonate 5%

Y-site administration: Incompatible with ampicillin, thiopental

Compatibility when admixed: Incompatible with aminophylline, hyaluronidase, mephentermine, sodium bicarbonate

Monitoring and Teaching Issues

Physical Assessment: Assess other medications patient may be taking for effectiveness and interactions (see Drug Interactions). See Warnings/Precautions and Contraindications for use cautions. Monitor therapeutic response (according to purpose for use) and adverse reactions (see Warnings/Precautions, Adverse Reactions, and Overdose/Toxicology). Assess knowledge/teach patient appropriate use, interventions to reduce side effects, and adverse symptoms to report (see Patient Education). I.V. central line with infusion pump and continuous cardiac/hemodynamic monitoring is necessary. **Pregnancy risk factor C** - benefits of use should outweigh possible risks. Note breast-feeding caution.

Patient Education: Use this medication exactly as directed; do not take more than recommended dosage. Avoid other stimulant prescriptive or OTC medications to avoid serious overdose reactions. You may experience dizziness, blurred vision, restlessness (use caution when driving or engaging in tasks requiring alertness until response to drug is known); or difficulty urinating (empty bladder immediately before taking this medication). Report excessive nervousness or excitation, inability to sleep, facial flushing, pounding heartbeat, muscle tremors or weakness, chest pain or palpitations, bronchial irritation or coughing, or increased sweating.

Ophthalmic: Wash hands before instilling. Sit or lie down to instill. Open eye, look at ceiling, and instill prescribed amount of medication. Close eye and roll eye in all directions, and apply gentle pressure to inner corner of eye. Do not let tip of applicator touch eye; do not contaminate tip of applicator (may cause eye infection, eye damage, or vision loss). Temporary stinging or burning may occur. Report persistent pain, burning, vision changes, swelling, itching, or worsening of condition.

Aerosol: Use aerosol or nebulizer as per instructions. Clear as much mucus as possible before use. Rinse mouth following each use. If more than one inhalation is necessary, wait 1 minute between inhalations. May cause restlessness or nervousness; use caution when driving or engaging in hazardous activities until response to medication is known. Report persistent nervousness, restlessness, sleeplessness, palpitations, tachycardia, chest pain, muscle tremors, dizziness, flushing, or if breathing difficulty persists.

Nasal: Instill 1 spray into each nostril 3-4 times a day. Report if symptoms worsen or nasal passages become irritated.

Pregnancy/breast-feeding precautions: Inform prescriber if you are or intend to become pregnant. Consult prescriber if breast-feeding.

Geriatric Considerations: The use of epinephrine in the treatment of acute exacerbations of asthma was studied in older adults. A dose of 0.3 mg S.C. every 20 minutes for three doses was well tolerated in older patients with no history of angina or recent myocardial infarction. There was no significant difference in the incidence of ventricular arrhythmias in older adults versus younger adults.

Pregnancy Issues: Crosses the placenta. Reported association with malformations in 1 study; may be secondary to severe maternal disease.

Related Information

Compatibility of Drugs *on page 1564*
Glaucoma Drug Comparison *on page 1575*
Inhalant (Asthma, Bronchospasm) Agents Comparison *on page 1577*
Inotropic and Vasoconstrictor Comparison *on page 1580*

Epinephrine *see* Ophthalmic Agents, Glaucoma *on page 1002*

Epinephrine and Lidocaine *see* Lidocaine and Epinephrine *on page 803*

Epinephrine and Pilocarpine *see* Pilocarpine and Epinephrine *on page 1083*

Epinephrine Bitartrate *see* Epinephrine *on page 470*

Epinephrine Hydrochloride *see* Epinephrine *on page 470*

EpiPen® *see* Epinephrine *on page 470*

EpiPen® Jr *see* Epinephrine *on page 470*

Epipodophyllotoxin *see* Etoposide *on page 536*

Epirubicin (ep i ROO bi sin)

U.S. Brand Names Ellence®

Generic Available No

Pharmacologic Category Antineoplastic Agent, Anthracycline

Pregnancy Risk Factor D

Lactation Excretion in breast milk unknown/contraindicated

Use As a component of adjuvant therapy following primary resection of primary breast cancer in patients with evidence of axillary node tumor involvement

Mechanism of Action/Effect Epirubicin inhibits DNA and RNA synthesis throughout the cell cycle.

Contraindications Hypersensitivity to epirubicin, other anthracyclines, or anthracenediones; baseline neutrophil count <1500 cells/mm^3; severe myocardial insufficiency; recent myocardial infarction; previous treatment with anthracyclines up to the maximum cumulative dose; severe hepatic dysfunction; pregnancy

Warnings/Precautions The U.S. Food and Drug Administration (FDA) currently recommends that procedures for proper handling and disposal of antineoplastic agents be considered. The primary toxicity is myelosuppression, especially of the granulocytic series, with less marked effects on platelets and erythroid series.

Cardiotoxicity may occur, particularly in patients who have received prior anthracyclines or pre-existing cardiac disease. Acute toxicity (primarily arrhythmias) and delayed toxicity (CHF) have been described. Reduce dosage and use with caution in mild to moderate hepatic impairment or in severe renal dysfunction (serum creatinine >5 mg/dL). May cause tumor lysis syndrome or radiation recall. Treatment with anthracyclines may increase the risk of secondary leukemias. May cause premature menopause in premenopausal women. For I.V. administration only, severe local tissue necrosis will result if extravasation occurs. Epirubicin is emetogenic.

Drug Interactions

Increased Effect/Toxicity: Cimetidine increased the blood levels of epirubicin (AUC increased by 50%).

Nutritional/Ethanol Interactions

Ethanol: Avoid ethanol (due to GI irritation).

Herb/Nutraceutical: St John's wort may decrease doxorubicin levels. Avoid black cohosh, dong quai in estrogen-dependent tumors.

Adverse Reactions

>10%:

Central nervous system: Lethargy (1% to 46%)
Dermatologic: Alopecia (69% to 95%)
Endocrine & metabolic: Amenorrhea (69% to 72%), hot flashes (5% to 39%)
Gastrointestinal: Nausea, vomiting (83% to 92%), mucositis (9% to 59%), diarrhea (7% to 25%)
Hematologic: Leukopenia (49% to 80%), neutropenia (54% to 80%), anemia (13% to 72%), thrombocytopenia (5% to 49%)
Local: Injection site reactions (3% to 20%)
Vesicant chemotherapy.
Ocular: Conjunctivitis (1% to 15%)
Miscellaneous: Infection (15% to 21%)

1% to 10%:

Cardiovascular: Congestive heart failure (0.4% to 1.5%), decreased LVEF (asymptomatic) (1.4% to 1.8%)
Central nervous system: Fever (1% to 5%)
Dermatologic: Rash (1% to 9%), skin changes (0.7% to 5%)
Gastrointestinal: Anorexia (2% to 3%)

Other reactions (percentage not specified): Acute lymphoid leukemia, acute myelogenous leukemia (0.2% at 3 years), anaphylaxis, hypersensitivity, increased transaminases, photosensitivity reaction, premature menopause, radiation recall, skin and nail hyperpigmentation, urticaria

Overdosage/Toxicology Symptoms of overdose are generally extensions of known cytotoxic effects, including myelosuppression, mucositis, gastrointestinal bleeding, lactic acidosis, multiple organ failure, and death. Delayed development of congestive heart failure may also occur. Treatment is supportive.

(Continued)

Epirubicin *(Continued)*

Pharmacodynamics/Kinetics

Half-Life Elimination: Triphasic; Mean terminal: 33 hours

Metabolism: Extensive via hepatic and extrahepatic (including RBCs) routes

Formulations Injection, solution [preservative free]: 2 mg/mL (25 mL, 100 mL)

Dosing

Adults:

Recommended starting dose: I.V.: 100-120 mg/m². Epirubicin is given in repeated 3- to 4-week cycles with the total dose given on day 1 of each cycle or divided equally and given on days 1 and 8 of each cycle. Patients receiving the 120 mg/m² regimen should also receive prophylactic antibiotics with TMP-SMX or a fluoroquinolone.

As a component of adjuvant therapy in patients with axillary-node positive breast cancer: I.V.:

CEF-120: 60 mg/m² on days 1 and 8 of cycle (in combination with cyclophosphamide and 5-fluorouracil); cycle is repeated every 28 days for 6 cycles

FEC-100: 100 mg/m² on day 1 of cycle (in combination with 5-fluorouracil and cyclophosphamide); cycle is repeated every 21 days for 6 cycles

Dosage adjustment in bone marrow dysfunction:

Patients with heavy pretreatment, pre-existing bone marrow depression, or the presence of neoplastic bone marrow infiltration: Consider lower starting doses of 75-90 mg/m²

Dosage modifications after the first treatment cycle: Nadir platelet counts <50,000/mm³, ANC <250/mm³, neutropenic fever, or grades 3/4 nonhematologic toxicity: Reduce day 1 dose in subsequent cycles to 75% of the current cycle. Day 1 chemotherapy in subsequent courses of treatment should be delayed until platelet counts are ≥100,000/mm³, ANC ≥1500/mm³, and nonhematologic toxicities have recovered to ≤ grade 1.

In addition, for patients receiving divided dose (day 1 and day 8) regimen:

Day 8 platelet counts 75,000-100,000/mm³ and ANC 1000-1499/mm³: Day 8 dose should be 75% of the day 1 dose.

Day 8 platelet counts <75,000/mm³, ANC <1000/mm³, or grade 3 or 4 nonhematologic toxicity: Omit day 8 dose.

Elderly: Plasma clearance of epirubicin in elderly female patients was noted to be reduced by 35%. Although no initial dosage reduction is specifically recommended, particular care should be exercised in monitoring toxicity and adjusting subsequent dosage in elderly patients (particularly females >70 years).

Renal Impairment: Severe renal impairment (serum creatinine >5 mg/dL): Lower doses should be considered.

Hepatic Impairment:

Bilirubin 1.2-3 mg/dL or AST 2-4 times the upper limit of normal: 50% of recommended starting dose.

Bilirubin >3 mg/dL or AST >4 times the upper limit of normal: 25% of recommended starting dose.

Administration

I.V.: Administer I.V. into the tubing of a freely flowing intravenous infusion (0.9% sodium chloride or 5% glucose solution) over 3-5 minutes. Avoid extravasation, associated with severe ulceration and soft tissue necrosis; flush with 5-10 mL of I.V. solution before and after drug administration. Should not be mixed with other drugs in the same syringe. Incompatible with heparin, fluorouracil, or any solution of alkaline pH.

Stability

Storage: Store refrigerated (2°C to 8°C/36°F to 46°F). Protect from light. Solution should be used within 24 hours of penetrating the rubber stopper.

Compatibility: Stable in D_5W, LR, NS; **incompatible** with any solution of alkaline pH

Incompatible with heparin, fluorouracil

Compatibility in syringe: Incompatible with fluorouracil, ifosfamide with mesna

Monitoring Laboratory Tests CBC with differential and platelet count, liver function tests, renal function, EKG, and left ventricular ejection fraction (baseline and repeated measurement). The method used for assessment of LVEF (echocardiogram or MUGA) should be consistent during routine monitoring.

Monitoring and Teaching Issues

Physical Assessment: This drug should be administered only under the supervision of a physician experienced in the use of chemotherapy. See Contraindications, Warnings/Precautions, and Dosing for use cautions. See Administration, Dosing, Reconstitution, and Compatibility for administration specifics. Premedication with an antiemetic may be ordered (emetogenic). Infusion site must be monitored closely to prevent extravasation (see Administration). Assess results of laboratory tests (see above) and patient response (see Adverse Reactions and Overdose/Toxicology) prior to each treatment and on a regular basis throughout therapy. Teach patient possible side effects and interventions (eg, importance of adequate hydration) and adverse symptoms to report (see Patient Education). **Pregnancy risk factor D** - determine that patient is not pregnant before beginning treatment. Instruct patients of childbearing age on appropriate barrier contraceptive measures. Breast-feeding is contraindicated.

Patient Education: Inform prescriber of all prescriptions, OTC medications, or herbal products you are taking, and any allergies you have. Do not take anything new during treatment unless approved by prescriber. This medication can only be administered by infusion. Report immediately any swelling, pain, burning, or redness at infusion site. Avoid alcohol. Maintain adequate hydration (2-3 L/day of fluids) unless advised by prescriber to restrict fluids, and adequate nutrition (small, frequent meals may help). You will be more susceptible to infection (avoid crowds and exposure to infection and do not have any vaccinations without consulting prescriber). May cause nausea or vomiting (small, frequent meals, frequent mouth care, sucking lozenges, or chewing gum may help); diarrhea (buttermilk, boiled milk, or yogurt may help); loss of hair (reversible); hyperpigmentation of skin or nails; mouth sores (frequent mouth care, soft toothbrush may help); or changes in menstrual cycle (consult prescriber). Report chest pain, swelling of extremities, palpitations, or rapid heartbeat; difficulty breathing or unusual cough; unresolved nausea, vomiting, or diarrhea; alterations in urinary pattern (increased or decreased); opportunistic infection (fever, chills, unusual bruising or bleeding, fatigue, purulent vaginal discharge, unhealed mouth sores); skin rash; abdominal pain; blood in urine or stool; or other unresolved reactions. **Pregnancy/breast-feeding precautions:** Do not get pregnant while taking this medication and for 1 month following therapy. Consult prescriber for appropriate barrier contraceptives. Do not breast-feed.

Breast-feeding Issues: Excretion in human breast milk is unknown, however, other anthracyclines are excreted. Breast-feeding is contraindicated.

Pregnancy Issues: Epirubicin is mutagenic and carcinogenic. If a pregnant woman is treated with epirubicin, or if a woman becomes pregnant while receiving this drug, she should be informed of the potential hazard to the fetus. Women of childbearing potential should be advised to avoid becoming pregnant.

Epitol® *see* Carbamazepine *on page 213*

Epivir® *see* Lamivudine *on page 768*

Epivir-HBV® *see* Lamivudine *on page 768*

Eplerenone (e PLER en one)

U.S. Brand Names Inspra™

Generic Available No

Pharmacologic Category Antihypertensive; Selective Aldosterone Blocker

Pregnancy Risk Factor B

Lactation Excretion in breast milk unknown/not recommended

Use Treatment of hypertension; may be used alone or in combination with other antihypertensive agents

Mechanism of Action/Effect Aldosterone increases blood pressure primarily by inducing sodium reabsorption. Eplerenone reduces blood pressure by blocking aldosterone binding at mineralocorticoid receptors found in the kidney, heart, blood vessels and brain.

Contraindications Hypersensitivity to eplerenone or any component of the formulation; serum potassium >5.5 mEq/L; type 2 diabetes mellitus (noninsulin dependent, NIDDM) with microalbuminuria; serum creatinine >2.0 mg/dL in males or >1.8 mg/dL in females; Cl_{cr} <50 mL/minute; concomitant use with potassium supplements or potassium-sparing diuretics, strong CYP3A4 inhibitors (see Drug Interactions for details)

Warnings/Precautions Dosage adjustment needed for patients on weak CYP3A4 inhibitors (see Drug Interactions for details). Monitor closely for hyperkalemia; increases in serum potassium were dose related during clinical trials and rates of hyperkalemia also increased with decreasing renal function. Safety and efficacy have not been established in pediatric patients or in patients with severe hepatic impairment.

Drug Interactions

Cytochrome P450 Effect: Substrate of **CYP3A4**

Decreased Effect: NSAIDs may decrease the antihypertensive effects of eplerenone.

Increased Effect/Toxicity: ACE inhibitors, angiotensin II receptor antagonists, NSAIDs, potassium supplements, and potassium-sparing diuretics increase the risk of hyperkalemia; concomitant use with potassium supplements and potassium sparing diuretics is contraindicated; monitor potassium levels with ACE inhibitors and angiotensin II receptor antagonists. Potent CYP3A3/4 inhibitors (ie, itraconazole, ketoconazole) lead to five-fold increase in eplerenone; concurrent use is contraindicated. Less potent CYP3A3/4 inhibitors (ie, erythromycin, fluconazole, saquinavir, verapamil) lead to approximately two-fold increase in eplerenone; starting dose should be decreased to 25 mg/day. Although interaction studies have not been conducted, monitoring of lithium levels is recommended.

Nutritional/Ethanol Interactions

Food: Grapefruit juice increases eplerenone AUC ~25%.

Herb/Nutraceutical: St John's wort decreases eplerenone AUC ~30%.

Adverse Reactions

>10%: Endocrine & metabolic: Hypertriglyceridemia (1% to 15%, dose related)

1% to 10%:

Central nervous system: Dizziness (3%), fatigue (2%)

Endocrine & metabolic: Hyponatremia (2%, dose related), hypercholesterolemia (<1% to 1%), hyperkalemia (dose related, up to 1% at maximum recommended dose), breast pain (males <1% to 1%), gynecomastia (males <1% to 1%)

Gastrointestinal: Diarrhea (2%), abdominal pain (1%)

Genitourinary: Abnormal vaginal bleeding (<1% to 2%)

Renal: Albuminuria (1%)

Respiratory: Cough (2%)

Miscellaneous: Flu-like syndrome (2%)

<1% (Limited to important or life-threatening): BUN increased, liver function tests increased, serum creatinine increased, uric acid increased

Overdosage/Toxicology Cases of human overdose have not been reported; hypotension or hyperkalemia would be expected. Treatment should be symptom-directed and supportive. Eplerenone is not removed by hemodialysis; binds extensively to charcoal.

Pharmacodynamics/Kinetics

Half-Life Elimination: 4-6 hours

Time to Peak: Plasma: 1.5 hours; may take up to 4 weeks for full therapeutic effect

Metabolism: Primarily hepatic via CYP3A4; metabolites inactive

Formulations Tablet, film-coated: 25 mg, 50 mg, 100 mg

Dosing

Adults: Hypertension: Oral: Initial: 50 mg once daily; may increase to 50 mg twice daily if response is not adequate; may take up to 4 weeks for full therapeutic response. Doses >100 mg/day are associated with increased risk of hyperkalemia and no greater therapeutic effect.

Concurrent use with weak CYP3A4 inhibitors: Initial: 25 mg once daily

(Continued)

Eplerenone *(Continued)*

Renal Impairment: Contraindicated with Cl_{cr} <50 mL/minute or serum creatinine >2.0 mg/dL in males or >1.8 md/dL in females. Risk of hyperkalemia increases with decreased renal function.

Hepatic Impairment: No dosage adjustment needed for mild to moderate impairment. Safety and efficacy not established for severe impairment.

Stability

Storage: Store at controlled room temperature of 25°C (77°F).

Monitoring Laboratory Tests Serum potassium (levels monitored every 2 weeks for the first 1-2 months, then monthly in clinical trials); renal function

Monitoring and Teaching Issues

Physical Assessment: See Contraindications, Warnings/Precautions, and Dosing for use cautions. Assess potential for interactions with other prescriptions, OTC medications, or herbal products patient may be taking (eg, hyperkalemia - see Drug Interactions). Assess results of laboratory tests (see above) prior to and at regular intervals during therapy. Assess therapeutic effectiveness and adverse response on a regular basis during therapy (see Adverse Reactions). Teach patient proper use, side effects and appropriate interventions, and adverse reactions to report (see Patient Education). Breast-feeding is not recommended.

Patient Education: Inform prescriber of all prescriptions, OTC medications, or herbal products you are taking, and any allergies you have. Do not take anything new during treatment without consulting prescriber. Do not use potassium supplement or salt substitutes without consulting prescriber. Take exactly as directed and do not discontinue without consulting prescriber. This drug does not eliminate need for diet or exercise regimen as recommended by prescriber. May cause dizziness or lightheadedness (use caution when driving or engaging in tasks that require alertness until response to drug is known); or diarrhea (boiled milk, buttermilk, or yogurt may help). Report chest pain, palpitations, or irregular heartbeat; unrelenting headache; persistent fatigue or flu-like symptoms; or other persistent adverse reactions. **Breast-feeding precaution:** Breast-feeding is not recommended.

Dietary Issues: May be taken with or without food. Do not use salt substitutes containing potassium.

EPO *see* Epoetin Alfa *on page 476*

Epoetin Alfa (e POE e tin AL fa)

U.S. Brand Names Epogen®; Procrit®

Synonyms EPO; Erythropoietin; *r*HuEPO-α

Generic Available No

Pharmacologic Category Colony Stimulating Factor

Pregnancy Risk Factor C

Lactation Excretion in breast milk unknown

Use

Treatment of anemia related to zidovudine therapy in HIV-infected patients; in patients when the endogenous erythropoietin level is ≤500 mU/mL and the dose of zidovudine is ≤4200 mg/week

Treatment of anemia in cancer patients on chemotherapy; in patients with nonmyeloid malignancies where anemia is caused by the effect of the concomitantly administered chemotherapy; to decrease the need for transfusions in patients who will be receiving chemotherapy for a minimum of 2 months

Reduction of allogeneic block transfusion in surgery patients scheduled to undergo elective, noncardiac, nonvascular surgery

Orphan drug: Epogen®: Treatment of anemia associated with end-stage renal disease; treatment of anemia associated with HIV infection or HIV treatment

Use - Unlabeled/Investigational Anemia associated with rheumatic disease; hypogenerative anemia of Rh hemolytic disease; sickle cell anemia; acute renal failure; Gaucher's disease; Castleman's disease; paroxysmal nocturnal hemoglobinuria

Mechanism of Action/Effect Induces red blood cell production in the bone marrow to be released into the blood stream where they mature to erythrocytes; results in rise in hematocrit and hemoglobin levels

Contraindications Hypersensitivity to albumin (human) or mammalian cell-derived products; uncontrolled hypertension

Warnings/Precautions Use with caution in patients with porphyria, hypertension, or a history of seizures; prior to and during therapy, iron stores must be evaluated. It is recommended that the epoetin dose be decreased if the hematocrit increase exceeds 4 points in any 2-week period. **Not** recommended for acute correction of severe anemia or as a substitute for transfusion. For patients receiving renal transplant, consider discontinuing at transplant or within 2 weeks of successful engraftment.

Pretherapy parameters:

Serum ferritin >100 ng/dL

Transferrin saturation (serum iron/iron binding capacity x 100) of 20% to 30%

Iron supplementation (usual oral dosing of 325 mg 2-3 times/day) should be given during therapy to provide for increased requirements during expansion of the red cell mass secondary to marrow stimulation by EPO unless iron stores are already in excess

For patients with endogenous serum EPO levels which are inappropriately low for hemoglobin level, documentation of the serum EPO level will help indicate which patients may benefit from EPO therapy. Serum EPO levels can be ordered routinely from Clinical Chemistry (red top serum separator tube). Refer to "Reference Range" for information on interpretation of EPO levels.

See table on following page.

Increased mortality has occurred when aggressive dosing is used in CHF or anginal patients undergoing hemodialysis. An Amgen-funded study determined that when patients were targeted for a hematocrit of 42% versus a less aggressive 30%, mortality was higher (35% versus 29%).

Pregnancy risk C.

Factors Limiting Response to Epoetin Alfa

Factor	Mechanism
Iron deficiency	Limits hemoglobin synthesis
Blood loss/hemolysis	Counteracts epoetin alfa-stimulated erythropoiesis
Infection/inflammation	Inhibits iron transfer from storage to bone marrow Suppresses erythropoiesis through activated macrophages
Aluminum overload	Inhibits iron incorporation into heme protein
Bone marrow replacement Hyperparathyroidsm Metastatic, neoplastic	Limits bone marrow volume
Folic acid/vitamin B_{12} deficiency	Limits hemoglobin synthesis
Patient compliance	Self-administered epoetin alfa or iron therapy

Adverse Reactions

>10%:

Cardiovascular: Hypertension

Central nervous system: Fatigue, headache, fever

1% to 10%:

Cardiovascular: Edema, chest pain, polycythemia

Central nervous system: Dizziness, seizures

Gastrointestinal: Nausea, vomiting, diarrhea

Hematologic: Clotted access

Neuromuscular & skeletal: Arthralgia, weakness

<1% (Limited to important or life-threatening): CVA/TIA, myocardial infarction

Overdosage/Toxicology Symptoms of overdose include erythrocytosis. Maintain adequate airway and provide other supportive measures and agents for treating anaphylaxis when the I.V. drug is given.

Pharmacodynamics/Kinetics

Bioavailability: S.C.: ~21% to 31%; Intraperitoneal epoetin: 3% (a few patients)

Half-Life Elimination: Circulating: Chronic renal failure: 4-13 hours; Healthy volunteers: 20% shorter

Time to Peak: Serum: S.C.: 2-8 hours

Metabolism: Some degradation does occur

Onset: Several days; Peak effect: 2-3 weeks

Formulations

Injection, solution [preservative free]: 2000 units/mL (1 mL); 3000 units/mL (1 mL); 4000 units/mL (1 mL); 10,000 units/mL (1 mL); 40,000 units/mL (1 mL) [contains human albumin]

Injection, solution [with preservative]: 10,000 units/mL (2 mL); 20,000 units/mL (2 mL) [contains human albumin and benzyl alcohol]

Dosing

Adults & Elderly: Individuals with anemia due to iron deficiency, sickle cell disease, autoimmune hemolytic anemia, and bleeding, generally have appropriate endogenous EPO levels to drive erythropoiesis and would not ordinarily be candidates for EPO therapy.

Chronic renal failure patients: I.V., S.C.:

Initial dose: 50-100 units/kg 3 times/week

Reduce dose by 25 units/kg when

1) hematocrit approaches 36% **or**

2) when hematocrit increases >4 points in any 2-week period

Increase dose if hematocrit does not increase by 5-6 points after 8 weeks of therapy and hematocrit is below suggested target range.

Suggested target hematocrit range: 30% to 36%

Maintenance dose: Individualize to target range.

Dialysis patients: Median dose: 75 units/kg 3 times/week

Nondialysis patients: Doses of 75-150 units/kg

Zidovudine-treated, HIV-infected patients: Patients with erythropoietin levels >500 mU/mL are **unlikely** to respond.

Initial dose: I.V., S.C.: 100 units/kg 3 times/week for 8 weeks

Increase dose by 50-100 units/kg 3 times/week if response is not satisfactory in terms of reducing transfusion requirements or increasing hematocrit after 8 weeks of therapy.

Evaluate response every 4-8 weeks thereafter and adjust the dose accordingly by 50-100 units/kg increments 3 times/week.

If patients have not responded satisfactorily to a 300 unit/kg dose 3 times/week, it is unlikely that they will respond to higher doses.

Stop dose if hematocrit exceeds 40% and resume treatment at a 25% dose reduction when hematocrit drops to 36%.

Cancer patients on chemotherapy: Treatment of patients with erythropoietin levels >200 mU/mL is **not recommended**

Initial dose: S.C.: 150 units/kg 3 times/week

Dose adjustment: If response is not satisfactory in terms of reducing transfusion requirement or increasing hematocrit after 8 weeks of therapy, the dose may be increased up to 300 units/kg 3 times/week. If patients do not respond, it is unlikely that they will respond to higher doses.

If hematocrit exceeds 40%, hold the dose until it falls to 36% and reduce the dose by 25% when treatment is resumed.

Surgery patients: Prior to initiating treatment, obtain a hemoglobin to establish that is >10 mg/dL or ≤13 mg/dL.

(Continued)

Epoetin Alfa *(Continued)*

Initial dose: S.C.: 300 units/kg/day for 10 days before surgery, on the day of surgery, and for 4 days after surgery

Alternative dose: S.C.: 600 units/kg in once weekly doses (21, 14, and 7 days before surgery) plus a fourth dose on the day of surgery

Renal Impairment:

Dialysis patient: Usually administered as I.V. bolus 3 times/week. While administration is independent of the dialysis procedure, it may be administered into the venous line at the end of the dialysis procedure to obviate the need for additional venous access.

Chronic renal failure patients not on dialysis: May be given either as an I.V. or S.C. injection.

Hemodialysis: Supplemental dose is not necessary.

Peritoneal dialysis: Supplemental dose is not necessary.

Stability

Storage: Vials should be stored at 2°C to 8°C (36°F to 46°F). **Do not freeze or shake.** Vials are stable 2 weeks at room temperature.

Single-dose 1 mL vial contains no preservative. Use one dose per vial. Do not re-enter vial. Discard unused portions.

Multidose 2 mL vial contains preservative. Store at 2°C to 8°C after initial entry and between doses. Discard 21 days after initial entry.

Reconstitution: For minimal dilution, mix with bacteriostatic 0.9% sodium chloride, containing 20 mL of 0.9% sodium chloride and benzyl alcohol as the bacteriostatic agent. Dilutions of 1:10 and 1:20 (1 part epoetin:19 parts sodium chloride) are stable for 18 hours at room temperature. Results showed no loss of epoetin alfa after a 1:20 dilution. 250 mcg/mL albumin remaining after a 1:10 dilution of formulated epoetin alfa should be sufficient to prevent it from binding to commonly encountered containers.

Compatibility: Stable in $D_{10}W$ with albumin 0.05%, $D_{10}W$ with albumin 0.1%; **incompatible** with $D_{10}W$ with albumin 0.01%, $D_{10}W$, NS

Monitoring Laboratory Tests Hematocrit should be determined twice weekly until stabilization within the target range (30% to 36%), and twice weekly for at least 2-6 weeks after a dose increase. See table.

Test	Initial Phase Frequency	Maintenance Phase Frequency
Hematocrit/hemoglobin*	2 x/week	2-4 x/month
Blood pressure	3 x/week	3 x/week
Serum ferritin	Monthly	Quarterly
Transferrin saturation	Monthly	Quarterly
Serum chemistries including CBC with differential, creatinine, blood urea nitrogen, potassium, phosphorous	Regularly per routine	Regularly per routine

Monitoring and Teaching Issues

Physical Assessment: See Contraindications, Warnings/Precautions, and Dosing for use cautions. Assess potential for interactions with other prescriptions, OTC medications, or herbal products patient may be taking (see Drug Interactions, eg, nutritional or supplemental iron). See Administration specifics. I.V. lines should be monitored for possible clotting. Assess results of laboratory tests (see above), therapeutic effectiveness, and adverse response (eg, hypovolemia, angioedema, postural hypotension - see Adverse Reactions and Overdose/Toxicology) on a regular basis during therapy. Teach patient appropriate use (injections technique and needle disposal), possible side effects and appropriate interventions, and adverse symptoms to report (see Patient Education). **Pregnancy risk factor C** - benefits of use should outweigh possible risks. Note breast-feeding caution.

Patient Education: Inform prescriber of all prescriptions, OTC medications, or herbal products you are taking, and any allergies you have. Do not take anything new without consulting prescriber. If self-administered, follow exact directions for injection and needle disposal. You will require frequent blood tests to determine appropriate dosage. Do not make significant changes in your dietary iron without consulting prescriber. Report signs or symptoms of edema (eg, swollen extremities, difficulty breathing, rapid weight gain); onset of severe headache; acute back pain; chest pain; or muscular tremors or seizure activity. **Pregnancy/breast-feeding precautions:** Inform prescriber if you are or intend to become pregnant. Consult prescriber if breast-feeding.

Geriatric Considerations: There is limited information about the use of epoetin alfa in the elderly. Endogenous erythropoietin secretion has been reported to be decreased in older adults with normocytic or iron-deficiency anemias or those with a serum hemoglobin concentration <12 g/dL; one study did not find such a relationship in the elderly with chronic anemia. A blunted erythropoietin response to anemia has been reported in patients with cancer, rheumatoid arthritis, and AIDS.

Pregnancy Issues: Epoetin alpha has been shown to have adverse effects in rats when given in doses 5 times the human dose. Use only if potential benefit justifies the potential risk to the fetus.

Additional Information Due to the delayed onset of erythropoiesis (7-10 days to ↑ reticulocyte count; 2-6 weeks to ↑ hemoglobin), erythropoietin is of no value in the acute treatment of anemia. Emergency/stat orders for erythropoietin are inappropriate.

Professional Services:

Amgen (Epogen®): 1-800-772-6436

Ortho Biotech (Procrit®): 1-800-325-7504

Reimbursement Assistance:

Amgen: 1-800-272-9376

Ortho Biotech: 1-800-553-3851

Epogen® *see* Epoetin Alfa *on page 476*

Epoprostenol (e poe PROST en ole)

U.S. Brand Names Flolan®

Synonyms Epoprostenol Sodium; PGI_2; PGX; Prostacyclin

Generic Available No

Pharmacologic Category Prostaglandin

Pregnancy Risk Factor B

Lactation Excretion in breast milk unknown

Use Orphan drug: Treatment of primary pulmonary hypertension; treatment of secondary pulmonary hypertension due to intrinsic precapillary pulmonary vascular disease

Use - Unlabeled/Investigational Other potential uses include pulmonary hypertension associated with ARDS, SLE, or CHF; neonatal pulmonary hypertension; cardiopulmonary bypass surgery; hemodialysis; atherosclerosis; peripheral vascular disorders; and neonatal purpura fulminans

Mechanism of Action/Effect Naturally occur ring prostacyclin (PG12) which acts as a strong vasodilator in all vascular beds; inhibits platelet aggregation

Contraindications Hypersensitivity to epoprostenol or to structurally-related compounds; chronic use in patients with CHF due to severe left ventricular systolic dysfunction

Warnings/Precautions Abrupt interruptions or large sudden reductions in dosage may result in rebound pulmonary hypertension. Some patients with primary pulmonary hypertension have developed pulmonary edema during dose ranging, which may be associated with pulmonary veno-occlusive disease. During chronic use, unless contraindicated, anticoagulants should be coadministered to reduce the risk of thromboembolism. Use cautiously with patients who have bleeding tendencies (inhibits platelet aggregation).

Drug Interactions

Increased Effect/Toxicity: The hypotensive effects of epoprostenol may be exacerbated by other vasodilators, diuretics, or by using acetate in dialysis fluids. Patients treated with anticoagulants (heparins, warfarin, thrombin inhibitors) or antiplatelet agents (ticlopidine, clopidogrel, IIb/IIIa antagonists, aspirin) and epoprostenol should be monitored for increased bleeding risk.

Adverse Reactions

>10%:

Cardiovascular: Flushing, tachycardia, shock, syncope, heart failure

Central nervous system: Fever, chills, anxiety, nervousness, dizziness, headache, hyperesthesia, pain

Gastrointestinal: Diarrhea, nausea, vomiting

Neuromuscular & skeletal: Jaw pain, myalgia, tremor, paresthesia

Respiratory: Hypoxia

Miscellaneous: Sepsis, flu-like symptoms

1% to 10%:

Cardiovascular: Bradycardia, hypotension, angina pectoris, edema, arrhythmias, pallor, cyanosis, palpitations, cerebrovascular accident, myocardial ischemia, chest pain

Central nervous system: Seizures, confusion, depression, insomnia

Dermatologic: Pruritus, rash

Endocrine & metabolic: Hypokalemia, weight change

Gastrointestinal: Abdominal pain, anorexia, constipation

Hematologic: Hemorrhage, disseminated intravascular coagulation

Hepatic: Ascites

Neuromuscular & skeletal: Arthralgias, bone pain, weakness

Ocular: Amblyopia

Respiratory: Cough increase, dyspnea, epistaxis, pleural effusion

Miscellaneous: Diaphoresis

<1% (Limited to important or life-threatening): Anemia, hypersplenism, hyperthyroidism, pancytopenia, splenomegaly

Overdosage/Toxicology Symptoms of overdose include headache, hypotension, tachycardia, nausea, vomiting, diarrhea, and flushing. If any of these symptoms occur, reduce the infusion rate until symptoms subside. If symptoms do not subside, consider drug discontinuation. No fatal events have been reported following overdose with epoprostenol.

Pharmacodynamics/Kinetics

Half-Life Elimination: 2.7-6 minutes; Continuous infusion: ~15 minutes

Metabolism: Rapidly hydrolyzed at neutral pH in blood and subject to some enzymatic degradation to one active metabolite and 13 inactive metabolites

Formulations Injection, powder for reconstitution, as sodium: 0.5 mg, 1.5 mg [provided with 50 mL sterile diluent]

Dosing

Adults & Elderly: Pulmonary hypertension associated with scleroderma: I.V.:

Acute dose ranging: The initial infusion rate should be 2 ng/kg/minute by continuous I.V. and increased in increments of 2 ng/kg/minute every 15 minutes or longer until dose-limiting effects are elicited (such as chest pain, anxiety, dizziness, changes in heart rate, dyspnea, nausea, vomiting, headache, hypotension and/or flushing).

Continuous chronic infusion: Initial: 4 ng/kg/minute **less** than the maximum-tolerated infusion rate determined during acute dose ranging.

If maximum-tolerated infusion rate is <5 ng/kg/minute the chronic infusion rate should be ½ the maximum-tolerated acute infusion rate.

Dosage adjustments: Dose adjustments in the chronic infusion rate should be based on persistence, recurrence, or worsening of patient symptoms of pulmonary hypertension. If symptoms persist or reoccur after improving, the infusion rate should be increased by 1-2 ng/kg/minute increments, every 15 minutes or more. Following establishment of a new chronic infusion rate, the patient should be observed and vital signs monitored.

(Continued)

Epoprostenol *(Continued)*

Stability

Storage: Refrigerate ampuls. Protect from freezing. Prepare fresh solutions every 24 hours.

Reconstitution: Prepare fresh solutions every 24 hours. Reconstitute with sterile diluent for epoprostenol. See table.

Preparation of Epoprostenol Infusion

To make 100 mL of solution with concentration:	Directions
3000 ng/mL	Dissolve one 0.5 mg vial with 5 mL supplied diluent, withdraw 3 mL, and add to sufficient diluent to make a total of 100 mL.
5000 ng/mL	Dissolve one 0.5 mg vial with 5 mL supplied diluent, withdraw entire vial contents, and add a sufficient volume of diluent to make a total of 100 mL.
10,000 ng/mL	Dissolve two 0.5 mg vials each with 5 mL supplied diluent, withdraw entire vial contents, and add a sufficient volume of diluent to make a total of 100 mL.
15,000 ng/mL	Dissolve one 1.5 mg vial with 5 mL supplied diluent, withdraw entire vial contents, and add a sufficient volume of diluent to make a total of 100 mL.

Compatibility: Stable in D_5W, $D_{10}W$, NS

Do not mix or administer with any other drugs prior to or during administration. Stable for 8 hours at room temperature.

Monitoring and Teaching Issues

Physical Assessment: **Institutional:** Continuous pulmonary and hemodynamic arterial monitoring, protimes. **Noninstitutional:** Avoid sudden rate reduction or abrupt withdrawal or interruption of therapy (see Warnings/Precautions). When adjustment in rate is made, monitor blood pressure (standing and supine) and pulse for several hours to ensure tolerance to new rate. Monitor for bleeding. Monitor (or teach appropriate caregiver or patient to monitor) vital signs on 3 times/day basis. Monitor for improved pulmonary function and improved quality of life. Be alert for any infusion pump malfunction. Assess for signs of overdose (eg, hypoxia, flushing, tachycardia, fever, chills, anxiety, acute headache, tremor, vomiting, diarrhea). Note breast-feeding caution.

Patient Education: Therapy on this drug will probably be prolonged, possibly for years. You may experience mild headache, nausea or vomiting, and some muscular pains (use of a mild analgesia may be recommended by your prescriber). Report immediately any signs or symptoms of acute or severe headache, back pain, increased difficult breathing, flushing, fever or chills, any unusual bleeding or bruising, or any onset of unresolved diarrhea. **Breast-feeding precaution:** Consult prescriber if breast-feeding.

Additional Information All orders for epoprostenol are distributed only by Olsten Health Services. To order the drug or to request reimbursement assistance, call 1-800-935-6526.

Epoprostenol Sodium *see* Epoprostenol *on page 479*

Eprosartan (ep roe SAR tan)

U.S. Brand Names Teveten®

Generic Available No

Pharmacologic Category Angiotensin II Receptor Blocker

Pregnancy Risk Factor C (1st trimester); D (2nd and 3rd trimesters)

Lactation Not recommended

Use Treatment of hypertension; may be used alone or in combination with other antihypertensives

Mechanism of Action/Effect Eprosartan is an angiotensin receptor antagonist which blocks the vasoconstriction and aldosterone-secreting effects of angiotensin II.

Contraindications Hypersensitivity to eprosartan or any component of the formulation; sensitivity to other A-II receptor antagonists; bilateral renal artery stenosis; primary hyperaldosteronism; pregnancy (2nd and 3rd trimesters)

Warnings/Precautions Avoid use or use a smaller dose in patients who are volume depleted; correct depletion first. Deterioration in renal function can occur with initiation. Use with caution in unilateral renal artery stenosis and pre-existing renal insufficiency; significant aortic/mitral stenosis. Safety and efficacy in pediatric patients has not established. Pregnancy risk C (1st trimester)/D (2nd and 3rd trimesters).

Drug Interactions

Cytochrome P450 Effect: Inhibits CYP2C8/9

Increased Effect/Toxicity: Eprosartan may increase risk of lithium toxicity. May increase risk of hyperkalemia with potassium-sparing diuretics (eg, amiloride, potassium, spironolactone, triamterene), potassium supplements, or high doses of trimethoprim.

Nutritional/Ethanol Interactions Herb/Nutraceutical: Avoid dong quai if using for hypertension (has estrogenic activity). Avoid ephedra, yohimbe, ginseng (may worsen hypertension). Avoid garlic (may have increased antihypertensive effect).

Adverse Reactions

1% to 10%:

Central nervous system: Fatigue (2%), depression (1%)

Endocrine & metabolic: Hypertriglyceridemia (1%)

Gastrointestinal: Abdominal pain (2%)

Genitourinary: Urinary tract infection (1%)

Respiratory: Upper respiratory tract infection (8%), rhinitis (4%), pharyngitis (4%), cough (4%)

Miscellaneous: Viral infection (2%), injury (2%)

<1% (Limited to important or life-threatening): Angina, arthritis, asthma, ataxia, BUN increased, creatinine increased, eczema, edema, esophagitis, ethanol intolerance, gingivitis, gout, influenza-like symptoms, leg cramps, leukopenia, maculopapular rash, migraine, neuritis, neutropenia, paresthesia, peripheral ischemia, purpura, renal calculus, somnolence, tendonitis, thrombocytopenia, tinnitus, tremor, urinary incontinence, vertigo

Overdosage/Toxicology The most likely manifestations of overdose would be hypotension and tachycardia. Initiate supportive care for symptomatic hypotension.

Pharmacodynamics/Kinetics

Bioavailability: 300 mg dose: 13%

Half-Life Elimination: Terminal: 5-9 hours

Time to Peak: Serum: Fasting: 1-2 hours

Metabolism: Minimally hepatic

Formulations Tablet, as mesylate: 400 mg, 600 mg

Dosing

Adults: Hypertension: Oral: Dosage must be individualized. Can administer once or twice daily with total daily doses of 400-800 mg. Usual starting dose is 600 mg once daily as monotherapy in patients who are euvolemic. Limited clinical experience with doses >800 mg.

Elderly: No starting dosage adjustment is necessary; however, carefully monitor the patient.

Renal Impairment: No starting dosage adjustment is necessary; however, carefully monitor the patient.

Hepatic Impairment: No starting dosage adjustment is necessary; however, carefully monitor the patient.

Monitoring Laboratory Tests Electrolytes, serum creatinine, BUN, urinalysis

Monitoring and Teaching Issues

Physical Assessment: See Contraindications, Warnings/Precautions, and Dosing for use cautions. Assess potential for interactions with other prescriptions, OTC medications, or herbal products patient may be taking (see Drug Interactions). Assess results of laboratory tests (see above), therapeutic effectiveness, and adverse response on a regular basis during therapy (eg, hypotension - see Adverse Reactions and Overdose/Toxicology). Teach patient appropriate use, possible side effects and appropriate interventions, and adverse symptoms to report (see Patient Education). **Pregnancy risk factor C/D** - see Pregnancy Risk Factor for use cautions. Instruct patient of childbearing age about appropriate use of barrier contraceptives. Breast-feeding is not recommended

Patient Education: Inform prescriber of all prescriptions, OTC medications, or herbal products you are taking, and any allergies you have. Do not take anything new during treatment unless approved by prescriber. Take exactly as directed and do not discontinue without consulting prescriber. This drug does not eliminate need for diet or exercise regimen as recommended by prescriber. May cause dizziness, fainting, or lightheadedness (use caution when driving or engaging in tasks that require alertness until response to drug is known); or postural hypotension (use caution when rising from lying or sitting position or climbing stairs). Report chest pain or palpitations; respiratory infection or cold symptoms; unusual cough; swelling of face, tongue, lips, or extremities; changes in urinary pattern; extreme fatigue; or other adverse response. **Pregnancy/breast-feeding precautions:** Inform prescriber if you are or intend to become pregnant. This drug should not be used in the 2nd or 3rd trimester of pregnancy. Consult prescriber for appropriate contraceptive measures if necessary. Consult prescriber if breast-feeding.

Related Information

Angiotensin Agents *on page 1547*

Epsom Salts (Magnesium Sulfate) *see* Magnesium Supplements *on page 831*

EPT *see* Teniposide *on page 1285*

Eptifibatide (ep TIF i ba tide)

U.S. Brand Names Integrilin®

Synonyms Intrifiban

Generic Available No

Pharmacologic Category Antiplatelet Agent, Glycoprotein IIb/IIIa Inhibitor

Pregnancy Risk Factor B

Lactation Excretion in breast milk unknown/not recommended

Use Treatment of patients with acute coronary syndrome (UA/NQMI), including patients who are to be managed medically and those undergoing percutaneous coronary intervention (PCI including PTCA; intracoronary stenting)

Mechanism of Action/Effect Eptifibatide is a IIb/IIa antagonist that reversibly blocks platelet aggregation and prevents thrombosis.

Contraindications Hypersensitivity to eptifibatide or any component of the product; active abnormal bleeding or a history of bleeding diathesis within the previous 30 days; history of CVA within 30 days or a history of hemorrhagic stroke; severe hypertension (systolic blood pressure >200 mm Hg or diastolic blood pressure >110 mm Hg) not adequately controlled on antihypertensive therapy; major surgery within the preceding 6 weeks; current or planned administration of another parenteral GP IIb/IIIa inhibitor; thrombocytopenia; serum creatinine >4 mg/dL; dependency on renal dialysis

Warnings/Precautions Bleeding is the most common complication. Most major bleeding occurs at the arterial access site where the cardiac catheterization was done. When bleeding can not be controlled with pressure, discontinue infusion and heparin. Use caution in patients with platelet counts <100,000/mm^3, hemorrhagic retinopathy, or with other drugs that affect hemostasis. Concurrent use with thrombolytics has not been established as safe. Minimize other procedures including arterial and venous punctures, I.M. injections, nasogastric tubes, etc. Prior to sheath removal, the aPTT or ACT should be checked (do not remove unless aPTT is <45 seconds or the ACT <150 seconds).

Drug Interactions

Increased Effect/Toxicity: Eptifibatide effect may be increased by other drugs which affect hemostasis include thrombolytics, oral anticoagulants, NSAIDs, dipyridamole,

(Continued)

Eptifibatide *(Continued)*

heparin, low molecular weight heparins, ticlopidine, and clopidogrel. Avoid concomitant use of other IIb/IIIa inhibitors. Cephalosporins which contain the MTT side chain may theoretically increase the risk of hemorrhage. Use with aspirin and heparin may increase bleeding over aspirin and heparin alone. However, aspirin and heparin were used concurrently in the majority of patients in the major clinical studies of eptifibatide.

Adverse Reactions Bleeding is the major drug-related adverse effect. Major bleeding was reported in 4.4% to 10.8%; minor bleeding was reported in 10.5% to 14.2%; requirement for transfusion was reported in 5.5% to 12.8%. Incidence of bleeding is also related to heparin intensity (aPTT goal 50-70 seconds). Patients weighing <70 kg may have an increased risk of major bleeding.

Cardiovascular: Hypotension
Local: Injection site reaction
Neuromuscular & skeletal: Back pain

1% to 10%: Hematologic: Thrombocytopenia (1.2% to 3.2%)
<1% (Limited to important or life-threatening): Anaphylaxis, GI hemorrhage, intracranial hemorrhage (0.5% to 0.7%), pulmonary hemorrhage

Overdosage/Toxicology Two cases of human overdose have been reported; neither case was eventful or associated with major bleeding. Symptoms of overdose in animal studies include loss of righting reflex, dyspnea, ptosis, decreased muscle tone, and petechial hemorrhage. Treatment is supportive.

Pharmacodynamics/Kinetics

Half-Life Elimination: 2.5 hours

Onset: Within 1 hour

Duration: Platelet function restored ~4 hours following discontinuation

Formulations Injection, solution: 0.75 mg/mL (100 mL); 2 mg/mL (10 mL, 100 mL)

Dosing

Adults & Elderly:

Acute coronary syndrome: I.V.: Bolus of 180 mcg/kg (maximum: 22.6 mg) over 1-2 minutes, begun as soon as possible following diagnosis, followed by a continuous infusion of 2 mcg/kg/minute (maximum: 15 mg/hour) until hospital discharge or initiation of CABG surgery, up to 72 hours. Concurrent aspirin (160-325 mg initially and daily thereafter) and heparin therapy (target aPTT 50-70 seconds) are recommended.

Percutaneous coronary intervention (PCI) with or without stenting: I.V.: Bolus of 180 mcg/kg (maximum: 22.6 mg) administered immediately before the initiation of PCI, followed by a continuous infusion of 2 mcg/kg/minute (maximum: 15 mg/hour). A second 180 mcg/kg bolus (maximum: 22.6 mg) should be administered 10 minutes after the first bolus. Infusion should be continued until hospital discharge or for up to 18-24 hours, whichever comes first; minimum of 12 hours of infusion is recommended. Concurrent aspirin (160-325 mg 1-24 hours before PCI and daily thereafter) and heparin therapy (ACT 200-300 seconds during PCI) are recommended. Heparin infusion after PCI is discouraged. In patients who undergo coronary artery bypass graft surgery, discontinue infusion prior to surgery.

Renal Impairment:

Acute coronary syndrome: I.V.: S_{cr} >2 mg/dL and <4 mg/dL: Use 180 mcg/kg bolus (maximum: 22.6 mg) and 1 mcg/kg/minute infusion (maximum: 7.5 mg/hour)

Percutaneous coronary intervention (PCI) with or without stenting: I.V.: S_{cr} >2 mg/dL and <4 mg/dL: Use 180 mcg/kg bolus (maximum: 22.6 mg) administered immediately before the initiation of PCI and followed by a continuous infusion of 1 mcg/kg/minute (maximum: 7.5 mg/hour). A second 180 mcg/kg (maximum: 22.6 mg) bolus should be administered 10 minutes after the first bolus.

Administration

I.V.: Administer bolus doses by I.V. push over 1-2 minutes. Begin continuous infusion immediately following bolus administration; administer directly from the 100 mL vial.

Stability

Storage: Vials should be stored refrigerated at 2°C to 8°C (36°F to 46°F). Vials can be kept at room temperature for 2 months. Protect from light until administration. Do not use beyond the expiration date. Discard any unused portion left in the vial.

Compatibility: Stable in NS (infusion may contain up to 60 mEq/L KCl), NS/D_5W (infusion may contain up to 60 mEq/L KCl)

Monitoring Laboratory Tests Laboratory tests at baseline and monitoring during therapy: hematocrit and hemoglobin, platelet count, serum creatinine, PT/aPTT (maintain aPTT between 50-70 seconds unless PCI is to be performed), and ACT with PCI (maintain ACT between 200-300 seconds during PCI). Prior to sheath removal, the aPTT or ACT should be checked (do not remove unless aPTT is <45 seconds or the ACT <150 seconds).

Monitoring and Teaching Issues

Physical Assessment: See Contraindications and Warnings/Precautions for use cautions. Assess other medications for possible interactions or additive effects (see Drug Interactions). Monitor vital signs and laboratory results prior to, during, and after therapy. Monitor closely for signs of excessive/unusual bleeding. Observe and teach patient bleeding precautions and adverse reactions to report. Breast-feeding is not recommended.

Patient Education: Emergency use may dictate depth of patient education. This medication can only be administered I.V. You will have a tendency to bleed easily following this medication. Use caution to prevent injury (use electric razor, use soft toothbrush, use caution with sharps). If bleeding occurs, apply pressure to bleeding spot until bleeding stops completely. Report unusual bruising or bleeding (eg, blood in urine, stool, or vomitus, bleeding gums), dizziness or vision changes, or back pain. **Breast-feeding precaution:** Breast-feeding is not recommended.

Equagesic® *see* Aspirin and Meprobamate *on page 125*
Equanil® *see* Meprobamate *on page 853*
Equilet® [OTC] *see* Calcium Supplements *on page 202*

Ergocalciferol (er goe kal SIF e role)

U.S. Brand Names Calciferol™; Drisdol®

Synonyms Activated Ergosterol; Viosterol; Vitamin D_2

Generic Available Yes

Pharmacologic Category Vitamin D Analog

Pregnancy Risk Factor A/C (dose exceeding RDA recommendation)

Lactation Enters breast milk/compatible

Use Treatment of refractory rickets, hypophosphatemia, hypoparathyroidism

Mechanism of Action/Effect Stimulates calcium and phosphate absorption from the small intestine, promotes secretion of calcium from bone to blood; promotes renal tubule phosphate resorption

Contraindications Hypersensitivity to ergocalciferol or any component of the formulation; hypercalcemia; malabsorption syndrome; evidence of vitamin D toxicity

Warnings/Precautions Administer with extreme caution in patients with impaired renal function, heart disease, renal stones, or arteriosclerosis. Must give concomitant calcium supplementation. Maintain adequate fluid intake. Avoid hypercalcemia. Renal function impairment with secondary hyperparathyroidism. Pregnancy risk A/C (dose exceeding RDA).

Drug Interactions

Decreased Effect: Cholestyramine, colestipol, mineral oil may decrease oral absorption.

Increased Effect/Toxicity: Thiazide diuretics may increase vitamin D effects. Cardiac glycosides may increase toxicity.

Adverse Reactions Generally well tolerated

Frequency not defined: Cardiac arrhythmias, hypertension (late), irritability, headache, psychosis (rare), somnolence, hyperthermia (late), pruritus, decreased libido (late), hypercholesterolemia, mild acidosis (late), polydipsia (late), nausea, vomiting, anorexia, pancreatitis, metallic taste, weight loss (rare), xerostomia, constipation, polyuria (late), increased BUN (late), increased LFTs (late), bone pain, myalgia, weakness, conjunctivitis, photophobia (late), vascular/nephrocalcinosis (rare)

Overdosage/Toxicology Symptoms of chronic overdose include hypercalcemia, weakness, fatigue, lethargy, and anorexia. Following withdrawal of the drug and oral decontamination, treatment consists of bedrest, liberal intake of fluids, reduced calcium intake, and cathartic administration. Severe hypercalcemia requires I.V. hydration and forced diuresis with I.V. furosemide. Urine output should be monitored and maintained at >3 mL/kg/hour during the acute treatment phase. I.V. saline can quickly and significantly increase excretion of calcium into urine. Calcitonin, mithramycin, and biphosphonates have all been used successfully to treat the more resistant cases of vitamin D-induced hypercalcemia.

Pharmacodynamics/Kinetics

Absorption: Readily; requires bile

Metabolism: Inactive until hydroxylated hepatically and renally to calcifediol and then to calcitriol (most active form)

Onset: Peak effect: ~1 month following daily doses

Formulations

Capsule (Drisdol®): 50,000 units [1.25 mg; contains tartrazine and soybean oil]

Injection, solution (Calciferol™): 500,000 units/mL [12.5 mg/mL] (1 mL) [contains sesame oil]

Liquid, drops (Calciferol™, Drisdol®): 8000 units/mL [200 mcg/mL] (60 mL) [OTC]

Dosing

Adults: Oral dosing is preferred; I.M. therapy is required with GI, liver, or biliary disease associated with malabsorption.

Dietary supplementation (each mcg = 40 USP units): Oral: 10 mcg/day (400 units)
Renal failure: Oral: 500 mcg/day (20,000 units)
Hypoparathyroidism: Oral: 625 mcg to 5 mg/day (25,000-200,000 units) and calcium supplements
Vitamin D-dependent rickets: Oral: 250 mcg to 1.5 mg/day (10,000-60,000 units)
Nutritional rickets and osteomalacia: Oral:
With normal absorption: 25-125 mcg/day (1000-5000 units)
With malabsorption: 250-7500 mcg/day (10,000-300,000 units)
Vitamin D-resistant rickets: Oral: 250-1500 mcg/day (10,000-60,000 units) with phosphate supplements

Elderly: Refer to adult dosing (see Geriatric Considerations and Additional Information).

Pediatrics: Oral dosing is preferred; I.M. therapy is required with GI, liver, or biliary disease associated with malabsorption.

Dietary supplementation (each mcg = 40 USP units):
Premature infants: 10-20 mcg/day (400-800 units), up to 750 mcg/day (30,000 units)
Infants and healthy children: 10 mcg/day (400 units)
Renal failure: Children: 100-1000 mcg/day (4000-40,000 units)
Hypoparathyroidism: Children: 1.25-5 mg/day (50,000-200,000 units) and calcium supplements
Vitamin D-dependent rickets: Children: 75-125 mcg/day (3000-5000 units); maximum: 1500 mcg/day
Nutritional rickets and osteomalacia:
Children with normal absorption: 25-125 mcg/day (1000-5000 units)
Children with malabsorption: 250-625 mcg/day (10,000-25,000 units)
Vitamin D-resistant rickets: Children: Initial: 1000-2000 mcg/day (40,000-80,000 units) with phosphate supplements; daily dosage is increased at 3- to 4-month intervals in 250-500 mcg (10,000-20,000 units) increments
Familial hypophosphatemia: 10,000-80,000 units daily plus 1-2 g/day elemental phosphorus

Administration

I.M.: Parenteral injection is for I.M. use only.

Stability

Storage: Protect from light.

Monitoring Laboratory Tests Serum calcium, BUN, phosphorus every 1-2 weeks

(Continued)

Ergocalciferol *(Continued)*

Monitoring and Teaching Issues

Physical Assessment: See Contraindications and Warnings/Precautions for use cautions. Assess effectiveness and interactions of other medications patient may be taking (see Drug Interactions). Monitor lab tests, effectiveness of therapy, and adverse effects at beginning of therapy and regularly with long-term use (see Adverse Reactions and Overdose/Toxicology). Assess knowledge/teach patient appropriate use (injection technique and needle disposal if I.M. self-administered), appropriate nutritional counseling, possible side effects/interventions, and adverse symptoms to report (see Patient Education). **Pregnancy risk factor A/C** - see Pregnancy Risk Factor for use cautions.

Patient Education: Take exact dose prescribed; do not take more than recommended. Your prescriber may recommend a special diet; do not increase calcium intake without consulting prescriber. Avoid magnesium supplements or magnesium-containing antacids. You may experience nausea, vomiting, or metallic taste (small, frequent meals, frequent mouth care, or sucking hard candy may help). Report chest pain or palpitations; acute headache, dizziness, or feeling of weakness; unresolved nausea or vomiting; persistent metallic taste; unrelieved muscle or bone pain; or CNS irritability. **Pregnancy precaution:** Inform prescriber if you are pregnant.

Geriatric Considerations: Recommended daily allowances (RDA) have not been developed for persons >65 years of age. Vitamin D, folate, and B_{12} (cyanocobalamin) have decreased absorption with age, but the clinical significance is yet unknown. Calorie requirements decrease with age and therefore, nutrient density must be increased to ensure adequate nutrient intake, including vitamins and minerals. Therefore, the use of a daily supplement with a multiple vitamin with minerals is recommended. Elderly consume less vitamin D, absorption may be decreased and many elderly have decreased sun exposure; therefore, elderly should receive supplementation with 800 units (20 mcg)/day. This is a recommendation of particular need to those with high risk for osteoporosis.

Additional Information 1.25 mg ergocalciferol provides 50,000 units of vitamin D activity.

Ergotamine Tartrate, Belladonna, and Phenobarbital *see* Belladonna, Phenobarbital, and Ergotamine *on page 152*

E•R•O Ear *see page 1519*

Ertapenem (er ta PEN em)

U.S. Brand Names Invanz®

Synonyms Ertapenem Sodium; L-749,345; MK-0826

Generic Available No

Pharmacologic Category Antibiotic, Carbapenem

Pregnancy Risk Factor B

Lactation Enters breast milk/use caution

Use Treatment of moderate-severe, complicated intra-abdominal infections, skin and skin structure infections, pyelonephritis, acute pelvic infections, and community-acquired pneumonia. Antibacterial coverage includes aerobic gram-positive organisms, aerobic gram-negative organisms, anaerobic organisms.

Methicillin-resistant *Staphylococcus*, *Enterococcus* spp, penicillin-resistant strains of *Streptococcus pneumoniae,* beta-lactamase-positive strains of *Haemophilus influenzae* are **resistant** to ertapenem, as are most *Pseudomonas aeruginosa*.

Mechanism of Action/Effect Inhibits cell wall biosynthesis; cell wall assembly is arrested and the bacteria eventually lyse.

Contraindications Hypersensitivity to ertapenem or any other component of the formulation; anaphylactic reactions to beta-lactam antibiotics. If using intramuscularly, known hypersensitivity to local anesthetics of the amide type (lidocaine is the diluent).

Warnings/Precautions Dosage adjustment required with impaired renal function; prolonged use may result in superinfection; use with caution in patients with CNS disorder (eg, brain lesions, history of seizures), compromised renal function, hypersensitivity to beta-lactams, the elderly; safety and efficacy in patients <18 years of age have not been established.

Drug Interactions

Increased Effect/Toxicity: Probenecid decreases the renal clearance of ertapenem.

Adverse Reactions

1% to 10%:

Cardiovascular: Swelling/edema (3%), chest pain (1%), hypertension (0.7% to 2%), hypotension (1% to 2%), tachycardia (1% to 2%)

Central nervous system: Headache (6% to 7%), altered mental status (ie, agitation, confusion, disorientation, decreased mental acuity, changed mental status, somnolence, stupor) (3% to 5%), fever (2% to 5%), insomnia (3%), dizziness (2%), fatigue (1%), anxiety (0.8% to 1%)

Dermatologic: Rash (2% to 3%), pruritus (1% to 2%), erythema (1% to 2%)

Gastrointestinal: Diarrhea (9% to 10%), nausea (6% to 9%), abdominal pain (4%), vomiting (4%), constipation (3% to 4%), acid regurgitation (1% to 2%), dyspepsia (1%), oral candidiasis (0.1% to 1%)

Genitourinary: Vaginitis (1% to 3%)

Hematologic: Platelet count increased (4% to 7%), eosinophils increased (1% to 2%)

Hepatic: Hepatic enzyme elevations (7% to 9%), alkaline phosphatase increase (4% to 7%)

Local: Infused vein complications (5% to 7%), phlebitis/thrombophlebitis (1.5% to 2%), extravasation (0.7% to 2%)

Neuromuscular & skeletal: Leg pain (0.4% to 1%)

Respiratory: Dyspnea (1% to 3%), cough (1% to 2%), pharyngitis (0.7% to 1%), rales/rhonchi (0.5% to 1%), respiratory distress (0.2% to 1%)

<1% (Limited to important or life-threatening): Arrhythmia, asthma, asystole, atrial fibrillation, bradycardia, cardiac arrest, cholelithiasis, epistaxis, gastrointestinal hemorrhage, gout, heart failure, heart murmur, hypoxemia, ileus, pancreatitis, pseudomembranous colitis,

pyloric stenosis, seizures (0.5%), subdural hemorrhage, syncope, urticaria, ventricular tachycardia, vertigo

Overdosage/Toxicology Treatment is symptom-directed and supportive. Removed by hemodialysis.

Pharmacodynamics/Kinetics

Absorption: I.M.: Almost complete

Bioavailability: I.M.: 90%

Half-Life Elimination: 4 hours

Time to Peak: I.M.: 2.3 hours

Metabolism: Hydrolysis to inactive metabolite

Formulations Injection, powder for reconstitution: 1 g

Dosing

Adults: Note: I.V. therapy may be administered for up to 14 days; I.M. for up to 7 days

Intra-abdominal infection: I.V., I.M.: 1 g/day for 5-14 days

Skin and skin structure infections: I.V., I.M.: 1 g/day for 7-14 days

Community-acquired pneumonia: I.V., I.M.: 1 g/day; duration of total antibiotic treatment: 10-14 days

Urinary tract infections/pyelonephritis: I.V., I.M.: 1 g/day; duration of total antibiotic treatment: 10-14 days

Acute pelvic infections: I.V., I.M.: 1 g/day for 3-10 days

Pediatrics: Safety and efficacy have not been established for pediatric patients.

Renal Impairment: Cl_{cr} <30 mL/minute: 500 mg/day

Hemodialysis: When the daily dose is given within 6 hours prior to hemodialysis, a supplementary dose of 150 mg is required following hemodialysis.

Hepatic Impairment: Adjustments cannot be recommended (lack of experience and research in this patient population).

Administration

I.M.: Avoid injection into a blood vessel. Make sure patient does not have an allergy to lidocaine or another anesthetic of the amide type. Administer by deep I.M. injection into a large muscle mass (eg, gluteal muscle or lateral part of the thigh). Do not administer I.M. preparation or drug reconstituted for I.M. administration intravenously.

I.V.: Infuse over 30 minutes

Stability

Storage: Before reconstitution store at ≤25°C (77°F). Reconstituted I.V. solution may be stored at room temperature and used within 6 hours **or** refrigerated, stored for up to 24 hours and used within 4 hours after removal from refrigerator. Do not freeze.

Reconstitution:

I.M.: Reconstitute 1 g vial with 3.2 mL of 1% lidocaine HCl injection (without epinephrine). Shake well. Use within 1 hour after preparation.

I.V.: Reconstitute 1 g vial with 10 mL of water for injection, 0.9% sodium chloride injection, or bacteriostatic water for injection. Shake well. Transfer to 50 mL of 0.9% sodium chloride injection.

Compatibility: Do not mix with other medications or use diluents containing dextrose.

Monitoring and Teaching Issues

Physical Assessment: Assess history of previous allergies or adverse drug reactions. See Contraindications and Warnings/Precautions for use cautions. See Administration directions. Monitor appropriate laboratory results (see Monitoring Laboratory Tests). Monitor closely for adverse reactions, especially CNS adverse effects (increased risk with patients who have history of seizures, head injuries, or other CNS events). Assess knowledge/teach patient appropriate use, interventions to reduce side effects, and adverse symptoms to report (see Patient Education). Note breast-feeding caution.

Patient Education: This medication can only be administered intravenously or by intramuscular injections; report warmth, swelling, irritation at infusion or injection site. Maintain adequate hydration (2-3 L/day of fluids) unless advised by prescriber to restrict fluids, and nutrition. Report unresolved nausea or vomiting (small, frequent meals, frequent mouth care, and sucking hard candy may help). Report immediately any CNS changes (eg, dizziness, disorientation, visual disturbances, headaches, confusion, or seizures). Report prolonged GI effects, diarrhea, vomiting, abdominal pain; change in respirations or difficulty breathing; chest pain or palpitations; skin rash; foul-smelling vaginal discharge; or white plaques in mouth. **Breast-feeding precaution:** Consult prescriber if breast-feeding.

Dietary Issues: Sodium content: 137 mg (~6 mEq) per gram of ertapenem

Breast-feeding Issues: The concentration in human breast milk within 24 hours of last dose (1 g I.V. for 3-10 days) ranged from <0.13 mcg/mL (lower limit of quantitation) to 0.38 mcg/mL. Five days after discontinuation of therapy, the ertapenem level was undetectable in 80% (4 of 5 women) and below the lower limit of quantitation in 20% (1 of 5 women).

Ertapenem Sodium *see* Ertapenem *on page 484*

***Erwinia* Asparaginase** *see* Asparaginase *on page 118*

Eryc® *see* Erythromycin (Systemic) *on page 486*

Erycette® *see* Erythromycin (Systemic) *on page 486*

Eryderm® *see* Erythromycin (Systemic) *on page 486*

Erygel® *see* Erythromycin (Systemic) *on page 486*

EryPed® *see* Erythromycin (Systemic) *on page 486*

Ery-Tab® *see* Erythromycin (Systemic) *on page 486*

Erythra-Derm™ *see* Erythromycin (Systemic) *on page 486*

Erythrocin® *see* Erythromycin (Systemic) *on page 486*

Erythromycin and Benzoyl Peroxide

(er ith roe MYE sin & BEN zoe il per OKS ide)

U.S. Brand Names Benzamycin®

Synonyms Benzoyl Peroxide and Erythromycin

Generic Available No

(Continued)

Erythromycin and Benzoyl Peroxide *(Continued)*

Pharmacologic Category Topical Skin Product; Topical Skin Product, Acne

Pregnancy Risk Factor C

Lactation Excretion in breast milk unknown/use caution

Use Topical control of acne vulgaris

Formulations Gel, topical: Erythromycin 30 mg and benzoyl peroxide 50 mg per g (47 g)

Dosing

Adults & Elderly: Acne: Topical: Apply twice daily, morning and evening.

Pediatrics: Adolescents: Refer to adult dosing.

Monitoring and Teaching Issues

Physical Assessment: See individual components listed in Related Information. **Pregnancy risk factor C** - benefits of use should outweigh possible risks. Note breast-feeding caution.

Patient Education: Also see Erythromycin (Systemic).

Based on Benzoyl Peroxide component: Cleanse and make sure skin is dry before applying; keep away from eyes, mouth, mucous membranes. If excessive redness or irritation occurs, discontinue use; avoid excessive sunlight, sun lamps, or other topical medication unless directed otherwise by a physician. May bleach color from fabrics; may be worn under make-up.

Pregnancy/breast-feeding precautions: Inform prescriber if you are or intend to become pregnant. Consult prescriber if breast-feeding.

Related Information

Erythromycin (Systemic) *on page 486*

Erythromycin and Sulfisoxazole (er ith roe MYE sin & sul fi SOKS a zole)

U.S. Brand Names Eryzole®; Pediazole®

Synonyms Sulfisoxazole and Erythromycin

Generic Available Yes

Pharmacologic Category Antibiotic, Macrolide; Antibiotic, Macrolide Combination; Antibiotic, Sulfonamide Derivative

Pregnancy Risk Factor C

Lactation Enters breast milk/compatible

Use Treatment of susceptible bacterial infections of the upper and lower respiratory tract, otitis media in children caused by susceptible strains of *Haemophilus influenzae*, and many other infections in patients allergic to penicillin

Formulations Suspension, oral: Erythromycin ethylsuccinate 200 mg and sulfisoxazole acetyl 600 mg per 5 mL (100 mL, 150 mL, 200 mL) [strawberry-banana flavor]

Dosing

Adults: Susceptible infections: Oral (dosage recommendation is based on the product's erythromycin content): 400 mg erythromycin and 1200 mg sulfisoxazole every 6 hours

Elderly: Not recommended for use in the elderly.

Pediatrics: Susceptible infections: Oral (dosage recommendation is based on the product's erythromycin content): ≥2 months: 50 mg/kg/day erythromycin and 150 mg/kg/day sulfisoxazole in divided doses every 6 hours; not to exceed 2 g erythromycin/day or 6 g sulfisoxazole/day for 10 days

Renal Impairment: Sulfisoxazole must be adjusted in renal impairment.

Cl_{cr} 10-50 mL/minute: Administer every 8-12 hours.

Cl_{cr} <10 mL/minute: Administer every 12-24 hours.

Monitoring and Teaching Issues

Physical Assessment: See individual components listed in Related Information. **Pregnancy risk factor C** - benefits of use should outweigh possible risks.

Patient Education: See individual components listed in Related Information. **Pregnancy precaution:** Inform prescriber if you are or intend to become pregnant.

Related Information

Erythromycin (Systemic) *on page 486*
SulfiSOXAZOLE *on page 1264*

Erythromycin Base *see* Erythromycin (Systemic) *on page 486*
Erythromycin Estolate *see* Erythromycin (Systemic) *on page 486*
Erythromycin Ethylsuccinate *see* Erythromycin (Systemic) *on page 486*
Erythromycin Gluceptate *see* Erythromycin (Systemic) *on page 486*
Erythromycin Lactobionate *see* Erythromycin (Systemic) *on page 486*
Erythromycin Stearate *see* Erythromycin (Systemic) *on page 486*

Erythromycin (er ith roe MYE sin)

U.S. Brand Names Akne-Mycin®; A/T/S®; E.E.S.®; Emgel®; Eryc®; Erycette®; Eryderm®; Erygel®; EryPed®; Ery-Tab®; Erythra-Derm™; Erythrocin®; PCE®; Romycin®; Staticin®; Theramycin Z®; T-Stat®

Synonyms Erythromycin Base; Erythromycin Estolate; Erythromycin Ethylsuccinate; Erythromycin Gluceptate; Erythromycin Lactobionate; Erythromycin Stearate

Generic Available Yes

Pharmacologic Category Antibiotic, Macrolide; Antibiotic, Ophthalmic; Antibiotic, Topical; Topical Skin Product; Topical Skin Product, Acne

Pregnancy Risk Factor B

Lactation Enters breast milk/compatible

Use

Systemic: Treatment of susceptible bacterial infections including *S. pyogenes*, some *S. pneumoniae*, some *S. aureus*, *M. pneumoniae*, *Legionella pneumophila*, diphtheria, pertussis, chancroid, *Chlamydia*, erythrasma, *N. gonorrhoeae*, *E. histolytica*, syphilis and nongonococcal urethritis, and *Campylobacter* gastroenteritis; used in conjunction with neomycin for decontaminating the bowel

Ophthalmic: Treatment of superficial eye infections involving the conjunctiva or cornea; neonatal ophthalmia

Topical: Treatment of acne vulgaris

Use - Unlabeled/Investigational Systemic: Treatment of gastroparesis

Mechanism of Action/Effect Inhibits RNA-dependent protein synthesis

Contraindications Hypersensitivity to erythromycin or any component of the formulation

Systemic: Pre-existing liver disease (erythromycin estolate); concomitant use with ergot derivatives, pimozide, astemizole, or cisapride; hepatic impairment

Warnings/Precautions Systemic: Hepatic impairment with or without jaundice has occurred, it may be accompanied by malaise, nausea, vomiting, abdominal colic, and fever; discontinue use if these occur; avoid using erythromycin lactobionate in neonates since formulations may contain benzyl alcohol which is associated with toxicity in neonates; observe for superinfections. Use in infants has been associated with infantile hypertrophic pyloric stenosis (IHPS). Macrolides have been associated with rare QT prolongation and ventricular arrhythmias, including torsade de pointes.

Drug Interactions

Cytochrome P450 Effect: Substrate of CYP2B6, **3A4**; Inhibits CYP1A2, **3A4**

Decreased Effect: Erythromycin may decrease the serum concentrations of zafirlukast. Erythromycin may antagonize the therapeutic effects of clindamycin and lincomycin.

Increased Effect/Toxicity: Avoid concomitant use of the following with erythromycin due to increased risk of malignant arrhythmias: Astemizole, cisapride, gatifloxacin, moxifloxacin, pimozide, sparfloxacin, thioridazine. Other agents that prolong the QT_c interval, including type Ia (eg, quinidine) and type III antiarrhythmic agents, and selected antipsychotic agents (eg, mesoridazine, thioridazine) should be used with extreme caution.

Erythromycin may increase the serum concentrations (and possibly the toxicity) of the following agents: Alfentanil (and possibly other narcotic analgesics), benzodiazepines (alprazolam, diazepam, midazolam, triazolam), buspirone, calcium channel blockers, dihydropyridine (felodipine), carbamazepine, cilostazol, clozapine, colchicine, cyclosporine, digoxin, disopyramide, ergot alkaloids (eg, bromocriptine), HMG-CoA reductase inhibitors (except fluvastatin, pravastatin), loratadine, methylprednisolone, rifabutin, tacrolimus, theophylline, sildenafil, valproate, vinblastine, vincristine, zopiclone.

The effects of neuromuscular-blocking agents and warfarin have been potentiated by erythromycin. Erythromycin serum concentrations may be increased by amprenavir (and possibly other protease inhibitors).

Nutritional/Ethanol Interactions

Ethanol: Avoid ethanol (may decrease absorption of erythromycin or enhance ethanol effects).

Food: Increased drug absorption with meals; erythromycin serum levels may be altered if taken with food.

Herb/Nutraceutical: St John's wort may decrease erythromycin levels.

Effects on Lab Values False-positive urinary catecholamines

Adverse Reactions

Systemic:

Cardiovascular: Ventricular arrhythmias, QT_c prolongation, torsade de pointes (rare), ventricular tachycardia (rare)

Central nervous system: Headache (8%), pain (2%), fever, seizures

Dermatitis: Rash (3%), pruritus (1%)

Gastrointestinal: Abdominal pain (8%), cramping, nausea (8%), oral candidiasis, vomiting (3%), diarrhea (7%), dyspepsia (2%), flatulence (2%), anorexia, pseudomembranous colitis, hypertrophic pyloric stenosis (including cases in infants or IHPS), pancreatitis

Hematologic: Eosinophilia (1%)

Hepatic: Cholestatic jaundice (most common with estolate), increased liver function tests (2%)

Local: Phlebitis at the injection site, thrombophlebitis

Neuromuscular & skeletal: Weakness (2%)

Respiratory: Dyspnea (1%), cough (3%)

Miscellaneous: Hypersensitivity reactions, allergic reactions

Topical: 1% to 10%: Dermatologic: Erythema, desquamation, dryness, pruritus

Overdosage/Toxicology Symptoms of overdose include nausea, vomiting, diarrhea, prostration, reversible pancreatitis, hearing loss with or without tinnitus or vertigo. Care is general and supportive only.

Pharmacodynamics/Kinetics

Absorption: Oral: Variable but better with salt forms than with base form; 18% to 45%; ethylsuccinate may be better absorbed with food

Half-Life Elimination: Peak: 1.5-2 hours; End-stage renal disease: 5-6 hours

Time to Peak: Serum: Base: 4 hours; Ethylsuccinate: 0.5-2.5 hours; delayed with food due to differences in absorption

Metabolism: Hepatic via demethylation

Formulations

Capsule, delayed release, enteric-coated pellets, as base (Eryc®): 250 mg

Gel, topical: 2% (30 g, 60 g)

A/T/S®: 2% (30 g)

Emgel®: 2% (27 g, 50 g)

Erygel®: 2% (30 g, 60 g)

Granules for oral suspension, as ethylsuccinate (E.E.S.®): 200 mg/5 mL (100 mL, 200 mL) [cherry flavor]

Injection, powder for reconstitution, as lactobionate (Erythrocin®): 500 mg, 1 g

Ointment, ophthalmic: 0.5% [5 mg/g] (1 g, 3.5 g)

Romycin®: 0.5% [5 mg/g] (3.5 g)

Ointment, topical (Akne-Mycin®): 2% (25 g)

Powder for oral suspension, as ethylsuccinate (Ery-Ped®): 200 mg/5 mL (5 mL, 100 mL, 200 mL) [fruit flavor]; 400 mg/5 mL (5 mL, 60 mL, 100 mL, 200 mL) [banana flavor]

(Continued)

Erythromycin (Systemic) *(Continued)*

Powder for oral suspension, as ethylsuccinate [drops] (Ery-Ped®): 100 mg/2.5 mL (50 mL) [fruit flavor]
Solution, topical: 1.5% (60 mL); 2% (60 mL)
A/T/S/®, Eryderm®, Erythra-Derm™, T-Stat®, Theramycin™ Z: 2% (60 mL)
Staticin®: 1.5% (60 mL)
Suspension, oral, as estolate: 125 mg/5 mL (480 mL); 250 mg/5 mL (480 mL) [orange flavor]
Suspension, oral, as ethylsuccinate: 200 mg/5 mL (480 mL); 400 mg/5 mL (480 mL)
E.E.S.®: 200 mg/5 mL (100 mL, 480 mL) [fruit flavor]; 400 mg/5 mL (100 mL, 480 mL) [orange flavor]
Swab (Erycette®, T-Stat®): 2% (60s)
Tablet, chewable, as ethylsuccinate (EryPed®): 200 mg [fruit flavor]
Tablet, delayed release, enteric coated, as base (Ery-Tab®): 250 mg, 333 mg, 500 mg
Tablet, film coated, as base: 250 mg, 500 mg
Tablet, film coated, as ethylsuccinate (E.E.S.®): 400 mg
Tablet, film coated, as stearate (Erythrocin®): 250 mg, 500 mg
Tablet, polymer-coated particles, as base (PCE®): 333 mg, 500 mg

Dosing

Adults & Elderly:

Susceptible infections (usual dose):
Oral:
Base: 250-500 mg every 6-12 hours
Ethylsuccinate: 400-800 mg every 6-12 hours
I.V.: Lactobionate: 15-20 mg/kg/day divided every 6 hours or 500 mg to 1 g every 6 hours, or given as a continuous infusion over 24 hours (maximum: 4 g/24 hours)
Ophthalmic infection: Ophthalmic: Instill ½" (1.25 cm) 2-6 times/day depending on the severity of the infection
Anti-infective: Topical: Apply over the affected area twice daily after the skin has been thoroughly washed and patted dry
Preop bowel preparation: 1 g erythromycin base at 1, 2, and 11 PM on the day before surgery combined with mechanical cleansing of the large intestine and oral neomycin
Gastrointestinal prokinetic (unlabeled use): I.V., Oral: Erythromycin has been used as a prokinetic agent to improve gastric emptying time and intestinal motility. In adults, 200 mg was infused I.V. initially followed by 250 mg orally 3 times/day 30 minutes before meals. Lower dosages have been used in some trials.

Pediatrics:

Neonates: Prophylaxis of neonatal gonococcal or chlamydial conjunctivitis: Ophthalmic: 0.5-1 cm ribbon of ointment should be instilled into each conjunctival sac
Infants and Children (**Note:** 400 mg ethylsuccinate = 250 mg base, stearate, or estolate salts):
Susceptible infections (systemic): Oral: 30-50 mg/kg/day divided every 6-8 hours; may double doses in severe infections
Antibiotic: I.V.: Lactobionate: 20-40 mg/kg/day divided every 6 hours
Ophthalmic infection: Ophthalmic: Refer to adult dosing.
Preop bowel preparation: 20 mg/kg erythromycin base at 1, 2, and 11 PM on the day before surgery combined with mechanical cleansing of the large intestine and oral neomycin
Topical: Refer to adult dosing.

Renal Impairment: Slightly dialyzable (5% to 20%); supplemental dose is not necessary in hemo- or peritoneal dialysis or in continuous arteriovenous or venovenous hemofiltration.

Administration

Oral: Do not crush enteric coated drug product. GI upset, including diarrhea, is common. May be administered with food to decrease GI upset. Do not give with milk or acidic beverages.

I.V.: Infuse 1 g over 20-60 minutes.

Other: Avoid contact of tip of ophthalmic ointment tube with affected eye.

Stability

Storage: Refrigerate oral suspension. Topical and ophthalmic formulations must be stored in a cool place, such as a refrigerator.

Reconstitution: Erythromycin lactobionate should be reconstituted with sterile water for injection without preservatives to avoid gel formation. The reconstituted solution is stable for 2 weeks when refrigerated or for 24 hours at room temperature.

Erythromycin I.V. infusion solution is stable at pH 6-8. Stability of lactobionate is pH dependent. I.V. form has the longest stability in 0.9% sodium chloride (NS) and should be prepared in this base solution whenever possible. Do not use D_5W as a diluent unless sodium bicarbonate is added to solution. If I.V. must be prepared in D_5W, 0.5 mL of the 8.4% sodium bicarbonate solution should be added per each 100 mL of D_5W.

Stability of parenteral admixture at room temperature (25°C) and at refrigeration temperature (4°C) is 24 hours.

Standard diluent: 500 mg/250 mL D_5W/NS; 750 mg/250 mL D_5W/NS; 1 g/250 mL D_5W/NS.

Compatibility: Erythromycin lactobionate: Stable in NS; **incompatible** with D_5LR, $D_{10}W$

Y-site administration: Incompatible with fluconazole
Compatibility in syringe: Incompatible with ampicillin, heparin
Compatibility when admixed: Incompatible with colistimethate, floxacillin, furosemide, heparin, metaraminol, metoclopramide, riboflavin, vitamin B complex with C

Monitoring Laboratory Tests Perform culture and sensitivity studies prior to initiating drug therapy.

Monitoring and Teaching Issues

Physical Assessment: Assess for previous allergy history prior to therapy. See Contraindications and Warnings/Precautions for use cautions. Assess potential for interactions with other prescriptions, OTC medications, or herbal products patient may be taking (see Drug Interactions). Note infusion specifics above. Assess therapeutic response and adverse reactions (see Adverse Reactions and Overdose/Toxicology). Teach patient proper use (according to formulation and purpose for use), possible side effects and interventions, and adverse symptoms to report (see Patient Education).

Patient Education: Inform prescriber of all prescriptions, OTC medications, or herbal products you are taking, and any allergies you have. Do not take anything new during treatment. Take as directed, around-the-clock, with a full glass of water (not juice or milk); may take with food to reduce GI upset. Do not chew or crush extended release capsules or tablets. Take complete prescription even if you are feeling better. Avoid alcohol (may cause adverse response). May cause nausea, vomiting, or mouth sores (small, frequent meals, frequent mouth care may help). Report immediately and unusual malaise, nausea, vomiting, abdominal colic, or fever; skin rash or itching; easy bruising or bleeding; vaginal itching or discharge; watery or bloody diarrhea; yellowing of skin or eyes, pale stool or dark urine; white plaques, sores, or fuzziness in mouth; or any change in hearing.

Dietary Issues: Systemic: Drug may cause GI upset; may take with food.

Sodium content of oral suspension (ethylsuccinate) 200 mg/5 mL: 29 mg (1.3 mEq)

Sodium content of base Filmtab® 250 mg: 70 mg (3 mEq)

Geriatric Considerations: Dose of erythromycin does not need to be adjusted in the elderly unless there is severe renal impairment or hepatic dysfunction. Elderly patients may be at an increased risk for torsade de pointes. Risk of ototoxicity may be increased in elderly, particularly when dose is ≥4 g/day in conjunction with renal or hepatic impairment.

Additional Information Due to differences in absorption, 400 mg erythromycin ethylsuccinate produces the same serum levels as 250 mg erythromycin base, stearate, or estolate. Do not use D_5W as a diluent unless sodium bicarbonate is added to solution; infuse over 20-60 minutes.

Related Information

Compatibility of Drugs *on page 1564*

Ophthalmic Agents *on page 1509*

Erythropoiesis Stimulating Protein *see* Darbepoetin Alfa *on page 365*

Erythropoietin *see* Epoetin Alfa *on page 476*

Eryzole® *see* Erythromycin and Sulfisoxazole *on page 486*

Escitalopram (es sye TAL oh pram)

U.S. Brand Names Lexapro™

Synonyms Escitalopram Oxalate; Lu-26-054; S-Citalopram

Generic Available No

Pharmacologic Category Antidepressant, Selective Serotonin Reuptake Inhibitor

Pregnancy Risk Factor C

Lactation Enters breast milk/not recommended

Use Treatment of major depressive disorder

Use - Unlabeled/Investigational Anxiety disorders

Mechanism of Action/Effect Escitalopram is the S-enantiomer of citalopram, which selectively inhibits the reuptake of serotonin with little to no effect on norepinephrine or dopamine reuptake.

Contraindications Hypersensitivity to escitalopram, citalopram, or any component of the formulation; concomitant use or within 2 weeks of MAO inhibitors

Warnings/Precautions Potential for severe reaction when used with MAO inhibitors; serotonin syndrome (hyperthermia, muscular rigidity, mental status changes/agitation, autonomic instability) may occur. May precipitate a shift to mania or hypomania in patients with bipolar disease. Has a low potential to impair cognitive or motor performance; caution operating hazardous machinery or driving. Use caution if suicidal risk may be present. Use caution with a previous seizure disorder or condition predisposing to seizures such as brain damage, alcoholism, or concurrent therapy with other drugs which lower the seizure threshold. May cause hyponatremia/SIADH. Use caution with other concurrent illness (due to limited experience). Use caution with renal or liver impairment; concomitant CNS depressants; pregnancy (high doses of citalopram has been associated with teratogenicity in animals). Safety and efficacy in pediatric patients have not been established. Pregnancy risk C.

Drug Interactions

Cytochrome P450 Effect: Substrate of **CYP2C19, 3A4**; Inhibits CYP2D6

Increased Effect/Toxicity:

MAO inhibitors: Escitalopram should not be used with nonselective MAO inhibitors (phenelzine, isocarboxazid) or other drugs with MAO inhibition (linezolid); fatal reactions have been reported. Wait 5 weeks after stopping escitalopram before starting a nonselective MAO inhibitor and 2 weeks after stopping an MAO inhibitor before starting escitalopram. Concurrent selegiline has been associated with mania, hypertension, or serotonin syndrome (risk may be reduced relative to nonselective MAO inhibitors).

Combined used of SSRIs and buspirone, meperidine, moclobemide, nefazodone, other SSRIs, tramadol, trazodone, and venlafaxine may increase the risk of serotonin syndrome. Escitalopram increases serum levels/effects of CYP2D6 substrates (tricyclic antidepressants)

Combined use of sumatriptan (and other serotonin agonists) may result in toxicity; weakness, hyper-reflexia, and incoordination have been observed with sumatriptan and SSRIs. In addition, concurrent use may theoretically increase the risk of serotonin syndrome; includes sumatriptan, naratriptan, rizatriptan, and zolmitriptan.

Nutritional/Ethanol Interactions

Ethanol: Avoid ethanol (may increase CNS depression).

Herb/Nutraceutical: Avoid valerian, St John's wort, SAMe, kava kava, and gotu kola (may increase CNS depression).

Adverse Reactions

>10%: Gastrointestinal: Nausea (15%)

1% to 10%:

Cardiovascular: Chest pain, hypertension, palpitation

(Continued)

Escitalopram *(Continued)*

Central nervous system: Insomnia (9%), somnolence (6%), dizziness (5%), fatigue (5%), dreaming abnormal, concentration impaired, fever, irritability, lethargy, lightheadedness, migraine, vertigo, yawning

Dermatologic: Rash

Endocrine & metabolic: Libido decreased (3%), anorgasmia (2%), hot flashes, menstrual cramps

Gastrointestinal: Diarrhea (8%), xerostomia (6%), appetite decreased (3%), constipation (3%), indigestion (3%), abdominal pain (2%), abdominal cramps, appetite increased, flatulence, gastroenteritis, gastroesophageal reflux, heartburn, toothache, vomiting, weight gain/loss

Genitourinary: Ejaculation disorder (9%), impotence (3%), urinary tract infection, urinary frequency

Neuromuscular & skeletal: Arthralgia, limb pain, muscle cramp, myalgia, neck/shoulder pain, paresthesia, tremor

Ocular: Blurred vision

Otic: Earache, tinnitus

Respiratory: Rhinitis (5%), sinusitis (3%), bronchitis, coughing, nasal or sinus congestion, sinus headache

Miscellaneous: Diaphoresis (5%), flu-like syndrome (5%), allergy

<1% (Limited to important or life-threatening): Anaphylaxis, anemia, anxiety attack, apathy, auditory hallucination, bilirubin increased, bradycardia, carbohydrate craving, chest tightness, confusion, depersonalization, depression aggravated, depression, EKG abnormal, emotional lability, excitability, hypercholesterolemia, hyperglycemia, hyper-reflexia, malaise, muscle contractions (involuntary), muscle weakness, panic reaction, suicidal tendency, suicide attempt, syncope, tachycardia, taste alteration, tics, vision abnormal, visual disturbance, weakness

Overdosage/Toxicology Treatment should be symptom-directed and supportive.

Pharmacodynamics/Kinetics

Bioavailability: ~80%

Half-Life Elimination: Escitalopram: 27-32 hours; S-desmethylcitalopram: 59 hours

Time to Peak: Escitalopram: 5 ± 1.5 hours; S-desmethylcitalopram: 14 hours

Metabolism: Hepatic via CYP2D6, 2C19, and 3A4 to an active metabolite, S-desmethylcitalopram (S-DCT); S-DCT is metabolized to S-didesmethylcitalopram (active) via CYP2D6

Onset: 1-2 weeks

Formulations Tablet: 5 mg, 10 mg, 20 mg

Dosing

Adults: Depression: Oral: Initial: 10 mg/day; dose may be increased to 20 mg/day after at least 1 week

Elderly: Depression: Oral: 10 mg/day

Renal Impairment:

Mild to moderate impairment: No dosage adjustment needed.

Severe impairment: Cl_{cr} <20 mL/minute: Use caution.

Hepatic Impairment: 10 mg/day

Administration

Oral: Administer once daily (morning or evening), with or without food.

Stability

Storage: Store at 25°C (77°F).

Monitoring and Teaching Issues

Physical Assessment: See Contraindications, Warnings/Precautions, and Dosing for use cautions. Assess potential for interactions with other prescriptions, OTC medications, or herbal products patient may be taking (eg, MAO inhibitors and other SSRIs - see Drug Interactions). Assess effectiveness of therapy and adverse reactions on a regular basis throughout therapy (eg, suicidal ideation, mania, or hypomania - see Warnings/Precautions, Adverse Reactions, and Overdose/Toxicology). Teach patient proper use, possible side effects and interventions, and adverse symptoms to report (see Patient Education). **Pregnancy risk factor C** - benefits of use should outweigh possible risks. Breast-feeding is not recommended.

Patient Education: Inform prescriber of all prescriptions, OTC medications, or herbal products you are taking, and any allergies you have. Do not take anything new during treatment without consulting prescriber. Take exactly as directed; do not alter dose or discontinue without consulting prescriber (effects of medication may take up to 3 weeks to occur). Avoid other stimulants: caffeine or alcohol. May cause dizziness, lightheadedness, insomnia, impaired concentration, headache (use caution when driving or engaging in tasks requiring alertness until response to drug is known); nausea, vomiting, loss or increase of appetite, indigestion, or heartburn (small, frequent meals, frequent mouth care, sucking lozenges, or chewing gum may help); constipation (increased dietary fluid, fruit, fiber, and increased exercise may help); sexual dysfunction (reversible when drug is discontinued); hot flashes or menstrual cramps; or muscle pain, cramps, or tremor (consult prescriber for approved analgesia). Report CNS changes (confusion, impaired concentration, severe headache, insomnia, nightmares, irritability); persistent GI changes; chest pain or palpitations; blurred vision or vision changes; ringing in ears; unusual cough; or other persistent adverse effects. **Pregnancy/breast-feeding precautions:** Inform prescriber if you are or intend to become pregnant. Breast-feeding is not recommended.

Dietary Issues: May be taken with or without food.

Breast-feeding Issues: Unsafe; somnolence, weight loss, and decreased feeding have been reported with citalopram use in breast-feeding infants. Bottle feeding is recommended.

Additional Information Escitalopram is the S-enantiomer of the racemic derivative citalopram; 20 mg escitalopram is equipotent to 40 mg citalopram.

Related Information
Antidepressant Agents *on page 1553*

Escitalopram Oxalate *see* Escitalopram *on page 489*
Esclim® *see* Estradiol *on page 494*
Eserine Salicylate *see* Physostigmine *on page 1079*
Eserine Sulfate *see* Ophthalmic Agents, Glaucoma *on page 1002*
Esgic® *see* Butalbital, Acetaminophen, and Caffeine *on page 192*
Esgic-Plus™ *see* Butalbital, Acetaminophen, and Caffeine *on page 192*
Eskalith® *see* Lithium *on page 810*
Eskalith CR® *see* Lithium *on page 810*

Esmolol (ES moe lol)

U.S. Brand Names Brevibloc®

Synonyms Esmolol Hydrochloride

Generic Available No

Pharmacologic Category Antiarrhythmic Agent, Class II; Beta Blocker, $Beta_1$ Selective

Pregnancy Risk Factor C (manufacturer); D (2nd and 3rd trimesters - expert analysis)

Lactation Excretion in breast milk unknown

Use Treatment of supraventricular tachycardia and atrial fibrillation/flutter (primarily to control ventricular rate); treatment of tachycardia and/or hypertension (especially intraoperative or postoperative)

Mechanism of Action/Effect Class II antiarrhythmic: $Beta_1$ adrenergic receptor blocking agent that competes with $beta_1$ adrenergic agonists for available beta receptor sites; it is a selective $beta_1$ antagonist with a very short duration of action; has little if any intrinsic sympathomimetic activity; and lacks membrane stabilizing action; it is administered intravenously and is used when beta blockade of short duration is desired or in critically ill patients in whom adverse effects of bradycardia, heart failure or hypotension may necessitate rapid withdrawal of the drug

Contraindications Hypersensitivity to esmolol or any component of the formulation; sinus bradycardia; heart block greater than first degree (except in patients with a functioning artificial pacemaker); cardiogenic shock; bronchial asthma; uncompensated cardiac failure; hypotension; pregnancy (2nd and 3rd trimesters)

Warnings/Precautions Hypotension is common; patients need close blood pressure monitoring. Administer cautiously in compensated heart failure and monitor for a worsening of the condition. Use caution in patients with PVD (can aggravate arterial insufficiency). Use caution with concurrent use of beta-blockers and either verapamil or diltiazem; bradycardia or heart block can occur. Avoid concurrent I.V. use of both agents. In general, beta-blockers should be avoided in patients with bronchospastic disease. Esmolol, a beta-1 selective beta-blocker, has been used cautiously in patients with bronchospastic disease with close monitoring of pulmonary status. Use with caution in patients with diabetes - may mask prominent hypoglycemic symptoms. May mask signs of thyrotoxicosis. May cause fetal bradycardia when administered in the 3rd trimester of pregnancy or at delivery. Use caution in patients with renal dysfunction (active metabolite retained). Do not use in the treatment of hypertension associated with vasoconstriction related to hypothermia. Extravasation can lead to skin necrosis and sloughing. Pregnancy risk C/D (2nd and 3rd trimesters).

Drug Interactions

Decreased Effect: Decreased effect of beta-blockers with aluminum salts, barbiturates, calcium salts, cholestyramine, colestipol, NSAIDs, penicillins (ampicillin), rifampin, salicylates, and sulfinpyrazone due to decreased bioavailability and plasma levels. Beta-blockers may decrease the effect of sulfonylureas. Xanthines (eg, theophylline, caffeine) may decrease effects of esmolol.

Increased Effect/Toxicity: Esmolol may increase the effect/toxicity of verapamil, and may increase potential for hypertensive crisis after or during withdrawal of either agent when combined with clonidine. Esmolol may extend the effect of neuromuscular blocking agents (succinylcholine). Esmolol may increase digoxin serum levels by 10% to 20% and may increase theophylline concentrations. Morphine may increase esmolol blood concentrations.

Effects on Lab Values ↑ cholesterol (S), glucose

Adverse Reactions

>10%:
- Cardiovascular: Asymptomatic hypotension (25%), symptomatic hypotension (12%)
- Miscellaneous: Diaphoresis (10%)

1% to 10%:
- Cardiovascular: Peripheral ischemia (1%)
- Central nervous system: Dizziness (3%), somnolence (3%), confusion (2%), headache (2%), agitation (2%), fatigue (1%)
- Gastrointestinal: Nausea (7%), vomiting (1%)
- Local: Pain on injection (8%)

<1% (Limited to important or life-threatening): Alopecia, bronchospasm, chest pain, CHF, depression, dyspnea, edema, exfoliative dermatitis, heart block, infusion site reactions, paresthesia, pruritus, pulmonary edema, rigors, seizures, severe bradycardia/asystole (rare), skin necrosis (from extravasation), syncope, thrombophlebitis, urinary retention

Overdosage/Toxicology Symptoms of overdose include hypotension, bradycardia, and heart block. Initially, fluids may be the best treatment for hypotension. Sympathomimetics (eg, epinephrine or dopamine), glucagon, or a pacemaker can be used to treat the toxic bradycardia, asystole, and/or hypotension.

Pharmacodynamics/Kinetics

Half-Life Elimination: Adults: 9 minutes

Metabolism: In blood by esterases

Onset: Beta-blockade: I.V.: 2-10 minutes (quickest when loading doses are administered)

Duration: 10-30 minutes; prolonged following higher cumulative doses, extended duration of use

(Continued)

Esmolol *(Continued)*

Formulations

Infusion [premixed in sodium chloride; preservative free]: 10 mg/mL (250 mL)

Injection, solution, as hydrochloride: 10 mg/mL (10 mL) [alcohol free]; 250 mg/mL (10 mL) [contains alcohol 25%]

Dosing

Adults & Elderly: Infusion requires an infusion pump (must be adjusted to individual response and tolerance):

Intraoperative tachycardia and/or hypertension (immediate control): I.V.: Initial bolus: 80 mg (~1 mg/kg) over 30 seconds, followed by a 150 mcg/kg/minute infusion, if necessary. Adjust infusion rate as needed to maintain desired heart rate and/or blood pressure, up to 300 mcg/kg/minute.

Supraventricular tachycardia or gradual control of postoperative tachycardia/hypertension: I.V.: Loading dose: 500 mcg/kg over 1 minute; follow with a 50 mcg/kg/minute infusion for 4 minutes; response to this initial infusion rate may be a rough indication of the responsiveness of the ventricular rate.

Infusion may be continued at 50 mcg/kg/minute or, if the response is inadequate, titrated upward in 50 mcg/kg/minute increments (increased no more frequently than every 4 minutes) to a maximum of 200 mcg/kg/minute.

To achieve more rapid response, following the initial loading dose and 50 mcg/kg/minute infusion, rebolus with a second 500 mcg/kg loading dose over 1 minute, and increase the maintenance infusion to 100 mcg/kg/minute for 4 minutes. If necessary, a third (and final) 500 mcg/kg loading dose may be administered, prior to increasing to an infusion rate of 150 mcg/minute. After 4 minutes of the 150 mcg/kg/minute infusion, the infusion rate may be increased to a maximum rate of 200 mcg/kg/minute (without a bolus dose).

Usual dosage range (SVT): 50-200 mcg/kg/minute with average dose of 100 mcg/kg/minute. For control of postoperative hypertension, as many as one-third of patients may require higher doses (250-300 mcg/kg/minute) to control blood pressure; the safety of doses >300 mcg/kg/minute has not been studied.

Guidelines for withdrawal of therapy:

Transfer to alternative antiarrhythmic drug (propranolol, digoxin, verapamil).

Infusion should be reduced by 50% 30 minutes following the first dose of the alternative agent.

Following the second dose of the alternative drug, patient's response should be monitored and if control is adequate for the first hours, esmolol may be discontinued.

Pediatrics:

Supraventricular tachycardias: I.V.: Children: A limited amount of information regarding esmolol use in pediatric patients is currently available. Some centers have utilized doses of 100-500 mcg/kg given over 1 minute for control of supraventricular tachycardias.

Postoperative hypertension: I.V.: Loading doses of 500 mcg/kg/minute over 1 minute with maximal doses of 50-250 mcg/kg/minute (mean = 173) have been used in addition to nitroprusside to treat postoperative hypertension after coarctation of aorta repair.

Renal Impairment: Not removed by hemo- or peritoneal dialysis. Supplemental dose is not necessary.

Administration

I.V.: The 250 mg/mL ampul is **not** for direct I.V. injection, but rather must first be diluted to a final concentration of 10 mg/mL (ie, 2.5 g in 250 mL or 5 g in 500 mL). Concentrations >10 mg/mL or infusion into small veins or through a butterfly catheter should be avoided (can cause thrombophlebitis).

Stability

Storage: Clear, colorless to light yellow solution should be stored at room temperature and protected from temperatures >40°C.

Reconstitution: Stability of parenteral admixture at room temperature (25°C) and at refrigeration temperature (4°C) is 24 hours.

Standard diluent: 5 g/500 mL NS

Compatibility: Stable in D_5LR, $D_5{}^1/_2NS$, D_5NS, D_5W, D_5W with KCl 40 mEq/L, LR, $^1/_2NS$, NS, sodium bicarbonate 5%

Y-site administration: Incompatible with amphotericin B cholesteryl sulfate complex, furosemide, warfarin

Compatibility when admixed: Incompatible with diazepam, procainamide, sodium bicarbonate, thiopental

Monitoring and Teaching Issues

Physical Assessment: Assess other medications patient may be taking for effectiveness and interactions (see Drug Interactions). See Warnings/Precautions and Contraindications for use cautions. See Dosing and Warnings/Precautions for withdrawal guidelines. Requires continuous cardiac, hemodynamic, and infusion site monitoring (extravasation). Monitor therapeutic response and adverse reactions (see Warnings/Precautions and Adverse Reactions). **Pregnancy risk factor C/D** - see Pregnancy Risk Factor for use cautions; benefits of use should outweigh possible risks. Note breast-feeding caution.

Patient Education: Esmolol is administered in emergencies, patient education should be appropriate to the situation. **Pregnancy precaution:** Inform prescriber if you are pregnant.

Geriatric Considerations: Due to alterations in the beta-adrenergic autonomic nervous system, beta-adrenergic blockade may result in less hemodynamic response than seen in younger adults.

Related Information

Antiarrhythmic Drugs *on page 1551*
Beta-Blockers *on page 1561*

Esmolol Hydrochloride *see* Esmolol *on page 491*

Esomeprazole (es oh ME pray zol)

U.S. Brand Names Nexium®

Synonyms Esomeprazole Magnesium

Generic Available No

Pharmacologic Category Proton Pump Inhibitor

Pregnancy Risk Factor B

Lactation Excretion in breast milk unknown/contraindicated

Use Short-term (4-8 weeks) treatment of erosive esophagitis; maintaining symptom resolution and healing of erosive esophagitis; treatment of symptomatic gastroesophageal reflux disease; as part of a multidrug regimen for *Helicobacter pylori* eradication in patients with duodenal ulcer disease (active or history of within the past 5 years)

Mechanism of Action/Effect Prevents gastric acid secretion

Contraindications Hypersensitivity to esomeprazole, lansoprazole, omeprazole, rabeprazole, or any component of the formulation

Warnings/Precautions Relief of symptoms does not preclude the presence of a gastric malignancy. Atrophic gastritis (by biopsy) has been noted with long-term omeprazole therapy; this may also occur with esomeprazole. No reports of enterochromaffin-like (ECL) cell carcinoids, dysplasia, or neoplasia has occurred. Safety and efficacy in pediatric patients have not been established.

Drug Interactions

Cytochrome P450 Effect: Substrate of **CYP2C19**, 3A4

Decreased Effect: Decreased absorption of dapsone, iron, itraconazole, ketoconazole and other drugs where an acidic stomach is required for absorption.

Increased Effect/Toxicity: Increased serum concentration of diazepam, digoxin, penicillins

Nutritional/Ethanol Interactions Food: Absorption is decreased by 33% to 53% when taken with food.

Adverse Reactions

1% to 10%:

Central nervous system: Headache (4% to 6%)

Gastrointestinal: Diarrhea (4%), nausea, flatulence, abdominal pain (4%), constipation, xerostomia

<1% (Limited to important or life-threatening): Allergic reactions, anaphylaxis, angina, angioedema, arthritis, asthma, confusion, depression, dyspnea; edema (facial, larynx, peripheral, tongue); goiter, hematuria, hypertension, hyponatremia, impotence, migraine, paresthesia, polymyalgia rheumatica, rash, thrombocytopenia, ulcerative stomatitis, urticaria, vertigo

Overdosage/Toxicology Treatment is symptom-directed and supportive; not dialyzable

Pharmacodynamics/Kinetics

Bioavailability: 90% with repeat dosing

Half-Life Elimination: 1-1.5 hours

Time to Peak: 1.5 hours

Metabolism: Hepatic via CYP2C19 and 3A4 enzymes to hydroxy, desmethyl, and sulfone metabolites (all inactive)

Formulations Capsule, delayed release: 20 mg, 40 mg

Dosing

Adults & Elderly:

Healing of erosive esophagitis: Oral: 20-40 mg once daily for 4-8 weeks; may consider an additional 4-8 weeks of treatment if patient is not healed

Maintenance of healing of erosive esophagitis: Oral: 20 mg once daily; clinical trials evaluated therapy for ≤6 months

Symptomatic gastroesophageal reflux: Oral: 20 mg once daily for 4 weeks; may consider an additional 4 weeks of treatment if symptoms do not resolve

Helicobacter pylori eradication: Oral: 40 mg once daily; requires combination therapy

Renal Impairment: No adjustment is necessary.

Hepatic Impairment:

Mild to moderate liver impairment (Child-Pugh Class A or B): No dosage adjustment needed.

Severe liver impairment (Child-Pugh Class C): Dose should not exceed 20 mg/day.

Administration

Oral: Capsule should be swallowed whole and taken at least 1 hour before eating. For patients with difficulty swallowing, open capsule and mix contents with 1 tablespoon of applesauce. Swallow immediately; mixture should not be chewed. The mixture should not be stored for future use.

Stability

Storage: Store at 15°C to 30°C (59°F to 86°F). Keep container tightly closed.

Compatibility: Contents of capsule remain intact when exposed to tap water, orange juice, apple juice, and yogurt.

Monitoring Laboratory Tests Susceptibility testing is recommended in patients who fail *H. pylori* eradication regimen (esomeprazole, clarithromycin, and amoxicillin).

Monitoring and Teaching Issues

Physical Assessment: Assess other medications patient may be taking for effectiveness and interactions (especially those dependent on cytochrome P450 metabolism or those dependent on a acid environment for absorption - see Drug Interactions). See Contraindications and Warnings/Precautions for use cautions. Monitor effectiveness of therapeutic response and adverse reactions at beginning of therapy and periodically throughout therapy (see Adverse Reactions and Overdose/Toxicology). Assess knowledge/teach appropriate use of this medication, interventions to reduce side effects, and adverse symptoms to report (see Patient Education). Breast-feeding is contraindicated.

Patient Education: Take as directed, 1 hour before eating at same time each day. Swallow capsule whole; do not crush or chew. If you cannot swallow capsule whole, open capsule, mix contents with 1 tablespoon of applesauce, and swallow immediately; do not chew mixture. Do not store for future use. You may experience headache; constipation (increased exercise, fluids, fruit, or fiber may help); diarrhea (boiled milk, yogurt, or buttermilk may help); or abdominal pain (should diminish with use). Report persistent headache, diarrhea, constipation, abdominal pain, changes in urination or pain on urination, chest pain or palpitations, changes in respiratory status, CNS changes, persistent muscular

(Continued)

Esomeprazole *(Continued)*

aches or pain, ringing in ears or visual changes, or other adverse reactions. **Breast-feeding precaution:** Do not breast-feed.

Dietary Issues: Take at least 1 hour before meals.

Additional Information Esomeprazole is the S-isomer of omeprazole.

Related Information

Helicobacter pylori Treatment *on page 1676*

Esomeprazole Magnesium *see* Esomeprazole *on page 492*

Esoterica® Regular [OTC] *see* Hydroquinone *on page 679*

Esterified Estrogens *see* Estrogens (Esterified) *on page 508*

Estinyl® *see* Ethinyl Estradiol *on page 514*

Estivin® II *see page 1509*

Estrace® *see* Estradiol *on page 494*

Estraderm® *see* Estradiol *on page 494*

Estradiol (es tra DYE ole)

U.S. Brand Names Alora®; Climara®; Delestrogen®; Depo®-Estradiol; Esclim®; Estrace®; Estraderm®; Estring®; Gynodiol®; Vagifem®; Vivelle®; Vivelle-Dot®

Synonyms Estradiol Cypionate; Estradiol Hemihydrate; Estradiol Transdermal; Estradiol Valerate

Generic Available Yes

Pharmacologic Category Estrogen Derivative

Pregnancy Risk Factor X

Lactation Enters breast milk/use caution

Use Treatment of moderate to severe vasomotor symptoms associated with menopause; treatment of vulvar and vaginal atrophy; hypoestrogenism (due to hypogonadism, castration, or primary ovarian failure); prostatic cancer (palliation), breast cancer (palliation), osteoporosis (prophylaxis); abnormal uterine bleeding due to hormonal imbalance; postmenopausal urogenital symptoms of the lower urinary tract (urinary urgency, dysuria)

Mechanism of Action/Effect Estrogens modulate the pituitary secretion of gonadotropins, luteinizing hormone, and follicle-stimulating hormone through a negative feedback system; estrogen replacement reduces elevated levels of these hormones in postmenopausal women.

Contraindications Hypersensitivity to estradiol or any component of the formulation; undiagnosed abnormal vaginal bleeding; history of or current thrombophlebitis or thromboembolic disorders; carcinoma of the breast, except in appropriately selected patients being treated for metastatic disease; estrogen-dependent tumor; porphyria; pregnancy

Warnings/Precautions Unopposed estrogens may increase the risk of endometrial carcinoma in postmenopausal women. Use with caution in patients with diseases which may be exacerbated by fluid retention, including asthma, epilepsy, migraine, diabetes, cardiac or renal dysfunction. Use with caution in patients with a history of hypercalcemia, hepatic disease, cardiovascular disease, and gallbladder disease. May increase blood pressure. May increase risk of venous thromboembolism. Estrogens may increase the risk of breast cancer (controversial/currently under study). Estrogen compounds are generally associated with lipid effects such as increased HDL-cholesterol and decreased LDL-cholesterol. Triglycerides may also be increased; use with caution in patients with familial defects of lipoprotein metabolism. Estrogens may cause premature closure of the epiphyses in young individuals. Safety and efficacy in pediatric patients have not been established. May increase size of pre-existing uterine leiomyomata. May increase the risk of benign hepatic adenoma, which may cause significant consequences in the event of rupture.

Use vaginal tablets with caution in patients with severely atrophic vaginal mucosa or following gynecological surgery due to possible trauma from the applicator. Oral therapy may be more convenient for vaginal atrophy and stress incontinence.

Before prescribing estrogen therapy to postmenopausal women, the risks and benefits must be weighed for each patient. Women should be informed of these risks and benefits, as well as possible effects of progestin when added to estrogen therapy.

Drug Interactions

Cytochrome P450 Effect: Substrate of **CYP1A2**, 2A6, 2B6, 2C8/9, 2C19, 2D6, 2E1, **3A4**; Inhibits CYP1A2; Induces CYP3A4

Decreased Effect: Rifampin, nelfinavir, and ritonavir decrease estradiol serum concentrations. Anticonvulsants which are enzyme inducers (barbiturates, carbamazepine, phenobarbital, phenytoin, primidone) may potentially decrease estrogen levels.

Increased Effect/Toxicity: Estradiol with hydrocortisone increases corticosteroid toxic potential. Anticoagulants and estradiol increase the potential for thromboembolic events.

Nutritional/Ethanol Interactions

Ethanol: Avoid ethanol (routine use increases estrogen level and risk of breast cancer).

Food: Folic acid absorption may be decreased

Herb/Nutraceutical: St John's wort may decrease estradiol levels. Avoid black cohosh, dong quai (has estrogenic activity). Avoid red clover, saw palmetto, ginseng.

Effects on Lab Values ↑ Prothrombin and factors VII, VIII, IX, X; ↑ platelet aggregability, thyroid-binding globulin, total thyroid hormone (T_4), serum triglycerides/phospholipids; ↓ antithrombin III, serum folate concentration

Adverse Reactions Frequency not defined.

Cardiovascular: Edema, hypertension, venous thromboembolism

Central nervous system: Dizziness, headache, mental depression, migraine

Dermatologic: Chloasma, erythema multiforme, erythema nodosum, hemorrhagic eruption, hirsutism, loss of scalp hair, melasma

Endocrine & metabolic: Breast enlargement, breast tenderness, changes in libido, increased thyroid-binding globulin, increased total thyroid hormone (T_4), increased serum triglycerides/phospholipids, increased HDL-cholesterol, decreased LDL-cholesterol, impaired glucose tolerance, hypercalcemia

Gastrointestinal: Abdominal cramps, bloating, cholecystitis, cholelithiasis, gallbladder disease, nausea, pancreatitis, vomiting, weight gain/loss

Genitourinary: Alterations in frequency and flow of menses, changes in cervical secretions, endometrial cancer, increased size of uterine leiomyomata, vaginal candidiasis

Vaginal: Trauma from applicator insertion may occur in women with severely atrophic vaginal mucosa

Hematologic: Aggravation of porphyria, decreased antithrombin III and antifactor Xa, increased levels of fibrinogen, increased platelet aggregability and platelet count; increased prothrombin and factors VII, VIII, IX, X

Hepatic: Cholestatic jaundice

Local: Transdermal patches: Burning, erythema, irritation, pruritus, rash

Neuromuscular & skeletal: Chorea

Ocular: Intolerance to contact lenses, steeping of corneal curvature

Respiratory: Pulmonary thromboembolism

Miscellaneous: Carbohydrate intolerance

Postmarketing events: Vivelle®; Anaphylaxis (isolated reports), elevated liver function tests (rare), leg pain

Overdosage/Toxicology Symptoms of overdose include fluid retention, jaundice, thrombophlebitis, nausea, and vomiting. Toxicity is unlikely following single exposure of excessive doses. Treatment following emesis and charcoal administration should be supportive and symptomatic.

Pharmacodynamics/Kinetics

Absorption: Oral, topical: Well absorbed

Metabolism: Oral: Hepatic via oxidation and conjugation in GI tract; hydroxylated via CYP3A4 to metabolites; first-pass effect; enterohepatic recirculation

Formulations

Cream, vaginal (Estrace®): 0.1 mg/g (12 g) [refill tube]: 0.1 mg/g (42.5 g) [tube with applicator]

Injection, oil, as cypionate (Depo®-Estradiol): 5 mg/mL (5 mL) [contains chlorobutanol; in cottonseed oil]

Injection, oil, as valerate (Delestrogen®):
- 10 mg/mL (5 mL) [contains chlorobutanol; in sesame oil]
- 20 mg/mL (5 mL) [contains benzyl alcohol; in castor oil]
- 40 mg/mL (5 mL) [contains benzyl alcohol; in castor oil]

Tablet, oral, micronized: 0.5 mg, 1 mg, 2 mg
- Estrace®: 0.5 mg, 1 mg, 2 mg [2 mg tablets contain tartrazine]
- Gynodiol®: 0.5 mg, 1 mg, 1.5 mg, 2 mg

Tablet, vaginal, as base (Vagifem®): 25 mcg

Transdermal system: 0.05 mg/24 hours (4s) [once-weekly patch]; 0.1 mg/24 hours (4s) [once-weekly patch]
- Alora® [twice-weekly patch]:
  - 0.05 mg/24 hours [18 cm^2, total estradiol 1.5 mg] (8s, 24s)
  - 0.075 mg/24 hours [27 cm^2, total estradiol 2.3 mg] (8s)
  - 0.1 mg/24 hours [36 cm^2, total estradiol 3 mg] (8s)
- Climara® [once-weekly patch]:
  - 0.025 mg/24 hours [6.5 cm^2, total estradiol 2.04 mg] (4s)
  - 0.05 mg/24 hours [12.5 cm^2, total estradiol 3.8 mg] (4s)
  - 0.075 mg/24 hours [18.75 cm^2, total estradiol 5.7 mg] (4s)
  - 0.1 mg/24 hours [25 cm^2, total estradiol 7.6 mg] (4s)
- Esclim® [twice-weekly patch]:
  - 0.025 mg/day [11 cm^2, total estradiol 5 mg] (8s)
  - 0.0375 mg/day [16.5 cm^2, total estradiol 7.5 mg] (8s)
  - 0.05 mg/day [22 cm^2, total estradiol 10 mg] (8s)
  - 0.075 mg/day [33 cm^2, total estradiol 15 mg] (8s)
  - 0.1 mg/day [44 cm^2, total estradiol 20 mg] (8s)
- Estraderm® [twice-weekly patch]:
  - 0.05 mg/24 hours [10 cm^2, total estradiol 4 mg] (8s)
  - 0.1 mg/24 hours [20 cm^2, total estradiol 8 mg] (8s)
- Vivelle® [twice-weekly patch]:
  - 0.025 mg/24 hours [7.25 cm^2, total estradiol 2.17 mg] (8s)
  - 0.0375 mg/24 hours [11 cm^2, total estradiol 3.28 mg] (8s)
  - 0.05 mg/24 hours [14.5 cm^2, total estradiol 4.33 mg] (8s)
  - 0.075 mg/24 hours [22 cm^2, total estradiol 6.57 mg] (8s)
  - 0.1 mg/24 hours [29 cm^2, total estradiol 8.66 mg] (8s)
- Vivelle-Dot® [twice-weekly patch]:
  - 0.0375 mg/day [3.75 cm^2, total estradiol 0.585 mg] (8s)
  - 0.05 mg/day [5 cm^2, total estradiol 0.78 mg] (8s)
  - 0.075 mg/day [7.5 cm^2, total estradiol 1.17 mg] (8s)
  - 0.1 mg/day [10 cm^2, total estradiol 1.56 mg] (8s)

Ring, vaginal (Estring®): 2 mg [gradually released over 90 days] (1s)

Dosing

Adults & Elderly: All dosage needs to be adjusted based upon the patient's response:

Atrophic vaginitis, vulvar/vaginal atrophy:

Intravaginal:

Vaginal cream: Atrophic vaginitis, kraurosis vulvae: Insert 2-4 g/day for 2 weeks then gradually reduce to 1/2 the initial dose for 2 weeks followed by a maintenance dose of 1 g 1-3 times/week

Vaginal ring (Estring®): Postmenopausal vaginal atrophy, urogenital symptoms: Following insertion, Estring® should remain in place for 90 days.

Vaginal tablets (Vagifem®); Atrophic vaginitis: Initial: Insert 1 tablet once daily for 2 weeks; maintenance: Insert 1 tablet twice weekly. Attempts to discontinue or taper medication should be made at 3- to 6-month intervals

Transdermal: Refer to product-specific dosing (below)

Breast cancer (females; inoperable, progressing): Oral: 10 mg 3 times/day for at least 3 months

(Continued)

Estradiol *(Continued)*

Hypogonadism:

Oral: 1-2 mg/day in a cyclic regimen for 3 weeks on drug, then 1 week off drug

I.M.: Cypionate: 1.5-2 mg monthly; Valerate: 10-20 mg every 4 weeks

Transdermal: Refer to product-specific dosing (below)

Osteoporosis prevention (females):

Oral: 0.5 mg/day in a cyclic regimen (3 weeks on and 1 week off of drug)

Transdermal: Refer to product-specific dosing (below)

Prostate cancer:

I.M. (valerate): ≥30 mg or more every 1-2 weeks

Oral (androgen-dependent, inoperable, progressing): 10 mg 3 times/day for at least 3 months

Moderate to severe vasomotor symptoms associated with menopause:

Oral (in addition to I.M. dosing): 1-2 mg daily, adjusted as necessary to limit symptoms. Administrations should be cyclic (3 weeks on, 1 week off). Patients should be re-evaluated at 3-6 month intervals to determine if treatment is still necessary

I.M.: Cypionate: 1-5 mg every 3-4 weeks; Valerate: 10-20 mg every 4 weeks

Transdermal: See product-specific dosing (below)

Transdermal product-specific dosing:

Note: Indicated dose may be used continuously in patients without an intact uterus. May be given continuously or cyclically (3 weeks on, 1 week off) in patients with an intact uterus. When changing patients from oral to transdermal therapy, start transdermal patch 1 week after discontinuing oral hormone (may begin sooner if symptoms reappear within 1 week):

Transdermal once-weekly patch (Climara®):

Moderate to severe vasomotor symptoms associated with menopause: Apply 0.025 mg/day patch once weekly. Adjust dose as necessary to control symptoms. Patients should be re-evaluated at 3- to 6-month intervals to determine if treatment is still necessary.

Prevention of osteoporosis in postmenopausal women: Apply patch once weekly; minimum effective dose 0.025 mg/day; adjust dosage based on response to therapy as indicated by biological markers and bone mineral density.

Transdermal twice-weekly patch (Alora®, Esclim®, Estraderm®, Vivelle®):

Moderate to severe vasomotor symptoms associated with menopause, vulvar/vaginal atrophy, female hypogonadism: Titrate to lowest dose possible to control symptoms, adjusting initial dose after the first month of therapy; re-evaluate therapy at 3- to 6-month intervals to taper or discontinue medication:

Alora®, Esclim®, Estraderm®, Vivelle-Dot®: Apply 0.05 mg patch twice weekly

Vivelle®: Apply 0.0375 mg patch twice weekly

Prevention of osteoporosis in postmenopausal women:

Alora®, Vivelle®, Vivelle-Dot®: Apply 0.025 mg patch twice weekly, increase dose as necessary

Estraderm®: Apply 0.05 mg patch twice weekly

Administration

I.M.: Injection for intramuscular administration only.

Topical: Aerosol topical corticosteroids applied under the patch may reduce allergic reactions. Do not apply transdermal system to breasts, but place on trunk of body (preferably abdomen). Rotate application sites.

Monitoring and Teaching Issues

Physical Assessment: See Contraindications, Warnings/Precautions, and Dosing for use cautions. Assess potential for interactions with other prescriptions, OTC medications, or herbal products patient may be taking (see Drug Interactions). Assess results of annual gynecological exam, therapeutic response (dependent on rationale for use), and adverse effects (eg, CNS, respiratory, fluid status changes, and thromboembolism - see Adverse Reactions) on a regular basis during therapy. Before prescribing estrogen therapy to postmenopausal women, the risks and benefits must be weighed for each patient. Women should be informed of these risks and benefits, as well as possible effects of progestin when added to estrogen therapy. Caution diabetic patients to monitor glucose levels closely (may impair glucose tolerance). Teach patient appropriate use (according to formulation), possible side effects and appropriate interventions (annual gynecological exam), and adverse symptoms to report (see Patient Education). **Pregnancy risk factor X** - determine that patient is not pregnant before starting therapy. Do not give to females of childbearing age unless patient is capable of complying with barrier contraceptive use. Advise patient about appropriate contraceptive measures as appropriate. Note breast-feeding caution.

Patient Education: Inform prescriber of all prescriptions, OTC medications, or herbal products you are taking, and any allergies you have. Do not take anything new without consulting prescriber. Use as prescribed; maintain prescribed cycles or term as prescribed. Avoid alcohol. Annual gynecologic and breast exams are important. If diabetic, monitor glucose levels closely (may impair glucose tolerance). May cause nausea or vomiting (small, frequent meals may help); abdominal pain, difficult/painful menstrual cycles; dizziness or mental depression (use caution when driving); rash; hair loss; headache; or breast pain, increased/decreased libido, or enlargement/tenderness of breasts. Report significant swelling of extremities; sudden acute pain in legs or calves, chest, or abdomen; shortness of breath; severe headache or vomiting; sudden blindness; weakness or numbness of arm or leg; unusual vaginal bleeding; yellowing of skin or eyes; or unusual bruising or bleeding. You may become intolerant to wearing contact lenses, notify prescriber if this occurs. **Pregnancy/breast-feeding precautions:** Inform prescriber if you are pregnant. Do not get pregnant while taking this medication. Consult prescriber for appropriate barrier contraceptive measures. This medication may cause fetal defects and should not be used during pregnancy. Consult prescriber if breast-feeding.

Transdermal patch: Apply to clean dry skin. Do not apply transdermal patch to breasts. Apply to trunk of body (preferably abdomen). Rotate application sites. Aerosol topical corticosteroids may reduce allergic skin reaction; report persistent skin reaction.

Intravaginal cream: Insert high in vagina. Wash hands and applicator before and after use.

Dietary Issues: Ensure adequate calcium and vitamin D intake when used for the prevention of osteoporosis.

Geriatric Considerations: Before prescribing estrogen therapy to postmenopausal women, the risks and benefits must be weighed for each patient. Data in women 80 years and older is minimal and it is unclear if reduced risk is applicable to women in this age group. Women should be informed of risks and benefits, as well as possible side effects and the return of menstrual bleeding (when cycled with a progestin), and should be involved in the prescribing options. Oral therapy may be more convenient for vaginal atrophy and urinary incontinence.

Breast-feeding Issues: The AAP considers ethinyl estradiol, an estrogen derivative, to be "usually compatible" with breast-feeding. Estrogen has been shown to decrease the quantity and quality of human milk; use only if clearly needed; monitor the growth of the infant closely.

Pregnancy Issues: Increased risk of fetal reproductive tract disorders and other birth defects; do not use during pregnancy.

Related Information

Estrogen Replacement Therapy *on page 1666*
Osteoporosis Management *on page 1696*

Estradiol and Medroxyprogesterone

(es tra DYE ole & me DROKS ee proe JES te rone)

U.S. Brand Names Lunelle™

Synonyms E_2C and MPA; Medroxyprogesterone Acetate and Estradiol Cypionate

Pharmacologic Category Contraceptive

Pregnancy Risk Factor X

Lactation Enters breast milk/not recommended

Use Prevention of pregnancy

Mechanism of Action/Effect Inhibits secretion of gonadotropins, leading to prevention of follicular maturation and ovulation. Also leads to thickening and reduction in volume of cervical mucus (decreases sperm penetration) and thinning of endometrium (reduces possibility of implantation).

Contraindications Hypersensitivity to estrogens, medroxyprogesterone, or any component of the formulation; undiagnosed abnormal vaginal bleeding; history of or current thrombophlebitis or thromboembolic disorders; severe hypertension; valvular heart disease with complications; cerebral vascular or coronary artery disease; carcinoma of the breast; estrogen-dependent tumor; hepatic disease or dysfunction; history of cholestatic jaundice during pregnancy or with prior hormonal contraceptive use, including severe pruritus of pregnancy; headaches with focal neurological symptoms; diabetes with vascular involvement; smoking ≥15 cigarettes/day and >35 years of age; pregnancy

Warnings/Precautions Risk of serious cardiovascular side effects increases in women >35 years of age who smoke cigarettes and in smokers and nonsmokers >40 years of age. Smoking is not advised; associated with an increased risk of thromboembolism, stroke, myocardial infarction, gallbladder disease, or liver tumor. Risk increases with a concurrent history of hypertension, hyperlipidemias (hypertriglyceridemia), obesity, or diabetes. Use with caution in patients with a history of gallbladder disease and patients with familial defects of lipoprotein metabolism. To decrease risk of thromboembolism, discontinue (if possible) 4 weeks prior to and for at least 2 weeks after elective surgery and following prolonged immobilization.

Use of combined oral contraceptives has been associated with a small increase in the frequency of breast cancer. Risk decreases over time after discontinuation. Some studies suggest an increased risk of intraepithelial neoplasia may be associated with oral contraceptive use. Increased risk of benign hepatic adenomas (extremely rare). There are case reports of retinal thrombosis. Discontinue if unexplained partial or complete vision loss, proptosis, diplopia, papilledema, or retinal vascular lesions. An ophthalmologist should evaluate contact lens wearers who develop changes in lens tolerance.

Efficacy is dependent upon adherence to dosing schedule (I.M. injections every 28-30 days, not to exceed 33 days). If injection is not received within 33 days, pregnancy must be ruled out prior to additional treatment. Does not protect against HIV infection or other sexually-transmitted diseases. Use with caution in patients with diseases which may be exacerbated by fluid retention, including asthma, epilepsy, migraine, diabetes, cardiac or renal dysfunction. Not for use prior to menarche or following menopause.

Drug Interactions

Cytochrome P450 Effect:

Estradiol: Substrate of **CYP1A2**, 2A6, 2B6, 2C8/9, 2C19, 2D6, 2E1, **3A4**; Inhibits CYP1A2; Induces CYP3A4

Medroxyprogesterone: Substrate of CYP3A4; Induces CYP3A4

Decreased Effect: Estradiol may decrease plasma levels of acetaminophen, clofibrate, morphine, salicylic acid, and temazepam. Enzyme inducers (carbamazepine, phenobarbital, phenytoin, and rifampin) may increase the metabolism of estradiol, resulting in decreased effect, leading to pregnancy. Griseofulvin, penicillins, and tetracyclines have been shown to alter pharmacokinetics of oral contraceptives leading to pregnancy; effects are not consistent with synthetic steroids. Aminoglutethimide and phenylbutazone may decrease contraceptive effectiveness and increase menstrual irregularities. St John's wort may induce hepatic enzymes resulting in decreased effect of contraceptive and breakthrough bleeding.

Increased Effect/Toxicity: Estradiol may inhibit metabolism of cyclosporine, prednisolone, and theophylline, leading to increased plasma levels.

(Continued)

Estradiol and Medroxyprogesterone *(Continued)*

Nutritional/Ethanol Interactions Herb/Nutraceutical: Ascorbic acid (>1 g/day) may increase serum levels of estradiol.

Effects on Lab Values Decreased antithrombin, increased prothrombin, and factors VII, VIII, IX, X; decreased serum folate concentration; increased platelet aggregability; increased thyroid-binding globulin; increased total thyroid hormone (T_4); increased triglycerides; impaired glucose tolerance; decreased plasma and urinary steroid levels; decreased gonadotropin levels; decreased sex hormone-binding globulin concentrations; increased sulfobromophthalein and other liver function tests

Adverse Reactions Frequency not defined.

Cardiovascular: Arterial thromboembolism, cerebral hemorrhage, cerebral thrombosis, edema, hypertension, mesenteric thrombosis, myocardial infarction

Central nervous system: Dizziness, emotional lability, headache, mental depression, migraine, nervousness, premenstrual syndrome

Dermatologic: Acne, alopecia, erythema multiforme, erythema nodosum, hirsutism, melasma, rash (allergic)

Endocrine & metabolic: Amenorrhea, breast enlargement, breast secretion, breast tenderness/pain, decreased lactation (immediately postpartum), decreased libido/libido changes, dysmenorrhea, menorrhagia, metrorrhagia, temporary infertility following discontinuation

Gastrointestinal: Abdominal pain, appetite changes, enlarged abdomen, colitis, gallbladder disease, nausea, weight gain/loss (weight gain was the most common reason for discontinuing medication)

Genitourinary: Cervical changes, cystitis-like syndrome, vaginal moniliasis, vaginitis, vulvovaginal disorder

Hematologic: Hemolytic uremic syndrome, hemorrhagic eruption, porphyria

Hepatic: Budd-Chiari syndrome, hepatic adenoma, benign hepatic tumor

Local: Thrombophlebitis

Neuromuscular & skeletal: Weakness

Ocular: Cataracts, intolerance to contact lenses, retinal thrombosis

Renal: Impaired renal function

Respiratory: Pulmonary thromboembolism

Miscellaneous: Anaphylaxis, carbohydrate intolerance

Overdosage/Toxicology Symptoms of estrogen/progestin overdose include nausea, vomiting, and vaginal bleeding or other menstrual irregularities. Treatment should be symptomatic.

Pharmacodynamics/Kinetics

Absorption: Prolonged

Half-Life Elimination: Mean: 17 β-estradiol: 8.4 days; MPA: 14.7 days

Time to Peak: 17 β-estradiol: 1-7 days; MPA: 1-10 days

Metabolism: Hepatic; estradiol via CYP1A2, 3A4, and 3A5-7 to estrone and estriol

Formulations Injection, suspension: Estradiol cypionate 5 mg and medroxyprogesterone acetate 25 mg per 0.5 mL (0.5 mL)

Dosing

Adults: Contraception (Female): I.M.: 0.5 mL

First dose: Within first 5 days of menstrual period or within 5 days of a complete 1st trimester abortion. Do not administer <4 weeks postpartum **if not breast-feeding** or <6 weeks postpartum **if breast-feeding**.

Maintenance dose: Monthly, every 28-30 days following previous injection; do not exceed 33 days. Pregnancy must be ruled out if >33 days have past between injections. Bleeding episodes cannot be used to guide injection schedule. Shortening schedule may lead to menstrual pattern changes.

Switching from other forms of contraception: First injection should be given within 7 days of last active oral contraceptive pill. When switching from other methods, timing of injection should ensure continuous contraceptive coverage.

Elderly: Not for postmenopausal use

Renal Impairment: Studies have not been conducted; however, dosage adjustment is not anticipated due to hepatic metabolism.

Hepatic Impairment: Contraindicated in hepatic dysfunction.

Stability

Storage: Store at controlled room temperature, 25°C (77°F).

Monitoring and Teaching Issues

Physical Assessment: Ascertain by laboratory tests that patient is not pregnant before administering this contraceptive. Assess other medications patient may be taking for interactions/effectiveness (see Drug Interactions). See Warnings/Precautions, Drug Interactions, and Monitoring Laboratory Tests for use cautions. See Administration information. Monitor closely for adverse reactions (see Adverse Reactions). Monitor diabetic patients for altered glucose tolerance. Assess knowledge/teach patient importance of regularly scheduled injections, adverse reactions to report, and interventions to reduce side-effects. Review all patient information before administering first dose. **Pregnancy risk factor X** - pregnancy must be excluded before administering each dose. Breast-feeding is not recommended.

Patient Education: This medication is used to prevent pregnancy and does not protect against HIV infection or other sexually transmitted disease. Periodic gynecologic exams and breast exams are important. In order for this medication to be effective you must have an injection every 28-30 days, regardless of bleeding pattern. If you miss an injection, pregnancy must be ruled out before additional treatment, and a barrier method of contraception should be used until treatment can be resumed. Inform prescriber prior to your first injection of all other medications, OTC products, herbal or dietary supplements that you are using. Avoid other medications, OTC products, herbal or dietary supplements unless approved by your prescriber. Maintain adequate hydration (2-3 L/day of fluids) unless advised by prescriber to restrict fluids. Your regular bleeding pattern may be change and you may eventually experience no bleeding at all. Notify prescriber if bleeding is unusually heavy or irregular. You may experience nausea or vomiting (small, frequent meals may help); dizziness or mental depression (use caution when driving or engaging in tasks requiring alertness until response to drug is known); photosensitivity (use sunscreen, wear protective clothing and eyewear, and avoid direct sunlight); rash; loss of hair; enlargement/tenderness of breasts; increased/decreased libido; or hot flashes (cool clothes and environment may help). Report sudden acute pain in legs or calves, chest, or abdomen; shortness of breath; severe headache or vomiting; weakness or numbness of arms or legs; unusual vaginal bleeding; yellowing of skin or eyes; change in color of urine or stool; easy bruising or bleeding; pain, swelling, or redness at injection site; breast lumps; or persistent and unresolved flu-like symptoms. **Pregnancy/breast-feeding precautions:** Contact your prescriber if you think you may become pregnant. Breast-feeding is not recommended.

Dietary Issues: Consider folic acid supplementation after discontinuing use, especially if patient is trying to conceive.

Breast-feeding Issues: Combination oral contraceptives decrease the quality and quantity of breast milk. Do not administer within 6 weeks of delivery if breast-feeding.

Pregnancy Issues: Should not be used during pregnancy; however, epidemiological studies do not indicate increased risk of birth defects when oral contraceptives were taken inadvertently in early pregnancy. May increase risk of hypospadias in the male fetus and virilization of the female fetus. Infants are at an increased risk of low birth weight, which is associated with increased risk of neonatal death. To decrease risk of thromboembolism in the mother, do not start treatment within 4 weeks of delivery (if not breast-feeding).

Additional Information Following discontinuation of treatment, ovulation would be expected to resume within 63-112 days. Fifty percent of women that stopped therapy in order to become pregnant achieved fertility within 6 months, 83% within 1 year. Thai women were found to have increased absorption and earlier return of ovulation following discontinuation of this medication during clinical trials. Efficacy was the same for women of all ethnic backgrounds. Dosing adjustment based on body weight is not needed.

Related Information

Estradiol *on page 494*
MedroxyPROGESTERone *on page 842*

Estradiol and Norethindrone (es tra DYE ole & nor eth IN drone)

U.S. Brand Names Activella™; CombiPatch®

Synonyms Norethindrone and Estradiol

Generic Available No

Pharmacologic Category Estrogen Derivative

Pregnancy Risk Factor X

Lactation Contraindicated

Use Women with an intact uterus:

Tablet: Treatment of moderate to severe vasomotor symptoms associated with menopause; treatment of vulvar and vaginal atrophy; prophylaxis for postmenopausal osteoporosis

Transdermal patch: Treatment of moderate to severe vasomotor symptoms associated with menopause; treatment of vulvar and vaginal atrophy; treatment of hypoestrogenism due to hypogonadism, castration, or primary ovarian failure

Contraindications Hypersensitivity to estrogens, progestins, or any components; carcinoma of the breast; estrogen-dependent tumor; undiagnosed abnormal vaginal bleeding; thrombophlebitis, thromboembolic disorders, or stroke; hysterectomy; pregnancy

Warnings/Precautions For use only in women with an intact uterus. Use with caution in patients with diseases that may be exacerbated by fluid retention, including asthma, epilepsy, migraine, diabetes, cardiac or renal dysfunction. Use with caution in patients with a history of hypercalcemia, cardiovascular disease, or gallbladder disease. May increase blood pressure. Use with caution in patients with liver dysfunction or disease. May increase risk of venous thromboembolism. Unopposed estrogens may increase the risk of endometrial carcinoma in postmenopausal women (incidence is less likely with the addition of progesterone). Estrogens may increase the risk of breast cancer; estrogen compounds are generally associated with lipid effects such as increased HDL-cholesterol, and decreased LDL-cholesterol; triglycerides may also be increased. Use with caution in patients with familial defects of lipoprotein metabolism. Safety and efficacy in children have not been established. May cause visual abnormalities. Discontinue if papilledema or renal vascular lesions develop.

Drug Interactions

Cytochrome P450 Effect:

Estradiol: Substrate of **CYP1A2**, 2A6, 2B6, 2C8/9, 2C19, 2D6, 2E1, **3A4**; Inhibits CYP1A2; Induces CYP3A4

Norethindrone: Substrate of **CYP3A4**; Induces CYP2C19

Adverse Reactions Frequency not defined.

Cardiovascular: Altered blood pressure, cardiovascular accident, edema, venous thromboembolism

Central nervous system: Dizziness, fatigue, headache, insomnia, mental depression, migraine, nervousness

Dermatologic: Chloasma, erythema multiforme, erythema nodosum, hemorrhagic eruption, hirsutism, itching, loss of scalp hair, melasma, pruritus, skin rash

Endocrine & metabolic: Breast enlargement, breast tenderness, breast pain, changes in libido

Gastrointestinal: Abdominal pain, bloating, changes in appetite, flatulence, gallbladder disease, nausea, pancreatitis, vomiting, weight gain/loss

Genitourinary: Alterations in frequency and flow of menses, changes in cervical secretions, cystitis-like syndrome, increased size of uterine leiomyomata, premenstrual-like syndrome, vaginal candidiasis, vaginitis

Hematologic: Aggravation of porphyria

Hepatic: Cholestatic jaundice

Local: Application site reaction (transdermal patch)

Neuromuscular & skeletal: Arthralgia, back pain, chorea, myalgia, weakness

Ocular: Intolerance to contact lenses, steeping of corneal curvature

Respiratory: Pharyngitis, pulmonary thromboembolism, rhinitis

Miscellaneous: Allergic reactions, carbohydrate intolerance, flu-like syndrome

(Continued)

Estradiol and Norethindrone *(Continued)*

Pharmacokinetic Note See individual agents.

Pharmacodynamics/Kinetics

Bioavailability: Activella™: Estradiol: 50%; Norethindrone: 100%

Half-Life Elimination:

Activella™: Estradiol: 12-14 hours; Norethindrone: 8-11 hours

Time to Peak: Activella™: Estradiol: 5-8 hours

Formulations

Tablet (Activella™): Estradiol 1 mg and norethindrone acetate 0.5 mg (28s)

Transdermal system (CombiPatch®):

0.05/0.14: Estradiol 0.05 mg and norethindrone acetate 0.14 mg per day (8s) [9 sq cm]

0.05/0.25: Estradiol 0.05 mg and norethindrone acetate 0.25 mg per day (8s) [16 sq cm]

Dosing

Adults & Elderly:

Hypoestrogenism: Transdermal (patch):

Continuous combined regimen: Apply one patch twice weekly

Continuous sequential regimen: Apply estradiol-only patch for first 14 days of cycle, followed by one CombiPatch™ applied twice weekly for the remaining 14 days of a 28-day cycle.

Menopause (moderate to severe vasomotor symptoms); vulvar and vaginal atrophy:

Oral (Activella™): 1 tablet daily

Transdermal (patch):

Continuous combined regimen: Apply one patch twice weekly

Continuous sequential regimen: Apply estradiol-only patch for first 14 days of cycle, followed by one CombiPatch™ applied twice weekly for the remaining 14 days of a 28-day cycle.

Osteoporosis, prevention in postmenopausal females (Activella™): Oral: 1 tablet daily

Administration

Other: Transdermal patch: Apply to clean dry skin. Do not apply transdermal patch to breasts; apply to lower abdomen, avoiding waistline. Rotate application sites.

Monitoring and Teaching Issues

Physical Assessment: See Contraindications, Warnings/Precautions, and Dosing for use cautions. Assess potential for interactions with other prescriptions, OTC medications, or herbal products patient may be taking (see Drug Interactions). Assess results of annual gynecological and breast exam, therapeutic effectiveness (according to purpose for use), and adverse response (eg, CNS changes, hypertension, thromboembolism, fluid retention, edema, CHF, respiratory changes - see Adverse Reactions and Overdose/Toxicology) on a regular basis during therapy. Before prescribing estrogen therapy to postmenopausal women, the risks and benefits must be weighed for each patient. Women should be informed of these risks and benefits, as well as possible effects of progestin when added to estrogen therapy. Caution diabetic patients to monitor glucose levels closely (may impair glucose tolerance). Teach patient appropriate use (according to formulation), possible side effects and appropriate interventions (annual gynecological and breast exam), and adverse symptoms to report (see Patient Education). **Pregnancy risk factor X** - determine that patient is not pregnant before starting therapy. Do not give to females of childbearing age unless patient is capable of complying with barrier contraceptive use. Advise patient about appropriate contraceptive measures as appropriate. Breast-feeding is contraindicated.

Patient Education: Inform prescriber of all prescriptions, OTC medications, or herbal products you are taking, and any allergies you have. Do not take anything new without consulting prescriber. Use as prescribed; maintain prescribed cycles or term as prescribed. Avoid alcohol. Annual gynecologic and breast exams are important. If diabetic, monitor glucose levels closely (may impair glucose tolerance). May cause nausea or vomiting (small, frequent meals may help); abdominal pain, difficult/painful menstrual cycles; dizziness or mental depression (use caution when driving); rash; hair loss; headache; or breast pain, increased/decreased libido, or tenderness/enlargement of breasts. Report significant swelling of extremities; sudden acute pain in legs or calves, chest, or abdomen; shortness of breath; severe headache or vomiting; sudden blindness; weakness or numbness of arm or leg; unusual vaginal bleeding; yellowing of skin or eyes; or unusual bruising or bleeding. You may become intolerant to wearing contact lenses, notify prescriber if this occurs. **Pregnancy/breast-feeding precautions:** Inform prescriber if you are pregnant or breast-feeding. Consult prescriber for appropriate barrier contraceptive measures. This medication may cause fetal defects and should not be used during pregnancy. Do not breast-feed.

Related Information

Estradiol *on page 494*

Norethindrone *on page 984*

Estradiol Cypionate *see* Estradiol *on page 494*

Estradiol Hemihydrate *see* Estradiol *on page 494*

Estradiol Transdermal *see* Estradiol *on page 494*

Estradiol Valerate *see* Estradiol *on page 494*

Estramustine (es tra MUS teen)

U.S. Brand Names Emcyt®

Synonyms Estramustine Phosphate Sodium

Generic Available No

Pharmacologic Category Antineoplastic Agent, Alkylating Agent

Pregnancy Risk Factor C

Lactation Excretion in breast milk unknown/contraindicated

Use Palliative treatment of prostatic carcinoma (progressive or metastatic)

Mechanism of Action/Effect Mechanism is not completely clear, thought to act as an alkylating agent and as estrogen

Contraindications Hypersensitivity to estramustine or any component, estradiol or nitrogen mustard; active thrombophlebitis or thromboembolic disorders

Warnings/Precautions The U.S. Food and Drug Administration (FDA) currently recommends that procedures for proper handling and disposal of antineoplastic agents be considered. Glucose tolerance may be decreased; elevated blood pressure may occur. Exacerbation of peripheral edema or congestive heart disease may occur. Use with caution in patients with impaired liver function, renal insufficiency, or metabolic bone diseases. Pregnancy risk C.

Drug Interactions

Decreased Effect: Milk products and calcium-rich foods/drugs may impair the oral absorption of estramustine phosphate sodium.

Nutritional/Ethanol Interactions Food: Estramustine serum levels may be decreased if taken with dairy products.

Adverse Reactions

>10%:

Cardiovascular: Edema

Endocrine & metabolic: Sodium retention, decreased libido, breast tenderness, breast enlargement

Gastrointestinal: Diarrhea, nausea

Hematologic: Thrombocytopenia

Respiratory: Dyspnea

1% to 10%:

Cardiovascular: Myocardial infarction

Central nervous system: Insomnia, lethargy

Gastrointestinal: Anorexia, flatulence, vomiting

Hematologic: Leukopenia

Local: Thrombophlebitis

Neuromuscular & skeletal: Leg cramps

Respiratory: Pulmonary embolism

<1% (Limited to important or life-threatening): Allergic reactions, anemia, angioedema, cardiac arrest, gynecomastia

Overdosage/Toxicology Symptoms of overdose include nausea, vomiting, and myelosuppression. There are no known antidotes; treatment is symptomatic and supportive.

Pharmacodynamics/Kinetics

Absorption: 75%

Half-Life Elimination: Terminal: 20-24 hours

Time to Peak: Serum: 2-3 hours

Metabolism: GI tract: Initial dephosphorylation; Hepatic: Oxidation and hydrolysis; metabolites include estramustine, estrone, estradiol, nitrogen mustard

Formulations Capsule, as phosphate sodium: 140 mg

Dosing

Adults & Elderly: Refer to individual protocols.

Prostate carcinoma:

Oral: 10-16 mg/kg/day (14 mg/kg/day is most common) or 140 mg 4 times/day (some patients have been maintained for >3 years on therapy) Refer to individual protocols.

I.V.: 300 mg/day for 3-4 weeks, then 300-450 mg/week for 3-8 weeks (investigational)

Stability

Storage: Refrigerate at 2°C to 8°C (36°F to 46°F). Capsules may be stored outside of refrigerator for up to 24-48 hours without affecting potency.

Monitoring and Teaching Issues

Physical Assessment: See Contraindications and Warnings/Precautions for use cautions. Assess potential for interactions with other prescriptions, OTC medications, or herbal products patient may be taking (see Drug Interactions). Assess results of laboratory tests, therapeutic effectiveness, and adverse response (eg, hypertension, CNS changes, thromboembolism - see Adverse Reactions and Overdose/Toxicology) on a regular basis during therapy. Teach patient appropriate use (injections technique and needle disposal), possible side effects and appropriate interventions, and adverse symptoms to report (see Patient Education). **Pregnancy risk factor C.**

Patient Education: Inform prescriber of all prescriptions, OTC medications, or herbal products you are taking, and any allergies you have. Do not take anything new without consulting prescriber. It may take several weeks to manifest effects of this medication. Store capsules in refrigerator. Do not take with milk or milk products. Preferable to take on empty stomach, 1 hour before or 2 hours after meals. May cause nausea or vomiting (small, frequent meals, frequent mouth care, chewing gum, or sucking lozenges may help); flatulence; diarrhea (buttermilk, boiled milk, or yogurt); decreased libido (reversible); or breast tenderness or enlargement. Report sudden acute pain or cramping in legs or calves, chest pain, shortness of breath, weakness or numbness of arms or legs, difficulty breathing, or edema (increased weight, swelling of legs or feet). **Pregnancy/breast-feeding precautions:** Male: Do not cause a female to become pregnant. Male/female: Consult prescriber for instruction on appropriate barrier contraceptive measures. This drug may cause severe fetal defects. Do not breast-feed.

Dietary Issues: Administer at least 1 hour before or 2 hours after eating.

Additional Information Although I.V. use is reported, no parenteral product is commercially available in the U.S.

Estramustine Phosphate Sodium *see* Estramustine *on page 500*

Estratab® [DSC] *see* Estrogens (Esterified) *on page 508*

Estring® *see* Estradiol *on page 494*

Estrogenic Substances, Conjugated *see* Estrogens (Conjugated/Equine) *on page 503*

Estrogen Replacement Therapy *see page 1666*

Estrogens (Conjugated A/Synthetic)

(ES troe jenz, KON joo gate ed aye sin THET ik)

U.S. Brand Names Cenestin®

Generic Available No

Pharmacologic Category Estrogen Derivative

Pregnancy Risk Factor X

Lactation Enters breast milk/use caution

Use Treatment of moderate to severe vasomotor symptoms of menopause; treatment of vulvar and vaginal atrophy

Mechanism of Action/Effect Estrogens modulate the pituitary secretion of gonadotropins, luteinizing hormone, and follicle-stimulating hormone through a negative feedback system; estrogen replacement reduces elevated levels of these hormones in postmenopausal women

Contraindications Hypersensitivity to estrogens or any component of the formulation; undiagnosed abnormal vaginal bleeding; history of or current thrombophlebitis or thromboembolic disorders; liver disease; carcinoma of the breast; estrogen dependent tumor; pregnancy

Warnings/Precautions Conjugated estrogens (alone or in combination with a progestin) should not be used to prevent coronary heart disease. Unopposed estrogens may increase the risk of endometrial carcinoma in postmenopausal women. Use with caution in patients with diseases which may be exacerbated by fluid retention, including asthma, epilepsy, migraine, diabetes, cardiac or renal dysfunction. Use with caution in patients with a history of hypercalcemia, cardiovascular disease, and gallbladder disease. May increase blood pressure. Use with caution in patients with hepatic disease. May increase risk of venous thromboembolism. Estrogens may increase the risk of breast cancer (controversial/currently under study). Estrogen compounds are generally associated with lipid effects such as increased HDL-cholesterol and decreased LDL-cholesterol. Triglycerides may also be increased; use with caution in patients with familial defects of lipoprotein metabolism. May exacerbate endometriosis. Before prescribing estrogen therapy to postmenopausal women, the risks and benefits must be weighed for each patient. Women should be informed of these risks and benefits, as well as possible effects of progestin when added to estrogen therapy. Use for shortest duration possible consistent with treatment goals. Conduct periodic risk:benefit assessments. When used solely for prevention of osteoporosis, carefully consider other treatment options. Safety and efficacy in pediatric patients have not been established.

Drug Interactions

Cytochrome P450 Effect: Based on estradiol and estrone: Substrate of **1A2**, 2A6, 2B6, 2C8/9, 2C19, 2D6, 2E1, **3A4**; Inhibits 1A2; Induces 3A4

Decreased Effect: CYP3A4 enzyme inducers may decrease estrogen plasma concentrations leading to decreased therapeutic effect or changes in uterine bleeding profile; examples of CYP3A4 enzyme inducers include carbamazepine, phenobarbital, and rifampin

Increased Effect/Toxicity: CYP3A4 enzyme inhibitors may increase estrogen plasma concentrations leading to increased incidence of adverse effects; examples of CYP3A4 enzyme inhibitors include clarithromycin, erythromycin, itraconazole, ketoconazole, and ritonavir. Anticoagulants increase the potential for thromboembolic events Estrogens may enhance the effects of hydrocortisone and prednisone

Nutritional/Ethanol Interactions

Ethanol: Avoid ethanol (routine use increases estrogen level and risk of breast cancer).

Food: Grapefruit juice may increase estrogen levels, leading to increased adverse effects.

Herb/Nutraceutical: St John's wort may decrease levels. Avoid black cohosh, dong quai (has estrogenic activity). Avoid red clover, saw palmetto, ginseng (due to potential hormonal effects).

Adverse Reactions Adverse effects associated with estrogen therapy; frequency not defined

Cardiovascular: Edema, hypertension, venous thromboembolism

Central nervous system: Dizziness, headache, mental depression, migraine

Dermatologic: Chloasma, erythema multiforme, erythema nodosum, hemorrhagic eruption, hirsutism, loss of scalp hair, melasma

Endocrine & metabolic: Breast enlargement, breast tenderness, changes in libido, thyroid-binding globulin increased, total thyroid hormone (T_4) increased, serum triglycerides/phospholipids increased, HDL-cholesterol increased, LDL-cholesterol decreased, impaired glucose tolerance, hypercalcemia

Gastrointestinal: Abdominal cramps, bloating, cholecystitis, cholelithiasis, gallbladder disease, nausea, pancreatitis, vomiting, weight gain/loss

Genitourinary: Alterations in frequency and flow of menses, changes in cervical secretions, endometrial cancer, increased size of uterine leiomyomata, vaginal candidiasis

Hematologic: Aggravation of porphyria, antithrombin III and antifactor Xa decreased, levels of fibrinogen decreased, platelet aggregability and platelet count increased; prothrombin and factors VII, VIII, IX, X increased

Hepatic: Cholestatic jaundice

Neuromuscular & skeletal: Chorea

Ocular: Intolerance to contact lenses, steeping of corneal curvature

Respiratory: Pulmonary thromboembolism

Miscellaneous: Carbohydrate intolerance

Overdosage/Toxicology Symptoms of overdose include nausea and vomiting; withdrawal bleeding may occur in females. Toxicity is unlikely following single exposures of excessive doses, any treatment following emesis and charcoal administration should be supportive and symptomatic.

Pharmacodynamics/Kinetics

Absorption: Readily absorbed

Time to Peak: 4-16 hours

Metabolism: Hepatic to metabolites

Formulations Tablet: 0.3 mg, 0.625 mg, 0.9 mg, 1.25 mg

Dosing

Adults & Elderly:

Moderate to severe vasomotor symptoms: Oral: 0.625 mg/day; may be titrated up to 1.25 mg/day; attempts to discontinue medication should be made at 3- to 6-month intervals

Vulvar and vaginal atrophy: Oral: 0.3 mg/day

Stability

Storage: Store at room temperature of 25°C (77°F).

Monitoring and Teaching Issues

Physical Assessment: See Contraindications, Warnings/Precautions, and Dosing for use cautions. Assess potential for interactions with other prescriptions, OTC medications, or herbal products patient may be taking (see Drug Interactions). Assess therapeutic effectiveness (according to purpose for use) and adverse response (eg, CNS changes, hypertension, thromboembolism, fluid retention, edema, CHF, respiratory changes - see Adverse Reactions and Overdose/Toxicology) on a regular basis during therapy. Before prescribing estrogen therapy to postmenopausal women, the risks and benefits must be weighed for each patient. Women should be informed of these risks and benefits, as well as possible effects of progestin when added to estrogen therapy. Caution diabetic patients to monitor glucose levels closely (may impair glucose tolerance). Teach patient appropriate use (according to formulation), possible side effects and appropriate interventions, and adverse symptoms to report (see Patient Education). **Pregnancy risk factor X** - determine that patient is not pregnant before starting therapy. Do not give to females of childbearing age unless patient is capable of complying with barrier contraceptive use. Advise patient about appropriate contraceptive measures as appropriate. Note breast-feeding caution.

Patient Education: Inform prescriber of all prescriptions, OTC medications, or herbal products you are taking, and any allergies you have. Do not take anything new without consulting prescriber. Use as prescribed; maintain prescribed cycles or term as prescribed. Avoid alcohol. Annual gynecologic and breast exams are important. If diabetic, monitor glucose levels closely (may impair glucose tolerance). May cause nausea or vomiting (small, frequent meals may help); abdominal pain, difficult/painful menstrual cycles; dizziness or mental depression (use caution when driving); rash; hair loss; headache; or breast pain, increased/decreased libido, or enlargement/tenderness of breasts. Report significant swelling of extremities; sudden acute pain in legs or calves, chest or abdomen; shortness of breath; severe headache or vomiting; sudden blindness; weakness or numbness of arm or leg; unusual vaginal bleeding; yellowing of skin or eyes; or unusual bruising or bleeding. You may become intolerant to wearing contact lenses, notify prescriber if this occurs. **Pregnancy/breast-feeding precautions:** Inform prescriber if you are pregnant or breast-feeding. Consult prescriber for appropriate barrier contraceptive measures. This medication may cause fetal defects and should not be used during pregnancy. Consult prescriber if breast-feeding.

Additional Information Not biologically equivalent to conjugated estrogens from equine source. Contains 9 unique estrogenic compounds (equine source contains at least 10 active estrogenic compounds).

Related Information

Estrogen Replacement Therapy *on page 1666*
Osteoporosis Management *on page 1696*
Pharmacotherapy of Urinary Incontinence *on page 1699*

Estrogens (Conjugated/Equine) (ES troe jenz KON joo gate ed EE kwine)

U.S. Brand Names Premarin®

Synonyms C.E.S.; Estrogenic Substances, Conjugated

Generic Available No

Pharmacologic Category Estrogen Derivative

Pregnancy Risk Factor X

Lactation Enters breast milk/use caution

Use Treatment of moderate to severe vasomotor symptoms associated with menopause; treatment of vulvar and vaginal atrophy; hypoestrogenism (due to hypogonadism, castration, or primary ovarian failure); prostatic cancer (palliation); breast cancer (palliation); osteoporosis (prophylaxis)

Use - Unlabeled/Investigational Uremic bleeding; abnormal uterine bleeding

Mechanism of Action/Effect Estrogens modulate the pituitary secretion of gonadotropins, luteinizing hormone, and follicle-stimulating hormone through a negative feedback system; estrogen replacement reduces elevated levels of these hormones in postmenopausal women

Contraindications Hypersensitivity to estrogens or any component of the formulation; undiagnosed abnormal vaginal bleeding; history of or current thrombophlebitis or thromboembolic disorders; carcinoma of the breast (except in appropriately selected patients being treated for metastatic disease); estrogen-dependent tumor; pregnancy

Warnings/Precautions Conjugated estrogens (alone or in combination with a progestin) should not be used to prevent coronary heart disease. Unopposed estrogens may increase the risk of endometrial carcinoma in postmenopausal women. Use with caution in patients with diseases which may be exacerbated by fluid retention, including asthma, epilepsy, migraine, diabetes, cardiac or renal dysfunction. Use with caution in patients with a history of hypercalcemia, cardiovascular disease, and gallbladder disease. May increase blood pressure. Use with caution in patients with hepatic disease. May increase risk of venous thromboembolism. Estrogens may increase the risk of breast cancer (controversial/currently under study). Estrogen compounds are generally associated with lipid effects such as increased HDL-cholesterol and decreased LDL-cholesterol. Triglycerides may also be increased; use with caution in patients with familial defects of lipoprotein metabolism. Estrogens may cause premature closure of the epiphyses in young individuals. May increase size of pre-existing uterine leiomyomata. Before prescribing estrogen therapy to postmenopausal women, the risks and benefits must be weighed for each patient. Women should be informed of these risks and benefits, as well as possible effects of progestin when added to estrogen therapy. Use for shortest duration possible consistent with treatment goals. Conduct periodic risk:benefit assessments. When used solely for prevention of osteoporosis, carefully consider other treatment options. Safety and efficacy in pediatric patients have not been established.
(Continued)

Estrogens (Conjugated/Equine) *(Continued)*

Drug Interactions

Cytochrome P450 Effect: Based on estradiol and estrone: Substrate of **1A2**, 2A6, 2B6, 2C8/9, 2C19, 2D6, 2E1, **3A4**; Inhibits 1A2; Induces 3A4

Decreased Effect: Rifampin, nelfinavir, and ritonavir decrease estradiol serum concentrations. Anticonvulsants which are enzyme inducers (barbiturates, carbamazepine, phenobarbital, phenytoin, primidone) may potentially decrease estrogen levels.

Increased Effect/Toxicity: Hydrocortisone taken with estrogen may cause corticosteroid-induced toxicity. Increased potential for thromboembolic events with anticoagulants.

Nutritional/Ethanol Interactions

Ethanol: Avoid ethanol (routine use increases estrogen level and risk of breast cancer).

Food: Folic acid absorption may be decreased.

Herb/Nutraceutical: St John's wort may decrease levels. Avoid black cohosh, dong quai (has estrogenic activity). Avoid red clover, saw palmetto, ginseng (due to potential hormonal effects).

Effects on Lab Values ↑ Prothrombin and factors VII, VIII, IX, X; ↑ platelet aggregability, thyroid-binding globulin, total thyroid hormone (T_4), serum triglycerides/phospholipids; ↓ antithrombin III, serum folate concentration

Adverse Reactions Frequency not defined.

Cardiovascular: Edema, hypertension, venous thromboembolism

Central nervous system: Dizziness, headache, mental depression, migraine

Dermatologic: Chloasma, erythema multiforme, erythema nodosum, hemorrhagic eruption, hirsutism, loss of scalp hair, melasma

Endocrine & metabolic: Breast enlargement, breast tenderness, changes in libido, increased thyroid-binding globulin, increased total thyroid hormone (T_4), increased serum triglycerides/phospholipids, increased HDL-cholesterol, decreased LDL-cholesterol, impaired glucose tolerance, hypercalcemia

Gastrointestinal: Abdominal cramps, bloating, cholecystitis, cholelithiasis, gallbladder disease, nausea, pancreatitis, vomiting, weight gain/loss

Genitourinary: Alterations in frequency and flow of menses, changes in cervical secretions, endometrial cancer, increased size of uterine leiomyomata, vaginal candidiasis

Hematologic: Aggravation of porphyria, decreased antithrombin III and antifactor Xa, increased levels of fibrinogen, increased platelet aggregability and platelet count; increased prothrombin and factors VII, VIII, IX, X

Hepatic: Cholestatic jaundice

Neuromuscular & skeletal: Chorea

Miscellaneous: Carbohydrate intolerance

Ocular: Intolerance to contact lenses, steeping of corneal curvature

Respiratory: Pulmonary thromboembolism

Overdosage/Toxicology Toxicity is unlikely following single exposures of excessive doses, any treatment following emesis and charcoal administration should be supportive and symptomatic. Effects noted after large doses include headache, nausea, and vomiting. Bleeding may occur in females.

Pharmacodynamics/Kinetics

Absorption: Well absorbed

Metabolism: Hepatic to inactive compounds

Formulations

Cream, vaginal: 0.625 mg/g (42.5 g)

Injection, powder for reconstitution: 25 mg [diluent contains benzyl alcohol]

Tablet: 0.3 mg, 0.625 mg, 0.9 mg, 1.25 mg, 2.5 mg

Dosing

Adults & Elderly:

Male and Female:

Breast cancer palliation, metastatic disease in selected patients: Oral: 10 mg 3 times/day for at least 3 months

Uremic bleeding: I.V.: 0.6 mg/kg/day for 5 days

Male: Androgen-dependent prostate cancer: Oral: 1.25-2.5 mg 3 times/day

Female:

Prevention of osteoporosis in postmenopausal women: Oral: 0.625 mg/day, cyclically* or daily, depending on medical assessment of patient

Moderate to severe vasomotor symptoms: Oral: 0.625 mg/day; lowest dose that will control symptoms should be used. Medication should be discontinued as soon as possible. May be given cyclically* or daily, depending on medical assessment of patient

Vulvar and vaginal atrophy:

Oral: 0.3-1.25 mg (or more) daily, depending on tissue response of the patient; lowest dose that will control symptoms should be used. Medication should be discontinued as soon as possible. May be given cyclically* or daily, depending on medical assessment of patient.

Vaginal cream: Intravaginal: ½ to 2 g/day given cyclically*

Female hypogonadism: Oral: 0.3-0.625 mg/day given cyclically*; adjust dose in response to symptoms and endometrium response; progestin treatment should be added to maintain bone mineral density

Female castration, primary ovarian failure: Oral: 1.25 mg/day given cyclically*; adjust according to severity of symptoms and patient response. For maintenance, adjust to the lowest effective dose.

Abnormal uterine bleeding:

Acute/heavy bleeding:

Oral: 1.25 mg, may repeat every 4 hours for 24 hours, followed by 1.25 mg once daily for 7-10 days

I.V.: 25 mg, may repeat every 4 hours up to 3 doses

Note: Oral/I.V.: Treatment should be followed by a low-dose oral contraceptive; medroxyprogesterone acetate along with or following estrogen therapy can also be given

Nonacute/lesser bleeding: Oral: 1.25 mg once daily for 7-10 days

***Cyclic administration:** Either 3 weeks on, 1 week off **or** 25 days on, 5 days off

Pediatrics: Adolescents: Refer to adult dosing.

Hepatic Impairment:

Mild to moderate liver impairment: Dosage reduction of estrogens is recommended.
Severe liver impairment: **Not recommended.**

Administration

Oral: Give at bedtime to minimize adverse effects.

I.M.: May be administered intramuscularly.

I.V.: Administer I.V. doses slowly to avoid a flushing reaction.

Stability

Storage: Refrigerate injection. At room temperature, the injection is stable for 24 months.

Reconstitution: Reconstituted solution is stable for 60 days at refrigeration.

Compatibility: Stable in D_5W and NS

Compatibility when admixed: Incompatible with ascorbic acid

Monitoring Laboratory Tests Yearly physical examination that includes blood pressure and Papanicolaou smear

Monitoring and Teaching Issues

Physical Assessment: See Contraindications, Warnings/Precautions, and Dosing for use cautions. Assess potential for interactions with other prescriptions, OTC medications, or herbal products patient may be taking (see Drug Interactions). Assess therapeutic effectiveness (according to purpose for use), and adverse response (eg, CNS changes, hypertension, thromboembolism, fluid retention, edema, CHF, respiratory changes - see Adverse Reactions and Overdose/Toxicology) on a regular basis during therapy. Before prescribing estrogen therapy to postmenopausal women, the risks and benefits must be weighed for each patient. Women should be informed of these risks and benefits, as well as possible effects of progestin when added to estrogen therapy. Caution patients with diabetes to monitor glucose levels closely (may impair glucose tolerance). Teach patient appropriate use (according to formulation), possible side effects and appropriate interventions, and adverse symptoms to report (see Patient Education). **Pregnancy risk factor X** - determine that patient is not pregnant before starting therapy. Do not give to females of childbearing age unless patient is capable of complying with barrier contraceptive use. Advise patient about appropriate contraceptive measures as appropriate. Note breast-feeding caution.

Patient Education: Inform prescriber of all prescriptions, OTC medications, or herbal products you are taking, and any allergies you have. Do not take anything new without consulting prescriber. Use as prescribed; maintain prescribed cycles or term as prescribed. Avoid alcohol. Annual gynecologic and breast exams are important. If diabetic, monitor glucose levels closely (may impair glucose tolerance). May cause nausea or vomiting (small, frequent meals may help); abdominal pain, difficult/painful menstrual cycles; dizziness or mental depression (use caution when driving); rash; hair loss; headache; or breast pain, increased/decreased libido, or tenderness/enlargement of breasts. Report significant swelling of extremities; sudden acute pain in legs or calves, chest, or abdomen; shortness of breath; severe headache or vomiting; sudden blindness; weakness or numbness of arm or leg; unusual vaginal bleeding; yellowing of skin or eyes; or unusual bruising or bleeding. You may become intolerant to wearing contact lenses, notify prescriber if this occurs. **Pregnancy/breast-feeding precautions:** Inform prescriber if you are pregnant. Consult prescriber for appropriate barrier contraceptive measures. This medication may cause fetal defects and should not be used during pregnancy. Consult prescriber if breast-feeding.

Dietary Issues: Ensure adequate calcium and vitamin D intake when used for the prevention of osteoporosis.

Geriatric Considerations: Before prescribing estrogen therapy to postmenopausal women, the risks and benefits must be weighed for each patient. Data in women 80 years and older is minimal and it is unclear if reduced risk is applicable to women in this age group. Women should be informed of risks and benefits, as well as possible side effects and the return of menstrual bleeding (when cycled with a progestin), and should be involved in prescribing options. Oral therapy may be more convenient for vaginal atrophy and urinary incontinence.

Breast-feeding Issues: The AAP considers ethinyl estradiol, an estrogen derivative, to be "usually compatible" with breast-feeding. Estrogen has been shown to decrease the quantity and quality of human milk. Use only if clearly needed. Monitor the growth of the infant closely.

Pregnancy Issues: Increased risk of fetal reproductive tract disorders and other birth defects; do not use during pregnancy.

Additional Information Contains 50% to 65% sodium estrone sulfate and 20% to 35% sodium equilin sulfate

Related Information

Estrogen Replacement Therapy *on page 1666*
Osteoporosis Management *on page 1696*
Pharmacotherapy of Urinary Incontinence *on page 1699*

Estrogens (Conjugated/Equine) and Medroxyprogesterone

(ES troe jenz KON joo gate ed EE kwine & me DROKS ee proe JES te rone)

U.S. Brand Names Premphase®; Prempro™

Synonyms Medroxyprogesterone and Estrogens (Conjugated); MPA and Estrogens (Conjugated)

Generic Available No

Pharmacologic Category Estrogen Derivative

Pregnancy Risk Factor X

(Continued)

Estrogens (Conjugated/Equine) and Medroxyprogesterone *(Continued)*

Lactation

Estrogens: Enters breast milk/use caution

Progestins: Enters breast milk/use caution

Use Women with an intact uterus: Treatment of moderate to severe vasomotor symptoms associated with menopause; treatment of atrophic vaginitis; osteoporosis (prophylaxis)

Mechanism of Action/Effect

Estrogens modulate the pituitary secretion of gonadotropins, luteinizing hormone, and follicle-stimulating hormone through a negative feedback system; estrogen replacement reduces elevated levels of these hormones in postmenopausal women.

In women with adequate estrogen, MPA transforms a proliferative endometrium into a secretory endometrium; when administered with conjugated estrogens, reduces the incidence of endometrial hyperplasia and risk of adenocarcinoma.

Contraindications Hypersensitivity to conjugated estrogens, medroxyprogesterone (MPA), or any component of the formulation; undiagnosed abnormal vaginal bleeding; history of or current thrombophlebitis or thromboembolic disorders; carcinoma of the breast; estrogen-dependent tumor; hepatic dysfunction or disease; pregnancy

Warnings/Precautions Conjugated estrogens (alone or in combination with a progestin) should not be used to prevent coronary heart disease. Use with caution in patients with diseases which may be exacerbated by fluid retention, including asthma, epilepsy, migraine, diabetes, cardiac or renal dysfunction. Use with caution in patients with a history of hypercalcemia, cardiovascular disease, and gallbladder disease. May increase blood pressure. May increase risk of venous thromboembolism. Unopposed estrogens may increase the risk of endometrial carcinoma in postmenopausal women. Risk may be decreased when estrogens are used in combination with MPA, monitor. Estrogens may increase the risk of breast cancer (controversial/currently under study). Estrogen compounds are generally associated with increased HDL-cholesterol and decreased LDL-cholesterol. Triglycerides may also be increased; use with caution in patients with familial defects of lipoprotein metabolism. Discontinue following visual disturbance which shows papilledema or retinal vascular lesions. Patients with a history of depression should be monitored; discontinue if depression recurs to a serious degree. Prior to therapy, the risks and benefits must be weighed for each patient. Women should be informed of these risks and benefits. Estrogens may cause premature closure of the epiphyses in young individuals. Use for shortest duration possible consistent with treatment goals. Conduct periodic risk:benefit assessments. When used solely for prevention of osteoporosis, carefully consider other treatment options. Safety and efficacy in pediatric patients have not been established.

Drug Interactions

Cytochrome P450 Effect:

Based on estradiol and estrone: Substrate of **1A2**, 2A6, 2B6, 2C8/9, 2C19, 2D6, 2E1, **3A4**; Inhibits 1A2; Induces 3A4

Medroxyprogesterone: Substrate of **CYP3A4**; Induces CYP3A4

Decreased Effect:

Conjugated estrogens:

Anticonvulsants which are enzyme inducers (barbiturates, carbamazepine, phenobarbital, phenytoin, primidone) may potentially decrease estrogen levels.

Rifampin, nelfinavir, and ritonavir decrease estradiol serum concentrations

MPA: Aminoglutethimide: May decrease effects by increasing hepatic metabolism

Increased Effect/Toxicity: Hydrocortisone taken with estrogen may cause corticosteroid-induced toxicity. Increased potential for thromboembolic events with anticoagulants.

Nutritional/Ethanol Interactions

Ethanol: Avoid ethanol (routine use increases estrogen level and risk of breast cancer).

Food: Folic acid absorption may be decreased.

Herb/Nutraceutical: St John's wort may decrease levels. Avoid black cohosh, dong quai (has estrogenic activity). Avoid red clover, saw palmetto, ginseng (due to potential hormonal effects).

Effects on Lab Values Accelerated PT, partial thromboplastin time, and platelet aggregation time; ↑ platelet count; ↑ HDL; ↑ factors II, VII antigen, VIII coagulant activity, IX, X, XII, XII-X complex, II-VII-X complex, and beta-thromboglobulin; ↑ levels of fibrinogen and fibrinogen activity; ↑ plasminogen antigen and activity; ↑ thyroid-binding globulin; ↑ triglycerides; impaired glucose tolerance; reduced response to metyrapone test; reduced serum folate concentration; other binding proteins may be elevated; ↓ LDL; ↓ levels of antifactor Xa and antithrombin III; ↓ antithrombin III activity

Adverse Reactions

>10%:

Central nervous system: Headache (28% to 37%), pain (11% to 13%), depression (6% to 11%)

Endocrine & metabolic: Breast pain (32% to 38%), dysmenorrhea (8% to 13%)

Gastrointestinal: Abdominal pain (16% to 23%), nausea (9% to 11%)

Neuromuscular & skeletal: Back pain (13% to 16%)

Respiratory: Pharyngitis (11% to 13%)

Miscellaneous: Infection (16% to 18%), flu-like syndrome (10% to 13%)

1% to 10%:

Cardiovascular: Peripheral edema (3% to 4%)

Central nervous system: Dizziness (3% to 5%)

Dermatologic: Pruritus (5% to 10%), rash (4% to 6%)

Endocrine & metabolic: Leukorrhea (5% to 9%)

Gastrointestinal: Flatulence (8% to 9%), diarrhea (5% to 6%), dyspepsia (5% to 6%)

Genitourinary: Vaginitis (5% to 7%), cervical changes (4% to 5%), vaginal hemorrhage (1% to 3%)

Neuromuscular & skeletal: Weakness (6% to 10%), arthralgia (7% to 9%), leg cramps (3% to 5%), hypertonia (3% to 4%)

Respiratory: Sinusitis (7% to 8%), rhinitis (6% to 8%)

Additional adverse effects reported with conjugated estrogens and/or progestins (limited): Abnormal vaginal bleeding, amenorrhea, anaphylactoid reactions, anaphylaxis, breast enlargement/tenderness, cerebral embolism/thrombosis, cholecystitis, cholelithiasis, cholestatic jaundice, chorea, coagulation factor changes, contact lens intolerance, decreased carbohydrate tolerance, endometrial hyperplasia, erythema multiforme, erythema nodosum, HDL-cholesterol increased, hirsutism, hypertension, increase in size of uterine leiomyomata, gallbladder disease, libido changes, LDL-cholesterol decreased, migraine, optic neuritis, pancreatitis, pulmonary embolism, retinal thrombosis, thrombophlebitis, triglycerides increased, urticaria

Overdosage/Toxicology Effects noted after large doses include nausea, vomiting; withdrawal bleeding may occur in females. Treatment should be supportive and symptomatic.

Pharmacokinetic Note See individual agents.

Pharmacodynamics/Kinetics

Half-Life Elimination:

Premphase®, Prempro™: 10-24 hours

Time to Peak:

Premphase®, Prempro™: 4-10 hours

Formulations Tablet:

Premphase® [therapy pack contains 2 separate tablet formulations]: Conjugated estrogens 0.625 mg [14 maroon tablets] and conjugated estrogen 0.625 mg/medroxyprogesterone acetate 5 mg [14 light blue tablets] (28s)

Prempro™:

0.625/2.5: Conjugated estrogens 0.625 mg and medroxyprogesterone acetate 2.5 mg (28s)

0.625/5: Conjugated estrogens 0.625 mg and medroxyprogesterone acetate 5 mg (28s)

Dosing

Adults & Elderly:

Treatment of moderate to severe vasomotor symptoms associated with menopause or treatment of atrophic vaginitis in females with an intact uterus: Oral:

Premphase®: One maroon conjugated estrogen 0.625 mg tablet daily on days 1 through 14 and one light blue conjugated estrogen 0.625 mg/MPA 5 mg tablet daily on days 15 through 28; re-evaluate patients at 3- and 6-month intervals to determine if treatment is still necessary; monitor patients for signs of endometrial cancer; rule out malignancy if unexplained vaginal bleeding occurs

Prempro™: One conjugated estrogen 0.625 mg/MPA 2.5 mg tablet daily; re-evaluate at 3-and 6-month intervals to determine if therapy is still needed; dose may be increased to one conjugated estrogen 0.625 mg/MPA 5 mg tablet daily in patients with bleeding or spotting, once malignancy has been ruled out

Osteoporosis prophylaxis in females with an intact uterus: Oral:

Premphase®: One maroon conjugated estrogen 0.625 tablet daily on days 1 through 14 and one light blue conjugated estrogen 0.625 mg/MPA 5 mg tablet daily on days 15 through 28; monitor patients for signs of endometrial cancer; rule out malignancy if unexplained vaginal bleeding occurs

Prempro™: One conjugated estrogen 0.625 mg/MPA 2.5 mg tablet daily; dose may be increased to one conjugated estrogen 0.625 mg/MPA 5 mg tablet daily; in patients with bleeding or spotting, once malignancy has been ruled out

Stability

Storage: Store at room temperature 20°C to 25°C (68°F to 77°F).

Monitoring Laboratory Tests Serum cholesterol, HDL, LDL triglycerides, Pap smear

Monitoring and Teaching Issues

Physical Assessment: See Contraindications, Warnings/Precautions, and Dosing for use cautions. Assess potential for interactions with other prescriptions, OTC medications, or herbal products patient may be taking (see Drug Interactions). Assess results of laboratory tests (see above), therapeutic effectiveness (according to purpose for use), and adverse response (eg, CNS changes, hypertension, thromboembolism, fluid retention, edema, CHF, respiratory changes - see Adverse Reactions and Overdose/Toxicology) on a regular basis during therapy. Caution diabetic patient to monitor glucose levels closely (may impair glucose tolerance). **Note:** Before prescribing estrogen therapy to postmenopausal women, the risks and benefits must be weighed for each patient. Women should be informed of these risks and benefits, as well as possible effects of progestin when added to estrogen therapy. Teach patient appropriate use, possible side effects and appropriate interventions, and adverse symptoms to report (see Patient Education). **Pregnancy risk factor X** - determine that patient is not pregnant before beginning treatment. Do not give to women of childbearing age unless patient is capable of complying with barrier contraceptive measures during therapy and for 1 month following therapy. Advise patient on appropriate contraceptive measures. Note breast-feeding caution.

Patient Education: Inform prescriber of all prescriptions, OTC medications, or herbal products you are taking, and any allergies you have. Do not take anything new without consulting prescriber. Take as prescribed at same time each day; maintain schedule. Avoid alcohol. Annual gynecologic and breast exams are important. If taking for prevention of osteoporosis, consult prescriber about calcium and vitamin D intake, and weight-bearing exercises. If diabetic, monitor glucose levels closely (may impair glucose tolerance). May cause nausea or vomiting (small, frequent meals may help); abdominal pain, difficult/painful menstrual cycles; dizziness or mental depression; rash; headache; or breast pain or increased/decreased libido. Report significant swelling of extremities; sudden acute pain in legs or calves, chest or abdomen; shortness of breath; severe headache or vomiting; sudden blindness; weakness or numbness of arm or leg; unusual vaginal bleeding; yellowing of skin or eyes; or unusual bruising or bleeding. You may become intolerant to wearing contact lenses, notify prescriber if this occurs. **Pregnancy/breast-feeding precautions:** This medication may cause fetal defects and should not be used during pregnancy. Consult prescriber if breast-feeding.

Dietary Issues: Administration with food decreases nausea, administer with food. Ensure adequate calcium and vitamin D intake when used for the prevention of osteoporosis.

(Continued)

Estrogens (Conjugated/Equine) and Medroxyprogesterone *(Continued)*

Breast-feeding Issues: The AAP considers ethinyl estradiol, an estrogen derivative, to be "usually compatible" with breast-feeding. Estrogen has been shown to decrease the quantity and quality of human milk. Monitor the growth of the infant closely. The AAP considers medroxyprogesterone to be "usually compatible" with breast-feeding.

Pregnancy Issues:

Estrogens: Increased risk of fetal reproductive tract disorders and other birth defects; do not use during pregnancy.

Progestins: Associated with fetal genital abnormalities when used during the 1st trimester; not recommended for use during pregnancy.

Related Information

MedroxyPROGESTERone *on page 842*

Estrogens (Esterified) (ES troe jenz es TER i fied)

U.S. Brand Names Estratab® [DSC]; Menest®

Synonyms Esterified Estrogens

Generic Available No

Pharmacologic Category Estrogen Derivative

Pregnancy Risk Factor X

Lactation Enters breast milk/use caution

Use Treatment of moderate to severe vasomotor symptoms associated with menopause; treatment of vulvar and vaginal atrophy; hypoestrogenism (due to hypogonadism, castration, or primary ovarian failure); prostatic cancer (palliation); breast cancer (palliation); osteoporosis (prophylaxis)

Mechanism of Action/Effect Esterified estrogens contain a mixture of estrogenic substances; the principle component is estrone. Estrogens modulate the pituitary secretion of gonadotropins, luteinizing hormone, and follicle-stimulating hormone through a negative feedback system; estrogen replacement reduces elevated levels of these hormones.

Contraindications Hypersensitivity to estrogens or any component of the formulation; undiagnosed abnormal vaginal bleeding; history of or current thrombophlebitis or thromboembolic disorders; carcinoma of the breast, except in appropriately selected patients being treated for metastatic disease; estrogen-dependent tumor; pregnancy

Warnings/Precautions Conjugated estrogens (alone or in combination with a progestin) should not be used to prevent coronary heart disease. Unopposed estrogens may increase the risk of endometrial carcinoma in postmenopausal women. Use with caution in patients with diseases which may be exacerbated by fluid retention, including asthma, epilepsy, migraine, diabetes, cardiac or renal dysfunction. Use with caution in patients with a history of hypercalcemia, cardiovascular disease, and gallbladder disease. May increase blood pressure. Use with caution in patients with hepatic disease. May increase risk of venous thromboembolism. Estrogens may increase the risk of breast cancer (controversial/currently under study). Estrogen compounds are generally associated with lipid effects such as increased HDL-cholesterol, and decreased LDL-cholesterol. Triglycerides may also be increased; use with caution in patients with familial defects of lipoprotein metabolism. May increase size of pre-existing uterine leiomyomata. Before prescribing estrogen therapy to postmenopausal women, the risks and benefits must be weighed for each patient. Women should be informed of these risks and benefits, as well as possible effects of progestin when added to estrogen therapy. Use for shortest duration possible consistent with treatment goals. Conduct periodic risk:benefit assessments. When used solely for prevention of osteoporosis, carefully consider other treatment options. Estrogens may cause premature closure of the epiphyses in young individuals. Safety and efficacy in pediatric patients have not been established.

Drug Interactions

Cytochrome P450 Effect: Based on estrone: Substrate of **1A2**, 2B6, 2C8/9, 2E1, **3A4**

Decreased Effect: Rifampin, nelfinavir, and ritonavir decrease estradiol serum concentrations. Anticonvulsants which are enzyme inducers (barbiturates, carbamazepine, phenobarbital, phenytoin, primidone) may potentially decrease estrogen levels.

Increased Effect/Toxicity: Hydrocortisone taken with estrogen may cause corticosteroid-induced toxicity. Increased potential for thromboembolic events with anticoagulants.

Nutritional/Ethanol Interactions

Ethanol: Avoid ethanol (routine use increases estrogen level and risk of breast cancer).

Food: Folic acid absorption may be decreased.

Herb/Nutraceutical: St John's wort may decrease levels. Avoid black cohosh, dong quai (has estrogenic activity). Avoid red clover, saw palmetto, ginseng (due to potential hormonal effects).

Effects on Lab Values Endocrine function test may be altered; ↑ prothrombin and factors VII, VIII, IX, X; ↑ platelet aggregability, thyroid-binding globulin, total thyroid hormone (T_4), serum triglycerides/phospholipids; ↓ antithrombin III, serum folate concentration

Adverse Reactions

Cardiovascular: Edema, hypertension, venous thromboembolism

Central nervous system: Dizziness, headache, mental depression, migraine

Dermatologic: Chloasma, erythema multiforme, erythema nodosum, hemorrhagic eruption, hirsutism, loss of scalp hair, melasma

Endocrine & metabolic: Breast enlargement, breast tenderness, changes in libido, increased thyroid-binding globulin, increased total thyroid hormone (T_4), increased serum triglycerides/phospholipids, increased HDL-cholesterol, decreased LDL-cholesterol, impaired glucose tolerance, hypercalcemia

Gastrointestinal: Abdominal cramps, bloating, cholecystitis, cholelithiasis, gallbladder disease, nausea, pancreatitis, vomiting, weight gain/loss

Genitourinary: Alterations in frequency and flow of menses, changes in cervical secretions, endometrial cancer, increased size of uterine leiomyomata, vaginal candidiasis

Hematologic: Aggravation of porphyria, decreased antithrombin III and antifactor Xa, increased levels of fibrinogen, increased platelet aggregability and platelet count; increased prothrombin and factors VII, VIII, IX, X

Hepatic: Cholestatic jaundice

Neuromuscular & skeletal: Chorea

Ocular: Intolerance to contact lenses, steeping of corneal curvature

Respiratory: Pulmonary thromboembolism

Miscellaneous: Carbohydrate intolerance

Overdosage/Toxicology Toxicity is unlikely following single exposures of excessive doses, any treatment following emesis and charcoal administration should be supportive and symptomatic. Effects noted after large doses include headache, nausea, and vomiting. Bleeding may occur in females.

Pharmacodynamics/Kinetics

Absorption: Readily

Metabolism: Rapidly hepatic to estrone sulfate, conjugated and unconjugated metabolites; first-pass effect

Formulations Tablet: 0.3 mg, 0.625 mg, 1.25 mg, 2.5 mg

Dosing

Adults & Elderly:

Prostate cancer (palliation): Oral: 1.25-2.5 mg 3 times/day

Female hypogonadism: Oral: 2.5-7.5 mg of estrogen daily for 20 days followed by a 10-day rest period. Administer cyclically (3 weeks on and 1 week off). If bleeding does not occur by the end of the 10-day period, repeat the same dosing schedule; the number of courses dependent upon the responsiveness of the endometrium. If bleeding occurs before the end of the 10-day period, begin an estrogen-progestin cyclic regimen of 2.5-7.5 mg esterified estrogens daily for 20 days. During the last 5 days of estrogen therapy, give an oral progestin. If bleeding occurs before regimen is concluded, discontinue therapy and resume on the fifth day of bleeding.

Moderate to severe vasomotor symptoms associated with menopause: Oral: 1.25 mg/day administered cyclically (3 weeks on and 1 week off). If patient has not menstruated within the last 2 months or more, cyclic administration is started arbitrary. If the patient is menstruating, cyclical administration is started on day 5 of the bleeding. For short-term use only and should be discontinued as soon as possible. Re-evaluate at 3- to 6-month intervals for tapering or discontinuation of therapy.

Atopic vaginitis and kraurosis vulvae: Oral: 0.3 to ≥1.25 mg/day, depending on the tissue response of the individual patient. Administer cyclically. For short-term use only and should be discontinued as soon as possible. Re-evaluate at 3- to 6-month intervals for tapering or discontinuation of therapy.

Breast cancer (palliation): Oral: 10 mg 3 times/day for at least 3 months

Osteoporosis in postmenopausal women: Oral: Initial: 0.3 mg/day and increase to a maximum daily dose of 1.25 mg/day; initiate therapy as soon as possible after menopause; cyclically or daily, depending on medical assessment of patient. Monitor patients with an intact uterus for signs of endometrial cancer; rule out malignancy if unexplained vaginal bleeding occurs

Female castration and primary ovarian failure: Oral: 1.25 mg/day, cyclically. Adjust dosage upward or downward, according to the severity of symptoms and patient response. For maintenance, adjust dosage to lowest level that will provide effective control.

Hepatic Impairment:

Mild to moderate liver impairment: Dosage reduction of estrogens is recommended.

Severe liver impairment: **Not recommended**.

Stability

Storage: Store below 30°C (86°F); protect from moisture

Monitoring and Teaching Issues

Physical Assessment: See Contraindications, Warnings/Precautions, and Dosing for use cautions. Assess potential for interactions with other prescriptions, OTC medications, or herbal products patient may be taking (see Drug Interactions). Assess results of laboratory tests, therapeutic effectiveness (according to purpose for use), and adverse response (eg, CNS changes, hypertension, thromboembolism, fluid retention, edema, CHF, respiratory changes - see Adverse Reactions and Overdose/Toxicology) on a regular basis during therapy. Caution diabetic patient to monitor glucose levels closely (may impair glucose tolerance). **Note:** Before prescribing estrogen therapy to postmenopausal women, the risks and benefits must be weighed for each patient. Women should be informed of these risks and benefits, as well as possible effects of progestin when added to estrogen therapy. Teach patient appropriate use, possible side effects and appropriate interventions, and adverse symptoms to report (see Patient Education). **Pregnancy risk factor X** - determine that patient is not pregnant before starting therapy. Do not give to females of childbearing age unless patient is capable of complying with barrier contraceptive use. Advise patient about appropriate contraceptive measures as appropriate. Note breast-feeding caution.

Patient Education: Inform prescriber of all prescriptions, OTC medications, or herbal products you are taking, and any allergies you have. Do not take anything new without consulting prescriber. Take as prescribed at same time each day; maintain prescribed schedule. Avoid alcohol. Annual gynecologic and breast exams are important. If taking for prevention of osteoporosis, ask prescriber about calcium and vitamin D intake, and weight-bearing exercises. If diabetic: monitor glucose levels closely (may impair glucose tolerance). May cause nausea or vomiting (small, frequent meals may help); abdominal pain, difficult/painful menstrual cycles; dizziness or mental depression; rash; headache; or breast pain or increased/decreased libido. Report significant swelling of extremities; sudden acute pain in legs or calves, chest or abdomen; shortness of breath; severe headache or vomiting; sudden blindness; weakness or numbness of arm or leg; unusual vaginal bleeding; yellowing of skin or eyes; or unusual bruising or bleeding. You may become intolerant to wearing contact lenses, notify prescriber if this occurs. **Pregnancy/breast-feeding precautions:** Inform prescriber if you are pregnant. Do not get pregnant while taking this drug; may cause fetal defects and should not be used during pregnancy. Consult prescriber if breast-feeding.

(Continued)

Estrogens (Esterified) *(Continued)*

Dietary Issues: Should be taken with food at same time each day. Ensure adequate calcium and vitamin D intake when used for the prevention of osteoporosis.

Breast-feeding Issues: The AAP considers ethinyl estradiol, an estrogen derivative, to be "usually compatible" with breast-feeding. Estrogen has been shown to decrease the quantity and quality of human milk; use only if clearly needed; monitor the growth of the infant closely.

Pregnancy Issues: Increased risk of fetal reproductive tract disorders and other birth defects; do not use during pregnancy.

Related Information

Estrogen Replacement Therapy *on page 1666*
Osteoporosis Management *on page 1696*

Estrostep® 21 [DSC] *see* Ethinyl Estradiol and Norethindrone *on page 527*
Estrostep® Fe *see* Ethinyl Estradiol and Norethindrone *on page 527*
ETAF *see* Aldesleukin *on page 54*

Etanercept (et a NER cept)

U.S. Brand Names Enbrel®

Generic Available No

Pharmacologic Category Antirheumatic, Disease Modifying

Pregnancy Risk Factor B

Lactation Excretion in breast milk unknown/not recommended

Use Reduction in signs and symptoms of moderately to severely active rheumatoid arthritis, moderately to severely active polyarticular juvenile arthritis, or psoriatic arthritis in patients who have had an inadequate response to one or more disease-modifying antirheumatic drugs (DMARDs)

Use - Unlabeled/Investigational Crohn's disease

Mechanism of Action/Effect Etanercept is a recombinant DNA-derived protein composed of tumor necrosis factor receptor (TNFR) linked to the Fc portion of human IgG1. Etanercept binds tumor necrosis factor (TNF) and blocks its interaction with cell surface receptors. TNF plays an important role in the inflammatory processes of rheumatoid arthritis (RA) and the resulting joint pathology.

Contraindications Hypersensitivity to etanercept or any component of the formulation; patients with sepsis (mortality may be increased); active infections (including chronic or local infection)

Warnings/Precautions Etanercept may affect defenses against infections and malignancies. Safety and efficacy in patients with immunosuppression or chronic infections have not been evaluated. Rare cases of tuberculosis have been reported. Discontinue administration if patient develops a serious infection. Do not start drug administration in patients with an active infection. Use caution in patients predisposed to infection, such as poorly-controlled diabetes.

Use caution in patients with pre-existing or recent-onset demyelinating CNS disorders or a history of significant hematologic abnormalities. Discontinue if significant hematologic abnormalities are confirmed.

The long-term immunogenicity, carcinogenic potential, or effect on fertility are unknown. The safety of etanercept has not been studied in children <4 years of age.

Allergic reactions may occur (<0.5%), but anaphylaxis has not been observed. If an anaphylactic reaction or other serious allergic reaction occurs, administration of etanercept should be discontinued immediately.

Patients should be brought up to date with all immunizations before initiating therapy. Live vaccines should not be given concurrently. Patients with a significant exposure to varicella virus should temporarily discontinue etanercept. Treatment with varicella zoster immune globulin should be considered.

Drug Interactions

Decreased Effect: Specific drug interaction studies have not been conducted with etanercept.

Increased Effect/Toxicity: Specific drug interaction studies have not been conducted with etanercept.

Adverse Reactions Events reported include those >3% with incidence higher than placebo.

>10%:
- Central nervous system: Headache (17%)
- Local: Injection site reaction (37%)
- Respiratory: Respiratory tract infection (38%), upper respiratory tract infection (29%), rhinitis (12%)
- Miscellaneous: Infection (35%), positive ANA (11%), positive antidouble-stranded DNA antibodies (15% by RIA, 3% by *Crithidia luciliae* assay)

≥3% to 10%:
- Central nervous system: Dizziness (7%)
- Dermatologic: Rash (5%)
- Gastrointestinal: Abdominal pain (5%), dyspepsia (4%), nausea (9%), vomiting (3%)
- Neuromuscular & skeletal: Weakness (5%)
- Respiratory: Pharyngitis (7%), respiratory disorder (5%), sinusitis (3%), cough (6%)

<3% (Limited to important or life-threatening): Alopecia, angioedema, aplastic anemia, cerebral ischemia, chest pain, cholecystitis, deep vein thrombosis, demyelinating CNS disorders, depression, dyspnea, flu syndrome, gastrointestinal hemorrhage, heart failure, infection (serious), malignancies, membranous glomerulopathy, myocardial infarction, myocardial ischemia, optic neuritis, pancreatitis, pancytopenia, paresthesia, polymyositis, pruritus, pulmonary disease, pulmonary embolism, seizures, stroke, thrombocytopenia, thrombophlebitis, tuberculosis, urticaria, vasculitis (cutaneous)

Pediatric patients (JRA): The percentages of patients reporting abdominal pain (17%) and vomiting (14.5%) was higher than in adult RA. Two patients developed varicella infection associated with aseptic meningitis which resolved without complications (see Warnings/Precautions).

Overdosage/Toxicology No dose-limiting toxicities have been observed during clinical trials. Single I.V. doses up to 60 mg/m^2 have been administered to healthy volunteers in an endotoxemia study without evidence of dose-limiting toxicities.

Pharmacodynamics/Kinetics

Half-Life Elimination: 115 hours (range: 98-300 hours)

Time to Peak: 72 hours (range: 48-96 hours)

Onset: ~2-3 weeks

Formulations Injection, powder for reconstitution: 25 mg [diluent contains benzyl alcohol]

Dosing

Adults: Rheumatoid arthritis, psoriatic arthritis: S.C.: 25 mg given twice weekly; if the physician determines that it is appropriate, patients may self-inject after proper training in injection technique.

Elderly: S.C.: Although greater sensitivity of some elderly patients cannot be ruled out, no overall differences in safety or effectiveness were observed.

Pediatrics: Juvenile rheumatoid arthritis: Children 4-17 years: S.C.: 0.4 mg/kg (maximum: 25 mg dose) twice weekly; doses should be separated by 72-96 hours

Administration

Other: Note: The needle cover of the diluent syringe contains dry natural rubber (latex), which should not be handled by persons sensitive to this substance. New injections should be given at least one inch from an old site and never into areas where the skin is tender, bruised, red, or hard.

Stability

Storage: The dose tray containing etanercept (sterile powder) must be refrigerated at 2°C to 8°C (36°F to 46°F). Do not freeze. Reconstituted solutions of etanercept should be administered as soon as possible after reconstitution. If not administered immediately after reconstitution, etanercept may be stored in the vial at 2°C to 8°C (36°F to 46°F) for up to 6 hours.

Reconstitution: Reconstitute aseptically with 1 mL sterile bacteriostatic water for injection, USP (supplied). Do not filter reconstituted solution during preparation or administration. Injection sites should be rotated. **Note:** The needle cover of the diluent syringe contains dry natural rubber (latex), which should not be handled by persons sensitive to this substance.

Monitoring and Teaching Issues

Physical Assessment: See Contraindications and Warnings/Precautions for use cautions. Monitor effectiveness of therapy (eg, pain, range of motion, mobility, ADL function, inflammation). Assess knowledge/teach patient appropriate administration (injection technique and needle disposal if self-administered), possible side effects/interventions, and adverse symptoms to report (see Patient Education). Breast-feeding is not recommended.

Patient Education: If self-injecting, follow instructions for injection and disposal of needles exactly. If redness, swelling, or irritation appears at the injection site, contact prescriber. Do not have any vaccinations while using this medication without consulting prescriber first. You may experience headache or dizziness (use caution when driving or engaging in tasks requiring alertness until response to drug is known). If stomach pain or cramping; unusual bleeding or bruising; persistent fever; paleness; blood in vomitus, stool, or urine occurs, stop medication and contact prescriber **immediately**. Also immediately report skin rash, unusual muscle or bone weakness, or signs of respiratory flu or other infection (eg, chills, fever, sore throat, easy bruising or bleeding, mouth sores, unhealed sores). **Breast-feeding precaution:** Breast-feeding is not recommended.

Breast-feeding Issues: It is not known whether etanercept is excreted in human milk or absorbed systemically after ingestion. Because many immunoglobulins are excreted in human milk, and because of the potential for serious adverse reactions in nursing infants from Enbrel®, a decision should be made whether to discontinue nursing or to discontinue the drug.

Pregnancy Issues: Developmental toxicity studies performed in animals have revealed no evidence of harm to the fetus. There are no studies in pregnant women; this drug should be used during pregnancy only if clearly needed.

Ethacrynate Sodium *see* Ethacrynic Acid *on page 511*

Ethacrynic Acid (eth a KRIN ik AS id)

U.S. Brand Names Edecrin® [DSC]

Synonyms Ethacrynate Sodium

Generic Available No

Pharmacologic Category Diuretic, Loop

Pregnancy Risk Factor B

Lactation Contraindicated (manufacturer)

Use Management of edema associated with congestive heart failure; hepatic cirrhosis or renal disease; short-term management of ascites due to malignancy, idiopathic edema, and lymphedema

Mechanism of Action/Effect Inhibits reabsorption of sodium and chloride in the ascending loop of Henle and distal renal tubule, interfering with the chloride-binding cotransport system, thus causing increased excretion of water, sodium, chloride, magnesium, and calcium

Contraindications Hypersensitivity to ethacrynic acid or any component of the formulation; anuria; history of severe watery diarrhea caused by this product; infants

Warnings/Precautions Adjust dose to avoid dehydration. In cirrhosis, avoid electrolyte and acid/base imbalances that might lead to hepatic encephalopathy. Ototoxicity is associated with rapid I.V. administration, renal impairment, excessive doses, and concurrent use of other ototoxins. Has been associated with a higher incidence of ototoxicity than other loop diuretics. Hypersensitivity reactions can rarely occur, however, ethacrynic acid has no cross-reactivity to sulfonamides or sulfonylureas. Monitor fluid status and renal function in an attempt to prevent oliguria, azotemia, and reversible increases in BUN and creatinine. Close

(Continued)

Ethacrynic Acid *(Continued)*

medical supervision of aggressive diuresis required. Watch for and correct electrolyte disturbances. Coadministration of antihypertensives may increase the risk of hypotension.

Drug Interactions

Decreased Effect: Probenecid decreases diuretic effects of ethacrynic acid. Glucose tolerance may be decreased by loop diuretics, requiring adjustment of hypoglycemic agents. Cholestyramine or colestipol may reduce bioavailability of ethacrynic acid. Indomethacin (and other NSAIDs) may reduce natriuretic and hypotensive effects of diuretics.

Increased Effect/Toxicity: Ethacrynic acid-induced hypokalemia may predispose to digoxin toxicity and may increase the risk of arrhythmia with drugs which may prolong QT interval, including type Ia and type III antiarrhythmic agents, cisapride, and some quinolones (sparfloxacin, gatifloxacin, and moxifloxacin). The risk of toxicity from lithium and salicylates (high dose) may be increased by loop diuretics. Hypotensive effects and/or adverse renal effects of ACE inhibitors and NSAIDs are potentiated by ethacrynic acid-induced hypovolemia. The effects of peripheral adrenergic-blocking drugs or ganglionic blockers may be increased by ethacrynic acid.

Ethacrynic acid may increase the risk of ototoxicity with other ototoxic agents (aminoglycosides, cis-platinum), especially in patients with renal dysfunction. Synergistic diuretic effects occur with thiazide-type diuretics. Diuretics tend to be synergistic with other antihypertensive agents, and hypotension may occur. Nephrotoxicity has been associated with concomitant use of cephaloridine or cephalexin.

Adverse Reactions Frequency not defined.

Central nervous system: Headache, fatigue, apprehension, confusion, fever, chills, encephalopathy (patients with pre-existing liver disease); vertigo

Dermatologic: Skin rash, Henoch-Schönlein purpura (in patient with rheumatic heart disease)

Endocrine & metabolic: Hyponatremia, hyperglycemia, variations in phosphorus, CO_2 content, bicarbonate, and calcium; reversible hyperuricemia, gout, hyperglycemia, hypoglycemia (occurred in two uremic patients who received doses above those recommended)

Gastrointestinal: Anorexia, malaise, abdominal discomfort or pain, dysphagia, nausea, vomiting, and diarrhea, gastrointestinal bleeding, acute pancreatitis (rare)

Genitourinary: Hematuria

Hepatic: Jaundice, abnormal liver function tests

Hematology: Agranulocytosis, severe neutropenia, thrombocytopenia

Local: Thrombophlebitis (with intravenous use), local irritation and pain,

Ocular: Blurred vision

Otic: Deafness, tinnitus, temporary or permanent deafness

Renal: Increased serum creatinine

Overdosage/Toxicology Symptoms of overdose include electrolyte depletion, volume depletion, dehydration, and circulatory collapse. Treatment is supportive.

Pharmacodynamics/Kinetics

Absorption: Oral: Rapid

Half-Life Elimination: Normal renal function: 2-4 hours

Metabolism: Hepatic (35% to 40%) to active cysteine conjugate

Onset: Diuresis: Oral: ~30 minutes; I.V.: 5 minutes; Peak effect: Oral: 2 hours; I.V.: 30 minutes

Duration: Oral: 12 hours; I.V.: 2 hours

Formulations

Injection, powder for reconstitution, as ethacrynate sodium: 50 mg

Tablet: 25 mg, 50 mg

Dosing

Adults: I.V. formulation should be diluted in D_5W or NS (1 mg/mL) and infused over several minutes.

Edema:

Oral: 50-100 mg/day in 1-2 divided doses; may increase in increments of 25-50 mg at intervals of several days to a maximum of 400 mg/24 hours.

I.V.: 0.5-1 mg/kg/dose (maximum: 100 mg/dose); repeat doses not routinely recommended; however, if indicated, repeat doses every 8-12 hours.

Elderly: Oral: Initial: 25-50 mg/day

Pediatrics:

Edema: Oral: Children: 1 mg/kg/dose once daily; increase at intervals of 2-3 days as needed, to a maximum of 3 mg/kg/day.

Renal Impairment:

Cl_{cr} <10 mL/minute: Avoid use.

Not removed by hemo- or peritoneal dialysis; supplemental dose is not necessary.

Administration

I.V.: Injection should **not** be given S.C. or I.M. due to local pain and irritation. Single I.V. doses should not exceed 100 mg. Administer each 10 mg over a minute.

Stability

Compatibility: Stable in D_5NS, D_5W, LR, NS

Incompatible whole blood or its derivatives

Compatibility when admixed: Incompatible with hydralazine, procainamide, ranitidine, tolazoline, triflupromazine

Monitoring Laboratory Tests Renal function, serum electrolytes

Monitoring and Teaching Issues

Physical Assessment: See Contraindications, Warnings/Precautions, and Dosing for use cautions. Assess potential for interactions with other prescriptions, OTC medications, or herbal products patient may be taking (see Drug Interactions). **Infusion:** See Administration. Assess results of laboratory tests (see above), therapeutic effectiveness (according to purpose for use), and adverse response (eg, dehydration, electrolyte imbalance, CNS changes - see Adverse Reactions and Overdose/Toxicology) on a regular basis during therapy. Caution diabetic patient to monitor glucose levels closely (may cause hyper/

hypoglycemia). Teach patient appropriate use, possible side effects and appropriate interventions, and adverse symptoms to report (see Patient Education). Breast-feeding is contraindicated.

Patient Education: Inform prescriber of all prescriptions, OTC medications, or herbal products you are taking, and any allergies you have. Do not take anything new without consulting prescriber. Take prescribed dose with food early in day. Include orange juice or bananas (or other potassium-rich foods) in your diet, but do not take potassium supplements without consulting prescriber. If diabetic: monitor serum glucose closely (this medication may alter glucose levels). May cause postural hypotension (use caution when rising from lying or sitting position, when climbing stairs, or when driving); lightheadedness, dizziness, or drowsiness (use caution driving or when engaging in hazardous activities); diarrhea (buttermilk, boiled milk, or yogurt may help); or decreased accommodation to heat (avoid excessive exercise in hot weather). Report hearing changes (ringing in ears); persistent headache; unusual confusion or nervousness; abdominal pain or blood stool (black stool); palpitations, chest pain, rapid heartbeat; flu-like symptoms; skin rash or itching; blurred vision; swelling of ankles or feet; weight changes of more than 3 lb/day; increased fatigue; or joint/muscle swelling, pain, cramping, or trembling. **Breast-feeding precaution:** Do not breast-feed.

Dietary Issues: This product may cause a potassium loss. Your healthcare provider may prescribe a potassium supplement, another medication to help prevent the potassium loss, or recommend that you eat foods high in potassium, especially citrus fruits. Do not change your diet on your own while taking this medication, especially if you are taking potassium supplements or medications to reduce potassium loss. Too much potassium can be as harmful as too little.

Geriatric Considerations: Ethacrynic acid is rarely used because of its increased incidence of ototoxicity as compared to the other loop diuretics (see Additional Information).

Related Information

Heart Failure *on page 1670*

Ethambutol (e THAM byoo tole)

U.S. Brand Names Myambutol®

Synonyms Ethambutol Hydrochloride

Generic Available Yes

Pharmacologic Category Antitubercular Agent

Pregnancy Risk Factor B

Lactation Enters breast milk/compatible

Use Treatment of tuberculosis and other mycobacterial diseases in conjunction with other antituberculosis agents

Mechanism of Action/Effect Suppresses mycobacteria multiplication by interfering with RNA synthesis

Contraindications Hypersensitivity to ethambutol or any component of the formulation; optic neuritis

Warnings/Precautions May cause optic neuritis, resulting in decreased visual acuity or other vision changes. Discontinue promptly in patients with changes in vision, color blindness, or visual defects (effects normally reversible, but reversal may require up to a year). Use only in children whose visual acuity can accurately be determined and monitored (not recommended for use in children <13 years of age). Dosage modification required in patients with renal insufficiency.

Drug Interactions

Decreased Effect: Ethambutol absorption is decreased when taken with aluminum salts.

Effects on Lab Values ↑ uric acid (S)

Adverse Reactions Frequency not defined.

Central nervous system: Headache, confusion, disorientation, malaise, mental confusion, fever

Dermatologic: Rash, pruritus

Endocrine & metabolic: Acute gout or hyperuricemia

Gastrointestinal: Abdominal pain, anorexia, nausea, vomiting

Hepatic: Abnormal LFTs

Neuromuscular & skeletal: Peripheral neuritis

Ocular: Optic neuritis; symptoms may include decreased acuity, scotoma, color blindness, or visual defects (usually reversible with discontinuation, irreversible blindness has been described)

Miscellaneous: Anaphylaxis

Overdosage/Toxicology Symptoms of overdose include decrease in visual acuity, anorexia, joint pain, and numbness of extremities. Treatment is supportive.

Pharmacodynamics/Kinetics

Absorption: ~80%

Half-Life Elimination: 2.5-3.6 hours; End-stage renal disease: 7-15 hours

Time to Peak: Serum: 2-4 hours

Metabolism: Hepatic (20%) to inactive metabolite

Formulations Tablet, as hydrochloride: 100 mg, 400 mg

Dosing

Adults & Elderly:

Note: A four-drug regimen (isoniazid, rifampin, pyrazinamide, and either streptomycin or ethambutol) is preferred for the initial, empiric treatment of TB. When the drug susceptibility results are available, the regimen should be altered as appropriate.

Tuberculosis: Oral:

Daily therapy: 15-25 mg/kg/day (maximum: 2.5 g/day)

Directly observed therapy (DOT): Twice weekly: 50 mg/kg (maximum: 2.5 g)

DOT: 3 times/week: 25-30 mg/kg (maximum: 2.5 g)

Disseminated *Mycobacterium avium* complex (MAC) in patients with advanced HIV infection: 15 mg/kg ethambutol in combination with azithromycin 600 mg daily

(Continued)

Ethambutol *(Continued)*

Pediatrics:

Ethambutol is generally not recommended in children whose visual acuity cannot be monitored. However, ethambutol should be considered for all children with organisms resistant to other drugs, when susceptibility to ethambutol has been demonstrated, or susceptibility is likely.

Tuberculosis: Oral: Children:

Daily therapy: 15-25 mg/kg/day (maximum: 2.5 g/day)

Directly observed therapy (DOT): Twice weekly: 50 mg/kg (maximum: 2.5 g)

DOT: 3 times/week: 25-30 mg/kg (maximum: 2.5 g)

Renal Impairment:

Cl_{cr} 10-50 mL/minute: Administer every 24-36 hours.

Cl_{cr} <10 mL/minute: Administer every 48 hours.

Slightly dialyzable (5% to 20%); administer dose postdialysis.

Peritoneal dialysis: Dose as for Cl_{cr} <10 mL/minute.

Continuous arteriovenous or venovenous hemofiltration: Administer every 24-36 hours.

Monitoring Laboratory Tests Periodic visual testing in patients receiving >15 mg/kg/day; periodic renal, hepatic, and hematopoietic tests

Monitoring and Teaching Issues

Physical Assessment: See Contraindications, Warnings/Precautions, Drug Interactions, and Dosing for use cautions. Assess results of laboratory tests (see above), therapeutic effectiveness, and adverse response (eg, CNS changes, neuritis, and ocular changes - see Adverse Reactions) on a regular basis during therapy. Teach patient appropriate use (need to adhere to dosing program), possible side effects and appropriate interventions, and adverse symptoms to report (see Patient Education).

Patient Education: Take as scheduled, with meals. Avoid missing doses and do not discontinue without consulting prescriber. May cause GI distress (small, frequent meals and good oral care may help), dizziness, disorientation, drowsiness (avoid driving or engaging in tasks that require alertness until response to drug is known). You will need to have frequent ophthalmic exams and periodic medical check-ups to evaluate drug effects. Report vision changes, numbness or tingling of extremities, or persistent loss of appetite.

Dietary Issues: May be taken with food as absorption is not affected, may cause gastric irritation.

Geriatric Considerations: Since most elderly patients acquired their tuberculosis before current antituberculin regimens were available, ethambutol is only indicated when patients are from areas where drug resistant *M. tuberculosis* is endemic, in HIV-infected elderly patients, and when drug resistant *M. tuberculosis* is suspected (see dose adjustments for renal impairment).

Related Information

Tuberculosis *on page 1705*

Ethambutol Hydrochloride *see* Ethambutol *on page 513*

Ethinyl Estradiol (ETH in il es tra DYE ole)

U.S. Brand Names Estinyl®

Generic Available No

Pharmacologic Category Estrogen Derivative

Pregnancy Risk Factor X

Lactation Enters breast milk/contraindicated (manufacturer)

Use Treatment of moderate to severe vasomotor symptoms associated with menopause; hypogonadism; prostatic cancer (palliation); breast cancer (palliation)

Mechanism of Action/Effect Ethinyl estradiol is a synthetic derivative of estradiol. Estrogens modulate the pituitary secretion of gonadotropins, luteinizing hormone and follicle stimulating hormone through a negative feedback system; estrogen replacement reduces elevated levels of these hormones.

Contraindications Hypersensitivity to estrogens or any component of the formulation; undiagnosed abnormal vaginal bleeding; history of or current thrombophlebitis or thromboembolic disorders; carcinoma of the breast, except in appropriately selected patients being treated for metastatic disease; estrogen-dependent tumor; pregnancy

Warnings/Precautions Unopposed estrogens may increase the risk of endometrial carcinoma in postmenopausal women. Use with caution in patients with diseases which may be exacerbated by fluid retention, including asthma, epilepsy, migraine, diabetes, cardiac or renal dysfunction. Use with caution in patients with a history of hypercalcemia, cardiovascular disease, and gallbladder disease. May increase blood pressure. Use with caution in patients with hepatic disease. May increase risk of venous thromboembolism. Estrogens may increase the risk of breast cancer (controversial/currently under study). Estrogen compounds are generally associated with lipid effects such as increased HDL-cholesterol, and decreased LDL-cholesterol; triglycerides may also be increased. Use with caution in patients with familial defects of lipoprotein metabolism. May increase size of pre-existing uterine leiomyomata. Patients with a history of depression should be monitored, discontinue if depression recurs to a serious degree. Before prescribing estrogen therapy to postmenopausal women, the risks and benefits must be weighed for each patient. Women should be informed of these risks and benefits, as well as possible effects of progestin when added to estrogen therapy. Estrogens may cause premature closure of the epiphyses in young individuals. Safety and efficacy in pediatric patients have not been established. Some tablet formulations contain tartrazine.

Drug Interactions

Cytochrome P450 Effect: Substrate of **CYP3A4**, 3A5-7; Inhibits CYP1A2, 2B6, 2C19, 3A4

Decreased Effect: Rifampin, nelfinavir, and ritonavir decrease estradiol serum concentrations. Anticonvulsants which are enzyme inducers (barbiturates, carbamazepine, phenobarbital, phenytoin, primidone) may potentially decrease estrogen levels.

Increased Effect/Toxicity: Hydrocortisone taken with estrogen may cause corticosteroid-induced toxicity. Increased potential for thromboembolic events with anticoagulants.

Nutritional/Ethanol Interactions

Ethanol: Routine use increases estrogen level and risk of breast cancer; avoid ethanol

Food: Folic acid absorption may be decreased

Herb/Nutraceutical: St John's wort may decrease levels. Avoid black cohosh, dong quai (has estrogenic activity). Avoid red clover, saw palmetto, ginseng (due to potential hormonal effects).

Effects on Lab Values ↑ prothrombin and factors VII, VIII, IX, X; ↑ platelet aggregability, thyroid-binding globulin, total thyroid hormone (T_4), serum triglycerides/phospholipids; ↓ antithrombin III, serum folate concentration

Adverse Reactions Frequency not defined.

Cardiovascular: Edema, hypertension, venous thromboembolism

Central nervous system: Dizziness, headache, mental depression, migraine

Dermatologic: Chloasma, erythema multiforme, erythema nodosum, hemorrhagic eruption, hirsutism, loss of scalp hair, melasma

Endocrine & metabolic: Breast enlargement, breast tenderness, changes in libido, increased thyroid-binding globulin, increased total thyroid hormone (T_4), increased serum triglycerides/phospholipids, increased HDL-cholesterol, decreased LDL-cholesterol, impaired glucose tolerance, hypercalcemia

Gastrointestinal: Abdominal cramps, bloating, cholecystitis, cholelithiasis, gallbladder disease, nausea, pancreatitis, vomiting, weight gain/loss

Genitourinary: Alterations in frequency and flow of menses, changes in cervical secretions, endometrial cancer, increased size of uterine leiomyomata, vaginal candidiasis

Hematologic: Aggravation of porphyria, decreased antithrombin III and antifactor Xa, increased levels of fibrinogen, increased platelet aggregability and platelet count; increased prothrombin and factors VII, VIII, IX, X

Hepatic: Cholestatic jaundice

Neuromuscular & skeletal: Chorea

Ocular: Intolerance to contact lenses, steeping of corneal curvature

Respiratory: Pulmonary thromboembolism

Miscellaneous: Carbohydrate intolerance

Overdosage/Toxicology Toxicity is unlikely following single exposures of excessive doses, any treatment following emesis and charcoal administration should be supportive and symptomatic. Effects noted after large doses include headache, nausea, and vomiting. Bleeding may occur in females.

Pharmacodynamics/Kinetics

Absorption: Oral: Rapid and complete

Bioavailability: 38% to 55%

Half-Life Elimination: ~8-25 hours

Time to Peak: Initial: 2-3 hours; Secondary: 12 hours

Metabolism: Primarily hepatic via CYP3A4; less first-pass effect than with estradiol; extensive enterohepatic recirculation; converted to estrone and estriol

Formulations Tablet: 0.02 mg [contains tartrazine], 0.05 mg

Dosing

Adults & Elderly:

Prostatic cancer (palliation): Oral: 0.15-2 mg/day

Female hypogonadism: Oral: 0.05 mg 1-3 times/day during the first 2 weeks of a theoretical menstrual cycle; follow with a progesterone during the last half of the arbitrary cycle; continue for 3-6 months. The patient should not be treated for the following 2 months to determine if additional therapy is needed.

Vasomotor symptoms associated with menopause: Oral: Usual dosage range: 0.02-0.05 mg/day; give cyclically for short-term use only and use the lowest dose that will control symptoms. Discontinue as soon as possible and administer cyclically (3 weeks on and 1 week off). Attempt to discontinue or taper medication at 3- to 6-month intervals. In severe cases (due to surgery or roentgenologic castration), doses of 0.05 mg 3 times/day may be needed initially. Clinical improvement may be seen within a few weeks, decrease to lowest dose which will control symptoms/

Breast cancer (palliation in appropriately selected postmenopausal women): Oral: 1 mg 3 times/day

Hepatic Impairment:

Mild to moderate liver impairment: Dosage reduction of estrogens is recommended.

Severe liver impairment: **Not recommended.**

Administration

Oral: Give at bedtime to minimize occurrence of adverse effects.

Stability

Storage: Store between 2°C and 30°C (36°F and 86°F)

Monitoring and Teaching Issues

Physical Assessment: See Contraindications, Warnings/Precautions and Dosing for use cautions. Assess potential for interactions with other prescriptions, OTC medications, or herbal products patient may be taking (see Drug Interactions). Assess results of laboratory tests, therapeutic effectiveness (according to purpose for use), and adverse response (eg, CNS changes, hypertension, thromboembolism, fluid retention, edema, CHF, respiratory changes - see Adverse Reactions and Overdose/Toxicology) on a regular basis during therapy. Caution diabetic patient to monitor glucose levels closely (may impair glucose tolerance). **Note:** Before prescribing estrogen therapy to postmenopausal women, the risks and benefits must be weighed for each patient. Women should be informed of these risks and benefits, as well as possible effects of progestin when added to estrogen therapy. Teach patient appropriate use, possible side effects and appropriate interventions, and adverse symptoms to report (see Patient Education). **Pregnancy risk factor X** - determine that patient is not pregnant before starting therapy. Do not give to childbearing age female unless capable of complying with barrier contraceptive use. Instruct patient on appropriate barrier contraceptive measures. Breast-feeding is contraindicated.

(Continued)

Ethinyl Estradiol *(Continued)*

Patient Education: Inform prescriber of all prescriptions, OTC medications, or herbal products you are taking, and any allergies you have. Do not take anything new without consulting prescriber. Take as prescribed at same time each day; maintain prescribed schedule. Avoid alcohol. Annual gynecologic and breast exams are important. If taking for prevention of osteoporosis, ask prescriber about calcium and vitamin D intake, and weight-bearing exercises. If diabetic, monitor glucose levels closely (may impair glucose tolerance). May cause nausea or vomiting (small, frequent meals may help); abdominal pain, difficult/painful menstrual cycles; dizziness or mental depression; rash; headache; or breast pain or increased/decreased libido. Report significant swelling of extremities; sudden acute pain in legs or calves, chest or abdomen; shortness of breath; severe headache or vomiting; sudden blindness; weakness or numbness of arm or leg; unusual vaginal bleeding; yellowing of skin or eyes; or unusual bruising or bleeding. You may become intolerant to wearing contact lenses, notify prescriber if this occurs. **Pregnancy/breast-feeding precautions:** Inform prescriber if you are pregnant or breast-feeding. Consult prescriber for appropriate barrier contraceptive measures. This medication may cause fetal defects and should not be used during pregnancy. Do not breast-feed.

Dietary Issues: Ensure adequate calcium and vitamin D intake when used for the prevention of osteoporosis.

Geriatric Considerations: Before prescribing estrogen therapy to postmenopausal women, the risks and benefits must be weighed for each patient. Data in women 80 years and older is minimal and it is unclear if the reduced risk is applicable to women in this age group. Women should be informed of these risks and benefits, as well as possible side effects and the return of menstrual bleeding (when cycled with a progestin), and be involved in the decision to prescribe. Oral therapy may be more convenient for vaginal atrophy and urinary incontinence.

Breast-feeding Issues: The AAP considers ethinyl estradiol, an estrogen derivative, to be "usually compatible" with breast-feeding. Estrogen has been shown to decrease the quantity and quality of human milk; use only if clearly needed and monitor the growth of the infant closely.

Ethinyl Estradiol and Desogestrel

(ETH in il es tra DYE ole & des oh JES trel)

U.S. Brand Names Apri®; Cyclessa®; Desogen®; Kariva™; Mircette®; Ortho-Cept®

Synonyms Desogestrel and Ethinyl Estradiol; Ortho Cept

Generic Available Yes

Pharmacologic Category Contraceptive; Estrogen and Progestin Combination

Pregnancy Risk Factor X

Lactation Enters breast milk/not recommended (AAP rates "compatible")

Use Prevention of pregnancy

Mechanism of Action/Effect Combination hormonal contraceptives inhibit ovulation and also produce changes in the cervical mucus and endometrium creating an unfavorable environment for sperm penetration and nidation.

Contraindications Hypersensitivity to ethinyl estradiol, etonogestrel, desogestrel, or any component of the formulation; thrombophlebitis or thromboembolic disorders (current or history of), cerebral vascular disease, coronary artery disease, valvular heart disease with complications, severe hypertension; diabetes mellitus with vascular involvement; severe headache with focal neurological symptoms; known or suspected breast carcinoma, endometrial cancer, estrogen-dependent neoplasms, undiagnosed abnormal genital bleeding; hepatic dysfunction or tumor, cholestatic jaundice of pregnancy, jaundice with prior combination hormonal contraceptive use; major surgery with prolonged immobilization; heavy smoking (≥15 cigarettes/day) in patients >35 years of age; pregnancy

Warnings/Precautions Combination hormonal contraceptives do not protect against HIV infection or other sexually-transmitted diseases. The risk of cardiovascular side effects increases in women who smoke cigarettes, especially those who are >35 years of age; women who use combination hormonal contraceptives should be strongly advised not to smoke. Combination hormonal contraceptives may lead to increased risk of myocardial infarction, use with caution in patients with risk factors for coronary artery disease. May increase the risk of thromboembolism. Combination hormonal contraceptives may have a dose-related risk of vascular disease, hypertension, and gallbladder disease. Women with hypertension should be encouraged to use another form of contraception. The use of combination hormonal contraceptives has been associated with a slight increase in frequency of breast cancer, however, studies are not consistent. Combination hormonal contraceptives may cause glucose intolerance. Retinal thrombosis has been reported (rarely). Use with caution in patients with renal disease, conditions that may be aggravated by fluid retention, depression, or history of migraine. Not for use prior to menarche.

The minimum dosage combination of estrogen/progestin that will effectively treat the individual patient should be used. New patients should be started on products containing <50 mcg of estrogen per tablet.

Drug Interactions

Cytochrome P450 Effect:

Ethinyl estradiol: Substrate of **CYP3A4**, 3A5-7; Inhibits CYP1A2, 2B6, 2C19, 3A4

Desogestrel: Substrate of **CYP2C19**

Decreased Effect: Combination hormonal contraceptives may decrease plasma levels of acetaminophen, clofibric acid, lorazepam, morphine, oxazepam, salicylic acid, temazepam. Contraceptive effect decreased by acitretin, aminoglutethimide, amprenavir, anticonvulsants, griseofulvin, lopinavir, nelfinavir, nevirapine, penicillins (effect not consistent), rifampin, ritonavir, tetracyclines (effect not consistent), troglitazone. Combination hormonal contraceptives may decrease (or increase) the effects of coumarin derivatives.

Increased Effect/Toxicity: Acetaminophen, ascorbic acid, and repaglinide may increase plasma levels of estrogen component. Atorvastatin and indinavir increase plasma levels of combination hormonal contraceptives. Combination hormonal contraceptives increase the plasma levels of alprazolam, chlordiazepoxide, cyclosporine, diazepam, prednisolone, selegiline, theophylline, tricyclic antidepressants. Combination hormonal contraceptives may increase (or decrease) the effects of coumarin derivatives.

Nutritional/Ethanol Interactions

Food: CNS effects of caffeine may be enhanced if combination hormonal contraceptives are used concurrently with caffeine. Grapefruit juice increases ethinyl estradiol concentrations and would be expected to increase progesterone serum levels as well; clinical implications are unclear.

Herb/Nutraceutical: St John's wort may decrease the effectiveness of combination hormonal contraceptives by inducing hepatic enzymes. Avoid dong quai and black cohosh (have estrogen activity). Avoid saw palmetto, red clover, ginseng.

Effects on Lab Values ↑ platelet aggregation, thyroid-binding globulin, total thyroid hormone (T_4), serum triglycerides/phospholipids; ↓ antithrombin III, serum folate concentration

Adverse Reactions Frequency not defined.

Cardiovascular: Arterial thromboembolism, cerebral hemorrhage, cerebral thrombosis, edema, hypertension, mesenteric thrombosis, myocardial infarction

Central nervous system: Depression, dizziness, headache, migraine, nervousness, premenstrual syndrome, stroke

Dermatologic: Acne, erythema multiforme, erythema nodosum, hirsutism, loss of scalp hair, melasma (may persist), rash (allergic)

Endocrine & metabolic: Amenorrhea, breakthrough bleeding, breast enlargement, breast secretion, breast tenderness, carbohydrate intolerance, lactation decreased (postpartum), glucose tolerance decreased, libido changes, menstrual flow changes, sex hormone-binding globulins (SHBG) increased, spotting, temporary infertility (following discontinuation), thyroid-binding globulin increased, triglycerides increased

Gastrointestinal: Abdominal cramps, appetite changes, bloating, cholestasis, colitis, gallbladder disease, jaundice, nausea, vomiting, weight gain/loss

Genitourinary: Cervical erosion changes, cervical secretion changes, cystitis-like syndrome, vaginal candidiasis, vaginitis

Hematologic: Antithrombin III decreased, folate levels decreased, hemolytic uremic syndrome, norepinephrine induced platelet aggregability increased, porphyria, prothrombin increased; factors VII, VIII, IX, and X

Hepatic: Benign liver tumors, Budd-Chiari syndrome, cholestatic jaundice, hepatic adenomas

Local: Thrombophlebitis

Ocular: Cataracts, change in corneal curvature (steepening), contact lens intolerance, optic neuritis, retinal thrombosis

Renal: Impaired renal function

Respiratory: Pulmonary thromboembolism

Miscellaneous: Hemorrhagic eruption

Overdosage/Toxicology Toxicity is unlikely following single exposures of excessive doses. May cause withdrawal bleeding in females. Any treatment following emesis and charcoal administration should be supportive and symptomatic.

Pharmacokinetic Note See Ethinyl Estradiol monograph.

Pharmacodynamics/Kinetics

Absorption:

Desogestrel: Rapid and complete

Half-Life Elimination:

Desogestrel: 37.1 hours

Metabolism:

Desogestrel: Hepatic via CYP2C9 to active metabolite etonogestrel (3-keto-desogestrel); etonogestrel metabolized via CYP3A4

Formulations Tablet:

Low-dose formulation:

Kariva™:

Day 1-21: Ethinyl estradiol 0.02 mg and desogestrel 0.15 mg [21 white tablets]

Day 22-23: 2 inactive light green tablets

Day 24-28: Ethinyl estradiol 0.01 mg [5 light blue tablets] (28s)

Mircette®:

Day 1-21: Ethinyl estradiol 0.02 mg and desogestrel 0.15 mg [21 white tablets]

Day 22-23: 2 inactive green tablets

Day 24-28: Ethinyl estradiol 0.01 mg [5 yellow tablets] (28s)

Monophasic formulations:

Apri® 28: Ethinyl estradiol 0.03 mg and desogestrel 0.15 mg [21 rose tablets and 7 white inactive tablets] (28s)

Desogen®: Ethinyl estradiol 0.03 mg and desogestrel 0.15 mg [21 white tablets and 7 green inactive tablets] (28s)

Ortho-Cept® 28: Ethinyl estradiol 0.03 mg and desogestrel 0.15 mg [21 orange tablets and 7 green inactive tablets] (28s)

Triphasic formulation: Cyclessa®:

Day 1-7:Ethinyl estradiol 0.025 mg and desogestrel 0.1 mg [7 light yellow tablets]

Day 8-14: Ethinyl estradiol 0.025 mg and desogestrel 0.125 mg [7 orange tablets]

Day 14-21: Ethinyl estradiol 0.025 mg and desogestrel 0.15 mg [7 red tablets]

Day 21-28: 7 green inactive tablets (28s)

Dosing

Adults: Female: Contraception: Oral:

Schedule 1 (Sunday starter): Dose begins on first Sunday after onset of menstruation; if the menstrual period starts on Sunday, take first tablet that very same day. **With a Sunday start, an additional method of contraception should be used until after the first 7 days of consecutive administration.**

For 21-tablet package: Dosage is 1 tablet daily for 21 consecutive days, followed by 7 days off of the medication; a new course begins on the 8th day after the last tablet is taken.

For 28-tablet package: Dosage is 1 tablet daily without interruption.

Schedule 2 (Day 1 starter): Dose starts on first day of menstrual cycle taking 1 tablet daily.

(Continued)

Ethinyl Estradiol and Desogestrel *(Continued)*

For 21-tablet package: Dosage is 1 tablet daily for 21 consecutive days, followed by 7 days off of the medication; a new course begins on the 8th day after the last tablet is taken.

For 28-tablet package: Dosage is 1 tablet daily without interruption.

If all doses have been taken on schedule and one menstrual period is missed, continue dosing cycle. If two consecutive menstrual periods are missed, pregnancy test is required before new dosing cycle is started.

Missed doses **monophasic formulations** (refer to package insert for complete information):

One dose missed: Take as soon as remembered or take 2 tablets next day

Two consecutive doses missed in the first 2 weeks: Take 2 tablets as soon as remembered or 2 tablets next 2 days. **An additional method of contraception should be used for 7 days after missed dose.**

Two consecutive doses missed in week 3 or three consecutive doses missed at any time: Schedule 1 (Sunday starter): Continue to take 1 tablet daily until Sunday, then discard the rest of the pack, and a new pack is started that same day. Schedule 2 (Day 1 starter): Current pack should be discarded, and a new pack started that same day. **An additional method of contraception should be used for 7 days after missed dose.**

Missed doses **biphasic/triphasic formulations** (refer to package insert for complete information):

One dose missed: Take as soon as remembered or take 2 tablets next day.

Two consecutive doses missed in week 1 or week 2 of the pack: Take 2 tablets as soon as remembered and 2 tablets the next day. Resume taking 1 tablet daily until the pack is empty. **An additional method of contraception should be used for 7 days after a missed dose.**

Two consecutive doses missed in week 3 of the pack; **an additional method of contraception must be used for 7 days after a missed dose**:

Schedule 1 (Sunday starter): Take 1 tablet every day until Sunday. Discard the remaining pack and start a new pack of pills on the same day.

Schedule 2 (Day 1 starter): Discard the remaining pack and start a new pack the same day.

Three or more consecutive doses missed; **an additional method of contraception must be used for 7 days after a missed dose**:

Schedule 1 (Sunday starter): Take 1 tablet every day until Sunday; on Sunday, discard the pack and start a new pack.

Schedule 2 (Day 1 starter): Discard the remaining pack and begin new pack of tablets starting on the same day.

Pediatrics: Female: Contraception: Oral: See adult dosing; not to be used prior to menarche.

Renal Impairment: Specific guidelines not available; use with caution.

Hepatic Impairment: Contraindicated in patients with hepatic impairment.

Administration

Oral: Administer at the same time each day.

Stability

Storage: Store at controlled room temperature of 25°C (77°F).

Monitoring and Teaching Issues

Physical Assessment: Monitor blood pressure on a regular basis. Assess for adverse reactions and potential drug interactions. Assess knowledge/teach importance of regular (monthly) blood pressure checks and annual physical assessment, Pap smear, and vision assessment. Teach importance of maintaining prescribed schedule of dosing (see Dosing for dosing and missed dose information). **Pregnancy risk factor X** - do not use if patient is pregnant. Breast-feeding is not recommended.

Patient Education: Oral contraceptives do not protect against HIV infection or other sexually-transmitted diseases. Take exactly as directed by prescriber (see package insert). You are at risk of becoming pregnant if doses are missed. Detailed and complete information on dosing and missed doses can be found in the package insert. Be aware that some medications may reduce the effectiveness of oral contraceptives; an alternate form of contraception may be needed. Check all medicines (prescription and over-the-counter), herbal and alternative products with prescriber. It is important that you check your blood pressure monthly (same day each month) and that you have an annual physical assessment, Pap smear, and vision exam while taking this medication. Avoid smoking while taking this medication; smoking increases risk of adverse effects, including thromboembolic events and heart attacks. You may experience loss of appetite (small, frequent meals will help); or constipation (increased exercise, fluids, fruit, fiber, or stool softeners may help). If diabetic, use accurate serum glucose testing to identify any changes in glucose tolerance; notify prescriber of significant changes so antidiabetic medication can be adjusted if necessary. Report immediately pain or muscle soreness; warmth, swelling, pain, or redness in calves; shortness of breath; sudden loss of vision; unresolved leg/foot swelling; change in menstrual pattern (unusual bleeding, amenorrhea, breakthrough spotting); breast tenderness that does not go away; acute abdominal cramping; signs of vaginal infection (drainage, pain, itching); CNS changes (blurred vision, confusion, acute anxiety, or unresolved depression); or significant weight gain (>5 lb/week). Notify prescriber of changes in contact lens tolerance. **Pregnancy/breast-feeding precautions:** This medication should not be used during pregnancy. If you suspect you may become pregnant, contact prescriber immediately. Breast-feeding is not recommended.

Dietary Issues: Should be taken at same time each day.

Breast-feeding Issues: Jaundice and breast enlargement in the nursing infant have been reported following the use of combination hormonal contraceptives. May decrease the quality and quantity of breast milk; a nonhormonal form of contraception is recommended.

Pregnancy Issues: Pregnancy should be ruled out prior to treatment and discontinued if pregnancy occurs. In general, the use of combination hormonal contraceptives when inadvertently taken early in pregnancy have not been associated with teratogenic effects. Due to increased risk of thromboembolism postpartum, combination hormonal contraceptives should not be started earlier than 4-6 weeks following delivery.

Related Information

Ethinyl Estradiol *on page 514*

Ethinyl Estradiol and Drospirenone

(ETH in il es tra DYE ole & droh SPYE re none)

U.S. Brand Names Yasmin®

Synonyms Drospirenone and Ethinyl Estradiol

Generic Available No

Pharmacologic Category Contraceptive

Pregnancy Risk Factor X

Lactation Enters breast milk/not recommended

Use Prevention of pregnancy

Mechanism of Action/Effect Combination oral contraceptives inhibit ovulation and also produce changes in the cervical mucus and endometrium creating an unfavorable environment for sperm penetration and nidation.

Contraindications Hypersensitivity to ethinyl estradiol, drospirenone, or to any component of the formulation; thrombophlebitis or thromboembolic disorders (current or history of), cerebral vascular disease, coronary artery disease; known or suspected breast carcinoma, endometrial cancer, estrogen-dependent neoplasms, undiagnosed abnormal genital bleeding; renal insufficiency, hepatic dysfunction or tumor, adrenal insufficiency, cholestatic jaundice of pregnancy, jaundice with prior oral contraceptive use; heavy smoking (≥15 cigarettes/day) in patients >35 years of age; pregnancy

Warnings/Precautions Oral contraceptives do not protect against HIV infection or other sexually-transmitted diseases. The risk of cardiovascular side effects increases in women who smoke cigarettes, especially those who are >35 years of age; women who use oral contraceptives should be strongly advised not to smoke. Oral contraceptives may lead to increased risk of myocardial infarction, use with caution in patients with risk factors for coronary artery disease. May increase the risk of thromboembolism. Oral contraceptives may have a dose-related risk of vascular disease (decreases HDL), hypertension, and gallbladder disease; a preparation with the lowest effective estrogen/progesterone combination should be used. Women with high blood pressure should be encouraged to use another form of contraception. Oral contraceptives may cause glucose intolerance. Retinal thrombosis has been reported (rarely) with oral contraceptive use. Use with caution in patients with conditions that may be aggravated by fluid retention, depression, or patients with history of migraine. Not for use prior to menarche.

Drospirenone has antimineralocorticoid activity that may lead to hyperkalemia in patients with renal insufficiency, hepatic dysfunction, or adrenal insufficiency. Use caution with medications that may increase serum potassium.

Drug Interactions

Cytochrome P450 Effect:

Ethinyl estradiol: Substrate of **CYP3A4**, 3A5-7; Inhibits CYP1A2, 2B6, 2C19, 3A4

Drospirenone: Substrate of CYP3A4; Inhibits CYP1A2, 2C8/9, 2C19, 3A4

Decreased Effect: Oral contraceptives may decrease the plasma concentration of acetaminophen, clofibric acid, morphine, salicylic acid, and temazepam. Aminoglutethimide, anticonvulsants (carbamazepine, felbamate, phenobarbital, phenytoin, topiramate), phenylbutazone, rifampin, and ritonavir may increase metabolism leading to decreased effect of oral contraceptives. Oral contraceptives may decrease (or increase) the effects of coumarin derivatives.

Increased Effect/Toxicity: ACE inhibitors, aldosterone antagonists, angiotensin II receptor antagonists, heparin, NSAIDs (when taken daily, long term), and potassium-sparing diuretics increase risk of hyperkalemia with concomitant use. Acetaminophen, ascorbic acid, and atorvastatin may increase plasma concentrations of oral contraceptives. Ethinyl estradiol may increase plasma concentrations of cyclosporine, prednisolone, selegiline, and theophylline. Oral contraceptives may increase (or decrease) the effects of coumarin derivatives.

Nutritional/Ethanol Interactions

Food: CNS effects of caffeine may be enhanced if oral contraceptives are used concurrently with caffeine. Grapefruit juice increases ethinyl estradiol concentrations; clinical implications are unclear.

Herb/Nutraceutical: St John's wort may decrease the effectiveness of oral contraceptives by inducing hepatic enzymes; may also result in breakthrough bleeding.

Adverse Reactions

>1%:

Central nervous system: Depression, dizziness, emotional lability, headache, migraine, nervousness

Dermatologic: Acne, pruritus, rash

Endocrine & metabolic: Amenorrhea, dysmenorrhea, intermenstrual bleeding, menstrual irregularities

Gastrointestinal: Abdominal pain, diarrhea, gastroenteritis, nausea, vomiting

Genitourinary: Cystitis, leukorrhea, vaginal moniliasis, vaginitis

Neuromuscular & skeletal: Back pain, weakness

Respiratory: Bronchitis, pharyngitis, sinusitis, upper respiratory infection

Miscellaneous: Allergic reaction, flu-like syndrome, infection

Adverse reactions reported with other oral contraceptives: Appetite changes, antithrombin III decreased, arterial thromboembolism, benign liver tumors, breast changes, Budd-Chiari syndrome, carbohydrate intolerance, cataracts, cerebral hemorrhage, cerebral thrombosis, cervical changes, change in corneal curvature (steepening), cholestatic jaundice, colitis, contact lens intolerance, decreased lactation (postpartum), deep vein thrombosis, diplopia, edema, erythema multiforme, erythema nodosum; factors VII, VIII, IX, X increased; folate serum concentrations decreased, gallbladder disease, glucose intolerance, hemorrhagic

(Continued)

Ethinyl Estradiol and Drospirenone *(Continued)*

eruption, hemolytic uremic syndrome, hepatic adenomas, hirsutism, hypercalcemia, hypertension, hyperglycemia, libido changes, melasma, mesenteric thrombosis, myocardial infarction, papilledema, platelet aggregability increased, porphyria, premenstrual syndrome, proptosis, prothrombin increased, pulmonary thromboembolism, renal function impairment, retinal thrombosis, sex hormone-binding globulin increased, thrombophlebitis, thyroid-binding globulin increased, total thyroid hormone (T_4) increased, triglycerides/phospholipids increased, vaginal candidiasis, weight changes

Overdosage/Toxicology May cause nausea; withdrawal bleeding may occur in females. Due to antimineralocorticoid properties of drospirenone, monitor potassium and sodium serum concentrations and evidence of metabolic acidosis.

Pharmacokinetic Note See Ethinyl Estradiol monograph.

Pharmacodynamics/Kinetics

Bioavailability:

Drospirenone: 76%

Half-Life Elimination:

Drospirenone: 30 hours

Time to Peak:

Drospirenone: 1-3 hours

Metabolism:

Drospirenone: To inactive metabolites; minor metabolism hepatically via CYP3A4

Formulations Tablet: Ethinyl estradiol 0.03 mg and drospirenone 3 mg [21 yellow active tablets and 7 white inactive tablets] (28s)

Dosing

Adults: Female: Contraception: Oral: Dosage is 1 tablet daily for 28 consecutive days. Dose should be taken at the same time each day, either after the evening meal or at bedtime. Dosing may be started on the first day of menstrual period (Day 1 starter) or on the first Sunday after the onset of the menstrual period (Sunday starter).

Day 1 starter: Dose starts on first day of menstrual cycle taking 1 tablet daily.

Sunday starter: Dose begins on first Sunday after onset of menstruation; if the menstrual period starts on Sunday, take first tablet that very same day. **With a Sunday start, an additional method of contraception should be used until after the first 7 days of consecutive administration.**

If all doses have been taken on schedule and one menstrual period is missed, continue dosing cycle. If two consecutive menstrual periods are missed, pregnancy test is required before new dosing cycle is started.

If doses have been missed during the first 3 weeks and the menstrual period is missed, pregnancy should be ruled out prior to continuing treatment.

Missed doses (monophasic formulations) (refer to package insert for complete information):

One dose missed: Take as soon as remembered or take 2 tablets next day

Two consecutive doses missed in the first 2 weeks: Take 2 tablets as soon as remembered or 2 tablets next 2 days. **An additional method of contraception should be used for 7 days after missed dose.**

Two consecutive doses missed in week 3 or three consecutive doses missed at any time: **An additional method of contraception must be used for 7 days after a missed dose.**

Day 1 starter: Current pack should be discarded, and a new pack should be started that same day.

Sunday starter: Continue dose of 1 tablet daily until Sunday, then discard the rest of the pack, and a new pack should be started that same day.

Any number of doses missed in week 4: Continue taking one pill each day until pack is empty; no back-up method of contraception is needed

Pediatrics: Female: Contraception: Oral: Refer to adult dosing; not to be used prior to menarche.

Renal Impairment: Contraindicated in patients with renal dysfunction (Cl_{cr} ≤50 mL/minute).

Hepatic Impairment: Contraindicated in patients with hepatic dysfunction.

Administration

Oral: To be taken at the same time each day, either after the evening meal or at bedtime

Stability

Storage: Store at 25°C (77°F).

Monitoring and Teaching Issues

Physical Assessment: See Warnings/Precautions, Contraindications, and Drug Interactions for extensive use cautions. Monitor or teach patient to monitor blood pressure on a regular (monthly) basis, and the importance of annual physical examinations (including Pap smear and vision exam). Assess knowledge/teach patient the importance of maintaining prescribed schedule of dosing (see Dosing), possible side effects, appropriate interventions, and adverse reactions to report (see Patient Education). **Pregnancy risk factor X** - determine patient is not pregnant prior to prescribing. Breast-feeding is not recommended.

Patient Education: Take exactly as directed by prescriber (see package insert). An additional form of contraception should be used until after the first 7 consecutive days of administration. You are at risk of becoming pregnant if doses are missed. If you miss a dose, take as soon as possible or double the dose the next day. If two or more consecutive doses are missed, contact prescriber for restarting directions. Detailed and complete information on dosing and missed doses can be found in the package insert. If any number of doses are missed in week 4, continue taking one pill each day until pack is empty; no back-up method of contraception is needed. Be aware that some medications may reduce the effectiveness of oral contraceptives; an alternate form of contraception may be needed (see Drug Interactions). It is important that you check your blood pressure monthly (on same day each month) and report any increased blood pressure to prescriber. Have an annual physical assessment, Pap smear, and vision exam while taking this medication.

Avoid smoking while taking this medication; smoking increases risk of adverse effects, including thromboembolic events and heart attacks. You may experience loss of appetite (small, frequent meals will help); or constipation (increased exercise, fluids, fruit, fiber, or stool softeners may help). If you are diabetic you should use accurate serum glucose testing to identify any changes in glucose tolerance; notify prescriber of significant changes so antidiabetic medication can be adjusted if necessary. Report immediately pain or muscle soreness; warmth, swelling, pain, or redness in calves; shortness of breath; sudden loss of vision; unresolved leg/foot swelling or weight gain (>5 lb); change in menstrual pattern (unusual bleeding, amenorrhea, breakthrough spotting); breast tenderness that does not go away; acute abdominal cramping; signs of vaginal infection (drainage, pain, itching); CNS changes (blurred vision, confusion, acute anxiety, or unresolved depression); or other persistent adverse effects. **Pregnancy/breast-feeding precautions:** Inform prescriber if you are pregnant. Consult prescriber if breast-feeding.

Breast-feeding Issues: The amount of drospirenone excreted in breast milk is ~0.02%, resulting in a maximum of ~3 mcg/day drospirenone to the infant. Jaundice and breast enlargement in the nursing infant have been reported following the use of other oral contraceptives. In addition, may decrease the quality and quantity of breast milk. Other forms of contraception are recommended while breast-feeding.

Pregnancy Issues: In general, the use of oral contraceptives when inadvertently taken early in pregnancy have not been associated with teratogenic effects. Esophageal atresia was reported in one infant with a single-cycle exposure to ethinyl estradiol and drospirenone *in utero* (association not known). Pregnancy should be ruled out prior to treatment and discontinued if pregnancy occurs. Due to increased risk of thromboembolism postpartum, do not start oral contraceptives earlier than 4-6 weeks following delivery.

Related Information

Ethinyl Estradiol *on page 514*

Ethinyl Estradiol and Ethynodiol Diacetate

(ETH in il es tra DYE ole & e thye noe DYE ole dye AS e tate)

U.S. Brand Names Demulen®; Zovia™

Synonyms Ethynodiol Diacetate and Ethinyl Estradiol

Generic Available Yes

Pharmacologic Category Contraceptive; Estrogen and Progestin Combination

Pregnancy Risk Factor X

Lactation Enters breast milk/not recommended (AAP rates "compatible")

Use Prevention of pregnancy

Use - Unlabeled/Investigational Treatment of hypermenorrhea, endometriosis, female hypogonadism

Mechanism of Action/Effect Combination hormonal contraceptives inhibit ovulation and also produce changes in the cervical mucus and endometrium creating an unfavorable environment for sperm penetration and nidation.

Contraindications Hypersensitivity to ethinyl estradiol, ethynodiol diacetate, or any component of the formulation; thrombophlebitis or thromboembolic disorders (current or history of), cerebral vascular disease, coronary artery disease, valvular heart disease with complications, severe hypertension; diabetes mellitus with vascular involvement; severe headache with focal neurological symptoms; known or suspected breast carcinoma, endometrial cancer, estrogen-dependent neoplasms, undiagnosed abnormal genital bleeding; hepatic dysfunction or tumor, cholestatic jaundice of pregnancy, jaundice with prior combination hormonal contraceptive use; major surgery with prolonged immobilization; heavy smoking (≥15 cigarettes/day) in patients >35 years of age; pregnancy

Warnings/Precautions Combination hormonal contraceptives do not protect against HIV infection or other sexually-transmitted diseases. The risk of cardiovascular side effects increases in women who smoke cigarettes, especially those who are >35 years of age; women who use combination hormonal contraceptives should be strongly advised not to smoke. Combination hormonal contraceptives may lead to increased risk of myocardial infarction, use with caution in patients with risk factors for coronary artery disease. May increase the risk of thromboembolism. Combination hormonal contraceptives may have a dose-related risk of vascular disease, hypertension, and gallbladder disease. Women with hypertension should be encouraged to use a nonhormonal form of contraception. The use of combination hormonal contraceptives has been associated with a slight increase in frequency of breast cancer, however, studies are not consistent. Combination hormonal contraceptives may cause glucose intolerance. Retinal thrombosis has been reported (rarely). Use with caution in patients with renal disease, conditions that may be aggravated by fluid retention, depression, or history of migraine. Not for use prior to menarche.

The minimum dosage combination of estrogen/progestin that will effectively treat the individual patient should be used. New patients should be started on products containing <50 mcg of estrogen per tablet.

Drug Interactions

Cytochrome P450 Effect: Ethinyl estradiol: Substrate of **CYP3A4**, 3A5-7; Inhibits CYP1A2, 2B6, 2C19, 3A4

Decreased Effect: Combination hormonal contraceptives may decrease plasma levels of acetaminophen, clofibric acid, lorazepam, morphine, oxazepam, salicylic acid, temazepam. Contraceptive effect decreased by acitretin, aminoglutethimide, amprenavir, anticonvulsants, griseofulvin, lopinavir, nelfinavir, nevirapine, penicillins (effect not consistent), rifampin, ritonavir, tetracyclines (effect not consistent). Combination hormonal contraceptives may decrease (or increase) the effects of coumarin derivatives.

Increased Effect/Toxicity: Acetaminophen and ascorbic acid may increase plasma levels of estrogen component. Atorvastatin and indinavir increase plasma levels of combination hormonal contraceptives. Combination hormonal contraceptives increase the plasma levels of alprazolam, chlordiazepoxide, cyclosporine, diazepam, prednisolone, selegiline, theophylline, tricyclic antidepressants. Combination hormonal contraceptives may increase (or decrease) the effects of coumarin derivatives.

(Continued)

Ethinyl Estradiol and Ethynodiol Diacetate *(Continued)*

Nutritional/Ethanol Interactions

Food: CNS effects of caffeine may be enhanced if combination hormonal contraceptives are used concurrently with caffeine. Grapefruit juice increases ethinyl estradiol concentrations and would be expected to increase progesterone serum levels as well; clinical implications are unclear.

Herb/Nutraceutical: St John's wort may decrease the effectiveness of combination hormonal contraceptives by inducing hepatic enzymes. Avoid dong quai and black cohosh (have estrogen activity). Avoid saw palmetto, red clover, ginseng.

Effects on Lab Values ↑ platelet aggregation, thyroid-binding globulin, total thyroid hormone (T_4), serum triglycerides/phospholipids; ↓ antithrombin III, serum folate concentration

Adverse Reactions Frequency not defined.

Cardiovascular: Arterial thromboembolism, cerebral hemorrhage, cerebral thrombosis, edema, hypertension, mesenteric thrombosis, myocardial infarction

Central nervous system: Depression, dizziness, headache, migraine, nervousness, premenstrual syndrome, stroke

Dermatologic: Acne, erythema multiforme, erythema nodosum, hirsutism, loss of scalp hair, melasma (may persist), rash (allergic)

Endocrine & metabolic: Amenorrhea, breakthrough bleeding, breast enlargement, breast secretion, breast tenderness, carbohydrate intolerance, lactation decreased (postpartum), glucose tolerance decreased, libido changes, menstrual flow changes, sex hormone-binding globulins (SHBG) increased, spotting, temporary infertility (following discontinuation), thyroid-binding globulin increased, triglycerides increased

Gastrointestinal: Abdominal cramps, appetite changes, bloating, cholestasis, colitis, gallbladder disease, jaundice, nausea, vomiting, weight gain/loss

Genitourinary: Cervical erosion changes, cervical secretion changes, cystitis-like syndrome, vaginal candidiasis, vaginitis

Hematologic: Antithrombin III decreased, folate levels decreased, hemolytic uremic syndrome, norepinephrine induced platelet aggregability increased, porphyria, prothrombin increased; factors VII, VIII, IX, and X increased

Hepatic: Benign liver tumors, Budd-Chiari syndrome, cholestatic jaundice, hepatic adenomas

Local: Thrombophlebitis

Ocular: Cataracts, change in corneal curvature (steepening), contact lens intolerance, optic neuritis, retinal thrombosis

Renal: Impaired renal function

Respiratory: Pulmonary thromboembolism

Miscellaneous: Hemorrhagic eruption

Overdosage/Toxicology Toxicity is unlikely following single exposures of excessive doses. May cause withdrawal bleeding in females. Any treatment following emesis and charcoal administration should be supportive and symptomatic.

Pharmacokinetic Note See Ethinyl Estradiol and Norethindrone monographs.

Pharmacodynamics/Kinetics

Half-Life Elimination:

Ethynodiol diacetate (converted to norethindrone) Terminal: 5-14 hours

Metabolism:

Ethynodiol diacetate (converted to norethindrone): Hepatic conjugation

Formulations Tablet, monophasic formulations:

Demulin® 1/35-21: Ethinyl estradiol 0.035 mg and ethynodiol diacetate 1 mg [white tablets] (21s)

Demulin® 1/35-28: Ethinyl estradiol 0.035 mg and ethynodiol diacetate 1 mg [21 white tablets and 7 blue inactive tablets] (28s)

Demulin® 1/50-21: Ethinyl estradiol 0.05 mg and ethynodiol diacetate 1 mg [white tablets] (21s)

Demulin® 1/50-28: Ethinyl estradiol 0.05 mg and ethynodiol diacetate 1 mg [21 white tablets and 7 pink inactive tablets] (28s)

Zovia™ 1/35-21: Ethinyl estradiol 0.035 mg and ethynodiol diacetate 1 mg [light pink tablets] (21s)

Zovia™ 1/35-28: Ethinyl estradiol 0.035 mg and ethynodiol diacetate 1 mg [21 light pink tablets and 7 white inactive tablets] (28s)

Zovia™ 1/50-21: Ethinyl estradiol 0.05 mg and ethynodiol diacetate 1 mg [pink tablets] (21s)

Zovia™ 1/50-28: Ethinyl estradiol 0.05 mg and ethynodiol diacetate 1 mg [21 pink tablets and 7 white inactive tablets] (28s)

Dosing

Adults:

Female: Contraception: Oral:

Schedule 1 (Sunday starter): Dose begins on first Sunday after onset of menstruation; if the menstrual period starts on Sunday, take first tablet that very same day. **With a Sunday start, an additional method of contraception should be used until after the first 7 days of consecutive administration:**

For 21-tablet package: 1 tablet/day for 21 consecutive days, followed by 7 days off of the medication; a new course begins on the 8th day after the last tablet is taken

For 28-tablet package: 1 tablet/day without interruption

Schedule 2 (Day-1 starter): Dose starts on first day of menstrual cycle taking 1 tablet/day:

For 21-tablet package: 1 tablet/day for 21 consecutive days, followed by 7 days off of the medication; a new course begins on the 8th day after the last tablet is taken

For 28-tablet package: 1 tablet/day without interruption

If all doses have been taken on schedule and one menstrual period is missed, continue dosing cycle. If two consecutive menstrual periods are missed, pregnancy test is required before new dosing cycle is started.

Missed doses **monophasic formulations** (refer to package insert for complete information):

One dose missed: Take as soon as remembered or take 2 tablets next day

Two consecutive doses missed in the first 2 weeks: Take 2 tablets as soon as remembered or 2 tablets next 2 days. **An additional method of contraception should be used for 7 days after missed dose.**

Two consecutive doses missed in week 3 or three consecutive doses missed at any time: **An additional method of contraception must be used for 7 days after a missed dose:**

Schedule 1 (Sunday starter): Continue dose of 1 tablet daily until Sunday, then discard the rest of the pack, and a new pack should be started that same day.

Schedule 2 (Day-1 starter): Current pack should be discarded, and a new pack should be started that same day.

Pediatrics: Female: Contraception: Oral: Refer to adult dosing; not to be used prior to menarche.

Renal Impairment: Specific guidelines not available; use with caution.

Hepatic Impairment: Contraindicated in patients with hepatic impairment.

Administration

Oral: Administer at the same time each day.

Stability

Storage: Store at controlled room temperature of 25°C (77°F).

Monitoring and Teaching Issues

Physical Assessment: Monitor or teach patient to monitor blood pressure on a regular basis. Monitor or teach patient to monitor for occurrence of adverse effects and symptoms to report (see Adverse Reactions). Assess knowledge/teach importance of regular (monthly) blood pressure checks and annual physical assessment, Pap smear, and vision assessment. Teach importance of maintaining prescribed schedule of dosing (see Dosing for dosing and missed dose information). **Pregnancy risk factor X** - do not use if patient is pregnant. Breast-feeding is not recommended.

Patient Education: Oral contraceptives do not protect against HIV or other sexually-transmitted diseases. Take exactly as directed by prescriber (also see package insert). You are at risk of becoming pregnant if doses are missed. Detailed and complete information on dosing and missed doses can be found in the package insert. Be aware that some medications may reduce the effectiveness of oral contraceptives; an alternate form of contraception may be needed. Check all medicines (prescription and OTC), herbal, and alternative products with prescriber. It is important that you check your blood pressure monthly (on same day each month) and that you have an annual physical assessment, Pap smear, and vision assessment while taking this medication. Avoid smoking while taking this medication; smoking increases risk of adverse effects, including thromboembolic events and heart attacks. You may experience loss of appetite (small, frequent meals will help); or constipation (increased exercise, fluids, fruit, fiber, or stool softeners may help). If diabetic, use accurate serum glucose testing to identify any changes in glucose tolerance; notify prescriber of significant changes so antidiabetic medication can be adjusted if necessary. Report immediately pain or muscle soreness; warmth, swelling, pain, or redness in calves; shortness of breath; sudden loss of vision; unresolved leg/foot swelling; change in menstrual pattern (unusual bleeding, amenorrhea, breakthrough spotting); breast tenderness that does not go away; acute abdominal cramping; signs of vaginal infection (drainage, pain, itching); CNS changes (blurred vision, confusion, acute anxiety, or unresolved depression); or significant weight gain (>5 lb/week). Notify prescriber of changes in contact lens tolerance. **Pregnancy/breast-feeding precautions:** This medication should not be used during pregnancy. If you suspect you may become pregnant, contact prescriber immediately. Breast-feeding is not recommended.

Dietary Issues: Should be taken with food at same time each day.

Breast-feeding Issues: Jaundice and breast enlargement in the nursing infant have been reported following the use of combination hormonal contraceptives. May decrease the quality and quantity of breast milk; a nonhormonal form of contraception is recommended.

Pregnancy Issues: Pregnancy should be ruled out prior to treatment and discontinued if pregnancy occurs. In general, the use of combination hormonal contraceptives when inadvertently taken early in pregnancy have not been associated with teratogenic effects. Due to increased risk of thromboembolism postpartum, combination hormonal contraceptives should not be started earlier than 4-6 weeks following delivery.

Related Information

Ethinyl Estradiol *on page 514*

Ethinyl Estradiol and Levonorgestrel

(ETH in il es tra DYE ole & LEE voe nor jes trel)

U.S. Brand Names Alesse®; Aviane™; Enpresse™; Lessina™; Levlen®; Levlite™; Levora®; Nordette®; Portia™; PREVEN™; Tri-Levlen®; Triphasil®; Trivora®

Synonyms Levonorgestrel and Ethinyl Estradiol

Generic Available Yes

Pharmacologic Category Contraceptive

Pregnancy Risk Factor X

Lactation Enters breast milk/not recommended

Use Prevention of pregnancy; postcoital contraception

Use - Unlabeled/Investigational Treatment of hypermenorrhea, endometriosis, female hypogonadism

Mechanism of Action/Effect Combination oral contraceptives inhibit ovulation and also produce changes in the cervical mucus and endometrium creating an unfavorable environment for sperm penetration and nidation

Contraindications Hypersensitivity to ethinyl estradiol, levonorgestrel, or any component of the formulation; thrombophlebitis or thromboembolic disorders (current or history of), cerebral vascular disease, coronary artery disease, valvular heart disease with complications, severe hypertension; diabetes mellitus with vascular involvement; severe headache with focal neurological symptoms; known or suspected breast carcinoma, endometrial cancer, estrogen-dependent neoplasms, undiagnosed abnormal genital bleeding; hepatic dysfunction

(Continued)

Ethinyl Estradiol and Levonorgestrel *(Continued)*

or tumor, cholestatic jaundice of pregnancy, jaundice with prior combination hormonal contraceptive use; major surgery with prolonged immobilization; heavy smoking (≥15 cigarettes/day) in patients >35 years of age; pregnancy

Warnings/Precautions Combination hormonal contraceptives do not protect against HIV infection or other sexually-transmitted diseases. The risk of cardiovascular side effects increases in women who smoke cigarettes, especially those who are >35 years of age; women who use combination hormonal contraceptives should be strongly advised not to smoke. Combination hormonal contraceptives may lead to increased risk of myocardial infarction, use with caution in patients with risk factors for coronary artery disease. May increase the risk of thromboembolism. Combination hormonal contraceptives may have a dose-related risk of vascular disease, hypertension, and gallbladder disease. Women with hypertension should be encouraged to use another form of contraception. The use of combination hormonal contraceptives has been associated with a slight increase in frequency of breast cancer, however, studies are not consistent. Combination hormonal contraceptives may cause glucose intolerance. Retinal thrombosis has been reported (rarely). Use with caution in patients with renal disease, conditions that may be aggravated by fluid retention, depression, or history of migraine. Not for use prior to menarche.

The minimum dosage combination of estrogen/progestin that will effectively treat the individual patient should be used. New patients should be started on products containing <50 mcg of estrogen per tablet.

Drug Interactions

Cytochrome P450 Effect:

Ethinyl estradiol: Substrate of **CYP3A4**, 3A5-7; Inhibits CYP1A2, 2B6, 2C19, 3A4

Levonorgestrel: Substrate of **CYP3A4**

Decreased Effect: Combination hormonal contraceptives may decrease plasma levels of acetaminophen, clofibric acid, lorazepam, morphine, oxazepam, salicylic acid, temazepam. Contraceptive effect decreased by acitretin, aminoglutethimide, amprenavir, anticonvulsants, griseofulvin, lopinavir, nelfinavir, nevirapine, penicillins (effect not consistent), rifampin, ritonavir, tetracyclines (effect not consistent). Combination hormonal contraceptives may decrease (or increase) the effects of coumarin derivatives.

Increased Effect/Toxicity: Acetaminophen and ascorbic acid may increase plasma levels of estrogen component. Atorvastatin and indinavir increase plasma levels of combination hormonal contraceptives. Combination hormonal contraceptives increase the plasma levels of alprazolam, chlordiazepoxide, cyclosporine, diazepam, prednisolone, selegiline, theophylline, tricyclic antidepressants. Combination hormonal contraceptives may increase (or decrease) the effects of coumarin derivatives.

Nutritional/Ethanol Interactions

Food: CNS effects of caffeine may be enhanced if combination hormonal contraceptives are used concurrently with caffeine. Grapefruit juice increases ethinyl estradiol concentrations and would be expected to increase progesterone serum levels as well; clinical implications are unclear.

Herb/Nutraceutical: St John's wort may decrease the effectiveness of combination hormonal contraceptives by inducing hepatic enzymes. Avoid dong quai and black cohosh (have estrogen activity). Avoid saw palmetto, red clover, ginseng.

Effects on Lab Values ↑ prothrombin and factors VII, VIII, IX, X; ↑ platelet aggregability, thyroid-binding globulin, total thyroid hormone (T_4), serum triglycerides/phospholipids ↓ antithrombin III, serum folate concentration

Adverse Reactions Frequency not defined.

Cardiovascular: Arterial thromboembolism, cerebral hemorrhage, cerebral thrombosis, edema, hypertension, mesenteric thrombosis, myocardial infarction

Central nervous system: Depression, dizziness, headache, migraine, nervousness, premenstrual syndrome, stroke

Dermatologic: Acne, erythema multiforme, erythema nodosum, hirsutism, loss of scalp hair, melasma (may persist), rash (allergic)

Endocrine & metabolic: Amenorrhea, breakthrough bleeding, breast enlargement, breast secretion, breast tenderness, carbohydrate intolerance, lactation decreased (postpartum), glucose tolerance decreased, libido changes, menstrual flow changes, sex hormone-binding globulins (SHBG) increased, spotting, temporary infertility (following discontinuation), thyroid-binding globulin increased, triglycerides increased

Gastrointestinal: Abdominal cramps, appetite changes, bloating, cholestasis, colitis, gallbladder disease, jaundice, nausea, vomiting, weight gain/loss

Genitourinary: Cervical erosion changes, cervical secretion changes, cystitis-like syndrome, vaginal candidiasis, vaginitis

Hematologic: Antithrombin III decreased, folate levels decreased, hemolytic uremic syndrome, norepinephrine induced platelet aggregability increased, porphyria, prothrombin increased; factors VII, VIII, IX, and X increased

Hepatic: Benign liver tumors, Budd-Chiari syndrome, cholestatic jaundice, hepatic adenomas

Local: Thrombophlebitis

Ocular: Cataracts, change in corneal curvature (steepening), contact lens intolerance, optic neuritis, retinal thrombosis

Renal: Impaired renal function

Respiratory: Pulmonary thromboembolism

Miscellaneous: Hemorrhagic eruption

Overdosage/Toxicology Toxicity is unlikely following single exposures of excessive doses. May cause withdrawal bleeding in females. Any treatment following emesis and charcoal administration should be supportive and symptomatic.

Pharmacokinetic Note See individual agents.

Formulations Tablet:

PREVEN™: Ethinyl estradiol 0.05 mg and levonorgestrel 0.25 mg (4s) [also available as a kit containing 4 tablets and a pregnancy test]

Low-dose formulations:

Alesse® 21: Ethinyl estradiol 0.02 mg and levonorgestrel 0.1 mg [pink tablets] (21s)

Alesse® 28: Ethinyl estradiol 0.02 mg and levonorgestrel 0.1 mg [21 pink tablets and 7 light green inactive tablets] (28s)
Aviane™ 28: Ethinyl estradiol 0.02 mg and levonorgestrel 0.1 mg [21 orange tablets and 7 light green inactive tablets] (28s)
Lessina™ 21, Levlite™ 21: Ethinyl estradiol 0.02 mg and levonorgestrel 0.1 mg [pink tablets] (21s)
Lessina™ 28, Levlite™ 28: Ethinyl estradiol 0.02 mg and levonorgestrel 0.1 mg [21 pink tablets and 7 white inactive tablets] (28s)

Monophasic formulations:
Levlen® 21: Ethinyl estradiol 0.03 mg and levonorgestrel 0.15 mg [light orange tablets] (21s)
Levlen® 28: Ethinyl estradiol 0.03 mg and levonorgestrel 0.15 mg [21 light orange tablets and 7 pink inactive tablets] (28s)
Levora® 21: Ethinyl estradiol 0.03 mg and levonorgestrel 0.15 mg [white tablets] (21s)
Levora® 28: Ethinyl estradiol 0.03 mg and levonorgestrel 0.15 mg [21 white tablets and 7 peach inactive tablets] (28s)
Nordette® 21: Ethinyl estradiol 0.03 mg and levonorgestrel 0.15 mg [light orange tablets] (21s)
Nordette® 28: Ethinyl estradiol 0.03 mg and levonorgestrel 0.15 mg [21 light orange tablets and 7 pink inactive tablets] (28s)
Portia™ 21: Ethinyl estradiol 0.03 mg and levonorgestrel 0.15 mg [pink tablets] (21s)
Portia™ 28: Ethinyl estradiol 0.03 mg and levonorgestrel 0.15 mg [21 pink tablets and 7 white inactive tablets] (28s)

Triphasic formulations:
Enpresse™:
Day 1-6: Ethinyl estradiol 0.03 mg and levonorgestrel 0.05 mg [6 pink tablets]
Day 7-11: Ethinyl estradiol 0.04 mg and levonorgestrel 0.075 mg [5 white tablets]
Day 12-21: Ethinyl estradiol 0.03 mg and levonorgestrel 0.125 mg [10 orange tablets]
Day 22-28: 7 light green inactive tablets (28s)
Tri-Levlen® 21, Triphasil® 21:
Day 1-6: Ethinyl estradiol 0.03 mg and levonorgestrel 0.05 mg [6 brown tablets]
Day 7-11: Ethinyl estradiol 0.04 mg and levonorgestrel 0.075 mg [5 white tablets]
Day 12-21: Ethinyl estradiol 0.03 mg and levonorgestrel 0.125 mg [10 light yellow tablets] (21s)
Trivora® 21:
Day 1-6: Ethinyl estradiol 0.03 mg and levonorgestrel 0.05 mg [6 blue tablets]
Day 7-11: Ethinyl estradiol 0.04 mg and levonorgestrel 0.075 mg [5 white tablets]
Day 12-21: Ethinyl estradiol 0.03 mg and levonorgestrel 0.125 mg [10 pink tablets] (21s)
Tri-Levlen® 28, Triphasil® 28:
Day 1-6: Ethinyl estradiol 0.03 mg and levonorgestrel 0.05 mg [6 brown tablets]
Day 7-11: Ethinyl estradiol 0.04 mg and levonorgestrel 0.075 mg [5 white tablets]
Day 12-21: Ethinyl estradiol 0.03 mg and levonorgestrel 0.125 mg [10 light yellow tablets]
Day 22-28: 7 light green inactive tablets (28s)
Trivora® 28:
Day 1-6: Ethinyl estradiol 0.03 mg and levonorgestrel 0.05 mg [6 blue tablets]
Day 7-11: Ethinyl estradiol 0.04 mg and levonorgestrel 0.075 mg [5 white tablets]
Day 12-21: Ethinyl estradiol 0.03 mg and levonorgestrel 0.125 mg [10 pink tablets]
Day 22-28: 7 peach inactive tablets (28s)

Dosing

Adults:

Female: Contraception: Oral:

Schedule 1 (Sunday starter): Dose begins on first Sunday after onset of menstruation; if the menstrual period starts on Sunday, take first tablet that very same day. With a Sunday start, an additional method of contraception should be used until after the first 7 days of consecutive administration:
For 21-tablet package: 1 tablet/day for 21 consecutive days, followed by 7 days off of the medication; a new course begins on the 8th day after the last tablet is taken
For 28-tablet package: 1 tablet/day without interruption

Schedule 2 (Day-1 starter): Dose starts on first day of menstrual cycle taking 1 tablet/day:
For 21-tablet package: 1 tablet/day for 21 consecutive days, followed by 7 days off of the medication; a new course begins on the 8th day after the last tablet is taken
For 28-tablet package: 1 tablet/day without interruption

If all doses have been taken on schedule and one menstrual period is missed, continue dosing cycle. If two consecutive menstrual periods are missed, pregnancy test is required before new dosing cycle is started.

Missed doses **monophasic formulations** (refer to package insert for complete information):
One dose missed: Take as soon as remembered or take 2 tablets next day
Two consecutive doses missed in the first 2 weeks: Take 2 tablets as soon as remembered or 2 tablets next 2 days. An additional method of contraception should be used for 7 days after missed dose.
Two consecutive doses missed in week 3 or three consecutive doses missed at any time: An additional method of contraception must be used for 7 days after a missed dose:
Schedule 1 (Sunday starter): Continue dose of 1 tablet daily until Sunday, then discard the rest of the pack, and a new pack should be started that same day.
Schedule 2 (Day-1 starter): Current pack should be discarded, and a new pack should be started that same day.

Missed doses **biphasic/triphasic formulations** (refer to package insert for complete information):
One dose missed: Take as soon as remembered or take 2 tablets next day.

(Continued)

Ethinyl Estradiol and Levonorgestrel *(Continued)*

Two consecutive doses missed in week 1 or week 2 of the pack: Take 2 tablets as soon as remembered and 2 tablets the next day. Resume taking 1 tablet daily until the pack is empty. An additional method of contraception should be used for 7 days after a missed dose.

Two consecutive doses missed in week 3 of the pack: An additional method of contraception must be used for 7 days after a missed dose.

Schedule 1 (Sunday starter): Take 1 tablet every day until Sunday. Discard the remaining pack and start a new pack of pills on the same day.

Schedule 2 (Day-1 starter): Discard the remaining pack and start a new pack the same day.

Three or more consecutive doses missed: An additional method of contraception must be used for 7 days after a missed dose.

Schedule 1 (Sunday starter): Take 1 tablet every day until Sunday; on Sunday, discard the pack and start a new pack.

Schedule 2 (Day-1 starter): Discard the remaining pack and begin new pack of tablets starting on the same day.

Female: Emergency contraception (PREVEN™): Oral: Initial: 2 tablets as soon as possible (but within 72 hours of unprotected intercourse), followed by a second dose of 2 tablets 12 hours later. Repeat dose or use antiemetic if vomiting occurs within 1 hour of dose.

Pediatrics: Female: Contraception or emergency contraception: Oral: Refer to adult dosing; not to be used prior to menarche.

Renal Impairment: Specific guidelines not available; use with caution.

Hepatic Impairment: Contraindicated in patients with hepatic impairment.

Administration

Oral: Administer at the same time each day.

Stability

Storage: Store at controlled room temperature of 25°C (77°F).

Monitoring and Teaching Issues

Physical Assessment: Monitor blood pressure on a regular basis. Assess for adverse reactions and potential drug interactions. Assess knowledge/teach importance of regular (monthly) blood pressure checks and annual physical assessment, Pap smear, and vision assessment. Teach importance of maintaining prescribed schedule of dosing (see Dosing for dosing and missed dose information). **Pregnancy risk factor X** - do not use if patient is pregnant. Breast-feeding is not recommended.

Patient Education: Oral contraceptives do not protect against HIV or other sexually-transmitted diseases. Take exactly as directed by prescriber (also see package insert). You are at risk of becoming pregnant if doses are missed. Detailed and complete information on dosing and missed doses can be found in the package insert. Be aware that some medications may reduce the effectiveness of oral contraceptives; an alternate form of contraception may be needed (see Drug Interactions). It is important that you check your blood pressure monthly (on same day each month) and that you have an annual physical assessment, Pap smear, and vision assessment while taking this medication. Avoid smoking while taking this medication; smoking increases risk of adverse effects, including thromboembolic events and heart attacks. You may experience loss of appetite (small, frequent meals will help); or constipation (increased exercise, fluids, fruit, fiber, or stool softeners may help). If diabetic, use accurate serum glucose testing to identify any changes in glucose tolerance; notify prescriber of significant changes so antidiabetic medication can be adjusted if necessary. Report immediately pain or muscle soreness; warmth, swelling, pain, or redness in calves; shortness of breath; sudden loss of vision; unresolved leg/foot swelling; change in menstrual pattern (unusual bleeding, amenorrhea, breakthrough spotting); breast tenderness that does not go away; acute abdominal cramping; signs of vaginal infection (drainage, pain, itching); CNS changes (blurred vision, confusion, acute anxiety, or unresolved depression); or significant weight gain (>5 lb/week). Notify prescriber of changes in contact lens tolerance. **Pregnancy/breast-feeding precautions:** This medication should not be used during pregnancy. If you suspect you may become pregnant, contact prescriber immediately. Breast-feeding is not recommended.

Emergency contraceptive kit (PREVEN™) is **not** recommended for ongoing pregnancy protection or as a routine form of contraception. PREVEN™ emergency contraceptive kit contains a pregnancy test. This test can be used to verify an existing pregnancy resulting from intercourse that occurred earlier in the concurrent menstrual cycle or the previous cycle. If a positive pregnancy result is obtained, the patient should **not** take the pills in the PREVEN™ kit. The patient should be instructed that if she vomits within 1 hour of taking either dose of the medication, she should contact her healthcare professional to discuss whether to repeat that dose or to take an antiemetic.

Dietary Issues: Should be taken at the same time each day.

Breast-feeding Issues: Jaundice and breast enlargement in the nursing infant have been reported following the use of combination hormonal contraceptives. May decrease the quality and quantity of breast milk; alternative form of contraception is recommended.

Pregnancy Issues: Pregnancy should be ruled out prior to treatment and discontinued if pregnancy occurs. In general, the use of combination hormonal contraceptives when inadvertently taken early in pregnancy have not been associated with teratogenic effects. Due to increased risk of thromboembolism postpartum, combination hormonal contraceptives should not be started earlier than 4-6 weeks following delivery.

Related Information

Ethinyl Estradiol *on page 514*
Levonorgestrel *on page 793*

Ethinyl Estradiol and NGM *see* Ethinyl Estradiol and Norgestimate *on page 530*

Ethinyl Estradiol and Norethindrone

(ETH in il es tra DYE ole & nor eth IN drone)

U.S. Brand Names Brevicon®; Estrostep® 21 [DSC]; Estrostep® Fe; femhrt®; Jenest™-28 [DSC]; Loestrin®; Loestrin® Fe; Microgestin™ Fe; Modicon®; Necon® 0.5/35; Necon® 1/35; Necon® 10/11; Norinyl® 1+35; Nortrel™; Ortho-Novum®; Ovcon®; Tri-Norinyl®

Synonyms Norethindrone Acetate and Ethinyl Estradiol; Ortho Novum

Generic Available Yes

Pharmacologic Category Contraceptive; Estrogen and Progestin Combination

Pregnancy Risk Factor X

Lactation Enters breast milk/not recommended

Use Prevention of pregnancy; treatment of acne; moderate to severe vasomotor symptoms associated with menopause; prevention of osteoporosis

Use - Unlabeled/Investigational Treatment of hypermenorrhea, endometriosis, female hypogonadism

Mechanism of Action/Effect Combination oral contraceptives inhibit ovulation, and also produce changes in the cervical mucus and the endometrium, creating an unfavorable environment for sperm penetration and nidation. In postmenopausal women, exogenous estrogen is used to replace decreased endogenous production. The addition of progestin reduces the incidence of endometrial hyperplasia and risk of adenocarcinoma in women with an intact uterus.

Contraindications Hypersensitivity to ethinyl estradiol, norethindrone, norethindrone acetate, or any component of the formulation; thrombophlebitis or thromboembolic disorders (current or history of), cerebral vascular disease, coronary artery disease, severe hypertension; diabetes mellitus with vascular involvement; severe headache with focal neurological symptoms; known or suspected breast carcinoma, endometrial cancer, estrogen-dependent neoplasms, undiagnosed abnormal genital bleeding; hepatic dysfunction or tumor, cholestatic jaundice of pregnancy, jaundice with prior combination hormonal contraceptive use; major surgery with prolonged immobilization; heavy smoking (≥15 cigarettes/day) in patients >35 years of age; pregnancy

Warnings/Precautions Combination hormonal contraceptives do not protect against HIV infection or other sexually-transmitted diseases. The risk of cardiovascular side effects increases in women who smoke cigarettes, especially those who are >35 years of age; women who use combination hormonal contraceptives should be strongly advised not to smoke. Combination hormonal contraceptives may lead to increased risk of myocardial infarction, use with caution in patients with risk factors for coronary artery disease. May increase the risk of thromboembolism. Combination hormonal contraceptives may have a dose-related risk of vascular disease, hypertension, and gallbladder disease. Women with hypertension should be encouraged to use another form of contraception. The use of combination hormonal contraceptives has been associated with a slight increase in frequency of breast cancer, however, studies are not consistent. Combination hormonal contraceptives may cause glucose intolerance. Retinal thrombosis has been reported (rarely). Use with caution in patients with renal disease, conditions that may be aggravated by fluid retention, depression, or history of migraine. Not for use prior to menarche.

The minimum dosage combination of estrogen/progestin that will effectively treat the individual patient should be used. New patients should be started on products containing <50 mcg of estrogen per tablet.

Acne: For use only in females ≥15 years, who also desire combination hormonal contraceptive therapy, are unresponsive to topical treatments, and have no contraindications to oral contraceptive use; treatment must continue for at least 6 months.

Vasomotor symptoms associated with menopause and prevention of osteoporosis: For use only in postmenopausal women with an intact uterus.

Drug Interactions

Cytochrome P450 Effect:

Ethinyl estradiol: Substrate of **CYP3A4**, 3A5-7; Inhibits CYP1A2, 2B6, 2C19, 3A4

Norethindrone: Substrate of **CYP3A4**; Induces 2C19

Decreased Effect: Combination hormonal contraceptives may decrease plasma levels of acetaminophen, clofibric acid, lorazepam, morphine, oxazepam, salicylic acid, temazepam. Contraceptive effect decreased by acitretin, aminoglutethimide, amprenavir, anticonvulsants, griseofulvin, lopinavir, nelfinavir, nevirapine, penicillins (effect not consistent), rifampin, ritonavir, tetracyclines (effect not consistent), troglitazone. Oral contraceptives may decrease (or increase) the effects of coumarin derivatives.

Increased Effect/Toxicity: Acetaminophen and ascorbic acid may increase plasma levels of estrogen component. Atorvastatin and indinavir increase plasma levels of combination hormonal contraceptives. Combination hormonal contraceptives increase the plasma levels of alprazolam, chlordiazepoxide, cyclosporine, diazepam, prednisolone, selegiline, theophylline, tricyclic antidepressants. Combination hormonal contraceptives may increase (or decrease) the effects of coumarin derivatives.

Nutritional/Ethanol Interactions

Food: CNS effects of caffeine may be enhanced if combination hormonal contraceptives are used concurrently with caffeine. Grapefruit juice increases ethinyl estradiol concentrations and would be expected to increase progesterone serum levels as well; clinical implications are unclear. Norethindrone absorption is increased by 27% following administration with food.

Herb/Nutraceutical: St John's wort may decrease the effectiveness of combination hormonal contraceptives by inducing hepatic enzymes. Avoid dong quai and black cohosh (have estrogen activity). Avoid saw palmetto, red clover, ginseng.

Effects on Lab Values ↑ prothrombin and factors VII, VIII, IX, X; ↑ platelet aggregability, thyroid-binding globulin, total thyroid hormone (T_4), serum triglycerides/phospholipids ↓ antithrombin III, serum folate concentration

Adverse Reactions As reported with oral contraceptive agents. Frequency not defined.

Cardiovascular: Arterial thromboembolism, cerebral hemorrhage, cerebral thrombosis, edema, hypertension, mesenteric thrombosis, myocardial infarction

(Continued)

Ethinyl Estradiol and Norethindrone *(Continued)*

Central nervous system: Depression, dizziness, headache, migraine, nervousness, premenstrual syndrome, stroke
Dermatologic: Acne, erythema multiforme, erythema nodosum, hirsutism, loss of scalp hair, melasma (may persist), rash (allergic)
Endocrine & metabolic: Amenorrhea, breakthrough bleeding, breast enlargement, breast secretion, breast tenderness, carbohydrate intolerance, lactation decreased (postpartum), glucose tolerance decreased, libido changes, menstrual flow changes, sex hormone-binding globulins (SHBG) increased, spotting, temporary infertility (following discontinuation), thyroid-binding globulin increased, triglycerides increased
Gastrointestinal: Abdominal cramps, appetite changes, bloating, cholestasis, colitis, gallbladder disease, jaundice, nausea, vomiting, weight gain/loss
Genitourinary: Cervical erosion changes, cervical secretion changes, cystitis-like syndrome, vaginal candidiasis, vaginitis
Hematologic: Antithrombin III decreased, folate levels decreased, hemolytic uremic syndrome, norepinephrine induced platelet aggregability increased, porphyria, prothrombin increased; factors VII, VIII, IX, and X
Hepatic: Benign liver tumors, Budd-Chiari syndrome, cholestatic jaundice, hepatic adenomas
Local: Thrombophlebitis
Ocular: Cataracts, change in corneal curvature (steepening), contact lens intolerance, optic neuritis, retinal thrombosis
Renal: Impaired renal function
Respiratory: Pulmonary thromboembolism
Miscellaneous: Hemorrhagic eruption

Overdosage/Toxicology Toxicity is unlikely following single exposures of excessive doses. May cause withdrawal bleeding in females. Any treatment following emesis and charcoal administration should be supportive and symptomatic.

Pharmacokinetic Note See individual agents.

Formulations Tablet:

femhrt® 1/5: Ethinyl estradiol 0.005 mg and norethindrone acetate 1 mg [white tablets]

Monophasic formulations:

- Brevicon®: Ethinyl estradiol 0.035 mg and norethindrone 0.5 mg [21 blue tablets and 7 orange inactive tablets] (28s)
- Loestrin® 21 1/20: Ethinyl estradiol 0.02 mg and norethindrone acetate 1 mg [white tablets] (21s)
- Loestrin® 21 1.5/30: Ethinyl estradiol 0.03 mg and norethindrone acetate 1.5 mg [green tablets] (21s)
- Loestrin® Fe 1/20, Microgestin™ Fe 1/20: Ethinyl estradiol 0.02 mg and norethindrone acetate 1 mg [21 white tablets] and ferrous fumarate 75 mg [7 brown tablets] (28s)
- Loestrin® Fe 1.5/30, Microgestin™ Fe 1.5/30: Ethinyl estradiol 0.03 mg and norethindrone acetate 1.5 mg [21 green tablets] and ferrous fumarate 75 mg [7 brown tablets] (28s)
- Modicon® 21: Ethinyl estradiol 0.035 mg and norethindrone 0.5 mg [white tablets] (21s)
- Modicon® 28: Ethinyl estradiol 0.035 mg and norethindrone 0.5 mg [21 white tablets and 7 green inactive tablets] (28s)
- Necon® 0.5/35-21: Ethinyl estradiol 0.035 mg and norethindrone 0.5 mg [light yellow tablets] (21s)
- Necon® 0.5/35-28: Ethinyl estradiol 0.035 mg and norethindrone 0.5 mg [21 light yellow tablets and 7 white inactive tablets] (28s)
- Necon® 1/35-21: Ethinyl estradiol 0.035 mg and norethindrone 1 mg [dark yellow tablets] (21s)
- Necon® 1/35-28: Ethinyl estradiol 0.035 mg and norethindrone 1 mg [21 dark yellow tablets and 7 white inactive tablets] (28s)
- Norinyl® 1+35: Ethinyl estradiol 0.035 mg and norethindrone 1 mg [21 yellow-green tablets and 7 orange inactive tablets] (28s)
- Nortrel™ 0.5/35 mg:
  - Ethinyl estradiol 0.035 mg and norethindrone 0.5 mg [light yellow tablets] (21s)
  - Ethinyl estradiol 0.035 mg and norethindrone 0.5 mg [21 light yellow tablets and 7 white inactive tablets] (28s)
- Nortrel™ 1/35 mg:
  - Ethinyl estradiol 0.035 mg and norethindrone 1 mg [yellow tablets] (21s)
  - Ethinyl estradiol 0.035 mg and norethindrone 1 mg [21 yellow tablets and 7 white inactive tablets] (28s)
- Ortho-Novum® 1/35 21: Ethinyl estradiol 0.035 mg and norethindrone 1 mg [peach tablets] (21s)
- Ortho-Novum® 1/35 28: Ethinyl estradiol 0.035 mg and norethindrone 1 mg [21 peach tablets and 7 green inactive tablets] (28s)
- Ovcon® 35 21-day: Ethinyl estradiol 0.035 mg and norethindrone 0.4 mg [peach tablets] (21s)
- Ovcon® 35 28-day: Ethinyl estradiol 0.035 mg and norethindrone 0.4 mg [21 peach tablets and 7 green inactive tablets] (28s)
- Ovcon® 50: Ethinyl estradiol 0.05 mg and norethindrone 1 mg [21 yellow tablets and 7 green inactive tablets] (28s)

Biphasic formulations:

- Jenest™-28 [DSC]:
  - Day 1-7: Ethinyl estradiol 0.035 mg and norethindrone 0.5 mg [7 white tablets]
  - Day 8-21: Ethinyl estradiol 0.035 mg and norethindrone 1 mg [14 peach tablets]
  - Day 22-28: 7 green inactive tablets (28s)
- Necon® 10/11-21:
  - Day 1-10: Ethinyl estradiol 0.035 mg and norethindrone 0.5 mg [10 light yellow tablets]
  - Day 11-21: Ethinyl estradiol 0.035 mg and norethindrone 1 mg [11 dark yellow tablets] (21s)
- Necon® 10/11-28:
  - Day 1-10: Ethinyl estradiol 0.035 mg and norethindrone 0.5 mg [10 light yellow tablets]

Day 11-21: Ethinyl estradiol 0.035 mg and norethindrone 1 mg [11 dark yellow tablets]
Day 22-28: 7 white inactive tablets (28s)

Ortho-Novum® 10/11-21:
Day 1-10: Ethinyl estradiol 0.035 mg and norethindrone 0.5 mg [10 white tablets]
Day 11-21: Ethinyl estradiol 0.035 mg and norethindrone 1 mg [11 peach tablet] (21s)

Ortho-Novum® 10/11-28:
Day 1-10: Ethinyl estradiol 0.035 mg and norethindrone 0.5 mg [10 white tablets]
Day 11-21: Ethinyl estradiol 0.035 mg and norethindrone 1 mg [11 peach tablet]
Day 22-28: 7 green inactive tablets (28s)

Triphasic formulations:

Estrostep® 21 [DSC]:
Day 1-5: Ethinyl estradiol 0.02 mg and norethindrone acetate 1mg [5 white triangular tablets]
Day 6-12: Ethinyl estradiol 0.03 mg and norethindrone acetate 1 mg [7 white square tablets]
Day 13-21: Ethinyl estradiol 0.035 mg and norethindrone acetate 1 mg [9 white round tablets] (21s)

Estrostep® Fe:
Day 1-5: Ethinyl estradiol 0.02 mg and norethindrone acetate 1 mg [5 white triangular tablets]
Day 6-12: Ethinyl estradiol 0.03 mg and norethindrone acetate 1 mg [7 white square tablets]
Day 13-21: Ethinyl estradiol 0.035 mg and norethindrone acetate 1 mg [9 white round tablets]
Day 22-28: Ferrous fumarate 75 mg [7 brown tablets] (28s)

Ortho-Novum® 7/7/7 21:
Day 1-7: Ethinyl estradiol 0.035 mg and norethindrone 0.5 mg [7 white tablets]
Day 8-14: Ethinyl estradiol 0.035 mg and norethindrone 0.75 mg [7 light peach tablets]
Day 15-21: Ethinyl estradiol 0.035 mg and norethindrone 1 mg [7 peach tablet] (21s)

Ortho-Novum® 7/7/7 28:
Day 1-7: Ethinyl estradiol 0.035 mg and norethindrone 0.5 mg [7 white tablets]
Day 8-14: Ethinyl estradiol 0.035 mg and norethindrone 0.75 mg [7 light peach tablets]
Day 15-21: Ethinyl estradiol 0.035 mg and norethindrone 1 mg [7 peach tablet]
Day 22-28: 7 green inactive tablets (28s)

Tri-Norinyl® 28:
Day 1-7: Ethinyl estradiol 0.035 mg and norethindrone 0.5 mg [7 blue tablets]
Day 8-16: Ethinyl estradiol 0.035 mg and norethindrone 1 mg [9 yellow-green tablets]
Day 17-21: Ethinyl estradiol 0.035 mg and norethindrone 0.5 mg [5 blue tablets]
Day 22-28: 7 orange inactive tablets (28s)

Dosing

Adults:

Adolescents ≥15 years and Adults: Female: Acne: Estrostep®: Oral: Refer to dosing for contraception

Moderate to severe vasomotor symptoms associated with menopause: femhrt® 1/5: Oral: 1 tablet daily; patients should be re-evaluated at 3- to 6-month intervals to determine if treatment is still necessary

Prevention of osteoporosis: femhrt® 1/5: Oral: 1 tablet daily

Contraception: Oral:

Schedule 1 (Sunday starter): Dose begins on first Sunday after onset of menstruation; if the menstrual period starts on Sunday, take first tablet that very same day. With a Sunday start, an additional method of contraception should be used until after the first 7 days of consecutive administration.

For 21-tablet package: Dosage is 1 tablet daily for 21 consecutive days, followed by 7 days off of the medication; a new course begins on the 8th day after the last tablet is taken.

For 28-tablet package: Dosage is 1 tablet daily without interruption.

Schedule 2 (Day 1 starter): Dose starts on first day of menstrual cycle taking 1 tablet daily.

For 21-tablet package: Dosage is 1 tablet daily for 21 consecutive days, followed by 7 days off of the medication; a new course begins on the 8th day after the last tablet is taken.

For 28-tablet package: Dosage is 1 tablet daily without interruption.

If all doses have been taken on schedule and one menstrual period is missed, continue dosing cycle. If two consecutive menstrual periods are missed, pregnancy test is required before new dosing cycle is started.

Missed doses **monophasic formulations** (refer to package insert for complete information):

One dose missed: Take as soon as remembered or take 2 tablets next day Two consecutive doses missed in the first 2 weeks: Take 2 tablets as soon as remembered or 2 tablets next 2 days. An additional method of contraception should be used for 7 days after missed dose.

Two consecutive doses missed in week 3 or three consecutive doses missed at any time: An additional method of contraception must be used for 7 days after a missed dose.

Schedule 1 (Sunday starter): Continue dose of 1 tablet daily until Sunday, then discard the rest of the pack, and a new pack should be started that same day.

Schedule 2 (Day 1 starter): Current pack should be discarded, and a new pack should be started that same day.

Missed doses **biphasic/triphasic formulations** (refer to package insert for complete information):

One dose missed: Take as soon as remembered or take 2 tablets next day.

Two consecutive doses missed in week 1 or week 2 of the pack: Take 2 tablets as soon as remembered and 2 tablets the next day. Resume taking 1 tablet daily until

(Continued)

Ethinyl Estradiol and Norethindrone *(Continued)*

the pack is empty. An additional method of contraception should be used for 7 days after a missed dose.

Two consecutive doses missed in week 3 of the pack: An additional method of contraception must be used for 7 days after a missed dose.

Schedule 1 (Sunday Starter): Take 1 tablet every day until Sunday. Discard the remaining pack and start a new pack of pills on the same day.

Schedule 2 (Day 1 starter): Discard the remaining pack and start a new pack the same day.

Three or more consecutive doses missed: An additional method of contraception must be used for 7 days after a missed dose.

Schedule 1 (Sunday Starter): Take 1 tablet every day until Sunday; on Sunday, discard the pack and start a new pack.

Schedule 2 (Day 1 Starter): Discard the remaining pack and begin new pack of tablets starting on the same day.

Pediatrics: Female:

Acne: Oral: Estrostep®: For use in females ≥15 years; refer to adult dosing for contraception

Contraception: Oral: Refer to adult dosing; not to be used prior to menarche.

Renal Impairment: Specific guidelines not available; use with caution.

Hepatic Impairment: Contraindicated in patients with hepatic impairment.

Administration

Oral: Administer at the same time each day.

Stability

Storage: Store at controlled room temperature of 25°C (77°F).

Estrostep®: Protect from light.

Monitoring and Teaching Issues

Physical Assessment: Monitor blood pressure on a regular basis. Monitor for adverse reactions and potential drug interactions. Assess knowledge/teach importance of regular (monthly) blood pressure checks and annual physical assessment, Pap smear, and vision assessment. Teach importance of maintaining prescribed schedule of dosing (see Dosing for dosing and missed dose information). **Pregnancy risk factor X** - do not use if patient is pregnant. Breast-feeding is not recommended.

Patient Education: Oral contraceptives do not protect against HIV infection or other sexually-transmitted diseases. Take exactly as directed by prescriber (also see package insert). You are at risk of becoming pregnant if doses are missed. Detailed and complete information on dosing and missed doses can be found in the package insert. Be aware that some medications may reduce the effectiveness of oral contraceptives; an alternate form of contraception may be needed (see Drug Interactions). It is important that you check your blood pressure monthly (on same day each month) and that you have an annual physical assessment, Pap smear, and vision assessment while taking this medication. Avoid smoking while taking this medication; smoking increases risk of adverse effects, including thromboembolic events and heart attacks. You may experience loss of appetite (small, frequent meals will help); or constipation (increased exercise, fluids, fruit, fiber, or stool softeners may help). If diabetic, use accurate serum glucose testing to identify any changes in glucose tolerance; notify prescriber of significant changes so antidiabetic medication can be adjusted if necessary. Report immediately pain or muscle soreness; warmth, swelling, pain, or redness in calves; shortness of breath; sudden loss of vision; unresolved leg/foot swelling; change in menstrual pattern (unusual bleeding, amenorrhea, breakthrough spotting); breast tenderness that does not go away; acute abdominal cramping; signs of vaginal infection (drainage, pain, itching); CNS changes (blurred vision, confusion, acute anxiety, or unresolved depression); or significant weight gain (>5 lb/week). Notify prescriber of changes in contact lens tolerance. **Pregnancy/breast-feeding precautions:** This medication should not be used during pregnancy. If you suspect you may become pregnant, contact prescriber immediately. Breast-feeding is not recommended.

femhrt®: In general, the above precautions are the same for women taking this medication for the prevention of osteoporosis or the treatment of "hot flashes." If taking for prevention of osteoporosis, ask prescriber about calcium and vitamin D intake, and weight-bearing exercises.

Dietary Issues: Should be taken at same time each day. May be taken with or without food.

Breast-feeding Issues: Jaundice and breast enlargement in the nursing infant have been reported following the use of combination hormonal contraceptives. May decrease the quality and quantity of breast milk; alternative form of contraception is recommended.

Pregnancy Issues: Pregnancy should be ruled out prior to treatment and discontinued if pregnancy occurs. In general, the use of combination hormonal contraceptives when inadvertently taken early in pregnancy have not been associated with teratogenic effects. Due to increased risk of thromboembolism postpartum, combination hormonal contraceptives should not be started earlier than 4-6 weeks following delivery.

Additional Information Norethindrone acetate 1 mg is equivalent to ethinyl estradiol 2.8 mcg.

Related Information

Ethinyl Estradiol *on page 514*

Ethinyl Estradiol and Norgestimate

(ETH in il es tra DYE ole & nor JES ti mate)

U.S. Brand Names Ortho-Cyclen®; Ortho Tri-Cyclen®; Ortho Tri-Cyclen® Lo

Synonyms Ethinyl Estradiol and NGM; Norgestimate and Ethinyl Estradiol; Ortho Cyclen; Ortho Tri Cyclen

Generic Available No

Pharmacologic Category Contraceptive; Estrogen and Progestin Combination

Pregnancy Risk Factor X

Lactation Enters breast milk/not recommended (AAP rates "compatible")

Use Prevention of pregnancy; treatment of acne

Mechanism of Action/Effect Combination hormonal contraceptives inhibit ovulation and also produce changes in the cervical mucus and endometrium creating an unfavorable environment for sperm penetration and nidation.

Contraindications Hypersensitivity to ethinyl estradiol, norgestimate, or any component of the formulation; thrombophlebitis or thromboembolic disorders (current or history of), cerebral vascular disease, coronary artery disease, valvular heart disease with complications, severe hypertension; severe headache with focal neurological symptoms; known or suspected breast carcinoma, endometrial cancer, estrogen-dependent neoplasms, undiagnosed abnormal genital bleeding; hepatic dysfunction or tumor, cholestatic jaundice of pregnancy, jaundice with prior combination hormonal contraceptive use; heavy smoking (≥15 cigarettes/day) in patients >35 years of age; pregnancy

Warnings/Precautions Combination hormonal contraceptives do not protect against HIV infection or other sexually-transmitted diseases. The risk of cardiovascular side effects increases in women who smoke cigarettes, especially those who are >35 years of age; women who use combination hormonal contraceptives should be strongly advised not to smoke. Combination hormonal contraceptives may lead to increased risk of myocardial infarction, use with caution in patients with risk factors for coronary artery disease. May increase the risk of thromboembolism. Combination hormonal contraceptives may have a dose-related risk of vascular disease, hypertension, and gallbladder disease. Women with hypertension should be encouraged to use a nonhormonal form of contraception. The use of combination hormonal contraceptives has been associated with a slight increase in frequency of breast cancer, however, studies are not consistent. Combination hormonal contraceptives may cause glucose intolerance. Retinal thrombosis has been reported (rarely). Use with caution in patients with renal disease, conditions that may be aggravated by fluid retention, depression, or history of migraine. Not for use prior to menarche.

The minimum dosage combination of estrogen/progestin that will effectively treat the individual patient should be used. New patients should be started on products containing <50 mcg of estrogen per tablet.

Acne: For use only in females ≥15 years, who also desire combination hormonal contraceptive therapy, are unresponsive to topical treatments, and have no contraindications to combination hormonal contraceptive use; treatment must continue for at least 6 months.

Drug Interactions

Cytochrome P450 Effect: Ethinyl estradiol: Substrate of **CYP3A4**, 3A5-7; Inhibits CYP1A2, 2B6, 2C19, 3A4

Decreased Effect: Combination hormonal contraceptives may decrease plasma levels of acetaminophen, clofibric acid, lorazepam, morphine, oxazepam, salicylic acid, temazepam. Contraceptive effect decreased by acitretin, aminoglutethimide, amprenavir, anticonvulsants, griseofulvin, lopinavir, nelfinavir, nevirapine, penicillins (effect not consistent), rifampin, ritonavir, tetracyclines (effect not consistent). Combination hormonal contraceptives may decrease (or increase) the effects of coumarin derivatives.

Increased Effect/Toxicity: Acetaminophen and ascorbic acid may increase plasma levels of estrogen component. Atorvastatin and indinavir increase plasma levels of combination hormonal contraceptives. Combination hormonal contraceptives increase the plasma levels of alprazolam, chlordiazepoxide, cyclosporine, diazepam, prednisolone, selegiline, theophylline, tricyclic antidepressants. Combination hormonal contraceptives may increase (or decrease) the effects of coumarin derivatives.

Nutritional/Ethanol Interactions

Food: CNS effects of caffeine may be enhanced if combination hormonal contraceptives are used concurrently with caffeine. Grapefruit juice increases ethinyl estradiol concentrations and would be expected to increase progesterone serum levels as well; clinical implications are unclear.

Herb/Nutraceutical: St John's wort may decrease the effectiveness of combination hormonal contraceptives by inducing hepatic enzymes. Avoid dong quai and black cohosh (have estrogen activity). Avoid saw palmetto, red clover, ginseng.

Effects on Lab Values ↑ amylase (S), cholesterol (S), iron (B), sodium (S), thyroxine (S); ↓ calcium (S), protein, prothrombin time

Adverse Reactions Frequency not defined.

Cardiovascular: Arterial thromboembolism, cerebral hemorrhage, cerebral thrombosis, edema, hypertension, mesenteric thrombosis, myocardial infarction

Central nervous system: Depression, dizziness, headache, migraine, nervousness, premenstrual syndrome, stroke

Dermatologic: Acne, erythema multiforme, erythema nodosum, hirsutism, loss of scalp hair, melasma (may persist), rash (allergic)

Endocrine & metabolic: Amenorrhea, breakthrough bleeding, breast enlargement, breast secretion, breast tenderness, carbohydrate intolerance, lactation decreased (postpartum), glucose tolerance decreased, libido changes, menstrual flow changes, sex hormone-binding globulins (SHBG) increased, spotting, temporary infertility (following discontinuation), thyroid-binding globulin increased, triglycerides increased

Gastrointestinal: Abdominal cramps, appetite changes, bloating, cholestasis, colitis, gallbladder disease, jaundice, nausea, vomiting, weight gain/loss

Genitourinary: Cervical erosion changes, cervical secretion changes, cystitis-like syndrome, vaginal candidiasis, vaginitis

Hematologic: Antithrombin III decreased, folate levels decreased, hemolytic uremic syndrome, norepinephrine induced platelet aggregability increased, porphyria, prothrombin increased; factors VII, VIII, IX, and X increased

Hepatic: Benign liver tumors, Budd-Chiari syndrome, cholestatic jaundice, hepatic adenomas

Local: Thrombophlebitis

Ocular: Cataracts, change in corneal curvature (steepening), contact lens intolerance, optic neuritis, retinal thrombosis

Renal: Impaired renal function

Respiratory: Pulmonary thromboembolism

Miscellaneous: Hemorrhagic eruption

(Continued)

Ethinyl Estradiol and Norgestimate *(Continued)*

Overdosage/Toxicology Toxicity is unlikely following single exposures of excessive doses. May cause withdrawal bleeding in females. Any treatment following emesis and charcoal administration should be supportive and symptomatic.

Pharmacokinetic Note See Ethinyl Estradiol monograph.

Pharmacodynamics/Kinetics

Absorption:

Norgestimate: Well absorbed

Half-Life Elimination:

Norgestimate: 17-deacetylnorgestimate: 12-30 hours

Metabolism:

Norgestimate: Hepatic; forms 17-deacetylnorgestimate (major active metabolite) and other metabolites

Formulations Tablet:

Monophasic formulation (Ortho-Cyclen®): Ethinyl estradiol 0.035 mg and norgestimate 0.25 mg [21 blue tablets and 7 green inactive tablets] (28s)

Triphasic formulations:

Ortho Tri-Cyclen®:

Day 1-7: Ethinyl estradiol 0.035 mg and norgestimate 0.18 mg [7 white tablets]
Day 8-14: Ethinyl estradiol 0.035 mg and norgestimate 0.215 mg [7 light blue tablets]
Day 15-21: Ethinyl estradiol 0.035 mg and norgestimate 0.25 mg [7 blue tablets]
Day 22-28: 7 green inactive tablets (28s)

Ortho Tri-Cyclen® Lo:

Day 1-7: Ethinyl estradiol 0.025 mg and norgestimate 0.18 mg [7 white tablets]
Day 8-14: Ethinyl estradiol 0.025 mg and norgestimate 0.215 mg [7 light blue tablets]
Day 15-21: Ethinyl estradiol 0.025 mg and norgestimate 0.25 mg [7 dark blue tablets]
Day 22-28: 7 green inactive tablets (28s)

Dosing

Adults: Female:

Acne (Ortho Tri-Cyclen®): Oral: Refer to dosing for contraception

Contraception: Oral:

Schedule 1 (Sunday starter): Dose begins on first Sunday after onset of menstruation; if the menstrual period starts on Sunday, take first tablet that very same day. **With a Sunday start, an additional method of contraception should be used until after the first 7 days of consecutive administration.**

For 21-tablet package: Dosage is 1 tablet daily for 21 consecutive days, followed by 7 days off of the medication; a new course begins on the 8th day after the last tablet is taken.

For 28-tablet package: Dosage is 1 tablet daily without interruption.

Schedule 2 (Day 1 starter): Dose starts on first day of menstrual cycle taking 1 tablet daily.

For 21-tablet package: Dosage is 1 tablet daily for 21 consecutive days, followed by 7 days off of the medication; a new course begins on the 8th day after the last tablet is taken.

For 28-tablet package: Dosage is 1 tablet daily without interruption.

If all doses have been taken on schedule and one menstrual period is missed, continue dosing cycle. If two consecutive menstrual periods are missed, pregnancy test is required before new dosing cycle is started.

Missed doses **monophasic formulations** (refer to package insert for complete information):

One dose missed: Take as soon as remembered or take 2 tablets next day

Two consecutive doses missed in the first 2 weeks: Take 2 tablets as soon as remembered or 2 tablets next 2 days. **An additional method of contraception should be used for 7 days after missed dose.**

Two consecutive doses missed in week 3 or three consecutive doses missed at any time: **An additional method of contraception must be used for 7 days after a missed dose:**

Schedule 1 (Sunday starter): Continue dose of 1 tablet daily until Sunday, then discard the rest of the pack, and a new pack should be started that same day.

Schedule 2 (Day 1 starter): Current pack should be discarded, and a new pack should be started that same day.

Missed doses **biphasic/triphasic formulations** (refer to package insert for complete information):

One dose missed: Take as soon as remembered or take 2 tablets next day.

Two consecutive doses missed in week 1 or week 2 of the pack: Take 2 tablets as soon as remembered and 2 tablets the next day. Resume taking 1 tablet daily until the pack is empty. **An additional method of contraception must be used for 7 days after a missed dose.**

Two consecutive doses missed in week 3 of the pack. **An additional method of contraception must be used for 7 days after a missed dose.**

Schedule 1 (Sunday starter): Take 1 tablet every day until Sunday. Discard the remaining pack and start a new pack of pills on the same day.

Schedule 2 (Day 1 starter): Discard the remaining pack and start a new pack the same day.

Three or more consecutive doses missed. **An additional method of contraception must be used for 7 days after a missed dose.**

Schedule 1 (Sunday starter): Take 1 tablet every day until Sunday; on Sunday, discard the pack and start a new pack.

Schedule 2 (Day 1 starter): Discard the remaining pack and begin new pack of tablets starting on the same day.

Pediatrics: Female:

Acne: Oral: Children ≥15 years; refer to adult dosing for contraception

Contraception: Oral: Refer to adult dosing; not to be used prior to menarche.

Renal Impairment: Specific guidelines not available; use with caution.

Hepatic Impairment: Contraindicated in patients with hepatic impairment.

Administration

Oral: Administer at the same time each day.

Stability

Storage: Store at controlled room temperature of 25°C (77°F).

Monitoring and Teaching Issues

Physical Assessment: Assess for adverse reactions and potential drug interactions. Emphasize importance of regular (monthly) blood pressure checks and annual physical assessment, Pap smear, and vision assessment. Teach importance of maintaining prescribed schedule of dosing (see Dosing for dosing and missed dose information). **Pregnancy risk factor X** - do not use if patient is pregnant. Breast-feeding is not recommended.

Patient Education: Oral contraceptives do not protect against HIV or other sexually-transmitted diseases. Take exactly as directed by prescriber (also see package insert). You are at risk of becoming pregnant if doses are missed. Detailed and complete information on dosing and missed doses can be found in the package insert. Be aware that some medications may reduce the effectiveness of oral contraceptives; an alternate form of contraception may be needed. Check all medicines (prescription and OTC), herbal, and alternative products with prescriber. It is important that you check your blood pressure monthly (on same day each month) and that you have an annual physical assessment, Pap smear, and vision assessment while taking this medication. Avoid smoking while taking this medication; smoking increases risk of adverse effects, including thromboembolic events and heart attacks. You may experience loss of appetite (small, frequent meals will help); or constipation (increased exercise, fluids, fruit, fiber, or stool softeners may help). If diabetic, use accurate serum glucose testing to identify any changes in glucose tolerance; notify prescriber of significant changes so antidiabetic medication can be adjusted if necessary. Report immediately pain or muscle soreness; warmth, swelling, pain, or redness in calves; shortness of breath; sudden loss of vision; unresolved leg/ foot swelling; change in menstrual pattern (unusual bleeding, amenorrhea, breakthrough spotting); breast tenderness that does not go away; acute abdominal cramping; signs of vaginal infection (drainage, pain, itching); CNS changes (blurred vision, confusion, acute anxiety, or unresolved depression); or significant weight gain (>5 lb/week). Notify prescriber of changes in contact lens tolerance. **Pregnancy/breast-feeding precautions:** This medication should not be used during pregnancy. If you suspect you may become pregnant, contact prescriber immediately. Breast-feeding is not recommended.

Dietary Issues: Should be taken at same time each day.

Breast-feeding Issues: Jaundice and breast enlargement in the nursing infant have been reported following the use of combination hormonal contraceptives. May decrease the quality and quantity of breast milk; a nonhormonal form of contraception is recommended.

Pregnancy Issues: Pregnancy should be ruled out prior to treatment and discontinued if pregnancy occurs. In general, the use of combination hormonal contraceptives when inadvertently taken early in pregnancy have not been associated with teratogenic effects. Due to increased risk of thromboembolism postpartum, combination hormonal contraceptives should not be started earlier than 4-6 weeks following delivery.

Related Information

Ethinyl Estradiol *on page 514*

Ethiofos *see* Amifostine *on page 74*

Ethmozine® *see* Moricizine *on page 925*

Ethosuximide (eth oh SUKS i mide)

U.S. Brand Names Zarontin®

Generic Available Yes

Pharmacologic Category Anticonvulsant, Succinimide

Pregnancy Risk Factor C

Lactation Enters breast milk/compatible

Use Management of absence (petit mal) seizures

Mechanism of Action/Effect Increases the seizure threshold and suppresses paroxysmal spike-and-wave pattern in absence seizures; depresses nerve transmission in the motor cortex

Contraindications Hypersensitivity to succinimides or any component of the formulation

Warnings/Precautions Use with caution in patients with hepatic or renal disease; abrupt withdrawal of the drug may precipitate absence status; ethosuximide may increase tonic-clonic seizures in patients with mixed seizure disorders; ethosuximide must be used in combination with other anticonvulsants in patients with both absence and tonic-clonic seizures. Succinimides have been associated with severe blood dyscrasias and cases of systemic lupus erythematosus. Consider evaluation of blood counts in patients with signs/ symptoms of infection. Safety and efficacy in patients <3 years of age have not been established. Pregnancy risk C.

Drug Interactions

Cytochrome P450 Effect: Substrate of **CYP3A4**

Decreased Effect: Enzyme inducers (phenobarbital, rifampin, phenytoin, valproic acid) may decrease levels of ethosuximide.

Increased Effect/Toxicity: Isoniazid may inhibit hepatic metabolism of ethosuximide with a resultant increase in ethosuximide serum concentrations. Ethosuximide may elevate phenytoin levels. Valproate acid has been reported to both increase and decrease ethosuximide levels.

Nutritional/Ethanol Interactions

Ethanol: Avoid ethanol (may increase CNS depression).

Herb/Nutraceutical: St John's wort may decrease ethosuximide levels.

Effects on Lab Values ↑ alkaline phosphatase (S); positive Coombs' [direct]; ↓ calcium (S)

Adverse Reactions Frequency not defined.

(Continued)

Ethosuximide *(Continued)*

Central nervous system: Ataxia, drowsiness, sedation, dizziness, lethargy, euphoria, headache, irritability, hyperactivity, fatigue, night terrors, disturbance in sleep, inability to concentrate, aggressiveness, mental depression (with cases of overt suicidal intentions), paranoid psychosis

Dermatologic: Stevens-Johnson syndrome, SLE, rash, hirsutism

Endocrine & metabolic: Increased libido

Gastrointestinal: Weight loss, gastric upset, cramps, epigastric pain, diarrhea, nausea, vomiting, anorexia, abdominal pain, gum hypertrophy, tongue swelling

Genitourinary: Vaginal bleeding, microscopic hematuria

Hematologic: Leukopenia, agranulocytosis, pancytopenia, eosinophilia

Ocular: Myopia

Miscellaneous: Hiccups

Overdosage/Toxicology Acute overdose can cause CNS depression, ataxia, stupor, coma, hypotension. Chronic overdose can cause skin rash, confusion, ataxia, proteinuria, hepatic dysfunction, and hematuria. Treatment is supportive. Hemoperfusion and hemodialysis may be useful.

Pharmacodynamics/Kinetics

Half-Life Elimination: Serum: Children: 30 hours; Adults: 50-60 hours

Time to Peak: Serum: Capsule: ~2-4 hours; Syrup: <2-4 hours

Metabolism: Hepatic (~80% to 3 inactive metabolites)

Formulations

Capsule: 250 mg

Syrup: 250 mg/5 mL (473 mL) [contains sodium benzoate; raspberry flavor]

Dosing

Adults & Elderly: Management of absence (petit mal) seizures: Oral: Initial: 250 mg twice daily; increase by 250 mg as needed every 4-7 days up to 1.5 g/day in 2 divided doses; usual maintenance dose: 20-40 mg/kg/day in 2 divided doses

Pediatrics: Absence (petit mal) seizures: Oral:

Children 3-6 years: Initial: 250 mg/day (or 15 mg/kg/day) in 2 divided doses; increase every 4-7 days; usual maintenance dose: 15-40 mg/kg/day in 2 divided doses.

Children >6 years: Refer to adult dosing.

Renal Impairment: Use with caution.

Hepatic Impairment: Use with caution.

Administration

Oral: Administer with food or milk to avoid GI upset.

Monitoring Laboratory Tests Trough serum concentrations, CBC, platelets, liver enzymes, urinalysis

Monitoring and Teaching Issues

Physical Assessment: Assess effectiveness and interactions of other medications patient may be taking (see Contraindications, Warnings/Precautions, and Drug Interactions). Monitor therapeutic response, laboratory values (see above), and adverse reactions (see Adverse Reactions) at beginning of therapy and periodically with long-term use. Observe and teach seizure/safety precautions. Taper dosage slowly when discontinuing. Assess knowledge/teach patient appropriate use, interventions to reduce side effects, and adverse symptoms to report (see Patient Education). **Pregnancy risk factor C** - benefits of use should outweigh possible risks.

Patient Education: Take exactly as directed; do not increase dose or frequency or discontinue without consulting prescriber. While using this medication, do not use alcohol and other prescription or OTC medications (especially pain medications, sedatives, antihistamines, or hypnotics) without consulting prescriber. Maintain adequate hydration (2-3 L/day of fluids) unless advised by prescriber to restrict fluids. You may experience drowsiness, dizziness, or blurred vision (use caution when driving or engaging in tasks requiring alertness until response to drug is known); nausea, vomiting, loss of appetite, or dry mouth (small, frequent meals, frequent mouth care, chewing gum, or sucking lozenges may help); or constipation (increased exercise, fluids, fruit, or fiber may help). Wear identification of epileptic status and medications. Report CNS changes, mentation changes, or changes in cognition; muscle cramping, weakness, tremors, or changes in gait; persistent GI symptoms (cramping, constipation, vomiting, anorexia); rash or skin irritations; unusual bruising or bleeding (mouth, urine, stool); or worsening of seizure activity or loss of seizure control. **Pregnancy precaution:** Inform prescriber if you are or intend to become pregnant.

Dietary Issues: Increase dietary intake of folate; may be administered with food or milk.

Geriatric Considerations: No specific studies with the use of this medication in the elderly. Consider renal function and proceed slowly with dosing increases; monitor closely.

Related Information

Peak and Trough Guidelines *on page 1544*

Seizure Treatment *on page 1700*

Ethoxynaphthamido Penicillin Sodium *see* Nafcillin *on page 941*

Ethyl Aminobenzoate *see* Benzocaine *on page 156*

Ethynodiol Diacetate and Ethinyl Estradiol *see* Ethinyl Estradiol and Ethynodiol Diacetate *on page 521*

Ethyol® *see* Amifostine *on page 74*

Etodolac (ee toe DOE lak)

U.S. Brand Names Lodine®; Lodine® XL

Synonyms Etodolic Acid

Generic Available Yes

Pharmacologic Category Nonsteroidal Anti-inflammatory Drug (NSAID)

Pregnancy Risk Factor C/D (3rd trimester)

Lactation Excretion in breast milk unknown/contraindicated

Use Acute and long-term use in the management of signs and symptoms of osteoarthritis and management of pain

Use - Unlabeled/Investigational Rheumatoid arthritis

Mechanism of Action/Effect Inhibits prostaglandin synthesis which results in decreased formation of prostaglandin precursors

Contraindications Hypersensitivity to etodolac, aspirin, other NSAIDs, or any component of the formulation; active gastric/duodenal ulcer disease; pregnancy (3rd trimester)

Warnings/Precautions Use with caution in patients with CHF, hypertension, dehydration, decreased renal or hepatic function, history of GI disease (bleeding or ulcers), or those receiving anticoagulants. Elderly are at a high risk for adverse effects from NSAIDs. As many as 60% of elderly can develop peptic ulceration and/or hemorrhage asymptomatically.

Use lowest effective dose for shortest period possible. Use of NSAIDs can compromise existing renal function especially when Cl_{cr} is <30 mL/minute. CNS adverse effects such as confusion, agitation, and hallucination are generally seen in overdose or high-dose situations; however, elderly may demonstrate these adverse effects at lower doses than younger adults. Withhold for at least 4-6 half-lives prior to surgical or dental procedures.

Pregnancy risk C/D (3rd trimester)

Drug Interactions

Decreased Effect: Decreased effect with aspirin. May reduce effect of some diuretics and antihypertensive effect of β-blockers.

Increased Effect/Toxicity: Etodolac may increase effect/toxicity of aspirin (GI irritation), lithium, methotrexate, digoxin, cyclosporine (nephrotoxicity), and warfarin (bleeding).

Nutritional/Ethanol Interactions

Ethanol: Avoid ethanol (may enhance gastric mucosal irritation).

Food: Etodolac peak serum levels may be decreased if taken with food.

Herb/Nutraceutical: Avoid cat's claw, dong quai, evening primrose, feverfew, garlic, ginger, ginkgo, red clover, horse chestnut, green tea, ginseng (all have additional antiplatelet activity)

Effects on Lab Values False-positive for urinary bilirubin and ketone increase bleeding time. Etodolac may cause a lowering of serum uric acid levels.

Adverse Reactions

1% to 10%:

Central nervous system: Depression (1% to 3%)

Dermatologic: Rash (1% to 3%), pruritus (1% to 3%)

Gastrointestinal: Abdominal cramps (3% to 9%), nausea (3% to 9%), vomiting (1% to 3%), dyspepsia (10%), diarrhea (3% to 9%), constipation (1% to 3%), flatulence (3% to 9%), melena (1% to 3%), gastritis (1% to 3%)

Genitourinary: Polyuria (1% to 3%)

Neuromuscular & skeletal: Weakness (3% to 9%)

Ocular: Blurred vision (1% to 3%)

Otic: Tinnitus (1% to 3%)

<1% (Limited to important or life-threatening): Acute renal failure, agranulocytosis, anemia, angioedema, arrhythmia, bone marrow suppression, CHF, dyspnea, erythema multiforme, exfoliative dermatitis, hemolytic anemia, hepatitis, hypertension, leukopenia, peripheral neuropathy, Stevens-Johnson syndrome, syncope, tachycardia, thrombocytopenia, toxic amblyopia, toxic epidermal necrolysis, urticaria

Overdosage/Toxicology Symptoms of overdose include acute renal failure, vomiting, drowsiness, leukocytosis. Management of NSAID intoxication is supportive and symptomatic.

Pharmacodynamics/Kinetics

Absorption: Well absorbed

Half-Life Elimination: 7 hours

Time to Peak: Serum: 1 hour

Metabolism: Hepatic

Onset: Analgesic: 2-4 hours; Maximum anti-inflammatory effect: A few days

Formulations

Capsule (Lodine®): 200 mg, 300 mg

Tablet (Lodine®): 400 mg, 500 mg

Tablet, extended release (Lodine® XL): 400 mg, 500 mg, 600 mg

Dosing

Adults:

Acute pain: Oral: 200-400 mg every 6-8 hours, as needed, not to exceed total daily doses of 1200 mg; for patients weighing <60 kg, total daily dose should not exceed 20 mg/kg/day.

Osteoarthritis and rheumatoid arthritis: Oral: Initial: 800-1200 mg/day given in divided doses: 400 mg 2 or 3 times/day; 300 mg 2, 3 or 4 times/day; 200 mg 3 or 4 times/day; total daily dose should not exceed 1200 mg; for patients weighing <60 kg, total daily dose should not exceed 20 mg/kg/day.

Lodine® XL: 400-1000 mg once daily

Note: A single dose of 76-100 mg is comparable to the analgesic effect of aspirin 650 mg

Elderly: In patients ≥65 years, no substantial differences in the pharmacokinetics or side-effects profile were seen compared with the general population.

Stability

Storage: Protect from moisture.

Monitoring Laboratory Tests CBC, liver enzymes; in patients receiving diuretics, monitor BUN/serum creatinine.

Monitoring and Teaching Issues

Physical Assessment: Systemic: Assess effectiveness and interactions of other medications patient may be taking (see Drug Interactions). See Warnings/Precautions and Contraindications for use cautions. Monitor laboratory tests (see above) and therapeutic and adverse reactions at beginning of therapy and periodically throughout therapy (see Warnings/Precautions, Adverse Reactions, and Overdose/Toxicology). Assess knowledge/teach patient appropriate use, interventions to reduce side effects, and adverse symptoms to

(Continued)

Etodolac *(Continued)*

report (see Patient Education). **Pregnancy risk factor C/D** - see Pregnancy Risk Factor for use cautions; benefits of use should outweigh possible risks. Breast-feeding is contraindicated.

Patient Education: Take this medication exactly as directed; do not increase dose without consulting prescriber. Do not crush tablets or break capsules. Take with food or milk to reduce GI distress. Maintain adequate hydration (2-3 L/day of fluids) unless advised by prescriber to restrict fluids. Do not use alcohol, aspirin or aspirin-containing medication, or any other anti-inflammatory medications without consulting prescriber. You may experience anorexia, nausea, vomiting, or heartburn (small, frequent meals, frequent mouth care, sucking lozenges, or chewing gum may help); drowsiness, dizziness, nervousness, or headache (use caution when driving or engaging in tasks requiring alertness until response to drug is known); or fluid retention (weigh yourself weekly and report unusual (3-5 lb/week) weight gain). GI bleeding, ulceration, or perforation can occur with or without pain; discontinue medication and contact prescriber if persistent abdominal pain or cramping, or blood in stool occurs. Report breathlessness, difficulty breathing, or unusual cough; chest pain, rapid heartbeat, palpitations; unusual bruising/bleeding; blood in urine, stool, mouth, or vomitus; swollen extremities; skin rash or itching; acute fatigue; or hearing changes (ringing in ears). **Pregnancy/breast-feeding precautions:** Inform prescriber if you are or intend to become pregnant. This drug should not be used in the 3rd trimester of pregnancy. Do not breast-feed.

Dietary Issues: May be taken with food to decrease GI distress.

Geriatric Considerations: Elderly are at high risk for adverse effects from NSAIDs. As much as 60% of elderly who experience GI side effects can develop peptic ulceration and/or hemorrhage asymptomatically.

Related Information

Nonsalicylate/Nonsteroidal Anti-inflammatory Comparison *on page 1587*

Etodolic Acid *see* Etodolac *on page 534*

Etopophos® *see* Etoposide Phosphate *on page 538*

Etoposide (e toe POE side)

U.S. Brand Names Toposar®; VePesid®

Synonyms Epipodophyllotoxin; VP-16; VP-16-213

Generic Available Yes

Pharmacologic Category Antineoplastic Agent, Podophyllotoxin Derivative

Pregnancy Risk Factor D

Lactation Enters breast milk/contraindicated

Use Treatment of lymphomas, ANLL, lung, testicular, bladder, and prostate carcinoma, hepatoma, rhabdomyosarcoma, uterine carcinoma, neuroblastoma, mycosis fungoides, Kaposi's sarcoma, histiocytosis, gestational trophoblastic disease, Ewing's sarcoma, Wilms' tumor, and brain tumors

Mechanism of Action/Effect Inhibits DNA synthesis leading to cell death.

Contraindications Hypersensitivity to etoposide or any component of the formulation; **intrathecal administration**; pregnancy

Warnings/Precautions The U.S. Food and Drug Administration (FDA) currently recommends that procedures for proper handling and disposal of antineoplastic agents be considered. Severe myelosuppression with resulting infection or bleeding may occur. Administer I.V. infusions over a period of at least 30-60 minutes. **Must be diluted - do not give IVP.** Dosage should be adjusted in patients with hepatic or renal impairment.

If etoposide contacts the skin, wash and flush thoroughly with water.

Drug Interactions

Cytochrome P450 Effect: Substrate of CYP1A2, 2E1, **3A4**; Inhibits CYP2C8/9, 3A4

Increased Effect/Toxicity: The effects of etoposide may be increased by calcium antagonists (increased effects noted *in vitro*). Cyclosporine may increase the levels of etoposide. Etoposide may increase the effects/toxicity of methotrexate and warfarin. There have been reports of frequent hepatic dysfunction with hyperbilirubinemia, ascites, and thrombocytopenia when etoposide is combined with carmustine.

Nutritional/Ethanol Interactions

Ethanol: Avoid ethanol (may increase GI irritation).

Food: Administration of food does not affect GI absorption with doses ≤200 mg of injection.

Herb/Nutraceutical: St John's wort may decrease etoposide levels.

Adverse Reactions

>10%:

- Dermatologic: Alopecia (reversible)
- Gastrointestinal: Diarrhea, nausea, vomiting severe mucositis (with BMT doses), anorexia
  - Emetic potential: Moderately low (10% to 30%)
- Hematologic: Anemia, leukopenia
  - WBC: Mild to severe
  - Platelets: Mild
  - Onset (days): 10
  - Nadir (days): granulocytes 7-14 days; platelets 9-16 days
  - Recovery (days): 21-28

1% to 10%:

- Cardiovascular: Hypotension: Related to drug infusion time; may be related to vehicle used in the I.V. preparation (polysorbate 80 plus polyethylene glycol). Best to administer the drug over 1 hour.
- Central nervous system: Unusual fatigue
- Gastrointestinal: Stomatitis, diarrhea, abdominal pain, hepatitic dysfunction

<1% (Limited to important or life-threatening): Tachycardia, neurotoxicity, peripheral neuropathy, toxic hepatitis (with high-dose therapy), flushing and bronchospasm (may be prevented by pretreatment with corticosteroids and antihistamines)

Irritant, thrombophlebitis has been reported

BMT:

Cardiovascular: Hypotension (infusion-related)
Dermatologic: Skin lesions resembling Stevens-Johnson syndrome, alopecia
Endocrine & metabolic: Metabolic acidosis
Gastrointestinal: Severe nausea and vomiting, mucositis
Hepatic: Hepatitis
Miscellaneous: Secondary malignancy, ethanol intoxication

Overdosage/Toxicology Symptoms of overdose include bone marrow suppression, leukopenia, thrombocytopenia, nausea, and vomiting. Treatment is supportive.

Pharmacodynamics/Kinetics

Absorption: Oral: 25% to 75%; significant inter- and intrapatient variation

Half-Life Elimination: Terminal: 4-15 hours; Children: Normal renal/hepatic function: 6-8 hours

Time to Peak: Serum: Oral: 1-1.5 hours

Metabolism: Hepatic to hydroxy acid and cislactone metabolites

Formulations

Capsule (VePesid®): 50 mg
Injection, solution: 20 mg/mL (5 mL, 25 mL, 50 mL) [contains benzyl alcohol]
Toposar®: 20 mg/mL (5 mL, 10 mL, 25 mL) [contains benzyl alcohol]
VePesid®: 20 mg/mL (5 mL, 7.5 mL, 25 mL, 50 mL) [contains benzyl alcohol

Dosing

Adults & Elderly: Refer to individual protocols.

Small cell lung cancer:
Oral: Twice the I.V. dose rounded to the nearest 50 mg given once daily if total dose ≤400 mg or in divided doses if >400 mg
I.V.: 35 mg/m^2/day for 4 days or 50 mg/m^2/day for 5 days every 3-4 weeks total dose ≤400 mg/day or in divided doses if >400 mg/day
IVPB: 200-250 mg/m^2 repeated every 7 weeks
Continuous intravenous infusion: 500 mg/m^2 over 24 hours every 3 weeks

Testicular cancer:
IVPB: 50-100 mg/m^2/day for 5 days repeated every 3-4 weeks
I.V.: 100 mg/m^2 every other day for 3 doses repeated every 3-4 weeks

BMT/relapsed leukemia: I.V.: 2.4-3.5 g/m^2 or 25-70 mg/kg administered over 4-36 hours
BMT high dose: I.V.: 750-2400 mg/m^2; 10-60 mg/kg; duration of infusion is 1-4 hours to 24 hours; generally combined with other high-dose chemotherapeutic drugs or total body irradiation (TBI).

Pediatrics: Refer to individual protocols.

Children: I.V.: 60-120 mg/m^2/day for 3-5 days every 3-6 weeks
AML: I.V.:
Remission induction: 150 mg/m^2/day for 2-3 days for 2-3 cycles
Intensification or consolidation: 250 mg/m^2/day for 3 days, courses 2-5
Brain tumor: I.V.: 150 mg/m^2/day on days 2 and 3 of treatment course
Neuroblastoma: I.V.: 100 mg/m^2/day over 1 hour on days 1-5 of cycle; repeat cycle every 4 weeks
BMT conditioning regimen used in patients with rhabdomyosarcoma or neuroblastoma: I.V. continuous infusion: 160 mg/m^2/day for 4 days
Conditioning regimen for allogenic BMT: I.V.: 60 mg/kg/dose as a single dose

Renal Impairment:

Cl_{cr} 10-50 mL/minute: Administer 75% of normal dose.
Cl_{cr} <10 mL minute: Administer 50% of normal dose.
Hemodialysis effects: Supplemental dose is not necessary.
CAPD effects: Unknown
CAVH effects: Unknown

Hepatic Impairment:

Bilirubin 1.5-3 mg/dL or AST 60-180 units: Reduce dose by 50%.
Bilirubin >3 mg/dL or AST >180 units: Reduce by 75%.

Administration

I.M.: Do not administer I.V. or S.C. (severe tissue necrosis).

I.V.: Irritant. Administer lower doses IVPB over at least 30 minutes to minimize the risk of hypotensive reactions.

Stability

Storage: Store intact vials of injection at room temperature and protected from light. Injection solution contains polyethylene glycol vehicle with absolute alcohol. Store oral capsules under refrigeration. Capsules are stable for 3 months at room temperature.

Reconstitution: VP-16 should be further diluted in D_5W or NS for administration. Diluted solutions have concentration-dependent stability: More concentrated solutions have shorter stability times.

At room temperature in D_5W or NS in polyvinyl chloride, the concentration is stable as follows:
0.2 mg/mL: 96 hours
0.4 mg/mL: 48 hours
0.6 mg/mL: 8 hours
1 mg/mL: 2 hours
2 mg/mL: 1 hour
20 mg/mL (undiluted): 24 hours

Standard I.V. dilution:

Lower dose regimens (<1 g/dose):

Doses may be diluted in 100-1000 mL of D_5W or NS
If the concentration is less than or equal to 0.6 mg/mL, the bag should be mixed with the appropriate expiration dating.
If the concentration is >0.6 mg/mL, the concentration is highly unstable and a syringe of undiluted etoposide accompanied with the appropriate volume of diluent will be sent to the nursing unit to be mixed at the bedside just prior to administration.

(Continued)

Etoposide *(Continued)*

High-dose regimens (>1g/dose):

Total dose should be drawn into an empty Viaflex® container and the appropriate amount of diluent (for a final concentration of 1 mg/mL) will be sent.

Use the **2-Channel Pump Method**: Instill all of the etoposide dose into one Viaflex® container (concentration = 20 mg/mL). Infuse this into one channel (Baxter Flow-Guard 6300 Dual Channel Volumetric Infusion Pump - or any 2-channel infusion pump that does not require a "hard" plastic cassette). Infuse the indicated diluent (ie, D_5W or NS) at a rate of at least 20 times the infusion rate of the etoposide to simulate a 1 mg/mL concentration in the line. The etoposide should be Y-sited into the port most proximal to the patient. A 0.22 micron filter should be attached to the line after the Y-site and before entry into the patient.

Compatibility: Stable in D_5W, LR

Y-site administration: Incompatible with cefepime, filgrastim, idarubicin

Monitoring Laboratory Tests CBC with differential, platelet count, bilirubin, renal function

Monitoring and Teaching Issues

Physical Assessment: See Contraindications, Warnings/Precautions, and Dosing for use cautions. Assess potential for interactions with other prescriptions, OTC medications, or herbal products patient may be taking (see Drug Interactions). See specific Administration, Dosing, Reconstitution, and Compatibility directions. Infusion site should be monitored closely to prevent extravasation (see Administration). Assess results of laboratory tests (see above), therapeutic effects, and adverse response (see Adverse Reactions) prior to each treatment and on a regular basis throughout therapy. Teach patient possible side effects and appropriate interventions and adverse symptoms to report (see Patient Education). **Pregnancy risk factor D** - determine that patient is not pregnant before beginning treatment. Instruct patients of childbearing age about appropriate barrier contraceptive measures. Breast-feeding contraindicated.

Patient Education: Inform prescriber of all prescriptions, OTC medications, or herbal products you are taking, and any allergies you have. Do not take anything new during treatment unless approved by prescriber. This medication may be administered by infusion. Report immediately any swelling, pain, burning, or redness at infusion site. Avoid alcohol. It is important to maintain adequate hydration (2-3 L/day of fluids) unless advised by prescriber to restrict fluids, and adequate nutrition (small, frequent meals may help). You will be more susceptible to infection (avoid crowds and exposure to infection and do not have any vaccinations without consulting prescriber). May cause nausea or vomiting (small, frequent meals, frequent mouth care, sucking lozenges, or chewing gum may help); diarrhea (buttermilk, boiled milk, or yogurt may help); loss of hair (reversible); or mouth sores (use soft toothbrush or cotton swabs for oral care and rinse mouth frequently). Report immediately chest pain, swelling of extremities, difficulty breathing, palpitations, or rapid heartbeat. Report extreme fatigue, pain or numbness in extremities, severe GI upset or diarrhea, bleeding or bruising, fever, chills, sore throat, vaginal discharge, difficulty breathing, yellowing of eyes or skin, or any changes in color of urine or stool. **Pregnancy/breast-feeding precautions:** Do not get pregnant while taking this medication. Consult prescriber for appropriate contraceptive measures to use during and for 1 month following therapy. Do not breast-feed.

Etoposide Phosphate (e toe POE side FOS fate)

U.S. Brand Names Etopophos®

Generic Available No

Pharmacologic Category Antineoplastic Agent, Podophyllotoxin Derivative

Pregnancy Risk Factor D

Lactation Enters breast milk/contraindicated

Use Treatment of refractory testicular tumors and small cell lung cancer

Mechanism of Action/Effect Etoposide phosphate is converted *in vivo* to the active moiety, etoposide, by dephosphorylation. Etoposide inhibits mitotic activity; inhibits cells from entering prophase; inhibits DNA synthesis. Initially thought to be mitotic inhibitors similar to podophyllotoxin, but actually have no effect on microtubule assembly. However, later shown to induce DNA strand breakage and inhibition of topoisomerase II (an enzyme which breaks and repairs DNA); etoposide acts in late S or early G2 phases.

Contraindications Hypersensitivity to etoposide, etoposide phosphate, or any component of the formulation; **intrathecal administration**; pregnancy

Warnings/Precautions The U.S. Food and Drug Administration (FDA) currently recommends that procedures for proper handling and disposal of antineoplastic agents be considered. Severe myelosuppression with resulting infection or bleeding may occur. Dosage should be adjusted in patients with hepatic or renal impairment.

If etoposide phosphate contacts the skin, wash and flush thoroughly with water.

Drug Interactions

Cytochrome P450 Effect: Substrate of CYP1A2, 2E1, **3A4**; Inhibits CYP2C8/9, 3A4

Increased Effect/Toxicity: Etoposide taken with warfarin may result in prolongation of bleeding times. Alteration of MTX transport has been found as a slow efflux of MTX and its polyglutamated form out of the cell, leading to intercellular accumulation of MTX. Calcium antagonists increase the rate of VP-16-induced DNA damage and cytotoxicity *in vitro*. Use with carmustine has shown reports of frequent hepatic dysfunction with hyperbilirubinemia, ascites, and thrombocytopenia. Cyclosporine may cause additive cytotoxic effects on tumor cells.

Nutritional/Ethanol Interactions

Ethanol: Avoid ethanol (may increase GI irritation).

Food: Administration of food does not affect GI absorption with doses ≤200 mg of injection.

Herb/Nutraceutical: St John's wort may decrease etoposide levels.

Adverse Reactions

>10%:

Dermatologic: Alopecia (reversible)

Gastrointestinal: Occasional diarrhea and infrequent nausea and vomiting at standard doses; severe mucositis occurs with high (BMT) doses, anorexia

Emetic potential: Moderately low (10% to 30%)

Hematologic: Myelosuppressive:

WBC: Mild to severe

Platelets: Mild

Onset (days): 10

Nadir (days): granulocytes 7-14 days; platelets 9-16 days

Recovery (days): 21-28

1% to 10%:

Cardiovascular: Hypotension: Related to drug infusion time; may be related to vehicle used in the I.V. preparation (polysorbate 80 plus polyethylene glycol)

Central nervous system: Unusual fatigue

Gastrointestinal: Stomatitis, abdominal pain, hepatic dysfunction

<1% (Limited to important or life-threatening): Tachycardia, neurotoxicity, fever, toxic hepatitis (with high-dose therapy), peripheral neuropathy, flushing and bronchospasm (may be prevented by pretreatment with corticosteroids and antihistamines)

BMT: Gastrointestinal: Nausea, vomiting, mucositis

Overdosage/Toxicology Symptoms of overdose include bone marrow suppression, leukopenia, thrombocytopenia, nausea, and vomiting. Treatment is supportive.

Pharmacodynamics/Kinetics

Half-Life Elimination: Terminal: 4-15 hours; Children: Normal renal/hepatic function: 6-8 hours

Metabolism: Hepatic (with a biphasic decay)

Formulations Injection, powder for reconstitution, as base: 100 mg

Dosing

Adults & Elderly: Refer to individual protocols.

Small cell lung cancer: I.V. (in combination with other approved chemotherapeutic drugs): **Equivalent doses of etoposide phosphate to an etoposide dosage** range of 35 mg/m^2/day for 4 days to 50 mg/m^2/day for 5 days. Courses are repeated at 3- to 4-week intervals after adequate recovery from any toxicity.

Testicular cancer: I.V. (in combination with other approved chemotherapeutic agents): **Equivalent dose of etoposide phosphate to etoposide dosage** range of 50-100 mg/m^2/day on days 1-5 to 100 mg/m^2/day on days 1, 3, and 5. Courses are repeated at 3- to 4-week intervals after adequate recovery from any toxicity.

BMT high dose: I.V.: 0.5-2 g/m^2 in 2 divided doses; maximum single-dose agent: 3.2 g/m^2; generally combined with other high-dose chemotherapeutic drugs.

Renal Impairment:

Cl_{cr} 15-50 mL/minute: Administer 75% of normal dose.

Cl_{cr} <15 mL minute: Data is not available and further dose reduction should be considered in these patients.

Hemodialysis: Supplemental dose is not necessary.

Peritoneal dialysis: Supplemental dose is not necessary.

CAPD effects: Unknown

CAVH effects: Unknown

Hepatic Impairment:

Bilirubin 1.5-3 mg/dL or AST 60-180 units: Reduce dose dose by 50%.

Bilirubin 3-5 mg/dL or AST >180 units: Reduce dose by 75%.

Bilirubin >5 mg/dL: Do not administer.

Administration

I.V.: Etoposide phosphate solutions should be administered over 30-60 minutes.

Stability

Storage: Store intact vials of injection under refrigeration 2°C to 8°C (36°F to 46°F). Protect from light. Store capsules in refrigerator.

Reconstitution: Reconstituted vials with 5 mL or 10 mL SWI, D_5W, NS, bacteriostatic SWI, or bacteriostatic NS to a concentration of 20 mg/mL or 10 mg/mL etoposide (22.7 mg/mL or 11.4 mg/mL etoposide phosphate), respectively. These solutions may be administered without further dilution or may be further diluted to a concentration as low as 0.1 mg/mL etoposide with either D_5W or NS. Solutions are stable in glass or plastic containers at room temperature 20°C to 25°C (68°F to 77°F) or under refrigeration 2°C to 8°C (36°F to 47°F) for up to 24 hours.

Compatibility: Stable in D_5W, NS, sterile water for injection

Y-site administration: Incompatible with amphotericin B, cefepime, chlorpromazine, imipenem/cilastatin, methylprednisolone sodium succinate, mitomycin, prochlorperazine edisylate

Monitoring Laboratory Tests CBC with differential, platelet count, bilirubin, renal function

Monitoring and Teaching Issues

Physical Assessment: See Contraindications, Warnings/Precautions, and Dosing for use cautions. Assess potential for interactions with other prescriptions, OTC medications, or herbal products patient may be taking (see Drug Interactions). See specific Administration, Dosing, Reconstitution, and Compatibility directions. Infusion site should be monitored closely to prevent extravasation. Assess therapeutic response, results of laboratory tests (see above), and adverse response (see Adverse Reactions) prior to each treatment and on a regular basis throughout therapy. Teach patient possible side effects and appropriate interventions and adverse symptoms to report (see Patient Education). **Pregnancy risk factor D** - determine that patient is not pregnant before beginning treatment. Do not give to women of childbearing unless patient is capable of complying with barrier contraceptive measures during therapy and for 1 month following therapy. Breast-feeding is contraindicated.

Patient Education: Inform prescriber of all prescriptions, OTC medications, or herbal products you are taking, and any allergies you have. Do not take anything new during treatment unless approved by prescriber. This medication may be administered by infusion. Report immediately any swelling, pain, burning, or redness at infusion site. Avoid alcohol. It is important to maintain adequate hydration (2-3 L/day of fluids) unless advised

(Continued)

Etoposide Phosphate *(Continued)*

by prescriber to restrict fluids, and adequate nutrition (small, frequent meals may help). You will be more susceptible to infection (avoid crowds and exposure to infection and do not have any vaccinations without consulting prescriber). May cause nausea or vomiting (small, frequent meals, frequent mouth care, sucking lozenges, or chewing gum may help); diarrhea (buttermilk, boiled milk, or yogurt may help); loss of hair (reversible); or mouth sores (use soft toothbrush or cotton swabs for oral care and rinse mouth frequently). Report immediately chest pain, swelling of extremities, difficulty breathing, palpitations, or rapid heartbeat. Report extreme fatigue, pain or numbness in extremities, severe GI upset or diarrhea, bleeding or bruising, fever, chills, sore throat, vaginal discharge, difficulty breathing, yellowing of eyes or skin, or changes in color of urine or stool. **Pregnancy/breast-feeding precautions:** Do not get pregnant while taking this medication. Consult prescriber for appropriate barrier contraceptive measures to use during and for 1 month following therapy. Do not breast-feed.

Eudal®-SR *see* Guaifenesin and Pseudoephedrine *on page 648*

Eulexin® *see* Flutamide *on page 587*

Eurax® Topical *see* Crotamiton *on page 336*

Evista® *see* Raloxifene *on page 1169*

Evoxac™ *see* Cevimeline *on page 265*

Exelon® *see* Rivastigmine *on page 1200*

Exemestane (ex e MES tane)

U.S. Brand Names Aromasin®

Generic Available No

Pharmacologic Category Antineoplastic Agent, Miscellaneous

Pregnancy Risk Factor D

Lactation Excretion in breast milk unknown/not recommended

Use Treatment of advanced breast cancer in postmenopausal women whose disease has progressed following tamoxifen therapy

Mechanism of Action/Effect Exemestane prevents conversion of androgens to estrogens (Aromatase inhibitor) and lowers circulating estrogen levels.

Contraindications Hypersensitivity to exemestane or any component of the formulation; pregnancy

Warnings/Precautions Not indicated for premenopausal women; not to be given with estrogen-containing agents. Use with caution in hepatic impairment or renal insufficiency.

Drug Interactions

Cytochrome P450 Effect: Substrate of CYP3A4

Increased Effect/Toxicity: Although exemestane is a CYP3A4 substrate, ketoconazole, a CYP3A4 inhibitor, did not change the pharmacokinetics of exemestane. No other potential drug interactions have been evaluated.

Nutritional/Ethanol Interactions

Food: Plasma levels increased by 40% when exemestane was taken with a fatty meal.

Herb/Nutraceutical: St John's wort may decrease exemestane levels. Avoid black cohosh, dong quai in estrogen-dependent tumors.

Adverse Reactions

>10%:

- Central nervous system: Fatigue (22%), pain (13%), depression (13%), insomnia (11%), anxiety (10%)
- Endocrine & metabolic: Hot flashes (13%)
- Gastrointestinal: Nausea (18%)

1% to 10%:

- Cardiovascular: Edema (7%), hypertension (5%), chest pain
- Central nervous system: Dizziness (8%), headache (8%), fever (5%), hypoesthesia, confusion
- Dermatologic: Rash, itching, alopecia
- Gastrointestinal: Vomiting (7%), abdominal pain (6%), anorexia (6%), constipation (5%), diarrhea (4%), increased appetite (3%), dyspepsia
- Genitourinary: Urinary tract infection
- Neuromuscular & skeletal: Weakness, paresthesia, pathological fracture, arthralgia
- Respiratory: Dyspnea (10%), cough (6%), bronchitis, sinusitis, pharyngitis, rhinitis
- Miscellaneous: Influenza-like symptoms (6%), diaphoresis (6%), lymphedema, infection

<1% (Limited to important or life-threatening): GGT increased, transaminases increased,

A dose-dependent decrease in sex hormone-binding globulin has been observed with daily doses of 25 mg or more. Serum luteinizing hormone and follicle-stimulating hormone levels have increased with this medicine.

Overdosage/Toxicology Daily doses as high as 800 mg have been used in healthy volunteers and 600 mg for 12 weeks in postmenopausal women with advanced breast cancer. If an overdose should occur, general supportive care would be indicated.

Pharmacodynamics/Kinetics

Absorption: Rapid

Half-Life Elimination: 24 hours

Time to Peak: Women with breast cancer: 1.2 hours

Metabolism: Extensively hepatic; oxidation (CYP3A4) of methylene group, reduction of 17-keto group with formation of many secondary metabolites; metabolites are inactive or inhibit aromatase with decreased potency compared to parent drug

Formulations Tablet: 25 mg

Dosing

Adults & Elderly: Breast cancer: Oral: 25 mg once daily after a meal; treatment should continue until tumor progression is evident.

Renal Impairment: Safety of chronic dosing in renal impairment has not been established.

Hepatic Impairment: Safety of chronic dosing in hepatic impairment has not been established.

Stability

Storage: Store at 25°C (77°F)

Monitoring and Teaching Issues

Physical Assessment: See Contraindications, Warnings/Precautions, and Dosing for use cautions. Assess patient response (see Adverse Reactions and Overdose/Toxicology) prior to each treatment and on a regular basis throughout therapy. Teach patient proper use, possible side effects and interventions (eg, importance of adequate hydration), and adverse symptoms to report (see Patient Education). **Pregnancy risk factor D** - determine that patient is not pregnant before beginning treatment. Instruct patients of childbearing age on appropriate barrier contraceptive measures. Breast-feeding is not recommended.

Patient Education: Take exactly as directed, after meals, at same time each day. If you have any history of hypertension, you should check your blood pressure frequently and notify prescriber of significant changes. May cause headache, dizziness, confusion, fatigue, anxiety, or insomnia (use caution when driving or engaging in tasks requiring alertness until response to medication is known); nausea, vomiting, or loss of appetite (small, frequent meals, good mouth care, chewing gum, or sucking hard candy may help); or hot flashes (cool dark room or cold compresses may help). Report chest pain or palpitations; acute headache or visual disturbances; unresolved GI problems; itching or burning on urination or vaginal discharge; acute joint, back, bone, or muscle pain; difficulty breathing, unusual cough, or respiratory infection; or other adverse response. **Pregnancy/breast-feeding precautions:** Do not get pregnant while taking this medication and for 1 month following therapy. Consult prescriber for appropriate contraceptive measures. Breast-feeding is not recommended.

Pregnancy Issues: Exemestane can cause fetal harm when administered to a pregnant woman. It is not indicated for premenopausal women, but if exposure occurred during pregnancy, risk to the fetus and potential risk for loss of the pregnancy should be discussed.

Ex-Lax® Stool Softener [OTC] *see* Docusate *on page 432*

Extendryl® Jr *see page 1522*

Extendryl® SR *see page 1522*

Eye-Sed® [OTC] *see* Zinc Supplements *on page 1423*

Eyesine® *see page 1509*

F_3T *see* Trifluridine *on page 1363*

Factor VIIa (Recombinant) (FAK ter SE ven aye ree KOM be nant)

U.S. Brand Names Novo-Seven®

Synonyms Coagulation Factor VIIa; rFVIIa

Generic Available No

Pharmacologic Category Antihemophilic Agent; Blood Product Derivative

Pregnancy Risk Factor C

Lactation Excretion in breast milk unknown/compatible

Use Treatment of bleeding episodes in patients with hemophilia A or B when inhibitors to factor VIII or factor IX are present

Mechanism of Action/Effect Promotes hemostasis by activating the extrinsic pathway of the coagulation cascade to promote formation of a fibrin-platelet hemostatic plug.

Contraindications Hypersensitivity to factor VII or any component of the formulation; hypersensitivity to mouse, hamster, or bovine proteins

Warnings/Precautions Patients should be monitored for signs and symptoms of activation of the coagulation system or thrombosis. Thrombotic events may be increased in patients with disseminated intravascular coagulation (DIC), advanced atherosclerotic disease, sepsis or crush injury. Decreased dosage or discontinuation is warranted in confirmed DIC. Efficacy with prolonged infusions and data evaluating this agent's long-term adverse effects are limited. Pregnancy risk C.

Adverse Reactions

1% to 10%:

Cardiovascular: Hypertension

Hematologic: Hemorrhage, decreased plasma fibrinogen

Musculoskeletal: Hemarthrosis

<1% (Limited to important or life-threatening): Abnormal renal function, allergic reactions, arthrosis, bradycardia, coagulation disorder, prothrombin decreased, disseminated intravascular coagulation (DIC), edema, headache, hypotension, increased fibrinolysis, injection-site reactions, pneumonia, pruritus, purpura, rash, vomiting

Overdosage/Toxicology Experience with overdose in humans is limited; an increased risk of thrombotic events may occur in overdosage. Treatment is symptomatic and supportive.

Pharmacodynamics/Kinetics

Half-Life Elimination: 2.3 hours (1.7-2.7)

Formulations Injection, powder for reconstitution: 1.2 mg, 2.4 mg, 4.8 mg

Dosing

Adults & Elderly: Hemophilia A or B (when inhibitors to Factor VIII or Factor IX are present): I.V. administration only: 90 mcg/kg every 2 hours until hemostasis is achieved or until the treatment is judged ineffective. The dose and interval may be adjusted based upon the severity of bleeding and the degree of hemostasis achieved. The duration of therapy following hemostasis has not been fully established; for patients experiencing severe bleeds, dosing should be continued at 3- to 6-hour intervals after hemostasis has been achieved and the duration of dosing should be minimized.

In clinical trials, dosages have ranged from 35-120 mcg/kg and a decision on the final therapeutic dosages was reached within 8 hours in the majority of patients.

(Continued)

Factor VIIa (Recombinant) *(Continued)*

Pediatrics: Refer to adult dosing.

Administration

I.V.: I.V. administration only; reconstitute only with the specified volume of sterile water for injection, USP; administer within 3 hours after reconstitution

Stability

Storage: Store under refrigeration (2°C to 8°C/36°F to 46°F). Reconstituted solutions may be stored at room temperature or under refrigeration, but must be infused within 3 hours of reconstitution.

Monitoring Laboratory Tests Monitor for evidence of hemostasis; although the prothrombin time, APTT, and factor VII clotting activity have no correlation with achieving hemostasis, these parameters may be useful as adjunct tests to evaluate efficacy and guide dose or interval adjustments

Monitoring and Teaching Issues

Physical Assessment: See Contraindications, Warnings/Precautions, and Dosing for use cautions. Assess potential for interactions with other prescriptions, OTC medications, herbal products patient may be taking - especially those medications that may affect coagulation or platelet function (see Drug Interactions). See infusion specifics above. Assess results of laboratory tests (see above). During and after therapy patient should be monitored closely (eg, vital signs, cardiac and CNS status, and adverse reactions (eg, acute hypersensitivity reaction) - see Adverse Reactions and Overdose/Toxicology). Provide patient education according to patient condition. **Pregnancy risk factor C** - benefits of use should outweigh possible risks.

Patient Education: This medication can only be administered I.V. Report swelling, pain, burning, or itching at infusion site. Report acute headache, visual changes, pain in joints or muscles, difficulty breathing, chills, back pain, dizziness, nausea, or other unusual effects. **Pregnancy precaution:** Inform prescriber if you are or intend to become pregnant.

Factor VIII (Human) *see* Antihemophilic Factor (Human) *on page 109*
Factor VIII (Porcine) *see* Antihemophilic Factor (Porcine) *on page 111*
Factor VIII (Recombinant) *see* Antihemophilic Factor (Recombinant) *on page 112*
Factrel® *see* Gonadorelin *on page 640*
Fahrenheit/Centigrade Conversion *see page 1534*

Famciclovir (fam SYE kloe veer)

U.S. Brand Names Famvir®

Generic Available No

Pharmacologic Category Antiviral Agent

Pregnancy Risk Factor B

Lactation Excretion in breast milk unknown/contraindicated

Use Management of acute herpes zoster (shingles) and recurrent episodes of genital herpes; treatment of recurrent herpes simplex in immunocompetent patients

Mechanism of Action/Effect The prodrug famciclovir undergoes rapid biotransformation to the active compound, penciclovir, then intracellular conversion to triphosphate which is active against HSV-1, HSV-2, VZV, and EBV infected cells.

Contraindications Hypersensitivity to famciclovir or any component of the formulation

Warnings/Precautions Has not been studied in immunocompromised patients or patients with ophthalmic or disseminated zoster. Dosage adjustment is required in patients with renal insufficiency (Cl_{cr} <60 mL/minute) and in patients with noncompensated hepatic disease. Safety and efficacy have not been established in children <18 years of age. May be carcinogenic/mutagenic.

Drug Interactions

Increased Effect/Toxicity:

Cimetidine: Penciclovir AUC may increase due to impaired metabolism.

Digoxin: C_{max} of digoxin increases by ~19%.

Probenecid: Penciclovir serum levels significantly increase.

Theophylline: Penciclovir AUC/C_{max} may increase and renal clearance decrease, although not clinically significant.

Nutritional/Ethanol Interactions Food: Rate of absorption and/or conversion to penciclovir and peak concentration are reduced with food, but bioavailability is not affected.

Adverse Reactions

1% to 10%:

Central nervous system: Fatigue (4% to 6%), fever (1% to 3%), dizziness (3% to 5%), somnolence (1% to 2%), headache

Dermatologic: Pruritus (1% to 4%)

Gastrointestinal: Diarrhea (4% to 8%), vomiting (1% to 5%), constipation (1% to 5%), anorexia (1% to 3%), abdominal pain (1% to 4%), nausea

Neuromuscular & skeletal: Paresthesia (1% to 3%)

Respiratory: Sinusitis/pharyngitis (2%)

<1% (Limited to important or life-threatening): Arthralgia, rigors, upper respiratory infection

Overdosage/Toxicology Supportive and symptomatic care is recommended. Hemodialysis may enhance elimination.

Pharmacodynamics/Kinetics

Absorption: Food decreases maximum peak concentration and delays time to peak; AUC remains the same

Bioavailability: 77%

Half-Life Elimination: Penciclovir: 2-3 hours (10, 20, and 7 hours in HSV-1, HSV-2, and VZV-infected cells respectively); prolonged with renal impairment

Time to Peak: 0.9 hours; C_{max} and T_{max} are decreased and prolonged with noncompensated hepatic impairment

Metabolism: Rapidly deacetylated and oxidized to penciclovir; not via CYP

Formulations Tablet: 125 mg, 250 mg, 500 mg

Dosing

Adults & Elderly: Initiate therapy as soon as herpes zoster is diagnosed:

Acute herpes zoster: Oral: 500 mg every 8 hours for 7 days

Genital herpes: Oral:

First episode: 250 mg 3 times/day for 7-10 days

Recurrent episodes: 125 mg twice daily for 5 days (500 mg twice daily for 7 days in HIV infected patients)

Prophylaxis: 250 mg twice daily

Severe (hospitalized patients): 250 mg twice daily

Recurrent herpes simplex in immunocompetent patients: Oral: 125 mg twice daily for 5 days

Recurrent orolabial herpes or genital herpes in HIV-infected patients: Oral: 500 mg twice daily for 7 days

Renal Impairment:

Herpes zoster:

Cl_{cr} ≥60 mL/minute: Administer 500 mg every 8 hours.

Cl_{cr} 40-59 mL/minute: Administer 500 mg every 12 hours.

Cl_{cr} 20-39 mL/minute: Administer 500 mg every 24 hours.

Cl_{cr} <20 mL/minute: Administer 250 mg every 24 hours.

Recurrent genital herpes:

Cl_{cr} ≥40 mL/minute: Administer 125 mg every 12 hours.

Cl_{cr} 20-39 mL/minute: Administer 125 mg every 24 hours.

Cl_{cr} <20 mL/minute: Administer 125 mg every 24 hours.

Suppression of recurrent genital herpes

Cl_{cr} ≥40 mL/minute: Administer 250 mg every 12 hours.

Cl_{cr} 20-39 mL/minute: Administer 125 mg every 12 hours.

Cl_{cr} <20 mL/minute: Administer 125 mg every 24 hours.

Recurrent orolabial or genital herpes in HIV-infected patients:

Cl_{cr} ≥40 mL/minute: Administer 500 mg every 12 hours.

Cl_{cr} 20-39 mL/minute: Administer 500 mg every 24 hours.

Cl_{cr} <20 mL/minute: Administer 250 mg every 24 hours.

Monitoring Laboratory Tests Periodic CBC during long-term therapy

Monitoring and Teaching Issues

Physical Assessment: See Contraindications, Warnings/Precautions, Drug Interactions, and Dosing for use cautions. Assess potential for interactions with other prescriptions, OTC medications, or herbal products patient may be taking (see Drug Interactions). Assess results of laboratory tests, therapeutic effects, and adverse response (see Adverse Reactions and Overdose/Toxicology). Teach patient proper use, possible side effects and appropriate interventions, and adverse symptoms to report (see Patient Education). Breast-feeding is contraindicated.

Patient Education: Inform prescriber of all prescriptions, OTC medications, or herbal products you are taking, and any allergies you have. Take for prescribed length of time, even if condition improves. Do not discontinue without consulting prescriber. This is not a cure for genital herpes. May cause mild GI disturbances (eg, nausea, vomiting, constipation, diarrhea), fatigue, headache, or muscle aches and pains. If these are severe, contact prescriber. **Breast-feeding precaution:** Do not breast-feed.

Dietary Issues: May be taken with food or on an empty stomach.

Geriatric Considerations: For herpes zoster (shingles) infections, famciclovir should be started within 72 hours of the appearance of the rash to be effective. Famciclovir has been shown to accelerate healing, reduce the duration of viral shedding, and resolve posthepatic neuralgia faster than placebo. Comparison trials to acyclovir or valacyclovir are not available. Adjust dose for estimated renal function.

Breast-feeding Issues: There is no specific data describing the excretion of famciclovir in breast milk and for its associated tumorigenicity. Discontinue nursing or the drug during lactation; however, acyclovir is a possible alternative for the nursing mother.

Additional Information Most effective if therapy is initiated within 72 hours of initial lesion.

Famotidine (fa MOE ti deen)

U.S. Brand Names Pepcid®; Pepcid® AC [OTC]

Generic Available Yes: Injection, tablets

Pharmacologic Category Histamine H_2 Antagonist

Pregnancy Risk Factor B

Lactation Enters breast milk/compatible

Use

Pepcid®: Therapy and treatment of duodenal ulcer, gastric ulcer, control gastric pH in critically ill patients, symptomatic relief in gastritis, gastroesophageal reflux, active benign ulcer, and pathological hypersecretory conditions

Pepcid® AC: Relief of heartburn, acid indigestion, and sour stomach

Use - Unlabeled/Investigational Part of a multidrug regimen for *H. pylori* eradication to reduce the risk of duodenal ulcer recurrence

Mechanism of Action/Effect Competitive inhibition of histamine at H_2 receptors of the gastric parietal cells, which inhibits gastric acid secretion

Contraindications Hypersensitivity to famotidine, other H_2 antagonists, or any component of the formulation

Warnings/Precautions Modify dose in patients with renal impairment; chewable tablets contain phenylalanine; multidose vials contain benzyl alcohol

Drug Interactions

Decreased Effect: Decreased serum levels of ketoconazole and itraconazole (reduced absorption).

Nutritional/Ethanol Interactions

Ethanol: Avoid ethanol (may cause gastric mucosal irritation).

Food: Famotidine bioavailability may be increased if taken with food.

(Continued)

Famotidine *(Continued)*

Adverse Reactions

Note: Agitation and vomiting have been reported in up to 14% of pediatric patients <1 year of age.

1% to 10%:

Central nervous system: Dizziness (1%), headache (5%)

Gastrointestinal: Constipation (1%), diarrhea (2%)

<1% (Limited to important or life-threatening): Agranulocytosis, bradycardia, bronchospasm, hypertension, AST/ALT increased, BUN/creatinine increased or proteinuria, neutropenia, palpitations, seizures, tachycardia, thrombocytopenia

Overdosage/Toxicology Symptoms of overdose include hypotension, tachycardia, vomiting, and drowsiness. Treatment is symptomatic and supportive.

Pharmacodynamics/Kinetics

Bioavailability: Oral: 40% to 50%

Half-Life Elimination: 2.5-3.5 hours, prolonged with renal impairment; Oliguria: 20 hours

Time to Peak: Serum: Oral: ~1-3 hours

Onset: GI: Oral: Within 1 hour

Duration: 10-12 hours

Formulations

Gelcap (Pepcid® AC): 10 mg

Infusion [premixed in NS] (Pepcid®): 20 mg (50 mL)

Injection, solution (Pepcid®): 10 mg/2 mL (4 mL, 20 mL) [contains benzyl alcohol]

Injection, solution [preservative free] (Pepcid®): 10 mg/2 mL (2 mL)

Powder for oral suspension (Pepcid®): 40 mg/5 mL (50 mL) [contains sodium benzoate; cherry-banana-mint flavor]

Tablet, chewable (Pepcid® AC): 10 mg [contains phenylalanine 1.4 mg/tablet; mint flavor]

Tablet: 10 mg [OTC], 20 mg, 40 mg

Pepcid®: 20 mg, 40 mg [film-coated]

Pepcid® AC: 10 mg

Dosing

Adults & Elderly:

Duodenal ulcer: Oral: Acute therapy: 40 mg/day at bedtime for 4-8 weeks; maintenance therapy: 20 mg/day at bedtime

Gastric ulcer: Oral: Acute therapy: 40 mg/day at bedtime

Hypersecretory conditions: Oral: Initial: 20 mg every 6 hours, may increase in increments up to 160 mg every 6 hours

GERD: Oral: 20 mg twice daily for 6 weeks

Esophagitis and accompanying symptoms due to GERD: Oral: 20 mg or 40 mg twice daily for up to 12 weeks

Helicobacter pylori eradication (unlabeled use): Oral: 40 mg once daily; requires combination therapy with antibiotics

Patients unable to take oral medication: I.V.: 20 mg every 12 hours

Heartburn, indigestion, sour stomach: Pepcid® AC [OTC]: Oral: 10 mg every 12 hours; dose may be taken 15-60 minutes before eating foods known to cause heartburn

Pediatrics: Treatment duration and dose should be individualized

Peptic ulcer: 1-16 years:

Oral: 0.5 mg/kg/day at bedtime or divided twice daily (maximum dose: 40 mg/day); doses of up to 1 mg/kg/day have been used in clinical studies

I.V.: 0.25 mg/kg every 12 hours (maximum dose: 40 mg/day); doses of up to 0.5 mg/kg have been used in clinical studies

GERD: Oral:

<3 months: 0.5 mg/kg once daily

3-12 months: 0.5 mg/kg twice daily

1-16 years: 1 mg/kg/day divided twice daily (maximum dose: 40 mg twice daily); doses of up to 2 mg/kg/day have been used in clinical studies

Renal Impairment:

Cl_{cr} <50 mL/minute: Manufacturer recommendation: Administer 50% of dose **or** increase the dosing interval to every 36-48 hours (to limit potential CNS adverse effects).

Cl_{cr} <10 mL/minute: Administer 50% of dose **or** increase dosing interval to every 36-48 hours.

Administration

I.V.: Administer over 15-30 minutes; may be given undiluted I.V. push (some centers dilute to a total volume of 5-10 mL). Inject no faster than 10 mg/minute.

Stability

Reconstitution:

I.V. Reconstituted I.V. solution is stable for 48 hours at room temperature. I.V. infusion in NS or D_5W solution is stable for 48 hours at room temperature.

Oral: Reconstituted oral suspension is stable for 30 days at room temperature. Do not freeze.

Compatibility: Stable in D_5W, $D_{10}W$, LR, fat emulsion 10%, NS, sodium bicarbonate 5%

Y-site administration: Incompatible with alatrofloxacin, amphotericin B cholesteryl sulfate complex, cefepime, piperacillin/tazobactam

Monitoring and Teaching Issues

Physical Assessment: See Contraindications and Warnings/Precautions for use cautions. Assess potential for interactions with other prescriptions, OTC medications, or herbal products patient may be taking (see Drug Interactions). Assess result of laboratory tests (see above) and patient response (see Adverse Reactions) prior to each treatment and on a regular basis throughout therapy. **I.V.:** See Administration specifics. Teach patient proper use, possible side effects and appropriate interventions, and adverse symptoms to report (see Patient Education).

Patient Education: Inform prescriber of all prescriptions, OTC medications, or herbal products you are taking, and any allergies you have. Do not take anything new without consulting prescriber. Take as directed; do not alter dose or frequency or discontinue without consulting prescriber. May cause some drowsiness or dizziness (use caution when driving or engaging in tasks that require alertness until response to drug is known); constipation (increased exercise, fluids, fruit, or fiber may help); or diarrhea (buttermilk, boiled milk, or yogurt may help). Report acute headache, unresolved constipation or diarrhea, palpitations, black tarry stools, abdominal pain, rash, worsening of condition being treated, or recurrence of symptoms after therapy is completed.

Oral suspension: Shake well before use.

Pepcid® AC: Do not use for more than 14 days unless recommended by prescriber.

Dietary Issues: Phenylalanine content: Pepcid® AC chewable: Each tablet contains 1.4 mg phenylalanine

Geriatric Considerations: H_2 blockers are the preferred drugs for treating PUD in the elderly due to cost and ease of administration. These agents are no less or more effective than any other therapy. Famotidine is on of the preferred agents (due to side effects, drug interaction profile, and pharmacokinetics). Treatment for PUD in the elderly is recommended for 12 weeks since their lesions are larger; therefore, take longer to heal. Always adjust dose based upon creatinine clearance.

Breast-feeding Issues: Famotidine is excreted in breast milk to a lesser degree than cimetidine another H_2-antagonist which is considered compatible with nursing.

Famvir® *see* Famciclovir *on page 542*

Fareston® *see* Toremifene *on page 1341*

Faslodex® *see* Fulvestrant *on page 611*

Fat Emulsion (fat e MUL shun)

U.S. Brand Names Intralipid®; Liposyn® III

Synonyms Intravenous Fat Emulsion

Generic Available No

Pharmacologic Category Caloric Agent

Pregnancy Risk Factor B/C

Lactation Excretion in breast milk unknown/compatible

Use Source of calories and essential fatty acids for patients requiring parenteral nutrition of extended duration

Mechanism of Action/Effect Essential for normal structure and function of cell membranes

Contraindications Hypersensitivity to fat emulsion or any component of the formulation; severe egg or legume (soybean) allergies; pathologic hyperlipidemia, lipoid nephrosis pancreatitis with hyperlipemia

Warnings/Precautions Use caution in patients with severe liver damage, pulmonary disease, anemia, or blood coagulation disorder. Use with caution in jaundiced, premature, and low birth weight children. Pregnancy risk B/C.

Adverse Reactions Frequency not defined.

Cardiovascular: Cyanosis, flushing, chest pain
Central nervous system: Headache, dizziness
Endocrine & metabolic: Hyperlipemia
Gastrointestinal: Nausea, vomiting, diarrhea
Hematologic: Hypercoagulability, thrombocytopenia in neonates (rare)
Hepatic: Hepatomegaly
Local: Thrombophlebitis
Respiratory: Dyspnea
Miscellaneous: Sepsis, diaphoresis

Overdosage/Toxicology Rapid administration results in fluid or fat overload causing dilution of serum electrolytes, overhydration, pulmonary edema, impaired pulmonary diffusion capacity, and metabolic acidosis. Treatment is supportive.

Pharmacodynamics/Kinetics

Half-Life Elimination: 0.5-1 hour

Metabolism: Undergoes lipolysis to free fatty acids which are utilized by reticuloendothelial cells

Formulations Injection, emulsion [soybean oil]:

Intralipid®: 10% [100 mg/mL] (100 mL, 250 mL, 500 mL); 20% [200 mg/mL] (50 mL, 100 mL, 250 mL, 500 mL, 1000 mL); 30% [300 mg/mL] (500 mL)

Liposyn® III: 10% [100 mg/mL] (200 mL, 500 mL); 20% [200 mg/mL] (200 mL, 500 mL); 30% [300 mg/mL] (500 mL)

Dosing

Adults & Elderly:

Caloric source: I.V. (fat emulsion should not exceed 60% of the total daily calories):

Initial: 1 g/kg/day, increase by 0.5-1 g/kg/day to a maximum of 2.5 g/kg/day of 10% and 3 g/kg/day of 20%; maximum rate of infusion: 0.25 g/kg/hour (1.25 mL/kg/hour of 20% solution); do not exceed 50 mL/hour (20%) or 100 mL/hour (10%)

Prevention of fatty acid deficiency (8% to 10% of total caloric intake): I.V.: 0.5-1 g/kg/24 hours

500 mL twice weekly at rate of 1 mL/minute for 30 minutes, then increase to 500 mL over 4-6 hours

Can be used on a daily basis as a caloric source in TPN

Pediatrics:

Caloric source: I.V. (fat emulsion should not exceed 60% of the total daily calories):

Premature Infants: Initial dose: 0.25-0.5 g/kg/day, increase by 0.25-0.5 g/kg/day to a maximum of 3 g/kg/day depending on needs/nutritional goals; limit to 1 g/kg/day if on phototherapy; maximum rate of infusion: 0.15 g/kg/hour (0.75 mL/kg/hour of 20% solution)

Infants and Children: Initial dose: 0.5-1 g/kg/day, increase by 0.5 g/kg/day to a maximum of 3 g/kg/day depending on needs/nutritional goals; maximum rate of infusion: 0.25 g/kg/hour (1.25 mL/kg/hour of 20% solution)

Adolescents: Refer to adult dosing.

(Continued)

Fat Emulsion *(Continued)*

Prevention of essential fatty acid deficiency (8% to 10% of total caloric intake): I.V.: 0.5-1 g/kg/24 hours

Children: 5-10 mL/kg/day at 0.1 mL/minute then up to 100 mL/hour

Administration

I.V.: At the onset of therapy, the patient should be observed for any immediate allergic reactions such as dyspnea, cyanosis, and fever. Infuse for 10-15 minutes at a slower rate. Infuse 10% at 1 mL/minute. If no untoward effects, may increase rate to 500 mL over 4-6 hours. Infuse 20% at 0.5 mL/minute initially; increase to rate of 250 mL over 4-6 hours.

Stability

Storage: May be stored at room temperature. Do not store partly used bottles for later use. Do not use if emulsion appears to be oiling out.

Monitoring Laboratory Tests Serum triglycerides before initiation of therapy and at least weekly during therapy. Frequent (some advise daily) platelet counts should be performed in neonatal patients receiving parenteral lipids.

Monitoring and Teaching Issues

Physical Assessment: See Contraindications and Warnings/Precautions for use cautions. Assess for allergy to eggs prior to initiating therapy (pruritic urticaria can occur in patients allergic to eggs). Inspect emulsion before administering. Do not administer if oil separation or oiliness is noted. Monitor closely for allergic reactions (see Administration), fluid overload, thrombosis or sepsis. **Pregnancy risk factor B/C.**

Patient Education: Report pain at infusion site, difficulty breathing, chest pain, calf pain, or excessive sweating. **Pregnancy precaution:** Inform prescriber if you are pregnant.

5-FC *see* Flucytosine *on page 567*

FC1157a *see* Toremifene *on page 1341*

FDA Name Differentiation Project: The Use of Tall-man Letters *see page 12*

FDA Pregnancy Categories *see page 16*

Federal OBRA Regulations Recommended Maximum Doses *see page 1610*

Feiba VH Immuno® *see* Anti-inhibitor Coagulant Complex *on page 113*

Felbamate (FEL ba mate)

U.S. Brand Names Felbatol®

Generic Available No

Pharmacologic Category Anticonvulsant, Miscellaneous

Pregnancy Risk Factor C

Lactation Enters breast milk/not recommended

Use Not as a first-line antiepileptic treatment; only in those patients who respond inadequately to alternative treatments and whose epilepsy is so severe that a substantial risk of aplastic anemia and/or liver failure is deemed acceptable in light of the benefits conferred by its use. Patient must be fully advised of risk and provide signed written informed consent. Felbamate can be used as either monotherapy or adjunctive therapy in the treatment of partial seizures (with and without generalization) and in adults with epilepsy.

Orphan drug: Adjunctive therapy in the treatment of partial and generalized seizures associated with Lennox-Gastaut syndrome in children

Mechanism of Action/Effect Mechanism of action is unknown but has properties in common with other marketed anticonvulsants. Has weak inhibitory effects on GABA-receptor binding, benzodiazepine receptor binding, and is devoid of activity at the MK-801 receptor binding site of the NMDA receptor-ionophore complex.

Contraindications Hypersensitivity to felbamate or any component of the formulation; use with caution in those patients who have demonstrated hypersensitivity reactions to other carbamates

Warnings/Precautions Use with caution in patients allergic to other carbamates (eg, meprobamate). Antiepileptic drugs should not be suddenly discontinued because of the possibility of increasing seizure frequency. **Reported 10 cases of aplastic anemia in the U.S. after 2½ to 6 months of therapy**. Carter Wallace and the FDA recommended the use of this agent be suspended unless withdrawal of the product would place a patient at greater risk as compared to the frequently fatal form of anemia. Pregnancy risk C.

Drug Interactions

Cytochrome P450 Effect: Substrate of CYP2E1, **3A4**; Inhibits CYP2C19; Induces CYP3A4

Decreased Effect: Carbamazepine, phenytoin may decrease serum felbamate concentrations. Felbamate may decrease carbamazepine levels and increase levels of the active metabolite of carbamazepine (10,11-epoxide) resulting in carbamazepine toxicity; monitor for signs of carbamazepine toxicity (dizziness, ataxia, nystagmus, drowsiness).

Increased Effect/Toxicity: Felbamate increases serum phenytoin, phenobarbital, and valproic acid concentrations which may result in toxicity; consider decreasing phenytoin or phenobarbital dosage by 25%. A decrease in valproic acid dosage may also be necessary.

Nutritional/Ethanol Interactions

Ethanol: Avoid ethanol (may increase CNS depression).

Food: Food does not affect absorption.

Herb/Nutraceutical: Avoid evening primrose (seizure threshold decreased).

Effects on Lab Values Blood urea nitrogen is slightly lower (1.25 mg/dL). May cause slightly elevated serum cholesterol level (about 7 mg/dL) in patients receiving about 2.6 g/day.

Adverse Reactions

>10%:

Central nervous system: Somnolence, headache, fatigue, dizziness

Gastrointestinal: Nausea, anorexia, vomiting, constipation

1% to 10%:

Cardiovascular: Chest pain, palpitations, tachycardia

Central nervous system: Depression or behavior changes, nervousness, anxiety, ataxia, stupor, malaise, agitation, psychological disturbances, aggressive reaction

Dermatologic: Skin rash, acne, pruritus
Gastrointestinal: Xerostomia, diarrhea, abdominal pain, weight gain, taste perversion
Neuromuscular & skeletal: Tremor, abnormal gait, paresthesia, myalgia
Ocular: Diplopia, abnormal vision
Respiratory: Sinusitis, pharyngitis
Miscellaneous: SGPT increase

<1% (Limited to important or life-threatening): Euphoria, hallucinations, leukocytosis, leukopenia, lymphadenopathy, migraine, suicide attempts, thrombocytopenia, urticaria

Overdosage/Toxicology Symptoms of overdose include sedation, gastrointestinal upset, and tachycardia. Provide general supportive care.

Pharmacodynamics/Kinetics

Absorption: Rapid and almost complete; food has no effect upon the tablet's absorption

Half-Life Elimination: 20-23 hours (average)

Time to Peak: Serum: ~3 hours

Formulations

Suspension, oral: 600 mg/5 mL (240 mL, 960 mL)
Tablet: 400 mg, 600 mg

Dosing

Adults:

Monotherapy: Oral:

Initial: 1200 mg/day in divided doses 3 or 4 times/day; titrate previously untreated patients under close clinical supervision, increasing the dosage in 600 mg increments every 2 weeks to 2400 mg/day based on clinical response and thereafter to 3600 mg/day as clinically indicated

Conversion to monotherapy: Initiate at 1200 mg/day in divided doses 3 or 4 times/day, reduce the dosage of the concomitant anticonvulsant(s) by 20% to 33% at the initiation of felbamate therapy; at week 2, increase the felbamate dosage to 2400 mg/day while reducing the dosage of the other anticonvulsant(s) up to an additional 33% of their original dosage; at week 3, increase the felbamate dosage up to 3600 mg/day and continue to reduce the dosage of the other anticonvulsant(s) as clinically indicated

Elderly: Refer to adult dosing; start at lowest dose (see Geriatric Considerations).

Pediatrics:

Monotherapy: Oral: Children >14 years: Refer to adult dosing.

Adjunctive therapy, Lennox-Gastaut (ages 2-14 years): Oral:

Week 1: Felbamate: 15 mg/kg/day divided 3-4 times/day
Concomitant anticonvulsant(s): Reduce original dosage by 20% to 30%.

Week 2: Felbamate: 30 mg/kg/day divided 3-4 times/day
Concomitant anticonvulsant(s): Reduce original dosage up to an additional 33%.

Week 3: Felbamate: 45 mg//kg/day divided 3-4 times/day
Concomitant anticonvulsant(s): Reduce dosage as clinically indicated.

Adjunctive therapy: Children >14 years and Adults:

Week 1: Felbamate: 1200 mg/day initial dose
Concomitant anticonvulsant(s): Reduce original dosage by 20% to 33%.

Week 2: Felbamate: 2400 mg/day (therapeutic range)
Concomitant anticonvulsant(s): Reduce original dosage by up to an additional 33%.

Week 3: Felbamate: 3600 mg/day (therapeutic range)
Concomitant anticonvulsant(s): Reduce original dosage as clinically indicated.

Administration

Oral: Administer on an empty stomach for best absorption.

Stability

Storage: Store medication in tightly closed container at room temperature away from excessive heat.

Monitoring Laboratory Tests Monitor serum levels of concomitant anticonvulsant therapy; monitor AST, ALT, and bilirubin on a weekly basis. Hematologic evaluations before therapy begins, frequently during therapy, and for a significant period after discontinuation.

Monitoring and Teaching Issues

Physical Assessment: Assess effectiveness and interactions of other medications patient may be taking (see Drug Interactions). See Warnings/Precautions and Contraindications for use cautions. Monitor therapeutic response (seizure activity, force, type, duration), laboratory values, and adverse reactions (see Adverse Reactions) at beginning of therapy and periodically with long-term use. Taper dosage slowly when discontinuing. Assess knowledge/teach patient safety and seizure precautions, appropriate use, interventions to reduce side effects, and adverse symptoms to report (see Patient Education). **Pregnancy risk factor C** - benefits of use should outweigh possible risks. Breast-feeding is not recommended.

Patient Education: Take exactly as directed; do not increase dose or frequency or discontinue without consulting prescriber. While using this medication, do not use alcohol and other prescription or OTC medications (especially pain medications, sedatives, antihistamines, or hypnotics) without consulting prescriber. Maintain adequate hydration (2-3 L/day of fluids) unless advised by prescriber to restrict fluids. You may experience drowsiness, dizziness, or blurred vision (use caution when driving or engaging in tasks requiring alertness until response to drug is known); or nausea, vomiting, loss of appetite, or dry mouth (small, frequent meals, frequent mouth care, chewing gum, or sucking lozenges may help). Wear identification of epileptic status and medications. Report CNS changes, mentation changes, or changes in cognition; muscle cramping, weakness, tremors, changes in gait; persistent GI symptoms (cramping, constipation, vomiting, anorexia); rash or skin irritations; unusual bruising or bleeding (mouth, urine, stool); cough, runny nose, sore throat, or difficulty breathing; or worsening of seizure activity or loss of seizure control. **Pregnancy/breast-feeding precautions:** Inform prescriber if you are or intend to become pregnant. Breast-feeding is not recommended.

Dietary Issues: May be taken without regard to meals.

Geriatric Considerations: Clinical studies have not included large numbers of patients >65 years of age. Due to decreased hepatic and renal function, dosing should start at the lower end of the dosage range.

(Continued)

Felbamate *(Continued)*

Additional Information Monotherapy has not been associated with gingival hyperplasia, impaired concentration, weight gain, or abnormal thinking. Because felbamate is the only drug shown effective in Lennox-Gastaut syndrome, it is considered an orphan drug for this indication.

Felbatol® *see* Felbamate *on page 546*

Feldene® *see* Piroxicam *on page 1094*

Felodipine (fe LOE di peen)

U.S. Brand Names Plendil®

Generic Available No

Pharmacologic Category Calcium Channel Blocker

Pregnancy Risk Factor C

Lactation Excretion in breast milk unknown

Use Treatment of hypertension, congestive heart failure

Mechanism of Action/Effect Inhibits calcium ions from entering the "slow channels" or select voltage-sensitive areas of vascular smooth muscle and myocardium during depolarization

Contraindications Hypersensitivity to felodipine, any component of the formulation, or other calcium channel blocker

Warnings/Precautions Use caution in patients with heart failure particularly with concurrent beta-blocker use. Elderly patients and patients with hepatic impairment should start off with a lower dose. Peripheral edema is the most common side effect (occurs within 2-3 weeks of starting therapy). May cause reflex tachycardia, hypotension, or syncope (rare). Safety and efficacy in children have not been established. Dosage titration should occur after 14 days on a given dose. Pregnancy risk C.

Drug Interactions

Cytochrome P450 Effect: Substrate of **CYP3A4**; Inhibits CYP2C8/9, 2D6, 3A4

Decreased Effect: Felodipine may decrease pharmacologic actions of theophylline. Calcium may reduce the calcium channel blocker's effects, particularly hypotension. Carbamazepine significantly reduces felodipine's bioavailability; avoid this combination. Nafcillin decreases plasma concentration of felodipine; avoid this combination. Rifampin increases the metabolism of felodipine. Felodipine may decrease pharmacologic actions of theophylline.

Increased Effect/Toxicity: Inhibitors of CYP3A4, including azole antifungals (ketoconazole, itraconazole) and erythromycin, may inhibit calcium channel blocker metabolism, increasing the effects of felodipine. Beta-blockers may have increased pharmacokinetic or pharmacodynamic interactions with felodipine. Cyclosporine increases felodipine's serum concentration. Ethanol increases felodipine's absorption; watch for a greater hypotensive effect.

Nutritional/Ethanol Interactions

Food: Increased therapeutic and vasodilator side effects, including severe hypotension and myocardial ischemia, may occur if felodipine is taken with grapefruit juice; avoid concurrent use. High-fat/carbohydrate meals will increase C_{max} by 60%; grapefruit juice will increase C_{max} by twofold.

Herb/Nutraceutical: St John's wort may decrease felodipine levels. Avoid dong quai if using for hypertension (has estrogenic activity). Avoid ephedra, yohimbe, ginseng (may worsen hypertension). Avoid garlic (may have increased antihypertensive effect).

Adverse Reactions

>10%: Central nervous system: Headache (11% to 15%)

2% to 10%: Cardiovascular: Peripheral edema (2% to 17%), tachycardia (0.4% to 2.5%), flushing (4% to 7%)

<1% (Limited to important or life-threatening): Angina, angioedema, anxiety, arrhythmia, CHF, CVA, libido decreased, depression, dizziness, gingival hyperplasia, dyspnea, dysuria, gynecomastia, hypotension, impotence, insomnia, irritability, leukocytoclastic vasculitis, myocardial infarction, nervousness, paresthesias, somnolence, syncope, urticaria, vomiting

Overdosage/Toxicology Primary cardiac symptoms of calcium blocker overdose include hypotension and bradycardia. Noncardiac symptoms include confusion, stupor, nausea, vomiting, metabolic acidosis, and hyperglycemia. Treat symptomatically.

Pharmacodynamics/Kinetics

Absorption: 100%; absolute: 20% due to first-pass effect

Half-Life Elimination: 11-16 hours

Metabolism: Hepatic; extensive first-pass effect

Onset: 2-5 hours

Duration: 16-24 hours

Formulations Tablet, extended release: 2.5 mg, 5 mg, 10 mg

Dosing

Adults: Hypertension: Oral: 5-10 mg once daily; increase by 5 mg at 2-week intervals, as needed, to a maximum of 20 mg/day.

Elderly: Oral: Initial 2.5 mg/day

Hepatic Impairment: Begin with 2.5 mg/day; do not use doses >10 mg/day.

Administration

Oral: Do not crush or chew extended release tablets; swallow whole.

Monitoring and Teaching Issues

Physical Assessment: See Warnings/Precautions for use cautions. Assess potential for interactions with prescription, OTC medications, or herbal products patient may be taking (eg, beta blockers or other drugs that effect blood pressure - see Drug Interactions). Assess for therapeutic effects and signs/symptoms of adverse reactions at beginning of therapy, when changing dosage, and periodically throughout long-term therapy (see Adverse Reactions and Overdose/Toxicology). When discontinuing, taper gradually (over 2 weeks). Teach patient proper use, possible side effects/interventions, and adverse symptoms to report (see Patient Education). **Pregnancy risk factor C** - benefits of use should outweigh possible risks. Note breast-feeding caution.

Patient Education: Inform prescriber of all prescriptions, OTC medications, or herbal products you are taking, and any allergies you have. Do not take anything new during treatment unless approved by prescriber. Take exactly as directed, without food. Avoid grapefruit juice. Swallow whole, do not crush or chew. Do not alter dose or stop taking without consulting prescriber. May cause headache (consult prescriber for analgesic); nausea or vomiting (small, frequent meals, frequent mouth care, chewing gum, or sucking lozenges may help); constipation (increased dietary bulk and fluids may help); or drowsiness (use caution when driving or engaging in tasks that require alertness until response to drug is known). Report persistent headache; vomiting; constipation; peripheral or facial swelling; weight gain >5 lb/week; or chest pain, palpitations, or respiratory changes. **Pregnancy/breast-feeding precautions:** Inform prescriber if you are or intend to become pregnant. Consult prescriber if breast-feeding.

Dietary Issues: Should be taken without food.

Geriatric Considerations: Elderly may experience a greater hypotensive response. Theoretically, constipation may be more of a problem in the elderly.

Additional Information Felodipine maintains renal and mesenteric blood flow during hemorrhagic shock in animals.

Related Information

Calcium Channel Blockers *on page 1563*

Felodipine and Enalapril *see* Enalapril and Felodipine *on page 466*

Femara® *see* Letrozole *on page 778*

femhrt® *see* Ethinyl Estradiol and Norethindrone *on page 527*

Femizol-M™ [OTC] *see* Miconazole *on page 899*

Fenesin™ *see* Guaifenesin *on page 646*

Fenesin™ DM *see* Guaifenesin and Dextromethorphan *on page 647*

Fenofibrate (fen oh FYE brate)

U.S. Brand Names TriCor®

Synonyms Procetofene; Proctofene

Generic Available No

Pharmacologic Category Antilipemic Agent, Fibric Acid

Pregnancy Risk Factor C

Lactation Excretion in breast milk unknown/not recommended

Use Adjunct to dietary therapy for the treatment of adults with very high elevations of serum triglyceride levels (types IV and V hyperlipidemia) who are at risk of pancreatitis and who do not respond adequately to a determined dietary effort; safety and efficacy may be greater than that of clofibrate; adjunct to dietary therapy for the reduction of low density lipoprotein cholesterol (LDL-C), total cholesterol (total-C), triglycerides, and apolipoprotein B (apo B) in adult patients with primary hypercholesterolemia or mixed dyslipidemia (Fredrickson types IIa and IIb); its efficacy can be enhanced by combination with other hypolipidemic agents that have a different mechanism of action

Mechanism of Action/Effect Fenofibric acid is believed to increase VLDL catabolism by enhancing the synthesis of lipoprotein lipase; as a result of a decrease in VLDL levels, total plasma triglycerides are reduced by 30% to 60%. Modest increase in HDL occurs in some hypertriglyceridemic patients.

Contraindications Hypersensitivity to fenofibrate or any component of the formulation; hepatic or severe renal dysfunction including primary biliary cirrhosis and unexplained persistent liver function abnormalities; pre-existing gallbladder disease

Warnings/Precautions Product reformulation has resulted in dosing changes; see Dosing. Hepatic transaminases can significantly elevate (dose-related). Regular monitoring of liver function tests is required. May cause cholelithiasis. Use caution when combining fenofibrate with HMG-CoA reductase inhibitors (may lead to myopathy, rhabdomyolysis). The effect of fenofibrate on coronary artery disease morbidity and mortality has not been established. Therapy should be withdrawn if an adequate response is not obtained after 2 months of therapy at the maximal daily dose. Rare hypersensitivity reactions may occur. Dose adjustment is required for renal impairment and elderly patients. Safety and efficacy in children have not been established. Pregnancy risk C.

Drug Interactions

Cytochrome P450 Effect: Substrate of CYP3A4

Decreased Effect: Rifampin (and potentially other enzyme inducers) may decrease levels of fenofibrate.

Increased Effect/Toxicity: The hypolipidemic effect of fenofibrate is increased when used with cholestyramine or colestipol. Fenofibrate may increase the effect of chlorpropamide and warfarin. Concurrent use of fenofibrate with HMG-CoA reductase inhibitors (atorvastatin, cerivastatin, fluvastatin, lovastatin, pravastatin, simvastatin) may increase the risk of myopathy and rhabdomyolysis. The manufacturer warns against concomitant use. However, combination therapy with statins has been used in some patients with resistant hyperlipidemias (with great caution).

Adverse Reactions

1% to 10%:

Gastrointestinal: Abdominal pain (5%), constipation (2%)

Hepatic: Abnormal liver function test (7%), creatine phosphokinase increased (3%), ALT increased (3%), AST increased (3%)

Neuromuscular & skeletal: Back pain (3%)

Respiratory: Respiratory disorder (6%), rhinitis (2%)

Frequency not defined (limited to important or life-threatening): Allergic reaction, alopecia, angina pectoris, anxiety, arrhythmias, asthma, atrial fibrillation, cholecystitis, cholelithiasis, colitis, depression, diabetes mellitus, dyspnea, eosinophilia, esophagitis, gastritis, gout, gynecomastia, hypoglycemia, kidney function abnormality, leukopenia, lymphadenopathy,

(Continued)

Fenofibrate *(Continued)*

myasthenia, myocardial infarction, neuralgia, paresthesia, photosensitivity reaction, rash, thrombocytopenia, urolithiasis, urticaria, vertigo, vomiting

Overdosage/Toxicology Symptoms of overdose include nausea, vomiting, diarrhea, and GI distress. Treatment is supportive. Hemodialysis has no effect on removal of fenofibric acid from the plasma.

Pharmacodynamics/Kinetics

Absorption: 60% to 90% with meals

Half-Life Elimination: 21 hours; Elderly: 30 hours; Hepatic impairment: 44-54 hours

Time to Peak: 4-6 hours

Metabolism: Tissue and plasma via esterases to active form, fenofibric acid; undergoes inactivation by glucuronidation hepatically or renally

Formulations

Capsule: 67 mg, 200 mg [DSC]

Tablet: 54 mg, 160 mg

Dosing

Adults: Note: As of September, 2001, a tablet formulation became available which will replace the capsules, as soon as existing supply is exhausted.

Hypertriglyceridemia: Oral: Initial:

Capsule: 67 mg/day with meals, up to 200 mg/day

Tablet: 54 mg/day with meals, up to 160 mg/day

Hypercholesterolemia or mixed hyperlipidemia: Oral: Initial:

Capsule: 200 mg/day with meals

Tablet: 160 mg/day with meals

Elderly: Initial: 67 mg/day (capsule) or 54 mg/day (tablet)

Renal Impairment: Decrease dose or increase dosing interval for patients with renal failure: Initial: 67 mg/day (capsule) or 54 mg/day (tablet)

Hemodialysis has no effect on removal of fenofibric acid from the plasma.

Administration

Oral: 6-8 weeks of therapy is required to determine efficacy.

Monitoring Laboratory Tests Total serum cholesterol and triglyceride concentration and CLDL, LDL, and HDL levels should be measured periodically; if only marginal changes are noted in 6-8 weeks, the drug should be discontinued. Serum transaminases should be measured every 3 months; if ALT values increase >100 units/L, therapy should be discontinued. Monitor LFTs prior to initiation, at 6 and 12 weeks after initiation or first dose, then periodically thereafter.

Monitoring and Teaching Issues

Physical Assessment: See Contraindications, Warnings/Precautions, Dosing, and Monitoring Laboratory Tests for use cautions. Assess potential for interactions with other prescriptions, OTC medications, or herbal products patient may be taking (see Drug Interactions). Assess result of laboratory tests and patient response (see Adverse Reactions) prior to each treatment and on a regular basis throughout therapy. Teach patient possible side effects and appropriate interventions and adverse symptoms to report (see Patient Education). **Pregnancy risk factor C** - benefits of use should outweigh possible risks. Breast-feeding is not recommended.

Patient Education: Inform prescriber of all prescriptions, OTC medications, or herbal products you are taking, and any allergies you have. Do not take anything new without consulting prescriber. Take as directed with food. Do not change dosage or dosage form or frequency without consulting prescriber. Maintain diet and exercise program as prescribed. May cause mild GI disturbances (eg, gas, diarrhea, constipation, nausea); inform prescriber if these are severe. Report immediately unusual muscle pain or weakness, skin rash or irritation, insomnia, or persistent dizziness. **Pregnancy/breast-feeding precautions:** Inform prescriber if you are or intend to become pregnant. Breast-feeding is not recommended.

Dietary Issues: Take with food.

Breast-feeding Issues: Tumor formation was observed in animal studies; nursing is not recommended if the medication cannot be discontinued.

Pregnancy Issues: Although teratogenicity and mutagenicity tests in animals have been negative, significant risk has been identified with clofibrate. Use should be avoided, if possible, in pregnant women since the neonatal glucuronide conjugation pathways are immature.

Additional Information In September, 2001, a tablet formulation of TriCor® was approved by the FDA. According to Abbott Laboratories, the tablet will replace the capsule formulation. It is important to note that the strengths of the tablet are not the same as the capsule. The tablet formulation has increased bioavailability, which produces equivalent plasma levels at lower doses. Patients previously taking the 200 mg capsule should be changed to the 160 mg tablet. Patients previously taking the 67 mg capsule should be changed to the 54 mg tablet. Tablets should be taken with food. Prescriptions for the capsules should be filled as written until the supply of capsules is depleted; at that time a new prescription for tablets should be requested from the prescriber.

Related Information

Hyperlipidemia Management *on page 1682*

Lipid-Lowering Agents *on page 1582*

Fenoprofen (fen oh PROE fen)

U.S. Brand Names Nalfon®

Synonyms Fenoprofen Calcium

Generic Available Yes: Tablet

Pharmacologic Category Nonsteroidal Anti-inflammatory Drug (NSAID)

Pregnancy Risk Factor B/D (3rd trimester)

Lactation Enters breast milk/not recommended

Use Symptomatic treatment of acute and chronic rheumatoid arthritis and osteoarthritis; relief of mild to moderate pain

Mechanism of Action/Effect Inhibits prostaglandin synthesis by decreasing the activity of the enzyme, cyclooxygenase, which results in decreased formation of prostaglandin precursors

Contraindications Hypersensitivity to fenoprofen, aspirin, or other NSAIDs; pregnancy (3rd trimester)

Warnings/Precautions Use with caution in patients with CHF, hypertension, dehydration, decreased renal or hepatic function, history of GI disease (bleeding or ulcers), or those receiving anticoagulants. Elderly are at a high risk for adverse effects from NSAIDs. As many as 60% of elderly can develop peptic ulceration and/or hemorrhage asymptomatically.

Use lowest effective dose for shortest period possible. Use of NSAIDs can compromise existing renal function especially when Cl_{cr} is <30 mL/minute. CNS adverse effects such as confusion, agitation, and hallucination are generally seen in overdose or high-dose situations; however, elderly may demonstrate these adverse effects at lower doses than younger adults. Withhold for at least 4-6 half-lives prior to surgical or dental procedures.

Pregnancy risk B/D (3rd trimester).

Drug Interactions

Decreased Effect: Decreased effect with phenobarbital.

Increased Effect/Toxicity: Increased effect/toxicity of phenytoin, sulfonamides, sulfonylureas, salicylates, and oral anticoagulants. Serum concentration/toxicity of methotrexate may be increased.

Nutritional/Ethanol Interactions

Ethanol: Avoid ethanol (may enhance gastric mucosal irritation).

Food: Fenoprofen peak serum levels may be decreased if taken with food.

Herb/Nutraceutical: Avoid cat's claw, dong quai, evening primrose, feverfew, garlic, ginger, ginkgo, red clover, horse chestnut, green tea, ginseng (all have additional antiplatelet activity).

Effects on Lab Values ↑ chloride (S), sodium (S)

Adverse Reactions

>10%:

- Central nervous system: Dizziness (7% to 15%), somnolence (9% to 15%)
- Gastrointestinal: Abdominal cramps (2% to 4%), heartburn, indigestion, nausea (8% to 14%), dyspepsia (10% to 14%), flatulence (14%), anorexia (14%), constipation (7% to 14%), occult blood in stool (14%), vomiting (3% to 14%), diarrhea (2% to 14%)

1% to 10%:

- Central nervous system: Headache (9%)
- Dermatologic: Itching
- Endocrine & metabolic: Fluid retention

<1% (Limited to important or life-threatening): Agranulocytosis, anemia, angioedema, arrhythmias, bone marrow depression, CHF, dyspnea, erythema multiforme, GI ulceration, hemolytic anemia, hepatitis, hypertension, leukopenia, polyuria, renal failure (acute), Stevens-Johnson syndrome, thrombocytopenia, tachycardia, toxic epidermal necrolysis

Overdosage/Toxicology Symptoms of overdose include acute renal failure, vomiting, drowsiness, and leukocytosis. Management of NSAID intoxication is supportive and symptomatic.

Pharmacodynamics/Kinetics

Absorption: Rapid, 80%

Half-Life Elimination: 2.5-3 hours

Time to Peak: Serum: ~2 hours

Metabolism: Extensively hepatic

Onset: A few days

Formulations

Capsule, as calcium (Nalfon®): 200 mg, 300 mg

Tablet, as calcium: 600 mg

Dosing

Adults & Elderly:

Rheumatoid arthritis and osteoarthritis: Oral: 300-600 mg 3-4 times/day up to 3.2 g/day

Mild to moderate pain: Oral: 200 mg every 4-6 hours as needed

Administration

Oral: Do not crush tablets. Swallow whole with a full glass of water. Take with food to minimize stomach upset.

Monitoring Laboratory Tests CBC, liver enzymes; urine output and BUN/serum creatinine in patients receiving diuretics

Monitoring and Teaching Issues

Physical Assessment: Assess effectiveness and interactions of other medications patient may be taking (see Contraindications and Drug Interactions). See Contraindications and Warnings/Precautions for use cautions. Monitor laboratory tests (see above), therapeutic response, and adverse reactions at beginning of therapy and periodically throughout therapy (see Warnings/Precautions, Adverse Reactions, and Overdose/Toxicology). Assess knowledge/teach patient appropriate use, interventions to reduce side effects, and adverse symptoms to report (see Patient Education). **Pregnancy risk factor B/D** - see Pregnancy Risk Factor for use cautions. Breast-feeding is not recommended. Ophthalmic absorption is probably minimal.

Patient Education: Take this medication exactly as directed; do not increase dose without consulting prescriber. Do not crush tablets or break capsules. Take with food or milk to reduce GI distress. Maintain adequate hydration (2-3 L/day of fluids) unless advised by prescriber to restrict fluids. Do not use alcohol, aspirin or aspirin-containing medication, or any other anti-inflammatory medications without consulting prescriber. You may experience drowsiness, dizziness, nervousness, or headache (use caution when driving or engaging in tasks requiring alertness until response to drug is known); anorexia, nausea, vomiting, or heartburn (small, frequent meals, frequent mouth care, sucking lozenges, or

(Continued)

Fenoprofen *(Continued)*

chewing gum may help); or fluid retention (weigh yourself weekly and report unusual (3-5 lb/week) weight gain). GI bleeding, ulceration, or perforation can occur with or without pain; discontinue medication and contact prescriber if persistent abdominal pain or cramping, or blood in stool occurs. Report breathlessness, difficulty breathing, or unusual cough; chest pain, rapid heartbeat, palpitations; unusual bruising/bleeding; blood in urine, stool, mouth, or vomitus; swollen extremities; skin rash or itching; acute fatigue; or hearing changes (ringing in ears). **Pregnancy/breast-feeding precautions:** Inform prescriber if you are or intend to become pregnant. This drug should not be used in the 3rd trimester of pregnancy. Breast-feeding is not recommended.

Dietary Issues: May be taken with food to decrease GI distress.

Geriatric Considerations: Elderly are at high risk for adverse effects from NSAIDs. As much as 60% of elderly can develop peptic ulceration and/or hemorrhage asymptomatically. The concomitant use of H_2 blockers, omeprazole, and sucralfate is not effective as prophylaxis with the exception of NSAID-induced duodenal ulcers which may be prevented by the use of ranitidine. Misoprostol is the only prophylactic agent proven effective. Also, concomitant disease and drug use contribute to the risk for GI adverse effects. Use lowest effective dose for shortest period possible. Consider renal function decline with age. Use of NSAIDs can compromise existing renal function especially when Cl_{cr} is ≤30 mL/minute. Tinnitus may be a difficult and unreliable indication of toxicity due to age-related hearing loss or eighth cranial nerve damage. CNS adverse effects such as confusion, agitation, and hallucination are generally seen in overdose or high-dose situations, but elderly may demonstrate these adverse effects at lower doses than younger adults.

Related Information

Nonsalicylate/Nonsteroidal Anti-inflammatory Comparison *on page 1587*

Fenoprofen Calcium *see* Fenoprofen *on page 550*

Fentanyl (FEN ta nil)

U.S. Brand Names Actiq®; Duragesic®; Sublimaze®

Synonyms Fentanyl Citrate

Restrictions C-II

Generic Available Yes: Injection only

Pharmacologic Category Analgesic, Narcotic; General Anesthetic

Pregnancy Risk Factor C/D (prolonged use or high doses at term)

Lactation Enters breast milk/use caution (AAP rates "compatible")

Use Sedation, relief of pain, preoperative medication, adjunct to general or regional anesthesia, management of chronic pain (transdermal product)

Actiq® is indicated only for management of breakthrough cancer pain in patients who are tolerant to and currently receiving opioid therapy for persistent cancer pain.

Mechanism of Action/Effect Binds with stereospecific receptors at many sites within the CNS, increases pain threshold, alters pain reception, inhibits ascending pain pathways

Contraindications Hypersensitivity to fentanyl or any component of the formulation; increased intracranial pressure; severe respiratory depression; severe liver or renal insufficiency; pregnancy (prolonged use or high doses near term)

Actiq® must not be used in patients who are intolerant to opioids. Patients are considered opioid-tolerant if they are taking at least 60 mg morphine/day, 50 mcg transdermal fentanyl/hour, or an equivalent dose of another opioid for ≥1 week.

Warnings/Precautions Fentanyl shares the toxic potentials of opiate agonists, and precautions of opiate agonist therapy should be observed. Use with caution in patients with bradycardia. Rapid I.V. infusion may result in skeletal muscle and chest wall rigidity → impaired ventilation → respiratory distress → apnea, bronchoconstriction, laryngospasm. Inject slowly over 3-5 minutes. Nondepolarizing skeletal muscle relaxant may be required. The elderly may be particularly susceptible to the CNS depressant and constipating effects of narcotics.

Topical patches: Serum fentanyl concentrations may increase approximately 33% for patients with a body temperature of 40°C secondary to a temperature-dependent increase in fentanyl release from the system and increased skin permeability. Patients who experience adverse reactions should be monitored for at least 12 hours after removal of the patch.

Pregnancy risk C/D (prolonged use or high doses at term).

Drug Interactions

Cytochrome P450 Effect: Substrate of **CYP3A4**; Inhibits CYP3A4

Decreased Effect: CYP3A4 inducers (including carbamazepine, phenytoin, phenobarbital, rifampin) may decrease serum levels of fentanyl by increasing metabolism.

Increased Effect/Toxicity: Increased sedation with CNS depressants, phenothiazines. Tricyclic antidepressants may potentiate fentanyl's adverse effects. Potential for serotonin syndrome if combined with other serotonergic drugs. CYP3A4 inhibitors (including erythromycin, clarithromycin, ketoconazole, itraconazole, and protease inhibitors) may increase serum concentration of fentanyl.

Nutritional/Ethanol Interactions

Ethanol: Avoid ethanol (may increase CNS depression).

Food: Glucose may cause hyperglycemia.

Herb/Nutraceutical: St John's wort may decrease fentanyl levels. Avoid valerian, St John's wort, kava kava, gotu kola (may increase CNS depression).

Adverse Reactions

>10%:

- Cardiovascular: Bradycardia, hypotension, peripheral vasodilation
- Central nervous system: Drowsiness, sedation, increased intracranial pressure
- Gastrointestinal: Nausea, vomiting
- Endocrine & metabolic: Antidiuretic hormone release
- Ocular: Miosis
- Neuromuscular & skeletal: Chest wall rigidity (high dose I.V.)

1% to 10%:
- Cardiovascular: Cardiac arrhythmias, orthostatic hypotension
- Central nervous system: Confusion, CNS depression
- Gastrointestinal: Constipation
- Ocular: Blurred vision
- Respiratory: Apnea, postoperative respiratory depression

<1% (Limited to important or life-threatening): Bronchospasm, convulsions, hypercarbia, laryngospasm, respiratory depression

Overdosage/Toxicology Symptoms of overdose include CNS depression, respiratory depression, and miosis. Treatment is supportive. Naloxone, 2 mg I.V. with repeat administration as necessary up to a total of 10 mg, can also be used to reverse toxic effects of the opiate.

Pharmacodynamics/Kinetics

Absorption: Transmucosal: Rapid, ~25% from the buccal mucosa; 75% swallowed with saliva and slowly absorbed from GI tract

Bioavailability: Transmucosal: ~50% (range: 36% to 71%)

Half-Life Elimination: 2-4 hours; Transmucosal: 6.6 hours (range: 5-15 hours)

Metabolism: Hepatic

Onset: Analgesic: I.M.: 7-15 minutes; I.V.: Almost immediate; Transmucosal: 5-15 minutes
Peak effect: Transmucosal: Analgesic: 20-30 minutes

Duration: I.M.: 1-2 hours; I.V.: 0.5-1 hour; Transmucosal: Related to blood level; respiratory depressant effect may last longer than analgesic effect

Formulations

Injection, solution, as citrate [preservative free]: 0.05 mg/mL (2 mL, 5 mL, 10 mL, 20 mL, 30 mL, 50 mL)
Sublimaze®: 0.05 mg/mL (2 mL, 5 mL, 10 mL, 20 mL)

Lozenge, oral transmucosal, as citrate [mounted on a plastic radiopaque handle] (Actiq®): 200 mcg, 400 mcg, 600 mcg, 800 mcg, 1200 mcg, 1600 mcg [raspberry flavor]

Transdermal system (Duragesic®): 25 mcg/hour [10 cm^2] (5s); 50 mcg/hour [20 cm^2] (5s); 75 mcg/hour [30 cm^2]; 100 mcg/hour [40 cm^2] (5s)

Dosing

Adults: Doses should be titrated to appropriate effects; wide range of doses, dependent upon desired degree of analgesia/anesthesia

Sedation for minor procedures/analgesia: I.M., I.V.: 0.5-1 mcg/kg/dose; higher doses are used for major procedures

Preoperative sedation, adjunct to regional anesthesia, postoperative pain: I.M., I.V.: 50-100 mcg/dose

Continuous sedation (including ICU settings): I.V.: Initial 25-50 mcg bolus; followed by continuous infusions at a rate of 1-3 mcg/kg/hour; titrate to response

Adjunct to general anesthesia: I.M., I.V.: 2-50 mcg/kg

General anesthesia without additional anesthetic agents: I.V. 50-100 mcg/kg with O_2 and skeletal muscle relaxant

Breakthrough cancer pain: Transmucosal: Actiq® dosing should be individually titrated to provide adequate analgesia with minimal side effects. It is indicated only for management of breakthrough cancer pain in patients who are tolerant to and currently receiving opioid therapy for persistent cancer pain. An initial starting dose of 200 mcg should be used for the treatment of breakthrough cancer pain. Patients should be monitored closely in order to determine the proper dose. If redosing for the same episode is necessary, the second dose may be started 15 minutes after completion of the first dose. Dosing should be titrated so that the patient's pain can be treated with one single dose. Generally, 1-2 days is required to determine the proper dose of analgesia with limited side effects. Once the dose has been determined, consumption should be limited to 4 units/day or less. Patients needing more than 4 units/day should have the dose of their long-term opioid re-evaluated. If signs of excessive opioid effects occur before a dose is complete, the unit should be removed from the patients mouth immediately, and subsequent doses decreased.

Pain control: Transdermal: Initial: 25 mcg/hour system; if currently receiving opiates, convert to fentanyl equivalent and administer equianalgesic dosage titrated to minimize the adverse effects and provide analgesia. To convert patients from oral or parenteral opioids to Duragesic®, the previous 24-hour analgesic requirement should be calculated. This analgesic requirement should be converted to the equianalgesic oral morphine dose. See tables.

Equianalgesic Doses of Opioid Agonists

Drug	Equianalgesic Dose (mg)	
	I.M.	P.O.
Codeine	130	200
Hydromorphone	1.5	7.5
Levorphanol	2	4
Meperidine	75	—
Methadone	10	20
Morphine	10	60
Oxycodone	15	30
Oxymorphone	1	10 (PR)

From *N Engl J Med*, 1985, 313:84-95.

The dosage should not be titrated more frequently than every 3 days after the initial dose or every 6 days thereafter. The majority of patients are controlled on every 72-hour administration, however, a small number of patients require every 48-hour administration.

(Continued)

Fentanyl *(Continued)*

Corresponding Doses of Oral/Intramuscular Morphine and Duragesic™

P.O. 24-Hour Morphine (mg/d)	I.M. 24-Hour Morphine (mg/d)	Duragesic™ Dose (mcg/h)
45-134	8-22	25
135-224	28-37	50
225-314	38-52	75
315-404	53-67	100
405-494	68-82	125
495-584	83-97	150
585-674	98-112	175
675-764	113-127	200
765-854	128-142	225
855-944	143-157	250
945-1034	158-172	275
1035-1124	173-187	300

Product information, Duragesic™ — Janssen Pharmaceutica, January, 1991.

Elderly: Elderly have been found to be twice as sensitive as younger patients to the effects of fentanyl. A wide range of doses may be used. When choosing a dose, take into consideration the following patient factors: age, weight, physical status, underlying disease states, other drugs used, type of anesthesia used, and the surgical procedure to be performed.

Transmucosal: Dose should be reduced to 2.5-5 mcg/kg. Suck on lozenge vigorously approximately 20-40 minutes before the start of procedure.

Pediatrics: Doses should be titrated to appropriate effects; wide range of doses, dependent upon desired degree of analgesia/anesthesia

Children 1-12 years:

Sedation for minor procedures/analgesia: I.M., I.V.: 1-2 mcg/kg/dose; may repeat at 30- to 60-minute intervals. **Note:** Children 18-36 months of age may require 2-3 mcg/kg/dose

Continuous sedation/analgesia: Initial I.V. bolus: 1-2 mcg/kg then 1 mcg/kg/hour; titrate upward; usual: 1-3 mcg/kg/hour

Pain control: Transdermal: Not recommended

Renal Impairment:

Cl_{cr} 10-50 mL/minute: Administer 75% of normal dose.

Cl_{cr} <10 mL/minute: Administer 50% of normal dose.

Administration

I.V.: Muscular rigidity may occur with rapid I.V. administration. During prolonged administration, dosage requirements may decrease.

Topical: Transdermal: Patients with an elevated temperature may have increased fentanyl absorption transdermally. Observe for adverse effects; dosage adjustment may be needed. Pharmacologic and adverse effects can be seen after discontinuation of transdermal system. Observe patients for at least 12 hours after transdermal product is removed. Keep transdermal product (both used and unused) out of the reach of children. Do **not** use soap, alcohol, or other solvents to remove transdermal gel if it accidentally touches skin, as they may increase transdermal absorption; use copious amounts of water.

Other: Transmucosal: Foil overwrap should be removed just prior to administration. Once removed, patient should place the unit in mouth and allow it to dissolve. Do **not** chew. Actiq® units may be occasionally moved from one side of the mouth to the other. The unit should be consumed over a period of 15 minutes. Unit should be removed after it is consumed or if patient has achieved an adequate response and/or shows signs of respiratory depression. For patients who have received transmucosal product within 6-12 hours, it is recommended that if other narcotics are required, they should be used at starting doses 1/4 to 1/3 those usually recommended.

Stability

Storage:

Injection formulation: Protect from light; **incompatible** when mixed in the same syringe with pentobarbital

Transmucosal: Store at controlled room temperature of 15°C to 30°C (59°F to 86°F)

Compatibility: Stable in D_5W, NS

Compatibility in syringe: Incompatible with pentobarbital

Compatibility when admixed: Incompatible with fluorouracil, methohexital, pentobarbital, thiopental

Monitoring and Teaching Issues

Physical Assessment: Assess other medications patient may be taking for additive or adverse interactions (see Drug Interactions). See Warnings/Precautions and Administration for use cautions. Monitor therapeutic effectiveness and signs of adverse or overdose reactions. Monitor blood pressure, CNS and respiratory status, and degree of sedation at beginning of therapy and at regular intervals with long-term use. Monitor closely for 12 hours after transdermal product is removed (see Administration - Topical). Order safety precautions for inpatient use. May cause physical and/or psychological dependence. Assess knowledge/teach patient appropriate use (if self-administered), adverse reactions to report (see Adverse Reactions), and appropriate interventions to reduce side effects. **Pregnancy risk factor C/D** - see Pregnancy Risk Factor for use cautions. Note breast-feeding caution.

Patient Education: While using this medication, do not use alcohol and other prescription or OTC medications (especially sedatives, tranquilizers, antihistamines, or pain medications) without consulting prescriber. If using Actiq® Oral Transmucosal, you may be at risk for dental carries due to the sugar content. Maintain good oral hygiene. Maintain adequate hydration (2-3 L/day of fluids) unless advised by prescriber to restrict fluids. May cause hypotension, dizziness, drowsiness, impaired coordination, or blurred vision (use caution when driving, climbing stairs, or changing position - rising from sitting or lying to standing, or when engaging in tasks requiring alertness until response to drug is known); nausea or vomiting (frequent mouth care, small, frequent meals, chewing gum, or sucking lozenges may help); or constipation (increased exercise, fluids, fruit, or fiber may help; if unresolved, consult prescriber about use of stool softeners). Report acute dizziness, chest pain, slow or rapid heartbeat, acute headache; confusion or changes in mentation; changes in voiding frequency or amount; swelling of extremities or unusual weight gain; shortness of breath or difficulty breathing; or vision changes. **Pregnancy/breast-feeding precautions:** Inform prescriber if you are or intend to become pregnant. Consult prescriber if breast-feeding.

Administration:

Transdermal: Apply to clean, dry skin, immediately after removing from package. Firmly press in place and hold for 20 seconds.

Actiq® transmucosal: Actiq® preparations contain an amount of medication that can be fatal to children. Keep all units out of the reach of children and discard any open units properly. Actiq® Welcome Kits are available which contain educational materials, safe storage and disposal instructions.

Dietary Issues: Glucose may cause hyperglycemia; monitor blood glucose concentrations. Actiq® contains 2 g sugar per unit.

Geriatric Considerations: The elderly may be particularly susceptible to the CNS depressant and constipating effects of narcotics; therefore, use with caution.

Additional Information Disposal of Actiq® units: After consumption of a complete unit, the handle may be disposed of in a trash container that is out of the reach of children. For a partially-consumed unit, or a unit that still has any drug matrix remaining on the handle, the handle should be placed under hot running tap water until the drug matrix has dissolved. Special child-resistant containers are available to temporarily store partially consumed units that cannot be disposed of immediately.

Fentanyl is 50-100 times as potent as morphine; morphine 10 mg I.M. is equivalent to fentanyl 0.1-0.2 mg I.M.; fentanyl has less hypotensive effects than morphine or meperidine due to minimal or no histamine release. Keep transdermal product (both used and unused) out of the reach of children. Do **not** use soap, alcohol, or other solvents to remove transdermal gel if it accidentally touches skin as they may increase transdermal absorption, use copious amounts of water.

Related Information

Compatibility of Drugs *on page 1564*
Compatibility of Drugs in Syringe *on page 1566*
Controlled Substances Comparison *on page 1568*
Narcotic/Opioid Analgesic Comparison *on page 1583*

Fentanyl Citrate *see* Fentanyl *on page 552*

Feosol® [OTC] *see* Iron Supplements *on page 744*

Feratab® [OTC] *see* Iron Supplements *on page 744*

Fer-Gen-Sol [OTC] *see* Iron Supplements *on page 744*

Fergon® [OTC] *see* Iron Supplements *on page 744*

Fer-In-Sol® [OTC] *see* Iron Supplements *on page 744*

Ferretts [OTC] *see* Iron Supplements *on page 744*

Ferric Gluconate (FER ik GLOO koe nate)

U.S. Brand Names Ferrlecit®

Synonyms Sodium Ferric Gluconate

Generic Available No

Pharmacologic Category Iron Salt

Pregnancy Risk Factor B

Lactation Excretion in breast milk unknown/use caution

Use Repletion of total body iron content in patients with iron-deficiency anemia who are undergoing hemodialysis in conjunction with erythropoietin therapy

Mechanism of Action/Effect Supplies a source to elemental iron necessary to the function of hemoglobin, myoglobin and specific enzyme systems; allows transport of oxygen via hemoglobin

Contraindications Hypersensitivity to ferric gluconate or any component of the formulation; use in any anemia not caused by iron deficiency; heart failure (of any severity); iron overload

Warnings/Precautions Potentially serious hypersensitivity reactions may occur. Fatal immediate hypersensitivity reactions have occurred with other iron carbohydrate complexes. Avoid rapid administration. Flushing and transient hypotension may occur. May augment hemodialysis-induced hypotension. Use with caution in elderly patients. Safety and efficacy in pediatric patients have not been established. Contains benzyl alcohol; do not use in neonates.

Drug Interactions

Decreased Effect: Chloramphenicol may decrease effect of ferric gluconate injection; ferric gluconate injection may decrease the absorption of oral iron

Adverse Reactions Major adverse reactions include hypotension and hypersensitivity reactions. Hypersensitivity reactions have included pruritus, chest pain, hypotension, nausea, abdominal pain, flank pain, fatigue and rash.

1% to 10%:

Cardiovascular: Hypotension (serious hypotension in 1%), chest pain, hypertension, syncope, tachycardia, angina, myocardial infarction, pulmonary edema, hypovolemia, peripheral edema

Central nervous system: Headache, fatigue, fever, malaise, dizziness, paresthesia, insomnia, agitation, somnolence, pain

(Continued)

Ferric Gluconate *(Continued)*

Dermatologic: Pruritus, rash
Endocrine & metabolic: Hyperkalemia, hypoglycemia, hypokalemia
Gastrointestinal: Abdominal pain, nausea, vomiting, diarrhea, rectal disorder, dyspepsia, flatulence, melena
Genitourinary: Urinary tract infection
Hematologic: Anemia, abnormal erythrocytes, lymphadenopathy
Local: Injection site reactions, injection site pain
Neuromuscular & skeletal: Weakness, back pain, leg cramps, myalgia, arthralgia, paresthesia
Ocular: Blurred vision, conjunctivitis
Respiratory: Dyspnea, cough, rhinitis, upper respiratory infection, pneumonia
Miscellaneous: Hypersensitivity reactions, infection, rigors, chills, flu-like syndrome, sepsis, carcinoma, diaphoresis (increased)

<1% (Limited to important or life-threatening): Dry mouth, epigastric pain, groin pain, hemorrhage, hypertonia, nervousness

Overdosage/Toxicology Symptoms of iron overdose include CNS toxicity, acidosis, hepatic and renal impairment, hematemesis, and lethargy. A serum iron level ≥300 µg/mL requires treatment due to severe toxicity. Treatment is generally symptomatic and supportive, but severe overdoses may be treated with deferoxamine. Deferoxamine may be administered I.V. (80 mg/kg over 24 hours) or I.M. (40-90 mg/kg every 8 hours). Usual toxic dose of elemental iron: ≥35 mg/kg.

Pharmacodynamics/Kinetics

Half-Life Elimination: Bound: 1 hour

Formulations Injection, solution: Elemental iron 12.5 mg/mL (5 mL) [contains benzyl alcohol 9 mg/mL]

Dosing

Adults & Elderly: A test dose of 2 mL diluted in 50 mL 0.9% sodium chloride over 60 minutes was previously recommended (not in current manufacturer labeling).

Repletion of iron in hemodialysis patients: I.V.: 125 mg elemental iron per 10 mL (either by I.V. infusion or slow I.V. injection). Most patients will require a cumulative dose of 1 g elemental iron over approximately 8 sequential dialysis treatments to achieve a favorable response.

Administration

I.V.: May be diluted prior to administration; avoid rapid administration. Infusion rate should not exceed 2.1 mg/minute. If administered undiluted, infuse slowly at a rate of up to 12.5 mg/minute. Monitor patient for hypotension or hypersensitivity reactions during infusion.

Stability

Storage: 20°C to 25°C (68°F to 77°F)

Reconstitution: For I.V. infusion, dilute 10 mL ferric gluconate in 100 mL 0.9% sodium chloride; use immediately after dilution

Compatibility: Stable in NS

Do not mix with parenteral nutrition solutions or other medications.

Monitoring Laboratory Tests Hemoglobin and hematocrit, serum ferritin, iron saturation

Monitoring and Teaching Issues

Physical Assessment: See Warnings/Precautions and Contraindications for use cautions. Monitor results of test dose (see Dosing), infusion rate, effectiveness of therapy (laboratory results), and adverse reactions at beginning of therapy and periodically during therapy (see Adverse Reactions and Overdose/Toxicology). Assess knowledge/teach patient adverse symptoms to report (see Patient Education). Note breast-feeding caution.

Patient Education: This medication will be administered by I.V. in conjunction with your dialysis treatment. Report chest pain, rapid heartbeat, or palpitations; difficulty breathing; headache, dizziness, agitation, or inability to sleep; nausea, vomiting, abdominal or flank pain; or skin rash, itching, or redness. **Breast-feeding precaution:** Consult prescriber if breast-feeding.

Additional Information Contains benzyl alcohol 9 mg/mL

Ferrlecit® *see* Ferric Gluconate *on page 555*
Ferro-Sequels® [OTC] *see* Iron Supplements *on page 744*
Ferrous Fumarate *see* Iron Supplements *on page 744*
Ferrous Gluconate *see* Iron Supplements *on page 744*
Ferrous Salts *see* Iron Supplements *on page 744*
Ferrous Sulfate *see* Iron Supplements *on page 744*
Ferrous Sulfate, Ascorbic Acid, Vitamin B Complex, and Folic Acid *see page 1522*
Fertinex® *see* Follitropins *on page 597*
$FeSO_4$ (Ferrous Sulfate) *see* Iron Supplements *on page 744*
Feverall® [OTC] *see* Acetaminophen *on page 35*
Fever Due to Drugs *see page 1526*

Fexofenadine (feks oh FEN a deen)

U.S. Brand Names Allegra®

Synonyms Fexofenadine Hydrochloride

Generic Available No

Pharmacologic Category Antihistamine, Nonsedating

Pregnancy Risk Factor C

Lactation Excretion in breast milk unknown/use caution (AAP rates "compatible")

Use Nonsedating antihistamine indicated for the relief of seasonal allergic rhinitis and chronic idiopathic urticaria

Mechanism of Action/Effect Fexofenadine is an active metabolite of terfenadine and like terfenadine it competes with histamine for H_1-receptor sites on effector cells in the GI tract, blood vessels, and respiratory tract; binds to lung receptors significantly greater than it binds to cerebellar receptors, resulting in a greatly reduced sedative potential

Contraindications Hypersensitivity to fexofenadine or any component of the formulation

Warnings/Precautions Safety and efficacy in children <6 years of age have not been established. Pregnancy risk C.

Drug Interactions

Cytochrome P450 Effect: Substrate of CYP3A4; Inhibits CYP2D6

Decreased Effect: Aluminum- and magnesium-containing antacids decrease plasma levels of fexofenadine; separate administration is recommended.

Increased Effect/Toxicity: Erythromycin and ketoconazole increased the levels of fexofenadine; however, no increase in adverse events or QT_c intervals was noted. The effect of other macrolide agents or azoles has not been investigated.

Nutritional/Ethanol Interactions

Ethanol: Avoid ethanol (although limited with fexofenadine, may increase risk of sedation).

Herb/Nutraceutical: St John's wort may decrease fexofenadine levels.

Adverse Reactions

>10%: Central nervous system: Headache 11% (with once-daily dosing)

1% to 10%:

Central nervous system: Fever (2%), dizziness (2%), pain (2%), drowsiness (1% to 2%), fatigue (1%)

Endocrine & metabolic: Dysmenorrhea (2%)

Gastrointestinal: Nausea (2%), dyspepsia (1%)

Neuromuscular & skeletal: Back pain (2% to 3%)

Otic: Otitis media (3%)

Respiratory: Cough (4%), upper respiratory tract infection (4%), sinusitis (2%)

Miscellaneous: Viral infection (3%)

<1% (Limited to important or life-threatening): Hypersensitivity reactions (anaphylaxis, angioedema, dyspnea, flushing, pruritus, rash, urticaria); insomnia, nervousness, sleep disorders, paroniria

Overdosage/Toxicology Limited information from overdose describes dizziness, drowsiness, and dry mouth. Not effectively removed by hemodialysis. Doses up to 690 mg twice daily were administered for 1 month without significant adverse effects. Treatment is supportive.

Pharmacodynamics/Kinetics

Half-Life Elimination: 14.4 hours

Time to Peak: Serum: ~2.6 hours

Metabolism: ~5% mostly by gut flora; 0.5% to 1.5% by CYP

Onset: 60 minutes

Duration: Antihistaminic effect: ≥12 hours

Formulations

Capsule, as hydrochloride: 60 mg [DSC]

Tablet, as hydrochloride: 30 mg, 60 mg, 180 mg

Dosing

Adults:

Seasonal allergic rhinitis: Oral: 60 mg twice daily **or** 180 mg once daily

Chronic idiopathic urticaria: Oral: 60 mg twice daily

Elderly: Starting dose: 60 mg once daily; adjust for renal impairment.

Pediatrics: Allergic rhinitis, idiopathic urticaria:

Children 6-11 years: Oral: 30 mg twice daily (once daily in children with impaired renal function).

Children ≥12 years: Refer to adult dosing.

Renal Impairment: Cl_{cr} <40 mL/minute: Administer 60 mg once daily; not effectively removed by hemodialysis.

Stability

Storage: Store at controlled room temperature of 20°C to 25°C (68°F to 77°F). Protect from excessive moisture.

Monitoring and Teaching Issues

Physical Assessment: Assess effectiveness and interactions of other medications patient may be taking (see Drug Interactions). Monitor effectiveness of therapy and adverse reactions (see Adverse Reactions) at beginning of therapy and periodically with long-term use. Assess knowledge/teach patient appropriate use, interventions to reduce side effects, and adverse symptoms to report (see Patient Education). **Pregnancy risk factor C** - benefits of use should outweigh possible risks. Note breast-feeding caution.

Patient Education: Take as directed; do not exceed recommended dose. Store at room temperature in a dry place. If taking antacids, separate administration of antacid and this medication. Avoid use of other depressants, alcohol, or sleep-inducing medications unless approved by prescriber. You may experience mild drowsiness or dizziness (use caution when driving or engaging in tasks requiring alertness until response to drug is known); or nausea (small, frequent meals, frequent mouth care, chewing gum, or sucking hard candy may help). Report persistent sedation or drowsiness, menstrual irregularities, or lack of improvement or worsening or condition. **Pregnancy/breast-feeding precautions:** Inform prescriber if you are or intend to become pregnant. Consult prescriber if breast-feeding.

Geriatric Considerations: Plasma levels in the elderly are generally higher than those observed in other age groups. Once daily dosing is recommended when starting therapy in elderly patients or patients with decreased renal function.

Fexofenadine and Pseudoephedrine

(feks oh FEN a deen & soo doe e FED rin)

U.S. Brand Names Allegra-D®

Synonyms Pseudoephedrine and Fexofenadine

Generic Available No

Pharmacologic Category Antihistamine/Decongestant Combination

Pregnancy Risk Factor C

(Continued)

Fexofenadine and Pseudoephedrine *(Continued)*

Lactation Enters breast milk/use caution (AAP rates "compatible")

Use Relief of symptoms associated with seasonal allergic rhinitis in adults and children 12 years of age and older. Symptoms treated effectively include sneezing, rhinorrhea, itchy nose/palate/ and/or throat, itchy/watery/red eyes, and nasal congestion.

Formulations Tablet, extended release: Fexofenadine hydrochloride 60 mg and pseudoephedrine hydrochloride 120 mg

Dosing

Adults & Elderly: Allergic symptoms and nasal congestion: Oral: One tablet twice daily. Avoid administration with food

Pediatrics: Children ≥12 years: Refer to adult dosing.

Renal Impairment: A dose of one tablet once daily is recommended as the starting dose in patients with decreased renal function.

Monitoring and Teaching Issues

Physical Assessment: See individual components listed in Related Information. **Pregnancy risk factor C** - benefits of use should outweigh possible risks. Note breast-feeding caution.

Patient Education: See individual components listed in Related Information. **Pregnancy/breast-feeding precautions:** Inform prescriber if you are pregnant. Consult prescriber if breast-feeding.

Related Information

Fexofenadine *on page 556*
Pseudoephedrine *on page 1150*

Fexofenadine Hydrochloride *see* Fexofenadine *on page 556*

Fiberall® Powder [OTC] *see* Psyllium *on page 1152*

Fiberall® Wafer [OTC] *see* Psyllium *on page 1152*

Fibrinolysin and Desoxyribonuclease

(fye brin oh LYE sin & des oks i rye boe NOO klee ase)

U.S. Brand Names Elase®; Elase-Chloromycetin®

Synonyms Desoxyribonuclease and Fibrinolysin

Generic Available No

Pharmacologic Category Enzyme

Pregnancy Risk Factor C

Lactation Excretion in breast milk unknown

Use Debriding agent; cervicitis; and irrigating agent in infected wounds

Formulations

Ointment (Elase®): Fibrinolysin 1 unit and desoxyribonuclease 666.6 units per g (10 g, 30 g)

Ointment (Elase-Chloromycetin®): Fibrinolysin 1 unit and desoxyribonuclease 666.6 units per g with chloramphenicol 10 mg per g (10 g, 30 g)

Dosing

Adults & Elderly: Wound cleansing: Topical:

Ointment: 2-3 times/day
Wet dressing: 3-4 times/day

Monitoring and Teaching Issues

Physical Assessment: Assess any allergy history prior to administering. Follow administration directions according to purpose. Assess knowledge/teach patient appropriate use, interventions to reduce side effects, and adverse symptoms to report (see Patient Education). **Pregnancy risk factor C** - benefits of use should outweigh possible risks. Note breast-feeding caution.

Patient Education: This medication is for topical use only. Do not swallow, apply anywhere other than instructed, or get near eyes. Follow exact instructions for use. As with any medication, keep out of the reach of children and do not share this medication with others.

Topical: Use as directed, one to three times daily. Wash hands prior to use. Use disposal gloves to apply. Clean wound as instructed. Apply thin layer to clean wound. Avoid putting ointment on skin surrounding wound. Cover with nonadhering dressing. Notify prescriber if wound worsens or rash, redness, or irritation occurs in area surrounding wound. Dispose of soiled dressings and gloves in sealed container.

Vaginal: Use as directed, at bedtime. Apply prescribed amount deep into vagina for 5 nights. Avoid getting ointment on genitalia (if this occurs, wash off immediately). Do not use more than recommended or stop treatment without consulting prescriber. Notify prescriber if unusual pain, itching, excessive discharge, or irritation of external genitalia occurs. Wash hands following administration.

Pregnancy/breast-feeding precautions: Inform prescriber if you are or intend to become pregnant. Consult prescriber if breast-feeding.

Filgrastim (fil GRA stim)

U.S. Brand Names Neupogen®

Synonyms G-CSF; Granulocyte Colony Stimulating Factor

Generic Available No

Pharmacologic Category Colony Stimulating Factor

Pregnancy Risk Factor C

Lactation Excretion in breast milk unknown/use caution

Use Stimulation of granulocyte production in patients with malignancies, including myeloid malignancies; receiving myelosuppressive therapy associated with a significant risk of neutropenia; severe chronic neutropenia (SCN); receiving bone marrow transplantation (BMT); undergoing peripheral blood progenitor cell (PBPC) collection

Mechanism of Action/Effect Stimulates the production, maturation, and activation of neutrophils, G-CSF activates neutrophils to increase both their migration and cytotoxicity. Natural proteins which stimulate hematopoietic stem cells to proliferate, prolong cell survival, stimulate cell differentiation, and stimulate functional activity of mature cells. CSFs are produced by a wide variety of cell types. Specific mechanisms of action are not yet fully understood, but possibly work by a second-messenger pathway with resultant protein production. See table.

Comparative Effects — G-CSF vs. GM-CSF

Proliferation/Differentiation	G-CSF (Filgrastim)	GM-CSF (Sargramostim)
Neutrophils	Yes	Yes
Eosinophils	No	Yes
Macrophages	No	Yes
Neutrophil migration	Enhanced	Inhibited

Contraindications Hypersensitivity to filgrastim, *E. coli*-derived proteins, or any component of the formulation; concurrent myelosuppressive chemotherapy or radiation therapy

Warnings/Precautions Complete blood count and platelet count should be obtained prior to chemotherapy. Do not use G-CSF in the period 24 hours before to 24 hours after administration of cytotoxic chemotherapy because of the potential sensitivity of rapidly dividing myeloid cells to cytotoxic chemotherapy. Precaution should be exercised in the usage of G-CSF in any malignancy with myeloid characteristics. G-CSF can potentially act as a growth factor for any tumor type, particularly myeloid malignancies. Tumors of nonhematopoietic origin may have surface receptors for G-CSF.

Allergic-type reactions have occurred in patients receiving G-CSF with first or later doses. Reactions tended to occur more frequently with intravenous administration and within 30 minutes of infusion. Most patients experience a 30% to 50% decrease in circulating leukocytes within 1-2 days following discontinuation of filgrastim.

Pregnancy risk C.

Drug Interactions

Increased Effect/Toxicity: Drugs which may potentiate the release of neutrophils (eg, lithium) should be used with caution.

Adverse Reactions Effects are generally mild and dose related

>10%:

- Central nervous system: Neutropenic fever, fever
- Dermatologic: Alopecia
- Gastrointestinal: Nausea, vomiting, diarrhea, mucositis, splenomegaly (more common in patients who prolonged (>14 days) treatment, usually subclinical)
- Neuromuscular & skeletal: Medullary bone pain (24%):

1% to 10%:

- Cardiovascular: Chest pain, fluid retention
- Central nervous system: Headache
- Dermatologic: Skin rash
- Gastrointestinal: Anorexia, stomatitis, constipation
- Hematologic: Leukocytosis
- Local: Pain at injection site
- Neuromuscular & skeletal: Weakness
- Respiratory: Dyspnea, cough, sore throat

<1% (Limited to important or life-threatening): Pericarditis, thrombophlebitis, transient supraventricular arrhythmia

Overdosage/Toxicology No clinical adverse effects have been seen with high doses producing ANC >10,000/mm^3. After discontinuing the drug there is a 50% decrease in circulating levels of neutrophils within 1-2 days, and return to pretreatment levels within 1-7 days.

Pharmacodynamics/Kinetics

Absorption: S.C.: 100%

Half-Life Elimination: 1.8-3.5 hours

Time to Peak: Serum: S.C.: 2-6 hours

Metabolism: Systemically degraded

Onset: ~24 hours; plateaus in 3-5 days

Duration: ANC decreases by 50% within 2 days after discontinuing G-CSF; white counts return to the normal range in 4-7 days; peak plasma levels can be maintained for up to 12 hours

Formulations

Injection, solution [preservative free, vial]: 300 mcg/mL (1 mL, 1.6 mL)

Injection, solution [preservative free, prefilled Singleject® syringe]: 600 mcg/mL (0.5 mL, 0.8 mL)

Dosing

Adults & Elderly: Refer to individual protocols.

Note: Dosing should be based on actual body weight (even in morbidly obese patients). Rounding doses to the nearest vial size often enhances patient convenience and reduces costs without compromising clinical response.

Myelosuppressive therapy: I.V., S.C.: 5 mcg/kg/day - doses may be increased by 5 mcg/kg according to the duration and severity of the neutropenia.

Bone marrow transplantation: I.V., S.C.: 5-10 mcg/kg/day - doses may be increased by 5 mcg/kg according to the duration and severity of neutropenia; recommended steps based on neutrophil response:

When ANC >1000/mm^3 for 3 consecutive days: Reduce filgrastim dose to 5 mcg/kg/day.

If ANC remains >1000/mm^3 for 3 more consecutive days: Discontinue filgrastim.

If ANC decreases to <1000/mm^3: Resume at 5 mcg/kg/day.

If ANC decreases <1000/mm^3 during the 5 mcg/kg/day dose, increase filgrastim to 10 mcg/kg/day and follow the above steps.

(Continued)

Filgrastim *(Continued)*

Peripheral blood progenitor cell (PBPC) collection: I.V., S.C.: 10 mcg/kg/day **or** 5-8 mcg/kg twice daily in donors. The optimal timing and duration of growth factor stimulation has not been determined.

Severe chronic neutropenia: S.C.:

Congenital: 6 mcg/kg twice daily

Idiopathic/cyclic: 5 mcg/kg/day

Pediatrics: Children: Refer to adult dosing.

Administration

I.V.: May be administered undiluted by S.C. or IVP administration. May also be administered by I.V. infusion over 15-60 minutes in D_5W.

Stability

Storage: Filgrastim is a clear, colorless solution and should be stored under refrigeration at 2°C to 8°C (36°F to 46°F) and protected from direct sunlight. Filgrastim should be protected from freezing and temperatures >30°C to avoid aggregation. The solution should not be shaken since bubbles and/or foam may form. If foaming occurs, the solution should be left undisturbed for a few minutes until bubbles dissipate.

Filgrastim is stable for 24 hours at 9°C to 30°C, however, the manufacturer recommends discarding after 6 hours because of microbiological concerns. The product is packaged as single-use vial without a preservative.

Undiluted filgrastim is stable for 24 hours at 15°C to 30°C and 7 days at 2°C to 8°C in tuberculin syringes. However, refrigeration and use within 24 hours are recommended because of concern for bacterial contamination.

Reconstitution: Filgrastim may be diluted in dextrose 5% in water to a concentration ≥15 mcg/mL for I.V. infusion administration. Minimum concentration is 15 mcg/mL Concentrations <15 mcg/mL require addition of albumin (1 mL of 5%) to the bag to prevent absorption to plastics/PVC. This diluted solution is stable for 7 days under refrigeration or at room temperature.

Compatibility: Standard diluent: ≥375 mcg/25 mL D_5W. Stable in D_5W; **incompatible** with NS

Y-site administration: Incompatible with amphotericin B, cefepime, cefoperazone, cefotaxime, cefoxitin, ceftizoxime, ceftriaxone, cefuroxime, clindamycin, dactinomycin, etoposide, fluorouracil, furosemide, heparin, mannitol, methylprednisolone sodium succinate, metronidazole, mitomycin, piperacillin, prochlorperazine edisylate, thiotepa

Monitoring Laboratory Tests CBC and platelet count should be obtained twice weekly. Leukocytosis (white blood cell counts ≥100,000/mm^3) has been observed in ~2% of patients receiving G-CSF at doses >5 mcg/kg/day. Monitor platelets and hematocrit regularly.

Monitoring and Teaching Issues

Physical Assessment: Assess for hypersensitivity to *E. coli* products prior to beginning therapy. See Contraindications, Warnings/Precautions, and Dosing for use cautions. Assess potential for interactions with prescriptions, OTC medications, or herbal products patient may be taking (see Drug Interactions). Assess results of laboratory tests (see above), therapeutic effects, and signs/symptoms of adverse reactions at beginning of therapy and periodically throughout therapy (eg, allergic-type reactions have occurred in patients receiving G-CSF with first or later doses - see Warnings/Precautions and Adverse Reactions). If self-administered, teach patient (or caregiver) proper storage, administration, and syringe/needle disposal. Teach patient (or caregiver) possible side effects and appropriate interventions and adverse symptoms to report (see Patient Education). **Pregnancy risk factor C** - benefits of use should outweigh possible risks. Note breast-feeding caution.

Patient Education: Inform prescriber of all prescriptions, OTC medications, or herbal products you are taking, and any allergies you have. Do not take anything new during treatment unless approved by prescriber. If self-administered, follow directions for proper storage and administration of S.C. medication. Never reuse syringes or needles. May cause bone pain (request analgesic); nausea or vomiting (small, frequent meals may help); hair loss (reversible); or sore mouth (frequent mouth care with soft toothbrush or cotton swab may help). Report unusual fever or chills; unhealed sores; severe bone pain; pain, redness, or swelling at injection site; unusual swelling of extremities or difficulty breathing; or chest pain and palpitations. **Pregnancy/breast-feeding precautions:** Inform prescriber if you are or intend to become pregnant. Consult prescriber if breast-feeding.

Additional Information

Reimbursement Hotline: 1-800-272-9376

Professional Services [Amgen]: 1-800-77-AMGEN

Finasteride (fi NAS teer ide)

U.S. Brand Names Propecia®; Proscar®

Generic Available No

Pharmacologic Category 5 Alpha-Reductase Inhibitor

Pregnancy Risk Factor X

Lactation Not indicated for use in women

Use

Propecia®: Treatment of male pattern hair loss in **men only**. Safety and efficacy were demonstrated in men between 18-41 years of age.

Proscar®: Treatment of symptomatic benign prostatic hyperplasia (BPH)

Use - Unlabeled/Investigational Adjuvant monotherapy after radical prostatectomy in the treatment of prostatic cancer; female hirsutism

Mechanism of Action/Effect Finasteride is a 4-azo analog of testosterone and is a competitive inhibitor of both tissue and hepatic 5-alpha reductase. This results in inhibition of the conversion of testosterone to dihydrotestosterone and markedly suppresses serum dihydrotestosterone levels. Depending on dose and duration, serum testosterone concentrations may or may not increase. Testosterone-dependent processes such as fertility, muscle strength, potency, and libido are not affected by finasteride.

Contraindications Hypersensitivity to finasteride or any component of the formulation; pregnancy; not for use in children

Warnings/Precautions A minimum of 6 months of treatment may be necessary to determine whether an individual will respond to finasteride. Use with caution in those patients with liver function abnormalities. Carefully monitor patients with a large residual urinary volume or severely diminished urinary flow for obstructive uropathy. These patients may not be candidates for finasteride therapy.

Drug Interactions

Cytochrome P450 Effect: Substrate of CYP3A4

Nutritional/Ethanol Interactions

Food: Administration with food may delay the rate and reduce the extent of oral absorption.

Herb/Nutraceutical: St John's wort may decrease finasteride levels. Avoid saw palmetto (concurrent use has not been adequately studied).

Adverse Reactions

1% to 10%:

Endocrine & metabolic: Libido decreased

Genitourinary: <4% incidence of erectile dysfunction, decreased volume of ejaculate

<1%, postmarketing and/or case reports: Hypersensitivity (pruritus, rash, urticaria, swelling of face/lips), testicular pain, breast tenderness, breast enlargement

Pharmacodynamics/Kinetics

Absorption: May be reduced with food

Bioavailability: Mean: 63%

Half-Life Elimination: Serum: Parent drug: ~5-17 hours (mean: 1.9 fasting, 4.2 with breakfast); Elderly: 8 hours; Adults: 6 hours (3-16); rate decreased in elderly, but no dosage adjustment needed

Time to Peak: Serum: 2-6 hours

Metabolism: Hepatic; two active metabolites identified

Onset: 3-6 months of ongoing therapy

Duration:

After a single oral dose as small as 0.5 mg: 65% depression of plasma dihydrotestosterone levels persists 5-7 days

After 6 months of treatment with 5 mg/day: Circulating dihydrotestosterone levels are reduced to castrate levels without significant effects on circulating testosterone; levels return to normal within 14 days of discontinuation of treatment

Formulations

Tablet, film coated:

Propecia®: 1 mg

Proscar®: 5 mg

Dosing

Adults & Elderly:

Benign prostatic hyperplasia (Proscar®): Oral: 5 mg/day as a single dose; clinical responses occur within 12 weeks to 6 months of initiation of therapy; long-term administration is recommended for maximal response

Male pattern baldness (Propecia®): Oral: 1 mg daily

Female hirsutism (unlabeled use): Oral: 5 mg/day

Renal Impairment: No adjustment is necessary.

Hepatic Impairment: Use with caution in patients with liver function abnormalities because finasteride is metabolized extensively in the liver

Administration

Oral: Administration with food may delay the rate and reduce the extent of oral absorption. Childbearing age women should not touch or handle this medication.

Monitoring Laboratory Tests Finasteride does not interfere with free PSA levels.

Monitoring and Teaching Issues

Physical Assessment: See Contraindications, Warnings/Precautions, and Dosing for use cautions. Assess potential for interactions with prescription, OTC medications, or herbal products patient may be taking (see Drug Interactions). Assess therapeutic effects and signs/symptoms of adverse reactions (see Adverse Reactions and Overdose/Toxicology). Teach patient proper use, possible side effects and appropriate interventions and adverse symptoms to report (see Patient Education). **Pregnancy risk factor X** - instruct patient on absolute need for barrier contraceptives. Childbearing age women should not touch or handle this medication.

Patient Education: Inform prescriber of all prescriptions, OTC medications, or herbal products you are taking, and any allergies you have. Do not take anything new during treatment unless approved by prescriber. Results of therapy may take several months. Take as directed, with fluids, 30 minutes before or 2 hours after meals. May cause decreased libido or impotence during therapy. Report any increase in urinary volume or voiding patterns occurs. **Pregnancy precautions:** This drug will cause fetal abnormalities - use barrier contraceptives and do not allow childbearing age women to touch or handle drug.

Geriatric Considerations: Clearance of finasteride is decreased in the elderly, but no dosage reductions are necessary.

Fioricet® *see* Butalbital, Acetaminophen, and Caffeine *on page 192*

Fioricet® with Codeine *see* Butalbital, Acetaminophen, Caffeine, and Codeine *on page 193*

Fiorinal® *see* Butalbital, Aspirin, and Caffeine *on page 194*

Fiorinal® With Codeine *see* Butalbital, Aspirin, Caffeine, and Codeine *on page 195*

Fisalamine *see* Mesalamine *on page 858*

FK506 *see* Tacrolimus *on page 1271*

Flagyl® *see* Metronidazole *on page 895*

Flagyl ER® *see* Metronidazole *on page 895*

Flarex® *see* Fluorometholone *on page 575*

Flecainide (fle KAY nide)

U.S. Brand Names Tambocor™

Synonyms Flecainide Acetate

Generic Available No

Pharmacologic Category Antiarrhythmic Agent, Class Ic

Pregnancy Risk Factor C

Lactation Enters breast milk/compatible

Use Prevention and suppression of documented life-threatening ventricular arrhythmias (eg, sustained ventricular tachycardia); controlling symptomatic, disabling supraventricular tachycardias in patients without structural heart disease in whom other agents fail

Mechanism of Action/Effect Class Ic antiarrhythmic; slows conduction in cardiac tissue by altering transport of ions across cell membranes; causes slight prolongation of refractory periods; decreases the rate of rise of the action potential without affecting its duration; increases electrical stimulation threshold of ventricle, His-Purkinje system; possesses local anesthetic and moderate negative inotropic effects

Contraindications Hypersensitivity to flecainide or any component of the formulation; pre-existing second- or third-degree AV block or with right bundle branch block when associated with a left hemiblock (bifascicular block) (except in patients with a functioning artificial pacemaker); cardiogenic shock; coronary artery disease (based on CAST study results); concurrent use of ritonavir or amprenavir

Warnings/Precautions Not recommend for patients with chronic atrial fibrillation. A worsening or new arrhythmia may occur (proarrhythmic effect). Use caution in heart failure (may precipitate or exacerbate CHF). Dose-related increases in PR, QRS, and QT intervals occur. Use with caution in sick sinus syndrome or with permanent pacemakers or temporary pacing wires (can increase endocardial pacing thresholds). Due to potential to exacerbate toxicity, pre-existing hypokalemia or hyperkalemia should be corrected before initiation of flecainide. Use caution in patients with significant hepatic impairment. Pregnancy risk C.

Drug Interactions

Cytochrome P450 Effect: Substrate of CYP1A2, **2D6**; Inhibits CYP2D6

Decreased Effect: Smoking and acid urine increase flecainide clearance.

Increased Effect/Toxicity: Flecainide concentrations may be increased by amiodarone (reduce flecainide 25% to 33%), amprenavir, cimetidine, digoxin, propranolol, quinidine, and ritonavir. Beta-adrenergic blockers, disopyramide, verapamil may enhance flecainide's negative inotropic effects. Alkalinizing agents (ie, high-dose antacids, cimetidine, carbonic anhydrase inhibitors, sodium bicarbonate) may decrease flecainide clearance, potentially increasing toxicity. Propranolol blood levels are increased by flecainide.

Nutritional/Ethanol Interactions Food: Clearance may be decreased in patients following strict vegetarian diets due to urinary pH ≥8. Dairy products (milk, infant formula, yogurt) may interfere with the absorption of flecainide in infants; there is one case report of a neonate (GA 34 weeks PNA >6 days) who required extremely large doses of oral flecainide when administered every 8 hours with feedings ("milk feeds"); changing the feedings from "milk feeds" to 5% glucose feeds alone resulted in a doubling of the flecainide serum concentration and toxicity.

Adverse Reactions

>10%:

- Central nervous system: Dizziness (19% to 30%)
- Ocular: Visual disturbances (16%)
- Respiratory: Dyspnea (~10%)

1% to 10%:

- Cardiovascular: Palpitations (6%), chest pain (5%), edema (3.5%), tachycardia (1% to 3%), proarrhythmic (4% to 12%), sinus node dysfunction (1.2%)
- Central nervous system: Headache (4% to 10%), fatigue (8%), nervousness (5%) additional symptoms occurring at a frequency between 1% and 3%: fever, malaise, hypoesthesia, paresis, ataxia, vertigo, syncope, somnolence, tinnitus, anxiety, insomnia, depression
- Dermatologic: Rash (1% to 3%)
- Gastrointestinal: Nausea (9%), constipation (1%), abdominal pain (3%), anorexia (1% to 3%), diarrhea (0.7% to 3%)
- Neuromuscular & skeletal: Tremor (5%), weakness (5%), paresthesias (1%)
- Ocular: Diplopia (1% to 3%), blurred vision

<1% (Limited to important or life-threatening): Alopecia, alters pacing threshold, amnesia, angina, AV block, bradycardia, bronchospasm, CHF, corneal deposits, depersonalization, euphoria, exfoliative dermatitis, granulocytopenia, heart block, increased P-R, leukopenia, metallic taste, neuropathy, paradoxical increase in ventricular rate in atrial fibrillation/flutter, paresthesia, photophobia, pneumonitis, pruritus, QRS duration, swollen lips/tongue/mouth, tardive dyskinesia, thrombocytopenia, urinary retention, urticaria, ventricular arrhythmias

Overdosage/Toxicology Flecainide has a narrow therapeutic index and severe toxicity may occur slightly above the therapeutic range, especially if combined with other antiarrhythmic drugs. (Acute single ingestion of twice the daily therapeutic dose is life-threatening). Symptoms of overdose include increase in P-R, QRS, or QT intervals and amplitude of the T wave, AV block, bradycardia, hypotension, ventricular arrhythmias (monomorphic or polymorphic ventricular tachycardia), and asystole. Other symptoms include dizziness, blurred vision, headache, and GI upset. Treatment is supportive.

Pharmacodynamics/Kinetics

Absorption: Oral: Rapid

Bioavailability: 85% to 90%

Half-Life Elimination: Infants: 11-12 hours; Children: 8 hours; Adults: 7-22 hours, increased with congestive heart failure or renal dysfunction; End-stage renal disease: 19-26 hours

Time to Peak: Serum: ~1.5-3 hours

Metabolism: Hepatic

Formulations Tablet, as acetate: 50 mg, 100 mg, 150 mg

Dosing

Adults & Elderly:

Life-threatening ventricular arrhythmias: Oral:

Initial: 100 mg every 12 hours; increase by 50-100 mg/day (given in 2 doses/day) every 4 days; maximum: 400 mg/day

For patients receiving 400 mg/day who are not controlled and have trough concentrations <0.6 μg/mL, dosage may be increased to 600 mg/day.

Prevention of paroxysmal supraventricular arrhythmias in patients with disabling symptoms but no structural heart disease: Oral:

Initial: 50 mg every 12 hours; increase by 50 mg twice daily at 4-day intervals; maximum: 300 mg/day

Pediatrics: Oral: Children:

Initial: 3 mg/kg/day or 50-100 mg/m^2/day in 3 divided doses

Usual: 3-6 mg/kg/day or 100-150 mg/m^2/day in 3 divided doses; up to 11 mg/kg/day or 200 mg/m^2/day for uncontrolled patients with subtherapeutic levels

Renal Impairment:

Cl_{cr} <10 mL/minute: Decrease usual dose by 25% to 50% in severe renal impairment.

Not dialyzable (0% to 5%) via hemo- or peritoneal dialysis; no supplemental dose is necessary.

Hepatic Impairment: Monitoring of plasma levels is recommended because half-life is significantly increased. When transferring from another antiarrhythmic agent, allow for 2-4 half-lives of the agent to pass before initiating flecainide therapy.

Administration

Oral: Administer around-the-clock to promote less variation in peak and trough serum levels.

Monitoring Laboratory Tests Periodic serum concentrations, especially in patients with renal or hepatic impairment

Monitoring and Teaching Issues

Physical Assessment: Assess other medications patient may be taking for effectiveness and interactions (see Drug Interactions). See Warnings/Precautions and Contraindications for use cautions. Monitor laboratory tests, therapeutic response, and adverse reactions (see Warnings/Precautions and Adverse Reactions) when beginning therapy, when titrating dosage, and periodically during long-term therapy. **Note:** Flecainide has a low toxic:therapeutic ratio and overdose may easily produce severe and life-threatening reactions (see Overdose/Toxicology). Assess knowledge/teach patient appropriate use, interventions to reduce side effects, and adverse symptoms to report (see Patient Education). **Pregnancy risk factor C** - benefits of use should outweigh possible risks.

Patient Education: Take exactly as directed, around-the-clock. Do not discontinue without consulting prescriber. You will require frequent monitoring while taking this medication. You may experience lightheadedness, nervousness, dizziness, visual disturbances (use caution when driving or engaging in tasks requiring alertness until response to drug is known); or nausea, vomiting, or loss of appetite (small, frequent meals may help). Report palpitations, chest pain, excessively slow or rapid heartbeat; acute nervousness, headache, or fatigue; unusual weight gain; unusual cough; difficulty breathing; swelling of hands or ankles; or muscle tremor, numbness, or weakness. **Pregnancy precaution:** Inform prescriber if you are or intend to become pregnant.

Related Information

Antiarrhythmic Drugs *on page 1551*

Flecainide Acetate *see* Flecainide *on page 562*

Fleet® Enema [OTC] *see* Phosphate Supplements *on page 1076*

Fleet® Phospho®-Soda [OTC] *see* Phosphate Supplements *on page 1076*

Fleet® Sof-Lax® [OTC] *see* Docusate *on page 432*

Flexeril® *see* Cyclobenzaprine *on page 338*

Flolan® *see* Epoprostenol *on page 479*

Flonase® *see* Fluticasone *on page 588*

Florical® [OTC] *see* Calcium Supplements *on page 202*

Florinef® *see* Fludrocortisone *on page 569*

Florone® *see* Topical Corticosteroids *on page 1334*

Floropryl® *see page 1509*

Flovent® *see* Fluticasone *on page 588*

Flovent® Rotadisk® *see* Fluticasone *on page 588*

Floxin® *see page 1519*

Floxin® *see* Ofloxacin *on page 993*

Floxuridine (floks YOOR i deen)

U.S. Brand Names FUDR®

Synonyms Fluorodeoxyuridine; FUDR

Generic Available Yes

Pharmacologic Category Antineoplastic Agent, Antimetabolite

Pregnancy Risk Factor D

Lactation Excretion in breast milk unknown/contraindicated

Use Management of hepatic metastases of colorectal and gastric cancers

Mechanism of Action/Effect Mechanism of action and pharmacokinetics are very similar to 5-FU; FUDR® is the deoxyribonucleotide of 5-FU. Inhibits DNA and RNA synthesis via formation of carbonium ions; cross-links strands of DNA, causing an imbalance of growth and cell death

Contraindications Hypersensitivity to floxuridine, fluorouracil, or any component of the formulation; pregnancy

Warnings/Precautions The U.S. Food and Drug Administration (FDA) currently recommends that procedures for proper handling and disposal of antineoplastic agents be considered.

(Continued)

Floxuridine *(Continued)*

Use caution in impaired kidney or liver function. Discontinue if intractable vomiting or diarrhea, precipitous fall in leukocyte or platelet counts, or myocardial ischemia occur. Use with caution in patients who have had high-dose pelvic radiation or previous use of alkylating agents. Patient should be hospitalized during initial course of therapy. Use of floxuridine with pentostatin has been associated with a high incidence of fatal pulmonary toxicity; this combination is not recommended.

If floxuridine contacts the skin, wash and flush thoroughly with water.

Drug Interactions

Decreased Effect: Patients may experience impaired immune response to vaccines; possible infection after administration of live vaccines in patients receiving immunosuppressants.

Increased Effect/Toxicity: Any form of therapy which adds to the stress of the patient, interferes with nutrition, or depresses bone marrow function will increase the toxicity of floxuridine. Pentostatin and floxuridine administered together has resulted in fatal pulmonary toxicity.

Nutritional/Ethanol Interactions Ethanol: Avoid ethanol (due to GI irritation).

Effects on Lab Values ↑ potassium (S)

Adverse Reactions

>10%:

- Central nervous system: Fever, chills, fatigue, pain
- Gastrointestinal: GI hemorrhage, stomatitis, esophagopharyngitis, diarrhea, gastritis, nausea, vomiting
- Hematologic: Severe hematologic toxicity, neutropenia, thrombocytopenia
  - Onset: 4-7 days
  - Nadir: 5-9 days
  - Recovery: 21 days
- Respiratory: Pneumonia

1% to 10%:

- Cardiovascular: Edema
- Central nervous system: Headache
- Dermatologic: Alopecia, dermatitis, rash
- Gastrointestinal: Anorexia, glossitis
  - Emetic potential: Very low (<10%)
- Genitourinary: Dysuria, urinary tract infection, hematuria, proteinuria
- Neuromuscular & skeletal: Myalgia, osteonecrosis, arthralgia
- Respiratory: Cough, dyspnea, sinusitis, epistaxis, hemoptysis, hypoxia, bronchitis, upper respiratory infection

<1% (Limited to important or life-threatening): Anaphylaxis, angina, hepatic necrosis, myocardial ischemia

Pharmacodynamics/Kinetics

Metabolism: Hepatic; Active metabolites: Floxuridine monophosphate (FUDR-MP) and fluorouracil; Inactive metabolites: Urea, CO_2, α-fluoro-β-alanine, α-fluoro-β-guanidopropionic acid, α-fluoro-β-ureidopropionic acid, and dihydrofluorouracil

Formulations Injection, powder for reconstitution: 500 mg

Dosing

Adults: Refer to individual protocols.

Colorectal or gastric metastases:

Intra-arterial: Primarily by an implantable pump: 0.1-0.6 mg/kg/day continuous intra-arterial administration for 14 days then heparinized saline is given for 14 days; toxicity requires dose reduction.

I.V.: Many regimens in use, examples:

- 0.15 mg/kg/day for 7-14 days
- 0.5-1 mg/kg/day for 6-15 days
- 30 mg/kg/day for 5 days, then 15 mg/kg/day every other day, up to 11 days

Elderly: Adjust dose since elderly patients are prone to toxicity.

Renal Impairment: Adjust dose relative to toxicity; patients with renal insufficiency are prone to toxicity.

Administration

I.V.: Infused for intra-arterial use, use infusion pump, either external or implanted.

Stability

Storage: Store intact vials at room temperature of 15°C to 30°C (59°F to 86°F). Reconstituted vials are stable for up to 2 weeks under refrigeration at 2°C to 8°C (36°C to 46°C). Solutions in 0.9% sodium chloride are stable in some ambulatory infusion pumps for up to 21 days.

Reconstitution: Dilute with 5 mL SWI for a final concentration of 100 mg/mL which is stable for 2 weeks under refrigeration (15°C to 30°C). Contains no preservative. Recommend use within 8 hours of reconstitution.

Compatibility: Stable in D_5W, NS, sterile water for injection

Y-site administration: Incompatible with allopurinol, cefepime

Monitoring Laboratory Tests CBC, platelet count, liver function

Monitoring and Teaching Issues

Physical Assessment: See Contraindications, Warnings/Precautions, and Dosing for use cautions. Assess potential for interactions with other prescriptions, OTC medications, or herbal products patient may be taking (see Drug Interactions). See specific Administration and Compatibility directions. Assess results of laboratory tests (see above), therapeutic effectiveness, and adverse response (eg, CNS changes, acute gastrointestinal reactions - see Adverse Reactions) on a regular basis throughout therapy. Teach patient (caregiver) care of implantable pump. Teach patient (caregiver) possible side effects and appropriate interventions and adverse symptoms to report (see Patient Education). **Pregnancy risk factor D** - determine that patient is not pregnant before beginning treatment. Instruct patients of childbearing age on appropriate barrier contraceptive measures. Breast-feeding is contraindicated.

Patient Education: Inform prescriber of all prescriptions, OTC medications, or herbal products you are taking, and any allergies you have. Do not take anything new during treatment unless approved by prescriber. This drug can only be administered by infusion. Follow instructions of prescriber for care of implantable pump. Avoid alcohol. It is important to maintain adequate hydration (2-3 L/day of fluids) unless advised by prescriber to restrict fluids, and nutrition (small, frequent meals may help). You will be more susceptible to infection (avoid crowds and exposure to infection and do not have any vaccinations without consulting prescriber). May cause nausea or vomiting (small, frequent meals, frequent mouth care, sucking lozenges, or chewing gum may help); loss of hair (reversible); diarrhea (buttermilk, boiled milk, or yogurt may help reduce diarrhea); mouth sores (use a soft toothbrush or cotton swabs for oral care); or sterility. Increased emotional or physical stress will adversely affect the response to this medication. Notify prescriber if you are experiencing unusual or elevated levels of stress. Report extreme fatigue; pain or numbness in extremities; severe GI upset or diarrhea; bleeding or bruising; fever, chills, or sore throat; vaginal discharge; or signs of fluid retention (eg, swelling extremities, difficulty breathing, unusual weight gain). **Pregnancy/breast-feeding precautions:** Do not get pregnant while taking this medication and for 1 month following therapy. Consult prescriber for appropriate barrier contraceptives. Do not breast-feed.

Flubenisolone *see* Betamethasone *on page 160*

Fluconazole (floo KOE na zole)

U.S. Brand Names Diflucan®

Generic Available No

Pharmacologic Category Antifungal Agent, Oral; Antifungal Agent, Parenteral

Pregnancy Risk Factor C

Lactation Excretion in breast milk unknown/use caution (AAP rates "compatible")

Use Treatment of oral or vaginal candidiasis unresponsive to nystatin or clotrimazole; nonlife-threatening *Candida* infections (eg, cystitis, esophagitis); treatment of hepatosplenic candidiasis; treatment of other *Candida* infections in persons unable to tolerate amphotericin B; treatment of cryptococcal infections; secondary prophylaxis for cryptococcal meningitis in persons with AIDS; antifungal prophylaxis in allogeneic bone marrow transplant recipients

Oral fluconazole should be used in persons able to tolerate oral medications; parenteral fluconazole should be reserved for patients who are both unable to take oral medications and are unable to tolerate amphotericin B (eg, due to hypersensitivity or renal insufficiency)

Mechanism of Action/Effect Interferes with cytochrome P450 activity, decreasing ergosterol synthesis (principal sterol in fungal cell membrane) and inhibiting cell membrane formation

Contraindications Hypersensitivity to fluconazole, other azoles, or any component of the formulation; concomitant administration with cisapride or astemizole

Warnings/Precautions Should be used with caution in patients with renal and hepatic dysfunction or previous hepatotoxicity from other azole derivatives. Patients who develop abnormal liver function tests during fluconazole therapy should be monitored closely and discontinued if symptoms consistent with liver disease develop. Pregnancy risk C.

Drug Interactions

Cytochrome P450 Effect: Inhibits CYP1A2, **2C8/9, 2C19, 3A4**

Decreased Effect: Rifampin decreases concentrations of fluconazole.

Increased Effect/Toxicity: Fluconazole may increase serum concentrations/effects of cyclosporine, phenytoin, rifabutin, tacrolimus, theophylline, rifabutin, sulfonylureas, warfarin, and zidovudine. Fluconazole may also increase cisapride or astemizole levels which has been associated with malignant arrhythmias. Hydrochlorothiazide may increase fluconazole levels.

Adverse Reactions Frequency not always defined.

Cardiovascular: Pallor, angioedema

Central nervous system: Headache (2% to 13%), seizures, dizziness

Dermatologic: Rash (2%), alopecia, toxic epidermal necrolysis, Stevens-Johnson syndrome

Endocrine & metabolic: Hypertriglyceridemia, hypokalemia

Gastrointestinal: Nausea (4% to 7%), vomiting (2%), abdominal pain (2% to 6%), diarrhea (2% to 3%), taste perversion

Hematologic: Leukopenia, thrombocytopenia

Hepatic: Hepatic failure (rare), hepatitis, cholestasis, jaundice, increased ALT/AST, increased alkaline phosphatase

Respiratory: Dyspnea

Miscellaneous: Anaphylactic reactions (rare)

Overdosage/Toxicology Symptoms of overdose include decreased lacrimation, salivation, respiration and motility, urinary incontinence, and cyanosis. Treatment includes supportive measures. A 3-hour hemodialysis will remove 50%.

Pharmacodynamics/Kinetics

Bioavailability: Oral: >90%

Half-Life Elimination: Normal renal function: 25-30 hours

Time to Peak: Serum: Oral: ~2-4 hours

Formulations

Infusion [premixed in sodium chloride or dextrose]: 2 mg/mL (100 mL, 200 mL)

Powder for oral suspension: 10 mg/mL (35 mL); 40 mg/mL (35 mL) [contains sodium benzoate; orange flavor]

Tablet: 50 mg, 100 mg, 150 mg, 200 mg

Dosing

Adults & Elderly: The daily dose of fluconazole is the same for both oral and I.V. administration

Fungal infections: Oral, I.V.: Once-daily dosing by indication: See table on next page.

(Continued)

Fluconazole *(Continued)*

Fluconazole — Once-Daily Dosing — Adults

Indication	Day 1	Daily Therapy	Minimum Duration of Therapy
Oropharyngeal candidiasis	200 mg	100 mg	14 d
Esophageal candidiasis	200 mg	100 mg	21 d and for at least 14 d following resolution of symptoms
Prevention of candidiasis in bone marrow transplant	400 mg	400 mg	3 d before neutropenia, 7 d after neutrophils >1000 cells/mm^3
Candidiasis UTIs, peritonitis	50-200 mg	50-200 mg	N/A
Systemic candidiasis	400 mg	200 mg	28 d
Cryptococcal meningitis			
acute	400 mg	200 mg	10-12 wk after CSF culture becomes negative
relapse suppression	200 mg	200 mg	N/A
Vaginal candidiasis	150 mg	Single dose	N/A

N/A = Not applicable

Pediatrics: Fungal infections: Oral, I.V.: Once-daily dosing by indication: See table.

Fluconazole — Once-Daily Dosing — Children

Indication	Day 1	Daily Therapy	Minimum Duration of Therapy
Oropharyngeal candidiasis	6 mg/kg	3 mg/kg	14 d
Esophageal candidiasis	6 mg/kg	3-12 mg/kg	21 d and for at least 2 wks following resolution of symptoms
Systemic candidiasis	—	6-12 mg/kg	28 d
Cryptococcal meningitis			
acute	12 mg/kg	6-12 mg/kg	10-12 wk after CSF culture becomes negative
relapse suppression	6 mg/kg	6 mg/kg	N/A

N/A = Not applicable

Renal Impairment:

Cl_{cr} 21-50 mL/minute: Administer 50% of recommended dose or administer every 48 hours.

Cl_{cr} <20 mL/minute: Administer 25% of recommended dose or administer every 72 hours.

Hemodialysis effects: 50% is removed by hemodialysis.

Continuous arteriovenous or venovenous hemofiltration: Dose as for Cl_{cr} 10-50 mL/minute.

Administration

I.M.: For I.V. only; do not administer I.M. or S.C.

I.V.: Administer maximum rate of infusion: 200 mg/hour.

Stability

Storage: Fluconazole for injection should be stored between 5°C to 30°C (glass bottles) or 5°C to 25°C (PVC).

Reconstitution: Standard diluent: 200 mg/100 mL NS (premixed); 400 mg/200 mL NS (premixed)

Compatibility: Stable in D_5W, LR, NS

Y-site administration: Incompatible with amphotericin B, amphotericin B cholesteryl sulfate complex, ampicillin, calcium gluconate, cefotaxime, ceftazidime, ceftriaxone, cefuroxime, chloramphenicol, clindamycin, co-trimoxazole, diazepam, digoxin, erythromycin lactobionate, furosemide, haloperidol, hydroxyzine, imipenem/cilastatin, pentamidine, piperacillin, ticarcillin

Compatibility when admixed: Incompatible with co-trimoxazole

Monitoring Laboratory Tests Culture prior to beginning therapy, periodic liver function (AST, ALT, alkaline phosphatase) and renal function, potassium

Monitoring and Teaching Issues

Physical Assessment: Assess allergy history prior to beginning therapy. See Contraindications, Warnings/Precautions, and Dosing for use cautions. Assess potential for interactions with other prescriptions, OTC medications, and herbal products patient may be taking (see Drug Interactions). See specific Administration and Compatibility directions. Assess results of laboratory tests (see above), therapeutic effects, and adverse response (see Adverse Reactions) on a regular basis throughout therapy. Teach patient use, possible side effects and appropriate interventions, and adverse symptoms to report (see Patient Education). **Pregnancy risk factor C** - benefits of use should outweigh possible risks. Note breast-feeding caution.

Patient Education: Inform prescriber of all prescriptions, OTC medications, or herbal products you are taking, and any allergies you have. Do not take anything new during treatment unless approved by prescriber. Take as directed, around-the-clock. Take full course of medication as ordered. Take with or without food. Follow good hygiene measures to prevent reinfection. Frequent blood tests may be required. Maintain adequate hydration (2-3 L/day of fluids) unless advised by prescriber to restrict fluids. May cause headache, dizziness, drowsiness (use caution when driving or engaging in tasks that require alertness until response to drug is known); or nausea, vomiting, or diarrhea (small, frequent meals, frequent mouth care, sucking lozenges, or chewing gum may help). Report skin rash, redness, or irritation; persistent GI upset; urinary pattern changes; excessively dry eyes or mouth; or changes in color of stool or urine. **Pregnancy/breast-feeding precautions:** Inform prescriber if you are or intend to become pregnant. Consult prescriber if breast-feeding.

Dietary Issues: Take with or without regard to food.

Geriatric Considerations: Fluconazole has not been specifically studied in the elderly population. Dose may need adjustment based on changes of renal function.

Flucytosine (floo SYE toe seen)

U.S. Brand Names Ancobon®

Synonyms 5-FC; 5-Flurocytosine

Generic Available No

Pharmacologic Category Antifungal Agent, Oral

Pregnancy Risk Factor C

Lactation Excretion in breast milk unknown/not recommended

Use Adjunctive treatment of susceptible fungal infections (usually *Candida* or *Cryptococcus*); synergy with amphotericin B for certain fungal infections (*Cryptococcus* spp., *Candida* spp.)

Mechanism of Action/Effect Penetrates fungal cells and interferes with fungal RNA and protein synthesis

Contraindications Hypersensitivity to flucytosine or any component

Warnings/Precautions Use with extreme caution in patients with renal impairment or bone marrow depression. Dosage modification is required in patients with impaired renal function. Pregnancy risk C.

Drug Interactions

Increased Effect/Toxicity: Increased effect with amphotericin B. Amphotericin B-induced renal dysfunction may predispose patient to flucytosine accumulation and myelosuppression.

Nutritional/Ethanol Interactions Food: Food decreases the rate, but not the extent of absorption.

Effects on Lab Values Flucytosine causes markedly false elevations in serum creatinine values when the Ektachem® analyzer is used.

Adverse Reactions Frequency not defined.

Central nervous system: Confusion, headache, hallucinations, dizziness, drowsiness, psychosis, parkinsonism, ataxia, sedation

Dermatologic: Rash, photosensitivity, pruritus, urticaria

Endocrine & metabolic: Temporary growth failure, hypoglycemia, hypokalemia

Gastrointestinal: Nausea, vomiting, diarrhea, abdominal pain, loss of appetite

Hematologic: Bone marrow suppression, anemia, leukopenia, thrombocytopenia

Hepatic: Elevated liver enzymes, hepatitis, jaundice, azotemia

Neuromuscular & skeletal: Peripheral neuropathy, paresthesia, weakness

Otic: Hearing loss

Renal: Elevated BUN and serum creatinine, renal failure

Respiratory: Respiratory arrest

Miscellaneous: Anaphylaxis

Overdosage/Toxicology Symptoms of overdose include nausea, vomiting, diarrhea, and bone marrow suppression. Treatment is supportive.

Pharmacodynamics/Kinetics

Absorption: 75% to 90%

Half-Life Elimination: 3-8 hours; Anuria: Up to 200 hours; End-stage renal disease: 75-200 hours

Time to Peak: Serum: ~2-6 hours

Metabolism: Minimally hepatic

Formulations Capsule: 250 mg, 500 mg

Dosing

Adults & Elderly: Fungal infections (adjunct): Oral: 50-150 mg/kg/day in divided doses every 6 hours

Pediatrics: Refer to adult dosing.

Renal Impairment: Use lower initial dose:

Cl_{cr} 20-40 mL/minute: Dose every 12 hours

Cl_{cr} 10-20 mL/minute: Dose every 24 hours

Cl_{cr} <10 mL/minute: Dose every 24-48 hours

Hemodialysis: Dialyzable (50% to 100%); administer dose posthemodialysis

Peritoneal dialysis: Adults: Administer 0.5-1 g every 24 hours

Continuous arteriovenous or venovenous hemodiafiltration effects: Dose as for Cl_{cr} 10-50 mL/minute

Administration

Oral: Administer around-the-clock to promote less variation in peak and trough serum levels.

Stability

Storage: Protect from light.

Monitoring Laboratory Tests Culture prior to first dose, serum creatinine, BUN, alkaline phosphatase, AST, ALT, CBC, serum flucytosine concentrations

Monitoring and Teaching Issues

Physical Assessment: See Contraindications, Warnings/Precautions, and Dosing for use cautions. Assess potential for interactions with other prescriptions, OTC medications, or herbal products patient may be taking (see Drug Interactions). Assess results of laboratory tests (see above), therapeutic effects, and adverse response (see Adverse Reactions) on a regular basis throughout therapy. Teach patient use, possible side effects and appropriate interventions, and adverse symptoms to report (see Patient Education). **Pregnancy risk factor C** - benefits of use should outweigh possible risks. Breast-feeding is not recommended.

Patient Education: Inform prescriber of all prescriptions, OTC medications, or herbal products you are taking, and any allergies you have. Do not take anything new during treatment unless approved by prescriber. Take capsules one at a time over a few minutes with food to reduce GI upset. Take full course of medication as ordered. Do not discontinue without consulting prescriber. Practice good hygiene measures to prevent reinfection. Frequent blood tests may be required. May cause nausea and vomiting (small, frequent

(Continued)

Flucytosine *(Continued)*

meals may help). Report rash; difficulty breathing; CNS changes (eg, confusion, hallucinations, ataxia, acute headache); yellowing of skin or eyes; changes in color of stool or urine; unresolved diarrhea or anorexia; or unusual bleeding, fatigue, or weakness. **Pregnancy/ breast-feeding precautions:** Inform prescriber if you are or intend to become pregnant. Breast-feeding is not recommended.

Geriatric Considerations: Adjust for renal function.

Fludara® *see* Fludarabine *on page 568*

Fludarabine (floo DARE a been)

U.S. Brand Names Fludara®

Synonyms Fludarabine Phosphate

Generic Available No

Pharmacologic Category Antineoplastic Agent, Antimetabolite

Pregnancy Risk Factor D

Lactation Excretion in breast milk unknown/contraindicated

Use Salvage therapy of non-Hodgkin's lymphoma and acute leukemias

Orphan drug: Treatment of chronic lymphocytic leukemia (CLL), including refractory CLL

Mechanism of Action/Effect Inhibits DNA synthesis by inhibition of DNA polymerase and ribonucleotide reductase.

Contraindications Hypersensitivity of fludarabine or any component of the formulation; pregnancy

Warnings/Precautions The U.S. Food and Drug Administration (FDA) currently recommends that procedures for proper handling and disposal of antineoplastic agents be considered. Use with caution with renal insufficiency, patients with a fever documented infection or pre-existing hematological disorders (particularly granulocytopenia) or in patients with pre-existing central nervous system disorder (epilepsy), spasticity, or peripheral neuropathy.

If fludarabine contacts the skin, wash and flush thoroughly with water.

Drug Interactions

Increased Effect/Toxicity: Cytarabine when administered with or prior to a fludarabine dose competes for deoxycytidine kinase decreasing the metabolism of F-ara-A to the active F-ara-ATP (inhibits the antineoplastic effect of fludarabine); however, administering fludarabine prior to cytarabine may stimulate activation of cytarabine.

Nutritional/Ethanol Interactions Ethanol: Avoid ethanol (due to GI irritation).

Adverse Reactions

>10%:

- Central nervous system: Fever, chills, fatigue, pain
- Dermatologic: Rash
- Gastrointestinal: Mild nausea, vomiting, diarrhea, stomatitis, GI bleeding
- Genitourinary: Urinary infection
- Hematologic: Anemia, thrombocytopenia, leukopenia; Myelosuppression: Dose-limiting toxicity; myelosuppression may not be related to cumulative dose
  - Granulocyte nadir: 13 days (3-25)
  - Platelet nadir: 16 days (2-32)
  - WBC nadir: 8 days
  - Recovery: 5-7 weeks
- Neuromuscular & skeletal: Paresthesia, myalgia, weakness
- Respiratory: Manifested as dyspnea and a nonproductive cough; lung biopsy has shown pneumonitis in some patients, pneumonia
- Miscellaneous: Infection

1% to 10%:

- Cardiovascular: Congestive heart failure, edema
- Central nervous system: Malaise, headache
- Dermatologic: Alopecia
- Endocrine & metabolic: Hyperglycemia
- Gastrointestinal: Anorexia
  - Emetic potential: Very low (<10%)
- Ocular: Blurred vision
- Otic: Hearing loss

<1% (Limited to important or life-threatening): Interstitial pneumonitis, life-threatening and sometimes fatal autoimmune hemolytic anemia (often recurs on rechallenge - steroid treatment may or may not be beneficial), metabolic acidosis, renal failure, reversible hepatotoxicity, severe neurotoxicity (reported with higher dose levels: most patients shown to have CNS demyelination; somnolence, blindness, coma, and death also occurred), tumor lysis syndrome

Overdosage/Toxicology There are clear dose-dependent toxic neurologic effects associated with fludarabine. Doses of 96 mg/m^2/day for 5-7 days are associated with a syndrome characterized by delayed blindness, coma, and death. Symptoms have appeared from 21-60 days following the last dose. Central nervous system toxicity has distinctive features of delayed onset and progressive encephalopathy resulting in fatality. CNS toxicity is reported at an incidence rate of 36% at high doses (≥96 mg/m^2/day for 5-7 days) and <0.2% for low doses (≤125 mg/m^2/course).

Pharmacodynamics/Kinetics

Bioavailability: 75%

Half-Life Elimination: 2-fluoro-vidarabine: 9 hours

Metabolism: I.V.: Fludarabine phosphate is rapidly dephosphorylated to 2-fluoro-vidarabine, which subsequently enters tumor cells and is phosphorylated to the active triphosphate derivative; rapidly dephosphorylated in the serum

Formulations Injection, powder for reconstitution, as phosphate: 50 mg

Dosing

Adults & Elderly:

Chronic lymphocytic leukemia: I.V.: 20-25 mg/m^2/day over a 30-minute period for 5 days; 5-day courses are repeated every 28-35 days days

Non-Hodgkin's lymphoma: I.V.: Loading dose: 20 mg/m^2 followed by 30 mg/m^2/day for 48 hours

Pediatrics:

Acute leukemia: I.V.: 10 mg/m^2 bolus over 15 minutes followed by continuous infusion of 30.5 mg/m^2/day over 5 days **or**

10.5 mg/m^2 bolus over 15 minutes followed by 30.5 mg/m^2/day over 48 hours followed by cytarabine has been used in clinical trials

Solid tumors: I.V.: 9 mg/m^2 bolus followed by 27 mg/m^2/day continuous infusion over 5 days

Renal Impairment:

Cl_{cr} 30-70 mL/minute: Reduce dose by 20%

Cl_{cr} <30 mL/minute: Not recommended

Administration

I.V.: Administer I.V. over 15-30 minutes or continuous infusion.

Stability

Storage: Store intact vials under refrigeration (2°C to 8°C).

Reconstitution: Reconstitute vials with 2 mL SWI to result in a concentration of 25 mg/mL. Solution is stable for 16 days at room temperature (22°C to 25°C) and under refrigeration (2°C to 8°C). Further dilution in 100 mL D_5W or NS is stable for 48 hours at room temperature or refrigeration.

Standard I.V. dilution: Dose/100 mL D_5W or NS

Stable for 48 hours at 4°C to 25°C

Compatibility: Stable in D_5W, NS, sterile water for injection

Y-site administration: Incompatible Acyclovir, amphotericin B, chlorpromazine, daunorubicin, ganciclovir, hydroxyzine, prochlorperazine edisylate

Monitoring Laboratory Tests CBC with differential, platelet count, AST, ALT, creatinine, serum albumin, uric acid

Monitoring and Teaching Issues

Physical Assessment: See Contraindications, Warnings/Precautions, and Dosing for use cautions. Assess potential for interactions with other prescriptions, OTC medications, or herbal products patient may be taking (see Drug Interactions). See specific Administration and Reconstitution directions. Assess results of laboratory tests (see above), therapeutic effects, and adverse response (see Adverse Reactions and Overdose/Toxicology) prior to each treatment and on a regular basis throughout therapy. Teach patient possible side effects and appropriate interventions and adverse symptoms to report (see Patient Education). **Pregnancy risk factor D** - determine that patient is not pregnant before beginning treatment. Instruct patients of childbearing age on appropriate barrier contraceptive measures. Breast-feeding is contraindicated.

Patient Education: Inform prescriber of all prescriptions, OTC medications, or herbal products you are taking, and any allergies you have. Do not take anything new during treatment unless approved by prescriber. This drug can only be administered by infusion. Avoid alcohol during treatment. It is important to maintain adequate hydration (2-3 L/day of fluids) unless advised by prescriber to restrict fluids, and nutrition (small, frequent meals may help). You will be more susceptible to infection (avoid crowds and exposure to infection and do not have any vaccinations without consulting prescriber). May cause mild nausea or vomiting (small, frequent meals, frequent mouth care, sucking lozenges, or chewing gum may help); loss of hair (reversible); diarrhea (buttermilk, boiled milk, or yogurt may help); or mouth sores (use soft toothbrush or cotton swabs for oral care). Report extreme fatigue; pain or numbness in extremities; severe GI upset or diarrhea; bleeding or bruising; fever, chills, or sore throat; vaginal discharge; difficulty or pain on urination; muscle pain or weakness; unusual cough or difficulty breathing; or other unusual side effects. **Pregnancy/breast-feeding precautions:** Inform prescriber if your are pregnant. Do not get pregnant while taking this medication and for 1 month following therapy. Consult prescriber for appropriate barrier contraceptives. Do not breast-feed.

Fludarabine Phosphate *see* Fludarabine *on page 568*

Fludrocortisone (floo droe KOR ti sone)

U.S. Brand Names Florinef®

Synonyms Fludrocortisone Acetate; Fluohydrisone Acetate; Fluohydrocortisone Acetate; 9α-Fluorohydrocortisone Acetate

Generic Available Yes

Pharmacologic Category Corticosteroid, Systemic

Pregnancy Risk Factor C

Lactation Excretion in breast milk unknown

Use Partial replacement therapy for primary and secondary adrenocortical insufficiency in Addison's disease; treatment of salt-losing adrenogenital syndrome

Mechanism of Action/Effect Promotes increased reabsorption of sodium and loss of potassium from renal distal tubules

Contraindications Hypersensitivity to fludrocortisone or any component of the formulation; systemic fungal infections

Warnings/Precautions Taper dose gradually when therapy is discontinued. Patients with Addison's disease are more sensitive to the action of the hormone and may exhibit side effects in an exaggerated degree. Pregnancy risk C.

Drug Interactions

Decreased Effect: Anticholinesterases effects are antagonized. Decreased corticosteroid effects by rifampin, barbiturates, and hydantoins. May decrease salicylate levels.

Adverse Reactions Frequency not defined.

Cardiovascular: Hypertension, edema, CHF

(Continued)

Fludrocortisone *(Continued)*

Central nervous system: Convulsions, headache, dizziness
Dermatologic: Acne, rash, bruising
Endocrine & metabolic: Hypokalemic alkalosis, suppression of growth, hyperglycemia, HPA suppression
Gastrointestinal: Peptic ulcer
Neuromuscular & skeletal: Muscle weakness
Ocular: Cataracts
Miscellaneous: Diaphoresis, anaphylaxis (generalized)

Overdosage/Toxicology Symptoms of overdose include hypertension, edema, hypokalemia, excessive weight gain. When consumed in excessive quantities, systemic hypercorticism and adrenal suppression may occur. In those cases, discontinuation of the corticosteroid should be done judiciously.

Pharmacodynamics/Kinetics

Absorption: Rapid and complete

Half-Life Elimination: Plasma: 30-35 minutes; Biological: 18-36 hours

Time to Peak: Serum: ~1.7 hours

Metabolism: Hepatic

Formulations Tablet, as acetate: 0.1 mg

Dosing

Adults & Elderly: Mineralocorticoid deficiency: Oral: 0.05-0.2 mg/day with ranges of 0.1 mg 3 times/week to 0.2 mg/day

Pediatrics: Mineralocorticoid deficiency: Oral: Infants and Children: 0.05-0.1 mg/day

Administration

Oral: Administration in conjunction with a glucocorticoid is preferable.

Monitoring Laboratory Tests Serum electrolytes, serum renin activity

Monitoring and Teaching Issues

Physical Assessment: Assess effectiveness and interactions of other medications patient may be taking (see Drug Interactions). See Contraindications and Warnings/Precautions for use cautions. Monitor for effectiveness of therapy and adverse reactions according to dose and length of therapy. Assess knowledge/teach patient appropriate use, possible side effects/interventions, and adverse symptoms to report (ie, opportunistic infection, adrenal suppression - see Adverse Reactions and Overdose/Toxicology). Instruct diabetics to monitor serum glucose levels closely; corticosteroids can alter glycemic response. Dose may need to be increased if patient is experiencing higher than normal levels of stress. When discontinuing, taper dose and frequency slowly. **Pregnancy risk factor C** - benefits of use should outweigh possible risks. Note breast-feeding caution.

Patient Education: Take exactly as directed. Do not take more than prescribed dose and do not discontinue abruptly; consult prescriber. Take with or after meals. Take once-a-day dose with food in the morning. Limit intake of caffeine or stimulants. Maintain adequate nutrition; consult prescriber for possibility of special dietary recommendations. If diabetic, monitor serum glucose closely and notify prescriber of changes; this medication can alter hypoglycemic requirements. Notify prescriber if you are experiencing higher than normal levels of stress; medication may need adjustment. Periodic ophthalmic examinations will be necessary with long-term use. You will be susceptible to infection (avoid crowds and exposure to infection). You may experience insomnia or nervousness; use caution when driving or engaging in tasks requiring alertness until response to drug is known. Report weakness, change in menstrual pattern, vision changes, signs of hyperglycemia, signs of infection (eg, fever, chills, mouth sores, perianal itching, vaginal discharge), other persistent side effects, or worsening of condition. **Pregnancy/breast-feeding precautions:** Inform prescriber if you are or intend to become pregnant. Consult prescriber if breast-feeding.

Dietary Issues: Systemic use of mineralocorticoids/corticosteroids may require a diet with increased potassium, vitamins A, B_6, C, D, folate, calcium, zinc, and phosphorus, and decreased sodium. With fludrocortisone, a decrease in dietary sodium is often not required as the increased retention of sodium is usually the desired therapeutic effect.

Geriatric Considerations: The most common use of fludrocortisone in the elderly is orthostatic hypotension that is unresponsive to more conservative measures. Attempt nonpharmacologic measures (hydration, support stockings etc) before starting drug therapy.

Additional Information In patients with salt-losing forms of congenital adrenogenital syndrome, use along with cortisone or hydrocortisone. Fludrocortisone 0.1 mg has sodium retention activity equal to DOCA® 1 mg.

Related Information

Corticosteroids Comparison, Systemic Equivalencies *on page 1572*

Fludrocortisone Acetate *see* Fludrocortisone *on page 569*

Flumadine® *see* Rimantadine *on page 1191*

Flumazenil (FLO may ze nil)

U.S. Brand Names Romazicon®

Generic Available No

Pharmacologic Category Antidote

Pregnancy Risk Factor C

Lactation Excretion in breast milk unknown/use caution

Use Benzodiazepine antagonist - reverses sedative effects of benzodiazepines used in general anesthesia; for management of benzodiazepine overdose; flumazenil does **not** antagonize the CNS effects of other GABA agonists (eg, ethanol, barbiturates, or general anesthetics), **does not** reverse narcotics

Mechanism of Action/Effect Competitively inhibits the activity at the benzodiazepine recognition site on the GABA/benzodiazepine receptor complex. Flumazenil does not antagonize the CNS effect of drugs affecting GABA-ergic neurons by means other than the benzodiazepine receptor (ethanol, barbiturates, general anesthetics) and does not reverse the effects of opioids.

Contraindications Hypersensitivity to flumazenil, benzodiazepines, or any component of the formulation; patients given benzodiazepines for control of potentially life-threatening conditions (eg, control of intracranial pressure or status epilepticus); patients who are showing signs of serious cyclic-antidepressant overdosage

Warnings/Precautions Patients at increased risk of seizures following flumazenil (high-risk patients): Patients receiving benzodiazepines for long-term sedation, tricyclic antidepressant overdose patients, concurrent major sedative-hypnotic drug withdrawal, recent therapy with repeated doses of parenteral benzodiazepines, and patients with myoclonic jerking or seizure activity prior to flumazenil administration.

Note: Does not reverse respiratory depression/hypoventilation or cardiac depression. Resedation occurs more frequently in patients where a large single dose or cumulative dose of a benzodiazepine is administered along with a neuromuscular blocking agent and multiple anesthetic agents. Flumazenil should be used with caution in the intensive care unit because of increased risk of unrecognized benzodiazepine dependence in such settings.

Pregnancy risk C.

Drug Interactions

Increased Effect/Toxicity: Use with caution in overdosage involving mixed drug overdose. Toxic effects may emerge (especially with cyclic antidepressants) with the reversal of the benzodiazepine effect by flumazenil.

Adverse Reactions

>10%: Gastrointestinal: Vomiting, nausea

1% to 10%:

Cardiovascular: Palpitations

Central nervous system: Headache, anxiety, nervousness, insomnia, abnormal crying, euphoria, depression, agitation, dizziness, emotional lability, ataxia, depersonalization, increased tears, dysphoria, paranoia

Endocrine & metabolic: Hot flashes

Gastrointestinal: Xerostomia

Local: Pain at injection site

Neuromuscular & skeletal: Tremor, weakness, paresthesia

Ocular: Abnormal vision, blurred vision

Respiratory: Dyspnea, hyperventilation

Miscellaneous: Diaphoresis

<1% (Limited to important or life-threatening): Bradycardia, chest pain, generalized convulsions, hypertension, tachycardia, ventricular extrasystoles, withdrawal syndrome

Pharmacodynamics/Kinetics

Half-Life Elimination: Adults: Alpha: 7-15 minutes; Terminal: 41-79 minutes

Metabolism: Hepatic; dependent upon hepatic blood flow

Onset: 1-3 minutes; 80% response within 3 minutes; Peak effect: 6-10 minutes

Duration: Resedation: ~1 hour; duration related to dose given and benzodiazepine plasma concentrations; reversal effects of flumazenil may wear off before effects of benzodiazepine

Formulations Injection, solution: 0.1 mg/mL (5 mL, 10 mL)

Dosing

Adults: See table.

Flumazenil

Adult dosage for **reversal of conscious sedation:** Intravenously through a freely running intravenous infusion into a large vein to minimize pain at the injection site	
Initial dose	0.2 mg intravenously over 15 seconds
Repeat doses	If desired level of consciousness is not obtained, 0.2 mg may be repeated at 1-minute intervals
Maximum total cumulative dose	1 mg (usual dose 0.6-1 mg) **In the event of resedation:** repeat doses may be given at 20-minute intervals with maximum of 1 mg/dose and 3 mg/hour
Adult dosage for **suspected benzodiazepine overdose:** Intravenously through a freely running intravenous infusion into a large vein to minimize pain at the injection site	
Initial dose	0.2 mg intravenously over 30 seconds
Repeat doses	0.5 mg over 30 seconds repeated at 1-minute intervals
Maximum total cumulative dose	3 mg (usual dose 1-3 mg) Patients with a partial response at 3 mg may require additional titration up to a total dose of 5 mg. If a patient has not responded 5 minutes after cumulative dose of 5 mg, the major cause of sedation is not likely due to benzodiazepines. **In the event of re-sedation:** may repeat doses at 20-minute intervals with maximum of 1 mg/dose and 3 mg/hour

Resedation: Repeated doses may be given at 20-minute intervals as needed; repeat treatment doses of 1 mg (at a rate of 0.5 mg/minute) should be given at any time and no more than 3 mg should be given in any hour. After intoxication with high doses of benzodiazepines, the duration of a single dose of flumazenil is not expected to exceed 1 hour; if desired, the period of wakefulness may be prolonged with repeated low intravenous doses of flumazenil, or by an infusion of 0.1-0.4 mg/hour. Most patients with benzodiazepine overdose will respond to a cumulative dose of 1-3 mg and doses >3 mg do not reliably produce additional effects. Rarely, patients with a partial response at 3 mg may require additional titration up to a total dose of 5 mg. **If a patient has not responded 5 minutes after receiving a cumulative dose of 5 mg, the major cause of sedation is not likely to be due to benzodiazepines.**

(Continued)

Flumazenil *(Continued)*

Elderly: Refer to adult dosing. No differences in safety or efficacy have been reported; however, increased sensitivity may occur in some elderly patients.

Pediatrics: I.V.: Children:

Reversal of benzodiazepine when used in conscious sedation or general anesthesia: Initial dose: 0.01 mg/kg (maximum dose: 0.2 mg) given over 15 seconds; may repeat 0.01 mg/kg (maximum dose: 0.2 mg) after 45 seconds, and then every minute to a maximum total cumulative dose of 0.05 mg/kg or 1 mg, whichever is lower; usual total dose: 0.08-1 mg (mean: 0.65 mg).

Management of benzodiazepine overdose: Minimal information available; initial dose: 0.01 mg/kg (maximum dose: 0.2 mg) with repeat doses of 0.01 mg/kg (maximum dose: 0.2 mg) given every minute to a maximum total cumulative dose of 1 mg. As an alternative to repeat bolus doses, follow-up continuous infusions of 0.005-0.01 mg/kg/hour have been used; further studies are needed.

Renal Impairment: Not significantly affected by renal failure (Cl_{cr} <10 mL/minute) or hemodialysis beginning 1 hour after drug administration.

Hepatic Impairment: Initial dose of flumazenil used for initial reversal of benzodiazepine effects is not changed; however, subsequent doses in liver disease patients should be reduced in amount or frequency.

Administration

I.V.: Administer in freely running I.V. into large vein. Inject over 15 seconds for general anesthesia and over 30 seconds for overdose.

Stability

Reconstitution: For I.V. use only. Once drawn up in the syringe or mixed with solution use within 24 hours. Discard any unused solution after 24 hours.

Compatibility: Stable in D_5W, LR, NS

Monitoring and Teaching Issues

Physical Assessment: Assess level of consciousness frequently. Monitor vital signs and airway closely. EKG monitoring and oxygenation via pulse oximetry is highly recommended. Observe continually for resedation, respiratory depression, preseizure activity, or other residual benzodiazepine effects. May require pain medication sooner after reversal. Assess for nausea and vomiting. **Pregnancy risk factor C** - benefits of use should outweigh possible risks. Note breast-feeding caution.

Patient Education: Flumazenil does not consistently reverse amnesia. Do not engage in activities requiring alertness for 18-24 hours after discharge. Resedation may occur in patients on long-acting benzodiazepines (such as diazepam). **Pregnancy/breast-feeding precautions:** Inform prescriber if you are or intend to become pregnant. Consult prescriber if breast-feeding.

Related Information

Antidotes, Antivenins, and Antitoxins *on page 1460*

Flunisolide (floo NIS oh lide)

U.S. Brand Names AeroBid®; AeroBid®-M; Nasalide®; Nasarel®

Generic Available No

Pharmacologic Category Corticosteroid, Inhalant (Oral); Corticosteroid, Nasal

Pregnancy Risk Factor C

Lactation Excretion in breast milk unknown/use caution

Use Steroid-dependent asthma; nasal solution is used for seasonal or perennial rhinitis

Mechanism of Action/Effect Decreases inflammation by suppression of migration of polymorphonuclear leukocytes and reversal of increased capillary permeability; does not depress hypothalamus

Contraindications Hypersensitivity to flunisolide or any component of the formulation; acute status asthmaticus; viral, tuberculosis, fungal, or bacterial respiratory infections; infections of the nasal mucosa

Warnings/Precautions Not to be used in status asthmaticus or for the relief of acute bronchospasm. May cause suppression of hypothalamic-pituitary-adrenal (HPA) axis, particularly in younger children or in patients receiving high doses for prolonged periods. Fatalities have occurred due to adrenal insufficiency in asthmatic patients during and after transfer from systemic corticosteroids to aerosol steroids; aerosol steroids do **not** provide the systemic steroid needed to treat patients having trauma, surgery, or infections. Withdrawal and discontinuation of the corticosteroid should be done slowly and carefully.

Controlled clinical studies have shown that orally-inhaled and intranasal corticosteroids may cause a reduction in growth velocity in pediatric patients, which appears to be related to dose and duration of exposure.

May suppress the immune system, patients may be more susceptible to infection. Use with caution in patients with systemic infections or ocular herpes simplex. Avoid exposure to chickenpox and measles.

Pregnancy risk C.

Drug Interactions

Increased Effect/Toxicity: Expected interactions similar to other corticosteroids

Salmeterol: The addition of salmeterol has been demonstrated to improve response to inhaled corticosteroids (as compared to increasing steroid dosage).

Adverse Reactions

>10%:

Cardiovascular: Pounding heartbeat

Central nervous system: Dizziness, headache, nervousness

Dermatologic: Itching, rash

Endocrine & metabolic: Adrenal suppression, menstrual problems

Gastrointestinal: GI irritation, anorexia, sore throat, bitter taste

Local: Nasal burning, *Candida* infections of the nose or pharynx, atrophic rhinitis

Respiratory: Sneezing, coughing, upper respiratory tract infection, bronchitis, nasal congestion, nasal dryness

Miscellaneous: Increased susceptibility to infections

1% to 10%:

Central nervous system: Insomnia, psychic changes

Dermatologic: Acne, urticaria

Gastrointestinal: Increase in appetite, dry mouth, dry throat, loss of taste perception

Ocular: Cataracts

Respiratory: Epistaxis

Miscellaneous: Diaphoresis, loss of smell

<1% (Limited to important or life-threatening): Bronchospasm, dyspnea, HPA axis suppression

Overdosage/Toxicology When consumed in high doses over prolonged periods, systemic hypercorticism and adrenal suppression may occur. In those cases, discontinuation of the corticosteroid should be done judiciously.

Pharmacodynamics/Kinetics

Absorption: Nasal inhalation: ~50%

Bioavailability: 40% to 50%

Half-Life Elimination: 1.8 hours

Metabolism: Rapidly hepatic to active metabolites

Formulations

Aerosol for oral inhalation:

AeroBid®: 250 mcg/actuation (7 g) [100 metered doses]

AeroBid-M®: 250 mcg/actuation (7 g) [100 metered doses; menthol flavor]

Solution, intranasal spray (Nasalide®, Nasarel®): 25 mcg/actuation (25 mL) [200 sprays]

Dosing

Adults & Elderly:

Asthma: Oral inhalation: 2 inhalations twice daily (morning and evening) up to 8 inhalations/day maximum

Seasonal allergic rhinitis: Nasal: 2 sprays in each nostril twice daily (morning and evening); maximum: 8 sprays/day in each nostril

Pediatrics: Children >6 years:

Asthma (Children >6 years): Oral inhalation: 2 inhalations twice daily (morning and evening) up to 4 inhalations/day

Seasonal allergic rhinitis (Children >6 years): Intranasal: 1 spray each nostril twice daily (morning and evening), not to exceed 4 sprays/day each nostril

Administration

Inhalation: Shake well before using. Do not use Nasalide® or Nasarel® orally. Throw out product after it has been opened for 3 months.

Monitoring and Teaching Issues

Physical Assessment: See Contraindications and Warnings/Precautions for use cautions. Not to be used to treat status asthmaticus or fungal infections of nasal passages. Monitor therapeutic effects and adverse reactions (see Warnings/Precautions, Adverse Reactions, and Overdose/Toxicology). When changing from systemic steroids to inhalational steroid, taper reduction of systemic medication slowly (see Warnings). Assess knowledge/teach patient appropriate use, interventions to reduce side effects, and adverse symptoms to report (see Patient Education). **Pregnancy risk factor C** - benefits of use should outweigh possible risks. Note breast-feeding caution.

Patient Education: Use as directed; do not use nasal preparations for oral inhalation. Do not increase dosage or discontinue abruptly without consulting prescriber. Review use of inhaler or spray with prescriber or follow package insert for directions. Keep oral inhaler clean and unobstructed. Always rinse mouth and throat after use of inhaler to prevent opportunistic infection. If you are also using an inhaled bronchodilator, wait 10 minutes before using this steroid aerosol. You may experience dizziness, anxiety, or blurred vision (rise slowly from sitting or lying position and use caution when driving or engaging in tasks requiring alertness until response to drug is known); or taste disturbance or aftertaste (frequent mouth care and mouth rinses may help). Report pounding heartbeat or chest pain; acute nervousness or inability to sleep; severe sneezing or nosebleed; difficulty breathing, sore throat, hoarseness, or bronchitis; difficulty breathing or bronchospasms; disturbed menstrual pattern; vision changes; loss of taste or smell perception; or worsening of condition or lack of improvement. **Pregnancy/breast-feeding precautions:** Inform prescriber if you are or intend to become pregnant. Consult prescriber if breast-feeding.

Inhaler: Sit when using. Take deep breaths for 3-5 minutes, and clear nasal passages before administration (use decongestant as needed). Hold breath for 5-10 seconds after use, and wait 1-3 minutes between inhalations. Follow package insert instructions for use. Do not exceed maximum dosage. If also using inhaled bronchodilator, use before flunisolide. Rinse mouth and throat after use to reduce aftertaste and prevent candidiasis.

Geriatric Considerations: Many elderly patients have difficulty using metered dose inhalers, which can limit their effectiveness. Assess technique in all older patients. A spacer device may be beneficial for the oral inhaler.

Additional Information Does not contain fluorocarbons; contains polyethylene glycol vehicle.

Effects of inhaled/intranasal steroids on growth have been observed in the absence of laboratory evidence of HPA axis suppression, suggesting that growth velocity is a more sensitive indicator of systemic corticosteroid exposure in pediatric patients than some commonly used tests of HPA axis function. The long-term effects of this reduction in growth velocity associated with orally-inhaled and intranasal corticosteroids, including the impact on final adult height, are unknown. The potential for "catch up" growth following discontinuation of treatment with inhaled corticosteroids has not been adequately studied.

Related Information

Inhalant (Asthma, Bronchospasm) Agents Comparison *on page 1577*

Fluocinolone *see* Topical Corticosteroids *on page 1334*

Fluocinolone, Hydroquinone, and Tretinoin

(floo oh SIN oh lone, HYE droe kwin one, & TRET i noyn)

U.S. Brand Names Tri-Luma™

Synonyms Hydroquinone, Fluocinolone Acetonide, and Tretinoin; Tretinoin, Fluocinolone Acetonide, and Hydroquinone

Generic Available No

Pharmacologic Category Corticosteroid, Topical; Depigmenting Agent; Retinoic Acid Derivative

Pregnancy Risk Factor C

Lactation Excretion in breast milk unknown/use caution

Use Short-term treatment of moderate to severe melasma of the face

Mechanism of Action/Effect Not clearly defined. Hydroquinone may interrupt melanin synthesis; reduces hyperpigmentation.

Contraindications Hypersensitivity to fluocinolone, hydroquinone, tretinoin, or any component of the formulation; TB of skin, herpes (including varicella); sulfite allergy

Warnings/Precautions For external use only. Should only be used along with measures for sun avoidance. Instruct patients to avoid UV exposure, including sunlight (protective clothing and sunscreen recommended). Local irritation, dryness, and pruritus may be expected following application. Avoid contact with abraded skin, mucous membranes, eyes, mouth, angles of the nose. Due to corticosteroid component, adverse systemic effects (including HPA axis suppression) may occur when used on large areas of the body, denuded areas, for prolonged periods of time, and/or with use of an occlusive dressing.

Hydroquinone may produce exogenous ochronosis (gradual blue/black darkening of skin); discontinuation is recommended. Contains sodium metabisulfite; may cause hypersensitivity reactions, including anaphylaxis, in individuals with sulfite allergy. Cutaneous hypersensitivity/contact dermatitis to individual ingredients has been reported; instruct patients to seek medical attention. Consider changing to nonhormonal contraceptive measures in patients who may be receiving hormonal contraceptives.

Has not been evaluated in skin types V and VI; excessive bleaching may occur in individuals with darker skin. Safety and efficacy have not been established in pediatric patients.

Pregnancy risk C.

Drug Interactions

Cytochrome P450 Effect: Tretinoin: Substrate of CYP2A6, 2B6, 2C8/9; Inhibits CYP2C8/9; Induces CYP2E1

Increased Effect/Toxicity: Avoid soaps/cosmetic preparations which are medicated, abrasive, irritating, or any product with strong drying effects (including alcohol, astringent, benzoyl peroxide, resorcinol, salicylic acid, sulfur). Drugs with photosensitizing effects should also be avoided (includes tetracyclines, thiazides, fluoroquinolones, phenothiazines, sulfonamides).

Nutritional/Ethanol Interactions

Food: Avoid excessive intake of vitamin A (cod liver oil, halibut fish oil).

Herb/Nutraceutical: Avoid dong quai, St John's wort (may also cause photosensitization). Avoid excessive amounts of vitamin A supplements.

Adverse Reactions

>10%

Dermatologic: Erythema (41%), desquamation (38%), burning (18%), dry skin (14%), pruritus (11%)

1% to 10%

Cardiovascular: Telangiectasia (3%)

Central nervous system: Paresthesia (3%), hyperesthesia (2%)

Dermatologic: Acne (5%), pigmentation change (2%), irritation (2%), papules (1%), rash (1%), rosacea (1%), vesicles (1%)

Gastrointestinal: Xerostomia (1%)

<1%: Other reactions reported with one or more components: Acneiform eruptions, allergic contact dermatitis, burning, Cushing's syndrome, folliculitis, HPA axis suppression, hypertrichosis, hypopigmentation, irritation, itching, miliaria, ochronosis (exogenous), perioral dermatitis, secondary infection, skin atrophy, striae

Overdosage/Toxicology Topically-applied products may be absorbed in sufficient amounts to produce systemic effects, particularly if applied to large surface area or to inflamed/damaged skin. Systemic hypercorticism and adrenal suppression may occur; in those cases, discontinuation and withdrawal of the corticosteroid should be done judiciously.

Pharmacodynamics/Kinetics

Absorption: Minimal

Metabolism: Hepatic for the small amount absorbed

Formulations Cream, topical: Hydroquinone 4%, tretinoin 0.05%, fluocinolone acetonide 0.01% (30 g) [contains sodium bisulfite]

Dosing

Adults & Elderly: Melasma: Topical: Apply a thin film once daily to hyperpigmented areas of melasma (including ½ inch of normal-appearing surrounding skin). Apply 30 minutes prior to bedtime; not indicated for use beyond 8 weeks. Do not use occlusive dressings.

Renal Impairment: No dosage adjustment required.

Administration

Topical: Apply 30 minutes before bedtime. Wash face with mild cleanser; rinse and pat dry. Apply to lesion and ½ inch of normal-appearing skin surrounding each lesion. Rub lightly and uniformly into the skin. Do not use occlusive dressings.

Stability

Storage: Store at 20°C to 25°C (68°F to 77°F).

Monitoring and Teaching Issues

Physical Assessment: See Contraindications and Warnings/Precautions for use cautions. Assess potential for interactions with other prescriptions, OTC medications, or herbal products patient may be taking (eg, anything with photosensitizing effect - see Drug

Interactions). Assess therapeutic effects and adverse response (see Adverse Reactions and Overdose/Toxicology). Teach patient use, possible side effects/interventions, and adverse symptoms to report (see Patient Education). **Pregnancy risk factor C** - benefits of use should outweigh possible risks. Note breast-feeding caution.

Patient Education: Inform prescriber of all prescriptions, OTC medications, or herbal products you are taking, and any allergies you have. This medication is for topical (skin) use only. Use exactly as directed (see below). Do not overuse or use for a longer period of time than prescribed. You will be sensitive to sunlight (avoid sunlight, wear sunscreen with SPF 30, and wear protective clothing); and sensitive to irritating skin products or cosmetics (avoid medicated preparations or agents with irritating or drying effects - you may use moisturizers and/or nonirritating cosmetics during the day). You may experience irritation and sensitivity to temperature changes, or excess bleaching effects. Report persistent burning, irritation, or eruptions on the skin; or if the condition being treated worsens or does not improve.

Application: Wash hands before beginning. Wash face with mild cleanser, rinse, and pat dry. Apply medication sparingly, in a very light film, rub in lightly. Avoid any contact with open or abraded skin, mucous membranes, eyes, mouth, or nose.

Pregnancy/breast-feeding precautions: Inform prescriber if you are or intend to become pregnant. Consult prescriber if breast-feeding.

Breast-feeding Issues: Avoid contact between nursing infant and cream.

Pregnancy Issues: There are no adequate and well-controlled studies in pregnant women. Tretinoin appears to have a low risk of teratogenicity when used topically since it is rapidly metabolized by the skin; however, there are rare reports of fetal defects. Risk may be greatest in 1st trimester. Use topically only if benefit to mother outweighs potential risk to fetus. In general, the use of topical corticosteroids during pregnancy is not considered to have significant risk, however, intrauterine growth retardation in the infant has been reported (rare). The use of large amounts or for prolonged periods of time should be avoided. Consider delaying treatment until after delivery.

Fluocinonide *see* Topical Corticosteroids *on page 1334*

Fluogen® *see page 1498*

Fluohydrisone Acetate *see* Fludrocortisone *on page 569*

Fluohydrocortisone Acetate *see* Fludrocortisone *on page 569*

Fluoracaine® Ophthalmic *see page 1461*

Fluorescein Sodium *see page 1461*

Fluorescite® Injection *see page 1461*

Fluorets® Ophthalmic Strips *see page 1461*

Fluor-I-Strip® *see page 1461*

Fluor-I-Strip-AT® *see page 1461*

Fluorodeoxyuridine *see* Floxuridine *on page 563*

9α-Fluorohydrocortisone Acetate *see* Fludrocortisone *on page 569*

Fluorometholone (flure oh METH oh lone)

U.S. Brand Names Eflone®; Flarex®; Fluor-Op®; FML®; FML® Forte

Generic Available Yes: Suspension (as base)

Pharmacologic Category Corticosteroid, Ophthalmic

Pregnancy Risk Factor C

Lactation Excretion in breast milk unknown/use caution

Use Treatment of steroid-responsive inflammatory conditions of the eye

Mechanism of Action/Effect Decreases inflammation by suppression of migration of polymorphonuclear leukocytes and reversal of increased capillary permeability

Contraindications Hypersensitivity to fluorometholone or any component of the formulation; viral diseases of the cornea and conjunctiva (including epithelial herpes simplex keratitis, vaccinia and varicella); mycobacterial or fungal infections of the eye; untreated eye infections which may be masked/enhanced by a steroid

Warnings/Precautions Not recommended in children <2 years of age. Prolonged use may result in glaucoma, elevated intraocular pressure, or other ocular damage. May exacerbate severity of viral infections, use caution in patients with history of herpes simplex. Re-evaluate after 2 days if symptoms have not improved. May delay healing following cataract surgery. Some products contain sulfites. Pregnancy risk C.

Adverse Reactions

Ocular: Anterior uveitis, burning upon application, cataract formation, conjunctival hyperemia, conjunctivitis, corneal ulcers, glaucoma with optic nerve damage, perforation of the globe, secondary ocular infection (bacterial, fungal, viral), intraocular pressure elevation, visual acuity and field defects, keratitis, mydriasis, stinging upon application, delayed wound healing

Miscellaneous: Systemic hypercorticoidism (rare) and taste perversion have also been reported

Overdosage/Toxicology When consumed in high doses over prolonged periods, systemic hypercorticism and adrenal suppression may occur. In those cases, discontinuation of the corticosteroid should be done judiciously.

Pharmacodynamics/Kinetics

Absorption: Into aqueous humor with slight systemic absorption

Formulations

Ointment, ophthalmic, as base (FML®): 0.1% (3.5 g)

Suspension, ophthalmic, as base: (5 mL, 10 mL, 15 mL)

Fluor-Op®: 0.1% (5 mL, 10 mL, 15 mL) [contains benzalkonium chloride and polyvinyl alcohol]

FML®: 0.1% (1 mL, 5 mL, 10 mL, 15 mL) [contains benzalkonium chloride]

FML® Forte: 0.25% (2 mL, 5 mL, 10 mL, 15 mL) [contains benzalkonium chloride and polyvinyl alcohol]

(Continued)

Fluorometholone *(Continued)*

Suspension, ophthalmic, as acetate:
Eflone®: 0.1% (5 mL, 10 mL)
Flarex®: 0.1% (5 mL, 10 mL) [contains benzalkonium chloride]

Dosing

Adults & Elderly:

Anti-inflammatory: Ophthalmic:

Ointment: Apply small amount (~½ inch ribbon) to conjunctival sac every 4 hours in severe cases; 1-3 times/day in mild to moderate cases.

Solution: Instill 1-2 drops into conjunctival sac every hour during day, every 2 hours at night until favorable response is obtained, then use 1 drop every 4 hours; for mild to moderate inflammation, instill 1-2 drops into conjunctival sac 2-4 times/day.

Note: Re-evaluate therapy if improvement is not seen within 2 days; use care not to discontinue prematurely; in chronic conditions, gradually decrease dosing frequency prior to discontinuing treatment.

Pediatrics: Children >2 years: Refer to adult dosing.

Stability

Storage: Store at room temperature.

Monitoring Laboratory Tests Intraocular pressure in patients with glaucoma or when used for ≥10 days; presence of secondary infections (including the development of fungal infections and exacerbation of viral infections)

Monitoring and Teaching Issues

Physical Assessment: See Contraindications, Warnings/Precautions, and Overdose/Toxicology for use cautions. Assess knowledge/teach patient appropriate use, interventions to reduce side effects, and adverse symptoms to report (see Patient Education). **Pregnancy risk factor C.** Note breast-feeding caution.

Patient Education: For ophthalmic use only. Apply prescribed amount as often as directed. Wash hands before using. Wipe away excess from skin around eye. Do not use any other eye preparation for at least 10 minutes. Do not touch tip of applicator to eye or any other surface. Do not share medication with anyone else. May cause sensitivity to bright light (dark glasses may help); temporary stinging or blurred vision may occur. Do not wear contacts during administration and for 15 minutes after. Inform prescriber if you experience eye pain, redness, burning, watering, dryness, double vision, puffiness around eye, vision changes, or other adverse eye response; worsening of condition or lack of improvement.

Ointment: Gently squeeze the tube to apply to inside of lower lid. Close eye for 1-2 minutes and roll eyeball in all directions.

Suspension: Shake well before using. Tilt head back and look upward. Gently pull down lower lid and put drop(s) in inner corner of eye. Close eye and roll eyeball in all directions. Do not blink for 30 seconds. Apply gentle pressure to inner corner of eye for 30 seconds.

Pregnancy/breast-feeding precautions: Inform prescriber if you are pregnant. Consult prescriber if breast-feeding.

Fluor-Op® *see* Fluorometholone *on page 575*
Fluoroplex® *see* Fluorouracil *on page 576*

Fluorouracil (flure oh YOOR a sil)

U.S. Brand Names Adrucil®; Carac™; Efudex®; Fluoroplex®

Synonyms 5-Fluorouracil; 5-FU

Generic Available Yes: Injection

Pharmacologic Category Antineoplastic Agent, Antimetabolite

Pregnancy Risk Factor D (injection); X (topical)

Lactation Excretion in breast milk unknown/not recommended

Use Treatment of carcinomas of the breast, colon, head and neck, pancreas, rectum, or stomach; topically for the management of actinic or solar keratoses and superficial basal cell carcinomas

Mechanism of Action/Effect Interferes with DNA synthesis by blocking the methylation of deoxyuricytic acid.

Contraindications Hypersensitivity to fluorouracil or any component of the formulation; poor nutritional status; depressed bone marrow function; thrombocytopenia; potentially serious infections; major surgery within the previous month; dihydropyrimidine dehydrogenase (DPD) enzyme deficiency; pregnancy

Warnings/Precautions The U.S. Food and Drug Administration (FDA) currently recommends that procedures for proper handling and disposal of antineoplastic agents be considered. Use with caution in patients who have had high-dose pelvic radiation or previous use of alkylating agents. Patient should be hospitalized during initial course of therapy. Use with caution in patients with impaired kidney or liver function. The drug should be discontinued if intractable vomiting or diarrhea, precipitous fall in leukocyte or platelet counts or myocardial ischemia occurs.

Preparation of fluorouracil should be performed in a Class II laminar flow biologic safety cabinet. Personnel should be wearing surgical gloves and a closed front surgical gown with knit cuffs. Appropriate safety equipment is recommended for preparation, administration, and disposal of antineoplastics. If fluorouracil contacts the skin, wash and flush thoroughly with water.

Drug Interactions

Decreased Effect: Methotrexate: This interaction is schedule dependent; **5-FU should be given following MTX, not prior to**. If 5-FU is given first: 5-FU inhibits the TS binding and thus the reduced folate pool is not depleted, thereby negating the effect of MTX.

Increased Effect/Toxicity: Leucovorin increases the folate pool and, in certain tumors, may promote TS inhibition and increase 5-FU activity. Leucovorin must be given before or with the 5-FU to prime the cells; it is not used as a rescue agent in this case. Allopurinol inhibits thymidine phosphorylase (an enzyme that activates 5-FU). The antitumor effect of

5-FU appears to be unaltered, but the toxicity is increased. Cimetidine results in increased plasma levels of 5-FU due to drug metabolism inhibition and reduction of liver blood flow induced by cimetidine.

Nutritional/Ethanol Interactions

Ethanol: Avoid ethanol (due to GI irritation).

Herb/Nutraceutical: Avoid black cohosh, dong quai in estrogen-dependent tumors.

Adverse Reactions Toxicity depends on route and duration of infusion

>10%:

Dermatologic: Dermatitis, pruritic maculopapular rash, alopecia

Gastrointestinal (route and schedule dependent): Heartburn, nausea, vomiting, anorexia, stomatitis, esophagitis, anorexia, stomatitis, and diarrhea

Emetic potential:

<1000 mg: Moderately low (10% to 30%)

≥1000 mg: Moderate (30% to 60%)

Hematologic: Leukopenia; Myelosuppressive (tends to be more pronounced in patients receiving bolus dosing of 5-FU):

WBC: Moderate

Platelets: Mild to moderate

Onset (days): 7-10

Nadir (days): 14

Recovery (days): 21

Local: **Irritant chemotherapy**

1% to 10%:

Dermatologic: Dry skin

Gastrointestinal: GI ulceration

<1% (Limited to important or life-threatening): Cardiac enzyme abnormalities, chest pain, coagulopathy, dyspnea, EKG changes similar to ischemic changes, hepatotoxicity; hyperpigmentation of nailbeds, face, hands, and veins used in infusion; hypotension, palmar-plantar syndrome (hand-foot syndrome), photosensitization

Cerebellar ataxia, headache, somnolence, ataxia are seen primarily in intracarotid arterial infusions for head and neck tumors.

Overdosage/Toxicology Symptoms of overdose include myelosuppression, nausea, vomiting, diarrhea, and alopecia. No specific antidote exists. Monitor hematologically for at least 4 weeks. Treatment is supportive.

Pharmacodynamics/Kinetics

Bioavailability: <75%, erratic and undependable

Half-Life Elimination: Biphasic: Initial: 6-20 minutes; doses of 400-600 mg/m^2 produce drug concentrations above the threshold for cytotoxicity for normal tissue and remain there for 6 hours; two metabolites, FdUMP and FUTP, have prolonged half-lives depending on the type of tissue; the clinical effect of these metabolites has not been determined

Metabolism: Hepatic (90%) via dehydrogenase enzyme; 5-FU must be metabolized to be active; dose may need to be omitted in patients with hepatic failure (bilirubin >5 mg/dL)

Duration: ~3 weeks

Formulations

Cream, topical:

Carac™: 0.5% (30 g)

Efudex®: 5% (25 g)

Fluoroplex®: 1% (30 g) [contains benzyl alcohol]

Injection, solution: 50 mg/mL (10 mL, 20 mL, 50 mL, 100 mL)

Adrucil®: 50 mg/mL (10 mL, 50 mL, 100 mL)

Solution, topical:

Efudex®: 2% (10 mL); 5% (10 mL)

Fluoroplex®: 1% (30 mL)

Dosing

Adults & Elderly:

Carcinoma of the breast, colon, pancreas, rectum, and stomach: Refer to individual protocols: All dosages are based on the patient's actual weight. However, the estimated lean body mass (dry weight) is used if the patient is obese or if there has been a spurious weight gain due to edema, ascites, or other forms of abnormal fluid retention.

I.V.: Manufacturers suggested dosing:

Initial sequence: 12 mg/kg once daily on days 1-4 (maximum daily dose: 800 mg); no treatment is given on day 5; if no toxicity is observed, administer 6 mg/kg on days 6, 8, 10, and 12; no treatment is given on days 7, 9, or 11

Poor risk patients/patients with poor nutritional status: 6 mg/kg once daily on days 1-3 (maximum dose: 400 mg); no therapy is given on day 4; if no toxicity is observed, administer 3 mg/kg on days 5, 7, and 9; no treatment is given on days 6 or 8

Maintenance: Repeat initial sequence every 30 days after last day of previous treatment **or** 10-15 mg/kg/week as a single dose (maximum 1 g/week, begin when toxic signs from initial course of treatment have subsided); further duration of treatment and dosage are dependent upon patient response; treatment has ranged from 9-45 courses over 12-60 months

Examples of other dosing regimens include:

Intermittent bolus dose in combination with other agents: 600 mg/m^2 every 3-4 weeks

Continuous infusion in combination with other agents: 1000 mg/m^2/day for 4-5 days every 3-4 weeks

Bolus dose in combination with leucovorin: 425 mg/m^2/day for 5 days every 4 weeks

Continuous protracted infusion: 200-300 mg/m^2/day

Actinic keratoses: Topical:

Carac™: Apply thin film to lesions once daily for up to 4 weeks, as tolerated

Efudex®: Apply cream or solution to lesions twice daily for 2-4 weeks; complete healing may not be evident for 1-2 months following treatment

Fluoroplex®: Apply to lesions twice daily for 2-6 weeks

Basal cell carcinoma: Topical: Efudex®: Apply 5% cream or solution to affected lesions twice daily for 3-6 weeks; treatment may be continued for up to 10-12 weeks

(Continued)

Fluorouracil *(Continued)*

Pediatrics: Refer to adult dosing.

Renal Impairment: Hemodialysis: Administer dose posthemodialysis.

Hepatic Impairment: Bilirubin >5 mg/dL: Omit use.

Administration

Oral: I.V. formulation may be given orally mixed in water, grape juice, or carbonated beverage.

I.V.: Irritant. Direct I.V. push injection (50 mg/mL solution needs no further dilution) or by I.V. infusion. Toxicity may be reduced by giving the drug as a constant infusion. Bolus doses may be administered by slow IVP or IVPB.

Topical: Wash hands immediately after topical application of the 5% cream; for external use only.

Stability

Storage: Store intact vials at room temperature and protect from light. Slight discoloration does not usually denote decomposition.

Reconstitution: Further dilution in D_5W or NS at concentrations of 0.5-10 mg/mL are stable for 72 hours at 4°C to 25°C.

Standard I.V. dilution:

I.V. push: Dose/syringe (concentration: 50 mg/mL)

Maximum syringe size for IVP is a 30 mL syringe and syringe should be <75% full.

Continuous intravenous infusion/IVPB: Dose/50-1000 mL D_5W or NS

Syringe and solution are stable for 72 hours at 4°C to 25°C.

Compatibility: Stable in D_5LR, D_5W, NS

Incompatible with concentrations >25 mg/mL of fluorouracil and >2 mg/mL of leucovorin (precipitation occurs)

Y-site administration: Incompatible with amphotericin B cholesteryl sulfate complex, droperidol, filgrastim, ondansetron, topotecan, vinorelbine

Compatibility in syringe: Incompatible with droperidol, epirubicin

Compatibility when admixed: Incompatible with carboplatin, cisplatin, cytarabine, diazepam, doxorubicin, fentanyl, leucovorin, metoclopramide, morphine

Monitoring Laboratory Tests CBC with differential, platelet count, renal and liver function

Monitoring and Teaching Issues

Physical Assessment: See Contraindications, Warnings/Precautions, and Dosing for use cautions. Assess potential for interactions with other prescriptions, OTC medications, or herbal products patient may be taking (see Drug Interactions). Assess results of laboratory tests prior to each infusion and regularly with topical use (patient should be hospitalized during initial course of therapy). Assess patient response (eg, cardiovascular, respiratory, and renal function - see Adverse Reactions and Overdose/Toxicology) prior to each infusion and on a regular basis throughout topical therapy. **Note:** The drug should be discontinued if intractable vomiting or diarrhea, precipitous fall in leukocyte or platelet counts, or myocardial ischemia occurs. Teach patient proper use (topical application), possible side effects and interventions (eg, importance of adequate hydration), and adverse symptoms to report (see Patient Education). **Pregnancy risk factor D/X** - determine that patient is not pregnant before starting therapy. Do not give to females of childbearing age unless patient is capable of complying with barrier contraceptive use. Male/female: Advise patient about appropriate contraceptive measures as appropriate. Breast-feeding is not recommended.

Patient Education: Inform prescriber of all prescriptions, OTC medications, or herbal products you are taking, and any allergies you have. Do not take anything new without consulting prescriber. Avoid alcohol. Maintain adequate hydration (2-3 L/day of fluids) unless advised by prescriber to restrict fluids, and nutrition (small, frequent meals may help). May cause sensitivity to sunlight (use sunblock, wear protective clothing, and avoid direct sunlight); susceptibility to infection (avoid crowds and exposure to infection); nausea, vomiting, diarrhea, or loss of appetite (small, frequent meals may help - request medication); weakness, lethargy, dizziness, decreased vision (use caution when driving or engaging in tasks requiring alertness until response to drug is known); or headache (request medication). Report signs and symptoms of infection (eg, fever, chills, sore throat, burning urination, vaginal itching or discharge, fatigue, mouth sores); bleeding (eg, black or tarry stools, easy bruising, unusual bleeding); vision changes; unremitting nausea, vomiting, or abdominal pain; CNS changes; difficulty breathing; chest pain or palpitations; severe skin reactions to topical application; or any other adverse reactions.

Topical: Use as directed; do not overuse. Wash hands thoroughly before and after applying medication. Avoid contact with eyes, nostrils, and mouth. Avoid occlusive dressings; use a porous dressing. May cause local reaction (pain, burning, or swelling); if severe contact prescriber.

Pregnancy/breast-feeding precautions: Inform prescriber if you are pregnant. Do not get pregnant during or for 1 month following therapy. Male: Do not cause a pregnancy. Male/female: Consult prescriber for instruction on appropriate contraceptive measures. This drug may cause severe fetal defects. Breast-feeding is not recommended.

Dietary Issues: Increase dietary intake of thiamine.

Pregnancy Issues: There are no adequate and well-controlled studies in pregnant women, however, fetal defects and miscarriages have been reported following use of topical and intravenous products. Use is contraindicated during pregnancy.

5-Fluorouracil *see* Fluorouracil *on page 576*

Fluoxetine (floo OKS e teen)

U.S. Brand Names Prozac®; Prozac® Weekly™; Sarafem™

Synonyms Fluoxetine Hydrochloride

Generic Available Yes: Excludes delayed release capsule

Pharmacologic Category Antidepressant, Selective Serotonin Reuptake Inhibitor

Pregnancy Risk Factor C

Lactation Enters breast milk/not recommended (AAP rates "of concern")

Use Treatment of major depressive disorder; treatment of binge-eating and vomiting in patients with moderate-to-severe bulimia nervosa; obsessive-compulsive disorder (OCD); premenstrual dysphoric disorder (PMDD); panic disorder with or without agoraphobia

Use - Unlabeled/Investigational Selective mutism

Mechanism of Action/Effect Inhibits CNS neuron serotonin reuptake; minimal or no effect on reuptake of norepinephrine or dopamine; does not significantly bind to alpha-adrenergic, histamine or cholinergic receptors

Contraindications Hypersensitivity to fluoxetine or any component of the formulation; patients receiving MAO inhibitors, thioridazine, or mesoridazine currently or within prior 14 days; MAO inhibitor, thioridazine, or mesoridazine should not be initiated until 5 weeks after the discontinuation of fluoxetine

Warnings/Precautions Potential for severe reaction when used with MAO inhibitors - serotonin syndrome (hyperthermia, muscular rigidity, mental status changes/agitation, autonomic instability) may occur. Fluoxetine use has been associated with occurrences of significant rash and allergic events. May precipitate a shift to mania or hypomania in patients with bipolar disease. May cause insomnia, anxiety, nervousness or anorexia. Use with caution in patients where weight loss is undesirable.

May impair cognitive or motor performance - caution operating hazardous machinery or driving. Use caution in patients with depression, particularly if suicidal risk may be present. Use caution in patients with a previous seizure disorder or condition predisposing to seizures or concurrent therapy with other drugs which lower the seizure threshold.

Use with caution in patients with hepatic or renal dysfunction and in elderly patients. May cause hyponatremia/SIADH. May increase the risks associated with electroconvulsive treatment. Use with caution in patients at risk of bleeding or receiving concurrent anticoagulant therapy - may cause impairment in platelet function. May alter glycemic control in patients with diabetes. Due to the long half-life of fluoxetine and its metabolites, the effects and interactions noted may persist for prolonged periods following discontinuation. May cause or exacerbate sexual dysfunction.

Pregnancy risk C.

Drug Interactions

Cytochrome P450 Effect: Substrate of 1A2, 2B6, **2C8/9**, 2C19, **2D6**, 2E1, 3A4; Inhibits 1A2, **2B6**, 2C8/9, 2C19, **2D6**, 3A4

Decreased Effect: Cyproheptadine may inhibit the effects of serotonin reuptake inhibitors. Lithium levels may be decreased by fluoxetine (in addition to reports of increased lithium levels).

Increased Effect/Toxicity:

MAO inhibitors: Fluoxetine should not be used with nonselective MAO inhibitors (phenelzine, isocarboxazid) or other drugs with MAO inhibition (linezolid); fatal reactions have been reported. Wait 5 weeks after stopping fluoxetine before starting a nonselective MAO inhibitor and 2 weeks after stopping an MAO inhibitor before starting fluoxetine. Concurrent selegiline has been associated with mania, hypertension, or serotonin syndrome (risk may be reduced relative to nonselective MAO inhibitors).

Phenothiazines: Fluoxetine may inhibit the metabolism of thioridazine or mesoridazine, resulting in increased plasma levels and increasing the risk of QT_c interval prolongation. This may lead to serious ventricular arrhythmias, such as torsade de pointes-type arrhythmias and sudden death. Do not use together. Wait at least 5 weeks after discontinuing fluoxetine prior to starting thioridazine.

Combined used of SSRIs and amphetamines, buspirone, meperidine, nefazodone, serotonin agonists (such as sumatriptan), sibutramine, other SSRIs, sympathomimetics, ritonavir, tramadol, and venlafaxine may increase the risk of serotonin syndrome. Fluoxetine may increase serum levels/effects of benzodiazepines (alprazolam and diazepam), beta-blockers (except atenolol or nadolol), carbamazepine, carvedilol, clozapine, cyclosporine (and possibly tacrolimus), dextromethorphan, digoxin, haloperidol, HMG-CoA reductase inhibitors (lovastatin and simvastatin - increasing the risk of rhabdomyolysis), phenytoin, propafenone, trazodone, tricyclic antidepressants, and valproic acid. Concurrent lithium may increase risk of neurotoxicity, and lithium levels may be increased. Risk of hyponatremia may increase with concurrent use of loop diuretics (bumetanide, furosemide, torsemide). Fluoxetine may increase the hypoprothrombinemic response to warfarin.

Combined use of sumatriptan (and other serotonin agonists) may result in toxicity; weakness, hyper-reflexia, and incoordination have been observed with sumatriptan and SSRIs. In addition, concurrent use may theoretically increase the risk of serotonin syndrome; includes sumatriptan, naratriptan, rizatriptan, and zolmitriptan.

Nutritional/Ethanol Interactions

Ethanol: Avoid ethanol (may increase CNS depression). Depressed patients should avoid/limit intake.

Herb/Nutraceutical: Avoid valerian, St John's wort, kava kava, gotu kola (may increase CNS depression).

Effects on Lab Values ↑ albumin in urine

Adverse Reactions Predominant adverse effects are CNS and GI

>10%:

Central nervous system: Headache (up to 21%), nervousness (7% to 14%), insomnia (9% to 24%), anxiety (12%), somnolence (12%)

Gastrointestinal: Nausea (22%), diarrhea (11%)

Neuromuscular & skeletal: Weakness (11%)

1% to 10%:

Cardiovascular: Vasodilation, palpitation, hypertension

Central nervous system: Amnesia, confusion, emotional lability, sleep disorder, dizziness, agitation, yawning, pain, fever, abnormal dreams, tremor

Dermatologic: Reactions may occur in up to 7%, including rash, urticaria, or pruritus

Systemic events, possibly related to vasculitis (including lupus-like syndrome), have occurred rarely in patients with rash; may include lung, kidney, and/or hepatic involvement. Death has been reported.

(Continued)

Fluoxetine *(Continued)*

Endocrine & metabolic: SIADH, hypoglycemia, hyponatremia (elderly or volume-depleted patients)

Gastrointestinal: Dyspepsia, increased appetite, constipation, vomiting, flatulence, weight gain/loss, abdominal pain, dyspepsia, xerostomia, anorexia (10%)

Genitourinary: Sexual dysfunction, urinary frequency

Ocular: Abnormal vision

Respiratory: Pharyngitis

Miscellaneous: Diaphoresis, fever, flu syndrome, infection, abnormal thinking

<1% (Limited to important or life-threatening): Allergies, alopecia, anaphylactoid reactions, angina, arrhythmia, asthma, cataract, CHF, cholelithiasis, cholestatic jaundice, colitis, dyskinesia, dysphagia, eosinophilic pneumonia, erythema nodosum, esophagitis, euphoria, exfoliative dermatitis, extrapyramidal symptoms (rare), gout, hallucinations, heart arrest, hepatic failure/necrosis, hemorrhage, hyperprolactinemia, immune-related hemolytic anemia, laryngospasm, lupus-like syndrome, myocardial infarction, neuroleptic malignant syndrome (NMS), optic neuritis, pancreatitis, pancytopenia, photosensitivity reaction, postural hypotension, priapism, pulmonary embolism, pulmonary hypertension, QT prolongation, renal failure, serotonin syndrome, Stevens-Johnson syndrome, syncope, thrombocytopenia, thrombocytopenic purpura, vasculitis, ventricular tachycardia (including torsade de pointes), vomiting

Overdosage/Toxicology Among 633 adult patients who overdosed on fluoxetine alone, 34 resulted in a fatal outcome. Symptoms of overdose include ataxia, sedation, coma, and EKG abnormalities (QT prolongation, torsade de pointes). Respiratory depression may occur, especially with coingestion of ethanol or other drugs. Seizures rarely occur. Treatment is supportive.

Pharmacokinetic Note Weekly formulation results in greater fluctuations between peak and trough concentrations of fluoxetine and norfluoxetine compared to once-daily dosing (24% daily/164% weekly; 17% daily/43% weekly, respectively). Trough concentrations are 76% lower for fluoxetine and 47% lower for norfluoxetine than the concentrations maintained by 20 mg once-daily dosing. Steady-state fluoxetine concentrations are ~50% lower following the once-weekly regimen compared to 20 mg once daily.

Pharmacodynamics/Kinetics

Absorption: Well absorbed; delayed 1-2 hours with weekly formulation

Half-Life Elimination: Adults:

Parent drug: 1-3 days (acute), 4-6 days (chronic), 7.6 days (cirrhosis); Metabolite (norfluoxetine): 9.3 days (range: 4-16 days), 12 days (cirrhosis)

Due to long half-life, resolution of adverse reactions after discontinuation may be slow

Time to Peak: 6-8 hours

Metabolism: Hepatic to norfluoxetine (active; equal to fluoxetine)

Formulations

Capsule, as hydrochloride: 10 mg, 20 mg, 40 mg

Prozac®: 10 mg, 20 mg, 40 mg

Sarafem™: 10 mg, 20 mg

Capsule, delayed release, as hydrochloride (Prozac® Weekly™): 90 mg

Solution, oral, as hydrochloride (Prozac®): 20 mg/5 mL (120 mL) [contains alcohol 0.23% and benzoic acid; mint flavor]

Tablet, as hydrochloride: 10 mg, 20 mg

Prozac®: 10 mg (scored)

Dosing

Adults: Depression, OCD, PMDD, bulimia: 20 mg/day in the morning; may increase after several weeks by 20 mg/day increments; maximum: 80 mg/day; doses >20 mg should be divided into morning and noon doses. **Note:** Lower doses of 5-10 mg/day have been used for initial treatment.

Usual dosage range:

Depression: 20-40 mg/day; patients maintained on Prozac® 20 mg/day may be changed to Prozac® Weekly™ 90 mg/week, starting dose 7 days after the last 20 mg/day dose

Obsessive compulsive disorder (OCD): 40-80 mg/day

Premenstrual dysphoric disorder (Sarafem™): 20 mg/day continuously, **or** 20 mg/day starting 14 days prior to menstruation and through first full day of menses (repeat with each cycle)

Obesity: 20-60 mg/day

Bulimia nervosa: 60-80 mg/day

Panic disorder: Initial: 10 mg/day; after 1 week, increase to 20 mg/day; may increase after several weeks; doses >60 mg/day have not been evaluated

Elderly: Oral: Some patients may require an initial dose of 10 mg/day with dosage increases of 10 mg and 20 mg every several weeks as tolerated; should not be taken at night unless patient experiences sedation.

Pediatrics: Selective mutism (unlabeled use): Oral:

<5 years: No dosing information available

5-18 years: Initial: 5-10 mg/day; titrate upwards as needed (usual maximum dose: 60 mg/day)

Renal Impairment:

Single dose studies: Pharmacokinetics of fluoxetine and norfluoxetine were similar among subjects with all levels of impaired renal function, including anephric patients on chronic hemodialysis.

Chronic administration: Additional accumulation of fluoxetine or norfluoxetine may occur in patients with severely impaired renal function.

Not removed by hemodialysis; use of lower dose or less frequent dosing is not usually necessary.

Hepatic Impairment: Elimination half-life of fluoxetine is prolonged in patients with hepatic impairment. A lower dose or less frequent dosing of fluoxetine should be used in these patients.

Cirrhosis patient: Administer a lower dose or less frequent dosing interval.

Compensated cirrhosis without ascites: Administer 50% of normal dose.

Stability

Storage: All dosage forms should be stored at controlled room temperature of 15°C to 30°C (50°F to 86°F); oral liquid should be dispensed in a light-resistant container

Monitoring Laboratory Tests Baseline liver and renal function before beginning drug therapy

Monitoring and Teaching Issues

Physical Assessment: Assess other medications patient may be taking for effectiveness and interactions (see Drug Interactions). See Contraindications and Warnings/Precautions for use cautions. Monitor laboratory tests, therapeutic response, and adverse reactions at beginning of therapy and periodically with long-term use (see Adverse Reactions and Overdose/Toxicology). Taper dosage slowly when discontinuing (see Warnings/Precautions about timing when discontinuing Prozac® and starting another antidepressant). Assess knowledge/teach patient appropriate use, interventions to reduce side effects and adverse symptoms to report (see Patient Education). **Pregnancy risk factor C** - benefits of use should outweigh possible risks. Breast-feeding is not recommended.

Patient Education: Take exactly as directed; do not increase dose or frequency. It may take 2-3 weeks to achieve desired results. Take once-a-day dose in the morning to reduce incidence of insomnia. Avoid alcohol, caffeine, and other prescription or OTC medications not approved by prescriber. Maintain adequate hydration (2-3 L/day of fluids) unless advised by prescriber to restrict fluids. You may experience drowsiness, lightheadedness, impaired coordination, dizziness, or blurred vision (use caution when driving or engaging in tasks requiring alertness until response to drug is known); constipation (increased exercise, fluids, fruit, or fiber may help); anorexia (maintain regular dietary intake to avoid excessive weight loss); or postural hypotension (use caution when climbing stairs or changing position from lying or sitting to standing). If diabetic, monitor serum glucose closely (may cause hypoglycemia). Report persistent CNS effects (nervousness, restlessness, insomnia, anxiety, excitation, headache, sedation); rash or skin irritation; muscle cramping, tremors, or change in gait; respiratory depression or difficulty breathing; or worsening of condition. **Pregnancy/breast-feeding precautions:** Inform prescriber if you are pregnant. Breast-feeding is not recommended.

Dietary Issues: May be taken with or without food.

Geriatric Considerations: Fluoxetine's favorable side effect profile makes it a useful alternative to the traditional tricyclic antidepressants. Its potential stimulating and anorexic effects may be bothersome to some patients. Has not been shown to be superior in efficacy to the traditional tricyclic antidepressants or other SSRIs. The long half-life in the elderly makes it less attractive compared to other SSRIs. Data from a clinical trial comparing fluoxetine to tricyclics suggests that fluoxetine is significantly less effective than nortriptyline in hospitalized elderly patients with unipolar major affective disorder, especially those with melancholia and concurrent cardiovascular diseases. As with other SSRIs, fluoxetine has been associated with hyponatremia in elderly patients.

Breast-feeding Issues: Colic, irritability, slow weight gain, feeding and sleep disorders have been reported in nursing infants.

Additional Information EKG may reveal S-T segment depression; not shown to be teratogenic in rodents; 15-60 mg/day, buspirone and cyproheptadine, may be useful in treatment of sexual dysfunction during treatment with a selective serotonin reuptake inhibitor.

Weekly capsules are a delayed release formulation containing enteric-coated pellets of fluoxetine hydrochloride, equivalent to 90 mg fluoxetine. Therapeutic equivalence of weekly formulation with daily formulation for delaying time to relapse has not been established.

Related Information

Antidepressant Agents *on page 1553*
Antidepressant Medication Guidelines *on page 1613*

Fluoxetine Hydrochloride *see* Fluoxetine *on page 578*

Fluphenazine (floo FEN a zeen)

U.S. Brand Names Prolixin®; Prolixin Decanoate®; Prolixin Enanthate® [DSC]

Synonyms Fluphenazine Decanoate; Fluphenazine Enanthate; Fluphenazine Hydrochloride

Generic Available Yes: Injection, tablet

Pharmacologic Category Antipsychotic Agent, Phenothiazine, Piperazine

Pregnancy Risk Factor C

Lactation Enters breast milk/not recommended

Use Management of manifestations of psychotic disorders and schizophrenia; depot formulation may offer improved outcome in individuals with psychosis who are nonadherent with oral antipsychotics

Use - Unlabeled/Investigational Pervasive developmental disorder

Mechanism of Action/Effect Blocks postsynaptic mesolimbic dopaminergic D_1 and D_2 receptors in the brain; depresses the release of hypothalamic and hypophyseal hormones; believed to depress the reticular activating system thus affecting basal metabolism, body temperature, wakefulness, vasomotor tone, and emesis

Contraindications Hypersensitivity to fluphenazine or any component of the formulation (cross-reactivity between phenothiazines may occur); severe CNS depression; coma; subcortical brain damage; blood dyscrasias; hepatic disease

Warnings/Precautions May be sedating, use with caution in disorders where CNS depression is a feature. Use with caution in Parkinson's disease. Caution in patients with hemodynamic instability; bone marrow suppression; predisposition to seizures; severe cardiac, renal, or respiratory disease. Esophageal dysmotility and aspiration have been associated with antipsychotic use - use with caution in patients at risk of pneumonia (ie, Alzheimer's disease). Caution in breast cancer or other prolactin-dependent tumors (may elevate prolactin levels). May alter temperature regulation or mask toxicity of other drugs due to antiemetic effects. May alter cardiac conduction; life-threatening arrhythmias have occurred with therapeutic doses of phenothiazines. Hypotension may occur, particularly with I.M. administration. May cause orthostatic hypotension - use with caution in patients at risk of this effect or those who

(Continued)

Fluphenazine *(Continued)*

would tolerate transient hypotensive episodes (cerebrovascular disease, cardiovascular disease, or other medications which may predispose). Adverse effects of depot injections may be prolonged.

Due to anticholinergic effects, use caution in patients with decreased gastrointestinal motility, urinary retention, BPH, xerostomia, visual problems, narrow-angle glaucoma (screening is recommended), and myasthenia gravis. Relative to other antipsychotics, fluphenazine has a low potency of cholinergic blockade.

May cause extrapyramidal symptoms, including pseudoparkinsonism, acute dystonic reactions, akathisia and tardive dyskinesia (risk of these reactions is high relative to other antipsychotics). May be associated with neuroleptic malignant syndrome (NMS) or pigmentary retinopathy.

Pregnancy risk C.

Drug Interactions

Cytochrome P450 Effect: Substrate of **CYP2D6**; Inhibits CYP1A2, 2D6, 2E1

Decreased Effect: Phenothiazines inhibit the activity of guanethidine, guanadrel, levodopa, and bromocriptine. Barbiturates and cigarette smoking may enhance the hepatic metabolism of fluphenazine. Fluphenazine and possibly other low potency antipsychotics may reverse the pressor effects of epinephrine.

Increased Effect/Toxicity: Effects on CNS depression may be additive when fluphenazine is combined with CNS depressants (narcotic analgesics, ethanol, barbiturates, cyclic antidepressants, antihistamines, sedative-hypnotics). Fluphenazine may increase the effects/toxicity of anticholinergics, antihypertensives, lithium (rare neurotoxicity), trazodone, or valproic acid. Concurrent use with TCA may produce increased toxicity or altered therapeutic response. Chloroquine and propranolol may increase chlorpromazine concentrations. Hypotension may occur when fluphenazine is combined with epinephrine. May increase the risk of arrhythmia when combined with antiarrhythmics, cisapride, pimozide, sparfloxacin, or other drugs which prolong QT interval. Metoclopramide may increase risk of extrapyramidal symptoms (EPS).

Nutritional/Ethanol Interactions

Ethanol: Avoid ethanol (may increase CNS depression).

Herb/Nutraceutical: Avoid dong quai, St John's wort (may also cause photosensitization). Avoid kava kava, gotu kola, valerian, St John's wort (may increase CNS depression).

Effects on Lab Values ↑ cholesterol (S), glucose; ↓ uric acid (S)

Adverse Reactions Frequency not defined.

Cardiovascular: Hypotension, tachycardia, fluctuations in blood pressure, hypertension, arrhythmias, edema

Central nervous system: Parkinsonian symptoms, akathisia, dystonias, tardive dyskinesia, dizziness, hyper-reflexia, headache, cerebral edema, drowsiness, lethargy, restlessness, excitement, bizarre dreams, EEG changes, depression, seizures, NMS, altered central temperature regulation

Dermatologic: Increased sensitivity to sun, rash, skin pigmentation, itching, erythema, urticaria, seborrhea, eczema, dermatitis

Endocrine & metabolic: Changes in menstrual cycle, breast pain, amenorrhea, galactorrhea, gynecomastia, changes in libido, elevated prolactin, SIADH

Gastrointestinal: Weight gain, loss of appetite, salivation, xerostomia, constipation, paralytic ileus, laryngeal edema

Genitourinary: Ejaculatory disturbances, impotence, polyuria, bladder paralysis, enuresis

Hematologic: Agranulocytosis, leukopenia, thrombocytopenia, nonthrombocytopenic purpura, eosinophilia, pancytopenia

Hepatic: Cholestatic jaundice, hepatotoxicity

Neuromuscular & skeletal: Trembling of fingers, SLE, facial hemispasm

Ocular: Pigmentary retinopathy, cornea and lens changes, blurred vision, glaucoma

Respiratory: Nasal congestion, asthma

Overdosage/Toxicology Symptoms of overdose include deep sleep, hypo- or hypertension, dystonia, seizures, extrapyramidal symptoms, and respiratory failure. Following initiation of essential overdose management, toxic symptom treatment and supportive treatment should be initiated.

Pharmacodynamics/Kinetics

Absorption: Oral: Erratic and variable

Half-Life Elimination: Derivative dependent: Enanthate: 84-96 hours; Hydrochloride: 33 hours; Decanoate: 163-232 hours

Metabolism: Hepatic

Onset: I.M., S.C. (derivative dependent): Hydrochloride salt: ~1 hour

Peak effect: Neuroleptic: Decanoate: 48-96 hours

Duration: Hydrochloride salt: 6-8 hours; Decanoate (lasts the longest): 24-72 hours

Formulations

Elixir, as hydrochloride (Prolixin®): 2.5 mg/5 mL (60 mL) [contains alcohol 14% and sodium benzoate]

Injection, as enanthate (Prolixin Enanthate®): 25 mg/mL (5 mL) [DSC] [contains benzyl alcohol, sesame oil]

Injection, oil, as decanoate: 25 mg/mL (1 mL, 5 mL) [may contain benzyl alcohol, sesame oil]

Prolixin Decanoate®: 25 mg/mL (1 mL, 5 mL) [contains benzyl alcohol, sesame oil]

Injection, solution, as hydrochloride (Prolixin®): 2.5 mg/mL (10 mL)

Solution, oral concentrate, as hydrochloride (Prolixin®): 5 mg/mL (120 mL) [contains alcohol 14%]

Tablet, as hydrochloride: 1 mg, 2.5 mg, 5 mg, 10 mg

Prolixin®: 1 mg, 2.5 mg, 5 mg [contains tartrazine], 10 mg

Dosing

Adults:

Psychosis:

Oral: 0.5-10 mg/day in divided doses at 6- to 8-hour intervals; some patients may require up to 40 mg/day

I.M.: 2.5-10 mg/day in divided doses at 6- to 8-hour intervals (parenteral dose is $^1/_3$ to $^1/_2$ the oral dose for the hydrochloride salts)

Maintenance injections (prolonged effect):

I.M., S.C. (decanoate): 12.5 mg every 3 weeks

Conversion from hydrochloride to decanoate I.M. 0.5 mL (12.5 mg) decanoate every 3 weeks is approximately equivalent to 10 mg hydrochloride/day

I.M. (enanthate): 12.5-25 mg every 3 weeks

Elderly: Initial (nonpsychotic patient, dementia behavior): 1-2.5 mg/day; increase dose at 4- to 7-day intervals by 1-2.5 mg/day. Increase dosing intervals (bid, tid) as necessary to control response or side effects. Maximum daily dose: 20 mg; gradual increases (titration) may prevent some side effects or decrease their severity.

Pediatrics: Childhood-onset pervasive developmental disorder (unlabeled use): Oral: 0.04 mg/kg/day

Renal Impairment: Use with caution; not dialyzable (0% to 5%).

Hepatic Impairment: Use with caution.

Administration

Oral: Avoid contact of oral solution or injection with skin (contact dermatitis). Oral liquid should be diluted in the following **only**: water, saline, 7-UP®, homogenized milk, carbonated orange beverages, pineapple, apricot, prune, orange, V8® juice, tomato, and grapefruit juices. Do **not** dilute in beverages containing caffeine, tannics, or pectinate.

I.M.: Watch for hypotension when administering I.M.

Monitoring Laboratory Tests Liver and kidney function, CBC prior to and regularly during therapy, ophthalmic screening

Monitoring and Teaching Issues

Physical Assessment: Assess other medications patient is taking for effectiveness and interactions (see Drug Interactions). See Contraindications and Warnings/Precautions for use cautions. Review ophthalmic screening and monitor laboratory tests (see above), therapeutic response, and adverse reactions at beginning of therapy and periodically with long-term use (see Adverse Reactions and Overdose/Toxicology). With I.M. or S.C. use, monitor closely for hypotension. Initiate at lower doses (see Dosing) and taper dosage slowly when discontinuing. Assess knowledge/teach patient appropriate use, interventions to reduce side effects, and adverse symptoms to report (see Patient Education). **Pregnancy risk factor C** - benefits of use should outweigh possible risks. Breast-feeding is not recommended.

Patient Education: Use exactly as directed; do not increase dose or frequency. Do not discontinue without consulting prescriber. Dilute with water, milk, orange or grapefruit juice; do not dilute with beverages containing caffeine, tannin, or pectinate (eg, coffee, colas, tea, or apple juice). Do not take within 2 hours of any antacid. Avoid alcohol or caffeine and other prescription or OTC medications not approved by prescriber. Avoid skin contact with medication; may cause contact dermatitis (wash immediately with warm, soapy water). Maintain adequate hydration (2-3 L/day of fluids) unless advised by prescriber to restrict fluids. You may experience excess drowsiness, lightheadedness, dizziness, or blurred vision (use caution driving or when engaging in tasks requiring alertness until response to drug is known); dry mouth, upset stomach, nausea, vomiting (small, frequent meals, frequent mouth care, chewing gum, or sucking lozenges may help); constipation (increased exercise, fluids, fruits, or fiber may help); postural hypotension (use caution climbing stairs or when changing position from lying or sitting to standing); urinary retention (void before taking medication); ejaculatory dysfunction (reversible); decreased perspiration (avoid strenuous exercise in hot environments); or photosensitivity (use sunscreen, wear protective clothing and eyewear, and avoid direct sunlight). Report persistent CNS effects (eg, trembling fingers, altered gait or balance, excessive sedation, seizures, unusual movements, anxiety, abnormal thoughts, confusion, personality changes); chest pain, palpitations, rapid heartbeat, severe dizziness; unresolved urinary retention or changes in urinary pattern; altered menstrual pattern, change in libido, swelling or pain in breasts (male or female); vision changes; skin rash or irritation or yellowing of skin; or worsening of condition. **Pregnancy/breast-feeding precautions:** Inform prescriber if you are or intend to become pregnant. Breast-feeding is not recommended.

Geriatric Considerations: (See Warnings/Precautions, Adverse Reactions, and Overdose/Toxicology.) Elderly patients have an increased risk of adverse response to side effects or adverse reactions to antipsychotics.

Additional Information Less sedative and hypotensive effects than chlorpromazine

Related Information

Antipsychotic Agents *on page 1558*
Antipsychotic Medication Guidelines *on page 1614*

Fluphenazine Decanoate *see* Fluphenazine *on page 581*
Fluphenazine Enanthate *see* Fluphenazine *on page 581*
Fluphenazine Hydrochloride *see* Fluphenazine *on page 581*
Flurandrenolide *see* Topical Corticosteroids *on page 1334*

Flurazepam (flure AZ e pam)

U.S. Brand Names Dalmane®

Synonyms Flurazepam Hydrochloride

Restrictions C-IV

Generic Available Yes

Pharmacologic Category Benzodiazepine

Pregnancy Risk Factor X

Lactation Excretion in breast milk unknown/not recommended

(Continued)

Flurazepam *(Continued)*

Use Short-term treatment of insomnia

Mechanism of Action/Effect Binds to stereospecific benzodiazepine receptors on the postsynaptic GABA neuron at several sites within the central nervous system, including the limbic system, reticular formation. Enhancement of the inhibitory effect of GABA on neuronal excitability results by increased neuronal membrane permeability to chloride ions. This shift in chloride ions results in hyperpolarization (a less excitable state) and stabilization.

Contraindications Hypersensitivity to flurazepam or any component of the formulation (cross-sensitivity with other benzodiazepines may exist); narrow-angle glaucoma; pregnancy

Warnings/Precautions As a hypnotic, should be used only after evaluation of potential causes of sleep disturbance. Failure of sleep disturbance to resolve after 7-10 days may indicate psychiatric or medical illness. Use is not recommended in patients with depressive disorders or psychoses. Avoid use in patients with sleep apnea. Use with caution in patients receiving concurrent CYP3A4 inhibitors, particularly when these agents are added to therapy. Use with caution in elderly or debilitated patients, patients with hepatic disease (including alcoholics), renal impairment, respiratory disease, impaired gag reflex, or obese patients.

Causes CNS depression (dose-related) which may impair physical and mental capabilities. Use with caution in patients receiving other CNS depressants or psychoactive agents. Benzodiazepines have been associated with falls and traumatic injury and should be used with extreme caution in patients who are at risk of these events (especially the elderly). May cause physical or psychological dependence - use with caution in patients with a history of drug dependence.

Benzodiazepines have been associated with anterograde amnesia. Paradoxical reactions, including hyperactive or aggressive behavior, have been reported with benzodiazepines, particularly in adolescent/pediatric or psychiatric patients. Does not have analgesic, antidepressant, or antipsychotic properties.

Drug Interactions

Cytochrome P450 Effect: Substrate of **CYP3A4**; Inhibits CYP2E1

Decreased Effect: Carbamazepine, rifampin, and rifabutin may enhance the metabolism of flurazepam and decrease its therapeutic effect; consider using an alternative sedative/hypnotic agent.

Increased Effect/Toxicity: Serum levels and response to flurazepam may be increased by amprenavir, cimetidine, ciprofloxacin, clarithromycin, clozapine, CNS depressants, diltiazem, disulfiram, digoxin, erythromycin, ethanol, fluconazole, fluoxetine, fluvoxamine, grapefruit juice, isoniazid, itraconazole, ketoconazole, labetalol, levodopa, loxapine, metoprolol, metronidazole, miconazole, nefazodone, nelfinavir, omeprazole, phenytoin, rifabutin, rifampin, ritonavir, troleandomycin, valproic acid, and verapamil.

Nutritional/Ethanol Interactions

Ethanol: Avoid ethanol (may increase CNS depression).

Food: Serum levels and response to flurazepam may be increased by grapefruit juice, but unlikely because of flurazepam's high oral bioavailability.

Herb/Nutraceutical: Avoid valerian, St John's wort, kava kava, gotu kola (may increase CNS depression).

Effects on Lab Values Elevated alkaline phosphatase, AST, ALT, and bilirubin (total and direct)

Adverse Reactions Frequency not defined.

Cardiovascular: Palpitations, chest pain

Central nervous system: Drowsiness, ataxia, lightheadedness, memory impairment, depression, headache, hangover effect, confusion, nervousness, dizziness, falling, apprehension, irritability, euphoria, slurred speech, restlessness, hallucinations, paradoxical reactions, talkativeness

Dermatologic: Rash, pruritus

Gastrointestinal: Xerostomia, constipation, increased/excessive salivation, heartburn, upset stomach, nausea, vomiting, diarrhea, increased or decreased appetite, bitter taste, weight gain/loss

Hematologic: Euphoria, granulocytopenia

Hepatic: Elevated SGOT/SGPT, total bilirubin, alkaline phosphatase; cholestatic jaundice

Neuromuscular & skeletal: Dysarthria, body/joint pain, reflex slowing, weakness

Ocular: Blurred vision, burning eyes, difficulty focusing

Otic: Tinnitus

Respiratory: Apnea, dyspnea

Miscellaneous: Diaphoresis, drug dependence

Overdosage/Toxicology Symptoms of overdose include respiratory depression, hypoactive reflexes, unsteady gait, and hypotension. Treatment for benzodiazepine overdose is supportive. Flumazenil has been shown to selectively block the binding of benzodiazepines to CNS receptors, resulting in a reversal of benzodiazepine-induced CNS depression. Respiratory depression may not be reversed.

Pharmacodynamics/Kinetics

Half-Life Elimination: Desalkylflurazepam:

Adults: Single dose: 74-90 hours; Multiple doses: 111-113 hours

Elderly (61-85 years): Single dose: 120-160 hours; Multiple doses: 126-158 hours

Metabolism: Hepatic to N-desalkylflurazepam (active)

Onset: Hypnotic: 15-20 minutes; Peak effect: 3-6 hours

Duration: 7-8 hours

Formulations Capsule, as hydrochloride: 15 mg, 30 mg

Dosing

Adults: Insomnia (short-term treatment): Oral: 15-30 mg at bedtime

Elderly: Oral: 15 mg at bedtime. Avoid use if possible.

Pediatrics: Hypnotic: Oral:

≤15 years: Dose not established

>15 years: 15 mg at bedtime

Administration

Oral: Give 30 minutes to 1 hour before bedtime on an empty stomach with full glass of water. Can be taken with food if GI distress occurs.

Stability

Storage: Store in light-resistant containers.

Monitoring and Teaching Issues

Physical Assessment: For short-term use. Assess effectiveness and interactions of other medications patient may be taking (see Drug Interactions). See Contraindications and Warnings/Precautions for use cautions. Assess for history of addiction; long-term use can result in dependence, abuse, or tolerance. Evaluate periodically for need for continued use. After long-term use, taper dosage slowly when discontinuing. Order safety precautions for inpatient use. Monitor therapeutic effectiveness and adverse reactions (see Adverse Reactions) at beginning of therapy and periodically with long-term use. Assess knowledge/teach patient appropriate use, interventions to reduce side effects, and adverse symptoms to report (see Patient Education). **Pregnancy risk factor X** - determine that patient is not pregnant before starting therapy. Do not give to sexually-active female patients unless capable of complying with barrier contraceptive use. Breast-feeding is not recommended.

Patient Education: Use exactly as directed; do not increase dose or frequency or discontinue without consulting prescriber. Drug may cause physical and/or psychological dependence. May take with food to decrease GI upset. While using this medication, do not use alcohol or other prescription or OTC medications (especially, pain medications, sedatives, antihistamines, or hypnotics) without consulting prescriber. Maintain adequate hydration (2-3 L/day of fluids) unless advised by prescriber to restrict fluids. You may experience drowsiness, dizziness, lightheadedness, or blurred vision (use caution when driving or engaging in tasks requiring alertness until response to drug is known); dry mouth, nausea, or vomiting (small, frequent meals, frequent mouth care, chewing gum, or sucking lozenges may help); difficulty urinating (void before taking medication); or altered libido (resolves when medication is discontinued). Report CNS changes (confusion, depression, increased sedation, excitation, headache, abnormal thinking, insomnia, or nightmares, memory impairment, impaired coordination); muscle pain or weakness; difficulty breathing; persistent dizziness, chest pain, or palpitations; alterations in normal gait; vision changes; ringing in ears; or ineffectiveness of medication. **Pregnancy/breast-feeding precautions:** Inform prescriber if you are pregnant. Do not get pregnant during or for 1 month following therapy. Consult prescriber for instruction on appropriate contraceptive measures. This drug may cause severe fetal defects. Breast-feeding is not recommended.

Geriatric Considerations: Due to its long-acting metabolite, flurazepam is not considered a drug of choice in the elderly. Long-acting benzodiazepines have been associated with falls in the elderly. Interpretive guidelines from the Health Care Financing. Administration (HCFA) discourage the use of this agent in residents of long-term care facilities.

Related Information

Anxiolytic/Hypnotic Use in Long-Term Care Facilities *on page 1608*
Benzodiazepines *on page 1560*

Flurazepam Hydrochloride *see* Flurazepam *on page 583*

Flurbiprofen (flure BI proe fen)

U.S. Brand Names Ansaid®; Ocufen®

Synonyms Flurbiprofen Sodium

Generic Available Yes

Pharmacologic Category Nonsteroidal Anti-inflammatory Drug (NSAID)

Pregnancy Risk Factor C/D (3rd trimester)

Lactation Excretion in breast milk unknown

Use

Oral: Acute or long-term treatment of signs and symptoms of rheumatoid arthritis and osteoarthritis

Ophthalmic: Inhibition of intraoperative miosis; prevention and management of postoperative ocular inflammation and postoperative cystoid macular edema remains to be determined

Mechanism of Action/Effect Inhibits prostaglandin synthesis by decreasing the activity of the enzyme, cyclooxygenase, which results in decreased formation of prostaglandin precursors

Contraindications Hypersensitivity to flurbiprofen or any component of the formulation; dendritic keratitis; pregnancy (3rd trimester)

Warnings/Precautions Use with caution in patients with CHF, hypertension, dehydration, decreased renal or hepatic function, history of GI disease (bleeding or ulcers), or those receiving anticoagulants. Elderly are at a high risk for adverse effects from NSAIDs. As many as 60% of elderly can develop peptic ulceration and/or hemorrhage asymptomatically.

Use lowest effective dose for shortest period possible. Use of NSAIDs can compromise existing renal function especially when Cl_{cr} is <30 mL/minute. The elderly may demonstrate CNS adverse effects at lower doses than younger adults. Withhold for at least 4-6 half-lives prior to surgical or dental procedures. Ophthalmic solution contains thimerosal.

Pregnancy risk C/D (3rd trimester).

Drug Interactions

Cytochrome P450 Effect: Substrate of CYP2C8/9; Inhibits CYP2C8/9

Decreased Effect: Ophthalmic: When used with concurrent administration of flurbiprofen, acetylcholine chloride and carbachol have been shown to be ineffective. Reports of acetylcholine chloride and carbachol being ineffective when used with flurbiprofen.

Increased Effect/Toxicity: Flurbiprofen may increase cyclosporine, digoxin, lithium, and methotrexate serum concentrations. The renal adverse effects of ACE inhibitors may be potentiated by NSAIDs. Corticosteroids may increase the risk of GI ulceration.

Nutritional/Ethanol Interactions

Ethanol: Avoid ethanol (may enhance gastric mucosal irritation).

Food: Food may decrease the rate but not the extent of absorption.

(Continued)

Flurbiprofen *(Continued)*

Herb/Nutraceutical: Avoid cat's claw, dong quai, evening primrose, feverfew, garlic, ginger, ginkgo, red clover, horse chestnut, green tea, ginseng (all have additional antiplatelet activity).

Adverse Reactions

Ophthalmic:

>10%: Ocular: Slowing of corneal wound healing, mild ocular stinging, itching and burning eyes, ocular irritation

1% to 10%: Ocular: Eye redness

Systemic:

1% to 10%:

Central nervous system: Headache, nervousness, dizziness

Dermatologic: Itching, rash

Endocrine & metabolic: Fluid retention

Gastrointestinal: Abdominal cramps, heartburn, indigestion, nausea, vomiting

Otic: Tinnitus

<1% (Limited to important or life-threatening): Acute renal failure, agranulocytosis, allergic reactions, angioedema, arrhythmias, aseptic meningitis, bone marrow suppression, CHF, dyspnea, erythema multiforme, GI ulceration, hallucinations, hemolytic anemia, hepatitis, hypertension, leukopenia, mental depression, peripheral neuropathy, Stevens-Johnson syndrome, thrombocytopenia, toxic amblyopia, toxic epidermal necrolysis, tachycardia, urticaria

Overdosage/Toxicology Symptoms of overdose include apnea, metabolic acidosis, coma, nystagmus, leukocytosis, and renal failure. Management of NSAID intoxication is supportive and symptomatic. Since many NSAIDs undergo enterohepatic cycling, multiple doses of charcoal may be needed to reduce the potential for delayed toxicities.

Pharmacodynamics/Kinetics

Half-Life Elimination: 5.7 hours

Time to Peak: 1.5 hours

Metabolism: Hepatic via CYP2C9

Onset: ~1-2 hours

Formulations

Solution, ophthalmic, as sodium (Ocufen®): 0.03% [contains thimerosal]

Tablet (Ansaid®): 50 mg, 100 mg

Dosing

Adults & Elderly:

Management of pain (including dental): Oral: 200-300 mg/day in 2, 3, or 4 divided doses

Rheumatoid arthritis and osteoarthritis: Oral: Initial: 50 mg 4 times/day to 100 mg 3 times/day; do not administer more than 100 mg for any single dose; maximum: 300 mg/day.

Ophthalmic anti-inflammatory/surgical aid: Ophthalmic: Instill 1 drop every 30 minutes, 2 hours prior to surgery (total of 4 drops to each affected eye).

Administration

Oral: Take with a full glass of water.

Monitoring and Teaching Issues

Physical Assessment: **Assess for allergic reaction to salicylate or other NSAIDs** (see Contraindications). See Warnings/Precautions for use cautions. Assess effectiveness and interactions of other medications patient may be taking (see Contraindications, Warnings/Precautions, and Drug Interactions). Monitor laboratory tests (see above), therapeutic response, and adverse reactions at beginning of therapy and periodically throughout therapy (see Warnings/Precautions, Adverse Reactions, and Overdose/Toxicology). Assess knowledge/teach patient appropriate use, interventions to reduce side effects, and adverse symptoms to report (see Patient Education). **Pregnancy risk factor C/D** - see Pregnancy Risk Factor for use cautions; benefits of use should outweigh possible risks. Note breast-feeding caution. Ophthalmic absorption is probably minimal.

Patient Education: Oral: Take this medication exactly as directed; do not increase dose without consulting prescriber. Do not crush tablets or break capsules. Take with food or milk to reduce GI distress. Maintain adequate hydration (2-3 L/day of fluids) unless advised by prescriber to restrict fluids. Do not use alcohol, aspirin or aspirin-containing medication, or any other anti-inflammatory medications without consulting prescriber. You may experience drowsiness, dizziness, nervousness, or headache (use caution when driving or engaging in tasks requiring alertness until response to drug is known); anorexia, nausea, vomiting, or heartburn (small, frequent meals, frequent mouth care, sucking lozenges, or chewing gum may help); fluid retention (weigh yourself weekly and report unusual (3-5 lb/week) weight gain). GI bleeding, ulceration, or perforation can occur with or without pain; discontinue medication and contact prescriber if persistent abdominal pain or cramping, or blood in stool occurs. Report breathlessness, difficulty breathing, or unusual cough; chest pain, rapid heartbeat, palpitations; unusual bruising/bleeding; blood in urine, stool, mouth, or vomitus; swollen extremities; skin rash or itching; acute fatigue; or hearing changes (ringing in ears). **Pregnancy/breast-feeding precautions:** Inform prescriber if you are or intend to become pregnant. This drug should not be used in the 3rd trimester of pregnancy. Consult prescriber if breast-feeding.

Ophthalmic: Wash hands before instilling. Sit or lie down to instill. Open eye, look at ceiling, and instill prescribed amount of medication. Close eye and roll eye in all directions, and apply gentle pressure to inner corner of eye. Do not let tip of applicator touch eye; do not contaminate tip of applicator (may cause eye infection, eye damage, or vision loss). Use protective dark eyewear until healed; avoid direct sunlight. Temporary stinging or burning may occur. Report persistent pain, burning, redness, vision changes, swelling, itching, or worsening of condition.

Dietary Issues: May be taken with food, milk, or antacid to decrease GI effects.

Geriatric Considerations: Elderly are at high risk for adverse effects from NSAIDs. As much as 60% of elderly can develop peptic ulceration and/or hemorrhage asymptomatically. The concomitant use of H_2 blockers, omeprazole, and sucralfate is not effective as prophylaxis with the exception of NSAID-induced duodenal ulcers which may be prevented by the use of ranitidine. Misoprostol is the only prophylactic agent proven effective. Also, concomitant disease and drug use contribute to the risk for GI adverse effects. Use lowest effective dose for shortest period possible. Consider renal function decline with age. Use of NSAIDs can compromise existing renal function especially when Cl_{cr} is ≤30 mL/minute. Tinnitus may be a difficult and unreliable indication of toxicity due to age-related hearing loss or eighth cranial nerve damage. CNS adverse effects such as confusion, agitation, and hallucination are generally seen in overdose or high-dose situations, but elderly may demonstrate these adverse effects at lower doses than younger adults.

Related Information

Nonsalicylate/Nonsteroidal Anti-inflammatory Comparison *on page 1587*

Ophthalmic Agents *on page 1509*

Flurbiprofen Sodium *see* Flurbiprofen *on page 585*

Fluress® Ophthalmic Solution *see page 1461*

5-Flurocytosine *see* Flucytosine *on page 567*

FluShield® *see page 1498*

Flutamide (FLOO ta mide)

U.S. Brand Names Eulexin®

Generic Available Yes

Pharmacologic Category Antineoplastic Agent, Antiandrogen

Pregnancy Risk Factor D

Lactation Not indicated for use in women

Use In combination therapy with LHRH agonist analogues in treatment of metastatic prostatic carcinoma. A study has shown that the addition of flutamide to leuprolide therapy in patients with advanced prostatic cancer increased median actuarial survival time to 34.9 months versus 27.9 months with leuprolide alone. To achieve benefit to combination therapy, both drugs need to be started simultaneously.

Use - Unlabeled/Investigational Female hirsutism

Mechanism of Action/Effect Nonsteroidal antiandrogen that inhibits androgen uptake or inhibits binding of androgen in target tissues

Contraindications Hypersensitivity to flutamide or any component of the formulation; severe hepatic impairment; pregnancy

Warnings/Precautions Product labeling states flutamide is not for use in women, particularly for nonlife-threatening conditions. Patients who have taken flutamide, with glucose-6 phosphate dehydrogenase deficiency or hemoglobin M disease or smokers are at risk of toxicities associated aniline exposure, including methemoglobinemia, hemolytic anemia, and cholestatic jaundice. Monitor methemoglobin levels. Severe and potentially fatal hepatic injury may occur (50% of cases within first 3 months of therapy). Serum transaminases should be monitored at baseline and monthly for the first four months of therapy, and periodically thereafter. These should also be repeated at the first sign and symptom of liver dysfunction. Use of flutamide is not recommended in patients with baseline elevation of transaminase levels (>2 times the upper limit of normal). Flutamide should be discontinued immediately at any time if the patient develops jaundice or elevation in serum transaminase levels (>2 times upper limit of normal).

Drug Interactions

Cytochrome P450 Effect: Substrate of **CYP1A2, 3A4**; Inhibits CYP1A2

Increased Effect/Toxicity: Warfarin effects may be increased.

Nutritional/Ethanol Interactions

Food: No effect on bioavailability of flutamide.

Herb/Nutraceutical: St John's wort may decrease flutamide levels.

Adverse Reactions

>10%:

Endocrine & metabolic: Gynecomastia, hot flashes, breast tenderness, galactorrhea (9% to 42%); impotence; decreased libido; tumor flare

Gastrointestinal: Nausea, vomiting (11% to 12%)

Hepatic: Increased AST (SGOT) and LDH levels, transient, mild

1% to 10%:

Cardiovascular: Hypertension (1%), edema

Central nervous system: Drowsiness, confusion, depression, anxiety, nervousness, headache, dizziness, insomnia

Dermatologic: Pruritus, ecchymosis, photosensitivity, herpes zoster

Gastrointestinal: Anorexia, increased appetite, constipation, indigestion, upset stomach (4% to 6%); diarrhea

Hematologic: Anemia (6%), leukopenia (3%), thrombocytopenia (1%)

Neuromuscular & skeletal: Weakness (1%)

<1% (Limited to important or life-threatening): Hepatic failure, hepatitis, jaundice, malignant breast neoplasm (male), myocardial infarction, pulmonary embolism, sulfhemoglobinemia, thrombophlebitis, yellow discoloration of the urine

Overdosage/Toxicology Symptoms of overdose include hypoactivity, ataxia, anorexia, vomiting, slow respiration, and lacrimation. Induce vomiting. Management is supportive. Dialysis is of no benefit.

Pharmacodynamics/Kinetics

Absorption: Rapid and complete

Half-Life Elimination: 5-6 hours

Metabolism: Extensively hepatic to more than 10 metabolites

Formulations Capsule: 125 mg

Dosing

Adults & Elderly: Refer to individual protocols.

Prostate carcinoma: Oral: 2 capsules every 8 hours for a total daily dose of 750 mg

Female hirsutism: Oral: 250 mg daily

(Continued)

Flutamide *(Continued)*

Administration

Oral: Contents of capsule may be opened and mixed with applesauce, pudding, or other soft foods. Mixing with a beverage is not recommended.

Stability

Storage: Store at room temperature.

Monitoring Laboratory Tests Serum transaminase levels should be obtained at baseline and repeated monthly for the first 4 months of therapy, and periodically thereafter. LFTs should be checked at the first sign or symptom of liver dysfunction. Other parameters include tumor reduction, testosterone/estrogen, prostate specific antigen, and phosphatase serum levels.

Monitoring and Teaching Issues

Physical Assessment: See Contraindications, Warnings/Precautions, and Dosing for use cautions. Assess potential for interactions with other prescriptions, OTC medications, or herbal products patient may be taking (see Drug Interactions). Assess results of laboratory tests (see above), therapeutic effects, and adverse response (see Adverse Reactions and Overdose/Toxicology) and on a regular basis throughout therapy. Teach patient proper use, possible side effects and appropriate interventions, and adverse symptoms to report (see Patient Education). **Pregnancy risk factor D** - determine that patient is not pregnant before beginning treatment. Instruct patients of childbearing age about appropriate barrier contraceptive measures. Note breast-feeding caution.

Patient Education: Inform prescriber of all prescriptions, OTC medications, or herbal products you are taking, and any allergies you have. Do not take anything new during treatment unless approved by prescriber. Take as directed; do not discontinue without consulting prescriber. May cause decreased libido, impotence, swelling of breasts, or decreased appetite (small, frequent meals may help). Report chest pain or palpitation; acute abdominal pain; pain, tingling, or numbness of extremities; swelling of extremities or unusual weight gain; difficulty breathing; or other persistent adverse effects. **Pregnancy/breast-feeding precautions:** Inform prescriber if you are pregnant and do not get pregnant during or for 1 month following therapy. Consult prescriber for instruction on appropriate barrier contraceptive measures. This drug may cause severe fetal defects. Consult prescriber about breast-feeding.

Geriatric Considerations: A study has shown that the addition of flutamide to leuprolide therapy in patients with advanced prostatic cancer increased median actuarial survival time to 34.9 months versus 27.9 months with leuprolide alone. No specific dose alterations are necessary in the elderly.

Flutex® *see* Topical Corticosteroids *on page 1334*
Flutex® *see* Triamcinolone *on page 1356*

Fluticasone (floo TIK a sone)

U.S. Brand Names Cutivate®; Flonase®; Flovent®; Flovent® Rotadisk®

Synonyms Fluticasone Propionate

Generic Available No

Pharmacologic Category Corticosteroid, Inhalant (Oral); Corticosteroid, Nasal; Corticosteroid, Topical; Corticosteroid, Topical (Medium Potency)

Pregnancy Risk Factor C

Lactation Excretion in breast milk unknown/use caution

Use

Inhalation: Maintenance treatment of asthma as prophylactic therapy. It is also indicated for patients requiring oral corticosteroid therapy for asthma to assist in total discontinuation or reduction of total oral dose. NOT indicated for the relief of acute bronchospasm.

Intranasal: Management of seasonal and perennial allergic rhinitis and nonallergic rhinitis in patients ≥4 years of age

Topical: Relief of inflammation and pruritus associated with corticosteroid-responsive dermatoses in patients ≥3 months of age

Mechanism of Action/Effect Fluticasone belongs to a new group of corticosteroids which utilizes a fluorocarbothioate ester linkage at the 17 carbon position; extremely potent vasoconstrictive and anti-inflammatory activity; has a weak HPA inhibitory potency when applied topically, which gives the drug a high therapeutic index. The effectiveness of inhaled fluticasone is due to its direct local effect. The mechanism of action for all topical corticosteroids is believed to be a combination of three important properties: anti-inflammatory activity, immunosuppressive properties, and antiproliferative actions.

Contraindications Hypersensitivity to fluticasone or any component of the formulation; primary treatment of status asthmaticus

Topical: Do not use if infection is present at treatment site, in the presence of skin atrophy, or for the treatment of rosacea or perioral dermatitis

Warnings/Precautions May cause suppression of hypothalamic-pituitary-adrenal (HPA) axis, particularly in younger children or in patients receiving high doses for prolonged periods. Fluticasone may cause less HPA axis suppression than therapeutically equivalent oral doses of prednisone. Particular care is required when patients are transferred from systemic corticosteroids to inhaled products due to possible adrenal insufficiency or withdrawal from steroids, including an increase in allergic symptoms. Patients receiving 20 mg per day of prednisone (or equivalent) may be most susceptible.

Controlled clinical studies have shown that orally-inhaled and intranasal corticosteroids may cause a reduction in growth velocity in pediatric patients. (In studies of orally-inhaled corticosteroids, the mean reduction in growth velocity was approximately 1 centimeter per year [range 0.3-1.8 cm per year] and appears to be related to dose and duration of exposure.) To minimize the systemic effects of orally-inhaled and intranasal corticosteroids, each patient should be titrated to the lowest effective dose.

May suppress the immune system, patients may be more susceptible to infection. Use with caution, if at all, in patients with systemic infections, active or quiescent tuberculosis infection, or ocular herpes simplex. Avoid exposure to chickenpox and measles.

Supplemental steroids (oral or parenteral) may be needed during stress or severe asthma attacks. Rare cases of vasculitis (Churg-Strauss syndrome) or other eosinophilic conditions can occur. Flovent® aerosol contains chlorofluorocarbons (CFCs).

Inhalation: Not to be used in status asthmaticus or for the relief of acute bronchospasm

Topical: May also cause suppression of HPA axis, especially when used on large areas of the body, denuded areas, for prolonged periods of time or with an occlusive dressing. Pediatric patients may be more susceptible to systemic toxicity. Safety and efficacy in pediatric patients <3 months of age have not been established.

Pregnancy risk C.

Drug Interactions

Cytochrome P450 Effect: Substrate of CYP3A4

Increased Effect/Toxicity:

CYP3A4 inhibitors: Serum level and/or toxicity of fluticasone may be increased; this effect was shown with ketoconazole, but not erythromycin. Other potential inhibitors include amiodarone, cimetidine, clarithromycin, delavirdine, diltiazem, dirithromycin, disulfiram, fluoxetine, fluvoxamine, grapefruit juice, indinavir, itraconazole, ketoconazole, nefazodone, nevirapine, propoxyphene, quinupristin-dalfopristin, ritonavir, saquinavir, verapamil, zafirlukast, zileuton.

Salmeterol: The addition of salmeterol has been demonstrated to improve response to inhaled corticosteroids (as compared to increasing steroid dosage).

Nutritional/Ethanol Interactions Herb/Nutraceutical: In theory, St John's wort may decrease serum levels of fluticasone by inducing CYP3A4 isoenzymes.

Adverse Reactions

Oral or nasal inhalation: Frequency depends upon population studied and dosing used. Reactions reported are representative of multiple oral formulations.

>3%:

Central nervous system: Headache (2% to 22%), fever (1% to 7%)

Gastrointestinal: Nausea/vomiting (1% to 8%)

Neuromuscular & skeletal: Muscle injury (1% to 5%), musculoskeletal pain (1% to 5%), back problems (<1% to 4%)

Respiratory: Upper respiratory tract infection (14% to 22%), throat irritation (3% to 22%), nasal congestion (4% to 16%), pharyngitis (6% to 14%), oral candidiasis (<1% to 11%), sinusitis/sinus infection (3% to 10%), rhinitis (1% to 9%), dysphonia (<1% to 8%),

Miscellaneous: Viral infection (2% to 5%)

<3% (Limited to important or life-threatening): Aggression, agitation, cataracts, cholecystitis, Churg-Strauss syndrome, Cushingoid features, depression, dyspnea, eosinophilic conditions, fungal skin infection, gastroenteritis, glaucoma, goiter, growth velocity reduction (in children/adolescents), increased intraocular pressure, lower respiratory infections, migraine, mood disorders, nasopharyngitis, nervousness, nose/throat polyps, oral ulcerations, paradoxical bronchospasm, paralysis of cranial nerves, photodermatitis, pruritus, skin rash, throat constriction, urticaria, vasculitis

Overdosage/Toxicology When consumed in high doses over prolonged periods, systemic hypercorticism and adrenal suppression may occur. In those cases, discontinuation of the corticosteroid should be done judiciously.

Pharmacodynamics/Kinetics

Absorption:

Cream: 5% (increased with inflammation)

Oral inhalation: Primarily via lungs; minimal GI absorption due to presystemic metabolism

Bioavailability: Oral inhalation: 14% to 30%

Metabolism: Hepatic via CYP3A4 to 17β-carboxylic acid (negligible activity)

Formulations

Aerosol for oral inhalation, as propionate (Flovent®):

44 mcg/inhalation (7.9 g) [60 metered doses], (13 g) [120 metered doses]

110 mcg/inhalation (7.9 g) [60 metered doses], (13 g) [120 metered doses]

220 mcg/inhalation (7.9 g) [60 metered doses], (13 g) [120 metered doses]

Cream, as propionate (Cutivate®): 0.05% (15 g, 30 g, 60 g)

Ointment, as propionate (Cutivate®): 0.005% (15 g, 30 g, 60 g)

Powder for oral inhalation, as propionate [4 blisters of the drug per Rotadisk®, 15 Rotadisks® per pack] (Flovent® Rotadisk®):

50 mcg (60s) [delivers 44 mcg/inhalation]

100 mcg (60s) [delivers 88 mcg/inhalation]

250 mcg (60s) [delivers 220 mcg/inhalation]

Suspension, intranasal spray, as propionate (Flonase®): 50 mcg/inhalation (16 g) [120 metered doses]

Dosing

Adults & Elderly:

Asthma: Inhalation, oral: **Note:** Titrate to the lowest effective dose once asthma stability is achieved

Flovent®: Dosing based on previous therapy

Bronchodilator alone: Recommended starting dose: 88 mcg twice daily; highest recommended dose: 440 mcg twice daily

Inhaled corticosteroids: Recommended starting dose: 88-220 mcg twice daily; highest recommended dose: 440 mcg twice daily; a higher starting dose may be considered in patients previously requiring higher doses of inhaled corticosteroids

Oral corticosteroids: Recommended starting dose: 880 mcg twice daily; highest recommended dose: 880 mcg twice daily; starting dose is patient dependent. In patients on chronic oral corticosteroids therapy, reduce prednisone dose no faster than 2.5 mg/day on a weekly basis; begin taper after ≥1 week of fluticasone therapy

Flovent® Diskus® and Rotadisk®: Dosing based on previous therapy

Bronchodilator alone: Recommended starting dose 100 mcg twice daily; highest recommended dose: 500 mcg twice daily

(Continued)

Fluticasone *(Continued)*

Inhaled corticosteroids: 100-250 mcg twice daily; highest recommended dose: 500 mcg twice daily; a higher starting dose may be considered in patients previously requiring higher doses of inhaled corticosteroids

Oral corticosteroids: 500-1000 mcg twice daily; highest recommended dose: 1000 mcg twice daily; starting dose is patient dependent. In patients on chronic oral corticosteroids therapy, reduce prednisone dose no faster than 2.5 mg/day on a weekly basis; begin taper after ≥1 week of fluticasone therapy

Inflammation/pruritus associated with corticosteroid-responsive dermatoses: Topical: Apply sparingly in a thin film twice daily; therapy should be discontinued when control is achieved. If no improvement is seen within 2 weeks, reassessment of diagnosis may be necessary.

Rhinitis: Intranasal: Initial: 2 sprays (50 mcg/spray) per nostril once daily; may also be divided into 100 mcg twice a day. After the first few days, dosage may be reduced to 1 spray per nostril once daily for maintenance therapy. Dosing should be at regular intervals.

Pediatrics:

Asthma: Inhalation, oral:

Flovent®: Children ≥12 years: Refer to adult dosing.

Flovent® Diskus® and Rotadisk®: **Note:** Titrate to the lowest effective dose once asthma stability is achieved; children previously maintained on Flovent® Rotadisk® may require dosage adjustments when transferred to Flovent® Diskus®

Children ≥4-11 years: Dosing based on previous therapy

Bronchodilator alone: Recommended starting dose: 50 mcg twice daily; highest recommended dose: 100 mcg twice daily

Inhaled corticosteroids: Recommended starting dose: 50 mcg twice daily; highest recommended dose: 100 mcg twice daily; a higher starting dose may be considered in patients previously requiring higher doses of inhaled corticosteroids

Children ≥11 years: Refer to adult dosing.

Inflammation/pruritus associated with corticosteroid-responsive dermatoses: Topical: Children ≥3 months: Apply sparingly in a thin film twice daily; therapy should be discontinued when control is achieved. If no improvement is seen within 2 weeks, reassessment of diagnosis may be necessary. Safety and efficacy for use in pediatric patients <3 months have not been established.

Rhinitis: Intranasal: Children ≥4 years and Adolescents: Initial: 1 spray (50 mcg/spray) per nostril once daily; patients not adequately responding or patients with more severe symptoms may use 2 sprays (100 mcg) per nostril. Depending on response, dosage may be reduced to 100 mcg daily. Total daily dosage should not exceed 2 sprays in each nostril (200 mcg)/day. Dosing should be at regular intervals.

Hepatic Impairment: Fluticasone is primarily cleared in the liver. Fluticasone plasma levels may be increased in patients with hepatic impairment, use with caution; monitor.

Administration

Inhalation:

Aerosol inhalation: Shake container thoroughly before using. Take 3-5 deep breaths. Use inhaler on inspiration. Allow 1 full minute between inhalations. Rinse mouth with water after use to reduce aftertaste and incidence of candidiasis.

Nasal spray: Shake bottle gently before using. Prime pump prior to first use (press 6 times until fine spray appears). Blow nose to clear nostrils. Insert applicator into nostril, keeping bottle upright, and close off the other nostril. Breathe in through nose. While inhaling, press pump to release spray. Nasal applicator may be removed and rinsed with warm water to clean.

Powder for oral inhalation: Flovent® Diskus®: Do not use with a spacer device. Do not exhale into Diskus®. Do not wash or take apart. Use in horizontal position.

Topical: Apply sparingly in a thin film of cream or ointment. Rub in lightly. Do not use for diaper dermatitis.

Stability

Storage:

Aerosol (oral inhalation), cream: Store between 2°C to 30°C (36°F to 86°F). Store aerosol with nozzle end down, protect from freezing and direct sunlight. Discard aerosol after labeled number of doses has been used.

Nasal spray: Store between 4°C to 30°C (39°F to 86°F). Discard after labeled number of doses has been used, even if bottle is not completely empty.

Powder for oral inhalation:

Flovent® Diskus®: Store at controlled room temperature, 20°C to 25°C (68°F to 77°F), in a dry place away from direct heat or sunlight. The 50 mcg strength should be discarded 6 weeks after opening protective wrap; the 100 mcg and 250 mcg strengths should be discarded 2 months after opening protective wrap (or when indicator reads "0", whichever comes first).

Flovent® Rotadisk®: Store at controlled room temperature, 20°C to 25°C (68°F to 77°F). Use blisters within 2 months of opening protective pouch.

Monitoring Laboratory Tests Growth (adolescents and children); signs/symptoms of HPA axis suppression/adrenal insufficiency; possible eosinophilic conditions (including Churg-Strauss syndrome)

Monitoring and Teaching Issues

Physical Assessment: Note Warnings/Precautions and Contraindications for use cautions. Monitor effectiveness of therapy and adverse reactions (see Adverse Reactions) at beginning of therapy and periodically with long-term use. Assess knowledge/teach patient appropriate use, interventions to reduce side effects, and adverse symptoms to report (see Patient Education). **Pregnancy risk factor C** - benefits of use should outweigh possible risks. Note breast-feeding caution.

Patient Education: Use as directed; do not overuse and use only for length of time prescribed. **Pregnancy/breast-feeding precautions:** Inform prescriber if you are or intend to become pregnant. Consult prescriber if breast-feeding.

Metered-dose inhalation: Sit when using. Take deep breaths for 3-5 minutes, and clear nasal passages before administration (use decongestant as needed). Hold breath for 5-10 seconds after use, and wait 1-3 minutes between inhalations. Follow package insert instructions for use. Do not exceed maximum dosage. If also using inhaled bronchodilator, use before fluticasone. Rinse mouth and throat after use to reduce aftertaste and prevent candidiasis.

Nasal spray: Shake gently before use. Use at regular intervals, no more frequently than directed. Report unusual cough or spasm; persistent nasal bleeding, burning, or irritation; or worsening of condition.

Powder for oral inhalation: Flovent® Diskus®: Do not attempt to take device apart. Do not use with a spacer device. Do not exhale into the Diskus®, use in a level horizontal position. Do not wash the mouthpiece.

Topical: For external use only. Apply thin film of cream to affected area only; rub in lightly. Do not apply occlusive covering unless advised by prescriber. Wash hand thoroughly after use; avoid contact with eyes. Notify prescriber if skin condition persists or worsens. Do not use for treatment of diaper dermatitis or under diapers or plastic pants.

Geriatric Considerations: No specific information for the elderly patient is available.

Pregnancy Issues: There are no adequate and well-controlled studies using inhaled fluticasone in pregnant women. Oral corticosteroid use has shown animals to be more prone to teratogenic effects than humans. Due to the natural increase in corticosteroid production during pregnancy, most women may require a lower steroid dose; use with caution.

Additional Information Effects of inhaled/intranasal steroids on growth have been observed in the absence of laboratory evidence of HPA axis suppression, suggesting that growth velocity is a more sensitive indicator of systemic corticosteroid exposure in pediatric patients than some commonly used tests of HPA axis function. The long-term effects of this reduction in growth velocity associated with orally-inhaled and intranasal corticosteroids, including the impact on final adult height, are unknown. The potential for "catch up" growth following discontinuation of treatment with inhaled corticosteroids has not been adequately studied.

Related Information

Inhalant (Asthma, Bronchospasm) Agents Comparison *on page 1577*

Fluticasone *see* Topical Corticosteroids *on page 1334*

Fluticasone and Salmeterol (floo TIK a sone & sal ME te role)

U.S. Brand Names Advair™ Diskus®

Synonyms Salmeterol and Fluticasone

Generic Available No

Pharmacologic Category $Beta_2$ Agonist; Corticosteroid, Inhalant (Oral)

Pregnancy Risk Factor C

Lactation

Fluticasone: Excretion in breast milk unknown/use caution

Salmeterol: Enters breast milk/use caution

Use Maintenance treatment of asthma in adults and children ≥12 years; **not** for use for relief of acute bronchospasm

Pharmacokinetic Note See individual agents.

Pharmacodynamics/Kinetics

Onset:

Advair™ Diskus®: 30-60 minutes; Peak effect: ≥1 week for full effect

Duration:

Advair™ Diskus®: 12 hours

Formulations Powder for oral inhalation:

100/50: Fluticasone propionate 100 mcg and salmeterol xinafoate 50 mcg (28s, 60s)

250/50: Fluticasone propionate 250 mcg and salmeterol xinafoate 50 mcg (28s, 60s)

500/50: Fluticasone propionate 500 mcg and salmeterol xinafoate 50 mcg (28s, 60s)

Dosing

Adults: Do not use to transfer patients from systemic corticosteroid therapy

Asthma (maintenance): Oral inhalation: One inhalation twice daily, morning and evening, 12 hours apart

Advair™ Diskus® is available in 3 strengths, initial dose prescribed should be based upon previous asthma therapy. Dose should be increased after 2 weeks if adequate response is not achieved. Patients should be titrated to lowest effective dose once stable. (Because each strength contains salmeterol 50 mcg/inhalation, dose adjustments should be made by changing inhaler strength. No more than 1 inhalation of any strength should be taken more than twice a day). Maximum dose: Fluticasone 500 mcg/salmeterol 50 mcg, one inhalation twice daily.

Patients not currently on inhaled corticosteroids: Fluticasone 100 mcg/salmeterol 50 mcg

Patients currently using inhaled beclomethasone dipropionate:

- ≤420 mcg/day: Fluticasone 100 mcg/salmeterol 50 mcg
- 462-840 mcg/day: Fluticasone 250 mcg/salmeterol 50 mcg

Patients currently using inhaled budesonide:

- ≤400 mcg/day: Fluticasone 100 mcg/salmeterol 50 mcg
- 800-1200 mcg/day: Fluticasone 250 mcg/salmeterol 50 mcg
- 1600 mcg/day: Fluticasone 500 mcg/salmeterol 50 mcg

Patients currently using inhaled flunisolide:

- ≤1000 mcg/day: Fluticasone 100 mcg/salmeterol 50 mcg
- 1250-2000 mcg/day: Fluticasone 250 mcg/salmeterol 50 mcg

Patients currently using inhaled fluticasone propionate aerosol:

- ≤176 mcg/day: Fluticasone 100 mcg/salmeterol 50 mcg

(Continued)

Fluticasone and Salmeterol *(Continued)*

440 mcg/day: Fluticasone 250 mcg/salmeterol 50 mcg
660-880 mcg/day: Fluticasone 500 mcg/salmeterol 50 mcg

Patients currently using inhaled fluticasone propionate powder:
≤200 mcg/day: Fluticasone 100 mcg/salmeterol 50 mcg
500 mcg/day: Fluticasone 250 mcg/salmeterol 50 mcg
1000 mcg/day: Fluticasone 500 mcg/salmeterol 50 mcg

Patients currently using inhaled triamcinolone acetonide:
≤1000 mcg/day: Fluticasone 100 mcg/salmeterol 50 mcg
1100-1600 mcg/day: Fluticasone 250 mcg/salmeterol 50 mcg

Elderly: No differences in safety or effectiveness have been seen in studies of patients ≥65 years of age. However, increased sensitivity may be seen in the elderly. Use with caution in patients with concomitant cardiovascular disease.

Pediatrics: Children ≥12 years: Refer to adult dosing.

Hepatic Impairment: Fluticasone is cleared by hepatic metabolism. No dosing adjustment suggested. Use with caution in patients with impaired liver function.

Monitoring and Teaching Issues

Physical Assessment: See individual components listed in Related Information. **Pregnancy risk factor C** - benefits of use should outweigh possible risks. Note breast-feeding caution.

Patient Education: See individual components listed in Related Information. **Pregnancy/breast-feeding precautions:** Inform prescriber if you are or intend to become pregnant. Consult prescriber if breast-feeding.

Related Information

Fluticasone *on page 588*
Salmeterol *on page 1210*

Fluticasone Propionate *see* Fluticasone *on page 588*

Fluvastatin (FLOO va sta tin)

U.S. Brand Names Lescol®; Lescol® XL

Generic Available No

Pharmacologic Category Antilipemic Agent, HMG-CoA Reductase Inhibitor

Pregnancy Risk Factor X

Lactation Enters breast milk/not recommended

Use To be used as a component of multiple risk factor intervention in patients at risk for atherosclerosis vascular disease due to hypercholesterolemia

Adjunct to dietary therapy to reduce elevated total cholesterol (total-C), LDL-C, triglyceride, and apolipoprotein B (apo-B) levels and to increase HDL-C in primary hypercholesterolemia and mixed dyslipidemia (Fredrickson types IIa and IIb); to slow the progression of coronary atherosclerosis in patients with coronary heart disease

Mechanism of Action/Effect Acts by competitively inhibiting 3-hydroxyl-3-methylglutaryl-coenzyme A (HMG-CoA) reductase, the enzyme that catalyzes the reduction of HMG-CoA to mevalonate; this is an early rate-limiting step in cholesterol biosynthesis. HDL is increased while total, LDL and VLDL cholesterols, apolipoprotein B, and plasma triglycerides are decreased.

Contraindications Hypersensitivity to fluvastatin or any component of the formulation; active liver disease; unexplained persistent elevations of serum transaminases; pregnancy; breast-feeding

Warnings/Precautions Secondary causes of hyperlipidemia should be ruled out prior to therapy. Liver function must be monitored by periodic laboratory assessment. Rhabdomyolysis with acute renal failure has occurred with fluvastatin and other HMG-CoA reductase inhibitors. Risk may be increased with concurrent use of other drugs which may cause rhabdomyolysis (including gemfibrozil, fibric acid derivatives, or niacin at doses ≥1 g/day). Temporarily discontinue in any patient experiencing an acute or serious condition predisposing to renal failure secondary to rhabdomyolysis. Use caution in patients with previous liver disease or heavy ethanol use. Treatment in patients <18 years of age is not recommended.

Drug Interactions

Cytochrome P450 Effect: Substrate of CYP2C8/9, 2D6, 3A4; Inhibits CYP1A2, **2C8/9**, 2D6, 3A4

Decreased Effect: Administration of cholestyramine at the same time with fluvastatin reduces absorption and clinical effect of fluvastatin. Separate administration times by at least 4 hours. Rifampin and rifabutin may decrease fluvastatin blood levels.

Increased Effect/Toxicity: Cimetidine, omeprazole, ranitidine, and ritonavir may increase fluvastatin blood levels. Clofibrate, erythromycin, gemfibrozil, fenofibrate, and niacin may increase the risk of myopathy and rhabdomyolysis. Anticoagulant effect of warfarin may be increased by fluvastatin. Cholestyramine effect will be additive with fluvastatin if administration times are separated. Fluvastatin may increase C_{max} and decrease clearance of digoxin.

Nutritional/Ethanol Interactions Food: Reduces rate but not the extent of absorption.

Effects on Lab Values ↑ serum transaminases, CPK, alkaline phosphatase, and bilirubin and thyroid function tests

Adverse Reactions As reported with fluvastatin capsules; in general, adverse reactions reported with fluvastatin extended release tablet were similar, but the incidence was less.

1% to 10%:
Central nervous system: Headache (9%), fatigue (3%), insomnia (3%)
Gastrointestinal: Dyspepsia (8%), diarrhea (5%), abdominal pain (5%), nausea (3%)
Genitourinary: Urinary tract infection (2%)
Neuromuscular & skeletal: Myalgia (5%)
Respiratory: Sinusitis (3%), bronchitis (2%)

<1% (Limited to important or life-threatening) including additional class-related events (not necessarily reported with fluvastatin therapy): Alopecia, anaphylaxis, angioedema, arthralgia, arthritis, cataracts, cholestatic jaundice, cirrhosis, depression, dermatomyositis, dyspnea, elevated transaminases, eosinophilia, erectile dysfunction, erythema multiforme, facial paresis, fatty liver, fever, fulminant hepatic necrosis, gynecomastia, hemolytic anemia, hepatitis, hepatoma, hypersensitivity reaction, impotence, increased CPK (>10x normal), increased ESR, leukopenia, memory loss, muscle cramps, myopathy, nodules, ophthalmoplegia, pancreatitis, paresthesia, peripheral nerve palsy, peripheral neuropathy, photosensitivity, polymyalgia rheumatica, positive ANA, pruritus, psychic disturbance, purpura, rash, renal failure (secondary to rhabdomyolysis), rhabdomyolysis, skin discoloration, Stevens-Johnson syndrome, systemic lupus erythematosus-like syndrome, taste alteration, thrombocytopenia, thyroid dysfunction, toxic epidermal necrolysis, tremor, urticaria, vasculitis, vertigo

Overdosage/Toxicology GI complaints and elevated SGOT and SGPT have been reported following large doses of the extended release tablets. In case of overdose, supportive measure should be instituted, as required; dialyzability is not known.

Pharmacodynamics/Kinetics

Bioavailability: Absolute: Capsule: 24%; Extended release tablet: 29%

Half-Life Elimination: Capsule: <3 hours; Extended release tablet: 9 hours

Metabolism: To inactive and active metabolites [oxidative metabolism via CYP2C9 (75%), 2C8 (~5%), and 3A4 (~20%) isoenzymes]; active forms do not circulate systemically; extensive first-pass hepatic extraction

Formulations

Capsule (Lescol®): 20 mg, 40 mg

Tablet, extended release (Lescol® XL): 80 mg

Dosing

Adults & Elderly: Dyslipidemia (also delay in progression of CAD): Oral:

Patients requiring ≥25% decrease in LDL-C: 40 mg capsule or 80 mg extended release tablet once daily in the evening; may also use 40 mg capsule twice daily

Patients requiring <25% decrease in LDL-C: 20 mg capsule once daily in the evening

Dosing range: 20-80 mg/day; adjust dose based on response to therapy; maximum response occurs within 4-6 weeks

Renal Impairment: Less than 6% is excreted renally. No dosage adjustment needed with mild to moderate renal impairment; use with caution in severe impairment.

Hepatic Impairment: Levels may accumulate in patients with liver disease (increased AUC and C_{max}). Use caution with severe hepatic impairment or heavy ethanol ingestion. Contraindicated in active liver disease or unexplained transaminase elevations. Decrease dose and monitor effects carefully in patients with hepatic insufficiency.

Administration

Oral: Patient should be placed on a standard cholesterol-lowering diet before and during treatment; fluvastatin may be taken without regard to meals; adjust dosage as needed in response to periodic lipid determinations during the first 4 weeks after a dosage change; lipid-lowering effects are additive when fluvastatin is combined with a bile-acid binding resin or niacin, however, it must be administered at least 2 hours following these drugs.

Stability

Storage: Store at 25°C (77°F); protect from light.

Monitoring Laboratory Tests Obtain baseline LFTs and total cholesterol profile. Repeat tests at 12 weeks after initiation of therapy or elevation in dose, and periodically thereafter. Monitor LDL-C at intervals no less than 4 weeks.

Monitoring and Teaching Issues

Physical Assessment: See Contraindications, Warnings/Precautions, Dosing, and Administration for use cautions. Assess potential for interactions with other prescriptions, OTC medications, or herbal products patient may be taking (see Drug Interactions). Assess results of laboratory tests (see above), therapeutic effects, and adverse response (see Adverse Reactions and Overdose/Toxicology) on a regular basis throughout therapy. Teach patient proper use, possible side effects and appropriate interventions, and adverse symptoms to report (see Patient Education). **Pregnancy risk factor X** - determine that patient is not pregnant before starting therapy. Do not give to sexually active female patients unless capable of complying with effective contraceptive use. Instruct patient in appropriate contraceptive measures. Breast-feeding is not recommended.

Patient Education: Inform prescriber of all prescriptions, OTC medications, or herbal products you are taking, and any allergies you have. Do not take anything new during treatment unless approved by prescriber. Take as directed, with or without food. Follow diet and exercise regimen as prescribed. You may experience nausea or dyspepsia (small, frequent meals, frequent mouth care, chewing gum, or sucking lozenges may help); diarrhea (buttermilk, boiled milk, or yogurt may help); or headache (consult prescriber for approved analgesic). Report muscle pain or cramping; tremor; or CNS changes (eg, memory loss, depression, personality changes; numbness, weakness, tingling or pain in extremities). **Pregnancy/breast-feeding precautions:** Inform prescriber if you are pregnant. Consult prescriber for instruction on appropriate contraceptive measures. This drug may cause severe fetal defects. Do not donate blood during or for 1 month following therapy (same reason). Breast-feeding is not recommended.

Dietary Issues: Before initiation of therapy, patients should be placed on a standard cholesterol-lowering diet for 3-6 months and the diet should be continued during drug therapy. May be taken without regard to meals.

Geriatric Considerations: The definition of and, therefore, when to treat hyperlipidemia in the elderly is a controversial issue. The National Cholesterol Education Program recommends that all adults 20 years of age and older maintain a plasma cholesterol <200 mg/dL. By this definition, 60% of all elderly would be considered to have a borderline high (200-239 mg/dL) or high (≥240 mg/dL) plasma cholesterol. However, plasma cholesterol has been shown to be a less reliable predictor of coronary heart disease in the elderly. Therefore, it is the authors' belief that pharmacologic treatment be reserved for those who are unable to obtain a desirable plasma cholesterol level by diet alone and for whom the

(Continued)

Fluvastatin *(Continued)*

benefits of treatment are believed to outweigh the potential adverse effects, drug interactions, and cost of treatment.

Breast-feeding Issues: Fluvastatin is excreted in human breast milk (milk plasma ratio 2:1); do not use in breast-feeding women.

Pregnancy Issues: Animal studies have shown delays in fetal skeletal development and fetal, neonatal, and maternal mortality. Congenital anomalies following use of other HMG-CoA reductase inhibitors in humans have been reported (rare). Use in women of childbearing potential only if they are highly unlikely to conceive; discontinue if pregnancy occurs.

Related Information

Hyperlipidemia Management *on page 1682*
Lipid-Lowering Agents *on page 1582*

Fluvirin® *see page 1498*

Fluvoxamine (floo VOKS ah meen)

U.S. Brand Names Luvox® [DSC]

Generic Available Yes

Pharmacologic Category Antidepressant, Selective Serotonin Reuptake Inhibitor

Pregnancy Risk Factor C

Lactation Enters breast milk/not recommended (AAP rates "of concern")

Use Treatment of obsessive-compulsive disorder (OCD) in children ≥8 years of age and adults

Use - Unlabeled/Investigational Treatment of major depression; panic disorder; anxiety disorders in children

Mechanism of Action/Effect Inhibits CNS neuron serotonin uptake; minimal or no effect on reuptake of norepinephrine or dopamine; does not significantly bind to alpha-adrenergic, histamine or cholinergic receptors

Contraindications Hypersensitivity to fluvoxamine or any component of the formulation; concurrent use with astemizole, pimozide, thioridazine, mesoridazine, or cisapride; use of MAO inhibitors within 14 days

Warnings/Precautions Potential for severe reaction when used with MAO inhibitors - serotonin syndrome (hyperthermia, muscular rigidity, mental status changes/agitation, autonomic instability) may occur. May precipitate a shift to mania or hypomania in patients with bipolar disease. Has a low potential to impair cognitive or motor performance - caution operating hazardous machinery or driving. Use caution in patients with depression, particularly if suicidal risk may be present. Use caution in patients with a previous seizure disorder or condition predisposing to seizures such as brain damage, alcoholism, or concurrent therapy with other drugs which lower the seizure threshold. Use with caution in patients with hepatic or renal dysfunction and in elderly patients. May cause hyponatremia/SIADH. Use with caution in patients with renal insufficiency or other concurrent illness (cardiovascular disease). Use with caution in patients at risk of bleeding or receiving concurrent anticoagulant therapy, although not consistently noted, fluvoxamine may cause impairment in platelet function. May cause or exacerbate sexual dysfunction. Pregnancy risk C.

Drug Interactions

Cytochrome P450 Effect: Substrate of **CYP1A2, 2D6**; Inhibits **CYP1A2, 2B6**, 2C8/9, **2C19**, 2D6, **3A4**

Decreased Effect: Cyproheptadine, a serotonin antagonist, may inhibit the effects of serotonin reuptake inhibitors (fluvoxamine); monitor for altered antidepressant response.

Increased Effect/Toxicity:

MAO inhibitors: Fluvoxamine should not be used with nonselective MAO inhibitors (phenelzine, isocarboxazid) and drugs with MAO inhibitor properties (linezolid); fatal reactions have been reported. Wait 5 weeks after stopping fluvoxamine before starting a nonselective MAO inhibitor and 2 weeks after stopping an MAO inhibitor before starting fluvoxamine. Concurrent selegiline has been associated with mania, hypertension, or serotonin syndrome (risk may be reduced relative to nonselective MAO inhibitors).

Phenothiazines: Fluvoxamine may inhibit the metabolism of thioridazine or mesoridazine, resulting in increased plasma levels and increasing the risk of QT_c interval prolongation. This may lead to serious ventricular arrhythmias, such as torsade de pointes-type arrhythmias and sudden death. Do not use together. Wait at least 5 weeks after discontinuing fluvoxamine prior to starting thioridazine.

Combined used of SSRIs and amphetamines, buspirone, meperidine, nefazodone, serotonin agonists (such as sumatriptan), sibutramine, other SSRIs, sympathomimetics, ritonavir, tramadol, and venlafaxine may increase the risk of serotonin syndrome. Fluvoxamine may increase serum levels/effects of benzodiazepines (alprazolam and diazepam), beta-blockers (except atenolol or nadolol), carbamazepine, carvedilol, clozapine, cyclosporin (and possibly tacrolimus), dextromethorphan, digoxin, haloperidol, HMG-CoA reductase inhibitors (lovastatin and simvastatin - increasing the risk of rhabdomyolysis), mexiletine, phenytoin, propafenone, quinidine, tacrine, theophylline, trazodone, tricyclic antidepressants, and valproic acid. Concurrent lithium may increase risk of nephrotoxicity. Risk of hyponatremia may increase with concurrent use of loop diuretics (bumetanide, furosemide, torsemide). Fluvoxamine may increase the hypoprothrombinemic response to warfarin.

Combined use of sumatriptan (and other serotonin agonists) may result in toxicity; weakness, hyper-reflexia, and incoordination have been observed with sumatriptan and SSRIs. In addition, concurrent use may theoretically increase the risk of serotonin syndrome; includes sumatriptan, naratriptan, rizatriptan, and zolmitriptan.

Nutritional/Ethanol Interactions

Ethanol: Avoid ethanol. Depressed patients should avoid/limit intake.

Food: The bioavailability of melatonin has been reported to be increased by fluvoxamine.

Herb/Nutraceutical: Avoid valerian, St John's wort, SAMe, kava kava (may increase risk of serotonin syndrome and/or excessive sedation).

Adverse Reactions

>10%:

Central nervous system: Headache, somnolence, insomnia, nervousness, dizziness

Gastrointestinal: Nausea, diarrhea, xerostomia

Neuromuscular & skeletal: Weakness

1% to 10%:

Cardiovascular: Palpitations

Central nervous system: Somnolence, headache, insomnia, dizziness, nervousness, mania, hypomania, vertigo, abnormal thinking, agitation, anxiety, malaise, amnesia, yawning, hypertonia, CNS stimulation, depression

Endocrine & metabolic: Decreased libido

Gastrointestinal: Abdominal pain, vomiting, dyspepsia, constipation, abnormal taste, anorexia, flatulence, weight gain

Genitourinary: Delayed ejaculation, impotence, anorgasmia, urinary frequency, urinary retention

Neuromuscular & skeletal: Tremors

Ocular: Blurred vision

Respiratory: Dyspnea

Miscellaneous: Diaphoresis

<1% (Limited to important or life-threatening): Acne, agranulocytosis, akinesia with fever, alopecia, anaphylaxis, anemia, angina, angioedema, aplastic anemia, ataxia, bradycardia, delayed menstruation, dermatitis, dry skin, dysuria, elevated liver transaminases, extrapyramidal reactions, Henoch-Schönlein purpura, hepatitis, lactation, leukocytosis, neuropathy, nocturia, pancreatitis, seizures, serotonin syndrome, SIADH, Stevens-Johnson syndrome, thrombocytopenia, torsade de pointes, toxic epidermal necrolysis, urticaria, vasculitis, ventricular tachycardia

Overdosage/Toxicology Symptoms of overdose include drowsiness, nausea, vomiting, abdominal pain, tremor, sinus bradycardia, and seizures. A specific antidote does not exist. Treatment is supportive.

Pharmacodynamics/Kinetics

Absorption: Steady-state plasma concentrations have been noted to be 2-3 times higher in children than those in adolescents; female children demonstrated a significantly higher AUC than males

Bioavailability: 53%; not significantly affected by food

Half-Life Elimination: ~15 hours

Time to Peak: Plasma: 3-8 hours

Metabolism: Hepatic

Formulations Tablet: 25 mg, 50 mg, 100 mg

Dosing

Adults: Obsessive-compulsive disorder: Oral: Initial: 50 mg at bedtime; adjust in 50 mg increments at 4- to 7-day intervals; usual dose range: 100-300 mg/day; divide total daily dose into 2 doses. Administer larger portion at bedtime.

Note: When total daily dose exceeds 50 mg, the dose should be given in 2 divided doses.

Elderly: Reduce dose, titrate slowly. See Geriatric Considerations.

Pediatrics: Obsessive-compulsive disorder: Oral:

Children 8-17 years: Initial: 25 mg at bedtime; adjust in 25 mg increments at 4- to 7-day intervals, as tolerated, to maximum therapeutic benefit: Range: 50-200 mg/day

Maximum: Children: 8-11 years: 200 mg/day, adolescents: 300 mg/day; lower doses may be effective in female versus male patients

Note: When total daily dose exceeds 50 mg, the dose should be given in 2 divided doses.

Hepatic Impairment: Reduce dose, titrate slowly.

Stability

Storage: Protect from high humidity and store at controlled room temperature 15°C to 30°C (59°F to 86°F); dispense in tight containers

Monitoring Laboratory Tests Liver and kidney function assessment prior to beginning drug therapy

Monitoring and Teaching Issues

Physical Assessment: Assess other medications patient may be taking for effectiveness and interactions (see Drug Interactions - P450 enzyme inhibitor). See Contraindications and Warnings/Precautions for use cautions. Monitor laboratory tests, therapeutic response, and adverse reactions at beginning of therapy and periodically with long-term use (see Adverse Reactions and Overdose/Toxicology). Taper dosage slowly when discontinuing (allow 3-4 weeks between discontinuing Luvox® and starting another antidepressant). Assess knowledge/teach patient appropriate use, interventions to reduce side effects, and adverse symptoms to report (see Patient Education). **Pregnancy risk factor C** - benefits of use should outweigh possible risks. Breast-feeding is not recommended.

Patient Education: Take exactly as directed; do not increase dose or frequency. It may take 2-3 weeks to achieve desired results. Avoid alcohol, caffeine, and other prescription or OTC medications unless approved by prescriber. Maintain adequate hydration (2-3 L/day of fluids) unless advised by prescriber to restrict fluids. You may experience drowsiness, lightheadedness, impaired coordination, dizziness, or blurred vision (use caution when driving or engaging in tasks requiring alertness until response to drug is known); nausea, vomiting, or anorexia (small, frequent meals, frequent mouth care, chewing gum, or sucking lozenges may help); constipation (increased exercise, fluids, fruits, or fiber may help); diarrhea (buttermilk, yogurt, or boiled milk may help); postural hypotension (use caution when climbing stairs or changing position from lying or sitting to standing); or decreased sexual function or libido (reversible). Report persistent CNS effects (nervousness, restlessness, insomnia, anxiety, excitation, headache, sedation, seizures, mania, abnormal thinking); rash or skin irritation; muscle cramping, tremors, or change in gait; chest pain or palpitations; change in urinary pattern; or worsening of condition. **Pregnancy/breast-feeding precautions:** Inform prescriber if you are or intend to become pregnant. Breast-feeding is not recommended.

(Continued)

Fluvoxamine *(Continued)*

Geriatric Considerations: Modify the initial dose and the subsequent dose titration in the elderly. It may be best to select a different agent when treating depression in the elderly.

Related Information

Antidepressant Agents *on page 1553*
Antidepressant Medication Guidelines *on page 1613*

Fluzone® *see page 1498*

FML® *see* Fluorometholone *on page 575*

FML® Forte *see* Fluorometholone *on page 575*

FML-S® *see page 1509*

Focalin™ *see* Dexmethylphenidate *on page 387*

Foille® [OTC] *see* Benzocaine *on page 156*

Foille® Medicated First Aid [OTC] *see* Benzocaine *on page 156*

Foille® Plus [OTC] *see* Benzocaine *on page 156*

Folacin *see* Folic Acid *on page 596*

Folate *see* Folic Acid *on page 596*

Folic Acid (FOE lik AS id)

Synonyms Folacin; Folate; Pteroylglutamic Acid

Generic Available Yes

Pharmacologic Category Vitamin, Water Soluble

Pregnancy Risk Factor A/C (dose exceeding RDA recommendation)

Lactation Enters breast milk/compatible

Use Treatment of megaloblastic and macrocytic anemias due to folate deficiency; dietary supplement to prevent neural tube defects

Mechanism of Action/Effect Folic acid is necessary for formation of a number of coenzymes in many metabolic systems, particularly for purine and pyrimidine synthesis; required for nucleoprotein synthesis and maintenance in erythropoiesis; stimulates WBC and platelet production in folate deficiency anemia

Contraindications Pernicious, aplastic, or normocytic anemias

Warnings/Precautions Doses >0.1 mg/day may obscure pernicious anemia with continuing irreversible nerve damage progression; the dose that masks anemia is controversial, but doses of 400 mg daily (or even less) have been reported. Resistance to treatment may occur with depressed hematopoiesis, alcoholism, deficiencies of other vitamins. Injection contains benzyl alcohol (1.5%) as preservative (use care in administration to neonates). Pregnancy risk A/C (dose exceeding RDA).

Drug Interactions

Decreased Effect: In folate-deficient patients, folic acid therapy may increase phenytoin metabolism which may lead to a decrease in the effect of phenytoin. Phenytoin, primidone, para-aminosalicylic acid, and sulfasalazine may decrease serum folate concentrations resulting in a folic acid deficiency. Concurrent administration of chloramphenicol and folic acid may result in antagonism of the hematopoietic response to folic acid.

Effects on Lab Values Falsely low serum concentrations may occur with the *Lactobacillus casei* assay method in patients on anti-infectives (eg, tetracycline).

Adverse Reactions <1% (Limited to important or life-threatening): Bronchospasm

Pharmacodynamics/Kinetics

Absorption: Proximal part of small intestine

Onset: Peak effect: Oral: 0.5-1 hour

Formulations

Injection, solution, as sodium folate: 5 mg/mL (10 mL) [contains benzyl alcohol]
Tablet: 0.4 mg, 0.8 mg, 1 mg

Dosing

Adults & Elderly: Folic acid supplementation: Oral, I.M., I.V., S.C.:
Initial: 1 mg/day; Deficiency: 1-3 mg/day
Maintenance dose: 0.5 mg/day
Women of childbearing age, pregnant, and lactating women: 0.8 mg/day

Pediatrics:
Infants: 0.1 mg/day
Children <4 years: Up to 0.3 mg/day
Children >4 years: 0.4 mg/day

Administration

Oral: A diluted solution for oral administration may be prepared by diluting 1 mL of folic acid injection (5 mg/mL), with 49 mL sterile water for injection. Resulting solution is 0.1 mg folic acid per 1 mL.

I.M.: May also be administered by deep I.M. injection.

I.V.: May also be administered by I.V. injection by diluting 1 mL of folic acid injection (5 mg/mL), with 49 mL sterile water for injection. Resulting solution is 0.1 mg folic acid per 1 mL.

Stability

Compatibility: Stable in D_5W, $D_{20}W$, NS, fat emulsion 10%; **incompatible** with $D_{40}W$, $D_{50}W$

Compatibility in syringe: Incompatible with doxapram

Compatibility when admixed: Incompatible with calcium gluconate

Monitoring and Teaching Issues

Physical Assessment: See Contraindications, Warnings/Precautions, Dosing, and Administration for use cautions. Assess potential for interactions with other prescriptions, OTC medications, or herbal products patient may be taking (see Drug Interactions). Assess therapeutic effects and adverse response (see Adverse Reactions) on a regular basis throughout therapy. Teach patient proper use, possible side effects and appropriate interventions, and adverse symptoms to report (see Patient Education). **Pregnancy risk factor A/C** - see Pregnancy Risk Factor for use cautions.

Patient Education: Inform prescriber of all prescriptions, OTC medications, or herbal products you are taking, and any allergies you have. Do not take anything new during treatment unless approved by prescriber. Take exactly as prescribed. Toxicity can occur from elevated doses. Increased intake of foods high in folic acid (eg, dried beans, nuts, bran, vegetables, fruits) may be recommended by prescriber. Excessive use of alcohol increases requirement for folic acid. May turn urine more intensely yellow. Report skin rash. **Pregnancy precaution:** Inform prescriber if you are pregnant.

Geriatric Considerations: Elderly frequently have combined nutritional deficiencies. Must rule out vitamin B_{12} deficiency before initiating folate therapy. Elderly RDA requirements from 1989 RDA are 200 mcg minimum (0.2 mg). Elderly, due to decreased nutrient intake, may benefit from daily intake of a multiple vitamin with minerals.

Folinic Acid *see* Leucovorin *on page 779*

Follistim® *see* Follitropins *on page 597*

Follitropin Alfa *see* Follitropins *on page 597*

Follitropin Alpha *see* Follitropins *on page 597*

Follitropin Beta *see* Follitropins *on page 597*

Follitropins (foe li TRO pins)

U.S. Brand Names Bravelle™; Fertinex®; Follistim®; Gonal-F®

Synonyms Follitropin Alfa; Follitropin Alpha; Follitropin Beta; Recombinant Human Follicle Stimulating Hormone; rFSH-alpha; rFSH-beta; rhFSH-alpha; rhFSH-beta; Urofollitropin

Generic Available No

Pharmacologic Category Gonadotropin; Ovulation Stimulator

Pregnancy Risk Factor X

Lactation Excretion in breast milk unknown/not recommended

Use

Urofollitropin:

Bravelle™: Ovulation induction in patients who previously received pituitary suppression

Fertinex®: Ovulation induction in patients with polycystic ovary syndrome and infertility who have not responded to clomiphene citrate therapy; Assisted Reproductive Technologies (ART)

Follitropin alfa (Gonal-F®), Follitropin beta (Follistim®): Ovulation induction in patients in whom the cause of infertility is functional and not caused by primary ovarian failure; ART; spermatogenesis induction

Mechanism of Action/Effect Urofollitropin is a preparation of highly purified follicle-stimulating hormone (FSH) extracted from the urine of postmenopausal women. Follitropin alfa and follitropin beta are human FSH preparations of recombinant DNA origin. Follitropins stimulate ovarian follicular growth in women who do not have primary ovarian failure. FSH is required for normal follicular growth, maturation, and gonadal steroid production.

Contraindications Hypersensitivity to follitropins or any component of the formulation; high levels of FSH indicating primary gonadal failure (ovarian or testicular); uncontrolled thyroid or adrenal dysfunction; the presence of any cause of infertility other than anovulation; tumor of the ovary, breast, uterus, hypothalamus, testis, or pituitary gland; abnormal vaginal bleeding of undetermined origin; ovarian cysts or enlargement not due to polycystic ovary syndrome; pregnancy

Warnings/Precautions These medications should only be used by physicians who are thoroughly familiar with infertility problems and their management. To minimize risks, use only at the lowest effective dose. Monitor ovarian response with serum estradiol and vaginal ultrasound on a regular basis.

Ovarian enlargement which may be accompanied by abdominal distention or abdominal pain, occurs in ~20% of those treated with urofollitropin and hCG, and generally regresses without treatment within 2-3 weeks. Ovarian hyperstimulation syndrome, characterized by severe ovarian enlargement, abdominal pain/distention, nausea, vomiting, diarrhea, dyspnea, and oliguria, and may be accompanied by ascites, pleural effusion, hypovolemia, electrolyte imbalance, hemoperitoneum, and thromboembolic events is reported in about 6% of patients. If hyperstimulation occurs, stop treatment and hospitalize patient. This syndrome develops rapidly within 24 hours to several days and generally occurs during the 7-10 days immediately following treatment. Hemoconcentration associated with fluid loss into the abdominal cavity has occurred and should be assessed by fluid intake & output, weight, hematocrit, serum & urinary electrolytes, urine specific gravity, BUN and creatinine, and abdominal girth. Determinations should be performed daily or more often if the need arises. Treatment is primarily symptomatic and consists of bed rest, fluid and electrolyte replacement and analgesics. The ascitic, pleural and pericardial fluids should never be removed because of the potential danger of injury.

Serious pulmonary conditions (atelectasis, acute respiratory distress syndrome and exacerbation of asthma) have been reported. Thromboembolic events, both in association with and separate from ovarian hyperstimulation syndrome, have been reported.

Multiple pregnancies have been associated with these medications, including triplet and quintuplet gestations. Advise patient of the potential risk of multiple births before starting the treatment.

Adverse Reactions Frequency varies by specific product and route of administration.

2% to 10%:

Central nervous system: Headache, dizziness, fever

Dermatologic: Acne (male), dermoid cyst (male), dry skin, body rash, hair loss, hives

Endocrine & metabolic: Ovarian hyperstimulation syndrome, adnexal torsion, mild to moderate ovarian enlargement, abdominal pain, ovarian cysts, breast tenderness, gynecomastia (male)

Gastrointestinal: Nausea, vomiting, diarrhea, abdominal cramps, bloating, flatulence, dyspepsia

Genitourinary: Urinary tract infection, menstrual disorder, intermenstrual bleeding, dysmenorrhea, cervical lesion

(Continued)

Follitropins *(Continued)*

Local: Pain, rash, swelling, or irritation at the site of injection
Neuromuscular & skeletal: Back pain, varicose veins (male)
Respiratory: Exacerbation of asthma, sinusitis, pharyngitis
Miscellaneous: Febrile reactions accompanied by chills, musculoskeletal, joint pains, malaise, headache, and fatigue; flu-like symptoms

<2% (Limited to important or life-threatening): Adnexal torsion, asthma, atelectasis, congenital abnormalities (incidence not greater than in general population), hemoperitoneum, hypotension, migraine, paresthesia, respiratory distress syndrome, somnolence, vaginal hemorrhage

Overdosage/Toxicology Aside from possible ovarian hyperstimulation and multiple gestations, little is known concerning the consequences of an acute overdose. Treatment is symptomatic.

Pharmacodynamics/Kinetics

Absorption: Rate limited: I.M., S.C.: Slower than elimination rate

Bioavailability: Ranges from ~66% to 82% depending on agent

Half-Life Elimination:

Mean: S.C.: Follitropin alfa: 24-32 hours; Follitropin beta: ~30 hours; Urofollitropin: 32-37 hours

Mean terminal: Multiple doses: I.M. follitropin alfa, S.C. follitropin beta: ~30 hours; I.M. urofollitropin: 15 hours, S.C. urofollitropin: 21 hours

Time to Peak:

Follitropin alfa: S.C.: 16 hours; I.M.: 25 hours
Follitropin beta: I.M.: 27 hours
Urofollitropin: Single dose: S.C.: 15-20 hours, I.M.: 10-17 hours; Multiple doses: I.M., S.C.: 10 hours

Metabolism: Total clearance of follitropin alfa was 0.6 L/hour following I.V. administration

Onset: Peak effect: Spermatogenesis, median: 165 days (range: 25-327 days); Follicle development: Within cycle

Formulations

Injection, powder for reconstitution [packaged with diluent]:
Follitropin alfa [rDNA origin, single-dose ampule] (Gonal-F®): 37.5 int. units, 75 int. units, 150 int. units
Follitropin alfa [rDNA origin, multidose vial] (Gonal-F®): 1200 int. units
Follitropin beta [rDNA origin] (Follistim®): 75 int. units
Urofollitropin [urine derived]:
Bravelle™ : 75 int. units
Fertinex®: 75 int. units, 150 int. units

Dosing

Adults: Note: Use the lowest dose consistent with the expectation of good results. Over the course of treatment, doses may vary depending on individual patient response. When used for ovulation induction, if response to follitropin is appropriate, hCG is given 1 day following the last dose. Withhold hCG if serum estradiol is >2000 pg/mL, if the ovaries are abnormally enlarged, or if abdominal pain occurs.

Urofollitropin: Female:

Bravelle™: Ovulation induction: I.M., S.C.: Initial: 150 int. units daily for the first 5 days of treatment. Dose adjustments of ≤75-150 int. units can be made every ≥2 days; maximum daily dose: 450 int. units; treatment >12 days is not recommended

Fertinex®: S.C.:

Ovulation induction: Initial: 75 int. units/day; consider dose adjustment after 5-7 days. Do not increase more than twice in any cycle or by more than 75 int. units per adjustment; dosage range: 75-300 int. units/day

ART: Initiate therapy in the early follicular phase (cycle day 2 or day 3) at a dose of 150 int. units/day, until sufficient follicular development is attained; in most cases, therapy should not exceed 10 days

Follitropin alfa: Gonal-F®: S.C.:

Ovulation induction: Female: Initial: 75 int. units/day; consider dose adjustment after 5-7 days; additional dose adjustments of up to 37.5 int. units may be considered after 14 days; further dose increases of the same magnitude can be made, if necessary, every 7 days (maximum dose: 300 int. units)

ART: Female: Initiate therapy with follitropin alfa in the early follicular phase (cycle day 2 or day 3) at a dose of 150 int. units/day, until sufficient follicular development is attained. In most cases, therapy should not exceed 10 days. In patients whose endogenous gonadotropin levels are suppressed, initiate follitropin alfa at a dose of 225 int. units/day. Continue treatment until adequate follicular development is indicated as determined by ultrasound in combination with measurement of serum estradiol levels. Consider adjustments to dose after 5 days based on the patient's response; adjust subsequent dosage every 3-5 days by ≤75-150 int. units additionally at each adjustment. Doses >450 int. units/day are not recommended. Once adequate follicular development is evident, administer hCG (5000-10,000 units) to induce final follicular maturation in preparation for oocyte.

Spermatogenesis induction: Male: Therapy should begin with hCG pretreatment until serum testosterone is in normal range, then 150 int. units 3 times/week with hCG 3 times/week; continue with lowest dose needed to induce spermatogenesis (maximum dose: 300 int. units 3 times/week); may be given for up to 18 months

Follitropin beta: Follistim®:

Female: I.M., S.C.:

Ovulation induction: Stepwise approach: Initiate therapy with 75 int. units/day for up to 14 days. Increase by 37.5 int. units at weekly intervals until follicular growth or serum estradiol levels indicate an adequate response. The maximum, individualized, daily dose that has been safely used for ovulation induction in patients during clinical trials is 300 int. units.

ART: A starting dose of 150-225 int. units of follitropin beta is recommended for at least the first 4 days of treatment. The dose may be adjusted for the individual patient based upon their ovarian response. Daily maintenance doses ranging from 75-300 int. units for 6-12 days are usually sufficient, although longer treatment may be necessary. Maintenance doses of up to 375-600 int. units may be necessary according to individual response. The maximum daily dose used in clinical studies is 600 int. units. When a sufficient number of follicles of adequate size are present, the final maturation of the follicles is induced by administering hCG at a dose of 5000-10,000 int. units. Oocyte retrieval is performed 34-36 hours later. Withhold hCG in cases where the ovaries are abnormally enlarged on the last day of follitropin beta therapy.

Male: S.C.: Spermatogenesis induction: **Note:** Begin therapy with hCG pretreatment to normalize serum testosterone levels. Once normal levels are reached, follitropin beta therapy is initiated, and must be administered concurrently with hCG treatment.

450 int. units/week given as 225 int. units twice weekly or 150 int. units 3 times/week with hCG; treatment response was noted at up to 12 months

Elderly: Refer to adult dosing. Clinical studies did not include patients >65 years of age.

Administration

I.M.:

Urofollitropin: Bravelle™: Administer I.M. or S.C.; gently massage site after administration. For S.C. injection, administer on lower abdomen; thigh is not recommended unless abdomen cannot be used. For I.M. injection, administer in upper quadrant of buttock near hip.

Follitropin beta: Follistim®: Administer I.M. or S.C. to female patients; administer S.C. only to males. The most convenient sites for S.C. injection are either in the abdomen around the navel or in the upper thigh. The best site for I.M. injection is the upper outer quadrant of the buttock muscle.

Other:

Urofollitropin:

Bravelle™: Administer S.C. or I.M.; gently massage site after administration. For S.C. injection, administer on lower abdomen; thigh is not recommended unless abdomen cannot be used. For I.M. injection, administer in upper quadrant of buttock near hip.

Fertinex®: Administer S.C.

Follitropin alpha: Gonal-F®: Administer S.C.

Follitropin beta: Follistim®: Administer S.C. or I.M. to female patients; administer S.C. only to males. The most convenient sites for S.C. injection are either in the abdomen around the navel or in the upper thigh. The best site for I.M. injection is the upper outer quadrant of the buttock muscle.

Stability

Storage:

Urofollitropin (Bravelle™, Fertinex®): Lyophilized powder may be stored in the refrigerator or at room temperature, 3°C to 25°C (37°F to 77°F). Protect from light; use immediately after reconstitution.

Follitropin alfa (Gonal-F®), Follitropin beta (Follistim®): Store powder refrigerated or at room temperature, 2°C to 25°C (36°F to 77°F). Protect from light.

Reconstitution:

Urofollitropin:

Bravelle™: Dissolve contents of vial in 1 mL **sterile saline**; gently swirl (do not shake); do not use if solution is not clear or contains particles. If more than 1 vial is required for a single dose, up to 6 vials can be reconstituted with 1 mL sterile saline and administered as a single injection. This is done by first reconstituting 1 vial with sterile saline as previously described, withdrawing the entire contents of the reconstituted vial and (using this as the diluent for the second vial) injecting into the second vial, etc. Use immediately after reconstitution.

Fertinex®: Dissolve the contents of 1 or more ampuls of urofollitropin in 0.5-1 mL of sterile saline (concentration should not exceed 225 int. units/0.5 mL). Use immediately after reconstitution.

Follitropin alfa: Gonal-F®:

Single-dose ampul: Dissolve the contents of one or more ampuls in 0.5-1 mL of sterile water for injection (concentration should not exceed 225 int. units/0.5 mL)

Multiple-dose vial: Dissolve the contents of the multidose vial with the contents of 1 prefilled syringe (bacteriostatic water for injection with 0.9% benzyl alcohol). **Do not shake.** Following reconstitution, store in refrigerator; protect from light; use within 28 days.

Follitropin beta: Follistim®: Inject 1 mL of 0.45% sodium chloride injection into vial of follitropin beta. **Do not shake**, but gently swirl until solution is clear; generally the follitropin beta dissolves immediately. Use immediately after reconstitution.

Monitoring Laboratory Tests Monitor sufficient follicular maturation. This may be directly estimated by sonographic visualization of the ovaries and endometrial lining or measuring serum estradiol levels. The combination of both ultrasonography and measurement of estradiol levels is useful for monitoring for the growth and development of follicles and timing hCG administration.

The clinical evaluation of estrogenic activity (changes in vaginal cytology and changes in appearance and volume of cervical mucus) provides an indirect estimate of the estrogenic effect upon the target organs and, therefore, it should only be used adjunctively with more direct estimates of follicular development (ultrasonography and serum estradiol determinations).

The clinical confirmation of ovulation is obtained by direct and indirect indices of progesterone production. The indices most generally used are: rise in basal body temperature, increase in serum progesterone, and menstruation following the shift in basal body temperature.

Spermatogenesis: Monitor serum testosterone levels, sperm count

(Continued)

Follitropins *(Continued)*

Monitoring and Teaching Issues

Physical Assessment: This medication should only be prescribed by a fertility specialist. See Warnings/Precautions and Contraindications for use cautions. Monitor laboratory tests and therapeutic response on a regular basis. Assess knowledge/teach patient appropriate use (injection technique and syringe disposal), interventions to reduce side effects, and adverse symptoms to report (see Patient Education). **Pregnancy risk factor X** - pregnancy must be excluded before starting medication. Breast-feeding is not recommended.

Patient Education: This medication can only be administered via injection. If you are using this medication at home, follow exact instruction for administering injections and disposal of syringes. Administer exact amount as instructed; do not alter dosage or miss a dose. If dose is missed, notify prescriber. Frequent laboratory tests will be required while you are on this therapy; do not miss appointments for laboratory tests or ultrasound. You may experience headache, dizziness, or fever (use caution when driving or engaging in tasks requiring alertness until response to drug is known); or nausea or vomiting (small, frequent meals, frequent oral care, sucking lozenges, or chewing gum may help). Report immediately abdominal pain/distension, bloating, persistent nausea, vomiting, diarrhea; dyspnea, difficulty breathing, exacerbation of asthma; swelling, pain, or redness of extremities; itching or burning on urination; menstrual irregularity, acute backache; rash, pain, or inflammation at injection site; or other adverse response. **Pregnancy/breast-feeding precautions:** Inform your prescriber if you are pregnant. Breast-feeding is not recommended.

Pregnancy Issues: Ectopic pregnancy, congenital abnormalities, and multiple births have been reported. The incidence of congenital abnormality is similar during natural conception.

Fomepizole *see page 1460*

Fondaparinux (fon da PARE i nuks)

U.S. Brand Names Arixtra®

Synonyms Fondaparinux Sodium

Generic Available No

Pharmacologic Category Factor Xa Inhibitor

Pregnancy Risk Factor B

Lactation Excretion in breast milk unknown/use caution

Use Prophylaxis of deep vein thrombosis (DVT) in patients undergoing surgery for hip fracture or hip or knee replacement

Use - Unlabeled/Investigational Treatment of DVT

Mechanism of Action/Effect Fondaparinux prevents factor Xa from binding with antithrombin III and inhibits thrombin formation and thrombus development.

Contraindications Hypersensitivity to fondaparinux or any component of the formulation; severe renal impairment (Cl_{cr} <30 mL/minute); body weight <50 kg; active major bleeding; bacterial endocarditis; thrombocytopenia associated with a positive *in vitro* test for antiplatelet antibody in the presence of fondaparinux

Warnings/Precautions Patients with recent or anticipated neuraxial anesthesia (epidural or spinal anesthesia) are at risk of spinal or epidural hematoma and subsequent paralysis. Not to be used interchangeably (unit-for-unit) with heparin, low molecular weight heparins (LMWHs), or heparinoids. Use caution in patients with moderate renal dysfunction (Cl_{cr} 30-50 mL/minute). Discontinue if severe dysfunction or labile function develops.

Use caution in congenital or acquired bleeding disorders; active ulcerative or angiodysplastic gastrointestinal disease; hemorrhagic stroke; shortly after brain, spinal, or ophthalmologic surgery; or in patients taking platelet inhibitors. Discontinue agents that may enhance the risk of hemorrhage if possible. If thrombocytopenia occurs discontinue fondaparinux. Use caution in the elderly, patients with a history of heparin-induced thrombocytopenia, patients with a bleeding diathesis, uncontrolled hypertension, recent gastrointestinal ulceration, diabetic retinopathy, and hemorrhage. Safety and efficacy in pediatric patients have not been established.

Drug Interactions

Increased Effect/Toxicity: Anticoagulants, antiplatelet agents, drotrecogin alfa, NSAIDs, salicylates, and thrombolytic agents may enhance the anticoagulant effect and/or increase the risk of bleeding.

Nutritional/Ethanol Interactions Herb/Nutraceutical: Avoid alfalfa, anise, bilberry, bladderwrack, bromelain, cat's claw, celery, coleus, cordyceps, dong quai, evening primrose oil, fenugreek, feverfew, garlic, ginger, ginkgo biloba, ginseng (American/Panax/Siberian), grape seed, green tea, guggul, horse chestnut seed, horseradish, licorice, prickly ash, red clover, reishi, sweet clover, turmeric, white willow (all possess anticoagulant or antiplatelet activity and as such, may enhance the anticoagulant effects of fondaparinux).

Adverse Reactions As with all anticoagulants, bleeding is the major adverse effect. Hemorrhage may occur at any site. Risk appears increased by a number of factors including renal dysfunction, age (>75 years), and weight (<50 kg).

>10%:

- Central nervous system: Fever (14%)
- Gastrointestinal: Nausea (11%)
- Hematologic: Anemia (20%)

1% to 10%:

- Cardiovascular: Edema (9%), hypotension (4%), confusion (3%)
- Central nervous system: Insomnia (5%), dizziness (4%), headache (2%), pain (2%)
- Dermatologic: Rash (8%), purpura (4%), bullous eruption (3%)
- Endocrine & metabolic: Hypokalemia (4%)
- Gastrointestinal: Constipation (9%), vomiting (6%), diarrhea (3%), dyspepsia (2%)
- Genitourinary: Urinary tract infection (4%), urinary retention (3%)
- Hematologic: Moderate thrombocytopenia (50,000-100,000/mm^3: 3%), major bleeding (2% to 3%), minor bleeding (3% to 4%), hematoma (3%)

Hepatic: SGOT increased (2%), SGPT increased (3%)
Local: Injection site reaction (bleeding, rash, pruritus)
Miscellaneous: Wound drainage increased (5%)
<1% (Limited to important or life-threatening): Severe thrombocytopenia (<50,000/mm³)

Overdosage/Toxicology Treatment is symptom-directed and supportive.

Pharmacodynamics/Kinetics

Absorption: Rapid and complete

Bioavailability: 100%

Half-Life Elimination: 17-21 hours; prolonged with worsening renal impairment

Time to Peak: 2-3 hours

Formulations Injection, solution, as sodium [prefilled syringe]: 2.5 mg/0.5 mL (0.5 mL)

Dosing

Adults: Adults ≥50 kg: DVT prophylaxis: S.C.: 2.5 mg once daily. **Note:** Initiate dose after hemostasis has been established, 6-8 hours postoperatively.

Elderly: Use caution, elimination may be prolonged; assess renal function before initiating therapy

Renal Impairment:

Cl_{cr} 30-50 mL/minute: Use caution
Cl_{cr} <30 mL/minute: Contraindicated

Administration

I.M.: Do not administer I.M.

Other: For S.C. administration only. Do not mix with other injections or infusions.

Stability

Storage: Store at 15°C to 30°C (59°F to 86°F).

Compatibility: Do not mix with other injections or infusions.

Monitoring and Teaching Issues

Physical Assessment: See Contraindications, Warnings/Precautions, and Dosing for use cautions. Assess potential for interactions with other prescriptions, OTC medications, or herbal products patient may be taking (especially anything that will affect coagulation or platelet function - see Drug Interactions). See administration specifics above. Bleeding precautions should be observed. Assess results of laboratory tests (see above), therapeutic effects, and adverse response (see Adverse Reactions and Overdose/Toxicology) regularly during therapy. Teach patient possible side effects and appropriate interventions (eg, bleeding precautions) and adverse symptoms to report (see Patient Education). Note breast-feeding caution.

Patient Education: Inform prescriber of all prescriptions, OTC medications, or herbal products you are taking, and any allergies you have. Do not take anything new during treatment without consulting prescriber. This drug can only be administered by injection. Report pain, burning, redness, or swelling at injection site. You may have a tendency to bleed easily while taking this drug (brush teeth with soft brush, floss with waxed floss, use electric razor, avoid scissors or sharp knives, and avoid potentially harmful activities). May cause nausea or vomiting (small, frequent meals, frequent mouth care, chewing gum, or sucking lozenges may help); or dizziness, headache, insomnia (use caution when driving or engaging in tasks that require alertness until response to drug is known). Report unusual bleeding or bruising (bleeding gums, nosebleed, blood in urine, dark stool); pain in joints or back; CNS changes (fever, confusion); unusual fever; persistent nausea or GI upset; changes in urinary pattern; or other persistent adverse response. **Breast-feeding precaution:** Consult prescriber if breast-feeding.

Fondaparinux Sodium *see* Fondaparinux *on page 600*
Foradil® Aerolizer™ *see* Formoterol *on page 601*

Formoterol (for MOH te rol)

U.S. Brand Names Foradil® Aerolizer™

Synonyms Formoterol Fumarate

Generic Available No

Pharmacologic Category $Beta_2$ Agonist

Pregnancy Risk Factor C

Lactation Excretion in breast milk unknown/use caution

Use Maintenance treatment of asthma and prevention of bronchospasm in patients ≥5 years of age with reversible obstructive airway disease, including patients with symptoms of nocturnal asthma, who require regular treatment with inhaled, short-acting $beta_2$ agonists; maintenance treatment of bronchoconstriction in patients with COPD; prevention of exercise-induced bronchospasm in patients ≥12 years of age

Mechanism of Action/Effect Relaxes bronchial smooth muscle

Contraindications Hypersensitivity to adrenergic amines, formoterol, or any component of the formulation; need for acute bronchodilation; within 2 weeks of MAO inhibitor use

Warnings/Precautions Formoterol is not meant to relieve acute asthmatic symptoms. Acute episodes should be treated with short-acting $beta_2$ agonist. Do not substitute for inhaled or oral corticosteroids. Short-acting beta agonists should only be used for acute asthma relief concurrently with formoterol. Increasing need for short-acting $beta_2$ agonists is a marker for deterioration in asthma. Re-evaluation is needed. Do not exceed recommended dose or dosing interval. Cardiovascular effects are not common with formoterol when used in recommended doses. All beta agonists may cause elevation in blood pressure, heart rate, and result in excitement (CNS). Use with caution in patients with cardiovascular disorders, convulsive disorders, thyrotoxicosis, or others who are sensitive to the effects of sympathomimetic amines. Paroxysmal bronchospasm (which can be fatal) has been reported with this and other inhaled agents. If this occurs, discontinue treatment. The elderly may be at greater risk of cardiovascular side effects; safety and efficacy have not been established in children <5 years of age. Pregnancy risk C.
(Continued)

Formoterol *(Continued)*

Drug Interactions

Cytochrome P450 Effect: Substrate of CYP2A6, 2C8/9, 2C19, 2D6

Increased Effect/Toxicity: Adrenergic agonists, antidepressants (tricyclic), beta-blockers, corticosteroids, diuretics, drugs that prolong QT_c interval, MAO inhibitors, theophylline derivatives

Adverse Reactions Children are more likely to have infection, inflammation, abdominal pain, nausea, and dyspepsia.

>10%: Miscellaneous: Viral infection (17%)

1% to 10%:

Cardiovascular: Chest pain (2%)

Central nervous system: Tremor (2%), dizziness (2%), insomnia (2%), dysphonia (1%)

Dermatologic: Rash (1%)

Respiratory: Bronchitis (5%), infection (3%), dyspnea (2%), tonsillitis (1%)

<1% (Limited to important or life-threatening): Anaphylactic reactions (severe hypotension, angioedema), asthma exacerbation

Overdosage/Toxicology Signs and symptoms would be those associated with excessive beta-adrenergic stimulation. Treatment would include symptomatic and supportive care. Prudent use of a cardioselective beta-adrenergic blocker (eg, atenolol or metoprolol) may help reduce the symptoms; keep in mind the potential for induction of bronchoconstriction in an asthmatic.

Pharmacodynamics/Kinetics

Absorption: Rapidly into plasma

Half-Life Elimination: ~10-14 hours

Time to Peak: Maximum improvement in FEV_1 in 1-3 hours

Metabolism: Hepatic via direct glucuronidation and O-demethylation; CYP2D6, CYP2C19, CYP2C8/9, CYP2A6 involved in O-demethylation

Duration: Improvement in FEV_1 observed for 12 hours in most patients

Formulations Powder for oral inhalation, as fumarate [capsule]: 12 mcg (12s, 60s) [contains lactose 25 mg]

Dosing

Adults & Elderly:

Asthma maintenance: Inhalation: 12 mcg capsule every 12 hours

Exercise-induced bronchospasm: Inhalation: 12 mcg capsule at least 15 minutes before exercise on an "as needed" basis; additional doses should not be used for another 12 hours. **Note:** If using for asthma maintenance, do not use additional doses for exercise-induced bronchospasm.

Maintenance treatment for COPD: Inhalation: 12 mcg capsule every 12 hours

Pediatrics:

Asthma maintenance: Inhalation: Children ≥5 years: 12 mcg capsule every 12 hours

Exercise-induced bronchospasm: Inhalation: Children ≥12 years: 12 mcg capsule at least 15 minutes before exercise on an "as needed" basis; additional doses should not be used for another 12 hours. **Note:** If using for asthma maintenance, do not use additional doses for exercise-induced bronchospasm.

Renal Impairment: Not studied

Administration

Inhalation: Remove capsule from foil blister **immediately** before use. Place capsule in the capsule-chamber in the base of the Aerolizer™ Inhaler. Must only use the Aerolizer™ Inhaler. Press both buttons **once only** and then release. Keep inhaler in a level, horizontal position. Exhale fully. Do not exhale into inhaler. Tilt head slightly back and inhale (rapidly, steadily and deeply). Hold breath as long as possible. If any powder remains in capsule, exhale and inhale again. Repeat until capsule is empty. Throw away empty capsule; do not leave in inhaler. Do not use a spacer with the Aerolizer™ Inhaler. Always keep capsules and inhaler dry.

Stability

Storage: Prior to dispensing, store in refrigerator at 2°C to 8°C (36°F to 46°F); after dispensing, store at room temperature at 20°C to 25°C (68°F to 77°F). Protect from heat and moisture. Capsules should always be stored in the blister and only removed immediately before use. Always check expiration date. Use within 4 months of purchase date or product expiration date, whichever comes first.

Monitoring Laboratory Tests Peak flow meter

Monitoring and Teaching Issues

Physical Assessment: Assess other medications patient may be taking for effectiveness and interactions (see Drug Interactions). See Contraindications, Warnings/Precautions, and Dosing for use cautions. Monitor therapeutic response and adverse reactions at beginning of therapy and periodically throughout period of therapy (see Adverse Reactions and Overdose/Toxicology). Assess knowledge/teach appropriate use of medication, interventions to reduce side effects, and adverse symptoms to report (see Patient Education). **Pregnancy risk factor C** - benefits of use should outweigh possible risks. Note breast-feeding caution.

Patient Education: Do not swallow capsules; this medication can only be used in the Aerolizer™ Inhaler. Use exactly as directed and do not use more often than recommended. Store capsules in blister and do not remove from blister until ready for treatment. Maintain adequate hydration (2-3 L/day of fluids) unless advised by prescriber to restrict fluids. It is recommended that you wear identification (Med-Alert bracelet) if you have an asthmatic condition. You may experience nervousness, dizziness, or insomnia (use caution when driving or engaging in hazardous activities until response to medication is known); dry mouth, nausea, or GI discomfort (small, frequent meals, good mouth care, sucking lozenges, or chewing gum may help); or difficulty voiding (always void before treatment). Report any unresolved GI upset, nervousness or dizziness, muscle cramping, chest pain or palpitations, skin rash, signs of infection, unusual cough, or worsening of condition. **Pregnancy/breast-feeding precautions:** Inform prescriber if you are or intend to become pregnant. Consult prescriber if breast-feeding.

Administration: Follow directions for use and storage of inhaler exactly. Wash hands prior to treatment and sit in comfortable position for treatment. Remove capsule from foil blister immediately before treatment and place capsule in the capsule-chamber in the base of the Aerolizer™ Inhaler. Press both buttons once only and then release. Hold inhaler in a level, horizontal position, exhale fully (do not exhale into inhaler). Tilt head slightly back and inhale from inhaler rapidly, steadily, and deeply. Hold breath as long as possible. If any powder remains in capsule, exhale and inhale again. Repeat until capsule is empty. Throw away empty capsule. Do not use a spacer with aerolizer. Do not wash inhaler; store in dry place.

Pregnancy Issues: When given orally to rats throughout organogenesis, formoterol caused delayed ossification and decreased fetal weight, but no malformations. There were no adverse events when given to pregnant rats in late pregnancy. Doses used were ≥70 times the recommended daily inhalation dose in humans. There are no adequate and well-controlled studies in pregnant women. Use only if benefit outweighs risk to the fetus. Beta agonists interfere with uterine contractility so use during labor only if benefit outweighs risk to the fetus.

Related Information

Inhalant (Asthma, Bronchospasm) Agents Comparison *on page 1577*

Formoterol Fumarate *see* Formoterol *on page 601*

5-Formyl Tetrahydrofolate *see* Leucovorin *on page 779*

Fortaz® *see* Ceftazidime *on page 249*

Fortovase® *see* Saquinavir *on page 1213*

Fosamax® *see* Alendronate *on page 56*

Foscarnet (fos KAR net)

U.S. Brand Names Foscavir®

Synonyms PFA; Phosphonoformate; Phosphonoformic Acid

Generic Available No

Pharmacologic Category Antiviral Agent

Pregnancy Risk Factor C

Lactation Excretion in breast milk unknown/contraindicated

Use

Herpes virus infections suspected to be caused by acyclovir - (HSV, VZV) or ganciclovir - (CMV) resistant strains (this occurs almost exclusively in immunocompromised persons, eg, with advanced AIDS), who have received prolonged treatment for a herpes virus infection

CMV retinitis in persons with AIDS; other CMV infections in persons unable to tolerate ganciclovir; may be given in combination with ganciclovir in patients who relapse after monotherapy with either drug

Mechanism of Action/Effect Pyrophosphate analogue which acts as a noncompetitive inhibitor of many viral RNA and DNA polymerases as well as HIV reverse transcriptase. Inhibitory effects occur at concentrations which do not affect host cellular DNA polymerases; however, some human cell growth suppression has been observed with high *in vitro* concentrations. Similar to ganciclovir, foscarnet is a virostatic agent. Foscarnet does not require activation by thymidine kinase.

Contraindications Hypersensitivity to foscarnet or any component of the formulation; Cl_{cr} <0.4 mL/minute/kg during therapy

Warnings/Precautions Renal impairment occurs to some degree in the majority of patients treated with foscarnet. Renal impairment may occur at any time (usually reversible within 1 week following dose adjustment or discontinuation, but some severe cases). Renal function should be closely monitored. Foscarnet may cause tooth disorders. Safety and effectiveness in children have not been studied. Monitor electrolytes carefully, particularly calcium, magnesium, phosphate, and potassium. Seizures have been experienced by up to 10% of AIDS patients. Risk factors for seizures include a low baseline absolute neutrophil count (ANC), impaired baseline renal function and low total serum calcium. Some patients who have experienced seizures have died, while others have been able to continue or resume foscarnet treatment after their mineral or electrolyte abnormality has been corrected, their underlying disease state treated, or their dose decreased. Foscarnet has been shown to be mutagenic *in vitro* and in mice at very high doses. Pregnancy risk C.

Drug Interactions

Increased Effect/Toxicity: Concurrent use with ciprofloxacin (or other fluoroquinolone) increases seizure potential. Acute renal failure (reversible) has been reported with cyclosporine due most likely to a synergistic toxic effect. Nephrotoxic drugs (amphotericin B, I.V. pentamidine, aminoglycosides, etc) should be avoided, if possible, to minimize additive renal risk with foscarnet. Concurrent use of pentamidine also increases the potential for hypocalcemia. Protease inhibitors (ritonavir, saquinavir) have been associated with an increased risk of renal impairment during concurrent use of foscarnet

Adverse Reactions

>10%:

Central nervous system: Fever, headache, seizures

Endocrine & metabolic: Electrolyte disorders (hyper- or hypocalcemia; hyper- or hypomagnesemia, hyper- or hypophosphatemia, or hypokalemia)

Gastrointestinal: Nausea, diarrhea, vomiting

Hematologic: Anemia

Renal: Nephrotoxicity (abnormal renal function, decreased creatinine clearance)

1% to 10%:

Central nervous system: Seizures (in up to 10% of HIV patients), fatigue, malaise, dizziness, hypoesthesia, depression, confusion, anxiety

Dermatologic: Rash

(Continued)

Foscarnet *(Continued)*

Gastrointestinal: Anorexia
Hematologic: Granulocytopenia, leukopenia
Local: Injection site pain
Neuromuscular & skeletal: Paresthesia, involuntary muscle contractions, rigors, neuropathy (peripheral), weakness
Ocular: Vision abnormalities
Respiratory: Coughing, dyspnea
Miscellaneous: Sepsis, diaphoresis (increased)

<1% (Limited to important or life-threatening): Arrhythmias, ascites, bradycardia, cardiac failure, cerebral edema, cholecystitis, cholelithiasis, hepatitis, hepatosplenomegaly, leg edema, peripheral edema, substernal chest pain, syncope, vocal cord paralysis

Overdosage/Toxicology Symptoms of overdose include seizures, renal dysfunction, perioral or limb paresthesia, and hypocalcemia. Treatment is supportive.

Pharmacodynamics/Kinetics

Half-Life Elimination: ~3 hours

Metabolism: Biotransformation does not occur

Formulations Injection, solution: 24 mg/mL (250 mL, 500 mL)

Dosing

Adults & Elderly:

CMV retinitis: I.V.:
Induction treatment: 60 mg/kg/dose every 8 hours for 14-21 days
Maintenance therapy: 90-120 mg/kg/day as a single infusion

Acyclovir-resistant HSV induction treatment: I.V.: 40 mg/kg/dose every 8-12 hours for 14-21 days

Pediatrics: Adolescents: Refer to adult dosing.

Renal Impairment: See tables.

Induction Dosing of Foscarnet in Patients with Abnormal Renal Function

Cl_{cr} (mL/min/kg)	HSV Equivalent to 40 mg/kg q12h	HSV Equivalent to 40 mg/kg q8h	CMV Equivalent to 60 mg/kg q8h	CMV Equivalent to 90 mg/kg q12h
<0.4	not recommended	not recommended	not recommended	not recommended
≥0.4-0.5	20 mg/kg every 24 hours	35 mg/kg every 24 hours	50 mg/kg every 24 hours	50 mg/kg every 24 hours
>0.5-0.6	25 mg/kg every 24 hours	40 mg/kg every 24 hours	60 mg/kg every 24 hours	60 mg/kg every 24 hours
>0.6-0.8	35 mg/kg every 24 hours	25 mg/kg every 12 hours	40 mg/kg every 12 hours	80 mg/kg every 24 hours
>0.8-1.0	20 mg/kg every 12 hours	35 mg/kg every 12 hours	50 mg/kg every 12 hours	50 mg/kg every 12 hours
>1.0-1.4	30 mg/kg every 12 hours	30 mg/kg every 8 hours	45 mg/kg every 8 hours	70 mg/kg every 12 hours
>1.4	40 mg/kg every 12 hours	40 mg/kg every 8 hours	60 mg/kg every 8 hours	90 mg/kg every 12 hours

Maintenance Dosing of Foscarnet in Patients with Abnormal Renal Function

Cl_{cr} (mL/min/kg)	CMV Equivalent to 90 mg/kg q24h	CMV Equivalent to 120 mg/kg q24h
<0.4	not recommended	not recommended
≥0.4-0.5	50 mg/kg every 48 hours	65 mg/kg every 48 hours
>0.5-0.6	60 mg/kg every 48 hours	80 mg/kg every 48 hours
>0.6-0.8	80 mg/kg every 48 hours	105 mg/kg every 48 hours
>0.8-1.0	50 mg/kg every 24 hours	65 mg/kg every 24 hours
>1.0-1.4	70 mg/kg every 24 hours	90 mg/kg every 24 hours
>1.4	90 mg/kg every 24 hours	120 mg/kg every 24 hours

Administration

I.V.: Use an infusion pump, at a rate not exceeding 1 mg/kg/minute. Adult induction doses of 60 mg/kg are administered over 1 hour. Adult maintenance doses of 90-120 mg/kg are infused over 2 hours.

Stability

Storage: Foscarnet injection is a clear, colorless solution. It should be stored at room temperature and protected from temperatures >40°C and from freezing.

Reconstitution: Foscarnet should be diluted in D_5W or NS and transferred to PVC containers. It is stable for 24 hours at room temperature or refrigeration. For peripheral line administration, foscarnet **must** be diluted to 12 mg/mL with D_5W or NS. For central line administration, foscarnet may be administered undiluted.

Compatibility: Stable in D_5W, NS; **incompatible** with LR, dextrose 30%, TPN, I.V. solutions containing calcium, magnesium, or vancomycin

Y-site administration: Incompatible with acyclovir, amphotericin B, diazepam, digoxin, diphenhydramine, dobutamine, droperidol, ganciclovir, haloperidol, leucovorin, midazolam, pentamidine, prochlorperazine edisylate, promethazine, trimetrexate

Monitoring Laboratory Tests Renal function, CBC, electrolytes, calcium, magnesium

Monitoring and Teaching Issues

Physical Assessment: See Contraindications, Warnings/Precautions, Drug Interactions, and Dosing for use cautions. Assess potential for interactions with other prescriptions, OTC medications, or herbal products patient may be taking (see Drug Interactions). See Administration, Reconstitution, and Compatibility for specific directions. Assess results of laboratory tests (see above), therapeutic effects, and adverse response (eg, nephrotoxicity, electrolyte imbalance, seizures - see Adverse Reactions and Overdose/Toxicology). Teach patient possible side effects and appropriate interventions and adverse symptoms to report (see Patient Education). **Pregnancy risk factor C** - benefits of use should outweigh possible risks. Use of barrier contraceptives has been recommended to reduce transmission of disease. Breast-feeding is contraindicated.

Patient Education: Inform prescriber of all prescriptions, OTC medications, or herbal products you are taking, and any allergies you have. Do not take anything new during treatment unless approved by prescriber. Foscarnet is not a cure for the disease; progression may occur during or following therapy. While on therapy, it is important to maintain adequate hydration (2-3 L/day of fluids) unless advised by prescriber to restrict fluids, and nutrition (small, frequent meals may help). Regular dental check-ups are recommended. May cause dizziness or confusion (use caution when driving or engaging in tasks that require alertness until response to drug is known); nausea and vomiting (small, frequent meals, frequent mouth care, chewing gum or sucking lozenges may help); or diarrhea (buttermilk, boiled milk, or yogurt may help). Report any change in sensorium or seizures; unresolved diarrhea or vomiting; unusual fever, chills, sore throat, unhealed sores, swollen lymph glands; or malaise. **Pregnancy/breast-feeding precautions:** Inform prescriber if you are pregnant. Barrier contraceptives are recommended to reduce transmission of disease. Do not breast-feed.

Geriatric Considerations: Information on the use of foscarnet is lacking in the elderly. Dose adjustments and proper monitoring must be performed because of the decreased renal function common in older patients.

Breast-feeding Issues: The CDC recommends **not** to breast-feed if diagnosed with HIV to avoid postnatal transmission of the virus.

Additional Information Sodium loading with 500 mL of 0.9% sodium chloride solution before and after foscarnet infusion helps to minimize the risk of nephrotoxicity.

Foscavir® *see* Foscarnet *on page 603*

Fosinopril (foe SIN oh pril)

U.S. Brand Names Monopril®

Generic Available No

Pharmacologic Category Angiotensin-Converting Enzyme (ACE) Inhibitor

Pregnancy Risk Factor C/D (2nd and 3rd trimesters)

Lactation Excretion in breast milk unknown

Use Treatment of hypertension, either alone or in combination with other antihypertensive agents; treatment of congestive heart failure, left ventricular dysfunction after myocardial infarction

Mechanism of Action/Effect Competitive inhibitor of angiotensin-converting enzyme (ACE); prevents conversion of angiotensin I to angiotensin II, a potent vasoconstrictor; results in lower levels of angiotensin II which causes an increase in plasma renin activity and a reduction in aldosterone secretion; a CNS mechanism may also be involved in hypotensive effect as angiotensin II increases adrenergic outflow from CNS; vasoactive kallikreins may be decreased in conversion to active hormones by ACE inhibitors, thus reducing blood pressure

Contraindications Hypersensitivity to fosinopril or any component of the formulation; angioedema related to previous treatment with an ACE inhibitor; idiopathic or hereditary angioedema; bilateral renal artery stenosis; primary hyperaldosteronism; pregnancy (2nd and 3rd trimesters)

Warnings/Precautions Anaphylactic reactions can occur. Angioedema can occur at any time during treatment (especially following first dose). Careful blood pressure monitoring (hypotension can occur especially in volume depleted patients). Dosage adjustment needed in severe renal impairment (Cl_{cr} <10 mL/minute). Use with caution in hypovolemia; collagen vascular diseases; valvular stenosis (particularly aortic stenosis); hyperkalemia; or before, during, or immediately after anesthesia. Avoid rapid dosage escalation which may lead to renal insufficiency. Hypersensitivity reactions may be seen during hemodialysis with high-flux dialysis membranes (eg, AN69). Hyperkalemia may rarely occur. Neutropenia/agranulocytosis with myeloid hyperplasia can rarely occur. Use with caution in unilateral renal artery stenosis and pre-existing renal insufficiency. Safety and efficacy in pediatric patients have not been established. Pregnancy risk C/D (2nd and 3rd trimesters).

Drug Interactions

Decreased Effect: Aspirin (high dose) may reduce the therapeutic effects of ACE inhibitors; at low dosages this does not appear to be significant. Rifampin may decrease the effect of ACE inhibitors. Antacids may decrease the bioavailability of ACE inhibitors (may be more likely to occur with captopril); separate administration times by 1-2 hours. NSAIDs, specifically indomethacin, may reduce the hypotensive effects of ACE inhibitors. More likely to occur in low renin or volume dependent hypertensive patients.

Increased Effect/Toxicity: Potassium supplements, co-trimoxazole (high dose), angiotensin II receptor antagonists (candesartan, losartan, irbesartan, etc), or potassium-sparing diuretics (amiloride, spironolactone, triamterene) may result in elevated serum potassium levels when combined with fosinopril. ACE inhibitor effects may be increased by phenothiazines or probenecid (increases levels of captopril). ACE inhibitors may increase serum concentrations/effects of digoxin, lithium, and sulfonlyureas.

Diuretics have additive hypotensive effects with ACE inhibitors, and hypovolemia increases the potential for adverse renal effects of ACE inhibitors. In patients with compromised renal function, coadministration with NSAIDs may result in further deterioration of renal function. Allopurinol and ACE inhibitors may cause a higher risk of hypersensitivity reaction when taken concurrently.

Nutritional/Ethanol Interactions Herb/Nutraceutical: Avoid dong quai if using for hypertension (has estrogenic activity). Avoid ephedra, garlic, yohimbe, ginseng (may worsen hypertension).

(Continued)

Fosinopril *(Continued)*

Effects on Lab Values Positive Coombs' (direct); may cause false-positive results in urine acetone determinations using sodium nitroprusside reagent; may cause false low serum digoxin levels with the Digi-Tab RIA kit for digoxin.

Adverse Reactions Note: Frequency ranges include data from hypertension and heart failure trials. Higher rates of adverse reactions have generally been noted in patients with CHF. However, the frequency of adverse effects associated with placebo is also increased in this population.

>10%: Central nervous system: Dizziness (1.6% to 11.9%)

1% to 10%:

Cardiovascular: Orthostatic hypotension (1.4% to 1.9%), palpitation (1.4%)

Central nervous system: Dizziness (1% to 2%; up to 12% in CHF patients), headache (3.2%), weakness (1.4%), fatigue (1% to 2%)

Endocrine & metabolic: Hyperkalemia (2.6%)

Gastrointestinal: Diarrhea (2.2%), nausea/vomiting (1.2% to 2.2%)

Hepatic: Increased transaminases

Neuromuscular & skeletal: Musculoskeletal pain (<1% to 3.3%), noncardiac chest pain (<1% to 2.2%)

Renal: Increased serum creatinine, worsening of renal function (in patients with bilateral renal artery stenosis or hypovolemia)

Respiratory: Cough (2.2% to 9.7%)

Miscellaneous: Upper respiratory infection (2.2%)

>1% but ≤ frequency in patients receiving placebo: Sexual dysfunction, fever, flu-like syndrome, dyspnea, rash, headache, insomnia

<1% (Limited to important or life-threatening): Anaphylactoid reaction, angina, angioedema, arthralgia, bronchospasm, cerebral infarction, cerebrovascular accident, eosinophilic vasculitis, gout, gynecomastia, hepatitis, hepatomegaly, myalgia, myocardial infarction, pancreatitis, paresthesia, photosensitivity, pleuritic chest pain, pruritus, rash, renal insufficiency, scleroderma, shock, sudden death, syncope, TIA, tinnitus, urticaria, vertigo. In a small number of patients, a symptom complex of cough, bronchospasm, and eosinophilia has been observed with fosinopril.

Other events reported with ACE inhibitors: Acute renal failure, agranulocytosis, anemia, aplastic anemia, bullous pemphigus, cardiac arrest, eosinophilic pneumonitis, exfoliative dermatitis, hemolytic anemia, hepatic failure, jaundice, neutropenia, pancytopenia, Stevens-Johnson syndrome, symptomatic hyponatremia, thrombocytopenia. In addition, a syndrome which may include fever, myalgia, arthralgia, interstitial nephritis, vasculitis, rash, eosinophilia and positive ANA, and elevated ESR has been reported for other ACE inhibitors.

Overdosage/Toxicology Mild hypotension has been the primary toxic effect seen with acute overdose. Bradycardia may also occur; hyperkalemia occurs even with therapeutic doses, especially in patients with renal insufficiency and those taking NSAIDs. Treatment is symptom-directed and supportive.

Pharmacodynamics/Kinetics

Absorption: 36%

Bioavailability: 36%

Half-Life Elimination: Serum (fosinoprilat): 12 hours

Time to Peak: Serum: ~3 hours

Metabolism: Prodrug, hydrolyzed to its active metabolite fosinoprilat by intestinal wall and hepatic esterases

Onset: 1 hour

Duration: 24 hours

Formulations Tablet: 10 mg, 20 mg, 40 mg

Dosing

Adults & Elderly:

Hypertension: Oral: Initial: 10 mg/day; increase to a maximum dose of 80 mg/day. Most patients are maintained on 20-40 mg/day. May need to divide the dose into two if trough effect is inadequate. Discontinue the diuretic, if possible 2-3 days before initiation of therapy. Resume diuretic therapy carefully, if needed.

Heart failure: Oral: Initial: 10 mg/day (5 mg if renal dysfunction present) and increase, as needed, to a maximum of 40 mg once daily over several weeks. Usual dose: 20-40 mg/day. If hypotension, orthostasis, or azotemia occurs during titration, consider decreasing concomitant diuretic dose, if any.

Renal Impairment: None needed since hepatobiliary elimination compensates adequately diminished renal elimination.

Hemodialysis: Moderately dialyzable (20% to 50%)

Hepatic Impairment: Decrease dose and monitor effects

Stability

Storage: Store at 25°C (77°F); excursions permitted to 15°C to 30°C (59°F to 86°F). Protect from moisture by keeping bottle tightly closed.

Monitoring Laboratory Tests CBC, renal function tests, electrolytes. If patient has renal impairment, then a baseline WBC with differential and serum creatinine should be evaluated and monitored closely during initial therapy.

Monitoring and Teaching Issues

Physical Assessment: See Contraindications, Warnings/Precautions, and Dosing for use cautions. Assess potential for interactions with other prescriptions, OTC medications, or herbal products patient may be taking (especially anything that may impact fluid balance or cardiac status - see Drug Interactions). Assess therapeutic effectiveness, laboratory tests (see above), and adverse response on a regular basis during therapy (eg, anaphylactic reactions, hypovolemia, angioedema, postural hypotension - see Adverse Reactions and Overdose/Toxicology). Teach patient appropriate use, possible side effects and appropriate interventions, and adverse symptoms to report (see Patient Education). **Pregnancy**

risk factor C/D - see Pregnancy Risk Factor for use cautions. Instruct patient in appropriate use of barrier contraceptives. Danger of use during pregnancy must outweigh risk to fetus - see Pregnancy Issues. Note breast-feeding caution.

Patient Education: Inform prescriber of all prescriptions, OTC medications, or herbal products you are taking, and any allergies you have. Do not take anything new during treatment unless approved by prescriber. Do not use potassium supplement or salt substitutes without consulting prescriber. Take exactly as directed; do not discontinue without consulting prescriber. This drug does not eliminate need for diet or exercise regimen as recommended by prescriber. May cause dizziness, fainting, or lightheadedness (use caution when driving or engaging in tasks that require alertness until response to drug is known); postural hypotension (use caution when rising from lying or sitting position or climbing stairs); or nausea, vomiting, abdominal pain, dry mouth, or loss of appetite (small, frequent meals, frequent mouth care, sucking lozenges, or chewing gum may help) - report if these persist. Report chest pain or palpitations; mouth sores; fever or chills; swelling of extremities, face, mouth, or tongue; skin rash; numbness, tingling, or pain in muscles; difficulty breathing; unusual cough; or other persistent adverse reactions. **Pregnancy/breast-feeding precautions:** Inform prescriber if you are or intend to become pregnant. This drug should not be used in the 2nd or 3rd trimester of pregnancy. Consult prescriber for appropriate contraceptive measures if necessary. Consult prescriber if breast-feeding.

Geriatric Considerations: Due to frequent decreases in glomerular filtration (also creatinine clearance) with aging, elderly patients may have exaggerated responses to ACE inhibitors. Differences in clinical response due to hepatic changes are not observed. ACE inhibitors may be preferred agents in elderly patients with congestive heart failure and diabetes mellitus. Diabetic proteinuria is reduced and insulin sensitivity is enhanced. In general, the side effect profile is favorable in the elderly and causes little or no CNS confusion; use lowest dose recommendations initially.

Pregnancy Issues: ACE inhibitors can cause fetal injury or death if taken during the 2nd or 3rd trimester. Discontinue ACE inhibitors as soon as pregnancy is detected.

Related Information

Angiotensin Agents *on page 1547*
Heart Failure *on page 1670*

Fosphenytoin (FOS fen i toyn)

U.S. Brand Names Cerebyx®

Synonyms Fosphenytoin Sodium

Generic Available No

Pharmacologic Category Anticonvulsant, Hydantoin

Pregnancy Risk Factor D

Lactation Enters breast milk/compatible (if serum level is within mother's therapeutic range)

Use Indicated for short-term parenteral administration when other means of phenytoin administration are unavailable, inappropriate or deemed less advantageous; the safety and effectiveness of fosphenytoin in this use has not been systematically evaluated for more than 5 days; may be used for the control of generalized convulsive status epilepticus and prevention and treatment of seizures occurring during neurosurgery

Mechanism of Action/Effect Diphosphate ester salt of phenytoin which acts as a water soluble prodrug of phenytoin; after administration, plasma esterases convert fosphenytoin to phosphate, formaldehyde and phenytoin as the active moiety; phenytoin works by stabilizing neuronal membranes and decreasing seizure activity by increasing efflux or decreasing influx of sodium ions across cell membranes in the motor cortex during generation of nerve impulses

Contraindications Hypersensitivity to phenytoin, other hydantoins, or any component of the formulation; patients with sinus bradycardia, sinoatrial block, second- and third-degree AV block, or Adams-Stokes syndrome; occurrence of rash during treatment (should not be resumed if rash is exfoliative, purpuric, or bullous); not recommended for use in children <4 years of age; pregnancy

Warnings/Precautions Doses of fosphenytoin are expressed as their phenytoin sodium equivalent. Antiepileptic drugs should not be abruptly discontinued. Hypotension may occur, especially after I.V. administration at high doses and high rates of administration. Administration of phenytoin has been associated with atrial and ventricular conduction depression and ventricular fibrillation. Careful cardiac monitoring is needed when administering I.V. loading doses of fosphenytoin. Use with caution in patients with hypotension and severe myocardial insufficiency. Discontinue if skin rash or lymphadenopathy occurs. Acute hepatotoxicity associated with a hypersensitivity syndrome characterized by fever, skin eruptions, and lymphadenopathy has been reported to occur within the first 2 months of treatment.

Drug Interactions

Cytochrome P450 Effect: As phenytoin: Substrate of **CYP2C8/9, 2C19**, 3A4; Induces **CYP2B6, 2C8/9, 2C19, 3A4**

Decreased Effect: No drugs are known to interfere with the conversion of fosphenytoin to phenytoin. Phenytoin may decrease the serum concentration or effectiveness of valproic acid, ethosuximide, felbamate, benzodiazepines, carbamazepine, lamotrigine, primidone, warfarin, oral contraceptives, corticosteroids, cyclosporine, theophylline, chloramphenicol, rifampin, doxycycline, quinidine, mexiletine, disopyramide, dopamine, or nondepolarizing skeletal muscle relaxants. Serum phenytoin concentrations may be decreased by rifampin, cisplatin, vinblastine, bleomycin, and folic acid.

Increased Effect/Toxicity: Phenytoin may increase phenobarbital and primidone levels. Protein binding of phenytoin can be affected by valproic acid or salicylates. Serum phenytoin concentrations may be increased by cimetidine, felbamate, ethosuximide, methsuximide, chloramphenicol, disulfiram, fluconazole, omeprazole, isoniazid, trimethoprim, or sulfonamides.

Effects on Lab Values May decrease serum concentrations of thyroxine; may produce artifactually low results in dexamethasone or metyrapone tests; may cause increased serum concentrations of glucose, alkaline phosphatase, and gamma glutamyl transpeptidase (GGT)

(Continued)

Fosphenytoin *(Continued)*

Adverse Reactions The more important adverse clinical events caused by the I.V. use of fosphenytoin or phenytoin are cardiovascular collapse and/or central nervous system depression. Hypotension can occur when either drug is administered rapidly by the I.V. route. Do not exceed a rate of 150 mg phenytoin equivalent/minute when administering fosphenytoin.

The adverse clinical events most commonly observed with the use of fosphenytoin in clinical trials were nystagmus, dizziness, pruritus, paresthesia, headache, somnolence, and ataxia. Paresthesia and pruritus were seen more often following fosphenytoin (versus phenytoin) administration and occurred more often with I.V. fosphenytoin than with I.M. administration. These events were dose- and rate-related (doses ≥15 mg/kg at a rate of 150 mg/minute). These sensations, generally described as itching, burning, or tingling are usually not at the infusion site. The location of the discomfort varied with the groin mentioned most frequently. The paresthesia and pruritus were transient events that occurred within several minutes of the start of infusion and generally resolved within 10 minutes after completion of infusion.

Transient pruritus, tinnitus, nystagmus, somnolence, and ataxia occurred 2-3 times more often at doses ≥15 mg/kg and rates ≥150 mg/minute.

I.V. administration (maximum dose/rate):

>10%:
- Central nervous system: Nystagmus, dizziness, somnolence, ataxia
- Dermatologic: Pruritus

1% to 10%:
- Cardiovascular: Hypotension, vasodilation, tachycardia
- Central nervous system: Stupor, incoordination, paresthesia, extrapyramidal syndrome, tremor, agitation, hypesthesia, dysarthria, vertigo, brain edema, headache
- Gastrointestinal: Nausea, tongue disorder, dry mouth, vomiting
- Ocular: Diplopia, amblyopia
- Otic: Tinnitus, deafness
- Neuromuscular & skeletal: Pelvic pain, muscle weakness, back pain
- Miscellaneous: Taste perversion

I.M. administration (substitute for oral phenytoin):

1% to 10%:
- Central nervous system: Nystagmus, tremor, ataxia, headache, incoordination, somnolence, dizziness, paresthesia, reflexes decreased
- Dermatologic: Pruritus
- Gastrointestinal: Nausea, vomiting
- Hematologic/lymphatic: Ecchymosis
- Neuromuscular & skeletal: Muscle weakness

<1% (Limited to important or life-threatening): Acidosis, acute hepatic failure, acute hepatotoxicity, alkalosis, anemia, atrial flutter, bundle branch block, cardiac arrest, cardiomegaly, cerebral hemorrhage, cerebral infarct, CHF, cyanosis, dehydration, hyperglycemia, hyperkalemia, hypertension, hypochromic anemia, hypokalemia, hypophosphatemia, ketosis, leukocytosis, leukopenia, lymphadenopathy, palpitations, postural hypotension, pulmonary embolus, QT interval prolongation, sinus bradycardia, syncope, thrombocytopenia, thrombophlebitis, ventricular extrasystoles

Overdosage/Toxicology Symptoms of fosphenytoin overdose include bradycardia, asystole, cardiac arrest, hypotension, vomiting, metabolic acidosis, and lethargy. Treatment is supportive for hypotension.

Pharmacokinetic Note See Phenytoin monograph for additional information.

Pharmacodynamics/Kinetics

Bioavailability: I.M.: 100%

Half-Life Elimination: Variable (mean: 12-29 hours); kinetics of phenytoin are saturable

Time to Peak: Conversion to phenytoin: Following I.V. administration conversion half-life is 15 minutes; following I.M. administration peak phenytoin levels are reached in 3 hours

Metabolism: Converted via hydrolysis to phenytoin

Onset: May be more rapid due to more rapid infusion

Formulations Injection, solution, as sodium: 75 mg/mL [equivalent to phenytoin sodium 50 mg/mL] (2 mL, 10 mL)

Dosing

Adults & Elderly:

Note: The dose, concentration in solutions, and infusion rates for fosphenytoin are expressed as phenytoin sodium equivalents. Fosphenytoin should always be prescribed and dispensed in phenytoin sodium equivalents.

Status epilepticus: I.V. **Only**: Loading dose: Phenytoin equivalent 15-20 mg/kg I.V. administered at 100-150 mg/minute

Nonemergent loading and maintenance dosing: I.V. or I.M.:
- Loading dose: Phenytoin equivalent 10-20 mg/kg I.V. or I.M. (max I.V. rate 150 mg/minute)
- Initial daily maintenance dose: Phenytoin equivalent 4-6 mg/kg/day I.V. or I.M.

Substitution for oral phenytoin therapy: I.V. or I.M.: May be substituted for oral phenytoin sodium at the same total daily dose, however, Dilantin® capsules are ~90% bioavailable by the oral route. Phenytoin, supplied as fosphenytoin, is 100% bioavailable by both the I.M. and I.V. routes. For this reason, plasma phenytoin concentrations may increase when I.M. or I.V. fosphenytoin is substituted for oral phenytoin sodium therapy. In clinical trials I.M. fosphenytoin was administered as a single daily dose utilizing either 1 or 2 injection sites. Some patients may require more frequent dosing.

Pediatrics:

Children 5-18 years: I.V.: A limited number of children have been studied. Seven children received a single I.V. loading dose of fosphenytoin 10-20 mg **PE**/kg for the treatment of acute generalized convulsive status epilepticus (Pellock, 1996). Some centers are using the phenytoin dosing guidelines in children and dosing fosphenytoin using **PE** doses equal to the phenytoin doses (ie, phenytoin 1 mg = fosphenytoin 1 mg **PE**). Further pediatric studies are needed.

Renal Impairment: Free phenytoin levels should be monitored closely in patients with renal disease or in those with hypoalbuminemia; furthermore, fosphenytoin clearance to phenytoin may be increased without a similar increase in phenytoin clearance in these patients leading to increase frequency and severity of adverse events.

Hepatic Impairment: Phenytoin clearance may be substantially reduced in cirrhosis and plasma level monitoring with dose adjustment advisable. Free phenytoin levels should be monitored closely in patients with hepatic disease or in those with hypoalbuminemia; furthermore, fosphenytoin clearance to phenytoin may be increased without a similar increase in phenytoin clearance in these patients leading to increase frequency and severity of adverse events.

Administration

I.M.: I.M. may be administered as a single daily dose using either 1 or 2 injection sites.

I.V.: I.V. administration rate should not exceed 150 mg/minute.

Stability

Storage: Refrigerate at 2°C to 8°C (36°F to 46°F). Do not store at room temperature for more than 48 hours. Do not use vials that develop particulate matter.

Compatibility: Stable in D_5LR, D_5½NS, D_5W, D_{10}W, hetastarch 6% in NS, mannitol 20%, LR, NS

Y-site administration: Incompatible with midazolam

Monitoring and Teaching Issues

Physical Assessment: See Use and Warnings/Precautions for use cautions. Assess all other medications patient may be taking (see Drug Interactions). Continuous monitoring is essential during infusion and for 30 minutes following infusion. Monitor closely for adverse or overdose reactions (See Adverse Reactions and Overdose/Toxicology) during and following infusion. **Pregnancy risk factor D** - determine that patient is not pregnant before beginning treatment.

Patient Education: Patients may not be in a position to evaluate their response. If conscious or alert, advise patient to report signs or symptoms of palpitations, racing or falling heartbeat, difficulty breathing, acute faintness, or CNS disturbances (eg, somnolence, ataxia), and visual disturbances. **Pregnancy precaution:** Inform prescriber if you are pregnant.

Geriatric Considerations: No significant changes in fosphenytoin pharmacokinetics with age have been noted. Phenytoin clearance is decreased in the elderly and lower doses may be needed. Elderly may have reduced hepatic clearance due to age decline in Phase I metabolism. Elderly may have low albumin which will increase free fraction and, therefore, pharmacologic response. Monitor closely in those who are hypoalbuminemic. Free fraction measurements advised, also elderly may display a higher incidence of adverse effects (cardiovascular) when using the I.V. loading regimen; therefore, recommended to decrease loading I.V. dose to 25 mg/minute.

Pregnancy Issues: Crosses placenta with fetal serum concentrations equal to those of mother. Eye, cardiac, cleft palate, and skeletal malformations have been noted. Fetal hydantoin syndrome associated with maternal ingestion of 100-800 mg/kg during 1st trimester.

Additional Information 1.5 mg fosphenytoin is approximately equivalent to 1 mg phenytoin. Equimolar fosphenytoin dose is 375 mg (75 mg/mL solution) to phenytoin 250 mg (50 mg/mL).

Fosphenytoin Sodium *see* Fosphenytoin *on page 607*

Fragmin® *see* Dalteparin *on page 357*

Frova® *see* Frovatriptan *on page 609*

Frovatriptan (froe va TRIP tan)

U.S. Brand Names Frova®

Synonyms Frovatriptan Succinate

Generic Available No

Pharmacologic Category Antimigraine Agent; Serotonin 5-$HT_{1B, 1D}$ Receptor Agonist

Pregnancy Risk Factor C

Lactation Excretion in breast milk unknown/use caution

Use Acute treatment of migraine with or without aura in adults

Mechanism of Action/Effect Blocks 5-HT_{1B} and 5-HT_{1D} receptors. Relieves symptoms of migraine by blocking vasoconstrictive and other effects of serotonin.

Contraindications Hypersensitivity to frovatriptan or any component of the formulation; patients with ischemic heart disease or signs or symptoms of ischemic heart disease (including Prinzmetal's angina, angina pectoris, myocardial infarction, silent myocardial ischemia); cerebrovascular syndromes (including strokes, transient ischemic attacks); peripheral vascular syndromes (including ischemic bowel disease); uncontrolled hypertension; use within 24 hours of ergotamine derivatives; use within 24 hours of another 5-HT_1 agonist; management of hemiplegic or basilar migraine; prophylactic treatment of migraine; severe hepatic impairment

Warnings/Precautions Not intended for migraine prophylaxis, or treatment of cluster headaches, hemiplegic or basilar migraines. Cardiac events, cerebral/subarachnoid hemorrhage, and stroke have been reported with 5-HT_1 agonist administration. Do not give to patients with risk factors for CAD until a cardiovascular evaluation has been performed. If the evaluation is satisfactory, the healthcare provider should administer the first dose and cardiovascular status should be periodically evaluated. Significant elevation in blood pressure has been reported on rare occasions in patients using other 5-HT_{1D} agonists with and without a history of hypertension. Vasospasm-related reactions have been reported other than coronary artery vasospasm. Peripheral vascular ischemia and colonic ischemia with abdominal pain and bloody diarrhea have occurred. Use with caution in patients with a history of seizure disorder. Safety and efficacy in pediatric patients have not been established. Pregnancy risk C.

(Continued)

Frovatriptan *(Continued)*

Drug Interactions

Cytochrome P450 Effect: Substrate of CYP1A2

Decreased Effect: The effects of frovatriptan may be decreased by CYP1A2 inducers (eg, carbamazepine, phenobarbital, phenytoin, ritonavir), ergotamine.

Increased Effect/Toxicity: The effects of frovatriptan may be increased by CYP1A2 inhibitors (eg, cimetidine, ciprofloxacin, erythromycin), estrogen derivatives, propranolol. Ergot derivatives may increase the effects of frovatriptan (do not use within 24 hours of each other). SSRIs may exhibit additive toxicity with frovatriptan or other serotonin agonists (eg, antidepressants, dextromethorphan, tramadol) leading to serotonin syndrome.

Nutritional/Ethanol Interactions Food: Food does not affect frovatriptan bioavailability.

Adverse Reactions

1% to 10%:

Cardiovascular: Chest pain (2%), flushing (4%), palpitation (1%)

Central nervous system: Dizziness (8%), fatigue (5%), headache (4%), hot or cold sensation (3%), anxiety (1%), dysesthesia (1%), hypoesthesia (1%), insomnia (1%), pain (1%)

Gastrointestinal: Hyposalivation (3%), dyspepsia (2%), abdominal pain (1%), diarrhea (1%), vomiting (1%)

Neuromuscular & skeletal: Paresthesia (4%), skeletal pain (3%)

Ocular: Visual abnormalities (1%)

Otic: Tinnitus (1%)

Respiratory: Rhinitis (1%), sinusitis (1%)

Miscellaneous: Diaphoresis (1%)

<1% (Limited to important or life-threatening): Abnormal dreaming, abnormal gait, abnormal lacrimation, abnormal reflexes, abnormal urine, agitation, amnesia, arthralgia, arthrosis, ataxia, back pain, bradycardia, bullous eruption, cheilitis, confusion, conjunctivitis, constipation, dehydration, depersonalization, depression, dysphagia, dyspnea, earache, EKG changes, emotional lability, epistaxis, eructation, esophagospasm, euphoria, eye pain, fever, gastroesophageal reflux, hiccup, hot flushes, hyperacusis, hyperesthesia, hypertonia, hyperventilation, hypocalcemia, hypoglycemia, hypotonia, impaired concentration, involuntary muscle contractions, laryngitis, leg cramps, malaise, micturition, muscle weakness, myalgia, nervousness, nocturia, peptic ulcer, personality disorder, pharyngitis, polyuria, pruritus, purpura, renal pain, rigors, saliva increased, salivary gland pain, speech disorder, stomatitis, syncope, tachycardia, taste perversion, thirst, tongue paralysis, toothache, tremor, unspecified pain, urinary frequency, vertigo, weakness

Overdosage/Toxicology Single oral doses of up to 100 mg have been reported without adverse effects. Treatment of overdose should be supportive and symptomatic. Monitor for at least 48 hours or until signs and symptoms subside. It is not known if hemodialysis or peritoneal dialysis is effective.

Pharmacodynamics/Kinetics

Bioavailability: 20% to 30%

Half-Life Elimination: 26 hours

Time to Peak: 2-4 hours

Metabolism: Primarily hepatic via CYP1A2

Formulations Tablet, as base: 2.5 mg

Dosing

Adults & Elderly: Migraine: Oral: 2.5 mg; if headache recurs, a second dose may be given if first dose provided some relief and at least 2 hours have elapsed since the first dose (maximum daily dose: 7.5 mg)

Renal Impairment: No adjustment necessary.

Hepatic Impairment: No adjustment necessary in mild to moderate hepatic impairment; use with caution in severe impairment

Administration

Oral: Take with fluids.

Stability

Storage: Store at room temperature of 25°C (77°F); protect from moisture and light.

Monitoring and Teaching Issues

Physical Assessment: See Contraindications, Warnings/Precautions (clear diagnosis of migraine), and Dosing for use cautions. Assess potential for interactions with other prescriptions, OTC medications, or herbal products patient may be taking (eg, ergot derivatives - see Drug Interactions). Cardiovascular status should be periodically evaluated and results of laboratory tests assessed. Assess effectiveness and adverse response (see Adverse Reactions and Overdose/Toxicology). Teach patient proper use, possible side effects and appropriate interventions, and adverse symptoms to report (see Patient Education). **Pregnancy risk factor C** - benefits of use should outweigh possible risks. Note breast-feeding caution.

Patient Education: Inform prescriber of all prescriptions (including oral contraceptives), OTC medications, or herbal products you are taking, and any allergies you have. This drug is to be used to reduce your migraine, not to prevent or reduce the number of attacks. Follow exact instructions for use. Do not take within 24 hours of any other migraine medication without first consulting prescriber. If first dose brings relief, a second dose may be taken anytime after 2 hours if migraine returns. Do not take more than three tablets (7.5 mg) in 24 hours without consulting prescriber. May cause dizziness, fatigue, insomnia, or drowsiness (use caution when driving or engaging in tasks requiring alertness until response to drug is known); dry mouth (frequent mouth care and sucking on lozenges may help); skin flushing or hot flashes (cool clothes or a cool environment may help); or mild abdominal discomfort or vomiting (small, frequent meals, good mouth care, chewing gum, or sucking lozenges may help). Report immediately any chest pain, palpitations, or irregular heartbeat; severe dizziness, acute headache, stiff or painful neck, facial swelling, muscle weakness or pain, changes in mental acuity, blurred vision, eye pain, or ringing in ears; changes in urinary pattern; difficulty breathing; or other persistent adverse effects. **Pregnancy/breast-feeding precautions:** Inform prescriber if you are or intend to become pregnant. Consult prescriber if breast-feeding.

Frovatriptan Succinate *see* Frovatriptan *on page 609*

Frusemide *see* Furosemide *on page 612*

FS Shampoo® [DSC] *see* Topical Corticosteroids *on page 1334*

5-FU *see* Fluorouracil *on page 576*

FUDR® *see* Floxuridine *on page 563*

Ful-Glo® Ophthalmic Strips *see page 1461*

Fulvestrant (fool VES trant)

U.S. Brand Names Faslodex®

Synonyms ICI 182,780

Generic Available No

Pharmacologic Category Antineoplastic Agent, Estrogen Receptor Antagonist

Pregnancy Risk Factor D

Lactation Excretion in breast milk unknown/contraindicated

Use Treatment of hormone receptor positive metastatic breast cancer in postmenopausal women with disease progression following anti-estrogen therapy.

Mechanism of Action/Effect Steroidal compound which competitively binds to estrogen receptors on tumors and other tissue targets; inhibits estrogen effects. Fulvestrant has no estrogen-receptor agonist activity. Causes down-regulation of estrogen receptors and inhibits tumor growth.

Contraindications Hypersensitivity to fulvestrant or any component of the formulation; contraindications to I.M. injections (bleeding diatheses, thrombocytopenia, or therapeutic anticoagulation); pregnancy

Warnings/Precautions Exclude pregnancy prior to use. Use caution in hepatic impairment; safety and efficacy in moderate to severe hepatic impairment have not been established. Vaginal bleeding is reported infrequently in patients receiving fulvestrant (after changing from existing hormonal therapy); if bleeding persists, consider further evaluation.

Drug Interactions

Cytochrome P450 Effect: Substrate of **CYP3A4**

Decreased Effect: Serum level of fulvestrant may be increased by enzyme-inducing agents, decreasing its therapeutic effect; potential inducers include phenobarbital, phenytoin, carbamazepine, rifampin, and rifabutin. However, a clinical study with rifampin did not demonstrate an effect on fulvestrant pharmacokinetics.

Increased Effect/Toxicity: Serum level and/or toxicity of fulvestrant may be increased by CYP3A4 inhibitors; inhibitors include amiodarone, cimetidine, clarithromycin, erythromycin, delavirdine, diltiazem, dirithromycin, disulfiram, fluoxetine, fluvoxamine, grapefruit juice, indinavir, itraconazole, ketoconazole, nefazodone, nevirapine, propoxyphene, quinupristin-dalfopristin, ritonavir, saquinavir, verapamil, zafirlukast, zileuton

Adverse Reactions

>10%:

Cardiovascular: Vasodilation (18%)

Central nervous system: Pain (19%), headache (15%)

Gastrointestinal: Nausea (26%), vomiting (13%), constipation (13%), diarrhea (12%), abdominal pain (12%)

Local: Injection site reaction (11%)

Neuromuscular & skeletal: Weakness (23%), bone pain (16%), back pain (14%)

Respiratory: Pharyngitis (16%), dyspnea (15%)

1% to 10%:

Cardiovascular: Edema (9%), chest pain (7%)

Central nervous system: Dizziness (7%), insomnia (7%), paresthesia (6%), fever (6%), depression (6%), anxiety (5%)

Dermatologic: Rash (7%)

Gastrointestinal: Anorexia (9%)

Genitourinary: Pelvic pain (10%), urinary tract infection (6%)

Hematologic: Anemia (5%)

Neuromuscular and skeletal: Arthritis (3%)

Respiratory: Cough (10%)

Miscellaneous: Increased diaphoresis (5%)

<1% (Limited to important or life-threatening): Leukopenia, myalgia, thrombosis, vaginal bleeding, vertigo

Overdosage/Toxicology No specific experience in overdose. Treatment is supportive.

Pharmacodynamics/Kinetics

Half-Life Elimination: ~40 days

Time to Peak: I.M.: ~7 days

Metabolism: Hepatic via multiple pathways (CYP3A4 substrate, relative contribution to metabolism unknown)

Duration: I.M.: Plasma levels maintained for at least 1 month

Formulations Injection, solution [prefilled syringe]: 50 mg/mL (2.5 mL, 5 mL) [contains alcohol, benzyl alcohol, benzyl stearate, castor oil]

Dosing

Adults: Metastatic breast cancer (postmenopausal women): I.M.: 250 mg at 1-month intervals

Renal Impairment: No dosage adjustment required.

Hepatic Impairment: Use in moderate to severe hepatic impairment has not been evaluated; use caution

Administration

I.M.: Administer by I.M. injection in the buttock; do not administer I.V., S.C., or intra-arterially. May be administered as a single 5 mL injection or two concurrent 2.5 mL injections.

(Continued)

Fulvestrant *(Continued)*

Stability

Storage: Store under refrigeration at 2°C to 8°C (36°F to 46°F).

Monitoring and Teaching Issues

Physical Assessment: Assess allergy history prior to beginning therapy. See Contraindications, Warnings/Precautions, and Dosing for use cautions. Assess potential for interactions with other prescriptions, OTC medications, or herbal products patient may be taking (see Drug Interactions). Assess therapeutic effects and adverse response (see Adverse Reactions and Overdose/Toxicology) on a regular basis throughout therapy. Teach patient use (if self-administered - injection technique and syringe/needle disposal), possible side effects and interventions, and adverse symptoms to report (see Patient Education). **Pregnancy risk factor D** - determine that female patient is not pregnant before beginning treatment. Do not give to women of childbearing age - approved for use only in postmenopausal women. Breast-feeding is contraindicated.

Patient Education: Inform prescriber of all prescriptions, OTC medications, or herbal products you are taking, and any allergies you have. Do not take anything new during treatment unless approved by prescriber. If self-administered, follow directions for injection and syringe/needle disposal. You may experience bone pain, back pain, or headache (consult prescriber for approved analgesic); nausea, vomiting, or loss of appetite (small, frequent meals, frequent mouth care, sucking lozenges, or chewing gum may help); dizziness (use caution when driving or engaging in tasks requiring alertness until response to drug is known); or increased perspiration. Report persistent pain; chest pain or palpitations; swelling of extremities or unusual weight gain (>5 lb/week); cough of difficulty breathing; burning on urination or changes in urinary pattern; or other persistent, unrelieved adverse effects. **Pregnancy/breast-feeding precautions**: Approved only for postmenopausal women. Severe fetal damage can occur with this drug. Do not breast-feed.

Breast-feeding Issues: Approved for use only in postmenopausal women

Pregnancy Issues: Antiestrogenic compounds have been associated with embryotoxicity, abnormalities in fetal development, and failure to maintain pregnancy in animal models. Approved for use only in postmenopausal women.

Fulvicin® P/G *see* Griseofulvin *on page 644*

Fulvicin-U/F® *see* Griseofulvin *on page 644*

Fungizone® *see* Amphotericin B (Conventional) *on page 94*

Fungoid® Tincture [OTC] *see* Miconazole *on page 899*

Furadantin® *see* Nitrofurantoin *on page 976*

Furazosin *see* Prazosin *on page 1111*

Furosemide (fyoor OH se mide)

U.S. Brand Names Lasix®

Synonyms Frusemide

Generic Available Yes

Pharmacologic Category Diuretic, Loop

Pregnancy Risk Factor C

Lactation Enters breast milk/use caution

Use Management of edema associated with congestive heart failure and hepatic or renal disease; alone or in combination with antihypertensives in treatment of hypertension

Mechanism of Action/Effect Inhibits reabsorption of sodium and chloride in the ascending loop of Henle and distal renal tubule, interfering with the chloride-binding cotransport system, thus causing increased excretion of water, sodium, chloride, magnesium, and calcium

Contraindications Hypersensitivity to furosemide, any component, or sulfonylureas; anuria; patients with hepatic coma or in states of severe electrolyte depletion until the condition improves or is corrected

Warnings/Precautions In cirrhosis, avoid electrolyte and acid/base imbalances that might lead to hepatic encephalopathy. Ototoxicity is associated with rapid I.V. administration, renal impairment, excessive doses, and concurrent use of other ototoxins. Hypersensitivity reactions can rarely occur. Monitor fluid status and renal function in an attempt to prevent oliguria, azotemia, electrolyte disturbances, dehydration, and reversible increases in BUN and creatinine. Coadministration of antihypertensives may increase the risk of hypotension. Avoid use of medications in which the toxicity is enhanced by hypokalemia (including quinolones with QT prolongation).

Chemical similarities are present among sulfonamides, sulfonylureas, carbonic anhydrase inhibitors, thiazides, and loop diuretics (except ethacrynic acid). Use in patients with sulfonylurea allergy is specifically contraindicated in product labeling, however, a risk of cross-reaction exists in patients with allergy to any of these compounds; avoid use when previous reaction has been severe.

Pregnancy risk C.

Drug Interactions

Decreased Effect: Indomethacin, aspirin, phenobarbital, phenytoin, and NSAIDs may reduce natriuretic and hypotensive effects of furosemide. Colestipol, cholestyramine, and sucralfate may reduce the effect of furosemide; separate administration by 2 hours. Furosemide may antagonize the effect of skeletal muscle relaxants (tubocurarine). Glucose tolerance may be decreased by furosemide, requiring an adjustment in the dose of hypoglycemic agents. Metformin may decrease furosemide concentrations.

Increased Effect/Toxicity: Furosemide-induced hypokalemia may predispose to digoxin toxicity and may increase the risk of arrhythmia with drugs which may prolong QT interval, including type Ia and type III antiarrhythmic agents, cisapride, and some quinolones (sparfloxacin, gatifloxacin, and moxifloxacin). The risk of toxicity from lithium and salicylates (high dose) may be increased by loop diuretics. Hypotensive effects and/or adverse renal effects of ACE inhibitors and NSAIDs are potentiated by furosemide-induced hypovolemia. The effects of peripheral adrenergic-blocking drugs or ganglionic blockers may be increased by furosemide.

Furosemide may increase the risk of ototoxicity with other ototoxic agents (aminoglycosides, cis-platinum), especially in patients with renal dysfunction. Synergistic diuretic effects occur with thiazide-type diuretics. Diuretics tend to be synergistic with other antihypertensive agents, and hypotension may occur.

Nutritional/Ethanol Interactions

Food: Furosemide serum levels may be decreased if taken with food.

Herb/Nutraceutical: Avoid dong quai if using for hypertension (has estrogenic activity). Avoid ephedra, yohimbe, ginseng (may worsen hypertension). Limit intake of natural licorice. Avoid garlic (may have increased antihypertensive effect).

Adverse Reactions Frequency not defined.

Cardiovascular: Orthostatic hypotension, necrotizing angiitis, thrombophlebitis, chronic aortitis, acute hypotension, sudden death from cardiac arrest (with I.V. or I.M. administration)

Central nervous system: Paresthesias, vertigo, dizziness, lightheadedness, headache, blurred vision, xanthopsia , fever, restlessness

Dermatologic: Exfoliative dermatitis, erythema multiforme, purpura, photosensitivity, urticaria, rash, pruritus, cutaneous vasculitis

Endocrine & metabolic: Hyperglycemia, hyperuricemia, hypokalemia, hypochloremia, metabolic alkalosis, hypocalcemia, hypomagnesemia, gout, hypernatremia

Gastrointestinal: Nausea, vomiting, anorexia, oral and gastric irritation, cramping, diarrhea, constipation, pancreatitis, intrahepatic cholestatic jaundice, ischemia hepatitis

Genitourinary: Urinary bladder spasm, urinary frequency

Hematological: Aplastic anemia (rare), thrombocytopenia, agranulocytosis (rare), hemolytic anemia, leukopenia, anemia, purpura

Neuromuscular & skeletal: Muscle spasm, weakness

Otic: Hearing impairment (reversible or permanent with rapid I.V. or I.M. administration), tinnitus, reversible deafness (with rapid I.V. or I.M. administration)

Renal: Vasculitis, allergic interstitial nephritis, glycosuria, fall in glomerular filtration rate and renal blood flow (due to overdiuresis), transient rise in BUN

Miscellaneous: Anaphylaxis (rare), exacerbate or activate systemic lupus erythematosus

Overdosage/Toxicology Symptoms of overdose include electrolyte depletion, volume depletion, hypotension, dehydration, and circulatory collapse. Treatment is supportive.

Pharmacodynamics/Kinetics

Absorption: Oral: 60% to 67%

Half-Life Elimination: Normal renal function: 0.5-1.1 hours; End-stage renal disease: 9 hours

Metabolism: Minimally hepatic

Onset: Diuresis: Oral: 30-60 minutes; I.M.: 30 minutes; I.V.: ~5 minutes; Peak effect: Oral: 1-2 hours

Duration: Oral: 6-8 hours; I.V.: 2 hours

Formulations

Injection, solution: 10 mg/mL (2 mL, 4 mL, 8 mL, 10 mL)

Solution, oral: 10 mg/mL (60 mL, 120 mL) [orange flavor]; 40 mg/5 mL (5 mL, 500 mL) [pineapple-peach flavor]

Tablet (Lasix®): 20 mg, 40 mg, 80 mg

Dosing

Adults:

Edema, CHF, or hypertension (diuresis):

Oral: 20-80 mg/dose initially increased in increments of 20-40 mg/dose at intervals of 6-8 hours; usual maintenance dose interval is twice daily or every day

I.M., I.V.: 20-40 mg/dose, may be repeated in 1-2 hours as needed and increased by 20 mg/dose with each succeeding dose up to 1000 mg/day; usual dosing interval: 6-12 hours

Continuous I.V. infusion: Initial I.V. bolus dose of 0.1 mg/kg followed by continuous I.V. infusion doses of 0.1 mg/kg/hour doubled every 2 hours to a maximum of 0.4 mg/kg/hour if urine output is <1 mL/kg/hour have been found to be effective and result in a lower daily requirement of furosemide than with intermittent dosing. Other studies have used 20-160 mg/hour continuous I.V. infusion.

Elderly: Oral, I.M., I.V.: Initial: 20 mg/day; increase slowly to desired response.

Pediatrics: Edema, CHF, or hypertension (diuresis): Infants and Children:

Oral: 1-2 mg/kg/dose increased in increments of 1 mg/kg/dose with each succeeding dose until a satisfactory effect is achieved to a maximum of 6 mg/kg/dose no more frequently than 6 hours

I.M., I.V.: 1 mg/kg/dose, increasing by each succeeding dose at 1 mg/kg/dose at intervals of 6-12 hours until a satisfactory response up to 6 mg/kg/dose

Renal Impairment:

Acute renal failure: Doses up to 1-3 g/day may be necessary to initiate desired response; avoid use in oliguric states.

Not removed by hemo- or peritoneal dialysis; supplemental dose is not necessary.

Hepatic Impairment: Diminished natriuretic effect with increased sensitivity to hypokalemia and volume depletion in cirrhosis. Monitor effects, particularly with high doses.

Administration

I.V.: I.V. injections should be given slowly over 1-2 minutes; maximum rate of administration for IVPB or infusion: 4 mg/minute; replace parenteral therapy with oral therapy as soon as possible

Stability

Storage: Furosemide injection should be stored at controlled room temperature and protected from light. Exposure to light may cause discoloration. Do not use furosemide solutions if they have a yellow color. Refrigeration may result in precipitation or crystallization, however, resolubilization at room temperature or warming may be performed without affecting the drugs stability.

Reconstitution: I.V. infusion solution mixed in NS or D_5W solution is stable for 24 hours at room temperature.

(Continued)

Furosemide *(Continued)*

Compatibility: Stable in D_5LR, D_5NS, D_5W, $D_{10}W$, $D_{20}W$, mannitol 20%, LR, NS

Y-site administration: Incompatible with alatrofloxacin, amiodarone, amsacrine, chlorpromazine, ciprofloxacin, clarithromycin, diltiazem, droperidol, esmolol, filgrastim, fluconazole, gatifloxacin, gemcitabine, gentamicin, hydralazine, idarubicin, levofloxacin, metoclopramide, midazolam, milrinone, netilmicin, nicardipine, ondansetron, quinidine gluconate, thiopental, vecuronium, vinblastine, vincristine, vinorelbine

Compatibility in syringe: Incompatible with doxapram, doxorubicin, droperidol, metoclopramide, milrinone, vinblastine, vincristine

Compatibility when admixed: Incompatible with buprenorphine, chlorpromazine, diazepam, dobutamine, erythromycin lactobionate, isoproterenol, meperidine, metoclopramide, netilmicin, prochlorperazine edisylate, promethazine

Monitoring Laboratory Tests Serum electrolytes, renal function

Monitoring and Teaching Issues

Physical Assessment: Assess for allergy to sulfonylurea before beginning therapy. See Contraindications, Warnings/Precautions, and Dosing for use cautions. Assess potential for interactions with other prescriptions, OTC medications, or herbal products patient may be taking (especially anything that may impact fluid balance or increase potential for ototoxicity or hypotension- see Drug Interactions). **I.V.:** See specific directions above. Assess results of laboratory tests, therapeutic effectiveness, and adverse response on a regular basis during therapy (eg, dehydration, electrolyte imbalance, postural hypotension - see Adverse Reactions and Overdose/Toxicology). Caution diabetics about closely monitoring glucose levels (glucose tolerance may be decreased). Teach patient appropriate use, possible side effects and appropriate interventions, and adverse symptoms to report (see Patient Education). **Pregnancy risk factor C** - benefits of use should outweigh possible risks. Note breast-feeding caution.

Patient Education: Inform prescriber of all prescriptions, OTC medications, or herbal products you are taking, and any allergies you have. Do not take anything new during treatment unless approved by prescriber. Take as directed with food or milk (to reduce GI distress) early in the day (daily), or if twice daily, take last dose in late afternoon in order to avoid sleep disturbance and achieve maximum therapeutic effect. Keep medication in original container, away from light; do not use discolored medication. Follow dietary advice of prescriber; include bananas or orange juice or other potassium-rich foods in daily diet. Do not take potassium supplements without advice of prescriber. Weigh yourself each day, at the same time, in the same clothes when beginning therapy and weekly on long-term therapy. Report unusual or unanticipated weight gain or loss. May cause dizziness, blurred vision, or drowsiness (use caution when driving or engaging in tasks that require alertness until response to drug is known); postural hypotension (use caution when rising from lying or sitting position or when climbing stairs); or sensitivity to sunlight (use sunblock or wear protective clothing and sunglasses). Report signs of edema (eg, weight gains, swollen ankles, feet or hands), trembling, numbness or fatigue, cramping or muscle weakness, palpitations, unresolved nausea or vomiting, or change in hearing. **Pregnancy/breast-feeding precautions:** Inform prescriber if you are or intend to become pregnant. Consult prescriber if breast-feeding.

Dietary Issues: This product may cause a potassium loss; your healthcare provider may prescribe a potassium supplement, another medication to help prevent the potassium loss, or recommend that you eat foods high in potassium, especially citrus fruits; do not change your diet on your own while taking this medication, especially if you are taking potassium supplements or medications to reduce potassium loss; too much potassium can be as harmful as too little; ideally, should be administered on an empty stomach; however, may be administered with food or milk if GI distress; do not mix with acidic solutions. Sodium content of 1 mL (injection): 0.162 mEq

Geriatric Considerations: Severe loss of sodium and/or increase in BUN can cause confusion. For any change in mental status in patients on furosemide, monitor electrolytes and renal function.

Breast-feeding Issues: Crosses into breast milk; may suppress lactation. AAP has NO RECOMMENDATION.

Related Information

Compatibility of Drugs *on page 1564*
Heart Failure *on page 1670*

Gabapentin (GA ba pen tin)

U.S. Brand Names Neurontin®

Generic Available No

Pharmacologic Category Anticonvulsant, Miscellaneous

Pregnancy Risk Factor C

Lactation Excretion in breast milk unknown/not recommended

Use Adjunct for treatment of partial seizures with and without secondary generalized seizures in patients >12 years of age with epilepsy; adjunct for treatment of partial seizures in pediatric patients 3-12 years of age; management of post-herpetic neuralgia (PHN) in adults

Use - Unlabeled/Investigational Bipolar disorder, social phobia; chronic pain

Mechanism of Action/Effect Exact mechanism of action is not known, but does have properties in common with other anticonvulsants; although structurally related to GABA, it does not interact with GABA receptors

Contraindications Hypersensitivity to gabapentin or any component of the formulation

Warnings/Precautions Avoid abrupt withdrawal, may precipitate seizures; may be associated with a slight incidence (0.6%) of status epilepticus and sudden deaths (0.0038 deaths/patient year); use cautiously in patients with severe renal dysfunction; rat studies demonstrated an association with pancreatic adenocarcinoma in male rats; clinical implication unknown. May cause CNS depression, which may impair physical or mental abilities. Patients must be cautioned about performing tasks which require mental alertness (ie, operating machinery or driving). Effects with other sedative drugs or ethanol may be potentiated. Pediatric patients (3-12 years of age) have shown increased incidence of CNS-related adverse effects, including emotional lability, hostility, thought disorder, and hyperkinesia. Safety and efficacy in children <3 years of age have not been established. Pregnancy risk C.

Drug Interactions

Decreased Effect: Gabapentin does not modify plasma concentrations of standard anticonvulsant medications (eg, valproic acid, carbamazepine, phenytoin, or phenobarbital). Antacids reduce the bioavailability of gabapentin by 20%.

Increased Effect/Toxicity: Cimetidine may increased gabapentin levels. Gabapentin may increase peak concentrations of norethindrone. Morphine may increase gabapentin serum concentrations.

Nutritional/Ethanol Interactions

Ethanol: Avoid ethanol (may increase CNS depression).

Food: Does not change rate or extent of absorption.

Herb/Nutraceutical: Avoid evening primrose (seizure threshold decreased). Avoid valerian, St John's wort, kava kava, gotu kola (may increase CNS depression).

Adverse Reactions

As reported in patients >12 years of age, unless otherwise noted

>10%:

Central nervous system: Somnolence (20%), dizziness (17%), ataxia (12%), fatigue (11% in adults)

Miscellaneous: Viral infection (11% in children 3-12 years)

1% to 10%:

Cardiovascular: Peripheral edema (2%)

Central nervous system: Fever (10% in children 3-12 years), hostility (8% in children 3-12 years), somnolence (8% in children 3-12 years), emotional lability (4% to 6% in children 3-12 years), fatigue (3% in children 3-12 years), abnormal thinking (2% in children and adults), amnesia (2%), depression (2%), dizziness (2% in children 3-12 years), dysarthria (2%), nervousness (2%), abnormal coordination (1%), twitching (1%)

Dermatologic: Pruritus (1%)

Gastrointestinal: Nausea/vomiting (8% in children 3-12 years), weight gain (3% in adults and children), dyspepsia (2%), dry throat (2%), xerostomia (2%), appetite stimulation (1%), constipation (1%), dental abnormalities (1%)

Genitourinary: Impotence (1%)

Hematologic: Leukopenia (1%), decreased WBC (1%)

Neuromuscular & skeletal: Tremor (7%), hyperkinesia (3% to 5% in children 3-12 years), back pain (2%), myalgia (2%)

Ocular: Nystagmus (8%), diplopia (6%), blurred vision (4%)

Respiratory: Rhinitis (4%), bronchitis (3% in children 3-12 years), pharyngitis (3%), coughing (2%), respiratory infection (2% in children 3-12 years)

<1% (Limited to important or life-threatening): Allergy, alopecia, angina pectoris, angioedema, erythema multiforme, ethanol intolerance, hepatitis, hyperlipidemia, hypertension, hyponatremia, intracranial hemorrhage, jaundice, new tumor formation/worsening of existing tumors, pancreatitis, peripheral vascular disorder, pneumonia, purpura, Stevens-Johnson syndrome, subdural hematoma, vertigo

Overdosage/Toxicology

Acute oral overdoses of up to 49 g have been reported; double vision, slurred speech, drowsiness, lethargy, and diarrhea were observed. Patients recovered with supportive care. Decontaminate using lavage/activated charcoal with cathartic. Multiple dosing of activated charcoal may be useful; hemodialysis may be useful.

Pharmacodynamics/Kinetics

Absorption: 50% to 60%

Half-Life Elimination: 5-6 hours

Formulations

Capsule: 100 mg, 300 mg, 400 mg

Solution, oral: 250 mg/5 mL (480 mL) [cool strawberry anise flavor]

Tablet: 600 mg, 800 mg

Dosing

Adults:

Anticonvulsant: Oral:

Initial: 300 mg 3 times/day, if necessary the dose may be increased up to 1800 mg/day

Maintenance: 900-1800 mg/day administered in 3 divided doses; doses of up to 2400 mg/day have been tolerated in long-term clinical studies; up to 3600 mg/day has been tolerated in short-term studies

Note: If gabapentin is discontinued or if another anticonvulsant is added to therapy, it should be done slowly over a minimum of 1 week.

Chronic pain: Oral: 300-1800 mg/day given in 3 divided doses has been the most common dosage range

Post-herpetic neuralgia: Day 1: 300 mg, Day 2: 300 mg twice daily, Day 3: 300 mg 3 times/day; dose may be titrated as needed for pain relief (range: 1800-3600 mg/day, daily doses >1800 mg do not generally show greater benefit)

Bipolar disorder: Oral: 300-3000 mg/day given in 3 divided doses

Elderly: Studies in elderly patients have shown a decrease in clearance as age increases. This is most likely due to age-related decreases in renal function; dose reductions may be needed.

Pediatrics: Anticonvulsant: Oral

Children 3-12 years: Initial: 10-15 mg/kg/day in 3 divided doses; titrate to effective dose over ~3 days; dosages of up to 50 mg/kg/day have been tolerated in clinical studies

Children 3-4 years: Effective dose: 40 mg/kg/day in 3 divided doses

Children ≥5-12 years: Effective dose: 25-35 mg/kg/day in 3 divided doses

Note: If gabapentin is discontinued or if another anticonvulsant is added to therapy, it should be done slowly over a minimum of 1 week

Children >12 years: Refer to adult dosing.

Renal Impairment: Children ≥12 years and Adults: See table on following page.

Administration

Oral: Administer first dose on first day at bedtime to avoid somnolence and dizziness. Dosage must be adjusted for renal function.

(Continued)

Gabapentin *(Continued)*

Neurontin® Dosing Adjustments in Renal Impairment

Creatinine Clearance (mL/min)	Total Daily Dose Range (mg/day)	Dosage Regimens Based on Renal Function (mg)				
≥60	900-3600	300 tid	400 tid	600 tid	800 tid	1200 tid
>30-59	400-1400	200 bid	300 bid	400 bid	500 bid	700 bid
>15-29	200-700	200 qd	300 qd	400 qd	500 qd	700 qd
15[1]	100-300	100 qd	125 qd	150 qd	200 qd	300 qd
Hemodialysis[2]		Post-Hemodialysis Supplemental Dose				
		125 mg	150 mg	200 mg	250 mg	350 mg

[1]Cl_{cr} <15 mL/minute: Reduce daily dose in proportion to creatinine clearance.

[2]Supplemental dose administered after each 4 hours of hemodialysis (maintenance doses based on renal function).

Stability

Storage: Store at 25°C (77°F); excursions permitted to 15°C to 30°C (59°F to 86°F).

Monitoring Laboratory Tests Monitor serum levels of concomitant anticonvulsant therapy. Routine monitoring of gabapentin levels is not mandatory.

Monitoring and Teaching Issues

Physical Assessment: Assess effectiveness and interactions of other medications patient may be taking (see Drug Interactions). Monitor therapeutic response, laboratory values, and adverse reactions (see Adverse Reactions) at beginning of therapy and periodically with long-term use. Taper dosage slowly when discontinuing. Assess knowledge/teach patient safety and seizure precautions, appropriate use, interventions to reduce side effects, and adverse symptoms to report (see Patient Education). **Pregnancy risk factor C** - benefits of use should outweigh possible risks. Breast-feeding is not recommended.

Patient Education: Take exactly as directed; do not increase dose or frequency. It may take 2-3 weeks to achieve desired results; may cause physical and/or psychological dependence. If prescribed once-a-day, take dose at bedtime. Do not stop medication abruptly, may lead to increased seizure activity. Avoid alcohol, caffeine, and other prescription or OTC medications not approved by prescriber. Maintain adequate hydration (2-3 L/day of fluids) unless advised by prescriber to restrict fluids. You may experience drowsiness, lightheadedness, impaired coordination, dizziness, or blurred vision (use caution when driving or engaging in tasks requiring alertness until response to drug is known); nausea, vomiting, or anorexia (small, frequent meals, frequent mouth care, chewing gum, or sucking lozenges may help); constipation (increased exercise, fluids, fruit, or fiber may help); diarrhea (buttermilk, yogurt, or boiled milk may help); postural hypotension (use caution when climbing stairs or changing position from lying or sitting to standing); or decreased sexual function or libido (reversible). Report persistent CNS effects (nervousness, restlessness, insomnia, anxiety, excitation, headache, sedation, seizures, mania, abnormal thinking); rash or skin irritation; muscle cramping, tremors, or change in gait; chest pain or palpitations; change in urinary pattern; or worsening of condition. **Pregnancy/breast-feeding precautions:** Inform prescriber if you are or intend to become pregnant. Breast-feeding is not recommended.

Dietary Issues: May be taken without regard to meals.

Geriatric Considerations: No clinical studies to specifically evaluate this drug in the elderly have been performed; however, in premarketing studies, patients >65 years of age did not demonstrate any difference in side effect profiles from younger adults. Since gabapentin is eliminated renally, dose **must** be adjusted for creatinine clearance in the elderly patient.

Breast-feeding Issues: Gabapentin is excreted in human breast milk. A nursed infant could be exposed to ~1 mg/kg/day of gabapentin; the effect on the child is not known. Use in breast-feeding women only if the benefits to the mother outweigh the potential risk to the infant.

Pregnancy Issues: No data on crossing the placenta; there have been reports of normal pregnancy outcomes, as well as respiratory distress, pyloric stenosis, and inguinal hernia following 1st trimester exposure to gabapentin plus carbamazepine; epilepsy itself, number of medications, genetic factors, or a combination of these probably influence the teratogenicity of anticonvulsant therapy. Use during pregnancy only if the potential benefit to the mother outweighs the potential risk to the fetus.

Gabitril® *see* Tiagabine *on page 1315*

Galantamine (ga LAN ta meen)

U.S. Brand Names Reminyl®

Synonyms Galantamine Hydrobromide

Generic Available No

Pharmacologic Category Acetylcholinesterase Inhibitor (Central)

Pregnancy Risk Factor B

Lactation Excretion in breast milk unknown/not recommended

Use Treatment of mild to moderate dementia of Alzheimer's disease

Mechanism of Action/Effect Increases the concentration of acetylcholine in the brain by slowing its metabolism.

Contraindications Hypersensitivity to galantamine or any component of the formulation; severe liver dysfunction (Child-Pugh score 10-15); severe renal dysfunction (Cl_{cr} <9 mL/minute)

Warnings/Precautions May exaggerate neuromuscular blockade effects of depolarizing neuromuscular-blocking agents like succinylcholine. Vagotonic effects on the SA and AV nodes may lead to bradycardia or AV block. Use caution in patients with supraventricular cardiac conduction delays (without a functional pacemaker in place) or patients taking concurrent medications that slow conduction through the SA or AV node. Use caution in peptic ulcer disease (or in patients at risk); seizure disorder; asthma; COPD; mild to moderate liver dysfunction; moderate renal dysfunction. May cause bladder outflow obstruction. Safety and efficacy in children have not been established.

Drug Interactions

Cytochrome P450 Effect: Substrate of CYP2D6, 3A4

Decreased Effect: Anticholinergic agents are antagonized by galantamine. CYP inducers may decrease galantamine levels.

Increased Effect/Toxicity: Succinylcholine: increased neuromuscular blockade. Amiodarone, beta-blockers without ISA activity, diltiazem, verapamil may increase bradycardia. NSAIDs increase risk of peptic ulcer. Cimetidine, ketoconazole, paroxetine, other CYP3A4 inhibitors, other CYP2D6 inhibitors increase levels of galantamine. Concurrent cholinergic agents may have synergistic effects. Digoxin may lead to AV block.

Nutritional/Ethanol Interactions

Ethanol: Avoid ethanol (may increase CNS adverse events).

Herb/Nutraceutical: St John's wort may decrease galantamine serum levels; avoid concurrent use.

Adverse Reactions

>10%: Gastrointestinal: Nausea (6% to 24%), vomiting (4% to 13%), diarrhea (6% to 12%)

1% to 10%:

Cardiovascular: Bradycardia (2% to 3%), syncope (0.4% to 2.2%: dose-related), chest pain (≥1%)

Central nervous system: Dizziness (9%), headache (8%), depression (7%), fatigue (5%), insomnia (5%), somnolence (4%), tremor (3%)

Gastrointestinal: Anorexia (7% to 9%), weight loss (5% to 7%), abdominal pain (5%), dyspepsia (5%), flatulence (≥1%)

Genitourinary: Urinary tract infection (8%), hematuria (<1% to 3%), incontinence (≥1%)

Hematologic: Anemia (3%)

Respiratory: Rhinitis (4%)

<1% (Limited to important or life-threatening): Alkaline phosphatase increased, aphasia, apraxia, ataxia, atrial fibrillation, AV block, bundle branch block, convulsions, delirium, diverticulitis, dysphagia, epistaxis, esophageal perforation, heart failure, hypokinesia, hypotension, melena, palpitations, paranoid reaction, paresthesia, paroniria, postural hypotension, purpura, QT prolongation, rectal hemorrhage, renal calculi, supraventricular tachycardia, T-wave inversion, thrombocytopenia, ventricular tachycardia, vertigo

Overdosage/Toxicology Symptoms of overdose may include bradycardia, collapse, convulsions, defecation, gastrointestinal cramping, hypotension, lacrimation, muscle fasciculations, muscle weakness, QT prolongation, respiratory depression, salivation, severe nausea, sweating, torsade de pointes, urination, ventricular tachycardia, vomiting. Treatment is symptom-directed and supportive. Atropine may be used as an antidote; initial dose 0.5-1 mg I.V. and titrate to effect. An atypical response in blood pressure and heart rate has been reported. Effects of hemodialysis are unknown.

Pharmacodynamics/Kinetics

Absorption: Rapid and complete

Bioavailability: 80% to 100%

Half-Life Elimination: 6-8 hours

Time to Peak: 1 hour

Metabolism: Hepatic; linear, CYP2D6 and 3A4; metabolized to epigalanthaminone and galanthaminone both of which have acetylcholinesterase inhibitory activity 130 times less than galantamine

Duration: 3 hours; maximum inhibition of erythrocyte acetylcholinesterase ~40% at 1 hour post 10 mg oral dose; levels return to baseline at 30 hours

Formulations

Solution, oral, as hydrobromide: 4 mg/mL (100 mL) [with calibrated pipette]

Tablet, as hydrobromide: 4 mg, 8 mg, 12 mg

Dosing

Adults: Note: Take with breakfast and dinner. If therapy is interrupted for ≥3 days, restart at the lowest dose and increase to current dose.

Mild to moderate dementia of Alzheimer's: Oral: Initial: 4 mg twice a day for 4 weeks

If 8 mg per day tolerated, increase to 8 mg twice daily for ≥4 weeks

If 16 mg per day tolerated, increase to 12 mg twice daily; range: 16-24 mg/day in 2 divided doses

Elderly: No dosage adjustment needed

Renal Impairment:

Moderate renal impairment: Maximum dose: 16 mg/day.

Severe renal dysfunction (Cl_{cr} <9 mL/minute): Use is not recommended

Hepatic Impairment:

Moderate liver dysfunction (Child-Pugh score 7-9): Maximum dose: 16 mg/day

Severe liver dysfunction (Child-Pugh score 10-15): Use is not recommended

Administration

Oral: Take with breakfast and dinner. If therapy is interrupted for ≥3 days, restart at the lowest dose and increase to current dose as patient tolerates. If using oral solution, mix dose with 3-4 ounces of any nonalcoholic beverage; mix well and drink immediately.

Stability

Storage: Store at 15°C to 30°C (59°F to 86°F). Do not freeze oral solution; protect from light.

Monitoring and Teaching Issues

Physical Assessment: Assess bladder and sphincter adequacy prior to starting therapy. Assess other medications patient may be taking for effectiveness and interactions (especially those dependent on cytochrome P450 metabolism - see Drug Interactions). See Contraindications and Warnings/Precautions for use cautions. Monitor effectiveness of therapeutic response and adverse reactions at beginning of therapy and periodically throughout therapy (eg, cholinergic crisis - see Adverse Reactions and Overdose/Toxicology). Assess knowledge/teach appropriate use, interventions to reduce side effects, and adverse symptoms to report (see Patient Education). Breast-feeding is not recommended.

(Continued)

Galantamine *(Continued)*

Patient Education: This medication will not cure Alzheimer's disease, but may help reduce symptoms. Use exactly as directed; do not increase dose or discontinue without consulting prescriber. Maintain adequate hydration (2-3 L/day of fluids) unless advised by prescriber to restrict fluids. May cause dizziness, sedation, hypotension, or tremor (use caution when driving or engaging in hazardous tasks, rise slowly from sitting or lying position, and use caution when climbing stairs until response to drug is known); diarrhea (boiled milk, yogurt, or buttermilk may help); or nausea or vomiting (small, frequent meals, good mouth care, sucking lozenges, or chewing gum may help). Report persistent GI disturbances; significantly increased salivation, sweating, or tearing; excessive fatigue, insomnia, dizziness, or depression; increased muscle, joint, or body pain or spasms; vision changes; respiratory changes, wheezing, or signs of dyspnea; chest pain or palpitations; or other adverse reactions. **Breast-feeding precaution:** Breast-feeding is not recommended.

Dietary Issues: Take with breakfast and dinner.

Pregnancy Issues: In animal studies, there was a slight increased in the incident of skeletal variations when given during organogenesis. Adequate, well-controlled studies in pregnant women do not exist. Should be used in pregnancy only if benefit outweighs potential risk to the fetus.

Galantamine Hydrobromide *see* Galantamine *on page 616*

Gamimune® N *see* Immune Globulin (Intravenous) *on page 703*

Gamma Benzene Hexachloride *see* Lindane *on page 805*

Gammagard® S/D *see* Immune Globulin (Intravenous) *on page 703*

Gammaphos *see* Amifostine *on page 74*

Gammar®-P I.V. *see* Immune Globulin (Intravenous) *on page 703*

Gamulin® Rh *see page 1498*

Ganciclovir (gan SYE kloe veer)

U.S. Brand Names Cytovene®; Vitrasert®

Synonyms DHPG Sodium; GCV Sodium; Nordeoxyguanosine

Generic Available No

Pharmacologic Category Antiviral Agent

Pregnancy Risk Factor C

Lactation Excretion in breast milk unknown/contraindicated

Use

Parenteral: Treatment of CMV retinitis in immunocompromised individuals, including patients with acquired immunodeficiency syndrome; prophylaxis of CMV infection in transplant patients; may be given in combination with foscarnet in patients who relapse after monotherapy with either drug

Oral: Alternative to the I.V. formulation for maintenance treatment of CMV retinitis in immunocompromised patients, including patients with AIDS, in whom retinitis is stable following appropriate induction therapy and for whom the risk of more rapid progression is balanced by the benefit associated with avoiding daily I.V. infusions.

Implant: Treatment of CMV retinitis

Mechanism of Action/Effect Ganciclovir is phosphorylated to a substrate which competitively inhibits the binding of deoxyguanosine triphosphate to DNA polymerase resulting in inhibition of viral DNA synthesis.

Contraindications Hypersensitivity to ganciclovir, acyclovir, or any component of the formulation; absolute neutrophil count $<500/mm^3$; platelet count $<25,000/mm^3$

Warnings/Precautions Dosage adjustment or interruption of ganciclovir therapy may be necessary in patients with neutropenia and/or thrombocytopenia and patients with impaired renal function. Use with extreme caution in children since long-term safety has not been determined and due to ganciclovir's potential for long-term carcinogenic and adverse reproductive effects. Ganciclovir may adversely affect spermatogenesis and fertility. Due to its mutagenic potential, contraceptive precautions for female and male patients need to be followed during and for at least 90 days after therapy with the drug. Take care to administer only into veins with good blood flow. Pregnancy risk C.

Drug Interactions

Decreased Effect: A decrease in blood levels of ganciclovir AUC may occur when used with didanosine.

Increased Effect/Toxicity: Immunosuppressive agents may increase hematologic toxicity of ganciclovir. Imipenem/cilastatin may increase seizure potential. Oral ganciclovir increases blood levels of zidovudine, although zidovudine decreases steady-state levels of ganciclovir. Since both drugs have the potential to cause neutropenia and anemia, some patients may not tolerate concomitant therapy with these drugs at full dosage. Didanosine levels are increased with concurrent ganciclovir. Other nephrotoxic drugs (eg, amphotericin and cyclosporine) may have additive nephrotoxicity with ganciclovir.

Adverse Reactions

>10%:

Central nervous system: Fever (38% to 48%)

Dermatologic: Rash (15% oral, 10% I.V.)

Gastrointestinal: Abdominal pain (17% to 19%), diarrhea (40%), nausea (25%), anorexia (15%), vomiting (13%)

Hematologic: Anemia (20% to 25%), leukopenia (30% to 40%)

1% to 10%:

Central nervous system: Confusion, neuropathy (8% to 9%), headache (4%)

Dermatologic: Pruritus (5%)

Hematologic: Thrombocytopenia (6%), neutropenia with ANC $<500/mm^3$ (5% oral, 14% I.V.)

Neuromuscular & skeletal: Paresthesia (6% to 10%), weakness (6%)

Ocular: Retinal detachment (8% oral, 11% I.V.; relationship to ganciclovir not established)

Miscellaneous: Sepsis (4% oral, 15% I.V.)

<1% (Limited to important or life-threatening): Alopecia, arrhythmia, ataxia, bronchospasm, coma, dyspnea, encephalopathy, eosinophilia, exfoliative dermatitis, extrapyramidal symptoms, hemorrhage, nervousness, pancytopenia, psychosis, renal failure, seizures, SIADH, Stevens-Johnson syndrome, torsade de pointes, urticaria, visual loss

Overdosage/Toxicology Symptoms of overdose include neutropenia, vomiting, hypersalivation, bloody diarrhea, cytopenia, and testicular atrophy. Treatment is supportive. Hemodialysis removes 50% of the drug. Hydration may be of some benefit.

Pharmacodynamics/Kinetics

Bioavailability: Oral: Fasting: 5%; Following food: 6% to 9%; Following fatty meal: 28% to 31%

Half-Life Elimination: 1.7-5.8 hours; prolonged with renal impairment; End-stage renal disease: 5-28 hours

Formulations

Capsule (Cytovene®): 250 mg, 500 mg

Implant, intravitreal (Vitrasert®): 4.5 mg [released gradually over 5-8 months]

Injection, powder for reconstitution, as sodium (Cytovene®): 500 mg

Dosing

Adults: Dosing is based on total body weight.

CMV retinitis:

I.V. (slow infusion):

Induction therapy: 5 mg/kg/dose every 12 hours for 14-21 days followed by maintenance therapy

Maintenance therapy: 5 mg/kg/day as a single daily dose for 7 days/week or 6 mg/kg/day for 5 days/week

Oral: 1000 mg 3 times/day with food **or** 500 mg 6 times/day with food

Prevention of CMV disease in patients with advanced HIV infection and normal renal function: Oral: 1000 mg 3 times/day with food

Prevention of CMV disease in transplant patients: Same initial and maintenance dose as CMV retinitis except duration of initial course is 7-14 days, duration of maintenance therapy is dependent on clinical condition and degree of immunosuppression

CMV implant: Intravitreally: One implant for 5- to 8-month period; following depletion of ganciclovir, as evidenced by progression of retinitis, implant may be removed and replaced

Elderly: Refer to adult dosing. In general, dose selection should be cautious, reflecting greater frequency of organ impairment.

Pediatrics: CMV retinitis: Children >3 months: Refer to adult dosing.

Renal Impairment:

I.V. (Induction):

Cl_{cr} 50-69 mL/minute: Administer 2.5 mg/kg/dose every 12 hours.

Cl_{cr} 25-49 mL/minute: Administer 2.5 mg/kg/dose every 24 hours.

Cl_{cr} 10-24 mL/minute: Administer 1.25 mg/kg/dose every 24 hours.

Cl_{cr} <10 mL/minute: Administer 1.25 mg/kg/dose 3 times/week following hemodialysis.

I.V. (Maintenance):

Cl_{cr} 50-69 mL/minute: Administer 2.5 mg/kg/dose every 24 hours.

Cl_{cr} 25-49 mL/minute: Administer 1.25 mg/kg/dose every 24 hours.

Cl_{cr} 10-24 mL/minute: Administer 0.625 mg/kg/dose every 24 hours

Cl_{cr} <10 mL/minute: Administer 0.625 mg/kg/dose 3 times/week following hemodialysis.

Oral:

Cl_{cr} 50-69 mL/minute: Administer 1500 mg/day or 500 mg 3 times/day.

Cl_{cr} 25-49 mL/minute: Administer 1000 mg/day or 500 mg twice daily.

Cl_{cr} 10-24 mL/minute: Administer 500 mg/day.

Cl_{cr} <10 mL/minute: Administer 500 mg 3 times/week following hemodialysis.

Hemodialysis effects: Dialyzable (50%) following hemodialysis; administer dose postdialysis. During peritoneal dialysis, dose as for Cl_{cr} <10 mL/minute. During continuous arteriovenous or venovenous hemofiltration, administer 2.5 mg/kg/dose every 24 hours.

Administration

Oral: Oral ganciclovir should be administered with food.

I.V.: The same precautions utilized with antineoplastic agents should be followed with ganciclovir administration. Ganciclovir should not be administered by I.M., S.C., or rapid IVP. Administer by slow I.V. infusion over at least 1 hour at a final concentration for administration not to exceed 10 mg/mL. Too rapid infusion can cause increased toxicity and excessive plasma levels.

Stability

Storage: Intact vials should be stored at room temperature and protected from temperatures >40°C.

Reconstitution: Preparation should take place in a vertical laminar flow hood with the same precautions as antineoplastic agents. Drug product should be reconstituted immediately before use and any unused portion should be discarded appropriately. Reconstitute powder with sterile water **not** bacteriostatic water because parabens may cause precipitation. Reconstituted solution is stable for 12 hours at room temperature, however, conflicting data indicates that reconstituted solution is stable for 60 days under refrigeration (4°C). Stability of parenteral admixture at room temperature (25°C) and at refrigeration temperature (4°C) is 5 days.

Compatibility: Stable in D_5W, LR, NS; **incompatible** with bacteriostatic water for injection (contains parabens and may cause precipitation)

Y-site administration: Incompatible with aldesleukin, amifostine, amsacrine, aztreonam, cefepime, cytarabine, doxorubicin, fludarabine, foscarnet, gemcitabine, ondansetron, piperacillin/tazobactam, sargramostim, vinorelbine

Monitoring Laboratory Tests CBC with differential and platelet count, serum creatinine before beginning therapy and on a regular basis thereafter; liver function tests

Monitoring and Teaching Issues

Physical Assessment: See Contraindications, Warnings/Precautions, Drug Interactions, and Dosing for use cautions. Assess potential for interactions with other prescriptions, OTC

(Continued)

Ganciclovir *(Continued)*

medications, or herbal products patient may be taking (see Drug Interactions). **I.V.:** See Administration, Reconstitution, and Compatibility. Assess results of laboratory tests (see Monitoring Lab Tests), therapeutic effects, and adverse response (eg, paresthesia, neutropenia, anemia, nephrotoxicity, retinal detachment - see Adverse Reactions and Overdose/ Toxicology). Teach possible side effects and appropriate interventions and adverse symptoms to report (see Patient Education). **Pregnancy risk factor C** - ganciclovir may adversely affect spermatogenesis and fertility. Due to its mutagenic potential, contraceptive precautions for both female and male patients need to be followed during and for at least 90 days after therapy with the drug. Instruct patients in appropriate barrier contraceptive measures. Breast-feeding is contraindicated.

Patient Education: Inform prescriber of all prescriptions, OTC medications, or herbal products you are taking, and any allergies you have. Do not take anything new during treatment unless approved by prescriber. Ganciclovir is not a cure for CMV retinitis. For oral administration, take as directed and maintain adequate hydration (2-3 L/day of fluids) unless advised by prescriber to restrict fluids. You will need frequent blood tests and regular ophthalmic exams while taking this drug. You may experience increased susceptibility to infection (avoid crowds and exposure to infection and do not have any vaccinations without consulting prescriber). You may experience confusion or headache (use cautions when driving or engaging in potentially hazardous tasks until response to drug is known); nausea, vomiting, or anorexia (small, frequent meals, frequent mouth care, chewing gum, or sucking lozenges may help); diarrhea (buttermilk, boiled milk, or yogurt may help); or photosensitivity (use sunscreen, wear protective clothing and eyewear, and avoid direct sunlight). Report rash, infection (fever, chills, unusual bleeding or bruising, infection, or unhealed sores or white plaques in mouth); abdominal pain; tingling, weakness, or pain in extremities; any vision changes; or pain, redness, swelling at injection site. **Pregnancy/ breast-feeding precautions**: Inform prescriber if you are pregnant. Males and females should use appropriate barrier contraceptive measures during and for 60-90 days following end of therapy. Consult prescriber for appropriate barrier contraceptive measures. Do not breast-feed.

Dietary Issues: Sodium content of 500 mg vial: 46 mg

Geriatric Considerations: Adjust dose based upon renal function.

Breast-feeding Issues: The CDC recommends **not** to breast-feed if diagnosed with HIV to avoid postnatal transmission of the virus.

Ganirelix (ga ni REL ix)

U.S. Brand Names Antagon®

Synonyms Ganirelix Acetate

Generic Available No

Pharmacologic Category Antigonadotropic Agent

Pregnancy Risk Factor X

Lactation Excretion in breast milk unknown/not recommended

Use Inhibits premature luteinizing hormone (LH) surges in women undergoing controlled ovarian hyperstimulation in fertility clinics.

Mechanism of Action/Effect Suppresses gonadotropin secretion and luteinizing hormone secretion to prevent ovulation until the follicles are of adequate size.

Contraindications Hypersensitivity to ganirelix or any component of the formulation; hypersensitivity to gonadotropin-releasing hormone or any other analog; known or suspected pregnancy

Warnings/Precautions Should only be prescribed by fertility specialists. The packaging contains natural rubber latex (may cause allergic reactions). Pregnancy must be excluded before starting medication.

Drug Interactions

Decreased Effect: No formal studies have been performed.

Increased Effect/Toxicity: No formal studies have been performed.

Adverse Reactions

1% to 10%:

Central nervous system: Headache (3%)

Endocrine & metabolic: Ovarian hyperstimulation syndrome (2%)

Gastrointestinal: Abdominal pain (5%), nausea (1%), and abdominal pain (1%)

Genitourinary: Vaginal bleeding (2%)

Local: Injection site reaction (1%)

<1% (Limited to important or life-threatening): Congenital abnormalities

Pharmacodynamics/Kinetics

Absorption: S.C.: Rapid

Bioavailability: 91.1%

Half-Life Elimination: 16.2 hours

Time to Peak: 1.1 hours

Metabolism: Hepatic to two primary metabolites (1-4 and 1-6 peptide)

Formulations Injection, solution, as acetate [prefilled glass syringe]: 250 mcg/0.5 mL [with 27-gauge x $^1/_2$ inch needle]

Dosing

Adults & Elderly: Adjunct to controlled ovarian hyperstimulation: S.C.: 250 mcg/day during the mid-to-late phase after initiating follicle-stimulating hormone on day 2 or 3 of cycle. Treatment should be continued daily until the day of chorionic gonadotropin administration.

Stability

Storage: Store at controlled room temperature of 15°C to 30°C (59°F to 86°F).

Monitoring Laboratory Tests Ultrasound to assess the follicle's size

Monitoring and Teaching Issues

Physical Assessment: This medication should only be prescribed by a fertility specialist. Assess/teach patient use (demonstrate injection procedures, syringe disposal), interventions to reduce side-effects, and adverse reactions to report (see Adverse Reactions).

Pregnancy risk factor X - pregnancy must be excluded before starting medication. Breast-feeding is not recommended.

Patient Education: This drug can only be given by injection as demonstrated. Use this and any other medications as directed by prescriber; do not skip any doses. You must keep all scheduled ultrasound appointments. You may experience headache (use of mild analgesic may help); or nausea (small, frequent meals, good mouth care, chewing gum, or sucking hard candy may help). Report immediately any sudden or acute abdominal pain; vaginal bleeding; or pain, itching, or signs of infection at injection site. **Note:** Packaging contains natural rubber latex; if you have a known latex allergy advise prescriber. **Pregnancy/breast-feeding precautions:** Do not get pregnant while taking this drug. Breast-feeding is not recommended.

Pregnancy Issues: Fetal resorption occurred in pregnant rats and rabbits. These effects are results of hormonal alterations and could result in fetal loss in humans. The drug should not be used in pregnant women.

Ganirelix Acetate *see* Ganirelix *on page 620*

Gani-Tuss® NR *see* Guaifenesin and Codeine *on page 647*

Gantanol® *see* Sulfamethoxazole *on page 1258*

Gantrisin® *see* SulfiSOXAZOLE *on page 1264*

Garamycin®*see page 1509*

Garamycin® *see* Gentamicin *on page 628*

Gastrocrom® *see* Cromolyn Sodium *on page 334*

Gatifloxacin (ga ti FLOKS a sin)

U.S. Brand Names Tequin®

Generic Available No

Pharmacologic Category Antibiotic, Quinolone

Pregnancy Risk Factor C

Lactation Excretion in breast milk unknown/not recommended

Use Treatment of the following infections when caused by susceptible bacteria: Acute bacterial exacerbation of chronic bronchitis due to *S. pneumoniae*, *H. influenzae*, *H. parainfluenzae*, *M. catarrhalis*, or *S. aureus*; acute sinusitis due to *S. pneumoniae*, *H. influenzae*; community-acquired pneumonia due to *S. pneumoniae*, *H. influenzae*, *H. parainfluenzae*, *M. catarrhalis*, *S. aureus*, *M. pneumoniae*, *C. pneumoniae*, or *L. pneumophilia*; uncomplicated skin and skin structure infection due to *S. aureus* or *S. pyogenes;* uncomplicated urinary tract infections (cystitis) due to *E. coli*, *K. pneumoniae*, or *P. mirabilis*; complicated urinary tract infections due to *E. coli*, *K. pneumoniae*, or *P. mirabilis*; pyelonephritis due to *E. coli*; uncomplicated urethral and cervical gonorrhea; acute, uncomplicated rectal infections in women due to *N. gonorrhoeae*

Mechanism of Action/Effect Inhibits bacterial DNA

Contraindications Hypersensitivity to gatifloxacin, other quinolone antibiotics, or any component of the formulation; known prolongation of QT interval, uncorrected hypokalemia, or concurrent administration of other medications known to prolong the QT interval (including Class Ia and Class III antiarrhythmics, cisapride, erythromycin, antipsychotics, and tricyclic antidepressants)

Warnings/Precautions Use with caution in patients with significant bradycardia (or receiving drugs which may cause bradycardia), acute myocardial ischemia, cardiovascular disease (especially with conduction disturbances), or individuals at risk of seizures (CNS disorders or concurrent therapy with medications which may lower seizure threshold). May cause increased CNS stimulation, increased intracranial pressure, convulsions, or psychosis. Discontinue in patients who experience significant CNS adverse effects (dizziness, hallucinations, suicidal ideation or actions), cardiovascular adverse effects (QT prolongation, arrhythmia) or hypersensitivity reactions. Use caution in renal dysfunction and severe hepatic insufficiency. Use caution in individuals with diabetes (glucose regulation may be altered); monitor closely and discontinue if hyper- or hypoglycemia occur. Quinolones may exacerbate myasthenia gravis.

Pseudomembranous colitis should be considered in all patients with diarrhea. Tendon inflammation and/or rupture has been reported with this and other quinolone antibiotics. Risk may be increased with concurrent corticosteroids, particularly in the elderly. Discontinue at first sign of tendon inflammation or pain. Safety and effectiveness in pediatric patients (<18 years) have not been established (animal data indicate a risk of permanent arthropathy).

Pregnancy risk C.

Drug Interactions

Decreased Effect: Metal cations (magnesium, aluminum, iron, and zinc) inhibit intestinal absorption of gatifloxacin (by up to 98%). Antacids, electrolyte supplements, sucralfate, quinapril, and some didanosine formulations should be avoided. Gatifloxacin should be administered 4 hours before or 8 hours after these agents. Calcium carbonate was not found to alter the absorption of gatifloxacin. Antineoplastic agents, H_2 antagonists, and proton pump inhibitors may also decrease absorption of some quinolones. Gatifloxacin may alter glucose control in patients receiving hypoglycemic agents with or without insulin.

Increased Effect/Toxicity: Drugs which prolong QT interval (including Class Ia and Class III antiarrhythmics, erythromycin, cisapride, antipsychotics, and cyclic antidepressants) are contraindicated with gatifloxacin. Drugs which may induce bradycardia (eg, beta-blockers, amiodarone) should be avoided, Probenecid, loop diuretics, and cimetidine (possibly other H_2 antagonists) may increase the serum concentrations of gatifloxacin (based on experience with other quinolones). Digoxin levels may be increased in some patients by gatifloxacin. NSAIDs and foscarnet have been associated with an increased risk of seizures with some quinolones (not reported with gatifloxacin). The hypoprothrombinemic effect of warfarin is enhanced by some quinolone antibiotics. Monitoring of the INR during concurrent therapy is recommended by the manufacturer. Gatifloxacin may alter glucose control in patients receiving hypoglycemic agents with or without insulin. Concurrent use of corticosteroids may increase risk of tendon rupture.

(Continued)

Gatifloxacin *(Continued)*

Nutritional/Ethanol Interactions Herb/Nutraceutical: Avoid dong quai, St John's wort (may also cause photosensitization).

Adverse Reactions

3% to 10%:

Central nervous system: Headache (3%), dizziness (3%)

Gastrointestinal: Nausea (8%), diarrhea (4%)

Genitourinary: Vaginitis (6%)

Local: Injection site reactions (5%)

<3% (Limited to important or life-threatening): Allergic reaction, anaphylactic reaction, angioneurotic edema, ataxia, bradycardia, bronchospasm, chest pain, colitis, depersonalization, depression, dysphagia, dyspnea, ethanol intolerance, euphoria, gastrointestinal hemorrhage, hallucination, hepatitis, hyper-/hypoglycemia (severe), increased INR, increased prothrombin time, myasthenia, nonketotic hyperglycemia, palpitation, paresthesia, pseudomembranous colitis, psychosis, rash, seizures, tendon rupture, thrombocytopenia, tinnitus, torsade de pointes, vertigo, vomiting

Overdosage/Toxicology Potential symptoms of overdose may include CNS excitation, seizures, QT prolongation, and arrhythmias (including torsade de pointes). Patients should be monitored by continuous EKG in the event of an overdose. Management is supportive and symptomatic. Not removed by dialysis.

Pharmacodynamics/Kinetics

Absorption: Oral: Well absorbed

Bioavailability: 96%

Half-Life Elimination: 7.1-13.9 hours; ESRD/CAPD: 30-40 hours

Time to Peak: Oral: 1 hour

Metabolism: Only 1%; no interaction with CYP

Formulations

Injection, solution: 10 mg/mL (20 mL, 40 mL)

Injection, infusion [premixed in D_5W]: 200 mg (100 mL); 400 mg (200 mL)

Tablet: 200 mg, 400 mg

Dosing

Adults:

Acute bacterial exacerbation of chronic bronchitis: Oral, I.V.: 400 mg every 24 hours for 5 days

Acute sinusitis: Oral, I.V.: 400 mg every 24 hours for 10 days

Community-acquired pneumonia: Oral, I.V.: 400 mg every 24 hours for 7-14 days

Uncomplicated skin/skin structure infections: Oral, I.V.: 400 mg every 24 hours for 7-10 days

Uncomplicated urinary tract infections (cystitis): Oral, I.V.: 400 mg single dose or 200 mg every 24 hours for 3 days

Complicated urinary tract infections: Oral, I.V.: 400 mg every 24 hours for 7-10 days

Acute pyelonephritis: Oral, I.V.: 400 mg every 24 hours for 7-10 days

Uncomplicated urethral gonorrhea in men, cervical or rectal gonorrhea in women: Oral, I.V.: 400 mg single dose

Elderly: No dosage adjustment is required based on age, however, assessment of renal function is particularly important in this population.

Pediatrics: Safety and efficacy not established

Renal Impairment: Creatinine clearance <40 mL/minute (or patients on hemodialysis/CAPD) should receive an initial dose of 400 mg, followed by a subsequent dose of 200 mg every 24 hours. Patients receiving single-dose or 3-day therapy for appropriate indications do not require dosage adjustment. Administer after hemodialysis.

Hepatic Impairment: No dosage adjustment is required in mild-moderate hepatic disease. No data are available in severe hepatic impairment (Child-Pugh Class C).

Administration

Oral: May be administered with or without food, milk, or calcium supplements. Gatifloxacin should be taken 4 hours before supplements (including multivitamins) containing iron, zinc, or magnesium.

I.V.: For I.V. infusion only. Concentrated injection (10 mg/mL) must be diluted to 2 mg/mL prior to administration. No further dilution is required for premixed 100 mL and 200 mL solutions. Infuse over 60 minutes. Avoid rapid or bolus infusions.

Stability

Storage: Store at 25°C (77°F). Do not freeze injection.

Reconstitution: Single-use vials must be diluted to a concentration of 2 mg/mL prior to administration; do not dilute with SWFI (a hypertonic solution results). May dilute with 5% dextrose in water, 0.9% sodium chloride, 5% dextrose in water and 0.9% sodium chloride injection, lactated Ringer's and 5% dextrose injection, 5% sodium bicarbonate injection, Plasma-Lyte® 56/5% dextrose injection, or M/6 sodium lactate. Also compatible with 5% dextrose or 0.45% sodium chloride containing up to 20 mEq/L potassium chloride.

Compatibility: Stable in D_5LR, D_5W, D_5NS, 5% dextrose or 0.45% sodium chloride containing up to 20 mEq/L potassium chloride, M/6 sodium lactate, NS, Plasma-Lyte® 56/5% dextrose injection, 5% sodium bicarbonate injection; **incompatible** with SWFI (results in a hypertonic solution)

Y-site administration: Incompatible with amphotericin B, amphotericin B cholesteryl sulfate complex, cefoperazone, cefoxitin, diazepam, furosemide, heparin, phenytoin, piperacillin, piperacillin/tazobactam, potassium phosphates, vancomycin

Monitoring Laboratory Tests WBC

Monitoring and Teaching Issues

Physical Assessment: Assess allergy history before initiating therapy. See Contraindications, Warnings/Precautions, and Dosing for use cautions. Assess potential for interactions with other prescriptions, OTC medications, or herbal products patient may be taking (see Drug Interactions). **I.V.:** See Administration, Reconstitution, and Compatibility. Patient must be monitored closely during and after infusion for immediate allergic reaction. Assess results of laboratory tests (see above), therapeutic effectiveness, and adverse effects (eg, changes in CNS, especially in elderly patients - see Adverse Reactions and Overdose/Toxicology) regularly during therapy. Teach patient appropriate use (oral), possible side effects and interventions, and adverse symptoms to report (see Patient Education). **Pregnancy risk factor C** - benefits of use should outweigh possible risks. Breast-feeding is not recommended.

Patient Education: Inform prescriber of all prescriptions, OTC medications, or herbal products you are taking, and any allergies you have. Do not take anything new without consulting prescriber. Avoid alcohol.

I.V.: Report any pain, itching, burning, or signs of irritation at infusion site.

Oral: Take exactly as directed with or without food. Take 4 hours before antacids or mineral supplements (iron, magnesium, or zinc). Do not miss a dose (take a missed dose as soon as possible unless it is almost time for next dose). Take entire prescription even if feeling better. Maintain adequate hydration (2-3 L/day of fluids) unless advised by prescriber to restrict fluids. May cause nausea, vomiting, taste perversion (small, frequent meals, good mouth care, chewing gum, or sucking hard candy may help); or headache, dizziness, insomnia, anxiety (use caution when driving or engaging in tasks requiring alertness until response is known). Report immediately any change in CNS (dizziness, insomnia, hallucinations, suicidal ideation or actions); rash or itching; difficulty breathing or swallowing; tendon pain; swelling of mouth, lips, tongue, or throat; chest pain or tightness; or back pain, Report changes in voiding pattern, vaginal itching, burning, or discharge; vision changes or hearing; abnormal bruising or bleeding or blood in urine; or other adverse reactions. **Pregnancy/breast-feeding precautions:** Inform prescriber if you are or intend to become pregnant. Breast-feeding is not recommended.

Dietary Issues: May take with or without food, milk, or calcium supplements. Gatifloxacin should be taken 4 hours before supplements (including multivitamins) containing iron, zinc, or magnesium.

G-CSF *see* Filgrastim *on page 558*

GCV Sodium *see* Ganciclovir *on page 618*

Gelatin, Absorbable *see page 1461*

Gelfilm® Ophthalmic *see page 1461*

Gelfoam® Topical *see page 1461*

Gemcitabine (jem SIT a been)

U.S. Brand Names Gemzar®

Synonyms Gemcitabine Hydrochloride

Generic Available No

Pharmacologic Category Antineoplastic Agent, Antimetabolite

Pregnancy Risk Factor D

Lactation Excretion in breast milk unknown/contraindicated

Use Adenocarcinoma of the pancreas; first-line therapy for patients with locally advanced (nonresectable stage II or stage III) or metastatic (stage IV) adenocarcinoma of the pancreas (indicated for patients previously treated with 5-FU); combination with cisplatin for the first-line treatment of patients with inoperable, locally advanced (stage IIIA or IIIB) or metastatic (stage IV) nonsmall-cell lung cancer

Mechanism of Action/Effect Nucleoside analogue that primarily kills cells undergoing DNA synthesis (S-phase) and blocks the progression of cells through the G1/S-phase boundary

Contraindications Hypersensitivity to gemcitabine or any component of the formulation; pregnancy

Warnings/Precautions The U.S. Food & Drug Administration (FDA) recommends that procedures for proper handling and disposal of antineoplastic agents be considered. Prolongation of the infusion time >60 minutes and more frequent than weekly dosing have been shown to increase toxicity. Gemcitabine can suppress bone marrow function manifested by leukopenia, thrombocytopenia and anemia, and myelosuppression is usually the dose-limiting ototoxicity. May cause fever in the absence of clinical infection. Use with caution in patients with pre-existing renal impairment and hepatic impairment Accidental exposure to skin should be thoroughly washed with soap and water immediately.

Drug Interactions

Decreased Effect: No confirmed interactions have been reported. No specific drug interaction studies have been conducted.

Nutritional/Ethanol Interactions Ethanol: Avoid ethanol (due to GI irritation).

Adverse Reactions

>10%:

Central nervous system: Fatigue, fever (40%), lethargy, pain (10% to 48%), somnolence (5% to 11%)

Dermatologic: Alopecia (15%); mild to moderate rashes (5% to 32%)

Endocrine & metabolic: Increased serum transaminase levels (~66%), mild, transient

Gastrointestinal: Mild nausea, vomiting, anorexia (20% to 70%); stomatitis (10% to 14%)

Hematologic: Myelosuppression (20% to 30%), primarily leukopenia, may be dose-limiting

Neuromuscular & skeletal: Weakness (15% to 25%)

Renal: Proteinuria, hematuria (45%), elevation of BUN

Respiratory: Mild to moderate dyspnea (10% to 23%)

Miscellaneous: Flu-like syndrome (myalgia, fever, chills, fatigue) (20% to 100%), may be dose-limiting

1% to 10%:

Dermatologic: Pruritus (8%)

Gastrointestinal: Mild diarrhea (7%), constipation (6%)

Hematologic: Thrombocytopenia (~10%), anemia (6%)

Hepatic: Elevated bilirubin (10%)

Neuromuscular & skeletal: Paresthesia (2% to 10%), peripheral neuropathies (paresthesias, decreased tendon reflexes) (3.5%)

Respiratory: Severe dyspnea (3%)

(Continued)

Gemcitabine *(Continued)*

Miscellaneous: Allergic reactions (4%), mild, usually edema, bronchospasm

<1% (Limited to important or life-threatening): Adult respiratory distress syndrome (ARDS), hemolytic-uremic syndrome, interstitial pneumonia, pulmonary edema

Overdosage/Toxicology Symptoms of overdose include myelosuppression, paresthesia, and severe rash. The principle toxicities were seen when a single dose as high as 5700 mg/m^2 was administered by I.V. infusion over 30 minutes every 2 weeks. Monitor blood counts and administer supportive therapy as needed.

Pharmacodynamics/Kinetics

Half-Life Elimination: Infusion time: ≤1 hour: 32-94 minutes; Infusion time: 3-4 hours: 4-10.5 hours

Time to Peak: 30 minutes

Metabolism: Hepatic, metabolites: di- and triphosphates (active); uridine derivative (inactive)

Formulations Injection, powder for reconstitution, as hydrochloride: 200 mg, 1 g

Dosing

Adults & Elderly: Refer to individual protocols.

Pancreatic cancer: I.V.: 1000 mg/m^2 over 30 minutes weekly for 7 weeks followed by 1 week rest; repeat cycles 3 out of every 4 weeks.

Nonsmall cell lung cancer (in combination with cisplatin): I.V.: 1000 mg/m^2 over 30 minutes on days 1, 8, 15; repeat every 28 days **or** 1250 mg/m^2 over 30 minutes on days 1, 8; repeat every 21 days.

Dosing reductions based on hematologic function: Patients who complete an entire 7-week initial cycle of gemcitabine therapy or a subsequent 3-week cycle at a dose of 1000 mg/m^2 may have the dose for subsequent cycles increased by 25% (1250 mg/m^2), provided that the absolute granulocyte count and platelet nadirs exceed 1500 x 10^6/L and 100,000 x 10^6/L, respectively, and if nonhematologic toxicity has not been more than World Health Organization Grade 1

For patients who tolerate the subsequent course, at a dose of 1250 mg/m^2, the dose for the next cycle can be increased to 1500 mg/m^2, provided again that the AGC and platelet nadirs exceed 1500 x 10^6/L and 100,000 x 10^6/L, respectively, and again, if nonhematologic toxicity has not been greater than WHO Grade 1

Renal Impairment: Use with caution; has not been studied in patients with significant renal dysfunction.

Hepatic Impairment: Use with caution; gemcitabine has not been studied in patients with significant hepatic dysfunction.

Administration

I.V.: Administer over 30 minutes.

Stability

Storage: Store intact vials at room temperature (20°C to 25°C/68°F to 77°F). When reconstituted with preservative-free sodium chloride, the resulting solution has a concentration of 38 mg/mL **(NOT 40 mg/mL as indicated on earlier labeling).** Reconstituted vials and infusion solutions diluted in 0.9% sodium chloride are stable up to 24 hours.

Reconstitution: Reconstitute with:

200 mg vial with 5 mL 0.9% NaCl
1000 mg vial with 25 mL 0.9% NaCl

Resulting solution is approximately 38 mg/mL, but is variable. A suggestion is to withdraw the entire solution into a syringe in order to determine the final concentration. The appropriate dose may be further diluted with 0.9% sodium chloride injection to concentrations as low as 0.1 mg/mL. Do not refrigerate.

Compatibility: Stable in D_5W, NS

Y-site administration: Incompatible with acyclovir, amphotericin B, cefoperazone, cefotaxime, furosemide, ganciclovir, imipenem/cilastatin, irinotecan, methotrexate, methylprednisolone sodium succinate, mitomycin, piperacillin, piperacillin/tazobactam, prochlorperazine edisylate

Monitoring Laboratory Tests Monitor CBC, including differential and platelet count, prior to each dose. Renal and hepatic function should be performed prior to initiation of therapy and periodically thereafter.

Monitoring and Teaching Issues

Physical Assessment: See Contraindications, Warnings/Precautions, and Dosing for use cautions. See specific Administration, Reconstitution, and Storage directions. Assess results of laboratory tests (see above), therapeutic effects, and adverse response (see Adverse Reactions and Overdose/Toxicology) prior to each treatment and on a regular basis throughout therapy. Teach patient possible side effects and appropriate interventions and adverse symptoms to report (see Patient Education). **Pregnancy risk factor D** - determine that patient is not pregnant before beginning treatment. Instruct patients of childbearing age on appropriate barrier contraceptive measures. Breast-feeding is contraindicated.

Patient Education: Inform prescriber of all prescriptions, OTC medications, or herbal products you are taking, and any allergies you have. Do not take anything new during treatment unless approved by prescriber. This drug can only be administered by infusion. During therapy, do not use alcohol. Maintain adequate hydration (2-3 L/day of fluids) unless advised by prescriber to restrict fluids, and nutrition (small, frequent meals may help). You will be more susceptible to infection (avoid crowds and exposure to infection and do not have any vaccinations without consulting prescriber). You may experience fatigue, lethargy, somnolence (use caution when driving or engaging in potentially hazardous tasks until response to drug is known); nausea or vomiting (small, frequent meals, frequent mouth care, sucking lozenges, or chewing gum may help); loss of hair (reversible); mouth sores (frequent mouth care and use of a soft toothbrush or cotton swabs may help); or diarrhea (buttermilk, boiled milk, or yogurt may help reduce diarrhea). This drug may cause sterility. Report extreme fatigue; severe GI upset or diarrhea; bleeding or bruising; fever, chills, sore throat; vaginal discharge; signs of fluid retention (swelling extremities, difficulty breathing, unusual weight gain); yellowing of skin or eyes; change in color of urine or stool; or muscle or skeletal pain or weakness. **Pregnancy/breast-feeding precautions**: Inform prescriber if you are pregnant. Do not get pregnant while taking this medication. Consult prescriber for appropriate barrier contraceptives measures. This drug may cause severe fetal birth defects. Do not breast-feed.

Geriatric Considerations: Clearance is affected by age. There is no evidence; however, that unusual dose adjustment is necessary in patients older than 65 years of age. In general, adverse reaction rates were similar to patients older and younger than 65 years. Grade 3/4 thrombocytopenia was more common in the elderly.

Pregnancy Issues: It is embryotoxic causing fetal malformations (cleft palate, incomplete ossification, fused pulmonary artery, absence of gallbladder) in animals. There are no studies in pregnant women. If patient becomes pregnant she should be informed of risks.

Gemcitabine Hydrochloride *see* Gemcitabine *on page 623*

Gemfibrozil (jem FI broe zil)

U.S. Brand Names Lopid®

Synonyms CI-719

Generic Available Yes

Pharmacologic Category Antilipemic Agent, Fibric Acid

Pregnancy Risk Factor C

Lactation Excretion in breast milk unknown/contraindicated

Use Treatment of hypertriglyceridemia in types IV and V hyperlipidemia for patients who are at greater risk for pancreatitis and who have not responded to dietary intervention

Mechanism of Action/Effect Inhibits lipolysis and decreases subsequent hepatic fatty acid uptake and hepatic secretion of VLDL; decreases serum levels of VLDL and increases HDL levels

Contraindications Hypersensitivity to gemfibrozil or any component of the formulation; significant hepatic or renal dysfunction; primary biliary cirrhosis; pre-existing gallbladder disease

Warnings/Precautions Possible increased risk of malignancy and cholelithiasis. No evidence of cardiovascular mortality benefit. Anemia and leukopenia have been reported. Elevations in serum transaminases can be seen. Discontinue if lipid response not seen. Be careful in patient selection; this is not a first- or second-line choice. Other agents may be more suitable. Adjustments in warfarin therapy may be required with concurrent use. Use caution when combining gemfibrozil with HMG-CoA reductase inhibitors (may lead to myopathy, rhabdomyolysis). Renal function deterioration has been seen when used in patients with a serum creatinine >2.0 mg/dL. Safety and efficacy in pediatric patients have not been established. Pregnancy risk C.

Drug Interactions

Cytochrome P450 Effect: Substrate of CYP3A4

Decreased Effect: Cyclosporine's blood levels may be reduced during concurrent therapy. Rifampin may decreased gemfibrozil blood levels.

Increased Effect/Toxicity: Gemfibrozil may potentiate the effects of bexarotene (avoid concurrent use), sulfonylureas (including glyburide, chlorpropamide), and warfarin. HMG-CoA reductase inhibitors (atorvastatin, fluvastatin, lovastatin, pravastatin, simvastatin) may increase the risk of myopathy and rhabdomyolysis. The manufacturer warns against the concurrent use of lovastatin (if unavoidable, limit lovastatin to <20 mg/day). Combination therapy with statins has been used in some patients with resistant hyperlipidemias (with great caution).

Nutritional/Ethanol Interactions Ethanol: Avoid ethanol to decrease triglycerides.

Adverse Reactions

>10% Gastrointestinal: Dyspepsia (20%)

1% to 10%:

Central nervous system: Fatigue (4%), vertigo (2%), headache (1%)

Dermatologic: Eczema (2%), rash (2%)

Gastrointestinal: Abdominal pain (10%), diarrhea (7%), nausea/vomiting (3%), constipation (1%)

<1% (Limited to important or life-threatening): Alopecia, anaphylaxis, angioedema, bone marrow hypoplasia, cataracts, depression, dermatomyositis/polymyositis, drug-induced lupus-like syndrome, eosinophilia, exfoliative dermatitis, hypokalemia, impotence, intracranial hemorrhage, jaundice, laryngeal edema, leukopenia, myasthenia, myopathy, nephrotoxicity, pancreatitis, paresthesia, peripheral neuritis, photosensitivity, positive ANA, rash, Raynaud's phenomenon, retinal edema, rhabdomyolysis, seizures, syncope, thrombocytopenia, urticaria, vasculitis

Overdosage/Toxicology Symptoms of overdose include abdominal pain, diarrhea, nausea, and vomiting. Treatment is supportive.

Pharmacodynamics/Kinetics

Absorption: Well absorbed

Half-Life Elimination: 1.4 hours

Time to Peak: Serum: 1-2 hours

Metabolism: Hepatic via oxidation to two inactive metabolites; undergoes enterohepatic recycling

Onset: May require several days

Formulations Tablet, film coated: 600 mg

Dosing

Adults & Elderly: Hyperlipidemia/hypertriglyceridemia: Oral: 1200 mg/day in 2 divided doses, 30 minutes before breakfast and dinner

Renal Impairment: Hemodialysis effects: Not removed by hemodialysis; supplemental dose is not necessary.

Monitoring Laboratory Tests Serum cholesterol, LFTs

Monitoring and Teaching Issues

Physical Assessment: See Contraindications, Warnings/Precautions, and Dosing for use cautions. Assess potential for interactions with other prescriptions, OTC medications, or

(Continued)

Gemfibrozil *(Continued)*

herbal products patient may be taking (see Drug Interactions). Assess results of laboratory tests (see Monitoring Lab Tests), therapeutic effects, and patient response (see Adverse Reactions and Overdose/Toxicology). Teach possible proper use, side effects and appropriate interventions, and adverse symptoms to report (see Patient Education). **Pregnancy risk factor C** - benefits of use should outweigh possible risks. Breast-feeding is contraindicated.

Patient Education: Inform prescriber of all prescriptions, OTC medications, or herbal products you are taking, and any allergies you have. Do not take anything new during treatment unless approved by prescriber. Should be taken 30 minutes before meals. Take with milk or meals if GI upset occurs. Avoid alcohol. Follow dietary recommendations of prescriber. You will need check-ups and blood work to assess effectiveness of therapy. You may experience loss of appetite and flatulence (small, frequent meals may help); or diarrhea (buttermilk, boiled milk, or yogurt may help). Report severe stomach pain, nausea, vomiting; headache; persistent diarrhea; or vision changes. **Pregnancy/breast-feeding precautions**: Inform prescriber if you are or intend to become pregnant. Do not breast-feed.

Dietary Issues: Before initiation of therapy, patients should be placed on a standard cholesterol-lowering diet for 3-6 months and the diet should be continued during drug therapy.

Geriatric Considerations: Gemfibrozil is the drug of choice for the treatment of hypertriglyceridemia and hypoalphaproteinemia in the elderly; it is usually well tolerated; myositis may be more common in patients with poor renal function.

Related Information

Hyperlipidemia Management *on page 1682*
Lipid-Lowering Agents *on page 1582*

Gemtuzumab Ozogamicin (gem TUZ yu mab oh zog a MY sin)

U.S. Brand Names Mylotarg®

Generic Available No

Pharmacologic Category Antineoplastic Agent, Monoclonal Antibody

Pregnancy Risk Factor D

Lactation Excretion in breast milk unknown/not recommended

Use Treatment of acute myeloid leukemia (CD33 positive) in first relapse in patients who are ≥60 years of age and who are not considered candidates for cytotoxic chemotherapy.

Mechanism of Action/Effect Antibody to CD33 antigen, which is expressed on leukemic blasts in 80% of patients with acute myeloid leukemia (AML), as well as normal myeloid cells. Binding results in internalization of the antibody-antigen complex. Following internalization, the calicheamicin derivative is released inside the myeloid cell. The calicheamicin derivative binds to DNA resulting in double strand breaks and cell death. Pluripotent stem cells and nonhematopoietic cells are not affected.

Contraindications Hypersensitivity to gemtuzumab ozogamicin, calicheamicin derivatives, or any component of the formulation; patients with anti-CD33 antibody; pregnancy

Warnings/Precautions The U.S. Food and Drug Administration (FDA) currently recommends that procedures for proper handling and disposal of antineoplastic agents be considered. Safety and efficacy in patients with poor performance status and organ dysfunction have not been established.

Infusion-related events are common, generally reported to occur with the first dose at the end of the 2-hour intravenous infusion. These symptoms usually resolved after 2-4 hours with a supportive therapy of acetaminophen, diphenhydramine, and intravenous fluids. Fewer infusion-related events were observed after the second dose. Postinfusion reactions, which may include fever, chills, hypotension, or dyspnea, may occur during the first 24 hours after administration. **Infusion-related reactions may be severe (including anaphylaxis, pulmonary edema, or ARDS).** Symptomatic intrinsic lung disease or high peripheral blast counts may increase the risk of severe reactions. Consider discontinuation in patients who develop severe infusion-related reactions.

Severe myelosuppression occurs in all patients at recommended dosages. Use caution in patients with renal impairment (no clinical experience) and hepatic impairment (no clinical experience in patients with bilirubin >2 mg/dL). Tumor lysis syndrome may occur as a consequence of leukemia treatment, adequate hydration and prophylactic allopurinol must be instituted prior to use. Other methods to lower WBC <30,000 cells/mm^3 may be considered (hydroxyurea or leukapheresis) to minimize the risk of tumor lysis syndrome, and/or severe infusion reactions. Has been associated with severe veno-occlusive disease or hepatotoxicity (risk may be increased by combination chemotherapy, previous hepatic disease, or hematopoietic stem cell transplant).

Drug Interactions

Decreased Effect: No formal drug interaction studies have been conducted.

Increased Effect/Toxicity: No formal drug interaction studies have been conducted.

Nutritional/Ethanol Interactions Ethanol: Avoid ethanol (due to GI irritation).

Adverse Reactions Percentages established in adults >60 years of age.

>10%:

- Cardiovascular: Peripheral edema (21%), hypertension (20%), hypotension (16%)
- Central nervous system: Chills (66%), fever (80%), headache (26%), pain (25%), dizziness (11%), insomnia (18%)
- Dermatologic: Rash (23%), petechiae (21%), ecchymosis (15%)
- Endocrine & metabolic: Hypokalemia (30%), hypokalemia
- Gastrointestinal: Nausea (64%), vomiting (55%), diarrhea (38%), anorexia (31%), abdominal pain (29%), constipation (28%), stomatitis/mucositis (25%), abdominal distention (11%), dyspepsia (11%)
- Hematologic: Neutropenia (98%; median recovery 40.5 days), thrombocytopenia (99%; median recovery 39 days); anemia (47%), bleeding (15%), lymphopenia

Hepatic: Hyperbilirubinemia (23%) increased LDH (18%), increased transaminases (9% to 17%)
Local: Local reaction (25%)
Neuromuscular & skeletal: Weakness (45%), back pain (18%)
Respiratory: Dyspnea (36%), epistaxis (29%; severe 3%), cough (19%), pharyngitis (14%)
Miscellaneous: Infection (28%), sepsis (24%), neutropenic fever (20%)

1% to 10%:
Cardiovascular: Tachycardia (10%)
Central nervous system: Depression (10%), cerebral hemorrhage (2%), intracranial hemorrhage (2%)
Endocrine & metabolic: Hypomagnesemia (4%), hyperglycemia (2%)
Genitourinary: Hematuria (10%; severe 1%), vaginal hemorrhage (7%)
Hematologic: Hemorrhage (8%), disseminated intravascular coagulation (DIC) (2%)
Hepatic: Elevated PT
Neuromuscular & skeletal: Arthralgia (10%)
Respiratory: Rhinitis (10%), hypoxia (6%), pneumonia (10%), rhinitis (10%)

<1% (Limited to important or life-threatening): Acute respiratory distress syndrome, anaphylaxis, hepatic failure, hepatosplenomegaly, hypersensitivity reactions, jaundice, noncardiogenic pulmonary edema, renal failure, veno-occlusive disease

Overdosage/Toxicology Symptoms are unknown. General supportive measures should be instituted. Gemtuzumab ozogamicin is not dialyzable.

Pharmacodynamics/Kinetics

Half-Life Elimination: Calicheamicin: Total: Initial: 45 hours, Repeat dose: 60 hours; Unconjugated: 100 hours (no change noted in repeat dosing)

Formulations Injection, powder for reconstitution: 5 mg

Dosing

Adults & Elderly: Refer to individual protocols.

AML (CD33 positive in patients ≥60 years): I.V.: 9 mg/m^2, infused over 2 hours. The patient should receive diphenhydramine 50 mg and acetaminophen 650-1000 mg orally 1 hour prior to administration of each dose. Acetaminophen dosage should be repeated as needed every 4 hours for two additional doses. A full treatment course is a total of two doses administered with 14 days between doses. Full hematologic recovery is not necessary for administration of the second dose. There has been only limited experience with repeat courses of gemtuzumab ozogamicin.

Administration

I.V.: Administer as infusion only, over at least 2 hours. Do not administer I.V. push (bolus). Infuse through a separate line equipped with a low protein-binding 1.2 micron terminal filter. May be infused peripherally or through a central line. Cover with UV protective bag during infusion. Premedication with acetaminophen and diphenhydramine should be administered prior to each infusion.

Stability

Storage: Light sensitive; protect from light. Store vials under refrigeration 2°C to 8°C or 36°F to 46°F.

Reconstitution: Prepare in biologic safety hood with the fluorescent light turned **off**. Allow to warm to room temperature prior to reconstitution. Reconstitute vial with 5 mL sterile water for injection, USP. Final concentration in vial is 1 mg/mL. Dilute desired dose in 100 mL of 0.9% sodium chloride injection. The resulting I.V. bag should be placed in a UV protectant bag and infused immediately. Reconstituted vials may be stored under refrigeration for up to 8 hours.

Compatibility: No information; infuse via separate line

Monitoring Laboratory Tests Monitor vital signs during the infusion and for 4 hours following the infusion. Monitor for signs/symptoms of postinfusion reaction. Monitor electrolytes, LFTs, CBC with differential, and platelet counts frequently.

Monitoring and Teaching Issues

Physical Assessment: Note Warnings/Precautions and Contraindications for extensive use cautions. Vital signs should be monitored during and for 4 hours after infusion. Laboratory tests and monitoring of laboratory results should be done on a regular basis (see Monitoring Lab Tests). Patient should be closely monitored for adverse reactions, including postinfusion reaction (see Adverse Reactions). Assess knowledge/teach patient purpose for use, adverse reactions and interventions, and adverse reactions to report (see Patient Education). **Pregnancy risk factor D** - determine that patient is not pregnant before beginning treatment. Instruct patients of childbearing age about appropriate barrier contraceptive measures. Breast-feeding is not recommended (see Pregnancy - Issues).

Patient Education: This medication can only be administered I.V. During infusion you will be closely monitored. You will need frequent laboratory tests during course of therapy. Do not use alcohol, aspirin-containing medications, or any prescription or OTC medications without consulting your prescriber. It is important to maintain adequate hydration (2-3 L/day of fluids) unless advised by prescriber to restrict fluids, and nutrition (small, frequent meals will help). You may experience nausea or vomiting (small, frequent meals, good mouth care, sucking lozenges or chewing gum may help); contact prescriber if nausea and vomiting persists. You will be highly susceptible to infection (avoid crowds and exposure to infection). Frequent mouth care with a soft toothbrush or soft swabs and avoidance of spicy or salty foods may reduce mouth sores. Report fever, chills; unusual bleeding or bruising; signs of infection (eg, sore throat, cough, white plaques in mouth or perianal area, burning on urination); respiratory difficulties; chest pain or palpitations; yellowing of the eyes or skin; or other persistent adverse effects. **Pregnancy/breast-feeding precautions:** Inform prescriber if you are or intend to become pregnant. Breast-feeding is not recommended.

Pregnancy Issues: May cause fetal harm when administered to a pregnant woman. Women of childbearing potential should avoid becoming pregnant while receiving treatment. If used in pregnancy or if patient becomes pregnant during treatment, the patients should be apprised of potential hazard to the fetus.

Gemzar® *see* Gemcitabine *on page 623*
Genahist® [OTC] *see* DiphenhydrAMINE *on page 422*

Genapap® [OTC] *see* Acetaminophen *on page 35*
Genapap® Children [OTC] *see* Acetaminophen *on page 35*
Genapap® Extra Strength [OTC] *see* Acetaminophen *on page 35*
Genapap® Infant [OTC] *see* Acetaminophen *on page 35*
Genaphed® [OTC] *see* Pseudoephedrine *on page 1150*
Genasoft® [OTC] *see* Docusate *on page 432*
Genatuss DM® [OTC] *see* Guaifenesin and Dextromethorphan *on page 647*
Gencalc® 600 [OTC] *see* Calcium Supplements *on page 202*
Genebs® [OTC] *see* Acetaminophen *on page 35*
Genebs® Extra Strength [OTC] *see* Acetaminophen *on page 35*
Generlac *see* Lactulose *on page 767*
Geneye® *see page 1509*
Gengraf™ *see* CycloSPORINE *on page 343*
Gen-K® *see* Potassium Supplements *on page 1106*
Genoptic® *see page 1509*
Genoptic® *see* Gentamicin *on page 628*
Genoptic® S.O.P. *see page 1509*
Genotropin® *see* Human Growth Hormone *on page 658*
Genotropin Miniquick® *see* Human Growth Hormone *on page 658*
Genpril® [OTC] *see* Ibuprofen *on page 688*
Gentacidin® *see page 1509*
Gentacidin® *see* Gentamicin *on page 628*
Gentak® *see page 1509*
Gentak® *see* Gentamicin *on page 628*

Gentamicin (jen ta MYE sin)

U.S. Brand Names Garamycin®; Genoptic®; Gentacidin®; Gentak®

Synonyms Gentamicin Sulfate

Generic Available Yes

Pharmacologic Category Antibiotic, Aminoglycoside; Antibiotic, Ophthalmic; Antibiotic, Topical

Pregnancy Risk Factor C

Lactation Enters breast milk (small amounts)/use caution (AAP rates "compatible")

Use Treatment of susceptible bacterial infections, normally gram-negative organisms including *Pseudomonas*, *Proteus*, *Serratia*, and gram-positive *Staphylococcus*; treatment of bone infections, respiratory tract infections, skin and soft tissue infections, as well as abdominal and urinary tract infections, endocarditis, and septicemia; used topically to treat superficial infections of the skin or ophthalmic infections caused by susceptible bacteria; prevention of bacterial endocarditis prior to dental or surgical procedures

Mechanism of Action/Effect Bactericidal; interferes with bacterial protein synthesis resulting in cell death

Contraindications Hypersensitivity to gentamicin or other aminoglycosides

Warnings/Precautions Not intended for long-term therapy due to toxic hazards associated with extended administration. Pre-existing renal insufficiency, vestibular or cochlear impairment, myasthenia gravis, hypocalcemia, conditions which depress neuromuscular transmission.

Parenteral aminoglycosides have been associated with significant nephrotoxicity or ototoxicity. Ototoxicity may be directly proportional to the amount of drug given and the duration of treatment and may not be reversible. Tinnitus or vertigo are indications of vestibular injury and impending hearing loss. Renal damage is usually reversible.

Pregnancy risk C.

Drug Interactions

Increased Effect/Toxicity: Penicillins, cephalosporins, amphotericin B, loop diuretics may increase nephrotoxic potential. Aminoglycosides may potentiate the effects of neuromuscular blocking agents.

Effects on Lab Values ↑ protein, BUN, AST, GPT, alkaline phosphatase, serum creatinine; ↓ magnesium potassium, sodium, calcium

Adverse Reactions

>10%:
- Central nervous system: Neurotoxicity (vertigo, ataxia)
- Neuromuscular & skeletal: Gait instability
- Otic: Ototoxicity (auditory), ototoxicity (vestibular)
- Renal: Nephrotoxicity, decreased creatinine clearance

1% to 10%:
- Cardiovascular: Edema
- Dermatologic: Skin itching, reddening of skin, rash

<1% (Limited to important or life-threatening): Agranulocytosis, allergic reaction, dyspnea, granulocytopenia, photosensitivity, pseudomotor cerebri, thrombocytopenia

Overdosage/Toxicology Symptoms of overdose include ototoxicity, nephrotoxicity, and neuromuscular toxicity. Serum level monitoring is recommended. The treatment of choice, following a single acute overdose, appears to be maintenance of urine output of at least 3 mL/kg/hour during the acute treatment phase. Dialysis is of questionable value in enhancing aminoglycoside elimination.

Pharmacodynamics/Kinetics

Absorption: Oral: None

Half-Life Elimination:
- Infants: <1 week old: 3-11.5 hours; 1 week to 6 months old: 3-3.5 hours
- Adults: 1.5-3 hours; End-stage renal disease: 36-70 hours

Time to Peak: Serum: I.M.: 30-90 minutes; I.V.: 30 minutes after 30-minute infusion

Formulations

Cream, topical, as sulfate (Garamycin®): 0.1% (15 g)

Infusion, as sulfate [premixed in NS]: 40 mg (50 mL); 60 mg (50 mL, 100 mL); 70 mg (50 mL); 80 mg (50 mL, 100 mL); 90 mg (100 mL); 100 mg (50 mL, 100 mL); 120 mg (100 mL)

Injection, solution, as sulfate [ADD-Vantage® vial]: 10 mg/mL (6 mL, 8 mL, 10 mL)

Injection, solution, as sulfate: 40 mg/mL (2 mL, 20 mL) [may contain sodium metabisulfite]

Garamycin®: 40 mg/mL (2 mL) [contains sodium bisulfite]

Injection, solution, pediatric, as sulfate: 10 mg/mL (2 mL) [may contain sodium metabisulfite]

Injection, solution, pediatric, as sulfate [preservative free]: 10 mg/mL (2 mL)

Ointment, ophthalmic, as sulfate: 0.3% [3 mg/g] (3.5 g)

Ointment, topical, as sulfate (Garamycin®): 0.1% (15 g)

Solution, ophthalmic, as sulfate: 0.3% (5 mL, 15 mL) [contains benzalkonium chloride]

Garamycin®, Gentacidin®: 0.3% (5 mL) [contains benzalkonium chloride]

Genoptic®: 0.3% (1 mL, 5 mL) [contains benzalkonium chloride]

Gentak®: 0.3% (5 mL, 15 mL) [contains benzalkonium chloride]

Dosing

Adults & Elderly: Individualization is critical because of the low therapeutic index.

Note: Use of ideal body weight (IBW) for determining the mg/kg/dose appears to be more accurate than dosing on the basis of total body weight (TBW). In morbid obesity, dosage requirement may best be estimated using a dosing weight of IBW + 0.4 (TBW - IBW). Initial and periodic peak and trough plasma drug levels should be determined, particularly in critically ill patients with serious infections or in disease states known to significantly alter aminoglycoside pharmacokinetics (eg, cystic fibrosis, burns, or major surgery)

Susceptible systemic infections: I.M., I.V.:

Severe life-threatening infections: 2-2.5 mg/kg/dose every 8 hours

Urinary tract infections: 1.5 mg/kg/dose every 8 hours

Synergy (for gram-positive infections): 1 mg/kg/dose every 8 hours

High-dose, once daily regimens: Some clinicians suggest 4-7 mg/kg (as a single daily dose) for all patients with normal renal function. This dose is at least as efficacious with similar, if not less, toxicity than conventional dosing.

CNS infections:

Intrathecal: 4-8 mg/day

Prevention of bacterial endocarditis:

Dental, oral, or upper respiratory procedures: 1.5 mg/kg not to exceed 80 mg with ampicillin (1-2 g) 30 minutes prior to procedure

GI/GU surgery: 1.5 mg/kg not to exceed 80 mg with ampicillin 2 g 30 minutes prior to procedure

Ocular infections: Ophthalmic:

Ointment: Instill ½" (1.25 cm) 2-3 times/day to every 3-4 hours.

Solution: Instill 1-2 drops every 2-4 hours, up to 2 drops every hour for severe infections.

Superficial dermatologic infections: Topical: Apply 3-4 times/day to affected area.

Pediatrics: Individualization is critical because of the low therapeutic index. **Use of ideal body weight (IBW) for determining the mg/kg/dose appears to be more accurate than dosing on the basis of total body weight (TBW).** In morbid obesity, dosage requirement may best be estimated using a dosing weight of IBW + 0.4 (TBW - IBW). Initial and periodic peak and trough plasma drug levels should be determined, particularly in critically ill patients with serious infections or in disease states known to significantly alter aminoglycoside pharmacokinetics (eg, cystic fibrosis, burns, or major surgery).

CNS infections: Intrathecal:

Newborns: 1 mg every day

Infants >3 months: 1-2 mg/day

Children: 4-8 mg/day

Susceptible systemic infections: I.M., I.V.:

Infants and Children <5 years: 2.5 mg/kg/dose every 8 hours*

Children >5 years: 1.5-2.5 mg/kg/dose every 8 hours*

Cystic fibrosis: 2.5 mg/kg/dose every 6 hours

Prevention of bacterial endocarditis: Dental, oral, upper respiratory procedures, GI/GU procedures: 2 mg/kg with ampicillin (50 mg/kg) 30 minutes prior to procedure

***Note:** Some patients may require larger or more frequent doses (eg, every 6 hours) if serum levels document the need (ie, cystic fibrosis or febrile granulocytopenic patients).

Ophthalmic, Dermatologic infections: Refer to adult dosing.

Renal Impairment:

Cl_{cr} ≥60 mL/minute: Administer every 8 hours.

Cl_{cr} 40-60 mL/minute: Administer every 12 hours.

Cl_{cr} 20-40 mL/minute: Administer every 24 hours.

Cl_{cr} 10-20 mL/minute: Administer every 48 hours.

Cl_{cr} <10 mL/minute: Administer every 72 hours.

Hemodialysis effects: Dialyzable; removal by hemodialysis: 30% removal of aminoglycosides occurs during 4 hours of HD. Administer dose after dialysis and follow levels.

Removal by continuous ambulatory peritoneal dialysis (CAPD):

Administration via CAPD fluid:

Gram-negative infection: 4-8 mg/L (4-8 mcg/mL) of CAPD fluid

Gram-positive infection (ie, synergy): 3-4 mg/L (3-4 mcg/mL) of CAPD fluid

Administration via I.V., I.M. route during CAPD: Dose as for Cl_{cr} <10 mL/minute and follow levels.

Removal via continuous arteriovenous or venovenous hemofiltration: Dose as for Cl_{cr} 10-40 mL/minute and follow levels.

(Continued)

Gentamicin *(Continued)*

Hepatic Impairment: Monitor plasma concentrations.

Administration

I.M.: Administer by deep I.M. route if possible. Slower absorption and lower peak concentrations, probably due to poor circulation in the atrophic muscle, may occur following I.M. injection; in paralyzed patients, suggest I.V. route.

I.V.: Administer other antibiotics at least 1 hour before or 1 hour after gentamicin.

Other: Administer any other ophthalmics 10 minutes before or after gentamicin preparations.

Stability

Storage: Gentamicin is a colorless to slightly yellow solution which should be stored between 2°C to 30°C, but refrigeration is not recommended.

Reconstitution: I.V. infusion solutions mixed in NS or D_5W solution are stable for 24 hours at room temperature and refrigeration.

Premixed bag: Manufacturer expiration date; remove from overwrap stability: 30 days

Compatibility: Stable in dextran 40, D_5W, $D_{10}W$, mannitol 20%, LR, NS; **incompatible** with fat emulsion 10%

Y-site administration: Incompatible with allopurinol, amphotericin B cholesteryl sulfate complex, cefamandole, furosemide, heparin, hetastarch, idarubicin, indomethacin, iodipamide meglumine, phenytoin, propofol, warfarin

Compatibility in syringe: Incompatible with ampicillin, cefamandole, heparin

Compatibility when admixed: Incompatible with amphotericin B, ampicillin, cefamandole, cefazolin with clindamycin, cefepime, heparin, nafcillin, ticarcillin

Monitoring Laboratory Tests Monitor urinalysis, BUN, serum creatinine, and hearing test before, during, and after treatment, particularly in those at risk for ototoxicity or those receiving prolonged therapy (>2 weeks). **Note:** Serum levels (peak and trough), aminoglycoside levels measured in blood taken from silastic central catheters have been known to give falsely high reading (draw via separate lumen or peripheral site, or flush well).

Monitoring and Teaching Issues

Physical Assessment: Assess effectiveness and interactions of other medications patient may be taking (see Contraindications and Drug Interactions). Assess kidney function and hearing before, during, and following therapy (see Warnings/Precautions). **Note:** This medication has a very low TI (see Dosing Instructions regarding body weight). Monitor therapeutic response, laboratory values (see above) and adverse reactions (see Warnings/Precautions, Adverse Reactions, and Overdose/Toxicology) at beginning of therapy and periodically throughout therapy. Assess knowledge/teach patient appropriate use, interventions to reduce side effects, and adverse symptoms to report (see Patient Education). **Pregnancy risk factor C** - benefits of use should outweigh possible risks. Note breast-feeding caution.

Patient Education: Take exactly as directed and when prescribed. Drink adequate amounts of water (2-3 L/day) unless advised by prescriber to restrict fluids. You may experience headaches, ringing in ears, dizziness, blurred vision (use caution when driving or engaging in tasks requiring alertness until response to drug is known); GI upset, loss of appetite (small, frequent meals and frequent mouth care may help); or photosensitivity (use sunscreen wear protective clothing and eyewear, and avoid direct sunlight). Report severe headache, changes in hearing acuity or ringing in ears, changes in urine pattern, difficulty breathing, rash, fever, unhealed sores, sores in mouth, vaginal drainage, muscle or bone pain, change in gait, or worsening of condition. **Pregnancy/breast-feeding precautions:** Inform prescriber if you are or intend to become pregnant. Consult prescriber if breast-feeding.

Ophthalmic: Wash hands before instilling. Sit or lie down to instill. Open eye, look at ceiling, and instill prescribed amount of solution (Ointment: Pull lower lid down gently, instill thin ribbon of ointment inside lid.) Close eye and roll eye in all directions, and apply gentle pressure to inner corner of eye. Do not let tip of applicator touch eye; do not contaminate tip of applicator (may cause eye infection, eye damage, or vision loss). Temporary stinging or blurred vision may occur. Report persistent pain, burning, vision changes, swelling, itching, or worsening of condition.

Topical: Apply thin film of ointment to affected area as often as recommended. May apply porous dressing. Report persistent burning, swelling, itching, worsening of condition, or lack of response to therapy.

Dietary Issues: Calcium, magnesium, potassium: Renal wasting may cause hypocalcemia, hypomagnesemia, and/or hypokalemia.

Geriatric Considerations: Aminoglycosides are important therapeutic interventions for susceptible organisms and as empiric therapy in seriously ill patients. Their use is not without risk of toxicity, however. Additional studies comparing high-dose, once-daily aminoglycosides to traditional dosing regimens in the elderly are needed before once-daily aminoglycoside dosing can be routinely adopted to this patient population.

Breast-feeding Issues: No data reported; however, gentamicin is not absorbed orally and other aminoglycosides may be taken while breast-feeding.

Related Information

Compatibility of Drugs *on page 1564*
Ophthalmic Agents *on page 1509*
Peak and Trough Guidelines *on page 1544*

Gentamicin Sulfate *see* Gentamicin *on page 628*

Gentran® *see* Dextran *on page 390*

Geocillin® *see* Carbenicillin *on page 216*

Geodon® *see* Ziprasidone *on page 1424*

Geref® Diagnostic *see page 1461*

Geref® Injection *see page 1461*

GG *see* Guaifenesin *on page 646*

Glatiramer Acetate (gla TIR a mer AS e tate)

U.S. Brand Names Copaxone®

Synonyms Copolymer-1

Generic Available No

Pharmacologic Category Biological, Miscellaneous

Pregnancy Risk Factor B

Lactation Excretion in breast milk unknown/use caution

Use Treatment of relapsing-remitting type multiple sclerosis; studies indicate that it reduces the frequency of attacks and the severity of disability; appears to be most effective for patients with minimal disability

Contraindications Previous hypersensitivity to any component of the copolymer formulation, glatiramer acetate, or mannitol

Warnings/Precautions For S.C. use only, **not for I.V. administration**. Glatiramer acetate is antigenic, and may possibly lead to the induction of untoward host responses. Systemic postinjection reactions occur in a substantial percentage of patients (~10% in premarketing studies). Safety and efficacy have not been established in patients <18 years of age.

Adverse Reactions Reported in >2% of patients in placebo-controlled trials:

>10%:

Cardiovascular: Chest pain (21%)

Central nervous system: Pain (28%), vasodilation (27%), anxiety (23%), palpitations (17%)

Dermatologic: Pruritus (18%), rash (18%), diaphoresis (15%)

Gastrointestinal: Nausea (22%), diarrhea (12%)

Local: Injection site reactions: Pain (73%), erythema (66%), inflammation (49%), pruritus (40%), mass (27%), induration (13%), welt (11%)

Neuromuscular & skeletal: Weakness (41%), arthralgia (24%), hypertonia (22%), back pain (16%)

Respiratory: Dyspnea (19%), rhinitis (14%)

Miscellaneous: Infection (50%), flu-like syndrome (19%), lymphadenopathy (12%)

1% to 10%:

Cardiovascular: Peripheral edema (7%), facial edema (6%), edema (3%), tachycardia (5%), hypertension (1%)

Central nervous system: Fever (8%), vertigo (6%), migraine (5%), syncope (5%), agitation (4%), chills (4%), confusion (2%), nervousness (2%), speech disorder (2%), abnormal dreams (1%), emotional lability (1%), stupor (1%)

Dermatologic: Bruising (8%), erythema (4%), urticaria (4%), skin nodule (2%), eczema, herpes zoster, pustular rash, skin atrophy

Endocrine & metabolic: Dysmenorrhea (6%), amenorrhea (1%), menorrhagia (1%), vaginal hemorrhage (1%)

Gastrointestinal: Anorexia (8%), vomiting (6%), gastrointestinal disorder (5%), gastroenteritis (3%), weight gain (3%), oral moniliasis (1%), ulcerative stomatitis (1%), salivary gland enlargement

Genitourinary: Urinary urgency (10%), vaginal moniliasis (8%), hematuria (1%), impotence (1%)

Local: Injection site reactions: Hemorrhage (5%), urticaria (5%), edema (1%), atrophy (1%), abscess (1%), hypersensitivity (1%)

Neuromuscular & skeletal: Tremor (7%), foot drop (3%)

Ocular: Eye disorder (4%), nystagmus (2%), visual field defect (1%)

Otic: Ear pain (7%)

Respiratory: Bronchitis (9%), laryngismus (5%)

Miscellaneous: Neck pain (8%), bacterial infection (5%), herpes simplex (4%), cyst (2%)

<1% (Limited to important or life-threatening): Anaphylactoid reaction, angina, angioedema, aphasia, arrhythmia, blindness, carcinoma (breast, bladder, lung), cardiomyopathy, cholecystitis, cholelithiasis, cirrhosis, coma, CHF, corneal ulcer, esophageal ulcer, esophagitis, ethanol intolerance, gastrointestinal hemorrhage, GI carcinoma, glaucoma, gout, hallucinations, hematemesis, hepatitis, hepatomegaly, hypotension, leukopenia, lupus erythematosus, mania, meningitis, myocardial infarction, neuralgia, optic neuritis, pancreatitis, pancytopenia, paraplegia, pericardial effusion, photosensitivity, postural hypotension, priapism, pulmonary embolism, rash, renal failure, rheumatoid arthritis, seizures, sepsis, serum sickness, splenomegaly, stomatitis, stroke, suicide attempt, thrombocytopenia, thrombosis

Overdosage/Toxicology Well tolerated; no serious toxicities can be anticipated

Pharmacodynamics/Kinetics

Metabolism: S.C.: Large percentage hydrolyzed locally

Formulations Injection, powder for reconstitution: 20 mg [contains mannitol 40 mg; packaged with sterile water for injection]

Dosing

Adults & Elderly: Multiple sclerosis (relapsing-remitting): S.C.: 20 mg daily

Administration

Other: If using glass prefilled syringe, **only** the auto*ject*® 2 *for glass syringe* device should be used (not the original Copaxone® autoject).

Stability

Storage: Store unreconstituted product in refrigerator at 2°C to 8°C (36°F to 46°F); excursions to room temperature for up to 1 week do not have a negative impact on potency. Diluent may be stored at room temperature

Reconstitution: Reconstituted product contains no preservative, use immediately.

Monitoring and Teaching Issues

Physical Assessment: See Contraindications, Warnings/Precautions, and Dosing for use cautions. Assess potential for interactions with other prescriptions, OTC medications, or herbal products patient may be taking (see Drug Interactions). Assess effectiveness and adverse response (eg, postinjection reactions: self-resolving flushing, chest tightness, dyspnea, palpitations - see Adverse Reactions). Teach patient proper use (reconstitution, injection technique, and syringe/needle disposal), possible side effects and appropriate

(Continued)

Glatiramer Acetate *(Continued)*

interventions, and adverse symptoms to report (see Patient Education). Note breast-feeding caution.

Patient Education: Inform prescriber of all prescriptions, OTC medications, or herbal products you are taking, and any allergies you have. This drug will not cure MS, but may help relieve the severity and frequency of attacks. This drug can only be given by subcutaneous injection; your prescriber will instruct you in how to prepare the medication, proper injection technique, and syringe/needle disposal. If using prefilled glass syringe, use **only** the auto*ject*® 2 *for glass syringe* device (not the original Copaxone® autoject). Do not stop or change doses without consulting your prescriber. May cause a transient reaction after injection, including flushing, chest tightness, dyspnea, or palpitations (usually last 30 minutes or less). May cause weakness, dizziness, confusion, nervousness, or anxiety (use caution when driving or engaging in tasks requiring alertness until response to drug is known); or nausea or vomiting (frequent mouth care and sucking on lozenges may help). Report chest pain or pounding heartbeat; persistent diarrhea or GI upset; infection (vaginal itching or drainage, sores in mouth, unusual fever or chills) or flu-like symptoms (swollen glands, chills, excessive sweating); bruising, rash, or skin irritation; joint pain or neck pain; swelling of puffiness of face; vision changes or ear pain; unusual cough or difficulty breathing; alterations in menstrual pattern; skin depression, hard lump, redness, pain, or swelling at injection site; or any other persistent adverse reactions. **Breast-feeding precaution:** Consult prescriber if breast-feeding.

Glaucoma Drug Comparison*see page 1575*

Gleevec™ *see* Imatinib *on page 695*

Gliadel® *see* Carmustine *on page 223*

Glibenclamide *see* GlyBURIDE *on page 636*

Glimepiride (GLYE me pye ride)

U.S. Brand Names Amaryl®

Generic Available No

Pharmacologic Category Antidiabetic Agent, Sulfonylurea

Pregnancy Risk Factor C

Lactation Excretion in breast milk unknown/contraindicated

Use Management of type 2 diabetes mellitus (noninsulin dependent, NIDDM) as an adjunct to diet and exercise to lower blood glucose or in combination with metformin; use in combination with insulin to lower blood glucose in patients whose hyperglycemia cannot be controlled by diet and exercise in conjunction with an oral hypoglycemic agent

Mechanism of Action/Effect Stimulates insulin release from the pancreatic beta cells; reduces glucose output from the liver; insulin sensitivity is increased at peripheral target sites

Contraindications Hypersensitivity to glimepiride, any component of the formulation, or sulfonamides; diabetic ketoacidosis (with or without coma)

Warnings/Precautions The administration of oral hypoglycemic drugs (eg, tolbutamide) has been reported to be associated with increased cardiovascular mortality as compared to treatment with diet alone or diet plus insulin. All sulfonylurea drugs are capable of producing severe hypoglycemia. Hypoglycemia is more likely to occur when caloric intake is deficient, after severe or prolonged exercise, when ethanol is ingested, or when more than one glucose-lowering drug is used.

Chemical similarities are present among sulfonamides, sulfonylureas, carbonic anhydrase inhibitors, thiazides, and loop diuretics (except ethacrynic acid). Use in patients with sulfonamide allergy is specifically contraindicated in product labeling, however, a risk of cross-reaction exists in patients with allergy to any of these compounds; avoid use when previous reaction has been severe.

Product labeling states oral hypoglycemic drugs may be associated with an increased cardiovascular mortality. Data to support this association are limited, and several studies (UKPDS) have not supported an association.

Pregnancy risk C.

Drug Interactions

Cytochrome P450 Effect: Substrate of **CYP2C8/9**

Decreased Effect: There may be a decreased effect of glimepiride with corticosteroids, cholestyramine, estrogens, oral contraceptives, phenytoin, rifampin, thiazide and other diuretics, phenothiazines, NSAIDs, thyroid products, nicotinic acid, isoniazid, sympathomimetics, urinary alkalinizers, and charcoal. **Note:** However, data from pooled data did **not** demonstrate drug interactions with calcium channel blockers, estrogens, NSAIDs, HMG-CoA reductase inhibitors, sulfonamides, or thyroid hormone.

Increased Effect/Toxicity: Anticoagulants, androgens, fluconazole, miconazole, salicylates, gemfibrozil, sulfonamides, tricyclic antidepressants, probenecid, MAO inhibitors, beta-blockers, methyldopa, digitalis glycosides, urinary acidifiers may increase the hypoglycemic effects of glimepiride.

Nutritional/Ethanol Interactions

Ethanol: Caution with ethanol (may cause hypoglycemia).

Herb/Nutraceutical: Caution with chromium, garlic, gymnema (may cause hypoglycemia).

Adverse Reactions

1% to 10%:

Central nervous system: Headache, dizziness

Gastrointestinal: Nausea

<1% (Limited to important or life-threatening): Agranulocytosis, aplastic anemia, blood dyscrasias, bone marrow suppression, cholestatic jaundice, hemolytic anemia, hepatitis, hypoglycemia, hyponatremia, thrombocytopenia

Other reactions reported with sulfonylureas: Porphyria, vasculitis

Overdosage/Toxicology Symptoms of overdose include low blood sugar, tingling of lips and tongue, nausea, yawning, confusion, agitation, tachycardia, sweating, convulsions, stupor, and coma. Intoxication with sulfonylureas can cause hypoglycemia and are best managed with glucose administration (oral for milder hypoglycemia or by injection in more severe forms). Patients should be monitored for a minimum of 24-48 hours after ingestion.

Pharmacodynamics/Kinetics

Absorption: 100%; delayed when given with food

Half-Life Elimination: 5-9 hours

Metabolism: Completely hepatic

Onset: Peak effect: Blood glucose reductions: 2-3 hours

Duration: 24 hours

Formulations Tablet: 1 mg, 2 mg, 4 mg

Dosing

Adults: Type 2 diabetes: Oral:

Initial: 1-2 mg once daily, administered with breakfast or the first main meal

Adjustment: Allow several days between dose titrations: usual maintenance dose: 1-4 mg once daily; after a dose of 2 mg once daily, increase in increments of 2 mg at 1- to 2-week intervals based upon the patient's blood glucose response to a maximum of 8 mg once daily

Combination with insulin therapy (fasting glucose level for instituting combination therapy is in the range of >150 mg/dL in plasma or serum depending on the patient): initial recommended dose: 8 mg once daily with the first main meal

After starting with low-dose insulin, upward adjustments of insulin can be done approximately weekly as guided by frequent measurements of fasting blood glucose. Once stable, combination-therapy patients should monitor their capillary blood glucose on an ongoing basis, preferably daily.

Elderly: Initial: 1 mg/day; dose titration and maintenance dosing should be conservative to avoid hypoglycemia

Renal Impairment: Cl_{cr} <22 mL/minute: Initial starting dose should be 1 mg and dosage increments should be based on fasting blood glucose levels.

Administration

Oral: May be taken with a meal or food.

Monitoring Laboratory Tests Urine for glucose and ketones, fasting blood glucose, hemoglobin A_{1c}, fructosamine

Monitoring and Teaching Issues

Physical Assessment: Assess any allergies prior to beginning therapy. See Contraindications, Warnings/Precautions, and Dosing for use cautions. Assess potential for interactions with other prescriptions, OTC medications, or herbal products patient may be taking (see Drug Interactions). Monitor laboratory tests (see Monitoring Lab Tests), therapeutic effects, and adverse response (see Adverse Reactions and Overdose/Toxicology) at regular intervals during therapy. Teach patient proper use (or refer patient to diabetic educator for instruction), possible side effects and appropriate interventions, and adverse symptoms to report (see Patient Education). **Pregnancy risk factor C** - benefits of use should outweigh possible risks. Breast-feeding is contraindicated.

Patient Education: Inform prescriber of all prescriptions, OTC medications, or herbal products you are taking, and any allergies you have. Do not take anything new during treatment unless approved by prescriber. This medication is used to control diabetes; it is not a cure. Monitor glucose as recommended by prescriber. Other important components of treatment plan may include prescribed diet and exercise regimen (consult prescriber or diabetic educator). Always carry quick source of sugar with you. Take exactly as directed with breakfast or the first main meal of the day. Do not change dose or discontinue without consulting prescriber. Avoid alcohol while taking this medication; could cause severe reaction. Do not take other medication within 2 hours of this medication unless advised by prescriber. If you experience hypoglycemic reaction, contact prescriber immediately. You may experience side effects during first weeks of therapy (eg, headache, nausea); consult prescriber if these persist. Report severe or persistent side effects (eg, hypoglycemia: palpitations, sweaty palms, lightheadedness; extended vomiting or flu-like symptoms; skin rash; easy bruising or bleeding; or change in color of urine or stool). **Pregnancy/breast-feeding precautions:** Inform prescriber if you are or intend to become pregnant. Do not breast-feed.

Dietary Issues: Administer with breakfast or the first main meal of the day. Dietary modification based on ADA recommendations is a part of therapy. Decreases blood glucose concentration. Hypoglycemia may occur. Must be able to recognize symptoms of hypoglycemia (palpitations, sweaty palms, lightheadedness).

Geriatric Considerations: Rapid and prolonged hypoglycemia (>12 hours) despite hypertonic glucose injections have been reported; age, hepatic, and renal impairment are independent risk factors for hypoglycemia; dosage titration should be made at weekly intervals. How "tightly" a geriatric patient's blood glucose should be controlled is controversial; however, a fasting blood sugar <150 mg/dL is now an acceptable end point. Such a decision should be based on the patient's functional and cognitive status, how well they recognize hypoglycemic or hyperglycemic symptoms, and how to respond to them and their other disease states.

Pregnancy Issues: Abnormal blood glucose levels are associated with a higher incidence of congenital abnormalities. Insulin is the drug of choice for the control of diabetes mellitus during pregnancy.

Related Information

Antidiabetic Oral Agents Comparison *on page 1556*

Diabetes Mellitus Management *on page 1661*

GlipiZIDE (GLIP i zide)

U.S. Brand Names Glucotrol®; Glucotrol® XL

Synonyms Glydiazinamide

Generic Available Yes: Not extended release formulation

Pharmacologic Category Antidiabetic Agent, Sulfonylurea

Pregnancy Risk Factor C

Lactation Excretion in breast milk unknown/contraindicated

(Continued)

GlipiZIDE *(Continued)*

Use Management of type 2 diabetes mellitus (noninsulin dependent, NIDDM)

Mechanism of Action/Effect Stimulates insulin release from the pancreatic beta cells; reduces glucose output from the liver; insulin sensitivity is increased at peripheral target sites

Contraindications Hypersensitivity to glipizide or any component of the formulation, other sulfonamides; type 1 diabetes mellitus (insulin dependent, IDDM)

Warnings/Precautions Use with caution in patients with severe hepatic disease; a useful agent since few drug to drug interactions and not dependent upon renal elimination of active drug.

Chemical similarities are present among sulfonamides, sulfonylureas, carbonic anhydrase inhibitors, thiazides, and loop diuretics (except ethacrynic acid). Use in patients with sulfonamide allergy is specifically contraindicated in product labeling, however, a risk of cross-reaction exists in patients with allergy to any of these compounds; avoid use when previous reaction has been severe.

Avoid use of extended release tablets (Glucotrol® XL) in patients with severe gastrointestinal narrowing or esophageal dysmotility.

Product labeling states oral hypoglycemic drugs may be associated with an increased cardiovascular mortality as compared to treatment with diet alone or diet plus insulin. Data to support this association are limited, and several studies, including a large prospective trial (UKPDS) have not supported an association.

Pregnancy risk C.

Drug Interactions

Cytochrome P450 Effect: Substrate of **2C8/9**

Decreased Effect: Decreased effect of glipizide with beta-blockers, cholestyramine, hydantoins, rifampin, thiazide diuretics, urinary alkalinizers, and charcoal.

Increased Effect/Toxicity: Increased effects/hypoglycemic effects of glipizide with H_2 antagonists, anticoagulants, androgens, cimetidine, fluconazole, salicylates, gemfibrozil, sulfonamides, tricyclic antidepressants, probenecid, MAO inhibitors, methyldopa, digitalis glycosides, and urinary acidifiers.

Nutritional/Ethanol Interactions

Ethanol: Caution with ethanol (may cause hypoglycemia or rare disulfiram reaction).

Food: A delayed release of insulin may occur if glipizide is taken with food. Should be administered 30 minutes before meals to avoid erratic absorption.

Herb/Nutraceutical: Caution with chromium, garlic, gymnema (may cause hypoglycemia).

Adverse Reactions Frequency not defined.

Cardiovascular: Edema

Central nervous system: Headache

Dermatologic: Rash, urticaria, photosensitivity

Endocrine & metabolic: Hypoglycemia, hyponatremia, SIADH (rare)

Gastrointestinal: Anorexia, nausea, vomiting, diarrhea, epigastric fullness, constipation, heartburn

Hematologic: Blood dyscrasias, aplastic anemia, hemolytic anemia, bone marrow suppression, thrombocytopenia, agranulocytosis

Hepatic: Cholestatic jaundice, hepatic porphyria

Renal: Diuretic effect (minor)

Miscellaneous: Disulfiram-like reaction

Overdosage/Toxicology Symptoms of overdose include low blood sugar, tingling of lips and tongue, nausea, yawning, confusion, agitation, tachycardia, sweating, convulsions, stupor, and coma. Intoxication with sulfonylureas can cause hypoglycemia and are best managed with glucose administration (oral for milder hypoglycemia or by injection in more severe forms).

Pharmacodynamics/Kinetics

Absorption: Delayed with food

Half-Life Elimination: 2-4 hours

Metabolism: Hepatic with metabolites

Onset: Peak effect: Blood glucose reductions: 1.5-2 hours

Duration: 12-24 hours

Formulations

Tablet (Glucotrol®): 5 mg, 10 mg

Tablet, extended release (Glucotrol® XL): 2.5 mg, 5 mg, 10 mg

Dosing

Adults: Type 2 diabetes: Oral:

Initial: 5 mg/day; give ~30 minutes before a meal to obtain the greatest reduction in postprandial hyperglycemia.

Adjustment: Adjust dosage at 2.5-5 mg daily increments as determined by blood glucose response at intervals of several days. Maximum recommended once-daily dose: 15 mg; maximum recommended total daily dose: 40 mg; extended release (Glucotrol® XL) maximum recommended dose: 20 mg.

Elderly: Initial: 2.5 mg/day; increase by 2.5-5 mg/day at 1- to 2-week intervals.

Renal Impairment: Cl_{cr} <10 mL/minute: Some investigators recommend not using.

Hepatic Impairment: Initial dosage should be 2.5 mg/day,

Administration

Oral: Administer 30 minutes before a meal to achieve greatest reduction in postprandial hyperglycemia. Patients who are NPO may need to have their dose held to avoid hypoglycemia.

Monitoring Laboratory Tests Urine for glucose and ketones, fasting blood glucose, hemoglobin A_{1c}, fructosamine

Monitoring and Teaching Issues

Physical Assessment: Assess allergy history prior to beginning therapy. See Contraindications, Warnings/Precautions, and Dosing for use cautions. Assess potential for interactions with other prescriptions, OTC medications, or herbal products patient may be taking (see Drug Interactions). Assess results of laboratory tests (see Monitoring Lab Tests), therapeutic effects, and adverse response (eg, hypoglycemia - see Adverse Reactions and Overdose/Toxicology) at regular intervals during therapy. Teach patient proper use (or refer patient to diabetic educator for instruction), possible side effects and appropriate interventions, and adverse symptoms to report (see Patient Education). **Pregnancy risk factor C** - benefits of use should outweigh possible risks. Breast-feeding is contraindicated.

Patient Education: Inform prescriber of all prescriptions, OTC medications, or herbal products you are taking, and any allergies you have. Do not take anything new during treatment unless approved by prescriber. This medication is used to control diabetes; it is not a cure. Monitor glucose as recommended by prescriber. Other important components of treatment plan may include prescribed diet and exercise regimen (consult prescriber or diabetic educator). Always carry quick source of sugar with you. Take exactly as directed, 30 minutes before meal(s), at the same time each day. Do not chew or crush extended release tablets. Do not change dose or discontinue without consulting prescriber. Avoid alcohol while taking this medication; could cause severe reaction. Do not take other medication within 2 hours of this medication unless advised by prescriber. If you experience hypoglycemic reaction, contact prescriber immediately. You may experience more sensitivity to sunlight (use sunscreen, wear protective clothing and eyewear, and avoid direct sunlight); or headache or nausea (consult prescriber if these persist). Report severe or persistent side effects (eg, hypoglycemia: palpitations, sweaty palms, lightheadedness; extended vomiting; diarrhea or constipation; flu-like symptoms; skin rash; easy bruising or bleeding; or change in color of urine or stool). **Pregnancy/breast-feeding precautions:** Inform prescriber if you are or intend to become pregnant. Do not breast-feed.

Dietary Issues: Take glipizide before meals. Dietary modification based on ADA recommendations is a part of therapy. Decreases blood glucose concentration. Hypoglycemia may occur. Must be able to recognize symptoms of hypoglycemia (palpitations, sweaty palms, lightheadedness).

Geriatric Considerations: Glipizide is a useful agent since there are few drug to drug interactions and elimination of the active drug is not dependent upon renal function. How "tightly" a geriatric patient's blood glucose should be controlled is controversial; however, a fasting blood sugar <150 mg/dL is now an acceptable end point. Such a decision should be based on the patient's functional and cognitive status, how well they recognize hypoglycemic or hyperglycemic symptoms, and how to respond to them and their other disease states.

Breast-feeding Issues: Due to risk of neonatal hypoglycemia, breast-feeding is contraindicated.

Pregnancy Issues: Crosses the placenta. Abnormal blood glucose levels are associated with a higher incidence of congenital abnormalities. Insulin is the drug of choice for the control of diabetes mellitus during pregnancy.

Related Information

Antidiabetic Oral Agents Comparison *on page 1556*
Diabetes Mellitus Management *on page 1661*
FDA Name Differentiation Project: The Use of Tall-man Letters *on page 12*

Glivec *see* Imatinib *on page 695*
GlucaGen® *see* Glucagon *on page 635*
GlucaGen® Diagnostic Kit *see* Glucagon *on page 635*

Glucagon (GLOO ka gon)

U.S. Brand Names GlucaGen®; GlucaGen® Diagnostic Kit; Glucagon Diagnostic Kit; Glucagon Emergency Kit

Generic Available No

Pharmacologic Category Antidote; Diagnostic Agent

Pregnancy Risk Factor B

Lactation Excretion in breast milk unknown/compatible

Use Management of hypoglycemia; diagnostic aid in the radiologic examination of GI tract when a hypnotic state is needed

Use - Unlabeled/Investigational Used with some success as a cardiac stimulant in management of severe cases of beta-adrenergic blocking agent overdosage

Mechanism of Action/Effect Stimulates adenylate cyclase to produce increased cyclic AMP, which promotes hepatic glycogenolysis and gluconeogenesis, causing a raise in blood glucose levels

Contraindications Hypersensitivity to glucagon or any component of the formulation

Warnings/Precautions Use with caution in patients with a history of insulinoma and/or pheochromocytoma.

Drug Interactions

Increased Effect/Toxicity: Glucagon and warfarin - hypoprothrombinemic effects may be increased, possibly with bleeding.

Adverse Reactions

Gastrointestinal: Nausea, vomiting (high incidence with rapid administration of high doses)
Miscellaneous: Hypersensitivity reactions (hypotension, respiratory distress, urticaria)

Overdosage/Toxicology Symptoms of overdose include hypokalemia, nausea, and vomiting.

Pharmacodynamics/Kinetics

Half-Life Elimination: Plasma: 3-10 minutes

Metabolism: Primarily hepatic; some inactivation occurring renally and in plasma

Onset: Peak effect: Blood glucose levels: Parenteral: 5-20 minutes

Duration: 60-90 minutes

Formulations

Injection, powder for reconstitution, as hydrochloride:
GlucaGen®, Glucagon: 1 mg [1 unit]
GlucaGen® Diagnostic Kit: 1 mg [1 unit] [packaged with sterile water]

(Continued)

Glucagon *(Continued)*

Glucagon Diagnostic Kit, Glucagon Emergency Kit: 1 mg [1 unit] [packaged with diluent syringe containing glycerin 12 mg/mL and water for injection]

Dosing

Adults & Elderly:

Hypoglycemia or insulin shock therapy: I.M., I.V., S.C.: 0.5-1 mg, may repeat in 20 minutes as needed. **If patient fails to respond to glucagon, I.V. dextrose must be given.**

Diagnostic aid: I.M., I.V.: 0.25-2 mg 10 minutes prior to procedure

Beta-blocker overdose (unlabeled use): I.V.: 3-10 mg **or** initial 0.5-5 mg bolus followed by continuous infusion 1-5 mg/hour

Pediatrics: Hypoglycemia or insulin shock therapy: I.M., I.V., S.C.: Children: 0.025-0.1 mg/kg/dose, not to exceed 1 mg/dose, repeated in 20 minutes as needed. **If patient fails to respond to glucagon, I.V. dextrose must be given.**

Administration

I.V.: Bolus may be associated with nausea and vomiting. Continuous infusions may be used in beta-blocker overdose/toxicity.

Stability

Reconstitution: Reconstitute powder for injection by adding 1 or 10 mL of sterile diluent to a vial containing 1 or 10 units of the drug, respectively, to provide solutions containing 1 mg of glucagon/mL. If dose to be administered is <2 mg of the drug, then use only the diluent provided by the manufacturer. If >2 mg, use sterile water for injection. Use immediately after reconstitution. After reconstitution, use immediately. May be kept at 5°C for up to 48 hours if necessary.

Monitoring Laboratory Tests Blood glucose

Monitoring and Teaching Issues

Physical Assessment: Arouse patient from hypoglycemic or insulin shock as soon as possible and administer carbohydrates. Evaluate insulin dosage and patient's ability to administer appropriate dose. Instruct patient (or significant other) in appropriate administration procedures for emergency use of glucagon. If home glucose monitoring device is available, check blood sugar as soon as possible.

Patient Education: Identify appropriate support person to administer glucagon if necessary. Follow prescribers instructions for administering glucagon. Review diet, insulin administration, and testing procedures with prescriber or diabetic educator.

Additional Information 1 unit = 1 mg

Glucagon Diagnostic Kit *see* Glucagon *on page 635*

Glucagon Emergency Kit *see* Glucagon *on page 635*

Glucocerebrosidase *see* Alglucerase *on page 58*

Glucophage® *see* Metformin *on page 866*

Glucophage® XR *see* Metformin *on page 866*

Glucotrol® *see* GlipiZIDE *on page 633*

Glucotrol® XL *see* GlipiZIDE *on page 633*

Glucovance® *see* Glyburide and Metformin *on page 638*

Glu-K® [OTC] *see* Potassium Supplements *on page 1106*

Glutethimide *see page 1568*

Glybenclamide *see* GlyBURIDE *on page 636*

Glybenzcyclamide *see* GlyBURIDE *on page 636*

GlyBURIDE (GLYE byoor ide)

U.S. Brand Names Diaβeta®; Glynase® PresTab®; Micronase®

Synonyms Glibenclamide; Glybenclamide; Glybenzcyclamide

Generic Available Yes

Pharmacologic Category Antidiabetic Agent, Sulfonylurea

Pregnancy Risk Factor C

Lactation Excretion in breast milk unknown/contraindicated

Use Management of type 2 diabetes mellitus (noninsulin dependent, NIDDM)

Use - Unlabeled/Investigational Alternative to insulin in women for the treatment of gestational diabetes (11-33 weeks gestation)

Mechanism of Action/Effect Stimulates insulin release from the pancreatic beta cells; reduces glucose output from the liver; insulin sensitivity is increased at peripheral target sites

Contraindications Hypersensitivity to glyburide, any component of the formulation, or other sulfonamides; type 1 diabetes mellitus (insulin dependent, IDDM), diabetic ketoacidosis with or without coma

Warnings/Precautions Elderly: Rapid and prolonged hypoglycemia (>12 hours) despite hypertonic glucose injections have been reported; age and hepatic and renal impairment are independent risk factors for hypoglycemia; dosage titration should be made at weekly intervals. Use with caution in patients with renal and hepatic impairment, malnourished or debilitated conditions, or adrenal or pituitary insufficiency.

Chemical similarities are present among sulfonamides, sulfonylureas, carbonic anhydrase inhibitors, thiazides, and loop diuretics (except ethacrynic acid). Use in patients with sulfonamide allergy is specifically contraindicated in product labeling, however, a risk of cross-reaction exists in patients with allergy to any of these compounds; avoid use when previous reaction has been severe.

Product labeling states oral hypoglycemic drugs may be associated with an increased cardiovascular mortality as compared to treatment with diet alone or diet plus insulin. Data to support this association are limited, and several studies, including a large prospective trial (UKPDS) have not supported an association.

Pregnancy risk C.

Drug Interactions

Decreased Effect: Thiazides and other diuretics, corticosteroids may decrease effectiveness of glyburide.

Increased Effect/Toxicity: Increased hypoglycemic effects of glyburide may occur with oral anticoagulants (warfarin), phenytoin, other hydantoins, salicylates, NSAIDs, sulfonamides, and beta-blockers. Ethanol ingestion may cause disulfiram reactions.

Nutritional/Ethanol Interactions

Ethanol: Caution with ethanol (may cause hypoglycemia).

Herb/Nutraceutical: Caution with chromium, garlic, gymnema (may cause hypoglycemia).

Adverse Reactions Frequency not defined.

Central nervous system: Headache, dizziness

Dermatologic: Pruritus, rash, urticaria, photosensitivity reaction

Gastrointestinal: Nausea, epigastric fullness, heartburn, constipation, diarrhea, anorexia

Endocrine & metabolic: Hypoglycemia, hyponatremia (SIADH reported with other sulfonylureas)

Genitourinary: Nocturia

Hematologic: Leukopenia, thrombocytopenia, hemolytic anemia, aplastic anemia, bone marrow suppression, agranulocytosis

Hepatic: Cholestatic jaundice, hepatitis

Neuromuscular & skeletal: Arthralgia, paresthesia

Ocular: Blurred vision

Renal: Diuretic effect (minor)

Overdosage/Toxicology Symptoms of overdose include severe hypoglycemia, seizures, cerebral damage, tingling of lips and tongue, nausea, yawning, confusion, agitation, tachycardia, sweating, convulsions, stupor, and coma. Intoxication with sulfonylureas can cause hypoglycemia and is best managed with glucose administration (oral for milder hypoglycemia or by injection in more severe forms).

Pharmacodynamics/Kinetics

Half-Life Elimination: 5-16 hours; may be prolonged with renal or hepatic impairment

Time to Peak: Serum: Adults: 2-4 hours

Metabolism: To one moderately active and several inactive metabolites

Onset: Serum insulin levels begin to increase 15-60 minutes after a single dose

Duration: ≤24 hours

Formulations

Tablet (Diaβeta®, Micronase®): 1.25 mg, 2.5 mg, 5 mg

Tablet, micronized (Glynase® PresTab®): 1.5 mg, 3 mg, 6 mg

Dosing

Adults: Type 2 diabetes: Oral:

Note: Regular tablets cannot be used interchangeably with micronized tablet formulations

Regular tablets (Diaβeta®, Micronase®):

Initial: 2.5-5 mg/day, administered with breakfast or the first main meal of the day. In patients who are more sensitive to hypoglycemic drugs, start at 1.25 mg/day.

Adjustment: Increase in increments of no more than 2.5 mg/day at weekly intervals based on the patient's blood glucose response

Maintenance: 1.25-20 mg/day given as single or divided doses; maximum: 20 mg/day

Micronized tablets (Glynase® PresTab™):

Initial: 1.5-3 mg/day, administered with breakfast or the first main meal of the day in patients who are more sensitive to hypoglycemic drugs, start at 0.75 mg/day. Increase in increments of no more than 1.5 mg/day in weekly intervals based on the patient's blood glucose response.

Maintenance: 0.75-12 mg/day given as a single dose or in divided doses. Some patients (especially those receiving >6 mg/day) may have a more satisfactory response with twice-daily dosing.

Elderly: Regular tablets (Diaβeta®, Micronase®): Oral: Initial: 1.25-2.5 mg/day, increase by 1.25-2.5 mg/day every 1-3 weeks. Refer to adult dosing.

Renal Impairment: Cl_{cr} <50 mL/minute: Not recommended

Hepatic Impairment: Use conservative initial and maintenance doses and avoid use in severe disease.

Administration

Oral: Administer with meals at the same time each day.

Monitoring Laboratory Tests Fasting blood glucose, hemoglobin A_{1c}, fructosamine

Monitoring and Teaching Issues

Physical Assessment: Assess allergy history prior to beginning therapy. See Contraindications, Warnings/Precautions, and Dosing for use cautions. Assess potential for interactions with other prescriptions, OTC medications, or herbal products patient may be taking (see Drug Interactions). Assess results of laboratory tests (see Monitoring Lab Tests), therapeutic effects, and adverse response (eg, hypoglycemia - see Adverse Reactions and Overdose/Toxicology) at regular intervals during therapy. Teach patient proper use (or refer patient to diabetic educator) for instruction, possible side effects and appropriate interventions, and adverse symptoms to report (see Patient Education). **Pregnancy risk factor C** - benefits of use should outweigh possible risks. Breast-feeding is contraindicated.

Patient Education: Inform prescriber of all prescriptions, OTC medications, or herbal products you are taking, and any allergies you have. Do not take anything new during treatment unless approved by prescriber. This medication is used to control diabetes; it is not a cure. Monitor glucose as recommended by prescriber. Other important components of treatment plan may include prescribed diet and exercise regimen (consult prescriber or diabetic educator). If you experience hypoglycemic reaction, contact prescriber immediately. Always carry quick source of sugar with you. Take exactly as directed, 30 minutes before meal(s) at the same time each day. Do not change dose or discontinue without consulting prescriber. Avoid alcohol while taking this medication; could cause severe reaction. Do not take other medication within 2 hours of this medication unless advised by

(Continued)

GlyBURIDE *(Continued)*

prescriber. You may experience more sensitivity to sunlight (use sunscreen, wear protective clothing and eyewear, and avoid direct sunlight); headache; or nausea (consult prescriber if these persist). Report severe or persistent side effects; hypoglycemia (palpitations, sweaty palms, lightheadedness); extended vomiting, diarrhea, or constipation; flu-like symptoms; skin rash; easy bruising or bleeding; or change in color of urine or stool. **Pregnancy/breast-feeding precautions:** Inform prescriber if you are or intend to become pregnant. Do not breast-feed.

Dietary Issues: Should be taken with meals at the same time each day. Dietary modification based on ADA recommendations is a part of therapy. Decreases blood glucose concentration. Hypoglycemia may occur. Must be able to recognize symptoms of hypoglycemia (palpitations, sweaty palms, lightheadedness).

Geriatric Considerations: Rapid and prolonged hypoglycemia (>12 hours) despite hypertonic glucose injections have been reported; age, hepatic, and renal impairment are independent risk factors for hypoglycemia; conservative initial dosing and slow titration are required to avoid hypoglycemic reactions; dosage titration should be made at weekly intervals.

Pregnancy Issues: Crosses the placenta. Hypoglycemia; ear defects reported; other malformations reported but may have been secondary to poor maternal glucose control/ diabetes. Insulin is the drug of choice for the control of diabetes mellitus during pregnancy.

Related Information

Antidiabetic Oral Agents Comparison *on page 1556*
Diabetes Mellitus Management *on page 1661*
FDA Name Differentiation Project: The Use of Tall-man Letters *on page 12*

Glyburide and Metformin (GLYE byoor ide & met FOR min)

U.S. Brand Names Glucovance®

Synonyms Glyburide and Metformin Hydrochloride

Generic Available No

Pharmacologic Category Antidiabetic Agent, Biguanide; Antidiabetic Agent, Sulfonylurea

Pregnancy Risk Factor B (manufacturer); C (expert analysis)

Lactation No data available/use caution

Use Initial therapy for management of type 2 diabetes mellitus (noninsulin dependent, NIDDM). Second-line therapy for management of type 2 diabetes (NIDDM) when hyperglycemia cannot be managed with a sulfonylurea or metformin; combination therapy with a thiazolidinedione may be required to achieve additional control.

Formulations

Tablet, film coated:

- 1.25 mg/250 mg: Glyburide 1.25 mg and metformin hydrochloride 250 mg
- 2.5 mg/500 mg: Glyburide 2.5 mg and metformin hydrochloride 500 mg
- 5 mg/500 mg: Glyburide 5 mg and metformin hydrochloride 500 mg

Dosing

Adults: Note: Dose must be individualized. All doses should be taken with a meal. Twice daily dosage should be taken with the morning and evening meals. Dosages expressed as glyburide/metformin components.

Type 2 diabetes: Oral:

Initial therapy (no prior treatment with sulfonylurea or metformin): 1.25 mg/250 mg once daily with a meal; patients with Hb A_{1c} >9% or fasting plasma glucose (FPG) >200 mg/ dL may start with 1.25 mg/250 mg twice daily

Dosage may be increased in increments of 1.25 mg/250 mg, at intervals of not less than 2 weeks; maximum daily dose: 10 mg/2000 mg (limited experience with higher doses)

Previously treated with a sulfonylurea or metformin alone: Initial: 2.5 mg/500 mg or 5 mg/ 500 mg twice daily; increase in increments no greater than 5 mg/500 mg; maximum daily dose: 20 mg/2000 mg

When switching patients previously on a sulfonylurea and metformin together, do not exceed the daily dose of glyburide (or glyburide equivalent) or metformin.

Note: May combine with a thiazolidinedione in patients with an inadequate response to glyburide/metformin therapy (risk of hypoglycemia may be increased).

Elderly: Refer to adult dosing. Conservative doses are recommended in the elderly due to potentially decreased renal function. **Do not titrate to maximum dose**. Should not be used in patients ≥80 years of age unless renal function is verified as normal.

Monitoring and Teaching Issues

Physical Assessment: See individual components listed in Related Information. **Pregnancy risk factor B/C** - see Pregnancy Risk Factor for use cautions; benefits of use should outweigh possible risks. Note breast-feeding caution.

Patient Education: See individual components listed in Related Information. **Pregnancy/ breast-feeding precautions:** Inform prescriber if you are or intend to become pregnant. Consult prescriber if breast-feeding.

Related Information

GlyBURIDE *on page 636*
Metformin *on page 866*

Glyburide and Metformin Hydrochloride *see* Glyburide and Metformin *on page 638*
Glycerin Suppository *see page 1581*
Glycerol Guaiacolate *see* Guaifenesin *on page 646*
Glycerol-T® *see* Theophylline and Guaifenesin *on page 1303*
Glyceryl Trinitrate *see* Nitroglycerin *on page 977*

Glycopyrrolate (glye koe PYE roe late)

U.S. Brand Names Robinul®; Robinul® Forte

Synonyms Glycopyrronium Bromide

Generic Available Yes: Injection

Pharmacologic Category Anticholinergic Agent

Pregnancy Risk Factor B

Lactation Excretion in breast milk unknown

Use Inhibit salivation and excessive secretions of the respiratory tract preoperatively; reversal of neuromuscular blockade; control of upper airway secretions; adjunct in treatment of peptic ulcer

Mechanism of Action/Effect Blocks the action of acetylcholine at parasympathetic sites in smooth muscle, secretory glands, and the CNS

Contraindications Hypersensitivity to glycopyrrolate or any component of the formulation; ulcerative colitis; narrow-angle glaucoma; acute hemorrhage; tachycardia; obstructive uropathy; paralytic ileus; obstructive disease of GI tract

Warnings/Precautions Not recommended in children <12 years of age for the management of peptic ulcer; infants, patients with Down syndrome, and children with spastic paralysis or brain damage may be hypersensitive to antimuscarine effects. Use caution in elderly, patients with autonomic neuropathy, hepatic or renal disease, ulcerative colitis may precipitate/aggravate toxic megacolon, hyperthyroidism, CAD, CHF, arrhythmias, tachycardia, BPH, hiatal hernia, with reflux. Caution should be used in individuals demonstrating decreased pigmentation (skin and iris coloration, dark versus light) since there has been some evidence that these individuals have an enhanced sensitivity to the anticholinergic response.

Drug Interactions

Decreased Effect: Decreased effect of levodopa.

Increased Effect/Toxicity: Increased toxicity with amantadine and cyclopropane. Effects of other anticholinergic agents may be increased by glycopyrrolate.

Adverse Reactions

>10%:
- Dermatologic: Dry skin
- Gastrointestinal: Constipation, dry throat, dry mouth
- Local: Irritation at injection site
- Respiratory: Dry nose
- Miscellaneous: Diaphoresis (decreased)

1% to 10%:
- Dermatologic: Increased sensitivity to light
- Endocrine & metabolic: Decreased flow of breast milk
- Gastrointestinal: Dysphagia

<1% (Limited to important or life-threatening): Increased intraocular pain, orthostatic hypotension, palpitations, tachycardia, ventricular fibrillation

Overdosage/Toxicology Symptoms of overdose include blurred vision, urinary retention, tachycardia, and absent bowel sounds. For anticholinergic overdose with severe life-threatening symptoms, physostigmine 1-2 mg S.C. or I.V. slowly, may be given to reverse these effects.

Pharmacodynamics/Kinetics

Absorption: Oral: Poor and erratic

Bioavailability: ~10%

Half-Life Elimination: 20-40 minutes

Metabolism: Hepatic (minimal)

Onset: Oral: 50 minutes; I.M.: 20-40 minutes; I.V.: ~1 minute; Peak effect: Oral: ~1 hour

Duration: Vagal effect: 2-3 hours; Inhibition of salivation: Up to 7 hours; Anticholinergic: Oral 8-12 hours

Formulations

Injection, solution (Robinul®): 0.2 mg/mL (1 mL, 2 mL, 5 mL, 20 mL) [contains benzyl alcohol]

Tablet:
- Robinul®: 1 mg
- Robinul® Forte: 2 mg

Dosing

Adults:

Control of secretions: I.M.:
- Preoperative: I.M.: 4.4 mcg/kg 30-60 minutes before procedure
- Intraoperative: I.V.: 0.1 mg repeated as needed at 2- to 3-minute intervals

Reversal of neuromuscular blockade: I.V.: 0.2 mg for each 1 mg of neostigmine or 5 mg of pyridostigmine administered or 5-15 mcg/kg glycopyrrolate with 25-70 mcg/kg of neostigmine or 0.1-0.3 mg/kg of pyridostigmine (agents usually administered simultaneously, but glycopyrrolate may be administered first if bradycardia is present)

Peptic ulcer:
- Oral: 1-2 mg 2-3 times/day
- I.M., I.V.: 0.1-0.2 mg 3-4 times/day

Reversal of neuromuscular blockade: I.V.: 0.2 mg for each 1 mg of neostigmine or 5 mg of pyridostigmine administered

Elderly: Refer to adult dosing and Special Geriatric Considerations.

Pediatrics:

Control of secretions
- Preoperative: I.M.:
  - <2 years: 4.4-8.8 mcg/kg 30-60 minutes before procedure
  - >2 years: 4.4 mcg/kg 30-60 minutes before procedure
- Intraoperative: I.V.: 4 mcg/kg not to exceed 0.1 mg; repeat at 2- to 3-minute intervals as needed.
- Chronic:
  - Oral: 40-100 mcg/kg/dose 3-4 times/day
  - I.M., I.V.: 4-10 mcg/kg/dose every 3-4 hours; maximum: 0.2 mg/dose or 0.8 mg/24 hours

Reversal of neuromuscular blockade: Refer to adult dosing.

(Continued)

Glycopyrrolate *(Continued)*

Administration

I.V.: Administer at a rate of 0.2 mg over 1-2 minutes.

Stability

Storage: Unstable at pH >6.

Compatibility: Stable in $D_5\frac{1}{2}NS$, D_5W, $D_{10}W$, LR, NS

Compatibility in syringe: Incompatible with chloramphenicol, dexamethasone sodium phosphate, diazepam, dimenhydrinate, methohexital, pentazocine, pentobarbital, secobarbital, sodium bicarbonate, thiopental

Compatibility when admixed: Incompatible with methylprednisolone sodium succinate

Monitoring and Teaching Issues

Physical Assessment: See Contraindications, Warnings/Precautions, and Dosing for use cautions. Assess potential for interactions with other prescriptions, OTC medications, or herbal products patient may be taking (eg, anything that may add to anticholinergic effects - see Drug Interactions). **I.V./I.M.:** See Administration specifics. Assess therapeutic effects, and adverse response (eg, excessive dryness: eyes, nose, mouth, throat - see Adverse Reactions and Overdose/Toxicology). Teach patient proper use (self-administered), possible side effects and appropriate interventions, and adverse symptoms to report (see Patient Education). Note breast-feeding caution.

Patient Education: Inform prescriber of all prescriptions, OTC medications, or herbal products you are taking, and any allergies you have. Do not take anything new during treatment unless approved by prescriber. Take as directed before meals; do not increase dose and do not discontinue without consulting prescriber. Void before taking medication. You may experience dizziness or blurred vision (use caution when driving or engaging in tasks that require alertness until response to drug is known); dry mouth (sucking on lozenges may help); photosensitivity (wear dark glasses in bright sunlight); decreased ability to sweat (use caution in hot weather or hot rooms or engaging in strenuous activity); or impotence (temporary). Report excessive and persistent anticholinergic effects (blurred vision, headache, flushing, tachycardia, nervousness, constipation, dizziness, insomnia, mental confusion or excitement, dry mouth, altered taste perception, dysphagia, palpitations, bradycardia, urinary hesitancy or retention, impotence, decreased sweating). **Breast-feeding precaution:** Consult prescriber if breast-feeding.

Geriatric Considerations: Anticholinergic agents are generally not well tolerated in the elderly and their use should be avoided when possible.

Related Information

Compatibility of Drugs *on page 1564*
Compatibility of Drugs in Syringe *on page 1566*

Glycopyrronium Bromide *see* Glycopyrrolate *on page 638*

Glydiazinamide *see* GlipiZIDE *on page 633*

Glynase® PresTab® *see* GlyBURIDE *on page 636*

Glyquin® *see* Hydroquinone *on page 679*

Glyset™ *see* Miglitol *on page 907*

Glytuss® [OTC] *see* Guaifenesin *on page 646*

GM-CSF *see* Sargramostim *on page 1215*

GnRH *see* Gonadorelin *on page 640*

GoLYTELY® *see* Polyethylene Glycol-Electrolyte Solution *on page 1098*

Gonadorelin (goe nad oh REL in)

U.S. Brand Names Factrel®

Synonyms GnRH; Gonadorelin Acetate; Gonadorelin Hydrochloride; Gonadotropin Releasing Hormone; LHRH; LRH; Luteinizing Hormone Releasing Hormone

Generic Available No

Pharmacologic Category Diagnostic Agent; Gonadotropin

Pregnancy Risk Factor B

Lactation Excretion in breast milk unknown

Use Evaluation of functional capacity and response of gonadotrophic hormones; evaluate abnormal gonadotropin regulation as in precocious puberty and delayed puberty.

Orphan drug: Lutrepulse®: Induction of ovulation in females with hypothalamic amenorrhea

Mechanism of Action/Effect Stimulates the release of luteinizing hormone (LH) from the anterior pituitary gland

Contraindications Hypersensitivity to gonadorelin or any component of the formulation; women with any condition that could be exacerbated by pregnancy; patients who have ovarian cysts or causes of anovulation other than those of hypothalamic origin; any condition that may worsened by reproductive hormones

Warnings/Precautions Hypersensitivity and anaphylactic reactions have occurred following multiple-dose administration. Use with caution in women in whom pregnancy could worsen pre-existing conditions (eg, pituitary prolactinemia). Multiple pregnancy is a possibility with gonadorelin.

Drug Interactions

Decreased Effect: Decreased levels/effect with oral contraceptives, digoxin, phenothiazines, and dopamine antagonists.

Increased Effect/Toxicity: Increased levels/effect with androgens, estrogens, progestins, glucocorticoids, spironolactone, and levodopa.

Adverse Reactions 1% to 10%: Local: Pain at injection site

Overdosage/Toxicology Symptoms of overdose include abdominal discomfort, nausea, headache, and flushing. Treatment is symptomatic.

Pharmacodynamics/Kinetics

Half-Life Elimination: 4 minutes

Onset: Peak effect: Maximal LH release: ~20 minutes

Duration: 3-5 hours

Formulations Injection, powder for reconstitution, as hydrochloride (Factrel®): 100 mcg [diluent contains benzyl alcohol]

Dosing

Adults:

Diagnostic test: I.V., S.C. (hydrochloride salt): 100 mcg administered in women during early phase of menstrual cycle (day 1-7)

Primary hypothalamic amenorrhea: I.V. (acetate): 5 mcg every 90 minutes via Lutrepulse® pump kit at treatment intervals of 21 days (pump will pulsate every 90 minutes for 7 days)

Pediatrics: Diagnostic test: Children >12 years: Refer to adult dosing.

Administration

I.V.:

Factrel®: Give I.V. push over 30 seconds.

Lutrepulse®: A presterilized reservoir bag with the infusion catheter set supplied with the kit should be filled with the reconstituted solution and administered I.V. using the Lutrepulse® pump. Set the pump to deliver 25-50 mL of solution, based upon the dose, over a pulse period of 1 minute and at a pulse frequency of 90 minutes.

Stability

Reconstitution:

Factrel®: Prepare immediately prior to use. After reconstitution, store at room temperature and use within 1 day. Discard unused portion.

Lutrepulse®: Reconstitute with diluent immediately prior to use and transfer to plastic reservoir. The solution will supply 90-minute pulsatile doses for 7 consecutive days (Lutrepulse® pump).

Monitoring Laboratory Tests LH, FSH

Monitoring and Teaching Issues

Physical Assessment: Assess other medications patient may be taking for effectiveness and interactions (see Drug Interactions). See Contraindications and Warnings/Precautions for use cautions. When used for induction of ovulation, monitor laboratory tests and therapeutic response. Assess knowledge/teach patient appropriate use (use of pulsating pump if applicable), interventions to reduce side effects, and adverse symptoms to report (see Patient Education). Note breast-feeding caution.

Patient Education: If receiving this drug via pulsating pump, check all procedures with prescriber, and use exactly as prescribed. Report any rash, pain, or inflammation at injection site, and any change in respiratory status.

Gonadorelin Acetate *see* Gonadorelin *on page 640*

Gonadorelin Hydrochloride *see* Gonadorelin *on page 640*

Gonadotropin Releasing Hormone *see* Gonadorelin *on page 640*

Gonak™ *see page 1461*

Gonal-F® *see* Follitropins *on page 597*

Gonic® *see* Chorionic Gonadotropin (Human) *on page 284*

Goniosol® *see page 1461*

Goserelin (GOE se rel in)

U.S. Brand Names Zoladex®

Synonyms Goserelin Acetate

Generic Available No

Pharmacologic Category Antineoplastic Agent, Miscellaneous; Gonadotropin Releasing Hormone Analog; Luteinizing Hormone-Releasing Hormone Analog

Pregnancy Risk Factor X

Lactation Enters breast milk/contraindicated

Use

Prostate carcinoma: Palliative treatment of advanced carcinoma of the prostate. An alternative treatment of prostatic cancer when orchiectomy or estrogen administration are either not indicated or unacceptable to the patient. Combination with flutamide for the management of locally confined stage T2b-T4 (stage B2-C) carcinoma of the prostate.

3.6 mg implant **only**:

Endometriosis: Management of endometriosis, including pain relief and reduction of endometriotic lesions for the duration of therapy

Advanced breast cancer: Palliative treatment of advanced breast cancer in pre- and perimenopausal women. Estrogen and progesterone receptor values may help to predict whether goserelin therapy is likely to be beneficial.

Note: The 10.8 mg implant is not indicated in women as the data are insufficient to support reliable suppression of serum estradiol

Mechanism of Action/Effect LHRH synthetic analog of luteinizing hormone-releasing hormone also known as gonadotropin-releasing hormone (GnRH)

Contraindications Hypersensitivity to goserelin or any component of the formulation; pregnancy (or potential to become pregnant)

Warnings/Precautions Initially, goserelin transiently increases serum levels of testosterone. Transient worsening of signs or symptoms, usually manifested by an increase in cancer-related pain which was managed symptomatically, may develop during the first few weeks of treatment. Isolated cases of ureteral obstruction and spinal cord compression have been reported. Patient's symptoms may initially worsen temporarily during first few weeks of therapy, cancer-related pain can usually be controlled by analgesics.

Effects on Lab Values Serum alkaline phosphatase, serum acid phosphatase, serum testosterone, serum LH and FSH, serum estradiol

Adverse Reactions Hormone replacement therapy may decrease vasomotor symptoms and loss of bone mineral density. Adverse reaction profile varies with gender and therapeutic use.

(Continued)

Goserelin *(Continued)*

>10%:

Central nervous system: Headache (11%)

Endocrine & metabolic: Hot flashes (53% to 62% of men, 100% of women), sexual dysfunction (15% to 21%), decreased libido, impotence, impaired erection (16% to 18%), tumor flare, bone pain (23% of women, 1% to 10% of men), vaginal dryness (10% to 14%)

1% to 10%:

Cardiovascular: Anginal pain, arrhythmias, hypertension, thromboembolic events, CHF, myocardial infarction (1% to 5%), edema

Central nervous system: Lethargy (5% to 8%), anxiety, depression, dizziness, insomnia

Dermatologic: Urticaria, maculopapular rashes (10%)

Endocrine & metabolic: Gynecomastia, breast swelling (3% to 5%), bone loss, diaphoresis

Gastrointestinal: Abdominal pain, taste disturbances, diarrhea, nausea, vomiting (5%), anorexia

<1% (Limited to important or life-threatening): Spinal cord compression, ovarian cyst formation, pituitary apoplexy (following initiation in patients with functional pituitary adenoma)

Changes in blood pressure (usually transient) have been associated with goserelin use. Osteoporosis, decreased bone mineral density, and fracture have been reported rarely in men treated with goserelin.

Overdosage/Toxicology Symptomatic management

Pharmacodynamics/Kinetics

Absorption: S.C.: Rapid and can be detected in serum in 10 minutes

Half-Life Elimination: S.C. dose: 5 hours; Renal impairment: 12 hours

Time to Peak: Serum: S.C.: 12-15 days

Formulations

Injection, solution, 1-month implant [disposable syringe; single-dose]: 3.6 mg [with 16-gauge hypodermic needle]

Injection, solution, 3-month implant [disposable syringe; single-dose]: 10.8 mg [with 14-gauge hypodermic needle]

Dosing

Adults & Elderly:

Prostate carcinoma: S.C.:

Monthly implant: 3.6 mg injected into upper abdomen every 28 days; while a delay of a few days is permissible, attempt to adhere to the 28-day schedule

3-month implant: 10.8 mg injected into the upper abdominal wall every 12 weeks; while a delay of a few days is permissible, attempt to adhere to the 12-week schedule

Note: Intended for long-term administration

Endometriosis: S.C.:

Monthly implant: 3.6 mg injected into upper abdomen every 28 days; while a delay of a few days is permissible, attempt to adhere to the 28-day schedule

3-month implant: 10.8 mg injected into the upper abdominal wall every 12 weeks; while a delay of a few days is permissible, attempt to adhere to the 12-week schedule

Note: Recommended duration of endometriosis treatment is 6 months; retreatment is not recommended since safety data is not available. If symptoms recur after a course of therapy, and further treatment is contemplated, consider monitoring bone mineral density. Currently, there are no clinical data on the effect of treatment of benign gynecological conditions with goserelin for periods >6 months.

Administration

Other: Subcutaneous: Do not remove the sterile syringe until immediately before use. Do not aspirate with goserelin syringe, if the needle is in a large vessel, blood will immediately appear in syringe chamber.

Stability

Storage: Zoladex® should be stored at room temperature not to exceed 25°C (77°F). Protect from light. Must be dispensed in an amber bag.

Monitoring and Teaching Issues

Physical Assessment: See Contraindications, Warnings/Precautions, and Dosing for use cautions. Assess potential for interactions with other prescriptions, OTC medications, or herbal products patient may be taking (see Drug Interactions). See Administration specifics. Assess therapeutic effects and adverse response (see Adverse Reactions and Overdose/Toxicology) periodically during therapy. Teach patient proper use, possible side effects and appropriate interventions, and adverse symptoms to report (see Patient Education). **Pregnancy risk factor X** - determine that patient is not pregnant before beginning treatment. Do not give to women of childbearing age unless female is capable of complying with barrier contraceptive measures 1 month prior to therapy, during therapy, and 1 month following therapy. Instruct patient in appropriate barrier contraceptive measures. Breast-feeding is contraindicated.

Patient Education: Inform prescriber of all prescriptions, OTC medications, or herbal products you are taking, and any allergies you have. Do not take anything new during treatment unless approved by prescriber. This drug must be implanted into your stomach every 28 days; it is important to maintain appointment schedule. Males or females - you may experience systemic hot flashes (cool clothes and temperatures may help); headache (consult prescriber for approved analgesic); constipation (increased bulk and water in diet or stool softener may help); sexual dysfunction (decreased libido, males - decreased erection, females - vaginal dryness); or bone pain (consult prescriber for approved analgesic). Symptoms may worsen temporarily during first weeks of therapy. Report chest pain, palpitations, or difficulty breathing; swelling of extremities; unusual persistent nausea, vomiting, or constipation; chest pain or difficulty breathing; unresolved dizziness; or skin rash. **Pregnancy/breast-feeding precautions:** Inform prescriber if you are pregnant; do not get pregnant 1 month before, during, or for 1 month following therapy. Consult prescriber for instruction on appropriate contraceptive measures. This drug may cause severe fetal defects. Do not donate blood during or for 1 month following therapy (same reason). Do not breast-feed.

Goserelin Acetate *see* Goserelin *on page 641*
GP 47680 *see* Oxcarbazepine *on page 1017*
G-Phed *see* Guaifenesin and Pseudoephedrine *on page 648*
G-Phed-PD *see* Guaifenesin and Pseudoephedrine *on page 648*

Granisetron (gra NI se tron)

U.S. Brand Names Kytril®

Generic Available No

Pharmacologic Category Selective 5-HT_3 Receptor Antagonist

Pregnancy Risk Factor B

Lactation Excretion in breast milk unknown/use caution

Use

Oral: Prophylaxis of chemotherapy-related emesis; prophylaxis of nausea and vomiting associated with radiation therapy, including total body irradiation and fractionated abdominal radiation

I.V.: Prophylaxis of chemotherapy-related emesis; prophylaxis and treatment of postoperative nausea and vomiting (PONV)

Mechanism of Action/Effect Selective 5-HT_3 receptor antagonist, blocking serotonin, both peripherally on vagal nerve terminals and centrally in the chemoreceptor trigger zone.

Contraindications Previous hypersensitivity to granisetron, other 5-HT_3 receptor antagonists, or any component of the formulation

Warnings/Precautions Chemotherapy-related emesis: May be prescribed for patients who are refractory to or have severe adverse reactions to standard antiemetic therapy or young patients (ie, <45 years of age who are more likely to develop extrapyramidal symptoms to high-dose metoclopramide) who are to receive highly emetogenic chemotherapeutic agents. Should not be prescribed for chemotherapeutic agents with a low emetogenic potential (eg, bleomycin, busulfan, cyclophosphamide <1000 mg, etoposide, 5-fluorouracil, vinblastine, vincristine).

Routine prophylaxis for PONV is not recommended. In patients where nausea and vomiting must be avoided postoperatively, administer to all patients even when expected incidence of nausea and vomiting is low. Use caution following abdominal surgery or in chemotherapy-induced nausea and vomiting; may mask progressive ileus or gastric distention. Use caution in patients with liver disease or in pregnancy.

Drug Interactions

Cytochrome P450 Effect: Substrate of CYP3A4

Nutritional/Ethanol Interactions Herb/Nutraceutical: St John's wort may decrease granisetron levels.

Adverse Reactions

>10%:
- Central nervous system: Headache (8% to 21%)
- Gastrointestinal: Constipation (3% to 18%)

1% to 10%:
- Cardiovascular: Hypertension (1% to 2%)
- Central nervous system: Dizziness, insomnia, anxiety, somnolence, fever (3% to 8%), pain (10%)
- Gastrointestinal: Abdominal pain, diarrhea (1% to 9%), dyspepsia
- Hepatic: Elevated liver enzymes (5% to 6%)
- Neuromuscular & skeletal: Weakness (5% to 18%)

<1% (Limited to important or life-threatening): Agitation, allergic reactions, anaphylaxis, angina, arrhythmias, atrial fibrillation, hot flashes, hypotension, syncope

Overdosage/Toxicology Treatment should be symptomatic and supportive.

Pharmacodynamics/Kinetics

Half-Life Elimination: Cancer patients: 10-12 hours; Healthy volunteers: 3-4 hours; PONV: 9 hours

Metabolism: Hepatic via N-demethylation, oxidation, and conjugation; some metabolites may have 5-HT_3 antagonist activity

Onset: Emesis: Controlled within 1-3 minutes

Duration: Generally up to 24 hours

Formulations

Injection, solution, as hydrochloride: 1 mg/mL (4 mL) [contains benzyl alcohol]
Injection, solution, as hydrochloride [preservative free]: 1 mg/mL (1 mL)
Tablet, as hydrochloride: 1 mg

Dosing

Adults & Elderly:

Prophylaxis of chemotherapy-related emesis:

Oral: 2 mg once daily up to 1 hour before chemotherapy or 1 mg twice daily; the first 1 mg dose should be given up to 1 hour before chemotherapy. **Note:** Administer granisetron on day(s) of chemotherapy.

I.V.:

Within U.S.: 10 mcg/kg/dose (or 1 mg/dose) administered IVPB over 5 minutes given within 30 minutes of chemotherapy: for some drugs (eg, carboplatin, cyclophosphamide) with a later onset of emetic action, 10 mcg/kg every 12 hours may be necessary.

Outside U.S.: 40 mcg/kg/dose (or 3 mg/dose); maximum: 9 mg/24 hours

Breakthrough: Repeat the dose 2-3 times within the first 24 hours as necessary (suggested by anecdotal information; not based on controlled trials, or generally recommended).

Note: Administer granisetron on the day(s) of chemotherapy

Prophylaxis of radiation therapy-associated emesis: Oral: 2 mg once daily given 1 hour before radiation therapy.

PONV: I.V.:

Prevention: 1 mg given undiluted over 30 seconds; administer before induction of anesthesia or before reversal of anesthesia

(Continued)

Granisetron *(Continued)*

Treatment: 1 mg given undiluted over 30 seconds

Pediatrics: Prophylaxis associated with cancer chemotherapy: Children >2 years: Refer to adult dosing.

Renal Impairment: No dosage adjustment required.

Hepatic Impairment: Kinetic studies in patients with hepatic impairment showed that total clearance was approximately halved; however, standard doses were very well tolerated.

Administration

Oral: Doses should be given up to 1 hour prior to initiation of chemotherapy/radiation

I.V.: Doses should be given within 30 minutes of initiation of chemotherapy. If diluted, can be administered over 5 minutes.

For prevention of PONV, administer before induction of anesthesia or before reversal of anesthesia.

For PONV, administer undiluted over 30 seconds.

Stability

Storage:

I.V.: Store at 15°C to 30°C (59°F to 86°F). Protect from light. Do not freeze vials.

Oral: Store tablet or oral solution at 15°C to 30°C (59°F to 86°F). Protect from light.

Reconstitution: I.V.: Stable when mixed in NS or D_5W for 24 hours at room temperature.

Compatibility: Stable in $D_5 1/2NS$, D_5NS, D_5W, NS, bacteriostatic water

Y-site administration: Incompatible with amphotericin B

Monitoring and Teaching Issues

Physical Assessment: See Contraindications, Warnings/Precautions, Dosing, and Administration for use cautions. Blood pressure and cardiac status should be monitored. Assess therapeutic effects (antiemetic) and adverse response (eg, acute headache - see Adverse Reactions) periodically during therapy. Teach patient possible side effects and appropriate interventions and adverse symptoms to report (see Patient Education). Note breast-feeding caution.

Patient Education: This drug will be administered on days when you receive chemotherapy to reduce nausea and vomiting. If outpatient chemotherapy, you may be given oral medication to take after return home; take as directed. May also be given to prevent or treat nausea and vomiting after surgery; take as directed. You may experience drowsiness (use caution when driving); persistent or acute headache (request analgesic from prescriber); or nausea (frequent mouth care, chewing gum, or sucking on lozenges may help). Report unrelieved headache, fever, diarrhea, or constipation. **Breast-feeding precaution:** Consult prescriber if breast-feeding.

Geriatric Considerations: Clinical trials with patients older than 65 years of age are limited; however, the data indicates that safety and efficacy are similar to that observed in younger adults. No adjustment in dose necessary for elderly.

Additional Information

Agents with high emetogenic potential (>90%) (dose/m^2):

Amifostine
Azacitidine
Carmustine ≥200 mg/m^2
Cisplatin ≥50 mg/m^2
Cyclophosphamide ≥1 g/m^2
Cytarabine ≥1500 mg/m^2
Dacarbazine ≥500 mg/m^2
Dactinomycin
Doxorubicin ≥60 mg/m^2
Lomustine ≥60 mg/m^2
Mechlorethamine
Melphalan ≥100 mg/m^2
Streptozocin
Thiotepa ≥100 mg/m^2

or two agents classified as having high or moderately high emetogenic potential as listed:

Agents with moderately high emetogenic potential (60% to 90%) (dose/m^2):

Carboplatin 200-400 mg/m^2
Carmustine <200 mg/m^2
Cisplatin <50 mg/m^2
Cyclophosphamide 600-999 mg/m^2
Dacarbazine <500 mg/m^2
Doxorubicin 21-59 mg/m^2
Hexamethyl melamine
Ifosfamide ≥5000 mg/m^2
Lomustine <60 mg/m^2
Methotrexate ≥250 mg/m^2
Pentostatin
Procarbazine

Related Information

Antiemetics for Chemotherapy-Induced Nausea and Vomiting *on page 1639*

Granulocyte Colony Stimulating Factor *see* Filgrastim *on page 558*

Granulocyte-Macrophage Colony Stimulating Factor *see* Sargramostim *on page 1215*

Grifulvin® V *see* Griseofulvin *on page 644*

Griseofulvin (gri see oh FUL vin)

U.S. Brand Names Fulvicin® P/G; Fulvicin-U/F®; Grifulvin® V; Gris-PEG®

Synonyms Griseofulvin Microsize; Griseofulvin Ultramicrosize

Generic Available Yes: Ultramicrosized product

Pharmacologic Category Antifungal Agent, Oral

Pregnancy Risk Factor C

Lactation Excretion in breast milk unknown

Use Treatment of susceptible tinea infections of the skin, hair, and nails

Mechanism of Action/Effect Inhibits fungal cell mitosis at metaphase; binds to human keratin making it resistant to fungal invasion

Contraindications Hypersensitivity to griseofulvin or any component of the formulation; severe liver disease; porphyria (interferes with porphyrin metabolism)

Warnings/Precautions Safe use in children ≤2 years of age has not been established; during long-term therapy, periodic assessment of hepatic, renal, and hematopoietic functions should be performed; may cause fetal harm when administered to pregnant women; avoid exposure to intense sunlight to prevent photosensitivity reactions; hypersensitivity cross reaction between penicillins and griseofulvin is possible. Pregnancy risk C.

Drug Interactions

Cytochrome P450 Effect: Induces CYP1A2, 2C8/9, 3A4

Decreased Effect: Barbiturates may decrease levels. Decreased warfarin activity. Decreased oral contraceptive effectiveness.

Increased Effect/Toxicity: Increased toxicity with ethanol, may cause tachycardia and flushing.

Nutritional/Ethanol Interactions

Ethanol: Avoid ethanol (may increase CNS depression). Ethanol will cause "disulfiram"-type reaction consisting of flushing, headache, nausea, and in some patients, vomiting and chest and/or abdominal pain.

Food: Griseofulvin concentrations may be increased if taken with food, especially with high-fat meals.

Effects on Lab Values False-positive urinary VMA levels

Adverse Reactions

Central nervous system: Headache, fatigue, dizziness, insomnia, mental confusion

Dermatologic: Rash (most common), urticaria (most common), photosensitivity, angioneurotic edema (rare)

Gastrointestinal: Nausea, vomiting, epigastric distress, diarrhea, GI bleeding

Genitourinary: Menstrual irregularities (rare)

Hematologic: Leukopenia

Neuromuscular & skeletal: Paresthesia (rare)

Renal: Hepatotoxicity, proteinuria, nephrosis

Miscellaneous: Oral thrush, drug-induced lupus-like syndrome (rare)

Overdosage/Toxicology Symptoms of overdose include lethargy, vertigo, blurred vision, nausea, vomiting, and diarrhea. Treatment is supportive.

Pharmacodynamics/Kinetics

Absorption: Ultramicrosize griseofulvin absorption is almost complete; absorption of microsize griseofulvin is variable (25% to 70% of an oral dose); enhanced by ingestion of a fatty meal (GI absorption of ultramicrosize is ~1.5 times that of microsize)

Half-Life Elimination: 9-22 hours

Metabolism: Extensively hepatic

Formulations

Suspension, oral, microsize (Grifulvin® V): 125 mg/5 mL (120 mL) [contains alcohol 0.2%]

Tablet, microsize (Fulvicin-U/F®): 250 mg, 500 mg

Tablet, ultramicrosize: 125 mg, 250 mg, 330 mg

Fulvicin® P/G: 125 mg, 165 mg, 250 mg, 330 mg

Gris-PEG®: 125 mg, 250 mg

Dosing

Adults & Elderly: Tinea infections: Oral:

Microsize: 500-1000 mg/day in single or divided doses

Ultramicrosize: 330-375 mg/day in single or divided doses; doses up to 750 mg/day have been used for infections more difficult to eradicate such as tinea unguium and tinea pedis.

Duration of therapy depends on the site of infection:

Tinea corporis: 2-4 weeks

Tinea capitis: 4-6 weeks or longer

Tinea pedis: 4-8 weeks

Tinea unguium: 4-6 months

Pediatrics: Tinea infections: Oral: Children >2 years:

Microsize: 10-15 mg/kg/day in single or divided doses

Ultramicrosize: 5.5-7.3 mg/kg/day in single or divided doses

Monitoring Laboratory Tests Periodic renal, hepatic, and hematopoietic function especially with long-term use

Monitoring and Teaching Issues

Physical Assessment: See Contraindications, Warnings/Precautions, and Dosing for use cautions. Assess results of laboratory tests (see above), therapeutic effects, and adverse response (see Adverse Reactions and Overdose/Toxicology) periodically during therapy. Teach patient possible side effects and appropriate interventions and adverse symptoms to report (see Patient Education). **Pregnancy risk factor C** - benefits of use should outweigh possible risks. **Note:** May cause fetal harm when administered to pregnant women. Oral contraceptives may have decreased effectiveness with griseofulvin. Note breast-feeding caution.

Patient Education: Inform prescriber of all prescriptions, OTC medications, or herbal products you are taking, and any allergies you have. Do not take anything new during treatment unless approved by prescriber. Take as directed, around-the-clock with food. Take full course of medication; do not discontinue without consulting prescriber. Avoid alcohol while taking this drug (disulfiram reactions). Practice good hygiene measures to prevent reinfection. Frequent blood tests may be required with prolonged therapy. You may experience nausea and vomiting (small, frequent meals may help); confusion, dizziness, drowsiness (use caution when driving or engaging in tasks that require alertness until response to drug is known); nausea, vomiting, or diarrhea (small, frequent meals, frequent mouth care, sucking lozenges, or chewing gum may help); or increased sensitivity to sun

(Continued)

Griseofulvin *(Continued)*

(use sunscreen, wear protective clothing and eyewear, and avoid excessive exposure to direct sunlight). Report skin rash; difficulty breathing; CNS changes (confusion, dizziness, acute headache); changes in color of stool or urine; white plaques in mouth; or worsening of condition. **Pregnancy/breast-feeding precautions:** Inform prescriber if you are or intend to become pregnant. Consult prescriber if breast-feeding.

Griseofulvin Microsize *see* Griseofulvin *on page 644*

Griseofulvin Ultramicrosize *see* Griseofulvin *on page 644*

Gris-PEG® *see* Griseofulvin *on page 644*

Growth Hormone *see* Human Growth Hormone *on page 658*

Guaifed® [OTC] *see* Guaifenesin and Pseudoephedrine *on page 648*

Guaifed-PD® *see* Guaifenesin and Pseudoephedrine *on page 648*

Guaifenesin (gwye FEN e sin)

U.S. Brand Names Amibid LA; Breonesin® [OTC] [DSC]; Diabetic Tussin® EX [OTC]; Duratuss-G®; Fenesin™; Glytuss® [OTC]; Guaifenex® G; Guaifenex® LA; Guiatuss® [OTC]; Humibid® L.A.; Humibid® Pediatric; Hytuss® [OTC]; Hytuss-2X® [OTC]; Liquibid®; Liquibid® 1200; Mucinex™ [OTC]; Organidin® NR; Phanasin [OTC]; Respa-GF®; Robitussin® [OTC]; Scot-Tussin® Sugar Free Expectorant [OTC]; Touro Ex®

Synonyms GG; Glycerol Guaiacolate

Generic Available Yes

Pharmacologic Category Expectorant

Pregnancy Risk Factor C

Lactation Excretion in breast milk unknown/use caution

Use Temporary control of cough due to minor throat and bronchial irritation

Mechanism of Action/Effect Thought to act as an expectorant by irritating the gastric mucosa and stimulating respiratory tract secretions, thereby increasing respiratory fluid volumes and decreasing phlegm viscosity

Contraindications Hypersensitivity to guaifenesin or any component of the formulation

Warnings/Precautions Do not use for persistent cough, such as occurs with smoking, asthma, or emphysema or cough accompanied by excessive secretions. Pregnancy risk C.

Drug Interactions

Increased Effect/Toxicity: May increase toxicity/effect of disulfiram, MAO inhibitors, metronidazole, and procarbazine.

Effects on Lab Values Possible color interference with determination of 5-HIAA and VMA

Adverse Reactions 1% to 10%:

Central nervous system: Drowsiness, headache

Dermatologic: Rash

Gastrointestinal: Nausea, vomiting, stomach pain

Overdosage/Toxicology Symptoms of overdose include vomiting, lethargy, coma, and respiratory depression. Treatment is supportive.

Pharmacodynamics/Kinetics

Absorption: Well absorbed

Half-Life Elimination: ~1 hour

Metabolism: Hepatic (60%)

Formulations

Caplet, sustained release (Touro Ex®): 575 mg

Capsule (Breonesin® [DSC], Hytuss-2X®): 200 mg

Capsule, sustained release (Humibid® Pediatric): 300 mg

Liquid: 100 mg/5 mL (120 mL, 240 mL, 480 mL)

- Diabetic Tussin EX®: 100 mg/5 mL (120 mL) [alcohol free, sugar free, dye free; contains phenylalanine 8.4 mg/5 mL]
- Organidin NR®: 100 mg/5 mL (480 mL) [contains sodium benzoate; raspberry flavor]

Syrup: 100 mg/5 mL (120 mL, 240 mL, 480 mL)

- Guiatuss®: 100 mg/5 mL (120 mL, 240 mL, 480 mL, 3840 mL) [alcohol free; fruit-mint flavor]
- Phanasin: 100 mg/5 mL (120 mL, 240 mL) [alcohol free, sugar free, sodium free]
- Robitussin®: 100 mg/5 mL (5 mL, 10 mL, 15 mL, 30 mL, 120 mL, 240 mL, 480 mL) [alcohol free]
- Scot-Tussin® Sugar Free Expectorant: 100 mg/5 mL (120 mL) [alcohol free, dye free; contains benzoic acid; grape flavor]

Tablet: 200 mg

- Glytuss®, Organidin® NR: 200 mg
- Hytuss®: 100 mg

Tablet, extended release (Mucinex™): 600 mg

Tablet, sustained release 600 mg, 1200 mg

- Amibid LA, Fenesin™; Guafenex® LA, Humibid® LA, Liquibid®, Respa-GF®: 600 mg
- Duratuss G, Liquibid® 1200: 1200 mg
- Guaifenex® G: 1200 mg [dye free, film coated]

Dosing

Adults & Elderly: Cough: Oral: 200-400 mg every 4 hours to a maximum of 2.4 g/day

Pediatrics: Cough: Oral:

- <2 years: 12 mg/kg/day in 6 divided doses
- 2-5 years: 50-100 mg every 4 hours, not to exceed 600 mg/day
- 6-11 years: 100-200 mg every 4 hours, not to exceed 1.2 g/day
- >12 years: Refer to adult dosing.

Stability

Storage: Protect from light.

Monitoring and Teaching Issues

Physical Assessment: Assess effectiveness of therapy and adverse reactions (see Adverse Reactions) at beginning of therapy and periodically with long-term use. Teach patient appropriate use, interventions to reduce side effects, and adverse symptoms to report (see Patient Education). **Pregnancy risk factor C** - benefits of use should outweigh possible risks. Note breast-feeding caution.

Patient Education: Inform prescriber of all prescriptions, OTC medications, or herbal products you are taking, and any allergies you have. Do not take anything new without consulting prescriber. Take as prescribed; do not exceed prescribed dose or frequency. Do not chew or crush timed-release capsule. Maintain adequate hydration (2-3 L/day of fluids) unless advised by prescriber to restrict fluids. You may experience some drowsiness (use caution when driving or engaging in tasks requiring alertness until response to drug is known). Report excessive drowsiness, difficulty breathing, or lack of improvement or worsening of condition. **Pregnancy/breast-feeding precautions:** Inform prescriber if you are or intend to become pregnant. Consult prescriber if breast-feeding.

Dietary Issues: Diabetic Tussin EX® contains phenylalanine 8.4 mg/5 mL.

Guaifenesin and Codeine (gwye FEN e sin & KOE deen)

U.S. Brand Names Brontex®; Cheracol®; Gani-Tuss® NR; Guaituss AC®; Mytussin® AC; Robafen® AC; Robitussin® A-C [DSC]; Romilar® AC; Tussi-Organidin® NR; Tussi-Organidin® S-NR

Synonyms Codeine and Guaifenesin

Restrictions C-V

Generic Available Yes

Pharmacologic Category Antitussive; Cough Preparation; Expectorant

Pregnancy Risk Factor C

Lactation Excretion in breast milk unknown/use caution

Use Temporary control of cough due to minor throat and bronchial irritation

Formulations

Liquid: Guaifenesin 100 mg and codeine phosphate 10 mg per 5 mL (120 mL, 480 mL)

- Brontex®: Guaifenesin 75 mg and codeine phosphate 2.5 mg per 5 mL (480 mL) [alcohol free; mint flavor]
- Gani-Tuss® NR: Guaifenesin 100 mg and codeine phosphate 10 mg per 5 mL (480 mL) [sugar free, alcohol free; raspberry flavor]
- Tussi-Organidin® NR: Guaifenesin 100 mg and codeine phosphate 10 mg per 5 mL (480 mL) [contains sodium benzoate; raspberry flavor]
- Tussi-Organidin® S-NR: Guaifenesin 100 mg and codeine phosphate 10 mg per 5 mL (120 mL) [contains sodium benzoate; raspberry flavor]

Syrup: Guaifenesin 100 mg and codeine phosphate 10 mg per 5 mL (120 mL, 480 mL)

- Cheracol®: Guaifenesin 100 mg and codeine phosphate 10 mg per 5 mL (120 mL) [contains alcohol 4.75% and benzoic acid]
- Guaituss AC®: Guaifenesin 100 mg and codeine phosphate 10 mg per 5 mL (120 mL, 480 mL, 3840 mL) [contains alcohol; sugar free; fruit-mint flavor]
- Mytussin® AC: Guaifenesin 100 mg and codeine phosphate 10 mg per 5 mL (120 mL, 480 mL, 3840 mL) [contains alcohol; sugar free; fruit flavor]
- Robafen AC: Guaifenesin 100 mg and codeine phosphate 10 mg per 5 mL (120 mL, 480 mL, 3840 mL)
- Robitussin® AC: Guaifenesin 100 mg and codeine phosphate 10 mg per 5 mL (120 mL) [contains alcohol 3.5%; contains sodium benzoate]
- Romilar® AC: Guaifenesin 100 mg and codeine phosphate 10 mg per 5 mL (480 mL) [contains phenylalanine; alcohol free, sugar free, dye free]

Tablet (Brontex®): Guaifenesin 300 mg and codeine phosphate 10 mg

Dosing

Adults & Elderly: Cough: Oral: 5-10 mL every 4-8 hours not to exceed 60 mL/24 hours

Pediatrics: Cough: Oral:

- 2-6 years: 1-1.5 mg/kg codeine/day divided into 4 doses administered every 4-6 hours (maximum: 30 mg/24 hours)
- 6-12 years: 5 mL every 4 hours, not to exceed 30 mL/24 hours
- >12 years: 10 mL every 4 hours, up to 60 mL/24 hours

Monitoring and Teaching Issues

Physical Assessment: See individual components listed in Related Information. **Pregnancy risk factor C** - benefits of use should outweigh possible risks. Note breast-feeding caution.

Patient Education: See individual components listed in Related Information. **Pregnancy/breast-feeding precautions:** Inform prescriber if you are or intend to become pregnant. Consult prescriber if breast-feeding.

Related Information

Codeine *on page 327*
Guaifenesin *on page 646*

Guaifenesin and Dextromethorphan

(gwye FEN e sin & deks troe meth OR fan)

U.S. Brand Names Aquatab® DM; Benylin® Expectorant [OTC]; Cheracol® D [OTC]; Cheracol® Plus [OTC]; Diabetic Tussin® DM [OTC]; Diabetic Tussin® DM Maximum Strength [OTC]; Duratuss® DM; Fenesin™ DM; Genatuss DM® [OTC]; Guaifenex® DM; Guiatuss-DM® [OTC]; Humibid® DM; Hydro-Tussin™ DM; Kolephrin® GG/DM [OTC]; Mytussin® DM [OTC]; Respa® DM; Robitussin® DM [OTC]; Robitussin® Sugar Free Cough [OTC]; Safe Tussin® 30 [OTC]; Silexin® [OTC]; Tolu-Sed® DM [OTC]; Touro® DM; Tussi-Organidin® DM NR; Vicks® 44E [OTC]; Vicks® Pediatric Formula 44E [OTC]

Synonyms Dextromethorphan and Guaifenesin

Generic Available Yes

Pharmacologic Category Antitussive; Cough Preparation; Expectorant

Pregnancy Risk Factor C

Lactation Excretion in breast milk unknown

Use Temporary control of cough due to minor throat and bronchial irritation

Pharmacokinetic Note See individual agents.

(Continued)

Guaifenesin and Dextromethorphan *(Continued)*

Pharmacodynamics/Kinetics

Onset: Oral: Antitussive: 15-30 minutes

Formulations

Liquid: Guaifenesin 100 mg and dextromethorphan hydrobromide 10 mg per 5 mL (120 mL, 240 mL)

Diabetic Tussin® DM: Guaifenesin 100 mg and dextromethorphan hydrobromide 10 mg per 5 mL (120 mL) [alcohol free, sugar free, dye free; contains phenylalanine 8.4 mg/5 mL]

Diabetic Tussin® DM Maximum Strength: Guaifenesin 200 mg and dextromethorphan hydrobromide 10 mg per 5 mL (120 mL) [alcohol free, sugar free, dye free; contains phenylalanine 8.4 mg/5 mL]

Duratuss® DM: Guaifenesin 200 mg and dextromethorphan hydrobromide 20 mg per 5 mL (480 mL, 3840 mL) [contains alcohol 5%, sodium benzoate; fruit flavor]

Hydro-Tussin™ DM: Guaifenesin 200 mg and dextromethorphan hydrobromide 20 mg per 5 mL (480 mL) [alcohol free, sugar free]

Robitussin® Sugar Free Cough: Guaifenesin 100 mg and dextromethorphan hydrobromide 10 mg per 5 mL (120 mL) [alcohol free, sugar free]

Safe Tussin® 30: Guaifenesin 100 mg and dextromethorphan hydrobromide 15 mg per 5 mL (120 mL) [alcohol free, sugar free, dye free; mint flavor]

Tussi-Organidin® DM NR: Guaifenesin 100 mg and dextromethorphan hydrobromide 10 mg per 5 mL (120 mL, 480 mL) [contains sodium benzoate; raspberry flavor]

Vicks® 44E: Guaifenesin 200 mg and dextromethorphan hydrobromide 20 mg per 15 mL (120 mL, 235 mL) [contains sodium 31 mg/15 mL, alcohol, sodium benzoate]

Vicks® Pediatric Formula 44E: Guaifenesin 100 mg and dextromethorphan hydrobromide 10 mg per 15 mL (120 mL) [alcohol free; contains sodium 30 mg/15 mL, sodium benzoate; cherry flavor]

Syrup: Guaifenesin 100 mg and dextromethorphan hydrobromide 10 mg per 5 mL (120 mL, 240 mL, 480 mL)

Benylin® Expectorant: Guaifenesin 100 mg and dextromethorphan hydrobromide 5 mg per 5 mL (120 mL) [alcohol free, sugar free; contains sodium benzoate; raspberry flavor]

Cheracol® D: Guaifenesin 100 mg and dextromethorphan hydrobromide 10 mg per 5 mL (120 mL, 180 mL) [contains alcohol, benzoic acid]

Cheracol® Plus: Guaifenesin 100 mg and dextromethorphan hydrobromide 10 mg per 5 mL (120 mL)

Genatuss DM®: Guaifenesin 100 mg and dextromethorphan hydrobromide 10 mg per 5 mL (120 mL) [cherry flavor]

Guiatuss® DM: Guaifenesin 100 mg and dextromethorphan hydrobromide 10 mg per 5 mL (120 mL, 240 mL, 480 mL, 3840 mL) [alcohol free; fruit-mint flavor]

Kolephrin® GG/DM: Guaifenesin 150 mg and dextromethorphan hydrobromide 10 mg per 5 mL (120 mL) [alcohol free; cherry flavor]

Mytussin® DM: Guaifenesin 100 mg and dextromethorphan hydrobromide 10 mg per 5 mL (120 mL, 480 mL) [alcohol free; cherry flavor]

Robitussin®-DM: Guaifenesin 100 mg and dextromethorphan hydrobromide 10 mg per 5 mL (5 mL, 120 mL, 360 mL, 480 mL) [alcohol free]

Silexin®: Guaifenesin 100 mg and dextromethorphan hydrobromide 10 mg per 5 mL (45 mL, 480 mL)

Tolu-Sed®: Guaifenesin 100 mg and dextromethorphan hydrobromide 10 mg per 5 mL (120 mL)

Tablet (Silexin®): Guaifenesin 100 mg and dextromethorphan hydrobromide 10 mg

Tablet, extended release: Guaifenesin 600 mg and dextromethorphan hydrobromide 30 mg

Aquatab® DM: Guaifenesin 1200 mg and dextromethorphan hydrobromide 60 mg

Fenesin™ DM, Guaifenex® DM, Humibid® DM, Respa DM®: Guaifenesin 600 mg and dextromethorphan hydrobromide 30 mg

Touro® DM: Guaifenesin 575 mg and dextromethorphan hydrobromide 30 mg

Dosing

Adults & Elderly: Cough: Oral: 5 mL every 4 hours or 10 mL every 6-8 hours not to exceed 40 mL/24 hours

Pediatrics: Cough: Oral:

Children: Dextromethorphan: 1-2 mg/kg/24 hours divided 3-4 times/day

Children >12 years: Refer to adult dosing.

Monitoring and Teaching Issues

Physical Assessment: See individual components listed in Related Information. **Pregnancy risk factor C** - benefits of use should outweigh possible risks. Note breast-feeding caution.

Patient Education: Also see Guaifenesin.

Based on Dextromethorphan component: Do not exceed recommended dosage; take with a large glass of water; if cough lasts more than 1 week or is accompanied by a rash, fever, or headache, notify physician.

Pregnancy/breast-feeding precautions: Inform prescriber if you are or intend to become pregnant. Consult prescriber if breast-feeding.

Related Information

Guaifenesin *on page 646*

Guaifenesin and Pseudoephedrine (gwye FEN e sin & soo doe e FED rin)

U.S. Brand Names Ami-Tex PSE; Anatuss LA; Aquatab®; Aquatab® D Dose Pack; Congestac®; Deconsal® II; Defen-LA®; Duratuss™; Duratuss™ GP; Entex® PSE; Eudal®-SR; G-Phed; G-Phed-PD; Guaifed® [OTC]; Guaifed-PD®; Guaifenex® GP; Guaifenex® PSE; Guaifen PSE; Guai-Vent™/PSE; Maxifed®; Maxifed-G®; Miraphen PSE; PanMist® Jr.; PanMist® LA; PanMist® S; Pseudo GG TR; Pseudovent™, Pseudovent™-Ped; Respa-1st®; Respaire®-60 SR; Respaire®-120 SR; Robitussin-PE® [OTC]; Robitussin® Severe Congestion [OTC]; Touro LA®; V-Dec-M®; Versacaps®; Zephrex®; Zephrex LA®

Synonyms Pseudoephedrine and Guaifenesin

Generic Available Yes

Pharmacologic Category Decongestant; Expectorant

Pregnancy Risk Factor C

Lactation Excretion in breast milk unknown

Use Enhance the output of respiratory tract fluid and reduce mucosal congestion and edema in the nasal passage

Formulations

Caplet (Congestac®): Guaifenesin 400 mg and pseudoephedrine hydrochloride 60 mg

Caplet, long acting (Touro LA®): Guaifenesin 500 mg and pseudoephedrine hydrochloride 120 mg

Capsule:

Pseudovent™: Guaifenesin 250 mg and pseudoephedrine hydrochloride 120 mg

Pseudovent™-Ped: Guaifenesin 300 mg and pseudoephedrine hydrochloride 60 mg

Robitussin® Severe Congestion: Guaifenesin 200 mg and pseudoephedrine hydrochloride 30 mg

Capsule, extended release:

G-Phed, Guaifed®, Respaire®-120 SR: Guaifenesin 250 mg and pseudoephedrine hydrochloride 120 mg

G-Phed-PD, Guaifed-PD®, Versacaps®: Guaifenesin 300 mg and pseudoephedrine hydrochloride 60 mg

Respaire®-60 SR: Guaifenesin 200 mg and pseudoephedrine hydrochloride 60 mg

Syrup:

PanMist®-S: Guaifenesin 200 mg and pseudoephedrine hydrochloride 45 mg per 5 mL (480 mL) [grape flavor]

Robitussin-PE®: Guaifenesin 100 mg and pseudoephedrine hydrochloride 30 mg per 5 mL (120 mL, 240 mL) [alcohol free]

Tablet: Zephrex®: Guaifenesin 400 mg and pseudoephedrine hydrochloride 60 mg

Tablet, extended release: Guaifenesin 600 mg and pseudoephedrine hydrochloride 60 mg; guaifenesin 600 mg and pseudoephedrine hydrochloride 120 mg; guaifenesin 1200 mg and pseudoephedrine hydrochloride 60 mg; guaifenesin 1200 mg and pseudoephedrine hydrochloride 120 mg

Amitex PSE, Duratuss®, Entex® PSE, Guaifen PSE, Guaifenex PSE® 120, Guai-Vent™/PSE, Miraphen PSE, Zephrex LA®: Guaifenesin 600 mg and pseudoephedrine hydrochloride 120 mg

Anatuss LA, Eudal®-SR: Guaifenesin 400 mg and pseudoephedrine hydrochloride 120 mg

Aquatab® D: Guaifenesin 1200 mg and pseudoephedrine hydrochloride 60 mg

Aquatab® D Dose Pack, Deconsal® II, Defen-LA®, Guaifenex PSE® 60, Respa-1st®: Guaifenesin 600 mg and pseudoephedrine hydrochloride 60 mg

Duratuss™ GP, Guaifenex® GP: Guaifenesin 1200 mg and pseudoephedrine hydrochloride 120 mg [dye free]

Maxifed®: Guaifenesin 700 mg and pseudoephedrine hydrochloride 80 mg

Maxifed-G®: Guaifenesin 550 mg and pseudoephedrine hydrochloride 60 mg

PanMist®-JR, Pseudo GG TR: Guaifenesin 600 mg and pseudoephedrine hydrochloride 45 mg

PanMist®-LA: Guaifenesin 800 mg and pseudoephedrine hydrochloride 80 mg

V-Dec-M®: Guaifenesin 500 mg and pseudoephedrine hydrochloride 120 mg

Dosing

Adults: Expectorant/decongestant: Oral: 10 mL syrup every 4 hours; maximum: 60 mL daily

Elderly: Refer to adult dosing; use with caution.

Monitoring and Teaching Issues

Physical Assessment: See individual components listed in Related Information. **Pregnancy risk factor C** - benefits of use should outweigh possible risks. Note breast-feeding caution.

Patient Education: See individual components listed in Related Information. **Pregnancy/breast-feeding precautions:** Inform prescriber if you are or intend to become pregnant. Consult prescriber if breast-feeding.

Related Information

Guaifenesin *on page 646*

Pseudoephedrine *on page 1150*

Guaifenesin and Theophylline *see* Theophylline and Guaifenesin *on page 1303*

Guaifenesin, Pseudoephedrine, and Codeine

(gwye FEN e sin, soo doe e FED rin, & KOE deen)

U.S. Brand Names Cheratussin DAC; Codafed® Expectorant; Codafed® Pediatric Expectorant; Dihistine® Expectorant; Guiatuss™ DAC®; Halotussin® DAC; Mytussin® DAC; Nucofed® Expectorant; Nucofed® Pediatric Expectorant; Nucotuss®; Robitussin®-DAC [DSC]

Synonyms Codeine, Guaifenesin, and Pseudoephedrine; Pseudoephedrine, Guaifenesin, and Codeine

Restrictions C-III; C-V

Generic Available Yes

Pharmacologic Category Antitussive/Decongestant/Expectorant

Pregnancy Risk Factor C

Lactation Excretion in breast milk unknown/use caution

Use Temporarily relieves nasal congestion and controls cough due to minor throat and bronchial irritation; helps loosen phlegm and thin bronchial secretions to make coughs more productive

Formulations

Liquid:

Cheratussin DAC: Guaifenesin 100 mg, pseudoephedrine hydrochloride 30 mg, and codeine phosphate 10 mg per 5 mL (480 mL) [sugar free]

Dihistine® Expectorant: Guaifenesin 100 mg, pseudoephedrine hydrochloride 30 mg, and codeine phosphate 10 mg per 5 mL (120 mL) [contains alcohol 7.5%; fruit flavor]

Halotussin DAC: Guaifenesin 100 mg, pseudoephedrine hydrochloride 30 mg, and codeine phosphate 10 mg per 5 mL (480 mL) [sugar free; cherry-raspberry flavor]

(Continued)

Guaifenesin, Pseudoephedrine, and Codeine *(Continued)*

Syrup:

Codafed® Expectorant: Guaifenesin 200 mg, pseudoephedrine hydrochloride 60 mg, and codeine phosphate 20 mg per 5 mL (480 mL) [wintergreen flavor]

Codafed® Pediatric Expectorant: Guaifenesin 100 mg, pseudoephedrine hydrochloride 30 mg, and codeine phosphate 10 mg per 5 mL (480 mL) [strawberry flavor]

Guiatuss™ DAC: Guaifenesin 100 mg, pseudoephedrine hydrochloride 30 mg, and codeine phosphate 10 mg per 5 mL (480 mL) [may contain codeine]

Robitussin®-DAC [DSC]: Guaifenesin 100 mg, pseudoephedrine hydrochloride 30 mg, and codeine phosphate 10 mg per 5 mL

Mytussin® DAC: Guaifenesin 100 mg, pseudoephedrine hydrochloride 30 mg, and codeine phosphate 10 mg per 5 mL (120 mL, 480 mL) [sugar free; contains alcohol 1.7%; strawberry-raspberry flavor]

Nucofed® Expectorant, Nucotuss® Expectorant: Guaifenesin 200 mg, pseudoephedrine hydrochloride 60 mg, and codeine phosphate 20 mg per 5 mL (480 mL) [contains alcohol 12.5%; cherry flavor]

Nucofed® Pediatric Expectorant: Guaifenesin 100 mg, pseudoephedrine hydrochloride 30 mg, and codeine phosphate 10 mg per 5 mL (480 mL) [contains alcohol 6%; strawberry flavor]

Dosing

Adults: Expectorant/decongestant/cough suppressant: Oral: 10 mL syrup every 4 hours

Elderly: Refer to adult dosing; use with caution.

Pediatrics: Expectorant/decongestant/cough suppressant: Oral:

Children 6-12 years: 5 mL every 4 hours, not to exceed 40 mL/24 hours

Children >12 years: Refer to adult dosing.

Monitoring and Teaching Issues

Physical Assessment: See individual components listed in Related Information. **Pregnancy risk factor C** - benefits of use should outweigh possible risks. Note breast-feeding caution.

Patient Education: See individual components listed in Related Information. **Pregnancy/breast-feeding precautions:** Inform prescriber if you are or intend to become pregnant. Consult prescriber if breast-feeding.

Related Information

Codeine *on page 327*
Guaifenesin *on page 646*
Pseudoephedrine *on page 1150*

Guaifenex® DM *see* Guaifenesin and Dextromethorphan *on page 647*
Guaifenex® G *see* Guaifenesin *on page 646*
Guaifenex® GP *see* Guaifenesin and Pseudoephedrine *on page 648*
Guaifenex® LA *see* Guaifenesin *on page 646*
Guaifenex® PSE *see* Guaifenesin and Pseudoephedrine *on page 648*
Guaifen PSE *see* Guaifenesin and Pseudoephedrine *on page 648*
Guaituss AC® *see* Guaifenesin and Codeine *on page 647*
Guai-Vent™/PSE *see* Guaifenesin and Pseudoephedrine *on page 648*
Guiatuss® [OTC] *see* Guaifenesin *on page 646*
Guiatuss™ DAC® *see* Guaifenesin, Pseudoephedrine, and Codeine *on page 649*
Guiatuss-DM® [OTC] *see* Guaifenesin and Dextromethorphan *on page 647*
Gynecort® [OTC] *see* Topical Corticosteroids *on page 1334*
Gyne-Lotrimin® [OTC] *see* Clotrimazole *on page 322*
Gyne-Lotrimin® 3 [OTC] *see* Clotrimazole *on page 322*
Gynix® [OTC] *see* Clotrimazole *on page 322*
Gynodiol® *see* Estradiol *on page 494*
Habitrol® *see* Nicotine *on page 968*
***Haemophilus* B Conjugate Vaccine** *see page 1498*
Halazepam *see page 1608*
Halcinonide *see* Topical Corticosteroids *on page 1334*
Halcion® *see* Triazolam *on page 1359*
Haldol® *see* Haloperidol *on page 650*
Haldol® Decanoate *see* Haloperidol *on page 650*
Haley's M-O® [OTC] *see* Magnesium Supplements *on page 831*
Halfprin® [OTC] *see* Aspirin *on page 121*
Hallucinogens *see page 1568*
Halobetasol *see* Topical Corticosteroids *on page 1334*
Halog® *see* Topical Corticosteroids *on page 1334*
Halog®-E *see* Topical Corticosteroids *on page 1334*

Haloperidol (ha loe PER i dole)

U.S. Brand Names Haldol®; Haldol® Decanoate

Synonyms Haloperidol Decanoate; Haloperidol Lactate

Generic Available Yes

Pharmacologic Category Antipsychotic Agent, Butyrophenone

Pregnancy Risk Factor C

Lactation Enters breast milk/not recommended (AAP rates "of concern")

Use Management of schizophrenia; control of tics and vocal utterances of Tourette's disorder in children and adults; severe behavioral problems in children

Use - Unlabeled/Investigational Treatment of psychosis; may be used for the emergency sedation of severely agitated or delirious patients; adjunctive treatment of ethanol dependence; antiemetic

Mechanism of Action/Effect Blocks postsynaptic mesolimbic dopaminergic D_1 and D_2 receptors in the brain; depresses the release of hypothalamic and hypophyseal hormones; believed to depress the reticular activating system thus affecting basal metabolism, body temperature, wakefulness, vasomotor tone, and emesis

Contraindications Hypersensitivity to haloperidol or any component of the formulation; Parkinson's disease; severe CNS depression; bone marrow suppression; severe cardiac or hepatic disease; coma

Warnings/Precautions May be sedating, use with caution in disorders where CNS depression is a feature. Caution in patients with hemodynamic instability, predisposition to seizures, subcortical brain damage, renal or respiratory disease. Esophageal dysmotility and aspiration have been associated with antipsychotic use - use with caution in patients at risk of pneumonia (ie, Alzheimer's disease). Caution in breast cancer or other prolactin-dependent tumors (may elevate prolactin levels). May alter temperature regulation or mask toxicity of other drugs due to antiemetic effects. Hypotension may occur, particularly with parenteral administration. Decanoate form should never be administered I.V. Adverse effects of decanoate may be prolonged. Avoid in thyrotoxicosis.

May alter cardiac conduction - life-threatening arrhythmias have occurred with therapeutic doses of antipsychotics. Use with caution in patients at risk of hypotension (orthostasis) or those who would tolerate transient hypotensive episodes (cerebrovascular disease, cardiovascular disease, or other medications which may predispose).

Use with caution in patients with decreased gastrointestinal motility, urinary retention, BPH, xerostomia, or visual problems. May exacerbate narrow-angle glaucoma (screening is recommended) or worsen myasthenia gravis. Relative to other neuroleptics, haloperidol has a low potency of cholinergic blockade.

May cause extrapyramidal symptoms, including pseudoparkinsonism, acute dystonic reactions, akathisia, and tardive dyskinesia (risk of these reactions is high relative to other neuroleptics). May be associated with neuroleptic malignant syndrome (NMS) or pigmentary retinopathy. Some tablets contain tartrazine.

Pregnancy risk C.

Drug Interactions

Cytochrome P450 Effect: Substrate of CYP1A2, **2D6, 3A4**; Inhibits **CYP2D6**

Decreased Effect: Haloperidol may inhibit the ability of bromocriptine to lower serum prolactin concentrations. Benztropine (and other anticholinergics) may inhibit the therapeutic response to haloperidol and excess anticholinergic effects may occur. Barbiturates, carbamazepine, and cigarette smoking may enhance the hepatic metabolism of haloperidol. Haloperidol may inhibit the antiparkinsonian effect of levodopa; avoid this combination.

Increased Effect/Toxicity: Haloperidol concentrations/effects may be increased by chloroquine, fluoxetine, paroxetine, propranolol, quinidine, and sulfadoxine-pyridoxine. Haloperidol may increase the effects of antihypertensives, CNS depressants (ethanol, narcotics, sedative-hypnotics), lithium, trazodone, and TCAs. Haloperidol in combination with indomethacin may result in drowsiness, tiredness, and confusion. Metoclopramide may increase risk of extrapyramidal symptoms (EPS).

Nutritional/Ethanol Interactions

Ethanol: Avoid ethanol (may increase CNS depression).

Herb/Nutraceutical: Avoid valerian, St John's wort, kava kava, gotu kola (may increase CNS depression).

Effects on Lab Values ↓ cholesterol (S)

Adverse Reactions Frequency not defined.

Cardiovascular: Hypotension, hypertension, tachycardia, arrhythmias, abnormal T waves with prolonged ventricular repolarization

Central nervous system: Restlessness, anxiety, extrapyramidal reactions, dystonic reactions, pseudoparkinsonian signs and symptoms, tardive dyskinesia, neuroleptic malignant syndrome (NMS), altered central temperature regulation, akathisia, tardive dystonia, insomnia, euphoria, agitation, drowsiness, depression, lethargy, headache, confusion, vertigo, seizures

Dermatologic: Hyperpigmentation, pruritus, rash, contact dermatitis, alopecia, photosensitivity (rare)

Endocrine & metabolic: Amenorrhea, galactorrhea, gynecomastia, sexual dysfunction, lactation, breast engorgement, mastalgia, menstrual irregularities, hyperglycemia, hypoglycemia, hyponatremia

Gastrointestinal: Nausea, vomiting, anorexia, constipation, diarrhea, hypersalivation, dyspepsia, xerostomia

Genitourinary: Urinary retention, priapism

Hematologic: Cholestatic jaundice, obstructive jaundice

Ocular: Blurred vision

Respiratory: Laryngospasm, bronchospasm

Miscellaneous: Heat stroke, diaphoresis

Overdosage/Toxicology Symptoms of overdose include deep sleep, dystonia, agitation, dysrhythmias, and extrapyramidal symptoms. Treatment is supportive and symptomatic.

Pharmacodynamics/Kinetics

Bioavailability: Oral: 60%

Half-Life Elimination: 20 hours

Time to Peak: Serum: 20 minutes

Metabolism: Hepatic to inactive compounds

Onset: Sedation: I.V.: ~1 hour

Duration: Decanoate: ~3 weeks

Formulations

Injection, oil, as decanoate (Haldol® Decanoate): 50 mg/mL (1 mL, 5 mL); 100 mg/mL (1 mL, 5 mL) [contains benzyl alcohol, sesame oil]

Injection, solution, as lactate (Haldol®): 5 mg/mL (1 mL, 10 mL)

Solution, oral concentrate, as lactate: 2 mg/mL (15 mL, 120 mL)

(Continued)

Haloperidol *(Continued)*

Tablet: 0.5 mg, 1 mg, 2 mg, 5 mg, 10 mg, 20 mg

Dosing

Adults:

Psychosis:

Oral: 0.5-5 mg 2-3 times/day; usual maximum: 30 mg/day

I.M. (as lactate): 2-5 mg every 4-8 hours as needed

I.M. (as decanoate): Initial: 10-20 times the daily oral dose administered at 4-week intervals

Maintenance dose: 10-15 times initial oral dose; used to stabilize psychiatric symptoms

Sedation in the intensive care unit:

I.M., IVP, IVPB: May repeat bolus doses after 30 minutes until calm achieved then administer 50% of the maximum dose every 6 hours.

Mild agitation: 0.5-2 mg

Moderate agitation: 2.5-5 mg

Severe agitation: 10-20 mg

Oral: Agitation: 5-10 mg

Continuous I.V. infusion (100 mg/100 mL D_5W): Rates of 1-40 mg/hour have been used

Rapid tranquilization of severely-agitated patient (administer every 30-60 minutes):

Oral: 5-10 mg

I.M.: 5 mg

Average total dose (oral or I.M.) for tranquilization: 10-20 mg

Elderly: Nonpsychotic patients, dementia behavior: Initial: Oral: 0.25-0.5 mg 1-2 times/day; increase dose at 4- to 7-day intervals by 0.25-0.5 mg/day. Increase dosing intervals (twice daily, 3 times/day, etc) as necessary to control response or side effects.

Pediatrics:

Children: 3-12 years (15-40 kg): Oral:

Initial: 0.05 mg/kg/day or 0.25-0.5 mg/day given in 2-3 divided doses; increase by 0.25-0.5 mg every 5-7 days; maximum: 0.15 mg/kg/day

Usual maintenance:

Agitation or hyperkinesia: 0.01-0.03 mg/kg/day once daily

Nonpsychotic disorders: 0.05-0.075 mg/kg/day in 2-3 divided doses

Psychotic disorders: 0.05-0.15 mg/kg/day in 2-3 divided doses

Children 6-12 years: Sedation/psychotic disorders: I.M. (as lactate): 1-3 mg/dose every 4-8 hours to a maximum of 0.15 mg/kg/day; change over to oral therapy as soon as able.

Renal Impairment: Hemodialysis/peritoneal dialysis: Supplemental dose is not necessary.

Administration

Oral: Dilute the oral concentrate with water or juice before administration. **Note:** Avoid skin contact with oral medication; may cause contact dermatitis.

I.M.: The decanoate injectable formulation should be administered I.M. only; **do not give decanoate I.V.**

I.V.:

Decanoate: Do **not** administer I.V.

Lactate: Although not an FDA-approved route of administration, Haldol® has been administered by this route in many acute care settings.

Stability

Storage: Protect oral dosage forms from light. Haloperidol lactate injection should be stored at controlled room temperature and protected from light, freezing, and temperatures >40°C. Exposure to light may cause discoloration and the development of a grayish-red precipitate over several weeks.

Reconstitution: Haloperidol lactate may be administered IVPB or I.V. infusion in D_5W solutions. NS solutions should not be used due to reports of decreased stability and incompatibility.

Standardized dose: 0.5-100 mg/50-100 mL D_5W

Stability of standardized solutions is 38 days at room temperature (24°C).

Compatibility: Stable in D_5W

Y-site administration: Incompatible with allopurinol, amphotericin B cholesteryl sulfate complex, cefepime, fluconazole, foscarnet, heparin, piperacillin/tazobactam, sargramostim

Compatibility in syringe: Incompatible with diphenhydramine, heparin, hydroxyzine, ketorolac

Monitoring Laboratory Tests Ophthalmic screening

Monitoring and Teaching Issues

Physical Assessment: Assess other medications patient is taking for effectiveness and interactions (especially drugs metabolized by P450 enzymes - see Drug Interactions). See Contraindications and Warnings/Precautions for use cautions. Review ophthalmic screening (see Monitoring Laboratory Tests) and monitor therapeutic response and adverse reactions at beginning of therapy and periodically with long-term use (see Adverse Reactions and Overdose/Toxicology). With I.M. or I.V. use, monitor for hypotension. Initiate at lower doses (see Dosing) and taper dosage slowly when discontinuing. Assess knowledge/teach patient appropriate use, interventions to reduce side effects, and adverse symptoms to report (see Patient Education). **Pregnancy risk factor C** - benefits of use should outweigh possible risks. Breast-feeding is not recommended.

Patient Education: Use exactly as directed; do not increase dose or frequency. It may take 2-3 weeks to achieve desired results; do not discontinue without consulting prescriber. Dilute oral concentration with water or juice. Do not take within 2 hours of any antacid. Store away from light. Avoid alcohol or caffeine and other prescription or OTC medications not approved by prescriber. Maintain adequate hydration (2-3 L/day of fluids) unless advised by prescriber to restrict fluids. Avoid skin contact with medication; may cause contact dermatitis (wash immediately with warm, soapy water). You may experience excess drowsiness, restlessness, dizziness, or blurred vision (use caution driving or when engaging in tasks requiring alertness until response to drug is known); nausea or vomiting (small, frequent meals, frequent mouth care, chewing gum, or sucking lozenges may help);

constipation (increased exercise, fluids, fruit, or fiber may help); postural hypotension (use caution climbing stairs or when changing position from lying or sitting to standing); urinary retention (void before taking medication); or decreased perspiration (avoid strenuous exercise in hot environments). Report persistent CNS effects (eg, trembling fingers, altered gait or balance, excessive sedation, seizures, unusual movements, anxiety, abnormal thoughts, confusion, personality changes); chest pain, palpitations, rapid heartbeat, severe dizziness; unresolved urinary retention or changes in urinary pattern; vision changes; skin rash or yellowing of skin; difficulty breathing; or worsening of condition. **Pregnancy/breast-feeding precautions:** Inform prescriber if you are or intend to become pregnant. Breast-feeding is not recommended.

Geriatric Considerations: (See Warnings/Precautions, Adverse Reactions, and Overdose/Toxicology.) Elderly patients have an increased risk of adverse response to side effects or adverse reactions to antipsychotics.

Breast-feeding Issues: Decline in developmental scores may be seen in nursing infants.

Related Information

Antiemetics for Chemotherapy-Induced Nausea and Vomiting *on page 1639*
Antipsychotic Agents *on page 1558*
Antipsychotic Medication Guidelines *on page 1614*

Haloperidol Decanoate *see* Haloperidol *on page 650*
Haloperidol Lactate *see* Haloperidol *on page 650*
Halotussin® DAC *see* Guaifenesin, Pseudoephedrine, and Codeine *on page 649*
Haltran® [OTC] *see* Ibuprofen *on page 688*
Hashish and Hashish Oil *see page 1568*
Havrix® *see page 1498*
hBNP *see* Nesiritide *on page 962*
HCFA Guidelines for Unnecessary Drugs in Long-Term Care Facilities *see page 1612*
hCG *see* Chorionic Gonadotropin (Human) *on page 284*
HCTZ *see* Hydrochlorothiazide *on page 664*
HCTZ and Telmisartan *see* Telmisartan and Hydrochlorothiazide *on page 1280*
HDA® Toothache [OTC] *see* Benzocaine *on page 156*
Healon® *see page 1509*
Healon® *see page 1461*
Healon® GV *see page 1509*
Healon® GV *see page 1461*
Heart Failure *see page 1670*
Hectorol® *see* Doxercalciferol *on page 445*
***Helicobacter pylori* Treatment** *see page 1676*
Helidac® *see* Bismuth Subsalicylate, Metronidazole, and Tetracycline *on page 170*
Helistat® *see page 1461*
Helixate® FS *see* Antihemophilic Factor (Recombinant) *on page 112*
Hemabate™ *see* Carboprost Tromethamine *on page 221*
Hemocyte™[OTC] *see* Iron Supplements *on page 744*
Hemofil® M *see* Antihemophilic Factor (Human) *on page 109*
Hemotene® *see page 1461*
Hemril-HC® *see* Hydrocortisone *on page 673*
Hemril-HC® Uniserts® *see* Topical Corticosteroids *on page 1334*

Heparin (HEP a rin)

U.S. Brand Names Hep-Lock®

Synonyms Heparin Calcium; Heparin Lock Flush; Heparin Sodium

Generic Available Yes

Pharmacologic Category Anticoagulant

Pregnancy Risk Factor C

Lactation Does not enter breast milk/compatible

Use Prophylaxis and treatment of thromboembolic disorders

Mechanism of Action/Effect Potentiates the action of antithrombin III and thereby inactivates thrombin (as well as activated coagulation factors IX, X, XI, XII, and plasmin) and prevents the conversion of fibrinogen to fibrin; heparin also stimulates release of lipoprotein lipase (lipoprotein lipase hydrolyzes triglycerides to glycerol and free fatty acids)

Contraindications Hypersensitivity to heparin or any component of the formulation; severe thrombocytopenia; uncontrolled active bleeding except when due to DIC; suspected intracranial hemorrhage; not for I.M. use; not for use when appropriate monitoring parameters cannot be obtained

Warnings/Precautions Hemorrhage is the most common complication. Risk factors for bleeding include bacterial endocarditis; congenital or acquired bleeding disorders; active ulcerative or angiodysplastic GI diseases; severe uncontrolled hypertension; hemorrhagic stroke; or use shortly after brain, spinal, or ophthalmology surgery; patient treated concomitantly with platelet inhibitors; conditions associated with increased bleeding tendencies (hemophilia, vascular purpura); recent GI bleeding; thrombocytopenia or platelet defects; severe liver disease; hypertensive or diabetic retinopathy; or in patients undergoing invasive procedures. A higher incidence of bleeding has been reported in women >60 years of age.

Patients who develop thrombocytopenia on heparin may be at risk of developing a new thrombus ("White-clot syndrome"). Hypersensitivity reactions can occur. Heparin should be used cautiously in patients with a documented hypersensitivity reaction and only in life-threatening situations. Osteoporosis can occur following long-term use (>6 months). May cause hyperkalemia due to effects on aldosterone. Discontinue therapy and consider alternatives if platelets are <100,000/mm^3. Patients >60 years of age may require lower doses of heparin.

(Continued)

Heparin *(Continued)*

Heparin does not possess fibrinolytic activity and, therefore, cannot lyse established thrombi; discontinue heparin if hemorrhage occurs; severe hemorrhage or overdosage may require protamine

Pregnancy risk C.

Drug Interactions

Decreased Effect: Nitroglycerin (I.V.) may decrease heparin's anticoagulant effect. This interaction has not been validated in some studies, and may only occur at high nitroglycerin dosages.

Increased Effect/Toxicity: The risk of hemorrhage associated with heparin may be increased by oral anticoagulants (warfarin), thrombolytics, dextran, and drugs which affect platelet function (eg, aspirin, NSAIDs, dipyridamole, ticlopidine, clopidogrel, IIb/IIIa antagonists). However, heparin is often used in conjunction with thrombolytic therapy or during the initiation of warfarin therapy to assure anticoagulation and to protect against possible transient hypercoagulability. Cephalosporins which contain the MTT side chain and parenteral penicillins (may inhibit platelet aggregation) may increase the risk of hemorrhage. Other drugs reported to increase heparin's anticoagulant effect include antihistamines, tetracycline, quinine, nicotine, and cardiac glycosides (digoxin).

Nutritional/Ethanol Interactions

Food: When taking for >6 months, may interfere with calcium absorption.

Herb/Nutraceutical: Avoid cat's claw, dong quai, evening primrose, feverfew, red clover, horse chestnut, garlic, green tea, ginseng, ginkgo (all have additional antiplatelet activity).

Effects on Lab Values ↑ thyroxine (S) (competitive protein binding methods), PT, PTT, bleeding time. A volume of at least 10 mL of blood should be removed and discarded from a heparinized line before blood samples are sent for coagulation testing.

Adverse Reactions

Cardiovascular: Chest pain, vasospasm (possibly related to thrombosis), hemorrhagic shock

Central nervous system: Fever, headache, chills

Dermatologic: Unexplained bruising, urticaria, alopecia, dysesthesia pedis, purpura, eczema, cutaneous necrosis (following deep S.C. injection), erythematous plaques (case reports)

Endocrine & metabolic: Hyperkalemia (supression of aldosterone), rebound hyperlipidemia on discontinuation

Gastrointestinal: Nausea, vomiting, constipation, hematemesis

Genitourinary: Frequent or persistent erection

Hematologic: Hemorrhage, blood in urine, bleeding from gums, epistaxis, adrenal hemorrhage, ovarian hemorrhage, retroperitoneal hemorrhage, thrombocytopenia (see note)

Hepatic: Elevated liver enzymes (AST/ALT) Local: Irritation, ulceration, cutaneous necrosis have been rarely reported with deep S.C. injections, I.M. injection (not recommended) is associated with a high incidence of these effects

Neuromuscular & skeletal: Peripheral neuropathy, osteoporosis (chronic therapy effect)

Respiratory: Hemoptysis, pulmonary hemorrhage, asthma, rhinitis, bronchospasm (case reports)

Ocular: Conjunctivitis (allergic reaction)

Miscellaneous: Allergic reactions, anaphylactoid reactions

Note: Thrombocytopenia has been reported to occur at an incidence between 0% and 30%. It is often of no clinical significance. However, immunologically mediated heparin-induced thrombocytopenia has been estimated to occur in 1% to 2% of patients, and is marked by a progressive fall in platelet counts and, in some cases, thromboembolic complications (skin necrosis, pulmonary embolism, gangrene of the extremities, stroke or myocardial infarction); daily platelet counts for 5-7 days at initiation of therapy may help detect the onset of this complication.

Overdosage/Toxicology The primary symptom of overdose is bleeding. Antidote is protamine; dose 1 mg neutralizes 1 mg (100 units) of heparin. Discontinue all heparin if evidence of progressive immune thrombocytopenia occurs.

Pharmacodynamics/Kinetics

Absorption: Oral, rectal, I.M.: Erratic at best from all these routes of administration; S.C. absorption is also erratic, but considered acceptable for prophylactic use

Half-Life Elimination: Mean: 1.5 hours; Range: 1-2 hours; affected by obesity, renal function, hepatic function, malignancy, presence of pulmonary embolism, and infections

Metabolism: Hepatic; may be partially metabolized in the reticuloendothelial system

Onset: Anticoagulation: I.V.: Immediate; S.C.: ~20-30 minutes

Formulations

Infusion, as sodium [premixed in NaCl 0.45%]: 12,500 units (250 mL); 25,000 units (250 mL, 500 mL)

Infusion, as sodium [preservative free; premixed in D_5W; porcine intestinal mucosa source]: 10,000 units (100 mL); 12,500 units (250 mL); 20,000 units (500 mL); 25,000 units (250 mL, 500 mL) [contains sodium bisulfite]

Infusion, as sodium [preservative free; premixed in NaCl 0.9%; porcine intestinal mucosa source]: 1000 units (500 mL); 2000 units (1000 mL)

Injection, solution, as sodium [beef lung source; multidose vial]: 1000 units/mL (10 mL, 30 mL); 5000 units/mL (10 mL), 10,000 units/mL (1 mL, 4 mL) [contains benzyl alcohol]

Injection, solution, as sodium [lock flush preparation; porcine intestinal mucosa source; multidose vial]: 10 units/mL (1 mL, 10 mL, 30 mL); 100 units/mL (1 mL, 5 mL)

Injection, solution, as sodium [lock flush preparation; porcine intestinal mucosa source; multidose vial]: 10 units/mL (10 mL, 30 mL); 100 units/mL (10 mL, 30 mL) [contains benzyl alcohol]

Injection, solution, as sodium [lock flush preparation; porcine intestinal mucosa source; prefilled syringe]: 10 units/mL (1 mL, 2 mL, 2.5 mL, 3 mL, 5 mL); 100 units/mL (1 mL, 2 mL, 2.5 mL, 3 mL, 5 mL) [contains benzyl alcohol]

Injection, solution, as sodium [preservative free; lock flush preparation; porcine intestinal mucosa source; prefilled syringe]: 10 units/mL (1 mL, 2 mL, 3 mL, 5 mL, 10 mL); 100 units/mL (1 mL, 2 mL, 3 mL, 5 mL, 10 mL)

Injection, solution, as sodium [porcine intestinal mucosa source; multidose vial]: 10,000 units/mL (5 mL) [contains benzyl alcohol]

Injection, solution, as sodium [porcine intestinal mucosa source; prefilled syringe]: 1000 units/mL (1 mL); 2500 units/mL (1 mL); 5000 units/mL (0.5 mL, 1 mL); 7500 units/mL (1 mL); 10,000 units/mL (1mL); 20,000 units/mL (1 mL) [contains benzyl alcohol]

Injection, solution, as sodium [preservative free; porcine intestinal mucosa source; prefilled syringe]: 10,000 units/mL (0.25 mL, 0.5 mL, 0.75 mL, 1 mL)

Injection, solution, as sodium [preservative free; porcine intestinal mucosa source; vial]: 1000 units/mL (2 mL); 2000 units/mL (5 mL, 10 mL); 2500 units/mL (5 mL, 10 mL)

Dosing

Adults:

DVT Prophylaxis (low-dose heparin): S.C.: 5000 units every 8-12 hours

Anticoagulation: I.V. infusion (weight-based dosing per institutional nomogram recommended):

Acute coronary syndromes: MI: Fibrinolytic therapy: I.V. infusion:

Alteplase or reteplase with first or second bolus: Concurrent bolus of 60 units/kg (maximum: 4000 units), then 12 units/kg/hour (maximum: 1000 units/hour) as continuous infusion. Check aPTT every 4-6 hours; adjust to target of 1.5-2 times the upper limit of control (50-70 seconds in clinical trials); usual range 10-30 units/kg/hour. Duration of heparin therapy depends on concurrent therapy and the specific patient risks for systemic or venous thromboembolism.

Streptokinase: Heparin use optional depending on concurrent therapy and specific patient risks for systemic or venous thromboembolism (anterior MI, CHF, previous embolus, atrial fibrillation, LV thrombus): If heparin is administered, start when aPTT <2 times the upper limit of control; do not use a bolus, but initiate infusion adjusted to a target aPTT of 1.5-2 times the upper limit of control (50-70 seconds in clinical trials). If heparin is not administered by infusion, 7500-12,500 units S.C. every 12 hours (when aPTT <2 times the upper limit of control) is recommended.

Percutaneous coronary intervention: Heparin bolus and infusion may be administered to an activated clotting time (ACT) of 300-350 seconds if no concurrent GPIIb/IIIa receptor antagonist is administered or 200-250 seconds if a GPIIb/IIIa receptor antagonist is administered.

Unstable angina (high-risk and some intermediate-risk patients): Initial bolus of 60-70 units/kg (maximum: 5000 units), followed by an initial infusion of 12-15 units/kg/hour (maximum: 1000 units/hour). The American College of Chest Physicians consensus conference has recommended dosage adjustments to correspond to a therapeutic range equivalent to heparin levels of 0.3-0.7 units/mL by antifactor Xa determinations, which correlates with aPTT values between 60 and 80 seconds

Venous thromboembolism (DVT/PE): 80 units/kg I.V. push followed by continuous infusion of 18 units/kg/hour

Anticoagulation: Intermittent I.V.: Initial: 10,000 units, then 50-70 units/kg (5000-10,000 units) every 4-6 hours

Line flushing: When using daily flushes of heparin to maintain patency of single and double lumen central catheters, 10 units/mL is commonly used for younger infants (eg, <10 kg) while 100 units/mL is used for older infants, children, and adults. Capped PVC catheters and peripheral heparin locks require flushing more frequently (eg, every 6-8 hours). Volume of heparin flush is usually similar to volume of catheter (or slightly greater). Additional flushes should be given when stagnant blood is observed in catheter, after catheter is used for drug or blood administration, and after blood withdrawal from catheter.

TPN: Addition of heparin (0.5-1 unit/mL) to peripheral and central TPN has been shown to increase duration of line patency. The final concentration of heparin used for TPN solutions may need to be decreased to 0.5 units/mL in small infants receiving larger amounts of volume in order to avoid approaching therapeutic amounts. Arterial lines are heparinized with a final concentration of 1 unit/mL.

Elderly: Patients >60 years of age may have higher serum levels and clinical response (longer aPTTs) as compared to younger patients receiving similar dosages. Lower dosages may be required.

Pediatrics:

Anticoagulation: Intermittent I.V.: Initial: 50-100 units/kg, then 50-100 units/kg every 4 hours

Anticoagulation: I.V. infusion: Initial: 50 units/kg, then 15-25 units/kg/hour; increase dose by 2-4 units/kg/hour every 6-8 hours as required

Note: Refer to adult dosing for notes on line flushing and TPN.

Administration

I.M.: Do not administer I.M. due to pain, irritation, and hematoma formation.

I.V.:

Continuous infusion: Infuse via infusion pump.

Heparin lock: Inject via injection cap using positive pressure flushing technique. Heparin lock flush solution is intended only to maintain patency of I.V. devices and is **not** to be used for anticoagulant therapy.

Stability

Storage: Heparin solutions are colorless to slightly yellow. Minor color variations do not affect therapeutic efficacy. Heparin should be stored at controlled room temperature and protected from freezing and temperatures >40°C.

Reconstitution: Stability at room temperature and refrigeration:

Prepared bag: 24 hours

Premixed bag: After seal is broken 4 days

Out of overwrap stability: 30 days

Standard diluent: 25,000 units/500 mL D_5W (premixed)

Minimum volume: 250 mL D_5W

Compatibility: Stable in dextran 6% in dextrose, dextran 6% in NS, D_5LR, $D_5{}^1/_4NS$, $D_5{}^1/_2NS$, $D_{25}W$, fat emulsion 10%, $^1/_2NS$, NS

(Continued)

Heparin *(Continued)*

Y-site administration: Incompatible with alatrofloxacin, alteplase, amiodarone, amphotericin B cholesteryl sulfate complex, amsacrine, ciprofloxacin, clarithromycin, diazepam, doxycycline, ergotamine, filgrastim, gatifloxacin, gentamicin, haloperidol, idarubicin, isosorbide dinitrate, levofloxacin, methotrimeprazine, nicardipine, phenytoin, tobramycin, triflupromazine, vancomycin

Compatibility in syringe: Incompatible with amikacin, amiodarone, chlorpromazine, diazepam, doxorubicin, droperidol, droperidol and fentanyl, erythromycin, erythromycin lactobionate, gentamicin, haloperidol, kanamycin, meperidine, methotrimeprazine, pentazocine, promethazine, streptomycin, tobramycin, triflupromazine, vancomycin, warfarin

Compatibility when admixed: Incompatible with alteplase, amikacin, atracurium, ciprofloxacin, cytarabine, daunorubicin, erythromycin lactobionate, gentamicin, hyaluronidase, kanamycin, levorphanol, meperidine, morphine, polymyxin B sulfate, promethazine, streptomycin

Monitoring Laboratory Tests Platelet counts, PTT, hemoglobin, hematocrit, signs of bleeding. For intermittent I.V. injections, PTT is measured 3.5-4 hours after I.V. injection. **Note:** Continuous I.V. infusion is preferred vs I.V. intermittent injections. For full-dose heparin (ie, nonlow-dose), the dose should be titrated according to PTT results. For anticoagulation, an APTT 1.5-2.5 times normal is usually desired. APTT is usually measured prior to heparin therapy, 6-8 hours after initiation of a continuous infusion (following a loading dose), and 6-8 hours after changes in the infusion rate; increase or decrease infusion by 2-4 units/kg/hour dependent on PTT.

Heparin infusion dose adjustment:

aPTT >3x control: Decrease infusion rate 50%.
aPTT 2-3x control: Decrease infusion rate 25%.
aPTT 1.5-2x control: No change.
aPTT <1.5x control: Increase rate of infusion 25%; max 2500 units/hour.

Monitoring and Teaching Issues

Physical Assessment: See Contraindications, Warnings/Precautions, and Dosing for use cautions. Assess potential for interactions with other prescriptions, OTC medications, or herbal products patient may be taking (especially anything that will affect coagulation or platelet function - see Drug Interactions). See Administration specifics. Bleeding precautions should be observed. Assess results of laboratory tests (see above), therapeutic effects, and adverse response (see Adverse Reactions and Overdose/Toxicology) regularly during therapy. Teach possible side effects and appropriate interventions (eg, bleeding precautions) and adverse symptoms to report (see Patient Education). **Pregnancy risk factor C** - benefits of use should outweigh possible risks.

Patient Education: Inform prescriber of all prescriptions, OTC medications, or herbal products you are taking, and any allergies you have. Do not take anything new during treatment unless approved by prescriber. This drug can only be administered by injection. You may have a tendency to bleed easily while taking this drug (brush teeth with soft brush, floss with waxed floss, use electric razor, avoid scissors or sharp knives, and potentially harmful activities). Report unusual bleeding or bruising (bleeding gums, nosebleed, blood in urine, dark stool); pain in joints or back; CNS changes (fever, confusion); unusual fever; persistent nausea or GI upset; or swelling or pain at injection site. **Pregnancy precaution:** Inform prescriber if you are pregnant.

Geriatric Considerations: At similar dosages, heparin levels tend to be higher in elderly patients (>60 years of age). In the clinical setting, age has not been shown to be a reliable predictor of a patient's anticoagulant response to heparin. However, it is common for older patients to have a "standard" response for the first 24-48 hours after a loading dose (5000 units) and a maintenance infusion of 800-1000 units/hour. After this period, they then have an exaggerated response (eg, elevated PTT), requiring a lower infusion rate. Hence, monitor closely during this period of therapy. Older women (>60 years of age) are more likely to have bleeding complications and osteoporosis may be a problem when used >3 months or total daily dose exceeds 30,000 units.

Related Information

Anticoagulant Therapy Guidelines *on page 1635*
Compatibility of Drugs *on page 1564*
Compatibility of Drugs in Syringe *on page 1566*
Heparins *on page 1576*
Protamine Sulfate *on page 1148*

Heparin Calcium *see* Heparin *on page 653*
Heparin Lock Flush *see* Heparin *on page 653*
Heparins *see page 1576*
Heparin Sodium *see* Heparin *on page 653*
Hepatitis A Vaccine *see page 1498*
Hepatitis B Immune Globulin *see page 1498*
Hepatitis B Vaccine *see page 1498*
Hep-Lock® *see* Heparin *on page 653*
Hepsera™ *see* Adefovir *on page 46*
Herbal and Nutritional Products *see page 1463*
Herceptin® *see* Trastuzumab *on page 1349*
Heroin *see page 1568*
HES *see* Hetastarch *on page 656*
Hespan® *see* Hetastarch *on page 656*

Hetastarch (HET a starch)

U.S. Brand Names Hespan®; Hextend®
Synonyms HES; Hydroxyethyl Starch
Generic Available Yes: Sodium chloride infusion

Pharmacologic Category Plasma Volume Expander, Colloid

Pregnancy Risk Factor C

Lactation Excretion in breast milk unknown/use caution

Use Blood volume expander used in treatment of hypovolemia

Hespan®: Adjunct in leukapheresis to improve harvesting and increasing the yield of granulocytes by centrifugal means

Use - Unlabeled/Investigational Hextend®: Priming fluid in pump oxygenators during cardiopulmonary bypass, and as a plasma volume expander during cardiopulmonary bypass

Mechanism of Action/Effect Produces plasma volume expansion by virtue of its highly colloidal starch structure, similar to albumin

Contraindications Hypersensitivity to hydroxyethyl starch or any component of the formulation; severe bleeding disorders, renal failure with oliguria or anuria, or severe congestive heart failure; per the manufacturer, Hextend® is also contraindicated in the treatment of lactic acidosis and in leukapheresis

Warnings/Precautions Anaphylactoid reactions have occurred; use caution in patients allergic to corn (may have cross allergy to hetastarch); use with caution in patients with thrombocytopenia (may interfere with platelet function); large volume may cause drops in hemoglobin concentrations; use with caution in patients at risk from overexpansion of blood volume, including the very young or aged patients, those with CHF or pulmonary edema; volumes >1500 mL may interfere with platelet function and prolong PT and PTT times; use with caution in patients with history of liver disease; note electrolyte content of Hextend® including calcium, lactate, and potassium; use caution in situations where electrolyte and/or acid-base disturbances may be exacerbated (renal impairment, respiratory alkalosis). Safety and efficacy in pediatric patients have not been established, but limited data available. Pregnancy risk C.

Adverse Reactions Frequency not defined.

Cardiovascular: Circulatory overload, heart failure, peripheral edema

Central nervous system: Chills, fever, headache, intracranial bleeding

Dermatologic: Itching, pruritus, rash

Endocrine & metabolic: Amylase levels increased, parotid gland enlargement, indirect bilirubin increased, metabolic acidosis

Gastrointestinal: Vomiting

Hematologic: Bleeding, factor VIII:C plasma levels decreased, decreased plasma aggregation decreased, von Willebrand factor decreased, dilutional coagulopathy; prolongation of PT, PTT, clotting time, and bleeding time; thrombocytopenia, anemia, disseminated intravascular coagulopathy (rare), hemolysis (rare)

Neuromuscular & skeletal: Myalgia

Miscellaneous: Anaphylactoid reactions, hypersensitivity, flu-like symptoms (mild)

Overdosage/Toxicology Symptoms of overdose include heart failure, nausea, vomiting, circulatory overload, and bleeding. Treatment is supportive. Hetastarch is not eliminated by hemodialysis.

Pharmacodynamics/Kinetics

Metabolism: Molecules >50,000 daltons require enzymatic degradation by the reticuloendothelial system or amylases in the blood

Onset: Volume expansion: I.V.: ~30 minutes

Duration: 24-36 hours

Formulations

Infusion [premixed in lactated electrolyte injection] (Hextend®): 6% (500 mL, 1000 mL)

Infusion, solution [premixed in NaCl 0.9%]: 6% (500 mL)

Dosing

Adults & Elderly:

Volume expansion: 500-1000 mL (up to 1500 mL/day) or 20 mL/kg/day (up to 1500 mL/day); larger volumes (15,000 mL/24 hours) have been used safely in small numbers of patients

Leukapheresis: 250-700 mL; **Note:** Citrate anticoagulant is added before use.

Pediatrics: Safety and efficacy have not been established.

Renal Impairment: Cl_{cr} <10 mL/minute: Initial dose is the same but subsequent doses should be reduced by 20% to 50% of normal.

Administration

I.V.: Administer I.V. only; infusion pump is required. May administer up to 1.2 g/kg/hour (20 mL/kg/hour). Change I.V. tubing or flush copiously with normal saline before administering blood through the same line. Change I.V. tubing at least every 24 hours. Do not administer Hextend® with blood through the same administration set. Anaphylactoid reactions can occur, have epinephrine and resuscitative equipment available.

Other: Leukapheresis: Mix Hespan® and citrate well. Administer to the input line of the centrifuge apparatus at a ration of 1:8 to 1:13 to venous whole blood.

Stability

Storage: Store at room temperature; do not freeze. In leukapheresis, admixtures of 500-560 mL of Hespan® with citrate concentrations up to 2.5% are compatible for 24 hours.

Reconstitution: Do not use if crystalline precipitate forms or is turbid deep brown.

Compatibility: Stable in NS

Y-site administration: Incompatible with amikacin, cefamandole, cefoperazone, cefotaxime, cefoxitin, gentamicin, ranitidine, theophylline, tobramycin

Monitoring Laboratory Tests If pulmonary artery catheter in place, monitor PCWP, SVR, and PVR; hemoglobin, hematocrit, cardiac index

Leukapheresis: CBC, total leukocyte and platelet counts, leukocyte differential count, hemoglobin, hematocrit, PT, PTT

Monitoring and Teaching Issues

Physical Assessment: See Use, Contraindications, Warnings/Precautions, and Dosing for use cautions. See Administration specifics. Patient must be monitored closely for hypersensitivity (anaphylactic reaction) and other major adverse reactions (see Adverse Reactions and Overdose/Toxicology). Blood pressure, pulse, central venous pressure, and

(Continued)

Hetastarch *(Continued)*

urine output should be monitored every 5-15 minutes for the first hour and closely thereafter (see above). Patient teaching should be appropriate to patient condition (see Patient Education). **Pregnancy risk factor C.**

Patient Education: Report immediately any difficulty breathing, acute headache, muscle pain, or abdominal cramping. **Pregnancy precaution:** Inform prescriber if you are pregnant.

Additional Information Hetastarch is a synthetic polymer derived from a waxy starch composed of amylopectin.

Hespan®: 6% hetastarch in 0.9% sodium chloride
- Molecular weight: 450,000
- Sodium: 154 mEq/L
- Chloride: 154 mEq/L

Hextend®: 6% hetastarch in lactated electrolyte injection
- Molecular weight: 670,000
- Sodium: 143 mEq/L
- Chloride: 124 mEq/L
- Calcium: 5 mEq/L
- Potassium: 3 mEq/L
- Magnesium: 0.9 mEq/L
- Lactate: 28 mEq/L
- Dextrose: 0.99 g/L

Hexachlorocyclohexane *see* Lindane *on page 805*

Hexadrol® *see* Topical Corticosteroids *on page 1334*

Hexadrol® Phosphate *see* Topical Corticosteroids *on page 1334*

Hexalen® *see* Altretamine *on page 70*

Hexamethylenetetramine *see* Methenamine *on page 870*

Hexamethylmelamine *see* Altretamine *on page 70*

HEXM *see* Altretamine *on page 70*

Hextend® *see* Hetastarch *on page 656*

HibTITER® *see page 1498*

Hi-Cor 1.0® *see* Topical Corticosteroids *on page 1334*

Hi-Cor 2.5® *see* Topical Corticosteroids *on page 1334*

Hiprex® *see* Methenamine *on page 870*

Histolyn-CYL® Injection *see page 1461*

Histoplasmin *see page 1461*

Hivid® *see* Zalcitabine *on page 1415*

HMM *see* Altretamine *on page 70*

HMS Liquifilm® *see* Medrysone *on page 843*

HN_2 *see* Mechlorethamine *on page 839*

Homatropine *see page 1509*

Horse Antihuman Thymocyte Gamma Globulin *see* Lymphocyte Immune Globulin *on page 829*

H.P. Acthar® Gel *see page 1461*

HTF919 *see* Tegaserod *on page 1278*

Humalog® *see* Insulin Preparations *on page 714*

Humalog® Mix 75/25™ *see* Insulin Preparations *on page 714*

Human Growth Hormone (HYU man grothe HOR mone)

U.S. Brand Names Genotropin®; Genotropin Miniquick®; Humatrope®; Norditropin®; Norditropin® Cartridges; Nutropin®; Nutropin AQ ®; Nutropin Depot®; Protropin®; Saizen®; Serostim®

Synonyms Growth Hormone; Somatrem; Somatropin

Generic Available No

Pharmacologic Category Growth Hormone

Pregnancy Risk Factor B/C (depending upon manufacturer)

Lactation Excretion in breast milk unknown/not recommended

Use

Children:
- Long-term treatment of growth failure due to lack of adequate endogenous growth hormone secretion (Genotropin®, Humatrope®, Norditropin®, Nutropin®, Nutropin AQ®, Nutropin® Depot™, Protropin®, Saizen®)
- Long-term treatment of short stature associated with Turner syndrome (Humatrope®, Nutropin®, Nutropin AQ®)
- Treatment of Prader-Willi syndrome (Genotropin®)
- Treatment of growth failure associated with chronic renal insufficiency (CRI) up until the time of renal transplantation (Nutropin®, Nutropin AQ®)
- Long-term treatment of growth failure in children born small for gestational age who fail to manifest catch-up growth by 2 years of age (Genotropin®)

Adults:
- AIDS wasting or cachexia with concomitant antiviral therapy (Serostim®)
- Replacement of endogenous growth hormone in patients with adult growth hormone deficiency who meet both of the following criteria (Genotropin®, Humatrope®, Nutropin®, Nutropin AQ®):
  - Biochemical diagnosis of adult growth hormone deficiency by means of a subnormal response to a standard growth hormone stimulation test (peak growth hormone ≤5 µg/L)
  - **and**

Adult-onset: Patients who have adult growth hormone deficiency whether alone or with multiple hormone deficiencies (hypopituitarism) as a result of pituitary disease, hypothalamic disease, surgery, radiation therapy, or trauma

or

Childhood-onset: Patients who were growth hormone deficient during childhood, confirmed as an adult before replacement therapy is initiated

Use - Unlabeled/Investigational Investigational: Congestive heart failure

Mechanism of Action/Effect Human growth hormone stimulates growth of linear bone, skeletal muscle, and organs; stimulates erythropoietin which increases red blood cell mass; exerts both insulin-like and diabetogenic effects.

Contraindications Hypersensitivity to growth hormone or any component of the formulation; growth promotion in pediatric patients with closed epiphyses; progression of any underlying intracranial lesion or actively growing intracranial tumor; acute critical illness due to complications following open heart or abdominal surgery; multiple accidental trauma or acute respiratory failure; evidence of active malignancy

Warnings/Precautions Use with caution in patients with diabetes or with risk factors for glucose intolerance; when administering to newborns, reconstitute with sterile water for injection; intracranial hypertension has been reported with growth hormone product, funduscopic examinations are recommended; progression of scoliosis may occur in children experiencing rapid growth; patients with growth hormone deficiency may develop slipped capital epiphyses more frequently, evaluate any child with new onset of a limp or with complaints of hip or knee pain; patients with Turner syndrome are at increased risk for otitis media and other ear/hearing disorders, cardiovascular disorders (including stroke, aortic aneurysm, hypertension), and thyroid disease, monitor carefully; products may contain benzyl alcohol, m-Cresol or glycerin, some products may be manufactured by recombinant DNA technology using *E. coli* as a precursor, consult specific product labeling. Not for I.V. injection. Pregnancy factor B/C (depending on manufacturer).

Drug Interactions

Decreased Effect: Glucocorticoid therapy may inhibit growth-promoting effects. Growth hormone may induce insulin resistance in patients with diabetes mellitus; monitor glucose and adjust insulin dose as necessary.

Adverse Reactions

Growth hormone deficiency: Antigrowth hormone antibodies, carpal tunnel syndrome (rare), fluid balance disturbances, glucosuria, gynocomastia (rare), headache, hematuria, hyperglycemia (mild), hypoglycemia, hypothyroidism, leukemia, lipoatrophy, muscle pain, increased growth of pre-existing nevi (rare), pain/ local reactions at the injection site, pancreatitis (rare), peripheral edema, exacerbation of psoriasis, seizures

Prader-Willi syndrome: Aggressiveness, arthralgia, edema, hair loss, headache, benign intracranial hypertension, myalgia

Turner syndrome: Humatrope®: Surgical procedures (45%), otitis media (43%), ear disorders (18%), hypothyroidism (13%), increased nevi (11%), peripheral edema (7%)

Adult growth hormone replacement: Increased ALT, increased AST, arthralgia, back pain, carpal tunnel syndrome, diabetes mellitus, fatigue, flu-like syndrome, generalized edema, gastritis, gynocomastia (rare), headache, hypoesthesia, joint disorder, myalgia, increased growth of pre-existing nevi, pain, pancreatitis (rare), paresthesia, peripheral edema, pharyngitis, rhinitis, stiffness in extremities, weakness

AIDS wasting or cachexia (limited): Serostim®: Musculoskeletal discomfort (54%), increased tissue turgor (27%), diarrhea (26%), neuropathy (26%), nausea (26%), fatigue (17%), albuminuria (15%), increased diaphoresis (14%), anorexia (12%), anemia (12%), increased AST (12%), insomnia (11%), tachycardia (11%), hyperglycemia (10%), increased ALT (10%)

Postmarketing and/or case reports: Diabetes, diabetic ketoacidosis, glucose intolerance

Small for gestational age: Mild, transient hyperglycemia; benign intracranial hypertension (rare); central precocious puberty; jaw prominence (rare); aggravation of pre-existing scoliosis (rare); injection site reactions; progression of pigmented nevi

Overdosage/Toxicology Symptoms of acute overdose may include initial hypoglycemia, hyperglycemia, fluid retention, headache, nausea, and vomiting. Long-term overdose may result in signs and symptoms of acromegaly.

Pharmacokinetic Note Somatrem and somatropin have equivalent pharmacokinetic properties.

Pharmacodynamics/Kinetics

Absorption: I.M., S.C.: Well absorbed

Half-Life Elimination: Preparation and route of administration dependent

Metabolism: Hepatic and renal (~90%)

Duration: Maintains supraphysiologic levels for 18-20 hours

Formulations

Injection, powder for reconstitution [rDNA origin]:

- Somatrem: Protropin® [diluent contains benzyl alcohol]: 5 mg [~15 int. units]; 10 mg [~30 int. units]
- Somatropin:
  - Genotropin® [preservative free]: 1.5 mg [4 int. units/mL] [delivers 1.3 mg/mL]
  - Genotropin® [with preservative]:
    - 5.8 mg [15 int. units/mL] [delivers 5 mg/mL]
    - 13.8 mg [36 int. units/mL] [delivers 12 mg/mL]
  - Genotropin Miniquick® [preservative free]: 0.2 mg, 0.4 mg, 0.6 mg, 0.8 mg, 1 mg, 1.2 mg, 1.4 mg, 1.6 mg, 1.8 mg, 2 mg [each strength delivers 0.25 mL]
  - Humatrope®: 5 mg [~15 int. units], 6 mg [18 int. units], 12 mg [36 int. units], 24 mg [72 int. units]
  - Norditropin® [diluent contains benzyl alcohol]: 4 mg [~12 int. units]; 8 mg [~24 int. units]
  - Nutropin® [diluent contains benzyl alcohol]: 5 mg [~15 int. units]; 10 mg [~30 int. units]
  - Nutropin Depot® [preservative free]: 13.5 mg, 18 mg, 22.5 mg
  - Saizen® [diluent contains benzyl alcohol]: 5 mg [~15 int. units]; 8.8 mg [~26.4 int. units]
  - Serostim®: 4 mg [12 int. units]; 5 mg [15 int. units]; 6 mg [18 int. units]

(Continued)

Human Growth Hormone *(Continued)*

Injection, solution [rDNA origin]: Somatropin:

Norditropin®: 5 mg/1.5 mL (1.5 mL); 10 mg/1.5 mL (1.5 mL); 15 mg/1.5 mL (1.5 mL) [cartridge]

Nutropin AQ®: 5 mg/mL [~30 int. units/2 mL] (2 mL) [vial or cartridge]

Dosing

Adults:

Growth hormone deficiency: To minimize adverse events in older or overweight patients, reduced dosages may be necessary. During therapy, dosage should be decreased if required by the occurrence of side effects or excessive IGF-I levels.

Somatropin:

Nutropin®, Nutropin® AQ: S.C.: ≤0.006 mg/kg/day; dose may be increased according to individual requirements, up to a maximum of 0.025 mg/kg/day in patients <35 years of age, or up to a maximum of 0.0125 mg/kg/day in patients ≥35 years of age

Humatrope®: S.C.: ≤0.006 mg/kg/day; dose may be increased according to individual requirements, up to a maximum of 0.0125 mg/kg/day

Genotropin®: S.C.: Weekly dosage: ≤0.04 mg/kg divided into 6-7 doses; dose may be increased at 4- to 8-week intervals according to individual requirements, to a maximum of 0.08 mg/kg/week

AIDS wasting or cachexia:

Serostim®: S.C.: Dose should be given once daily at bedtime; patients who continue to lose weight after 2 weeks should be re-evaluated for opportunistic infections or other clinical events; rotate injection sites to avoid lipodystrophy

Daily dose based on body weight:

<35 kg: 0.1 mg/kg
35-45 kg: 4 mg
45-55 kg: 5 mg
>55 kg: 6 mg

Elderly: Patients ≥65 years of age may be more sensitive to the action of growth hormone and more prone to adverse effects; in general, dosing should be cautious, beginning at low end of dosing range.

Pediatrics:

Growth hormone deficiency:

Somatrem: Protropin®: I.M., S.C.: Weekly dosage: 0.3 mg/kg divided into daily doses

Somatropin:

Genotropin®: S.C.: Weekly dosage: 0.16-0.24 mg/kg divided into 6-7 doses

Humatrope®: I.M., S.C.: Weekly dosage: 0.18 mg/kg; maximum replacement dose: 0.3 mg/kg/week; dosing should be divided into equal doses given 3 times/week on alternating days, 6 times/week, or daily

Norditropin®: S.C.: Weekly dosage: 0.024-0.034 mg/kg administered in the evening, divided into doses 6-7 times/week; cartridge and vial formulations are bioequivalent; cartridge formulation does not need to be reconstituted prior to use; cartridges must be administered using the corresponding color-coded NordiPen® injection pen

Nutropin® Depot™: S.C.:

Once-monthly injection: 1.5 mg/kg administered on the same day of each month; patients >15 kg will require more than 1 injection per dose

Twice-monthly injection: 0.75 mg/kg administered twice each month on the same days of each month (eg, days 1 and 15 of each month); patients >30 kg will require more than 1 injection per dose

Nutropin®, Nutropin® AQ: S.C.: Weekly dosage: 0.3 mg/kg divided into daily doses; pubertal patients: ≤0.7 mg/kg/week divided daily

Saizen®: I.M., S.C.: Weekly dosage: 0.06 mg/kg administered 3 times/week

Note: Therapy should be discontinued when patient has reached satisfactory adult height, when epiphyses have fused, or when the patient ceases to respond. Growth of 5 cm/year or more is expected, if growth rate does not exceed 2.5 cm in a 6-month period, double the dose for the next 6 months; if there is still no satisfactory response, discontinue therapy

Chronic renal insufficiency (CRI): Nutropin®, Nutropin® AQ: S.C.: Weekly dosage: 0.35 mg/kg divided into daily injections; continue until the time of renal transplantation

Dosage recommendations in patients treated for CRI who require dialysis:

Hemodialysis: Administer dose at night prior to bedtime or at least 3-4 hours after hemodialysis to prevent hematoma formation from heparin

CCPD: Administer dose in the morning following dialysis

CAPD: Administer dose in the evening at the time of overnight exchange

Turner syndrome: Humatrope®, Nutropin®, Nutropin® AQ: S.C.: Weekly dosage: ≤0.375 mg/kg divided into equal doses 3-7 times per week

Prader-Willi syndrome: Genotropin®: S.C.: Weekly dosage: 0.24 mg/kg divided into 6-7 doses

Small for gestational age: Genotropin®: S.C.: Weekly dosage: 0.48 mg/kg divided into 6-7 doses

Renal Impairment: Reports indicate patients with chronic renal failure tend to have decreased clearance; specific dosing suggestions not available

Hepatic Impairment: Clearance may be reduced in patients with severe hepatic dysfunction; specific dosing suggestions are not available.

Administration

I.M.: Do not shake; administer S.C. or I.M.; refer to product labeling; when administering to newborns, reconstitute with sterile water for injection

Stability

Storage:

Somatrem: Protropin®: Before and after reconstitution, store at 2°C to 8°C (36°F to 46°F), avoid freezing; when reconstituted with bacteriostatic water for injection; use within 14 days; when reconstituted with sterile water for injection, use immediately (only one dose per vial) and discard unused portion

Somatropin:

Genotropin®: Store at 2°C to 8°C (36°F to 46°F), do not freeze, protect from light

1.5 mg cartridge: Following reconstitution, store under refrigeration and use within 24 hours; discard unused portion

5.8 mg and 13.8 mg cartridge: Following reconstitution, store under refrigeration and use within 21 days

Miniquick®: Store in refrigerator prior to dispensing, but may be stored ≤25°C (77°F) for up to 3 months after dispensing; once reconstituted, solution must be refrigerated and used within 24 hours; discard unused portion

Humatrope®:

Vial: Before and after reconstitution, store at 2°C to 8°C (36°F to 46°F), avoid freezing; when reconstituted with bacteriostatic water for injection, use within 14 days; when reconstituted with sterile water for injection, use within 24 hours and discard unused portion

Cartridge: Before and after reconstitution, store at 2°C to 8°C (36°F to 46°F), avoid freezing; following reconstitution, stable for 14 days under refrigeration. Dilute with solution provided with cartridges **ONLY**; do not use diluent provided with vials

Norditropin®: Store at 2°C to 8°C (36°F to 46°F), do not freeze; avoid direct light

Cartridge: Must be used within 4 weeks once inserted into pen

Powder for injection: Must be used within 14 days of reconstitution

Nutropin®: Before and after reconstitution, store at 2°C to 8°C (36°F to 46°F), avoid freezing

Vial: Reconstitute with bacteriostatic water for injection; use reconstituted vials within 14 days; when reconstituted with sterile water for injection, use immediately and discard unused portion

AQ formulation: Use within 28 days following initial use

Depot™: Before suspension, store at 2°C to 8°C (36°F to 46°F), avoid freezing; use suspended solution immediately; dilute only with diluent provided

Saizen®: Prior to reconstitution, store at room temperature 15°C to 30°C (59°F to 86°F); following reconstitution with bacteriostatic water for injection, reconstituted solution should be refrigerated and used within 14 days; when reconstituted with sterile water for injection, use immediately and discard unused portion

Serostim®: Prior to reconstitution, store at room temperature 15°C to 30°C (59°F to 86°F); reconstitute with sterile water for injection; store reconstituted solution under refrigeration and use within 24 hours, avoid freezing. Do not use if cloudy

Reconstitution:

Somatrem: Protropin®: Vial:

5 mg: Reconstitute with 1-5 mL bacteriostatic water for injection.

10 mg: Reconstitute with 1-10 mL bacteriostatic water for injection.

Somatropin:

Genotropin®: Reconstitute with diluent provided.

Genotropin MiniQuick®: Reconstitute with diluent provided. Consult the instructions provided with the reconstitution device.

Humatrope®:

Cartridge: Consult HumatroPen™ User Guide for complete instructions for reconstitution. **Do not use diluent provided with vials.**

Vial: 5 mg: Reconstitute with 1.5-5 mL diluent provided.

Norditropin®: Vial: Reconstitute with 2 mL of diluent provided.

Nutropin®: Vial:

5 mg: Reconstitute with 1-5 mL bacteriostatic water for injection.

10 mg: Reconstitute with 1-10 mL bacteriostatic water for injection.

Nutropin® Depot™: Reconstitute with diluent provided **only**.

Saizen®: VialL: 5 mg: Reconstitute with 1-3 mL bacteriostatic water for injection or sterile water for injection.

Serostim®: Vial: Reconstitute with 0.5-1 mL sterile water for injection.

Monitoring Laboratory Tests Growth curve, periodic thyroid function tests, bone age (annually), periodical urine testing for glucose, somatomedin C (IGF-I) levels; funduscopic examinations at initiation of therapy and periodically during treatment; serum phosphorus, alkaline phosphatase and parathyroid hormone. If growth deceleration is observed in children treated for growth hormone deficiency, and not due to other causes, evaluate for presence of antibody formation. Strict blood glucose monitoring in diabetic patients.

Somatrem (Protropin®): Consider changing to somatropin if antibody binding capacity is >2 mg/L

Monitoring and Teaching Issues

Physical Assessment: See Contraindications, Warnings/Precautions, and Dosing for use cautions. Assess potential for interactions with other prescriptions, OTC medications, or herbal products patient may be taking (see Drug Interactions). Assess results of laboratory tests. Assess patient response (according to purpose for use) and adverse reactions (see Adverse Reactions and Overdose/Toxicology). Instruct patients with diabetes to monitor glucose levels closely (may induce insulin intolerance). Instruct patient in proper use if self-administered (storage, reconstitution, injection techniques, and syringe/needle disposal), possible side effects and appropriate interventions, and adverse symptoms to report (see Patient Education). **Pregnancy risk factor B/C** - see Pregnancy Risk Factor for use cautions; benefits of use should outweigh possible risks. Note breast-feeding caution.

Patient Education: Inform prescriber of all prescriptions, OTC medications, or herbal products you are taking, and any allergies you have. This drug can only be administered by injection. If self-administered, you will be instructed by prescriber on proper storage, reconstitution, injection technique, and syringe/needle disposal. Use exactly as prescribed; do not discontinue or alter dose without consulting prescriber. Report immediately any pain, redness, burning, drainage, or swelling at injection site. If diabetic, you should monitor glucose levels closely; this medication may cause an alteration in your insulin levels. May cause side effects which are particular to purpose for use and formulation prescribed; your prescriber will instruct you in particular side effects for your medication. Report immediately unusual or persistent bleeding, excessive fatigue or swelling (edema) of extremities, joint

(Continued)

Human Growth Hormone *(Continued)*

or muscle pain or headache, nausea or vomiting, personality changes, or other persistent adverse effects. **Pregnancy/breast-feeding precaution:** Inform prescriber if you are or intend to become pregnant. Consult prescriber if breast-feeding.

Humate-P® *see* Antihemophilic Factor (Human) *on page 109*
Humatrope® *see* Human Growth Hormone *on page 658*
Humegon™ *see* Menotropins *on page 850*
Humibid® DM *see* Guaifenesin and Dextromethorphan *on page 647*
Humibid® L.A. *see* Guaifenesin *on page 646*
Humibid® Pediatric *see* Guaifenesin *on page 646*
Humorsol® *see* Ophthalmic Agents, Glaucoma *on page 1002*
Humulin® 50/50 *see* Insulin Preparations *on page 714*
Humulin® 70/30 *see* Insulin Preparations *on page 714*
Humulin® L *see* Insulin Preparations *on page 714*
Humulin® N *see* Insulin Preparations *on page 714*
Humulin® R *see* Insulin Preparations *on page 714*
Humulin® R (Concentrated) U-500 *see* Insulin Preparations *on page 714*
Humulin® U *see* Insulin Preparations *on page 714*
Hurricaine® *see* Benzocaine *on page 156*
HXM *see* Altretamine *on page 70*
Hyate:C® *see* Antihemophilic Factor (Porcine) *on page 111*
Hycamptamine *see* Topotecan *on page 1339*
Hycamtin™ *see* Topotecan *on page 1339*
Hycort® *see* Topical Corticosteroids *on page 1334*

HydrALAZINE (hye DRAL a zeen)

Synonyms Apresoline [DSC]; Hydralazine Hydrochloride

Generic Available Yes

Pharmacologic Category Vasodilator

Pregnancy Risk Factor C

Lactation Enters breast milk/compatible

Use Management of moderate to severe hypertension, congestive heart failure, hypertension secondary to pre-eclampsia/eclampsia; treatment of primary pulmonary hypertension

Mechanism of Action/Effect Direct vasodilation of arterioles (with little effect on veins) with decreased systemic resistance

Contraindications Hypersensitivity to hydralazine or any component of the formulation; mitral valve rheumatic heart disease

Warnings/Precautions May cause a drug-induced lupus-like syndrome (more likely on larger doses, longer duration). Adjust dose in severe renal dysfunction. Use with caution in CAD (increase in tachycardia may increase myocardial oxygen demand). Use with caution in pulmonary hypertension (may cause hypotension). Titrate cautiously to response. Hypotensive effect after I.V. administration may be delayed and unpredictable in some patients. Hydralazine-induced fluid and sodium retention may require addition or increased dosage of a diuretics. Pregnancy risk C.

Drug Interactions

Cytochrome P450 Effect: Inhibits CYP3A4

Decreased Effect: NSAIDs (eg, indomethacin) may decrease the hemodynamic effects of hydralazine.

Increased Effect/Toxicity: Hydralazine may increase levels of beta-blockers (metoprolol, propranolol). Some beta-blockers (acebutolol, atenolol, and nadolol) are unlikely to be affected due to limited hepatic metabolism. Concurrent use of hydralazine with MAO inhibitors may cause a significant decrease in blood pressure. Propranolol may increase hydralazine serum concentrations.

Nutritional/Ethanol Interactions

Ethanol: Avoid ethanol (may increase CNS depression).

Food: Food enhances bioavailability of hydralazine.

Herb/Nutraceutical: Avoid dong quai if using for hypertension (has estrogenic activity). Avoid ephedra, yohimbe, ginseng (may worsen hypertension). Avoid garlic (may have increased antihypertensive effect).

Adverse Reactions Frequency not defined.

Cardiovascular: Tachycardia, angina pectoris, orthostatic hypotension (rare), dizziness (rare), paradoxical hypertension, peripheral edema, vascular collapse (rare), flushing

Central nervous system: Increased intracranial pressure (I.V., in patient with pre-existing increased intracranial pressure), fever (rare), chills (rare), anxiety*, disorientation*, depression*, coma*

Dermatologic: Rash (rare), urticaria (rash), pruritus (rash)

Gastrointestinal: Anorexia, nausea, vomiting, diarrhea, constipation, adynamic ileus

Genitourinary: Difficulty in micturition, impotence

Hematologic: Hemolytic anemia (rare), eosinophilia (rare), decreased hemoglobin concentration (rare), reduced erythrocyte count (rare), leukopenia (rare), agranulocytosis (rare), thrombocytopenia (rare)

Neuromuscular & skeletal: Rheumatoid arthritis, muscle cramps, weakness, tremors, peripheral neuritis (rare)

Ocular: Lacrimation, conjunctivitis

Respiratory: Nasal congestion, dyspnea

Miscellaneous: Drug-induced lupus-like syndrome (dose-related; fever, arthralgia, splenomegaly, lymphadenopathy, asthenia, myalgia, malaise, pleuritic chest pain, edema, positive ANA, positive LE cells, maculopapular facial rash, positive direct Coombs' test, pericarditis, pericardial tamponade), diaphoresis

*Seen in uremic patients and severe hypertension where rapidly escalating doses may have caused hypotension leading to these effects.

Overdosage/Toxicology Symptoms of overdose include hypotension, tachycardia, and shock. Treatment is supportive and symptomatic.

Pharmacodynamics/Kinetics

Bioavailability: 30% to 50%; increased with food

Half-Life Elimination: Normal renal function: 2-8 hours; End-stage renal disease: 7-16 hours

Metabolism: Hepatically acetylated; extensive first-pass effect (oral)

Onset: Oral: 20-30 minutes; I.V.: 5-20 minutes

Duration: Oral: 2-4 hours; I.V.: 2-6 hours

Formulations

Injection, solution, as hydrochloride: 20 mg/mL (1 mL)

Tablet, as hydrochloride: 10 mg, 25 mg, 50 mg, 100 mg

Dosing

Adults:

Hypertension: Oral:

Initial: 10 mg 4 times/day

Increase by 10-25 mg/dose every 2-5 days

Maximum: 300 mg/day

Acute hypertension: I.M., I.V.: Initial: 10-20 mg/dose every 4-6 hours as needed, may increase to 40 mg/dose; change to oral therapy as soon as possible.

Congestive heart failure: Oral:

Initial dose: 10-25 mg 3-4 times/day

Adjustment: Dosage must be adjusted based on individual response.

Target dose: 75 mg 4 times/day in combination with isosorbide dinitrate (40 mg 4 times a day)

Range: Typically 200-600 mg daily in 2-4 divided doses. Dosages as high as 3 g/day have been used in some patients for symptomatic and hemodynamic improvement. Hydralazine 75 mg 4 times a day combined with isosorbide dinitrate 40 mg 4 times a day were shown in clinical trials to provide a mortality benefit in the treatment of CHF. Higher doses may be used for symptomatic and hemodynamic improvement following optimization of standard therapy.

Pre-eclampsia/eclampsia: I.M., I.V.: 5 mg/dose then 5-10 mg every 20-30 minutes as needed

Elderly: Oral: Initial: 10 mg 2-3 times/day; increase by 10-25 mg/day every 2-5 days.

Pediatrics:

Hypertension: Oral: Initial: 0.75-1 mg/kg/day in 2-4 divided doses; increase over 3-4 weeks to maximum of 7.5 mg/kg/day in 2-4 divided doses; maximum daily dose: 200 mg/day

Acute hypertension: I.M., I.V.: 0.1-0.2 mg/kg/dose (not to exceed 20 mg) every 4-6 hours as needed, up to 1.7-3.5 mg/kg/day in 4-6 divided doses

Renal Impairment:

Cl_{cr} 10-50 mL/minute: Administer every 8 hours.

Cl_{cr} <10 mL/minute: Administer every 8-16 hours in fast acetylators and every 12-24 hours in slow acetylators.

Hemodialysis effects: Supplemental dose is not necessary.

Peritoneal dialysis effects: Supplemental dose is not necessary.

Administration

I.V.: Inject over 1 minute. Hypotensive effect may be delayed and unpredictable in some patients.

Stability

Storage: Intact ampuls/vials of hydralazine should not be stored under refrigeration because of possible precipitation or crystallization.

Reconstitution: Hydralazine should be diluted in NS for IVPB administration due to decreased stability in D_5W. Stability of IVPB solution in NS is 4 days at room temperature.

Compatibility: Stable in dextran 6% in dextrose, dextran 6% in NS, D_5LR, $D_5{}^1/_4NS$, $D_5{}^1/_2NS$, D_5NS, $D_{10}W$, LR, $^1/_2NS$, NS; **incompatible** with D_5W

Y-site administration: Incompatible with aminophylline, ampicillin, diazoxide, furosemide

Compatibility when admixed: Incompatible with aminophylline, ampicillin, chlorothiazide, edetate calcium disodium, ethacrynate, hydrocortisone sodium succinate, mephentermine, methohexital, nitroglycerin, phenobarbital, verapamil

Monitoring Laboratory Tests ANA titer

Monitoring and Teaching Issues

Physical Assessment: See Contraindications, Warnings/Precautions, and Dosing for use cautions. Assess potential for interactions with other prescriptions, OTC medications, or herbal products patient may be taking (see Drug Interactions). **I.V.:** See Administration specifics. Orthostatic precautions should be observed and patient monitored closely during and following infusion. Assess results of laboratory tests, therapeutic response (decreased blood pressure), and adverse response (eg, hypotension, fluid retention - see Adverse Reactions and Overdose/Toxicology) periodically during therapy. Teach patient proper use, possible side effects and appropriate interventions, and adverse symptoms to report (see Patient Education). **Pregnancy risk factor C** - benefits of use should outweigh possible risks.

Patient Education: Inform prescriber of all prescriptions, OTC medications, or herbal products you are taking, and any allergies you have. Do not take anything new during treatment unless approved by prescriber. Take as directed, with meals. Avoid alcohol. This medication does not replace other antihypertensive interventions; follow prescriber's instructions for diet and lifestyle changes. Weigh daily at the same time, in the same clothes for the first 2 weeks and weekly thereafter. Report weight gain >5 lb/week, swelling of feet or ankles. May cause dizziness or weakness (change position slowly when rising from sitting or lying position, climbing stairs, and avoid driving or activities requiring alertness until response to drug is known); nausea or vomiting (small, frequent meals, frequent mouth care, chewing gum, or sucking lozenges may help); impotence (reversible); diarrhea

(Continued)

HydrALAZINE *(Continued)*

(boiled milk, buttermilk, or yogurt may help); or constipation (increased exercise, fluids, fruit, or fiber may help). Report chest pain, rapid heartbeat, or palpitations; flu-like symptoms; difficulty breathing; skin rash; numbness and tingling of extremities; muscle cramps, weakness, or tremors; or unresolved GI problems. **Pregnancy precaution:** Inform prescriber if you are or intend to become pregnant

Dietary Issues: Administer with meals.

Breast-feeding Issues: Crosses into breast milk in extremely small amounts. Available evidence suggests safe use during breast-feeding. AAP considers **compatible** with breast-feeding.

Pregnancy Issues: Crosses the placenta. One report of fetal arrhythmia; transient neonatal thrombocytopenia and fetal distress reported following late 3rd trimester use. A large amount of clinical experience with the use of this drug for management of hypertension during pregnancy is available.

Related Information

FDA Name Differentiation Project: The Use of Tall-man Letters *on page 12*

Heart Failure *on page 1670*

Hydralazine and Hydrochlorothiazide

(hye DRAL a zeen & hye droe klor oh THYE a zide)

Synonyms Apresazide [DSC]; Hydrochlorothiazide and Hydralazine

Generic Available Yes

Pharmacologic Category Antihypertensive Agent Combination

Pregnancy Risk Factor C

Lactation Enters breast milk/compatible

Use Management of moderate to severe hypertension and treatment of congestive heart failure

Formulations

Capsule:

25/25: Hydralazine hydrochloride 25 mg and hydrochlorothiazide 25 mg

50/50: Hydralazine hydrochloride 50 mg and hydrochlorothiazide 50 mg

100/50: Hydralazine hydrochloride 100 mg and hydrochlorothiazide 50 mg

Dosing

Adults: Hypertension: Oral: 1 capsule twice daily

Elderly: Refer to dosing in individual monographs.

Monitoring and Teaching Issues

Physical Assessment: See individual components listed in Related Information. **Pregnancy risk factor C** - benefits of use should outweigh possible risks.

Patient Education: See individual components listed in Related Information. **Pregnancy precaution:** Inform prescriber if you are or intend to become pregnant.

Related Information

HydrALAZINE *on page 662*

Hydrochlorothiazide *on page 664*

Hydralazine Hydrochloride *see* HydrALAZINE *on page 662*

Hydramine® [OTC] *see* DiphenhydrAMINE *on page 422*

Hydramine® Cough [OTC] *see* DiphenhydrAMINE *on page 422*

Hydrated Chloral *see* Chloral Hydrate *on page 268*

Hydrea® *see* Hydroxyurea *on page 682*

Hydrocet® *see* Hydrocodone and Acetaminophen *on page 667*

Hydrochlorothiazide (hye droe klor oh THYE a zide)

U.S. Brand Names Aquazide® H; Hydrocot®; Microzide™; Oretic®

Synonyms HCTZ

Generic Available Yes

Pharmacologic Category Diuretic, Thiazide

Pregnancy Risk Factor B (manufacturer); D (expert analysis)

Lactation Enters breast milk/use caution (AAP rates "compatible")

Use Management of mild to moderate hypertension; treatment of edema in congestive heart failure and nephrotic syndrome

Use - Unlabeled/Investigational Treatment of lithium-induced diabetes insipidus

Mechanism of Action/Effect Inhibits sodium reabsorption in the distal tubules causing increased excretion of sodium and water as well as potassium and hydrogen ions

Contraindications Hypersensitivity to hydrochlorothiazide or any component of the formulation, thiazides, or sulfonamide-derived drugs; anuria; renal decompensation; pregnancy

Warnings/Precautions Avoid in severe renal disease (ineffective as a diuretic). Electrolyte disturbances (hypokalemia, hypochloremic alkalosis, hyponatremia) can occur. Use with caution in severe hepatic dysfunction; hepatic encephalopathy can be caused by electrolyte disturbances. Gout may be precipitated in patients with a history of gout, a familial predisposition to gout, or chronic renal failure. Use caution in patients with diabetes; may alter glucose control. May cause SLE exacerbation or activation. Use with caution in patients with moderate or high cholesterol concentrations. Photosensitization may occur. Correct hypokalemia before initiating therapy.

Chemical similarities are present among sulfonamides, sulfonylureas, carbonic anhydrase inhibitors, thiazides, and loop diuretics (except ethacrynic acid). Use in patients with sulfonamide allergy is specifically contraindicated in product labeling, however, a risk of cross-reaction exists in patients with allergy to any of these compounds; avoid use when previous reaction has been severe.

Drug Interactions

Decreased Effect: Effects of oral hypoglycemics may be decreased. Decreased absorption of hydrochlorothiazide with cholestyramine and colestipol. NSAIDs can decrease the efficacy of thiazides, reducing the diuretic and antihypertensive effects.

Increased Effect/Toxicity: Increased effect of hydrochlorothiazide with furosemide and other loop diuretics. Increased hypotension and/or renal adverse effects of ACE inhibitors may result in aggressively diuresed patients. Beta-blockers increase hyperglycemic effects of thiazides in type 2 diabetes mellitus. Cyclosporine and thiazides can increase the risk of gout or renal toxicity. Digoxin toxicity can be exacerbated if a thiazide induces hypokalemia or hypomagnesemia. Lithium toxicity can occur with thiazides due to reduced renal excretion of lithium. Thiazides may prolong the duration of action with neuromuscular blocking agents.

Nutritional/Ethanol Interactions

Food: Hydrochlorothiazide peak serum levels may be decreased if taken with food. This product may deplete potassium, sodium, and magnesium.

Herb/Nutraceutical: Avoid dong quai if using for hypertension (has estrogenic activity). Dong quai may also cause photosensitization. Avoid ephedra, ginseng, yohimbe (may worsen hypertension). Avoid garlic (may have increased antihypertensive effect).

Effects on Lab Values ↑ creatine phosphokinase [CPK] (S), ammonia (B), amylase (S), calcium (S), chloride (S), cholesterol (S), glucose, acid (S); ↓ chloride (S), magnesium, potassium (S), sodium (S); tyramine and phentolamine tests; histamine tests for pheochromocytoma

Adverse Reactions

1% to 10%:

- Cardiovascular: Orthostatic hypotension, hypotension
- Dermatologic: Photosensitivity
- Endocrine & metabolic: Hypokalemia
- Gastrointestinal: Anorexia, epigastric distress

<1% (Limited to important or life-threatening): Agranulocytosis, allergic myocarditis, allergic reactions (possibly with life-threatening anaphylactic shock), alopecia, aplastic anemia, eosinophilic pneumonitis, erythema multiforme, exfoliative dermatitis, hemolytic anemia, hepatic function impairment, hypercalcemia, interstitial nephritis, leukopenia, pancreatitis, renal failure, respiratory distress, Stevens-Johnson syndrome, thrombocytopenia, toxic epidermal necrolysis

Overdosage/Toxicology Symptoms of overdose include hypermotility, diuresis, lethargy, confusion, and muscle weakness. Treatment is supportive.

Pharmacodynamics/Kinetics

Absorption: ~50% to 80%

Bioavailability: 50% to 80%

Half-Life Elimination: 5.6-14.8 hours

Time to Peak: 1-2.5 hours

Metabolism: Not metabolized

Onset: Diuresis: ~2 hours; Peak effect: 4-6 hours

Duration: 6-12 hours

Formulations

Capsule (Microzide™): 12.5 mg

Solution, oral: 50 mg/5 mL (500 mL) [contains sodium benzoate; mint flavor]

Tablet: 25 mg, 50 mg, 100 mg

- Aquazide® H: 50 mg
- Oretic®: 25 mg, 50 mg

Dosing

Adults: Hypertension, edema (diuretic): Oral (effect of drug may be decreased when used every day): 25-100 mg/day in 1-2 doses; maximum: 200 mg/day; minimal increase in response and more electrolyte disturbances are seen with doses >50 mg/day

Elderly: Oral: 12.5-25 mg once daily; minimal increase in response and more electrolyte disturbances are seen with doses >50 mg/day (see Special Geriatric Considerations).

Pediatrics: Hypertension, edema (diuretic): Oral (effect of drug may be decreased when used every day):

- <6 months: 2-3 mg/kg/day in 2 divided doses
- >6 months: 2 mg/kg/day in 2 divided doses

Note: In pediatric patients, chlorothiazide may be preferred over hydrochlorothiazide as there are more dosage formulations (eg, suspension) available.

Renal Impairment: Cl_{cr} <30 mL/minute: Dosing adjustment not effective, therefore not generally recommended.

Administration

Oral: May be taken with food or milk. Take early in day to avoid nocturia. Take the last dose of multiple doses no later than 6 PM unless instructed otherwise.

Monitoring Laboratory Tests Serum electrolytes, BUN, creatinine

Monitoring and Teaching Issues

Physical Assessment: Assess allergy history prior to beginning therapy. See Contraindications, Warnings/Precautions, and Dosing for use cautions. Assess potential for interactions with other prescriptions, OTC medications, or herbal products patient may be taking (see Drug Interactions). Assess results of laboratory tests (see above), therapeutic effects (according to purpose for use), and adverse response (see Adverse Reactions and Overdose/Toxicology) regularly during therapy. Caution diabetic patients to monitor glucose levels closely; may alter glucose control. Teach proper use, possible side effects and appropriate interventions, and adverse symptoms to report (see Patient Education). **Pregnancy risk factor B/D** - see Pregnancy Risk Factor for use cautions. Note breast-feeding caution.

Patient Education: Inform prescriber of all prescriptions, OTC medications, or herbal products you are taking, and any allergies you have. Do not take anything new during treatment unless approved by prescriber. This medication does not replace other antihypertensive interventions; follow prescriber's instructions for diet and lifestyle changes. Take as directed, with meals, early in the day to avoid nocturia. Your prescriber may prescribe a potassium supplement or recommend that you eat foods high in potassium (include bananas and/or orange juice in daily diet). Do not change your diet on your own while taking this medication, especially if you are taking potassium supplements or medications

(Continued)

Hydrochlorothiazide *(Continued)*

to reduce potassium loss; too much potassium can be as harmful as too little. If diabetic, monitor serum glucose closely; this medication may increase serum glucose levels. May cause dizziness or postural hypotension (use caution when rising from sitting or lying position, when driving, climbing stairs, or engaging in tasks that require alertness until response to drug is known); nausea or vomiting (small, frequent meals, frequent mouth care, sucking lozenges, or chewing gum may help); impotence (reversible); constipation (increased exercise, fluids, fruit, or fiber may help); or photosensitivity (use sunscreen, wear protective clothing and eyewear, and avoid direct sunlight). Report persistent flu-like symptoms, chest pain, palpitations, muscle cramping, difficulty breathing, skin rash or itching, unusual bruising or easy bleeding, or excessive fatigue. **Pregnancy/ breast-feeding precautions:** Inform prescriber if you are pregnant. Consult prescriber if breast-feeding.

Geriatric Considerations: Hydrochlorothiazide is not effective in patients with a Cl_{cr} <30 mL/minute, therefore, it may not be a useful agent in many elderly patients.

Additional Information If given the morning of surgery it may render the patient volume depleted and blood pressure may be labile during general anesthesia. Effect of drug may be decreased when used every day.

Related Information

Heart Failure *on page 1670*

Hydrochlorothiazide and Amiloride *see* Amiloride and Hydrochlorothiazide *on page 78*

Hydrochlorothiazide and Benazepril *see* Benazepril and Hydrochlorothiazide *on page 155*

Hydrochlorothiazide and Bisoprolol *see* Bisoprolol and Hydrochlorothiazide *on page 172*

Hydrochlorothiazide and Captopril *see* Captopril and Hydrochlorothiazide *on page 213*

Hydrochlorothiazide and Enalapril *see* Enalapril and Hydrochlorothiazide *on page 466*

Hydrochlorothiazide and Hydralazine *see* Hydralazine and Hydrochlorothiazide *on page 664*

Hydrochlorothiazide and Irbesartan *see* Irbesartan and Hydrochlorothiazide *on page 736*

Hydrochlorothiazide and Lisinopril *see* Lisinopril and Hydrochlorothiazide *on page 810*

Hydrochlorothiazide and Losartan *see* Losartan and Hydrochlorothiazide *on page 826*

Hydrochlorothiazide and Methyldopa *see* Methyldopa and Hydrochlorothiazide *on page 881*

Hydrochlorothiazide and Moexipril *see* Moexipril and Hydrochlorothiazide *on page 923*

Hydrochlorothiazide and Propranolol *see* Propranolol and Hydrochlorothiazide *on page 1146*

Hydrochlorothiazide and Quinapril *see* Quinapril and Hydrochlorothiazide *on page 1162*

Hydrochlorothiazide and Reserpine

(hye droe klor oh THYE a zide & re SER peen)

Synonyms Reserpine and Hydrochlorothiazide

Restrictions Not available in U.S.

Generic Available Yes

Pharmacologic Category Antihypertensive Agent Combination

Pregnancy Risk Factor C

Lactation Enters breast milk/compatible

Use Management of mild to moderate hypertension; treatment of edema in congestive heart failure and nephrotic syndrome

Formulations

Tablet:

25: Hydrochlorothiazide 25 mg and reserpine 0.125 mg

50: Hydrochlorothiazide 50 mg and reserpine 0.125 mg

Dosing

Adults: Hypertension: Oral: 1-2 tablets once or twice daily

Elderly: Refer to dosing in individual monographs.

Monitoring and Teaching Issues

Physical Assessment: See individual components listed in Related Information. **Pregnancy risk factor C** - benefits of use should outweigh possible risks.

Patient Education: See individual components listed in Related Information. **Pregnancy precaution:** Inform prescriber if you are or intend to become pregnant.

Related Information

Hydrochlorothiazide *on page 664*

Reserpine *on page 1178*

Hydrochlorothiazide and Spironolactone

(hye droe klor oh THYE a zide & speer on oh LAK tone)

U.S. Brand Names Aldactazide®

Synonyms Spironolactone and Hydrochlorothiazide

Generic Available Yes

Pharmacologic Category Antihypertensive Agent Combination

Pregnancy Risk Factor C

Lactation Enters breast milk/use caution

Use Management of mild to moderate hypertension; treatment of edema in congestive heart failure and nephrotic syndrome, and cirrhosis of the liver accompanied by edema and/or ascites

Formulations Tablet: Hydrochlorothiazide 25 mg and spironolactone 25 mg

Aldactazide®:

25/25: Hydrochlorothiazide 25 mg and spironolactone 25 mg

50/50: Hydrochlorothiazide 50 mg and spironolactone 50 mg

Dosing

Adults: Hypertension, edema: Oral:

Hydrochlorothiazide 25 mg and spironolactone 25 mg: ½-8 tablets daily

Hydrochlorothiazide 50 mg and spironolactone 50 mg: ½-4 tablets daily in 1-2 doses

Elderly: Oral: Initial: 1 tablet/day; increase as necessary.

Renal Impairment: Efficacy of hydrochlorothiazide is limited in patients with Cl_{cr} <30 mL/minute.

Monitoring and Teaching Issues

Physical Assessment: See individual components listed in Related Information. **Pregnancy risk factor C** - benefits of use should outweigh possible risks. Note breast-feeding caution.

Patient Education: See individual components listed in Related Information. **Pregnancy/breast-feeding precautions:** Inform prescriber if you are or intend to become pregnant. Consult prescriber if breast-feeding.

Related Information

Hydrochlorothiazide *on page 664*

Spironolactone *on page 1244*

Hydrochlorothiazide and Telmisartan *see* Telmisartan and Hydrochlorothiazide *on page 1280*

Hydrochlorothiazide and Triamterene

(hye droe klor oh THYE a zide & trye AM ter een)

U.S. Brand Names Dyazide®; Maxzide®; Maxzide®-25

Synonyms Triamterene and Hydrochlorothiazide

Generic Available Yes

Pharmacologic Category Antihypertensive Agent Combination; Diuretic, Potassium Sparing; Diuretic, Thiazide

Pregnancy Risk Factor C (per manufacturer)

Lactation Excretion in breast milk unknown/use caution

Use Management of mild to moderate hypertension; treatment of edema in congestive heart failure and nephrotic syndrome

Formulations

Capsule (Dyazide®): Hydrochlorothiazide 25 mg and triamterene 37.5 mg

Tablet:

Maxzide®: Hydrochlorothiazide 50 mg and triamterene 75 mg

Maxzide®-25: Hydrochlorothiazide 25 mg and triamterene 37.5 mg

Dosing

Adults & Elderly: Hypertension, edema: Oral:

Triamterene 37.5 mg and hydrochlorothiazide 25 mg: 1-2 tablets/capsules once daily

Triamterene 75 mg and hydrochlorothiazide 50 mg: ½-1 tablet daily

Monitoring and Teaching Issues

Physical Assessment: See individual components listed in Related Information. **Pregnancy risk factor C** - benefits of use should outweigh possible risks. Note breast-feeding caution.

Patient Education: See also Hydrochlorothiazide.

Triamterene component: Does not cause potassium loss; avoid excessive potassium intake (eg, salt substitutes, low-salt foods, bananas, nuts). Weigh yourself daily at the same time, in the same clothes, and report weight loss greater than 5 lb/week. Urine may appear blue (normal). You may experience dizziness, drowsiness, headache (use caution when driving or engaging in tasks requiring alertness until response to drug is known); nausea (small, frequent meals, frequent mouth care, sucking lozenges, or chewing gum may help); decreased sexual ability (reversible with discontinuing of medication); or postural hypotension (change position slowly when rising from sitting or lying). Report persistent fatigue, muscle weakness, paresthesia, confusion, anorexia, headaches, lethargy, hyper-reflexia, seizures, swelling of extremities or difficulty breathing (eg, chest pain, rapid heartbeat or palpitations).

Pregnancy/breast-feeding precautions: Inform prescriber if you are or intend to become pregnant. Consult prescriber if breast-feeding.

Related Information

Hydrochlorothiazide *on page 664*

Hydrochlorothiazide and Valsartan *see* Valsartan and Hydrochlorothiazide *on page 1388*

Hydrocil® [OTC] *see* Psyllium *on page 1152*

Hydrocodone *see page 1583*

Hydrocodone *see page 1568*

Hydrocodone and Acetaminophen

(hye droe KOE done & a seet a MIN oh fen)

U.S. Brand Names Anexsia®; Bancap HC®; Ceta-Plus®; Co-Gesic®; Hydrocet®; Hydrogesic® [DSC]; Lorcet® 10/650; Lorcet®-HD; Lorcet® Plus; Lortab®; Margesic® H; Maxidone™; Norco®; Stagesic®; Vicodin®; Vicodin® ES; Vicodin® HP; Zydone®

Synonyms Acetaminophen and Hydrocodone

Restrictions C-III

Generic Available Yes

Pharmacologic Category Analgesic Combination (Narcotic)

Pregnancy Risk Factor C

Lactation Excretion in breast milk unknown/contraindicated

Use Relief of moderate to severe pain; antitussive (hydrocodone)

Contraindications Hypersensitivity to hydrocodone, acetaminophen, or any component of the formulation; CNS depression; severe respiratory depression

(Continued)

Hydrocodone and Acetaminophen *(Continued)*

Warnings/Precautions Use with caution in patients with hypersensitivity reactions to other phenanthrene derivative opioid agonists (morphine, hydrocodone, hydromorphone, levorphanol, oxycodone, oxymorphone). Tablets contain metabisulfite which may cause allergic reactions. Pregnancy risk C.

Drug Interactions

Cytochrome P450 Effect:

Hydrocodone: Substrate of **CYP2D6**

Acetaminophen: Substrate of CYP1A2, 2A6, 2C8/9, 2D6, 2E1, 3A4

Decreased Effect: Decreased effect with phenothiazines

Increased Effect/Toxicity: Hydrocodone with other narcotic analgesics, CNS depressants, antianxiety agents, or antipsychotics may cause enhanced CNS depression. MAO inhibitors or tricyclic antidepressants with hydrocodone may increase the effect of either agent.

Nutritional/Ethanol Interactions

Ethanol: Avoid ethanol or limit to <3 drinks/day.

Food: Rate of absorption of acetaminophen may be decreased when administered with food high in carbohydrates.

Herb/Nutraceutical: Avoid valerian, St John's wort, SAMe, kava kava (may increase risk excessive sedation).

Adverse Reactions

Cardiovascular: Hypotension, bradycardia

Central nervous system: Lightheadedness, dizziness, sedation, drowsiness, fatigue, confusion

Gastrointestinal: Nausea, vomiting

Genitourinary: Decreased urination

Neuromuscular & skeletal: Weakness

Respiratory: Dyspnea

<1% (Limited to important or life-threatening): Biliary tract spasm, hallucinations, histamine release, physical and psychological dependence with prolonged use, urinary tract spasm

Overdosage/Toxicology Symptoms of overdose include hepatic necrosis, blood dyscrasias, and respiratory depression. Treatment consists of acetylcysteine 140 mg/kg orally (loading) followed by 70 mg/kg every 4 hours for 17 doses; therapy should be initiated based upon laboratory analysis suggesting a high probability for hepatotoxic potential. Naloxone, 2 mg I.V. with repeat administration as necessary up to a total of 10 mg, can also be used to reverse toxic effects of the opiate. Activated charcoal is effective at binding certain chemicals, and this is especially true for acetaminophen.

Pharmacokinetic Note See Acetaminophen monograph.

Pharmacodynamics/Kinetics

Half-Life Elimination:

Hydrocodone: 3.3-4.4 hours

Metabolism:

Hydrocodone: Hepatic; O-demethylation; N-demethylation and 6-ketosteroid reduction

Onset:

Hydrocodone: Narcotic analgesic: 10-20 minutes

Duration:

Hydrocodone: 4-8 hours

Formulations

Capsule (Bancap HC®, Ceta-Plus®, Hydrocet®, Hydrogesic®, Lorcet®-HD, Margesic® H, Stagesic®): Hydrocodone bitartrate 5 mg and acetaminophen 500 mg

Elixir (Lortab®): Hydrocodone bitartrate 2.5 mg and acetaminophen 167 mg per 5 mL (480 mL) [contains alcohol 7%; tropical fruit punch flavor]

Tablet:
- Hydrocodone bitartrate 2.5 mg and acetaminophen 500 mg
- Hydrocodone bitartrate 5 mg and acetaminophen 500 mg
- Hydrocodone bitartrate 7.5 mg and acetaminophen 500 mg
- Hydrocodone bitartrate 7.5 mg and acetaminophen 650 mg
- Hydrocodone bitartrate 7.5 mg and acetaminophen 750 mg
- Hydrocodone bitartrate 10 mg and acetaminophen 325 mg
- Hydrocodone bitartrate 10 mg and acetaminophen 500 mg
- Hydrocodone bitartrate 10 mg and acetaminophen 650 mg
- Anexsia®:
  - 5/325: Hydrocodone bitartrate 5 mg and acetaminophen 325 mg
  - 5/500: Hydrocodone bitartrate 5 mg and acetaminophen 500 mg
  - 7.5/325: Hydrocodone bitartrate 7.5 mg and acetaminophen 325 mg
  - 7.5/650: Hydrocodone bitartrate 7.5 mg and acetaminophen 650 mg
  - 10/660: Hydrocodone bitartrate 10 mg and acetaminophen 660 mg
- Co-Gesic® 5/500: Hydrocodone bitartrate 5 mg and acetaminophen 500 mg
- Lorcet® 10/650: Hydrocodone bitartrate 10 mg and acetaminophen 650 mg
- Lorcet® Plus: Hydrocodone bitartrate 7.5 mg and acetaminophen 650 mg
- Lortab®:
  - 2.5/500: Hydrocodone bitartrate 2.5 mg and acetaminophen 500 mg
  - 5/500: Hydrocodone bitartrate 5 mg and acetaminophen 500 mg
  - 7.5/500: Hydrocodone bitartrate 7.5 mg and acetaminophen 500 mg
  - 10/500: Hydrocodone bitartrate 10 mg and acetaminophen 500 mg
- Maxidone™: Hydrocodone bitartrate 10 mg and acetaminophen 750 mg
- Norco®:
  - Hydrocodone bitartrate 5 mg and acetaminophen 325 mg
  - Hydrocodone bitartrate 7.5 mg and acetaminophen 325 mg
  - Hydrocodone bitartrate 10 mg and acetaminophen 325 mg
- Vicodin®: Hydrocodone bitartrate 5 mg and acetaminophen 500 mg
- Vicodin® ES: Hydrocodone bitartrate 7.5 mg and acetaminophen 750 mg
- Vicodin® HP: Hydrocodone bitartrate 10 mg and acetaminophen 660 mg

Zydone®:

Hydrocodone bitartrate 5 mg and acetaminophen 400 mg
Hydrocodone bitartrate 7.5 mg and acetaminophen 400 mg
Hydrocodone bitartrate 10 mg and acetaminophen 400 mg

Dosing

Adults: Oral (doses should be titrated to appropriate analgesic effect); for children ≥12 years of age and adults, the dosage of acetaminophen should be limited to ≤4 g/day (and possibly less in patients with hepatic impairment or ethanol use)

Analgesic: 1-2 tablets or capsules every 4-6 hours or 5-10 mL solution every 4-6 hours as needed for pain

Hydrocodone 2.5-5 mg and acetaminophen 400-500 mg; maximum: 8 tablets/capsules per day

Hydrocodone 7.5 mg and acetaminophen: 400-650 mg; maximum: 6 tablets/capsules per day

Hydrocodone 2.5 mg and acetaminophen: 167 mg/5 mL (elixir/solution); maximum: 6 Tbsp/day

Hydrocodone 7.5 mg and acetaminophen 750 mg; maximum: 5 tablets/capsules per day

Hydrocodone 10 mg and acetaminophen: 350-660 mg; maximum: 6 tablets/day per product labeling

Elderly: Doses should be titrated to appropriate analgesic effect; 2.5-5 mg of the hydrocodone component every 4-6 hours. Do not exceed 4 g/day of acetaminophen.

Pediatrics: Doses should be titrated to appropriate analgesic effect. For children ≥12 years of age and adults, the dosage of acetaminophen should be limited to ≤4 g/day (and possibly less in patients with hepatic impairment or ethanol use). Oral:

Antitussive (hydrocodone): 0.6 mg/kg/day in 3-4 divided doses; even though dosing by hydrocodone, make sure to keep within age-specific acetaminophen doses as well.

A single dose should not exceed 10 mg in children >12 years, 5 mg in children 2-12 years, and 1.25 mg in children <2 years of age.

Analgesic (acetaminophen): Refer to Acetaminophen monograph.

Hepatic Impairment: Use with caution. Limited, low-dose therapy usually well tolerated in hepatic disease/cirrhosis; however, cases of hepatotoxicity at daily acetaminophen dosages <4 g/day have been reported. Avoid chronic use in hepatic impairment.

Monitoring and Teaching Issues

Physical Assessment: **Assess patient for history of liver disease or ethanol abuse** (acetaminophen and excessive ethanol may have adverse liver effects). Assess other medications patient may be taking for additive or adverse interactions (see Drug Interactions). See Contraindications and Warnings/Precautions for use cautions. Monitor therapeutic effectiveness and signs of adverse reactions (see Adverse Reactions and Overdose/Toxicology) at beginning of therapy and at regular intervals with long-term use. Order safety precautions for inpatient use. May cause physical and/or psychological dependence. Discontinue slowly after long-term use. Assess knowledge/teach patient appropriate use, adverse reactions to report, and appropriate interventions to reduce side effects. **Pregnancy risk factor C** - benefits of use should outweigh possible risks. Breast-feeding is contraindicated.

Patient Education: If self-administered, use exactly as directed; do not increase dose or frequency. Drug may cause physical and/or psychological dependence. Take with food or milk. While using this medication, do not use alcohol and other prescription or OTC medications (especially sedatives, tranquilizers, antihistamines, or pain medications) without consulting prescriber. Maintain adequate hydration (2-3 L/day of fluids) unless advised by prescriber to restrict fluids. May cause dizziness, lightheadedness, confusion, or drowsiness (use caution when driving, climbing stairs, or changing position - rising from sitting or lying to standing, or when engaging in tasks requiring alertness until response to drug is known); or nausea or vomiting (frequent mouth care, frequent sips of fluids, chewing gum, or sucking lozenges may help). Report chest pain or palpitations; persistent dizziness, shortness of breath, or difficulty breathing; unusual bleeding or bruising; or unusual fatigue and weakness. **Pregnancy/breast-feeding precautions:** Inform prescriber if you are or intend to become pregnant. Do not breast-feed.

Geriatric Considerations: The elderly may be particularly susceptible to the CNS depressant action (sedation, confusion) and constipating effects of narcotics. If 1 tablet/dose is used, it may be useful to add an additional 325 mg of acetaminophen to maximize analgesic effect and minimize additional risk of narcotic related adverse effects.

Breast-feeding Issues:

Hydrocodone: No data reported.
Acetaminophen: May be taken while breast-feeding.

Additional Information Acetaminophen dosing for pediatric patients: 10-15 mg/kg/dose **or alternatively,**

Up to 3 months: 40 mg
4-11 months: 80 mg
1-2 years: 120 mg
2-3 years: 160 mg
4-5 years: 240 mg
6-8 years: 320 mg
9-10 years: 400 mg
11 years: 480 mg

Related Information

Acetaminophen *on page 35*

Hydrocodone and Aspirin (hye droe KOE done & AS pir in)

U.S. Brand Names Damason-P®

Synonyms Aspirin and Hydrocodone

Restrictions C-III

Generic Available No

(Continued)

Hydrocodone and Aspirin *(Continued)*

Pharmacologic Category Analgesic Combination (Narcotic)

Pregnancy Risk Factor D

Lactation Enters breast milk/contraindicated

Use Relief of moderate to moderately severe pain

Mechanism of Action/Effect

Based on **hydrocodone** component: Binds to opiate receptors in the CNS, altering the perception of and response to pain; suppresses cough in medullary center; produces generalized CNS depression

Based on **aspirin** component: Inhibits prostaglandin synthesis, acts on the hypothalamus heat-regulating center to reduce fever, blocks prostaglandin synthetase action which prevents formation of the platelet-aggregating substance thromboxane A_2

Contraindications

Based on **hydrocodone** component: Hypersensitivity to hydrocodone or any component of the formulation

Based on **aspirin** component: Hypersensitivity to salicylates, other NSAIDs, or any component of the formulation; asthma; rhinitis; nasal polyps; inherited or acquired bleeding disorders (including factor VII and factor IX deficiency); pregnancy (in 3rd trimester especially); do not use in children (<16 years) for viral infections (chickenpox or flu symptoms), with or without fever, due to a potential association with Reye's syndrome

Warnings/Precautions Use with caution in patients with impaired renal function, erosive gastritis, or peptic ulcer disease. Children and teenagers should not use for chickenpox or flu symptoms before a physician is consulted about Reye's syndrome.

Drug Interactions

Cytochrome P450 Effect:

Hydrocodone: Substrate of **CYP2D6**

Aspirin: Substrate of CYP2C8/9

Decreased Effect: Based on **aspirin** component: The effects of ACE inhibitors may be blunted by aspirin administration (may be significant only at higher aspirin dosages). Aspirin may decrease the effects of beta-blockers, loop diuretics (furosemide), thiazide diuretics, and probenecid. Aspirin may cause a decrease in NSAIDs serum concentration and decrease the effects of probenecid. Increased serum salicylate levels when taken with with urine acidifiers (ammonium chloride, methionine).

Increased Effect/Toxicity:

Based on **hydrocodone** component: CNS depressants, MAO inhibitors, general anesthetics, and tricyclic antidepressants may potentiate the effects of opiate agonists; dextroamphetamine may enhance the analgesic effect of opiate agonists.

Based on **aspirin** component: May increase methotrexate serum levels/toxicity and may displace valproic acid from binding sites which can result in toxicity. NSAIDs and aspirin increase GI adverse effects (ulceration). Aspirin with oral anticoagulants (warfarin), thrombolytic agents, heparin, low molecular weight heparins, and antiplatelet agents (ticlopidine, clopidogrel, dipyridamole, NSAIDs, and IIb/IIIa antagonists) may increase risk of bleeding. Bleeding times may be additionally prolonged with verapamil. The effects of older sulfonylurea agents (tolazamide, tolbutamide) may be potentiated due to displacement from plasma proteins. This effect does not appear to be clinically significant for newer sulfonylurea agents (glyburide, glipizide, glimepiride).

Nutritional/Ethanol Interactions

Based on **hydrocodone** component: Ethanol: Avoid or limit ethanol (may increase CNS depression). Watch for sedation.

Based on **aspirin** component:

Ethanol: Avoid ethanol (may enhance gastric mucosal damage).

Food: Food may decrease the rate but not the extent of oral absorption. Take with food or or large volume of water or milk to minimize GI upset.

Herb/Nutraceutical: Avoid cat's claw, dong quai, evening primrose, feverfew, garlic, ginger, ginkgo, red clover, horse chestnut, green tea, ginseng (all have additional antiplatelet activity).

Effects on Lab Values Urine glucose, urinary 5-HIAA, serum uric acid

Adverse Reactions

>10%:

Cardiovascular: Hypotension

Central nervous system: Lightheadedness, dizziness, sedation, drowsiness, fatigue

Gastrointestinal: Nausea, heartburn, stomach pains, heartburn, epigastric discomfort

Neuromuscular & skeletal: Weakness

1% to 10%:

Cardiovascular: Bradycardia

Central nervous system: Confusion

Dermatologic: Rash

Gastrointestinal: Vomiting, gastrointestinal ulceration

Genitourinary: Decreased urination

Hematologic: Hemolytic anemia

Respiratory: Dyspnea

Miscellaneous: Anaphylactic shock

<1% (Limited to important or life-threatening): Biliary tract spasm, bronchospasm, hallucinations, hepatotoxicity, histamine release, leukopenia, occult bleeding, physical and psychological dependence with prolonged use, prolongated bleeding time, thrombocytopenia, urinary tract spasm

Overdosage/Toxicology Naloxone is the antidote for hydrocodone. Naloxone, 2 mg I.V. with repeat administration as necessary up to a total of 10 mg, can also be used to reverse toxic effects of the opiate. Nomograms, such as the "Done" nomogram, can be very helpful for estimating the severity of aspirin poisoning and for directing treatment using serum salicylate levels. Treatment can also be based upon symptomatology; symptoms of aspirin overdose include tinnitus, headache, dizziness, confusion, metabolic acidosis, hyperpyrexia, hypoglycemia, and coma.

Pharmacokinetic Note See Aspirin monograph.

Pharmacodynamics/Kinetics

Half-Life Elimination:

Hydrocodone: 3.3-4.4 hours

Metabolism:

Hydrocodone: Hepatic; O-demethylation; N-demethylation and 6-ketosteroid reduction

Onset:

Hydrocodone: Narcotic analgesic: 10-20 minutes

Duration:

Hydrocodone: 4-8 hours

Formulations Tablet: Hydrocodone bitartrate 5 mg and aspirin 500 mg

Dosing

Adults: Analgesic: Oral: 1-2 tablets every 4-6 hours as needed for pain

Elderly: Refer to dosing in individual monographs.

Administration

Oral: Administer with food or a full glass of water to minimize GI distress.

Monitoring and Teaching Issues

Physical Assessment: **Do not use for persons with allergic reaction to aspirin or aspirin-containing medications.** Assess other medications patient may be taking for additive or adverse interactions (see Drug Interactions). Monitor therapeutic effectiveness and adverse reactions (see Adverse Reactions) at beginning of therapy and at regular intervals with long-term use. May cause physical and/or psychological dependence. Discontinue slowly after long-term use. Assess knowledge/teach patient appropriate use if self-administered. Teach patient to monitor for adverse reactions, adverse reactions to report, and appropriate interventions to reduce side effects. **Pregnancy risk factor D** - determine that patient is not pregnant before beginning treatment. Instruct patients of childbearing age about appropriate barrier contraceptive measures. Breast-feeding is contraindicated.

Patient Education: If self-administered, use exactly as directed; do not increase dose or frequency. Drug may cause physical and/or psychological dependence. Take with food or milk. While using this medication, do not use alcohol, excessive amounts of vitamin C, or salicylate-containing foods (curry powder, prunes, raisins, tea, or licorice), other aspirin- or salicylate-containing medications, and other prescription or OTC medications (especially sedatives, tranquilizers, antihistamines, or pain medications) without consulting prescriber. Maintain adequate hydration (2-3 L/day of fluids) unless advised by prescriber to restrict fluids. May cause hypotension, dizziness, drowsiness, impaired coordination, or blurred vision (use caution when driving, climbing stairs, or changing position - rising from sitting or lying to standing, or when engaging in tasks requiring alertness until response to drug is known); nausea, vomiting, or dry mouth (frequent mouth care, small, frequent meals, chewing gum, or sucking lozenges may help); or constipation (increased exercise, fluids, fruit, or fiber may help; if unresolved, consult prescriber about use of stool softeners). Report ringing in ears; persistent stomach pain; unresolved nausea or vomiting; difficulty breathing or shortness of breath; yellowing of skin or eyes; changes in color of stool or urine; or unusual bruising or bleeding. **Pregnancy/breast-feeding precautions:** Use appropriate contraceptive measures; do not get pregnant while taking this drug. Do not breast-feed.

Breast-feeding Issues:

Hydrocodone: No data reported.

Aspirin: Cautious use due to potential adverse effects in nursing infants.

Related Information

Aspirin *on page 121*

Hydrocodone and Ibuprofen (hye droe KOE done & eye byoo PROE fen)

U.S. Brand Names Vicoprofen®

Synonyms Ibuprofen and Hydrocodone

Restrictions C-III

Generic Available No

Pharmacologic Category Analgesic, Narcotic

Pregnancy Risk Factor C/D (3rd trimester)

Lactation Excretion in breast milk unknown/contraindicated

Use Short-term (generally <10 days) management of moderate to severe acute pain; is not indicated for treatment of such conditions as osteoarthritis or rheumatoid arthritis

Mechanism of Action/Effect

Based on **hydrocodone** component: Binds to opiate receptors in the CNS, altering the perception of and response to pain; suppresses cough in medullary center; produces generalized CNS depression

Based on **ibuprofen** component: Inhibits prostaglandin synthesis by decreasing the activity of the enzyme, cyclooxygenase, which results in decreased formation of prostaglandin precursors

Contraindications Hypersensitivity to hydrocodone, ibuprofen, aspirin, other NSAIDs, or any component of the formulation; pregnancy (3rd trimester)

Warnings/Precautions Use with caution in patients with asthma or in patients who have experienced hypersensitivity reactions to opioids due to cross sensitivity to hydrocodone. Hydrocodone may produce drug dependence. Pregnancy risk factor C/D (3rd trimester).

Drug Interactions

Cytochrome P450 Effect:

Hydrocodone: Substrate of **CYP2D6**

Ibuprofen: Substrate of CYP2C8/9, 2C19; Inhibits CYP2C8/9

Decreased Effect: Based on **ibuprofen** component: Aspirin may decrease ibuprofen serum concentrations. Ibuprofen may decrease the effect of some antihypertensive agents (including ACE inhibitors and angiotensin antagonists) and diuretics.

Increased Effect/Toxicity: Anticholinergic agents taken with hydrocodone may cause paralytic ileus. Aspirin taken concomitantly may enhance adverse effects. Other CNS

(Continued)

Hydrocodone and Ibuprofen *(Continued)*

depressants (eg, antihistamines, alcohol, antipsychotics, etc) taken concomitantly may exhibit additive CNS toxicity. Warfarin taken with ibuprofen may result in additional risk of bleeding. Methotrexate taken with ibuprofen may enhance methotrexate toxicity. Furosemide taken with ibuprofen may reduce the effect of furosemide. Lithium taken with ibuprofen may elevate lithium serum levels.

Nutritional/Ethanol Interactions

Based on **hydrocodone** component: Ethanol: Avoid or limit ethanol (may increase CNS depression). Watch for sedation.

Based on **ibuprofen** component:

Ethanol: Avoid ethanol (may enhance gastric mucosal irritation).

Food: Ibuprofen peak serum levels may be decreased if taken with food.

Herb/Nutraceutical: Avoid cat's claw, dong quai, evening primrose, feverfew, garlic, ginger, ginkgo, red clover, horse chestnut, green tea, ginseng (all have additional antiplatelet activity).

Adverse Reactions

>10%:

Central nervous system: Headache (27%), dizziness (14%), sedation (22%)

Dermatologic: Rash, urticaria

Gastrointestinal: Constipation (22%), nausea (21%), dyspepsia (12%)

1% to 10%:

Cardiovascular: Bradycardia, palpitations (<3%), vasodilation (<3%), edema (3% to 9%)

Central nervous system: Headache, nervousness, confusion, fever (<3%), pain (3% to 9%), anxiety (3% to 9%), thought abnormalities

Dermatologic: Itching (3% to 9%)

Endocrine & metabolic: Fluid retention

Gastrointestinal: Vomiting (3% to 9%), anorexia, diarrhea (3% to 9%), xerostomia (3% to 9%), flatulence (3% to 9%), gastritis (<3%), melena (<3%), mouth ulcers (<3%)

Genitourinary: Polyuria (<3%)

Neuromuscular & skeletal: Weakness (3% to 9%)

Otic: Tinnitus

Respiratory: Dyspnea, hiccups, pharyngitis, rhinitis

Miscellaneous: Flu syndrome (<3%), infection (3% to 9%)

<1% (Limited to important or life-threatening): Acute renal failure, agranulocytosis, anemia, arrhythmias, aseptic meningitis, biliary tract spasm, bone marrow suppression, CHF, depression, diplopia, erythema multiforme, hallucinations, hemolytic anemia, hepatitis, histamine release, inhibition of platelet aggregation, leukopenia, neutropenia, peripheral neuropathy, physical and psychological dependence with prolonged use, Stevens-Johnson syndrome, thrombocytopenia, toxic amblyopia, toxic epidermal necrolysis, urinary tract spasm, urticaria

Overdosage/Toxicology Symptoms of toxicity may include respiratory depression, CNS depression, metabolic acidosis, seizures, hypotension, blood loss, coma, meiosis, and renal failure. Naloxone is the antidote for hydrocodone. Naloxone, 2 mg I.V. with repeat administration as necessary up to a total of 10 mg, can also be used to reverse toxic effects of the opiate. Treatment of NSAID overdose is supportive with symptomatic management as necessary.

Pharmacokinetic Note See Ibuprofen monograph.

Pharmacodynamics/Kinetics

Half-Life Elimination:

Hydrocodone: 3.3-4.4 hours

Time to Peak:

Hydrocodone: 1.7 hours

Metabolism:

Hydrocodone: Hepatic; O-demethylation; N-demethylation and 6-ketosteroid reduction

Onset:

Hydrocodone: Narcotic analgesic: 10-20 minutes

Duration:

Hydrocodone: 4-8 hours

Formulations Tablet: Hydrocodone bitartrate 7.5 mg and ibuprofen 200 mg

Dosing

Adults: Analgesic: Oral (Short-term use is recommended, not to exceed 10 days): 1 tablet every 4-6 hours, do not exceed 5 tablets during a 24-hour period.

Elderly: Refer to dosing in individual monographs.

Monitoring and Teaching Issues

Physical Assessment: Assess other medications patient may be taking for additive or adverse interactions (see Drug Interactions). Monitor for effectiveness of pain relief and monitor for signs of overdose (see Overdose/Toxicology). Monitor vital signs and signs of adverse reactions (see Adverse Reactions) at beginning of therapy and at regular intervals with long-term use. May cause physical and/or psychological dependence. Discontinue slowly after long-term use. For inpatients, implement safety measures (eg, side rails up, call light within reach, instructions to call for assistance, etc). Assess knowledge/teach patient appropriate use if self-administered. Teach patient to monitor for adverse reactions, adverse reactions to report, and appropriate interventions to reduce side effects. **Pregnancy risk factor C/D** - see Pregnancy Risk Factor for use cautions; benefits of use should outweigh possible risks. Breast-feeding is contraindicated.

Patient Education: If self-administered, use exactly as directed; do not increase dose or frequency. Drug may cause physical and/or psychological dependence. Take with food or milk. While using this medication, do not use alcohol and other prescription or OTC medications (especially sedatives, tranquilizers, antihistamines, or pain medications) without consulting prescriber. Maintain adequate hydration (2-3 L/day of fluids) unless advised by prescriber to restrict fluids. May cause dizziness, drowsiness, confusion, nervousness, or anxiety (use caution when driving, climbing stairs, or changing position - rising from sitting or lying to standing, or when engaging in tasks requiring alertness until response to drug is known); nausea, dry mouth, decreased appetite, or gastric distress (frequent mouth care, frequent sips of fluids, chewing gum, or sucking lozenges may help); or constipation (increased exercise, fluids, fruit, or fiber may help; if unresolved, consult prescriber about use of stool softeners). Report chest pain or palpitations; persistent dizziness, shortness of breath, or difficulty breathing; unusual bleeding (stool, mouth, urine) or bruising; unusual fatigue and weakness; change in elimination patterns; or change in color of urine or stool. **Pregnancy/breast-feeding precautions:** Inform prescriber if you are or intend to become pregnant. Do not breast-feed.

Geriatric Considerations: Elderly patients have been reported to have a higher incidence of constipation and may be more sensitive to the renal effects of ibuprofen. Therefore, consider using lower doses or longer intervals between doses if alternative agents cannot be used.

Pregnancy Issues: As with other NSAID-containing products, this agent should be avoided in late pregnancy because it may cause premature closure of the ductus arteriosus.

Additional Information The antipyretic and anti-inflammatory activity of ibuprofen may reduce fever and inflammation, thus diminishing their utility as diagnostic signs in detecting complications of presumed noninfectious, noninflammatory painful conditions.

Related Information

Ibuprofen *on page 688*

Hydrocort® *see* Topical Corticosteroids *on page 1334*

Hydrocortisone (hye droe KOR ti sone)

U.S. Brand Names A-hydroCort®; Anucort-HC®; Anusol-HC®; Anusol® HC-1 [OTC]; Aquanil™ HC [OTC]; CaldeCORT® [OTC]; Cetacort®; Clocort™; CortaGel® Maximum Strength [OTC]; Cortaid® Intensive Therapy [OTC]; Cortaid® Maximum Strength [OTC]; Cortaid® Sensitive Skin With Aloe [OTC]; Cortef®; Corticool® [OTC]; Cortifoam®; Cortizone®-5 [OTC]; Cortizone®-10 Maximum Strength [OTC]; Cortizone®-10 Plus Maximum Strength [OTC]; Cortizone® 10 Quick Shot [OTC]; Cortizone® for Kids [OTC]; Dermarest Dricort® [OTC]; Dermtex® HC [OTC]; EarSol® HC; Hemril-HC®; Hydrocortone®; Hydrocortone® Phosphate; Hytone®; LactiCare-HC®; Locoid®; Locoid Lipocream®; Nupercainal® Hydrocortisone Cream [OTC]; Nutracort®; Pandel®; Post Peel Healing Balm [OTC]; Preparation H® Hydrocortisone [OTC]; Proctocort®; ProctoCream® HC; Proctosol-HC®; Sarnol®-HC [OTC]; Solu-Cortef®; Summer's Eve® SpecialCare™ Medicated Anti-Itch Cream [OTC]; Texacort®; Theracort® [OTC]; Westcort®

Synonyms Compound F; Cortisol; Hydrocortisone Acetate; Hydrocortisone Buteprate; Hydrocortisone Butyrate; Hydrocortisone Cypionate; Hydrocortisone Sodium Phosphate; Hydrocortisone Sodium Succinate; Hydrocortisone Valerate

Generic Available Yes

Pharmacologic Category Corticosteroid, Rectal; Corticosteroid, Systemic; Corticosteroid, Topical

Pregnancy Risk Factor C

Lactation Excretion in breast milk unknown

Use Management of adrenocortical insufficiency; relief of inflammation of corticosteroid-responsive dermatoses (low and medium potency topical corticosteroid); adjunctive treatment of ulcerative colitis

Mechanism of Action/Effect Decreases inflammation by suppression of migration of polymorphonuclear leukocytes and reversal of increased capillary permeability

Contraindications Hypersensitivity to hydrocortisone or any component of the formulation; serious infections, except septic shock or tuberculous meningitis; viral, fungal, or tubercular skin lesions

Warnings/Precautions Use with caution in patients with hyperthyroidism, cirrhosis, nonspecific ulcerative colitis, hypertension, osteoporosis, thromboembolic tendencies, CHF, convulsive disorders, myasthenia gravis, thrombophlebitis, peptic ulcer, diabetes, glaucoma, cataracts, or tuberculosis. Use caution in hepatic impairment. Acute adrenal insufficiency may occur with abrupt withdrawal after long-term therapy or with stress. Young pediatric patients may be more susceptible to adrenal axis suppression from topical therapy. Because of the risk of adverse effects, systemic corticosteroids should be used cautiously in the elderly, in the smallest possible dose, and for the shortest possible time. Pregnancy risk C.

Drug Interactions

Cytochrome P450 Effect: Substrate of CYP3A4; Induces CYP3A4

Decreased Effect: Hydrocortisone may decrease the hypoglycemic effect of insulin. Phenytoin, phenobarbital, ephedrine, and rifampin increase metabolism of hydrocortisone resulting in a decreased steroid blood level.

Increased Effect/Toxicity: Hydrocortisone in combination with oral anticoagulants may increase prothrombin time. Potassium-depleting diuretics increase risk of hypokalemia. Cardiac glycosides increase risk of arrhythmias or digitalis toxicity secondary to hypokalemia.

Nutritional/Ethanol Interactions

Ethanol: Avoid ethanol (may enhance gastric mucosal irritation).

Food: Hydrocortisone interferes with calcium absorption.

Herb/Nutraceutical: St John's wort may decrease hydrocortisone levels. Avoid cat's claw, echinacea (have immunostimulant properties).

Adverse Reactions

Systemic:

>10%:

Central nervous system: Insomnia, nervousness

Gastrointestinal: Increased appetite, indigestion

1% to 10%:

Central nervous system: Dizziness, lightheadedness, headache

Dermatologic: Hirsutism, hypopigmentation

Endocrine & metabolic: Diabetes mellitus

Neuromuscular & skeletal: Arthralgia

Ocular: Cataracts, glaucoma

(Continued)

Hydrocortisone *(Continued)*

Respiratory: Epistaxis
Miscellaneous: Diaphoresis
<1% (Limited to important or life-threatening): Alkalosis, amenorrhea, sodium and water retention, Cushing's syndrome, glucose intolerance, growth suppression, hyperglycemia, hypokalemia, pituitary-adrenal axis suppression, pseudotumor cerebri, seizures

Topical:
1% to 10%:
Dermatologic: Itching, allergic contact dermatitis, erythema, dryness papular rashes, folliculitis, furunculosis, pustules, pyoderma, vesiculation, hyperesthesia, skin infection (secondary)
Local: Burning, irritation
<1% (Limited to important or life-threatening): Cataracts (posterior subcapsular), Cushing's syndrome, glaucoma, hypokalemic syndrome

Overdosage/Toxicology When consumed in high doses for prolonged periods, systemic hypercorticism and adrenal suppression may occur. In those cases, discontinuation of the corticosteroid should be done judiciously.

Pharmacodynamics/Kinetics

Absorption: Rapid by all routes, except rectally
Half-Life Elimination: Biologic: 8-12 hours
Metabolism: Hepatic
Onset:
Hydrocortisone acetate: Slow
Hydrocortisone sodium phosphate (water soluble): Rapid
Hydrocortisone sodium succinate (water soluble): Rapid
Duration:
Hydrocortisone acetate: Long
Hydrocortisone sodium phosphate (water soluble): Short

Formulations

Aerosol, rectal, as acetate (Cortifoam®): 10% (15 g) [90 mg/applicator]
Aerosol, topical spray, as base
Cortizone® 10 Quick Shot: 1% (44 mL) [contains benzyl alcohol]
Dermtex® HC: 1% (52 mL) [contains menthol 1%]
Cream, rectal, as acetate (Nupercainal® Hydrocortisone Cream): 1% (30 g)
Cream, rectal, as base:
Cortizone®-10: 1% (30g) [contains aloe]
Preparation H® Hydrocortisone: 1% (27 g)
Cream, topical, as acetate: 0.5% (30 g) [available with aloe]; 1% (30 g) [available with aloe]
Cortaid® Maximum Strength: 1% (15 g, 30 g, 40 g)
Cortaid® Sensitive Skin With Aloe: 0.5% (15 g) [contains aloe vera gel]
Cream, topical, as base: 0.5% (30 g); 1% (1.5 g, 30 g, 454 g); 2.5% (20 g, 30 g, 454 g)
Anusol-HC®: 2.5% (30 g) [contains benzyl alcohol]
CaldeCORT®: 1% (15 g, 30 g)[contains aloe vera gel and benzyl alcohol]
Cortaid® Intensive Therapy: 1% (60 g)
Cortaid® Maximum Strength: 1% (15 g, 30 g, 40 g, 60 g) [contains aloe vera gel and benzyl alcohol]
Cortizone®-5: 0.5% (30 g, 60 g) [contains aloe]
Cortizone®-10 Maximum Strength: 1% (15 g, 30 g, 60 g) [contains aloe]
Cortizone®-10 Plus Maximum Strength: 1% (30 g, 60 g) [contains vitamins A, D, E and aloe]
Cortizone® for Kids: 0.5% (30 g) [contains aloe]
Dermarest® Dri-Cort: 1% (15 g, 30 g)
Hytone®: 2.5% (30 g, 60 g)
Post Peel Healing Balm: 1% (23 g)
ProctoCream® HC: 2.5% (30 g) [contains benzyl alcohol]
Proctocort®: 1% (30 g)
Proctosol-HC®: 2.5% (30 g)
Summer's Eve® SpecialCare™ Medicated Anti-Itch Cream: 1% (30 g)
Cream, topical, as butyrate (Locoid®, Locoid Lipocream®): 0.1% (15 g, 45 g)
Cream, topical, as probutate (Pandel®): 0.1% (15 g, 45 g, 80 g)
Cream, topical, as valerate (Westcort®): 0.2% (15 g, 45 g, 60 g)
Gel, topical, as base
Corticool®: 1% (45 g)
Cortagel® Maximum Strength: 1% (15 g, 30 g) [contains aloe vera gel]
Injection, powder for reconstitution, as sodium succinate:
A-Hydrocort®: 100 mg, 250 mg [diluent contains benzyl alcohol]
Solu-Cortef®: 100 mg, 250 mg, 500 mg, 1 g [diluent contains benzyl alcohol]
Injection, solution, as sodium phosphate (Hydrocortone® Phosphate): 50 mg/mL (2 mL) [contains sodium bisulfite]
Lotion, topical, as base: 1% (120 mL); 2.5% (60 mL)
Aquanil™ HC: 1% (120 mL)
Cetacort®, Sarnol®-HC: 1% (60 mL)
Hytone®: 1% (30 mL, 120 mL); 2.5% (60 mL)
LactiCare-HC®: 1% (120 mL); 2.5% (60 mL, 120 mL)
Nutracort®: 1% (60 mL, 120 mL); 2.5% (60 mL, 120 mL)
Theracort®: 1% (120 mL)
Ointment, topical, as acetate: 1% (30 g) [available with aloe]
Anusol® HC-1: 1% (21 g)
Cortaid® Maximum Strength: 1% (15 g, 30 g)
Ointment, topical, as base: 0.5% (30 g); 1% (30 g, 454 g); 2.5% (20 g, 30 g, 454 g)
Cortizone®-5: 0.5% (30 g) [contains aloe]
Cortizone®-10 Maximum Strength: 1% (30 g, 60 g)
Hytone®: 2.5% (30 g)
Ointment, topical, as base [in Orabase®]: 1% (25 g, 110 g, 454 g)

Ointment, topical, as butyrate (Locoid®): 0.1% (15 g, 45 g)
Ointment, topical, as valerate (Westcort®): 0.2% (15 g, 45 g, 60 g)
Solution, otic, as base (EarSol® HC): 1% (30 mL) [contains alcohol 44%, benzyl benzoate, yerba santa]
Solution, rectal, as base (Colocort™): 100 mg/60 mL (7s) [packaged as single-dose enemas]
Solution, topical, as base (Texacort®): 1% (30 mL) [DSC]; 2.5% (30 mL) [contains alcohol]
Solution, topical, as butyrate (Locoid®): 0.1% (20 mL, 60 mL) [contains alcohol 50%]
Suppository, rectal, as acetate: 25 mg (12s, 24s)
  Anucort™ HC: 25 mg (12s, 24s, 100s)
  Anusol-HC®: 25 mg (12s, 24s)
  Hemril® HC: 25 mg (12s)
  Proctocort®: 30 mg (12s, 24s)
  Proctosol-HC®: 25 mg (12s, 24s)
Suspension, oral, as cypionate (Cortef®): 10 mg/5 mL (120 mL) [contains benzoic acid] [DSC]
Tablet, as base: 20 mg
  Cortef®: 5 mg, 10 mg, 20 mg
  Hydrocortone®: 10 mg

Dosing

Adults: Dose should be based on severity of disease and patient response.

Acute adrenal insufficiency: I.M., I.V.: Succinate: 100 mg I.V. bolus, then 300 mg/day in divided doses every 8 hours or as a continuous infusion for 48 hours. Once patient is stable change to oral, 50 mg every 8 hours for 6 doses, then taper to 30-50 mg/day in divided doses.

Chronic adrenal corticoid insufficiency: Oral: 20-30 mg/day

Anti-inflammatory or immunosuppressive: Oral, I.M., I.V.: Succinate: 15-240 mg every 12 hours

Congenital adrenal hyperplasia: Oral: Initial: 10-20 mg/m^2/day in 3 divided doses; a variety of dosing schedules have been used. **Note:** Inconsistencies have occurred with liquid formulations; tablets may provide more reliable levels. Doses must be individualized by monitoring growth, bone age, and hormonal levels. Mineralocorticoid and sodium supplementation may be required based upon electrolyte regulation and plasma renin activity.

Shock: I.M., I.V.: Succinate: 500 mg to 2 g every 2-6 hours

Status asthmaticus: I.V.: Succinate: 1-2 mg/kg/dose every 6 hours for 24 hours, then maintenance of 0.5-1 mg/kg every 6 hours

Stress dosing (surgery) in patients known to be adrenally-suppressed or on chronic systemic steroids: I.V.:

  Minor stress (ie, inguinal herniorrhaphy): 25 mg/day for 1 day

  Moderate stress (ie, joint replacement, cholecystectomy): 50-75 mg/day (25 mg every 8-12 hours) for 1-2 days

  Major stress (pancreatoduodenectomy, esophagogastrectomy, cardiac surgery): 100-150 mg/day (50 mg every 8-12 hours) for 2-3 days

Rheumatic diseases:

  Intralesional, intra-articular, soft tissue injection: Acetate:
    Large joints: 25 mg (up to 37.5 mg)
    Small joints: 10-25 mg
  Tendon sheaths: 5-12.5 mg
  Soft tissue infiltration: 25-50 mg (up to 75 mg)
  Bursae: 25-37.5 mg
  Ganglia: 12.5-25 mg

Dermatosis: Topical: Apply to affected area 3-4 times/day.

Ulcerative colitis: Rectal: 10-100 mg 1-2 times/day for 2-3 weeks

Elderly: Because of the risk of adverse effects, systemic corticosteroids should be used cautiously in the elderly, in the smallest possible dose, and for the shortest possible time.

Pediatrics: Dose should be based on severity of disease and patient response.

Acute adrenal insufficiency: I.M., I.V.:

  Infants and young Children: Succinate: 1-2 mg/kg/dose bolus, then 25-150 mg/day in divided doses every 6-8 hours

  Older Children: Succinate: 1-2 mg/kg bolus then 150-250 mg/day in divided doses every 6-8 hours

Anti-inflammatory or immunosuppressive:

  Infants and Children:
    Oral: 2.5-10 mg/kg/day **or** 75-300 mg/m^2/day every 6-8 hours
    I.M., I.V.: Succinate: 1-5 mg/kg/day **or** 30-150 mg/m^2/day divided every 12-24 hours
  Adolescents: Oral, I.M., I.V.: Succinate: 15-240 mg every 12 hours

Congenital adrenal hyperplasia: Oral: Initial: 10-20 mg/m^2/day in 3 divided doses; a variety of dosing schedules have been used. **Note:** Inconsistencies have occurred with liquid formulations; tablets may provide more reliable levels. Doses must be individualized by monitoring growth, bone age, and hormonal levels. Mineralocorticoid and sodium supplementation may be required based upon electrolyte regulation and plasma renin activity

Physiologic replacement: Children:
  Oral: 0.5-0.75 mg/kg/day **or** 20-25 mg/m^2/day every 8 hours
  I.M.: Succinate: 0.25-0.35 mg/kg/day **or** 12-15 mg/m^2/day once daily

Shock: I.M., I.V.: Succinate:
  Children: Initial: 50 mg/kg, then repeated in 4 hours and/or every 24 hours as needed
  Adolescents: 500 mg to 2 g every 2-6 hours

Status asthmaticus: Children: I.V.: Succinate: 1-2 mg/kg/dose every 6 hours for 24 hours, then maintenance of 0.5-1 mg/kg every 6 hours.

Dermatosis: Topical: Children >2 years: Apply to affected area 3-4 times/day (Buteprate: Apply once or twice daily).

(Continued)

Hydrocortisone *(Continued)*

Administration

Oral: Administer with food or milk to decrease GI upset.

I.V.:

Parenteral: Hydrocortisone sodium succinate may be administered by I.M. or I.V. routes.

I.V. bolus: Dilute to 50 mg/mL and give over 30 seconds to several minutes (depending on the dose).

I.V. intermittent infusion: Dilute to 1 mg/mL and give over 20-30 minutes.

Note: Should be administered in a 0.1-1 mg/mL concentration due to stability problems.

Topical: Apply a thin film sparingly to clean, dry skin and rub in gently.

Stability

Storage: Hydrocortisone sodium phosphate and hydrocortisone sodium succinate are clear, light yellow solutions which are heat labile.

Reconstitution: After initial reconstitution, hydrocortisone sodium succinate solutions are stable for 3 days at room temperature and refrigeration if protected from light. Stability of parenteral admixture (Solu-Cortef®) at room temperature (25°C) and at refrigeration temperature (4°C) is concentration dependent.

Minimum volume: Concentration should not exceed 1 mg/mL.
Stability of concentration ≤1 mg/mL: 24 hours
Stability of concentration >1 mg/mL to <25 mg/mL: Unpredictable, 4-6 hours
Stability of concentration ≥25 mg/mL: 3 days
Standard diluent (Solu-Cortef®): 50 mg/50 mL D_5W; 100 mg/100 mL D_5W

Compatibility:

Hydrocortisone sodium phosphate:

Stable in D_5W, NS, fat emulsion 10%

Y-site administration: Incompatible with sargramostim

Compatibility in syringe: Incompatible with doxapram

Hydrocortisone sodium succinate:

Stable in dextran 6% in dextrose, dextran 6% in NS, D_5LR, $D_5{}^1/_4NS$, $D_5{}^1/_2NS$, D_5NS, D_5W, $D_{10}W$, $D_{20}W$, LR, $^1/_2NS$, NS, fat emulsion 10%

Y-site administration: Incompatible with ciprofloxacin, diazepam, ergotamine, idarubicin, midazolam, phenytoin, sargramostim

Compatibility in syringe: Incompatible with doxapram

Compatibility when admixed: Incompatible with aminophylline with cephalothin, bleomycin, colistimethate, ephedrine, hydralazine, nafcillin, pentobarbital, phenobarbital, prochlorperazine edisylate, promethazine

Monitoring Laboratory Tests Serum glucose, electrolytes

Monitoring and Teaching Issues

Physical Assessment: Monitor laboratory results, effects and interactions of other medications patient may be taking, response to therapy and adverse effects according to diagnosis, formulation of hydrocortisone, dosage, and extent of time used (see Drug Interactions, Adverse Reactions, Dosage Forms, and Dosing). Systemic administration and long-term use will require close and frequent monitoring, especially for Cushing's syndrome. Assess/teach patient appropriate use, interventions for possible adverse reactions, and symptoms to report (see Patient Education). **Pregnancy risk factor C** - benefits of use should outweigh possible risks. (Topical absorption may be minimal.) Note breast-feeding caution.

Patient Education: Systemic: Take as directed; do not increase doses and do not stop abruptly without consulting prescribed. Dosage of systemic hydrocortisone is usually tapered off gradually. Take oral dose with food to reduce GI upset. Avoid alcohol. Hydrocortisone may cause immunosuppression and mask symptoms of infection; avoid exposure to contagion and notify prescriber of any signs of infection (eg, fever, chills, sore throat, injury) and notify dentist or surgeon (if necessary) that you are taking this medication. You may experience increased appetite, indigestion, or increased nervousness. Report any sudden weight gain (>5 lb/week), swelling of extremities or difficulty breathing, abdominal pain, severe vomiting, black or tarry stools, fatigue, anorexia, weakness, or unusual mood swings. **Pregnancy/breast-feeding precautions:** Inform prescriber if you are or intend to become pregnant. Consult prescriber if breast-feeding.

Topical: Before applying, wash area gently and thoroughly. Apply a thin film to cleansed area and rub in gently until medication vanishes. Avoid exposing affected area to sunlight; you will be more sensitive and severe sunburn may occur. Consult prescriber if breast-feeding.

Rectal: Gently insert suppository as high as possible with gloved finger while lying down. Avoid injury with long or sharp fingernails. Remain in resting position for 10 minutes after insertion.

Dietary Issues: Systemic use of corticosteroids may require a diet with increased potassium, vitamins A, B_6, C, D, folate, calcium, zinc, phosphorus, and decreased sodium. Sodium content of 1 g (sodium succinate injection): 47.5 mg (2.07 mEq)

Additional Information Hydrocortisone base topical cream, lotion, and ointments in concentrations of 0.25%, 0.5%, and 1% may be OTC or prescription depending on the product labeling.

Related Information

Compatibility of Drugs *on page 1564*
Corticosteroids Comparison, Systemic Equivalencies *on page 1572*

Hydrocortisone *see* Topical Corticosteroids *on page 1334*

Hydrocortisone Acetate *see* Hydrocortisone *on page 673*

Hydrocortisone and Benzoyl Peroxide *see* Benzoyl Peroxide and Hydrocortisone *on page 158*

Hydrocortisone and Iodoquinol *see* Iodoquinol and Hydrocortisone *on page 732*

Hydrocortisone and Lidocaine *see* Lidocaine and Hydrocortisone *on page 803*

Hydrocortisone, Bacitracin, Neomycin, and Polymyxin B *see* Bacitracin, Neomycin, Polymyxin B, and Hydrocortisone *on page 145*

Hydrocortisone Buteprate *see* Hydrocortisone *on page 673*

Hydrocortisone Butyrate *see* Hydrocortisone *on page 673*

Hydrocortisone Cypionate *see* Hydrocortisone *on page 673*

Hydrocortisone Sodium Phosphate *see* Hydrocortisone *on page 673*

Hydrocortisone Sodium Succinate *see* Hydrocortisone *on page 673*

Hydrocortisone Valerate *see* Hydrocortisone *on page 673*

Hydrocortone® *see* Hydrocortisone *on page 673*

Hydrocortone® Phosphate *see* Hydrocortisone *on page 673*

Hydrocot® *see* Hydrochlorothiazide *on page 664*

Hydrogesic® [DSC] *see* Hydrocodone and Acetaminophen *on page 667*

Hydromagnesium Aluminate *see* Magaldrate *on page 830*

Hydromorphone (hye droe MOR fone)

U.S. Brand Names Dilaudid®; Dilaudid-HP®

Synonyms Dihydromorphinone; Hydromorphone Hydrochloride

Restrictions C-II

Generic Available Yes

Pharmacologic Category Analgesic, Narcotic

Pregnancy Risk Factor B/D (prolonged use or high doses at term)

Lactation Excretion in breast milk unknown/not recommended

Use Management of moderate to severe pain; antitussive at lower doses

Mechanism of Action/Effect Binds to opiate receptors in the CNS, causing inhibition of ascending pain pathways, altering the perception of and response to pain; causes cough supression by direct central action in the medulla; produces generalized CNS depression

Contraindications Hypersensitivity to hydromorphone, any component of the formulation, or other phenanthrene derivative; pregnancy (prolonged use or high doses at term)

Warnings/Precautions Tablet and cough syrup contain tartrazine which may cause allergic reactions; hydromorphone shares toxic potential of opiate agonists, and precaution of opiate agonist therapy should be observed; extreme caution should be taken to avoid confusing the highly concentrated injection with the less concentrated injectable product, injection contains benzyl alcohol; use with caution in patients with hypersensitivity to other phenanthrene opiates, in patients with respiratory disease, or severe liver or renal failure; tolerance or drug dependence may result from extended use.

An opioid-containing analgesic regimen should be tailored to each patient's needs and based upon the type of pain being treated (acute, versus chronic), the route of administration, degree of tolerance for opioids (naive versus chronic user), age, weight, and medical condition. The optimal analgesic dose varies widely among patients. Doses should be titrated to pain relief/prevention. I.M. use may result in variable absorption and a lag time to peak effect.

Drug Interactions

Increased Effect/Toxicity: CNS depressants, phenothiazines, and tricyclic antidepressants may potentiate the adverse effects of hydromorphone.

Nutritional/Ethanol Interactions

Ethanol: Avoid ethanol (may increase CNS depression).

Herb/Nutraceutical: Avoid valerian, St John's wort, kava kava, gotu kola (may increase CNS depression).

Effects on Lab Values ↑ aminotransferase [ALT (SGPT)/AST (SGOT)] (S)

Adverse Reactions Frequency not defined.

Cardiovascular: Palpitations, hypotension, peripheral vasodilation, tachycardia, bradycardia, flushing of face

Central nervous system: CNS depression, increased intracranial pressure, fatigue, headache, nervousness, restlessness, dizziness, lightheadedness, drowsiness, hallucinations, mental depression, seizures

Dermatologic: Pruritus, rash, urticaria

Endocrine & metabolic: Antidiuretic hormone release

Gastrointestinal: Nausea, vomiting, constipation, stomach cramps, xerostomia, anorexia, biliary tract spasm, paralytic ileus

Genitourinary: Decreased urination, ureteral spasm, urinary tract spasm

Hepatic: LFTs increased, AST increased, ALT increased

Local: Pain at injection site (I.M.)

Neuromuscular & skeletal: Trembling, weakness, myoclonus

Ocular: Miosis

Respiratory: Respiratory depression, dyspnea

Miscellaneous: Histamine release, physical and psychological dependence

Overdosage/Toxicology Symptoms of overdose include CNS depression, respiratory depression, miosis, apnea, pulmonary edema, and convulsions. Along with supportive measures, naloxone, 2 mg I.V. with repeat administration as necessary up to a total of 10 mg, can also be used to reverse toxic effects of the opiate.

Pharmacodynamics/Kinetics

Absorption: I.M.: Variable and delayed

Bioavailability: 62%

Half-Life Elimination: 1-3 hours

Metabolism: Hepatic; no active metabolites

Onset: Analgesic: Oral: 15-30 minutes; Peak effect: Oral: 30-60 minutes

Duration: 4-5 hours

Formulations

Injection, powder for reconstitution, as hydrochloride (Dilaudid-HP®): 250 mg

Injection, solution, as hydrochloride: 1 mg/mL (1 mL); 2 mg/mL (1 mL, 20 mL); 4 mg/mL (1 mL)

Dilaudid®: 1 mg/mL (1 mL); 2 mg/mL (1 mL, 20 mL); 4 mg/mL (1 mL)

(Continued)

Hydromorphone *(Continued)*

Dilaudid-HP®: 10 mg/mL (1 mL, 5 mL, 50 mL)
Liquid, oral, as hydrochloride (Dilaudid®): 1 mg/mL (480 mL) [may contain trace amounts of sodium bisulfite]
Suppository, rectal, as hydrochloride (Dilaudid®): 3 mg (6s)
Tablet, as hydrochloride (Dilaudid®): 2 mg, 4 mg, 8 mg (8 mg tablets may contain trace amounts of sodium bisulfite)

Dosing

Adults:

Acute pain (moderate to severe): **Note:** These are guidelines and do not represent the maximum doses that may be required in all patients. Doses should be titrated to pain relief/prevention.

Oral:

Initial: Opiate-naive: 2-4 mg every 3-4 hours as needed; patients with prior opiate exposure may require higher initial doses

Usual dosage range: 2-8 mg every 3-4 hours as needed

I.V.: Initial: Opiate-naive: 0.2-0.6 mg every 2-3 hours as needed; patients with prior opiate exposure may tolerate higher initial doses

Note: More frequent dosing may be needed.

Mechanically-ventilated patients (based on 70 kg patient): 0.7-2 mg every 1-2 hours as needed; infusion (based on 70 kg patient): 0.5-1 mg/hour

Patient-controlled analgesia (PCA): (Opiate-naive: Consider lower end of dosing range)

Usual concentration: 0.2 mg/mL
Demand dose: Usual: 0.1-0.2 mg; range: 0.05-0.5 mg
Lockout interval: 5-15 minutes
4-hour limit: 4-6 mg

Epidural:

Bolus dose: 1-1.5 mg
Infusion concentration: 0.05-0.075 mg/mL
Infusion rate: 0.04-0.4 mg/hour
Demand dose: 0.15 mg
Lockout interval: 30 minutes

I.M., S.C.: **Note:** I.M. use may result in variable absorption and a lag time to peak effect.

Initial: Opiate-naive: 0.8-1 mg every 4-6 hours as needed; patients with prior opiate exposure may require higher initial doses

Usual dosage range: 1-2 mg every 3-6 hours as needed

Rectal: 3 mg every 4-8 hours as needed

Chronic pain: Patients taking opioids chronically may become tolerant and require doses higher than the usual dosage range to maintain the desired effect. Tolerance can be managed by appropriate dose titration. There is no optimal or maximal dose for hydromorphone in chronic pain. The appropriate dose is one that relieves pain throughout its dosing interval without causing unmanageable side effects.

Antitussive: Oral: 1 mg every 3-4 hours as needed

Note: Doses should be titrated to appropriate analgesic effects; when changing routes of administration, note that oral doses are <50% as effective as parenteral doses (may be only one-fifth as effective).

Elderly: Doses should be titrated to appropriate analgesic effects. When changing routes of administration, note that oral doses are less than half as effective as parenteral doses (may be only 20% as effective).

Pain: Oral: 1-2 mg every 4-6 hours
Antitussive: Refer to adult dosing.

Pediatrics:

Acute pain (moderate to severe): **Note:** These are guidelines and do not represent the maximum doses that may be required in all patients. Doses should be titrated to pain relief/prevention.

Young Children ≥6 months and <50 kg:

Oral: 0.03-0.08 mg/kg/dose every 3-4 hours as needed
I.V.: 0.015 mg/kg/dose every 3-6 hours as needed

Older Children >50 kg: Refer to adult dosing.

Antitussive: Oral:

Children 6-12 years: 0.5 mg every 3-4 hours as needed
Children >12 years: 1 mg every 3-4 hours as needed

Hepatic Impairment: Dose adjustment should be considered.

Administration

I.M.: May be given S.C. or I.M.; for IVP, must be given slowly over 2-3 minutes (rapid IVP has been associated with an increase in side effects, especially respiratory depression and hypotension). Vial stopper contains latex.

Stability

Storage: Store injection and oral dosage forms at 25°C (77°F). Protect tablets from light. A slightly yellowish discoloration has not been associated with a loss of potency.

Compatibility: Stable in D_5LR, D_5W, $D_5{}^1\!/_2NS$, D_5NS, LR, ½NS, NS

Y-site administration: Incompatible with amphotericin B cholesteryl sulfate complex, diazepam, minocycline, phenobarbital, phenytoin, sargramostim, tetracycline, thiopental

Compatibility in syringe: Incompatible with ampicillin, diazepam, hyaluronidase, phenobarbital, phenytoin

Compatibility when admixed: Incompatible with sodium bicarbonate, thiopental

Monitoring and Teaching Issues

Physical Assessment: Assess other medications patient may be taking for additive or adverse interactions (see Drug Interactions). Monitor for effectiveness of pain relief, adverse reactions, and signs of overdose (see Overdose/Toxicology) at beginning of therapy and periodically during long-term use. May cause physical and/or psychological dependence. For inpatients, implement safety measures. Assess knowledge/teach patient appropriate use (if self-administered). Teach patient to monitor for adverse reactions (see Adverse Reactions), adverse reactions to report, and appropriate interventions to reduce side effects. Discontinue slowly after prolonged use. **Pregnancy risk factor B/D** - see Pregnancy Risk Factor for use cautions. Breast-feeding is not recommended.

Patient Education: If self-administered, use exactly as directed; do not increase dose or frequency. Drug may cause physical and/or psychological dependence. While using this medication, do not use alcohol and other prescription or OTC medications (especially sedatives, tranquilizers, antihistamines, or pain medications) without consulting prescriber. Maintain adequate hydration (2-3 L/day of fluids) unless advised by prescriber to restrict fluids. May cause dizziness, drowsiness, impaired coordination, or blurred vision (use caution when driving, climbing stairs, or changing position - rising from sitting or lying to standing, or when engaging in tasks requiring alertness until response to drug is known); loss of appetite, nausea, or vomiting (frequent mouth care, small, frequent meals, chewing gum, or sucking lozenges may help); or constipation (increased exercise, fluids, fruit, or fiber may help; if unresolved, consult prescriber about use of stool softeners). Report chest pain, slow or rapid heartbeat, acute dizziness, or persistent headache; swelling of extremities or unusual weight gain; changes in urinary elimination; acute headache; back or flank pain or spasms; or other adverse reactions. **Pregnancy/breast-feeding precautions:** Inform prescriber if you are or intend to become pregnant. Breast-feeding is not recommended.

Geriatric Considerations: Elderly may be particularly susceptible to the CNS depressant and constipating effects of narcotics.

Additional Information Equianalgesic doses: Morphine 10 mg I.M. = hydromorphone 1.5 mg I.M.

Related Information

Controlled Substances Comparison *on page 1568*

Narcotic/Opioid Analgesic Comparison *on page 1583*

Hydromorphone Hydrochloride *see* Hydromorphone *on page 677*

Hydroquinol *see* Hydroquinone *on page 679*

Hydroquinone (HYE droe kwin one)

U.S. Brand Names Alphaquin HP; Alustra™; Claripel™; Eldopaque® [OTC]; Eldopaque Forte®; Eldoquin® [OTC]; Eldoquin Forte®; Esoterica® Regular [OTC]; Glyquin®; Lustra®; Lustra-AF™; Melanex®; Melpaque HP®; Melquin-3® [OTC]; Melquin HP®; NeoStrata AHA [OTC]; Nuquin HP®; Palmer's® Skin Success Fade Cream™ [OTC]; Solaquin® [OTC]; Solaquin Forte®

Synonyms Hydroquinol; Quinol

Generic Available Yes: 4% cream

Pharmacologic Category Depigmenting Agent

Pregnancy Risk Factor C

Lactation Excretion in breast milk unknown

Use Gradual bleaching of hyperpigmented skin conditions

Mechanism of Action/Effect Produces reversible depigmentation of the skin by suppression of melanocyte metabolic processes, in particular the inhibition of the enzymatic oxidation of tyrosine to DOPA (3,4-dihydroxyphenylalanine); sun exposure reverses this effect and will cause repigmentation.

Contraindications Hypersensitivity to hydroquinone or any component of the formulation; sunburn, depilatory usage

Warnings/Precautions Limit application to area no larger than face and neck or hands and arms. Pregnancy risk C.

Adverse Reactions Frequency not defined.

Dermatologic: Dermatitis, dryness, erythema, stinging, inflammatory reaction, sensitization

Local: Irritation

Pharmacodynamics/Kinetics

Onset: Onset of depigmentation produced by hydroquinone varies among individuals

Duration: Onset and duration of depigmentation produced by hydroquinone varies among individuals

Formulations

Cream, topical: 4% (30 g) [may contain sodium metabisulfite]
- Alphaquin HP, Alustra™: 4% (30 g)
- Eldopaque®: 2% (15 g, 30 g)
- Eldopaque Forte®, Eldoquin Forte®: 4% (30 g) [contains sodium metabisulfite]
- Esoterica® Regular: 2% (85 g) [contains sodium bisulfite]
- Lustra®: 4% (30 g, 60 g) [contains sodium metabisulfite]
- Melquin HP®: 4% (15 g, 30 g) [contains sodium metabisulfite]
- Nuquin HP: 4% (15 g, 30 g, 60 g) [contains sodium metabisulfite]
- Palmer's® Skin Success Fade Cream™: 2% (81 g, 132 g) [contains sodium sulfite; available in regular, oily skin, and dry skin formulas]

Cream, topical [with sunscreen]: 4% (30 g) [may contain sodium metabisulfite]
- Claripel™: 4% (45 g) [contains sodium metabisulfite]
- Glyquin®: 4% (30 g)
- Solaquin®: 2% (30 g)
- Solaquin Forte®: 4% (30 g) [contains sodium metabisulfite]
- Lustra-AF™: 4% (30 g, 60 g) [contains sodium metabisulfite]
- Melpaque HP®: 4% (15 g, 30 g) [contains sodium metabisulfite; sunblocking cream base]

Gel, topical (NeoStrata AHA): 2% (45 g) [contains sodium bisulfite and sodium sulfite]

Gel, topical [with sunscreen]:
- Nuquin HP: 4% (15 g, 30 g) [contains sodium bisulfite]
- Solaquin Forte®: 4% (30 g) [contains sodium metabisulfite]

Solution, topical (Melanex®, Melquin-3®): 3% (30 mL)

(Continued)

Hydroquinone *(Continued)*

Dosing

Adults & Elderly: Bleaching: Topical: Apply a thin layer and rub in twice daily.

Pediatrics: Refer to adult dosing.

Administration

Topical: For external use only; avoid contact with eyes

Monitoring and Teaching Issues

Physical Assessment: See Contraindications and Warnings/Precautions for use cautions. See application directions above. When applied to large areas or for extensive periods of time, monitor for adverse reactions. Assess knowledge/teach patient appropriate application and use and adverse symptoms to report (see Patient Education). **Pregnancy risk factor C** - systemic absorption may be minimal with appropriate use. Note breast-feeding caution.

Patient Education: Use exactly as directed; do not overuse. Therapeutic effect may take several weeks. Test response by applying to small area of unbroken skin and check in 24 hours; if irritation or blistering occurs do not use. Avoid contact with eyes. Do not apply to open wounds or weeping areas. Before using, wash and dry area gently. Apply a thin film to affected area and rub in gently. Avoid direct sunlight or use sunblock or protective clothing to prevent repigmentation. Report swelling, redness, rash, itching, signs of infection, worsening of condition, or lack of healing. **Pregnancy/breast-feeding precautions:** Inform prescriber if you are or intend to become pregnant. Consult prescriber if breast-feeding.

Hydroquinone, Fluocinolone Acetonide, and Tretinoin *see* Fluocinolone, Hydroquinone, and Tretinoin *on page 574*

HydroTex® [OTC] *see* Topical Corticosteroids *on page 1334*

Hydro-Tussin™-CBX *see* Carbinoxamine and Pseudoephedrine *on page 217*

Hydro-Tussin™ DM *see* Guaifenesin and Dextromethorphan *on page 647*

Hydroxocobalamin (hye droks oh koe BAL a min)

Synonyms Vitamin B_{12}

Generic Available Yes

Pharmacologic Category Vitamin, Water Soluble

Pregnancy Risk Factor A/C (dose exceeding RDA recommendation)

Lactation Enters breast milk/compatible

Use Treatment of pernicious anemia, vitamin B_{12} deficiency, increased B_{12} requirements due to pregnancy, thyrotoxicosis, hemorrhage, malignancy, liver or kidney disease

Use - Unlabeled/Investigational Neuropathies, multiple sclerosis

Mechanism of Action/Effect Coenzyme for various metabolic functions, including fat and carbohydrate metabolism and protein synthesis, used in cell replication and hematopoiesis

Contraindications Hypersensitivity to cyanocobalamin or any component of the formulation, cobalt; patients with hereditary optic nerve atrophy

Warnings/Precautions Some products contain benzoyl alcohol. Avoid use in premature infants. An intradermal test dose should be performed for hypersensitivity. Use only if oral supplementation not possible or when treating pernicious anemia. Pregnancy risk A/C (dose exceeding RDA).

Adverse Reactions

1% to 10%:

Dermatologic: Itching

Gastrointestinal: Diarrhea

<1% (Limited to important or life-threatening): Peripheral vascular thrombosis

Formulations Injection, solution: 1000 mcg/mL (30 mL)

Dosing

Adults & Elderly: Vitamin B_{12} deficiency: I.M.: 30 mcg/day for 5-10 days, followed by 100-200 mcg/month

Pediatrics: Vitamin B_{12} deficiency: I.M.: 1-5 mg given in single doses of 100 mcg over 2 or more weeks, followed by 30-50 mcg/month.

Administration

I.M.: Administer I.M. only. May require coadministration of folic acid.

Stability

Storage: Clear pink to red solutions are stable at room temperature; protect from light; incompatible with chlorpromazine, phytonadione, prochlorperazine, warfarin, ascorbic acid, dextrose, heavy metals, oxidizing or reducing agents; avoid freezing

Monitoring Laboratory Tests Reticulocyte count, Hct, iron and folic acid, and serum levels before treatment, after first week of treatment, and routinely thereafter

Monitoring and Teaching Issues

Physical Assessment: See Contraindications and Warnings/Precautions for use cautions. Monitor laboratory tests at beginning of therapy and periodically with long-term therapy. Assess knowledge/teach patient appropriate administration (injection technique and needle disposal), appropriate nutrition, and adverse symptoms to report (see Patient Education). **Pregnancy risk factor A/C** - see Pregnancy Risk Factor for use cautions.

Patient Education: Use exactly as directed. Pernicious anemia may require monthly injections for life. Report skin rash; swelling, pain, or redness in extremities; or acute persistent diarrhea. **Pregnancy precaution:** Inform prescriber if you are pregnant.

Geriatric Considerations: Evidence exists that people, particularly elderly, whose serum cobalamin concentrations are <500 pg/mL, should receive replacement parenteral therapy. This recommendation is based upon neuropsychiatric disorders and cardiovascular disorders associated with lower sodium cobalamin concentrations.

Hydroxyamphetamine and Tropicamide *see page 1461*

Hydroxycarbamide *see* Hydroxyurea *on page 682*

Hydroxychloroquine (hye droks ee KLOR oh kwin)

U.S. Brand Names Plaquenil®

Synonyms Hydroxychloroquine Sulfate

Generic Available Yes

Pharmacologic Category Aminoquinoline (Antimalarial)

Pregnancy Risk Factor C

Lactation Enters breast milk/compatible

Use Suppression and treatment of acute attacks of malaria; treatment of systemic lupus erythematosus and rheumatoid arthritis

Use - Unlabeled/Investigational Porphyria cutanea tarda, polymorphous light eruptions

Mechanism of Action/Effect Interferes with digestive vacuole function within sensitive malarial parasites by increasing the pH and interfering with lysosomal degradation of hemoglobin; inhibits locomotion of neutrophils and chemotaxis of eosinophils; impairs complement-dependent antigen-antibody reactions

Contraindications Hypersensitivity to hydroxychloroquine, 4-aminoquinoline derivatives, or any component of the formulation; retinal or visual field changes attributable to 4-aminoquinolines

Warnings/Precautions Use with caution in patients with hepatic disease, G6PD deficiency, psoriasis, and porphyria. Long-term use in children is not recommended. Perform baseline and periodic (6 months) ophthalmologic examinations. Test periodically for muscle weakness. Pregnancy risk C.

Drug Interactions

Decreased Effect: Chloroquine and other 4-aminoquinolones absorption may be decreased due to GI binding with kaolin or magnesium trisilicate.

Increased Effect/Toxicity: Cimetidine increases levels of chloroquine and probably other 4-aminoquinolones.

Nutritional/Ethanol Interactions Ethanol: Avoid ethanol (due to GI irritation).

Adverse Reactions Frequency not defined.

Cardiovascular: Cardiomyopathy (rare, relationship to hydroxychloroquine unclear)

Central nervous system: Irritability, nervousness, emotional changes, nightmares, psychosis, headache, dizziness, vertigo, seizures, ataxia, lassitude

Dermatologic: Bleaching of hair, alopecia, pigmentation changes (skin and mucosal; black-blue color), rash (urticarial, morbilliform, lichenoid, maculopapular, purpuric, erythema annulare centrifugum, Stevens-Johnson syndrome, acute generalized exanthematous pustulosis, and exfoliative dermatitis)

Endocrine & metabolic: Weight loss

Gastrointestinal: Anorexia, nausea, vomiting, diarrhea, abdominal cramping

Hematologic: Aplastic anemia, agranulocytosis, leukopenia, thrombocytopenia, hemolysis (in patients with glucose-6-phosphate deficiency)

Hepatic: Abnormal liver function/hepatic failure (isolated cases)

Neuromuscular & skeletal: Myopathy, palsy, or neuromyopathy leading to progressive weakness and atrophy of proximal muscle groups (may be associated with mild sensory changes, loss of deep tendon reflexes, and abnormal nerve conduction)

Ocular: Disturbance in accommodation, keratopathy, corneal changes/deposits (visual disturbances, blurred vision, photophobia - reversible on discontinuation), macular edema, atrophy, abnormal pigmentation, retinopathy (early changes reversible - may progress despite discontinuation if advanced), optic disc pallor/atrophy, attenuation of retinal arterioles, pigmentary retinopathy, scotoma, decreased visual acuity, nystagmus

Otic: Tinnitus, deafness

Miscellaneous: Exacerbation of porphyria and nonlight sensitive psoriasis

Overdosage/Toxicology Symptoms of overdose include headache, drowsiness, visual changes, cardiovascular collapse, and seizures followed by respiratory and cardiac arrest. Treatment is symptomatic. Urinary alkalinization will enhance renal elimination.

Pharmacodynamics/Kinetics

Absorption: Complete

Half-Life Elimination: 32-50 days

Time to Peak: Rheumatic disease: Several months

Metabolism: Hepatic

Onset: Rheumatic disease: May require 4-6 weeks to respond

Formulations Tablet, as sulfate: 200 mg [equivalent to 155 mg base]

Dosing

Adults & Elderly:

Note: Hydroxychloroquine sulfate 200 mg is equivalent to 155 mg hydroxychloroquine base and 250 mg chloroquine phosphate.

Chemoprophylaxis of malaria: 310 mg base weekly on same day each week; begin 2 weeks before exposure. Continue for 4-6 weeks after leaving endemic area; if suppressive therapy is not begun prior to the exposure, double the initial dose and give in 2 doses, 6 hours apart.

Malaria, acute attack: 620 mg first dose day 1; 310 mg in 6 hours day 1; 310 mg in 1 dose day 2; and 310 mg in 1 dose on day 3

Rheumatoid arthritis: 310-465 mg/day to start taken with food or milk; increase dose until optimum response level is reached; usually after 4-12 weeks dose should be reduced by ½ and a maintenance dose of 155-310 mg/day given

Lupus erythematosus: 310 mg every day or twice daily for several weeks depending on response; 155-310 mg/day for prolonged maintenance therapy

Pediatrics:

Note: Hydroxychloroquine sulfate 200 mg is equivalent to 155 mg hydroxychloroquine base and 250 mg chloroquine phosphate.

Chemoprophylaxis of malaria: Oral: 5 mg/kg (base) once weekly; should not exceed the recommended adult dose. Begin 2 weeks before exposure and continue for 4-6 weeks after leaving endemic area. If suppressive therapy is not begun prior to the exposure, double the initial dose and give in 2 doses, 6 hours apart.

(Continued)

Hydroxychloroquine *(Continued)*

Malaria, acute attack: Oral: 10 mg/kg (base) initial dose; followed by 5 mg/kg at 6, 24, and 48 hours.

JRA or SLE: Oral: 3-5 mg/kg/day divided 1-2 times/day; avoid exceeding 7 mg/kg/day.

Hepatic Impairment: Use with caution; dosage adjustment may be necessary.

Administration

Oral: Take with food or milk.

Monitoring Laboratory Tests CBC, liver function

Monitoring and Teaching Issues

Physical Assessment: See Contraindications and Warnings/Precautions for use cautions. Assess potential for interactions with other prescriptions, OTC medications, or herbal products patient may be taking (see Drug Interactions). Assess effectiveness of therapy (according to purpose for therapy), laboratory tests (see above), and adverse response (eg, deep tendon reflexes, muscle weakness - see Adverse Reactions and Overdose/Toxicology). Teach patient appropriate use, possible side effects/interventions, and adverse symptoms to report (see Patient Education). **Pregnancy risk factor C** - benefits of use should outweigh possible risks.

Patient Education: Inform prescriber of all prescriptions, OTC medications, or herbal products you are taking, and any allergies you have. Do not take anything new during treatment unless approved by prescriber. It is important to complete full course of therapy, which may take up to 6 months for full effect. May be taken with meals to decrease GI upset and bitter aftertaste. Avoid alcohol. You should have regular ophthalmic exams (every 4-6 months) if using this medication over extended periods. You may experience skin discoloration (blue/black), hair bleaching, or skin rash. If you have psoriasis, you may experience exacerbation. You may experience dizziness, headache, nervousness, or light-headedness (use caution when driving or engaging in tasks requiring alertness until response to drug is known); nausea, vomiting, or loss of appetite (small, frequent meals, frequent mouth care, sucking lozenges, or chewing gum may help); or increased sensitivity to sunlight (wear dark glasses and protective clothing, use sunblock, and avoid direct exposure to sunlight). Report weakness, numbness, tingling or tremors in muscles; vision changes; rash or itching; persistent diarrhea or GI disturbances; change in hearing acuity or ringing in the ears; chest pain or palpitation; CNS changes; unusual fatigue; easy bruising or bleeding, or any other persistent adverse reactions. **Pregnancy precaution:** Inform prescriber if you are or intend to become pregnant.

Dietary Issues: May be taken with food or milk.

Hydroxychloroquine Sulfate *see* Hydroxychloroquine *on page 681*

Hydroxydaunomycin Hydrochloride *see* DOXOrubicin *on page 446*

Hydroxyethyl Starch *see* Hetastarch *on page 656*

Hydroxypropyl Methylcellulose *see page 1461*

Hydroxyurea (hye droks ee yoor EE a)

U.S. Brand Names Droxia™; Hydrea®; Mylocel™

Synonyms Hydroxycarbamide

Generic Available Yes: Capsule

Pharmacologic Category Antineoplastic Agent, Antimetabolite

Pregnancy Risk Factor D

Lactation Enters breast milk/contraindicated

Use CML in chronic phase; radiosensitizing agent in the treatment of primary brain tumors, head and neck tumors, uterine cervix and nonsmall cell lung cancer, and psoriasis; treatment of hematologic conditions such as essential thrombocythemia, polycythemia vera, hypereosinophilia, and hyperleukocytosis due to acute leukemia. Has shown activity against renal cell cancer, melanoma, ovarian cancer, head and neck cancer (excluding lip cancer), and prostate cancer.

Orphan drug: Droxia™: Sickle cell anemia: Specifically for patients >18 years of age who have had at least three "painful crises" in the previous year - to reduce frequency of these crises and the need for blood transfusions

Mechanism of Action/Effect Interferes with synthesis of DNA, without interfering with RNA synthesis

Contraindications Hypersensitivity to hydroxyurea or any component of the formulation; severe anemia; severe bone marrow suppression; WBC <2500/mm^3 or platelet count <100,000/mm^3; pregnancy

Warnings/Precautions Use with caution in patients with renal impairment, in patients who have received prior irradiation therapy with exacerbation of postirradiation erythema, bone marrow suppression, erythrocytic abnormalities, mucositis, and in the elderly. The U.S. Food and Drug Administration (FDA) currently recommends that procedures for proper handling and disposal of antineoplastic agents be considered. May cause pancreatitis, neuropathy, or hepatotoxicity; risk is increased in HIV-infected patients receiving didanosine and/or stavudine. Secondary leukemias have been reported with long-term use.

Drug Interactions

Increased Effect/Toxicity: Zidovudine, zalcitabine, didanosine may increase synergy. The potential for neurotoxicity may increase with concomitant administration with fluorouracil. Hydroxyurea modulates the metabolism and cytotoxicity of cytarabine; dose reduction is recommended. Hydroxyurea may precipitate didanosine- or stavudine-induced pancreatitis, hepatotoxicity, or neuropathy; concomitant use is not recommended.

Adverse Reactions Frequency not defined.

Cardiovascular: Edema

Central nervous system: Drowsiness (with high doses), hallucinations, headache, dizziness, disorientation, seizures, fever, chills

Dermatologic: Erythema of the hands and face, maculopapular rash, pruritus, dry skin, dermatomyositis-like skin changes, hyperpigmentation, atrophy of skin and nails, scaling and violet papules (long-term use), nail banding, skin cancer

Endocrine & metabolic: Hyperuricemia

Gastrointestinal: Nausea, vomiting, stomatitis, anorexia, diarrhea, constipation, mucositis (potentiated in patients receiving radiation), pancreatitis, ulceration of buccal mucosa and GI epithelium (severe intoxication)

Emetic potential: Low (10% to 30%)

Genitourinary: Dysuria

Hematologic: Myelosuppression (primarily leukopenia); Dose-limiting toxicity, causes a rapid drop in leukocyte count (seen in 4-5 days in nonhematologic malignancy and more rapidly in leukemia); thrombocytopenia and anemia occur less often

Onset: 24-48 hours

Nadir: 10 days

Recovery: 7 days after stopping drug (reversal of WBC count occurs rapidly but the platelet count may take 7-10 days to recover)

Other hematologic effects include megaloblastic erythropoiesis, macrocytosis, hemolysis, decreased serum iron, persistent cytopenias, secondary leukemias (long-term use)

Hepatic: Elevation of hepatic enzymes, hepatotoxicity, hyperbilirubinemia (polycythemia vera)

Neuromuscular & skeletal: Weakness, peripheral neuropathy

Renal: Increased creatinine and BUN due to impairment of renal tubular function

Respiratory: Acute diffuse pulmonary infiltrates (rare), dyspnea, pulmonary fibrosis

Overdosage/Toxicology Symptoms of overdose include myelosuppression, facial swelling, hallucinations, and disorientation. Treatment is supportive.

Pharmacodynamics/Kinetics

Absorption: Readily (≥80%)

Half-Life Elimination: 3-4 hours

Time to Peak: ~2 hours

Metabolism: Hepatic and via GI tract; 50% degradation by enzymes of intestinal bacteria

Formulations

Capsule: 500 mg

Droxia™: 200 mg, 300 mg, 400 mg

Hydrea®: 500 mg

Tablet (Mylocel™): 1000 mg

Dosing

Adults & Elderly: Refer to individual protocols.

Note: Dose should always be titrated to patient response and WBC counts; usual oral doses range from 10-30 mg/kg/day or 500-3000 mg/day; if WBC count falls to <2500 cells/mm^3, or the platelet count to <100,000/mm^3, therapy should be stopped for at least 3 days and resumed when values rise toward normal.

Solid tumors: Oral:

Intermittent therapy: 80 mg/kg as a single dose every third day

Continuous therapy: 20-30 mg/kg/day given as a single dose/day

Concomitant therapy with irradiation: 80 mg/kg as a single dose every third day starting at least 7 days before initiation of irradiation

Resistant chronic myelocytic leukemia: Oral: Continuous therapy: 20-30 mg/kg as a single daily dose

HIV (in combination with antiretroviral agents): 1000-1500 mg daily in single or divided doses

Sickle cell anemia (moderate/severe disease): Initial: 15 mg/kg/day, increased by 5 mg/kg every 12 weeks if blood counts are in an acceptable range until the maximum tolerated dose of 35 mg/kg/day is achieved or the dose that does not produce toxic effects

Pediatrics: Refer to individual protocols. All dosage should be based on ideal or actual body weight, whichever is less: Children:

No FDA-approved dosage regimens have been established; dosages of 1500-3000 mg/m^2 as a single dose in combination with other agents every 4-6 weeks have been used in the treatment of pediatric astrocytoma, medulloblastoma, and primitive neuroectodermal tumors

CML: Oral: Initial: 10-20 mg/kg/day once daily; adjust dose according to hematologic response

Renal Impairment:

Cl_{cr} 10-50 mL/minute: Administer 50% of normal dose.

Cl_{cr} <10 mL/minute: Administer 20% of normal dose.

Hemodialysis effects: Supplemental dose is not necessary.

CAPD effects: Unknown

CAVH effects: Dose for GFR 10-50 mL/minute.

Administration

Oral: Capsules may be opened and emptied into water (will not dissolve completely).

Stability

Storage: Store capsules at room temperature. Capsules may be opened and emptied into water (will not dissolve completely).

Monitoring Laboratory Tests CBC with differential, platelets, renal and liver function, serum uric acid

Sickle cell disease: Monitor for toxicity every 2 weeks. If toxicity occurs, stop treatment until the bone marrow recovers; restart at 2.5 mg/kg/day less than the dose at which toxicity occurs. If no toxicity occurs over the next 12 weeks, then the subsequent dose should be increased by 2.5 mg/kg/day. Reduced dosage of hydroxyurea alternating with erythropoietin may decrease myelotoxicity and increase levels of fetal hemoglobin in patients who have not been helped by hydroxyurea alone.

Acceptable range: Neutrophils ≥2500 cells/mm^3, platelets ≥95,000/mm^3, hemoglobin >5.3 g/dL, and reticulocytes ≥95,000/mm^3 if the hemoglobin concentration is <9 g/dL

Toxic range: Neutrophils <2000 cells/mm^3, platelets <80,000/mm^3, hemoglobin <4.5 g/dL, and reticulocytes <80,000/mm^3 if the hemoglobin concentration is <9 g/dL

Monitoring and Teaching Issues

Physical Assessment: See Contraindications, Warnings/Precautions, and Dosing for use cautions. Assess potential for interactions with other prescriptions, OTC medications, or

(Continued)

Hydroxyurea *(Continued)*

herbal products patient may be taking (see Drug Interactions). Hydroxyurea therapy requires close supervision. Assess results of laboratory tests (see Monitoring Lab Tests), therapeutic effects, and adverse response (see Adverse Reactions and Overdose/Toxicology) frequently during treatment. Teach proper use and need for frequent monitoring, possible side effects and appropriate interventions, and adverse symptoms to report (see Patient Education). **Pregnancy risk factor D** - determine that patient is not pregnant before beginning treatment. Instruct patients of childbearing about appropriate barrier contraceptive measures. Breast-feeding is contraindicated.

Patient Education: Inform prescriber of all prescriptions, OTC medications, or herbal products you are taking, and any allergies you have. Do not take anything new during treatment unless approved by prescriber. Take capsules exactly as directed by prescriber (dosage and timing will be specific to purpose of therapy). Contents of capsule may be emptied into a glass of water and taken immediately. You will require frequent monitoring and blood tests while taking this medication to assess effectiveness and monitor adverse reactions. You will be susceptible to infection (avoid crowds and exposure to infection and do not have any vaccinations without consulting prescriber). You may experience nausea, vomiting, or loss of appetite (small, frequent meals, frequent mouth care, sucking lozenges, or chewing gum may help); constipation (increased exercise, fluid, fruit, or fiber may help); diarrhea (buttermilk, boiled milk, or yogurt may help); or mouth sores (frequent mouth care will help). Report persistent vomiting, diarrhea, constipation, stomach pain, or mouth sores; skin rash, redness, irritation, or sores; painful or difficult urination; CNS changes (increased confusion, depression, hallucinations, lethargy, or seizures); opportunistic infection (persistent fever or chills, unusual fatigue, white plaques in mouth, vaginal discharge, or unhealed sores); unusual lassitude, weakness, or muscle tremors; easy bruising/bleeding; or blood in vomitus, stool, or urine. **Note:**People not taking hydroxyurea should not be exposed to it. If powder from capsule is spilled, wipe up with damp, disposable towel immediately, and discard the towel in a closed container, such as a plastic bag. Wash hands thoroughly. **Pregnancy/breast-feeding precautions:** Do not get pregnant while taking this medication. Consult prescriber for appropriate barrier contraceptive measures. Do not breast-feed.

Geriatric Considerations: Elderly may be more sensitive to the effects of this drug. Advance dose slowly and adjust dose for renal function with careful monitoring.

Pregnancy Issues: Hydroxyurea is teratogenic and fetotoxic in animals; data on use during human pregnancy is limited. Effective contraception is recommended in women of childbearing potential.

Additional Information Although I.V. use is reported, no parenteral product is commercially available in the U.S.

If WBC decreases to <2500/mm^3 or platelet count to <100,000/mm^3, interrupt therapy until values rise significantly toward normal. Treat anemia with whole blood replacement; do not interrupt therapy. Adequate trial period to determine effectiveness is 6 weeks. Almost all patients receiving hydroxyurea in clinical trials needed to have their medication stopped for a time to allow their low blood count to return to acceptable levels.

HydrOXYzine (hye DROKS i zeen)

U.S. Brand Names Atarax®; Vistaril®

Synonyms Hydroxyzine Hydrochloride; Hydroxyzine Pamoate

Generic Available Yes

Pharmacologic Category Antiemetic; Antihistamine

Pregnancy Risk Factor C

Lactation Enters breast milk/contraindicated

Use Treatment of anxiety; preoperative sedative; antipruritic

Use - Unlabeled/Investigational Antiemetic; ethanol withdrawal symptoms

Mechanism of Action/Effect Competes with histamine for H_1-receptor sites on effector cells in the gastrointestinal tract, blood vessels, and respiratory tract. Possesses skeletal muscle relaxing, bronchodilator, antihistamine, antiemetic, and analgesic properties.

Contraindications Hypersensitivity to hydroxyzine or any component of the formulation

Warnings/Precautions Causes sedation, caution must be used in performing tasks which require alertness (ie, operating machinery or driving). Sedative effects of CNS depressants or ethanol are potentiated. S.C., intra-arterial, and I.V. administration are not recommended since thrombosis and digital gangrene can occur; extravasation can result in sterile abscess and marked tissue induration; should be used with caution in patients with narrow-angle glaucoma, prostatic hyperplasia, and bladder neck obstruction; should also be used with caution in patients with asthma or COPD. Not recommended for use as a sedative or anxiolytic in the elderly. Pregnancy risk C.

Drug Interactions

Cytochrome P450 Effect: Inhibits CYP2D6

Increased Effect/Toxicity: CNS depressants, anticholinergics, used in combination with hydroxyzine may result in additive effects.

Nutritional/Ethanol Interactions

Ethanol: Avoid ethanol (may increase CNS depression).

Herb/Nutraceutical: Avoid valerian, St John's wort, kava kava, gotu kola (may increase CNS depression).

Adverse Reactions Frequency not defined.

Central nervous system: Drowsiness, headache, fatigue, nervousness, dizziness

Gastrointestinal: Xerostomia

Neuromuscular & skeletal: Tremor, paresthesia, seizure

Ocular: Blurred vision

Respiratory: Thickening of bronchial secretions

Overdosage/Toxicology Symptoms of overdose include seizures, sedation, and hypotension. There is no specific treatment for antihistamine overdose. Clinical toxicity is due to blockade of cholinergic receptors. For anticholinergic overdose with severe life-threatening symptoms, physostigmine 1-2 mg I.V. slowly, may be given to reverse these effects.

Pharmacodynamics/Kinetics

Absorption: Oral: Rapid

Half-Life Elimination: 3-7 hours

Time to Peak: ~2 hours

Metabolism: Exact fate unknown

Onset: 15-30 minutes

Duration: 4-6 hours

Formulations

Capsule, as pamoate (Vistaril®): 25 mg, 50 mg, 100 mg

Injection, solution, as hydrochloride: 25 mg/mL (1 mL); 50 mg/mL (1 mL, 2 mL, 10 mL)
Vistaril®: 50 mg/mL (10 mL) [contains benzyl alcohol]

Suspension, oral, as pamoate (Vistaril®): 25 mg/5 mL (120 mL, 480 mL) [lemon flavor]

Syrup, as hydrochloride: 10 mg/5 mL (120 mL, 480 mL, 4000 mL)
Atarax®: 10 mg/5 mL (480 mL) [contains alcohol, sodium benzoate; mint flavor]

Tablet, as hydrochloride: 10 mg, 25 mg, 50 mg
Atarax®: 10 mg, 25 mg, 50 mg, 100 mg

Dosing

Adults:

Antiemetic: I.M.: 25-100 mg/dose every 4-6 hours as needed

Anxiety: Oral: 25-100 mg 4 times/day; maximum: 600 mg/day

Preoperative sedation:
Oral: 50-100 mg
I.M.: 25-100 mg

Management of pruritus: Oral: 25 mg 3-4 times/day

Elderly: Management of pruritus: 10 mg 3-4 times/day; increase to 25 mg 3-4 times/day if necessary.

Pediatrics: Children:
Oral: 0.6 mg/kg/dose every 6 hours
I.M.: 0.5-1 mg/kg/dose every 4-6 hours as needed

Hepatic Impairment: Change dosing interval to every 24 hours in patients with primary biliary cirrhosis.

Administration

I.M.: Administer deep in large muscle.

I.V.: Irritant. Use caution when administering I.V.

Stability

Storage: Protect from light. Store at 15°C to 30°C and protected from freezing.

Compatibility:

Y-site administration: Incompatible with allopurinol, amifostine, amphotericin B cholesteryl sulfate complex, cefepime, doxorubicin liposome, fluconazole, fludarabine, paclitaxel, piperacillin/tazobactam, sargramostim

Compatibility in syringe: Incompatible with dimenhydrinate, haloperidol, ketorolac, pentobarbital, ranitidine

Compatibility when admixed: Incompatible with aminophylline, amobarbital, chloramphenicol, penicillin G potassium, penicillin G sodium, pentobarbital, phenobarbital

Monitoring and Teaching Issues

Physical Assessment: Assess other medications patient may be taking for effectiveness and possible interactions (see Warnings/Precautions and Drug Interactions). **Systemic:** Monitor therapeutic response and adverse reactions (see Adverse Reactions); ensure patient safety by having patient void prior to administration; and ensure adequate hydration and environmental temperature control. **Oral:** Monitor therapeutic response according to purpose for use, adverse reactions (see Warnings/Precautions, Adverse Reactions, and Overdose/Toxicology). Assess knowledge/teach patient appropriate use, interventions to reduce side effects, and adverse symptoms to report (see Patient Education). **Pregnancy risk factor C** - benefits of use should outweigh possible risks. Breast-feeding is contraindicated.

Patient Education: Will cause drowsiness, avoid alcohol and other CNS depressants. Avoid driving and other hazardous tasks until the CNS effects are known. **Pregnancy/breast-feeding precautions:** Inform prescriber if you are or intend to become pregnant. Do not breast-feed.

Geriatric Considerations: Anticholinergic effects are not well tolerated in the elderly. Hydroxyzine may be useful as a short-term antipruritic, but it is not recommended for use as a sedative or anxiolytic in the elderly.

Additional Information Although not recommended in the product labeling due to the possibility of arterial and venous spasms, intravascular hemolysis, and orthostatic hypotension, hydroxyzine can be administered as a short (15- to 30-minute) I.V. infusion.

Hydroxyzine hydrochloride: Anxanil®, Atarax®, Hydroxacen®, Quiess®, Vistaril® injection, Vistazine®

Hydroxyzine pamoate: Hy-Pam®, Vistaril® capsule and suspension

Related Information

Anxiolytic/Hypnotic Use in Long-Term Care Facilities *on page 1608*
Compatibility of Drugs *on page 1564*
FDA Name Differentiation Project: The Use of Tall-man Letters *on page 12*

Hydroxyzine Hydrochloride *see* HydrOXYzine *on page 684*
Hydroxyzine Pamoate *see* HydrOXYzine *on page 684*
Hygroton [DSC] *see* Chlorthalidone *on page 279*
Hyoscine *see* Scopolamine *on page 1218*

Hyoscyamine (hye oh SYE a meen)

U.S. Brand Names Anaspaz®; Cystospaz®; Cystospaz-M®; Hyosine; Levbid®; Levsin®; Levsinex®; Levsin/SL®; NuLev™; Spacol; Spacol T/S; Symax SL; Symax SR

Synonyms Hyoscyamine Sulfate; *l*-Hyoscyamine Sulfate

Generic Available Yes

(Continued)

Hyoscyamine *(Continued)*

Pharmacologic Category Anticholinergic Agent

Pregnancy Risk Factor C

Lactation Excreted in breast milk/not recommended

Use

Oral: Adjunctive therapy for peptic ulcers, irritable bowel, neurogenic bladder/bowel; treatment of infant colic, GI tract disorders caused by spasm; to reduce rigidity, tremors, sialorrhea, and hyperhidrosis associated with parkinsonism; as a drying agent in acute rhinitis

Injection: Preoperative antimuscarinic to reduce secretions and block cardiac vagal inhibitory reflexes; to improve radiologic visibility of the kidneys; symptomatic relief of biliary and renal colic; reduce GI motility to facilitate diagnostic procedures (ie, endoscopy, hypotonic duodenography); reduce pain and hypersecretion in pancreatitis, certain cases of partial heart block associated with vagal activity; reversal of neuromuscular blockade

Mechanism of Action/Effect Blocks the action of acetylcholine at parasympathetic sites in smooth muscle, secretory glands, and the CNS; increases cardiac output, dries secretions, antagonizes histamine and serotonin

Contraindications Hypersensitivity to belladonna alkaloids or any component of the formulation; glaucoma; obstructive uropathy; myasthenia gravis; obstructive GI tract disease, paralytic ileus, intestinal atony of elderly or debilitated patients, severe ulcerative colitis, toxic megacolon complicating ulcerative colitis; unstable cardiovascular status in acute hemorrhage, myocardial ischemia

Warnings/Precautions Heat prostration may occur in hot weather. Diarrhea may be a sign of incomplete intestinal obstruction, treatment should be discontinued if this occurs. May produce side effects as seen with other anticholinergic medications including drowsiness, dizziness, blurred vision, or psychosis. Children and the elderly may be more susceptible to these effects. Use with caution in children with spastic paralysis. Use with caution in patients with autonomic neuropathy, coronary heart disease, CHF, cardiac arrhythmias, prostatic hyperplasia, hyperthyroidism, hypertension, chronic lung disease, renal disease, and hiatal hernia associated with reflux esophagitis. Use with caution in the elderly, may precipitate undiagnosed glaucoma and/or severely impair memory function (especially in those patients with previous memory problems). NuLev™ contains phenylalanine. Pregnancy risk C.

Drug Interactions

Decreased Effect: Decreased effect with antacids.

Increased Effect/Toxicity: Increased toxicity with amantadine, antihistamines, antimuscarinics, haloperidol, phenothiazines, tricyclic antidepressants, and MAO inhibitors.

Adverse Reactions Frequency not defined.

Cardiovascular: Palpitations, tachycardia

Central nervous system: Ataxia, dizziness, drowsiness, headache, insomnia, mental confusion/excitement, nervousness, speech disorder, weakness

Dermatologic: Urticaria

Endocrine & metabolic: Lactation suppression

Gastrointestinal: Bloating, constipation, dry mouth, loss of taste, nausea, vomiting

Genitourinary: Impotence, urinary hesitancy, urinary retention

Ocular: Blurred vision, cycloplegia, increased ocular tension, mydriasis

Miscellaneous: Allergic reactions, sweating decreased

Overdosage/Toxicology Symptoms of overdose include dilated, unreactive pupils; blurred vision; hot, dry flushed skin; CNS stimulation; dryness of mucous membranes; difficulty swallowing; foul breath; diminished or absent bowel sounds; urinary retention; tachycardia; hyperthermia; hypertension; and increased respiratory rate. For anticholinergic overdose with severe life-threatening symptoms, physostigmine 0.5-2 mg S.C. or I.V. slowly, may be given to reverse these effects; may repeat as necessary to reverse the effects, up to total of 5 mg. Hyoscyamine sulfate is dialyzable.

Pharmacodynamics/Kinetics

Absorption: Well absorbed

Half-Life Elimination: 3-5 hours

Metabolism: Hepatic

Onset: 2-3 minutes

Duration: 4-6 hours

Formulations

Capsule, timed release, as sulfate (Cystospaz-M®, Levsinex®): 0.375 mg

Elixir, as sulfate: 0.125 mg/5 mL (480 mL)

Hyosine: 0.125 mg/5 mL (480 mL) [contains alcohol 20% and sodium benzoate; orange flavor]

Levsin®: 0.125 mg/5 mL (480 mL) [contains alcohol 20%; orange flavor]

Injection, solution, as sulfate (Levsin®): 0.5 mg/mL (1 mL)

Liquid, as sulfate (Spacol): 0.125 mg/5 mL (120 mL) [sugar free, alcohol free, simethicone based, bubblegum flavor]

Solution, oral drops, as sulfate: 0.125 mg/mL (15 mL)

Hyosine: 0.125 mg/mL (15 mL) [contains alcohol 5% and sodium benzoate; orange flavor]

Levsin®: 0.125 mg/mL (15 mL) [contains alcohol 5%; orange flavor]

Tablet (Cystospaz®): 0.15 mg

Tablet, as sulfate (Anaspaz®, Levsin®, Spacol): 0.125 mg

Tablet, extended release, as sulfate (Levbid®, Symax SR, Spacol T/S): 0.375 mg

Tablet, orally-disintegrating, as sulfate (NuLev™): 0.125 mg [contains phenylalanine 1.7 mg/tablet, mint flavor]

Tablet, sublingual, as sulfate: 0.125 mg

Levsin/SL®: 0.125 mg [peppermint flavor]

Symax SL: 0.125 mg

Dosing

Adults & Elderly:

Gastrointestinal spasms:

Oral or S.L.: 0.125-0.25 mg every 4 hours or as needed (before meals or food); maximum: 1.5 mg/24 hours

Cystospaz®: 0.15-0.3 mg up to 4 times/day

Oral, timed release: 0.375-0.75 mg every 12 hours; maximum: 1.5 mg/24 hours

I.M., I.V., S.C.: 0.25-0.5 mg; may repeat as needed up to 4 times/day, at 4-hour intervals

Diagnostic procedures: I.V.: 0.25-0.5 mg given 5-10 minutes prior to procedure

Preanesthesia: I.V.: 5 mcg/kg given 30-60 minutes prior to induction of anesthesia or at the time preoperative narcotics or sedatives are administered

To reduce drug-induced bradycardia during surgery: I.V.: 0.125 mg; repeat as needed

Reverse neuromuscular blockade: I.V.: 0.2 mg for every 1 mg neostigmine (or the physostigmine/pyridostigmine equivalent)

Pediatrics:

Children <2 years: Gastrointestinal disorders: Oral: Dose as listed, based on age and weight (kg) using the 0.125 mg/mL drops. Repeat dose every 4 hours as needed:

3.4 kg: 4 drops; maximum: 24 drops/24 hours

5 kg: 5 drops; maximum: 30 drops/24 hours

7 kg: 6 drops; maximum: 36 drops/24 hours

10 kg: 8 drops; maximum: 48 drops/24 hours

Children 2-12 years:Gastrointestinal disorders: Oral or S.L.: Dose as listed, based on age and weight (kg); repeat dose every 4 hours as needed:

10 kg: 0.031-0.033 mg; maximum: 0.75 mg/24 hours

20 kg: 0.0625 mg; maximum: 0.75 mg/24 hours

40 kg: 0.0938 mg; maximum: 0.75 mg/24 hours

50 kg: 0.125 mg; maximum: 0.75 mg/24 hours

Children >2 years: Preanesthesia: I.V.: Refer to adult dosing.

Administration

Oral: Oral: Tablets should be administered before meals or food.

Levbid®: Tablets are scored and may be broken in half for dose titration; do not crush or chew.

Levsin/SL®: Tablets may be used sublingually, chewed, or swallowed whole.

NuLev™: Tablet is placed on tongue and allowed to disintegrate before swallowing; may take with or without water.

Symax SL: Tablets may be used sublingually or swallowed whole.

I.M.: May be administered without dilution.

I.V.: Inject over at least 1 minute. May be administered without dilution.

Stability

Storage: Store at controlled room temperature. Protect NuLev™ from moisture.

Monitoring and Teaching Issues

Physical Assessment: See Contraindications, Warnings/Precautions, and Dosing for use cautions. Assess potential for interactions with other prescriptions, OTC medications, or herbal products patient may be taking (eg, anything that may add to anticholinergic effects - see Drug Interactions). **I.V./I.M.:** See Administration specifics and have patient void before administration. Assess therapeutic effects and adverse response (eg, excessive dryness - eyes, nose, mouth, throat - see Adverse Reactions and Overdose/Toxicology). Teach patient proper use (according to formulations prescribed), possible side effects and appropriate interventions, and adverse symptoms to report (see Patient Education). **Pregnancy risk factor C** - benefits of use should outweigh possible risks. Breast-feeding is not recommended.

Patient Education: Inform prescriber of all prescriptions, OTC medications, or herbal products you are taking, and any allergies you have. Do not take anything new during treatment unless approved by prescriber. Take as directed before meals; do not increase dose and do not discontinue without consulting prescriber. Void immediately before taking medication. Do not crush or chew (swallow whole) extended release form. Levbid® and Levsinex® may not completely disintegrate and may be excreted. You may experience dizziness or blurred vision (use caution when driving or engaging in tasks that require alertness until response to drug is known); dry mouth (sucking on lozenges may help); photosensitivity (wear dark glasses in bright sunlight); decreased ability to sweat (use caution in hot weather or hot rooms or when engaging in strenuous activity); or impotence (temporary). Report excessive and persistent anticholinergic effects (blurred vision, headache, flushing, tachycardia, nervousness, constipation, dizziness, insomnia, mental confusion or excitement, dry mouth, altered taste perception, dysphagia, palpitations, bradycardia, urinary hesitancy or retention, impotence, decreased sweating). **Pregnancy/breast-feeding precautions:** Inform prescriber if you are or intend to become pregnant. Breast-feeding is not recommended.

Sublingual tablets: Place tablet under tongue and allow to dissolve.

Orally-disintegrating tablet (Nu-Lev™): Place tablet on tongue and allow to disintegrate before swallowing. Take with or without food.

Dietary Issues: Should be taken before meals or food; NuLev™ contains phenylalanine

Geriatric Considerations: Avoid long-term use. The potential for toxic reactions is higher than the potential benefit, elderly are particularly prone to CNS side effects of anticholinergics (eg, confusion, delirium, hallucinations). Side effects often occur before clinical response is obtained. Generally not recommended because of the side effects.

Breast-feeding Issues: Excreted in breast milk in trace amounts. May also suppress lactation. Breast-feeding is not recommended.

Hyoscyamine, Atropine, Scopolamine, and Phenobarbital

(hye oh SYE a meen, A troe peen, skoe POL a meen & fee noe BAR bi tal)

U.S. Brand Names Donnatal® [DSC]

Synonyms Atropine, Hyoscyamine, Scopolamine, and Phenobarbital; Phenobarbital, Hyoscyamine, Atropine, and Scopolamine; Scopolamine, Hyoscyamine, Atropine, and Phenobarbital

(Continued)

Hyoscyamine, Atropine, Scopolamine, and Phenobarbital *(Continued)*

Generic Available No

Pharmacologic Category Anticholinergic Agent; Antispasmodic Agent, Gastrointestinal

Pregnancy Risk Factor C

Lactation Excretion in breast milk unknown/use caution

Use Adjunct in treatment of peptic ulcer disease, irritable bowel, spastic colitis, spastic bladder, and renal colic

Pharmacodynamics/Kinetics

Absorption: Well absorbed

Formulations

Capsule (Donnatal®): Hyoscyamine sulfate 0.1037 mg, atropine sulfate 0.0194 mg, scopolamine hydrobromide 0.0065 mg, and phenobarbital 16.2 mg

Elixir (Donnatal®): Hyoscyamine sulfate 0.1037 mg, atropine sulfate 0.0194 mg, scopolamine hydrobromide 0.0065 mg, and phenobarbital 16.2 mg per 5 mL (120 mL, 480 mL, 4000 mL) [contains alcohol 23%; citrus flavor]

Tablet (Donnatal®): Hyoscyamine sulfate 0.1037 mg, atropine sulfate 0.0194 mg, scopolamine hydrobromide 0.0065 mg, and phenobarbital 16.2 mg

Dosing

Adults & Elderly: Spasmolytic: Oral: 1-2 capsules or tablets 3-4 times/day; or 1 Donnatal® Extentab® in sustained release form every 12 hours; or 5-10 mL elixir 3-4 times/day or every 8 hours

Pediatrics: Oral:

Children 2-12 years: Kinesed® dose: ½ to 1 tablet 3-4 times/day

Children: Donnatal® elixir: 0.1 mL/kg/dose every 4 hours; maximum dose: 5 mL **or** alternatively, dose (mL) based on weight (kg):

4.5 kg: 0.5 mL every 4 hours OR 0.75 mL every 6 hours
10 kg: 1 mL every 4 hours OR 1.5 mL every 6 hours
14 kg: 1.5 mL every 4 hours OR 2 mL every 6 hours
23 kg: 2.5 mL every 4 hours OR 3.8 mL every 6 hours
34 kg: 3.8 mL every 4 hours OR 5 mL every 6 hours
≥45 kg: 5 mL every 4 hours OR 7.5 mL every 6 hours

Monitoring and Teaching Issues

Physical Assessment: See individual components listed in Related Information. **Pregnancy risk factor C** - benefits of use should outweigh possible risks. Note breast-feeding caution.

Patient Education: See individual components listed in Related Information. **Pregnancy/breast-feeding precautions:** Inform prescriber if you are or intend to become pregnant. Consult prescriber if breast-feeding.

Related Information

Atropine *on page 134*
Hyoscyamine *on page 685*
Phenobarbital *on page 1067*
Scopolamine *on page 1218*

Hyoscyamine Sulfate *see* Hyoscyamine *on page 685*
Hyosine *see* Hyoscyamine *on page 685*
Hyperlipidemia Management *see page 1677*
Hypertension *see page 1682*
Hyrexin-50® *see* DiphenhydrAMINE *on page 422*
Hytone® *see* Hydrocortisone *on page 673*
Hytone® *see* Topical Corticosteroids *on page 1334*
Hytrin® *see* Terazosin *on page 1288*
Hytuss® [OTC] *see* Guaifenesin *on page 646*
Hytuss-2X® [OTC] *see* Guaifenesin *on page 646*
Hyzaar® *see* Losartan and Hydrochlorothiazide *on page 826*
Iberet-Folic-500® CR Tablet *see page 1522*
Ibidomide Hydrochloride *see* Labetalol *on page 764*

Ibuprofen (eye byoo PROE fen)

U.S. Brand Names Advil® [OTC]; Advil® Children's [OTC]; Advil® Infants' Concentrated Drops [OTC]; Advil® Junior [OTC]; Advil® Migraine [OTC]; Genpril® [OTC]; Haltran® [OTC]; Ibu-Tab®; I-Prin [OTC]; Menadol® [OTC]; Midol® Maximum Strength Cramp Formula [OTC]; Motrin®; Motrin® Children's [OTC]; Motrin® IB [OTC]; Motrin® Infants' [OTC]; Motrin® Junior Srength [OTC]; Motrin® Migraine Pain [OTC]

Synonyms *p*-Isobutylhydratropic Acid

Generic Available Yes: Caplet, suspension, tablet

Pharmacologic Category Nonsteroidal Anti-inflammatory Drug (NSAID)

Pregnancy Risk Factor B/D (3rd trimester)

Lactation Enters breast milk (minimal)/use caution (AAP rates "compatible")

Use Inflammatory diseases and rheumatoid disorders including juvenile rheumatoid arthritis, mild to moderate pain, fever, dysmenorrhea, gout, ankylosing spondylitis, acute migraine headache

Use - Unlabeled/Investigational Cystic fibrosis

Mechanism of Action/Effect Inhibits prostaglandin synthesis by decreasing the activity of the enzyme, cyclooxygenase, which results in decreased formation of prostaglandin precursors

Contraindications Hypersensitivity to ibuprofen, any component of the formulation, aspirin, or other NSAIDs; patients with "aspirin triad" (bronchial asthma, aspirin intolerance, rhinitis); pregnancy (3rd trimester)

Warnings/Precautions Use with caution in patients with CHF, hypertension, dehydration, decreased renal or hepatic function, history of GI disease (bleeding or ulcers), or those receiving anticoagulants. Elderly are at a high risk for adverse effects from NSAIDs. As many as 60% of elderly can develop peptic ulceration and/or hemorrhage asymptomatically. Fatal asthmatic and anaphylactoid reactions have occurred in patients with "aspirin triad" (see Contraindications).

Use lowest effective dose for shortest period possible. Use of NSAIDs can compromise existing renal function especially when Cl_{cr} is <30 mL/minute. CNS adverse effects such as confusion, agitation, and hallucination are generally seen in overdose or high-dose situations; however, elderly may demonstrate these adverse effects at lower doses than younger adults. Do not exceed 3200 mg/day. Withhold for at least 4-6 half-lives prior to surgical or dental procedures.

Drug Interactions

Cytochrome P450 Effect: Substrate of CYP2C8/9, 2C19; Inhibits CYP2C8/9

Decreased Effect: Aspirin may decrease ibuprofen serum concentrations. Ibuprofen may decrease the effect of some antihypertensive agents (including ACE inhibitors and angiotensin antagonists) and diuretics.

Increased Effect/Toxicity: Ibuprofen may increase cyclosporine, digoxin, lithium, and methotrexate serum concentrations. The renal adverse effects of ACE inhibitors may be potentiated by NSAIDs. Corticosteroids may increase the risk of GI ulceration.

Nutritional/Ethanol Interactions

Ethanol: Avoid ethanol (may enhance gastric mucosal irritation).

Food: Ibuprofen peak serum levels may be decreased if taken with food.

Herb/Nutraceutical: Avoid cat's claw, dong quai, evening primrose, feverfew, garlic, ginger, ginkgo, red clover, horse chestnut, green tea, ginseng (all have additional antiplatelet activity).

Effects on Lab Values ↑ chloride (S), sodium (S), bleeding time

Adverse Reactions

1% to 10%:

- Central nervous system: Headache (1% to 3%), nervousness (<3%), fatigue (<3%)
- Dermatologic: Itching (1% to 3%), rash (3% to 9%), urticaria
- Endocrine & metabolic: Fluid retention
- Gastrointestinal: Dyspepsia (1% to 3%), vomiting (1% to 3%), abdominal pain/cramps/distress (1% to 3%), peptic ulcer, GI bleed, GI perforation, heartburn, nausea (3% to 9%), diarrhea (1% to 3%), constipation (1% to 3%), flatulence (1% to 3%), indigestion (1% to 3%)
- Otic: Tinnitus

<1% (Limited to important or life-threatening): Acute renal failure, agranulocytosis, angioedema, aplastic anemia, arrhythmias, aseptic meningitis with fever and coma, bone marrow depression, CHF, dyspnea, eosinophilia, erythema multiforme, hemolytic anemia, Henoch-Schönlein vasculitis, hepatitis, hypertension, leukopenia, lupus erythematosus syndrome, neutropenia, Stevens-Johnson syndrome, thrombocytopenia, toxic epidermal necrolysis

Overdosage/Toxicology Symptoms of overdose include apnea, metabolic acidosis, coma, nystagmus, seizures, leukocytosis, and renal failure. Management of NSAID intoxication is supportive and symptomatic. Since many NSAIDs undergo enterohepatic cycling, multiple doses of charcoal may be needed to reduce the potential for delayed toxicities.

Pharmacodynamics/Kinetics

Absorption: Oral: Rapid (85%)

Half-Life Elimination: 2-4 hours; End-stage renal disease: Unchanged

Time to Peak: ~1-2 hours

Metabolism: Hepatic via oxidation

Onset: Analgesic: 30-60 minutes; Anti-inflammatory: ≤7 days; Peak effect: 1-2 weeks

Duration: 4-6 hours

Formulations

Caplet: 200 mg [OTC]
- Advil®: 200 mg [contains sodium benzoate]
- Menadol®, Motrin® IB, Motrin® Migraine Pain: 200 mg
- Motrin® Junior Strength: 100 mg [contains tartrazine]

Capsule, liqui-gel:
- Advil®: 200 mg
- Advil® Migraine: 200 mg [solubilized ibuprofen]

Gelcap:
- Advil®: 200 mg
- Motrin® IB: 200 mg [contains benzyl alcohol]

Suspension, oral: 100 mg/5 mL (5 mL, 120 mL, 480 mL)
- Advil® Children's: 100 mg/5 mL (60 mL, 120 mL) [contains sodium benzoate; blue raspberry, fruit, and grape flavors]
- Motrin® Children's: 100 mg/5 mL (60 mL, 120 mL) [contains sodium benzoate; berry, dye-free berry, bubble gum, and grape flavors]

Suspension, oral drops:
- Advil® Infants' Concentrated Drops: 40 mg/mL (15 mL) [contains sodium benzoate; fruit and grape flavors]
- Motrin® Infants': 40 mg/mL (15 mL) [contains sodium benzoate; berry and dye-free berry flavors]

Tablet: 200 mg [OTC], 400 mg, 600 mg, 800 mg
- Advil®: 200 mg [contains sodium benzoate]
- Advil® Junior: 100 mg [contains sodium benzoate; coated tablets]
- Genpril®, Haltran®, I-Prin, Midol® Maximum Strength Cramp Formula, Motrin® IB: 200 mg
- Ibu-Tab®, Motrin®: 400 mg, 600 mg, 800 mg

Tablet, chewable:
- Advil® Children's: 50 mg [contains phenylalanine 2.1 mg; fruit and grape flavors]
- Advil® Junior: 100 mg [contains phenylalanine 2.1 mg; fruit and grape flavors]

(Continued)

Ibuprofen *(Continued)*

Motrin® Children's: 50 mg [contains phenylalanine 1.4 mg; orange flavor]
Motrin® Junior Strength: 100 mg [contains phenylalanine 2.1 mg; grape and orange flavors]

Dosing

Adults & Elderly:

Inflammatory disease: Oral: 400-800 mg/dose 3-4 times/day; maximum: 3.2 g/day

Analgesia/pain/fever/dysmenorrhea: oral: 200-400 mg/dose every 4-6 hours; maximum daily dose: 1.2 g (unless directed by physician)

Pediatrics:

Antipyretic: Oral: 6 months to 12 years: Temperature <102.5°F (39°C): 5 mg/kg/dose; temperature >102.5°F: 10 mg/kg/dose given every 6-8 hours; maximum daily dose: 40 mg/kg/day

Juvenile rheumatoid arthritis: Oral: 30-70 mg/kg/24 hours divided every 6-8 hours
<20 kg: Maximum: 400 mg/day
20-30 kg: Maximum: 600 mg/day
30-40 kg: Maximum: 800 mg/day
>40 kg: Refer to adult dosing.
Start at lower end of dosing range and titrate upward; maximum: 2.4 g/day

Analgesic: Oral: 4-10 mg/kg/dose every 6-8 hours

Hepatic Impairment: Avoid use in severe hepatic impairment.

Administration

Oral: Administer with food.

Monitoring Laboratory Tests CBC, periodic liver function, renal function (serum BUN, and creatinine)

Monitoring and Teaching Issues

Physical Assessment: Assess patient for allergic reaction to salicylates or other NSAIDs (see Contraindications). Assess other medications patient may be taking for additive or adverse interactions (see Warnings/Precautions and Drug Interactions). Monitor therapeutic effectiveness, and signs of adverse reactions or overdose (see Overdose/Toxicology and Adverse Reactions) at beginning of therapy and periodically during long-term therapy. With long-term therapy, periodic ophthalmic exams are recommended. Assess knowledge/teach patient appropriate use. Teach patient to monitor for adverse reactions, adverse reactions to report, and appropriate interventions to reduce side effects. **Pregnancy risk factor B/D** - see Pregnancy Risk Factor for use cautions; benefits of use should outweigh possible risks. Note breast-feeding caution.

Patient Education: If self-administered, use exactly as directed; do not increase dose or frequency. Adverse reactions can occur with overuse. Consult your prescriber before use if you have hypertension or heart failure. Do not take longer than 3 days for fever, or 10 days for pain without consulting medical advisor. Take with food or milk. While using this medication, do not use alcohol, excessive amounts of vitamin C, or salicylate containing foods (curry powder, prunes, raisins, tea, or licorice), other prescription or OTC medications containing aspirin or salicylate, or other NSAIDs without consulting prescriber. Maintain adequate hydration (2-3 L/day of fluids) unless advised by prescriber to restrict fluids. May discolor urine (red/pink). You may experience nausea, vomiting, gastric discomfort (frequent mouth care, small, frequent meals, chewing gum, sucking lozenges may help). GI bleeding, ulceration, or perforation can occur with or without pain. Stop taking medication and report ringing in ears; persistent cramping or stomach pain; unresolved nausea or vomiting; difficulty breathing or shortness of breath; unusual bruising or bleeding (mouth, urine, stool); skin rash; unusual swelling of extremities; chest pain; or palpitations. **Pregnancy/breast-feeding precautions:** Inform prescriber if you are or intend to become pregnant. This drug should not be used in the 3rd trimester of pregnancy. Consult prescriber if breast-feeding.

Dietary Issues: Should be taken with food; sucrose content of 5 mL (suspension): 2.5 g

Geriatric Considerations: Elderly are at a high risk for adverse effects from NSAIDs. As much as 60% of elderly can develop peptic ulceration and/or hemorrhage asymptomatically. The concomitant use of H_2 blockers, omeprazole, and sucralfate is not effective as prophylaxis with the exception of NSAID-induced duodenal ulcers which may be prevented by the use of ranitidine. Misoprostol is the only prophylactic agent proven effective. Also, concomitant disease and drug use contribute to the risk for GI adverse effects. Use lowest effective dose for shortest period possible. Consider renal function decline with age. Use of NSAIDs can compromise existing renal function especially when Cl_{cr} is ≤30 mL/minute. Tinnitus may be a difficult and unreliable indication of toxicity due to age-related hearing loss or eighth cranial nerve damage. CNS adverse effects such as confusion, agitation, and hallucination are generally seen in overdose or high-dose situations, but elderly may demonstrate these adverse effects at lower doses than younger adults.

Breast-feeding Issues: Limited data suggests minimal excretion in breast milk.

Related Information

Nonsalicylate/Nonsteroidal Anti-inflammatory Comparison *on page 1587*

Ibuprofen and Hydrocodone *see* Hydrocodone and Ibuprofen *on page 671*
Ibu-Tab® *see* Ibuprofen *on page 688*

Ibutilide (i BYOO ti lide)

U.S. Brand Names Corvert®

Synonyms Ibutilide Fumarate

Generic Available No

Pharmacologic Category Antiarrhythmic Agent, Class III

Pregnancy Risk Factor C

Lactation Enters breast milk/contraindicated

Use Acute termination of atrial fibrillation or flutter of recent onset; the effectiveness of ibutilide has not been determined in patients with arrhythmias >90 days in duration

Mechanism of Action/Effect Exact mechanism of action is unknown; prolongs the action potential in cardiac tissue

Contraindications Hypersensitivity to ibutilide or any component of the formulation; QT_c >440 msec

Warnings/Precautions Potentially fatal arrhythmias (eg, polymorphic ventricular tachycardia) can occur with ibutilide, **usually** in association with torsade de pointes (QT prolongation). The drug should be given in a setting of continuous EKG monitoring and by personnel trained in treating arrhythmias particularly polymorphic ventricular tachycardia. Patients with chronic atrial fibrillation often revert after conversion; the risks of treatment may not be justified when compared to alternative management. Safety and efficacy in children have not been established. Use caution in elderly patients. Avoid concurrent use of any drug that can prolong QT interval. Correct hyperkalemia and hypomagnesemia before using. Monitor for heart block. Pregnancy risk C.

Drug Interactions

Increased Effect/Toxicity: Class Ia antiarrhythmic drugs (disopyramide, quinidine, and procainamide) and other class III drugs such as amiodarone and sotalol should not be given concomitantly with ibutilide due to their potential to prolong refractoriness. Signs of digoxin toxicity may be masked when coadministered with ibutilide. Toxicity of ibutilide is potentiated by concurrent administration of other drugs which may prolong QT interval: phenothiazines, tricyclic and tetracyclic antidepressants, cisapride, sparfloxacin, gatifloxacin, moxifloxacin, erythromycin, and astemizole.

Adverse Reactions

1% to 10%:

Cardiovascular: Sustained polymorphic ventricular tachycardia (ie, torsade de pointes) (2%, often requiring cardioversion), nonsustained polymorphic ventricular tachycardia (3%), nonsustained monomorphic ventricular tachycardia (5%), ventricular extrasystoles (5%), nonsustained monomorphic VT (5%), tachycardia/supraventricular tachycardia (3%), hypotension (2%), bundle branch block (2%), AV block (2%), bradycardia (1%), QT segment prolongation, hypertension (1%), palpitations (1%)

Central nervous system: Headache (4%)

Gastrointestinal: Nausea (>1%)

<1% (Limited to important or life-threatening): Congestive heart failure, erythematous bullous lesions, idioventricular rhythm, nodal arrhythmia, renal failure, supraventricular extrasystoles, sustained monomorphic ventricular tachycardia, syncope (0.3%, not > placebo)

Overdosage/Toxicology Symptoms of overdose include CNS depression, rapid gasping breathing, and convulsions. Arrhythmias occur. Treatment is supportive. Antiarrhythmics are generally avoided.

Pharmacodynamics/Kinetics

Half-Life Elimination: 2-12 hours (average: 6 hours)

Metabolism: Extensively hepatic; oxidation

Onset: ~90 minutes after start of infusion (1/2 of conversions to sinus rhythm occur during infusion)

Formulations Injection, solution, as fumarate: 0.1 mg/mL (10 mL)

Dosing

Adults: Atrial fibrillation/flutter: I.V.:

<60 kg: 0.01 mg/kg over 10 minutes

≥60 kg: 1 mg over 10 minutes

If the arrhythmia does not terminate within 10 minutes after the end of the initial infusion, a second infusion of equal strength may be infused over a 10-minute period.

Elderly: Refer to adult dosing. Dose selection should be cautious, usually starting at the lower end of the dosing range.

Administration

I.V.: May be administered undiluted or diluted in 50 mL diluent (0.9% NS or D_5W). Infuse over 10 minutes.

Stability

Reconstitution: May be administered undiluted or diluted in 50 mL diluent (0.9% NS or D_5W). Admixtures are chemically and physically stable for 24 hours at room temperature and for 48 hours at refrigerated temperatures.

Monitoring Laboratory Tests Electrolytes

Monitoring and Teaching Issues

Physical Assessment: Assess other medications patient may be taking for effectiveness and interactions (see Drug Interactions). See Warnings/Precautions for use cautions. Requires infusion pump and continuous cardiac and hemodynamic monitoring during and for 4 hours following infusion (see Administration). Monitor laboratory tests (see above), therapeutic response, and adverse reactions (see Warnings/Precautions and Adverse Reactions). Teach patient adverse symptoms to report (see Patient Education). **Pregnancy risk factor C** - benefits of use should outweigh possible risks. Breast-feeding is contraindicated.

Patient Education: This drug is only given I.V. and you will be on continuous cardiac monitoring during and for several hours following administration. You may experience headache or irregular heartbeat during infusion. Report chest pain or difficulty breathing immediately. **Pregnancy/breast-feeding precautions:** Inform prescriber if you are or intend to become pregnant. Do not breast-feed.

Pregnancy Issues: Teratogenic and embryocidal in rats; avoid use in pregnancy.

Related Information

Antiarrhythmic Drugs *on page 1551*

Ibutilide Fumarate *see* Ibutilide *on page 690*

ICI 182,780 *see* Fulvestrant *on page 611*

ICI 204, 219 *see* Zafirlukast *on page 1413*

ICRF-187 *see* Dexrazoxane *on page 389*

Idamycin® [DSC] *see* Idarubicin *on page 692*

Idamycin PFS® *see* Idarubicin *on page 692*

Idarubicin (eye da ROO bi sin)

U.S. Brand Names Idamycin® [DSC]; Idamycin PFS®

Synonyms 4-demethoxydaunorubicin; 4-dmdr; Idarubicin Hydrochloride

Generic Available No

Pharmacologic Category Antineoplastic Agent, Anthracycline

Pregnancy Risk Factor D

Lactation Excretion in breast milk unknown

Use Treatment of acute leukemias (AML, ANLL, ALL), accelerated phase or blast crisis of chronic myelogenous leukemia (CML), breast cancer

Mechanism of Action/Effect Similar to daunorubicin, idarubicin exhibits inhibitory effects on DNA and RNA polymerase.

Contraindications Hypersensitivity to idarubicin, daunorubicin, or any component of the formulation; bilirubin >5 mg/dL; pregnancy

Warnings/Precautions The U.S. Food and Drug Administration (FDA) currently recommends that procedures for proper handling and disposal of antineoplastic agents be considered. Give I.V. slowly into a freely flowing I.V. infusion. Do not give I.M. or S.C.; severe necrosis can result if extravasation occurs. Can cause myocardial toxicity and is more common in patients who have previously received anthracyclines or have pre-existing cardiac disease. Reduce dose in patients with impaired hepatic function. Irreversible myocardial toxicity may occur as total dosage approaches 137.5 mg/m^2. Severe myelosuppression is also possible.

Idarubicin preparation should be performed in a Class II laminar flow biologic safety cabinet. Personnel should be wearing surgical gloves and a closed front surgical gown with knit cuffs. Appropriate safety equipment is recommended for preparation, administration, and disposal of antineoplastics. If idarubicin contacts the skin, wash and flush thoroughly with water.

Drug Interactions

Decreased Effect: Patients may experience impaired immune response to vaccines; possible infection after administration of live vaccines in patients receiving immunosuppressants.

Adverse Reactions

>10%:

Cardiovascular: Transient EKG abnormalities (supraventricular tachycardia, S-T wave changes, atrial or ventricular extrasystoles); generally asymptomatic and self-limiting. Congestive heart failure, dose-related. The relative cardiotoxicity of idarubicin compared to doxorubicin is unclear. Some investigators report no increase in cardiac toxicity at cumulative oral idarubicin doses up to 540 mg/m^2; other reports suggest a maximum cumulative intravenous dose of 150 mg/m^2.

Central nervous system: Headache

Dermatologic: Alopecia (25% to 30%), radiation recall, skin rash (11%), urticaria

Gastrointestinal: Nausea, vomiting (30% to 60%); diarrhea (9% to 22%); stomatitis (11%); GI hemorrhage (30%)

Emetic potential: Moderate (30% to 60%)

Genitourinary: Discoloration of urine (reddish)

Hematologic: Myelosuppression, primarily leukopenia; thrombocytopenia and anemia. Effects are generally less severe with oral dosing.

Nadir: 10-15 days

Recovery: 21-28 days

Hepatic: Elevations of bilirubin and transaminases (44%)

Local: Tissue necrosis upon extravasation, erythematous streaking

Vesicant chemotherapy

1% to 10%:

Central nervous system: Seizures

Neuromuscular & skeletal: Peripheral neuropathy

<1% (Limited to important or life-threatening): Hyperuricemia

Overdosage/Toxicology Symptoms of overdose include severe myelosuppression and increased GI toxicity. Treatment is supportive. It is unlikely that therapeutic efficacy or toxicity would be altered by conventional peritoneal or hemodialysis.

Pharmacodynamics/Kinetics

Half-Life Elimination: I.V.: 12-27 hours

Time to Peak: Serum: ~2-4 hours; varies considerably

Metabolism: Hepatic to idarubicinol (pharmacologically active)

Formulations

Injection, powder for reconstitution, as hydrochloride (Idamycin®): 20 mg [DSC]

Injection, solution, as hydrochloride [preservative free] (Idamycin PFS®): 1 mg/mL (5 mL, 10 mL, 20 mL)

Dosing

Adults & Elderly: Refer to individual protocols.

Leukemia: I.V.:

Induction: 12 mg/m^2/day for 3 days

Consolidation: 10-12 mg/m^2/day for 2 days

Pediatrics:

Leukemia: I.V.: 10-12 mg/m^2 once daily for 3 days every 3 weeks.

Solid tumors: I.V.: 5 mg/m^2 once daily for 3 days every 3 weeks.

Renal Impairment: Dose reduction is recommended.

Serum creatinine ≥2 mg/dL: Reduce dose by 25%.

Hepatic Impairment:

Bilirubin 1.5-5.0 mg/dL or AST 60-180 units: Reduce dose 50%.

Bilirubin >5 mg/dL or AST >180 units: Do not administer.

Administration

I.V.: Vesicant. Administer by intermittent infusion over 10-15 minutes.

Stability

Storage: Store intact vials of lyophilized powder at room temperature and protect from light.

Reconstitution: Dilute powder with NS to a concentration of 1 mg/mL as follows: Solution is stable for 72 hours at room temperature and 7 days under refrigeration.

5 mg = 5 mL

10 mg = 10 mL

Further dilution in D_5W or NS is stable for 4 weeks at room temperature and protected from light.

Standard I.V. dilution:

I.V. push: Dose/syringe (concentration is 1 mg/mL)

Maximum syringe size for IVP is 30 mL syringe and syringe should be ≤75% full.

IVPB: Dose/100 mL D_5W or NS

Syringe and IVPB solutions are stable for 72 hours at room temperature and 7 days under refrigeration.

Compatibility: Stable in D_5NS, D_5W, LR, NS, sterile water for injection; **incompatible** with bacteriostatic water

Y-site administration: Incompatible with acyclovir, allopurinol, ampicillin/sulbactam, cefazolin, cefepime, ceftazidime, clindamycin, dexamethasone sodium phosphate, etoposide, fluorouracil, furosemide, gentamicin, heparin, hydrocortisone sodium succinate, lorazepam, meperidine, methotrexate, piperacillin/tazobactam, sodium bicarbonate, teniposide, vancomycin, vincristine

Compatibility when admixed: Incompatible with heparin

Monitoring Laboratory Tests CBC with differential, platelet count, ECHO, EKG, serum electrolytes, creatinine, uric acid, ALT, AST, bilirubin

Monitoring and Teaching Issues

Physical Assessment: See Contraindications, Warnings/Precautions, and Dosing for use cautions. Assess potential for interactions with other prescriptions, OTC medications, or herbal products patient may be taking (see Drug Interactions). See Administration, Dosing, Reconstitution, and Compatibility for administration specifics. Infusion site must be closely monitored; extravasation can cause severe cellulitis or tissue necrosis (see Administration). Assess therapeutic response, results of laboratory tests (see above), and monitor adverse response (especially cardiac toxicity - see Adverse Reactions and Overdose/Toxicology) prior to each infusion and on a regular basis throughout therapy. Teach patient possible side effects and appropriate interventions and adverse symptoms to report (see Patient Education). **Pregnancy risk factor D** - determine that patient is not pregnant before beginning treatment. Instruct patients of childbearing age about appropriate barrier contraceptive measures. Note breast-feeding caution.

Patient Education: Inform prescriber of all prescriptions, OTC medications, or herbal products you are taking, and any allergies you have. Do not take anything new during treatment unless approved by prescriber. This medication can only be administered I.V. Report immediately any swelling, pain, burning, or redness at infusion site. Avoid alcohol. It is important to maintain adequate hydration (2-3 L/day of fluids) unless advised by prescriber to restrict fluids, and nutrition (small, frequent meals). You will be more susceptible to infection (avoid crowds and exposure to infection and do not have any vaccinations without consulting prescriber). You may experience nausea or vomiting (small, frequent meals, frequent mouth care, sucking lozenges, or chewing gum may help); diarrhea (buttermilk, boiled milk, or yogurt may help); or loss of hair (reversible). Urine may turn red-pink urine (normal). Report immediately chest pain, swelling of extremities, difficulty breathing, palpitations, or rapid heartbeat. Report unresolved nausea, vomiting, or diarrhea; alterations in urinary pattern (increased or decreased); opportunistic infection (eg, fever, chills, unusual bruising or bleeding, signs of infection fatigue, purulent vaginal discharge, unhealed mouth sores); abdominal pain or blood in stools; excessive fatigue; yellowing of eyes or skin; swelling of extremities; difficulty breathing; or unresolved diarrhea. **Pregnancy/breast-feeding precautions:** Do not get pregnant while taking this medication. Consult prescriber for use appropriate contraceptive measures to use during and for 1 month following therapy. Consult prescriber if breast-feeding.

Idarubicin Hydrochloride *see* Idarubicin *on page 692*

Ideal Body Weight Calculation *see page 1531*

Ifex® *see* Ifosfamide *on page 693*

IFLrA *see* Interferon Alfa-2a *on page 717*

Ifosfamide (eye FOSS fa mide)

U.S. Brand Names Ifex®

Generic Available No

Pharmacologic Category Antineoplastic Agent, Alkylating Agent

Pregnancy Risk Factor D

Lactation Enters breast milk/contraindicated

Use Treatment of lung cancer, Hodgkin's and non-Hodgkin's lymphoma, breast cancer, acute and chronic lymphocytic leukemias, ovarian cancer, sarcomas, pancreatic and gastric carcinomas

Orphan drug: Treatment of testicular cancer

Mechanism of Action/Effect Inhibits protein synthesis and DNA synthesis; an analogue of cyclophosphamide, and like cyclophosphamide, it undergoes activation by microsomal enzymes in the liver. Ifosfamide is metabolized to active compounds, ifosfamide mustard, and acrolein.

Contraindications Hypersensitivity to ifosfamide or any component of the formulation; patients with severely depressed bone marrow function; pregnancy

Warnings/Precautions The U.S. Food and Drug Administration (FDA) currently recommends that procedures for proper handling and disposal of antineoplastic agents be considered. Used in combination with mesna as a prophylactic agent to protect against hemorrhagic cystitis. Use with caution in patients with impaired renal function or those with compromised

(Continued)

Ifosfamide *(Continued)*

bone marrow reserve. May require therapy cessation if confusion or coma occurs; carcinogenic in rats.

Preparation of ifosfamide should be performed in a Class II laminar flow biologic safety cabinet. Personnel should be wearing surgical gloves and a closed front surgical gown with knit cuffs. Appropriate safety equipment is recommended for preparation, administration, and disposal of antineoplastics. If ifosfamide contacts the skin, wash and flush thoroughly with water.

Drug Interactions

Cytochrome P450 Effect: Substrate of CYP2A6, **2B6, 2C8/9, 2C19, 3A4**; Induces CYP2C8/9

Increased Effect/Toxicity: Activation by microsomal enzymes may be enhanced during therapy with enzyme inducers such as phenobarbital, carbamazepine, and phenytoin.

Nutritional/Ethanol Interactions Herb/Nutraceutical: St John's wort may decrease ifosfamide levels.

Adverse Reactions

>10%:

Central nervous system: Somnolence, confusion, hallucinations (12%)
Dermatologic: Alopecia (75% to 100%)
Endocrine & metabolic: Metabolic acidosis (31%)
Gastrointestinal: Nausea and vomiting (58%), may be more common with higher doses or bolus infusions; constipation
Genitourinary: Hemorrhagic cystitis (40% to 50%), patients should be vigorously hydrated (at least 2 L/day) and receive mesna
Hematologic: Myelosuppression, leukopenia (65% to 100%), thrombocytopenia (10%) - dose-related
Onset: 7-14 days
Nadir: 21-28 days
Recovery: 21-28 days
Renal: Hematuria (6% to 92%)

1% to 10%:

Central nervous system: Hallucinations, depressive psychoses, polyneuropathy
Dermatologic: Dermatitis, nail banding/ridging, hyperpigmentation
Endocrine & metabolic: SIADH, sterility, elevated transaminases (3%)
Hematologic: Anemia
Local: Phlebitis
Renal: Increased creatinine/BUN (6%)
Respiratory: Nasal stuffiness

<1% (Limited to important or life-threatening): Acute tubular necrosis, anorexia, cardiotoxicity, diarrhea, pulmonary fibrosis, stomatitis

Overdosage/Toxicology Symptoms of overdose include myelosuppression, nausea, vomiting, diarrhea, and alopecia; direct extensions of the drug's pharmacologic effect. Treatment is supportive.

Pharmacokinetic Note Pharmacokinetics are dose dependent.

Pharmacodynamics/Kinetics

Half-Life Elimination: Beta: High dose: 11-15 hours (3800-5000 mg/m^2); Lower dose: 4-7 hours (1800 mg/m^2)

Time to Peak: Plasma: Oral: Within 1 hour

Metabolism: Hepatic to active metabolites; requires biotransformation before it can act as an alkylating agent; metabolite acrolein is the toxic agent implicated in development of hemorrhagic cystitis

Formulations Injection, powder for reconstitution: 1 g, 3 g [packaged with Mesnex® (mesna) 1 g]

Dosing

Adults & Elderly: Refer to individual protocols.

Antineoplastic: I.V.:
50 mg/kg/day or 700-2000 mg/m^2 for 5 days every 3-4 weeks
Alternatives: 2400 mg/m^2/day for 3 days or 5000 mg/m^2 as a single dose every 3-4 weeks

Note: To prevent bladder toxicity, ifosfamide should be given with extensive hydration consisting of at least 2 L of oral or I.V. fluid per day. The dose-limiting toxicity is hemorrhagic cystitis and, therefore, ifosfamide should be used in conjunction with a uroprotective agent, such as mesna.

Pediatrics: Refer to individual protocols.

Antineoplastic: I.V.:
1200-1800 mg/m^2/day for 3-5 days every 21-28 days **or**
5 g/m^2 once every 21-28 days **or**
3 g/m^2/day for 2 days every 21-28 days
See note in adult dosing.

Renal Impairment:

Cl_{cr} 10-50 mL/minute: Administer 75% of normal dose.
Cl_{cr} <10 mL/minute: Administer 50% of normal dose.

Hepatic Impairment: Although no specific guidelines are available, it is possible that adjusted doses are indicated in hepatic disease. One study (Falkson G, Hunt M, Borden EC, et al, "An Extended Phase II Trial of Ifosfamide Plus Mesna in Malignant Mesothelioma," *Invest New Drugs*, 1992, 10:337-43) recommended the following dosage adjustments: AST >300 or bilirubin >3.0 mg/dL: Decrease ifosfamide dose by 75%.

Administration

I.V.: Administer slow I.V. push, IVPB over 30 minutes or continuous intravenous infusion over 5 days. Mesna should be administered concomitantly (20% of the ifosfamide dose 15 minutes before, 4 hours after and 8 hours after ifosfamide administration).

Stability

Storage: Store intact vials at room temperature or under refrigeration. Syringe and IVPB are stable for 7 days at room temperature and 6 weeks under refrigeration.

Reconstitution: Dilute powder with SWI or NS to a concentration of 50 mg/mL as follows. Incompatible with bacteriostatic SWI or NS. Solution is stable for 7 days at room temperature and 3 weeks under refrigeration.

1 g vial = 20 mL

3 g vial = 60 mL

Further dilution in NS, D_5W or LR is stable for 7 days at room temperature

Compatible with mesna in NS for up to 9 days at room temperature.

Standard I.V. dilution:

I.V. push: Dose/syringe (concentration = 50 mg/mL)

Maximum syringe size for IVP is a 30 mL syringe and syringe should be ≤75% full

IVPB: Dose/100-1000 mL D_5W or NS

Compatibility: Incompatible with bacteriostatic SWI or bacteriostatic NS. Stable in D_5LR, D_5NS, D_5W, LR, ½NS, NS

Y-site administration: Incompatible Cefepime, methotrexate

Compatibility in syringe: Incompatible with mesna with epirubicin

Compatibility when admixed: Incompatible with mesna with epirubicin

Monitoring Laboratory Tests CBC with differential, platelet count, urinalysis, liver and renal function

Monitoring and Teaching Issues

Physical Assessment: See Warnings/Precautions, Contraindications, and Dosing for extensive use cautions. Assess potential for interactions with other prescriptions, OTC medications, or herbal products patient may be taking (eg, increased nephrotoxicity - see Drug Interactions). **I.V.:** See Administration and Compatibility information. Maintain adequate hydration for 72 hours prior to infusion to minimize risk of hemorrhagic cystitis (2-3 L/day) unless advised by prescriber to restrict fluids. Premedicate with antiemetic prior to each infusion. Infusion site should be monitored closely prevent extravasation. Assess results of laboratory tests (see above), therapeutic effectiveness (according to purpose for use), and adverse response (see Adverse Reactions and Overdose/Toxicology) prior to each infusion and regularly during therapy. Teach patient (or caregiver) possible side effects and appropriate interventions (eg, importance of adequate hydration) and adverse symptoms to report (see Patient Education). **Pregnancy risk factor D** - determine that patient is not pregnant before beginning treatment. Instruct patients of childbearing age about use of appropriate barrier contraceptive measures during therapy and for 1 month following therapy. Breast-feeding contraindicated.

Patient Education: Inform prescriber of all prescriptions, OTC medications, or herbal products you are taking, and any allergies you have. Do not take anything new during treatment unless approved by prescriber. This drug can only be administered by infusion. Report immediately any swelling, redness, or pain at infusion site. Maintain adequate hydration (3-4 L/day of fluids unless instructed to restrict fluid intake) for at least 3 days prior to infusion and each day of therapy. You will be more susceptible to infection (avoid crowds and exposure to infection and do not have any vaccinations without consulting prescriber). May cause loss of hair (reversible, although regrowth hair may be different color or texture); fertility or amenorrhea; nausea or vomiting (small, frequent meals, good mouth care, chewing gum, or sucking lozenges may help - if persistent consult prescriber for antiemetic); headache (consult prescriber for analgesic); or mouth sores (use soft toothbrush or cotton swab for oral care). Report any difficulty or pain with urination; chest pain, rapid heartbeat, or palpitations; CNS changes (eg, hallucinations, confusion, somnolence); unusual rash; persistent nausea or vomiting; swelling of extremities; difficulty breathing; unusual fatigue; or opportunistic infection (eg, fever, chills, easy bruising or unusual bleeding). **Pregnancy/breast-feeding precautions:** Inform prescriber if you are pregnant. Do not get pregnant during or for 1 month following therapy. Male: Do not cause a female to become pregnant. Male/female: Consult prescriber for instruction on appropriate contraceptive measures. This drug may cause severe fetal defects. Do not breast-feed.

Related Information

Mesna *on page 860*

IL-2 *see* Aldesleukin *on page 54*

Ilotycin® *see page 1509*

Imatinib (eye MAT eh nib)

U.S. Brand Names Gleevec™

Synonyms CGP 57148B; Glivec; Imatinib Mesylate; STI571

Generic Available No

Pharmacologic Category Antineoplastic, Tyrosine Kinase Inhibitor

Pregnancy Risk Factor D

Lactation Excretion in breast milk unknown/not recommended

Use Treatment of patients with chronic myeloid leukemia (CML) in blast crisis, accelerated phase, or in chronic phase after failure of interferon-alpha therapy; treatment of Kit-positive (CD117) unresectable and/or (metastatic) malignant gastrointestinal stromal tumors (GIST)

Use - Unlabeled/Investigational Philadelphia chromosome-positive leukemias

Mechanism of Action/Effect Inhibits a specific enzyme (Bcr-Abl tyrosine kinase) produced by the Philadelphia chromosome found in many patients with chronic myeloid leukemia (CML). Inhibition of this enzyme blocks proliferation and induces cell death in leukemic cells. Also inhibits tyrosine kinase for platelet-derived growth factor (SCF), c-kit, and events mediated by PDGF and SCF.

Contraindications Hypersensitivity to imatinib or any component of the formulation; pregnancy

Warnings/Precautions Often associated with fluid retention, weight gain, and edema; occasionally leading to significant complications, including pleural effusion, pericardial effusion, pulmonary edema, and ascites. Use caution in patients where fluid accumulation may be

(Continued)

Imatinib *(Continued)*

poorly tolerated, such as in cardiovascular disease (CHF or hypertension) and pulmonary disease. Use with caution in renal impairment, hematologic impairment, or hepatic disease. May cause GI irritation, hematologic toxicity (neutropenia, or thrombocytopenia), or hepatotoxicity. Hepatotoxic reactions may be severe. Has been associated with development of opportunistic infections. Use with caution in patients receiving concurrent therapy with drugs which alter cytochrome P450 activity or require metabolism by these isoenzymes. Safety and efficacy in patients <18 years of age have not been established.

Drug Interactions

Cytochrome P450 Effect: Substrate of CYP1A2, 2D6, 2C8/9, 2C19, **3A4**, Inhibits CYP2C8/9, 2D6, **3A4**

Decreased Effect: Metabolism of imatinib may be increased by CYP3A4 enzyme inducers, decreasing its therapeutic effect. An interaction has been established with phenytoin; other potential inducers include phenobarbital, carbamazepine, rifampin, and rifabutin.

Increased Effect/Toxicity: Note: Drug interaction data is limited. Few clinical studies have been conducted. Many interactions listed below are derived by extrapolation from *in vitro* inhibition of cytochrome P450 isoenzymes.

Acetaminophen: Chronic use may increase potential for hepatotoxic reaction with imatinib (case report of hepatic failure with concurrent therapy).

Due to potent CYP3A4 inhibition, imatinib should not be used with cisapride, pimozide, thioridazine, and/or mesoridazine, may result in potential life-threatening toxicities. Imatinib may also inhibit the metabolism of benzodiazepines (alprazolam, diazepam, and triazolam), some beta-blockers, carbamazepine, carvedilol, clozapine, dextromethorphan, haloperidol, HMG-CoA reductase inhibitors (except pravastatin and fluvastatin), immunosuppressants (cyclosporine, sirolimus, and tacrolimus), methadone, nefazodone, phenothiazines (thioridazine and mesoridazine should be avoided), phenytoin, propafenone, quinidine, sibutramine, sildenafil, tramadol, SSRIs, tricyclic antidepressants, trazodone, vinca alkaloids (vincristine, vinblastine), and warfarin. Increased toxicity leading to liver failure has been reported with regular concomitant acetaminophen use (case report).

Serum concentrations and/or toxicity of imatinib may be increased by drugs which inhibit CYP3A4. Established with ketoconazole; other inhibitors include amiodarone, cimetidine, clarithromycin, delavirdine, diltiazem, dirithromycin, disulfiram, erythromycin, fluoxetine, fluvoxamine, grapefruit juice, indinavir, itraconazole, nefazodone, nevirapine, propoxyphene, quinupristin-dalfopristin, ritonavir, saquinavir, verapamil, zafirlukast, and zileuton.

Nutritional/Ethanol Interactions

Ethanol: Avoid ethanol.

Food: Food may reduce gastrointestinal irritation.

Herb/Nutraceutical: Avoid St John's wort (may increase metabolism and decrease imatinib plasma concentration).

Adverse Reactions Adverse effect profile is based on limited data, established in patients with a wide variation in level of illness. Patients in blast crisis or accelerated disease reported a higher frequency of symptoms. In many cases, other medications were used concurrently.

>10%:

Cardiovascular: Fluid retention (superficial, 51% to 66%; other 2% to 16%)

Central nervous system: Headache (24% to 28%, severe <1% to 4%), fatigue (24% to 33%, severe <1% to 3%), fever (14% to 38%)

Dermatologic: Rash (32% to 39%, severe 3% to 4%)

Endocrine & metabolic: Hypokalemia (2% to 12%)

Gastrointestinal: Nausea (55% to 68%), diarrhea (33% to 49%, severe <1% to 4%), vomiting (28% to 54%, severe <1% to 3%), dyspepsia (9% to 19%), abdominal pain (20% to 26%), constipation (4% to 13%), weight gain (4% to 14%), anorexia (3% to 14%)

Hematologic: Hematologic toxicity (neutropenia, thrombocytopenia, anemia) is common (higher in blast crisis or accelerated phase in CML, up to 30% to 46%) and may require dosage adjustment, interruption, or discontinuation of therapy

Neuromuscular & skeletal: Muscle cramps (25% to 46%, severe <1%), musculoskeletal pain (27% to 39%, severe 1% to 8%), arthralgia (21% to 26%), myalgia (7% to 18%)

Respiratory: Cough (9% to 22%), dyspnea (5% to 16%), epistaxis (3% to 12%)

Miscellaneous: Night sweats (8% to 10%)

1% to 10%:

Cardiovascular: Edema (severe 1% to 5%; includes pleural effusion, pulmonary edema, pericardial effusion, anasarca, and ascites)

Central nervous system: CNS hemorrhage (<1% to 4%)

Dermatologic: Pruritus (6% to 10%), petechiae (<1% to 10%)

Gastrointestinal: Gastrointestinal hemorrhage (<1% to 5%), intratumoral hemorrhage

Hepatic: Hepatotoxicity (1% to 4%); elevated transaminases, bilirubin, and alkaline phosphatase

Neuromuscular & skeletal: Weakness (5% to 10%)

Renal: Increased serum creatinine

Respiratory: Nasopharyngitis (5% to 10%), pneumonia (1% to 10%)

Miscellaneous: Tumor lysis syndrome

Overdosage/Toxicology Experience with overdose is limited (>800 mg/day). Hematologic adverse effects are more common at dosages >750 mg/day. Treatment is symptomatic and supportive.

Pharmacodynamics/Kinetics

Bioavailability: 98%

Half-Life Elimination: Parent drug: 18 hours; N-demethyl metabolite: 40 hours

Time to Peak: 2-4 hours

Metabolism: Hepatic via CYP3A4 (minor metabolism via CYP1A2, CYP2D6, CYP2C9, CYP2C19); primary metabolite (active): N-demethylated piperazine derivative

Formulations Capsule, as mesylate: 100 mg

Dosing

Adults & Elderly: Note: Dose should be taken with food and large glass of water:

Chronic myeloid leukemia (CML): Oral:

Chronic phase: 400 mg once daily; may be increased to 600 mg daily in the event of disease progression, loss of previously achieved response, or failure to achieve response after at least 3 months of therapy (in absence of toxic effects)

Accelerated phase or blast crisis: 600 mg once daily; may be increased to 800 mg daily (400 mg twice daily) in the event of disease progression, loss of previously achieved response, or failure to achieve response after at least 3 months of therapy (in absence of toxic effects)

Gastrointestinal stromal tumors: 400-600 mg/day

Dosage adjustment for hepatotoxicity or other nonhematologic adverse reactions:

Withhold therapy for any severe nonhematologic event (severe hepatotoxicity or severe fluid retention). May resume treatment, as appropriate, following resolution of acute event, depending on the initial severity of the event.

If elevations of bilirubin >3 times upper limit of normal (ULN) or transaminases (ALT/AST) >5 times ULN occur, withhold until bilirubin <1.5 times ULN or transaminases <2.5 times ULN. Resume treatment at reduced dose (if initial dose 400 mg/day, reduce to 300 mg/day, if initial dose 600 mg/day then reduce to 400 mg/day).

Dosage adjustment for hematologic adverse reactions:

Chronic phase (initial dose 400 mg/day): If ANC $<1.0 \times 10^9$/L and/or platelets $<50 \times 10^9$/L: Discontinue until ANC $\geq 1.5 \times 10^9$/L and platelets $\geq 75 \times 10^9$/L, resume treatment at 400 mg/day; if depression in neutrophils or platelets recurs, withhold until recovery (as above), and re-institute treatment at 300 mg/day

Accelerated phase or blast crisis (initial dose 600 mg/day): If ANC $<0.5 \times 10^9$/L and/or platelets $<10 \times 10^9$/L: Check to establish whether cytopenia is related to leukemia (bone marrow aspirate). If unrelated to leukemia, reduce dose of imatinib to 400 mg daily. If cytopenia persists for an additional 2 weeks, further reduce dose to 300 mg/day. If cytopenia persists for 4 weeks and is still unrelated to leukemia, stop treatment until ANC $\geq 1.0 \times 10^9$/L and platelets $\geq 20 \times 10^9$/L, resume treatment at 300 mg/day.

Hepatic Impairment: Withhold therapy for any severe nonhematologic event (severe hepatotoxicity or severe fluid retention). May resume treatment, as appropriate, following resolution of acute event, depending on the initial severity of the event. If elevations of bilirubin >3 times upper limit of normal (ULN) or transaminases (ALT/AST) >5 times ULN occur, withhold until bilirubin <1.5 times ULN or transaminases <2.5 times ULN. Resume treatment at reduced dose (if initial dose 400 mg/day, reduce to 300 mg/day; if initial dose 600 mg/day then reduce to 400 mg/day).

Administration

Oral: Should be administered with food and a large glass of water; vigorous hydration and administration of allopurinol are recommended.

Stability

Storage: Store at 25°C (77°F); excursions permitted to 15°C to 30°C (59°F to 86°F).

Monitoring Laboratory Tests CBC (weekly for first month, biweekly for second month, then periodically thereafter), liver function tests (at baseline and monthly or as clinically indicated), and renal function.

Monitoring and Teaching Issues

Physical Assessment: Monitor closely any other medication patient may be taking for effectiveness and possible interactions prior to beginning therapy (especially those drugs affected by cytochrome P450 actions - see Drug Interactions). See Warnings/Precautions and Dosing for use cautions. Monitor laboratory results (see Monitoring Lab Tests), therapeutic response, and adverse reactions (see Adverse Reactions) at beginning of therapy and periodically during therapy. Monitor weight and fluid status on a regular basis. Teach appropriate use, interventions to reduce side effects, and symptoms to report (see Patient Educations). **Pregnancy risk factor D** - determine that patient is not pregnant before beginning treatment. Instruct patients of childbearing age about appropriate barrier contraceptive measures. Breast-feeding is not recommended.

Patient Education: Take exactly as directed; do not alter or discontinue dose without consulting prescriber. Take with food or a large glass of water. Avoid alcohol, chronic use of acetaminophen or aspirin, OTC or prescription medications, or herbal products unless approved by prescriber. Maintain adequate hydration (2-3 L/day of fluids) unless advised by prescriber to restrict fluids. You will be required to have regularly scheduled laboratory tests while on this medication. You will be more susceptible to infection (avoid crowds and exposure to infection and do not receive any vaccination unless approved by prescriber). You may experience headache or fatigue (use caution when driving or engaging in tasks requiring alertness until response to drug in known); loss of appetite, nausea, vomiting, or mouth sores (small, frequent meals, frequent mouth care, chewing gum, or sucking lozenges may help); constipation (increased exercise, fluids, fruit, or fiber may help); or diarrhea (buttermilk, boiled milk, or yogurt may reduce diarrhea). Report chest pain, palpitations, or swelling of extremities; cough, difficulty breathing, or wheezing; weight gain >5 lb; skin rash; muscle or bone pain, tremors, or cramping; persistent fatigue or weakness; easy bruising or unusual bleeding (eg, tarry stools, blood in vomitus, stool, urine, or mouth); persistent GI problems or pain; or other adverse effects. **Pregnancy/breast-feeding precautions:** Inform prescriber if you are pregnant. Do not get pregnant. Use appropriate contraception while on this medication. Breast-feeding is not recommended.

Dietary Issues: Should be taken with food and a large glass of water to decrease gastrointestinal irritation.

Geriatric Considerations: Incidence of edema and edema-related adverse effects is increased in elderly patients.

Additional Information Median time to hematologic response was one month; only short-term studies have been completed. Follow-up is insufficient to estimate duration of cytogenic response.

Imatinib Mesylate *see* Imatinib *on page 695*

Imdur® *see* Isosorbide Mononitrate *on page 750*
Imidazole Carboxamide *see* Dacarbazine *on page 353*
Imipemide *see* Imipenem and Cilastatin *on page 698*

Imipenem and Cilastatin (i mi PEN em & sye la STAT in)

U.S. Brand Names Primaxin®
Synonyms Imipemide
Generic Available No
Pharmacologic Category Antibiotic, Carbapenem
Pregnancy Risk Factor C
Lactation Enters breast milk (small amounts)/use caution
Use Treatment of respiratory tract, urinary tract, intra-abdominal, gynecologic, bone and joint, skin structure, and polymicrobic infections as well as bacterial septicemia and endocarditis. Antibacterial activity includes resistant gram-negative bacilli (*Pseudomonas aeruginosa* and *Enterobacter* sp), gram-positive bacteria (methicillin-sensitive *Staphylococcus aureus* and *Streptococcus* sp) and anaerobes.

Note: I.M. administration is not intended for severe or life-threatening infections (eg, septicemia, endocarditis, shock)

Mechanism of Action/Effect A carbapenem with broad-spectrum antibacterial activity including resistant gram-negative bacilli (*Pseudomonas aeruginosa* and *Enterococcus* sp), gram-positive bacteria (methicillin-sensitive *Staphylococcus aureus* and *Enterococcus* sp) and anaerobes; inhibits cell wall synthesis; cilastatin prevents renal metabolism of imipenem
Contraindications Hypersensitivity to imipenem/cilastatin or any component of the formulation; consult information on Lidocaine for contraindications associated with I.M. dosing
Warnings/Precautions Dosage adjustment is required in patients with impaired renal function. Prolonged use may result in superinfection. Has been associated with CNS adverse events. Use with caution in patients with a history of seizures or hypersensitivity to beta-lactams. Elderly patients often require lower doses (adjust carefully to renal function). Refer to Lidocaine monograph for warnings/precautions associated with I.M. dosing. Pregnancy risk C.
Drug Interactions

Increased Effect/Toxicity: Beta-lactam antibiotics and probenecid may increase potential for toxicity.

Effects on Lab Values Interferes with urinary glucose determination using Clinitest®
Adverse Reactions

1% to 10%:
- Gastrointestinal: Nausea/diarrhea/vomiting (1% to 2%)
- Local: Phlebitis (3%), pain at I.M. injection site (1%)

<1% (Limited to important or life-threatening): Anaphylaxis, angioneurotic edema, confusion (acute), drug fever, dyspnea, emergence of resistant strains of *P. aeruginosa*, encephalopathy, eosinophilia, erythema multiforme, hallucinations, hemolytic anemia, hemorrhagic colitis, hepatitis, hypersensitivity, hypotension, increased PT, jaundice, leukopenia, neutropenia (including agranulocytosis), pancytopenia, paresthesia, positive Coombs' test, pruritus, pseudomembranous colitis, psychic disturbances, rash, renal failure (acute), seizures, somnolence, Stevens-Johnson syndrome, thrombocytopenia, toxic epidermal necrolysis, urticaria, vertigo

Overdosage/Toxicology Symptoms of overdose include neuromuscular hypersensitivity and seizures. Hemodialysis may be helpful to aid in removal of the drug from blood; otherwise, treatment is supportive or symptom-directed.
Pharmacodynamics/Kinetics

Absorption: I.M.: Imipenem: 60% to 75%; cilastatin: 95% to 100%
Half-Life Elimination: Both drugs: 60 minutes; prolonged with renal impairment
Metabolism: Renally by dehydropeptidase; activity is blocked by cilastatin; cilastatin is partially metabolized renally

Formulations

Injection, powder for reconstitution [I.M.]: Imipenem 500 mg and cilastatin 500 mg
Injection, powder for reconstitution [I.V.]: Imipenem 250 mg and cilastatin 250 mg; imipenem 500 mg and cilastatin 500 mg

Dosing

Adults & Elderly: Dosage based on **imipenem** content:
- Mild infections:
  - I.M.: 500 mg every 12 hours; intra-abdominal infections: 750 mg every 12 hours
  - I.V.:
    - Fully-susceptible organisms: 250 mg every 6 hours (1g/day)
    - Moderately-susceptible organisms: 500 mg every 6 hours (2 g/day)
- Moderate infections:
  - I.M.: 750 mg every 12 hours
  - I.V.:
    - Fully-susceptible organisms: 500 mg every 6-8 hours (1.5-2 g/day)
    - Moderately-susceptible organisms: 500 mg every 6 hours or 1 g every 8 hours (2-3 g/day)
- Severe infections: I.V.: **Note:** I.M. administration is not intended for severe or life-threatening infections (eg, septicemia, endocarditis, shock):
  - Fully-susceptible organisms: 500 mg every 6 hours (2 g/day)
  - Moderately-susceptible organisms: 1 g every 6-8 hours (3-4 g/day)
  - Maximum daily dose should not exceed 50 mg/kg or 4 g/day, whichever is lower
- Urinary tract infection, uncomplicated: I.V.: 250 mg every 6 hours (1 g/day)
- Urinary tract infection, complicated: I.V.: 500 mg every 6 hours (2 g/day)

Pediatrics: Dosage based on **imipenem** content:
- Non-CNS infections: I.V.:
  - Neonates:
    - <1 week: 25 mg/kg every 12 hours
    - 1-4 weeks: 25 mg/kg every 8 hours

4 weeks to 3 months: 25 mg/kg every 6 hours

Children: >3 months: 15-25 mg/kg every 6 hours

Maximum dosage: Susceptible infections: 2 g/day; moderately susceptible organisms: 4 g/day

Cystic fibrosis: I.V.: Children: Doses up to 90 mg/kg/day have been used

Renal Impairment: I.V.: **Note:** Adjustments have not been established for I.M. dosing:

Patients with a Cl_{cr} <5 mL/minute/1.73 m^2 should not receive imipenem/cilastatin unless hemodialysis is instituted within 48 hours.

Patients weighing <30 kg with impaired renal function should not receive imipenem/cilastatin.

Hemodialysis: Use the dosing recommendation for patients with a Cl_{cr} 6-20 mL/minute.

Peritoneal dialysis: Dose as for Cl_{cr} <10 mL/minute.

Continuous arteriovenous or venovenous hemofiltration: Dose as for Cl_{cr} 20-30 mL/minute; monitor for seizure activity. Imipenem is well removed by CAVH but cilastatin is not; removes 20 mg of imipenem per liter of filtrate per day.

See table.

Imipenem and Cilastatin Dosage in Renal Impairment

Reduced I.V. Dosage Regimen Based on Creatinine Clearance (mL/minute/1.73 m^2) and Body Weight (kg)					
	Body Weight (kg)				
	≥70	60	50	40	30
Total daily dose for normal renal function: 1 g/day					
Cl_{cr} ≥71	250 mg q6h	250 mg q8h	125 mg q6h	125 mg q6h	125 mg q8h
Cl_{cr} 41-70	250 mg q8h	125 mg q6h	125 mg q6h	125 mg q8h	125 mg q8h
Cl_{cr} 21-40	250 mg q12h	250 mg q12h	125 mg q8h	125 mg q12h	125 mg q12h
Cl_{cr} 6-20	250 mg q12h	125 mg q12h	125 mg q12h	125 mg q12h	125 mg q12h
Total daily dose for normal renal function: 1.5 g/day					
Cl_{cr} ≥71	500 mg q8h	250 mg q6h	250 mg q6h	250 mg q8h	125 mg q6h
Cl_{cr} 41-70	250 mg q6h	250 mg q8h	250 mg q8h	125 mg q6h	125 mg q8h
Cl_{cr} 21-40	250 mg q8h	250 mg q8h	250 mg q12h	125 mg q8h	125 mg q8h
Cl_{cr} 6-20	250 mg q12h	250 mg q12h	250 mg q12h	125 mg q12h	125 mg q12h
Total daily dose for normal renal function: 2 g/day					
Cl_{cr} ≥71	500 mg q6h	500 mg q8h	250 mg q6h	250 mg q6h	250 mg q8h
Cl_{cr} 41-70	500 mg q8h	250 mg q6h	250 mg q6h	250 mg q8h	125 mg q6h
Cl_{cr} 21-40	250 mg q6h	250 mg q8h	250 mg q8h	250 mg q12h	125 mg q8h
Cl_{cr} 6-20	250 mg q12h	250 mg q12h	250 mg q12h	250 mg q12h	125 mg q12h
Total daily dose for normal renal function: 3 g/day					
Cl_{cr} ≥71	1000 mg q8h	750 mg q8h	500 mg q6h	500 mg q8h	250 mg q6h
Cl_{cr} 41-70	500 mg q6h	500 mg q8h	500 mg q8h	250 mg q6h	250 mg q8h
Cl_{cr} 21-40	500 mg q8h	500 mg q8h	250 mg q6h	250 mg q8h	250 mg q8h
Cl_{cr} 6-20	500 mg q12h	500 mg q12h	250 mg q12h	250 mg q12h	250 mg q12h
Total daily dose for normal renal function: 4 g/day					
Cl_{cr} ≥71	1000 mg q6h	1000 mg q8h	750 mg q8h	500 mg q6h	500 mg q8h
Cl_{cr} 41-70	750 mg q8h	750 mg q8h	500 mg q6h	500 mg q8h	250 mg q6h
Cl_{cr} 21-40	500 mg q6h	500 mg q8h	500 mg q8h	250 mg q6h	250 mg q8h
Cl_{cr} 6-20	500 mg q12h	500 mg q12h	500 mg q12h	250 mg q12h	250 mg q12h

Administration

I.M.: Prepare 500 mg vial with 2 mL 1% lidocaine; prepare 750 mg vial with 3 mL 1% lidocaine **(do not use lidocaine with epinephrine)**. Administer by deep injection into a large muscle (gluteal or lateral thigh). Aspiration is necessary to avoid inadvertent injection into a blood vessel.

I.V.: Do not administer I.V. push. Final concentration should not exceed 5 mg/mL. Infuse over 30-60 minutes.

Stability

Storage: Imipenem/cilastatin powder for injection should be stored at <30°C.

Reconstitution: All IVPB should be prepared fresh. Do not use dextrose as a diluent due to limited stability. Reconstituted solutions are stable 10 hours at room temperature and 48 hours at refrigeration (4°C) with NS. If reconstituted with 5% or 10% dextrose injection, 5% dextrose and sodium bicarbonate, 5% dextrose and 0.9% sodium chloride, is stable for 4 hours at room temperature and 24 hours when refrigerated. Imipenem is inactivated at acidic or alkaline pH.

Standard diluent: 500 mg/100 mL NS; 1 g/250 mL NS

Compatibility: Y-site administration: Incompatible with allopurinol, amphotericin B cholesteryl sulfate complex, etoposide phosphate, fluconazole, gemcitabine, lorazepam, meperidine, midazolam, sargramostim, sodium bicarbonate

Monitoring Laboratory Tests Perform culture and sensitivity studies prior to initiating therapy. Periodically monitor renal, hepatic, and hematologic function.

(Continued)

Imipenem and Cilastatin *(Continued)*

Monitoring and Teaching Issues

Physical Assessment: See Contraindications, Warnings/Precautions, and Dosing for use cautions. See Administration and Reconstitution. Patient should be monitored for renal, hepatic, hematologic and CNS status. Assess results of laboratory tests (see above), therapeutic effects, and adverse response (see Adverse Reactions and Overdose/Toxicology) periodically during therapy. Note caution about glucose monitoring (interferes with urinary glucose determination using Clinitest®). Teach patient possible side effects and appropriate interventions and adverse symptoms to report (see Patient Education). **Pregnancy risk factor C** - benefits of use should outweigh possible risks. Note breast-feeding caution.

Patient Education: Inform prescriber of all prescriptions, OTC medications, or herbal products you are taking, and any allergies you have. Do not take anything new during treatment unless approved by prescriber. This medication can only be administered by injection or infusion. Report immediately any warmth, swelling, pain, or redness at infusion or injection site. Maintain adequate hydration (2-3 L/day of fluids) unless advised by prescriber to restrict fluids, and nutrition (small, frequent meals). If diabetic, drug may cause false test results with Clinitest® urine glucose monitoring; use of another type of glucose monitoring is preferable. Report immediately any CNS changes (dizziness, hallucinations, anxiety, visual disturbances); swelling of throat, tongue, lips, or face; chills or fever; or unusual discharge or foul-smelling urine. **Pregnancy/breast-feeding precautions:** Inform prescriber if you are or intend to become pregnant. Consult prescriber if breast-feeding.

Dietary Issues: Sodium content of 1 g injection:

I.M.: 64.4 mg (2.8 mEq)

I.V.: 73.6 mg (3.2 mEq)

Geriatric Considerations: Many of the seizures attributed to imipenem/cilastatin were in elderly patients. Dose must be carefully adjusted for creatinine clearance.

Imipramine (im IP ra meen)

U.S. Brand Names Tofranil®; Tofranil-PM®

Synonyms Imipramine Hydrochloride; Imipramine Pamoate

Generic Available Yes: Tablet

Pharmacologic Category Antidepressant, Tricyclic (Tertiary Amine)

Pregnancy Risk Factor D

Lactation Enters breast milk/not recommended (AAP rates "of concern")

Use Treatment of various forms of depression

Use - Unlabeled/Investigational Enuresis in children; analgesic for certain chronic and neuropathic pain; panic disorder; attention-deficit/hyperactivity disorder (ADHD)

Mechanism of Action/Effect Traditionally believed to increase the synaptic concentration of serotonin and/or norepinephrine in the central nervous system by inhibition of their reuptake by the presynaptic neuronal membrane. However, additional receptor effects have been found including desensitization of adenyl cyclase, down regulation of beta-adrenergic receptors, and down regulation of serotonin receptors.

Contraindications Hypersensitivity to imipramine (cross-reactivity with other dibenzodiazepines may occur) or any component of the formulation; concurrent use of MAO inhibitors (within 14 days); in a patient during acute recovery phase of MI; pregnancy

Warnings/Precautions May cause drowsiness/sedation, resulting in impaired performance of tasks requiring alertness (ie, operating machinery or driving). Sedative effects may be additive with other CNS depressants and/or ethanol. May worsen psychosis in some patients or precipitate a shift to mania or hypomania in patients with bipolar disease. May cause hyponatremia/SIADH. May increase the risks associated with electroconvulsive therapy. Discontinue, when possible, prior to elective surgery. Therapy should not be abruptly discontinued in patients receiving high doses for prolonged periods.

Use with caution in patients at risk of hypotension (high risk of orthostasis) or in patients where transient hypotensive episodes would be poorly tolerated (cardiovascular disease or cerebrovascular disease). Use with caution in elderly patients, patients with diabetes, thyroid disease (or patients receiving thyroid supplements), hepatic dysfunction, renal dysfunction, urinary retention, benign prostatic hyperplasia, narrow-angle glaucoma, xerostomia, visual problems, constipation, or a history of bowel obstruction.

Use caution in patients with depression, particularly if suicidal risk may be present. Use with caution in patients with a history of cardiovascular disease (including previous MI, stroke, tachycardia, or conduction abnormalities). Use caution in patients with a previous seizure disorder or condition predisposing to seizures such as brain damage, alcoholism, or concurrent therapy with other drugs which lower the seizure threshold. Has been associated with photosensitization.

Drug Interactions

Cytochrome P450 Effect: Substrate of CYP1A2, 2B6, **2C19, 2D6**, 3A4; Inhibits CYP1A2, 2C19, 2D6, 2E1

Decreased Effect: Carbamazepine, phenobarbital, and rifampin may increase the metabolism of imipramine resulting in decreased effect of imipramine. Imipramine inhibits the antihypertensive response to bethanidine, clonidine, debrisoquin, guanadrel, guanethidine, guanabenz, and guanfacine. Cholestyramine and colestipol may bind TCAs and reduce their absorption; monitor for altered response.

Increased Effect/Toxicity: Imipramine increases the effects of amphetamines, anticholinergics, other CNS depressants (sedatives, hypnotics, or ethanol), chlorpropamide, tolazamide, and warfarin. When used with MAO inhibitors, hyperpyrexia, hypertension, tachycardia, confusion, seizures, and **deaths have been reported** (serotonin syndrome). Serotonin syndrome has also been reported with ritonavir (rare). The SSRIs (to varying degrees), cimetidine, grapefruit juice, indinavir, methylphenidate, ritonavir, quinidine, diltiazem, and verapamil inhibit the metabolism of TCAs and clinical toxicity may result. Use of lithium with a TCA may increase the risk for neurotoxicity. Phenothiazines may increase concentration of some TCAs and TCAs may increase concentration of phenothiazines. Pressor response to I.V. epinephrine, norepinephrine, and phenylephrine may be enhanced in patients receiving TCAs (**Note:** Effect is unlikely with epinephrine or levonordefrin dosages typically administered as infiltration in combination with local anesthetics). Combined use of beta-agonists or drugs which prolong QT_c (including quinidine, procainamide, disopyramide, cisapride, sparfloxacin, gatifloxacin, moxifloxacin) with TCAs may predispose patients to cardiac arrhythmias.

Nutritional/Ethanol Interactions

Ethanol: Avoid ethanol (may increase CNS depression).

Food: Grapefruit juice may inhibit the metabolism of some TCAs and clinical toxicity may result.

Herb/Nutraceutical: St John's wort may decrease imipramine levels. Avoid valerian, St John's wort, SAMe, kava kava (may increase risk of serotonin syndrome and/or excessive sedation).

Effects on Lab Values ↑ glucose

Adverse Reactions Frequency not defined.

Cardiovascular: Orthostatic hypotension, arrhythmias, tachycardia, hypertension, palpitations, myocardial infarction, heart block, EKG changes, CHF, stroke

Central nervous system: Dizziness, drowsiness, headache, agitation, insomnia, nightmares, hypomania, psychosis, fatigue, confusion, hallucinations, disorientation, delusions, anxiety, restlessness, seizures

Endocrine & metabolic: Gynecomastia, breast enlargement, galactorrhea, increase or decrease in libido, increase or decrease in blood sugar, SIADH

Gastrointestinal: Nausea, unpleasant taste, weight gain/loss, xerostomia, constipation, ileus, stomatitis, abdominal cramps, vomiting, anorexia, epigastric disorders, diarrhea, black tongue

Genitourinary: Urinary retention, impotence

Neuromuscular & skeletal: Weakness, numbness, tingling, paresthesias, incoordination, ataxia, tremor, peripheral neuropathy, extrapyramidal symptoms

Ocular: Blurred vision, disturbances of accommodation, mydriasis

Otic: Tinnitus

Miscellaneous: Diaphoresis

<1% (Limited to important or life-threatening): Agranulocytosis, alopecia, cholestatic jaundice, eosinophilia, increased liver enzymes, itching, petechiae, photosensitivity, purpura, rash, thrombocytopenia, urticaria

Overdosage/Toxicology Symptoms of overdose include confusion, hallucinations, constipation, cyanosis, tachycardia, urinary retention, ventricular tachycardia, and seizures. Following initiation of essential overdose management, toxic symptoms should be treated. Ventricular arrhythmias often respond to concurrent systemic alkalinization (sodium bicarbonate 0.5-2 mEq/kg I.V.) Physostigmine (1-2 mg I.V. slowly for adults) may be indicated to reverse life-threatening cardiac arrhythmias.

Pharmacodynamics/Kinetics

Absorption: Well absorbed

Half-Life Elimination: 6-18 hours

Metabolism: Hepatic via CYP to desipramine (active) and other metabolites; significant first-pass effect

Onset: Peak antidepressant effect: Usually after ≥2 weeks

Formulations

Capsule, as pamoate (Tofranil-PM®): 75 mg, 100 mg, 125 mg, 150 mg

Tablet, as hydrochloride (Tofranil®): 10 mg, 25 mg, 50 mg [generic tablets may contain sodium benzoate]

Dosing

Adults: Antidepressant:

Oral: Initial: 25 mg 3-4 times/day; increase dose gradually, total dose may be given at bedtime; maximum: 300 mg/day.

Note: Maximum antidepressant effect may not be seen for 2 or more weeks after initiation of therapy.

Elderly: Initial dose: 10-25 mg at bedtime; increase by 10-25 mg every 3 days for inpatients and weekly for outpatients if tolerated. Average daily dose to achieve a therapeutic concentration: 100 mg/day; range: 50-150 mg/day.

Pediatrics:

Depression: Oral:

Children: 1.5 mg/kg/day with dosage increments of 1 mg/kg every 3-4

Adolescents: Oral: Initial: 25-50 mg/day; increase gradually; maximum: 100 mg/day in single or divided doses. days to a maximum dose of 5 mg/kg/day in 1-4 divided doses; monitor carefully especially with doses ≥3.5 mg/kg/day.

Enuresis: Oral: Children ≥6 years: Initial: 10-25 mg at bedtime, if inadequate response still seen after 1 week of therapy, increase by 25 mg/day; dose should not exceed 2.5 mg/kg/day or 50 mg at bedtime if 6-12 years of age or 75 mg at bedtime if ≥12 years of age.

Adjunct in the treatment of cancer pain: Oral: Initial: 0.2-0.4 mg/kg at bedtime; dose may be increased by 50% every 2-3 days up to 1-3 mg/kg/dose at bedtime.

Monitoring Laboratory Tests EKG, CBC

Monitoring and Teaching Issues

Physical Assessment: Assess other medications patient may be taking for effectiveness and interactions (see Drug Interactions). See Contraindications and Warnings/Precautions for use cautions. Monitor laboratory tests, therapeutic response, and adverse reactions at beginning of therapy and periodically with long-term use (see Adverse Reactions and Overdose/Toxicology). Taper dosage slowly when discontinuing (allow 3-4 weeks between discontinuing Tofranil® and starting another antidepressant). Assess knowledge/teach patient appropriate use, interventions to reduce side effects, and adverse symptoms to report (see Patient Education). **Pregnancy risk factor D** - determine that patient is not pregnant before beginning treatment. Instruct patients of childbearing age about appropriate barrier contraceptive measures. Breast-feeding is not recommended.

(Continued)

Imipramine *(Continued)*

Patient Education: Take exactly as directed; do not increase dose or frequency. It may take 2-3 weeks to achieve desired results. Take in the evening. Avoid alcohol, caffeine, and other prescription or OTC medications not approved by prescriber. Maintain adequate hydration (2-3 L/day of fluids) unless advised by prescriber to restrict fluids. You may experience drowsiness, lightheadedness, impaired coordination, dizziness, or blurred vision (use caution when driving or engaging in tasks requiring alertness until response to drug is known); nausea, vomiting, altered taste, dry mouth (small, frequent meals, frequent mouth care, chewing gum, or sucking lozenges may help); constipation (increased exercise, fluids, fruit, or fiber may help); diarrhea (buttermilk, yogurt, or boiled milk may help); postural hypotension (use caution when climbing stairs or changing position from lying or sitting to standing); or urinary retention (void before taking medication). Report persistent insomnia; muscle cramping or tremors; chest pain, palpitations, rapid heartbeat, swelling of extremities, or severe dizziness; unresolved urinary retention; rash or skin irritation; yellowing of eyes or skin; pale stools/dark urine; or worsening of condition. **Pregnancy/breast-feeding precautions:** Do not get pregnant while taking this medication; use appropriate barrier contraceptive measures. Breast-feeding is not recommended.

Geriatric Considerations: Orthostatic hypotension is a concern with this agent, especially in patients taking other medications that may affect blood pressure. May precipitate arrhythmias in predisposed patients; may aggravate seizures. A less anticholinergic antidepressant may be a better choice. Data from a clinical trial comparing fluoxetine to tricyclics suggests that fluoxetine is significantly less effective than nortriptyline in hospitalized elderly patients with unipolar major affective disorder, especially those with melancholia and concurrent cardiovascular diseases.

Related Information

Antidepressant Agents *on page 1553*
Antidepressant Medication Guidelines *on page 1613*
Peak and Trough Guidelines *on page 1544*
Pharmacotherapy of Urinary Incontinence *on page 1699*

Imipramine Hydrochloride *see* Imipramine *on page 700*

Imipramine Pamoate *see* Imipramine *on page 700*

Imiquimod (i mi KWI mod)

U.S. Brand Names Aldara™

Generic Available No

Pharmacologic Category Skin and Mucous Membrane Agent; Topical Skin Product

Pregnancy Risk Factor B

Lactation Excretion in breast milk unknown/consult prescriber

Use Treatment of external genital and perianal warts/condyloma acuminata in children ≥12 years of age and adults

Mechanism of Action/Effect Mechanism of action is unknown; however, induces cytokines, including interferon-alfa and others

Contraindications Hypersensitivity to imiquimod or any component of the formulation

Warnings/Precautions Imiquimod has not been evaluated for the treatment of urethral, intravaginal, cervical, rectal, or intra-anal human papilloma viral disease and is not recommended for these conditions. Topical imiquimod is not intended for ophthalmic use. Topical imiquimod administration is not recommended until genital/perianal tissue is healed from any previous drug or surgical treatment. Imiquimod has the potential to exacerbate inflammatory conditions of the skin. Safety and efficacy in patients <12 years of age have not been established.

Drug Interactions

Cytochrome P450 Effect: Substrate of CYP1A2, 3A4

Adverse Reactions

>10%: Local, mild/moderate: Erythema (54% to 61%), itching (22% to 32%), erosion (21% to 32%), burning (9% to 26%), excoriation/flaking (18% to 25%), edema (12% to 17%), scabbing (9% to 13%)

1% to 10%:

- Central nervous system: Pain (2% to 8%), headache (4% to 5%)
- Local, severe: Erythema (4%), erosion (1%), edema (1%)
- Local, mild/moderate: Pain, induration, ulceration (5% to 7%), vesicles (2% to 3%), soreness (<1% to 3%)
- Neuromuscular & skeletal: Myalgia (1%)
- Miscellaneous: Influenza-like symptoms (1% to 3%), fungal infections (2% to 11%)

Overdosage/Toxicology Overdosage is unlikely because of minimal percutaneous absorption. Persistent topical overdosing of imiquimod could result in severe local skin reactions. The most clinically serious adverse event reported following multiple oral imiquimod doses of ≥200 mg was hypotension that resolved following oral or I.V. fluid administration. Treat symptomatically

Pharmacodynamics/Kinetics

Absorption: Minimal

Formulations Cream: 5% (12s) [contains benzyl alcohol; single-dose packets]

Dosing

Adults & Elderly: Perianal warts/condyloma acuminata: Topical: Apply 3 times/week on alternative days prior to normal sleeping hours and leave on the skin for 6-10 hours. Following treatment period, remove cream by washing the treated area with mild soap and water. Continue imiquimod treatment until there is total clearance of the genital/perianal warts for ≤16 weeks. A rest period of several days may be taken if required by the patient's discomfort or severity of the local skin reaction. Treatment may resume once the reaction subsides.

Pediatrics: Children ≥12 years: Refer to adult dosing.

Administration

Topical: Nonocclusive dressings such as cotton gauze or cotton underwear may be used in the management of skin reactions. Handwashing before and after cream application is recommended. Imiquimod is packaged in single-use packets that contain sufficient cream to cover a wart area of up to 20 cm^2; avoid use of excessive amounts of cream. Instruct patients to apply imiquimod to external or perianal warts; not for vaginal use. Apply a thin layer to the wart area and rub in until the cream is no longer visible. Do not occlude the application site.

Stability

Storage: Do not store at <25°C (7°F); avoid freezing.

Monitoring and Teaching Issues

Physical Assessment: See Warnings/Precautions and Dosing for use cautions. Teach patient appropriate use, possible side effects and appropriate interventions, and adverse symptoms to report (see Patient Education). **Pregnancy risk factor B** - this medication may weaken condoms and vaginal diaphragms; advice patient on appropriate forms of protection. Note breast-feeding caution.

Patient Education: This medication will not eliminate nor prevent the transmission of the virus. For external use only; avoid contact with eyes, mouth, or vagina. Use only as frequently as directed and apply as instructed. May cause pain, itching, redness, burning, flaking, swelling, or scabbing in treated area. If these effects persist or become severe or open sores develop, stop treatment and notify prescriber. Prescriber may recommend a rest period of several days before resuming treatment. **Pregnancy/breast-feeding precautions:** This medication may weaken condoms or vaginal diaphragms; consult prescriber for appropriate forms of protection. Inform prescriber if you are or intend to become pregnant. Consult prescriber if breast-feeding.

Apply treatment just prior to sleeping and leave on 6-10 hours. Wash hands thoroughly before and after application. Wash and dry area to be treated before applying cream. After treatment period, remove cream with mild soap and water. Apply a thin layer to external warts and rub in until cream is no longer visible. Avoid use of excessive cream. May cover area with light gauze dressing or cotton underwear; do not apply occlusive dressing.

Imitrex® *see* Sumatriptan Succinate *on page 1267*

Immune Globulin, Intramuscular *see page 1498*

Immune Globulin (Intravenous) (i MYUN GLOB yoo lin IN tra VEE nus)

U.S. Brand Names Carimune™; Gamimune® N; Gammagard® S/D; Gammar®-P I.V.; Iveegam EN; Panglobulin®; Polygam® S/D; Venoglobulin®-S

Synonyms IVIG

Generic Available No

Pharmacologic Category Immune Globulin

Pregnancy Risk Factor C

Lactation Excretion in breast milk unknown

Use

Treatment of primary immunodeficiency syndromes (congenital agammaglobulinemia, severe combined immunodeficiency syndromes [SCIDS], common variable immunodeficiency, X-linked immunodeficiency, Wiskott-Aldrich syndrome); idiopathic thrombocytopenic purpura (ITP); Kawasaki disease (in combination with aspirin)

Prevention of bacterial infection in B-cell chronic lymphocytic leukemia (CLL); pediatric HIV infection; bone marrow transplant (BMT)

Use - Unlabeled/Investigational Autoimmune diseases (myasthenia gravis, SLE, bullous pemphigoid, severe rheumatoid arthritis), Guillain-Barré syndrome; used in conjunction with appropriate anti-infective therapy to prevent or modify acute bacterial or viral infections in patients with iatrogenically-induced or disease-associated immunodepression; autoimmune hemolytic anemia or neutropenia, refractory dermatomyositis/polymyositis

Mechanism of Action/Effect Replacement therapy for primary and secondary immunodeficiencies; interference with F_c receptors on the cells of the reticuloendothelial system for autoimmune cytopenias and ITP; possible role of contained antiviral-type antibodies

Contraindications Hypersensitivity to immune globulin or any component of the formulation; selective IgA deficiency

Warnings/Precautions Anaphylactic hypersensitivity reactions can occur, especially in IgA-deficient patients; studies indicate that the currently available products have no discernible risk of transmitting HIV or hepatitis B; aseptic meningitis may occur with high doses (≥2 g/kg). Use with caution in the elderly, patients with renal disease, diabetes mellitus, volume depletion, sepsis, paraproteinemia, and nephrotoxic medications due to risk of renal dysfunction. Patients should be adequately hydrated prior to therapy. Acute renal dysfunction (increased serum creatinine, oliguria, acute renal failure) can rarely occur; usually within 7 days of use (more likely with products stabilized with sucrose). Use caution in patients with a history of thrombotic events or cardiovascular disease; there is clinical evidence of a possible association between thrombotic events and administration of intravenous immune globulin. For intravenous administration only. Pregnancy risk C.

Drug Interactions

Decreased Effect: Decreased effect of live virus vaccines (measles, mumps, rubella); separate administration by at least 3 months

Adverse Reactions Frequency not defined.

Cardiovascular: Flushing of the face, tachycardia, hypertension, hypotension, chest tightness, angioedema, lightheadedness, chest pain, myocardial infarction, CHF, pulmonary embolism

Central nervous system: Anxiety, chills, dizziness, drowsiness, fatigue, fever, headache, irritability, lethargy, malaise, aseptic meningitis syndrome

Dermatologic: Pruritus, rash, urticaria

Gastrointestinal: Abdominal cramps, nausea, vomiting

Hematologic: Autoimmune hemolytic anemia, mild hemolysis

(Continued)

Immune Globulin (Intravenous) *(Continued)*

Local: Pain or irritation at the infusion site

Neuromuscular & skeletal: Arthralgia, back or hip pain, myalgia, nuchal rigidity

Ocular: Photophobia, painful eye movements

Renal: Acute renal failure, acute tubular necrosis, anuria, BUN elevated, creatinine elevated, nephrotic syndrome, oliguria, proximal tubular nephropathy, osmotic nephrosis

Respiratory: Dyspnea, wheezing, infusion-related lung injury

Miscellaneous: Diaphoresis, hypersensitivity reactions, anaphylaxis

Pharmacodynamics/Kinetics

Half-Life Elimination: IgG (variable among patients): Healthy subjects: 14-24 days; Patients with congenital humoral immunodeficiencies: 26-35 days; hypermetabolism associated with fever and infection have coincided with a shortened half-life

Onset: I.V.: Provides immediate antibody levels

Duration: Immune effects: 3-4 weeks (variable)

Formulations

Injection, solution [preservative free; solvent detergent-treated]:

Gamimune® N: 10% [100 mg/mL] (10 mL, 50 mL, 100 mL, 200 mL)

Venoglobulin® S: 5% [50 mg/mL] (50 mL, 100 mL, 200 mL); 10% [100 mg/mL] (50 mL, 100 mL, 200 mL) [stabilized with human albumin]

Injection, powder for reconstitution [preservative free]:

Carimune™, Panglobulin®: 1 g, 3 g, 6 g, 12 g

Gammar®-P I.V.: 1 g, 2.5 g, 5 g, 10 g [stabilized with human albumin and sucrose]

Iveegam EN: 0.5 g, 1 g, 2.5 g, 5 g [stabilized with glucose]

Injection, powder for reconstitution [preservative free, solvent detergent treated] (Gammagard® S/D): 2.5 g, 5 g, 10 g [stabilized with human albumin, glycine, glucose, and polyethylene glycol]

Dosing

Adults & Elderly: Approved doses and regimens may vary between brands; check manufacturer guidelines. **Note:** Some clinicians dose IVIG on ideal body weight or an adjusted ideal body weight in morbidly obese patients. The volume of distribution of IVIG preparations in healthy subjects is similar to that observed with endogenous IgG. IVIG remains primarily in the intravascular space. Patients with congenital humoral immunodeficiencies appear to have about 70% of the IVIG available in the intravascular space.

Primary immunodeficiency disorders: I.V.: 200-400 mg/kg every 4 weeks or as per monitored serum IgG concentrations

B-cell chronic lymphocytic leukemia (CLL): I.V.: 400 mg/kg/dose every 3 weeks

Idiopathic thrombocytopenic purpura (ITP): I.V.:

Acute: 400 mg/kg/day for 5 days or 1000 mg/kg/day for 1-2 days

Chronic: 400 mg/kg as needed to maintain platelet count >30,000/mm^3; may increase dose to 800 mg/kg (1000 mg/kg if needed)

Kawasaki disease: Initiate therapy within 10 days of disease onset: I.V.: 2 g/kg as a single dose administered over 10 hours, or 400 mg/kg/day for 4 days. **Note:** Must be used in combination with aspirin: 80-100 mg/kg/day in 4 divided doses for 14 days; when fever subsides, dose aspirin at 3-5 mg/kg once daily for ≥6-8 weeks

Acquired immunodeficiency syndrome (patients must be symptomatic) (unlabeled use): I.V.:

200-250 mg/kg/dose every 2 weeks

400-500 mg/kg/dose every month or every 4 weeks

Autoimmune hemolytic anemia and neutropenia (unlabeled use): I.V.: 1000 mg/kg/dose for 2-3 days

Autoimmune diseases (unlabeled use): I.V.: 400 mg/kg/day for 4 days

Bone marrow transplant: I.V.: 500 mg/kg beginning on days 7 and 2 pretransplant, then 500 mg/kg/week for 90 days post-transplant

Adjuvant to severe cytomegalovirus infections (unlabeled use): I.V.: 500 mg/kg/dose every other day for 7 doses

Guillain-Barré syndrome (unlabeled use): I.V.:

400 mg/kg/day for 4 days

1000 mg/kg/day for 2 days

2000 mg/kg/day for one day

Refractory dermatomyositis (unlabeled use): I.V.: 2 g/kg/dose every month x 3-4 doses

Refractory polymyositis (unlabeled use): I.V.: 1 g/kg/day x 2 days every month x 4 doses

Chronic inflammatory demyelinating polyneuropathy (unlabeled use): I.V.:

400 mg/kg/day for 5 doses once each month

800 mg/kg/day for 3 doses once each month

1000 mg/kg/day for 2 days once each month

Pediatrics: Approved doses and regimens may vary between brands; check manufacturer guidelines. **Note:** Some clinicians dose IVIG on ideal body weight or an adjusted ideal body weight in morbidly obese patients. The volume of distribution of IVIG preparations in healthy subjects is similar to that observed with endogenous IgG. IVIG remains primarily in the intravascular space. Patients with congenital humoral immunodeficiencies appear to have about 70% of the IVIG available in the intravascular space.

Pediatric HIV: I.V.: 400 mg/kg every 28 days

Severe systemic viral and bacterial infections: Children: I.V.: 500-1000 mg/kg/week

Prevention of gastroenteritis: Infants and Children: Oral: 50 mg/kg/day divided every 6 hours

For additional indications, refer to adult dosing.

Renal Impairment: Cl_{cr} <10 mL/minute: Avoid use.

Administration

I.V.: For I.V. use only. For initial treatment, a lower concentration and/or a slower rate of infusion should be used.

Stability

Storage: Stability and dilution is dependent upon the manufacturer and brand; do not freeze:

Gamimune® N, Iveegam EN: Store at 2°C to 8°C (35°F to 46°F).

Gammar® P I.V.,Gammagard® S/D, Polygam® S/D, Venoglobulin®-S: Store below 25°C (77°F).

Panglobulin®, Sandoglobulin®: Store at room temperature, below 30°C (86°F).

Reconstitution: Dilution is dependent upon the manufacturer and brand; do not shake, avoid foaming; discard unused portion:

Iveegam EN: Reconstitute with sterile water for injection; use immediately after reconstitution

Gammagard® S/D, Polygam® S/D: Reconstitute with sterile water for injection; when diluted aseptically in a sterile laminar air flow hood, may store diluted solution under refrigeration for up to 24 hours. If reconstituted outside of laminar flow hood, use within 2 hours

Panglobulin®, Sandoglobulin®: Reconstitute with NS, D_5W or sterile water for injection; when diluted aseptically in a sterile laminar flow hood, may store diluted solution under refrigeration for up to 24 hours.

Gammar®-P I.V.: Reconstitute with sterile water for injection.

Compatibility: Stable in D_5W, $D_{15}W$, $D_5{}^1/_4NS$

Monitoring and Teaching Issues

Physical Assessment: Assess for history of previous allergic reactions (see Contraindications). See Administration for safe infusion. Patient should be monitored during infusion for vital sign changes and adverse or allergic reactions (see Adverse Reactions). Teach patient adverse symptoms to report (see Patient Education). **Pregnancy risk factor C** - benefits of use should outweigh possible risks. Note breast-feeding caution.

Patient Education: This medication can only be administered by infusion. You will be monitored closely during the infusion. If you experience nausea ask for assistance, do not get up alone. Do not have any vaccinations for the next 3 months without consulting prescriber. Immediately report chills; chest pain, tightness, or rapid heartbeat; acute back pain; or difficulty breathing. **Pregnancy/breast-feeding precautions:** Inform prescriber if you are or intend to become pregnant. Consult prescriber if breast-feeding.

Additional Information

Intravenous Immune Globulin Product Comparison:

Gamimune®N:

FDA indication: Primary immunodeficiency, ITP
Contraindication: IgA deficiency
IgA content: 270 mcg/mL
Adverse reactions (%): 5.2
Plasma source: >2000 paid donors
Half-life: 21 days
IgG subclass (%):
IgG_1 (60-70): 60
IgG_2 (19-31): 29.4
IgG_3 (5-8.4): 6.5
IgG_4 (0.7-4): 4.1
Monomers (%): >95
Gamma globulin (%): >98
Storage: Refrigerate
Recommendations for **initial** infusion rate: 0.01-0.02 mL/kg/minute
Maximum infusion rate: 0.08 mL/kg/minute
Maximum concentration for infusion (%):10

Gammagard®SD:

FDA indication: Primary immunodeficiency, ITP, CLL prophylaxis
Contraindication: None (caution with IgA deficiency)
IgA content: 0.92-1.6 mcg/mL
Adverse reactions (%): 6
Plasma source: 4000-5000 paid donors
Half-life: 24 days
IgG subclass (%):
IgG_1 (60-70): 67 (66.8)*
IgG_2 (19-31): 25 (25.4)
IgG_3 (5-8.4): 5 (7.4)
IgG_4 (0.7-4): 3 (0.3)
Monomers (%): >95
Gamma globulin (%): >90
Storage: Room temperature
Recommendations for **initial** infusion rate: 0.5 mL/kg/hour
Maximum infusion rate: 4 mL/kg/hour
Maximum concentration for infusion (%): 5

Gammar®-P I.V.:

FDA indication: Primary immunodeficiency
Contraindication: IgA deficiency
IgA content: <20 mcg/mL
Adverse reactions (%): 15
Plasma source: >8000 paid donors
Half-life: 21-24 days
IgG subclass (%):
IgG_1 (60-70): 69
IgG_2 (19-31): 23
IgG_3 (5-8.4): 6
IgG_4 (0.7-4): 2
Monomers (%): >98
Gamma globulin (%): >98

(Continued)

Immune Globulin (Intravenous) *(Continued)*

Storage: Room temperature
Recommendations for **initial** infusion rate: 0.01-0.02 mL/kg/minute
Maximum infusion rate: 0.06 mL/kg/minute
Maximum concentration for infusion (%): 5

Polygram®:
FDA indication: Primary immunodeficiency, ITP, CLL
Contraindication: None (caution with IgA deficiency)
IgA content: 0.74 ± 0.33 mcg/mL
Adverse reactions (%): 6
Plasma source: 50,000 voluntary donors
Half-life: 21-25 days
IgG subclass (%):
IgG_1 (60-70): 67
IgG_2 (19-31): 25
IgG_3 (5-8.4): 5
IgG_4 (0.7-4): 3
Monomers (%): >95
Gamma globulin (%): >90
Storage: Room temperature
Recommendations for **initial** infusion rate: 0.5 mL/kg/hour
Maximum infusion rate: 4 mL/kg/hour
Maximum concentration for infusion (%): 10

Sandoglobulin®:
FDA indication: Primary immunodeficiency, ITP
Contraindication: IgA deficiency
IgA content: 720 mcg/mL
Adverse reactions (%): 2.5-6.6
Plasma source: 8000-15,000 voluntary donors
Half-life: 21-23 days
IgG subclass (%):
IgG_1 (60-70): 60.5 (55.3)*
IgG_2 (19-31): 30.2 (35.7)
IgG_3 (5-8.4): 6.6 (6.3)
IgG_4 (0.7-4): 2.6 (2.6)
Monomers (%): >92
Gamma globulin (%): >96
Storage: Room temperature
Recommendations for **initial** infusion rate: 0.01-0.03 mL/kg/minute
Maximum infusion rate: 2.5 mL/minute
Maximum concentration for infusion (%): 12

Venoglobulin®-I:
FDA indication: Primary immunodeficiency, ITP
Contraindication: IgA deficiency
IgA content: 20-24 mcg/mL
Adverse reactions (%): 6
Plasma source: 6000-9000 paid donors
Half-life: 29 days
IgG subclass (%):
IgG_1 (60-70): 62.3**
IgG_2 (19-31): 32.8
IgG_3 (5-8.4): 2.9
IgG_4 (0.7-4): 2
Monomers (%): >98
Gamma globulin (%): >98
Storage: Room temperature
Recommendations for **initial** infusion rate: 0.01-0.02 mL/kg/minute
Maximum infusion rate: 0.04 mL/kg/minute
Maximum concentration for infusion (%):10

*Skvaril F and Gardi A, "Differences Among Available Immunoglobulin Preparations for Intravenous Use," *Pediatr Infect Dis J*, 1988, 7:543-48.

**Roomer J, Morgenthaler JJ, Scherz R, et al, "Characterization of Various Immunoglobulin Preparations for Intravenous Application," *Vox Sang*, 1982, 42:62-73.

Immunization Recommendations *see page 1481*
Immunizations (Vaccines) *see page 1498*
Imodium® A-D [OTC] *see* Loperamide *on page 815*
Imogam® *see page 1498*
Imovax® Rabies ID Vaccine *see page 1498*
Imovax® Rabies Vaccine *see page 1498*
Imuran® *see* Azathioprine *on page 138*
Inamrinone *see page 1580*
I-Naphline® *see page 1509*
Inapsine® *see* Droperidol *on page 453*

Indapamide (in DAP a mide)

U.S. Brand Names Lozol®
Generic Available Yes
Pharmacologic Category Diuretic, Thiazide-Related
Pregnancy Risk Factor B (manufacturer); D (expert analysis)
Lactation Excretion in breast milk unknown

Use Management of mild to moderate hypertension; treatment of edema in congestive heart failure and nephrotic syndrome

Mechanism of Action/Effect Enhances sodium, chloride, and water excretion by interfering with the transport of sodium ions across the renal tubular epithelium

Contraindications Hypersensitivity to indapamide or any component of the formulation, thiazides, or sulfonamide-derived drugs; anuria; renal decompensation; pregnancy (based on expert analysis)

Warnings/Precautions Use with caution in severe renal disease. Use with caution in severe hepatic dysfunction; hepatic encephalopathy can be caused by electrolyte disturbances. Gout may be precipitated in patients with a history of gout, a familial predisposition to gout, or chronic renal failure. Use caution in patients with diabetes; may alter glucose control. May cause SLE exacerbation or activation. Use with caution in patients with moderate or high cholesterol concentrations. Photosensitization may occur. Correct hypokalemia before initiating therapy. Electrolyte disturbances (hypokalemia, hypochloremic alkalosis, hyponatremia) may occur with use.

Chemical similarities are present among sulfonamides, sulfonylureas, carbonic anhydrase inhibitors, thiazides, and loop diuretics (except ethacrynic acid). Use in patients with thiazide or sulfonamide allergy is specifically contraindicated in product labeling, however, a risk of cross-reaction exists in patients with allergy to any of these compounds; avoid use when previous reaction has been severe.

Drug Interactions

Decreased Effect: Effects of oral hypoglycemics may be decreased. Decreased absorption of indapamide with cholestyramine and colestipol. NSAIDs can decrease the efficacy of thiazide-type diuretics, reducing the diuretic and antihypertensive effects.

Increased Effect/Toxicity: The diuretic effect of indapamide is synergistic with furosemide and other loop diuretics. Increased hypotension and/or renal adverse effects of ACE inhibitors may result in aggressively diuresed patients. Cyclosporine and thiazide-type diuretics can increase the risk of gout or renal toxicity. Digoxin toxicity can be exacerbated if a diuretic induces hypokalemia or hypomagnesemia. Lithium toxicity can occur with thiazide-type diuretics due to reduced renal excretion of lithium. Thiazide-type diuretics may prolong the duration of action of neuromuscular blocking agents.

Nutritional/Ethanol Interactions Herb/Nutraceutical: Avoid dong quai if using for hypertension (has estrogenic activity). Avoid ephedra, yohimbe, ginseng (may worsen hypertension). Avoid garlic (may have increased antihypertensive effect).

Adverse Reactions

1% to 10%:

Cardiovascular: Orthostatic hypotension, palpitations, flushing

Central nervous system: Dizziness, lightheadedness, vertigo, headache, weakness, restlessness, drowsiness, fatigue, lethargy, malaise, lassitude, anxiety, agitation, depression, nervousness

Gastrointestinal: Anorexia, gastric irritation, nausea, vomiting, abdominal pain, cramping, bloating, diarrhea, constipation, dry mouth, weight loss

Genitourinary: Nocturia, frequent urination, polyuria

Neuromuscular & skeletal: Muscle cramps, spasm

Ocular: Blurred vision

Respiratory: Rhinorrhea

<1% (Limited to important or life-threatening): Cutaneous vasculitis, glycosuria, hypercalcemia, hyperglycemia, hyperuricemia, impotency, necrotizing angiitis, pancreatitis, purpura, reduced libido, vasculitis

Overdosage/Toxicology Symptoms of overdose include lethargy, diuresis, hypermotility, confusion, and muscle weakness. Treatment is supportive.

Pharmacodynamics/Kinetics

Absorption: Complete

Half-Life Elimination: 14-18 hours

Time to Peak: 2-2.5 hours

Metabolism: Extensively hepatic

Onset: 1-2 hours

Duration: ≤36 hours

Formulations Tablet: 1.25 mg, 2.5 mg

Dosing

Adults & Elderly:

Edema: Oral: 2.5-5 mg/day. **Note:** There is little therapeutic benefit to increasing the dose >5 mg/day; there is, however, an increased risk of electrolyte disturbances.

Hypertension: Oral: 1.25 mg in the morning, may increase to 5 mg/day by increments of 1.25-2.5 mg; consider adding another antihypertensive and decreasing the dose if response is not adequate.

Administration

Oral: May be taken with food or milk. Take early in day to avoid nocturia. Take the last dose of multiple doses no later than 6 PM unless instructed otherwise.

Monitoring Laboratory Tests Serum electrolytes, renal function

Monitoring and Teaching Issues

Physical Assessment: Assess allergy history prior to beginning therapy. See Contraindications, Warnings/Precautions, and Dosing for use cautions. Assess potential for interactions with other prescriptions, OTC medications, or herbal products patient may be taking (see Drug Interactions). Assess results of laboratory tests (see Monitoring Lab Tests), therapeutic effects, and adverse response (see Adverse Reactions and Overdose/Toxicology) at regular intervals during therapy. Instruct diabetic patient to monitor glucose levels closely; may interfere with oral hypoglycemic medications. Teach patient proper use, possible side effects (eg, orthostatic hypotension, electrolyte imbalance) and appropriate interventions, and adverse symptoms to report (see Patient Education). **Pregnancy risk factor B/D** - see Pregnancy Risk Factor for use cautions; benefits of use should outweigh possible risks. Note breast-feeding caution.

(Continued)

Indapamide *(Continued)*

Patient Education: Inform prescriber of all prescriptions, OTC medications, or herbal products you are taking, and any allergies you have. Do not take anything new during treatment unless approved by prescriber. Take as directed, early in the day. Do not exceed recommended dosage. This medication does not replace other antihypertensive interventions; follow prescriber's instructions for diet and lifestyle changes. If diabetic, monitor serum glucose closely (medication may decrease effect of oral hypoglycemics). Monitor weight on a regular basis. Report sudden or excessive weight gain (>5 lb/week), swelling of ankles or hands, or difficulty breathing. You may experience dizziness, weakness, or drowsiness (use caution when rising from sitting or lying position, when climbing stairs and when driving or engaging in tasks that require alertness until response to drug is known); sensitivity to sunlight (use sunblock, wear protective clothing or sunglasses); impotence (reversible); or dry mouth or thirst (frequent mouth care, chewing gum, or sucking lozenges may help). Report any changes in visual acuity; unusual bleeding; chest pain or palpitations; or numbness, tingling, cramping of muscles. **Breast-feeding precaution:** Consult prescriber if breast-feeding.

Dietary Issues: May be taken with food or milk to decrease GI adverse effects.

Geriatric Considerations: Thiazide diuretics lose efficacy when Cl_{cr} is <30-35 mL/minute. Many elderly may have Cl_{cr} below this limit. Calculate Cl_{cr} for elderly before initiating therapy. Indapamide has the advantage over thiazide diuretics in that it is effective when Cl_{cr} is <30 mL/minute.

Inderal® *see* Propranolol *on page 1143*

Inderal® LA *see* Propranolol *on page 1143*

Inderide® *see* Propranolol and Hydrochlorothiazide *on page 1146*

Inderide® LA *see* Propranolol and Hydrochlorothiazide *on page 1146*

Indinavir (in DIN a veer)

U.S. Brand Names Crixivan®

Generic Available No

Pharmacologic Category Antiretroviral Agent, Protease Inhibitor

Pregnancy Risk Factor C

Lactation Excretion in breast milk unknown/contraindicated

Use Treatment of HIV infection; should always be used as part of a multidrug regimen (at least three antiretroviral agents)

Mechanism of Action/Effect Indinavir is a protease inhibitor which prevents cleavage of protein precursors essential for HIV infection of new cells and viral replication.

Contraindications Hypersensitivity to indinavir or any component of the formulation; concurrent use of astemizole, cisapride, triazolam, midazolam, pimozide, or ergot alkaloids

Warnings/Precautions Because indinavir may cause nephrolithiasis/urolithiasis the drug should be discontinued if signs and symptoms occur. Indinavir should not be administered concurrently with lovastatin or simvastatin (caution with atorvastatin and cerivastatin) because of competition for metabolism of these drugs through the CYP3A4 system, and potential serious or life-threatening events. Use caution with other drugs metabolized by this enzyme (particular caution with sildenafil). Avoid concurrent use of St John's wort. Patients with hepatic insufficiency due to cirrhosis should have dose reduction. Warn patients about fat redistribution that can occur. Indinavir has been associated with hemolytic anemia (discontinue if diagnosed), hepatitis, and hyperglycemia (exacerbation or new-onset diabetes). Pregnancy risk C.

Drug Interactions

Cytochrome P450 Effect: Substrate of CYP2D6, **3A4**; Inhibits CYP2C8/9, 2C19, 2D6, **3A4**

Decreased Effect: Concurrent use of efavirenz, rifampin, and rifabutin may decrease the effectiveness of indinavir (dosage increase of indinavir is recommended); concurrent use of rifampin is not recommended; dosage decrease of rifabutin is recommended. The efficacy of protease inhibitors may be decreased when given with nevirapine. Gastric pH is lowered and absorption may be decreased when didanosine and indinavir are taken <1 hour apart. Fluconazole may decrease serum concentration of indinavir.

Increased Effect/Toxicity: Levels of indinavir are increased by delavirdine, itraconazole, ketoconazole, nelfinavir, sildenafil, and ritonavir. Cisapride, pimozide, and astemizole should be avoided with indinavir due to life-threatening cardiotoxicity. Concurrent use of indinavir with lovastatin and simvastatin may increase the risk of myopathy or rhabdomyolysis. Cautious use of atorvastatin and cerivastatin may be possible. Benzodiazepines with indinavir may result in prolonged sedation and respiratory depression (midazolam and triazolam are contraindicated). Concurrent use of ergot alkaloids is contraindicated. Amprenavir and rifabutin concentrations are increased during concurrent therapy with indinavir. Other medications metabolized by cytochrome P450 isoenzyme 3A4 (including calcium channel blockers) may be affected. Concurrent sildenafil is associated with increased risk of hypotension, visual changes, and priapism. Clarithromycin and quinidine may increase serum concentrations of indinavir. Serum concentrations of these drugs may also be increased. Other CYP3A4 inhibitors may have similar effects.

Nutritional/Ethanol Interactions

Food: Indinavir bioavailability may be decreased if taken with food. Meals high in calories, fat, and protein result in a significant decrease in drug levels. Indinavir serum concentrations may be decreased by grapefruit juice.

Herb/Nutraceutical: St John's wort *(Hypericum)* appears to induce CYP3A enzymes and has lead to 57% reductions in indinavir AUCs and 81% reductions in trough serum concentrations, which may lead to treatment failures; concurrent use is contraindicated.

Adverse Reactions Protease inhibitors cause dyslipidemia which includes elevated cholesterol and triglycerides and a redistribution of body fat centrally to cause "protease paunch", buffalo hump, facial atrophy, and breast enlargement. These agents also cause hyperglycemia (exacerbation or new-onset diabetes).

>10%:

Hepatic: Hyperbilirubinemia (14%)

Renal: Nephrolithiasis/urolithiasis (29%, pediatric patients)

1% to 10%:

Central nervous system: Headache (6%), insomnia (3%)

Gastrointestinal: Abdominal pain (9%), nausea (12%), diarrhea/vomiting (4% to 5%), taste perversion (3%)

Neuromuscular & skeletal: Weakness (4%), flank pain (3%)

Renal: Nephrolithiasis/urolithiasis (12%, adult patients), hematuria

<1% (Limited to important or life-threatening): Acute renal failure, alopecia, anaphylactoid reactions, angina, anorexia, crystalluria, decreased hemoglobin, depression, dizziness, dysuria, erythema multiforme, fever, hemolytic anemia, hepatic failure, hepatitis, hyperglycemia, increased serum cholesterol, interstitial nephritis, malaise, myocardial infarction, new-onset diabetes, pancreatitis, paresthesia (oral), pruritus, pyelonephritis, somnolence, Stevens-Johnson syndrome, urticaria, vasculitis, xerostomia

Pharmacodynamics/Kinetics

Absorption: Administration with a high fat, high calorie diet resulted in a reduction in AUC and in maximum serum concentration (77% and 84% respectively); lighter meal resulted in little or no change in these parameters.

Bioavailability: Good

Half-Life Elimination: 1.8 ± 0.4 hour

Time to Peak: 0.8 ± 0.3 hour

Metabolism: Hepatic via CYP3A4 enzymes; seven metabolites of indinavir identified

Formulations Capsule, as sulfate: 100 mg, 200 mg, 333 mg, 400 mg

Dosing

Adults & Elderly: HIV: Oral: 800 mg every 8 hours

Note: Dosage adjustments for indinavir when administered in combination therapy:

Delavirdine, itraconazole, or ketoconazole: Reduce indinavir dose to 600 mg every 8 hours

Efavirenz: Increase indinavir dose to 1000 mg every 8 hours

Lopinavir and ritonavir (Kaletra™): Indinavir 600 mg twice daily

Nevirapine: Increase indinavir dose to 1000 mg every 8 hours

Rifabutin: Reduce rifabutin to ½ the standard dose plus increase indinavir to 1000 mg every 8 hours

Ritonavir: Adjustments necessary for both agents:

Ritonavir 100-200 mg twice daily plus indinavir 800 mg twice daily **or**

Ritonavir 400 mg twice daily plus indinavir 400 mg twice daily

Pediatrics: HIV: Investigational: 500 mg/m^2 every 8 hours (patients with smaller BSA may require lower doses of 300-400 mg/m^2 every 8 hours)

Hepatic Impairment: 600 mg every 8 hours with mild/medium impairment due to cirrhosis or with ketoconazole coadministration

Administration

Oral: Drink at least 48 oz of water daily. Administer with water, 1 hour before or 2 hours after a meal. Administer around-the-clock to avoid significant fluctuation in serum levels.

Stability

Storage: Capsules are sensitive to moisture; medication should be stored and used in the original container and the desiccant should remain in the bottle

Monitoring Laboratory Tests Monitor viral load, CD4 count, triglycerides, cholesterol, glucose, liver function tests, CBC

Monitoring and Teaching Issues

Physical Assessment: See Contraindications, Warnings/Precautions, and Dosing for use cautions. Assess potential for interactions with other prescriptions, OTC medications, or herbal products patient may be taking (see Drug Interactions). Assess results of laboratory tests (see Monitoring Laboratory Tests), therapeutic effects, and adverse response (see Adverse Reactions and Overdose/Toxicology) at regular intervals during therapy. Teach patient proper use, possible side effects and appropriate interventions (eg, glucose testing; protease inhibitors may cause hyperglycemia [exacerbation or new-onset diabetes]), and adverse symptoms to report (see Patient Education). **Pregnancy risk factor C** - benefits of use should outweigh possible risks. Breast-feeding is contraindicated.

Patient Education: Inform prescriber of all prescriptions, OTC medications, or herbal products you are taking, and any allergies you have. Do not take anything new during treatment unless approved by prescriber. Indinavir is not a cure for AIDS. Take as directed, around-the-clock, with a large glass of water, preferably 1 hour before or 2 hours after meals. May take with light meal (eg, dry toast, skim milk, corn flakes) to reduce GI upset. Capsules are sensitive to moisture medication should be stored and used in the original container and the desiccant should remain in the bottle. Maintain adequate hydration (2-3 L/day of fluids) unless advised by prescriber to restrict fluids. Indinavir may be prescribed with a combination of other medications; time these medications as directed by prescriber. You may be advised to check your glucose levels (this drug can cause exacerbation or new-onset diabetes). You may experience body changes due to redistribution of body fat, facial atrophy, or breast enlargement (normal effects of drug); nausea or vomiting (small, frequent meals, frequent mouth care, chewing gum, or sucking lozenges may help); muscle weakness or flank pain (consult prescriber for approved analgesic); or headache or insomnia (consult prescriber for medication). Report chest pain or palpitations, difficult or painful urination, persistent diarrhea or vomiting, or other persistent adverse effects. **Pregnancy/breast-feeding precautions:** Inform prescriber if you are or intend to become pregnant. Do not breast-feed.

Dietary Issues: Should be taken without food but with water 1 hour before or 2 hours after a meal. Administration with lighter meals (eg, dry toast, skim milk, corn flakes) resulted in little/no change in indinavir concentration. If taking with ritonavir, may take with food. Patient should drink at least 48 oz of water daily.

Breast-feeding Issues: HIV-infected mothers are discouraged from breast-feeding to decrease potential transmission of HIV.

(Continued)

Indinavir *(Continued)*

Pregnancy Issues: Safety and pharmacokinetic studies are currently underway in pregnant women; hyperbilirubinemia may be exacerbated in neonates. Pregnancy and protease inhibitors are both associated with an increased risk of hyperglycemia. Glucose levels should be closely monitored. Healthcare professionals are encouraged to contact the antiretroviral pregnancy registry to monitor outcomes of pregnant women exposed to antiretroviral medications (1-800-258-4263).

Related Information

Tuberculosis *on page 1705*

Indocin® *see* Indomethacin *on page 710*

Indocin® I.V. *see* Indomethacin *on page 710*

Indocin® SR *see* Indomethacin *on page 710*

Indocyanine Green *see page 1461*

Indometacin *see* Indomethacin *on page 710*

Indomethacin (in doe METH a sin)

U.S. Brand Names Indocin®; Indocin® I.V.; Indocin® SR

Synonyms Indometacin; Indomethacin Sodium Trihydrate

Generic Available Yes: Capsule, suspension

Pharmacologic Category Nonsteroidal Anti-inflammatory Drug (NSAID)

Pregnancy Risk Factor B/D (3rd trimester)

Lactation Enters breast milk/use caution (AAP rates "compatible")

Use Management of inflammatory diseases and rheumatoid disorders; moderate pain; acute gouty arthritis, acute bursitis/tendonitis, moderate to severe osteoarthritis, rheumatoid arthritis, ankylosing spondylitis; I.V. form used as alternative to surgery for closure of patent ductus arteriosus in neonates

Mechanism of Action/Effect Inhibits prostaglandin synthesis by decreasing the activity of the enzyme, cyclooxygenase, which results in decreased formation of prostaglandin precursors

Contraindications Hypersensitivity to indomethacin, any component of the formulation, aspirin, or other NSAIDs; patients in whom asthma, urticaria, or rhinitis are precipitated by NSAIDs/aspirin; active GI bleeding or ulcer disease; premature neonates with necrotizing enterocolitis; impaired renal function; active bleeding; thrombocytopenia; pregnancy (3rd trimester)

Warnings/Precautions Use with caution in patients with CHF, hypertension, dehydration, decreased renal or hepatic function, history of GI disease (bleeding or ulcers), or those receiving anticoagulants. Elderly are at a high risk for adverse effects from NSAIDs. As many as 60% of elderly can develop peptic ulceration and/or hemorrhage asymptomatically.

Use lowest effective dose for shortest period possible. Use of NSAIDs can compromise existing renal function especially when Cl_{cr} is <30 mL/minute. Discontinue if signs/symptoms of hepatic injury occur. Elderly may demonstrate adverse CNS effects at lower doses than younger adults. Use caution in patients with depression or other psychiatric disorder, epilepsy, or parkinsonism; discontinue if severe CNS adverse effects occur. Inhibits platelet aggregation. Withhold for at least 4-6 half-lives prior to surgical or dental procedures.

Drug Interactions

Cytochrome P450 Effect: Substrate of CYP2C8/9, 2C19; Inhibits CYP2C8/9, 2C19

Decreased Effect: May decrease antihypertensive effects of beta-blockers, hydralazine, ACE inhibitors, and angiotensin II antagonists. Indomethacin may decrease the antihypertensive and diuretic effect of thiazides (hydrochlorothiazide, etc) and loop diuretics (furosemide, bumetanide).

Increased Effect/Toxicity: Indomethacin may increase serum potassium with potassium-sparing diuretics. Probenecid may increase indomethacin serum concentrations. Other NSAIDs may increase GI adverse effects. May increase nephrotoxicity of cyclosporine and increase renal adverse effects of ACE inhibitors. Indomethacin may increase serum concentrations of digoxin, methotrexate, lithium, and aminoglycosides (reported with I.V. use in neonates).

Nutritional/Ethanol Interactions

Ethanol: Avoid ethanol (may enhance gastric mucosal irritation).

Food: Food may decrease the rate but not the extent of absorption. Indomethacin peak serum levels may be delayed if taken with food.

Herb/Nutraceutical: Avoid cat's claw, dong quai, evening primrose, feverfew, garlic, ginger, ginkgo, red clover, horse chestnut, green tea, ginseng (all have additional antiplatelet activity).

Effects on Lab Values Positive Coombs' [direct]; ↑ sodium, chloride, bleeding time

Adverse Reactions

>10%: Central nervous system: Headache (12%)

1% to 10%:

Central nervous system: Dizziness (3% to 9%), drowsiness (<1%), fatigue (<3%), vertigo (<3%), depression (<3%), malaise (<3%), somnolence (<3%)

Gastrointestinal: Nausea (3% to 9%), epigastric pain (3% to 9%), abdominal pain/cramps/distress (<3%), anorexia (<1%), GI bleeding (<1%), ulcers (<1%), perforation (<1%), heartburn (3% to 9%), indigestion (3% to 9%), constipation (<3%), diarrhea (<3%), dyspepsia (3% to 9%)

Hematologic: Inhibition of platelet aggregation (3% to 9%)

Otic: Tinnitus (<3%)

<1% (Limited to important or life-threatening): Acute respiratory distress, agranulocytosis, anaphylaxis, angioedema, arrhythmias, aseptic meningitis, asthma, bone marrow suppression, bronchospasm, cholestatic jaundice, CHF, depression, dyspnea/bronchospasm, erythema multiforme, exfoliative dermatitis, GI ulceration, hallucinations, hemolytic anemia, hepatitis (including fatal cases), hypersensitivity reactions, hypertension, hypoglycemia (I.V.), inhibition of platelet aggregation, interstitial nephritis, nephrotic syndrome, peripheral

neuropathy, proctitis, psychic disturbances, psychosis, rash, renal failure, retinal/macular disturbances, shock, somnolence, Stevens-Johnson syndrome, thrombocytopenia, toxic amblyopia, toxic epidermal necrolysis, urticaria

Overdosage/Toxicology Symptoms of overdose include drowsiness, lethargy, nausea, vomiting, seizures, paresthesia, headache, dizziness, GI bleeding, cerebral edema, tinnitus, leukocytosis, and renal failure. Management of NSAID intoxication is supportive and symptomatic.

Pharmacodynamics/Kinetics

Absorption: Prompt and extensive

Half-Life Elimination: 4.5 hours; prolonged with neonates

Time to Peak: Oral: ~3-4 hours

Metabolism: Hepatic; significant enterohepatic recirculation

Onset: ~30 minutes

Duration: 4-6 hours

Formulations

Capsule (Indocin®): 25 mg, 50 mg

Capsule, sustained release (Indocin® SR): 75 mg

Injection, powder for reconstitution, as sodium trihydrate (Indocin® I.V.): 1 mg

Suspension, oral (Indocin®): 25 mg/5 mL (237 mL) [contains alcohol 1%; pineapple-coconut-mint flavor]

Dosing

Adults & Elderly: Inflammatory/rheumatoid disorders: Oral: 25-50 mg/dose 2-3 times/day; maximum dose: 200 mg/day; extended release capsule should be given on a 1-2 times/day schedule

Pediatrics:

Patent ductus arteriosus:

Neonates: I.V.: Initial: 0.2 mg/kg, followed by 2 doses depending on postnatal age (PNA):

PNA **at time of first dose** <48 hours: 0.1 mg/kg at 12- to 24-hour intervals

PNA **at time of first dose** 2-7 days: 0.2 mg/kg at 12- to 24-hour intervals

PNA **at time of first dose** >7 days: 0.25 mg/kg at 12- to 24-hour intervals

In general, may use 12-hour dosing interval if urine output >1 mL/kg/hour after prior dose; use 24-hour dosing interval if urine output is <1 mL/kg/hour but >0.6 mL/kg/hour; doses should be withheld if patient has oliguria (urine output <0.6 mL/kg/hour) or anuria

Inflammatory/rheumatoid disorders: Children: Oral: 1-2 mg/kg/day in 2-4 divided doses; maximum dose: 4 mg/kg/day; not to exceed 150-200 mg/day

Administration

Oral: Administer with food, milk, or antacids to decrease GI adverse effects. Extended release capsules must be swallowed whole, do not crush.

I.V.: Administer over 20-30 minutes at a concentration of 0.5-1 mg/mL in preservative-free sterile water for injection or normal saline. Reconstitute I.V. formulation just prior to administration; discard any unused portion; avoid I.V. bolus administration or infusion via an umbilical catheter into vessels near the superior mesenteric artery as these may cause vasoconstriction and can compromise blood flow to the intestines. Do not administer intra-arterially.

Stability

Storage: I.V.: Store below 30°C (86°F). Protect from light.

Reconstitution: Reconstitute just prior to administration; discard any unused portion. Do not use preservative-containing diluents for reconstitution.

Compatibility: Stable in NS

Y-site administration: Incompatible with amino acid injection, calcium gluconate, cimetidine, dobutamine, dopamine, gentamicin, levofloxacin, tobramycin, tolazoline

Monitoring Laboratory Tests Renal function (serum creatinine, BUN), CBC, liver function

Monitoring and Teaching Issues

Physical Assessment: See Contraindications, Warnings/Precautions, and Dosing for use cautions. Assess potential for interactions with other prescriptions, OTC medications, or herbal products patient may be taking (see Drug Interactions). Assess results of laboratory tests (see above), therapeutic effectiveness (according to rationale for use), and adverse response when beginning therapy and at regular intervals during treatment (see Warnings/Precautions, Adverse Reactions, and Overdose/Toxicology). Teach patient proper use, side effects and interventions (regular ophthalmic evaluations with long-term use), and adverse symptoms to report (see Patient Education). **Pregnancy risk factor B/D** - see Pregnancy Risk Factor for use cautions. Note breast-feeding caution.

Patient Education: Inform prescriber of all prescriptions, OTC medications, or herbal products you are taking, and any allergies you have. Do not take anything new during treatment without consulting prescriber. Use exactly as directed; do not increase dose without consulting prescriber. Do not crush, break, or chew capsules. Take with food or milk to reduce GI distress. Maintain adequate hydration (2-3 L/day of fluids) unless advised to restrict fluids. May cause drowsiness, dizziness, nervousness, or headache (use caution when driving or engaging in tasks that require alertness until response to drug is known); anorexia, nausea, vomiting, or heartburn (small, frequent meals, frequent mouth care, chewing gum, or sucking lozenges may help): fluid retention (weigh yourself weekly and report unusually weight gain >3-5 lb/week); or may turn urine green (normal). GI bleeding, ulceration, or perforation can occur with or without pain; discontinue medication and contact prescriber if persistent abdominal pain or cramping or blood in stool occurs. Report difficult breathing or unusual cough; chest pain, rapid heartbeat, or palpitations; unusual bruising or bleeding; blood in urine, gums, or vomitus; swollen extremities; skin rash, irritation, or itching; acute persistent fatigue; or vision changes or ringing in ears. **Pregnancy/breast-feeding precautions:** Inform prescriber if you are or intend to become pregnant. This drug should not be used in the 3rd trimester of pregnancy. Consult prescriber if breast-feeding.

(Continued)

Indomethacin *(Continued)*

Dietary Issues: May cause GI upset, bleeding, ulceration, perforation; take with food or milk to minimize GI upset.

Geriatric Considerations: Elderly are at high risk for adverse effects from NSAIDs. As much as 60% of elderly can develop peptic ulceration and/or hemorrhage asymptomatically. The concomitant use of H_2 blockers, omeprazole, and sucralfate is not effective as prophylaxis with the exception of NSAID-induced duodenal ulcers which may be prevented by the use of ranitidine. Misoprostol is the only prophylactic agent proven effective. Also, concomitant disease and drug use contribute to the risk for GI adverse effects. Use lowest effective dose for shortest period possible. Consider renal function decline with age. Use of NSAIDs can compromise existing renal function especially when Cl_{cr} is ≤30 mL/minute. Tinnitus may be a difficult and unreliable indication of toxicity due to age-related hearing loss or eighth cranial nerve damage. CNS adverse effects such as confusion, agitation, and hallucination are generally seen in overdose or high-dose situations, but elderly may demonstrate these adverse effects at lower doses than younger adults. Indomethacin frequently causes confusion at recommended doses in the elderly.

Related Information

Nonsalicylate/Nonsteroidal Anti-inflammatory Comparison *on page 1587*

Indomethacin Sodium Trihydrate *see* Indomethacin *on page 710*

INF-alpha 2 *see* Interferon Alfa-2b *on page 719*

Infanrix™ *see page 1498*

Infantaire [OTC] *see* Acetaminophen *on page 35*

INFeD® *see* Iron Dextran Complex *on page 741*

Infergen® *see* Interferon Alfacon-1 *on page 725*

Inflamase® Forte *see* PrednisoLONE *on page 1113*

Inflamase® Mild *see page 1509*

Inflamase® Mild *see* PrednisoLONE *on page 1113*

Infliximab (in FLIKS e mab)

U.S. Brand Names Remicade®

Synonyms Infliximab, Recombinant

Generic Available No

Pharmacologic Category Antirheumatic, Disease Modifying; Gastrointestinal Agent, Miscellaneous; Monoclonal Antibody

Pregnancy Risk Factor B (manufacturer)

Lactation Excretion in breast milk unknown/not recommended

Use

Crohn's disease: Reduce the signs and symptoms of moderate to severe disease in patients who have an inadequate response to conventional therapy; reduce the number of draining enterocutaneous fistulas in fistulizing disease

Rheumatoid arthritis: Used with methotrexate in patients who have had an inadequate response to methotrexate alone; used with methotrexate to inhibit the progression of structural damage and improve physical function in patients with moderate to severe disease

Mechanism of Action/Effect Infliximab is a monoclonal antibody that binds to human tumor necrosis factor alpha (TNFα) receptor sites, thereby decreasing inflammatory and other responses.

Contraindications Hypersensitivity to murine proteins or any component of the formulation; congestive heart failure

Warnings/Precautions Medications for the treatment of hypersensitivity reactions should be available for immediate use. Discontinue the drug if a reaction occurs. Autoimmune antibodies and a lupus-like syndrome have been reported. If antibodies to double-stranded DNA are confirmed in a patient with lupus-like symptoms, treatment should be discontinued. Rare cases of demyelinating disease have been reported, use with caution in patients with pre-existing or recent onset CNS demyelinating disorders. Treatment may lead to antibody development to infliximab. Chronic exposure to immunosuppressants in patients with Crohn's disease or rheumatoid arthritis has been associated with the increased risk of developing lymphomas; the effect of infliximab is not known.

Serious infections, including sepsis and fatal infections, have been reported in patients receiving TNF-blocking agents. Many of the serious infections in patients treated with infliximab have occurred in patients on concomitant immunosuppressive therapy. Caution should be exercised when considering the use of infliximab in patients with a chronic infection or history of recurrent infection. Infliximab should not be given to patients with a clinically-important, active infection. Patients should be tested for latent tuberculosis (positive reaction to PPD but no evidence of active tuberculosis) with a tuberculin skin test before infliximab is started. Treatment of latent tuberculosis should be initiated before infliximab is used. Other opportunistic infections (eg, invasive fungal infections, listeriosis, *Pneumocystis*) have occurred during therapy. The risk/benefit ratio should be weighed in patients who have resided in regions where histoplasmosis is prevalent. Patients who develop a new infection while undergoing treatment with infliximab should be monitored closely. If a patient develops a serious infection or sepsis, infliximab should be discontinued.

Safety and efficacy for use in juvenile rheumatoid arthritis and in pediatric patients with Crohn's disease have not been established.

Increased mortality and hospitalization were seen in clinical trials where infliximab was used to treat CHF. As a result, infliximab is not recommended to treat Crohn's disease or rheumatoid arthritis in patients with existing CHF. The manufacturer recommends re-evaluation of patients with CHF who started treatment with infliximab for Crohn's disease or rheumatoid arthritis prior to this information, and treatment should be stopped if CHF worsens. In addition, consider discontinuing infliximab if significant clinical response is not attained, and monitor cardiac status closely if treatment is continued.

Drug Interactions

Decreased Effect: Specific drug interaction studies have not been conducted.

Decreased toxicity: Immunosuppressants: When used with infliximab, may decrease the risk of infusion related reactions, and may decrease development of anti-double-stranded DNA antibodies

Increased Effect/Toxicity: Specific drug interaction studies have not been conducted.

Adverse Reactions Note: Although profile is similar, frequency of effects may be different in specific populations (Crohn's disease vs rheumatoid arthritis).

>10%:

Central nervous system: Headache (22% to 23%), fatigue (8% to 11%), fever (8% to 10%)

Dermatologic: Rash (6% to 12%)

Gastrointestinal: Nausea (17%), diarrhea (3% to 13%), abdominal pain (10% to 12%)

Local: Infusion reactions (19%)

Respiratory: Upper respiratory tract infection (16% to 26%), cough (5% to 13%), sinusitis (5% to 13%), pharyngitis (9% to 11%)

Miscellaneous: Development of antinuclear antibodies (34%); infections (32%); Crohn's patients with fistulizing disease: Development of new abscess (12%, 8-16 weeks after the last infusion)

2% to 10%:

Cardiovascular: Chest pain (5% to 6%, similar to placebo)

Central nervous system: Pain (8% to 9%), dizziness (8% to 10%, similar to placebo)

Dermatologic: Pruritus (5% to 6%)

Gastrointestinal: Vomiting (7% to 9%), dyspepsia (5% to 6%)

Genitourinary: Urinary tract infection (3% to 8%, similar to placebo)

Neuromuscular & skeletal: Arthralgia (5% to 6%), back pain (5% to 6%)

Respiratory: Bronchitis (6% to 7%), rhinitis (6% to 9%)

Miscellaneous: Development of antibodies to double-stranded DNA (9%)

<2% (Limited to important or life-threatening): Arrhythmia, AV block, azotemia, basal cell carcinoma, bradycardia, brain infarction, breast cancer, cardiac arrest, cardiac failure, cholecystitis, cholelithiasis, delirium; demyelinating disorders (multiple sclerosis, optic neuritis); depression, dyspnea, encephalopathy, gastrointestinal hemorrhage, Guillain-Barré syndrome, hemarthrosis, hepatitis, hydronephrosis, hypertension, hypotension, injection site inflammation, interstitial fibrosis, interstitial pneumonitis, intestinal obstruction, intestinal perforation, intestinal stenosis, kidney infarction, latent tuberculosis reactivation, leukopenia, lupus erythematosus syndrome, lymphangitis, lymphoma, myocardial ischemia, neuropathy, pancreatitis, peripheral ischemia, peritonitis, pleural effusion, pneumothorax, pulmonary edema, pulmonary embolism, pyelonephritis, renal failure, respiratory insufficiency, sepsis, splenic infarction, spinal stenosis, splenomegaly, syncope, thrombocytopenia, thrombophlebitis (deep), upper motor neuron lesion, worsening CHF

Overdosage/Toxicology Doses of up to 20 mg/kg have been given without toxic effects. In case of overdose, treatment should be symptom-directed and supportive.

Pharmacodynamics/Kinetics

Half-Life Elimination: 8-9.5 days

Onset: Crohn's disease: ~2 weeks

Formulations Injection, powder for reconstitution: 100 mg

Dosing

Adults & Elderly:

Crohn's disease:

Moderately- to severely-active: I.V.: 5 mg/kg as a single infusion over a minimum of 2 hours

Fistulizing: I.V.: 5 mg/kg as an infusion over a minimum of 2 hours; dose repeated at 2- and 6 weeks after the initial infusion

Rheumatoid arthritis: I.V. (in combination with methotrexate therapy): 3 mg/kg followed by an additional 3 mg/kg at 2- and 6 weeks after the first dose; then repeat every 8 weeks thereafter; doses have ranged from 3-10 mg/kg intravenous infusion repeated at 4-week intervals or 8-week intervals

Pediatrics: Safety and efficacy have not been established

Renal Impairment: No adjustment is recommended.

Hepatic Impairment: No adjustment necessary.

Administration

I.V.: Infuse over at least 2 hours

Stability

Storage: Store vials at 2°C to 8°C (36°F to 46°F); do not freeze; does not contain preservative

Reconstitution: Reconstitute vials with 10 mL sterile water for injection; swirl vial gently to dissolve powder, do not shake, allow solution to stand for 5 minutes; total dose of reconstituted product should be further diluted to 250 mL of 0.9% sodium chloride injection; infusion of dose should begin within 3 hours of preparation

Compatibility: Do not infuse with other agents.

Monitoring and Teaching Issues

Physical Assessment: Monitor therapeutic response (reduction of signs and symptoms of Crohn's disease or reduction in number of Crohn's-related fistulas), adverse reactions (see Warnings/Precautions and Adverse Reactions). Place and read PPD before initiation. Treatment of latent TB infection should be initiated prior to treatment with infliximab. Teach patient appropriate interventions to reduce side effects and adverse symptoms to report (see Patient Education). Breast-feeding is not recommended.

Patient Education: This drug can only be administered by infusion. Report headache or unusual fatigue; increased nausea or abdominal pain; cough, runny nose, difficulty breathing; chest pain or persistent dizziness; fatigue, muscle pain or weakness, back pain; fever or chills; mouth sores; vaginal itching or discharge; sore throat; unhealed sores; or frequent infections. **Breast-feeding precaution:** Breast-feeding is not recommended.

(Continued)

Infliximab *(Continued)*

Breast-feeding Issues: It is not known whether infliximab is secreted in human milk. Because many immunoglobulins are secreted in milk and the potential for serious adverse reactions exists, a decision should be made whether to discontinue nursing or discontinue the drug, taking into account the importance of the drug to the mother.

Infliximab, Recombinant *see* Infliximab *on page 712*

Influenza Virus Vaccine *see page 1498*

Infumorph® *see* Morphine Sulfate *on page 926*

INH *see* Isoniazid *on page 746*

Inhalant (Asthma, Bronchospasm) Agents Comparison *see page 1577*

Innohep® *see* Tinzaparin *on page 1324*

Inotropic and Vasoconstrictor Comparison *see page 1580*

Insect Sting Kit *see page 1460*

Inspra™ *see* Eplerenone *on page 475*

Insulin Preparations (IN su lin prep a RAY shuns)

U.S. Brand Names Humalog®; Humalog® Mix 75/25™; Humulin® 50/50; Humulin® 70/30; Humulin® L; Humulin® N; Humulin® R; Humulin® R (Concentrated) U-500; Humulin® U; Lantus®; Lente® Iletin® II; Novolin® 70/30; Novolin® L; Novolin® N; Novolin® R; NovoLog®; NPH Iletin® II; Regular Iletin® II; Velosulin® BR (Buffered)

Generic Available No

Pharmacologic Category Antidiabetic Agent, Insulin; Antidote

Pregnancy Risk Factor B; C (insulin glargine [Lantus®]; insulin aspart [NovoLog®])

Lactation Does not enter breast milk/compatible

Use Treatment of type 1 diabetes mellitus (insulin dependent, IDDM); type 2 diabetes mellitus (noninsulin dependent, NIDDM) unresponsive to treatment with diet and/or oral hypoglycemics; adjunct to parenteral nutrition; hyperkalemia (regular insulin only; use with glucose to shift potassium into cells to lower serum potassium levels)

Mechanism of Action/Effect The principal hormone required for proper glucose utilization in normal metabolic processes; it is obtained from beef or pork pancreas or a biosynthetic process converting pork insulin to human insulin; insulins are categorized into 3 groups related to promptness, duration, and intensity of action

Warnings/Precautions Any change of insulin should be made cautiously. Changing manufacturers, type and/or method of manufacture, may result in the need for a change of dosage. Human insulin differs from animal-source insulin. Hypoglycemia may result from increased work or exercise without eating. Use with caution in patients with a previous hypersensitivity reaction. S.C. doses used in insulin-resistant patients must be reduced if given I.V. (only regular insulin should be given I.V.). Safety and efficacy of NovoLog® in children has not been established. Pregnancy risk B/C.

Drug Interactions

Cytochrome P450 Effect: Induces CYP1A2

Decreased Effect: Decreased hypoglycemic effect of insulin with corticosteroids, dextrothyroxine, diltiazem, dobutamine, epinephrine, niacin, oral contraceptives, thiazide diuretics, thyroid hormone, and smoking.

Increased Effect/Toxicity: Increased hypoglycemic effect of insulin with alcohol, alpha-blockers, anabolic steroids, beta-blockers (nonselective beta-blockers may delay recovery from hypoglycemic episodes and mask signs/symptoms of hypoglycemia; cardioselective beta-blocker agents may be alternatives), clofibrate, guanethidine, MAO inhibitors, pentamidine, phenylbutazone, salicylates, sulfinpyrazone, and tetracyclines.

Insulin increases the risk of hypoglycemia associated with oral hypoglycemic agents (including sulfonylureas, metformin, pioglitazone, rosiglitazone, and troglitazone).

Nutritional/Ethanol Interactions

Ethanol: Caution with ethanol (may increase hypoglycemia).

Food: Insulin shifts potassium from extracellular to intracellular space. Decreases potassium serum concentration.

Herb/Nutraceutical: Use caution with chromium, garlic, gymnema (may increase hypoglycemia).

Adverse Reactions Frequency not defined.

Cardiovascular: Palpitation, tachycardia, pallor

Central nervous system: Fatigue, mental confusion, loss of consciousness, headache, hypothermia

Dermatologic: Urticaria, redness

Endocrine & metabolic: Hypoglycemia

Gastrointestinal: Hunger, nausea, numbness of mouth

Local: Itching, edema, stinging, pain or warmth at injection site; atrophy or hypertrophy of S.C. fat tissue

Neuromuscular & skeletal: Muscle weakness, paresthesia, tremors

Ocular: Transient presbyopia or blurred vision

Miscellaneous: Diaphoresis, anaphylaxis

Overdosage/Toxicology Symptoms of overdose include tachycardia, anxiety, hunger, tremor, pallor, headache, motor dysfunction, speech disturbances, sweating, palpitations, coma, and death. Antidote is glucose and glucagon, if necessary.

Pharmacodynamics/Kinetics

Absorption: Biosynthetic regular human insulin is absorbed from the S.C. injection site more rapidly than insulins of animal origin (60-90 minutes peak vs 120-150 minutes peak respectively) and lowers the initial blood glucose much faster. Human Ultralente® insulin is absorbed about twice as quickly as its bovine equivalent, and bioavailability is also improved. Human Lente® insulin preparations are also absorbed more quickly than their animal equivalents. Insulin glargine (Lantus®) is designed to form microprecipitates when injected subcutaneously. Small amounts of insulin glargine are then released over a 24-hour period, with no pronounced peak. Insulin glargine (Lantus®) for the treatment of type 1 diabetes (insulin dependent, IDDM) and type 2 diabetes mellitus (noninsulin dependent, NIDDM) in patients who require basal (long-acting) insulin.

Bioavailability: Medium-acting S.C. Lente®-type human insulins did not differ from the corresponding porcine insulins

Onset: Biosynthetic NPH human insulin is more rapid than corresponding porcine insulins; human insulin and purified porcine regular insulin are similarly efficacious following S.C. administration. Medium-acting S.C. Lente®-type human insulins did not differ from the corresponding porcine insulins

Lispro (Humalog®): 0.25 hours; Peak effect: 0.5-1.5 hours
Insulin aspart (NovoLog®): 0.5 hours; Peak effect: 1-3 hours
Insulin, regular (Novolin® R): 0.5-1 hours; Peak effect: 2-3 hours
Isophane insulin suspension (NPH) (Novolin® N): 1-1.5 hours; Peak effect: 4-12 hours
Insulin zinc suspension (Lente®): 1-2.5 hours; Peak effect: 8-12 hours
Isophane insulin suspension and regular insulin injection (Novolin® 70/30): 0.5 hours; Peak effect: 2-12 hours
Extended insulin zinc suspension (Ultralente®): 4-8 hours; Peak effect: 16-18 hours

Duration: Biosynthetic NPH human insulin shows a shorter duration of action than corresponding porcine insulins; human insulin and purified porcine regular insulin are similarly efficacious following S.C. administration. The duration of action of highly purified porcine insulins is shorter than that of conventional insulin equivalents. Duration depends on type of preparation and route of administration as well as patient-related variables. In general, the larger the dose of insulin, the longer the duration of activity.

Lispro (Humalog®): 6-8 hours
Insulin aspart (NovoLog®): 3-5 hours
Insulin, regular (Novolin® R): 8-12 hours
Isophane insulin suspension (NPH) (Novolin® N): 24 hours
Insulin zinc suspension (Lente®): 18-24 hours
Isophane insulin suspension and regular insulin injection (Novolin® 70/30): 24 hours
Extended insulin zinc suspension (Ultralente®): >36 hours
Insulin glargine (Lantus®): 24 hours

Formulations

RAPID-ACTING:
Injection, solution, aspart, human:
NovoLog®: 100 units/mL (10 mL vial)
NovoLog® [PenFill®]: 100 units/mL (3 mL cartridge)
Injection, solution, lispro, human (Humalog®): 100 units/mL (1.5 mL cartridge, 3 mL disposable pen, 10 mL vial)

SHORT-ACTING:
Injection, solution, regular, human:
Humlin® R: 100 units/mL (10 mL vial)
Novolin® R: 100 units/mL (1.5 mL prefilled syringe, 10 mL vial)
Novolin® R [PenFill®]: 100 units/mL (1.5 mL cartridge, 3 mL cartridge)
Injection, solution, regular, human, buffered (Velosulin® BR): 100 units/mL (10 mL vial)
Injection, solution, regular, human, concentrate (Humulin® R U-500): 500 units/mL (20 mL vial)
Injection, solution, regular, purified pork (Regular Iletin® II): 100 units/mL (10 mL vial)

INTERMEDIATE-ACTING:
Injection, suspension, lente, human [zinc] (Humulin® L, Novolin® L): 100 units/mL (10 mL vial)
Injection, suspension, lente, purified pork [zinc] (Lente® Iletin II): 100 units/mL (10 mL vial)
Injection, suspension, NPH, human [isophane]:
Humulin® N: 100 units/mL (3 mL disposable pen, 10 mL vial)
Novolin® N: 100 units/mL (1.5 mL prefilled syringe, 10 mL vial)
Novolin® N [PenFill®]: 100 units/mL (1.5 mL cartridge, 3 mL cartridge)
Injection, suspension, NPH, purified pork [isophane] (NPH Iletin® II): 100 units/mL (10 mL vial)

LONG-ACTING:
Injection, suspension, Ultralente®, human [zinc] (Humulin U Ultralente®): 100 units/mL (10 mL vial)
Injection, solution, glargine, human (Lantus®): 100 unit/mL (10 mL vial)

COMBINATION, INTERMEDIATE-ACTING:
Injection, lispro human suspension 75% and rapid-acting lispro human solution 25% (Humalog® Mix 75/25™): 100 units/mL (3 mL disposable pen, 10 mL vial)
Injection, NPH human insulin suspension 50% and short-acting regular human insulin solution 50% (Humulin® 50/50): 100 units/mL (10 mL vial)
Injection, NPH human insulin suspension 70% and short-acting regular human insulin solution 30%:
Humulin® 70/30: 100 units/mL (3 mL disposable pen, 10 mL vial)
Novolin® 70/30: 100 units/mL (1.5 mL prefilled syringe, 10 mL vial)
Novolin® 70/30 [PenFill®]: 100 units/mL (1.5 mL cartridge, 3 mL cartridge)

Dosing

Adults & Elderly:

Diabetes mellitus: I.V. (Regular insulin), I.M., S.C.:

Note: The number and size of daily doses, time of administration, and diet and exercise require continuous medical supervision. In addition, specific formulations may require distinct administration procedures.

Rapid-acting (Lispro or aspart) should be given within 10-15 minutes before the start of a meal. Lispro may be given immediately after a meal.
Human regular insulin should be given within 30-60 minutes before a meal.
Intermediate-acting insulins may be administered 1-2 times/day.
Long-acting insulins may be administered once daily.

(Continued)

Insulin Preparations *(Continued)*

Insulin glargine (Lantus®) should be administered subcutaneously once daily at bedtime. Maintenance doses should be administered subcutaneously and sites should be rotated to prevent lipodystrophy.

Usual initial dose: Adults: 0.5-1 units/kg/day in divided doses; Adolescents (growth spurts): 0.8-1.2 units/kg/day in divided doses

Adjust dose to maintain premeal and bedtime blood glucose of 80-140 mg/dL (children <5 years: 100-200 mg/dL)

Insulin glargine (Lantus®):

Type 2 diabetes (patient not already on insulin): 10 units once daily, adjusted according to patient response (range in clinical study 2-100 units/day)

Patients already receiving insulin: In clinical studies, when changing to insulin glargine from once-daily NPH or Ultralente® insulin, the initial dose was not changed; when changing from twice-daily NPH to once daily insulin glargine, the total daily dose was reduced by 20% and adjusted according to patient response

Hyperkalemia: I.V. (Regular insulin): Administer calcium gluconate and $NaHCO_3$ first then 50% dextrose at 0.5-1 mL/kg and insulin 1 unit for every 4-5 g dextrose given

Diabetic ketoacidosis: Children and Adults: I.V. (Regular insulin): Loading dose: 0.1 unit/kg, then maintenance continuous infusion: 0.1 unit/kg/hour (range: 0.05-0.2 units/kg/hour depending upon the rate of decrease of serum glucose - too rapid decrease of serum glucose may lead to cerebral edema).

Optimum rate of decrease (serum glucose): 80-100 mg/dL/hour

Note: Newly diagnosed patients with IDDM presenting in DKA and patients with blood sugars <800 mg/dL may be relatively "sensitive" to insulin and should receive loading and initial maintenance doses approximately 1/2 of those indicated above.

Infusion should continue until reversal of acid-base derangement/ketonemia. Serum glucose is not a direct indicator of these abnormalities, and may decrease more rapidly than correction of the range of metabolic abnormalities.

Pediatrics: Refer to adult dosing. Adolescents (growth spurts): 0.8-1.2 units/kg/day in divided doses.

Renal Impairment: Insulin requirements are reduced due to changes in insulin clearance or metabolism.

Cl_{cr} 10-50 mL/minute: Administer 75% of normal dose.

Cl_{cr} <10 mL/minute: Administer 25% to 50% of normal dose and monitor glucose closely.

Hemodialysis: Because of a large molecular weight (6000 daltons), insulin is not significantly removed by either peritoneal or hemodialysis.

Supplemental dose is not necessary.

Peritoneal dialysis: Supplemental dose is not necessary.

Continuous arteriovenous or venovenous hemofiltration effects: Supplemental dose is not necessary.

Administration

I.V.: Regular insulin may be administered by S.C., I.M., or I.V. routes. Buffered insulin (Velosulin® BR) should not be administered with any other form of insulin.

I.V. administration (requires use of an infusion pump): **Only regular insulin** may be administered I.V.

To be ordered as units/hour: Example: Standard diluent of regular insulin only: 100 units/100 mL NS (can be given as a more diluted solution, ie, 100 units/250 mL NS)

Other: Cold injections should be avoided. S.C. administration is usually made into the thighs, arms, buttocks, or abdomen, with sites rotated. When mixing regular insulin with other preparations of insulin, regular insulin should be drawn into syringe first.

Buffered insulin (Velosulin® BR) should not be mixed with any other form of insulin

Insulin aspart (NovoLog®): Can be infused S.C. by external insulin pump; do not dilute or mix with other insulins when used in an external pump for S.C. infusion; should replace insulin in reservoir every 48 hours.

Insulin glargine (Lantus®): Cannot be diluted or mixed with any other insulin or solution; should be administered S.C. only; use only if solution is clear and colorless

Insulin lispro (Humalog®): May be administered within 15 minutes before or immediately after a meal

Stability

Storage:

Newer neutral formulation of regular insulin is stable at room temperature up to one month (studies indicate up to 24-30 months)

Insulin aspart (NovoLog®): Can be infused S.C. by external insulin pump; do not dilute or mix with other insulins when used in an external pump for S.C. infusion; insulin in reservoir should be replaced every 48 hours. Do not expose to temperatures ≥37°C (98.6°F).

Insulin glargine (Lantus®): When refrigeration is unavailable, 10 mL vials and 3 mL cartridges may be stored at room temperature for up to 28 days, 5 mL vials may be stored at room temperature for 14 days; solution not used within these times must be discarded

Freezing causes more damage to insulin than room temperatures up to 100°F. Avoid direct sunlight.

Reconstitution: Standard diluent: 100 units/100 mL NS; **Note:** All bags should be prepared fresh; tubing should be flushed 30 minutes prior to administration to allow adsorption as time permits

Compatibility: Buffered insulin (Velosulin® BR) should not be mixed with any other form of insulin. Isophane insulin suspension (NPH) is **compatible** with regular insulin. Protamine zinc insulin suspension is **compatible** with regular insulin.

Y-site administration: Incompatible with dopamine, nafcillin, norepinephrine, ranitidine

Compatibility when admixed: Incompatible with aminophylline, amobarbital, chlorothiazide, cytarabine, dobutamine, methylprednisolone sodium succinate, octreotide, pentobarbital, phenobarbital, phenytoin, thiopental

Monitoring Laboratory Tests Urine sugar and acetone, serum glucose, electrolytes, Hb A_{1c}, lipid profile

Monitoring and Teaching Issues

Physical Assessment: See Contraindications, Warnings/Precautions, and Dosing for use cautions. Assess potential for interactions with other prescriptions, OTC medications, or herbal products patient may be taking (see Drug Interactions). See Administration, and Compatibility for I.V. specifics. Assess results of laboratory tests (see Monitoring Laboratory Tests), therapeutic effects, and adverse response (eg, hypoglycemia - see Adverse Reactions and Overdose/Toxicology) at regular intervals during therapy. Teach patient proper use, including appropriate injection technique and syringe/needle disposal and monitoring requirements (or refer to diabetic educator), possible side effects and appropriate interventions, and adverse symptoms to report (see Patient Education). **Pregnancy risk factor B/C** - see Pregnancy Risk Factor for use cautions; benefits of use should outweigh possible risks.

Patient Education: Inform prescriber of all prescriptions, OTC medications, or herbal products you are taking, and any allergies you have. Do not take anything new during treatment unless approved by prescriber. This medication is used to control diabetes; it is not a cure. It is imperative to follow other components of prescribed treatment (eg, diet and exercise regimen). Take exactly as directed. Do not change dose or discontinue unless advised by prescriber. With insulin aspart (NovoLog®), you must start eating within 5-10 minutes after injection. If you experience hypoglycemic reaction, contact prescriber immediately. Always carry quick source of sugar with you. Monitor glucose levels as directed by prescriber. Report adverse side effects, including chest pain or palpitations; persistent fatigue, confusion, headache; skin rash or redness; numbness of mouth, lips, or tongue; muscle weakness or tremors; vision changes; difficulty breathing; or nausea, vomiting, or flu-like symptoms. **Pregnancy precaution:** Inform prescriber if you are or intend to become pregnant.

Dietary Issues: Dietary modification based on ADA recommendations is a part of therapy. Monitor potassium serum concentration.

Geriatric Considerations: How "tightly" a geriatric patient's blood glucose should be controlled is controversial; however, a fasting blood sugar <150 mg/dL is now an acceptable end point. Such a decision should be based on the patient's functional and cognitive status, how well they recognize hypoglycemic or hyperglycemic symptoms, and how to respond to them and their other disease states. Patients who are unable to accurately draw up their dose will need assistance such as prefilled syringes. Initial doses may require considerations for renal function in the elderly with dosing adjusted subsequently based on blood glucose monitoring.

Breast-feeding Issues: The gastrointestinal tract destroys insulin when administered orally and therefore would not be expected to be absorbed intact by the breast-feeding infant.

Pregnancy Issues: Does not cross the placenta. Insulin is the drug of choice for the control of diabetes mellitus during pregnancy. There are no well-controlled studies using insulin glargine (Lantus®) during pregnancy; use during pregnancy only if clearly needed.

Additional Information The term "purified" refers to insulin preparations containing no more than 10 ppm proinsulin (purified and human insulins are less immunogenic). Buffering agent in Velosulin® BR may alter the activity of other insulin products.

Related Information

Diabetes Mellitus Management *on page 1661*

Intal® *see* Cromolyn Sodium *on page 334*

Integrilin® *see* Eptifibatide *on page 481*

α-2-interferon *see* Interferon Alfa-2b *on page 719*

Interferon Alfa-2a (in ter FEER on AL fa too aye)

U.S. Brand Names Roferon-A®

Synonyms IFLrA; rIFN-A

Generic Available No

Pharmacologic Category Interferon

Pregnancy Risk Factor C

Lactation Enters breast milk/contraindicated (AAP rates "compatible")

Use

Patients >18 years of age: Hairy cell leukemia, AIDS-related Kaposi's sarcoma, chronic hepatitis C

Children and Adults: Chronic myelogenous leukemia (CML), Philadelphia chromosome positive, within 1 year of diagnosis (limited experience in children)

Use - Unlabeled/Investigational Adjuvant therapy for malignant melanoma, AIDS-related thrombocytopenia, cutaneous ulcerations of Behçet's disease, brain tumors, metastatic ileal carcinoid tumors, cervical and colorectal cancers, genital warts, idiopathic mixed cryoglobulinemia, hemangioma, hepatitis D, hepatocellular carcinoma, idiopathic hypereosinophilic syndrome, mycosis fungoides, Sézary syndrome, low-grade non-Hodgkin's lymphoma, macular degeneration, multiple myeloma, renal cell carcinoma, basal and squamous cell skin cancer, essential thrombocythemia, cutaneous T-cell lymphoma

Mechanism of Action/Effect Alpha interferons are a family of proteins that have antiviral, antiproliferative, and immune-regulating activity. Inhibits cell growth and proliferation and enhances immune response.

Contraindications Hypersensitivity to alfa interferon, benzyl alcohol, or any component of the formulation; autoimmune disorders, including autoimmune hepatitis; transplant patients receiving therapeutic immunosuppression; visceral AIDS-related Kaposi's sarcoma associated with rapidly-progressing or life-threatening disease

Warnings/Precautions Use with caution in patients with seizure disorders, brain metastases, compromised CNS, multiple sclerosis, and patients with pre-existing cardiac disease (ischemic or thromboembolic), arrhythmias, renal impairment (Cl_{cr} <50 mL/minute) or hepatic impairment, or myelosuppression; may cause severe psychiatric adverse events (psychosis,

(Continued)

Interferon Alfa-2a *(Continued)*

mania, depression, suicidal behavior/ideation) in patients with and without previous psychiatric symptoms, avoid use in severe psychiatric disorders or in patients with a history of depression; careful neuropsychiatric monitoring is required during therapy. May cause thyroid dysfunction or hyperglycemia, use caution in patients with diabetes. Use caution in patients with pulmonary dysfunction. Treatment should be discontinued in patients with worsening or persistently severe signs/symptoms of autoimmune, infectious, ischemic (including radiographic changes or worsening hepatic function), or neuropsychiatric disorders (including depression and/or suicidal thoughts/behavior). Safety and efficacy in children <18 years of age have not been established. Higher doses in the elderly or in malignancies other than hairy cell leukemia may result in severe obtundation. Ophthalmologic disorders (including retinal hemorrhages, cotton wool spots, and retinal artery or vein obstruction) have occurred in patients receiving alpha interferons. **Due to differences in dosage, patients should not change brands of interferons.** Injection solution contains benzyl alcohol, do not use in neonates or infants. Pregnancy risk C.

Drug Interactions

Cytochrome P450 Effect: Induces CYP1A2

Decreased Effect: Prednisone may decrease the therapeutic effects of interferon alpha. A decreased response to erythropoietin has been reported (case reports) in patients receiving interferons. Interferon alpha may decrease the serum concentrations of melphalan (may or may not decrease toxicity of melphalan).

Increased Effect/Toxicity: Cimetidine may augment the antitumor effects of interferon in melanoma. Theophylline clearance has been reported to be decreased in hepatitis patients receiving interferon. Vinblastine enhances interferon toxicity in several patients; increased incidence of paresthesia has also been noted. Interferons may increase the adverse/toxic effects of ACE inhibitors, specifically the development of granulocytopenia. Agranulocytosis has been reported with concurrent use of clozapine (case report). Interferons may increase the anticoagulant effects of warfarin, and interferons may increase serum levels of zidovudine.

Adverse Reactions Flu-like symptoms are common (up to 92%).

>10%:

Cardiovascular: Chest pain (4% to 11%), edema (11%), hypertension (11%)

Central nervous system: Psychiatric disturbances (including depression and suicidal behavior/ideation; reported incidence highly variable, generally >15%), fatigue (90%), headache (52%), dizziness (21%), irritability (15%), insomnia (14%), somnolence, lethargy, confusion, mental impairment, and motor weakness (most frequently seen at high doses [>100 million units], usually reverses within a few days); vertigo (19%); mental status changes (12%)

Dermatologic: Rash (usually maculopapular) on the trunk and extremities (7% to 18%), alopecia (19% to 22%), pruritus (13%), dry skin

Endocrine & metabolic: Hypocalcemia (10% to 51%), hyperglycemia (33% to 39%), elevation of transaminase levels (25% to 30%), elevation of alkaline phosphatase (48%)

Gastrointestinal: Loss of taste, anorexia (30% to 70%), nausea (28% to 53%), vomiting (10% to 30%, usually mild), diarrhea (22% to 34%, may be severe), taste change (13%), dry throat, xerostomia, abdominal cramps, abdominal pain

Hematologic (often due to underlying disease): Myelosuppression; neutropenia (32% to 70%); thrombocytopenia (22% to 70%); anemia (24% to 65%, may be dose-limiting, usually seen only during the first 6 months of therapy)

Onset: 7-10 days

Nadir: 14 days, may be delayed 20-40 days in hairy cell leukemia

Recovery: 21 days

Hepatic: Elevation of AST (SGOT) (77% to 80%), LDH (47%), bilirubin (31%)

Local: Injection site reaction (29%)

Neuromuscular & skeletal: Weakness (may be severe at doses >20,000,000 units/day); arthralgia and myalgia (5% to 73%, usually during the first 72 hours of treatment); rigors

Renal: Proteinuria (15% to 25%)

Respiratory: Cough (27%), irritation of oropharynx (14%)

Miscellaneous: Flu-like syndrome (up to 92% of patients), loss of taste, diaphoresis (15%)

1% to 10%:

Cardiovascular: Hypotension (6%), supraventricular tachyarrhythmias, palpitations (<3%), acute myocardial infarction (<1% to 1%)

Central nervous system: Confusion (10%), delirium

Dermatologic: Erythema (diffuse), urticaria

Endocrine & metabolic: Hyperphosphatemia (2%)

Gastrointestinal: Stomatitis, pancreatitis (<5%), flatulence, liver pain

Genitourinary: Impotence (6%), menstrual irregularities

Neuromuscular & skeletal: Leg cramps; peripheral neuropathy, paresthesias (7%), and numbness (4%) are more common in patients previously treated with vinca alkaloids or receiving concurrent vinblastine

Ocular: Conjunctivitis (4%)

Respiratory: Dyspnea (7.5%), epistaxis (4%), rhinitis (3%)

Miscellaneous: Antibody production to interferon (10%)

<1% (Limited to important or life-threatening): Acute renal failure, aplastic anemia, autoimmune reaction with worsening of liver disease, bronchospasm, cardiomyopathy, coma, CHF, GI hemorrhage, hallucinations, hemolytic anemia, hyponatremia (SIADH), mania, pneumonia, seizures, stroke, syncope, vasculitis

Overdosage/Toxicology Symptoms of overdose include CNS depression, obtundation, flu-like symptoms, and myelosuppression. Treatment is supportive.

Pharmacodynamics/Kinetics

Absorption: Filtered and absorbed at the renal tubule

Bioavailability: I.M.: 83%; S.C.: 90%

Half-Life Elimination: I.V.: 3.7-8.5 hours (mean: ~5 hours)

Time to Peak: Serum: I.M., S.C.: ~6-8 hours

Metabolism: Primarily renal; filtered through glomeruli and undergoes rapid proteolytic degradation during tubular reabsorption

Formulations

Injection, solution [multidose vial]: 6 million units/mL (3 mL) [contains benzyl alcohol]

Injection, solution, [single-dose prefilled syringe; S.C. use only]: 3 million units/0.5 mL (0.5 mL); 6 million units/0.5 mL (0.5 mL); 9 million units/0.5 mL (0.5 mL) [contains benzyl alcohol]

Injection, solution [single-dose vial]: 36 million units/mL (1 mL) [contains benzyl alcohol]

Dosing

Adults & Elderly: Refer to individual protocols.

Hairy cell leukemia: S.C., I.M.: 3 million units/day for 16-24 weeks, then 3 million units 3 times/week for up to 6-24 months

Chronic myelogenous leukemia (CML): S.C., I.M.: 9 million units/day, continue treatment until disease progression

AIDS-related Kaposi's sarcoma: S.C., I.M.: 36 million units/day for 10-12 weeks, then 36 million units 3 times/week; to minimize adverse reactions, can use escalating dose (3-, 9-, then 18 million units each day for 3 days, then 36 million units daily thereafter). If severe reactions occur, reduce dose by 50% or discontinue until reaction subsides.

Hepatitis C: S.C., I.M.: 3 million units 3 times/week for 12 months

Dosage adjustment for toxicity: If severe adverse reactions occur, modify dosage (reduce dose by 50%) or temporarily discontinue treatment until reaction subsides.

Pediatrics: Refer to individual protocols. Children (limited data):

Chronic myelogenous leukemia (CML): I.M.: 2.5-5 million units/m^2/day. **Note:** In juveniles, higher dosages (30 million units/m^2/day) have been associated with severe adverse events, including death.

Renal Impairment: Not removed by hemodialysis

Administration

I.M.: Reconstitute with recommended amount of bacteriostatic water and agitate gently; do not shake. **Note:** Different vial strengths require different amounts of diluent.

Other: S.C. administration is suggested for those who are at risk for bleeding or are thrombocytopenic. Rotate S.C. injection site. Patient should be well hydrated. Reconstitute with recommended amount of bacteriostatic water and agitate gently; do not shake. **Note:** Different vial strengths require different amounts of diluent.

Stability

Storage: Refrigerate (2°C to 8°C/36°F to 46°F); do not freeze; do not shake; after reconstitution, the solution is stable for 24 hours at room temperature and for 1 month when refrigerated

Monitoring Laboratory Tests Baseline chest x-ray, EKG, CBC with differential, liver function, electrolytes, platelets, weight; patients with pre-existing cardiac abnormalities, or in advanced stages of cancer should have EKGs taken before and during treatment.

Monitoring and Teaching Issues

Physical Assessment: Monitor laboratory results on a regular basis (see Monitoring Laboratory Tests). Monitor for effectiveness of therapy and possible adverse reactions (see Warnings/Precautions and Adverse Reactions). Assess knowledge/instruct patient/caregiver on appropriate reconstitution, injection and needle disposal, possible side effects, and symptoms to report (see Patient Education). **Pregnancy risk factor C** - barrier contraceptive teaching may be appropriate. Breast-feeding is contraindicated.

Patient Education: Use as directed; do not change dosage or schedule of administration without consulting prescriber. Maintain adequate hydration (2-3 L/day of fluids) unless advised by prescriber to restrict fluids. You may experience flu-like syndrome (acetaminophen may help); nausea, vomiting, dry mouth, or metallic taste (small, frequent meals, frequent mouth care, sucking lozenges, or chewing gum may help); or drowsiness, dizziness, agitation, abnormal thinking (use caution when driving or engaging in tasks requiring alertness until response to drug is known). Inform prescriber **immediately** if you feel depressed or have any thoughts of suicide. Report unusual bruising or bleeding; persistent abdominal disturbances; unusual fatigue; muscle pain or tremors; chest pain or palpitation; swelling of extremities or unusual weight gain; difficulty breathing; pain, swelling, or redness at injection site; or other unusual symptoms. **Pregnancy/breast-feeding precautions:** Inform prescriber if you are or intend to become pregnant. Do not breast-feed.

Geriatric Considerations: No specific data is available for the elderly; however, pay close attention to Warnings/Precautions.

Breast-feeding Issues: Women with hepatitis C should be instructed that there is a theoretical risk the virus may be transmitted in breast milk. HIV-infected mothers are discouraged from breast-feeding to decrease potential transmission of HIV.

Pregnancy Issues: Safety and efficacy for use during pregnancy have not been established. Interferon alpha has been shown to decrease serum estradiol and progesterone levels in humans. Menstrual irregularities and abortion have been reported in animals. Effective contraception is recommended during treatment.

Interferon Alfa-2b (in ter FEER on AL fa too bee)

U.S. Brand Names Intron® A

Synonyms INF-alpha 2; α-2-interferon; rLFN-α2

Generic Available No

Pharmacologic Category Interferon

Pregnancy Risk Factor C

Lactation Enters breast milk/not recommended (AAP rates "compatible")

Use

Patients >1 year of age: Chronic hepatitis B

(Continued)

Interferon Alfa-2b *(Continued)*

Patients >18 years of age: Condyloma acuminata, chronic hepatitis C, hairy cell leukemia, malignant melanoma, AIDS-related Kaposi's sarcoma, follicular non-Hodgkin's lymphoma

Use - Unlabeled/Investigational AIDS-related thrombocytopenia, cutaneous ulcerations of Behçet's disease, carcinoid syndrome, cervical cancer, lymphomatoid granulomatosis, genital herpes, hepatitis D, chronic myelogenous leukemia (CML), non-Hodgkin's lymphomas (other than follicular lymphoma, see approved use), polycythemia vera, medullary thyroid carcinoma, multiple myeloma, renal cell carcinoma, basal and squamous cell skin cancers, essential thrombocytopenia, thrombocytopenic purpura

Investigational: West Nile virus

Mechanism of Action/Effect Alpha interferons are a family of proteins that have antiviral, antiproliferative, and immune-regulating activity. Inhibits cell growth and proliferation and enhances immune response.

Contraindications Hypersensitivity to interferon alfa or any component of the formulation; patients with visceral AIDS-related Kaposi's sarcoma associated with rapidly-progressing or life-threatening disease; decompensated liver disease; autoimmune hepatitis; history of autoimmune disease; immunocompromised or transplant patients

Warnings/Precautions Use with caution in patients with a history of seizures, brain metastases, multiple sclerosis, cardiac disease (ischemic or thromboembolic), arrhythmias, myelosuppression, hepatic impairment, or renal dysfunction. Use caution in patients with a history of pulmonary disease, coagulopathy, thyroid disease, hypertension, or diabetes mellitus (particularly if prone to DKA). Avoid use in patient with autoimmune disorders; worsening of psoriasis and/or development of autoimmune disorders has been associated with alpha interferons. May cause severe psychiatric adverse events (psychosis, mania, depression, suicidal behavior/ideation) in patients with and without previous psychiatric symptoms, avoid use in severe psychiatric disorders or in patients with a history of depression; careful neuropsychiatric monitoring is required during therapy. Higher doses in elderly patients, or diseases other than hairy cell leukemia, may result in increased CNS toxicity. Ophthalmologic disorders (including retinal hemorrhages, cotton wool spots, and retinal artery or vein obstruction) have occurred in patients receiving alpha interferons.

A transient increase in SGOT (>2x baseline) is common in patients treated with interferon alfa-2b for chronic hepatitis. Therapy generally may continue, however, functional indicators (albumin, prothrombin time, bilirubin) should be monitored at 2-week intervals. Treatment should be discontinued in patients who develop severe pulmonary symptoms with chest x-ray changes, autoimmune disorders, worsening of hepatic function, psychiatric symptoms (including depression and/or suicidal thoughts/behaviors), severe or persistent infectious or ischemic disorders. Safety and efficacy in children <18 years of age have not been established (except in chronic hepatitis B). **Due to differences in dosage, patients should not change brands of interferons.**

Pregnancy risk C.

Drug Interactions

Cytochrome P450 Effect: Induces CYP1A2

Increased Effect/Toxicity: Cimetidine may augment the antitumor effects of interferon in melanoma. Theophylline clearance has been reported to be decreased in hepatitis patients receiving interferon. Vinblastine enhances interferon toxicity in several patients; increased incidence of paresthesia has also been noted. Interferons may increase the adverse/toxic effects of ACE inhibitors, specifically the development of granulocytopenia. Agranulocytosis has been reported with concurrent use of clozapine (case report). Interferons may increase the anticoagulant effects of warfarin, and interferons may increase serum levels of zidovudine.

Adverse Reactions Flu-like symptoms are common (up to 79%)

>10%:

Cardiovascular: Chest pain (2% to 28%)

Central nervous system: Fatigue (8% to 96%), headache (21% to 62%), fever (34% to 94%), depression (4% to 40%), somnolence (1% to 33%), irritability (1% to 22%), paresthesia (1% to 21%, more common in patients previously treated with vinca alkaloids or receiving concurrent vinblastine), dizziness (7% to 23%), confusion (1% to 12%), malaise (3% to 14%), pain (3% to 15%), insomnia (1% to 12%), impaired concentration (1% to 14%, usually reverses within a few days), amnesia (1% to 14%), chills (45% to 54%),

Dermatologic: Alopecia (8% to 38%), rash (usually maculopapular) on the trunk and extremities (1% to 25%), pruritus (3% to 11%), dry skin (1% to 10%)

Endocrine & metabolic: Hypocalcemia (10% to 51%), hyperglycemia (33% to 39%), amenorrhea (up to 12% in lymphoma)

Gastrointestinal: Anorexia (1% to 69%), nausea (19% to 66%), vomiting (2% to 32%, usually mild), diarrhea (2% to 45%, may be severe), taste change (2% to 24%), xerostomia (1% to 28%), abdominal pain (2% to 23%), gingivitis (2% to 14%), constipation (1% to 14%)

Hematologic: Myelosuppression; neutropenia (30% to 66%); thrombocytopenia (5% to 15%); anemia (15% to 32%, may be dose-limiting, usually seen only during the first 6 months of therapy)

Onset: 7-10 days

Nadir: 14 days, may be delayed 20-40 days in hairy cell leukemia

Recovery: 21 days

Hepatic: Increased transaminases (increased SGOT in up to 63%), elevation of alkaline phosphatase (48%), right upper quadrant pain (15% in hepatitis C)

Local: Injection site reaction (1% to 20%)

Neuromuscular & skeletal: Weakness (5% to 63%) may be severe at doses >20,000,000 units/day; mild arthralgia and myalgia (5% to 75% - usually during the first 72 hours of treatment), rigors (2% to 42%), back pain (1% to 19%), musculoskeletal pain (1% to 21%), paresthesia (1% to 21%)

Renal: Urinary tract infection (up to 5% in hepatitis C)

Respiratory: Dyspnea (1% to 34%), cough (1% to 31%), pharyngitis (1% to 31%),
Miscellaneous: Loss of smell, flu-like symptoms (5% to 79%), diaphoresis (2% to 21%)

5% to 10%:

Cardiovascular: Hypertension (9% in hepatitis C)
Central nervous system: Anxiety (1% to 9%), nervousness (1% to 3%), vertigo (up to 8% in lymphoma)
Dermatologic: Dermatitis (1% to 8%)
Endocrine & metabolic: Decreased libido (1% to 5%)
Gastrointestinal: Loose stools (1% to 21%), dyspepsia (2% to 8%)
Neuromuscular & skeletal: Hypoesthesia (1% to 10%)
Respiratory: Nasal congestion (1% to 10%)

<5% (Limited to important or life-threatening): Acute hypersensitivity reactions, allergic reactions, angina, aphasia, arrhythmia, ataxia, atrial fibrillation, Bell's palsy, bronchospasm, cardiomyopathy, CHF, coma, depression, epidermal necrolysis, extrapyramidal disorder, gastrointestinal hemorrhage, gingival hyperplasia, granulocytopenia, hallucinations, hemolytic anemia, hemoptysis, hepatic encephalopathy (rare), hepatic failure (rare), hepatotoxic reaction, hypoventilation, jaundice, lupus erythematosus, mania, myocardial infarction, nephrotic syndrome, pancreatitis, polyarteritis nodosa, psychosis, pulmonary embolism, pulmonary fibrosis, Raynaud's phenomenon, renal failure, seizures, stroke, suicidal ideation, suicide attempt, syncope, tendonitis, thrombocytopenic purpura, thrombosis, vasculitis

Overdosage/Toxicology Symptoms of overdose include CNS depression, obtundation, flu-like symptoms, and myelosuppression. Treatment is supportive.

Pharmacodynamics/Kinetics

Bioavailability: I.M.: 83%; S.C.: 90%

Half-Life Elimination: I.M., I.V.: 2 hours; S.C.: 3 hours

Time to Peak: Serum: I.M., S.C.: ~3-12 hours

Metabolism: Primarily renal

Formulations

Injection, powder for reconstitution: 3 million units; 5 million units; 10 million units; 18 million units; 25 million units; 50 million units [contains human albumin; diluent contains benzyl alcohol]

Injection, solution [multidose prefilled pen]:
Delivers 3 million units/0.2 mL (1.5 mL) [delivers 6 doses; 18 million units]
Delivers 5 million units/0.2 mL (1.5 mL) [delivers 6 doses; 30 million units]
Delivers 10 million units/0.2 mL (1.5 mL) [delivers 6 doses; 60 million units]

Injection, solution [multidose vial]: 6 million units/mL (3 mL); 10 million units/mL (2.5 mL)

Injection, solution [single-dose vial]: 3 million units/ 0.5 mL (0.5 mL); 5 million units/0.5 mL (0.5 mL); 10 million units/ mL (1 mL)

See also Interferon Alfa-2b and Ribavirin Combination Pack monograph.

Dosing

Adults & Elderly: Refer to individual protocols.

Hairy cell leukemia: I.M., S.C.: 2 million units/m^2 3 times/week for 2-6 months

Lymphoma (follicular): S.C.: 5 million units 3 times/week for up to 18 months

Malignant melanoma: 20 million units/m^2 I.V. for 5 consecutive days per week for 4 weeks, then 10 million units/m^2 S.C. 3 times/week for 48 weeks

AIDS-related Kaposi's sarcoma: I.M., S.C.: 30 million units/m^2 3 times/week

Chronic hepatitis B: I.M., S.C.: 5 million units/day or 10 million units 3 times/week for 16 weeks

Chronic hepatitis C: I.M., S.C.: 3 million units 3 times/week for 16 weeks. In patients with normalization of ALT at 16 weeks, continue treatment for 18-24 months; consider discontinuation if normalization does not occur at 16 weeks. **Note:** May be used in combination therapy with ribavirin in previously untreated patients or in patients who relapse following alpha interferon therapy; refer to Interferon Alfa-2b and Ribavirin Combination Pack monograph.

Condyloma acuminata: Intralesionally: 1 million units/lesion (maximum: 5 lesions/treatment) 3 times/week (on alternate days) for 3 weeks. Use 1 million unit per 0.1 mL concentration.

Pediatrics: Refer to individual protocols.

Chronic hepatitis B: S.C.: Children 1-17 years: 3 million units/m^2 3 times/week for 1 week; then 6 million units/m^2 3 times/week; maximum: 10 million units 3 times/week; total duration of therapy 16-24 weeks

Administration

Other: S.C. administration is suggested for those who are at risk for bleeding or are thrombocytopenic. Rotate S.C. injection site. Patient should be well hydrated. Reconstitute with recommended amount of bacteriostatic water and agitate gently; do not shake. **Note:** Different vial strengths require different amounts of diluent. Do not use 3-, 5-, 18-, and 25 million unit strengths intralesionally, solutions are hypertonic; 50 million unit strength is not for use in condylomata, hairy cell leukemia, or chronic hepatitis.

Stability

Storage: Store intact vials at refrigeration (2°C to 8°C); powder and premixed solutions are stable at room temperature for 7 days. Reconstitute vials with diluent; reconstituted solution is stable for 30 days under refrigeration (2°C to 8°C).

Reconstitution: Reconstitute vials with diluent. Solution is stable for 30 days under refrigeration (2°C to 8°C).

Compatibility: Stable in LR, NS; **incompatible** with D_5W

Monitoring Laboratory Tests Baseline chest x-ray, EKG, CBC with differential, liver function, electrolytes, platelets; patients with pre-existing cardiac abnormalities, or in advanced stages of cancer should have EKGs taken before and during treatment. Discontinue if neutrophils <0.5 x 10^9/L, platelets <25 x 10^9/L.

Monitoring and Teaching Issues

Physical Assessment: Monitor laboratory results on a regular basis (see Monitoring Laboratory Tests). Monitor for effectiveness of therapy and possible adverse reactions (see

(Continued)

Interferon Alfa-2b *(Continued)*

Warnings/Precautions and Adverse Reactions). Assess knowledge/instruct patient/caregiver on appropriate reconstitution, injection and needle disposal, possible side effects, and symptoms to report (see Patient Education). **Pregnancy risk factor C** - barrier contraceptive teaching may be appropriate. Breast-feeding is not recommended.

Patient Education: Use as directed; do not change dosage or schedule of administration without consulting prescriber. Maintain adequate hydration (2-3 L/day of fluids) unless advised by prescriber to restrict fluids. You may experience flu-like syndrome (acetaminophen may help); nausea, vomiting, dry mouth, or metallic taste (small, frequent meals, frequent mouth care, sucking lozenges, or chewing gum may help); fatigue, drowsiness, insomnia, dizziness, agitation, abnormal thinking (use caution when driving or engaging in tasks requiring alertness until response to drug is known). Inform prescriber **immediately** if you feel depressed or have any thoughts of suicide. Report unusual bruising or bleeding; persistent abdominal disturbances; unusual fatigue; muscle pain or tremors; chest pain or palpitation; swelling of extremities or unusual weight gain; difficulty breathing; pain, swelling, or redness at injection site; or other unusual symptoms. **Pregnancy/breast-feeding precautions:** Inform prescriber if you are or intend to become pregnant. Breast-feeding is not recommended.

Breast-feeding Issues: Women with hepatitis C should be instructed that there is a theoretical risk the virus may be transmitted in breast milk. HIV-infected mothers are discouraged from breast-feeding to decrease potential transmission of HIV.

Pregnancy Issues: Safety and efficacy for use during pregnancy have not been established. Interferon alpha has been shown to decrease serum estradiol and progesterone levels in humans. Menstrual irregularities and abortion have been reported in animals. Effective contraception is recommended during treatment.

Interferon Alfa-2b and Ribavirin

(in ter FEER on AL fa too bee & rye ba VYE rin)

U.S. Brand Names Rebetron®

Synonyms Interferon Alfa-2b and Ribavirin Combination Pack; Ribavirin and Interferon Alfa-2b Combination Pack

Generic Available No

Pharmacologic Category Antiviral Agent; Interferon

Pregnancy Risk Factor X

Lactation Excretion in breast milk unknown/not recommended

Use The combination therapy of oral ribavirin with interferon alfa-2b, recombinant (Intron® A) injection is indicated for the treatment of chronic hepatitis C in patients with compensated liver disease who have relapsed after alpha interferon therapy.

Mechanism of Action/Effect

Interferon Alfa-2b: Alpha interferons are a family of proteins, produced by nucleated cells, that have antiviral, antiproliferative, and immune-regulating activity. There are 16 known subtypes of alpha interferons. Interferons interact with cells through high affinity cell surface receptors. Following activation, multiple effects can be detected including induction of gene transcription. Inhibits cellular growth, alters the state of cellular differentiation, interferes with oncogene expression, alters cell surface antigen expression, increases phagocytic activity of macrophages, and augments cytotoxicity of lymphocytes for target cells

Ribavirin: Inhibits replication of RNA and DNA viruses; inhibits influenza virus RNA polymerase activity and inhibits the initiation and elongation of RNA fragments resulting in inhibition of viral protein synthesis

Contraindications Hypersensitivity to interferon alfa-2b, ribavirin, or any component of the formulation; autoimmune hepatitis; males with a pregnant female partner; pregnancy

Warnings/Precautions

Interferon alfa-2b: Use with caution in patients with a history of seizures, brain metastases, multiple sclerosis, cardiac disease (ischemic or thromboembolic), arrhythmias, myelosuppression, hepatic impairment, or renal dysfunction (Cl_{cr} <50 mL/minute). Use caution in patients with a history of pulmonary disease, coagulopathy, thyroid disease, hypertension, or diabetes mellitus (particularly if prone to DKA). Caution in patients receiving drugs that may cause lactic acidosis (eg, nucleoside analogues). May cause severe psychiatric adverse events in patients with and without previous psychiatric symptoms, avoid use in severe psychiatric disorders or in patients with a history of depression; careful neuropsychiatric monitoring is required during therapy. Avoid use in patient with autoimmune disorders. Higher doses in elderly patients, or diseases other than hairy cell leukemia, may result in increased CNS toxicity. Treatment should be discontinued in patients who develop severe pulmonary symptoms with chest x-ray changes, autoimmune disorders, worsening of hepatic function, psychiatric symptoms (including depression and/or suicidal thoughts/behaviors), ischemic and/or infectious disorders. Ophthalmologic disorders (including retinal hemorrhages, cotton wool spots and retinal artery or vein obstruction) have occurred in patients receiving alpha interferons. Hypertriglyceridemia has been reported (discontinue if severe).

Safety and efficacy in children <18 years of age have not been established. Do not treat patients with visceral AIDS-related Kaposi's sarcoma associated with rapidly-progressing or life-threatening disease. A transient increase in SGOT (>2x baseline) is common in patients treated with interferon alfa-2b for chronic hepatitis. Therapy generally may continue, however, functional indicators (albumin, prothrombin time, bilirubin) should be monitored at 2-week intervals. **Due to differences in dosage, patients should not change brands of interferons.**

Intron® A may cause bone marrow suppression, including very rarely, aplastic anemia. Hemolytic anemia (hemoglobin <10 g/dL) was observed in 10% of treated patients in clinical trials; anemia occurred within 1-2 weeks of initiation of therapy.

Ribavirin: Oral: Anemia has been observed in patients receiving the interferon/ribavirin combination. Severe psychiatric events have also occurred including depression and suicidal behavior during combination therapy; avoid use in patients with a psychiatric history. Hemolytic anemia is a significant toxicity; usually occurring within 1-2 weeks. Assess cardiac disease before initiation. Anemia may worsen underlying cardiac disease; use caution. If any deterioration in cardiovascular status occurs, discontinue therapy. Negative pregnancy test is required before initiation and monthly thereafter. Avoid pregnancy in female patients and female partners of patients during therapy by using two effective forms of contraception; continue contraceptive measures for at least 6 months after completion of therapy. If patient or female partner becomes pregnant during treatment, she should be counseled about potential risks of exposure. Discontinue therapy in suspected/confirmed pancreatitis. Use caution in elderly patients; higher frequency of anemia; take renal function into consideration before initiating. Safety and efficacy have not been established in organ transplant patients, decompensated liver disease, concurrent hepatitis B virus or HIV exposure, or pediatric patients. Use caution in patients receiving concurrent medications which may cause lactic acidosis (ie, nucleoside analogues).

Drug Interactions

Decreased Effect:

Interferon alpha: Prednisone may decrease the therapeutic effects of interferon alpha. A decreased response to erythropoietin has been reported (case reports) in patients receiving interferons. Interferon alpha may decrease the serum concentrations of melphalan (may or may not decrease toxicity of melphalan).

Ribavirin: Decreased effect of zidovudine.

Increased Effect/Toxicity: Interferon alpha: Cimetidine may augment the antitumor effects of interferon in melanoma. Theophylline clearance has been reported to be decreased in hepatitis patients receiving interferon. Vinblastine enhances interferon toxicity in several patients; increased incidence of paresthesia has also been noted. Interferons may increase the adverse/toxic effects of ACE inhibitors, specifically the development of granulocytopenia. Agranulocytosis has been reported with concurrent use of clozapine (case report). Interferons may increase the anticoagulant effects of warfarin, and interferons may increase serum levels of zidovudine. Concomitant use of ribavirin and nucleoside analogues may increase the risk of developing lactic acidosis.

Adverse Reactions Note: Adverse reactions listed are specific to combination regimen in previously untreated hepatitis patients. See individual agents for additional adverse reactions reported with each agent during therapy for other diseases.

>10%

Central nervous system: Fatigue (68%), headache (63%), insomnia (39%), fever (37%), depression (32%), irritability (23%), dizziness (17%), impaired concentration (11%)

Dermatologic: Alopecia (28%), pruritus (21%), rash (20%)

Gastrointestinal: Nausea (38%), anorexia (27%), dyspepsia (14%), vomiting (11%)

Hematologic: Leukopenia, neutropenia (usually recovers within 4 weeks of treatment discontinuation), anemia

Hepatic: Hyperbilirubinemia (27% - only 0.9% >3.0 mg/dL)

Local: Injection site inflammation (13%)

Neuromuscular & skeletal: Myalgia (61%), rigors (40%), arthralgia (30%), musculoskeletal pain (20%)

Respiratory: Dyspnea (19%)

Miscellaneous: Flu-like syndrome (14%)

1% to 10%:

Cardiovascular: Chest pain (5%)

Central nervous system: Emotional lability (7%), nervousness (4%)

Endocrine & metabolic: Thyroid abnormalities (hyper- or hypothyroidism), increased serum uric acid, hyperglycemia

Gastrointestinal; taste perversion (7%)

Hematologic: Hemolytic anemia (10%), thrombocytopenia, anemia

Local: Injection site reaction (7%)

Neuromuscular & skeletal: Weakness (9%)

Respiratory: Sinusitis (9%)

<1% (Limited to important or life-threatening): Acute hypersensitivity reactions, anaphylaxis, angioedema, aplastic anemia (very rare), arrhythmia, bronchoconstriction, cardiomyopathy, cotton wool spots, diabetes, hallucinations, hearing loss, hepatotoxic reactions, hypertriglyceridemia, hypotension, myocardial infarction, nephrotic syndrome, pancreatitis, pneumonia, pneumonitis, renal failure, retinal hemorrhages, retinal artery or vein obstruction, severe psychiatric reactions, suicidal behavior, suicidal ideation, tinnitus, urticaria; rare cases of autoimmune diseases including vasculitis, polyarteritis reaction, rheumatoid arthritis, lupus erythematosus, and Raynaud's phenomenon

Overdosage/Toxicology Interferon Alfa-2b: Signs and symptoms of overdose include CNS depression, obtundation, flu-like symptoms, myelosuppression; treatment is supportive.

Pharmacokinetic Note See individual agents.

Formulations

Combination package for patients ≥75 kg:

Injection, solution: Interferon alfa-2b (Intron® A): 3 million int. units/0.5 mL (0.5 mL) [6 vials (3 million int. units/vial), 6 syringes and alcohol swabs]

Capsules: Ribavirin (Rebetol®): 200 mg (70s)

Injection, solution: Interferon alfa-2b (Intron® A): 3 million int. units/0.5 mL (3.8 mL) [1 multidose vial (18 million int. units/vial), 6 syringes and alcohol swabs]

Capsules: Ribavirin (Rebetol®): 200 mg (70s)

Injection, solution: Interferon alfa-2b (Intron® A): 3 million int. units/0.2 mL (1.5 mL) [1 multidose pen (18 million int. units/pen), 6 needles and alcohol swabs]

Capsules: Ribavirin (Rebetol®): 200 mg (70s)

Combination package for patients >75 kg:

Injection, solution: Interferon alfa-2b (Intron® A): 3 million int. units/0.5 mL (0.5 mL) [6 vials (3 million int. units/vial), 6 syringes and alcohol swabs]

Capsules: Ribavirin (Rebetol®): 200 mg (84s)

(Continued)

Interferon Alfa-2b and Ribavirin *(Continued)*

Injection, solution: Interferon alfa-2b (Intron® A): 3 million int. units/0.5 mL (3.8 mL) [1 multidose vial (18 million int. units/vial), 6 syringes and alcohol swabs]
Capsules: Ribavirin (Rebetol®): 200 mg (84s)

Injection, solution: Interferon alfa-2b (Intron® A): 3 million int. units/0.2 mL (1.5 mL) [1 multidose pen (18 million int. units/pen), 6 needles and alcohol swabs]
Capsules: Ribavirin (Rebetol®): 200 mg (84s)

Combination package for Rebetol® dose reduction:
Injection, solution: Interferon alfa-2b (Intron® A): 3 million int. units/0.5 mL (0.5 mL) [6 vials (3 million int. units/vial), 6 syringes and alcohol swabs]
Capsules: Ribavirin (Rebetol®): 200 mg (42s)

Injection, solution: Interferon alfa-2b (Intron® A): 3 million int. units/0.5 mL (3.8 mL) [1 multidose vial (18 million int. units/vial), 6 syringes and alcohol swabs]
Capsules: Ribavirin (Rebetol®): 200 mg (42s)

Injection, solution: Interferon alfa-2b (Intron® A): 3 million int. units/0.2 mL (1.5 mL) [1 multidose pen (18 million int. units/pen), 6 needles and alcohol swabs]
Capsules: Ribavirin (Rebetol®): 200 mg (42s)

Dosing

Adults & Elderly: Chronic hepatitis C: Recommended dosage of combination therapy:
Intron® A: S.C.: 3 million int. units 3 times/week **and**
Rebetrol® capsule: Oral: Range: 1000-1200 mg in a divided daily (morning and evening) dose for 24 weeks
≤75 kg (165 pounds): 1000 mg/day (two 200 mg capsules in the morning and three 200 mg capsules in the evening)
>75 kg: 1200 mg/day (three 200 mg capsules in the morning and three 200 mg capsules in the evening)

Pediatrics: Chronic hepatitis C: **Note:** Safety and efficacy have not been established; dosing based on pharmacokinetic profile: Recommended dosage of combination therapy (Intron® A with Rebetrol®):
Intron® A: S.C.:
25-61 kg: 3 million int. units/m^2 3 times/week
>61 kg: Refer to adult dosing
Rebetrol® capsule: Oral:
25-36 kg: 400 mg/day (200 mg twice daily)
37-49 kg: 600 mg/day (200 mg in morning and 400 mg in evening)
50-61 kg: 800 mg/day (400 mg twice daily)
>61 kg: Refer to adult dosing

Stability

Storage: Store the Rebetol® capsules plus Intron® A injection combination package refrigerated between 2°C and 8°C (36°F and 46°F)
When separated, the individual carton of Rebetol® capsules should be stored refrigerated between 2°C and 8°C (36°F and 46°F) or at 25°C (77°F); excursions are permitted between 15°C and 30°C (59°F and 86°F)
When separated, the individual carton or vial of Intron® A injection and the Intron® A multidose pen should be stored refrigerated between 2°C and 8°C (36°F and 46°F)

Monitoring Laboratory Tests Obtain pretreatment CBC, liver function tests, TSH, and electrolytes and monitor routinely throughout therapy (at 2 weeks and 4 weeks, more frequently if indicated); discontinue if WBC <1.0 x 10^9/L, neutrophils <0.5 x 10^9/L, platelets <25 x 10^9/L, or if hemoglobin <8.5 g/dL (in cardiac patients, discontinue if hemoglobin <12 g/dL after 4 weeks of dosage reduction). Baseline chest x-ray, EKG, weight; patients with pre-existing cardiac abnormalities, or in advanced stages of cancer should have EKGs taken before and during treatment; reticulocyte count, I & O

Monitoring and Teaching Issues

Physical Assessment: Assess other medications patient may be taking for increased risk of drug/drug interactions (see Drug Interactions). See Warnings/Precautions, Contraindications, and Adverse Reactions for use cautions. Monitor laboratory results and adverse reactions (see Adverse Reactions) on a frequent and regular basis during therapy. (See monographs for Interferon Alfa-2b and Ribavirin). See specific Administration directions. Assess knowledge/teach patient appropriate use (including appropriate injection technique and needle disposal), interventions to reduce side effects, and adverse symptoms to report (see Patient Education). **Pregnancy risk factor X** - determine that patient is not pregnant before beginning treatment and do not give to women of childbearing age or to males who may have intercourse with women of childbearing ages unless both male and female are capable of complying with barrier contraceptive measures for 6 months prior to therapy and for 1 month following therapy. Breast-feeding is not recommended.

Patient Education: This a combination therapy. Both the injections and the oral capsules are necessary for effective therapy. Follow administration directions exactly and dispose of needles as instructed. Do not discontinue, alter dose or frequency without consulting prescriber. Take at the same times each day. Maintain adequate hydration (2-3 L/day of fluids) unless advised by prescriber to restrict fluids. You may experience flu-like symptoms (consult prescriber for relief); nausea, vomiting, or GI upset (small, frequent meals, frequent mouth care, sucking lozenges, or chewing gum may help); or insomnia, drowsiness, lethargy, fatigue, dizziness, abnormal thinking (use caution when driving or engaging in tasks that require alertness until response to drug is known). Report unusual bruising or bleeding, inflammation or pain at injection site, persistent GI disturbances, muscle pain or tremors, chest pain or palpitations, swelling of extremities, unusual weight gain, or rash. Contact prescriber immediately if you experience unusual agitation, nervousness, feelings of depression, or have thoughts of suicide. **Pregnancy/breast-feeding precautions:** This drug will cause severe fetal defects. Inform prescriber if you are pregnant. Females must not get pregnant or males must not cause a pregnancy during therapy, and for 6 months after therapy is completed. Pregnancy tests are required for females. Consult prescriber for instruction on appropriate barrier contraceptive measures. Breast-feeding is not recommended.

Dietary Issues: Take oral formulation without regard to food, but always in a consistent manner with respect to food intake (ie, always take with food or always take on an empty stomach).

Breast-feeding Issues: Women with hepatitis C should be instructed that there is a theoretical risk the virus may be transmitted in breast milk.

Pregnancy Issues: Abortifacient and teratogenic effects have been reported. Women of childbearing potential should not be treated unless 2 reliable forms of contraception are used. In addition, male patients and their female partners must also use 2 reliable forms of contraception. Pregnancy must be avoided for 6 months following therapy.

Additional Information

Rebetron™ - Guidelines for Dosing Modifications

Hemoglobin:

<10 g/dL: Reduce dose of Rebetol® to 600 mg/day

<8.5 d/dL: Permanently discontinue Rebetol®/Intron® A combination therapy

Hemoglobin in patients with cardiac history:

≥2 g/dL decrease during any 4-week period during therapy: Reduce of Rebetol® to 600 mg/day, reduce dose of Intron® A to 1.5 million int. units 3 times/week

<12 g/dL after 4 weeks on reduced dose: Permanently discontinue Rebetol®/Intron® A combination therapy

White blood count:

<1.5 x 10^9/L: Reduce Intron® A dose to 1.5 million int. units 3 times/week

<1.0 x 10^9/L: Permanently discontinue Rebetol®/Intron® A combination therapy

Neutrophil count:

<0.75 x 10^9/L: Reduce Intron® A dose to 1.5 million int. units 3 times/week

<0.5 x 10^9/L: Permanently discontinue Rebetol®/Intron® A combination therapy

Platelet count:

<50 x 10^9/L: Reduce Intron® A dose to 1.5 million int. units 3 times/week

<25 x 10^9/L: Permanently discontinue Rebetol®/Intron® A combination therapy

Interferon Alfa-2b and Ribavirin Combination Pack *see* Interferon Alfa-2b and Ribavirin *on page 722*

Interferon Alfacon-1 (in ter FEER on AL fa con one)

U.S. Brand Names Infergen®

Generic Available No

Pharmacologic Category Interferon

Pregnancy Risk Factor C

Lactation Excretion in breast milk unknown/use caution (AAP rates "compatible")

Use Treatment of chronic hepatitis C virus (HCV) infection in patients ≥18 years of age with compensated liver disease and anti-HCV serum antibodies or HCV RNA.

Mechanism of Action/Effect Alpha interferons are a family of proteins, produced by nucleated cells, that have antiviral, antiproliferative, and immune-regulating activity. There are at least 25 alpha interferons identified. Interferons interact with cells through high affinity cell surface receptors. Following activation, multiple effects can be detected. Interferons induce gene transcription, inhibit cellular growth, alter the state of cellular differentiation, interfere with oncogene expression, alter cell surface antigen expression, increase phagocytic activity of macrophages, and augment cytotoxicity of lymphocytes for target cells. Although all alpha interferons share similar properties, the actual biological effects vary between subtypes.

Contraindications Hypersensitivity to interferon alfacon-1 or any component of the formulation, other alpha interferons, or *E. coli*-derived products

Warnings/Precautions Severe psychiatric adverse effects, including depression, suicidal ideation, and suicide attempt, may occur. Avoid use in severe psychiatric disorders. Use with caution in patients with a history of depression. Use with caution in patients with prior cardiac disease (ischemic or thromboembolic), arrhythmias, patients who are chronically immunosuppressed, and patients with endocrine disorders. Do not use in patients with hepatic decompensation. Ophthalmologic disorders (including retinal hemorrhages, cotton wool spots and retinal artery or vein obstruction) have occurred in patients using other alpha interferons. Prior to start of therapy, visual exams are recommended for patients with diabetes mellitus or hypertension. Treatment should be discontinued in patients with worsening or persistently severe signs/symptoms of autoimmune, infectious, ischemic (including radiographic changes or worsening hepatic function), or neuropsychiatric disorders (including depression and/or suicidal thoughts/behavior). Use caution in patients with autoimmune disorders; type-1 interferon therapy has been reported to exacerbate autoimmune diseases. Do not use interferon alfacon-1 in patients with autoimmune hepatitis. Use caution in patients with low peripheral blood counts or myelosuppression, including concurrent use of myelosuppressive therapy. Safety and efficacy have not been determined for patients <18 years of age. Pregnancy risk C.

Drug Interactions

Decreased Effect: Prednisone may decrease the therapeutic effects of interferon alpha. A decreased response to erythropoietin has been reported (case reports) in patients receiving interferons. Interferon alpha may decrease the serum concentrations of melphalan (may or may not decrease toxicity of melphalan).

Increased Effect/Toxicity: Cimetidine may augment the antitumor effects of interferon in melanoma. Theophylline clearance has been reported to be decreased in hepatitis patients receiving interferon. Vinblastine enhances interferon toxicity in several patients; increased incidence of paresthesia has also been noted. Interferons may increase the adverse/toxic effects of ACE inhibitors, specifically the development of granulocytopenia. Agranulocytosis has been reported with concurrent use of clozapine (case report). Interferons may increase the anticoagulant effects of warfarin, and interferons may increase serum levels of zidovudine.

Adverse Reactions Adverse reactions reported using 9 mcg/dose interferon alfacon-1 3 times/week. Reactions listed were reported in ≥5% of patients treated.

(Continued)

Interferon Alfacon-1 *(Continued)*

>10%:

Central nervous system: Headache (82%), fatigue (69%), fever (61%), insomnia (39%), nervousness (31%), depression (26%), dizziness (22%), anxiety (19%), noncardiac chest pain (13%), emotional lability (12%), malaise (11%)

Dermatologic: Alopecia (14%), pruritus (14%), rash (13%)

Endocrine & metabolic: Hot flashes (13%)

Gastrointestinal: Abdominal pain (41%), nausea (40%), diarrhea (29%), anorexia (24%), dyspepsia (21%), vomiting (12%)

Hematologic: Granulocytopenia (23%), thrombocytopenia (19%), leukopenia (15%)

Local: Injection site erythema (23%)

Neuromuscular & skeletal: Myalgia (58%), body pain (54%), arthralgia (51%), back pain (42%), limb pain (26%), neck pain (14%), skeletal pain (14%), paresthesia (13%)

Respiratory: Pharyngitis (34%), upper respiratory tract infection (31%), cough (22%), sinusitis (17%), rhinitis (13%), respiratory tract congestion (12%)

Miscellaneous: Flu-like syndrome (15%), increased diaphoresis (12%)

1% to 10%:

Cardiovascular: Peripheral edema (9%), hypertension (5%), tachycardia (4%), palpitations (3%)

Central nervous system: Amnesia (10%), hypoesthesia (10%), abnormal thinking (8%), agitation (6%), confusion (4%), somnolence (4%)

Dermatologic: Bruising (6%), erythema (6%), dry skin (6%), wound (4%)

Endocrine & metabolic: Thyroid test abnormalities (9%), dysmenorrhea (9%), increased triglycerides (6%), menstrual disorder (6%), decreased libido (5%), hypothyroidism (4%)

Gastrointestinal: Constipation (9%), flatulence (8%), toothache (7%), decreased salivation (6%), hemorrhoids (6%), weight loss (5%), taste perversion (3%)

Genitourinary: Vaginitis (8%), genital moniliasis (2%)

Hepatic: Hepatomegaly (5%), liver tenderness (5%), increased prothrombin time (3%)

Local: Injection site pain (9%), access pain (8%), injection site bruising (6%)

Neuromuscular & skeletal: Weakness (9%), hypertonia (7%), musculoskeletal disorder (4%)

Ocular: Conjunctivitis (8%), eye pain (5%), vision abnormalities (3%)

Otic: Tinnitus (6%), earache (5%), otitis (2%)

Respiratory: Upper respiratory tract congestion (10%), epistaxis (8%), dyspnea (7%), bronchitis (6%)

Miscellaneous: Allergic reaction (7%), lymphadenopathy (6%), lymphocytosis (5%), infection (3%)

Flu-like symptoms, which included headache, fatigue, fever, myalgia, rigors, arthralgia, and increased diaphoresis, were the most commonly reported adverse reaction. This was reported separately from flu-like syndrome. Most patients were treated symptomatically.

Other adverse reactions associated with interferon therapy include arrhythmia, autoimmune disorders, chest pain, hepatotoxic reactions, lupus erythematosus, myocardial infarction, neuropsychiatric disorders (including suicidal thoughts/behavior), pneumonia, pneumonitis, severe hypersensitivity reactions (rare), vasculitis

Overdosage/Toxicology One overdose has been reported. A patient received ten times the prescribed dose (150 mcg) for 3 days. In addition to an increase in anorexia, chills, fever, and myalgia, there was also an increase in ALT, AST, and LDH. Laboratory values reportedly returned to baseline within 30 days.

Pharmacokinetic Note Pharmacokinetic studies have not been conducted on patients with chronic hepatitis C.

Pharmacodynamics/Kinetics

Time to Peak: Healthy volunteers: 24-36 hours

Formulations Injection, solution [preservative free; prefilled syringe or single-dose vial]; 30 mcg/mL (0.3 mL, 0.5 mL)

Dosing

Adults & Elderly:

Chronic HCV infection: S.C.: 9 mcg 3 times/week for 24 weeks; allow 48 hours between doses.

Patients who have previously tolerated interferon therapy but did not respond or relapsed: S.C.: 15 mcg 3 times/week for 6 months

Dose reduction for toxicity: Dose should be held in patients who experience a severe adverse reaction, and treatment should be stopped or decreased if the reaction does not become tolerable.

Doses were reduced from 9 mcg to 7.5 mcg in the pivotal study.

For patients receiving 15 mcg/dose, doses were reduced in 3 mcg increments. Efficacy is decreased with doses <7.5 mcg.

Pediatrics: Not indicated for patients <18 years of age.

Hepatic Impairment: Avoid use in decompensated hepatic disease.

Administration

I.V.: Interferon alfacon-1 is given by S.C. injection, 3 times/week, with at least 48 hours between doses.

Stability

Storage: Store in refrigerator 2°C to 8°C (36°F to 46°F). Do not freeze. Avoid exposure to direct sunlight. Do not shake vigorously.

Monitoring Laboratory Tests Hemoglobin and hematocrit, white blood cell count, platelets, triglycerides, and thyroid function. Laboratory tests should be taken 2 weeks prior to therapy, after therapy has begun, and periodically during treatment. HCV RNA, and ALT to determine success/response to therapy.

The following guidelines were used during the clinical studies as acceptable baseline values:

Platelet count ≥75 x 10^9/L

Hemoglobin ≥100 g/L

ANC ≥1500 x 10^6/L

S_{cr} <180 μmol/L (<2 mg/dL) or Cl_{cr} >0.83 mL/second (>50 mL/minute)

Serum albumin ≥25 g/L
Bilirubin WNL
TSH and T_4 WNL

Patients should also be monitored for signs of depression. Patients with pre-existing diabetes mellitus or hypertension should have an ophthalmologic exam prior to treatment.

Monitoring and Teaching Issues

Physical Assessment: See Warnings/Precautions and Contraindications for extensive use cautions. Assess other medications patient may be taking for effectiveness and interactions (see Drug Interactions). Laboratory tests must be monitored closely on a regular basis during therapy (see Monitoring Lab Tests). Patient with pre-existing diabetes mellitus or hypertension should have an ophthalmic exam prior to beginning treatment. Patient must be monitored closely for adverse reactions (see Adverse Reactions). If self-administered, instruct patient in appropriate storage, injection technique, and syringe disposal. Assess knowledge/teach patient purpose for use, adverse reactions and interventions, and adverse reactions to report (see Patient Education). **Pregnancy risk factor C** - benefits of use should outweigh possible risks. Note breast-feeding caution.

Patient Education: Use exactly as directed (if self-administered, follow exact instructions for injection and syringe disposal). Do not alter dosage or brand of medication without consulting prescriber. You will need frequent laboratory tests during course of therapy. If you have diabetes or hypertension you should have ophthalmic exam prior to beginning therapy. You may experience headache, dizziness, nervousness, anxiety (use caution when driving or engaging in dangerous tasks until response to medication is known); nausea, vomiting, diarrhea, or loss of appetite (small, frequent meals, frequent mouth care, sucking hard candy or chewing gum may help); flu-like symptoms such as headache, fatigue, muscle or joint pain, increased perspiration (mild non-narcotic analgesic may help); or hair lose (will probably grow back when treatment is completed). Promptly report any persistent GI upset; insomnia, depression, anxiety, nervousness; chest pain or palpitations; muscle, bone, or joint pain; respiratory difficulties or congestion; vision changes; or other persistent adverse effects. **Pregnancy/breast-feeding precautions:** Inform prescriber if you are or intend to become pregnant. Consult prescriber if breast-feeding.

Breast-feeding Issues: Women with hepatitis C should be instructed that there is a theoretical risk the virus may be transmitted in breast milk.

Pregnancy Issues: There have been no well-controlled studies in pregnant women. Animal studies have shown embryolethal or abortifacient effects. Males and females who are being treated with interferon alfacon-1 should use effective contraception.

Interferon Beta-1a (in ter FEER on BAY ta won aye)

U.S. Brand Names Avonex®; Rebif®

Synonyms rIFN beta-1a

Generic Available No

Pharmacologic Category Interferon

Pregnancy Risk Factor C

Lactation Excretion in breast milk unknown/not recommended

Use Treatment of relapsing forms of multiple sclerosis (MS), to slow the accumulation of physical disability and decrease the frequency of clinical exacerbations

Mechanism of Action/Effect Interferon beta differs from naturally occurring human protein by a single amino acid substitution and the lack of carbohydrate side chains; alters the expression and response to surface antigens and can enhance immune cell activities. Properties of interferon beta that modify biologic responses are mediated by cell surface receptor interactions; mechanism in the treatment of MS is unknown.

Contraindications Hypersensitivity to natural or recombinant interferons, human albumin, or any other component of the formulation

Warnings/Precautions Interferons have been associated with severe psychiatric adverse events (psychosis, mania, depression, suicidal behavior/ideation) in patients with and without previous psychiatric symptoms, avoid use in severe psychiatric disorders and use caution in patients with a history of depression; patients exhibiting depressive symptoms should be closely monitored and discontinuation of therapy should be considered. Due to high incidence of flu-like adverse effects, use caution in patients with pre-existing cardiovascular disease, pulmonary disease, seizure disorders, myelosuppression, renal impairment or hepatic impairment. Suspend treatment if jaundice or symptoms of hepatic dysfunction occur. Safety and efficacy in patients <18 years of age have not been established. Pregnancy risk C.

Drug Interactions

Increased Effect/Toxicity: Interferons may increase the adverse/toxic effects of ACE inhibitors, specifically the development of granulocytopenia. Agranulocytosis has been reported with concurrent use of clozapine (case report). Interferons may increase the anticoagulant effects of warfarin, and interferons may increase serum levels of zidovudine.

Adverse Reactions Note: Flu-like symptoms (including headache, fever, myalgia, and weakness) are the most common adverse reaction (up to 61%) and may diminish with repeated dosing. Frequencies noted here indicate the highest reported frequency for either product, either from placebo-controlled trials or comparative studies (some effects reported for only one product).

In a comparative study, the adverse effect profiles of Avonex® and Rebif® were noted to be similar; with the exception of three adverse events noted to occur more frequently in the Rebif® group: Transaminase elevations, local reactions, and reductions in white blood cell counts.

>10%:

Central nervous system: Headache (30% to 70%), fever (23% to 28%), chills (21%), sleep disturbance (19%), dizziness (15%), depression (11% to 13%), insomnia (10% to 13%)

Gastrointestinal: Nausea (33%), abdominal pain (9% to 22%) diarrhea (16%), dyspepsia (11%)

Hematologic: Leukopenia (up to 36% in Rebif® patients), lymphadenopathy (12%)

(Continued)

Interferon Beta-1a *(Continued)*

Hepatic: Transaminases increased (up to 27% with Rebif®; hepatic dysfunction noted in <10%)
Local: Injection site disorders: A comparative trial noted events in 80% with Rebif® versus 24% with Avonex® (includes inflammation, pain, bruising, or site reaction)
Neuromuscular & skeletal: Myalgia (25% to 34%), back pain (23% to 25%), skeletal pain (15%), weakness (21%)
Ocular: Visual abnormalities (13%)
Respiratory: Upper respiratory tract infection (31%), sinusitis (18%), rhinitis (15% to 17%)
Miscellaneous; Flu-like symptoms (61%), infection (11%)

1% to 10%:
Cardiovascular: Chest pain (8%), syncope (4%), vasodilation (4%)
Central nervous system: Somnolence (5%), suicidal tendency (4%), malaise (5%), seizure (5%), ataxia (5%)
Dermatologic: Urticaria (5%), alopecia (4%), rash (7%)
Endocrine & metabolic: Thyroid abnormalities (up to 6% with Rebif®)
Gastrointestinal: Abdominal pain (9%), anorexia (7%), xerostomia (5%)
Genitourinary: Vaginitis (4%), ovarian cyst (3%), urinary frequency (7%), incontinence (4%)
Hematologic: Thrombocytopenia (8%), anemia (8%), eosinophilia (5%)
Hepatic: Hepatic function abnormalities (9%), hyperbilirubinemia (3%)
Neuromuscular & skeletal: Arthralgia (9%), muscle spasm (7%), rigors (13%)
Ocular: Dry eyes (3%)
Otic: Otitis media (6%), hearing decreased (3%)
Respiratory: Dyspnea (6%)
Miscellaneous: Herpesvirus infection (3%), hypersensitivity reaction (3%)

<1% (Limited to important or life-threatening): Amnesia, anaphylaxis, arrhythmia, basal cell carcinoma, Bell's palsy, cardiac arrest, colitis, erythema multiforme, gastrointestinal hemorrhage, hepatic failure, hypothyroidism, injection site necrosis, intestinal perforation, myasthenia, osteonecrosis, pharyngeal edema, photosensitivity, psychosis, pulmonary embolism, rash, sepsis, Stevens-Johnson syndrome, vaginal hemorrhage

Overdosage/Toxicology

Symptoms of overdose include CNS depression, obtundation, flu-like symptoms, myelosuppression

Treatment is supportive

Pharmacokinetic Note Limited data due to small doses used.

Pharmacodynamics/Kinetics

Half-Life Elimination: Avonex®: 10 hours; Rebif®: 69 hours

Time to Peak: Serum: Avonex® (I.M.): 3-15 hours; Rebif® (S.C.): 14 hours

Formulations

Injection, powder for reconstitution (Avonex®): 33 mcg [6.6 million units] [contains albumin; packaged with diluent, alcohol wipes, and access pin and needle]

Injection, solution [preservative free; prefilled syringe] (Rebif®): 22 mcg/mL (0.5 mL); 44 mcg/mL (0.5 mL) [contains albumin]

Dosing

Adults & Elderly: Multiple sclerosis:
I.M. (Avonex®): 30 mcg once weekly
S.C. (Rebif®): Initial: 8.8 mcg 3 times/week, increasing over a 4-week period to the recommended dose of 44 mcg 3 times/week; doses should be separated by at least 48 hours

Administration

I.M.: Avenox®: Must be given by I.M. injection. Reconstitute with 1.1 mL of diluent and swirl gently to dissolve.

Other: Rebif®: Administer S.C. at the same time of day on the same 3 days each week (ie, late afternoon/evening Mon, Wed, Fri).

Stability

Storage:
Avonex®: Store unreconstituted vial or reconstituted vial at 2°C to 8°C (36°F to 46°F). If refrigeration is not available, may be stored at 25°C (77°F) for up to 30 days. Do not freeze.
Rebif®: Store at 2°C to 8°C (36°F to 46°F). Do not freeze. Protect from light.

Reconstitution: Avonex®: The reconstituted product contains no preservative and is for single-use only; discard unused portion. Use the reconstituted product within 6 hours.

Monitoring Laboratory Tests Liver function, blood chemistries, complete blood count and differential, BUN, creatinine

Rebif®: CBC and liver function testing at 1-, 3-, and 6 months, then periodically thereafter. Thyroid function every 6 months (in patients with pre-existing abnormalities and/or clinical indications)

Monitoring and Teaching Issues

Physical Assessment: Monitor laboratory results on a regular a basis (see Monitoring Laboratory Tests). Monitor for effectiveness of therapy and possible adverse reactions (see Warnings/Precautions and Adverse Reactions). Assess knowledge/instruct patient/caregiver on appropriate reconstitution, injection and needle disposal, possible side effects, and symptoms to report (see Patient Education). **Pregnancy risk factor C** - barrier contraceptive teaching may be appropriate. Breast-feeding is not recommended.

Patient Education: This is not a cure for MS; you will continue to receive regular treatment and follow-up for MS. Use as directed; do not change dosage or schedule of administration without consulting prescriber. If self-injecting and you miss a dose, take it as soon as you remember, but two injections should not be given within 48 hours of each other. Maintain adequate hydration (2-3 L/day of fluids) unless advised by prescriber to restrict fluids. You may experience flu-like syndrome (acetaminophen may help); nausea, vomiting, or loss of appetite (small, frequent meals, frequent mouth care, sucking lozenges, or chewing gum may help); or drowsiness, sleep disturbances, dizziness, agitation, or abnormal thinking (use caution when driving or engaging in tasks requiring alertness until response to drug is known). Inform prescriber **immediately** if you feel depressed or have any thoughts of suicide. Report unusual bruising or bleeding; persistent abdominal disturbances; unusual fatigue; muscle pain or tremors; chest pain or palpitations; swelling of extremities; visual disturbances; pain, swelling, or redness at injection site; or other unusual symptoms. **Pregnancy/breast-feeding precautions:** Inform prescriber if you are or intend to become pregnant. Breast-feeding is not recommended.

Breast-feeding Issues: Potential for serious adverse reactions. Because its use has not been evaluated during lactation, breast-feeding is not recommended

Pregnancy Issues: Safety and efficacy in pregnant women have not been established. Treatment should be discontinued if a woman becomes pregnant, or plans to become pregnant during therapy. A dose-related abortifacient activity was reported in Rhesus monkeys.

Interferon Beta-1b (in ter FEER on BAY ta won bee)

U.S. Brand Names Betaseron®

Synonyms rIFN beta-1b

Generic Available No

Pharmacologic Category Interferon

Pregnancy Risk Factor C

Lactation Excretion in breast milk unknown/contraindicated

Use Reduces the frequency of clinical exacerbations in ambulatory patients with relapsing-remitting multiple sclerosis (MS)

Mechanism of Action/Effect Alters the expression and response to cell surface antigens and can enhance immune cell activities; mechanism in MS in unknown

Contraindications Hypersensitivity to *E. coli* derived products, natural or recombinant interferon beta, albumin human or any other component of the formulation

Warnings/Precautions Interferons have been associated with severe psychiatric adverse events (psychosis, mania, depression, suicidal behavior/ideation) in patients with and without previous psychiatric symptoms, avoid use in severe psychiatric disorders and use caution in patients with a history of depression; patients exhibiting symptoms of depression should be closely monitored and discontinuation of therapy should be considered. Due to high incidence of flu-like adverse effects, use caution in patients with pre-existing cardiovascular disease, pulmonary disease, seizure disorders, myelosuppression, renal impairment or hepatic impairment. Severe injection site reactions (necrosis) may occur; patient and/or caregiver competency in injection technique should be confirmed and periodically re-evaluated. Safety and efficacy in patients with chronic progressive MS and in patients <18 years of age have not been established. Pregnancy risk C.

Drug Interactions

Increased Effect/Toxicity: Interferons may increase the adverse/toxic effects of ACE inhibitors, specifically the development of granulocytopenia. Risk: Monitor A case report of agranulocytosis has been reported with concurrent use of clozapine. Case reports of decreased hematopoietic effect with erythropoietin. Interferon alpha may decrease the P450 isoenzyme metabolism of theophylline. Interferons may increase the anticoagulant effects of warfarin. Interferons may decrease the metabolism of zidovudine.

Adverse Reactions Note: Flu-like symptoms are reported in the majority of patients (76%).

>10%:

Central nervous system: Headache (84%), fever (59%), pain (52%), chills (46%), dizziness (35%), malaise (15%), anxiety (15%), migraine (12%)

Endocrine & metabolic: Dysmenorrhea (18%), menstrual disorder (17%), metrorrhagia (15%), hypoglycemia (15%)

Gastrointestinal: Diarrhea (35%), abdominal pain (32%), constipation (24%), vomiting (21%)

Hematologic: Lymphopenia (82%), neutropenia (18%), leukopenia (16%), lymphadenopathy (14%)

Hepatic: SGPT increased >5x baseline (19%), SGOT increased >5x baseline (4%)

Local: injection site reaction (85%)

Neuromuscular & skeletal: Weakness (49%), myalgia (44%). Hypertonia (26%), myasthenia (13%)

Ocular: Conjunctivitis (12%)

Respiratory: Sinusitis (36%)

Miscellaneous: Flu-like symptoms (76%), increased diaphoresis (23%)

1% to 10% (Limited to important or life-threatening):

Cardiovascular: Hypertension (7%), peripheral vascular disorder (5%), hemorrhage (3%)

Central nervous system: Somnolence (6%), confusion (4%), seizure (2%), suicide attempt (2%), amnesia (2%)

Dermatologic: Alopecia (4%)

Endocrine & metabolic: Menorrhagia (6%), fibrocystic breast (3%), breast neoplasm (2%), goiter (2%)

Hepatic: Bilirubin increased >2.5x baseline (6%), SGOT increased >5x baseline (4%)

Local: Injection site necrosis (5%)

Renal: Proteinuria (5%)

Respiratory: Dyspnea (8%), laryngitis (6%)

<1% (Limited to important or life-threatening): Apnea, arrhythmia, cardiac arrest, cardiomegaly, cerebral hemorrhage, coma, delirium, erythema nodosum, ethanol intolerance, exfoliative dermatitis, GI hemorrhage, hallucinations, heart failure, hematemesis, hepatitis, mania, myocardial infarction, pancreatitis, pericardial effusion, photosensitivity, psychosis, pulmonary embolism, rash, sepsis, shock, SIADH, skin necrosis, syncope, thrombocytopenia, vaginal hemorrhage

Overdosage/Toxicology Symptoms of overdose include CNS depression, obtundation, flu-like symptoms, and myelosuppression. Treatment is supportive.

Pharmacokinetic Note Limited data due to small doses used.

(Continued)

Interferon Beta-1b *(Continued)*

Pharmacodynamics/Kinetics

Half-Life Elimination: 8 minutes to 4.3 hours

Time to Peak: 1-8 hours

Formulations Injection, powder for reconstitution: 0.3 mg [9.6 million units] [contains albumin; packaged with diluent]

Dosing

Adults & Elderly: Multiple sclerosis (relapsing-remitting): S.C.: 0.25 mg (8 million units) every other day

Pediatrics: Not recommended in children <18 years of age

Administration

Other: S.C.: Withdraw 1 mL of reconstituted solution from the vial into a sterile syringe fitted with a 27-gauge needle and inject the solution subcutaneously. Sites for self-injection include arms, abdomen, hips, and thighs. S.C. administration is suggested for those who are at risk for bleeding or are thrombocytopenic. Rotate S.C. injection site. Patient should be well hydrated. Reconstitute with recommended amount of bacteriostatic water and agitate gently; do not shake. **Note:** Different vial strengths require different amounts of diluent.

Stability

Storage: Store at room temperature of 25°C (77°F); excursions permitted to 15°C to 30°C (59°F to 86°F). If not used immediately following reconstitution, refrigerate at 2°C to 8°C (36°F to 46°F); do not freeze or shake solution.

Reconstitution: Use product within 3 hours of reconstitution.

Monitoring Laboratory Tests Hemoglobin, liver function, blood chemistries

Monitoring and Teaching Issues

Physical Assessment: Monitor laboratory results (see above). Monitor closely for adverse reactions (see Adverse Reactions), especially patients with psychiatric or suicidal histories. Assess patient/caregiver knowledge and teach proper administration for S.C. injections and disposal of needles if appropriate. Teach the need for adequate hydration. Monitor for opportunistic infection. **Pregnancy risk factor C** - benefits of use should outweigh possible risks. Breast-feeding is contraindicated.

Patient Education: This is not a cure for MS; you will continue to receive regular treatment and follow-up for MS. Use as directed; do not change dosage or schedule of administration without consulting prescriber. Maintain adequate hydration (2-3 L/day of fluids) unless advised by prescriber to restrict fluids. You may experience flu-like syndrome (acetaminophen may help); nausea, vomiting, or loss of appetite (small, frequent meals, frequent mouth care, sucking lozenges, or chewing gum may help); or drowsiness, sleep disturbances, dizziness, agitation, or abnormal thinking (use caution when driving or engaging in tasks requiring alertness until response to drug is known). Inform prescriber **immediately** if you feel depressed or have any thoughts of suicide. Report any broken skin or black-blue discoloration around the injection site. Report unusual bruising or bleeding; persistent abdominal disturbances; unusual fatigue; muscle pain or tremors; chest pain or palpitations, swelling of extremities; visual disturbances; pain, swelling, or redness at injection site; or other unusual symptoms. **Pregnancy/breast-feeding precautions:** Inform prescriber if you are or intend to become pregnant. Do not breast-feed.

Breast-feeding Issues: Because its use has not been evaluated during lactation, breast-feeding is not recommended

Pregnancy Issues: Safety and efficacy in pregnant women has not been established. Treatment should be discontinued if a woman becomes pregnant, or plans to become pregnant during therapy. A dose-related abortifacient activity was reported in Rhesus monkeys.

Additional Information May be available only in small supplies; for information on availability and distribution, call the patient information line at 800-580-3837.

Interferon Gamma-1b (in ter FEER on GAM ah won bee)

U.S. Brand Names Actimmune®

Generic Available No

Pharmacologic Category Interferon

Pregnancy Risk Factor C

Lactation Excretion in breast milk unknown/contraindicated

Use Reduce frequency and severity of serious infections associated with chronic granulomatous disease; delay time to disease progression in patients with severe, malignant osteopetrosis

Contraindications Hypersensitivity to interferon gamma, *E. coli* derived proteins, or any component of the formulation

Warnings/Precautions Patients with pre-existing cardiac disease, seizure disorders, CNS disturbances, or myelosuppression should be carefully monitored; long-term effects on growth and development are unknown; safety and efficacy in children <1 year of age have not been established. Pregnancy risk C.

Drug Interactions

Cytochrome P450 Effect: Inhibits CYP2E1

Increased Effect/Toxicity: Interferon gamma-1b may increase hepatic enzymes or enhance myelosuppression when taken with other myelosuppressive agents. May decrease cytochrome P450 concentrations leading to increased serum concentrations of drugs metabolized by this pathway.

Nutritional/Ethanol Interactions Herb/Nutraceutical: Dietary supplements containing aristolochic acid (found most often in Chinese medicines/herbal therapies); cases of nephropathy and ESRD associated with their use.

Adverse Reactions Based on 50 mcg/m^2 dose administered 3 times weekly for chronic granulomatous disease

>10%:

Central nervous system: Fever (52%), headache (33%), chills (14%), fatigue (14%)

Dermatologic: Rash (17%)
Gastrointestinal: Diarrhea (14%), vomiting (13%)
Local: Injection site erythema or tenderness (14%)

1% to 10%:
Central nervous system: Depression (3%)
Gastrointestinal: Nausea (10%), abdominal pain (8%)
Neuromuscular & skeletal: Myalgia (6%), arthralgia (2%), back pain (2%)

Pharmacodynamics/Kinetics

Absorption: I.M., S.C.: Slowly

Half-Life Elimination: I.V.: 38 minutes; I.M., S.C.: 3-6 hours

Time to Peak: Plasma: I.M.: 4 hours (1.5 ng/mL); S.C.: 7 hours (0.6 ng/mL)

Formulations Injection, solution [preservative free]: 100 mcg [2 million int. units] (0.5 mL)
Previously, 100 mcg was expressed as 3 million units. This is equivalent to 2 million int. units.

Dosing

Adults & Elderly: If severe reactions occur, modify dose (50% reduction) or therapy should be discontinued until adverse reactions abate.

Chronic granulomatous disease: S.C.:
BSA ≤0.5 m^2: 1.5 mcg/kg/dose 3 times/week
BSA >0.5 m^2: 50 mcg/m^2 (1 million int. units/m^2) 3 times/week

Severe, malignant osteopetrosis: Children >1 year: S.C.:
BSA ≤0.5 m^2: 1.5 mcg/kg/dose 3 times/week
BSA >0.5 m^2: 50 mcg/m^2 (1 million int. units/m^2) 3 times/week

Note: Previously expressed as 1.5 million units/m^2; 50 mcg is equivalent to 1 million int. units/m^2.

Pediatrics: Children >1 year: Refer to adult dosing.

Stability

Storage: Store in refrigerator. Do not freeze. Do not shake. Discard if left unrefrigerated for >12 hours.

Monitoring Laboratory Tests CBC, platelet counts, renal and liver function, urinalysis (at 3-month intervals during treatment)

Monitoring and Teaching Issues

Physical Assessment: Monitor closely for effectiveness and/or interactions (see Drug Interactions). Monitor laboratory results on a regular basis (see Monitoring Laboratory Tests). Monitor for effectiveness of therapy and possible adverse reactions (see Warnings/Precautions and Adverse Reactions). Assess knowledge and instruct patient/caregiver on appropriate reconstitution, injection and needle disposal, possible side effects, and symptoms to report (see Patient Education). **Pregnancy risk factor C** - benefits of use should outweigh possible risks. Breast-feeding is contraindicated.

Patient Education: This is not a cure for MS; you will continue to receive regular treatment and follow-up for MS. Use as directed; do not change the dosage or schedule of administration without consulting prescriber. Maintain adequate hydration (2-3 L/day of fluids) unless advised by prescriber to restrict fluids. You may experience flu-like syndrome (acetaminophen may help); nausea, vomiting, or loss of appetite (small, frequent meals, frequent mouth care, sucking lozenges, or chewing gum may help); or drowsiness, dizziness, agitation, or abnormal thinking (use caution when driving or engaging in tasks requiring alertness until response to drug is known). Report unusual bruising or bleeding; persistent abdominal disturbances; unusual fatigue; muscle pain or tremors; chest pain or palpitations; swelling of extremities; visual disturbances; pain, swelling, or redness at injection site; or other unusual symptoms. **Pregnancy/breast-feeding precautions:** Inform prescriber if you are or intend to become pregnant. Do not breast-feed.

Breast-feeding Issues: Potential for serious adverse reactions. Because its use has not been evaluated during lactation, breast-feeding is not recommended

Pregnancy Issues: Safety and efficacy in pregnant women has not been established. Treatment should be discontinued if a woman becomes pregnant, or plans to become pregnant during therapy. A dose-related abortifacient activity was reported in Rhesus monkeys.

Interleukin-2 *see* Aldesleukin *on page 54*

Intralipid® *see* Fat Emulsion *on page 545*

Intravenous Fat Emulsion *see* Fat Emulsion *on page 545*

Intrifiban *see* Eptifibatide *on page 481*

Intron® A *see* Interferon Alfa-2b *on page 719*

Invanz® *see* Ertapenem *on page 484*

Invirase® *see* Saquinavir *on page 1213*

Iodoquinol (eye oh doe KWIN ole)

U.S. Brand Names Yodoxin®

Synonyms Diiodohydroxyquin

Generic Available No

Pharmacologic Category Amebicide

Pregnancy Risk Factor C

Lactation Excretion in breast milk unknown

Use Treatment of acute and chronic intestinal amebiasis; asymptomatic cyst passers; *Blastocystis hominis* infections; ineffective for amebic hepatitis or hepatic abscess

Mechanism of Action/Effect Contact amebicide that works in the lumen of the intestine by an unknown mechanism

Contraindications Hypersensitivity to iodine or iodoquinol or any component of the formulation; hepatic damage; pre-existing optic neuropathy

Warnings/Precautions Optic neuritis, optic atrophy, and peripheral neuropathy have occurred following prolonged use. Avoid long-term therapy. Use with caution in patients with thyroid disease. Pregnancy risk C.

(Continued)

Iodoquinol *(Continued)*

Effects on Lab Values May increase protein-bound serum iodine concentrations reflecting a decrease in ^{131}I uptake; false-positive ferric chloride test for phenylketonuria

Adverse Reactions Frequency not defined.

Central nervous system: Fever, chills, agitation, retrograde amnesia, headache
Dermatologic: Rash, urticaria, pruritus
Endocrine & metabolic: Thyroid gland enlargement
Gastrointestinal: Diarrhea, nausea, vomiting, stomach pain, abdominal cramps
Neuromuscular & skeletal: Peripheral neuropathy, weakness
Ocular: Optic neuritis, optic atrophy, visual impairment
Miscellaneous: Itching of rectal area

Overdosage/Toxicology Chronic overdose can result in vomiting, diarrhea, abdominal pain, metallic taste, paresthesia, paraplegia, and loss of vision. Can lead to destruction of long fibers of the spinal cord and optic nerve. Acute overdose may cause delirium, stupor, coma, and amnesia. Treatment is symptomatic.

Pharmacodynamics/Kinetics

Absorption: Poor and erratic

Metabolism: Hepatic

Formulations

Powder: 25 g, 100 g
Tablet: 210 mg, 650 mg

Dosing

Adults: Treatment of susceptible infections: Oral: 650 mg 3 times/day after meals for 20 days; not to exceed 2 g/day

Elderly: This agent is no longer a drug of choice; use only if other therapy is contraindicated or has failed. Due to optic nerve damage, use cautiously in the elderly.

Pediatrics: Treatment of susceptible infections: Oral: Children: 30-40 mg/kg/day (maximum: 650 mg/dose) in 3 divided doses for 20 days; not to exceed 1.95 g/day

Administration

Oral: Tablets may be crushed and mixed with applesauce or chocolate syrup. May take with food or milk to reduce stomach upset. Complete full course of therapy.

Monitoring Laboratory Tests Ophthalmologic exam

Monitoring and Teaching Issues

Physical Assessment: Check allergy history (iodine) prior to beginning therapy. See Contraindications, Warnings/Precautions, and Drug Interactions for use cautions. Teach patient appropriate use, reinfection prevention, possible side effects/interventions, and adverse symptoms to report (see Adverse Reactions, Overdose/Toxicology, and Patient Education). **Pregnancy risk factor C** - benefits of use should outweigh possible risks. Note breast-feeding caution.

Patient Education: Inform prescriber of all prescriptions, OTC medications, or herbal products you are taking, and any allergies you have. Do not take anything new during treatment unless approved by prescriber. Take as directed; complete full course of therapy. Maintain adequate hydration (2-3 L/day of fluids) unless advised by prescriber to restrict fluids, and nutrition (small, frequent meals may help). You may experience GI upset (small, frequent meals, frequent mouth care, sucking lozenges, or chewing gum may help). Report unresolved or severe nausea or vomiting, skin rash, fever, or fatigue. **Pregnancy/breast-feeding precautions:** Inform prescriber if you are or intend to become pregnant. Consult prescriber if breast-feeding.

Dietary Issues: Should be taken after meals.

Iodoquinol and Hydrocortisone

(eye oh doe KWIN ole & hye droe KOR ti sone)

U.S. Brand Names Dermazene®; Vytone®

Synonyms Hydrocortisone and Iodoquinol

Generic Available Yes

Pharmacologic Category Antifungal Agent, Topical; Corticosteroid, Topical

Pregnancy Risk Factor C

Lactation Excretion in breast milk unknown

Use Treatment of eczema; infectious dermatitis; chronic eczematoid otitis externa; mycotic dermatoses

Formulations Cream: Iodoquinol 1% and hydrocortisone acetate 1% (30 g)

Dermazene®: Iodoquinol 1% and hydrocortisone acetate 1% (30 g, 45 g)
Vytone®: Iodoquinol 1% and hydrocortisone acetate 1% (30 g)

Dosing

Adults & Elderly: Eczema, dermatoses: Topical: Apply 3-4 times/day

Monitoring and Teaching Issues

Physical Assessment: See individual components listed in Related Information. **Pregnancy risk factor C** - benefits of use should outweigh possible risks. Note breast-feeding caution.

Patient Education: See individual components listed in Related Information. **Pregnancy/breast-feeding precautions:** Inform prescriber if you are or intend to become pregnant. Consult prescriber if breast-feeding.

Related Information

Hydrocortisone *on page 673*
Iodoquinol *on page 731*

Iopidine® *see page 1461*

Iopidine® *see* Ophthalmic Agents, Glaucoma *on page 1002*

Iosopan® Plus *see* Magaldrate and Simethicone *on page 831*

I-Paracaine® *see page 1461*

Ipecac Syrup (IP e kak SIR up)

Generic Available Yes

Pharmacologic Category Antidote

Pregnancy Risk Factor C

Lactation Excretion in breast milk unknown/use caution

Use Treatment of acute oral drug overdosage and in certain poisonings

Mechanism of Action/Effect Irritates the gastric mucosa and stimulates the medullary chemoreceptor trigger zone to induce vomiting

Contraindications Hypersensitivity to ipecac or any component of the formulation; do not use in unconscious patients; patients with no gag reflex; following ingestion of strong bases, acids, or volatile oils; when seizures are likely

Warnings/Precautions Do not confuse ipecac syrup with ipecac fluid extract, which is 14 times more potent. Use with caution in patients with cardiovascular disease and bulimics. May not be effective in antiemetic overdose. Pregnancy risk C.

Drug Interactions

Decreased Effect: Activated charcoal, milk, carbonated beverages decrease the effect of ipecac syrup.

Increased Effect/Toxicity: Phenothiazines (chlorpromazine has been associated with serious dystonic reactions).

Nutritional/Ethanol Interactions Food: Milk, carbonated beverages may decrease effectiveness.

Adverse Reactions Frequency not defined.

Cardiovascular: Cardiotoxicity
Central nervous system: Lethargy
Gastrointestinal: Protracted vomiting, diarrhea
Neuromuscular & skeletal: Myopathy

Overdosage/Toxicology Contains cardiotoxin. Symptoms of overdose include tachycardia, CHF, atrial fibrillation, depressed myocardial contractility, myocarditis, diarrhea, persistent vomiting, and hypotension. Treatment is activated charcoal and gastric lavage.

Pharmacodynamics/Kinetics

Absorption: Significant amounts, mainly when it does not produce emesis

Onset: 15-30 minutes

Duration: 20-25 minutes; 60 minutes in some cases

Formulations Syrup: 70 mg/mL (30 mL) [contains alcohol]

Dosing

Adults & Elderly: Emetic: Oral: 15-30 mL followed by 200-300 mL of water; repeat dose one time if vomiting does not occur within 20 minutes.

Pediatrics: Emetic: Oral:

6-12 months: 5-10 mL followed by 10-20 mL/kg of water; repeat dose one time if vomiting does not occur within 20 minutes.

1-12 years: 15 mL followed by 10-20 mL/kg of water; repeat dose one time if vomiting does not occur within 20 minutes.

If emesis does not occur within 30 minutes after second dose, ipecac must be removed from stomach by gastric lavage.

Administration

Oral: Do **not** administer to unconscious patients. Patients should be kept active and moving following administration of ipecac. If vomiting does not occur after second dose, gastric lavage may be considered to remove ingested substance.

Monitoring and Teaching Issues

Physical Assessment: The Poison Control Center should be contacted before administration. Administer only to conscious patients. If vomiting does not occur within 30 minutes, contact the Poison Control Center (or prescriber) again. Assess patient's knowledge for home use. Note breast-feeding caution.

Patient Education: The Poison Control Center should be contacted before administration. Take only as directed; do not take more than recommended or more often than recommended. Follow with 8 oz of water. If vomiting does not occur within 30 minutes, contact the Poison Control Center or emergency services again. Do not administer if vomiting. If vomiting occurs after taking, do not eat or drink until vomiting subsides. **Breast-feeding precaution:** Consult prescriber if breast-feeding.

I-Pentolate® *see page 1509*
I-Pentolate® *see page 1461*
I-Phrine® *see page 1509*
IPOL™ *see page 1498*

Ipratropium (i pra TROE pee um)

U.S. Brand Names Atrovent®

Synonyms Ipratropium Bromide

Generic Available Yes: Solution for nebulization

Pharmacologic Category Anticholinergic Agent

Pregnancy Risk Factor B

Lactation Excretion in breast milk unknown/use caution

Use Anticholinergic bronchodilator used in bronchospasm associated with COPD, bronchitis, and emphysema; symptomatic relief of rhinorrhea associated with the common cold and allergic and nonallergic rhinitis

Mechanism of Action/Effect Blocks the action of acetylcholine at parasympathetic sites in bronchial smooth muscle causing bronchodilation

Contraindications Hypersensitivity to atropine, its derivatives, or any component of the formulation

Warnings/Precautions Not indicated for the initial treatment of acute episodes of bronchospasm. Use with caution in patients with narrow-angle glaucoma, prostatic hyperplasia, or
(Continued)

Ipratropium *(Continued)*

bladder neck obstruction. Ipratropium has not been specifically studied in the elderly, but it is poorly absorbed from the airways and appears to be safe in this population.

Drug Interactions

Increased Effect/Toxicity: Increased therapeutic effect with albuterol. Increased toxicity with anticholinergics or drugs with anticholinergic properties and dronabinol.

Adverse Reactions

Inhalation aerosol and inhalation solution:

1% to 10%:

Cardiovascular: Palpitations (2%)

Central nervous system: Nervousness (3%), dizziness (2%), fatigue, headache (6%), pain (4%)

Dermatologic: Rash (1%)

Gastrointestinal: Nausea, xerostomia, stomach upset, dry mucous membranes

Respiratory: Nasal congestion, dyspnea (10%), increased sputum (1%), bronchospasm (2%), pharyngitis (3%), rhinitis (2%), sinusitis (5%)

Miscellaneous: Influenza-like symptoms

<1% (Limited to important or life-threatening): Hypersensitivity reactions

Nasal spray: Epistaxis (8%) nasal, dryness (5%), nausea (2%)

Overdosage/Toxicology Symptoms of overdose include dry mouth, drying of respiratory secretions, cough, nausea, GI distress, blurred vision or impaired visual accommodation, headache, and nervousness. Acute overdose with ipratropium by inhalation is unlikely since it is so poorly absorbed. However, if poisoning occurs, it can be treated like any other anticholinergic toxicity. An anticholinergic overdose with severe life-threatening symptoms may be treated with physostigmine 1-2 mg S.C. or I.V. slowly.

Pharmacodynamics/Kinetics

Absorption: Negligible

Onset: Bronchodilation: 1-3 minutes; Peak effect: 1.5-2 hours

Duration: ≤4-6 hours

Formulations

Solution for nebulization, as bromide: 0.02% (2.5 mL)

Solution for oral inhalation, as bromide: 18 mcg/actuation (14 g)

Solution, intranasal spray, as bromide: 0.03% (30 mL); 0.06% (15 mL)

Dosing

Adults & Elderly:

Bronchospasm:

Nebulization: 500 mcg (one unit-dose vial) 3-4 times/day with doses 6-8 hours apart

Metered dose inhaler: 2 inhalations 4 times/day, up to 12 inhalations/24 hours

Colds (symptomatic relief of rhinorrhea): Safety and efficacy of use beyond 4 days not established: Nasal spray (0.06%): 2 sprays in each nostril 3-4 times/day

Allergic/nonallergic rhinitis: Nasal spray (0.03%): 2 sprays in each nostril 2-3 times/day

Pediatrics:

Bronchospasm:

Nebulization:

Infants and Children ≤12 years: 125-250 mcg 3 times/day

Children >12 years: Refer to adult dosing.

Metered dose inhaler:

Children 3-12 years: 1-2 inhalations 3 times/day, up to 6 inhalations/24 hours

Children >12 years: Refer to adult dosing.

Colds (symptomatic relief of rhinorrhea): Intranasal: Safety and efficacy of use beyond 4 days in patients with the common cold have not been established:

Children 5-11 years: 0.06%: 2 sprays in each nostril 3 times/day

Children ≥5 years and Adults: 0.06%: 2 sprays in each nostril 3-4 times/day

Allergic/nonallergic rhinitis: Intranasal: Children ≥6 years: Refer to adult dosing.

Monitoring and Teaching Issues

Physical Assessment: See Contraindications, Warnings/Precautions, and Dosing for use cautions. Assess potential for interactions with other prescriptions, OTC medications, or herbal products patient may be taking (especially anything that may have anticholinergic properties - see Drug Interactions). Assess patient response (see Adverse Reactions and Overdose/Toxicology) on a regular basis throughout therapy. Teach patient proper use, possible side effects and interventions (eg, importance of adequate hydration), and adverse symptoms to report (see Patient Education). Note breast-feeding caution.

Patient Education: Inform prescriber of all prescriptions, OTC medications, or herbal products you are taking, and any allergies you have. Do not take anything new without consulting prescriber. Use exactly as directed (see below). Do not use more often than recommended. Store solution away from light. Maintain adequate hydration (2-3 L/day of fluids) unless advised by prescriber to restrict fluids. May cause sensitivity to heat (avoid extremes in temperature); nervousness, dizziness, or fatigue (use caution when driving or engaging in tasks requiring alertness until response to drug is known); dry mouth, unpleasant taste, stomach upset (small, frequent meals, frequent mouth care, chewing gum, or sucking hard candy may help); or difficulty urinating (always void before treatment). Report unresolved GI upset, dizziness or fatigue, vision changes, palpitations, persistent inability to void, nervousness, or insomnia. **Breast-feeding precaution:** Consult prescriber if breast-feeding.

Inhaler: Follow instructions for use accompanying the product. Close eyes when administering ipratropium; blurred vision may result if sprayed into eyes. Effects are enhanced by holding breath 10 seconds after inhalation; wait at least 1 full minute between inhalations.

Nebulizer: Wash hands before and after treatment. Wash and dry nebulizer after each treatment. Twist open the top of one unit dose vial and squeeze the contents into the nebulizer reservoir. Connect the nebulizer reservoir to the mouthpiece or face mask. Connect nebulizer to compressor. Sit in a comfortable, upright position. Place mouthpiece in your mouth or put on the face mask and turn on the compressor. If a face mask is used, avoid leakage around the mask (temporary blurring of vision, worsening of narrow-angle glaucoma, or eye pain may occur if mist gets into eyes). Breathe calmly and deeply until no more mist is formed in the nebulizer (about 5 minutes). At this point, treatment is finished.

Geriatric Considerations: Older patients may find it difficult to use the metered dose inhaler. A spacer device may be useful. Ipratropium has not been specifically studied in the elderly, but it is poorly absorbed from the airways and appears to be safe in this population.

Related Information

Inhalant (Asthma, Bronchospasm) Agents Comparison *on page 1577*

Ipratropium and Albuterol (i pra TROE pee um & al BYOO ter ole)

U.S. Brand Names Combivent®; DuoNeb™

Synonyms Albuterol and Ipratropium

Generic Available No

Pharmacologic Category Bronchodilator

Pregnancy Risk Factor C

Lactation Excretion in breast milk unknown

Use Treatment of COPD in those patients that are currently on a regular bronchodilator who continue to have bronchospasms and require a second bronchodilator

Formulations

Aerosol for oral inhalation (Combivent®): Ipratropium bromide 18 mcg and albuterol sulfate 103 mcg per actuation [200 doses] (14.7 g)

Solution for oral inhalation (DuoNeb™): Ipratropium bromide 0.5 mg [0.017%] and albuterol base 2.5 mg [0.083%] per 3 mL vial (30s, 60s)

Dosing

Adults & Elderly: COPD:

Inhalation: 2 metered-dose inhalations 4 times/day; may receive additional doses as necessary, but total number of doses in 24 hours should not exceed 12 inhalations.

Inhalation via nebulization: Initial: 3 mL every 6 hours (maximum: 3 mL every 4 hours)

Monitoring and Teaching Issues

Physical Assessment: See individual components listed in Related Information. **Pregnancy risk factor C** - benefits of use should outweigh possible risks. Note breast-feeding caution.

Patient Education: See individual components listed in Related Information. **Pregnancy/breast-feeding precautions:** Inform prescriber if you are or intend to become pregnant. Consult prescriber if breast-feeding.

Related Information

Albuterol *on page 52*

Ipratropium *on page 733*

Ipratropium Bromide *see* Ipratropium *on page 733*

I-Prin [OTC] *see* Ibuprofen *on page 688*

Iproveratril Hydrochloride *see* Verapamil *on page 1396*

Irbesartan (ir be SAR tan)

U.S. Brand Names Avapro®

Generic Available No

Pharmacologic Category Angiotensin II Receptor Blocker

Pregnancy Risk Factor C/D (2nd and 3rd trimesters)

Lactation Excretion in breast milk unknown/contraindicated

Use Treatment of hypertension alone or in combination with other antihypertensives; treatment of diabetic nephropathy in patients with type 2 diabetes mellitus (noninsulin dependent, NIDDM) and hypertension

Mechanism of Action/Effect Irbesartan is an angiotensin receptor antagonist. Angiotensin II acts as a vasoconstrictor and stimulates the release of aldosterone, which results in reabsorption of sodium and water. These effects result in an elevation in blood pressure. Irbesartan blocks the AT1 angiotensin II receptor, thereby blocking the vasoconstriction and the aldosterone secreting effects of angiotensin II.

Contraindications Hypersensitivity to irbesartan or any component of the formulation; hypersensitivity to other A-II receptor antagonists; primary hyperaldosteronism; bilateral renal artery stenosis; pregnancy (2nd and 3rd trimesters)

Warnings/Precautions Avoid use or use smaller doses in patients who are volume depleted; correct depletion first. Deterioration in renal function can occur with initiation. Use with caution in unilateral renal artery stenosis and pre-existing renal insufficiency; significant aortic/mitral stenosis. Safety and efficacy have not been established in pediatric patients <6 years of age. Pregnancy risk C/D (2nd and 3rd trimesters).

Drug Interactions

Cytochrome P450 Effect: Substrate of CYP2C8/9; Inhibits CYP2C8/9, 3A4

Increased Effect/Toxicity: Potassium salts/supplements, co-trimoxazole (high dose), ACE inhibitors, and potassium-sparing diuretics (amiloride, spironolactone, triamterene) may increase the risk of hyperkalemia.

Nutritional/Ethanol Interactions Herb/Nutraceutical: Avoid dong quai if using for hypertension (has estrogenic activity). Avoid ephedra, yohimbe, ginseng (may worsen hypertension). Avoid garlic (may have increased antihypertensive effect).

Adverse Reactions Unless otherwise indicated, percentage of incidence is reported for patients with hypertension.

>10%: Endocrine & metabolic: Hyperkalemia (19%, diabetic nephropathy)

1% to 10%:

Cardiovascular: Orthostatic hypotension (5%, diabetic nephropathy)

Central nervous system: Fatigue (4%), dizziness (10%, diabetic nephropathy)

Gastrointestinal: Diarrhea (3%), dyspepsia (2%)

Respiratory: Upper respiratory infection (9%), cough (2.8% versus 2.7% in placebo)

<1% (Limited to important or life-threatening): Angina, angioedema, arrhythmia, cardiopulmonary arrest, conjunctivitis, decreased libido, depression, dyspnea, ecchymosis, edema,

(Continued)

Irbesartan *(Continued)*

epistaxis, gout, heart failure, hyperkalemia, hypotension, increased transaminases, jaundice, myocardial infarction, orthostatic hypotension, paresthesia, sexual dysfunction, stroke, urticaria. May be associated with worsening of renal function in patients dependent on renin-angiotensin-aldosterone system.

Overdosage/Toxicology Likely manifestations of overdose include hypotension and tachycardia. Treatment is supportive. Not removed by hemodialysis.

Pharmacodynamics/Kinetics

Bioavailability: 60% to 80%

Half-Life Elimination: Terminal: 11-15 hours

Time to Peak: Serum: 1.5-2 hours

Metabolism: Hepatic, primarily CYP2C9

Onset: Peak levels in 1-2 hours

Duration: >24 hours

Formulations Tablet: 75 mg, 150 mg, 300 mg

Dosing

Adults:

Hypertension: Oral: 150 mg once daily; patients may be titrated to 300 mg once daily. **Note:** Starting dose in volume-depleted patients should be 75 mg.

Nephropathy in patients with type 2 diabetes and hypertension: Oral: Target dose: 300 mg once daily

Elderly: Although AUC and C_{max} values are higher in elderly patients, no specific dosage reduction is recommended. Refer to adult dosing.

Pediatrics: Hypertension: Oral:

<6 years: Safety and efficacy have not been established.

≥6-12 years: Initial: 75 mg once daily; may be titrated to a maximum of 150 mg once daily

13-16 years: Refer to adult dosing.

Renal Impairment: No dosage adjustment necessary with mild to severe impairment unless the patient is also volume depleted.

Stability

Storage: Store at room temperature of 15°C to 30°C (59°F to 86°F).

Monitoring Laboratory Tests Electrolytes, serum creatinine, BUN, urinalysis

Monitoring and Teaching Issues

Physical Assessment: See Contraindications, Warnings/Precautions, and Dosing for use cautions. Assess potential for interactions with other prescriptions, OTC medications, or herbal products patient may be taking (see Drug Interactions). Assess results of laboratory tests (see Monitoring Lab Tests), therapeutic effects, and adverse response (see Adverse Reactions and Overdose/Toxicology) at regular intervals during therapy. Teach patient proper use, possible side effects and appropriate interventions, and adverse symptoms to report (see Patient Education). **Pregnancy risk factor C/D** - see Pregnancy Risk Factor for use cautions; benefits of use should outweigh possible risks. Instruct patients of childbearing age about appropriate barrier contraceptive measures. Breast-feeding is contraindicated.

Patient Education: Inform prescriber of all prescriptions, OTC medications, or herbal products you are taking, and any allergies you have. Do not take anything new during treatment unless approved by prescriber. Take exactly as directed; do not discontinue without consulting prescriber. May be taken with or without food. Take first dose at bedtime. This medication does not replace other antihypertensive interventions; follow prescriber's instructions for diet and lifestyle changes.. May cause dizziness, fainting, or lightheadedness (use caution when driving or engaging in tasks that require alertness until response to drug is known); nausea, vomiting, or abdominal pain (small, frequent meals, frequent mouth care, sucking lozenges, or chewing gum may help); or diarrhea (buttermilk, boiled milk, yogurt may help). Report chest pain or palpitations, skin rash, fluid retention (swelling of extremities), difficulty breathing or unusual cough, or other persistent adverse reactions. **Pregnancy/breast-feeding precautions:** Inform prescriber if you are or intend to become pregnant. This drug should not be used in the 2nd or 3rd trimester of pregnancy. Consult prescriber for appropriate contraceptive measures if necessary. Consult prescriber if breast-feeding.

Dietary Issues: May be taken with or without food.

Pregnancy Issues: The drug should be discontinued as soon as possible after detection of pregnancy. Drugs which act directly on the renin-angiotensin system can cause fetal and neonatal morbidity and death.

Related Information

Angiotensin Agents *on page 1547*

Irbesartan and Hydrochlorothiazide

(ir be SAR tan & hye droe klor oh THYE a zide)

U.S. Brand Names Avalide®

Synonyms Avapro® HCT; Hydrochlorothiazide and Irbesartan

Generic Available No

Pharmacologic Category Antihypertensive Agent Combination

Pregnancy Risk Factor C/D (2nd and 3rd trimesters)

Lactation Enters breast milk/contraindicated

Use Combination therapy for the management of hypertension

Formulations

Tablet:

Irbesartan 150 mg and hydrochlorothiazide 12.5 mg

Irbesartan 300 mg and hydrochlorothiazide 12.5 mg

Dosing

Adults & Elderly:

Hypertension: Oral: Dose must be individualized. A patient who is not controlled with either agent alone may be switched to the combination product. Mean effect increases with the dose of each component. The lowest dosage available is irbesartan 150 mg/hydrochlorothiazide 12.5 mg. Dose increases should be made not more frequently than every 2-4 weeks.

Pediatrics: Refer to adult dosing.

Monitoring and Teaching Issues

Physical Assessment: See individual components listed in Related Information. **Pregnancy risk factor C/D** - see Pregnancy Risk Factor for use cautions; benefits of use should outweigh possible risks. Breast-feeding is contraindicated.

Patient Education: See individual components listed in Related Information. **Pregnancy/breast-feeding precautions:** Inform prescriber if you are or intend to become pregnant. Do not breast-feed.

Related Information

Hydrochlorothiazide *on page 664*
Irbesartan *on page 735*

Ircon® [OTC] *see* Iron Supplements *on page 744*

Irinotecan (eye rye no TEE kan)

U.S. Brand Names Camptosar®

Synonyms Camptothecin-11; CPT-11

Generic Available No

Pharmacologic Category Antineoplastic Agent, Natural Source (Plant) Derivative

Pregnancy Risk Factor D

Lactation Enters breast milk/contraindicated

Use A component of first-line therapy in combination with 5-fluorouracil and leucovorin for the treatment of metastatic carcinoma of the colon or rectum; treatment of metastatic carcinoma of the colon or rectum which has recurred or progressed following fluorouracil-based therapy

Use - Unlabeled/Investigational Lung cancer (small cell and nonsmall cell), cervical cancer, gastric cancer, pancreatic cancer, leukemia, lymphoma, breast cancer

Mechanism of Action/Effect Irinotecan and its active metabolite (SN-38) bind reversibly to topoisomerase I and stabilize the cleavable complex so that religation of the cleaved DNA strand cannot occur. This results in the accumulation of cleavable complexes and single-strand DNA breaks. This interaction results in double-stranded DNA breaks and cell death consistent with S-phase cell cycle specificity.

Contraindications Hypersensitivity to irinotecan or any component of the formulation; pregnancy

Warnings/Precautions The U.S. Food and Drug Administration (FDA) currently recommends that procedures for proper handling and disposal of antineoplastic agents be considered. Irinotecan can induce both early and late forms of diarrhea (mediated by different mechanisms). The administration of irinotecan should be delayed until the patient recovers and subsequent doses should be decreased. Premedication with loperamide is not recommended.

Deaths due to sepsis following severe myelosuppression have been reported. Therapy should be discontinued if neutropenic fever occurs or if the absolute neutrophil count is <500/mm^3. The dose of irinotecan should be reduced if there is a clinically significant decrease in the total WBC (<200/mm^3), neutrophil count (<1000/mm^3), hemoglobin (<8 g/dL), or platelet count (<100,000/mm^3). Routine administration of a colony-stimulating factor is generally not necessary. Avoid extravasation.

Patients with even modest elevations in total serum bilirubin levels (1.0-2.0 mg/dL) have a significantly greater likelihood of experiencing first-course grade 3 or 4 neutropenia than those with bilirubin levels that were <1.0 mg/dL. Patients with abnormal glucuronidation of bilirubin, such as those with Gilbert's syndrome, may also be at greater risk of myelosuppression when receiving therapy with irinotecan.

Patients with diarrhea should be carefully monitored and treated promptly. Two severe (life-threatening) forms of diarrhea may occur. Early diarrhea occurs during or within 24 hours of receiving irinotecan; is characterized by cholinergic symptoms (eg, increased salivation, diaphoresis, abdominal cramping); and is usually responsive to atropine. Late diarrhea occurs more than 24 hours after treatment; may lead to dehydration, electrolyte imbalance, or sepsis; and is usually responsive to loperamide. Patients should receive fluid and electrolyte replacement as indicated, or antibiotics if ileus, fever, or neutropenia develop.

Use caution in patients who previously received pelvic/abdominal radiation, elderly patients with comorbid conditions, or baseline performance status of 2; close monitoring is recommended.

Drug Interactions

Cytochrome P450 Effect: Substrate of **CYP2B6, 3A4**

Increased Effect/Toxicity: Hold diuretics during dosing due to potential risk of dehydration secondary to vomiting and/or diarrhea induced by irinotecan. Prophylactic dexamethasone as an antiemetic may enhance lymphocytopenia. Prochlorperazine may increase incidence of akathisia. Adverse reactions such as myelosuppression and diarrhea would be expected to be exacerbated by other antineoplastic agents.

Adverse Reactions

>10%:

Cardiovascular: Vasodilation

Central nervous system: Insomnia, dizziness, fever (45.4%)

Dermatologic: Alopecia (60.5%), rash

Gastrointestinal: Irinotecan therapy may induce two different forms of diarrhea. Onset, symptoms, proposed mechanisms and treatment are different. Overall, 56.9% of patients treated experience abdominal pain and/or cramping during therapy. Anorexia, constipation, flatulence, stomatitis, and heartburn have also been reported.

Diarrhea: Dose-limiting toxicity with weekly dosing regimen

(Continued)

Irinotecan *(Continued)*

Early diarrhea (50.7% incidence) usually occurs during or within 24 hours of administration. May be accompanied by symptoms of cramping, vomiting, flushing, and diaphoresis. It is thought to be mediated by cholinergic effects which can be successfully managed with atropine (refer to Warnings/Precautions).

Late diarrhea (87.8% incidence) usually occurs >24 hours after treatment. National Cancer Institute (NCI) grade 3 or 4 diarrhea occurs in 30.6% of patients. Late diarrhea generally occurs with a median of 11 days after therapy and lasts approximately 3 days. Patients experiencing grade 3 or 4 diarrhea were noted to have symptoms a total of 7 days. Correlated with irinotecan or SN-38 levels in plasma and bile. Due to the duration, dehydration and electrolyte imbalances are significant clinical concerns. Loperamide therapy is recommended. The incidence of grade 3 or 4 late diarrhea is significantly higher in patients ≥ 65 years of age: close monitoring and prompt initiation of high-dose loperamide therapy is prudent (refer to Warnings/Precautions).

Emetic potential: Moderately high (86.2% incidence, however, only 12.5% grade 3 or 4 vomiting)

Hematologic: Myelosuppressive: Dose-limiting toxicity with 3 week dosing regimen

Grade 1-4 neutropenia occurred in 53.9% of patients. Patients who had previously received pelvic or abdominal radiation therapy or a bilirubin of ≥1.0 mg/dL were noted to have a significantly increased incidence of grade 3 or 4 neutropenia. White blood cell count nadir is 15 days after administration and is more frequent than thrombocytopenia. Recovery is usually within 24-28 days and cumulative toxicity has not been observed.

WBC: Mild to severe
Platelets: Mild
Onset: 10 days
Nadir: 14-16 days
Recovery: 21-28 days

Neuromuscular & skeletal: Weakness (75.7%)
Respiratory: Dyspnea (22%), coughing, rhinitis
Miscellaneous: Diaphoresis

1% to 10%: Local: **Irritant chemotherapy**; thrombophlebitis has been reported

<1% (Limited to important or life-threatening): Anaphylactoid reaction, anaphylaxis, bleeding, colitis, ileus, renal failure (acute), renal impairment; pulmonary toxicity (dyspnea, fever, reticulonodular infiltrates on chest x-ray)

Overdosage/Toxicology Symptoms of overdose include bone marrow suppression, leukopenia, thrombocytopenia, nausea, and vomiting. Treatment is supportive.

Pharmacodynamics/Kinetics

Half-Life Elimination: Parent drug: Alpha: 0.2 hours, Beta: 2.5 hours, Gamma: 14.2 hours; SN-38: 3-23.9 hours

Time to Peak: SN-38: 30-minute infusion: ~1 hour

Metabolism: Via intestinal mucosa, plasma, hepatic, and perhaps in some tumors; converted to SN-38 by carboxylesterase enzymes; undergoes glucuronidation, the metabolites having much less activity than SN-38. Enterohepatic recirculation results in a second peak in the concentration of SN-38. The lactones of both irinotecan and SN-38 undergo hydrolysis to inactive hydroxy acid forms.

Formulations Injection, solution, as hydrochloride: 20 mg/mL (2 mL, 5 mL)

Dosing

Adults & Elderly: Refer to individual protocols.

Single-agent therapy:

I.V.: Weekly regimen: 125 mg/m^2 over 90 minutes on days 1, 8, 15, and 22, followed by a 2-week rest
Adjusted dose level -1: 100 mg/m^2
Adjusted dose level -2: 75 mg/m^2

I.V.: Once-every-3-week regimen: 350 mg/m^2 over 90 minutes, once every 3 weeks
Adjusted dose level -1: 300 mg/m^2
Adjusted dose level -2: 250 mg/m^2

Note: A reduction in the starting dose by one dose level may be considered for patients ≥65 years of age, prior pelvic/abdominal radiotherapy, performance status of 2, or increased bilirubin (dosing for patients with a bilirubin >2 mg/dL cannot be recommended based on lack of data per manufacturer)

Depending on the patient's ability to tolerate therapy, doses should be adjusted in increments of 25-50 mg/m^2. Irinotecan doses may range 50-150 mg/m^2.

Combination therapy with 5-FU and leucovorin: Six-week (42-day) cycle (next cycle beginning on day 45):

I.V.: 125 mg/m^2 over 90 minutes on days 1, 8, 15, and 22; to be given in combination with bolus leucovorin and 5-FU (leucovorin administered immediately following irinotecan; 5-FU immediately following leucovorin)
Adjusted dose level -1: 100 mg/m^2
Adjusted dose level -2: 75 mg/m^2

180 mg/m^2 over 90 minutes on days 1, 15, and 22; to be given in combination with infusional leucovorin and bolus/infusion 5-FU (leucovorin administered immediately following irinotecan; 5-FU immediately following leucovorin)
Adjusted dose level -1: 150 mg/m^2
Adjusted dose level -2: 120 mg/m^2

Note: For all regimens: It is recommended that new courses begin only after the granulocyte count recovers to ≥1500/mm^3, the platelet count recovers to ≥100,000/mm^3, and treatment-related diarrhea has fully resolved. Treatment should be delayed 1-2 weeks to allow for recovery from treatment-related toxicities. If the patient has not recovered after a 2-week delay, consideration should be given to discontinuing irinotecan.

Dosing adjustment for toxicities: A decrease in dose level corresponds to a decrease in irinotecan dosage by 25-50 mg/m^2; specific dose levels corresponding to individual protocols should be consulted. Single-agent schedules and combination schedules: See tables.

Single-Agent Schedule: Recommended Dosage Modifications[1]

Toxicity NCI Grade[2] (Value)	During a Cycle of Therapy	At the Start of Subsequent Cycles of Therapy (After Adequate Recovery), Compared to the Starting Dose in the Previous Cycle[1]	
	Weekly	Weekly	Once Every 3 Weeks
No toxicity	Maintain dose level	↑ 25 mg/m² up to a maximum dose of 150 mg/m²	Maintain dose level
Neutropenia			
1 (1500-1999/mm³)	Maintain dose level	Maintain dose level	Maintain dose level
2 (1000-1499/mm³)	↓ 25 mg/m²	Maintain dose level	Maintain dose level
3 (500-999/mm³)	Omit dose until resolved to ≤ grade 2, then ↓ 25 mg/m²	↓ 25 mg/m²	↓ 50 mg/m²
4 (<500/mm³)	Omit dose until resolved to ≤ grade 2, then ↓ 50 mg/m²	↓ 50 mg/m²	↓ 50 mg/m²
Neutropenic Fever (grade 4 neutropenia and ≥ grade 2 fever)	Omit dose until resolved, then ↓ 50 mg/m²	↓ 50 mg/m²	↓ 50 mg/m²
Other Hematologic Toxicities	Dose modifications for leukopenia, thrombocytopenia, and anemia during a course of therapy and at the start of subsequent courses of therapy are also based on NCI toxicity criteria and are the same as recommended for neutropenia above.		
Diarrhea			
1 (2-3 stools/day > pretreatment)	Maintain dose level	Maintain dose level	Maintain dose level
2 (4-6 stools/day > pretreatment)	↓ 25 mg/m²	Maintain dose level	Maintain dose level
3 (7-9 stools/day > pretreatment)	Omit dose until resolved to ≤ grade 2, then ↓ 25 mg/m²	↓ 25 mg/m²	↓ 50 mg/m²
4 (≥10 stools/day > pretreatment)	Omit dose until resolved to ≤ grade 2, then ↓ 50 mg/m²	↓ 50 mg/m²	↓ 50 mg/m²
Other Nonhematologic Toxicities[3]			
1	Maintain dose level	Maintain dose level	Maintain dose level
2	↓ 25 mg/m²	↓ 25 mg/m²	↓ 50 mg/m²
3	Omit dose until resolved to ≤ grade 2, then ↓ 25 mg/m²	↓ 25 mg/m²	↓ 50 mg/m²
4	Omit dose until resolved to ≤ grade 2, then ↓ 50 mg/m²	↓ 50 mg/m²	↓ 50 mg/m²

[1]All dose modifications should be based on the worst preceding toxicity.
[2]National Cancer Institute Common Toxicity Criteria (version 1.0)
[3]Excludes alopecia, anorexia, asthenia

Combination Schedules: Recommended Dosage Modifications[1]

Toxicity NCI[2] Grade (Value)	**During a Cycle of Therapy**	**At the Start of Subsequent Cycles of Therapy (After Adequate Recovery), Compared to the Starting Dose in the Previous Cycle[1]**
No toxicity	Maintain dose level	Maintain dose level
Neutropenia		
1 (1500-1999/mm³)	Maintain dose level	Maintain dose level
2 (1000-1499/mm³)	↓ 1 dose level	Maintain dose level
3 (500-999/mm³)	Omit dose until resolved to ≤ grade 2, then ↓ 1 dose level	↓ 1 dose level
4 (<500/mm³)	Omit dose until resolved to ≤ grade 2, then ↓ 2 dose levels	↓ 2 dose levels
Neutropenic Fever (grade 4 neutropenia and ≥ grade 2 fever)	Omit dose until resolved, then ↓ 2 dose levels	
Other Hematologic Toxicities	Dose modifications for leukopenia or thrombocytopenia during a course of therapy and at the start of subsequent courses of therapy are also based on NCI toxicity criteria and are the same as recommended for neutropenia above.	
Diarrhea		
1 (2-3 stools/day > pretreatment)	Delay dose until resolved to baseline, then give same dose	Maintain dose level
2 (4-6 stools/day > pretreatment)	Omit dose until resolved to baseline, then ↓ 1 dose level	Maintain dose level
3 (7-9 stools/day > pretreatment)	Omit dose until resolved to baseline, then ↓ by 1 dose level	↓ 1 dose level
4 (≥10 stools/day > pretreatment)	Omit dose until resolved to baseline, then ↓ 2 dose levels	↓ 2 dose levels
Other Nonhematologic Toxicities[3]		
1	Maintain dose level	Maintain dose level
2	Omit dose until resolved to ≤ grade 1, then ↓ 1 dose level	Maintain dose level
3	Omit dose until resolved to ≤ grade 2, then ↓ 1 dose level	↓ 1 dose level
4	Omit dose until resolved to ≤ grade 2, then ↓ 2 dose levels	↓ 2 dose levels
Mucositis and/or stomatitis	Decrease only 5-FU, not irinotecan	Decrease only 5-FU, not irinotecan

[1]All dose modifications should be based on the worst preceding toxicity.
[2]National Cancer Institute Common Toxicity Criteria (version 1.0)
[3]Excludes alopecia, anorexia, asthenia

(Continued)

Irinotecan *(Continued)*

Hepatic Impairment: AUC of irinotecan and SN-38 have been reported to be higher in patients with known hepatic tumor involvement. The manufacturer recommends that no change in dosage or administration be made for patients with liver metastases and normal hepatic function. In patients with a combined history of prior pelvic/abdominal irradiation and modestly elevated total serum bilirubin levels (1.0-2.0 mg/dL) prior to treatment with irinotecan, there may be substantially increased likelihood of grade 3 or 4 neutropenia. Consideration may be given to starting irinotecan at a lower dose (eg, 100 mg/m^2) in such patients. Definite recommendations regarding the most appropriate starting dose in patients who have pretreatment total serum bilirubin elevations >2.0 mg/dL are not available, but it is likely that lower starting doses will need to be considered in such patients.

Administration

I.V.: Irritant. Infuse over 90 minutes. If administered in combination with fluorouracil and leucovorin, administer leucovorin immediately after irinotecan, and administer fluorouracil immediately after leucovorin. Premedication with antiemetics (dexamethasone plus ondansetron/granisetron) is recommended, at least 30 minutes prior to irinotecan. Atropine should be considered in patients experiencing cholinergic symptoms.

Stability

Storage: Store at controlled room temperature 15°C to 30°C (59°F to 86°F). Protect from light. Solutions diluted in 5% dextrose injection and stored at refrigerated temperatures approximately 2°C to 8°C and protected from light are physically and chemically stable for 48 hours.

Reconstitution: Dose of irinotecan is diluted in D_5W to a final concentration of 0.12-2.8 mg/mL (most commonly in 500 mL D_5W) and infused over 90 minutes. 0.9% NaCl can be used, but precipitation of irinotecan under refrigeration is more likely to occur with the latter solution, and D_5W is generally preferred.

Compatibility: Stable in D_5W, NS

Y-site administration: Incompatible with gemcitabine

Compatibility when admixed: Incompatible with methylprednisolone sodium succinate

Monitoring Laboratory Tests CBC with differential and platelet count

Monitoring and Teaching Issues

Physical Assessment: See Contraindications, Warnings/Precautions, and Dosing for use cautions. Assess potential for interactions with other prescriptions, OTC medications, or herbal products patient may be taking (see Drug Interactions). Premedicate with antiemetic (emetic potential moderately high). Infusion site must be monitored to prevent extravasation. Assess results of laboratory tests (see Monitoring Lab Tests), therapeutic effects, and adverse response (eg, acute diarrhea, sepsis - see Adverse Reactions, Overdose/Toxicology, and Warnings/Precautions) at regular intervals during therapy. Teach patient proper use, possible side effects and appropriate interventions, and adverse symptoms to report (see Patient Education). **Pregnancy risk factor D** - determine that patient is not pregnant before beginning treatment. Instruct patients of childbearing age about appropriate barrier contraceptive measures. Breast-feeding is contraindicated.

Patient Education: Inform prescriber of all prescriptions, OTC medications, or herbal products you are taking, and any allergies you have. Do not take anything new during treatment unless approved by prescriber. This drug can only be administered by infusion. Report immediately any burning, pain, redness, or swelling at infusion site. Maintain adequate hydration (3-4 L/day of fluids unless instructed to restrict fluid intake) during therapy. May cause severe diarrhea: report immediately any diarrhea or signs of dehydration (eg, fainting, dizziness, lightheadedness). You will be more susceptible to infection (avoid crowds and exposure to infection and do not have any vaccinations without consulting prescriber). You may experience nausea or vomiting (small, frequent meals, frequent mouth care, sucking lozenges, or chewing gum may help); hair loss (will regrow after treatment is completed). Report unresolved nausea, or vomiting, alterations in urinary pattern (increased or decreased); opportunistic infection (fever, chills, unusual bruising or bleeding, fatigue, purulent vaginal discharge, unhealed mouth sores), chest pain or difficulty breathing. **Pregnancy/breast-feeding precautions:** Inform prescriber if you are pregnant, Do not get pregnant or cause a pregnancy (males) while taking this medication. Consult prescriber for use appropriate contraceptive measures to use (may cause severe fetal defects), Do not breast-feed.

Pregnancy Issues: Has shown to be teratogenic in animals. Teratogenic effects include a variety of external, visceral, and skeletal abnormalities. The patient should be warned of potential hazards to the fetus.

Other Issues: Diarrhea is dose related. High doses of loperamide can increase tolerated dose of irinotecan.

Additional Information Irinotecan can induce both early and late forms of diarrhea that appear to be mediated by different mechanisms. Early diarrhea (during or within 24 hours of administration) is cholinergic in nature. It can be preceded by complaints of diaphoresis and abdominal cramping and may be ameliorated by the administration of atropine. The elderly (≥65 years of age) are at particular risk for diarrhea. Late diarrhea (occurring >24 hours after administration) can be prolonged and may lead to dehydration and electrolyte imbalance, and can be life-threatening. Late diarrhea should be treated promptly with loperamide. If grade 3 diarrhea (7-9 stools daily, incontinence, or severe cramping) or grade 4 diarrhea (≥10 stools daily, grossly bloody stool, or need for parenteral support), the administration of irinotecan should be delayed until the patient recovers and subsequent doses should be decreased.

Early diarrhea treatment: 0.25-1 mg of intravenous atropine should be considered (unless clinically contraindicated) in patients experiencing diaphoresis, abdominal cramping, or early diarrhea

Late diarrhea treatment: High-dose loperamide: Oral: 4 mg at the first onset of late diarrhea and then 2 mg every 2 hours until the patient is diarrhea-free for at least 12 hours. During the night, the patient may take 4 mg of loperamide every 4 hours. **Premedication with loperamide is not recommended.**

Iron Dextran Complex (EYE ern DEKS tran KOM pleks)

U.S. Brand Names Dexferrum®; INFeD®

Generic Available No

Pharmacologic Category Iron Salt

Pregnancy Risk Factor C

Lactation Enters breast milk/contraindicated

Use Treatment of microcytic hypochromic anemia resulting from iron deficiency in patients in whom oral administration is infeasible or ineffective

Mechanism of Action/Effect The released iron, from the plasma, eventually replenishes the depleted iron stores in the bone marrow where it is incorporated into hemoglobin

Contraindications Hypersensitivity to iron dextran or any component of the formulation; all anemias that are not involved with iron deficiency; hemochromatosis; hemolytic anemia

Warnings/Precautions Use with caution in patients with history of asthma, hepatic impairment, or rheumatoid arthritis. Not recommended in children <4 months of age. Deaths associated with parenteral administration following anaphylactic-type reactions have been reported. Use only in patients where the iron deficient state is not amenable to oral iron therapy. A test dose of 0.5 mL I.V. or I.M. should be given to observe for adverse reactions. I.V. administration of iron dextran is often preferred. Pregnancy risk C.

Drug Interactions

Decreased Effect: Decreased effect with chloramphenicol.

Nutritional/Ethanol Interactions Food: Iron bioavailability may be decreased if taken with dairy products.

Effects on Lab Values May cause falsely elevated values of serum bilirubin and falsely decreased values of serum calcium.

Adverse Reactions

>10%:

- Cardiovascular: Flushing
- Central nervous system: Dizziness, fever, headache, pain
- Gastrointestinal: Nausea, vomiting, metallic taste
- Local: Staining of skin at the site of I.M. injection
- Miscellaneous: Diaphoresis

1% to 10%:

- Cardiovascular: Hypotension (1% to 2%)
- Dermatologic: Urticaria (1% to 2%), phlebitis (1% to 2%)
- Gastrointestinal: Diarrhea
- Genitourinary: Discoloration of urine

<1% (Limited to important or life-threatening): Anaphylactoid reaction, anaphylaxis, shock (cardiovascular collapse, respiratory difficulty; most frequently within minutes of administration)

Note: Diaphoresis, urticaria, arthralgia, fever, chills, dizziness, headache, and nausea may be delayed 24-48 hours after I.V. administration or 3-4 days after I.M. administration.

Overdosage/Toxicology Symptoms of overdose include erosion of GI mucosa, pulmonary edema, hyperthermia, convulsions, tachycardia, hepatic and renal impairment, coma, hematemesis, lethargy, tachycardia, and acidosis. Serum iron level >300 μg/mL requires treatment of overdose due to severe toxicity. If severe iron overdose (when the serum iron concentration exceeds the total iron-binding capacity) occurs, it may be treated with deferoxamine. Deferoxamine may be administered I.V. (80 mg/kg over 24 hours) or I.M. (40-90 mg/kg every 8 hours).

Pharmacodynamics/Kinetics

Absorption:

I.M.: 50% to 90% promptly absorbed; balance slowly absorbed over month

I.V.: Uptake of iron by the reticuloendothelial system appears to be constant at about 10-20 mg/hour

Milliliters of Iron Dextran (50 mg/mL)
Required for Hemoglobin Restoration and Replacement of Iron Stores

Patient's IBW (kg)	Observed Hemoglobin							
	3 g/dL	4 g/dL	5 g/dL	6 g/dL	7 g/dL	8 g/dL	9 g/dL	10 g/dL
5	3	3	3	3	2	2	2	2
10	7	6	6	5	5	4	4	3
15	10	9	9	8	7	7	6	5
20	16	15	14	13	12	11	10	9
25	20	18	17	16	15	14	13	12
30	23	22	21	19	18	17	15	14
35	27	26	24	23	21	20	18	17
40	31	29	28	26	24	22	21	19
45	35	33	31	29	27	25	23	21
50	39	37	35	32	30	28	26	24
55	43	41	38	36	33	31	28	26
60	47	44	42	39	36	34	31	28
65	51	48	45	42	39	36	34	31
70	55	52	49	45	42	39	36	33
75	59	55	52	49	45	42	39	35
80	63	59	55	52	48	45	41	38
85	66	63	59	55	51	48	44	40
90	70	66	62	58	54	50	46	42
95	74	70	66	62	57	53	49	45
100	78	74	69	65	60	56	52	47

Iron dextran doses calculated for normal adult hemoglobin of 14.8 g/dL for IBW >15 kg, and normal hemoglobin of 12.0 g/dL for IBW ≤15 kg.

(Continued)

Iron Dextran Complex *(Continued)*

Formulations Injection, solution:
Dexferrum®: 50 mg/mL (1 mL, 2 mL)
INFeD®: 50 mg/mL (2 mL)

Dosing

Adults & Elderly:

Note: A 0.5 mL test dose (0.25 mL in infants) should be given prior to starting iron dextran therapy; total dose should be divided into a daily schedule for I.M., total dose may be given as a single continuous infusion. A Z-track administration method should be used for all I.M. injections

Iron-deficiency anemia: I.M., I.V.:

Dose (mL) = 0.0476 x LBW (kg) x (normal Hgb - observed Hgb) + (1 mL/5 kg) of LBW to a maximum of 14 mL for iron stores (LBW = lean body weight)

Adults and children >15 kg: Dose (mL) = 0.0442 (desired Hgb - observed Hgb) x IBW + [0.26 x IBW (kg)]; see table on previous page.

IBW (male) = 50 kg + (2.3 kg x inches over 60")
IBW (female) = 45.5 kg + (2.3 kg x inches over 60")

Iron replacement therapy for blood loss: I.M., I.V.: Replacement iron (mg) = blood loss (mL) x Hct

Maximum daily dose (can administer total dose at one time I.V.): >50 kg: 100 mg iron (2 mL)

Pediatrics:

A 0.5 mL test dose (0.25 mL in infants) should be given prior to starting iron dextran therapy. Total dose should be divided into a daily schedule for I.M.; total dose may be given as a single continuous infusion.

Iron-deficiency anemia: Refer to adult dosing.

Iron replacement therapy for blood loss: Refer to adult dosing.

Maximum daily dose (can administer total dose at one time I.V.):

Infants <5 kg: 25 mg iron (0.5 mL)

Children:

5-10 kg: 50 mg iron (1 mL)
10-50 kg: 100 mg iron (2 mL)

Administration

I.M.: Use Z-track technique for I.M. administration (deep into the upper outer quadrant of buttock).

I.V.: May be administered I.V. bolus at rate ≤50 mg/minute or diluted in 250-1000 mL NS and infused over 1-6 hours. Infuse initial 25 mL slowly, observe for allergic reactions. Have epinephrine nearby.

Stability

Storage: Store at room temperature.

Reconstitution: Stability of parenteral admixture at room temperature (25°C) is 3 months.
Standard diluent: Dose/250-1000 mL NS
Minimum volume: 250 mL NS

Compatibility: Stable in D_5W, NS

Monitoring Laboratory Tests Hemoglobin, hematocrit, reticulocyte count, serum ferritin

Monitoring and Teaching Issues

Physical Assessment: Monitor laboratory tests regularly. Monitor patient for adverse reactions (see Adverse Reactions). Note that adverse response may occur some time (1-4 days) after administration. Assess patients with rheumatoid arthritis for exacerbated swelling and joint pain; adjust medications as needed. **Pregnancy risk factor C.** Breast-feeding is contraindicated.

Patient Education: You will need frequent blood tests while on this therapy. If you have rheumatoid arthritis you may experience increased swelling or joint pain; consult prescriber for medication adjustment. If you experience dizziness or severe headache, use caution when driving or engaging in tasks that require alertness until response to drug is known. Small frequent meals, frequent mouth care, sucking lozenges, or chewing gum may relieve nausea and metallic taste. You may experience increased sweating. Report acute GI problems, fever, difficulty breathing, rapid heartbeat, yellowing of skin or eyes, or swelling of hands and feet. **Pregnancy/breast-feeding precautions:** Inform prescriber if you are or intend to become pregnant. Do not breast-feed.

Geriatric Considerations: Anemia in the elderly is most often caused by "anemia of chronic disease", a result of aging effect in bone marrow, or associated with inflammation rather than blood loss. Iron stores are usually normal or increased, with a serum ferritin >50 ng/mL and a decreased total iron binding capacity. Hence, the anemia is not secondary to iron deficiency but the inability of the reticuloendothelial system to use available iron stores. I.V. administration of iron dextran is often preferred over I.M. in the elderly secondary to a decreased muscle mass and the need for daily injections.

Iron Sucrose (EYE ern SOO krose)

U.S. Brand Names Venofer®

Generic Available No

Pharmacologic Category Iron Salt

Pregnancy Risk Factor B

Lactation Excretion in breast milk unknown/use caution

Use Treatment of iron-deficiency anemia in patients undergoing chronic hemodialysis who are receiving supplemental erythropoietin therapy

Mechanism of Action/Effect Iron sucrose is dissociated by the reticuloendothelial system into iron and sucrose. The released iron increases serum iron concentrations and is incorporated into hemoglobin.

Contraindications Hypersensitivity to iron sucrose or any component of the formulation; evidence of iron overload; anemia not caused by iron deficiency

Warnings/Precautions **Fatal and potentially fatal hypersensitivity reactions (characterized by anaphylactic shock, loss of consciousness, collapse, hypotension, dyspnea, and convulsion) have been reported.** Facilities for cardiopulmonary resuscitation must be available during administration. Hypotension has been reported frequently in patients receiving intravenous iron, may be related to total dose or rate of administration (avoid rapid I.V. injection), follow recommended guidelines. Withhold iron in the presence of tissue iron overload, periodic monitoring of hemoglobin, hematocrit, serum ferritin, and transferrin saturation is recommended. Safety and efficacy in children has not been established.

Drug Interactions

Decreased Effect: Chloramphenicol may diminish the therapeutic effects of iron sucrose injection. Iron sucrose injection may reduce the absorption of oral iron preparations.

Adverse Reactions Fatal and life-threatening anaphylactoid reactions (characterized by anaphylactic shock, loss of consciousness, collapse, hypotension, dyspnea, or convulsion) have been reported; hypotension may be related to total dose or rate of administration.

>5%:

Cardiovascular: Hypotension (36%)
Central nervous system: Headache
Gastrointestinal: Nausea, vomiting, diarrhea
Neuromuscular & skeletal: Leg cramps (23%)

1% to 5%:

Cardiovascular: Chest pain, hypertension, hypervolemia
Central nervous system: Fever, malaise, dizziness
Dermatologic: Pruritus
Gastrointestinal: Abdominal pain
Hepatic: Elevated enzymes
Local: Application site reaction
Neuromuscular & skeletal: Musculoskeletal pain, weakness
Respiratory: Dyspnea, pneumonia, cough

<1% (Limited to important or life-threatening): Anaphylactoid reactions, anaphylactic shock, facial rash, loss of consciousness, necrotizing enterocolitis (reported in premature infants, no causal relationship established), seizures, urticaria

Overdosage/Toxicology Symptoms associated with overdose or rapid infusion include hypotension, headache, vomiting, nausea, dizziness, joint aches, paresthesia, abdominal and muscle pain, edema, and cardiovascular collapse. Reducing rate of infusion can alleviate some symptoms. Most symptoms can be treated with I.V. fluids, hydrocortisone, and/or antihistamines.

Although rare, if a severe iron overdose (serum iron concentration exceeds TIBC) occurs, deferoxamine may be administered intravenously.

Pharmacodynamics/Kinetics

Half-Life Elimination: Healthy adults: 6 hours

Metabolism: Dissociated into iron and sucrose by the reticuloendothelial system

Formulations Injection, solution [preservative free]: 20 mg of elemental iron/mL (5 mL)

Dosing

Adults: Doses expressed in mg of **elemental** iron.

Iron-deficiency anemia: I.V.: 100 mg (5 mL of iron sucrose injection) administered 1-3 times/week during dialysis, to a total dose of 1000 mg (10 doses); administer no more than 3 times/week; may continue to administer at lowest dose necessary to maintain target hemoglobin, hematocrit, and iron storage parameters

Test dose: Product labeling does not indicate need for a test dose in product-naive patients; test doses were administered in some clinical trials as 50 mg (2.5 mL) in 50 mL 0.9% NaCl administered over 3-10 minutes

Elderly: Insufficient data to identify differences between elderly and other adults; use caution.

Administration

I.V.: Not for rapid (bolus) I.V. injection; administer through dialysis line. Do not mix with other medications or parenteral nutrient solutions.

Slow I.V. injection: 1 mL (20 mg iron) of undiluted solution per minute (5 minutes/vial)

Infusion: Dilute 1 vial (5 mL) in maximum of 100 mL 0.9% NaCl; infuse over at least 15 minutes.

Stability

Storage: Store vials at room temperature.

Reconstitution: May be administered via the dialysis line as an undiluted solution or by diluting 100 mg (5 mL) in 100 mL normal saline. Solution is stable for 48 hours at room temperature or under refrigeration. Do not mix with other medications.

Monitoring Laboratory Tests Hematocrit, hemoglobin, serum ferritin, transferrin, percent transferrin saturation, TIBC; takes about 4 weeks of treatment to see increased serum iron and ferritin, and decreased TIBC. Serum iron concentrations should be drawn 48 hours after last dose.

Monitoring and Teaching Issues

Physical Assessment: Assess other medications patient may be taking for effectiveness and interactions (see Drug Interactions). See Contraindications and Warnings/Precautions for use cautions. See Administration directions and Warnings/Precautions for I.V. use (facilities for cardiopulmonary resuscitation must be available during administration). Monitor laboratory tests, therapeutic response, and adverse reactions at beginning of therapy and periodically throughout therapy (see Adverse Reactions and Overdose/Toxicology). Assess knowledge/teach patient appropriate use according to product and purpose (dangers of iron overdosing), interventions to reduce side effects, and adverse symptoms to report (see Patient Education). Note breast-feeding caution.

Patient Education: I.V.: You will be watched closely during infusion. You will need frequent blood tests while on this therapy. You may experience hypotension (use caution when driving or climbing stairs or engaging in tasks requiring alertness until response to drug is

(Continued)

Iron Sucrose *(Continued)*

known); black tarry stools (normal), nausea, vomiting (taking with meals will reduce this), constipation (adequate fluids and exercise may help, may need a stool softener); or diarrhea (buttermilk, boiled milk, or yogurt may help). Report immediately severe unresolved GI irritation (cramping, nausea, vomiting, diarrhea, constipation); headache, lethargy, fatigue, dizziness, or other CNS changes; rapid respiration; leg cramps; chest pain or palpations; vision changes; choking sensation; loss of consciousness; or convulsions. **Breast-feeding precaution:** Consult prescriber if breast-feeding.

Iron Sulfate (Ferrous Sulfate) *see* Iron Supplements *on page 744*

Iron Supplements (EYE ern SUP la ments)

U.S. Brand Names Feosol® [OTC]; Feratab® [OTC]; Fer-Gen-Sol [OTC]; Fergon® [OTC]; Fer-In-Sol® [OTC]; Ferretts [OTC]; Ferro-Sequels® [OTC]; Hemocyte™[OTC]; Ircon® [OTC]; Nephro-Fer® [OTC]; Slow FE® [OTC]

Synonyms Ferrous Fumarate; Ferrous Gluconate; Ferrous Salts; Ferrous Sulfate; $FeSO_4$ (Ferrous Sulfate); Iron Sulfate (Ferrous Sulfate)

Generic Available Yes

Pharmacologic Category Iron Salt; Mineral, Oral; Mineral, Parenteral

Pregnancy Risk Factor A

Lactation Enters breast milk/compatible

Use Prevention and treatment of iron deficiency anemias; supplemental therapy for patients receiving epoetin alfa

Mechanism of Action/Effect Iron is released from the plasma and eventually replenishes the depleted iron stores in the bone marrow where it is incorporated into hemoglobin; allows the transportation of oxygen via hemoglobin

Contraindications Hypersensitivity to iron salts; hemochromatosis; hemolytic anemia

Warnings/Precautions Avoid using for longer than 6 months, except in patients with conditions that require prolonged therapy. Avoid in patients with peptic ulcer, enteritis, or ulcerative colitis; those receiving frequent blood transfusions; use in premature infants (until the vitamin E stores, deficient at birth, are replenished); some products contain sulfites and/or tartrazine which may cause allergic reactions in susceptible individuals

Drug Interactions

Decreased Effect: Absorption of oral preparation of iron and tetracyclines is decreased when both of these drugs are given together. Absorption of quinolones may be decreased due to formation of a ferric ion-quinolone complex. Concurrent administration of antacids and cimetidine may decrease iron absorption. Iron may decrease absorption of penicillamine, methyldopa, and levodopa when given at the same time. Response to iron therapy may be delayed in patients receiving chloramphenicol.

Increased Effect/Toxicity: Concurrent administration ≥200 mg vitamin C per 30 mg elemental iron increases absorption of oral iron.

Nutritional/Ethanol Interactions Milk, cereals, dietary fiber, tea, coffee, or eggs decrease absorption of iron.

Effects on Lab Values False-positive for blood in stool by the guaiac test

Adverse Reactions Frequency not defined:

Gastrointestinal: GI irritation, epigastric pain, nausea, diarrhea, dark stools, constipation
Genitourinary: Discoloration of urine (black or dark)
Miscellaneous: Liquid preparations may temporarily stain the teeth

Pharmacodynamics/Kinetics

Absorption: Oral: Iron is absorbed in the duodenum and upper jejunum. In persons with normal iron stores 10% of an oral dose is absorbed, this is increased to 20% to 30% in persons with inadequate iron stores. Food and achlorhydria will decrease absorption.

Half-Life Elimination: Iron is largely bound to serum transferrin and excreted in the urine, sweat, sloughing of intestinal mucosa, and by menses.

Time to Peak: Peak reticulocytosis occurs in 5-10 days, and hemoglobin values increase within 2-4 weeks

Onset: Hematologic response to either oral or parenteral iron salts is essentially the same; red blood cell form and color changes within 3-10 days

Formulations Elemental iron listed in brackets:

Ferrous fumarate:

Tablet: 325 mg [106 mg]
- Ferretts: 325 mg [106 mg]
- Hemocyte®: 324 mg [106 mg]
- Ircon®: 200 mg [66 mg]
- Nephro-Fer™: 350 mg [115 mg]

Tablet, chewable (Feostat®): 100 mg [33 mg] [chocolate flavor]
Tablet, timed release (Ferro-Sequels®): 150 mg [50 mg] with docusate sodium 100 mg

Ferrous gluconate:

Tablet: 240 mg [27 mg]; 246 mg [28 mg]; 300 mg [34 mg]; 324 mg [37 mg]; 325 mg [38 mg]
- Fergon®: 320 mg [37 mg]

Ferrous sulfate:

Drops, oral: 75 mg/0.6 mL (50 mL) [15 mg/0.6 mL]
- Fer-Gen-Sol: 75 mg/0.6 mL (50 mL) [15 mg/0.6 mL] [lemon-lime flavor]
- Fer-In-Sol®: 75 mg/0.6 mL (50 mL) [15 mg/0.6 mL] [contains 0.2% alcohol and sodium bisulfite]

Tablet: 324 mg [65 mg]; 325 mg [65 mg]
- Feratab®: 300 mg [60 mg]

Tablet, exsiccated (Feosol®): 200 mg [65 mg]
Tablet, exsiccated, timed release (Slow FE®): 160 mg [50 mg]

Dosing

Adults: Multiple salt forms of iron exist; close attention must be paid to the salt form when ordering and administering iron; incorrect selection or substitution of one salt for another without proper dosage adjustment may result in serious over- or underdosing.

Oral (Dose expressed in terms of **elemental** iron):
Recommended Daily Allowance (RDA): See table
Iron deficiency: 60-100 mg elemental iron twice daily up to 60 mg elemental iron 4 times/day, or 50 mg elemental iron (extended release) 1-2 times/day
Prophylaxis: 60-100 mg elemental iron/day (see table)

Elemental Iron Content of Iron Salts

Iron Salt	Elemental Iron Content (% of salt form)	Approximate Equivalent Doses (mg of iron salt)
Ferrous fumarate	33	197
Ferrous gluconate	11.6	560
Ferrous sulfate	20	324

Elderly: Refer to adult dosing and Special Geriatric Considerations.
Pediatrics: Multiple salt forms of iron exist; close attention must be paid to the salt form when ordering and administering iron; incorrect selection or substitution of one salt for another without proper dosage adjustment may result in serious over- or underdosing.
Oral (dose expressed in terms of **elemental** iron):
Recommended Daily Allowance, see table.

Recommended Daily Allowance of Iron (dosage expressed as elemental iron)

Age	RDA (mg)
<5 months	5
5 months to 10 years	10
Male	
11-18 years	12
>18 years	10
Female	
11-50 years	15
>50 years	10

Premature neonates: 2-4 mg elemental iron/kg/day divided every 12-24 hours (maximum dose: 15 mg/day)
Infants and Children:
Severe iron deficiency anemia: 4-6 mg elemental iron/kg/day in 3 divided doses
Mild to moderate iron deficiency anemia: 3 mg elemental iron/kg/day in 1-2 divided doses
Prophylaxis: 1-2 mg elemental iron/kg/day up to a maximum of 15 mg elemental iron/day

Administration
Oral: Do not chew or crush sustained release preparations. Administer with water or juice between meals for maximum absorption; may administer with food if GI upset occurs. Do not administer with milk or milk products.

Monitoring Laboratory Tests Serum iron, total iron binding capacity, reticulocyte count, hemoglobin, ferritin

Monitoring and Teaching Issues
Physical Assessment: Assess other medications patient may be taking; instruct patient accordingly about timing of medications and dangers of iron overdosing. Monitor for adverse side effects and indications of overdose.
Patient Education: Take this drug as prescribed; do not increase dose. Take at the same time each day. Do not take within 1 hour of other medications or antacids. May be taken with food, but not with milk, eggs, caffeine-containing drinks, cereals, or foods containing dietary fiber. If mixed with liquid (juice or water) use a straw to prevent staining of teeth. You may experience black tarry stools and black or dark urine (normal); nausea, vomiting (taking with meals will reduce this); or constipation (adequate fluids and exercise may help, may need a stool softener). Report severe unresolved GI irritation, lethargy, rapid respiration, CNS changes, and unrelieved constipation. Keep out of reach of children.
Geriatric Considerations: Anemia in the elderly is often caused by "anemia of chronic disease", a result of aging changes in the bone marrow, or associated with inflammation rather than blood loss. Iron stores are usually normal or increased, with a serum ferritin >50 ng/mL and a decreased total iron binding capacity. Hence, the anemia is not secondary to iron deficiency but the inability of the reticuloendothelial system to use available iron stores. Timed release iron preparations should be avoided due to their erratic absorption. Products combined with a laxative or stool softener should not be used unless the need for the combination is demonstrated.

Additional Information When treating iron deficiency anemias, treat for 3-4 months after hemoglobin/hematocrit return to normal in order to replenish total body stores. Elemental iron dosages as high as 15 mg/kg/day have been used to supplement neonates receiving concomitant epoetin alpha in the treatment of anemia of prematurity.

ISD *see* Isosorbide Dinitrate *on page 749*
ISDN *see* Isosorbide Dinitrate *on page 749*
ISMN *see* Isosorbide Mononitrate *on page 750*
Ismo® *see* Isosorbide Mononitrate *on page 750*
Ismotic® *see page 1509*
Isobamate *see* Carisoprodol *on page 221*
Isocarboxazid *see page 1553*

Isoflurophate *see page 1509*

Isoflurophate *see page 1575*

Isometheptene, Acetaminophen, and Dichloralphenazone *see* Acetaminophen, Isometheptene, and Dichloralphenazone *on page 38*

Isometheptene, Dichloralphenazone, and Acetaminophen *see* Acetaminophen, Isometheptene, and Dichloralphenazone *on page 38*

Isoniazid (eye soe NYE a zid)

U.S. Brand Names Nydrazid®

Synonyms INH; Isonicotinic Acid Hydrazide

Generic Available Yes

Pharmacologic Category Antitubercular Agent

Pregnancy Risk Factor C

Lactation Enters breast milk/compatible

Use Treatment of susceptible tuberculosis infections; prophylactically in those individuals exposed to tuberculosis

Mechanism of Action/Effect Unknown, but may include the inhibition of myocolic acid synthesis resulting in disruption of the bacterial cell wall

Contraindications Hypersensitivity to isoniazid or any component of the formulation; acute liver disease; previous history of hepatic damage during isoniazid therapy

Warnings/Precautions Use with caution in patients with renal impairment and chronic liver disease. Severe and sometimes fatal hepatitis may occur or develop even after many months of treatment. Patients must report any prodromal symptoms of hepatitis, such as fatigue, weakness, malaise, anorexia, nausea, or vomiting. Periodic ophthalmic examinations are recommended even when usual symptoms do not occur. Pyridoxine (10-50 mg/day) is recommended in individuals likely to develop peripheral neuropathies. Pregnancy risk C.

Drug Interactions

Cytochrome P450 Effect: Substrate of **CYP2E1**; Inhibits CYP1A2, 2C8/9, 2C19, 2D6, 2E1, 3A4; Induces CYP2E1 (after discontinuation)

Decreased Effect: Decreased effect/levels of isoniazid with aluminum salts.

Increased Effect/Toxicity: Increased toxicity/levels of oral anticoagulants, carbamazepines, cycloserine, hydantoins, and hepatically metabolized benzodiazepines. Reaction with disulfiram.

Nutritional/Ethanol Interactions

Ethanol: Avoid ethanol (increases the risk of hepatitis).

Food: Isoniazid serum levels may be decreased if taken with food. Clinically severe elevated blood pressure may occur if isoniazid is taken with tyramine-containing foods. Avoid foods with histamine or tyramine (cheese, broad beans, dry sausage, salami, nonfresh meat, liver pate, soy bean, liquid and powdered protein supplements, wine). Isoniazid decreases folic acid absorption. Isoniazid alters pyridoxine metabolism.

Effects on Lab Values False-positive urinary glucose with Clinitest®

Adverse Reactions

>10%:

Gastrointestinal: Loss of appetite, nausea, vomiting, stomach pain

Hepatic: Mild increased LFTs (10% to 20%)

Neuromuscular & skeletal: Weakness, peripheral neuropathy (dose-related incidence, 10% to 20% incidence with 10 mg/kg/day)

1% to 10%:

Central nervous system: Dizziness, slurred speech, lethargy

Hepatic: Progressive liver damage (increases with age; 2.3% in patients >50 years)

Neuromuscular & skeletal: Hyper-reflexia

<1% (Limited to important or life-threatening): Blood dyscrasias, depression, psychosis, seizures

Overdosage/Toxicology Symptoms of overdose include nausea, vomiting, slurred speech, dizziness, blurred vision, hallucinations, stupor, coma, and intractable seizures. The onset of metabolic acidosis is within 30 minutes to 3 hours. Because of high morbidity and mortality rates with isoniazid overdose, patients who are asymptomatic after an overdose should be monitored for 4-6 hours. Pyridoxine has been shown to be effective in the treatment of intoxication, especially when seizures occur. Pyridoxine I.V. is administered on a milligram to milligram dose. If the amount of isoniazid ingested is unknown, 5 g of pyridoxine should be given over 3-5 minutes and may be followed by an additional 5 g in 30 minutes. Treatment is supportive. Forced diuresis and hemodialysis can result in more rapid removal.

Pharmacodynamics/Kinetics

Absorption: Rapid and complete; rate can be slowed with food

Half-Life Elimination: Fast acetylators: 30-100 minutes; Slow acetylators: 2-5 hours; may be prolonged with hepatic or severe renal impairment

Time to Peak: Serum: 1-2 hours

Metabolism: Hepatic with decay rate determined genetically by acetylation phenotype

Formulations

Injection, solution (Nydrazid®): 100 mg/mL (10 mL)

Syrup: 50 mg/5 mL (473 mL) [orange flavor]

Tablet: 100 mg, 300 mg

Dosing

Adults & Elderly: Recommendations often change due to resistant strains and newly developed information; consult *MMWR* for current CDC recommendations. Intramuscular is available in patients who are unable to either take or absorb oral therapy.

TB prophylaxis: Oral: 300 mg/day for 6 months in patients who do not have HIV infection and 12 months in patients who have HIV infection

TB treatment: Oral:

Daily therapy: 5 mg/kg/day given daily (usual dose: 300 mg/day); 10 mg/kg/day in 1-2 divided doses in patients with disseminated disease

Directly observed therapy (DOT): Twice weekly therapy: 15 mg/kg (maximum: 900 mg); 3 times/week therapy: 15 mg/kg (maximum: 900 mg)

Note: A four-drug regimen (isoniazid, rifampin, pyrazinamide, and either streptomycin or ethambutol) is preferred for the initial, empiric treatment of TB. When the drug susceptibility results are available, the regimen should be altered as appropriate.

Note: Concomitant administration of 6-50 mg/day pyridoxine is recommended in malnourished patients or those prone to neuropathy (eg, alcoholics, diabetics).

Pediatrics: Recommendations often change due to resistant strains and newly developed information; consult *MMWR* for current CDC recommendations. Intramuscular is available in patients who are unable to either take or absorb oral therapy.

TB prophylaxis: Oral: Infants and Children: 10 mg/kg/day in 1-2 divided doses (maximum: 300 mg/day) 6 months in patients who do not have HIV infection and 12 months in patients who have HIV infection

TB treatment: Oral: Infants and Children:

Daily therapy: 10-20 mg/kg/day in 1-2 divided doses (maximum: 300 mg/day)

Directly observed therapy (DOT): Twice weekly therapy: 20-40 mg/kg (maximum: 900 mg/day); 3 times/week therapy: 20-40 mg/kg (maximum: 900 mg)

Note: A four-drug regimen (isoniazid, rifampin, pyrazinamide, and either streptomycin or ethambutol) is preferred for the initial, empiric treatment of TB. When the drug susceptibility results are available, the regimen should be altered as appropriate.

Renal Impairment:

Cl_{cr} <10 mL/minute: Administer 50% of normal dose.

Hemodialysis: Dose after dialysis.

Dialyzable (50% to 100%)

Hepatic Impairment: Dose should be reduced in severe hepatic disease.

Administration

Oral: Should be administered 1 hour before or 2 hours after meals on an empty stomach.

Stability

Storage: Protect oral dosage forms from light.

Monitoring Laboratory Tests Transaminase levels at baseline 1, 3, 6, and 9 months

Monitoring and Teaching Issues

Physical Assessment: See Contraindications and Warnings/Precautions for use cautions. Assess potential for interactions with other prescriptions, OTC medications, or herbal products patient may be taking (see Drug Interactions). Assess results of laboratory tests (see Monitoring Lab Tests), therapeutic effects, and adverse response (see Adverse Reactions and Overdose/Toxicology) at regular intervals during therapy. Caution diabetic patients about using Clinitest®. Teach patient proper use, possible side effects and appropriate interventions (eg, diet [see Tyramine Foods List] and ophthalmic examinations), and adverse symptoms to report (see Patient Education). **Pregnancy risk factor C** - benefits of use should outweigh possible risks.

Patient Education: Inform prescriber of all prescriptions, OTC medications, or herbal products you are taking, and any allergies you have. Do not take anything new during treatment unless approved by prescriber. Best if taken on an empty stomach, 1 hour before or 2 hours after meals. Avoid missing any dose and do not discontinue without notifying prescriber. Avoid alcohol and tyramine-containing foods (eg, aged cheese, broad beans, dry sausage, preserved meats or sausages, liver pate, fish, soy bean, protein supplements, wine) and increase dietary intake of folate, niacin, magnesium. If diabetic, use serum testing (isoniazid may affect Clinitest® results). You will need to have frequent ophthalmic exams and periodic medical check-ups to evaluate drug effects. You may experience nausea or vomiting (small, frequent meals, frequent mouth care, chewing gum, or sucking lozenges may help). Report tingling or numbness in hands or feet, loss of sensation, unusual weakness, fatigue, nausea or vomiting, dark colored urine, change in urinary pattern, yellowing skin or eyes, or change in color of stool. **Pregnancy precaution:** Inform prescriber if you are or intend to become pregnant.

Dietary Issues: Should be taken 1 hour before or 2 hours after meals on an empty stomach; increase dietary intake of folate, niacin, magnesium.

Geriatric Considerations: Age has not been shown to affect the pharmacokinetics of INH since acetylation phenotype determines clearance and half-life, acetylation rate does not change significantly with age. Most strains of *M. tuberculosis* found the elderly should be susceptible to INH since most acquired their initial infection prior to INH's introduction.

Related Information

Tuberculosis *on page 1705*

Tyramine Foods List *on page 1601*

Isoniazid and Rifampin *see* Rifampin and Isoniazid *on page 1187*

Isoniazid, Rifampin, and Pyrazinamide *see* Rifampin, Isoniazid, and Pyrazinamide *on page 1188*

Isonicotinic Acid Hydrazide *see* Isoniazid *on page 746*

Isonipecaine Hydrochloride *see* Meperidine *on page 851*

Isopropyl Alcohol *see page 1519*

Isoproterenol (eye soe proe TER e nole)

U.S. Brand Names Isuprel®

Synonyms Isoproterenol Hydrochloride

Generic Available Yes

Pharmacologic Category $Beta_1$/$Beta_2$ Agonist

Pregnancy Risk Factor C

Lactation Excretion in breast milk unknown

Use Ventricular arrhythmias due to AV nodal block; hemodynamically compromised bradyarrhythmias or atropine- and dopamine-resistant bradyarrhythmias (when transcutaneous/venous pacing is not available); temporary use in third-degree AV block until pacemaker insertion

(Continued)

Isoproterenol *(Continued)*

Use - Unlabeled/Investigational Temporizing measure before transvenous pacing for torsade de pointes; diagnostic aid (vasovagal syncope)

Mechanism of Action/Effect Stimulates $beta_1$- and $beta_2$-receptors resulting in relaxation of bronchial, GI, and uterine smooth muscle, increased heart rate and contractility, vasodilation of peripheral vasculature

Contraindications Hypersensitivity to sulfites or isoproterenol, any component of the formulation, or other sympathomimetic amines; angina, pre-existing cardiac arrhythmias (ventricular); tachycardia or AV block caused by cardiac glycoside intoxication

Warnings/Precautions Use with extreme caution; not currently a treatment of choice. Use with caution in elderly patients, diabetics, renal or cardiovascular disease, hyperthyroidism. Excessive or prolonged use may result in decreased effectiveness of isoproterenol. Pregnancy risk C.

Drug Interactions

Increased Effect/Toxicity: Sympathomimetic agents may cause headaches and elevate blood pressure. General anesthetics may cause arrhythmias.

Nutritional/Ethanol Interactions Herb/Nutraceutical: Avoid ephedra, yohimbe (may cause CNS stimulation).

Adverse Reactions Frequency not defined.

Cardiovascular: Premature ventricular beats, bradycardia, hypertension, hypotension, chest pain, palpitations, tachycardia, ventricular arrhythmias, myocardial infarction size increased

Central nervous system: Headache, nervousness or restlessness

Gastrointestinal: Nausea, vomiting

Respiratory: Dyspnea

Overdosage/Toxicology Symptoms of overdose include tremor, nausea, vomiting, and hypotension. Beta-adrenergic stimulation can cause increased heart rate, decreased blood pressure, and CNS excitation. Treat symptomatically.

Pharmacodynamics/Kinetics

Half-Life Elimination: 2.5-5 minutes

Metabolism: Via conjugation in many tissues including hepatic and pulmonary

Onset: Bronchodilation: I.V.: Immediate

Duration: I.V.: 10-15 minutes

Formulations Injection, solution, as hydrochloride: 0.02 mg/mL (10 mL); 0.2 mg/mL (1:5000) (1 mL, 5 mL) [contains sodium metabisulfite]

Dosing

Adults: Cardiac arrhythmias: I.V.: Initial: 2 mcg/minute; titrate to patient response (2-10 mcg/minute)

Elderly: Refer to adult dosing. Start at the low end of the dosing range, reflecting the frequency of decreased hepatic, renal, or cardiac function and of concomitant diseases of other drug therapies.

Pediatrics: Cardiac arrhythmias: I.V.: Start 0.1 mcg/kg/minute (usual effective dose 0.2-2 mcg/kg/minute)

Administration

I.V.: I.V. infusion administration requires the use of an infusion pump.

To prepare for infusion: 1 mg isoproterenol to 500 mL D_5W, final concentration 2 mcg/mL

Stability

Storage: Isoproterenol solution should be stored at room temperature. It should not be used if a color or precipitate is present. Exposure to air, light, or increased temperature may cause a pink to brownish pink color to develop.

Reconstitution: Stability of parenteral admixture at room temperature (25°C) or at refrigeration (4°C) is 24 hours.

Standard diluent: 2 mg/500 mL D_5W; 4 mg/500 mL D_5W

Minimum volume: 1 mg/100 mL D_5W

Compatibility: Stable in dextran 6% in dextrose, dextran 6% in NS, D_5LR, $D_5{}^1/_4$ NS, $D_5{}^1/_2$NS, D_5NS, D_5W, $D_{10}W$, LR, $^1/_2$NS, NS; **incompatible** with sodium bicarbonate 5%, and alkaline solutions

Compatibility when admixed: Incompatible with aminophylline, furosemide, sodium bicarbonate

Monitoring Laboratory Tests EKG, arterial blood gas, arterial blood pressure, CVP

Monitoring and Teaching Issues

Physical Assessment: Monitor laboratory tests, cardiac, respiratory, and hemodynamic status when used in acute or emergency situations. Assess knowledge/teach patient appropriate use and administration procedures and adverse reactions to report. **Pregnancy risk factor C** - benefits of use should outweigh possible risks. Note breast-feeding caution.

Patient Education: You may experience nervousness, dizziness, or fatigue (use caution when driving or engaging in tasks requiring alertness until response to drug is known); or dry mouth, nausea, or vomiting (small, frequent meals may reduce the incidence of nausea or vomiting). Report chest pain, rapid heartbeat or palpitations, unresolved/persistent GI upset, dizziness, fatigue, trembling, increased anxiety, sleeplessness, or difficulty breathing. **Pregnancy/breast-feeding precautions:** Inform prescriber if you are pregnant. Consult prescriber if breast-feeding.

Related Information

Inotropic and Vasoconstrictor Comparison *on page 1580*

Isoproterenol Hydrochloride *see* Isoproterenol *on page 747*

Isoptin® SR *see* Verapamil *on page 1396*

Isopto® Atropine *see page 1509*

Isopto® Atropine *see* Atropine *on page 134*

Isopto® Carbachol *see* Ophthalmic Agents, Glaucoma *on page 1002*

Isopto® Carpine *see* Ophthalmic Agents, Glaucoma *on page 1002*

Isopto® Carpine *see* Pilocarpine *on page 1082*

Isopto® Cetapred® *see page 1509*

Isopto® Homatropine *see page 1509*

Isopto® Hyoscine *see page 1509*

Isopto® Hyoscine *see* Scopolamine *on page 1218*

Isordil® *see* Isosorbide Dinitrate *on page 749*

Isosorbide *see page 1509*

Isosorbide Dinitrate (eye soe SOR bide dye NYE trate)

U.S. Brand Names Dilatrate®-SR; Isordil®

Synonyms ISD; ISDN

Generic Available Yes: Tablet

Pharmacologic Category Vasodilator

Pregnancy Risk Factor C

Lactation Excretion in breast milk unknown

Use Prevention and treatment of angina pectoris; for congestive heart failure; to relieve pain, dysphagia, and spasm in esophageal spasm with GE reflux

Mechanism of Action/Effect Relaxes vascular smooth muscles, decreases arterial resistance and venous return which reduces cardiac oxygen demand. Additionally, coronary artery dilation improves collateral flow to ischemic regions; esophageal smooth muscle is relaxed via the same mechanism.

Contraindications Hypersensitivity to isosorbide dinitrate or any component of the formulation; hypersensitivity to organic nitrates; concurrent use with sildenafil; angle-closure glaucoma (intraocular pressure may be increased); head trauma or cerebral hemorrhage (increase intracranial pressure); severe anemia

Warnings/Precautions Use with caution in volume depletion, hypotension, and right ventricular infarctions. Paradoxical bradycardia and increased angina pectoris can accompany hypotension. Postural hypotension may also occur; ethanol may potentiate this effect. Tolerance does develop to nitrates and appropriate dosing is needed to minimize this. Safety and efficacy have not been established in pediatric patients. Nitrate may aggravate angina caused by hypertrophic cardiomyopathy. Pregnancy risk C.

Drug Interactions

Cytochrome P450 Effect: Substrate of **CYP3A4**

Increased Effect/Toxicity: Combinations of sildenafil and nitrates has been associated with severe hypotensive reactions and death.

Nutritional/Ethanol Interactions Ethanol: Caution with ethanol (may increase risk of hypotension).

Effects on Lab Values ↓ cholesterol (S)

Adverse Reactions Frequency not defined.

Cardiovascular: Hypotension (infrequent), postural hypotension, crescendo angina (uncommon), rebound hypertension (uncommon), pallor, cardiovascular collapse, tachycardia, shock, flushing, peripheral edema

Central nervous system: Headache (most common), lightheadedness (related to blood pressure changes), syncope (uncommon), dizziness, restlessness

Gastrointestinal: Nausea, vomiting, bowel incontinence, xerostomia

Genitourinary: Urinary incontinence

Hematologic: Methemoglobinemia (rare, overdose)

Neuromuscular & skeletal: Weakness

Ocular: Blurred vision

Miscellaneous: Cold sweat

The incidence of hypotension and adverse cardiovascular events may be increased when used in combination with sildenafil (Viagra®).

Overdosage/Toxicology Symptoms of overdose include hypotension, throbbing headache, palpitations, visual disturbances, tachycardia, methemoglobinemia, flushing, diaphoresis, metabolic acidosis, and coma. High levels or methemoglobinemia can cause signs or symptoms of hypoxemia. Treat symptomatically.

Pharmacodynamics/Kinetics

Half-Life Elimination: Parent drug: 1-4 hours; Metabolite (5-mononitrate): 4 hours

Metabolism: Extensively hepatic to conjugated metabolites, including isosorbide 5-mononitrate (active) and 2-mononitrate (active)

Onset: Sublingual tablet: 2-10 minutes; Chewable tablet: 3 minutes; Oral tablet: 45-60 minutes

Duration: Sublingual tablet: 1-2 hours; Chewable tablet: 0.5-2 hours; Oral tablet: 4-6 hours

Formulations

Capsule, sustained release (Dilatrate®-SR): 40 mg

Tablet: 5 mg, 10 mg, 20 mg, 30 mg,

Isordil®: 5 mg, 10 mg, 20 mg, 30mg, 40 mg

Tablet, chewable: 5 mg, 10 mg

Tablet, sublingual (Isordil®): 2.5 mg, 5 mg, 10 mg

Dosing

Adults:

Angina: Oral: 5-40 mg 4 times/day or 40 mg every 8-12 hours in sustained released dosage form

Congestive heart failure:

Oral:

Initial: 10 mg 3 times/day

Target: 40 mg 3 times/day

Maximum: 80 mg 3 times/day

Sublingual: 2.5-10 mg every 4-6 hours

Chewable tablet: 5-10 mg every 2-3 hours

(Continued)

Isosorbide Dinitrate *(Continued)*

Note: Tolerance to nitrate effects develops with chronic exposure. Dose escalation does not overcome this effect. Short periods (10-14 hours) of nitrate withdrawal help minimize tolerance.

Elderly: Elderly patients should be given lowest recommended adult daily doses initially and titrate upward.

Renal Impairment: Hemodialysis: During hemodialysis, administer dose postdialysis or administer supplemental 10-20 mg dose. During peritoneal dialysis, supplemental dose is not necessary.

Administration

Oral: Do not crush sublingual tablets. Do not administer around-the-clock. The first dose of nitrates should be administered in a prescriber's office to observe for maximal cardiovascular dynamic effects and adverse effects (orthostatic blood pressure drop, headache).

Monitoring and Teaching Issues

Physical Assessment: See Contraindications, Warnings/Precautions, and Drug Interactions for use cautions. Assess potential for interactions with other prescriptions, OTC medications, or herbal products patient may be taking (see Drug Interactions). See Administration warning. Assess results of laboratory tests (see Monitoring Lab Tests), therapeutic effects, and adverse response (eg, hypotension - see Adverse Reactions and Overdose/Toxicology) at regular intervals during therapy. When discontinuing, reduce dosage gradually. Teach patient proper use, possible side effects and appropriate interventions, and adverse symptoms to report (see Patient Education). **Pregnancy risk factor C** - benefits of use should outweigh possible risks. Note breast-feeding caution.

Patient Education: Inform prescriber of all prescriptions, OTC medications, or herbal products you are taking, and any allergies you have. Do not take anything new during treatment unless approved by prescriber. Take as directed, at the same time each day. Do not chew or swallow sublingual tablets; allow them to dissolve under your tongue. Do not crush or chew sustained release capsules, swallow whole with 8 oz water. Do not change brands without consulting prescriber. Do not discontinue abruptly. Keep medication in original container, tightly closed. Avoid alcohol; combination may cause severe hypotension. May cause postural hypotension (take medication while sitting down and use caution when rising from sitting or lying position or climbing stairs); dizziness, weakness, or blurred vision (use caution when driving or engaging in hazardous activities until response to drug is known); or nausea or vomiting (small, frequent meals, frequent mouth care, chewing gum, or sucking lozenges may help). If chest pain occurs, seek emergency medical help at once. Report acute headache, rapid heartbeat, unusual restlessness or dizziness, muscular weakness, or blurring vision. **Pregnancy/breast-feeding precautions:** Inform prescriber if you are or intend to become pregnant. Consult prescriber if breast-feeding.

Related Information

Heart Failure *on page 1670*

Isosorbide Mononitrate (eye soe SOR bide mon oh NYE trate)

U.S. Brand Names Imdur®; Ismo®; Monoket®

Synonyms ISMN

Generic Available Yes

Pharmacologic Category Vasodilator

Pregnancy Risk Factor C

Lactation Excretion in breast milk unknown

Use Long-acting metabolite of the vasodilator isosorbide dinitrate used for the prophylactic treatment of angina pectoris

Mechanism of Action/Effect Systemic venodilation, decreasing preload and increasing ejection fractions; improves congestive symptoms in heart failure and improves the myocardial perfusion in patients with coronary artery disease

Contraindications Hypersensitivity to isosorbide or any component of the formulation; hypersensitivity to organic nitrates; concurrent use with sildenafil; angle-closure glaucoma (intraocular pressure may be increased); head trauma or cerebral hemorrhage (increase intracranial pressure); severe anemia

Warnings/Precautions Use with caution in volume depletion, hypotension, and right ventricular infarctions. Paradoxical bradycardia and increased angina pectoris can accompany hypotension. Orthostatic hypotension can also occur; ethanol can accentuate this. Tolerance does develop to nitrates and appropriate dosing is needed to minimize this (drug-free interval). Safety and efficacy have not been established in pediatric patients. Nitrates may aggravate angina caused by hypertrophic cardiomyopathy. Pregnancy risk C.

Drug Interactions

Cytochrome P450 Effect: Substrate of **CYP3A4**

Increased Effect/Toxicity: Combinations of sildenafil and nitrates has been associated with severe hypotensive reactions and death. CYP3A4 inhibitors may increase hypotensive response.

Nutritional/Ethanol Interactions Ethanol: Caution with ethanol (may increase risk of hypotension).

Adverse Reactions

>10%: Central nervous system: Headache (19% to 38%)

1% to 10%:

Central nervous system: Dizziness (3% to 5%)

Gastrointestinal: Nausea/vomiting (2% to 4%)

<1% (Limited to important or life-threatening): Angina pectoris, arrhythmias, atrial fibrillation, impotence, methemoglobinemia (rare), pruritus, rash, supraventricular tachycardia, syncope, vomiting

The incidence of hypotension and adverse cardiovascular events may be increased when used in combination with sildenafil (Viagra®).

Overdosage/Toxicology Symptoms of overdose include hypotension, throbbing headache, palpitations, visual disturbances, tachycardia, methemoglobinemia, flushing, diaphoresis, metabolic acidosis, and coma. High levels or methemoglobinemia can cause signs or symptoms of hypoxemia. Treat symptomatically.

Pharmacodynamics/Kinetics

Absorption: Nearly complete and low intersubject variability in its pharmacokinetic parameters and plasma concentrations

Half-Life Elimination: Mononitrate: ~4 hours

Metabolism: Hepatic

Onset: 30-60 minutes

Formulations

Tablet: 10 mg, 20 mg

Ismo®: 20 mg

Monoket®: 10 mg, 20 mg

Tablet, extended release (Imdur®): 30 mg, 60 mg, 120 mg

Dosing

Adults: Angina: Oral:

Regular tablet: 5-10 mg twice daily with the two doses given 7 hours apart (eg, 8 AM and 3 PM) to decrease tolerance development; then titrate to 10 mg twice daily in first 2-3 days.

Extended release tablet: Initial: 30-60 mg given in morning as a single dose; titrate upward as needed, giving at least 3 days between increases; maximum daily single dose: 240 mg

Tolerance to nitrate effects develops with chronic exposure. Dose escalation does not overcome this effect. Tolerance can only be overcome by short periods of nitrate absence from the body. Short periods (10-12 hours) of nitrate withdrawal help minimize tolerance. Recommended dosage regimens incorporate this interval. General recommendations are to take the last dose of short-acting agents no later than 7 PM; administer 2 times/day rather than 4 times/day. Administer sustained release tablet once daily in the morning.

Elderly: Start with lowest recommended adult dose.

Renal Impairment: Not necessary for elderly or patients with altered renal or hepatic function. Tolerance to nitrate effects develops with chronic exposure.

Administration

Oral: The first dose of nitrates (ie, sublingual, chewable, oral) should be taken in a prescriber's office to observe for maximal cardiovascular dynamic effects and adverse effects (eg, orthostatic blood pressure drop, headache). Daily dose should be taken in the morning upon arising. Asymmetrical dosing regimen of 7 AM and 3 PM or 9 AM and 5 PM to allow for a nitrate-free dosing interval to minimize nitrate tolerance. Do not administer around-the-clock, an 8- to 12-hour nitrate-free interval is needed each day to prevent tolerance. Extended release tablets should not be chewed or crushed. Should be swallowed with a half-glassful of fluid.

Stability

Storage: Tablets should be stored in a tight container at room temperature of 15°C to 30°C (59°F to 86°F).

Monitoring Laboratory Tests Orthostasis

Monitoring and Teaching Issues

Physical Assessment: See Contraindications, Warnings/Precautions, and Dosing for use cautions. Assess potential for interactions with other prescriptions, OTC medications, or herbal products patient may be taking (see Drug Interactions). See specific Administration directions. Assess results of laboratory tests (see Monitoring Lab Tests), therapeutic effects, and adverse response (see Adverse Reactions and Overdose/Toxicology) at regular intervals during therapy. When discontinuing, reduce dosage gradually. Teach patient proper use, possible side effects and appropriate interventions, and adverse symptoms to report (see Patient Education). **Pregnancy risk factor C** - benefits of use should outweigh possible risks. Note breast-feeding caution.

Patient Education: Inform prescriber of all prescriptions, OTC medications, or herbal products you are taking, and any allergies you have. Do not take anything new during treatment unless approved by prescriber. Take exactly as directed, at the same time each day. Take last dose in early evening. Do not chew or crush extended forms; swallow whole with 8 oz of water. Do not change brands without consulting prescriber. Do not discontinue abruptly. Keep medication in original container, tightly closed. Avoid alcohol; combination may cause severe hypotension. May cause postural hypotension (take medication while sitting down and use caution when rising from sitting or lying position or climbing stairs); dizziness, weakness, or blurred vision (use caution when driving or engaging in hazardous activities until response to drug is known); or nausea or vomiting (small, frequent meals, frequent mouth care, chewing gum, or sucking lozenges may help). If chest pain occurs, seek emergency medical help at once. Report acute headache, rapid heartbeat, unusual restlessness or dizziness, muscular weakness, or blurring vision. **Pregnancy/breast-feeding precautions:** Inform prescriber if you are or intend to become pregnant. Consult prescriber if breast-feeding.

Geriatric Considerations: The first dose of nitrates (sublingual, chewable, oral) should be taken in a physician's office to observe for maximal cardiovascular dynamic effects and adverse effects (orthostatic blood pressure drop, headache). The use of nitrates for angina may occasionally promote reflux esophagitis. This may require dose adjustments or changing therapeutic agents to correct this adverse effect.

Isotretinoin (eye soe TRET i noyn)

U.S. Brand Names Accutane®

Synonyms 13-*cis*-Retinoic Acid

Restrictions Prescriptions for Accutane® may not be dispensed unless they are affixed with a yellow self-adhesive Accutane® qualification sticker filled out by the prescriber. Telephone, fax, or computer-generated prescriptions are no longer valid. Prescriptions may not be written for more than a 1-month supply and must be dispensed with a patient education guide every month. In addition, prescriptions for females must be filled within 7 days of the date noted on the yellow sticker; prescriptions filled after 7 days of the noted date are considered to be

(Continued)

Isotretinoin *(Continued)*

expired and cannot be honored. Pharmacists may call the manufacturer to confirm the prescriber's authority to write for this medication, however, this is not mandatory.

Prescribers will be provided with Accutane® qualification stickers after they have read the details of the S.M.A.R.T. program and have signed and mailed to the manufacturer their agreement to participate. A half-day continuing education program is also available. Audits of pharmacies will be conducted to monitor program compliance.

Generic Available No

Pharmacologic Category Retinoic Acid Derivative

Pregnancy Risk Factor X

Lactation Excretion in breast milk unknown/contraindicated

Use Treatment of severe recalcitrant nodular acne unresponsive to conventional therapy

Use - Unlabeled/Investigational Investigational: Treatment of children with metastatic neuroblastoma or leukemia that does not respond to conventional therapy

Mechanism of Action/Effect Reduces sebaceous gland size and reduces sebum production; regulates cell proliferation and differentiation

Contraindications Hypersensitivity to isotretinoin or any component of the formulation; sensitivity to parabens, vitamin A, or other retinoids; pregnancy

Warnings/Precautions This medication should only be prescribed by prescribers competent in treating severe recalcitrant nodular acne, are experienced in the use of systemic retinoids and are participating in the pregnancy prevention programs authorized by the FDA and product manufacturer. Use with caution in patients with diabetes mellitus, hypertriglyceridemia; acute pancreatitis and fatal hemorrhagic pancreatitis (rare) have been reported; not to be used in women of childbearing potential unless woman is capable of complying with effective contraceptive measures; therapy is begun after two negative pregnancy tests; effective contraception must be used for at least 1 month before beginning therapy, during therapy, and for 1 month after discontinuation of therapy. Prescriptions should be written for no more than a 1-month supply, and pregnancy testing and counseling should be repeated monthly. Because of the high likelihood of teratogenic effects (~20%), do not prescribe isotretinoin for women who are or who are likely to become pregnant while using the drug (see Additional Information for details). Male and female patients must be enrolled in the manufacturer sponsored and FDA approved monitoring programs. Depression, psychosis, aggressive or violent behavior, and rarely suicidal thoughts and actions have been reported during isotretinoin usage. Discontinuation of treatment alone may not be sufficient, further evaluation may be necessary. Cases of pseudotumor cerebri (benign intracranial hypertension) have been reported, some with concomitant use of tetracycline (avoid using together). Patients with papilledema, headache, nausea, vomiting, and visual disturbances should be referred to a neurologist and treatment with isotretinoin discontinued. Hearing impairment, which can continue after therapy is discontinued, may occur. Clinical hepatitis, elevated liver enzymes, inflammatory bowel disease, skeletal hyperostosis, premature epiphyseal closure, vision impairment, corneal opacities, and decreased night vision have also been reported with the use of isotretinoin. Bone mineral density may decrease; use caution in patients with a genetic predisposition to bone disorders (ie osteoporosis, osteomalacia) and with disease states or concomitant medications that can induce bone disorders. Patients may be at risk when participating in activities with repetitive impact (such as sports). Safety of long-term use is not established and is not recommended.

Drug Interactions

Decreased Effect: Isotretinoin may increase clearance of carbamazepine resulting in reduced carbamazepine levels. Microdosed progesterone preparations ("mini-pills") may not be an adequate form of contraception.

Increased Effect/Toxicity: Increased toxicity: Corticosteroids may cause osteoporosis; interactive effect with isotretinoin unknown; use with caution. Phenytoin may cause osteomalacia; interactive effect with isotretinoin unknown; use with caution. Cases of pseudotumor cerebri have been reported in concurrent use with tetracycline; avoid combination.

Nutritional/Ethanol Interactions

Ethanol: Avoid or limit ethanol (may increase triglyceride levels if taken in excess).

Food: Isotretinoin bioavailability increased if taken with food or milk.

Herb/Nutraceutical: Avoid dong quai, St John's Wort (may also cause photosensitization and may decrease the effectiveness of birth control pills). Additional vitamin A supplements may lead to vitamin A toxicity (dry skin, irritation, arthralgias, myalgias, abdominal pain, hepatic changes); avoid use.

Adverse Reactions Frequency not defined.

Cardiovascular: Palpitation, tachycardia, vascular thrombotic disease, stroke, chest pain, syncope, flushing

Central nervous system: Edema, fatigue, pseudotumor cerebri, dizziness, drowsiness, headache, insomnia, lethargy, malaise, nervousness, paresthesias, seizures, stroke, suicidal ideation, suicide attempts, suicide, depression, psychosis, aggressive or violent behavior, emotional instability

Dermatologic: Cutaneous allergic reactions, purpura, acne fulminans, alopecia, bruising, cheilitis, dry mouth, dry nose, dry skin, epistaxis, eruptive xanthomas, fragility of skin, hair abnormalities, hirsutism, hyperpigmentation, hypopigmentation, peeling of palms, peeling of soles, photoallergic reactions, photosensitizing reactions, pruritus, rash, dystrophy, paronychia, facial erythema, seborrhea, eczema, increased sunburn susceptibility, diaphoresis, urticaria, abnormal wound healing

Endocrine & metabolic: Increased triglycerides (25%), elevated blood glucose, increased HDL, increased cholesterol, abnormal menses

Gastrointestinal: Weight loss, inflammatory bowel disease, regional ileitis, pancreatitis, bleeding and inflammation of the gums, colitis, nausea, nonspecific gastrointestinal symptoms

Genitourinary: Nonspecific urogenital findings

Hematologic: Anemia, thrombocytopenia, neutropenia, agranulocytosis, pyogenic granuloma

Hepatic: Hepatitis

Neuromuscular & skeletal: Skeletal hyperostosis, calcification of tendons and ligaments, premature epiphyseal closure, arthralgia, CPK elevations, arthritis, tendonitis, bone abnormalities, weakness, back pain (29% in pediatric patients), rhabdomyolysis (rare), bone mineral density decreased

Ocular: Corneal opacities, decreased night vision, cataracts, color vision disorder, conjunctivitis, dry eyes, eyelid inflammation, keratitis, optic neuritis, photophobia, visual disturbances

Otic: Hearing impairment, tinnitus

Renal: Vasculitis, glomerulonephritis,

Respiratory: Bronchospasms, respiratory infection, voice alteration, Wegener's granulomatosis

Miscellaneous: Allergic reactions, anaphylactic reactions, lymphadenopathy, infection, disseminated herpes simplex, diaphoresis

Overdosage/Toxicology Symptoms of overdose include headache, vomiting, flushing, abdominal pain, cheilosis, dizziness, and ataxia. All signs or symptoms have been transient. Patients should not donate blood for at least 30 days following overdose. Male patients should use a condom or avoid sexual activity for 30 days following overdose.

Pharmacodynamics/Kinetics

Half-Life Elimination: Terminal: Parent drug: 21 hours; Metabolite: 21-24 hours

Time to Peak: Serum: 3-5 hours

Metabolism: Hepatic via CYP2B6, 2C8, 2C9, 2D6, 3A4; forms metabolites; major metabolite: 4-oxo-isotretinoin (active)

Formulations Capsule: 10 mg, 20 mg, 40 mg

Dosing

Adults & Elderly: Severe recalcitrant nodular acne: Oral: 0.5-2 mg/kg/day in 2 divided doses (dosages as low as 0.05 mg/kg/day have been reported to be beneficial) for 15-20 weeks or until the total cyst count decreases by 70%, whichever is sooner. A second course of therapy may be initiated after a period of ≥2 months off therapy.

Pediatrics:

Neuroblastoma (investigational): Oral: Children: Maintenance therapy for neuroblastoma: 100-250 mg/m^2/day in 2 divided doses

Acne (severe recalcitrant nodular): Children: Refer to adult dosing.

Hepatic Impairment: Empiric dose reductions are recommended in patient with hepatitis.

Administration

Oral: Administer with food. Capsules can be swallowed, or chewed and swallowed. The capsule may be opened with a large needle and the contents placed on applesauce or ice cream for patients unable to swallow the capsule. Whole capsules should be swallowed with a full glass of liquid.

Stability

Storage: Store at room temperature and protect from light.

Monitoring Laboratory Tests Must have pregnancy test prior to beginning therapy, CBC with differential and platelet count, baseline sedimentation rate, serum triglycerides, liver enzymes

Monitoring and Teaching Issues

Physical Assessment: See Contraindications and Warnings/Precautions for use cautions. Assess effectiveness and interactions of other medications patient may be taking (see Drug Interactions). Monitor lab tests, effectiveness of therapy, and adverse effects at beginning of therapy and regularly with long-term use (see Adverse Reactions and Overdose/Toxicology). Monitor diabetic patients closely. Assess knowledge/teach patient appropriate use, possible side effects/interventions, and adverse symptoms to report (see Patient Education). **Pregnancy risk factor X** - determine that patient is not pregnant before beginning treatment and do not give to women of childbearing age unless female is capable of complying with barrier contraceptive measures 1 month prior to therapy, during therapy, and 1 month following therapy. Breast-feeding is contraindicated.

Patient Education: A patient information/consent form must be signed before this medication is prescribed. Do not sign (and do not take this medication) if you do not understand any information on the form. Use exactly as directed; do not take more than recommended. Prescriptions will be written for a 1-month supply and must be filled within 7 days; they will not be honored if filled after that time or if they do not have the appropriate yellow qualification sticker attached. Capsule can be chewed and swallowed, swallowed, or opened with a large needle and contents sprinkled on applesauce or ice cream. Whole capsules should be swallowed with a full glass of liquid. Do not take any other vitamin A products, limit vitamin A intake, and increase exercise during therapy. Limit or avoid alcohol intake. Exacerbations of acne may occur during first weeks of therapy. You may experience headache, loss of night vision, lethargy, or visual disturbances (use caution when driving or engaging in tasks requiring alertness until response to drug is known); photosensitivity (use sunscreen, wear protective clothing and eyewear, and avoid direct sunlight); dry mouth or nausea (small, frequent meals, sucking hard candy, or chewing gum may may help); or dryness, redness, or itching of skin, eye irritation, or increased sensitivity to contact lenses (wear regular glasses). Discontinue therapy and report acute vision changes, rectal bleeding, abdominal cramping, or unresolved diarrhea. **Pregnancy/breast-feeding precautions:** Inform prescriber if you are pregnant. Do not get pregnant 1 month before, during, or for 1 month following therapy. This drug may cause severe fetal defects. Two forms of contraception and monthly tests to rule out pregnancy are required during therapy. It is important to note that any type of contraception may fail, it is the responsibility of the patient to be compliant with contraceptive therapy. Do not donate blood during or for 1 month following therapy (same reason). Breast-feeding is contraindicated.

Dietary Issues: Should be taken with food. Limit intake of vitamin A; avoid use of other vitamin A products

Pregnancy Issues: Major fetal abnormalities (both internal and external), spontaneous abortion, premature births and low IQ scores in surviving infants have been reported. This medication is contraindicated in females of childbearing potential unless they are able to comply with the guidelines of pregnancy prevention programs put in place by the FDA and the manufacturer of Accutane®.

(Continued)

Isotretinoin *(Continued)*

Additional Information Females of childbearing potential must receive oral and written information reviewing the hazards of therapy and the effects that isotretinoin can have on a fetus. Therapy should not begin without two negative pregnancy tests, one to be performed in the physician's office when qualifying the patient for treatment, the second test performed on the second day of the next normal menstrual period or 11 days after the last unprotected intercourse, whichever is last. Two forms of contraception (a primary and secondary form as described in the pregnancy prevention program materials) must be used during treatment and limitations to their use must be explained. Prescriptions should be written for no more than a 1-month supply, and pregnancy testing and counseling should be repeated monthly. Urine pregnancy test kits (for monthly pregnancy testing) and a Pregnancy Prevention Program kit (to be given to the patient prior to therapy) are provided by the manufacturer. Any cases of accidental pregnancy should be reported to the manufacturer or the FDA MedWatch Program. All patients (male and female) must read and sign the informed consent material provided in the pregnancy prevention program. Prescriptions will not be honored unless they have the yellow qualification sticker affixed.

Isradipine (iz RA di peen)

U.S. Brand Names DynaCirc®; DynaCirc® CR

Generic Available No

Pharmacologic Category Calcium Channel Blocker

Pregnancy Risk Factor C

Lactation Excretion in breast milk unknown/not recommended

Use Treatment of hypertension

Mechanism of Action/Effect Inhibits calcium ion from entering the "slow channels" or select voltage-sensitive areas of vascular smooth muscle and myocardium during depolarization

Contraindications Hypersensitivity to isradipine or any component of the formulation; hypotension (<90 mm Hg systolic)

Warnings/Precautions Use cautiously in CHF, hypertropic cardiomyopathy (IHSS), and in hepatic dysfunction. Safety and efficacy have not been established in pediatric patients. Adjust doses at 2- to 4-week intervals. Pregnancy risk C.

Drug Interactions

Cytochrome P450 Effect: Substrate of **CYP3A4**

Decreased Effect: NSAIDs (diclofenac) may decrease the antihypertensive response of isradipine. Isradipine may cause a decrease in lovastatin effect. Rifampin may reduce blood levels and effects of isradipine due to enzyme induction (other enzyme inducers may share this effect).

Increased Effect/Toxicity: Isradipine may increase cardiovascular adverse effects of beta-blockers. Isradipine may minimally increase cyclosporine levels. Azole antifungals (and potentially other inhibitors of CYP3A4) may increase levels of isradipine; avoid this combination.

Nutritional/Ethanol Interactions

Food: Administration with food delays absorption, but does not affect availability

Herb/Nutraceutical: St John's wort may decrease isradipine levels. Avoid dong quai if using for hypertension (has estrogenic activity). Avoid ephedra, yohimbe, ginseng (may worsen hypertension). Avoid garlic (may have increased antihypertensive effect).

Adverse Reactions

>10%: Central nervous system: Headache (dose-related 1.9% to 22%)

1% to 10%:

- Cardiovascular: Edema (dose-related 1.2% to 8.7%), palpitations (dose-related 0.8% to 5.1%), flushing (dose-related 0.8% to 5.1%), tachycardia (1% to 3.4%), chest pain (1.7% to 2.7%)
- Central nervous system: Dizziness (1.6% to 8%), fatigue (dose-related 0.4% to 8.5%), flushing (9%)
- Dermatologic: Rash (1.5% to 2%)
- Gastrointestinal: Nausea (1% to 5.1%), abdominal discomfort (0% to 3.3%), vomiting (0% to 1.3%), diarrhea (0% to 3.4%)
- Renal: Urinary frequency (1.3% to 3.4%)
- Respiratory: Dyspnea (0.5% to 3.4%)

0.5% to 1% (Limited to important or life-threatening): Atrial fibrillation, cough, cramps of legs and feet, depression, dyspnea, gingival hyperplasia (incidence unknown), heart failure, hypotension, impotence, insomnia, lethargy, leukopenia, myocardial infarction, paresthesias, pruritus, stroke, syncope, urticaria, ventricular fibrillation

Overdosage/Toxicology Primary cardiac symptoms of calcium blocker overdose include hypotension and bradycardia. Hypotension is caused by peripheral vasodilation, myocardial depression, and bradycardia. Bradycardia results from sinus bradycardia, second- or third-degree atrioventricular block, or sinus arrest with junctional rhythm. Intraventricular conduction is usually not affected so QRS duration is normal (verapamil does prolong the PR interval and bepridil prolongs the QT interval and may cause ventricular arrhythmias, including torsade de pointes).

Noncardiac symptoms include confusion, stupor, nausea, vomiting, metabolic acidosis and hyperglycemia. Repeated calcium administration may promptly reverse the depressed cardiac contractility (but not sinus node depression or peripheral vasodilation).

Pharmacodynamics/Kinetics

Absorption: 90% to 95%

Bioavailability: 15% to 24%

Half-Life Elimination: 8 hours

Time to Peak: Serum: 1-1.5 hours

Metabolism: Hepatic; extensive first-pass effect

Duration: 8-16 hours

Formulations

Capsule (DynaCirc®): 2.5 mg, 5 mg

Tablet, controlled release (DynaCirc® CR): 5 mg, 10 mg

Dosing

Adults: Hypertension: Oral: 2.5 mg twice daily; antihypertensive response is seen in 2-3 hours; maximal response in 2-4 weeks; increase dose at 2- to 4-week intervals at 2.5-5 mg increments; usual dose range: 5-20 mg/day. **Note:** Most patients show no improvement with doses >10 mg/day except adverse reaction rate increases.

Elderly: Maximum dose in the elderly should be 10 mg/day. Antihypertensive response is seen in 2-3 hours; maximal response in 2-4 weeks. Increase dose at 2- to 4-week intervals at 2.5-5 mg increments; usual dose range: 5-20 mg/day. **Note:** Most patients show no improvement with doses >10 mg/day except adverse reaction rate increases.

Administration

Oral: May open capsule; avoid crushing contents

Monitoring and Teaching Issues

Physical Assessment: See Contraindications, Warnings/Precautions, and Dosing for use cautions. Assess potential for interactions with other prescriptions, OTC medications, or herbal products patient may be taking (see Drug Interactions). Assess results of laboratory tests (see Monitoring Lab Tests), therapeutic effects, and adverse response (eg, cardiac status, blood pressure, fluid balance - see Adverse Reactions and Overdose/Toxicology) at regular intervals during therapy. Teach patient proper use, possible side effects and appropriate interventions, and adverse symptoms to report (see Patient Education). **Pregnancy risk factor C** - benefits of use should outweigh possible risks. Note breast-feeding caution.

Patient Education: Inform prescriber of all prescriptions, OTC medications, or herbal products you are taking, and any allergies you have. Do not take anything new during treatment unless approved by prescriber. Take as prescribed, with or without food. Do not stop abruptly without consulting prescriber. Do not crush extended release tablets. This medication does not replace other antihypertensive interventions; follow prescriber's instructions for diet and lifestyle changes. You may experience headache (if unrelieved, consult prescriber for approved analgesic); nausea or vomiting (small, frequent meals, frequent mouth care, chewing gum, or sucking lozenges may help); constipation (increased dietary bulk and fluids may help); or dizziness, fatigue, confusion (use caution when driving or engaging in potentially hazardous tasks until response to drug is known). Report unrelieved headache, vomiting, or constipation; chest pain, palpitations, or rapid heartbeat; swelling of hands or feet or sudden weight gain (>5 lb/week); or unusual cramps in legs or feet. **Pregnancy/breast-feeding precautions:** Inform prescriber if you are or intend to become pregnant. Consult prescriber if breast-feeding.

Dietary Issues: May be taken without regard to meals.

Geriatric Considerations: Elderly may experience a greater hypotensive response. Constipation may be more of a problem in the elderly.

Related Information

Calcium Channel Blockers *on page 1563*

Isuprel® *see* Isoproterenol *on page 747*

Itraconazole (i tra KOE na zole)

U.S. Brand Names Sporanox®

Generic Available No

Pharmacologic Category Antifungal Agent, Oral

Pregnancy Risk Factor C

Lactation Enters breast milk/not recommended

Use Treatment of susceptible fungal infections in immunocompromised and immunocompetent patients including blastomycosis and histoplasmosis; indicated for aspergillosis, and onychomycosis of the toenail; treatment of onychomycosis of the fingernail without concomitant toenail infection via a pulse-type dosing regimen; has activity against *Aspergillus*, *Candida*, *Coccidioides*, *Cryptococcus*, *Sporothrix*, tinea unguium

Oral: Useful in superficial mycoses including dermatophytoses (eg, tinea capitis), pityriasis versicolor, sebopsoriasis, vaginal and chronic mucocutaneous candidiases; systemic mycoses including candidiasis, meningeal and disseminated cryptococcal infections, paracoccidioidomycosis, coccidioidomycoses; miscellaneous mycoses such as sporotrichosis, chromomycosis, leishmaniasis, fungal keratitis, alternariosis, zygomycosis

Oral solution (not capsules): Marketed for oral and esophageal candidiasis

Intravenous solution: Indicated in the treatment of blastomycosis, histoplasmosis (nonmeningeal), and aspergillosis (in patients intolerant or refractory to amphotericin B therapy)

Mechanism of Action/Effect Interferes with cytochrome P450 activity, decreasing ergosterol synthesis (principal sterol in fungal cell membrane) and inhibiting cell membrane formation

Contraindications Hypersensitivity to itraconazole, any component of the formulation, or to other azoles; concurrent administration with astemizole, cisapride, dofetilide, ergot derivatives, lovastatin, midazolam, pimozide, quinidine, or simvastatin; treatment of onychomycosis in patients with evidence of left ventricular dysfunction, CHF, or a history of CHF

Warnings/Precautions Rare cases of serious cardiovascular adverse events, including death, ventricular tachycardia and torsade de pointes have been observed due to increased cisapride concentrations induced by itraconazole. Not recommended for use in patients with active liver disease, elevated liver enzymes, or prior hepatotoxic reactions to other drugs. Itraconazole has been associated with rare cases of serious hepatotoxicity (including fatal cases and cases within the first week of treatment); treatment should be discontinued in patients who develop clinical symptoms or abnormal liver function tests during itraconazole therapy except in cases where expected benefit exceeds risk. Use with caution in patients with left ventricular dysfunction or a history of CHF or neuropathy when itraconazole is being used for indications other than onychomycosis. Discontinue if signs or symptoms of CHF occur during treatment. Due to differences in bioavailability, oral capsules and oral solution **cannot** be used interchangeably. Pregnancy risk C.

(Continued)

Itraconazole *(Continued)*

Drug Interactions

Cytochrome P450 Effect: Substrate of **CYP3A4**; Inhibits **CYP3A4**

Decreased Effect: Decreased serum levels with carbamazepine, didanosine (oral solution only), isoniazid, phenobarbital, phenytoin, rifabutin, and rifampin. **Should not be administered concomitantly with rifampin.** Absorption requires gastric acidity; therefore, antacids, H_2 antagonists (cimetidine, famotidine, nizatidine, and ranitidine), proton pump inhibitors (omeprazole, lansoprazole, rabeprazole), and sucralfate may significantly reduce bioavailability resulting in treatment failures and should not be administered concomitantly. Oral contraceptive efficacy may be reduced (limited data).

Increased Effect/Toxicity: Due to inhibition of hepatic CYP3A4, itraconazole use is contraindicated with astemizole, cisapride, dofetilide, lovastatin, midazolam, pimozide, quinidine, simvastatin, and triazolam due to large substantial increases in the toxicity of these agents. Itraconazole may also increase the levels of benzodiazepines (alprazolam, diazepam, and others), buspirone, busulfan, calcium channel blockers (felodipine, nifedipine, verapamil), cyclosporine, digoxin, docetaxel, HMG-CoA reductase inhibitors (except fluvastatin, pravastatin), oral hypoglycemics (sulfonylureas), methylprednisolone, phenytoin, sirolimus, tacrolimus, trimetrexate, vincristine, vinblastine, warfarin, and zolpidem. Other medications metabolized by CYP3A4 should be used with caution. Amprenavir (and possibly other protease inhibitors), clarithromycin, and erythromycin may increase itraconazole concentrations.

Nutritional/Ethanol Interactions

Food: Capsules: Enhanced by food and possibly by gastric acidity; avoid grapefruit juice. Solution: Decreased by food, time to peak concentration prolonged by food. Absorption of both products is increased when taken with a cola beverage.

Herb/Nutraceutical: St John's wort may decrease itraconazole levels.

Adverse Reactions Listed incidences are for higher doses appropriate for systemic fungal infections.

>10%: Gastrointestinal: Nausea (11%)

1% to 10%:

- Cardiovascular: Edema (4%), hypertension (3%)
- Central nervous system: Headache (4%), fatigue (2% to 3%), malaise (1%), fever (3%), dizziness (2%)
- Dermatologic: Rash (9%), pruritus (3%)
- Endocrine & metabolic: Decreased libido (1%), hypertriglyceridemia, hypokalemia (2%)
- Gastrointestinal: Abdominal pain (2%), anorexia (1%), vomiting (5%), diarrhea (3%)
- Hepatic: Abnormal LFTs (3%), hepatitis
- Renal: Albuminuria (1%)

<1% (Limited to important or life-threatening): Adrenal suppression, allergic reactions (urticaria, angioedema), alopecia, anaphylaxis, arrhythmia, CHF, constipation, gastritis, gynecomastia, hepatic failure, impotence, neutropenia, peripheral neuropathy, pulmonary edema, somnolence, Stevens-Johnson syndrome, tinnitus

Overdosage/Toxicology Overdoses are well tolerated. Treatment is supportive. Dialysis is not effective.

Pharmacodynamics/Kinetics

Absorption: Requires gastric acidity; capsule better absorbed with food, solution better absorbed on empty stomach; hypochlorhydria has been reported in HIV-infected patients; therefore, oral absorption in these patients may be decreased

Bioavailability: 55%; Fasting: 40%; Postprandial: 100%

Half-Life Elimination: Oral: After single 200 mg dose: 21 ± 5 hours; 64 hours at steady-state; I.V.: steady-state: 35 hours; steady-state concentrations are achieved in 13 days with multiple administration of itraconazole 100-400 mg/day.

Metabolism: Extensively hepatic into >30 metabolites including hydroxy-itraconazole (major metabolite); appears to have *in vitro* antifungal activity. Main metabolic pathway is oxidation; may undergo saturation metabolism with multiple dosing.

Formulations

Capsule: 100 mg

Injection, solution: 10 mg/mL (25 mL) [packaged in a kit containing sodium chloride 0.9% (50 mL); filtered infusion set (1)]

Solution, oral: 100 mg/10 mL (150 mL) [cherry flavor]

Dosing

Adults & Elderly:

Blastomycosis/histoplasmosis:

- Oral: 200 mg once daily, if no obvious improvement or there is evidence of progressive fungal disease, increase the dose in 100 mg increments to a maximum of 400 mg/day. Doses >200 mg/day are given in 2 divided doses. Length of therapy varies from 1 day to >6 months depending on the condition and mycological response.
- I.V.: 200 mg twice daily for 4 doses, followed by 200 mg daily

Aspergillosis:

- Oral: 200-400 mg/day
- I.V.: 200 mg twice daily for 4 doses, followed by 200 mg daily

Onychomycosis: Oral: 200 mg once daily for 12 consecutive weeks

Life-threatening infections:

- Oral: Loading dose: 200 mg 3 times/day (600 mg/day) should be given for the first 3 days of therapy.
- I.V.: 200 mg twice daily for 4 doses, followed by 200 mg daily

Oropharyngeal and esophageal candidiasis: Oral solution: 100-200 mg once daily

Pediatrics: Efficacy and safety have not been established; a small number of patients 3-16 years of age have been treated with 100 mg/day for systemic fungal infections with no serious adverse effects reported.

Renal Impairment: Not necessary. Itraconazole injection is not recommended in patients with a creatinine clearance <30 mL/minute.

Not dialyzable

Hepatic Impairment: May be necessary, but specific guidelines are not available. Risk-to-benefit evaluation should be undertaken in patients who develop liver function abnormalities during treatment.

Administration

Oral: Doses >200 mg/day are given in 2 divided doses; do not administer with antacids. Capsule absorption is best if taken with food, therefore, it is best to administer itraconazole after meals; solution should be taken on an empty stomach. Absorption of both products is increased when taken with a cola beverage.

I.V.: Using a flow control device, infuse 60 mL of the dilute solution (3.33 mg/mL = 200 mg itraconazole, pH ~4.8) intravenously over 60 minutes, using an extension line and the infusion set provided. After administration, flush the infusion set with 15-20 mL of 0.9% sodium chloride over 30 seconds to 15 minutes, via the two-way stopcock. Do not use bacteriostatic sodium chloride injection, USP. The compatibility of Sporanox® injection with flush solutions other than 0.9% sodium chloride (normal saline) is not known. Discard the entire infusion line.

Stability

Storage: Dilute with 0.9% sodium chloride only. Do not use dextrose or lactated Ringer's. Stable for 48 hours at room temperature or under refrigeration.

Reconstitution: A precise mixing ratio is required to maintain stability (3.33:1) and avoid precipitate formation. Add 25 mL (1 ampul) to 50 mL 0.9% sodium chloride. Mix and withdraw 15 mL of solution before infusing.

Monitoring Laboratory Tests Left ventricular function in patients with pre-existing hepatic dysfunction, and in all patients being treated for longer than 1 month.

Monitoring and Teaching Issues

Physical Assessment: See Contraindications, Warnings/Precautions, and Dosing for use cautions. Assess potential for interactions with other prescriptions, OTC medications, or herbal products patient may be taking (see Drug Interactions). See specific Administration instructions. Assess results of laboratory tests (see Monitoring Lab Tests), therapeutic effects, and adverse response (see Adverse Reactions and Overdose/Toxicology) at regular intervals during therapy. Teach patient proper use, possible side effects and appropriate interventions, and adverse symptoms to report (see Patient Education). **Pregnancy risk factor C** - benefits of use should outweigh possible risks. Caution patients - Oral contraceptive efficacy may be reduced. Breast-feeding is not recommended.

Patient Education: Inform prescriber of all prescriptions, OTC medications, or herbal products you are taking, and any allergies you have. Do not take anything new during treatment unless approved by prescriber. Use exactly as directed. Stop therapy and report any signs and symptoms that may suggest liver dysfunction immediately so that the appropriate laboratory testing can be done; signs and symptoms may include unusual fatigue, anorexia, nausea and/or vomiting, jaundice, dark urine, or pale stool. Take full course of medication, do not discontinue without consulting prescriber. Take capsule with food; solution on empty stomach, 1 hour before or 2 hours after meals. Observe good hygiene measures to prevent reinfection. If diabetic, test serum glucose regularly (may affect response to oral hypoglycemics). Frequent blood tests may be required with prolonged therapy. You may experience dizziness or drowsiness (use caution when driving or engaging in tasks that require alertness until response to drug is known); nausea, vomiting, or anorexia (small, frequent meals, frequent mouth care, sucking lozenges, or chewing gum may help); or skin rash or other persistent adverse reactions. **Pregnancy/breast-feeding precautions:** Inform prescriber if you are or intend to become pregnant. Consult prescriber about oral contraceptive use - efficacy may be reduced. Breast-feeding is not recommended.

Dietary Issues:

Capsule: Administer with food.

Solution: Take without food, if possible.

Additional Information Due to potential toxicity, the manufacturer recommends confirmation of diagnosis testing of nail specimens prior to treatment of onychomycosis.

I-Tropine® *see page 1509*

Iveegam EN *see* Immune Globulin (Intravenous) *on page 703*

IVIG *see* Immune Globulin (Intravenous) *on page 703*

I.V. to Oral Conversion *see page 1691*

Japanese Encephalitis Virus Vaccine, Inactivated *see page 1498*

Jenest™-28 [DSC] *see* Ethinyl Estradiol and Norethindrone *on page 527*

JE-VAX® *see page 1498*

K+® 10 *see* Potassium Supplements *on page 1106*

Kadian® *see* Morphine Sulfate *on page 926*

Kala® [OTC] *see Lactobacillus on page 766*

Kaletra™ *see* Lopinavir and Ritonavir *on page 817*

Kaochlor® *see* Potassium Supplements *on page 1106*

Kaochlor® SF *see* Potassium Supplements *on page 1106*

Kaon® *see* Potassium Supplements *on page 1106*

Kaon-Cl® *see* Potassium Supplements *on page 1106*

Kaon-Cl-10® *see* Potassium Supplements *on page 1106*

Kariva™ *see* Ethinyl Estradiol and Desogestrel *on page 516*

Kay Ciel® *see* Potassium Supplements *on page 1106*

Kayexalate® *see* Sodium Polystyrene Sulfonate *on page 1236*

K+ Care® *see* Potassium Supplements *on page 1106*

K+ Care® ET *see* Potassium Supplements *on page 1106*

KCl (Potassium Chloride) *see* Potassium Supplements *on page 1106*

K-Dur-10® *see* Potassium Supplements *on page 1106*

K-Dur-20® *see* Potassium Supplements *on page 1106*

Keflex® *see* Cephalexin *on page 259*

Keftab® *see* Cephalexin *on page 259*

Kefurox® *see* Cefuroxime *on page 255*

Kefzol® *see* Cefazolin *on page 234*

Kemadrin® *see* Procyclidine *on page 1129*

Kenacort® *see* Triamcinolone *on page 1356*

Kenaject-40® *see* Triamcinolone *on page 1356*

Kenalog® *see* Topical Corticosteroids *on page 1334*

Kenalog® *see* Triamcinolone *on page 1356*

Kenalog-10® *see* Triamcinolone *on page 1356*

Kenalog-40® *see* Triamcinolone *on page 1356*

Kenalog® H *see* Topical Corticosteroids *on page 1334*

Kenalog® H *see* Triamcinolone *on page 1356*

Kenalog® in Orabase® *see* Topical Corticosteroids *on page 1334*

Kenalog® in Orabase® *see* Triamcinolone *on page 1356*

Kenonel® *see* Topical Corticosteroids *on page 1334*

Kenonel® *see* Triamcinolone *on page 1356*

Keoxifene Hydrochloride *see* Raloxifene *on page 1169*

Keppra® *see* Levetiracetam *on page 784*

Kerlone® *see* Betaxolol *on page 163*

Kerlone®: Lumigan™ *see* Ophthalmic Agents, Glaucoma *on page 1002*

Ketoconazole (kee toe KOE na zole)

U.S. Brand Names Nizoral®; Nizoral® A-D [OTC]

Generic Available Yes

Pharmacologic Category Antifungal Agent, Oral; Antifungal Agent, Topical

Pregnancy Risk Factor C

Lactation Enters breast milk/not recommended

Use Treatment of susceptible fungal infections, including candidiasis, oral thrush, blastomycosis, histoplasmosis, paracoccidioidomycosis, coccidioidomycosis, chromomycosis, candiduria, chronic mucocutaneous candidiasis, as well as certain recalcitrant cutaneous dermatophytoses; used topically for treatment of tinea corporis, tinea cruris, tinea versicolor, and cutaneous candidiasis, seborrheic dermatitis

Mechanism of Action/Effect Inhibits several fungal enzymes that results in a build-up of toxic concentrations of hydrogen peroxide resulting in cell death

Contraindications Hypersensitivity to ketoconazole or any component of the formulation; CNS fungal infections (due to poor CNS penetration); coadministration with ergot derivatives, astemizole, or cisapride is contraindicated due to risk of potentially fatal cardiac arrhythmias

Warnings/Precautions Use with caution in patients with impaired hepatic function; has been associated with hepatotoxicity, including some fatalities; perform periodic liver function tests; high doses of ketoconazole may depress adrenocortical function. Pregnancy risk C.

Drug Interactions

Cytochrome P450 Effect: Substrate of **CYP3A4**; Inhibits CYP1A2, 2A6, 2B6, 2C8/9, 2C19, 2D6, **3A4**

Decreased Effect: Oral: Decreased serum levels with carbamazepine, didanosine (oral solution only), isoniazid, phenobarbital, phenytoin, rifabutin, and rifampin. **Should not be administered concomitantly with rifampin.** Absorption requires gastric acidity; therefore, antacids, H_2 antagonists (cimetidine, famotidine, nizatidine, and ranitidine), proton pump inhibitors (omeprazole, lansoprazole, rabeprazole), and sucralfate may significantly reduce bioavailability resulting in treatment failures and should not be administered concomitantly. Oral contraceptive efficacy may be reduced (limited data).

Increased Effect/Toxicity: Due to inhibition of hepatic CYP3A4, ketoconazole use is contraindicated with astemizole, cisapride, lovastatin, midazolam, simvastatin, and triazolam due to large substantial increases in the toxicity of these agents. Ketoconazole may also increase the levels of benzodiazepines (alprazolam. diazepam, and others), buspirone, busulfan, calcium channel blockers (felodipine, nifedipine, verapamil), cyclosporine, digoxin, docetaxel, HMG-CoA reductase inhibitors (except fluvastatin, pravastatin), oral hypoglycemics (sulfonylureas), methylprednisolone, phenytoin, quinolone, sirolimus, tacrolimus, trimetrexate, vincristine, vinblastine, warfarin, and zolpidem. Other medications metabolized by CYP3A4 should be used with caution. Amprenavir (and possibly other protease inhibitors), clarithromycin, and erythromycin may increase ketoconazole concentrations.

Nutritional/Ethanol Interactions

Food: Ketoconazole peak serum levels may be prolonged if taken with food.

Herb/Nutraceutical: St John's wort may decrease ketoconazole levels.

Adverse Reactions

Oral:

1% to 10%:

Dermatologic: Pruritus (2%)

Gastrointestinal: Nausea/vomiting (3% to 10%), abdominal pain (1%)

<1% (Limited to important or life-threatening): Bulging fontanelles, chills, depression, diarrhea, dizziness, fever, gynecomastia, headache, hemolytic anemia, hepatotoxicity, impotence, leukopenia, photophobia, somnolence, thrombocytopenia

Cream: Severe irritation, pruritus, stinging (~5%)

Shampoo: Increases in normal hair loss, irritation (<1%), abnormal hair texture, scalp pustules, mild dryness of skin, itching, oiliness/dryness of hair

Overdosage/Toxicology Oral: Symptoms of overdose include dizziness, headache, nausea, vomiting, diarrhea. Overdoses are well tolerated. Treatment includes supportive measures and gastric decontamination.

Pharmacodynamics/Kinetics

Absorption: Oral: Rapid (~75%); Shampoo: None

Bioavailability: Decreases as gastric pH increases

Half-Life Elimination: Biphasic: Initial: 2 hours; Terminal: 8 hours

Time to Peak: Serum: 1-2 hours

Metabolism: Partially hepatic via CYP3A4 to inactive compounds

Formulations

Cream, topical (Nizoral®): 2% (15 g, 30 g, 60 g)
Shampoo, topical (Nizoral® A-D): 1% (6 mL, 120 mL, 207 mL)
Tablet (Nizoral®): 200 mg

Dosing

Adults & Elderly: Fungal infections:

Oral: 200-400 mg/day as a single daily dose
Shampoo: Apply twice weekly for 4 weeks with at least 3 days between each shampoo.
Topical: Rub gently into the affected area once daily to twice daily.

Pediatrics: Oral: Children ≥2 years: 3.3-6.6 mg/kg/day as a single dose for 1-2 weeks for candidiasis, for at least 4 weeks in recalcitrant dermatophyte infections, and for up to 6 months for other systemic mycoses

Renal Impairment: Not dialyzable (0% to 5%)

Hepatic Impairment: Dose reductions should be considered in patients with severe liver disease.

Administration

Oral: Do not take with antacids; take at least 2 hours before antacids.

Topical: Cream and shampoo: External use only.

Monitoring Laboratory Tests Liver function

Monitoring and Teaching Issues

Physical Assessment: See Contraindications, Warnings/Precautions, and Dosing for use cautions. Assess potential for interactions with other prescriptions, OTC medications, or herbal products patient may be taking (see Drug Interactions). Assess results of laboratory tests. Assess patient response (see Adverse Reactions and Overdose/Toxicology) on a regular basis throughout therapy. Teach patient proper use, possible side effects and interventions (eg, importance of adequate hydration), and adverse symptoms to report (see Patient Education). **Pregnancy risk factor C** - benefits of use should outweigh possible risks. Breast-feeding is not recommended.

Patient Education: Inform prescriber of all prescriptions, OTC medications, or herbal products you are taking, and any allergies you have. Do not take anything new without consulting prescriber. Oral formulation may be taken with food, at least 2 hours before any antacids. Take full course of medication as directed; some infections may require long periods of therapy. If diabetic, test serum glucose regularly; may impact effectiveness of oral hypoglycemics. May cause nausea and vomiting (small, frequent meals, frequent mouth care, sucking lozenges, or chewing gum may help); headache (mild analgesic may be necessary); or dizziness (use caution when driving). Report unresolved headache, rash or itching, yellowing of eyes or skin, changes in color of urine or stool, chest pain or palpitations, or sense of fullness or ringing in ears. **Pregnancy/breast-feeding precautions:** Inform prescriber if you are or intend to become pregnant. Breast-feeding is not recommended.

Topical: Wash and dry area before applying medication thinly. Do not cover with occlusive dressing. Report severe skin irritation or if condition does not improve.

Shampoo: Allow 3 days between shampoos. You may experience some hair loss, scalp irritations, itching change in hair texture, or scalp pustules. Report severe side effects or if infestation persists.

Dietary Issues: May be taken with food or milk to decrease GI adverse effects.

Ketoprofen (kee toe PROE fen)

U.S. Brand Names Orudis® [DSC]; Orudis® KT [OTC]; Oruvail®

Generic Available Yes: Capsule

Pharmacologic Category Nonsteroidal Anti-inflammatory Drug (NSAID)

Pregnancy Risk Factor B/D (3rd trimester)

Lactation Excretion in breast milk unknown/use caution

Use Acute and long-term treatment of rheumatoid arthritis and osteoarthritis; primary dysmenorrhea; mild to moderate pain

Mechanism of Action/Effect Inhibits prostaglandin synthesis by decreasing the activity of the enzyme, cyclooxygenase, which results in decreased formation of prostaglandin precursors

Contraindications Hypersensitivity to ketoprofen, any component of the formulation, or other NSAIDs/aspirin; pregnancy (3rd trimester)

Warnings/Precautions Use with caution in patients with CHF, hypertension, dehydration, decreased renal or hepatic function, history of GI disease (bleeding or ulcers), or those receiving anticoagulants. Elderly are at a high risk for adverse effects from NSAIDs. As many as 60% of elderly can develop peptic ulceration and/or hemorrhage asymptomatically.

Use lowest effective dose for shortest period possible. Use of NSAIDs can compromise existing renal function especially when Cl_{cr} is <30 mL/minute. CNS adverse effects (confusion, hallucinations) are generally seen in overdose or high-dose situations; however, elderly may demonstrate these adverse effects at lower doses than younger adults. Withhold for at least 4-6 half-lives prior to surgical or dental procedures. Safety and efficacy in pediatric patients have not been established (per manufacturer).

Pregnancy risk B/D (3rd trimester).

Drug Interactions

Cytochrome P450 Effect: Inhibits CYP2C8/9

Decreased Effect: Decreased effect of diuretics (loop and thiazides). May decrease effects of antihypertensives.

(Continued)

Ketoprofen *(Continued)*

Increased Effect/Toxicity: Increased effect/toxicity with probenecid, lithium, anticoagulants, and methotrexate.

Nutritional/Ethanol Interactions

Ethanol: Avoid ethanol (due to GI irritation).

Food: Although food affects the bioavailability of ketoprofen, analgesic efficacy is not significantly diminished; food slows rate of absorption resulting in delayed and reduced peak serum concentrations.

Effects on Lab Values ↑ chloride (S), sodium (S), bleeding time

Adverse Reactions

>10%:

Central nervous system: Headache (11%)

Gastrointestinal: Dyspepsia (11%)

1% to 10%:

Central nervous system: Nervousness

Dermatologic: Rash, itching

Endocrine & metabolic: Fluid retention

Gastrointestinal: Vomiting (>1%), diarrhea (3% to 9%), nausea (3% to 9%), constipation (3% to 9%), abdominal distress/cramping/pain (3% to 9%), flatulence (3% to 9%), anorexia (>1%), stomatitis (>1%)

Genitourinary: Urinary tract infection (>1%)

Otic: Tinnitus

<1% (Limited to important or life-threatening): Agranulocytosis, anemia, bronchospasm, bullous rash, CHF, dyspnea, exfoliative dermatitis, hematuria, hemolysis, hepatic dysfunction, hypercoagulability, hypertension, interstitial nephritis, nephrotic syndrome, palpitation, purpura, renal failure, tachycardia, thrombocytopenia

Overdosage/Toxicology Symptoms of overdose include apnea, metabolic acidosis, coma, nystagmus, seizures, leukocytosis, and renal failure. Management of NSAID intoxication is supportive and symptomatic. Since many NSAIDs undergo enterohepatic cycling, multiple doses of charcoal may be needed to reduce the potential for delayed toxicities.

Pharmacodynamics/Kinetics

Absorption: Almost complete

Half-Life Elimination: 1-4 hours

Time to Peak: Serum: 0.5-2 hours

Metabolism: Hepatic

Onset: Peak effect: 1-2 hours

Formulations

Capsule (Orudis® [DSC]): 50 mg, 75 mg

Capsule, extended release (Oruvail®): 100 mg, 150 mg, 200 mg

Tablet (Orudis® KT): 12.5 mg

Dosing

Adults:

Rheumatoid arthritis or osteoarthritis: Oral: 50-75 mg 3-4 times/day up to a maximum of 300 mg/day

Mild to moderate pain: Oral: 25-50 mg every 6-8 hours up to a maximum of 300 mg/day

Elderly: Oral: Initial: 25-50 mg 3-4 times/day; increase up to 150-300 mg/day (maximum daily dose: 300 mg).

Pediatrics: Note: Safety and efficacy in pediatric patients have not been established (per manufacturer)

Fever: Oral: Children 3 months to 14 years: 0.5-1 mg/kg every 6-8 hours

Mild to moderate pain, rheumatoid arthritis: Children >12 years: Refer to adult dosing.

Administration

Oral: May take with food to reduce GI upset.

Monitoring Laboratory Tests CBC, occult blood loss, periodic liver function; renal function (urine output, serum BUN, creatinine)

Monitoring and Teaching Issues

Physical Assessment: Assess effectiveness and interactions of other medications patient may be taking (see Contraindications and Drug Interactions). Monitor laboratory tests (see above), therapeutic response, and adverse or overdose reactions (see Adverse Reactions) at beginning of therapy and periodically throughout therapy. Schedule ophthalmic evaluations for patients who develop eye complaints during long-term NSAID therapy. Assess knowledge/teach patient appropriate use, interventions to reduce side effects, and adverse symptoms to report (see Patient Education). **Pregnancy risk factor B/D** - see Pregnancy Risk Factor for use cautions. Note breast-feeding caution.

Patient Education: Take this medication exactly as directed; do not increase dose without consulting prescriber. Do not crush tablets or break capsules. Take with food or milk to reduce GI distress. Maintain adequate hydration (2-3 L/day of fluids) unless advised by prescriber to restrict fluids. Do not use alcohol, aspirin or aspirin-containing medication, or any other anti-inflammatory medications without consulting prescriber. You may experience drowsiness, dizziness, nervousness, or headache (use caution when driving or engaging in tasks requiring alertness until response to drug is known); anorexia, nausea, vomiting, or heartburn (small, frequent meals, frequent mouth care, sucking lozenges, or chewing gum may help); fluid retention (weigh yourself weekly and report unusual (3-5 lb/week) weight gain). GI bleeding, ulceration, or perforation can occur with or without pain; discontinue medication and contact prescriber if persistent abdominal pain or cramping, or blood in stool occurs. Report breathlessness, difficulty breathing, or unusual cough; chest pain, rapid heartbeat, palpitations; unusual bruising/bleeding; blood in urine, stool, mouth, or vomitus; swollen extremities; skin rash or itching; acute fatigue; or hearing changes (ringing in ears). **Pregnancy/breast-feeding precautions:** Inform prescriber if you are or intend to become pregnant. This drug should not be used in the 3rd trimester of pregnancy. Consult prescriber if breast-feeding.

Dietary Issues: In order to minimize gastrointestinal effects, ketoprofen can be prescribed to be taken with food or milk.

Geriatric Considerations: Elderly are at high risk for adverse effects from NSAIDs. As much as 60% of elderly can develop peptic ulceration and/or hemorrhage asymptomatically. The concomitant use of H_2 blockers, omeprazole, and sucralfate is not effective as prophylaxis with the exception of NSAID-induced duodenal ulcers which may be prevented by the use of ranitidine. Misoprostol is the only prophylactic agent proven effective. Also, concomitant disease and drug use contribute to the risk for GI adverse effects. Use lowest effective dose for shortest period possible. Consider renal function decline with age. Use of NSAIDs can compromise existing renal function especially when Cl_{cr} is ≤30 mL/minute. Tinnitus may be a difficult and unreliable indication of toxicity due to age-related hearing loss or eighth cranial nerve damage. CNS adverse effects such as confusion, agitation, and hallucination are generally seen in overdose or high-dose situations, but elderly may demonstrate these adverse effects at lower doses than younger adults.

Related Information

Nonsalicylate/Nonsteroidal Anti-inflammatory Comparison *on page 1587*

Ketorolac (KEE toe role ak)

U.S. Brand Names Acular®; Acular® PF; Toradol®

Synonyms Ketorolac Tromethamine

Generic Available Yes: Injection, tablet

Pharmacologic Category Nonsteroidal Anti-inflammatory Drug (NSAID)

Pregnancy Risk Factor C/D (3rd trimester); ophthalmic: C

Lactation Enters breast milk/contraindicated (AAP rates "compatible")

Use

Oral, injection: Short-term (≤5 days) management of moderately-severe acute pain requiring analgesia at the opioid level

Ophthalmic: Temporary relief of ocular itching due to seasonal allergic conjunctivitis; postoperative inflammation following cataract extraction; reduction of ocular pain and photophobia following incisional refractive surgery

Mechanism of Action/Effect A potent NSAID; provides analgesia by inhibiting the synthesis of prostaglandin

Contraindications Hypersensitivity to ketorolac, aspirin, other NSAIDs, or any component of the formulation; patients who have developed nasal polyps, angioedema, or bronchospastic reactions to other NSAIDs; active or history of peptic ulcer disease; recent or history of GI bleeding or perforation; patients with advanced renal disease or risk of renal failure; labor and delivery; nursing mothers; prophylaxis before major surgery; suspected or confirmed cerebrovascular bleeding; hemorrhagic diathesis; concurrent ASA or other NSAIDs; epidural or intrathecal administration; concomitant probenecid; pregnancy (3rd trimester)

Warnings/Precautions

Systemic: Treatment should be started with I.V./I.M. administration then changed to oral only as a continuation of treatment. Total therapy is not to exceed 5 days. Should not be used for minor or chronic pain. Hypersensitivity reactions have occurred flowing the first dose of ketorolac injection, including patients without prior exposure to ketorolac, aspirin, or other NSAIDs. Use extra caution and reduce dosages in the elderly because it is cleared renally somewhat slower, and the elderly are also more sensitive to the renal effects of NSAIDs and have a greater risk of GI perforation and bleeding; use with caution in patients with CHF, hypertension, dehydration, decreased renal or hepatic function, or those receiving anticoagulants. May prolong bleeding time; do not use when hemostasis is critical. Patients should be euvolemic prior to treatment. Low doses of narcotics may be needed for breakthrough pain. Withhold for at least 4-6 half-lives prior to surgical or dental procedures.

Ophthalmic: May increase bleeding time associated with ocular surgery. Use with caution in patients with known bleeding tendencies or those receiving anticoagulants. Do not administer while wearing soft contact lenses. Safety and efficacy in pediatric patients <3 years of age have not been established.

Pregnancy risk C/D (3rd trimester).

Drug Interactions

Decreased Effect: Decreased effect: Decreased antihypertensive effect seen with ACE inhibitors and angiotensin II antagonists; decreased antiepileptic effect seen with carbamazepine, phenytoin

Increased Effect/Toxicity: Increased toxicity: Lithium, methotrexate, probenecid increased drug level; increased effect/toxicity with salicylates, probenecid, anticoagulants, nondepolarizing muscle relaxants, alprazolam, fluoxetine, thiothixene

Nutritional/Ethanol Interactions

Ethanol: Avoid ethanol (may enhance gastric mucosal irritation).

Food: Oral: High-fat meals may delay time to peak (by ~1 hour) and decrease peak concentrations.

Herb/Nutraceutical: Avoid cat's claw, dong quai, evening primrose, feverfew, garlic, ginger, ginkgo, red clover, horse chestnut, green tea, ginseng (all have additional antiplatelet activity).

Effects on Lab Values ↑ chloride (S), sodium (S), bleeding time

Adverse Reactions

>10%:

Systemic:

Central nervous system: Headache (17%)

Gastrointestinal: Gastrointestinal pain (13%), dyspepsia (12%), nausea (12%)

Ophthalmic solution: Ocular: Transient burning/stinging (Acular®: 40%; Acular® PF: 20%)

>1% to 10%:

Systemic:

Cardiovascular: Edema (4%), hypertension

Central nervous system: Dizziness (7%), drowsiness (6%)

Dermatologic: Pruritus, purpura, rash

Gastrointestinal: Diarrhea (7%), constipation, flatulence, gastrointestinal fullness, vomiting, stomatitis

Local: Injection site pain (2%)

(Continued)

Ketorolac *(Continued)*

Miscellaneous: Diaphoresis

Ophthalmic solution: Ocular: Ocular irritation, allergic reactions, superficial ocular infection, superficial keratitis, iritis, ocular inflammation

≤1% (Limited to important or life-threatening): Acute renal failure, anaphylactoid reaction, anaphylaxis, bronchospasm, convulsions, dyspnea, eosinophilia, extrapyramidal symptoms, GI hemorrhage, GI perforation, hemolytic uremic syndrome, hepatitis, hypersensitivity reactions, laryngeal edema, liver failure, rash, nephritis, peptic ulceration, pulmonary edema, stupor, syncope, Stevens-Johnson syndrome, thrombocytopenia, urinary retention, vertigo, toxic epidermal necrolysis, wound hemorrhage (postoperative)

Overdosage/Toxicology Symptoms of overdose include abdominal pain, peptic ulcers, and metabolic acidosis. Management of NSAID intoxication is supportive and symptomatic. Dialysis is not effective.

Pharmacodynamics/Kinetics

Absorption: Oral: Well absorbed

Half-Life Elimination: 2-8 hours; increased 30% to 50% in elderly

Time to Peak: Serum: I.M.: 30-60 minutes

Metabolism: Hepatic

Onset: Analgesic: I.M.: ~10 minutes; Peak effect: Analgesic: 2-3 hours

Duration: Analgesic: 6-8 hours

Formulations

Injection, solution, as tromethamine: 15 mg/mL (1 mL); 30 mg/mL (1 mL, 2 mL) [contains alcohol]

Solution, ophthalmic, as tromethamine:

Acular®: 0.5% (3 mL, 5 mL, 10 mL) [contains benzalkonium chloride]

Acular® P.F. [preservative free]: 0.5% (0.4 mL)

Tablet, as tromethamine (Toradol®): 10 mg

Dosing

Adults:

Moderately-severe acute pain: Children ≥16 years and Adults: **The maximum combined duration of treatment (for parenteral and oral) is 5 days**; do not increase dose or frequency; supplement with low dose opioids if needed for breakthrough pain. For patients <50 kg and/or ≥65 years of age, see Elderly dosing.

I.M.: 60 mg as a single dose or 30 mg every 6 hours (maximum daily dose: 120 mg)

I.V.: 30 mg as a single dose or 30 mg every 6 hours (maximum daily dose: 120 mg)

Oral: 20 mg, followed by 10 mg every 4-6 hours; do not exceed 40 mg/day; oral dosing is intended to be a continuation of I.M. or I.V. therapy only

Ophthalmic uses:

Seasonal allergic conjunctivitis (relief of ocular itching): Children ≥3 years and Adults: Ophthalmic: Instill 1 drop (0.25 mg) 4 times/day for seasonal allergic conjunctivitis

Inflammation following cataract extraction: Children ≥12 years and Adults: Ophthalmic: Instill 1 drop (0.25 mg) to affected eye(s) 4 times/day beginning 24 hours after surgery; continue for 2 weeks

Pain and photophobia following incisional refractive surgery: Children ≥12 years and Adults: Ophthalmic: Instill 1 drop (0.25 mg) 4 times/day to affected eye for up to 3 days

Elderly: Elderly >65 years: Renal insufficiency or weight <50 kg: **Note:** Ketorolac has decreased clearance and increased half-life in the elderly. In addition, the elderly have reported increased incidence of GI bleeding, ulceration, and perforation. The maximum combined duration of treatment (for parenteral and oral) is 5 days.

I.M.: 30 mg as a single dose or 15 mg every 6 hours (maximum daily dose: 60 mg)

I.V.: 15 mg as a single dose or 15 mg every 6 hours (maximum daily dose: 60 mg)

Oral: 10 mg every 4-6 hours; do not exceed 40 mg/day; oral dosing is intended to be a continuation of I.M. or I.V. therapy only

Pediatrics: Note: The use of ketorolac in children <16 years of age is outside of product labeling. For children 2-16 years: Dosing guidelines are not established; **do not exceed adult doses**.

Anti-inflammatory, single-dose treatment:

I.M., I.V.: 0.4-1 mg/kg as a single dose; **Note:** Limited information exists. Single I.V. doses of 0.5 mg/kg, 0.75 mg/kg, 0.9 mg/kg and 1 mg/kg have been studied in children 2-16 years of age for postoperative analgesia. One study (Maunuksela, 1992) used a titrating dose starting with 0.2 mg/kg up to a total of 0.5 mg/kg (median dose required: 0.4 mg/kg).

Oral: One study used 1 mg/kg as a single dose for analgesia in 30 children (mean ± SD age: 3 ± 2.5 years) undergoing bilateral myringotomy

Anti-inflammatory, multiple-dose treatment: I.M., I.V., Oral: No pediatric studies exist; one report (Buck, 1994) of the clinical experience with ketorolac in 112 children, 6 months to 19 years of age (mean: 9 years), described usual I.V. maintenance doses of 0.5 mg/kg every 6 hours (mean dose: 0.52 mg/kg; range: 0.17-1 mg/kg)

Seasonal allergic conjunctivitis: Ophthalmic: Children ≥3 years: Refer to adult dosing.

Renal Impairment: Do not use in patients with advanced renal impairment. Patients with moderately-elevated serum creatinine should use half the recommended dose, not to exceed 60 mg/day I.M./I.V.

Hepatic Impairment: Use with caution, may cause elevation of liver enzymes

Administration

Oral: May take with food to reduce GI upset.

I.M.: Administer slowly and deeply into the muscle. Analgesia begins in 30 minutes and maximum effect within 2 hours.

I.V.: Administer I.V. bolus over a minimum of 15 seconds; onset within 30 minutes; peak analgesia within 2 hours.

Other: Ophthalmic solution: Contact lenses should be removed before instillation.

Stability

Storage: Ketorolac injection and ophthalmic solution should be stored at controlled room temperature and protected from light. Injection is clear and has a slight yellow color. Precipitation may occur at relatively low pH values. Store tablets at controlled room temperature.

Compatibility: Stable in D_5NS, D_5W, LR, NS

Compatibility when admixed: Incompatible with hydroxyzine, meperidine, morphine, promethazine

Monitoring Laboratory Tests Renal function (serum creatinine, BUN, urine output), CBC, liver function, platelets

Monitoring and Teaching Issues

Physical Assessment: Assess allergy history prior to beginning therapy. See Contraindications, Warnings/Precautions, and Dosing for use cautions. Assess potential for interactions with other prescriptions, OTC medications, or herbal products patient may be taking (see Drug Interactions). **I.V./I.M.:** See Administration and Dosing. Vital signs should be monitored on a regular basis during infusion or following injection. Assess results of laboratory tests (see above) and patient response (see Adverse Reactions and Overdose/Toxicology) on a regular basis throughout therapy. Teach patient proper use, possible side effects and interventions (eg, importance of adequate hydration), and adverse symptoms to report (see Patient Education). **Pregnancy risk factor C/D** - see Pregnancy Risk Factor for use cautions. Instruct patient of childbearing age about appropriate use of barrier contraceptives. Breast-feeding is contraindicated.

Patient Education: Inform prescriber of all prescriptions, OTC medications, or herbal products you are taking, and any allergies you have. Do not take anything new without consulting prescriber (especially aspirin-containing products or other NSAIDs or any other NSAIDs). Use exactly as directed; do not increase dose or frequency. Adverse reactions can occur with overuse. Oral doses may be taken with food or milk. Avoid alcohol. Maintain adequate hydration (2-3 L/day of fluids) unless advised by prescriber to restrict fluids. May cause nausea or vomiting (frequent mouth care, small, frequent meals, chewing gum, or sucking lozenges may help). Report GI bleeding, ulceration or perforation with or without pain (stop medication and report abdominal pain or blood in urine or stool); ringing in ears; unresolved nausea or vomiting; difficulty breathing or shortness of breath; skin rash; unusual swelling of extremities; chest pain; or palpitations. **Pregnancy/breast-feeding precautions:** Inform prescriber if you are or intend to become pregnant. This drug should not be used in the 2nd or 3rd trimester of pregnancy. Consult prescriber for appropriate contraceptive measures if necessary. Consult prescriber if breast-feeding.

Ophthalmic: Instill drops as often as recommended. Wash hands before instilling. Sit or lie down to instill. Open eye, look at ceiling, and instill prescribed amount of solution. Close eye and roll eye in all directions. Apply gentle pressure to inner corner of eye for 1-2 minutes after instillation. Do not let tip of applicator touch eye; do not contaminate tip of applicator (may cause eye infection, eye damage, or vision loss). Temporary stinging or blurred vision may occur. Do not wear soft contact lenses. Report persistent pain, burning, double vision, swelling, itching, or worsening of condition.

Dietary Issues: Administer tablet with food or milk to decrease gastrointestinal distress.

Geriatric Considerations: Ketorolac is eliminated more slowly in the elderly. It is recommended to use lower doses in the elderly. The elderly are at high risk for adverse effects from NSAIDs. As much as 60% of elderly can develop peptic ulceration and/or hemorrhage asymptomatically. The concomitant use of H_2 blockers, omeprazole, and sucralfate is not effective as prophylaxis with the exception of NSAID-induced duodenal ulcers which may be prevented by the use of ranitidine. Misoprostol is the only prophylactic agent proven effective. Also, concomitant disease and drug use contribute to the risk for GI adverse effects. Use lowest effective dose for shortest period possible. Consider renal function decline with age. Use of NSAIDs can compromise existing renal function especially when Cl_{cr} is ≤30 mL/minute. Tinnitus may be a difficult and unreliable indication of toxicity due to age-related hearing loss or eighth cranial nerve damage. CNS adverse effects such as confusion, agitation, and hallucination are generally seen in overdose or high-dose situations, but elderly may demonstrate these adverse effects at lower doses than younger adults.

Pregnancy Issues: Ketorolac is contraindicated during labor and delivery (may inhibit uterine contractions and adversely affect fetal circulation). Avoid use of ketorolac ophthalmic solution during late pregnancy.

Additional Information First parenteral NSAID for analgesia; 30 mg provides the analgesia comparable to 12 mg of morphine or 100 mg of meperidine.

Related Information

Nonsalicylate/Nonsteroidal Anti-inflammatory Comparison *on page 1587*

Ophthalmic Agents *on page 1509*

Labetalol (la BET a lole)

U.S. Brand Names Normodyne®; Trandate®

Synonyms Ibidomide Hydrochloride; Labetalol Hydrochloride

Generic Available Yes

Pharmacologic Category Beta Blocker With Alpha-Blocking Activity

Pregnancy Risk Factor C (manufacturer); D (2nd and 3rd trimesters - expert analysis)

Lactation Enters breast milk/use caution (AAP rates "compatible")

Use Treatment of mild to severe hypertension; I.V. for hypertensive emergencies

Mechanism of Action/Effect Blocks alpha-, $beta_1$-, and $beta_2$-adrenergic receptor sites; elevated renins are reduced

Contraindications Hypersensitivity to labetalol or any component of the formulation; sinus bradycardia; heart block greater than first degree (except in patients with a functioning artificial pacemaker); cardiogenic shock; bronchial asthma; uncompensated cardiac failure; pregnancy (2nd and 3rd trimesters)

Warnings/Precautions Use only with extreme caution in compensated heart failure and monitor for a worsening of the condition. Use caution with concurrent use of beta-blockers and either verapamil or diltiazem; bradycardia or heart block can occur. Avoid concurrent I.V. use of both agents. Patients with bronchospastic disease should not receive beta-blockers. Labetalol may be used with caution in patients with nonallergic bronchospasm (chronic bronchitis, emphysema). Use cautiously in diabetics because it can mask prominent hypoglycemic symptoms. Can mask signs of thyrotoxicosis. Can cause fetal harm when administered in pregnancy. Use cautiously in hepatic impairment. Use caution when using I.V. labetalol and inhalational anesthetics concurrently (significant myocardial depression). Avoid abrupt discontinuation in patients with a history of CAD. Pregnancy risk C/D (2nd and 3rd trimesters).

Drug Interactions

Cytochrome P450 Effect: Substrate of **CYP2D6**; Inhibits CYP2D6

Decreased Effect: Decreased effect of beta-blockers with aluminum salts, barbiturates, calcium salts, cholestyramine, colestipol, NSAIDs, penicillins (ampicillin), rifampin, salicylates, and sulfinpyrazone due to decreased bioavailability and plasma levels. Beta-blockers may decrease the effect of sulfonylureas.

Increased Effect/Toxicity: Inhibitors of CYP2D6 including quinidine, paroxetine, and propafenone are likely to increase blood levels of labetalol. Cimetidine increases the bioavailability of labetalol. Labetalol has additive hypotensive effects with other antihypertensive agents. Concurrent use with alpha-blockers (prazosin, terazosin) and beta-blockers increases the risk of orthostasis. Concurrent use with diltiazem, verapamil, or digoxin may increase the risk of bradycardia with beta-blocking agents. Halothane, enflurane, isoflurane, and potentially other inhalation anesthetics may cause synergistic hypotension. Beta-blockers may affect the action or levels of ethanol, disopyramide, nondepolarizing muscle relaxants, and theophylline although the effects are difficult to predict.

Nutritional/Ethanol Interactions

Food: Labetalol serum concentrations may be increased if taken with food.

Herb/Nutraceutical: Avoid dong quai if using for hypertension (has estrogenic activity). Avoid ephedra, yohimbe, ginseng (may worsen hypertension). Avoid natural licorice (causes sodium and water retention and increases potassium loss). Avoid garlic (may have increased antihypertensive effect).

Effects on Lab Values False-positive urine catecholamines, VMA if measured by fluorometric or photometric methods; use HPLC or specific catecholamine radioenzymatic technique

Adverse Reactions

>10%:

Central nervous system: Dizziness (1% to 16%)

Gastrointestinal: Nausea (0% to 19%)

1% to 10%:

Cardiovascular: Edema (0% to 2%), hypotension (1% to 5%); with IV use, hypotension may occur in up to 58%

Central nervous system: Fatigue (1% to 10%), paresthesia (1% to 5%), headache (2%), vertigo (2%), weakness (1%)

Dermatologic: Rash (1%), scalp tingling (1% to 5%)

Gastrointestinal: Vomiting (<1% to 3%), dyspepsia (1% to 4%)

Genitourinary: Ejaculatory failure (0% to 5%), impotence (1% to 4%)

Hepatic: Increased transaminases (4%)

Respiratory: Nasal congestion (1% to 6%), dyspnea (2%)

Miscellaneous: Taste disorder (1%), abnormal vision (1%)

<1% (Limited to important or life-threatening): Alopecia (reversible), anaphylactoid reaction, angioedema, bradycardia, bronchospasm, cholestatic jaundice, CHF, diabetes insipidus, heart block, hepatic necrosis, hepatitis, hypersensitivity, hypotension, Peyronie's disease, positive ANA, pruritus, Raynaud's syndrome, syncope, systemic lupus erythematosus, toxic myopathy, urinary retention, urticaria, ventricular arrhythmias (I.V.)

Other adverse reactions noted with beta-adrenergic blocking agents include mental depression, catatonia, short-term memory loss, emotional lability, intensification of pre-existing AV block, laryngospasm, respiratory distress, agranulocytosis, thrombocytopenic purpura, nonthrombocytopenic purpura, mesenteric artery thrombosis, and ischemic colitis.

Overdosage/Toxicology Symptoms of intoxication include cardiac disturbances, CNS toxicity, bronchospasm, hypoglycemia, and hyperkalemia. The most common cardiac symptoms include hypotension and bradycardia. Atrioventricular block, intraventricular conduction disturbances, cardiogenic shock, and asystole may occur with severe overdose, especially with membrane-depressant drugs (eg, propranolol). CNS effects include convulsions, coma, and respiratory arrest and are commonly seen with propranolol and other membrane-depressant and lipid-soluble drugs. Treatment is symptomatic. Glucagon may be administered to improve cardiac function.

Pharmacodynamics/Kinetics

Bioavailability: Oral: 25%; increased with liver disease, elderly, and concurrent cimetidine

Half-Life Elimination: Normal renal function: 2.5-8 hours

Metabolism: Hepatic, primarily via glucuronide conjugation; extensive first-pass effect

Onset: Oral: 20 minutes to 2 hours; I.V.: 2-5 minutes; Peak effect: Oral: 1-4 hours; I.V.: 5-15 minutes

Duration: Oral (dose dependent): 8-24 hours; I.V.: 2-4 hours

Formulations

Injection, solution, as hydrochloride (Normodyne®): 5 mg/mL (20 mL, 40 mL)

Injection, solution, as hydrochloride [prefilled syringe]: 5 mg/mL (4 mL)

Normodyne®: 5 mg/mL (4 mL, 8 mL)

Tablet, as hydrochloride: 100 mg, 200 mg, 300 mg

Normodyne®: 100 mg, 200 mg, 300 mg

Trandate®: 100 mg, 200 mg [contains sodium benzoate], 300 mg

Dosing

Adults:

Hypertension: Oral: Initial: 100 mg twice daily, may increase as needed every 2-3 days by 100 mg until desired response is obtained; usual dose: 200-400 mg twice daily; not to exceed 2.4 g/day

Acute hypertension (hypertensive urgency/emergency):

I.V. bolus: 20 mg or 1-2 mg/kg whichever is lower, IVP over 2 minutes, may give 40-80 mg at 10-minute intervals, up to 300 mg total dose

I.V. infusion: Initial: 2 mg/minute; titrate to response up to 300 mg total dose. Administration requires the use of an infusion pump.

Note: Continuous infusion at low rates (2-4 mg/hour) have been used in some settings for patients unable to transition rapidly to oral medication.

Elderly: Oral: Initial: 100 mg 1-2 times/day increasing as needed

Pediatrics: Note: Due to limited documentation of its use, labetalol should be initiated cautiously in pediatric patients with careful dosage adjustment and blood pressure monitoring.

Hypertension:

Oral: Limited information regarding labetalol use in pediatric patients is currently available in literature. Some centers recommend initial oral doses of 4 mg/kg/day in 2 divided doses. Reported oral doses have started at 3 mg/kg/day and 20 mg/kg/day and have increased up to 40 mg/kg/day.

I.V., intermittent bolus doses of 0.3-1 mg/kg/dose have been reported.

For treatment of pediatric hypertensive emergencies, initial continuous infusions of 0.4-1 mg/kg/hour with a maximum of 3 mg/kg/hour have been used; administration requires the use of an infusion pump.

Renal Impairment: Not removed by hemo- or peritoneal dialysis; supplemental dose is not necessary.

Hepatic Impairment: Dosage reduction may be necessary.

Administration

I.V.: Bolus administered over 2 minutes.

Stability

Storage: Labetalol should be stored at room temperature or under refrigeration and should be protected from light and freezing. The solution is clear to slightly yellow.

Reconstitution: Stability of parenteral admixture at room temperature (25°C) and refrigeration temperature (4°C) is 3 days.

Standard diluent: 500 mg/250 mL D_5W

Minimum volume: 250 mL D_5W

(Continued)

Labetalol *(Continued)*

Compatibility: Stable in D_5LR, $D_5{}^1/_4NS$, $D_5{}^1/_3NS$, D_5NS, D_5W, LR, NS; most stable at pH of 2-4. **Incompatible** with sodium bicarbonate 5% and alkaline solutions.

Y-site administration: Incompatible with amphotericin B cholesteryl sulfate complex, cefoperazone, ceftriaxone, nafcillin, thiopental, warfarin

Compatibility when admixed: Incompatible with sodium bicarbonate

Monitoring and Teaching Issues

Physical Assessment: See Contraindications, Warnings/Precautions, and Dosing for use cautions. Assess potential for interactions with other prescriptions, OTC medications, or herbal products patient may be taking (especially anything that will effect blood pressure - see Drug Interactions). For I.V. specifics, see Dosing and Administration. Blood pressure and heart rate should be assessed prior to and following first dose and any change in dosage. Caution diabetic patients to monitor glucose levels closely; beta-blockers may alter glucose tolerance. Assess results of laboratory tests (see above), therapeutic effectiveness, and adverse response (eg, CHF - see Adverse Reactions and Overdose/Toxicology). Teach patient proper use, possible side effects and appropriate interventions, and adverse symptoms to report (see Patient Education). **Pregnancy risk factor C/D** - see Pregnancy Risk Factor for use cautions; benefits of use should outweigh possible risks. Instruct patients of childbearing age about appropriate barrier contraceptive measures. Note breast-feeding caution.

Patient Education: Inform prescriber of all prescriptions, OTC medications, or herbal products you are taking, and any allergies you have. Do not take anything new during treatment unless approved by prescriber. Take as directed, with meals. Do not skip dose or discontinue without consulting prescriber. This medication does not replace other antihypertensive interventions; follow prescriber's instructions for diet and lifestyle changes. If diabetic, monitor serum glucose closely and notify prescriber of changes (this medication can alter hypoglycemic requirements). You may experience drowsiness, dizziness, or impaired judgment (use caution when driving or engaging in tasks that require alertness until response to drug is known); postural hypotension (use caution when rising from sitting or lying position or when climbing stairs); dry mouth, nausea, or loss of appetite (frequent mouth care or sucking lozenges may help); or sexual dysfunction (reversible, may resolve with continued use). Report altered CNS status (eg, fatigue, depression, numbness or tingling of fingers, toes, or skin); palpitations or slowed heartbeat; difficulty breathing; edema or cold extremities; or other persistent side effects. **Pregnancy/breast-feeding precautions:** Inform prescriber if you are or intend to become pregnant. Consult prescriber if breast-feeding.

Geriatric Considerations: Due to alterations in the beta-adrenergic autonomic nervous system, beta-adrenergic blockade may result in less hemodynamic response than seen in younger adults.

Breast-feeding Issues: Available evidence suggests safe use during breast-feeding. Monitor breast-fed infant for symptoms of beta-blockade.

Pregnancy Issues: Crosses the placenta. Bradycardia, hypotension, hypoglycemia, intrauterine growth rate (IUGR). IUGR probably related to maternal hypertension. Available evidence suggests safe use during pregnancy.

Related Information

Beta-Blockers *on page 1561*

Labetalol Hydrochloride *see* Labetalol *on page 764*

Laboratory Reference Values for Adults *see page 1535*

Laboratory Reference Values for Children *see page 1539*

LactiCare-HC® *see* Hydrocortisone *on page 673*

LactiCare-HC® *see* Topical Corticosteroids *on page 1334*

Lactinex® [OTC] *see Lactobacillus on page 766*

Lactobacillus (lak toe ba SIL us)

U.S. Brand Names Bacid® [OTC]; Kala® [OTC]; Lactinex® [OTC]; Megadophilus® [OTC]; MoreDophilus® [OTC]; Probiotica® [OTC]; Superdophilus® [OTC]

Synonyms *Lactobacillus acidophilus*; *Lactobacillus acidophilus* and *Lactobacillus bulgaricus*; *Lactobacillus reuteri*

Generic Available Yes

Pharmacologic Category Antidiarrheal

Pregnancy Risk Factor Not available

Lactation Excretion in breast milk unknown/use caution

Use Treatment of uncomplicated diarrhea particularly that caused by antibiotic therapy; re-establish normal physiologic and bacterial flora of the intestinal tract

Mechanism of Action/Effect Creates an environment unfavorable to potentially pathogenic fungi or bacteria through the production of lactic acid, and favors establishment of an aciduric flora, thereby suppressing the growth of pathogenic microorganisms; helps re-establish normal intestinal flora

Contraindications Allergy to milk or lactose

Warnings/Precautions Discontinue if high fever is present. Do not use in children <2 years of age.

Adverse Reactions No data reported

Pharmacodynamics/Kinetics

Absorption: Oral: None

Formulations

Capsule: *Lactobacillus acidophilus* 100 million units

Bacid®: *Lactobacillus acidophilus* 500 million units

Megadophilus®, Superdophilus®: *Lactobacillus acidophilus* 2 billion units [available in dairy based or dairy free formulations]

Granules (Lactinex®): Mixed culture *L. acidophilus, L. bulgaricus* per 1 g packet (12s)

Powder:

Megadophilus®, Superdophilus®: *Lactobacillus acidophilus* 2 billion units per half-teaspoon (49 g) [available in dairy based or dairy free formulations]

MoreDophilus®: *Lactobacillus acidophilus* 12.4 billion units per teaspoon [carrot derived] (30 g, 120 g)

Tablet (Kala®): *Lactobacillus acidophilus* 200 million units [soy based]

Tablet, chewable:

Lactinex®: Mixed culture *L. acidophilus, L. bulgaricus*

Probiotica®: *L. reuteri* 100 million units (30s, 60s) [lemon flavor]

Dosing

Adults & Elderly: Diarrhea: Oral:

Capsules: 2 capsules 2-4 times/day

Granules: 1 packet added to or taken with cereal, food, milk, fruit juice, or water, 3-4 times/day

Powder: 1 teaspoonful daily with liquid

Tablet, chewable: 4 tablets 3-4 times/day; may follow each dose with a small amount of milk, fruit juice, or water

Pediatrics: Children >2 years: Refer to adult dosing.

Stability

Storage: Store in refrigerator.

Monitoring and Teaching Issues

Physical Assessment: See Warnings/Precautions and Contraindications for use cautions. Instruct patient to discontinue and notify prescriber if high fever develops. Note breast-feeding caution.

Patient Education: Granules may be added to or taken with cereal, food, milk, fruit juice, or water. You may experience increased flatus while taking this medication. Discontinue and notify prescriber if a high fever develops. Refrigerate Lactinex® and Bacid®. **Breast-feeding precaution:** Consult prescriber if breast-feeding.

Dietary Issues: Granules or contents of capsules may be added to or administered with cereal, food, milk, fruit juice, or water.

Lactobacillus acidophilus *see Lactobacillus on page 766*

Lactobacillus acidophilus* and *Lactobacillus bulgaricus *see Lactobacillus on page 766*

Lactobacillus reuteri *see Lactobacillus on page 766*

Lactoflavin *see* Riboflavin *on page 1183*

Lactulose (LAK tyoo lose)

U.S. Brand Names Cholac®; Constilac®; Constulose®; Enulose®; Generlac; Kristalose™

Generic Available Yes

Pharmacologic Category Ammonium Detoxicant; Laxative, Miscellaneous

Pregnancy Risk Factor B

Lactation Excretion in breast milk unknown

Use Adjunct in the prevention and treatment of portal-systemic encephalopathy; treatment of chronic constipation

Mechanism of Action/Effect The bacterial degradation of lactulose resulting in an acidic pH inhibits the diffusion of NH_3 into the blood by causing the conversion of NH_3 to NH_4+; also enhances the diffusion of NH_3 from the blood into the gut where conversion to NH_4+ occurs; produces an osmotic effect in the colon with resultant distention promoting peristalsis

Contraindications Hypersensitivity to lactulose or any component of the formulation; galactosemia (or patients requiring a low galactose diet)

Warnings/Precautions Use with caution in patients with diabetes mellitus; monitor periodically for electrolyte imbalance when lactulose is used >6 months or in patients predisposed to electrolyte abnormalities (eg, elderly); patients receiving lactulose and an oral anti-infective agent should be monitored for possible inadequate response to lactulose

Drug Interactions

Decreased Effect: Oral neomycin, laxatives, antacids

Adverse Reactions Frequency not defined: Gastrointestinal: Flatulence, diarrhea (excessive dose), abdominal discomfort, nausea, vomiting, cramping

Overdosage/Toxicology Symptoms of overdose include diarrhea, abdominal pain, hypochloremic alkalosis, dehydration, hypotension, and hypokalemia. Treatment includes supportive care.

Pharmacodynamics/Kinetics

Absorption: Not appreciable

Metabolism: Via colonic flora to lactic acid and acetic acid; requires colonic flora for drug activation

Formulations

Crystals for reconstitution (Kristalose™): 10 g/packet (30s), 20 g/packet (30s)

Syrup: 10 g/15 mL (15 mL, 30 mL, 237 mL, 473 mL, 946 mL, 1000 mL, 1890 mL)

Cholac®, Constilac®: 10 g/15 mL (30 mL, 240 mL, 480 mL, 960 mL, 1920 mL, 3875 mL)

Constulose®: 10 g/15 mL (240 mL, 960 mL)

Enulose®: 10 g/15 mL (480 mL, 1900 mL)

Generlac: 10 g/15 mL (480 mL, 1920 mL)

Dosing

Adults & Elderly:

Note: Diarrhea may indicate overdosage and responds to dose reduction.

Acute portal-systemic encephalopathy (PSE):

Oral: 20-30 g (30-45 mL) every 1-2 hours to induce rapid laxation; adjust dosage daily to produce 2-3 soft stools; doses of 30-45 mL may be given hourly to cause rapid laxation, then reduce to recommended dose; usual daily dose: 60-100 g (90-150 mL) daily

Rectal: 200 g (300 mL) diluted with 700 mL of $H_2$0 or NS; administer rectally via rectal balloon catheter and retain 30-60 minutes every 4-6 hours.

Constipation: Oral: 10-20 g/day (15-30 mL/day) increased to 60 mL/day if necessary

(Continued)

Lactulose *(Continued)*

Pediatrics: Diarrhea may indicate overdosage and responds to dose reduction.

Prevention of portal systemic encephalopathy (PSE): Oral:

Infants: 2.5-10 mL/day divided 3-4 times/day; adjust dosage to produce 2-3 stools/day.

Older Children: Daily dose of 40-90 mL divided 3-4 times/day; if initial dose causes diarrhea, then reduce it immediately; adjust dosage to produce 2-3 stools/day.

Constipation: 5 g/day (7.5 mL) after breakfast

Administration

Oral: Dilute lactulose in water, usually 60-120 mL, prior to administering through a gastric or feeding tube.

Other: Syrup formulation has been used in preparation of rectal solution.

Stability

Storage: Keep solution at room temperature to reduce viscosity. Discard solution if cloudy or very dark.

Monitoring Laboratory Tests Serum potassium, serum ammonia

Monitoring and Teaching Issues

Physical Assessment: See Contraindications, Warnings/Precautions, and Dosing for use cautions. Assess results of laboratory tests (see above), therapeutic effectiveness, and adverse response (eg, CHF - see Adverse Reactions and Overdose/Toxicology). Teach patient proper use, possible side effects and appropriate interventions, and adverse symptoms to report (see Patient Education). Note breast-feeding caution.

Patient Education: Not for long-term use. Take as directed, alone, or diluted with water, juice or milk, or take with food. Laxative results may not occur for 24-48 hours; do not take more often than recommended or for a longer time than recommended. Do not use any other laxatives while taking lactulose. Increased fiber, fluids, and exercise may also help reduce constipation. Do not use if experiencing abdominal pain, nausea, or vomiting. Diarrhea may indicate overdose. May cause flatulence, belching, or abdominal cramping. Report persistent or severe diarrhea or abdominal cramping. **Breast-feeding precaution:** Consult prescriber if breast-feeding.

Dietary Issues: Contraindicated in patients on galactose-restricted diet; may be mixed with fruit juice, milk, water, or citrus-flavored carbonated beverages.

Geriatric Considerations: Elderly are more likely to show CNS signs of dehydration and electrolyte loss than younger adults. Therefore, monitor closely for fluid and electrolyte loss with chronic use. Sorbitol is equally effective as a laxative and less expensive. However, sorbitol **cannot be substituted** in the treatment of hepatic encephalopathy.

Related Information

Laxatives: Classification and Properties *on page 1581*

L-AmB *see* Amphotericin B (Liposomal) *on page 98*

Lamictal® *see* Lamotrigine *on page 770*

Lamisil® *see* Terbinafine *on page 1289*

Lamisil® AT™ *see* Terbinafine *on page 1289*

Lamisil® Dermgel *see* Terbinafine *on page 1289*

Lamisil® Solution *see* Terbinafine *on page 1289*

Lamivudine (la MI vyoo deen)

U.S. Brand Names Epivir®; Epivir-HBV®

Synonyms 3TC

Generic Available No

Pharmacologic Category Antiretroviral Agent, Reverse Transcriptase Inhibitor (Nucleoside)

Pregnancy Risk Factor C

Lactation Enters breast milk/contraindicated

Use

Epivir®: Treatment of HIV infection when antiretroviral therapy is warranted; should always be used as part of a multidrug regimen (at least three antiretroviral agents)

Epivir-HBV®: Treatment of chronic hepatitis B associated with evidence of hepatitis B viral replication and active liver inflammation

Use - Unlabeled/Investigational Prevention of HIV following needlesticks (with or without protease inhibitor)

Mechanism of Action/Effect *In vitro*, lamivudine is phosphorylated to its active 5′-triphosphate metabolite (L-TP), which inhibits HIV reverse transcription via viral DNA chain termination; L-TP also inhibits the RNA- and DNA-dependent DNA polymerase activities of reverse transcriptase. The monophosphate form is incorporated into viral DNA by hepatitis B polymerase, resulting in DNA chain termination.

Contraindications Hypersensitivity to lamivudine or any component of the formulation

Warnings/Precautions A decreased dosage is recommended in patients with renal dysfunction since AUC, C_{max}, and half-life increased with diminishing renal function; use with extreme caution in children with history of pancreatitis or risk factors for development of pancreatitis. Do not use as monotherapy in treatment of HIV. Treatment of HBV in patients with unrecognized/untreated HIV may lead to rapid HIV resistance. Treatment of HIV in patients with unrecognized/untreated HBV may lead to rapid HBV resistance. Patients with HIV infection should receive only dosage forms appropriate for treatment of HIV.

Lactic acidosis and severe hepatomegaly with steatosis have been reported, including fatal cases. Use caution in hepatic impairment. Pregnancy, obesity, and/or prolonged therapy may increase the risk of lactic acidosis and liver damage.

Monitor patients closely for several months following discontinuation of therapy for chronic hepatitis B; clinical exacerbations may occur.

Pregnancy risk C.

Drug Interactions

Decreased Effect: Zalcitabine and lamivudine may inhibit the intracellular phosphorylation of each other; concomitant use should be avoided.

Increased Effect/Toxicity: Zidovudine concentrations increase significantly (~39%) with lamivudine coadministration. Trimethoprim/sulfamethoxazole increases lamivudine's blood levels. Concomitant use of ribavirin and nucleoside analogues may increase the risk of developing lactic acidosis (includes adefovir, didanosine, lamivudine, stavudine, zalcitabine, zidovudine).

Nutritional/Ethanol Interactions Food: Food decreases the rate of absorption and C_{max}; however, there is no change in the systemic AUC. Therefore, may be taken with or without food.

Adverse Reactions (As reported in adults treated for HIV infection)

>10%:

Central nervous system: Headache, fatigue

Gastrointestinal: Nausea, diarrhea, vomiting, pancreatitis (range: 0.5% to 18%; higher percentage in pediatric patients)

Neuromuscular & skeletal: Peripheral neuropathy, paresthesia, musculoskeletal pain

1% to 10%:

Central nervous system: Dizziness, depression, fever, chills, insomnia

Dermatologic: Rash

Gastrointestinal: Anorexia, abdominal pain, heartburn, elevated amylase

Hematologic: Neutropenia

Hepatic: Elevated AST, ALT

Neuromuscular & skeletal: Myalgia, arthralgia

Respiratory: Nasal signs and symptoms, cough

<1% (Limited to important or life-threatening): Alopecia, anaphylaxis, anemia, hepatomegaly, hyperbilirubinemia, hyperglycemia, increased CPK, lactic acidosis, lymphadenopathy, peripheral neuropathy, pruritus, red cell aplasia, rhabdomyolysis, splenomegaly, steatosis, stomatitis, thrombocytopenia, urticaria, weakness

Overdosage/Toxicology Limited information is available, although there have been no clinical signs or symptoms noted, and hematologic tests remained normal in overdose. No antidote is available. Unknown dialyzability.

Pharmacodynamics/Kinetics

Absorption: Rapid

Bioavailability: Absolute: Cp_{max} decreased with food although AUC not significantly affected

Children: 66%

Adults: 87%

Half-Life Elimination: Children: 2 hours; Adults: 5-7 hours

Metabolism: 5.6% to trans-sulfoxide metabolite

Formulations

Solution, oral:

Epivir®: 10 mg/mL (240 mL) [strawberry-banana flavor]

Epivir-HBV®: 5 mg/mL (240 mL) [strawberry-banana flavor]

Tablet:

Epivir®: 150 mg, 300 mg

Epivir-HBV®: 100 mg

Dosing

Adults & Elderly: Note: The formulation and dosage of Epivir-HBV® are not appropriate for patients infected with both HBV and HIV.

HIV: Oral (use with at least two other antiretroviral agents): 150 mg twice daily **or** 300 mg once daily

Prevention of HIV following needlesticks (unlabeled use): Oral: 150 mg twice daily (with zidovudine with or without a protease inhibitor, depending on risk)

Treatment of hepatitis B (Epivir-HBV®): Oral: 100 mg/day

Pediatrics: Note: The formulation and dosage of Epivir-HBV® are not appropriate for patients infected with both HBV and HIV.

HIV: Oral (Use with at least two other antiretroviral agents)

3 months to 16 years: 4 mg/kg twice daily (maximum: 150 mg twice daily)

>16 years: Refer to adult dosing.

Treatment of hepatitis B: Oral: Children 2-17 years: 3 mg/kg once daily (maximum: 100 mg/day)

Renal Impairment: Oral:

Pediatric patients: Insufficient data; however, dose reduction should be considered.

Treatment of HIV patients >16 years:

Cl_{cr} 30-49 mL/minute: Administer 150 mg once daily.

Cl_{cr} 15-29 mL/minute: Administer 150 mg first dose, then 100 mg once daily.

Cl_{cr} 5-14 mL/minute: Administer 150 mg first dose, then 50 mg once daily.

Cl_{cr} <5 mL/minute: Administer 50 mg first dose, then 25 mg once daily.

Dialysis: No data available.

Treatment of hepatitis B patients: Adults:

Cl_{cr} 30-49 mL/minute: Administer 100 mg first dose, then 50 mg once daily.

Cl_{cr} 15-29 mL/minute: Administer 100 mg first dose, then 25 mg once daily.

Cl_{cr} 5-14 mL/minute: Administer 35 mg first dose, then 15 mg once daily.

Cl_{cr} <5 mL/minute: Administer 35 mg first dose, then 25 mg once daily.

Dialysis: No additional dosing is required after routine hemodialysis.

Administration

Oral: May be taken with or without food. Adjust dosage in renal failure.

Stability

Storage: Store at 2°C to 25°C (68°F to 77°F) tightly closed.

Monitoring Laboratory Tests Amylase, bilirubin, liver enzymes, CBC

Monitoring and Teaching Issues

Physical Assessment: See Contraindications, Warnings/Precautions, Drug Interactions, and Dosing for use cautions. Assess results of laboratory tests (see above), therapeutic response, and adverse reactions (see Adverse Reactions and Overdose/Toxicology) on a regular basis throughout therapy. Teach patient proper use (see Administration), possible

(Continued)

Lamivudine *(Continued)*

side effects and appropriate interventions, and adverse symptoms to report (see Patient Education). **Pregnancy Risk Factor C** - benefits of use should outweigh possible risks. Breast-feeding is contraindicated.

Patient Education: Inform prescriber of all prescriptions, OTC medications, or herbal products you are taking, and any allergies you have. Do not take anything new during treatment unless approved by prescriber. Lamivudine is not a cure for HIV or hepatitis B, nor has it been found to reduce transmission. Long-term effects are unknown. You will need frequent blood tests to adjust dosage for maximum therapeutic effect. Take as directed for full course of therapy; do not discontinue (even if feeling better). Take with or without food. Do not take antacids within 1 hour of lamivudine. Mix four tablets in 3-5 oz water, allow to stand a few minutes, and stir; drink immediately. You may experience loss of appetite; change in taste (sucking on lozenges, chewing gum, or small, frequent meals may help); dizziness or numbness (use caution when driving or engaging in tasks that require alertness until response to drug is known); or headache, fever, or muscle pain (an analgesic may be recommended). Report persistent lethargy, acute headache, severe nausea or vomiting, difficulty breathing, loss of sensation, or rash. **Pregnancy/ breast-feeding precautions:** Inform prescriber if you are or intend to become pregnant. Do not breast-feed.

Dietary Issues: May be taken with or without food.

Breast-feeding Issues: HIV-infected mothers are discouraged from breast-feeding to decrease potential transmission of HIV.

Pregnancy Issues: Lamivudine crosses the placenta. It may be used in combination with zidovudine in HIV-infected women who are in labor, but have had no prior antiretroviral therapy, in order to reduce the maternal-fetal transmission of HIV. Cases of lactic acidosis/ hepatic steatosis syndrome have been reported in pregnant women receiving nucleoside analogues. It is not known if pregnancy itself potentiates this known side effect; however, pregnant women may be at increased risk of lactic acidosis and liver damage. Hepatic enzymes and electrolytes should be monitored frequently during the 3rd trimester of pregnancy in women receiving nucleoside analogues. Health professionals are encouraged to contact the antiretroviral pregnancy registry to monitor outcomes of pregnant women exposed to antiretroviral medications (1-800-258-4263).

Additional Information Lamivudine has been well studied in the treatment of chronic hepatitis B infection. Potential compliance problems, frequency of administration, and adverse effects should be discussed with patients before initiating therapy to help prevent the emergence of resistance.

Lamivudine, Abacavir, and Zidovudine *see* Abacavir, Lamivudine, and Zidovudine *on page 31*

Lamivudine and Zidovudine *see* Zidovudine and Lamivudine *on page 1421*

Lamotrigine (la MOE tri jeen)

U.S. Brand Names Lamictal®

Synonyms BW-430C; LTG

Generic Available No

Pharmacologic Category Anticonvulsant, Miscellaneous

Pregnancy Risk Factor C

Lactation Enters breast milk/not recommended (AAP rates "of concern")

Use Adjunctive therapy in the treatment of partial seizures in adults with epilepsy (safety and effectiveness in children <16 years of age have not been established); conversion to monotherapy in adults with partial seizures who are receiving treatment with a single enzyme-inducing antiepileptic drug

Orphan drug: Adjunctive therapy in the generalized seizures of Lennox-Gastaut syndrome in pediatrics and adults

Use - Unlabeled/Investigational Bipolar disorder

Mechanism of Action/Effect A triazine derivative which inhibits release of glutamate (an excitatory amino acid) and inhibits voltage-sensitive sodium channels, which stabilizes neuronal membranes. Lamotrigine has weak inhibitory effect on the $5HT_3$ receptor; *in vitro* inhibits dihydrofolate reductase.

Contraindications Hypersensitivity to lamotrigine or any component of the formulation

Warnings/Precautions Use with caution in patients with impaired renal, hepatic, or cardiac function. Avoid abrupt cessation, taper over at least 2 weeks if possible. Severe and potentially life-threatening skin rashes have been reported; this appears to occur most frequently in pediatric patients. Discontinue at first sign of rash unless rash is clearly not drug related. May cause CNS depression, which may impair physical or mental abilities. Patients must be cautioned about performing tasks which require mental alertness (ie, operating machinery or driving). Effects with other sedative drugs or ethanol may be potentiated. **Use caution in writing and/or interpreting prescriptions/orders; medication dispensing errors have occurred with similar-sounding medications (Lamisil®, Ludiomil®, lamivudine, labetalol, and Lomotil®).** Pregnancy risk C.

Drug Interactions

Decreased Effect: Acetaminophen, carbamazepine, phenytoin, phenobarbital may decrease concentrations of lamotrigine. Lamotrigine enhances the metabolism of valproic acid.

Increased Effect/Toxicity: Lamotrigine may increase the epoxide metabolite of carbamazepine resulting in toxicity. Valproic acid increases blood levels of lamotrigine. Toxicity has been reported following addition of sertraline (limited documentation).

Nutritional/Ethanol Interactions

Ethanol: Avoid ethanol (may increase CNS depression).

Food: Has no effect on absorption.

Herb/Nutraceutical: Avoid evening primrose (seizure threshold decreased).

Adverse Reactions

>10%:

Central nervous system: Headache (29%), dizziness (7% to 38%), ataxia (7% to 22%), somnolence

Gastrointestinal: Nausea (7% to 19%)

Ocular: Diplopia (28%), blurred vision (16%)

Respiratory: Rhinitis (7% to 14%)

1% to 10%:

Central nervous system: Depression (4%), anxiety (4%), irritability, confusion, speech disorder, difficulty concentrating, emotional lability, malaise, seizure (3% to 4%), incoordination, insomnia (5% to 6%)

Dermatologic: Hypersensitivity rash (10%), pruritus (3%)

Gastrointestinal: Abdominal pain, vomiting (9%), diarrhea (6%), dyspepsia (5% to 7%), constipation (4%), anorexia (2%)

Genitourinary: Vaginitis (4%), dysmenorrhea (7%)

Neuromuscular & skeletal: Tremor (6%), arthralgia, joint pain

Ocular: Nystagmus (2%)

Miscellaneous: Flu syndrome (7%), fever (2% to 6%)

<1% (Limited to important or life-threatening): Acute renal failure, agranulocytosis, allergic reactions, alopecia, amnesia, angina, angioedema, aplastic anemia, apnea, atrial fibrillation, bronchospasm, depersonalization, disseminated intravascular coagulation (DIC), dysarthria, dysphagia, dyspnea, eosinophilia, erythema multiforme, esophagitis, GI hemorrhage, gingival hyperplasia, hemolytic anemia, hemorrhage, hepatitis, hypersensitivity reactions (including rhabdomyolysis), immunosuppression (progressive), impotence, leukopenia, lupus-like reaction, mania, movement disorder, multiorgan failure, neutropenia, pancreatitis, pancytopenia, paralysis, Parkinson's disease exacerbation, rash, red cell aplasia, Stevens-Johnson syndrome, stroke, suicidal ideation, urticaria, vasculitis

Overdosage/Toxicology Symptoms of overdose include QRS prolongation, AV block, dizziness, drowsiness, sedation, and ataxia. Enhancement of elimination: Multiple dosing of activated charcoal may be useful.

Pharmacodynamics/Kinetics

Half-Life Elimination: 24 hours; Concomitant valproic acid therapy: 59 hours; Concomitant phenytoin or carbamazepine therapy: 15 hours

Time to Peak: 1-4 hours

Metabolism: Hepatic and renal

Formulations

Tablet: 25 mg, 100 mg, 150 mg, 200 mg

Tablet, dispersible/chewable: 2 mg, 5 mg, 25 mg [black currant flavor]

Dosing

Adults & Elderly:

Lennox-Gastaut (adjunctive) or treatment of partial seizures (adjunctive): Oral:

Patients receiving AED regimens containing valproic acid:

Initial dose: 25 mg every other day for 2 weeks, then 25 mg every day for 2 weeks

Maintenance dose: 100-400 mg/day in 1-2 divided doses (usual range 100-200 mg/day). Dose may be increased by 25-50 mg every day for 1-2 weeks in order to achieve maintenance dose.

Patients receiving enzyme-inducing AED regimens without valproic acid:

Initial dose: 50 mg/day for 2 weeks, then 100 mg in 2 doses for 2 weeks; thereafter, daily dose can be increased by 100 mg every 1-2 weeks to be given in 2 divided doses

Usual maintenance dose: 300-500 mg/day in 2 divided doses; doses as high as 700 mg/day have been reported

Partial seizures (monotherapy) conversion from single enzyme-inducing AED regimen: Oral: Initial dose: 50 mg/day for 2 weeks, then 100 mg in 2 doses for 2 weeks; thereafter, daily dose should be increased by 100 mg every 1-2 weeks to be given in 2 divided doses until reaching a dose of 500 mg/day. Concomitant enzyme inducing AED should then be withdrawn by 20% decrements each week over a 4-week period. Patients should be monitored for rash.

Bipolar disorder (unlabeled use): Oral: 25 mg/day for 2 weeks, followed by 50 mg/day for 2 weeks, followed by 100 mg/day for 1 week; thereafter, daily dosage may be increased by 100 mg/week, up to a maximum of 500 mg/day as clinically indicated

Pediatrics: Note: Only whole tablets should be used for dosing, rounded down to the nearest whole tablet.

Partial seizures: Oral: Children >16 years: Refer to adult dosing.

Lennox-Gastaut (adjunctive): Oral:

Children <6.7 kg: Not recommended; therapy cannot be initiated using the dosing guidelines (smallest available strength is 2 mg chewable, dispersible tablet)

Children 2-12 years: **Note:** Children 2-6 years will likely require maintenance doses at the higher end of recommended range

Patients receiving AED regimens containing valproic acid: Weeks 1 and 2: 0.15 mg/kg/day in 1-2 divided doses; round dose down to the nearest whole tablet. For patients >6.7 kg and <14 kg, dosing should be 2 mg every other day.

Weeks 3 and 4: 0.3 mg/kg/day in 1-2 divided doses; round dose down to the nearest whole tablet

Maintenance dose: Titrate dose to effect; after week 4, increase dose every 1-2 weeks by a calculated increment; calculate increment as 0.3 mg/kg/day rounded down to the nearest whole tablet; add this amount to the previously administered daily dose; usual maintenance: 1-5 mg/kg/day in 1-2 divided doses; maximum: 200 mg/day

Patients receiving enzyme-inducing AED regimens without valproic acid:

Weeks 1 and 2: 0.6 mg/kg/day in 2 divided doses; round dose down to the nearest whole tablet

Weeks 3 and 4: 1.2 mg/kg/day in 2 divided doses; round dose down to the nearest whole tablet

(Continued)

Lamotrigine *(Continued)*

Maintenance dose: Titrate dose to effect; after week 4, increase dose every 1-2 weeks by a calculated increment; calculate increment as 1.2 mg/kg/day rounded down to the nearest whole tablet; add this amount to the previously administered daily dose; usual maintenance: 5-15 mg/kg/day in 2 divided doses; maximum: 400 mg/day

Children >12 years: Refer to adult dosing.

Renal Impairment: Decreased dosage may be effective in patients with significant renal impairment; use with caution.

Administration

Oral: Doses should be rounded down to the nearest whole tablet. Dispersible tablets may be chewed, dispersed in water or swallowed whole. To disperse tablets, add to a small amount of liquid (just enough to cover tablet); let sit ~1 minute until dispersed; swirl solution and consume immediately. Do not administer partial amounts of liquid. If tablets are chewed, a small amount of water or diluted fruit juice should be used to aid in swallowing.

Stability

Storage: Store at 25°C (77°F). Excursions are permitted to 15°C to 30°C (59°F to 86°F). Protect from light.

Monitoring Laboratory Tests Serum levels of concurrent anticonvulsants, LFTs, renal function

Monitoring and Teaching Issues

Physical Assessment: Assess effectiveness and interactions of other medications patient may be taking (see Drug Interactions). Monitor therapeutic response, laboratory values, and adverse reactions (see Adverse Reactions) at beginning of therapy and periodically with long-term use. Taper dosage slowly when discontinuing. Observe and teach seizure/safety precautions. Use caution in writing and/or interpreting prescriptions/orders. Confusion between Lamictal® (lamotrigine) and Lamisil® (terbinafine) has occurred. Assess knowledge/teach patient appropriate use, interventions to reduce side effects, and adverse symptoms to report (see Patient Education). **Pregnancy risk factor C** - benefits of use should outweigh possible risks. Breast-feeding is not recommended.

Patient Education: Take exactly as directed; do not increase dose or frequency or discontinue without consulting prescriber. Only whole tablets should be used for dosing, rounded down to the nearest whole tablet. When having the prescription refilled, contact the prescriber if the medicine looks different or the label name has changed. While using this medication, do not use alcohol and other prescription or OTC medications (especially pain medications, sedatives, antihistamines, or hypnotics) without consulting prescriber. Maintain adequate hydration (2-3 L/day of fluids) unless advised by prescriber to restrict fluids. You may experience drowsiness, dizziness, or blurred vision (use caution when driving or engaging in tasks requiring alertness until response to drug is known); or nausea, vomiting, loss of appetite, heartburn, or dry mouth (small, frequent meals, frequent mouth care, chewing gum, or sucking lozenges may help). Wear identification of epileptic status and medications. Report CNS changes, mentation changes, or changes in cognition; persistent GI symptoms (cramping, constipation, vomiting, anorexia); skin rash; swelling of face, lips, or tongue; easy bruising or bleeding (mouth, urine, stool); vision changes; worsening of seizure activity, or loss of seizure control. **Pregnancy/breast-feeding precautions:** Inform prescriber if you are or intend to become pregnant. Breast-feeding is not recommended.

Dietary Issues: Take without regard to meals; drug may cause GI upset.

Geriatric Considerations: Use with caution in the elderly with significant renal impairment.

Lamprene® *see* Clofazimine *on page 309*

Lanacane® [OTC] *see* Benzocaine *on page 156*

Lanacort® [OTC] *see* Topical Corticosteroids *on page 1334*

Lanoxicaps® *see* Digoxin *on page 411*

Lanoxin® *see* Digoxin *on page 411*

Lansoprazole (lan SOE pra zole)

U.S. Brand Names Prevacid®

Generic Available No

Pharmacologic Category Proton Pump Inhibitor

Pregnancy Risk Factor B

Lactation Excretion in breast milk unknown/contraindicated

Use Short-term treatment of active duodenal ulcers; maintenance treatment of healed duodenal ulcers; as part of a multidrug regimen for *H. pylori* eradication to reduce the risk of duodenal ulcer recurrence; short-term treatment of active benign gastric ulcer; treatment of NSAID-associated gastric ulcer; to reduce the risk of NSAID-associated gastric ulcer in patients with a history of gastric ulcer who require an NSAID; short-term treatment of symptomatic GERD; short-term treatment for all grades of erosive esophagitis; to maintain healing of erosive esophagitis; long-term treatment of pathological hypersecretory conditions, including Zollinger-Ellison syndrome

Mechanism of Action/Effect A proton pump inhibitor which decreases acid secretion in gastric parietal cells

Contraindications Hypersensitivity to lansoprazole or any component of the formulation

Warnings/Precautions Severe liver dysfunction may require dosage reductions. Symptomatic response does not exclude malignancy. Safety and efficacy have not been established in children <1 year of age.

Drug Interactions

Cytochrome P450 Effect: Substrate of CYP2C8/9, **2C19, 3A4**; Inhibits CYP2C8/9, **2C19**, 2D6, 3A4; Induces CYP1A2

Decreased Effect: Lansoprazole may decrease blood levels/absorption of ketoconazole, itraconazole, ampicillin esters, iron salts, digoxin and other drugs dependent upon acid for absorption. Lansoprazole may decrease theophylline levels (slightly). Sucralfate delays and reduces lansoprazole absorption by 30%.

Nutritional/Ethanol Interactions

Ethanol: Avoid ethanol (may cause gastric mucosal irritation).

Food: Lansoprazole serum concentrations may be decreased if taken with food.

Adverse Reactions

1% to 10%: Gastrointestinal: Abdominal pain (2%), diarrhea (4%, more likely at doses of 60 mg/day), constipation (1%), nausea (1%)

<1% (Limited to important or life-threatening): Abnormal vision, agitation, allergic reaction, ALT increased, anaphylactoid reaction, anemia, angina, anxiety, aplastic anemia, arrhythmia, AST increased, chest pain, convulsion, depression, dizziness, dry eyes, dry mouth, esophagitis, gastrin levels increased, gastrointestinal disorder, glucocorticoids increased, globulins increased, hemolysis, hepatotoxicity, hyperglycemia, LDH increased, maculopapular rash, photophobia, rash, RBC abnormal, taste perversion, tinnitus, tremor, vertigo, visual field defect, vomiting, WBC abnormal

Overdosage/Toxicology No symptoms of toxicity were observed in animal studies; limited human experience in overdose. Treatment is symptomatic and supportive.

Pharmacodynamics/Kinetics

Absorption: Rapid

Bioavailability: 80%; decreased 50% if given 30 minutes following food

Half-Life Elimination: 2 hours; Elderly: 2.9 hours; Hepatic impairment: ≤7 hours

Time to Peak: Plasma: 1.7 hours

Metabolism: Hepatic and in parietal cells to two inactive metabolites

Duration: >1 day

Formulations

Capsule, delayed release: 15 mg, 30 mg

Granules, oral suspension, delayed release: 15 mg/packet (30s), 30 mg/packet (30s)

Dosing

Adults & Elderly:

Symptomatic GERD: Oral: Short-term treatment: 15 mg once daily for up to 8 weeks

Erosive esophagitis: Oral: Short-term treatment: 30 mg once daily for up to 8 weeks; continued treatment for an additional 8 weeks may be considered for recurrence or for patients that do not heal after the first 8 weeks of therapy; maintenance therapy: 15 mg once daily

Hypersecretory conditions: Oral: Initial: 60 mg once daily; adjust dose based upon patient response and to reduce acid secretion to <10 mEq/hour (5 mEq/hour in patients with prior gastric surgery); doses of 90 mg twice daily have been used; administer doses >120 mg/day in divided doses

Duodenal ulcer: Oral: Short-term treatment: 15 mg once daily for 4 weeks; maintenance therapy: 15 mg once daily

Helicobacter pylori eradication: Currently accepted recommendations (may differ from product labeling): Oral: Dose varies with regimen: 30 mg once daily or 60 mg/day in 2 divided doses; requires combination therapy with antibiotics

Gastric ulcer: Oral: Short-term treatment: 30 mg once daily for up to 8 weeks

NSAID-associated gastric ulcer (healing): Oral: 30 mg once daily for 8 weeks; controlled studies did not extend past 8 weeks

NSAID-associated gastric ulcer (to reduce risk): Oral: 15 mg once daily for up to 12 weeks; controlled studies did not extend past 12 weeks

Pediatrics: GERD, erosive esophagitis: Oral: Children 1-11 years:

≤30 kg: 15 mg once daily

>30 kg: 30 mg once daily

Renal Impairment: No adjustment is necessary.

Hepatic Impairment: May require a dose reduction.

Administration

Oral: Administer before food. The intact granules should not be chewed or crushed; however, in addition to oral suspension, several options are available for those patients unable to swallow capsules:

Capsules may be opened and the intact granules sprinkled on 1 tablespoon of applesauce, Ensure® pudding, cottage cheese, yogurt, or strained pears. The granules should then be swallowed immediately.

Capsules may be opened and emptied into ~60 mL orange juice, apple juice, or tomato juice; mix and swallow immediately. Rinse the glass with additional juice and swallow to assure complete delivery of the dose.

Capsule granules may be mixed with apple, cranberry, grape, orange, pineapple, prune, tomato and V-8® juice and stored for up to 30 minutes.

Other: Nasogastric tube administration: Capsules can be opened, the granules mixed (not crushed) with 40 mL of apple juice and then injected through the NG tube into the stomach, then flush tube with additional apple juice.

Stability

Storage: Store at 15°C to 30°C (59°F to 86°F); protect from light and moisture.

Reconstitution: Oral suspension: Empty packet into container with 2 tablespoons of water. Do **not** mix with other liquids or food. Stir well and drink immediately.

Monitoring Laboratory Tests Patients with Zollinger-Ellison syndrome should be monitored for gastric acid output, which should be maintained at ≤10 mEq/hour during the last hour before the next lansoprazole dose. Lab monitoring should include CBC, liver function, renal function, and serum gastrin levels.

Monitoring and Teaching Issues

Physical Assessment: Assess periodic laboratory results. Assess effectiveness of medications that require an acid medium for absorption (eg, ketoconazole, itraconazole). Monitor effectiveness of ulcer symptom relief. Breast-feeding is contraindicated.

Patient Education: Take as directed, before eating. Do not crush or chew granules. Patients who may have difficulty swallowing capsules may open the delayed-release capsules and sprinkle the contents on applesauce, pudding, cottage cheese, yogurt, or

(Continued)

Lansoprazole *(Continued)*

Ensure. Avoid alcohol. Report unresolved diarrhea. **Breast-feeding precaution:** Do not breast-feed.

Dietary Issues: Should be taken before eating.

Geriatric Considerations: The clearance of lansoprazole is decreased in the elderly; however, the half-life is only increased by 50% to 100%. This still results in a short half-life and no accumulation is seen in the elderly. The rate of healing and side effects is similar to younger adults; no dosage adjustment is necessary.

Related Information

Helicobacter pylori Treatment *on page 1676*

Lansoprazole, Amoxicillin, and Clarithromycin

(lan SOE pra zole, a moks i SIL in, & kla RITH roe mye sin)

U.S. Brand Names Prevpac®

Synonyms Amoxicillin, Lansoprazole, and Clarithromycin; Clarithromycin, Lansoprazole, and Amoxicillin

Generic Available No

Pharmacologic Category Antibiotic, Macrolide Combination; Antibiotic, Penicillin; Gastrointestinal Agent, Miscellaneous

Pregnancy Risk Factor C (clarithromycin)

Lactation Excretion in breast milk unknown/contraindicated

Use Eradication of *H. pylori* to reduce the risk of recurrent duodenal ulcer

Formulations Combination package (Prevpac®) [14-day supply; each administration card contains]:

Capsule (Trimox®): Amoxicillin 500 mg (4 capsules/day)

Capsule, delayed release (Prevacid®): Lansoprazole 30 mg (2 capsules/day)

Tablet (Biaxin®): Clarithromycin 500 mg (2 tablets/day)

Dosing

Adults & Elderly: *H. pylori* eradication: Oral: Lansoprazole 30 mg, amoxicillin 1 g, and clarithromycin 500 mg taken together twice daily

Monitoring and Teaching Issues

Physical Assessment: See individual components listed in Related Information. **Pregnancy risk factor C** (clarithromycin) - benefits of use should outweigh possible risks. Breast-feeding is contraindicated.

Patient Education: See individual components listed in Related Information. **Pregnancy/breast-feeding precautions:** Inform prescriber if you are or intend to become pregnant. Do not breast-feed.

Related Information

Amoxicillin *on page 88*

Clarithromycin *on page 304*

Lansoprazole *on page 772*

Lantus® *see* Insulin Preparations *on page 714*

Lariam® *see* Mefloquine *on page 843*

Lasix® *see* Furosemide *on page 612*

L-asparaginase *see* Asparaginase *on page 118*

Latanoprost *see page 1575*

Latanoprost *see* Ophthalmic Agents, Glaucoma *on page 1002*

Latrodectus mactans *see page 1460*

Lavacol® *see page 1460*

Laxatives: Classification and Properties *see page 1581*

L-Carnitine *see* Levocarnitine *on page 787*

LCR *see* VinCRIStine *on page 1401*

L-Deprenyl *see* Selegiline *on page 1221*

Leflunomide (le FLU no mide)

U.S. Brand Names Arava™

Generic Available No

Pharmacologic Category Antirheumatic, Disease Modifying

Pregnancy Risk Factor X

Lactation Excretion in breast milk unknown/contraindicated

Use Treatment of active rheumatoid arthritis to reduce signs and symptoms and to retard structural damage as evidenced by x-ray erosions and joint space narrowing

Mechanism of Action/Effect Inhibits pyrimidine synthesis, resulting in antiproliferative and anti-inflammatory effects

Contraindications Hypersensitivity to leflunomide or any component of the formulation; pregnancy

Warnings/Precautions Leflunomide has been associated with rare reports of hepatotoxicity, hepatic failure, and death. Hepatic disease (including seropositive hepatitis B or C patients) may increase risk of hepatotoxicity. Immunosuppression may increase the risk of lymphoproliferative disorders or other malignancies. Women of childbearing potential should not receive leflunomide until pregnancy has been excluded, patients have been counseled concerning fetal risk, and reliable contraceptive measures have been confirmed. Caution in renal impairment, immune deficiency, bone marrow dysplasia or severe uncontrolled infection. Discontinue if evidence of bone marrow suppression occurs, and begin procedure for accelerated removal (cholestyramine and activated charcoal, see Toxicology/Overdose). The use of live vaccines is not recommended. Leflunomide will increase uric acid excretion.

Drug Interactions

Cytochrome P450 Effect: Inhibits CYP2C8/9

Decreased Effect: Administration of cholestyramine and activated charcoal enhance the elimination of leflunomide's active metabolite.

Increased Effect/Toxicity: Theoretically, concomitant use of drugs metabolized by this enzyme, including many NSAIDs, may result in increased serum concentrations and possible toxic effects. Coadministration with methotrexate increases the risk of hepatotoxicity. Leflunomide may also enhance the hepatotoxicity of other drugs. Tolbutamide free fraction may be increased. Rifampin may increase serum concentrations of leflunomide. Leflunomide has uricosuric activity and may enhance activity of other uricosuric agents.

Nutritional/Ethanol Interactions Food: No interactions with food have been noted.

Adverse Reactions

>10%:

Gastrointestinal: Diarrhea (17%)

Respiratory: Respiratory tract infection (15%)

1% to 10% (Limited to important or life-threatening):

Cardiovascular: Hypertension (10%), chest pain (2%), vasculitis, edema (peripheral)

Central nervous system: Headache (7%), dizziness (4%) paresthesia (2%), fever, neuralgia, neuritis, sleep disorder

Dermatologic: Alopecia (10%), rash (10%), pruritus (4%), dry skin (2%), eczema (2%), dermatitis, hair discoloration, subcutaneous nodule, skin disorder/discoloration

Endocrine & metabolic: Hypokalemia (1%), diabetes mellitus, hyperlipidemia, hyperthyroidism

Gastrointestinal: Nausea (9%), weight loss (4%), anorexia (3%), gastroenteritis (3%), stomatitis (3%), vomiting (3%), cholelithiasis, colitis, esophagitis, gingivitis, melena, candidiasis (oral)

Genitourinary: Urinary tract infection (5%), albuminuria, cystitis, dysuria, hematuria

Hematologic: Anemia

Neuromuscular & skeletal: Tenosynovitis (3%), arthralgia (1%), muscle cramps (1%), neck pain, pelvic pain, arthrosis, bursitis, myalgia, bone necrosis, bone pain, tendon rupture

Ocular: Cataract, conjunctivitis

Respiratory: Bronchitis (7%), cough (3%), pharyngitis (3%), pneumonia (2%), rhinitis (2%), sinusitis (2%), asthma, dyspnea

Miscellaneous: Infection (4%), allergic reactions (2%)

<1% (Limited to important or life-threatening): Anaphylaxis, eosinophilia, hepatotoxicity, hepatic failure, leukopenia, thrombocytopenia, urticaria

Overdosage/Toxicology There is no human experience with overdose. Leflunomide is not dialyzable. Cholestyramine and/or activated charcoal enhance elimination of leflunomide's active metabolite (MI). In cases of significant overdose or toxicity, cholestyramine 8 g every 8 hours for 1-3 days may be administered to enhance elimination. Plasma levels are reduced by approximately 40% in 24 hours and 49% to 65% after 48 hours of cholestyramine dosing.

Pharmacodynamics/Kinetics

Bioavailability: 80%

Half-Life Elimination: Mean: 14-15 days; enterohepatic recycling appears to contribute to the long half-life of this agent, since activated charcoal and cholestyramine substantially reduce plasma half-life

Time to Peak: 6-12 hours

Metabolism: Hepatic to A77 1726 (MI) which accounts for nearly all pharmacologic activity; further metabolism to multiple inactive metabolites; undergoes enterohepatic recirculation

Formulations Tablet: 10 mg, 20 mg

Dosing

Adults: Rheumatoid arthritis: Oral: Initial: 100 mg/day for 3 days, followed by 20 mg/day; dosage may be decreased to 10 mg/day in patients who have difficulty tolerating the 20 mg dose. Due to the long half-life of the active metabolite, plasma levels may require a prolonged period to decline after dosage reduction.

Elderly: Although hepatic function may decline with age, no specific dosage adjustment is recommended. Patients should be monitored closely for adverse effects which may require dosage adjustment.

Renal Impairment: No specific dosage adjustment is recommended. There is no clinical experience in the use of leflunomide in patients with renal impairment. The free fraction of MI is doubled in dialysis patients. Patients should be monitored closely for adverse effects requiring dosage adjustment.

Hepatic Impairment: No specific dosage adjustment is recommended. Since the liver is involved in metabolic activation and subsequent metabolism/elimination of leflunomide, patients with hepatic impairment should be monitored closely for adverse effects requiring dosage adjustment.

Guidelines for dosage adjustment or discontinuation based on the severity and persistence of ALT elevation have been developed. For ALT elevations >2 times the upper limit of normal, dosage reduction to 10 mg/day may allow continued administration (consider increased monitoring frequency - ie, weekly). Cholestyramine 8 g 3 times/day for 1-3 days may be administered to decrease plasma levels. If elevations >2 times but less than or equal to 3 times the upper limit of normal persist, liver biopsy is recommended. If elevations >3 times the upper limit of normal persist despite cholestyramine administration and dosage reduction, leflunomide should be discontinued and drug elimination should be enhanced with additional cholestyramine as indicated.

Stability

Storage: Protect from light; store at 25°C (77°F).

Monitoring Laboratory Tests Serum transaminase determinations at baseline and monthly during the initial phase of treatment; if stable, monitoring frequency may be decreased to intervals determined by the individual clinical situation. Monitor for abnormalities in hepatic function tests or symptoms of hepatotoxicity.

Monitoring and Teaching Issues

Physical Assessment: Assess other medications patient may be taking for effectiveness and interactions (see Warnings/Precautions and Drug Interactions). Monitor laboratory tests (see above), therapeutic effects, and adverse reactions (see Warnings/Precautions and Adverse Reactions). Assess knowledge/teach patient appropriate use, interventions to reduce side effects, and adverse symptoms to report (see Patient Education). **Pregnancy**

(Continued)

Leflunomide *(Continued)*

risk factor X - determine that patient is not pregnant before starting therapy. Do not give to sexually-active female patients unless capable of complying with barrier contraceptive use. Breast-feeding is contraindicated.

Patient Education: Take as directed; do not increase dose without consulting prescriber. Maintain adequate hydration (2-3 L/day of fluids) unless advised by prescriber to restrict fluids. Store medication away from light. You may experience diarrhea (buttermilk, boiled milk, or yogurt may help); nausea, vomiting, loss of appetite, and flatulence (small, frequent meals, frequent mouth care, chewing gum, or sucking lozenges may help); or dizziness (use caution when driving or engaging in tasks requiring alertness until response to drug is known). If diabetic, monitor blood sugars closely; this medication may alter glucose levels. If you experience symptoms such as nausea, vomiting, stomach pain or swelling, jaundice, dark urine, or unusual tiredness, report these to your prescriber **immediately.** Report chest pain, palpitations, rapid heartbeat, or swelling of extremities; persistent GI problems; skin rash, redness, irritation, acne, ulcers, or easy bruising; frequent, painful, or difficult urination, or genital itching or irritation; depression, acute headache, anxiety, or difficulty sleeping; weakness, muscle tremors, cramping or weakness, back pain, or altered gait; cough, cold symptoms, wheezing, or difficulty breathing; easy bruising/bleeding; blood in vomitus, stool, urine; or other unusual effects related to this medication. **Pregnancy/ breast-feeding precautions:** Inform prescriber if you are pregnant. Do not get pregnant or have sex unless using appropriate contraception while on this medication. This drug may cause severe fetal defects. Do not breast-feed.

Dietary Issues: Administer without regard to meals.

Breast-feeding Issues: It is not known whether leflunomide is secreted in human milk. Because many immunoglobulins are secreted in milk, and the potential for serious adverse reactions exists, a decision should be made whether to discontinue nursing or discontinue the drug, taking into account the importance of the drug to the mother.

Pregnancy Issues: Has been associated with teratogenic and embryolethal effects in animal models at low doses. Leflunomide is contraindicated in pregnant women or women of childbearing potential who are not using reliable contraception. Pregnancy must be excluded prior to initiating treatment. Following treatment, pregnancy should be avoided until the drug elimination procedure is completed.

Additional Information To enhance elimination, a drug elimination procedure has been developed. Without this procedure, it may take up to 2 years to reach plasma concentrations <0.02 mg/L (a concentration expected to have minimal risk of teratogenicity based on animal models). The procedure consists of the following steps: Administer cholestyramine 8 g 3 times/day for 11 days (the 11 days do not need to be consecutive). Plasma levels <0.02 mg/L should be verified by two separate tests performed at least 14 days apart. If plasma levels are >0.02 mg/L, additional cholestyramine treatment should be considered.

Lente® Iletin® II *see* Insulin Preparations *on page 714*

Lepirudin (leh puh ROO din)

U.S. Brand Names Refludan®

Synonyms Lepirudin (rDNA); Recombinant Hirudin

Generic Available No

Pharmacologic Category Anticoagulant, Thrombin Inhibitor

Pregnancy Risk Factor B

Lactation Enters breast milk/consult prescriber

Use Indicated for anticoagulation in patients with heparin-induced thrombocytopenia (HIT) and associated thromboembolic disease in order to prevent further thromboembolic complications

Use - Unlabeled/Investigational Investigational: Prevention or reduction of ischemic complications associated with unstable angina

Mechanism of Action/Effect Lepirudin is a highly specific direct thrombin inhibitor. Each molecule is capable of binding one molecule of thrombin and inhibiting its thrombogenic activity.

Contraindications Hypersensitivity to hirudins or any component of the formulation

Warnings/Precautions Discontinue therapy if platelets are <100,000/mm^3. Cautiously administer after a thrombolytic episode; risk of intracranial bleeding. Hemorrhage is the most common complication. Patients at increased risk of bleeding include: bacterial endocarditis; congenital or acquired bleeding disorders; recent puncture of large vessels or organ biopsy; recent CVA, stroke, intracerebral surgery, or other neuraxial procedure; severe uncontrolled hypertension; advanced renal impairment; recent major surgery; recent major bleeding (intracranial, GI, intraocular, or pulmonary). Reduce dose in severe renal impairment (Cl_{cr} <15 mL/ minute and on hemodialysis). Strict monitoring of aPTT is required; formation of antihirudin antibodies can increase the anticoagulant effect of lepirudin. Use cautiously in cirrhosis. Allergic reactions may occur frequently in patients treated concomitantly with streptokinase; caution is warranted during re-exposure due to limited clinical experience. Potentially may cause hyperkalemia by affecting aldosterone (similar to heparin).

Drug Interactions

Increased Effect/Toxicity: Thrombolytics may enhance anticoagulant properties of lepirudin on aPTT and can increase the risk of bleeding complications. Bleeding risk may also be increased by oral anticoagulants (warfarin) and platelet function inhibitors (NSAIDs, dipyridamole, ticlopidine, clopidogrel, IIb/IIIa antagonists, and aspirin).

Nutritional/Ethanol Interactions Herb/Nutraceutical: Avoid cat's claw, dong quai, evening primrose, feverfew, garlic, ginger, ginkgo, red clover, horse chestnut, green tea, ginseng (all have additional antiplatelet activity)

Adverse Reactions As with all anticoagulants, bleeding is the most common adverse event associated with lepirudin. Hemorrhage may occur at virtually any site. Risk is dependent on multiple variables.

HIT patients:

>10%: Hematologic: Anemia (12%), bleeding from puncture sites (11%), hematoma (11%)

1% to 10%:

Cardiovascular: Heart failure (3%), pericardial effusion (1%), ventricular fibrillation (1%)
Central nervous system: Fever (7%)
Dermatologic: Eczema (3%), maculopapular rash (4%)
Gastrointestinal: GI bleeding/rectal bleeding (5%)
Genitourinary: Vaginal bleeding (2%)
Hepatic: Increased transaminases (6%)
Renal: Hematuria (4%)
Respiratory: Epistaxis (4%)

<1% (Limited to important or life-threatening): Hemoperitoneum, hemoptysis, injection site reactions, liver bleeding, mouth bleeding, pruritus, pulmonary bleeding, retroperitoneal bleeding, thrombocytopenia, urticaria

Non-HIT populations (including those receiving thrombolytics and/or contrast media):

1% to 10%: Respiratory: Bronchospasm/stridor/dyspnea/cough

<1% (Limited to important or life-threatening): Allergic reactions (unspecified), anaphylactoid reactions, anaphylaxis, angioedema, intracranial bleeding (0.6%), laryngeal edema, thrombocytopenia, tongue edema

Overdosage/Toxicology Risk of bleeding is increased, and therefore management is directed towards control of bleeding.

Pharmacodynamics/Kinetics

Half-Life Elimination: Initial: ~10 minutes: Terminal: Healthy volunteers: 1.3 hours; Significant renal impairment (Cl_{cr} <15 mL/minute and on hemodialysis): ≤2 days

Metabolism: Via release of amino acids via catabolic hydrolysis of parent drug

Formulations Injection, powder for reconstitution: 50 mg

Dosing

Adults & Elderly: Note: Maximum dose: Do not exceed 0.21 mg/kg/hour unless an evaluation of coagulation abnormalities limiting response has been completed. **Dosing is weight-based, however, patients weighing >110 kg should not receive doses greater than the recommended dose for a patient weighing 110 kg (44 mg bolus and initial maximal infusion rate of 16.5 mg/hour).**

Heparin-induced thrombocytopenia: I.V.: Bolus dose: 0.4 mg/kg IVP (over 15-20 seconds), followed by continuous infusion at 0.15 mg/kg/hour; bolus and infusion must be reduced in renal insufficiency

Concomitant use with thrombolytic therapy: I.V.: Bolus dose: 0.2 mg/kg IVP (over 15-20 seconds), followed by continuous infusion at 0.1 mg/kg/hour

Dosing adjustments during infusions: Monitor first aPTT 4 hours after the start of the infusion. Subsequent determinations of aPTT should be obtained at least once daily during treatment. More frequent monitoring is recommended in renally impaired patients. Any aPTT ratio measurement out of range (1.5-2.5) should be confirmed prior to adjusting dose, unless a clinical need for immediate reaction exists. If the aPTT is below target range, increase infusion by 20%. If the aPTT is in excess of the target range, decrease infusion rate by 50%. A repeat aPTT should be obtained 4 hours after any dosing change.

Use in patients scheduled for switch to oral anticoagulants: Reduce lepirudin dose gradually to reach aPTT ratio just above 1.5 before starting warfarin therapy; as soon as INR reaches 2.0, lepirudin therapy should be discontinued.

Renal Impairment: All patients with Cl_{cr} <60 or serum creatinine >1.5 mg/dL require dosage reduction.

Initial: Bolus dose: 0.2 mg/kg IVP (over 15-20 seconds); see table. Additional bolus doses of 0.1 mg/kg may be administered every other day (only if aPTT falls below lower therapeutic limit).

Lepirudin Infusion Rates in Patients With Renal Impairment

Creatinine Clearance (mL/minute)	Serum Creatinine (mg/dL)	Adjusted Infusion Rate	
		% of Standard Initial Infusion Rate	mg/kg/hour
45-60	1.6-2.0	50%	0.075
30-44	2.1-3.0	30%	0.045
15-29	3.1-6.0	15%	0.0225
<15	>6.0	Avoid or STOP infusion	

Administration

Oral: Administer **only** intravenously

I.V.: I.V. bolus: Inject slowly for continuous infusion; solutions with 0.2 or 0.4 mg/mL may be used.

Stability

Reconstitution: Reconstitute 50 mg vials with 1 mL water for injection or 0.9% sodium chloride injection. Bolus dose: Prepare 5 mg/mL solution by transferring contents of 1 reconstituted vial to single use, sterile syringe. Dilute to total volume of 10 mL with 0.9 sodium chloride or 5% dextrose injection. To prepare continuous infusion solutions, either 0.9% sodium chloride or 5% dextrose may be used. Add contents of two reconstituted vials to either 250 mL (to prepare 0.4 mg/mL solution) or 500 mL (to prepare 0.2 mg/mL solution). Once reconstituted, use immediately. Reconstituted solutions remain stable for 24 hours (duration of infusion).

Monitoring Laboratory Tests The aPTT ratio should be maintained between 1.5 and 2.5. Ratio is calculated by patient's value at a given time divided by reference value (commonly the median of a laboratory normal range).

Monitoring and Teaching Issues

Physical Assessment: See Contraindications, Warnings/Precautions, and Dosing for use cautions. Assess potential for interactions with other prescriptions, OTC medications, or

(Continued)

Lepirudin *(Continued)*

herbal products patient may be taking (especially anything that will affect coagulation or platelet function - see Drug Interactions). See Administration specifics. Bleeding precautions should be observed. Assess results of laboratory tests (see above), therapeutic effects, and adverse response (see Adverse Reactions and Overdose/Toxicology) regularly during therapy. Teach possible side effects and appropriate interventions (eg, bleeding precautions) and adverse symptoms to report (see Patient Education). Note breast-feeding caution.

Patient Education: Inform prescriber of all prescriptions, OTC medications, or herbal products you are taking, and any allergies you have. Do not take anything new during treatment unless approved by prescriber. This drug can only be administered by infusion. Report immediately any pain, swelling, burning, or bleeding at infusion site. You may have a tendency to bleed easily while taking this drug (brush teeth with soft brush, floss with waxed floss, use electric razor, avoid scissors or sharp knives, and avoid potentially harmful activities). Report unusual bleeding or bruising (bleeding gums, nosebleed, blood in urine, dark stool); pain in joints or back; CNS changes (fever, confusion); unusual fever; persistent nausea or GI upset; or swelling or pain at injection site. **Breast-feeding precaution:** Consult prescriber if breast-feeding.

Lepirudin (rDNA) *see* Lepirudin *on page 776*

Lescol® *see* Fluvastatin *on page 592*

Lescol® XL *see* Fluvastatin *on page 592*

Lessina™ *see* Ethinyl Estradiol and Levonorgestrel *on page 523*

Letrozole (LET roe zole)

U.S. Brand Names Femara®

Generic Available No

Pharmacologic Category Antineoplastic Agent, Aromatase Inhibitor

Pregnancy Risk Factor D

Lactation Excretion in breast milk unknown/not recommended

Use First-line treatment of hormone receptor positive or hormone receptor unknown, locally advanced, or metastatic breast cancer in postmenopausal women; treatment of advanced breast cancer in postmenopausal women with disease progression following antiestrogen therapy

Mechanism of Action/Effect Nonsteroidal, competitive inhibitor of the aromatase enzyme system, which catalyzes conversion of androgens to estrogens. Inhibition leads to a significant reduction in plasma estrogen levels. Does not affect synthesis of adrenal or thyroid hormones, aldosterone, or androgens.

Contraindications Hypersensitivity to letrozole or any component of the formulation; pregnancy

Warnings/Precautions Dose-related effects on hematologic or chemistry parameters have not been observed. Moderate decreases in lymphocyte counts may be seen and are transient in about 50% of affected patients. Increases in transaminases ≥5 times the upper limit of normal and of bilirubin ≥1.5 times the upper limit of normal were most often, but not always, associated with metastatic liver disease. Safety and efficacy have not been established in pediatric patients.

Drug Interactions

Cytochrome P450 Effect: Substrate of CYP2A6, 3A4; Inhibits CYP2A6, 2C19

Increased Effect/Toxicity: Inhibitors of this enzyme may, in theory, increase letrozole blood levels. Letrozole inhibits cytochrome P450 isoenzyme 2A6 and 2C19 *in vitro* and may increase blood levels of drugs metabolized by these enzymes. Specific drug interaction studies have not been reported.

Adverse Reactions

>10% :

Cardiovascular: Hot flushes (5% to 18%)

Central nervous system: Headache (8% to 12%), fatigue (6% to 11%)

Gastrointestinal: Nausea (13% to 15%)

Neuromuscular & skeletal: Musculoskeletal pain, bone pain (20%), back pain (17%), arthralgia (8% to 14%),

Respiratory: Dyspnea (7% to 14%), cough (5% to 11%)

2% to 10%:

Cardiovascular: Chest pain (3% to 8%), peripheral edema (5%), hypertension (5% to 7%)

Central nervous system: Pain (5%), insomnia (6%), dizziness (3% to 5%), somnolence (2% to 3%), depression (<5%), anxiety (<5%), vertigo (<5%)

Dermatologic: Rash (5%), alopecia (<5% to 5%), pruritus (1%)

Endocrine & metabolic: Breast pain (5%), hypercholesterolemia (3%)

Gastrointestinal: Vomiting (7%), constipation (6% to 9%), diarrhea (5% to 7%), abdominal pain (4% to 6%), anorexia (4%), dyspepsia (3% to 4%), weight loss (6%), weight gain (2%)

Neuromuscular & skeletal: Weakness (4% to 5%)

Miscellaneous: Flu (5% to 6%)

<2% (Limited to important or life-threatening): Angina, cardiac ischemia, coronary artery disease, hemiparesis, hemorrhagic stroke, myocardial infarction, portal vein thrombosis, pulmonary embolism, thrombocytopenia, thrombotic stroke, transient ischemic attack, venous thrombosis

Overdosage/Toxicology Firm recommendations for treatment are not possible; emesis could be induced if the patient is alert. In general, supportive care and frequent monitoring of vital signs are appropriate.

Pharmacodynamics/Kinetics

Absorption: Well absorbed; not affected by food

Half-Life Elimination: Terminal: ~2 days

Time to Peak: Steady state, plasma: 2-6 weeks

Metabolism: Hepatic via CYP3A4 and CYP2A6 to an inactive carbinol metabolite

Formulations Tablet: 2.5 mg

Dosing

Adults & Elderly: Refer to individual protocols.

Breast cancer in postmenopausal women: Oral: 2.5 mg once daily without regard to meals; continue treatment until tumor progression is evident. Patients treated with letrozole do not require glucocorticoid or mineralocorticoid replacement therapy.

Renal Impairment: No dosage adjustment is required in patients with renal impairment if Cl_{cr} is ≥10 mL/minute.

Hepatic Impairment: No dosage adjustment is recommended for patients with mild-to-moderate hepatic impairment. Patients with severe impairment of liver function have not been studied; dose patients with severe impairment of liver function with caution.

Stability

Storage: Store at 15°C to 30°C (59°F to 86°F)

Monitoring Laboratory Tests CBC, thyroid function tests, serum electrolytes, serum transaminases, serum creatinine

Monitoring and Teaching Issues

Physical Assessment: See Contraindications, Warnings/Precautions, and Dosing for use cautions. Assess potential for interactions with other prescriptions, OTC medications, or herbal products patient may be taking (see Drug Interactions). Assess results of laboratory tests (see above), therapeutic response, and adverse reactions (see Adverse Reactions and Overdose/Toxicology) on a regular basis throughout therapy. Teach patient proper use (see Administration), possible side effects and appropriate interventions, and adverse symptoms to report (see Patient Education). **Pregnancy risk factor D** - determine that patient is not pregnant before beginning treatment. Instruct patients of childbearing age about appropriate barrier contraceptive measures. Breast-feeding is not recommended.

Patient Education: Inform prescriber of all prescriptions, OTC medications, or herbal products you are taking, and any allergies you have. Do not take anything new during treatment unless approved by prescriber. Take as directed, without regard to food. You may experience nausea, vomiting, hot flashes, or loss of appetite (frequent mouth care, small, frequent meals, chewing gum, or sucking lozenges may help); musculoskeletal pain or headache (mild analgesics may offer relief); sleepiness, fatigue, or dizziness (use caution when driving, climbing stairs, or engaging in tasks that require alertness until response to drug is known); constipation (increased exercise, or dietary fruit or fluids may help); diarrhea (buttermilk, boiled milk, or yogurt may help); or loss of hair (will grow back). Report chest pain, pressure, palpitations, or swollen extremities; weakness, severe headache, numbness, or loss of strength in any part of the body; difficulty speaking; vaginal bleeding; unusual signs of bleeding or bruising; difficulty breathing; severe nausea; or muscle pain; or skin rash. **Pregnancy/breast-feeding precautions:** Do not get pregnant while taking this medication; consult prescriber for appropriate barrier contraceptive measures. (May cause fetal harm). Breast-feeding is not recommended.

Dietary Issues: May be taken without regard to meals.

Pregnancy Issues: Letrozole may cause fetal harm when administered to pregnant women. Letrozole is embryotoxic and fetotoxic when administered to rats. There are no studies in pregnant women and letrozole is indicated for postmenopausal women.

Leucovorin (loo koe VOR in)

Synonyms Calcium Leucovorin; Citrovorum Factor; Folinic Acid; 5-Formyl Tetrahydrofolate; Leucovorin Calcium

Generic Available Yes

Pharmacologic Category Antidote; Vitamin, Water Soluble

Pregnancy Risk Factor C

Lactation Enters breast milk/compatible

Use Antidote for folic acid antagonists (methotrexate >100 mg/m^2, trimethoprim, pyrimethamine); treatment of megaloblastic anemias when folate is deficient as in infancy, sprue, pregnancy, and nutritional deficiency when oral folate therapy is not possible; in combination with fluorouracil in the treatment of malignancy

Mechanism of Action/Effect A reduced form of folic acid, but does not require a reduction reaction by an enzyme for activation, allows for purine and thymidine synthesis, a necessity for normal erythropoiesis; leucovorin supplies the necessary cofactor blocked by MTX, enters the cells via the same active transport system as MTX

Contraindications Hypersensitivity to leucovorin or any component of the formulation; pernicious anemia or vitamin B_{12} deficient megaloblastic anemias; should **NOT** be administered intrathecally/intraventricularly

Warnings/Precautions Pregnancy risk C.

Drug Interactions

Decreased Effect: May decrease efficacy of co-trimoxazole against *Pneumocystis carinii* pneumonitis

Increased Effect/Toxicity: Increased toxicity of fluorouracil

Adverse Reactions Limited to important or life-threatening symptoms: Seizures, thrombocytosis, wheezing, anaphylactoid reactions

Pharmacodynamics/Kinetics

Absorption: Oral, I.M.: Rapid and well absorbed

Bioavailability: 31% (following 200 mg dose)

Half-Life Elimination: Leucovorin: 15 minutes; 5MTHF: 33-35 minutes

Metabolism: Intestinal mucosa and hepatically to 5-methyl-tetrahydrofolate (5MTHF; active)

(Continued)

Leucovorin *(Continued)*

Onset: Oral: ~30 minutes; I.V.: ~5 minutes

Formulations

Injection, powder for reconstitution, as calcium: 50 mg, 100 mg, 200 mg, 350 mg
Injection, solution, as calcium: 10 mg/mL (50 mL)
Tablet, as calcium: 5 mg, 10 mg, 15 mg, 25 mg

Dosing

Adults & Elderly:

Treatment of folic acid antagonist overdosage (eg, pyrimethamine or trimethoprim): Oral: 2-15 mg/day for 3 days or until blood counts are normal or 5 mg every 3 days; doses of 6 mg/day are needed for patients with platelet counts <100,000/mm^3.

Folate-deficient megaloblastic anemia: I.M.: 1 mg/day

Megaloblastic anemia secondary to congenital deficiency of dihydrofolate reductase: I.M.: 3-6 mg/day

Rescue dose (rescue therapy should start within 24 hours of MTX therapy): I.V.: 10 mg/m^2 to start, then 10 mg/m^2 every 6 hours orally for 72 hours until serum MTX concentration is <10^{-8} molar. If serum creatinine 24 hours after methotrexate is elevated 50% or more above the pre-MTX serum creatinine **or** the serum MTX concentration is >5×10^{-6} molar (see graph), increase dose to 100 mg/m^2/dose every 3 hours until serum methotrexate level is <1×10^{-8} molar.

Investigational: Post I.T. methotrexate: Oral, I.V.: 12 mg/m^2 as a single dose; post high-dose methotrexate: 100-1000 mg/m^2/dose until the serum methotrexate level is less than 1×10^{-7} molar.

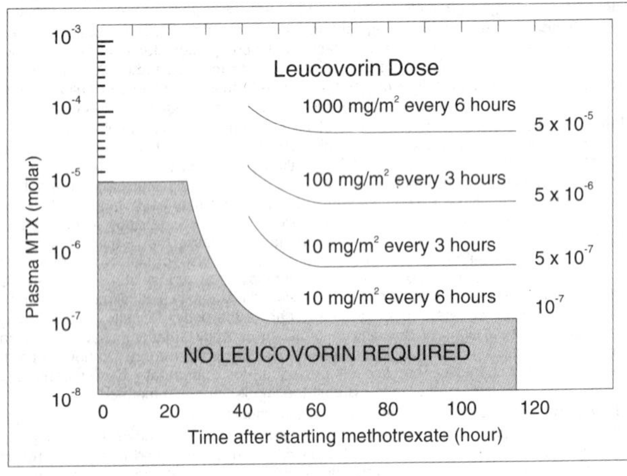

Note: The drug should be given parenterally instead of orally in patients with GI toxicity, nausea, vomiting, and when individual doses are >25 mg.

Pediatrics: Refer to adult dosing.

Administration

Oral: Maximum oral dose: 25 mg

I.V.: Leucovorin calcium should be administered I.M. or I.V. I.V. infusion should not exceed 160 mg/minute of leucovorin.

Stability

Storage: Leucovorin injection should be stored at room temperature and protected from light.

Reconstitution: Reconstituted solution is stated to be chemically stable for 7 days. Stability of parenteral admixture at room temperature (25°C) is 24 hours. Stability of parenteral admixture at refrigeration temperature (4°C) is 4 days.

Standard diluent: 50-100 mg/50 mL D_5W
Minimum volume: 50 mL D_5W

Compatibility: Stable in $D_{10}NS$, D_5W, $D_{10}W$, LR, sterile water for injection, bacteriostatic water

Y-site administration: Incompatible with amphotericin B cholesteryl sulfate complex, droperidol, foscarnet, sodium bicarbonate

Compatibility in syringe: Incompatible with droperidol

Compatibility when admixed: Incompatible with concentrations >2 mg/mL of leucovorin and >25 mg/mL of fluorouracil

Monitoring Laboratory Tests Plasma MTX concentration as a therapeutic guide to high-dose MTX therapy with leucovorin factor rescue. Leucovorin is continued until the plasma MTX level is <1×10^{-7} molar. Each dose of leucovorin is increased if the plasma MTX concentration is excessively high (see graph). With 4- to 6-hour high-dose MTX infusions, plasma drug values in excess of 5×10^{-5} and 10^{-6} molar at 24 and 48 hours after starting the infusion, respectively, are often predictive of delayed MTX clearance; see graph.

Monitoring and Teaching Issues

Physical Assessment: Monitor for adverse reactions (see Adverse Reactions). **Pregnancy risk factor C** - benefits of use should outweigh possible risks.

Patient Education: Take as directed, at evenly spaced intervals around-the-clock. Maintain hydration (2-3 L of water/day while taking for rescue therapy). For folic acid deficiency, eat foods high in folic acid (eg, meat proteins, bran, dried beans, asparagus, green leafy vegetables). Report difficulty breathing, lethargy, or rash or itching. **Pregnancy precaution:** Inform prescriber if you are or intend to become pregnant.

Related Information

Fluorouracil *on page 576*
Methotrexate *on page 874*

Leucovorin Calcium *see* Leucovorin *on page 779*

Leukeran® *see* Chlorambucil *on page 270*

Leukine™ *see* Sargramostim *on page 1215*

Leuprolide (loo PROE lide)

U.S. Brand Names Eligard™; Lupron®; Lupron Depot®; Lupron Depot-Ped®; Viadur®

Synonyms Leuprolide Acetate; Leuprorelin Acetate

Generic Available Yes: Injection (solution)

Pharmacologic Category Antineoplastic Agent, Miscellaneous; Luteinizing Hormone-Releasing Hormone Analog

Pregnancy Risk Factor X

Lactation Excretion in breast milk unknown/contraindicated

Use Palliative treatment of advanced prostate carcinoma; combination therapy with flutamide for treating metastatic prostatic carcinoma; management of endometriosis as initial treatment and/or treatment of recurrent symptoms; preoperative treatment of anemia caused by uterine leiomyomata (fibroids); central precocious puberty

Use - Unlabeled/Investigational Treatment of breast, ovarian, and endometrial cancer; infertility; prostatic hyperplasia

Mechanism of Action/Effect Potent inhibitor of gonadotropin secretion; continuous daily administration results in suppression of ovarian and testicular steroidogenesis due to decreased levels of LH and FSH with subsequent decrease in testosterone (male) and estrogen (female) levels

Contraindications Hypersensitivity to leuprolide, GnRH, GnRH-agonist analogs, or any component of the formulation; spinal cord compression (orchiectomy suggested); undiagnosed abnormal vaginal bleeding; pregnancy; breast-feeding

Warnings/Precautions Transient increases in testosterone serum levels occur at the start of treatment. Tumor flare, bone pain, urinary tract obstruction or spinal cord compression have been reported when used for prostate cancer; closely observe patients for weakness, paresthesias, and urinary tract obstruction in first few weeks of therapy. Observe patients with metastatic vertebral lesions or urinary obstruction closely. Exacerbation of endometriosis or uterine leiomyomata may occur initially. Decreased bone density has been reported when used for ≥6 months. Use caution in patients with a history of psychiatric illness; alteration in mood, memory impairment, and depression have been associated with use.

Effects on Lab Values Interferes with pituitary gonadotropic and gonadal function tests during and up to 3 months after therapy

Adverse Reactions

Children:

1% to 10%

Central nervous system: Pain (2%)

Dermatologic: Acne (2%), rash (2%), seborrhea (2%)

Genitourinary: Vaginitis (2%), vaginal bleeding (2%), vaginal discharge (2%)

Local: Injection site reaction (5%)

<1%: Alopecia, cervix disorder, dysphagia, emotional lability, epistaxis, fever, gingivitis, gynecomastia, headache, nausea, nervousness, peripheral edema, personality disorder, sexual maturity accelerated, skin striae, somnolence, syncope, urinary incontinence, vasodilation, vomiting, weight gain

Adults (frequency dependent upon formulation and indication):

Cardiovascular: Angina, atrial fibrillation, CHF, deep vein thrombosis, edema, hot flashes, hypertension, tachycardia

Central nervous system: Abnormal thinking, agitation, amnesia, confusion, convulsion, dementia, depression, dizziness, fever, headache, insomnia, pain, vertigo

Dermatologic: Alopecia, bruising, cellulitis

Endocrine & metabolic: Breast enlargement, breast tenderness, dehydration, hyperglycemia, hyperlipidemia, hyperphosphatemia, libido decreased, menstrual disorders, potassium decreased

Gastrointestinal: Anorexia, appetite increased, diarrhea, dysphagia, eructation, GI hemorrhage, gingivitis, gum hemorrhage, intestinal obstruction, peptic ulcer

Genitourinary: Balanitis, impotence, testicular atrophy, urinary disorder, vaginitis

Hematologic: Platelets decreased, PT prolonged, WBC increased

Hepatic: Hepatomegaly, liver function tests abnormal

Local: Abscess, injection site reaction

Neuromuscular & skeletal: Leg cramps, myalgia, paresthesia, weakness

Renal: BUN increased

Respiratory: Allergic reaction, emphysema, hemoptysis, hypoxia, lung edema

Miscellaneous: Body odor, flu-like syndrome, neoplasm, voice alteration

Children and Adults: Postmarketing/case reports: Anaphylactic reactions, asthmatic reactions, bone density decreased, hypotension, induration at the injection site, peripheral neuropathy, photosensitivity, prostate pain, pulmonary embolism, rash, spinal fracture/paralysis, tenosynovitis-like symptoms, urticaria, WBC decreased

Overdosage/Toxicology Treatment is supportive.

(Continued)

Leuprolide *(Continued)*

Pharmacodynamics/Kinetics

Bioavailability: Oral: None; S.C.: 94%

Half-Life Elimination: 3 hours

Metabolism: Not well defined; forms smaller, inactive peptides and metabolites

Onset: Following transient increase, testosterone suppression occurs in ~2-4 weeks of continued therapy

Formulations

Implant, as acetate (Viadur®): 65 mg [released over 12 months]

Injection, solution, as acetate (Lupron®): 5 mg/mL (2.8 mL) [contains benzyl alcohol]

Injection, powder for reconstitution, as acetate [depot formulation]:
- Eligard™: 7.5 mg
- Lupron Depot®: 3.75 mg, 7.5 mg
- Lupron Depot®-3 Month: 11.25 mg, 22.5 mg
- Lupron Depot®-4 Month: 30 mg
- Lupron Depot-Ped®: 7.5 mg, 11.25 mg, 15 mg

Dosing

Adults & Elderly:

Advanced prostatic carcinoma:

S.C.:
- Eligard™: 7.5 mg monthly **or** 22.5 mg every 3 months
- Lupron®: 1 mg/day
- Viadur®: 65 mg implanted subcutaneously every 12 months

I.M.:
- Lupron Depot®: 7.5 mg/dose given monthly (every 28-33 days) **or**
- Lupron Depot-3®: 22.5 mg every 3 months **or**
- Lupron Depot-4®: 30 mg every 4 months

Endometriosis: I.M.: Initial therapy may be with leuprolide alone or in combination with norethindrone; if retreatment for an additional 6 months is necessary, norethindrone should be used. Retreatment is not recommended for longer than one additional 6-month course.
- Lupron Depot®: 3.75 mg/month for up to 6 months **or**
- Lupron Depot-3®: 11.25 mg every 3 months for up to 2 doses (6 months total duration of treatment)

Uterine leiomyomata (fibroids): I.M. (in combination with iron):
- Lupron Depot®: 3.75 mg/month for up to 3 months **or**
- Lupron Depot-3®: 11.25 mg as a single injection

Pediatrics: Precocious puberty (consider discontinuing by age 11 for females and by age 12 for males):

S.C. (Lupron®): 20-45 mcg/kg/day; titrate dose upward by 10 mcg/kg/day if down-regulation is not achieved

I.M. (Lupron Depot-Ped®): 0.3 mg/kg/dose given every 28 days (minimum dose: 7.5 mg)
- ≤25 kg: 7.5 mg
- >25-37.5 kg: 11.25 mg
- >37.5 kg: 15 mg

Titrate dose upward in 3.75 mg every 4 weeks if down-regulation is not achieved.

Administration

I.M.:

Eligard™: Packaged in two syringes; one contains the Atrigel® polymer system, and the second contains leuprolide acetate powder; follow instructions for mixing; must be administered within 30 minutes of mixing

Lupron Depot®: Do not use needles smaller than 22 gauge; reconstitute only with diluent provided

Other: Viadur® implant: Requires surgical implantation (subcutaneous) and removal at 12-month intervals

Stability

Storage:

Lupron®: Store unopened vials of injection in refrigerator, vial in use can be kept at room temperature of ≤30°C (86°F) for several months with minimal loss of potency. Protect from light and store vial in carton until use. Do not freeze.

Eligard™: Store at 2°C to 8°C (36°F to 46°C). Allow to reach room temperature prior to using; once mixed, must be administered within 30 minutes.

Lupron Depot® may be stored at room temperature of 25°C, excursions permitted to 15°C to 30°C (59°F to 86°F). Upon reconstitution, the suspension does not contain a preservative and should be used immediately.

Viadur® may be stored at room temperature of 15°C to 30°C (59°F and 86°F).

Monitoring Laboratory Tests Precocious puberty: GnRH testing (blood LH and FSH levels), testosterone in males and estradiol in females

Monitoring and Teaching Issues

Physical Assessment: See Contraindications, Warnings/Precautions, and Dosing for use cautions. Assess results of laboratory tests (see above), therapeutic response, and adverse reactions (eg, urinary tract obstruction, weakness, paresthesias, and urinary tract obstruction in first few weeks of therapy - see Adverse Reactions and Overdose/Toxicology) on a regular basis throughout therapy. Teach patient (or caregiver) proper use (eg, storage, injection technique, syringe/needle disposal), possible side effects and appropriate interventions, and adverse symptoms to report (see Patient Education). **Pregnancy risk factor X** - determine that patient is not pregnant before beginning treatment and do not give to females of childbearing age unless capable of complying with barrier contraceptive measures 1 month prior to therapy, during therapy, and 1 month following therapy. Instruct patient in appropriate contraceptive measures. Breast-feeding is contraindicated.

Patient Education: Use as directed. Do not discontinue without consulting prescriber. You may experience disease flare (increased bone pain) and urinary retention during early treatment (usually resolves); dizziness, headache, lethargy, or faintness (use caution when driving or engaging in tasks that require alertness until response to drug is known); nausea or vomiting (small, frequent meals or analgesics may help); hot flashes, flushing, or redness (cold clothes and cool environment may help); breast swelling or tenderness; or decreased libido. Report irregular or rapid heartbeat, palpitations, chest pain; inability to void or changes in urinary pattern; unresolved nausea or vomiting; numbness of extremities; breast swelling or pain, difficulty breathing, or redness, swelling or pain at injection sites. **Pregnancy/breast-feeding precautions:** Inform prescriber if you are pregnant. Do not get pregnant. Consult prescriber for appropriate barrier contraceptive use during and for a time following therapy. Do not breast-feed.

Geriatric Considerations: Leuprolide has the advantage of not increasing risk of atherosclerotic vascular disease, causing swelling of breasts, fluid retention, and thromboembolism as compared to estrogen therapy.

Pregnancy Issues: Pregnancy must be excluded prior to the start of treatment. Although leuprolide usually inhibits ovulation and stops menstruation, contraception is not ensured and a nonhormonal contraceptive should be used.

Additional Information

Eligard™ Atrigel®: A nongelatin-based, biodegradable, polymer matrix

Viadur®: Leuprolide acetate implant containing 72 mg of leuprolide acetate, equivalent to 65 mg leuprolide free base. One Viadur® implant delivers 120 mcg of leuprolide/day over 12 months.

Leuprolide Acetate *see* Leuprolide *on page 781*

Leuprorelin Acetate *see* Leuprolide *on page 781*

Leurocristine *see* VinCRIStine *on page 1401*

Leustatin™ *see* Cladribine *on page 303*

Levalbuterol (leve al BYOO ter ole)

U.S. Brand Names Xopenex®

Synonyms R-albuterol

Generic Available No

Pharmacologic Category $Beta_2$ Agonist

Pregnancy Risk Factor C

Lactation Excretion in breast milk unknown/contraindicated

Use Treatment or prevention of bronchospasm in adults and adolescents ≥6 years of age with reversible obstructive airway disease

Mechanism of Action/Effect Relaxes bronchial smooth muscle by action on beta-2 receptors with little effect on heart rate

Contraindications Hypersensitivity to levalbuterol, albuterol, or any component of the formulation

Warnings/Precautions Use with caution in patients with cardiovascular disease, including coronary artery disease, hypertension, or history of arrhythmias (may increase heart rate, blood pressure or other symptoms, including EKG changes). Fatalities have been associated with excessive use of sympathomimetics. Use with caution in diabetic patients and in patients with hypokalemia. Use with caution during labor and delivery. May cause paradoxical bronchospasm and/or hypersensitivity reactions. Safety and efficacy in patients <6 years of age has not been established. Pregnancy risk C.

Drug Interactions

Decreased Effect: Beta-blockers (particularly nonselective agents) block the effect of levalbuterol. Digoxin levels may be decreased.

Increased Effect/Toxicity: May add to effects of medications which deplete potassium (eg, loop or thiazide diuretics). Cardiac effects of levalbuterol may be potentiated in patients receiving MAO inhibitors, tricyclic antidepressants, sympathomimetics (eg, amphetamine, dobutamine), or inhaled anesthetics (eg, enflurane).

Adverse Reactions Immediate hypersensitivity reactions have occurred, including angioedema, oropharyngeal edema, urticaria, rash, and anaphylaxis. Events reported include those ≥2% with incidence higher than placebo in patients ≥12 years of age.

>10%:

Endocrine & metabolic: Increased serum glucose, decreased serum potassium

Respiratory: Viral infection (7% to 12%), rhinitis (3% to 11%)

>2% to <10%:

Central nervous system: Nervousness (3% to 10%), tremor (≤7%), anxiety (≤3%), dizziness (1% to 3%), migraine (≤3%), pain (1% to 3%)

Cardiovascular: Tachycardia (~3%)

Gastrointestinal: Dyspepsia (1% to 3%)

Neuromuscular & skeletal: Leg cramps (≤3%%)

Respiratory: Cough (1% to 4%), nasal edema (1% to 3%), sinusitis (1% to 4%)

Miscellaneous: Flu-like syndrome (1% to 4%), accidental injury (≤3%)

<2% (Limited to important or life-threatening): Abnormal EKG, anaphylaxis, angioedema, arrhythmias, asthma exacerbation, bronchospasm (paradoxical), hypesthesia (hand), paresthesia, rash, syncope, urticaria, vomiting, wheezing; immediate hypersensitivity reactions have occurred (including angioedema, oropharyngeal edema, urticaria, rash, and anaphylaxis)

Overdosage/Toxicology Symptoms of overdose include tachycardia, tremor, hypertension, angina, and seizures. Hypokalemia also may occur. Cardiac arrest and death may be associated with abuse of beta-agonist bronchodilators. Treatment includes immediate discontinuation and symptomatic and supportive therapies. Cautions use of beta-adrenergic blocking agents may be considered in severe cases.

(Continued)

Levalbuterol *(Continued)*

Pharmacodynamics/Kinetics

Absorption: A portion of inhaled dose is absorbed to systemic circulation

Half-Life Elimination: 3.3-4 hours

Time to Peak: Serum: 0.2 hours

Onset: 10-17 minutes (measured as a 15% increase in FEV_1); Peak effect: 1.5 hours

Duration: 5-6 hours (up to 8 hours in some patients)

Formulations Solution for nebulization: 0.31 mg/3 mL (24s); 0.63 mg/3 mL (24s); 1.25 mg/3 mL (24s)

Dosing

Adults: Bronchospasm: Inhalation: 0.63 mg 3 times/day at intervals of 6-8 hours, via nebulization. Dosage may be increased to 1.25 mg 3 times/day with close monitoring for adverse effects. Most patients gain optimal benefit from regular use.

Elderly: Only a small number of patients have been studied. Although greater sensitivity of some elderly patients cannot be ruled out, no overall differences in safety or effectiveness were observed. An initial dose of 0.63 mg should be used in all patients >65 years of age.

Pediatrics: Bronchospasm:

Children 6-11 years: 0.31 mg 3 times/day via nebulization (maximum dose: 0.63 mg 3 times/day)

Children >12 years: Refer to adult dosing.

Administration

Inhalation: Administered **only** via nebulization. Safety and efficacy were established when administered with the following nebulizers: PARI LC Jet™, PARI LC Plus™, as well as the following compressors: PARI Master®, Dura-Neb® 2000, and Dura-Neb® 3000.

Stability

Storage: Store in protective foil pouch at room temperature of 20°C to 25°C (68°F to 77°F). Protect from light and excessive heat. Vials should be used within 2 weeks after opening protective pouch. Use within 1 week and protect from light if removed from pouch.

Monitoring Laboratory Tests FEV_1 and/or peak expiratory flow rate, arterial blood gases (if condition warrants); in selected patients, serum, glucose, and potassium.

Monitoring and Teaching Issues

Physical Assessment: Assess effectiveness and interactions of other medications patient may be taking (see Drug Interactions). See Contraindications and Warnings/Precautions for use cautions. Monitor therapeutic effectiveness (patient response and lab values), adverse reactions (eg, anaphylaxis or hypertension, first dose administered under supervision), or overdose (see Adverse Reaction, and Overdose/Toxicology). Diabetics should monitor serum glucose on a regular basis (possibility of hyperglycemia). Assess knowledge/teach patient appropriate use (safe use of nebulizer), interventions to reduce side effects, and adverse reactions to report (see Patient Education). **Pregnancy risk factor C** - benefits of use should outweigh possible risks. Breast-feeding is contraindicated.

Patient Education: Use only when necessary or as prescribed; tolerance may develop with overuse. Do not administer more frequently than prescribed. First dose should not be used when you are alone. Avoid OTC medications without consulting prescriber. Maintain adequate hydration (2-3 L/day of fluids) unless advised by prescriber to restrict fluids. Stress or excessive exercising may exacerbate wheezing or bronchospasm (controlled breathing or relaxation techniques may help). If diabetic, you will need to monitor serum glucose levels closely until response is known; notify diabetic advisor if hyperglycemia occurs. You may experience tremor, anxiety, dizziness (use caution when driving or engaging in hazardous activities until response to drug is known); or temporarily upset stomach, nausea, or vomiting (small, frequent meals, frequent mouth care, chewing gum, or sucking hard candy may help). Paradoxical bronchospasm can occur. Stop drug immediately and notify prescriber if any of the following occur: chest pain, tightness, palpitations; severe headache; difficulty breathing; increased nervousness, restlessness, or trembling; muscle cramps or weakness; or seizures. Report unusual signs of flu or infection, leg or muscle cramps, unusual cough, persistent GI problems, vision changes, or other adverse effects. **Pregnancy/breast-feeding precautions:** Inform prescriber if you are or intend to become pregnant. Do not breast-feed.

Administration: Wash hands, sit to administer. Shake container, exhale slowly and completely through nose, inhale deeply through mouth while administering aerosol. Hold breath for 2-3 seconds, then exhale slowly. Allow 1 minute between inhalations. Wash mouthpiece with soap and water after each use. Rinse mouth to remove any unpleasant taste.

Breast-feeding Issues: It is not known whether levalbuterol is excreted in human milk. Breast-feeding should be avoided or the drug should be discontinued.

Related Information

Inhalant (Asthma, Bronchospasm) Agents Comparison *on page 1577*

Levaquin® *see* Levofloxacin *on page 790*

Levarterenol Bitartrate *see* Norepinephrine *on page 983*

Levbid® *see* Hyoscyamine *on page 685*

Levetiracetam (lev e tir AS e tam)

U.S. Brand Names Keppra®

Generic Available No

Pharmacologic Category Anticonvulsant, Miscellaneous

Pregnancy Risk Factor C

Lactation Enters breast milk/not recommended

Use Indicated as adjunctive therapy in the treatment of partial onset seizures in adults with epilepsy

Mechanism of Action/Effect Precise mechanism has not been defined. Does not appear to bind receptors or increase second messengers currently known to be involved in inhibitory or excitatory neurotransmission. Anticonvulsant activity is related to protection from secondary generalization from focal seizure activity. May selectively prevent hypersynchronization of epileptiform activity, inhibiting propagation of seizure activity.

Contraindications Hypersensitivity to levetiracetam or any component of the formulation

Warnings/Precautions May cause CNS adverse events, including somnolence and fatigue (treated by discontinuation, reduction, or hospitalization) or coordination difficulty (usually treated by reduction). Behavioral abnormalities, such as psychosis, hallucinations, psychotic depression and other behavioral symptoms (agitation, anger, aggression, irritability, hostility, anxiety, apathy, emotional lability, depersonalization, and depression) have been treated by reduction of dose and in some cases hospitalization. Levetiracetam should be withdrawn gradually to minimize the potential of increased seizure frequency. Pregnancy risk C.

Drug Interactions

Increased Effect/Toxicity: No interaction was observed in pharmacokinetic trials with other anticonvulsants, including phenytoin, carbamazepine, valproic acid, phenobarbital, lamotrigine, gabapentin, and primidone.

Nutritional/Ethanol Interactions

Ethanol: Avoid ethanol (may increase CNS depression).

Food: Food may delay, but does not affect the extent of absorption.

Adverse Reactions

>10%:

Central nervous system: Somnolence (15% vs 8% with placebo)

Neuromuscular & skeletal: Weakness (15% vs 9% with placebo)

<10%:

Central nervous system: Psychotic symptoms (1%), amnesia (2% vs 1% with placebo), ataxia (3% vs 1% with placebo), depression (4% vs 2% with placebo), dizziness (9% vs 4% with placebo), emotional lability (2%), nervousness (4% vs 2% with placebo), vertigo (3% vs 1% with placebo); other behavioral symptoms (agitation, anger, aggression, irritability, hostility, anxiety, apathy, depersonalization)

Hematologic: Decreased erythrocyte counts (3%), decreased leukocytes (2% to 3%)

Neuromuscular & skeletal: Ataxia and other coordination difficulties (3% vs 2% with placebo), pain (7% vs 6% with placebo)

Ocular: Diplopia (2% vs 1% with placebo)

Postmarketing and/or case reports: Leukopenia, neutropenia, pancytopenia, thrombocytopenia

Overdosage/Toxicology Limited experience. Symptoms would be expected to include drowsiness, somnolence and ataxia. Treatment is symptomatic and supportive. Hemodialysis may be effective.

Pharmacodynamics/Kinetics

Absorption: Rapid and complete

Bioavailability: 100%

Half-Life Elimination: 6-8 hours

Metabolism: Not extensive; primarily by enzymatic hydrolysis

Onset: Peak effect: 1 hour

Formulations Tablet: 250 mg, 500 mg, 750 mg

Dosing

Adults: Partial onset seizures (adjunctive): Oral: Initial: 500 mg twice daily; additional dosing adjustments should be made at 2 week intervals. The maximum daily dose is 3000 mg/day.

Elderly: No dosage adjustment is recommended based solely on age, however, renal function should be evaluated closely in this population

Renal Impairment:

Cl_{cr} >80 mL/minute: Administer 500-1500 mg every 12 hours.

Cl_{cr} 50-80 mL/minute: Administer 500-1000 mg every 12 hours.

Cl_{cr} 30-50 mL/minute: Administer 250-750 mg every 12 hours.

Cl_{cr} <30 mL/minute: Administer 250-500 mg every 12 hours. Patients with ESRD receiving dialysis may receive 500-1000 mg every 24 hours, with a supplemental dose of 250-500 mg given after each dialysis.

Hepatic Impairment: No adjustment necessary.

Stability

Storage: Store at 25°C (77°F).

Monitoring and Teaching Issues

Physical Assessment: Assess effectiveness and interactions of other medications patient may be taking (see Contraindications, Warnings/Precautions, and Drug Interactions). Monitor therapeutic response, laboratory values, and adverse reactions (see Adverse Reactions) at beginning of therapy and periodically with long-term use. Taper dosage slowly when discontinuing. Observe and teach seizure/safety precautions. Assess knowledge/teach patient appropriate use, interventions to reduce side effects, and adverse symptoms to report (see Patient Education). **Pregnancy risk factor C** - benefits of use should outweigh possible risks. Breast-feeding is not recommended.

Patient Education: Take exactly as directed; do not increase dose or frequency or discontinue without consulting prescriber. While using this medication, do not use alcohol and other prescription or OTC medications (especially pain medications, sedatives, antihistamines, or hypnotics) without consulting prescriber. Maintain adequate hydration (2-3 L/day of fluids) unless advised by prescriber to restrict fluids. You may experience drowsiness, dizziness, or blurred vision (use caution when driving or engaging in tasks requiring alertness until response to drug is known); or nausea, vomiting, loss of appetite, or dry mouth (small, frequent meals, frequent mouth care, chewing gum, or sucking lozenges may help). Wear identification of epileptic status and medications. Report CNS changes, mentation changes, or changes in cognition; muscle cramping, weakness, tremors, changes in gait; persistent GI symptoms (cramping, constipation, vomiting, anorexia); rash or skin irritations; unusual bruising or bleeding (mouth, urine, stool); or worsening of seizure activity or loss of seizure control. **Pregnancy/breast-feeding precautions:** Inform prescriber if you are or intend to become pregnant or are breast-feeding.

Breast-feeding Issues: Excreted in breast milk. Breast-feeding is not recommended (per manufacturer).

Levlen® *see* Ethinyl Estradiol and Levonorgestrel *on page 523*
Levlite™ *see* Ethinyl Estradiol and Levonorgestrel *on page 523*
Levobetaxolol *see page 1575*
Levobetaxolol *see* Ophthalmic Agents, Glaucoma *on page 1002*
Levobunolol *see page 1575*
Levobunolol *see* Ophthalmic Agents, Glaucoma *on page 1002*

Levobupivacaine (LEE voe byoo PIV a kane)

U.S. Brand Names Chirocaine®

Generic Available No

Pharmacologic Category Local Anesthetic

Pregnancy Risk Factor B

Lactation Excretion in breast milk unknown/use caution

Use Production of local or regional anesthesia for surgery and obstetrics, and for postoperative pain management

Mechanism of Action/Effect Blocks both the initiation and transmission of nerve impulses

Contraindications Hypersensitivity to levobupivacaine, any component of the formulation, bupivacaine, or any local anesthetic of the amide type

Warnings/Precautions Local anesthetics should be administered only by clinicians familiar with the use of local anesthetic agents, procedures, and management of drug-related toxicity and other acute emergencies. Resuscitative equipment and medications should be readily available. Not for intravenous injection (cardiac arrest may occur) or obstetrical paracervical block. Risk of cardiac toxicity increases with higher concentration solutions. Avoid use of 0.75% solution with obstetrical patients. Use with caution in patients with hypotension, hypovolemia, heart block, hepatic impairment, cardiac impairment, or those receiving other local anesthetics or structurally-related agents.

Drug Interactions

Cytochrome P450 Effect: Substrate of CYP1A2, 3A4

Increased Effect/Toxicity: Although not specifically studies, inhibitors of CYP3A4 and CYP1A2 may increase levels/toxicity of levobupivacaine.

Nutritional/Ethanol Interactions Herb/Nutraceutical: St John's wort may decrease levobupivacaine levels.

Adverse Reactions

>10%:

Cardiovascular: Hypotension (20% to 31%)

Central nervous system: Pain (postoperative) (7% to 18%), fever (7% to 17%)

Gastrointestinal: Nausea (12% to 21%), vomiting (8% to 14%)

Hematologic: Anemia (10% to 12%)

1% to 10%:

Central nervous system: Pain (4% to 8%), headache (5% to 7%), dizziness (5% to 6%), hypoesthesia (3%), somnolence (1%), anxiety (1%), hypothermia (2%)

Cardiovascular: Abnormal EKG (3%), bradycardia (2%), tachycardia (2%), hypertension (1%)

Dermatologic: Pruritus (4% to 9%), purpura (1%)

Endocrine & metabolic: Breast pain - female (1%)

Gastrointestinal: Constipation (3% to 7%), enlarged abdomen (3%), flatulence (2%), abdominal pain (2%), dyspepsia (2%), diarrhea (1%)

Genitourinary: Urinary incontinence (1%), urine flow decreased (1%), urinary tract infection (1%)

Hematologic: Leukocytosis (1%)

Local: Anesthesia (1%)

Neuromuscular & skeletal: Back pain (6%), rigors (3%), paresthesia (2%)

Ocular: Diplopia (3%)

Renal: Albuminuria (3%), hematuria (2%)

Respiratory: Cough (1%)

Miscellaneous: Fetal distress (5% to 10%), delayed delivery (6%), hemorrhage in pregnancy (2%), uterine abnormality (2%), increased wound drainage (1%)

<1% (Limited to important or life-threatening): Apnea, arrhythmia, atrial fibrillation, bronchospasm, cardiac arrest, confusion, dyspnea, generalized spasm, ileus, involuntary muscle contraction, pulmonary edema, skin discoloration, syncope

Overdosage/Toxicology Related to local concentration or due to unintended intrathecal or intravenous injection. Symptoms may include restlessness, anxiety, incoherent speech, lightheadedness, numbness and tingling of the mouth and lips, metallic taste, tinnitus, dizziness, blurred vision, tremors, respiratory arrest, twitching, depression or drowsiness. In addition, cardiac toxicity, including AV block, bradycardia, arrhythmia, and hypotension may occur. Treatment is symptomatic.

Pharmacodynamics/Kinetics

Absorption: Dependent on route of administration and dose

Half-Life Elimination: 1.3 hours

Time to Peak: Epidural: 30 minutes

Metabolism: Extensively hepatic via CYP3A4 and CYP1A2

Onset: Epidural: 10-14 minutes

Duration: Dose dependent: 1-8 hours

Formulations Injection, solution [preservative free]: 2.5 mg/mL (10 mL, 30 mL); 5 mg/mL (10 mL, 30 mL); 7.5 mg/mL (10 mL, 30 mL)

Dosing

Adults & Elderly: Note: Rapid injection of a large volume of local anesthetic solution should be avoided. Fractional (incremental) doses are recommended.

Guidelines (individual response varies): See table on following page.

Maximum dosage: Epidural doses up to 375 mg have been administered incrementally to patients during a surgical procedure.

Intraoperative block and postoperative pain: 695 mg in 24 hours

Postoperative epidural infusion over 24 hours: 570 mg
Single-fractionated injection for brachial plexus block: 300 mg

	Concentration	Volume	Dose	Motor Block
Surgical Anesthesia				
Epidural for surgery	0.5%-0.75%	10-20 mL	50-150 mg	Moderate to complete
Epidural - C-section	0.5%	20-30 mL	100-150 mg	Moderate to complete
Peripheral nerve	0.25%-0.5%	0.4 mL/kg (30 mL)	1-2 mg/kg (75-150 mg)	Moderate to complete
Ophthalmic	0.75%	5-15 mL	37.5-112.5 mg	Moderate to complete
Local infiltration	0.25%	60 mL	150 mg	Not applicable
Pain Management				
Labor analgesia (epidural bolus)	0.25%	10-20 mL	25-50 mg	Minimal to moderate
Postoperative pain (epidural infusion)	0.125%*-0.25%	4-10 mL/h	5-25 mg/h	Minimal to moderate

* 0.125%: Adjunct therapy with fentanyl or clonidine

Administration

Other: Isopropyl or ethyl alcohol are recommended to disinfect the surface of the vial. Disinfectants containing heavy metals should not be used for mucous membrane disinfection since they have been related to incidents of swelling and edema. Prior to administration, it is essential that aspiration for blood or cerebrospinal fluid (where applicable) be performed prior to injecting any local anesthetic, both before the original dosage and at all subsequent doses (to avoid intravascular or intrathecal injection). A negative aspiration does not ensure against intrathecal or intravascular injection. Rapid injection of a large volume of local anesthetic solution should be avoided. Fractional (incremental) doses are recommended. Monitor patient during and after injection for symptoms of CNS or cardiac toxicity.

Stability

Storage: Store at room temperature (20°C to 25°C/68°F to 77°F). Disinfectants containing heavy metals should not be used for mucous membrane disinfection since they have been related to incidents of swelling and edema. Isopropyl or ethyl alcohol is recommended. Stability of solution in vial has been demonstrated following an autoclave cycle at 121°C for 15 minutes.

Compatibility: Stable in 0.9% NS USP. Stable for 24 hours in PVC bags at room temperature when diluted to 0.625-2.5 mg levobupivacaine per mL.

Incompatible with alkaline pH solutions (pH >8.5)

Monitoring and Teaching Issues

Physical Assessment: Monitor for effectiveness of anesthesia according to purpose for use. Monitor closely during and after injection for symptoms of CNS or cardiac toxicity (see Adverse reactions). Monitor for return of sensation. Use appropriate patient safety measures until full return of sensation. Teach patient adverse symptoms to report (see Patient Education). Note breast-feeding caution.

Patient Education: This medication is given to reduce sensation and pain. You will experience decreased sensation to pain, heat, or cold in the area and/or decreased muscle strength (depending on area of application). Until sensation returns, use caution to prevent injury (eg, avoid extremes of heat or cold to area, do not use sharp objects, avoid driving, climbing stairs, or sudden moves if muscle strength is affected). Immediately report chest pain or palpitations; increased restlessness, anxiety, dizziness or lightheadedness; sensation of sudden muscle weakness; swelling or tingling of mouth or lips; metallic taste; vision changes or hearing. Consult prescriber if breast-feeding.

Pregnancy Issues: Local anesthetics rapidly cross the placenta and may cause varying degrees of maternal, fetal, and neonatal toxicity. Close maternal and fetal monitoring (heart rate and electronic fetal monitoring advised) are required during obstetrical use.

Levocabastine *see page 1509*

Levocarnitine (lee voe KAR ni teen)

U.S. Brand Names Carnitor®

Synonyms L-Carnitine

Generic Available Yes

Pharmacologic Category Dietary Supplement

Pregnancy Risk Factor B

Lactation Excretion in breast milk unknown/use caution

Use Orphan drug:

Oral: Primary systemic carnitine deficiency; acute and chronic treatment of patients with an inborn error of metabolism which results in secondary carnitine deficiency

I.V.: Acute and chronic treatment of patients with an inborn error of metabolism which results in secondary carnitine deficiency; prevention and treatment of carnitine deficiency in patients with end-stage renal disease (ESRD) who are undergoing hemodialysis.

Mechanism of Action/Effect Carnitine is a naturally occurring metabolic compound which facilitates energy production

Warnings/Precautions Caution in patients with seizure disorders or in those at risk of seizures (CNS mass or medications which may lower seizure threshold). Both new-onset seizure activity as well as an increased frequency of seizures has been observed. Safety and efficacy of oral carnitine have not been established in ESRD. Chronic administration of high oral doses to patients with severely compromised renal function or ESRD patients on dialysis may result in accumulation of metabolites.

Effects on Lab Values Normal carnitine levels are 40-50 μmol/L; levels should be maintained on therapy between 35-60 μmol/L. therapy between 35-60 μmol/L.

Adverse Reactions Frequencies noted with I.V. therapy (hemodialysis patients):

Cardiovascular: Hypertension (18% to 21%), peripheral edema (3% to 6%)

(Continued)

Levocarnitine *(Continued)*

Central nervous system: Dizziness (10% to 18%), fever (5% to 12%), paresthesia (3% to 12%), depression (5% to 6%)
Endocrine & metabolic: Hypercalcemia (6% to 15%)
Gastrointestinal: Diarrhea (9% to 35%), abdominal pain (5% to 21%), vomiting (9% to 21%), nausea (5% to 12%)
Neuromuscular & skeletal: Weakness (9% to 12%)
Miscellaneous: Allergic reaction (2% to 6%)

Overdosage/Toxicology No reports of overdose. Easily removed by dialysis.

Pharmacodynamics/Kinetics
Bioavailability: Tablet/solution: 15% to 16%
Half-Life Elimination: 17.4 hours
Time to Peak: Tablet/solution: 3.3 hours
Metabolism: Hepatic (limited with moderate renal impairment), to trimethylamine (TMA) and trimethylamine N-oxide (TMAO)

Formulations
Capsule: 250 mg
Injection, solution (Carnitor®): 200 mg/mL (5 mL)
Solution, oral (Carnitor®): 100 mg/mL (118 mL) [cherry flavor]
Tablet: 500 mg
Carnitor®: 330 mg

Dosing
Adults & Elderly:
Carnitine supplementation: Oral: 990 mg (oral tablets) 2-3 times/day or 1-3 g/day (oral solution)
Metabolic disorders: I.V.: 50 mg/kg as a slow 2- to 3-minute I.V. bolus or by I.V. infusion
Severe metabolic crisis: I.V.:
A loading dose of 50 mg/kg over 2-3 minutes followed by an equivalent dose over the following 24 hours administered as every 3 hours or every 4 hours (never less than every 6 hours either by infusion or by intravenous injection)
All subsequent daily doses are recommended to be in the range of 50 mg/kg or as therapy may require.
The highest dose administered has been 300 mg/kg.
It is recommended that a plasma carnitine concentration be obtained prior to beginning parenteral therapy accompanied by weekly and monthly monitoring.
ESRD patients on hemodialysis: I.V.:
Predialysis levocarnitine concentrations below normal (40-50 μmol/L): 10-20 mg/kg dry body weight as a slow 2- to 3-minute bolus after each dialysis session
Dosage adjustments should be guided by predialysis trough levocarnitine concentrations and downward dose adjustments (to 5 mg/kg after dialysis) may be made as early as every 3rd or 4th week of therapy.
Pediatrics: Carnitine supplementation:
Oral: Infants/Children: Initial: 50 mg/kg/day; titrate to 50-100 mg/kg/day in divided doses with a maximum dose of 3 g/day
I.V.: Refer to adult dosing.

Administration
Oral: Solution may be dissolved in either drink or liquid food. The oral solution should be consumed slowly and spaced evenly throughout the day to improve tolerance. Doses should be spaced every 3 to 4 hours throughout the day, preferably during or following meals.
I.V.: Hemodialysis patients: Injection should be given over 2-3 minutes into the venous return line after each dialysis session.

Stability
Storage: Store at 25°C (77°F). Compatible at concentrations between 0.5-8 mg/mL in 0.9% sodium chloride or lactated Ringer's solution. Stable in PVC bags for 24 hours.

Monitoring Laboratory Tests Plasma concentrations should be obtained prior to beginning parenteral therapy, and should be monitored weekly to monthly. In metabolic disorders: monitor blood chemistry, vital signs, and plasma carnitine levels (maintain between 35-60 μmol/L). In ESRD patients on dialysis: Plasma levels below the normal range should prompt initiation of therapy. Monitor predialysis (trough) plasma carnitine levels.

Monitoring and Teaching Issues
Physical Assessment: **I.V.:** Monitor therapeutic response according to rational for therapy and adverse reactions (eg, CNS, hypertension, see Adverse Reactions). **Oral:** Monitor therapeutic response and assess severity. Assess knowledge and teach patient appropriate use, interventions to reduce side effects, and adverse reactions to report. Note breast-feeding caution.
Patient Education: I.V.: Report immediately any dizziness, loss of feeling, acute headache, tremors, or nausea.

Oral: Take exactly as directed; do not alter dose or frequency except as directed by prescriber. Dissolve solution in any liquid and drink with or following meals. The oral solution should be consumed slowly and spaced evenly throughout the day to improve tolerance. You may experience abdominal pain, nausea, or vomiting (small, frequent meals, chewing gum, or sucking hard candy); diarrhea (yogurt, boiled milk, or buttermilk may help); or dizziness (use caution driving or engaging in hazardous activities until response to drug is known). Report acute headache, chest pain, tremors, or visual changes; muscle or skeletal weakness; skin rash; swelling of extremities; or other adverse effects. **Breast-feeding precaution:** Consult prescriber if breast-feeding.
Breast-feeding Issues: In breast-feeding women, use must be weighed against the potential exposure of the infant to increased carnitine intake. Use caution in breast-feeding women.
Pregnancy Issues: No adequate or well controlled studies in pregnant women. However, carnitine is a naturally occurring substance in mammalian metabolism.

Additional Information Although supplemental carnitine has been shown to increase carnitine concentrations, effects on the signs and symptoms of carnitine deficiency have not been determined.

Levodopa and Carbidopa (lee voe DOE pa & kar bi DOE pa)

U.S. Brand Names Sinemet®; Sinemet® CR

Synonyms Carbidopa and Levodopa

Generic Available Yes

Pharmacologic Category Anti-Parkinson's Agent, Dopamine Agonist

Pregnancy Risk Factor C

Lactation Excretion in breast milk unknown

Use Idiopathic Parkinson's disease; postencephalitic parkinsonism; symptomatic parkinsonism

Use - Unlabeled/Investigational Restless leg syndrome

Mechanism of Action/Effect Parkinson's symptoms are due to a lack of striatal dopamine; levodopa circulates in the plasma to the blood-brain-barrier (BBB), where it crosses, to be converted by striatal enzymes to dopamine; carbidopa inhibits the peripheral plasma breakdown of levodopa by inhibiting its decarboxylation, and thereby increases available levodopa at the BBB

Contraindications Hypersensitivity to levodopa, carbidopa, or any component of the formulation; narrow-angle glaucoma; use of MAO inhibitors within prior 14 days (however, may be administered concomitantly with the manufacturer's recommended dose of an MAO inhibitor with selectivity for MAO type B); history of melanoma or undiagnosed skin lesions

Warnings/Precautions Use with caution in patients with history of cardiovascular disease (including myocardial infarction and arrhythmias); pulmonary diseases such as asthma, psychosis, wide-angle glaucoma, peptic ulcer disease; as well as in renal, hepatic, or endocrine disease. Sudden discontinuation of levodopa may cause a worsening of Parkinson's disease. Elderly may be more sensitive to CNS effects of levodopa. May cause or exacerbate dyskinesias. May cause orthostatic hypotension; Parkinson's disease patients appear to have an impaired capacity to respond to a postural challenge; use with caution in patients at risk of hypotension (such as those receiving antihypertensive drugs) or where transient hypotensive episodes would be poorly tolerated (cardiovascular disease or cerebrovascular disease). Observe patients closely for development of depression with concomitant suicidal tendencies. Some products may contain tartrazine. Has been associated with a syndrome resembling neuroleptic malignant syndrome on withdrawal or significant dosage reduction after long-term use. Toxic reactions have occurred with dextromethorphan. Protein in the diet should be distributed throughout the day to avoid fluctuations in levodopa absorption. Pregnancy risk C.

Drug Interactions

Decreased Effect: Antipsychotics, benzodiazepines, L-methionine, phenytoin, pyridoxine, spiramycin, and tacrine may inhibit the antiparkinsonian effects of levodopa; monitor for reduced effect. Antipsychotics may inhibit the antiparkinsonian effects of levodopa via dopamine receptor blockade. Use antipsychotics with low dopamine blockade (clozapine, olanzapine, quetiapine). High-protein diets may inhibit levodopa's efficacy; avoid high protein foods. Iron binds levodopa and reduces its bioavailability; separate doses of iron and levodopa.

Increased Effect/Toxicity: Concurrent use of levodopa with nonselective MAO inhibitors may result in hypertensive reactions via an increased storage and release of dopamine, norepinephrine, or both. Use with carbidopa to minimize reactions if combination is necessary; otherwise avoid combination.

Nutritional/Ethanol Interactions

Ethanol: Avoid ethanol (due to CNS depression).

Food: Avoid high protein diets and high intakes of vitamin B_6.

Herb/Nutraceutical: Avoid kava kava (may decrease effects). Pyridoxine in doses >10-25 mg (for levodopa alone) or higher doses >200 mg/day (for levodopa/carbidopa) may decrease efficacy.

Effects on Lab Values False-positive reaction for urinary glucose with Clinitest®; false-negative reaction using Clinistix®; false-positive urine ketones with Acetest®, Ketostix®, Labstix®

Adverse Reactions Frequency not defined.

Cardiovascular: Orthostatic hypotension, arrhythmias, chest pain, hypertension, syncope, palpitations, phlebitis

Central nervous system: Dizziness, anxiety, confusion, nightmares, headache, hallucinations, on-off phenomenon, decreased mental acuity, memory impairment, disorientation, delusions, euphoria, agitation, somnolence, insomnia, gait abnormalities, nervousness, ataxia, EPS, falling, psychosis, peripheral neuropathy, seizures (causal relationship not established)

Dermatologic: Rash, alopecia, malignant melanoma, hypersensitivity (angioedema, urticaria, pruritus, bullous lesions, Henoch-Schönlein purpura)

Endocrine & metabolic: Increased libido

Gastrointestinal: Anorexia, nausea, vomiting, constipation, GI bleeding, duodenal ulcer, diarrhea, dyspepsia, taste alterations, sialorrhea, heartburn

Genitourinary: Discoloration of urine, urinary frequency

Hematologic: Hemolytic anemia, agranulocytosis, thrombocytopenia, leukopenia; decreased hemoglobin and hematocrit; abnormalities in AST and ALT, LDH, bilirubin, BUN, Coombs' test

Neuromuscular & skeletal: Choreiform and involuntary movements, paresthesia, bone pain, shoulder pain, muscle cramps, weakness

Ocular: Blepharospasm, oculogyric crises (may be associated with acute dystonic reactions)

Renal: Difficult urination

Respiratory: Dyspnea, cough

Miscellaneous: Hiccups, discoloration of sweat, diaphoresis (increased)

Overdosage/Toxicology Symptoms of overdose include palpitations, arrhythmias, spasms; may cause hypertension or hypotension. Treatment is supportive. EKG monitoring is warranted. May precipitate a variety of arrhythmias.

(Continued)

Levodopa and Carbidopa *(Continued)*

Pharmacokinetic Note See individual agents.

Formulations

Tablet (Sinemet®):

10/100: Carbidopa 10 mg and levodopa 100 mg

25/100: Carbidopa 25 mg and levodopa 100 mg

25/250: Carbidopa 25 mg and levodopa 250 mg

Tablet, sustained release (Sinemet® CR):

Carbidopa 25 mg and levodopa 100 mg

Carbidopa 50 mg and levodopa 200 mg

Dosing

Adults:

Parkinson's disease: Oral: Initial: Carbidopa 25 mg/levodopa 100 mg 2-4 times/day, increase as necessary to a maximum of carbidopa 200 mg/levodopa 2000 mg per day

Conversion from Sinemet® to Sinemet® CR (50/200): (Sinemet® [total daily dose of levodopa] / Sinemet® CR)

300-400 mg / 1 tablet twice daily

500-600 mg / 1½ tablets twice daily or one 3 times/day

700-800 mg / 4 tablets in 3 or more divided doses

900-1000 mg / 5 tablets in 3 or more divided doses

Intervals between doses of Sinemet® CR should be 4-8 hours while awake.

Restless leg syndrome (unlabeled use): Oral: Carbidopa 25 mg/levodopa 100 mg given 30-60 minutes before bedtime; may repeat dose once

Elderly: Initial dose: 25/100 twice daily, increase as necessary. Sinemet® CR may be used as initial therapy.

Administration

Oral: Space doses evenly over the waking hours. Give with meals to decrease GI upset. Sustained release product should not be crushed.

Monitoring and Teaching Issues

Physical Assessment: Assess effectiveness and interactions of other medications patient may be taking (see Contraindications and Drug Interactions). Monitor therapeutic response and adverse reactions (including levodopa toxicity) at beginning of therapy and periodically throughout therapy (see Warnings/Precautions, Adverse Reactions, and Overdose/Toxicology). Assess knowledge/teach patient appropriate use, interventions to reduce side effects, and adverse symptoms to report (see Patient Education). **Pregnancy risk factor C** - benefits of use should outweigh possible risks. Note breast-feeding caution.

Patient Education: Take exactly as directed; do not change dosage or discontinue without consulting prescriber. Do not crush sustained release form. Therapeutic effects may take several weeks or months to achieve and you may need frequent monitoring during first weeks of therapy. Take with meals if GI upset occurs, before meals if dry mouth occurs, after eating if drooling or if nausea occurs. Take at the same time each day. Maintain adequate hydration (2-3 L/day of fluids) unless advised by prescriber to restrict fluids; void before taking medication. Do not use alcohol and prescription or OTC sedatives or CNS depressants without consulting prescriber. Urine or perspiration may appear darker. You may experience drowsiness, dizziness, confusion, or vision changes (use caution when driving, climbing stairs, or engaging in tasks requiring alertness until response to drug is known); orthostatic hypotension (use caution when changing position - rising to standing from sitting or lying); increased susceptibility to heat stroke, decreased perspiration (use caution in hot weather - maintain adequate fluids and reduce exercise activity); constipation (increased exercise, fluids, fruit, or fiber may help); dry skin or nasal passages (consult prescriber for appropriate relief); or nausea, vomiting, loss of appetite, or stomach discomfort (small, frequent meals, frequent mouth care, chewing gum, or sucking lozenges may help). Report unresolved constipation or vomiting; chest pain or irregular heartbeat; difficulty breathing; acute headache or dizziness; CNS changes (hallucination, loss of memory, nervousness, etc); painful or difficult urination; abdominal pain or blood in stool; increased muscle spasticity or rigidity; skin rash; or significant worsening of condition. **Pregnancy/breast-feeding precautions:** Inform prescriber if you are or intend to become pregnant. Consult prescriber if breast-feeding.

Dietary Issues: Levodopa peak serum concentrations may be decreased if taken with food. High protein diets (>2 g/kg) may decrease the efficacy of levodopa via competition with amino acids in crossing the blood-brain barrier.

Geriatric Considerations: The elderly may be more sensitive to the CNS effects of levodopa.

Additional Information 50-100 mg/day of carbidopa is needed to block the peripheral conversion of levodopa to dopamine. "On-off" (a clinical syndrome characterized by sudden periods of drug activity/inactivity), can be managed by giving smaller, more frequent doses of Sinemet® or adding a dopamine agonist or selegiline; when adding a new agent, doses of Sinemet® can usually be decreased. Protein in the diet should be distributed throughout the day to avoid fluctuations in levodopa absorption. Levodopa is the drug of choice when rigidity is the predominant presenting symptom.

Levo-Dromoran® *see* Levorphanol *on page 795*

Levofloxacin (lee voe FLOKS a sin)

U.S. Brand Names Levaquin®; Quixin™

Generic Available No

Pharmacologic Category Antibiotic, Quinolone

Pregnancy Risk Factor C

Lactation Enters breast milk/contraindicated

Use

Systemic:

Acute bacterial exacerbation of chronic bronchitis due to *S. aureus, S. pneumoniae* (including penicillin-resistant strains), *H. influenzae, H. parainfluenzae,*or *M. catarrhalis*

Acute maxillary sinusitis due to *S. pneumoniae, H. influenzae,* or *M. catarrhalis*
Acute pyelonephritis caused by *E. coli*
Community-acquired pneumonia due to *S. aureus, S. pneumoniae* (including penicillin-resistant strains), *H. influenzae, H. parainfluenzae, M. catarrhalis, C. pneumoniae, L. pneumophila,* or *M. pneumoniae*
Nosocomial pneumonia due to methicillin-susceptible *S. aureus, Pseudomonas aeruginosa, Serratia marcescens, E. coli, K. pneumoniae, H. influenzae,* or *S. pneumoniae*
Skin or skin structure infections:
Complicated, due to methicillin-susceptible *S. aureus, Enterococcus faecalis, S. pyogenes,* or *Proteus mirabilis*
Uncomplicated, due to *S. aureus* or *S. pyogenes*
Urinary tract infections:
Complicated, due to gram-negative bacteria (*E. coli, Enterobacter cloacae, Klebsiella pneumoniae, Proteus mirabilis, Enterococcus faecalis,* or *Pseudomonas aeruginosa*)
Uncomplicated, due to *E. coli, K. pneumoniae,* or *S. saprophyticus*
Ophthalmic: Bacterial conjunctivitis due to *S. aureus, S. epidermidis, S. pneumoniae, Streptococcus* (groups C/F), *Streptococcus* (group G), Viridans group streptococci, *Corynebacterium* spp, *H. influenzae, Acinetobacter lwoffii,* or *Serratia marcescens*

Mechanism of Action/Effect Levofloxacin, a fluorinated quinolone, is a pyridine carboxylic acid derivative which exerts a broad spectrum bactericidal effect. It inhibits DNA gyrase inhibitor, an essential bacterial enzyme that maintains the superhelical structure of DNA. DNA gyrase is required for DNA replication and transcription, DNA repair, recombination, and transposition within the bacteria.

Contraindications Hypersensitivity to levofloxacin, any component of the formulation, or other quinolones

Warnings/Precautions Systemic: Not recommended in children <18 years of age; CNS stimulation may occur (tremor, restlessness, confusion, and very rarely hallucinations or seizures); use with caution in patients with known or suspected CNS disorders or renal dysfunction; use caution to avoid possible photosensitivity reactions during and for several days following fluoroquinolone therapy

Rare cases of torsade de pointes have been reported in patients receiving levofloxacin. Risk may be minimized by avoiding use in patients with bradycardia, hypokalemia, hypomagnesemia, cardiomyopathy, or in those receiving concurrent therapy with Class Ia or Class III antiarrhythmics.

Severe hypersensitivity reactions, including anaphylaxis, have occurred with quinolone therapy. If an allergic reaction occurs (itching, urticaria, dyspnea or facial edema, loss of consciousness, tingling, cardiovascular collapse), discontinue drug immediately. Prolonged use may result in superinfection; pseudomembranous colitis may occur and should be considered in all patients who present with diarrhea. Tendon inflammation and/or rupture has been reported; discontinue at first sign of tendon inflammation or pain. Risk may be increased with concurrent corticosteroids, particularly in the elderly. Quinolones may exacerbate myasthenia gravis.

Ophthalmic solution: For topical use only. Do not inject subconjunctivally or introduce into anterior chamber of the eye. Contact lenses should not be worn during treatment for bacterial conjunctivitis. Safety and efficacy in children <1 year of age have not been established.

Pregnancy risk C.

Drug Interactions

Cytochrome P450 Effect: Inhibits **CYP1A2**

Decreased Effect: Metal cations (magnesium, aluminum, iron, and zinc) bind quinolones in the gastrointestinal tract and inhibit absorption (by up to 98%). Due to electrolyte content, antacids, electrolyte supplements, sucralfate, quinapril, and some didanosine formulations should be avoided. Levofloxacin should be administered 2 hours before or 2 hours after these agents. Antineoplastic agents may decrease the absorption of quinolones.

Increased Effect/Toxicity: Quinolones may cause increased levels of azlocillin, cyclosporine, and caffeine/theophylline (effect of levofloxacin on theophylline metabolism appears limited). Azlocillin, cimetidine, loop diuretics (furosemide, torsemide), and probenecid increase quinolone levels (decreased renal secretion). An increased incidence of seizures may occur with foscarnet or NSAIDs. The hypoprothrombinemic effect of warfarin is enhanced by some quinolone antibiotics. QT_c-prolonging agents (including Class Ia and Class III antiarrhythmics, erythromycin, cisapride, antipsychotics, and cyclic antidepressants) should be avoided with levofloxacin. Levofloxacin does not alter warfarin levels, but may alter the gastrointestinal flora. Monitor INR closely during therapy. Concurrent use of corticosteroids may increase risk of tendon rupture.

Adverse Reactions

1% to 10%:
Central nervous system: Dizziness, fever, headache, insomnia
Gastrointestinal: Nausea, vomiting, diarrhea, constipation
Ocular (with ophthalmic solution use): Decreased vision (transient), foreign body sensation, transient ocular burning, ocular pain or discomfort, photophobia
Respiratory: Pharyngitis

<1% (Limited to important or life-threatening):
Systemic: Acute renal failure; allergic reaction (including pneumonitis rash, pneumonitis, and anaphylaxis); anaphylactoid reaction, arrhythmias (including ventricular tachycardia and torsade de pointes), arthralgia, bradycardia, cardiac failure, dysphonia, eosinophilia, erythema multiforme, granulocytopenia, hemolytic anemia, hepatic failure, hypertension, intracranial hypertension, jaundice, leukocytosis, leukopenia, leukorrhea, photosensitivity (<0.1%), pseudomembraneous colitis, pulmonary embolism, QT_c prolongation, seizures, Stevens-Johnson syndrome, tachycardia, tendon rupture, transaminases increased, thrombocytopenia, tremor
Ophthalmic solution: Allergic reaction, lid edema, ocular dryness, ocular itching

Overdosage/Toxicology

Symptoms of overdose include acute renal failure, seizures

(Continued)

Levofloxacin *(Continued)*

Treatment should include GI decontamination and supportive care; not removed by peritoneal or hemodialysis

Pharmacodynamics/Kinetics

Absorption: Well absorbed

Bioavailability: 100%

Half-Life Elimination: 6 hours

Time to Peak: Serum: 1 hour

Metabolism: Minimally hepatic

Formulations

Infusion [premixed in D_5W] (Levaquin®): 5 mg/mL (50 mL, 100 mL, 150 mL)
Injection, solution [preservative free] (Levaquin®): 25 mg/mL (20 mL, 30 mL)
Solution, ophthalmic (Quixen™): 0.5% (5 mL) [contains benzalkonium chloride]
Tablet (Levaquin®): 250 mg, 500 mg, 750 mg

Dosing

Adults & Elderly:

Acute bacterial exacerbation of chronic bronchitis: Oral, I.V.: 500 mg every 24 hours for at least 7 days
Nosocomial pneumonia: Oral, I.V.: 750 mg every 24 hours for 7-14 days
Community-acquired pneumonia: Oral, I.V.: 500 mg every 24 hours for 7-14 days
Acute maxillary sinusitis: Oral, I.V.: 500 mg every 24 hours for 10-14 days
Uncomplicated skin infections: Oral, I.V.: 500 mg every 24 hours for 7-10 days
Complicated skin infections: Oral, I.V.: 750 mg every 24 hours for 7-14 days
Uncomplicated urinary tract infections: Oral, I.V.: 250 mg once daily for 3 days
Complicated urinary tract infections, including acute pyelonephritis: Oral, I.V.: 250 mg every 24 hours for 10 days
Conjunctivitis (bacterial): Ophthalmic:
Treatment day 1 and day 2: Instill 1-2 drops into affected eye(s) every 2 hours while awake, up to 8 times/day
Treatment day 3 through day 7: Instill 1-2 drops into affected eye(s) every 4 hours while awake, up to 4 times/day

Pediatrics: Not for systemic use.
Conjunctivitis (bacterial): Ophthalmic: Children ≥1 year: Refer to adult dosing.

Renal Impairment:

Chronic bronchitis, acute maxillary sinusitis, uncomplicated skin infection, community-acquired pneumonia:
Cl_{cr} 20-49 mL/minute: Administer 250 mg every 24 hours (initial: 500 mg)
Cl_{cr} 10-19 mL/minute: Administer 250 mg every 48 hours (initial: 500 mg)
Complicated UTI, acute pyelonephritis:
Cl_{cr} 20-49 mL/minute: No dosage adjustment required required
Cl_{cr} 10-19 mL/minute: Administer 250 mg every 48 hours
Uncomplicated UTI: No dosage adjustment required
Complicated skin infection or nosocomial pneumonia:
Cl_{cr} 20-49 mL/minute: Administer 750 mg every 48 hours mg
Cl_{cr} 10-19 mL/minute: Administer 500 mg every 48 hours (initial: 750 mg)
Hemodialysis/CAPD: 250 mg every 48 hours (initial: 500 mg for most infections; initial: 750 mg for complicated skin/soft tissue infections followed by 500 mg every 48 hours)

Administration

Oral: May be administered without regard to meals.

I.V.: Infuse I.V. solution over 60 minutes. Too rapid of infusion can lead to hypotension. Avoid administration through an intravenous line with a solution containing multivalent cations (ie, magnesium, calcium).

Stability

Storage: Stable for 72 hours when diluted to 5 mg/mL in a compatible I.V. fluid and stored at room temperature. Stable for 14 days when stored under refrigeration. Stable for 6 months when frozen; do not refreeze. Do not thaw in microwave or by bath immersion. Ophthalmic solution should be stored at 15°C to 25°C (59°F to 77°F).

Compatibility: Stable in D_5LR, D_5NS, D_5W, NS; **incompatible** with mannitol 20%, sodium bicarbonate 5%

Y-site administration: Incompatible with acyclovir, alprostadil, furosemide, heparin, indomethacin, nitroglycerin, sodium nitroprusside

Monitoring Laboratory Tests Perform culture and sensitivity studies prior to initiating drug therapy. Monitor CBC periodically during therapy. Monitor renal or hepatic function if therapy is prolonged.

Monitoring and Teaching Issues

Physical Assessment: Assess allergy history before initiating therapy. See Contraindications, Warnings/Precautions, and Dosing for use cautions. Assess potential for interactions with other prescriptions, OTC medications, or herbal products patient may be taking (see Drug Interactions). **I.V.:** See specifics above and monitor closely for severe hypersensitivity reactions, including anaphylaxis. If an allergic reaction occurs drug should be discontinued immediately. Assess results of laboratory tests (see above), therapeutic effectiveness, and adverse effects (eg, hypersensitivity reactions can occur days after therapy has started - see Adverse Reactions and Overdose/Toxicology) regularly during therapy. Teach patient appropriate use (according to formulation), possible side effects and interventions, and adverse symptoms to report (see Patient Education). **Pregnancy risk factor C** - benefits of use should outweigh possible risks. Breast-feeding is contraindicated.

Patient Education: Inform prescriber of all prescriptions, OTC medications, or herbal products you are taking, and any allergies you have. Do not take anything new during treatment unless approved by prescriber. Take exactly as directed; at least 2 hours before or 2 hours after antacids or other drug products containing calcium, iron, or zinc. Take entire prescription even if feeling better. Maintain adequate hydration (2-3 L/day of fluids) unless advised by prescriber to restrict fluid intake. You may experience dizziness, lightheadedness, or confusion (use caution when driving or engaging in tasks that require alertness until response to drug is known); nausea or vomiting (small, frequent meals, frequent mouth care, sucking lozenges, or chewing gum may help); or photosensitivity (use sunscreen, wear protective clothing and eyewear, and avoid direct sunlight). If signs of inflammation or tendon pain occur, discontinue use immediately and report to prescriber. If allergic reaction occurs (itching, urticaria, difficulty breathing, facial edema, difficulty swallowing, loss of consciousness, tingling, chest pain, palpitations), discontinue use immediately and report to prescriber. Report persistent diarrhea or constipation; signs of infection (unusual fever or chills); vaginal itching or foul-smelling vaginal discharge; or easy bruising or bleeding. **Pregnancy/breast-feeding precautions:** Inform prescriber if you are or intend to become pregnant. Do not breast-feed.

Ophthalmic: Wash hands before instilling solution. Sit or lie down to instill. Open eye, look at ceiling, and instill prescribed amount of solution. Close eye and roll eye in all directions, and apply gentle pressure to inner corner of eye. Do not let tip of applicator touch eye; do not contaminate tip of applicator (may cause eye infection, eye damage, or vision loss). Temporary stinging or blurred vision may occur. Report persistent pain, burning, vision changes, swelling, itching, or worsening of condition. Discontinue medication and contact prescriber immediately if you develop a rash or allergic reaction. Do not wear contact lenses.

Dietary Issues: May be taken without regard to meals.

Geriatric Considerations: Expanded spectra and once daily dosing. Adjust dose for renal function.

Breast-feeding Issues: Quinolones are known to distribute well into breast milk; consequently, use during lactation should be avoided, if possible.

Additional Information Ophthalmic solution contains benzalkonium chloride 0.005% as a preservative.

Related Information

Tuberculosis *on page 1705*

Levonorgestrel (LEE voe nor jes trel)

U.S. Brand Names Mirena®; Norplant® Implant [DSC]; Plan B®

Synonyms LNg 20

Generic Available No

Pharmacologic Category Contraceptive

Pregnancy Risk Factor X

Lactation Enters breast milk/use caution (AAP rates "compatible")

Use Prevention of pregnancy

Mechanism of Action/Effect Ovulation is inhibited and an insufficient luteal phase has also been demonstrated with levonorgestrel administration.

Contraindications Hypersensitivity to levonorgestrel or any component of the formulation; undiagnosed abnormal uterine bleeding, active hepatic disease or malignant tumors, active thrombophlebitis, or thromboembolic disorders (current or history of), known or suspected carcinoma of the breast; history of intracranial hypertension; renal impairment; pregnancy

Additional product-specific contraindications: Intrauterine system: Congenital or acquired uterine anomaly, acute pelvic inflammatory disease, history of pelvic inflammatory disease (unless there has been a subsequent intrauterine pregnancy), postpartum endometritis, infected abortion within past 3 months, known or suspected uterine or cervical neoplasia, unresolved/abnormal Pap smear, untreated acute cervicitis or vaginitis, patient or partner with multiple sexual partners, conditions which increase susceptibility to infections (ie, leukemia, AIDS, I.V. drug abuse), unremoved IUD, history of ectopic pregnancy, conditions which predispose to ectopic pregnancy

Warnings/Precautions Menstrual bleeding patterns may be altered, missed menstrual periods should not be used to identify early pregnancy. These products do not protect against HIV infection or other sexually-transmitted diseases. Patients presenting with lower abdominal pain should be evaluated for follicular atresia and ectopic pregnancy. Patients receiving enzyme-inducing medications should be evaluated for an alternative method of contraception. Levonorgestrel may affect glucose tolerance, monitor serum glucose in patients with diabetes. Safety and efficacy for use in renal or hepatic impairment have not been established. Use with caution in conditions that may be aggravated by fluid retention, depression, or history of migraine. Only for use in women of reproductive age.

Use of combination hormonal contraceptives increases the risk of cardiovascular side effects in women who smoke cigarettes, especially those who are >35 years of age; although this may be an estrogen-related effect, the risk with progestin-only contraceptives is not known and women should be strongly advised not to smoke. Combination hormonal contraceptives may lead to increased risk of myocardial infarction and should be used with caution in patients with risk factors for coronary artery disease; the actual risk with progestin-only contraceptives is not known, however, there have been postmarketing reports of myocardial infarction in women using levonorgestrel-only contraception. May increase the risk of thromboembolism; discontinue therapy if this occurs. Combination hormonal contraceptives may have a dose-related risk of vascular disease and hypertension; strokes have also been reported with postmarketing use of levonorgestrel-only contraception. Women with hypertension should be encouraged to use a nonhormonal form of contraception. The use of combination hormonal contraceptives has been associated with a slight increase in frequency of breast cancer (studies are not consistent); studies with progestin only contraceptives have been similar. Retinal thrombosis has been reported (rarely) with combination hormonal contraceptives and may be related to the estrogen component, however, progestin-only therapy should also be discontinued with unexplained partial or complete loss of vision.

Additional formulation-specific warnings:

Intrauterine system: Increased incidence of group A streptococcal sepsis and pelvic inflammatory disease (may be asymptomatic); may perforate uterus or cervix; risk of perforation is increased in lactating women; partial penetration or embedment in the myometrium may decrease effectiveness and lead to difficult removal; postpartum insertion should be delayed

(Continued)

Levonorgestrel *(Continued)*

until uterine involution is complete; use caution in patients with coagulopathy or receiving anticoagulants

Oral tablet: Not intended to be used for routine contraception and will not terminate an existing pregnancy

Subdermal capsules: Insertion-related complications may occur; expulsion of capsules, capsule displacement, thrombophlebitis, and superficial phlebitis have been reported. Insertion and removal are surgical procedures. To decrease risk of thromboembolic disease, consider removing capsules with prolonged immobilization. Idiopathic intracranial hypertension has been reported and may be more likely to occur in obese females.

Drug Interactions

Cytochrome P450 Effect: Substrate of **CYP3A4**

Decreased Effect: Enzyme inducers: May increase the metabolism of levonorgestrel resulting in decreased effect; includes carbamazepine, phenobarbital, phenytoin, and rifampin; additional contraceptive measures may be needed with use of enzyme inducers or following their withdrawal

Nutritional/Ethanol Interactions Herb/Nutraceutical: St John's wort (an enzyme inducer) may decrease serum levels of levonorgestrel.

Effects on Lab Values ↑ triiodothyronine uptake; ↓ concentrations of sex hormone-binding globulin, thyroxine concentrations (slight)

Adverse Reactions

Intrauterine system:

>5%:

Cardiovascular: Hypertension

Central nervous system: Headache, depression, nervousness

Dermatologic: Acne

Endocrine & metabolic: Breast pain, dysmenorrhea, decreased libido, abnormal Pap smear, amenorrhea (20% at 1 year), enlarged follicles (12%)

Gastrointestinal: Abdominal pain, nausea, weight gain

Genitourinary: Leukorrhea, vaginitis

Neuromuscular & skeletal: Back pain

Respiratory: Upper respiratory tract infection, sinusitis

<3%: Alopecia, anemia, cervicitis, dyspareunia, eczema, failed insertion, migraine, sepsis, vomiting

Oral tablets:

>10%:

Central nervous system: Fatigue (17%), headache (17%), dizziness (11%)

Endocrine & metabolic: Heavier menstrual bleeding (14%), lighter menstrual bleeding (12%), breast tenderness (11%)

Gastrointestinal: Nausea (23%), abdominal pain (18%),

1% to 10%: Gastrointestinal: Vomiting (6%), diarrhea (5%)

Subdermal capsules:

>10%: Endocrine & metabolic: Increased/prolonged bleeding (28%), spotting (17%)

1% to 10%:

Endocrine & metabolic: Breast discharge (≥5%), menstrual irregularities

Gastrointestinal: Abdominal discomfort (≥5%)

Genitourinary: Cervicitis (≥5%), leukorrhea (≥5%), vaginitis (≥5%)

Local: Pain/itching at implant site (4%, usually transient)

Neuromuscular & skeletal: Musculoskeletal pain (≥5%)

Miscellaneous: Removal difficulties (6%); these may include multiple incisions, remaining capsule fragments, pain, multiple visits, deep placement, lengthy procedure

<1% (Limited to important or life-threatening): Alopecia, breast cancer, deep vein thrombosis, emotional lability, hirsutism, hyperpigmentation, idiopathic intracranial hypertension, infection at implant site, myocardial infarction, pulmonary embolism, rash, stroke, superficial venous thrombosis, thrombotic thrombocytopenic purpura (TTP), urticaria, vomiting

Overdosage/Toxicology Can result if >6 capsules are *in situ*. Symptoms include uterine bleeding irregularities and fluid retention. Treatment includes removal of all implanted capsules.

Pharmacodynamics/Kinetics

Absorption: Rapid and complete

Bioavailability: 100%

Half-Life Elimination: Oral tablet: ~24 hours

Metabolism: To inactive metabolites

Duration: Subdermal capsules/intrauterine system: Up to 5 years

Formulations

Implant, subdermal capsule (Norplant® [DSC]): 36 mg (6s)

Intrauterine device (Mirena®): 52 mg levonorgestrel/unit

Tablet (Plan B®): 0.75 mg

Dosing

Adults & Elderly:

Long-term prevention of pregnancy:

Subdermal capsules (Norplant®): Total administration doses (implanted): 216 mg in 6 capsules which should be implanted during the first 7 days of onset of menses subdermally in the upper arm. Each Norplant® silastic capsule releases 80 mcg of levonorgestrel/day for 6-18 months, following which a rate of release of 25-30 mcg/day is maintained for ≤5 years. Capsules should be removed by end of 5th year.

Intrauterine system (Mirena®): To be inserted into uterine cavity; should be inserted within 7 days of onset of menstruation or immediately after 1st trimester abortion. Releases 20 mcg levonorgestrel/day over 5 years. May be removed and replaced with a new unit at anytime during menstrual cycle. Do not leave any one system in place for >5 years.

Emergency contraception: Oral tablet (Plan B™): One 0.75 mg tablet as soon as possible within 72 hours of unprotected sexual intercourse. A second 0.75 mg tablet should be taken 12 hours after the first dose; may be used at any time during menstrual cycle.

Administration

Other:

Intrauterine system: Inserted in the uterine cavity, to a depth of 6-9 cm, with the provided insertion device; should not be forced into the uterus

Subdermal capsules: Six capsules are subdermally inserted to the medial aspect of the upper arm (under local anesthetic). Capsules are inserted in a fanlike manner, ~8-10 cm above the elbow crease, with the instruments provided. Prior to removal, palpate the area to locate all 6 capsules. The removal may take more time and may be more painful than the insertion.

Stability

Storage: Store at room temperature of 25°C (77°F).

Monitoring and Teaching Issues

Physical Assessment: Monitor for prolonged menstrual bleeding, amenorrhea, irregularity of menses, and other adverse effects (see Adverse Reactions). Caution patient about need for annual medical exams. **Pregnancy risk factor X** - determine pregnancy status before inserting Norplant®. Note breast-feeding caution.

Patient Education: This drug does not protect against HIV infection or other sexually-transmitted diseases. Cigarette smoking is not recommended. You may experience cramping, headache, abdominal discomfort, hair loss, weight changes, or unusual menses (breakthrough bleeding, irregularity, excessive bleeding). Report sudden acute headache or visual disturbance, unusual nausea or vomiting, any loss of feeling in arms or legs, or lower abdominal pain. **Pregnancy/breast-feeding precautions:** Inform prescriber if you are pregnant. Consult prescriber if breast-feeding.

Intrauterine system: This method provides up to 5 years of birth control from a T-shaped device inserted into the uterus. It will be inserted and removed by your prescriber. Notify your prescriber if the system comes out by itself, if you have long-lasting or heavy bleeding, unusual vaginal discharge, low abdominal pain, painful sexual intercourse, chills or fever. There is an increased risk of ectopic pregnancy with this product. Thread placement should be checked following each menstrual cycle; do not pull thread.

Tablet: This method provides emergency contraception. It is used after your normal form of birth control has failed, or following unprotected sexual intercourse. It should be used within 72 hours. Contact prescriber if you vomit within 1 hour of taking either dose.

Subdermal capsules: This method consists of 6 capsules, which will be placed under the skin, on the inside of your upper arm. They can provide up to 5 years of birth control. The capsules must be inserted and removed by your prescriber, do not attempt to remove implants yourself. Following insertion, keep area dry and avoid heavy lifting for 2-3 days. Report irritation at insertion site.

Breast-feeding Issues: Enters breast milk (infant serum levels of ~7% have been found when using the intrauterine system, 1% to 6% with the oral tablets), use caution; not considered contraception method of first choice for breast-feeding women (AAP considers **compatible** with breast-feeding)

Pregnancy Issues: Epidemiologic studies have not shown an increased risk of birth defects when used prior to pregnancy or inadvertently during early pregnancy, although rare reports of congenital anomalies have been reported.

Intrauterine system: Women who become pregnant with an IUD in place risk septic abortion (septic shock and death may occur), removal of IUD may result in pregnancy loss. In addition, miscarriage, premature labor, and premature delivery may occur if pregnancy is continued with IUD in place.

Additional Information

Intrauterine system: The cumulative 5-year pregnancy rate is ~0.7 pregnancies/100 users. Over 70% of women in the trials had previously used IUDs. The reported pregnancy rate after 12 months was ≤0.2 pregnancies/100 users. Approximately 80% of women who wish to conceive have become pregnant within 12 months of device removal. The recommended patient profile for this product: A woman who has at least one child, is in a stable and mutually-monogamous relationship, no history of pelvic inflammatory disease, and no history of ectopic pregnancy or predisposition to ectopic pregnancy.

Oral tablet: When used as directed for emergency contraception, the expected pregnancy rate is decreased from 8% to 1%. Approximately 87% of women have their next menstrual period at approximately the expected time. A rapid return to fertility following use is expected.

Subdermal capsules: The net cumulative 5-year pregnancy rate for levonorgestrel implant use has been reported to be from 1.5-3.9 pregnancies/100 users. This compares to a cumulative rate of 4.9 pregnancies/100 women with an IUD after 5 years. At the end of the first year of use, the pregnancy rate with levonorgestrel implants has been reported to be from 0.2-0.6 pregnancies/100 users. This compares quite favorably with the 2.3 pregnancies/100 users of oral contraceptives during the first year of use and 2.4 pregnancies/100 women with an IUD during the first year. Norplant® is a very efficient, yet reversible, method of contraception. The long duration of action may be particularly advantageous in women who desire an extended period of contraceptive protection without sacrificing the possibility of future fertility.

Levonorgestrel and Ethinyl Estradiol *see* Ethinyl Estradiol and Levonorgestrel *on page 523*

Levophed® *see* Norepinephrine *on page 983*

Levora® *see* Ethinyl Estradiol and Levonorgestrel *on page 523*

Levorphanol (lee VOR fa nole)

U.S. Brand Names Levo-Dromoran®

Synonyms Levorphanol Tartrate; Levorphan Tartrate

Restrictions C-II

Generic Available Yes: Tablet

(Continued)

Levorphanol *(Continued)*

Pharmacologic Category Analgesic, Narcotic

Pregnancy Risk Factor B/D (prolonged use or high doses at term)

Lactation Excretion in breast milk unknown/not recommended

Use Relief of moderate to severe pain, also used parenterally for preoperative sedation and an adjunct to nitrous oxide/oxygen anesthesia; 2 mg levorphanol produces analgesia comparable to that produced by 10 mg of morphine

Mechanism of Action/Effect Levorphanol tartrate is a synthetic opioid agonist that is classified as a morphinan derivative. Opioids interact with stereospecific opioid receptors in various parts of the central nervous system and other tissues.

Contraindications Hypersensitivity to levorphanol or any component of the formulation; pregnancy B/D (prolonged use or high doses at term)

Warnings/Precautions Use with caution in patients with hypersensitivity reactions to other phenanthrene derivative opioid agonists (morphine, hydrocodone, hydromorphone, levorphanol, oxycodone, oxymorphone); respiratory diseases including asthma, emphysema, COPD, or severe liver or renal insufficiency. Some preparations contain sulfites which may cause allergic reactions. May be habit-forming. Dextromethorphan has equivalent antitussive activity but has much lower toxicity in accidental overdose. Elderly may be particularly susceptible to the CNS depressant and constipating effects of narcotics.

Drug Interactions

Increased Effect/Toxicity: CNS depression is enhanced with coadministration of other CNS depressants.

Nutritional/Ethanol Interactions

Ethanol: Avoid or limit ethanol (may increase CNS depression). Watch for sedation.

Herb/Nutraceutical: Avoid valerian, St John's wort, kava kava, gotu kola (may increase CNS depression).

Adverse Reactions Frequency not defined.

Cardiovascular: Palpitations, hypotension, bradycardia, peripheral vasodilation, cardiac arrest, shock, tachycardia

Central nervous system: CNS depression, fatigue, drowsiness, dizziness, nervousness, headache, restlessness, anorexia, malaise, confusion, coma, convulsion, insomnia, amnesia, mental depression, hallucinations, paradoxical CNS stimulation, intracranial pressure (increased),

Dermatologic: Pruritus, urticaria, rash

Endocrine & metabolic: Antidiuretic hormone release

Gastrointestinal: Nausea, vomiting, dyspepsia, stomach cramps, xerostomia, constipation, abdominal pain, dry mouth, biliary tract spasm, paralytic ileus

Genitourinary: Decreased urination, urinary tract spasm, urinary retention

Local: Pain at injection site

Neuromuscular & skeletal: Weakness

Ocular: Miosis, diplopia

Respiratory: Respiratory depression, apnea, hypoventilation, cyanosis

Miscellaneous: Histamine release, physical and psychological dependence

Overdosage/Toxicology Symptoms of overdose include CNS depression, respiratory depression, miosis, apnea, pulmonary edema, and convulsions. Naloxone, 2 mg I.V. with repeat administration as necessary up to a total dose of 10 mg, can be used to reverse opiate effects.

Pharmacodynamics/Kinetics

Half-Life Elimination: 11-16 hours

Metabolism: Hepatic

Onset: Oral: 10-60 minutes

Duration: 4-8 hours

Formulations

Injection, solution, as tartrate: 2 mg/mL (1 mL, 10 mL)

Tablet, as tartrate: 2 mg

Dosing

Adults & Elderly: Analgesia/sedation:

Oral: 2 mg every 6-24 hours as needed

S.C.: 2 mg, up to 3 mg if necessary, every 6-8 hours

I.V.: Not recommended (if no alternative; dilute to 10 mL with NS and inject no faster than 1 mg/min)

Hepatic Impairment: Reduce dose in patients with liver disease.

Administration

Oral: For lactating women, administer 4-6 hours prior to breast-feeding.

I.V.: Inject 3 mg over 4-5 minutes

Stability

Storage: Store at room temperature. Protect from freezing.

Compatibility: when admixed: Incompatible with aminophylline, ammonium chloride, amobarbital, chlorothiazide, heparin, pentobarbital, phenobarbital, phenytoin, sodium bicarbonate, thiopental

Monitoring and Teaching Issues

Physical Assessment: Assess other medications patient may be taking for additive or adverse interactions (see Drug Interactions). Monitor therapeutic effectiveness, adverse reactions and signs of overdose (see Overdose/Toxicology). Monitor vital signs, CNS and respiratory status, at beginning of therapy and at regular intervals with long-term use. May cause physical and/or psychological dependence. Safety measures required for inpatients. Assess knowledge/teach patient appropriate use (if self-administered). Teach patient to monitor for adverse reactions (see Adverse Reactions), adverse reactions to report, and appropriate interventions to reduce side effects. Discontinue slowly after prolonged use. **Pregnancy risk factor B/D** - see Pregnancy Risk Factor for use cautions. Breast-feeding is not recommended.

Patient Education: If self-administered, use exactly as directed; do not increase dose or frequency. Drug may cause physical and/or psychological dependence. While using this medication, do not use alcohol and other prescription or OTC medications (especially sedatives, tranquilizers, antihistamines, or pain medications) without consulting prescriber. Maintain adequate hydration (2-3 L/day of fluids) unless advised by prescriber to restrict fluids. May cause hypotension, dizziness, drowsiness, impaired coordination, or blurred vision (use caution when driving, climbing stairs, or changing position - rising from sitting or lying to standing, or when engaging in tasks requiring alertness until response to drug is known); loss of appetite, nausea, or vomiting (frequent mouth care, small, frequent meals, chewing gum, or sucking lozenges may help); or constipation (increased exercise, fluids, fruit, or fiber may help; if unresolved, consult prescriber about use of stool softeners). Report chest pain, slow or rapid heartbeat, acute dizziness, or persistent headache; swelling of extremities or unusual weight gain; changes in urinary elimination; acute headache; back or flank pain or spasms; blurred vision; skin rash; or shortness of breath. **Pregnancy/breast-feeding precautions:** Inform prescriber if you are or intend to become pregnant. Breast-feeding is not recommended.

Geriatric Considerations: The elderly may be particularly susceptible to the CNS depressant and constipating effects of narcotics.

Related Information

Narcotic/Opioid Analgesic Comparison *on page 1583*

Levorphanol Tartrate *see* Levorphanol *on page 795*

Levorphan Tartrate *see* Levorphanol *on page 795*

Levothroid® *see* Levothyroxine *on page 797*

Levothyroxine (lee voe thye ROKS een)

U.S. Brand Names Levothroid®; Levoxyl®; Novothyrox; Synthroid®; Unithroid®

Synonyms Levothyroxine Sodium; *L*-Thyroxine Sodium; T_4

Generic Available Yes: Injection

Pharmacologic Category Thyroid Product

Pregnancy Risk Factor A

Lactation Enters breast milk/compatible

Use Replacement or supplemental therapy in hypothyroidism; pituitary TSH suppression

Mechanism of Action/Effect It is believed the thyroid hormone exerts its many metabolic effects through control of DNA transcription and protein synthesis

Contraindications Hypersensitivity to levothyroxine sodium or any component of the formulation; recent MI or thyrotoxicosis; uncorrected adrenal insufficiency

Warnings/Precautions Ineffective and potentially toxic for weight reduction. High doses may produce serious or even life-threatening toxic effects particularly when used with some anorectic drugs. Use with caution and reduce dosage in patients with angina pectoris or other cardiovascular disease. Use cautiously in the elderly since they may be more likely to have compromised cardiovascular functions. Patients with adrenal insufficiency, myxedema, diabetes mellitus and insipidus may have symptoms exaggerated or aggravated. Thyroid replacement requires periodic assessment of thyroid status. Chronic hypothyroidism predisposes patients to coronary artery disease.

Drug Interactions

Decreased Effect: Also refer to Additional Information. Some medications may decrease absorption of levothyroxine: Cholestyramine, colestipol (separate administration by at least 2 hours); aluminum- and magnesium-containing antacids, iron preparations, sucralfate, Kayexalate® (separate administration by at least 4 hours). Enzyme inducers (phenytoin, phenobarbital, carbamazepine, and rifampin/rifabutin) may decrease levothyroxine levels. Levothyroxine may decrease effect of oral sulfonylureas. Serum levels of digoxin and theophylline may be altered by thyroid function. Estrogens may decrease serum free-thyroxine concentrations.

Increased Effect/Toxicity: Also refer to Additional Information. Levothyroxine may potentiate the hypoprothrombinemic effect of warfarin (and other oral anticoagulants). Tricyclic antidepressants (TCAs) coadministered with levothyroxine may increase potential for toxicity of both drugs. Coadministration with ketamine may lead to hypertension and tachycardia.

Nutritional/Ethanol Interactions Food: Taking levothyroxine with enteral nutrition may cause reduced bioavailability and may lower serum thyroxine levels leading to signs or symptoms of hypothyroidism. Limit intake of goitrogenic foods (eg, asparagus, cabbage, peas, turnip greens, broccoli, spinach, Brussels sprouts, lettuce, soybeans). Soybean flour (infant formula), cottonseed meal, walnuts, and dietary fiber may decrease absorption of levothyroxine from the GI tract.

Effects on Lab Values Many drugs may have effects on thyroid function tests: para-aminosalicylic acid, aminoglutethimide, amiodarone, barbiturates, carbamazepine, chloral hydrate, clofibrate, colestipol, corticosteroids, danazol, diazepam, estrogens, ethionamide, fluorouracil, I.V. heparin, insulin, lithium, methadone, methimazole, mitotane, nitroprusside, oxyphenbutazone, phenylbutazone, PTU, perphenazine, phenytoin, propranolol, salicylates, sulfonylureas, and thiazides.

Adverse Reactions Frequency not defined.

Cardiovascular: Angina, arrhythmias, blood pressure increased, cardiac arrest, flushing, heart failure, MI, palpitations, pulse increased, tachycardia

Central nervous system: Anxiety, emotional lability, fatigue, fever, headache, hyperactivity, insomnia, irritability, nervousness, pseudotumor cerebri (children), seizures (rare)

Dermatologic: Alopecia

Endocrine & metabolic: Fertility impaired, menstrual irregularities

Gastrointestinal: Abdominal cramps, appetite increased, diarrhea, vomiting, weight loss

Hepatic: Liver function tests increased

Neuromuscular & skeletal: Bone mineral density decreased, muscle weakness, tremors, slipped capital femoral epiphysis (children)

Respiratory: Dyspnea

(Continued)

Levothyroxine *(Continued)*

Miscellaneous: Diaphoresis, heat intolerance, hypersensitivity (to inactive ingredients, symptoms include urticaria, pruritus, rash, flushing, angioedema, GI symptoms, fever, arthralgia, serum sickness, wheezing)

Overdosage/Toxicology

Chronic: Chronic overdose may cause hyperthyroidism, weight loss, nervousness, sweating, tachycardia, insomnia, heat intolerance, menstrual irregularities, palpitations, psychosis, and fever. Overtreatment of children may result in premature closure of epiphyses or craniosynostosis (infants). Reduce dose or temporarily discontinue therapy. Hypothalamic-pituitary-thyroid axis will return to normal in 6-8 weeks. Serum T_4 levels do not correlate well with toxicity. Provide general supportive care

Acute: Acute overdose may cause fever, hypoglycemia, CHF, and unrecognized adrenal insufficiency. Acute massive overdose may be life-threatening; treatment should be symptomatic and supportive. Massive overdose may be a require beta-blockers for increased sympathomimetic activity.

Pharmacodynamics/Kinetics

Absorption: Oral: Erratic (40% to 80%); decreases with age

Half-Life Elimination: Euthyroid: 6-7 days; Hypothyroid: 9-10 days; Hyperthyroid: 3-4 days

Time to Peak: Serum: 2-4 hours

Metabolism: Hepatic to triiodothyronine (active)

Onset: Therapeutic: Oral: 3-5 days; I.V. 6-8 hours; Peak effect: I.V.: ~24 hours

Formulations

Injection, powder for reconstitution, as sodium (Synthroid®): 0.2 mg, 0.5 mg

Tablet, as sodium:

Levothroid®, Levoxyl®, Synthroid®: 25 mcg, 50 mcg, 75 mcg, 88 mcg, 100 mcg, 112 mcg, 125 mcg, 137 mcg, 150 mcg, 175 mcg, 200 mcg, 300 mcg

Novothyrox: 25 mcg, 50 mcg, 75 mcg, 88 mcg, 100 mcg, 112 mcg, 125 mcg, 137 mcg, 150 mcg, 175 mcg, 200 mcg, 300 mcg [dye free]

Unithroid®: 25 mcg, 50 mcg, 75 mcg, 88 mcg, 100 mcg, 112 mcg, 125 mcg, 150 mcg, 175 mcg, 200 mcg, 300 mcg

Dosing

Adults: Doses should be adjusted based on clinical response and laboratory parameters.

Hypothyroidism:

Oral: 1.7 mcg/kg/day in otherwise healthy adults <50 years old, children in whom growth and puberty are complete, and older adults who have been recently treated for hyperthyroidism or who have been hypothyroid for only a few months. Titrate dose every 6 weeks. Average starting dose ~100 mcg; usual doses are ≤200 mcg/day; doses ≥300 mcg/day are rare (consider poor compliance, malabsorption, and/or drug interactions). **Note:** For patients >50 years or patients with cardiac disease, refer to elderly dosing.

I.M., I.V.: 50% of the oral dose

Severe hypothyroidism: Oral: Initial: 12.5-25 mcg/day; adjust dose by 25 mcg/day every 2-4 weeks as appropriate

Subclinical hypothyroidism (if treated): Oral: 1 mcg/kg/day

TSH suppression: Oral:

Well-differentiated thyroid cancer: Highly individualized; Doses >2 mcg/kg/day may be needed to suppress TSH to <0.1 mU/L.

Benign nodules and nontoxic multinodular goiter: Goal TSH suppression: 0.1-0.3 mU/L

Myxedema coma or stupor: I.V.: 200-500 mcg, then 100-300 mcg the next day if necessary; smaller doses should be considered in patients with cardiovascular disease

Elderly: Doses should be adjusted based on clinical response and laboratory parameters.

Hypothyroidism:

Oral:

>50 years without cardiac disease **or** <50 years with cardiac disease: Initial: 25-50 mcg/day; adjust dose at 6- to 8-week intervals as needed

>50 years with cardiac disease: Initial: 12.5-25 mcg/day; adjust dose by 12.5-25 mcg increments at 4- to 6-week intervals

Note: Elderly patients may require <1 mcg/kg/day

I.M., I.V.: 50% of the oral dose

Myxedema coma: I.V.: Refer to adult dosing; lower doses may be needed

Pediatrics: Doses should be adjusted based on clinical response and laboratory parameters.

Hypothyroidism:

Oral:

Newborns: Initial: 10-15 mcg/kg/day. Lower doses of 25 mcg/day should be considered in newborns at risk for cardiac failure. Newborns with T_4 levels <5 mcg/dL should be started at 50 mcg/day. Adjust dose at 4- to 6-week intervals.

Infants and Children: Dose based on body weight and age as listed below. Children with severe or chronic hypothyroidism should be started at 25 mcg/day; adjust dose by 25 mcg every 2-4 weeks. In older children, hyperactivity may be decreased by starting with 1/4 of the recommended dose and increasing by 1/4 dose each week until the full replacement dose is reached. Refer to adult dosing once growth and puberty are complete.

0-3 months: 10-15 mcg/kg/day
3-6 months: 8-10 mcg/kg/day
6-12 months: 6-8 mcg/kg/day
1-5 years: 5-6 mcg/kg/day
6-12 years: 4-5 mcg/kg/day
12 years: 2-3 mcg/kg/day

I.M., I.V.: 50% of the oral dose

Administration

Oral: Administer in the morning on an empty stomach, at least 30 minutes before food. Tablets may be crushed and suspended in 1-2 teaspoonfuls of water; suspension should be used immediately.

I.V.: Dilute vial with 5 mL normal saline; use immediately after reconstitution; do not mix with other IV fluids

Stability

Storage: Store tablets and injection at room temperature of 15°C to 30°C (59°F to 86°F). Protect tablets from light and moisture.

Reconstitution: Dilute vial with 5 mL normal saline. Shake well and use immediately after reconstitution; discard any unused portions.

Compatibility: Do not mix I.V. solution with other I.V. infusion solutions.

Monitoring Laboratory Tests Thyroid function (serum thyroxine, thyrotropin concentrations), resin triiodothyronine uptake (RT_3U), free thyroxine index (FTI), T_4, TSH, TSH may be elevated during the first few months of thyroid replacement despite patients being clinically euthyroid. In cases where T_4 remains low and TSH is within normal limits, an evaluation of "free" (unbound) T_4 is needed to evaluate further increase in dosage.

Monitoring and Teaching Issues

Physical Assessment: See Contraindications, Warnings/Precautions, and Dosing for use cautions. Assess potential for interactions with other prescriptions, OTC medications, or herbal products patient may be taking (eg, high doses may produce serious or even life-threatening toxic effects particularly when used with some anorectic drugs - see extensive list of Drug Interactions). See I.V. Administration. Assess results of laboratory tests (see above) and adverse effects (eg, hypo/hyperthyroidism - see Adverse Reactions and Overdose/Toxicology) regularly during therapy. **Important:** Many drugs may have effects on thyroid function tests (see Effects on Lab Values) when assessing results of thyroid function tests. Teach patient appropriate use, possible side effects and interventions, and adverse symptoms to report (see Patient Education).

Patient Education: Inform prescriber of all prescriptions, OTC medications, or herbal products you are taking, and any allergies you have. Do not take anything new during treatment unless approved by prescriber. Thyroid replacement therapy is generally for life. Take as directed, in the morning before breakfast. Do not take antacids or iron preparations within 8 hours of thyroid medication. Do not change brands and do not discontinue without consulting prescriber. Consult prescriber if drastically increasing or decreasing intake of goitrogenic food (eg, asparagus, cabbage, peas, turnip greens, broccoli, spinach, Brussels sprouts, lettuce, soybeans). Report chest pain, rapid heart rate, palpitations, heat intolerance, excessive sweating, increased nervousness, agitation, or lethargy.

Dietary Issues: Should be taken on an empty stomach, at least 30 minutes before food.

Geriatric Considerations: The elderly do not have a change in serum thyroxine (T_4) associated with aging; however, plasma T_3 concentrations are decreased 25% to 40% in the elderly. There is not a compensatory rise in thyrotropin suggesting that lower T_3 is not reacted upon as a deficiency by the pituitary. This indicates a slightly lower than normal dosage of thyroid hormone replacement is usually sufficient in older patients than in younger adult patients. TSH must be monitored since insufficient thyroid replacement (elevated TSH) is a risk for coronary artery disease and excessive replacement (low TSH) may cause signs of hyperthyroidism and excessive bone loss. Some clinicians suggest levothyroxine is the drug of choice for replacement therapy.

Breast-feeding Issues: Minimally excreted in human milk; adequate levels are needed to maintain normal lactation

Pregnancy Issues: Untreated maternal hypothyroidism may have adverse effects on fetal growth and development and is associated with higher rate of complications (spontaneous abortion, pre-eclampsia, stillbirth, premature delivery). Treatment should not be discontinued during pregnancy. TSH levels should be monitored during each trimester and 6-8 weeks postpartum. Increased doses may be needed during pregnancy.

Additional Information Equivalent doses: Thyroid USP 60 mg ~ levothyroxine 0.05-0.06 mg ~ liothyronine 0.015-0.0375 mg

50-60 mg thyroid ~ 50-60 mcg levothyroxine and 12.5-15 mcg liothyronine Liotrix®

Note: Several medications have effects on thyroid production or conversion. The impact in thyroid replacement has not been specifically evaluated, but patient response should be monitored:

Methimazole: Decreases thyroid hormone secretion, while propylthiouracil decrease thyroid hormone secretion and decreases conversion of T_4 to T_3.

Beta-adrenergic antagonists: Decrease conversion of T_4 to T_3 (dose related, propranolol ≥160 mg/day); patients may be clinically euthyroid.

Iodide, iodine-containing radiographic contrast agents may decrease thyroid hormone secretion; may also increase thyroid hormone secretion, especially in patients with Graves' disease.

Other agents reported to impact on thyroid production/conversion include aminoglutethimide, amiodarone, chloral hydrate, diazepam, ethionamide, interferon-alpha, interleukin-2, lithium, lovastatin (case report), glucocorticoids (dose-related), 6-mercaptopurine, sulfonamides, thiazide diuretics, and tolbutamide.

In addition, a number of medications have been noted to cause transient depression in TSH secretion, which may complicate interpretation of monitoring tests for levothyroxine, including corticosteroids, octreotide, and dopamine. Metoclopramide may increase TSH secretion

Related Information

Thyroid *on page 1313*

Levothyroxine Sodium *see* Levothyroxine *on page 797*

Levoxyl® *see* Levothyroxine *on page 797*

Levsin® *see* Hyoscyamine *on page 685*

Levsinex® *see* Hyoscyamine *on page 685*

Levsin/SL® *see* Hyoscyamine *on page 685*

Lexapro™ *see* Escitalopram *on page 489*

Lexxel® *see* Enalapril and Felodipine *on page 466*

LHRH *see* Gonadorelin *on page 640*

***l*-Hyoscyamine Sulfate** *see* Hyoscyamine *on page 685*

Lidocaine (LYE doe kane)

U.S. Brand Names Anestacon®; Band-Aid® Hurt-Free™ Antiseptic Wash [OTC]; Burnamycin [OTC]; Burn Jel [OTC]; Burn-O-Jel [OTC]; ELA-Max® [OTC]; ELA-Max® 5 [OTC]; Lida-Mantle®; Lidoderm®; Premjact® [OTC]; Solarcaine® Aloe Extra Burn Relief [OTC]; Topicaine® [OTC]; Xylocaine®; Xylocaine® MPF; Xylocaine® Viscous; Zilactin-L® [OTC]

Synonyms Lidocaine Hydrochloride; Lignocaine Hydrochloride

Generic Available Yes: Gel, injection, ointment, solution

Pharmacologic Category Analgesic, Topical; Antiarrhythmic Agent, Class Ib; Local Anesthetic

Pregnancy Risk Factor B (manufacturer); C (expert analysis)

Lactation Enters breast milk (small amounts)/compatible

Use Local anesthetic and acute treatment of ventricular arrhythmias from myocardial infarction, cardiac manipulation, digitalis intoxication; drug of choice for ventricular ectopy, ventricular tachycardia (VT), ventricular fibrillation (VF); for pulseless VT or VF preferably administer **after** defibrillation and epinephrine; control of premature ventricular contractions, wide-complex paroxysmal supraventricular tachycardia (PSVT); control of hemodynamically compromising PVCs; hemodynamically stable VT

ELA-Max® is a topical local anesthetic for use in laser, cosmetic, and outpatient surgeries; minor burns, cuts, and abrasions of the skin

Orphan drug: Lidoderm® Patch: Relief of allodynia (painful hypersensitivity) and chronic pain in postherpetic neuralgia

Mechanism of Action/Effect Class Ib antiarrhythmic; suppresses automaticity of conduction tissue by increasing electrical stimulation threshold of ventricles, His-Purkinje system, and spontaneous depolarization of ventricles during diastole by direct action on tissues; blocks both initiation and conduction of nerve impulses by decreasing the neuronal membrane's permeability to sodium ions, which results in inhibition of depolarization with resultant blockade of conduction

Contraindications Hypersensitivity to lidocaine or any component of the formulation; hypersensitivity to another local anesthetic of the amide type; Adam-Stokes syndrome; severe degrees of SA, AV, or intraventricular heart block (except in patients with a functioning artificial pacemaker)

Warnings/Precautions

Intravenous: Constant EKG monitoring is necessary during I.V. administration. Use cautiously in hepatic impairment, any degree of heart block, Wolff-Parkinson-White syndrome, CHF, marked hypoxia, severe respiratory depression, hypovolemia, history of malignant hyperthermia, or shock. Increased ventricular rate may be seen when administered to a patient with atrial fibrillation. Correct any underlying causes of ventricular arrhythmias. Monitor closely for signs and symptoms of CNS toxicity. The elderly may be prone to increased CNS and cardiovascular side effects. Reduce dose in hepatic dysfunction and CHF.

Injectable anesthetic: Follow appropriate administration techniques so as not to administer any intravascularly. Solutions containing antimicrobial preservatives should not be used for epidural or spinal anesthesia. Some solutions contain a bisulfite; avoid in patients who are allergic to bisulfite. Resuscitative equipment, medicine and oxygen should be available in case of emergency. Use products containing epinephrine cautiously in patients with significant vascular disease, compromised blood flow, or during or following general anesthesia (increased risk of arrhythmias). Adjust the dose for the elderly, pediatric, acutely ill, and debilitated patients.

Topical: ELA-Max® cream: Do not leave on large body areas for >2 hours. Observe young children closely to prevent accidental ingestion. Not for use ophthalmic use or for use on mucous membranes.

Pregnancy risk B/C.

Drug Interactions

Cytochrome P450 Effect: Substrate of CYP1A2, 2A6, 2B6, 2C8/9, **2D6, 3A4**; Inhibits CYP1A2, 2D6

Increased Effect/Toxicity: Concomitant cimetidine or propranolol may result in increased serum concentrations of lidocaine resulting in toxicity. Serum concentrations/toxicity of lidocaine may be increased by inhibitors of CYP3A4, including amprenavir, cimetidine, ciprofloxacin, clarithromycin, clozapine, diltiazem, disulfiram, digoxin, erythromycin, ethanol, fluconazole, fluoxetine, fluvoxamine, grapefruit juice, isoniazid, itraconazole, ketoconazole, labetalol, levodopa, loxapine, metoprolol, metronidazole, miconazole, nefazodone, nelfinavir, omeprazole, phenytoin, rifabutin, rifampin, ritonavir, troleandomycin, valproic acid, and verapamil. Effect of succinylcholine may be enhanced by lidocaine.

Nutritional/Ethanol Interactions Herb/Nutraceutical: St John's wort may decrease lidocaine levels; avoid concurrent use.

Adverse Reactions Effects vary with route of administration. Many effects are dose-related.

Frequency not defined:

Cardiovascular: Bradycardia, hypotension, heart block, arrhythmias, cardiovascular collapse, sinus node supression, increase defibrillator threshold, vascular insufficiency (periarticular injections), arterial spasms

Central nervous system: Drowsiness after administration is usually a sign of a high blood level. Other effects may include lightheadedness, dizziness, tinnitus, blurred vision,

vomiting, twitching, tremors, lethargy, coma, agitation, slurred speech, seizures, anxiety, euphoria, hallucinations, paresthesia, psychosis
Dermatologic: Itching, rash, edema of the skin, contact dermatitis
Gastrointestinal: Nausea, vomiting, taste disorder
Local:Thrombophlebitis
Neuromuscular & skeletal: Transient radicular pain (subarachnoid administration; up to 1.9%)
Ocular: Blurred vision, diplopia
Respiratory: Dyspnea, respiratory depression or arrest, bronchospasm
Miscellaneous: Allergic reactions, urticaria, edema, anaphylactoid reaction

Following spinal anesthesia positional headache (3%), shivering (2%) nausea, peripheral nerve symptoms, respiratory inadequacy and double vision (<1%), hypotension, cauda equina syndrome

Postmarketing and/or case reports: ARDS (inhalation), asystole, methemoglobinemia, severe back pain

Overdosage/Toxicology Lidocaine has a narrow therapeutic index. Severe toxicity may occur at doses slightly above the therapeutic range, especially in conjunction with other antiarrhythmic drugs. Symptoms of overdose include sedation, confusion, coma, seizures, respiratory arrest, and cardiac toxicity (sinus arrest, AV block, asystole, and hypotension). QRS and QT intervals are usually normal, although they may be prolonged after massive overdose. Other effects include dizziness, paresthesia, tremor, ataxia, and GI disturbance. Treatment is supportive.

Pharmacodynamics/Kinetics

Half-Life Elimination: Biphasic: Prolonged with congestive heart failure, liver disease, shock, severe renal disease; Initial: 7-30 minutes; Terminal: Infants, premature: 3.2 hours, Adults: 1.5-2 hours

Metabolism: 90% hepatic; active metabolites monoethylglycinexylidide (MEGX) and glycinexylidide (GX) can accumulate and may cause CNS toxicity

Onset: Single bolus dose: 45-90 seconds

Duration: 10-20 minutes

Formulations

Cream, rectal (ELA-Max® 5): 5% (30 g) [contains benzyl alcohol]
Cream, topical (ELA-Max®): 4% (5 g, 30 g) [contains benzyl alcohol]
Cream, topical, as hydrochloride (LidaMantle®): 3% (30 g)
Gel, topical:
  Burn-O-Jel: 0.5% (90 g)
  Topicaine®: 4% (1 g, 10 g, 30 g, 113 g) [contains benzyl alcohol, aloe vera, and jojoba]
Gel, topical, as hydrochloride: 2% (30 g)
  Burn Jel: 2% (3.5 g, 120 g)
  Solarcaine® Aloe Extra Burn Relief: 0.5% (226 g) [contains aloe vera gel and tartrazine]
Infusion, as hydrochloride [premixed in D_5W]: 0.4% [4 mg/mL] (250 mL, 500 mL); 0.8% [8 mg/mL] (250 mL, 500 mL)
Injection, solution, as hydrochloride: 0.5% [5 mg/mL] (50 mL); 1% [10 mg/mL] (5 mL, 20 mL, 30 mL, 50 mL); 1.5% [15 mg/mL] (20 mL); 2% [20 mg/mL] (2 mL, 5 mL, 20 mL, 30 mL, 50 mL)
  Xylocaine®: 0.5% [5 mg/mL] (50 mL); 1% [10 mg/mL] (10 mL, 20 mL, 50 mL); 2% [20 mg/mL] (1.8 mL, 10 mL, 20 mL, 50 mL); 4% [40 mg/mL] (5 mL)
Injection, solution, as hydrochloride [preservative free]: 0.5% [5 mg/mL] (50 mL); 1% [10 mg/mL] (2 mL, 5 mL, 30 mL); 1.5% [15 mg/mL] (20 mL); 2% [20 mg/mL] (5 mL, 10 mL); 4% [40 mg/mL] (5 mL); 10% [100 mg/mL] (10 mL); 20% [200 mg/mL] (10 mL)
  Xylocaine® MPF: 0.5% [5 mg/mL] (50 mL); 1% [10 mg/mL] (2 mL, 5 mL, 10 mL, 20 mL, 30 mL); 1.5% [15 mg/mL] (10 mL, 20 mL); 2% [2 mg/mL] (2 mL, 5 mL, 10 mL); 4% [40 mg/mL] (5 mL)
Injection, solution, as hydrochloride [premixed in $D_{7.5}W$, preservative free]: 5% (2 mL)
  Xylocaine®-MPF: 1.5% (2 mL)
Jelly, topical, as hydrochloride:
  Anestacon®: 2% (15 mL, 240 mL) [contains benzalkonium chloride]
  Xylocaine®: 2% (5 mL, 10 mL, 20 mL, 30 mL)
Liquid, topical (Zilactin®-L): 2.5% (7.5 mL)
Ointment, topical: 5% (37 g)
  Xylocaine®: 2.5% (35 g) [OTC]; 5% (3.5 g, 35 g) [mint or unflavored]
Patch, transdermal (Lidoderm®): 5% (30s)
Solution, topical, as hydrochloride: 2% [20 mg/mL] (15 mL, 240 mL); 4% [40 mg/mL] (50 mL)
  Band-Aid® Hurt-Free™ Antiseptic Wash: 2% (180 mL)
  Xylocaine®: 4% [40 mg/mL] (50 mL)
Solution, viscous, as hydrochloride: 2% [20 mg/mL] (20 mL, 100 mL)
  Xylocaine® Viscous: 2% [20 mg/mL] (20 mL, 100 mL, 450 mL)
Spray, topical:
  Burnamycin: 0.5% (60 mL) [contains aloe vera gel]
  Premjact®: 9.6% (13 mL)
  Solarcaine® Aloe Extra Burn Relief: 0.5% (127 g) [contains aloe vera]

Dosing

Adults:

Topical local anesthetic: Topical: Apply to affected area as needed; maximum: 3 mg/kg/dose; do not repeat within 2 hours.
  ELA-Max® cream; Apply ¼ inch thick layer to intact skin. Leave on until adequate anesthetic effect is obtained. Remove cream and cleanse area before beginning procedure.
Injectable local anesthetic: Varies with procedure, degree of anesthesia needed, vascularity of tissue, duration of anesthesia required, and physical condition of patient; maximum: 4.5 mg/kg/dose; do not repeat within 2 hours.
Postherpetic neuralgia: Patch: Postherpetic neuralgia: Apply patch to most painful area. Up to 3 patches may be applied in a single application. Patch may remain in place for up to 12 hours in any 24-hour period.

(Continued)

Lidocaine *(Continued)*

Antiarrhythmic:

I.V.: 1-1.5 mg/kg bolus over 2-3 minutes; may repeat doses of 0.5-0.75 mg/kg in 5-10 minutes up to a total of 3 mg/kg; continuous infusion: 1-4 mg/minute

I.V. (2 g/250 mL D_5W) infusion rates (infusion pump should be used for I.V. infusion administration):

1 mg/minute: 7 mL/hour
2 mg/minute: 15 mL/hour
3 mg/minute: 21 mL/hour
4 mg/minute: 30 mL/hour

Ventricular fibrillation (after defibrillation and epinephrine):

I.V.: Initial: 1.5 mg/kg, may repeat boluses as above; follow with continuous infusion after return of perfusion.

Prevention of ventricular fibrillation: Initial bolus: 0.5 mg/kg; repeat every 5-10 minutes to a total dose of 2 mg/kg

Refractory ventricular fibrillation: Repeat 1.5 mg/kg bolus may be given 3-5 minutes after initial dose.

Endotracheal: 2-2.5 times the I.V. dose

Note: Decrease dose in patients with CHF, shock, or hepatic disease.

Elderly: Refer to adult dosing. Patients >65 years of age may benefit from weight-based dosing.

Pediatrics:

Topical local anesthetic: Refer to adult dosing.

Injectable local anesthetic: Refer to adult dosing.

Antiarrhythmic: Endotracheal, I.O., I.V.: Children: Loading dose: 1 mg/kg; may repeat in 10-15 minutes x 2 doses; after loading dose, start I.V. continuous infusion 20-50 mcg/kg/minute (300 mcg/kg/minute per American Heart Association).

Use 20 mcg/kg/minute in patients with shock, hepatic disease, mild congestive heart failure (CHF).

Moderate to severe CHF may require $^1/_2$ loading dose and lower infusion rates to avoid toxicity.

Renal Impairment: Not dialyzable (0% to 5%) by hemo- or peritoneal dialysis; supplemental dose is not necessary.

Hepatic Impairment: Reduce dose in acute hepatitis and decompensated cirrhosis by 50%.

Administration

I.V.: Use microdrip (60 drops/mL) or infusion pump to administer an accurate dose.

Topical: Patch may be cut to appropriate size. Remove immediately if burning sensation occurs. Wash hands after application.

Other: Endotracheal doses should be diluted to 10 mL with normal saline prior to E.T. administration

Stability

Storage: Lidocaine injection is stable at room temperature. Stability of parenteral admixture at room temperature (25°C) is the expiration date on premixed bag; out of overwrap stability is 30 days.

Reconstitution: Standard diluent: 2 g/250 mL D_5W

Compatibility: Stable in D_5LR, $D_5{}^1/_2NS$, D_5NS, D_5W, LR, $^1/_4NS$, NS

Y-site administration: Incompatible with amphotericin B cholesteryl sulfate complex, thiopental

Compatibility in syringe: Incompatible with cefazolin

Compatibility when admixed: Incompatible Amphotericin B, dacarbazine, methohexital, phenytoin

Monitoring Laboratory Tests I.V.: Serum lidocaine levels. Therapeutic levels range from 1.5-5 mcg/mL; >6 mcg/mL is associated with toxicity.

Monitoring and Teaching Issues

Physical Assessment: Assess other medications patient may be taking for adverse interactions (see Drug Interactions). **Local anesthetic:** Monitor for effectiveness of anesthesia, and adverse reactions (see Adverse Reactions). **Dermatologic:** Monitor for return of sensation. **Oral:** Use caution to prevent gagging or choking. Avoid food or drink for 1 hour. Teach patient adverse reactions to report; use and teach appropriate interventions to promote safety. **Antiarrhythmic: I.V.:** EKG and vital signs must be closely and continually monitored. Keep patient supine to reduce hypotensive effects. Assess frequently for adverse reactions or signs of toxicity (see Adverse Reactions and Overdose/Toxicology). Teach patient adverse reactions to report and appropriate interventions to promote safety. **Pregnancy risk factor B/C** - see Pregnancy Risk Factor for use cautions; benefits of use should outweigh possible risks.

Patient Education: I.V.: You will be monitored during infusion. Do not get up without assistance. Report dizziness, numbness, double vision, nausea, pain or burning at infusion site, nightmares, hearing strange noises, seeing unusual visions, or difficulty breathing.

Dermatologic: You will experience decreased sensation to pain, heat, or cold in the area and/or decreased muscle strength (depending on area of application) until effects wear off; use necessary caution to reduce incidence of possible injury until full sensation returns. Report irritation, pain, persistent numbness, tingling, swelling; restlessness, dizziness, acute weakness; blurred vision; ringing in ears; or difficulty breathing.

Oral: Lidocaine can cause numbness of tongue, cheeks, and throat. Do not eat or drink for 1 hour after use. Take small sips of water at first to ensure that you can swallow without difficulty. Your tongue and mouth may be numb; use caution avoid biting yourself. Immediately report swelling of face, lips, or tongue.

Transdermal patch: Patch may be cut to appropriate size. Apply patch to most painful area. Up to 3 patches may be applied in a single application. Patch may remain in place for up to 12 hours in any 24-hour period. Remove immediately if burning sensation occurs. Wash hands after application.

Pregnancy precaution: Inform prescriber if you are pregnant.

Geriatric Considerations: Due to decreases in Phase I metabolism and possibly decrease in splanchnic perfusion with age, there may be a decreased clearance or increased half-life in the elderly and increased risk for CNS side effects and cardiac effects.

Related Information

Antiarrhythmic Drugs *on page 1551*

Peak and Trough Guidelines *on page 1544*

Lidocaine and Epinephrine (LYE doe kane & ep i NEF rin)

U.S. Brand Names Xylocaine® MPF With Epinephrine; Xylocaine® With Epinephrine

Synonyms Epinephrine and Lidocaine

Generic Available Yes

Pharmacologic Category Local Anesthetic

Pregnancy Risk Factor B

Lactation Enters breast milk/compatible

Use Local infiltration anesthesia; AVS for nerve block

Pharmacokinetic Note See individual agents.

Pharmacodynamics/Kinetics

Onset: Peak effect: ~5 minutes

Duration: Dose and anesthetic procedure dependent: ~2 hours

Formulations

Injection, solution, as hydrochloride, with epinephrine 1:50,000 (Xylocaine® with Epinephrine): Lidocaine 2% [20 mg/mL] (1.8 mL) [contains sodium metabisulfite]

Injection, solution, as hydrochloride, with epinephrine 1:100,000: Lidocaine 1% [10 mg/mL] (20 mL, 30 mL, 50 mL); Lidocaine 2% (20 mL, 30 mL, 50 mL)

Xylocaine® with Epinephrine: Lidocaine 1% [10 mg/mL] (10 mL 20 mL, 50 mL); Lidocaine 2% (1.8 mL, 10 mL, 20 mL, 50 mL) [contains sodium metabisulfite]

Injection, solution, as hydrochloride, with epinephrine 1:200,000: Lidocaine 0.5% [5 mg/mL] (50 mL)

Xylocaine® with Epinephrine: Lidocaine 0.5% [5 mg/mL] (50 mL) [contains sodium metabisulfite]

Injection, solution, as hydrochloride, with epinephrine 1:200,000 [methylparaben free]: Lidocaine 1% [10 mg/mL] (30 mL); Lidocaine 1.5% (5 mL, 30 mL); Lidocaine 2% (20 mL) [contains sodium metabisulfite]

Xylocaine® MPF with Epinephrine: Lidocaine 1% [10 mg/mL] (5 mL, 10 mL, 30 mL); 1.5% [15 mg/mL] (5 mL, 10 mL, 30 mL); Lidocaine 2% [20 mg/mL] (5 mL, 10 mL, 20 mL) [contains sodium metabisulfite]

Dosing

Adults & Elderly: Local anesthetic: Infiltration: Dosage varies with the anesthetic procedure, degree of anesthesia needed, vascularity of tissue, duration of anesthesia required, and physical condition of patient.

Pediatrics: Local anesthetic: Infiltration: Children: Use lidocaine concentrations of 0.5% to 1% (or even more diluted) to decrease possibility of toxicity. Lidocaine dose should not exceed 7 mg/kg/dose; do not repeat within 2 hours.

Monitoring and Teaching Issues

Physical Assessment: See individual components listed in Related Information.

Patient Education: See individual components listed in Related Information.

Related Information

Epinephrine *on page 470*

Lidocaine *on page 800*

Lidocaine and Hydrocortisone (LYE doe kane & hye droe KOR ti sone)

U.S. Brand Names Lida-Mantle HC®

Synonyms Hydrocortisone and Lidocaine

Generic Available No

Pharmacologic Category Anesthetic/Corticosteroid

Pregnancy Risk Factor B (lidocaine); C (hydrocortisone)

Lactation For topical use

Use Topical anti-inflammatory and anesthetic for skin disorders

Formulations Cream, topical: Lidocaine 3% and hydrocortisone 0.5% (30 g, 85 g)

Dosing

Adults & Elderly: Anti-inflammatory/anesthetic: Topical: Apply 2-4 times/day.

Monitoring and Teaching Issues

Physical Assessment: See individual components listed in Related Information. **Pregnancy risk factor B/C** - see Pregnancy Risk Factor for use cautions; benefits of use should outweigh possible risks.

Patient Education: See individual components listed in Related Information. **Pregnancy precaution:** Inform prescriber if you are or intend to become pregnant.

Related Information

Hydrocortisone *on page 673*

Lidocaine *on page 800*

Lidocaine and Prilocaine (LYE doe kane & PRIL oh kane)

U.S. Brand Names EMLA®

Synonyms Prilocaine and Lidocaine

Generic Available No

Pharmacologic Category Local Anesthetic

Pregnancy Risk Factor B

Lactation Enters breast milk/compatible

Use Topical anesthetic for use on normal intact skin to provide local analgesia for minor procedures such as I.V. cannulation or venipuncture; has also been used for painful procedures such as lumbar puncture and skin graft harvesting; for superficial minor surgery of

(Continued)

Lidocaine and Prilocaine *(Continued)*

genital mucous membranes and as an adjunct for local infiltration anesthesia in genital mucous membranes.

Mechanism of Action/Effect Local anesthetic action occurs by stabilization of neuronal membranes and inhibiting the ionic fluxes required for the initiation and conduction of impulses

Contraindications

Hypersensitivity to amide type anesthetic agents [ie, lidocaine, prilocaine, dibucaine, mepivacaine, bupivacaine, etidocaine]; hypersensitivity to any component of the formulation selected; application on mucous membranes or broken or inflamed skin; infants <1 month of age if gestational age is <37 weeks; infants <12 months of age receiving therapy with methemoglobin-inducing agents; children with congenital or idiopathic methemoglobinemia, or in children who are receiving medications associated with drug-induced methemoglobinemia [ie, acetaminophen (overdosage), benzocaine, chloroquine, dapsone, nitrofurantoin, nitroglycerin, nitroprusside, phenazopyridine, phenelzine, phenobarbital, phenytoin, quinine, sulfonamides]

Warnings/Precautions Use with caution in patients receiving class I antiarrhythmic drugs, since systemic absorption occurs and synergistic toxicity is possible. Although the incidence of systemic adverse reactions with EMLA® is very low, caution should be exercised, particularly when applying over large areas and leaving on for longer than 2 hours.

Drug Interactions

Cytochrome P450 Effect: Lidocaine: Substrate of CYP1A2, 2A6, 2B6, 2C8/9, **2D6, 3A4**; Inhibits CYP1A2, 2D6

Increased Effect/Toxicity: Class I antiarrhythmic drugs (tocainide, mexiletine): Effects are additive and potentially synergistic. Prilocaine may enhance the effect of other drugs known to induce methemoglobinemia.

Adverse Reactions Frequency not defined.

Cardiovascular: Hypotension, angioedema
Central nervous system: Shock
Dermatologic: Hyperpigmentation, erythema, itching, rash, burning, urticaria
Genitourinary: Blistering of foreskin (rare)
Local: Burning, stinging, edema
Respiratory: Bronchospasm
Miscellaneous: Alteration in temperature sensation, hypersensitivity reactions

Pharmacokinetic Note See individual agents.

Pharmacodynamics/Kinetics

Absorption:

EMLA®: Related to duration of application and area where applied
3-hour application: 3.6% lidocaine and 6.1% prilocaine
24-hour application: 16.2% lidocaine and 33.5% prilocaine

Onset:

EMLA®: 1 hour; Peak effect: 2-3 hours

Duration:

EMLA®: 1-2 hours after removal

Formulations

Cream, topical: Lidocaine 2.5% and prilocaine 2.5% (5 g, 30 g) [each 5 g tube is packaged with two Tegaderm® dressings]

Disc, topical: 1 g (2s, 10s) [contains lidocaine 25 mg and prilocaine 25 mg per 10 cm^2 disc]

Dosing

Adults & Elderly:

Anesthetic: Topical: EMLA® cream and EMLA® anesthetic disc: A thick layer of EMLA® cream is applied to intact skin and covered with an occlusive dressing, or alternatively, an EMLA® anesthetic disc is applied to intact skin

Note: Dermal analgesia can be expected to increase for up to 3 hours under occlusive dressing and persist for 1-2 hours after removal of the cream

Minor dermal procedures (eg, I.V. cannulation or venipuncture): Topical: Apply 2.5 g of cream (1/2 of the 5 g tube) over 20-25 cm of skin surface area, or 1 anesthetic disc (1 g over 10 cm^2) for at least 1 hour. **Note:** In clinical trials, 2 sites were usually prepared in case there was a technical problem with cannulation or venipuncture at the first site.

Major dermal procedures (eg, more painful dermatological procedures involving a larger skin area such as split thickness skin graft harvesting): Topical: Apply 2 g of cream per 10 cm^2 of skin and allow to remain in contact with the skin for at least 2 hours.

Adult male genital skin (eg, pretreatment prior to local anesthetic infiltration): Apply a thick layer of cream (1 g/10 cm^2) to the skin surface for 15 minutes. Local anesthetic infiltration should be performed immediately after removal of EMLA® cream.

Adult females: Genital mucous membranes: Minor procedures (eg, removal of condylomata acuminata, pretreatment for local anesthetic infiltration): Apply 5-10 g (thick layer) of cream for 5-10 minutes

Pediatrics:

Local anesthetic (procedures): Topical:

Note: Dosing is based on child's age and weight: Although the incidence of systemic adverse effects with EMLA® is very low, caution should be exercised, particularly when applying over large areas and leaving on for >2 hours

Children (intact skin): EMLA® should **not** be used in neonates with a gestational age <37 weeks nor in infants <12 months of age who are receiving treatment with methemoglobin-inducing agents

Dosing is based on child's age and weight:

Age 0-3 months or <5 kg: Apply a maximum of 1 g over no more than 10 cm^2 of skin; leave on for no longer than 1 hour.

Age 3 months to 12 months and >5 kg: Apply no more than a maximum 2 g total over no more than 20 cm^2 of skin; leave on for no longer than 4 hours.

Age 1-6 years and >10 kg: Apply no more than a maximum of 10 g total over no more than 100 cm^2 of skin; leave on for no longer than 4 hours.

Age 7-12 years and >20 kg: Apply no more than a maximum 20 g total over no more than 200 cm^2 of skin; leave on for no longer than 4 hours.

Note: If a patient greater than 3 months old does not meet the minimum weight requirement, the maximum total dose should be restricted to the corresponding maximum based on patient weight.

Renal Impairment: Smaller areas of treatment are recommended for patients with renal dysfunction.

Hepatic Impairment: Smaller areas of treatment are recommended for patients with hepatic dysfunction.

Administration

Topical: For external use only. Choose two application sites available for intravenous access. Apply a thick layer (2.5 g/site ~1/2 of a 5 g tube) of cream to each designated site of intact skin. Cover each site with the occlusive dressing (Tegaderm®). Mark the time on the dressing. **Allow at least 1 hour for optimum therapeutic effect.** Remove the dressing and wipe off excess EMLA® cream (gloves should be worn). **Smaller areas of treatment are recommended for debilitated patients.**

Stability

Storage: Store at room temperature.

Monitoring and Teaching Issues

Physical Assessment: Use on intact skin only (see Administration - Topical). Monitor for effectiveness of anesthesia and adverse reactions (see Adverse Reactions). Monitor for return of sensation.

Patient Education: This drug will block sensation to the applied area. Report irritation, pain, burning at application site.

Breast-feeding Issues: Usual infiltration doses of lidocaine and prilocaine given to nursing mothers has not been shown to affect the health of the nursing infant.

Related Information

Lidocaine *on page 800*

Lidocaine Hydrochloride *see* Lidocaine *on page 800*

Lidoderm® *see* Lidocaine *on page 800*

Lignocaine Hydrochloride *see* Lidocaine *on page 800*

Lindane (LIN dane)

Synonyms Benzene Hexachloride; Gamma Benzene Hexachloride; Hexachlorocyclohexane

Generic Available Yes

Pharmacologic Category Antiparasitic Agent, Topical; Pediculocide; Scabicidal Agent

Pregnancy Risk Factor B

Lactation Enters breast milk/compatible

Use Treatment of scabies (*Sarcoptes scabiei*), *Pediculus capitis* (head lice), and *Pediculus pubis* (crab lice); FDA recommends reserving lindane as a second-line agent or with inadequate response to other therapies

Mechanism of Action/Effect Directly absorbed by parasites and ova through the exoskeleton; stimulates the nervous system resulting in seizures and death of parasitic arthropods

Contraindications Hypersensitivity to lindane or any component of the formulation; premature neonates; acutely inflamed skin or raw, weeping surfaces

Warnings/Precautions Use with caution in infants and small children, and patients with a history of seizures. Avoid contact with face, eyes, mucous membranes, and urethral meatus. Because of the potential for systemic absorption and CNS side effects, lindane should be used with caution. Not considered a drug of first choice; consider permethrin or crotamiton agent first.

Drug Interactions

Increased Effect/Toxicity: Oil-based hair dressing may increase potential for toxicity of lindane.

Adverse Reactions <1% (Limited to important or life-threatening): Aplastic anemia, ataxia, burning and stinging, cardiac arrhythmia, contact dermatitis, dizziness, eczematous eruptions, headache, hematuria, hepatitis, nausea, pulmonary edema, restlessness, seizures, skin and adipose tissue may act as repositories, vomiting

Overdosage/Toxicology Symptoms of overdose include vomiting, restlessness, ataxia, seizures, arrhythmias, pulmonary edema, hematuria, and hepatitis. The drug is absorbed through the skin, mucous membranes, and GI tract, and has occasionally caused serious CNS, hepatic, and renal toxicity when used excessively for prolonged periods, or with accidental ingestion. If ingested, perform gastric lavage and general supportive measures.

Pharmacodynamics/Kinetics

Absorption: ≤13% systemically

Half-Life Elimination: Children: 17-22 hours

Time to Peak: Serum: Children: 6 hours

Metabolism: Hepatic

Formulations

Lotion, topical: 1% (60 mL, 473 mL)

Shampoo, topical: 1% (60 mL, 473 mL)

Dosing

Adults:

Scabies: Topical: Apply a thin layer of lotion and massage it on skin from the neck to the toes (head to toe in infants). For adults, bathe and remove the drug after 8-12 hours; repeat treatment in 7 days if lice or nits are still present. For infants, wash off 6 hours after application.

Pediculosis, capitis and pubis: Topical: 15-30 mL of shampoo is applied and lathered for 4-5 minutes. Rinse hair thoroughly and comb with a fine tooth comb to remove nits. Repeat treatment in 7 days if lice or nits are still present.

(Continued)

Lindane *(Continued)*

Elderly: Refer to adult dosing; use with caution (see Geriatric Considerations).

Pediatrics: Refer to adult dosing.

Administration

Oral: Never administer orally.

Topical: For topical use only. Apply to dry, cool skin; do not apply to face or eyes.

Monitoring and Teaching Issues

Physical Assessment: Assess head, hair, and skin surfaces for presence of lice and nits. Assess knowledge/teach patient appropriate application and use and adverse symptoms (see Adverse Reactions) to report.

Patient Education: For external use only. Do not apply to face and avoid getting in eyes. Do not apply immediately after hot soapy bath. Apply from neck to toes. Bathe to remove drug after 8-12 hours. Repeat in 7 days if lice or nits are still present. Clothing and bedding must be washed in hot water or dry cleaned to kill nits. Wash combs and brushes with lindane shampoo and thoroughly rinse. May need to treat all members of household and all sexual contacts concurrently. Report if condition persists or infection occurs.

Geriatric Considerations: Because of the potential for systemic absorption and CNS side effects, lindane should be used with caution. Not considered a drug of first choice; consider permethrin or crotamiton agent first.

Breast-feeding Issues: Small amounts are excreted in breast milk; however, the amounts are approximately equal to the amounts absorbed by an infant treated topically.

Pregnancy Issues: There are no well-controlled studies in pregnant women; treat no more than twice during a pregnancy.

Linezolid (li NE zoh lid)

U.S. Brand Names Zyvox™

Generic Available No

Pharmacologic Category Antibiotic, Oxazolidinone

Pregnancy Risk Factor C

Lactation Excretion in breast milk unknown/use caution

Use Treatment of vancomycin-resistant *Enterococcus faecium* (VRE) infections, nosocomial pneumonia caused by *Staphylococcus aureus* including MRSA or *Streptococcus pneumoniae* (penicillin-susceptible strains only), complicated and uncomplicated skin and skin structure infections, and community-acquired pneumonia caused by susceptible gram-positive organisms.

Mechanism of Action/Effect Inhibits bacterial protein synthesis by binding to bacterial 23S ribosomal RNA of the 50S subunit. This prevents the formation of a functional 70S initiation complex that is essential for the bacterial translation process. Linezolid is bacteriostatic against enterococci and staphylococci and bactericidal against most strains of streptococci.

Contraindications Hypersensitivity to linezolid or any other component of the formulation

Warnings/Precautions Myelosuppression has been reported and may be dependent on duration of therapy (generally >2 weeks of treatment); use with caution in patients with pre-existing myelosuppression, in patients receiving other drugs which may cause bone marrow suppression, or in chronic infection (previous or concurrent antibiotic therapy). Weekly CBC monitoring is recommended. Discontinue linezolid in patients developing myelosuppression (or in whom myelosuppression worsens during treatment).

Linezolid has mild MAO inhibitor properties and has the potential to have the same interactions as other MAO inhibitors; use with caution in uncontrolled hypertension, pheochromocytoma, carcinoid syndrome, or untreated hyperthyroidism; avoid use with serotonergic agents such as TCAs, venlafaxine, trazodone, sibutramine, meperidine, dextromethorphan, and SSRIs; consider alternatives before initiating outpatient treatment (unnecessary use may lead the development of resistance to linezolid).

Pregnancy risk C.

Drug Interactions

Increased Effect/Toxicity: Linezolid is a reversible, nonselective inhibitor of MAO. Serotonergic agents (eg, TCAs, venlafaxine, trazodone, sibutramine, meperidine, dextromethorphan, and SSRIs) may cause a serotonin syndrome (eg, hyperpyrexia, cognitive dysfunction) when used concomitantly. Adrenergic agents (eg, phenylpropanolamine, pseudoephedrine, sympathomimetic agents, vasopressor or dopaminergic agents) may cause hypertension. Tramadol may increase the risk of seizures when used concurrently with linezolid. Myelosuppressive medications may increase risk of myelosuppression when used concurrently with linezolid.

Nutritional/Ethanol Interactions

Ethanol: Avoid ethanol (may contain tyramine, hypertensive crisis may result).

Food: Avoid foods (eg, cheese) and beverages containing tyramine in patients receiving linezolid (hypertensive crisis may result).

Adverse Reactions

1% to 10%:

- Cardiovascular: Hypertension (1% to 3%)
- Central nervous system: Headache (0.5% to 11%), insomnia (3%), dizziness (0.4% to 2%), fever (2%)
- Dermatologic: Rash (2%)
- Gastrointestinal: Nausea (3% to 10%), diarrhea (3% to 11%), vomiting (1% to 4%), constipation (2%), taste alteration (1% to 2%), tongue discoloration (0.2% to 1%), oral moniliasis (0.4% to 1%), pancreatitis
- Genitourinary: Vaginal moniliasis (1% to 2%)
- Hematologic: Thrombocytopenia (0.3% to 10%), anemia, leukopenia, neutropenia
- Hepatic: Abnormal LFTs (0.4% to 1%)
- Miscellaneous: Fungal infections (0.1% to 2%)

<1% (Limited to important or life-threatening): *C. difficile*-related complications, creatinine increased, dyspepsia, localized abdominal pain, pruritus. In addition to hematologic effects observed in trials, myelosuppression (including anemia, leukopenia, pancytopenia, and

thrombocytopenia) has been reported, and may be more common in patients receiving linezolid for >2 weeks.

Overdosage/Toxicology Treatment includes supportive care. Hemodialysis may improve elimination (30% of a dose is removed during a 3-hour hemodialysis session).

Pharmacodynamics/Kinetics

Absorption: Rapid and extensive

Bioavailability: 100%

Half-Life Elimination: 4-5 hours

Time to Peak: 1-2 hours

Metabolism: Hepatic via oxidation of the morpholine ring, resulting in two inactive metabolites (aminoethoxyacetic acid, hydroxyethyl glycine); does not involve CYP

Formulations

Infusion [premixed]: 200 mg (100 mL); 400 mg (200 mL); 600 mg (300 mL)

Suspension, oral: 20 mg/mL (150 mL) [orange flavor]

Tablet: 400 mg, 600 mg

Dosing

Adults & Elderly:

VRE infections: Oral, I.V.: 600 mg every 12 hours for 14-28 days

Nosocomial pneumonia, complicated skin and skin structure infections, community-acquired pneumonia including concurrent bacteremia: Oral, I.V.: 600 mg every 12 hours for 10-14 days

Uncomplicated skin and skin structure infections: Oral: 400 mg every 12 hours for 10-14 days

Renal Impairment: No adjustment is recommended. The two primary metabolites may accumulate in patients with renal impairment but the clinical significance is unknown. Weigh the risk of accumulation of metabolites versus the benefit of therapy. Both linezolid and the two metabolites are eliminated by dialysis. Linezolid should be given after hemodialysis.

Hepatic Impairment: No dosage adjustment required for mild to moderate hepatic insufficiency (Child-Pugh class A or B). Use in severe hepatic insufficiency has not been adequately evaluated.

Stability

Storage: Store at 25°C (77°F). Protect from light. Keep infusion bags in overwrap until ready for use. Protect infusion bags from freezing.

Reconstitution: Use reconstituted suspension within 21 days.

Compatibility: Stable in dextran 6% in NS, D_5NS, D_{10}NS, D_5W, D_{10}W, NS

Compatibility in syringe: Incompatible with ampicillin

Compatibility when admixed: Incompatible with kanamycin, phenytoin

Monitoring Laboratory Tests At least weekly CBC and platelet counts, particularly in patients at increased risk of bleeding, with pre-existing myelosuppression, on concomitant medications that cause bone marrow suppression, in those who require >2 weeks of therapy, or in those with chronic infection who have received previous or concomitant antibiotic therapy.

Monitoring and Teaching Issues

Physical Assessment: Assess for previous drug allergies before administering first dose. See Contraindications and Warnings/Precautions for use cautions. Assess other medications patient may be taking for effectiveness and interactions (see Drug Interactions). Monitor laboratory tests (see above), therapeutic effect, and adverse reactions (see Adverse Reactions and Overdose/Toxicology) on a regular basis during therapy. Assess knowledge/teach patient appropriate use of oral medication. **Oral/I.V.:** Assess knowledge/teach patient interventions to reduce side effects (including tyramine-free diet - see Tyramine Foods List *on page 1601*) and adverse reactions to report (see Patient Education). **Pregnancy risk factor C** - benefits of use should outweigh possible risks. Note breast-feeding caution.

Patient Education: Oral: Take exactly as directed. Do not alter dosage without consulting prescriber. Complete full course of therapy even if condition appears controlled. Maintain adequate hydration (2-3 L/day of fluids) unless advised by prescriber to restrict fluids. Avoid alcohol. Avoid tyramine-containing foods (eg, pickles, aged cheese, wine).

Oral/I.V.: You may experience GI discomfort, nausea, vomiting, taste alteration (small, frequent meals, frequent mouth care, sucking lozenges, or chewing gum may help); mild headache (analgesic may help); or constipation (increase exercise, fluids, fruit, or fiber may help). Report immediately unresolved, liquid diarrhea; white plaques in mouth; skin rash or irritation; acute headache, dizziness, blurred vision; or other persistent adverse reactions. **Pregnancy/breast-feeding precautions:** Inform prescriber if you are or intend to become pregnant. Consult prescriber if breast-feeding.

Dietary Issues: Take with or without food. Suspension contains 20 mg phenylalanine per teaspoonful.

Lioresal® *see* Baclofen *on page 145*

Liovistin™ *see page 1509*

Lipancreatin *see* Pancrelipase *on page 1029*

Lipid-Lowering Agents *see page 1582*

Lipitor® *see* Atorvastatin *on page 128*

Liposyn® III *see* Fat Emulsion *on page 545*

Lipram® *see* Pancrelipase *on page 1029*

Lipram® 4500 *see* Pancrelipase *on page 1029*

Lipram-CR® *see* Pancrelipase *on page 1029*

Lipram-PN® *see* Pancrelipase *on page 1029*

Lipram-UL® *see* Pancrelipase *on page 1029*

Liquibid® *see* Guaifenesin *on page 646*

Liquibid® 1200 *see* Guaifenesin *on page 646*

Liqui-Char® [OTC] *see* Charcoal *on page 266*

Liquid Antidote *see* Charcoal *on page 266*

Liquid Pred® *see* PredniSONE *on page 1115*

Liquiprin® for Children [OTC] *see* Acetaminophen *on page 35*

Lisinopril (lyse IN oh pril)

U.S. Brand Names Prinivil®; Zestril®

Generic Available Yes

Pharmacologic Category Angiotensin-Converting Enzyme (ACE) Inhibitor

Pregnancy Risk Factor C/D (2nd and 3rd trimesters)

Lactation Excretion in breast milk unknown (similar drug captopril is compatible)

Use Treatment of hypertension, either alone or in combination with other antihypertensive agents; adjunctive therapy in treatment of CHF (afterload reduction); treatment of hemodynamically stable patients within 24 hours of acute myocardial infarction, to improve survival; treatment of acute myocardial infarction within 24 hours in hemodynamically stable patients to improve survival; treatment of left ventricular dysfunction after myocardial infarction

Mechanism of Action/Effect Competitive inhibitor of angiotensin-converting enzyme (ACE); prevents conversion of angiotensin I to angiotensin II, a potent vasoconstrictor; results in lower levels of angiotensin II which causes an increase in plasma renin activity and a reduction in aldosterone secretion

Contraindications Hypersensitivity to lisinopril or any component of the formulation; angioedema related to previous treatment with an ACE inhibitor; bilateral renal artery stenosis; primary hyperaldosteronism; pregnancy (2nd and 3rd trimesters)

Warnings/Precautions Angioedema can occur at any time during treatment (especially following first dose). Careful blood pressure monitoring with first dose (hypotension can occur especially in volume depleted patients). Dosage adjustment required in renal impairment. Use with caution in hypovolemia; collagen vascular diseases; valvular stenosis (particularly aortic stenosis); hyperkalemia; or before, during, or immediately after anesthesia. Avoid rapid dosage escalation, which may lead to renal insufficiency. Anaphylactic reactions, and neutropenia/agranulocytosis with myeloid hyperplasia may occur (rare). Hypersensitivity reactions may be seen during hemodialysis with high-flux dialysis membranes (eg, AN69). Deterioration in renal function can occur with initiation. Use with caution in unilateral renal artery stenosis and pre-existing renal insufficiency. Pregnancy risk C/D (2nd and 3rd trimesters).

Drug Interactions

Decreased Effect: Aspirin (high dose) may reduce the therapeutic effects of ACE inhibitors; at low dosages this does not appear to be significant. Rifampin may decrease the effect of ACE inhibitors. Antacids may decrease the bioavailability of ACE inhibitors (may be more likely to occur with captopril); separate administration times by 1-2 hours. NSAIDs, specifically indomethacin, may reduce the hypotensive effects of ACE inhibitors. More likely to occur in low renin or volume dependent hypertensive patients.

Increased Effect/Toxicity: Potassium supplements, co-trimoxazole (high dose), angiotensin II receptor antagonists (candesartan, losartan, irbesartan, etc), or potassium-sparing diuretics (amiloride, spironolactone, triamterene) may result in elevated serum potassium levels when combined with lisinopril. ACE inhibitor effects may be increased by phenothiazines or probenecid (increases levels of captopril). ACE inhibitors may increase serum concentrations/effects of digoxin, lithium, and sulfonlyureas.

Diuretics have additive hypotensive effects with ACE inhibitors, and hypovolemia increases the potential for adverse renal effects of ACE inhibitors. In patients with compromised renal function, coadministration with NSAIDs may result in further deterioration of renal function. Allopurinol and ACE inhibitors may cause a higher risk of hypersensitivity reaction when taken concurrently.

Nutritional/Ethanol Interactions Herb/Nutraceutical: Avoid dong quai if using for hypertension (has estrogenic activity). Avoid ephedra, yohimbe, ginseng (may worsen hypertension). Avoid garlic (may have increased antihypertensive effect).

Effects on Lab Values May cause false-positive results in urine acetone determinations using sodium nitroprusside reagent; ↑ potassium (S), serum creatinine/BUN

Adverse Reactions Note: Frequency ranges include data from hypertension and heart failure trials. Higher rates of adverse reactions have generally been noted in patients with CHF. However, the frequency of adverse effects associated with placebo is also increased in this population.

1% to 10%:

Cardiovascular: Orthostatic effects (1%), hypotension (1% to 4%)

Central nervous system: Headache (4% to 6%), dizziness (5% to 12%), fatigue (3%), weakness (1%)

Dermatologic: Rash (1% to 2%)

Endocrine & metabolic: Hyperkalemia (2% to 5%)

Gastrointestinal: Diarrhea (3% to 4%), nausea (2%), vomiting (1%), abdominal pain (2%)

Genitourinary: Impotence (1%)

Hematologic: Decreased hemoglobin (small)

Neuromuscular & skeletal: Chest pain (3%)

Renal: Increased serum creatinine (often transient), increased BUN (2%); deterioration in renal function (in patients with bilateral renal artery stenosis or hypovolemia)

Respiratory: Cough (4% to 9%), upper respiratory infection (2% to 2%)

<1% (Limited to important or life-threatening): Acute renal failure, alopecia, anaphylactoid reactions, angioedema, anuria, arrhythmia, arthralgia, asthma, ataxia, azotemia, bone marrow suppression, bronchospasm, cardiac arrest, decreased libido, gout, hepatitis, hyperkalemia, hyponatremia, increased bilirubin, increased transaminases, infiltrates, jaundice (cholestatic), myocardial infarction, neutropenia, oliguria, orthostatic hypotension, pancreatitis, paresthesia, pemphigus, peripheral neuropathy, photosensitivity, pleural effusion, pulmonary embolism, Stevens-Johnson syndrome, stroke, systemic lupus erythematosus, thrombocytopenia, TIA, toxic epidermal necrolysis, tremor, urticaria, vasculitis, vertigo, vision loss. In addition, a syndrome which may include fever, myalgia, arthralgia,

interstitial nephritis, vasculitis, rash, eosinophilia and positive ANA, and elevated ESR has been reported with ACE inhibitors.

Overdosage/Toxicology Mild hypotension has been the primary toxic effect seen with acute overdose. Bradycardia may also occur; hyperkalemia occurs even with therapeutic doses, especially in patients with renal insufficiency and those taking NSAIDs. Treatment and is symptomatic and supportive.

Pharmacodynamics/Kinetics

Absorption: Well absorbed; unaffected by food

Half-Life Elimination: 11-12 hours

Onset: 1 hour; Peak effect: Hypotensive: Oral: ~6 hours

Duration: 24 hours

Formulations Tablet: 2.5 mg, 5 mg, 10 mg, 20 mg, 30 mg, 40 mg

Dosing

Adults:

Hypertension: Oral: Initial: 10 mg/day; increase doses 5-10 mg/day at 1- to 2-week intervals; maximum daily dose: 40 mg

Patients taking diuretics should have them discontinued 2-3 days prior to initiating lisinopril if possible. Restart diuretic after blood pressure is stable if needed. If diuretic cannot be discontinued prior to therapy, begin with 5 mg with close supervision until stable blood pressure. In patients with hyponatremia (<130 mEq/L), start dose at 2.5 mg/day,

Congestive heart failure: Oral: Initial: 5 mg; then increase by no more than 10 mg increments at intervals no less than 2 weeks to a maximum daily dose of 40 mg. Usual maintenance: 5-40 mg/day as a single dose. Patients should start/continue standard therapy, including diuretics, beta-blockers, and digoxin, as indicated.

Acute myocardial infarction (within 24 hours in hemodynamically stable patients): Oral: 5 mg immediately, then 5 mg at 24 hours, 10 mg at 48 hours, and 10 mg every day thereafter for 6 weeks. Patients should continue to receive standard treatments such as thrombolytics, aspirin, and beta-blockers.

Elderly: Oral:

Initial: 2.5-5 mg/day; increase doses 2.5-5 mg/day at 1- to 2-week intervals; maximum daily dose: 40 mg

Patients taking diuretics should have them discontinued 2-3 days prior to initiating lisinopril if possible. Restart diuretic after blood pressure is stable if needed. In patients with hyponatremia (<130 mEq/L), start dose at 2.5 mg/day (see Renal Impairment).

Renal Impairment:

Cl_{cr} 10-50 mL/minute: Administer 50% to 75% of normal dose.

Cl_{cr} <10 mL/minute: Administer 25% to 50% of normal dose.

Dialyzable (50%)

Administration

Oral: Watch for hypotensive effects within 1-3 hours of first dose or new higher dose.

Monitoring Laboratory Tests CBC, renal function tests, electrolytes. If patient has renal impairment, a baseline WBC with differential and serum creatinine should be evaluated and monitored closely during the first 3 months of therapy.

Monitoring and Teaching Issues

Physical Assessment: See Contraindications, Warnings/Precautions, and Dosing for use cautions. Assess potential for interactions with other prescriptions, OTC medications, or herbal products patient may be taking (especially anything that may impact fluid balance or cardiac status - see Drug Interactions). Assess results of laboratory tests (see above), therapeutic effectiveness, and adverse response on a regular basis during therapy (eg, hypovolemia, angioedema, postural hypotension - see Adverse Reactions and Overdose/Toxicology). Teach patient appropriate use, possible side effects and appropriate interventions, and adverse symptoms to report (see Patient Education). **Pregnancy risk factor C/D** - see Pregnancy Risk Factor for use cautions. Instruct patient of childbearing age about use of appropriate barrier contraception (see Pregnancy Issues).

Patient Education: Inform prescriber of all prescriptions, OTC medications, or herbal products you are taking, and any allergies you have. Do not take anything new during treatment unless approved by prescriber. Do not use potassium supplement or salt substitutes without consulting prescriber. Take exactly as directed; do not discontinue without consulting prescriber. Take first dose at bedtime. Take all doses on an empty stomach, 1 hour before or 2 hours after meals. This drug does not eliminate need for diet or exercise regimen as recommended by prescriber. May cause dizziness, fainting, or lightheadedness (use caution when driving or engaging in tasks that require alertness until response to drug is known); postural hypotension (use caution when rising from lying or sitting position or climbing stairs); or nausea, vomiting, abdominal pain, dry mouth, or transient loss of appetite (small, frequent meals, frequent mouth care, sucking lozenges, or chewing gum may help) - report if these persist. Report chest pain or palpitations; mouth sores; fever or chills; swelling of extremities, face, mouth, or tongue; skin rash; numbness, tingling, or pain in muscles; difficulty breathing or unusual cough; other persistent adverse reactions. **Pregnancy/breast-feeding precautions:** Inform prescriber if you are or intend to become pregnant. This drug should not be used in the 2nd or 3rd trimester of pregnancy. Consult prescriber for appropriate contraceptive measures if necessary. Consult prescriber if breast-feeding.

Geriatric Considerations: Due to frequent decreases in glomerular filtration (also creatinine clearance) with aging, elderly patients may have exaggerated responses to ACE inhibitors. Differences in clinical response due to hepatic changes are not observed. ACE inhibitors may be preferred agents in elderly patients with congestive heart failure and diabetes mellitus. Diabetic proteinuria is reduced and insulin sensitivity is enhanced. In general, the side effect profile is favorable in the elderly and causes little or no CNS confusion. Use lowest dose recommendations initially.

Breast-feeding Issues: Crosses into breast milk; AAP considers **compatible** with breast-feeding.

Pregnancy Issues: ACE inhibitors can cause fetal injury or death if taken during the 2nd or 3rd trimester. Discontinue ACE inhibitors as soon as pregnancy is detected.

(Continued)

Lisinopril *(Continued)*

Related Information

Angiotensin Agents *on page 1547*
Heart Failure *on page 1670*

Lisinopril and Hydrochlorothiazide

(lyse IN oh pril & hye droe klor oh THYE a zide)

U.S. Brand Names Prinzide®; Zestoretic®

Synonyms Hydrochlorothiazide and Lisinopril

Generic Available No

Pharmacologic Category Antihypertensive Agent Combination

Pregnancy Risk Factor C/D (2nd and 3rd trimesters)

Lactation

Hydrochlorothiazide: Compatible
Lisinopril: Excretion in breast milk unknown

Use Treatment of hypertension

Formulations Tablet:

Lisinopril 10 mg and hydrochlorothiazide 12.5 mg
Lisinopril 20 mg and hydrochlorothiazide 12.5 mg
Lisinopril 20 mg and hydrochlorothiazide 25 mg

Dosing

Adults & Elderly: Hypertension: Oral: Initial: Lisinopril 10 mg/hydrochlorothiazide 12.5 mg or lisinopril 20 mg/hydrochlorothiazide 12.5 mg with further increases of either or both components could depend on clinical response. Doses >80 mg/day lisinopril or >50 mg/day hydrochlorothiazide are not recommended.

Renal Impairment: Dosage adjustments should be made with caution. Usual regimens of therapy need not be adjusted as long as patient's Cl_{cr} >30 mL/minute. In patients with more severe renal impairment, loop diuretics are preferred.

Monitoring and Teaching Issues

Physical Assessment: See individual components listed in Related Information. **Pregnancy risk factor C/D** - see Pregnancy Risk Factor for use cautions. Assess knowledge/instruct patient on need to use appropriate contraceptive measures and the need to avoid pregnancy. Note breast-feeding caution.

Patient Education: See individual components listed in Related Information. **Pregnancy/breast-feeding precautions:** Inform prescriber if you are or intend to become pregnant. Consult prescriber if breast-feeding.

Related Information

Hydrochlorothiazide *on page 664*
Lisinopril *on page 808*

Lithium (LITH ee um)

U.S. Brand Names Eskalith®; Eskalith CR®; Lithobid®

Synonyms Lithium Carbonate; Lithium Citrate

Generic Available Yes

Pharmacologic Category Lithium

Pregnancy Risk Factor D

Lactation Enters breast milk/contraindicated

Use Management of bipolar disorders

Use - Unlabeled/Investigational Potential augmenting agent for antidepressants; aggression, post-traumatic stress disorder, conduct disorder in children

Mechanism of Action/Effect Stabilizes mood by actions on nerve cells of the central nervous system; involves serotonin, phosphatidylinositol cycle, and dopamine receptor sensitivity

Contraindications Hypersensitivity to lithium or any component of the formulation; avoid use in patients with severe cardiovascular or renal disease, or with severe debilitation, dehydration, or sodium depletion; pregnancy

Warnings/Precautions Lithium toxicity is closely related to serum levels and can occur at therapeutic doses; serum lithium determinations are required to monitor therapy. Use with caution in patients with thyroid disease, mild-moderate renal impairment, or mild-moderate cardiovascular disease. Use caution in patients receiving medications which alter sodium excretion (eg, diuretics, ACE inhibitors, NSAIDs), or in patients with significant fluid loss (protracted sweating, diarrhea, or prolonged fever); temporary reduction or cessation of therapy may be warranted. Some elderly patients may be extremely sensitive to the effects of lithium, see Usual Dosage and Reference Range. Chronic therapy results in diminished renal concentrating ability (nephrogenic DI). Changes in renal function should be monitored, and re-evaluation of treatment may be necessary. Use caution in patients at risk of suicide (suicidal thoughts or behavior).

Use with caution in patients receiving neuroleptic medications - a syndrome resembling NMS has been associated with concurrent therapy. Lithium may impair the patient's alertness, affecting the ability to operate machinery or driving a vehicle. Neuromuscular-blocking agents should be administered with caution; the response may be prolonged.

Higher serum concentrations may be required and tolerated during an acute manic phase; however, the tolerance decreases when symptoms subside. Normal fluid and salt intake must be maintained during therapy.

Drug Interactions

Decreased Effect: Combined use of lithium and chlorpromazine may lower serum concentrations of both drugs. Sodium bicarbonate and high sodium intake may reduce serum lithium concentrations via enhanced excretion. Lithium may blunt the pressor response to sympathomimetics (epinephrine, norepinephrine).

Increased Effect/Toxicity: Concurrent use of lithium with carbamazepine, diltiazem, SSRIs (fluoxetine, fluvoxamine), haloperidol, methyldopa, metronidazole (rare), phenothiazines, phenytoin, TCAs, and verapamil may increase the risk for neurotoxicity. Lithium concentrations/toxicity may be increased by diuretics, NSAIDs (sulindac and aspirin may be exceptions), ACE inhibitors, angiotensin receptor antagonists (losartan), tetracyclines, or COX-2 inhibitors (celecoxib).

Lithium and MAO inhibitors should generally be avoided due to use reports of fatal malignant hyperpyrexia; risk with selective MAO type B inhibitors (selegiline) appears to be lower. Potassium iodide may enhance the hypothyroid effects of lithium. Combined use of lithium with tricyclic antidepressants or sibutramine may increase the risk of serotonin syndrome; this combination is best avoided. Lithium may potentiate effect of neuromuscular blockers.

Nutritional/Ethanol Interactions Food: Lithium serum concentrations may be increased if taken with food. Limit caffeine.

Effects on Lab Values ↑ calcium (S), glucose, magnesium, potassium (S); ↓ thyroxine (S)

Adverse Reactions Frequency not defined.

Cardiovascular: Cardiac arrhythmias, hypotension, sinus node dysfunction, flattened or inverted T waves (reversible), edema, bradycardia, syncope

Central nervous system: Dizziness, vertigo, slurred speech, blackout spells, seizures, sedation, restlessness, confusion, psychomotor retardation, stupor, coma, dystonia, fatigue, lethargy, headache, pseudotumor cerebri, slowed intellectual functioning, tics

Dermatologic: Dry or thinning of hair, folliculitis, alopecia, exacerbation of psoriasis, rash

Endocrine & metabolic: Euthyroid goiter and/or hypothyroidism, hyperthyroidism, hyperglycemia, diabetes insipidus

Gastrointestinal: Polydipsia, anorexia, nausea, vomiting, diarrhea, xerostomia, metallic taste, weight gain

Genitourinary: Incontinence, polyuria, glycosuria, oliguria, albuminuria

Hematologic: Leukocytosis

Neuromuscular & skeletal: Tremor, muscle hyperirritability, ataxia, choreoathetoid movements, hyperactive deep tendon reflexes, myasthenia gravis (rare)

Ocular: Nystagmus, blurred vision, transient scotoma

Miscellaneous: Discoloration of fingers and toes

Overdosage/Toxicology Symptoms of overdose include sedation, confusion, tremor, joint pain, visual changes, seizures, and coma. There is no specific antidote for lithium poisoning. For acute ingestion following initiation of essential overdose management, begin correction of fluid and electrolyte imbalance. Hemodialysis and whole bowel irrigation is the treatment of choice for severe intoxications; charcoal is ineffective.

Pharmacodynamics/Kinetics

Absorption: Rapid and complete

Half-Life Elimination: 18-24 hours; can increase to more than 36 hours in elderly or with renal impairment

Time to Peak: Serum: Nonsustained release: ~0.5-2 hours

Metabolism: Not metabolized

Formulations

Capsule, as carbonate: 150 mg, 300 mg, 600 mg

Eskalith®: 300 mg [contains benzyl alcohol]

Syrup, as citrate: 300 mg/5 mL (5 mL, 10 mL, 480 mL) [contains alcohol]

Tablet, as carbonate: 300 mg

Tablet, controlled release, as carbonate (Eskalith CR®): 450 mg

Tablet, slow release, as carbonate (Lithobid®): 300 mg

Dosing

Adults: Bipolar disorders: Oral: 900-2400 mg/day in 3-4 divided doses or 900-1800 mg/day in two divided doses of sustained release

Note: Monitor serum concentrations and clinical response (efficacy and toxicity) to determine proper dose

Elderly: Bipolar disorders: Oral: Initial: 300 mg twice daily; increase weekly in increments of 300 mg/day, monitoring levels; rarely need to go >900-1200 mg/day.

Pediatrics:

Bipolar disorders: Oral: Children 6-12 years: 15-60 mg/kg/day in 3-4 divided doses; dose not to exceed usual adult dosage. **Note:** Monitor serum concentrations and clinical response (efficacy and toxicity) to determine proper dose.

Conduct disorder (unlabeled use): Oral: Children 6-12 years: 15-30 mg/kg/day in 3-4 divided doses; dose not to exceed usual adult dosage

Renal Impairment:

Cl_{cr} 10-50 mL/minute: Administer 50% to 75% of normal dose.

Cl_{cr} <10 mL/minute: Administer 25% to 50% of normal dose.

Dialyzable (50% to 100%)

Administration

Oral: Give with meals to decrease GI upset.

Monitoring Laboratory Tests Serum lithium every 3-4 days during initial therapy. Monitor renal, hepatic, thyroid, and cardiovascular function; fluid status; serum electrolytes; CBC with differential, urinalysis.

Levels should be obtained twice weekly until both patient's clinical status and levels are stable then levels may be obtained every 1-2 months.

Timing of serum samples: Draw trough just before next dose.

Therapeutic levels:

Acute mania: 0.6-1.2 mEq/L (SI: 0.6-1.2 mmol/L)

Protection against future episodes in most patients with bipolar disorder: 0.8-1 mEq/L (SI: 0.8-1.0 mmol/L); a higher rate of relapse is described in subjects who are maintained at <0.4 mEq/L (SI: 0.4 mmol/L).

Elderly patients can usually be maintained at lower end of therapeutic range (0.6-0.8 mEq/L).

Toxic concentration: >2 mEq/L (SI: >2 mmol/L)

(Continued)

Lithium *(Continued)*

Adverse effect levels:
GI complaints/tremor: 1.5-2 mEq/L
Confusion/somnolence: 2-2.5 mEq/L
Seizures/death: >2.5 mEq/L

Monitoring and Teaching Issues

Physical Assessment: Assess effectiveness and interactions of other medications patient may be taking (see Drug Interactions). See Contraindications and Warnings/Precautions for use cautions. Monitor laboratory results at beginning of therapy, when adjusting dose, and periodically thereafter (see above). Monitor effectiveness of therapy and adverse reactions at beginning of therapy and periodically with long-term use. (**Note:** Lithium has a very small window of safety (TI) - see Adverse Reactions). Assess knowledge/teach patient appropriate use, interventions to reduce side effects, and importance of reporting adverse symptoms promptly. **Pregnancy risk factor D** - determine that patient is not pregnant before beginning treatment. Instruct patients of childbearing age about appropriate barrier contraceptive measures. Breast-feeding is contraindicated.

Patient Education: Take exactly as directed; do not change dosage without consulting prescriber. Do not crush or chew tablets or capsules. Maintain adequate hydration (2-3 L/day of fluids) unless advised by prescriber to restrict fluids (especially in summer). Avoid changes in sodium content (eg, low sodium diets); reduction of sodium can increase lithium toxicity. Limit caffeine intake (diuresis can increase lithium toxicity). Frequent blood test and monitoring will be necessary. You may experience decreased appetite or altered taste sensation (small, frequent meals may help maintain nutrition); or drowsiness or dizziness, especially during early therapy (use caution when driving or engaging in tasks requiring alertness until response to drug is known). Immediately report unresolved diarrhea, abrupt changes in weight, muscular tremors or lack of coordination, fever, or changes in urinary volume. **Pregnancy/breast-feeding precautions:** Do not get pregnant while taking this medication; use appropriate contraceptive measures. Do not breast-feed.

Dietary Issues: May be taken with meals to avoid GI upset; have patient drink 2-3 L of water daily.

Geriatric Considerations: Some elderly patients may be extremely sensitive to the effects of lithium. Initial doses need to be adjusted for renal function in the elderly; thereafter, adjust doses based upon serum concentrations and response.

Pregnancy Issues: Cardiac malformations in the infant, including Ebstein's anomaly, are associated with use of lithium during the first trimester of pregnancy. Nontoxic effects to the newborn include shallow respiration, hypotonia, lethargy, cyanosis, diabetes insipidus, thyroid depression, and nontoxic goiter when lithium is used near term. Efforts should be made to avoid lithium use during the first trimester; if an alternative therapy is not appropriate, the lowest possible dose of lithium should be used throughout the pregnancy. Fetal echocardiography and ultrasound to screen for anomalies should be conducted between 16-20 weeks of gestation. Lithium levels should be monitored in the mother and may need adjusted following delivery.

Related Information

Peak and Trough Guidelines *on page 1544*

Lithium Carbonate *see* Lithium *on page 810*
Lithium Citrate *see* Lithium *on page 810*
Lithobid® *see* Lithium *on page 810*
LMD® *see* Dextran *on page 390*
LNg 20 *see* Levonorgestrel *on page 793*
LoCHOLEST® *see* Cholestyramine Resin *on page 282*
LoCHOLEST® Light *see* Cholestyramine Resin *on page 282*
Locoid® *see* Hydrocortisone *on page 673*
Locoid® *see* Topical Corticosteroids *on page 1334*
Locoid Lipocream® *see* Hydrocortisone *on page 673*
Lodine® *see* Etodolac *on page 534*
Lodine® XL *see* Etodolac *on page 534*
Lodoxamide Tromethamine *see page 1509*
Loestrin® *see* Ethinyl Estradiol and Norethindrone *on page 527*
Loestrin® Fe *see* Ethinyl Estradiol and Norethindrone *on page 527*
L-OHP *see* Oxaliplatin *on page 1012*

Lomefloxacin (loe me FLOKS a sin)

U.S. Brand Names Maxaquin®

Synonyms Lomefloxacin Hydrochloride

Generic Available No

Pharmacologic Category Antibiotic, Quinolone

Pregnancy Risk Factor C

Lactation Excretion in breast milk unknown/contraindicated

Use Lower respiratory infections, acute bacterial exacerbation of chronic bronchitis, and urinary tract infections caused by *E. coli*, *K. pneumoniae*, *P. mirabilis*, *P. aeruginosa*; also has gram-positive activity including *S. pneumoniae* and some staphylococci; surgical prophylaxis (transrectal prostate biopsy or transurethral procedures)

Use - Unlabeled/Investigational Skin infections, sexually-transmitted diseases

Mechanism of Action/Effect Inhibits DNA-gyrase in susceptible organisms thereby inhibits relaxation of supercoiled DNA and promotes breakage of DNA strands. DNA gyrase (topoisomerase II), is an essential bacterial enzyme that maintains the superhelical structure of DNA and is required for DNA replication and transcription, DNA repair, recombination, and transposition.

Contraindications Hypersensitivity to lomefloxacin, any component of the formulation, or other members of the quinolone group (such as, nalidixic acid, oxolinic acid, cinoxacin, norfloxacin, and ciprofloxacin); avoid use in children <18 years of age due to association of other quinolones with transient arthropathies

Warnings/Precautions Not recommended in children <18 years of age; CNS stimulation may occur (tremor, restlessness, confusion, and very rarely hallucinations or seizures); use with caution in patients with known or suspected CNS disorders or renal dysfunction; use caution to avoid possible photosensitivity reactions during and for several days following fluoroquinolone therapy. Quinolones may exacerbate myasthenia gravis.

Severe hypersensitivity reactions, including anaphylaxis, have occurred with quinolone therapy. If an allergic reaction occurs (itching, urticaria, dyspnea or facial edema, loss of consciousness, tingling, cardiovascular collapse), discontinue drug immediately. Prolonged use may result in superinfection; pseudomembranous colitis may occur and should be considered in all patients who present with diarrhea. Tendon inflammation and/or rupture has been reported. Risk may be increased with concurrent corticosteroids, particularly in the elderly. Discontinue at first sign of tendon inflammation or pain.

Pregnancy risk C.

Drug Interactions

Cytochrome P450 Effect: Inhibits **CYP1A2**

Decreased Effect: Decreased absorption with antacids containing aluminum, magnesium, and/or calcium (by up to 98% if given at the same time). Antineoplastic agents may decrease quinolone absorption.

Increased Effect/Toxicity: Quinolones can cause elevated levels of caffeine, warfarin, cyclosporine, and theophylline. Azlocillin, imipenem, cimetidine, loop diuretics, and probenecid may increase lomefloxacin serum levels. Increased CNS stimulation may occur with caffeine, theophylline, NSAIDs. Foscarnet has been associated with seizures in patients receiving quinolones. Concurrent use of corticosteroids may increase risk of tendon rupture.

Nutritional/Ethanol Interactions

Food: Lomefloxacin peak serum levels may be prolonged if taken with food.

Herb/Nutraceutical: Avoid dong quai, St John's wort (may cause photosensitization).

Adverse Reactions

1% to 10%:

Central nervous system: Headache (3%), dizziness (2%)

Dermatologic: Photosensitivity (2%)

Gastrointestinal: Nausea (4%)

<1% (Limited to important or life-threatening): Abdominal pain, abnormal taste, allergic reaction, angina pectoris, anuria, arrhythmia, back pain, bradycardia, cardiac failure, chest pain, chills, coma, constipation, convulsions, cough, cyanosis, decreased heat tolerance, diaphoresis (increased), discoloration of tongue, dyspnea, dysuria, earache, edema, epistaxis, extrasystoles, facial edema, fatigue, flatulence, flu-like symptoms, flushing, gout, hematuria, hyperkinesia, hypertension, hypoglycemia, hypotension, increased fibrinolysis, leg cramps, malaise, myalgia, myocardial infarction; paresthesia, purpura, rash, syncope, tachycardia, thirst, thrombocytopenia, tremor, urinary disorders, vertigo, vomiting, weakness, xerostomia; quinolones have been associated with tendon rupture and tendonitis

Overdosage/Toxicology Symptoms of overdose include acute renal failure and seizures. Treatment is supportive; not removed by peritoneal or hemodialysis.

Pharmacodynamics/Kinetics

Absorption: Well absorbed

Half-Life Elimination: 5-7.5 hours

Formulations Tablet, as hydrochloride: 400 mg

Dosing

Adults:

Lower respiratory and urinary tract infections (UTI): Oral: 400 mg once daily for 10-14 days

Urinary tract infection (UTI) due to susceptible organisms:

Uncomplicated cystitis caused by *E. coli*: Oral: Female: 400 mg once daily for 3 successive days

Uncomplicated cystitis caused by *Klebsiella pneumoniae, Proteus mirabilis*, or *Staphylococcus saprophyticus*: Oral: Female: 400 mg once daily for 10 successive days

Complicated UTI caused by *E. coli, Klebsiella pneumoniae, Proteus mirabilis*, or *Pseudomonas aeruginosa*: Oral: 400 mg once daily for 14 successive days

Surgical prophylaxis: Oral: 400 mg 2-6 hours before surgery

Uncomplicated gonorrhea: Oral: 400 mg as a single dose

Elderly: No adjustment necessary for Cl_{cr} ≥40 mL/minute. Follow renal adjustments for patients with reduced renal function.

Renal Impairment:

Cl_{cr} 10-40 mL/minute: Initial loading dose = 400 mg; followed by 200 mg once daily maintenance dose

Hemodialysis: Use loading dose of 400 mg; followed by 200 mg once daily for treatment duration.

Administration

Oral: Take 1 hour before or 2 hours after meals.

Monitoring Laboratory Tests Perform culture and sensitivity studies prior to initiating therapy to determine the causative organism and its susceptibility to lomefloxacin. Monitor CBC, renal and hepatic function periodically if therapy is prolonged.

Monitoring and Teaching Issues

Physical Assessment: Assess allergy history before initiating therapy. See Contraindications, Warnings/Precautions, and Dosing for use cautions. Assess potential for interactions with other prescriptions, OTC medications, or herbal products patient may be taking (see Drug Interactions). **I.V.:** See Administration specifics and monitor closely for severe hypersensitivity reactions. If an allergic reaction occurs drug should be discontinued immediately. Assess results of laboratory tests (see above), therapeutic effectiveness, and adverse effects (eg, hypersensitivity reactions which can occur days after therapy has started and opportunistic infection - see Adverse Reactions and Overdose/Toxicology) regularly during therapy. Teach patient appropriate use (according to formulation), possible

(Continued)

Lomefloxacin *(Continued)*

side effects and interventions, and adverse symptoms to report (see Patient Education). **Pregnancy risk factor C** - benefits of use should outweigh possible risks. Breast-feeding is contraindicated.

Patient Education: Inform prescriber of all prescriptions, OTC medications, or herbal products you are taking, and any allergies you have. Do not take anything new during treatment unless approved by prescriber. Take exactly as directed: at least 4 hours before or 8 hours after antacids or other drug products containing calcium, iron, or zinc. Take entire prescription even if feeling better. Maintain adequate hydration (2-3 L/day of fluids) unless advised by prescriber to restrict fluids. You may experience dizziness, lightheadedness, or confusion (use caution when driving or engaging in tasks that require alertness until response to drug is known); nausea or vomiting (small, frequent meals, frequent mouth care, sucking lozenges, or chewing gum may help); or photosensitivity (use sunscreen, wear protective clothing and eyewear, and avoid direct sunlight). Discontinue use immediately and report to prescriber if inflammation, tendon pain, or allergic reaction occurs (itching urticaria, difficulty breathing, facial edema, difficulty swallowing, loss of consciousness, tingling, chest pain, palpitations). Report palpitations or chest pain; CNS changes (excitability, seizures); persistent diarrhea or constipation; signs of infection (unusual fever or chills, vaginal itching or foul-smelling vaginal discharge, easy bruising or bleeding). **Pregnancy/breast-feeding precautions:** Inform prescriber if you are or intend to become pregnant. Do not breast-feed.

Dietary Issues: May be taken without regard to meals.

Geriatric Considerations: Dosage adjustment is not necessary in patients with normal renal function, Cl_{cr} ≥40 mL/minute; otherwise, follow dosage guidelines for renal impairment. Age-associated increase in half-life and decrease in clearance are thought to be secondary to age-related changes in renal function.

Lomefloxacin Hydrochloride *see* Lomefloxacin *on page 812*

Lomocot® *see* Diphenoxylate and Atropine *on page 424*

Lomotil® *see* Diphenoxylate and Atropine *on page 424*

Lomustine (loe MUS teen)

U.S. Brand Names CeeNU®

Synonyms CCNU

Generic Available No

Pharmacologic Category Antineoplastic Agent, Alkylating Agent

Pregnancy Risk Factor D

Lactation Enters breast milk/contraindicated

Use Treatment of brain tumors and Hodgkin's disease, non-Hodgkin's lymphoma, melanoma, renal carcinoma, lung cancer, colon cancer

Mechanism of Action/Effect Inhibits DNA and RNA synthesis via carbamylation of DNA polymerase, alkylation of DNA, and alteration of RNA, proteins, and enzymes

Contraindications Hypersensitivity to lomustine, any component of the formulation, or other nitrosoureas; pregnancy

Warnings/Precautions The U.S. Food and Drug Administration (FDA) currently recommends that procedures for proper handling and disposal for antineoplastic agents be considered. Use with caution in patients with depressed platelet, leukocyte or erythrocyte counts. Bone marrow depression, notably thrombocytopenia and leukopenia, may lead to bleeding and overwhelming infections in an already compromised patient; will last for at least 6 weeks after a dose, do not give courses more frequently than every 6 weeks because the toxicity is cumulative. Use with caution in patients with liver function abnormalities.

Drug Interactions

Cytochrome P450 Effect: Substrate of **CYP2D6**; Inhibits CYP2D6, 3A4

Decreased Effect: Decreased effect with phenobarbital, resulting in reduced efficacy of both drugs.

Increased Effect/Toxicity: Increased toxicity with cimetidine, reported to cause bone marrow depression or to potentiate the myelosuppressive effects of lomustine.

Nutritional/Ethanol Interactions Ethanol: Avoid ethanol (due to GI irritation).

Effects on Lab Values Liver function tests

Adverse Reactions

>10%:
- Gastrointestinal: Nausea, vomiting
  - Emetic potential:
  - <60 mg: Moderately high (60% to 90%)
  - ≥60 mg: High (>90%)
  - Time course of nausea/vomiting: Onset: 2-6 hours; Duration: 4-6 hours
- Hematologic: Leukopenia; Thrombocytopenia; Myelosuppression: Anemia; effects occur 4-6 weeks after a dose and may persist for 1-2 weeks
  - WBC: Moderate
  - Platelets: Severe
  - Onset (days): 14
  - Nadir (weeks): 4-5
  - Recovery (weeks): 6

1% to 10%:
- Central nervous system: Neurotoxicity
- Dermatologic: Skin rash, alopecia
- Gastrointestinal: Stomatitis, diarrhea
- Hematologic: Anemia
- Renal: Renal failure

<1% (Limited to important or life-threatening): Hepatotoxicity, pulmonary fibrosis with cumulative doses >600 mg

Overdosage/Toxicology Symptoms of overdose include nausea, vomiting, and leukopenia. There are no known antidotes. Treatment is symptomatic and supportive.

Pharmacodynamics/Kinetics

Absorption: Complete; appears in plasma within 3 minutes after administration

Half-Life Elimination: Parent drug: 16-72 hours; Active metabolite: Terminal: 1.3-2 days

Time to Peak: Serum: Active metabolite: ~3 hours

Metabolism: Rapidly hepatic via hydroxylation producing at least two active metabolites; enterohepatically recycled

Duration: Marrow recovery: ≤6 weeks

Formulations

Capsule: 10 mg, 40 mg, 100 mg

Capsule [dose pack]: 10 mg (2s); 40 mg (2s); 100 mg (2s)

Dosing

Adults & Elderly: Refer to individual protocols.

Chemotherapy: Oral: 100-130 mg/m^2 as a single dose every 6 weeks; readjust after initial treatment according to platelet and leukocyte counts

With compromised marrow function: Initial dose: 100 mg/m^2 as a single dose every 6 weeks

Repeat courses should only be administered after adequate recovery: WBC >4000 and platelet counts >100,000

Subsequent dosing adjustment based on nadir:

Leukocytes 2000-2900/mm^3, platelets 25,000-74,999/mm^3: Administer 70% of prior dose

Leukocytes <2000/mm^3, platelets <25,000/mm^3: Administer 50% of prior dose

Pediatrics: Chemotherapy: Oral (refer to individual protocols): Children: 75-150 mg/m^2 as a single dose every 6 weeks; subsequent doses are readjusted after initial treatment according to platelet and leukocyte counts.

Renal Impairment:

Cl_{cr} 10-50 mL/minute: Administer 75% of normal dose.

Cl_{cr} <10 mL/minute: Administer 50% of normal dose.

Hemodialysis effects: Supplemental dose is not necessary.

Administration

Oral: Take with fluids on an empty stomach; no food or drink for 2 hours after administration.

Stability

Storage: Refrigerate (<40°C/<104°F).

Monitoring Laboratory Tests CBC with differential, platelet count, hepatic and renal function, pulmonary function

Monitoring and Teaching Issues

Physical Assessment: See Contraindications, Warnings/Precautions, Drug Interactions, and Dosing for use cautions. Assess results of laboratory tests (see above), therapeutic effects, and adverse response (see Adverse Reactions and Overdose/Toxicology) prior to each treatment and on a regular basis throughout therapy. Teach patient possible side effects and appropriate interventions and adverse symptoms to report (see Patient Education). **Pregnancy risk factor D** - determine that patient is not pregnant before beginning treatment. Instruct patients of childbearing age about use of appropriate barrier contraceptive measures during therapy and for 1 month following therapy. Breast-feeding is contraindicated.

Patient Education: Inform prescriber of all prescriptions, OTC medications, or herbal products you are taking, and any allergies you have. Do not take anything new during treatment unless approved by prescriber. Take with fluids on an empty stomach; do not eat or drink for 2 hours prior to or following administration to reduce nausea and vomiting. During therapy, do not use alcohol. It is important to maintain adequate hydration (2-3 L/day of fluids) unless advised by prescriber to restrict fluids, and nutrition (small, frequent meals may help). You will be more susceptible to infection (avoid crowds and exposure to infection and do not have any vaccinations without consulting prescriber). You may experience hair loss (reversible); nausea or vomiting (small, frequent meals, frequent mouth care, sucking lozenges, or chewing gum may help or consult prescriber for approved antiemetic); mouth sores (frequent mouth care and use of a soft toothbrush or cotton swabs may help); or diarrhea (buttermilk, boiled milk, or yogurt may help reduce diarrhea - consult prescriber for approved medication). Report persistent nausea, vomiting, or diarrhea; bleeding or bruising; fever, chills, sore throat; vaginal discharge; rash; blood in urine, stool, or vomitus; delayed healing of any wounds; yellowing of skin or eyes; or changes in color of urine of stool. **Pregnancy/breast-feeding precautions:** Do not get pregnant while taking this medication. Consult prescriber for appropriate barrier contraceptives measures. This drug may cause severe fetal birth defects. Do not breast-feed.

Dietary Issues: Should be taken with fluids on an empty stomach; no food or drink for 2 hours after administration to decrease nausea.

Pregnancy Issues: May cause fetal harm when administered to a pregnant woman. Women of childbearing potential should be advised to avoid pregnancy and should be advised of the potential harm to the fetus.

Lonox® *see* Diphenoxylate and Atropine *on page 424*

Loperamide (loe PER a mide)

U.S. Brand Names Imodium® A-D [OTC]

Synonyms Loperamide Hydrochloride

Generic Available Yes

Pharmacologic Category Antidiarrheal

Pregnancy Risk Factor B

Lactation Enters breast milk/compatible

Use Treatment of acute diarrhea and chronic diarrhea associated with inflammatory bowel disease; chronic functional diarrhea (idiopathic), chronic diarrhea caused by bowel resection or organic lesions; to decrease the volume of ileostomy discharge

Use - Unlabeled/Investigational Treatment of traveler's diarrhea in combination with trimethoprim-sulfamethoxazole (co-trimoxazole) (3-day therapy)

(Continued)

Loperamide *(Continued)*

Mechanism of Action/Effect Acts directly on intestinal muscles to inhibit peristalsis and prolongs transit time enhancing fluid and electrolyte movement through intestinal mucosa; reduces fecal volume, increases viscosity, and diminishes fluid and electrolyte loss; demonstrates antisecretory activity; exhibits peripheral action

Contraindications Hypersensitivity to loperamide or any component of the formulation; bloody diarrhea; patients who must avoid constipation; diarrhea resulting from some infections; pseudomembranous colitis

Warnings/Precautions Large first-pass metabolism, use with caution in hepatic dysfunction. Should not be used if diarrhea accompanied by high fever, blood in stool.

Drug Interactions

Increased Effect/Toxicity: Loperamide may potentiate the adverse effects of CNS depressants, phenothiazines, tricyclic antidepressants.

Adverse Reactions Frequency not defined.

Cardiovascular: Shock

Central nervous system: Dizziness, drowsiness, fatigue, sedation

Dermatologic: Rash, toxic epidermal necrolysis

Gastrointestinal: Abdominal cramping, abdominal distention, constipation, dry mouth, nausea, paralytic ileus, vomiting

Miscellaneous: Anaphylaxis

Overdosage/Toxicology Symptoms of overdose include CNS and respiratory depression, GI cramping, constipation, GI irritation, nausea, and vomiting. Overdose is noted when daily doses approximate 60 mg of loperamide. Treatment of overdose includes gastric lavage followed by 100 g activated charcoal through a nasogastric tube. Naloxone, 2 mg I.V. with repeat administration as necessary up to a total dose of 10 mg, can be used to reverse opiate effects.

Pharmacodynamics/Kinetics

Absorption: <40%

Half-Life Elimination: 7-14 hours

Metabolism: Hepatic (>50%) to inactive compounds

Onset: 0.5-1 hour

Formulations

Caplet, as hydrochloride (Imodium® A-D): 2 mg

Capsule, as hydrochloride: 2 mg

Liquid, oral, as hydrochloride: 1 mg/5 mL (5 mL, 10 mL, 120 mL)

Imodium® A-D: 1 mg/5 mL (60 mL, 120 mL) [contains sodium benzoate, benzoic acid; cherry mint flavor]

Tablet, as hydrochloride: 2 mg

Dosing

Adults & Elderly:

Acute diarrhea: Oral: Initial: 4 mg (2 capsules), followed by 2 mg after each loose stool, up to 16 mg/day (8 capsules)

Chronic diarrhea: Oral: Initial: Follow acute diarrhea; maintenance dose should be slowly titrated downward to minimum required to control symptoms (typically, 4-8 mg/day in divided doses)

Traveler's diarrhea: Oral: Treat for no more than 2 days: 4 mg after first loose stool followed by 2 mg after each subsequent stool; maximum dose: 8 mg/day

Pediatrics:

Acute diarrhea: Oral: Initial doses (in first 24 hours):

2-6 years: 1 mg 3 times/day

6-8 years: 2 mg twice daily

8-12 years: 2 mg 3 times/day

Maintenance: After initial dosing, 0.1 mg/kg doses after each loose stool, but not exceeding initial dosage

Chronic diarrhea: Oral: 0.08-0.24 mg/kg/day divided 2-3 times/day, maximum: 2 mg/dose

Traveler's diarrhea: Treat for no more than 2 days

6-8 years: 1 mg after first loose stool followed by 1 mg after each subsequent stool; maximum dose: 4 mg/day

9-11 years: 2 mg after first loose stool followed by 1 mg after each subsequent stool; maximum dose: 6 mg/day

12 years to Adults: Refer to adult dosing.

Administration

Oral: Therapy for chronic diarrhea should not exceed 10 days.

Monitoring and Teaching Issues

Physical Assessment: Assess for cause of diarrhea before administering first dose. See Contraindications, Warnings/Precautions, and Drug Interactions for use cautions. Teach patient proper use, possible side effects and appropriate interventions, and adverse symptoms to report (see Patient Education).

Patient Education: Adults should not take more than 8 capsules or 80 mL in 24 hours. May cause drowsiness; use caution. Increased exercise, identifying and avoiding foods that cause diarrhea, safe food preparation and storage, use of buttermilk, yogurt, or boiled milk may help reduce diarrhea. If acute diarrhea lasts longer than 48 hours, consult prescriber. Do not take if diarrhea is bloody.

Geriatric Considerations: Elderly are particularly sensitive to fluid and electrolyte loss. This generally results in lethargy, weakness, and confusion. Repletion and maintenance of electrolytes and water are essential in the treatment of diarrhea. Drug therapy must be limited in order to avoid toxicity with this agent.

Loperamide Hydrochloride *see* Loperamide *on page 815*

Lopid® *see* Gemfibrozil *on page 625*

Lopinavir *see* Lopinavir and Ritonavir *on page 817*

Lopinavir and Ritonavir (loe PIN a veer & rit ON uh veer)

U.S. Brand Names Kaletra™

Synonyms Lopinavir

Generic Available No

Pharmacologic Category Antiretroviral Agent, Protease Inhibitor

Pregnancy Risk Factor C

Lactation Excretion in breast milk unknown/contraindicated

Use Treatment of HIV infection in combination with other antiretroviral agents

Mechanism of Action/Effect A coformulation of lopinavir and ritonavir. The lopinavir component is the active inhibitor of HIV protease. Lopinavir inhibits HIV protease and renders the enzyme incapable of processing polyprotein precursor which leads to production of noninfectious immature HIV particles. The ritonavir component inhibits the CYP3A metabolism of lopinavir, allowing increased plasma levels of lopinavir.

Contraindications Hypersensitivity to lopinavir, ritonavir, or any component of the formulation; administration with medications highly dependent upon CYP3A or CYP2D6 for clearance for which increased levels are associated with serious and/or life-threatening events. Ritonavir is contraindicated with astemizole, cisapride, dihydroergotamine, ergonovine, ergotamine, flecainide, lovastatin, methylergonovine, midazolam, pimozide, propafenone, simvastatin, triazolam.

Warnings/Precautions Cases of pancreatitis, some fatal, have been associated with lopinavir/ritonavir; use caution in patients with a history of pancreatitis. Patients with signs or symptoms of pancreatitis should be evaluated and therapy suspended as clinically appropriate. Diabetes mellitus and exacerbation of diabetes mellitus have been reported in patients taking protease inhibitors. Use caution in patients with hepatic impairment; patients with hepatitis or elevations in transaminases prior to the start of therapy may be at increased risk for further increases in transaminases. Large increases in total cholesterol and triglycerides have been reported; screening should be done prior to therapy and periodically throughout treatment. Avoid concurrent use of St John's wort (may lead to loss of virologic response and/or resistance). Hemophilia type A and type B have been reported with protease inhibitor use. Redistribution or accumulation of body fat has been observed in patients using antiretroviral therapy. The potential for cross-resistance with other protease inhibitors is currently under study. Safety and efficacy have not been established for children <6 months of age. Pregnancy risk C.

Drug Interactions

Cytochrome P450 Effect:

Lopinavir: Substrate of 3A4

Ritonavir: Substrate of CYP1A2, 2B6, **2D6, 3A4**; Inhibits CYP2C8/9, 2C19, **2D6**, 2E1, **3A4**; Induces CYP1A2, 2C8/9, 3A4

Decreased Effect: Carbamazepine, dexamethasone, phenobarbital, phenytoin, and rifampin may decrease levels of lopinavir. Non-nucleoside reverse transcriptase inhibitors: Efavirenz, nevirapine may decrease levels of lopinavir. To avoid incompatibility with didanosine, administer didanosine 1 hour before or 2 hours after lopinavir/ritonavir. Decreased levels of ethinyl estradiol may result from concurrent use. Lopinavir/ritonavir may decrease levels of abacavir, atovaquone, or zidovudine.

Increased Effect/Toxicity:

Contraindicated drugs: Life-threatening arrhythmias may result from concurrent use of flecainide or propafenone. Concurrent use is contraindicated. Concurrent use of cisapride, pimozide, astemizole is also contraindicated. Some benzodiazepines (midazolam and triazolam) are contraindicated, due to the potential for increased response/respiratory depression. Concurrent use of ergot alkaloids is contraindicated, due to potential toxicity.

Serum levels of other antiarrhythmics, including amiodarone, bepridil, lidocaine (systemic), and quinidine may be increased with concurrent use. Serum levels of calcium channel blockers (including felodipine, nicardipine, and nifedipine), clarithromycin, immunosuppressants (cyclosporin, tacrolimus, sirolimus), HMG-CoA reductase inhibitors (lovastatin and simvastatin are not recommended, atorvastatin and cerivastatin should be used at lowest possible dose), itraconazole, ketoconazole, methadone, and rifabutin (decreased dose recommended) may be increased. Serum levels of protease inhibitors may be altered during concurrent therapy. Ritonavir may increase serum concentrations of amprenavir, indinavir, or saquinavir. Serum levels of sildenafil may be substantially increased (use caution at decreased dose of sildenafil, maximum of 25 mg in 48 hours). Warfarin serum levels may also be increased.

Delavirdine increases levels of lopinavir; dosing recommendations are not yet established.

Lopinavir/ritonavir solution contains alcohol, concurrent use with disulfiram or metronidazole should be avoided. May cause disulfiram-like reaction.

Nutritional/Ethanol Interactions Herb/Nutraceutical: St John's wort may decrease levels of protease inhibitors and lead to possible resistance; concurrent use in not recommended.

Adverse Reactions Protease inhibitors cause dyslipidemia which includes elevated cholesterol and triglycerides and a redistribution of body fat centrally to cause "protease paunch," buffalo hump, facial atrophy, and breast enlargement. These agents also cause hyperglycemia.

>10%:

- Endocrine & metabolic: Hypercholesterolemia (9% to 28%), triglycerides increased (9% to 28%)
- Gastrointestinal: Diarrhea (16% to 24%), nausea (3% to 15%)
- Hepatic: GGT increased (4% to 25%)

2% to 10%:

- Central nervous system: Headache (2% to 7%), pain (0% to 2%), insomnia (1% to 2%)
- Dermatologic: Rash (1% to 4%)
- Endocrine & metabolic: Hyperglycemia (1% to 4%), hyperuricemia (up to 4%), sodium decreased (3% children), organic phosphorus decreased (up to 2%), amylase increased (2% to 10%)

(Continued)

Lopinavir and Ritonavir *(Continued)*

Gastrointestinal: Abnormal stools (up to 6%), abdominal pain (2% to 4%), vomiting (2% to 5%), dyspepsia (0.5% to 2%)
Hematologic: Platelets decreased (4% children), neutrophils decreased (1% to 3%)
Hepatic: AST increased (2% to 9%), ALT increased (4% to 8%), bilirubin increased (children 3%)
Neuromuscular & skeletal: Weakness (4% to 7%)

<2% (Limited to important or life-threatening): Alopecia, amnesia, ataxia, avitaminosis, cholecystitis, Cushing's syndrome, deep vein thrombosis, depression, diabetes mellitus, dyskinesia, dyspnea, exfoliative dermatitis, facial paralysis, flu-like syndrome, hepatic dysfunction, lactic hemorrhagic colitis, maculopapular rash, migraine, neuritis, pancreatitis, paresthesia, peripheral neuropathy, pulmonary edema, renal calculus, somnolence, tinnitus, vasculitis

Overdosage/Toxicology Solution contains 42.4% alcohol; overdosage in a child may cause alcohol-related toxicity and may be potentially lethal. Treatment should be symptomatic and supportive. Activated charcoal may aid in the removal of unabsorbed medication.

Pharmacokinetic Note See Ritonavir monograph.

Pharmacodynamics/Kinetics

Half-Life Elimination:

Lopinavir: 5-6 hours

Metabolism:

Lopinavir: Hepatic via CYP3A; 13 metabolites identified

Formulations

Capsule: Lopinavir 133.3 mg and ritonavir 33.3 mg
Solution, oral: Lopinavir 80 mg and ritonavir 20 mg per mL (160 mL) [contains alcohol 42.4%]

Dosing

Adults: HIV infection (as a component of combination therapy): Oral (take with food): Lopinavir 400 mg/ritonavir 100 mg twice daily

Dosage adjustment when taken with efavirenz or nevirapine: Oral (take with food): Lopinavir 533 mg/ritonavir 133 mg twice daily

Elderly: Initial studies did not include enough elderly patients to determine effects based on age. Use with caution due to possible decreased hepatic, renal, and cardiac function.

Pediatrics: HIV infection (component of combination therapy): Oral (take with food):

Children 6 months to 12 years: Dosage based on weight, presented based on mg of lopinavir (maximum dose: Lopinavir 400 mg/ritonavir 100 mg)
- 7-<15 kg: 12 mg/kg twice daily
- 15-40 kg: 10 mg/kg twice daily
- >40 kg: Refer to adult dosing.

Children >12 years: Refer to adult dosing.

Dosage adjustment when taken with efavirenz or nevirapine:

Children 6 months to 12 years:
- 7-<15 kg: 13 mg/kg twice daily
- 15-50 kg: 11 mg/kg twice daily
- >50 kg: Refer to adult dosing

Children >12 years: Refer to adult dosing.

Renal Impairment: Has not been studied in patients with renal impairment; however, a decrease in clearance is not expected.

Hepatic Impairment: No specific guidelines available - plasma levels may be increased in patients with hepatic impairment.

Administration

Oral: Take with food; if using didanosine, take didanosine 1 hour before or 2 hours after lopinavir/ritonavir

Stability

Storage: Oral solution and gelatin capsules: Store at 2°C to 8°C (36°F to 46°F). Avoid exposure to excessive heat. If stored at room temperature (25°C or 77°F), use within 2 months.

Monitoring and Teaching Issues

Physical Assessment: See Contraindications, Warnings/Precautions, and Dosing for use cautions. Assess potential for interactions with other prescriptions, OTC medications, or herbal products patient may be taking (see Drug Interactions). Assess patient response at regular intervals during therapy (see Adverse Reactions and Overdose/Toxicology). Teach patient proper use, possible side effects and appropriate interventions (eg, glucose testing; protease inhibitors may cause hyperglycemia - exacerbation or new-onset diabetes), and adverse symptoms to report (see Patient Education). **Pregnancy risk factor C** - benefits of use should outweigh possible risks. May decrease effects of ethinyl estradiol containing contraceptives. Advise patient about alternative contraceptive measures. Breast-feeding is contraindicated.

Patient Education: Inform prescriber of all prescriptions, OTC medications, or herbal products you are taking, and any allergies you have. Do not take anything new during treatment unless approved by prescriber. This is not a cure for HIV, nor has it been shown to reduce transmission of HIV. Take as directed, with meals. Maintain adequate hydration (2-3 L/day of fluids) unless advised by prescriber to restrict fluids. This drug may be prescribed with a combination of other medications; time these medications as directed by prescriber. You may be advised to check your glucose levels (this drug can cause exacerbation or new-onset diabetes). May cause body changes due to redistribution of body fat, facial atrophy, or breast enlargement (normal effects of drug); dizziness, insomnia, abnormal thinking (use caution when driving or engaging in potentially hazardous tasks until response to drug is known); nausea, vomiting, or taste perversion (small, frequent meals, frequent mouth care, chewing gum, or sucking lozenges may help); muscle weakness (consult prescriber for approved analgesic); headache or insomnia (consult prescriber for medication); gynecomastia, hypogonadism (male), decreased libido, or abnormal ejaculation; muscle weakness; or hair loss. Report chest pain, calf pain, redness or swelling, facial edema, palpitations; difficulty breathing; unresolved and persistent GI effects; rash or skin breakdown or discoloration; or any other persistent adverse effects. **Pregnancy/breast-feeding precautions:** Inform prescriber if you are or intend to become pregnant. May reduce effectiveness of some contraceptives. Consult prescriber for appropriate contraceptive measures. Do not breast-feed.

Dietary Issues: Should be taken with food.

Breast-feeding Issues: HIV-infected mothers are discouraged from breast-feeding to decrease potential transmission of HIV.

Pregnancy Issues: It is not known if lopinavir crosses the placenta; transfer of ritonavir is minimal based on preliminary data. Pregnancy and protease inhibitors are both associated with an increased risk of hyperglycemia. Glucose levels should be closely monitored. Health professionals are encouraged to contact the antiretroviral pregnancy registry to monitor outcomes of pregnant women exposed to antiretroviral medications (1-800-258-4263).

Related Information

Ritonavir *on page 1196*

Lopressor® *see* Metoprolol *on page 893*

Lorabid® *see* Loracarbef *on page 819*

Loracarbef (lor a KAR bef)

U.S. Brand Names Lorabid®

Generic Available No

Pharmacologic Category Antibiotic, Carbacephem

Pregnancy Risk Factor B

Lactation Excretion in breast milk unknown/use caution

Use Infections caused by susceptible organisms involving the respiratory tract, acute otitis media, sinusitis, skin and skin structure, bone and joint, and urinary tract and gynecologic

Mechanism of Action/Effect Inhibits bacterial cell wall synthesis by binding to one or more of the penicillin binding proteins (PBPs); inhibits the final transpeptidation step of peptidoglycan synthesis in bacterial cell walls, thus inhibiting cell wall biosynthesis.

Contraindications Hypersensitivity to loracarbef, any component of the formulation, or cephalosporins

Warnings/Precautions Modify dosage in patients with severe renal impairment; prolonged use may result in superinfection; use with caution in patients with a previous history of hypersensitivity to other beta-lactam antibiotics (eg, penicillins, cephalosporins)

Drug Interactions

Increased Effect/Toxicity: Loracarbef serum levels are increased with coadministered probenecid.

Nutritional/Ethanol Interactions Food: Administration with food decreases and delays the peak plasma concentration.

Adverse Reactions

≥1%:

Central nervous system: Headache (1% to 3%), somnolence (<2%)

Dermatologic: Rash (1% to 3%)

Gastrointestinal: Diarrhea (4% to 6%), nausea (2%), vomiting (1% to 3%), anorexia (<2%), abdominal pain (1%)

Genitourinary: Vaginitis (1%)

Respiratory: Rhinitis (2% to 6%)

<1%: Anaphylaxis, arthralgia, candidiasis, cholestasis, eosinophilia, hemolytic anemia, interstitial nephritis, jaundice, nephrotoxicity with transient elevations of BUN/creatinine, nervousness, neutropenia, positive Coombs' test, pruritus, pseudomembranous colitis, seizures (with high doses and renal dysfunction), serum sickness-like reaction, slightly increased AST/ALT, Stevens-Johnson syndrome, thrombocytopenia, urticaria

Overdosage/Toxicology Symptoms of overdose include abdominal discomfort and diarrhea. Treatment is supportive.

Pharmacodynamics/Kinetics

Absorption: Rapid

Half-Life Elimination: ~1 hour

Time to Peak: Serum: ~1 hour

Formulations

Capsule: 200 mg, 400 mg

Powder for oral suspension: 100 mg/5 mL (100 mL); 200 mg/5 mL (100 mL) [strawberry bubblegum flavor]

Dosing

Adults & Elderly:

Uncomplicated urinary tract infections: Oral: 200 mg once daily for 7 days

Skin and soft tissue: Oral: 200 mg every 12 hours for 7 days

Uncomplicated pyelonephritis: Oral: 400 mg every 12 hours for 14 days

Pharyngitis/tonsillitis: Oral: 200 mg every 12 hours for 10 days

Sinusitis: Oral: 400 mg every 12 hours for 10 days

Upper/lower respiratory tract infection: Oral: 400 mg every 12 hours for 7-14 days

Pediatrics:

Acute otitis media: Oral: Children: 15 mg/kg twice daily for 10 days

Pharyngitis and impetigo: Oral: Children: 7.5-15 mg/kg twice daily for 10 days

Renal Impairment:

Cl_{cr} ≥50 mL/minute: Administer usual dose.

Cl_{cr} 10-49 mL/minute: Administer 50% of usual dose at usual interval or usual dose given half as often.

Cl_{cr} <10 mL/minute: Administer usual dose every 3-5 days.

Hemodialysis: Doses should be administered after dialysis sessions.

Administration

Oral: Take on an empty stomach at least 1 hour before or 2 hours after meals. Finish all medication. Shake suspension well before using.

(Continued)

Loracarbef *(Continued)*

Stability

Storage: Suspension may be kept at room temperature for 14 days.

Monitoring Laboratory Tests Perform culture and sensitivity studies prior to initiating therapy.

Monitoring and Teaching Issues

Physical Assessment: Assess previous history of allergies. See Contraindications, Warnings/Precautions, and Dosing for use cautions. Assess results of laboratory tests (see above), therapeutic effectiveness, and adverse response on a regular basis during therapy (see Adverse Reactions and Overdose/Toxicology). Teach patient appropriate use, possible side effects and appropriate interventions, and adverse symptoms to report (see Patient Education). Note breast-feeding caution.

Patient Education: Inform prescriber of all prescriptions, OTC medications, or herbal products you are taking, and any allergies you have. Do not take anything new during treatment unless approved by prescriber. Take as directed, preferably on an empty stomach, 1 hour before or 2 hours after meals. Take entire prescription even if feeling better. Shake suspension well before using. Maintain adequate hydration (2-3 L/day of fluids) unless advised by prescriber to restrict fluids. You may experience nausea, vomiting, or anorexia (small, frequent meals, frequent mouth care, sucking lozenges, or chewing gum may help). Report immediately any signs of skin rash, joint or back pain, or difficulty breathing. Report unusual fever, chills, vaginal itching or foul-smelling vaginal discharge, or easy bruising or bleeding. **Breast-feeding precaution:** Consult prescriber if breast-feeding.

Dietary Issues: Should be taken on an empty stomach at least 1 hour before or 2 hours after meals.

Geriatric Considerations: Half-life is slightly prolonged with age, presumably due to the reduced creatinine clearance related to aging. Adjust dose for renal function.

Loratadine (lor AT a deen)

U.S. Brand Names Claritin®

Generic Available No

Pharmacologic Category Antihistamine, Nonsedating

Pregnancy Risk Factor B

Lactation Enters breast milk/not recommended (AAP rates "compatible")

Use Relief of nasal and non-nasal symptoms of seasonal allergic rhinitis; treatment of chronic idiopathic urticaria

Mechanism of Action/Effect Long-acting tricyclic antihistamine with selective peripheral histamine H_1 receptor antagonistic properties; management of idiopathic chronic urticaria

Contraindications Hypersensitivity to loratadine or any component of the formulation

Warnings/Precautions Patients with liver or renal impairment should start with a lower dose (10 mg every other day), since their ability to clear the drug will be reduced. Safety in children <6 years of age has not been established.

Drug Interactions

Cytochrome P450 Effect: Substrate of CYP2D6, 3A4

Increased Effect/Toxicity: Increased plasma concentrations of loratadine and its active metabolite with ketoconazole and erythromycin, however, no change in QT_c interval was seen. Increased toxicity with procarbazine, other antihistamines, alcohol. Protease inhibitors (amprenavir, ritonavir, nelfinavir) may increase the serum levels of loratadine.

Nutritional/Ethanol Interactions

Ethanol: Avoid ethanol (although sedation is limited with loratadine, may increase risk of CNS depression).

Food: Increases bioavailability and delays peak.

Herb/Nutraceutical: St John's wort may decrease loratadine levels.

Adverse Reactions

Adults:

Central nervous system: Headache (12%), somnolence (8%), fatigue (4%)

Gastrointestinal: Xerostomia (3%)

Children:

Central nervous system: Nervousness (4% ages 6-12 years), fatigue (3% ages 6-12 years, 2% to 3% ages 2-5 years), malaise (2% ages 6-12 years)

Dermatologic: Rash (2% to 3% ages 2-5 years)

Gastrointestinal: Abdominal pain (2% ages 6-12 years), stomatitis (2% to 3% ages 2-5 years)

Neuromuscular & skeletal: Hyperkinesia (3% ages 6-12 years)

Ocular: Conjunctivitis (2% ages 6-12 years)

Respiratory: Wheezing (4% ages 6-12 years), dysphonia (2% ages 6-12 years), upper respiratory infection (2% ages 6-12 years), epistaxis (2% to 3% ages 2-5 years), pharyngitis (2% to 3% ages 2-5 years), flu-like symptoms (2% to 3% ages 2-5 years)

Miscellaneous: Viral infection (2% to 3% ages 2-5 years)

Adults and Children: <2% (Limited to important or life-threatening): Abnormal hepatic function, agitation, alopecia, altered lacrimation, altered micturition, altered salivation, altered taste, amnesia, anaphylaxis, angioneurotic edema, anorexia, arthralgia, back pain, blepharospasm, blurred vision, breast enlargement, breast pain, bronchospasm, chest pain, confusion, depression, dizziness, dysmenorrhea, dyspnea, erythema multiforme, hemoptysis, hepatic necrosis, hepatitis, hypotension, impaired concentration, impotence, insomnia, irritability, jaundice, menorrhagia, migraine, nausea, palpitations, paresthesia, paroniria, peripheral edema, photosensitivity, pruritus, purpura, rigors, seizures, supraventricular tachyarrhythmia, syncope, tachycardia, tremor, urinary discoloration, urticaria, thrombocytopenia, vaginitis, vertigo, vomiting, weight gain

Overdosage/Toxicology Symptoms of overdose include somnolence, tachycardia, and headache. No specific antidote is available. Treatment is symptomatic and supportive. Loratadine is not eliminated by dialysis.

Pharmacodynamics/Kinetics

Absorption: Rapid

Half-Life Elimination: 12-15 hours

Metabolism: Extensively hepatic via CYP2D6 and 3A4 to active metabolite

Onset: 1-3 hours; Peak effect: 8-12 hours

Duration: >24 hours

Formulations

Syrup (Claritin®): 1 mg/mL (480 mL) [contains sodium benzoate]
Tablet (Claritin®): 10 mg
Tablet, rapidly-disintegrating (Claritin® RediTabs®): 10 mg [mint flavor]

Dosing

Adults & Elderly: Seasonal allergic rhinitis, chronic idiopathic urticaria: Oral: 10 mg/day

Pediatrics:

Children 2-5 years: Seasonal allergic rhinitis, chronic idiopathic urticaria: Oral: 5 mg once daily
Children ≥6 years: Refer to adult dosing.

Hepatic Impairment: 10 mg every other day to start

Administration

Oral: Take on an empty stomach.

Stability

Storage: Store at 2°C to 25°C (36°F to 77°F).

Rapidly disintegrating tablets: Use within 6 months of opening foil pouch, and immediately after opening individual tablet blister. Store in a dry place.

Monitoring and Teaching Issues

Physical Assessment: Assess effectiveness and interactions of other medications patient may be taking (see Drug Interactions). See Warnings/Precautions for use cautions. Monitor effectiveness of therapy and adverse reactions (see Adverse Reactions) at beginning of therapy and periodically with long-term use. Assess knowledge/teach patient appropriate use, interventions to reduce side effects, and adverse symptoms to report (see Patient Education). Breast-feeding is not recommended.

Patient Education: Take as directed; do not exceed recommended dose. Avoid use of other depressants, alcohol, or sleep-inducing medications unless approved by prescriber. You may experience drowsiness or dizziness (use caution when driving or engaging in tasks requiring alertness until response to drug is known); or dry mouth or nausea (small, frequent meals, frequent mouth care, chewing gum, or sucking hard candy may help). Report persistent dizziness, sedation, or seizures; chest pain, rapid heartbeat, or palpitations; swelling of face, mouth, lips, or tongue; difficulty breathing; changes in urinary pattern; yellowing of skin or eyes; dark urine or pale stool; or lack of improvement or worsening or condition. **Breast-feeding precaution:** Breast-feeding is not recommended.

Rapidly-disintegrating tablets: Place tablet on tongue; it dissolves rapidly. May be used with or without water. Use within 6 months of opening foil pouch, and immediately after opening individual tablet blister.

Dietary Issues: Take on an empty stomach.

Geriatric Considerations: Loratadine is one of the newer, nonsedating antihistamines. Because of its low incidence of side effects, it seems to be a good choice in the elderly. However, there is a wide variation in loratadine half-life reported in the elderly and this should be kept in mind when initiating dosing.

Loratadine and Pseudoephedrine (lor AT a deen & soo doe e FED rin)

U.S. Brand Names Claritin-D® 12-Hour; Claritin-D® 24-Hour

Synonyms Pseudoephedrine and Loratadine

Generic Available No

Pharmacologic Category Antihistamine/Decongestant Combination

Pregnancy Risk Factor B

Lactation Enters breast milk/not recommended

Use Temporary relief of symptoms of seasonal allergic rhinitis and nasal congestion

Formulations Tablet, extended release:

Claritin-D® 12-hour: Loratadine 5 mg and pseudoephedrine sulfate 120 mg
Claritin-D® 24-hour: Loratadine 10 mg and pseudoephedrine sulfate 240 mg

Dosing

Adults & Elderly: Seasonal allergic rhinitis/nasal congestion:

Oral: 1 tablet every 12 hours
Extended release: 1 tablet daily

Renal Impairment: Cl_{cr} <30 mL/minute: Administer lower initial dose (1 tablet/day) because of reduced clearance.

Hepatic Impairment: Should be avoided.

Monitoring and Teaching Issues

Physical Assessment: See individual components listed in Related Information. Breast-feeding is not recommended.

Patient Education: See individual components listed in Related Information. Do not crush, break, or chew tablet. Take with a full glass of water. **Breast-feeding precaution:** Breast-feeding is not recommended.

Related Information

Loratadine *on page 820*
Pseudoephedrine *on page 1150*

Lorazepam (lor A ze pam)

U.S. Brand Names Ativan®; Lorazepam Intensol®

Restrictions C-IV

Generic Available Yes

Pharmacologic Category Benzodiazepine

Pregnancy Risk Factor D

(Continued)

Lorazepam *(Continued)*

Lactation Enters breast milk/contraindicated (AAP rates "of concern")

Use

Oral: Management of anxiety disorders or short-term relief of the symptoms of anxiety or anxiety associated with depressive symptoms

I.V.: Status epilepticus, preanesthesia for desired amnesia, antiemetic adjunct

Use - Unlabeled/Investigational Ethanol detoxification; insomnia; psychogenic catatonia; partial complex seizures

Mechanism of Action/Effect Binds to stereospecific benzodiazepine receptors on the postsynaptic GABA neuron at several sites within the central nervous system, including the limbic system, reticular formation. Enhancement of the inhibitory effect of GABA on neuronal excitability results by increased neuronal membrane permeability to chloride ions. This shift in chloride ions results in hyperpolarization (a less excitable state) and stabilization.

Contraindications Hypersensitivity to lorazepam or any component of the formulation (cross-sensitivity with other benzodiazepines may exist); acute narrow-angle glaucoma; sleep apnea (parenteral); intra-arterial injection of parenteral formulation; severe respiratory insufficiency (except during mechanical ventilation); pregnancy

Warnings/Precautions Causes CNS depression (dose-related) which may impair physical and mental capabilities. Use with caution in patients receiving other CNS depressants or psychoactive agents. Benzodiazepines have been associated with falls and traumatic injury and should be used with extreme caution in patients who are at risk of these events (especially the elderly). Use with caution in patients with a history of drug dependence.

Use with caution in elderly or debilitated patients, patients with hepatic disease (including alcoholics), renal impairment, respiratory disease, impaired gag reflex, or obese patients. Prolonged lorazepam use may have a possible relationship to GI disease, including esophageal dilation. Use is not recommended in patients with depressive disorders or psychoses. Avoid use in patients with sleep apnea.

The parenteral formulation of lorazepam contains polyethylene glycol and propylene glycol. Toxicity reported with prolonged infusion. Also contains benzyl alcohol - avoid rapid injection in neonates or prolonged infusions. Intra-arterial injection or extravasation should be avoided.

Benzodiazepines have been associated with anterograde amnesia. Paradoxical reactions, including hyperactive or aggressive behavior, have been reported with benzodiazepines, particularly in adolescent/pediatric or psychiatric patients. Does not have analgesic, antidepressant, or antipsychotic properties.

Drug Interactions

Decreased Effect: Oral contraceptives may increase the clearance of lorazepam. Lorazepam may decrease the antiparkinsonian efficacy of levodopa. Theophylline and other CNS stimulants may antagonize the sedative effects of lorazepam.

Increased Effect/Toxicity: Ethanol and other CNS depressants may increase the CNS effects of lorazepam. Scopolamine in combination with parenteral lorazepam may increase the incidence of sedation, hallucinations, and irrational behavior. There are rare reports of significant respiratory depression, stupor, and/or hypotension with concomitant use of loxapine and lorazepam. Use caution if concomitant administration of loxapine and CNS drugs is required.

Nutritional/Ethanol Interactions

Ethanol: Avoid or limit ethanol (may increase CNS depression).

Herb/Nutraceutical: Avoid valerian, St John's wort, kava kava, gotu kola (may increase CNS depression).

Effects on Lab Values May result in elevated liver function tests

Adverse Reactions

>10%:

Central nervous system: Sedation

Respiratory: Respiratory depression

1% to 10%:

Cardiovascular: Hypotension

Central nervous system: Confusion, dizziness, akathisia, unsteadiness, headache, depression, disorientation, amnesia

Dermatologic: Dermatitis, rash

Gastrointestinal: Weight gain/loss, nausea, changes in appetite

Neuromuscular & skeletal: Weakness

Respiratory: Nasal congestion, hyperventilation, apnea

<1% (Limited to important or life-threatening): Menstrual irregularities, increased salivation, blood dyscrasias, reflex slowing, physical and psychological dependence with prolonged use, polyethylene glycol or propylene glycol poisoning (prolonged I.V. infusion)

Overdosage/Toxicology Symptoms of overdose include confusion, coma, hypoactive reflexes, dyspnea, labored breathing. **Note:** Prolonged infusions have been associated with toxicity from propylene glycol and/or polyethylene glycol. Treatment for benzodiazepine overdose is supportive. Flumazenil has been shown to selectively block the binding of benzodiazepines to CNS receptors, resulting in a reversal of benzodiazepine-induced CNS depression but not respiratory depression

Pharmacodynamics/Kinetics

Absorption: Oral, I.M.: Prompt

Half-Life Elimination: Neonates: 40.2 hours; Older children: 10.5 hours; Adults: 12.9 hours; Elderly: 15.9 hours; End-stage renal disease: 32-70 hours

Metabolism: Hepatic to inactive compounds

Onset: Hypnosis: I.M.: 20-30 minutes; Sedation, anticonvulsant: I.V.: 5 minutes; oral: 0.5-1 hour

Duration: 6-8 hours

Formulations

Injection, solution (Ativan®): 2 mg/mL (1 mL, 10 mL); 4 mg/mL (1 mL, 10 mL) [contains benzyl alcohol]

Solution, oral concentrate (Lorazepam Intensol®): 2 mg/mL (30 mL) [alcohol free, dye free]

Tablet (Ativan®): 0.5 mg, 1 mg, 2 mg

Dosing

Adults:

Antiemetic: Oral, I.V. (**Note:** May be administered sublingually; not a labeled route): 0.5-2 mg every 4-6 hours as needed

Anxiety and sedation: Oral: 1-10 mg/day in 2-3 divided doses; usual dose: 2-6 mg/day in divided doses; initial dose should not exceed 2 mg in debilitated patients

Insomnia: Oral: 2-4 mg at bedtime

Preoperative:

I.M.: 0.05 mg/kg administered 2 hours before surgery; maximum: 4 mg/dose

I.V.: 0.044 mg/kg 15-20 minutes before surgery; usual maximum: 2 mg/dose

Operative amnesia: I.V.: Up to 0.05 mg/kg; maximum: 4 mg/dose

Status epilepticus: I.V.: 4 mg/dose given slowly over 2-5 minutes; may repeat in 10-15 minutes; usual maximum dose: 8 mg

Rapid tranquilization of agitated patient (administer every 30-60 minutes):

Oral: 1-2 mg

I.M.: 0.5-1 mg

Average total dose for tranquilization: 4-8 mg

Elderly: Anxiety and sedation: Oral, I.V.: 0.5-4 mg/day; refer to adult dosing for other indications. Dose selection should generally be on the low end of the dosage range (ie, initial dose not to exceed 2 mg)

Pediatrics:

Antiemetic: Children 2-15 years: I.V.: 0.05 mg/kg (up to 2 mg/dose) prior to chemotherapy

Anxiety and sedation: Infants and Children: Oral, I.V.: Usual: 0.05 mg/kg/dose (range: 0.02-0.09 mg/kg) every 4-8 hours

Sedation (preprocedure): Infants and Children:

Oral, I.M., I.V.: Usual: 0.05 mg/kg; range: 0.02-0.09 mg/kg

I.V.: May use smaller doses (eg, 0.01-0.03 mg/kg) and repeat every 20 minutes, as needed to titrate to effect

Status epilepticus: I.V.:

Infants and Children: 0.1 mg/kg slow I.V. over 2-5 minutes, do not exceed 4 mg/single dose; may repeat second dose of 0.05 mg/kg slow I.V. in 10-15 minutes if needed

Adolescents: 0.07 mg/kg slow I.V. over 2-5 minutes; maximum: 4 mg/dose; may repeat in 10-15 minutes

Administration

I.M.: Should be administered deep into the muscle mass.

I.V.: Inadvertent intra-arterial injection may produce arteriospasm resulting in gangrene which may require amputation.

Stability

Storage: Intact vials should be refrigerated and protected from light. Do not use discolored or precipitate containing solutions. Injectable vials may be stored at room temperature for up to 60 days.

Reconstitution: Stability of parenteral admixture at room temperature (25°C) is 24 hours. Standard diluent: 1 mg/100 mL D_5W

Compatibility:

Y-site administration: Incompatible with aldesleukin, aztreonam, floxacillin, foscarnet, idarubicin, imipenem/cilastatin, omeprazole, ondansetron, sargramostim, sufentanil

Compatibility in syringe: Incompatible with sufentanil

Compatibility when admixed: Incompatible with buprenorphine, dexamethasone sodium phosphate with diphenhydramine and metoclopramide

Monitoring and Teaching Issues

Physical Assessment: Assess other medications the patient may be taking for effectiveness and interactions (see Drug Interactions). See Contraindications and Warnings/Precautions for use cautions. **Oral:** Assess for history of addiction; long-term use can result in dependence, abuse, or tolerance; periodically evaluate need for continued use. Monitor therapeutic response, adverse reactions and overdose at beginning of therapy and periodically with long-term use (see Adverse Reactions and Overdose/Toxicology). Taper dosage slowly when discontinuing. Assess knowledge/teach patient appropriate use, interventions to reduce side effects, and adverse symptoms to report (see Patient Education). **I.V./I.M.:** Monitor vital signs and CNS status (possible retrograde amnesia I.V.), and ability to void. Maintain bedrest for 2-3 hours, and observe when up. **Pregnancy risk factor D** - determine that patient is not pregnant before beginning treatment. Instruct patients of childbearing age about appropriate barrier contraceptive measures. Breast-feeding is contraindicated.

Patient Education: Oral: Take exactly as directed; do not increase dose or frequency. Drug may cause physical and/or psychological dependence. Do not use alcohol or other prescription or OTC medications (especially pain medications, sedatives, antihistamines, or hypnotics) without consulting prescriber. Maintain adequate hydration (2-3 L/day of fluids) unless advised by prescriber to restrict fluids. You may experience drowsiness, lightheadedness, impaired coordination, dizziness, or blurred vision (use caution when driving or engaging in tasks requiring alertness until response to drug is known); nausea, vomiting, or dry mouth (small, frequent meals, frequent mouth care, chewing gum, or sucking lozenges may help); constipation (increased exercise, fluids, fruit, or fiber may help); altered sexual drive or ability (reversible); or photosensitivity (use sunscreen, wear protective clothing and eyewear, and avoid direct sunlight). Report persistent CNS effects (eg, confusion, depression, increased sedation, excitation, headache, agitation, insomnia or nightmares, dizziness, fatigue, impaired coordination, changes in personality, or changes in cognition); changes in urinary pattern; chest pain, palpitations, or rapid heartbeat; muscle cramping, weakness, tremors, or rigidity; ringing in ears or visual disturbances; excessive perspiration; excessive GI symptoms (cramping, constipation, vomiting, anorexia); or worsening of condition. **Pregnancy/breast-feeding precautions:** Do not get pregnant while taking this medication; use appropriate contraceptive measures. Do not breast-feed.

(Continued)

Lorazepam *(Continued)*

Geriatric Considerations: Because lorazepam is relatively short-acting with an inactive metabolite, it is a preferred agent to use in elderly patients when a benzodiazepine is indicated. Use with caution since elderly patients have decreased pulmonary reserve and are more prone to hypoxia.

Breast-feeding Issues: Crosses into breast milk and no data on clinical effects on the infant. AAP states MAY BE OF CONCERN.

Pregnancy Issues: Crosses the placenta. Respiratory depression or hypotonia if administered near time of delivery.

Other Issues: Taper dosage gradually after long-term therapy, especially in epileptic patients. Abrupt withdrawal may cause tremors, nausea, vomiting, abdominal and/or muscle cramps.

Additional Information Oral doses >0.09 mg/kg produced ↑ ataxia without ↑ sedative benefit vs lower doses; preferred anxiolytic when I.M. route needed. Abrupt discontinuation after sustained use (generally >10 days) may cause withdrawal symptoms.

Related Information

Antiemetics for Chemotherapy-Induced Nausea and Vomiting *on page 1639*
Anxiolytic/Hypnotic Use in Long-Term Care Facilities *on page 1608*
Benzodiazepines *on page 1560*

Lorazepam Intensol® *see* Lorazepam *on page 821*

Lorcet® 10/650 *see* Hydrocodone and Acetaminophen *on page 667*

Lorcet®-HD *see* Hydrocodone and Acetaminophen *on page 667*

Lorcet® Plus *see* Hydrocodone and Acetaminophen *on page 667*

Lortab® *see* Hydrocodone and Acetaminophen *on page 667*

Losartan (loe SAR tan)

U.S. Brand Names Cozaar®

Synonyms DuP 753; Losartan Potassium; MK594

Generic Available No

Pharmacologic Category Angiotensin II Receptor Blocker

Pregnancy Risk Factor C/D (2nd and 3rd trimesters)

Lactation Excretion in breast milk unknown/not recommended

Use Treatment of hypertension; treatment of diabetic nephropathy in patients with type 2 diabetes mellitus (noninsulin dependent, NIDDM) and a history of hypertension

Mechanism of Action/Effect As a selective and competitive, nonpeptide angiotensin II receptor antagonist, losartan blocks the vasoconstrictor and aldosterone-secreting effects of angiotensin II. Losartan increases urinary flow rate and in addition to being natriuretic and kaliuretic, increases excretion of chloride, magnesium, uric acid, calcium, and phosphate.

Contraindications Hypersensitivity to losartan or any component of the formulation; hypersensitivity to other A-II receptor antagonists; primary hyperaldosteronism; bilateral renal artery stenosis; pregnancy (2nd and 3rd trimesters)

Warnings/Precautions Avoid use or use a smaller dose in patients who are volume depleted. Deterioration in renal function can occur with initiation. Use with caution in unilateral renal artery stenosis and pre-existing renal insufficiency; significant aortic/mitral stenosis. Safety and efficacy in pediatric patients have not been established. Pregnancy risk C/D (2nd and 3rd trimesters).

Drug Interactions

Cytochrome P450 Effect: Substrate of **CYP2C8/9, 3A4**; Inhibits CYP1A2, 2C8/9, 2C19, 3A4

Decreased Effect: Phenobarbital (CYP3A4 and 2C8/9 inducer) caused a reduction of losartan in serum by 20%, clinical effect is unknown. Other enzyme inducers may affect serum concentrations of losartan. Rifampin may reduce antihypertensive efficacy of losartan. NSAIDs may decrease the efficacy of losartan.

Increased Effect/Toxicity: Cimetidine may increase the absorption of losartan by 18% (clinical effect is unknown). Blood levels of losartan may be increased by inhibitors of CYP2C9 (amiodarone, fluoxetine, isoniazid, ritonavir, sulfonamides) and 3A4 (diltiazem, erythromycin, verapamil, ketoconazole, itraconazole). Potassium salts/supplements, co-trimoxazole (high dose), ACE inhibitors, and potassium-sparing diuretics (amiloride, spironolactone, triamterene) may increase the risk of hyperkalemia. Risk of lithium toxicity may be increased by losartan.

Nutritional/Ethanol Interactions Herb/Nutraceutical: St John's wort may decrease levels. Avoid dong quai if using for hypertension (has estrogenic activity). Avoid ephedra, yohimbe, ginseng (may worsen hypertension). Avoid garlic (may have increased antihypertensive effect).

Adverse Reactions

>10%:

- Cardiovascular: Chest pain (12% diabetic nephropathy)
- Central nervous system: Fatigue (14% diabetic nephropathy)
- Endocrine: Hypoglycemia (14% diabetic nephropathy)
- Gastrointestinal: Diarrhea (2% hypertension to 15% diabetic nephropathy)
- Genitourinary: Urinary tract infection (13% diabetic nephropathy)
- Hematology: Anemia (14% diabetic nephropathy)
- Neuromuscular & skeletal: Weakness (14% diabetic nephropathy), back pain (2% hypertension to 12% diabetic nephropathy)
- Respiratory: Cough (11% diabetic nephropathy; 17% to 29% hypertension but similar to that associated with hydrochlorothiazide or placebo therapy)

1% to 10%:

- Cardiovascular: Hypotension (7% diabetic nephropathy), orthostatic hypotension (4% hypertension to 4% diabetic nephropathy), first-dose hypotension (dose-related: <1% with 50 mg, 2% with 100 mg)
- Central nervous system: Dizziness (4%), hypoesthesia (5% diabetic nephropathy), fever (4% diabetic nephropathy), insomnia (1%)

Dermatology: Cellulitis (7% diabetic nephropathy)

Endocrine: Hyperkalemia (<1% hypertension to 7% diabetic nephropathy)

Gastrointestinal: Gastritis (5% diabetic nephropathy), weight gain (4% diabetic nephropathy), dyspepsia (1% to 4%), abdominal pain (2%), nausea (2%)

Neuromuscular & skeletal: Muscular weakness (7% diabetic nephropathy), knee pain (5% diabetic nephropathy), leg pain (1% to 5%), muscle cramps (1%), myalgia (1%),

Respiratory: Bronchitis (10% diabetic nephropathy), upper respiratory infection (8%), nasal congestion (2%), sinusitis (1% hypertension to 6% diabetic nephropathy)

Miscellaneous: Infection (5% diabetic nephropathy), flu-like syndrome (10% diabetic nephropathy)

>1% but frequency ≤ placebo: Edema, abdominal pain, nausea, headache, pharyngitis

<1% (Limited to important or life-threatening): Acute psychosis with paranoid delusions, ageusia, alopecia, anemia, angina, angioedema, arrhythmias, AV block (second degree), depression, dysgeusia, dyspnea, gout, Henoch-Schönlein purpura, hepatitis, hyperkalemia, hyponatremia, impotence, maculopapular rash, myocardial infarction, panic disorder, pancreatitis, paresthesia, peripheral neuropathy, photosensitivity, renal impairment (patients dependent on renin-angiotensin-aldosterone system), stroke, syncope, urticaria, vasculitis, vertigo

Overdosage/Toxicology Hypotension and tachycardia may occur with significant overdose. Treatment should be supportive.

Pharmacodynamics/Kinetics

Bioavailability: 25% to 33%; AUC of E-3174 is four times greater than that of losartan

Half-Life Elimination: Losartan: 1.5-2 hours; E-3174: 6-9 hours

Time to Peak: Serum: Losartan: 1 hour; E-3174: 3-4 hours

Metabolism: Hepatic (14%) via CYP2C9 and 3A4 to an active metabolite E-3174 (40 times more potent than losartan); extensive first-pass effect

Onset: 6 hours

Formulations Tablet, film coated, as potassium: 25 mg, 50 mg, 100 mg

Dosing

Adults & Elderly:

Hypertension: Oral: Initial: 25-50 mg once daily; can be administered once or twice daily with total daily doses ranging from 25-100 mg

Usual initial doses in patients receiving diuretics or those with intravascular volume depletion: 25 mg

Nephropathy in patients with type 2 diabetes and hypertension: Oral: Initial: 50 mg once daily; can be increased to 100 mg once daily based on blood pressure response

Renal Impairment:

No adjustment is necessary.

Hemodialysis effects: Not removed via hemodialysis.

Hepatic Impairment: Reduce the initial dose to 25 mg/day; divide dosage intervals into two.

Administration

Oral: May be administered with or without food.

Stability

Storage: Store at 15°C to 30°C (59°F to 86°F). Protect from light.

Monitoring Laboratory Tests Electrolytes, serum creatinine, BUN, urinalysis, CBC

Monitoring and Teaching Issues

Physical Assessment: See Contraindications and Warnings/Precautions for use cautions. Assess potential for interactions with other prescriptions, OTC medications, or herbal products patient may be taking (see Drug Interactions). Assess results of laboratory tests (see above), therapeutic effectiveness, and adverse response on a regular basis during therapy (eg, hypotension - see Adverse Reactions and Overdose/Toxicology). Teach patient appropriate use, possible side effects and appropriate interventions, and adverse symptoms to report (see Patient Education). **Pregnancy risk factor C/D** - see Pregnancy Risk Factor for use cautions. Instruct patients of childbearing age about appropriate use of barrier contraceptives (see Pregnancy Issues). Breast-feeding is contraindicated.

Patient Education: Inform prescriber of all prescriptions, OTC medications, or herbal products you are taking, and any allergies you have. Do not take anything new during treatment unless approved by prescriber. Do not use potassium supplement or salt substitutes without consulting prescriber. Take exactly as directed and do not discontinue without consulting prescriber. Preferable to take on an empty stomach, 1 hour before or 2 hours after meals. This drug does not eliminate need for diet or exercise regimen as recommended by prescriber. May cause dizziness, fainting, or lightheadedness (use caution when driving or engaging in tasks that require alertness until response to drug is known); postural hypotension (use caution when rising from lying or sitting position or climbing stairs); diarrhea (boiled milk, buttermilk, or yogurt may help). Report chest pain or palpitations; unrelenting headache; back or muscle pain or weakness, CNS changes (delusions or depression); swelling of face mouth, tongue or throat; or other persistent adverse reactions. **Pregnancy/breast-feeding precautions:** Inform prescriber if you are or intend to become pregnant. This drug should not be used in the 2nd or 3rd trimester of pregnancy. Consult prescriber for appropriate contraceptive measures if necessary. Consult prescriber if breast-feeding.

Dietary Issues: May be taken with or without food.

Geriatric Considerations: Serum concentrations of losartan and its metabolites are not significantly different in the elderly patient and no initial dose adjustment is necessary even in low creatinine clearance states (<30 mL/minute).

Breast-feeding Issues: Avoid use in the nursing mother, if possible, since it is postulated that losartan is excreted in breast milk. Recommend discontinuing drug or discontinuing nursing based on the importance of the drug to the mother.

Related Information

Angiotensin Agents *on page 1547*

Losartan and Hydrochlorothiazide

(loe SAR tan & hye droe klor oh THYE a zide)

U.S. Brand Names Hyzaar®

Synonyms Hydrochlorothiazide and Losartan

Generic Available No

Pharmacologic Category Antihypertensive Agent Combination

Pregnancy Risk Factor C/D (2nd and 3rd trimesters)

Lactation Enters breast milk/contraindicated

Use Treatment of hypertension

Formulations Tablet, film coated:

50-12.5: Losartan potassium 50 mg and hydrochlorothiazide 12.5 mg

100-25: Losartan potassium 100 mg and hydrochlorothiazide 25 mg

Dosing

Adults: Hypertension: Oral: 1 tablet/day

Titration by clinical effect: Patients not controlled on losartan alone may be switched to losartan/hydrochlorothiazide once daily. If the blood pressure remains uncontrolled after 3 weeks, the dose may be increased to 2 tablets of losartan 50 mg/hydrochlorothiazide 12.5 mg or 1 tablet of losartan 100 mg/hydrochlorothiazide 25 mg once daily.

More than 2 tablets/day of losartan 50 mg/hydrochlorothiazide 12.5 mg or more than 1 tablet of losartan 100 mg/hydrochlorothiazide 25 mg are not recommended. Maximum antihypertensive effect is attained in about 3 weeks.

Elderly: Refer to dosing in individual monographs.

Renal Impairment: Usual regimens may be followed as long as Cl_{cr} is ≥30 mL/minute. In patients with more severe renal impairment, loop diuretics are preferred.

Hepatic Impairment: Not recommended for titration in patients with hepatic impairment.

Monitoring and Teaching Issues

Physical Assessment: See individual components listed in Related Information. **Pregnancy risk factor C/D** - see Pregnancy Risk Factor for use cautions. Assess knowledge/instruct patient on need to use appropriate contraceptive measures and the need to avoid pregnancy. Breast-feeding is contraindicated.

Patient Education: See individual components listed in Related Information. **Pregnancy/breast-feeding precautions:** Inform prescriber if you are or intend to become pregnant. Do not breast-feed.

Related Information

Hydrochlorothiazide *on page 664*
Losartan *on page 824*

Losartan Potassium *see* Losartan *on page 824*

Lotemax® *see page 1509*

Lotensin® *see* Benazepril *on page 154*

Lotensin® HCT *see* Benazepril and Hydrochlorothiazide *on page 155*

Loteprednol *see page 1509*

Lotrel® *see* Amlodipine and Benazepril *on page 87*

Lotrimin® *see* Clotrimazole *on page 322*

Lotrimin® AF [OTC] *see* Clotrimazole *on page 322*

Lotrimin® AF Powder/Spray [OTC] *see* Miconazole *on page 899*

Lotrisone® *see* Betamethasone and Clotrimazole *on page 162*

Lovastatin (LOE va sta tin)

U.S. Brand Names Altocor™; Mevacor®

Synonyms Mevinolin; Monacolin K

Generic Available Yes: Immediate release tablet

Pharmacologic Category Antilipemic Agent, HMG-CoA Reductase Inhibitor

Pregnancy Risk Factor X

Lactation Enters breast milk/contraindicated

Use

Adjunct to dietary therapy to decrease elevated serum total and LDL-cholesterol concentrations in primary hypercholesterolemia

Primary prevention of coronary artery disease (patients without symptomatic disease with average to moderately elevated total and LDL-cholesterol and below average HDL-cholesterol); slow progression of coronary atherosclerosis in patients with coronary heart disease

Adjunct to dietary therapy in adolescent patients (10-17 years of age, females >1 year post-menarche) with heterozygous familial hypercholesterolemia having LDL >189 mg/dL, **or** LDL >160 mg/dL with positive family history of premature cardiovascular disease (CVD), **or** LDL >160 mg/dL with the presence of at least two other CVD risk factors

Mechanism of Action/Effect Lovastatin acts by competitively inhibiting 3-hydroxyl-3-methylglutaryl-coenzyme A (HMG-CoA) reductase, the enzyme that catalyzes the rate-limiting step in cholesterol biosynthesis.

Contraindications Hypersensitivity to lovastatin or any component of the formulation; active liver disease; unexplained persistent elevations of serum transaminases; pregnancy; breast-feeding

Warnings/Precautions Liver function must be monitored by periodic laboratory assessment. Rhabdomyolysis with acute renal failure has occurred. Risk is dose-related and is increased with concurrent use of lipid-lowering agents which may cause rhabdomyolysis (gemfibrozil, fibric acid derivatives, or niacin at doses ≥1 g/day) or during concurrent use with potent CYP3A4 inhibitors (including amiodarone, clarithromycin, cyclosporine, erythromycin, itraconazole, ketoconazole, nefazodone, grapefruit juice in large quantities, verapamil, or protease inhibitors such as indinavir, nelfinavir, or ritonavir). Weigh the risk versus benefit when combining any of these drugs with lovastatin. Temporarily discontinue in any patient experiencing an acute or serious condition predisposing to renal failure secondary to rhabdomyolysis. Use with caution in patients who consume large amounts of ethanol or have a history of liver disease. Safety and efficacy of the immediate release tablet have not been evaluated in prepubertal patients, patients <10 years of age, or doses >40 mg/day in appropriately-selected adolescents; extended release tablets have not been studied in patients <20 years of age.

Drug Interactions

Cytochrome P450 Effect: Substrate of **CYP3A4**; Inhibits CYP2C8/9, 2D6

Decreased Effect: Cholestyramine taken with lovastatin reduces lovastatin absorption and effect.

Increased Effect/Toxicity: Inhibitors of CYP3A4 (amiodarone, amprenavir, clarithromycin, cyclosporine, diltiazem, fluvoxamine, erythromycin, fluconazole, indinavir, itraconazole, ketoconazole, miconazole, nefazodone, nelfinavir, ritonavir, troleandomycin, and verapamil) increase lovastatin blood levels and may increase the risk of myopathy and rhabdomyolysis. Limit dose to ≤40 mg with amiodarone or verapamil. Suspend lovastatin therapy during concurrent clarithromycin, erythromycin, itraconazole, or ketoconazole therapy. Cyclosporine, clofibrate, fenofibrate, gemfibrozil, and niacin also may increase the risk of myopathy and rhabdomyolysis. Limit dose to ≤20 mg with concurrent gemfibrozil. The effect/toxicity of warfarin (elevated PT) and levothyroxine may be increased by lovastatin. Digoxin, norethindrone, and ethinyl estradiol levels may be increased. Effects are additive with other lipid-lowering therapies.

Nutritional/Ethanol Interactions

Food: The therapeutic effect of lovastatin may be decreased if taken with food. Lovastatin serum concentrations may be increased if taken with grapefruit juice; avoid concurrent intake of large quantities (>1 quart/day).

Herb/Nutraceutical: St John's wort may decrease lovastatin levels.

Effects on Lab Values ↑ liver transaminases (S), altered thyroid function tests

Adverse Reactions Percentages as reported with immediate release tablets; similar adverse reactions seen with extended release tablets.

>10%: Neuromuscular & skeletal: Increased CPK (>2x normal) (11%)

1% to 10%:

Central nervous system: Headache (2% to 3%), dizziness (0.5% to 1%)

Dermatologic: Rash (0.8% to 1%)

Gastrointestinal: Abdominal pain (2% to 3%), constipation (2% to 4%), diarrhea (2% to 3%), dyspepsia (1% to 2%), flatulence (4% to 5%), nausea (2% to 3%)

Neuromuscular & skeletal: Myalgia (2% to 3%), weakness (1% to 2%), muscle cramps (0.6% to 1%)

Ocular: Blurred vision (0.8% to 1%)

<1% (Limited to important or life-threatening): Acid regurgitation, alopecia, arthralgia, chest pain, dermatomyositis, eye irritation, insomnia, leg pain, paresthesia, pruritus, vomiting, xerostomia

Additional class-related events or case reports (not necessarily reported with lovastatin therapy): Alopecia, alteration in taste, anaphylaxis, angioedema, anorexia, anxiety, arthritis, cataracts, chills, cholestatic jaundice, cirrhosis, decreased libido, depression, dryness of skin/mucous membranes, dyspnea, elevated transaminases, eosinophilia, erectile dysfunction, erythema multiforme, facial paresis, fatty liver, fever, flushing, fulminant hepatic necrosis, gynecomastia, hemolytic anemia, hepatitis, hepatoma, hyperbilirubinemia, hypersensitivity reaction, impaired extraocular muscle movement, impotence, increased alkaline phosphatase, increased CPK (>10x normal), increased ESR, increased GGT, leukopenia, malaise, memory loss, myopathy, nail changes, nodules, ophthalmoplegia, pancreatitis, paresthesia, peripheral nerve palsy, peripheral neuropathy, photosensitivity, polymyalgia rheumatica, positive ANA, pruritus, psychic disturbance, purpura, rash, renal failure (secondary to rhabdomyolysis), rhabdomyolysis, skin discoloration, Stevens-Johnson syndrome, systemic lupus erythematosus-like syndrome, thrombocytopenia, thyroid dysfunction, toxic epidermal necrolysis, tremor, urticaria, vasculitis, vertigo, vomiting

Overdosage/Toxicology Few adverse events have been reported. Treatment is symptomatic.

Pharmacodynamics/Kinetics

Absorption: 30%; increased with extended release tablets

Bioavailability: Increased with extended release tablets

Half-Life Elimination: 1.1-1.7 hours

Time to Peak: Serum: 2-4 hours

Metabolism: Hepatic; extensive first-pass effect; hydrolyzed to B-hydroxy acid (active)

Onset: LDL-cholesterol reductions: 3 days

Formulations

Tablet (Mevacor®): 10 mg, 20 mg, 40 mg

Tablet, extended release (Altocor™): 10 mg, 20 mg, 40 mg, 60 mg

Dosing

Adults & Elderly: Dyslipidemia and primary prevention of CAD: Oral: Initial: 20 mg with evening meal, then adjust at 4-week intervals; maximum: 80 mg/day immediate release tablet **or** 60 mg/day extended release tablet. Before initiation of therapy, patients should be placed on a standard cholesterol-lowering diet for 3-6 months and the diet should be continued during drug therapy. Patients receiving immunosuppressant drugs should start at 10 mg/day and not exceed 20 mg/day. Patients receiving concurrent therapy with niacin or fibrates should not exceed 20 mg lovastatin. Patients receiving amiodarone or verapamil should not exceed 40 mg lovastatin daily.

Pediatrics: Adolescents 10-17 years: Heterozygous familial hypercholesterolemia: Oral (immediate release tablet):

LDL reduction <20%: Initial: 10 mg/day with evening meal

LDL reduction ≥20%: Initial: 20 mg/day with evening meal

Usual range: 10-40 mg with evening meal, then adjust dose at 4-week intervals

Renal Impairment: Cl_{cr} <30 mL/minute: Use with caution and carefully consider doses >20 mg/day.

(Continued)

Lovastatin *(Continued)*

Administration

Oral: Administer with meals. Do not crush or chew extended release tablets.

Stability

Storage:

Tablet, immediate release: Store between 5°C to 30°C (41°F to 86°F). Protect from light.

Tablet, extended release: Store between 20°C to 25°C (68°F to 77°F). Avoid excessive heat and humidity.

Monitoring Laboratory Tests Obtain baseline LFTs and total cholesterol profile. LFTs should be performed before initiation of therapy, at 6 and 12 weeks after initiation or first dose, and periodically thereafter.

Monitoring and Teaching Issues

Physical Assessment: See Contraindications and Warnings/Precautions for use cautions. Assess potential for interactions with other prescriptions, OTC medications, or herbal products patient may be taking (see Drug Interactions). Monitor laboratory tests (see above) and patient response (see Adverse Reactions and Overdose/Toxicology) on a regular basis throughout therapy. Teach patient proper use, possible side effects and appropriate interventions, and adverse symptoms to report (see Patient Education). **Pregnancy risk factor X** - determine that patient is not pregnant before starting therapy. Do not give to women of childbearing age unless they are capable of complying with effective contraceptive use. Instruct patient in appropriate contraceptive measures. Breast-feeding is contraindicated.

Patient Education: Inform prescriber of all prescriptions, OTC medications, or herbal products you are taking, and any allergies you have. Do not take anything new during treatment unless approved by prescriber. Take as directed, with food at evening meal. Follow diet and exercise regimen as prescribed. You will have periodic blood tests to assess effectiveness and you should arrange for periodic ophthalmic exams while taking lovastatin (check for cataracts). You may experience nausea or dyspepsia (small, frequent meals, frequent mouth care, chewing gum, or sucking lozenges may help); diarrhea (buttermilk, boiled milk, or yogurt may help); or headache (see prescriber for analgesic). Report muscle pain or cramping; tremor; CNS changes (eg, memory loss, depression, personality changes; numbness, weakness, tingling or pain in extremities). **Pregnancy/breast-feeding precautions:** Inform prescriber if you are pregnant. Consult prescriber for appropriate barrier contraceptive measures to use during and for 1 month following therapy. This drug may cause severe fetal defects. Do not donate blood during or for 1 month following therapy. Do not breast-feed.

Dietary Issues: Before initiation of therapy, patients should be placed on a standard cholesterol-lowering diet for 6 weeks and the diet should be continued during drug therapy. Avoid intake of large quantities of grapefruit juice (≥1 quart/day)

Geriatric Considerations: The definition of and, therefore, when to treat hyperlipidemia in the elderly is a controversial issue. The National Cholesterol Education Program recommends that all adults 20 years of age and older maintain a plasma cholesterol <200 mg/dL. By this definition, 60% of all elderly would be considered to have a borderline high (200-239 mg/dL) or high (≥240 mg/dL) plasma cholesterol. However, plasma cholesterol has been shown to be a less reliable predictor of coronary heart disease in the elderly. Therefore, it is the authors' belief that pharmacologic treatment be reserved for those who are unable to obtain a desirable plasma cholesterol level by diet alone and for whom the benefits of treatment are believed to outweigh the potential adverse effects, drug interactions, and cost of treatment.

Pregnancy Issues: Safety and efficacy have not been established for use during pregnancy (treatment should be discontinued if pregnancy is recognized). Administer to women of childbearing potential only if conception is unlikely; females should be counseled on appropriate contraceptive methods.

Related Information

Hyperlipidemia Management *on page 1682*
Lipid-Lowering Agents *on page 1582*

Lovenox® *see* Enoxaparin *on page 467*

Lowsium® Plus *see* Magaldrate and Simethicone *on page 831*

Lozol® *see* Indapamide *on page 706*

L-PAM *see* Melphalan *on page 848*

LRH *see* Gonadorelin *on page 640*

L-Sarcolysin *see* Melphalan *on page 848*

LSD *see page 1568*

LTG *see* Lamotrigine *on page 770*

***L*-Thyroxine Sodium** *see* Levothyroxine *on page 797*

Lu-26-054 *see* Escitalopram *on page 489*

Lugol's Solution *see* Potassium Iodide *on page 1105*

Luminal® Sodium *see* Phenobarbital *on page 1067*

Lunelle™ *see* Estradiol and Medroxyprogesterone *on page 497*

Lupron® *see* Leuprolide *on page 781*

Lupron Depot® *see* Leuprolide *on page 781*

Lupron Depot-Ped® *see* Leuprolide *on page 781*

Lustra® *see* Hydroquinone *on page 679*

Lustra-AF™ *see* Hydroquinone *on page 679*

Luteinizing Hormone Releasing Hormone *see* Gonadorelin *on page 640*

Luvox® [DSC] *see* Fluvoxamine *on page 594*

Luxiq™ *see* Betamethasone *on page 160*

Luxiq™ *see* Topical Corticosteroids *on page 1334*

LY170053 *see* Olanzapine *on page 995*

LYMErix™ *see page 1498*

Lymphocyte Immune Globulin (LIM foe site i MYUN GLOB yoo lin)

U.S. Brand Names Atgam®

Synonyms Antithymocyte Globulin (Equine); Antithymocyte Immunoglobulin; ATG; Horse Antihuman Thymocyte Gamma Globulin

Generic Available No

Pharmacologic Category Immunosuppressant Agent

Pregnancy Risk Factor C

Lactation Excretion in breast milk unknown

Use Prevention and treatment of acute renal and other solid organ allograft rejection; treatment of moderate to severe aplastic anemia in patients not considered suitable candidates for bone marrow transplantation; prevention of graft-versus-host disease following bone marrow transplantation

Mechanism of Action/Effect May involve elimination of antigen-reactive T lymphocytes (killer cells) in peripheral blood or alteration of T-cell function

Contraindications Hypersensitivity to lymphocytic immune globulin, any component of the formulation, thimerosal, or other equine gamma globulins; severe, unremitting leukopenia and/or thrombocytopenia

Warnings/Precautions For I.V. use only. Must be administered via central line due to chemical phlebitis. Should only be used by physicians experienced in immunosuppressive therapy or management of solid organ or bone marrow transplant patients. Adequate laboratory and supportive medical resources must be readily available in the facility for patient management. Rash, dyspnea, hypotension, or anaphylaxis precludes further administration of the drug. Dose must be administered over at least 4 hours. Patient may need to be pretreated with an antipyretic, antihistamine, and/or corticosteroid. Pregnancy risk C.

Adverse Reactions

>10%:

- Central nervous system: Fever, chills
- Dermatologic: Rash
- Hematologic: Leukopenia, thrombocytopenia
- Miscellaneous: Systemic infection

1% to 10%:

- Cardiovascular: Hypotension, hypertension, tachycardia, edema, chest pain
- Central nervous system: Headache, malaise, pain
- Gastrointestinal: Diarrhea, nausea, stomatitis, GI bleeding
- Local: Edema or redness at injection site, thrombophlebitis
- Neuromuscular & skeletal: Myalgia, back pain
- Renal: Abnormal renal function tests
- Respiratory: Dyspnea
- Miscellaneous: Sensitivity reactions: Anaphylaxis may be indicated by hypotension, respiratory distress, serum sickness, viral infection

<1% (Limited to important or life-threatening): Acute renal failure, anemia, hemolysis, lymphadenopathy, seizures

Pharmacodynamics/Kinetics

Half-Life Elimination: Plasma: 1.5-12 days

Formulations Injection, solution: 50 mg/mL (5 mL)

Dosing

Adults & Elderly: Note: An intradermal skin test is recommended prior to administration of the initial dose of ATG; use 0.1 mL of a 1:1000 dilution of ATG in normal saline. A positive skin reaction consists of a wheal ≥10 mm in diameter. If a positive skin test occurs, the first infusion should be administered in a controlled environment with intensive life support immediately available. A systemic reaction precludes further administration of the drug. The absence of a reaction does **not** preclude the possibility of an immediate sensitivity reaction.

First dose: Premedicate with diphenhydramine 50 mg orally 30 minutes prior to and hydrocortisone 100 mg I.V. 15 minutes prior to infusion and acetaminophen 650 mg 2 hours after start of infusion.

Aplastic anemia protocol: I.V.: 10-20 mg/kg/day for 8-14 days, then give every other day for 7 more doses **or** 40 mg/kg/day for 4 days.

Renal allograft rejection, prevention: I.V.: 15 mg/kg/day for 14 days, then give every other day for 7 more doses for a total of 21 doses in 28 days; initial dose should be administered within 24 hours before or after transplantation.

Renal allograft rejection, treatment: I.V.: 10-15 mg/kg/day for 14 days, then give every other day for 7 more doses.

Pediatrics: Note; An intradermal skin test is recommended prior to administration of the initial dose of ATG; use 0.1 mL of a 1:1000 dilution of ATG in normal saline. A positive skin reaction consists of a wheal ≥10 mm in diameter. If a positive skin test occurs, the first infusion should be administered in a controlled environment with intensive life support immediately available. A systemic reaction precludes further administration of the drug. The absence of a reaction does **not** preclude the possibility of an immediate sensitivity reaction.

First dose: Premedicate with diphenhydramine 50 mg orally 30 minutes prior to and hydrocortisone 100 mg I.V. 15 minutes prior to infusion and acetaminophen 650 mg 2 hours after start of infusion.

Children: I.V.:

Aplastic anemia protocol: 10-20 mg/kg/day for 8-14 days; then administer every other day for 7 more doses; addition doses may be given every other day for 21 total doses in 28 days.

Renal allograft: 5-25 mg/kg/day

Administration

I.V.: Infuse dose over at least 4 hours. Any severe systemic reaction to the skin test such as generalized rash, tachycardia, dyspnea, hypotension, or anaphylaxis should preclude further therapy. **Epinephrine and resuscitative equipment should be nearby.** Patient

(Continued)

Lymphocyte Immune Globulin *(Continued)*

may need to be pretreated with an antipyretic, antihistamine, and/or corticosteroid. Mild itching and erythema can be treated with antihistamines.

Stability

Storage: Ampuls must be refrigerated.

Reconstitution: Dose must be diluted in 0.45% or 0.9% sodium chloride. Diluted solution is stable for 12 hours (including infusion time) at room temperature and 24 hours (including infusion time) at refrigeration. **The use of dextrose solutions is not recommended (precipitation may occur).**

Standard diluent: Dose/1000 mL NS or 0.45% sodium chloride

Minimum volume: Concentration should not exceed 1 mg/mL for a peripheral line or 4 mg/mL for a central line.

Monitoring Laboratory Tests Lymphocyte profile, CBC with differential, platelet count

Monitoring and Teaching Issues

Physical Assessment: Assess for history of previous allergic reactions (see Contraindications). See Warnings/Precautions and Administration for safe infusion and pretreatment recommendations. Monitor vital signs during infusion and observe for adverse or allergic reactions (see Adverse Reactions). Teach patient adverse symptoms to report (see Patient Education). **Pregnancy risk factor C** - benefits of use should outweigh possible risks. Note breast-feeding caution.

Patient Education: This medication can only be administered by infusion. You will be monitored closely during the infusion. Do not get up alone; ask for assistance if you must get up or change position. Do not have any vaccinations for the next 3 months without consulting prescriber. Immediately report chills; persistent dizziness or nausea; itching or stinging; acute back pain; chest pain, tightness, or rapid heartbeat; or difficulty breathing. **Pregnancy/breast-feeding precautions:** Inform prescriber if you are pregnant. Consult prescriber if breast-feeding.

Lymphocyte Mitogenic Factor *see* Aldesleukin *on page 54*

Lysodren® *see* Mitotane *on page 915*

Macrobid® *see* Nitrofurantoin *on page 976*

Macrodantin® *see* Nitrofurantoin *on page 976*

Magaldrate (MAG al drate)

U.S. Brand Names Riopan® [OTC]

Synonyms Hydromagnesium Aluminate

Generic Available Yes

Pharmacologic Category Antacid

Pregnancy Risk Factor C

Lactation Excretion in breast milk unknown/compatible

Use Symptomatic relief of hyperacidity associated with peptic ulcer, gastritis, peptic esophagitis and hiatal hernia

Contraindications Colostomy or ileostomy; appendicitis; ulcerative colitis; diverticulitis

Warnings/Precautions Pregnancy risk C.

Drug Interactions

Decreased Effect: Tetracyclines, digoxin, iron salts, isoniazid or quinolones; indomethacin absorption can be decreased by the aluminum, or increased by the magnesium (appears to be insignificant).

Adverse Reactions Frequency not defined.

Central nervous system: Encephalopathy

Endocrine & metabolic: Aluminum intoxication, hypophosphatemia, hypermagnesemia, milk-alkali syndrome

Gastrointestinal: Constipation, chalky taste, stomach cramps, fecal impaction, diarrhea, nausea, vomiting, discoloration of feces (white speckles), rebound hyperacidity

Neuromuscular & skeletal: Osteomalacia

Overdosage/Toxicology

Serious, potentially life-threatening electrolyte disturbances may occur with long-term use or overdosage due to diarrhea; hypermagnesemia may occur. CNS depression, confusion, hypotension, muscle weakness, blockage of peripheral neuromuscular transmission.

Serum level >4 mEq/L (4.8 mg/dL): Deep tendon reflexes may be depressed

Serum level ≥10 mEq/L (12 mg/dL): Deep tendon reflexes may disappear, respiratory paralysis may occur, heart block may occur

I.V. calcium (5-10 mEq) will reverse respiratory depression or heart block; in extreme cases, peritoneal dialysis or hemodialysis may be required.

Serum level >12 mEq/L may be fatal, serum level ≥10 mEq/L may cause complete heart block

Formulations Suspension, oral: 540 mg/5 mL (360 mL)

Dosing

Adults & Elderly: The recommended dietary allowance (RDA) of magnesium is 4.5 mg/kg which is a total daily allowance of 350-400 mg for adult men and 280-300 mg for adult women. During pregnancy the RDA is 300 mg and during lactation the RDA is 355 mg.

Hyperacidity: Oral: 480-1080 mg between meals (1-2 hours after meals and at bedtime)

Renal Impairment: Cl_{cr} <30 mL/minute: Not recommended due to risk of hypermagnesemia.

Monitoring and Teaching Issues

Physical Assessment: See Contraindications, Warnings/Precautions, and Drug Interactions for use cautions. See Adverse Reactions and Overdose/Toxicology. Teach patient appropriate use, possible side effects and appropriate interventions, and adverse symptoms to report (see Patient Education). **Pregnancy risk factor C** - benefits of use should outweigh possible risks.

Patient Education: Inform prescriber of all prescriptions, OTC medications, or herbal products you are taking, and any allergies you have. Do not take anything new during

treatment unless approved by prescriber. Take as directed; do not increase dose. Serious electrolyte imbalance can occur with overuse. Report persistent nausea, vomiting, abdominal pain, constipation, diarrhea, or blood in urine. **Pregnancy precaution:** Inform prescriber if you are or intend to become pregnant.

Dietary Issues: Should be taken on empty stomach.

Geriatric Considerations: Elderly, due to disease or drug therapy, may be predisposed to diarrhea or constipation. Diarrhea may result in electrolyte imbalance. Decreased renal function (Cl_{cr} <30 mL/minute) may result in toxicity of aluminum or magnesium. Drug interactions must be considered. If possible, administer antacid 1-2 hours apart from other drugs. When treating ulcers, consider buffer capacity (mEq/mL) antacid.

Magaldrate and Simethicone (MAG al drate & sye METH i kone)

U.S. Brand Names Iosopan® Plus; Lowsium® Plus; Riopan Plus® [OTC]; Riopan Plus® Double Strength [OTC]

Synonyms Simethicone and Magaldrate

Generic Available Yes

Pharmacologic Category Antacid; Antiflatulent

Pregnancy Risk Factor C

Lactation Excretion in breast milk unknown/compatible

Use Relief of hyperacidity associated with peptic ulcer, gastritis, peptic esophagitis and hiatal hernia which are accompanied by symptoms of gas

Formulations

Suspension, oral:

Magaldrate 540 mg and simethicone 20 mg per 5 mL (360 mL, 420 mL)

Magaldrate 540 mg and simethicone 40 mg per 5 mL (360 mL)

Magaldrate 1080 mg and simethicone 40 mg per 5 mL (360 mL)

Tablet, chewable:

Magaldrate 540 mg and simethicone 20 mg

Magaldrate 1080 mg and simethicone 20 mg

Dosing

Adults & Elderly: Hyperacidity/gas: Oral: 5-10 mL between meals and at bedtime

Monitoring and Teaching Issues

Physical Assessment: See individual components listed in Related Information. **Pregnancy risk factor C** - benefits of use should outweigh possible risks.

Patient Education: Also see Magaldrate. **Pregnancy precaution:** Inform prescriber if you are or intend to become pregnant.

Related Information

Magaldrate *on page 830*

Mag-Carb® *see* Magnesium Supplements *on page 831*

Mag Delay® *see* Magnesium Supplements *on page 831*

Mag-Gel® 600 *see* Magnesium Supplements *on page 831*

Maginex™ *see* Magnesium Supplements *on page 831*

Maginex™ DS *see* Magnesium Supplements *on page 831*

Magnesia Magma (Magnesium Hydroxide) *see* Magnesium Supplements *on page 831*

Magnesium Carbonate *see* Magnesium Supplements *on page 831*

Magnesium Chloride *see* Magnesium Supplements *on page 831*

Magnesium Citrate *see* Magnesium Supplements *on page 831*

Magnesium Gluconate *see* Magnesium Supplements *on page 831*

Magnesium Hydroxide *see* Magnesium Supplements *on page 831*

Magnesium Hydroxide and Mineral Oil Emulsion *see* Magnesium Supplements *on page 831*

Magnesium Lactate *see* Magnesium Supplements *on page 831*

Magnesium Oxide *see* Magnesium Supplements *on page 831*

Magnesium Sulfate *see* Magnesium Supplements *on page 831*

Magnesium Supplements (mag NEE zee um SUP la ments)

U.S. Brand Names Chloromag®; Haley's M-O® [OTC]; Mag-Carb®; Mag Delay®; Mag-Gel® 600; Maginex™; Maginex™ DS; Magonate® [OTC]; Mag-Ox 400® [OTC]; Mag-SR®; Mag-Tab SR®; Phillips'® Milk of Magnesia [OTC]; Slow-Mag® [OTC]; Uro-Mag® [OTC]

Synonyms Citrate of Magnesia (Magnesium Citrate); Epsom Salts (Magnesium Sulfate); Magnesia Magma (Magnesium Hydroxide); Magnesium Carbonate; Magnesium Chloride; Magnesium Citrate; Magnesium Gluconate; Magnesium Hydroxide; Magnesium Hydroxide and Mineral Oil Emulsion; Magnesium Lactate; Magnesium Oxide; Magnesium Sulfate; Milk of Magnesia (Magnesium Hydroxide); MOM (Magnesium Hydroxide)

Generic Available Yes

Pharmacologic Category Electrolyte Supplement

Pregnancy Risk Factor B

Lactation Enters breast milk/compatible

Use

Treatment and prevention of hypomagnesemia **(magnesium chloride, magnesium lactate, magnesium carbonate, magnesium sulfate, magnesium gluconate, and magnesium oxide)**

Treatment of hypertension **(magnesium sulfate)**

Treatment of encephalopathy and seizures associated with acute nephritis **(magnesium sulfate)**

Short-term treatment of constipation **(magnesium citrate, magnesium hydroxide, magnesium sulfate, and magnesium oxide)**

Treatment of hyperacidity symptoms **(magnesium hydroxide and magnesium oxide)**

Adjunctive treatment in moderate to severe acute asthma **(magnesium sulfate)**

Mechanism of Action/Effect Magnesium is important as a cofactor in many enzymatic reactions in the body. There are at least 300 enzymes which are dependent upon magnesium

(Continued)

Magnesium Supplements *(Continued)*

for normal functioning. Actions on lipoprotein lipase have been found to be important in reducing serum cholesterol. Magnesium is necessary for the maintaining of serum potassium and calcium levels due to its effect on the renal tubule. In the heart, magnesium acts as a calcium channel blocker. It also activates sodium potassium ATPase in the cell membrane to promote resting polarization and produce arrhythmias. Promotes bowel evacuation by causing osmotic retention of fluid which distends the colon and produces increased peristaltic activity when taken orally. To reduce stomach acidity, it reacts with hydrochloric acid in the stomach to form magnesium chloride.

Contraindications Hypersensitivity to formulation; serious renal impairment; myocardial damage or heart block; colostomy or ileostomy; intestinal obstruction, impaction, or perforation; appendicitis; abdominal pain

Warnings/Precautions Use with caution in patients with impaired renal function (accumulation of magnesium may lead to magnesium intoxication) and digitalized patients (may alter cardiac conduction leading to heart block). Magnesium chloride injection contains benzyl alcohol which may cause allergic reactions in susceptible individuals; large amounts of benzyl alcohol (99 mg/kg/day) have been associated with a potentially fatal toxicity ("gasping syndrome") in neonates (metabolic acidosis, respiratory distress, gasping respirations, CNS dysfunction [convulsions, intracranial hemorrhage], hypotension and cardiovascular collapse); avoid or use magnesium chloride injection with caution in neonates. Avoid use of Magonate® solution in neonates; contains sodium benzoate and *in vitro* and animal studies have shown that benzoate, a metabolite of benzyl alcohol, displaces bilirubin from protein binding sites.

Drug Interactions

Decreased Effect: Magnesium salts, when given orally, may decrease the absorption of the following: H_2 antagonists, phenytoin, iron salts, penicillamine, tetracycline, ciprofloxacin, benzodiazepines, chloroquine, steroids, and glyburide. Systemic magnesium may enhance the effects of calcium channel blockers and neuromuscular blockers. May share additive CNS depressant effects with CNS depressants. If sufficient alkalinization of the urine by magnesium salts occurs, the excretion of salicylates is enhanced and the tubular reabsorption of quinidine is enhanced (increased effect).

Adverse Reactions Adverse effects with magnesium therapy are related to the magnesium serum level.

>3 mg/dL: Depressed CNS, blocked peripheral neuromuscular transmission leading to anticonvulsant effects
>5 mg/dL: Depressed deep tendon reflexes, flushing, somnolence
>12 mg/dL: Respiratory paralysis, complete heart block

Other effects (frequency not defined):
Cardiovascular: Hypotension
Endocrine & metabolic: Hypermagnesemia
Gastrointestinal: Diarrhea, abdominal cramps, gas formation
Neuromuscular & skeletal: Muscle weakness

Overdosage/Toxicology See Adverse Reactions.

Pharmacodynamics/Kinetics

Absorption: Oral: Up to 30%

Half-Life Elimination: Renal with unabsorbed drug excreted in feces

Onset: Anticonvulsant: I.M.: 60 minutes; I.V.: Immediately; Laxative: Oral: 4-8 hours

Duration: Anticonvulsant: I.M.: 3-4 hours; I.V.: 30 minutes

Formulations Elemental magnesium listed in brackets:

Magnesium carbonate: Capsule, gelatin (Mag-Carb™): 250 mg [5.8 mEq; 70 mg]

Magnesium chloride:
Injection: 200 mg/mL [1.97 mEq/mL] (50 mL)
Tablet, extended release: 535 mg [64 mg]

Magnesium citrate: Solution, oral: 300 mL (1.75 g/30 mL)

Magnesium gluconate:
Liquid: 326 mg [17.6 mg] per 5 mL; 1000 mg [54 mg] per 5 mL
Tablet: 500 mg [27 mg]

Magnesium hydroxide:
Liquid, oral: 400 mg/5 mL (15 mL, 30 mL, 100 mL, 120 mL, 180 mL, 360 mL, 720 mL)
Liquid, oral concentrate: 800 mg/5 mL (240 mL) [10 mL equivalent to 30 mL milk of magnesia USP]
Tablet, chewable: 300 mg, 600 mg

Magnesium hydroxide and mineral oil:
Suspension, oral (Haley's M-O®): Magnesium hydroxide 300 mg and mineral oil 1.25 mL per 5 mL (12 oz, 29 oz) [equivalent to magnesium hydroxide 24 mL/mineral oil emulsion 6 mL]

Magnesium lactate: Caplet, sustained release (Mag-Tab SR®): 835 mg [7 mEq; 84 mg]

Magnesium L-aspartate hydrochloride:
Granules (MaginexTM DS): 1230 mg [10 mEq; 122 mg] per packet [lemon flavor]
Tablet, enteric coated (MaginexTM): 615 mg [5 mEq; 61 mg]

Magnesium oxide:
Capsule: 140 mg [84 mg]
Tablet: 400 mg [241.3 mg]

Magnesium sulfate:
Granules: ~40 mEq magnesium/5 g (120 g, 240 g)
Injection: 100 mg/mL (20 mL); 125 mg/mL (8 mL); 200 mg/mL (50 mL); 500 mg/mL (2 mL, 5 mL, 10 mL, 50 mL)

Dosing

Adults: Multiple salt forms of magnesium exist; close attention must be paid to the salt form when ordering and administering magnesium; incorrect selection or substitution of one salt for another without proper dosage adjustment may result in serious over- or underdosing.

Recommended daily allowance (RDA): See table.

Magnesium - Recommended Daily Allowance (RDA) (in terms of elemental magnesium)

Age	RDA (mg/day)
<5 months	40
5-12 months	60
1-3 years	80
4-6 years	120
7-10 years	170
Male	
11-14 years	270
15-18 years	400
>19 years	350
Female	
11-14 years	280
15-18 years	300
>19 years	280

HYPOMAGNESEMIA:

Magnesium gluconate: Oral: 500-1000 mg 3 times/day

Magnesium sulfate:

I.M., I.V.: 1 g every 6 hours for 4 doses, or 250 mg/kg over a 4-hour period; for severe hypomagnesemia: 8-12 g/day in divided doses has been used

Oral: 3 g every 6 hours for 4 doses

DAILY MAINTENANCE MAGNESIUM: I.V.:

Magnesium sulfate or magnesium chloride: 0.2-0.5 mEq/kg/day or 3-10 mEq/1000 kcal/day (maximum 8-16 mEq/day)

MANAGEMENT OF SEIZURES AND HYPERTENSION: I.M., I.V.:

Magnesium sulfate: 1 g every 6 hours for 4 doses as needed

BRONCHODILATION (adjunctive treatment in moderate to severe acute asthma; unlabeled use): I.V.:

Magnesium sulfate: 2 g as a single dose

Note: Literature evaluating magnesium sulfate's efficacy in the relief of bronchospasm has utilized single dosages in patient's with acute symptomatology who have received aerosol β-agonist therapy.

CATHARTIC: Oral:

Magnesium citrate (Citrate of magnesia): 150-300 mL

Magnesium hydroxide (Milk of magnesia, MOM): 30-60 mL/day once or in divided doses

Magnesium hydroxide and mineral oil (Haley's M-O) (pediatric dosage to provide equivalent dosage of magnesium hydroxide) 30-45 mL once or in divided doses

Magnesium sulfate: 10-30 g

Magnesium oxide: Adults: 2-4 g at bedtime with full glass of water

ANTACID Oral:

Magnesium hydroxide:

Liquid: 5-15 mL/dose, up to 4 times/day

Liquid concentrate: 2.5-7.5 mL/dose, up to 4 times/day

Tablet: 622-1244 mg/dose, up to 4 times/day

Magnesium oxide: 140 mg 3-4 times/day or 400-840 mg/day

Pediatrics: Multiple salt forms of magnesium exist; close attention must be paid to the salt form when ordering and administering magnesium; incorrect selection or substitution of one salt for another without proper dosage adjustment may result in serious over- or underdosing.

Recommended daily allowance of magnesium: See table.

HYPOMAGNESEMIA:

Neonates: I.V.:

Magnesium sulfate: 25-50 mg/kg/dose (0.2-0.4 mEq/kg/dose) every 8-12 hours for 2-3 doses

Magnesium chloride: 0.2-0.4 mEq/kg/dose every 8-12 hours for 2-3 doses

Children:

I.M., I.V.:

Magnesium sulfate: 25-50 mg/kg/dose (0.2-0.4 mEq/kg/dose) every 4-6 hours for 3-4 doses; maximum single dose: 2000 mg (16 mEq)

Magnesium chloride: 0.2-0.4 mEq/kg/dose every 4-6 hours for 3-4 doses; maximum single dose 16 mEq

Oral:

Magnesium chloride, gluconate, lactate, carbonate, oxide, or sulfate salts: 10-20 mg/kg **elemental magnesium** per dose 4 times/day

DAILY MAINTENANCE MAGNESIUM: I.V.:

Magnesium sulfate or magnesium chloride:

Neonates, Infants, and Children ≤45 kg: 0.25-0.5 mEq/kg/day

Adolescents >45 kg: 0.2-0.5 mEq/kg/day or 3-10 mEq/1000 kcal/day (maximum 8-16 mEq/day)

(Continued)

Magnesium Supplements *(Continued)*

MANAGEMENT OF SEIZURES AND HYPERTENSION: I.M., I.V.:

Magnesium sulfate: Children: 20-100 mg/kg/dose every 4-6 hours as needed; in severe cases doses as high as 200 mg/kg/dose have been used

BRONCHODILATION (adjunctive treatment in moderate to severe acute asthma; unlabeled use): I.V.:

Magnesium sulfate:

Children: 25 mg/kg/dose (maximum dose 2 g) as a single dose

Note: Literature evaluating magnesium sulfate's efficacy in the relief of bronchospasm has utilized single dosages in patient's with acute symptomatology who have received aerosol β-agonist therapy.

CATHARTIC: Oral:

Magnesium citrate (Citrate of magnesia):

<6 years: 2-4 mL/kg given once or in divided doses
6-12 years: 100-150 mL
≥12 years: 150-300 mL

Magnesium hydroxide (Milk of magnesia, MOM):

<2 years: 0.5 mL/kg/dose
2-5 years: 5-15 mL/day once or in divided doses
6-11 years: 15-30 mL/day once or in divided doses
≥12 years: 30-60 mL/day once or in divided doses

Magnesium hydroxide and mineral oil (Haley's M-O) (pediatric dosage to provide equivalent dosage of magnesium hydroxide)

<2 years: 0.6 mL/kg/dose
2-5 years: 6-18 mL/day once or in divided doses
6-11 years: 18-36 mL/day once or in divided doses
≥12 years: 30-45 mL once or in divided doses

Magnesium sulfate: Children: 0.25 g/kg/dose once or in divided doses

ANTACID Oral:

Magnesium hydroxide: Children: Liquid: 2.5-5 mL/dose, up to 4 times/day

Renal Impairment: Patients in severe renal failure should not receive magnesium due to toxicity from accumulation. Patients with a Cl_{cr} <25 mL/minute receiving magnesium should have serum magnesium levels monitored.

Administration

Oral:

Solution: Mix with water and administer on an empty stomach; chill **magnesium citrate** prior to administration to improve palatability.

Tablet: Take with full glass of water; chew **magnesium hydroxide** chewable tablets thoroughly; do not chew or crush sustained release formulations.

Granules: Mix each packet in 4 ounces water or juice prior to administration.

I.V.: Intermittent infusion: Dilute to a concentration of 0.5 mEq/mL (60 mg/mL of **magnesium sulfate**) (maximum concentration: 1.6 mEq/mL, 200 mg/mL of **magnesium sulfate**) and infuse over 2-4 hours. Do not exceed 1 mEq/kg/hour (125 mg/kg/hour of **magnesium sulfate**). In severe circumstances, half of the dosage to be administered may be infused over the first 15-20 minutes. For I.M. administration, dilute **magnesium sulfate** to a maximum concentration of 200 mg/mL prior to injection. Rapid infusions (utilized for treatment of severe asthma or torsade de pointes VT) over 10-20 minutes may be used (magnesium sulfate).

Monitoring Laboratory Tests Serum magnesium, deep tendon reflexes, renal function

Monitoring and Teaching Issues

Physical Assessment: See Contraindications and Warnings/Precautions for use cautions. Assess other medications patient is taking for adverse interactions (see Drug Interactions).

I.V.: Administration of high doses (continuous infusions) requires monitoring of EKG, vital signs, muscle strength, respiratory effort, CNS status, and deep tendon reflexes. See Administration - I.V. for infusion directions. In many institutions, smaller intermittent doses (1-2 g infused over 0.5-2 hours) do not require continuous EKG monitoring (consult institutional policies), however, monitoring of physical signs/symptoms should be conducted.

Oral: Monitor I & O ratio and edema.

Note: MOM concentrate is 3 times as potent as regular strength product. Assess knowledge/teach patient appropriate and use and adverse symptoms (see Adverse Reactions) to report.

Patient Education: Take as directed, with water or juice. Shake liquid well before using. Take 1 hour prior to or after other medications. You may experience excessive diarrhea, gastric cramping, dizziness (use fall precautions). Report rectal bleeding, tarry stools, unresolved abdominal cramps, or unrelieved constipation.

Geriatric Considerations: Elderly, due to disease or drug therapy, may be predisposed to diarrhea. Diarrhea may result in electrolyte imbalance. Decreased renal function (Cl_{cr} <30 mL/minute) may result in toxicity; monitor for toxicity (see Warnings/Precautions and Contraindications).

Additional Information 1 g elemental magnesium = 83.3 mEq = 41.1 mmol

Related Information

Antiarrhythmic Drugs *on page 1551*
Laxatives: Classification and Properties *on page 1581*

Magonate® [OTC] *see* Magnesium Supplements *on page 831*
Mag-Ox 400® [OTC] *see* Magnesium Supplements *on page 831*
Mag-SR® *see* Magnesium Supplements *on page 831*
Mag-Tab SR® *see* Magnesium Supplements *on page 831*
Malarone™ *see* Atovaquone and Proguanil *on page 131*
Mallamint® [OTC] *see* Calcium Supplements *on page 202*
Mallazine® *see page 1509*
Malt Soup Extract *see page 1581*

Mandol® *see* Cefamandole *on page 232*
Mandrake *see* Podophyllum Resin *on page 1097*

Mannitol (MAN i tole)

U.S. Brand Names Osmitrol®; Resectisol® Irrigation Solution

Synonyms *D*-Mannitol

Generic Available Yes

Pharmacologic Category Diuretic, Osmotic

Pregnancy Risk Factor C

Lactation Excretion in breast milk unknown

Use Reduction of increased intracranial pressure associated with cerebral edema; promotion of diuresis in the prevention and/or treatment of oliguria or anuria due to acute renal failure; reduction of increased intraocular pressure; promoting urinary excretion of toxic substances; genitourinary irrigant in transurethral prostatic resection or other transurethral surgical procedures

Mechanism of Action/Effect Increases the osmotic pressure of glomerular filtrate, which inhibits tubular reabsorption of water and electrolytes and increases urinary output

Contraindications Hypersensitivity to mannitol or any component or the formulation; severe renal disease (anuria); dehydration; active intracranial bleeding; severe pulmonary edema or congestion

Warnings/Precautions Should not be administered until adequacy of renal function and urine flow is established. Cardiovascular status should also be evaluated. Do not administer electrolyte-free mannitol solutions with blood. Pregnancy risk C.

Drug Interactions

Increased Effect/Toxicity: Lithium toxicity (with diuretic-induced hyponatremia).

Adverse Reactions Frequency not defined.

Cardiovascular: Circulatory overload, CHF

Central nervous system: Headache, convulsions, headache, chills, dizziness

Dermatologic: Rash

Endocrine & metabolic: Fluid and electrolyte imbalance, water intoxication, dehydration and hypovolemia secondary to rapid diuresis, hyponatremia

Gastrointestinal: Nausea, vomiting, xerostomia

Genitourinary: Polyuria, dysuria

Local: Tissue necrosis

Ocular: Blurred vision

Respiratory: Pulmonary edema

Miscellaneous: Allergic reactions

Overdosage/Toxicology Symptoms of overdose include polyuria, hypotension, cardiovascular collapse, pulmonary edema, hyponatremia, hypokalemia, oliguria, and seizures. Increased electrolyte excretion and fluid overload can occur. Hemodialysis will clear mannitol and reduce osmolality.

Pharmacodynamics/Kinetics

Half-Life Elimination: 1.1-1.6 hours

Metabolism: Minimally hepatic to glycogen

Onset: Diuresis: Injection: 1-3 hours; Reduction in intracerebral pressure: ~15 minutes

Duration: Reduction in intracerebral pressure: 3-6 hours

Formulations

Injection: 5% [50 mg/mL] (1000 mL); 10% [100 mg/mL] (500 mL, 1000 mL); 15% [150 mg/mL] (500 mL); 20% [200 mg/mL] (250 mL, 500 mL); 25% [250 mg/mL] (50 mL)

Solution, urogenital: 0.5% [5 mg/mL] (2000 mL); 0.54% [5.4 mg/mL] (1500 mL, 3000 mL) [with sorbitol 2.7 g/mL]

Dosing

Adults & Elderly:

Test dose (to assess adequate renal function): I.V.: 12.5 g (200 mg/kg) over 3-5 minutes to produce a urine flow of at least 30-50 mL of urine per hour over the next 2-3 hours.

Diuretic: Initial: 0.5-1 g/kg; Maintenance: 0.25-0.5 g/kg every 4-6 hours; usual adult dose: 20-200 g/24 hours

Intracranial pressure/Cerebral edema: I.V.: 1.5-2 g/kg/dose as a 15% to 20% solution over ≥30 minutes; maintain serum osmolality 310-320 mOsm/kg.

Preoperative for neurosurgery: I.V.: 1.5-2 g/kg administered 1-1.5 hours prior to surgery.

Transurethral: Irrigation: Use urogenital solution as required for irrigation.

Pediatrics:

Test dose (to assess adequate renal function): I.V.: Children: 200 mg/kg over 3-5 minutes to produce a urine flow of at least 1 mL/kg for 1-3 hours

Diuretic: I.V.: Children: Initial: 0.5-1 g/kg; Maintenance: 0.25-0.5 g/kg given every 4-6 hours

Administration

I.V.: Vesicant. Do not administer with blood. Crenation and agglutination of red blood cells may occur if administered with whole blood.

Stability

Storage: Should be stored at room temperature (15°C to 30°C) and protected from freezing. Crystallization may occur at low temperatures. Do not use solutions that contain crystals, heating in a hot water bath and vigorous shaking may be utilized for resolubilization. Cool solutions to body temperature before using.

Compatibility:

Y-site administration: Incompatible with cefepime, doxorubicin liposome, filgrastim

Compatibility when admixed: Incompatible with imipenem/cilastatin, meropenem

Monitoring Laboratory Tests Renal function, serum electrolytes, serum and urine osmolality; for treatment of elevated intracranial pressure, maintain serum osmolality 310-320 mOsm/kg

Monitoring and Teaching Issues

Physical Assessment: See Contraindications, Warnings/Precautions, and Dosing for use cautions. Assess effects and interactions of other prescriptions, OTC medications, or

(Continued)

Mannitol *(Continued)*

herbal products patient may be taking (see Drug Interactions). See specifics for Administration and Storage. Infusion site must be monitored for extravasation. Assess results of laboratory tests (see above), therapeutic effectiveness (according to purpose for use, eg, cerebral edema or trauma - ICP and neurological status; reducing intraocular pressure - eye pain, decreased visual acuity; renal failure - urine specific gravity and urinary output), and adverse response (see Adverse Reactions and Overdose/Toxicology). Patient teaching should be appropriate to patient condition (see Patient Education). **Pregnancy risk factor C** - benefits of use should outweigh possible risks. Note breast-feeding caution.

Patient Education: This medication can only be given by infusion. Report immediately any muscle weakness, numbness, tingling, acute headache, nausea, dizziness, blurred vision, eye pain, difficulty breathing, chest pain, or pain at infusion site. **Pregnancy/ breast-feeding precautions:** Inform prescriber if you are pregnant. Consult prescriber if breast-feeding.

Additional Information May autoclave or heat to redissolve crystals; mannitol 20% has an approximate osmolarity of 1100 mOsm/L and mannitol 25% has an approximate osmolarity of 1375 mOsm/L

Mapap® [OTC] *see* Acetaminophen *on page 35*
Mapap® Children's [OTC] *see* Acetaminophen *on page 35*
Mapap® Extra Strength [OTC] *see* Acetaminophen *on page 35*
Mapap® Infants [OTC] *see* Acetaminophen *on page 35*
Maprotiline *see page 1553*
Marcillin® *see* Ampicillin *on page 101*
Margesic® H *see* Hydrocodone and Acetaminophen *on page 667*
Marijuana *see page 1568*
Marinol® *see* Dronabinol *on page 452*

Masoprocol (ma SOE pro kole)

U.S. Brand Names Actinex®

Generic Available Yes

Pharmacologic Category Topical Skin Product, Acne

Pregnancy Risk Factor B

Lactation Excretion in breast milk unknown

Use Treatment of actinic keratosis

Mechanism of Action/Effect Antiproliferative activity against keratinocytes

Contraindications Hypersensitivity to masoprocol or any component of the formulation

Warnings/Precautions Occlusive dressings should not be used. For external use only.

Adverse Reactions

>10%:
- Dermatologic: Erythema, flaking, dryness, itching
- Local: Burning

1% to 10%:
- Dermatologic: Soreness, rash, blistering, excoriation, skin roughness, wrinkling
- Neuromuscular & skeletal: Paresthesia
- Ocular: Eye irritation

Pharmacodynamics/Kinetics

Absorption: Topical: <1% to 2%

Formulations Cream: 10% (30 g)

Dosing

Adults & Elderly: Actinic keratosis: Topical: Wash and dry area. Gently massage into affected area every morning and evening for 28 days.

Administration

Topical: For external use only. Avoid contact with eyes and mucous membranes. Do not use occlusive dressings. Wash hands immediately after use.

Monitoring and Teaching Issues

Physical Assessment: Monitor effectiveness of therapy and adverse reactions at beginning and periodically during therapy. Assess knowledge/teach patient appropriate use and adverse symptoms to report (see Patient Education). Note breast-feeding caution.

Patient Education: For external use only. Apply with gloves in thin film to thoroughly clean/ dry skin; avoid area around eyes or mouth. Do not cover with occlusive dressing. Results make take some time to appear. May stain clothing or fabrics. You may experience transient stinging or burning after application. Report worsening of condition; eye irritation; or skin redness, dryness, peeling, or burning that persists between applications. **Breast-feeding precaution:** Consult prescriber if breast-feeding.

Maternal/Fetal Medications *see page 1602*
Maternal/Fetal Toxicology *see page 1605*
Matulane® *see* Procarbazine *on page 1125*
Mavik® *see* Trandolapril *on page 1345*
Maxair™ *see* Pirbuterol *on page 1093*
Maxair™ Autohaler™ *see* Pirbuterol *on page 1093*
Maxalt® *see* Rizatriptan *on page 1201*
Maxalt-MLT® *see* Rizatriptan *on page 1201*
Maxaquin® *see* Lomefloxacin *on page 812*
Maxidex® *see* Dexamethasone *on page 382*
Maxidone™ *see* Hydrocodone and Acetaminophen *on page 667*
Maxifed® *see* Guaifenesin and Pseudoephedrine *on page 648*
Maxifed-G® *see* Guaifenesin and Pseudoephedrine *on page 648*
Maxiflor® *see* Topical Corticosteroids *on page 1334*
Maxipime® *see* Cefepime *on page 238*

Maxitrol® *see page 1509*

Maxivate® *see* Betamethasone *on page 160*

Maxivate® *see* Topical Corticosteroids *on page 1334*

Maxzide® *see* Hydrochlorothiazide and Triamterene *on page 667*

Maxzide®-25 *see* Hydrochlorothiazide and Triamterene *on page 667*

May Apple *see* Podophyllum Resin *on page 1097*

Mazanor® *see* Mazindol *on page 837*

Mazindol (MAY zin dole)

U.S. Brand Names Mazanor®; Sanorex®

Restrictions C-IV

Generic Available No

Pharmacologic Category Anorexiant

Pregnancy Risk Factor C

Lactation Enters breast milk/not recommended

Use Short-term adjunct in exogenous obesity

Mechanism of Action/Effect An isoindole with pharmacologic activity similar to amphetamine; produces CNS stimulation in humans and animals and appears to work primarily in the limbic system

Contraindications Hypersensitivity to mazindol or any component of the formulation; agitated states; history of drug abuse; MAO inhibitors

Warnings/Precautions Tolerance may develop within a few weeks. If this occurs, discontinue drug. Do not increase dose. Not recommended for severe hypertensive patients or patients with symptomatic cardiovascular disease including arrhythmias. Stimulants may unmask tics in individuals with coexisting Tourette's syndrome.

Serious, potentially life-threatening toxicities may occur when thyroid hormones (at dosages above usual daily hormonal requirements) are used in combination with sympathomimetic amines to induce weight loss. Treatment of obesity is not an approved use for thyroid hormone.

Pregnancy risk C.

Drug Interactions

Decreased Effect: Mazindol may decrease the hypotensive effect of guanethidine; monitor.

Increased Effect/Toxicity: Mazindol enhances the pressor effect of exogenous catecholamines (norepinephrine) and potential blood pressure increases in patients taking sympathomimetic medications.

Nutritional/Ethanol Interactions Ethanol: Avoid ethanol (may increase CNS depression).

Adverse Reactions Frequency not defined.

Cardiovascular: Palpitation, tachycardia, edema

Central nervous system: Insomnia, overstimulation, dizziness, dysphoria, drowsiness, depression, headache, restlessness

Dermatologic: Rash, clamminess

Endocrine & metabolic: Changes in libido

Gastrointestinal: Nausea, constipation, vomiting, xerostomia, unpleasant taste, diarrhea, abdominal cramps

Genitourinary: Dysuria, polyuria, impotence

Neuromuscular & skeletal: Tremor, weakness

Ocular: Blurred vision, corneal opacities

Miscellaneous: Diaphoresis (excessive)

Overdosage/Toxicology Symptoms of overdose include hypertension, tachycardia, and hyperthermia. Treatment is supportive.

Pharmacodynamics/Kinetics

Half-Life Elimination: 33-55 hours

Formulations

Tablet:

Mazanor®: 1 mg

Sanorex®: 1 mg, 2 mg

Dosing

Adults & Elderly: Obesity (short-term treatment): Oral: Initial: 1 mg once daily and adjust to patient response; usual dose is 1 mg 3 times daily, 1 hour before meals, or 2 mg once daily, 1 hour before lunch. Take with meals to avoid GI discomfort.

Stability

Storage: Store below 77°F (25°C).

Monitoring and Teaching Issues

Physical Assessment: Assess effectiveness and interactions of other medications patient may be taking (see Drug Interactions). Assess for history of psychopathology, homicidal or suicidal tendencies, or addiction; long-term use can result in dependence, abuse, or tolerance. Periodically evaluate the need for continued use. Monitor vital signs, and adverse reactions at start of therapy, when changing dosage, and at regular intervals during therapy (see Adverse Reactions). Monitor serum glucose closely with diabetic patients (may alter antidiabetic requirements). Taper dosage slowly when discontinuing. Assess knowledge/teach patient appropriate use, possible side effects, and symptoms to report (see Patient Education). **Pregnancy risk factor C** - benefits of use should outweigh possible risks (see Pregnancy Issues). Breast-feeding is not recommended.

Patient Education: Take exactly as directed; do not increase dose or frequency without consulting prescriber. Take 1 hour before meals; if gastric distress occurs may be taken with meals (do not take at bedtime). Avoid alcohol, caffeine, or OTC medications that act as stimulants. You may experience restlessness, false sense of euphoria, or impaired judgment (use caution when driving or engaging in tasks requiring alertness until response to drug is known); nausea or vomiting (small, frequent meals, frequent mouth care may help); constipation (increased exercise, fluids, fruit, or fiber may help); diarrhea (buttermilk,

(Continued)

Mazindol *(Continued)*

boiled milk, or yogurt may help); or altered libido (reversible). Diabetics need to monitor serum glucose closely (may alter antidiabetic medication requirements). Report chest pain, palpitations, or irregular heartbeat; muscle weakness or tremors; CNS changes (aggressiveness, restlessness, euphoria, sleep disturbances); testicular pain or changes in sexual activity; blurred vision; or changes in urinary patterns. **Pregnancy/breast-feeding precautions:** Inform prescriber if you are or intend to become pregnant. Breast-feeding is not recommended.

Related Information

Obesity Treatment Guidelines for Adults *on page 1693*

Measles and Rubella Vaccines, Combined *see page 1498*

Measles, Mumps, and Rubella Vaccines, Combined *see page 1498*

Measles Virus Vaccine, Live *see page 1498*

Mebendazole (me BEN da zole)

U.S. Brand Names Vermox®

Generic Available No

Pharmacologic Category Anthelmintic

Pregnancy Risk Factor C

Lactation Excretion in breast milk unknown/use caution

Use Treatment of pinworms (*Enterobius vermicularis*), whipworms (*Trichuris trichiura*), roundworms (*Ascaris lumbricoides*), and hookworms (*Ancylostoma duodenale*)

Mechanism of Action/Effect Selectively and irreversibly blocks glucose uptake and other nutrients in susceptible adult intestine-dwelling helminths

Contraindications Hypersensitivity to mebendazole or any component of the formulation

Warnings/Precautions Pregnancy and children <2 years of age are relative contraindications since safety has not been established. Not effective for hydatid disease. Pregnancy risk C.

Drug Interactions

Decreased Effect: Anticonvulsants such as carbamazepine and phenytoin may increase metabolism of mebendazole

Nutritional/Ethanol Interactions Food: Mebendazole serum levels may be increased if taken with food.

Effects on Lab Values ↑ LFTs

Adverse Reactions Frequency not defined.

Cardiovascular: Angioedema
Central nervous system: Fever, dizziness, headache, seizures
Dermatologic: Rash, itching, alopecia (with high doses)
Gastrointestinal: Abdominal pain, diarrhea, nausea, vomiting
Hematologic: Neutropenia (sore throat, unusual fatigue)
Neuromuscular & skeletal: Unusual weakness

Overdosage/Toxicology Symptoms of overdose include abdominal pain and altered mental status. Treatment is supportive.

Pharmacodynamics/Kinetics

Absorption: 2% to 10%
Half-Life Elimination: 1-11.5 hours
Time to Peak: Serum: 2-4 hours
Metabolism: Extensively hepatic

Formulations Tablet, chewable: 100 mg

Dosing

Adults & Elderly:

Pinworms: Oral: 100 mg as a single dose; may need to repeat after 2 weeks; treatment should include family members in close contact with patient.

Whipworms, roundworms, hookworms: Oral: 1 tablet twice daily, morning and evening on 3 consecutive days; if patient is not cured within 3-4 weeks, a second course of treatment may be administered.

Capillariasis: Oral: 200 mg twice daily for 20 days

Pediatrics: Refer to adult dosing.

Renal Impairment: Not dialyzable (0% to 5%)

Hepatic Impairment: Dosage reduction may be necessary in patients with liver dysfunction.

Administration

Oral: Tablets may be chewed, swallowed whole, or crushed and mixed with food.

Monitoring Laboratory Tests Check for helminth ova in feces within 3-4 weeks following the initial therapy. Periodically assess hematologic and hepatic function.

Monitoring and Teaching Issues

Physical Assessment: See Contraindications, Warnings/Precautions, Drug Interactions, and Dosing for use cautions. Since worm infestations are easily transmitted, all persons sharing same household should be treated. Teach proper use, transmission prevention, side effects and appropriate interventions, and adverse reactions to report (see Patient Education). **Pregnancy risk factor C** - benefits of use should outweigh possible risks. Note breast-feeding caution.

Patient Education: Inform prescriber of all prescriptions, OTC medications, or herbal products you are taking, and any allergies you have. Do not take anything new during treatment unless approved by prescriber. Take exactly as directed for full course of medication. Tablets may be chewed, swallowed whole, or crushed and mixed with food. Increase dietary intake of fruit juices. All family members and close friends should also be treated. To reduce possibility of reinfection, wash hands and scrub nails carefully with soap and hot water before handling food, before eating, and before and after toileting. Keep hands out of mouth. Disinfect toilet daily and launder bed linens, undergarments, and nightclothes daily with hot water and soap. Do not go barefoot and do not sit directly on grass or ground. May cause abdominal pain, nausea, or vomiting (small, frequent meals, frequent mouth care, sucking lozenges, or chewing gum may help); or hair loss (reversible). Report skin rash or itching, unusual fatigue or sore throat, unresolved diarrhea or vomiting, or CNS changes. **Pregnancy/breast-feeding precautions:** Inform prescriber if you are or intend to become pregnant. Consult prescriber if breast-feeding.

Dietary Issues: Tablet can be crushed and mixed with food, swallowed whole, or chewed.

Breast-feeding Issues: Since only 2% to 10% of mebendazole is absorbed, it is unlikely that it is excreted in breast milk in significant quantities.

Mechlorethamine (me klor ETH a meen)

U.S. Brand Names Mustargen®

Synonyms HN_2; Mechlorethamine Hydrochloride; Mustine; Nitrogen Mustard

Generic Available No

Pharmacologic Category Antineoplastic Agent, Alkylating Agent

Pregnancy Risk Factor D

Lactation Excretion in breast milk unknown/not recommended

Use Combination therapy of Hodgkin's disease and malignant lymphomas; non-Hodgkin's lymphoma; palliative treatment of bronchogenic, breast and ovarian carcinoma; may be used by intracavitary injection for treatment of metastatic tumors; pleural and other malignant effusions; topical treatment of mycosis fungoides

Mechanism of Action/Effect Alkylating agent that inhibits DNA and RNA synthesis via formation of carbonium ions; produces interstrand and intrastrand cross-links in DNA resulting in miscoding, breakage, and failure of replication

Contraindications Hypersensitivity to mechlorethamine or any component of the formulation; pre-existing profound myelosuppression or infection; pregnancy

Warnings/Precautions The U.S. Food and Drug Administration (FDA) currently recommends that procedures for proper handling and disposal of antineoplastic agents be considered. Appropriate safety equipment is recommended for preparation, administration, and disposal of antineoplastics. If mechlorethamine contacts the skin, wash and flush thoroughly with water. Extravasation of the drug into subcutaneous tissues results in painful inflammation and induration; sloughing may occur. Patients with lymphomas should receive prophylactic allopurinol 2-3 days prior to therapy to prevent complications resulting from tumor lysis.

Drug Interactions

Decreased Effect: Patients may experience impaired immune response to vaccines; possible infection after administration of live vaccines in patients receiving immunosuppressants.

Nutritional/Ethanol Interactions Ethanol: Avoid ethanol (due to GI irritation).

Adverse Reactions

>10%:

- Endocrine & metabolic: Delayed menses, oligomenorrhea, temporary or permanent amenorrhea, impaired spermatogenesis; spermatogenesis may return in patients in remission several years after the discontinuation of chemotherapy, chromosomal abnormalities
- Gastrointestinal: Nausea and vomiting usually occur in nearly 100% of patients and onset is within 30 minutes to 2 hours after administration
  - Emetic potential: High (>90%)
  - Time course of nausea/vomiting: Onset: 1-3 hours; duration 2-8 hours
- Genitourinary: Azoospermia
- Hematologic: Myelosuppressive: Leukopenia and thrombocytopenia can be severe; caution should be used with patients who are receiving radiotherapy, secondary leukemia
  - WBC: Severe
  - Platelets: Severe
  - Onset (days): 4-7
  - Nadir (days): 14
  - Recovery (days): 21
- Otic: Ototoxicity
- Miscellaneous: Precipitation of herpes zoster

1% to 10%:

- Central nervous system: Fever, vertigo
- Dermatologic: Alopecia
- Endocrine & metabolic: Hyperuricemia
- Gastrointestinal: Diarrhea, anorexia, metallic taste
- Local: Thrombophlebitis/extravasation: May cause local vein discomfort which may be relieved by warm soaks and pain medication. A brown discoloration of veins may occur. Mechlorethamine is a strong vesicant and can cause tissue necrosis and sloughing.
  Vesicant chemotherapy
- Secondary malignancies: Have been reported after several years in 1% to 6% of patients treated
- Neuromuscular & skeletal: Weakness
- Otic: Tinnitus
- Miscellaneous: Hypersensitivity, anaphylaxis

<1% (Limited to important or life-threatening): Hemolytic anemia, hepatotoxicity, myelosuppression, peripheral neuropathy

Overdosage/Toxicology Suppression of all formed elements of blood, uric acid crystals, nausea, vomiting, and diarrhea. Sodium thiosulfate is the specific antidote for nitrogen mustard extravasations. Treatment of systemic overdose is supportive.

Pharmacodynamics/Kinetics

Absorption: Intracavitary administration: Incomplete secondary to rapid deactivation by body fluids

Half-Life Elimination: <1 minute

Metabolism: Rapid hydrolysis and demethylation, possibly in plasma

Duration: Unchanged drug is undetectable in blood within a few minutes

Formulations Injection, powder for reconstitution, as hydrochloride: 10 mg

(Continued)

Mechlorethamine *(Continued)*

Dosing

Adults & Elderly: Refer to individual protocols. Dosage should be based on ideal dry weight. The presence of edema or ascites must be considered so that dosage will be based on actual weight unaugmented by these conditions.

MOPP: I.V.: 6 mg/m^2 on days 1 and 8 of a 28-day cycle

Typical dose: I.V.: 0.4 mg/kg **or** 12-16 mg/m^2 for one dose **or** divided into 0.1 mg/kg/day for 4 days, repeated at 4- to 6-week intervals

Intracavitary: 10-20 mg diluted in 10 mL of SWI or 0.9% sodium chloride

Intrapericardially: 0.2-0.4 mg/kg diluted in up to 100 mL of 0.9% sodium chloride

Topical mechlorethamine has been used in the treatment of cutaneous lesions of mycosis fungoides. A skin test should be performed prior to treatment with the topical preparation to detect sensitivity and possible irritation (use fresh mechlorethamine 0.1 mg/mL and apply over a 3 x 5 cm area of normal skin).

Pediatrics: Refer to individual protocols. Dosage should be based on ideal dry weight; the presence of edema or ascites must be considered so that dosage will be based on actual weight unaugmented by these conditions.

Children: MOPP: I.V.: 6 mg/m^2 on days 1 and 8 of a 28-day cycle

Renal Impairment:

Hemodialysis: Not removed; supplemental dosing is not necessary.

Peritoneal dialysis: Not removed; supplemental dosing is not necessary.

Administration

I.V.: Vesicant. Margin of error is very slight. Check dosage carefully before administration. Administer with caution. Administer I.V. push through a free flowing I.V. over 1-3 minutes at a concentration not to exceed 1 mg/mL.

Stability

Storage:

Store intact vials at room temperature

Solutions are usually reconstituted at 1 mg/mL with SWI, D_5W, or NS. The manufacturer reports that reconstituted solutions are stable for 15 minutes and should be prepared immediately before use. Other sources suggest the drug may be stable for 1-4 hours, particularly in nonacidic solutions.

Reconstitution: Must be prepared fresh - solution is stable for only 1 hour after dilution and must be administered within 1 hour. Dilute powder with 10 mL SWI to a final concentration of 1 mg/mL. May be diluted in up to 100 mL NS for intracavitary administration.

Standard I.V. dilution: I.V. push: Dose/syringe (concentration is 1 mg/mL)

Maximum syringe for IVP is 30 mL and syringe should be ≤75% full.

Compatibility: Stable in sterile water for injection; **incompatible** with D_5W

Y-site administration: Incompatible with allopurinol, cefepime

Compatibility when admixed: Incompatible with methohexital

Monitoring Laboratory Tests CBC with differential and platelet count

Monitoring and Teaching Issues

Physical Assessment: See Contraindications, Warnings/Precautions, and Dosing for use cautions. Assess potential for interactions with other prescriptions, OTC medications, or herbal products patient may be taking (see Drug Interactions). See Administration, Dosing, Reconstitution, and Compatibility for administration specifics. Premedication with antiemetic recommended. Infusion site must be closely monitored; extravasation can cause sloughing or tissue necrosis (see Administration). Assess results of laboratory tests (see above), therapeutic effects, and adverse response, which can be severe and involve several systems (see Adverse Reactions and Overdose/Toxicology) prior to each treatment and on a regular basis throughout therapy. Teach patient possible side effects and appropriate interventions (eg, importance of adequate hydration) and adverse symptoms to report (see Patient Education). **Pregnancy risk factor D** - determine that patient is not pregnant before beginning treatment. Instruct patients of childbearing age appropriate barrier contraceptive measures. Breast-feeding is not recommended.

Patient Education: Inform prescriber of all prescriptions, OTC medications, or herbal products you are taking, and any allergies you have. Do not take anything new during treatment unless approved by prescriber. This medication can only be given by infusion. Report immediately any swelling, redness, pain, or burning at infusion site. Do not use alcohol during treatment. Maintain adequate fluid balance (2-3 L/day) unless advised by prescriber to restrict fluids, and adequate nutrition (small, frequent meals, frequent mouth care, sucking lozenges, or chewing gum may reduce anorexia and nausea). May cause discoloration (brown color) of veins used for infusion; hair loss (reversible); easy bleeding or bruising (use soft toothbrush or cotton swabs and frequent mouth care, use electric razor, avoid sharp knives or scissors); or increased susceptibility to infection (avoid crowds and exposure to infection and do not have any vaccinations unless approved by prescriber). This drug may cause menstrual irregularities, permanent sterility, and birth defects. Report changes in auditory or visual acuity; unusual bleeding or bruising or persistent fever or sore throat; blood in urine, stool, or vomitus; delayed healing of any wounds; skin rash; yellowing of skin or eyes; changes in color of urine of stool; acute or unresolved nausea or vomiting; diarrhea; or loss of appetite. **Pregnancy/breast-feeding precautions:** Inform prescriber if you are pregnant. Do not get pregnant while taking this medication and for 1 month following therapy; consult prescriber for appropriate barrier contraceptives. Breast-feeding is not recommended.

Mechlorethamine Hydrochloride *see* Mechlorethamine *on page 839*

Meclizine (MEK li zeen)

U.S. Brand Names Antivert®; Antrizine®; Bonine® [OTC]; Dizmiss® [OTC]; Dramamine® II [OTC]; Meni-D®; Vergon® [OTC]

Synonyms Meclizine Hydrochloride; Meclozine Hydrochloride

Generic Available Yes

Pharmacologic Category Antiemetic; Antihistamine

Pregnancy Risk Factor B

Lactation Excretion in breast milk unknown/not recommended

Use Prevention and treatment of symptoms of motion sickness; management of vertigo with diseases affecting the vestibular system

Mechanism of Action/Effect Has central anticholinergic action by blocking chemoreceptor trigger zone; decreases excitability of the middle ear labyrinth and blocks conduction in the middle ear vestibular-cerebellar pathways

Contraindications Hypersensitivity to meclizine or any component of the formulation

Warnings/Precautions Use with caution in patients with angle-closure glaucoma, prostatic hyperplasia, pyloric or duodenal obstruction, or bladder neck obstruction. Use with caution in hot weather, and during exercise. Elderly may be at risk for anticholinergic side effects such as glaucoma, prostatic hyperplasia, constipation, GI obstructive disease. If vertigo does not respond in 1-2 weeks, it is advised to discontinue use.

Drug Interactions

Increased Effect/Toxicity: Increased toxicity with CNS depressants, neuroleptics, and anticholinergics.

Nutritional/Ethanol Interactions Ethanol: Avoid ethanol (may increase CNS depression).

Adverse Reactions

>10%:

Central nervous system: Slight to moderate drowsiness

Respiratory: Thickening of bronchial secretions

1% to 10%:

Central nervous system: Headache, fatigue, nervousness, dizziness

Gastrointestinal: Appetite increase, weight gain, nausea, diarrhea, abdominal pain, dry mouth

Neuromuscular & skeletal: Arthralgia

Respiratory: Pharyngitis

<1% (Limited to important or life-threatening): Bronchospasm, hepatitis, hypotension, palpitations

Overdosage/Toxicology Symptoms of overdose include CNS depression, confusion, nervousness, hallucinations, dizziness, blurred vision, nausea, vomiting, and hyperthermia. There is no specific treatment for antihistamine overdose. Clinical toxicity is due to blockade of cholinergic receptors. For anticholinergic overdose with severe life-threatening symptoms, physostigmine 1-2 mg I.V. slowly, may be given to reverse these effects.

Pharmacodynamics/Kinetics

Half-Life Elimination: 6 hours

Metabolism: Hepatic

Onset: ~1 hour

Duration: 8-24 hours

Formulations

Capsule, as hydrochloride: 25 mg, 30 mg

Tablet, as hydrochloride: 12.5 mg, 25 mg, 50 mg

Tablet, chewable, as hydrochloride: 25 mg

Dosing

Adults:

Motion sickness: Oral: 12.5-25 mg 1 hour before travel, repeat dose every 12-24 hours if needed; doses up to 50 mg may be needed

Vertigo: Oral: 25-100 mg/day in divided doses

Elderly: Refer to adult dosing; start at lowest dose.

Pediatrics: Children >12 years: Refer to adult dosing.

Monitoring and Teaching Issues

Physical Assessment: Determine cause of vomiting before beginning therapy. Assess effectiveness and interactions of other medications patient may be taking (see Drug Interactions). See Warnings/Precautions and Contraindications for use cautions. Monitor effectiveness of therapy and adverse response (see Adverse Reactions and Overdose/Toxicology). Assess knowledge/teach patient possible side effects and appropriate interventions and adverse symptoms to report (see Patient Education). Breast-feeding is not recommended.

Patient Education: Take exactly as prescribed; do not increase dose. Avoid alcohol, other CNS depressants, sleeping aids without consulting prescriber. You may experience dizziness, drowsiness, or blurred vision (use caution when driving or engaging in tasks that require alertness until response to drug is known); dry mouth (frequent mouth care, sucking lozenges, or chewing gum may help); constipation (increased exercise, fluids, fruit, or may help); or heat intolerance (avoid excessive exercise, hot environments, maintain adequate hydration). Report CNS change (hallucination, confusion, nervousness); sudden or unusual weight gain; unresolved nausea or diarrhea; chest pain or palpitations; muscle pain; or changes in urinary pattern. **Breast-feeding precaution:** Breast-feeding is not recommended.

Geriatric Considerations: Due to anticholinergic action, use lowest dose in divided doses to avoid side effects and their inconvenience. Limit use if possible. May cause confusion or aggravate symptoms of confusion in those with dementia.

Meclizine Hydrochloride *see* Meclizine *on page 840*

Meclofenamate *see page 1587*

Meclozine Hydrochloride *see* Meclizine *on page 840*

Medicinal Carbon *see* Charcoal *on page 266*

Medicinal Charcoal *see* Charcoal *on page 266*

Medralone® *see* MethylPREDNISolone *on page 885*

Medrol® *see* MethylPREDNISolone *on page 885*

MedroxyPROGESTERone (me DROKS ee proe JES te rone)

U.S. Brand Names Depo-Provera®; Provera®

Synonyms Acetoxymethylprogesterone; Medroxyprogesterone Acetate; Methylacetoxyprogesterone

Generic Available Yes

Pharmacologic Category Contraceptive; Progestin

Pregnancy Risk Factor X

Lactation Enters breast milk/compatible

Use Endometrial carcinoma or renal carcinoma as well as secondary amenorrhea or abnormal uterine bleeding due to hormonal imbalance; reduction of endometrial hyperplasia in postmenopausal women receiving 0.625 mg conjugated estrogens for 12-14 consecutive days per month; Depo-Provera® injection is used for the prevention of pregnancy

Use - Unlabeled/Investigational Hypoventilation disorders, advanced breast cancer

Mechanism of Action/Effect Inhibits secretion of pituitary gonadotropins, which prevents follicular maturation and ovulation, stimulates growth of mammary tissue

Contraindications Hypersensitivity to medroxyprogesterone or any component of the formulation; cerebral apoplexy, undiagnosed vaginal bleeding, liver dysfunction; thrombophlebitis; pregnancy

Warnings/Precautions Use with caution in patients with depression, diabetes, epilepsy, asthma, migraines, renal or cardiac dysfunction. Pretreatment exams should include Pap smear, physical exam of breasts and pelvic areas. May increase serum cholesterol, LDL, decrease HDL and triglycerides. Use of any progestin (progesterone and derivatives ie, medroxyprogesterone) during the first 4 months of pregnancy is not recommended. Monitor patient closely for loss of vision, sudden onset of proptosis, diplopia, migraine, and signs or symptoms of thromboembolic disorders.

Drug Interactions

Cytochrome P450 Effect: Substrate of **CYP3A4**; Induces CYP3A4

Decreased Effect: Aminoglutethimide may decrease effects by increasing hepatic metabolism.

Effects on Lab Values Altered thyroid and liver function tests

Adverse Reactions Frequency not defined.

Cardiovascular: Edema, embolism, central thrombosis

Central nervous system: Mental depression, fever, insomnia, somnolence, headache (rare), dizziness

Dermatologic: Melasma or chloasma, allergic rash with or without pruritus, acne, hirsutism, angioneurotic edema

Endocrine & metabolic: Breakthrough bleeding, spotting, changes in menstrual flow, amenorrhea, increased breast tenderness, changes in cervical erosion and secretions

Gastrointestinal: Weight gain/loss, anorexia, nausea

Hepatic: Cholestatic jaundice

Local: Pain at injection site, sterile abscess, thrombophlebitis

Neuromuscular & skeletal: Weakness

Respiratory: Pulmonary embolism

Miscellaneous: Anaphylaxis

Overdosage/Toxicology Toxicity is unlikely following single exposure of excessive doses. Supportive treatment is adequate in most cases.

Pharmacodynamics/Kinetics

Absorption: Oral: Well absorbed; I.M.: Slow

Bioavailability: 0.6% to 10%

Half-Life Elimination: Oral: 38-46 hours; I.M.: Acetate: 50 days

Time to Peak: Oral: 2-4 hours

Metabolism: Oral: Hepatic via hydroxylated and conjugated

Formulations

Injection, suspension, as acetate (Depot-Provera®): 150 mg/mL (1 mL); 400 mg/mL (1 mL, 2.5 mL, 10 mL)

Tablet, as acetate (Provera®): 2.5 mg, 5 mg, 10 mg

Dosing

Adults & Elderly:

Amenorrhea: Oral: 5-10 mg/day or 2.5 mg/day for 5-10 days

Abnormal uterine bleeding: Oral: 5-10 mg for 5-10 days starting on day 16 or 21 of cycle

Accompanying cyclic estrogen therapy, postmenopausal: Oral: 2.5-10 mg the last 10-13 days of estrogen dosing each month

Contraception: I.M.: 150 mg every 3 months

Endometrial or renal carcinoma: I.M.: 400-1000 mg/week

Hypoventilation syndromes (unlabeled use): Oral: 20 mg 3 times/day

Pediatrics: Adolescents: Refer to adult dosing.

Hepatic Impairment: Dose needs to be lowered in patients with alcoholic cirrhosis.

Monitoring Laboratory Tests Must have pregnancy test prior to beginning therapy.

Monitoring and Teaching Issues

Physical Assessment: Monitor for effectiveness of therapy and adverse effects (see Adverse Reactions). Instruct patient on appropriate dose scheduling (according to purpose of therapy), possible side effects, and symptoms to report (see Patient Education). **Pregnancy risk factor X** - determine that patient is not pregnant before starting therapy. Do not give to sexually-active female patients unless capable of complying with barrier contraceptive use.

Patient Education: Follow dosage schedule and do not take more than prescribed. You may experience sensitivity to sunlight (use sunblock, wear protective clothing and eyewear, and avoid extensive exposure to direct sunlight); dizziness, anxiety, depression (use caution when driving or engaging in tasks that require alertness until response to drug is known); changes in appetite (maintain adequate hydration and diet - 2-3 L/day of fluids unless advised by prescriber to restrict fluids); decreased libido or increased body hair (reversible when drug is discontinued); hot flashes (cool clothes and environment may help). May cause discoloration of stool (green). Report swelling of face, lips, or mouth; absence or altered menses; abdominal pain; vaginal itching, irritation, or discharge; heat, warmth, redness, or swelling of extremities; or sudden onset change in vision. **Pregnancy precaution:** Inform prescriber if you are pregnant. Do not get pregnant during or for 1 month following therapy. Consult prescriber for instruction on appropriate barrier contraceptive measures. This drug may cause severe fetal defects.

Geriatric Considerations: No specific recommendations for dosage adjustments. Monitor closely for adverse effects when starting therapy.

Related Information

Estrogen Replacement Therapy *on page 1666*
FDA Name Differentiation Project: The Use of Tall-man Letters *on page 12*

Medroxyprogesterone Acetate *see* MedroxyPROGESTERone *on page 842*

Medroxyprogesterone Acetate and Estradiol Cypionate *see* Estradiol and Medroxyprogesterone *on page 497*

Medroxyprogesterone and Estrogens (Conjugated) *see* Estrogens (Conjugated/Equine) and Medroxyprogesterone *on page 505*

Medrysone (ME dri sone)

U.S. Brand Names HMS Liquifilm®

Generic Available No

Pharmacologic Category Corticosteroid, Ophthalmic

Pregnancy Risk Factor C

Lactation Excretion in breast milk unknown/use caution

Use Treatment of allergic conjunctivitis, vernal conjunctivitis, episcleritis, ophthalmic epinephrine sensitivity reaction

Mechanism of Action/Effect Decreases inflammation by suppression of migration of polymorphonuclear leukocytes and reversal of increased capillary permeability

Contraindications Hypersensitivity to medrysone or any component of the formulation; fungal, viral, or untreated pus-forming bacterial ocular infections; not for use in iritis and uveitis

Warnings/Precautions Prolonged use has been associated with the development of corneal or scleral perforation and posterior subcapsular cataracts. May mask or enhance the establishment of acute purulent untreated infections of the eye. Use caution in patients with glaucoma. Medrysone is a synthetic corticosteroid; structurally related to progesterone; if no improvement after several days of treatment, discontinue medrysone and institute other therapy. Duration of therapy: 3-4 days to several weeks dependent on type and severity of disease. Taper dose to avoid disease exacerbation. Safety and efficacy have not been established in children <3 years of age. Pregnancy risk C.

Adverse Reactions Frequency not defined: Ocular: Acute anterior uveitis, allergic reactions, blurred vision (mild, temporary), burning, cataracts, conjunctivitis, corneal thinning, corneal ulcers, delayed wound healing, foreign body sensation, glaucoma, IOP increased, keratitis, mydriasis, optic nerve damage, ptosis, secondary ocular infection stinging, visual activity defects

Overdosage/Toxicology Systemic toxicity is unlikely from the ophthalmic preparation.

Pharmacodynamics/Kinetics

Absorption: Through aqueous humor

Metabolism: Hepatic if absorbed

Formulations Solution, ophthalmic: 1% (5 mL, 10 mL) [contains benzalkonium chloride]

Dosing

Adults & Elderly: Conjunctivitis: Ophthalmic: Instill 1 drop in conjunctival sac 2-4 times/day up to every 4 hours; may use every 1-2 hours during first 1-2 days.

Pediatrics: Children ≥3 years: Refer to adult dosing.

Administration

Other: Ophthalmic: Shake well before using. Do not touch dropper to the eye.

Stability

Storage: Store at room temperature of 25°C (77°F). Protect from freezing.

Monitoring and Teaching Issues

Physical Assessment: See Contraindications, Warnings/Precautions, and Adverse Reactions for use cautions. Assess knowledge/teach patient appropriate use, possible side effects and appropriate interventions, and adverse symptoms to report (see Patient Education). **Pregnancy risk factor C** - systemic absorption is unlikely or minimal. Note breast-feeding caution.

Patient Education: This medication is only for use in your eyes. Use exactly as directed (see below). May cause sensitivity to light (dark glasses may help); or temporary stinging, burning, or blurred vision. Report pain, swelling, scratchiness, itching, watering, or dryness of eye; drainage, redness, or sign of eye infection; change in vision (eg, double vision, reduced visual field, halo around lights); or worsening of condition or lack of improvement in 3-4 days. **Pregnancy/breast-feeding precautions:** Inform prescriber if you are pregnant. Consult prescriber if breast-feeding.

Wash hands thoroughly before using. Shake well before using. Do not allow applicator tip to touch eye. Gently pull down lower lid and put drop(s) into inner corner of eye. Close eye and roll eyeball in all directions. Do not blink for 30 seconds. Apply gently pressure to inner corner of eye for 30 seconds. Gently wipe away any excess from skin around eye. Do not use any other eye medication for 10-15 minutes.

Mefenamic Acid *see page 1587*

Mefloquine (ME floe kwin)

U.S. Brand Names Lariam®

Synonyms Mefloquine Hydrochloride

Generic Available No

Pharmacologic Category Antimalarial Agent

(Continued)

Mefloquine *(Continued)*

Pregnancy Risk Factor C

Lactation Enters breast milk/not recommended

Use Treatment of acute malarial infections and prevention of malaria

Mechanism of Action/Effect Mefloquine is a quinoline-methanol compound structurally similar to quinine; mefloquine's effectiveness in the treatment and prophylaxis of malaria is due to the destruction of the asexual blood forms of the malarial pathogens that affect humans, *Plasmodium falciparum*, *P. vivax*, *P. malariae*, *P. ovale*

Contraindications Hypersensitivity mefloquine or any component of the formulation; epilepsy; cardiac conduction abnormalities; severe psychiatric disorder (including active or recent history of depression, generalized anxiety disorder, psychosis, or schizophrenia)

Warnings/Precautions Discontinue if unexplained neuropsychiatric disturbances occur. Use caution in epilepsy patients or in patients with significant cardiac disease. If mefloquine is to be used for a prolonged period, periodic evaluations including liver function tests and ophthalmic examinations should be performed. (Retinal abnormalities have not been observed with mefloquine in humans; however, it has with long-term administration to rats). In cases of life-threatening, serious, or overwhelming malaria infections due to *Plasmodium falciparum*, patients should be treated with intravenous antimalarial drug. Mefloquine may be given orally to complete the course. Caution should be exercised with regard to driving, piloting airplanes, and operating machines since dizziness, disturbed sense of balance.

Use with caution in patients with a previous history of depression (see contraindications regarding psychiatric illness including active/recent depression). May cause a range of psychiatric symptoms, including psychosis (symptoms occasionally reported to persist long after discontinuation). Rare cases of suicidal ideation and suicide have been reported (no causal relationship established). The appearance of psychiatric symptoms such as acute anxiety, depression, restlessness or confusion may be a prodrome to more serious events; when used as prophylaxis, substitute an alternative medication.

Pregnancy risk C.

Drug Interactions

Cytochrome P450 Effect: Substrate of **CYP3A4**; Inhibits CYP3A4

Decreased Effect: Mefloquine may decrease the effect of valproic acid.

Increased Effect/Toxicity: Increased bradycardia possible with beta-blockers; caution with other drugs that alter cardiac conduction; increased toxicity with chloroquine, quinine, and quinidine (hold treatment until at least 12 hours after these later drugs)

Adverse Reactions

1% to 10%:

Central nervous system: Difficulty concentrating, headache, insomnia, lightheadedness, vertigo

Gastrointestinal: Vomiting (3%), diarrhea, stomach pain, nausea

Ocular: Visual disturbances

Otic: Tinnitus

<1% (Limited to important or life-threatening): Ataxia, aggressive behavior, anxiety, AV block, bradycardia, depression, erythema multiforme, hallucinations, hypotension, panic attacks, paranoia, paresthesia, psychosis, Stevens-Johnson syndrome, suicidal ideation and behavior (causal relationship not established), syncope, thrombocytopenia, tremor

Overdosage/Toxicology Cardiotoxic symptoms of overdose include vomiting and diarrhea. Treatment is supportive.

Pharmacodynamics/Kinetics

Absorption: Well absorbed

Half-Life Elimination: 21-22 days

Metabolism: Extensively hepatic

Formulations Tablet, as hydrochloride: 250 mg

Dosing

Adults & Elderly:

Malaria, treatment of mild to moderate infection: Oral: 5 tablets (1250 mg) as a single dose with at least 8 oz of water

Malaria prophylaxis: Oral: 1 tablet (250 mg) weekly starting 1 week before travel, continuing weekly during travel and for 4 weeks after leaving endemic area

Pediatrics: Malaria prophylaxis: Oral: Children:

15-19 kg: ¼ tablet

20-30 kg: ½ tablet

31-45 kg: ¾ tablet

>45 kg: 1 tablet

Administer weekly starting 1 week before travel, continuing weekly during travel and for 4 weeks after leaving endemic area.

Administration

Oral: Do not take drug on an empty stomach. Take with food and at least 8 oz of water.

Monitoring Laboratory Tests When use is prolonged, periodically monitor liver function tests.

Monitoring and Teaching Issues

Physical Assessment: See Contraindications, Warnings/Precautions, and Dosing (eg, treatment vs prophylaxis) for use cautions. Assess potential for interactions with other prescriptions, OTC medications, or herbal products patient may be taking (see Drug Interactions). Assess results of laboratory tests, effectiveness of therapy, and adverse response (eg, CNS changes - see Adverse Reactions and Overdose/Toxicology). Teach patient appropriate use, possible side effects/interventions (eg, need for ophthalmic exams), and adverse symptoms to report (see Patient Education). **Pregnancy risk factor C** - benefits of use should outweigh possible risks. Breast-feeding is not recommended.

Patient Education: Inform prescriber of all prescriptions, OTC medications, or herbal products you are taking, and any allergies you have. Do not take anything new during treatment unless approved by prescriber. Take as directed; full course of treatment may take several months. For prophylaxis, begin 1 week before traveling to endemic areas, continue during travel period and for 4 weeks following return. Take with 8 oz of water. Avoid alcohol. You should have regular ophthalmic exams (every 4-6 months) if using this medication over extended periods. May cause dizziness, changes in mentation, insomnia, headache, visual disturbances, disturbed sense of balance (use caution when driving or engaging in tasks requiring alertness until response to drug is known); or nausea, vomiting, loss of appetite (small, frequent meals, frequent mouth care, sucking lozenges, or chewing gum may help). Report vision changes, persistent GI disturbances, change in hearing acuity or ringing in the ears, CNS changes, unusual fatigue, or any other persistent adverse reactions. If you are taking this for prophylaxis of malaria and experience symptoms of anxiety, confusion, depression, nervousness, or restlessness, report these symptoms **immediately** to the prescriber (symptoms may worsen) and stop taking this medication. **Pregnancy/breast-feeding precautions:** Inform prescriber if you are pregnant. Use reliable contraception during and for 2 months following treatment. Breast-feeding is not recommended.

Mefloquine Hydrochloride *see* Mefloquine *on page 843*

Mefoxin® *see* Cefoxitin *on page 245*

Megace® *see* Megestrol *on page 845*

Megadophilus® [OTC] *see Lactobacillus on page 766*

Megestrol (me JES trole)

U.S. Brand Names Megace®

Synonyms Megestrol Acetate

Generic Available Yes

Pharmacologic Category Antineoplastic Agent, Miscellaneous; Progestin

Pregnancy Risk Factor X

Lactation Enters breast milk/contraindicated

Use Palliative treatment of breast and endometrial carcinoma

Orphan drug: Treatment of anorexia, cachexia, or significant weight loss (≥10% baseline body weight); treatment of AIDS

Mechanism of Action/Effect A synthetic progestin with antiestrogenic properties which disrupt the estrogen receptor cycle. May also have a direct effect on the endometrium. Megestrol is an antineoplastic progestin thought to act through an antileutenizing effect mediated via the pituitary.

Contraindications Hypersensitivity to megestrol or any component of the formulation; pregnancy

Warnings/Precautions The U.S. Food and Drug Administration (FDA) currently recommends that procedures for proper handling and disposal of antineoplastic agents be considered. Use with caution in patients with a history of thrombophlebitis. Elderly females may have vaginal bleeding or discharge and need to be forewarned of this side effect and inconvenience.

May suppress hypothalamic-pituitary-adrenal (HPA) axis during chronic administration. Consider the possibility of adrenal suppression in any patient receiving or being withdrawn from chronic therapy when signs/symptoms suggestive of hypoadrenalism are noted (during stress or in unstressed state). Laboratory evaluation and replacement/stress doses of rapid-acting glucocorticoid should be considered.

Nutritional/Ethanol Interactions Herb/Nutraceutical: Avoid black cohosh, dong quai in estrogen-dependent tumors.

Effects on Lab Values Altered thyroid and liver function tests

Adverse Reactions

Cardiovascular: Edema, hypertension (≤8%), cardiomyopathy, palpitations

Central nervous system: Insomnia, depression (≤6%), fever (2% to 6%), headache (≤10%), pain (≤6%, similar to placebo), confusion (1% to 3%), convulsions (1% to 3%), depression (1% to 3%)

Dermatologic: Allergic rash (2% to 12%) with or without pruritus, alopecia

Endocrine & metabolic: Breakthrough bleeding and amenorrhea, spotting, changes in menstrual flow, changes in cervical erosion and secretions, increased breast tenderness, changes in vaginal bleeding pattern, edema, fluid retention, hyperglycemia (≤6%), diabetes, HPA axis suppression, adrenal insufficiency, Cushing's syndrome

Gastrointestinal: Weight gain (not attributed to edema or fluid retention), nausea (≤5%, less than placebo), vomiting, diarrhea (8% to 15%, similar to placebo), flatulence (≤10%), constipation (1% to 3%)

Genitourinary: Impotence (4% to 14%), decreased libido (≤5%)

Hepatic: Cholestatic jaundice, hepatotoxicity, hepatomegaly (1% to 3%)

Local: Thrombophlebitis

Neuromuscular & skeletal: Carpal tunnel syndrome, weakness, paresthesia (1% to 3%)

Respiratory: Hyperpnea, dyspnea (1% to 3%), cough (1% to 3%)

Miscellaneous: Diaphoresis

Overdosage/Toxicology Toxicity is unlikely following single exposure of excessive doses.

Pharmacodynamics/Kinetics

Absorption: Well absorbed

Half-Life Elimination: 15-20 hours

Time to Peak: Serum: 1-3 hours

Metabolism: Completely hepatic to free steroids and glucuronide conjugates

Onset: ≥2 months of continuous therapy

Formulations

Suspension, oral, as acetate: 40 mg/mL (240 mL) [contains alcohol 0.06%]

Tablet, as acetate: 20 mg, 40 mg

Dosing

Adults & Elderly: Refer to individual protocols.

Breast carcinoma (female): Oral: 40 mg 4 times/day

Endometrial carcinoma: Oral: 40-320 mg/day in divided doses; use for 2 months to determine efficacy; maximum doses used have been up to 800 mg/day.

(Continued)

Megestrol *(Continued)*

Uterine bleeding: Oral: 40 mg 2-4 times/day

HIV-related cachexia (male/female): Oral: Initial: 800 mg/day; daily doses of 400 and 800 mg/day were found to be clinically effective.

Renal Impairment: No data available; however, the urinary excretion of megestrol acetate administered in doses of 4-90 mg ranged from 56% to 78% within 10 days.

Hemodialysis: Megestrol acetate has not been tested for dialyzability; however, due to its low solubility, it is postulated that dialysis would not be an effective means of treating an overdose.

Stability

Storage: Store at 25°C (77°F), excursions permitted at 15°C to 30°C (59°F to 86°F)

Compatibility: Megestrol acetate (Megace®) oral suspension is stable in water, orange juice, apple juice, or Sustacal H.C. for immediate consumption.

Monitoring and Teaching Issues

Physical Assessment: See Contraindications, Warnings/Precautions and Dosing for use cautions. Assess potential for interactions with other prescriptions, OTC medications, or herbal products patient may be taking (see Drug Interactions). See Administration, Dosing, and Compatibility for I.V. administration specifics. Assess therapeutic effects and adverse response (see Adverse Reactions and Overdose/Toxicology) on a regular basis throughout therapy. Teach patient proper use (oral), possible side effects and appropriate interventions (eg, importance of adequate hydration), and adverse symptoms to report (see Patient Education). **Pregnancy risk factor X** - determine that patient is not pregnant before beginning treatment. Do not give to women of childbearing age unless they are capable of complying with barrier contraceptives. Instruct patients about appropriate barrier contraceptive measures. Breast-feeding is contraindicated.

Patient Education: Inform prescriber of all prescriptions, OTC medications, or herbal products you are taking, and any allergies you have. Do not take anything new during treatment unless approved by prescriber. Follow dosage schedule and do not take more than prescribed. May cause sensitivity to sunlight (use sunblock, wear protective clothing, and avoid extended exposure to direct sunlight); dizziness, anxiety, depression (use caution when driving or engaging in tasks that require alertness until response to drug is known); change in appetite (maintain adequate hydration and diet - 2-3 L/day of fluids unless advised by prescriber to restrict fluids); decreased libido or increased body hair (reversible when drug is discontinued); or hot flashes (cool clothes and environment may help). Report swelling of face, lips, or mouth; absent or altered menses; abdominal pain; vaginal itching, irritation, or discharge; heat, warmth, redness, or swelling of extremities; or sudden onset change in vision. **Pregnancy/breast-feeding precautions:** Do not get pregnant while taking this medication and for 1 month following therapy; consult prescriber for appropriate barrier contraceptives. This drug may cause fetal defects. Do not donate blood during or for 1 month following therapy. Do not breast-feed.

Geriatric Considerations: Elderly females may have vaginal bleeding or discharge and need to be forewarned of this side effect and inconvenience. No specific changes in dose are required for elderly. Megestrol has been used in the treatment of the failure to thrive syndrome in cachectic elderly in addition to proper nutrition.

Megestrol Acetate *see* Megestrol *on page 845*

Melanex® *see* Hydroquinone *on page 679*

Mellaril® *see* Thioridazine *on page 1306*

Meloxicam (mel OX ee cam)

U.S. Brand Names MOBIC®

Generic Available No

Pharmacologic Category Nonsteroidal Anti-inflammatory Drug (NSAID)

Pregnancy Risk Factor C/D (3rd trimester)

Lactation Excretion in breast milk unknown/contraindicated

Use Relief of signs and symptoms of osteoarthritis

Mechanism of Action/Effect Inhibits prostaglandin synthesis by decreasing the activity of the enzyme, cyclooxygenase, which results in decreased formation of prostaglandin precursors

Contraindications Hypersensitivity to meloxicam or any component of the formulation, aspirin, or other NSAIDs; pregnancy C/D (3rd trimester)

Warnings/Precautions Gastrointestinal irritation, ulceration, bleeding, and perforation may occur with NSAIDs. Serious complications may occur without prior symptoms of gastrointestinal distress. Use with caution in patients with a history of GI disease (bleeding or ulcers), decreased renal function, hepatic disease, CHF, dehydration, hypertension, or asthma. Use with caution in elderly patients. Anaphylactoid reactions may occur, even with no prior exposure to meloxicam. Use in advanced renal disease is not recommended. May alter platelet function; use with caution in patients receiving anticoagulants or with hemostatic disorders. Safety and efficacy in pediatric patients have not been established. Withhold for at least 4-6 half-lives prior to surgical or dental procedures. Pregnancy risk C/D (3rd trimester).

Drug Interactions

Cytochrome P450 Effect: Substrate of CYP2C8/9, 3A4; Inhibits CYP2C8/9

Decreased Effect: Cholestyramine (and possibly colestipol) increases the clearance of meloxicam. Hydralazine's antihypertensive effect is decreased; avoid concurrent use. Loop diuretic efficacy (diuretic and antihypertensive effect) may be reduced by NSAIDs. Antihypertensive effects of thiazide diuretics are decreased; avoid concurrent use.

Increased Effect/Toxicity: Anticoagulants (warfarin, heparin, LMWHs) in combination with NSAIDs can cause increased risk of bleeding. Antiplatelet drugs (ticlopidine, clopidogrel, aspirin, abciximab, dipyridamole, eptifibatide, tirofiban) can cause an increased risk of bleeding. Aspirin increases serum concentrations (AUC) of meloxicam (in addition to potential for additive adverse effects); concurrent use is not recommended. Corticosteroids may increase the risk of GI ulceration; avoid concurrent use. NSAIDs may increase serum creatinine, potassium, blood pressure, and cyclosporine levels; monitor cyclosporine levels and renal function carefully. Lithium levels can be increased; avoid concurrent use if possible or monitor lithium levels and adjust dose. When NSAID is stopped, lithium will need adjustment again. Serum concentration/toxicity of methotrexate may be increased. Warfarin INRs may be increased by meloxicam. Monitor INR closely, particularly during initiation or change in dose. May increase risk of bleeding. Use lowest possible dose for shortest duration possible.

Nutritional/Ethanol Interactions Ethanol: Avoid ethanol (may enhance gastric mucosal irritation).

Adverse Reactions

1% to 10%:

Cardiovascular: Edema (2% to 5%)

Central nervous system: Headache and dizziness occurred in 2% to 8% of patients, but occurred less frequently than placebo in controlled trials

Dermatologic: Rash (1% to 3%)

Gastrointestinal: Diarrhea (3% to 8%), dyspepsia (5%), nausea (4%), flatulence (3%), abdominal pain (2% to 3%)

Respiratory: Upper respiratory infection (2% to 3%), pharyngitis (1% to 3%)

Miscellaneous: Flu-like symptoms (4% to 5%), falls (3%)

<2% (Limited to important or life-threatening): Agranulocytosis, allergic reaction, alopecia, anaphylactic reaction, angina, angioedema, anxiety, arrhythmia, bronchospasm, bullous eruption, cardiac failure, colitis, confusion, depression, duodenal perforation, duodenal ulcer, dyspnea, erythema multiforme, gastric perforation, gastric ulcer, gastritis, gastroesophageal reflux, gastrointestinal hemorrhage, hematemesis, hematuria, hepatic failure, hepatitis, hypertension, hypotension, interstitial nephritis, intestinal perforation, jaundice, leukopenia, melena, myocardial infarction, pancreatitis, paresthesia, photosensitivity reaction, pruritus, purpura, renal failure, seizures, shock, somnolence, Stevens-Johnson syndrome, syncope, thrombocytopenia, tinnitus, toxic epidermal necrolysis, tremor, ulcerative stomatitis, urticaria, vasculitis, vertigo

Overdosage/Toxicology Symptoms of overdose include lethargy, drowsiness, nausea, vomiting, and epigastric pain. Rarely, severe symptoms have been associated with NSAID overdose including apnea, metabolic acidosis, coma, nystagmus, seizures, leukocytosis, and renal failure. Management of NSAID intoxication is supportive and symptomatic. Since meloxicam undergoes enterohepatic cycling, multiple doses of charcoal may be needed to reduce the potential for delayed toxicities. Cholestyramine has been shown to increase meloxicam clearance.

Pharmacodynamics/Kinetics

Bioavailability: 89%

Half-Life Elimination: 15-20 hours

Time to Peak: 5-10 hours

Metabolism: Hepatic via CYP2C9 and CYP3A4 (minor)

Formulations Tablet: 7.5 mg, 15 mg

Dosing

Adults: Osteoarthritis: Oral: Initial: 7.5 mg once daily; some patients may receive additional benefit from an increased dose of 15 mg once daily.

Elderly: Refer to adult dosing. Increased concentrations may occur in elderly patients (particularly in females); however, no specific dosage adjustment is recommended.

Renal Impairment: No specific dosage adjustment is recommended for mild to moderate renal impairment. Avoid use in significant renal impairment.

Hepatic Impairment: No specific adjustment is recommended in hepatic impairment. Patients with severe hepatic impairment have not been adequately studied.

Stability

Storage: Store at 25°C (77°F).

Monitoring Laboratory Tests CBC, periodic liver function, renal function (serum BUN, and creatinine)

Monitoring and Teaching Issues

Physical Assessment: Assess effectiveness and interactions of other medications patient may be taking (see extensive Drug Interactions). See Warnings/Precautions and Contraindications for use cautions. Monitor laboratory tests (see above) and therapeutic and adverse reactions at beginning of therapy and periodically throughout therapy (see Warnings/Precautions, Adverse Reactions, and Overdose/Toxicology). Assess knowledge/teach patient appropriate use, interventions to reduce side effects, and adverse symptoms to report. **Pregnancy risk factor C/D** - note Pregnancy Risk Factor for use cautions; benefits of use should outweigh possible risks. Breast-feeding is contraindicated.

Patient Education: Take this medication exactly as directed; do not increase dose without consulting prescriber. Take with food or milk to reduce GI distress. Maintain adequate hydration (2-3 L/day of fluids) unless advised by prescriber to restrict fluids. Avoid alcohol, excessive vitamin C intake, or salicylate-containing foods (eg, curry powder, prunes, raisins, tea, or licorice). Do not use aspirin or aspirin-containing medication, or any other anti-inflammatory medications without consulting prescriber. You may experience anorexia, nausea, vomiting, or heartburn (small, frequent meals, frequent mouth care, sucking lozenges, or chewing gum may help); drowsiness, dizziness, nervousness, or headache (use caution when driving or engaging in tasks requiring alertness until response to drug is known); or fluid retention (weigh yourself weekly and report unusual (3-5 lb/week) weight gain). GI bleeding, ulceration, or perforation can occur with or without pain; discontinue medication and contact prescriber if persistent abdominal pain or cramping, or blood in stool occurs. Report breathlessness, difficulty breathing, or unusual cough; chest pain, rapid heartbeat, palpitations; unusual bruising/bleeding; blood in urine, stool, mouth, or vomitus; swollen extremities; skin rash or itching; acute fatigue, hearing changes (ringing in ears); or other adverse reactions. **Pregnancy/breast-feeding precautions:** Inform prescriber if you are or intend to become pregnant. This drug should not be used in the 3rd trimester of pregnancy. Do not breast-feed.

(Continued)

Meloxicam *(Continued)*

Dietary Issues: Should be taken with food or milk to minimize gastrointestinal irritation.

Breast-feeding Issues: It is not known whether meloxicam is excreted in human milk. Due to a potential for serious adverse reactions, the manufacturer recommends that a decision be made whether to discontinue nursing or discontinue the drug, taking into account the importance of the drug to the mother.

Pregnancy Issues: May cause premature closure of the ductus arteriosus in the 3rd trimester of pregnancy.

Related Information

Nonsalicylate/Nonsteroidal Anti-inflammatory Comparison *on page 1587*

Melpaque HP® *see* Hydroquinone *on page 679*

Melphalan (MEL fa lan)

U.S. Brand Names Alkeran®

Synonyms L-PAM; L-Sarcolysin; Phenylalanine Mustard

Generic Available No

Pharmacologic Category Antineoplastic Agent, Alkylating Agent

Pregnancy Risk Factor D

Lactation Excretion in breast milk unknown/not recommended

Use Palliative treatment of multiple myeloma and nonresectable epithelial ovarian carcinoma; neuroblastoma, rhabdomyosarcoma, breast cancer

Mechanism of Action/Effect Alkylating agent which is a derivative of mechlorethamine that inhibits DNA and RNA synthesis via formation of carbonium ions; cross-links strands of DNA

Contraindications Hypersensitivity to melphalan or any component of the formulation; severe bone marrow suppression; patients whose disease was resistant to prior therapy; pregnancy

Warnings/Precautions The U.S. Food and Drug Administration (FDA) currently recommends that procedures for proper handling and disposal of antineoplastic agents be considered. Appropriate safety equipment is recommended for preparation, administration, and disposal of antineoplastics. If melphalan injection contacts the skin, wash and flush thoroughly with water. Melphalan is potentially mutagenic, carcinogenic, and teratogenic; produces amenorrhea. Reduce dosage or discontinue therapy if leukocyte count is <3000/ mm^3 or platelet count is <100,000/mm^3; use with caution in patients with bone marrow suppression, impaired renal function, or who have received prior chemotherapy or irradiation; will cause amenorrhea. Toxicity to immunosuppressives is increased in the elderly. Start with lowest recommended adult doses. Signs of infection, such as fever and WBC rise, may not occur. Lethargy and confusion may be more prominent signs of infection.

Drug Interactions

Decreased Effect: Cimetidine and other H_2 antagonists: The reduction in gastric pH has been reported to decrease bioavailability of melphalan by 30%.

Increased Effect/Toxicity: Cyclosporine: Risk of nephrotoxicity is increased by melphalan.

Nutritional/Ethanol Interactions

Ethanol: Avoid ethanol (due to GI irritation).

Food: Food interferes with oral absorption.

Effects on Lab Values False-positive Coombs' test [direct]

Adverse Reactions

>10%: Hematologic: Myelosuppressive: Leukopenia and thrombocytopenia are the most common effects of melphalan. Irreversible bone marrow failure has been reported.

- WBC: Moderate
- Platelets: Moderate
- Onset (days): 7
- Nadir (days): 8-10 and 27-32
- Recovery (days): 42-50

1% to 10%:

- Cardiovascular: Vasculitis
- Dermatologic: Vesiculation of skin, alopecia, pruritus, rash
- Endocrine & metabolic: SIADH, sterility and amenorrhea
- Gastrointestinal: Nausea and vomiting are mild; stomatitis and diarrhea are infrequent
  - Emetic potential: Low (<10%): <100 mg/m^2; high (>90%): >100 mg/m^2
- Genitourinary: Bladder irritation, hemorrhagic cystitis
- Hematologic: Anemia, agranulocytosis, hemolytic anemia
- Hepatic: Transaminases increased (hepatitis, jaundice have been reported)
- Respiratory: Pulmonary fibrosis, interstitial pneumonitis
- Miscellaneous: Hypersensitivity, secondary malignancies

BMT:

- Dermatologic: Alopecia
- Gastrointestinal: Mucositis (severity increases with Cl_{cr} ≤40 mL/minute), nausea and vomiting (moderate), diarrhea
- Hematologic: Myelosuppression, secondary leukemia
- Renal: Increased serum creatinine and azotemia possible without adequate hydration
- Rare side effects: Abnormal LFTs, interstitial pneumonitis, secondary leukemia, SIADH, vasculitis

Overdosage/Toxicology Symptoms of overdose include hypocalcemia, pulmonary fibrosis, nausea and vomiting, and bone marrow suppression. Treatment is symptomatic and supportive.

Pharmacodynamics/Kinetics

Absorption: Oral: Variable and incomplete

Bioavailability: Unpredictable, decreasing from 85% to 58% with repeated doses

Half-Life Elimination: Terminal: 1.5 hours

Time to Peak: Serum: ~2 hours

Formulations

Injection, powder for reconstitution: 50 mg

Tablet: 2 mg

Dosing

Adults & Elderly: Refer to individual protocols; dose should always be adjusted to patient response and weekly blood counts.

Multiple myeloma:

Oral: 6 mg/day initially adjusted as indicated **or** 0.15 mg/kg/day for 7 days **or** 0.25 mg/kg/day for 4 days; repeat at 4- to 6-week intervals.

Multiple myeloma: I.V.: 16 mg/m^2 administered at 2-week intervals for 4 doses, then repeat monthly as per protocol for multiple myeloma.

Ovarian carcinoma: Oral: 0.2 mg/kg/day for 5 days, repeat every 4-5 weeks

High dose BMT: I.V.: 140-240 mg/m^2 as a single dose or divided into 2-5 daily doses. Infuse over 20-60 minutes.

Pediatrics: Oral (refer to individual protocols); dose should always be adjusted to patient response and weekly blood counts.

Various protocols: Oral: 4-20 mg/m^2/day for 1-21 days

Pediatric rhabdomyosarcoma: I.V.: 10-35 mg/m^2/dose every 21-28 days

High-dose melphalan with bone marrow transplantation for neuroblastoma: I.V.: 70-100 mg/m^2/day on day 7 and 6 before BMT **or** 140-220 mg/m^2 single dose before BMT **or** 50 mg/m^2/day for 4 days **or** 70 mg/m^2/day for 3 days.

Renal Impairment:

Cl_{cr} 10-50 mL/minute: Administer 75% of normal dose.

Cl_{cr} <10 mL/minute: Administer 50% of normal dose.

or

BUN <30 mg/dL: Reduce dose by 50%.

Serum creatinine <1.5 mg/dL: Reduce dose by 50%.

Hemodialysis effects: Unknown

CAPD effects: Unknown

CAVH effects: Unknown

Hepatic Impairment: BUN <30 mg/dL: Reduce dose by 50%.

Administration

Oral: Administer on an empty stomach.

I.V.: Due to limited stability, complete administration of I.V. dose should occur within 60 minutes of reconstitution

I.V. infusion: I.V. dose is FDA-approved for administration as a single infusion over 15-20 minutes

I.V. bolus: I.V. may be administered via central line and via peripheral vein as a rapid I.V. bolus; there have not been any unexpected or serious adverse events specifically related to rapid I.V. bolus administration; the most common adverse events were transient mild symptoms of hot flush and tingling sensation over the body

Central line: I.V. bolus doses of 17-200 mg/m^2 (reconstituted and not diluted) have been infused over 2-20 minutes

Peripheral line: I.V. bolus doses of 2-23 mg/m^2 (reconstituted and not diluted) have been infused over 1-4 minutes

Stability

Storage: Tablets/injection: Protect from light. Store at room temperature (15°C to 30°C).

Reconstitution:

Injection: Preparation: **The time between reconstitution/dilution and administration of parenteral melphalan must be kept to a minimum (<60 minutes) because reconstituted and diluted solutions are unstable**. Dissolve powder initially with 10 mL of diluent to a concentration of 5 mg/mL. **Immediately** dilute dose in NS to a concentration ≤0.45 mg/mL. If the solution is **highly unstable**, administration should occur within 1 hour of dissolution. Do not refrigerate solution; precipitation occurs.

Standard I.V. dilution:

Dose/250-500 mL NS (concentration ≤0.45 mg/mL)

Must be prepared fresh; solution is stable for 1 hour after dilution and must be administered within that time period.

Compatibility: Incompatible with D_5W, LR

Y-site administration: Incompatible with amphotericin B, chlorpromazine

Monitoring Laboratory Tests CBC with differential, platelet count, serum electrolytes, serum uric acid

Monitoring and Teaching Issues

Physical Assessment: Monitoring See Contraindications, Warnings/Precautions, and Dosing for use cautions. Assess potential for interactions with other prescriptions, OTC medications, or herbal products patient may be taking (see Drug Interactions). See Administration and Reconstitution. Infusion/injection site should be monitored closely to prevent extravasation. Assess results of laboratory tests (see above), therapeutic effects, and adverse response (see Adverse Reactions and Overdose/Toxicology) regularly during therapy. Teach patient proper use (oral), possible side effects and appropriate interventions, and adverse symptoms to report (see Patient Education). **Pregnancy risk factor D** - determine that patient is not pregnant before beginning treatment. Instruct patient in appropriate use of barrier contraceptive measures during therapy and for 1 month following therapy. Breast-feeding is not recommended.

Patient Education: Inform prescriber of all prescriptions, OTC medications, or herbal products you are taking, and any allergies you have. Do not take anything new during treatment unless approved by prescriber.

(Continued)

Melphalan *(Continued)*

I.V.: Report immediately any pain, burning, swelling at infusion site.

Oral: Take on an empty stomach, if possible, 1 hour before or 2 hours after meals. Avoid alcohol. It is important that you maintain adequate nutrition (small, frequent meals may help) and adequate hydration (2-3 L/day of fluids) unless advised by prescriber to restrict fluids. You may be more susceptible to infection (avoid crowds and exposure to infection and do not have any vaccinations unless approved by prescriber). May cause hair loss (reversible); easy bleeding or bruising (use soft toothbrush or cotton swabs and frequent mouth care, use electric razor, avoid sharp knives or scissors); or nausea or vomiting (small, frequent meals, frequent mouth care, chewing gum, or sucking lozenges may help). Report chest pain or palpitations; unusual fatigue; difficulty or pain on urination; unusual bruising/bleeding; difficulty breathing; pain or redness.

Pregnancy/breast-feeding precautions: Inform prescriber if you are pregnant. Do not get pregnant during or for 1 month following therapy. Consult prescriber for instruction on appropriate contraceptive measures. This drug may cause severe fetal defects. Breast-feeding is not recommended.

Dietary Issues: Should be taken on an empty stomach (1 hour prior to or 2 hours after meals).

Geriatric Considerations: Toxicity to immunosuppressives is increased in the elderly. Start with lowest recommended adult doses. Signs of infection, such as fever and WBC rise, may not occur. Lethargy and confusion may be more prominent signs of infection.

Melquin-3® [OTC] *see* Hydroquinone *on page 679*

Melquin HP® *see* Hydroquinone *on page 679*

Menadol® [OTC] *see* Ibuprofen *on page 688*

Menest® *see* Estrogens (Esterified) *on page 508*

Meni-D® *see* Meclizine *on page 840*

Meningococcal Polysaccharide Vaccine, Groups A, C, Y, and W-135 *see page 1498*

Menomune®-A/C/Y/W-135 *see page 1498*

Menotropins (men oh TROE pins)

U.S. Brand Names Humegon™; Pergonal®; Repronex®

Generic Available No

Pharmacologic Category Gonadotropin; Ovulation Stimulator

Pregnancy Risk Factor X

Lactation Excretion in breast milk unknown/contraindicated (not likely to be used)

Use Sequentially with hCG to induce ovulation and pregnancy in the infertile woman with functional anovulation or in patients who have previously received pituitary suppression; stimulation of multiple follicle development in ovulatory patients as part of an *in vitro* fertilization program; used with hCG in men to stimulate spermatogenesis in those with primary hypogonadotropic hypogonadism

Mechanism of Action/Effect Actions occur as a result of both follicle stimulating hormone (FSH) effects and luteinizing hormone (LH) effects; menotropins stimulate the development and maturation of the ovarian follicle (FSH), cause ovulation (LH), and stimulate the development of the corpus luteum (LH); in males it stimulates spermatogenesis (LH)

Contraindications Hypersensitivity to menotropins or any component of the formulation; primary ovarian failure as indicated by a high follicle-stimulating hormone (FSH) level; uncontrolled thyroid and adrenal dysfunction; abnormal bleeding of undetermined origin; intracranial lesion (ie, pituitary tumor); ovarian cyst or enlargement not due to polycystic ovary syndrome; infertility due to any cause other than anovulation (except candidates for *in vitro* fertilization); men with normal urinary gonadotropin concentrations, elevated gonadotropin levels indicating primary testicular failure; pregnancy

Warnings/Precautions Advise patient of frequency and potential hazards of multiple pregnancy. To minimize the hazard of abnormal ovarian enlargement, use the lowest possible dose.

Drug Interactions

Increased Effect/Toxicity: Clomiphene may decrease the amount of human menopausal gonadotropin (HMG) needed to induce ovulation (Gonadorelin, Factrel®); should not be used with drugs that stimulate ovulation.

Adverse Reactions

Male:

>10%: Endocrine & metabolic: Gynecomastia

1% to 10%: Erythrocytosis (dyspnea, dizziness, anorexia, syncope, epistaxis)

Female:

1% to 10%:

- Central nervous system: Headache
- Endocrine & metabolic: Breast tenderness
- Gastrointestinal: Abdominal cramping, abdominal pain, diarrhea, enlarged abdomen, nausea, vomiting
- Genitourinary: Ectopic pregnancy, OHSS (% is dose related), ovarian disease, vaginal hemorrhage
- Local: Injection site edema/reaction
- Miscellaneous: Infection, pelvic pain

Frequency not defined:

- Cardiovascular: Stroke, tachycardia, thrombosis (venous or arterial)
- Central nervous system: Dizziness
- Dermatologic: Angioedema, urticaria
- Genitourinary: Adnexal torsion, hemoperitoneum, ovarian enlargement
- Neuromuscular & skeletal: Limb necrosis
- Respiratory: Acute respiratory distress syndrome, atelectasis, dyspnea, embolism, laryngeal edema pulmonary infarction tachypnea
- Miscellaneous: Allergic reactions, anaphylaxis, rash

Overdosage/Toxicology Symptoms of overdose include ovarian hyperstimulation.

Formulations

Injection:

Follicle stimulating hormone activity 75 units and luteinizing hormone activity 75 units per 2 mL ampul

Follicle stimulating hormone activity 150 units and luteinizing hormone activity 150 units per 2 mL ampul

Dosing

Adults:

Spermatogenesis (Male): I.M.: Following pretreatment with hCG, 1 ampul 3 times/week and hCG 2000 units twice weekly until sperm is detected in the ejaculate (4-6 months) then may be increased to 2 ampuls of menotropins (150 units FSH/150 units LH) 3 times/week

Induction of ovulation (Female): I.M.: 1 ampul/day (75 units of FSH and LH) for 9-12 days followed by 10,000 units hCG 1 day after the last dose; repeated at least twice at same level before increasing dosage to 2 ampuls (150 units FSH/150 units LH)

Infertile patients with oligo-anovulation (Repronex®): I.M., S.C.: Initial: 150 int. units daily for the first 5 days of treatment. Adjustments should not be made more frequently than once every 2 days and should not exceed 75-150 int. units per adjustment. Maximum daily dose should not exceed 450 int. units and dosing beyond 12 days is not recommended. If patient's response to Repronex® is appropriate, hCG 5000-10,000 units should be given one day following the last dose of Repronex®.

Assisted reproductive technologies (Repronex®): I.M., S.C.: Initial (in patients who have received GnRH agonist or antagonist pituitary suppression): 225 int. units; adjustments in dose should not be made more frequently than once every 2 days and should not exceed more than 75-50 int. units per adjustment. The maximum daily doses of Repronex® given should not exceed 450 int. units and dosing beyond 12 days is not recommended. Once adequate follicular development is evident, hCG (5000-10,000 units) should be administered to induce final follicular maturation in preparation for oocyte retrieval.

Administration

I.M.: I.M. administration only.

Stability

Storage: Lyophilized powder may be refrigerated or stored at room temperature.

Reconstitution: After reconstitution inject immediately, discard any unused portion.

Monitoring and Teaching Issues

Physical Assessment: Female: Assess knowledge/teach appropriate method for measuring basal body temperature to indicate ovulation. Stress importance of following prescriber's instructions for timing intercourse. If self-administered, assess/teach appropriate injection technique and needle disposal. **Pregnancy risk factor X** - determine pregnancy status prior to beginning therapy.

Patient Education: Self injection: Follow prescriber's recommended schedule for injections. Multiple ovulations resulting in multiple pregnancies have been reported. Male infertility and/or breast enlargement may occur. Report pain at injection site; enlarged breasts (male); difficulty breathing; nosebleeds; acute abdominal discomfort; fever; or warmth, swelling, pain, or redness in calves.

Pregnancy Issues: Ectopic pregnancy and congenital abnormalities have been reported. The incidence of congenital abnormality is similar during natural conception.

Meperidine (me PER i deen)

U.S. Brand Names Demerol®; Meperitab®

Synonyms Isonipecaine Hydrochloride; Meperidine Hydrochloride; Pethidine Hydrochloride

Restrictions C-II

Generic Available Yes

Pharmacologic Category Analgesic, Narcotic

Pregnancy Risk Factor B/D (prolonged use or high doses at term)

Lactation Enters breast milk/contraindicated (AAP rates "compatible")

Use Management of moderate to severe pain; adjunct to anesthesia and preoperative sedation

Mechanism of Action/Effect Binds to opiate receptors in the CNS, causing inhibition of ascending pain pathways, altering the perception of and response to pain; produces generalized CNS depression

Contraindications Hypersensitivity to meperidine or any component of the formulation; patients receiving MAO inhibitors presently or in the past 14 days; pregnancy (prolonged use or high doses near term)

Warnings/Precautions Use with caution in patients with pulmonary, hepatic, renal disorders, or increased intracranial pressure; use with caution in patients with renal failure or seizure disorders or those receiving high-dose meperidine; normeperidine (an active metabolite and CNS stimulant) may accumulate and precipitate twitches, tremors, or seizures; some preparations contain sulfites which may cause allergic reaction; not recommended as a drug of first choice for the treatment of chronic pain in the elderly due to the accumulation of normeperidine; for acute pain, its use should be limited to 1-2 doses; tolerance or drug dependence may result from extended use

Drug Interactions

Decreased Effect: Phenytoin may decrease the analgesic effects of meperidine.

Increased Effect/Toxicity: Meperidine may aggravate the adverse effects of isoniazid. MAO inhibitors, fluoxetine, and other serotonin uptake inhibitors greatly potentiate the effects of meperidine, severe toxic reactions may occur. CNS depressants, tricyclic antidepressants, and phenothiazines may potentiate the effects of meperidine. Ritonavir may increase the risk of CNS toxicity and seizures of meperidine (increased formation of normeperidine).

Nutritional/Ethanol Interactions

Ethanol: Avoid or limit ethanol (may increase CNS depression). Watch for sedation.

Food: Glucose may cause hyperglycemia; monitor blood glucose concentrations.

(Continued)

Meperidine *(Continued)*

Herb/Nutraceutical: Avoid valerian, St John's wort, kava kava, gotu kola (may increase CNS depression).

Effects on Lab Values ↑ amylase (S), BSP retention, CPK (I.M. injections)

Adverse Reactions Frequency not defined.

Cardiovascular: Hypotension

Central nervous system: Fatigue, drowsiness, dizziness, nervousness, headache, restlessness, malaise, confusion, mental depression, hallucinations, paradoxical CNS stimulation, increased intracranial pressure, seizures (associated with metabolite accumulation)

Dermatologic: Rash, urticaria

Gastrointestinal: Nausea, vomiting, constipation, anorexia, stomach cramps, xerostomia, biliary spasm, paralytic ileus

Genitourinary: Ureteral spasms, decreased urination

Local: Pain at injection site

Neuromuscular & skeletal: Weakness

Respiratory: Dyspnea

Miscellaneous: Histamine release, physical and psychological dependence

Overdosage/Toxicology Symptoms of overdose include CNS depression, respiratory depression, mydriasis, bradycardia, pulmonary edema, chronic tremor, CNS excitability, and seizures. Treatment is symptomatic. Naloxone, 2 mg I.V. with repeat administration as necessary up to a total dose of 10 mg, can be used to reverse opiate effects. Naloxone should not be used to treat meperidine-induced seizures.

Pharmacodynamics/Kinetics

Bioavailability: ~50% to 60%; increased with liver disease

Half-Life Elimination:

Parent drug: Terminal phase: Neonates: 23 hours (range: 12-39 hours); Adults: 2.5-4 hours, Liver disease: 7-11 hours

Normeperidine (active metabolite): 15-30 hours; can accumulate with high doses or renal impairment

Metabolism: Hepatic; active metabolite (normeperidine)

Onset: Analgesic: Oral, S.C., I.M.: 10-15 minutes; I.V.: ~5 minutes; Peak effect: Oral, S.C., I.M.: ~1 hour

Duration: Oral, S.C., I.M.: 2-4 hours

Formulations

Infusion, as hydrochloride: 10 mg/mL (30 mL) [via compatible infusion device only]

Injection, as hydrochloride [multidose vial]: 50 mg/mL (30 mL); 100 mg/mL (20 mL)

Injection, as hydrochloride [single-dose]: 25 mg/dose (1 mL); 50 mg/dose (1 mL); 75 mg/dose (1 mL); 100 mg/dose (1 mL)

Syrup, as hydrochloride: 50 mg/5 mL (500 mL)

Tablet, as hydrochloride: 50 mg, 100 mg

Dosing

Adults: Analgesic: Oral, I.M., I.V.: S.C.: 50-150 mg/dose every 3-4 hours as needed; oral therapy is discouraged.

Note: Doses should be titrated to necessary analgesic effect. When changing route of administration, note that oral doses are about half as effective as parenteral dose. Oral route not recommended for chronic pain.

Elderly: Doses should be titrated to necessary analgesic effect, with adjustments for renal impairment. When changing route of administration, note that oral doses are about half as effective as parenteral dose.

Oral: 50 mg every 4 hours

I.M.: 25 mg every 4 hours

Pediatrics: Analgesic: Oral, I.M., I.V., S.C.: Children: 1-1.5 mg/kg/dose every 3-4 hours as needed; 1-2 mg/kg as a single dose preoperative medication may be used; maximum 100 mg/dose. Oral therapy is discouraged.

Note: Doses should be titrated to necessary analgesic effect. When changing route of administration, note that oral doses are about half as effective as parenteral dose. Oral route not recommended for chronic pain.

Renal Impairment:

Cl_{cr} 10-50 mL/minute: Administer 75% of normal dose.

Cl_{cr} <10 mL/minute: Administer 50% of normal dose.

Note: Repeated use in renal impairment **should be avoided** due to potential accumulation of neuroexcitatory metabolite.

Hepatic Impairment: Increased narcotic effect in cirrhosis; reduction in dose is more important for oral than I.V. route.

Administration

I.V.: Meperidine may be administered I.M. (preferably), S.C., or I.V. IVP should be given slowly, use of a 10 mg/mL concentration has been recommended.

Stability

Storage: Meperidine injection should be stored at room temperature and protected from light and freezing. Protect oral dosage forms from light.

Compatibility: Stable in dextran 6% in dextrose, dextran 6% in NS, D_5LR, $D_5{}^1/_4NS$, $D_5{}^1/_2NS$, D_5NS, D_5W, $D_{10}W$, LR, $^1/_2NS$, NS

Y-site administration: Incompatible with allopurinol, amphotericin B cholesteryl sulfate complex, cefepime, cefoperazone, doxorubicin liposome, idarubicin, imipenem/cilastatin, minocycline

Compatibility in syringe: Incompatible with heparin, morphine, pentobarbital

Compatibility when admixed: Incompatible with aminophylline, amobarbital, floxacillin, furosemide, heparin, morphine, phenobarbital, phenytoin, thiopental

Monitoring and Teaching Issues

Physical Assessment: Assess other medications patient may be taking for additive or adverse interactions (see Drug Interactions). Monitor therapeutic effectiveness and adverse reactions or overdose at beginning of therapy and at regular intervals with long-term use (see Adverse Reactions and Overdose/Toxicology). Monitor frequently for need, may cause physical and/or psychological dependence. For inpatients, implement safety measures. Assess knowledge/teach patient appropriate use (if self-administered), adverse reactions to report, and appropriate interventions to reduce side effects. Discontinue slowly after prolonged use. **Pregnancy risk factor B/D** - see Pregnancy Risk Factor for use cautions. Breast-feeding is contraindicated.

Patient Education: If self-administered, use exactly as directed; do not increase dose or frequency. Drug may cause physical and/or psychological dependence. While using this medication, do not use alcohol and other prescription or OTC medications (especially sedatives, tranquilizers, antihistamines, or pain medications) without consulting prescriber. Maintain adequate hydration (2-3 L/day of fluids) unless advised by prescriber to restrict fluids. May cause hypotension, dizziness, drowsiness, impaired coordination, or blurred vision (use caution when driving, climbing stairs, or changing position - rising from sitting or lying to standing, or when engaging in tasks requiring alertness until response to drug is known); loss of appetite, nausea, or vomiting (frequent mouth care, small, frequent meals, chewing gum, or sucking lozenges may help); or constipation (increased exercise, fluids, fruit, or fiber may help; if unresolved, consult prescriber about use of stool softeners). Report chest pain, slow or rapid heartbeat, acute dizziness or persistent headache; changes in mental status; swelling of extremities or unusual weight gain; changes in urinary elimination; acute headache; back or flank pain or muscle spasms; blurred vision; skin rash; or shortness of breath. **Pregnancy/breast-feeding precautions:** Inform prescriber if you are or intend to become pregnant. Do not breast-feed.

Geriatric Considerations: Meperidine is not recommended as a drug of first choice for the treatment of chronic pain in the elderly due to the accumulation of its metabolite, normeperidine, which leads to serious CNS side effects (eg, tremor, seizures, etc). For acute pain, its use should be limited to 1-2 doses.

Related Information

Compatibility of Drugs *on page 1564*
Compatibility of Drugs in Syringe *on page 1566*
Narcotic/Opioid Analgesic Comparison *on page 1583*

Meperidine Hydrochloride *see* Meperidine *on page 851*
Meperitab® *see* Meperidine *on page 851*
Mephentermine *see page 1461*
Mephentermine *see page 1580*
Mephyton® *see* Phytonadione *on page 1080*

Meprobamate (me proe BA mate)

U.S. Brand Names Equanil®; Miltown®

Restrictions C-IV

Generic Available Yes

Pharmacologic Category Antianxiety Agent, Miscellaneous

Pregnancy Risk Factor D

Lactation Enters breast milk/not recommended

Use Management of anxiety disorders

Use - Unlabeled/Investigational Demonstrated value for muscle contraction, headache, premenstrual tension, external sphincter spasticity, muscle rigidity, opisthotonos-associated with tetanus

Mechanism of Action/Effect Affects the thalamus and limbic system; also appears to inhibit multineuronal spinal reflexes

Contraindications Hypersensitivity to meprobamate, related compounds (including carisoprodol), or any component of the formulation; acute intermittent porphyria; pre-existing CNS depression; narrow-angle glaucoma; severe uncontrolled pain; pregnancy

Warnings/Precautions Physical and psychological dependence and abuse may occur; abrupt cessation may precipitate withdrawal. Use with caution in patients with depression or suicidal tendencies, or in patients with a history of drug abuse. May cause CNS depression, which may impair physical or mental abilities. Patients must be cautioned about performing tasks which require mental alertness (ie, operating machinery or driving). Effects with other sedative drugs or ethanol may be potentiated. Not recommended in children <6 years of age; allergic reaction may occur in patients with history of dermatological condition (usually by fourth dose). Use with caution in patients with renal or hepatic impairment, or with a history of seizures. Use caution in the elderly as it may cause confusion, cognitive impairment, or excessive sedation.

Drug Interactions

Increased Effect/Toxicity: CNS depressants (ethanol) may increase CNS depression.

Nutritional/Ethanol Interactions

Ethanol: Avoid ethanol (may increase CNS depression).

Herb/Nutraceutical: Avoid valerian, St John's wort, kava kava, gotu kola (may increase CNS depression).

Adverse Reactions Frequency not defined.

Cardiovascular: Syncope, peripheral edema, palpitations, tachycardia, arrhythmia

Central nervous system: Drowsiness, ataxia, dizziness, paradoxical excitement, confusion, slurred speech, headache, euphoria, chills, vertigo, paresthesia, overstimulation

Dermatologic: Rashes, purpura, dermatitis, Stevens-Johnson syndrome, petechiae, ecchymosis

Gastrointestinal: Diarrhea, vomiting, nausea

Hematologic: Leukopenia, eosinophilia, agranulocytosis, aplastic anemia

Neuromuscular & skeletal: Weakness

Ocular: Blurred vision, impairment of accommodation

Renal: Renal failure

Respiratory: Wheezing, dyspnea, bronchospasm, angioneurotic edema

Overdosage/Toxicology Symptoms of overdose include drowsiness, lethargy, ataxia, coma, hypotension, shock, and death. Treatment is supportive following attempts to enhance drug elimination.

(Continued)

Meprobamate *(Continued)*

Pharmacodynamics/Kinetics

Half-Life Elimination: 10 hours

Metabolism: Hepatic

Onset: Sedation: ~1 hour

Formulations Tablet: 200 mg, 400 mg

Dosing

Adults: Oral: 400 mg 3-4 times/day, up to 2400 mg/day

Elderly: Oral (use lowest effective dose): Initial: 200 mg 2-3 times/day

Pediatrics: Oral: 6-12 years: 100-200 mg 2-3 times/day

Renal Impairment:

Cl_{cr} 10-50 mL/minute: Administer every 9-12 hours.

Cl_{cr} <10 mL/minute: Administer every 12-18 hours.

Moderately dialyzable (20% to 50%)

Hepatic Impairment: Probably necessary in patients with liver disease; no specific recommendations.

Monitoring and Teaching Issues

Physical Assessment: Assess other medications the patient may be taking for effectiveness and interactions (see Drug Interactions). See Contraindications and Warnings/Precautions for use cautions. Assess for history of addiction; long-term use can result in dependence, abuse, or tolerance; periodically evaluate need for continued use. Monitor therapeutic response and adverse reactions or overdose at beginning of therapy and periodically with long-term use (see Adverse Reactions and Overdose/Toxicology). Taper dosage slowly when discontinuing. Assess knowledge/teach patient appropriate use, interventions to reduce side effects, and adverse symptoms to report (see Patient Education). **Pregnancy risk factor D** - determine that patient is not pregnant before beginning treatment. Instruct patients of childbearing age about appropriate barrier contraceptive measures. Breast-feeding is not recommended.

Patient Education: Take exactly as directed; do not increase dose or frequency. Drug may cause physical and/or psychological dependence. Do not use alcohol or other prescription or OTC medications (especially pain medications, sedatives, antihistamines, or hypnotics) without consulting prescriber. Maintain adequate hydration (2-3 L/day of fluids) unless advised by prescriber to restrict fluids. You may experience drowsiness, lightheadedness, impaired coordination, dizziness, or blurred vision (use caution when driving or engaging in tasks requiring alertness until response to drug is known); nausea, vomiting, or dry mouth (small, frequent meals, frequent mouth care, chewing gum, or sucking lozenges may help); or diarrhea (boiled milk, yogurt, or buttermilk may help). Report persistent CNS effects, skin rash or irritation, changes in urinary pattern, wheezing or difficulty breathing, or worsening of condition. **Pregnancy/breast-feeding precautions:** Do not get pregnant while taking this medication; use appropriate contraceptive measures. Breast-feeding is not recommended.

Geriatric Considerations: Meprobamate is not considered a drug of choice in the elderly because of its potential to cause physical and psychological dependence. Interpretive guidelines from the Health Care Financing Administration (HCFA) strongly discourage the use of meprobamate in residents of long-term care facilities.

Breast-feeding Issues: Breast milk concentrations are higher than plasma; effects are unknown.

Additional Information Withdrawal should be gradual over 1-2 weeks. Benzodiazepine and buspirone are better choices for treatment of anxiety disorders.

Meprobamate and Aspirin *see* Aspirin and Meprobamate *on page 125*

Mepron® *see* Atovaquone *on page 130*

Mequinol and Tretinoin (ME kwi nol & TRET i noyn)

U.S. Brand Names Solagé™

Synonyms Tretinoin and Mequinol

Generic Available No

Pharmacologic Category Retinoic Acid Derivative; Vitamin A Derivative; Vitamin, Topical

Pregnancy Risk Factor X

Lactation Excretion in breast milk unknown/use caution

Use Treatment of solar lentigines; the efficacy of using Solagé™ daily for >24 weeks has not been established. The local cutaneous safety of Solagé™ in non-Caucasians has not been adequately established.

Mechanism of Action/Effect Solar lentigines are localized, pigmented, macular lesions of the skin on areas of the body chronically exposed to the sun. Mequinol is a substrate for the enzyme tyrosinase and acts as a competitive inhibitor of the formation of melanin precursors. The mechanisms of depigmentation for both drugs is unknown.

Contraindications Hypersensitivity to mequinol, tretinoin, or any component of the formulation; pregnancy, women of childbearing potential

Warnings/Precautions Discontinue if hypersensitivity is noted. Use extreme caution in eczematous skin conditions. Safety and efficacy have not been established in moderately or heavily pigmented skin. Not to be taken with photosensitizing drugs (eg, thiazides, tetracyclines, fluoroquinolones, phenothiazines, sulfonamides). Do not use in sunburned patients until they have fully recovered. Use extreme caution in patients who have significant exposure to the sun through their occupation. Use caution in patient with history or family history of vitiligo. Weather extremes (wind, cold) may be irritating to users of Solagé™. Do not use in pediatric patients. No bathing or showering for at least 6 hours after application. Effects of chronic use (>52 weeks) are unknown.

Drug Interactions

Cytochrome P450 Effect: Tretinoin: Substrate of CYP2A6, 2B6, 2C8/9; Inhibits CYP2C8/9; Induces CYP2E1

Increased Effect/Toxicity:

Topical products with skin drying effects (eg, those containing alcohol, astringents, spices, or lime; medicated soaps or shampoos; permanent wave solutions; hair depilatories or waxes; and others) may increase skin irritation. Avoid concurrent use.

Photosensitizing drugs (eg, thiazides, tetracyclines, fluoroquinolones, phenothiazines, sulfonamides) can further increase sun sensitivity. Avoid concurrent use.

Adverse Reactions

>10%: Dermatologic: Erythema (49%), burning, stinging or tingling (26%), desquamation (14%), pruritus (12%),

1% to 10%: Dermatologic: Skin irritation (5%), hypopigmentation (5%), halo hypopigmentation (7%), rash (3%), dry skin (3%), crusting (3%), vesicular bullae rash (2%), contact allergic reaction (1%)

Overdosage/Toxicology Excessive topical application will lead to marked redness, peeling, discomfort or hypopigmentation. Oral ingestion may lead to the adverse events seen in vitamin A overdose. If oral ingestion occurs, the patient should be monitored and appropriate supportive measures used as necessary. In rats who ingested 5 mL/kg, the signs of toxicity were of ethanol (high ethanol content in formulation).

Pharmacodynamics/Kinetics

Absorption: Percutaneous absorption was 4.4% of tretinoin when applied as 0.8 mL of Solagé™ to a 400 cm^2 area of the back

Time to Peak: Mequinol: 2 hours

Formulations Liquid, topical: Mequinol 2% and tretinoin 0.01% (30 mL)

Dosing

Adults & Elderly: Solar lentigines: Topical: Apply twice daily to solar lentigines using the applicator tip while avoiding application to the surrounding skin. Separate application by at least 8 hours or as directed by physician.

Administration

Topical: Use applicator tip. Avoid application to surrounding skin, eyes, mouth, paranasal creases, or mucous membranes.

Stability

Storage: Store at controlled room temperature of 15°C to 30°C (59°F to 86°F); flammable, keep away from heat and open flame

Monitoring and Teaching Issues

Physical Assessment: See Contraindications and Warnings/Precautions for use cautions. Assess effectiveness and interactions of other medications (see Drug Interactions). Monitor effectiveness of therapy and adverse effects at beginning of therapy and regularly with long-term use (see Adverse Reactions and Overdose/Toxicology). Assess knowledge/teach patient appropriate use, possible side effects/interventions, and adverse symptoms to report (See Patient Education). **Pregnancy risk factor X** - determine that patient is not pregnant before beginning treatment and do not give to women of childbearing age unless female is capable of complying with barrier contraceptive measures 1 month prior to therapy, during therapy, and 1 month following therapy. Note breast-feeding caution.

Patient Education: Use exactly as directed (use applicator tip, avoid application to surrounding skin, eyes, mouth, nose creases, or mucous membranes. Separate applications by at least 8 hours. Wait 30 minutes after application before applying make-up and do not bath or shower for 6 hours after application). Do not use more frequently than recommended. Do not use other vitamin A topical products; limit vitamin A intake. Avoid topical products with skin drying effects (eg, those containing alcohol, astringents, spices, lime, medicated soaps or shampoos, permanent wave solutions, depilatories or other hair removal products, etc). You will be very sensitive to direct sunlight or sunlamps (use sunscreen, wear protective clothing and eyewear, and avoid direct exposure to sunlight or sunlamps). You may experience stinging, burning, or irritation after application. If skin reactions are severe or persistent, discontinue use and contact prescriber. **Pregnancy/breast-feeding precautions:** Inform prescriber if you are pregnant. Do not get pregnant 1 month before, during, or for 1 month following therapy. Consult prescriber for instruction on appropriate contraceptive measures. This drug may cause severe fetal defects. Do not donate blood during or for 1 month following therapy (same reason). Consult prescriber if breast-feeding.

Related Information

Selected Prescription Combination Products *on page 1522*

Mercaptopurine (mer kap toe PYOOR een)

U.S. Brand Names Purinethol®

Synonyms 6-Mercaptopurine; 6-MP

Restrictions Note: I.V. formulation is not commercially available in the U.S.

Generic Available No

Pharmacologic Category Antineoplastic Agent, Antimetabolite

Pregnancy Risk Factor D

Lactation Enters breast milk/contraindicated

Use Maintenance therapy in acute lymphoblastic leukemia (ALL); other (less common) uses include chronic granulocytic leukemia, induction therapy in ALL, and treatment of non-Hodgkin's lymphomas

Mechanism of Action/Effect Purine antagonist which inhibits DNA and RNA synthesis

Contraindications Hypersensitivity to mercaptopurine or any component of the formulation; patients whose disease showed prior resistance to mercaptopurine or thioguanine; severe liver disease, severe bone marrow suppression; pregnancy

Warnings/Precautions The U.S. Food and Drug Administration (FDA) currently recommends that procedures for proper handling and disposal of antineoplastic agents be considered. Mercaptopurine is potentially carcinogenic, and may be teratogenic; use with caution in patients with prior bone marrow suppression. Common signs of infection, such as fever and leukocytosis may not occur; lethargy and confusion may be more prominent signs of infection.

(Continued)

Mercaptopurine *(Continued)*

To avoid potentially serious dosage errors, the terms "6-mercaptopurine" or "6-MP" should be avoided; use of these terms has been associated with sixfold overdosages.

Drug Interactions

Decreased Effect: 6-MP inhibits the anticoagulation effect of warfarin by an unknown mechanism.

Increased Effect/Toxicity:

Allopurinol can cause increased levels of 6-MP by inhibition of xanthine oxidase. Decrease dose of 6-MP by 75% when both drugs are used concomitantly. Seen only with oral 6-MP usage, not with I.V. May potentiate effect of bone marrow suppression (reduce 6-MP to 25% of dose).

Doxorubicin: Synergistic liver toxicity with 6-MP in >50% of patients, which resolved with discontinuation of the 6-MP.

Hepatotoxic drugs: Any agent which could potentially alter the metabolic function of the liver could produce higher drug levels and greater toxicities from either 6-MP or thioguanine (6-TG).

Aminosalicylates (olsalazine, mesalamine, sulfasalazine): May inhibit TPMT, increasing toxicity/myelosuppression of mercaptopurine.

Adverse Reactions

>10%:

Hematologic: Myelosuppression; leukopenia, thrombocytopenia, anemia

Onset: 7-10 days

Nadir: 14-16 days

Recovery: 21-28 days

Hepatic: Intrahepatic cholestasis and focal centralobular necrosis (40%), characterized by hyperbilirubinemia, increased alkaline phosphatase and AST, jaundice, ascites, encephalopathy; more common at doses >2.5 mg/kg/day. Usually occurs within 2 months of therapy but may occur within 1 week, or be delayed up to 8 years.

1% to 10%:

Central nervous system: Drug fever

Dermatologic: Hyperpigmentation, rash

Endocrine & metabolic: Hyperuricemia

Gastrointestinal: Nausea, vomiting, diarrhea, stomatitis, anorexia, stomach pain, mucositis

Renal: Renal toxicity

<1% (Limited to important or life-threatening): Dry and scaling rash, eosinophilia, glossitis, tarry stools

Overdosage/Toxicology Symptoms of overdose include nausea and vomiting (immediate); bone marrow suppression, hepatic necrosis, and gastroenteritis (delayed). Treatment is supportive.

Pharmacodynamics/Kinetics

Absorption: Variable and incomplete (16% to 50%)

Half-Life Elimination: Age dependent: Children: 21 minutes; Adults: 47 minutes

Time to Peak: Serum: ~2 hours

Metabolism: Hepatic and via GI mucosa; hepatically via xanthine oxidase and methylation to sulfate conjugates, 6-thiouric acid, and other inactive compounds; first-pass effect

Formulations Tablet, scored: 50 mg

Dosing

Adults: Refer to individual protocols.

Induction: Oral: 2.5-5 mg/kg/day (100-200 mg)

Maintenance: Oral: 1.5-2.5 mg/kg/day **OR** 80-100 mg/m^2/day given once daily

Elderly: Due to renal decline with age, start with lower recommended doses for adults.

Pediatrics: Refer to individual protocols: Maintenance: Oral: Children: 75 mg/m^2/day given once daily

Renal Impairment: Dose should be reduced to avoid accumulation, but specific guidelines are not available.

Hemodialysis: Removed; supplemental dosing is usually required

Hepatic Impairment: Dose should be reduced to avoid accumulation, but specific guidelines are not available.

Administration

I.V.: Further dilute the 10 mg/mL reconstituted solution in normal saline or D_5W to a final concentration for administration of 1-2 mg/mL; administer by slow I.V. continuous infusion.

Stability

Storage: Store at room temperature.

Monitoring Laboratory Tests CBC with differential, platelet count, liver function, uric acid, renal function

Monitoring and Teaching Issues

Physical Assessment: See Contraindications, Warnings/Precautions (eg, prescription writing warning), and Dosing for use cautions. Assess potential for interactions with other prescriptions, OTC medications, or herbal products patient may be taking (see Drug Interactions). Assess results of laboratory tests (see above), therapeutic effects, and adverse response (eg, hepatic function, nutritional status, blood dyscrasias, and renal status - see Adverse Reactions and Overdose/Toxicology) on a regular basis throughout therapy. Teach patient proper use, possible side effects and appropriate interventions (eg, importance of adequate hydration), and adverse symptoms to report (see Patient Education). **Pregnancy risk factor D** - determine that patient is not pregnant before beginning treatment. Instruct patient in appropriate use of barrier contraceptive measures during therapy and for 1 month following therapy. Breast-feeding is contraindicated.

Patient Education: Inform prescriber of all prescriptions, OTC medications, or herbal products you are taking, and any allergies you have. Do not take anything new during treatment unless approved by prescriber. Take daily dose at the same time each day. Preferable to take an on empty stomach, 1 hour before or 2 hours after meals. Maintain adequate hydration (2-3 L/day of fluids) unless advised by prescriber to restrict fluids. You may be more susceptible to infection (avoid crowds and exposure to infection and do not have any vaccinations without consulting prescriber). May cause nausea and vomiting, diarrhea, or loss of appetite (small, frequent meals may help/request medication); weakness or lethargy (use caution when driving or engaging in tasks that require alertness until response to drug is known); mouth sores; or headache (consult prescriber for approved medications). Report signs of persistent fever; opportunistic infection (eg, fever, chills, sore throat, burning urination, fatigue); bleeding (eg, tarry stools, easy bruising); unresolved mouth sores; nausea or vomiting; swelling of extremities; difficulty breathing; unusual weight gain; or changes in urinary pattern. **Pregnancy/breast-feeding precautions:** Inform prescriber if you are pregnant. Do not get pregnant while taking this medication. Consult prescriber for appropriate contraceptive measures. Do not breast-feed.

Dietary Issues: Should not be administered with meals.

Geriatric Considerations: Toxicity to immunosuppressives is increased in the elderly. Start with lowest recommended adult doses. Signs of infection, such as fever and WBC rise, may not occur. Lethargy and confusion may be more prominent signs of infection.

6-Mercaptopurine *see* Mercaptopurine *on page 855*

Mercapturic Acid *see* Acetylcysteine *on page 40*

Meridia® *see* Sibutramine *on page 1226*

Meropenem (mer oh PEN em)

U.S. Brand Names Merrem® I.V.

Generic Available No

Pharmacologic Category Antibiotic, Carbapenem

Pregnancy Risk Factor B

Lactation Excretion in breast milk unknown/use caution

Use Intra-abdominal infections (complicated appendicitis and peritonitis) caused by viridans group streptococci, *E. coli*, *K. pneumoniae*, *P. aeruginosa*, *B. fragilis*, *B. thetaiotaomicron*, and *Peptostreptococcus* sp; also indicated for bacterial meningitis in pediatric patients >3 months of age caused by *S. pneumoniae*, *H. influenzae*, and *N. meningitidis*; meropenem has also been used to treat soft tissue infections, febrile neutropenia, and urinary tract infections

Mechanism of Action/Effect Inhibits cell wall synthesis in susceptible bacteria

Contraindications Hypersensitivity to meropenem, any component of the formulation, or other carbapenems (eg, imipenem); patients who have experienced anaphylactic reactions to other beta-lactams

Warnings/Precautions Pseudomembranous colitis and hypersensitivity reactions have occurred and often require immediate drug discontinuation. Thrombocytopenia has been reported in patients with significant renal dysfunction. Seizures have occurred in patients with underlying neurologic disorders (less frequent than with Primaxin®). Safety and efficacy have not been established for children <3 months of age. Superinfection possible with long courses of therapy.

Drug Interactions

Decreased Effect: Serum concentrations of valproic acid may be reduced during meropenem therapy (potentially to subtherapeutic levels).

Increased Effect/Toxicity: Probenecid interferes with renal excretion of meropenem.

Effects on Lab Values ↑ SGPT, SGOT, alkaline phosphatase, LDH, bilirubin, platelets, eosinophils, BUN, creatinine; ↓ platelets, hemoglobin/hematocrit, WBC; prolonged or shortened PT; prolonged PTT; positive direct or indirect Coombs' test; presence of urine red blood cells

Adverse Reactions

1% to 10%:

Central nervous system: Headache (2%)

Dermatologic: Rash (2% to 3%, includes diaper-area moniliasis in pediatrics), pruritus (1%)

Gastrointestinal: Diarrhea (4% to 5%), nausea/vomiting (1% to 4%), constipation (1%), oral moniliasis (up to 2% in pediatric patients), glossitis

Local: Inflammation at the injection site (2%), phlebitis/thrombophlebitis (1%), injection site reaction (1%)

Respiratory: Apnea (1%)

Miscellaneous: Sepsis (2%), septic shock (1%)

<1% (Limited to important or life-threatening): Agitation/delirium, agranulocytosis, angioedema, anorexia, arrhythmias, cholestatic jaundice/jaundice, decreased prothrombin time, dyspepsia, dyspnea, eosinophilia, epistaxis, erythema multiforme, gastrointestinal hemorrhage, hallucinations, heart failure, hemoperitoneum, hepatic failure, hypotension, ileus, leukopenia, melena, myocardial infarction, neutropenia, paresthesia, pleural effusion, pulmonary edema, renal failure, seizures, Stevens-Johnson syndrome, toxic epidermal necrolysis, urticaria, vaginal moniliasis

Overdosage/Toxicology No cases of acute overdose with resultant symptoms have been reported. Supportive therapy is recommended. Meropenem and metabolite are removable by dialysis.

Pharmacodynamics/Kinetics

Half-Life Elimination:

Normal renal function: 1-1.5 hours

Cl_{cr} 30-80 mL/minute: 1.9-3.3 hours

Cl_{cr} 2-30 mL/minute: 3.82-5.7 hours

Time to Peak: Tissue: 1 hour following infusion

Metabolism: Hepatic; metabolized to open beta-lactam form (inactive)

Formulations

Injection, powder for reconstitution: 500 mg, 1 g

ADD-Vantage®: 500 mg, 1 g

Dosing

Adults:

Susceptible infections: I.V.: 1 g every 8 hours

(Continued)

Meropenem *(Continued)*

Elderly: Refer to adult dosing. No differences in safety or efficacy have been reported, however, increased sensitivity may occur in some elderly patients. Adjust dose based on renal function; see Warnings/Precautions.

Pediatrics:

Intra-abdominal infections: I.V.:

Children >3 months (<50 kg): 20 mg/kg every 8 hours (maximum dose: 1 g every 8 hours)

Children >50 kg: 1 g every 8 hours

Meningitis: I.V.:

Children >3 months (<50 kg): 40 mg/kg every 8 hours (maximum dose: 2 g every 8 hours)

Children >50 kg: 2 g every 8 hours

Renal Impairment:

Cl_{cr} 26-50 mL/minute: Administer 1 g every 12 hours.

Cl_{cr} 10-25 mL/minute: Administer 500 mg every 12 hours.

Cl_{cr} <10 mL/minute: Administer 500 mg every 24 hours.

Meropenem and its metabolites are readily dialyzable.

Continuous arteriovenous hemofiltration: Dose as for Cl_{cr} 10-50 mL/minute.

Administration

I.V.: Administer I.V. infusion over 15-30 minutes; I.V. bolus injection over 3-5 minutes.

Stability

Storage: Dry powder should be stored at controlled room temperature 20°C to 25°C (68°F to 77°F).

Reconstitution: Meropenem infusion vials reconstituted with sodium chloride are stable for up to 2 hours at room temperature or for 18 hours refrigerated; reconstituted with dextrose 5% injections are stable for 1 hour at room temperature and 8 hours refrigerated. Mini bags with normal saline are stable for up to 24 hours refrigerated; with dextrose stable for 6 hours.

Compatibility:

Y-site administration: Incompatible with amphotericin B, diazepam, metronidazole

Compatibility when admixed: Incompatible with amphotericin B, metronidazole, multivitamins

Monitoring Laboratory Tests Perform culture and sensitivity testing prior to initiating therapy. Monitor renal function, liver function, CBC.

Monitoring and Teaching Issues

Physical Assessment: Assess previous history of allergies. See Contraindications, Warnings/Precautions, Drug Interactions, and Dosing for use cautions. See Administration, Reconstitution, and Compatibility for infusion specifics. Infusion site must be monitored for phlebitis/thrombophlebitis. Assess results of laboratory tests (see above), therapeutic response, and adverse response (eg, hypersensitivity and CNS events, opportunistic infection - see Adverse Reactions and Overdose/Toxicology) on a regular basis throughout therapy. Teach patient proper use, possible side effects and appropriate interventions (eg, importance of adequate hydration), and adverse symptoms to report (see Patient Education). Note breast-feeding caution.

Patient Education: Inform prescriber of all prescriptions, OTC medications, or herbal products you are taking, and any allergies you have. Do not take anything new during treatment unless approved by prescriber. This medication can only be given by infusion. Report immediately any burning, pain, swelling, or redness at infusion site. Maintain adequate hydration (2-3 L/day of fluids) unless advised by prescriber to restrict fluids. May cause nausea or vomiting (small, frequent meals, frequent mouth care, chewing gum, or sucking lozenges may help); diarrhea (boiled milk, buttermilk, or yogurt may help); or headache. Report persistent GI distress, diarrhea, mouth sores, difficulty breathing, headache, or CNS changes (agitation, delirium). **Breast-feeding precaution:** Consult prescriber if breast-feeding.

Dietary Issues: 1 g of meropenem contains 90.2 mg of sodium as sodium carbonate (3.92 mEq)

Geriatric Considerations: Adjust dose based on renal function.

Breast-feeding Issues: Although no teratogenic or infant harm has been found in studies, excretion in breast milk is not known and this drug should be used during lactation only if clearly indicated.

Merrem® I.V. *see* Meropenem *on page 857*

Meruvax II *see page 1498*

Mesalamine (me SAL a meen)

U.S. Brand Names Asacol®; Canasa™; Pentasa®; Rowasa®

Synonyms 5-Aminosalicylic Acid; 5-ASA; Fisalamine; Mesalazine

Generic Available No

Pharmacologic Category 5-Aminosalicylic Acid Derivative

Pregnancy Risk Factor B

Lactation Enters breast milk/use caution

Use

Oral: Treatment and maintenance of remission of mildly to moderately active ulcerative colitis

Rectal: Treatment of active mild to moderate distal ulcerative colitis, proctosigmoiditis, or proctitis

Mechanism of Action/Effect Mesalamine (5-aminosalicylic acid) is the active component of sulfasalazine; the specific mechanism of action of mesalamine is unknown; however, it is thought that it modulates local chemical mediators of the inflammatory response, especially leukotrienes; action appears topical rather than systemic

Contraindications Hypersensitivity to mesalamine, sulfasalazine, salicylates, or any component of the formulation

Warnings/Precautions May cause an acute intolerance syndrome. Pericarditis should be considered in patients with chest pain; pancreatitis should be considered in patients with new abdominal complaints. Use with caution in patients with impaired hepatic or renal function. Postmarketing reports suggest an increased incidence of blood dyscrasias in patients >65 years of age. In addition, elderly may have difficulty administering and retaining rectal suppositories and decreased renal function; use with caution and monitor. Safety and efficacy in pediatric patients have not been established.

Rowasa® enema: Contains potassium metabisulfite; may cause anaphylactic reactions in patients with sulfite allergies.

Drug Interactions

Decreased Effect: Decreased digoxin bioavailability.

Increased Effect/Toxicity: Mesalamine may increase the risk of myelosuppression from azathioprine, mercaptopurine, and thioguanine.

Nutritional/Ethanol Interactions Food: Oral: Mesalamine serum levels may be decreased if taken with food.

Adverse Reactions Adverse effects vary depending upon dosage form. Effects as reported with tablets, unless otherwise noted:

>10%:

Central nervous system: Pain (14%)

Gastrointestinal: Abdominal pain (18%; enema: 8%)

Genitourinary: Eructation (16%)

Respiratory: Pharyngitis (11%)

1% to 10%:

Cardiovascular: Chest pain (3%), peripheral edema (3%)

Central nervous system: Chills (3%), dizziness (suppository: 3%), fever (enema: 3%; suppository: 1%), insomnia (2%), malaise (2%)

Dermatologic: Rash (6%; suppository: 1%), pruritus (3%; enema: 1%), acne (2%; suppository: 1%)

Gastrointestinal: Dyspepsia (6%), constipation (5%), vomiting (5%), colitis exacerbation (3%; suppository: 1%), nausea (capsule: 3%), flatulence (enema: 6%), hemorrhoids (enema: 1%), nausea and vomiting (capsule: 1%), rectal pain (enema: 1%; suppository: 2%)

Local: Pain on insertion of enema tip (enema: 1%)

Neuromuscular & skeletal: Back pain (7%; enema: 1%), arthralgia (5%), hypertonia (5%), myalgia (3%), arthritis (2%), leg/joint pain (enema: 2%),

Ocular: Conjunctivitis (2%)

Respiratory: Flu-like syndrome (3%; enema: 5%), diaphoresis (3%), cough increased (2%)

<1% (Limited to important or life-threatening): Agranulocytosis, alopecia, aplastic anemia, cholestatic jaundice, cholecystitis, edema, elevated liver enzymes, erythema nodosum, fibrosing alveolitis, gout, Guillain-Barré syndrome, hepatitis, hepatocellular damage, hepatotoxicity, interstitial nephritis, Kawasaki-like syndrome, liver failure, liver necrosis, lupus-like syndrome, minimal change nephrotic syndrome, myocarditis, nephropathy, pancreatitis, pancytopenia, pericarditis, thrombocytopenia, vertigo

Overdosage/Toxicology Symptoms of overdose include decreased motor activity, diarrhea, vomiting, and renal function impairment. Treatment is supportive; emesis, gastric lavage, and follow with activated charcoal slurry.

Pharmacodynamics/Kinetics

Absorption: Rectal: Variable and dependent upon retention time, underlying GI disease, and colonic pH; Oral: Tablet: ~28%, Capsule: ~20% to 30%

Half-Life Elimination: 5-ASA: 0.5-1.5 hours; acetyl-5-ASA: 5-10 hours

Time to Peak: Serum: 4-7 hours

Metabolism: Hepatic and via GI tract to acetyl-5-aminosalicylic acid

Formulations

Capsule, controlled release (Pentasa®): 250 mg

Suppository, rectal (Canasa™, Rowasa®): 500 mg

Suspension, rectal (Rowasa®): 4 g/60 mL [contains potassium metabisulphite] (7s)

Tablet, delayed release, enteric coated (Asacol®): 400 mg

Dosing

Adults:

Treatment of ulcerative colitis: Oral:

Capsule: 1 g 4 times/day

Tablet: 800 mg 3 times/day for 6 weeks

Maintenance of remission of ulcerative colitis: Oral:

Capsule: 1 g 4 times/day

Tablet: 1.6 g/day in divided doses

Distal ulcerative colitis, proctosigmoiditis, or proctitis: Rectal: Retention enema: 60 mL (4 g) at bedtime, retained overnight, approximately 8 hours

Active ulcerative proctitis: Rectal:

Rectal suppository: Insert 1 suppository in rectum twice daily; retain suppositories for at least 1-3 hours to achieve maximum benefit

Canasa™: May increase to 3 times/day if inadequate response is seen after 2 weeks.

Note: Some patients may require rectal and oral therapy concurrently.

Elderly: Refer to adult dosing. Use with caution.

Administration

Oral: Swallow capsules or tablets whole, do not chew or crush.

Other:

Rectal enema: Shake bottle well. Retain enemas for 8 hours or as long as practical.

Suppository: Remove foil wrapper; avoid excessive handling. Should be retained for at least 1-3 hours to achieve maximum benefit.

(Continued)

Mesalamine *(Continued)*

Stability

Storage:

Enema: Store at controlled room temperature. Use promptly once foil wrap is removed; contents may darken with time (do not use if dark brown)

Suppository: Store at controlled room temperature away from direct heat, light, and humidity; do not refrigerate

Tablet: Store at controlled room temperature

Monitoring Laboratory Tests CBC and renal function, particularly in elderly patients

Monitoring and Teaching Issues

Physical Assessment: Assess history of allergies prior to beginning treatment. See Contraindications, Warnings/Precautions, Drug Interactions, and Dosing for use cautions. Assess results of laboratory tests (see above), therapeutic response, and adverse response (see Adverse Reactions and Overdose/Toxicology). Teach patient proper use (according to formulation), possible side effects and appropriate interventions (eg, importance of adequate hydration), and adverse symptoms to report (see Patient Education). Note breast-feeding caution.

Patient Education: Inform prescriber of all prescriptions, OTC medications, or herbal products you are taking, and any allergies you have. Do not take anything new during treatment unless approved by prescriber. Take as directed.

Oral: Do not chew or break tablets or capsules. Notify prescriber if whole or partial tablets are repeatedly found in stool.

Enemas: Shake well before using, retain for 8 hours or as long as possible.

Suppository: Do not refrigerate. After removing foil wrapper, insert high in rectum without excessive handling (warmth will melt suppository). Retain suppositories for at least 1-3 hours to achieve maximum benefit. Report severe abdominal pain, unresolved diarrhea, jaundice, severe headache, any unusual pain (back, joint, muscle, swelling of extremities, or chest pain).

Enema and suppository: May cause staining of clothing, undergarments; lubricating gel may be used if needed to assist insertion.

Pregnancy/breast-feeding precautions: Consult prescriber if breast-feeding.

Geriatric Considerations: Elderly may have difficulty administering and retaining rectal suppositories. Given renal function decline with aging, monitor serum creatinine often during therapy.

Breast-feeding Issues: Adverse effects (diarrhea) in a nursing infant have been reported while the mother received rectal administration of mesalamine within 12 hours after the first dose. The AAP recommends to monitor the infant stool for consistency and to use with caution.

Mesalazine *see* Mesalamine *on page 858*
Mescaline and Peyote *see page 1568*

Mesna (MES na)

U.S. Brand Names Mesnex™

Synonyms Sodium 2-Mercaptoethane Sulfonate

Generic Available No

Pharmacologic Category Antidote

Pregnancy Risk Factor B

Lactation Excretion in breast milk unknown/contraindicated

Use Orphan drug: Mesna is a uroprotectant used to prevent hemorrhagic cystitis induced by ifosfamide and cyclophosphamide; mesna is always given in conjunction with ifosfamide, and is often given in conjunction with cyclophosphamide

Mechanism of Action/Effect Binds with and detoxifies urotoxic metabolites of ifosfamide and cyclophosphamide to prevent hemorrhagic cystitis induced by ifosfamide and cyclophosphamide

Contraindications Hypersensitivity to mesna or other thiol compounds, or any component of the formulation

Warnings/Precautions Examine morning urine specimen for hematuria prior to ifosfamide or cyclophosphamide treatment; if hematuria (>50 RBC/HPF) develops, reduce the ifosfamide/cyclophosphamide dose or discontinue the drug; will not prevent or alleviate other toxicities associated with ifosfamide or cyclophosphamide and will not prevent hemorrhagic cystitis in all patients. Allergic reactions have been reported; patients with autoimmune disorders may be at increased risk. Symptoms ranged from mild hypersensitivity to systemic anaphylactic reactions. I.V. formulation contains benzyl alcohol; do not use in neonates or infants.

Drug Interactions

Decreased Effect: Warfarin: Questionable alterations in coagulation control.

Effects on Lab Values False-positive urinary ketones with Multistix® or Labstix®

Adverse Reactions It is difficult to distinguish reactions from those caused by concomitant chemotherapy.

>10%: Gastrointestinal: Bad taste in mouth with oral administration (100%), vomiting (secondary to the bad taste after oral administration, or with high I.V. doses)

<1% (Limited to important or life-threatening): Anaphylaxis, hypersensitivity, hypertonia, injection site reaction, limb pain, myalgia, platelet count decreased, tachycardia, tachypnea

Pharmacodynamics/Kinetics

Bioavailability: Oral: 45% to 79%

Half-Life Elimination: Parent drug: 24 minutes; Mesna disulfide: 72 minutes

Time to Peak: Plasma: 2-3 hours

Metabolism: Rapidly oxidized intravascularly to mesna disulfide; mesna disulfide is reduced in renal tubules back to mesna following glomerular filtration.

Formulations

Injection: 100 mg/mL (2 mL, 4 mL, 10 mL)

Tablet: 400 mg

Dosing

Adults & Elderly: Refer to individual protocols.

I.V. regimen: Recommended dose is 60% of the ifosfamide dose given in 3 divided doses, with ifosfamide, and 4 hours and 8 hours after the ifosfamide dose.

Note: Other I.V. doses/regimens include 4 divided doses of mesna (0, 3, 6, and 9 hours after the start of ifosfamide) and continuous infusions. Continuous infusions commonly employ doses equal to the dose of ifosfamide or cyclophosphamide. It has been suggested that continuous infusions provide more consistent urinary free thiol levels. Infusions are continued for 8-24 hours after completion of ifosfamide or cyclophosphamide.

I.V./Oral regimen: Commonly, the first dose is I.V. and the 2-hour and 6-hour doses are oral. I.V. dose is 20% of the ifosfamide dose at the time of ifosfamide dosing. Oral doses are 40% of the ifosfamide dose and are given 2 hours and 6 hours after the ifosfamide dose.

Note: Total dose equal 100% of the ifosfamide dose.

Pediatrics: Refer to adult dosing.

Administration

Oral: For oral administration (if tablets are not used), injection may be diluted in 1:1, 1:2, 1:10, 1:100 concentrations in carbonated beverages (cola, ginger ale, Pepsi®, Sprite®, Dr Pepper®, etc), juices (apple or orange), or whole milk (chocolate or white), and is stable 24 hours at refrigeration; used in conjunction with ifosfamide; examine morning urine specimen for hematuria prior to ifosfamide or cyclophosphamide treatment. Patients who vomit within 2 hours of taking oral mesna should repeat the dose or receive I.V. mesna.

I.V.: Administer by I.V. infusion over 15-30 minutes or per protocol. Mesna can be diluted in D_5W or NS to a final concentration of 1-20 mg/mL.

Stability

Storage: Store unopened vials at controlled room temperature of 20°C to 25°C (68°F to 77°F). The opened ampuls will be oxidized to dimesna upon exposure to air. Solutions of mesna in D_5W, D_5W/NaCl, 0.9% NaCl, or lactated Ringer's are reported to be stable for at least 48 hours. A solution of ifosfamide and mesna in lactated Ringer's was reported to be stable for 7 days in an ambulatory infusion pump. Mesna is reported to be stable in glass or plastic syringes at refrigerator, room, or body temperature for at least 9 days. Stability in syringes decreases with exposure to air and the resultant oxidation to dimesna. Mesna is stable for at least 7 days when diluted 1:2 or 1:5 with grape and orange flavored syrups or 1:1 to 1:100 in carbonated drinks for oral administration.

Reconstitution: Standard dose: Dose/100-1000 mL D_5W or NS to a final concentration of 1-20 mg/mL

Compatibility: Stable in $D_5{}^1/_4$NS, $D_5{}^1/_3$NS, $D_5{}^1/_2$NS, D_5W, LR, NS

Y-site administration: Incompatible with amphotericin B cholesteryl sulfate complex

Compatibility in syringe: Incompatible with ifosfamide/epirubicin

Compatibility when admixed: Incompatible with carboplatin, cisplatin, ifosfamide/epirubicin

Monitoring Laboratory Tests Urinalysis

Monitoring and Teaching Issues

Physical Assessment: See Contraindications and Warnings/Precautions for use cautions. Monitor laboratory results (see above) and assess frequently for bladder hemorrhage. Breast-feeding is contraindicated.

Patient Education: This drug is given to help prevent side effects of other chemotherapeutic agents you are taking. **Breast-feeding precaution:** Do not breast-feed.

Related Information

Ifosfamide *on page 693*

Mesnex™ *see* Mesna *on page 860*

Mesoridazine (mez oh RID a zeen)

U.S. Brand Names Serentil®

Synonyms Mesoridazine Besylate

Generic Available No

Pharmacologic Category Antipsychotic Agent, Phenothiazine, Piperidine

Pregnancy Risk Factor C

Lactation Enters breast milk/contraindicated (AAP rates "of concern")

Use Management of schizophrenic patients who fail to respond adequately to treatment with other antipsychotic drugs, either because of insufficient effectiveness or the inability to achieve an effective dose due to intolerable adverse effects from these drugs

Use - Unlabeled/Investigational Psychosis

Mechanism of Action/Effect Blockade of postsynaptic CNS dopamine$_2$ receptors in the mesolimbic and mesocortical areas

Contraindications Hypersensitivity to mesoridazine or any component of the formulation (cross-reactivity between phenothiazines may occur); severe CNS depression and coma; prolonged QT interval (>450 msec), including prolongation due to congenital causes; history of arrhythmias; concurrent use of medications which prolong QT_c (including type Ia and type III antiarrhythmics, cyclic antidepressants, some fluoroquinolones, cisapride)

Warnings/Precautions Has been shown to prolong QT_c interval in a dose-dependent manner (associated with an increased risk of torsade de pointes). Patients should have a baseline EKG prior to initiation, and should not receive mesoridazine if baseline QT_c >450 msec. Mesoridazine should be discontinued in patients with a QT_c interval >500 msec. Potassium levels must be evaluated and normalized prior to and throughout treatment.

May cause hypotension, particularly with I.M. administration. Highly sedating, use with caution in disorders where CNS depression is a feature. Use with caution in Parkinson's disease. Caution in patients with hemodynamic instability; bone marrow suppression; predisposition to seizures; subcortical brain damage; severe cardiac, hepatic, renal, or respiratory disease. Esophageal dysmotility and aspiration have been associated with antipsychotic use;

(Continued)

Mesoridazine *(Continued)*

use with caution in patients at risk of pneumonia (ie, Alzheimer's disease). Caution in breast cancer or other prolactin-dependent tumors (may elevate prolactin levels). May alter temperature regulation or mask toxicity of other drugs due to antiemetic effects. May cause orthostatic hypotension - use with caution in patients at risk of this effect or those who would tolerate transient hypotensive episodes (cerebrovascular disease, cardiovascular disease, or other medications which may predispose).

Phenothiazines may cause anticholinergic effects (confusion, agitation, constipation, xerostomia, blurred vision, urinary retention). Therefore, they should be used with caution in patients with decreased gastrointestinal motility, urinary retention, BPH, xerostomia, or visual problems. Conditions which also may be exacerbated by cholinergic blockade include narrow-angle glaucoma (screening is recommended) and worsening of myasthenia gravis. Relative to other antipsychotics, mesoridazine has a high potency of cholinergic blockade.

May cause extrapyramidal symptoms, including pseudoparkinsonism, acute dystonic reactions, akathisia, and tardive dyskinesia (risk of these reactions is low relative to other neuroleptics). May be associated with neuroleptic malignant syndrome (NMS) or pigmentary retinopathy (particularly at doses >1 g/day).

Pregnancy risk C.

Drug Interactions

Decreased Effect: Mesoridazine may inhibit the activity of bromocriptine and levodopa. Benztropine (and other anticholinergics) may inhibit the therapeutic response to mesoridazine and excess anticholinergic effects may occur. Mesoridazine and possibly other low potency antipsychotic may reverse the pressor effects of epinephrine.

Increased Effect/Toxicity: Use of mesoridazine with other agents known to prolong QT_c may increase the risk of malignant arrhythmias; concurrent use is contraindicated - includes type I and type III antiarrhythmics, TCAs, and some quinolone antibiotics (sparfloxacin, moxifloxacin, gatifloxacin). Mesoridazine may increase the effect and/or toxicity of antihypertensives, anticholinergics, lithium, CNS depressants (ethanol, narcotics), and trazodone. Metoclopramide may increase risk of extrapyramidal symptoms (EPS).

Nutritional/Ethanol Interactions

Ethanol: Avoid ethanol (may increase CNS depression).

Herb/Nutraceutical: Avoid valerian, St John's wort, kava kava, gotu kola (may increase CNS depression).

Effects on Lab Values ↑ cholesterol (S), glucose; ↓ uric acid (S)

Adverse Reactions Frequency not defined.

Cardiovascular: Hypotension, orthostatic hypotension, tachycardia, QT prolongation (dose dependent, up to 100% of patients at higher dosages), syncope, edema

Central nervous system: Pseudoparkinsonism, akathisia, dystonias, tardive dyskinesia, dizziness, drowsiness, restlessness, ataxia, slurred speech, neuroleptic malignant syndrome (NMS), impairment of temperature regulation, lowering of seizure threshold

Dermatologic: Increased sensitivity to sun, rash, itching, angioneurotic edema, dermatitis, discoloration of skin (blue-gray)

Endocrine & metabolic: Changes in menstrual cycle, changes in libido, gynecomastia, lactation, galactorrhea

Gastrointestinal: Constipation, xerostomia, weight gain, nausea, vomiting, stomach pain

Genitourinary: Difficulty in urination, ejaculatory disturbances, impotence, enuresis, incontinence, priapism, urinary retention

Hematologic: Agranulocytosis, leukopenia, eosinophilia, thrombocytopenia, anemia, aplastic anemia

Hepatic: Cholestatic jaundice, hepatotoxicity

Neuromuscular & skeletal: Weakness, tremor, rigidity

Ocular: Pigmentary retinopathy, photophobia, blurred vision, cornea and lens changes

Respiratory: Nasal congestion

Miscellaneous: Diaphoresis (decreased), lupus-like syndrome

Overdosage/Toxicology Symptoms of overdose include deep sleep, coma, extrapyramidal symptoms, abnormal involuntary muscle movements, and hypotension. Monitor for cardiac arrhythmias and avoid use of drugs which prolong QT interval. Treatment is symptomatic and supportive.

Pharmacodynamics/Kinetics

Absorption: Tablet: Erratic; Liquid: More dependable

Half-Life Elimination: 24-48 hours

Time to Peak: Serum: 2-4 hours; Steady-state serum: 4-7 days

Duration: 4-6 hours

Formulations

Injection, as besylate: 25 mg/mL (1 mL)

Liquid, oral, as besylate: 25 mg/mL (118 mL)

Tablet, as besylate: 10 mg, 25 mg, 50 mg, 100 mg

Dosing

Adults:

Schizophrenia/psychoses:

Oral: 25-50 mg 3 times/day; maximum: 100-400 mg/day

Note: Concentrate may be diluted just prior to administration with distilled water, acidified tap water, orange or grape juice. Do not prepare and store bulk dilutions.

I.M.: Initial: 25 mg, repeat in 30-60 minutes as needed; optimal dosage range: 25-200 mg/day

Elderly: Behavioral symptoms associated with dementia:

Oral: Initial: 10 mg 1-2 times/day; if <10 mg/day is desired, consider administering 10 mg every other day (qod). Increase dose at 4- to 7-day intervals by 10-25 mg/day; increase dose intervals (bid, tid, etc) as necessary to control response or side effects. Maximum daily dose: 250 mg. Gradual increases (titration) may prevent some side effects or decrease their severity.

I.M.: Initial: 25 mg; repeat doses in 30-60 minutes if necessary. Dose range: 25-200 mg/day. Elderly usually require less than maximal daily dose.

Renal Impairment: Not dialyzable (0% to 5%)

Administration

Oral: Dilute oral concentrate just prior to administration with distilled water, acidified tap water, orange or grape juice. Do not prepare and store bulk dilutions. Do not mix oral solutions of mesoridazine and lithium, these oral liquids are incompatible when mixed. **Note:** Avoid skin contact with oral medication; may cause contact dermatitis.

I.M.: Watch for hypotension when administering I.M.

I.V.: Watch for hypotension when administering I.V.

Stability

Storage: Protect all dosage forms from light; clear or slightly yellow solutions may be used; should be dispensed in amber or opaque vials/bottles.

Reconstitution: Solutions may be diluted or mixed with fruit juices or other liquids but must be administered immediately after mixing; do not prepare bulk dilutions or store bulk dilutions.

Monitoring Laboratory Tests Baseline liver and kidney function, CBC prior to and periodically during therapy, ophthalmic screening; Baseline (and periodic) EKG and serum potassium; do not initiate if QT_c >450 msec (discontinue in QT_c 500 msec)

Monitoring and Teaching Issues

Physical Assessment: Assess other medications patient is taking for effectiveness and interactions (see Drug Interaction). See Contraindications and Warnings/Precautions for use cautions. Review ophthalmic screening and monitor laboratory results, therapeutic response, and adverse reactions at beginning of therapy and periodically with long-term use (see Adverse Reactions and Overdose/Toxicology). With I.M. or I.V. use, monitor closely for hypotension. **Note:** Avoid skin contact with oral or injection medication; may cause contact dermatitis (wash immediately with warm, soapy water). Initiate at lower doses (see Dosing) and taper dosage slowly when discontinuing. Assess knowledge/teach patient appropriate use, interventions to reduce side effects, and adverse symptoms to report (see Patient Education). **Pregnancy risk factor C** - instruct patient about appropriate contraceptive use. Breast-feeding is contraindicated.

Patient Education: Use exactly as directed; do not increase dose or frequency. It may take 2-3 weeks to achieve desired results; do not discontinue without consulting prescriber. Dilute oral concentration with water, orange or grape juice. Do not take within 2 hours of any antacid. Avoid alcohol or caffeine and other prescription or OTC medications not approved by prescriber. Maintain adequate hydration (2-3 L/day of fluids) unless advised by prescriber to restrict fluids. Avoid skin contact with medication; may cause contact dermatitis (wash immediately with warm, soapy water). You may experience excess drowsiness, restlessness, dizziness, or blurred vision (use caution driving or when engaging in tasks requiring alertness until response to drug is known); dry mouth, nausea, vomiting (small, frequent meals, frequent mouth care, chewing gum, or sucking lozenges may help); constipation (increased exercise, fluids, fruit, or fiber may help); postural hypotension (use caution climbing stairs or when changing position from lying or sitting to standing); urinary retention (void before taking medication); photosensitivity (use sunscreen, wear protective clothing and eyewear, and avoid direct sunlight); decreased perspiration (avoid strenuous exercise in hot environments); or changes in menstrual cycle, libido, ejaculation (will resolve when medication is discontinued). Report persistent CNS effects (eg, trembling fingers, altered gait or balance, excessive sedation, seizures, unusual movements, anxiety, abnormal thoughts, confusion, personality changes); chest pain, palpitations, rapid heartbeat, severe dizziness; unresolved urinary retention or changes in urinary pattern; menstrual pattern, change in libido, swelling or pain in breasts (male or female); vision changes; skin rash or yellowing of skin; difficulty breathing; or worsening of condition. **Pregnancy/breast-feeding precautions:** Inform prescriber if you are or intend to become pregnant. Do not breast-feed.

Geriatric Considerations: (See Warnings/Precautions, Adverse Reactions, and Overdose/Toxicology.) Elderly patients have an increased risk of adverse response to side effects or adverse reactions to antipsychotics.

Additional Information Coadministration of two or more antipsychotics does not improve clinical response and may increase the potential for adverse effects.

Related Information

Antipsychotic Agents *on page 1558*

Antipsychotic Medication Guidelines *on page 1614*

Mesoridazine Besylate *see* Mesoridazine *on page 861*

Mestinon® *see* Pyridostigmine *on page 1154*

Mestinon® Timespan® *see* Pyridostigmine *on page 1154*

Mestranol and Norethindrone (MES tra nole & nor eth IN drone)

U.S. Brand Names Necon® 1/50; Norinyl® 1+50; Ortho-Novum® 1/50

Synonyms Norethindrone and Mestranol; Ortho Novum 1/50

Generic Available Yes

Pharmacologic Category Contraceptive; Estrogen and Progestin Combination

Pregnancy Risk Factor X

Lactation Enters breast milk/not recommended (AAP rates "compatible")

Use Prevention of pregnancy

Use - Unlabeled/Investigational Treatment of hypermenorrhea, endometriosis, female hypogonadism

Mechanism of Action/Effect Combination hormonal contraceptives inhibit ovulation and also produce changes in the cervical mucus and endometrium creating an unfavorable environment for sperm penetration and nidation.

Contraindications Hypersensitivity to mestranol, norethindrone, or any component of the formulation; thrombophlebitis or thromboembolic disorders (current or history of), cerebral vascular disease, coronary artery disease, valvular heart disease with complications, severe (Continued)

Mestranol and Norethindrone *(Continued)*

hypertension; diabetes mellitus with vascular involvement; severe headache with focal neurological symptoms; known or suspected breast carcinoma, endometrial cancer, estrogen-dependent neoplasms, undiagnosed abnormal genital bleeding; hepatic dysfunction or tumor, cholestatic jaundice of pregnancy, jaundice with prior combination hormonal contraceptive use; major surgery with prolonged immobilization; heavy smoking (≥15 cigarettes/day) in patients >35 years of age; pregnancy

Warnings/Precautions Use with caution in patients with a history of thromboembolism, stroke, myocardial infarction, liver tumor, hypertension, cardiac, renal or hepatic insufficiency; use of any progestin during the first 4 months of pregnancy is not recommended; risk of cardiovascular side effects increases in those women who smoke cigarettes and in women >35 years of age. Use of oral contraceptives has been associated with a small increase in the frequency of breast cancer. Some studies suggest an increased risk of intraepithelial neoplasia may also be associated with oral contraceptive use. Not for use prior to menarche. Combination hormonal contraceptives do not protect against HIV infection or other sexually-transmitted diseases. The risk of cardiovascular side effects increases in women who smoke cigarettes, especially those who are >35 years of age; women who use combination hormonal contraceptives should be strongly advised not to smoke. Combination hormonal contraceptives may lead to increased risk of myocardial infarction, use with caution in patients with risk factors for coronary artery disease. May increase the risk of thromboembolism. Combination hormonal contraceptives may have a dose-related risk of vascular disease, hypertension, and gallbladder disease. Women with hypertension should be encouraged to use a nonhormonal form of contraception. The use of combination hormonal contraceptives has been associated with a slight increase in frequency of breast cancer, however, studies are not consistent. Combination hormonal contraceptives may cause glucose intolerance. Retinal thrombosis has been reported (rarely). Use with caution in patients with renal disease, conditions that may be aggravated by fluid retention, depression, or history of migraine. Not for use prior to menarche.

The minimum dosage combination of estrogen/progestin that will effectively treat the individual patient should be used. New patients should be started on products containing <50 mcg of estrogen per tablet.

Drug Interactions

Cytochrome P450 Effect:

Mestranol: Substrate of **CYP2C19**; Based on active metabolite ethinyl estradiol: Substrate of **CYP3A4**, 3A5-7; Inhibits CYP1A2, 2B6, 2C19, 3A4

Norethindrone: Substrate of **CYP3A4**; Induces CYP2C19

Decreased Effect: Combination hormonal contraceptives may decrease plasma levels of acetaminophen, clofibric acid, lorazepam, morphine, oxazepam, salicylic acid, temazepam. Contraceptive effect decreased by acitretin, aminoglutethimide, amprenavir, anticonvulsants, griseofulvin, lopinavir, nelfinavir, nevirapine, penicillins (effect not consistent), rifampin, ritonavir, tetracyclines (effect not consistent) troglitazone. Combination hormonal contraceptives may decrease (or increase) the effects of coumarin derivatives.

Increased Effect/Toxicity: Acetaminophen and ascorbic acid may increase plasma levels of estrogen component. Atorvastatin and indinavir increase plasma levels of combination hormonal contraceptives. Combination hormonal contraceptives increase the plasma levels of alprazolam, chlordiazepoxide, cyclosporine, diazepam, prednisolone, selegiline, theophylline, tricyclic antidepressants. Combination hormonal contraceptives may increase (or decrease) the effects of coumarin derivatives.

Nutritional/Ethanol Interactions

Food: CNS effects of caffeine may be enhanced if oral contraceptives are used concurrently with caffeine. Grapefruit juice increases ethinyl estradiol concentrations and would be expected to increase progesterone serum levels as well; clinical implications are unclear.

Herb/Nutraceutical: St John's wort may decrease the effectiveness of combination hormonal contraceptives by inducing hepatic enzymes. Avoid dong quai and black cohosh (have estrogen activity). Avoid saw palmetto, red clover, ginseng.

Adverse Reactions Frequency not defined.

Cardiovascular: Arterial thromboembolism, cerebral hemorrhage, cerebral thrombosis, edema, hypertension, mesenteric thrombosis, myocardial infarction

Central nervous system: Depression, dizziness, headache, migraine, nervousness, premenstrual syndrome, stroke

Dermatologic: Acne, erythema multiforme, erythema nodosum, hirsutism, loss of scalp hair, melasma (may persist), rash (allergic)

Endocrine & metabolic: Amenorrhea, breakthrough bleeding, breast enlargement, breast secretion, breast tenderness, carbohydrate intolerance, lactation decreased (postpartum), glucose tolerance decreased, libido changes, menstrual flow changes, sex hormone-binding globulins (SHBG) increased, spotting, temporary infertility (following discontinuation), thyroid-binding globulin increased, triglycerides increased

Gastrointestinal: Abdominal cramps, appetite changes, bloating, cholestasis, colitis, gallbladder disease, jaundice, nausea, vomiting, weight gain/loss

Genitourinary: Cervical erosion changes, cervical secretion changes, cystitis-like syndrome, vaginal candidiasis, vaginitis

Hematologic: Antithrombin III decreased, folate levels decreased, hemolytic uremic syndrome, norepinephrine induced platelet aggregability increased, porphyria, prothrombin increased; factors VII, VIII, IX, and X increased

Hepatic: Benign liver tumors, Budd-Chiari syndrome, cholestatic jaundice, hepatic adenomas

Local: Thrombophlebitis

Ocular: Cataracts, change in corneal curvature (steepening), contact lens intolerance, optic neuritis, retinal thrombosis

Renal: Impaired renal function

Respiratory: Pulmonary thromboembolism

Miscellaneous: Hemorrhagic eruption

Overdosage/Toxicology Toxicity is unlikely following single exposures of excessive doses. May cause withdrawal bleeding in females. Any treatment following emesis and charcoal administration should be supportive and symptomatic.

Pharmacokinetic Note See Norethindrone monograph and Ethinyl Estradiol monograph for additional information.

Pharmacodynamics/Kinetics

Metabolism:

Mestranol: Hepatic via demethylation to ethinyl estradiol

Formulations Tablet, monophasic formulations:

Necon® 1/50-21: Norethindrone 1 mg and mestranol 0.05 mg [light blue tablets] (21s)

Necon® 1/50-28: Norethindrone 1 mg and mestranol 0.05 mg [21 light blue tablets and 7 white inactive tablets] (28s)

Norinyl® 1+50: Norethindrone 1 mg and mestranol 0.05 mg [21 white tablets and 7 orange inactive tablets] (28s)

Ortho-Novum® 1/50: Norethindrone 1 mg and mestranol 0.05 mg [21 yellow tablets and 7 green inactive tablets] (28s)

Dosing

Adults: Female: Contraception: Oral:

Schedule 1 (Sunday starter): Dose begins on first Sunday after onset of menstruation; if the menstrual period starts on Sunday, take first tablet that very same day. **With a Sunday start, an additional method of contraception should be used until after the first 7 days of consecutive administration.**

For 21-tablet package: Dosage is 1 tablet daily for 21 consecutive days, followed by 7 days off of the medication; a new course begins on the 8th day after the last tablet is taken.

For 28-tablet package: Dosage is 1 tablet daily without interruption.

Schedule 2 (Day 1 starter): Dose starts on first day of menstrual cycle taking 1 tablet daily.

For 21-tablet package: Dosage is 1 tablet daily for 21 consecutive days, followed by 7 days off of the medication; a new course begins on the 8th day after the last tablet is taken.

For 28-tablet package: Dosage is 1 tablet daily without interruption.

If all doses have been taken on schedule and one menstrual period is missed, continue dosing cycle. If two consecutive menstrual periods are missed, pregnancy test is required before new dosing cycle is started.

Missed doses **monophasic formulations** (refer to package insert for complete information):

One dose missed: Take as soon as remembered or take 2 tablets next day

Two consecutive doses missed in the first 2 weeks: Take 2 tablets as soon as remembered or 2 tablets next 2 days. **An additional method of contraception should be used for 7 days after missed dose.**

Two consecutive doses missed in week 3 or three consecutive doses missed at any time: **An additional method of contraception must be used for 7 days after a missed dose:**

Schedule 1 (Sunday starter): Continue dose of 1 tablet daily until Sunday, then discard the rest of the pack, and a new pack should be started that same day.

Schedule 2 (Day 1 starter): Current pack should be discarded, and a new pack should be started that same day.

Pediatrics: Female: Contraception: Oral: See adult dosing; not to be used prior to menarche.

Renal Impairment: Specific guidelines not available; use with caution.

Hepatic Impairment: Contraindicated in patients with hepatic impairment.

Administration

Oral: Administer at the same time each day.

Stability

Storage: Store at controlled room temperature of 25°C (77°F).

Monitoring and Teaching Issues

Physical Assessment: Monitor or teach patient to monitor blood pressure on a regular basis. Monitor or teach patient to monitor for occurrence of adverse effects and symptoms to report (see Adverse Reactions). Assess knowledge/teach importance of regular (monthly) blood pressure checks and annual physical assessment, Pap smear, and vision assessment. Teach importance of maintaining prescribed schedule of dosing (see Dosing for dosing and missed dose information). **Pregnancy risk factor X** - do not use if patient is pregnant. Breast-feeding is not recommended.

Patient Education: Oral contraceptives do not protect against HIV or other sexually-transmitted disease. Take exactly as directed by prescriber (also see package insert). Take at the same time each day. You are at risk of becoming pregnant if doses are missed. Detailed and complete information on dosing and missed doses can be found in the package insert. Be aware that some medications may reduce the effectiveness of oral contraceptives; an alternate form of contraception may be needed. Check all medicines (prescription and OTC), herbal, and alternative products with prescriber. It is important that you check your blood pressure monthly (on same day each month) and that you have an annual physical assessment, Pap smear, and vision assessment while taking this medication. Avoid smoking while taking this medication; smoking increases risk of adverse effects, including thromboembolic events and heart attacks. You may experience loss of appetite (small, frequent meals will help); or constipation (increased exercise, fluids, fruit, fiber, or stool softeners may help). If diabetic, use accurate serum glucose testing to identify any changes in glucose tolerance; notify prescriber of significant changes so antidiabetic medication can be adjusted if necessary. Report immediately pain or muscle soreness; warmth, swelling, pain, or redness in calves; shortness of breath; sudden loss of vision; unresolved leg or foot swelling; change in menstrual pattern (unusual bleeding, amenorrhea, breakthrough spotting); breast tenderness that does not go away; acute abdominal cramping; signs of vaginal infection (drainage, pain, itching); CNS changes (blurred vision, confusion, acute anxiety, or unresolved depression); or significant weight gain (>5 lb/week). Notify prescriber of changes in contact lens tolerance. **Pregnancy/breast-feeding precautions:**

(Continued)

Mestranol and Norethindrone *(Continued)*

This medication should not be used during pregnancy. If you suspect you may become pregnant, contact prescriber immediately. Breast-feeding is not recommended.

Dietary Issues: Should be taken at same time each day.

Breast-feeding Issues: Jaundice and breast enlargement in the nursing infant have been reported following the use of combination hormonal contraceptives. May decrease the quality and quantity of breast milk; a nonhormonal form of contraception is recommended.

Pregnancy Issues: Pregnancy should be ruled out prior to treatment and discontinued if pregnancy occurs. In general, the use of combination hormonal contraceptives when inadvertently taken early in pregnancy have not been associated with teratogenic effects. Due to increased risk of thromboembolism postpartum, combination hormonal contraceptives should not be started earlier than 4-6 weeks following delivery.

Related Information

Norethindrone *on page 984*

Metacortandralone *see* PrednisoLONE *on page 1113*

Metadate® CD *see* Methylphenidate *on page 882*

Metadate™ ER *see* Methylphenidate *on page 882*

Metamucil® [OTC] *see* Psyllium *on page 1152*

Metamucil® Smooth Texture [OTC] *see* Psyllium *on page 1152*

Metaraminol *see page 1580*

Metformin (met FOR min)

U.S. Brand Names Glucophage®; Glucophage® XR

Synonyms Metformin Hydrochloride

Generic Available Yes: Regular release only

Pharmacologic Category Antidiabetic Agent, Biguanide

Pregnancy Risk Factor B

Lactation Excretion in breast milk unknown/not recommended

Use Management of type 2 diabetes mellitus (noninsulin dependent, NIDDM) as monotherapy when hyperglycemia cannot be managed on diet alone. May be used concomitantly with a sulfonylurea or insulin to improve glycemic control.

Use - Unlabeled/Investigational Treatment of HIV lipodystrophy syndrome

Mechanism of Action/Effect Decreases hepatic glucose production, decreasing intestinal absorption of glucose and improves insulin sensitivity (increases peripheral glucose uptake and utilization)

Contraindications Hypersensitivity to metformin or any component of the formulation; renal disease or renal dysfunction (serum creatinine ≥1.5 mg/dL in males or ≥1.4 mg/dL in females or abnormal clearance); clinical situations predisposing to hypoxemia, including conditions such as cardiovascular collapse, respiratory failure, acute myocardial infarction, acute congestive heart failure, and septicemia; acute or chronic metabolic acidosis with or without coma (including diabetic ketoacidosis); should be temporarily discontinued for 48 hours in patients undergoing radiologic studies involving the intravascular administration of iodinated contrast materials (potential for acute alteration in renal function).

Warnings/Precautions Administration of oral antidiabetic drugs has been reported to be associated with increased cardiovascular mortality. Metformin does not appear to share this risk. Lactic acidosis is a rare, but potentially severe consequence of therapy with metformin. Withhold therapy in hypoxemia, dehydration, or sepsis. The risk of lactic acidosis is increased in any patient with CHF requiring pharmacologic management. This risk is particularly high during acute or unstable CHF because of the risk of hypoperfusion and hypoxemia. The risk of accumulation and lactic acidosis also increases with the degree of impairment of renal function. Patients with renal function below the limit of normal for their age should not receive metformin. In elderly patients, renal function should be monitored regularly; should not be used in any patient ≥80 years of age unless measurement of creatinine clearance verifies normal renal function. Use of concomitant medications that may affect renal function (ie, affect tubular secretion) may also affect metformin disposition. Therapy should be suspended for any surgical procedures (resume only after normal intake resumed and normal renal function is verified). Avoid use in patients with impaired liver function. Patient must be instructed to avoid excessive acute or chronic ethanol use. Lactic acidosis should be suspected in any diabetic patient receiving metformin who has evidence of acidosis when evidence of ketoacidosis is lacking. Safety and efficacy of metformin have been established for use in children ≥10 years of age; the extended release preparation is for use in patients ≥17 years of age.

Drug Interactions

Decreased Effect: Drugs which tend to produce hyperglycemia (eg, diuretics, corticosteroids, phenothiazines, thyroid products, estrogens, oral contraceptives, phenytoin, nicotinic acid, sympathomimetics, calcium channel blocking drugs, isoniazid) may lead to a loss of glucose control.

Increased Effect/Toxicity: Furosemide and cimetidine may increase metformin blood levels. Cationic drugs (eg, amiloride, digoxin, morphine, procainamide, quinidine, quinine, ranitidine, triamterene, trimethoprim, and vancomycin) which are eliminated by renal tubular secretion have the potential to increase metformin levels by competing for common renal tubular transport systems.

Nutritional/Ethanol Interactions

Ethanol: Avoid or limit ethanol (incidence of lactic acidosis may be increased; may cause hypoglycemia).

Food: Food decreases the extent and slightly delays the absorption. May decrease absorption of vitamin B_{12} and/or folic acid.

Herb/Nutraceutical: Caution with chromium, garlic, gymnema (may cause hypoglycemia).

Adverse Reactions

>10%:

Gastrointestinal: Nausea/vomiting (6% to 25%), diarrhea (10% to 53%), flatulence (12%)

Neuromuscular & skeletal: Weakness (9%)

1% to 10%:

Cardiovascular: Chest discomfort, flushing, palpitation

Central nervous system: Headache (6%), chills, dizziness, lightheadedness

Dermatologic: Rash

Endocrine & metabolic: Hypoglycemia

Gastrointestinal: Indigestion (7%), abdominal discomfort (6%), abdominal distention, abnormal stools, constipation, dyspepsia/ heartburn, taste disorder

Neuromuscular & skeletal: Myalgia

Respiratory: Dyspnea, upper respiratory tract infection

Miscellaneous: Decreased vitamin B_{12} levels (7%), increased diaphoresis, flu-like syndrome, nail disorder

<1% (Limited to important or life-threatening): Lactic acidosis, megaloblastic anemia

Overdosage/Toxicology Hypoglycemia has not been observed with ingestion up to 85 g of metformin, although lactic acidosis has occurred in such circumstances. Metformin is dialyzable with a clearance of up to 170 mL/minute. Hemodialysis may be useful for removal of accumulated drug from patients in whom metformin overdose is suspected. Treatment is supportive.

Pharmacodynamics/Kinetics

Bioavailability: Absolute: Fasting: 50% to 60%

Half-Life Elimination: Plasma: 6.2 hours

Onset: Within days; maximum effects up to 2 weeks

Formulations

Tablet, as hydrochloride: 500 mg, 850 mg, 1000 mg

Tablet, extended release, as hydrochloride: 500 mg

Dosing

Adults: Note: Oral (allow 1-2 weeks between dose titrations): Generally, clinically significant responses are not seen at doses <1500 mg daily; however, a lower recommended starting dose and gradual increased dosage is recommended to minimize gastrointestinal symptoms

Adults ≥17 years: Management of type 2 diabetes mellitus: Oral:

500 mg tablets: Initial: 500 mg twice daily (give with the morning and evening meals); dosage increases should be made in increments of 1 tablet every week, given in divided doses, up to a maximum of 2500 mg/day. Doses of up to 2000 mg/day may be given twice daily; if a dose of 2500 mg/day is required, it may be better tolerated 3 times/day (with meals).

850 mg tablets: Initial: 850 mg once daily (give with the morning meal); dosage increases should be made in increments of 1 tablet every **other** week, given in divided doses, up to a maximum of 2550 mg/day. Usual maintenance dose: 850 mg twice daily (with the morning and evening meals). Some patients may be given 850 mg 3 times/day (with meals).

Extended release tablets: Initial: 500 mg once daily (with the evening meal); dosage may be increased by 500 mg weekly; maximum dose: 2000 mg once daily. If glycemic control is not achieved at maximum dose, may divide dose to 1000 mg twice daily; if doses >2000 mg/day are needed, switch to regular release tablets and titrate to maximum dose of 2550 mg/day

Transfer from other antidiabetic agents: No transition period is generally necessary except when transferring from chlorpropamide. When transferring from chlorpropamide, care should be exercised during the first 2 weeks because of the prolonged retention of chlorpropamide in the body, leading to overlapping drug effects and possible hypoglycemia.

Concomitant metformin and oral sulfonylurea therapy: If patients have not responded to 4 weeks of the maximum dose of metformin monotherapy, consider a gradual addition of an oral sulfonylurea, even if prior primary or secondary failure to a sulfonylurea has occurred. Continue metformin at the maximum dose.

Failed sulfonylurea therapy: Patients with prior failure on glyburide may be treated by gradual addition of metformin. Initiate with glyburide 20 mg and metformin 500 mg daily. Metformin dosage may be increased by 500 mg/day at weekly intervals, up to a maximum of 2500 mg/day (dosage of glyburide maintained at 20 mg/day).

Concomitant metformin and insulin therapy: Initial: 500 mg metformin once daily, continue current insulin dose; increase by 500 mg metformin weekly until adequate glycemic control is achieved

Maximum dose: 2500 mg metformin; 2000 mg metformin extended release

Decrease insulin dose 10% to 25% when FPG <120 mg/dL; monitor and make further adjustments as needed

Elderly: The initial and maintenance dosing should be conservative, due to the potential for decreased renal function. Generally, elderly patients should **not** be titrated to the maximum dose of metformin.

Pediatrics: Note: Allow 1-2 weeks between dose titrations: Generally, clinically significant responses are not seen at doses <1500 mg daily; however, a lower recommended starting dose and gradual increased dosage is recommended to minimize gastrointestinal symptoms

Children 10-16 years: Management of type 2 diabetes mellitus: Oral: 500 mg tablets: Initial: 500 mg twice daily (give with the morning and evening meals); dosage increases should be made in increments of 1 tablet every week, given in divided doses, up to a maximum of 2000 mg/day

Renal Impairment: The plasma and blood half-life of metformin is prolonged and the renal clearance is decreased in proportion to the decrease in creatinine clearance. Metformin is contraindicated in the presence of renal dysfunction defined as a serum creatinine >1.5 mg/dL in males or >1.4 mg/dL in females or a creatinine clearance <60 mL/minute.

Hepatic Impairment: Avoid metformin; liver disease is a risk factor for the development of lactic acidosis during metformin therapy.

(Continued)

Metformin *(Continued)*

Administration

Oral: Extended release dosage form should be swallowed whole; do not crush, break, or chew

Stability

Storage: Store at 20°C to 25°C (68°F to 77°F).

Monitoring Laboratory Tests Urine for glucose and ketones, fasting blood glucose, hemoglobin A_{1c}, and fructosamine. Initial and periodic monitoring of hematologic parameters (eg, hemoglobin/hematocrit and red blood cell indices) and renal function should be performed, at least annually. While megaloblastic anemia has been rarely seen with metformin, if suspected, vitamin B_{12} deficiency should be excluded.

Monitoring and Teaching Issues

Physical Assessment: See Contraindications, Warnings/Precautions, and Dosing for use cautions. Assess potential for interactions with other prescriptions, OTC medications, or herbal products patient may be taking (eg, anything that may effect glucose levels - see Drug Interactions). Assess results of laboratory tests (see above), therapeutic effects, and adverse response (eg, assess for signs and symptoms of vitamin B_{12} and/or folic acid deficiency; supplementation may be required - see Adverse Reactions and Overdose/Toxicology) during therapy. Teach patient (or refer patient to diabetic educator for instruction) in appropriate use, possible side effects and appropriate interventions, and adverse symptoms to report (see Patient Education). Breast-feeding is not recommended.

Patient Education: Inform prescriber of all prescriptions, OTC medications, or herbal products you are taking, and any allergies you have. Do not take anything new during treatment unless approved by prescriber. Take as directed (may take with food to decrease GI upset). Do not chew or crush tablets. Parts of extended-release tablets may be excreted in the stool (normal). Do not change dosage or discontinue without consulting prescriber. Avoid overuse of alcohol (could cause severe reaction). It is important to follow dietary and lifestyle recommendations of prescriber. You will be instructed in signs of hypo- or hyperglycemia by prescriber or diabetic educator. May cause drowsiness or dizziness (use caution driving or engaging in potentially hazardous tasks until response to drug is known); nausea or vomiting (taking with meals, eating small, frequent meals, frequent mouth care, or sucking lozenges may help); or abdominal distention, flatulence, diarrhea, constipation, or heartburn (if these persist consult prescriber for approved medication). Report immediately unusual weakness or fatigue; unusual muscle pain; persistent GI discomfort; dizziness or lightheadedness; sudden difficulty breathing, chest discomfort, slow or irregular heartbeat; or other adverse reactions. **Breast-feeding precaution:** Breast-feeding is not recommended.

Dietary Issues: Drug may cause GI upset; take with food (to decrease GI upset). Take at the same time each day. Dietary modification based on ADA recommendations is a part of therapy. Monitor for signs and symptoms of vitamin B_{12} and/or folic acid deficiency; supplementation may be required.

Geriatric Considerations: Limited data suggests that metformin's total body clearance may be decreased and AUC and half-life increased in older patients; presumably due to decreased renal clearance. Metformin has been well tolerated by the elderly but lower doses and frequent monitoring are recommended.

Breast-feeding Issues: It is not known if metformin is excreted in human breast milk (excretion occurs in animal models); insulin therapy should be considered in breast-feeding women.

Pregnancy Issues: Abnormal blood glucose levels are associated with a higher incidence of congenital abnormalities. Insulin is the drug of choice for the control of diabetes mellitus during pregnancy.

Related Information

Antidiabetic Oral Agents Comparison *on page 1556*
Diabetes Mellitus Management *on page 1661*

Metformin Hydrochloride *see* Metformin *on page 866*
Methacholine *see page 1461*

Methadone (METH a done)

U.S. Brand Names Dolophine®; Methadose®

Synonyms Methadone Hydrochloride

Restrictions C-II

Generic Available Yes

Pharmacologic Category Analgesic, Narcotic

Pregnancy Risk Factor B/D (prolonged use or high doses at term)

Lactation Enters breast milk/use caution (AAP rates "compatible")

Use Management of severe pain; detoxification and maintenance treatment of narcotic addiction (if used for detoxification and maintenance treatment of narcotic addiction, it must be part of an FDA-approved program)

Mechanism of Action/Effect Binds to opiate receptors in the CNS, causing inhibition of ascending pain pathways, altering the perception of and response to pain; produces generalized CNS depression

Contraindications Hypersensitivity to methadone or any component of the formulation; pregnancy (prolonged use or high doses near term)

Warnings/Precautions Because methadone's effects on respiration last much longer than its analgesic effects, the dose must be titrated slowly; not considered a drug of first choice in the elderly, who may be particularly susceptible to its CNS depressant and constipating effects. May cause respiratory depression - use caution in patients with respiratory disease or pre-existing respiratory depression. Potential for drug dependency exists, abrupt cessation may precipitate withdrawal. Use caution in elderly, debilitated, or pediatric patients.

Use with caution in patients with depression or suicidal tendencies, or in patients with a history of drug abuse. Tolerance or psychological and physical dependence may occur with prolonged use. Use with caution in patients with hepatic, pulmonary, or renal function impairment. May cause CNS depression, which may impair physical or mental abilities. Effects with other sedative drugs or ethanol may be potentiated. Elderly may be more sensitive to CNS depressant and constipating effects. Use with caution in patients with head injury or increased ICP, biliary tract dysfunction or pancreatitis; history of ileus or bowel obstruction, glaucoma, hyperthyroidism, adrenal insufficiency, prostatic hyperplasia or urinary stricture, CNS depression, toxic psychosis, alcoholism, delirium tremens, or kyphoscoliosis. Tablets are to be used only for oral administration and must not be used for injection.

Drug Interactions

Cytochrome P450 Effect: Substrate of CYP2C8/9, 2C19, 2D6, **3A4**; Inhibits **CYP2D6**, 3A4

Decreased Effect: Barbiturates, carbamazepine, nevirapine, phenytoin, primidone, rifampin and ritonavir may decrease serum methadone concentrations via enhanced hepatic metabolism; monitor for methadone withdrawal. Larger doses of methadone may be required.

Increased Effect/Toxicity: Fluconazole, itraconazole, and ketoconazole increase serum methadone concentrations via CYP3A4 inhibition; an increased narcotic effect may be experienced. Similar effects may be seen with ritonavir, nelfinavir, amiodarone, erythromycin, clarithromycin, diltiazem, verapamil, paroxetine, fluoxetine, and other inhibitors of CYP2D6 or CYP3A4.

Nutritional/Ethanol Interactions

Ethanol: Avoid ethanol (may increase CNS effects). Watch for sedation.

Herb/Nutraceutical: Avoid St John's wort (may decrease methadone levels; may increase CNS depression). Avoid valerian, kava kava, gotu kola (may increase CNS depression). Methadone is metabolized by CYP3A4 in the intestines; avoid concurrent use of grapefruit juice.

Effects on Lab Values ↑ thyroxine (S), aminotransferase [ALT (SGPT)/AST (SGOT)] (S)

Adverse Reactions Frequency not defined.

Cardiovascular: Bradycardia, peripheral vasodilation, cardiac arrest, syncope, faintness

Central nervous system: Euphoria, dysphoria, headache, insomnia, agitation, disorientation, drowsiness, dizziness, lightheadedness, sedation

Dermatologic: Pruritus, urticaria, rash

Endocrine & metabolic: Decreased libido

Gastrointestinal: Nausea, vomiting, constipation, anorexia, stomach cramps, xerostomia, biliary tract spasm

Genitourinary: Urinary retention or hesitancy, antidiuretic effect, impotence

Neuromuscular & skeletal: Weakness

Ocular: Miosis, visual disturbances

Respiratory: Respiratory depression, respiratory arrest

Miscellaneous: Physical and psychological dependence

Overdosage/Toxicology Symptoms of overdose include respiratory depression, CNS depression, miosis, hypothermia, circulatory collapse, and convulsions. Treatment is supportive. Naloxone, 2 mg I.V. with repeat administration as necessary up to a total of 10 mg, can also be used to reverse toxic effects of the opiate.

Pharmacodynamics/Kinetics

Half-Life Elimination: 15-29 hours; may be prolonged with alkaline pH

Metabolism: Hepatic via N-demethylation

Onset: Oral: Analgesic: 0.5-1 hour; Parenteral: 10-20 minutes; Peak effect: Parenteral: 1-2 hours

Duration: Oral: 6-8 hours, increases to 22-48 hours with repeated doses

Formulations

Injection, as hydrochloride: 10 mg/mL (20 mL)

Solution, oral, as hydrochloride: 5 mg/5 mL (5 mL, 500 mL); 10 mg/5 mL (500 mL)

Solution, oral concentrate, as hydrochloride: 10 mg/mL (30 mL)

Tablet, as hydrochloride: 5 mg, 10 mg

Tablet, dispersible, as hydrochloride: 40 mg

Dosing

Adults: Important note: Methadone accumulates with repeated doses and dosage may need to be adjusted downward after 3-5 days to prevent toxic effects. Some patients may benefit from every 8- to 12-hour dosing interval (pain control). Doses should be titrated to appropriate effects.

Analgesia: Oral, I.M., S.C.: 2.5-10 mg every 3-8 hours as needed, up to 5-20 mg every 6-8 hours. Higher doses may be required in patients with severe, debilitating pain or in patients who have become narcotic tolerant.

Detoxification: Oral: 15-40 mg/day; should not exceed 21 days and may not be repeated earlier than 4 weeks after completion of preceding course

Maintenance of opiate dependence: Oral: 20-120 mg/day

Elderly: Important note: Methadone accumulates with repeated doses and dosage may need to be adjusted downward after 3-5 days to prevent toxic effects. Some patients may benefit from every 8- to 12-hour dosing interval (pain control). Doses should be titrated to appropriate effects: Oral, I.M.: 2.5 mg every 8-12 hours (see Geriatrics Considerations).

Pediatrics: Important note: Methadone accumulates with repeated doses and dosage may need to be adjusted downward after 3-5 days to prevent toxic effects. Some patients may benefit from every 8- to 12-hour dosing interval (pain control). Doses should be titrated to appropriate effects. Children: Analgesia:

Oral, I.M., S.C.: 0.7 mg/kg/24 hours divided every 4-6 hours as needed or 0.1-0.2 mg/kg every 4-12 hours as needed; maximum: 10 mg/dose

I.V.: 0.1 mg/kg every 4 hours initially for 2-3 doses, then every 6-12 hours as needed; maximum: 10 mg/dose

Renal Impairment:

Cl_{cr} <10 mL/minute: Administer 50% to 75% of normal dose. **Important note:** Methadone accumulates with repeated doses and dosage may need to be adjusted downward after

(Continued)

Methadone *(Continued)*

3-5 days to prevent toxic effects. Some patients may benefit from every 8- to 12-hour dosing interval (pain control).

Hepatic Impairment: Avoid in severe liver disease.

Stability

Compatibility: Stable in NS; highly **incompatible** with all other I.V. agents when mixed together

Monitoring and Teaching Issues

Physical Assessment: Assess other medications patient may be taking for additive or adverse interactions (see Drug Interactions). Monitor therapeutic effectiveness adverse reactions of overdose at beginning of therapy and at regular intervals with long-term use (see Adverse Reactions and Overdose/Toxicology). May cause physical and/or psychological dependence. For inpatients, implement safety measures. Assess knowledge/teach patient appropriate use (if self-administered) adverse reactions to report, and appropriate interventions to reduce side effects. Discontinue slowly after prolonged use. **Pregnancy risk factor B/D** - see Pregnancy Risk Factor for use cautions. Note breast-feeding caution.

Patient Education: If self-administered, use exactly as directed; do not increase dose or frequency. Drug may cause physical and/or psychological dependence. While using this medication, do not use alcohol and other prescription or OTC medications (especially sedatives, tranquilizers, antihistamines, or pain medications) without consulting prescriber. Maintain adequate hydration (2-3 L/day of fluids) unless advised by prescriber to restrict fluids. May cause hypotension, dizziness, drowsiness, impaired coordination, or blurred vision (use caution when driving, climbing stairs, or changing position - rising from sitting or lying to standing, or when engaging in tasks requiring alertness until response to drug is known); loss of appetite, nausea, or vomiting (frequent mouth care, small, frequent meals, chewing gum, or sucking lozenges may help); or constipation (increased exercise, fluids, fruit, or fiber may help; if unresolved, consult prescriber about use of stool softeners). Report chest pain, slow or rapid heartbeat, acute dizziness or persistent headache; changes in mental status; swelling of extremities or unusual weight gain; changes in urinary elimination; acute headache; back or flank pain or muscle spasms; blurred vision; skin rash; or shortness of breath. **Pregnancy/breast-feeding precautions:** Inform prescriber if you are or intend to become pregnant. If you are breast-feeding, take medication immediately after breast-feeding or 3-4 hours prior to next feeding.

Geriatric Considerations: Because of its long half-life and risk of accumulation, methadone is not considered a drug of first choice in the elderly. The elderly may be particularly susceptible to the CNS depressant and constipating effects of narcotics. Adjust dose for renal function.

Additional Information Methadone accumulates with repeated doses and dosage may need to be adjusted downward after 3-5 days to prevent toxic effects. Some patients may benefit from every 8- to 12-hour dosing interval (pain control). Oral dose for detoxification and maintenance may be administered in Tang®, Kool-Aid®, apple juice, grape Crystal Light®.

Related Information

Controlled Substances Comparison *on page 1568*
Narcotic/Opioid Analgesic Comparison *on page 1583*

Methadone Hydrochloride *see* Methadone *on page 868*
Methadose® *see* Methadone *on page 868*
Methaminodiazepoxide Hydrochloride *see* Chlordiazepoxide *on page 273*
Methamphetamine *see page 1693*

Methenamine (meth EN a meen)

U.S. Brand Names Hiprex®; Urex®

Synonyms Hexamethylenetetramine; Methenamine Hippurate; Methenamine Mandelate

Generic Available Yes

Pharmacologic Category Antibiotic, Miscellaneous

Pregnancy Risk Factor C

Lactation Enters breast milk/compatible

Use Prophylaxis or suppression of recurrent urinary tract infections; urinary tract discomfort secondary to hypermotility

Mechanism of Action/Effect Methenamine is hydrolyzed to formaldehyde and ammonia in acidic urine; formaldehyde has nonspecific bactericidal action

Contraindications Hypersensitivity to methenamine or any component of the formulation; severe dehydration, renal insufficiency, hepatic insufficiency in patients receiving hippurate salt; patients receiving sulfonamides

Warnings/Precautions Use with caution in patients with hepatic disease, gout, and the elderly; doses of 8 g/day for 3-4 weeks may cause bladder irritation, some products may contain tartrazine; methenamine should not be used to treat infections outside of the lower urinary tract. Use care to maintain an acid pH of the urine, especially when treating infections due to urea splitting organisms (eg, *Proteus* and strains of *Pseudomonas*); reversible increases in LFTs have occurred during therapy especially in patients with hepatic dysfunction. Pregnancy risk C.

Drug Interactions

Decreased Effect: Sodium bicarbonate and acetazolamide will decrease effect secondary to alkalinization of urine.

Increased Effect/Toxicity: Sulfonamides may precipitate in the urine.

Nutritional/Ethanol Interactions Food: Foods/diets which alkalinize urine pH >5.5 decrease therapeutic effect of methenamine.

Effects on Lab Values ↑ catecholamines and VMA (U); ↓ HIAA (U)

Adverse Reactions

1% to 10%:

- Dermatologic: Rash (4%)
- Gastrointestinal: Nausea, dyspepsia (4%)
- Genitourinary: Dysuria (4%)

<1% (Limited to important or life-threatening): Bladder irritation, crystalluria (especially with large doses), increased AST/ALT (reversible, rare)

Overdosage/Toxicology The drug is well tolerated. Treatment is supportive.

Pharmacodynamics/Kinetics

Absorption: Readily

Half-Life Elimination: 3-6 hours

Metabolism: Gastric juices: Hydrolyze 10% to 30% unless protected via enteric coating; Hepatic: ~10% to 25%

Formulations

Suspension, oral, as mandelate: 0.5 g/5 mL (480 mL)

Tablet, as hippurate (Hiprex®, Urex®): 1 g [Hiprex® contains tartrazine dye]

Tablet, enteric coated, as mandelate: 500 mg, 1 g

Dosing

Adults & Elderly: Urinary tract infection: Oral:

Hippurate: 0.5 to 1 g twice daily

Mandelate: 1 g 4 times/day after meals and at bedtime

Pediatrics: Oral:

<6 years: 0.25 g/30 lb 4 times/day

6-12 years:

Hippurate: 25-50 mg/kg/day divided every 12 hours or 0.5-1 g twice daily

Mandelate: 50-75 mg/kg/day divided every 6 hours or 0.5 g 4 times/day

>12 years: Refer to adult dosing.

Renal Impairment: Cl_{cr} <50 mL/minute: Avoid use.

Administration

Oral: Administer around-the-clock to promote less variation in effect. Foods/diets which alkalinize urine pH >5.5 decrease activity of methenamine.

Stability

Storage: Protect from excessive heat

Monitoring Laboratory Tests Urinalysis, periodic liver function

Monitoring and Teaching Issues

Physical Assessment: See Contraindications and Warnings/Precautions for use cautions. Assess potential for interactions with other prescriptions, OTC medications, or herbal products patient may be taking (see Drug Interactions). Assess results of laboratory tests (see above), therapeutic effects, and adverse response (see Adverse Reactions and Overdose/Toxicology) during therapy. Teach patient proper use, possible side effects and appropriate interventions, and adverse symptoms to report (see Patient Education). **Pregnancy risk factor C** - benefits of use should outweigh possible risks.

Patient Education: Inform prescriber of all prescriptions, OTC medications, or herbal products you are taking, and any allergies you have. Do not take anything new during treatment unless approved by prescriber. Take per recommended schedule, at regular intervals around-the-clock. Complete full course of therapy; do not skip doses. Maintain adequate hydration (2-3 L/day of fluids) unless advised by prescriber to restrict fluids. Avoid excessive citrus fruits, milk, or alkalizing medications. May cause nausea or vomiting or GI upset (small, frequent meals, frequent mouth care, sucking lozenges, or chewing gum may help). Report pain on urination or blood in urine, skin rash, other persistent adverse effects, or if condition does not improve. **Pregnancy precaution:** Inform prescriber if you are or intend to become pregnant.

Dietary Issues: Foods/diets which alkalinize urine pH >5.5 decrease activity of methenamine; cranberry juice can be used to acidify urine and increase activity of methenamine. Hiprex® contains tartrazine dye.

Geriatric Considerations: Methenamine has little, if any, role in the treatment or prevention of infections in patients with indwelling urinary (Foley®) catheters. Furthermore, in noncatheterized patients, more effective antibiotics are available for the prevention or treatment of urinary tract infections. The influence of decreased renal function on the pharmacologic effects of methenamine results are unknown.

Additional Information Should not be used to treat infections outside of the lower urinary tract. Methenamine has little, if any, role in the treatment or prevention of infections in patients with indwelling urinary (Foley) catheters. Furthermore, in noncatheterized patients, more effective antibiotics are available for the prevention or treatment of urinary tract infections. The influence of decreased renal function on the pharmacologic effects of methenamine results are unknown.

Methenamine Hippurate *see* Methenamine *on page 870*

Methenamine Mandelate *see* Methenamine *on page 870*

Methergine® *see* Methylergonovine *on page 881*

Methimazole (meth IM a zole)

U.S. Brand Names Tapazole®

Synonyms Thiamazole

Generic Available Yes

Pharmacologic Category Antithyroid Agent

Pregnancy Risk Factor D

Lactation Enters breast milk/contraindicated (manufacturer) (AAP rates "compatible")

Use Palliative treatment of hyperthyroidism, return the hyperthyroid patient to a normal metabolic state prior to thyroidectomy, and to control thyrotoxic crisis that may accompany thyroidectomy. The use of antithyroid thioamides is as effective in elderly as they are in younger adults; however, the expense, potential adverse effects, and inconvenience (compliance, monitoring) make them undesirable. The use of radioiodine due to ease of administration and less concern for long-term side effects and reproduction problems (some older males) makes it a more appropriate therapy.

Mechanism of Action/Effect Inhibits the synthesis of thyroid hormones by blocking the oxidation of iodine in the thyroid gland, blocking iodine's ability to combine with tyrosine to form thyroxine and triiodothyronine (T_3), does not inactivate circulating T_4 and T_3

(Continued)

Methimazole *(Continued)*

Contraindications Hypersensitivity to methimazole or any component of the formulation; nursing mothers (per manufacturer; however, expert analysis and the AAP state this drug may be used with caution in nursing mothers); pregnancy

Warnings/Precautions Use with extreme caution in patients receiving other drugs known to cause myelosuppression particularly agranulocytosis, patients >40 years of age. Avoid doses >40 mg/day (↑ myelosuppression). May cause acneiform eruptions or worsen the condition of the thyroid.

Drug Interactions

Cytochrome P450 Effect: Inhibits CYP1A2, 2A6, 2B6, 2C8/9, 2C19, 2D6, 2E1, 3A4

Increased Effect/Toxicity: Increased toxicity with lithium or potassium iodide. Anticoagulant effect of warfarin may be increased. Dosage of some drugs (including beta-blockers, digoxin, and theophylline) require adjustment during treatment of hyperthyroidism.

Adverse Reactions Frequency not defined.

Cardiovascular: Edema

Central nervous system: Headache, vertigo, drowsiness, CNS stimulation, depression

Dermatologic: Skin rash, urticaria, pruritus, erythema nodosum, skin pigmentation, exfoliative dermatitis, alopecia

Endocrine & metabolic: Goiter

Gastrointestinal: Nausea, vomiting, stomach pain, abnormal taste, constipation, weight gain, salivary gland swelling

Hematologic: Leukopenia, agranulocytosis, granulocytopenia, thrombocytopenia, aplastic anemia, hypoprothrombinemia

Hepatic: Cholestatic jaundice, jaundice, hepatitis

Neuromuscular & skeletal: Arthralgia, paresthesia

Renal: Nephrotic syndrome

Miscellaneous: SLE-like syndrome

Overdosage/Toxicology Symptoms of overdose include nausea, vomiting, epigastric distress, headache, fever, arthralgia, pruritus, edema, pancytopenia, and signs of hypothyroidism. Management of overdose is supportive.

Pharmacodynamics/Kinetics

Bioavailability: 80% to 95%

Half-Life Elimination: 4-13 hours

Metabolism: Hepatic

Onset: Antithyroid: Oral: 12-18 hours

Duration: 36-72 hours

Formulations Tablet: 5 mg, 10 mg

Dosing

Adults & Elderly: Hyperthyroidism: Oral: Administer in 3 equally divided doses at approximately 8-hour intervals

Initial: 15 mg/day for mild hyperthyroidism; 30-40 mg/day in moderately severe hyperthyroidism; 60 mg/day in severe hyperthyroidism; maintenance: 5-15 mg/day

Adjust dosage as required to achieve and maintain serum T_3, T_4, and TSH levels in the normal range. An elevated T_3 may be the sole indicator of inadequate treatment. An elevated TSH indicates excessive antithyroid treatment.

Pediatrics: Oral: Administer in 3 equally divided doses at ~8-hour intervals.

Children: Initial: 0.4 mg/kg/day in 3 divided doses; maintenance: 0.2 mg/kg/day in 3 divided doses up to 30 mg/24 hours maximum

Alternatively: Initial: 0.5-0.7 mg/kg/day **or** 15-20 mg/m^2/day in 3 divided doses

Maintenance: $^1/_3$ to $^2/_3$ of the initial dose beginning when the patient is euthyroid

Maximum: 30 mg/24 hours

Stability

Storage: Protect from light.

Monitoring Laboratory Tests T_4, T_3, CBC with differential, liver function (baseline and as needed), serum thyroxine, free thyroxine index

Monitoring and Teaching Issues

Physical Assessment: See Contraindications, Warnings/Precautions, and Dosing for use cautions. Assess potential for interactions with other prescriptions, OTC medications, or herbal products patient may be taking (see Drug Interactions). Assess results of laboratory tests (see above), therapeutic effects, and patient response (eg, hyper/hypothyroidism - see Adverse Reactions and Overdose/Toxicology) during therapy. Teach patient proper use, possible side effects and appropriate interventions, and adverse symptoms to report (see Patient Education). **Pregnancy risk factor D** - determine that patient is not pregnant before beginning treatment. Instruct patient in appropriate use of barrier contraceptive measures during therapy. Breast-feeding is contraindicated.

Patient Education: Inform prescriber of all prescriptions, OTC medications, or herbal products you are taking, and any allergies you have. Do not take anything new during treatment unless approved by prescriber. Take as directed, at the same time each day, around-the-clock (eg, every 8 hours). Do not miss doses or make up missed doses. This drug will need to be taken for an extended period of time to achieve appropriate results. May cause nausea or vomiting (small, frequent meals may help); or dizziness or drowsiness (use caution when driving or engaging in tasks that require alertness until response to drug is known). Report rash, fever, unusual bleeding or bruising, unresolved headache, yellowing of eyes or skin, changes in color of urine or feces, or unresolved malaise. **Pregnancy/breast-feeding precautions:** Inform prescriber if you are pregnant and do not get pregnant while taking this medicine. Consult prescriber for appropriate barrier contraceptive measures. Do not breast-feed.

Dietary Issues: Should be taken consistently in relation to meals every day.

Geriatric Considerations: The use of antithyroid thioamides is as effective in the elderly as in younger adults; however, the expense, potential adverse effects, and inconvenience (compliance, monitoring) make them undesirable.

Breast-feeding Issues: Use with caution; consider monitoring thyroid function in the infant (weekly or biweekly)

Methocarbamol (meth oh KAR ba mole)

U.S. Brand Names Robaxin®

Generic Available Yes

Pharmacologic Category Skeletal Muscle Relaxant

Pregnancy Risk Factor C

Lactation Enters breast milk/compatible

Use Treatment of muscle spasm associated with acute painful musculoskeletal conditions, supportive therapy in tetanus

Mechanism of Action/Effect Causes skeletal muscle relaxation by reducing the transmission of impulses from the spinal cord to skeletal muscle

Contraindications Hypersensitivity to methocarbamol or any component of the formulation; renal impairment

Warnings/Precautions Rate of injection should not exceed 3 mL/minute. Solution is hypertonic. Avoid extravasation. Use with caution in patients with a history of seizures. Pregnancy risk C.

Drug Interactions

Increased Effect/Toxicity: Increased effect/toxicity with CNS depressants.

Nutritional/Ethanol Interactions

Ethanol: Avoid ethanol (may increase CNS depression).

Herb/Nutraceutical: Avoid valerian, St John's wort, kava kava, gotu kola (may increase CNS depression).

Adverse Reactions Frequency not defined.

Cardiovascular: Flushing of face, bradycardia, hypotension

Central nervous system: Drowsiness, dizziness, lightheadedness, syncope, convulsion, vertigo, headache, fever

Dermatologic: Allergic dermatitis, urticaria, pruritus, rash

Gastrointestinal: Nausea, vomiting, metallic taste

Hematologic: Leukopenia

Local: Pain at injection site, thrombophlebitis

Ocular: Nystagmus, blurred vision, diplopia, conjunctivitis

Renal: Renal impairment

Respiratory: Nasal congestion

Miscellaneous: Allergic manifestations, anaphylactic reaction

Overdosage/Toxicology Symptoms of overdose include cardiac arrhythmias, nausea, vomiting, drowsiness, and coma. Treatment is supportive.

Pharmacodynamics/Kinetics

Half-Life Elimination: 1-2 hours

Time to Peak: Serum: ~2 hours

Metabolism: Hepatic

Onset: Muscle relaxation: Oral: ~30 minutes

Formulations

Injection: 100 mg/mL [in polyethylene glycol 50%] (10 mL)

Tablet: 500 mg, 750 mg

Dosing

Adults: Muscle spasm:

Oral: 1.5 g 4 times/day for 2-3 days, then decrease to 4-4.5 g/day in 3-6 divided doses

I.M., I.V.: 1 g every 8 hours if oral not possible

Elderly: Oral: Initial: 500 mg 4 times/day; titrate to response.

Pediatrics: Tetanus (recommended **only** for use in tetanus): I.V.: 15 mg/kg/dose or 500 mg/m^2/dose, may repeat every 6 hours if needed; maximum dose: 1.8 g/m^2/day for 3 days only

Renal Impairment: Do not administer parenteral formulation to patients with renal dysfunction.

Administration

Oral: Tablets may be crushed and mixed with food or liquid if needed. Avoid alcohol.

I.V.: Maximum rate is 3 mL/minute.

Stability

Storage: Injection when diluted to 4 mg/mL in sterile water, 5% dextrose, or 0.9% saline is stable for 6 days at room temperature; do **not** refrigerate after dilution

Monitoring and Teaching Issues

Physical Assessment: Assess other medications for excess CNS depression. See Contraindications and Warnings/Precautions for use cautions. Monitor effectiveness of therapy (according to rational for therapy) and adverse reactions (see Adverse Reactions) at beginning and periodically during therapy. Monitor I.V. site closely to prevent extravasation. Assess knowledge/teach patient appropriate use, interventions to reduce side effects, and adverse symptoms to report (see Patient Education). **Pregnancy risk factor C** - benefits of use should outweigh possible risks.

Patient Education: Take exactly as directed. Do not increase dose or discontinue without consulting prescriber. Do not use alcohol, prescriptive or OTC antidepressants, sedatives, or pain medications without consulting prescriber. You may experience drowsiness, dizziness, lightheadedness (avoid driving or engaging in tasks requiring alertness until response to drug is known); or nausea or vomiting (small, frequent meals, frequent mouth care, or sucking hard candy may help). Report excessive drowsiness or mental agitation, chest pain, skin rash, swelling of mouth/face, difficulty speaking, or vision changes. **Pregnancy precaution:** Inform prescriber if you are or intend to become pregnant.

Geriatric Considerations: There is no specific information on the use of skeletal muscle relaxants in the elderly. Methocarbamol has a short half-life, so it may be considered one of the safer agents in this class.

Methocarbamol and Aspirin (meth oh KAR ba mole & AS pir in)

U.S. Brand Names Robaxisal®

Synonyms Aspirin and Methocarbamol

Generic Available Yes

Pharmacologic Category Skeletal Muscle Relaxant

Pregnancy Risk Factor C/D (full-dose aspirin in 3rd trimester)

Lactation Enters breast milk/use caution due to aspirin content

Use Adjunct to rest, physical therapy, and other measures for the relief of discomfort associated with acute, painful musculoskeletal disorders

Formulations Tablet: Methocarbamol 400 mg and aspirin 325 mg

Dosing

Adults: Muscle spasm/pain: Oral: 2 tablets 4 times/day

Elderly: Refer to dosing in individual monographs.

Monitoring and Teaching Issues

Physical Assessment: See individual components listed in Related Information. **Pregnancy risk factor C/D** - see Pregnancy Risk Factor for use cautions. Assess knowledge/ instruct patient on need to use appropriate contraceptive measures and the need to avoid pregnancy. Note breast-feeding caution.

Patient Education: See individual components listed in Related Information. **Pregnancy/ breast-feeding precautions:** Inform prescriber if you are or intend to become pregnant. Consult prescriber if breast-feeding.

Related Information

Aspirin *on page 121*
Methocarbamol *on page 873*

Methotrexate (meth oh TREKS ate)

U.S. Brand Names Rheumatrex®; Trexall™

Synonyms Amethopterin; Methotrexate Sodium; MTX

Generic Available Yes

Pharmacologic Category Antineoplastic Agent, Antimetabolite

Pregnancy Risk Factor D

Lactation Enters breast milk/contraindicated

Use Treatment of trophoblastic neoplasms; leukemias; psoriasis; rheumatoid arthritis (RA), including polyarticular-course juvenile rheumatoid arthritis (JRA); breast, head and neck, and lung carcinomas; osteosarcoma; sarcomas; carcinoma of gastric, esophagus, testes; lymphomas; mycosis fungoides (cutaneous T-cell lymphoma)

Mechanism of Action/Effect An antimetabolite that inhibits DNA synthesis and cell reproduction in cancerous cells

Folates must be in the reduced form (FH_4) to be active

Folates are activated by dihydrofolate reductase (DHFR)

DHFR is inhibited by MTX (by binding irreversibly), causing an increase in the intracellular dihydrofolate pool (the inactive cofactor) and inhibition of both purine and thymidylate synthesis (TS)

MTX enters the cell through an energy-dependent and temperature-dependent process which is mediated by an intramembrane protein; this carrier mechanism is also used by naturally occurring reduced folates, including folinic acid (leucovorin), making this a competitive process

At high drug concentrations (>20 μM), MTX enters the cell by a second mechanism which is not shared by reduced folates; the process may be passive diffusion or a specific, saturable process, and provides a rationale for high-dose MTX

A small fraction of MTX is converted intracellularly to polyglutamates, which leads to a prolonged inhibition of DHFR

Contraindications Hypersensitivity to methotrexate or any component of the formulation; severe renal or hepatic impairment; pre-existing profound bone marrow suppression in patients with psoriasis or rheumatoid arthritis, alcoholic liver disease, AIDS, pre-existing blood dyscrasias; pregnancy

Warnings/Precautions The U.S. Food and Drug Administration (FDA) currently recommends that procedures for proper handling and disposal of antineoplastic agents be considered. Appropriate safety equipment is recommended for preparation, administration, and disposal of antineoplastics. If methotrexate contacts the skin, wash and flush thoroughly with water.

May cause photosensitivity type reaction; reduce dosage in patients with renal or hepatic impairment, ascites, and pleural effusion. Use with caution in patients with peptic ulcer disease, ulcerative colitis, or pre-existing bone marrow suppression. Monitor closely for pulmonary disease; use with caution in the elderly. Methotrexate given concomitantly with radiotherapy may increase the risk of soft tissue necrosis and osteonecrosis. Safety and efficacy in pediatric patients have been established only in cancer chemotherapy and polyarticular-course JRA.

Because of the possibility of severe toxic reactions, fully inform patient of the risks involved. May cause hepatotoxicity, fibrosis and cirrhosis, along with marked bone marrow depression. Death from intestinal perforation may occur. Use caution when used with other hepatotoxic agents (azathioprine, retinoids, sulfasalazine).

Severe bone marrow suppression, aplastic anemia, and GI toxicity have occurred during concomitant administration with NSAIDs.

Toxicity from methotrexate or any immunosuppressive is increased in the elderly. Must monitor carefully. For rheumatoid arthritis and psoriasis, immunosuppressive therapy should only be used when disease is active and less toxic; traditional therapy is ineffective. Recommended doses should be reduced when initiating therapy in the elderly due to possible decreased metabolism, reduced renal function, and presence of interacting diseases and drugs.

Methotrexate penetrates slowly into 3rd space fluids, such as pleural effusions or ascites, and exits slowly from these compartments (slower than from plasma). The potential for toxicity may be increased under these conditions. Methotrexate formulations and/or diluents containing preservatives should not be used for intrathecal or high-dose therapy. Methotrexate injection may contain benzyl alcohol and should not be used in neonates.

Drug Interactions

Decreased Effect: Corticosteroids have been reported to decrease methotrexate entry into leukemia cells. Administration should be separated by 12 hours. Dexamethasone has been reported to not affect methotrexate entry. May decrease phenytoin and 5-FU activity.

Increased Effect/Toxicity:

Live virus vaccines → vaccinia infections.

Vincristine: Inhibits MTX efflux from the cell, leading to increased and prolonged MTX levels in the cell; the dose of VCR needed to produce this effect is not achieved clinically.

Organic acids: Salicylates, sulfonamides, probenecid, and high doses of penicillins compete with MTX for transport and reduce renal tubular secretion. Salicylates and sulfonamides may also displace MTX from plasma proteins, increasing MTX levels.

Ara-C: Increased formation of the Ara-C nucleotide can occur when MTX precedes Ara-C, thus promoting the action of Ara-C.

Cyclosporine: CSA and MTX interfere with each other's renal elimination, which may result in increased toxicity.

Nonsteroidal anti-inflammatory drugs (NSAIDs): Severe bone marrow suppression, aplastic anemia, and GI toxicity have been reported with concomitant therapy. Should not be used during moderate or high-dose methotrexate due to increased and prolonged methotrexate levels (may increase toxicity). NSAID use during treatment of rheumatoid arthritis has not been fully explored, but continuation of prior regimen has been allowed in some circumstances, with cautious monitoring.

Patients receiving concomitant therapy with methotrexate and other potential hepatotoxins (eg, azathioprine, retinoids, sulfasalazine) should be closely monitored for possible increased risk of hepatotoxicity.

Nutritional/Ethanol Interactions

Ethanol: Avoid ethanol (may be associated with increased liver injury).

Food: Methotrexate peak serum levels may be decreased if taken with food. Milk-rich foods may decrease MTX absorption. Folate may decrease drug response.

Herb/Nutraceutical: Avoid echinacea (has immunostimulant properties).

Adverse Reactions Frequencies vary widely with dose (chemotherapy versus immune modulation).

>10%:

Cardiovascular: Vasculitis

Central nervous system (with I.T. administration only):

Arachnoiditis: Acute reaction manifested as severe headache, nuchal rigidity, vomiting, and fever; may be alleviated by reducing the dose

Subacute toxicity: 10% of patients treated with 12-15 mg/m^2 of I.T. MTX may develop this in the second or third week of therapy; consists of motor paralysis of extremities, cranial nerve palsy, seizures, or coma. This has also been seen in pediatric cases receiving very high-dose I.V. MTX (when enough MTX can get across into the CSF).

Demyelinating encephalopathy: Seen months or years after receiving MTX; usually in association with cranial irradiation or other systemic chemotherapy

Dermatologic: Reddening of skin

Endocrine & metabolic: Hyperuricemia, defective oogenesis or spermatogenesis

Gastrointestinal: Ulcerative stomatitis, glossitis, gingivitis, nausea, vomiting, diarrhea, anorexia, intestinal perforation, mucositis (dose dependent; appears in 3-7 days after therapy, resolving within 2 weeks)

Emetic potential:

<100 mg: Moderately low (10% to 30%)

≥100 mg or <250 mg: Moderate (30% to 60%)

≥250 mg: Moderately high (60% to 90%)

Hematologic: Leukopenia, thrombocytopenia

Renal: Renal failure, azotemia, nephropathy

Respiratory: Pharyngitis

1% to 10%:

Central nervous system: Dizziness, malaise, encephalopathy, seizures, fever, chills

Dermatologic: Alopecia, rash, photosensitivity, depigmentation or hyperpigmentation of skin

Endocrine & metabolic: Diabetes

Genitourinary: Cystitis

Hematologic: Hemorrhage

Myelosuppressive: This is the primary dose-limiting factor (along with mucositis) of MTX; occurs about 5-7 days after MTX therapy, and should resolve within 2 weeks

WBC: Mild

Platelets: Moderate

Onset: 7 days

Nadir: 10 days

Recovery: 21 days

Hepatic: Cirrhosis and portal fibrosis have been associated with chronic MTX therapy; acute elevation of liver enzymes are common after high-dose MTX, and usually resolve within 10 days.

Neuromuscular & skeletal: Arthralgia

Ocular: Blurred vision

Renal: Renal dysfunction: Manifested by an abrupt rise in serum creatinine and BUN and a fall in urine output; more common with high-dose MTX, and may be due to precipitation of the drug. The best treatment is prevention: Aggressively hydrate with 3 L/m^2/day starting 12 hours before therapy and continue for 24-36 hours; alkalinize the urine by adding 50 mEq of bicarbonate to each liter of fluid; keep urine flow over 100 mL/hour and urine pH >7.

(Continued)

Methotrexate *(Continued)*

Respiratory: Pneumonitis: Associated with fever, cough, and interstitial pulmonary infiltrates; treatment is to withhold MTX during the acute reaction; interstitial pneumonitis has been reported to occur with an incidence of 1% in patients with RA (dose 7.5-15 mg/week)

<1% (Limited to important or life-threatening): Anaphylaxis, decreased resistance to infection, osteonecrosis and soft tissue necrosis (with radiotherapy), plaque erosions (psoriasis)

Overdosage/Toxicology Symptoms of overdose include nausea, vomiting, alopecia, melena, and renal failure.

Antidote: Leucovorin; administer as soon as toxicity is seen. Administer 10 mg/m² orally or parenterally. Follow with 10 mg/m² orally every 6 hours for 72 hours. After 24 hours following methotrexate administration, if the serum creatinine is ≥50% premethotrexate serum creatinine, increase leucovorin dose to 100 mg/m² every 3 hours until serum MTX level is <5 x 10^{-8} M. Hydration and alkalinization may be used to prevent precipitation of MTX or MTX metabolites in the renal tubules. Toxicity in low dose range is negligible, but may present mucositis and mild bone marrow suppression; severe bone marrow toxicity can result from overdose. Generally, neither peritoneal nor hemodialysis have been shown to increase elimination. However, effective clearance of methotrexate has been reported with acute, intermittent hemodialysis using a high-flux dialyzer. Leucovorin should be administered intravenously, never intrathecally, for overdoses of intrathecal methotrexate.

Pharmacodynamics/Kinetics

Absorption: Oral: Rapid; well absorbed at low doses (<30 mg/m²), incomplete after large doses; I.M. injection: Complete

Half-Life Elimination: Low dose: 3-10 hours; High dose: 8-12 hours

Time to Peak: Serum: Oral: 1-2 hours; Parenteral: 30-60 minutes

Metabolism: <10%; degraded by intestinal flora to DAMPA by carboxypeptidase; hepatic aldehyde oxidase converts MTX to 7-OH MTX; polyglutamates are produced intracellularly and are just as potent as MTX; their production is dose- and duration-dependent and they are slowly eliminated by the cell once formed

Onset: Antirheumatic: 3-6 weeks; additional improvement may continue longer than 12 weeks

Formulations

Injection, as sodium: 25 mg/mL (2 mL, 10 mL) [with benzyl alcohol 0.9%]
Injection, as sodium [preservative free]: 25 mg/mL (2 mL, 4 mL, 8 mL, 10 mL)
Injection, powder for reconstitution: 20 mg, 1 g
Tablet, as sodium: 2.5 mg
Rheumatrex®: 25 mg
Trexall™: 5 mg, 7.5 mg, 10 mg, 15 mg
Tablet, as sodium [dose pack] (Rheumatrex® Dose Pack): 2.5 mg (4 cards with 2, 3, 4, 5, or 6 tablets each)

Dosing

Adults: Refer to individual protocols. May be administered orally, I.M., intra-arterially, intrathecally, I.V., or S.C.

Leucovorin may be administered concomitantly or within 24 hours of methotrexate.

I.V.: Range is wide from 30-40 mg/m²/week to 100-7500 mg/m² with leucovorin rescue.

Doses not requiring leucovorin rescue range from 30-40 mg/m² I.V. or I.M. repeated weekly, or oral regimens of 10 mg/m² twice weekly.

High-dose MTX is considered to be >100 mg/m² and can be as high as 1500-7500 mg/m². These doses require leucovorin rescue. Patients receiving doses ≥1000 mg/m² should have their urine alkalinized with bicarbonate or Bicitra® prior to and following MTX therapy.

Trophoblastic neoplasms: Oral, I.M.: 15-30 mg/day for 5 days; repeat in 7 days for 3-5 courses

Head and neck cancer: Oral, I.M., I.V.: 25-50 mg/m² once weekly

Mycosis fungoides (cutaneous T-cell lymphoma): Oral, I.M.: Initial (early stages): 5-50 mg once weekly; dose reduction/cessation should be guided by response and hematologic monitoring. In patients with poor response to weekly therapy, MTX has also been given twice weekly in doses ranging from 15-37.5 mg.

Rheumatoid arthritis: Oral: 7.5 mg once weekly **or** 2.5 mg every 12 hours for 3 doses/week generally; not to exceed 20 mg/week

Bone marrow suppression is increased at dosages >20 mg/week; absorption and GI effects may be improved with I.M. administration at higher end of dosage range.

Psoriasis: Oral: 2.5-5 mg/dose every 12 hours for 3 doses given once weekly **or** Oral, I.M.: 10-25 mg/dose given once weekly

Ectopic pregnancy: I.M./I.V.: 50 mg/m² single-dose without leucovorin rescue

Elderly: Refer to individual protocols; adjust for renal impairment.

Rheumatoid arthritis/psoriasis: Oral: Initial: 5 mg once weekly

If nausea occurs, split dose to 2.5 mg every 12 hours for the day of administration.

Dose may be increased to 7.5 mg/week based on response, not to exceed 20 mg/week.

Neoplastic disease: Refer to specific disease protocols.

Pediatrics: Refer to individual protocols. May be administered orally, I.M., intra-arterially, intrathecally, or I.V.

Note: Leucovorin may be administered concomitantly or within 24 hours of methotrexate.

Dermatomyositis: Oral: 15-20 mg/m²/week as a single dose once weekly or 0.3-1 mg/kg/dose once weekly

Juvenile rheumatoid arthritis: Oral, I.M.: Recommended starting dose: 10 mg/m² once weekly (at higher doses, gastrointestinal side effects may be decreased with I.M. administration); 5-15 mg/m²/week as a single dose **or** as 3 divided doses given 12 hours apart

Antineoplastic dosage range:

Oral, I.M.: 7.5-30 mg/m²/week **or** every 2 weeks

I.V.: 10-18,000 mg/m² bolus dosing **or** continuous infusion over 6-42 hours; see table.

Methotrexate Dosing Schedules

Dose	Route	Frequency
Conventional		
15-20 mg/m^2	P.O.	Twice weekly
30-50 mg/m^2	P.O., I.V.	Weekly
15 mg/day for 5 days	P.O., I.M.	Every 2-3 weeks
Intermediate		
50-150 mg/m^2	I.V. push	Every 2-3 weeks
240 mg/m^2*	I.V. infusion	Every 4-7 days
0.5-1 g/m^2*	I.V. infusion	Every 2-3 weeks
High		
1-12 g/m^2*	I.V. infusion	Every 1-3 weeks

*Followed with leucovorin rescue - refer to Leucovorin monograph for details.

Pediatric solid tumors (high-dose): I.V.:
- <12 years: 12 g/m^2 (dosage range: 12-18 g)
- ≥12 years: 8 g/m^2 (maximum: 18 g)

Acute lymphocytic leukemia (intermediate-dose): I.V.: Loading: 100 mg/m^2 over 1 hour, followed by a 35-hour infusion of 900 mg/m^2/day

Meningeal leukemia: I.T.: 10-15 mg/m^2 (maximum dose: 15 mg) **or**
- ≤3 months: 3 mg/dose
- 4-11 months: 6 mg/dose
- 1 year: 8 mg/dose
- 2 years: 10 mg/dose
- ≥3 years: 12 mg/dose
- I.T. doses are prepared with preservative-free MTX only. Hydrocortisone may be added to the I.T. preparation; total volume should range from 3-6 mL. Doses should be repeated at 2- to 5-day intervals until CSF counts return to normal followed by a dose once weekly for 2 weeks then monthly thereafter.

Renal Impairment:

Cl_{cr} 61-80 mL/minute: Reduce dose to 75%.
Cl_{cr} 51-60 mL/minute: Reduce dose to 70%.
Cl_{cr} 10-50 mL/minute: Reduce dose to 30% to 50%.
Cl_{cr} <10 mL/minute: Avoid use.
Hemodialysis effects: Not dialyzable (0% to 5%)
Supplemental dose is not necessary.
Peritoneal dialysis effects: Supplemental dose is not necessary.
CAVH effects: Unknown

Hepatic Impairment:

Bilirubin 3.1-5 mg/dL or AST >180 units: Administer 75% of dose.
Bilirubin >5 mg/dL: Do not use.

Administration

I.V.: Methotrexate may be administered I.M., I.V., or I.T.; refer to Stability section for I.V. administration recommendations based on dosage.

Stability

Storage: Store intact vials at room temperature (15°C to 25°C) and protect from light.

Reconstitution: Dilute powder with D_5W or NS to a concentration ≤25 mg/mL (20 mg and 50 mg vials) and 50 mg/mL (1 g vial) as follows. Solution is stable for 7 days at room temperature.
- 20 mg = 20 mL (1 mg/mL)
- 50 mg = 5 mL (10 mg/mL)
- 1 g = 19.4 mL (50 mg/mL)

Further dilution in D_5W or NS is stable for 24 hours at room temperature (21°C to 25°C).

Standard I.V. dilution: Maximum syringe size for IVP is a 30 mL syringe and syringe should be ≤75% full.
- Doses <149 mg: Administer slow I.V. push
  - Dose/syringe (concentration ≤25 mg/mL)
- Doses of 150-499 mg: Administer IVPB over 20-30 minutes
  - Dose/50 mL D_5W or NS
- Doses of 500-1500 mg: Administer IVPB over ≥60 minutes
  - Dose/250 mL D_5W or NS
- Doses >1500 mg: Administer IVPB over 1-6 hours
  - Dose/1000 mL D_5W or NS

Standard I.M. dilution: Dose/syringe (concentration = 25 mg/mL)

I.V. dilutions are stable for 8 days at room temperature (25°C).

Standard intrathecal dilution:
- Use preservative-free preparations for high-dose and intrathecal administration.
- Dose/3-5 mL LR ± methotrexate (12 mg) ± hydrocortisone (15-25 mg)
- Intrathecal dilutions are stable for 7 days at room temperature (25°C) but due to sterility issues, use within 24 hours.

Compatibility: Stable in D_5NS, D_5W, NS

Y-site administration: Incompatible with chlorpromazine, gemcitabine, idarubicin, ifosfamide, midazolam, nalbuphine, promethazine, propofol

Compatibility when admixed: Incompatible with bleomycin

Monitoring Laboratory Tests For prolonged use (especially rheumatoid arthritis, psoriasis) a baseline liver biopsy, repeated at each 1-1.5 g cumulative dose interval, should be performed; WBC and platelet counts every 4 weeks; CBC and creatinine, LFTs every 3-4 months; chest x-ray

(Continued)

Methotrexate *(Continued)*

Monitoring and Teaching Issues

Physical Assessment: See Contraindications, Warnings/Precautions, and Dosing for use cautions. Assess potential for interactions with other prescriptions, OTC medications, or herbal products patient may be taking (see Drug Interactions). Assess results of laboratory tests (see above), therapeutic effects, and patient response (eg, hyper/hypothyroidism - see Adverse Reactions and Overdose/Toxicology) during therapy. Teach patient proper use, possible side effects and appropriate interventions, and adverse symptoms to report (see Patient Education). **Pregnancy risk factor D** - determine that patient is not pregnant before beginning treatment. Instruct patient in appropriate use of barrier contraceptive measures during therapy. Breast-feeding is contraindicated.

Patient Education: Inform prescriber of all prescriptions, OTC medications, or herbal products you are taking, and any allergies you have. Do not take anything new during treatment unless approved by prescriber. **Infusion/injection:** Report immediately any redness, swelling, pain, or burning at infusion/injection site. It is very important to maintain adequate hydration (2-3 L/day of fluids) unless instructed to restrict fluid intake, and nutrition (small, frequent meals may help). Avoid alcohol to prevent serious side effects. You will be more susceptible to infection (avoid crowds and exposure to infection and do not have any vaccinations without consulting prescriber). May cause sensitivity to sunlight (use sunscreen, wear protective clothing, and eyewear); nausea or vomiting (small, frequent meals, frequent mouth care, sucking lozenges, or chewing gum may help - if unresolved, contact prescriber); drowsiness, dizziness, numbness, or blurred vision (use caution when driving or engaging in tasks that require alertness until response to drug is known); loss of hair (may be reversible); color change of skin; permanent sterility; or mouth sores (frequent mouth care with soft toothbrush or cotton swabs and frequent rinses may help). Report immediately any rash, excessive or unusual fatigue, or difficulty breathing. Report rapid heartbeat or palpitations, black or tarry stools, fever, chills, unusual bleeding or bruising, shortness of breath, persistent GI disturbances, diarrhea, constipation, pain on urination or change in urinary patterns, or any other persistent adverse effects. **Pregnancy/breast-feeding precautions:** Do not get pregnant while taking this medication. Consult prescriber for appropriate barrier contraceptive measures. This drug may cause birth defects. Do not breast-feed.

Dietary Issues:

Sodium content of 100 mg injection: 20 mg (0.86 mEq)

Sodium content of 100 mg (low sodium) injection: 15 mg (0.65 mEq)

Geriatric Considerations: Toxicity to methotrexate or any immunosuppressive is increased in the elderly. Must monitor carefully. For rheumatoid arthritis and psoriasis, immunosuppressive therapy should only be used when disease is active and less toxic, traditional therapy is ineffective. Recommended doses should be reduced when initiating therapy in the elderly due to possible decreased metabolism, reduced renal function, and presence of interacting diseases and drugs. Adjust dose as needed for renal function (Cl_{cr}).

Additional Information Latex-free products: 50 mg/2 mL, 100 mg/4 mL, and 250 mg/10 mL vials with and without preservatives by Immunex

Related Information

Leucovorin *on page 779*

Methotrexate Sodium *see* Methotrexate *on page 874*

Methoxamine *see page 1580*

Methoxsalen (meth OKS a len)

U.S. Brand Names 8-MOP®; Oxsoralen®; Oxsoralen-Ultra®; Uvadex®

Synonyms Methoxypsoralen; 8-Methoxypsoralen; 8-MOP

Generic Available No

Pharmacologic Category Psoralen

Pregnancy Risk Factor C

Lactation Excretion in breast milk unknown

Use

Oral: Symptomatic control of severe, recalcitrant disabling psoriasis, not responsive to other therapy when the diagnosis has been supported by biopsy. Administer only in conjunction with a schedule of controlled doses of long wave ultraviolet (UV) radiation; also used with long wave ultraviolet (UV) radiation for repigmentation of idiopathic vitiligo.

Topical: Repigmenting agent in vitiligo, used in conjunction with controlled doses of UVA or sunlight

Orphan drug: Uvadex®: Palliative treatment of skin manifestations of cutaneous T-cell lymphoma

Mechanism of Action/Effect Bonds covalently to pyrimidine bases in DNA, inhibits the synthesis of DNA, and suppresses cell division. The augmented sunburn reaction involves excitation of the methoxsalen molecule by radiation in the long-wave ultraviolet light (UVA), resulting in transference of energy to the methoxsalen molecule producing an excited state ("triplet electronic state"). The molecule, in this "triplet state", then reacts with cutaneous DNA.

Contraindications Hypersensitivity to methoxsalen (psoralens) or any component of the formulation; children <12 years of age; diseases associated with photosensitivity; cataract; invasive squamous cell cancer

Warnings/Precautions Family history of sunlight allergy or chronic infections. Lotion should only be applied under direct supervision of a physician and should not be dispensed to the patient. For use only if inadequate response to other forms of therapy; serious burns may occur from UVA or sunlight even through glass if dose and or exposure schedule is not maintained. Some products may contain tartrazine. Use caution in patients with hepatic or cardiac disease. Pregnancy risk C.

Drug Interactions

Cytochrome P450 Effect: Substrate of CYP2A6; Inhibits **CYP1A2, 2A6**, 2C8/9, 2C19, 2D6, 2E1, 3A4

Increased Effect/Toxicity: Concomitant therapy with other photosensitizing agents such as anthralin, coal tar, griseofulvin, phenothiazines, nalidixic acid, sulfanilamides, tetracyclines, and thiazide diuretics.

Nutritional/Ethanol Interactions Food: Methoxsalen serum concentrations may be increased if taken with food. Avoid furocoumarin-containing foods (limes, figs, parsley, celery, cloves, lemon, mustard, carrots).

Adverse Reactions Frequency not always defined.

Cardiovascular: Severe edema, hypotension

Central nervous system: Nervousness, vertigo, depression

Dermatologic: Painful blistering, burning, and peeling of skin; pruritus (10%), freckling, hypopigmentation, rash, cheilitis, erythema, itching

Gastrointestinal: Nausea (10%)

Neuromuscular & skeletal: Loss of muscle coordination

Overdosage/Toxicology Symptoms of overdose include nausea and severe burns. Follow accepted treatment of severe burns. Keep room darkened until reaction subsides (8-24 hours or more).

Pharmacodynamics/Kinetics

Bioavailability: May be less with capsule than with gelcap

Time to Peak: Serum: Oral: 2-4 hours

Metabolism: Hepatic

Formulations

Capsule (8-MOP®): 10 mg

Gelcap (Oxsoralen-Ultra®): 10 mg

Lotion (Oxsoralen®): 1% (30 mL)

Solution, sterile (Uvadex®): 20 mcg/mL (10 mL) **[not for injection]**

Dosing

Adults & Elderly:

Psoriasis: Oral: 10-70 mg 1½-2 hours before exposure to ultraviolet light, 2-3 times at least 48 hours apart; dosage is based upon patient's body weight and skin type.

Vitiligo:

Oral: 20 mg 2-4 hours before exposure to UVA light or sunlight; limit exposure to 15-40 minutes based on skin basic color and exposure.

Topical: Apply lotion 1-2 hours before exposure to UVA light, no more than once weekly.

Pediatrics: Vitiligo: Children >12 years: Refer to adult dosing.

Monitoring and Teaching Issues

Physical Assessment: See Contraindications, Warnings/Precautions, and Drug Interactions for use cautions. **Note:** This drug is administered in conjunction with ultraviolet light or ultraviolet radiation therapy. Teach patient proper use, side effects and interventions (eg, sunlight precautions), and adverse reactions to report (see Patient Education). **Pregnancy risk factor C** - benefits of use should outweigh possible risks. Note breast-feeding caution.

Patient Education: Inform prescriber of all prescriptions, OTC medications, or herbal products you are taking, and any allergies you have. Do not take anything new during treatment unless approved by prescriber. This medication is used in conjunction with specific ultraviolet treatment. Take as directed, with food or milk to reduce nausea. Consult prescriber for specific dietary instructions. Avoid use of any other skin treatments unless approved by prescriber. Control exposure to direct sunlight as per prescriber's instructions. If sunlight cannot be avoided, use sunblock (consult prescriber for specific SPF level); wear protective clothing and wraparound protective eyewear. Consult prescriber immediately if burning, blistering, or skin irritation occur. **Pregnancy/breast-feeding precautions:** Inform prescriber if you are or intend to become pregnant. Consult prescriber if breast-feeding.

Dietary Issues: To reduce nausea, oral drug can be administered with food or milk or in 2 divided doses 30 minutes apart.

Methoxypsoralen *see* Methoxsalen *on page 878*

8-Methoxypsoralen *see* Methoxsalen *on page 878*

Methylacetoxyprogesterone *see* MedroxyPROGESTERone *on page 842*

Methyldopa (meth il DOE pa)

U.S. Brand Names Aldomet®

Synonyms Methyldopate Hydrochloride

Generic Available Yes

Pharmacologic Category Alpha-Adrenergic Inhibitor

Pregnancy Risk Factor B

Lactation Enters breast milk/compatible

Use Management of moderate to severe hypertension

Mechanism of Action/Effect Stimulation of central alpha-adrenergic receptors by a false transmitter that results in a decreased sympathetic outflow to the heart, kidneys, and peripheral vasculature

Contraindications Hypersensitivity to methyldopa or any component of the formulation; active hepatic disease; liver disorders previously associated with use of methyldopa; on MAO inhibitors; bisulfite allergy if using oral suspension or injectable

Warnings/Precautions Monitor for hemolytic anemia, positive Coombs' test, and liver dysfunction. A diuretic may be needed for weight gain or edema management. Its CNS side effects prevent it from being used frequently. It is the drug of choice for treatment of hypertension in pregnancy. Do not use oral suspension or injectable if bisulfite allergy.

Drug Interactions

Decreased Effect: Iron supplements can interact and cause a significant **increase** in blood pressure. Ferrous sulfate and ferrous gluconate decrease bioavailability. Barbiturates and TCAs may reduce response to methyldopa.

Increased Effect/Toxicity: Beta-blockers, MAO inhibitors, phenothiazines, and sympathomimetics (including epinephrine) may result in hypertension (sometimes severe) when combined with methyldopa. Methyldopa may increase lithium serum levels resulting in lithium toxicity. Levodopa may cause enhanced blood pressure lowering; methyldopa may

(Continued)

Methyldopa *(Continued)*

also potentiate the effect of levodopa. Tolbutamide, haloperidol, and anesthetics effects/toxicity are increased with methyldopa.

Nutritional/Ethanol Interactions Herb/Nutraceutical: Avoid dong quai if using for hypertension (has estrogenic activity). Avoid ephedra, yohimbe, ginseng (may worsen hypertension). Avoid valerian, St John's wort, kava kava, gotu kola (may increase CNS depression). Avoid natural licorice (causes sodium and water retention and increases potassium loss). Avoid garlic (may have increased antihypertensive effect).

Effects on Lab Values Methyldopa interferes with the following laboratory tests: urinary uric acid, serum creatinine (alkaline picrate method), AST (colorimetric method), and urinary catecholamines (falsely high levels)

Adverse Reactions

>10%: Cardiovascular: Peripheral edema

1% to 10%:

Central nervous system: Drug fever, mental depression, anxiety, nightmares, drowsiness, headache

Gastrointestinal: Dry mouth

<1% (Limited to important or life-threatening): Bradycardia (sinus), cholestasis or hepatitis and heptocellular injury, cirrhosis, dyspnea, gynecomastia, hemolytic anemia, hyperprolactinemia, increased liver enzymes, jaundice, leukopenia, orthostatic hypotension, positive Coombs' test, sexual dysfunction, SLE-like syndrome, sodium retention, thrombocytopenia, transient leukopenia or granulocytopenia

Overdosage/Toxicology Symptoms of overdose include hypotension, sedation, bradycardia, dizziness, constipation or diarrhea, flatus, nausea, and vomiting. Treatment is supportive and symptomatic. Can be removed by hemodialysis.

Pharmacodynamics/Kinetics

Half-Life Elimination: 75-80 minutes; End-stage renal disease: 6-16 hours

Metabolism: Intestinal and hepatic

Onset: Peak effect: Hypotensive: Oral/parenteral: 3-6 hours

Duration: 12-24 hours

Formulations

Injection, as methyldopate hydrochloride: 50 mg/mL (5 mL, 10 mL)

Suspension, oral: 250 mg/5 mL (5 mL, 473 mL)

Tablet: 125 mg, 250 mg, 500 mg

Dosing

Adults: Hypertension:

Oral: Initial: 250 mg 2-3 times/day; increase every 2 days as needed; usual dose: 1-1.5 g/day in 2-4 divided doses; maximum: 3 g/day

I.V.: 250-1000 mg every 6-8 hours; maximum: 1 g every 6 hours

Elderly: Oral: Initial: 125 mg 1-2 times/day; increase by 125 mg every 2-3 days as needed. Adjust for renal impairment. See Geriatric Considerations.

Pediatrics: Hypertension:

Oral: Children: Initial: 10 mg/kg/day in 2-4 divided doses; increase every 2 days as needed to maximum dose of 65 mg/kg/day. Do not exceed 3 g/day.

I.V.: Children: 5-10 mg/kg/dose every 6-8 hours up to a total dose of 65 mg/kg/24 hours or 3 g/24 hours

Renal Impairment:

Cl_{cr} >50 mL/minute: Administer every 8 hours.

Cl_{cr} 10-50 mL/minute: Administer every 8-12 hours.

Cl_{cr} <10 mL/minute: Administer every 12-24 hours.

Slightly dialyzable (5% to 20%)

Administration

I.V.: Infuse over 30 minutes.

Stability

Storage: Injectable dosage form is most stable at acid to neutral pH. Stability of parenteral admixture at room temperature (25°C) is 24 hours. Stability of parenteral admixture at refrigeration temperature (4°C) is 4 days.

Standard diluent: 250-500 mg/100 mL D_5W

Compatibility: Stable in dextran 6% in NS, D_5NS, D_5W, sodium bicarbonate 5%, NS

Compatibility when admixed: Incompatible with amphotericin B, methohexital

Monitoring Laboratory Tests CBC, liver enzymes, Coombs' test (direct)

Monitoring and Teaching Issues

Physical Assessment: See Contraindications, Warnings/Precautions, and Dosing for use cautions. Assess potential for interactions with other prescriptions, OTC medications, or herbal products patient may be taking (eg, anything that affects blood pressure - see Drug Interactions). See Administration and Storage for infusion specifics. Continuous monitoring is recommended for I.V. infusion. Assess results of laboratory tests (see above), therapeutic effects, and adverse reactions (see Adverse Reactions and Overdose/Toxicology) regularly during therapy. Teach patient use, possible side effects and appropriate interventions, and adverse symptoms to report (see Patient Education).

Patient Education: Inform prescriber of all prescriptions, OTC medications, or herbal products you are taking, and any allergies you have. Do not take anything new during treatment unless approved by prescriber (especially any cough or cold remedies, diet pills, stay-awake medications). Oral: Take as directed. Do not skip dose or discontinue without consulting prescriber. Follow recommended diet and exercise program. This medication may cause altered color of urine (normal); drowsiness, dizziness, or impaired judgment (use caution when driving or engaging in tasks that require alertness until response to drug is known); postural hypotension (use caution when rising from sitting or lying position or when climbing stairs); or dry mouth or nausea (frequent mouth care or sucking lozenges may help). Report altered CNS status (eg, nightmares, depression, anxiety, increased nervousness); sudden weight gain (weigh yourself in the same clothes at the same time of day once a week); unusual or persistent swelling of ankles, feet, or extremities; palpitations or rapid heartbeat; persistent weakness, fatigue, or unusual bleeding; or other persistent side effects.

Dietary Issues: Dietary requirements for vitamin B_{12} and folate may be increased with high doses of methyldopa.

Geriatric Considerations: Because of its CNS effects, methyldopa is not considered a drug of first choice in the elderly.

Breast-feeding Issues: Crosses into breast milk at extremely low levels. AAP considers **compatible** with breast-feeding.

Pregnancy Issues: Crosses the placenta. Hypotension reported. A large amount of clinical experience with the use of these drugs for the management of hypertension during pregnancy is available. Available evidence suggests safe use during pregnancy.

Methyldopa and Hydrochlorothiazide

(meth il DOE pa & hye droe klor oh THYE a zide)

U.S. Brand Names Aldoril®

Synonyms Hydrochlorothiazide and Methyldopa

Generic Available Yes

Pharmacologic Category Antihypertensive Agent Combination

Pregnancy Risk Factor C

Lactation Enters breast milk/compatible

Use Management of moderate to severe hypertension

Formulations

Tablet:

Aldoril® 15: Methyldopa 250 mg and hydrochlorothiazide 15 mg
Aldoril® 25: Methyldopa 250 mg and hydrochlorothiazide 25 mg
Aldoril® D30: Methyldopa 500 mg and hydrochlorothiazide 30 mg
Aldoril® D50: Methyldopa 500 mg and hydrochlorothiazide 50 mg

Dosing

Adults: Hypertension: Oral: 1 tablet 2-3 times/day for first 48 hours, then decrease or increase at intervals of not less than 2 days until an adequate response is achieved. Patients requiring higher doses may receive Aldoril® D30 or D50 once daily. Hydrochlorothiazide doses greater than 50 mg daily should be avoided.

Elderly: Refer to dosing in individual monographs.

Renal Impairment: Cl_{cr} 30 mL/minute: Thiazides are recommended; loop diuretics are preferred.

Monitoring and Teaching Issues

Physical Assessment: See individual components listed in Related Information. **Pregnancy risk factor C** - benefits of use should outweigh possible risks.

Patient Education: See individual components listed in Related Information. **Pregnancy precaution:** Inform prescriber if you are or intend to become pregnant.

Related Information

Hydrochlorothiazide *on page 664*
Methyldopa *on page 879*

Methyldopate Hydrochloride *see* Methyldopa *on page 879*
Methylene Blue *see page 1461*
Methylergometrine Maleate *see* Methylergonovine *on page 881*

Methylergonovine (meth il er goe NOE veen)

U.S. Brand Names Methergine®

Synonyms Methylergometrine Maleate; Methylergonovine Maleate

Generic Available No

Pharmacologic Category Ergot Derivative

Pregnancy Risk Factor C

Lactation Excretion in breast milk unknown/not recommended

Use Prevention and treatment of postpartum and postabortion hemorrhage caused by uterine atony or subinvolution

Mechanism of Action/Effect Similar smooth muscle actions as seen with ergotamine; however, it affects primarily uterine smooth muscles producing sustained contractions and thereby shortens the third stage of labor

Contraindications Hypersensitivity to methylergonovine or any component of the formulation; induction of labor; threatened spontaneous abortion; hypertension; toxemia

Warnings/Precautions Use caution in patients with sepsis, obliterative vascular disease, hepatic or renal involvement, or hypertension. Give with extreme caution if using I.V. Pregnancy risk C.

Drug Interactions

Cytochrome P450 Effect: Substrate of **CYP3A4**

Increased Effect/Toxicity: Avoid use of 5-HT_1 receptor antagonists (sumatriptan) within 24 hours (per manufacturer). Erythromycin, clarithromycin, and troleandomycin may increase levels of ergot alkaloids, resulting in toxicity (ischemia, vasospasm). Rare toxicity (peripheral vasoconstriction) has been reported with propranolol. Ritonavir, amprenavir, and nelfinavir increase blood levels of ergot alkaloids; avoid concurrent use. Concurrent use of sibutramine may cause serotonin syndrome; avoid concurrent use. Rarely, weakness and incoordination have been noted when SSRIs are used concurrently with 5-HT_1 agonists. The effects of vasoconstrictors may be increased by ergot derivatives.

Adverse Reactions Frequency not defined.

Cardiovascular: Hypertension, temporary chest pain, palpitations
Central nervous system: Hallucinations, dizziness, seizures, headache
Endocrine & metabolic: Water intoxication
Gastrointestinal: Nausea, vomiting, diarrhea, foul taste
Local: Thrombophlebitis
Neuromuscular & skeletal: Leg cramps
Otic: Tinnitus

(Continued)

Methylergonovine *(Continued)*

Renal: Hematuria
Respiratory: Dyspnea, nasal congestion
Miscellaneous: Diaphoresis

Overdosage/Toxicology Symptoms of overdose include prolonged gangrene, numbness in extremities, acute nausea, vomiting, abdominal pain, respiratory depression, hypotension, and seizures. Treatment is symptomatic and supportive.

Pharmacodynamics/Kinetics

Absorption: Rapid

Half-Life Elimination: Biphasic: Initial: 1-5 minutes; Terminal: 0.5-2 hours

Time to Peak: Serum: 0.5-3 hours

Metabolism: Hepatic

Onset: Oxytocic: Oral: 5-10 minutes; I.M.: 2-5 minutes; I.V.: Immediately

Duration: Oral: ~3 hours; I.M.: ~3 hours; I.V.: 45 minutes

Formulations

Injection, as maleate: 0.2 mg/mL (1 mL)
Tablet, as maleate: 0.2 mg

Dosing

Adults & Elderly: Prevention of hemorrhage:

Oral: 0.2 mg 3-4 times/day for 2-7 days

I.M.: 0.2 mg after delivery of anterior shoulder, after delivery of placenta, or during puerperium; may be repeated as required at intervals of 2-4 hours

I.V.: Same dose as I.M., but should not be routinely administered I.V. because of possibility of inducing sudden hypertension and cerebrovascular accident

Administration

I.V.: Ampuls containing discolored solution should not be used. Administer over no less than 60 seconds.

Stability

Storage: Ampuls must be protected from light and stored at temperatures 25°C (<77°F).

Compatibility: Stable in NS

Monitoring and Teaching Issues

Physical Assessment: See Contraindications, Warnings/Precautions, Dosing, and Drug Interactions for use cautions. Blood pressure, vaginal bleeding, CNS status, and patient response should be monitored on a regular basis - especially with infusion or injection. Assess therapeutic effectiveness and adverse reactions (eg, ergotamine toxicity: headache, ringing in ears, nausea and vomiting, diarrhea, numbness or coldness of extremities, confusion, hallucinations, dyspnea, chest pain, convulsions - see Adverse Reactions and Overdose/Toxicology). Teach patient proper use when self-administered, possible side effects, and appropriate interventions (see Patient Education). **Pregnancy risk factor C**. Breast-feeding is not recommended.

Patient Education: This drug will generally not be needed for more than a week. May cause nausea and vomiting (small, frequent meals may help), dizziness, headache, or ringing in the ears (will reverse when drug is discontinued). Report any difficulty breathing, acute headache, numb cold extremities, or severe abdominal cramping. **Breast-feeding precaution:** Breast-feeding is not recommended.

Pregnancy Issues: Prolonged constriction of the uterine vessels and/or increased myometrial tone may lead to reduced placental blood flow. This has contributed to fetal growth retardation in animals.

Methylergonovine Maleate *see* Methylergonovine *on page 881*
Methylin™ *see* Methylphenidate *on page 882*
Methylin™ ER *see* Methylphenidate *on page 882*
Methylmorphine *see* Codeine *on page 327*

Methylphenidate (meth il FEN i date)

U.S. Brand Names Concerta™; Metadate® CD; Metadate™ ER; Methylin™; Methylin™ ER; Ritalin®; Ritalin® LA; Ritalin-SR®

Synonyms Methylphenidate Hydrochloride

Restrictions C-II

Generic Available Yes

Pharmacologic Category Central Nervous System Stimulant

Pregnancy Risk Factor C

Lactation Excretion in breast milk unknown/use caution

Use Treatment of attention-deficit/hyperactivity disorder (ADHD); symptomatic management of narcolepsy

Use - Unlabeled/Investigational Depression (especially elderly or medically ill)

Mechanism of Action/Effect Mild CNS stimulant; blocks the reuptake mechanism of dopaminergic neurons; appears to stimulate the cerebral cortex and subcortical structures similar to amphetamines

Contraindications Hypersensitivity to methylphenidate, any component of the formulation, or idiosyncrasy to sympathomimetic amines; marked anxiety, tension, and agitation; glaucoma; use during or within 14 days following MAO inhibitor therapy; Tourette's syndrome or tics

Warnings/Precautions Has demonstrated value as part of a comprehensive treatment program for ADHD. Safety and efficacy in children <6 years of age not established. Use with caution in patients with bipolar disorder, diabetes mellitus, cardiovascular disease, hyperthyroidism, seizure disorders, insomnia, porphyria, or hypertension. Use caution in patients with history of ethanol or drug abuse. May exacerbate symptoms of behavior and thought disorder in psychotic patients. Do not use to treat severe depression or fatigue states. Potential for drug dependency exists - avoid abrupt discontinuation in patients who have received for prolonged periods. Visual disturbances have been reported (rare). Stimulant use has been associated with growth suppression. Stimulants may unmask tics in individuals with coexisting Tourette's syndrome. Concerta™ should not be used in patients with esophageal motility disorders or pre-existing severe gastrointestinal narrowing (small bowel disease, short gut syndrome, history of peritonitis, cystic fibrosis, chronic intestinal pseudo-obstruction, Meckel's diverticulum). Pregnancy risk C.

Drug Interactions

Cytochrome P450 Effect: Substrate of **CYP2D6**; Inhibits CYP2D6

Decreased Effect: Effectiveness of antihypertensive agents may be decreased. Carbamazepine may decrease the effect of methylphenidate.

Increased Effect/Toxicity: Methylphenidate may cause hypertensive effects when used in combination with MAO inhibitors or drugs with MAO-inhibiting activity (linezolid). Risk may be less with selegiline (MAO type B selective at low doses); it is best to avoid this combination. NMS has been reported in a patient receiving methylphenidate and venlafaxine. Methylphenidate may increase levels of phenytoin, phenobarbital, TCAs, and warfarin. Increased toxicity with clonidine and sibutramine.

Nutritional/Ethanol Interactions

Ethanol: Avoid ethanol (may cause CNS depression).

Food: Food may increase oral absorption; Concerta™ formulation is not affected. Food delays early peak and high-fat meals increase C_{max} and AUC of Metadate® CD formulation.

Herb/Nutraceutical: Avoid ephedra (may cause hypertension or arrhythmias) and yohimbe (also has CNS stimulatory activity).

Adverse Reactions Frequency not defined.

Cardiovascular: Angina, cardiac arrhythmias, cerebral arteritis, cerebral occlusion, hypertension, hypotension, palpitations, pulse increase/decrease, tachycardia

Central nervous system: Depression, dizziness, drowsiness, fever, headache, insomnia, nervousness, neuroleptic malignant syndrome (NMS), Tourette's syndrome, toxic psychosis

Dermatologic: Erythema multiforme, exfoliative dermatitis, hair loss, rash, urticaria

Endocrine & metabolic: Growth retardation

Gastrointestinal: Abdominal pain, anorexia, nausea, vomiting, weight loss

Hematologic: Anemia, leukopenia, thrombocytopenic purpura

Hepatic: Abnormal liver function tests, hepatic coma, transaminase elevation

Neuromuscular & skeletal: Arthralgia, dyskinesia

Ocular: Blurred vision

Renal: Necrotizing vasculitis

Respiratory: Cough increased, pharyngitis, sinusitis, upper respiratory tract infection

Miscellaneous: Hypersensitivity reactions

Overdosage/Toxicology Symptoms of overdose include vomiting, agitation, tremor, hyperpyrexia, muscle twitching, hallucinations, tachycardia, mydriasis, sweating, and palpitations. There is no specific antidote; treatment is supportive.

Pharmacodynamics/Kinetics

Absorption: Readily

Half-Life Elimination: 2-4 hours

Time to Peak: C_{max}: 6-8 hours

Metabolism: Hepatic via de-esterification to active metabolite

Onset: Peak effect:

Immediate release tablet: Cerebral stimulation: ~2 hours

Extended release capsule (Metadate® CD): Biphasic; initial peak similar to immediate release product, followed by second rising portion (corresponding to extended release portion)

Sustained release tablet: 4-7 hours

Osmotic release tablet (Concerta™): Initial: 1-2 hours

Duration: Immediate release tablet: 3-6 hours; Sustained release tablet: 8 hours

Formulations

Capsule, extended release, as hydrochloride

Metadate® CD: 20 mg

Ritalin® LA: 20 mg, 30 mg, 40 mg

Tablet, as hydrochloride: 5 mg, 10 mg, 20 mg

Methylin™, Ritalin®: 5 mg, 10 mg, 20 mg

Tablet, extended release, as hydrochloride (Metadate™ ER): 10 mg, 20 mg

Tablet, osmotic controlled release, as hydrochloride (Concerta™): 18 mg, 27 mg, 36 mg, 54 mg

Tablet, sustained release, as hydrochloride: 20 mg

Methylin™ ER: 10 mg, 20 mg

Ritalin-SR®: 20 mg

Dosing

Adults & Elderly:

Narcolepsy: Oral: 10 mg 2-3 times/day, up to 60 mg/day

Depression: Oral: Initial: 2.5 mg every morning before 9 AM; dosage may be increased by 2.5-5 mg every 2-3 days as tolerated to a maximum of 20 mg/day. May be divided (eg, 7 AM and 12 noon), but should not be given after noon. Do not use sustained release product.

ADHD: Oral: Refer to pediatric dosing.

Note: Discontinue periodically to re-evaluate or if no improvement occurs within 1 month.

Pediatrics: Note: Oral: Discontinue periodically to re-evaluate or if no improvement occurs within 1 month.

ADHD: Oral: Children ≥6 years: Initial: 0.3 mg/kg/dose or 2.5-5 mg/dose given before breakfast and lunch; increase by 0.1 mg/kg/dose or by 5-10 mg/day at weekly intervals; usual dose: 0.5-1 mg/kg/day; maximum dose: 2 mg/kg/day or 90 mg/day

Extended release:

Metadate™ ER, Methylin™ ER, Ritalin® SR: Duration of action is 8 hours. May be given in place of regular tablets, once the daily dose is titrated using the regular tablets and the titrated 8-hour dosage corresponds to sustained release tablet size.

(Continued)

Methylphenidate *(Continued)*

Concerta™:

Children not currently taking methylphenidate:

Initial: 18 mg once daily in the morning

Adjustment: May increase to maximum of 54 mg/day in increments of 18 mg/day; dose may be adjusted at weekly intervals

Children currently taking methylphenidate: **Note:** Dosing based on current regimen and clinical judgment; suggested dosing listed below:

Patients taking methylphenidate 5 mg 2-3 times/day or 20 mg/day sustained release formulation: Initial dose: 18 mg once every morning (maximum: 54 mg/day)

Patients taking methylphenidate 10 mg 2-3 times/day or 40 mg/day sustained release formulation: Initial dose: 36 mg once every morning (maximum: 54 mg/day)

Patients taking methylphenidate 15 mg 2-3 times/day or 60 mg/day sustained release formulation: Initial dose: 54 mg once every morning (maximum: 54 mg/day)

Note: A 27 mg dosage strength is available for situations in which a dosage between 18 mg and 36 mg is desired.

Metadate® CD, Ritalin® LA: Initial: 20 mg once daily; may be adjusted in 10-20 mg increments at weekly intervals; maximum: 60 mg/day

Administration

Oral: Do not crush or allow patient to chew sustained release dosage form. To effectively avoid insomnia, dosing should be completed by noon.

Concerta™: Administer dose once daily in the morning. May be taken with or without food, but must be taken with water, milk, or juice.

Metadate® CD, Ritalin® LA: Capsules may be opened and the contents sprinkled onto a small amount (equal to 1 tablespoon) of applesauce. Swallow applesauce without chewing. Do not crush or chew capsule contents.

Stability

Storage:

Immediate release tablet: Do not store above 30°C (86°F); protect from light

Extended release capsule: Store in dose pack provided at 25°C (77°F)

Sustained release tablet: Do not store above 30°C (86°F); protect from moisture

Osmotic controlled release tablet (Concerta™): Store at 25°C (77°F); protect from humidity

Monitoring and Teaching Issues

Physical Assessment: Assess effectiveness and interactions of other medications patient may be taking (see Drug Interactions). See Contraindications and Warnings/Precautions for use cautions. Assess for history of addiction; long-term use can result in dependence, abuse, or tolerance. Evaluate periodically for need for continued use. After long-term use, taper dosage slowly when discontinuing. Monitor laboratory tests, effectiveness of therapy, and adverse reactions at beginning of therapy and periodically with long-term use. Assess knowledge/teach patient appropriate use, interventions to reduce side effects, and importance of reporting adverse symptoms promptly. **Pregnancy risk factor C** - benefits of use should outweigh possible risks. Note breast-feeding caution.

Patient Education: Take exactly as directed, 30-45 minutes before meals with a full glass of water. Do not change dosage or discontinue without consulting prescriber. Response may take some time. Do not crush or chew sustained release dosage forms. Tablets and sustained release tablets should be taken 30-45 minutes before meals. Concerta™ may be taken with or without food, but must be taken with water, milk, or juice. Metadate® CD and Ritalin® LA capsules may be opened and the contents sprinkled onto a small amount (equal to 1 tablespoon) of applesauce. Swallow applesauce without chewing. Do not crush or chew capsule contents. Avoid alcohol, caffeine, or other stimulants. Maintain adequate hydration (2-3 L/day of fluids) unless advised by prescriber to restrict fluids. You may experience decreased appetite or weight loss (small, frequent meals may help maintain adequate nutrition); or restlessness, impaired judgment, or dizziness, especially during early therapy (use caution when driving or engaging in tasks requiring alertness until response to drug is known). Report unresolved rapid heartbeat; excessive agitation, nervousness, insomnia, tremors, or dizziness; blackened stool; skin rash or irritation; or altered gait or movement. Concerta™ tablet shell may appear intact in stool; this is normal. **Pregnancy/breast-feeding precautions:** Inform prescriber if you are or intend to become pregnant. Consult prescriber if breast-feeding.

Dietary Issues: Should be taken 30-45 minutes before meals. Concerta™ is not affected by food and should be taken with water, milk, or juice. Metadate® CD should be taken before breakfast. Metadate™ ER should be taken before breakfast and lunch.

Geriatric Considerations: Methylphenidate is often useful in treating elderly patients who are discouraged, withdrawn, apathetic, or disinterested in their activities. In particular, it is useful in patients who are starting a rehabilitation program but have resigned themselves to fail; these patients may not have a major depressive disorder; will not improve memory or cognitive function; use with caution in patients with dementia who may have increased agitation and confusion (see Dosage and Adverse Reactions).

Additional Information Treatment with methylphenidate may include "drug holidays" or periodic discontinuation in order to assess the patient's requirements and to decrease tolerance and limit suppression of linear growth and weight. Specific patients may require 3 doses/day for treatment of ADHD (ie, additional dose at 4 PM).

Concerta™ is an osmotic controlled release formulation (OROS®) of methylphenidate. The tablet has an immediate-release overcoat that provides an initial dose of methylphenidate within 1 hour. The overcoat covers a trilayer core. The trilayer core is composed of two layers containing the drug and excipients, and one layer of osmotic components. As water from the gastrointestinal tract enters the core, the osmotic components expand and methylphenidate is released.

Metadate® CD capsules contain a mixture of immediate release and extended release beads, designed to release 30% of the dose (6 mg) immediately and 70% (14 mg) over an extended period.

Ritalin® LA uses a combination of immediate release and enteric coated, delayed release beads.

Related Information

Controlled Substances Comparison *on page 1568*

Methylphenidate Hydrochloride *see* Methylphenidate *on page 882*

Methylphytyl Napthoquinone *see* Phytonadione *on page 1080*

MethylPREDNISolone (meth il pred NIS oh lone)

U.S. Brand Names A-methaPred®; depMedalone®; Depoject®; Depo-Medrol®; Depopred®; Duralone®; Medralone®; Medrol®; M-Prednisol®; Solu-Medrol®

Synonyms 6-α-Methylprednisolone; Methylprednisolone Acetate; Methylprednisolone Sodium Succinate

Generic Available Yes

Pharmacologic Category Corticosteroid, Systemic

Pregnancy Risk Factor C

Lactation Excretion in breast milk unknown

Use Primarily as an anti-inflammatory or immunosuppressant agent in the treatment of a variety of diseases including those of hematologic, allergic, inflammatory, neoplastic, and autoimmune origin. Prevention and treatment of graft-versus-host disease following allogeneic bone marrow transplantation.

Use - Unlabeled/Investigational Treatment of fibrosing-alveolitis phase of adult respiratory distress syndrome (ARDS)

Mechanism of Action/Effect In a tissue-specific manner, corticosteroids regulate gene expression subsequent to binding specific intracellular receptors and translocation into the nucleus. Corticosteroids exert a wide array of physiologic effects, including modulation of carbohydrate, protein, and lipid metabolism, and maintenance of fluid and electrolyte homeostasis. Moreover, cardiovascular, immunologic, musculoskeletal, endocrine, and neurologic physiology are influenced by corticosteroids.

Contraindications Hypersensitivity to methylprednisolone or any component of the formulation; viral, fungal, or tubercular skin lesions; administration of live virus vaccines; serious infections, except septic shock or tuberculous meningitis. Methylprednisolone formulations containing benzyl alcohol preservative are contraindicated in infants.

Warnings/Precautions Use with caution in patients with hyperthyroidism, cirrhosis, nonspecific ulcerative colitis, hypertension, osteoporosis, thromboembolic tendencies, CHF, convulsive disorders, myasthenia gravis, thrombophlebitis, peptic ulcer, diabetes, glaucoma, cataracts, or tuberculosis. Use caution in hepatic impairment. Acute adrenal insufficiency may occur with abrupt withdrawal after long-term therapy or with stress. Because of the risk of adverse effects, systemic corticosteroids should be used cautiously in the elderly, in the smallest possible dose, and for the shortest possible time. Pregnancy risk C.

Drug Interactions

Cytochrome P450 Effect: Substrate of CYP3A4; Inhibits CYP3A4

Decreased Effect: Phenytoin, phenobarbital, rifampin increase clearance of methylprednisolone. Potassium-depleting diuretics enhance potassium depletion. Skin test antigens, immunizations decrease antibody response and increase potential infections.

Increased Effect/Toxicity: Methylprednisolone may increase circulating glucose levels; may need adjustments of insulin or oral hypoglycemics. Methylprednisolone increases cyclosporine and tacrolimus blood levels. Itraconazole increases corticosteroid levels.

Nutritional/Ethanol Interactions

Ethanol: Avoid ethanol (may increase gastric mucosal irritation).

Food: Methylprednisolone interferes with calcium absorption. Limit caffeine.

Herb/Nutraceutical: St John's wort may decrease methylprednisolone levels. Avoid cat's claw, echinacea (have immunostimulant properties).

Effects on Lab Values Interferes with skin tests

Adverse Reactions Frequency not defined.

Cardiovascular: Edema, hypertension, arrhythmias

Central nervous system: Insomnia, nervousness, vertigo, seizures, psychoses, pseudotumor cerebri, headache, mood swings, delirium, hallucinations, euphoria

Dermatologic: Hirsutism, acne, skin atrophy, bruising, hyperpigmentation

Endocrine & metabolic: Diabetes mellitus, adrenal suppression, hyperlipidemia, Cushing's syndrome, pituitary-adrenal axis suppression, growth suppression, glucose intolerance, hypokalemia, alkalosis, amenorrhea, sodium and water retention, hyperglycemia

Gastrointestinal: Increased appetite, indigestion, peptic ulcer, nausea, vomiting, abdominal distention, ulcerative esophagitis, pancreatitis

Hematologic: Transient leukocytosis

Neuromuscular & skeletal: Arthralgia, muscle weakness, osteoporosis, fractures

Ocular: Cataracts, glaucoma

Miscellaneous: Infections, hypersensitivity reactions, avascular necrosis, secondary malignancy, intractable hiccups

Overdosage/Toxicology When consumed in high doses for prolonged periods, systemic hypercorticism and adrenal suppression may occur. In these cases, discontinuation should be done judiciously. Arrhythmias and cardiovascular collapse are possible with rapid intravenous infusion of high-dose methylprednisolone. May mask signs and symptoms of infection.

Pharmacodynamics/Kinetics

Half-Life Elimination: 3-3.5 hours; reduced in obese

Onset: Peak effect (route dependent): Oral: 1-2 hours; I.M.: 4-8 days; Intra-articular: 1 week; methylprednisolone sodium succinate is highly soluble and has a rapid effect by I.M. and I.V. routes

Duration: Route dependent: Oral: 30-36 hours; I.M.: 1-4 weeks; Intra-articular: 1-5 weeks; methylprednisolone acetate has a low solubility and has a sustained I.M. effect

(Continued)

MethylPREDNISolone *(Continued)*

Formulations

Injection, as acetate: 20 mg/mL (5 mL, 10 mL); 40 mg/mL (1 mL, 5 mL, 10 mL); 80 mg/mL (1 mL, 5 mL)

Injection, as sodium succinate: 40 mg (1 mL, 3 mL); 125 mg (2 mL, 5 mL); 500 mg (1 mL, 4 mL, 8 mL, 20 mL); 1000 mg (1 mL, 8 mL, 50 mL); 2000 mg (30.6 mL)

Tablet: 2 mg, 4 mg, 8 mg, 16 mg, 24 mg, 32 mg

Tablet [dose pack]: 4 mg (21s)

Dosing

Adults: Only sodium succinate may be given I.V.; methylprednisolone sodium succinate is highly soluble and has a rapid effect by I.M. and I.V. routes. Methylprednisolone acetate has a low solubility and has a sustained I.M. effect.

Anti-inflammatory or immunosuppressive:

Oral: 2-60 mg/day in 1-4 divided doses to start, followed by gradual reduction in dosage to the lowest possible level consistent with maintaining an adequate clinical response.

I.M. (sodium succinate): 10-80 mg/day once daily

I.M. (acetate): 10-80 mg every 1-2 weeks

I.V. (sodium succinate): 10-40 mg over a period of several minutes and repeated I.V. or I.M. at intervals depending on clinical response; when high dosages are needed, give 30 mg/kg over a period ≥30 minutes and may be repeated every 4-6 hours for 48 hours.

Status asthmaticus: I.V. (sodium succinate): Loading dose: 2 mg/kg/dose, then 0.5-1 mg/kg/dose every 6 hours for up to 5 days

High-dose therapy for acute spinal cord injury: I.V. bolus: 30 mg/kg over 15 minutes, followed 45 minutes later by an infusion of 5.4 mg/kg/hour for 23 hours

Acute spinal cord injury: I.V. (sodium succinate): 30 mg/kg over 15 minutes, followed in 45 minutes by a continuous infusion of 5.4 mg/kg/hour for 23 hours

Lupus nephritis: High-dose "pulse" therapy: I.V. (sodium succinate): 1 g/day for 3 days

Aplastic anemia: I.V. (sodium succinate): 1 mg/kg/day or 40 mg/day (whichever dose is higher), for 4 days. After 4 days, change to oral and continue until day 10 or until symptoms of serum sickness resolve, then rapidly reduce over approximately 2 weeks.

Pneumocystis pneumonia in AIDs patients: I.V.: 40-60 mg every 6 hours for 7-10 days

Intra-articular (acetate): Administer every 1-5 weeks.

Large joints: 20-80 mg

Small joints: 4-10 mg

Intralesional (acetate): 20-60 mg every 1-5 weeks

Elderly: Only sodium succinate salt may be given I.V. Use the lowest effective adult dose.

Pediatrics: Dosing should be based on the lesser of ideal body weight or actual body weight. **Only sodium succinate may be given I.V.;** methylprednisolone sodium succinate is highly soluble and has a rapid effect by I.M. and I.V. routes. Methylprednisolone acetate has a low solubility and has a sustained I.M. effect.

Anti-inflammatory or immunosuppressive: Oral, I.M., I.V. (sodium succinate): Children: 0.5-1.7 mg/kg/day **or** 5-25 mg/m^2/day in divided doses every 6-12 hours; "Pulse" therapy: 15-30 mg/kg/dose over ≥30 minutes given once daily for 3 days

Status asthmaticus: Children: I.V. (sodium succinate): Loading dose: 2 mg/kg/dose, then 0.5-1 mg/kg/dose every 6 hours for up to 5 days

Acute spinal cord injury: I.V. (sodium succinate): 30 mg/kg over 15 minutes, followed in 45 minutes by a continuous infusion of 5.4 mg/kg/hour for 23 hours

Lupus nephritis: I.V. (sodium succinate): 30 mg/kg over ≥30 minutes every other day for 6 doses

Renal Impairment:

Hemodialysis effects: Slightly dialyzable (5% to 20%)

Administer dose posthemodialysis.

Administration

Oral: Give oral formulation with meals to decrease GI upset. Give daily dose in the morning to mimic normal peak blood levels.

I.V.: Only sodium succinate formulation may be given I.V. Acetate salt should not be given I.V.

Parenteral: Methylprednisolone sodium succinate may be administered I.M. or I.V.; I.V. administration may be IVP over one to several minutes or IVPB or continuous I.V. infusion.

I.V.: Succinate:

Low dose: ≤1.8 mg/kg or ≤125 mg/dose: I.V. push over 3-15 minutes

Moderate dose: ≥2 mg/kg or 250 mg/dose: I.V. over 15-30 minutes

High dose: 15 mg/kg or ≥500 mg/dose: I.V. over ≥30 minutes

Doses >15 mg/kg or ≥1 g: Administer over 1 hour

Do **not** administer high-dose I.V. push; hypotension, cardiac arrhythmia, and sudden death have been reported in patients given high-dose methylprednisolone I.V. push over <20 minutes. Intermittent infusion over 15-60 minutes; maximum concentration: I.V. push 125 mg/mL.

Topical: For external use only. Apply sparingly.

Stability

Storage: Intact vials of methylprednisolone sodium succinate should be stored at controlled room temperature.

Reconstitution: Reconstituted solutions of methylprednisolone sodium succinate should be stored at room temperature (15°C to 30°C) and used within 48 hours. Stability of parenteral admixture at room temperature (25°C) and at refrigeration temperature (4°C) is 48 hours.

Standard diluent (Solu-Medrol®): 40 mg/50 mL D_5W; 125 mg/50 mL D_5W

Minimum volume (Solu-Medrol®): 50 mL D_5W

Compatibility: Incompatible with $D_5{}^1/_2NS$

Y-site administration: Incompatible with allopurinol, amsacrine, ciprofloxacin, docetaxel, etoposide phosphate, filgrastim, gemcitabine, ondansetron, paclitaxel, propofol, sargramostim, vinorelbine

Compatibility in syringe: Incompatible with doxapram

Compatibility when admixed: Incompatible with calcium gluconate, glycopyrrolate, insulin (regular), metaraminol, nafcillin, penicillin G sodium

Monitoring Laboratory Tests Blood glucose, electrolytes

Monitoring and Teaching Issues

Physical Assessment: Assess effectiveness and interactions of other medications patient may be taking (see Drug Interactions). See Contraindications and Warnings/Precautions for use cautions. Monitor for effectiveness of therapy and adverse reactions according to dose, route, and length of therapy (especially with systemic administration - see above). Assess knowledge/teach patient appropriate use, possible side effects/interventions, and adverse symptoms to report (ie, opportunistic infection, adrenal suppression - see Adverse Reactions, Overdose/Toxicology, and Patient Education). Instruct diabetics to monitor serum glucose levels closely; corticosteroids can alter glycemic response. Dose may need to be increased if patient is experiencing higher than normal levels of stress. When discontinuing, taper dose and frequency slowly. **Pregnancy risk factor C** - benefits of use should outweigh possible risks. Note breast-feeding caution.

Patient Education: Maintain adequate nutritional intake; consult prescriber for possibility of special dietary instructions. If diabetic, monitor serum glucose closely and notify prescriber of any changes; this medication can alter hypoglycemic requirements. Avoid alcohol. Inform prescriber if you are experiencing unusual stress; dosage may need to be adjusted. You will be susceptible to infection (avoid crowds and and exposure to infection). You may experience insomnia or nervousness; use caution when driving or engaging in tasks requiring alertness until response to drug is known. Report increased pain, swelling, or redness in area being treated; excessive or sudden weight gain; swelling of extremities; difficulty breathing; muscle pain or weakness; change in menstrual pattern; vision changes; signs of hyperglycemia; signs of infection (eg, fever, chills, mouth sores, perianal itching, vaginal discharge); blackened stool; other persistent side effects; or worsening of condition. **Pregnancy/breast-feeding precautions:** Inform prescriber if you are or intend to become pregnant. Consult prescriber if breast-feeding.

Oral: Take as directed, with food or milk. Take once-a-day dose in the morning. Do not take more than prescribed or discontinue without consulting prescriber.

Intra-articular: Refrain from excessive use of joint following therapy, even if pain is gone.

Dietary Issues: Should be taken after meals or with food or milk; need diet rich in pyridoxine, vitamin C, vitamin D, folate, calcium, phosphorus, and protein.

Sodium content of 1 g sodium succinate injection: 2.01 mEq; 53 mg of sodium succinate salt is equivalent to 40 mg of methylprednisolone base

Methylprednisolone acetate: Depo-Medrol®

Methylprednisolone sodium succinate: Solu-Medrol®

Geriatric Considerations: Because of the risk of adverse effects, systemic corticosteroids should be used cautiously in the elderly, in the smallest possible dose, and for the shortest possible time.

Additional Information Sodium content of 1 g sodium succinate injection: 2.01 mEq; 53 mg of sodium succinate salt is equivalent to 40 mg of methylprednisolone base

Methylprednisolone acetate: Depo-Medrol®

Methylprednisolone sodium succinate: Solu-Medrol®

Related Information

Antiemetics for Chemotherapy-Induced Nausea and Vomiting *on page 1639*

Corticosteroids Comparison, Systemic Equivalencies *on page 1572*

FDA Name Differentiation Project: The Use of Tall-man Letters *on page 12*

6-α-Methylprednisolone *see* MethylPREDNISolone *on page 885*

Methylprednisolone Acetate *see* MethylPREDNISolone *on page 885*

Methylprednisolone Sodium Succinate *see* MethylPREDNISolone *on page 885*

MethylTESTOSTERone (meth il tes TOS te rone)

U.S. Brand Names Android®; Oreton® Methyl; Testred®; Virilon®

Restrictions C-III

Generic Available Yes

Pharmacologic Category Androgen

Pregnancy Risk Factor X

Lactation Excretion in breast milk unknown/contraindicated

Use

Male: Hypogonadism; delayed puberty; impotence and climacteric symptoms

Female: Palliative treatment of metastatic breast cancer

Mechanism of Action/Effect Male: Stimulates receptors in organs and tissues to promote growth and development of male sex organs and maintains secondary sex characteristics in androgen-deficient males.

Contraindications Hypersensitivity to methyltestosterone or any component of the formulation; in males, known or suspected carcinoma of the breast or the prostate; pregnancy

Warnings/Precautions Use with extreme caution in patients with liver or kidney disease or serious heart disease. May accelerate bone maturation without producing compensatory gain in linear growth.

Drug Interactions

Decreased Effect: Decreased oral anticoagulant effect

Increased Effect/Toxicity: Effects of oral anticoagulants and hypoglycemic agents may be increased. Toxicity may occur with cyclosporine; avoid concurrent use.

Adverse Reactions Frequency not defined.

Male: Virilism, priapism, prostatic hyperplasia, prostatic carcinoma, impotence, testicular atrophy, gynecomastia

(Continued)

MethylTESTOSTERone *(Continued)*

Female: Virilism, menstrual problems (amenorrhea), breast soreness, hirsutism (increase in pubic hair growth) atrophy
Cardiovascular: Edema
Central nervous system: Headache, anxiety, depression
Dermatologic: Acne, "male pattern" baldness, seborrhea
Endocrine & metabolic: Hypercalcemia, hypercholesterolemia
Gastrointestinal: GI irritation, nausea, vomiting
Hematologic: Leukopenia, polycythemia
Hepatic: Hepatic dysfunction, hepatic necrosis, cholestatic hepatitis
Miscellaneous: Hypersensitivity reactions

Overdosage/Toxicology Abnormal liver function tests

Pharmacodynamics/Kinetics

Metabolism: Hepatic

Formulations

Capsule: 10 mg
Tablet: 10 mg, 25 mg

Dosing

Adults: Note: Buccal absorption produces twice the androgenic activity of oral tablets.

Male (Hypogonadism; delayed puberty; impotence and climacteric symptoms):
Oral: 10-40 mg/day
Buccal: 5-25 mg/day
Breast pain/engorgement (Female):
Oral: 80 mg/day for 3-5 days
Buccal: 40 mg/day for 3-5 days
Breast cancer (Female):
Oral: 50-200 mg/day
Buccal: 25-100 mg/day

Elderly: Refer to adult dosing (buccal absorption produces twice the androgenic activity of oral tablets).

Monitoring and Teaching Issues

Physical Assessment: (For use in children see pediatric reference). See Contraindications, Warnings/Precautions, and Dosing for use cautions. Assess potential for interactions with other prescriptions, OTC medications, or herbal products patient may be taking (see Drug Interactions). Assess therapeutic effects (according to purpose for use) and adverse reactions (see Adverse Reactions and Overdose/Toxicology) regularly during therapy. Caution diabetic patients; effects of hypoglycemic agents may be increased. Teach patient proper use, possible side effects and appropriate interventions, and adverse symptoms to report (see Patient Education). **Pregnancy risk factor X** - determine that patient is not pregnant before beginning treatment. Instruct patients of childbearing age or males who may have intercourse with women of childbearing age on appropriate barrier contraceptive measures. Breast-feeding is contraindicated.

Patient Education: Inform prescriber of all prescriptions, OTC medications, or herbal products you are taking, and any allergies you have. Do not take anything new during treatment unless approved by prescriber. Take as directed; do not discontinue without consulting prescriber. If diabetic, monitor serum glucose closely and notify prescriber of changes; this medication can alter hypoglycemic requirements. May cause acne, growth of body hair, loss of libido, impotence, or menstrual irregularity (usually reversible); or nausea or vomiting (small, frequent meals, frequent mouth care, sucking lozenges, or chewing gum may help). Report changes in menstrual pattern; deepening of voice or unusual growth of body hair; fluid retention (swelling of ankles, feet, or hands, difficulty breathing, or sudden weight gain); change in color of urine or stool; yellowing of eyes or skin; unusual bruising or bleeding; or other adverse reactions. **Pregnancy/breast-feeding precautions:** Inform prescriber if you are pregnant. Do not get pregnant or cause a pregnancy (males) during or for 1 month following therapy. Consult prescriber for instruction on appropriate barrier contraceptive measures. This drug may cause severe fetal defects. Do not breast-feed.

Geriatric Considerations: Since elderly males have prostate changes with age, it would be best to obtain a PSA initially and periodically. Retention of sodium and water could be a problem in patients with CHF and hypertension.

Related Information

FDA Name Differentiation Project: The Use of Tall-man Letters *on page 12*

Methysergide (meth i SER jide)

U.S. Brand Names Sansert®

Synonyms Methysergide Maleate

Generic Available No

Pharmacologic Category Ergot Derivative

Pregnancy Risk Factor X

Lactation Enters breast milk/contraindicated

Use Prophylaxis of vascular headache

Mechanism of Action/Effect Ergotamine congener, however, actions appear to differ; methysergide has minimal ergotamine-like oxytocic or vasoconstrictive properties, and has significantly greater serotonin-like properties

Contraindications Hypersensitivity to methysergide, tartrazine, or any component of the formulation; acute migraine attack; peripheral vascular disease; severe arteriosclerosis; collagen diseases or fibrotic processes; impairment of renal or hepatic function; valvular heart disease; debilitated states; pulmonary disease; severe hypertension; phlebitis; serious infections; pregnancy

Warnings/Precautions Patients receiving long-term therapy may develop retroperitoneal fibrosis, pleuropulmonary fibrosis and fibrotic thickening of the cardiac valves. Continuous administration should not exceed 6 months (reduce dose gradually in last 2-3 weeks of each treatment course). Fibrosis occurs rarely when therapy is interrupted for 3-4 weeks every 6 months. Not recommended for use in pediatric patients. Some products may contain tartrazine.

Drug Interactions

Cytochrome P450 Effect: Substrate of **CYP3A4**

Increased Effect/Toxicity: Serotonin agonists may produce excessive vasoconstriction; avoid concurrent use with 24 hours; includes sumatriptan, naratriptan, rizatriptan, zolmitriptan. Concurrent use of beta-blockers may cause peripheral ischemia. Erythromycin and clarithromycin may increase ergot alkaloid toxicity; avoid concurrent use. Protease inhibitors may increase ergot alkaloid toxicity; avoid concurrent use (amprenavir, ritonavir, saquinavir). Concurrent use of vasoconstrictors may produce excessive vasoconstriction and should be avoided.

Adverse Reactions Frequency not defined.

Cardiovascular: Postural hypotension, peripheral ischemia, peripheral edema, tachycardia, bradycardia, edema

Central nervous system: Insomnia, drowsiness, euphoria, dizziness, seizures, fever

Dermatologic: Rash, telangiectasia, flushing

Gastrointestinal: Nausea, vomiting, abdominal pain, diarrhea, heartburn, weight gain

Hematologic: Neutropenia, eosinophilia, thrombocytopenia

Neuromuscular & skeletal: Weakness, myalgia, arthralgia

Note: Fibrotic complications: Retroperitoneal, pleuropulmonary, cardiac (aortic root, aortic valve, mitral valve) fibrosis, and Peyronie's disease have been reported.

Overdosage/Toxicology Symptoms of overdose include hyperactivity, limb spasms, impaired mental function, and impaired circulation. Treatment is supportive.

Pharmacodynamics/Kinetics

Half-Life Elimination: ~10 hours

Metabolism: Hepatic to methylergonovine and glucuronide metabolite

Formulations Tablet, as maleate: 2 mg

Dosing

Adults: Vascular headache (prophylaxis): Oral: 4-8 mg/day with meals; if no improvement is noted after 3 weeks, drug is unlikely to be beneficial. Must not be given continuously for longer than 6 months, and a drug-free interval of 3-4 weeks must follow each 6-month course.

Elderly: Refer to adult dosing; use with caution.

Monitoring and Teaching Issues

Physical Assessment: See Contraindications, Warnings/Precautions, and Dosing for use cautions. Assess potential for interactions with other prescriptions, OTC medications, or herbal products patient may be taking (see Drug Interactions). Assess therapeutic effects and adverse reactions (see Adverse Reactions and Overdose/Toxicology) regularly during and following therapy. When discontinuing, reduce dosage gradually to prevent "rebound" headache. Teach patient proper use, possible side effects and appropriate interventions, and adverse symptoms to report (see Patient Education). **Pregnancy risk factor X** - determine that patient is not pregnant before beginning treatment. Do not give to women of childbearing age unless they are capable of complying with barrier contraceptives. Instruct patients about appropriate barrier contraceptive measures. Breast-feeding is contraindicated.

Patient Education: Inform prescriber of all prescriptions, OTC medications, or herbal products you are taking, and any allergies you have. Do not take anything new during treatment unless approved by prescriber. This drug is meant to prevent migraine headaches, not treat acute attacks. Take as directed with food; do not take more than recommended and do not discontinue without consulting prescriber (must be discontinued slowly). May cause weight gain (monitor dietary intake and exercise); dizziness or vertigo (use caution when driving or engaging in tasks that require alertness until response to drug is known); nausea or vomiting (small frequent meal, frequent mouth care, chewing gum, or sucking lozenges may help); or diarrhea (should lessen with continued use - try buttermilk, boiled milk, or yogurt). Report cold, numb, tingling, or painful extremities or leg cramps; chest pain, difficulty breathing, or shortness of breath; or pain on urination. **Pregnancy/breast-feeding precautions:** Inform prescriber if you are pregnant. Do not get pregnant during or for 1 month following therapy. Consult prescriber for instruction on appropriate barrier contraceptive measures. This drug may cause severe fetal defects. Do not breast-feed.

Dietary Issues: May be taken with food or milk.

Geriatric Considerations: Use cautiously in the elderly, particularly since many elderly have cardiovascular disease which would put them at risk for cardiovascular adverse effects.

Methysergide Maleate *see* Methysergide *on page 888*

Meticorten® *see* PredniSONE *on page 1115*

Metimyd® *see page 1509*

Metipranolol *see page 1575*

Metipranolol *see* Ophthalmic Agents, Glaucoma *on page 1002*

Metoclopramide (met oh kloe PRA mide)

U.S. Brand Names Reglan®

Generic Available Yes

Pharmacologic Category Gastrointestinal Agent, Prokinetic

Pregnancy Risk Factor B

Lactation Enters breast milk/not recommended (AAP rates "of concern")

Use Prevention and/or treatment of nausea and vomiting associated with chemotherapy, radiation therapy, or postsurgery; symptomatic treatment of diabetic gastric stasis; gastroesophageal reflux; facilitation of intubation of the small intestine

Mechanism of Action/Effect Blocks dopamine receptors in chemoreceptor trigger zone of the CNS; enhances the response to acetylcholine of tissue in upper GI tract causing

(Continued)

Metoclopramide *(Continued)*

enhanced motility and accelerated gastric emptying without stimulating gastric, biliary, or pancreatic secretions

Contraindications Hypersensitivity to metoclopramide or any component of the formulation; GI obstruction, perforation or hemorrhage; pheochromocytoma; history of seizure disorder

Warnings/Precautions Use with caution in patients with Parkinson's disease and in patients with a history of mental illness; has been associated with extrapyramidal symptoms and depression; may exacerbate seizures; neuroleptic malignant syndrome (NMS) has rarely been reported. Use lowest recommended doses initially; may cause transient increase in serum aldosterone; use caution in patients who are at risk of fluid overload (CHF, cirrhosis); dosage and/or frequency of administration should be modified in response to degree of renal impairment.

Drug Interactions

Cytochrome P450 Effect: Substrate of CYP1A2, 2D6; Inhibits CYP2D6

Decreased Effect: Anticholinergic agents antagonize metoclopramide's actions.

Increased Effect/Toxicity: Opiate analgesics may increase CNS depression. Metoclopramide may increase extrapyramidal symptoms (EPS) or risk when used concurrently with antipsychotic agents.

Nutritional/Ethanol Interactions Ethanol: Avoid ethanol (may increase CNS depression).

Effects on Lab Values ↑ aminotransferase [ALT (SGPT)/AST (SGOT)] (S), amylase (S)

Adverse Reactions Adverse reactions are more common/severe at dosages used for prophylaxis of chemotherapy-induced emesis.

>10%:
- Central nervous system: Restlessness, drowsiness, extrapyramidal symptoms (high-dose, up to 34%)
- Gastrointestinal: Diarrhea (may be dose-limiting)
- Neuromuscular & skeletal: Weakness

1% to 10%:
- Central nervous system: Insomnia, depression
- Dermatologic: Rash
- Endocrine & metabolic: Breast tenderness, prolactin stimulation
- Gastrointestinal: Nausea, xerostomia

<1% (Limited to important or life-threatening): Agranulocytosis, allergic reaction, AV block, CHF, gynecomastia, hepatotoxicity, hypertension or hypotension, jaundice, methemoglobinemia, neuroleptic malignant syndrome (NMS), sulfhemoglobinemia, tachycardia, tardive dyskinesia

Overdosage/Toxicology Symptoms of overdose include drowsiness, ataxia, extrapyramidal symptoms, seizures, methemoglobinemia (in infants). Disorientation, muscle hypertonia, irritability, and agitation are common. Metoclopramide often causes extrapyramidal symptoms (eg, dystonic reactions) requiring management with diphenhydramine 1-2 mg/kg (adults) up to a maximum of 50 mg I.M. or I.V. slow push followed by a maintenance dose for 48-72 hours. When these reactions are unresponsive to diphenhydramine, benztropine mesylate I.V. 1-2 mg (adults) may be effective. These agents are generally effective within 2-5 minutes.

Pharmacodynamics/Kinetics

Half-Life Elimination: May be dose dependent: Normal renal function: 4-7 hours

Onset: Oral: 0.5-1 hour; I.V.: 1-3 minutes

Duration: Therapeutic: 1-2 hours, regardless of route

Formulations

Injection: 5 mg/mL (2 mL, 10 mL, 30 mL, 50 mL, 100 mL)
Solution, oral concentrate: 10 mg/mL (10 mL, 30 mL)
Syrup: 5 mg/5 mL (10 mL, 480 mL) [sugar free]
Tablet: 5 mg, 10 mg

Dosing

Adults:

Antiemetic (chemotherapy-induced emesis): I.V.: 1-2 mg/kg 30 minutes before chemotherapy and every 2-4 hours to every 4-6 hours (and usually given with diphenhydramine 25-50 mg I.V./oral)

Gastroesophageal reflux: Oral: 10-15 mg/dose up to 4 times/day 30 minutes before meals or food and at bedtime. Single doses of 20 mg are occasionally needed for provoking situations. Efficacy of continuing metoclopramide beyond 12 weeks in reflux has not been determined.

Gastrointestinal hypomotility (gastroparesis):
- Oral: 10 mg 30 minutes before each meal and at bedtime for 2-8 weeks
- I.V. (for severe symptoms): 10 mg over 1-2 minutes; 10 days of I.V. therapy may be necessary for best response.

Postoperative nausea and vomiting: I.M.: 10 mg near end of surgery; 20 mg doses may be used

Facilitate intubation: I.V.: 10 mg

Elderly:

Antiemetic (chemotherapy-induced emesis):
- I.V.: 1-2 mg/kg/dose every 2-4 hours or (postsurgery); direct I.V. administration should be given slowly over 1-2 minutes.
- I.M.: 10-20 mg (near end of surgery)

Diabetic gastroparesis:
- Oral: Initial: 5 mg 30 minutes before meals and at bedtime for 2-8 weeks; increase if necessary to 10 mg doses.
- I.V.: Initiate at 5 mg over 1-2 minutes; increase to 10 mg if necessary.

Gastroesophageal reflux: Oral: 5 mg 4 times/day, 30 minutes before meals and at bedtime; increase dose to 10 mg 4 times/day if no response at lower dose.

Postoperative nausea and vomiting: I.M.: 5 mg near end of surgery; may repeat dose if necessary.

Pediatrics:

Gastroesophageal reflux: Oral: Children: 0.1-0.2 mg/kg/dose up to 4 times/day; efficacy of continuing metoclopramide beyond 12 weeks in reflux has not been determined. Total daily dose should not exceed 0.5 mg/kg/day.

Gastrointestinal hypomotility (gastroparesis): Oral, I.M., I.V.: Children: 0.1 mg/kg/dose up to 4 times/day, not to exceed 0.5 mg/kg/day.

Antiemetic (chemotherapy-induced emesis): I.V.: Children: 1-2 mg/kg 30 minutes before chemotherapy and every 2-4 hours

Facilitate intubation: I.V.: Children:

<6 years: 0.1 mg/kg

6-14 years: 2.5-5 mg

Renal Impairment:

Cl_{cr} 10-40 mL/minute: Administer 50% of normal dose.

Cl_{cr} <10 mL/minute: Administer 25% of normal dose.

Not dialyzable (0% to 5%); supplemental dose is not necessary.

Administration

I.V.: Lower doses of metoclopramide can be given I.V. push undiluted over 1-2 minutes. Parenteral doses of up to 10 mg should be given I.V. push. Higher doses to be given IVPB. Infuse over at least 15 minutes.

Stability

Storage: Injection is a clear, colorless solution and should be stored at controlled room temperature and protected from freezing. Injection is photosensitive and should be protected from light during storage. Dilutions do not require light protection if used within 24 hours.

Reconstitution: Stability of parenteral admixture at room temperature (25°C) and at refrigeration temperature (4°C) is 24 hours.

Standard diluent: 10-150 mg/50 mL D_5W or NS

Minimum volume: 50 mL D_5W or NS; send 10 mg unmixed to nursing unit

Compatibility: Stable in $D_5\frac{1}{2}NS$, D_5W, mannitol 20%, LR, NS

Y-site administration: Incompatible with allopurinol, amphotericin B cholesteryl sulfate complex, amsacrine, cefepime, doxorubicin liposome, furosemide, propofol

Compatibility in syringe: Incompatible with ampicillin, calcium gluconate, chloramphenicol, furosemide, penicillin G potassium, sodium bicarbonate

Compatibility when admixed: Incompatible with dexamethasone sodium phosphate with lorazepam and diphenhydramine, erythromycin lactobionate, floxacillin, fluorouracil, furosemide

Monitoring Laboratory Tests Periodic renal function

Monitoring and Teaching Issues

Physical Assessment: See Contraindications, Warnings/Precautions, and Dosing for use cautions. Assess potential for interactions with other prescriptions, OTC medications, or herbal products patient may be taking (see Drug Interactions). **I.V.:** See Administration and Reconstitution; vital signs should be monitored during infusion. Inpatients should use safety measures (eg, side rails up, call light within reach) and caution patient to call for assistance with ambulation. Assess results of laboratory tests (see above), therapeutic effects (according to purpose for use), and adverse reactions (see Adverse Reactions and Overdose/Toxicology - eg, extrapyramidal effects, parkinsonian-like reactions, adverse CNS changes). Teach patient proper use, possible side effects and appropriate interventions, and adverse symptoms to report (see Patient Education). Breast-feeding is not recommended.

Patient Education: Inform prescriber of all prescriptions, OTC medications, or herbal products you are taking, and any allergies you have. Do not take anything new during treatment unless approved by prescriber. Oral: Take this drug as prescribed, 30 minutes prior to eating. Do not increase dosage. Avoid alcohol. May cause dizziness, drowsiness, or blurred vision (use caution when driving or engaging in tasks that require alertness until response to drug is known); cause restlessness, anxiety, depression, or insomnia (will reverse when medication is discontinued). Report any CNS changes, spasticity or involuntary movements, unresolved diarrhea. **Breast-feeding precaution:** Breast-feeding is not recommended.

Geriatric Considerations: Elderly are more likely to develop tardive dyskinesia syndrome (especially elderly females) reactions than younger adults. Use lowest recommended doses initially. Must consider renal function (estimate creatinine clearance). It is recommended to do involuntary movement assessments on elderly using this medication at high doses and for long-term therapy.

Breast-feeding Issues: Enters breast milk; increased milk production; 2 reports of mild intestinal discomfort; AAP states MAY BE OF CONCERN.

Related Information

Antiemetics for Chemotherapy-Induced Nausea and Vomiting *on page 1639*

Metocurine Iodide *see page 1461*

Metolazone (me TOLE a zone)

U.S. Brand Names Mykrox®; Zaroxolyn®

Generic Available No

Pharmacologic Category Diuretic, Thiazide-Related

Pregnancy Risk Factor B (manufacturer); D (expert analysis)

Lactation Enters breast milk/use caution

Use Management of mild to moderate hypertension; treatment of edema in congestive heart failure and nephrotic syndrome, impaired renal function

Mechanism of Action/Effect Inhibits sodium reabsorption in the distal tubules causing increased excretion of sodium and water, as well as, potassium and hydrogen ions

Contraindications Hypersensitivity to metolazone, any component of the formulation, other thiazides, and sulfonamide derivatives; anuria; hepatic coma; pregnancy

(Continued)

Metolazone *(Continued)*

Warnings/Precautions Electrolyte disturbances (hypokalemia, hypochloremic alkalosis, hyponatremia) can occur. Use with caution in severe hepatic dysfunction; hepatic encephalopathy can be caused by electrolyte disturbances. Gout can be precipitate in certain patients with a history of gout, a familial predisposition to gout, or chronic renal failure. Cautious use in diabetics; may see a change in glucose control. Hypersensitivity reactions can occur. Can cause SLE exacerbation or activation. Use caution in severe renal impairment. Orthostatic hypotension may occur (potentiated by alcohol, barbiturates, narcotics, other antihypertensive drugs). Mykrox® tablets are not interchangeable with Zaroxolyn® tablets. Use with caution in patients with moderate or high cholesterol concentrations. Photosensitization may occur.

Chemical similarities are present among sulfonamides, sulfonylureas, carbonic anhydrase inhibitors, thiazides, and loop diuretics (except ethacrynic acid). Use in patients with thiazide or sulfonamide allergy is specifically contraindicated in product labeling, however, a risk of cross-reaction exists in patients with allergy to any of these compounds; avoid use when previous reaction has been severe.

Drug Interactions

Decreased Effect: Decreased absorption of metolazone with cholestyramine and colestipol. NSAIDs can decrease the efficacy of thiazide-type diuretics, reducing the diuretic and antihypertensive effects.

Increased Effect/Toxicity: Increased diuretic effect of metolazone with furosemide and other loop diuretics. Increased hypotension and/or renal adverse effects of ACE inhibitors may result in aggressively diuresed patients. Cyclosporine and thiazide-type diuretics can increase the risk of gout or renal toxicity. Digoxin toxicity can be exacerbated if a diuretic induces hypokalemia or hypomagnesemia. Lithium toxicity can occur with thiazide-type diuretics due to reduced renal excretion of lithium. Thiazide-type diuretics may prolong the duration of action of neuromuscular blocking agents.

Nutritional/Ethanol Interactions Herb/Nutraceutical: Avoid dong quai if using for hypertension (has estrogenic activity). Avoid dong quai, St John's wort (may also cause photosensitization). Avoid ephedra, yohimbe, ginseng (may worsen hypertension). Avoid natural licorice. Avoid garlic (may have increased antihypertensive effect).

Adverse Reactions

>10%: Central nervous system: Dizziness

1% to 10%:

- Cardiovascular: Orthostatic hypotension, palpitations, chest pain, cold extremities (rapidly acting), edema (rapidly acting), venous thrombosis (slow acting), syncope (slow acting)
- Central nervous system: Headache, fatigue, lethargy, malaise, lassitude, anxiety, depression, nervousness, "weird" feeling (rapidly acting), chills (slow acting)
- Dermatologic: Rash, pruritus, dry skin (rapidly acting)
- Endocrine & metabolic: Hypokalemia, impotence, reduced libido, excessive volume depletion (slow acting), hemoconcentration (slow acting), acute gouty attach (slow acting), weakness
- Gastrointestinal: Nausea, vomiting, abdominal pain, cramping, bloating, diarrhea or constipation, dry mouth
- Genitourinary: Nocturia
- Neuromuscular & skeletal: Muscle cramps, spasm
- Ocular: Eye itching (rapidly acting)
- Otic: Tinnitus (rapidly acting)
- Respiratory: Cough (rapidly acting), epistaxis (rapidly acting), sinus congestion (rapidly acting), sore throat (rapidly acting),

<1% (Limited to important or life-threatening): Agranulocytosis, aplastic anemia, glycosuria, hepatitis, hypercalcemia, hyperglycemia, leukopenia, pancreatitis, purpura, Stevens-Johnson syndrome, thrombocytopenia, toxic epidermal necrolysis

Overdosage/Toxicology Symptoms of overdose include orthostatic hypotension, dizziness, drowsiness, syncope, hemoconcentration and hemodynamic changes due to plasma volume depletion. Treatment is symptomatic and supportive.

Pharmacodynamics/Kinetics

Absorption: Incomplete

Bioavailability: Mykrox® reportedly has highest

Half-Life Elimination: Dependent upon renal function: 6-20 hours

Metabolism: Undergoes enterohepatic recirculation

Onset: Diuresis: ~60 minutes

Duration: 12-24 hours

Formulations

Tablet, rapid acting (Mykrox®): 0.5 mg

Tablet, slow acting (Zaroxolyn®): 2.5 mg, 5 mg, 10 mg

Dosing

Adults:

- Edema: Oral: 5-20 mg/dose every 24 hours
- Hypertension: Oral: 2.5-5 mg/dose every 24 hours
- Hypertension (Mykrox®): Oral: 0.5 mg/day; if response is not adequate, increase dose to maximum of 1 mg/day.

Elderly: Oral:

- Zaroxolyn®: Initial: 2.5 mg/day or every other day
- Mykrox®: 0.5 mg once daily; may increase to 1 mg if response is inadequate; do not use more than 1 mg/day.

Pediatrics: Limited experience in pediatric patients. Doses used have generally ranged from 0.05 to 0.1 mg/kg administered once daily. Prolonged use is not recommended.

Renal Impairment: Not dialyzable (0% to 5%)

Administration

Oral: May be taken with food or milk. Take early in day to avoid nocturia. Take the last dose of multiple doses no later than 6 PM unless instructed otherwise.

Monitoring Laboratory Tests Serum electrolytes (potassium, sodium, chloride, bicarbonate), renal function

Monitoring and Teaching Issues

Physical Assessment: Assess allergy history prior to beginning therapy. See Contraindications, Warnings/Precautions, and Dosing for use cautions. Assess potential for interactions with other prescriptions, OTC medications, or herbal products patient may be taking (see Drug Interactions). Assess results of laboratory tests (see above), therapeutic effects, and adverse reactions (see Adverse Reactions and Overdose/Toxicology - eg, electrolyte imbalance, hypotension). Caution diabetics (may see a change in glucose control). Teach patient proper use, possible side effects and appropriate interventions, and adverse symptoms to report (see Patient Education). **Pregnancy risk factor B/D** - see Pregnancy Risk Factor for use cautions; benefits of use should outweigh possible risks. Note breast-feeding caution.

Patient Education: Inform prescriber of all prescriptions, OTC medications, or herbal products you are taking, and any allergies you have. Do not take anything new during treatment unless approved by prescriber. Take exactly as directed, after breakfast. Include bananas or orange juice in daily diet but do not take dietary supplements without advice of prescriber. This medication does not replace other antihypertensive interventions; follow prescriber's instructions for diet and lifestyle changes. Weigh yourself weekly at the same time, in the same clothes. Report weight gain >5 lb/week. May cause dizziness or weakness (change position slowly when rising from sitting or lying, avoid driving or tasks requiring alertness until response to drug is known); nausea or loss of appetite (small, frequent meals, frequent mouth care, chewing gum, or sucking lozenges may help); impotence (reversible); constipation (increased exercise, fluids, fruit, or fiber may help); or photosensitivity (use sunscreen, wear protective clothing and eyewear, and avoid direct sunlight). Report flu-like symptoms, headache, joint soreness or weakness, difficulty breathing, skin rash, excessive fatigue, swelling of extremities, or difficulty breathing. **Pregnancy/breast-feeding precautions:** Inform prescriber if you are pregnant. Do not get pregnant while taking this medication. Consult prescriber for appropriate contraceptives. Consult prescriber if breast-feeding.

Dietary Issues: Should be taken after breakfast; may require potassium supplementation

Geriatric Considerations: When metolazone is used in combination with other diuretics, there is an increased risk of azotemia and electrolyte depletion, particularly in the elderly, monitor closely. May be effective in patients with glomerular filtration rate <20 mL/minute. Metolazone is often used in combination with a loop diuretic in patients who are unresponsive to the loop diuretic alone.

Additional Information Metolazone 5 mg is approximately equivalent to hydrochlorothiazide 50 mg. When taken the day of surgery, it may cause hypovolemia and the hypertensive patient undergoing general anesthesia to have labile blood pressure; use with caution prior to surgery or perioperatively.

Related Information

Heart Failure *on page 1670*

Metoprolol (me toe PROE lole)

U.S. Brand Names Lopressor®; Toprol-XL®

Synonyms Metoprolol Tartrate

Generic Available Yes: Except sustained release product

Pharmacologic Category Beta Blocker, $Beta_1$ Selective

Pregnancy Risk Factor C (manufacturer); D (2nd and 3rd trimesters - expert analysis)

Lactation Enters breast milk/use caution (AAP rates "compatible")

Use Treatment of hypertension and angina pectoris; prevention of myocardial infarction, atrial fibrillation, flutter, symptomatic treatment of hypertrophic subaortic stenosis; to reduce mortality/hospitalization in patients with congestive heart failure (stable NYHA Class II or III) in patients already receiving ACE inhibitors, diuretics, and/or digoxin (sustained-release only)

Use - Unlabeled/Investigational Treatment of ventricular arrhythmias, atrial ectopy, migraine prophylaxis, essential tremor, aggressive behavior

Mechanism of Action/Effect Selective inhibitor of $beta_1$-adrenergic receptors; competitively blocks $beta_1$-receptors, with little or no effect on $beta_2$-receptors at doses <100 mg; does not exhibit any membrane stabilizing or intrinsic sympathomimetic activity

Contraindications Hypersensitivity to metoprolol or any component of the formulation; sinus bradycardia; heart block greater than first degree (except in patients with a functioning artificial pacemaker); cardiogenic shock; uncompensated cardiac failure; pregnancy (2nd and 3rd trimesters)

Warnings/Precautions Use with caution in compensated heart failure; monitor closely for a worsening of the condition (efficacy has been demonstrated for metoprolol). Use caution in patients with PVD (can aggravate arterial insufficiency). Use caution with concurrent use of beta-blockers and either verapamil or diltiazem; bradycardia or heart block can occur. Avoid concurrent I.V. use of both agents. In general, beta-blockers should be avoided in patients with bronchospastic disease. Metoprolol, with B1 selectivity, should be used cautiously in bronchospastic disease with close monitoring. Use cautiously in diabetics because it can mask prominent hypoglycemic symptoms. Can mask signs of thyrotoxicosis. Can cause fetal harm when administered in pregnancy. Use cautiously in the hepatically impaired. Use care with anesthetic agents which decrease myocardial function. Beta-blocker therapy should not be withdrawn abruptly (particularly in patients with CAD), but gradually tapered to avoid acute tachycardia, hypertension, and/or ischemia. Pregnancy risk C/D (2nd and 3rd trimesters).

Drug Interactions

Cytochrome P450 Effect: Substrate of CYP2C19, **2D6**; Inhibits CYP2D6

Decreased Effect: Decreased effect of beta-blockers with aluminum salts, barbiturates, calcium salts, cholestyramine, colestipol, NSAIDs, penicillins (ampicillin), rifampin, salicylates, and sulfinpyrazone due to decreased bioavailability and plasma levels. Beta-blockers may decrease the effect of sulfonylureas.

Increased Effect/Toxicity: Metoprolol may increase the effects of other drugs which slow AV conduction (digoxin, verapamil, diltiazem), alpha-blockers (prazosin, terazosin), and

(Continued)

Metoprolol *(Continued)*

alpha-adrenergic stimulants (epinephrine, phenylephrine). Metoprolol may mask the tachycardia from hypoglycemia caused by insulin and oral hypoglycemics. In patients receiving concurrent therapy, the risk of hypertensive crisis is increased when either clonidine or the beta-blocker is withdrawn. Reserpine has been shown to enhance the effect of beta-blockers. Beta-blockers may increase the action or levels of ethanol, disopyramide, nondepolarizing muscle relaxants, and theophylline although the effects are difficult to predict.

Nutritional/Ethanol Interactions

Food: Food increases absorption. Metoprolol serum levels may be increased if taken with food.

Herb/Nutraceutical: Avoid dong quai if using for hypertension (has estrogenic activity). Avoid ephedra, yohimbe, ginseng (may worsen hypertension). Avoid garlic (may have increased antihypertensive effect).

Adverse Reactions

>10%:

Central nervous system: Drowsiness, insomnia
Endocrine & metabolic: Decreased sexual ability

1% to 10%:

Cardiovascular: Bradycardia, palpitations, edema, CHF, reduced peripheral circulation
Central nervous system: Mental depression
Gastrointestinal: Diarrhea or constipation, nausea, vomiting, stomach discomfort
Respiratory: Bronchospasm
Miscellaneous: Cold extremities

<1% (Limited to important or life-threatening): Arrhythmias, arthralgia, chest pain, confusion (especially in the elderly), depression, dyspnea, hallucinations, headache, hepatic dysfunction, hepatitis, jaundice, leukopenia, nervousness, orthostatic hypotension, thrombocytopenia

Overdosage/Toxicology Symptoms of intoxication include cardiac disturbances, CNS toxicity, bronchospasm, hypoglycemia and hyperkalemia. The most common cardiac symptoms include hypotension and bradycardia. Atrioventricular block, intraventricular conduction disturbances, cardiogenic shock, and asystole may occur with severe overdose, especially with membrane-depressant drugs (eg, propranolol). CNS effects include convulsions, coma, and respiratory arrest. Treatment is symptom-directed and supportive.

Pharmacodynamics/Kinetics

Absorption: 95%
Bioavailability: Oral: 40% to 50%
Half-Life Elimination: 3-4 hours; End-stage renal disease: 2.5-4.5 hours
Metabolism: Extensively hepatic; significant first-pass effect
Onset: Peak effect: Antihypertensive: Oral: 1.5-4 hours
Duration: 10-20 hours

Formulations

Injection, as tartrate: 1 mg/mL (5 mL)
Tablet, as tartrate: 25 mg, 50 mg, 100 mg
Tablet, sustained release, as succinate [equivalent to tartrate]: 25 mg, 50 mg, 100 mg, 200 mg

Dosing

Adults:

Hypertension, angina, SVT, MI prophylaxis:

Oral: 100-450 mg/day in 2-3 divided doses, begin with 50 mg twice daily and increase doses at weekly intervals to desired effect

Extended release: Same daily dose administered as a single dose

I.V.: Hypertension: Has been given in dosages 1.25-5 mg every 6-12 hours in patients unable to take oral medications

Congestive heart failure: Oral (extended release): Initial: 25 mg once daily (reduce to 12.5 mg once daily in NYHA class higher than class II); may double dosage every 2 weeks as tolerated, up to 200 mg/day

Myocardial infarction (acute): I.V.: 5 mg every 2 minutes for 3 doses in early treatment of myocardial infarction; thereafter give 50 mg orally every 6 hours 15 minutes after last I.V. dose and continue for 48 hours; then administer a maintenance dose of 100 mg twice daily.

Elderly: Oral: Initial: 25 mg/day; usual dose range: 25-300 mg/day; increase at 1- to 2-week intervals.

Extended release: 25-50 mg/day initially as a single dose; increase at 1- to 2-week intervals.

Pediatrics: Hypertension, arrhythmia: Oral: Children: 1-5 mg/kg/24 hours divided twice daily; allow 3 days between dose adjustments.

Renal Impairment: Hemodialysis: Administer dose posthemodialysis or administer 50 mg supplemental dose. Supplemental dose is not necessary following peritoneal dialysis.

Hepatic Impairment: Reduced dose is probably necessary.

Administration

Oral: Do not crush or chew sustained release tablets.
I.M.: Administer I.V. push: inject slowly over 1 minute
I.V.: Administer I.V. push, inject slowly over 1 minute.

Stability

Compatibility: Stable in D_5W, NS

Y-site administration: Incompatible with amphotericin B cholesteryl sulfate complex

Monitoring and Teaching Issues

Physical Assessment: See Contraindications, Warnings/Precautions, and Dosing for use cautions. Assess potential for interactions with other prescriptions, OTC medications, or herbal products patient may be taking (see Drug Interactions). **I.V.:** See specifics above and monitor blood pressure and cardiac status. Assess therapeutic effectiveness and adverse reactions (see Adverse Reactions and Overdose/Toxicology - eg, fluid balance, CHF, postural hypotension). Caution diabetics (may decrease the effect of sulfonylureas and can mask prominent hypoglycemic symptoms). Teach patient proper use (oral), possible side effects and appropriate interventions, and adverse symptoms to report (see Patient Education). **Pregnancy risk factor C/D** - see Pregnancy Risk Factor for use cautions; benefits of use should outweigh possible risks. Instruct patient in appropriate contraceptive measures. Note breast-feeding caution.

Patient Education: I.V. use in emergency situations: Patient information is appropriate to patient condition.

Oral: Inform prescriber of all prescriptions, OTC medications, or herbal products you are taking, and any allergies you have. Do not take anything new during treatment unless approved by prescriber. Take exactly as directed. Do not change dosage or discontinue without consulting prescriber. Take pulse daily, prior to medication and follow prescriber's instruction about holding medication. Do not take with antacids. If diabetic, monitor serum sugar closely (drug may alter glucose tolerance or mask signs of hypoglycemia). May cause fatigue, dizziness, or postural hypotension (use caution when changing position from lying or sitting to standing, when driving, or when climbing stairs until response to medication is known); or alteration in sexual performance (reversible). Report unresolved swelling of extremities, difficulty breathing or new cough, unresolved fatigue, unusual weight gain, unresolved constipation, or unusual muscle weakness. **Pregnancy/breast-feeding precautions:** Inform prescriber if you are or intend to become pregnant. Consult prescriber if breast-feeding.

Dietary Issues: Regular tablets should be taken with food. Sustained release tablets may be taken without regard to meals.

Geriatric Considerations: Due to alterations in the beta-adrenergic autonomic nervous system, beta-adrenergic blockade may result in less hemodynamic response than seen in younger adults.

Breast-feeding Issues: Metoprolol is considered compatible by the AAP. However, monitor the infant for signs of beta-blockade (hypotension, bradycardia, etc) with long-term use.

Pregnancy Issues: Crosses the placenta. None; mild IUGR probably secondary to maternal hypertension. Available evidence suggests safe use during pregnancy.

Related Information

Beta-Blockers *on page 1561*
Heart Failure *on page 1670*

Metoprolol Tartrate *see* Metoprolol *on page 893*

MetroCream® *see* Metronidazole *on page 895*

MetroGel® Topical *see* Metronidazole *on page 895*

MetroGel®-Vaginal *see* Metronidazole *on page 895*

Metro I.V.® *see* Metronidazole *on page 895*

MetroLotion® *see* Metronidazole *on page 895*

Metronidazole (me troe NI da zole)

U.S. Brand Names Flagyl®; Flagyl ER®; MetroCream®; MetroGel® Topical; MetroGel®-Vaginal; Metro I.V.®; MetroLotion®; Noritate™; Protostat® Oral

Synonyms Metronidazole Hydrochloride

Generic Available Yes

Pharmacologic Category Amebicide; Antibiotic, Topical; Antibiotic, Miscellaneous; Antiprotozoal

Pregnancy Risk Factor B (may be contraindicated in 1st trimester)

Lactation Enters breast milk/not recommended (AAP rates "of concern")

Use Treatment of susceptible anaerobic bacterial and protozoal infections in the following conditions: Amebiasis, symptomatic and asymptomatic trichomoniasis; skin and skin structure infections; CNS infections; intra-abdominal infections (as part of combination regimen); systemic anaerobic infections; treatment of antibiotic-associated pseudomembranous colitis (AAPC), bacterial vaginosis; as part of a multidrug regimen for *H. pylori* eradication to reduce the risk of duodenal ulcer recurrence; also used in Crohn's disease and hepatic encephalopathy

Orphan drug: MetroGel® Topical: Treatment of acne rosacea

Mechanism of Action/Effect Inhibits DNA synthesis in susceptible organisms

Contraindications Hypersensitivity to metronidazole or any component of the formulation; pregnancy (1st trimester - found to be carcinogenic in rats)

Warnings/Precautions Use with caution in patients with liver impairment due to potential accumulation, blood dyscrasias; history of seizures, CHF, or other sodium retaining states; reduce dosage in patients with severe liver impairment, CNS disease, and severe renal failure (Cl_{cr} <10 mL/minute); if *H. pylori* is not eradicated in patients being treated with metronidazole in a regimen, it should be assumed that metronidazole-resistance has occurred and it should not again be used; seizures and neuropathies have been reported especially with increased doses and chronic treatment; if this occurs, discontinue therapy

Drug Interactions

Cytochrome P450 Effect: Inhibits CYP2C8/9, 3A4

Decreased Effect: Phenytoin, phenobarbital (potentially other enzyme inducers) may decrease metronidazole half-life and effects.

Increased Effect/Toxicity: Ethanol may cause a disulfiram-like reaction. Warfarin and metronidazole may increase bleeding times (PT) which may result in bleeding. Cimetidine may increase metronidazole levels. Metronidazole may inhibit metabolism of cisapride, causing potential arrhythmias; avoid concurrent use. Metronidazole may increase lithium levels/toxicity.

Nutritional/Ethanol Interactions

Ethanol: Metronidazole inhibits ethanol's usual metabolism. Avoid all ethanol or any ethanol-containing drugs (may cause disulfiram-like reaction characterized by flushing,

(Continued)

Metronidazole *(Continued)*

headache, nausea, vomiting, sweating or tachycardia). Patients should be warned to avoid ethanol during and 72 hours after therapy.

Food: Peak antibiotic serum concentration lowered and delayed, but total drug absorbed not affected.

Effects on Lab Values May cause falsely decreased AST and ALT levels.

Adverse Reactions

Systemic:

>10%:

Central nervous system: Dizziness, headache

Gastrointestinal (12%): Nausea, diarrhea, loss of appetite, vomiting

<1% (Limited to important or life-threatening): Ataxia, change in taste sensation, dark urine, disulfiram-type reaction with ethanol, furry tongue, hypersensitivity, leukopenia, metallic taste, neuropathy, pancreatitis, seizures, thrombophlebitis, vaginal candidiasis, xerostomia

Vaginal:

>10%: Genitourinary: *Candida* cervicitis or vaginitis

1% to 10%:

Central nervous system: Dry mouth, furry tongue, diarrhea, nausea, vomiting, anorexia

Gastrointestinal: Altered taste sensation

Genitourinary: Burning or irritation of penis of sexual partner; burning or increased frequency of urination, vulvitis, dark urine

Overdosage/Toxicology Symptoms of overdose include nausea, vomiting, ataxia, seizures, and peripheral neuropathy. Treatment is symptomatic and supportive.

Pharmacodynamics/Kinetics

Absorption: Oral: Well absorbed; Topical: Concentrations achieved systemically after application of 1 g topically are 10 times less than those obtained after a 250 mg oral dose

Half-Life Elimination: Neonates: 25-75 hours; Others: 6-8 hours, prolonged with hepatic impairment; End-stage renal disease: 21 hours

Time to Peak: Serum: Oral: Immediate release: 1-2 hours

Metabolism: Hepatic (30% to 60%)

Formulations

Capsule: 375 mg

Cream: 0.75% (45 g), 1% (30 g)

Gel: 0.75% [7.5 mg/mL] (30 g)

Gel, vaginal: 0.75% [5 g applicator delivering 37.5 mg] (70 g tube)

Injection, powder for reconstitution, as hydrochloride: 500 mg

Injection [ready-to-use]: 5 mg/mL (100 mL)

Lotion: 0.75%

Tablet: 250 mg, 500 mg

Tablet, extended release: 750 mg

Dosing

Adults:

Amebiasis: Oral: 500-750 mg every 8 hours for 5-10 days

Trichomoniasis: Oral: 250 mg every 8 hours for 7 days or 2 g as a single dose

Anaerobic infections: Oral, I.V.: 500 mg every 6-8 hours, not to exceed 4 g/day

Antibiotic-associated pseudomembranous colitis: Oral: 250-500 mg 3-4 times/day for 10-14 days

Helicobacter pylori eradication: Oral: 250 mg with meals and at bedtime for 14 days; requires combination therapy with at least one other antibiotic and an acid-suppressing agent (proton pump inhibitor or H_2 blocker)

Vaginosis: Intravaginal: 1 applicatorful (~37.5 mg metronidazole) once or twice daily for 5 days; apply once in morning and evening if using twice daily, if daily, use at bedtime

Acne rosacea: Topical: Apply and rub a thin film twice daily, morning and evening, to entire affected areas after washing. Significant therapeutic results should be noticed within 3 weeks. Clinical studies have demonstrated continuing improvement through 9 weeks of therapy.

Elderly: Use the lower end of the dosing recommendations for adults; do not administer as single dose as efficacy has not been established.

Pediatrics:

Anaerobic infections: Oral, I.V.:

Postnatal age >7 days:

1200-2000 g: 15 mg/kg/day in divided doses every 12 hours

>2000 g: 30 mg/kg/day in divided doses every 12 hours

Infants and Children:

Oral: 15-35 mg/kg/day in divided doses every 8 hours

I.V.: 30 mg/kg/day in divided doses every 6 hours

Clostridium difficile (antibiotic-associated colitis): Oral: 20 mg/kg/day divided every 6 hours

Maximum dose: 2 g/day

Amebiasis: Infants and Children: Oral: 35-50 mg/kg/day in divided doses every 8 hours for 10 days

Trichomoniasis: Infants and Children: Oral: 15-30 mg/kg/day in divided doses every 8 hours for 7 days

Renal Impairment:

Cl_{cr} <10 mL/minute: Administer 50% of dose or every 12 hours.

Hemodialysis effects: Extensively removed by hemodialysis and peritoneal dialysis (50% to 100%). Administer dose posthemodialysis. During peritoneal dialysis, dose as for Cl_{cr} <10 mL/minute.

Continuous arteriovenous or venovenous hemofiltration: Dose as for normal renal function

Hepatic Impairment: Unchanged in mild liver disease; reduce dosage in severe liver disease.

Administration

Oral: May be taken with food to minimize stomach upset.

I.V.: Avoid contact between the drug and aluminum in the infusion set.

Topical: No disulfiram-like reactions have been reported after **topical** application, although metronidazole can be detected in the blood.

Stability

Storage: Metronidazole injection should be stored at 15°C to 30°C and protected from light. Product may be refrigerated but crystals may form; crystals redissolve on warming to room temperature. Prolonged exposure to light will cause a darkening of the product. However, short-term exposure to normal room light does not adversely affect metronidazole stability. Direct sunlight should be avoided. Stability of parenteral admixture at room temperature (25°C): Out of overwrap stability: 30 days.

Reconstitution: Standard diluent: 500 mg/100 mL NS

Compatibility: Stable in D_5W, NS

Y-site administration: Incompatible with amphotericin B cholesteryl sulfate complex, aztreonam, filgrastim, meropenem, warfarin

Compatibility when admixed: Incompatible with aztreonam, dopamine, meropenem

Monitoring and Teaching Issues

Physical Assessment: Assess effectiveness and interactions of other medications patient may be taking (see Drug Interactions). Monitor laboratory tests, therapeutic response and adverse, reactions (see Warnings/Precautions and Adverse Reactions) according to dose, route of administration, and purpose of therapy. Assess knowledge/teach patient appropriate use, interventions to reduce side effects, and adverse symptoms to report (see Patient Education). **Pregnancy risk factor B** - see Pregnancy Risk Factor for use cautions. Breast-feeding is not recommended.

Patient Education: Take exactly as directed. May take with or without food. Take with food if medication causes upset stomach. Avoid alcohol during and for 72 hours after last dose. With alcohol you may experience severe flushing, headache, nausea, vomiting, or chest and abdominal pain. May discolor urine (brown/black/dark) (normal). You may experience "metallic" taste disturbance or nausea or vomiting (small, frequent meals, frequent mouth care, chewing gum, or sucking lozenges may help). Refrain from intercourse or use a barrier contraceptive if being treated for trichomoniasis. Report unresolved or severe fatigue; weakness; fever or chills; mouth or vaginal sores; numbness, tingling, or swelling of extremities; difficulty breathing; or lack of improvement or worsening of condition. **Pregnancy/breast-feeding precautions:** Inform prescriber if you are pregnant. Breast-feeding is not recommended.

Topical: Wash hands and area before applying. Apply medication thinly. Wash hands after applying. Avoid contact with eyes. Do not cover with occlusive dressing. Report severe skin irritation or if condition does not improve.

Dietary Issues: Take on an empty stomach. Drug may cause GI upset; if GI upset occurs, take with food. Sodium content of 500 mg (I.V.): 322 mg (14 mEq).

Geriatric Considerations: Adjust dose based on renal function.

Breast-feeding Issues: It is suggested to stop breast-feeding for 12-24 hours following single dose therapy to allow excretion of dose.

Pregnancy Issues: Crosses the placenta (carcinogenic in rats); contraindicated for the treatment of trichomoniasis during the first trimester of pregnancy, unless alternative treatment is inadequate. Until safety and efficacy for other indications have been established, use only during pregnancy when the benefit to the mother outweighs the potential risk to the fetus.

Related Information

Helicobacter pylori Treatment *on page 1676*

Metronidazole, Bismuth Subsalicylate, and Tetracycline *see* Bismuth Subsalicylate, Metronidazole, and Tetracycline *on page 170*

Metronidazole Hydrochloride *see* Metronidazole *on page 895*

Metronidazole, Tetracycline, and Bismuth Subsalicylate *see* Bismuth Subsalicylate, Metronidazole, and Tetracycline *on page 170*

Metubine® Iodide *see page 1461*

Mevacor® *see* Lovastatin *on page 826*

Mevinolin *see* Lovastatin *on page 826*

Mexiletine (MEKS i le teen)

U.S. Brand Names Mexitil®

Generic Available Yes

Pharmacologic Category Antiarrhythmic Agent, Class Ib

Pregnancy Risk Factor C

Lactation Enters breast milk/compatible

Use Management of serious ventricular arrhythmias; suppression of PVCs

Use - Unlabeled/Investigational Diabetic neuropathy

Mechanism of Action/Effect Class IB antiarrhythmic, structurally related to lidocaine, which inhibits inward sodium current, decreases rate of rise of Phase 0, increases effective refractory period/action potential duration ratio

Contraindications Hypersensitivity to mexiletine or any component of the formulation; cardiogenic shock; second- or third-degree AV block (except in patients with a functioning artificial pacemaker)

Warnings/Precautions Can be proarrhythmic. May cause acute hepatic injury. Use cautiously in patients with first-degree block, pre-existing sinus node dysfunction, intraventricular conduction delays, significant hepatic dysfunction, hypotension, or severe CHF. Electrolytes disturbances alter response. Alterations in urinary pH may change urinary excretion. Rare hepatic toxicity may occur. Electrolyte abnormalities should be corrected before initiating therapy (can worsen CHF). Pregnancy risk C.

(Continued)

Mexiletine *(Continued)*

Drug Interactions

Cytochrome P450 Effect: Substrate of **CYP1A2, 2D6**; Inhibits CYP1A2

Decreased Effect: Decreased mexiletine plasma levels when used with phenobarbital, phenytoin, rifampin, cimetidine, or other hepatic enzyme inducers. Urinary acidifying agents may decrease mexiletine levels.

Increased Effect/Toxicity: Mexiletine and caffeine or theophylline may result in elevated levels of theophylline and caffeine. Quinidine, fluvoxamine, and urinary alkalinizers (antacids, sodium bicarbonate, acetazolamide) may increase mexiletine blood levels.

Nutritional/Ethanol Interactions Food: Food may decrease the rate, but not the extent of oral absorption; diets which affect urine pH can increase or decrease excretion of mexiletine. Avoid dietary changes that alter urine pH.

Effects on Lab Values Abnormal liver function test, positive ANA, thrombocytopenia

Adverse Reactions

>10%:

Central nervous system: Lightheadedness (11% to 25%), dizziness (20% to 25%), nervousness (5% to 10%), incoordination (10%)

Gastrointestinal: GI distress (41%), nausea/vomiting (40%)

Neuromuscular & skeletal: Trembling, unsteady gait, tremor (13%), ataxia (10% to 20%)

1% to 10%:

Cardiovascular: Chest pain (3% to 8%), premature ventricular contractions (1% to 2%), palpitations (4% to 8%), angina (2%), proarrhythmic (10% to 15% in patients with malignant arrhythmias)

Central nervous system: Confusion, headache, insomnia (5% to 7%), depression (2%)

Dermatologic: Rash (4%)

Gastrointestinal: Constipation or diarrhea (4% to 5%), xerostomia (3%), abdominal pain (1%)

Neuromuscular & skeletal: Weakness (5%), numbness of fingers or toes (2% to 4%), paresthesias (2%), arthralgias (1%)

Ocular: Blurred vision (5% to 7%), nystagmus (6%)

Otic: Tinnitus (2% to 3%)

Respiratory: Dyspnea (3%)

<1% (Limited to important or life-threatening): Agranulocytosis, alopecia, AV block, cardiogenic shock, CHF, dysphagia, exfoliative dermatitis, hallucinations, hepatic necrosis, hepatitis, hypotension, impotence, leukopenia, myelofibrosis, pancreatitis (rare), psychosis, pulmonary fibrosis, seizures, sinus arrest, SLE syndrome, Stevens-Johnson syndrome, syncope, thrombocytopenia, torsade de pointes, upper GI bleeding, urinary retention, urticaria

Overdosage/Toxicology Has a narrow therapeutic index and severe toxicity may occur slightly above the therapeutic range, especially with other antiarrhythmic drugs. Acute ingestion of twice the daily therapeutic dose is potentially life-threatening. Symptoms of overdose include sedation, confusion, coma, seizures, respiratory arrest and cardiac toxicity (sinus arrest, AV block, asystole, and hypotension). The QRS and QT intervals are usually normal, although they may be prolonged after massive overdose. Other effects include dizziness, paresthesia, tremor, ataxia, and GI disturbance. Treatment is symptomatic and supportive.

Pharmacodynamics/Kinetics

Absorption: Elderly have a slightly slower rate, but extent of absorption is the same as young adults

Half-Life Elimination: Adults: 10-14 hours (average: 14.4 hours elderly, 12 hours younger adults); prolonged with hepatic impairment or heart failure

Time to Peak: 2-3 hours

Metabolism: Hepatic; low first-pass effect

Formulations Capsule: 150 mg, 200 mg, 250 mg

Dosing

Adults & Elderly: Arrhythmias: Oral: Initial: 200 mg every 8 hours (may load with 400 mg if necessary); adjust dose every 2-3 days; usual dose: 200-300 mg every 8 hours; maximum: 1.2 g/day (some patients respond to every 12-hour dosing). When switching from another antiarrhythmic, initiate a 200 mg dose 6-12 hours after stopping former agents, 3-6 hours after stopping procainamide.

Hepatic Impairment: Patients with hepatic impairment or CHF may require dose reduction; reduce dose to 25% to 30% of usual dose

Administration

Oral: Take with food. Administer around-the-clock to promote less variation in peak and trough serum levels.

Monitoring Laboratory Tests Regular serum levels

Monitoring and Teaching Issues

Physical Assessment: Assess other medications patient may be taking for effectiveness and interactions (see Drug Interactions). See Warnings/Precautions for use cautions. Monitor laboratory tests, therapeutic response, and adverse reactions (see Warnings/Precautions and Adverse Reactions) at beginning of therapy, when titrating dosage, and on a regular basis with long-term therapy. **Note:** Mexiletine has a low toxic:therapeutic ratio and overdose may easily produce severe and life-threatening reactions (see Overdose/Toxicology). Assess knowledge/teach patient appropriate use, interventions to reduce side effects, and adverse symptoms to report (see Patient Education). **Pregnancy risk factor C** - benefits of use should outweigh possible risks.

Patient Education: Take exactly as directed with food or antacids, around-the-clock. Do not take additional doses or discontinue without consulting prescriber. Do not change diet without consulting prescriber. You will need regular cardiac checkups and blood tests while taking this medication. You may experience drowsiness or dizziness, numbness, or visual changes (use caution when driving or engaging in tasks requiring alertness until response to drug is known); nausea, vomiting, or heartburn (small, frequent meals, frequent mouth care, chewing gum, or sucking lozenges may help); or headaches or sleep disturbances (usually temporary, if persistent consult prescriber). Report chest pain, palpitation, or erratic heartbeat; increased weight or swelling of hands or feet; chills, fever, or persistent sore throat; numbness, weakness, trembling, or unsteady gait; blurred vision or ringing in ears; or difficulty breathing. **Pregnancy precaution:** Inform prescriber if you are or intend to become pregnant.

Related Information

Antiarrhythmic Drugs *on page 1551*

Mexitil® *see* Mexiletine *on page 897*

Miacalcin® *see* Calcitonin *on page 199*

Micanol® *see* Anthralin *on page 108*

Micarderm® *see* Miconazole *on page 899*

Micardis® *see* Telmisartan *on page 1279*

Micardis® HCT *see* Telmisartan and Hydrochlorothiazide *on page 1280*

Micatin® [OTC] *see* Miconazole *on page 899*

Miconazole (mi KON a zole)

U.S. Brand Names Aloe Vesta® 2-n-1 Antifungal [OTC]; Baza® Antifungal [OTC]; Carrington Antifungal [OTC]; Femizol-M™ [OTC]; Fungoid® Tincture [OTC]; Lotrimin® AF Powder/Spray [OTC]; Micarderm®; Micatin® [OTC]; Micro-Guard® [OTC]; Mitrazol™ [OTC]; Monistat® 1 Combination Pack [OTC]; Monistat® 3 [OTC]; Monistat® 7 [OTC]; Monistat-Derm®; Triple Care® Antifungal [OTC]; Zeasorb®-AF [OTC]

Synonyms Miconazole Nitrate

Generic Available Yes

Pharmacologic Category Antifungal Agent, Topical; Antifungal Agent, Vaginal

Pregnancy Risk Factor C

Lactation Excretion in breast milk unknown/use caution

Use Treatment of vulvovaginal candidiasis and a variety of skin and mucous membrane fungal infections

Mechanism of Action/Effect Inhibits biosynthesis of ergosterol, damaging the fungal cell wall membrane, which increases permeability causing leaking of nutrients

Contraindications Hypersensitivity to miconazole or any component of the formulation

Warnings/Precautions For external use only; discontinue if sensitivity or irritation develop. Petrolatum-based vaginal products may damage rubber or latex condoms or diaphragms. Separate use by 3 days. Pregnancy risk C.

Drug Interactions

Cytochrome P450 Effect: Substrate of **CYP3A4**; Inhibits CYP2A6, 2C8/9, 2E1, 3A4

Decreased Effect: Amphotericin B may decrease antifungal effect of both agents.

Increased Effect/Toxicity: **Note:** The majority of reported drug interactions were observed following intravenous miconazole administration. Although systemic absorption following topical and/or vaginal administration is low, potential interactions due to CYP isoenzyme inhibition may occur (rarely). This may be particularly true in situations where topical absorption may be increased (ie, inflamed tissue).

Miconazole coadministered with warfarin has increased the anticoagulant effect of warfarin (including reports associated with vaginal miconazole therapy of as little as 3 days). Phenytoin levels may be increased. Miconazole may inhibit the metabolism of oral sulfonylureas. Concurrent administration of cisapride is contraindicated due to an increased risk of cardiotoxicity.

Nutritional/Ethanol Interactions Herb/Nutraceutical: St John's wort may decrease miconazole levels.

Effects on Lab Values ↑ protein

Adverse Reactions Frequency not defined.

Topical: Allergic contact dermatitis, burning, maceration

Vaginal: Abdominal cramps, burning, irritation, itching

Pharmacodynamics/Kinetics

Absorption: Topical: Negligible

Half-Life Elimination: Multiphasic: Initial: 40 minutes; Secondary: 126 minutes; Terminal: 24 hours

Metabolism: Hepatic

Formulations

Combination products: Miconazole nitrate vaginal suppository 200 mg (3s) and miconazole nitrate external cream 2%; Miconazole nitrate vaginal suppository 100 mg (7s) and miconazole nitrate external cream 2%

Monistat® 1 Combination Pack: Miconazole nitrate vaginal insert 1200 mg (1) and miconazole external cream 2% (5 g) [Note: Do not confuse with 1-Day™ (formerly Monistat® 1) which contains tioconazole]

Monistat® 3 Combination Pack: Miconazole nitrate vaginal suppository 200 mg (3s) and miconazole nitrate external cream 2%

Monistat® 3 Cream Combination Pack: Miconazole nitrate vaginal cream 4% and miconazole nitrate external cream 2%

Monistat® 7 Combination Pack: Miconazole nitrate vaginal suppository 100 mg (7s) and miconazole nitrate external cream 2%

Monistat® 7 Combination Pack: Miconazole nitrate vaginal cream 2% (7 prefilled applicators) and miconazole nitrate external cream 2%

Cream, topical, as nitrate: 2% (15 g, 30 g, 45 g)

Baza® Antifungal: 2% (4 g, 57 g, 142 g) [zinc oxide based formula]

Carrington Antifungal: 2% (150 g)

Micaderm®: 2% (30 g)

Micatin®: 2% (15 g)

Micro-Guard®, Mitrazol™: 2% (60 g)

Monistat-Derm®: 2% (15 g, 30 g, 85 g)

Triple Care® Antifungal: 2% (60 g, 98 g)

Cream, vaginal, as nitrate [available in prefilled or with single refillable applicator]: 2% (45 g)

Femizol-M™: 2% (47 g)

(Continued)

Miconazole *(Continued)*

Monistat® 3: 4% (15 g, 25 g)
Monistat® 7: 2% (45 g)
Liquid, spray, as nitrate (Micatin®): 2% (90 mL, 105 mL)
Lotion, powder, as nitrate (Zeasorb®-AF): 2% (56 g) [contains alcohol 70%]
Ointment, topical, as nitrate: (Aloe Vesta® 2-n-1 Antifungal): 2% (60 g, 150 g)
Powder, topical, as nitrate:
Lotrimin® AF, Micatin®, Micro-Guard®: 2% (90 g)
Mitrazol™: 2% (30 g)
Zeasorb®-AF: 2% (70 g)
Powder spray, topical, as nitrate (Lotrimin® AF): 2% (100 g)
Suppository, vaginal, as nitrate: 100 mg (7s); 200 mg (3s)
Monistat® 3: 200 mg (3s)
Monistat® 7: 100 mg (7s)
Tincture, topical, as nitrate (Fungoid®): 2% (30 mL, 473 mL) [contains isopropyl alcohol 30%]

Dosing

Adults & Elderly:
Tinea pedis and tinea corporis: Topical: Apply twice daily for 4 weeks
Tinea cruris: Topical: Apply twice daily for 2 weeks
Vulvovaginal candidiasis: Vaginal:
Cream, 2%: Insert 1 applicatorful at bedtime for 7 days
Cream, 4%: Insert 1 applicatorful at bedtime for 3 days
Suppository, 100 mg: Insert 1 suppository at bedtime for 7 days
Suppository, 200 mg: Insert 1 suppository at bedtime for 3 days
Suppository, 1200 mg: Insert 1 suppository at bedtime (a one-time dose)

Note: Many products are available as a combination pack, with a suppository for vaginal instillation and cream to relieve external symptoms.

Pediatrics: Refer to adult dosing. **Note:** Not for OTC use in children <2 years.

Monitoring and Teaching Issues

Physical Assessment: See Contraindications and Warnings/Precautions for use cautions. Assess potential for interactions with other prescriptions, OTC medications, or herbal products patient may be taking (see Drug Interactions). Caution patients with diabetes to test serum glucose regularly (may inhibit the metabolism of oral sulfonylureas). Teach proper use, possible side effects and appropriate interventions (eg, bleeding precautions), and adverse symptoms to report (see Patient Education). **Pregnancy risk factor C** - benefits of use should outweigh possible risks. Note breast-feeding caution.

Patient Education: Inform prescriber of all prescriptions, OTC medications, or herbal products you are taking, and any allergies you have. Do not take anything new during treatment. Use full course of therapy as directed; do not discontinue without consulting prescriber. Some infections may require long periods of therapy. Practice good hygiene measures to prevent reinfection. If you are diabetic, you should test serum glucose regularly - this medication may inhibit the metabolism of oral sulfonylureas. Report persistent burning, itching, or irritation to healthcare provider. **Pregnancy/breast-feeding precautions:** Inform prescriber if you are or intend to become pregnant. Consult prescriber if breast-feeding.

Topical: Wash and dry area before applying medication; apply thinly. Do not get in or near eyes. Not for OTC use in children <2 years of age.

Vaginal: Consult with healthcare provider if using for a vaginal yeast infection for the first time. Insert high in vagina. Refrain from intercourse during treatment. Condoms and diaphragms may not be effective during therapy. Do not use tampons, douches, spermicides, or other vaginal products during treatment.

Geriatric Considerations: Assess patient's ability to self administer, may be difficult in patients with arthritis or limited range of motion.

Miconazole Nitrate *see* Miconazole *on page 899*
MICRhoGAM™ *see page 1498*
Microfibrillar Collagen Hemostat *see page 1461*
Microgestin™ Fe *see* Ethinyl Estradiol and Norethindrone *on page 527*
Micro-Guard® [OTC] *see* Miconazole *on page 899*
Micro-K® 10 Entencaps *see* Potassium Supplements *on page 1106*
Micro-K® Entencaps *see* Potassium Supplements *on page 1106*
Micro-K® LS *see* Potassium Supplements *on page 1106*
Micronase® *see* GlyBURIDE *on page 636*
Micronor® *see* Norethindrone *on page 984*
Microzide™ *see* Hydrochlorothiazide *on page 664*
Micrurus fluvius *see page 1460*
Midamor® *see* Amiloride *on page 77*

Midazolam (MID aye zoe lam)

U.S. Brand Names Versed® [DSC]
Synonyms Midazolam Hydrochloride
Restrictions C-IV
Generic Available Yes
Pharmacologic Category Benzodiazepine
Pregnancy Risk Factor D
Lactation Enters breast milk/not recommended (AAP rates "of concern")
Use Preoperative sedation and provides conscious sedation prior to diagnostic or radiographic procedures; ICU sedation (continuous infusion); intravenous anesthesia (induction); intravenous anesthesia (maintenance)
Use - Unlabeled/Investigational Anxiety, status epilepticus

Mechanism of Action/Effect Binds to stereospecific benzodiazepine receptors on the postsynaptic GABA neuron at several sites within the central nervous system, including the limbic system, reticular formation. Enhancement of the inhibitory effect of GABA on neuronal excitability results by increased neuronal membrane permeability to chloride ions. This shift in chloride ions results in hyperpolarization (a less excitable state) and stabilization.

Contraindications Hypersensitivity to midazolam or any component of the formulation, including benzyl alcohol (cross-sensitivity with other benzodiazepines may exist); parenteral form is not for intrathecal or epidural injection; narrow-angle glaucoma; pregnancy

Warnings/Precautions May cause severe respiratory depression, respiratory arrest, or apnea. Use with extreme caution, particularly in noncritical care settings. Appropriate resuscitative equipment and qualified personnel must be available for administration and monitoring. Initial dosing must be cautiously titrated and individualized, particularly in elderly or debilitated patients, hepatic impairment, or renal impairment, particularly if other CNS depressants (including opiates) are used concurrently. Initial doses in elderly or debilitated patients should not exceed 2.5 mg. Use with caution in patients with respiratory disease or impaired gag reflex. Use during upper airway procedures may increase risk of hypoventilation. Prolonged responses have been noted following extended administration by continuous infusion (possibly due to metabolite accumulation) or in the presence of drugs which inhibit midazolam metabolism.

May cause hypotension - hemodynamic events are more common in pediatric patients or patients with hemodynamic instability. Hypotension and/or respiratory depression may occur more frequently in patients who have received narcotic analgesics. Use with caution in obese patients, chronic renal failure, and CHF. Parenteral form contains benzyl alcohol - avoid rapid injection in neonates or prolonged infusions. Should not be used in shock, coma, or acute alcohol intoxication. Avoid intra-arterial administration or extravasation of parenteral formulation.

Causes CNS depression (dose-related) resulting in sedation, dizziness, confusion, or ataxia which may impair physical and mental capabilities. A minimum of 1 day should elapse after midazolam administration before attempting to drive or operate machinery. Use with caution in patients receiving other CNS depressants or psychoactive agents. Effects with other sedative drugs or ethanol may be potentiated. Benzodiazepines have been associated with falls and traumatic injury and should be used with extreme caution in patients who are at risk of these events (especially the elderly).

Midazolam causes anterograde amnesia. Paradoxical reactions, including hyperactive or aggressive behavior have been reported with benzodiazepines, particularly in adolescent/pediatric or psychiatric patients. Does not have analgesic, antidepressant, or antipsychotic properties.

Benzodiazepines have been associated with dependence and acute withdrawal symptoms on discontinuation or reduction in dose. Acute withdrawal, including seizures, may be precipitated after administration of flumazenil to patients receiving long-term benzodiazepine therapy.

Drug Interactions

Cytochrome P450 Effect: Substrate of CYP2B6, **3A4**; Inhibits CYP2C8/9, 3A4

Decreased Effect: Carbamazepine, phenytoin, and rifampin may reduce the effects of midazolam.

Increased Effect/Toxicity: Midazolam levels/effects may be increased by inhibitors of CYP3A4, including delavirdine, indinavir, saquinavir, quinupristin-dalfopristin, zafirlukast, zileuton, verapamil, troleandomycin, miconazole, itraconazole, nifedipine, grapefruit juice, diltiazem, fluconazole, ketoconazole, clarithromycin, and erythromycin. Use is contraindicated with amprenavir and ritonavir. **If narcotics or other CNS depressants are administered concomitantly, the midazolam dose should be reduced by 30% if <65 years of age, or by at least 50% if >65 years of age.**

Nutritional/Ethanol Interactions

Ethanol: Avoid ethanol (may increase CNS depression).

Food: Grapefruit juice may increase serum concentrations of midazolam; avoid concurrent use with oral form.

Herb/Nutraceutical: Avoid concurrent use with St John's wort (may decrease midazolam levels, may increase CNS depression). Avoid concurrent use with valerian, kava kava, gotu kola (may increase CNS depression).

Adverse Reactions As reported in adults unless otherwise noted:

>10%: Respiratory: Decreased tidal volume and/or respiratory rate decrease, apnea (3% children)

1% to 10%:

Cardiovascular: Hypotension (3% children)

Central nervous system: Drowsiness (1%), oversedation, headache (1%), seizure-like activity (1% children)

Gastrointestinal: Nausea (3%), vomiting (3%)

Local: Pain and local reactions at injection site (4% I.M., 5% I.V.; severity less than diazepam)

Ocular: Nystagmus (1% children)

Respiratory: Cough (1%)

Miscellaneous: Physical and psychological dependence with prolonged use, hiccups (4%, 1% children), paradoxical reaction (2% children)

<1% (Limited to important or life-threatening): Agitation, amnesia, bigeminy, bronchospasm, emergence delirium, euphoria, hallucinations, laryngospasm, rash

Overdosage/Toxicology Symptoms of overdose include respiratory depression, hypotension, coma, stupor, confusion, and apnea. Treatment for benzodiazepine overdose is supportive. Flumazenil has been shown to selectively block the binding of benzodiazepines to its receptor, resulting in reversal of CNS depression but not always respiratory depression.

(Continued)

Midazolam *(Continued)*

Pharmacodynamics/Kinetics

Absorption: Oral: Rapid

Bioavailability: Mean: 45%

Half-Life Elimination: 1-4 hours; prolonged with cirrhosis, congestive heart failure, obesity, elderly

Metabolism: Extensively hepatic via CYP3A4

Onset: I.M.: Sedation: ~15 minutes; I.V.: 1-5 minutes; Peak effect: I.M.: 0.5-1 hour

Duration: I.M.: Up to 6 hours; Mean: 2 hours

Formulations

Injection, as hydrochloride: 1 mg/mL (2 mL, 5 mL, 10 mL); 5 mg/mL (1 mL, 2 mL, 5 mL, 10 mL)

Syrup, as hydrochloride: 2 mg/mL (118 mL)

Dosing

Adults: The dose of midazolam needs to be individualized based on the patient's age, underlying diseases, and concurrent medications. Decrease dose (by ~30%) if narcotics or other CNS depressants are administered concomitantly. **Personnel and equipment needed for standard respiratory resuscitation should be immediately available during midazolam administration.**

Preoperative sedation:
- I.M.: 0.07-0.08 mg/kg 30-60 minutes prior to surgery/procedure; usual dose: 5 mg; **Note:** Reduce dose in patients with COPD, high-risk patients, patients ≥60 years of age, and patients receiving other narcotics or CNS depressants
- I.V.: 0.02-0.04 mg/kg; repeat every 5 minutes as needed to desired effect or up to 0.1-0.2 mg/kg
- Intranasal (not an approved route): 0.2 mg/kg (up to 0.4 mg/kg in some studies); administer 30-45 minutes prior to surgery/procedure

Conscious sedation: I.V.: Initial: 0.5-2 mg slow I.V. over at least 2 minutes; slowly titrate to effect by repeating doses every 2-3 minutes if needed; usual total dose: 2.5-5 mg; use decreased doses in elderly.
- Healthy Adults <60 years:
  - Initial: Some patients respond to doses as low as 1 mg; no more than 2.5 mg should be administered over a period of 2 minutes. Additional doses of midazolam may be administered after a 2-minute waiting period and evaluation of sedation after each dose increment. A total dose >5 mg is generally not needed. If narcotics or other CNS depressants are administered concomitantly, the midazolam dose should be reduced by 30%. Refer to elderly dosing for patients ≥60 years, debilitated, or chronically ill.
  - Maintenance: 25% of dose used to reach sedative effect

Anesthesia: I.V.:
- Induction:
  - Unpremedicated patients: 0.3-0.35 mg/kg (up to 0.6 mg/kg in resistant cases)
  - Premedicated patients: 0.15-0.35 mg/kg
- Maintenance: 0.05-0.3 mg/kg as needed, or continuous infusion 0.25-1.5 mcg/kg/minute

Sedation in mechanically-ventilated patients: I.V. continuous infusion: 100 mg in 250 mL D_5W or NS (if patient is fluid-restricted, may concentrate up to a maximum of 0.5 mg/mL); initial dose: 0.01-0.05 mg/kg (~0.5-4 mg for a typical adult) initially and either repeated at 10-15 minute intervals until adequate sedation is achieved or continuous infusion rates of 0.02-0.1 mg/kg/hour (1-7 mg/hour) and titrate to reach desired level of sedation

Elderly: The dose of midazolam needs to be individualized based on the patient's age, underlying diseases, and concurrent medications. Decrease dose (by ~30%) if narcotics or other CNS depressants are administered concomitantly. **Personnel and equipment needed for standard respiratory resuscitation should be immediately available during midazolam administration.**

I.V.: Conscious sedation: Initial: 0.5 mg slow I.V.; give no more than 1.5 mg in a 2-minute period. If additional titration is needed, give no more than 1 mg over 2 minutes, waiting another 2 or more minutes to evaluate sedative effect. A total dose >3.5 mg is rarely necessary.

Pediatrics: The dose of midazolam needs to be individualized based on the patient's age, underlying diseases, and concurrent medications. Decrease dose (by ~30%) if narcotics or other CNS depressants are administered concomitantly. **Personnel and equipment needed for standard respiratory resuscitation should be immediately available during midazolam administration.**

Children <6 years may require higher doses and closer monitoring than older children; calculate dose on ideal body weight

Conscious sedation for procedures or preoperative sedation:
- Oral: 0.25-0.5 mg/kg as a single dose preprocedure, up to a maximum of 20 mg; administer 30-40 minutes prior to procedure. Children <6 years, or less cooperative patients may require as much as 1 mg/kg as a single dose; 0.25 mg/kg may suffice for children 6-16 years of age.
- Intranasal (not an approved route): 0.2 mg/kg (up to 0.4 mg/kg in some studies), administered 30-45 minutes prior to procedure
- I.M.: 0.1-0.15 mg/kg 30-60 minutes before surgery or procedure; range 0.05-0.15 mg/kg; doses up to 0.5 mg/kg have been used in more anxious patients; maximum total dose: 10 mg
- I.V.:
  - Infants <6 months: Limited information is available in nonintubated infants; dosing recommendations not clear; infants <6 months are at higher risk for airway obstruction and hypoventilation; titrate dose in small increments to desired effect; monitor carefully

Infants 6 months to Children 5 years: Initial: 0.05-0.1 mg/kg; titrate dose carefully; total dose of 0.6 mg/kg may be required; usual maximum total dose: 6 mg

Children 6-12 years: Initial: 0.025-0.05 mg/kg; titrate dose carefully; total doses of 0.4 mg/kg may be required; usual maximum total dose: 10 mg

Children 12-16 years: Dose as adults; usual maximum total dose: 10 mg

Conscious sedation during mechanical ventilation: I.V.:

Neonates: I.V. continuous infusion: 0.05-1 mcg/kg/minute. Use smallest dose possible; use lower doses (up to 0.5 mcg/kg/minute) for preterm neonates

Children: Loading dose: 0.05-0.2 mg/kg, followed by initial continuous infusion: 1-2 mcg/kg/minute; titrate to the desired effect; usual range: 0.4-6 mcg/kg/minute

Status epilepticus refractory to standard therapy: I.V.: Infants >2 months and Children: Loading dose: 0.15 mg/kg followed by a continuous infusion of 1 mcg/kg/minute; titrate dose upward very 5 minutes until clinical seizure activity is controlled; mean infusion rate required in 24 children was 2.3 mcg/kg/minute with a range of 1-18 mcg/kg/minute

Renal Impairment:

Hemodialysis: Supplemental dose is not necessary.

Peritoneal dialysis: Significant drug removal is unlikely based on physiochemical characteristics.

Administration

Oral: Do not mix with any liquid (such as grapefruit juice) prior to administration.

I.M.: Give deep I.M. into large muscle.

I.V.: Administer by slow I.V. injection over at least 2-5 minutes at a concentration of 1-5 mg/mL or by I.V. infusion. Continuous infusions should be administered via an infusion pump.

Other: Intranasal: Administer using a 1 mL needleless syringe into the nares over 15 seconds; use the 5 mg/mL injection; ½ of the dose may be administered to each nare

Stability

Storage: Stable for 24 hours at room temperature/refrigeration; at a final concentration of 0.5 mg/mL, stable for up to 24 hours when diluted with D_5W or NS, or for up to 4 hours when diluted with lactated Ringer's; admixtures do not require protection from light for short-term storage

Compatibility: Stable in D_5NS, D_5W, NS; **incompatible** with LR

Y-site administration: Incompatible with albumin, amphotericin B cholesteryl sulfate complex, ampicillin, bumetanide, butorphanol, ceftazidime, cefuroxime, clonidine, dexamethasone sodium succinate, floxacillin, foscarnet, fosphenytoin, furosemide, hydrocortisone sodium succinate, imipenem/cilastatin, methotrexate, nafcillin, omeprazole, sodium bicarbonate, thiopental, trimethoprim/sulfamethoxazole

Compatibility in syringe: Incompatible with dimenhydrinate, pentobarbital, perphenazine, prochlorperazine edisylate, ranitidine

Monitoring and Teaching Issues

Physical Assessment: Assess other medications the patient may be taking for effectiveness and interactions (see Drug Interactions). See Contraindications and Warnings for use cautions. I.V. monitor cardiac and respiratory status continuously (see Dosing). Monitor I.V. infusion site carefully for extravasation. **I.V./I.M.:** Monitor closely following administration. Bedrest and assistance with ambulation necessary for several hours. **Note:** Full recovery usually occurs within 2-3 hours, but may take 6 hours.

Pregnancy risk factor D - determine pregnancy status. Benefits of use should outweigh possible risks for fetus. Breast-feeding is not recommended.

Patient Education: Avoid use of alcohol or prescription or OTC sedatives or hypnotics for a minimum of 24 hours after administration. Avoid driving or engaging in any tasks that require alertness for 24 hours following administration. You may experience some loss of memory following administration. **Pregnancy/breast-feeding precautions:** Advise prescriber if you are pregnant; this medication is contraindicated for pregnant women. Breast-feeding is not recommended.

Dietary Issues: Injection: Sodium content of 1 mL: 0.14 mEq

Geriatric Considerations: If concomitant CNS depressant medications are used in the elderly, the midazolam dose will be at least 50% less than doses used in healthy, young, unpremedicated patients (see Warnings/Precautions and Pharmacokinetics).

Additional Information Abrupt discontinuation after sustained use (generally >10 days) may cause withdrawal symptoms. For neonates, since both concentrations of the injection contain 1% benzyl alcohol, use the 5 mg/mL injection and dilute to 0.5 mg/mL with SWI without preservatives to decrease the amount of benzyl alcohol delivered to the neonate; with continuous infusion, midazolam may accumulate in peripheral tissues; use lowest effective infusion rate to reduce accumulation effects; midazolam is 3-4 times as potent as diazepam; paradoxical reactions associated with midazolam use in children (eg, agitation, restlessness, combativeness) have been successfully treated with flumazenil (see Massanari, 1997).

Related Information

Benzodiazepines *on page 1560*

Compatibility of Drugs in Syringe *on page 1566*

Midazolam Hydrochloride *see* Midazolam *on page 900*

Midodrine (MI doe dreen)

U.S. Brand Names ProAmatine®

Synonyms Midodrine Hydrochloride

Generic Available No

Pharmacologic Category $Alpha_1$ Agonist

Pregnancy Risk Factor C

Lactation No data available

Use Orphan drug: Treatment of symptomatic orthostatic hypotension

Use - Unlabeled/Investigational Investigational: Management of urinary incontinence

Mechanism of Action/Effect Midodrine forms an active metabolite, desglymidodrine that is an $alpha_1$-agonist. This agent increases arteriolar and venous tone resulting in a rise in

(Continued)

Midodrine *(Continued)*

standing, sitting, and supine systolic and diastolic blood pressure in patient with orthostatic hypotension.

Contraindications Hypersensitivity to midodrine or any component of the formulation; severe organic heart disease; urinary retention; pheochromocytoma; thyrotoxicosis; persistent and significant supine hypertension; concurrent use of fludrocortisone

Warnings/Precautions Only indicated for patients for whom orthostatic hypotension significantly impairs their daily life. Use is not recommended with supine hypertension and caution should be exercised in patients with diabetes, visual problems, urinary retention (reduce initial dose), or hepatic dysfunction. Monitor renal and hepatic function prior to and periodically during therapy. Safety and efficacy has not been established in children. Discontinue and re-evaluate therapy if signs of bradycardia occur. Pregnancy risk C.

Drug Interactions

Increased Effect/Toxicity: Concomitant fludrocortisone results in hypernatremia or an increase in intraocular pressure and glaucoma. Bradycardia may be accentuated with concomitant administration of cardiac glycosides, psychotherapeutics, and beta-blockers. Alpha agonists may increase the pressure effects and alpha antagonists may negate the effects of midodrine.

Adverse Reactions

>10%:

Dermatologic: Piloerection (13%), pruritus (12%)
Genitourinary: Urinary urgency, retention, or polyuria, dysuria (up to 13%)
Neuromuscular & skeletal: Paresthesia (18.3%)

1% to 10%:

Cardiovascular: Supine hypertension (7%), facial flushing
Central nervous system: Confusion, anxiety, dizziness, chills (5%)
Dermatologic: Rash, dry skin (2%)
Gastrointestinal: Xerostomia, nausea, abdominal pain
Neuromuscular & skeletal: Pain (5%)

<1% (Limited to important or life-threatening): Headache, insomnia

Overdosage/Toxicology

Symptoms of overdose include hypertension, piloerection, urinary retention

Treatment is symptomatic following gastric decontamination; alpha-sympatholytics and/or dialysis may be helpful

Pharmacodynamics/Kinetics

Absorption: Rapid
Bioavailability: Absolute: 93%
Half-Life Elimination: Active drug: ~3-4 hours; Prodrug: 25 minutes
Time to Peak: Serum: Active drug: 1-2 hours; Prodrug: 30 minutes
Metabolism: Hepatic; rapid deglycination to desglymidodrine occurs in many tissues and plasma
Onset: ~1 hour
Duration: 2-3 hours

Formulations Tablet, as hydrochloride: 2.5 mg, 5 mg, 10 mg

Dosing

Adults & Elderly: Orthostatic hypotension: Oral: 10 mg 3 times/day during daytime hours (every 3-4 hours) when patient is upright (maximum: 40 mg/day)

Renal Impairment: 2.5 mg 3 times/day; gradually increase as tolerated.

Administration

Oral: Doses may be given in approximately 3- to 4-hour intervals (eg, shortly before or upon rising in the morning, at midday, in the late afternoon not later than 6 PM). Avoid dosing after the evening meal or within 4 hours of bedtime. Continue therapy only in patients who appear to attain symptomatic improvement during initial treatment. Standing systolic blood pressure may be elevated 15-30 mm Hg at 1 hour after a 10 mg dose. Some effect may persist for 2-3 hours.

Monitoring Laboratory Tests Kidney and liver function tests

Monitoring and Teaching Issues

Physical Assessment: See Contraindications, Warnings/Precautions, and Dosing for use cautions (eg, use only for patients for whom orthostatic hypotension significantly impairs their daily life). Assess potential for interactions with other prescriptions, OTC medications, or herbal products patient may be taking (see Drug Interactions). See Administration specifics. Assess results of laboratory tests (see above), therapeutic effectiveness and adverse reactions (see Adverse Reactions and Overdose/Toxicology) at beginning of therapy and on a regular basis with long-term therapy. Teach patient possible side effects and appropriate interventions, and adverse symptoms to report (see Patient Education). **Pregnancy risk factor C** - benefits of use should outweigh possible risks. Note breast-feeding caution.

Patient Education: Inform prescriber of all prescriptions, OTC medications, or herbal products you are taking, and any allergies you have. Do not take anything new during treatment unless approved by prescriber. Take exactly as directed when upright; do not take within 4 hours of bedtime or when lying down at any time. May cause urinary urgency or retention (void before taking or consult prescriber if difficulty persists); or dizziness, drowsiness, or headache (use caution when driving or engaging in tasks that require alertness until response to drug is known). Report skin rash, severe gastric upset or pain, muscle weakness or pain, or other persistent side effects. **Pregnancy/breast-feeding precautions:** Inform prescriber if you are or intend to become pregnant. Consult prescriber if breast-feeding.

Breast-feeding Issues: No studies are available. Use during lactation should be avoided unless the potential benefit outweighs the risk to the fetus.

Midodrine Hydrochloride *see* Midodrine *on page 903*

Midol® Maximum Strength Cramp Formula [OTC] *see* Ibuprofen *on page 688*

Midrin® *see* Acetaminophen, Isometheptene, and Dichloralphenazone *on page 38*

Mifeprex® *see* Mifepristone *on page 905*

Mifepristone (mi fe PRIS tone)

U.S. Brand Names Mifeprex®

Synonyms RU-486; RU-38486

Restrictions There are currently no clinical trials with mifepristone in oncology open in the U.S.; investigators wishing to obtain the agent for use in oncology patients must apply for a patient-specific IND from the FDA. Mifepristone will be supplied only to licensed physicians who sign and return a "Prescriber's Agreement." Distribution of mifepristone will be subject to specific requirements imposed by the distributor. Mifepristone will **not** be available to the public through licensed pharmacies.

Generic Available No

Pharmacologic Category Abortifacient; Antineoplastic Agent, Hormone Antagonist; Antiprogestin

Pregnancy Risk Factor X

Lactation Excretion in breast milk unknown/contraindicated

Use Medical termination of intrauterine pregnancy, through day 49 of pregnancy. Patients may need treatment with misoprostol and possibly surgery to complete therapy

Use - Unlabeled/Investigational Treatment of unresectable meningioma; has been studied in the treatment of breast cancer, ovarian cancer, and adrenal cortical carcinoma

Mechanism of Action/Effect Mifepristone, a synthetic steroid, competitively binds to the intracellular progesterone receptor, blocking the effects of progesterone. When used for the termination of pregnancy, this leads to contraction-inducing activity in the myometrium. In the absence of progesterone, mifepristone acts as a partial progesterone agonist. Mifepristone also has weak antiglucocorticoid and antiandrogenic properties; it blocks the feedback effect of cortisol on corticotropin secretion.

Contraindications Hypersensitivity to mifepristone, misoprostol, other prostaglandins, or any component of the formulation; chronic adrenal failure; porphyrias; hemorrhagic disorder or concurrent anticoagulant therapy; pregnancy termination >49 days; intrauterine device (IUD) in place; ectopic pregnancy or undiagnosed adnexal mass; concurrent long-term corticosteroid therapy; inadequate or lack of access to emergency medical services; inability to understand effects and/or comply with treatment

Warnings/Precautions Patient must be instructed of the treatment procedure and expected effects. A signed agreement form must be kept in the patient's file. Physicians may obtain patient agreement forms, physician enrollment forms, and medical consultation directly from Danco Laboratories at 1-877-432-7596. Adverse effects (including blood transfusions, hospitalization, ongoing pregnancy, and other major complications) must be reported in writing to the medication distributor. To be administered only by physicians who can date pregnancy, diagnose ectopic pregnancies, provide access to surgical abortion (if needed), and can provide access to emergency care. Medication will be distributed directly to these physicians following signed agreement with the distributor. Must be administered under supervision by the qualified physician. Pregnancy is dated from day 1 of last menstrual period (presuming a 28-day cycle, ovulation occurring midcycle). Pregnancy duration can be determined using menstrual history and clinical examination. Ultrasound should be used if an ectopic pregnancy is suspected or if duration of pregnancy is uncertain. Bleeding occurs and should be expected (average 9-16 days, may be ≥30 days). Bleeding may require blood transfusion (rare), curettage, saline infusions, and/or vasoconstrictors. Use caution in patients with severe anemia. Confirmation of pregnancy termination by clinical exam or ultrasound must be made 14 days following treatment. Manufacturer recommends surgical termination of pregnancy when medical termination fails or is not complete. Prescriber should determine in advance whether they will provide such care themselves or through other providers. Preventative measures to prevent rhesus immunization must be taken prior to surgical abortion. Prescriber should also give the patient clear instructions on whom to call and what to do in the event of an emergency following administration of mifepristone.

Safety and efficacy have not been established for use in women with chronic cardiovascular, hypertensive, respiratory, or renal disease, diabetes mellitus, severe anemia, or heavy smokers. Women >35 years of age and smokers (>10 cigarettes/day) were excluded from clinical trials. Safety and efficacy in pediatric patients have not been established.

Drug Interactions

Cytochrome P450 Effect: Substrate of CYP3A4; Inhibits CYP2D6, 3A4

Decreased Effect: Enzyme inducers may increase the metabolism of mifepristone resulting in decreased effect; includes carbamazepine, dexamethasone, phenobarbital, phenytoin, and rifampin. St John's wort may induce mifepristone metabolism, leading to decreased levels.

Increased Effect/Toxicity: There are no reported interactions. It might be anticipated that the effects of one or both agents would be minimized if mifepristone were administered concurrently with a progestin (exogenous). During concurrent use of CYP3A4 inhibitors, serum level and/or toxicity of mifepristone may be increased; inhibitors include amiodarone, cimetidine, clarithromycin, erythromycin, delavirdine, diltiazem, dirithromycin, disulfiram, fluoxetine, fluvoxamine, grapefruit juice, indinavir, itraconazole, ketoconazole, nefazodone, nevirapine, propoxyphene, quinupristin-dalfopristin, ritonavir, saquinavir, verapamil, zafirlukast, zileuton; monitor for altered response

Nutritional/Ethanol Interactions

Food: Do not take with grapefruit juice; grapefruit juice may inhibit mifepristone metabolism leading to increased levels.

Herb/Nutraceutical: Avoid St John's wort (may induce mifepristone metabolism, leading to decreased levels).

Effects on Lab Values hCG levels will not be useful to confirm pregnancy termination until at least 10 days following mifepristone treatment.

Adverse Reactions Vaginal bleeding and uterine cramping are expected to occur when this medication is used to terminate a pregnancy; 90% of women using this medication for this purpose also report adverse reactions

(Continued)

Mifepristone *(Continued)*

>10%:

- Central nervous system: Headache (2% to 31%), dizziness (1% to 12%)
- Gastrointestinal: Abdominal pain (cramping) (96%), nausea (43% to 61%), vomiting (18% to 26%), diarrhea (12% to 20%)
- Genitourinary: Uterine cramping (83%)

1% to 10%:

- Cardiovascular: Syncope (1%)
- Central nervous system: Fatigue (10%), fever (4%), insomnia (3%), anxiety (2%), fainting (2%)
- Gastrointestinal: Dyspepsia (3%)
- Genitourinary: Uterine hemorrhage (5%), vaginitis (3%), pelvic pain (2%)
- Hematologic: Decreased hemoglobin >2 g/dL (6%), anemia (2%), leukorrhea (2%)
- Neuromuscular & skeletal: Back pain (9%), rigors (3%), leg pain (2%), weakness (2%)
- Respiratory: Sinusitis (2%)
- Miscellaneous: Viral infection (4%)

<1% (Limited to important or life-threatening): Bacterial infection, significant elevations of hepatic enzymes (rare), myocardial infarction, ruptured ectopic pregnancy

In trials for unresectable meningioma, the most common adverse effects included fatigue, hot flashes, gynecomastia or breast tenderness, hair thinning, and rash. In premenopausal women, vaginal bleeding may be seen shortly after beginning therapy and cessation of menses is common. Thyroiditis and effects related to antiglucocorticoid activity have also been noted.

Overdosage/Toxicology In studies using 3 times the recommended dose for termination of pregnancy, no serious maternal adverse effects were reported. This medication is supplied in single-dose containers to be given under physician supervision, therefore, the risk of overdose should be low. In case of massive ingestion, treat symptomatically and monitor for signs of adrenal failure.

Pharmacodynamics/Kinetics

Bioavailability: 69%

Half-Life Elimination: Terminal: 18 hours following a slower phase where 50% eliminated between 12-72 hours

Time to Peak: 90 minutes

Metabolism: Hepatic via CYP3A4 to three metabolites (may possess some antiprogestin and antiglucocorticoid activity)

Formulations Tablet: 200 mg

Dosing

Adults:

Termination of pregnancy: Oral: Treatment consists of three office visits by the patient; the patient must read medication guide and sign patient agreement prior to treatment:

- Day 1: 600 mg (three 200 mg tablets) taken as a single dose under physician supervision
- Day 3: Patient must return to the healthcare provider 2 days following administration of mifepristone; if termination of pregnancy cannot be confirmed using ultrasound or clinical examination: 400 mcg (two 200 mcg tablets) of misoprostol; patient may need treatment for cramps or gastrointestinal symptoms at this time
- Day 14: Patient must return to the healthcare provider ~14 days after administration of mifepristone; confirm complete termination of pregnancy by ultrasound or clinical exam. Surgical termination is recommended to manage treatment failures.

Unlabeled use: Refer to individual protocols. The dose used in meningioma is usually 200 mg/day, continued based on toxicity and response.

Elderly: Safety and efficacy have not been established.

Renal Impairment: Safety and efficacy have not been established.

Hepatic Impairment: Safety and efficacy have not been established; use with caution due to CYP3A4 metabolism.

Stability

Storage: Store at room temperature of 25°C (77°F).

Monitoring and Teaching Issues

Physical Assessment: May only be administered under supervision of a qualified physician. Patient must be instructed in procedure and sign patient agreement forms. See Restrictions, Contraindications, Warnings/Precautions for extensive use cautions/directions. Monitor response (see Monitoring Laboratory Tests) and adverse reactions (see Adverse Reactions and Monitoring Lab Tests). Assess knowledge/teach patient interventions to reduce side effects, and adverse reactions to report (see Patient Education). **Pregnancy risk factor X** - this medication is used to terminate pregnancy. Breast-feeding is contraindicated.

Patient Education: This medication is used to terminate pregnancy under 7 weeks. It must be administered under direction of a qualified physician. You will need follow-up visits as directed by your prescriber (approximately 3 days and 14 days after treatment). Surgical termination of pregnancy may be required if medication fails; there is a risk of fetal malformation if treatment fails. You may experience vaginal bleeding and cramping that is heavier than a normal menstrual period; report immediately if severe or persistent. You may experience nausea, vomiting, and diarrhea. It is possible to get pregnant before your next period. Once the pregnancy has proved to be ended, contraception should be started before having sexual intercourse. Read carefully all information about this medication provided by your prescriber. **Pregnancy/breast-feeding precautions:** Your physician will give you a phone number to call for problems, questions, or emergencies; you should not use this medication if you do not have access to emergency care. You will be given a medication guide to help you understand this medication and its effects. It is important to review this carefully. Ask any questions you may have. You will also be required to sign a form saying that you understand the effects of this treatment and are able to return to the physician for follow-up appointments. Do not breast-feed. Discard breast milk for a few days following use of this medication.

Breast-feeding Issues: Breast milk should be discarded for a few days following use of this medication.

Pregnancy Issues: This medication is used to terminate pregnancy; there are no approved treatment indications for its use during pregnancy. Prostaglandins (including mifepristone and misoprostol) may have teratogenic effects when used during pregnancy.

Additional Information Medication will be distributed directly to qualified physicians following signed agreement with the distributor, Danco Laboratories. It will not be available through pharmacies.

Miglitol (MIG li tol)

U.S. Brand Names Glyset™

Generic Available No

Pharmacologic Category Antidiabetic Agent, Alpha-Glucosidase Inhibitor

Pregnancy Risk Factor B

Lactation Enters breast milk (small amounts)/not recommended

Use Type 2 diabetes mellitus (noninsulin-dependent, NIDDM):

Monotherapy adjunct to diet to improve glycemic control in patients with type 2 diabetes mellitus (noninsulin-dependent, NIDDM) whose hyperglycemia cannot be managed with diet alone

Combination therapy with a sulfonylurea when diet plus either miglitol or a sulfonylurea alone do not result in adequate glycemic control. The effect of miglitol to enhance glycemic control is additive to that of sulfonylureas when used in combination.

Mechanism of Action/Effect In contrast to sulfonylureas, miglitol does not enhance insulin secretion. The antihyperglycemic action of miglitol results from a reversible inhibition of membrane-bound intestinal alpha-glucosidases which hydrolyze oligosaccharides and disaccharides to glucose and other monosaccharides in the brush border of the small intestine. In diabetic patients, this enzyme inhibition results in delayed glucose absorption and lowering of postprandial hyperglycemia.

Contraindications Hypersensitivity to miglitol or any of component of the formulation; diabetic ketoacidosis; inflammatory bowel disease; colonic ulceration; partial intestinal obstruction or predisposition to intestinal obstruction; chronic intestinal diseases associated with marked disorders of digestion or absorption or with conditions that may deteriorate as a result of increased gas formation in the intestine

Warnings/Precautions GI symptoms are the most common reactions. The incidence of abdominal pain and diarrhea tend to diminish considerably with continued treatment. Long-term clinical trials in diabetic patients with significant renal dysfunction (serum creatinine >2 mg/dL) have not been conducted. Treatment of these patients is not recommended. Because of its mechanism of action, miglitol administered alone should not cause hypoglycemia in the fasting of postprandial state. In combination with a sulfonylurea will cause a further lowering of blood glucose and may increase the hypoglycemic potential of the sulfonylurea.

Drug Interactions

Decreased Effect: Miglitol may decrease the absorption and bioavailability of digoxin, propranolol, and ranitidine. Digestive enzymes (amylase, pancreatin, charcoal) may reduce the effect of miglitol and should **not** be taken concomitantly.

Adverse Reactions

>10%: Gastrointestinal: Flatulence (41.5%), diarrhea (28.7%), abdominal pain (11.7%)

1% to 10%: Dermatologic: Rash (4.3%)

Overdosage/Toxicology An overdose of miglitol will not result in hypoglycemia. An overdose may result in transient increases in flatulence, diarrhea, and abdominal discomfort. No serious systemic reactions are expected in the event of an overdose.

Pharmacodynamics/Kinetics

Absorption: Saturable at high doses: 25 mg dose: Completely absorbed; 100 mg dose: 50% to 70% absorbed

Half-Life Elimination: ~2 hours

Time to Peak: 2-3 hours

Metabolism: None

Formulations Tablet: 25 mg, 50 mg, 100 mg

Dosing

Adults & Elderly: Type 2 diabetes (noninsulin dependent, NIDDM): Oral: 25 mg 3 times/day with the first bite of food at each meal; the dose may be increased to 50 mg 3 times/day after 4-8 weeks; maximum recommended dose: 100 mg 3 times/day

Renal Impairment: Miglitol is primarily excreted by the kidneys; there is little information of miglitol in patients with a Cl_{cr} <25 mL/minute.

Hepatic Impairment: No adjustment necessary.

Administration

Oral: Should be taken orally at the start (with the first bite) of each main meal.

Monitoring Laboratory Tests Monitor therapeutic response by periodic blood glucose tests; measurement of glycosylated hemoglobin is recommended for the monitoring of long-term glycemic control.

Monitoring and Teaching Issues

Physical Assessment: See Contraindications, Warnings/Precautions, and Drug Interactions for use cautions. Assess results of laboratory tests (see above), therapeutic effects, and adverse response (see Adverse Reactions and Overdose/Toxicology) on a regular basis throughout therapy. Teach patient proper use (or refer patient to diabetic educator), possible side effects and appropriate interventions (eg, importance of adequate hydration), and adverse symptoms to report (see Patient Education). Breast-feeding is not recommended.

Patient Education: Inform prescriber of all prescriptions, OTC medications, or herbal products you are taking, and any allergies you have. Do not take anything new during treatment unless approved by prescriber. Take exactly as directed, with the first bite of each main meal. Do not change dosage or discontinue without first consulting prescriber. Do not take other medications with or within 2 hours of this medication unless advised by

(Continued)

Miglitol *(Continued)*

prescriber. Avoid alcohol. It is important to follow dietary and lifestyle recommendations of prescriber. You will be instructed in signs of hypo- or hyperglycemia by prescriber or diabetic educator. If combining this medication with other diabetic medication (eg, sulfonylureas, insulin), keep source of glucose (sugar) on hand in case hypoglycemia occurs. May cause mild side effects during first weeks of therapy (eg, bloating, flatulence, diarrhea, abdominal discomfort); these should diminish over time. Report severe or persistent side effects, fever, extended vomiting or flu, or change in color of urine or stool. **Breast-feeding precaution:** Breast-feeding is not recommended.

Pregnancy Issues: Abnormal blood glucose levels are associated with a higher incidence of congenital abnormalities. Insulin is the drug of choice for the control of diabetes mellitus during pregnancy.

Related Information

Antidiabetic Oral Agents Comparison *on page 1556*
Diabetes Mellitus Management *on page 1661*

Migranal® *see* Dihydroergotamine *on page 416*

Migratine® *see* Acetaminophen, Isometheptene, and Dichloralphenazone *on page 38*

Milk of Magnesia (Magnesium Hydroxide) *see* Magnesium Supplements *on page 831*

Milliequivalent Conversions *see page 1541*

Milophene® *see* ClomiPHENE *on page 312*

Milrinone (MIL ri none)

U.S. Brand Names Primacor®

Synonyms Milrinone Lactate

Generic Available Yes

Pharmacologic Category Phosphodiesterase Enzyme Inhibitor

Pregnancy Risk Factor C

Lactation Excretion in breast milk unknown

Use Short-term I.V. therapy of congestive heart failure; calcium antagonist intoxication

Mechanism of Action/Effect Phosphodiesterase inhibitor resulting in vasodilation

Contraindications Hypersensitivity to milrinone, inamrinone, or any component of the formulation; concurrent use of inamrinone

Warnings/Precautions Avoid in severe obstructive aortic or pulmonic valvular disease. Milrinone may aggravate outflow tract obstruction in hypertrophic subaortic stenosis. Supraventricular and ventricular arrhythmias have developed in high-risk patients. Ensure that ventricular rate controlled in atrial fibrillation/flutter prior to initiating milrinone. Not recommended for use in acute MI patients. Monitor and correct fluid and electrolyte problems. Adjust dose in renal dysfunction. Has not been demonstrated to be safe or effective for longer than 48 hours. Pregnancy risk C.

Adverse Reactions

1% to 10%:

Cardiovascular: Arrhythmias, hypotension

Central nervous system: Headache

<1% (Limited to important or life-threatening): Atrial fibrillation, chest pain, hypokalemia, myocardial infarction, thrombocytopenia, ventricular fibrillation

Overdosage/Toxicology Treatment is supportive and symptomatic.

Pharmacodynamics/Kinetics

Half-Life Elimination: I.V.: 136 minutes in patients with congestive heart failure (CHF); patients with severe CHF have a more prolonged half-life, with values ranging from 1.7-2.7 hours. Patients with CHF have a reduction in the systemic clearance of milrinone, resulting in a prolonged elimination half-life. Alternatively, one study reported that 1 month of therapy with milrinone did not change the pharmacokinetic parameters for patients with CHF despite improvement in cardiac function.

Metabolism: Hepatic (12%)

Onset: I.V.: 5-15 minutes

Serum level: I.V.: Following a 125 mcg/kg dose, peak plasma concentrations ~1000 ng/mL were observed at 2 minutes postinjection, decreasing to <100 ng/mL in 2 hours

Drug concentration levels:

Therapeutic:

Serum levels of 166 ng/mL, achieved during I.V. infusions of 0.25-1 mcg/kg/minute, were associated with sustained hemodynamic benefit in severe congestive heart failure patients over a 24-hour period

Maximum beneficial effects on cardiac output and pulmonary capillary wedge pressure following I.V. infusion have been associated with plasma milrinone concentrations of 150-250 ng/mL

Toxic: Serum concentrations >250-300 ng/mL have been associated with marked reductions in mean arterial pressure and tachycardia; however, more studies are required to determine the toxic serum levels for milrinone

Formulations

Infusion, as lactate [in D_5W]: 200 mcg/mL (100 mL, 200 mL)
Injection, as lactate: 1 mg/mL (5 mL, 10 mL, 20 mL, 50 mL)

Maintenance Dosage	Dose Rate (mcg/kg/min)	Total Dose (mg/kg/24 h)
Minimum	0.375	0.59
Standard	0.500	0.77
Maximum	0.750	1.13

Dosing

Adults & Elderly: CHF/Hemodynamic support: I.V.: Loading dose: 50 mcg/kg administered over 10 minutes followed by a maintenance dose titrated according to the hemodynamic and clinical response, see table on previous page.

Renal Impairment:

Cl_{cr} 50 mL/minute/1.73 m^2: Administer 0.43 mcg/kg/minute.
Cl_{cr} 40 mL/minute/1.73 m^2: Administer 0.38 mcg/kg/minute.
Cl_{cr} 30 mL/minute/1.73 m^2: Administer 0.33 mcg/kg/minute.
Cl_{cr} 20 mL/minute/1.73 m^2: Administer 0.28 mcg/kg/minute.
Cl_{cr} 10 mL/minute/1.73 m^2: Administer 0.23 mcg/kg/minute.
Cl_{cr} 5 mL/minute/1.73 m^2: Administer 0.2 mcg/kg/minute.

Administration

I.V.: Infuse via infusion pump.

Stability

Storage: Colorless to pale yellow solution. Store at room temperature and protect from light.

Reconstitution: Stable at 0.2 mg/mL in 0.9% sodium chloride or D_5W for 72 hours at room temperature in normal light.

Standardized dose: 20 mg in 80 mL of 0.9% sodium chloride or D_5W (0.2 mg/mL)

Compatibility: Stable in D_5W, LR, ½NS, NS

Y-site administration: Incompatible with furosemide, procainamide

Compatibility in syringe: Incompatible with furosemide

Compatibility when admixed: Incompatible with bumetanide, furosemide, procainamide

Monitoring Laboratory Tests Serum potassium

Monitoring and Teaching Issues

Physical Assessment: Use infusion pump. Monitor cardiac/hemodynamic status continuously during therapy and serum potassium at regular intervals. **Pregnancy risk factor C.** Note breast-feeding caution.

Patient Education: This drug can only be given intravenously. If you experience increased voiding call for assistance. Report pain at infusion site, numbness or tingling of extremities, or difficulty breathing. **Pregnancy/breast-feeding precautions:** Inform prescriber if you are pregnant. Consult prescriber if breast-feeding.

Related Information

Inotropic and Vasoconstrictor Comparison *on page 1580*

Milrinone Lactate *see* Milrinone *on page 908*

Miltown® *see* Meprobamate *on page 853*

Mineral Oil *see page 1581*

Mini-Gamulin® Rh *see page 1498*

Minipress® *see* Prazosin *on page 1111*

Minitran™ *see* Nitroglycerin *on page 977*

Minizide® *see* Prazosin and Polythiazide *on page 1113*

Minocin® *see* Minocycline *on page 909*

Minocycline (mi noe SYE kleen)

U.S. Brand Names Dynacin®; Minocin®; Vectrin® [DSC]

Synonyms Minocycline Hydrochloride

Generic Available Yes

Pharmacologic Category Antibiotic, Tetracycline Derivative

Pregnancy Risk Factor D

Lactation Enters breast milk/not recommended (AAP rates "compatible")

Use Treatment of susceptible bacterial infections of both gram-negative and gram-positive organisms; treatment of anthrax (inhalational, cutaneous, and gastrointestinal); acne, meningococcal carrier state

Mechanism of Action/Effect Inhibits bacterial protein synthesis by binding with the 30S and possibly the 50S ribosomal subunit(s) of susceptible bacteria; cell wall synthesis is not affected

Contraindications Hypersensitivity to minocycline, other tetracyclines, or any component of the formulation; pregnancy

Warnings/Precautions Avoid use during tooth development (children ≤8 years of age) unless other drugs are not likely to be effective or are contraindicated. May be associated with increases in BUN secondary to anti-anabolic effects. Avoid in renal insufficiency (associated with hepatotoxicity). CNS effects (lightheadedness, vertigo) may occur, potentially affecting a patient's ability to drive or operate heavy machinery. Has been associated (rarely) with pseudotumor cerebri. May cause photosensitivity.

Drug Interactions

Decreased Effect: Decreased effect with antacids (aluminum, calcium, zinc, or magnesium), bismuth salts, sodium bicarbonate, barbiturates, carbamazepine, hydantoins. Although anecdotal reports suggest oral contraceptive efficacy could be reduced by tetracyclines, this has been refuted by more rigorous scientific and clinical data.

Increased Effect/Toxicity: Minocycline may increase the effect of warfarin.

Nutritional/Ethanol Interactions

Food: Minocycline serum concentrations are not altered if taken with dairy products.

Herb/Nutraceutical: Avoid dong quai, St John's wort (may also cause photosensitization).

Adverse Reactions

>10%: Miscellaneous: Discoloration of teeth (in children)

1% to 10%:

Central nervous system: Lightheadedness, vertigo
Dermatologic: Photosensitivity
Gastrointestinal: Nausea, diarrhea

<1%: Acute renal failure, anaphylaxis, angioedema, diabetes insipidus, eosinophilia, erythema multiforme, esophagitis, exfoliative dermatitis, hemolytic anemia, hepatitis, hepatic failure, neutropenia, paresthesia, pericarditis, pigmentation of nails, pseudotumor

(Continued)

Minocycline *(Continued)*

cerebri, rash, Stevens-Johnson syndrome, superinfections, thrombocytopenia, thyroid dysfunction (extremely rare), tinnitus, vomiting

Overdosage/Toxicology Symptoms of overdose include diabetes insipidus, nausea, anorexia, and diarrhea. Treatment is supportive.

Pharmacodynamics/Kinetics

Absorption: Well absorbed

Half-Life Elimination: 15 hours

Formulations

Capsule, as hydrochloride: 50 mg, 75 mg, 100 mg

Dynacin®: 50 mg, 75 mg, 100 mg

Vectrin® [DSC]: 50 mg, 100 mg

Capsule, pellet-filled, as hydrochloride (Minocin®): 50 mg, 100 mg

Injection, powder for reconstitution, as hydrochloride (Minocin®): 100 mg

Dosing

Adults & Elderly:

Infection: Oral, I.V.: 200 mg stat, 100 mg every 12 hours not to exceed 400 mg/24 hours

Acne: Oral: 50 mg 1-3 times/day

Pediatrics: Children >8 years: Oral, I.V.: Initial: 4 mg/kg followed by 2 mg/kg/dose every 12 hours

Renal Impairment: Not dialyzable (0% to 5%)

Administration

Oral: May be taken with food or milk.

I.V.: Infuse I.V. minocycline slowly, usually over a 4- to 6-hour period.

Stability

Compatibility: Stable in D_5NS, D_5W, LR, NS

Y-site administration: Incompatible with allopurinol, amifostine, hydromorphone, meperidine, morphine, piperacillin/tazobactam, propofol, thiotepa

Compatibility in syringe: Incompatible with doxapram

Compatibility when admixed: Incompatible with rifampin

Monitoring Laboratory Tests Perform culture and sensitivity testing prior to initiating therapy.

Monitoring and Teaching Issues

Physical Assessment: Assess allergy history before beginning therapy. See Contraindications, Warnings/Precautions, and Dosing for use cautions. Assess potential for interactions with other prescriptions, OTC medications, or herbal products patient may be taking (see Drug Interactions). **Infusion:** See Administration; infusion site must be closely monitored to prevent extravasation. Assess results of laboratory tests (see above), therapeutic effectiveness, and adverse reactions (see Adverse Reactions and Overdose/Toxicology) on a regular basis throughout therapy. Teach patient proper use, possible side effects and interventions (eg, importance of adequate hydration), and adverse symptoms to report (see Patient Education). **Pregnancy risk factor D** - determine that patient is not pregnant before beginning treatment. Instruct patients of childbearing age on appropriate barrier contraceptive measures. Breast-feeding is not recommended.

Patient Education: Inform prescriber of all prescriptions, OTC medications, or herbal products you are taking, and any allergies you have. Do not take anything new during treatment unless approved by prescriber. Take at intervals around-the-clock; may be taken with food. Complete full course of therapy; do not discontinue even if condition is resolved. May cause photosensitivity reaction (avoid sun, use sunblock, or wear protective clothing); nausea (small, frequent meals, frequent mouth care, chewing gum, or sucking lozenges may help); or diarrhea (boiled milk, buttermilk, or yogurt may help). Report rash or itching, unresolved nausea or diarrhea, change in urinary output (excess); or opportunistic infection (eg, fever, chills, sore throat, burning urination, fatigue). **Pregnancy/breast-feeding precautions:** Do not get pregnant while taking this medication. Consult prescriber for appropriate barrier contraceptive measures. Breast-feeding is not recommended

Dietary Issues: May be taken with food or milk.

Geriatric Considerations: Minocycline has not been studied in the elderly but its CNS effects may limit its use (see Adverse Reactions). Dose reduction for renal function not necessary.

Breast-feeding Issues: Although tetracyclines are excreted in limited amounts, the potential for staining of unerupted teeth has led some experts to recommend against breast-feeding. The AAP identified tetracyclines as "compatible" with breast-feeding.

Pregnancy Issues: May cause permanent discoloration (brown-grey) of teeth. Animal studies indicate possible embryotoxicity.

Minocycline Hydrochloride *see* Minocycline *on page 909*

Mintezol® *see* Thiabendazole *on page 1303*

Miochol-E® *see page 1509*

Miostat® Intraocular *see* Ophthalmic Agents, Glaucoma *on page 1002*

MiraLax™ *see* Polyethylene Glycol-Electrolyte Solution *on page 1098*

Mirapex® *see* Pramipexole *on page 1108*

Miraphen PSE *see* Guaifenesin and Pseudoephedrine *on page 648*

Mircette® *see* Ethinyl Estradiol and Desogestrel *on page 516*

Mirena® *see* Levonorgestrel *on page 793*

Mirtazapine (mir TAZ a peen)

U.S. Brand Names Remeron®; Remeron® SolTab™

Generic Available No

Pharmacologic Category Antidepressant, Alpha-2 Antagonist

Pregnancy Risk Factor C

Lactation Excretion in breast milk unknown/not recommended

Use Treatment of depression

Mechanism of Action/Effect Mirtazapine is a tetracyclic antidepressant that works by its central presynaptic $alpha_2$-adrenergic antagonist effects, which results in increased release of norepinephrine and serotonin. It is also a potent antagonist of $5\text{-}HT_2$ and $5\text{-}HT_3$ serotonin receptors and H1 histamine receptors and a moderate peripheral $alpha_1$-adrenergic and muscarinic antagonist; it does not inhibit the reuptake of norepinephrine or serotonin.

Contraindications Hypersensitivity to mirtazapine or any component of the formulation; use of MAO inhibitors within 14 days

Warnings/Precautions Discontinue immediately if signs and symptoms of neutropenia/agranulocytosis occur. May cause sedation, resulting in impaired performance of tasks requiring alertness (ie, operating machinery or driving). Sedative effects may be additive with other CNS depressants and/or ethanol. The degree of sedation is moderate-high relative to other antidepressants. May worsen psychosis in some patients or precipitate a shift to mania or hypomania in patients with bipolar disease. The risks of orthostatic hypotension or anticholinergic effects are low relative to other antidepressants. The incidence of sexual dysfunction with mirtazapine is generally lower than with SSRIs.

May increase appetite and stimulate weight gain, may increase serum cholesterol and triglyceride levels. Use caution in patients with depression, particularly if suicidal risk may be present. Use caution in patients with a previous seizure disorder or condition predisposing to seizures such as brain damage, alcoholism, or concurrent therapy with other drugs which lower the seizure threshold. Use with caution in patients with hepatic or renal dysfunction and in elderly patients.

SolTab™ formulation contains phenylalanine.

Pregnancy risk C.

Drug Interactions

Cytochrome P450 Effect: Substrate of **CYP1A2**, 2C8/9, **2D6, 3A4**; Inhibits CYP1A2, 3A4

Decreased Effect: Decreased effect seen with clonidine, CYP inducers

Increased Effect/Toxicity: Increased sedative effect seen with CNS depressants, CYP inhibitors, linezolid, MAO inhibitors, selegiline, sibutramine

Nutritional/Ethanol Interactions

Ethanol: Avoid ethanol (may increase CNS depression).

Herb/Nutraceutical: Avoid St John's wort (may decrease mirtazapine levels). Avoid valerian, St John's wort, SAMe, kava kava (may increase CNS depression).

Adverse Reactions

>10%:

- Central nervous system: Somnolence (54%)
- Endocrine & metabolic: Cholesterol increased
- Gastrointestinal: Constipation (13%), xerostomia (25%), appetite increased (17%), weight gain (12%; weight gain of >7% reported in 8% of adults, ≤49% of pediatric patients)

1% to 10%:

- Cardiovascular: Hypertension, vasodilatation, peripheral edema (2%), edema (1%)
- Central nervous system: Dizziness (7%), abnormal dreams (4%), abnormal thoughts (3%), confusion (2%), malaise
- Endocrine & metabolic: Triglycerides increased
- Gastrointestinal: Vomiting, anorexia, abdominal pain
- Genitourinary: Urinary frequency (2%)
- Neuromuscular & skeletal: Myalgia (2%), back pain (2%), arthralgias, tremor (2%), weakness (8%)
- Respiratory: Dyspnea (1%)
- Miscellaneous: Flu-like symptoms (5%), thirst (<1%)

<1% (Limited to important or life-threatening): Agranulocytosis, dehydration, liver function test increases, lymphadenopathy, neutropenia, orthostatic hypotension, seizures (1 case reported), torsade de pointes (1 case reported), weight loss

Overdosage/Toxicology Experience with overdose is limited. Signs and symptoms have included disorientation, drowsiness, impaired memory, and tachycardia. Treatment should be symptomatic and supportive. Activated charcoal should be administered. Emesis is not recommended; however, gastric lavage with airway protection may be used in symptomatic patients or if performed soon after ingestion. Consider the possibility of multiple drug involvement.

Pharmacodynamics/Kinetics

Bioavailability: 50%

Half-Life Elimination: 20-40 hours; hampered with renal or hepatic impairment

Time to Peak: Serum: 2 hours

Metabolism: Extensively hepatic via CYP1A2, 2C9, 2D6, 3A4 and via demethylation and hydroxylation

Formulations

Tablet: 15 mg, 30 mg, 45 mg

Tablet, orally-disintegrating:

- 15 mg [phenylalanine 2.6 mg/tablet] [orange flavor]
- 30 mg [phenylalanine 5.2 mg/tablet] [orange flavor]
- 45 mg [phenylalanine 7.8 mg/tablet] [orange flavor]

Dosing

Adults: Depression: Oral: Initial: 15 mg nightly, titrate up to 15-45 mg/day with dose increases made no more frequently than every 1-2 weeks. There is an inverse relationship between dose and sedation.

Elderly: Decreased clearance seen (40% males, 10% females); no specific dosage adjustment recommended by manufacturer.

Renal Impairment:

Cl_{cr} 11-39 mL/minute: 30% decreased clearance

Cl_{cr} <10 mL/minute: 50% decreased clearance

(Continued)

Mirtazapine *(Continued)*

Hepatic Impairment: Clearance is decreased by 30%.

Stability

Storage: Store at controlled room temperature

SolTab™: Protect from light and moisture; use immediately upon opening tablet blister

Monitoring and Teaching Issues

Physical Assessment: Assess other medications patient may be taking for effectiveness and interactions (see Drug Interactions). See Warnings/Precautions for use cautions. Has potential for psychological or physiological dependence, abuse, or tolerance. Monitor therapeutic response and adverse reactions at beginning of therapy and periodically with long-term use (see Adverse Reactions and Overdose/Toxicology). Taper dosage slowly when discontinuing. Assess knowledge/teach patient appropriate use, interventions to reduce side effects, and adverse symptoms to report (see Patient Education). **Pregnancy risk factor C** - benefits of use should outweigh possible risks. Breast-feeding is not recommended.

Patient Education: Take exactly as directed; do not increase dose or frequency. It may take 2-3 weeks to achieve desired results. Take once-a-day dose at bedtime. Avoid alcohol, caffeine, and other prescription or OTC medications not approved by prescriber. Maintain adequate hydration (2-3 L/day of fluids) unless advised by prescriber to restrict fluids. You may experience drowsiness, dizziness, or lightheadedness (use caution when driving or engaging in tasks requiring alertness until response to drug is known); nausea, vomiting, anorexia, or dry mouth (small, frequent meals, frequent mouth care, chewing gum, or sucking lozenges may help); or orthostatic hypotension (use caution when climbing stairs or changing position from lying or sitting to standing). Report persistent insomnia, agitation, or confusion; muscle cramping, tremors, weakness, or change in gait; breathlessness or difficulty breathing; chest pain, palpitations, or rapid heartbeat; change in urinary pattern; vision changes or eye pain; yellowing of eyes or skin; pale stools/dark urine; or worsening of condition.

SolTab™: Open blister pack and place tablet on the tongue. Do not split tablet. Tablet is formulated to dissolve on the tongue without water.

Pregnancy/breast-feeding precautions: Inform prescriber if you are or intend to become pregnant. Breast-feeding is not recommended.

Dietary Issues: Remeron® SolTab™ contains phenylalanine: 2.6 mg per 15 mg tablet; 5.2 mg per 30 mg tablet; 7.8 mg per 45 mg tablet

Additional Information Note: At least 14 days should elapse between discontinuation of an MAO inhibitor and initiation of therapy with mirtazapine; at least 14 days should be allowed after discontinuing mirtazapine before starting an MAO inhibitor.

Related Information

Antidepressant Agents *on page 1553*
Antidepressant Medication Guidelines *on page 1613*

Misoprostol (mye soe PROST ole)

U.S. Brand Names Cytotec®

Generic Available Yes

Pharmacologic Category Prostaglandin

Pregnancy Risk Factor X

Lactation Excretion in breast milk unknown/contraindicated

Use Prevention of NSAID-induced gastric ulcers; medical termination of pregnancy of ≤49 days (in conjunction with mifepristone)

Use - Unlabeled/Investigational Cervical ripening and labor induction; NSAID-induced nephropathy; fat malabsorption in cystic fibrosis

Mechanism of Action/Effect Misoprostol is a synthetic prostaglandin E_1 analog that replaces the protective prostaglandins consumed with prostaglandin-inhibiting therapies (eg, NSAIDs); has been shown to induce uterine contractions

Contraindications Hypersensitivity to misoprostol, prostaglandins, or any component of the formulation; pregnancy (when used to reduce NSAID-induced ulcers)

Warnings/Precautions Safety and efficacy have not been established in children <18 years of age. Use with caution in patients with renal impairment and the elderly. Not to be used in pregnant women or women of childbearing potential unless woman is capable of complying with effective contraceptive measures; therapy is normally begun on the second or third day of next normal menstrual period. Uterine perforation and/or rupture have been reported in association with intravaginal use to induce labor or with combined oral/intravaginal use to induce abortion. The manufacturer states that Cytotec® should not be used as a cervical-ripening agent for induction of labor. However, The American College of Obstetricians and Gynecologists (ACOG) continues to support this off-label use.

Drug Interactions

Decreased Effect: Antacids may diminish absorption (not clinically significant)

Nutritional/Ethanol Interactions Food: Misoprostol peak serum concentrations may be decreased if taken with food (not clinically significant).

Adverse Reactions

>10%: Gastrointestinal: Diarrhea, abdominal pain

1% to 10%:

Central nervous system: Headache

Gastrointestinal: Constipation, flatulence, nausea, dyspepsia, vomiting

<1% (Limited to important or life-threatening): Anaphylaxis, anxiety, appetite changes, arrhythmia, bronchospasm, confusion, depression, drowsiness, edema, fetal or infant death (when used during pregnancy), fever, GI bleeding, GI inflammation, gingivitis, gout, hypertension, hypotension, impotence, loss of libido, neuropathy, neurosis, purpura, rash, reflux, rigors, thrombocytopenia, uterine rupture, weakness, weight changes

Overdosage/Toxicology Symptoms of overdose include sedation, tremor, convulsions, dyspnea, abdominal pain, diarrhea, hypotension, and bradycardia. Treatment is symptom-directed and supportive.

Pharmacodynamics/Kinetics

Absorption: Rapid

Half-Life Elimination: Metabolite: 20-40 minutes

Time to Peak: Serum: Active metabolite: Fasting: 15-30 minutes

Metabolism: Hepatic; rapidly de-esterified to misoprostol acid (active)

Formulations Tablet: 100 mcg, 200 mcg

Dosing

Adults:

Prevention of NSAID-inducer ulcers: Oral: 200 mcg 4 times/day with food; if not tolerated, may decrease dose to 100 mcg 4 times/day with food or 200 mcg twice daily with food. Last dose of the day should be taken at bedtime.

Labor induction or cervical ripening (unlabeled use): Intravaginal: 25 mcg (1/4 of 100 mcg tablet); may repeat at intervals no more frequent than every 3-6 hours. Do not use in patients with previous cesarean delivery or prior major uterine surgery.

Medical termination of pregnancy: Oral: Refer to Mifepristone monograph.

Elderly: Oral: 100-200 mcg 4 times/day with food; if 200 mcg 4 times/day not tolerated, reduce to 100 mcg 4 times/day or 200 mcg twice daily with food. **Note:** To avoid the diarrhea potential, doses can be initiated at 100 mcg/day and increased 100 mcg/day at 3-day intervals until desired dose is achieved; also, recommend administering with food to decrease diarrhea incidence.

Pediatrics: Children 8-16 years: Oral: Fat absorption in cystic fibrosis (unlabeled use): 100 mcg 4 times/day

Administration

Oral: Incidence of diarrhea may be lessened by having patient take dose right after meals. Therapy is usually begun on the second or third day of the next normal menstrual period.

Stability

Storage: Store at or below 25°C (77°F).

Monitoring and Teaching Issues

Physical Assessment: Assess knowledge/teach appropriate antiulcer diet and lifestyle. Monitor renal function and fluid balance. **Pregnancy risk factor X** - determine that patient is not pregnant before beginning treatment and do not give to women of childbearing age or to males who may have intercourse with women of childbearing age unless both male and female are capable of complying with barrier contraceptive measures during therapy and for 1 month following therapy. Breast-feeding is contraindicated.

Patient Education: Take as directed; continue taking your NSAIDs while taking this medication. Take with meals or after meals to prevent nausea, diarrhea, and flatulence. Avoid using antacids. You may experience increased menstrual pain, or cramping; request analgesics. Report abnormal menstrual periods, spotting (may occur even in postmenstrual women), or severe menstrual bleeding. **Pregnancy/breast-feeding precautions:** When used to prevent NSAID-induced ulcers: Inform prescriber if you are pregnant. Do not get pregnant during or for 1 month following therapy. Male: Do not cause a female to become pregnant. Male/female: Consult prescriber for instruction on appropriate contraceptive measures. This drug may cause severe fetal defects, miscarriage, or abortion; do not share medication with others. Do not breast-feed.

Dietary Issues: Should be taken with food; incidence of diarrhea may be lessened by having patient take dose right after meals.

Geriatric Considerations: Elderly, due to extensive use of NSAIDs and the high percentage of asymptomatic hemorrhage and perforation from NSAIDs, are at risk for NSAID-induced ulcers and may be candidates for misoprostol use. However, routine use for prophylaxis is not justified. Patients must be selected upon demonstration that they are at risk for NSAID-induced lesions. Misoprostol should not be used as a first-line therapy for gastric or duodenal ulcers.

Breast-feeding Issues: It is not known if misoprostol is excreted in human milk, however, because significant diarrhea may occur in a nursing infant, breast-feeding is contraindicated

Pregnancy Issues: Misoprostol is an abortifacient. During pregnancy, use to prevent NSAID-induced ulcers is contraindicated. Reports of fetal death, congenital anomalies, uterine perforation, and abortion have been received after the use of misoprostol in pregnancy.

Misoprostol and Diclofenac *see* Diclofenac and Misoprostol *on page 402*

Mithracin® *see* Plicamycin *on page 1096*

Mithramycin *see* Plicamycin *on page 1096*

Mitomycin (mye toe MYE sin)

U.S. Brand Names Mutamycin®

Synonyms Mitomycin-C; MTC

Generic Available Yes

Pharmacologic Category Antineoplastic Agent, Antibiotic

Pregnancy Risk Factor D

Lactation Enters breast milk/contraindicated

Use Therapy of disseminated adenocarcinoma of stomach or pancreas in combination with other approved chemotherapeutic agents; bladder cancer, colorectal cancer

Mechanism of Action/Effect Isolated from *Streptomyces caespitosus*; acts primarily as an alkylating agent and produces DNA cross-linking (primarily with guanine and cytosine pairs); cell-cycle nonspecific; inhibits DNA and RNA synthesis by alkylation and cross-linking the strands of DNA

Contraindications Hypersensitivity to mitomycin or any component of the formulation; platelet counts <75,000/mm^3; leukocyte counts <3000/mm^3 or serum creatinine >1.7 mg/dL; thrombocytopenia; pregnancy

Warnings/Precautions The U.S. Food and Drug Administration (FDA) currently recommends that procedures for proper handling and disposal of antineoplastic agents be considered. Use with caution in patients who have received radiation therapy or in the presence of

(Continued)

Mitomycin *(Continued)*

hepatobiliary dysfunction; reduce dosage in patients who are receiving radiation therapy simultaneously. Hemolytic-uremic syndrome, potentially fatal, occurs in some patients receiving long-term therapy. It is correlated with total dose (single doses ≥60 mg or cumulative doses ≥50 mg/m^2) and total duration of therapy (>5-11 months). **Mitomycin is a potent vesicant, may cause ulceration, necrosis, cellulitis, and tissue sloughing if infiltrated.**

Drug Interactions

Increased Effect/Toxicity: *Vinca* alkaloids or doxorubicin may enhance cardiac toxicity when coadministered with mitomycin.

Nutritional/Ethanol Interactions Herb/Nutraceutical: Avoid black cohosh, dong quai in estrogen-dependent tumors.

Adverse Reactions

>10%:
- Cardiovascular: Congestive heart failure (3% to 15%) (doses >30 mg/m^2)
- Dermatologic: Alopecia, nail banding/discoloration
- Gastrointestinal: Nausea, vomiting and anorexia (14%)
- Hematologic: Anemia (19% to 24%); myelosuppression, common, dose-limiting, delayed
  - Onset: 3 weeks
  - Nadir: 4-6 weeks
  - Recovery: 6-8 weeks

1% to 10%:
- Dermatologic: Rash
- Gastrointestinal: Stomatitis
- Neuromuscular: Paresthesias
- Respiratory: Interstitial pneumonitis, infiltrates, dyspnea, cough (7%)

<1% (Limited to important or life-threatening): Extravasation reactions, fever, hemolytic uremic syndrome, malaise, pruritus, renal failure

Overdosage/Toxicology Symptoms of overdose include bone marrow suppression, nausea, vomiting, and alopecia. Treatment is symptom-directed and supportive.

Pharmacodynamics/Kinetics

Half-Life Elimination: 23-78 minutes; Terminal: 50 minutes

Metabolism: Hepatic

Formulations Injection, powder for reconstitution: 5 mg, 20 mg, 40 mg

Dosing

Adults & Elderly: Refer to individual protocols. I.V.:
- Single-agent therapy: I.V.: 20 mg/m^2 every 6-8 weeks
- Combination therapy: I.V.: 10 mg/m^2 every 6-8 weeks
- Bone marrow transplant: I.V.:
  - 40-50 mg/m^2
  - 2-40 mg/m^2/day for 3 days
- Total cumulative dose should not exceed 50 mg/m^2; see table.

Mitomycin

Nadir After Prior Dose per mm^3		% of Prior Dose to Be Given
Leukocytes	Platelets	
4000	>100,000	100
3000-3999	75,000-99,999	100
2000-2999	25,000-74,999	70
2000	<25,000	50

Bladder carcinoma: Intravesicular instillations: 20-40 mg/dose (1 mg/mL in sterile aqueous solution) instilled into the bladder for 3 hours repeated up to 3 times/week for up to 20 procedures per course.

Pediatrics: Refer to adult dosing.

Renal Impairment: Varying approaches to dosing adjustments have been published. Consult individual protocols.

Cl_{cr} <10 mL/minute: Administer 75% of normal dose

Note: The manufacturer states that Mutamycin® should not be given to patients with serum creatinine >1.7 mg/dL.

Hemodialysis: Unknown

CAPD effects: Unknown

CAVH effects: Unknown

Hepatic Impairment: Although some mitomycin may be excreted in the bile, no specific guidelines regarding dosage adjustment in hepatic impairment can be made.

Administration

I.V.: Vesicant. Administer slow I.V. push by central line only.

Stability

Storage: Store intact vials of lyophilized powder at room temperature.

Reconstitution:

Store intact vials of lyophilized powder at room temperature

Dilute powder with SWI to a concentration of 0.5 mg/mL as follows: Solution is stable for 7 days at room temperature and 14 days at refrigeration if protected from light
- 5 mg = 10 mL
- 20 mg = 40 mL
- 40 mg = 80 mL
- Further dilution to 20-40 mcg/mL:
  - In normal saline: Stable for 12 hours at room temperature
  - In D_5: Stable for 3 hours at room temperature
  - In sodium lactate: Stable for 12 hours at room temperature

Standard I.V. dilution:

I.V. push: Dose/syringe (concentration = 0.5 mg/mL)

Maximum syringe size for IVP is a 30 mL syringe and syringe should be ≤75% full

Syringe is stable for 7 days at room temperature and 14 days at refrigeration if protected from light

IVPB: Dose/100 mL NS

IVPB solution is stable for 24 hours at room temperature

Compatibility: Stable in LR

Y-site administration: Incompatible with aztreonam, cefepime, etoposide phosphate, filgrastim, gemcitabine, piperacillin/tazobactam, sargramostim, topotecan, vinorelbine

Compatibility when admixed: Incompatible with bleomycin

Monitoring Laboratory Tests Platelet count, CBC with differential, prothrombin time, renal and pulmonary function

Monitoring and Teaching Issues

Physical Assessment: See Contraindications, Warnings/Precautions, and Dosing for use cautions. Assess potential for interactions with other prescriptions, OTC medications, or herbal products patient may be taking (see Drug Interactions). **Infusion:** See Administration; infusion site must be closely monitored to prevent extravasation (eg, mitomycin is a potent vesicant, may cause ulceration, necrosis, cellulitis, and tissue sloughing if infiltrated - see Administration). Assess results of laboratory tests (see above), therapeutic effectiveness, and adverse reactions (eg, signs of CHF, hydration, nutritional status, and opportunistic infection - see Adverse Reactions and Overdose/Toxicology) on a regular basis throughout therapy. Teach patient possible side effects and interventions and adverse symptoms to report (see Patient Education). **Pregnancy risk factor D** - determine that patient is not pregnant before beginning treatment. Instruct patients of childbearing age about appropriate barrier contraceptive measures. Breast-feeding is contraindicated.

Patient Education: Inform prescriber of all prescriptions, OTC medications, or herbal products you are taking, and any allergies you have. Do not take anything new during treatment unless approved by prescriber. This drug can only be given intravenously. Report immediately any redness, swelling, burning, or pain at infusion site. Maintain adequate hydration (2-3 L/day of fluids) unless advised by prescriber to restrict fluids, and nutrition. May cause nausea, vomiting, or anorexia (small, frequent meals, frequent mouth care, chewing gum, or sucking lozenges may help); mouth sores (use soft toothbrush, waxed dental floss, and frequent mouth rinses); or loss of hair or discoloration of nails (may be reversible when therapy is discontinued). Report rash or itching, unresolved nausea or diarrhea; difficulty breathing, swelling of extremities, sudden weight gain, or unusual cough; any numbness, tingling, or loss of sensation; or opportunistic infection (fever, chills, sore throat, burning urination, fatigue). **Pregnancy/breast-feeding precautions:** Do not get pregnant while taking this medication. Consult prescriber for appropriate barrier contraceptive measures. Do not breast-feed.

Mitomycin-C *see* Mitomycin *on page 913*

Mitotane (MYE toe tane)

U.S. Brand Names Lysodren®

Synonyms o,p′-DDD

Generic Available No

Pharmacologic Category Antineoplastic Agent, Miscellaneous

Pregnancy Risk Factor C

Lactation Enters breast milk/contraindicated

Use Treatment of adrenocortical carcinoma

Use - Unlabeled/Investigational Treatment of Cushing's syndrome

Mechanism of Action/Effect Causes adrenal cortical atrophy; drug affects mitochondria in adrenal cortical cells and decreases production of cortisol; also alters the peripheral metabolism of steroids

Contraindications Hypersensitivity to mitotane or any component of the formulation

Warnings/Precautions The U.S. Food and Drug Administration (FDA) currently recommends that procedures for proper handling and disposal of antineoplastic agents be considered. Steroid replacement with glucocorticoid, and sometimes mineralocorticoid, is necessary. It has been recommended that replacement therapy be initiated at the start of therapy, rather than waiting for evidence of adrenal insufficiency. Because mitotane can increase the metabolism of hydrocortisone, higher than usual replacement doses of the latter may be required. Acute adrenal insufficiency may occur in the face of shock, trauma, or infection. Mitotane should be discontinued temporarily in this setting and appropriate steroid coverage should be administered. Pregnancy risk C.

Drug Interactions

Decreased Effect: Mitotane may enhance the clearance of barbiturates and warfarin by induction of the hepatic microsomal enzyme system resulting in a decreased effect. Coadministration of spironolactone has resulted in negation of mitotane's effect. Mitotane may increase clearance of phenytoin by microsomal enzyme stimulation.

Increased Effect/Toxicity: CNS depressants taken with mitotane may enhance CNS depression.

Nutritional/Ethanol Interactions Ethanol: Avoid ethanol (may increase CNS depression).

Adverse Reactions The following reactions are reversible:

Central nervous system: CNS depression (32%), dizziness (15%), headache (5%), confusion (3%)

Dermatologic: Skin rash (12%)

Gastrointestinal: Anorexia (24%), nausea (39%), vomiting (37%), diarrhea (13%)

Neuromuscular & skeletal: Muscle tremor (3%), weakness (12%)

Overdosage/Toxicology Symptoms of overdose include diarrhea, vomiting, numbness of limbs, and weakness. Treatment is symptom-directed and supportive.

(Continued)

Mitotane *(Continued)*

Pharmacodynamics/Kinetics

Absorption: Oral: ~35% to 40%

Half-Life Elimination: 18-159 days

Time to Peak: Serum: 3-5 hours

Metabolism: Hepatic and other tissues

Formulations Tablet, scored: 500 mg

Dosing

Adults & Elderly: Adrenal carcinoma: Oral: Start at 1-6 g/day in divided doses, then increase incrementally to 8-10 g/day in 3-4 divided doses; dose is changed on basis of side effect with aim of giving as high a dose as tolerated; maximum daily dose: 18 g

Pediatrics: Adrenal carcinoma: Oral: Children: 0.1-0.5 mg/kg or 1-2 g/day in divided doses increasing gradually to a maximum of 5-7 g/day

Hepatic Impairment: Dose may need to be decreased in patients with liver disease.

Stability

Storage: Protect from light. Store at room temperature.

Monitoring and Teaching Issues

Physical Assessment: See Contraindications, Warnings/Precautions, and Dosing for use cautions. Assess potential for interactions with other prescriptions, OTC medications, or herbal products patient may be taking (see Drug Interactions). Assess therapeutic effectiveness and adverse response (see Adverse Reactions and Overdose/Toxicology). Teach patient proper use, possible side effects and appropriate interventions, and adverse symptoms to report (see Patient Education). **Pregnancy risk factor C** - benefits of use should outweigh possible risks. Breast-feeding is contraindicated.

Patient Education: Inform prescriber of all prescriptions, OTC medications, or herbal products you are taking, and any allergies you have. Do not take anything new during treatment unless approved by prescriber. Take as directed; do not alter dose or discontinue without consulting prescriber. Desired effects of this drug may not be seen for 2-3 months. Wear identification that alerts medical personnel that you are taking this drug in event of shock or trauma. Maintain adequate hydration (2-3 L/day of fluids) unless advised by prescriber to restrict fluids, and nutrition. Avoid alcohol. May cause dizziness, headache, confusion (avoid driving or performing tasks requiring alertness until response to drug is known); nausea, vomiting, or loss of appetite (small, frequent meals, frequent mouth care, sucking lozenges, or chewing gum may help); or diarrhea (buttermilk, boiled milk, or yogurt may help). Report severe vomiting or diarrhea; or muscular twitching, tremor, numbness, or weakness. **Pregnancy/breast-feeding precautions:** Inform prescriber if you are or intend to become pregnant. Do not breast-feed.

Mitoxantrone (mye toe ZAN trone)

U.S. Brand Names Novantrone®

Synonyms DHAD; Mitoxantrone Hydrochloride

Generic Available No

Pharmacologic Category Antineoplastic Agent, Antibiotic

Pregnancy Risk Factor D

Lactation Enters breast milk/contraindicated

Use Treatment of acute nonlymphocytic leukemia (ANLL) in adults in combination with other agents; very active against various leukemias, lymphoma, and breast cancer; moderately active against pediatric sarcoma; treatment of secondary (chronic) progressive, progressive relapsing, or worsening relapsing-remitting multiple sclerosis; treatment of pain related to advanced hormone-refractory prostate cancer (in combination with corticosteroids)

Mechanism of Action/Effect Analogue of the anthracyclines, but different in mechanism of action, cardiac toxicity, and potential for tissue necrosis; inhibits DNA and RNA synthesis

Contraindications Hypersensitivity to mitoxantrone or any component of the formulation; multiple sclerosis with left ventricular ejection fraction (LVEF) <50% or clinically significant decrease in LVEF; pregnancy

Warnings/Precautions The FDA currently recommends that procedures for proper handling and disposal of antineoplastic agents be considered. Appropriate safety equipment is recommended for preparation, administration, and disposal of antineoplastics. If mitoxantrone contacts the skin, wash and flush thoroughly with water.

Dosage should be reduced in patients with impaired hepatobiliary function; not for treatment of multiple sclerosis in patients with concurrent hepatic impairment. Treatment may lead to severe myelosuppression; use with caution in patients with pre-existing myelosuppression. Do not use if baseline neutrophil count <1500 cells/mm^3 (except for treatment of ANLL). May cause myocardial toxicity and potentially-fatal CHF; risk increases with cumulative dosing. Predisposing factors for mitoxantrone-induced cardiotoxicity include prior anthracycline therapy, prior cardiovascular disease, and mediastinal irradiation. The risk of developing cardiotoxicity is <3% when the cumulative doses are <100-120 mg/m^2 in patients with predisposing factors and <160 mg/m^2 in patients with no predisposing factors. Monitor for cardiac toxicity throughout treatment and prior to each dose once cumulative dose of 100 mg/m^2 is reached in patients with multiple sclerosis, and once cumulative dose of 140 mg/m^2 is reached for patients with cancer. Not for treatment of primary progressive multiple sclerosis. Has been associated with the development of secondary acute myelogenous leukemia and myelodysplasia when used in combination with other antineoplastic agents. For I.V. use only (not for intra-arterial or intrathecal injection). May cause urine, saliva, tears, and sweat to turn blue-green for 24 hours postinfusion. Whites of eyes may have blue-green tinge (this is normal).

Drug Interactions

Cytochrome P450 Effect: Inhibits CYP3A4

Decreased Effect: Patients may experience impaired immune response to vaccines; possible infection after administration of live vaccines in patients receiving immunosuppressants.

Nutritional/Ethanol Interactions Herb/Nutraceutical: Avoid black cohosh, dong quai in estrogen-dependent tumors.

Adverse Reactions

>10%:

Central nervous system: Headache

Dermatologic: Alopecia

Gastrointestinal: Nausea, vomiting, diarrhea, abdominal pain, mucositis, stomatitis, GI bleeding

Emetic potential: Moderate (31% to 72%)

Genitourinary: Discoloration of urine (blue-green)

Hepatic: Abnormal LFTs

Respiratory: Coughing, dyspnea

1% to 10%:

Cardiovascular: Cardiotoxicity (primarily in patients who have received prior anthracycline therapy), CHF, hypotension

Central nervous system: Seizures, fever

Dermatologic: Pruritus, skin desquamation

Hematologic: Myelosuppressive effects of chemotherapy:

WBC: Mild

Platelets: Mild

Onset: 7-10 days

Nadir: 14 days

Recovery: 21 days

Hepatic: Transient elevation of liver enzymes, jaundice

Ocular: Conjunctivitis

Renal: Renal failure

Miscellaneous: Development of secondary leukemia (~1% to 2%)

<1% (Limited to important or life-threatening): Anaphylactoid reactions, anaphylaxis, interstitial pneumonitis (has occurred during combination chemotherapy), **irritant chemotherapy** with blue skin discoloration, tissue necrosis following extravasation, pain or redness at injection site, phlebitis

Overdosage/Toxicology Symptoms of overdose include leukopenia, tachycardia, and marrow hypoplasia. No known antidote. Treatment is symptom-directed and supportive.

Pharmacodynamics/Kinetics

Half-Life Elimination: Terminal: 23-215 hours; may be prolonged with hepatic impairment

Metabolism: Hepatic; pathway not determined

Formulations Injection, as base: 2 mg/mL (10 mL, 12.5 mL, 15 mL)

Dosing

Adults & Elderly: Refer to individual protocols. I.V. (may dilute in D_5W or NS):

ANLL leukemias: I.V.: 12 mg/m^2/day once daily for 3 days; acute leukemia in relapse: 8-12 mg/m^2/day once daily for 4-5 days

Solid tumors: I.V.: 12-14 mg/m^2 every 3-4 weeks **or** 2-4 mg/m^2/day for 5 days

Maximum total dose: 80-120 mg/m^2 in patients with predisposing factor and <160 mg in patients with no predisposing factor

BMT high dose: I.V.: 24-48 mg/m^2 as a single dose; duration of infusion is 1-4 hours; generally combined with other high-dose chemotherapeutic drugs.

Hormone-refractory prostate cancer: I.V.: 12-14 mg/m^2 over 5-15 minutes via intravenous infusion every 21 days

Multiple sclerosis: I.V.: 12 mg/m^2 over 5-15 minutes via intravenous infusion every 3 months; do **not** use if LVEF <50% (or following significant reduction); cumulative lifetime dose should not exceed ≥140 mg/m^2

Dose modifications are based on degree of leukopenia or thrombocytopenia. See table.

Granulocyte Count Nadir (cells/mm^2)	Platelet Count Nadir (cells/mm^2)	Total Bilirubin (mg/dL)	Dose Adjustment
>2000	>150,000	<1.5	Increase by 1 mg/m^2
1000-2000	75,000-150,000	<1.5	Maintain same dose
<1000	<75,000	1.5-3	Decrease by 1 mg/m^2

Pediatrics: Refer to individual protocols.

ANLL leukemias: I.V. (may dilute in D_5W or NS):

Children ≤2 years: 0.4 mg/kg/day once daily for 3-5 days

Children >2 years: Refer to adult dosing.

Solid tumors: I.V.: Children: 18-20 mg/m^2 every 3-4 weeks **OR** 5-8 mg/m^2 every week

Hepatic Impairment: Official dosage adjustment recommendations have not been established.

Moderate dysfunction (bilirubin 1.5-3 mg/dL): Some clinicians recommend a 50% dosage reduction.

Severe dysfunction (bilirubin >3.0 mg/dL) have a lower total body clearance and may require a dosage adjustment to 8 mg/m^2; some clinicians recommend a dosage reduction to 25% of dose.

Dose modifications based on degree of leukopenia or thrombocytopenia; see table.

Administration

I.V.: Irritant. Do **not** give I.V. bolus over <3 minutes; can be administered I.V. intermittent infusion over 15-30 minutes.

Stability

Storage: Store intact vials at room temperature or refrigeration.

Reconstitution: Dilute in at least 50 mL of NS or D_5W. Solution is stable for 7 days at room temperature or refrigeration.

Standard I.V. dilution: IVPB: Dose/100 mL D_5W or NS

Solution is stable for 7 days at room temperature and refrigeration.

(Continued)

Mitoxantrone *(Continued)*

Compatibility: Stable in in D_5NS, D_5W, NS

Y-site administration: Incompatible with amphotericin B cholesteryl sulfate complex, aztreonam, cefepime, doxorubicin liposome, paclitaxel, piperacillin/tazobactam, propofol

Compatibility when admixed: Incompatible with heparin

Monitoring Laboratory Tests CBC, serum uric acid, liver function, echocardiogram

Monitoring and Teaching Issues

Physical Assessment: See Contraindications, Warnings/Precautions, and Dosing for use cautions. Assess potential for interactions with other prescriptions, OTC medications, or herbal products patient may be taking (see Drug Interactions). See infusion specifics above; infusion site must be monitored closely to prevent extravasation. Assess results of laboratory tests (see above), therapeutic effectiveness, and adverse response (see Adverse Reactions and Overdose/Toxicology). Teach patient possible side effects and appropriate interventions and adverse symptoms to report (see Patient Education). **Pregnancy risk factor D** - determine that patient is not pregnant before beginning treatment. Instruct patients of childbearing age about appropriate barrier contraceptive measures. Breast-feeding is contraindicated.

Patient Education: Inform prescriber of all prescriptions, OTC medications, or herbal products you are taking, and any allergies you have. Do not take anything new during treatment unless approved by prescriber. This drug can only be given by infusion. Report immediately any redness, swelling, burning, or pain at infusion site. Maintain adequate hydration (2-3 L/day of fluids) unless advised by prescriber to restrict fluids, and nutrition. You will be more susceptible to infection (avoid crowds and exposure to infection and do not have any vaccinations without consulting prescriber). May cause urine, saliva, tears, sweat, and whites of eyes to turn blue-green for 24 hours postinfusion (this is normal); nausea, vomiting, or GI upset (small, frequent meals, frequent mouth care, chewing gum, or sucking lozenges may help); mouth sores (use soft toothbrush or cotton swabs, waxed dental floss, and frequent mouth rinses); headache, dizziness, or blurred vision (use caution when driving or engaging in tasks that are potentially hazardous until response to drug is known); or loss of hair (may be reversible). Report chest pain or palpitations; difficulty breathing or constant cough; swelling of extremities or sudden weight gain; persistent fever or chills; or opportunistic infection (eg, fever, chills, sore throat, burning urination, fatigue). **Pregnancy/breast-feeding precautions:** Do not get pregnant while taking this medication. Consult prescriber for appropriate barrier contraceptive measures. Breast-feeding is not recommended.

Breast-feeding Issues: Mitoxantrone is excreted in human milk and significant concentrations (180 mg/mL) have been reported for 28 days after the last administration. Because of the potential for serious adverse reactions in infants from mitoxantrone, breast-feeding should be discontinued before starting treatment.

Pregnancy Issues: May cause fetal harm if administered to a pregnant woman. Women with multiple sclerosis and who are biologically capable of becoming pregnant should have a pregnancy test prior to each dose. Mitoxantrone is excreted in human milk and significant concentrations (180 mg/mL) have been reported for 28 days after the last administration.

Mitoxantrone Hydrochloride *see* Mitoxantrone *on page 916*

Mitrazol™ [OTC] *see* Miconazole *on page 899*

Mivacron® *see* Mivacurium *on page 918*

Mivacurium (mye va KYOO ree um)

U.S. Brand Names Mivacron®

Synonyms Mivacurium Chloride

Generic Available No

Pharmacologic Category Neuromuscular Blocker Agent, Nondepolarizing

Pregnancy Risk Factor C

Lactation Excretion in breast milk unknown/use caution

Use Adjunct to general anesthesia to facilitate endotracheal intubation and to relax skeletal muscles during surgery; to facilitate mechanical ventilation in ICU patients; does not relieve pain or produce sedation

Contraindications Hypersensitivity to mivacurium chloride, any component of the formulation, or other benzylisoquinolinium agents; use of multidose vials in patients with allergy to benzyl alcohol; pre-existing tachycardia

Warnings/Precautions Ventilation must be supported during neuromuscular blockade; does not counteract bradycardia produced by anesthetics/vagal stimulation; prolonged neuromuscular block may be seen in patients with reduced or atypical plasma cholinesterase activity (eg, pregnancy, liver or kidney disease, infections, peptic ulcer, anemia); patients homozygous for the atypical plasma cholinesterase gene are extremely sensitive to the neuromuscular blocking effect of mivacurium (use extreme caution if at all in those patients); duration prolonged in patients with renal and/or hepatic impairment; reduce initial dosage and inject slowly (over 60 seconds) in patients in whom substantial histamine release would be potentially hazardous; certain clinical conditions may result in potentiation or antagonism of neuromuscular blockade (such as, potentiation by electrolyte abnormalities, neuromuscular diseases, or acidosis; antagonism with demyelinating lesions).

Increased sensitivity in patients with myasthenia gravis, Eaton-Lambert syndrome, resistance in burn patients (>30% of body) for period of 5-70 days postinjury; resistance in patients with muscle trauma, denervation, immobilization, infection.

Pregnancy risk C.

Drug Interactions

Decreased Effect: Effect of nondepolarizing neuromuscular blockers may be reduced by carbamazepine (chronic use), corticosteroids (also associated with myopathy - see increased effect), phenytoin (chronic use), sympathomimetics, and theophylline.

Increased Effect/Toxicity: Increased effects are possible with aminoglycosides, beta-blockers, clindamycin, calcium channel blockers, halogenated anesthetics, imipenem, ketamine, lidocaine, loop diuretics (furosemide), macrolides (case reports), magnesium sulfate, procainamide, quinidine, quinolones, tetracyclines, and vancomycin. May increase risk of myopathy when used with high-dose corticosteroids for extended periods. Drugs which inhibit acetylcholinesterase may prolong effect of mivacurium.

Adverse Reactions

>10%: Cardiovascular: Flushing of face

1% to 10%: Cardiovascular: Hypotension

<1% (Limited to important or life-threatening): Anaphylactoid reaction, anaphylaxis, bradycardia, bronchospasm, cutaneous erythema, dizziness, endogenous histamine release, hypersensitivity reactions, hypoxemia, injection site reaction, muscle spasms, rash, tachycardia, wheezing

Pharmacodynamics/Kinetics

Half-Life Elimination: 2 minutes (more active isomers only)

Metabolism: Via plasma cholinesterase

Onset: Neuromuscular blockade: I.V. (dose dependent): 1.5-3 minutes

Duration: Short due to rapid hydrolysis by plasma cholinesterases; clinically effective block may last for 12-20 minutes; spontaneous recovery may be 95% complete in 25-30 minutes; duration shorter in children and may be slightly longer in elderly

Formulations

Infusion, as chloride [in D_5W]: 0.5 mg/mL (50 mL)

Injection, as chloride: 2 mg/mL (5 mL, 10 mL)

Dosing

Adults & Elderly: Note: Continuous infusion requires an infusion pump; dose should be based on ideal body weight

Neuromuscular blockade: Initial: I.V.: 0.15-0.25 mg/kg bolus followed by maintenance doses of 0.1 mg/kg at approximately 15-minute intervals; for prolonged neuromuscular block, initial infusion of 9-10 mcg/kg/minute is used upon evidence of spontaneous recovery from initial dose, usual infusion rate of 6-7 mcg/kg/minute (1-15 mcg/kg/minute) under balanced anesthesia; initial dose after succinylcholine for intubation (balanced anesthesia): Adults: 0.1 mg/kg

Pretreatment/priming: 10% of intubating dose given 3-5 minutes before initial dose

Pediatrics: Note: Continuous infusion requires an infusion pump; dose should be based on ideal body weight

Neuromuscular blockade: I.V.: Children 2-12 years (duration of action is shorter and dosage requirements are higher): 0.2 mg/kg followed by average infusion rate of 14 mcg/kg/minute (range: 5-31 mcg/kg/minute) upon evidence of spontaneous recovery from initial dose

Renal Impairment: 150 mcg/kg I.V. bolus; duration of action of blockade: 1.5 times longer in ESRD, may decrease infusion rates by as much as 50%, dependent on degree of renal impairment.

Hepatic Impairment: 150 mcg/kg I.V. bolus; duration of blockade: 3 times longer in ESLD, may decrease rate of infusion by as much as 50% in ESLD, dependent on the degree of impairment

Administration

I.V.: Children require higher mivacurium infusion rates than adults; during opioid/nitrous oxide/oxygen anesthesia, the infusion rate required to maintain 89% to 99% neuromuscular block averages 14 mcg/kg/minute (range: 5-31). For adults and children, the amount of infusion solution required per hour depends upon the clinical requirements of the patient, the concentration of mivacurium in the infusion solution, and the patient's weight. The contribution of the infusion solution to the fluid requirements of the patient must be considered.

Stability

Storage: Store at room temperature of 15°C to 25°C (59°F to 77°F); protect from direct ultraviolet light.

Compatibility: Stable in D_5LR, D_5NS, D_5W, LR, NS

Monitoring and Teaching Issues

Physical Assessment: Only clinicians experienced in the use of neuromuscular blocking agents should administer and/or manage the use of mivacurium. See Contraindications, Warnings/Precautions, and Dosing for use cautions. Assess potential for interactions with other prescriptions, OTC medications, or herbal products patient may be taking (eg, other drugs that affect neuromuscular activity may increase/decrease neuromuscular block induced by mivacurium - see Drug Interactions). Dosage and rate of administration should be individualized and titrated to the desired effect, according to relevant clinical factors, premedication, concomitant medication, age, and general condition of the patient. Ventilatory support must be instituted and maintained until adequate respiratory muscle function and/or airway protection are assured. This drug does not cause anesthesia or analgesia; pain must be treated with appropriate agents. Continuous monitoring of vital signs, cardiac and respiratory status, and neuromuscular block (objective assessment with peripheral external nerve stimulator) are mandatory until full muscle tone has returned (see Adverse Reactions). Safety precautions must be maintained until full muscle tone has returned. **Note:** It may take longer for return of muscle tone in elderly persons or patients with myasthenia gravis, myopathy, other neuromuscular diseases, dehydration, electrolyte imbalance, or severe acid/base imbalance. Provide appropriate teaching/support prior to, during, and following administration.

Long-term use: Vital signs and fluid levels must be monitored regularly during treatment. Every 2- to 3-hour repositioning, and skin, mouth, and eye care is necessary while patient is sedated. Emotional and sensory support (auditory and environmental) should be provided.

Pregnancy risk factor C - benefits of use should outweigh possible risks. Note breast-feeding caution.

(Continued)

Mivacurium *(Continued)*

Patient Education: Patient education should be appropriate for patient condition. Reassurance of constant monitoring and emotional support should precede and follow administration. Patients should be reminded as muscle tone returns not to attempt to change position or rise from bed without assistance and to report and skin rash, hives, pounding heartbeat, difficulty breathing, or muscle tremors. **Pregnancy/breast-feeding precaution:** Inform prescriber if you are pregnant. Consult prescriber if breast-feeding.

Additional Information Mivacurium is classified as a short-duration neuromuscular-blocking agent. Do not mix with barbiturates in the same syringe. Mivacurium does not appear to have a cumulative effect on the duration of blockade. It does not relieve pain or produce sedation.

Mivacurium Chloride *see* Mivacurium *on page 918*

MK383 *see* Tirofiban *on page 1327*

MK462 *see* Rizatriptan *on page 1201*

MK594 *see* Losartan *on page 824*

MK-0826 *see* Ertapenem *on page 484*

MMR *see page 1498*

M-M-R® II *see page 1498*

MOBIC® *see* Meloxicam *on page 846*

Modafinil (moe DAF i nil)

U.S. Brand Names Provigil®

Restrictions C-IV

Generic Available No

Pharmacologic Category Stimulant

Pregnancy Risk Factor C

Lactation Excretion in breast milk unknown/use caution

Use Improve wakefulness in patients with excessive daytime sleepiness associated with narcolepsy

Use - Unlabeled/Investigational Attention-deficit/hyperactivity disorder (ADHD); treatment of fatigue in MS and other disorders

Mechanism of Action/Effect The exact mechanism of action is unclear, it does not appear to alter the release of dopamine or norepinephrine, it may exert its stimulant effects by decreasing GABA-mediated neurotransmission, although this theory has not yet been fully evaluated; several studies also suggest that an intact central alpha-adrenergic system is required for modafinil's activity; the drug increases high-frequency alpha waves while decreasing both delta and theta wave activity, and these effects are consistent with generalized increases in mental alertness

Contraindications Hypersensitivity to modafinil or any component of the formulation

Warnings/Precautions History of angina, ischemic EKG changes, left ventricular hypertrophy, or clinically significant mitral valve prolapse in association with CNS stimulant use; caution should be exercised when modafinil is given to patients with a history of psychosis, recent history of myocardial infarction, and because it has not yet been adequately studied in patients with hypertension, periodic monitoring of hypertensive patients receiving modafinil may be appropriate; caution is warranted when operating machinery or driving, although functional impairment has not been demonstrated with modafinil, all CNS-active agents may alter judgment, thinking and/or motor skills. Efficacy of oral contraceptives may be reduced, therefore, use of alternative contraception should be considered. Pregnancy risk C.

Drug Interactions

Cytochrome P450 Effect: Substrate of **CYP3A4**; Inhibits CYP2C8/9, 2C19; Induces CYP1A2, 2B6, 3A4

Decreased Effect: Modafinil may decrease serum concentrations of oral contraceptives, cyclosporine, and to a lesser degree, theophylline. Agents that induce CYP3A4, including phenobarbital, carbamazepine, and rifampin may result in decreased modafinil levels. There is also evidence to suggest that modafinil may induce its own metabolism.

Increased Effect/Toxicity: Modafinil may increase levels of diazepam, mephenytoin, phenytoin, propranolol, and warfarin. In populations deficient in the CYP2D6 isoenzyme, where CYP2C19 acts as a secondary metabolic pathway, concentrations of tricyclic antidepressants and selective serotonin reuptake inhibitors may be increased during coadministration.

Adverse Reactions Limited to reports equal to or greater than placebo-related events.

<10%:

Cardiovascular: Chest pain (2%), hypertension (2%), hypotension (2%), vasodilation (1%), arrhythmia (1%), syncope (1%)

Central nervous system: Headache (50%, compared to 40% with placebo), nervousness (8%), dizziness (5%), depression (4%), anxiety (4%), cataplexy (3%), insomnia (3%), chills (2%), fever (1%), confusion (1%), amnesia (1%), emotional lability (1%), ataxia (1%)

Dermatologic: Dry skin (1%)

Endocrine & metabolic: Hyperglycemia (1%), albuminuria (1%)

Gastrointestinal: Diarrhea (8%), nausea (13%, compared to 4% with placebo), xerostomia (5%), anorexia (5%), vomiting (1%), mouth ulceration (1%), gingivitis (1%)

Genitourinary: Abnormal urine (1%), urinary retention (1%), ejaculatory disturbance (1%)

Hematologic: Eosinophilia (1%)

Hepatic: Abnormal LFTs (3%)

Neuromuscular & skeletal: Paresthesias (3%), dyskinesia (2%), neck pain (2%), hypertonia (2%), neck rigidity (1%), joint disorder (1%), tremor (1%)

Ocular: Amblyopia (2%), abnormal vision (2%)

Respiratory: Pharyngitis (6%), rhinitis (11%, compared to 8% with placebo), lung disorder (4%), dyspnea (2%), asthma (1%), epistaxis (1%)

Overdosage/Toxicology Symptoms of overdose include agitation, irritability, aggressiveness, confusion, nervousness, tremor, insomnia, palpitations, and elevations in hemodynamic parameters. Treatment is symptomatic and supportive. Cardiac monitoring is warranted.

Pharmacokinetic Note Modafinil is a racemic compound (10% *d*-isomer and 90% *l*-isomer at steady state), whose enantiomers have different pharmacokinetics.

Pharmacodynamics/Kinetics

Half-Life Elimination: Effective half-life: 15 hours; Steady-state: 2-4 days

Time to Peak: Serum: 2-4 hours

Metabolism: Hepatic; multiple pathways including CYP3A4

Formulations Tablet: 100 mg, 200 mg

Dosing

Adults:

ADHD (unlabeled use): Oral: 100-300 mg once daily

Narcolepsy: Oral: Initial: 200 mg as a single daily dose in the morning

Doses of 400 mg/day, given as a single dose, have been well tolerated, but there is no consistent evidence that this dose confers additional benefit.

Elderly: Elimination of modafinil and its metabolites may be reduced as a consequence of aging and as a result, lower doses should be considered.

Pediatrics: ADHD (unlabeled use): Oral: 50-100 mg once daily

Renal Impairment: Inadequate data to determine safety and efficacy in severe renal impairment.

Hepatic Impairment: Dose should be reduced to one-half of that recommended for patients with normal liver function.

Monitoring and Teaching Issues

Physical Assessment: See Contraindications and Warnings/Precautions for use cautions. Assess effectiveness and interactions of other medications, especially those that are metabolized by P450 enzymes (see Drug Interactions). Note that modafinil has potential for abuse; caution patient about inappropriate or overuse. Assess knowledge/teach patient appropriate use, adverse symptoms to report (see Patient Education), and interventions to reduce side effects. **Pregnancy risk factor C** - benefits of use should outweigh possible risks. Note breast-feeding caution.

Patient Education: Take exactly as prescribed; do not exceed recommended dosage without consulting prescriber. Maintain healthy sleep hygiene. Do not share medication with anyone else. Void before taking medication. You may experience headache, nervousness, confusion, or dizziness (use caution when driving or engaging in tasks requiring alertness until response to drug is known); diarrhea (yogurt or buttermilk may help); or dry mouth or sore mouth, loss of appetite, or vomiting (small, frequent meals, frequent mouth care, chewing gum, or sucking lozenges may help). If diabetic, monitor glucose levels closely. Report chest pain or palpitations; difficulty breathing; excessive insomnia, CNS agitation, depression, or memory disturbances; vision changes; changes in urinary pattern or ejaculation disturbances; or persistent joint pain or stiffness. **Pregnancy/breast-feeding precautions:** Inform prescriber if you are or intend to become pregnant. Consult prescriber if breast-feeding.

Pregnancy Issues: Currently, there are no studies in humans evaluating its teratogenicity. Embryotoxicity of modafinil has been observed in animal models at dosages above those employed therapeutically. As a result, it should be used cautiously during pregnancy and should be used only when the potential risk of drug therapy is outweighed by the drug's benefits.

Modane® Bulk [OTC] *see* Psyllium *on page 1152*

Modicon® *see* Ethinyl Estradiol and Norethindrone *on page 527*

Modified Shohl's Solution *see* Sodium Citrate and Citric Acid *on page 1236*

Moduretic® *see* Amiloride and Hydrochlorothiazide *on page 78*

Moexipril (mo EKS i pril)

U.S. Brand Names Univasc®

Synonyms Moexipril Hydrochloride

Generic Available No

Pharmacologic Category Angiotensin-Converting Enzyme (ACE) Inhibitor

Pregnancy Risk Factor C/D (2nd and 3rd trimesters)

Lactation Excretion in breast milk unknown/use caution

Use Treatment of hypertension, alone or in combination with thiazide diuretics; treatment of left ventricular dysfunction after myocardial infarction

Mechanism of Action/Effect Competitive inhibitor of angiotensin-converting enzyme (ACE); prevents conversion of angiotensin I to angiotensin II, a potent vasoconstrictor; results in lower levels of angiotensin II which causes an increase in plasma renin activity and a reduction in aldosterone secretion

Contraindications Hypersensitivity to moexipril, moexiprilat, or any component of the formulation; hypersensitivity or allergic reactions or angioedema related to previous treatment with an ACE inhibitor; pregnancy (2nd or 3rd trimester)

Warnings/Precautions Anaphylactic reactions can occur. Angioedema can occur at any time during treatment (especially following first dose). Careful blood pressure monitoring with first dose (hypotension can occur especially in volume depleted patients). Dosage adjustment needed in renal impairment. Use with caution in hypovolemia; collagen vascular diseases; valvular stenosis (particularly aortic stenosis); hyperkalemia; or before, during, or immediately after anesthesia. Avoid rapid dosage escalation which may lead to renal insufficiency. Neutropenia/agranulocytosis with myeloid hyperplasia can rarely occur. Hypersensitivity reactions may be seen during hemodialysis with high-flux dialysis membranes (eg, AN69). Deterioration in renal function can occur with initiation. Use with caution in unilateral renal artery stenosis and pre-existing renal insufficiency. Pregnancy risk C/D (2nd and 3rd trimesters).

(Continued)

Moexipril *(Continued)*

Drug Interactions

Decreased Effect: Aspirin (high dose) may reduce the therapeutic effects of ACE inhibitors; at low dosages this does not appear to be significant. Rifampin may decrease the effect of ACE inhibitors. Antacids may decrease the bioavailability of ACE inhibitors (may be more likely to occur with captopril); separate administration times by 1-2 hours. NSAIDs, specifically indomethacin, may reduce the hypotensive effects of ACE inhibitors. More likely to occur in low renin or volume dependent hypertensive patients.

Increased Effect/Toxicity: Potassium supplements, co-trimoxazole (high dose), angiotensin II receptor antagonists (candesartan, losartan, irbesartan, etc), or potassium-sparing diuretics (amiloride, spironolactone, triamterene) may result in elevated serum potassium levels when combined with moexipril. ACE inhibitor effects may be increased by probenecid (increases levels of captopril). ACE inhibitors may increase serum concentrations/effects of digoxin, lithium, and sulfonlyureas.

Diuretics have additive hypotensive effects with ACE inhibitors, and hypovolemia increases the potential for adverse renal effects of ACE inhibitors. In patients with compromised renal function, coadministration with NSAIDs may result in further deterioration of renal function. Allopurinol and ACE inhibitors may cause a higher risk of hypersensitivity reaction when taken concurrently.

Nutritional/Ethanol Interactions

Food: Food may delay and reduce peak serum levels.

Herb/Nutraceutical: Avoid dong quai if using for hypertension (has estrogenic activity). Avoid ephedra, yohimbe, ginseng (may worsen hypertension). Avoid garlic (may have increased antihypertensive effect).

Effects on Lab Values ↑ BUN, creatinine, potassium, positive Coombs' [direct]; ↓ cholesterol (S); may cause false-positive results in urine acetone determinations using sodium nitroprusside reagent

Adverse Reactions

1% to 10%:

- Cardiovascular: Hypotension, peripheral edema
- Central nervous system: Headache, dizziness, fatigue
- Dermatologic: Rash, alopecia, flushing, rash
- Endocrine & metabolic: Hyperkalemia, hyponatremia
- Gastrointestinal: Diarrhea, nausea, heartburn
- Genitourinary: Polyuria
- Neuromuscular & skeletal: Myalgia
- Renal: Reversible increases in creatinine or BUN
- Respiratory: Cough, pharyngitis, upper respiratory infection, sinusitis

<1% (Limited to important or life-threatening): Alopecia, anemia, arrhythmias, bronchospasm, cerebrovascular accident, chest pain, dyspnea, elevated LFTs, eosinophilic pneumonitis, hepatitis, hypercholesterolemia, myocardial infarction, oliguria, orthostatic hypotension, palpitations, proteinuria, syncope

Overdosage/Toxicology Mild hypotension has been the primary toxic effect seen with acute overdose. Bradycardia may also occur. Hyperkalemia occurs even with therapeutic doses, especially in patients with renal insufficiency and those taking NSAIDs. Treatment is symptom-directed and supportive.

Pharmacodynamics/Kinetics

Bioavailability: Moexiprilat: 13%; reduced with food (AUC decreased by ~40%)

Half-Life Elimination: Moexipril: 1 hour; Moexiprilat: 2-9 hours

Time to Peak: 1.5 hours

Metabolism: Parent drug: Hepatic and via GI tract to moexiprilat, 1000 times more potent than parent

Onset: Peak effect: 1-2 hours

Duration: >24 hours

Formulations Tablet, as hydrochloride: 7.5 mg, 15 mg

Dosing

Adults: Hypertension, LV dysfunction (post MI): Oral: Initial: 7.5 mg once daily (in patients **not** receiving diuretics), 1 hour prior to a meal **or** 3.75 mg once daily (when combined with thiazide diuretics); maintenance dose: 7.5-30 mg/day in 1 or 2 divided doses 1 hour before meals

Elderly: Dose the same as adults; adjust for renal impairment. Tablet may be cut in half (3.75 mg) for starting therapy (see Renal Impairment and Additional Information).

Renal Impairment: Cl_{cr} ≤40 mL/minute: Patients may be cautiously placed on 3.75 mg once daily, then upwardly titrated to a maximum of 15 mg/day.

Administration

Oral: Food may delay and reduce peak serum levels; take on an empty stomach, if possible.

Monitoring Laboratory Tests Electrolytes, CBC, renal function. If patient has renal impairment, a baseline WBC with differential and serum creatinine should be evaluated and monitored closely during the first 3 months of therapy.

Monitoring and Teaching Issues

Physical Assessment: See Contraindications and Warnings/Precautions for use cautions. Assess potential for interactions with other prescriptions, OTC medications, or herbal products patient may be taking (see Drug Interactions). Assess results of laboratory tests (see above), therapeutic effectiveness, and adverse responses (see Adverse Reactions and Overdose/Toxicology) on a regular basis. Teach patient appropriate use, possible side effects and interventions, and adverse symptoms to report (see Patient Education). **Pregnancy risk factor C/D** - see Pregnancy Risk Factor for use cautions. Instruct patient in appropriate use of barrier contraceptives (see Pregnancy Issues). Note breast-feeding caution.

Patient Education: Inform prescriber of all prescriptions, OTC medications, or herbal products you are taking, and any allergies you have. Do not take anything new without consulting prescriber. Take as directed on an empty stomach, 1 hour before or 2 hours after meals. Do not alter dose or discontinue without consulting prescriber. Take first dose at bedtime. Do not take potassium supplements or salt substitutes containing potassium without consulting prescriber. This drug does not eliminate need for diet or exercise regimen as recommended by prescriber. May cause dizziness, fainting, or lightheadedness (use caution when driving or engaging in tasks that require alertness until response to drug is known); postural hypotension (use caution when rising from lying or sitting position or climbing stairs); nausea or heartburn (small, frequent meals, frequent mouth care, sucking lozenges, or chewing gum may help); diarrhea (buttermilk, boiled milk, or yogurt may help); or loss of hair (may be reversible when drug is discontinued). Report difficulty breathing or unusual cough, painful muscles, rash, excessive urination, or other persistent adverse reactions. **Pregnancy/breast-feeding precautions:** Do not get pregnant while taking this medication. Consult prescriber for appropriate contraceptive measures. Consult prescriber if breast-feeding.

Dietary Issues: Administer on an empty stomach.

Geriatric Considerations: Due to frequent decreases in glomerular filtration (also creatinine clearance) with aging, elderly patients may have exaggerated responses to ACE inhibitors. Differences in clinical response due to hepatic changes are not observed.

Pregnancy Issues: ACE inhibitors can cause fetal injury or death if taken during the 2nd or 3rd trimester. Discontinue ACE inhibitors as soon as pregnancy is detected.

Related Information

Angiotensin Agents *on page 1547*

Moexipril and Hydrochlorothiazide

(mo EKS i pril & hye droe klor oh THYE a zide)

U.S. Brand Names Uniretic®

Synonyms Hydrochlorothiazide and Moexipril

Generic Available No

Pharmacologic Category Antihypertensive Agent Combination

Pregnancy Risk Factor C/D (2nd and 3rd trimesters)

Lactation Enters breast milk/use caution

Use Combination therapy for hypertension, however, not indicated for initial treatment of hypertension; replacement therapy in patients receiving separate dosage forms (for patient convenience); when monotherapy with one component fails to achieve desired antihypertensive effect, or when dose-limiting adverse effects limit upward titration of monotherapy

Formulations Tablet:

Moexipril hydrochloride 7.5 mg and hydrochlorothiazide 12.5 mg
Moexipril hydrochloride 15 mg and hydrochlorothiazide 12.5 mg
Moexipril hydrochloride 15 mg and hydrochlorothiazide 25 mg

Dosing

Adults: Adults: Oral: 7.5-30 mg of moexipril, taken either in a single or divided dose one hour before meals; hydrochlorothiazide dose should be ≤50 mg/day

Elderly: Overall safety and efficacy are not different in elderly patients, although a higher moexipril AUC was observed in elderly patients. Greater sensitivity to effects may be observed in some older individuals. Refer to adult dosing.

Monitoring and Teaching Issues

Physical Assessment: See individual components listed in Related Information. **Pregnancy risk factor C/D** - see Pregnancy Risk Factor for use cautions. Assess knowledge/instruct patient on need to use appropriate contraceptive measures and the need to avoid pregnancy. Note breast-feeding caution.

Patient Education: See individual components listed in Related Information. **Pregnancy/breast-feeding precautions:** Inform prescriber if you are or intend to become pregnant. Consult prescriber if breast-feeding.

Related Information

Hydrochlorothiazide *on page 664*
Moexipril *on page 921*

Moexipril Hydrochloride *see* Moexipril *on page 921*
Mollifene® Ear Wax Removal Formula *see page 1519*
Mometasone *see* Topical Corticosteroids *on page 1334*
MOM (Magnesium Hydroxide) *see* Magnesium Supplements *on page 831*
Monacolin K *see* Lovastatin *on page 826*
Monarc® M *see* Antihemophilic Factor (Human) *on page 109*
Monistat® 1 Combination Pack [OTC] *see* Miconazole *on page 899*
Monistat® 3 [OTC] *see* Miconazole *on page 899*
Monistat® 7 [OTC] *see* Miconazole *on page 899*
Monistat-Derm® *see* Miconazole *on page 899*
Monoclate-P® *see* Antihemophilic Factor (Human) *on page 109*
Monoclonal Antibody *see* Muromonab-CD3 *on page 932*
Monodox® *see* Doxycycline *on page 450*
Mono-Gesic® *see* Salsalate *on page 1212*
Monoket® *see* Isosorbide Mononitrate *on page 750*
Monopril® *see* Fosinopril *on page 605*

Montelukast

(mon te LOO kast)

U.S. Brand Names Singulair®

Synonyms Montelukast Sodium

Restrictions Singulair® oral granules received FDA approval July, 2002. A formal marketing date has not been announced.

Generic Available No

Pharmacologic Category Leukotriene Receptor Antagonist

Pregnancy Risk Factor B

(Continued)

Montelukast *(Continued)*

Lactation Excretion in breast milk unknown/use caution (zafirlukast is contraindicated)

Use Prophylaxis and chronic treatment of asthma in adults and children ≥1 year of age

Mechanism of Action/Effect Montelukast is a selective leukotriene receptor antagonist which inhibits cysteinyl leukotriene that is responsible for edema, smooth muscle contraction that is felt to be associated with the signs and symptoms of asthma.

Contraindications Hypersensitivity to montelukast or any component of the formulation

Warnings/Precautions Inform phenylketonuric patients that the chewable tablet contains phenylalanine. Montelukast is only for prophylactic treatment and should **not** be used for acute asthma attacks, including status asthmaticus; neither should it be used as monotherapy for exercise-induced asthma. Has been associated with eosinophilic vasculitis (Churg-Strauss syndrome), usually following reduction or withdrawal of oral corticosteroids. Health care providers should be alert to eosinophilia, vasculitic rash, worsening pulmonary symptoms, cardiac complications, and/or neuropathy presenting in their patients. A casual association between montelukast and these underlying conditions has not been established. Safety and efficacy in children <1 year of age have not been established.

Drug Interactions

Cytochrome P450 Effect: Substrate of **CYP2C8/9, 3A4**; Inhibits CYP2C8/9

Decreased Effect: Phenobarbital decreases montelukast area under the curve by 40%. Clinical significance is uncertain. Rifampin may increase the metabolism of montelukast similar to phenobarbital. No dosage adjustment is recommended when taking phenobarbital with montelukast.

Nutritional/Ethanol Interactions Herb/Nutraceutical: St John's wort may decrease montelukast levels.

Adverse Reactions (As reported in adults)

>10%: Central nervous system: Headache (18%)

1% to 10%:

- Central nervous system: Dizziness (2%), fatigue (2%), fever (2%)
- Dermatologic: Rash (2%)
- Gastrointestinal: Dyspepsia (2%), dental pain (2%), gastroenteritis (2%), abdominal pain (3%)
- Neuromuscular & skeletal: Weakness (2%)
- Respiratory: Cough (3%), nasal congestion (2%)
- Miscellaneous: Flu-like symptoms (4%), trauma (1%)

<1% (Limited to important or life-threatening): Anaphylaxis, angioedema, Churg-Strauss syndrome (systemic eosinophilia vasculitis), hepatic eosinophilic infiltration (rare), myalgia, pancreatitis, pruritus, seizures

Overdosage/Toxicology No specific antidote

Remove unabsorbed material from the GI tract, employ clinical monitoring and institute supportive therapy if required

Pharmacodynamics/Kinetics

Absorption: Rapid

Bioavailability: Tablet: 10 mg: Mean: 64%; 5 mg: 63% to 73%

Half-Life Elimination: Plasma: Mean: 2.7-5.5 hours

Time to Peak: Serum: Tablet: 10 mg: 3-4 hours; 5 mg: 2-2.5 hours; 4 mg: 2 hours

Metabolism: Extensively hepatic via CYP3A4 and 2C8/9

Duration: >24 hours

Formulations

Granules, as sodium: 4 mg/packet

Tablet, as sodium: 10 mg

Tablet, chewable, as sodium: 4 mg [cherry flavor; contains phenylalanine 0.674 mg]; 5 mg [cherry flavor; contains phenylalanine 0.842 mg]

Dosing

Adults & Elderly: Asthma: Oral: One 10 mg tablet daily in the evening

Pediatrics: Asthma: Oral:

- <1 year: Safety and efficacy have not been established
- 12-23 months: 4 mg (oral granules) once daily, taken in the evening
- 2-5 years: 4 mg (chewable tablet or oral granules) once daily, taken in the evening
- 6-14 years: Chew one 5 mg chewable tablet/day, taken in the evening
- ≥15 years: Refer to adult dosing.

Renal Impairment: No adjustment is necessary.

Hepatic Impairment: No adjustment necessary in mild to moderate hepatic disease. Patients with severe hepatic disease were **not** studied.

Administration

Oral: Take dose in the evening. Granules may be administered directly in the mouth or mixed with applesauce, carrots, rice, or ice cream. Administer within 15 minutes of opening packet. Do not mix in liquids.

Stability

Storage: Store at room temperature of 15°C to 30°C (59°F to 86°F). Protect from moisture and light.

Granules: Use within 15 minutes of opening packet.

Monitoring and Teaching Issues

Physical Assessment: Not for use in acute asthma attacks, including status asthmaticus. Assess effectiveness and interactions of other medications patient may be taking (see Drug Interactions). See Contraindications and Warnings/Precautions for use cautions. Monitor effectiveness of therapy and adverse reactions (see Adverse Reactions) at beginning of therapy and periodically with long-term use. Assess knowledge/teach patient appropriate use, interventions to reduce side effects, and adverse symptoms to report (see Patient Education). Note breast-feeding caution.

Patient Education: This medication is not for an acute asthmatic attack; in acute attack, follow instructions of prescriber. Do not stop other asthma medication unless advised by prescriber. Chewable tablet contains phenylalanine. Take every evening on a continuous basis; do not discontinue even if feeling better (this medication may help reduce incidence of acute attacks). Granules may be administered directly in the mouth or mixed with applesauce, carrots, rice, or ice cream (do not mix in liquids); administer within 15 minutes of opening packet. You may experience mild headache (mild analgesic may help); or fatigue or dizziness (use caution when driving). Report skin rash or itching, abdominal pain or persistent GI upset, unusual cough or congestion, or worsening of asthmatic condition. **Breast-feeding precaution:** Consult prescriber if breast-feeding.

Dietary Issues: Tablet, chewable: 4 mg strength contains phenylalanine 0.674 mg; 5 mg strength contains phenylalanine 0.842 mg

Montelukast Sodium *see* Montelukast *on page 923*
8-MOP® *see* Methoxsalen *on page 878*
MoreDophilus® [OTC] *see Lactobacillus on page 766*

Moricizine (mor I siz een)

U.S. Brand Names Ethmozine®

Synonyms Moricizine Hydrochloride

Generic Available No

Pharmacologic Category Antiarrhythmic Agent, Class I

Pregnancy Risk Factor B

Lactation Enters breast milk/not recommended

Use Treatment of ventricular tachycardia and life-threatening ventricular arrhythmias

Use - Unlabeled/Investigational PVCs, complete and nonsustained ventricular tachycardia, atrial arrhythmias

Mechanism of Action/Effect Class I antiarrhythmic agent; reduces the fast inward current carried by sodium ions, shortens Phase I and Phase II repolarization, resulting in decreased action potential duration and effective refractory period

Contraindications Hypersensitivity to moricizine or any component of the formulation; pre-existing second- or third-degree AV block (except in patients with a functioning artificial pacemaker); right bundle branch block when associated with left hemiblock or bifascicular block (unless functional pacemaker in place); cardiogenic shock

Warnings/Precautions Can be proarrhythmic; watch for new rhythm disturbances or existing arrhythmias that worsen. Use cautiously in CAD, previous history of MI, CHF, and cardiomegaly. The CAST II trial demonstrated a decreased trend in survival for patients receiving moricizine. Dose-related increases in PR and QRS intervals occur. Use cautiously in patients with pre-existing conduction abnormalities, and significant hepatic impairment. Safety and efficacy have not been established in pediatric patients.

Drug Interactions

Cytochrome P450 Effect: Substrate of **CYP3A4**; Induces CYP1A2, 3A4

Decreased Effect: Moricizine may decrease levels of theophylline (50%) and diltiazem.

Increased Effect/Toxicity: Moricizine levels may be increased by cimetidine and diltiazem. Digoxin may result in additive prolongation of the PR interval when combined with moricizine (but not rate of second- and third-degree AV block). Drugs which may prolong QT interval (including cisapride, erythromycin, phenothiazines, cyclic antidepressants, and some quinolones) are contraindicated with type Ia antiarrhythmics. Moricizine has some type Ia activity, and caution should be used.

Nutritional/Ethanol Interactions Food: Moricizine peak serum concentrations may be decreased if taken with food.

Adverse Reactions

>10%: Central nervous system: Dizziness

1% to 10%:

Cardiovascular: Proarrhythmia, palpitations, cardiac death, EKG abnormalities, CHF
Central nervous system: Headache, fatigue, insomnia
Endocrine & metabolic: Decreased libido
Gastrointestinal: Nausea, diarrhea, ileus
Ocular: Blurred vision, periorbital edema
Respiratory: Dyspnea

<1% (Limited to important or life-threatening): Apnea, cardiac chest pain, hypotension or hypertension, myocardial infarction, supraventricular arrhythmias, syncope, ventricular tachycardia

Overdosage/Toxicology Has a narrow therapeutic index and severe toxicity may occur slightly above the therapeutic range, especially if combined with other antiarrhythmic drugs. Acute single ingestion of twice the daily therapeutic dose is life-threatening. Symptoms of overdose include increases in PR, QRS, QT intervals and amplitude of the T wave, AV block, bradycardia, hypotension, ventricular arrhythmias (monomorphic or polymorphic ventricular tachycardia), and asystole. Other symptoms include dizziness, blurred vision, headache, and GI upset.

Treatment is symptom-directed and supportive. **Note:** Type Ia antiarrhythmic agents should not be used to treat cardiotoxicity caused by type Ic drugs.

Pharmacodynamics/Kinetics

Bioavailability: 38%

Half-Life Elimination: Healthy volunteers: 3-4 hours; Cardiac disease: 6-13 hours

Metabolism: Significant first-pass effect; some enterohepatic recycling

Formulations Tablet, as hydrochloride: 200 mg, 250 mg, 300 mg

Dosing

Adults & Elderly: Ventricular arrhythmias: Oral: 200-300 mg every 8 hours, adjust dosage at 150 mg/day at 3-day intervals. See table on following page for dosage recommendations of transferring from other antiarrhythmic agents to Ethmozine®. Hospitalization is required to start therapy.

Renal Impairment: Start at 600 mg/day or less.

Hepatic Impairment: Start at 600 mg/day or less.

(Continued)

Moricizine *(Continued)*

Transferred From	Start Ethmozine®
Encainide, propafenone, tocainide, or mexiletine	8-12 hours after last dose
Flecainide	12-24 hours after last dose
Procainamide	3-6 hours after last dose
Quinidine, disopyramide	6-12 hours after last dose

Monitoring Laboratory Tests Electrolytes (correct any imbalance) prior to beginning therapy

Monitoring and Teaching Issues

Physical Assessment: Assess other medications patient may be taking for effectiveness and interactions (see Drug Interactions). See Warnings/Precautions for use cautions. Monitor laboratory tests (see above), therapeutic response, and adverse reactions (see Warnings/Precautions and Adverse Reactions) at beginning of therapy, when titrating dosage, and on a regular basis with long-term therapy. **Note:** Moricizine has a low toxic:therapeutic ratio and overdose may easily produce severe and life-threatening reactions (see Overdose/Toxicology). Assess knowledge/teach patient appropriate use, interventions to reduce side effects, and adverse symptoms to report (see Patient Education). Breast-feeding is not recommended.

Patient Education: Take exactly as directed; do not take additional doses or discontinue without consulting prescriber. You will need regular cardiac checkups and blood tests while taking this medication. You may experience dizziness or visual changes (use caution when driving or engaging in tasks requiring alertness until response to drug is known); nausea or vomiting (small, frequent meals, frequent mouth care, chewing gum, or sucking lozenges may help); or headaches, sleep disturbances, or decreased libido (usually temporary, if persistent consult prescriber). Report chest pain, palpitation, or erratic heartbeat; increased weight or swelling of hands or feet; blurred vision or facial swelling; acute diarrhea; changes in bowel or bladder patterns; or difficulty breathing. **Breast-feeding precaution:** Breast-feeding is not recommended.

Dietary Issues: Best if taken on an empty stomach.

Geriatric Considerations: Due to moricizine binding to plasma albumin and alpha-glycoprotein, other highly bound drugs may displace moricizine. Since elderly may require multiple drugs, caution with highly bound drugs is necessary. Consider changes in renal and hepatic function with age and monitor closely since half-life may be prolonged.

Related Information

Antiarrhythmic Drugs *on page 1551*

Moricizine Hydrochloride *see* Moricizine *on page 925*

Morphine Sulfate (MOR feen SUL fate)

U.S. Brand Names Astramorph™ PF; Avinza™; Duramorph®; Infumorph®; Kadian®; MS Contin®; MSIR®; Oramorph SR®; RMS®; Roxanol®; Roxanol 100®; Roxanol®-T

Synonyms MS

Restrictions C-II

Generic Available Yes

Pharmacologic Category Analgesic, Narcotic

Pregnancy Risk Factor B/D (prolonged use or high doses at term)

Lactation Enters breast milk/use caution (AAP rates "compatible")

Use Relief of moderate to severe acute and chronic pain; relief of pain of myocardial infarction; relief of dyspnea of acute left ventricular failure and pulmonary edema; preanesthetic medication

Orphan drug: Infumorph™: Used in microinfusion devices for intraspinal administration in treatment of intractable chronic pain

Mechanism of Action/Effect Binds to opiate receptors in the CNS, causing inhibition of ascending pain pathways, altering the perception of and response to pain; produces generalized CNS depression

Contraindications Hypersensitivity to morphine sulfate or any component of the formulation; increased intracranial pressure; severe respiratory depression (in absence of resuscitative equipment or ventilatory support); acute or severe asthma; known or suspected paralytic ileus (sustained release products only); sustained release products are not recommended in acute/postoperative pain; pregnancy (prolonged use or high doses at term)

Warnings/Precautions Infants <3 months of age are more susceptible to respiratory depression, use with caution and generally in reduced doses in this age group; use with caution in patients with impaired respiratory function or severe hepatic dysfunction and in patients with hypersensitivity reactions to other phenanthrene derivative opioid agonists (codeine, hydrocodone, hydromorphone, levorphanol, oxycodone, oxymorphone). May cause hypotension in patients with acute myocardial infarction. Tolerance or drug dependence may result from extended use.

Use caution in CNS depression, toxic psychosis, delirium tremens, or convulsive disorders. Sedation and psychomotor impairment are likely, and are additive with other CNS depressants or ethanol. Extended or sustained release dosage forms should not be crushed or chewed. Controlled-, extended-, or sustained-release products are not intended for "as needed (PRN)" use.

Use caution in renal impairment (metabolite accumulation); use caution in gastrointestinal motility disturbances (particularly with sustained release preparations), thyroid disorders (Addison's disease, myxedema, or hypothyroidism), prostatic hyperplasia, or urethral stricture.

Elderly and/or debilitated may be particularly susceptible to the CNS depressant and constipating effects of narcotics. May mask diagnosis or clinical course in patients with acute abdominal conditions.

Drug Interactions

Cytochrome P450 Effect: Substrate of CYP2D6

Decreased Effect: Diuretic effects may be decreased (due to antidiuretic hormone release).

Increased Effect/Toxicity: CNS depressants (phenothiazines, tranquilizers, anxiolytics, sedatives, hypnotics, or alcohol), tricyclic antidepressants may potentiate the effects of morphine and other opiate agonists. Dextroamphetamine may enhance the analgesic effect of morphine and other opiate agonists. Concurrent use of MAO inhibitors and meperidine has been associated with significant adverse effects. Use caution with morphine. Some manufacturers recommend avoiding use within 14 days of MAO inhibitors.

Nutritional/Ethanol Interactions

Ethanol: Avoid ethanol (may increase CNS depression).

Food: Administration of oral morphine solution with food may increase bioavailability (ie, a report of 34% increase in morphine AUC when morphine oral solution followed a high-fat meal). The bioavailability of Oramorph SR® does not appear to be affected by food.

Herb/Nutraceutical: Avoid valerian, St John's wort, kava kava, gotu kola (may increase CNS depression).

Effects on Lab Values ↑ aminotransferase [ALT (SGPT)/AST (SGOT)] (S)

Adverse Reactions Note: Percentages are based on a study in 19 chronic cancer pain patients (*J Pain Symptom Manage*, 1995, 10:416-22). Chronic use of various opioids in cancer pain is accompanied by similar adverse reactions; individual patient differences are unpredictable, and percentage may differ in acute pain (surgical) treatment.

Frequency not defined: Flushing, CNS depression, sedation, antidiuretic hormone release, physical and psychological dependence, diaphoresis

>10%:

- Cardiovascular: Palpitations, hypotension, bradycardia
- Central nervous system: Drowsiness (48%, tolerance usually develops to drowsiness with regular dosing for 1-2 weeks); dizziness (20%); confusion
- Dermatologic: Pruritus (may be secondary to histamine release)
- Gastrointestinal: Nausea (28%, tolerance usually develops to nausea and vomiting with chronic use); vomiting (9%); constipation (40%, tolerance develops very slowly if at all); xerostomia (78%)
- Genitourinary: Urinary retention (16%)
- Local: Pain at injection site
- Neuromuscular & skeletal: Weakness
- Miscellaneous: Histamine release

1% to 10%:

- Central nervous system: Restlessness, headache, false feeling of well being
- Gastrointestinal: Anorexia, GI irritation, paralytic ileus
- Genitourinary: Decreased urination
- Neuromuscular & skeletal: Trembling
- Ocular: Vision problems
- Respiratory: Respiratory depression, dyspnea

<1% (Limited to important or life-threatening): Anaphylaxis, biliary tract spasm, hallucinations, insomnia, intestinal obstruction, intracranial pressure increased, increased liver function tests, mental depression, miosis, muscle rigidity, paradoxical CNS stimulation, peripheral vasodilation, urinary tract spasm

Overdosage/Toxicology Symptoms of overdose include respiratory depression, miosis, hypotension, bradycardia, apnea, and pulmonary edema. Treatment is symptomatic. Naloxone, 2 mg I.V. with repeat administration as necessary up to a total dose of 10 mg, can be used to reverse opiate effects.

Pharmacodynamics/Kinetics

Absorption: Oral: Variable

Bioavailability: Oral: 17% to 33% (first-pass effect limits oral bioavailability; oral:parenteral effectiveness reportedly varies from 1:6 in opioid naive patients to 1:3 with chronic use)

Half-Life Elimination: Adults: 2-4 hours (not sustained/controlled/extended release forms)

Metabolism: Hepatic via conjugation with glucuronic acid to morphine-3-glucuronide (inactive), morphine-6-glucuronide (active), and in lesser amounts, morphine-3-6-diglucuronide; other minor metabolites include normorphine (active) and the 3-ethereal sulfate

Onset: Oral: 1 hour; I.V.: 5-10 minutes

Duration: Pain relief (not sustained/controlled/extended release): 4 hours

Formulations

Capsule (MSIR®): 15 mg, 30 mg

Capsule, extended release (Avinza™): 30 mg, 60 mg, 90 mg, 120 mg

Capsule, sustained release (Kadian®): 20 mg, 30 mg, 50 mg, 60 mg, 100 mg

Infusion [premixed in dextrose]: 0.2 mg/mL (250 mL, 500 mL); 1 mg/mL (100 mL, 250 mL, 500 mL)

Injection, solution: 0.5 mg/mL (10 mL); 1 mg/mL (10 mL, 30 mL, 50 mL); 2 mg/mL (1 mL); 4 mg/mL (1 mL); 5 mg/mL (1 mL, 30 mL, 50 mL); 8 mg/mL (1 mL); 10 mg/mL (1 mL, 2 mL, 10 mL); 15 mg/mL (1 mL, 20 mL); 25 mg/mL (4 mL, 10 mL, 20 mL, 40 mL, 50 mL); 50 mg/mL (10 mL, 20 mL, 40 mL, 50 mL)

- Astramorph™ PF [preservative free]: 0.5 mg/mL (2 mL, 10 mL); 1 mg/mL (2 mL, 10 mL)
- Infumorph® [preservative free]: 10 mg/mL (20 mL); 25 mg/mL (20 mL)
- Duramorph® [preservative free]: 0.5 mg/mL (10 mL); 1 mg/mL (10 mL)

Solution, oral: 10 mg/5 mL (5 mL, 100 mL, 500 mL); 20 mg/mL (30 mL, 120 mL, 240 mL); 20 mg/5 mL (5 mL, 100 mL, 120 mL, 500 mL)

- MSIR®: 10 mg/5 mL (120 mL); 20 mg/mL (30 mL, 120 mL) [contains sodium benzoate]
- Roxanol®: 20 mg/mL (30 mL, 120 mL)
- Roxanol® T: 20 mg/mL (30 mL, 120 mL) [flavored; tinted]
- Roxanol 100®: 100 mg/5 mL (240 mL) [with calibrated spoon]

Suppository, rectal (RMS®): 5 mg, 10 mg, 20 mg, 30 mg

Tablet: 15 mg, 30 mg

- MSIR®: 15 mg, 30 mg

Tablet, controlled release: MS Contin®: 15 mg, 30 mg, 60 mg, 100 mg, 200 mg

(Continued)

Morphine Sulfate *(Continued)*

Tablet, extended release: 15 mg, 30 mg, 60 mg, 100 mg, 200 mg
Tablet, sustained release (Oramorph SR®): 15 mg, 30 mg, 60 mg, 100 mg

Dosing

Adults: Doses should be titrated to appropriate effect; when changing routes of administration in chronically treated patients, please note that **oral doses are approximately 50% as effective as parenteral dose.**

Analgesia/sedation:

Oral:

Prompt release formulations: 10-30 mg every 4 hours as needed

Controlled-, extended-, or sustained release formulations: **Note:** A patient's morphine requirement is usually established using prompt-release formulations. Conversion to long-acting products may be considered for continuous treatment for several days. Higher dosages (MS Contin® 200 mg or Avinza™ 60 mg, 90 mg, 120 mg) should be reserved for use only in opioid-tolerant patients.

Tablets, controlled release (MS Contin®), sustained release (Oramorph SR®) or extended release: Daily dose divided and administered every 8 or every 12 hours

Capsules, sustained release (Kadian®): Daily dose administered once daily or in two divided doses daily (every 12 hours)

Capsules, extended release (Avinza™): Daily dose administer once daily (for best results, administer at same time each day).

I.M., I.V., S.C.: 2.5-20 mg/dose every 2-6 hours as needed; usual: 10 mg/dose every 4 hours as needed

I.V., S.C. continuous infusion: 0.8-10 mg/hour; may increase depending on pain relief/adverse effects; usual range: up to 80 mg/hour

Epidural: Initial: 5 mg in lumbar region; if inadequate pain relief within 1 hour, give 1-2 mg; maximum: 10 mg/24 hours.

Intrathecal ($^1/_{10}$ of epidural dose): 0.2-1 mg/dose; repeat doses are **not** recommended.

Rectal: 10-20 mg every 4 hours

Elderly: Refer to adult dosing. Use with caution; may require reduced dosage in the elderly and debilitated patients.

Pediatrics: Doses should be titrated to appropriate effect. When changing routes of administration in chronically treated patients, please note that oral doses are approximately $^1/_2$ as effective as parenteral dose.

Analgesia: Infants and Children:

Oral: Tablet and solution (prompt release): 0.2-0.5 mg/kg/dose every 4-6 hours as needed; tablet (controlled release): 0.3-0.6 mg/kg/dose every 12 hours

I.M., I.V., S.C.: 0.1-0.2 mg/kg/dose every 2-4 hours as needed; usual maximum: 15 mg/dose; may initiate at 0.05 mg/kg/dose

I.V., S.C. continuous infusion: Sickle cell or cancer pain: 0.025-2 mg/kg/hour; postoperative pain: 0.01-0.04 mg/kg/hour

Sedation/analgesia for procedures: I.V.: 0.05-0.1 mg/kg 5 minutes before the procedure

Adolescents >12 years: Sedation/analgesia for procedures: I.V.: 3-4 mg and repeat in 5 minutes if necessary.

Renal Impairment:

Cl_{cr} 10-50 mL/minute: Administer 75% of normal dose.

Cl_{cr} <10 mL/minute: Administer 50% of normal dose.

Hepatic Impairment: Unchanged in mild liver disease; substantial extrahepatic metabolism may occur. Excessive sedation may occur in cirrhosis.

Administration

Oral: Do not crush controlled release drug product, swallow whole. Kadian® can be opened and sprinkled on applesauce. Avinza™ can also be opened and sprinkled on applesauce; do not crush or chew the beads. Administration of oral morphine solution with food may increase bioavailability (not observed with Oramorph SR®).

I.V.: When giving morphine I.V. push, it is best to first dilute in 4-5 mL of sterile water, and then to administer slowly (eg, 15 mg over 3-5 minutes). Use preservative-free solutions for intrathecal or epidural use.

Stability

Storage:

Suppositories: Refrigerate suppositories; do not freeze.

Injection: Degradation depends on pH and presence of oxygen; relatively stable in pH ≤4; darkening of solutions indicate degradation.

Reconstitution: Usual concentration for continuous I.V. infusion = 0.1-1 mg/mL in D_5W.

Compatibility: Stable in dextran 6% in dextrose, dextran 6% in NS, D_5LR, $D_5{}^1/_4NS$, $D_5{}^1/_2NS$, D_5NS, D_5W, $D_{10}W$, LR, $^1/_2NS$, NS

Y-site administration: Incompatible with alatrofloxacin, amphotericin B cholesteryl sulfate complex, cefepime, doxorubicin liposome, minocycline, sargramostim

Compatibility in syringe: Incompatible with meperidine, thiopental

Compatibility when admixed: Incompatible with aminophylline, amobarbital, chlorothiazide, floxacillin, fluorouracil, heparin, meperidine, phenobarbital, phenytoin, sodium bicarbonate, thiopental

Monitoring and Teaching Issues

Physical Assessment: Assess other medications patient may be taking for additive or adverse interactions (see Drug Interactions). Monitor vital signs, respiratory and CNS status, therapeutic effectiveness, and adverse reactions or overdose at regular intervals with long-term use (see Adverse Reactions and Overdose/Toxicology). May cause physical and/or psychological dependence. For inpatients, implement safety measures. Assess knowledge/teach patient appropriate use (if self-administered), adverse reactions to report, and appropriate interventions to reduce side effects. Discontinue slowly after prolonged use. **Pregnancy risk factor B/D** - see Pregnancy Risk Factor for use cautions. Note breast-feeding caution.

Patient Education: If self-administered, use exactly as directed; do not increase dose or frequency. Do not crush or chew controlled release tablets. May cause physical and/or psychological dependence. While using this medication, do not use alcohol and other prescription or OTC medications (especially sedatives, tranquilizers, antihistamines, or pain medications) without consulting prescriber. Maintain adequate hydration (2-3 L/day of fluids) unless advised by prescriber to restrict fluids. May cause hypotension, dizziness, drowsiness, impaired coordination, or blurred vision (use caution when driving, climbing stairs, or changing position - rising from sitting or lying to standing, or when engaging in tasks requiring alertness until response to drug is known); loss of appetite, nausea, or vomiting (frequent mouth care, small, frequent meals, chewing gum, or sucking lozenges may help); or constipation (increased exercise, fluids, fruit, or fiber may help; if unresolved, consult prescriber about use of stool softeners and/or laxatives). Report chest pain, slow or rapid heartbeat, acute dizziness, or persistent headache; changes in mental status; swelling of extremities or unusual weight gain; changes in urinary elimination or pain on urination; acute headache; back or flank pain; muscle spasms; blurred vision; skin rash; or shortness of breath. **Pregnancy/breast-feeding precautions:** Inform prescriber if you are or intend to become pregnant. If you are breast-feeding, take medication immediately after breast-feeding or 3-4 hours prior to next feeding.

Dietary Issues: Morphine may cause GI upset; take with food if GI upset occurs. Be consistent when taking morphine with or without meals.

Geriatric Considerations: The elderly may be particularly susceptible to the CNS depressant and constipating effects of narcotics. For chronic administration of narcotic analgesics, morphine is preferable in the elderly due to its pharmacokinetics and side effect profile as compared to meperidine and methadone.

Breast-feeding Issues: If patient is breast-feeding, morphine sulfate should be administered immediately after breast-feeding or 3-4 hours prior to next feeding.

Related Information

Compatibility of Drugs *on page 1564*
Compatibility of Drugs in Syringe *on page 1566*
Controlled Substances Comparison *on page 1568*
Narcotic/Opioid Analgesic Comparison *on page 1583*

Motofen® *see* Difenoxin and Atropine *on page 408*
Motrin® *see* Ibuprofen *on page 688*
Motrin® Children's [OTC] *see* Ibuprofen *on page 688*
Motrin® IB [OTC] *see* Ibuprofen *on page 688*
Motrin® Infants' [OTC] *see* Ibuprofen *on page 688*
Motrin® Junior Srength [OTC] *see* Ibuprofen *on page 688*
Motrin® Migraine Pain [OTC] *see* Ibuprofen *on page 688*

Moxifloxacin (mox i FLOKS a sin)

U.S. Brand Names ABC Pack™ (Avelox®); Avelox®

Synonyms Moxifloxacin Hydrochloride

Generic Available No

Pharmacologic Category Antibiotic, Quinolone

Pregnancy Risk Factor C

Lactation Excretion in breast milk unknown/not recommended

Use Treatment of mild to moderate community-acquired pneumonia, acute bacterial exacerbation of chronic bronchitis, acute bacterial sinusitis, uncomplicated skin infections

Mechanism of Action/Effect Moxifloxacin is a quinolone antibiotic with bactericidal activity against susceptible gram negative and gram positive microorganisms.

Contraindications Hypersensitivity to moxifloxacin, other quinolone antibiotics, or any component of the formulation

Warnings/Precautions Use with caution in patients with significant bradycardia or acute myocardial ischemia. Moxifloxacin causes a dose-dependent QT prolongation. Coadministration of moxifloxacin with other drugs that also prolong the QT interval or induce bradycardia (eg, beta-blockers, amiodarone) should be avoided. Careful consideration should be given in the use of moxifloxacin in patients with cardiovascular disease, particularly in those with conduction abnormalities. Use with caution in individuals at risk of seizures (CNS disorders or concurrent therapy with medications which may lower seizure threshold). Discontinue in patients who experience significant CNS adverse effects (dizziness, hallucinations, suicidal ideation or actions). Not recommended in patients with moderate to severe hepatic insufficiency. Use with caution in diabetes; glucose regulation may be altered. Tendon inflammation and/or rupture has been reported with quinolone antibiotics. Risk may be increased with concurrent corticosteroids, particularly in the elderly. Discontinue at first signs or symptoms of tendon pain.

Severe hypersensitivity reactions, including anaphylaxis, have occurred with quinolone therapy. If an allergic reaction occurs (itching, urticaria, dyspnea or facial edema, loss of consciousness, tingling, cardiovascular collapse) discontinue drug immediately. Prolonged use may result in superinfection; pseudomembranous colitis may occur and should be considered in all patients who present with diarrhea. Quinolones may exacerbate myasthenia gravis, use with caution (rare, potentially life-threatening weakness of respiratory muscles may occur).

Pregnancy risk C.

Drug Interactions

Decreased Effect: Metal cations (magnesium, aluminum, iron, and zinc) bind quinolones in the gastrointestinal tract and inhibit absorption (by up to 98%). Antacids, multivitamins with minerals, sucralfate, and some didanosine formulations should be avoided. Moxifloxacin should be administered 4 hours before or 8 hours (a minimum of 2 hours before and 2 hours after) after these agents. Antineoplastic agents may decrease the absorption of quinolones.

Increased Effect/Toxicity: Drugs which prolong QT interval (including Class Ia and Class III antiarrhythmics, erythromycin, cisapride, antipsychotics, and cyclic antidepressants) are

(Continued)

Moxifloxacin *(Continued)*

contraindicated with moxifloxacin. Cimetidine and probenecid increase quinolone levels. An increased incidence of seizures may occur with foscarnet or NSAIDs. Serum levels of some quinolones are increased by loop diuretic administration. Digoxin levels may be increased in some patients by quinolones. The hypoprothrombinemic effect of warfarin is enhanced by some quinolone antibiotics. Monitoring of the INR during concurrent therapy is recommended by the manufacturer. Concurrent use of corticosteroids may increase risk of tendon rupture.

Nutritional/Ethanol Interactions Food: Absorption is not affected by administration with a high-fat meal or yogurt.

Adverse Reactions

3% to 10%:

Central nervous system: Dizziness (3%)

Gastrointestinal: Nausea (7%), diarrhea (6%)

<3% (Limited to important or life-threatening): Allergic reactions, anaphylactic reaction, anaphylactic shock, anxiety, confusion, convulsions, EKG abnormalities, hallucinations, hyperglycemia, hypoglycemia, hypertension, hypotension, injection site reaction, peripheral edema, prothrombin time increased/decreased, QT prolongation, tachycardia, tendon disorders, tongue discoloration, tremor, vertigo, vision abnormalities, ventricular tachycardia

Overdosage/Toxicology Potential symptoms of overdose may include CNS excitation, seizures, QT prolongation, and arrhythmias (including torsade de pointes). Patients should be monitored by continuous EKG in the event of an overdose. Management is supportive and symptomatic.

Pharmacodynamics/Kinetics

Absorption: Well absorbed; not affected by high fat meal or yogurt

Bioavailability: 90%

Half-Life Elimination: Oral: 12 hours; I.V.: 15 hours

Metabolism: Hepatic via glucuronide (14%) and sulfate (38%) conjugation

Formulations

Solution for infusion, as hydrochloride [premixed in sodium chloride 0.8%]: 400 mg/250 mL

Tablet, as hydrochloride: 400 mg

Tablet, as hydrochloride [dose pack] (Avelox® ABC Pack™): 400 mg (5/card)

Dosing

Adults & Elderly:

Acute bacterial sinusitis: Oral, I.V.: 400 mg every 24 hours for 10 days

Chronic bronchitis, acute bacterial exacerbation: Oral, I.V.: 400 mg every 24 hours for 5 days

Note: Avelox® ABC Pack™ (Avelox® Bronchitis Course) contains five tablets of 400 mg each.

Community-acquired pneumonia: Oral, I.V.: 400 mg every 24 hours for 7-14 days

Uncomplicated skin infections: Oral, I.V.: 400 mg every 24 hours for 7 days

Renal Impairment: No adjustment is necessary.

Hepatic Impairment: No dosage adjustment is required in mild to moderate hepatic insufficiency (Child-Pugh Classes A and B). Not recommended in patients with severe hepatic insufficiency.

Administration

I.V.: I.V.: Infuse over 60 minutes; do not infuse by rapid or bolus intravenous infusion

Stability

Storage: Store at 25°C (77°F). I.V.: Do not refrigerate.

Compatibility: Stable in 0.9% NS, 1M sodium chloride, D_5W, $D_{10}W$, sterile water for injection, LR

Do not add other medications to intravenous solution

Monitoring Laboratory Tests WBC, signs of infection

Monitoring and Teaching Issues

Physical Assessment: Assess allergy history before initiating therapy. See Contraindications, Warnings/Precautions, and Dosing for use cautions. Assess potential for interactions with other prescriptions, OTC medications, or herbal products patient may be taking (see Drug Interactions). Assess results of laboratory tests (see above), therapeutic effectiveness, and adverse effects (see Adverse Reactions and Overdose/Toxicology) regularly during therapy. Discontinue at first sign of hypersensitivity reaction or tendon inflammation or pain. Teach patient appropriate use, possible side effects and interventions, and adverse symptoms to report (see Patient Education). **Pregnancy risk factor C** - benefits of use should outweigh possible risks. Breast-feeding is not recommended.

Patient Education: Inform prescriber of all prescriptions, OTC medications, or herbal products you are taking, and any allergies you have. Do not take anything new during treatment unless approved by prescriber. Take exactly as directed with or without food. Do not take antacids 4 hours before or 8 hours after taking this medication. Do not miss a dose (take a missed dose as soon as possible, unless it is almost time for your next dose). Take entire prescription even if feeling better. Maintain adequate hydration (2-3 L/day of fluids) unless advised by prescriber to restrict fluids. May cause nausea, vomiting, taste perversion (small, frequent meals, good mouth care, chewing gum, or sucking hard candy may help); headache, dizziness, insomnia, anxiety (use caution when driving or engaging in tasks requiring alertness until response to drug is known). Report immediately any swelling of mouth, lips, tongue or throat; chest pain or tightness; difficulty breathing; back pain; itching; skin rash; tingling; tendon pain; confusion, dizziness, abnormal thinking, or anxiety; or insomnia. Report changes in voiding pattern; vaginal itching, burning, or discharge; vision changes or hearing; abnormal bruising or bleeding or blood in urine; or other adverse reactions. **Pregnancy/breast-feeding precautions:** Inform prescriber if you are or intend to become pregnant. Breast-feeding is not recommended.

Dietary Issues: May be taken with or without food. Take 4 hours before or 8 hours after multiple vitamins, antacids, or other products containing magnesium, aluminum, iron, or zinc.

Moxifloxacin Hydrochloride *see* Moxifloxacin *on page 929*
Moxilin® *see* Amoxicillin *on page 88*
6-MP *see* Mercaptopurine *on page 855*
MPA and Estrogens (Conjugated) *see* Estrogens (Conjugated/Equine) and Medroxyprogesterone *on page 505*
M-Prednisol® *see* MethylPREDNISolone *on page 885*
M-R-VAX® II *see page 1498*
MS *see* Morphine Sulfate *on page 926*
MS Contin® *see* Morphine Sulfate *on page 926*
MSIR® *see* Morphine Sulfate *on page 926*
MTC *see* Mitomycin *on page 913*
MTX *see* Methotrexate *on page 874*
Mucinex™ [OTC] *see* Guaifenesin *on page 646*
Mucomyst® *see* Acetylcysteine *on page 40*
Mucosil™ *see* Acetylcysteine *on page 40*
Multitest CMI® *see page 1461*
Mumps Skin Test Antigen *see page 1461*
Mumps Virus Vaccine *see page 1498*

Mupirocin (myoo PEER oh sin)

U.S. Brand Names Bactroban®; Bactroban® Nasal

Synonyms Mupirocin Calcium; Pseudomonic Acid A

Generic Available No

Pharmacologic Category Antibiotic, Topical

Pregnancy Risk Factor B

Lactation Excretion in breast milk unknown/use caution

Use

Intranasal: Eradication of nasal colonization with MRSA in adult patients and healthcare workers

Topical treatment of impetigo due to *Staphylococcus aureus*, beta-hemolytic *Streptococcus*, and *S. pyogenes*

Mechanism of Action/Effect Binds to bacterial isoleucyl transfer-RNA synthetase resulting in the inhibition of protein and RNA synthesis

Contraindications Hypersensitivity to mupirocin, polyethylene glycol, or any component of the formulation

Warnings/Precautions Potentially toxic amounts of polyethylene glycol contained in the vehicle may be absorbed percutaneously in patients with extensive burns or open wounds. Prolonged use may result in over growth of nonsusceptible organisms. For external use only. Not for treatment of pressure sores.

Adverse Reactions Frequency not defined.

Central nervous system: Dizziness, headache
Dermatologic: Pruritus, rash, erythema, dry skin, cellulitis, dermatitis
Gastrointestinal: Nausea, taste perversion
Local: Burning, stinging, tenderness, edema, pain
Respiratory: Rhinitis, upper respiratory tract infection, pharyngitis, cough

Pharmacodynamics/Kinetics

Absorption: Topical: Penetrates outer layers of skin; systemic absorption minimal through intact skin

Half-Life Elimination: 17-36 minutes

Metabolism: Skin: 3% to monic acid

Formulations

Cream, as calcium: 2% (15 g, 30 g)
Ointment: 2% (22 g)
Ointment, as calcium: 2% (15 g, 30 g)
Ointment, intranasal, as calcium [single-use tube]: 2% (1 g)

Dosing

Adults & Elderly:

Impetigo: Topical: Apply small amount to affected area 2-5 times/day for 5-14 days.

Elimination of MRSA colonization: Nasal: In adults (12 years of age and older), approximately one-half of the ointment from the single-use tube should be applied into one nostril and the other half into the other nostril twice daily for 5 days.

Pediatrics:

Topical: Children: Refer to adult dosing.
Nasal: ≥12 years: Refer to adult dosing.

Administration

Topical: For external use only.

Stability

Compatibility: Do not mix with Aquaphor®, coal tar solution, or salicylic acid.

Monitoring and Teaching Issues

Physical Assessment: See Warnings/Precautions and Contraindications for use cautions. Assess for effectiveness of therapy and symptoms of infection. Assess knowledge/teach patient appropriate application and use and adverse symptoms (see Adverse Reactions) to report. Note breast-feeding caution.

Patient Education: For external use only. Wash hands before and after application. Apply thin film over affected areas exactly as directed. Avoid getting in eyes. Report rash, persistent burning, stinging, swelling, itching, or pain. Contact prescriber if no improvement is seen in 3-5 days. **Breast-feeding precaution:** Consult prescriber if breast-feeding.

Additional Information Not for treatment of pressure sores; contains polyethylene glycol vehicle.

Mupirocin Calcium *see* Mupirocin *on page 931*

Murine® Ear Drops *see page 1519*
Murine® Plus *see page 1509*

Muromonab-CD3 (myoo roe MOE nab see dee three)

U.S. Brand Names Orthoclone OKT® 3

Synonyms Monoclonal Antibody; OKT3

Generic Available No

Pharmacologic Category Immunosuppressant Agent

Pregnancy Risk Factor C

Lactation Excretion in breast milk unknown/contraindicated

Use Treatment of acute allograft rejection in renal transplant patients; treatment of acute hepatic, kidney, and pancreas rejection episodes resistant to conventional treatment. Acute graft-versus-host disease following bone marrow transplantation resistant to conventional treatment.

Mechanism of Action/Effect Reverses graft rejection by binding to T cells and interfering with their function

Contraindications Hypersensitivity to OKT3 or any murine product; patients in fluid overload or those with >3% weight gain within 1 week prior to start of OKT3; mouse antibody titers >1:1000

Warnings/Precautions It is imperative, especially prior to the first few doses, that there be no clinical evidence of volume overload, uncontrolled hypertension, or uncompensated heart failure, including a clear chest x-ray and weight restriction of ≤3% above the patient's minimum weight during the week prior to injection.

May result in an increased susceptibility to infection; dosage of concomitant immunosuppressants should be reduced during OKT3 therapy; cyclosporine should be decreased to 50% usual maintenance dose and maintenance therapy resumed about 4 days before stopping OKT3.

Severe pulmonary edema has occurred in patients with fluid overload.

First dose effect (flu-like symptoms, anaphylactic-type reaction): may occur within 30 minutes to 6 hours up to 24 hours after the first dose and may be minimized by using the recommended regimens. See table.

Suggested Prevention/Treatment of Muromonab-CD3 First-Dose Effects

Adverse Reaction	Effective Prevention or Palliation	Supportive Treatment
Severe pulmonary edema	Clear chest x-ray within 24 hours preinjection; weight restriction to ≤3% gain over 7 days preinjection	Prompt intubation and oxygenation 24 hours close observation
Fever, chills	15 mg/kg methylprednisolone sodium succinate 1 hour preinjection; fever reduction to <37.8°C (100°F) 1 hour preinjection; acetaminophen (1 g orally) and diphenhydramine (50 mg orally) 1 hour preinjection	Cooling blanket Acetaminophen prn
Respiratory effects	100 mg hydrocortisone sodium succinate 30 minutes postinjection	Additional 100 mg hydrocortisone sodium succinate prn for wheezing; if respiratory distress, give epinephrine 1:1000 (0.3 mL S.C.)

Cardiopulmonary resuscitation may be needed. If the patient's temperature is >37.8°C, reduce before administering OKT3

Pregnancy risk C.

Drug Interactions

Decreased Effect: Decreased effect with immunosuppressive drugs.

Increased Effect/Toxicity: Recommend decreasing dose of prednisone to 0.5 mg/kg, azathioprine to 0.5 mg/kg (approximate 50% decrease in dose), and discontinuing cyclosporine while patient is receiving OKT3.

Adverse Reactions First-dose effect (cytokine release syndrome), onset 1-3 hours after dose, duration 12-16 hours, severity mild to life-threatening, signs and symptoms include fever, chilling, dyspnea, wheezing, chest pain, chest tightness, nausea, vomiting, and diarrhea. Hypervolemic pulmonary edema, nephrotoxicity, meningitis, and encephalopathy are possible. Reactions tend to decrease with repeated doses.

>10%:
- Cardiovascular: Tachycardia (including ventricular)
- Central nervous system: Dizziness, faintness
- Gastrointestinal: Diarrhea, nausea, vomiting
- Hematologic: Transient lymphopenia
- Neuromuscular & skeletal: Trembling
- Respiratory: Dyspnea

1% to 10%:
- Central nervous system: Headache
- Neuromuscular & skeletal: Stiff neck
- Ocular: Photophobia
- Respiratory: Pulmonary edema

<1% (Limited to important or life-threatening): BUN increased, chest pain or tightness, creatinine increased, dyspnea, hypertension, hypotension, pancytopenia, secondary lymphoproliferative disorder or lymphoma, thrombosis of major vessels in renal allograft, wheezing

Pharmacodynamics/Kinetics

Time to Peak: Steady-state: Trough: 3-14 days

Duration: 7 days after discontinuation

Formulations Injection: 1 mg/mL (5 mL)

Dosing

Adults & Elderly: Treatment of acute allograft rejection or acute graft-versus-host disease: I.V. (refer to individual protocols): 5 mg/day once daily for 10-14 days

Pediatrics: Refer to individual protocols. Treatment of acute allograft rejection or acute graft-versus-host disease: I.V.

Children <30 kg: 2.5 mg/day once daily for 7-14 days

Children >30 kg: 5 mg/day once daily for 7-14 days

or

Children <12 years: 0.1 mg/kg/day once daily for 10-14 days

Children ≥12 years: Refer to adult dosing.

Renal Impairment: Removal by dialysis: Molecular size of OKT3 is 150,000 daltons. Not dialyzed by most standard dialyzers; however, may be dialyzed by high flux dialysis. OKT3 will be removed by plasmapheresis. Administer following dialysis treatments.

Administration

I.V.: Give I.V. push over <1 minute at a final concentration of 1 mg/mL; **do not give I.M.**. Methylprednisolone sodium succinate 1 mg/kg I.V. given prior to first muromonab-CD3 administration, and I.V. hydrocortisone sodium succinate 50-100 mg, given 30 minutes after administration are strongly recommended to decrease the incidence of reactions to the first dose.

Stability

Storage: Refrigerate; do not shake or freeze. Stable in Becton Dickinson syringe for 16 hours at room temperature or refrigeration.

Monitoring Laboratory Tests Chest x-ray, CBC with differential, immunologic monitoring of T cells, serum levels of OKT3

Monitoring and Teaching Issues

Physical Assessment: Note Drug Interactions information. Monitor pretreatment laboratory results prior to beginning therapy. Monitor closely for acute adverse pulmonary and cardiac effects, and anaphylactic-type effects during and for 24 hours following first infusion (see Warnings/Precautions). Monitor vital signs, cardiac status, respiratory status, and adverse reactions on a regular basis. Assess knowledge/instruct patient about adverse reactions to report (eg, opportunistic infection) and appropriate interventions to reduce side effects. **Pregnancy risk factor C.** Breast-feeding is contraindicated.

Patient Education: There may be a severe reaction to the first infusion of this medication. You may experience high fever, chills, difficulty breathing, or congestion. You will be closely monitored and comfort measures provided. Effects are substantially reduced with subsequent infusions. During the period of therapy and for some time after the regimen of infusions you will be susceptible to infection. People may wear masks and gloves while caring for you to protect you as much as possible from infection (avoid crowds and exposure to infection). You may experience dizziness, faintness, or trembling (use caution until response to medication is known); nausea or vomiting (small, frequent meals, frequent mouth care); or sensitivity to direct sunlight (wear dark glasses, and protective clothing, use sunscreen, or avoid exposure to direct sunlight). Report chest pain or tightness; symptoms of respiratory infection, wheezing, or difficulty breathing; vision change; or muscular trembling. **Pregnancy/breast-feeding precautions:** Inform prescriber if you are or intend to become pregnant. Do not breast-feed.

Muro's Opcon® *see page 1509*

Muse® Pellet *see* Alprostadil *on page 65*

Mustargen® *see* Mechlorethamine *on page 839*

Mustine *see* Mechlorethamine *on page 839*

Mutamycin® *see* Mitomycin *on page 913*

Myambutol® *see* Ethambutol *on page 513*

Mycelex® *see* Clotrimazole *on page 322*

Mycelex®-3 *see* Clotrimazole *on page 322*

Mycelex®-7 [OTC] *see* Clotrimazole *on page 322*

Mycelex® Twin Pack [OTC] *see* Clotrimazole *on page 322*

Myciguent [OTC] *see* Neomycin *on page 958*

Mycinettes® [OTC] *see* Benzocaine *on page 156*

Mycitracin® [OTC] *see* Bacitracin, Neomycin, and Polymyxin B *on page 144*

Mycobutin® *see* Rifabutin *on page 1184*

Mycolog®-II *see* Nystatin and Triamcinolone *on page 990*

Mycophenolate (mye koe FEN oh late)

U.S. Brand Names CellCept®

Synonyms Mycophenolate Mofetil

Generic Available No

Pharmacologic Category Immunosuppressant Agent

Pregnancy Risk Factor C (manufacturer)

Lactation Excretion in breast milk unknown/not recommended

Use Prophylaxis of organ rejection concomitantly with cyclosporine and corticosteroids in patients receiving allogenic renal, cardiac, or hepatic transplants. Intravenous formulation is an alternative dosage form to oral capsules, suspension, and tablets.

Use - Unlabeled/Investigational Treatment of rejection in liver transplant patients unable to tolerate tacrolimus or cyclosporine due to neurotoxicity; mild rejection in heart transplant patients; treatment of moderate-severe psoriasis

Mechanism of Action/Effect Inhibition of purine synthesis of human lymphocytes and proliferation of human lymphocytes

(Continued)

Mycophenolate *(Continued)*

Contraindications Hypersensitivity to mycophenolate mofetil, mycophenolic acid, or any component of the formulation; intravenous is contraindicated in patients who are allergic to polysorbate 80

Warnings/Precautions Increased risk for infection and development of lymphoproliferative disorders. Patients should be monitored appropriately and given supportive treatment should these conditions occur. Increased toxicity in patients with renal impairment. Should be used with caution in patients with active peptic ulcer disease.

Mycophenolate mofetil is a potential teratogen; tablets should not be crushed, and capsules should not be opened or crushed. Avoid inhalation or direct contact with skin or mucous membranes of the powder contained in the capsules and the powder for oral suspension. Caution should be exercised in the handling and preparation of solutions of intravenous mycophenolate. Avoid skin contact with the intravenous solution and reconstituted suspension. If such contact occurs, wash thoroughly with soap and water, rinse eyes with plain water.

Theoretically, use should be avoided in patients with the rare hereditary deficiency of hypoxanthine-guanine phosphoribosyltransferase (such as Lesch-Nyhan or Kelley-Seegmiller syndrome). Oral suspension contains 0.56 mg phenylalanine/mL, use caution if administered to patients with phenylketonuria. Intravenous solutions should be given over at least 2 hours; **never** administer intravenous solution by rapid or bolus injection.

Pregnancy risk C.

Drug Interactions

Decreased Effect: Antacids decrease serum levels (C_{max} and AUC); **do not administer together**. Cholestyramine resin decreases serum levels; **do not administer together**. Avoid use of live vaccines; vaccinations may be less effective. During concurrent use of oral contraceptives, progesterone levels are not significantly affected, however, effect on estrogen component varies; an additional form of contraception should be used.

Increased Effect/Toxicity: Acyclovir and ganciclovir levels may increase due to competition for tubular secretion of these drugs. Probenecid may increase mycophenolate levels due to inhibition of tubular secretion. High doses of salicylates may increase free fraction of mycophenolic acid. Azathioprine's bone marrow suppression may be potentiated; do not administer together.

Nutritional/Ethanol Interactions

Food: Decreases C_{max} of MPA by 40% however, the extent of absorption is not changed

Herb/Nutraceutical: Avoid cat's claw, echinacea (have immunostimulant properties)

Adverse Reactions Reported following oral dosing of mycophenolate alone in renal, cardiac, and hepatic allograft rejection studies. In general, lower doses used in renal rejection patients had less adverse effects than higher doses. Rates of adverse effects were similar for each indication, except for those unique to the specific organ involved.

>10%:

Cardiovascular: Hypertension (28% to 77%), peripheral edema (27% to 64%), hypotension (18% to 32%), edema (12% to 28%), cardiovascular disorder (26%), chest pain (13% to 26%), tachycardia (20% to 22%), arrhythmia (19%), bradycardia (17%), hypervolemia (17%), pericardial effusion (16%), heart failure (12%)

Central nervous system: Pain (31% to 76%), headache (16% to 54%), fever (21% to 52%), insomnia (9% to 52%), tremor (11% to 34%), anxiety (19% to 28%), dizziness (6% to 28%), depression (16% to 17%), confusion (13% to 17%), agitation (13%), chills (11%), somnolence (11%), nervousness (10% to 11%)

Dermatologic: Rash (18% to 22%), pruritus (14%), skin disorder (12%), diaphoresis (11%), acne (10% to 12%)

Endocrine & metabolic: Hyperglycemia (9% to 47%), hypercholesterolemia (8% to 41%), hypomagnesemia (18% to 39%), hypokalemia (10% to 37%), hypocalcemia (30%), elevated LDH (23%), hyperkalemia (9% to 22%), elevated AST (17%), elevated ALT (16%), hyperuricemia (16%), hypophosphatemia (12% to 16%), acidosis (14%), hypoproteinemia (13%), hyponatremia (11%)

Gastrointestinal: Abdominal pain (25% to 62%), nausea (20% to 54%), diarrhea (31% to 51%), constipation (18% to 41%), vomiting (12% to 34%), anorexia (25%), dyspepsia (13% to 22%), abdominal enlargement (19%), weight gain (16%), flatulence (13% to 14%), oral moniliasis (10% to 12%), nausea and vomiting (10% to 11%)

Genitourinary: Urinary tract infection (13% to 37%), urinary tract disorder

Hematologic: Leukopenia (23% to 46%), anemia (26% to 43%), leukocytosis (7% to 40%), thrombocytopenia (8% to 38%), hypochromic anemia (7% to 25%), ecchymosis (17%)

Hepatic: Abnormal liver function tests (25%), ascites (24%), bilirubinemia (14% to 18%), cholangitis (14%), hepatitis (13%), cholestatic jaundice (12%)

Neuromuscular & skeletal: Back pain (12% to 47%), weakness (14% to 43%), paresthesia (15% to 21%), leg cramps (17%), hypertonia (16%), myasthenia (12%), myalgia (12%)

Ocular: Amblyopia (15%)

Renal: Elevated creatinine (20% to 40%), elevated BUN (10% to 35%), abnormal kidney function (22% to 27%), oliguria (14% to 17%), hematuria (12% to 14%), kidney tubular necrosis (6% to 10%)

Respiratory: Respiratory infection (16% to 37%), dyspnea (15% to 37%), pleural effusion (17% to 34%), increased cough (13% to 31%), lung disorder (22% to 30%), sinusitis (11% to 26%), rhinitis (19%), pharyngitis (9% to 18%), pneumonia (11% to 14%), atelectasis (13%), asthma (11%), bronchitis

Miscellaneous: Infection (18% to 27%), sepsis (18% to 27%), herpes simplex (10% to 21%), accidental injury (11% to 19%), mucocutaneous *Candida* (15% to 18%), CMV viremia/syndrome (12% to 14%), hernia (12%), CMV tissue invasive disease (6% to 11%), herpes zoster cutaneous disease (6% to 11%)

1% to 10%:

Cardiovascular: I.V.: Thrombosis (4%)

Dermatologic: Nonmelanoma skin carcinomas (2% to 4%)

Endocrine & metabolic: Hypoglycemia (10%)

Hematologic: Severe neutropenia (2% to 4%), lymphoproliferative disease/lymphoma (0.4% to 1%)

Local: I.V.: Phlebitis (4%)

Miscellaneous: Abnormal healing (10%), peritonitis (10%), fatal sepsis (2% to 5%), other systemic/opportunistic infections (see above), malignancy (0.7% to 2%)

<1% (Limited to important or life-threatening): Colitis, infectious endocarditis, interstitial lung disorders, meningitis, pancreatitis, pulmonary fibrosis (rare, fatalities reported)

Overdosage/Toxicology There are no reported overdoses with mycophenolate. At plasma concentrations >100 mcg/mL, small amounts of the inactive metabolite MPAG are removed by hemodialysis. Excretion of the active metabolite, MPA, may be increased by using bile acid sequestrants (cholestyramine).

Pharmacodynamics/Kinetics

Absorption: AUC values for MPA are lower in the early post-transplant period versus later (>3 months) post-transplant period. The extent of absorption in pediatrics is similar to that seen in adults, although there was wide variability reported.

Bioavailability: Oral: 94%

Half-Life Elimination: Oral: 17 hours; I.V.: 18 hours

Metabolism: Hepatic and via GI tract; hydrolyzed to mycophenolic acid (MPA; active metabolite); enterohepatic recirculation of MPA may occur; MPA is glucuronidated to MPAG (inactive metabolite)

Onset: Peak effect: Correlation of toxicity or efficacy is still being developed, however, one study indicated that 12-hour AUCs >40 mcg/mL/hour were correlated with efficacy and decreased episodes of rejection

Formulations

Capsule, as mofetil: 250 mg

Injection: 500 mg

Suspension, oral, as mofetil: 200 mg/mL (225 mL)

Tablet, film coated, as mofetil: 500 mg

Dosing

Adults:

Renal transplantation:

I.V.: 1 g twice daily

Oral: 1 g twice daily; doses >2 g/day are not recommended in these patients because of the possibility for enhanced immunosuppression as well as toxicities. The initial dose should be given as soon as possible following transplantation. The intravenous solution may be given until the oral medication can be tolerated (up to 14 days). Although a dose of 1.5 g twice daily was used in clinical trials and shown to be effective, no efficacy advantage was established. Patients receiving 2 g/day demonstrated an overall better safety profile than patients receiving 3 g/day.

Cardiac transplantation:

I.V.: 1.5 g twice daily

Oral: 1.5 g twice daily

Hepatic transplantation:

I.V.: 1 g twice daily

Oral: 1.5 g twice daily

Dosing adjustment for toxicity (neutropenia): ANC <1.3 x 10^3/µL: Dosing should be interrupted or the dose reduced, appropriate diagnostic tests performed and patients managed appropriately.

Elderly: Dosage is the same as younger patients, however, dosing should be cautious due to possibility of increased hepatic, renal, or cardiac dysfunction. Elderly patients may be at an increased risk of certain infections, gastrointestinal hemorrhage, and pulmonary edema, as compared to younger patients.

Pediatrics:

Renal transplant: Oral: Children:

Suspension: 600 mg/m^2/dose twice daily; maximum dose: 1 g twice daily

Alternatively, may use solid dosage forms according to BSA as follows:

BSA 1.25-1.5 m^2: 750 mg capsule twice daily

BSA >1.5 m^2: 1 g capsule or tablet twice daily

Renal Impairment:

Renal transplant: GFR <25 mL/minute in patients outside the immediate post-transplant period: Doses >1 g administered twice daily should be avoided. Patients should be carefully observed. No dose adjustments are needed in renal transplant patients experiencing delayed graft function postoperatively.

Cardiac or liver transplant: No data available; mycophenolate may be used in cardiac or hepatic transplant patients with severe chronic renal impairment if the potential benefit outweighs the potential risk.

Hemodialysis: Not removed; supplemental dose is not necessary.

Peritoneal dialysis: Supplemental dose is not necessary.

Hepatic Impairment: No dosage adjustment is recommended for renal patients with severe hepatic parenchymal disease; however, it is not currently known whether dosage adjustments are necessary for hepatic disease with other etiologies.

Administration

I.V.: Intravenous solutions should be given over at least 2 hours. Do not administer intravenous solution by rapid or bolus injection. The oral suspension cannot be mixed with other medications.

Stability

Storage: Tablets/capsules/powder for oral suspension should be stored at room temperature (15°C to 39°C/59°F to 86°F). Tablets should also be protected from light. Intact vials of injection should be stored at room temperature (15°C to 30°C/59°F to 86°F).

Stability of the infusion solution: 4 hours from reconstitution and dilution of the product. Store solutions at 15°C to 30°C (59°F to 86°F)

Once reconstituted, the oral solution may be stored at room temperature or under refrigeration. Do not freeze. The mixed solution is stable for 60 days.

(Continued)

Mycophenolate *(Continued)*

Reconstitution: Mycophenolate injection does not contain an antibacterial preservative; therefore, reconstitution and dilution of the product must be done under aseptic conditions. Preparation of intravenous formulation should take place in a vertical laminar flow hood with the same precautions as antineoplastic agents.

Intravenous preparation procedure:

Step 1:

a. Two vials of mycophenolate injection are used for preparing a 1 g dose, whereas 3 vials are needed for each 1.5 g dose. Reconstitute the contents of each vial by injecting 14 mL of 5% dextrose injection.
b. Gently shake the vial to dissolve the drug
c. Inspect the resulting slightly yellow solution for particulate matter and discoloration prior to further dilution. Discard the vial if particulate matter or discoloration is observed.

Step 2:

a. To prepare a 1 g dose, further dilute the contents of the two reconstituted vials into 140 mL of 5% dextrose in water. To prepare a 1.5 g dose, further dilute the contents of the three reconstituted vials into 210 mL of 5% dextrose in water. The final concentration of both solutions is 6 mg mycophenolate mofetil per mL.
b. Inspect the infusion solution for particulate matter or discoloration. Discard the infusion solution if particulate matter or discoloration is observed.

Oral Suspension: Should be constituted by a pharmacist prior to dispensing to the patient and **not** mixed with any other medication. Closed bottle should be tapped to loosen the powder. Add 47 mL of water to the bottle and shake well for ~1 minute. Add another 47 mL of water to the bottle and shake well for an additional minute. Remove child-resistant cap and push bottle adapter into neck of the bottle; close bottle with child-resistant cap tightly to assure proper placement of adapter and status of child-resistant cap. Final concentration is 200 mg/mL of mycophenolate mofetil.

Monitoring Laboratory Tests Renal and liver function, CBC

Monitoring and Teaching Issues

Physical Assessment: Assess other medications patient may be taking for effectiveness and interactions (see Drug Interactions). See Warnings/Precautions and Contraindications for use cautions. Monitor laboratory tests, response to therapy, and adverse reactions (see Warnings/Precautions and Adverse Reactions). Diabetic patients should monitor glucose levels closely (this medication may alter glucose levels). Monitor/instruct patient on appropriate interventions to reduce side effects, to monitor for signs of opportunistic infection, and adverse reactions to report. **Pregnancy risk factor C** - benefits of use should outweigh possible risks. Breast-feeding is not recommended.

Patient Education: Take oral formulations as directed, preferably 1 hour before or 2 hours after meals. Do not take within 1 hour before or 2 hours after antacids or cholestyramine medications. Do not alter dose and do not discontinue without consulting prescriber. Maintain adequate hydration (2-3 L/day of fluids) during entire course of therapy unless advised by prescriber to restrict fluids. You will be susceptible to infection (avoid crowds and exposure to infection). May be at increased risk for skin cancer, wear protective clothing and use sunscreen with high protective factor to help limit exposure to sunlight and UV light. If you are diabetic, monitor glucose levels closely (drug may alter glucose levels). You may experience dizziness or trembling (use caution until response to medication is known); nausea or vomiting (small, frequent meals, frequent mouth care may help); diarrhea (boiled milk, yogurt, or buttermilk may help); sores or white plaques in mouth (frequent rinsing of mouth and frequent mouth care may help); or muscle or back pain (mild analgesics may be recommended). Report chest pain; acute headache or dizziness; symptoms of respiratory infection, cough, or difficulty breathing; unresolved GI effects; fatigue, chills, fever unhealed sores, white plaques in mouth; irritation in genital area or unusual discharge; unusual bruising or bleeding; or other unusual effects related to this medication. **Pregnancy/breast-feeding precautions:** Inform prescriber if you are or intend to become pregnant. Two reliable forms of contraception should be used prior to, during, and for 6 weeks after therapy. Breast-feeding is not recommended.

Dietary Issues: Oral dosage formulations should be taken on an empty stomach. However, in stable renal transplant patients, may be administered with food if necessary.

Breast-feeding Issues: It is unknown if mycophenolate is excreted in human milk. Due to potentially serious adverse reactions, the decision to discontinue the drug or discontinue breast-feeding should be considered.

Pregnancy Issues: There are no adequate and well-controlled studies using mycophenolate in pregnant women, however, it may cause fetal harm. Women of childbearing potential should have a negative pregnancy test prior to beginning therapy. Two reliable forms of contraception should be used prior to, during, and for 6 weeks after therapy.

Mycophenolate Mofetil *see* Mycophenolate *on page 933*

Mycostatin® *see* Nystatin *on page 989*

Mydfrin® *see page 1509*

Mydfrin® Ophthalmic *see* Phenylephrine *on page 1071*

Mydriacyl® *see page 1509*

Mydriacyl® *see page 1461*

Mykrox® *see* Metolazone *on page 891*

Myleran® *see* Busulfan *on page 190*

Mylocel™ *see* Hydroxyurea *on page 682*

Mylotarg® *see* Gemtuzumab Ozogamicin *on page 626*

Mysoline® *see* Primidone *on page 1119*

Mytelase® *see* Ambenonium *on page 73*

Mytrex® *see* Nystatin and Triamcinolone *on page 990*

Mytussin® AC *see* Guaifenesin and Codeine *on page 647*

Mytussin® DAC *see* Guaifenesin, Pseudoephedrine, and Codeine *on page 649*

Mytussin® DM [OTC] *see* Guaifenesin and Dextromethorphan *on page 647*

Nabi-HB® *see page 1498*

Nabumetone (na BYOO me tone)

U.S. Brand Names Relafen®

Generic Available Yes

Pharmacologic Category Nonsteroidal Anti-inflammatory Drug (NSAID)

Pregnancy Risk Factor C/D (3rd trimester)

Lactation Enters breast milk/not recommended

Use Management of osteoarthritis and rheumatoid arthritis

Use - Unlabeled/Investigational Sunburn, mild to moderate pain

Mechanism of Action/Effect Nabumetone is a nonacidic NSAID that inhibits the production of inflammation and pain during arthritis. The active metabolite of nabumetone is felt to be the compound primarily responsible for therapeutic effect. Comparatively, the parent drug is a poor inhibitor of prostaglandin synthesis.

Contraindications Hypersensitivity to NSAIDs including aspirin, or any component of the formulation; should not be administered to patients with active peptic ulceration and those with severe hepatic impairment or in patients in whom nabumetone, aspirin, or other NSAIDs have induced asthma, urticaria, or other allergic-type reactions; fatal asthmatic reactions have occurred following NSAID administration; pregnancy (3rd trimester)

Warnings/Precautions Use with caution in patients with CHF, hypertension, dehydration, decreased renal or hepatic function, history of GI disease (bleeding or ulcers), or those receiving anticoagulants. Elderly are at a high risk for adverse GI and CNS effects from NSAIDs. As many as 60% of elderly can develop peptic ulceration and/or hemorrhage asymptomatically.

Use lowest effective dose for shortest period possible. Use of NSAIDs can compromise existing renal function especially when Cl_{cr} is <30 mL/minute. Withhold for at least 4-6 half-lives prior to surgical or dental procedures. May have adverse effects on fetus. Use with caution with dehydration. Use in children is not recommended.

Pregnancy risk C/D (3rd trimester).

Drug Interactions

Decreased Effect: NSAIDs may decrease the effect of some antihypertensive agents, including ACE inhibitors, angiotensin receptor antagonists, and hydralazine. The efficacy of diuretics (loop and/or thiazide) may be decreased.

Increased Effect/Toxicity: NSAIDs may increase digoxin, methotrexate, and lithium serum concentrations. The renal adverse effects of ACE inhibitors may be potentiated by NSAIDs. Potential for bleeding may be increased with anticoagulants or antiplatelet agents. Concurrent use of corticosteroids may increase the risk of GI ulceration.

Nutritional/Ethanol Interactions

Ethanol: Avoid ethanol (may enhance gastric mucosal irritation).

Food: Nabumetone peak serum concentrations may be increased if taken with food or dairy products.

Herb/Nutraceutical: Avoid cat's claw, dong quai, evening primrose, feverfew, garlic, ginger, ginkgo, red clover, horse chestnut, green tea, ginseng (all have additional antiplatelet activity).

Adverse Reactions

>10%:

Central nervous system: Dizziness

Dermatologic: Rash

Gastrointestinal: Abdominal cramps, abdominal pain (12%), diarrhea (14%), dyspepsia (13%), heartburn, indigestion, nausea

1% to 10%:

Cardiovascular: Edema

Central nervous system: Dizziness, headache, fatigue, insomnia, nervousness, somnolence

Dermatologic: Pruritus, rash

Gastrointestinal: Constipation, flatulence, nausea, guaiac postive stool, stomatitis, gastritis, dry mouth, vomiting

Otic: Tinnitus

<1% (Limited to important or life-threatening): Albuminuria, alopecia, anaphylactoid reaction, anaphylaxis, angina, angioneurotic edema, arrhythmia, asthma, azotemia, bullous eruptions, cholestatic jaundice, confusion, CHF, depression, duodenal ulcer, dysphagia, dyspnea, eosinophilic pneumonia, erythema multiforme, gastric ulcer, GI bleeding, granulocytopenia, hepatic failure, hepatitis, hypersensitivity pneumonitis, hypertension, hyperuricemia, impotence, interstitial nephritis, interstitial pneumonitis, leukopenia, myocardial infarction, nephrotic syndrome, nightmares, pancreatitis, paresthesia, photosensitivity, pseudoporphyria cutanea tarda, renal failure, Stevens-Johnson syndrome, syncope, thrombocytopenia, toxic epidermal necrolysis, urticaria, vasculitis

Overdosage/Toxicology Symptoms of overdose include apnea, metabolic acidosis, coma, nystagmus, leukocytosis, and renal failure. Management of NSAID intoxication is supportive and symptomatic.

Pharmacodynamics/Kinetics

Half-Life Elimination: Major metabolite: 24 hours

Time to Peak: Serum: Metabolite: Oral: 3-6 hours; Synovial fluid: 4-12 hours

Metabolism: Prodrug, rapidly metabolized to an active metabolite (6-methoxy-2-naphthylacetic acid); extensive first-pass effect

Onset: Several days

Formulations Tablet: 500 mg, 750 mg

(Continued)

Nabumetone *(Continued)*

Dosing

Adults: Osteoarthritis, rheumatoid arthritis: Oral: 1000 mg/day; an additional 500-1000 mg may be needed in some patients to obtain more symptomatic relief; may be administered once or twice daily.

Elderly: Refer to adult dosing; do not exceed 2000 mg/day.

Renal Impairment: None necessary; however, adverse effects due to accumulation of inactive metabolites of nabumetone that are renally excreted have not been studied and should be considered.

Monitoring Laboratory Tests Patients with renal insufficiency: Baseline renal function followed by repeat test within weeks (to determine if renal function has deteriorated)

Monitoring and Teaching Issues

Physical Assessment: Assess effectiveness and interactions of other medications patient may be taking (see Contraindications and Drug Interactions). Monitor laboratory tests (see above) and therapeutic response, and adverse reactions (eg, GI effects, hepatotoxicity, or ototoxicity) at beginning of therapy and periodically throughout therapy (see Warnings/Precautions, Adverse Reactions, and Overdose/Toxicology). Schedule ophthalmic evaluations for patients who develop eye complaints during long-term NSAID therapy. Assess knowledge/teach patient appropriate use, interventions to reduce side effects, and adverse symptoms to report (see Patient Education). **Pregnancy risk factor C.** Breast-feeding is not recommended.

Patient Education: Take this medication exactly as directed; do not increase dose without consulting prescriber. Do not crush tablets. Take with food or milk to reduce GI distress. Maintain adequate hydration (2-3 L/day of fluids) unless advised by prescriber to restrict fluids. Do not use alcohol, aspirin or aspirin-containing medication, or any other anti-inflammatory medications without consulting healthcare prescriber. You may experience drowsiness, dizziness, nervousness, or headache (use caution when driving or engaging in tasks requiring alertness until response to drug is known); anorexia, nausea, vomiting, or heartburn (small, frequent meals, frequent oral care, sucking lozenges, or chewing gum may help); fluid retention (weigh yourself weekly and report unusual (3-5 lb/week) weight gain). GI bleeding, ulceration, or perforation can occur with or without pain; discontinue medication and contact prescriber if persistent abdominal pain or cramping, or blood in stool occurs. Report breathlessness, difficulty breathing, or unusual cough; chest pain, rapid heartbeat, palpitations; unusual bruising/bleeding; blood in urine, stool, mouth, or vomitus; swollen extremities; skin rash or itching; acute fatigue; or hearing changes (ringing in ears). **Pregnancy/breast-feeding precautions:** Inform prescriber if you are pregnant. Breast-feeding is not recommended.

Geriatric Considerations: In trials with nabumetone, no significant differences were noted between young and elderly in regards to efficacy and safety. However, elderly are at high risk for adverse effects from NSAIDs. As much as 60% of elderly can develop peptic ulceration and/or hemorrhage asymptomatically. The concomitant use of H_2 blockers, omeprazole, and sucralfate is not effective as prophylaxis with the exception of NSAID-induced duodenal ulcers which may be prevented by the use of ranitidine. Misoprostol is the only prophylactic agent proven effective. Also, concomitant disease and drug use contribute to the risk for GI adverse effects. Use lowest effective dose for shortest period possible. Consider renal function decline with age. Use of NSAIDs can compromise existing renal function especially when Cl_{cr} is ≤30 mL/minute. Tinnitus may be a difficult and unreliable indication of toxicity due to age-related hearing loss or eighth cranial nerve damage. CNS adverse effects such as confusion, agitation, and hallucination are generally seen in overdose or high-dose situations, but elderly may demonstrate these adverse effects at lower doses than younger adults.

Related Information

Nonsalicylate/Nonsteroidal Anti-inflammatory Comparison *on page 1587*

NAC *see* Acetylcysteine *on page 40*

***N*-Acetylcysteine** *see* Acetylcysteine *on page 40*

***N*-Acetyl-L-cysteine** *see* Acetylcysteine *on page 40*

N-Acetyl-P-Aminophenol *see* Acetaminophen *on page 35*

Nadolol (nay DOE lole)

U.S. Brand Names Corgard®

Generic Available Yes

Pharmacologic Category Beta Blocker, Nonselective

Pregnancy Risk Factor C

Lactation Enters breast milk/use caution (AAP rates "compatible")

Use Treatment of hypertension and angina pectoris; prophylaxis of migraine headaches

Mechanism of Action/Effect Competitively blocks response to $beta_1$- and $beta_2$-adrenergic stimulation; does not exhibit any membrane stabilizing or intrinsic sympathomimetic activity

Contraindications Hypersensitivity to nadolol or any component of the formulation; bronchial asthma; sinus bradycardia; sinus node dysfunction; heart block greater than first degree (except in patients with a functioning artificial pacemaker); cardiogenic shock; uncompensated cardiac failure

Warnings/Precautions Administer only with extreme caution in patients with compensated heart failure, monitor for a worsening of the condition. Efficacy in heart failure has not been established for nadolol. Use caution with concurrent use of beta-blockers and either verapamil or diltiazem; bradycardia or heart block can occur. In general, patients with bronchospastic disease should not receive beta-blockers. Nadolol, if used at all, should be used cautiously in bronchospastic disease with close monitoring. Use cautiously in diabetics because it can mask prominent hypoglycemic symptoms. Can mask signs of thyrotoxicosis. Can cause fetal harm when administered in pregnancy. Use cautiously in the renally impaired (dosage adjustments are required). Use care with anesthetic agents which decrease myocardial function. Beta-blocker therapy should not be withdrawn abruptly (particularly in patients with CAD), but gradually tapered to avoid acute tachycardia, hypertension, and/or ischemia. Pregnancy risk C.

Drug Interactions

Decreased Effect: Decreased effect of beta-blockers with aluminum salts, barbiturates, calcium salts, cholestyramine, colestipol, NSAIDs, penicillins (ampicillin), rifampin, salicylates, and sulfinpyrazone due to decreased bioavailability and plasma levels. Beta-blockers may decrease the effect of sulfonylureas (possibly hyperglycemia). Nonselective beta-blockers blunt the effect of beta-2 adrenergic agonists (albuterol).

Increased Effect/Toxicity: The heart rate lowering effects of nadolol are additive with other drugs which slow AV conduction (digoxin, verapamil, diltiazem). Concurrent use of alpha-blockers (prazosin, terazosin) with beta-blockers may increase risk of orthostasis. Nadolol may mask the tachycardia from hypoglycemia caused by insulin and oral hypoglycemics. In patients receiving concurrent therapy, the risk of hypertensive crisis is increased when either clonidine or the beta-blocker is withdrawn. Reserpine has been shown to enhance the effect of beta-blockers. Avoid using with alpha-adrenergic stimulants (phenylephrine, epinephrine, etc) which may have exaggerated hypertensive responses. Beta-blockers may affect the action or levels of ethanol, disopyramide, nondepolarizing muscle relaxants, and theophylline although the effects are difficult to predict. The vasoconstrictive effects of ergot alkaloids may be enhanced.

Nutritional/Ethanol Interactions Herb/Nutraceutical: Avoid dong quai if using for hypertension (has estrogenic activity). Avoid ephedra, garlic, yohimbe, ginseng (may worsen hypertension). Avoid natural licorice (causes sodium and water retention and increases potassium loss).

Adverse Reactions

>10%:

Central nervous system: Drowsiness, insomnia

Endocrine & metabolic: Decreased sexual ability

1% to 10%:

Cardiovascular: Bradycardia, palpitations, edema, CHF, reduced peripheral circulation

Central nervous system: Mental depression

Gastrointestinal: Diarrhea or constipation, nausea, vomiting, stomach discomfort

Respiratory: Bronchospasm

Miscellaneous: Cold extremities

<1% (Limited to important or life-threatening): Arrhythmias, chest pain, confusion (especially in the elderly), depression, dyspnea, hallucinations, leukopenia, orthostatic hypotension, thrombocytopenia

Overdosage/Toxicology Symptoms of intoxication include cardiac disturbances, CNS toxicity, bronchospasm, hypoglycemia and hyperkalemia. The most common cardiac symptoms include hypotension and bradycardia. Atrioventricular block, intraventricular conduction disturbances, cardiogenic shock, and asystole may occur with severe overdose. CNS effects include convulsions, coma, and respiratory arrest. Treatment is symptom-directed and supportive. Glucagon has been used to reverse cardiac depression.

Pharmacodynamics/Kinetics

Absorption: 30% to 40%

Half-Life Elimination: Adults: 10-24 hours, prolonged with renal impairment; End-stage renal disease: 45 hours

Time to Peak: Serum: 2-4 hours

Duration: 17-24 hours

Formulations Tablet: 20 mg, 40 mg, 80 mg, 120 mg, 160 mg

Dosing

Adults: Hypertension, angina: Oral: Initial: 40-80 mg/day, increase dosage gradually by 40-80 mg increments at 3- to 7-day intervals until optimum clinical response is obtained with profound slowing of heart rate. Doses up to 160-240 mg/day in angina and 240-320 mg/day in hypertension may be necessary. Doses as high as 640 mg/day have been used.

Elderly: Oral: Initial: 20 mg/day; increase doses by 20 mg increments at 3- to 7-day intervals; usual dosage range: 20-240 mg/day. Adjust for renal impairment.

Renal Impairment:

Cl_{cr} 31-40 mL/minute: Administer every 24-36 hours or administer 50% of normal dose.

Cl_{cr} 10-30 mL/minute: Administer every 24-48 hours or administer 50% of normal dose.

Cl_{cr} <10 mL/minute: Administer every 40-60 hours or administer 25% of normal dose.

Hemodialysis effects: Moderately dialyzable (20% to 50%) via hemodialysis. Administer dose postdialysis or administer 40 mg supplemental dose. Supplemental dose is not necessary following peritoneal dialysis.

Hepatic Impairment: Reduced dose is probably necessary.

Monitoring and Teaching Issues

Physical Assessment: Assess other medications the patient may taking for effectiveness and interactions (see Drug Interactions). Assess blood pressure and heart rate prior to and following first dose, any change in dosage, and periodically thereafter. Monitor or advise patient to monitor weight and fluid balance, assess for signs of CHF, and assess therapeutic effectiveness. Monitor serum glucose levels of diabetic patients since beta-blockers may alter glucose tolerance. Use/teach postural hypotension precautions. **Pregnancy risk factor C** - benefits of use should outweigh possible risks. Note breast-feeding caution.

Patient Education: Check pulse daily prior to taking medication. If pulse is <50, hold medication and consult prescriber. Take exactly as directed; do not adjust dosage or discontinue without consulting prescriber. May cause dizziness, fatigue, blurred vision; change position slowly (lying/sitting to standing) and use caution when driving or engaging in tasks that require alertness until response to drug is known. Exercise and increasing bulk or fiber in diet may help resolve constipation. If diabetic, monitor serum glucose closely (the drug may mask symptoms of hypoglycemia). Report swelling in feet or legs, difficulty breathing or persistent cough, unresolved fatigue, unusual weight gain >5 lb/week, or unresolved constipation. **Pregnancy/breast-feeding precautions:** Inform prescriber if you are or intend to become pregnant. Consult prescriber if breast-feeding.

(Continued)

Nadolol *(Continued)*

Dietary Issues: May be taken without regard to meals.

Geriatric Considerations: Due to alterations in the beta-adrenergic autonomic nervous system, beta-adrenergic blockade may result in less hemodynamic response than seen in younger adults. Studies indicate that despite decreased sensitivity to the chronotropic effects of beta blockade with age, there appears to be an increased myocardial sensitivity to the negative inotropic effect during stress (eg, exercise). See Warnings/Precautions.

Breast-feeding Issues: Considered compatible by the AAP. However, monitor the infant for signs of beta-blockade (hypotension, bradycardia, etc) with long-term use.

Pregnancy Issues: Bradycardia, hypotension, hypoglycemia, respiratory depression, hypothermia, IUGR reported. IUGR probably related to maternal hypertension. Alternative beta-blockers are preferred for use during pregnancy due to limited data.

Related Information

Beta-Blockers *on page 1561*

Nafarelin (NAF a re lin)

U.S. Brand Names Synarel®

Synonyms Nafarelin Acetate

Generic Available No

Pharmacologic Category Hormone, Posterior Pituitary; Luteinizing Hormone-Releasing Hormone Analog

Pregnancy Risk Factor X

Lactation Enters breast milk/contraindicated

Use Treatment of endometriosis, including pain and reduction of lesions; treatment of central precocious puberty (gonadotropin-dependent precocious puberty) in children of both sexes

Mechanism of Action/Effect Potent synthetic decapeptide analogue of gonadotropin-releasing hormone (GnRH; LHRH) which is approximately 200 times more potent than GnRH in terms of pituitary release of luteinizing hormone (LH) and follicle-stimulating hormone (FSH)

Contraindications Hypersensitivity to GnRH, GnRH-agonist analogs, or any component of the formulation; undiagnosed abnormal vaginal bleeding; pregnancy

Warnings/Precautions Use with caution in patients with risk factors for decreased bone mineral content. Nafarelin therapy may pose an additional risk. Hypersensitivity reactions occur in 0.2% of the patients.

Adverse Reactions

>10%:

- Central nervous system: Headache, emotional lability
- Dermatologic: Acne
- Endocrine & metabolic: Hot flashes, breakthrough bleeding, spotting, menorrhagia, decreased libido, decreased breast size, amenorrhea, hypoestrogenism
- Genitourinary: Vaginal dryness
- Neuromuscular & skeletal: Myalgia
- Respiratory: Nasal irritation

1% to 10%:

- Cardiovascular: Edema, chest pain
- Central nervous system: Insomnia, mental depression
- Dermatologic: Urticaria, rash, pruritus, seborrhea
- Respiratory: Dyspnea, rhinitis

<1% (Limited to important or life-threatening): Libido increased, weight loss

Pharmacodynamics/Kinetics

Time to Peak: Serum: 10-45 minutes

Formulations Solution, intranasal spray, as acetate: 2 mg/mL (8 mL) [200 mcg/spray: 60 metered doses]

Dosing

Adults & Elderly: Endometriosis: Nasal: 1 spray (200 mcg) in 1 nostril each morning and the other nostril each evening starting on days 2-4 of menstrual cycle for 6 months

Pediatrics: Central precocious puberty: Nasal: 2 sprays (400 mcg) into each nostril in the morning 2 sprays (400 mcg) into each nostril in the evening. If inadequate suppression, may increase dose to 3 sprays (600 mcg) into alternating nostrils 3 times/day.

Administration

Inhalation: Nasal spray: Do not give to pregnant or breast-feeding patients. Do not use topical nasal decongestant for at least 30 minutes after nafarelin use.

Stability

Storage: Store at room temperature. Protect from light.

Monitoring and Teaching Issues

Physical Assessment: (For treatment of precocious puberty, consult appropriate pediatric reference.) See Contraindications, Warnings/Precautions, and Dosing for use cautions. Assess therapeutic effectiveness and adverse response (see Adverse Reactions and Overdose/Toxicology). Teach patient (caregiver) proper use (correct timing and administration of nasal spray), possible side effects and appropriate interventions, and adverse symptoms to report (see Patient Education). **Pregnancy risk factor X** - determine that female patient is not pregnant before beginning therapy. Do not give to childbearing age female unless capable of complying with barrier contraceptive use. Breast-feeding is contraindicated.

Patient Education: Endometriosis: You will begin this treatment between days 2-4 of your regular menstrual cycle. Use as directed - daily at the same time (arising and bedtime), and rotate nostrils. Maintain regular follow-up schedule. May cause hot flashes, flushing, or redness (cold clothes and cool environment may help); decreased or increased libido; emotional lability; weight gain; decreased breast size; or hirsutism. Report any breakthrough bleeding or continuing menstruation or musculoskeletal pain. Do not use a nasal decongestant within 30 minutes after nafarelin. **Pregnancy/breast-feeding precautions:** Inform prescriber if you are pregnant. Do not get pregnancy while taking this medication.

Consult prescriber for instruction on appropriate contraceptive measures. Consult prescriber if breast-feeding.

Additional Information Each spray delivers 200 mcg

Nafarelin Acetate *see* Nafarelin *on page 940*

Nafazair® *see page 1509*

Nafcillin (naf SIL in)

Synonyms Ethoxynaphthamido Penicillin Sodium; Nafcillin Sodium; Nallpen; Sodium Nafcillin

Generic Available Yes

Pharmacologic Category Antibiotic, Penicillin

Pregnancy Risk Factor B

Lactation Enters breast milk/use caution

Use Treatment of infections such as osteomyelitis, septicemia, endocarditis, and CNS infections caused by susceptible strains of staphylococci species

Mechanism of Action/Effect Interferes with bacterial cell wall synthesis during active multiplication, causing cell wall death and resultant bactericidal activity against susceptible bacteria

Contraindications Hypersensitivity to nafcillin, or any component of the formulation, or penicillins

Warnings/Precautions Extravasation of I.V. infusions should be avoided. Modification of dosage is necessary in patients with both severe renal and hepatic impairment. Elimination rate will be slow in neonates.

Drug Interactions

Cytochrome P450 Effect: Induces **CYP3A4**

Decreased Effect: Chloramphenicol may decrease nafcillin efficacy. If taken concomitantly with warfarin, nafcillin may inhibit the anticoagulant response to warfarin. This effect may persist for up to 30 days after nafcillin has been discontinued. Subtherapeutic cyclosporine levels may result when taken concomitantly with nafcillin. Although anecdotal reports suggest oral contraceptive efficacy could be reduced by penicillins, this has been refuted by more rigorous scientific and clinical data.

Increased Effect/Toxicity: Probenecid may cause an increase in nafcillin levels.

Effects on Lab Values Positive Coombs' test (direct)

Adverse Reactions Frequency not defined.

Central nervous system: Pain, fever

Dermatologic: Rash

Gastrointestinal: Nausea, diarrhea

Hematologic: Agranulocytosis, bone marrow depression, neutropenia

Local: Pain, swelling, inflammation, phlebitis, skin sloughing, and thrombophlebitis at the injection site; oxacillin (less likely to cause phlebitis) is often preferred in pediatric patients

Renal: Interstitial nephritis (acute)

Miscellaneous: Hypersensitivity reactions

Overdosage/Toxicology Symptoms of penicillin overdose include neuromuscular hypersensitivity (eg, agitation, hallucinations, asterixis, encephalopathy, confusion, and seizures). Electrolyte imbalance may occur if the preparation contains potassium or sodium salts, especially in renal failure. Treatment is supportive or symptom-directed.

Pharmacodynamics/Kinetics

Half-Life Elimination:

Neonates: <3 weeks: 2.2-5.5 hours; 4-9 weeks: 1.2-2.3 hours

Children 3 months to 14 years: 0.75-1.9 hours

Adults: Normal renal/hepatic function: 30 minutes to 1.5 hours

Time to Peak: Serum: I.M.: 30-60 minutes

Metabolism: Primarily hepatic; undergoes enterohepatic recirculation

Formulations

Infusion [premixed iso-osmotic dextrose solution]: 1 g (50 mL); 2 g (100 mL)

Injection, powder for reconstitution, as sodium: 1 g, 2 g, 10 g

Dosing

Adults & Elderly: Susceptible infections:

I.M.: 500 mg every 4-6 hours

I.V.: 500-2000 mg every 4-6 hours

Pediatrics:

Susceptible infections: Children:

I.M.: 25 mg/kg twice daily

I.V.:

Mild to moderate infections: 50-100 mg/kg/day in divided doses every 6 hours

Severe infections: 100-200 mg/kg/day in divided doses every 4-6 hours

Maximum dose: 12 g/day

Renal Impairment: No adjustment is necessary.

Hemodialysis effects: Not dialyzable (0% to 5%) via hemodialysis. Supplemental dose is not necessary with hemo- or peritoneal dialysis or continuous arteriovenous or venovenous hemofiltration.

Hepatic Impairment: In patients with both hepatic and renal impairment, modification of dosage may be necessary; no data available.

Administration

I.M.: Rotate injection sites.

I.V.: Vesicant. Administer around-the-clock to promote less variation in peak and trough serum levels. Infuse over 30-60 minutes.

Stability

Storage: Reconstituted parenteral solution is stable for 3 days at room temperature, 7 days when refrigerated, or 12 weeks when frozen. For I.V. infusion in NS or D_5W, solution is stable for 24 hours at room temperature and 96 hours when refrigerated.

Compatibility: Stable in dextran 40 10% in dextrose, D_5LR, $D_5{}^1/_4NS$, $D_5{}^1/_2NS$, D_5NS, D_5W, $D_{10}NS$, $D_{10}W$, LR, NS

(Continued)

Nafcillin *(Continued)*

Y-site administration: Incompatible with droperidol, fentanyl and droperidol, insulin (regular), labetalol, midazolam, nalbuphine, pentazocine, verapamil

Compatibility when admixed: Incompatible with ascorbic acid injection, aztreonam, bleomycin, cytarabine, gentamicin, hydrocortisone sodium succinate, methylprednisolone sodium succinate, promazine

Monitoring Laboratory Tests Perform culture and sensitivity studies prior to initiating drug therapy. Monitor renal, hepatic, CBC with prolonged therapy.

Monitoring and Teaching Issues

Physical Assessment: Assess for allergy history prior to starting therapy. See Contraindications and Warnings/Precautions for use cautions. Assess potential for interactions with other prescriptions, OTC medications, or herbal products patient may be taking (see Drug Interactions). Infusion/Injection site must be monitored closely to prevent extravasation (see Administration). Assess for therapeutic effect and adverse reactions (eg, opportunistic infection (eg, fever, chills, unhealed sores, white plaques in mouth or vagina, purulent vaginal discharge, fatigue) - see Adverse Reactions and Overdose/Toxicology). Teach patient possible side effects and interventions and adverse symptoms to report (see Patient Education). Note breast-feeding caution.

Patient Education: Inform prescriber of all prescriptions, OTC medications, or herbal products you are taking, and any allergies you have. Do not take anything new during treatment unless approved by prescriber. This medication can only be administered by infusion or injection. Report immediately any redness, swelling, burning, or pain at injection/infusion site; difficulty breathing or swallowing; chest pain; or rash. May cause nausea (small, frequent meals, frequent mouth care, chewing gum, or sucking lozenges may help); or opportunistic infection (eg, fever, chills, sore throat, burning urination, fatigue). Report persistent side effects or if condition does not respond to treatment. **Breast-feeding precaution:** Consult prescriber if breast-feeding.

Dietary Issues: Sodium content of 1 g: 76.6 mg (3.33 mEq)

Geriatric Considerations: Nafcillin has not been studied exclusively in the elderly, however, given its route of elimination, dosage adjustments based upon age and renal function are not necessary. Consider sodium content in patients who may be sensitive to volume expansion (ie, CHF).

Nafcillin Sodium *see* Nafcillin *on page 941*

$NaHCO_3$ *see* Sodium Bicarbonate *on page 1234*

Nalbuphine (NAL byoo feen)

U.S. Brand Names Nubain®

Synonyms Nalbuphine Hydrochloride

Generic Available Yes

Pharmacologic Category Analgesic, Narcotic

Pregnancy Risk Factor B/D (prolonged use or high doses at term)

Lactation Excretion in breast milk unknown/use caution

Use Relief of moderate to severe pain; preoperative analgesia, postoperative and surgical anesthesia, and obstetrical analgesia during labor and delivery

Mechanism of Action/Effect Binds to opiate receptors in the CNS, causing inhibition of ascending pain pathways, altering the perception of and response to pain; produces generalized CNS depression

Contraindications Hypersensitivity to nalbuphine or any component, including sulfites; pregnancy (prolonged use or high dosages at term)

Warnings/Precautions Use with caution in patients with recent myocardial infarction, biliary tract surgery, or sulfite sensitivity; may produce respiratory depression; use with caution in women delivering premature infants; use with caution in patients with a history of drug dependence, head trauma or increased intracranial pressure, decreased hepatic or renal function, or pregnancy; tolerance or drug dependence may result from extended use

Drug Interactions

Increased Effect/Toxicity: Barbiturate anesthetics may increase CNS depression.

Nutritional/Ethanol Interactions

Ethanol: Avoid ethanol (may increase CNS depression).

Herb/Nutraceutical: Avoid valerian, St John's wort, kava kava, gotu kola (may increase CNS depression).

Adverse Reactions

>10%:

Central nervous system: Fatigue, drowsiness

Miscellaneous: Histamine release

1% to 10%:

Cardiovascular: Hypotension

Central nervous system: Headache, nightmares, dizziness

Gastrointestinal: Anorexia, nausea, vomiting, dry mouth

Local: Pain at injection site

Neuromuscular & skeletal: Weakness

<1% (Limited to important or life-threatening): Bradycardia, dyspnea, hypertension, narcotic withdrawal, pulmonary edema, tachycardia

Overdosage/Toxicology Symptoms of overdose include CNS depression, respiratory depression, miosis, hypotension, and bradycardia. Treatment is symptomatic. Naloxone, 2 mg I.V. with repeat administration as necessary up to a total dose of 10 mg, can be used to reverse opiate effects.

Pharmacodynamics/Kinetics

Half-Life Elimination: 3.5-5 hours

Metabolism: Hepatic

Onset: Peak effect: I.M.: 30 minutes; I.V.: 1-3 minutes

Formulations Injection, solution, as hydrochloride: 10 mg/mL (1 mL, 10 mL); 20 mg/mL (1 mL, 10 mL)

Dosing

Adults: Analgesic: I.M., I.V., S.C.: 10 mg/70 kg every 3-6 hours; maximum single dose: 20 mg; maximum daily dose: 160 mg

Elderly: Refer to adult dosing; use with caution.

Pediatrics: I.M., I.V., S.C.: Children 10 months to 14 years: Premedication: 0.2 mg/kg; maximum: 20 mg/dose

Renal Impairment: Use with caution and reduce dose.

Hepatic Impairment: Use with caution and reduce dose.

Stability

Compatibility: Stable in D_5NS, $D_{10}W$, LR, NS

Y-site administration: Incompatible with allopurinol, amphotericin B cholesteryl sulfate complex, cefepime, docetaxel, methotrexate, nafcillin, piperacillin/tazobactam, sargramostim, sodium bicarbonate

Compatibility in syringe: Incompatible with diazepam, ketorolac, pentobarbital

Monitoring and Teaching Issues

Physical Assessment: Assess effectiveness and interactions of other medications patient may be taking (see Contraindications and Drug Interactions). Monitor therapeutic response (eg, pain relief) and adverse reactions at beginning of therapy and periodically throughout therapy (see Warnings/Precautions, Adverse Reactions, and Overdose/Toxicology). For inpatients, implement safety measures. Generally used in conjunction with surgical anesthesia or during labor and delivery; however, if self-administered for relief of pain, assess knowledge/teach patient appropriate use, adverse reactions to report (see Adverse Reactions), and appropriate interventions to reduce side effects (see Patient Education). **Pregnancy risk factor B/D** - see Pregnancy Risk Factor for use cautions. Note breast-feeding caution.

Patient Education: If self-administered, use exactly as directed; do not increase dose or frequency. Drug may cause physical and/or psychological dependence. While using this medication, do not use alcohol and other prescription or OTC medications (especially sedatives, tranquilizers, antihistamines, or pain medications) without consulting prescriber. Maintain adequate hydration (2-3 L/day of fluids) unless advised by prescriber to restrict fluids. May cause hypotension, dizziness, drowsiness, impaired coordination, or blurred vision (use caution when driving, climbing stairs, or changing position - rising from sitting or lying to standing, or when engaging in tasks requiring alertness until response to drug is known); loss of appetite, nausea, or vomiting (frequent mouth care, small, frequent meals, chewing gum, or sucking lozenges may help); or constipation (increased exercise, fluids, fruit, or fiber may help; if unresolved, consult prescriber about use of stool softeners). Report chest pain, slow or rapid heartbeat, acute dizziness or persistent headache; changes in mental status; swelling of extremities or unusual weight gain; changes in urinary elimination or pain on urination; acute headache; back or flank pain or muscle spasms; blurred vision; skin rash; or shortness of breath. **Pregnancy/breast-feeding precautions:** Inform prescriber if you are or intend to become pregnant. If you are breast-feeding, take medication immediately after breast-feeding or 3-4 hours prior to next feeding.

Geriatric Considerations: The elderly may be particularly susceptible to CNS effects; monitor closely.

Related Information

Compatibility of Drugs in Syringe *on page 1566*
Narcotic/Opioid Analgesic Comparison *on page 1583*

Nalbuphine Hydrochloride *see* Nalbuphine *on page 942*
Nalfon® *see* Fenoprofen *on page 550*
Nallpen *see* Nafcillin *on page 941*
***N*-allylnoroxymorphine Hydrochloride** *see* Naloxone *on page 944*

Nalmefene (NAL me feen)

U.S. Brand Names Revex®

Synonyms Nalmefene Hydrochloride

Generic Available No

Pharmacologic Category Antidote

Pregnancy Risk Factor B

Lactation Enters breast milk/use caution

Use Complete or partial reversal of opioid drug effects, including respiratory depression induced by natural or synthetic opioids; reversal of postoperative opioid depression; management of known or suspected opioid overdose

Mechanism of Action/Effect Nalmefene acts as a competitive antagonist at opioid receptor sites, preventing or reversing the respiratory depression, sedation, and hypotension induced by opiates; no pharmacologic activity of its own (eg, opioid agonist activity) has been demonstrated

Contraindications Hypersensitivity to nalmefene, naltrexone, or any component of the formulation

Warnings/Precautions May induce symptoms of acute withdrawal in opioid-dependent patients; recurrence of respiratory depression is possible if the opioid involved is long-acting; observe patients until there is no reasonable risk of recurrent respiratory depression. Safety and efficacy have not been established in children. Avoid abrupt reversal of opioid effects in patients of high cardiovascular risk or who have received potentially cardiotoxic drugs. Pulmonary edema and cardiovascular instability have been reported in association with abrupt reversal with other narcotic antagonists. Animal studies indicate nalmefene may not completely reverse buprenorphine-induced respiratory depression.

Drug Interactions

Increased Effect/Toxicity: Potential increased risk of seizures may exist with use of flumazenil and nalmefene coadministration.

Adverse Reactions

>10%: Gastrointestinal: Nausea

(Continued)

Nalmefene *(Continued)*

1% to 10%:
Cardiovascular: Tachycardia, hypertension, hypotension, vasodilation
Central nervous system: Fever, dizziness, headache, chills
Gastrointestinal: Vomiting
Miscellaneous: Postoperative pain

<1% (Limited to important or life-threatening): Agitation, arrhythmia, bradycardia, confusion, depression, diarrhea, myoclonus, nervousness, pharyngitis, pruritus, somnolence, tremor, urinary retention, xerostomia

Overdosage/Toxicology No reported symptoms with significant overdose. Large doses of opioids administered to overcome a full blockade of opioid antagonists, however, have resulted in adverse respiratory and circulatory reactions.

Pharmacodynamics/Kinetics

Bioavailability: I.M., I.V., S.C.: 100%

Half-Life Elimination: 10.8 hours

Time to Peak: Serum: I.M.: 2.3 hours; I.V.: <2 minutes; S.C.: 1.5 hours

Metabolism: Hepatic via glucuronide conjugation to metabolites with little or no activity

Onset: I.M., S.C.: 5-15 minutes

Formulations Injection, solution, as hydrochloride: 100 mcg/mL [blue label] (1 mL); 1000 mcg/mL [green label] (2 mL)

Dosing

Adults & Elderly:

Reversal of postoperative opioid depression: I.V.: Blue labeled product (100 mcg/mL): Titrate to reverse the undesired effects of opioids; initial dose for nonopioid dependent patient: 0.25 mcg/kg followed by 0.25 mcg/kg incremental doses at 2- to 5-minute intervals. After a total dose >1 mcg/kg, further therapeutic response is unlikely.

Management of known/suspected opioid overdose: I.V.: Green labeled product (1000 mcg/mL): Initial: 0.5 mg/70 kg; may repeat with 1 mg/70 kg in 2-5 minutes. Further increase beyond a total dose of 1.5 mg/70 kg will not likely result in improved response and may result in cardiovascular stress and precipitated withdrawal syndrome. (If opioid dependency is suspected, administer a challenge dose of 0.1 mg/70 kg; if no withdrawal symptoms are observed in 2 minutes, the recommended doses can be administered).

Note: If recurrence of respiratory depression is noted, dose may again be titrated to clinical effect using incremental doses.

Note: If I.V. access is lost or not readily obtainable, a single S.C. or I.M. dose of 1 mg may be effective in 5-15 minutes.

Renal Impairment: Not necessary with single uses, however, slow administration (over 60 seconds) of incremental doses is recommended to minimize hypertension and dizziness.

Hepatic Impairment: Not necessary with single uses, however, slow administration (over 60 seconds) of incremental doses is recommended to minimize hypertension and dizziness.

Administration

I.M.: If I.V. access is lost or not readily obtainable, a single S.C. or I.M. dose of 1 mg may be effective in 5-15 minutes.

I.V.: Slow administration (over 60 seconds) of incremental doses is recommended to minimize hypertension and dizziness.

Stability

Compatibility: Stable in D_5LR, $D_5{}^1/_2NS$, D_5W, LR, sodium bicarbonate 5%, $^1/_2NS$, NS

Monitoring and Teaching Issues

Physical Assessment: Assess patient for opioid dependency (see Warnings/Precautions). Monitor vital signs and cardiac status carefully during infusion and for some time thereafter (effects may continue for several days, use nonopioid analgesics for pain). Note breast-feeding caution.

Patient Education: This drug can only be administered I.V. You may experience drowsiness, dizziness, or blurred vision for several days; use caution when driving or engaging in tasks requiring alertness until response to drug is known. Small frequent meals and good mouth care may reduce any nausea or vomiting. Report yellowing of eyes or skin, unusual bleeding, dark or tarry stools, acute headache, or palpitations. **Breast-feeding precaution:** Wait 4 hours before breast-feeding.

Breast-feeding Issues: Limited information available; do not use in lactating women if possible.

Pregnancy Issues: Limited information available

Additional Information Proper steps should be used to prevent use of the incorrect dosage strength. The goal of treatment in the postoperative setting is to achieve reversal of excessive opioid effects without inducing a complete reversal and acute pain.

If opioid dependence is suspected, nalmefene should only be used in opioid overdose if the likelihood of overdose is high based on history or the clinical presentation of respiratory depression with concurrent pupillary constriction is present.

Nalmefene Hydrochloride *see* Nalmefene *on page 943*

Naloxone (nal OKS one)

U.S. Brand Names Narcan®

Synonyms *N*-allylnoroxymorphine Hydrochloride; Naloxone Hydrochloride

Generic Available Yes

Pharmacologic Category Antidote

Pregnancy Risk Factor C

Lactation Excretion in breast milk unknown/not recommended

Use

Complete or partial reversal of opioid depression, including respiratory depression, induced by natural and synthetic opioids, including propoxyphene, methadone, and certain mixed agonist-antagonist analgesics: nalbuphine, pentazocine, and butorphanol

Diagnosis of suspected opioid tolerance or acute opioid overdose

Adjunctive agent to increase blood pressure in the management of septic shock

Use - Unlabeled/Investigational PCP and ethanol ingestion

Mechanism of Action/Effect Pure opioid antagonist that competes and displaces narcotics at opioid receptor sites

Contraindications Hypersensitivity to naloxone or any component of the formulation

Warnings/Precautions Due to an association between naloxone and acute pulmonary edema, use with caution in patients with cardiovascular disease or in patients receiving medications with potential adverse cardiovascular effects (eg, hypotension, pulmonary edema or arrhythmias). Excessive dosages should be avoided after use of opiates in surgery. Abrupt postoperative reversal may result in nausea, vomiting, sweating, tachycardia, hypertension, seizures, and other cardiovascular events (including pulmonary edema and arrhythmias). May precipitate withdrawal symptoms in patients addicted to opiates, including pain, hypertension, sweating, agitation, irritability; in neonates: shrill cry, failure to feed. Recurrence of respiratory depression is possible if the opioid involved is long-acting; observe patients until there is no reasonable risk of recurrent respiratory depression. Pregnancy risk C.

Drug Interactions

Decreased Effect: Decreased effect of narcotic analgesics.

Adverse Reactions Frequency not defined.

Cardiovascular: Hypertension, hypotension, tachycardia, ventricular arrhythmias, cardiac arrest

Central nervous system: Irritability, anxiety, narcotic withdrawal, restlessness, seizures

Gastrointestinal: Nausea, vomiting, diarrhea

Neuromuscular & skeletal: Tremulousness

Respiratory: Dyspnea, pulmonary edema, runny nose, sneezing

Miscellaneous: Diaphoresis

Overdosage/Toxicology Naloxone is the drug of choice for respiratory depression that is known or suspected to be caused by overdose of an opiate or opioid. **Caution:** Naloxone's effects are due to its action on narcotic reversal, not due to any direct effect upon opiate receptors. Therefore, adverse events occur secondarily to reversal (withdrawal) of narcotic analgesia and sedation, which can cause severe reactions.

Pharmacodynamics/Kinetics

Half-Life Elimination: Neonates: 1.2-3 hours; Adults: 1-1.5 hours

Metabolism: Primarily hepatic via glucuronidation

Onset: Endotracheal, I.M., S.C.: 2-5 minutes; I.V.: ~2 minutes

Duration: 20-60 minutes; since shorter than that of most opioids, repeated doses are usually needed

Formulations

Injection, neonatal solution, as hydrochloride: 0.02 mg/mL (2 mL)

Injection, solution, as hydrochloride: 0.4 mg/mL (1 mL, 10 mL); 1 mg/mL (2 mL, 10 mL)

Dosing

Adults & Elderly: Narcotic overdose: I.M., I.V. (preferred), intratracheal, S.C.:

I.V.: 0.4-2 mg every 2-3 minutes as needed; may need to repeat doses every 20-60 minutes. If no response is observed after 10 mg, question the diagnosis. **Note:** Use 0.1-0.2 mg increments in patients who are opioid dependent and in postoperative patients to avoid large cardiovascular changes.

Continuous infusion: I.V.: If continuous infusion is required, calculate dosage/hour based on effective intermittent dose used and duration of adequate response seen, titrate dose 0.04-0.16 mg/kg/hour for 2-5 days in children, adult dose typically 0.25-6.25 mg/hour (short-term infusions as high as 2.4 mg/kg/hour have been tolerated in adults during treatment for septic shock); alternatively, continuous infusion utilizes $^2/_3$ of the initial naloxone bolus on an hourly basis; add 10 times this dose to each liter of D_5W and infuse at a rate of 100 mL/hour; $^1/_2$ of the initial bolus dose should be readministered 15 minutes after initiation of the continuous infusion to prevent a drop in naloxone levels; increase infusion rate as needed to assure adequate ventilation

Pediatrics:

Postanesthesia narcotic reversal: I.M., I.V. (preferred), intratracheal, S.C.: Infants and Children: 0.01 mg/kg; may repeat every 2-3 minutes as needed based on response

Narcotic overdose:

I.M., I.V. (preferred), intratracheal, S.C.:

Birth (including premature infants) to 5 years or <20 kg: 0.1 mg/kg; repeat every 2-3 minutes if needed; may need to repeat doses every 20-60 minutes

>5 years or ≥20 kg: 2 mg/dose; if no response, repeat every 2-3 minutes; may need to repeat doses every 20-60 minutes

Continuous infusion: I.V.: Refer to adult dosing.

Administration

I.V.:

I.V. push: Administer over 30 seconds as undiluted preparation

I.V. continuous infusion: Dilute to 4 mcg/mL in D_5W or normal saline

Other: Intratracheal: Dilute to 1-2 mL with normal saline

Stability

Storage: Store at 25°C (77°F). Protect from light.

Reconstitution: Stable in 0.9% sodium chloride and D_5W at 4 mcg/mL for 24 hours.

Compatibility: Stable in D_5W, NS

Y-site administration: Incompatible with amphotericin B cholesteryl sulfate complex

Monitoring and Teaching Issues

Physical Assessment: Assess patient for opioid dependency (see Warnings/Precautions). Monitor vital signs and cardiorespiratory status continuously during infusion, maintain patent airway. **Pregnancy risk factor C** - benefits of use should outweigh possible risks. Breast-feeding is not recommended.

(Continued)

Naloxone *(Continued)*

Patient Education: If patient is responsive, instructions are individualized. This drug can only be administered I.V. Report difficulty breathing, palpitations, or tremors. **Breast-feeding precaution:** Breast-feeding is not recommended.

Geriatric Considerations: In small trials, naloxone has shown temporary improvement in Alzheimer's disease; however, is not recommended for treatment.

Breast-feeding Issues: No data reported. Since naloxone is used for opiate reversal the concern should be on opiate drug levels in a breast-feeding mother and transfer to the infant rather than naloxone exposure. The safest approach would be **not** to breast-feed.

Pregnancy Issues: Consider benefit to the mother and the risk to the fetus before administering to a pregnant woman who is known or suspected to be opioid dependent. May precipitate withdrawal in both the mother and fetus.

Additional Information May contain methyl and propylparabens

Naloxone and Buprenorphine *see* Buprenorphine and Naloxone *on page 186*

Naloxone Hydrochloride *see* Naloxone *on page 944*

Naloxone Hydrochloride Dihydrate and Buprenorphine Hydrochloride *see* Buprenorphine and Naloxone *on page 186*

Naltrexone (nal TREKS one)

U.S. Brand Names ReVia®

Synonyms Naltrexone Hydrochloride

Generic Available Yes

Pharmacologic Category Antidote

Pregnancy Risk Factor C

Lactation Excretion in breast milk unknown

Use Treatment of ethanol dependence; blockade of the effects of exogenously administered opioids

Mechanism of Action/Effect Naltrexone (a pure opioid antagonist) is a cyclopropyl derivative of oxymorphone similar in structure to naloxone and nalorphine (a morphine derivative); it acts as a competitive antagonist at opioid receptor sites

Contraindications Hypersensitivity to naltrexone or any component of the formulation; narcotic dependence or current use of opioid analgesics; acute opioid withdrawal; failure to pass Narcan® challenge or positive urine screen for opioids; acute hepatitis; liver failure

Warnings/Precautions Dose-related hepatocellular injury is possible; the margin of separation between the apparent safe and hepatotoxic doses appear to be only fivefold or less. May precipitate withdrawal symptoms in patients addicted to opiates, including pain, hypertension, sweating, agitation, irritability; in neonates: shrill cry, failure to feed. Use with caution in patients with hepatic or renal impairment.

Patients who had been treated with naltrexone may respond to lower opioid doses than previously used. This could result in potentially life-threatening opioid intoxication. Patients should be aware that they may be more sensitive to lower doses of opioids after naltrexone treatment is discontinued. Use of naltrexone does not eliminate or diminish withdrawal symptoms.

Pregnancy risk C.

Drug Interactions

Decreased Effect: Naltrexone decreases effects of opioid-containing products.

Increased Effect/Toxicity: Lethargy and somnolence have been reported with the combination of naltrexone and thioridazine.

Adverse Reactions

>10%:

Central nervous system: Insomnia, nervousness, headache, low energy

Gastrointestinal: Abdominal cramping, nausea, vomiting

Neuromuscular & skeletal: Arthralgia

1% to 10%:

Central nervous system: Increased energy, feeling down, irritability, dizziness, anxiety, somnolence

Dermatologic: Rash

Endocrine & metabolic: Polydipsia

Gastrointestinal: Diarrhea, constipation

Genitourinary: Delayed ejaculation, impotency

<1% (Limited to important or life-threatening): Depression, disorientation, hallucinations, narcotic withdrawal, paranoia, restlessness, suicide attempts

Overdosage/Toxicology Symptoms of overdose include clonic-tonic convulsions and respiratory failure. Patients receiving up to 800 mg/day for 1 week have shown no toxicity. Seizures and respiratory failure have been seen in animals.

Pharmacodynamics/Kinetics

Absorption: Almost complete

Half-Life Elimination: 4 hours; 6-β-naltrexol: 13 hours

Time to Peak: Serum: ~60 minutes

Metabolism: Extensive first-pass effect to 6-β-naltrexol

Duration: 50 mg: 24 hours; 100 mg: 48 hours; 150 mg: 72 hours

Formulations Tablet, as hydrochloride: 50 mg

Dosing

Adults & Elderly: Opioid dependence or alcoholism (Do not give until patient is opioid-free for 7-10 days as required by urine analysis): Oral: 25 mg; if no withdrawal signs within 1 hour give another 25 mg; maintenance regimen is flexible, variable and individualized (50 mg/day to 100-150 mg 3 times/week).

Renal Impairment: Use caution.

Hepatic Impairment: Use caution. An increase in naltrexone AUC of approximately five- and tenfold in patients with compensated or decompensated liver cirrhosis respectively, compared with normal liver function has been reported.

Monitoring Laboratory Tests Periodic LFTs

Monitoring and Teaching Issues

Physical Assessment: Do not use until patient has been opioid-free for 7-10 days. Assess carefully for several days following start of therapy for narcotic withdrawal symptoms or severe adverse reactions (see Adverse Reactions). Use non-narcotic analgesics for pain. **Pregnancy risk factor C** - benefits should outweigh possible risks. Note breast-feeding caution.

Patient Education: This medication will help you achieve abstinence from opiates if taken as directed. Do not increase or change dose. Do not use opiates or any medications not approved by your prescriber during naltrexone therapy. You may experience drowsiness, dizziness, or blurred vision (use caution when driving or engaging in tasks requiring alertness until response to drug is known); nausea or vomiting (small, frequent meals, frequent mouth care, chewing gum, or sucking lozenges may help); or decreased sexual function (reversible when drug is discontinued). Report yellowing of skin or eyes, change in color of stool or urine, increased perspiration or chills, acute headache, palpitations, or unusual joint pain. **Pregnancy/breast-feeding precautions:** Inform prescriber if you are or intend to become pregnant. Consult prescriber if breast-feeding.

Naltrexone Hydrochloride *see* Naltrexone *on page 946*

Nandrolone (NAN droe lone)

U.S. Brand Names Deca-Durabolin® [DSC]

Synonyms Nandrolone Decanoate; Nandrolone Phenpropionate

Restrictions C-III

Generic Available Yes

Pharmacologic Category Androgen

Pregnancy Risk Factor X

Lactation Excretion in breast milk unknown/contraindicated

Use Control of metastatic breast cancer; management of anemia of renal insufficiency

Mechanism of Action/Effect Promotes tissue-building processes, increases production of erythropoietin, causes protein anabolism; increases hemoglobin and red blood cell volume

Contraindications Hypersensitivity to nandrolone or any component of the formulation; carcinoma of breast or prostate; nephrosis; pregnancy; not for use in infants

Warnings/Precautions Monitor diabetic patients carefully. Anabolic steroids may cause peliosis hepatis, liver cell tumors, and blood lipid changes with increased risk of arteriosclerosis. Use with caution in elderly patients, they may be at greater risk for prostatic hyperplasia. Use with caution in patients with cardiac, renal, or hepatic disease or epilepsy.

Drug Interactions

Increased Effect/Toxicity: Nandrolone may increase the effect of oral anticoagulants, insulin, oral hypoglycemic agents, adrenal steroids, or ACTH when taken together.

Effects on Lab Values Altered glucose tolerance tests

Adverse Reactions

Male: Postpubertal:

>10%:

Dermatologic: Acne
Endocrine & metabolic: Gynecomastia
Genitourinary: Bladder irritability, priapism

1% to 10%:

Central nervous system: Insomnia, chills
Endocrine & metabolic: Decreased libido, hepatic dysfunction,
Gastrointestinal: Nausea, diarrhea
Genitourinary: Prostatic hyperplasia (elderly)
Hematologic: Iron-deficiency anemia, suppression of clotting factors

<1% (Limited to important or life-threatening): Hepatic necrosis, hepatocellular carcinoma

Male: Prepubertal:

>10%:

Dermatologic: Acne
Endocrine & metabolic: Virilism

1% to 10%:

Central nervous system: Chills, insomnia, factors
Dermatologic: Hyperpigmentation
Gastrointestinal: Diarrhea, nausea
Hematologic: Iron deficiency anemia, suppression of clotting

<1% (Limited to important or life-threatening): Hepatocellular carcinoma, necrosis

Female:

>10%: Endocrine & metabolic: Virilism

1% to 10%:

Central nervous system: Chills, insomnia
Endocrine & metabolic: Hypercalcemia
Gastrointestinal: Nausea, diarrhea
Hematologic: Iron deficiency anemia, suppression of clotting factors
Hepatic: Hepatic dysfunction

<1% (Limited to important or life-threatening): Hepatic necrosis, hepatocellular carcinoma

Pharmacodynamics/Kinetics

Absorption: I.M.: 77%

Metabolism: Hepatic

Onset: 3-6 months

Duration: Up to 30 days

Formulations Injection, solution, as decanoate [in sesame oil]: 100 mg/mL (2 mL); 200 mg/mL (1 mL) [contains benzyl alcohol]

(Continued)

Nandrolone *(Continued)*

Dosing

Adults & Elderly:

Breast cancer, male/female (phenpropionate): I.M.: 50-100 mg/week

Anemia of renal insufficiency (decanoate): I.M.:

Male: 100-200 mg/week

Female: 50-100 mg/week

Note: Deep I.M. (into gluteal muscle):

Pediatrics: Deep I.M. (into gluteal muscle): Children 2-13 years (decanoate): 25-50 mg every 3-4 weeks

Administration

I.M.: Inject deeply I.M., preferably into the gluteal muscle.

Monitoring Laboratory Tests LFTs on a regular basis

Monitoring and Teaching Issues

Physical Assessment: See Contraindications, Warnings/Precautions, and Dosing for use cautions. Assess potential for interactions with other prescriptions, OTC medications, or herbal products patient may be taking (see Drug Interactions). Assess results of laboratory tests (see above), therapeutic effectiveness (according to purpose of use), and adverse response (see Adverse Reactions and Overdose/Toxicology). Caution diabetic patients to monitor serum glucose closely (may increase the effect of insulin and oral hypoglycemic agents). Teach patient possible side effects and appropriate interventions and adverse symptoms to report (eg, adverse reactions may differ according to age/gender of patient - see Patient Education). **Pregnancy risk factor X** - determine that patient is not pregnant before starting therapy. Do not give to females of childbearing age unless patient is capable of complying with barrier contraceptive use. Breast-feeding is contraindicated.

Patient Education: Inform prescriber of all prescriptions, OTC medications, or herbal products you are taking, and any allergies you have. Do not take anything new during treatment unless approved by prescriber. This drug can only be given injection. Report immediately any redness, swelling, burning, or pain at injection site. If diabetic, monitor serum glucose closely and notify prescriber of significant changes (nandrolone may increase the effect of insulin and oral hypoglycemic agents). May cause nausea or vomiting (small, frequent meals, frequent mouth care, sucking lozenges, or chewing gum may help); diarrhea (buttermilk, boiled milk, yogurt may help). **Male:** acne, swelling of breasts, loss of libido, impotence. **Female:** virilism, menstrual irregularity (usually reversible). Report changes in menstrual pattern; enlarged or painful breasts; deepening of voice or unusual growth of body hair; fluid retention (eg, swelling of ankles, feet, or hands, difficulty breathing, or sudden weight gain); bladder irritability; unresolved CNS changes (eg, nervousness, chills, insomnia); change in color of urine or stool; yellowing of eyes or skin; unusual bruising or bleeding; or other adverse reactions. **Pregnancy/breast-feeding precautions:** Inform prescriber if you are pregnant. Do not get pregnant during or for 1 month following therapy. Consult prescriber for instruction on appropriate contraceptive measures. This drug may cause severe fetal defects. Do not breast-feed.

Additional Information Both phenpropionate and decanoate are injections in oil.

Related Information

Controlled Substances Comparison *on page 1568*

Nandrolone Decanoate *see* Nandrolone *on page 947*

Nandrolone Phenpropionate *see* Nandrolone *on page 947*

Naphazoline *see page 1509*

Naphazoline and Antazoline *see page 1509*

Naphazoline and Pheniramine *see page 1509*

Naphcon-A® [OTC] *see page 1509*

Naphcon Forte® *see page 1509*

Naprelan® *see* Naproxen *on page 948*

Naprosyn® *see* Naproxen *on page 948*

Naproxen (na PROKS en)

U.S. Brand Names Aleve® [OTC]; Anaprox®; Anaprox® DS; EC-Naprosyn®; Naprelan®; Naprosyn®

Synonyms Naproxen Sodium

Generic Available Yes

Pharmacologic Category Nonsteroidal Anti-inflammatory Drug (NSAID)

Pregnancy Risk Factor B/D (3rd trimester)

Lactation Enters breast milk/compatible

Use Management of inflammatory disease and rheumatoid disorders (including juvenile rheumatoid arthritis); acute gout; mild to moderate pain; dysmenorrhea; fever, migraine headache

Mechanism of Action/Effect Inhibits prostaglandin synthesis by decreasing the activity of the enzyme, cyclooxygenase, which results in decreased formation of prostaglandin precursors

Contraindications Hypersensitivity to naproxen, aspirin, other NSAIDs, or any component of the formulation; pregnancy (3rd trimester)

Warnings/Precautions Use with caution in patients with GI disease (bleeding or ulcers), cardiovascular disease (CHF, hypertension), dehydration, renal or hepatic impairment, and patients receiving anticoagulants. Perform ophthalmologic evaluation for those who develop eye complaints during therapy (blurred vision, diminished vision, changes in color vision, retinal changes); NSAIDs may mask signs/symptoms of infections; photosensitivity reported. Elderly are at a high risk for adverse effects (including gastrointestinal and CNS adverse effects) from NSAIDs. As many as 60% of elderly can develop peptic ulceration and/or hemorrhage asymptomatically.

Use lowest effective dose for shortest period possible. Use of NSAIDs can compromise existing renal function especially when Cl_{cr} is <30 mL/minute. Withhold for at least 4-6 half-lives prior to surgical or dental procedures.

Pregnancy risk B/D (3rd trimester).

Drug Interactions

Cytochrome P450 Effect: Substrate of CYP1A2, 2C8/9

Decreased Effect: NSAIDs may decrease the effect of some antihypertensive agents, including ACE inhibitors, angiotensin receptor antagonists, and hydralazine. The efficacy of diuretics (loop and/or thiazide) may be decreased.

Increased Effect/Toxicity: Naproxen could displace other highly protein-bound drugs, increasing the effect of oral anticoagulants, hydantoins, salicylates, sulfonamides, and first-generation sulfonylureas. Naproxen and warfarin may cause a slight increase in free warfarin. Naproxen and probenecid may cause increased levels of naproxen. Naproxen and methotrexate may significantly increase and prolong blood methotrexate concentration, which may be severe or fatal. May increase lithium or cyclosporine levels. Corticosteroids may increase risk of GI ulceration.

Nutritional/Ethanol Interactions

Ethanol: Avoid or limit ethanol (may enhance gastric mucosal irritation).

Food: Naproxen absorption rate may be decreased if taken with food.

Herb/Nutraceutical: Avoid cat's claw, dong quai, evening primrose, feverfew, garlic, ginger, ginkgo, red clover, horse chestnut, green tea, ginseng (all have additional antiplatelet activity).

Effects on Lab Values ↑ chloride (S), sodium (S), bleeding time

Adverse Reactions

1% to 10%:

Central nervous system: Headache (11%), nervousness, malaise (<3%), somnolence (3% to 9%)

Dermatologic: Itching, pruritus, rash, ecchymosis (3% to 9%)

Endocrine & metabolic: Fluid retention (3% to 9%)

Gastrointestinal: Abdominal discomfort, nausea (3% to 9%), heartburn, constipation (3% to 9%), GI bleeding, ulcers, perforation, indigestion, diarrhea (<3%), abdominal distress/cramps/pain (3% to 9%), dyspepsia (<3%), stomatitis (<3%), heartburn (<3%)

Hematologic: Hemolysis (3% to 9%), ecchymosis (3% to 9%)

Otic: Tinnitus (3% to 9%)

Respiratory: Dyspnea (3% to 9%)

<1% (Limited to important or life-threatening): Acute renal failure, agranulocytosis, allergic rhinitis, anemia, angioedema, arrhythmias, aseptic meningitis, bone marrow suppression, bronchospasm, CHF, erythema multiforme, GI ulceration, hallucinations, hemolytic anemia, hepatitis, hypertension, leukopenia, mental depression, peripheral neuropathy, renal dysfunction, Stevens-Johnson syndrome, thrombocytopenia, toxic amblyopia, toxic epidermal necrolysis, urticaria, vomiting

Overdosage/Toxicology Symptoms of overdose include drowsiness, heartburn, vomiting, CNS depression, leukocytosis, and renal failure. Management is supportive and symptomatic. Seizures tend to be very short-lived and often do not require drug treatment.

Pharmacodynamics/Kinetics

Absorption: Almost 100%

Half-Life Elimination: Normal renal function: 12-15 hours; End-stage renal disease: Unchanged

Time to Peak: Serum: 1-2 hours

Onset: Analgesic: 1 hour; Anti-inflammatory: ~2 weeks; Peak effect: Anti-inflammatory: 2-4 weeks

Duration: Analgesic: ≤7 hours; Anti-inflammatory: ≤12 hours

Formulations

Caplet, as sodium (Aleve®): 220 mg [equivalent to naproxen 200 mg and sodium 20 mg]

Gelcap, as sodium (Aleve®): 220 mg [equivalent to naproxen 200 mg and sodium 20 mg]

Suspension, oral (Naprosyn®): 125 mg/5 mL (480 mL) [contains sodium 0.3 mEq/mL; orange-pineapple flavor]

Tablet (Naprosyn®): 250 mg, 375 mg, 500 mg

Tablet, as sodium: 220 mg [equivalent to naproxen 200 mg and sodium 20 mg]; 275 mg [equivalent to naproxen 250 mg and sodium 25 mg]; 550 mg [equivalent to naproxen 500 mg and sodium 50 mg]

Aleve®: 220 mg [equivalent to naproxen 200 mg and sodium 20 mg]

Anaprox®: 275 mg [equivalent to naproxen 250 mg and sodium 25 mg]

Anaprox® DS: 550 mg [equivalent to naproxen 500 mg and sodium 50 mg]

Tablet, controlled release, as sodium: 550 mg [equivalent to naproxen 500 mg and sodium 50 mg]

Naprelan®: 421.5 mg [equivalent to naproxen 375 mg and sodium 37.5 mg]; 550 mg [equivalent to naproxen 500 mg and sodium 50 mg]

Tablet, delayed release (EC-Naprosyn®): 375 mg, 500 mg

Dosing

Adults:

Rheumatoid arthritis, osteoarthritis, and ankylosing spondylitis: 500-1000 mg/day in 2 divided doses; may increase to 1.5 g/day of naproxen base for limited time period

Mild to moderate pain or dysmenorrhea: Oral: Initial: 500 mg, then 250 mg every 6-8 hours; maximum: 1250 mg/day naproxen base

Elderly: Refer to adult dosing and Geriatric Considerations.

Pediatrics:

Fever: Oral: Children >2 years: 2.5-10 mg/kg/dose; maximum: 10 mg/kg/day

Juvenile arthritis: Oral: Children >2 years: 10 mg/kg/day in 2 divided doses

Hepatic Impairment: Reduce dose to 50%.

Administration

Oral: Suspension: Shake well before administration. Administer with food, milk, or antacids to decrease GI adverse effects.

Monitoring Laboratory Tests Periodic liver function, CBC, BUN, serum creatinine

(Continued)

Naproxen *(Continued)*

Monitoring and Teaching Issues

Physical Assessment: Assess effectiveness and interactions of other medications patient may be taking (see Contraindications and Drug Interactions). Monitor laboratory tests (see above), therapeutic response, and adverse reactions (eg, GI effects, hepatotoxicity, or ototoxicity) at beginning of therapy and periodically throughout therapy (see Warnings/Precautions, Adverse Reactions, and Overdose/Toxicology). Schedule ophthalmic evaluations for patients who develop eye complaints during long-term NSAID therapy (see Warnings/Precautions). Assess knowledge/teach patient appropriate use, interventions to reduce side effects, and adverse symptoms to report (see Patient Education). **Pregnancy risk factor B/D** - see Pregnancy Risk Factor for use cautions.

Patient Education: Take this medication exactly as directed; do not increase dose without consulting prescriber. Do not crush tablets. Take with food or milk to reduce GI distress. Maintain adequate hydration (2-3 L/day of fluids) unless advised by prescriber to restrict fluids. Do not use alcohol, aspirin or aspirin-containing medication, or any other anti-inflammatory medications without consulting prescriber. You may experience drowsiness, dizziness, lightheadedness, or headache (use caution when driving or engaging in tasks requiring alertness until response to drug is known); anorexia, nausea, vomiting, or heartburn (small, frequent meals, frequent mouth care, sucking lozenges, or chewing gum may help); or fluid retention (weigh yourself weekly and report unusual (3-5 lb/week) weight gain). GI bleeding, ulceration, or perforation can occur with or without pain; or discontinue medication and contact prescriber if persistent abdominal pain or cramping, or blood in stool occurs. Report breathlessness, difficulty breathing, or unusual cough; chest pain, rapid heartbeat, palpitations; unusual bruising/bleeding; blood in urine, stool, mouth, or vomitus; swollen extremities; skin rash or itching; acute fatigue; or changes in eyesight (double vision, color changes, blurred vision), hearing, or ringing in ears. **Pregnancy/breast-feeding precautions:** Notify prescriber if you are or intend to become pregnant. Do not take this drug during last trimester of pregnancy.

Dietary Issues: Drug may cause GI upset, bleeding, ulceration, perforation; take with food or milk to minimize GI upset.

Geriatric Considerations: Elderly are at high risk for adverse effects from NSAIDs. As much as 60% of elderly can develop peptic ulceration and/or hemorrhage asymptomatically. The concomitant use of H_2 blockers, omeprazole, and sucralfate is not effective as prophylaxis with the exception of NSAID-induced duodenal ulcers which may be prevented by the use of ranitidine. Misoprostol is the only prophylactic agent proven effective. Also, concomitant disease and drug use contribute to the risk for GI adverse effects. Use lowest effective dose for shortest period possible. Consider renal function decline with age. Use of NSAIDs can compromise existing renal function especially when Cl_{cr} is ≤30 mL/minute. Tinnitus may be a difficult and unreliable indication of toxicity due to age-related hearing loss or eighth cranial nerve damage. CNS adverse effects such as confusion, agitation, and hallucination are generally seen in overdose or high-dose situations, but elderly may demonstrate these adverse effects at lower doses than younger adults.

Additional Information Naproxen: Naprosyn®; naproxen sodium: Anaprox®; 275 mg of Anaprox® equivalent to 250 mg of Naprosyn®

Related Information

Nonsalicylate/Nonsteroidal Anti-inflammatory Comparison *on page 1587*

Naproxen Sodium *see* Naproxen *on page 948*

Naratriptan (NAR a trip tan)

U.S. Brand Names Amerge®

Synonyms Naratriptan Hydrochloride

Generic Available No

Pharmacologic Category Serotonin 5-HT_{1D} Receptor Agonist

Pregnancy Risk Factor C

Lactation Excretion in breast milk unknown/not recommended

Use Treatment of acute migraine headache with or without aura

Mechanism of Action/Effect The therapeutic effect for migraine is due to serotonin agonist activity.

Contraindications Hypersensitivity to naratriptan or any component of the formulation; cerebrovascular, peripheral vascular disease (ischemic bowel disease), ischemic heart disease (angina pectoris, history of myocardial infarction, or proven silent ischemia); or in patients with symptoms consistent with ischemic heart disease, coronary artery vasospasm, or Prinzmetal's angina; uncontrolled hypertension or patients who have received within 24 hours another 5-HT agonist (sumatriptan, zolmitriptan) or ergotamine-containing product; patients with known risk factors associated with coronary artery disease; patients with severe hepatic or renal disease (Cl_{cr} <15 mL/minute); do not administer naratriptan to patients with hemiplegic or basilar migraine

Warnings/Precautions Use only if there is a clear diagnosis of migraine. Patients who are at risk of CAD but have had a satisfactory cardiovascular evaluation may receive naratriptan but with extreme caution (ie, in a physician's office where there are adequate precautions in place to protect the patient). Blood pressure may increase with the administration of naratriptan. Monitor closely, especially with the first administration of the drug. If the patient does not respond to the first dose, re-evaluate the diagnosis of migraine before trying a second dose. Pregnancy risk C.

Drug Interactions

Decreased Effect: Smoking increases the clearance of naratriptan.

Increased Effect/Toxicity: Ergot-containing drugs (dihydroergotamine or methysergide) may cause vasospastic reactions when taken with naratriptan. Avoid concomitant use with ergots; separate dose of naratriptan and ergots by at least 24 hours. Oral contraceptives taken with naratriptan reduced the clearance of naratriptan ~30% which may contribute to adverse effects. Selective serotonin reuptake inhibitors (SSRIs) (eg, fluoxetine, fluvoxamine, paroxetine, sertraline) may cause lack of coordination, hyper-reflexia, or weakness and should be avoided when taking naratriptan.

Adverse Reactions

1% to 10%:

Central nervous system: Dizziness, drowsiness, malaise/fatigue

Gastrointestinal: Nausea, vomiting

Neuromuscular & skeletal: Paresthesias

Miscellaneous: Pain or pressure in throat or neck

<1% (Limited to important or life-threatening): Allergic reaction, atrial fibrillation, atrial flutter, coronary artery vasospasm, hallucinations, myocardial infarction, PR prolongation, premature ventricular contractions, QT_c prolongation, seizure, ventricular fibrillation, ventricular tachycardia

Pharmacodynamics/Kinetics

Absorption: Well absorbed

Bioavailability: 70%

Time to Peak: 2-3 hours

Metabolism: Hepatic via CYP

Onset: 30 minutes

Formulations Tablet: 1 mg, 2.5 mg

Dosing

Adults: Migraine: Oral: 1 mg to 2.5 mg at the onset of headache. It is recommended to use the lowest possible dose to minimize adverse effects. If headache returns or dose not fully resolve, the dose may be repeated after 4 hours. Do not exceed 5 mg in 24 hours.

Elderly: Not recommended for use in the elderly.

Renal Impairment:

Cl_{cr}: 18-39 mL/minute: Initial: 1 mg; do not exceed 2.5 mg in 24 hours.

Cl_{cr}: <15 mL/minute: Do not use.

Hepatic Impairment: Contraindicated in patients with severe liver failure. The maximum dose is 2.5 mg in 24 hours for patients with mild or moderate liver failure. The recommended starting dose is 1 mg.

Administration

Oral: Do **not** crush or chew tablet; swallow whole with water.

Monitoring and Teaching Issues

Physical Assessment: See Contraindications, Warnings/Precautions (clear diagnosis of migraine), and Dosing for use cautions. Assess potential for interactions with other prescriptions, OTC medications, or herbal products patient may be taking (eg, oral contraceptives - see Drug Interactions). Assess therapeutic effectiveness and adverse response (see Adverse Reactions and Overdose/Toxicology). Teach patient proper use, possible side effects and appropriate interventions, and adverse symptoms to report (see Patient Education). **Pregnancy risk factor C** - benefits of use should outweigh possible risks. Breast-feeding is not recommended.

Patient Education: Inform prescriber of all prescriptions, OTC medications, or herbal products you are taking, and any allergies you have. Do not take anything new during treatment unless approved by prescriber. This drug is to be used to reduce your migraine, not to prevent or reduce the number of attacks. If headache returns or is not fully resolved, the dose may be repeated after 4 hours. If you have no relief with first dose, do not take a second dose without consulting prescriber. **Do not exceed 5 mg in 24 hours. Do not take within 24 hours of any other migraine medication without first consulting prescriber.** May cause dizziness, fatigue, or drowsiness (use caution when driving or engaging in tasks that require alertness until response to drug is known); or nausea or vomiting (small, frequent meals, frequent mouth care, chewing gum, or sucking lozenges may help). Report immediately any chest pain, palpitations, or rapid heartbeat; tightness in throat or neck; or rash, itching, or hives. **Pregnancy/breast-feeding precautions:** Inform prescriber if you are or intend to become pregnant. Consult prescriber if breast-feeding.

Geriatric Considerations: Naratriptan was not studied in patients >65 years of age. Use in elderly patients is not recommended because of the presence of risk factors associated with adverse effects. These include the presence of coronary artery disease, decreased liver or renal function, and the risk of pronounced blood pressure increases.

Related Information

Antimigraine Drugs *on page 1557*

Naratriptan Hydrochloride *see* Naratriptan *on page 950*

Narcan® *see* Naloxone *on page 944*

Narcotic/Opioid Analgesic Comparison *see page 1583*

Nardil® *see* Phenelzine *on page 1065*

Nasacort® *see* Triamcinolone *on page 1356*

Nasacort® AQ *see* Triamcinolone *on page 1356*

Nasalcrom® [OTC] *see* Cromolyn Sodium *on page 334*

Nasalide® *see* Flunisolide *on page 572*

Nasarel® *see* Flunisolide *on page 572*

Nascobal® *see* Cyanocobalamin *on page 337*

Nasonex® *see* Topical Corticosteroids *on page 1334*

Natagrelide *see page 1661*

Nateglinide (na TEG li nide)

U.S. Brand Names Starlix®

Generic Available No

Pharmacologic Category Antidiabetic Agent, Miscellaneous

Pregnancy Risk Factor C

Lactation Excretion in breast milk unknown/not recommended

(Continued)

Nateglinide *(Continued)*

Use Management of type 2 diabetes mellitus (noninsulin dependent, NIDDM) as monotherapy when hyperglycemia cannot be managed by diet and exercise alone; in combination with metformin to lower blood glucose in patients whose hyperglycemia cannot be controlled by exercise, diet, and metformin alone.

Mechanism of Action/Effect Increases insulin release from pancreatic beta cells; decreases postprandial hyperglycemia; not a sulfonylurea

Contraindications Hypersensitivity to nateglinide or any component of the formulation; diabetic ketoacidosis, with or without coma (treat with insulin); type 1 diabetes mellitus (insulin dependent, IDDM); patients not adequately controlled on oral agents which stimulate insulin release (eg, glyburide)

Warnings/Precautions Use with caution in patients with moderate to severe hepatic impairment. All oral hypoglycemic agents are capable of producing hypoglycemia. Proper patient selection, dosage, and instructions to the patients are important to avoid hypoglycemic episodes. It may be necessary to discontinue nateglinide and administer insulin if the patient is exposed to stress (ie, fever, trauma, infection, surgery). Indicated for adjunctive therapy with metformin; not to be used as a substitute for metformin monotherapy. Combination treatment with sulfonylureas is not recommended (no additional benefit). Safety and efficacy in pediatric patients have not been established. Pregnancy risk C.

Drug Interactions

Cytochrome P450 Effect: Substrate of **CYP2C8/9, 3A4**; Inhibits CYP2C8/9

Decreased Effect: Decreased hypoglycemic effect: Possible decreased hypoglycemic effect may be seen with thiazides, corticosteroids, thyroid products, and sympathomimetic drugs. Monitor glucose closely when agents are initiated, modified, or discontinued.

Increased Effect/Toxicity: Increased hypoglycemic effect: Possible increased hypoglycemic effect may be seen with NSAIDs, salicylates, MAO inhibitors, and nonselective beta-adrenergic blocking agents. Monitor glucose closely when agents are initiated, modified, or discontinued. Drugs which are highly protein bound may increase effect (theoretical, *in vitro* studies have not documented this effect)

Nutritional/Ethanol Interactions

Ethanol: Avoid ethanol (increased risk of hypoglycemia).

Food: Rate of absorption is decreased and time to T_{max} is delayed when taken with food. Food does not affect AUC. Multiple peak plasma concentrations may be observed if fasting. Not affected by composition of meal.

Adverse Reactions As reported with nateglinide monotherapy:

1% to 10%:

Central nervous system: Dizziness (4%)
Endocrine & metabolic: Hypoglycemia (2%), increased uric acid
Gastrointestinal: Weight gain
Neuromuscular & skeletal: Arthropathy (3%)
Respiratory: Upper respiratory infection (10%)
Miscellaneous: Flu-like symptoms (4%)

Overdosage/Toxicology In case of overdose, hypoglycemic symptoms would be expected. Severe hypoglycemic reactions should be treated with intravenous glucose. Dialysis is not effective.

Pharmacodynamics/Kinetics

Absorption: Rapid

Bioavailability: 73%

Half-Life Elimination: 1.5 hours

Time to Peak: ≤1 hour

Metabolism: Hepatic via hydroxylation followed by glucuronide conjugation via CYP2C9 (70%) and CYP3A4 (30%) to metabolites

Onset: Insulin secretion: ~20 minutes; Peak effect: 1 hour

Duration: 4 hours

Formulations Tablet: 60 mg, 120 mg

Dosing

Adults: Management of type 2 diabetes mellitus: Oral: Initial and maintenance dose: 120 mg 3 times/day, 1-30 minutes before meals; may be given alone or in combination with metformin; patients close to Hb A_{1c} goal may be started at 60 mg 3 times/day

Elderly: No changes in safety and efficacy were seen in patients ≥65 years; however, some elderly patients may show increased sensitivity to dosing,

Renal Impairment: No specific dosage adjustment is recommended for patients with mild to severe renal disease. Patients on dialysis showed reduced medication exposure and plasma protein binding.

Hepatic Impairment: Increased serum levels are seen with mild hepatic insufficiency; no dosage adjustment is needed. Has not been studied in patients with moderate to severe liver disease; use with caution.

Stability

Storage: Store at 25°C (77°F).

Monitoring Laboratory Tests Glucose and Hb A_{1c} levels, weight, lipid profile

Monitoring and Teaching Issues

Physical Assessment: See Contraindications, Warnings/Precautions, and Dosing for use cautions. Assess potential for interactions with other prescriptions, OTC medications, or herbal products patient may be taking (see Drug Interactions). Assess results of laboratory tests (see above), therapeutic effects, and adverse response (see Adverse Reactions and Overdose/Toxicology) on a regular basis throughout therapy. Teach patient proper use (or refer patient to diabetic educator), possible side effects and appropriate interventions (eg, importance of adequate hydration), and adverse symptoms to report (see Patient Education). **Pregnancy risk factor C** - benefits of use should outweigh possible risks. Breast-feeding is not recommended.

Patient Education: Inform prescriber of all prescriptions, OTC medications, or herbal products you are taking, and any allergies you have. Do not take anything new during

treatment unless approved by prescriber. Take this medication exactly as directed, 1-30 minutes before a meal. If you skip a meal (or add an extra meal) skip (or add) a dose for that meal. Do not change dosage or discontinue without first consulting prescriber. Follow dietary and lifestyle recommendations of provider. You will be instructed in signs of hypo- or hyperglycemia by healthcare provide or diabetic educator; be alert for adverse hypoglycemia (tachycardia, profuse perspiration, tingling of lips and tongue, seizures, or change in sensorium) and follow prescriber's instructions for intervention. Note that unusual strenuous exercise, excessive alcohol intake, or acute reduction in caloric intake may increase risk of hypoglycemia. Persistent nausea or vomiting, or severely decreased dietary intake may increase risk of hyperglycemia. May cause mild side effects during first weeks of therapy (dizziness, weight gain, mild muscle aches or pain, or flu-like symptoms); if these do not diminish, notify prescriber. Report signs of respiratory infection or other persistent adverse effects. **Pregnancy/breast-feeding precautions:** Inform prescriber if you are or intend to become pregnant. Breast-feeding is not recommended.

Dietary Issues: Nateglinide should be taken 1-30 minutes prior to meals. Scheduled dose should not be taken if meal is missed. Dietary modification based on ADA recommendations is a part of therapy. Decreases blood glucose concentration. Hypoglycemia may occur. Must be able to recognize symptoms of hypoglycemia (palpitations, sweaty palms, lightheadedness).

Pregnancy Issues: Safety and efficacy in pregnant women have not been established. Do not use during pregnancy. Abnormal blood glucose levels are associated with a higher incidence of congenital abnormalities. Insulin is the drug of choice for the control of diabetes mellitus during pregnancy.

Additional Information An increase in weight was seen in nateglinide monotherapy, which was not seen when used in combination with metformin.

Natrecor® *see* Nesiritide *on page 962*
Natriuretic Peptide *see* Nesiritide *on page 962*
Nature-Throid® NT *see* Thyroid *on page 1313*
Navane® *see* Thiothixene *on page 1311*
Navelbine® *see* Vinorelbine *on page 1403*
Nebcin® *see* Tobramycin *on page 1329*
NebuPent™ *see* Pentamidine *on page 1049*
Necon® 0.5/35 *see* Ethinyl Estradiol and Norethindrone *on page 527*
Necon® 1/35 *see* Ethinyl Estradiol and Norethindrone *on page 527*
Necon® 1/50 *see* Mestranol and Norethindrone *on page 863*
Necon® 10/11 *see* Ethinyl Estradiol and Norethindrone *on page 527*
Nedocromil *see page 1509*

Nedocromil (ne doe KROE mil)

U.S. Brand Names Alocril™; Tilade®

Synonyms Nedocromil Sodium

Generic Available No

Pharmacologic Category Mast Cell Stabilizer

Pregnancy Risk Factor B

Lactation Excretion in breast milk unknown/use caution

Use

Aerosol: Maintenance therapy in patients with mild to moderate bronchial asthma

Ophthalmic: Treatment of itching associated with allergic conjunctivitis

Mechanism of Action/Effect Inhibits the activation of and mediator release from a variety of inflammatory cell types associated with asthma including eosinophils, neutrophils, macrophages, mast cells, monocytes, and platelets; it inhibits the release of histamine, leukotrienes, and slow-reacting substance of anaphylaxis; it inhibits the development of early and late bronchoconstriction responses to inhaled antigen

Contraindications Hypersensitivity to nedocromil or any component of the formulation

Warnings/Precautions

Aerosol: Safety and efficacy in children <6 years of age have not been established. If systemic or inhaled steroid therapy is at all reduced, monitor patients carefully. Nedocromil is **not** a bronchodilator and, therefore, should not be used for reversal of acute bronchospasm.

Ophthalmic solution: Users of contact lenses should not wear them during periods of symptomatic allergic conjunctivitis

Adverse Reactions

Inhalation:

>10%: Gastrointestinal: Unpleasant taste after inhalation

1% to 10%:

- Cardiovascular: Chest pain
- Central nervous system: Dizziness, dysphonia, headache, fatigue
- Dermatologic: Rash
- Gastrointestinal: Nausea, vomiting, heartburn, diarrhea, abdominal pain, dry mouth
- Hepatic: Increased ALT
- Neuromuscular & skeletal: Arthritis, tremor
- Respiratory: Cough, pharyngitis, rhinitis, bronchitis, upper respiratory infection, bronchospasm, increased sputum production

Ophthalmic solution

>10%:

- Central nervous system: Headache
- Gastrointestinal: Unpleasant taste
- Ocular: Burning, irritation, stinging
- Respiratory: nasal congestion

1% to 10%

- Ocular: Conjunctivitis, eye redness, photophobia
- Respiratory: Asthma, rhinitis

(Continued)

Nedocromil *(Continued)*

Pharmacodynamics/Kinetics

Bioavailability: 7% to 9%

Half-Life Elimination: 1.5-2 hours

Duration: Therapeutic effect: 2 hours

Formulations

Aerosol for inhalation, as sodium (Tilade®): 1.75 mg/activation (16.2 g)

Solution, ophthalmic, as sodium (Alocril™): 2% (5 mL) [contains benzalkonium chloride]

Dosing

Adults & Elderly:

Asthma: Inhalation: 2 inhalations 4 times/day; may reduce dosage to 2-3 times/day once desired clinical response to initial dose is observed. Drug has no known therapeutic systemic activity when delivered by inhalation.

Allergic conjunctivitis: Ophthalmic: 1-2 drops in each eye twice daily

Pediatrics: Children ≥6 years: Refer to adult dosing.

Stability

Storage: Store at 2°C to 30°C/36°F to 86°F. Do not freeze.

Monitoring and Teaching Issues

Physical Assessment: Not for use during acute bronchospasm. Monitor effectiveness of therapy and adverse reactions (see Adverse Reactions) at beginning of therapy and periodically with long-term use. Assess knowledge/teach patient appropriate use, interventions to reduce side effects, and adverse symptoms to report (see Patient Education). Note breast-feeding caution.

Patient Education: Aerosol: Do not use during acute bronchospasm. Use exactly as directed; do not use more often than instructed or discontinue without consulting prescriber. You may experience drowsiness, dizziness, fatigue, especially during early therapy (use caution when driving or engaging in tasks requiring alertness until response to drug is known); dry mouth, nausea, or vomiting (small, frequent meals, frequent mouth care, chewing gum, or sucking lozenges may help). Report persistent runny nose, cough, cold symptoms; unresolved GI effects; skin rash; joint pain or tremor; or if breathing difficulty persists or worsens. **Breast-feeding precaution:** Consult prescriber if breast-feeding.

Inhaler: Review use with prescriber or follow package insert for directions. Prime with 3 activations prior to first use or if unused more than 7 days. Keep inhaler clean and unobstructed. Always rinse mouth and throat after use of inhaler to prevent advantageous infection. If you are also using a steroid bronchodilator, wait 10 minutes before using this aerosol.

Ophthalmic: Do not wear contact lenses with allergic conjunctivitis. For the eye only. Open eyes, look up, and pull lower lid down. Squeeze medicine into lower eyelid and close eye. Do not touch bottle tip to eye, eyelid, or other skin.

Geriatric Considerations: Elderly may have difficulty using inhaler delivery system, especially if they have physical or medical impairment (ie, Parkinson's disease, stroke, etc). If this prophylactic modality is desired but patient cannot tolerate nedocromil inhalations, consider cromolyn sodium solution for nebulizer use.

Additional Information Nedocromil has no known therapeutic systemic activity when delivered by inhalation.

Related Information

Inhalant (Asthma, Bronchospasm) Agents Comparison *on page 1577*

Nedocromil Sodium *see* Nedocromil *on page 953*

Nefazodone (nef AY zoe done)

U.S. Brand Names Serzone®

Synonyms Nefazodone Hydrochloride

Generic Available No

Pharmacologic Category Antidepressant, Serotonin Reuptake Inhibitor/Antagonist

Pregnancy Risk Factor C

Lactation Enters breast milk/not recommended

Use Treatment of depression

Use - Unlabeled/Investigational Post-traumatic stress disorder

Mechanism of Action/Effect Inhibits neuronal reuptake of serotonin and norepinephrine; also blocks $5\text{-}HT_2$ and $alpha_1$ receptors; has no significant affinity for $alpha_2$, beta-adrenergic, $5\text{-}HT_{1A}$, cholinergic, dopaminergic, or benzodiazepine receptors

Contraindications Hypersensitivity to nefazodone, related compounds (phenylpiperazines), or any component of the formulation; liver injury due to previous nefazodone treatment, active liver disease, or elevated serum transaminases; concurrent use or use of MAO inhibitors within previous 14 days; use in a patient during the acute recovery phase of MI; concurrent use with astemizole, carbamazepine, cisapride, or pimozide; concurrent therapy with triazolam or alprazolam is generally contraindicated (dosage must be reduced by 75% for triazolam and 50% for alprazolam; such reductions may not be possible with available dosage forms).

Warnings/Precautions Cases of life-threatening hepatic failure have been reported; discontinue if clinical signs or symptoms suggest liver failure. Nefazodone should not be initiated within 1 week of discontinuing a MAO inhibitor. May cause sedation, resulting in impaired performance of tasks requiring alertness (ie, operating machinery or driving). Sedative effects may be additive with other CNS depressants. Does not potentiate ethanol but use is not advised. The degree of sedation is low relative to other antidepressants. May worsen psychosis in some patients or precipitate a shift to mania or hypomania in patients with bipolar disease. May increase the risks associated with electroconvulsive therapy. This agent should be discontinued, when possible, prior to elective surgery. Therapy should not be abruptly discontinued in patients receiving high doses for prolonged periods. Rare reports of priapism have occurred. The incidence of sexual dysfunction with nefazodone is generally lower than with SSRIs.

Use with caution in patients at risk of hypotension or in patients where transient hypotensive episodes would be poorly tolerated (cardiovascular disease or cerebrovascular disease). The risk of postural hypotension is low relative to other antidepressants. Use with caution in patients with urinary retention, benign prostatic hyperplasia, narrow-angle glaucoma, xerostomia, visual problems, constipation, or history of bowel obstruction (due to anticholinergic effects). The degree of anticholinergic blockade produced by this agent is very low relative to other cyclic antidepressants.

Use caution in patients with depression, particularly if suicidal risk may be present. Use caution in patients with a previous seizure disorder or condition predisposing to seizures such as brain damage, alcoholism, or concurrent therapy with other drugs which lower the seizure threshold. Use with caution in patients with renal dysfunction and in elderly patients. Use with caution in patients with a history of cardiovascular disease (including previous MI, stroke, tachycardia, or conduction abnormalities). However, the risk of conduction abnormalities with this agent is very low relative to other antidepressants.

Pregnancy risk C.

Drug Interactions

Cytochrome P450 Effect: Substrate of **CYP2D6, 3A4**; Inhibits CYP1A2, 2B6, 2D6, **3A4**

Decreased Effect: Carbamazepine may reduce serum concentrations of nefazodone - concurrent administration should be avoided.

Increased Effect/Toxicity:

CYP3A4 substrates: Serum concentrations of drugs metabolized by CYP3A4 may be elevated by nefazodone; cisapride, pimozide, and triazolam are contraindicated. Nefazodone may increase the serum levels/effects of antiarrhythmics (amiodarone, lidocaine, propafenone, quinidine), some antipsychotics (clozapine, haloperidol, mesoridazine, quetiapine, and risperidone), some benzodiazepines (triazolam is contraindicated; decrease alprazolam dose by 50%), buspirone (limit buspirone dose to <2.5 mg/day), calcium channel blockers, cyclosporine, digoxin, donepezil, HMG-CoA reductase inhibitors (lovastatin, simvastatin - increased risk of myositis), methadone, oral contraceptives, protease inhibitors (ritonavir, saquinavir), sibutramine, sildenafil, tacrolimus, tricyclic antidepressants, vinca alkaloids, and zolpidem.

CYP3A4 inhibitors: Serum level and/or toxicity of nefazodone may be increased; inhibitors include amiodarone, cimetidine, clarithromycin, erythromycin, delavirdine, diltiazem, dirithromycin, disulfiram, fluoxetine, fluvoxamine, grapefruit juice, indinavir, itraconazole, ketoconazole, metronidazole, nevirapine, propoxyphene, quinupristin-dalfopristin, ritonavir, saquinavir, verapamil, zafirlukast, zileuton

MAO inhibitors: Concurrent use may lead to serotonin syndrome; avoid concurrent use or use within 14 days (includes phenelzine, isocarboxazid, and linezolid). Selegiline may increase the risk of serotonin syndrome, particularly at higher doses (>10 mg/day, where selectivity for MAO type B is decreased).

Theoretically, concurrent use of buspirone, meperidine, serotonin agonists (sumatriptan, rizatriptan), SSRIs, and venlafaxine may result in serotonin syndrome.

Nutritional/Ethanol Interactions

Ethanol: Avoid ethanol (may increase CNS depression).

Food: Nefazodone absorption may be delayed and bioavailability may be decreased if taken with food.

Herb/Nutraceutical: Avoid valerian, St John's wort, SAMe, kava kava (may increase risk of serotonin syndrome and/or excessive sedation).

Adverse Reactions

>10%:

Central nervous system: Headache, drowsiness, insomnia, agitation, dizziness

Gastrointestinal: Xerostomia, nausea, constipation

Neuromuscular & skeletal: Weakness

1% to 10%:

Cardiovascular: Bradycardia, hypotension, peripheral edema, postural hypotension, vasodilation

Central nervous system: Chills, fever, incoordination, lightheadedness, confusion, memory impairment, abnormal dreams, decreased concentration, ataxia, psychomotor retardation, tremor

Dermatologic: Pruritus, rash

Endocrine & metabolic: Breast pain, impotence, libido decreased

Gastrointestinal: Gastroenteritis, vomiting, dyspepsia, diarrhea, increased appetite, thirst, taste perversion

Genitourinary: Urinary frequency, urinary retention

Hematologic: Hematocrit decreased

Neuromuscular & skeletal: Arthralgia, hypertonia, paresthesia, neck rigidity, tremor

Ocular: Blurred vision (9%), abnormal vision (7%), eye pain, visual field defect

Otic: Tinnitus

Respiratory: Bronchitis, cough, dyspnea, pharyngitis

Miscellaneous: Flu syndrome, infection

<1% (Limited to important or life-threatening): Allergic reaction, angioedema, AV block, galactorrhea, gynecomastia, hallucinations, hepatic failure, hepatic necrosis, hepatitis, hyponatremia, impotence, increased prolactin, leukopenia, liver function tests (abnormal), photosensitivity, priapism, rhabdomyolysis (with lovastatin/simvastatin), seizures, serotonin syndrome, Stevens-Johnson syndrome, thrombocytopenia

Overdosage/Toxicology Symptoms of overdose include drowsiness, vomiting, hypotension, tachycardia, incontinence, and coma. Following initiation of essential overdose management, toxic symptoms should be treated.

(Continued)

Nefazodone *(Continued)*

Pharmacodynamics/Kinetics

Bioavailability: 20% (variable)

Half-Life Elimination: Parent drug: 2-4 hours; active metabolites persist longer

Time to Peak: Serum: 1 hour, prolonged in presence of food

Metabolism: Hepatic to three active metabolites: Triazoledione, hydroxynefazodone, and m-chlorophenylpiperazine (mCPP)

Onset: Therapeutic: Up to 6 weeks

Formulations Tablet, as hydrochloride: 50 mg, 100 mg, 150 mg, 200 mg, 250 mg

Dosing

Adults: Depression: Oral: 200 mg/day, administered in two divided doses initially, with a range of 300-600 mg/day in two divided doses thereafter.

Elderly: Oral: Initial: 50 mg twice daily; increase dose to 100 mg twice daily in 2 weeks; usual maintenance dose: 200-400 mg/day

Pediatrics: Children and Adolescents: Depression: Oral: Target dose: 300-400 mg/day (mean: 3.4 mg/kg)

Administration

Oral: Dosing after meals may decrease lightheadedness and postural hypotension, but may also decrease absorption and therefore effectiveness.

Stability

Storage: Store at room temperature, below 40°C (104°F) in a tight container.

Monitoring Laboratory Tests If AST/ALT increase beyond 3 times ULN, the drug should be discontinued and not reintroduced.

Monitoring and Teaching Issues

Physical Assessment: Assess other medications patient may be taking for effectiveness and interactions (see Drug Interactions). See Warnings/Precautions for use cautions. Monitor therapeutic response and adverse reactions at beginning of therapy and periodically with long-term use (see Adverse Reactions and Overdose/Toxicology). Taper dosage slowly when discontinuing. Assess knowledge/teach patient appropriate use, interventions to reduce side effects, and adverse symptoms to report (see Patient Education). **Pregnancy risk factor C** - benefits of use should outweigh possible risks. Breast-feeding is not recommended.

Patient Education: Take exactly as directed; do not increase dose or frequency. It may take 2-3 weeks to achieve desired results. Avoid alcohol, caffeine, and other prescription or OTC medications not approved by prescriber. Maintain adequate hydration (2-3 L/day of fluids) unless advised by prescriber to restrict fluids. You may experience drowsiness, dizziness, or lightheadedness (use caution when driving or engaging in tasks requiring alertness until response to drug is known); nausea or vomiting (small, frequent meals, frequent mouth care, chewing gum, or sucking lozenges may help); or orthostatic hypotension (use caution when climbing stairs or changing position from lying or sitting to standing). Report persistent insomnia or excessive daytime sedation; muscle cramping, tremors, weakness, tiredness, or change in gait; chest pain, palpitations, or rapid heartbeat; vision changes or eye pain; difficulty breathing or breathlessness; malaise, loss of appetite, GI complaints, abdominal pain, or blood in stool; yellowing of skin or eyes (jaundice); or worsening of condition. **Pregnancy/breast-feeding precautions:** Inform prescriber if you are or intend to become pregnant. Breast-feeding is not recommended.

Geriatric Considerations: Data on nefazodone in the elderly is limited, specifically regarding efficacy. Clinical trials in adult patients have found it superior to placebo and similar to imipramine. Nefazodone's C_{max} and AUC have been reported to be increased twofold in the elderly and women after a single dose compared to younger patients, however, these differences were markedly reduced with multiple dosing.

Breast-feeding Issues: Drowsiness, lethargy, poor feeding, and failure to maintain body temperature have been reported in a nursing infant.

Additional Information May cause less sexual dysfunction than other antidepressants. Women and elderly receiving single doses attain significant higher peak concentrations than male volunteers.

Related Information

Antidepressant Agents *on page 1553*
Antidepressant Medication Guidelines *on page 1613*

Nefazodone Hydrochloride *see* Nefazodone *on page 954*

Nelfinavir (nel FIN a veer)

U.S. Brand Names Viracept®

Generic Available No

Pharmacologic Category Antiretroviral Agent, Protease Inhibitor

Pregnancy Risk Factor B

Lactation Excretion in breast milk unknown/contraindicated

Use In combination with other antiretroviral therapy in the treatment of HIV infection

Mechanism of Action/Effect Inhibits HIV-1 protease enzyme; inhibition of the viral protease prevents cleavage of the gag-pol polyprotein resulting in the production of immature, noninfectious virions; cross-resistance with other protease inhibitors is possible, although, not known at this time

Contraindications Hypersensitivity to nelfinavir or any component of the formulation; phenylketonuria; concurrent therapy with amiodarone, astemizole, cisapride, ergot derivatives, lovastatin, midazolam, quinidine, simvastatin, triazolam

Warnings/Precautions Avoid use of powder formulation in patients with phenylketonuria since it contains 11.2 mg phenylalanine per gram of powder. Use extreme caution when administered to patients with hepatic insufficiency since nelfinavir is metabolized in the liver and excreted predominantly in the feces. Avoid concurrent use of St John's wort. Concurrent use with some anticonvulsants may significantly limit nelfinavir's effectiveness. Spontaneous bleeding episodes have been reported in patients with hemophilia A and B. New onset diabetes mellitus, exacerbation of diabetes, and hyperglycemia have been reported in HIV-infected patients receiving protease inhibitors.

Drug Interactions

Cytochrome P450 Effect: Substrate of CYP2C8/9, **2C19**, 2D6, **3A4**; Inhibits CYP1A2, 2B6, 2C8/9, 2C19, 2D6, **3A4**

Decreased Effect: Rifampin decreases nelfinavir's blood levels (AUC decreased by ~82%); the two drugs should not be administered concurrently. Serum levels of ethinyl estradiol and norethindrone (including many oral contraceptives) may decrease significantly with administration of nelfinavir. Patients should use alternative methods of contraceptives during nelfinavir therapy. Phenobarbital, phenytoin, and carbamazepine may decrease serum levels and consequently effectiveness of nelfinavir. Delavirdine concentrations may be decreased by up to 50% during nelfinavir treatment. Nelfinavir's effectiveness may be decreased with concomitant nevirapine use.

Increased Effect/Toxicity: Nelfinavir inhibits the metabolism of cisapride, astemizole, amiodarone, quinidine, lovastatin, simvastatin - should not be administered concurrently due to risk of life-threatening cardiac arrhythmias. Concentrations of atorvastatin and cerivastatin may be increased by nelfinavir. Do not administer with ergot alkaloids. Rifabutin plasma levels (AUC) are increased when coadministered with nelfinavir (decrease rifabutin dose by 50%). Nelfinavir increases levels of ketoconazole and indinavir. An increase in midazolam and triazolam serum levels may occur resulting in significant oversedation when administered with nelfinavir. Indinavir and ritonavir may increase nelfinavir plasma concentrations resulting in potential increases in side effects (the safety of these combinations have not been established). Concentrations of nelfinavir may be doubled during therapy with delavirdine. Sildenafil serum concentration may be substantially increased (do not exceed single doses of 25 mg in 48 hours).

Nutritional/Ethanol Interactions

Food: Nelfinavir taken with food increases plasma concentration time curve (AUC) by two- to threefold. Do not administer with acidic food or juice (orange juice, apple juice, or applesauce) since the combination may have a bitter taste.

Herb/Nutraceutical: St John's wort may decrease nelfinavir serum concentrations; avoid concurrent use.

Adverse Reactions Protease inhibitors cause hyperglycemia and dyslipidemia (elevated cholesterol/triglycerides) and a redistribution of fat (protease paunch, buffalo hump, facial atrophy and breast engorgement)

>10%: Gastrointestinal: Diarrhea

1% to 10%:

- Central nervous system: Impaired concentration
- Dermatologic: Rash
- Gastrointestinal: Nausea, flatulence, abdominal pain
- Neuromuscular & skeletal: Weakness

<1% (Limited to important or life-threatening): Allergic reaction, arthralgia, dyspnea, elevated LFTs, fever, GI bleeding, hepatitis, hyperlipidemia, hyperuricemia, hypoglycemia, kidney calculus, leukopenia, migraine, pancreatitis, seizures, suicidal ideation, thrombocytopenia, vomiting

Overdosage/Toxicology No data available; however, unabsorbed drug should be removed via gastric lavage and activated charcoal; significant symptoms beyond gastrointestinal disturbances are likely following acute overdose; hemodialysis will not be effective due to high protein binding of nelfinavir

Pharmacodynamics/Kinetics

Absorption: Food increases plasma concentration-time curve (AUC) by two- to threefold

Half-Life Elimination: 3.5-5 hours

Time to Peak: Serum: 2-4 hours

Metabolism: Hepatic via CYP3A4; major metabolite has activity comparable to parent drug

Formulations

Powder, oral: 50 mg/g (144 g) [contains phenylalanine 11.2 mg]

Tablet, film coated: 250 mg

Dosing

Adults & Elderly: HIV infection: Oral: 1250 mg (5 tablets of 250 mg each) twice daily with food or 750 mg (3 tablets of 250 mg each) 3 times/day with food

Note: Dosage adjustments for nelfinavir when administered in combination with ritonavir: Nelfinavir 500-750 mg twice daily plus ritonavir 400 mg twice daily

Pediatrics: HIV infection: Oral: Children 2-13 years (labeled dose): 20-30 mg/kg 3 times/day with a meal or light snack; if tablets are unable to be taken, use oral powder in small amount of water, milk, formula, or dietary supplements. Do not use acidic food/juice or store for >6 hours.

Note: Clinically, dosages as high as 45 mg/kg every 8 hours are used. Twice-daily dosages of 50-55 mg/kg are under investigation in older children (>6 years).

Renal Impairment: No adjustment is necessary.

Hepatic Impairment: Use caution when administering to patients with hepatic impairment since nelfinavir is predominantly eliminated by the liver.

Administration

Oral: Oral powder: Mix powder or tablets in a small amount of water, milk, formula, soy milk, soy formula, or dietary supplement. Be sure entire contents is consumed to receive full dose. Do not use acidic food/juice to dilute due to bitter taste. Do not store dilution for longer than 6 hours.

Stability

Storage: Store at room temperature. Oral powder (or dissolved tablets) diluted in nonacidic liquid is stable for 6 hours at room temperature.

Monitoring Laboratory Tests Liver function tests, blood glucose levels, CBC with differential, CD4 cell count, plasma levels of HIV RNA

Monitoring and Teaching Issues

Physical Assessment: See Contraindications and Warnings/Precautions (clear diagnosis of migraine) for use cautions. Assess potential for interactions with other prescriptions,

(Continued)

Nelfinavir *(Continued)*

OTC medications, or herbal products patient may be taking (eg, oral contraceptives - see Drug Interactions). Assess therapeutic effectiveness and adverse response (see Adverse Reactions and Overdose/Toxicology). Teach patient proper use, possible side effects and appropriate interventions, and adverse symptoms to report (eg, adverse reactions may differ according to age/gender of patient - see Patient Education). Breast-feeding is contraindicated.

Patient Education: Inform prescriber of all prescriptions, OTC medications, or herbal products you are taking, and any allergies you have. Do not take anything new during treatment unless approved by prescriber. This drug is not a cure for HIV and has not been shown to reduce the risk of transmitting HIV to others. The long-term effects of use are not known. Take exactly as directed with food. Mix powder with nonacid, noncitric fluids, and do not store reconstituted powder mixture for longer than 6 hours. If unable to swallow tablets whole, the tablet may be dissolved in water or crushed in food. Mixed or dissolved tablets must be consumed within 6 hours. If you miss a dose, take as soon as possible and return to your regular schedule (never take a double dose). Frequent blood tests may be required with prolonged therapy. May cause nausea or vomiting (small, frequent meals, frequent mouth care, chewing gum, or sucking lozenges may help). Report rash; difficulty breathing; CNS changes (migraine, confusion, suicidal ideation); muscular or skeletal pain, weakness, or tremors; or other adverse reactions. **Pregnancy/breast-feeding precautions:** Use appropriate barrier contraceptive measures (as alternative to oral contraceptives) to reduce risk of transmitting infection and potential pregnancy. Inform prescriber if you are or intend to become pregnant.

Dietary Issues: Should be taken as scheduled with food.

Breast-feeding Issues: HIV-infected mothers are discouraged from breast-feeding to decrease potential transmission of HIV.

Pregnancy Issues: Preliminary data show that nelfinavir pharmacokinetics may be affected by pregnancy; studies are not yet complete. Pregnancy and protease inhibitors are both associated with an increased risk of hyperglycemia. Glucose levels should be closely monitored. Health professionals are encouraged to contact the antiretroviral pregnancy registry to monitor outcomes of pregnant women exposed to antiretroviral medications (1-800-258-4263).

Related Information

Tuberculosis *on page 1705*

Nembutal® *see* Pentobarbital *on page 1053*

Neo-Calglucon® [OTC] *see* Calcium Supplements *on page 202*

NeoDecadron® *see* Neomycin and Dexamethasone *on page 959*

NeoDexadron® *see page 1509*

Neo-Dexameth® *see page 1509*

Neo-Fradin™ *see* Neomycin *on page 958*

Neomycin (nee oh MYE sin)

U.S. Brand Names Myciguent [OTC]; Neo-Fradin™; Neo-Rx

Synonyms Neomycin Sulfate

Generic Available Yes

Pharmacologic Category Ammonium Detoxicant; Antibiotic, Aminoglycoside; Antibiotic, Topical

Pregnancy Risk Factor C

Lactation Excretion in breast milk unknown

Use Orally to prepare GI tract for surgery; topically to treat minor skin infections; treatment of diarrhea caused by *E. coli*; adjunct in the treatment of hepatic encephalopathy

Mechanism of Action/Effect Interferes with bacterial protein synthesis by binding to 30S ribosomal subunits

Contraindications Hypersensitivity to neomycin or any component of the formulation, or other aminoglycosides; intestinal obstruction

Warnings/Precautions Use with caution in patients with renal impairment, pre-existing hearing impairment (ototoxicity), neuromuscular disorders. Topical neomycin is a contact sensitizer with sensitivity occurring in 5% to 15% of patients treated with the drug. Symptoms include itching, reddening, edema, and failure to heal. Do not use as peritoneal lavage. Pregnancy risk C.

Drug Interactions

Decreased Effect: May decrease GI absorption of digoxin and methotrexate.

Increased Effect/Toxicity: Oral neomycin may potentiate the effects of oral anticoagulants. Neomycin may increase the adverse effects with other neurotoxic, ototoxic, or nephrotoxic drugs.

Adverse Reactions

Oral:

>10%: Gastrointestinal: Nausea, diarrhea, vomiting, irritation or soreness of the mouth or rectal area

<1% (Limited to important or life-threatening): Dyspnea, eosinophilia, nephrotoxicity, neurotoxicity, ototoxicity (auditory), ototoxicity (vestibular)

Topical: >10%: Dermatologic: Contact dermatitis

Overdosage/Toxicology Symptoms of overdose (rare due to poor oral bioavailability) include ototoxicity, nephrotoxicity, and neuromuscular toxicity. The treatment of choice following a single acute overdose appears to be maintenance of urine output of at least 3 mL/kg/hour during the acute treatment phase. Dialysis is of questionable value in enhancing aminoglycoside elimination. If required, hemodialysis is preferred over peritoneal dialysis in patients with normal renal function. Chelation with penicillin may be of benefit.

Pharmacodynamics/Kinetics

Absorption: Oral, percutaneous: Poor (3%)

Half-Life Elimination: Age and renal function dependent: 3 hours

Time to Peak: Serum: Oral: 1-4 hours; I.M.: ~2 hours

Metabolism: Slightly hepatic

Formulations

Ointment, topical, as sulfate (Myciguent): 3.5 mg/g (15 g, 30 g)

Powder, micronized, as sulfate [for prescription compounding] (Neo-Rx): (10 g, 100 g)

Solution, oral, as sulfate (Neo-Fradin™): 125 mg/5 mL (480 mL) [contains benzoic acid; cherry flavor]

Tablet, as sulfate: 500 mg

Dosing

Adults & Elderly:

Dermatologic infections: Topical: Apply ointment 1-4 times/day; topical solutions containing 0.1% to 1% neomycin have been used for irrigation

Preoperative intestinal antisepsis: Oral: 1 g each hour for 4 doses then 1 g every 4 hours for 5 doses; or 1 g at 1 PM, 2 PM, and 11 PM on day preceding surgery as an adjunct to mechanical cleansing of the bowel and oral erythromycin; or 6 g/day divided every 4 hours for 2-3 days

Hepatic coma: Oral: 500-2000 mg every 6-8 hours or 4-12 g/day divided every 4-6 hours for 5-6 days

Chronic hepatic insufficiency: Oral: 4 g/day for an indefinite period

Pediatrics:

Preoperative intestinal antisepsis: Oral: Children: 90 mg/kg/day divided every 4 hours for 2 days; or 25 mg/kg at 1 PM, 2 PM, and 11 PM on the day preceding surgery as an adjunct to mechanical cleansing of the intestine and in combination with erythromycin base

Hepatic coma: Oral: Children: 50-100 mg/kg/day in divided doses every 6-8 hours or 2.5-7 g/m^2/day divided every 4-6 hours for 5-6 days not to exceed 12 g/day

Dermatologic infections: Topical: Children: Refer to adult dosing.

Monitoring Laboratory Tests Renal function; perform culture and sensitivity prior to initiating therapy.

Monitoring and Teaching Issues

Physical Assessment: Assess effectiveness and interactions of other medications patient may be taking (see Drug Interactions). See Contraindications and Warnings/Precautions for use cautions. Monitor effectiveness of therapy, laboratory tests (see Monitoring Laboratory Tests), and adverse response (eg, ototoxicity, nephrotoxicity, neurotoxicity - see Adverse Reactions and Overdose/Toxicology). Assess knowledge/teach patient appropriate use (application of cream/ointment), possible side effects/interventions, and adverse symptoms to report (see Patient Education). **Pregnancy risk factor C** - benefits of use should outweigh possible risks. Minimal absorption across GI mucosa or skin surfaces, however with ulceration, open or burned surfaces (especially large surfaces) absorption is possible. Note breast-feeding caution.

Patient Education: Oral: Take as directed. Maintain adequate hydration (2-3 L/day of fluids) unless advised by prescriber to restrict fluids. You may experience nausea or vomiting (small, frequent meals, frequent mouth care, sucking lozenges, or chewing gum may help); constipation (increased exercise, fluids, fruit, or fiber may help, or consult prescriber); or diarrhea (buttermilk, boiled milk, or yogurt may help). Report immediately any change in hearing; ringing or sense of fullness in ears; persistent diarrhea; changes in voiding patterns; or numbness, tingling, or pain in any extremity. **Pregnancy/breast-feeding precautions:** Inform prescriber if you are or intend to become pregnant. Consult prescriber if breast-feeding.

Topical: Apply a thin film of cream or ointment; do not overuse. Report rash, itching, redness, or failure of condition to improve.

Neomycin and Dexamethasone (nee oh MYE sin & deks a METH a sone)

U.S. Brand Names NeoDecadron®

Synonyms Dexamethasone and Neomycin

Generic Available No

Pharmacologic Category Antibiotic/Corticosteroid, Ophthalmic

Pregnancy Risk Factor C

Lactation Excretion in breast milk unknown

Use Treatment of steroid responsive inflammatory conditions of the palpebral and bulbar conjunctiva, lid, cornea, and anterior segment of the globe

Formulations Solution, ophthalmic: Neomycin sulfate 0.35% [3.5 mg/mL] and dexamethasone sodium phosphate 0.1% [1 mg/mL] (5 mL) [contains benzalkonium chloride and sodium bisulfite]

Dosing

Adults & Elderly: Inflammation/infection: Ophthalmic: Instill 1-2 drops in eye(s) every 3-4 hours

Monitoring and Teaching Issues

Physical Assessment: See individual components listed in Related Information. **Pregnancy risk factor C** - benefits of use should outweigh possible risks. Note breast-feeding caution.

Patient Education: See individual components listed in Related Information. **Pregnancy/breast-feeding precautions:** Inform prescriber if you are or intend to become pregnant. Consult prescriber if breast-feeding.

Related Information

Dexamethasone *on page 382*
Neomycin *on page 958*
Ophthalmic Agents *on page 1509*

Neomycin and Polymyxin B (nee oh MYE sin & pol i MIKS in bee)

U.S. Brand Names Neosporin® G.U. Irrigant

Synonyms Polymyxin B and Neomycin

Generic Available No

Pharmacologic Category Antibiotic, Topical

Pregnancy Risk Factor C/D (for G.U. irrigant)

Lactation Excretion in breast milk unknown

Use Short-term as a continuous irrigant or rinse in the urinary bladder to prevent bacteriuria and gram-negative rod septicemia associated with the use of indwelling catheters; to help prevent infection in minor cuts, scrapes, and burns

Pharmacokinetic Note See individual agents.

Pharmacodynamics/Kinetics

Absorption: Topical: Not absorbed following application to intact skin; absorbed through denuded or abraded skin, peritoneum, wounds, or ulcers

Formulations Solution, irrigant: Neomycin sulfate 40 mg and polymyxin B sulfate 200,000 units per mL (1 mL, 20 mL)

Dosing

Adults & Elderly:

Bladder irrigation: **Not for I.V. injection**; add 1 mL irrigant to 1 liter isotonic saline solution and connect container to the inflow of lumen of 3-way catheter. Continuous irrigant or rinse in the urinary bladder for up to a maximum of 10 days with administration rate adjusted to patient's urine output; usually no more than 1 L of irrigant is used per day.

Dermatologic conditions: Topical: Apply cream 1-4 times/day to affected area.

Pediatrics: Refer to adult dosing.

Monitoring and Teaching Issues

Physical Assessment: See individual components listed in Related Information. **Pregnancy risk factor C/D** - see Pregnancy Risk Factor for use cautions. Assess knowledge/instruct patient on need to use appropriate contraceptive measures and the need to avoid pregnancy. Note breast-feeding caution.

Patient Education: See individual components listed in Related Information. **Pregnancy/breast-feeding precautions:** Inform prescriber if you are or intend to become pregnant. Consult prescriber if breast-feeding.

Related Information

Neomycin *on page 958*

Polymyxin B *on page 1100*

Neomycin, Bacitracin, and Polymyxin B *see* Bacitracin, Neomycin, and Polymyxin B *on page 144*

Neomycin, Bacitracin, Polymyxin B, and Hydrocortisone *see* Bacitracin, Neomycin, Polymyxin B, and Hydrocortisone *on page 145*

Neomycin, Polymyxin B, and Dexamethasone *see page 1509*

Neomycin, Polymyxin B, and Gramicidin *see page 1509*

Neomycin, Polymyxin B, and Hydrocortisone *see page 1519*

Neomycin, Polymyxin B, and Hydrocortisone *see page 1509*

Neomycin, Polymyxin B, and Prednisolone *see page 1509*

Neomycin Sulfate *see* Neomycin *on page 958*

Neoral® *see* CycloSPORINE *on page 343*

Neo-Rx *see* Neomycin *on page 958*

Neosar® *see* Cyclophosphamide *on page 339*

Neosporin® G.U. Irrigant *see* Neomycin and Polymyxin B *on page 960*

Neosporin® Ophthalmic Ointment *see page 1509*

Neosporin® Ophthalmic Ointment *see* Bacitracin, Neomycin, and Polymyxin B *on page 144*

Neosporin® Ophthalmic Solution *see page 1509*

Neosporin® Topical [OTC] *see* Bacitracin, Neomycin, and Polymyxin B *on page 144*

Neostigmine (nee oh STIG meen)

U.S. Brand Names Prostigmin®

Synonyms Neostigmine Bromide; Neostigmine Methylsulfate

Generic Available Yes: Injection

Pharmacologic Category Acetylcholinesterase Inhibitor

Pregnancy Risk Factor C

Lactation Excretion in breast milk unknown/not recommended

Use Diagnosis and treatment of myasthenia gravis; prevention and treatment of postoperative bladder distention and urinary retention; reversal of the effects of nondepolarizing neuromuscular-blocking agents after surgery

Mechanism of Action/Effect Inhibits destruction of acetylcholine by acetylcholinesterase which facilitates transmission of impulses across myoneural junction

Contraindications Hypersensitivity to neostigmine, bromides, or any component of the formulation; GI or GU obstruction

Warnings/Precautions Does **not** antagonize and may prolong the Phase I block of depolarizing muscle relaxants (eg, succinylcholine). Use with caution in patients with epilepsy, asthma, bradycardia, hyperthyroidism, cardiac arrhythmias, or peptic ulcer. Adequate facilities should be available for cardiopulmonary resuscitation when testing and adjusting dose for myasthenia gravis. Have atropine and epinephrine ready to treat hypersensitivity reactions. Overdosage may result in cholinergic crisis, this must be distinguished from myasthenic crisis. Anticholinesterase insensitivity can develop for brief or prolonged periods. Pregnancy risk C.

Drug Interactions

Decreased Effect: Antagonizes effects of nondepolarizing muscle relaxants (eg, pancuronium, tubocurarine). Atropine antagonizes the muscarinic effects of neostigmine.

Increased Effect/Toxicity: Neuromuscular blocking agent effects are increased when combined with neostigmine.

Effects on Lab Values ↑ aminotransferase [ALT (SGPT)/AST (SGOT)] (S), amylase (S)

Adverse Reactions Frequency not defined.

Cardiovascular: Arrhythmias (especially bradycardia), hypotension, decreased carbon monoxide, tachycardia, AV block, nodal rhythm, nonspecific EKG changes, cardiac arrest, syncope, flushing

Central nervous system: Convulsions, dysarthria, dysphonia, dizziness, loss of consciousness, drowsiness, headache

Dermatologic: Skin rash, thrombophlebitis (I.V.), urticaria

Gastrointestinal: Hyperperistalsis, nausea, vomiting, salivation, diarrhea, stomach cramps, dysphagia, flatulence

Genitourinary: Urinary urgency

Neuromuscular & skeletal: Weakness, fasciculations, muscle cramps, spasms, arthralgias

Ocular: Small pupils, lacrimation

Respiratory: Increased bronchial secretions, laryngospasm, bronchiolar constriction, respiratory muscle paralysis, dyspnea, respiratory depression, respiratory arrest, bronchospasm

Miscellaneous: Diaphoresis (increased), anaphylaxis, allergic reactions

Overdosage/Toxicology Symptoms of overdose include muscle weakness, blurred vision, excessive sweating, tearing and salivation, nausea, vomiting, diarrhea, hypertension, bradycardia, muscle weakness, and paralysis. Atropine sulfate injection should be readily available as an antagonist for the effects of neostigmine.

Pharmacodynamics/Kinetics

Absorption: Oral: Poor, <2%

Half-Life Elimination: Normal renal function: 0.5-2.1 hours; End-stage renal disease: Prolonged

Metabolism: Hepatic

Onset: I.M.: 20-30 minutes; I.V.: 1-20 minutes

Duration: I.M.: 2.5-4 hours; I.V.: 1-2 hours

Formulations

Injection, solution, as methylsulfate: 0.5 mg/mL (1 mL, 10 mL); 1 mg/mL (10 mL)

Tablet, as bromide: 15 mg

Dosing

Adults & Elderly:

Myasthenia gravis, diagnosis: I.M.: 0.02 mg/kg as a single dose

Myasthenia gravis, treatment:

- Oral: 15 mg/dose every 3-4 hours up to 375 mg/day maximum
- I.M., I.V., S.C.: 0.5-2.5 mg every 1-3 hours up to 10 mg/24 hours maximum

Reversal of nondepolarizing neuromuscular blockade after surgery in conjunction with atropine: I.V.: 0.5-2.5 mg; total dose not to exceed 5 mg

Bladder atony: I.M., S.C.:

- Prevention: 0.25 mg every 4-6 hours for 2-3 days
- Treatment: 0.5-1 mg every 3 hours for 5 doses after bladder has emptied

Pediatrics:

Myasthenia gravis:

- Diagnosis: I.M.: Children: 0.04 mg/kg as a single dose
- Treatment: Children:
  - Oral: 2 mg/kg/day divided every 3-4 hours
  - I.M., I.V., S.C.: 0.01-0.04 mg/kg every 2-4 hours

Reversal of nondepolarizing neuromuscular blockade after surgery in conjunction with atropine: I.V.:

- Infants: 0.025-0.1 mg/kg/dose
- Children: 0.025-0.08 mg/kg/dose

Renal Impairment:

Cl_{cr} 10-50 mL/minute: Administer 50% of normal dose.

Cl_{cr} <10 mL/minute: Administer 25% of normal dose.

Administration

I.M.: In the diagnosis of myasthenia gravis, all anticholinesterase medications should be discontinued for at least 8 hours before administering neostigmine.

Stability

Compatibility: Stable in NS

Monitoring and Teaching Issues

Physical Assessment: Used for MG diagnosis by physicians. For bladder atony, assess bladder adequacy prior to administering medication. Monitor therapeutic response and adverse effects (including cholinergic crisis - see Adverse Reactions and Overdose/Toxicology). Teach patient symptoms to report (see Patient Education). **Pregnancy risk factor C** - benefits of use should outweigh possible risks. Breast-feeding is not recommended.

Patient Education: Take this drug exactly as prescribed. You may experience visual difficulty (eg, blurring and dark adaptation - use caution at night) or urinary frequency. Promptly report any muscle weakness, difficulty breathing, severe or unresolved diarrhea, persistent abdominal cramping or vomiting, sweating, or tearing. **Pregnancy/breast-feeding precautions:** Inform prescriber if you are pregnant. Breast-feeding is not recommended.

Geriatric Considerations: Many elderly will have diseases which may influence the use of neostigmine. Also, many elderly will need doses reduced 50% due to creatinine clearances in the 10-50 mL/minute range (common in the aged). Side effects or concomitant disease may warrant use of pyridostigmine.

Neostigmine Bromide *see* Neostigmine *on page 960*

Neostigmine Methylsulfate *see* Neostigmine *on page 960*

NeoStrata AHA [OTC] *see* Hydroquinone *on page 679*

Neo-Synephrine® *see page 1509*

Neo-Synephrine® Injection *see* Phenylephrine *on page 1071*

Neo-Synephrine® Nasal [OTC] *see* Phenylephrine *on page 1071*
Neo-Synephrine® Ophthalmic *see* Phenylephrine *on page 1071*
Neotricin HC® Ophthalmic Ointment *see page 1509*
Nephro-Calci® [OTC] *see* Calcium Supplements *on page 202*
Nephro-Fer® [OTC] *see* Iron Supplements *on page 744*

Nesiritide (ni SIR i tide)

U.S. Brand Names Natrecor®

Synonyms B-type Natriuretic Peptide (Human); hBNP; Natriuretic Peptide

Generic Available No

Pharmacologic Category Natriuretic Peptide, B-type, Human; Vasodilator

Pregnancy Risk Factor C

Lactation Excretion in breast milk unknown/use caution

Use Treatment of acutely decompensated congestive heart failure (CHF) in patients with dyspnea at rest or with minimal activity

Mechanism of Action/Effect Binds to cell surface receptors in vasculature, resulting in smooth muscle cell relaxation. Has been shown to produce dose-dependent reductions in pulmonary capillary wedge pressure (PCWP) and systemic arterial pressure providing symptomatic improvements (dyspnea decreased) for several days.

Contraindications Hypersensitivity to natriuretic peptide or any component of the formulation; cardiogenic shock (when used as primary therapy); hypotension (systolic blood pressure <90 mm Hg)

Warnings/Precautions May cause hypotension; administer in clinical situations when blood pressure may be closely monitored. Use caution in patients systolic blood pressure <100 mm Hg (contraindicated if <90 mm Hg); more likely to experience hypotension. Effects may be additive with other agents capable of causing hypotension. Hypotensive effects may last for several hours.

Should not be used in patients with low filling pressures, or in patients with conditions which depend on venous return including significant valvular stenosis, restrictive or obstructive cardiomyopathy, constrictive pericarditis, and pericardial tamponade. May be associated with development of azotemia; use caution in patients with renal impairment or in patients where renal perfusion is dependent on renin-angiotensin-aldosterone system.

Monitor for allergic or anaphylactic reactions. Use caution with prolonged infusions; limited experience for infusions >48 hours. Safety and efficacy in pediatric patients have not been established.

Pregnancy risk C.

Drug Interactions

Increased Effect/Toxicity: An increased frequency of symptomatic hypotension was observed with concurrent administration of ACE inhibitors. Other hypotensive agents are likely to have additive effects on hypotension. In patients receiving diuretic therapy leading to depletion of intravascular volume, the risk of hypotension and/or renal impairment may be increased. Nesiritide should be avoided in patients with low filling pressures.

Adverse Reactions Note: Frequencies cited below were recorded in VMAC trial at dosages similar to approved labeling. Higher frequencies have been observed in trials using higher dosages of nesiritide.

>10%:
- Cardiovascular: Hypotension (total: 11%; symptomatic: 4% at recommended dose, up to 17% at higher doses)
- Renal: Increased serum creatinine (28% with >0.5 mg/dL increase over baseline)

1% to 10%:
- Cardiovascular: Ventricular tachycardia (3%)*, ventricular extrasystoles (3%)*, angina (2%)*, bradycardia (1%), tachycardia, atrial fibrillation, AV node conduction abnormalities
- Central nervous system: Headache (8%)*, dizziness (3%)*, insomnia (2%), anxiety (3%), fever, confusion, paresthesia, somnolence, tremor
- Dermatologic: Pruritus, rash
- Gastrointestinal: Nausea (4%)*, abdominal pain (1%)*, vomiting (1%)*
- Hematologic: Anemia
- Local: Injection site reaction
- Neuromuscular & skeletal: Back pain (4%), leg cramps
- Ocular: Amblyopia
- Respiratory: Cough (increased), hemoptysis, apnea
- Miscellaneous: Increased diaphoresis

*Frequency less than or equal to placebo or other standard therapy

Overdosage/Toxicology No data. Symptoms of overdose would be expected to include excessive and/or prolonged hypotension. Treatment is symptomatic and supportive. Drug discontinuation and/or dosage reduction may be required.

Pharmacodynamics/Kinetics

Half-Life Elimination: Initial (distribution) 2 minutes; Terminal: 18 minutes

Time to Peak: 1 hour

Metabolism: Proteolytic cleavage by vascular endopeptidases and proteolysis following receptor binding and cellular internalization

Onset: 15 minutes (60% of 3-hour effect achieved)

Duration: >60 minutes (up to several hours) for systolic blood pressure; hemodynamic effects persist longer than serum half-life would predict

Formulations Injection, powder for reconstitution: 1.5 mg

Dosing

Adults: Congestive heart failure: I.V.: Initial: 2 mcg/kg (bolus); followed by continuous infusion at 0.01 mcg/kg/minute; **Note:** Should not be initiated at a dosage higher than initial recommended dose. At intervals of ≥3 hours, the dosage may be increased by 0.005 mcg/kg/minute (preceded by a bolus of 1 mcg/kg), up to a maximum of 0.03 mcg/kg/minute.

Increases beyond the initial infusion rate should be limited to selected patients and accompanied by hemodynamic monitoring.

Patients experiencing hypotension during the infusion: Infusion should be interrupted. May attempt to restart at a lower dose (reduce initial infusion dose by 30% and omit bolus).

Renal Impairment: No adjustment required

Administration

I.V.: Do not administer through a heparin-coated catheter (concurrent administration of heparin via a separate catheter is acceptable, per manufacturer).

Stability

Storage: Vials may be stored at controlled room temperature of 20°C to 25°C (68°F to 77 °F) or under refrigeration at 2°C to 8°C (36°F to 46°F). Following reconstitution, vials are stable under these conditions for up to 24 hours.

Reconstitution: Reconstitute 1.5 mg vial with 5 mL of diluent removed from a premixed plastic I.V. bag (compatible with 5% dextrose, 0.9% sodium chloride, 5% dextrose and 0.45% sodium chloride, or 5% dextrose and 0.2% sodium chloride). Do not shake vial to dissolve (roll gently). Withdraw entire contents of vial and add to 250 mL I.V. bag. Resultant concentration of solution approximately 6 mcg/mL.

Compatibility: Incompatible with heparin, insulin, ethacrynate sodium, bumetanide, enalaprilat, hydralazine, and furosemide. Do not administer through the same catheter. Do not administer with any solution containing sodium metabisulfite. Catheter must be flushed between administration of nesiritide and physically incompatible drugs.

Monitoring and Teaching Issues

Physical Assessment: See Contraindications, Warnings/Precautions, and Dosing for use cautions. Assess potential for interactions with other prescriptions, OTC medications, or herbal products patient may be taking (eg, other hypotensive agents or diuretics - see Drug Interactions). See I.V. Administration specifics. Blood pressure should be monitored before and at frequent intervals during and for 24 hours following infusion (hemodynamic monitoring with larger doses). Assess results of laboratory tests and patient response on a regular basis throughout therapy (eg, hypersensitivity, hypotension - see Adverse Reactions and Overdose/Toxicology). Teach patient possible side effects and interventions and adverse symptoms to report (see Patient Education). **Pregnancy risk factor C** - benefits of use should outweigh possible risks. Note breast-feeding caution.

Patient Education: Inform prescriber of all prescriptions, OTC medications, or herbal products you are taking, and any allergies you have. This medication can only be administered by infusion; you will be monitored closely during and following infusion. Report immediately any pain, burning, swelling at infusion site, or any signs of allergic reaction (eg, difficulty breathing or swallowing, back pain, chest tightness, rash, hives, swelling of lips or mouth). Remain in bed until advised otherwise; call for assistance with turning or changing position. Report any chest pain, difficulty breathing, confusion, nausea, leg cramps, or any other adverse effects. **Pregnancy/breast-feeding precautions:** Inform prescriber if you are or intend to become pregnant. Consult prescriber if breast-feeding.

Additional Information The duration of symptomatic improvement with nesiritide following discontinuation of the infusion has been limited (generally lasting several days). Atrial natriuretic peptide, which is related to nesiritide, has been associated with increased vascular permeability. This has not been observed in clinical trials with nesiritide, but patients should be monitored for this effect.

Related Information

Heart Failure *on page 1670*

Nestrex® [OTC] *see* Pyridoxine *on page 1156*

Neupogen® *see* Filgrastim *on page 558*

Neurontin® *see* Gabapentin *on page 614*

Neut® *see* Sodium Bicarbonate *on page 1234*

Neutra-Phos® [OTC] *see* Phosphate Supplements *on page 1076*

Neutra-Phos®-K [OTC] *see* Phosphate Supplements *on page 1076*

Neutrexin® *see* Trimetrexate Glucuronate *on page 1367*

Nevirapine (ne VYE ra peen)

U.S. Brand Names Viramune®

Generic Available No

Pharmacologic Category Antiretroviral Agent, Reverse Transcriptase Inhibitor (Non-nucleoside)

Pregnancy Risk Factor C

Lactation Enters breast milk/contraindicated

Use In combination therapy with other antiretroviral agents for the treatment of HIV-1 in adults

Mechanism of Action/Effect Blocks the RNA-dependent DNA polymerase activity

Contraindications Hypersensitivity to nevirapine or any component of the formulation; manufacturer recommends against concurrent administration of ketoconazole or oral contraceptives

Warnings/Precautions Resistant HIV virus emerges rapidly and uniformly when nevirapine is administered as monotherapy. Therefore, always administer in combination with at least 1 additional antiretroviral agent. Consider alteration of antiretroviral therapies if disease progression occurs while patients are receiving nevirapine. Safety and efficacy have not been established in neonates.

Nevirapine must be initiated with a 14-day lead-in dosing period to decrease the incidence of adverse effects. Severe hepatotoxic reactions may also occur (fulminant and cholestatic hepatitis, hepatic necrosis), and in some cases have resulted in hepatic failure and death. Intensive monitoring is required during the initial 12 weeks of therapy to detect potentially life-threatening dermatologic, hypersensitivity, and hepatic reactions. Patients with a history of chronic hepatitis (B or C) or increased transaminase levels (AST or ALT) may be at increased risk of hepatotoxic reactions.

(Continued)

Nevirapine *(Continued)*

Severe life-threatening skin reactions (eg, Stevens-Johnson syndrome, toxic epidermal necrolysis, hypersensitivity reactions with rash and organ dysfunction) have occurred. If a severe dermatologic or hypersensitivity reaction occurs, or if signs and symptoms of hepatitis occur, nevirapine should be permanently discontinued.

Pregnancy risk C.

Drug Interactions

Cytochrome P450 Effect: Substrate of CYP2B6, 2D6, **3A4**; Inhibits CYP1A2, 2D6, 3A4; Induces **CYP2B6, 3A4**

Decreased Effect: Rifampin and rifabutin may decrease nevirapine concentrations due to induction of CYP3A; since nevirapine may decrease concentrations of protease inhibitors (eg, indinavir, saquinavir), they should not be administered concomitantly or doses should be increased. Nevirapine may decrease the effectiveness of oral contraceptives - suggest alternate method of birth control. Nevirapine also decreases the effect of ketoconazole and methadone. Nevirapine may decrease serum concentrations of some protease inhibitors (AUC of indinavir and saquinavir may be decreased - no effect noted with ritonavir), specific dosage adjustments have not been recommended (no adjustment recommended for ritonavir).

Increased Effect/Toxicity: Cimetidine, itraconazole, ketoconazole, and some macrolide antibiotics may increase nevirapine plasma concentrations. Increased toxicity when used concomitantly with protease inhibitors or oral contraceptives. Ketoconazole should NOT be coadministered. Concurrent administration of prednisone for the initial 14 days of nevirapine therapy was associated with an increased incidence and severity of rash.

Nutritional/Ethanol Interactions Herb/Nutraceutical: Nevirapine serum concentration may be decreased by St John's wort; avoid concurrent use.

Adverse Reactions

>10%:

Central nervous system: Headache (11%), fever (8% to 11%)
Dermatologic: Rash (15% to 20%)
Gastrointestinal: Diarrhea (15% to 20%)
Hematologic: Neutropenia (10% to 11%)

1% to 10%:

Gastrointestinal: Ulcerative stomatitis (4%), nausea, abdominal pain (2%)
Hematologic: Anemia
Hepatic: Hepatitis, increased LFTs (2% to 4%)
Neuromuscular & skeletal: Peripheral neuropathy, paresthesia (2%), myalgia

<1% (Limited to important or life-threatening): Hepatic necrosis, hepatotoxicity, severe hypersensitivity/dermatologic reactions (may include severe rash, fever, blisters, oral lesions, conjunctivitis, facial edema, muscle or joint aches, general malaise, hepatitis, eosinophilia, granulocytopenia, lymphadenopathy, or renal dysfunction), Stevens-Johnson syndrome. If a severe hypersensitivity reaction occurs, nevirapine should be permanently discontinued.

Overdosage/Toxicology No toxicities have been reported with acute ingestion of large sums of tablets.

Pharmacodynamics/Kinetics

Absorption: >90%

Half-Life Elimination: Decreases over 2- to 4-week time with chronic dosing due to autoinduction (ie, half-life = 45 hours initially and decreases to 23 hours)

Time to Peak: Serum: 2-4 hours

Metabolism: Extensively hepatic via CYP3A4 (hydroxylation to inactive compounds); may undergo enterohepatic recycling

Formulations

Suspension, oral: 50 mg/5 mL (240 mL)
Tablet: 200 mg

Dosing

Adults & Elderly: HIV infection: Oral: Initial: 200 mg once daily for 14 days; maintenance: 200 mg twice daily (in combination with an additional antiretroviral agents). **Note:** If a therapy is interrupted for >7 days, restart with initial dose for 14 days.

Pediatrics: HIV infection: Oral:

Children 2 months to <8 years: Initial: 4 mg/kg/dose once daily for 14 days; increase dose to every 12 hours if no rash or other adverse effects occur; maintenance dose: 7 mg/kg/dose every 12 hours; maximum dose: 200 mg/dose every 12 hours

Children ≥8 years: Initial: 4 mg/kg/dose once daily for 14 days; increase dose to 4 mg/kg/dose every 12 hours if no rash or other adverse effects occur; maximum dose: 200 mg/dose every 12 hours

Alternative pediatric dosing (unlabeled): 120-200 mg/m^2 every 12 hours; this dosing has been proposed due to the fact that dosing based on mg/kg may result in an abrupt decrease in dose at the 8th birthday, which may be inappropriate.

Note: If a therapy is interrupted for >7 days, restart with initial dose for 14 days

Administration

Oral: May be administered with or without food. May be administered with an antacid or didanosine. Shake suspension gently prior to administration.

Monitoring Laboratory Tests Perform CBC. Liver function tests should be monitored at baseline, and intensively during the first 12 weeks of therapy (optimal frequency not established, recommendations recommend more often than once a month, including prior to dose escalation, and at 2 weeks following dose escalation), then periodically throughout therapy; observe for CNS side effects.

Monitoring and Teaching Issues

Physical Assessment: See Contraindications, Warnings/Precautions, and Dosing for use cautions. Assess potential for interactions with other prescriptions, OTC medications, or herbal products patient may be taking (see Drug Interactions). Assess results of laboratory tests (see above) prior to beginning therapy, at any dose changes, and at regular intervals during long-term therapy. Assess therapeutic effectiveness and adverse response (see

Adverse Reactions and Overdose/Toxicology). Teach patient proper use, possible side effects and appropriate interventions, and adverse symptoms to report (see Patient Education). **Pregnancy risk factor C** - benefits of use should outweigh possible risks. Nevirapine may decrease the effectiveness of oral contraceptives - instruct about alternate method of birth control. Breast-feeding is contraindicated.

Patient Education: Inform prescriber of all prescriptions, OTC medications, or herbal products you are taking, and any allergies you have. Do not take anything new during treatment unless approved by prescriber. This is not a cure for HIV and has not been shown to reduce the risk of transmitting HIV to others. The long-term effects of use are not known. Take as directed, with food. If unable to swallow tablets whole, the tablet may be dissolved in water or crushed in food. Shake suspension gently prior to use. Use oral syringe for volumes of 5 mL or less. When using dosing cups, rinse cup with water and drink. If you miss a dose, take as soon as possible and return to regular schedule (never take a double dose). Frequent blood tests may be required with prolonged therapy. May cause diarrhea (buttermilk, boiled milk, or yogurt may help); or headache (consult prescriber for approved analgesic). If rash develops, stop medicine and contact prescriber immediately. Report fever, blisters, facial edema, muscle or joint pain, general malaise, difficulty breathing, persistent diarrhea or nausea, or pain or irritation in eyes. **Pregnancy/breast-feeding precautions:** Inform prescriber if you are or intend to become pregnant. Consult prescriber for appropriate barrier contraceptives (nevirapine may decrease the effectiveness of oral contraceptives) to reduce risk of transmitting infection and possible pregnancy. Do not breast-feed.

Breast-feeding Issues: HIV-infected mothers are discouraged from breast-feeding to decrease potential transmission of HIV.

Pregnancy Issues: Nevirapine crosses the placenta. It may be used in combination with zidovudine in HIV-infected women who are in labor, but have had no prior antiretroviral therapy, in order to reduce the maternal-fetal transmission of HIV. Health professionals are encouraged to contact the antiretroviral pregnancy registry to monitor outcomes of pregnant women exposed to antiretroviral medications (1-800-258-4263).

Additional Information Potential compliance problems, frequency of administration, and adverse effects should be discussed with patients before initiating therapy to help prevent the emergence of resistance.

Related Information

Tuberculosis *on page 1705*

Nexium® *see* Esomeprazole *on page 492*

Niacin (NYE a sin)

U.S. Brand Names Niacor®; Niaspan®; Nicotinex [OTC]; Slo-Niacin® [OTC]

Synonyms Nicotinic Acid; Vitamin B_3

Generic Available Yes

Pharmacologic Category Antilipemic Agent, Miscellaneous; Vitamin, Water Soluble

Pregnancy Risk Factor A/C (dose exceeding RDA recommendation)

Lactation Enters breast milk/consult healthcare provider

Use Adjunctive treatment of hyperlipidemias; peripheral vascular disease and circulatory disorders; treatment of pellagra; dietary supplement; use in elevating HDL in patients with dyslipidemia

Mechanism of Action/Effect Component of two coenzymes which is necessary for tissue respiration, lipid metabolism, and glycogenolysis; inhibits the synthesis of very low density lipoproteins

Contraindications Hypersensitivity to niacin, niacinamide, or any component of the formulation; liver disease; active peptic ulcer; severe hypotension; arterial hemorrhage

Warnings/Precautions Monitor liver function tests, blood glucose. May elevate uric acid levels; use with caution in patients predisposed to gout. Large doses should be administered with caution to patients with gallbladder disease, jaundice, liver disease, or diabetes. Some products may contain tartrazine. Pregnancy risk A/C (dose exceeding RDA).

Drug Interactions

Decreased Effect: The effect of oral hypoglycemics may be decreased by niacin. Niacin may inhibit uricosuric effects of sulfinpyrazone and probenecid. Aspirin (or other NSAIDs) decreases niacin-induced flushing.

Increased Effect/Toxicity: Niacin increase the potential for myopathy and/or rhabdomyolysis with lovastatin (and possibly other HMG-CoA reductase inhibitors). Use with adrenergic blocking agents may result in additive vasodilating effect and postural hypotension.

Effects on Lab Values False elevations in some fluorometric determinations of urinary catecholamines; false-positive urine glucose (Benedict's reagent)

Adverse Reactions

1% to 10%:

- Cardiovascular: Generalized flushing
- Central nervous system: Headache
- Gastrointestinal: Bloating, flatulence, nausea
- Hepatic: Abnormalities of hepatic function tests, jaundice
- Neuromuscular & skeletal: Paresthesia in extremities
- Miscellaneous: Increased sebaceous gland activity, sensation of warmth

<1% (Limited to important or life-threatening): Blurred vision, dizziness, liver damage (dose-related incidence), rash, syncope, tachycardia, vasovagal attacks, wheezing

Overdosage/Toxicology Symptoms of acute overdose include flushing, GI distress, and pruritus. Chronic excessive use has been associated with hepatitis. Antihistamines may relieve niacin-induced histamine release; otherwise treatment is symptomatic.

Pharmacodynamics/Kinetics

Half-Life Elimination: 45 minutes

Time to Peak: Serum: ~45 minutes

Metabolism: Niacin converts to niacinamide (dose dependent); niacinamide (30%) hepatically metabolized

(Continued)

Niacin *(Continued)*

Formulations

Capsule, extended release: 125 mg, 250 mg, 400 mg, 500 mg
Capsule, timed release: 250 mg
Elixir (Nicotinex): 50 mg/5 mL (473 mL) [contains alcohol 10% (sherry wine)]
Tablet: 50 mg, 100 mg, 250 mg, 500 mg
Niacor®: 500 mg
Tablet, controlled release (Slo-Niacin®): 250 mg, 500 mg, 750 mg
Tablet, extended release (Niaspan®): 500 mg, 750 mg, 1000 mg
Tablet, timed release: 250 mg, 500 mg, 750 mg, 1000 mg

Dosing

Adults & Elderly:

Recommended daily allowances:
Male: 25-50 years: 19 mg/day; >51 years: 15 mg/day
Female: 25-50 years: 15 mg/day; >51 years: 13 mg/day

Hyperlipidemia: Oral: Usual target dose: 1.5-6 g/day in 3 divided doses with or after meals using a dosage titration schedule; extended release: 375 mg to 2 g once daily at bedtime

Regular release formulation (Niacor®): Initial: 250 mg once daily (with evening meal); increase frequency and/or dose every 4-7 days to desired response or first-level therapeutic dose (1.5-2 g/day in 2-3 divided doses); after 2 months, may increase at 2- to 4-week intervals to 3 g/day in 3 divided doses

Extended release formulation (Niaspan®): 500 mg at bedtime for 4 weeks, then 1 g at bedtime for 4 weeks; adjust dose to response and tolerance; can increase to a maximum of 2 g/day, but only at 500 mg/day at 4-week intervals

Pellagra: Oral: 50-100 mg 3-4 times/day, maximum: 500 mg/day
Niacin deficiency: Oral: 10-20 mg/day, maximum: 100 mg/day

Pediatrics:

Pellagra: Oral: Children: 50-100 mg/dose 3 times/day
Recommended daily allowances:
0-0.5 years: 5 mg/day
0.5-1 year: 6 mg/day
1-3 years: 9 mg/day
4-6 years: 12 mg/day
7-10 years: 13 mg/day

Children and Adolescents: Oral: Recommended daily allowances:
Male:
11-14 years: 17 mg/day
15-18 years: 20 mg/day
19-24 years: 19 mg/day
Female: 11-24 years: 15 mg/day

Monitoring Laboratory Tests Blood glucose, liver function tests (with large doses or prolonged therapy), serum cholesterol

Monitoring and Teaching Issues

Physical Assessment: Assess other medications patient may be taking for increased risk of drug/drug interactions (see Drug Interactions). See Warnings/Precautions and Adverse Reactions for use cautions. Assess knowledge/teach patient appropriate use (including appropriate injection technique and needle disposal), interventions to reduce side effects, and adverse symptoms to report (see Patient Education). **Pregnancy risk factor A/C** - see Pregnancy Risk Factor for use cautions. Note breast-feeding caution.

Patient Education: Take exactly as directed; do not exceed recommended dosage. Take with food to reduce incidence of GI upset. Do not crush sustained release capsules. You may experience flushing, sensation of heat, or headache; these reactions may be decreased by increasing dose slowly or by taking aspirin (consult prescriber) 30 minutes prior to taking niacin. You may experience dizziness, lightheadedness (use caution when driving or engaging in tasks requiring alertness until response to drug is known). Report persistent GI disturbance or changes in color of urine or stool. **Pregnancy/breast-feeding precautions:** Inform prescriber if you are pregnant. Consult prescriber if breast-feeding.

Dietary Issues: Should be taken after meals.

Related Information

Hyperlipidemia Management *on page 1682*
Lipid-Lowering Agents *on page 1582*

Niacor® *see* Niacin *on page 965*

Niaspan® *see* Niacin *on page 965*

NiCARdipine (nye KAR de peen)

U.S. Brand Names Cardene®; Cardene® I.V.; Cardene® SR

Synonyms Nicardipine Hydrochloride

Generic Available Yes: Capsule

Pharmacologic Category Calcium Channel Blocker

Pregnancy Risk Factor C

Lactation Enters breast milk/not recommended

Use Chronic stable angina (immediate-release product only); management of essential hypertension (immediate and sustained release; parenteral only for short time that oral treatment is not feasible)

Use - Unlabeled/Investigational Congestive heart failure

Mechanism of Action/Effect Inhibits calcium ion from entering the "slow channels" or select voltage-sensitive areas of vascular smooth muscle and myocardium during depolarization, producing a relaxation of coronary vascular smooth muscle and coronary vasodilation; increases myocardial oxygen delivery in patients with vasospastic angina

Contraindications Hypersensitivity to nicardipine or any component of the formulation; advanced aortic stenosis; severe hypotension; cardiogenic shock; ventricular tachycardia

Warnings/Precautions Blood pressure lowering should be done at a rate appropriate for the patient's condition. Rapid drops in blood pressure can lead to arterial insufficiency. Use with caution in CAD (can cause increase in angina), CHF (can worsen heart failure symptoms), and pheochromocytoma (limited clinical experience). Peripheral infusion sites (for I.V. therapy) should be changed ever 12 hours. Titrate I.V. dose cautiously in patients with CHF, renal, or hepatic dysfunction. Use the I.V. form cautiously in patients with portal hypertension (can cause increase in hepatic pressure gradient). Safety and efficacy have not been demonstrated in pediatric patients. Abrupt withdrawal may cause rebound angina in patients with CAD. Pregnancy risk C.

Drug Interactions

Cytochrome P450 Effect: Substrate of CYP1A2, 2C8/9, 2D6, 2E1, **3A4**; Inhibits CYP2C8/9, 2C19, 2D6, 3A4

Decreased Effect: Rifampin (and potentially other enzyme inducers) increase the metabolism of calcium channel blockers.

Increased Effect/Toxicity: H_2 blockers (cimetidine) may increase the bioavailability of nicardipine. Serum concentrations/toxicity of nicardipine may be increased by inhibitors of CYP3A4, including amprenavir, cimetidine, ciprofloxacin, clarithromycin, clozapine, diltiazem, disulfiram, digoxin, erythromycin, ethanol, fluconazole, fluoxetine, fluvoxamine, grapefruit juice, isoniazid, itraconazole, ketoconazole, labetalol, levodopa, loxapine, metoprolol, metronidazole, miconazole, nefazodone, nelfinavir, omeprazole, phenytoin, propranolol, rifabutin, rifampin, ritonavir, troleandomycin, valproic acid, and verapamil. Calcium may reduce the calcium channel blocker's effects, particularly hypotension. Cyclosporine levels (and possibly tacrolimus) may be increased by nicardipine. May increase effect of vecuronium (reduce dose 25%) and increase serum levels of metoprolol.

Nutritional/Ethanol Interactions

Ethanol: Avoid ethanol (may increase CNS depression).

Food: Nicardipine average peak concentrations may be decreased if taken with food. Serum concentrations/toxicity of nicardipine may be increased by grapefruit juice; avoid concurrent use.

Herb/Nutraceutical: St John's wort may decrease levels. Avoid dong quai if using for hypertension (has estrogenic activity). Avoid ephedra, yohimbe, ginseng (may worsen hypertension). Avoid garlic (may have increased antihypertensive effect).

Adverse Reactions

1% to 10%:

Cardiovascular: Flushing (6% to 10%), palpitations (3% to 4%), tachycardia (1% to 3%), peripheral edema (dose-related 7% to 8%), increased angina (dose-related 5.6%)

Central nervous system: Headache (6% to 8%), dizziness (4% to 7%), somnolence (4% to 6%), paresthesia (1%)

Dermatologic: Rash (1%)

Gastrointestinal: Nausea (2% to 5%), dry mouth (1%)

Neuromuscular & skeletal: Weakness (4% to 6%), myalgia (1%)

<1% (Limited to important or life-threatening): Abnormal EKG, dyspnea, gingival hyperplasia, nervousness, parotitis, sustained tachycardia, syncope

Overdosage/Toxicology The primary cardiac symptoms of calcium blocker overdose include hypotension and bradycardia. Noncardiac symptoms include confusion, stupor, nausea, vomiting, metabolic acidosis, and hyperglycemia. Following initial gastric decontamination, if possible, repeated calcium administration may promptly reverse the depressed cardiac contractility (but not sinus node depression or peripheral vasodilation). Glucagon and epinephrine may treat refractory hypotension. Glucagon and epinephrine also increase the heart rate (outside the U.S., 4-aminopyridine may be available as an antidote). Dialysis and hemoperfusion are not effective in enhancing elimination although repeat-dose activated charcoal may serve as an adjunct with sustained-release preparations.

Pharmacodynamics/Kinetics

Absorption: Oral: ~100%

Bioavailability: 35%

Half-Life Elimination: 2-4 hours

Time to Peak: Serum: 20-120 minutes

Metabolism: Hepatic; extensive first-pass effect

Onset: Oral: 1-2 hours; I.V.: 10 minutes; Hypotension: ~20 minutes

Duration: 2-6 hours

Formulations

Capsule (Cardene®): 20 mg, 30 mg

Capsule, sustained release (Cardene® SR): 30 mg, 45 mg, 60 mg

Injection, solution (Cardene® IV): 2.5 mg/mL (10 mL)

Dosing

Adults & Elderly: The total daily dose of immediate-release product may not automatically be equivalent to the daily sustained-release dose; use caution in converting.

Hypertension: Oral:

Immediate release: Initial: 20 mg 3 times/day; usual: 20-40 mg 3 times/day (allow 3 days between dose increases)

Sustained release: Initial: 30 mg twice daily, titrate up to 60 mg twice daily

Acute hypertension: I.V. (dilute to 0.1 mg/mL): Initial: 5 mg/hour increased by 2.5 mg/hour every 15 minutes to a maximum of 15 mg/hour

Note: Oral to I.V. dose equivalents:

20 mg every 8 hours orally = 0.5 mg/hour I.V.

30 mg every 8 hours orally = 1.2 mg/hour I.V.

40 mg every 8 hours orally = 2.2 mg/hour I.V.

Renal Impairment: Titrate dose beginning with 20 mg 3 times/day (immediate release) or 30 mg twice daily (sustained release).

Hepatic Impairment: Starting dose: 20 mg twice daily (immediate release) with titration. Refer to "Note" in adult dosing.

(Continued)

NiCARdipine *(Continued)*

Administration

Oral: Do not chew or crush the sustained release formulation, swallow whole. Do not open or cut capsules.

I.V.: Ampuls must be diluted before use. Administer as a slow continuous infusion.

Stability

Storage: I.V.: Store at room temperature and protect from light. Freezing does not affect stability.

Compatibility: Stable in D_5W with KCl 40 mEq, $D_5{}^1/_2NS$, D_5NS, D_5W, $^1/_2NS$, NS; **incompatible** with sodium bicarbonate 5%, LR

Y-site administration: Incompatible with furosemide, heparin, thiopental

Monitoring and Teaching Issues

Physical Assessment: See Contraindications, Warnings/Precautions, and Dosing for use cautions. Assess potential for interactions with other prescriptions, OTC medications, or herbal products patient may be taking (see Drug Interactions). See infusion specifics above; infusion site must be monitored closely to prevent extravasation and peripheral infusion sites (for I.V. therapy) should be changed ever 12 hours. Assess therapeutic effectiveness and adverse response (eg, cardiac status and blood pressure when starting, adjusting dose, or discontinuing - see Adverse Reactions and Overdose/Toxicology). Teach patient proper use, possible side effects and appropriate interventions (eg, orthostatic precautions), and adverse symptoms to report (see Patient Education). **Pregnancy risk factor C** - benefits of use should outweigh possible risks. Breast-feeding is not recommended.

Patient Education: Inform prescriber of all prescriptions, OTC medications, or herbal products you are taking, and any allergies you have. Do not take anything new during treatment unless approved by prescriber.

I.V.: Report immediately any swelling, redness, burning, or pain at infusion site.

Oral: Take as directed; do not alter dose or decrease without consulting prescriber. Do not crush or chew sustained release forms; swallow whole. Take with nonfatty food. Avoid caffeine and alcohol. Consult prescriber before increasing exercise routine (decreased angina does not mean it is safe to increase exercise). May cause orthostatic hypotension (change position slowly from sitting or lying to standing, or when climbing stairs); sore mouth (inspect gums for swelling or redness - use soft toothbrush, waxed dental floss, and frequent mouth rinses); dizziness or fatigue (use caution when driving or engaging in tasks that require alertness until response to drug is known); or nausea and dry mouth (small, frequent meals, frequent mouth care, chewing gum, or sucking lozenges may help). Report chest pain, palpitations, rapid heartbeat; swelling of extremities; muscle weakness or pain; difficulty breathing; or nervousness. **Pregnancy/breast-feeding precautions:** Inform prescriber if you are or intend to become pregnant. Breast-feeding is not recommended.

Geriatric Considerations: Elderly may experience a greater hypotensive response. Constipation may be more of a problem in the elderly.

Related Information

Calcium Channel Blockers *on page 1563*
FDA Name Differentiation Project: The Use of Tall-man Letters *on page 12*

Nicardipine Hydrochloride *see* NiCARdipine *on page 966*

NicoDerm® CQ® [OTC] *see* Nicotine *on page 968*

Nicorette® [OTC] *see* Nicotine *on page 968*

Nicotine (nik oh TEEN)

U.S. Brand Names NicoDerm® CQ® [OTC]; Nicorette® [OTC]; Nicotrol® Inhaler; Nicotrol® NS; Nicotrol® Patch [OTC]

Synonyms Habitrol®

Generic Available Yes: Transdermal patch and gum

Pharmacologic Category Smoking Cessation Aid

Pregnancy Risk Factor D (transdermal); X (chewing gum)

Lactation Excretion in breast milk unknown/contraindicated

Use Treatment to aid smoking cessation for the relief of nicotine withdrawal symptoms (including nicotine craving)

Use - Unlabeled/Investigational Management of ulcerative colitis (transdermal)

Mechanism of Action/Effect Nicotine is one of two naturally-occurring alkaloids which exhibit their primary effects via autonomic ganglia stimulation. Nicotine is a potent ganglionic and central nervous system stimulant, the actions of which are mediated via nicotine-specific receptors. Stimulation of the central nervous system (CNS) is characterized by tremors and respiratory excitation. However, convulsions may occur with higher doses, along with respiratory failure secondary to both central paralysis and peripheral blockade to respiratory muscles.

Contraindications Hypersensitivity to nicotine or any component of the formulation; patients who are smoking during the postmyocardial infarction period; patients with life-threatening arrhythmias, or severe or worsening angina pectoris; active temporomandibular joint disease (gum); pregnancy; not for use in nonsmokers

Warnings/Precautions The risk versus the benefits must be weighed for each of these groups: patients with CAD, serious cardiac arrhythmias, vasospastic disease. Use caution in patients with hyperthyroidism, pheochromocytoma, or insulin-dependent diabetes. Use with caution in oropharyngeal inflammation and in patients with history of esophagitis, peptic ulcer, coronary artery disease, vasospastic disease, angina, hypertension, hyperthyroidism, pheochromocytoma, diabetes, severe renal dysfunction, and hepatic dysfunction. The inhaler should be used with caution in patients with bronchospastic disease (other forms of nicotine replacement may be preferred). Safety and efficacy have not been established in pediatric patients. Cautious use of topical nicotine in patients with certain skin diseases. Hypersensitivity to the topical products can occur. Dental problems may be worsened by chewing the gum. Urge patients to stop smoking completely when initiating therapy.

Drug Interactions

Cytochrome P450 Effect: Substrate of CYP1A2, 2A6, 2B6, 2C8/9, 2C19, 2D6, 2E1, 3A4; Inhibits CYP2A6

Increased Effect/Toxicity: Nicotine increases the hemodynamic and AV blocking effects of adenosine; monitor. Cimetidine increases nicotine concentrations; therefore, may decrease amount of gum or patches needed. Monitor for treatment-emergent hypertension in patients treated with the combination of nicotine patch and bupropion.

Adverse Reactions

Chewing gum:

>10%:

Cardiovascular: Tachycardia

Central nervous system: Headache (mild)

Gastrointestinal: Nausea, vomiting, indigestion, excessive salivation, belching, increased appetite

Miscellaneous: Mouth or throat soreness, jaw muscle ache, hiccups

1% to 10%:

Central nervous system: Insomnia, dizziness, nervousness

Endocrine & metabolic: Dysmenorrhea

Gastrointestinal: GI distress, eructation

Neuromuscular & skeletal: Muscle pain

Respiratory: Hoarseness

Miscellaneous: Hiccups

<1% (Limited to important or life-threatening): Atrial fibrillation, erythema, hypersensitivity reactions, itching

Transdermal systems:

>10%:

Central nervous system: Insomnia, abnormal dreams

Dermatologic: Pruritus, erythema

Local: Application site reaction

Respiratory: Rhinitis, cough, pharyngitis, sinusitis

1% to 10%:

Cardiovascular: Chest pain

Central nervous system: Dysphoria, anxiety, difficulty concentrating, dizziness, somnolence

Dermatologic: Rash

Gastrointestinal: Diarrhea, dyspepsia, nausea, xerostomia, constipation, anorexia, abdominal pain

Neuromuscular & skeletal: Arthralgia, myalgia

<1% (Limited to important or life-threatening): Atrial fibrillation, hypersensitivity reactions, itching, nervousness, taste perversion, thirst, tremor

Overdosage/Toxicology Symptoms of overdose include nausea, vomiting, abdominal pain, mental confusion, diarrhea, salivation, tachycardia, respiratory and cardiovascular collapse. Treatment is symptomatic and supportive. Remove patch, rinse area with water, and dry. Do not use soap as this may increase absorption.

Pharmacodynamics/Kinetics

Absorption: Transdermal: Slow

Half-Life Elimination: 4 hours

Time to Peak: Serum: Transdermal: 8-9 hours

Metabolism: Hepatic, primarily to cotinine ($^1/_5$ as active)

Onset: Intranasal: More closely approximate the time course of plasma nicotine levels observed after cigarette smoking than other dosage forms

Duration: Transdermal: 24 hours

Formulations

Gum, chewing, as polacrilex (Nicorette®): 2 mg/square (48s, 108s, 168s); 4 mg/square (48s, 108s, 168s) [mint, orange, and original flavors]

Oral inhalation system (Nicotrol® Inhaler): 10 mg cartridge [delivering 4 mg nicotine] (42s) [each unit consists of 1 mouthpiece, 7 storage trays each containing 6 cartridges, and 1 storage case]

Patch, transdermal: 7 mg/24 (7s, 30s); 14 mg/24 hours (7s, 14s, 30s); 21 mg/24 hours (7s, 14s, 30s)

Kit: Step 1: 21 mg/24 hours (28s); Step 2: 14 mg/24 hours (14s); Step 3: 7 mg/24 hours (14s) [kit also contains support material]

NicoDerm® CQ® [clear patch]: 7 mg/24 hours (14s); 14 mg/24 hours (14s); 21 mg/24 hours (14s)

NicoDerm® CQ® [tan patch]: 7 mg/24 hours (14s); 14 mg/24 hours (14s); 21 mg/24 hours (7s, 14s)

Nicotrol®: 15 mg/16 hours (7s)

Solution, intranasal spray (Nicotrol® NS): 10 mg/mL (10 mL) [delivers 0.5 mg/spray; 200 sprays]

Dosing

Adults:

Tobacco cessation:

Gum: Chew 1 piece of gum when urge to smoke, up to 30 pieces/day; most patients require 10-12 pieces of gum/day

Inhaler: Usually 6 to 16 cartridges per day; best effect was achieved by frequent continuous puffing (20 minutes); recommended duration of treatment is 3 months, after which patients may be weaned from the inhaler by gradual reduction of the daily dose over 6-12 weeks

Transdermal patch: (patients should be advised to completely stop smoking upon initiation of therapy): Apply new patch every 24 hours to nonhairy, clean, dry skin on the upper body or upper outer arm; each patch should be applied to a different site. **Note:** Adjustment may be required during initial treatment (move to higher dose if experiencing withdrawal symptoms; lower dose if side effects are experienced).

(Continued)

Nicotine *(Continued)*

Habitrol®, Nicoderm CQ®:

Patients smoking ≥10 cigarettes/day: Begin with step 1 (21 mg/day) for 4-6 weeks, **followed by** step 2 (14 mg/day) for 2 weeks; **finish with** step 3 (7 mg/day) for 2 weeks

Patients smoking <10 cigarettes/day: Begin with step 2 (14 mg/day) for 6 weeks, **followed by** step 3 (7 mg/day) for 2 weeks

Note: Initial starting dose for patients <100 pounds, history of cardiovascular disease: 14 mg/day for 4-6 weeks, **followed by** 7 mg/day for 2-4 weeks

Note: Patients who are receiving >600 mg/day of cimetidine: Decrease to the next lower patch size

Nicotrol®: One patch daily for 6 weeks

Prostep®:

Patients smoking >15 cigarettes/day: One 22 mg patch daily for 6 weeks

Patients smoking ≤15 cigarettes/day: One 11 mg patch daily for 6 weeks

Benefits of use of nicotine transdermal patches beyond 3 months have not been demonstrated

Spray: 1-2 sprays/hour; do not exceed more than 5 doses (10 sprays) per hour; each dose (2 sprays) contains 1 mg of nicotine. **Warning:** A dose of 40 mg can cause fatalities

Ulcerative colitis: Transdermal: Titrated to 22-25 mg/day

Elderly: Refer to adult dosing; use with caution.

Administration

Oral: Patients should be instructed to chew slowly to avoid jaw ache and to maximize benefit.

Topical: Patches cannot be cut. Use of an aerosol corticosteroid may diminish local irritation under patches.

Stability

Storage: Store inhaler cartridge at room temperature not to exceed 30°C (86°F); protect cartridges from light

Monitoring and Teaching Issues

Physical Assessment: See Contraindications and Warnings/Precautions for use cautions. Monitor cardiac status and vital signs prior to, when beginning, and periodically during therapy. Monitor effectiveness of therapy (according to rational for therapy), and adverse reactions (see extensive list of Adverse Reactions) at beginning and periodically during therapy. Assess knowledge/teach patient appropriate use, interventions to reduce side effects, and adverse symptoms to report for prescribed form of drug (see Patient Education). **Pregnancy risk factor D/X** - see Pregnancy Risk Factor for use cautions. Determine that patient is not pregnant before beginning treatment and do not give to women of childbearing age unless female is capable of complying with barrier contraceptive measures. Breast-feeding is contraindicated.

Patient Education: Use exactly as directed; do not use more often than prescribed. Stop smoking completely during therapy. Do not smoke, chew tobacco, use snuff, nicotine gum, or any other form of nicotine. Nicotine overdose could occur.

Gum: Chew slowly for 30 minutes. Discard chewed gum away from access by children.

Transdermal patch: Follow directions in package for dosing schedule and use. Do not cut patches or wear more than one patch at a time. Remove backing from patch and press immediately on skin. Hold for 10 seconds. Apply to clean, dry skin in different site each day. Do not touch eyes; wash hands after application. You may experience vivid dreams and sleep disturbances, dizziness or lightheadedness (use caution driving or when engaging in tasks requiring alertness until response to drug is known). For nausea, vomiting or GI upset, small, frequent meals, chewing gum, and frequent oral care may help. Report persistent vomiting, diarrhea, chills, sweating, chest pain or palpitations, or burning or redness at application site.

Spray: Follow directions in package. Blow nose gently before use. Use 1-2 sprays/hour; do not exceed 5 doses (10 sprays) per hour. Excessive use can result in severe (even life-threatening) reactions. You may experience temporary stinging or burning after spray.

Pregnancy/breast-feeding precautions: Inform prescriber if you are pregnant. Do not get pregnant during or for 1 month following therapy. Consult prescriber for instruction on appropriate contraceptive measures. This drug may cause severe fetal defects. Do not breast-feed.

Geriatric Considerations: Must evaluate benefit in the elderly who may have chronic diseases mentioned (see Warnings/Precautions and Contraindications). The transdermal systems are as effective in the elderly as they are in younger adults; however, complaints of body aches, dizziness, and asthenia were reported more often in the elderly.

Additional Information A cigarette has 10-25 mg nicotine. Use of an aerosol corticosteroid may diminish local irritation under patches.

Nicotinex [OTC] *see* Niacin *on page 965*

Nicotinic Acid *see* Niacin *on page 965*

Nicotrol® Inhaler *see* Nicotine *on page 968*

Nicotrol® NS *see* Nicotine *on page 968*

Nicotrol® Patch [OTC] *see* Nicotine *on page 968*

Nifedical™ XL *see* NIFEdipine *on page 970*

NIFEdipine (nye FED i peen)

U.S. Brand Names Adalat® CC; Nifedical™ XL; Procardia®; Procardia XL®

Generic Available Yes

Pharmacologic Category Calcium Channel Blocker

Pregnancy Risk Factor C

Lactation Enters breast milk/compatible

Use Angina and hypertension (sustained release only), pulmonary hypertension

Mechanism of Action/Effect Inhibits calcium ion from entering the "slow channels" or select voltage-sensitive areas of vascular smooth muscle and myocardium during depolarization, producing a relaxation of coronary vascular smooth muscle and coronary vasodilation; increases myocardial oxygen delivery in patients with vasospastic angina

Contraindications Hypersensitivity to nifedipine or any component of the formulation; immediate release preparation for treatment of urgent or emergent hypertension; acute MI

Warnings/Precautions **The use of sublingual short-acting nifedipine in hypertensive emergencies and pseudoemergencies is neither safe nor effective and SHOULD BE ABANDONED!** Serious adverse events (cerebrovascular ischemia, syncope, heart block, stroke, sinus arrest, severe hypotension, acute myocardial infarction, EKG changes, and fetal distress) have been reported in relation to such use.

Blood pressure lowering should be done at a rate appropriate for the patient's condition. Rapid drops in blood pressure can lead to arterial insufficiency. Increased angina and/or MI has occurred with initiation or dosage titration of calcium channel blockers. Use caution in severe aortic stenosis. Use caution in patients with severe hepatic impairment (may need dosage adjustment). Abrupt withdrawal may cause rebound angina in patients with CAD. Use caution in CHF (may cause worsening of symptoms). Avoid grapefruit juice during treatment with nifedipine.

Pregnancy risk C.

Drug Interactions

Cytochrome P450 Effect: Substrate of CYP2D6, **3A4**; Inhibits CYP1A2, 2C8/9, 2D6, 3A4

Decreased Effect: Phenobarbital and nifedipine may decrease nifedipine levels. Quinidine and nifedipine may decrease quinidine serum levels. Rifampin and nifedipine may decrease nifedipine serum levels. Calcium may reduce the hypotension from of calcium channel blockers.

Increased Effect/Toxicity: H_2-blockers may increase bioavailability and serum concentrations of nifedipine. Serum concentrations/toxicity of nifedipine may be increased by inhibitors of CYP3A4, including amprenavir, cimetidine, ciprofloxacin, clarithromycin, clozapine, diltiazem, disulfiram, digoxin, erythromycin, ethanol, fluconazole, fluoxetine, fluvoxamine, grapefruit juice, isoniazid, itraconazole, ketoconazole, labetalol, levodopa, loxapine, metoprolol, metronidazole, miconazole, nefazodone, nelfinavir, omeprazole, phenytoin, rifabutin, rifampin, ritonavir, troleandomycin, valproic acid, and verapamil. Nifedipine may increase serum levels of digoxin, phenytoin, theophylline, and vincristine.

Nutritional/Ethanol Interactions

Ethanol: Avoid ethanol (may increase CNS depression).

Food: Nifedipine serum levels may be decreased if taken with food. Food may decrease the rate but not the extent of absorption of Procardia XL®. Increased therapeutic and vasodilator side effects, including severe hypotension and myocardial ischemia, may occur if nifedipine is taken by patients ingesting grapefruit.

Herb/Nutraceutical: St John's wort may decrease nifedipine levels. Avoid dong quai if using for hypertension (has estrogenic activity). Avoid ephedra, yohimbe, ginseng (may worsen hypertension). Avoid garlic (may have increased antihypertensive effect).

Adverse Reactions

>10%:

Cardiovascular: Flushing (10% to 25%), peripheral edema (dose-related 7% to 10%; up to 50%)

Central nervous system: Dizziness/lightheadedness/giddiness (10% to 27%), headache (10% to 23%)

Gastrointestinal: Nausea/heartburn (10% to 11%)

Neuromuscular & skeletal: Weakness (10% to 12%)

≥1% to 10%:

Cardiovascular: Palpitations (≤2% to 7%), transient hypotension (dose-related 5%), CHF (2%)

Central nervous system: Nervousness/mood changes (≤2% to 7%), shakiness (≤2%), jitteriness (≤2%), sleep disturbances (≤2%), difficulties in balance (≤2%), fever (≤2%), chills (≤2%)

Dermatologic: Dermatitis (≤2%), pruritus (≤2%), urticaria (≤2%)

Endocrine & metabolic: Sexual difficulties (≤2%)

Gastrointestinal: Diarrhea (≤2%), constipation (≤2%), cramps (≤2%), flatulence (≤2%), gingival hyperplasia (≤10%)

Neuromuscular & skeletal: Muscle cramps/tremor (≤2% to 8%), weakness (10%), inflammation (≤2%), joint stiffness (≤2%)

Ocular: Blurred vision (≤2%)

Respiratory: Cough/wheezing (6%), nasal congestion/sore throat (≤2% to 6%), chest congestion (≤2%), dyspnea (≤2%)

Miscellaneous: Diaphoresis (≤2%)

<1% (Limited to important or life-threatening): Agranulocytosis, allergic hepatitis, angina, angioedema, aplastic anemia, arthritis with positive ANA, bezoars (sustained-release preparations), cerebral ischemia, depression, erythema multiforme, erythromelalgia, exfoliative dermatitis, extrapyramidal symptoms, fever, gingival hyperplasia, gynecomastia, leukopenia, memory dysfunction, paranoid syndrome, phototoxicity, purpura, Stevens-Johnson syndrome, syncope, thrombocytopenia, tinnitus, transient blindness

Reported with use of sublingual short-acting nifedipine: Acute myocardial infarction, cerebrovascular ischemia, EKG changes, fetal distress, heart block, severe hypotension, sinus arrest, stroke, syncope

Overdosage/Toxicology Primary cardiac symptoms of calcium blocker overdose include hypotension and bradycardia. Noncardiac symptoms include confusion, stupor, nausea, vomiting, metabolic acidosis, and hyperglycemia. Following initial gastric decontamination, treat symptomatically.

(Continued)

NIFEdipine *(Continued)*

Pharmacodynamics/Kinetics

Bioavailability: Capsule: 45% to 75%; Sustained release: 65% to 86%

Half-Life Elimination: Adults: Healthy: 2-5 hours, Cirrhosis: 7 hours; Elderly: 6.7 hours

Metabolism: Hepatic to inactive metabolites

Onset: ~20 minutes

Formulations

Capsule, liquid-filled (Procardia®): 10 mg, 20 mg

Tablet, extended release: 30 mg, 60 mg, 90 mg

Adalat® CC, Procardia XL®: 30 mg, 60 mg, 90 mg

Nifedical™ XL: 30 mg, 60 mg

Dosing

Adults & Elderly:

Hypertension: Oral: Initial: 10 mg 3 times/day as capsules or 30 mg once daily as sustained release

Usual dose: 10-30 mg 3 times/day as capsules or 30-60 mg once daily as sustained release

Maximum: 120-180 mg/day

Increase sustained release at 7- to 14-day intervals

Pediatrics:

Hypertrophic cardiomyopathy: Oral: Children: 0.6-0.9 mg/kg/24 hours in 3-4 divided doses

Hypertension: Oral: Adolescents: Refer to adult dosing.

Hepatic Impairment: Reduce oral dose by 50% to 60% in patients with cirrhosis.

Administration

Oral: Extended release tablets should be swallowed whole; do not crush or chew.

Monitoring and Teaching Issues

Physical Assessment: See Contraindications, Warnings/Precautions (eg, avoid sublingual use), and Dosing for use cautions. Assess potential for interactions with other prescriptions, OTC medications, or herbal products patient may be taking (see Drug Interactions). Assess therapeutic effectiveness and adverse response (eg, cardiac status and blood pressure when starting, adjusting dose, or discontinuing - see Adverse Reactions and Overdose/Toxicology). Teach patient proper use, possible side effects and appropriate interventions (eg, orthostatic precautions), and adverse symptoms to report (see Patient Education). **Pregnancy risk factor C** - benefits of use should outweigh possible risks.

Patient Education: Inform prescriber of all prescriptions, OTC medications, or herbal products you are taking, and any allergies you have. Do not take anything new during treatment unless approved by prescriber. Take as directed; do not alter dose or decrease without consulting prescriber. Do not crush or chew sustained release forms, swallow whole. Take with nonfatty food. Avoid caffeine, alcohol, and grapefruit juice. Consult prescriber before increasing exercise routine (decreased angina does not mean it is safe to increase exercise). May cause orthostatic hypotension (change position slowly from sitting or lying to standing, or when climbing stairs); sore mouth (inspect gums for swelling or redness - use soft toothbrush, waxed dental floss, and frequent mouth rinses); dizziness, difficulties in balance, or fatigue (use caution when driving or engaging in tasks that require alertness until response to drug is known); or nausea or heartburn (small, frequent meals, frequent mouth care, chewing gum, or sucking lozenges may help). Report chest pain, palpitations, rapid heartbeat; swelling of extremities; muscle weakness or pain; difficulty breathing; nervousness or mood change, rash; or vision changes. **Pregnancy/breast-feeding precautions:** Inform prescriber if you are or intend to become pregnant.

Dietary Issues: Capsule is rapidly absorbed orally if it is administered without food, but may result in vasodilator side effects; administration with low-fat meals may decrease flushing. Avoid grapefruit juice.

Geriatric Considerations: Elderly may experience a greater hypotensive response. Theoretically, constipation may be more of a problem in elderly patients. The half-life of nifedipine is extended in elderly patients (6.7 hours) as compared to younger subjects (3.8 hours).

Breast-feeding Issues: Crosses into breast milk. Available evidence suggests safe use during breast-feeding. AAP considers **compatible** with breast-feeding.

Pregnancy Issues: Hypotension, IUGR reported. IUGR probably related to maternal hypertension. May exhibit tocolytic effects.

Additional Information When measuring smaller doses from the liquid-filled capsules, consider the following concentrations (for Procardia®) 10 mg capsule = 10 mg/0.34 mL; 20 mg capsule = 20 mg/0.45 mL; may be used preoperative to treat hypertensive urgency.

Considerable attention has been directed to potential increases in mortality and morbidity when short-acting nifedipine is used in treating hypertension. The rapid reduction in blood pressure may precipitate adverse cardiovascular events. At this time, there is no indication for the use of short-acting calcium channel blocker therapy. Nifedipine also has potent negative inotropic effects and can worsen heart failure.

Related Information

Calcium Channel Blockers *on page 1563*

FDA Name Differentiation Project: The Use of Tall-man Letters *on page 12*

Nilandron® *see* Nilutamide *on page 972*

Nilutamide (ni LU ta mide)

U.S. Brand Names Nilandron®

Generic Available No

Pharmacologic Category Antineoplastic Agent, Antiandrogen

Pregnancy Risk Factor C

Lactation Not indicated for use in women

Use Treatment of metastatic prostate cancer

Mechanism of Action/Effect Nonsteroidal antiandrogen that inhibits androgen uptake or inhibits binding of androgen in target tissues

Contraindications Hypersensitivity to nilutamide or any component of the formulation; severe hepatic impairment; severe respiratory insufficiency

Warnings/Precautions May cause interstitial pneumonitis; the suggestive signs of pneumonitis most often occurred within the first 3 months of nilutamide treatment. Has been associated with severe hepatitis, which has resulted in fatality. In addition, foreign postmarketing surveillance has revealed isolated cases of aplastic anemia (a causal relationship with nilutamide could not be ascertained).

May alter time for visual adaptation to darkness, ranging from seconds to a few minutes. This effect sometimes does not abate as drug treatment is continued. Caution patients who experience this effect about driving at night or through tunnels. This effect can be alleviated by wearing tinted glasses.

Pregnancy risk C.

Drug Interactions

Cytochrome P450 Effect: Substrate of **CYP2C19**; Inhibits CYP2C19

Nutritional/Ethanol Interactions

Ethanol: Avoid ethanol. Up to 5% of patients may experience a systemic reaction (flushing, hypotension, malaise) when combined with nilutamide.

Herb/Nutraceutical: St John's wort may decrease nilutamide levels.

Adverse Reactions

>10%:

- Central nervous system: Headache, insomnia
- Endocrine & metabolic: Hot flashes (30% to 67%), gynecomastia (10%)
- Gastrointestinal: Nausea (mild - 10% to 32%), abdominal pain (10%), constipation, anorexia
- Genitourinary: Testicular atrophy (16%), libido decreased
- Hepatic: Transient elevation in serum transaminases (8% to 13%)
- Ocular: Impaired dark adaptation (13% to 57%), usually reversible with dose reduction, may require discontinuation of the drug in 1% to 2% of patients
- Respiratory: Dyspnea (11%)

1% to 10%:

- Cardiovascular: Chest pain, edema, heart failure, hypertension, syncope
- Central nervous system: Dizziness, drowsiness, malaise, hypesthesia, depression
- Dermatologic: Pruritus, alopecia, dry skin, rash
- Endocrine & metabolic: Disulfiram-like reaction (hot flashes, rashes) (5%); Flu-like syndrome, fever
- Gastrointestinal: Vomiting, diarrhea, dyspepsia, GI hemorrhage, melena, weight loss, xerostomia
- Genitourinary: Hematuria, nocturia
- Hematologic: Anemia
- Hepatic: Hepatitis (1%)
- Neuromuscular & skeletal: Arthritis, paresthesia
- Ocular: Chromatopsia (9%), abnormal vision (6% to 7%), cataracts, photophobia
- Respiratory: Interstitial pneumonitis (2% - typically exertional dyspnea, cough, chest pain, and fever; most often occurring within the first 3 months of treatment); rhinitis
- Miscellaneous: Diaphoresis

<1% (Limited to important or life-threatening): Aplastic anemia

Overdosage/Toxicology Symptoms of overdose may include nausea, vomiting, malaise, headache, dizziness, and elevated liver enzymes. Management is supportive. Dialysis is of no benefit.

Pharmacodynamics/Kinetics

Absorption: Rapid and complete

Half-Life Elimination: Terminal: 23-87 hours; Metabolites: 35-137 hours

Metabolism: Hepatic, forms active metabolites

Formulations Tablet: 150 mg

Dosing

Adults & Elderly: Refer to individual protocols. Prostate cancer: Oral: 300 mg daily for 30 days starting the same day or day after surgical castration, then 150 mg/day

Stability

Storage: Store at room temperature of 15°C to 30°C (59°F to 86°F). Protect from light.

Monitoring Laboratory Tests Chest x-rays prior to and regularly during treatment. Measure serum hepatic enzyme levels at baseline and at regular intervals (3 months). If transaminases increase over 2-3 times the upper limit of normal, discontinue treatment. Perform appropriate laboratory testing at the first symptom/sign of liver injury (eg, jaundice, dark urine, fatigue, abdominal pain, or unexplained GI symptoms).

Monitoring and Teaching Issues

Physical Assessment: See Contraindications, Warnings/Precautions, and Dosing for use cautions. Assess potential for interactions with other prescriptions, OTC medications, or herbal products patient may be taking (see Drug Interactions). Assess results of laboratory tests (see above) prior to and regularly during therapy. Assess therapeutic effectiveness and adverse response (see Adverse Reactions and Overdose/Toxicology). Teach patient proper use, possible side effects and appropriate interventions (eg, orthostatic precautions), and adverse symptoms to report (see Patient Education). **Pregnancy risk factor C.**

Patient Education: Inform prescriber of all prescriptions, OTC medications, or herbal products you are taking, and any allergies you have. Do not take anything new during treatment unless approved by prescriber. Take as prescribed; do not change dosing schedule or stop taking without consulting prescriber. Avoid alcohol while taking this medication; may cause severe reaction. Periodic laboratory tests are necessary while taking this medication. May cause loss of light accommodation (avoid night driving and use caution in poorly lighted or changing light situations such as tunnels); dizziness, confusion, or blurred vision (avoid driving or engaging in tasks that are potentially hazardous until response to drug is known); nausea or anorexia (small, frequent meals, frequent mouth

(Continued)

Nilutamide *(Continued)*

care, chewing gum, or sucking lozenges may help); or hot flashes, gynecomastia, decreased libido, impotence or sexual dysfunction (consult prescriber). Report any decreased respiratory function (eg, dyspnea, increased cough); difficulty or painful voiding or blood in urine; or other persistent adverse effects.

Dietary Issues: May be taken without regard to food.

Nimbex® *see* Cisatracurium *on page 296*

Nimodipine (nye MOE di peen)

U.S. Brand Names Nimotop®

Generic Available No

Pharmacologic Category Calcium Channel Blocker

Pregnancy Risk Factor C

Lactation Enters breast milk/not recommended

Use Spasm following subarachnoid hemorrhage from ruptured intracranial aneurysms regardless of the patients neurological condition postictus (Hunt and Hess grades I-V)

Mechanism of Action/Effect Nimodipine shares the pharmacology of other calcium channel blockers; animal studies indicate that nimodipine has a greater effect on cerebral arterials than other arterials; inhibits calcium ion from entering the "slow channels" or select voltage sensitive areas of vascular smooth muscle and myocardium during depolarization

Contraindications Hypersensitivity to nimodipine or any component of the formulation

Warnings/Precautions May cause reductions in blood pressure. Use caution in hepatic impairment. Intestinal pseudo-obstruction and ileus have been reported during the use of nimodipine. Use caution in patients with decreased GI motility of a history of bowel obstruction. Use caution when treating patients with increased intracranial pressure. Pregnancy risk C.

Drug Interactions

Cytochrome P450 Effect: Substrate of **CYP3A4**

Decreased Effect: Rifampin (and potentially other enzyme inducers) increase the metabolism of calcium channel blockers.

Increased Effect/Toxicity: Calcium channel blockers and nimodipine may result in enhanced cardiovascular effects of other calcium channel blockers. Cimetidine, omeprazole, and valproic acid may increase serum nimodipine levels. The effects of antihypertensive agents may be increased by nimodipine. Azole antifungals (itraconazole, ketoconazole, fluconazole), erythromycin, protease inhibitors (amprenavir, nelfinavir, ritonavir) and other inhibitors of cytochrome P450 isoenzyme 3A4 may inhibit calcium channel blocker metabolism.

Nutritional/Ethanol Interactions

Food: Nimodipine has shown a 1.5 fold increase in bioavailability when taken with grapefruit juice; avoid concurrent use.

Herb/Nutraceutical: St John's wort may decrease levels. Avoid dong quai if using for hypertension (has estrogenic activity). Avoid ephedra, yohimbe, ginseng (may worsen hypertension). Avoid garlic (may have increased antihypertensive effect).

Adverse Reactions

1% to 10%:

Cardiovascular: Reductions in systemic blood pressure (1% to 8%)

Central nervous system: Headache (1% to 4%)

Dermatologic: Rash (1% to 2%)

Gastrointestinal: Diarrhea (2% to 4%), abdominal discomfort (2%)

<1% (Limited to important or life-threatening): Anemia, CHF, deep vein thrombosis, depression, disseminated intravascular coagulation, dyspnea, EKG abnormalities, GI hemorrhage, hemorrhage, hepatitis, jaundice, neurological deterioration, rebound vasospasm, thrombocytopenia, vomiting

Overdosage/Toxicology Primary cardiac symptoms of calcium blocker overdose include hypotension and bradycardia. Noncardiac symptoms include confusion, stupor, nausea, vomiting, metabolic acidosis and hyperglycemia. Treat symptomatically.

Pharmacodynamics/Kinetics

Bioavailability: 13%

Half-Life Elimination: 3 hours; prolonged with renal impairment

Time to Peak: Serum: ~1 hour

Metabolism: Extensively hepatic

Formulations Capsule, liquid filled: 30 mg

Dosing

Adults & Elderly: Subarachnoid hemorrhage: Oral: 60 mg every 4 hours for 21 days, start therapy within 96 hours after subarachnoid hemorrhage.

Renal Impairment: Not removed by hemo- or peritoneal dialysis; supplemental dose is not necessary.

Hepatic Impairment: Reduce dosage to 30 mg every 4 hours in patients with liver failure.

Administration

Oral: If the capsules cannot be swallowed, the liquid may be removed by making a hole in each end of the capsule with an 18-gauge needle and extracting the contents into a syringe. If given via NG tube, follow with a flush of 30 mL NS.

Monitoring and Teaching Issues

Physical Assessment: See Contraindications, Warnings/Precautions, and Dosing for use cautions. Assess potential for interactions with other prescriptions, OTC medications, or herbal products patient may be taking (eg, other antihypertensives - see Drug Interactions). See Administration specifics. Assess therapeutic effectiveness and adverse response (eg, cardiac status and blood pressure when starting or adjusting dose and periodically during long-term therapy - see Adverse Reactions and Overdose/Toxicology). Teach patient proper use, possible side effects and appropriate interventions, and adverse symptoms to report (see Patient Education). **Pregnancy risk factor C** - benefits of use should outweigh possible risks. Breast-feeding is not recommended.

Patient Education: Inform prescriber of all prescriptions, OTC medications, or herbal products you are taking, and any allergies you have. Do not take anything new during treatment unless approved by prescriber. Take as directed; do not alter dose or decrease without consulting prescriber. Avoid grapefruit juice. May cause orthostatic hypotension (change position slowly from sitting or lying to standing, or when climbing stairs); headache (consult prescriber for approved analgesic); or diarrhea (buttermilk, boiled milk, or yogurt may help). Report chest pain, palpitations, slow heartbeat, difficulty breathing, or other persistent adverse effects. **Pregnancy/breast-feeding precautions:** Inform prescriber if you are or intend to become pregnant. Consult prescriber if breast-feeding.

Geriatric Considerations: Elderly may experience a greater hypotensive response. Constipation may be more of a problem in the elderly.

Pregnancy Issues: Teratogenic and embryotoxic effects have been demonstrated in small animals. No well controlled studies have been conducted in pregnant women.

Nimotop® *see* Nimodipine *on page 974*

Nipent® *see* Pentostatin *on page 1056*

Nisoldipine (NYE sole di peen)

U.S. Brand Names Sular®

Generic Available No

Pharmacologic Category Calcium Channel Blocker

Pregnancy Risk Factor C

Lactation Excretion in breast milk unknown

Use Management of hypertension, alone or in combination with other antihypertensive agents

Mechanism of Action/Effect As a dihydropyridine calcium channel blocker, structurally similar to nifedipine, nisoldipine impedes the movement of calcium ions into vascular smooth muscle and cardiac muscle. Dihydropyridines are potent vasodilators and are not as likely to suppress cardiac contractility and slow cardiac conduction as other calcium antagonists such as verapamil and diltiazem; nisoldipine is 5-10 times as potent a vasodilator as nifedipine.

Contraindications Hypersensitivity to nisoldipine, any component of the formulation, or other dihydropyridine calcium channel blockers

Warnings/Precautions May cause increased angina and/or myocardial infarction in patients with coronary artery disease (rare). Use with caution in patients with hypotension, CHF, and hepatic impairment. Blood pressure lowering must be done at a rate appropriate for the patient's condition. Pregnancy risk C.

Drug Interactions

Cytochrome P450 Effect: Substrate of **CYP3A4**; Inhibits CYP1A2, 3A4

Decreased Effect: Rifampin, phenytoin, and potentially other enzyme inducers decrease the levels of nisoldipine. Calcium may decrease the hypotension from calcium channel blockers.

Increased Effect/Toxicity: H_2-antagonists or omeprazole may cause an increase in the serum concentrations of nisoldipine. Digoxin and nisoldipine may increase digoxin effect. Azole antifungals (itraconazole, ketoconazole, fluconazole), erythromycin, and other inhibitors of cytochrome P450 isoenzyme 3A4 may inhibit calcium channel blocker metabolism. Calcium may reduce the calcium channel blocker's effects, particularly hypotension.

Nutritional/Ethanol Interactions

Food: Nisoldipine bioavailability may be increased if taken with high-lipid foods or with grapefruit juice. Avoid grapefruit products before and after dosing.

Herb/Nutraceutical: St John's wort may decrease nisoldipine levels. Avoid dong quai if using for hypertension (has estrogenic activity). Avoid ephedra, yohimbe, ginseng (may worsen hypertension). Avoid garlic (may have increased antihypertensive effect).

Adverse Reactions

>10%:

Cardiovascular: Peripheral edema (dose-related 7% to 29%)

Central nervous system: Headache (22%)

1% to 10%:

Cardiovascular: Chest pain (2%), palpitations (3%), vasodilation (4%)

Central nervous system: Dizziness (3% to 10%)

Dermatologic: Rash (2%)

Gastrointestinal: Nausea (2%)

Respiratory: Pharyngitis (5%), sinusitis (3%), dyspnea (3%), cough (5%)

<1% (Limited to important or life-threatening): Alopecia, amblyopia, angina, anxiety, ataxia, atrial fibrillation, cerebral ischemia, cholestatic jaundice, confusion, CHF, depression, dyspnea, exfoliative dermatitis, first-degree AV block, GI hemorrhage, gingival hyperplasia, gout, impotence, leukopenia, migraine, myasthenia, myocardial infarction, paresthesia, pruritus, pulmonary edema, rash, somnolence, stroke, supraventricular tachycardia, syncope, temporary unilateral loss of vision, tinnitus, T-wave abnormalities on EKG (flattening, inversion, nonspecific changes), urticaria, vaginal hemorrhage, ventricular extrasystoles, vertigo

Overdosage/Toxicology Primary cardiac symptoms of calcium blocker overdose include hypotension and bradycardia. Noncardiac symptoms include confusion, stupor, nausea, vomiting, metabolic acidosis and hyperglycemia. Treat symptomatically.

Pharmacodynamics/Kinetics

Absorption: Well absorbed

Bioavailability: 5%

Half-Life Elimination: 7-12 hours

Time to Peak: 6-12 hours

Metabolism: Extensively hepatic to inactive metabolites; first-pass effect

Duration: >24 hours

Formulations Tablet, extended release: 10 mg, 20 mg, 30 mg, 40 mg

(Continued)

Nisoldipine *(Continued)*

Dosing

Adults: Hypertension: Oral: Initial: 20 mg once daily, then increase by 10 mg/week (or longer intervals) to attain adequate control of blood pressure; doses >60 mg once daily are not recommended.

Elderly: Initial dose: 10 mg/day, increase by 10 mg/week (or longer intervals) to attain adequate blood pressure control. Those with hepatic disease should be started with 10 mg/day.

Hepatic Impairment: A starting dose not exceeding 10 mg/day is recommended for patients with hepatic impairment.

Administration

Oral: Administer at the same time each day to ensure minimal fluctuation of serum levels. Avoid high-fat diet.

Monitoring and Teaching Issues

Physical Assessment: See Contraindications, Warnings/Precautions, and Dosing for use cautions. Assess potential for interactions with other prescriptions, OTC medications, or herbal products patient may be taking (eg, other antihypertensives - see Drug Interactions). Assess therapeutic effectiveness and adverse response (eg, cardiac status and blood pressure when starting or adjusting dose and periodically during long-term therapy - see Adverse Reactions and Overdose/Toxicology). Taper dose gradually (over 2 weeks) when discontinuing. Teach patient proper use, possible side effects and appropriate interventions, and adverse symptoms to report (see Patient Education). **Pregnancy risk factor C** - benefits of use should outweigh possible risks. Note breast-feeding caution.

Patient Education: Inform prescriber of all prescriptions, OTC medications, or herbal products you are taking, and any allergies you have. Do not take anything new during treatment unless approved by prescriber. Take exactly as directed; do not alter dose or decrease without consulting prescriber. Do not crush or chew capsules; swallow whole. Take with food, but avoid fatty food and grapefruit juice. This drug does not replace diet and other exercise recommendations of prescriber. May cause orthostatic hypotension (change position slowly when rising from sitting or lying, or when climbing stairs); headache (consult prescriber for approved analgesic); dizziness (use caution when driving or engaging in tasks that require alertness until response to drug is known); or nausea (small, frequent meals, frequent mouth care, chewing gum, or sucking lozenges may help). Report chest pain, palpitations, irregular heartbeat; difficulty breathing; unusual cough; rash; vision changes; anxiety, confusion, depression, or other CNS changes; or other persistent adverse reactions. **Pregnancy/breast-feeding precautions:** Inform prescriber if you are or intend to become pregnant. Consult prescriber if breast-feeding.

Geriatric Considerations: Elderly may experience a greater hypotensive response. Constipation may be more of a problem in the elderly. Calcium channel blockers are no more effective in the elderly than other therapies; however, they do not cause significant CNS effects which is an advantage over some antihypertensive agents.

Related Information

Calcium Channel Blockers *on page 1563*

Nitalapram *see* Citalopram *on page 301*
Nitrek® *see* Nitroglycerin *on page 977*
Nitro-Bid® *see* Nitroglycerin *on page 977*
Nitro-Dur® *see* Nitroglycerin *on page 977*

Nitrofurantoin (nye troe fyoor AN toyn)

U.S. Brand Names Furadantin®; Macrobid®; Macrodantin®

Generic Available Yes: Capsule, macrocrystal

Pharmacologic Category Antibiotic, Miscellaneous

Pregnancy Risk Factor B

Lactation Enters breast milk/compatible

Use Prevention and treatment of urinary tract infections caused by susceptible gram-negative and some gram-positive organisms; *Pseudomonas*, *Serratia*, and most species of *Proteus* are generally resistant to nitrofurantoin

Mechanism of Action/Effect Inhibits several bacterial enzyme systems including acetyl coenzyme A interfering with metabolism and possibly cell wall synthesis

Contraindications Hypersensitivity to nitrofurantoin or any component of the formulation; renal impairment; infants <1 month (due to the possibility of hemolytic anemia)

Warnings/Precautions Use with caution in patients with G6PD deficiency, patients with anemia, vitamin B deficiency, diabetes mellitus, or electrolyte abnormalities. Therapeutic concentrations of nitrofurantoin are not attained in urine of patients with Cl_{cr} <40 mL/minute (elderly). Use with caution if prolonged therapy is anticipated due to possible pulmonary toxicity.

Drug Interactions

Decreased Effect: Antacids decrease absorption of nitrofurantoin.

Increased Effect/Toxicity: Probenecid decreases renal excretion of nitrofurantoin.

Nutritional/Ethanol Interactions

Ethanol: Avoid ethanol (may increase CNS depression).

Food: Nitrofurantoin serum concentrations may be increased if taken with food.

Effects on Lab Values False-positive urine glucose with Clinitest®

Adverse Reactions Frequency not defined.

Cardiovascular: Chest pains

Central nervous system: Chills, dizziness, drowsiness, fatigue, fever, headache

Dermatologic: Exfoliative dermatitis, itching, rash

Gastrointestinal: *C. difficile*-colitis, diarrhea, loss of appetite/vomiting/nausea (most common), sore throat, stomach upset

Hematologic: Hemolytic anemia

Hepatic: Hepatitis, increased LFTs

Neuromuscular & skeletal: Arthralgia, numbness, paresthesia, weakness

Respiratory: Cough, dyspnea, pneumonitis, pulmonary fibrosis
Miscellaneous: Hypersensitivity, lupus-like syndrome

Overdosage/Toxicology Symptoms of overdose include vomiting. Treatment is supportive.

Pharmacodynamics/Kinetics

Absorption: Well absorbed; macrocrystalline is absorbed more slowly due to slower dissolution (causes less GI distress)

Bioavailability: Increased with food

Half-Life Elimination: 20-60 minutes; prolonged with renal impairment

Metabolism: Body tissues (except plasma) metabolize 60% of drug to inactive metabolites

Formulations

Capsule, macrocrystal: 50 mg, 100 mg
Macrodantin®: 25 mg, 50 mg, 100 mg
Capsule, macrocrystal/monohydrate (Macrobid®): 100 mg
Suspension, oral (Furadantin®): 25 mg/5 mL (470 mL)

Dosing

Adults:

UTI Treatment: Oral: 50-100 mg/dose every 6 hours (not to exceed 400 mg/24 hours)
Prophylaxis of UTI: Oral: 50-100 mg/dose at bedtime

Elderly: Refer to adult dosing (see Geriatric Considerations).

Pediatrics:

UTI Treatment: Oral: Children >1 month: 5-7 mg/kg/day in divided doses every 6 hours; maximum: 400 mg/day

Chronic therapy: Oral: 1-2 mg/kg/day in divided doses every 12-24 hours; maximum dose: 100 mg/day

Renal Impairment:

Cl_{cr} <50 mL/minute: Avoid use.

Avoid use in hemo- and peritoneal dialysis and continuous arteriovenous or venovenous hemofiltration.

Administration

Oral: Suspension: Shake well before use. Higher peak serum levels may cause increased GI upset. Give with meals to slow the rate of absorption and decrease adverse effects.

Monitoring Laboratory Tests CBC, periodic liver function. Perform culture and sensitivity prior to initiating therapy.

Monitoring and Teaching Issues

Physical Assessment: See Contraindications, Warnings/Precautions, and Drug interactions for use cautions. Assess results of laboratory tests (see above), therapeutic effectiveness, and adverse response (see Adverse Reactions and Overdose/Toxicology). Caution diabetic patients about altered response to Clinitest® (may cause false-positive urine glucose). Teach patient proper use, possible side effects and appropriate interventions, and adverse symptoms to report (see Patient Education).

Patient Education: Inform prescriber of all prescriptions, OTC medications, or herbal products you are taking, and any allergies you have. Do not add anything new during treatment unless approved by prescriber. Take entire prescription, even if you are feeling better. Take at equal intervals around-the-clock; preferably on an empty stomach with a full glass of water (1 hour before or 2 hours after meals). Maintain adequate hydration (2-3 L/day of fluids) unless advised by prescriber to restrict fluids. If diabetic, drug may cause false test results with Clinitest® urine glucose monitoring; use of another type of glucose monitoring is preferable. May cause nausea or vomiting (small, frequent meals, frequent mouth care, sucking lozenges, or chewing gum may help); or diarrhea (buttermilk, boiled milk, or yogurt may help). Report immediately and rash; swelling of face, tongue, mouth, or throat; or chest tightness. Report if condition being treated worsens or does not improve by the time prescription is completed. **Pregnancy precaution:** This drug may interfere with oral contraceptives. Consult prescriber for an alternate form of birth control.

Geriatric Considerations: Because of nitrofurantoin's decreased efficacy in patients with a Cl_{cr} <40 mL/minute and its side effect profile, it is not an antibiotic of choice for acute or prophylactic treatment of urinary tract infections in the elderly.

Additional Information Nitrofurantoin macrocrystal/monohydrate is Macrobid®

Nitrogard® *see* Nitroglycerin *on page 977*

Nitrogen Mustard *see* Mechlorethamine *on page 839*

Nitroglycerin (nye troe GLI ser in)

U.S. Brand Names Deponit® [DSC]; Minitran™; Nitrek®; Nitro-Bid®; Nitro-Dur®; Nitrogard®; Nitrol®; Nitrolingual®; NitroQuick®; Nitrostat®; Nitro-Tab®; NitroTime®

Synonyms Glyceryl Trinitrate; Nitroglycerol; NTG

Generic Available Yes: Capsule, injection, patch, tablet

Pharmacologic Category Vasodilator

Pregnancy Risk Factor C

Lactation Excretion in breast milk unknown

Use Treatment of angina pectoris; I.V. for congestive heart failure (especially when associated with acute myocardial infarction); pulmonary hypertension; hypertensive emergencies occurring perioperatively (especially during cardiovascular surgery)

Mechanism of Action/Effect Reduces cardiac oxygen demand by decreasing left ventricular pressure and systemic vascular resistance; dilates coronary arteries and improves collateral flow to ischemic regions; esophageal smooth muscle is relaxed by same mechanism

Contraindications Hypersensitivity to organic nitrates; hypersensitivity to isosorbide, nitroglycerin, or any component of the formulation; concurrent use with sildenafil; angle-closure glaucoma (intraocular pressure may be increased); head trauma or cerebral hemorrhage (increase intracranial pressure); severe anemia; allergy to adhesive (transdermal product)

I.V. product: Hypotension; uncorrected hypovolemia; inadequate cerebral circulation; increased intracranial pressure; constrictive pericarditis; pericardial tamponade
(Continued)

Nitroglycerin *(Continued)*

Warnings/Precautions Severe hypotension can occur. Use with caution in volume depletion, hypotension, and right ventricular infarctions. Paradoxical bradycardia and increased angina pectoris can accompany hypotension. Orthostatic hypotension can also occur. Ethanol can accentuate this. Tolerance does develop to nitrates and appropriate dosing is needed to minimize this (drug-free interval). Safety and efficacy have not been established in pediatric patients. Avoid use of long-acting agents in acute MI or CHF; cannot easily reverse. Nitrate may aggravate angina caused by hypertrophic cardiomyopathy. Pregnancy risk C.

Drug Interactions

Decreased Effect: I.V. nitroglycerin may antagonize the anticoagulant effect of heparin (possibly only at high nitroglycerin dosages); monitor closely. May need to decrease heparin dosage when nitroglycerin is discontinued. Alteplase (tissue plasminogen activator) has a lesser effect when used with I.V. nitroglycerin; avoid concurrent use. Ergot alkaloids may cause an increase in blood pressure and decrease in antianginal effects; avoid concurrent use.

Increased Effect/Toxicity: Has been associated with severe reactions and death when sildenafil is given concurrently with nitrites. Ethanol can cause hypotension when nitrates are taken 1 hour or more after ethanol ingestion.

Adverse Reactions

Spray or patch:

>10%: Central nervous system: Headache (patch 63%, spray 50%)

1% to 10%:

Cardiovascular: Hypotension (patch 4%), increased angina (patch 2%)

Central nervous system: Lightheadedness (patch 6%), syncope (patch 4%)

<1% (Limited to important or life-threatening): Allergic reactions, application site irritation (patch), collapse, dizziness, exfoliative dermatitis, methemoglobinemia (rare, overdose), pallor, palpitations, perspiration, rash, restlessness, vertigo, weakness

Topical, sublingual, intravenous: Frequency not defined:

Cardiovascular: Hypotension (infrequent), postural hypotension, crescendo angina (uncommon), rebound hypertension (uncommon), pallor, cardiovascular collapse, tachycardia, shock, flushing, peripheral edema

Central nervous system: Headache (most common), lightheadedness (related to blood pressure changes), syncope (uncommon), dizziness, restlessness

Gastrointestinal: Nausea, vomiting, bowel incontinence, xerostomia

Genitourinary: Urinary incontinence

Hematologic: Methemoglobinemia (rare, overdose)

Neuromuscular & skeletal: Weakness

Ocular: Blurred vision

Miscellaneous: Cold sweat

Overdosage/Toxicology Symptoms of overdose include hypotension, throbbing headache, palpitations, bloody diarrhea, bradycardia, cyanosis, tissue hypoxia, metabolic acidosis, clonic convulsions, circulatory collapse, and methemoglobinemia with extremely large overdoses. Treatment is supportive and symptomatic.

Pharmacodynamics/Kinetics

Half-Life Elimination: 1-4 minutes

Metabolism: Extensive first-pass effect

Onset: Sublingual tablet: 1-3 minutes; Translingual spray: 2 minutes; Buccal tablet: 2-5 minutes; Sustained release: 20-45 minutes; Topical: 15-60 minutes; Transdermal: 40-60 minutes; I.V. drip: Immediate

Peak effect: Sublingual tablet: 4-8 minutes; Translingual spray: 4-10 minutes; Buccal tablet: 4-10 minutes; Sustained release: 45-120 minutes; Topical: 30-120 minutes; Transdermal: 60-180 minutes; I.V. drip: Immediate

Duration: Sublingual tablet: 30-60 minutes; Translingual spray: 30-60 minutes; Buccal tablet: 2 hours; Sustained release: 4-8 hours; Topical: 2-12 hours; Transdermal: 18-24 hours; I.V. drip: 3-5 minutes

Formulations

Aerosol, translingual spray (Nitrolingual®): 0.4 mg/metered spray (12 g) [contains alcohol 20%; 200 metered sprays]

Capsule, extended release (Nitro-Time®): 2.5 mg, 6.5 mg, 9 mg

Infusion [premixed in D_5W]: 0.1 mg/mL (250 mL, 500 mL); 0.2 mg/mL (250 mL); 0.4 mg/mL (250 mL, 500 mL)

Injection, solution: 5 mg/mL (5 mL, 10 mL) [contains alcohol and propylene glycol]

Ointment, topical:

Nitro-Bid®: 2% [20 mg/g] (30 g, 60 g)

Nitrol®: 2% [20 mg/g] (3 g, 60 g)

Tablet, buccal, extended release (Nitrogard®): 2 mg, 3 mg

Tablet, sublingual (NitroQuick®, Nitrostat®, Nitro-Tab®): 0.3 mg, 0.4 mg, 0.6 mg

Transdermal system [once daily patch]: 0.1 mg/hour (30s); 0.2 mg/hour (30s); 0.4 mg/hour (30s); 0.6 mg/hour (30s)

Deponit®: 0.1 mg/hour (30s); 0.2 mg/hour (30s); 0.4 mg/hour (30s) [DSC]

Minitran™: 0.1 mg/hour (30s); 0.2 mg/hour (30s); 0.4 mg/hour (30s); 0.6 mg/hour (30s)

Nitrek®: 0.2 mg/hour (30s); 0.4 mg/hour (30s); 0.6 mg/hour (30s)

Nitro-Dur®: 0.1 mg/hour (30s); 0.2 mg/hour (30s); 0.3 mg/hour (30s); 0.4 mg/hour (30s); 0.6 mg/hour (30s); 0.8 mg/hour (30s)

Dosing

Adults & Elderly: Note: Hemodynamic and antianginal tolerance often develop within 24-48 hours of continuous nitrate administration.

Angina/coronary artery disease:

Buccal: Initial: 1 mg every 3-5 hours while awake (3 times/day); titrate dosage upward if angina occurs with tablet in place.

Oral: 2.5-9 mg 2-4 times/day (up to 26 mg 4 times/day)

I.V.: 5 mcg/minute, increase by 5 mcg/minute every 3-5 minutes to 20 mcg/minute. If no response at 20 mcg/minute increase by 10 mcg/minute every 3-5 minutes, up to 200 mcg/minute.

Ointment: Include a nitrate free interval, ~10 to 12 hours; Apply 0.5" to 2" every 6 hours with a nitrate free interval.

Patch, transdermal: 0.2-0.4 mg/hour initially and titrate to doses of 0.4-0.8 mg/hour. Tolerance is minimized by using a patch-on period of 12-14 hours and patch-off period of 10-12 hours.

Sublingual: 0.2-0.6 mg every 5 minutes for maximum of 3 doses in 15 minutes; may also use prophylactically 5-10 minutes prior to activities which may provoke an attack.

Translingual: 1-2 sprays into mouth under tongue every 3-5 minutes for maximum of 3 doses in 15 minutes, may also be used 5-10 minutes prior to activities which may provoke an attack prophylactically.

Note: May need to use nitrate-free interval (10-12 hours/day) to avoid tolerance development. Tolerance may possibly be reversed with acetylcysteine. Gradually decrease dose in patients receiving NTG for prolonged period to avoid withdrawal reaction.

Pediatrics: Note: Hemodynamic and antianginal tolerance often develop within 24-48 hours of continuous nitrate administration.

Pulmonary hypertension: I.V. Continuous infusion: Children: Start 0.25-0.5 mcg/kg/minute and titrate by 1 mcg/kg/minute at 20- to 60-minute intervals to desired effect; usual dose: 1-3 mcg/kg/minute; maximum: 5 mcg/kg/minute

Administration

Oral: Do not crush sublingual drug product.

I.V.: I.V. must be prepared in glass bottles and use special sets intended for nitroglycerin. glass I.V. bottles and administration sets provided by manufacturer.

Topical: Transdermal patches are labeled as mg/hour.

Stability

Storage: Doses should be made in glass bottles, Excel® or PAB® containers. Adsorption occurs to soft plastic (eg, PVC). Premixed bottles are stable according to the manufacturer's expiration dating. Store sublingual tablets and ointment in tightly closed containers at 15°C to 30°C. Store spray at 25°C (excursions permitted to 15°C to 30°C (59°F to 86°F)).

Reconstitution: Doses should be made in glass bottles, Excel® or PAB® containers; adsorption occurs to soft plastic (eg, PVC). Nitroglycerin diluted in D_5W or NS in glass containers is physically and chemically stable for 48 hours at room temperature and 7 days under refrigeration. In D_5W or NS in Excel®/PAB® containers is physically and chemically stable for 24 hours at room temperature and 14 days under refrigeration.

Standard diluent: 50 mg/250 mL D_5W; 50 mg/500 mL D_5W

Minimum volume: 100 mg/250 mL D_5W; concentration should not exceed 400 mcg/mL.

Compatibility: Stable in D_5LR, $D_5{}^1/_2NS$, D_5NS, LR, $^1/_2NS$

Y-site administration: Incompatible with alteplase, levofloxacin

Compatibility when admixed: Dose is variable and may require titration, therefore it is not advisable to mix with other agents. **Incompatible** with hydralazine, phenytoin

Monitoring and Teaching Issues

Physical Assessment: See Contraindications, Warnings/Precautions, and Dosing for use cautions. Assess potential for interactions with other prescriptions, OTC medications, or herbal products patient may be taking (see Drug Interactions). See Administration specifics for different formulations above. Assess therapeutic effectiveness (cardiac status) and adverse response (eg, hypotension and arrhythmias - see Adverse Reactions and Overdose/Toxicology). Dose should be reduced gradually when discontinuing after long-term therapy. Teach patient proper use (according to purpose and formulation), possible side effects and appropriate interventions (eg, drug-free intervals), and adverse symptoms to report (see Patient Education). **Pregnancy risk factor C** - benefits of use should outweigh possible risks. Note breast-feeding caution.

Patient Education: Inform prescriber of all prescriptions, OTC medications, or herbal products you are taking, and any allergies you have. Do not add anything new during treatment unless approved by prescriber. Take as per directions (see below). Do not change brands without consulting prescriber. Do not discontinue abruptly. Keep medication in original container, tightly closed. If anginal chest pain is unresolved in 15 minutes, seek emergency medical help at once. Daily use may cause dizziness or lightheadedness (use caution when driving or engaging in hazardous activities until response to drug is known); headache (consult prescriber for approved analgesic); hypotension (use care when changing position from sitting or lying to standing, when climbing stairs or when engaging in tasks that are potentially hazardous until response to drug is known); GI disturbances (small, frequent meals, frequent mouth care, chewing gum, or sucking lozenges may help). Report acute headache, rapid heartbeat, unusual restlessness or dizziness, muscular weakness, or blurred vision or seeing abnormal colors. **Pregnancy/breast-feeding precautions:** Inform prescriber if you are or intend to become pregnant. Consult prescriber if breast-feeding.

Oral: Take as directed. Do not chew or swallow sublingual tablets; allow to dissolve under tongue. Sit down before using sublingual or buccal tablet or spray form. Do not chew or crush extended release capsules; swallow with 8 oz of water.

Spray: Spray directly on mucous membranes; do not inhale.

Topical: Spread prescribed amount thinly on applicator; rotate application sites.

Transdermal: Use as directed; place on hair-free area of skin, rotate sites (usually, patches will be removed for a period each day)

Geriatric Considerations: Caution should be used when using nitrate therapy in the elderly due to hypotension. Hypotension is enhanced in the elderly due to decreased baroreceptor response, decreased venous tone, and often hypovolemia (dehydration) or other hypotensive drugs.

(Continued)

Nitroglycerin *(Continued)*

Additional Information I.V. preparations contain alcohol and/or propylene glycol; may need to use nitrate-free interval (10-12 hours/day) to avoid tolerance development. Tolerance may possibly be reversed with acetylcysteine; gradually decrease dose in patients receiving NTG for prolonged period to avoid withdrawal reaction.

Concomitant use of sildenafil (Viagra®) may precipitate acute hypotension, myocardial infarction, or death. Nitrates used in right ventricular infarction may induce acute hypotension. Nitrate use in severe pericardial effusion may reduce cardiac filling pressure and precipitate cardiac tamponade. In the management of heart failure, the combination of isosorbide dinitrate and hydralazine confers beneficial effects on disease progression and cardiac outcomes.

Related Information

Compatibility of Drugs *on page 1564*

Nitroglycerol *see* Nitroglycerin *on page 977*

Nitrol® *see* Nitroglycerin *on page 977*

Nitrolingual® *see* Nitroglycerin *on page 977*

Nitropress® *see* Nitroprusside *on page 980*

Nitroprusside (nye troe PRUS ide)

U.S. Brand Names Nitropress®

Synonyms Nitroprusside Sodium; Sodium Nitroferricyanide; Sodium Nitroprusside

Generic Available Yes: Solution

Pharmacologic Category Vasodilator

Pregnancy Risk Factor C

Lactation Excretion in breast milk unknown

Use Management of hypertensive crises; congestive heart failure; used for controlled hypotension to reduce bleeding during surgery

Mechanism of Action/Effect Causes peripheral vasodilation by direct action on venous and arteriolar smooth muscle, thus reducing peripheral resistance; will increase cardiac output by decreasing afterload; reduces aortal and left ventricular impedance

Contraindications Hypersensitivity to nitroprusside or any component of the formulation; treatment of compensatory hypertension (aortic coarctation, arteriovenous shunting); high output failure; congenital optic atrophy or tobacco amblyopia

Warnings/Precautions Except when used briefly or at low (<2 mcg/kg/minute) infusion rates, nitroprusside gives rise to large cyanide quantities. Do not use the maximum dose for more than 10 minutes. Use with extreme caution in patients with elevated intracranial pressure. Use extreme caution in patients with hepatic or renal dysfunction. Watch for cyanide toxicity in patients with impaired hepatic function. Use the lowest end of the dosage range with renal impairment. Thiocyanate toxicity occurs in patients with renal impairment or those on prolonged infusions. Continuous blood pressure monitoring is needed. Pregnancy risk C.

Adverse Reactions 1% to 10%:

Cardiovascular: Excessive hypotensive response, palpitations, substernal distress
Central nervous system: Disorientation, psychosis, headache, restlessness
Endocrine & metabolic: Thyroid suppression
Gastrointestinal: Nausea, vomiting
Neuromuscular & skeletal: Weakness, muscle spasm
Otic: Tinnitus
Respiratory: Hypoxia
Miscellaneous: Diaphoresis, thiocyanate toxicity

Overdosage/Toxicology Symptoms of overdose include hypotension, vomiting, hyperventilation, tachycardia, muscular twitching, hypothyroidism, cyanide or thiocyanate toxicity. Thiocyanate toxicity includes psychosis, hyper-reflexia, confusion, weakness, tinnitus, seizures, and coma; cyanide toxicity includes acidosis (decreased HCO_3, decreased pH, increased lactate), increase in mixed venous blood oxygen tension, tachycardia, altered consciousness, coma, convulsions, and almond smell on breath.

Nitroprusside has been shown to release cyanide *in vivo* with hemoglobin. Cyanide toxicity does not usually occur because of the rapid uptake of cyanide by erythrocytes and its eventual incorporation into thiocyanate in the liver. However, high doses, prolonged administration of nitroprusside, or reduced elimination can lead to cyanide poisoning or thiocyanate intoxication. Anemia and liver impairment pose a risk for cyanide accumulation, while renal impairment predisposes thiocyanate accumulation. If toxicity develops, airway support with oxygen therapy is appropriate, followed closely with antidotal therapy of amyl nitrate perles, sodium nitrate 300 mg I.V. for adults (range based on hemoglobin concentration: 6-12 mg/kg for children) and sodium thiosulfate 12.5 g I.V. for adults (range based on hemoglobin concentration: 0.95-1.95 mL/kg of the 25% solution for children); nitrates should not be administered to neonates and small children. Thiocyanate is dialyzable. May be mixed with sodium thiosulfate in I.V. to prevent cyanide toxicity.

Pharmacodynamics/Kinetics

Half-Life Elimination: Parent drug: <10 minutes; Thiocyanate: 2.7-7 days

Metabolism: Nitroprusside is converted to cyanide ions in the bloodstream; decomposes to prussic acid which in the presence of sulfur donor is converted to thiocyanate (hepatic and renal rhodanase systems)

Onset: BP reduction <2 minutes

Duration: 1-10 minutes

Formulations

Injection, powder for reconstitution, as sodium: 50 mg
Injection, solution, as sodium: 25 mg/mL (2 mL)

Dosing

Adults & Elderly:

Acute hypertension: I.V.: Initial: 0.3-0.5 mcg/kg/minute; increase in increments of 0.5 mcg/kg/minute, titrating to the desired hemodynamic effect or the appearance of headache or nausea; usual dose: 3 mcg/kg/minute; rarely need >4 mcg/kg/minute; maximum: 10 mcg/kg/minute. When >500 mcg/kg is administered by prolonged infusion of faster than 2 mcg/kg/minute, cyanide is generated faster than an unaided patient can handle.

Note: Administration requires the use of an infusion pump. Average dose: 5 mcg/kg/minute.

Pediatrics:

Pulmonary hypertension: I.V.: Children: Initial: 1 mcg/kg/minute by continuous I.V. infusion; increase in increments of 1 mcg/kg/minute at intervals of 20-60 minutes; titrating to the desired response; usual dose: 3 mcg/kg/minute, rarely need >4 mcg/kg/minute; maximum: 5 mcg/kg/minute.

Note: Administration requires the use of an infusion pump. Average dose: 5 mcg/kg/minute.

Renal Impairment: Limit use; accumulation of thiocyanate may occur.

Hepatic Impairment: Limit use; risk of cyanide toxicity.

Administration

I.V.: I.V. infusion only, use only as an infusion with 5% dextrose in water. Infusion pump required. Not for direct injection.

Stability

Storage:

Use only clear solutions; solutions of nitroprusside exhibit a color described as brownish, brown, brownish-pink, light orange, and straw. Solutions are highly sensitive to light. Exposure to light causes decomposition, resulting in a highly colored solution of orange, dark brown or blue. **A blue color indicates almost complete degradation and breakdown to cyanide.**

Solutions should be wrapped with aluminum foil or other opaque material to protect from light (do as soon as possible)

Stability of parenteral admixture at room temperature (25°C) and at refrigeration temperature (4°C): 24 hours

Reconstitution: Brownish solution is usable, discard if bluish in color. Nitroprusside sodium should be reconstituted freshly by diluting 50 mg in 250-1000 mL of D_5W. Use only clear solutions; solutions of nitroprusside exhibit a color described as brownish, brown, brownish-pink, light orange, and straw. Solutions are highly sensitive to light. Exposure to light causes decomposition, resulting in a highly colored solution of orange, dark brown or blue. **A blue color indicates almost complete degradation and breakdown to cyanide. Solutions should be wrapped with aluminum foil or other opaque material to protect from light (do as soon as possible)**. Stability of parenteral admixture at room temperature (25°C) and at refrigeration temperature (4°C) is 24 hours.

Compatibility: Stable in LR

Y-site administration: Incompatible with levofloxacin

Compatibility when admixed: Incompatible with atracurium

Monitoring and Teaching Issues

Physical Assessment: See Contraindications, Warnings/Precautions, and Dosing for use cautions. Assess potential for interactions with other prescriptions, OTC medications, or herbal products patient may be taking (see Drug Interactions). See Administration, Storage, and Reconstitution for infusion specifics. Infusion site must be monitored closely to prevent extravasation. Continuous blood pressure monitoring is needed. Assess therapeutic effectiveness and adverse response (see Adverse Reactions and Overdose/Toxicology - eg, acid/base balance, metabolic acidosis is early sign of cyanide toxicity). Provide patient teaching according to patient condition (see Patient Education). **Pregnancy risk factor C** - benefits of use should outweigh possible risks. Note breast-feeding caution.

Patient Education: Patient condition should indicate extent of education and instruction needed. This drug can only be given I.V. You will be monitored at all times during infusion. Promptly report any chest pain or pain/burning at site of infusion. **Breast-feeding precaution:** Consult prescriber if breast-feeding.

Geriatric Considerations: Elderly patients may have an increased sensitivity to nitroprusside possibly due to a decreased baroreceptor reflex, altered sensitivity to vasodilating effects or a resistance of cardiac adrenergic receptors to stimulation by catecholamines.

Nitroprusside Sodium *see* Nitroprusside *on page 980*

NitroQuick® *see* Nitroglycerin *on page 977*

Nitrostat® *see* Nitroglycerin *on page 977*

Nitro-Tab® *see* Nitroglycerin *on page 977*

NitroTime® *see* Nitroglycerin *on page 977*

Nix® [OTC *see* Permethrin *on page 1061*

Nizatidine (ni ZA ti deen)

U.S. Brand Names Axid®; Axid® AR [OTC]

Generic Available Yes: Capsule

Pharmacologic Category Histamine H_2 Antagonist

Pregnancy Risk Factor C

Lactation Enters breast milk/may be compatible

Use Treatment and maintenance of duodenal ulcer; treatment of benign gastric ulcer; treatment of gastroesophageal reflux disease (GERD); OTC tablet used for the prevention of meal-induced heartburn, acid indigestion, and sour stomach

Use - Unlabeled/Investigational Part of a multidrug regimen for *H. pylori* eradication to reduce the risk of duodenal ulcer recurrence

Mechanism of Action/Effect Nizatidine is an H_2-receptor antagonist.

Contraindications Hypersensitivity to nizatidine or any component of the formulation; hypersensitivity to other H_2 antagonists (cross-sensitivity has been observed)

Warnings/Precautions Use with caution in children <12 years of age. Use with caution in patients with liver and renal impairment. Dosage modification required in patients with renal impairment. Pregnancy risk C.

(Continued)

Nizatidine *(Continued)*

Drug Interactions

Decreased Effect: May decrease the absorption of itraconazole or ketoconazole.

Nutritional/Ethanol Interactions Ethanol: Avoid ethanol (may cause gastric mucosal irritation).

Effects on Lab Values False-positive urine protein using Multistix®, gastric acid secretion test, skin tests allergen extracts, serum creatinine and serum transaminase concentrations, urine protein test

Adverse Reactions

>10%: Central nervous system: Headache (16%)

1% to 10%:

Central nervous system: Dizziness, insomnia, somnolence, nervousness, anxiety

Dermatologic: Rash, pruritus

Gastrointestinal: Abdominal pain, constipation, diarrhea, nausea, flatulence, vomiting, heartburn, dry mouth, anorexia

<1% (Limited to important or life-threatening): Alkaline phosphatase increased, anemia, AST/ALT increased, bronchospasm, eosinophilia, hepatitis, jaundice, laryngeal edema, thrombocytopenic purpura, ventricular tachycardia

Overdosage/Toxicology Symptoms of overdose include muscular tremor, vomiting, and rapid respiration. LD_{50} ~80 mg/kg. Treatment is symptomatic and supportive.

Pharmacodynamics/Kinetics

Absorption: >70%

Bioavailability: >70%

Half-Life Elimination: 1-2 hours; prolonged with renal impairment

Time to Peak: Plasma: 0.5-3.0 hours

Metabolism: Partially hepatic

Formulations

Capsule (Axid®): 150 mg, 300 mg

Tablet (Axid® AR): 75 mg

Dosing

Adults & Elderly:

Duodenal ulcer, acute treatment: Oral: 300 mg at bedtime or 150 mg twice daily

Duodenal ulcer, maintenance therapy: Oral: 150 mg/day

Gastric ulcer: Oral: 150 mg twice daily or 300 mg at bedtime

GERD: Oral: 150 mg twice daily

Meal-induced heartburn, acid indigestion, and sour stomach: Oral: 75 mg tablet [OTC] twice daily, 30-60 minutes prior to consuming food or beverages

Helicobacter pylori eradication (unlabeled use): Oral: 150 mg twice daily; requires combination therapy

Renal Impairment:

Cl_{cr} 50-80 mL/minute: Administer 75% of normal dose.

Cl_{cr} 10-50 mL/minute: Administer 50% of normal dose or 150 mg/day for active treatment and 150 mg every other day for maintenance treatment.

Cl_{cr} <10 mL/minute: Administer 25% of normal dose or 150 mg every other day for treatment and 150 mg every 3 days for maintenance treatment.

Administration

Oral: Giving dose at 6 PM may better suppress nocturnal acid secretion than taking dose at 10 PM.

Monitoring and Teaching Issues

Physical Assessment: See Contraindications, Warnings/Precautions, Drug Interactions, and Dosing for use cautions. Assess therapeutic effectiveness and adverse response (see Adverse Reactions and Overdose/Toxicology). Teach patient proper use, possible side effects and appropriate interventions, and adverse symptoms to report (see Patient Education). **Pregnancy risk factor C** - benefits of use should outweigh possible risks.

Patient Education: Inform prescriber of all prescriptions, OTC medications, or herbal products you are taking, and any allergies you have. Do not add anything new during treatment unless approved by prescriber. Take as directed; do not change dose or discontinue without consulting prescriber. Do not take within 1 hour of any antacids. Follow diet instructions of prescriber. May cause drowsiness; use caution when driving or engaging in tasks that require alertness until response to drug is known. Report fever, sore throat, tarry stools, CNS changes, or muscle or joint pain. **Pregnancy precaution:** Inform prescriber if you are or intend to become pregnant.

Geriatric Considerations: H_2 blockers are the preferred drugs for treating peptic ulcer disorder (PUD) in the elderly due to cost and ease of administration. These agents are no less or more effective than any other therapy. The preferred agents (due to side effects and drug interaction profile and pharmacokinetics) are ranitidine, famotidine, and nizatidine. Treatment for PUD in the elderly is recommended for 12 weeks since their lesions are larger, and therefore, take longer to heal. Always adjust dose based upon creatinine clearance.

Nizoral® *see* Ketoconazole *on page 758*

Nizoral® A-D [OTC] *see* Ketoconazole *on page 758*

N-Methylhydrazine *see* Procarbazine *on page 1125*

Nolvadex® *see* Tamoxifen *on page 1274*

Nonsalicylate/Nonsteroidal Anti-inflammatory Comparison *see page 1587*

Noradrenaline *see* Norepinephrine *on page 983*

Noradrenaline Acid Tartrate *see* Norepinephrine *on page 983*

Norco® *see* Hydrocodone and Acetaminophen *on page 667*

Norcuron® *see* Vecuronium *on page 1393*

Nordeoxyguanosine *see* Ganciclovir *on page 618*

Nordette® *see* Ethinyl Estradiol and Levonorgestrel *on page 523*

Norditropin® *see* Human Growth Hormone *on page 658*

Norditropin® Cartridges *see* Human Growth Hormone *on page 658*

Norepinephrine (nor ep i NEF rin)

U.S. Brand Names Levophed®

Synonyms Levarterenol Bitartrate; Noradrenaline; Noradrenaline Acid Tartrate; Norepinephrine Bitartrate

Generic Available No

Pharmacologic Category Alpha/Beta Agonist

Pregnancy Risk Factor C

Lactation Excretion in breast milk unknown

Use Treatment of shock which persists after adequate fluid volume replacement

Mechanism of Action/Effect Stimulates $beta_1$-adrenergic receptors and alpha-adrenergic receptors causing increased contractility and heart rate as well as vasoconstriction, thereby increasing systemic blood pressure and coronary blood flow; clinically alpha effects (vasoconstriction) are greater than beta effects (inotropic and chronotropic effects)

Contraindications Hypersensitivity to norepinephrine, bisulfites (contains metabisulfite), or any component of the formulation; hypotension from hypovolemia except as an emergency measure to maintain coronary and cerebral perfusion until volume could be replaced; mesenteric or peripheral vascular thrombosis unless it is a lifesaving procedure; during anesthesia with cyclopropane or halothane anesthesia (risk of ventricular arrhythmias)

Warnings/Precautions Assure adequate circulatory volume to minimize need for vasoconstrictors. Avoid hypertension; monitor blood pressure closely and adjust infusion rate. Infuse into a large vein if possible. Avoid infusion into leg veins. Watch I.V. site closely. Avoid extravasation. Never use leg veins for infusion sites. Pregnancy risk C.

Drug Interactions

Decreased Effect: Alpha blockers may blunt response to norepinephrine.

Increased Effect/Toxicity: The effects of norepinephrine may be increased by tricyclic antidepressants, MAO inhibitors, antihistamines (diphenhydramine, tripelennamine), beta-blockers (nonselective), guanethidine, ergot alkaloids, reserpine, and methyldopa. Atropine sulfate may block the reflex bradycardia caused by norepinephrine and enhances the vasopressor response.

Adverse Reactions Frequency not defined.

Cardiovascular: Bradycardia, arrhythmias, peripheral (digital) ischemia
Central nervous system: Headache (transient), anxiety
Local: Skin necrosis (with extravasation)
Respiratory: Dyspnea, respiratory difficulty

Overdosage/Toxicology Symptoms of overdose include hypertension, sweating, cerebral hemorrhage, and convulsions. Infiltrate the area of extravasation with phentolamine 5-10 mg in 10-15 mL of saline solution.

Pharmacodynamics/Kinetics

Metabolism: Via catechol-o-methyltransferase (COMT) and monoamine oxidase (MAO)

Onset: I.V.: Very rapid-acting

Duration: Limited

Formulations Injection, solution, as bitartrate: 1 mg/mL (4 mL) [contains sodium metabisulfite]

Dosing

Adults & Elderly: Note: Norepinephrine dosage is stated in terms of norepinephrine base and intravenous formulation is norepinephrine bitartrate.

Norepinephrine bitartrate 2 mg = norepinephrine base 1 mg

Hypotension/shock: Continuous I.V. infusion:

Initiate at 4 mcg/minute and titrate to desired response; 8-12 mcg/minute is usual range
ACLS dosing range: 0.5-30 mcg/minute

Rate of infusion: 4 mg in 500 mL D_5W

2 mcg/minute = 15 mL/hour
4 mcg/minute = 30 mL/hour
6 mcg/minute = 45 mL/hour
8 mcg/minute = 60 mL/hour
10 mcg/minute = 75 mL/hour

Pediatrics: Administration requires the use of an infusion pump

Note: Norepinephrine dosage is stated in terms of norepinephrine base and intravenous formulation is norepinephrine bitartrate.

Norepinephrine bitartrate 2 mg = Norepinephrine base 1 mg
Hypotension/shock: Continuous I.V. infusion: Children: Initial: 0.05-0.1 mcg/kg/minute; titrate to desired effect; maximum dose: 1-2 mcg/kg/minute

Administration

I.V.: Administer into large vein to avoid the potential for extravasation; potent drug, must be diluted prior to use. Rate (mL/hour) = dose (mcg/kg/minute) x weight (kg) x 60 minutes/hour divided by concentration (mcg/mL). Central line administration is required. Do not administer $NaHCO_3$ through an I.V. line containing norepinephrine.

Stability

Storage: Readily oxidized; protect from light. Do not use if brown coloration.

Reconstitution: Dilute with D_5W or D_5NS, but not recommended to dilute in normal saline. Stability of parenteral admixture at room temperature (25°C) is 24 hours.

Compatibility: Stable in alkaline solutions; D_5NS, D_5W, LR; may dilute with D_5W or D_5NS, but not recommended to dilute in normal saline. Stability of parenteral admixture at room temperature (25°C) is 24 hours.

Y-site administration: Incompatible with insulin (regular), thiopental

Compatibility when admixed: Incompatible with aminophylline, amobarbital, chlorothiazide, chlorpheniramine, pentobarbital, phenobarbital, phenytoin, sodium bicarbonate, streptomycin, thiopental

Monitoring and Teaching Issues

Physical Assessment: Assess other medications patient may be taking (see Drug Interactions). Monitor blood pressure and cardiac status, CNS status, skin temperature and color

(Continued)

Norepinephrine *(Continued)*

during and following infusion. Monitor fluid status. Assess infusion site frequently for extravasation. Blanching along vein pathway is a preliminary sign of extravasation. **Pregnancy risk factor C.** Note breast-feeding caution.

Patient Education: This drug is used in emergency situations. Patient information is based on patient condition.

Related Information

Compatibility of Drugs *on page 1564*
Inotropic and Vasoconstrictor Comparison *on page 1580*

Norepinephrine Bitartrate *see* Norepinephrine *on page 983*

Norethindrone (nor eth IN drone)

U.S. Brand Names Aygestin®; Micronor®; Nor-QD®

Synonyms Norethindrone Acetate; Norethisterone

Generic Available Yes: Tablet, as acetate

Pharmacologic Category Contraceptive; Progestin

Pregnancy Risk Factor X

Lactation Enters breast milk/use caution

Use Treatment of amenorrhea; abnormal uterine bleeding; endometriosis, oral contraceptive; **higher rate of failure with progestin only contraceptives**

Mechanism of Action/Effect Inhibits secretion of pituitary gonadotropin (LH) which prevents follicular maturation and ovulation; in the presence of adequate endogenous estrogen, transforms a proliferative endometrium to a secretory one

Contraindications Hypersensitivity to norethindrone or any component of the formulation; thromboembolic disorders; severe hepatic disease; breast cancer; undiagnosed vaginal bleeding; pregnancy

Warnings/Precautions Use of any progestin during the first 4 months of pregnancy is not recommended. Discontinue if sudden partial or complete loss of vision, proptosis, diplopia, or migraine occur. **There is a higher rate of failure with progestin only contraceptives.** Progestin-induced withdrawal bleeding occurs within 3-7 days after discontinuation of drug. Use with caution in patients with asthma, diabetes, seizure disorder, hyperlipidemias, migraine, cardiac or renal dysfunction, or psychic depression.

Drug Interactions

Cytochrome P450 Effect: Substrate of **CYP3A4**; Induces CYP2C19

Decreased Effect: Rifampin (potentially other enzyme inducers) and nelfinavir decrease the pharmacologic effect of norethindrone.

Nutritional/Ethanol Interactions

Food: Limit caffeine.

Herb/Nutraceutical: High-dose vitamin C (1 g/day) may increase adverse effects. Avoid St John's wort.

Effects on Lab Values Thyroid function test, metyrapone test, liver function tests, coagulation tests (prothrombin time, factors VII, VIII, IX, X)

Adverse Reactions

>10%:
- Cardiovascular: Edema
- Endocrine & metabolic: Breakthrough bleeding, spotting, changes in menstrual flow, amenorrhea
- Gastrointestinal: Anorexia
- Local: Pain at injection site
- Neuromuscular & skeletal: Weakness

1% to 10%:
- Cardiovascular: Edema
- Central nervous system: Mental depression, fever, insomnia
- Dermatologic: Melasma or chloasma, allergic rash with or without pruritus
- Endocrine & metabolic: Increased breast tenderness
- Gastrointestinal: Weight gain/loss
- Genitourinary: Changes in cervical erosion and secretions
- Hepatic: Cholestatic jaundice

Pharmacodynamics/Kinetics

Absorption: Oral, transdermal: Rapidly absorbed

Bioavailability: 64%

Half-Life Elimination: 5-14 hours

Time to Peak: 1-2 hours

Metabolism: Oral: Hepatic via reduction and conjugation; first-pass effect

Formulations

Tablet (Micronor®, Nor-QD®): 0.35 mg
Tablet, as acetate (Aygestin®): 5 mg

Dosing

Adults:

Contraception (Females): Oral: Progesterone only: Norethindrone 0.35 mg every day of the year starting on first day of menstruation; if one dose is missed take as soon as remembered; then next tablet at regular time; if two doses are missed, take one of the missed doses, discard the other, and take daily dose at usual time; if three doses are missed, use another form of birth control until menses appear or pregnancy is ruled out

Amenorrhea and abnormal uterine bleeding: Oral:
- Norethindrone: 5-20 mg/day on days 5-25 of menstrual cycle
- Acetate salt: 2.5-10 mg on days 5-25 of menstrual cycle

Endometriosis: Oral:
- Norethindrone: 10 mg/day for 2 weeks; increase at increments of 5 mg/day every 2 weeks until 30 mg/day; continue for 6-9 months or until breakthrough bleeding demands temporary termination

Acetate salt: 5 mg/day for 14 days; increase at increments of 2.5 mg/day every 2 weeks up to 15 mg/day; continue for 6-9 months or until breakthrough bleeding demands temporary termination

Pediatrics: Adolescents: Refer to adult dosing

Administration

Oral: Take with food.

Monitoring Laboratory Tests Long-term therapy, annual Pap tests, mammogram

Monitoring and Teaching Issues

Physical Assessment: Assess patient knowledge/teach appropriate administration schedule, adverse signs to report. Teach appropriate breast self-exam and the need for regular breast self-exam and necessity of annual physical check-up with long-term use. **Pregnancy risk factor X** - determine that patient is not pregnant before beginning treatment. Note breast-feeding caution.

Patient Education: Take according to prescribed schedule. Follow instructions for regular self-breast exam. You may experience dizziness or lightheadedness; use caution when driving or engaging in tasks that require alertness until response to drug is known. Limit intake of caffeine. Avoid high-dose vitamin C. You may experience photosensitivity; use sunscreen, wear protective clothing and eyewear, and avoid direct sunlight. You may experience loss of hair (reversible), weight gain or loss. Report sudden severe headache or vomiting, disturbances of vision or speech, sudden blindness, numbness of weakness in an extremity, chest pain, calf pain, difficulty breathing, depression or acute fatigue, unusual bleeding, spotting, or changes in menstrual flow. **Pregnancy/breast-feeding precautions:** Inform prescriber if you are pregnant. Consult prescriber if breast-feeding.

Dietary Issues: Should be taken with food at same time each day.

Breast-feeding Issues: Norethindrone can cause changes in milk production in the mother. Monitor infant growth. Use lowest possible dose of norethindrone for less effect on milk production.

Related Information

Estrogen Replacement Therapy *on page 1666*

Norethindrone Acetate *see* Norethindrone *on page 984*

Norethindrone Acetate and Ethinyl Estradiol *see* Ethinyl Estradiol and Norethindrone *on page 527*

Norethindrone and Estradiol *see* Estradiol and Norethindrone *on page 499*

Norethindrone and Mestranol *see* Mestranol and Norethindrone *on page 863*

Norethisterone *see* Norethindrone *on page 984*

Norflex™ *see* Orphenadrine *on page 1009*

Norgesic™ *see* Orphenadrine, Aspirin, and Caffeine *on page 1010*

Norgesic™ Forte *see* Orphenadrine, Aspirin, and Caffeine *on page 1010*

Norgestimate *see page 1666*

Norgestimate and Ethinyl Estradiol *see* Ethinyl Estradiol and Norgestimate *on page 530*

Norgestrel (nor JES trel)

U.S. Brand Names Ovrette®

Generic Available No

Pharmacologic Category Contraceptive

Pregnancy Risk Factor X

Lactation Enters breast milk/use caution

Use Prevention of pregnancy; **progestin only products have higher risk of failure in contraceptive use**

Mechanism of Action/Effect Inhibits secretion of pituitary gonadotropin (LH) which prevents follicular maturation and ovulation

Contraindications Hypersensitivity to norgestrel or any component of the formulation; hypersensitivity to tartrazine; thromboembolic disorders; severe hepatic disease; breast cancer; undiagnosed vaginal bleeding; pregnancy

Warnings/Precautions Discontinue if sudden loss of vision or if diplopia or proptosis occur. Use with caution in patients with a history of mental depression.

Drug Interactions

Cytochrome P450 Effect: Substrate of **CYP3A4**

Decreased Effect: Azole antifungals (ketoconazole, itraconazole, fluconazole), barbiturates, hydantoins (phenytoin), carbamazepine, and rifampin decrease oral contraceptive efficacy due to increased metabolism. Antibiotics (penicillins, tetracyclines, griseofulvin) may decrease efficacy of oral contraceptives.

Increased Effect/Toxicity: Oral contraceptives may increase toxicity of acetaminophen, anticoagulants, benzodiazepines, caffeine, corticosteroids, metoprolol, theophylline, and tricyclic antidepressants.

Nutritional/Ethanol Interactions

Food: CNS effects of caffeine may be enhanced if oral contraceptives are used concurrently with caffeine.

Herb/Nutraceutical: St John's wort may decrease levels. Avoid dong quai and black cohosh (have estrogen activity). Avoid saw palmetto, red clover, ginseng.

Effects on Lab Values Thyroid function tests, metyrapone test, liver function tests

Adverse Reactions Frequency not defined.

Cardiovascular: Embolism, cerebral thrombosis, edema

Central nervous system: Mental depression, fever, insomnia

Dermatologic: Melasma or chloasma, allergic rash with or without pruritus

Endocrine & metabolic: Breakthrough bleeding, spotting, changes in menstrual flow, amenorrhea, changes in cervical erosion and secretions, increased breast tenderness

Gastrointestinal: Weight gain/loss, anorexia

Hepatic: Cholestatic jaundice

Local: Thrombophlebitis

Neuromuscular & skeletal: Weakness

(Continued)

Norgestrel *(Continued)*

Overdosage/Toxicology
Toxicity is unlikely following single exposures of excessive doses.
Supportive treatment is adequate in most cases.

Pharmacodynamics/Kinetics
Absorption: Oral: Well absorbed
Half-Life Elimination: ~20 hours
Metabolism: Primarily hepatic via reduction and conjugation

Formulations Tablet: 0.075 mg [contains tartrazine]

Dosing
Adults: Contraception: Oral: Administer daily, starting the first day of menstruation, take 1 tablet at the same time each day, every day of the year. If one dose is missed, take as soon as remembered, then next tablet at regular time; if two doses are missed, take 1 tablet as soon as it is remembered, followed by an additional dose that same day at the usual time. When one or two doses are missed, additional contraceptive measures should be used until 14 consecutive tablets have been taken. If three doses are missed, discontinue norgestrel and use an additional form of birth control until menses or pregnancy is ruled out.

Monitoring and Teaching Issues
Physical Assessment: Monitor or teach patient to monitor blood pressure on a regular basis. Monitor or teach patient to monitor for occurrence of adverse effects and symptoms to report (see Adverse Reactions). Assess knowledge/teach importance of regular (monthly) blood pressure checks and annual physical assessment, Pap smear, and vision assessment. Teach importance of maintaining prescribed schedule of dosing (see Dosing for dosing and missed dose information). **Pregnancy risk factor X** - do not use if patient is pregnant. Note breast-feeding caution.

Patient Education: Take exactly as directed by prescriber (also see package insert). You are at risk of becoming pregnant if doses are missed. If you miss a dose, take as soon as possible or double the dose next day. If more than three doses are missed, contact prescriber for restarting directions. Use additional form of contraception during first week of taking this medication. Detailed and complete information on dosing and missed doses can be found in the package insert. Be aware that some medications may reduce the effectiveness of oral contraceptives; an alternate form of contraception may be needed (see Drug Interactions). It is important that you check your blood pressure monthly (on same day each month) and that you have an annual physical assessment, Pap smear, and vision assessment while taking this medication. Avoid smoking while taking this medication; smoking increases risk of adverse effects, including thromboembolic events and heart attacks. You may experience loss of appetite (small, frequent meals will help); or constipation (increased exercise, fluids, fruit, fiber, or stool softeners may help). If diabetic, use accurate serum glucose testing to identify any changes in glucose tolerance; notify prescriber of significant changes so antidiabetic medication can be adjusted if necessary. Report immediately pain or muscle soreness; warmth, swelling, or redness in calves; shortness of breath; sudden loss of vision; unresolved leg or foot swelling; change in menstrual pattern (unusual bleeding, amenorrhea, breakthrough spotting); breast tenderness that does not go away; acute abdominal cramping; signs of vaginal infection (drainage, pain, itching); CNS changes (blurred vision, confusion, acute anxiety, or unresolved depression); or significant weight gain (>5 lb/week). **Pregnancy/breast-feeding precautions:** This drug may cause severe fetal complication. If you suspect you may become pregnant, contact prescriber immediately. Consult prescriber if breast-feeding.

Dietary Issues: Should be taken with food at same time each day.

Norinyl® 1+35 *see* Ethinyl Estradiol and Norethindrone *on page 527*
Norinyl® 1+50 *see* Mestranol and Norethindrone *on page 863*
Noritate™ *see* Metronidazole *on page 895*
Normal Human Serum Albumin *see* Albumin *on page 50*
Normal Serum Albumin (Human) *see* Albumin *on page 50*
Normodyne® *see* Labetalol *on page 764*
Norplant® Implant [DSC] *see* Levonorgestrel *on page 793*
Norpramin® *see* Desipramine *on page 377*
Nor-QD® *see* Norethindrone *on page 984*
Nortrel™ *see* Ethinyl Estradiol and Norethindrone *on page 527*

Nortriptyline (nor TRIP ti leen)

U.S. Brand Names Aventyl® HCl; Pamelor®

Synonyms Nortriptyline Hydrochloride

Generic Available Yes

Pharmacologic Category Antidepressant, Tricyclic (Secondary Amine)

Pregnancy Risk Factor D

Lactation Enters breast milk/contraindicated (AAP rates "of concern")

Use Treatment of symptoms of depression

Use - Unlabeled/Investigational Chronic pain, anxiety disorders, enuresis, attention-deficit/hyperactivity disorder (ADHD)

Mechanism of Action/Effect Traditionally believed to increase the synaptic concentration of serotonin and/or norepinephrine in the central nervous system by inhibition of their reuptake by the presynaptic neuronal membrane. However, additional receptor effects have been found including desensitization of adenyl cyclase, down regulation of beta-adrenergic receptors, and down regulation of serotonin receptors.

Contraindications Hypersensitivity to nortriptyline and similar chemical class, or any component of the formulation; use of MAO inhibitors within 14 days; use in a patient during the acute recovery phase of MI; pregnancy

Warnings/Precautions May cause sedation, resulting in impaired performance of tasks requiring alertness (ie, operating machinery or driving). Sedative effects may be additive with other CNS depressants and/or ethanol. May worsen psychosis in some patients or precipitate a shift to mania or hypomania in patients with bipolar disease. May increase the risks associated with electroconvulsive therapy. This agent should be discontinued, when possible, prior to elective surgery. Therapy should not be abruptly discontinued in patients receiving high doses for prolonged periods. May alter glucose regulation - use caution in patients with diabetes.

May cause orthostatic hypotension (risk is low relative to other antidepressants); use caution in cardiovascular or cerebrovascular disease. Use caution in patients with urinary retention, benign prostatic hyperplasia, narrow-angle glaucoma, xerostomia, visual problems, constipation, or history of bowel obstruction.

Use caution in patients with depression, particularly if suicidal risk may be present. Use with caution in patients with a history of cardiovascular disease (including previous MI, stroke, tachycardia, or conduction abnormalities). The risk conduction abnormalities with this agent is moderate relative to other antidepressants. Use caution in patients with a previous seizure disorder or condition predisposing to seizures such as brain damage, alcoholism, or concurrent therapy with other drugs which lower the seizure threshold. Use with caution in hyperthyroid patients or those receiving thyroid supplementation. Use with caution in patients with hepatic or renal dysfunction and in elderly patients.

Drug Interactions

Cytochrome P450 Effect: Substrate of CYP1A2, 2C19, **2D6**, 3A4; Inhibits CYP2D6, 2E1

Decreased Effect: Carbamazepine, phenobarbital, and rifampin may increase the metabolism of nortriptyline resulting in decreased effect of nortriptyline. Nortriptyline inhibits the antihypertensive response to bethanidine, clonidine, debrisoquin, guanadrel, guanethidine, guanabenz, or guanfacine. Cholestyramine and colestipol may bind TCAs and reduce their absorption; monitor for altered response.

Increased Effect/Toxicity: Nortriptyline increases the effects of amphetamines, anticholinergics, other CNS depressants (sedatives, hypnotics, ethanol), chlorpropamide, tolazamide, and warfarin. When used with MAO inhibitors, hyperpyrexia, hypertension, tachycardia, confusion, seizures, and **deaths have been reported** (serotonin syndrome). Serotonin syndrome has also been reported with ritonavir (rare). The SSRIs (to varying degrees), cimetidine, grapefruit juice, indinavir, methylphenidate, ritonavir, quinidine, diltiazem, and verapamil inhibit the metabolism of TCAs and clinical toxicity may result. Use of lithium with a TCA may increase the risk for neurotoxicity. Phenothiazines may increase concentration of some TCAs and TCAs may increase concentration of phenothiazines. Pressor response to I.V. epinephrine, norepinephrine, and phenylephrine may be enhanced in patients receiving TCAs (**Note:** Effect is unlikely with epinephrine or levonordefrin dosages typically administered as infiltration in combination with local anesthetics). Combined use of beta-agonists or drugs which prolong QT_c (including quinidine, procainamide, disopyramide, cisapride, sparfloxacin, gatifloxacin, moxifloxacin) with TCAs may predispose patients to cardiac arrhythmias. Use with altretamine may cause orthostatic hypotension.

Nutritional/Ethanol Interactions

Ethanol: Avoid ethanol (may increase CNS depression).

Food: Grapefruit juice may inhibit the metabolism of some TCAs and clinical toxicity may result.

Herb/Nutraceutical: Avoid valerian, St John's wort, SAMe, kava kava (may increase risk of serotonin syndrome and/or excessive sedation).

Effects on Lab Values ↑ glucose

Adverse Reactions Frequency not defined.

Cardiovascular: Postural hypotension, arrhythmias, hypertension, heart block, tachycardia, palpitations, myocardial infarction

Central nervous system: Confusion, delirium, hallucinations, restlessness, insomnia, disorientation, delusions, anxiety, agitation, panic, nightmares, hypomania, exacerbation of psychosis, incoordination, ataxia, extrapyramidal symptoms, seizures

Dermatologic: Alopecia, photosensitivity, rash, petechiae, urticaria, itching

Endocrine & metabolic: Sexual dysfunction, gynecomastia, breast enlargement, galactorrhea, increase or decrease in libido, increase in blood sugar, SIADH

Gastrointestinal: Xerostomia, constipation, vomiting, anorexia, diarrhea, abdominal cramps, black tongue, nausea, unpleasant taste, weight gain/loss

Genitourinary: Urinary retention, delayed micturition, impotence, testicular edema

Hematologic: Rarely agranulocytosis, eosinophilia, purpura, thrombocytopenia

Hepatic: Increased liver enzymes, cholestatic jaundice

Neuromuscular & skeletal: Tremor, numbness, tingling, paresthesias, peripheral neuropathy

Ocular: Blurred vision, eye pain, disturbances in accommodation, mydriasis

Otic: Tinnitus

Miscellaneous: Diaphoresis (excessive), allergic reactions

Overdosage/Toxicology Symptoms of overdose include agitation, confusion, hallucinations, urinary retention, hypothermia, hypotension, seizures, and ventricular tachycardia. Treatment is symptomatic and supportive. Alkalinization by sodium bicarbonate and/or hyperventilation may limit cardiac toxicity.

Pharmacodynamics/Kinetics

Half-Life Elimination: 28-31 hours

Time to Peak: Serum: 7-8.5 hours

Metabolism: Primarily hepatic; extensive first-pass effect

Onset: Therapeutic: 1-3 weeks

Formulations

Capsule, as hydrochloride: 10 mg, 25 mg, 50 mg, 75 mg

Aventyl® HCl: 10 mg, 25 mg

Pamelor®: 10 mg, 25 mg, 50 mg, 75 mg [may contain benzyl alcohol; 50 mg may also contain sodium bisulfite]

Solution, as hydrochloride (Aventyl® HCl, Pamelor®): 10 mg/5 mL (473 mL) [contains alcohol 4% and benzoic acid]

(Continued)

Nortriptyline *(Continued)*

Dosing

Adults: Depression: Oral: 25 mg 3-4 times/day up to 150 mg/day

Elderly: Note: Nortriptyline is one of the best tolerated TCAs in the elderly.

Initial: 10-25 mg at bedtime

Dosage can be increased by 25 mg every 3 days for inpatients and weekly for outpatients if tolerated.

Usual maintenance dose: 75 mg as a single bedtime dose or 2 divided doses; however, lower or higher doses may be required to stay within the therapeutic window.

Pediatrics:

Nocturnal enuresis: Oral: Children:

6-7 years (20-25 kg): 10 mg/day

8-11 years (25-35 kg): 10-20 mg/day

>11 years (35-54 kg): 25-35 mg/day

Depression and/or ADHD (unlabeled use): Oral:

Children 6-12 years: 1-3 mg/kg/day or 10-20 mg/day in 3-4 divided doses

Adolescents: 30-100 mg/day in divided doses

Hepatic Impairment: Lower doses and slower titration are recommended dependent on individualization of dosage.

Stability

Storage: Protect from light.

Monitoring and Teaching Issues

Physical Assessment: See Contraindications, Warnings/Precautions, and Dosing for use cautions. Assess potential for interactions with other prescriptions, OTC medications, or herbal products patient may be taking (see extensive list of Drug Interactions). Assess for suicidal tendencies before beginning therapy. May cause physiological or psychological dependence, tolerance, or abuse; periodically evaluate need for continued use. Assess therapeutic response (mental status, mood, affect) and adverse reactions (eg, suicidal ideation - see Adverse Reactions and Overdose/Toxicology) at beginning of therapy and periodically with long-term use. Taper dosage slowly when discontinuing (allow 3-4 weeks between discontinuing this medication and starting another antidepressant). Caution patients with diabetes to monitor glucose levels closely; may increase or decrease serum glucose levels. Teach patient appropriate use, interventions to reduce side effects, and adverse symptoms to report (see Patient Education). **Pregnancy risk factor D** - determine that patient is not pregnant before beginning treatment. Instruct patients of childbearing age on appropriate barrier contraceptive measures. Breast-feeding is contraindicated.

Patient Education: Inform prescriber of all prescriptions, OTC medications, or herbal products you are taking, and any allergies you have. Do not take anything new during treatment unless approved by prescriber. Take exactly as directed; take once-a-day dose at bedtime. Do not increase dose or frequency; may take 2-3 weeks to achieve desired results. This drug may cause physical and/or psychological dependence. Avoid alcohol and grapefruit juice. Maintain adequate hydration (2-3 L/day of fluids) unless advised by prescriber to restrict fluids. May cause drowsiness, lightheadedness, impaired coordination, dizziness, or blurred vision (use caution when driving or engaging in tasks requiring alertness until response to drug is known); nausea, vomiting, loss of appetite, or disturbed taste (small, frequent meals, good mouth care, chewing gum, or sucking lozenges may help); constipation (increased exercise, fluids, fruit, or fiber may help); urinary retention (void before taking medication); postural hypotension (use caution climbing stairs or when changing position from lying or sitting to standing); altered sexual drive or ability (reversible); or photosensitivity (use sunscreen, wear protective clothing and eyewear, and avoid direct sunlight). Report chest pain, palpitations, or rapid heartbeat; persistent CNS effects (eg, nervousness, restlessness, insomnia, anxiety, excitation, headache, agitation, impaired coordination, changes in cognition); muscle cramping, weakness, tremors, or rigidity; blurred vision or eye pain; breast enlargement or swelling; yellowing of skin or eyes; or worsening of condition. **Pregnancy/breast-feeding precautions:** Inform prescriber if you pregnant. Do not get pregnant while taking this medication. Consult prescriber for appropriate contraceptive measures. Do not breast-feed.

Geriatric Considerations: Since nortriptyline is the least likely of the tricyclic antidepressants (TCAs) to cause orthostatic hypotension and one of the least anticholinergic and sedating TCAs, it is a preferred agent when a TCA is indicated. Data from a clinical trial comparing fluoxetine to tricyclics suggests that fluoxetine is significantly less effective than nortriptyline in hospitalized elderly patients with unipolar affective disorder, especially those with melancholia and concurrent cardiovascular disease.

Related Information

Antidepressant Agents *on page 1553*

Antidepressant Medication Guidelines *on page 1613*

Peak and Trough Guidelines *on page 1544*

Pharmacotherapy of Urinary Incontinence *on page 1699*

Nortriptyline Hydrochloride *see* Nortriptyline *on page 986*

Norvasc® *see* Amlodipine *on page 86*

Norvir® *see* Ritonavir *on page 1196*

Nostril® Nasal [OTC] *see* Phenylephrine *on page 1071*

Novacet® Topical *see page 1522*

Novantrone® *see* Mitoxantrone *on page 916*

Novarel™ *see* Chorionic Gonadotropin (Human) *on page 284*

Novocain® *see* Procaine *on page 1124*

Novolin® 70/30 *see* Insulin Preparations *on page 714*

Novolin® L *see* Insulin Preparations *on page 714*

Novolin® N *see* Insulin Preparations *on page 714*

Novolin® R *see* Insulin Preparations *on page 714*

NovoLog® *see* Insulin Preparations *on page 714*

Novo-Seven® *see* Factor VIIa (Recombinant) *on page 541*
Novothyrox *see* Levothyroxine *on page 797*
NPH Iletin® II *see* Insulin Preparations *on page 714*
NSC-13875 *see* Altretamine *on page 70*
NSC-26271 *see* Cyclophosphamide *on page 339*
NSC-106977 (*Erwinia*) *see* Asparaginase *on page 118*
NSC-109229 (*E. coli*) *see* Asparaginase *on page 118*
NSC-125066 *see* Bleomycin *on page 174*
NSC-373364 *see* Aldesleukin *on page 54*
NTG *see* Nitroglycerin *on page 977*
Nubain® *see* Nalbuphine *on page 942*
Nucofed® Expectorant *see* Guaifenesin, Pseudoephedrine, and Codeine *on page 649*
Nucofed® Pediatric Expectorant *see* Guaifenesin, Pseudoephedrine, and Codeine *on page 649*
Nucotuss® *see* Guaifenesin, Pseudoephedrine, and Codeine *on page 649*
NuLev™ *see* Hyoscyamine *on page 685*
NuLytely® *see* Polyethylene Glycol-Electrolyte Solution *on page 1098*
Numorphan® *see* Oxymorphone *on page 1023*
Nupercainal® Hydrocortisone Cream [OTC] *see* Hydrocortisone *on page 673*
Nuquin HP® *see* Hydroquinone *on page 679*
Nuromax® *see* Doxacurium *on page 440*
Nutracort® *see* Hydrocortisone *on page 673*
Nutracort® *see* Topical Corticosteroids *on page 1334*
Nutritional and Herbal Products *see page 1463*
Nutropin® *see* Human Growth Hormone *on page 658*
Nutropin AQ ® *see* Human Growth Hormone *on page 658*
Nutropin Depot® *see* Human Growth Hormone *on page 658*
Nydrazid® *see* Isoniazid *on page 746*

Nystatin (nye STAT in)

U.S. Brand Names Bio-Statin®; Mycostatin®; Nystat-Rx®; Nystop®; Pedi-Dri®

Generic Available Yes: Cream, ointment, suspension, tablet

Pharmacologic Category Antifungal Agent, Oral Nonabsorbed; Antifungal Agent, Topical; Antifungal Agent, Vaginal

Pregnancy Risk Factor B/C (oral)

Lactation Does not enter breast milk/compatible (not absorbed orally)

Use Treatment of susceptible cutaneous, mucocutaneous, and oral cavity fungal infections normally caused by the *Candida* species

Mechanism of Action/Effect Binds to sterols in fungal cell membrane, changing the cell wall permeability allowing for leakage of cellular contents and cell death

Contraindications Hypersensitivity to nystatin or any component of the formulation

Warnings/Precautions Pregnancy risk B/C (oral)

Adverse Reactions

Frequency not defined: Dermatologic: Contact dermatitis, Stevens-Johnson syndrome
1% to 10%: Gastrointestinal: Nausea, vomiting, diarrhea, stomach pain
<1% (Limited to important or life-threatening): Hypersensitivity reactions

Overdosage/Toxicology Symptoms of overdose include nausea, vomiting, and diarrhea. Treatment is supportive.

Pharmacodynamics/Kinetics

Absorption: Topical: None through mucous membranes or intact skin; Oral: Poorly absorbed

Onset: Symptomatic relief from candidiasis: 24-72 hours

Formulations

Capsule (Bio-Statin®): 500,000 units, 1 million units
Cream: 100,000 units/g (15 g, 30 g)
  Mycostatin®: 100,000 units/g (30 g)
Lozenge (Mycostatin®): 200,000 units
Ointment, topical: 100,000 units/g (15 g, 30 g)
Powder, for prescription compounding: 50 million units (10 g); 150 million units (30 g); 500 million units (100 g); 2 billion units (400 g)
  Nystat-Rx®: 50 million units (10 g); 150 million units (30 g); 500 million units (100 g); 1 billion units (190 g); 2 billion units (350 g)
Powder, topical:
  Mycostatin®, Nystop®: 100,000 units/g (15 g)
  Pedi-Dri®: 100,000 units/g (56.7 g)
Suspension, oral: 100,000 units/mL (5 mL, 60 mL, 480 mL)
  Mycostatin®: 100,000 units/mL (60 mL, 480 mL) [contains alcohol ≤1%; cherry-mint flavor]
Tablet (Mycostatin®): 500,000 units
Tablet, vaginal: 100,000 units (15s) [packaged with applicator]

Dosing

Adults & Elderly:

Oral candidiasis: Suspension (swish and swallow orally): 400,000-600,000 units 4 times/day; troche: 200,000-400,000 units 4-5 times/day

Mucocutaneous infections: Topical: Apply 2-3 times/day to affected areas; very moist topical lesions are treated best with powder.

Intestinal infections: Oral tablets: 500,000-1,000,000 units every 8 hours

Vaginal infections: Vaginal tablets: Insert 1 tablet/day at bedtime for 2 weeks. (May also be given orally.)

Note: Powder for compounding: Children and Adults: $^1/_8$ teaspoon (500,000 units) to equal approximately $^1/_2$ cup of water; give 4 times/day

(Continued)

Nystatin *(Continued)*

Pediatrics:

Oral candidiasis:

Suspension (swish and swallow orally):

Premature infants: 100,000 units 4 times/day

Infants: 200,000 units 4 times/day or 100,000 units to each side of mouth 4 times/day

Children: 400,000-600,000 units 4 times/day

Troche: Children: Refer to adult dosing.

Powder for compounding: Children: Refer to adult dosing.

Mucocutaneous infections: Children: Refer to adult dosing.

Administration

Oral:

Suspension: Shake well before using. Should be swished about the mouth and retained in the mouth for as long as possible (several minutes) before swallowing.

Troches: Must be allowed to dissolve slowly and should not be chewed or swallowed whole.

Stability

Storage: Keep vaginal inserts in refrigerator. Protect from temperature extremes, moisture, and light.

Monitoring and Teaching Issues

Physical Assessment: Determine that cause of infection is fungal. Avoid skin contact when applying. Monitor therapeutic response, adverse reactions (see Adverse Reactions) at beginning of therapy and periodically throughout therapy. Assess knowledge/teach patient appropriate use, interventions to reduce side effects, and adverse symptoms to report (see Patient Education). **Pregnancy risk factor B/C** - benefits of use should outweigh possible risks.

Patient Education: Take as directed. Maintain adequate hydration (2-3 L/day of fluids) unless advised by prescriber to restrict fluids. Do not allow medication to come in contact with eyes. Report persistent nausea, vomiting, or diarrhea; or if condition being treated worsens or does not improve. **Pregnancy precaution:** Inform prescriber if you are pregnant.

Oral tablets: Swallow whole; do not crush or chew.

Oral suspension: Shake well before using. Remove dentures, clean mouth (do not replace dentures until after using medications). Swish suspension in mouth for several minutes before swallowing.

Oral troches: Remove dentures, clean mouth (do not replace dentures until after using medication). Allow troche to dissolve in mouth; do not chew or swallow whole.

Topical: Wash and dry area before applying (do not reuse towels without washing, apply clean clothing after use). Report unresolved burning, redness, or swelling in treated areas.

Vaginal tablets: Wash hands before using. Lie down to insert high into vagina at bedtime.

Geriatric Considerations: For oral infections, patients who wear dentures must have them removed and cleaned in order to eliminate source of reinfection.

Nystatin and Triamcinolone (nye STAT in & trye am SIN oh lone)

U.S. Brand Names Mycolog®-II; Mytrex®

Synonyms Triamcinolone and Nystatin

Generic Available Yes

Pharmacologic Category Antifungal Agent, Topical; Corticosteroid, Topical

Pregnancy Risk Factor C

Lactation Excretion in breast milk unknown

Use Treatment of cutaneous candidiasis

Formulations

Cream (Mycolog®-II, Mytrex®): Nystatin 100,000 units and triamcinolone acetonide 0.1% (15 g, 30 g, 60 g)

Ointment: Nystatin 100,000 units and triamcinolone acetonide 0.1% (15 g, 30 g, 60 g)

Mycolog®-II: Nystatin 100,000 units and triamcinolone acetonide 0.1% (15 g, 30 g, 60 g)

Mytrex®: Nystatin 100,000 units and triamcinolone acetonide 0.1% (15 g, 30 g)

Dosing

Adults & Elderly: Cutaneous *Candida*: Topical: Apply sparingly 2-4 times/day,

Pediatrics: Refer to adult dosing.

Monitoring and Teaching Issues

Physical Assessment: See individual components listed in Related Information. **Pregnancy risk factor C** - benefits of use should outweigh possible risks. Note breast-feeding caution.

Patient Education: See individual components listed in Related Information. **Pregnancy/breast-feeding precautions:** Inform prescriber if you are or intend to become pregnant. Consult prescriber if breast-feeding.

Related Information

Nystatin *on page 989*

Triamcinolone *on page 1356*

Nystat-Rx® *see* Nystatin *on page 989*

Nystop® *see* Nystatin *on page 989*

Nytol® [OTC] *see* DiphenhydrAMINE *on page 422*

Nytol® Maximum Strength [OTC] *see* DiphenhydrAMINE *on page 422*

Obesity Treatment Guidelines for Adults *see page 1693*

OCL® *see* Polyethylene Glycol-Electrolyte Solution *on page 1098*

Octreotide (ok TREE oh tide)

U.S. Brand Names Sandostatin®; Sandostatin LAR®

Synonyms Octreotide Acetate

Generic Available No

Pharmacologic Category Antidiarrheal; Somatostatin Analog

Pregnancy Risk Factor B

Lactation Enters breast milk/contraindicated

Use Control of symptoms in patients with metastatic carcinoid and vasoactive intestinal peptide-secreting tumors (VIPomas); pancreatic tumors, gastrinoma, secretory diarrhea, acromegaly

Use - Unlabeled/Investigational AIDS-associated secretory diarrhea, control of bleeding of esophageal varices, breast cancer, cryptosporidiosis, Cushing's syndrome, insulinomas, small bowel fistulas, postgastrectomy dumping syndrome, chemotherapy-induced diarrhea, graft-versus-host disease (GVHD) induced diarrhea, Zollinger-Ellison syndrome, congenital hyperinsulinism

Mechanism of Action/Effect Mimics natural somatostatin by inhibiting serotonin release, and the secretion of gastrin, VIP, insulin, glucagon, secretin, motilin, and pancreatic polypeptide. Decreases growth hormone and IGF-1 in acromegaly.

Contraindications Hypersensitivity to octreotide or any component of the formulation

Warnings/Precautions Dosage adjustment may be required to maintain symptomatic control. Insulin requirements may be reduced as well as sulfonylurea requirements. Monitor patients for cholelithiasis, hyper- or hypoglycemia. Use with caution in patients with renal impairment. Do not administer Sandostatin LAR® intravenously or subcutaneously.

Drug Interactions

Decreased Effect: Octreotide may lower cyclosporine serum levels (case report of a transplant rejection due to reduction of serum cyclosporine levels). Codeine effect may be reduced.

Increased Effect/Toxicity: Octreotide may increase the effect of insulin or sulfonylurea agents which may result in hypoglycemia.

Adverse Reactions

>10%:

Cardiovascular: Sinus bradycardia (19% to 25%)

Endocrine & metabolic: Hyperglycemia (15% acromegaly, 27% carcinoid)

Gastrointestinal: Diarrhea (36% to 58% acromegaly), abdominal pain (30% to 44% acromegaly), flatulence (13% to 26% acromegaly), constipation (9% to 19% acromegaly), nausea (10% to 30%)

1% to 10%:

Cardiovascular: Flushing, edema, conduction abnormalities (9% to 10%), arrhythmias (3% to 9%)

Central nervous system: Fatigue, headache, dizziness, vertigo, anorexia, depression

Endocrine & metabolic: Hypoglycemia (2% acromegaly, 4% carcinoid), hyperglycemia (1%), hypothyroidism, galactorrhea

Gastrointestinal: Nausea, vomiting, diarrhea, constipation, abdominal pain, cramping, discomfort, fat malabsorption, loose stools, flatulence, tenesmus

Hepatic: Jaundice, hepatitis, increase LFTs, cholelithiasis has occurred, presumably by altering fat absorption and decreasing the motility of the gallbladder

Local: Pain at injection site (dose-related)

Neuromuscular & skeletal: Weakness

<1% (Limited to important or life-threatening): Alopecia, Bell's palsy, chest pain, dyspnea, gallstones, hypertensive reaction, thrombophlebitis

Overdosage/Toxicology Symptoms of overdose include hypo- or hyperglycemia, blurred vision, dizziness, drowsiness, and loss of motor function. Well tolerated bolus doses up to 1000 mcg have failed to produce adverse effects.

Pharmacodynamics/Kinetics

Absorption: S.C.: Rapid

Bioavailability: S.C.: 100%

Half-Life Elimination: 60-110 minutes

Metabolism: Extensively hepatic

Duration: S.C.: 6-12 hours

Formulations

Injection, microspheres for suspension, as acetate [depot formulation] (Sandostatin LAR®): 10 mg, 20 mg, 30 mg [with diluent and syringe]

Injection, solution, as acetate (Sandostatin®): 0.05 mg/mL (1 mL); 0.1 mg/mL (1 mL); 0.2 mg/mL (5 mL); 0.5 mg/mL (1 mL); 1 mg/mL (5 mL)

Dosing

Adults & Elderly:

Carcinoid tumors:

S.C., I.V.: Initial: 50 mcg 1-2 times/day; titrate dose based on response/tolerance. Range: 100-600 mcg/day in 2-4 divided doses

I.M. Depot injection: Patients must be stabilized on subcutaneous octreotide for at least 2 weeks before switching to the long-acting depot: Upon switch: 20 mg I.M. intragluteally every 4 weeks for 2-3 months, then the dose may be modified based upon response

Dosage adjustment: See dosing for VIPomas.

VIPomas:

S.C., I.V.: Initial 2 weeks: 200-300 mcg/day in 2-4 divided doses; titrate dose based on response/tolerance. Range: 150-750 mcg/day (doses >450 mcg/day are rarely required)

I.M. Depot injection: Patients must be stabilized on subcutaneous octreotide for at least 2 weeks before switching to the long-acting depot: Upon switch: 20 mg I.M. intragluteally every 4 weeks for 2-3 months, then the dose may be modified based upon response

Dosage adjustment for carcinoid tumors and VIPomas: After 2 months of depot injections the dosage may be continued or modified as follows:

Increase to 30 mg I.M. every 4 weeks if symptoms are inadequately controlled

(Continued)

Octreotide *(Continued)*

Decrease to 10 mg I.M. every 4 weeks, for a trial period, if initially responsive to 20 mg dose

Dosage >30 mg is not recommended

Diarrhea: I.V.: Initial: 50-100 mcg every 8 hours; increase by 100 mcg/dose at 48-hour intervals; maximum dose: 500 mcg every 8 hours

Esophageal varices bleeding: I.V. bolus: 25-50 mcg followed by continuous I.V. infusion of 25-50 mcg/hour

Acromegaly:

S.C., I.V.: Initial: 50 mcg three times daily; titrate to achieve growth hormone levels less than 5 ng/mL or IGF-I (somatomedin C) levels <1.9 U/mL in males and <2.2 U/mL in females. Usual effective dose 100 mcg three times/day. Range 300-1500 mcg/day

Note: Should be withdrawn yearly for a 4 week interval in patients who have received irradiation. Resume if levels increase and signs/symptoms recur.

I.M. Depot injection: Patients must be stabilized on subcutaneous octreotide for at least 2 weeks before switching to the long-acting depot: Upon switch: 20 mg I.M. intragluteally every 4 weeks for 2-3 months, then the dose may be modified based upon response

Dosage adjustment for acromegaly: After 3 months of depot injections the dosage may be continued or modified as follows:

GH ≤1 ng/mL, IGF-1 is normal, symptoms controlled: Reduce octreotide LAR® to 10 mg I.M. every 4 weeks

GH ≤2.5 ng/mL, IGF-1 is normal, symptoms controlled: Maintain octreotide LAR® at 20 mg I.M. every 4 weeks

GH >2.5 ng/mL, IGF-1 is elevated, or symptoms uncontrolled: Increase octreotide LAR® to 30 mg I.M. every 4 weeks

Dosages >40 mg are not recommended

Pediatrics: Infants and Children:

Diarrhea: I.V., S.C.: Doses of 1-10 mcg/kg every 12 hours have been used in children beginning at the low end of the range and increasing by 0.3 mcg/kg/dose at 3-day intervals. Suppression of growth hormone (animal data) is of concern when used as long-term therapy.

Congenital hyperinsulinism (unlabeled): S.C.: Doses of 3-40 mcg/kg/day have been used.

Renal Impairment: Half-life may be increased, requiring adjustment of maintenance dose.

Administration

I.M.: Depot formulation (Sandostatin LAR®): Administer immediately after reconstitution; administer in gluteal muscle, avoid deltoid administration

I.V.: Regular injection only (not suspension): IVP should be administered undiluted over 3 minutes. IVPB should be administered over 15-30 minutes. Continuous I.V. infusion rates have ranged from 25-50 mcg/hour for the treatment of esophageal variceal bleeding.

Other: Regular injection formulation (not depot) can be administered S.C.

Stability

Storage: Octreotide is a clear solution and should be stored under refrigeration. Ampuls may be stored at room temperature for up to 14 days when protected from light.

Reconstitution: Stability of parenteral admixture in NS at room temperature (25°C) and at refrigeration temperature (4°C) is 48 hours.

Common diluent: 50-100 mcg/50 mL NS; common diluent for continuous I.V. infusion: 1200 mcg/250 mL NS

Minimum volume: 50 mL NS

Compatibility: Stable in D_5W, NS; **incompatible** with fat emulsion 10%

Monitoring Laboratory Tests Vitamin B_{12} levels with chronic therapy

Monitoring and Teaching Issues

Physical Assessment: See Contraindications, Warnings/Precautions, and Dosing for use cautions. Assess potential for interactions with other prescriptions, OTC medications, or herbal products patient may be taking (see extensive list of Drug Interactions). See Administration specifics. Assess results of laboratory tests (see above), therapeutic effectiveness, and adverse effects (see Adverse Reactions and Overdose/Toxicology). Caution diabetic patients to monitor serum glucose closely; may increase the effect of insulin or sulfonylureas, which may result in hypoglycemia. Teach patient use if self-administered (injection technique and syringe/needle disposal) the possible side effects and interventions and adverse symptoms to report (see Patient Education). Breast-feeding is contraindicated.

Patient Education: Inform prescriber of all prescriptions, OTC medications, or herbal products you are taking, and any allergies you have. Do not take anything new during treatment unless approved by prescriber. If self-administered, follow instructions for injection and syringe/needle disposal. Schedule injections between meals to decrease GI effects. Consult prescriber about appropriate diet. Diabetic patients should monitor serum glucose closely and notify prescriber of significant changes (this drug may increase the effects of insulin or sulfonylureas). May cause skin flushing; nausea or vomiting (small, frequent meals, frequent mouth care, sucking lozenges, or chewing gum may help); or dizziness, fatigue, or drowsiness (use caution when driving or engaging in tasks that require alertness until response to drug is known). Report unusual weight gain, swelling of extremities, or difficulty breathing; acute or persistent GI distress (eg, diarrhea, vomiting, constipation, abdominal pain); muscle weakness or tremors or loss of motor function; chest pain or palpitations; blurred vision; depression; or redness, swelling, burning, or pain at injection site. **Breast-feeding precaution:** Do not breast-feed.

Dietary Issues: Schedule injections between meals to decrease GI effects.

Octreotide Acetate *see* Octreotide *on page 991*

Ocu-Chlor® *see page 1509*

Ocu-Chlor® *see* Chloramphenicol *on page 271*

Ocufen® *see page 1509*

Ocufen® *see* Flurbiprofen *on page 585*

Ocuflox™ *see page 1509*

Ocuflox® *see* Ofloxacin *on page 993*
Ocupress® Ophthalmic *see* Ophthalmic Agents, Glaucoma *on page 1002*
Ocusert Pilo-20® [DSC] *see* Ophthalmic Agents, Glaucoma *on page 1002*
Ocusert Pilo-20® [DSC] *see* Pilocarpine *on page 1082*
Ocusert Pilo-40® [DSC] *see* Ophthalmic Agents, Glaucoma *on page 1002*
Ocusert Pilo-40® [DSC] *see* Pilocarpine *on page 1082*
Ocu-Sul® *see* Sulfacetamide *on page 1256*

Ofloxacin (oh FLOKS a sin)

U.S. Brand Names Floxin®; Ocuflox®

Generic Available No

Pharmacologic Category Antibiotic, Quinolone

Pregnancy Risk Factor C

Lactation Enters breast milk/contraindicated (AAP rates "compatible")

Use Quinolone antibiotic for skin and skin structure, lower respiratory, and urinary tract infections and sexually-transmitted diseases. Active against many gram-positive and gram-negative aerobic bacteria.

Ophthalmic: Treatment of superficial ocular infections involving the conjunctiva or cornea due to strains of susceptible organisms

Otic: Otitis externa, chronic suppurative otitis media (patients >12 years of age); acute otitis media

Mechanism of Action/Effect Ofloxacin, a fluorinated quinolone, is a pyridine carboxylic acid derivative which exerts a broad spectrum bactericidal effect. It inhibits DNA gyrase inhibitor, an essential bacterial enzyme that maintains the superhelical structure of DNA. DNA gyrase is required for DNA replication and transcription, DNA repair, recombination, and transposition within the bacteria.

Contraindications Hypersensitivity to ofloxacin or other members of the quinolone group such as nalidixic acid, oxolinic acid, cinoxacin, norfloxacin, and ciprofloxacin; hypersensitivity to any component of the formulation

Warnings/Precautions Use with caution in patients with epilepsy or other CNS diseases which could predispose seizures. Use with caution in patients with renal impairment. Failure to respond to an ophthalmic antibiotic after 2-3 days may indicate the presence of resistant organisms, or another causative agent. Insomnia may be more common with ofloxacin than with other quinolones. Use caution with systemic preparation in children <18 years of age due to association of other quinolones with transient arthropathy. Has been associated with rare tendonitis or ruptured tendons (discontinue immediately with signs of inflammation or tendon pain). Risk may be increased with concurrent corticosteroids, particularly in the elderly. Discontinue at first signs or symptoms of tendon pain. Quinolones may exacerbate myasthenia gravis.

Severe hypersensitivity reactions, including anaphylaxis, have occurred with quinolone therapy. Discontinue immediately if an allergic reaction occurs. Prolonged use may result in superinfection; pseudomembranous colitis may occur and should be considered in all patients who present with diarrhea.

Pregnancy risk C.

Drug Interactions

Cytochrome P450 Effect: Inhibits CYP1A2

Decreased Effect: Metal cations (magnesium, aluminum, iron, and zinc) bind quinolones in the gastrointestinal tract and inhibit absorption (as much as 98%). Antacids, electrolyte supplements, sucralfate, quinapril, and some didanosine formulations should be avoided. Ofloxacin should be administered 4 hours before or 8 hours after these agents. Antineoplastic agents may decrease the absorption of quinolones.

Increased Effect/Toxicity: Quinolones can cause increased caffeine, warfarin, cyclosporine, and theophylline levels (unlikely to occur with ofloxacin). Azlocillin, cimetidine, and probenecid may increase ofloxacin serum levels. Foscarnet and NSAIDs have been associated with an increased risk of seizures with some quinolones. Serum levels of some quinolones are increased by loop diuretic administration. The hypoprothrombinemic effect of warfarin is enhanced by some quinolone antibiotics. Ofloxacin does not alter warfarin levels, but may alter the gastrointestinal flora which may increase warfarin's effect. Concurrent use of corticosteroids may increase risk of tendon rupture.

Nutritional/Ethanol Interactions

Food: Ofloxacin average peak serum concentrations may be decreased by 20% if taken with food.

Herb/Nutraceutical: Avoid dong quai, St John's wort (may also cause photosensitization).

Adverse Reactions

Ophthalmic:

>10%: Ocular: Burning or other discomfort of the eye, crusting or crystals in corner of eye

1% to 10%:

Gastrointestinal: Bad taste instillation

Ocular: Foreign body sensation, conjunctival hyperemia, itching of eye, ocular or facial edema, redness, stinging, photophobia

<1% (Limited to important or life-threatening): Dizziness, nausea

Otic: Local reactions (3%), earache (1%), tinnitus, otorrhagia

Systemic:

1% to 10%:

Cardiovascular: Chest pain (1% to 3%)

Central nervous system: Headache (1% to 9%), insomnia (3% to 7%), dizziness (1% to 5%), fatigue (1% to 3%), somnolence (1% to 3%), sleep disorders, nervousness (1% to 3%), pyrexia (1% to 3%), pain

Dermatologic: Rash/pruritus (1% to 3%)

Gastrointestinal: Diarrhea (1% to 4%), vomiting (1% to 3%), GI distress, cramps, abdominal cramps (1% to 3%), flatulence (1% to 3%), abnormal taste (1% to 3%), xerostomia (1% to 3%), decreased appetite, nausea (3% to 10%)

(Continued)

Ofloxacin *(Continued)*

Genitourinary: Vaginitis (1% to 3%), external genital pruritus in women
Local: Pain at injection site
Ocular: Superinfection (ophthalmic), photophobia, lacrimation, dry eyes, stinging, visual disturbances (1% to 3%)
Miscellaneous: Trunk pain

<1% (Limited to important or life-threatening): Anxiety, cognitive change, depression, euphoria, hallucinations, hepatitis, interstitial nephritis, paresthesia, photosensitivity, seizures, Stevens-Johnson syndrome, syncope, tinnitus, Tourette's syndrome, vasculitis, vertigo; quinolones have been associated with tendonitis and tendon rupture

Overdosage/Toxicology Symptoms of overdose include acute renal failure, seizures, nausea, and vomiting. Treatment includes GI decontamination, if possible, and supportive care. Not removed by peritoneal or hemodialysis.

Pharmacodynamics/Kinetics

Absorption: Well absorbed; food causes only minor alterations

Half-Life Elimination: 5-7.5 hours; prolonged with renal impairment

Formulations

Infusion [premixed in D_5W] (Floxin®): 200 mg (50 mL); 400 mg (100 mL)
Injection, solution [single-dose vial] (Floxin®): 40 mg/mL (10 mL)
Solution, ophthalmic (Ocuflox®): 0.3% (5 mL, 10 mL) [contains benzalkonium chloride]
Solution, otic (Floxin®[): 0.3% (5 mL, 10 mL)
Tablet (Floxin®): 200 mg, 300 mg, 400 mg

Dosing

Adults:

Susceptible systemic infections (except prostatitis): Oral, I.V.: 200-400 mg every 12 hours for 7-10 days for most infections
Prostatitis: Oral, I.V.: 200-400 mg every 12 hours for 6 weeks
Conjunctivitis: Ophthalmic: Instill 1-2 drops in affected eye(s) every 2-4 hours for the first 2 days, then use 4 times/day for an additional 5 days.
Corneal ulcer: Ophthalmic: Instill 1-2 drops every 30 minutes while awake and every 4-6 hours after retiring for the first 2 days; beginning on day 3, instill 1-2 drops every hour while awake for 4-6 additional days; thereafter, 1-2 drops 4 times/day until clinical cure.
Otitis externa: Otic: 10 drops into affected ear twice daily for 10 days
Chronic otitis media with perforated tympanic membranes: Otic: 10 drops into affected ear twice daily for 14 days

Elderly: Oral, I.V.: 200-400 mg every 12-24 hours (based on estimated renal function) for 7 days to 6 weeks depending on indication.

Pediatrics: Not for systemic use

Conjunctivitis: Ophthalmic: Children ≥1 year: Refer to adult dosing.
Corneal ulcer: Ophthalmic: Children ≥1 year: Refer to adult dosing.
Otitis externa: Otic: Children >1-12 years: Instill 5 drops into affected ear twice daily for 10 days.
Acute otitis media with tympanotomy tubes: Otic: Children >1-12 years: Instill 5 drops into affected ear twice daily for 10 days.

Renal Impairment:

Cl_{cr} 10-50 mL/minute: Administer 50% of normal dose or administer every 24 hours.
Cl_{cr} <10 mL/minute: Administer 25% of normal dose or administer 50% of normal dose every 24 hours.
Continuous arteriovenous or venovenous hemofiltration: 300 mg every 24 hours

Administration

Oral: Do not take within 2 hours of food or any antacids which contain zinc, magnesium, or aluminum.

I.V.: Administer over at least 60 minutes. Infuse separately. Do not infuse though lines containing solutions with magnesium or calcium.

Stability

Compatibility: Stable in D_5LR, D_5NS, D_5W, mannitol 20%, sodium bicarbonate 5%, NS

Y-site administration: Incompatible with amphotericin B cholesteryl sulfate complex, cefepime, doxorubicin liposome

Monitoring Laboratory Tests Perform culture and sensitivity studies before initiating therapy. Monitor CBC, renal and hepatic function periodically if therapy is prolonged.

Monitoring and Teaching Issues

Physical Assessment: Assess allergy history before initiating therapy. See Contraindications and Warnings/Precautions for use cautions. Assess potential for interactions with other prescriptions, OTC medications, or herbal products patient may be taking (see extensive list of Drug Interactions). See administration specifics for different formulations above. Assess results of laboratory tests (see above) therapeutic effectiveness, and adverse effects (see Adverse Reactions and Overdose/Toxicology). Teach patient appropriate use (according to formulation), possible side effects and interventions, and adverse symptoms to report (see Patient Education). **Pregnancy risk factor C** - benefits of use should outweigh possible risks. Breast-feeding is contraindicated.

Patient Education: Inform prescriber of all prescriptions, OTC medications, or herbal products you are taking, and any allergies you have. Do not take anything new during treatment unless approved by prescriber.

I.V.: Immediately report any stinging, burning, pain, redness, or swelling at infusion site.

Oral: Take per recommended schedule; complete full course of therapy and do not skip doses. Take on an empty stomach (1 hour before or 2 hours after meals, dairy products, antacids, or other medication). Oral/I.V.: Maintain adequate hydration (2-3 L/day of fluids) unless advised by prescriber to restrict fluids. May cause dizziness, lightheadedness, or headache (use caution when driving or engaging in tasks that require alertness until response to drug is known); nausea, vomiting, or taste perversion (small, frequent meals, frequent mouth care, sucking lozenges, or chewing gum may help); photosensitivity (use sunscreen, wear protective clothing and eyewear, and avoid direct sunlight). If inflammation or tendon pain occurs discontinue use immediately and report to prescriber. If sign of allergic reaction (eg, itching, urticaria, difficulty breathing, facial edema or difficulty swallowing, loss of consciousness, tingling, chest pain, palpitations) occurs, discontinue use immediately and report to prescriber. Report GI disturbances; CNS changes (eg, excessive sleepiness, agitation, or tremors); skin rash; vision changes; difficulty breathing; signs of opportunistic infection (eg, sore throat, chills, fever, burning, itching on urination, vaginal discharge, white plaques in mouth); or worsening of condition.

Pregnancy/breast-feeding precautions: Inform prescriber if you are or intend to become pregnant. Do not breast-feed.

Ophthalmic: Tilt head back, instill 1-2 drops in affected eye as frequently as prescribed. Do not let tip of applicator touch eye; do not contaminate tip of applicator (may cause eye infection, eye damage, or vision loss). May cause some stinging or burning or a bad taste in you mouth after instillation. Report persistent pain, burning, swelling, or visual disturbances.

Otic: Shake suspension well before using. Wash hands before and after applying drops. Lie with affected ear up and instill prescribed number of drops into ear. Remain on side with ear up for 5 minutes.

Geriatric Considerations: Dosage must be carefully adjusted to renal function. The half-life of ofloxacin may be prolonged, and serum concentrations are elevated in elderly patients even in the absence of overt renal impairment.

Breast-feeding Issues: Theoretically, may affect cartilage in weight-bearing joints.

Related Information

Ophthalmic Agents *on page 1509*
Otic Agents *on page 1519*
Tuberculosis *on page 1705*

OKT3 *see* Muromonab-CD3 *on page 932*

Olanzapine (oh LAN za peen)

U.S. Brand Names Zyprexa®; Zyprexa® Zydis®

Synonyms LY170053

Generic Available No

Pharmacologic Category Antipsychotic Agent, Thienobenzodiazepine

Pregnancy Risk Factor C

Lactation Enters breast milk/contraindicated

Use Treatment of the manifestations of schizophrenia; short-term treatment of acute mania episodes associated with bipolar mania

Use - Unlabeled/Investigational Treatment of psychotic symptoms

Mechanism of Action/Effect Olanzapine is a thienobenzodiazepine neuroleptic; thought to work by antagonizing dopamine and serotonin activities. It is a selective monoaminergic antagonist with high affinity binding to serotonin 5-HT_{2A} and 5-HT_{2C}, dopamine D_{1-4}, muscarinic M_{1-5}, histamine H_1 and alpha$_1$-adrenergic receptor sites. Olanzapine binds weakly to GABA-A, BZD, and beta-adrenergic receptors.

Contraindications Hypersensitivity to olanzapine or any component of the formulation

Warnings/Precautions Moderate to highly sedating, use with caution in disorders where CNS depression is a feature. Use with caution in Parkinson's disease. Caution in patients with hemodynamic instability; bone marrow suppression; predisposition to seizures; subcortical brain damage; severe cardiac, hepatic, renal, or respiratory disease. Esophageal dysmotility and aspiration have been associated with antipsychotic use - use with caution in patients at risk of pneumonia (ie, Alzheimer's disease). Caution in breast cancer or other prolactin-dependent tumors (may elevate prolactin levels). May alter temperature regulation or mask toxicity of other drugs due to antiemetic effects. Life-threatening arrhythmias have occurred with therapeutic doses of some neuroleptics. Significant weight gain may occur.

May cause anticholinergic effects (constipation, xerostomia, blurred vision, urinary retention); therefore, they should be used with caution in patients with decreased gastrointestinal motility, urinary retention, BPH, xerostomia, or visual problems. Conditions which also may be exacerbated by cholinergic blockade include narrow-angle glaucoma (screening is recommended) and worsening of myasthenia gravis. Relative to other neuroleptics, olanzapine has a moderate potency of cholinergic blockade.

May cause extrapyramidal symptoms, including pseudoparkinsonism, acute dystonic reactions, akathisia, and tardive dyskinesia (risk of these reactions is very low relative to other neuroleptics). May be associated with neuroleptic malignant syndrome (NMS). May cause hyperglycemia - use with caution in patients with diabetes or other disorders of glucose regulation.

Pregnancy risk C.

Drug Interactions

Cytochrome P450 Effect: Substrate of CYP1A2, 2D6; Inhibits CYP1A2, 2C8/9, 2C19, 2D6, 3A4

Decreased Effect: Olanzapine levels may be decreased by cytochrome P450 enzyme inducers such as rifampin, omeprazole, and carbamazepine (also cigarette smoking). Olanzapine may antagonize the effects of levodopa and dopamine agonists.

Increased Effect/Toxicity: Olanzapine levels may be increased by CYP1A2 inhibitors such as cimetidine and fluvoxamine. Sedations from olanzapine is increased with ethanol or other CNS depressants. The risk of hypotension and orthostatic hypotension from olanzapine is increased by concurrent antihypertensives. Metoclopramide may increase risk of extrapyramidal symptoms (EPS).

Nutritional/Ethanol Interactions

Ethanol: Avoid ethanol (may increase CNS depression).

Herb/Nutraceutical: Avoid dong quai, St John's wort (may also cause photosensitization). Avoid kava kava, gotu kola, valerian, St John's wort (may increase CNS depression).

(Continued)

Olanzapine *(Continued)*

Adverse Reactions

>10%: Central nervous system: Headache, somnolence, insomnia, agitation, nervousness, hostility, dizziness

1% to 10%:

Cardiovascular: Postural hypotension, tachycardia, hypotension, peripheral edema

Central nervous system: Dystonic reactions, parkinsonian events, amnesia, euphoria, stuttering, akathisia, anxiety, personality changes, fever

Dermatologic: Rash

Gastrointestinal: Xerostomia, constipation, abdominal pain, weight gain, increased appetite

Genitourinary: Premenstrual syndrome

Neuromuscular & skeletal: Arthralgia, neck rigidity, twitching, hypertonia, tremor

Ocular: Amblyopia

Respiratory: Rhinitis, cough, pharyngitis

<1% (Limited to important or life-threatening): Diabetes mellitus, hyperglycemia, neuroleptic malignant syndrome, priapism, seizures, tardive dyskinesia

Pharmacokinetic Note Tablets and orally-disintegrating tablets are bioequivalent.

Pharmacodynamics/Kinetics

Absorption: Well absorbed; not affected by food; tablets and orally-disintegrating tablets are bioequivalent

Half-Life Elimination: 21-54 hours; approximately 1.5 times greater in elderly

Time to Peak: ~6 hours

Metabolism: Highly metabolized via direct glucuronidation and cytochrome P450 mediated oxidation (CYP1A2, CYP2D6)

Formulations

Tablet (Zyprexa®): 2.5 mg, 5 mg, 7.5 mg, 10 mg, 15 mg, 20 mg

Tablet, orally-disintegrating (Zyprexa® Zydis®): 5 mg [contains phenylalanine 0.34 mg/tablet], 10 mg [contains phenylalanine 0.45 mg/tablet], 15 mg [contains phenylalanine 0.67 mg/tablet], 20 mg [contains phenylalanine 0.9 mg/tablet]

Dosing

Adults:

Schizophrenia: Oral: Usual starting dose: 5-10 mg once daily; increase to 10 mg once daily within 5-7 days, thereafter adjust by 5 mg/day at 1-week intervals, up to a maximum of 20 mg/day. Doses as high as 30-50 mg per day have been used.

Acute mania associated with bipolar disorder: Oral: Initial: 10-15 mg once daily; increase by 5 mg/day at intervals of not less than 24 hours; maximum dose: 20 mg/day

Elderly: Schizophrenia: Usual starting dose: 2.5 mg/day, increase as clinically indicated and monitor blood pressure; typical dosage range: 2.5-10 mg/day

Pediatrics: Schizophrenia/bipolar disorder: Oral: Initial: 2.5 mg/day; titrate as necessary to 20 mg/day (0.12-0.29 mg/kg/day)

Renal Impairment: Not removed by dialysis

Hepatic Impairment: Dosage adjustment may be necessary, however, there are no specific recommendations. Monitor closely.

Administration

Oral: Orally-disintegrating tablets: Remove from foil blister by peeling back (do not push tablet through the foil). Place tablet in mouth immediately upon removal. Tablet dissolves rapidly in saliva and may be swallowed with or without liquid.

Stability

Storage: Store at room temperature (20°C to 25°C); protect from light

Monitoring Laboratory Tests Ophthalmic screening

Monitoring and Teaching Issues

Physical Assessment: Assess other medications patient is taking for effectiveness and interactions (especially with drugs that alter P450 enzymes - see Drug Interactions). See Contraindications and Warnings/Precautions for use cautions. Review ophthalmic screening (see Monitoring Laboratory Tests). Monitor therapeutic response and adverse reactions at beginning of therapy and periodically with long-term (see Adverse Reactions and Overdose/Toxicology). Initiate at lower doses (see Dosing) and taper dosage slowly when discontinuing. Assess knowledge/teach patient appropriate use, interventions to reduce side effects, and adverse symptoms to report (see Patient Education). **Pregnancy risk factor C** - benefits of use should outweigh possible risks. Breast-feeding is contraindicated.

Patient Education: Use exactly as directed; do not increase dose or frequency. It may take 2-3 weeks to achieve desired results; do not discontinue without consulting prescriber. For orally-disintegrating tablets, remove from foil blister by peeling back (do not push tablet through the foil). Place tablet in mouth immediately upon removal. Tablet dissolves rapidly in saliva and may be swallowed with or without liquid. Avoid alcohol or caffeine and other prescription or OTC medications not approved by prescriber. Maintain adequate hydration (2-3 L/day of fluids) unless advised by prescriber to restrict fluids. You may experience excess drowsiness, restlessness, dizziness, or blurred vision (use caution driving or when engaging in tasks requiring alertness until response to drug is known); or constipation (increased exercise, fluids, fruit, or fiber may help). Report persistent CNS effects (eg, trembling fingers, altered gait or balance, excessive sedation, seizures, unusual movements, anxiety, abnormal thoughts, confusion, personality changes); unresolved constipation or GI effects; vision changes; difficulty breathing; unusual cough or flu-like symptoms; or worsening of condition. **Pregnancy/breast-feeding precautions:** Inform prescriber if you are or intend to become pregnant. Do not breast-feed.

Dietary Issues: Zyprexa® Zydis®: 5 mg tablet contains phenylalanine 0.34 mg; 10 mg tablet contains phenylalanine 0.45 mg; 15 mg tablet contains phenylalanine 0.67 mg; 20 mg tablet contains phenylalanine 0.9 mg

Geriatric Considerations: (See Warnings/Precautions, Adverse Reactions, and Overdose/Toxicology.) Elderly patients have an increased risk of adverse response to side effects or adverse reactions to antipsychotics.

Related Information

Antipsychotic Agents *on page 1558*
Antipsychotic Medication Guidelines *on page 1614*

Olmesartan (ole me SAR tan)

U.S. Brand Names Benicar™

Synonyms Olmesartan Medoxomil

Generic Available No

Pharmacologic Category Angiotensin II Receptor Blocker

Pregnancy Risk Factor C/D (2nd and 3rd trimesters)

Lactation Excretion in breast milk unknown/contraindicated

Use Treatment of hypertension with or without concurrent use of other antihypertensive agents

Mechanism of Action/Effect As a selective and competitive, nonpeptide angiotensin II receptor antagonist, olmesartan blocks the vasoconstrictor and aldosterone-secreting effects of angiotensin II. Olmesartan increases urinary flow rate and in addition to being natriuretic and kaliuretic, increases excretion of chloride, magnesium, uric acid, calcium, and phosphate.

Contraindications Hypersensitivity to olmesartan or any component of the formulation; hypersensitivity to other A-II receptor antagonists; primary hyperaldosteronism; bilateral renal artery stenosis; pregnancy (2nd and 3rd trimesters)

Warnings/Precautions Avoid use or use a smaller dose in patients who are volume depleted; correct depletion first. Deterioration in renal function can occur with initiation. Use with caution in unilateral renal artery stenosis and pre-existing renal insufficiency; significant aortic/mitral stenosis. Safety and efficacy in pediatric patients have not been established. Pregnancy risk C/D (2nd and 3rd trimesters).

Drug Interactions

Decreased Effect: NSAIDs may decrease the efficacy of olmesartan.

Increased Effect/Toxicity: The risk of hyperkalemia may be increased during concomitant use with potassium-sparing diuretics, potassium supplements, and trimethoprim; may increase risk of lithium toxicity.

Nutritional/Ethanol Interactions

Food: Does not affect olmesartan bioavailability.

Herb/Nutraceutical: Avoid ephedra, yohimbe, ginseng (may worsen hypertension). Avoid garlic (may have increased antihypertensive effect).

Adverse Reactions

1% to 10%:

Central nervous system: Dizziness (3%), headache
Endocrine & metabolic: Hyperglycemia, hypertriglyceridemia
Gastrointestinal: Diarrhea
Neuromuscular & skeletal: Back pain, CPK increased
Renal: Hematuria
Respiratory: Bronchitis, pharyngitis, rhinitis, sinusitis, upper respiratory tract infection
Miscellaneous: Flu-like syndrome

<1% (Limited to important or life-threatening): Abdominal pain, arthralgia, arthritis, bilirubin increased, chest pain, dyspepsia, facial edema, fatigue, gastroenteritis, hypercholesterolemia, hyperlipidemia, hyperuricemia, insomnia, liver enzymes increased, myalgia, nausea, pain, peripheral edema, rash, skeletal pain, tachycardia, urinary tract infection, vertigo

Overdosage/Toxicology Hypotension and tachycardia may occur with significant overdose. Bradycardia is possible if vagal stimulation occurs. Treatment should be supportive.

Pharmacodynamics/Kinetics

Bioavailability: 26%

Half-Life Elimination: Terminal: 13 hours

Time to Peak: 1-2 hours

Metabolism: Olmesartan medoxomil is hydrolyzed in the GI tract to active olmesartan. No further metabolism occurs.

Formulations Tablet, film coated, as medoxomil: 5 mg, 20 mg, 40 mg

Dosing

Adults & Elderly: Antihypertensive: Oral: Initial: Usual starting dose is 20 mg once daily; if initial response is inadequate, may be increased to 40 mg once daily after 2 weeks. May administer with other antihypertensive agents if blood pressure inadequately controlled with olmesartan. Consider lower starting dose in patients with possible depletion of intravascular volume (eg, patients receiving diuretics).

Renal Impairment: No specific guidelines for dosage adjustment; patients undergoing hemodialysis have not been studied.

Hepatic Impairment: No adjustment necessary.

Administration

Oral: May be administered with or without food.

Stability

Storage: Store at 20°C to 25°C (68°F to 77°F).

Monitoring and Teaching Issues

Physical Assessment: See Contraindications, Warnings/Precautions, and Dosing for use cautions. Assess potential for interactions with other prescriptions, OTC medications, or herbal products patient may be taking (see Drug Interactions). Assess result of laboratory tests (see Monitoring Laboratory Tests), therapeutic effects, and adverse response (see Adverse Reactions and Overdose/Toxicology) on a regular basis throughout therapy. Instruct diabetic patients to monitor glucose levels closely (may cause hyperglycemia). Teach patient proper use, possible side effects and interventions, and adverse symptoms to report (see Patient Education). **Pregnancy risk factor C/D** - instruct female patients on appropriate barrier contraceptive measures. Breast-feeding is contraindicated.

Patient Education: Inform prescriber of all prescriptions, OTC medications, or herbal products you are taking, and any allergies you have. Do not take anything new during treatment unless approved by prescriber. Take exactly as directed. Do not alter dose or discontinue without consulting prescriber. May be taken with or without food. This drug

(Continued)

Olmesartan *(Continued)*

does not eliminate the need for diet or exercise regimen as recommended by prescriber. If diabetic, check glucose levels closely (drug may alter glucose levels). You may experience headache or dizziness (use caution when driving or engaging in tasks that require alertness until response to drug is known); diarrhea (boiled milk, buttermilk, or yogurt may help); or back or joint pain (consult prescriber for approved analgesic). Report chest pain or palpitations; unrelieved headache; flu-like symptoms or upper respiratory infection; or other persistent adverse reactions. **Pregnancy/breast-feeding precautions:** Inform prescriber if you are or intend to become pregnant. This drug should not be used in the 2nd or 3rd trimester of pregnancy. Consult prescriber for appropriate contraceptive measures if necessary. Consult prescriber if breast-feeding.

Dietary Issues: May be taken with or without food.

Olmesartan Medoxomil *see* Olmesartan *on page 997*

Olopatadine *see page 1509*

Olsalazine (ole SAL a zeen)

U.S. Brand Names Dipentum®

Synonyms Olsalazine Sodium

Generic Available No

Pharmacologic Category 5-Aminosalicylic Acid Derivative

Pregnancy Risk Factor C

Lactation Enters breast milk/use caution (monitor for diarrhea)

Use Maintenance of remission of ulcerative colitis in patients intolerant to sulfasalazine

Mechanism of Action/Effect The mechanism of action appears to be localized in the colon rather than systemic

Contraindications Hypersensitivity to olsalazine, salicylates, or any component of the formulation

Warnings/Precautions Diarrhea is a common adverse effect of olsalazine. Use with caution in patients with hypersensitivity to salicylates, sulfasalazine, or mesalamine. Pregnancy risk C.

Drug Interactions

Increased Effect/Toxicity: Olsalazine has been reported to increase the prothrombin time in patients taking warfarin. Olsalazine may increase the risk of myelosuppression with azathioprine, mesalamine, or sulfasalazine.

Effects on Lab Values ↑ ALT, AST (S)

Adverse Reactions

>10%: Gastrointestinal: Diarrhea, cramps, abdominal pain

1% to 10%:

Central nervous system: Headache, fatigue, depression

Dermatologic: Rash, itching

Gastrointestinal: Nausea, heartburn, bloating, anorexia

Neuromuscular & skeletal: Arthralgia

<1% (Limited to important or life-threatening): Blood dyscrasias, cholestatic jaundice, cirrhosis, hepatic necrosis, hepatitis, jaundice, Kawasaki-like syndrome

Overdosage/Toxicology Symptoms of overdose include decreased motor activity and diarrhea. Treatment is supportive.

Pharmacodynamics/Kinetics

Absorption: <3%; very little intact olsalazine is systemically absorbed

Half-Life Elimination: 56 minutes

Time to Peak: ~1 hour

Metabolism: Primarily via colonic bacteria to active drug, 5-aminosalicylic acid

Formulations Capsule, as sodium: 250 mg

Dosing

Adults & Elderly: Ulcerative colitis: Oral: 1 g/day in 2 divided doses

Administration

Oral: Take with food in evenly divided doses.

Monitoring and Teaching Issues

Physical Assessment: Assess allergy history before initiating therapy. See Contraindications, Warnings/Precautions, and Drug Interactions for use cautions. Assess therapeutic effectiveness and adverse effects (see Adverse Reactions and Overdose/Toxicology). Teach patient appropriate use (according to formulation), possible side effects and interventions, and adverse symptoms to report (see Patient Education). **Pregnancy risk factor C** - benefits of use should outweigh possible risks. Note breast-feeding caution.

Patient Education: Inform prescriber of all prescriptions, OTC medications, or herbal products you are taking, and any allergies you have. Do not take anything new during treatment unless approved by prescriber. Take as directed, with meals, in evenly divided doses. May cause flu-like symptoms or muscle pain (consult prescriber for approved analgesic); diarrhea (buttermilk, boiled milk, or yogurt may help); or nausea or loss of appetite (small, frequent meals, frequent mouth care, sucking lozenges, or chewing gum may help). Report persistent diarrhea or abdominal cramping, skin rash or itching, or other adverse reactions. **Pregnancy/breast-feeding precautions:** Inform prescriber if you are or intend to become pregnant. Consult prescriber if breast-feeding.

Dietary Issues: Administer with food, increases residence of drug in body.

Geriatric Considerations: No specific data is available on elderly to suggest the drug needs alterations in dose. Since so little is absorbed, dosing should not be changed for reasons of age. Diarrhea may pose a serious problem for elderly in that it may cause dehydration, electrolyte imbalance, hypotension, and confusion.

Olsalazine Sodium *see* Olsalazine *on page 998*

Olux™ *see* Topical Corticosteroids *on page 1334*

Omeprazole (oh ME pray zol)

U.S. Brand Names Prilosec®

Generic Available No

Pharmacologic Category Proton Pump Inhibitor

Pregnancy Risk Factor C

Lactation Excretion in breast milk unknown/use caution

Use Short-term (4-8 weeks) treatment of active duodenal ulcer disease or active benign gastric ulcer; treatment of heartburn and other symptoms associated with gastroesophageal reflux disease (GERD); short-term (4-8 weeks) treatment of endoscopically-diagnosed erosive esophagitis; maintenance healing of erosive esophagitis; long-term treatment of pathological hypersecretory conditions; as part of a multidrug regimen for *H. pylori* eradication to reduce the risk of duodenal ulcer recurrence

Use - Unlabeled/Investigational Healing NSAID-induced ulcers; prevention of NSAID-induced ulcers

Mechanism of Action/Effect Suppresses gastric acid secretion by inhibiting the parietal cell H+/K+ ATP pump

Contraindications Hypersensitivity to omeprazole or any component of the formulation

Warnings/Precautions In long-term (2-year) studies in rats, omeprazole produced a dose-related increase in gastric carcinoid tumors. While available endoscopic evaluations and histologic examinations of biopsy specimens from human stomachs have not detected a risk from short-term exposure to omeprazole, further human data on the effect of sustained hypochlorhydria and hypergastrinemia is needed to rule out the possibility of an increased risk for the development of tumors in humans receiving long-term therapy. Bioavailability may be increased in the elderly. Safety and efficacy have not been established in children <2 years of age. Pregnancy risk C.

Drug Interactions

Cytochrome P450 Effect: Substrate of CYP2A6, 2C8/9, **2C19**, 2D6, 3A4; Inhibits CYP2C8/9, **2C19**, 2D6, **3A4**; Induces CYP1A2

Decreased Effect: The clinical effect of ketoconazole, itraconazole, and other drugs dependent upon acid for absorption is reduced; voriconazole not affected. Theophylline clearance is increased slightly.

Increased Effect/Toxicity: Omeprazole may increase the half-life of diazepam, digoxin, phenytoin, warfarin, and other drugs metabolized by the liver. Voriconazole may significantly increase serum levels of omeprazole (for omeprazole dosages >40 mg/day, reduce omeprazole dose by 50%). Serum levels of other proton pump inhibitors may also be increased.

Nutritional/Ethanol Interactions

Ethanol: Avoid ethanol (may cause gastric mucosal irritation).

Food: Food delays absorption.

Herb/Nutraceutical: St John's wort may decrease omeprazole levels.

Adverse Reactions

1% to 10%:

Central nervous system: Headache (7%), dizziness (2%)

Dermatologic: Rash (2%)

Gastrointestinal: Diarrhea (3%), abdominal pain (2%), nausea (2%), vomiting (2%), constipation (1%)

Neuromuscular & skeletal: Weakness (1%), back pain (1%)

Respiratory: Upper respiratory infection (2%), cough (1%)

<1% (Limited to important or life-threatening): Agranulocytosis, alopecia, angina, angioedema, atrophic gastritis, erythema multiforme, esophageal candidiasis, gynecomastia, hallucinations, hemifacial dysesthesia, hemolytic anemia, hepatic encephalopathy, hepatic failure, hepatic necrosis, hyponatremia, interstitial nephritis, jaundice, leukocytosis, mucosal atrophy (tongue), neutropenia, pancreatitis, pancytopenia, paresthesia, psychic disturbance, somnolence, Stevens-Johnson syndrome, thrombocytopenia, toxic epidermal necrolysis, urticaria, vertigo

Overdosage/Toxicology Limited experience with overdose in humans. Symptoms include confusion, drowsiness, blurred vision, tachycardia, nausea, flushing, diaphoresis, headache, dry mouth. Treatment is symptom-directed and supportive.

Pharmacodynamics/Kinetics

Half-Life Elimination: 0.5-1 hour

Metabolism: Extensively hepatic

Onset: Antisecretory: ~1 hour; Peak effect: 2 hours

Duration: 72 hours

Formulations Capsule, delayed release: 10 mg, 20 mg, 40 mg

Dosing

Adults & Elderly:

Active duodenal ulcer: Oral: 20 mg/day for 4-8 weeks

Gastric ulcers: Oral: 40 mg/day for 4-8 weeks

Symptomatic GERD: Oral: 20 mg/day for up to 4 weeks

Erosive esophagitis: Oral: 20 mg/day for 4-8 weeks

Helicobacter pylori eradication: Oral: Dose varies with regimen: 20 mg once daily **or** 40 mg/day as single dose or in 2 divided doses; requires combination therapy with antibiotics

Pathological hypersecretory conditions: Oral: Initial: 60 mg once daily; doses up to 120 mg 3 times/day have been administered; administer daily doses >80 mg in divided doses

Pediatrics: GERD or other acid-related disorders: Oral: Children ≥2 years:

<20 kg: 10 mg once daily

≥20 kg: 20 mg once daily

Renal Impairment: No adjustment is necessary.

Hepatic Impairment: No adjustment necessary.

Administration

Oral: Capsule should be swallowed whole. Do not chew, crush, or open. May be opened and contents added to applesauce. Administration via NG tube should be in an acidic juice.

(Continued)

Omeprazole *(Continued)*

Other: The manufacturer recommends the use of an acidic juice for preparation to administer via nasogastric (NG) tube. Alternative methods have been described as follows. NG tube administration for the prevention of stress-related mucosal damage in ventilated, critically-ill patients. The manufacturer makes no judgment regarding the safety or efficacy of these practices.

The contents of one or two 20 mg omeprazole capsules were poured into a syringe; 10-20 mL of an 8.4% sodium bicarbonate solution was withdrawn in the syringe; 30 minutes were allowed for the enteric-coated omeprazole granules to break down. The resulting milky substance was shaken prior to administration. The NG tube was then flushed with 5-10 mL of water then clamped for at least 1 hour. Patients received omeprazole 40 mg once, then 40 mg 6-8 hours later, then 20 mg once daily using this technique.

Another study used a different technique. The omeprazole capsule (20 mg or 40 mg) was opened; then the intact granules were poured into a container holding 30 mL of water. With the plunger removed, $^1/_3$ to $^1/_2$ of the granules were then poured into a 30 mL syringe which was attached to a nasogastric tube (NG). The plunger was replaced with 1 cm of air between the granules and the plunger top while the plunger was depressed. This process was repeated until all the granules were flushed, then a final 15 mL of water was flushed through the tube. Patients who received omeprazole 40 mg in this manner had a more predictable increase in intragastric pH than patients who received omeprazole 20 mg.

Stability

Storage: Omeprazole stability is a function of pH; it is rapidly degraded in acidic media, but has acceptable stability under alkaline conditions. Prilosec® is supplied as capsules for oral administration; each capsule contains omeprazole in the form of enteric coated granules to inhibit omeprazole degradation by gastric acidity; therefore, the manufacturer recommends against extemporaneously preparing it in an oral liquid form for administration via an NG tube.

Monitoring and Teaching Issues

Physical Assessment: Assess other medications patient may be taking for effectiveness and interactions (especially those dependent on cytochrome P450 metabolism or those dependent on a acid environment for absorption - see Drug Interactions). See Contraindications and Warnings/Precautions for use cautions. Monitor effectiveness of therapeutic response and adverse reactions at beginning of therapy and periodically throughout therapy (see Adverse Reactions and Overdose/Toxicology). Assess knowledge/teach appropriate use of this medication, interventions to reduce side effects, and adverse symptoms to report (see Patient Education). **Pregnancy risk factor C** - benefits of use should outweigh possible risks. Note breast-feeding caution.

Patient Education: Take as directed, before eating. Do not crush or chew capsules. Capsule may be opened and contents added to applesauce. Avoid alcohol. You may experience anorexia; small, frequent meals may help to maintain adequate nutrition. Report changes in urination or pain on urination, unresolved severe diarrhea, testicular pain, or changes in respiratory status. **Pregnancy/breast-feeding precautions:** Inform prescriber if you are or intend to become pregnant. Inform prescriber if breast-feeding.

Dietary Issues: Should be taken on an empty stomach.

Geriatric Considerations: The incidence of side effects in the elderly is no different than that of younger adults (≤65 years) despite slight decrease in elimination and increase in bioavailability. Bioavailability may be increased in the elderly (≥65 years of age), however, dosage adjustments are not necessary.

Related Information

Helicobacter pylori Treatment *on page 1676*

Omnicef® *see* Cefdinir *on page 235*

Oncaspar® *see* Pegaspargase *on page 1040*

Oncovin® [DSC] *see* VinCRIStine *on page 1401*

Ondansetron (on DAN se tron)

U.S. Brand Names Zofran®; Zofran® ODT

Synonyms Ondansetron Hydrochloride

Generic Available No

Pharmacologic Category Selective 5-HT_3 Receptor Antagonist

Pregnancy Risk Factor B

Lactation Excretion in breast milk unknown/opportunity for use is minimal

Use Prevention of nausea and vomiting associated with moderately to highly emetogenic cancer chemotherapy; radiotherapy in patients receiving total body irradiation or fractions to the abdomen; postoperatively, when nausea and vomiting should be avoided

Use - Unlabeled/Investigational Treatment of early-onset alcoholism

Mechanism of Action/Effect Selective 5-HT_3 receptor antagonist, blocking serotonin, both peripherally on vagal nerve terminals and centrally in the chemoreceptor trigger zone

Contraindications Hypersensitivity to ondansetron, other selective 5-HT_3 antagonists, or any component of the formulation

Warnings/Precautions Ondansetron should be used on a scheduled basis, not on an "as needed" (PRN) basis, since data supports the use of this drug in the prevention of nausea and vomiting and not in the rescue of nausea and vomiting. Ondansetron should only be used in the first 24-48 hours of receiving chemotherapy. Data does not support any increased efficacy of ondansetron in delayed nausea and vomiting. Does not stimulate gastric or intestinal peristalsis; may mask progressive ileus and/or gastric distension. Orally-disintegrating tablets contain phenylalanine.

Drug Interactions

Cytochrome P450 Effect: Substrate of CYP1A2, 2C8/9, 2D6, 2E1, **3A4**; Inhibits CYP1A2, 2C8/9, 2D6

Decreased Effect: Decreased effect: CYP1A2, 2D6, 2E1, and 3A4 enzyme inducers (eg, barbiturates, carbamazepine, rifampin, phenytoin, and phenylbutazone) may change the clearance of ondansetron; monitor

Increased Effect/Toxicity: Increased toxicity: CYP1A2, 2D6, 2E1, and 3A4 enzyme inhibitors (eg, cimetidine, allopurinol, and disulfiram) may change the clearance of ondansetron; monitor

Nutritional/Ethanol Interactions

Food: Food increases the extent of absorption. The C_{max} and T_{max} do not change much.

Herb/Nutraceutical: St John's wort may decrease ondansetron levels.

Adverse Reactions

>10%:

Cardiovascular: Malaise/fatigue (9% to 13%)

Central nervous system: Headache (9% to 27%)

1% to 10%:

Central nervous system: Drowsiness (8%), fever (2% to 8%), dizziness (4% to 7%), anxiety (6%), cold sensation (2%)

Dermatologic: Pruritus (2% to 5%), rash (1%)

Gastrointestinal: Constipation (6% to 9%), diarrhea (3% to 7%)

Genitourinary: Gynecological disorder (7%), urinary retention (5%)

Hepatic: Increased ALT/AST (1% to 2%)

Local: Injection site reaction (4%)

Neuromuscular & skeletal: Paresthesia (2%)

Respiratory: Hypoxia (9%)

<1% (Limited to important or life-threatening): Angioedema, anaphylaxis, angina, bronchospasm, cardiopulmonary arrest, dyspnea, dystonic reactions, EKG changes, extrapyramidal reactions, grand mal seizures, hiccups, hypersensitivity reactions, hypokalemia, hypotension, laryngeal edema, laryngospasm, oculogyric crisis, shock, stridor, tachycardia, vascular occlusive events

Overdosage/Toxicology Sudden transient blindness, severe constipation, hypotension, and vasovagal episode with transient secondary heart block have been reported in some cases of overdose. I.V. doses of up to 252 mg/day have been inadvertently given without adverse effects. There is no specific antidote. Treatment is symptom-directed and supportive.

Pharmacodynamics/Kinetics

Bioavailability: Oral: 56%

Half-Life Elimination: Children <15 years: 2-3 hours; Adults: 3-6 hours

Time to Peak: Oral: ~2 hours

Metabolism: Extensively hepatic via hydroxylation, followed by glucuronide or sulfate conjugation; CYP1A2, CYP2D6, and CYP3A4 substrate

Onset: ~30 minutes

Formulations

Injection, solution, as hydrochloride (Zofran®): 2 mg/mL (2 mL, 20 mL)

Infusion, as hydrochloride [premixed in D_5W] (Zofran®): 32 mg (50 mL)

Solution, as hydrochloride (Zofran®): 4 mg/5 mL (50 mL) [contains sodium benzoate; strawberry flavor]

Tablet, as hydrochloride (Zofran®): 4 mg, 8 mg, 24 mg

Tablet, orally-disintegrating (Zofran® ODT): 4 mg, 8 mg [each strength contains phenylalanine <0.03 mg/tablet; strawberry flavor]

Dosing

Adults & Elderly:

Chemotherapy-induced emesis:

I.V.: Administer either three 0.15 mg/kg doses or a single 32 mg dose:

Three-dose regimen: Initial dose is given 30 minutes prior to chemotherapy with subsequent doses administered 4 and 8 hours after the first dose

Single-dose regimen: 32 mg is infused over 15 minutes beginning 30 minutes before the start of emetogenic chemotherapy

Highly-emetogenic agents/single-day therapy: Oral: 24 mg given 30 minutes prior to the start of therapy

Moderately-emetogenic agents: Oral: 8 mg every 8 hours for 2 doses beginning 30 minutes before chemotherapy, then 8 mg every 12 hours for 1-2 days after chemotherapy completed

Total body irradiation: Oral: 8 mg 1-2 hours before each fraction of radiotherapy administered each day

Single high-dose fraction radiotherapy to abdomen: Oral: 8 mg 1-2 hours before irradiation, then 8 mg every 8 hours after first dose for 1-2 days after completion of radiotherapy

Daily fractionated radiotherapy to abdomen: Oral: 8 mg 1-2 hours before irradiation, then 8 mg every 8 hours after first dose for each day of radiotherapy

Postoperative nausea and vomiting:

Oral: 16 mg given one hour prior to induction of anesthesia

I.M., I.V.: 4 mg as a single dose immediately before induction of anesthesia, or shortly following procedure if vomiting occurs

Pediatrics:

Chemotherapy-induced emesis:

I.V.: Children 4-18 years: 0.15 mg/kg/dose administered 30 minutes prior to chemotherapy, 4 and 8 hours after the first dose

Oral:

4-11 years: 4 mg 30 minutes before chemotherapy; repeat 4 and 8 hours after initial dose, then 4 mg every 8 hours for 1-2 days after chemotherapy completed

≥12 years: Refer to adult dosing.

Postoperative nausea and vomiting: I.V.: Children 2-12 years:

≤40 kg: 0.1 mg/kg; >40 kg: 4 mg

Renal Impairment: No adjustment is necessary.

Hepatic Impairment: Maximum daily dose: 8 mg in patients with severe liver disease (Child-Pugh score ≥10)

(Continued)

Ondansetron *(Continued)*

Administration

Oral: Oral dosage forms should be given 30 minutes prior to chemotherapy; 1-2 hours before radiotherapy; 1 hour prior to the induction of anesthesia

Orally-disintegrating tablets: Do not remove from blister until needed. Peel backing off the blister, do not push tablet through. Using dry hands, place tablet on tongue and allow to dissolve. Swallow with saliva.

The I.V. preparation has been successful when administered orally.

I.M.: Should be given undiluted

I.V.: Give first dose 30 minutes prior to beginning chemotherapy; the I.V. preparation has been successful when administered orally

I.V. push: Inject over 2-5 minutes

IVPB: Infuse over 15 minutes

Stability

Storage:

Oral solution: Store between 15°C and 30°C (59°F and 86°F); protect from light

Tablet: Store between 2°C and 30°C (36°F and 86°F)

Vial: Store between 2°C and 30°C (36°F and 86°F); protect from light

Reconstitution: Stable when mixed in 5% dextrose or 0.9% sodium chloride for 48 hours at room temperature. Does not need protection from light.

Compatibility: Stable in $D_5{}^1/_2NS$, D_5NS, D_5W, mannitol 10%, LR, NS, NS 3%; do not mix injection with alkaline solutions

Y-site administration: Incompatible with acyclovir, allopurinol, aminophylline, amphotericin B, amphotericin B cholesteryl sulfate complex, ampicillin, ampicillin/sulbactam, amsacrine, cefepime, cefoperazone, furosemide, ganciclovir, lorazepam, methylprednisolone sodium succinate, piperacillin, sargramostim, sodium bicarbonate

Monitoring and Teaching Issues

Physical Assessment: See Contraindications, Warnings/Precautions, and Dosing for use cautions. Assess potential for interactions with other prescriptions, OTC medications, or herbal products patient may be taking (see extensive list of Drug Interactions). See Administration specifics. Assess therapeutic effectiveness and adverse effects (see Adverse Reactions and Overdose/Toxicology). Teach patient appropriate use (according to formulation), possible side effects and interventions, and adverse symptoms to report (see Patient Education).

Patient Education: Inform prescriber of all prescriptions, OTC medications, or herbal products you are taking, and any allergies you have. Do not take anything new during treatment unless approved by prescriber. If self-administered, take as directed. May cause drowsiness or dizziness (use caution when driving or engaging in tasks that require alertness until response to drug is known): or fatigue, diarrhea, constipation, or headache (request appropriate treatment from prescriber). Do not change position rapidly (rise slowly). Report persistent headache, excessive drowsiness, fever, numbness or tingling, or changes in elimination patterns (constipation or diarrhea); or chest pain or palpitations.

Orally-disintegrating tablets: Do not remove from blister until needed. Peel backing off the blister, do not push tablet through. Using dry hands, place tablet on tongue and allow to dissolve. Swallow with saliva. Contains <0.03 mg phenylalanine/tablet.

Dietary Issues: Take without regard to meals.

Potassium: Hypokalemia; monitor potassium serum concentration

Orally-disintegrating tablet contains <0.03 mg phenylalanine

Geriatric Considerations: Elderly have a slightly decreased hepatic clearance rate. This does not, however, require a dose adjustment.

Related Information

Antiemetics for Chemotherapy-Induced Nausea and Vomiting *on page 1639*

Ondansetron Hydrochloride *see* Ondansetron *on page 1000*

ONTAK® *see* Denileukin Diftitox *on page 375*

Onxol™ *see* Paclitaxel *on page 1025*

OPC13013 *see* Cilostazol *on page 288*

Opcon® *see page 1509*

o,p′-DDD *see* Mitotane *on page 915*

Ophthalmic Agents *see page 1509*

Ophthalmic Agents, Glaucoma (op THAL mik AY gents, glaw COE ma)

U.S. Brand Names AKBeta®; AKPro®; Alphagan® [DSC]; Alphagan® P; Azopt™; Betagan® Liquifilm®; Betaxon®; Betoptic® S; Carbastat®; Carboptic®; Epifrin®, Glaucon®; Epinal®; Humorsol®; Iopidine®; Isopto® Carbachol; Isopto® Carpine; Kerlone®: Lumigan™; Miostat® Intraocular; Ocupress® Ophthalmic; Ocusert Pilo-20® [DSC]; Ocusert Pilo-40® [DSC]; OptiPranolol®; Phospholine Iodide®; Pilocar®; Pilopine HS®; Piloptic®; Propine®; Timoptic®; Timoptic® OcuDose®; Timoptic-XE®; Travatan™ Trusopt®; Xalatan®; Zaditor™

Synonyms Apraclonidine; Betaxolol; Bimatoprost; Brimonidine; Brinzolamide; Carbachol; Carteolol; Demecarium; Dipivefrin; Dorzolamide; Echothiophate; Epinephrine; Eserine Sulfate; Ketotifen; Latanoprost; Levobetaxolol; Levobunolol; Metipranolol; Physostigmine; Pilocarpine; Timolol; Travoprost

Pharmacologic Category Ophthalmic Agent

Pregnancy Risk Factor C/B (sympathomimetics)

Use Lowering intraocular pressure in patients with chronic, open-angle glaucoma or ocular hypertension

Mechanism of Action/Effect

Direct-acting cholinergic agents: Direct-acting cholinergic stimulation resulting in increased outflow of aqueous humor, and possibly some decrease in production. These effects decrease intraocular pressure.

Acetylcholinesterase inhibitors: Inhibition of acetylcholinesterase increases the persistence of local acetylcholine concentrations, resulting in cholinergic effects. These effects include an increase in the outflow of aqueous humor, reducing intraocular pressure.

Sympathomimetics: Stimulate alpha- or beta-adrenoreceptors to increase outflow of aqueous humor, reducing intraocular pressure.

Carbonic anhydrase inhibitors: Inhibition of carbonic anhydrase decreases production of aqueous humor secretion and results in a reduction in intraocular pressure.

Beta-blockers: Lowers intraocular pressure by reducing production of aqueous humor and possibly increases outflow of aqueous humor.

Prostaglandins and/or prostinoid agonists: Increase outflow of aqueous humor.

Contraindications Hypersensitivity to the individual drug or any component; individual formulations may contain sulfites or benzalkonium chloride

Direct-acting cholinergic agents and acetylcholinesterase inhibitors: Acute inflammatory disease of the anterior chamber, acute iritis

Sympathomimetics: Angle-closure glaucoma

Beta-blockers: Second and third degree A-V block, severe asthma, severe congestive heart failure, cardiogenic shock, severe COPD

Prostaglandins and/or prostinoid agonists: Pregnancy

Warnings/Precautions Systemic absorption may lead to hypersensitivity reactions and/or systemic effects. Do not administer while wearing contact lenses.

Direct-acting cholinergic agents and acetylcholinesterase inhibitors: Use with caution in the presence of corneal abrasion or in patients undergoing general anesthesia, peptic ulcer, narrow-angle glaucoma, Parkinson's disease, or urinary tract obstruction.

Sympathomimetics: Use with caution in patients with hypertension, dysrhythmias, or cardiac disease. Dipivefrin contains sodium metabisulfite.

Carbonic anhydrase inhibitors: Use with caution in renal or hepatic impairment (agents and metabolites may accumulate), sulfonamide allergy (due to cross-reactivity). Use with oral carbonic anhydrase inhibitors is not recommended. Dorzolamide contains benzalkonium chloride.

Beta-blockers: Use with caution in patients with congestive heart failure, asthma, diabetes mellitus, heart block, bradycardia, thyroid disease, or peripheral vascular disease. Travaprost may permanently change/increase brown pigmentation of the iris, the eyelid skin, and eyelashes. In addition, may increase the length and/or number of eyelashes (may vary between eyes); changes occur slowly and may not be noticeable for months or years. Bacterial keratitis, caused by inadvertent contamination of multiple-dose ophthalmic solutions, has been reported. Use caution in patients with intraocular inflammation, aphakic patients, pseudophakic patients with a torn posterior lens capsule, or patients with risk factors for macular edema. Contains benzalkonium chloride which may be adsorbed by contact lenses; remove contacts prior to administration and wait 15 minutes before reinserting. Contact with contents of vial should be avoided in women who are pregnant or attempting to become pregnant; in case of accidental exposure to the skin, wash the exposed area with soap and water immediately. Safety and efficacy have not been determined for use in patients with renal or hepatic impairment, angle-closure-, inflammatory-, or neovascular glaucoma. Safety and efficacy in pediatric patients have not been established.

Prostaglandins and/or prostinoid agonists: May permanently change/increase brown pigmentation of the iris, the eyelid skin, and eyelashes. In addition, may increase the length and/or number of eyelashes (may vary between eyes); changes occur slowly and may not be noticeable for months or years. Bacterial keratitis, caused by inadvertent contamination of multiple-dose ophthalmic solutions, has been reported. Use caution in patients with intraocular inflammation, aphakic patients, pseudophakic patients with a torn posterior lens capsule, or patients with risk factors for macular edema. Some products may contain benzalkonium chloride which may be adsorbed by contact lenses; remove contacts prior to administration and wait 15 minutes before reinserting. Contact with contents of vial should be avoided in women who are pregnant or attempting to become pregnant; in case of accidental exposure to the skin, wash the exposed area with soap and water immediately.

Adverse Reactions Representative profiles of adverse effects are listed by pharmacologic category. Consult complete product prescribing information for individual products.

Direct-acting cholinergic agents and acetylcholinesterase inhibitors:

>10%:
- Ocular: Blurred vision

1% to 10%:
- Central nervous system: Headache
- Genitourinary: Polyuria
- Ocular: Burning, stinging, ciliary spasm, retinal detachment, photophobia, acute iritis, lacrimation, conjunctival and ciliary congestion (early in therapy)

<1% (limited to important or life-threatening symptoms): Hypertension, tachycardia, nausea, vomiting, diarrhea, salivation, diaphoresis

Sympathomimetic agents:

>10%:
- Central nervous system: Headache, fatigue, drowsiness
- Gastrointestinal: Dry mouth
- Ocular: Burning, stinging, ocular hyperemia, blurring, ocular allergic reactions, ocular pruritus

1% to 10%:
- Central nervous system: Dizziness
- Gastrointestinal: Taste disturbances
- Ocular: Blepharitis, ocular irritation, corneal staining, photophobia, eyelid erythema, eyelid edema, ocular pain, ocular dryness, tearing, abnormal vision, lid crusting, conjunctival hemorrhage, ocular discharge, bulbar conjunctival follicles
- Respiratory: Upper respiratory symptoms

<1% (limited to important or life-threatening symptoms): Allergic reactions, diarrhea, tachycardia, hypotension, arrhythmias

(Continued)

Ophthalmic Agents, Glaucoma *(Continued)*

Carbonic anhydrase inhibitors:

1% to 10%:

Gastrointestinal: Bitter taste

Ocular: Burning, stinging, discomfort, blurred vision, tearing, dryness, photophobia, superficial punctate, keratitis, ocular allergic irritation

<1% (limited to important or life-threatening symptoms): Headache, fatigue, rash, nausea, urolithiasis, weakness, iridocyclitis, electrolyte disturbance

Beta-blockers:

>10%: Ocular: Burning, stinging

1% to 10%:

Cardiovascular: Bradycardia, arrhythmia, hypotension

Central nervous system: Dizziness, headache

Dermatologic: Alopecia, erythema

Ocular: Blepharoconjunctivitis, conjunctivitis

Respiratory: Bronchospasm

<1% (limited to important or life-threatening symptoms): Rash, pruritus, visual disturbances, keratitis

Prostaglandins and/or prostinoid agonists:

>10%: Ocular: Hyperemia

1% to 10%:

Cardiovascular: Angina, bradycardia

Central nervous system: Headache, depression

Ocular: Iris discoloration, keratitis, pigmentation of periocular skin (eyelid), visual disturbance, elongation of eyelashes

Respiratory: Sinusitis, bronchitis

<1% (limited to important or life-threatening symptoms): Bacterial conjunctivitis (due to solution contamination)

Pharmacodynamics/Kinetics

Absorption: Most agents are absorbed into the systemic circulation, however, detailed absorption characteristics and pharmacokinetic data are unavailable (see Warnings/Precautions and Drug Interactions).

Half-Life Elimination:

Betaxolol: 12-22 hours (after oral administration)

Carteolol: 6 hours (after oral administration)

Dorzolamide: Terminal RBC half-life of 147 days

Latanoprost: 17 minutes

Levobetaxolol: 20 hours

Metipranolol: ~3 hours

Physostigmine: 15-40 minutes

Timolol: 2-2.7 hours; prolonged with reduced renal function

Onset:

Apraclonidine: Ophthalmic: 1 hour; maximum IOP: 3-5 hours

Betaxolol: Ophthalmic: 30 minutes

Bimatoprost: Onset 4 hours; max effect: 8-12 hours

Brimonidine: 1-4 hours

Carbachol: Ophthalmic instillation: Onset of miosis: 10-20 minutes; Intraocular administration: Onset of miosis: Within 2-5 minutes

Dipivefrin: Ocular pressure effect: Within 30 minutes; Mydriasis: May occur within 30 minutes

Dorzolamide: Peak effect: 2 hours

Echothiophate: Miosis: 10-30 minutes; Intraocular pressure decrease: 4-8 hours; Peak intraocular pressure decrease: 24 hours

Epinephrine: Conjunctival instillation: Intraocular pressure falls within 1 hour; Peak effect: Within 4-8 hours

Ketotifen: Within minutes

Latanoprost: 3-4 hours; Maximum effect: 8-12 hours

Levobunolol: Decrease in intraocular pressure (IOP) can be noted within 1 hour; Peak effect: 2-6 hours

Metipranolol: ≤30 minutes; Maximum effect: ~2 hours

Pilocarpine:

Ophthalmic instillation: Miosis: Within 10-30 minutes; Intraocular pressure reduction: 1 hour required

Physostigmine: Within 2 minutes

Travoprost: Onset 2 hours; maximal effect after 12 hours

Duration:

Betaxolol: 12 hours

Brimonidine: 12 hours

Brinzolamide: 8-12 hours

Carbachol: Duration of reduction in intraocular pressure: 4-8 hours; Intraocular administration: 24 hours

Carteolol: 12 hours

Dipivefrin: Ocular pressure effect: ≥12 hours; Mydriasis: Several hours

Dorzolamide: 8-12 hours

Echothiophate: Up to 1-4 weeks

Epinephrine: Conjunctival instillation: Duration of ocular effect: 12-24 hours

Ketotifen: 8-12 hours

Levobunolol: 1-7 days

Metipranolol: Intraocular pressure reduction has persisted for 24 hours following ocular instillation.

Pilocarpine:

Ophthalmic instillation: Miosis: 4-8 hours; Intraocular pressure reduction: 4-12 hours

Physostigmine: 12-48 hours

Timolol: ~4 hours; intraocular effects persist for 24 hours after ophthalmic instillation

Formulations

Apraclonidine: Solution, ophthalmic, as hydrochloride: 0.5% (5 mL); 1% (0.1 mL)

Betaxolol:

Solution, ophthalmic, as hydrochloride: 0.5% (5 mL, 10 mL, 15 mL) [contains benzalkonium chloride]

Suspension, ophthalmic, as hydrochloride (Betoptic® S): 0.25% (2.5 mL, 10 mL, 15 mL) [contains benzalkonium chloride]

Bimatoprost: Solution, ophthalmic: 0.03% (2.5 mL, 5 mL) [contains benzalkonium chloride]

Brimonidine: Solution, ophthalmic, as tartrate: Alphagan® [DSC]: 0.2% (5 mL, 10 mL, 15 mL) [contains benzalkonium chloride]; Alphagan® P: 0.15% (5 mL, 10 mL, 15 mL) [contains Purite® 0.005% as preservative]

Brinzolamide: Suspension, ophthalmic: 1% (5 mL, 10 mL, 15 mL) [contains benzalkonium chloride]

Carbachol:

Solution, intraocular (Carbastat®, Miostat®): 0.01% (1.5 mL)

Solution, ophthalmic: Carboptic®: 3% (15 mL); Isopto® Carbachol: 0.75% (15 mL, 30 mL); 1.5% (15 mL, 30 mL); 2.25% (15 mL); 3% (15 mL, 30 mL)

Carteolol: Solution, ophthalmic, as hydrochloride (Ocupress®): 1% (5 mL, 10 mL)

Demecarium: Solution, ophthalmic, as bromide: 0.125% (5 mL); 0.25% (5 mL)

Dipivefrin: Solution, ophthalmic, as hydrochloride: 0.1% (5 mL, 10 mL, 15 mL)

Dorzolamide: Solution, ophthalmic, as hydrochloride: 2%

Echothiophate: Powder, ophthalmic: 1.5 mg [0.03%] (5 mL); 3 mg [0.06%] (5 mL); 6.25 mg [0.125%] (5 mL); 12.5 mg [0.25%] (5 mL)

Epinephrine:

Solution, ophthalmic, as borate (Epinal®): 0.5% (7.5 mL); 1% (7.5 mL)

Solution, ophthalmic, as hydrochloride (Epifrin®, Glaucon®): 0.1% (1 mL); 0.5% (15 mL); 1% (10 mL, 15 mL); 2% (10 mL, 15 mL)

Ketotifen: Solution, ophthalmic, as fumarate: 0.025% (5 mL) [contains benzalkonium chloride]

Latanoprost: Solution, ophthalmic: 0.005% (2.5 mL)

Levobetaxolol: Solution, ophthalmic: 0.05% (5 mL, 10 mL, 15 mL)

Levobunolol: Solution, ophthalmic, as hydrochloride: 0.25% (5 mL, 10 mL, 15 mL); 0.5% (2 mL, 5 mL, 10 mL, 15 mL)

Metipranolol: Solution, ophthalmic, as hydrochloride: 0.3% (5 mL, 10 mL)

Physostigmine: Ointment, ophthalmic, as sulfate: 0.25% (3.5 g, 3.7 g)

Pilocarpine:

Gel, ophthalmic, as hydrochloride (Pilopine HS®): 4% (3.5 g) [contains benzalkonium chloride]

Ocular therapeutic system: Ocusert Pilo-2-® [DSC]: Releases 20 mcg/hour for 1 week (8s); Ocusert Pilo-40® [DSC]: Releases 40 mcg/hour for 1 week (8s)

Solution, ophthalmic, as hydrochloride: 1% (15 mL), 2% (15 mL), 4% (15 mL), 6% (15 mL) [may contain benzalkonium chloride]

Isopto® Carpine: 1% (15 mL); 2% (15 mL, 30 mL); 4% (15 mL, 30 mL); 6% (15 mL); 8% (15 mL) [contains benzalkonium chloride]

Pilocar®: 0.5% (15 mL); 1% (1 mL, 15 mL); 2% (1 mL, 15 mL); 3% (15 mL); 4% (1 mL, 15 mL); 6% (15 mL) [contains benzalkonium chloride]

Piloptic®: 0.5% (15 mL); 1% (15 mL); 2% (15 mL); 3% (15 mL); 4% (15 mL); 6% (15 mL) [contains benzalkonium chloride]

Timolol:

Gel-forming solution, ophthalmic, as maleate (Timoptic-XE®): 0.25% (2.5 mL, 5 mL); 0.5% (2.5 mL, 5 mL)

Solution, ophthalmic, as hemihydrate (Betimol®): 0.25% (5 mL, 10 mL, 15 mL); 0.5% (5 mL, 10 mL, 15 mL) [contains benzalkonium chloride]

Solution, ophthalmic, as maleate: 0.25% (5 mL, 10 mL, 15 mL); 0.5% (5 mL, 10 mL, 15 mL) [contains benzalkonium chloride]

Timoptic®: 0.25% (5 mL, 10 mL); 0.5% (5 mL, 10 mL) [contains benzalkonium chloride]

Solution, ophthalmic, as maleate [preservative free] (Timoptic® OcuDose®): 0.25% (0.2 mL);0.5% (0.2 mL) [single use]

Travoprost: Solution, ophthalmic: 0.004% (2.5 mL) [contains benzalkonium chloride]

Dosing

Adults:

Apraclonidine: Instill 1 drop in operative eye 1 hour prior to laser surgery, second drop in eye upon completion of procedure.

Bimatoprost: Instill 1 into affected eyes once daily (in evening).

Betaxolol: Instill 1 drop twice daily.

Brimonidine: Instill 1 drop in affected eye(s) 3 times/day (approximately every 8 hours).

Brinzolamide: Instill 1 drop in affected eye(s) 3 times/day.

Carbachol:

Ophthalmic: Instill 1-2 drops up to 3 times/day.

Intraocular: Instill 0.5 mL into anterior chamber before or after securing sutures.

Carteolol: Instill 1 drop in affected eye(s) twice daily.

Demecarium:

Glaucoma: Instill 1 drop into eyes twice weekly to a maximum dosage of 1 or 2 drops twice daily for up to 4 months.

Strabismus:

Diagnosis: Instill 1 drop daily for 2 weeks, then 1 drop every 2 days for 2-3 weeks. If eyes become straighter, an accommodative factor is demonstrated.

Therapy: Instill not more than 1 drop at a time in both eyes every day for 2-3 weeks. Then reduce dosage to 1 drop every other day for 3-4 weeks and re-evaluate. Continue at 1 drop every 2 days to 1 drop twice a week and evaluate the patient's condition every 4-12 weeks. If improvement continues, reduce dose to 1 drop once a week and eventually stop medication. Discontinue therapy after 4 months if control of the condition still requires 1 drop every 2 days.

Dipivefrin: Instill 1 drop every 12 hours into the eyes.

Dorzolamide: Glaucoma: Instill 1 drop in the affected eye(s) 3 times/day.

(Continued)

Ophthalmic Agents, Glaucoma *(Continued)*

Echothiophate:

Glaucoma: Instill 1 drop twice daily into eyes with 1 dose just prior to bedtime. Some patients have been treated with 1 dose/day or every other day

Accommodative esotropia:

Diagnosis: Instill 1 drop of 0.125% once daily into both eyes at bedtime for 2-3 weeks.

Treatment: Use lowest concentration and frequency which gives satisfactory response, with a maximum dose of 0.125% once daily, although more intensive therapy may be used for short periods of time.

Epinephrine: Instill 1-2 drops in eye(s) once or twice daily.

Ketotifen: Instill 1 drop in the affected eye(s) every 8-12 hours.

Latanoprost: Instill 1 drop in the affected eye(s) once daily in the evening.

Levobetaxolol: Instill 1 drop in the affected eye(s) twice daily.

Levobunolol: Instill 1 drop in the affected eye(s) 1-2 times/day.

Metipranolol: Instill 1 drop in the affected eye(s) twice daily.

Physostigmine:

Ointment (eserine sulfate): Instill a small quantity to lower fornix up to 3 times/day.

Solution (Isopto® Eserine): Instill 1-2 drops into eye(s) up to 4 times/day.

Pilocarpine:

Nitrate solution: Shake well before using; instill 1-2 drops 2-4 times/day.

Hydrochloride solution:

Instill 1-2 drops up to 6 times/day; adjust the concentration and frequency as required to control elevated intraocular pressure.

To counteract the mydriatic effects of sympathomimetic agents: Instill 1 drop of a 1% solution in the affected eye.

Gel: Instill 0.5" ribbon into lower conjunctival sac once daily at bedtime.

Timolol: Initial: 0.25% solution, instill 1 drop twice daily; increase to 0.5% solution if response not adequate; decrease to 1 drop/day if controlled; do not exceed 1 drop twice daily of 0.5% solution.

Travoprost: Instill 1 into affected eyes once daily (in evening).

Elderly: Refer to adult dosing and Special Geriatric Considerations.

Administration

Other: After instillation, apply finger pressure over nasolacrimal duct to decrease systemic absorption.

Stability

Storage: Store solutions at room temperature. Refrigerate pilocarpine gel.

Monitoring and Teaching Issues

Physical Assessment: See Drug Interactions, Contraindications, and Warnings/Precautions for use cautions. Monitor therapeutic effectiveness (ie, periodic intraocular pressure, fundoscopic exam, or visual field testing) at regular intervals with long-term therapy. Assess knowledge/teach patient appropriate use, interventions to reduce side effects, and adverse symptoms to report (see Adverse Reactions, Overdose/Toxicology, and Patient Education). **Pregnancy risk factor C/B** - benefits of use should outweigh possible risks.

Patient Education: For ophthalmic use only. Apply prescribed amount as often as directed. Wash hands before using and do not touch tip of applicator to eye or contaminate tip of applicator. Tilt head back and look upward. Gently pull down lower lid and put drop(s) inside lower eyelid at inner corner. Close eye and roll eyeball in all directions. Do not blink for 1/2 minute. Apply gentle pressure to inner corner of eye for 30 seconds. Wipe away excess from skin around eye. Do not use any other eye preparation for at least 10 minutes. Do not share medication with anyone else. Temporary stinging or blurred vision may occur. Immediately report any adverse cardiac or CNS effects (usually signifies overdose). Report persistent eye pain, redness, burning, watering, dryness, double vision, puffiness around eye, vision disturbances, other adverse eye response, or worsening of condition or lack of improvement. **Pregnancy/breast-feeding precautions:** Inform prescriber if you are or intend to become pregnant.

Geriatric Considerations: Because systemic absorption does occur with ophthalmic administration, the elderly with other disease states or syndromes that may be affected by an individual agent (cholinergic drugs with Parkinson's, beta-blockers in bradycardia, CHF, COPD, etc) should be monitored closely.

Related Information

Glaucoma Drug Comparison *on page 1575*

Ophthetic® *see page 1461*

Opium and Belladonna *see* Belladonna and Opium *on page 151*

Opium Tincture (OH pee um TING chur)

Synonyms DTO; Opium Tincture, Deodorized

Restrictions C-II

Generic Available Yes

Pharmacologic Category Analgesic, Narcotic; Antidiarrheal

Pregnancy Risk Factor B/D (prolonged use or high doses at term)

Lactation Enters breast milk/use caution

Use Treatment of diarrhea or relief of pain

Mechanism of Action/Effect Contains many narcotic alkaloids including morphine; its mechanism for gastric motility inhibition is primarily due to this morphine content; it results in a decrease in digestive secretions, an increase in GI muscle tone, and therefore a reduction in GI propulsion

Contraindications Hypersensitivity to morphine sulfate or any component of the formulation; increased intracranial pressure; severe respiratory depression; severe hepatic or renal insufficiency; pregnancy (prolonged use or high dosages near term)

Warnings/Precautions Opium shares the toxic potential of opiate agonists, and usual precautions of opiate agonist therapy should be observed; some preparations contain sulfites which may cause allergic reactions; infants <3 months of age are more susceptible to respiratory depression, use with caution and generally in reduced doses in this age group; this is **not** paregoric, dose accordingly

Drug Interactions

Increased Effect/Toxicity: Opium tincture and CNS depressants, MAO inhibitors, tricyclic antidepressants may potentiate the effects of opiate agonists (eg, codeine, morphine, etc). Dextroamphetamine may enhance the analgesic effect of opiate agonists.

Nutritional/Ethanol Interactions Ethanol: Avoid ethanol (may increase CNS depression).

Effects on Lab Values ↑ aminotransferase [ALT (SGPT)/AST (SGOT)] (S)

Adverse Reactions Frequency not defined.

Cardiovascular: Palpitations, hypotension, bradycardia, peripheral vasodilation,

Central nervous system: Drowsiness, dizziness, restlessness, headache, malaise, CNS depression, increased intracranial pressure, insomnia, mental depression

Gastrointestinal: Nausea, vomiting, constipation, anorexia, stomach cramps, biliary tract spasm

Genitourinary: Decreased urination, urinary tract spasm

Neuromuscular & skeletal: Weakness

Ocular: Miosis

Respiratory: Respiratory depression

Miscellaneous: Histamine release, physical and psychological dependence

Overdosage/Toxicology Primary attention should be directed to ensuring adequate respiratory exchange. Naloxone, 2 mg I.V. with repeat administration as necessary up to a total of 10 mg, can also be used to reverse toxic effects of the opiate.

Pharmacodynamics/Kinetics

Absorption: Variable

Metabolism: Hepatic

Duration: 4-5 hours

Formulations Liquid: 10% (120 mL, 480 mL) [0.6 mL equivalent to morphine 6 mg; contains alcohol 19%]

Dosing

Adults & Elderly:

Diarrhea: Oral: 0.3-1 mL/dose every 2-6 hours to maximum of 6 mL/24 hours

Analgesia: Oral: 0.6-1.5 mL/dose every 3-4 hours

Pediatrics:

Diarrhea: Oral: Children: 0.005-0.01 mL/kg/dose every 3-4 hours for a maximum of 6 doses/24 hours

Analgesia: Oral: Children: 0.01-0.02 mL/kg/dose every 3-4 hours

Stability

Storage: Protect from light

Monitoring and Teaching Issues

Physical Assessment: Assess other medications patient may be taking for additive or adverse interactions (see Drug Interactions). Monitor vital signs, effectiveness of pain relief, adverse reactions, and signs of overdose (see above) at beginning of therapy and at regular intervals with long-term use. May cause physical and/or psychological dependence. For inpatients, implement safety measures. Assess knowledge/teach patient appropriate use (if self-administered). Teach patient to monitor for adverse reactions (see Adverse Reactions), adverse reactions to report, and appropriate interventions to reduce side effects (see Patient Education). Discontinue slowly after prolonged use. **Pregnancy risk factor B/D** - see Pregnancy Risk Factor for use cautions. Note breast-feeding caution.

Patient Education: If self-administered, use exactly as directed; do not increase dose or frequency. Drug may cause physical and/or psychological dependence. While using this medication, do not use alcohol and other prescription or OTC medications (especially sedatives, tranquilizers, antihistamines, or pain medications) without consulting prescriber. Maintain adequate hydration (2-3 L/day of fluids) May cause hypotension, dizziness, drowsiness, impaired coordination, or blurred vision (use caution when driving, climbing stairs, or changing position - rising from sitting or lying to standing, or when engaging in tasks requiring alertness until response to drug is known); or dry mouth (frequent mouth care, small, frequent meals, chewing gum, or sucking lozenges may help). Report slow or rapid heartbeat, acute dizziness, or persistent headache; changes in mental status; swelling of extremities or unusual weight gain; changes in urinary elimination or pain on urination; acute headache; trembling or muscle spasms; blurred vision; skin rash; or shortness of breath. **Pregnancy/breast-feeding precautions:** Inform prescriber if you are or intend to become pregnant. If you are breast-feeding, take medication immediately after breast-feeding or 3-4 hours prior to next feeding.

Opium Tincture, Deodorized *see* Opium Tincture *on page 1006*

Opticrom® *see page 1509*

Opticrom® *see* Cromolyn Sodium *on page 334*

Opticyl® *see page 1509*

Opticyl® *see page 1461*

Optigene® Tetrasine® Extra *see page 1509*

Optimine® *see* Azatadine *on page 137*

OptiPranolol® *see* Ophthalmic Agents, Glaucoma *on page 1002*

Orabase®-B [OTC] *see* Benzocaine *on page 156*

Orabase® HCA *see* Topical Corticosteroids *on page 1334*

Oracit® *see* Sodium Citrate and Citric Acid *on page 1236*

Orajel® [OTC] *see* Benzocaine *on page 156*

Orajel® Baby [OTC] *see* Benzocaine *on page 156*

Orajel® Baby Nighttime [OTC] *see* Benzocaine *on page 156*

Orajel® Maximum Strength [OTC] *see* Benzocaine *on page 156*

Oramorph SR® *see* Morphine Sulfate *on page 926*

Orap™ *see* Pimozide *on page 1085*

Orapred® *see* PrednisoLONE *on page 1113*

Orasol® [OTC] *see* Benzocaine *on page 156*

Orasone® *see* PredniSONE *on page 1115*

Orazinc® [OTC] *see* Zinc Supplements *on page 1423*

Oretic® *see* Hydrochlorothiazide *on page 664*

Oreton® Methyl *see* MethylTESTOSTERone *on page 887*

ORG 946 *see* Rocuronium *on page 1203*

Organidin® NR *see* Guaifenesin *on page 646*

Orgaran® [DSC] *see* Danaparoid *on page 359*

ORG NC 45 *see* Vecuronium *on page 1393*

Orlistat (OR li stat)

U.S. Brand Names Xenical®

Generic Available No

Pharmacologic Category Lipase Inhibitor

Pregnancy Risk Factor B

Lactation Excretion in breast milk unknown/not recommended

Use Management of obesity, including weight loss and weight management when used in conjunction with a reduced-calorie diet; reduce the risk of weight regain after prior weight loss; indicated for obese patients with an initial body mass index (BMI) ≥30 kg/m^2 or ≥27 kg/m^2 in the presence of other risk factors

Mechanism of Action/Effect Inhibits gastric and pancreatic lipases, thus inhibiting the absorption of dietary fats (by 30% at doses of 120 mg 3 times/day)

Contraindications Hypersensitivity to orlistat or any component of the formulation; chronic malabsorption syndrome or cholestasis

Warnings/Precautions Patients should be advised to adhere to dietary guidelines; gastrointestinal adverse events may increase if taken with a diet high in fat (>30% total daily calories from fat). The daily intake of fat should be distributed over three main meals. If taken with any one meal very high in fat, the possibility of gastrointestinal effects increases. Patients should be counseled to take a multivitamin supplement that contains fat-soluble vitamins to ensure adequate nutrition because orlistat has been shown to reduce the absorption of some fat-soluble vitamins and beta-carotene. The supplement should be taken once daily at least 2 hours before or after the administration of orlistat (ie, bedtime). Some patients may develop increased levels of urinary oxalate following treatment; caution should be exercised when prescribing it to patients with a history of hyperoxaluria or calcium oxalate nephrolithiasis. As with any weight-loss agent, the potential exists for misuse in appropriate patient populations (eg, patients with anorexia nervosa or bulimia). **Note:** Dispensing errors have been made between Xenical® (orlistat) and Xeloda® (capecitabine).

Drug Interactions

Decreased Effect: Vitamin K absorption may be decreased when taken with orlistat. Coadministration with cyclosporine may decrease plasma levels of cyclosporine.

Adverse Reactions

>10%

Central nervous system: Headache (31%)

Gastrointestinal: Oily spotting (27%), abdominal pain/discomfort (26%), flatus with discharge (24%), fatty/oily stool (20%), fecal urgency (22%), oily evacuation (12%), increased defecation (11%)

Neuromuscular & skeletal: Back pain (14%)

Respiratory: Upper respiratory infection (38%)

1% to 10%

Central nervous system: Fatigue (7%), anxiety (5%), sleep disorder (4%)

Dermatologic: Dry skin (2%)

Endocrine & metabolic: Menstrual irregularities (10%)

Gastrointestinal: Fecal incontinence (8%), nausea (8%), infectious diarrhea (5%), rectal pain/discomfort (5%), vomiting (4%)

Neuromuscular & skeletal: Arthritis (5%), myalgia (4%)

Otic: Otitis (4%)

<1% (Limited to important or life-threatening): Allergic reactions, anaphylaxis, angioedema, pruritus, rash, urticaria

Overdosage/Toxicology Single doses of 800 mg and multiple doses of up to 400 mg 3 times daily for 15 days have been studied in normal weight and obese patients without significant adverse findings. In case of significant overdose, it is recommended that the patient be observed for 24 hours.

Formulations Capsule: 120 mg

Dosing

Adults & Elderly: Obesity: Oral: 120 mg 3 times daily with each main meal containing fat (during or up to 1 hour after the meal); omit dose if meal is occasionally missed or contains no fat. **Note:** A once-daily multivitamin containing the fat-soluble vitamins (A, D, E, and K) should be administered at least 2 hours prior to orlistat.

Monitoring Laboratory Tests Changes in coagulation parameters

Monitoring and Teaching Issues

Physical Assessment: Assess effectiveness of other medications patient may be taking (especially anticoagulants - see Drug Interactions). Monitor effectiveness of therapy, laboratory results, and adverse reactions at beginning of therapy and periodically during therapy (see Adverse Reactions). Assess knowledge/teach patient appropriate use, possible side effects and interventions, and adverse symptoms to report (see Patient Education). Breast-feeding is not recommended.

Patient Education: Take this medication exactly as ordered; do not alter prescribed dose without consulting prescriber. Maintain prescribed diet (high-fat meals may result in GI distress), exercise regimen, and vitamin supplements as prescribed. You may experience dizziness or lightheadedness (use caution when driving or engaging in tasks requiring alertness until response to drug is known) or increased flatus and fecal urgency (this may lessen with continued use). Report persistent back, muscle, or joint pain; signs of respiratory tract infection or flu-like symptoms; skin rash or irritation; or other reactions. **Breast-feeding precaution:** Breast-feeding is not recommended.

Pregnancy Issues: There are no adequate and well-controlled studies of orlistat in pregnant women. Because animal reproductive studies are not always predictive of human response, orlistat is not recommended for use during pregnancy. Teratogenicity studies were conducted in rats and rabbits at doses up to 800 mg/kg/day. Neither study showed embryotoxicity or teratogenicity. This dose is 23 and 47 times the daily human dose calculated on a body surface area basis for rats and rabbits, respectively.

Related Information

Obesity Treatment Guidelines for Adults *on page 1693*

Orphenadrine (or FEN a dreen)

U.S. Brand Names Norflex™

Synonyms Orphenadrine Citrate

Generic Available Yes

Pharmacologic Category Anti-Parkinson's Agent, Anticholinergic; Skeletal Muscle Relaxant

Pregnancy Risk Factor C

Lactation Excretion in breast milk unknown

Use Treatment of muscle spasm associated with acute painful musculoskeletal conditions; supportive therapy in tetanus

Mechanism of Action/Effect Indirect skeletal muscle relaxant thought to work by central atropine-like effects; has some euphorogenic and analgesic properties

Contraindications Hypersensitivity to orphenadrine or any component of the formulation; glaucoma; GI obstruction; cardiospasm; myasthenia gravis

Warnings/Precautions Use with caution in patients with CHF or cardiac arrhythmias. Some products contain sulfites. Pregnancy risk C.

Drug Interactions

Cytochrome P450 Effect: Substrate of CYP1A2, 2B6, 2D6, 3A4; Inhibits CYP1A2, 2A6, 2B6, 2C8/9, 2C19, 2D6, 2E1, **3A4**

Increased Effect/Toxicity: Orphenadrine may increase potential for anticholinergic adverse effects of anticholinergic agents; includes drugs with high anticholinergic activity (diphenhydramine, TCAs, phenothiazines). Sedative effects of may be additive in concurrent use of orphenadrine and CNS depressants (monitor). Effects of levodopa may be decreased by orphenadrine. Monitor.

Nutritional/Ethanol Interactions

Ethanol: Avoid ethanol (may increase CNS depression).

Herb/Nutraceutical: St John's wort may decrease orphenadrine levels. Avoid valerian, St John's wort, kava kava, gotu kola (may increase CNS depression).

Adverse Reactions

>10%:

Central nervous system: Drowsiness, dizziness

Ocular: Blurred vision

1% to 10%:

Cardiovascular: Flushing of face, tachycardia, syncope

Dermatologic: Rash

Gastrointestinal: Nausea, vomiting, constipation

Genitourinary: Decreased urination

Neuromuscular & skeletal: Weakness

Ocular: Nystagmus, increased intraocular pressure

Respiratory: Nasal congestion

<1% (Limited to important or life-threatening): Aplastic anemia, hallucinations

Overdosage/Toxicology Symptoms of overdose include blurred vision, tachycardia, confusion, seizures, respiratory arrest, and dysrhythmias. There is no specific treatment for antihistamine overdose. Clinical toxicity is due to blockade of cholinergic receptors. Lethal dose is 2-3 g; treatment is generally symptomatic. For anticholinergic overdose with severe life-threatening symptoms, physostigmine 1-2 mg I.V. slowly, may be given to reverse these effects.

Pharmacodynamics/Kinetics

Half-Life Elimination: 14-16 hours

Metabolism: Extensively hepatic

Onset: Peak effect: Oral: Within 2-4 hours

Duration: 4-6 hours

Formulations

Injection, solution, as citrate: 30 mg/mL (2 mL) [contains sodium bisulfite]

Tablet, extended release, as citrate: 100 mg

Dosing

Adults: Muscle spasms:

Oral: 100 mg twice daily

I.M., I.V.: 60 mg every 12 hours

Elderly: Not recommended for use in the elderly (see Geriatric Considerations).

Administration

Oral: Do not crush sustained release drug product.

Monitoring and Teaching Issues

Physical Assessment: See Warnings/Precautions and Contraindications for use cautions. Monitor effectiveness of therapy (according to rational for therapy), and adverse reactions (see Adverse Reactions) at beginning of therapy and periodically with long-term use. Do not discontinue abruptly; taper dosage slowly. Assess knowledge/teach patient appropriate use, interventions to reduce side effects, and adverse symptoms to report (see Patient Education). **Pregnancy risk factor C** - benefits of use should outweigh possible risks. Note breast-feeding caution.

(Continued)

Orphenadrine *(Continued)*

Patient Education: Take exactly as directed. Do not increase dose or discontinue without consulting prescriber. Do not chew or crush sustained release tablets. Do not use alcohol, prescriptive or OTC antidepressants, sedatives, or pain medications without consulting prescriber. You may experience drowsiness, dizziness, lightheadedness (avoid driving or engaging in tasks requiring alertness until response to drug is known); nausea or vomiting (small, frequent meals, frequent mouth care, or sucking hard candy may help); constipation (increased exercise, fluids, fruit, or fibers may help); or decreased urination (void before taking medication). Report excessive drowsiness or mental agitation, chest pain, skin rash, swelling of mouth/face, difficulty speaking, or vision changes. **Pregnancy/breast-feeding precautions:** Inform prescriber if you are or intend to become pregnant. Consult prescriber if breast-feeding.

Geriatric Considerations: Because of its anticholinergic side effects, orphenadrine is not a drug of choice in the elderly.

Orphenadrine, Aspirin, and Caffeine

(or FEN a dreen, AS pir in, & KAF een)

U.S. Brand Names Norgesic™; Norgesic™ Forte; Orphengesic; Orphengesic Forte

Synonyms Aspirin, Orphenadrine, and Caffeine; Caffeine, Orphenadrine, and Aspirin

Generic Available Yes

Pharmacologic Category Skeletal Muscle Relaxant

Pregnancy Risk Factor D

Lactation Enters breast milk/use caution due to aspirin content

Use Relief of discomfort associated with skeletal muscular conditions

Formulations

Tablet: Orphenadrine citrate 25 mg, aspirin 385 mg, and caffeine 30 mg; orphenadrine citrate 50 mg, aspirin 770 mg, and caffeine 60 mg

Norgesic™, Orphengesic: Orphenadrine citrate 25 mg, aspirin 385 mg, and caffeine 30 mg

Norgesic™ Forte, Orphengesic Forte: Orphenadrine citrate 50 mg, aspirin 770 mg, and caffeine 60 mg

Dosing

Adults: Muscular pain/spasms: Oral: 1-2 tablets 3-4 times/day

Elderly: Not recommended for use in the elderly; see individual agents

Monitoring and Teaching Issues

Physical Assessment: See individual components listed in Related Information. **Pregnancy risk factor D** - determine that patient is not pregnant before beginning treatment. Instruct patients of childbearing age about appropriate barrier contraceptive measures. Note breast-feeding caution.

Patient Education: See individual components listed in Related Information. **Pregnancy/breast-feeding precautions:** Inform prescriber if you are or intend to become pregnant. Consult prescriber if breast-feeding.

Related Information

Aspirin *on page 121*
Orphenadrine *on page 1009*

Orphenadrine Citrate *see* Orphenadrine *on page 1009*
Orphengesic *see* Orphenadrine, Aspirin, and Caffeine *on page 1010*
Orphengesic Forte *see* Orphenadrine, Aspirin, and Caffeine *on page 1010*
Ortho-Cept® *see* Ethinyl Estradiol and Desogestrel *on page 516*
Orthoclone OKT® 3 *see* Muromonab-CD3 *on page 932*
Ortho-Cyclen® *see* Ethinyl Estradiol and Norgestimate *on page 530*
Ortho-Novum® *see* Ethinyl Estradiol and Norethindrone *on page 527*
Ortho-Novum® 1/50 *see* Mestranol and Norethindrone *on page 863*
Ortho Tri-Cyclen® *see* Ethinyl Estradiol and Norgestimate *on page 530*
Ortho Tri-Cyclen® Lo *see* Ethinyl Estradiol and Norgestimate *on page 530*
Orudis® [DSC] *see* Ketoprofen *on page 759*
Orudis® KT [OTC] *see* Ketoprofen *on page 759*
Oruvail® *see* Ketoprofen *on page 759*
Os-Cal® 500 [OTC] *see* Calcium Supplements *on page 202*

Oseltamivir (o sel TAM e veer)

U.S. Brand Names Tamiflu®

Generic Available No

Pharmacologic Category Antiviral Agent; Neuraminidase Inhibitor

Pregnancy Risk Factor C

Lactation Excretion in breast milk unknown/not recommended

Use Treatment of uncomplicated acute illness due to influenza (A or B) infection in adults and children >1 year of age who have been symptomatic for no more than 2 days; prophylaxis against influenza (A or B) infection in adults and adolescents ≥13 years of age

Mechanism of Action/Effect Thought to inhibit influenza virus by altering virus particle aggregation and release

Contraindications Hypersensitivity to oseltamivir or any component of the formulation

Warnings/Precautions Oseltamivir is not a substitute for the flu shot. Dosage adjustment is required for creatinine clearance between 10-30 mL/minute. Safety and efficacy in children (<18 years) have not been established for treatment regimens. Safety and efficacy have not been established for prophylactic use in patients <13 years of age. Also consider primary or concomitant bacterial infections. Safety and efficacy for treatment or prophylaxis in immunocompromised patients have not been established. Pregnancy risk C.

Drug Interactions

Increased Effect/Toxicity: Cimetidine and amoxicillin have no effect on plasma concentrations. Probenecid increases oseltamivir carboxylate serum concentration by twofold. Dosage adjustments are not required.

Adverse Reactions

As seen with **treatment** doses: 1% to 10%:

Central nervous system: Insomnia (adults 1%), vertigo (1%)

Gastrointestinal: Nausea (10%), vomiting (9%)

Similar adverse effects were seen in **prophylactic** use, however, the incidence was generally less. The following reactions were seen more commonly with prophylactic use: Headache (20%), fatigue (8%), cough (6%), diarrhea (3%)

<1% (Limited to important or life-threatening): Aggravation of diabetes, arrhythmia, confusion, hepatitis, pseudomembranous colitis, pyrexia, rash, seizure, swelling of face or tongue, toxic epidermal necrolysis, unstable angina,

Overdosage/Toxicology Single doses of 1000 mg resulted in nausea and vomiting.

Pharmacodynamics/Kinetics

Absorption: Well absorbed

Bioavailability: 75% reaches systemic circulation in active form

Half-Life Elimination: Oseltamivir carboxylate: 6-10 hours; similar in geriatrics (68-78 years)

Time to Peak: C_{max}: Oseltamivir: 65 ng/mL; Oseltamivir carboxylate: 348 ng/mL

Metabolism: Hepatic (90%) to oseltamivir carboxylate; neither the parent drug nor active metabolite has any effect on CYP.

Formulations

Capsule, as phosphate: 75 mg

Powder for oral suspension: 12 mg/mL (25 mL) [contains sodium benzoate; tutti-frutti flavor]

Dosing

Adults & Elderly:

Influenza treatment: Oral: 75 mg twice daily initiated within 2 days of onset of symptoms; duration of treatment: 5 days

Influenza prophylaxis: Oral: 75 mg once daily for at least 7 days; treatment should begin within 2 days of contact with an infected individual. During community outbreaks, dosing is 75 mg once daily. May be used for up to 6 weeks; duration of protection lasts for length of dosing period

Pediatrics:

Influenza treatment: Oral:

Note: Initiate treatment within 2 days of onset of symptoms; duration of treatment: 5 days:

Children: 1-12 years:

≤15 kg: 30 mg twice daily

>15 kg - ≤23 kg: 45 mg twice daily

>23 kg - ≤40 kg: 60 mg twice daily

>40 kg: 75 mg twice daily

Adolescents: Refer to adult dosing.

Influenza prophylaxis: Adolescents: Oral: 75 mg once daily for at least 7 days; treatment should begin within 2 days of contact with an infected individual. During community outbreaks, dosing is 75 mg once daily. May be used for up to 6 weeks; duration of protection lasts for length of dosing period.

Renal Impairment:

Cl_{cr} 10-30 mL/minute:

Treatment: Reduce dose to 75 mg once daily for 5 days.

Prophylaxis: Administer 75 mg every other day.

Cl_{cr} <10 mL/minute: Has not been studied.

Hepatic Impairment: Has not been evaluated

Stability

Storage: Capsules and powder for suspension: Store at 25°C (77°F). Once reconstituted, the suspension may be stored at room temperature or under refrigeration (2°C to 8°C / 36°F to 46°F); do not freeze; use within 10 days of preparation

Reconstitution: Oral suspension: Reconstitute with 23 mL of water (to make 25 mL total suspension).

Monitoring and Teaching Issues

Physical Assessment: This is **not** a substitute for the influenza vaccine. Teach patient appropriate use, interventions to reduce side effects, and adverse reactions to report (see Adverse Reactions and Patient Education). **Pregnancy risk factor C** - benefits of use should outweigh possible risks. Breast-feeding is not recommended.

Patient Education: This is not a substitute for the flu shot. Must be taken within 2 days of onset of flu symptoms (eg, fever, cough, headache, fatigue, muscular weakness, and sore throat). Take as directed; do not increase dose or frequency, and do not miss a dose. You may experience nausea or vomiting (small, frequent meals, good mouth care, chewing gum, or sucking hard candy may help). Report significant adverse effects to your prescriber. **Pregnancy/breast-feeding precautions:** Not recommended for pregnant or nursing women. Inform prescriber if you are or intend to become pregnant or are breast-feeding.

Dietary Issues: Take with or without food; take with food to improve tolerance.

Breast-feeding Issues: Oseltamivir and its metabolite are excreted in the breast milk of lactating rats. It is unknown if they appear in human milk.

Pregnancy Issues: There are insufficient human data to determine the risk to a pregnant woman or developing fetus. Studies evaluating the effects on embryo-fetal development in rats and rabbits showed a dose-dependent increase in the rates of minor skeleton abnormalities in exposed offspring. The rate of each abnormality remained within the background rate of occurrence in the species studied.

Osmitrol® *see* Mannitol *on page 835*

Osteoporosis Management *see page 1696*

Otic Agents *see page 1519*

Oticair® *see page 1519*
Otic-Care® Otic *see page 1519*
Otic Domeboro® *see page 1519*
Otobiotic® Otic *see page 1519*
Otocalm® Ear *see page 1519*
Otocalm® Ear *see page 1522*
Otocort® Otic *see page 1519*
Otosporin® Otic *see page 1519*
Ovcon® *see* Ethinyl Estradiol and Norethindrone *on page 527*
Overdose and Toxicology *see page 1617*
Ovidrel® *see* Chorionic Gonadotropin (Recombinant) *on page 285*
Ovrette® *see* Norgestrel *on page 985*

Oxaliplatin (ox AL i pla tin)

U.S. Brand Names Eloxatin™

Synonyms Diaminocyclohexane Oxalatoplatinum; L-OHP

Generic Available No

Pharmacologic Category Antineoplastic Agent, Alkylating Agent

Pregnancy Risk Factor D

Lactation Excretion in breast milk unknown/not recommended

Use Treatment of metastatic colon or rectal carcinoma, in combination with fluorouracil (5-FU) and leucovorin, in patients whose disease has recurred or progressed during or within 6 months of completing therapy with 5-FU/leucovorin and irinotecan

Use - Unlabeled/Investigational Orphan drug: Ovarian cancer

Mechanism of Action/Effect Oxaliplatin is an alkylating agent. It binds to DNA, RNA, or proteins, disrupting DNA function.

Contraindications Hypersensitivity to oxaliplatin, other platinum-containing compounds, or any component of the formulation; pregnancy

Warnings/Precautions The U.S. Food and Drug Administration (FDA) currently recommends that procedures for proper handling and disposal of antineoplastic agents be considered. Anaphylactic-like reaction may occur within minutes of oxaliplatin administration. Two different types of neuropathy may occur: 1) Acute (within first 2 days), reversible (resolves within 14 days), primarily peripheral symptoms that are often exacerbated by cold; and 2) a more persistent (>14 days) presentation that often interferes with daily activities (eg, writing, buttoning, swallowing), these symptoms may improve upon discontinuing treatment. May cause pulmonary fibrosis. Caution in renal dysfunction. Safety and efficacy in pediatric patients have not been established.

Drug Interactions

Increased Effect/Toxicity: Taxane derivatives may increase oxaliplatin toxicity if administered before the platin as a sequential infusion; nephrotoxic agents (aminoglycosides) may increase oxaliplatin toxicity

Adverse Reactions Based on clinical trial data using oxaliplatin alone. Some adverse effects may be increased when therapy is combined with 5-FU/leucovorin.

>10%:

Central nervous system: Fatigue (61%), fever (25%), pain (14%), headache (13%), insomnia (11%)
Gastrointestinal: Nausea (64%), diarrhea (46%), vomiting (37%), abdominal pain (31%), constipation (31%), anorexia (20%), stomatitis (14%)
Hematologic: Anemia (64%), thrombocytopenia (30%), leukopenia (13%)
Hepatic: SGOT increased (54%), SGPT increased (36%); total bilirubin increased (13%)
Neuromuscular & skeletal: Neuropathy, peripheral (acute 65%, persistent 43%), back pain (11%)
Respiratory: Dyspnea (13%), coughing (11%)

1% to 10%:

Cardiovascular: Edema (10%), chest pain (5%), flushing (3%), thromboembolism (2%)
Central nervous system: Rigors (9%), dizziness (7%), hand-foot syndrome (1%)
Dermatologic: Rash (5%), alopecia (3%)
Endocrine & metabolic: Dehydration (5%), hypokalemia (3%)
Gastrointestinal: Dyspepsia (7%), taste perversion (5%), flatulence (3%), mucositis (2%), gastroesophageal reflux (1%)
Genitourinary: Dysuria (1%)
Hematologic: Neutropenia (7%)
Local: Injection site reaction (9%)
Neuromuscular & skeletal: Arthralgia (7%)
Ocular: Abnormal lacrimation (1%)
Renal: Serum creatinine increased (10%)
Respiratory: URI (7%), rhinitis (6%), epistaxis (2%), pharyngitis (2%)
Miscellaneous: Allergic reactions (3%), hiccup (2%)

Postmarketing and/or case reports: Anaphylactic shock, angioedema, cranial nerve palsies, deep tendon reflex loss, deafness, decreased visual acuity, dysarthria, fasciculations, hemolytic uremia syndrome, ileus, immuno-allergic thrombocytopenia, interstitial lung diseases, intestinal obstruction, Lhermittes' sign, metabolic acidosis, optic neuritis, pancreatitis, pulmonary fibrosis, visual field disturbance

Overdosage/Toxicology Overdose symptoms are extensions of known side effects (eg, thrombocytopenia, myelosuppression, nausea, vomiting, neurotoxicity, respiratory symptoms). Treatment should be supportive.

Pharmacodynamics/Kinetics

Half-Life Elimination: Distribution: 0.4-16.8 hours; elimination: 391 hours

Metabolism: Nonenzymatic (rapid and extensive), forms active and inactive derivatives

Formulations Injection, powder for reconstitution: 50 mg, 100 mg

Dosing

Adults: I.V.: Dosed in combination with 5-FU/leucovorin on day 1 of a 2-day treatment protocol that is repeated on a 2-week cycle; premedication with antiemetics is recommended.

Day 1: 85 mg/m² oxaliplatin infused over 2 hours (administered simultaneously with leucovorin via a Y-line), followed by a 5-FU bolus and 22-hour infusion of 5-FU

Day 2: Leucovorin and 5-FU administered as on Day 1.

Dosage adjustment for toxicity: Prolongation of oxaliplatin infusion time from 2 hours to 6 hours may reduce some acute toxicities.

Persistent grade 2 neuropathy: Consider reducing dose to 65 mg/m²

Persistent grade 3 neuropathy: Consider discontinuing therapy

Patients recovering from grade 3/4 gastrointestinal or hematologic toxicity: Consider reduced dose (65 mg/m²)

Elderly: No dosing adjustment recommended.

Renal Impairment: Use with caution; specific guidelines not established.

Administration

I.V.: Administer as a diluted solution (in D_5W) over 2 hours.

Stability

Storage: Store lyophilized powder at room temperature of 25°C (77°F) and under normal lighting; excursions permitted to 15°C to 30°C (59°F to 86°F). Reconstituted solution may be stored up to 24 hours under refrigeration at 2°C to 8°C (36°F to 46°F). Diluted solution is stable up to 6 hours at room temperature of 20°C to 25°C (68°F to 77°F) or up to 24 hours under refrigeration at 2°C to 8°C (36°F to 46°F).

Reconstitution: Do not reconstitute using a chloride-containing solution (eg, NaCl). Reconstitute with water for injection USP or D_5W (10 mL for 50 mg vial, 20 mL for 100 mg vial). Further dilution with D_5W (250 or 500 mL) is required prior to administration.

Compatibility: Incompatible with alkaline solutions (eg, 5-FU) and chloride-containing solutions. Flush infusion line with D_5W prior to, and following, administration of concomitant medications via same I.V. line.

Monitoring and Teaching Issues

Physical Assessment: See Contraindications, Warnings/Precautions, and Dosing for use cautions. Assess potential for interactions with other prescriptions, OTC medications, or herbal products patient may be taking (see Drug Interactions). See I.V. Administration specifics. Patient must be observed closely for hypersensitivity reaction (which can occur within minutes of administration). Assess results of laboratory tests, therapeutic effectiveness, and adverse reactions (eg, neuropathy - see Adverse Reactions and Overdose/ Toxicology) prior to initiating therapy and on a regular basis throughout therapy. Teach patient possible side effects and interventions and adverse symptoms to report (see Patient Education). **Pregnancy risk factor D** - determine that patient is not pregnant before beginning treatment. Instruct patients of childbearing age about appropriate barrier contraceptive measures during therapy and for 1 month following therapy. Breast-feeding is not recommended.

Patient Education: Inform prescriber of all prescriptions, OTC medications, or herbal products you are taking, and any allergies you have. Do not take anything new during treatment without consulting prescriber. This medication can only be administered by infusion; you will be monitored closely during and following infusion. Report immediately any pain, burning, swelling at infusion site, or any signs of allergic reaction (eg, difficulty breathing or swallowing, back pain, chest tightness, rash, hives, swelling of lips or mouth). It is important that you maintain adequate nutrition (small, frequent meals may help) and adequate hydration (2-3 L/day of fluids) unless instructed to restrict fluid intake. You will be susceptible to infection (avoid crowds and exposure to infection and do not have any vaccinations without consulting prescriber). May cause nausea, vomiting, loss of appetite, or taste perversion (small, frequent meals, frequent mouth care, chewing gum, or sucking lozenges may help - if nausea/vomiting is unresolved, consult prescriber for approved antiemetic); mouth sores (use soft toothbrush or cotton swabs for mouth care); diarrhea (boiled milk, buttermilk, or yogurt may help); or loss of hair (reversible). Report any numbness, pain, tingling, or loss of sensation of extremities; chest pain or palpitations; swelling, pain, or hot areas in legs; unusual fatigue; unusual bruising or bleeding; difficulty breathing; muscle cramps or twitching; change in hearing acuity; or other persistent adverse effects. **Pregnancy/breast-feeding precautions:** Do not get pregnant while taking this medication; use appropriate barrier contraceptive measures. Breast-feeding is not recommended.

Oxaprozin (oks a PROE zin)

U.S. Brand Names Daypro®

Generic Available No

Pharmacologic Category Nonsteroidal Anti-inflammatory Drug (NSAID)

Pregnancy Risk Factor C/D (3rd trimester)

Lactation Excretion in breast milk unknown/not recommended

Use Acute and long-term use in the management of signs and symptoms of osteoarthritis and rheumatoid arthritis; juvenile rheumatoid arthritis

Mechanism of Action/Effect Inhibits prostaglandin synthesis by decreasing the activity of the enzyme, cyclooxygenase, which results in decreased formation of prostaglandin precursors

Contraindications Hypersensitivity to oxaprozin, aspirin, other NSAIDs, or any component of the formulation; advanced kidney disease; pregnancy (3rd trimester)

Warnings/Precautions GI toxicity (bleeding, ulceration, perforation) may occur at any time without symptoms. Use caution with history of ulcer disease, gastrointestinal bleeding, elderly, or debilitated patients; use lowest effective dose for shortest period possible. Anaphylactoid reactions have been reported with NSAID use, even without prior exposure; may be more common in patients with the aspirin triad. Use caution in patients with pre-existing asthma. Use caution with decreased renal or hepatic function, congestive heart failure, dehydration, hypertension, coagulation disorders, anticoagulants. Rare cases of severe hepatic reactions (including necrosis, jaundice, fulminant hepatitis) have been reported. Use

(Continued)

Oxaprozin *(Continued)*

of NSAIDs can compromise existing renal function especially when Cl_{cr} is <30 mL/minute; renal toxicity, renal papillary necrosis may occur. May cause mild photosensitivity reactions. Elderly are at a high risk for adverse effects from NSAIDs. As much as 60% of elderly can develop peptic ulceration and/or hemorrhage asymptomatically. Withhold for at least 4-6 half-lives prior to surgical or dental procedures. Safety and efficacy have not been established in children <6 years of age. Pregnancy risk C/D (3rd trimester).

Drug Interactions

Decreased Effect: Oxaprozin may decrease the effect of some antihypertensive agents (including ACE inhibitors and angiotensin antagonists) and diuretics.

Increased Effect/Toxicity: Oxaprozin may increase cyclosporine, digoxin, lithium, and methotrexate serum concentrations. The renal adverse effects of ACE inhibitors may be potentiated by NSAIDs. Corticosteroids may increase the risk of GI ulceration. The risk of bleeding with anticoagulants (warfarin, antiplatelet agents, low molecular weight heparins) may be increased.

Nutritional/Ethanol Interactions

Ethanol: Avoid ethanol (may enhance gastric mucosal irritation).

Herb/Nutraceutical: Avoid cat's claw, dong quai, evening primrose, feverfew, garlic, ginger, ginkgo, red clover, horse chestnut, green tea, ginseng (all have additional antiplatelet activity).

Adverse Reactions

1% to 10%:

Cardiovascular: Edema

Central nervous system: Confusion, depression, dizziness, headache, sedation, sleep disturbance, somnolence

Dermatologic: Pruritus, rash

Gastrointestinal: Abdominal distress, abdominal pain, anorexia, constipation, diarrhea, flatulence, gastrointestinal ulcer, gross bleeding with perforation, heartburn, nausea, vomiting

Hematologic: Anemia, bleeding time increased

Hepatic: Liver enzyme elevation

Otic: Tinnitus

Renal: Dysuria, renal function abnormal, urinary frequency

<1% (Limited to important or life-threatening; effects reported with oxaprozin or other NSAIDs): Acute interstitial nephritis, acute renal failure, agranulocytosis, anaphylaxis, angioedema, asthma, bruising, CHF, erythema multiforme, exfoliative dermatitis, gastritis, gastrointestinal bleeding, hearing decreased, hematemesis, hematuria, hemorrhoidal bleeding, hepatitis, hypersensitivity reaction, hypertension, jaundice, leukopenia, nephrotic syndrome, pancreatitis, peptic ulcer, photosensitivity, rectal bleeding, renal insufficiency, Stevens-Johnson syndrome, toxic epidermal necrolysis, thrombocytopenia

Overdosage/Toxicology Symptoms of overdose include acute renal failure, vomiting, drowsiness, and leukocytes. Management of NSAID intoxication is supportive and symptomatic. Since many NSAIDs undergo enterohepatic cycling, multiple doses of charcoal may be needed to reduce the potential for delayed toxicities.

Pharmacodynamics/Kinetics

Absorption: Almost complete

Half-Life Elimination: 40-50 hours

Time to Peak: 2-4 hours

Metabolism: Hepatic, forms metabolites

Onset: Steady-state 4-7 days

Formulations Tablet: 600 mg

Dosing

Adults & Elderly:

Osteoarthritis: Oral: 600-1200 mg once daily

Rheumatoid arthritis: Oral: 1200 mg once daily; a one-time loading dose of up to 1800 mg/day or 26 mg/kg (whichever is lower) may be given

Note: Maximum: 1800 mg/day or 26 mg/kg (whichever is lower) in divided doses

Pediatrics: Juvenile rheumatoid arthritis: Oral: Individualize to lowest effective dose.

Children 6-16 years:

22-31 kg: 600 mg once daily

32-54 kg: 900 mg once daily

≥55 kg: 1200 mg once daily

Renal Impairment: 600 mg once daily; dose may be increased to 1200 mg with close monitoring.

Hepatic Impairment: Use caution in patients with severe dysfunction.

Stability

Storage: Store at 25°C (77°F). Protect from light. Keep bottle tightly closed.

Monitoring Laboratory Tests CBC; hepatic, renal function

Monitoring and Teaching Issues

Physical Assessment: Assess effectiveness and interactions of other medications patient may be taking (see Contraindications and Drug Interactions). Monitor laboratory tests (see above), therapeutic response, and adverse reactions at beginning of therapy and periodically throughout therapy (see Warnings/Precautions, Adverse Reactions, and Overdose/Toxicology). Schedule ophthalmic evaluations for patients who develop eye complaints during long-term NSAID therapy. Assess knowledge/teach patient appropriate use, interventions to reduce side effects, and adverse symptoms to report (see Patient Education). **Pregnancy risk factor C/D** - see Pregnancy Risk Factor for use cautions; benefits of use should outweigh possible risks. Breast-feeding is not recommended.

Patient Education: Take this medication exactly as directed; do not increase dose without consulting prescriber. Do not crush tablets. Take with food or milk to reduce GI distress. Maintain adequate hydration (2-3 L/day of fluids) unless advised by prescriber to restrict fluids. Do not use alcohol, aspirin or aspirin-containing medication, or any other anti-inflammatory medications without consulting prescriber. You may experience drowsiness, dizziness, or nervousness (use caution when driving or engaging in tasks requiring alertness until response to drug is known); anorexia, nausea, vomiting, or heartburn (small, frequent meals, frequent mouth care, sucking lozenges, or chewing gum may help). GI bleeding, ulceration, or perforation can occur with or without pain. Discontinue medication and contact prescriber if persistent abdominal pain, cramping, or blood in stool occurs. Report vaginal bleeding; breathlessness, difficulty breathing, or unusual cough; chest pain, rapid heartbeat, palpitations; unusual bruising or bleeding (blood in urine, mouth, or vomitus); swollen extremities; skin rash or itching; acute fatigue; or swelling of face, lips, tongue, or throat. **Pregnancy/breast-feeding precautions:** Inform prescriber if you are or intend to become pregnant. This drug should not be used in the 3rd trimester of pregnancy. Breast-feeding is not recommended.

Geriatric Considerations: Elderly are at high risk for adverse effects from NSAIDs. As much as 60% of elderly can develop peptic ulceration and/or hemorrhage asymptomatically. The concomitant use of H_2 blockers, omeprazole, and sucralfate is not generally effective as prophylaxis with the exception of NSAID-induced duodenal ulcers which may be prevented by the use of ranitidine. Misoprostol is the only prophylactic agent proven effective. Also, concomitant disease and drug use contribute to the risk for GI adverse effects. Use lowest effective dose for shortest period possible. Consider renal function decline with age. Use of NSAIDs can compromise existing renal function especially when Cl_{cr} is ≤30 mL/minute. Tinnitus may be a difficult and unreliable indication of toxicity due to age-related hearing loss or eighth cranial nerve damage. CNS adverse effects such as confusion, agitation, and hallucination are generally seen in overdose or high-dose situations, but elderly may demonstrate these adverse effects at lower doses than younger adults.

Pregnancy Issues: Safety and efficacy in pregnant women have not been established. Exposure late in pregnancy may lead to premature closure of the ductus arteriosus and may inhibit uterine contractions.

Related Information

Nonsalicylate/Nonsteroidal Anti-inflammatory Comparison *on page 1587*

Oxazepam (oks A ze pam)

U.S. Brand Names Serax®

Restrictions C-IV

Generic Available Yes: Capsule

Pharmacologic Category Benzodiazepine

Pregnancy Risk Factor D

Lactation Enters breast milk/not recommended

Use Treatment of anxiety; management of ethanol withdrawal

Use - Unlabeled/Investigational Anticonvulsant in management of simple partial seizures; hypnotic

Mechanism of Action/Effect Binds to stereospecific benzodiazepine receptors on the postsynaptic GABA neuron at several sites within the central nervous system, including the limbic system, reticular formation. Enhancement of the inhibitory effect of GABA on neuronal excitability results by increased neuronal membrane permeability to chloride ions. This shift in chloride ions results in hyperpolarization (a less excitable state) and stabilization.

Contraindications Hypersensitivity to oxazepam or any component of the formulation (cross-sensitivity with other benzodiazepines may exist); narrow-angle glaucoma (not in product labeling, however, benzodiazepines are contraindicated); not indicated for use in the treatment of psychosis; pregnancy

Warnings/Precautions May cause hypotension (rare) - use with caution in patients with cardiovascular or cerebrovascular disease, or in patients who would not tolerate transient decreases in blood pressure. Serax® 15 mg tablet contains tartrazine; use is not recommended in pediatric patients <6 years of age; dose has not been established between 6-12 years of age.

Use with caution in elderly or debilitated patients, patients with hepatic disease (including alcoholics), or renal impairment. Use with caution in patients with respiratory disease or impaired gag reflex. Avoid use in patients with sleep apnea.

Causes CNS depression (dose-related) resulting in sedation, dizziness, confusion, or ataxia which may impair physical and mental capabilities. Use with caution in patients receiving other CNS depressants or psychoactive agents. Benzodiazepines have been associated with falls and traumatic injury and should be used with extreme caution in patients who are at risk of these events (especially the elderly).

Use caution in patients with depression, particularly if suicidal risk may be present. Use with caution in patients with a history of drug dependence. Benzodiazepines have been associated with dependence and acute withdrawal symptoms on discontinuation or reduction in dose.

Benzodiazepines have been associated with anterograde amnesia. Paradoxical reactions, including hyperactive or aggressive behavior have been reported with benzodiazepines, particularly in adolescent/pediatric or psychiatric patients. Does not have analgesic, antidepressant, or antipsychotic properties.

Drug Interactions

Decreased Effect: Oral contraceptives may increase the clearance of oxazepam. Theophylline and other CNS stimulants may antagonize the sedative effects of oxazepam. Phenytoin may increase the clearance of oxazepam.

Increased Effect/Toxicity: Ethanol and other CNS depressants may increase the CNS effects of oxazepam. Oxazepam may decrease the antiparkinsonian efficacy of levodopa. Flumazenil may cause seizures if administered following long-term benzodiazepine treatment.

Nutritional/Ethanol Interactions

Ethanol: Avoid ethanol (may increase CNS depression).

(Continued)

Oxazepam *(Continued)*

Herb/Nutraceutical: Avoid valerian, St John's wort, kava kava, gotu kola (may increase CNS depression).

Adverse Reactions Frequency not defined.

Cardiovascular: Syncope (rare), edema

Central nervous system: Drowsiness, ataxia, dizziness, vertigo, memory impairment, headache, paradoxical reactions (excitement, stimulation of effect), lethargy, amnesia, euphoria

Dermatologic: Rash

Endocrine & metabolic: Decreased libido, menstrual irregularities

Genitourinary: Incontinence

Hematologic: Leukopenia, blood dyscrasias

Hepatic: Jaundice

Neuromuscular & skeletal: Dysarthria, tremor, reflex slowing

Ocular: Blurred vision, diplopia

Miscellaneous: Drug dependence

Overdosage/Toxicology Symptoms of overdose include somnolence, confusion, coma, hypoactive reflexes, dyspnea, hypotension, slurred speech, and impaired coordination. Treatment for benzodiazepine overdose is supportive. Flumazenil has been shown to selectively block the binding of benzodiazepines to CNS receptors, resulting in a reversal of benzodiazepine-induced CNS depression, but not respiratory depression due to toxicity.

Pharmacodynamics/Kinetics

Absorption: Almost complete

Half-Life Elimination: 2.8-5.7 hours

Time to Peak: Serum: 2-4 hours

Metabolism: Hepatic to inactive compounds (primarily as glucuronides)

Formulations

Capsule: 10 mg, 15 mg, 30 mg

Tablet: 15 mg

Dosing

Adults:

Anxiety: Oral: 10-30 mg 3-4 times/day

Ethanol withdrawal: Oral: 15-30 mg 3-4 times/day

Hypnotic: Oral: 15-30 mg

Elderly: Oral: Anxiety: 10 mg 2-3 times/day; increase gradually as needed to a total of 30-45 mg/day. Dose titration should be slow to evaluate sensitivity.

Pediatrics: Anxiety: Oral: Children: 1 mg/kg/day has been administered

Renal Impairment: Not dialyzable (0% to 5%)

Administration

Oral: Give orally in divided doses

Monitoring and Teaching Issues

Physical Assessment: Assess other medications the patient may be taking for effectiveness and interactions (see Drug Interactions). See Contraindications and Warnings/Precautions for use cautions. Assess for history of addiction; long-term use can result in dependence, abuse, or tolerance; periodically evaluate need for continued use. Monitor therapeutic response and adverse reactions at beginning of therapy and periodically with long-term use (see Adverse Reactions and Overdose/Toxicology). Taper dosage slowly when discontinuing. Assess knowledge/teach patient appropriate use, interventions to reduce side effects, and adverse symptoms to report (see Patient Education). **Pregnancy risk factor D** - determine that patient is not pregnant before beginning treatment. Instruct patients of childbearing age about appropriate barrier contraceptive measures. Breast-feeding is not recommended.

Patient Education: Take exactly as directed; do not increase dose or frequency. It may take 2-3 weeks to achieve desired results. Drug may cause physical and/or psychological dependence. Do not use alcohol or other prescription or OTC medications (especially pain medications, sedatives, antihistamines, or hypnotics) without consulting prescriber. Maintain adequate hydration (2-3 L/day of fluids) unless advised by prescriber to restrict fluids. You may experience drowsiness, lightheadedness, impaired coordination, dizziness, or blurred vision (use caution when driving or engaging in tasks requiring alertness until response to drug is known); nausea, vomiting, or dry mouth (small, frequent meals, frequent mouth care, chewing gum, or sucking lozenges may help); constipation (increased exercise, fluids, fruit, or fiber may help); altered sexual drive or ability (reversible); or photosensitivity (use sunscreen, wear protective clothing and eyewear, and avoid direct sunlight). Report persistent CNS effects (eg, confusion, depression, increased sedation, excitation, headache, agitation, insomnia or nightmares, dizziness, fatigue, impaired coordination, changes in personality, or changes in cognition); changes in urinary pattern; muscle cramping, weakness, tremors, or rigidity; ringing in ears or visual disturbances; chest pain, palpitations, or rapid heartbeat; excessive perspiration, excessive GI symptoms (cramping, constipation, vomiting, anorexia); or worsening of condition. **Pregnancy/breast-feeding precautions:** Do not get pregnant while taking this medication; use appropriate barrier contraceptive measures. Breast-feeding is not recommended.

Geriatric Considerations: Because of its relatively short half-life and its lack of active metabolites, oxazepam is recommended for use in the elderly when a benzodiazepine is indicated.

Other Issues: Taper dosage gradually after long-term therapy, especially in epileptic patients. Abrupt withdrawal may cause tremors, nausea, vomiting, abdominal and/or muscle cramps.

Additional Information Not intended for management of anxieties and minor distresses associated with everyday life. Treatment longer than 4 months should be re-evaluated to determine the patient's need for the drug. Abrupt discontinuation after sustained use (generally >10 days) may cause withdrawal symptoms.

Related Information

Anxiolytic/Hypnotic Use in Long-Term Care Facilities *on page 1608*

Benzodiazepines *on page 1560*

Oxcarbazepine (ox car BAZ e peen)

U.S. Brand Names Trileptal®

Synonyms GP 47680

Generic Available No

Pharmacologic Category Anticonvulsant, Miscellaneous

Pregnancy Risk Factor C

Lactation Enters breast milk/contraindicated

Use Monotherapy or adjunctive therapy in the treatment of partial seizures in adults with epilepsy; adjunctive therapy in the treatment of partial seizures in children (4-16 years of age) with epilepsy

Use - Unlabeled/Investigational Antimanic

Mechanism of Action/Effect Precise mechanism of action has not been determined. Believed to prevent the spread of seizures by decreasing propagation of synaptic impulses.

Contraindications Hypersensitivity to oxcarbazepine or any component of the formulation

Warnings/Precautions Clinically significant hyponatremia (sodium <125 mmol/L) can develop during oxcarbazepine use; monitor serum sodium, particularly during the first 3 months of therapy or in patients at risk for hyponatremia. As with all antiepileptic drugs, oxcarbazepine should be withdrawn gradually to minimize the potential of increased seizure frequency. Use of oxcarbazepine has been associated with CNS related adverse events, most significant of these were cognitive symptoms including psychomotor slowing, difficulty with concentration, and speech or language problems, somnolence or fatigue, and coordination abnormalities, including ataxia and gait disturbances. Use caution in patients with previous hypersensitivity to carbamazepine (cross-sensitivity occurs in 25% to 30%). May reduce the efficacy of oral contraceptives (nonhormonal contraceptive measures are recommended). Pregnancy risk C.

Drug Interactions

Cytochrome P450 Effect: Inhibits CYP2C19; Induces **CYP3A4**

Decreased Effect: Oxcarbazine serum concentrations may be reduced by carbamazepine, phenytoin, phenobarbital, valproic acid and verapamil (decreases levels of active oxcarbazepine metabolite). Oxcarbazepine reduces the serum concentrations of felodipine (similar effects may be anticipated with other dihydropyridines), oral contraceptives (use alternative contraceptive measures), and verapamil.

Increased Effect/Toxicity: Serum concentrations of phenytoin and phenobarbital are increased by oxcarbazepine.

Nutritional/Ethanol Interactions

Ethanol: Avoid ethanol (may increase CNS depression).

Herb/Nutraceutical: St John's wort may decrease oxcarbazepine levels. Avoid evening primrose (seizure threshold decreased). Avoid valerian, St John's wort, kava kava, gotu kola.

Effects on Lab Values Thyroid function tests may depress serum T_4 without affecting T_3 levels or TSH.

Adverse Reactions As reported in adults with doses of up to 2400 mg/day (includes patients on monotherapy, adjunctive therapy, and those not previously on AEDs); incidence in children was similar.

>10%:

Central nervous system: Dizziness (22% to 49%), somnolence (20% to 36%), headache (13% to 32%, placebo 23%), ataxia (5% to 31%), fatigue (12% to 15%), vertigo (6% to 15%)

Gastrointestinal: Vomiting (7% to 36%), nausea (15% to 29%), abdominal pain (10% to 13%)

Neuromuscular & skeletal: Abnormal gait (5% to 17%), tremor (3% to 16%)

Ocular: Diplopia (14% to 40%), nystagmus (7% to 26%), abnormal vision (4% to 14%)

1% to 10%:

Cardiovascular: Hypotension (1% to 2%)

Central nervous system: Nervousness (2% to 5%), amnesia (4%), agitation (1% to 2%),

Dermatologic: Rash (4%)

Endocrine & metabolic: Hyponatremia (1% to 3%)

Gastrointestinal: Diarrhea (5% to 7%), gastritis (1% to 2%)

Neuromuscular & skeletal: Weakness (3% to 6%), back pain (4%), falls (4%), abnormal coordination (1% to 4%), muscle weakness (1% to 2%)

Ocular: Abnormal accommodation (2%)

Respiratory: Upper respiratory tract infection (7%)

<1% (Limited to important or life-threatening): Aggressive reaction, alopecia, amnesia, angioedema, aphasia, asthma, blood in stool, cardiac failure, cataract, cerebral hemorrhage, cholelithiasis, convulsions aggravated, delirium, duodenal ulcer, dysphagia, dysphonia, dyspnea, dystonia, erythema multiforme, eosinophilia, extrapyramidal disorder, gastric ulcer, genital pruritus, gingival hyperplasia, hematemesis, hematuria, hemianopia, hemiplegia, hypersensitivity reaction, intermenstrual bleeding, laryngismus, leukopenia, maculopapular rash, malaise, manic reaction, menorrhagia, migraine, muscle contractions (involuntary), neuralgia, oculogyric crisis, paralysis, photosensitivity reaction, postural hypotension, priapism, purpura, psychosis, scotoma, sialoadenitis, Stevens-Johnson syndrome, stupor, syncope, systemic lupus erythematosus, tetany, thrombocytopenia, toxic epidermal necrolysis, urticaria

Overdosage/Toxicology Symptoms may include CNS depression (somnolence, ataxia). Treatment is symptomatic and supportive.

Pharmacodynamics/Kinetics

Absorption: Complete; food has no affect on rate or extent

Bioavailability: Decreased in children <8 years; increased in elderly >60 years

Half-Life Elimination: Parent drug: 2 hours; MHD: 9 hours; Cl_{cr} 30 mL/minute: 19 hours

Time to Peak: Serum: 4.5 hours (3-13 hours)

Metabolism: Hepatic to 10-monohydroxy metabolite (active); MHD which is further conjugated to DHD (inactive)

(Continued)

Oxcarbazepine *(Continued)*

Formulations

Suspension, oral: 300 mg/5 mL (250 mL) [contains ethanol]

Tablet: 150 mg, 300 mg, 600 mg

Dosing

Adults & Elderly:

Adjunctive therapy, partial seizures (epilepsy): Oral: Initial: 300 mg twice daily; dosage may be increased by 600 mg/day at approximate weekly intervals. Recommended daily dose is 1200 mg/day in 2 divided doses. Although daily doses >1200 mg/day demonstrated greater efficacy, most patients were unable to tolerate 2400 mg/day (due to CNS effects).

Conversion to monotherapy, partial seizures (epilepsy): Oral: Patients receiving concomitant antiepileptic drugs (AEDs): Initial: 300 mg twice daily while simultaneously reducing the dose of concomitant AEDs. Withdraw concomitant AEDs completely over 3-6 weeks, while increasing the oxcarbazine dose in increments of 600 mg/day at weekly intervals, reaching the maximum oxcarbazine dose (2400 mg/day) in about 2-4 weeks (lower doses have been effective in patients in whom monotherapy has been initiated).

Initiation of monotherapy, partial seizures (epilepsy): Oral: Patients not receiving prior AEDs: 300 mg twice daily (total dose 600 mg/day). Increase dose by 300 mg/day every third day to a dose of 1200 mg/day. Higher dosages (2400 mg/day) have been shown to be effective in patients converted to monotherapy from other AEDs.

Pediatrics: Adjunctive treatment, partial seizures (epilepsy): Oral: Children 4-16 years: Initial 8-10 mg/kg/day (not to exceed 600 mg/day) given in a twice daily regimen. Maintenance: The target maintenance dose should be achieved over 2 weeks, and depends on weight of the child:

20-29 kg: 900 mg/day in 2 divided doses
29.1-39 kg: 1200 mg/day in 2 divided doses
>39 kg: 1800 mg/day in 2 divided doses

Renal Impairment: Initial dose should be reduced by 50%, and the dosage increased slowly to achieve the desired clinical response.

Hepatic Impairment: No dosage adjustment recommended in mild to moderate hepatic impairment. Patients with severe hepatic impairment have not been evaluated.

Administration

Oral: Suspension: Prior to using for the first time, firmly insert the plastic adapter provided with the bottle. Cover adapter with child-resistant cap when not in use. Shake bottle for at least 10 seconds, remove child-resistant cap and insert the oral dosing syringe provided to withdraw appropriate dose. Dose may be taken directly from oral syringe or may be mixed in a small glass of water immediately prior to swallowing. Rinse syringe with warm water after use and allow to dry thoroughly. Discard any unused portion after 7 weeks of first opening bottle.

Stability

Storage: Store tablets and suspension at 25°C (77°F). Use suspension within 7 weeks of first opening container.

Monitoring Laboratory Tests Seizure frequency, serum sodium (particularly during first 3 months of therapy), symptoms of CNS depression (dizziness, headache, somnolence). Additional serum sodium monitoring is recommended during maintenance treatment in patients receiving other medications known to decrease sodium levels, in patients with signs/symptoms of hyponatremia, and in patients with an increase in seizure frequency or severity.

Monitoring and Teaching Issues

Physical Assessment: Assess complete allergy history (carbamazepine). Assess effectiveness and interactions of other medications (see Drug Interactions). See Warnings/Precautions and Contraindications for use cautions. Monitor therapeutic effectiveness (seizure activity, frequency, duration, type), laboratory results (see above), and adverse reactions (see Adverse Reactions). Dosage should be tapered when discontinuing to reduce risk of increased seizures. Assess knowledge/teach patient appropriate use, interventions to reduce side effects, and adverse reactions to report (see Patient Education). **Pregnancy risk factor C** - benefits of use should outweigh possible risks. **Note:** Oxcarbazepine may reduce the effectiveness of oral contraceptives, nonhormonal contraception is recommended. Breast-feeding is contraindicated.

Patient Education: Take exactly as directed. Do not increase dose or frequency or discontinue without consulting prescriber. While using the medication do not use alcohol and other prescription or OTC medications (especially medications to relieve pain, induce sleep, reduce anxiety, treat or prevent cold, coughs, or allergies) unless approved by prescriber. Maintain adequate hydration (2-3 L/day of fluids) unless advised by prescriber to restrict fluids. You may experience drowsiness, dizziness, or blurred vision (use caution when driving or engaging in tasks requiring alertness until response to drug is known); nausea or vomiting (small, frequent meals, good mouth care, chewing gum, or sucking hard candy may help, or contact prescriber). Report CNS changes, increase in seizure frequency or severity, mentation changes, changes in cognition or memory, acute fatigue or weakness, or insomnia; muscle cramping, weakness, or pain; rash or skin irritations; unusual bruising or bleeding (mouth, urine, stool); swelling of extremities; or other adverse response. **Pregnancy/breast-feeding precautions:** Inform prescriber if you are or intend to become pregnant. **Note:** Oxcarbazepine may reduce the effectiveness of oral contraceptives, nonhormonal contraception is recommended. Do not breast-feed.

Dietary Issues: May be taken with or without food.

Breast-feeding Issues: Oxcarbazepine and its active metabolite (MHD) are excreted in human breast milk. A milk-to-plasma concentration ratio of 0.5 was found for both. Because of the potential for serious adverse reactions to oxcarbazepine in nursing infants, a decision should be made whether to discontinue nursing or to discontinue the drug in nursing women.

Pregnancy Issues: Although many epidemiological studies of congenital anomalies in infants born to women treated with various anticonvulsants during pregnancy have been reported, none of these investigations includes enough women treated with oxcarbazepine to assess possible teratogenic effects of this drug. Given that teratogenic effects have been observed in animal studies, and that oxcarbazepine is structurally related to carbamazepine (teratogenic in humans), use during pregnancy only if the benefit to the mother outweighs the potential risk to the fetus. Nonhormonal forms of contraception should be used during therapy.

Oxpentifylline *see* Pentoxifylline *on page 1057*

Oxsoralen® *see* Methoxsalen *on page 878*

Oxsoralen-Ultra® *see* Methoxsalen *on page 878*

Oxybutynin (oks i BYOO ti nin)

U.S. Brand Names Ditropan®; Ditropan® XL

Synonyms Oxybutynin Chloride

Generic Available Yes: Not extended release formulation

Pharmacologic Category Antispasmodic Agent, Urinary

Pregnancy Risk Factor B

Lactation Enters breast milk/contraindicated

Use Antispasmodic for neurogenic bladder (urgency, frequency, urge incontinence) and uninhibited bladder

Mechanism of Action/Effect Direct antispasmodic effect on smooth muscle, also inhibits the action of acetylcholine on smooth muscle (exhibits $^1/_5$ the anticholinergic activity of atropine, but is 4-10 times the antispasmodic activity); does not block effects at skeletal muscle or at autonomic ganglia; increases bladder capacity, decreases uninhibited contractions, and delays desire to void; therefore, decreases urgency and frequency

Contraindications Hypersensitivity to oxybutynin or any component of the formulation; glaucoma, myasthenia gravis; partial or complete GI obstruction; GU obstruction; ulcerative colitis; intestinal atony; megacolon; toxic megacolon

Warnings/Precautions Use with caution in patients with urinary tract obstruction, hyperthyroidism, reflux esophagitis, heart disease, hepatic or renal disease, prostatic hyperplasia, autonomic neuropathy, hypertension, hiatal hernia. Caution should be used in the elderly due to anticholinergic activity (eg, confusion, constipation, blurred vision, and tachycardia).

Drug Interactions

Cytochrome P450 Effect: Substrate of CYP3A4; Inhibits CYP2D6, 3A4

Increased Effect/Toxicity: Additive sedation with CNS depressants and alcohol. Additive anticholinergic effects with antihistamines and anticholinergic agents.

Effects on Lab Values May suppress the wheal and flare reactions to skin test antigens.

Adverse Reactions

>10%:

- Central nervous system: Drowsiness
- Gastrointestinal: Dry mouth, constipation
- Miscellaneous: Diaphoresis (decreased)

1% to 10%:

- Cardiovascular: Tachycardia, palpitations
- Central nervous system: Dizziness, insomnia, fever, headache
- Dermatologic: Rash
- Endocrine & metabolic: Decreased flow of breast milk, decreased sexual ability, hot flashes
- Gastrointestinal: Nausea, vomiting
- Genitourinary: Urinary hesitancy or retention
- Neuromuscular & skeletal: Weakness
- Ocular: Blurred vision, mydriatic effect

<1% (Limited to important or life-threatening): Increased intraocular pressure

Overdosage/Toxicology Symptoms of overdose include hypotension, circulatory failure, psychotic behavior, flushing, respiratory failure, paralysis, tremor, irritability, seizures, delirium, hallucinations, and coma. Treatment is symptomatic and supportive. For anticholinergic overdose with severe life-threatening symptoms, physostigmine 1-2 mg I.V. slowly, may be given to reverse these effects.

Pharmacodynamics/Kinetics

Absorption: Rapid and well absorbed

Half-Life Elimination: 1-2.3 hours

Time to Peak: Serum: ~60 minutes

Metabolism: Hepatic

Onset: 30-60 minutes; Peak effect: 3-6 hours

Duration: 6-10 hours

Formulations

Syrup, as chloride (Ditropan®): 5 mg/5 mL (473 mL)

Tablet, as chloride (Ditropan®): 5 mg

Tablet, extended release, as chloride (Ditropan® XL): 5 mg, 10 mg, 15 mg

Dosing

Adults: Bladder spasms: Oral:

Regular release: 5 mg 2-3 times/day up to maximum of 5 mg 4 times/day

Extended release: Initial: 5 mg once daily, may increase in 5-10 mg increments; maximum: 30 mg daily

Note: Should be discontinued periodically to determine whether the patient can manage without the drug and to minimize resistance to the drug.

Elderly: Oral: 2.5-5 mg twice daily; increase by 2.5 mg increments every 1-2 days. **Note:** Should be discontinued periodically to determine whether the patient can manage without the drug and to minimize resistance to the drug.

Pediatrics: Bladder spasms: Oral: Children:

1-5 years: 0.2 mg/kg/dose 2-4 times/day

>5 years: 5 mg twice daily, up to 5 mg 4 times/day maximum

(Continued)

Oxybutynin *(Continued)*

Administration

Oral: Should be administered on an empty stomach with water.

Monitoring and Teaching Issues

Physical Assessment: See Contraindications and Warnings/Precautions. Assess other medications patient may be taking for interactions (see Drug Interactions). Assess voiding pattern, incontinent episodes, frequency, urgency, distention, and urinary retention prior to beginning therapy and periodically with long-term use. Assess knowledge/teach patient appropriate use, possible side effects, and symptoms to report (see Patient Education). Breast-feeding is contraindicated.

Patient Education: Take prescribed dose preferably on an empty stomach, 1 hour before or 2 hours after meals. Swallow extended-release tablets whole, do not chew or crush. You may experience dizziness, lightheadedness, or drowsiness (use caution when driving or engaging in tasks requiring alertness until response to drug is known); dry mouth or changes in appetite (small, frequent meals, frequent mouth care, sucking lozenges, or chewing gum may help); constipation (increased exercise, fluids, fruit, fiber, or stool softener may help); decreased sexual ability (reversible with discontinuance of drug); or decreased sweating (use caution in hot weather, avoid extreme exercise or activity). Report rapid heartbeat, palpitations, or chest pain; difficulty voiding; or vision changes. **Breast-feeding precaution:** Do not breast-feed.

Dietary Issues: Should be taken on an empty stomach with water.

Geriatric Considerations: Caution should be used in the elderly due to anticholinergic activity (eg, confusion, constipation, blurred vision, and tachycardia). Start with lower doses. Oxybutynin may cause memory problems in the elderly. A study of 12 health volunteers with an average age of 69 showed cognitive decline while taking the drug (*J Am Geriatr Soc*, 1998, L46:8-13).

Related Information

Pharmacotherapy of Urinary Incontinence *on page 1699*

Oxybutynin Chloride *see* Oxybutynin *on page 1019*

Oxycel® *see page 1461*

Oxycodone (oks i KOE done)

U.S. Brand Names OxyContin®; Oxydose™; OxyFast®; OxyIR®; Percolone® [DSC]; Roxicodone™; Roxicodone™ Intensol™

Synonyms Dihydrohydroxycodeinone; Oxycodone Hydrochloride

Restrictions C-II

Generic Available Yes

Pharmacologic Category Analgesic, Narcotic

Pregnancy Risk Factor B/D (prolonged use or high doses at term)

Lactation Enters breast milk/use caution

Use Management of moderate to severe pain, normally used in combination with non-narcotic analgesics

OxyContin® is indicated for around-the-clock management of moderate to severe pain when an analgesic is needed for an extended period of time. **Note:** OxyContin® is not intended for use as an "as needed" analgesic or for immediately-postoperative pain management (should be used postoperatively only if the patient has received it prior to surgery or if severe, persistent pain is anticipated).

Mechanism of Action/Effect Binds to opiate receptors in the CNS, causing inhibition of ascending pain pathways, altering the perception of and response to pain; produces generalized CNS depression

Contraindications Hypersensitivity to oxycodone or any component of the formulation; significant respiratory depression; hypercarbia; acute or severe bronchial asthma; OxyContin® is also contraindicated in paralytic ileus (known or suspected); pregnancy (prolonged use or high doses at term)

Warnings/Precautions Use with caution in patients with hypersensitivity reactions to other phenanthrene derivative opioid agonists (morphine, hydrocodone, hydromorphone, levorphanol, oxycodone, oxymorphone), respiratory diseases including asthma, emphysema, or COPD. Use with caution in pancreatitis or biliary tract disease, acute alcoholism (including delirium tremens), adrenocortical insufficiency, CNS depression/coma, kyphoscoliosis (or other skeletal disorder which may alter respiratory function), hypothyroidism (including myxedema), prostatic hyperplasia, urethral stricture, and toxic psychosis.

Use with caution in the elderly, debilitated, severe hepatic or renal function. Hemodynamic effects (hypotension, orthostasis) may be exaggerated in patients with hypovolemia, concurrent vasodilating drugs, or in patients with head injury. Respiratory depressant effects and capacity to elevate CSF pressure may be exaggerated in presence of head injury, other intracranial lesion, or pre-existing intracranial pressure. Tolerance or drug dependence may result from extended use. Healthcare provider should be alert to problems of abuse, misuse, and diversion. Do **not** crush controlled-release tablets. Some preparations contain sulfites which may cause allergic reactions. OxyContin® 80 mg and 160 mg strengths are for use only in opioid-tolerant patients requiring high daily dosages >160 mg (80 mg formulation) or >320 mg (160 mg formulation).

Drug Interactions

Cytochrome P450 Effect: Substrate of **CYP2D6**

Increased Effect/Toxicity: MAO inhibitors may increase adverse symptoms. Cimetidine may increase narcotic analgesic serum levels resulting in toxicity. CNS depressants (barbiturates, ethanol) and TCAs may potentiate the sedative and respiratory depressive effects of morphine and other opiate agonists. Dextroamphetamine may enhance the analgesic effect of morphine and other opiate agonists.

Nutritional/Ethanol Interactions

Ethanol: Avoid ethanol (may increase CNS depression).

Herb/Nutraceutical: Avoid valerian, St John's wort, kava kava, gotu kola (may increase CNS depression).

Adverse Reactions

>10%:

Cardiovascular: Hypotension
Central nervous system: Fatigue, drowsiness, dizziness
Gastrointestinal: Nausea, vomiting
Neuromuscular & skeletal: Weakness

1% to 10%:

Central nervous system: Nervousness, headache, restlessness, malaise
Gastrointestinal: Stomach cramps, dry mouth, biliary spasm, constipation
Genitourinary: Ureteral spasms, decreased urination
Ocular: Blurred vision
Miscellaneous: Histamine release

<1% (Limited to important or life-threatening): Dyspnea

Note: Deaths due to overdose have been reported due to misuse/abuse after crushing the sustained release tablets.

Overdosage/Toxicology Symptoms of toxicity include CNS depression, respiratory depression, and miosis. Naloxone, 2 mg I.V. with repeat administration as necessary up to a total of 10 mg, can also be used to reverse toxic effects of the opiate.

Pharmacodynamics/Kinetics

Half-Life Elimination: 2-3 hours

Metabolism: Hepatic

Onset: Pain relief: 10-15 minutes; Peak effect: 0.5-1 hour

Duration: 3-6 hours; Controlled release: ≤12 hours

Formulations

Capsule, immediate release, as hydrochloride (OxyIR®): 5 mg
Solution, oral, as hydrochloride (Roxicodone™): 5 mg/5 mL (5 mL, 500 mL) [contains alcohol]
Solution, oral concentrate, as hydrochloride:
Oxydose™: 20 mg/mL (30 mL) [contains sodium benzoate; berry flavor]
OxyFast®: 20 mg/mL (30 mL) [contains sodium benzoate]
Roxicodone™ Intensol™: 20 mg/mL (30 mL) [contains sodium benzoate]
Tablet, as hydrochloride: 5 mg
Percolone® [DSC]: 5 mg
Roxicodone™: 5 mg, 15 mg, 30 mg
Tablet, controlled release, as hydrochloride (OxyContin®): 10 mg, 20 mg, 40 mg, 80 mg, 160 mg

Dosing

Adults & Elderly:

Management of pain: Oral:
Regular or immediate release formulations: 2.5-5 mg every 6 hours as needed
Controlled release:
Opioid naive (not currently on opioid): 10 mg every 12 hours
Currently on opioid/ASA or acetaminophen or NSAID combination:
1-5 tablets: 10-20 mg every 12 hours
6-9 tablets: 20-30 mg every 12 hours
10-12 tablets: 30-40 mg every 12 hours
May continue the nonopioid as a separate drug.
Currently on opioids: Use standard conversion chart to convert daily dose to oxycodone equivalent. Divide daily dose in 2 (for every 12-hour dosing) and round down to nearest dosage form.

Pediatrics: Oral: Regular or immediate release formulations:
6-12 years: 1.25 mg every 6 hours as needed
>12 years: 2.5 mg every 6 hours as needed

Hepatic Impairment: Reduce dosage in patients with severe liver disease.

Administration

Oral: Do not crush controlled-release tablets.

Stability

Storage: Tablets should be stored at room temperature.

Monitoring and Teaching Issues

Physical Assessment: Assess other medications patient may be taking for additive or adverse interactions (see Drug Interactions). Monitor for effectiveness of pain relief and monitor for signs of overdose (see above). Monitor vital signs and CNS status at beginning of therapy and at regular intervals with long-term use. May cause physical and/or psychological dependence. For inpatients, implement safety measures. Assess knowledge/teach patient appropriate use (if self-administered). Teach patient to monitor for adverse reactions (see Adverse Reactions), adverse reactions to report, and appropriate interventions to reduce side effects (see Patient Education). Taper dosage slowly when discontinuing. **Pregnancy risk factor B/D** - see Pregnancy Risk Factor for use cautions. Note breast-feeding caution.

Patient Education: If self-administered, use exactly as directed; do not increase dose or frequency. Drug may cause physical and/or psychological dependence. Do not crush or chew controlled-release tablets. While using this medication, do not use alcohol and other prescription or OTC medications (especially sedatives, tranquilizers, antihistamines, or pain medications) without consulting prescriber. Maintain adequate hydration (2-3 L/day of fluids) unless advised by prescriber to restrict fluids. May cause hypotension, dizziness, drowsiness, impaired coordination, or blurred vision (use caution when driving, climbing stairs, or changing position - rising from sitting or lying to standing, or when engaging in tasks requiring alertness until response to drug is known); nausea, vomiting, or dry mouth (frequent mouth care, small, frequent meals, chewing gum, or sucking lozenges may help); or constipation (increased exercise, fluids, fruit, or fiber may help; if unresolved, consult prescriber about use of stool softeners). Report persistent dizziness or headache; excessive fatigue or sedation; changes in mental status; changes in urinary elimination or pain on urination; weakness or trembling; blurred vision; or shortness of breath. **Pregnancy/**

(Continued)

Oxycodone *(Continued)*

breast-feeding precautions: Inform prescriber if you are or intend to become pregnant. If you are breast-feeding, take medication immediately after breast-feeding or 3-4 hours prior to next feeding.

Geriatric Considerations: The elderly may be particularly susceptible to the CNS depressant and constipating effects of narcotics. Serum levels at a given dose may also be increased relative to concentrations in younger patients.

Additional Information Prophylactic use of a laxative should be considered. OxyContin® 80 mg and 160 mg tablets are for use in opioid-tolerant patients only.

Related Information

Controlled Substances Comparison *on page 1568*
Narcotic/Opioid Analgesic Comparison *on page 1583*

Oxycodone and Acetaminophen (oks i KOE done & a seet a MIN oh fen)

U.S. Brand Names Endocet®; Percocet® 2.5/325; Percocet® 5/325; Percocet® 7.5/325; Percocet® 7.5/500; Percocet® 10/325; Percocet® 10/650; Roxicet®; Roxicet® 5/500; Tylox®

Synonyms Acetaminophen and Oxycodone

Restrictions C-II

Generic Available Yes

Pharmacologic Category Analgesic, Narcotic

Pregnancy Risk Factor C/D (prolonged periods or high doses at term)

Lactation Enters breast milk/use caution

Use Management of moderate to severe pain

Formulations

Caplet (Roxicet® 5/500): Oxycodone hydrochloride 5 mg and acetaminophen 500 mg

Capsule: Oxycodone hydrochloride 5 mg and acetaminophen 500 mg

Tylox®: Oxycodone hydrochloride 5 mg and acetaminophen 500 mg [contains sodium benzoate and sodium metabisulfite]

Solution, oral (Roxicet®): Oxycodone hydrochloride 5 mg and acetaminophen 325 mg per 5 mL (5 mL, 500 mL) [contains alcohol <0.5%]

Tablet: Oxycodone hydrochloride 5 mg and acetaminophen 325 mg; oxycodone hydrochloride 7.5 mg and acetaminophen 500 mg; oxycodone hydrochloride 10 mg and acetaminophen 650 mg

Endocet®: Oxycodone hydrochloride 5 mg and acetaminophen 325 mg
Percocet® 2.5/325: Oxycodone hydrochloride 2.5 mg and acetaminophen 325 mg
Percocet® 5/325: Oxycodone hydrochloride 5 mg and acetaminophen 325 mg
Percocet® 7.5/325: Oxycodone hydrochloride 7.5 mg and acetaminophen 325 mg
Percocet® 7.5/500: Oxycodone hydrochloride 7.5 mg and acetaminophen 500 mg
Percocet® 10/325: Oxycodone hydrochloride 10 mg and acetaminophen 325 mg
Percocet® 10/650: Oxycodone hydrochloride 10 mg and acetaminophen 650 mg
Roxicet®: Oxycodone hydrochloride 5 mg and acetaminophen 325 mg

Dosing

Adults: Doses should be given every 4-6 hours as needed and titrated to appropriate analgesic effects. **Note:** Initial dose is based on the **oxycodone** content; however, the maximum daily dose is based on the **acetaminophen** content.

Maximum daily dose, **based on acetaminophen content:** Oral: 4 g/day.
Mild to moderate pain: Oral: Initial dose, **based on oxycodone content:** 5 mg
Severe pain: Oral: Initial dose, **based on oxycodone content:** 15-30 mg

Elderly: Doses should be titrated to appropriate analgesic effects: Oral: Initial dose, **based on oxycodone content:** 2.5-5 mg every 6 hours. Do not exceed 4 g/day of acetaminophen.

Pediatrics: Doses should be given every 4-6 hours as needed and titrated to appropriate analgesic effects. **Note:** Initial dose is based on the **oxycodone** content; however, the maximum daily dose is based on the **acetaminophen** content.

Maximum dose, **based on acetaminophen content**: Oral: Children <45 kg: 90 mg/kg/day; children >45 kg: 4 g/day
Mild to moderate pain: Oral: Initial dose, **based on oxycodone content:** 0.05-0.1 mg/kg/dose
Severe pain: Oral: Initial dose, **based on oxycodone content:** 0.3 mg/kg/dose

Hepatic Impairment: Dose should be reduced in patients with severe liver disease.

Monitoring and Teaching Issues

Physical Assessment: See individual components listed in Related Information. **Pregnancy risk factor C/D** - see Pregnancy Risk Factor for use cautions; benefits of use should outweigh possible risks. Note breast-feeding caution.

Patient Education: See individual components listed in Related Information. **Pregnancy/breast-feeding precautions:** Inform prescriber if you are or intend to become pregnant. Consult prescriber if breast-feeding.

Related Information

Acetaminophen *on page 35*
Oxycodone *on page 1020*

Oxycodone and Aspirin (oks i KOE done & AS pir in)

U.S. Brand Names Endodan®; Percodan®; Percodan®-Demi [DSC]

Synonyms Aspirin and Oxycodone

Restrictions C-II

Generic Available Yes

Pharmacologic Category Analgesic, Narcotic

Pregnancy Risk Factor D

Lactation Enters breast milk/use caution due to aspirin content

Use Management of moderate to severe pain

Formulations

Tablet: Oxycodone hydrochloride 4.5 mg, oxycodone terephthalate 0.38 mg, and aspirin 325 mg

Endodan®, Percodan®: Oxycodone hydrochloride 4.5 mg, oxycodone terephthalate 0.38 mg, and aspirin 325 mg

Percodan®-Demi [DSC]: Oxycodone hydrochloride 2.25 mg, oxycodone terephthalate 0.19 mg, and aspirin 325 mg

Dosing

Adults & Elderly: Analgesic: Oral (based on oxycodone combined salts): Percodan®: 1 tablet every 6 hours as needed for pain or Percodan®-Demi: 1-2 tablets every 6 hours as needed for pain

Hepatic Impairment: Dose should be reduced in patients with severe liver disease.

Monitoring and Teaching Issues

Physical Assessment: See individual components listed in Related Information. **Pregnancy risk factor D** - determine that patient is not pregnant before beginning treatment. Instruct patients of childbearing age about appropriate barrier contraceptive measures. Note breast-feeding caution.

Patient Education: See individual components listed in Related Information. **Pregnancy/breast-feeding precautions:** Inform prescriber if you are or intend to become pregnant. Consult prescriber if breast-feeding.

Related Information

Aspirin *on page 121*
Oxycodone *on page 1020*

Oxycodone Hydrochloride *see* Oxycodone *on page 1020*
OxyContin® *see* Oxycodone *on page 1020*
Oxydose™ *see* Oxycodone *on page 1020*
OxyFast® *see* Oxycodone *on page 1020*
OxyIR® *see* Oxycodone *on page 1020*

Oxymorphone (oks i MOR fone)

U.S. Brand Names Numorphan®

Synonyms Oxymorphone Hydrochloride

Restrictions C-II

Generic Available No

Pharmacologic Category Analgesic, Narcotic

Pregnancy Risk Factor B/D (prolonged use or high doses at term)

Lactation Excretion in breast milk unknown/use caution

Use Management of moderate to severe pain and preoperatively as a sedative and a supplement to anesthesia

Mechanism of Action/Effect Oxymorphone hydrochloride (Numorphan®) is a potent narcotic analgesic with uses similar to those of morphine. The drug is a semisynthetic derivative of morphine (phenanthrene derivative) and is closely related to hydromorphone chemically (Dilaudid®).

Contraindications Hypersensitivity to oxymorphone or any component of the formulation; increased intracranial pressure; severe respiratory depression; pregnancy (prolonged use or high doses at term)

Warnings/Precautions Some preparations contain sulfites which may cause allergic reactions; infants <3 months of age are more susceptible to respiratory depression, use with caution and generally in reduced doses in this age group; use with caution in patients with impaired respiratory function or severe hepatic dysfunction and in patients with hypersensitivity reactions to other phenanthrene derivative opioid agonists (codeine, hydrocodone, hydromorphone, levorphanol, oxycodone, oxymorphone); tolerance or drug dependence may result from extended use

Drug Interactions

Decreased Effect: Decreased effect with phenothiazines.

Increased Effect/Toxicity: Increased effect/toxicity with CNS depressants (phenothiazines, tranquilizers, anxiolytics, sedatives, hypnotics, alcohol), tricyclic antidepressants, and dextroamphetamine.

Nutritional/Ethanol Interactions

Ethanol: Avoid ethanol (may increase CNS depression).

Herb/Nutraceutical: Avoid valerian, St John's wort, kava kava, gotu kola (may increase CNS depression).

Adverse Reactions

>10%:

- Cardiovascular: Hypotension
- Central nervous system: Fatigue, drowsiness, dizziness
- Gastrointestinal: Nausea, vomiting, constipation
- Neuromuscular & skeletal: Weakness
- Miscellaneous: Histamine release

1% to 10%:

- Central nervous system: Nervousness, headache, restlessness, malaise, confusion
- Gastrointestinal: Anorexia, stomach cramps, xerostomia, biliary spasm
- Genitourinary: Decreased urination, ureteral spasms
- Local: Pain at injection site
- Respiratory: Dyspnea

<1% (Limited to important or life-threatening): Mental depression, hallucinations, paradoxical CNS stimulation, increased intracranial pressure, rash, urticaria, paralytic ileus, histamine release, physical and psychological dependence

Overdosage/Toxicology Symptoms of overdose include respiratory depression, miosis, hypotension, bradycardia, apnea, and pulmonary edema. Treatment of overdose includes maintaining patent airway and establishing an I.V. line. Naloxone, 2 mg I.V., with repeat

(Continued)

Oxymorphone *(Continued)*

administration as necessary up to a total of 10 mg, can also be used to reverse toxic effects of the opiate.

Pharmacodynamics/Kinetics

Metabolism: Hepatic via glucuronidation

Onset: Analgesic: I.V., I.M., S.C.: 5-10 minutes; Rectal: 15-30 minutes

Duration: Analgesic: Parenteral, rectal: 3-4 hours

Formulations

Injection, solution, as hydrochloride: 1 mg (1 mL); 1.5 mg/mL (10 mL)

Suppository, rectal, as hydrochloride: 5 mg

Dosing

Adults & Elderly: Analgesia:

I.M., S.C.: 0.5 mg initially, 1-1.5 mg every 4-6 hours as needed

I.V.: 0.5 mg initially

Rectal: 5 mg every 4-6 hours

Stability

Storage: Refrigerate suppository.

Monitoring and Teaching Issues

Physical Assessment: Assess other medications patient may be taking for additive or adverse interactions (see Drug Interactions). Monitor therapeutic effectiveness, adverse reactions, and signs of overdose (see above) at beginning of therapy and at regular intervals with long-term use. May cause physical and/or psychological dependence. For inpatients, implement safety measures. Assess knowledge/teach patient appropriate use (if self-administered). Teach patient to monitor for adverse reactions (see Adverse Reactions), adverse reactions to report, and appropriate interventions to reduce side effects (see Patient Education). **Pregnancy risk factor B/D** - see Pregnancy Risk Factor for use cautions. Note breast-feeding caution.

Patient Education: If self-administered, use exactly as directed; do not increase dose or frequency or discontinue without consulting prescriber. Drug may cause physical and/or psychological dependence. While using this medication, do not use alcohol and other prescription or OTC medications (especially sedatives, tranquilizers, antihistamines, or pain medications) without consulting prescriber. Maintain adequate hydration (2-3 L/day of fluids) unless advised by prescriber to restrict fluids. May cause hypotension, dizziness, drowsiness, impaired coordination, or blurred vision (use caution when driving, climbing stairs, or changing position - rising from sitting or lying to standing, or when engaging in tasks requiring alertness until response to drug is known); nausea, vomiting or dry mouth (frequent mouth care, small, frequent meals, chewing gum, or sucking lozenges may help); or constipation (increased exercise, fluids, fruit, or fiber may help; if unresolved, consult prescriber about use of stool softeners). Report persistent dizziness or headache; excessive fatigue or sedation; changes in mental status; changes in urinary elimination or pain on urination; weakness or trembling; blurred vision; or shortness of breath. **Pregnancy/breast-feeding precautions:** Inform prescriber if you are or intend to become pregnant. If you are breast-feeding, take medication immediately after breast-feeding or 3-4 hours prior to next feeding.

Geriatric Considerations: The elderly may be particularly susceptible to the CNS depressant and constipating effects of narcotics.

Related Information

Narcotic/Opioid Analgesic Comparison *on page 1583*

Oxymorphone Hydrochloride *see* Oxymorphone *on page 1023*

Oxytetracycline and Hydrocortisone *see page 1509*

Oxytocin (oks i TOE sin)

U.S. Brand Names Pitocin®

Synonyms Pit

Generic Available Yes

Pharmacologic Category Oxytocic Agent

Pregnancy Risk Factor X

Lactation Excretion in breast milk unknown/contraindicated

Use Induces labor at term; controls postpartum bleeding

Mechanism of Action/Effect Produces rhythmic uterine contractions characteristic of delivery and stimulates breast milk flow during nursing

Contraindications Hypersensitivity to oxytocin or any component of the formulation; significant cephalopelvic disproportion; unfavorable fetal positions; fetal distress; hypertonic or hyperactive uterus; contraindicated vaginal delivery; prolapse, total placenta previa, and vasa previa

Warnings/Precautions To be used for medical rather than elective induction of labor. May produce antidiuretic effect (ie, water intoxication and excess uterine contractions). High doses or hypersensitivity to oxytocin may cause uterine hypertonicity, spasm, tetanic contraction, or rupture of the uterus. Severe water intoxication with convulsions, coma, and death has been associated with a slow oxytocin infusion over 24 hours.

Adverse Reactions

Fetal: <1% (Limited to important or life-threatening): Arrhythmias, bradycardia, brain damage, death, hypoxia, intracranial hemorrhage, neonatal jaundice

Maternal: <1% (Limited to important or life-threatening): Anaphylactic reactions, arrhythmias, coma, death, fatal afibrinogenemia, hypotension, increased blood loss, increased uterine motility, nausea, pelvic hematoma, postpartum hemorrhage, premature ventricular contractions, seizures, SIADH with hyponatremia, tachycardia, vomiting

Overdosage/Toxicology Symptoms of overdose include tetanic uterine contractions, impaired uterine blood flow, amniotic fluid embolism, uterine rupture, SIADH, and seizures. Treatment is symptom-directed and supportive.

Pharmacodynamics/Kinetics

Half-Life Elimination: 1-5 minutes

Metabolism: Rapidly hepatic and via plasma (by oxytocinase) and to a smaller degree the mammary gland

Onset: Uterine contractions: I.V.: ~1 minute

Duration: <30 minutes

Formulations

Injection, solution: 10 units/mL (1 mL, 10 mL)
Pitocin®: 10 units/mL (1 mL)

Dosing

Adults: I.V. administration requires the use of an infusion pump.

Induction of labor: I.V.: 0.001-0.002 units/minute; increase by 0.001-0.002 units every 15-30 minutes until contraction pattern has been established; maximum dose should not exceed 20 milliunits/minute.

Postpartum bleeding:
I.M.: Total dose of 10 units after delivery
I.V.: 10-40 units by I.V. infusion in 1000 mL of intravenous fluid at a rate sufficient to control uterine atony

Administration

I.V.: Sodium chloride 0.9% (NS) and dextrose 5% in water (D_5W) have been recommended as diluents; dilute 10-40 units to 1 L in NS, LR, or D_5W.

Stability

Storage: Oxytocin should be stored at 2°C to 8°C and protected from freezing.

Compatibility: Stable in dextran 6% in dextrose, dextran 6% in NS, D_5LR, $D_5{}^1/_4NS$, $D_5{}^1/_2NS$, D_5NS, D_5W, $D_{10}W$, LR, $^1/_2NS$, NS

Compatibility when admixed: Incompatible with fibrinolysin (human), norepinephrine, prochlorperazine edisylate, warfarin

Monitoring and Teaching Issues

Physical Assessment: I.V., I.M.: Monitor blood pressure, fluid intake and output, and labor closely if using oxytocin for induction; fetal monitoring is strongly recommended (see Adverse Reactions). **Pregnancy risk factor X.** Breast-feeding is contraindicated.

Patient Education: I.V./I.M.: Generally used in emergency situations. Drug teaching should be incorporated in other situational teaching. **Breast-feeding precaution:** Do not breast-feed.

Oyst-Cal 500 [OTC] *see* Calcium Supplements *on page 202*
Oystercal® 500 *see* Calcium Supplements *on page 202*
P-071 *see* Cetirizine *on page 263*
Pacerone® *see* Amiodarone *on page 81*

Paclitaxel (PAK li taks el)

U.S. Brand Names Onxol™; Taxol®

Generic Available Yes

Pharmacologic Category Antineoplastic Agent, Natural Source (Plant) Derivative

Pregnancy Risk Factor D

Lactation Enters breast milk/contraindicated

Use Treatment of advanced carcinoma of the ovary in combination with cisplatin; treatment of metastatic carcinoma of the ovary after failure of first-line or subsequent chemotherapy; adjuvant treatment of node-positive breast cancer administered sequentially to standard doxorubicin-containing chemotherapy; treatment of metastatic breast cancer after failure of combination chemotherapy or relapse within 6 months of adjuvant chemotherapy; treatment of nonsmall cell lung cancer; second-line treatment of AIDS-related Kaposi's sarcoma

Mechanism of Action/Effect Paclitaxel exerts its effects on microtubules and their protein subunits, tubulin dimers. Paclitaxel promotes microtubule assembly by enhancing the action of tubulin dimers, stabilizing existing microtubules, and inhibiting their disassembly. Maintaining microtubule assembly inhibits mitosis and affecting cell death. The G_2- and M-phases of the cell cycle are affected. In addition, the drug can distort mitotic spindles, resulting in the breakage of chromosomes.

Contraindications Hypersensitivity to paclitaxel or any component of the formulation; pregnancy

Warnings/Precautions The FDA currently recommends that procedures for proper handling and disposal of antineoplastic agents be considered. All patients should be premedicated prior to Taxol® administration to prevent severe hypersensitivity reactions. Current evidence indicates that prolongation of the infusion (to ≥6 hours) plus premedication may minimize this effect.

Appropriate safety equipment is recommended for preparation, administration, and disposal of antineoplastics. If paclitaxel contacts the skin, wash and flush thoroughly with water.

When administered as sequential infusions, taxane derivatives (docetaxel, paclitaxel) should be administered before platinum derivatives (carboplatin, cisplatin) to limit myelosuppression and to enhance efficacy.

Elderly patients have an increased risk of toxicity (neutropenia, neuropathy).

Drug Interactions

Cytochrome P450 Effect: Substrate of **CYP2C8/9, 3A4**; Induces CYP3A4

Decreased Effect: Paclitaxel metabolism is dependent on cytochrome P450 isoenzymes. Inducers of these enzymes may decrease the effect of paclitaxel.

Increased Effect/Toxicity: In Phase I trials, myelosuppression was more profound when given after cisplatin than with alternative sequence. Pharmacokinetic data demonstrates a decrease in clearance of ~33% when administered following cisplatin. Possibility of an inhibition of metabolism in patients treated with ketoconazole. When administered as sequential infusions, observational studies indicate a potential for increased toxicity when platinum derivatives (carboplatin, cisplatin) are administered before taxane derivatives (docetaxel, paclitaxel).

(Continued)

Paclitaxel *(Continued)*

Nutritional/Ethanol Interactions Herb/Nutraceutical: Avoid black cohosh, dong quai in estrogen-dependent tumors. Avoid valerian, St John's wort, kava kava, gotu kola (may increase CNS depression).

Adverse Reactions

>10%:

Allergic: Appear to be primarily nonimmunologically mediated release of histamine and other vasoactive substances; almost always seen within the first hour of an infusion (~75% occur within 10 minutes of starting the infusion); incidence is significantly reduced by premedication

Cardiovascular: Bradycardia (transient, 25%)

Hematologic: Myelosuppression, leukopenia, neutropenia (6% to 21%), thrombocytopenia

Onset: 8-11 days

Nadir: 15-21 days

Recovery: 21 days

Dermatologic: Alopecia (87%), venous erythema, tenderness, discomfort, phlebitis (2%)

Neurotoxicity: Sensory and/or autonomic neuropathy (numbness, tingling, burning pain), myopathy or myopathic effects (25% to 55%), and central nervous system toxicity. May be cumulative and dose-limiting.

Gastrointestinal: Severe, potentially dose-limiting mucositis, stomatitis (15%), most common at doses >390 mg/m^2

Hepatic: Mild increases in liver enzymes

Neuromuscular & skeletal: Arthralgia, myalgia

1% to 10%:

Cardiovascular: Myocardial infarction

Gastrointestinal: Mild nausea and vomiting (5% to 6%), diarrhea (5% to 6%)

Hematologic: Anemia

<1% (Limited to important or life-threatening): Ataxia, atrial fibrillation, enterocolitis, hepatic encephalopathy, intestinal obstruction, interstitial pneumonia, necrotic changes and ulceration following extravasation, neuroencephalopathy, ototoxicity (tinnitus and hearing loss), pancreatitis, paralytic ileus, pruritus, pulmonary fibrosis, radiation recall, radiation pneumonitis, rash, seizures, Stevens-Johnson syndrome, toxic epidermal necrolysis, visual disturbances (scintillating scotomata)

Pharmacodynamics/Kinetics

Half-Life Elimination: Mean: Terminal: 5.3-17.4 hours after 1- and 6-hour infusions at dosing levels of 15-275 mg/m^2

Metabolism: Hepatic in animals; evidence suggests similar in humans

Formulations

Injection, solution: 6 mg/mL (5 mL, 16.7 mL, 50 mL)

Onxol™: 6 mg/mL (5 mL, 25 mL, 50 mL) [contains alcohol]

Taxol®: 6 mg/mL (5 mL, 16.7 mL, 50 mL) [contains alcohol]

Dosing

Adults & Elderly: Premedication with dexamethasone (20 mg orally or I.V. at 12 and 6 hours **or** 14 and 7 hours before the dose), diphenhydramine (50 mg I.V. 30-60 minutes prior to the dose), and cimetidine, famotidine or ranitidine (I.V. 30-60 minutes prior to the dose) is recommended

Ovarian carcinoma: I.V.:

First-line therapy: 175 mg/m^2 over 3 hours every 3 weeks

or 135 mg/m^2 over 24 hours every 3 weeks

After failure of first-line therapy: 135-175 mg/m^2 over 3 hours every 3 weeks (doses up to 350 mg/m^2 have been studied, but are not generally recommended)

or 50-80 mg/m^2 over 1-3 hours weekly

or 1.4-4 mg/m^2/day continuous infusion for 14 days every 4 weeks

Metastatic breast cancer: I.V.:

Adjuvant treatment of node-positive breast cancer: 175 mg/m^2 over 3 hours every 3 weeks for 4 courses

Metastatic or recurrent disease: 175 mg/m^2 over 3 hours every 3 weeks

Nonsmall cell lung carcinoma: I.V.: 135 mg/m^2 over 24 hours, followed by cisplatin 75 mg/m^2; repeat every 3 weeks

AIDS-related Kaposi's sarcoma: I.V.: 135 mg/m^2 over 3 hours every 3 weeks **or** 100 mg/m^2 over 3 hours every 2 weeks

Dosage modification for toxicity (solid tumors, including ovary, breast, and lung carcinoma): Courses of paclitaxel should not be repeated until the neutrophil count is ≥1500 cells/mm^3 and the platelet count is ≥100,000 cells/mm^3; reduce dosage by 20% for patients experiencing severe peripheral neuropathy or severe neutropenia (neutrophil <500 cells/mm^3 for a week or longer)

Dosage modification for immunosuppression in advanced HIV disease: Paclitaxel should not be given to patients with HIV if the baseline or subsequent neutrophil count is <1000 cells/mm^3. Additional modifications include: Reduce dosage of dexamethasone in premedication to 10 mg orally; reduce dosage by 20% in patients experiencing severe peripheral neuropathy or severe neutropenia (neutrophil <500 cells/mm^3 for a week or longer); initiate concurrent hematopoietic growth factor (G-CSF) as clinically indicated

Renal Impairment:

Hemodialysis: Significant drug removal is unlikely based on physiochemical characteristics.

Peritoneal dialysis: Significant drug removal is unlikely based on physiochemical characteristics.

Hepatic Impairment:

Total bilirubin ≤1.5 mg/dL and AST >2x normal limits: Total dose <135 mg/m^2

Total bilirubin 1.6-3.0 mg/dL: Total dose ≤75 mg/m^2

Total bilirubin ≥3.1 mg/dL: Total dose ≤50 mg/m^2

Administration

I.V.: Irritant. Manufacturer recommends administration over 1-24 hours. Other routes are being studied. When administered as sequential infusions, taxane derivatives should be administered before platinum derivatives (cisplatin, carboplatin) to limit myelosuppression and to enhance efficacy.

Anaphylactoid-like reactions have been reported: Corticosteroids (dexamethasone), H_1-antagonists (diphenhydramine), and H_2-antagonists (famotidine), should be administered prior to paclitaxel administration to minimize potential for anaphylaxis

Administer I.V. infusion over 1-24 hours; use of a 0.22 micron in-line filter is recommended during the infusion

Nonpolyvinyl (non-PVC) tubing (eg, polyethylene) should be used to minimize leaching. Formulated in a vehicle known as Cremophor® EL (polyoxyethylated castor oil). Cremophor® EL has been found to leach the plasticizer DEHP from polyvinyl chloride infusion bags or administration sets. Contact of the undiluted concentrate with plasticized polyvinyl chloride (PVC) equipment or devices is not recommended. Administer through I.V. tubing containing an in-line (NOT >0.22 μ) filter; administration through IVEX-2® filters (which incorporate short inlet and outlet polyvinyl chloride-coated tubing) has not resulted in significant leaching of DEHP.

Stability

Storage: Store intact vials at room temperature of 20°C to 25°C (68°F to 77°F).

Reconstitution: Further dilution in NS or D_5W to a concentration of 0.3-1.2 mg/mL is stable for up to 27 hours at room temperature (25°C) and ambient light conditions.

Standard I.V. dilution: IVPB: Dose/500-1000 mL D_5W or NS

Solutions are stable for 27 hours at room temperature (25°C).

Paclitaxel should be dispensed in either glass or Excel™/PAB™ containers. Should also use **nonpolyvinyl** (non-PVC) tubing (eg, polyethylene) to minimize leaching.

Compatibility: Stable in D_5LR, D_5NS, NS

Y-site administration: Incompatible with amphotericin B, amphotericin B cholesteryl sulfate complex, chlorpromazine, doxorubicin liposome, hydroxyzine, methylprednisolone sodium succinate, mitoxantrone

Monitoring Laboratory Tests CBC with differential and platelet count, liver and kidney function

Monitoring and Teaching Issues

Physical Assessment: See Contraindications, Warnings/Precautions, and Dosing for use cautions. Assess potential for interactions with other prescriptions, OTC medications, or herbal products patient may be taking (see Drug Interactions). See above for infusion specifics. Premedication prior to infusion is recommended (see Dosing). Infusion site should be monitored to prevent extravasation. Assess results of laboratory tests (see above) prior to and regularly during therapy. Assess therapeutic effectiveness and adverse response (eg, peripheral neuropathy, myelosuppression, opportunistic infection, and hypersensitivity - see Adverse Reactions and Overdose/Toxicology). Teach patient possible side effects and appropriate interventions and adverse symptoms to report (see Patient Education). **Pregnancy risk factor D** - determine that patient is not pregnant before beginning treatment. Instruct patients of childbearing age about appropriate barrier contraceptive measures. Breast-feeding is contraindicated.

Patient Education: Inform prescriber of all prescriptions, OTC medications, or herbal products you are taking, and any allergies you have. Do not take anything new during treatment unless approved by prescriber. This drug can only be given by infusion. Report immediately any redness, swelling, burning, pain at infusion site or signs of allergic reaction (eg, difficulty breathing or swallowing, chest tightness, rash, hives, swelling of lips or mouth). Maintain adequate hydration (2-3 L/day of fluids) unless advised by prescriber to restrict fluids, and nutrition. You will be more susceptible to infection (avoid crowds and exposure to infection and do not have any vaccinations without consulting prescriber). May cause loss of hair (will grow back after therapy); experience nausea or vomiting (consult prescriber for approved antiemetic); feel weak or lethargic (use caution when driving or engaging in tasks that require alertness until response to drug is known); or mouth sores (use good oral care, bush with soft toothbrush and use waxed dental floss). Report numbness or tingling in fingers or toes (use care to prevent injury); signs of opportunistic infection (fever, chills, sore throat, burning urination, fatigue); unusual bleeding (tarry stools, easy bruising, or blood in stool, urine, or mouth); unresolved mouth sores; nausea or vomiting; or skin rash or itching. **Pregnancy/breast-feeding precautions:** Do not get pregnant while taking this medication. Consult prescriber for appropriate barrier contraceptive measures. Do not breast-feed.

Geriatric Considerations: Elderly patients may have a higher incidence of severe neuropathy, severe myelosuppression, or cardiovascular events as compared to younger patients.

Breast-feeding Issues: Antineoplastic agents are generally contraindicated.

Additional Information Sensory neuropathy is almost universal at doses >250 mg/m^2; motor neuropathy is uncommon at doses <250 mg/m^2. Myopathic effects are common with doses >200 mg/m^2, generally occur within 2-3 days of treatment, and resolve over 5-6 days. Patients with pre-existing neuropathies from chemotherapy or coexisting conditions (eg, diabetes mellitus) may be at a higher risk.

Palgic®-D *see* Carbinoxamine and Pseudoephedrine *on page 217*

Palgic®-DS *see* Carbinoxamine and Pseudoephedrine *on page 217*

Palmer's® Skin Success Fade Cream™ [OTC] *see* Hydroquinone *on page 679*

Pamelor® *see* Nortriptyline *on page 986*

Pamidronate (pa mi DROE nate)

U.S. Brand Names Aredia®

Synonyms Pamidronate Disodium

Generic Available Yes

Pharmacologic Category Antidote; Bisphosphonate Derivative

(Continued)

Pamidronate *(Continued)*

Pregnancy Risk Factor D

Lactation Excretion in breast milk unknown/use caution

Use Treatment of hypercalcemia associated with malignancy; treatment of osteolytic bone lesions associated with multiple myeloma or metastatic breast cancer; moderate to severe Paget's disease of bone

Mechanism of Action/Effect A biphosphonate which inhibits bone resorption via actions on osteoclasts or on osteoclast precursors. Does not appear to produce any significant effects on renal tubular calcium handling and is poorly absorbed following oral administration (high oral doses have been reported effective); therefore, I.V. therapy is preferred.

Contraindications Hypersensitivity to pamidronate, other biphosphonates, or any component of the formulation; pregnancy

Warnings/Precautions May cause deterioration in renal function. Use caution in patients with renal impairment and avoid in severe renal impairment. Assess serum creatinine prior to each dose; withhold dose in patients with bone metastases who experience deterioration in renal function. Leukopenia has been observed with oral pamidronate and monitoring of white blood cell counts is suggested. Vein irritation and thrombophlebitis may occur with infusions. In elderly patients, monitor serum electrolytes periodically since elderly are often receiving diuretics which can result in decreases in serum calcium, potassium, and magnesium.

Adverse Reactions As reported with hypercalcemia of malignancy; percentage of adverse effect varies upon dose and duration of infusion.

>10%:
- Central nervous system: Fever (18% to 26%), fatigue (12%)
- Endocrine & metabolic: Hypophosphatemia (9% to 18%), hypokalemia (4% to 18%), hypomagnesemia (4% to 12%), hypocalcemia (1% to 12%)
- Gastrointestinal: Nausea (up to 18%), anorexia (1% to 12%)
- Local: Infusion site reaction (up to 18%)

1% to 10%:
- Cardiovascular: Atrial fibrillation (0% to 6%), hypertension (up to 6%), syncope (up to 6%), tachycardia (up to 6%), atrial flutter (up to 1%), cardiac failure (up to 1%)
- Central nervous system: Somnolence (1% to 6%), psychosis (up to 4%), insomnia (up to 1%)
- Endocrine & metabolic: Hypothyroidism (6%)
- Gastrointestinal: Constipation (4% to 6%), stomatitis (up to 1%)
- Hematologic: Leukopenia (up to 4%), neutropenia (up to 1%), thrombocytopenia (up to 1%)
- Neuromuscular & skeletal: Myalgia (up to 1%)
- Renal: Uremia (up to 4%)
- Respiratory: Rales (up to 6%), rhinitis (up to 6%), upper respiratory tract infection (up to 3%)

<1% (Limited to important or life-threatening): Allergic reaction, anaphylactic shock, angioedema, episcleritis, hypotension, iritis, scleritis, uveitis

Overdosage/Toxicology Symptoms of overdose include hypocalcemia, EKG changes, seizures, bleeding, paresthesia, carpopedal spasm, and fever. Treat with I.V. calcium gluconate, and general supportive care; fever and hypotension can be treated with corticosteroids.

Pharmacodynamics/Kinetics

Absorption: Poor; pharmacokinetic studies lacking

Half-Life Elimination: 21-35 hours; Bone: Terminal: ~300 days

Metabolism: Not metabolized

Onset: 24-48 hours; Peak effect: Maximum: 5-7 days

Formulations Injection, powder for reconstitution: 30 mg, 90 mg

Dosing

Adults & Elderly: Drug must be diluted properly before administration and infused intravenously slowly. Due to risk of nephrotoxicity, doses should not exceed 90 mg.

Hypercalcemia of malignancy: I.V.:

Moderate cancer-related hypercalcemia (corrected serum calcium: 12-13.5 mg/dL): 60-90 mg, as a single dose, given as a slow infusion over 2-24 hours; dose should be diluted in 1000 mL 0.45% NaCl, 0.9% NaCl, or D_5W

Severe cancer-related hypercalcemia (corrected serum calcium: >13.5 mg/dL): 90 mg, as a single dose, as a slow infusion over 2-24 hours; dose should be diluted in 1000 mL 0.45% NaCl, 0.9% NaCl, or D_5W

A period of 7 days should elapse before the use of second course; repeat infusions every 2-3 weeks have been suggested, however, could be administered every 2-3 months according to the degree and of severity of hypercalcemia and/or the type of malignancy.

Note: Some investigators have suggested a lack of a dose-response relationship. Courses of pamidronate for hypercalcemia may be repeated at varying intervals, depending on the duration of normocalcemia (median 2-3 weeks), but the manufacturer recommends a minimum interval between courses of 7 days. Oral etidronate at a dose of 20 mg/kg/day has been used to maintain the calcium lowering effect following I.V. bisphosphonates, although it is of limited effectiveness.

Osteolytic bone lesions with multiple myeloma: I.V.: 90 mg in 500 mL D_5W, 0.45% NaCl or 0.9% NaCl administered over 4 hours on a monthly basis

Osteolytic bone lesions with metastatic breast cancer: I.V.: 90 mg in 250 mL D_5W, 0.45% NaCl or 0.9% NaCl administered over 2 hours, repeated every 3-4 weeks

Paget's disease: I.V.: 30 mg in 500 mL 0.45% NaCl, 0.9% NaCl or D_5W administered over 4 hours for 3 consecutive days

Renal Impairment: Not recommended in severe renal impairment (patients with bone metastases).

Dosing adjustment in renal toxicity: In patients with bone metastases, treatment should be withheld in patients who experience deterioration in renal function (increase of serum creatinine ≥0.5 mg/dL in patients with normal baseline or ≥1.0 mg/dL in patients with abnormal baseline). Resumption of therapy may be considered when serum creatinine returns to within 10% of baseline.

Administration

I.V.: Drug must be properly diluted before administration and slowly infused intravenously (over at least 2 hours).

Stability

Storage: Do not store powder for reconstitution at temperatures above 30°C (86°F).

Reconstitution: Reconstitute by adding 10 mL of sterile water for injection to each vial of lyophilized pamidronate disodium powder, the resulting solution will be 30 mg/10 mL or 90 mg/10 mL. The reconstituted solution is stable under refrigeration at 2°C to 8°C (36°F to 46°F) for 24 hours.

Pamidronate may be further diluted in 250-1000 mL of 0.45% or 0.9% sodium chloride or 5% dextrose; pamidronate should not be mixed with calcium-containing solutions (eg, Ringer's solution). Pamidronate solution for infusion is stable at room temperature for up to 24 hours.

Compatibility: Incompatible with calcium-containing infusion solutions such as lactated Ringer's

Monitoring Laboratory Tests Serum electrolytes, monitor for hypocalcemia for at least 2 weeks after therapy; serum calcium, phosphate, magnesium, CBC with differential; monitor serum creatinine prior to each dose

Monitoring and Teaching Issues

Physical Assessment: Monitor laboratory results (see above) and assess for signs of hypocalcemia. Ensure adequate hydration. **Pregnancy risk factor D** - assess knowledge/instruct patient on need to use appropriate contraceptive measures and the need to avoid pregnancy. Note breast-feeding caution.

Patient Education: This medication can only be administered intravenously. Avoid foods high in calcium or vitamins with minerals during infusion or for 2-3 hours after completion. You may experience nausea or vomiting (small, frequent meals and good mouth care may help); or recurrent bone pain (consult prescriber for analgesic). Report unusual muscle twitching or spasms, severe diarrhea/constipation, or acute bone pain. **Pregnancy/breast-feeding precautions:** Inform prescriber if you are or intend to become pregnant. Consult prescriber if breast-feeding.

Geriatric Considerations: Has not been studied exclusively in the elderly. Monitor serum electrolytes periodically since elderly are often receiving diuretics which can result in decreases in serum calcium, potassium, and magnesium.

Pregnancy Issues: Pamidronate has been shown to cross the placenta and cause embryo/fetal effects in animals. There are no adequate and well-controlled studies in pregnant women; use is not recommended during pregnancy.

Pamidronate Disodium *see* Pamidronate *on page 1027*

Pancrease® *see* Pancrelipase *on page 1029*

Pancrease® MT *see* Pancrelipase *on page 1029*

Pancrecarb MS® *see* Pancrelipase *on page 1029*

Pancrelipase (pan kre LI pase)

U.S. Brand Names Creon®; Ku-Zyme® HP; Lipram®; Lipram® 4500; Lipram-CR®; Lipram-PN®; Lipram-UL®; Pancrease®; Pancrease® MT; Pancrecarb MS®; Pangestyme™ CN; Pangestyme™ EC; Pangestyme™ MT; Pangestyme™ UL; Ultrase®; Ultrase® MT; Viokase®; Zymase® [DSC]

Synonyms Lipancreatin

Generic Available Yes

Pharmacologic Category Enzyme

Pregnancy Risk Factor B/C (product specific)

Lactation Excretion in breast milk unknown/use caution

Use Replacement therapy in symptomatic treatment of malabsorption syndrome caused by pancreatic insufficiency

Use - Unlabeled/Investigational Treatment of occluded feeding tubes

Mechanism of Action/Effect Replaces endogenous pancreatic enzymes to assist in digestion of protein, starch and fats

Contraindications Hypersensitivity to pork protein or any component of the formulation; acute pancreatitis or acute exacerbations of chronic pancreatic disease

Warnings/Precautions Pancrelipase is inactivated by acids. Use microencapsulated products whenever possible, since these products permit better dissolution of enzymes in the duodenum and protect the enzyme preparations from acid degradation in the stomach. Fibrotic strictures in the colon, some requiring surgery, have been reported with high doses; use caution, especially in children with cystic fibrosis. Use caution when adjusting doses or changing brands. Avoid inhalation of powder, may cause nasal and respiratory tract irritation. Pregnancy risk B/C (product specific).

Nutritional/Ethanol Interactions Food: Avoid placing contents of opened capsules on alkaline food (pH >5.5); pancrelipase may impair absorption of oral iron and folic acid.

Adverse Reactions Frequency not defined; occurrence of events may be dose related.

Central nervous system: Pain

Dermatologic: Rash

Endocrine & metabolic: Hyperuricemia

Gastrointestinal: Nausea, cramps, constipation, diarrhea, perianal irritation/inflammation (large doses), irritation of the mouth, abdominal pain, intestinal obstruction, vomiting, flatulence, melena, weight loss, fibrotic strictures, greasy stools

Ocular: Lacrimation

Renal: Hyperuricosuria

Respiratory: Sneezing, dyspnea, bronchospasm

Miscellaneous: Allergic reactions

Overdosage/Toxicology Symptoms of overdose include diarrhea, other transient intestinal upset, hyperuricosuria, and hyperuricemia. Treatment is supportive.

(Continued)

Pancrelipase *(Continued)*

Pharmacodynamics/Kinetics

Absorption: None; acts locally in GI tract

Formulations

Capsule: Ku-Zyme® HP: Lipase 8000 units, protease 30,000 units, amylase 30,000 units

Capsule, delayed release:
- Lipram 4500: Lipase 4500 units, protease 25000 units, amylase 20000 units
- Pangestyme™ CN-10: Lipase 10,000 units, protease 37,500 units, amylase 33,200 units
- Pangestyme™ CN-20: Lipase 20,000 units, protease 75,000 units, amylase 66,400 units

Capsule, delayed release, enteric coated microspheres:
- Creon® 5: Lipase 5000 units, protease 18,750 units, amylase 16,600 units
- Creon® 10, Lipram-CR10®: Lipase 10,000 units, protease 37,500 units, amylase 33,200 units
- Creon® 20, Lipram-CR20®: Lipase 20,000 units, protease 75,000 units, amylase 66,400 units
- Lipram-PN10®: Lipase 10,000 units, protease 30,000 units, amylase 39,000 units
- Lipram-PN16®: Lipase 16,000 units, protease 48,000 units, amylase 48,000 units
- Lipram-UL12®: Lipase 12,000 units, protease 39,000 units, amylase 39,000 units
- Lipram-UL18®: Lipase 18,000 units, protease 58,500 units, amylase 58,500 units
- Lipram-UL20®: Lipase 20,000 units, protease 65,000 units, amylase 65,000 units
- Pancrecarb MS-4®: Lipase 4000 units, protease 25,000 units, amylase 25,000 units
- Pancrecarb MS-8®: Lipase 8000 units, protease 45,000 units, amylase 40,000 units

Capsule, delayed release, enteric coated spheres: Zymase®: Lipase 12,000 units, protease 24,000 units, amylase 24,000 units [DSC]

Capsule, enteric-coated microspheres
- Pancrease®, Pangestyme™ EC: Lipase 4500 units, protease 25,000 units, amylase 20,000 units
- Ultrase®: Lipase 4500 units, protease 25,000 units, amylase 20,000 units

Capsule, enteric coated microtablets:
- Pancrease® MT 4: Lipase 4000 units, protease 12,000 units, amylase 12,000 units
- Pancrease® MT 10: Lipase 10,000 units, protease 30,000 units, amylase 30,000 units
- Pancrease® MT 16, Pangestyme™ MT 16: Lipase 16,000 units, protease 48,000 units, amylase 48,000 units
- Pancrease® MT 20: Lipase 20,000 units, protease 44,000 units, amylase 56,000 units
- Pangestyme™ UL 12: Lipase 12,000 units, protease 39,000 units, amylase 39,000 units
- Pangestyme™ UL 18: Lipase 18,000 units, protease 58,500 units, amylase 58,500 units
- Pangestyme™ UL 20: Lipase 20,000 units, protease 65,000 units, amylase 65,000 units

Capsule, enteric coated minitablets:
- Ultrase® MT12: Lipase 12,000 units, protease 39,000 units, amylase 39,000 units
- Ultrase® MT18: Lipase 18,000 units, protease 58,500 units, amylase 58,500 units
- Ultrase® MT20: Lipase 20,000 units, protease 65,000 units, amylase 65,000 units

Powder (Viokase®): Lipase 16,800 units, protease 70,000 units, amylase 70,000 units per 0.7 g (227 g)

Tablet:
- Viokase® 8: Lipase 8000 units, protease 30,000 units, amylase 30,000 units
- Viokase® 16: Lipase 16,000 units, protease 60,000 units, amylase 60,000 units

Dosing

Adults & Elderly:

Malabsorption: Oral:

Powder: Actual dose depends on the condition being treated and the digestive requirements of the patient: 0.7 g (1/4 teaspoonful) with meals

Capsules/tablets: The following dosage recommendations are only an approximation for initial dosages. The actual dosage will depend on the condition being treated and the digestive requirements of the individual patient. Adjust dose based on body weight and stool fat content. Total daily dose reflects ~3 meals/day and 2-3 snacks/day, with half the mealtime dose given with a snack. Older patients may need less units/kg due to increased weight, but decreased ingestion of fat/kg. Maximum dose: 2500 units of lipase/kg/meal (10,000 units of lipase/kg/day): 4000-48,000 units of lipase with meals and with snacks

Occluded feeding tubes: One tablet of Viokase® crushed with one 325 mg tablet of sodium bicarbonate (to activate the Viokase®) in 5 mL of water can be instilled into the nasogastric tube and clamped for 5 minutes; then, flushed with 50 mL of tap water

Pediatrics: Malabsorption: Oral:

Powder: Actual dose depends on the condition being treated and the digestive requirements of the patient: Children <1 year: Start with 1/8 teaspoonful with feedings

Capsules/tablets: The following dosage recommendations are only an approximation for initial dosages. The actual dosage will depend on the condition being treated and the digestive requirements of the individual patient. Adjust dose based on body weight and stool fat content. Total daily dose reflects ~3 meals/day and 2-3 snacks/day, with half the mealtime dose given with a snack.

Children:
- <1 year: 2000 units of lipase with meals
- 1-6 years: 4000-8000 units of lipase with meals and 4000 units with snacks
- 7-12 years: 4000-12,000 units of lipase with meals and snacks

Administration

Oral: Oral: Administer with meals or snacks and swallow whole with a generous amount of liquid. Do not crush or chew; retention in the mouth before swallowing may cause mucosal irritation and stomatitis. Delayed-release capsules containing enteric-coated microspheres or microtablets may also be opened and the contents sprinkled on soft food with a low pH that does not require chewing, such as applesauce, gelatin; apricot, banana, or sweet potato baby food; baby formula. Dairy products such as milk, custard, or ice cream may have a high pH and should be avoided. Avoid inhalation of powder, may cause nasal and respiratory tract irritation.

Stability

Storage: Store between 15°C to 25°C (59°F to 77°F). Keep in a dry place. Do not refrigerate.

Monitoring and Teaching Issues

Physical Assessment: See Contraindications, Warnings/Precautions, Drug Interactions, and Dosing for use cautions. If powder spills on skin, wash off immediately, do not inhale powder when preparing. Assess patient response (see Adverse Reactions and Overdose/Toxicology). Teach patient proper use, possible side effects and appropriate interventions and adverse symptoms to report (see Patient Education). **Pregnancy risk factor B/C** - see Pregnancy Risk Factor for use cautions; benefits of use should outweigh possible risks. Note breast-feeding caution.

Patient Education: Inform prescriber of all prescriptions, OTC medications, or herbal products you are taking, and any allergies you have. Do not take anything new during treatment unless approved by prescriber. Take right before or with meals. Avoid taking with alkaline food. Do not chew, crush, or dissolve delayed release capsules; swallow whole. If powder spills on skin, wash off immediately, do not inhale powder when preparing. You may experience some gastric discomfort. Report unusual rash, persistent GI upset; or difficulty breathing. **Pregnancy/breast-feeding precautions:** Inform prescriber if you are or intend to become pregnant. Consult prescriber if breast-feeding.

Dietary Issues: Should be used as part of a high-calorie diet, appropriate for age and clinical status. Administer with meals or snacks and swallow whole with a generous amount of liquid. Do not crush or chew. Delayed-release capsules containing enteric coated microspheres or microtablets may also be opened and the contents sprinkled on soft food with a low pH such as applesauce, gelatin; apricot, banana, or sweet potato baby food; baby formula. Dairy products such as milk, custard or ice cream may have a high pH and should be avoided.

Geriatric Considerations: No special considerations are necessary since drug is dosed to response; however, drug-induced diarrhea can result in unwanted side effects (confusion, hypotension, lethargy, fluid and electrolyte loss).

Breast-feeding Issues: Systemic absorption and concentration in the breast milk is unlikely, but unknown.

Pancuronium (pan kyoo ROE nee um)

U.S. Brand Names Pavulon®

Synonyms Pancuronium Bromide

Generic Available Yes

Pharmacologic Category Neuromuscular Blocker Agent, Nondepolarizing

Pregnancy Risk Factor C

Lactation Excretion in breast milk unknown/not recommended

Use Adjunct to general anesthesia to facilitate endotracheal intubation and to relax skeletal muscles during surgery; to facilitate mechanical ventilation in ICU patients; does not relieve pain or produce sedation

Drug of choice for neuromuscular blockade except in patients with renal failure, hepatic failure, or cardiovascular instability or in situations not suited for pancuronium's long duration of action

Mechanism of Action/Effect Blocks neural transmission at the myoneural junction by binding with cholinergic receptor sites

Contraindications Hypersensitivity to pancuronium, bromide, or any component of the formulation

Warnings/Precautions Ventilation must be supported during neuromuscular blockade; use with caution in patients with renal and/or hepatic impairment (adjust dose appropriately); certain clinical conditions may result in potentiation or antagonism of neuromuscular blockade:

Potentiation: Electrolyte abnormalities, severe hyponatremia, severe hypocalcemia, severe hypokalemia, hypermagnesemia, neuromuscular diseases, acidosis, acute intermittent porphyria, renal failure, hepatic failure

Antagonism: Alkalosis, hypercalcemia, demyelinating lesions, peripheral neuropathies, diabetes mellitus

Increased sensitivity in patients with myasthenia gravis, Eaton-Lambert syndrome; resistance in burn patients (>30% of body) for period of 5-70 days postinjury; resistance in patients with muscle trauma, denervation, immobilization, infection.

Pregnancy risk C.

Drug Interactions

Decreased Effect: Effect of nondepolarizing neuromuscular blockers may be reduced by carbamazepine (chronic use), corticosteroids (also associated with myopathy - see increased effect), phenytoin (chronic use), sympathomimetics, and theophylline.

Increased Effect/Toxicity: Increased effects are possible with aminoglycosides, beta-blockers, clindamycin, calcium channel blockers, halogenated anesthetics, imipenem, ketamine, lidocaine, loop diuretics (furosemide), macrolides (case reports), magnesium sulfate, procainamide, quinidine, quinolones, tetracyclines, and vancomycin. May increase risk of myopathy when used with high-dose corticosteroids for extended periods.

Adverse Reactions Frequency not defined.

Cardiovascular: Elevation in pulse rate, elevated blood pressure and cardiac output, tachycardia, edema, skin flushing, circulatory collapse

Dermatologic: Rash, itching, erythema, burning sensation along the vein

Gastrointestinal: Excessive salivation

Neuromuscular & skeletal: Profound muscle weakness

Respiratory: Wheezing, bronchospasm

Miscellaneous: Hypersensitivity reaction

Overdosage/Toxicology Symptoms of overdose include apnea, respiratory depression, and cardiovascular collapse. Pyridostigmine, neostigmine, or edrophonium in conjunction with atropine will usually antagonize the action of pancuronium.

(Continued)

Pancuronium *(Continued)*

Pharmacodynamics/Kinetics

Half-Life Elimination: 110 minutes

Metabolism: Hepatic (30% to 45%)

Onset: Peak effect: I.V.: 2-3 minutes

Duration: Dose dependent: 40-60 minutes

Formulations Injection, as bromide: 1 mg/mL (10 mL); 2 mg/mL (2 mL, 5 mL)

Dosing

Adults & Elderly: Administer I.V.; dose to effect; doses will vary due to interpatient variability; use ideal body weight for obese patients

Neuromuscular blockade: Initial: 0.06-0.1 mg/kg or 0.05 mg/kg after initial dose of succinylcholine for intubation; maintenance dose: 0.01 mg/kg 60-100 minutes after initial dose and then 0.01 mg/kg every 25-60 minutes

Pretreatment/priming: 10% of intubating dose given 3-5 minutes before initial dose

ICU: 0.05-0.1 mg/kg bolus followed by 0.8-1.7 mcg/kg/minute once initial recovery from bolus observed or 0.1-0.2 mg/kg every 1-3 hours

Pediatrics: Infants >1 month and Children: Refer to adult dosing.

Renal Impairment: Elimination half-life is doubled, plasma clearance is reduced, and rate of recovery is sometimes much slower.

Cl_{cr} 10-50 mL/minute: Administer 50% of normal dose.

Cl_{cr} <10 mL/minute: Do not use.

Hepatic Impairment: Elimination half-life is doubled, plasma clearance is doubled, recovery time is prolonged, volume of distribution is increased (50%) and results in a slower onset, higher total dosage, and prolongation of neuromuscular blockade. Patients with liver disease may develop slow resistance to nondepolarizing muscle relaxant. Large doses may be required and problems may arise in antagonism.

Administration

I.V.: May be administered undiluted by rapid I.V. injection.

Stability

Storage: Refrigerate; however, is stable for up to 6 months at room temperature.

Compatibility: Stable in D_5NS, D_5W, LR, NS

Y-site administration: Incompatible with diazepam, thiopental

Monitoring and Teaching Issues

Physical Assessment: Only clinicians experienced in the use of neuromuscular blocking drugs should administer and/or manage the use of pancuronium. Dosage and rate of administration should be individualized and titrated to the desired effect, according to relevant clinical factors, premedication, concomitant medications, age, and general condition of the patient. See Use, Contraindications, and Warnings/Precautions for appropriate use cautions. Ventilatory support must be instituted and maintained until adequate respiratory muscle function and/or airway protection are assured. Assess other medications for effectiveness and safety. Other drugs that affect neuromuscular activity may increase/decrease neuromuscular block induced by pancuronium. This drug does not cause anesthesia or analgesia; pain must be treated with appropriate analgesic agents. Continuous monitoring of vital signs, cardiac status, respiratory status, and degree of neuromuscular block (objective assessment with peripheral external nerve stimulator) is mandatory and until full muscle tone has returned (see Adverse Reactions). Muscle tone returns in a predictable pattern, starting with diaphragm, abdomen, chest, limbs, and finally muscles of the neck, face, and eyes. Safety precautions must be maintained until full muscle tone has returned. **Note:** It may take longer for return of muscle tone in obese or elderly patients or patients with renal or hepatic disease, myasthenia gravis, myopathy, other neuromuscular disease, dehydration, electrolyte imbalance, or severe acid/base imbalance. Provide appropriate patient teaching/support prior to and following administration.

Long-term use: Monitor fluid levels (intake and output) during and following infusion. Reposition patient and provide appropriate skin care, mouth care, and care of patient's eyes every 2-3 hours while sedated. Provide appropriate emotional and sensory support (auditory and environmental).

Pregnancy risk factor C. Note breast-feeding caution.

Patient Education: Patient will usually be unconscious prior to administration. Patient education should be appropriate to individual situation. Reassurance of constant monitoring and emotional support to reduce fear and anxiety should precede and follow administration. Following return of muscle tone, do not attempt to change position or rise from bed without assistance. Report immediately any skin rash or hives, pounding heartbeat, difficulty breathing, or muscle tremors. **Pregnancy/breast-feeding precautions:** Inform prescriber if you are pregnant. Consult prescriber if breast-feeding.

Additional Information Pancuronium is classified as a long-duration neuromuscular-blocking agent. Neuromuscular blockade will be prolonged in patients with decreased renal function. Pancuronium does not relieve pain or produce sedation. It may produce cumulative effect on duration of blockade. It produces tachycardia secondary to vagolytic activity and sympathetic stimulation.

Pancuronium Bromide *see* Pancuronium *on page 1031*

Pandel® *see* Hydrocortisone *on page 673*

Pandel® *see* Topical Corticosteroids *on page 1334*

Pangestyme™ CN *see* Pancrelipase *on page 1029*

Pangestyme™ EC *see* Pancrelipase *on page 1029*

Pangestyme™ MT *see* Pancrelipase *on page 1029*

Pangestyme™ UL *see* Pancrelipase *on page 1029*

Panglobulin® *see* Immune Globulin (Intravenous) *on page 703*

PanMist® Jr. *see* Guaifenesin and Pseudoephedrine *on page 648*

PanMist® LA *see* Guaifenesin and Pseudoephedrine *on page 648*

PanMist® S *see* Guaifenesin and Pseudoephedrine *on page 648*

Panretin® *see* Alitretinoin *on page 59*

Pantoprazole (pan TOE pra zole)

U.S. Brand Names Protonix®

Generic Available No

Pharmacologic Category Proton Pump Inhibitor

Pregnancy Risk Factor B

Lactation Excretion in breast milk unknown/contraindicated

Use

Oral: Treatment and maintenance of healing of erosive esophagitis associated with GERD; reduction in relapse rates of daytime and nighttime heartburn symptoms in GERD; hypersecretory disorders associated with Zollinger-Ellison syndrome or other neoplastic disorders

I.V.: As an alternative to oral therapy in patients unable to continue oral pantoprazole; hypersecretory disorders associated with Zollinger-Ellison syndrome or other neoplastic disorders

Use - Unlabeled/Investigational Peptic ulcer disease, active ulcer bleeding with parenterally-administered pantoprazole; adjunct treatment with antibiotics for *Helicobacter pylori* eradication

Mechanism of Action/Effect Suppresses gastric acid secretion by inhibiting the parietal cell H^+/K^+ ATP pump

Contraindications Hypersensitivity to pantoprazole or any component of the formulation

Warnings/Precautions Symptomatic response does not preclude gastric malignancy. Not indicated for maintenance therapy. Safety and efficacy for use beyond 16 weeks have not been established. Safety and efficacy in pediatric patients have not been established.

Drug Interactions

Cytochrome P450 Effect: Substrate of **CYP2C19**, 3A4; Induces CYP1A2, 3A4

Decreased Effect: Drugs (eg, itraconazole, ketoconazole, and other azole antifungals, ampicillin esters, iron salts) where absorption is determined by an acidic gastric pH, may have decreased absorption when used concurrently. Monitor for change in effectiveness.

Nutritional/Ethanol Interactions Ethanol: Avoid ethanol (may cause gastric mucosal irritation).

Adverse Reactions

1% to 10%:

Cardiovascular: Chest pain (I.V. ≤6%)

Central nervous system: Pain, migraine, anxiety, dizziness, headache (I.V. >1%)

Dermatologic: Rash (I.V. 6%), pruritus (I.V. 4%)

Endocrine & metabolic: Hyperglycemia (1%), hyperlipidemia

Gastrointestinal: Diarrhea (4%), constipation, dyspepsia, gastroenteritis, nausea, rectal disorder, vomiting, abdominal pain (I.V. 12%)

Genitourinary: Urinary frequency, urinary tract infection

Hepatic: Liver function test abnormality, increased SGPT

Local: Injection site pain (>1%)

Neuromuscular & skeletal: Weakness, back pain, neck pain, arthralgia, hypertonia

Respiratory: Bronchitis, increased cough, dyspnea, pharyngitis, rhinitis, sinusitis, upper respiratory tract infection

Miscellaneous: Flu syndrome, infection

<1% (Limited to important or life-threatening): Allergic reaction, anaphylaxis, anemia, angina pectoris, angioedema, anterior ischemic optic neuropathy, arrhythmia, asthma, blurred vision, cholecystitis, cholelithiasis, cholestatic jaundice, CHF, convulsion, depression, diabetes mellitus, erythema multiforme, extraocular palsy, gastrointestinal carcinoma, gastrointestinal hemorrhage, glaucoma, gout, hepatic failure, hepatitis, hypokinesia, hypotension, increased salivation, myocardial ischemia, pancreatitis, pancytopenia, retinal vascular disorder, rhabdomyolysis, speech disorder, Stevens-Johnson syndrome, syncope, thrombophlebitis (I.V.), thrombosis, tinnitus, toxic epidermal necrolysis

Overdosage/Toxicology Treatment of an overdose would include appropriate supportive treatment. No adverse events were seen with ingestions of 400 and 600 mg doses. Pantoprazole is not removed by hemodialysis.

Pharmacodynamics/Kinetics

Absorption: Well absorbed

Bioavailability: 77%

Half-Life Elimination: 1 hour

Time to Peak: Oral: 2.5 hours

Metabolism: Extensively hepatic; CYP2C19 (demethylation), CYP3A4; no evidence that metabolites have pharmacologic activity

Formulations

Injection, powder for reconstitution: 40 mg

Tablet, enteric coated: 20 mg, 40 mg

Dosing

Adults & Elderly:

Erosive esophagitis associated with GERD:

Oral:

Treatment: 40 mg once daily for up to 8 weeks; an additional 8 weeks may be used in patients who have not healed after an 8-week course

Maintenance of healing: 40 mg once daily

Note: Lower doses (20 mg once daily) have been used successfully in mild GERD treatment and maintenance of healing

I.V.: 40 mg once daily (infused over 15 minutes) for 7-10 days

Helicobacter pylori eradication (unlabeled use): I.V.: Doses up to 40 mg twice daily have been used as part of combination therapy

Hypersecretory disorders (including Zollinger-Ellison):

Oral: Initial: 40 mg twice daily; adjust dose based on patient needs; doses up to 240 mg/day have been administered

(Continued)

Pantoprazole *(Continued)*

I.V.: 80 mg twice daily; adjust dose based on acid output measurements; 160-240 mg/day in divided doses has been used for a limited period (up to 7 days)

Renal Impairment: No adjustment is required. Pantoprazole is not removed by hemodialysis.

Hepatic Impairment: No adjustment is required.

Administration

Oral: Tablets should be swallowed whole, do not crush or chew. Do not administer via nasogastric or feeding tube.

I.V.: Infuse over 15 minutes at a rate not to exceed 3 mg/minute; use in-line filter (positioned below Y-site if used)

Stability

Storage:

Oral: Store tablet at 15°C to 30°C (59°F to 77°F)

I.V.: Store at 2°C to 8°C (36°F to 46°F)

Reconstitution: Reconstitute with 10 mL 0.9% sodium chloride; add to 100 mL D_5W or 0.9% sodium chloride; use within 12 hours

Monitoring and Teaching Issues

Physical Assessment: See Warnings/Precautions for use cautions. Assess other medications for effectiveness and interactions (cytochrome P450 enzyme substrate), especially those drugs where absorption is determined by an acidic gastric pH (see Drug Interactions). Monitor therapeutic effectiveness and adverse effects at beginning of therapy and regularly with long-term use (see Adverse Reactions and Overdose/Toxicology). Assess knowledge/teach patient appropriate use, possible side effects/interventions, and adverse symptoms to report (See Patient Education). Breast-feeding is contraindicated.

Patient Education: Take as directed; do not alter dosage without consulting prescriber. Take at similar time each day. Swallow tablet whole (do not crush or chew). Avoid alcohol. You may experience dizziness, headache, or anxiety (use caution when driving or engaging in dangerous activities until response to medication is known); vomiting or loss of appetite (small, frequent meals, frequent mouth care, sucking lozenges, or chewing gum may help); or diarrhea (boiled milk, yogurt, or buttermilk may help). Report persistent abdominal discomfort; chest pain or palpitations; acute headache; unresolved diarrhea; excessive fatigue; increased muscle, joint, or body pain; shortness of breath or wheezing; cold or flu symptoms; changes in urinary pattern; or other persistent adverse reactions. **Pregnancy/breast-feeding precautions:** Inform prescriber if you are pregnant. Do not breast-feed.

Dietary Issues: Oral: May be taken with or without food.

Breast-feeding Issues: Pantoprazole and its metabolites are excreted in the milk of rats. It is unknown if pantoprazole is excreted in human milk. Do not use in women who are breast-feeding.

Papacon® *see* Papaverine *on page 1034*

Papaverine (pa PAV er een)

U.S. Brand Names Papacon®; Para-Time S.R.®; Pavacot®

Synonyms Papaverine Hydrochloride; Pavabid [DSC]

Generic Available Yes

Pharmacologic Category Vasodilator

Pregnancy Risk Factor C

Lactation Excretion in breast milk unknown/not recommended

Use Oral: Relief of peripheral and cerebral ischemia associated with arterial spasm and myocardial ischemia complicated by arrhythmias

Use - Unlabeled/Investigational Investigational: Parenteral: Various vascular spasms associated with muscle spasms as in myocardial infarction, angina, peripheral and pulmonary embolism, peripheral vascular disease, angiospastic states, and visceral spasm (ureteral, biliary, and GI colic); testing for impotence

Mechanism of Action/Effect Smooth muscle spasmolytic producing a generalized smooth muscle relaxation including: vasodilatation, GI sphincter relaxation, bronchiolar muscle relaxation, and potentially a depressed myocardium (with large doses); muscle relaxation may occur due to inhibition or cyclic nucleotide phosphodiesterase, increasing cyclic AMP; muscle relaxation is unrelated to nerve innervation; papaverine increases cerebral blood flow in normal subjects; oxygen uptake is unaltered

Contraindications Hypersensitivity to papaverine or any component of the formulation

Warnings/Precautions Use with caution in patients with glaucoma. Administer I.V. cautiously since apnea and arrhythmias may result. May, in large doses, depress cardiac conduction (eg, AV node) leading to arrhythmias. May interfere with levodopa therapy of Parkinson's disease. Hepatic hypersensitivity has been noted with jaundice, eosinophilia, and abnormal LFTs. Pregnancy risk C.

Drug Interactions

Decreased Effect: Papaverine decreases the effects of levodopa.

Nutritional/Ethanol Interactions Ethanol: Avoid ethanol (may increase CNS depression).

Adverse Reactions Frequency not defined.

Cardiovascular: Arrhythmias (with rapid I.V. use), flushing of the face, mild hypertension, tachycardias

Central nervous system: Drowsiness, headache, lethargy, sedation, vertigo

Gastrointestinal: Abdominal distress, anorexia, constipation, diarrhea, nausea

Hepatic: Chronic hepatitis, hepatic hypersensitivity

Respiratory: Apnea (with rapid I.V. use)

Overdosage/Toxicology Symptoms of overdose include nausea, vomiting, weakness, gastric distress, ataxia, hepatic dysfunction, drowsiness, nystagmus, hyperventilation, hypotension, and hypokalemia. Treatment is supportive.

Pharmacodynamics/Kinetics

Half-Life Elimination: 0.5-1.5 hours

Metabolism: Rapidly hepatic

Onset: Oral: Rapid

Formulations

Capsule, sustained release, as hydrochloride: 150 mg

Injection, as hydrochloride: 30 mg/mL (2 mL, 10 mL)

Dosing

Adults & Elderly: Arterial spasm:

Oral, sustained release: 150-300 mg every 12 hours; in difficult cases: 150 mg every 8 hours

I.M., I.V.: 30-65 mg (rarely up to 120 mg); may repeat every 3 hours

Pediatrics: Arterial spasm: I.M., I.V.: 6 mg/kg/day in 4 divided doses

Administration

I.V.: Rapid I.V. administration may result in arrhythmias and fatal apnea; administer no faster than over 1-2 minutes.

Stability

Storage: Protect from heat or freezing. Refrigerate injection at 2°C to 8°C (35°F to 46°F).

Reconstitution: Solutions should be clear to pale yellow. Precipitates with lactated Ringer's.

Compatibility: Stable in dextran 6% in dextrose, dextran 6% in NS, D_5LR, $D_5{}^1/_4NS$, $D_5{}^1/_2NS$, D_5NS, D_5W, $D_{10}W$, $^1/_2NS$, NS; **incompatible** with LR

Compatibility in syringe: Incompatible with diatrizoate meglumine 52%, diatrizoate sodium 8%

Compatibility when admixed: Incompatible with aminophylline with trimecaine

Monitoring and Teaching Issues

Physical Assessment: See Contraindications, Warnings/Precautions, Drug Interactions, and Dosing for use cautions. **I.V., I.M.:** Blood pressure and heart rate should be monitored. **Oral:** Blood pressure and heart rate should be monitored prior to therapy and at frequent intervals thereafter. Assess therapeutic effectiveness and adverse response (see Adverse Reactions and Overdose/Toxicology). Teach patient proper use, possible side effects and appropriate interventions and adverse symptoms to report (see Patient Education). **Pregnancy risk factor C** - benefits of use should outweigh possible risks. Breast-feeding is not recommended.

Patient Education: Inform prescriber of all prescriptions, OTC medications, or herbal products you are taking, and any allergies you have. Do not take anything new during treatment unless approved by prescriber. Take as directed; do not alter dose or discontinue without consulting prescriber. Swallow extended release capsules whole; do not chew, crush, or dissolve. May cause dizziness, confusion, or blurred vision (avoid driving or engaging in tasks that require alertness until response to drug is known); or constipation (increased exercise, fluids, fruit, or fiber may help). Report rapid heartbeat or palpitations and CNS changes (eg, depression, persistent sedation or lethargy, or acute headache). **Pregnancy/breast-feeding precautions:** Inform prescriber if you are or intend to become pregnant. Breast-feeding is not recommended.

Dietary Issues: May be taken with food.

Geriatric Considerations: Vasodilators have been used to treat dementia upon the premise that dementia is secondary to a cerebral blood flow insufficiency. The hypothesis is that if blood flow could be increased, cognitive function would be increased. This hypothesis is no longer valid. The use of vasodilators for cognitive dysfunction is not recommended or proven by appropriate scientific study.

Papaverine Hydrochloride *see* Papaverine *on page 1034*

Para-Aminosalicylate Sodium *see* Aminosalicylate Sodium *on page 80*

Paracetamol *see* Acetaminophen *on page 35*

Parafon Forte® DSC *see* Chlorzoxazone *on page 281*

Paraplatin® *see* Carboplatin *on page 218*

Parathar™ Injection *see page 1461*

Para-Time S.R.® *see* Papaverine *on page 1034*

Paregoric (par e GOR ik)

Synonyms Camphorated Tincture of Opium

Restrictions C-III

Generic Available Yes

Pharmacologic Category Analgesic, Narcotic

Pregnancy Risk Factor B/D (prolonged use or high doses)

Lactation Enters breast milk/use caution

Use Treatment of diarrhea or relief of pain; neonatal opiate withdrawal

Mechanism of Action/Effect Increases smooth muscle tone in GI tract, decreases motility and peristalsis, diminishes digestive secretions

Contraindications Hypersensitivity to opium or any component of the formulation; diarrhea caused by poisoning until the toxic material has been removed; pregnancy (prolonged use or high doses)

Warnings/Precautions Use with caution in patients with respiratory, hepatic or renal dysfunction, severe prostatic hyperplasia, or history of narcotic abuse. Opium shares the toxic potential of opiate agonists, and usual precautions of opiate agonist therapy should be observed. Some preparations contain sulfites which may cause allergic reactions.

Drug Interactions

Increased Effect/Toxicity: Increased effect/toxicity with CNS depressants (eg, alcohol, narcotics, benzodiazepines, tricyclic antidepressants, MAO inhibitors, phenothiazine).

Nutritional/Ethanol Interactions Ethanol: Avoid ethanol (may increase CNS depression).

Effects on Lab Values ↑ aminotransferase [ALT (SGPT)/AST (SGOT)] (S)

Adverse Reactions Frequency not defined.

(Continued)

Paregoric *(Continued)*

Cardiovascular: Hypotension, peripheral vasodilation
Central nervous system: Drowsiness, dizziness, insomnia, CNS depression, mental depression, increased intracranial pressure, restlessness, headache, malaise
Gastrointestinal: Constipation, anorexia, stomach cramps, nausea, vomiting, biliary tract spasm
Genitourinary: Ureteral spasms, decreased urination, urinary tract spasm
Hepatic: Increased liver function tests
Neuromuscular & skeletal: Weakness
Ocular: Miosis
Respiratory: Respiratory depression
Miscellaneous: Physical and psychological dependence, histamine release

Overdosage/Toxicology Symptoms of overdose include hypotension, drowsiness, seizures, and respiratory depression. Naloxone, 2 mg I.V. with repeat administration as necessary up to a total of 10 mg, can be used to reverse opiate effects.

Pharmacodynamics/Kinetics

Metabolism: In terms of opium: Hepatic

Formulations Liquid: 2 mg morphine equivalent/5 mL [equivalent to 20 mg opium powder] (473 mL)

Dosing

Adults & Elderly: Diarrhea: Oral: 5-10 mL 1-4 times/day

Pediatrics:

Neonatal opiate withdrawal: Oral: 3-6 drops every 3-6 hours as needed, or initially 0.2 mL every 3 hours; increase dosage by approximately 0.05 mL every 3 hours until withdrawal symptoms are controlled; it is rare to exceed 0.7 mL/dose. Stabilize withdrawal symptoms for 3-5 days, then gradually decrease dosage over a 2- to 4-week period.
Diarrhea: Oral: Children: 0.25-0.5 mL/kg 1-4 times/day

Stability

Storage: Store in light-resistant, tightly closed container

Monitoring and Teaching Issues

Physical Assessment: Monitor for excessive sedation, respiratory depression, or hypotension. Has potential for psychological or physiological dependence. **Pregnancy risk factor B/D** - see Pregnancy Risk Factor for use cautions. Note breast-feeding caution.

Patient Education: Take exactly as directed; do not increase dosage. May cause dependence with prolonged or excessive use. Avoid alcohol or any other prescription and OTC medications that may cause sedation (sleeping medications, some cough/cold remedies, antihistamines, etc). You may experience drowsiness, dizziness, or impaired judgment (use caution when driving or engaging in tasks that require alertness until response to drug is known) or postural hypotension (use caution when rising from sitting or lying position or when climbing stairs). You may experience nausea or loss of appetite (small, frequent meals may help) or constipation (a laxative may be necessary). Report unresolved nausea, vomiting, difficulty breathing (shortness of breath or decreased respirations), chest pain, or palpitations. **Pregnancy/breast-feeding precautions:** Inform prescriber if you are pregnant. If nursing, take immediately after feeding or 4-6 hour before next feeding.

Breast-feeding Issues: Information regarding use while breast-feeding is based on experience with morphine. Probably safe with low doses and by administering dose after breast-feeding to further minimize exposure to the drug. Monitor the infant for possible side effects related to opiates.

Additional Information Contains morphine 0.4 mg/mL and alcohol 45%. Do **not** confuse this product with opium tincture which is 25 times **more** potent; each 5 mL of paregoric contains 2 mg morphine equivalent, 0.02 mL anise oil, 20 mg benzoic acid, 20 mg camphor, 0.2 mL glycerin and alcohol; final alcohol content 45%; paregoric also contains papaverine and noscapine; because all of these additives may be harmful to neonates, **a 25-fold dilution of opium tincture** is often preferred for treatment of neonatal abstinence syndrome (opiate withdrawal).

Paremyd® Ophthalmic *see page 1461*

Paricalcitol (par eh CAL ci tol)

U.S. Brand Names Zemplar™

Generic Available No

Pharmacologic Category Vitamin D Analog

Pregnancy Risk Factor C

Lactation Excretion in breast milk unknown/use caution

Use Prevention and treatment of secondary hyperparathyroidism associated with chronic renal failure. Has been evaluated only in hemodialysis patients.

Mechanism of Action/Effect Synthetic vitamin D analog which has been shown to reduce PTH serum concentrations

Contraindications Hypersensitivity to paricalcitol or any component of the formulation; patients with evidence of vitamin D toxicity; hypercalcemia

Warnings/Precautions Chronic administration can place patients at risk of hypercalcemia, elevated calcium-phosphorus product, and metastatic calcification. It should not be used in patients with evidence of hypercalcemia or vitamin D toxicity. Pregnancy risk C.

Drug Interactions

Increased Effect/Toxicity: Phosphate or vitamin D-related compounds should not be taken concurrently. Digitalis toxicity is potentiated by hypercalcemia.

Adverse Reactions The three most frequently reported events in clinical studies were nausea, vomiting, and edema, which are commonly seen in hemodialysis patients.

>10%: Gastrointestinal: Nausea (13%)
1% to 10%:
Cardiovascular: Palpitations, peripheral edema (7%)
Central nervous system: Chills, malaise, fever, lightheadedness (5%)

Gastrointestinal: Vomiting (8%), GI bleeding (5%), xerostomia (3%)
Respiratory: Pneumonia (5%)
Miscellaneous: Flu-like symptoms, sepsis

Overdosage/Toxicology Acute overdose may cause hypercalcemia. Monitor serum calcium and phosphorus closely during titration of paricalcitol. Dosage reduction/interruption may be required if hypercalcemia develops. Chronic use may predispose to metastatic calcification. Bone lesions may develop if parathyroid hormone is suppressed below normal.

Formulations Injection: 5 mcg/mL (1 mL, 2 mL, 5 mL)

Dosing

Adults & Elderly: Hyperparathyroidism, secondary (prevention and treatment): I.V.: 0.04-0.1 mcg/kg (2.8-7 mcg) given as a bolus dose no more frequently than every other day at any time during dialysis; dose as high as 0.24 mcg/kg (16.8 mcg) have been administered safely. Usually start with 0.04 mcg/kg 3 times/week by I.V. bolus, increased by 0.04 mcg/kg every 2 weeks.

Renal Impairment: Refer to adult dosing.

Hepatic Impairment: Kinetics have not been investigated in hepatically impaired patients.

Monitoring Laboratory Tests Serum calcium and phosphorus should be monitored closely (eg, twice weekly) during dose titration. Monitor serum PTH. In trials, a mean PTH level reduction of 30% was achieved within 6 weeks.

Monitoring and Teaching Issues

Physical Assessment: Monitor laboratory results (see Monitoring Laboratory Tests). See Warnings/Precautions and Drug Interactions. Monitor patient response and adverse effects. Monitor for signs and symptoms of vitamin D intoxication. Assess knowledge/instruct patient on safe and appropriate use of paricalcitol and dietary requirements (see Patient Education). **Pregnancy risk factor C** - benefits of use should outweigh possible risks. Note breast-feeding caution.

Patient Education: Take as directed; do not increase dosage without consulting prescriber. Adhere to diet as recommended (do not take any other phosphate or vitamin D related compounds while taking paricalcitol). You may experience nausea or vomiting (small, frequent meals, frequent mouth care, chewing gums, or sucking lozenges may help); swelling of extremities (elevate feet when sitting); or lightheadedness or dizziness (use caution when driving or engaging in tasks requiring alertness until response to drug is known). Report persistent fever, gastric disturbances, abdominal pain or blood in stool, chest pain or palpitations, or signs of respiratory infection or flu. **Pregnancy/breast-feeding precautions:** Inform prescriber if you are or intend to become pregnant. Consult prescriber if breast-feeding.

Geriatric Considerations: Kinetics have not been investigated in geriatric patients.

Pariprazole *see* Rabeprazole *on page 1168*
Parlodel® *see* Bromocriptine *on page 177*
Parnate® *see* Tranylcypromine *on page 1348*

Paroxetine (pa ROKS e teen)

U.S. Brand Names Paxil®; Paxil® CR™

Generic Available No

Pharmacologic Category Antidepressant, Selective Serotonin Reuptake Inhibitor

Pregnancy Risk Factor C

Lactation Enters breast milk/use caution (AAP rates "of concern")

Use Treatment of depression in adults; treatment of panic disorder with or without agoraphobia; obsessive-compulsive disorder (OCD) in adults; social anxiety disorder (social phobia); generalized anxiety disorder (GAD); post-traumatic stress disorder (PTSD)

Paxil® CR™: Treatment of depression; treatment of panic disorder

Use - Unlabeled/Investigational May be useful in eating disorders, impulse control disorders, self-injurious behavior; premenstrual disorders, vasomotor symptoms of menopause; treatment of depression and obsessive-compulsive disorder (OCD) in children

Mechanism of Action/Effect Paroxetine is a selective serotonin reuptake inhibitor, chemically unrelated to tricyclic, tetracyclic, or other antidepressants; presumably, the inhibition of serotonin reuptake from brain synapse stimulated serotonin activity in the brain

Contraindications Hypersensitivity to paroxetine or any component of the formulation; use of MAO inhibitors or within 14 days; concurrent use with thioridazine or mesoridazine

Warnings/Precautions Potential for severe reaction when used with MAO inhibitors - serotonin syndrome (hyperthermia, muscular rigidity, mental status changes/agitation, autonomic instability) may occur. May precipitate a shift to mania or hypomania in patients with bipolar disease. Has a low potential to impair cognitive or motor performance - caution operating hazardous machinery or driving. Low potential for sedation or anticholinergic effects relative to cyclic antidepressants. Use caution in patients with depression, particularly if suicidal risk may be present. Use caution in patients with a previous seizure disorder or condition predisposing to seizures such as brain damage, alcoholism, or concurrent therapy with other drugs which lower the seizure threshold. Use with caution in patients with hepatic or dysfunction and in elderly patients. May cause hyponatremia/SIADH. Use with caution in patients at risk of bleeding or receiving anticoagulant therapy - may cause impairment in platelet aggregation. Use with caution in patients with renal insufficiency or other concurrent illness (due to limited experience). May cause or exacerbate sexual dysfunction. Upon discontinuation of paroxetine therapy, gradually taper dose. Pregnancy risk C.

Drug Interactions

Cytochrome P450 Effect: Substrate of **CYP2D6**; Inhibits CYP1A2, **2B6**, 2C8/9, 2C19, **2D6**, 3A4

Decreased Effect: Cyproheptadine, a serotonin antagonist, may inhibit the effects of serotonin reuptake inhibitors (paroxetine).

Increased Effect/Toxicity:

MAO inhibitors: Paroxetine should not be used with nonselective MAO inhibitors (phenelzine, isocarboxazid) or other drugs with MAO inhibition (linezolid); fatal reactions have been reported. Wait 5 weeks after stopping fluoxetine before starting a nonselective

(Continued)

Paroxetine *(Continued)*

MAO inhibitor and 2 weeks after stopping an MAO inhibitor before starting paroxetine. Concurrent selegiline has been associated with mania, hypertension, or serotonin syndrome (risk may be reduced relative to nonselective MAO inhibitors).

Phenothiazines: Paroxetine may inhibit the metabolism of thioridazine or mesoridazine, resulting in increased plasma levels and increasing the risk of QT_c interval prolongation. This may lead to serious ventricular arrhythmias, such as torsade de pointes-type arrhythmias and sudden death. Do not use together. Wait at least 5 weeks after discontinuing paroxetine prior to starting thioridazine.

Combined used of SSRIs and amphetamines, buspirone, meperidine, nefazodone, serotonin agonists (such as sumatriptan), sibutramine, other SSRIs, sympathomimetics, ritonavir, tramadol, and venlafaxine may increase the risk of serotonin syndrome. Paroxetine may increase serum levels/effects of benzodiazepines (alprazolam and diazepam), carbamazepine, carvedilol, clozapine, cyclosporine (and possibly tacrolimus), dextromethorphan, digoxin, haloperidol, HMG-CoA reductase inhibitors (lovastatin and simvastatin - increasing the risk of rhabdomyolysis), phenytoin, propafenone, theophylline, trazodone, tricyclic antidepressants, and valproic acid. Concurrent lithium may increase risk of nephrotoxicity. Risk of hyponatremia may increase with concurrent use of loop diuretics (bumetanide, furosemide, torsemide). Paroxetine may increase the hypoprothrombinemic response to warfarin.

Combined use of sumatriptan (and other serotonin agonists) may result in toxicity; weakness, hyper-reflexia, and incoordination have been observed with sumatriptan and SSRIs. In addition, concurrent use may theoretically increase the risk of serotonin syndrome; includes sumatriptan, naratriptan, rizatriptan, and zolmitriptan.

Nutritional/Ethanol Interactions

Ethanol: Avoid ethanol.

Food: Peak concentration is increased, but bioavailability is not significantly altered by food.

Herb/Nutraceutical: Avoid valerian, St John's wort, SAMe, kava kava.

Effects on Lab Values ↑ LFTs

Adverse Reactions

>10%:

Central nervous system: Headache, somnolence, dizziness, insomnia
Gastrointestinal: Nausea, xerostomia, constipation, diarrhea
Genitourinary: Ejaculatory disturbances
Neuromuscular & skeletal: Weakness
Miscellaneous: Diaphoresis

1% to 10%:

Cardiovascular: Palpitations, vasodilation, postural hypotension
Central nervous system: Nervousness, anxiety, yawning, abnormal dreams
Dermatologic: Rash
Endocrine & metabolic: Decreased libido, delayed ejaculation
Gastrointestinal: Anorexia, flatulence, vomiting, dyspepsia, taste perversion
Genitourinary: Urinary frequency, impotence
Neuromuscular & skeletal: Tremor, paresthesia, myopathy, myalgia

<1% (Limited to important or life-threatening): Acute renal failure, agranulocytosis, akinesia, allergic alveolitis, alopecia, amenorrhea, anaphylactoid reaction, anaphylaxis, angioedema, aplastic anemia, asthma, atrial fibrillation, bone marrow aplasia, bruxism, bundle branch block, colitis, dysphasia, eclampsia, EPS, erythema multiforme, exfoliative dermatitis, Guillain-Barré syndrome, hemolytic anemia, hepatic necrosis, hypotension, laryngismus, leukopenia, mania, migraine, myasthenia, neuroleptic malignant syndrome (NMS), optic neuritis, pancreatitis, pancytopenia, porphyria, priapism, pulmonary hypertension, seizures (including status epilepticus), serotonin syndrome, SIADH, thrombocytopenia, torsade de pointes, toxic epidermal necrolysis, ventricular fibrillation, ventricular tachycardia, withdrawal reactions (dizziness; sensory disturbances - eg, paresthesias such as electric shock sensations; agitation; anxiety; nausea; diaphoresis - particularly following abrupt withdrawal)

Overdosage/Toxicology Symptoms of overdose include somnolence, nausea, vomiting, hepatic dysfunction, drowsiness, sinus tachycardia, urinary retention, renal failure (acute), and dilated pupils. Convulsions, status epilepticus, and ventricular arrhythmias (including torsade de pointes) have been reported, as well as serotonin syndrome and manic reaction. There are no specific antidotes, following attempts at decontamination, treatment is supportive and symptomatic. Forced diuresis, dialysis, and hemoperfusion are unlikely to be beneficial.

Pharmacodynamics/Kinetics

Half-Life Elimination: 21 hours

Time to Peak: 5.2 hours

Metabolism: Extensively hepatic via CYP

Formulations

Suspension, oral (Paxil®): 10 mg/5 mL (250 mL) [orange flavor]
Tablet (Paxil®): 10 mg, 20 mg, 30 mg, 40 mg
Tablet, controlled release (Paxil® CR™): 12.5 mg, 25 mg, 37.5 mg

Dosing

Adults:

Depression: Oral: Initial: 20 mg given once daily preferably in the morning; increase if needed by 10 mg/day increments at intervals of at least 1 week; maximum dose: 50 mg/day

Paxil® CR™: Oral: Initial: 25 mg given once daily; increase if needed by 12.5 mg/day increments at intervals of at least 1 week; maximum dose: 62.5 mg/day

Obsessive-compulsive disorder: Oral: Initial: 20 mg given once daily preferably in the morning; increase if needed by 10 mg/day increments at intervals of at least 1 week; recommended dose: 40 mg/day; range: 20-60 mg/day; maximum dose: 60 mg/day

Panic disorder: Oral: Initial: 10 mg given once daily preferably in the morning; increase if needed by 10 mg/day increments at intervals of at least 1 week; recommended dose: 40 mg/day; range: 10-60 mg/day; maximum dose: 60 mg/day

Paxil® CR™: Oral: Initial: 12 mg given once daily; increase if needed by 12.5 mg/day at intervals of at least 1 week; maximum dose: 75 mg/day

Social anxiety disorder: Oral: Initial: 20 mg given once daily preferably in the morning; recommended dose: 20 mg/day; range: 20-60 mg/day; doses >20 mg may not have additional benefit

Generalized anxiety disorder (GAD): Oral: Initial: 20 mg once daily preferably administered in the morning; doses of 20-50 mg/day were used in clinical trials, however, no greater benefit was seen with doses >20 mg. If dose is increased, adjust in increments of 10 mg/day at 1-week intervals.

Post-traumatic stress disorder (PTSD): Oral: Initial: 20 mg given once daily, preferably in the morning; if needed, dosage may by increased in increments of 10 mg/day at intervals of at least 1 week; range: 20-50 mg

Note: Upon discontinuation of paroxetine therapy, gradually taper dose (taper-phase regimen used in PTSD/GAD clinical trials involved an incremental decrease in the daily dose by 10 mg/day at weekly intervals; when 20 mg/day dose was reached, this dose was continued for 1 week before treatment was stopped).

Elderly: Depression, obsessive compulsive disorder, panic attack, social anxiety disorder: Oral: Initial: 10 mg/day; increase if needed by 10 mg/day increments at intervals of at least 1 week; maximum dose: 40 mg/day

Paxil® CR™; Initial: 12.5 mg/day; increase if needed by 12.5 mg/day increments at intervals of at least 1 week; maximum dose: 50 mg/day

Pediatrics:

Depression (unlabeled use): Oral: Initial: 10 mg/day and adjusted upward on an individual basis to 20 mg/day

OCD (unlabeled use): Oral: Initial: 10 mg/day and titrate up as necessary to 60 mg/day

Self-Injurious behavior (unlabeled use): Oral: 20 mg/day

Renal Impairment: Adults: Initial: 10 mg/day; increase if needed by 10 mg/day increments at intervals of at least 1 week; maximum dose: 40 mg/day

Paxil® CR™; Initial: 12.5 mg/day; increase if needed by 12.5 mg/day increments at intervals of at least 1 week; maximum dose: 50 mg/day

Hepatic Impairment: Adults: Initial: 10 mg/day; increase if needed by 10 mg/day increments at intervals of at least 1 week; maximum dose: 40 mg/day

Paxil® CR™; Initial: 12.5 mg/day; increase if needed by 12.5 mg/day increments at intervals of at least 1 week; maximum dose: 50 mg/day

Administration

Oral: May be administered with or without food. Do not crush, break, or chew controlled release tablets.

Stability

Storage:

Suspension: Store at ≤25°C (≤77°F)

Tablet: Store at 15°C to 30°C (59°F to 86°F)

Monitoring Laboratory Tests Hepatic and renal function

Monitoring and Teaching Issues

Physical Assessment: Assess other medications patient may be taking for effectiveness and interactions (see Drug Interactions). See Warnings/Precautions for use cautions. Monitor laboratory tests, therapeutic response, and adverse reactions at beginning of therapy and periodically with long-term use (see Adverse Reactions and Overdose/Toxicology). Taper dosage slowly when discontinuing. Assess knowledge/teach patient appropriate use, interventions to reduce side effects, and adverse symptoms to report (see Patient Education). **Pregnancy risk factor C** - benefits of use should outweigh possible risks. Note breast-feeding caution.

Patient Education: Take exactly as directed; do not increase dose or frequency or discontinue without consulting prescriber. It may take 2-3 weeks to achieve desired results. Take in the morning to reduce the incidence of insomnia (may be taken with or without food). Do not crush, break, or chew controlled release (Paxil® CR™) tablets. Avoid alcohol, caffeine, and other prescription or OTC medications not approved by prescriber. Maintain adequate hydration (2-3 L/day of fluids) unless advised by prescriber to restrict fluids. You may experience drowsiness, dizziness, or lightheadedness (use caution when driving or engaging in tasks requiring alertness until response to drug is known); nausea, vomiting, anorexia, or dry mouth (small, frequent meals, frequent mouth care, chewing gum, or sucking lozenges may help); or orthostatic hypotension (use caution when climbing stairs or changing position from lying or sitting to standing). Report persistent insomnia or excessive daytime sedation; muscle cramping, tremors, weakness, or change in gait; chest pain, palpitations, or rapid heartbeat; vision changes or eye pain; difficulty breathing or breathlessness; abdominal pain or blood in stool; or worsening of condition. **Pregnancy/breast-feeding precautions:** Inform prescriber if you are or intend to become pregnant. Inform prescriber if breast-feeding.

Dietary Issues: May be taken with or without food.

Geriatric Considerations: Paroxetine's favorable side effect profile make it a useful alternative to traditional tricyclic antidepressants. Paroxetine is the most sedating of the currently available selective serotonin reuptake inhibitors. Paroxetine's half-life is approximately 21 hours and it has no active metabolites.

Additional Information Has properties similar to fluvoxamine maleate; buspirone (15-60 mg/day) may be useful in treatment of sexual dysfunction during treatment with a selective serotonin reuptake inhibitor. Paxil® CR™ incorporates a multi-layer formulation (Geomatrix™) to control dissolution and absorption.

Related Information

Antidepressant Agents *on page 1553*

Antidepressant Medication Guidelines *on page 1613*

PAS *see* Aminosalicylate Sodium *on page 80*

Patanol™ *see page 1509*
Patient Education for Management of Common Side Effects *see page 27*
Patient Factors That Influence Drug Therapy *see page 25*
Pavabid [DSC] *see* Papaverine *on page 1034*
Pavacot® *see* Papaverine *on page 1034*
Pavulon® *see* Pancuronium *on page 1031*
Paxil® *see* Paroxetine *on page 1037*
Paxil® CR™ *see* Paroxetine *on page 1037*
PCA *see* Procainamide *on page 1122*
PC-Cap® *see* Propoxyphene and Aspirin *on page 1142*
PCE® *see* Erythromycin (Systemic) *on page 486*
Peak and Trough Guidelines *see page 1544*
PediaCare® Decongestant Infants [OTC] *see* Pseudoephedrine *on page 1150*
Pediapred® *see* PrednisoLONE *on page 1113*
Pediatric Dosage Estimation *see page 1546*
Pediazole® *see* Erythromycin and Sulfisoxazole *on page 486*
Pedi-Dri® *see* Nystatin *on page 989*
PediOtic® Otic *see page 1519*
PedvaxHIB™ *see page 1498*

Pegaspargase (peg AS par jase)

U.S. Brand Names Oncaspar®

Synonyms PEG-L-asparaginase

Generic Available No

Pharmacologic Category Antineoplastic Agent, Miscellaneous

Pregnancy Risk Factor C

Lactation Enters breast milk/contraindicated

Use Treatment of acute lymphocytic leukemia, blast crisis of chronic lymphocytic leukemia (CLL), salvage therapy of non-Hodgkin's lymphoma; may be used in some patients who have had hypersensitivity reactions to *E. coli* asparaginase

Mechanism of Action/Effect

Pegaspargase is a modified version of the enzyme L-asparaginase; the L-asparaginase used in the manufacture of pegaspargase is derived from *Escherichia coli*

Some malignant cells (ie, lymphoblastic leukemia cells and those of lymphocyte derivation) must acquire the amino acid asparagine from surrounding fluid such as blood, whereas normal cells can synthesize their own asparagine. asparaginase is an enzyme that deaminates asparagine to aspartic acid and ammonia in the plasma and extracellular fluid and therefore deprives tumor cells of the amino acid for protein synthesis.

Contraindications Hypersensitivity to pegaspargase or any component of the formulation; pancreatitis or a history of pancreatitis; patients who have had significant hemorrhagic events associated with prior asparaginase therapy; previous serious allergic reactions, such as generalized urticaria, bronchospasm, laryngeal edema, hypotension, or other unacceptable adverse reactions to pegaspargase

Warnings/Precautions The U.S. Food and Drug Administration (FDA) currently recommends that procedures for proper handling and disposal of antineoplastic agents be considered.

Monitor for severe allergic reactions. Use cautiously in patients with an underlying coagulopathy or previous hematologic complications from asparaginase, hepatic dysfunction, hyperglycemia or diabetes, or pancreatitis. May be used cautiously in patients who have had hypersensitivity reactions to *E. coli* asparaginase; however, up to 33% of patients who have an allergic reaction to *E. coli* asparaginase will also react to pegaspargase.

Pregnancy risk C.

Drug Interactions

Decreased Effect: Asparaginase terminates methotrexate action by inhibition of protein synthesis and prevention of cell entry into the S Phase.

Increased Effect/Toxicity:

Aspirin, dipyridamole, heparin, warfarin, NSAIDs: Imbalances in coagulation factors have been noted with the use of pegaspargase - use with caution.

Vincristine and prednisone: An increased toxicity has been noticed when asparaginase is administered with VCR and prednisone.

Cyclophosphamide (decreased metabolism)

Mercaptopurine (increased hepatotoxicity)

Vincristine (increased neuropathy)

Prednisone (hyperglycemia)

Adverse Reactions In general, pegaspargase toxicities tend to be less frequent and appear somewhat later than comparable toxicities of asparaginase. Intramuscular rather than intravenous injection may decrease the incidence of coagulopathy; GI, hepatic, and renal toxicity.

>10%:

Cardiovascular: Edema

Central nervous system: Fatigue, disorientation (10%)

Gastrointestinal: Nausea, vomiting (50% to 60%), generally mild to moderate, but may be severe and protracted in some patients; anorexia (33%); abdominal pain (38%); diarrhea (28%); increased serum lipase and amylase

Hematologic: Hypofibrinogenemia and depression of clotting factors V and VII, variable decreases in factors VII and IX, severe protein C deficiency and decrease in antithrombin III - overt bleeding is uncommon, but may be dose-limiting, or fatal in some patients

Neuromuscular & skeletal: Weakness (33%)

Miscellaneous: Acute allergic reactions, including fever, rash, urticaria, arthralgia, hypotension, angioedema, bronchospasm, anaphylaxis (10% to 30%) - dose-limiting in some patients

1% to 10%:

Cardiovascular: Hypotension, tachycardia, thrombosis

Dermatologic: Urticaria, erythema, lip edema

Endocrine & metabolic: Hyperglycemia (3%)

Gastrointestinal: Acute pancreatitis (1%)

<1% (Limited to important or life-threatening): Agitation, bronchospasm, coma, convulsions, depression, dyspnea, hallucinations, paresthesias, parkinsonian symptoms (tremor, increased muscle tone), seizures, somnolence; transient elevations of transaminases, bilirubin, and alkaline phosphatase

Mild to moderate myelosuppression, leukopenia, anemia, thrombocytopenia; onset: 7 days, nadir: 14 days, recovery: 21 days

Overdosage/Toxicology Symptoms of overdose include nausea and diarrhea.

Pharmacodynamics/Kinetics

Half-Life Elimination: 5.73 days; unaffected by age, renal or hepatic function

Metabolism: Systemically degraded

Duration: Asparaginase was measurable for at least 15 days following initial treatment with pegaspargase

Formulations Injection [preservative free]: 750 units/mL

Dosing

Adults & Elderly: Refer to individual protocols. Dose must be individualized based upon clinical response and tolerance of the patient. I.M. administration is **preferred** over I.V. administration. I.M. administration may decrease the incidence of hepatotoxicity, coagulopathy, and GI and renal disorders.

Acute lymphoblastic leukemia (ALL): I.M., I.V.: 2500 units/m^2 every 14 days

Pediatrics: Refer to individual protocols. Dose must be individualized based upon clinical response and tolerance of the patient. I.M. administration is **preferred** over I.V. administration. I.M. administration may decrease the incidence of hepatotoxicity, coagulopathy, and GI and renal disorders.

Acute lymphoblastic leukemia: I.M., I.V.:

Body surface area <0.6 m^2: 82.5 IU/kg every 14 days

Body surface area ≥0.6 m^2: 2500 IU/m^2 every 14 days

Administration

I.M.: Must only be given as a deep intramuscular injection into a large muscle.

I.M.: limit the volume of a single injection site to 2 mL. If the volume to be administered is >2 mL, use multiple injection sites.

I.V.:

May be given as a 1- to 2-hour I.V. infusion; **do not give I.V. push**. Some institutions recommend the following precautions for pegaspargase administration:

Have parenteral epinephrine, diphenhydramine, and hydrocortisone available at the bedside

Have a freely running I.V. in place

Have a physician readily accessible

Monitor the patient closely for 30-60 minutes

Stability

Storage: Refrigerate at 2°C to 8°C (36°F to 46°F). Do not use of cloudy or if precipitate is present. Do not use if stored at room temperature for >48 hours. Do **not** freeze. Do not use product if it is known to have been frozen. Single-use vial; discard unused portions.

Reconstitution: Avoid excessive agitation; do **not** shake.

Standard I.M. dilution: Do not exceed 2 mL volume per injection site

Standard I.V. dilution: Dose/100 mL NS or D_5W; stable for 48 hours at room temperature.

Monitoring Laboratory Tests CBC, urinalysis, amylase, liver enzymes, prothrombin time, renal function, blood glucose

Monitoring and Teaching Issues

Physical Assessment: See Contraindications, Warnings/Precautions, and Dosing for use cautions. Assess potential for interactions with other prescriptions, OTC medications, or herbal products patient may be taking (see Drug Interactions). Note infusion cautions above (see I.V. Administration for anaphylactic cautions); patient should be closely observed during and for 1 hour following each infusion (anaphylactic reactions can occur with each dose). Assess results of laboratory tests (see above) and therapeutic effectiveness. Monitor closely for adverse response (see Adverse Reactions and Overdose/Toxicology). Teach patient possible side effects and appropriate interventions and adverse symptoms to report (see Patient Education). **Pregnancy risk factor C** - benefits of use should outweigh possible risk (see Pregnancy Issues). Breast-feeding is contraindicated.

Patient Education: Inform prescriber of all prescriptions, OTC medications, or herbal products you are taking, and any allergies you have. Do not take anything new during treatment unless approved by prescriber. This drug can only be given by infusion or injection; report immediately any redness, swelling, burning, or pain at infusion site or any signs of allergic reaction (eg, difficulty breathing or swallowing, chest tightness, rash, hives, swelling of lips or mouth). Maintain adequate hydration (2-3 L/day of fluids) unless advised by prescriber to restrict fluids, and nutrition. You may be more susceptible to infection (avoid crowds and exposure to infection and do not have vaccinations without consulting prescriber). May cause nausea, vomiting, or loss of appetite (small, frequent meals, frequent mouth care, chewing gum, or sucking lozenges may help); mouth sores (use soft toothbrush, waxed dental floss, and frequent mouth rinses); diarrhea (buttermilk, boiled milk, or yogurt may help); dizziness, drowsiness, syncope, or blurred vision (use caution when driving or engaging in tasks that require alertness until response to drug is known); increased sweating; decreased sexual drive; or cough. Report edema (eg, swelling of extremities or sudden weight gain); persistent nausea, vomiting, or diarrhea; unusual bleeding or bruising; black tarry stools; blood in urine or stool, pinpoint red spots on your

(Continued)

Pegaspargase *(Continued)*

skin; or weakness or fatigue. **Pregnancy/breast-feeding precautions:** Inform prescriber if you are or intend to become pregnant. Do not breast-feed.

Pregnancy Issues: Based on limited reports in humans, the use of asparaginase does not seem to pose a major risk to the fetus when used in the 2nd and 3rd trimesters, or when exposure occurs prior to conception in either females or males. Because of the teratogenicity observed in animals and the lack of human data after 1st trimester exposure, asparaginase should be used cautiously, if at all, during this period.

Additional Information Not commercially available in the U.S.; obtain from Olsten Health Services 1-888-276-2217.

PEG-L-asparaginase *see* Pegaspargase *on page 1040*

PemADD® *see* Pemoline *on page 1042*

PemADD® CT *see* Pemoline *on page 1042*

Pemoline (PEM oh leen)

U.S. Brand Names Cylert®; PemADD®; PemADD® CT

Synonyms Phenylisohydantoin; PIO

Restrictions C-IV

Generic Available Yes

Pharmacologic Category Stimulant

Pregnancy Risk Factor B

Lactation Excretion in breast milk unknown/not recommended

Use Treatment of attention-deficit/hyperactivity disorder (ADHD) (not first-line)

Use - Unlabeled/Investigational Narcolepsy

Mechanism of Action/Effect Blocks the reuptake mechanism of dopaminergic neurons, appears to act at the cerebral cortex and subcortical structures; CNS and respiratory stimulant with weak sympathomimetic effects; actions may be mediated via increase in CNS dopamine

Contraindications Hypersensitivity to pemoline or any component of the formulation; hepatic impairment (including abnormalities on baseline liver function tests); children <6 years of age; Tourette's syndrome; psychosis

Warnings/Precautions Not considered first-line therapy for ADHD due to association with hepatic failure. The manufacturer has recommended that signed informed consent following a discussion of risks and benefits must or should be obtained prior to the initiation of therapy. Therapy should be discontinued if a response is not evident after 3 weeks of therapy. Pemoline should not be started in patients with abnormalities in baseline liver function tests, and should be discontinued if clinically significant liver function test abnormalities are revealed at any time during therapy. Use with caution in patients with renal dysfunction or psychosis. In general, stimulant medications should be used with caution in patients with bipolar disorder, diabetes mellitus, cardiovascular disease, seizure disorders, insomnia, porphyria, or hypertension (although pemoline has been demonstrated to have a low potential to elevate blood pressure relative to other stimulants). May exacerbate symptoms of behavior and thought disorder in psychotic patients. Potential for drug dependency exists - avoid abrupt discontinuation in patients who have received for prolonged periods. Stimulant use has been associated with growth suppression, and careful monitoring is recommended.

Drug Interactions

Decreased Effect: Pemoline in combination with antiepileptic medications may decrease seizure threshold.

Increased Effect/Toxicity: Use caution when pemoline is used with other CNS-acting medications.

Nutritional/Ethanol Interactions Ethanol: Avoid ethanol (may increase CNS depression).

Adverse Reactions Frequency not defined.

Central nervous system: Insomnia, dizziness, drowsiness, mental depression, increased irritability, seizures, precipitation of Tourette's syndrome, hallucinations, headache, movement disorders

Dermatologic: Rash

Endocrine & metabolic: Suppression of growth in children

Gastrointestinal: Anorexia, weight loss, stomach pain, nausea

Hematologic: Aplastic anemia

Hepatic: Increased liver enzyme (usually reversible upon discontinuation), hepatitis, jaundice, hepatic failure

Overdosage/Toxicology Symptoms of overdose include tachycardia, hallucinations, and agitation. There is no specific antidote for intoxication and treatment is primarily supportive.

Pharmacodynamics/Kinetics

Half-Life Elimination: Children: 7-8.6 hours; Adults: 12 hours

Time to Peak: Serum: 2-4 hours

Metabolism: Partially hepatic

Onset: Peak effect: 4 hours

Duration: 8 hours

Formulations

Tablet: 18.75 mg, 37.5 mg, 75 mg

Tablet, chewable: 37.5 mg

Dosing

Adults & Elderly: ADHD: Oral: Initial: 37.5 mg given once daily in the morning, increase by 18.75 mg/day at weekly intervals; usual effective dose range: 56.25-75 mg/day; maximum: 112.5 mg/day; dosage range: 0.5-3 mg/kg/24 hours; significant benefit may not be evident until third or fourth week of administration.

Pediatrics: Children ≥6 years: Refer to adult dosing.

Renal Impairment: Cl_{cr} <50 mL/minute: Avoid use.

Administration

Oral: Administer medication in the morning.

Monitoring Laboratory Tests Liver enzymes (baseline and every 2 weeks)

Monitoring and Teaching Issues

Physical Assessment: Assess effectiveness and interactions of other medications patient may be taking (see Drug Interactions). See Contraindications and Warnings/Precautions for use cautions. After long-term use, taper dosage slowly when discontinuing. Monitor laboratory results (see above), effectiveness of therapy, and adverse reactions at beginning of therapy and periodically with long-term use. Assess knowledge/teach patient appropriate use, interventions to reduce side effects, and adverse symptoms to report (see Patient Education). Breast-feeding is not recommended.

Patient Education: Take exactly as directed; do not change dosage or discontinue without consulting prescriber. Response may some time. Avoid alcohol, caffeine, or other stimulants. Maintain adequate hydration (2-3 L/day of fluids) unless advised by prescriber to restrict fluids. You may experience nausea, decreased appetite, or altered taste sensation (small, frequent meals may help maintain adequate nutrition); or drowsiness, dizziness, or mental depression, especially during early therapy (use caution when driving or engaging in tasks requiring alertness until response to drug is known). Report unresolved rapid heartbeat; excessive agitation, nervousness, insomnia, tremors, dizziness, or seizures; skin rash or irritation; altered gait or movement; unusual mouth movements or vocalizations (Tourette's syndrome); yellowing of skin or eyes; or dark urine or pale stools. **Breast-feeding precaution:** Breast-feeding is not recommended.

Additional Information Treatment of ADHD should include "Drug Holidays" or periodic discontinuation of stimulant medication in order to assess the patient's requirements and to decrease tolerance and limit suppression of linear growth and weight. The labeling for Cylert® includes recommendations for liver function monitoring and a Patient Information Consent Form.

Penciclovir (pen SYE kloe veer)

U.S. Brand Names Denavir™

Generic Available No

Pharmacologic Category Antiviral Agent

Pregnancy Risk Factor B

Lactation Excretion in breast milk unknown

Use Topical treatment of herpes simplex labialis (cold sores); potentially used for Epstein-Barr virus infections

Mechanism of Action/Effect Phosphorylated in the virus-infected cells to penciclovir triphosphate, which competitively inhibits DNA polymerase in HSV-1 and HSV-2 strains. This prevents viral replication by inhibition of viral DNA synthesis. Some activity has been demonstrated against Epstein-Barr and varicella-zoster virus (VZV).

Contraindications Hypersensitivity to the penciclovir or any component of the formulation; previous and significant adverse reactions to famciclovir

Warnings/Precautions Apply only to herpes labialis on lips and face. Application to mucous membranes is not recommended. Effect has not been evaluated in immunocompromised patients.

Adverse Reactions

>10%: Dermatologic: Erythema (mild) (50%)

1% to 10%: Central nervous system: Headache (5.3%)

<1% (Limited to important or life-threatening): Local anesthesia

Overdosage/Toxicology Penciclovir is poorly absorbed if ingested orally. Adverse reactions related to oral ingestion are unlikely.

Pharmacodynamics/Kinetics

Absorption: Topical: None

Formulations Cream: 1% [10 mg/g] (1.5 g)

Dosing

Adults & Elderly: Herpes simplex labialis (cold sores): Topical: Apply cream at the first sign or symptom of cold sore (eg, tingling, swelling); apply every 2 hours during waking hours for 4 days.

Stability

Storage: Store at or below 30°C. Do not freeze.

Monitoring and Teaching Issues

Physical Assessment: See Contraindications and Warnings/Precautions for use cautions. Assess for effectiveness of therapy. Teach patient appropriate application and use and adverse symptoms (see Adverse Reactions) to report (see Patient Education). Note breast-feeding caution.

Patient Education: This is not a cure for herpes (recurrences tend to appear within 3 months of original infection), nor will this medication reduce the risk of transmission to others when lesions are present. For external use only. Wash hands before and after application. Apply this film over affected areas at first sign of cold sore. Avoid use of other topical creams, lotions, or ointments unless approved by prescriber. You may experience headache, mild rash, or taste disturbances. **Breast-feeding precaution:** Consult prescriber if breast-feeding.

Additional Information Penciclovir is the active metabolite of the prodrug famciclovir. Penciclovir is an alternative to topical acyclovir for HSV-1 and HSV-2 infections. Neither drug will prevent recurring HSV attacks.

Penecort® *see* Topical Corticosteroids *on page 1334*

Penicillin G Benzathine (pen i SIL in jee BENZ a theen)

U.S. Brand Names Bicillin® L-A; Permapen® Isoject®

Synonyms Benzathine Benzylpenicillin; Benzathine Penicillin G; Benzylpenicillin Benzathine

(Continued)

Penicillin G Benzathine *(Continued)*

Generic Available No

Pharmacologic Category Antibiotic, Penicillin

Pregnancy Risk Factor B

Lactation Enters breast milk/compatible

Use Active against some gram-positive organisms, few gram-negative organisms such as *Neisseria gonorrhoeae*, and some anaerobes and spirochetes; used in the treatment of syphilis; used only for the treatment of mild to moderately severe infections caused by organisms susceptible to low concentrations of penicillin G or for prophylaxis of infections caused by these organisms

Mechanism of Action/Effect Interferes with bacterial cell wall synthesis during active multiplication, causing cell wall death and resultant bactericidal activity against susceptible bacteria

Contraindications Hypersensitivity to penicillin or any component of the formulation

Warnings/Precautions Use with caution in patients with impaired renal function, seizure disorder. CDC and AAP do not currently recommend the use of penicillin G benzathine to treat congenital syphilis or neurosyphilis due to reported treatment failures and lack of published clinical data on its efficacy.

Drug Interactions

Decreased Effect: Tetracyclines may decrease penicillin effectiveness. Although anecdotal reports suggest oral contraceptive efficacy could be reduced by penicillins, this has been refuted by more rigorous scientific and clinical data.

Increased Effect/Toxicity: Probenecid increases penicillin levels. Aminoglycosides may lead to synergistic efficacy.

Effects on Lab Values Positive Coombs' [direct], false-positive urinary and/or serum proteins; false-positive or negative urinary glucose using Clinitest®

Adverse Reactions Frequency not defined.

Central nervous system: Convulsions, confusion, drowsiness, myoclonus, fever

Dermatologic: Rash

Endocrine & metabolic: Electrolyte imbalance

Hematologic: Positive Coombs' reaction, hemolytic anemia

Local: Pain, thrombophlebitis

Renal: Acute interstitial nephritis

Miscellaneous: Anaphylaxis, hypersensitivity reactions, Jarisch-Herxheimer reaction

Overdosage/Toxicology Symptoms of penicillin overdose include neuromuscular hypersensitivity (eg, agitation, hallucinations, asterixis, encephalopathy, confusion, and seizures). Electrolyte imbalance may occur if the preparation contains potassium or sodium salts, especially in renal failure. Hemodialysis may be helpful to aid in removal of the drug from blood; otherwise, treatment is supportive or symptom-directed.

Pharmacodynamics/Kinetics

Absorption: I.M.: Slow

Time to Peak: Serum: 12-24 hours

Duration: Dose dependent: 1-4 weeks; larger doses result in more sustained levels

Formulations Injection, suspension [prefilled syringe]:

Bicillin® L-A: 600,000 units/mL (1 mL, 2 mL, 4 mL)

Permapen® Isoject®: 600,000 units/mL (2 mL)

Dosing

Adults: Administer I.M. as undiluted injection; higher doses result in more sustained rather than higher levels. Use a penicillin G benzathine-penicillin G procaine combination to achieve early peak levels in acute infections.

Group A streptococcal upper respiratory infection: I.M.: 1.2 million units as a single dose

Prophylaxis of recurrent rheumatic fever: I.M.: 1.2 million units every 3-4 weeks or 600,000 units twice monthly

Early syphilis: I.M.: 2.4 million units as a single dose in 2 injection sites

Syphilis of more than 1-year duration: I.M.: 2.4 million units in 2 injection sites once weekly for 3 doses

Note: Not indicated as single drug therapy for neurosyphilis, but may be given 1 time/week for 3 weeks following I.V. treatment (refer to Penicillin G monograph for dosing)

Elderly: Not indicated as single drug therapy for neurosyphilis, but may be given 1 time/week for 3 weeks following I.V. treatment (see Penicillin G for dosing). No adjustment for renal function or age is necessary. Following equal, simple I.M. injections, the elderly have serum penicillin concentrations approximately twice that of younger adults 48, 96, and 144 hours postadministration.

Pediatrics: Administer I.M. as undiluted injection; higher doses result in more sustained rather than higher levels. Use a penicillin G benzathine-penicillin G procaine combination to achieve early peak levels in acute infections. Dosage frequency depends on infection being treated.

Asymptomatic congenital syphilis: I.M.: Neonates >1200g: 50,000 units/kg for 1 dose

Group A streptococcal upper respiratory infection: I.M.: Infants and Children: 25,000-50,000 units/kg as a single dose; maximum: 1.2 million units

Prophylaxis of recurrent rheumatic fever: I.M.: Infants and Children: 25,000-50,000 units/kg every 3-4 weeks; maximum: 1.2 million units/dose

Early syphilis: I.M.: Infants and Children: 50,000 units/kg as a single injection; maximum: 2.4 million units

Syphilis of more than 1-year duration: I.M.: Infants and Children: 50,000 units/kg every week for 3 doses; maximum: 2.4 million units/dose

Administration

I.M.: Administer by deep I.M. injection in the upper outer quadrant of the buttock. Do **not** give I.V., intra-arterially, or S.C. When doses are repeated, rotate the injection site.

Stability

Storage: Store in refrigerator.

Monitoring Laboratory Tests Perform culture and sensitivity before administering first dose.

Monitoring and Teaching Issues

Physical Assessment: Assess for allergy history prior to starting therapy. See Contraindications and Warnings/Precautions for use cautions. Assess potential for interactions with other prescriptions, OTC medications, or herbal products patient may be taking (see Drug Interactions). Caution diabetic patients about altered response to Clinitest®. Assess for therapeutic effectiveness and adverse reactions (eg, hypersensitivity reactions, opportunistic infection - see Adverse Reactions and Overdose/Toxicology). Teach patient possible side effects and interventions, and adverse symptoms to report (see Patient Education).

Patient Education: Inform prescriber of all prescriptions, OTC medications, or herbal products you are taking, and any allergies you have. Do not take anything new during treatment unless approved by prescriber. This drug can only be given by injection. Report immediately any redness, swelling, burning, or pain at infusion site or any signs of allergic reaction (eg, difficulty breathing or swallowing, chest tightness, rash, hives, swelling of lips or mouth). Maintain adequate hydration (2-3 L/day of fluids) unless advised by prescriber to restrict fluids. If being treated for sexually-transmitted disease, partner will also need to be treated. If diabetic, drug may cause false test results with Clinitest®; consult prescriber for alternative method of glucose monitoring. May cause confusion or drowsiness (use caution when driving or engaging in tasks that require alertness until response to drug is known). Report persistent adverse effects or signs of opportunistic infection (eg, fever, chills, unhealed sores, white plaques in mouth or vagina, purulent vaginal discharge, fatigue).

Penicillin G (Parenteral/Aqueous)

(pen i SIL in jee pa REN ter al AYE kwee us)

U.S. Brand Names Pfizerpen®

Synonyms Benzylpenicillin Potassium; Benzylpenicillin Sodium; Crystalline Penicillin; Penicillin G Potassium; Penicillin G Sodium

Generic Available Yes

Pharmacologic Category Antibiotic, Penicillin

Pregnancy Risk Factor B

Lactation Enters breast milk/compatible

Use Active against some gram-positive organisms, generally not *Staphylococcus aureus*; some gram-negative organisms such as *Neisseria gonorrhoeae*, and some anaerobes and spirochetes

Mechanism of Action/Effect Interferes with bacterial cell wall synthesis during active multiplication, causing cell wall death and resultant bactericidal activity against susceptible bacteria

Contraindications Hypersensitivity to penicillin or any component of the formulation

Warnings/Precautions Avoid intravascular or intra-arterial administration or injection into or near major peripheral nerves or blood vessels since such injections may cause severe and/or permanent neurovascular damage. Use with caution in patients with renal impairment (dosage reduction required), pre-existing seizure disorders.

Drug Interactions

Decreased Effect: Tetracyclines may decrease penicillin effectiveness. Although anecdotal reports suggest oral contraceptive efficacy could be reduced by penicillins, this has been refuted by more rigorous scientific and clinical data.

Increased Effect/Toxicity: Probenecid increases penicillin levels. Aminoglycosides may lead to synergistic efficacy.

Effects on Lab Values False-positive or negative urinary glucose determination using Clinitest®; positive Coombs' [direct]; false-positive urinary and/or serum proteins

Adverse Reactions Frequency not defined.

Central nervous system: Convulsions, confusion, drowsiness, myoclonus, fever
Dermatologic: Rash
Endocrine & metabolic: Electrolyte imbalance
Hematologic: Positive Coombs' reaction, hemolytic anemia
Local: Thrombophlebitis
Renal: Acute interstitial nephritis
Miscellaneous: Anaphylaxis, hypersensitivity reactions, Jarisch-Herxheimer reaction

Overdosage/Toxicology Symptoms of penicillin overdose include neuromuscular hypersensitivity (eg, agitation, hallucinations, asterixis, encephalopathy, confusion, and seizures). Electrolyte imbalance may occur if the preparation contains potassium or sodium salts, especially in renal failure. Treatment is supportive or symptom-directed.

Pharmacodynamics/Kinetics

Half-Life Elimination:

Neonates: <6 days old: 3.2-3.4 hours; 7-13 days old: 1.2-2.2 hours; >14 days old: 0.9-1.9 hours
Children and Adults: Normal renal function: 20-50 minutes
End-stage renal disease: 3.3-5.1 hours

Time to Peak: Serum: I.M.: ~30 minutes; I.V. ~1 hour

Metabolism: Hepatic (30%) to penicilloic acid

Formulations

Injection, penicillin G potassium [premixed, frozen]: 1 million units, 2 million units, 3 million units
Injection, penicillin G sodium: 5 million units
Injection, powder for reconstitution, penicillin G potassium: 1 million units, 5 million units, 10 million units, 20 million units

Dosing

Adults & Elderly:

Susceptible infections: I.M., I.V.: 2-24 million units/day in divided doses every 4 hours depending on sensitivity of the organism and severity of the infection

(Continued)

Penicillin G (Parenteral/Aqueous) *(Continued)*

Neurosyphilis: 18-24 million units/day in divided doses every 3-4 hours for 10-14 days

Pediatrics:

Neonatal infections: I.M., I.V.: Neonates:

Postnatal age ≤7 days:

≤2000 g: 50,000 units/kg/day in divided doses every 12 hours

Meningitis: 100,000 units/kg/day in divided doses every 12 hours

>2000 g: 75,000 units/kg/day in divided doses every 8 hours

Meningitis: 150,000 units/kg/day in divided doses every 8 hours

Congenital syphilis: 100,000 units/kg/day in divided doses every 12 hours

Group B streptococcal meningitis: 250,000-450,000 units/kg/day in divided doses every 8 hours

Postnatal age >7 days:

<1200 g: 50,000 units/kg/day in divided doses every 12 hours

Meningitis: 100,000 units/kg/day in divided doses every 12 hours

1200-2000 g: 75,000 units/kg/day in divided doses every 8 hours

Meningitis: 150,000 units/kg/day in divided doses every 8 hours

>2000 g: 100,000 units/kg/day in divided doses every 6 hours

Meningitis: 200,000 units/kg/day in divided doses every 6 hours

Congenital syphilis: 150,000 units/kg/day in divided doses every 8 hours

Group B streptococcal meningitis: I.V.: 450,000 units/kg/day in divided doses every 6 hours

Moderate infections: I.M., I.V.: Infants and Children: 100,000 to 250,000 units/kg/day in divided doses every 4-6 hours

Severe infections: I.M., I.V.: Infants and Children: 250,000-400,000 units/kg/day in divided doses every 4-6 hours; maximum dose: 24 million units/day

Renal Impairment: Dosage modification is required in patients with renal insufficiency.

Cl_{cr} 30-50 mL/minute: Administer every 6 hours.

Cl_{cr} 10-30 mL/minute: Administer every 8 hours.

Cl_{cr} <10 mL/minute: Administer every 12 hours.

Moderately dialyzable (20% to 50%)

Continuous arteriovenous or venovenous hemofiltration: Dose as for Cl_{cr} 10-50 mL/minute.

Administration

I.M.: Administer I.M. by deep injection in the upper outer quadrant of the buttock. Administer injection around-the-clock to promote less variation in peak and trough levels.

I.V.: While I.M. route is preferred route of administration, large doses should be administered by continuous I.V. infusion. Determine volume and rate of fluid administration required in a 24-hour period. Add appropriate daily dosage to this fluid. Rapid administration or excessive dosage can cause electrolyte imbalance, cardiac arrhythmias, and/or seizures.

Stability

Storage: Penicillin G potassium is stable at room temperature.

Reconstitution: Reconstituted parenteral solution is stable for 7 days when refrigerated (2°C to 15°C). Penicillin G potassium for I.V. infusion in NS or D_5W, solution is stable for 24 hours at room temperature.

Compatibility: Inactivated in acidic or alkaline solutions

Penicillin G potassium:

Stable in dextran 6% in dextrose, dextran 6% in NS, D_5LR, $D_5{}^1/_4NS$, $D_5{}^1/_2NS$, D_5NS, D_5W, $D_{10}W$, LR, $^1/_2NS$, NS, hetastarch 6%; **incompatible** with dextran 70 6% in dextrose, dextran 40 10% in dextrose

Compatibility in syringe: Incompatible with metoclopramide

Compatibility when admixed: Incompatible with aminoglycosides, aminophylline, amphotericin B, chlorpromazine, dopamine, floxacillin, hydroxyzine, metaraminol, pentobarbital, phenytoin, prochlorperazine mesylate, promazine, thiopental, vancomycin, vitamin B complex with C with oxytetracycline

Penicillin G sodium:

Stable in dextran 40 10%; **incompatible** with fat emulsion 10%

Compatibility when admixed: Incompatible with amphotericin B, bleomycin, chlorpromazine, cytarabine, floxacillin, hydroxyzine, methylprednisolone sodium succinate, prochlorperazine mesylate, promethazine, vancomycin

Monitoring Laboratory Tests Perform culture and sensitivity before administering first dose.

Monitoring and Teaching Issues

Physical Assessment: Assess for allergy history prior to starting therapy. See Contraindications and Warnings/Precautions for use cautions. Assess potential for interactions with other prescriptions, OTC medications, or herbal products patient may be taking (see Drug Interactions). Caution diabetic patients about altered response to Clinitest®. Assess therapeutic effectiveness and adverse reactions (eg, hypersensitivity reactions, opportunistic infection - see Adverse Reactions and Overdose/Toxicology). Teach patient possible side effects and interventions, and adverse symptoms to report (see Patient Education).

Patient Education: Inform prescriber of all prescriptions, OTC medications, or herbal products you are taking, and any allergies you have. Do not take anything new during treatment unless approved by prescriber. This drug can only be given by injection or infusion. Report immediately any redness, swelling, burning, or pain at infusion site or any signs of allergic reaction (eg, difficulty breathing or swallowing, chest tightness, rash, hives, swelling of lips or mouth). Maintain adequate hydration (2-3 L/day of fluids) unless advised by prescriber to restrict fluids. If being treated for sexually-transmitted disease, partner will also need to be treated. If diabetic, drug may cause false test results with Clinitest®, consult prescriber for alternative method of glucose monitoring. May cause confusion or drowsiness (use caution when driving or engaging in tasks that require alertness until response to drug is known). Report persistent adverse effects or signs of opportunistic infection (eg, fever, chills, unhealed sores, white plaques in mouth or vagina, purulent vaginal discharge, fatigue).

Geriatric Considerations: Despite a reported prolonged half-life, it is usually not necessary to adjust the dose of penicillin G or VK in the elderly to account for renal function changes with age, however, it is advised to calculate an estimated creatinine clearance and adjust dose accordingly. Consider sodium content in patients who may be sensitive to volume expansion (ie, CHF).

Additional Information 1 million units is approximately equal to 625 mg.

Penicillin G potassium injection:

Potassium content per million units: 65.6 mg (1.7 mEq)

Sodium content per million units: 23.5 mg (1.02 mEq)

Penicillin G Potassium *see* Penicillin G (Parenteral/Aqueous) *on page 1045*

Penicillin G Procaine (pen i SIL in jee PROE kane)

U.S. Brand Names Wycillin®

Synonyms APPG; Aqueous Procaine Penicillin G; Procaine Benzylpenicillin; Procaine Penicillin G

Generic Available Yes

Pharmacologic Category Antibiotic, Penicillin

Pregnancy Risk Factor B

Lactation Enters breast milk/compatible

Use Moderately severe infections due to *Treponema pallidum* and other penicillin G-sensitive microorganisms that are susceptible to low, but prolonged serum penicillin concentrations; anthrax due to *Bacillus anthracis* (postexposure) to reduce the incidence or progression of disease following exposure to aerolized *Bacillus anthracis*

Mechanism of Action/Effect Inhibits bacterial cell wall synthesis by binding to one or more of the penicillin binding proteins (PBPs); which in turn inhibits the final transpeptidation step of peptidoglycan synthesis in bacterial cell walls, thus inhibiting cell wall biosynthesis. Bacteria eventually lyse due to ongoing activity of cell wall autolytic enzymes (autolysins and murein hydrolases) while cell wall assembly is arrested.

Contraindications Hypersensitivity to penicillin, procaine, or any component of the formulation

Warnings/Precautions May need to modify dosage in patients with severe renal impairment, seizure disorders. Avoid I.V., intravascular, or intra-arterial administration of penicillin G procaine since severe and/or permanent neurovascular damage may occur. Use of penicillin for longer than 2 weeks may be associated with an increased risk for some adverse reactions (neutropenia, serum sickness).

Drug Interactions

Decreased Effect: Tetracyclines may decrease penicillin effectiveness. Although anecdotal reports suggest oral contraceptive efficacy could be reduced by penicillins, this has been refuted by more rigorous scientific and clinical data.

Increased Effect/Toxicity: Probenecid increases penicillin levels. Aminoglycosides may lead to synergistic efficacy.

Effects on Lab Values Positive Coombs' [direct], false-positive urinary and/or serum proteins

Adverse Reactions Frequency not defined.

Cardiovascular: Myocardial depression, vasodilation, conduction disturbances

Central nervous system: Confusion, drowsiness, myoclonus, CNS stimulation, seizures

Hematologic: Positive Coombs' reaction, hemolytic anemia, neutropenia

Local: Pain at injection site, thrombophlebitis, sterile abscess at injection site

Renal: Interstitial nephritis

Miscellaneous: Pseudoanaphylactic reactions, hypersensitivity reactions, Jarisch-Herxheimer reaction, serum sickness

Overdosage/Toxicology Symptoms of penicillin overdose include neuromuscular hypersensitivity (eg, agitation, hallucinations, asterixis, encephalopathy, confusion, and seizures). Electrolyte imbalance may occur if the preparation contains potassium or sodium salts, especially in renal failure. Hemodialysis may be helpful to aid in removal of the drug from blood; otherwise, treatment is supportive or symptom-directed.

Pharmacodynamics/Kinetics

Absorption: I.M.: Slow

Time to Peak: Serum: 1-4 hours

Metabolism: ~30% hepatically inactivated

Duration: Therapeutic: 15-24 hours

Formulations Injection, suspension: 300,000 units/mL (10 mL); 600,000 units/mL (1 mL, 2 mL, 4 mL)

Dosing

Adults & Elderly:

Anthrax:

Inhalational (postexposure prophylaxis): I.M.: 1,200,000 units every 12 hours

Note: Overall treatment duration should be 60 days. Available safety data suggest continued administration of penicillin G procaine for longer than 2 weeks may incur additional risk of adverse reactions. Clinicians may consider switching to effective alternative treatment for completion of therapy beyond 2 weeks.

Cutaneous (treatment): I.M.: 600,000-1,200,000 units/day; alternative therapy is recommended in severe cutaneous or other forms of anthrax infection

Uncomplicated gonorrhea: I.M.: 1 g probenecid orally, then 4.8 million units procaine penicillin divided into 2 injection sites 30 minutes later

Endocarditis caused by susceptible viridans *Streptococcus* (when used in conjunction with an aminoglycoside): I.M.: 1.2 million units every 6 hours for 2-4 weeks

Neurosyphilis: I.M.: 2-4 million units/day with 500 mg probenecid by mouth 4 times/day for 10-14 days; **penicillin G aqueous I.V. is the preferred agent**

Pediatrics:

Susceptible infections: I.M.: Infants and Children: 25,000-50,000 units/kg/day in divided doses every 12-24 hours; not to exceed 4.8 million units/24 hours

Anthrax, inhalational (postexposure prophylaxis): I.M.: 25,000 units/kg every 12 hours (maximum: 1,200,000 units every 12 hours).

(Continued)

Penicillin G Procaine *(Continued)*

Note: Overall treatment duration should be 60 days. Available safety data suggest continued administration of penicillin G procaine for longer than 2 weeks may incur additional risk for adverse reactions. Clinicians may consider switching to effective alternative treatment for completion of therapy beyond 2 weeks.

Congenital syphilis: I.M.: 50,000 units/kg/day once daily for 10 days; if more than 1 day of therapy is missed, the entire course should be restarted

Renal Impairment:

Cl_{cr} 10-30 mL/minute: Administer every 8-12 hours.

Cl_{cr} <10 mL/minute: Administer every 12-18 hours.

Moderately dialyzable (20% to 50%)

Administration

I.M.: Procaine suspension is for deep I.M. injection only. Rotate the injection site.

Stability

Storage: Store in refrigerator.

Monitoring Laboratory Tests Periodic renal and hematologic function with prolonged therapy; WBC count; perform culture and sensitivity before administering first dose.

Monitoring and Teaching Issues

Physical Assessment: Assess for allergy history prior to starting therapy. See Contraindications and Warnings/Precautions for use cautions. Assess potential for interactions with other prescriptions, OTC medications, or herbal products patient may be taking (see Drug Interactions). Caution diabetic patients about altered response to Clinitest®. Assess results of laboratory tests (see above), therapeutic effectiveness, and adverse reactions (eg, hypersensitivity reactions, opportunistic infection - see Adverse Reactions and Overdose/Toxicology). Teach patient possible side effects and interventions, and adverse symptoms to report (see Patient Education).

Patient Education: Inform prescriber of all prescriptions, OTC medications, or herbal products you are taking, and any allergies you have. Do not take anything new during treatment unless approved by prescriber. This drug can only be given by injection. Report immediately any redness, swelling, burning, or pain at infusion site or any signs of allergic reaction (eg, difficulty breathing or swallowing, chest tightness, rash, hives, swelling of lips or mouth). Maintain adequate hydration (2-3 L/day of fluids) unless advised by prescriber to restrict fluids. May cause confusion or drowsiness (use caution when driving or engaging in tasks that require alertness until response to drug is known). Report chest pain, palpitations, or irregular heartbeat; persistent adverse effects; or signs of opportunistic infection (eg, fever, chills, unhealed sores, white plaques in mouth or vagina, purulent vaginal discharge, fatigue). If diabetic, drug may cause false test results with Clinitest® urine glucose monitoring; use of glucose oxidase methods (Clinistix®) or serum glucose monitoring is preferable.

Geriatric Considerations: Dosage does not usually need to be adjusted in the elderly, however, if multiple doses are to be given, adjust dose for renal function.

Penicillin G Sodium *see* Penicillin G (Parenteral/Aqueous) *on page 1045*

Penicillin V Potassium (pen i SIL in vee poe TASS ee um)

U.S. Brand Names Suspen®; Truxcillin®; Veetids®

Synonyms Pen VK; Phenoxymethyl Penicillin

Generic Available Yes

Pharmacologic Category Antibiotic, Penicillin

Pregnancy Risk Factor B

Lactation Enters breast milk (other penicillins are compatible with breast-feeding)

Use Treatment of infections caused by susceptible organisms involving the respiratory tract, otitis media, sinusitis, skin, and urinary tract; prophylaxis in rheumatic fever

Mechanism of Action/Effect Inhibits bacterial cell wall synthesis by binding to one or more of the penicillin binding proteins (PBPs); which in turn inhibits the final transpeptidation step of peptidoglycan synthesis in bacterial cell walls, thus inhibiting cell wall biosynthesis. Bacteria eventually lyse due to ongoing activity of cell wall autolytic enzymes (autolysins and murein hydrolases) while cell wall assembly is arrested.

Contraindications Hypersensitivity to penicillin or any component of the formulation

Warnings/Precautions Use with caution in patients with severe renal impairment (modify dosage).

Drug Interactions

Decreased Effect: Tetracyclines may decrease penicillin effectiveness. Although anecdotal reports suggest oral contraceptive efficacy could be reduced by penicillins, this has been refuted by more rigorous scientific and clinical data.

Increased Effect/Toxicity: Probenecid increases penicillin levels. Aminoglycosides may cause synergistic efficacy.

Nutritional/Ethanol Interactions Food: Decreases drug absorption rate; decreases drug serum concentration.

Effects on Lab Values False-positive or negative urinary glucose determination using Clinitest®; positive Coombs' [direct]; false-positive urinary and/or serum proteins

Adverse Reactions

>10%: Gastrointestinal: Mild diarrhea, vomiting, nausea, oral candidiasis

<1% (Limited to important or life-threatening): Acute interstitial nephritis, convulsions, hemolytic anemia, positive Coombs' reaction

Overdosage/Toxicology Symptoms of penicillin overdose include neuromuscular hypersensitivity (eg, agitation, hallucinations, asterixis, encephalopathy, confusion, and seizures). Electrolyte imbalance may occur if the preparation contains potassium or sodium salts, especially in renal failure. Hemodialysis may be helpful to aid in removal of the drug from blood; otherwise, treatment is supportive or symptom-directed.

Pharmacodynamics/Kinetics

Absorption: 60% to 73%

Half-Life Elimination: 30 minutes; prolonged with renal impairment

Time to Peak: Serum: 0.5-1 hour

Formulations 250 mg = 400,000 units

Powder for oral solution: 125 mg/5 mL (80 mL, 100 mL, 150 mL, 200 mL); 250 mg/5 mL (80 mL, 100 mL, 150 mL, 200 mL)

Tablet: 250 mg, 500 mg

Dosing

Adults & Elderly:

Systemic infections: Oral: 125-500 mg every 6-8 hours

Prophylaxis of pneumococcal infections: Oral: 250 mg twice daily

Prophylaxis of recurrent rheumatic fever: Oral: 250 mg twice daily

Pediatrics:

Systemic infections: Oral:

<12 years: 25-50 mg/kg/day in divided doses every 6-8 hours; maximum dose: 3 g/day

≥12 years: 125-500 mg every 6-8 hours

Prophylaxis of pneumococcal infections: Oral:

<5 years: 125 mg twice daily

≥5 years: 250 mg twice daily

Prophylaxis of recurrent rheumatic fever: Oral:

<5 years: 125 mg twice daily

≥5 years: 250 mg twice daily

Renal Impairment:

Cl_{cr} 10-50 mL/minute: Administer every 8-12 hours.

Cl_{cr} <10 mL/minute: Administer every 12-16 hours.

Administration

Oral: Administer around-the-clock to promote less variation in peak and trough serum levels. Take on an empty stomach 1 hour before or 2 hours after meals, to enhance absorption, take until gone, do not skip doses.

Stability

Storage: Refrigerate suspension after reconstitution; discard after 14 days.

Monitoring Laboratory Tests Periodic renal and hematologic function during prolonged therapy; perform culture and sensitivity before administering first dose.

Monitoring and Teaching Issues

Physical Assessment: Assess for allergy history prior to starting therapy. See Contraindications and Warnings/Precautions for use cautions. Assess potential for interactions with other prescriptions, OTC medications, or herbal products patient may be taking (see Drug Interactions). Caution diabetic patients about altered response to Clinitest®. Assess results of laboratory tests (see above), therapeutic effectiveness, and adverse reactions (see Adverse Reactions and Overdose/Toxicology). Teach patient proper use, possible side effects and interventions, and adverse symptoms to report (see Patient Education).

Patient Education: Inform prescriber of all prescriptions, OTC medications, or herbal products you are taking, and any allergies you have. Do not take anything new during treatment unless approved by prescriber. Take as directed at intervals around-the-clock, preferable on an empty stomach (1 hour before or 2 hours after a meal). Take entire prescription; do not skip doses or discontinue without consulting prescriber. Take a missed dose as soon as possible. If almost time for next dose, skip the missed dose and return to your regular schedule. Do not take a double dose. Maintain adequate hydration (2-3 L/day of fluids) unless advised by prescriber to restrict fluids. If diabetic, drug may cause false test results with Clinitest®, consult prescriber for alternative method of glucose monitoring. May cause nausea or vomiting (small, frequent meals, frequent mouth care, chewing gum, or sucking lozenges may help); or diarrhea (buttermilk, boiled milk, or yogurt may help). Report persistent adverse effects; signs of opportunistic infection (eg, fever, chills, unhealed sores, white plaques in mouth or vagina, purulent vaginal discharge, fatigue); or signs of hypersensitivity reaction (rash, hives, itching, swelling of lips, tongue, mouth, or throat).

Dietary Issues: Take on an empty stomach 1 hour before or 2 hours after meals.

Breast-feeding Issues: No data reported; however, other penicillins may be taken while breast-feeding.

Additional Information 0.7 mEq of potassium per 250 mg penicillin V; 250 mg equals 400,000 units of penicillin

Pentacarinat® *see* Pentamidine *on page 1049*

Pentagastrin *see page 1461*

Pentam-300® *see* Pentamidine *on page 1049*

Pentamidine (pen TAM i deen)

U.S. Brand Names NebuPent™; Pentacarinat®; Pentam-300®

Synonyms Pentamidine Isethionate

Generic Available Yes

Pharmacologic Category Antibiotic, Miscellaneous

Pregnancy Risk Factor C

Lactation Excretion in breast milk unknown/contraindicated

Use Treatment and prevention of pneumonia caused by *Pneumocystis carinii*; treatment of trypanosomiasis and visceral leishmaniasis

Mechanism of Action/Effect Interferes with RNA/DNA synthesis and phospholipids leading to cell death in protozoa.

Contraindications Hypersensitivity to pentamidine isethionate or any component of the formulation (inhalation and injection)

Warnings/Precautions Use with caution in patients with diabetes mellitus, renal or hepatic dysfunction, hyper-/hypotension, leukopenia, thrombocytopenia, asthma, or hypo-/hyperglycemia. Pregnancy risk C.

(Continued)

Pentamidine *(Continued)*

Drug Interactions

Cytochrome P450 Effect: Substrate of **CYP2C19**; Inhibits CYP2D6

Increased Effect/Toxicity: Pentamidine may potentiate the effect of other drugs which prolong QT interval (cisapride, astemizole, sparfloxacin, gatifloxacin, moxifloxacin, and type Ia and type III antiarrhythmics).

Nutritional/Ethanol Interactions Ethanol: Avoid ethanol (may increase CNS depression or aggravate hypoglycemia).

Adverse Reactions

Inhalation:

>10%:
- Cardiovascular: Chest pain
- Dermatologic: Rash
- Respiratory: Wheezing, dyspnea, coughing, pharyngitis

1% to 10%: Gastrointestinal: Bitter or metallic taste

<1% (Limited to important or life-threatening): Hypoglycemia, renal insufficiency

Systemic:

>10%:
- Cardiovascular: Hypotension
- Dermatologic: Rash
- Endocrine & metabolic: Hyperglycemia or hypoglycemia
- Gastrointestinal: Nausea, vomiting, anorexia, diarrhea
- Hematologic: Leukopenia or neutropenia, thrombocytopenia
- Hepatic: Elevated LFTs
- Renal: Nephrotoxicity

1% to 10%:
- Hematologic: Anemia
- Cardiovascular: Cardiac arrhythmias
- Gastrointestinal: Pancreatitis, metallic taste
- Local: Local reactions at injection site

<1% (Limited to important or life-threatening): Arrhythmias

Overdosage/Toxicology Symptoms of overdose include hypotension, hypoglycemia, and cardiac arrhythmias. Treatment is supportive.

Pharmacodynamics/Kinetics

Absorption: I.M.: Well absorbed; Inhalation: Limited systemic absorption

Half-Life Elimination: Terminal: 6.4-9.4 hours; may be prolonged with severe renal impairment

Formulations

Injection, powder for reconstitution, as isethionate: 300 mg

Powder for nebulization, as isethionate: 300 mg

Dosing

Adults & Elderly:

Treatment of PCP: I.M., I.V. (I.V. preferred): 4 mg/kg/day once daily for 14 days

Prevention of PCP: Inhalation: 300 mg every 4 weeks via Respirgard® II nebulizer

Pediatrics:

Treatment of PCP pneumonia: I.M., I.V. (I.V. preferred): Children: 4 mg/kg/day once daily for 10-14 days

Prevention of PCP pneumonia: Children:
- I.M., I.V.: 4 mg/kg monthly or every 2 weeks
- Inhalation (aerosolized pentamidine in children ≥5 years): 300 mg/dose given every 3-4 weeks via Respirgard® II inhaler (8 mg/kg dose has also been used in children <5 years)

Treatment of trypanosomiasis: I.V.: 4 mg/kg/day once daily for 10 days

Renal Impairment:

Cl_{cr} 10-50 mL/minute: Administer dose every 24-36 hours.

Cl_{cr} <10 mL/minute: Administer dose every 48 hours.

Not removed by hemo- or peritoneal dialysis or continuous arteriovenous or venovenous hemofiltration. Supplemental dose is not necessary.

Administration

I.M.: Deep I.M.

I.V.: Do not use NS as a diluent. Infuse I.V. slowly over a period of at least 60 minutes or administer deep I.M.

Inhalation: Virtually undetectable amounts are transferred to healthcare personnel during aerosol administration.

Stability

Storage: Do not refrigerate due to the possibility of crystallization.

Reconstitution: Reconstituted solutions (60-100 mg/mL) are stable for 48 hours at room temperature and do not require light protection. Diluted solutions (1-2.5 mg/mL) in D_5W are stable for at least 24 hours at room temperature.

Compatibility: Stable in D_5W, NS, sterile water for injection

Y-site administration: Incompatible with aldesleukin, cefazolin, cefoperazone, cefotaxime, cefoxitin, ceftazidime, ceftriaxone, fluconazole, foscarnet, linezolid

Monitoring Laboratory Tests Liver and renal function, blood glucose, serum potassium and calcium, EKG, CBC with platelets

Monitoring and Teaching Issues

Physical Assessment: Assess for allergy history prior to starting therapy. See Contraindications and Warnings/Precautions for use cautions. Assess potential for interactions with other prescriptions, OTC medications, or herbal products patient may be taking (see Drug Interactions). **I.V./I.M.:** Patients should be lying down. Blood pressure, cardiac status, and respiratory function should be monitored closely during I.V. administration or following I.M. injection. Assess results of laboratory tests (see above), therapeutic effectiveness, and adverse reactions (see Adverse Reactions and Overdose/Toxicology). Teach patient proper use, possible side effects and interventions, and adverse symptoms to report (see

Patient Education). **Pregnancy risk factor C** - benefits of use should outweigh possible risks. Breast-feeding is contraindicated.

Patient Education: Inform prescriber of all prescriptions, OTC medications, or herbal products you are taking, and any allergies you have. Do not take anything new without consulting prescriber. I.V. or I.M. preparations must be given every day. Inhalant drug must be prepared and used with a nebulizer as directed once every 4 weeks. Frequent blood tests and blood pressure checks will be required while using this drug. PCP pneumonia may still occur despite pentamidine use. Maintain adequate hydration (2-3 L/day of fluids) unless instructed to restrict fluid intake. Avoid alcohol. If diabetic, monitor glucose levels closely and frequently. May cause hypotension (use caution when rising from sitting or lying position or when climbing stairs); or metallic taste, nausea, vomiting, or anorexia (small, frequent meals, frequent mouth care, chewing gum, or sucking lozenges may help). Report chest pain or irregular heartbeat; unusual confusion or hallucinations; rash; or unusual wheezing, coughing, or difficulty breathing. **Pregnancy/breast-feeding precautions:** Inform prescriber if you are or intend to become pregnant. Do not breast-feed.

Geriatric Considerations: Ten percent of acquired immunodeficiency syndrome (AIDS) cases are in the elderly and this figure is expected to increase. Pentamidine has not as yet been studied exclusively in this population. Adjust dose for renal function.

Pentamidine Isethionate *see* Pentamidine *on page 1049*

Pentasa® *see* Mesalamine *on page 858*

Pentazocine (pen TAZ oh seen)

U.S. Brand Names Talwin®; Talwin® NX

Synonyms Pentazocine Hydrochloride; Pentazocine Lactate

Restrictions C-IV

Generic Available Yes

Pharmacologic Category Analgesic, Narcotic

Pregnancy Risk Factor B/D (prolonged use or high doses at term)

Lactation Enters breast milk/use caution

Use Relief of moderate to severe pain; has also been used as a sedative prior to surgery and as a supplement to surgical anesthesia

Mechanism of Action/Effect Binds to opiate receptors in the CNS, causing inhibition of ascending pain pathways, altering the perception of and response to pain; produces generalized CNS depression; partial agonist-antagonist

Contraindications Hypersensitivity to pentazocine or any component of the formulation; increased intracranial pressure (unless the patient is mechanically ventilated); pregnancy (prolonged use or high doses at term)

Warnings/Precautions Use with caution in seizure-prone patients, acute myocardial infarction, patients undergoing biliary tract surgery, patients with renal and hepatic dysfunction, head trauma, increased intracranial pressure, and patients with a history of prior opioid dependence or abuse; pentazocine may precipitate opiate withdrawal symptoms in patients who have been receiving opiates regularly; injection contains sulfites which may cause allergic reaction; tolerance or drug dependence may result from extended use. Severe vascular complications have resulted from misuse (injection) of Talwin® tablet formulations.

Drug Interactions

Decreased Effect: May potentiate or reduce analgesic effect of opiate agonist (eg, morphine) depending on patients tolerance to opiates; can precipitate withdrawal in narcotic addicts.

Increased Effect/Toxicity: Increased effect/toxicity with tripelennamine (can be lethal), CNS depressants (eg, phenothiazines, tranquilizers, anxiolytics, sedatives, hypnotics, alcohol).

Nutritional/Ethanol Interactions Ethanol: Avoid ethanol (may increase CNS depression).

Adverse Reactions Frequency not defined.

Cardiovascular: Hypotension, palpitations, peripheral vasodilation

Central nervous system: Malaise, headache, restlessness, nightmares, insomnia, CNS depression, sedation, hallucinations, confusion, disorientation, dizziness, euphoria, drowsiness

Dermatologic: Rash, pruritus

Gastrointestinal: Nausea, vomiting, xerostomia, constipation, anorexia, diarrhea, GI irritation, biliary tract spasm

Genitourinary: Urinary tract spasm

Local: Tissue damage and irritation with I.M./S.C. use

Neuromuscular & skeletal: Weakness

Ocular: Blurred vision, miosis

Respiratory: Dyspnea, respiratory depression (rare)

Miscellaneous: Histamine release, physical and psychological dependence

Overdosage/Toxicology Symptoms of overdose include drowsiness, sedation, respiratory depression, and coma. Naloxone, 2 mg I.V., with repeat administration as necessary up to a total of 10 mg, can also be used to reverse toxic effects of the opiate.

Pharmacodynamics/Kinetics

Bioavailability: Oral: ~20%; increased to 60% to 70% with cirrhosis

Half-Life Elimination: 2-3 hours; prolonged with hepatic impairment

Metabolism: Hepatic via oxidative and glucuronide conjugation pathways; extensive first-pass effect

Onset: Oral, I.M., S.C.: 15-30 minutes; I.V.: 2-3 minutes

Duration: Oral: 4-5 hours; Parenteral: 2-3 hours

Formulations

Injection, as lactate: 30 mg/mL (1 mL, 1.5 mL, 2 mL, 10 mL)

Tablet: Pentazocine hydrochloride 50 mg and naloxone hydrochloride 0.5 mg

(Continued)

Pentazocine *(Continued)*

Dosing

Adults: Analgesic:

Oral: 50 mg every 3-4 hours; may increase to 100 mg/dose if needed, but should not exceed 600 mg/day

I.M., S.C.: 30-60 mg every 3-4 hours, not to exceed total daily dose of 360 mg

I.V.: 30 mg every 3-4 hours; do **not** exceed 30 mg/dose.

Elderly: Elderly patients may be more sensitive to the analgesic and sedating effects. The elderly may also have impaired renal function. If needed, dosing should be started at the lower end of dosing range and adjust dose for renal function (see Geriatric Considerations).

Pediatrics: Analgesic:

Children: I.M., S.C.:

5-8 years: 15 mg

8-14 years: 30 mg

Children >12 years: Oral: 50 mg every 3-4 hours; may increase to 100 mg/dose if needed, but should not exceed 600 mg/day

Renal Impairment:

Cl_{cr} 10-50 mL/minute: Administer 75% of normal dose.

Cl_{cr} <10 mL/minute: Administer 50% of normal dose.

Hepatic Impairment: Reduce dose or avoid use in patients with liver disease.

Administration

I.V.: Rotate injection site for I.M., S.C. use; avoid intra-arterial injection.

Stability

Storage: Injection: Store at room temperature, protect from heat and from freezing.

Compatibility:

Y-site administration: Incompatible with nafcillin

Compatibility in syringe: Incompatible with glycopyrrolate, heparin, pentobarbital

Compatibility when admixed: Incompatible with aminophylline, amobarbital, pentobarbital, phenobarbital, sodium bicarbonate

Monitoring and Teaching Issues

Physical Assessment: Assess other medications patient may be taking for additive or adverse interactions (see Drug Interactions). Monitor therapeutic effectiveness, adverse reactions, and overdose (see Overdose/Toxicology) at beginning of therapy and at regular intervals with long-term use. May cause physical and/or psychological dependence. For inpatients, implement safety measures. Assess knowledge/teach patient appropriate use (if self-administered), adverse reactions to report (see Adverse Reactions), and appropriate interventions to reduce side effects (see Patient Education). **Pregnancy risk factor B/D** - see Pregnancy Risk Factor for use cautions. Note breast-feeding caution.

Patient Education: If self-administered, use exactly as directed; do not increase dose or frequency. Drug may cause physical and/or psychological dependence. While using this medication, do not use alcohol and other prescription or OTC medications (especially sedatives, tranquilizers, antihistamines, or pain medications) without consulting prescriber. Maintain adequate hydration (2-3 L/day of fluids) unless advised by prescriber to restrict fluids. May cause hypotension, dizziness, drowsiness, impaired coordination, or blurred vision (use caution when driving, climbing stairs, or changing position - rising from sitting or lying to standing, or when engaging in tasks requiring alertness until response to drug is known); nausea, vomiting, loss of appetite, or dry mouth (frequent mouth care, small, frequent meals, chewing gum, or sucking lozenges may help); or constipation (increased exercise, fluids, fruit, or fiber may help; if unresolved, consult prescriber about use of stool softeners). Report persistent dizziness or headache; excessive fatigue or sedation; changes in mental status; changes in urinary elimination or pain on urination; weakness or trembling; blurred vision; or shortness of breath. **Pregnancy/breast-feeding precautions:** Inform prescriber if you are or intend to become pregnant. Consult prescriber if breast-feeding.

Geriatric Considerations: Pentazocine is not recommended for use in the elderly because of its propensity to cause delirium and agitation. If pentazocine must be used, be sure to adjust dose for renal function.

Additional Information Pentazocine hydrochloride: Talwin® NX tablet (with naloxone); naloxone is used to prevent abuse by dissolving tablets in water and using as injection.

Related Information

Compatibility of Drugs in Syringe *on page 1566*

Narcotic/Opioid Analgesic Comparison *on page 1583*

Pentazocine Compound (pen TAZ oh seen KOM pownd)

U.S. Brand Names Talacen®; Talwin® Compound

Generic Available Yes

Pharmacologic Category Analgesic Combination (Narcotic)

Pregnancy Risk Factor D/C (Talacen®)

Lactation Enters breast milk/contraindicated

Use Relief of moderate to severe pain; sedative prior to surgery; supplement to surgical anesthesia

Contraindications Hypersensitivity to pentazocine, aspirin, acetaminophen, or any component of the formulation; pregnancy

Warnings/Precautions Contains sodium metasulfite as sulfite that may cause allergic-type reactions; potential for elevating CSF pressure due to respiratory effects which may be exaggerated in presence of head injury, intracranial lesions, or pre-existing increase in intracranial lesions. May experience hallucinations, disorientation, and confusion. May cause psychological and physical dependence. Use with caution in patients with myocardial infarction who have nausea or vomiting, patients with respiratory depression, severely limited respiratory reserve, severe bronchial asthma, other obstructive respiratory conditions or cyanosis, impaired renal or hepatic function, patients prone to seizures. Talwin® Compound:

Use with caution in patients with peptic ulcer or patients on anticoagulation therapy. Pregnancy risk D/C (Talacen®).

Nutritional/Ethanol Interactions

Ethanol: Avoid ethanol (may increase CNS depression).

Herb/Nutraceutical: Avoid valerian, St John's wort, kava kava, gotu kola (may increase CNS depression).

Adverse Reactions Frequency not defined.

Cardiovascular: Tachycardia or bradycardia, hypertension or hypotension

Central nervous system: Nervousness, headache, restlessness, malaise, dizziness, fatigue, drowsiness, false sense of well-being, convulsions, increased intracranial pressure

Dermatologic: Rash, urticaria, erythema multiforme, Stevens-Johnson syndrome

Gastrointestinal: Nausea, vomiting, dry mouth, biliary spasm, constipation

Genitourinary: Ureteral spasms, decreased urination

Local: Pain at injection site

Neuromuscular & skeletal: Weakness

Ocular: Blurred vision

Respiratory: Dyspnea

Miscellaneous: Histamine release

Pharmacokinetic Note See individual agents.

Pharmacodynamics/Kinetics

Half-Life Elimination: Pentazocine: 3.6 hours; acetaminophen: 2.8 hours

Onset: Pentazocine: 15-30 minutes; acetaminophen: 30 minutes

Formulations

Tablet:

Talacen®: Pentazocine hydrochloride 25 mg and acetaminophen 650 mg

Talwin® Compound: Pentazocine hydrochloride 12.5 mg and aspirin 325 mg

Dosing

Adults & Elderly: Analgesic: Oral:

Talwin®: 2 tablets 3-4 times/day

Talacen®: 1 caplet every 4 hours up to maximum of 6 caplets

Stability

Storage: Controlled room temperature 15°C to 30°C (59°F to 86°F)

Monitoring and Teaching Issues

Physical Assessment: Assess patient for history of liver disease or ethanol abuse (acetaminophen and excessive ethanol may have adverse liver effects). Assess other medications patient may be taking for additive or adverse interactions (see Drug Interactions). Monitor therapeutic effectiveness, adverse reactions (see Adverse Reactions), and signs of overdose at beginning of therapy and at regular intervals with long-term use. May cause physical and/or psychological dependence. For inpatients, implement safety measures. Assess knowledge/teach patient appropriate use (if self-administered), adverse reactions to report, and appropriate interventions to reduce side effects (see Patient Education). **Pregnancy risk factor C/D** - see Pregnancy Risk Factor for use cautions; benefits of use should outweigh possible risks. Breast-feeding is contraindicated.

Patient Education: If self-administered, use exactly as directed; do not increase dose or frequency. Drug may cause physical and/or psychological dependence. Take with food or milk. While using this medication, do not use alcohol and other prescription or OTC medications (especially sedatives, tranquilizers, antihistamines, or pain medications) without consulting prescriber. Maintain adequate hydration (2-3 L/day of fluids) unless advised by prescriber to restrict fluids. May cause hypotension, dizziness, drowsiness, confusion, or nervousness (use caution when driving, climbing stairs, or changing position - rising from sitting or lying to standing, or when engaging in tasks requiring alertness until response to drug is known); nausea, dry mouth, decreased appetite, or gastric distress (frequent mouth care, frequent sips of fluids, chewing gum, or sucking lozenges may help); or constipation (increased exercise, fluids, fruit, or fiber may help; if unresolved, consult prescriber about use of stool softeners). Report chest pain, rapid heartbeat, or palpitations; persistent dizziness; change in mental status; shortness of breath or difficulty breathing; unusual bleeding (stool, mouth, urine) or bruising; unusual fatigue and weakness; pain on urination; change in elimination patterns or change in color of urine or stool; or unresolved nausea or vomiting. **Pregnancy/breast-feeding precautions:** Inform prescriber if you are or intend to become pregnant. Do not breast-feed.

Pregnancy Issues: Not known whether affects fetus. Use only if clearly needed.

Pentazocine Hydrochloride *see* Pentazocine *on page 1051*

Pentazocine Lactate *see* Pentazocine *on page 1051*

Pentobarbital (pen toe BAR bi tal)

U.S. Brand Names Nembutal®

Synonyms Pentobarbital Sodium

Restrictions C-II (capsules, injection); C-III (suppositories)

Generic Available Yes

Pharmacologic Category Anticonvulsant, Barbiturate; Barbiturate

Pregnancy Risk Factor D

Lactation Enters breast milk/contraindicated

Use Sedative/hypnotic; preanesthetic; high-dose barbiturate coma for treatment of increased intracranial pressure or status epilepticus unresponsive to other therapy

Use - Unlabeled/Investigational Tolerance test during withdrawal of sedative hypnotics

Mechanism of Action/Effect Short-acting barbiturate with sedative, hypnotic, and anticonvulsant properties. Barbiturates depress the sensory cortex, decrease motor activity, alter cerebellar function, and produce drowsiness, sedation, and hypnosis. In high doses, barbiturates exhibit anticonvulsant activity; barbiturates produce dose-dependent respiratory depression.

Contraindications Hypersensitivity to barbiturates or any component of the formulation; marked hepatic impairment; dyspnea or airway obstruction; porphyria; pregnancy

(Continued)

Pentobarbital *(Continued)*

Warnings/Precautions Tolerance to hypnotic effect can occur; do not use for >2 weeks to treat insomnia. Potential for drug dependency exists, abrupt cessation may precipitate withdrawal, including status epilepticus in epileptic patients. Do not administer to patients in acute pain. Use caution in elderly, debilitated, renally impaired, hepatic dysfunction, or pediatric patients. May cause paradoxical responses, including agitation and hyperactivity, particularly in acute pain and pediatric patients. Use with caution in patients with depression or suicidal tendencies, or in patients with a history of drug abuse. Tolerance, psychological and physical dependence may occur with prolonged use.

May cause CNS depression, which may impair physical or mental abilities. Patients must cautioned about performing tasks which require mental alertness (ie, operating machinery or driving). Effects with other sedative drugs or ethanol may be potentiated. Use of this agent as a hypnotic in the elderly is not recommended due to its long half-life and potential for physical and psychological dependence.

May cause respiratory depression or hypotension, particularly when administered intravenously. Use with caution in hemodynamically unstable patients or patients with respiratory disease. High doses (loading doses of 15-35 mg/kg given over 1-2 hours) have been utilized to induce pentobarbital coma, but these higher doses often cause hypotension requiring vasopressor therapy.

Drug Interactions

Cytochrome P450 Effect: Induces **CYP2A6, 3A4**

Decreased Effect: Barbiturates such as pentobarbital are hepatic enzyme inducers, and (only with chronic use) may increase the metabolism of antipsychotics, some beta-blockers (unlikely with atenolol and nadolol), calcium channel blockers, chloramphenicol, cimetidine, corticosteroids, cyclosporine, disopyramide, doxycycline, ethosuximide, felbamate, furosemide, griseofulvin, lamotrigine, phenytoin, propafenone, quinidine, tacrolimus, TCAs, and theophylline. Barbiturates may increase the metabolism of estrogens and reduce the efficacy of oral contraceptives; an alternative method of contraception should be considered. Barbiturates inhibit the hypoprothrombinemic effects of oral anticoagulants via increased metabolism. Barbiturates may enhance the metabolism of methadone resulting in methadone withdrawal.

Increased Effect/Toxicity: When combined with other CNS depressants, ethanol, narcotic analgesics, antidepressants, or benzodiazepines, additive respiratory and CNS depression may occur. Chronic use of barbiturates may enhance the hepatotoxic potential of acetaminophen overdoses. Chloramphenicol, MAO inhibitors, valproic acid, and felbamate may inhibit barbiturate metabolism. Barbiturates may impair the absorption of griseofulvin, and may enhance the nephrotoxic effects of methoxyflurane.

Nutritional/Ethanol Interactions

Ethanol: Avoid ethanol (may increase CNS depression).

Food: Food may decrease the rate but not the extent of oral absorption.

Effects on Lab Values ↑ ammonia (B); ↓ bilirubin (S)

Adverse Reactions Frequency not defined.

Cardiovascular: Bradycardia, hypotension, syncope

Central nervous system: Drowsiness, lethargy, CNS excitation or depression, impaired judgment, "hangover" effect, confusion, somnolence, agitation, hyperkinesia, ataxia, nervousness, headache, insomnia, nightmares, hallucinations, anxiety, dizziness

Dermatologic: Rash, exfoliative dermatitis, Stevens-Johnson syndrome

Gastrointestinal: Nausea, vomiting, constipation

Hematologic: Agranulocytosis, thrombocytopenia, megaloblastic anemia

Local: Pain at injection site, thrombophlebitis with I.V. use

Renal: Oliguria

Respiratory: Laryngospasm, respiratory depression, apnea (especially with rapid I.V. use), hypoventilation, apnea

Miscellaneous: Gangrene with inadvertent intra-arterial injection

Overdosage/Toxicology Symptoms of overdose include unsteady gait, slurred speech, confusion, jaundice, hypothermia, hypotension, respiratory depression, and coma. Treat symptomatically. Charcoal hemoperfusion may be beneficial in stage IV coma due to high serum concentration.

Pharmacodynamics/Kinetics

Half-Life Elimination: Terminal: Children: 25 hours; Adults, healthy: 22 hours (range: 35-50 hours)

Metabolism: Extensively hepatic via hydroxylation and oxidation pathways

Onset: Oral, rectal: 15-60 minutes; I.M.: 10-15 minutes; I.V.: ~1 minute

Duration: Oral, rectal: 1-4 hours; I.V.: 15 minutes

Formulations

Capsule, as sodium (C-II): 50 mg, 100 mg

Injection, as sodium (C-II): 50 mg/mL (20 mL, 50 mL)

Suppository, rectal (C-III): 60 mg, 200 mg

Dosing

Adults:

Hypnotic:

Oral: 100-200 mg at bedtime or 20 mg 3-4 times/day for daytime sedation

I.M.: 150-200 mg

I.V.: Initial: 100 mg, may repeat every 1-3 minutes up to 200-500 mg total dose

Rectal: 120-200 mg at bedtime

Preoperative sedation: I.M.: 150-200 mg

Barbiturate coma in head injury patients or status epilepticus: I.V.: Loading dose: 5-10 mg/kg given slowly over 1-2 hours; monitor blood pressure and respiratory rate; maintenance infusion: initial: 1 mg/kg/hour; may increase to 2-3 mg/kg/hour; maintain burst suppression on EEG

Status epilepticus: **Note**: Intubation required; monitor hemodynamics: I.V.: Loading dose: 2-15 mg/kg given slowly over 1-2 hours; maintenance infusion: 0.5-3 mg/kg/hour

Tolerance testing (unlabeled use): 200 mg every 2 hours until signs of intoxication are exhibited at any time during the 2 hours after the dose; maximum dose: 1000 mg

Elderly: Not recommended for use in the elderly (see Geriatric Considerations).

Pediatrics:

Children:

Sedative: Oral: 2-6 mg/kg/day divided in 3 doses; maximum: 100 mg/day

Hypnotic: I.M.: 2-6 mg/kg; maximum: 100 mg/dose

Rectal:

2 months to 1 year (10-20 lb): 30 mg

1-4 years (20-40 lb): 30-60 mg

5-12 years (40-80 lb): 60 mg

12-14 years (80-110 lb): 60-120 mg

or

<4 years: 3-6 mg/kg/dose

>4 years: 1.5-3 mg/kg/dose

Preoperative/preprocedure sedation: ≥6 months:

Note: Limited information is available for infants <6 months of age.

Oral, I.M., rectal: 2-6 mg/kg; maximum: 100 mg/dose

I.V.: 1-3 mg/kg to a maximum of 100 mg until asleep

Children 5-12 years: Conscious sedation prior to a procedure: I.V.: 2 mg/kg 5-10 minutes before procedures, may repeat one time

Adolescents: Conscious sedation: Oral, I.V.: 100 mg prior to a procedure

Barbiturate coma in head injury patients: I.V.: Loading dose: 5-10 mg/kg given slowly over 1-2 hours; monitor blood pressure and respiratory rate; Maintenance infusion: Initial: 1 mg/kg/hour; may increase to 2-3 mg/kg/hour; maintain burst suppression on EEG

Status epilepticus: I.V.: **Note**: Intubation required; monitor hemodynamics: Loading dose: 5-15 mg/kg given slowly over 1-2 hours; maintenance infusion: 0.5-5 mg/kg/hour

Hepatic Impairment: Reduce dosage in patients with severe liver dysfunction.

Administration

I.M.: Pentobarbital may be administered by deep I.M.: No more than 5 mL (250 mg) should be injected at any one site because of possible tissue irritation.

I.V.: Pentobarbital must be administered by slow I.V. injection. I.V. push doses can be given undiluted, but should be administered no faster than 50 mg/minute. Avoid intra-arterial injection. Has many incompatibilities when given I.V.

Stability

Storage: Protect from freezing. Aqueous solutions are not stable; a commercially available vehicle (containing propylene glycol) is more stable. When mixed with an acidic solution, precipitate may form. Use only clear solution.

Compatibility: Stable in dextran 6% in dextrose, dextran 6% in NS, D_5LR, $D_5{}^1/_4NS$, $D_5{}^1/_2NS$, D_5NS, $D_{10}W$, LR, $^1/_2NS$

Y-site administration: Incompatible with amphotericin B cholesteryl sulfate complex

Compatibility in syringe: Incompatible with atropine with cimetidine, butorphanol, chlorpromazine, cimetidine, dimenhydrinate, diphenhydramine, droperidol, fentanyl, glycopyrrolate, hydroxyzine, meperidine, midazolam, nalbuphine, pentazocine, perphenazine, prochlorperazine edisylate, promazine, promethazine, ranitidine

Compatibility when admixed: Incompatible with cefazolin, chlorpheniramine, cimetidine, clindamycin, droperidol, ephedrine, fentanyl, hydrocortisone sodium succinate, hydroxyzine, insulin (regular), levorphanol, norepinephrine, pancuronium, penicillin G potassium, pentazocine, phenytoin, promazine, promethazine, streptomycin, triflupromazine, vancomycin

Monitoring and Teaching Issues

Physical Assessment: Assess effectiveness and interactions of other medications patient may be taking (see Contraindications, Warnings/Precautions, and Drug Interactions). Assess for history of addiction; long-term use can result in dependence, abuse, or tolerance. Periodically evaluate the need for continued use. **I.V.** (see Administration): Keep patient under observation. Monitor cardio/respiratory status and institute patient safety precautions. Monitor effectiveness of therapy and adverse reactions (see Adverse Reactions). **Oral:** Monitor therapeutic response and adverse reactions (see Adverse Reactions) at beginning of therapy and periodically with long-term use. Assess knowledge/teach patient appropriate use, possible side effects, and symptoms to report (see Patient Education). **Pregnancy risk factor D** - determine that patient is not pregnant before beginning treatment. Instruct patients of childbearing age about appropriate barrier contraceptive measures. Breast-feeding is contraindicated.

Patient Education: I.M./I.V.: Patient instructions and information are determined by patient condition and therapeutic purpose. If self-administered, use exactly as directed; do not increase dose or frequency. Drug may cause physical and/or psychological dependence. While using this medication, do not use alcohol and other prescription or OTC medications (especially pain medications, sedatives, antihistamines, or hypnotics) without consulting prescriber. Maintain adequate hydration (2-3 L/day of fluids) unless advised by prescriber to restrict fluids. You may experience drowsiness, dizziness, or blurred vision (use caution when driving or engaging in tasks requiring alertness until response to drug is known); nausea, vomiting, or loss of appetite (small, frequent meals, frequent mouth care, chewing gum, or sucking lozenges may help); or constipation (increased exercise, fluids, fruit, or fiber may help). Report skin rash or irritation; CNS changes (confusion, depression, increased sedation, excitation, headache, insomnia, or nightmares); difficulty breathing or shortness of breath; changes in urinary pattern or menstrual pattern; muscle weakness or tremors; or difficulty swallowing or feeling of tightness in throat. **Pregnancy/breast-feeding precautions:** Do not get pregnant; use appropriate contraceptive measures to prevent possible harm to the fetus. Do not breast-feed.

Geriatric Considerations: Use of this agent as a hypnotic in the elderly is not recommended due to its long half-life and addiction potential.

Additional Information Sodium content of 1 mL injection: 5 mg (0.2 mEq)

Related Information

Compatibility of Drugs in Syringe *on page 1566*

Pentobarbital Sodium *see* Pentobarbital *on page 1053*

Pentostatin (PEN toe stat in)

U.S. Brand Names Nipent®

Synonyms DCF; Deoxycoformycin; 2′-deoxycoformycin

Generic Available No

Pharmacologic Category Antineoplastic Agent, Antibiotic

Pregnancy Risk Factor D

Lactation Enters breast milk/contraindicated

Use Treatment of adult patients with alpha-interferon-refractory hairy cell leukemia; non-Hodgkin's lymphoma, cutaneous T-cell lymphoma

Mechanism of Action/Effect Results in cell death, probably through inhibiting DNA or RNA synthesis. Following a single dose, pentostatin has the ability to inhibit ADA for periods exceeding 1 week.

Contraindications Hypersensitivity to pentostatin or any component; pregnancy

Warnings/Precautions The FDA currently recommends that procedures for proper handling and disposal of antineoplastic agents be considered. Use extreme caution in the presence of renal insufficiency. Use with caution in patients with signs or symptoms of impaired hepatic function.

Preparation of pentostatin should be performed in a Class II laminar flow biologic safety cabinet. Appropriate safety equipment is recommended for preparation, administration, and disposal of antineoplastics. If pentostatin contacts the skin, wash and flush thoroughly with water.

Drug Interactions

Increased Effect/Toxicity: Increased toxicity with vidarabine, fludarabine, and allopurinol.

Adverse Reactions

>10%:

- Central nervous system: Fever, chills, infection (57%), severe, life-threatening (35%); headache, lethargy, seizures, coma (10% to 15%), potentially dose-limiting, uncommon at doses 4 mg/m^2
- Dermatologic: Skin rashes (25% to 30%), alopecia (10%)
- Gastrointestinal: Mild to moderate nausea, vomiting (60%), controlled with non-5-HT_3 antagonist antiemetics; stomatitis, diarrhea (13%), anorexia
- Genitourinary: Acute renal failure (35%)
- Hematologic: Thrombocytopenia (50%), dose-limiting in 25% of patients; anemia (40% to 45%), neutropenia, mild to moderate, not dose-limiting (11%)
  - Nadir: 7 days
  - Recovery: 10-14 days
- Hepatic: Mild to moderate increases in transaminase levels (30%), usually transient; hepatitis (19%), usually reversible
- Respiratory: Pulmonary edema (15%), may be exacerbated by fludarabine

1% to 10%:

- Cardiovascular: Chest pain, arrhythmia, peripheral edema
- Central nervous system: Opportunistic infections (8%); anxiety, confusion, depression, dizziness, insomnia, nervousness, somnolence, myalgias, malaise
- Dermatologic: Dry skin, eczema, pruritus
- Gastrointestinal: Constipation, flatulence, weight loss
- Neuromuscular & skeletal: Paresthesia, weakness
- Ocular: Moderate to severe keratoconjunctivitis, abnormal vision, eye pain
- Otic: Ear pain
- Respiratory: Dyspnea, pneumonia, bronchitis, pharyngitis, rhinitis, epistaxis, sinusitis (3% to 7%)

<1% (Limited to important or life-threatening): Dysuria, hematuria, hypersensitivity reactions, increased BUN, thrombophlebitis

Overdosage/Toxicology Symptoms of overdose include severe renal, hepatic, pulmonary, and CNS toxicity. Treatment is supportive.

Pharmacodynamics/Kinetics

Half-Life Elimination: Terminal: 5-15 hours

Formulations Injection, powder for reconstitution: 10 mg/vial

Dosing

Adults & Elderly: Refer to individual protocols.

Refractory hairy cell leukemia: 4 mg/m^2 every other week; I.V. bolus over ≥3-5 minutes in D_5W or NS at concentrations ≥2 mg/mL

Renal Impairment:

Cl_{cr} <60 mL/minute: Use extreme caution.

Cl_{cr} 50-60 mL/minute: Administer 2 mg/m^2/dose.

Hepatic Impairment:

Bilirubin 1.5-3 mg/dL or AST 60-180 units/L: Administer 75% of normal dose.

Bilirubin 3-5 mg/dL or AST >180 units/L: Administer 50% of normal dose.

Bilirubin >5 mg/dL: Do not administer.

Administration

I.V.: I.V. bolus over ≥3-5 minutes in D_5W or NS at concentrations ≥2 mg/mL

Stability

Storage: Vials are stable under refrigeration at 2°C to 8°C.

Reconstitution: Reconstituted vials or further dilutions, may be stored at room temperature exposed to ambient light. Diluted solutions are stable for 24 hours in D_5W or 48 hours in NS or lactated Ringer's at room temperature. Infusion with 5% dextrose injection USP or 0.9% sodium chloride injection USP does not interact with PVC-containing administration sets or containers.

Compatibility: Stable in LR, NS

Monitoring Laboratory Tests CBC with differential, platelet count, liver function, serum uric acid, renal function

Monitoring and Teaching Issues

Physical Assessment: See Contraindications, Warnings/Precautions, and Dosing for use cautions. Note Drug Interactions (above). See above for infusion specifics. Assess results of laboratory tests (see above) prior to and regularly during therapy. Assess therapeutic effectiveness and adverse response (eg, nutritional status, renal function, myelosuppression, pulmonary edema, opportunistic infection - see Adverse Reactions and Overdose/Toxicology). Teach patient possible side effects and appropriate interventions and adverse symptoms to report (see Patient Education). **Pregnancy risk factor D** - determine that patient is not pregnant before beginning treatment. Instruct patients of childbearing age about appropriate barrier contraceptive measures. Breast-feeding is contraindicated.

Patient Education: Inform prescriber of all prescriptions, OTC medications, or herbal products you are taking, and any allergies you have. Do not take anything new during treatment unless approved by prescriber. This drug can only be given by infusion on a specific schedule. Report immediately any redness, swelling, burning, or pain at infusion site; or signs of hypersensitivity (eg, difficulty breathing or swallowing, chest tightness, rash, hives, swelling of lips or mouth). Maintain adequate hydration (2-3 L/day of fluids) unless advised by prescriber to restrict fluids. You may be more susceptible to infection (avoid crowds and exposure to infection and do not have any vaccinations without consulting prescriber). May cause nausea and vomiting, or loss of appetite (small, frequent meals or frequent mouth care may help - or request medication from prescriber); headache (consult prescriber for approved analgesic); dizziness, confusion or lethargy (use caution when driving); or mouth sores (use frequent oral care with soft toothbrush or cotton swabs). Report signs of infection (eg, fever, chills, sore throat, mouth sores, burning urination, perianal itching, or vaginal discharge); unusual bruising or bleeding (eg, tarry stools, blood in urine, stool, or vomitus); vision changes or hearing; muscle tremors, weakness, or pain; CNS changes (eg, hallucinations, confusion, insomnia, seizures); or difficulty breathing. **Pregnancy/breast-feeding precautions:** Do not get pregnant while taking this medication. Consult prescriber for appropriate contraceptive measures. Do not breast-feed.

Pentoxifylline (pen toks I fi leen)

U.S. Brand Names Trental®

Synonyms Oxpentifylline

Generic Available Yes

Pharmacologic Category Blood Viscosity Reducer Agent

Pregnancy Risk Factor C

Lactation Enters breast milk/effect on infant unknown

Use Treatment of intermittent claudication on the basis of chronic occlusive arterial disease of the limbs; may improve function and symptoms, but not intended to replace more definitive therapy

Use - Unlabeled/Investigational AIDS patients with increased TNF, CVA, cerebrovascular diseases, diabetic atherosclerosis, diabetic neuropathy, gangrene, hemodialysis shunt thrombosis, vascular impotence, cerebral malaria, septic shock, sickle cell syndromes, and vasculitis

Mechanism of Action/Effect Mechanism of action remains unclear; is thought to reduce blood viscosity and improve blood flow by altering the rheology of red blood cells

Contraindications Hypersensitivity to pentoxifylline, xanthines, or any component of the formulation; recent cerebral and/or retinal hemorrhage

Warnings/Precautions Use with caution in patients with renal impairment or chronic occlusive arterial disease of the limbs. Pregnancy risk C.

Drug Interactions

Cytochrome P450 Effect: Inhibits CYP1A2

Decreased Effect: Blood pressure changes (decreases) have been observed with the addition of pentoxifylline therapy in patients receiving antihypertensives.

Increased Effect/Toxicity: Pentoxifylline levels may be increased with cimetidine and other H_2 antagonists. May increase anticoagulation with warfarin. Pentoxifylline may increase the serum levels of theophylline.

Nutritional/Ethanol Interactions Food: Food may decrease rate but not extent of absorption. Pentoxifylline peak serum levels may be decreased if taken with food.

Effects on Lab Values ↓ calcium (S), magnesium (S); false-positive theophylline levels

Adverse Reactions

1% to 10%:

Central nervous system: Dizziness, headache

Gastrointestinal: Heartburn, nausea, vomiting

<1% (Limited to important or life-threatening): Angioedema, arrhythmias, chest pain, cholecystitis, congestion, dyspnea, hallucinations, hepatitis, jaundice, rash, tremor

Overdosage/Toxicology Symptoms of overdose include hypotension, flushing, convulsions, deep sleep, agitation, bradycardia, and AV block. Treatment is supportive.

Pharmacodynamics/Kinetics

Absorption: Well absorbed

Half-Life Elimination: Parent drug: 24-48 minutes; Metabolites: 60-96 minutes

Time to Peak: Serum: 2-4 hours

Metabolism: Hepatic and via erythrocytes; extensive first-pass effect

Formulations Tablet, controlled release: 400 mg

Dosing

Adults & Elderly: Peripheral vascular disease: Oral: 400 mg 3 times/day with meals; may reduce to 400 mg twice daily if GI or CNS side effects occur

Monitoring and Teaching Issues

Physical Assessment: See Contraindications and Warnings/Precautions for use cautions. Assess potential for interactions with other prescriptions, OTC medications, or herbal products patient may be taking (see Drug Interactions). Assess therapeutic effectiveness, and adverse reactions at regular intervals during therapy (eg, cardiac status and blood pressure - see Adverse Reactions and Overdose/Toxicology). Teach patient proper use, possible side effects and interventions, and adverse symptoms to report (see Patient

(Continued)

Pentoxifylline *(Continued)*

Education). **Pregnancy risk factor C** - benefits of use should outweigh possible risks. Note breast-feeding caution.

Patient Education: Inform prescriber of all prescriptions, OTC medications, or herbal products you are taking, and any allergies you have. Do not take anything new during treatment unless approved by prescriber. This may relieve pain of claudication, but additional therapy may be recommended. Take as prescribed for full length of prescription. May cause dizziness (use caution when driving or engaging in tasks that are potentially hazardous until response to drug is known); or heartburn, nausea, or vomiting (small, frequent meals, frequent mouth care, chewing gum, or sucking lozenges may help). Report chest pain; swelling of lips, mouth, or tongue; persistent headache; difficulty breathing; rash; or unrelieved nausea or vomiting. **Pregnancy/breast-feeding precautions:** Inform prescriber if you are or intend to become pregnant. Consult prescriber if breast-feeding.

Dietary Issues: May be taken with meals or food.

Geriatric Considerations: Pentoxifylline's value in the treatment of intermittent claudication is controversial. Walking distance improved statistically in some clinical trials, but the actual distance was minimal when applied to improving physical activity (see Usual Dosage and Monitoring Parameters).

Pen VK *see* Penicillin V Potassium *on page 1048*

Pepcid® *see* Famotidine *on page 543*

Pepcid® AC [OTC] *see* Famotidine *on page 543*

Peptavlon® *see page 1461*

Pepto-Bismol® [OTC] *see* Bismuth *on page 169*

Pepto-Bismol® Maximum Strength [OTC] *see* Bismuth *on page 169*

Percocet® 2.5/325 *see* Oxycodone and Acetaminophen *on page 1022*

Percocet® 5/325 *see* Oxycodone and Acetaminophen *on page 1022*

Percocet® 7.5/325 *see* Oxycodone and Acetaminophen *on page 1022*

Percocet® 7.5/500 *see* Oxycodone and Acetaminophen *on page 1022*

Percocet® 10/325 *see* Oxycodone and Acetaminophen *on page 1022*

Percocet® 10/650 *see* Oxycodone and Acetaminophen *on page 1022*

Percodan® *see* Oxycodone and Aspirin *on page 1022*

Percodan®-Demi [DSC] *see* Oxycodone and Aspirin *on page 1022*

Percolone® [DSC] *see* Oxycodone *on page 1020*

Perdiem® Plain [OTC] *see* Psyllium *on page 1152*

Pergolide (PER go lide)

U.S. Brand Names Permax®

Synonyms Pergolide Mesylate

Generic Available No

Pharmacologic Category Anti-Parkinson's Agent, Dopamine Agonist; Ergot Derivative

Pregnancy Risk Factor B

Lactation Excretion in breast milk unknown/not recommended

Use Adjunctive treatment to levodopa/carbidopa in the management of Parkinson's disease

Use - Unlabeled/Investigational Tourette's disorder, chronic motor or vocal tic disorder

Mechanism of Action/Effect Pergolide is a semisynthetic ergot alkaloid similar to bromocriptine but stated to be more potent (10-1000 times) and longer-acting; it is a centrally-active dopamine agonist stimulating both D_1 and D_2 receptors. Pergolide is believed to exert its therapeutic effect by directly stimulating postsynaptic dopamine receptors in the nigrostriatal system.

Contraindications Hypersensitivity to pergolide mesylate, other ergot derivatives, or any component of the formulation

Warnings/Precautions Symptomatic hypotension occurs in 10% of patients. Use with caution in patients with a history of cardiac arrhythmias, hallucinations, or mental illness.

Drug Interactions

Cytochrome P450 Effect: Inhibits **CYP2D6**, 3A4

Decreased Effect: Dopamine antagonists (ie, antipsychotics, metoclopramide) may diminish the effects of pergolide; these combinations should generally be avoided.

Increased Effect/Toxicity: Use caution with other highly plasma protein bound drugs.

Nutritional/Ethanol Interactions Ethanol: Avoid ethanol (may cause CNS depression).

Adverse Reactions

>10%:

Central nervous system: Dizziness, somnolence, confusion, hallucinations, dystonia

Gastrointestinal: Nausea, constipation

Neuromuscular & skeletal: Dyskinesia

Respiratory: Rhinitis

1% to 10%:

Cardiovascular: Myocardial infarction, postural hypotension, syncope, arrhythmias, peripheral edema, vasodilation, palpitations, chest pain, hypertension

Central nervous system: Chills, insomnia, anxiety, psychosis, EPS, incoordination

Dermatologic: Rash

Gastrointestinal: Diarrhea, abdominal pain, xerostomia, anorexia, weight gain, dyspepsia, taste perversion

Hematologic: Anemia

Neuromuscular & skeletal: Weakness, myalgia, tremor, NMS (with rapid dose reduction), pain

Ocular: Abnormal vision, diplopia

Respiratory: Dyspnea, epistaxis

Miscellaneous: Flu syndrome, hiccups

<1% (Limited to important or life-threatening): Pericarditis, pericardial effusion, pleural effusion, pleural fibrosis, pleuritis, pneumothorax, retroperitoneal fibrosis, vasculitis

Overdosage/Toxicology Symptoms of overdose include vomiting, hypotension, agitation, hallucinations, ventricular extrasystoles, and possible seizures. Data on overdose is limited. Treatment is supportive.

Pharmacodynamics/Kinetics

Absorption: Well absorbed

Half-Life Elimination: 27 hours

Metabolism: Extensively hepatic

Formulations Tablet, as mesylate: 0.05 mg, 0.25 mg, 1 mg

Dosing

Adults:

Parkinson's disease: Oral: Start with 0.05 mg/day for 2 days, then increase dosage by 0.1 or 0.15 mg/day every 3 days over next 12 days, increase dose by 0.25 mg/day every 3 days until optimal therapeutic dose is achieved, up to 5 mg/day maximum; usual dosage range: 2-3 mg/day in 3 divided doses

Note: When adding pergolide to levodopa/carbidopa, the dose of the latter can usually and should be decreased. Patients no longer responsive to bromocriptine may benefit by being switched to pergolide.

Elderly: Refer to Geriatric Considerations.

Pediatrics: Children and Adolescents: Tourette's disorder, chronic motor or vocal disorder (unlabeled uses): Oral: Up to 300 mcg/day

Monitoring and Teaching Issues

Physical Assessment: Assess effectiveness and interactions of other medications patient may be taking (see Contraindications and Drug Interactions). Monitor therapeutic response and adverse reactions at beginning of therapy and periodically throughout therapy (see Warnings/Precautions, Adverse Reactions, and Overdose/Toxicology). Assess knowledge/ teach patient appropriate use, interventions to reduce side effects, and adverse symptoms to report (see Patient Education). Breast-feeding is not recommended.

Patient Education: Take exactly as directed (may be prescribed in conjunction with levodopa/carbidopa); do not change dosage or discontinue without consulting prescriber. Therapeutic effects may take several weeks or months to achieve and you may need frequent monitoring during first weeks of therapy. Take with meals if GI upset occurs, before meals if dry mouth occurs, after eating if drooling or if nausea occurs. Take at the same time each day. Maintain adequate hydration (2-3 L/day of fluids) unless advised by prescriber to restrict fluids; void before taking medication. Do not use alcohol and prescription or OTC sedatives or CNS depressants without consulting prescriber. You may experience drowsiness, dizziness, confusion, or vision changes (use caution when driving, climbing stairs, or engaging in tasks requiring alertness until response to drug is known); orthostatic hypotension (use caution when changing position - rising to standing from sitting or lying); constipation (increased exercise, fluids, fruit, or fiber may help); runny nose or flu-like symptoms (consult prescriber for appropriate relief); nausea, vomiting, loss of appetite, or stomach discomfort (small, frequent meals, frequent mouth care, chewing gum, or sucking lozenges may help); or photosensitivity (use sunscreen, wear protective clothing and eyewear, and avoid direct sunlight). Report unresolved constipation or vomiting; chest pain, palpitations, irregular heartbeat; ringing in ears; CNS changes (hallucination, loss of memory, seizures, acute headache, nervousness, etc); painful or difficult urination; increased muscle spasticity, rigidity, or involuntary movements; skin rash; or significant worsening of condition. **Breast-feeding precaution:** Breast-feeding is not recommended.

Geriatric Considerations: High incidence of syncope and orthostatic hypotension upon initiation of therapy. Use with caution in patients prone to cardiac dysrhythmias and in patients with a history of confusion or hallucinations.

Pergolide Mesylate *see* Pergolide *on page 1058*

Pergonal® *see* Menotropins *on page 850*

Periactin® *see* Cyproheptadine *on page 347*

Perindopril Erbumine (per IN doe pril er BYOO meen)

U.S. Brand Names Aceon®

Generic Available No

Pharmacologic Category Angiotensin-Converting Enzyme (ACE) Inhibitor

Pregnancy Risk Factor D (especially 2nd and 3rd trimesters)

Lactation Enters breast milk (small amounts)/effect on infant unknown

Use Treatment of stage I or II hypertension and congestive heart failure; treatment of left ventricular dysfunction after myocardial infarction

Mechanism of Action/Effect Competitive inhibitor of angiotensin-converting enzyme (ACE); prevents conversion of angiotensin I to angiotensin II, a potent vasoconstrictor; results in lower levels of angiotensin II which, in turn, causes an increase in plasma renin activity and a reduction in aldosterone secretion

Contraindications Hypersensitivity to perindopril or any component of the formulation; angioedema related to previous treatment with an ACE inhibitor; bilateral renal artery stenosis; primary hyperaldosteronism; pregnancy (2nd and 3rd trimesters)

Warnings/Precautions Angioedema can occur at any time during treatment (especially following first dose). Careful blood pressure monitoring with first dose (hypotension can occur especially in volume depleted patients). Dosage adjustment needed in renal impairment. Use with caution in hypovolemia; collagen vascular diseases; valvular stenosis (particularly aortic stenosis); hyperkalemia; or before, during, or immediately after anesthesia. Avoid rapid dosage escalation, which may lead to renal insufficiency. Neutropenia/agranulocytosis with myeloid hyperplasia can rarely occur. Hypersensitivity reactions may be seen during hemodialysis with high-flux dialysis membranes (eg, AN69). Use with caution in unilateral renal artery stenosis and pre-existing renal insufficiency.

Drug Interactions

Decreased Effect: Aspirin (high dose) may reduce the therapeutic effects of ACE inhibitors; at low dosages this does not appear to be significant. Rifampin may decrease the effect of ACE inhibitors. Antacids may decrease the bioavailability of ACE inhibitors (may

(Continued)

Perindopril Erbumine *(Continued)*

be more likely to occur with captopril); separate administration times by 1-2 hours. NSAIDs, specifically indomethacin, may reduce the hypotensive effects of ACE inhibitors. More likely to occur in low renin or volume dependent hypertensive patients.

Increased Effect/Toxicity: Potassium supplements, co-trimoxazole (high dose), angiotensin II receptor antagonists (candesartan, losartan, irbesartan, etc), or potassium-sparing diuretics (amiloride, spironolactone, triamterene) may result in elevated serum potassium levels when combined with perindopril. ACE inhibitor effects may be increased by phenothiazines or probenecid (increases levels of captopril). ACE inhibitors may increase serum concentrations/effects of digoxin, lithium, and sulfonlyureas.

Diuretics have additive hypotensive effects with ACE inhibitors, and hypovolemia increases the potential for adverse renal effects of ACE inhibitors. In patients with compromised renal function, coadministration with NSAIDs may result in further deterioration of renal function. Allopurinol and ACE inhibitors may cause a higher risk of hypersensitivity reaction when taken concurrently.

Nutritional/Ethanol Interactions

Food: Perindopril active metabolite concentrations may be lowered if taken with food.

Herb/Nutraceutical: Avoid dong quai if using for hypertension (has estrogenic activity). Avoid ephedra, yohimbe, ginseng (may worsen hypertension). Avoid garlic (may have increased antihypertensive effect).

Adverse Reactions

>10% Central nervous system: Headache (23%)

1% to 10%:

- Cardiovascular: edema (4%), chest pain (2%)
- Central nervous system: Dizziness (8%), sleep disorders (3%), depression (2%), fever (2%), weakness (8%), nervousness (1%)
- Dermatologic: Rash (2%)
- Endocrine & metabolic: Hyperkalemia (1%), increased triglycerides (1%)
- Gastrointestinal: Nausea (2%), diarrhea (4%), vomiting (2%), dyspepsia (2%), abdominal pain (3%), flatulence (1%)
- Genitourinary: Sexual dysfunction (male: 1%)
- Hepatic: Increased ALT (2%)
- Neuromuscular & skeletal: Back pain (6%), upper extremity pain (3%), lower extremity pain (5%), paresthesia (2%), joint pain (1%), myalgia (1%), arthritis (1%)
- Renal: Proteinuria (2%)
- Respiratory: Cough (incidence is higher in women, 3:1) (12%), sinusitis (5%), rhinitis (5%), pharyngitis (3%)
- Otic: Tinnitus (2%)
- Miscellaneous: Viral infection (3%)

Note: Some reactions occurred at an incidence >1% but ≤ placebo.

<1% (Limited to important or life-threatening): Amnesia, anaphylaxis, angioedema, anxiety, dyspnea, erythema, gout, migraine, myocardial infarction, nephrolithiasis, orthostatic hypotension, pruritus, psychosocial disorder, pulmonary fibrosis, purpura, stroke, syncope, urinary retention, vertigo

Additional adverse effects associated with **ACE inhibitors** include agranulocytosis, neutropenia, decreases in creatinine clearance in some elderly hypertensive patients or those with chronic renal failure, and worsening of renal function in patients with bilateral renal artery stenosis or hypovolemic patients (diuretic therapy). In addition, a syndrome which may include fever, myalgia, arthralgia, interstitial nephritis, vasculitis, rash, eosinophilia and positive ANA, and elevated ESR has been reported with ACE inhibitors.

Overdosage/Toxicology Mild hypotension has been the primary toxic effect seen with acute overdose. Bradycardia may also occur. Hyperkalemia occurs even with therapeutic doses, especially in patients with renal insufficiency and those taking NSAIDs. Treatment is symptom-directed and supportive.

Pharmacodynamics/Kinetics

Bioavailability: Perindopril: 65% to 95%

Half-Life Elimination: Parent drug: 1.5-3 hours; Metabolite: Effective: 3-10 hours, Terminal: 30-120 hours

Time to Peak: Chronic therapy: Perindopril: 1 hour; Perindoprilat: 3-4 hours (maximum perindoprilat serum levels are 2-3 times higher and T_{max} is shorter following chronic therapy); CHF: Perindoprilat: 6 hours

Metabolism: Hydrolyzed hepatically to active metabolite, perindoprilat (~17% to 20% of a dose) and other inactive metabolites

Onset: Peak effect: 1-2 hours

Formulations Tablet: 2 mg, 4 mg, 8 mg

Dosing

Adults:

Congestive heart failure: Oral: 4 mg once daily

Hypertension: Oral: Initial: 4 mg/day but may be titrated to response; usual range: 4-8 mg/day, maximum: 16 mg/day

Elderly: Due to greater bioavailability and lower renal clearance of the drug in elderly subjects, dose reduction of 50% is recommended.

Renal Impairment:

Cl_{cr} >60 mL/minute: Administer 4 mg/day.

Cl_{cr} 30-60 mL/minute: Administer 2 mg/day.

Cl_{cr} 15-29 mL/minute: Administer 2 mg every other day.

Cl_{cr} <15 mL/minute: Administer 2 mg on the day of dialysis.

Perindopril and its metabolites are dialyzable.

Monitoring Laboratory Tests Serum creatinine, electrolytes, and WBC with differential initially and repeated at 2-week intervals for at least 90 days (particularly important in patients with renal impairment at baseline).

Monitoring and Teaching Issues

Physical Assessment: See Contraindications, Warnings/Precautions, and Dosing for use cautions. Assess potential for interactions with other prescriptions, OTC medications, or herbal products patient may be taking (see Drug Interactions). Suggested that first dose be administered in prescriber's office with careful blood pressure monitoring (hypotension can occur especially with first dose and angioedema can occur at any time during treatment, especially following first dose). Assess results of laboratory tests (see above) and patient response at beginning of therapy, when adjusting dose, and periodically with long-term therapy (eg, BP (standing and sitting), cardiac status and fluid balance - see Adverse Reactions and Overdose/Toxicology). Teach patient appropriate use, possible side effects and interventions, and adverse symptoms to report (see Patient Education). **Pregnancy risk factor D** - determine that patient is not pregnant prior to beginning therapy. Instruct patient in appropriate use of barrier contraceptives (see Pregnancy Issues). Note breast-feeding caution.

Patient Education: Inform prescriber of all prescriptions, OTC medications, or herbal products you are taking, and any allergies you have. Do not take anything new without consulting prescriber. Take as directed; do not alter dose or discontinue without consulting prescriber. Take first dose at bedtime. Do not take potassium supplements or salt substitutes containing potassium without consulting prescriber. This drug does not eliminate need for diet or exercise regimen as recommended by prescriber. May cause increased cough (if persistent or bothersome, contact prescriber); headache (consult prescriber for approved analgesic); postural hypotension (use caution when rising from lying or sitting position or climbing stairs); dizziness (use caution when driving or engaging in tasks that require alertness until response to drug is known); nausea or vomiting (small, frequent meals, frequent mouth care, sucking lozenges, or chewing gum may help); or diarrhea (buttermilk, boiled milk, or yogurt may help). Report chest pain, difficulty breathing or persistent cough, painful muscles or joints, rash, ringing in ears, or other persistent adverse reactions. **Pregnancy/breast-feeding precautions:** Inform prescriber if you are or intend to become pregnant. This drug should not be used in the 2nd or 3rd trimester of pregnancy. Consult prescriber for appropriate contraceptive measures if necessary. Consult prescriber if breast-feeding.

Pregnancy Issues: ACE inhibitors can cause fetal injury or death if taken during the 2nd or 3rd trimester. Discontinue ACE inhibitors as soon as pregnancy is detected.

Related Information

Angiotensin Agents *on page 1547*

Periostat® *see* Doxycycline *on page 450*

Permapen® Isoject® *see* Penicillin G Benzathine *on page 1043*

Permax® *see* Pergolide *on page 1058*

Permethrin (per METH rin)

U.S. Brand Names A200® Lice [OTC]; Acticin®; Elimite®; Nix® [OTC; R&C® Lice [DSC]; RID® Spray [OTC]

Generic Available Yes

Pharmacologic Category Antiparasitic Agent, Topical; Scabicidal Agent

Pregnancy Risk Factor B

Lactation Effect on infant unknown

Use Single-application treatment of infestation with *Pediculus humanus capitis* (head louse) and its nits or *Sarcoptes scabiei* (scabies); indicated for prophylactic use during epidemics of lice

Mechanism of Action/Effect Inhibits sodium ion influx through nerve cell membrane channels in parasites resulting in delayed repolarization and thus paralysis and death of the pest

Contraindications Hypersensitivity to pyrethyroid, pyrethrin, chrysanthemums, or any component of the formulation; lotion is contraindicated for use in infants <2 months of age

Warnings/Precautions Treatment may temporarily exacerbate the symptoms of itching, redness, and swelling. For external use only.

Adverse Reactions 1% to 10%:

Dermatologic: Pruritus, erythema, rash of the scalp

Local: Burning, stinging, tingling, numbness or scalp discomfort, edema

Pharmacodynamics/Kinetics

Absorption: <2%

Metabolism: Hepatic via ester hydrolysis to inactive metabolites

Formulations

Cream, topical (Acticin®, Elimite®): 5% (60 g) [contains coconut oil]

Liquid, topical (Nix®): 1% (60 mL) [contains isopropyl alcohol 20%; creme rinse formulation]

Lotion, topical: 1% (59 mL)

Shampoo (A200® Lice): 0.33% (60 mL, 120 mL) [contains benzyl alcohol]

Solution, spray [for bedding and furniture]

- A200® Lice: 0.5% (180 mL)
- Nix®: 0.25% (148 mL)
- RID®: 0.5% (150 mL)

Dosing

Adults & Elderly:

Head lice: Topical: After hair has been washed with shampoo, rinsed with water and towel dried, apply a sufficient volume of creme rinse to saturate the hair and scalp; also apply behind the ears and at the base of the neck; leave on hair for 10 minutes before rinsing off with water; remove remaining nits. May repeat in 1 week if lice or nits still present; in areas of head lice resistance to 1% permethrin, 5% permethrin has been applied to clean, dry hair and left on overnight (8-14 hours) under a shower cap.

Scabies: Topical: Apply cream from head to toe; leave on for 8-14 hours before washing off with water; for infants, also apply on the hairline, neck, scalp, temple, and forehead; may reapply in 1 week if live mites appear. Permethrin 5% cream was shown to be safe and effective when applied to an infant <1 month of age with neonatal scabies; time of application was limited to 6 hours before rinsing with soap and water.

(Continued)

Permethrin *(Continued)*

Pediatrics:

Head lice and scabies: Topical: Children >2 months: Refer to adult dosing.

Administration

Topical: Avoid contact with eyes and mucous membranes during application.

Cream rinse/lotion: Shake cream rinse well before using. Apply immediately after hair is shampooed, rinsed, and towel-dried. Apply enough to saturate hair and scalp (especially behind ears and on nape of neck). Leave on hair for 10 minutes before rinsing with water. Remove nits with fine-tooth comb. May repeat in 1 week if lice or nits are still present.

Cream: Apply from neck to toes. Bathe to remove drug after 8-14 hours. Repeat in 7 days if lice or nits are still present. Report if condition persists or infection occurs.

Monitoring and Teaching Issues

Physical Assessment: See Warnings/Precautions and Contraindications for use cautions. Assess head, hair, and skin surfaces for presence of lice and nits. Assess knowledge/teach patient appropriate application and use and adverse symptoms (see Adverse Reactions above) to report (see Patient Education). Note breast-feeding caution.

Patient Education: For external use only. Do not apply to face and avoid contact with eyes or mucous membrane. Clothing and bedding must be washed in hot water or dry cleaned to kill nits. May need to treat all members of household and all sexual contacts concurrently. Wash all combs and brushes with permethrin and thoroughly rinse. **Breast-feeding precaution:** Consult prescriber if breast-feeding.

Cream rinse/lotion: Apply immediately after hair is shampooed, rinsed, and towel-dried. Apply enough to saturate hair and scalp (especially behind ears and on nape of neck). Leave on hair for 10 minutes before rinsing with water. Remove nits with fine-tooth comb. May repeat in 1 week if lice or nits are still present.

Cream: Apply from neck to toes. Bathe to remove drug after 8-14 hours. Repeat in 7 days if lice or nits are still present. Report if condition persists or infection occurs.

Geriatric Considerations: Because of its minimal absorption, permethrin is a drug of choice and is preferred over lindane.

Perphenazine (per FEN a zeen)

U.S. Brand Names Trilafon®

Generic Available Yes

Pharmacologic Category Antipsychotic Agent, Phenothiazine, Piperazine

Pregnancy Risk Factor C

Lactation Enters breast milk/not recommended (AAP rates "of concern")

Use Treatment of severe schizophrenia; nausea and vomiting

Use - Unlabeled/Investigational Ethanol withdrawal; dementia in elderly; Tourette's syndrome; Huntington's chorea; spasmodic torticollis; Reye's syndrome; psychosis

Mechanism of Action/Effect Blocks postsynaptic mesolimbic dopaminergic receptors in the brain; exhibits alpha-adrenergic blocking effect and depresses the release of hypothalamic and hypophyseal hormones

Contraindications Hypersensitivity to perphenazine or any component of the formulation (cross-reactivity between phenothiazines may occur); severe CNS depression; subcortical brain damage; bone marrow suppression; blood dyscrasias; coma

Warnings/Precautions May cause hypotension, particularly with parenteral administration. May be sedating, use with caution in disorders where CNS depression is a feature. Use with caution in Parkinson's disease. Caution in patients with hemodynamic instability; predisposition to seizures; severe cardiac, hepatic, renal, or respiratory disease. Esophageal dysmotility and aspiration have been associated with antipsychotic use - use with caution in patients at risk of pneumonia (ie, Alzheimer's disease). Caution in breast cancer or other prolactin-dependent tumors (may elevate prolactin levels). May alter temperature regulation or mask toxicity of other drugs due to antiemetic effects. May alter cardiac conduction - life-threatening arrhythmias have occurred with therapeutic doses of phenothiazines. May cause orthostatic hypotension - use with caution in patients at risk of this effect or those who would tolerate transient hypotensive episodes (cerebrovascular disease, cardiovascular disease, or other medications which may predispose).

Due to anticholinergic effects, use with caution in patients with decreased gastrointestinal motility, urinary retention, BPH, xerostomia, visual problems, narrow-angle glaucoma (screening is recommended) and myasthenia gravis. Relative to other neuroleptics, perphenazine has a low potency of cholinergic blockade.

May cause extrapyramidal symptoms, including pseudoparkinsonism, acute dystonic reactions, akathisia, and tardive dyskinesia (risk of these reactions is moderate-high relative to other neuroleptics). May be associated with neuroleptic malignant syndrome (NMS) or pigmentary retinopathy.

Pregnancy risk C.

Drug Interactions

Cytochrome P450 Effect: Substrate of CYP1A2, 2C8/9, 2C19, **2D6**, 3A4; Inhibits CYP1A2, **2D6**

Decreased Effect: Phenothiazines inhibit the ability of bromocriptine to lower serum prolactin concentrations. Benztropine (and other anticholinergics) may inhibit the therapeutic response to perphenazine and excess anticholinergic effects may occur. Cigarette smoking and barbiturates may enhance the hepatic metabolism of chlorpromazine. Antihypertensive effects of guanethidine and guanadrel may be inhibited by perphenazine. Perphenazine may inhibit the antiparkinsonian effect of levodopa. Perphenazine and possibly other low potency antipsychotics may reverse the pressor effects of epinephrine.

Increased Effect/Toxicity: Effects on CNS depression may be additive when perphenazine is combined with CNS depressants (narcotic analgesics, ethanol, barbiturates, cyclic antidepressants, antihistamines, or sedative-hypnotics). Perphenazine may increase the effects/toxicity of anticholinergics, antihypertensives, lithium (rare neurotoxicity), trazodone, or valproic acid. Concurrent use with TCA may produce increased toxicity or altered therapeutic response. Chloroquine and propranolol may increase perphenazine concentrations. Hypotension may occur when perphenazine is combined with epinephrine. May increase the risk of arrhythmia when combined with antiarrhythmics, cisapride, pimozide, sparfloxacin, or other drugs which prolong QT interval. Metoclopramide may increase risk of extrapyramidal symptoms (EPS). Drugs which inhibit CYP2D6 may increase serum concentrations of perphenazine (includes amiodarone, cimetidine, delavirdine, fluoxetine, paroxetine, propafenone, quinidine, ritonavir, and sertraline).

Nutritional/Ethanol Interactions

Ethanol: Avoid ethanol (may increase CNS depression).

Herb/Nutraceutical: Avoid kava kava, gotu kola, valerian, St John's wort (may increase CNS depression).

Effects on Lab Values ↑ cholesterol (S), glucose; ↓ uric acid (S)

Adverse Reactions Frequency not defined.

Cardiovascular: Hypotension, orthostatic hypotension, hypertension, tachycardia, bradycardia, dizziness, cardiac arrest

Central nervous system: Extrapyramidal symptoms (pseudoparkinsonism, akathisia, dystonias, tardive dyskinesia), dizziness, cerebral edema, seizures, headache, drowsiness, paradoxical excitement, restlessness, hyperactivity, insomnia, neuroleptic malignant syndrome (NMS), impairment of temperature regulation

Dermatologic: Increased sensitivity to sun, rash, discoloration of skin (blue-gray)

Endocrine & metabolic: Hypoglycemia, hyperglycemia, galactorrhea, lactation, breast enlargement, gynecomastia, menstrual irregularity, amenorrhea, SIADH, changes in libido

Gastrointestinal: Constipation, weight gain, vomiting, stomach pain, nausea, xerostomia, salivation, diarrhea, anorexia, ileus

Genitourinary: Difficulty in urination, ejaculatory disturbances, incontinence, polyuria, ejaculating dysfunction, priapism

Hematologic: Agranulocytosis, leukopenia, eosinophilia, hemolytic anemia, thrombocytopenic purpura, pancytopenia

Hepatic: Cholestatic jaundice, hepatotoxicity

Neuromuscular & skeletal: Tremor

Ocular: Pigmentary retinopathy, blurred vision, cornea and lens changes

Respiratory: Nasal congestion

Miscellaneous: Diaphoresis

Overdosage/Toxicology Symptoms of overdose include deep sleep, dystonia, agitation, coma, abnormal involuntary muscle movements, hypotension, and arrhythmias (QT_c prolongation, AV block, torsade de pointes, ventricular tachycardia/fibrillation). Children may have convulsive seizures.

Treatment is symptom-directed and supportive. Induction of emesis is not recommended. Peritoneal dialysis and hemodialysis are of no value. Gastric lavage and administration of activated charcoal together with a laxative should be considered. Cardiac function should be monitored for at least 5 days. Norepinephrine may be used to treat hypotension, but epinephrine should **not** be used.

Pharmacodynamics/Kinetics

Absorption: Oral: Well absorbed

Half-Life Elimination: Perphenazine: 9-12 hours; 7-hydroxyperphenazine: 11.3 hours

Time to Peak: Serum: Perphenazine: 1-3 hours; 7-hydroxyperphenazine: 2-4 hours

Metabolism: Extensively hepatic to metabolites via sulfoxidation, hydroxylation, dealkylation, and glucuronidation

Formulations

Injection: 5 mg/mL (1 mL)

Solution, oral concentrate: 16 mg/5 mL (118 mL) [berry flavor]

Tablet: 2 mg, 4 mg, 8 mg, 16 mg

Dosing

Adults:

Schizophrenia/psychoses:

Oral: 4-16 mg 2-4 times/day not to exceed 64 mg/day

I.M.: 5 mg every 6 hours up to 15 mg/day in ambulatory patients and 30 mg/day in hospitalized patients

Nausea/vomiting:

Oral: 8-16 mg/day in divided doses up to 24 mg/day

I.M.: 5-10 mg every 6 hours as necessary up to 15 mg/day in ambulatory patients and 30 mg/day in hospitalized patients

I.V. (severe): 1 mg at 1- to 2-minute intervals up to a total of 5 mg

Elderly: Behavioral symptoms associated with dementia: Oral: Initial: 2-4 mg 1-2 times/day; increase at 4- to 7-day intervals by 2-4 mg/day. Increase dose intervals (bid, tid, etc) as necessary to control behavior response or side effects. Maximum daily dose: 32 mg; gradual increase (titration) and bedtime administration may prevent some side effects or decrease their severity.

Pediatrics:

Schizophrenia/psychoses: Oral:

1-6 years: 4-6 mg/day in divided doses

6-12 years: 6 mg/day in divided doses

>12 years: 4-16 mg 2-4 times/day

I.M.: 5 mg every 6 hours

Nausea/vomiting: I.M.: 5 mg every 6 hours

Renal Impairment: Not dialyzable (0% to 5%)

Hepatic Impairment: Dosage reductions should be considered in patients with liver disease although no specific guidelines are available.

Administration

Oral: Dilute oral concentration to at least 2 oz with water, juice, or milk only. Do not mix with liquids containing caffeine (coffee, cola), tannins (tea), or pectins (apple juice). Use

(Continued)

Perphenazine *(Continued)*

approximately 60 mL diluent for each 5 mL of concentrate. Take immediately. **Note:** Avoid skin contact with oral medication; may cause contact dermatitis.

I.V.: I.V. use, injection should be diluted to at least 0.5 mg/mL with NS and given at a rate of 1 mg/minute.

Stability

Storage: Store at 2°C to 25°C (36°F to 77°F). Protect all dosage forms from light; clear or slightly yellow solutions may be used; should be dispensed in amber or opaque vials/bottles. Do not prepare bulk dilutions or store bulk dilutions.

Reconstitution: Do not mix with beverages containing caffeine (coffee, cola), tannins (tea), or pectinates (apple juice) since physical incompatibility exists; use ~60 mL diluent for each 5 mL of concentrate; protect all dosage forms from light; clear or slightly yellow solutions may be used; should be dispensed in amber or opaque vials/bottles. Solutions may be diluted or mixed with fruit juices or other liquids but must be administered immediately after mixing; do not prepare bulk dilutions or store bulk dilutions.

Compatibility: Stable in NS

Y-site administration: Incompatible with cefoperazone

Compatibility in syringe: Incompatible with midazolam, pentobarbital, thiethylperazine

Monitoring Laboratory Tests Baseline liver and kidney function, CBC prior to and periodically during therapy, ophthalmic screening

Monitoring and Teaching Issues

Physical Assessment: Assess other medications patient is taking for effectiveness and interactions (see Drug Interactions). See Contraindications and Warnings/Precautions for use cautions. Monitor ophthalmic screening, laboratory results (see above), therapeutic response, and adverse reactions at beginning of therapy and periodically with long-term use (see Adverse Reactions and Overdose/Toxicology). With I.M. or I.V. use, monitor closely for hypotension. **Note:** Skin contact with oral or injection medication may cause contact dermatitis. Initiate at lower doses (see Dosing) and taper dosage slowly when discontinuing. Assess knowledge/teach patient appropriate use, interventions to reduce side effects, and adverse symptoms to report (see Patient Education). **Pregnancy risk factor C** - instruct patient about appropriate contraceptive use. Breast-feeding is not recommended.

Patient Education: Use exactly as directed; do not increase dose or frequency. It may take 2-3 weeks to achieve desired results; do not discontinue without consulting prescriber. Dilute oral concentration with milk, water, or citrus; do not dilute with liquids containing coffee, tea, or apple juice. Do not take within 2 hours of any antacid. Avoid alcohol or caffeine and other prescription or OTC medications not approved by prescriber. Maintain adequate hydration (2-3 L/day of fluids) unless advised by prescriber to restrict fluids. Avoid skin contact with medication; may cause contact dermatitis (wash immediately with warm, soapy water). You may experience excess drowsiness, restlessness, dizziness, or blurred vision (use caution driving or when engaging in tasks requiring alertness until response to drug is known); dry mouth, nausea, vomiting (small, frequent meals, frequent mouth care, chewing gum, or sucking lozenges may help); constipation (increased exercise, fluids, fruit, or fiber may help); postural hypotension (use caution climbing stairs or when changing position from lying or sitting to standing); urinary retention (void before taking medication); photosensitivity (use sunscreen, wear protective clothing and eyewear, and avoid direct sunlight); or decreased perspiration (avoid strenuous exercise in hot environments). Report persistent CNS effects (eg, trembling fingers, altered gait or balance, excessive sedation, seizures, unusual movements, anxiety, abnormal thoughts, confusion, personality changes); chest pain, palpitations, rapid heartbeat, severe dizziness; unresolved urinary retention or changes in urinary pattern; menstrual pattern, change in libido, or ejaculatory difficulty; vision changes; skin rash or yellowing of skin; difficulty breathing; or worsening of condition. **Pregnancy/breast-feeding precautions:** Inform prescriber if you are or intend to become pregnant. Breast-feeding is not recommended.

Geriatric Considerations: (See Warnings/Precautions, Adverse Reactions, and Overdose/Toxicology.) Elderly patients have an increased risk of adverse response to side effects or adverse reactions to antipsychotics. Plasma levels at a given dose are increased in elderly patients. Older patients are also at higher risk of tardive dyskinesia, and prescribing should be approached in a manner which minimizes the development of this effect.

Related Information

Antiemetics for Chemotherapy-Induced Nausea and Vomiting *on page 1639*
Antipsychotic Agents *on page 1558*
Antipsychotic Medication Guidelines *on page 1614*

Persantine® *see* Dipyridamole *on page 426*

Pethidine Hydrochloride *see* Meperidine *on page 851*

PFA *see* Foscarnet *on page 603*

Pfizerpen® *see* Penicillin G (Parenteral/Aqueous) *on page 1045*

PGE$_1$ *see* Alprostadil *on page 65*

PGE$_2$ *see* Dinoprostone *on page 421*

PGI$_2$ *see* Epoprostenol *on page 479*

PGX *see* Epoprostenol *on page 479*

Phanasin [OTC] *see* Guaifenesin *on page 646*

Pharmacokinetics, Pharmacodynamics, Pharmacotherapeutics *see page 21*

Pharmacotherapy of Urinary Incontinence *see page 1699*

Phenameth® DM *see* Promethazine and Dextromethorphan *on page 1135*

Phenaphen® With Codeine *see* Acetaminophen and Codeine *on page 37*

Phenazopyridine (fen az oh PEER i deen)

U.S. Brand Names Azo-Dine® [OTC]; Azo-Gesic® [OTC]; Azo-Standard®; Baridium®; Prodium™ [OTC]; Pyridiate®; Pyridium®; Uristat® [OTC]; Urodol® [OTC]; Urofemme® [OTC]; Urogesic®

Synonyms Phenazopyridine Hydrochloride; Phenylazo Diamino Pyridine Hydrochloride

Generic Available Yes

Pharmacologic Category Analgesic, Urinary

Pregnancy Risk Factor B

Lactation Excretion in breast milk unknown

Use Symptomatic relief of urinary burning, itching, frequency and urgency in association with urinary tract infection or following urologic procedures

Mechanism of Action/Effect An azo dye which exerts local anesthetic or analgesic action on urinary tract mucosa through an unknown mechanism

Contraindications Hypersensitivity to phenazopyridine or any component of the formulation; kidney or liver disease; patients with a Cl_{cr} <50 mL/minute

Warnings/Precautions Does not treat infection, acts only as an analgesic; drug should be discontinued if skin or sclera develop a yellow color; use with caution in patients with renal impairment. Use of this agent in the elderly is limited since accumulation of phenazopyridine can occur in patients with renal insufficiency. Use is contraindicated in patients with a Cl_{cr} <50 mL/minute.

Effects on Lab Values Phenazopyridine may cause delayed reactions with glucose oxidase reagents (Clinistix®); cupric sulfate tests (Clinitest®) are not affected; interference may also occur with urine ketone tests (Acetest®, Ketostix®) and urinary protein tests; tests for urinary steroids and porphyrins may also occur

Adverse Reactions

1% to 10%:

- Central nervous system: Headache, dizziness
- Gastrointestinal: Stomach cramps

<1% (Limited to important or life-threatening): Acute renal failure, hemolytic anemia, hepatitis, methemoglobinemia

Overdosage/Toxicology Symptoms of overdose include methemoglobinemia, hemolytic anemia, skin pigmentation, and renal and hepatic impairment. For methemoglobinemia, the antidote is methylene blue 1-2 mg/kg I.V.

Pharmacodynamics/Kinetics

Metabolism: Hepatic and via other tissues

Formulations Tablet, as hydrochloride: 95 mg, 97.2 mg, 100 mg, 200 mg

Dosing

Adults & Elderly: Urinary analgesic: Oral: 100-200 mg 3 times/day after meals for 2 days when used concomitantly with an antibacterial agent

Pediatrics: Urinary analgesic: Oral: Children: 12 mg/kg/day in 3 divided doses administered after meals for 2 days

Renal Impairment:

Cl_{cr} 50-80 mL/minute: Administer every 8-16 hours.

Cl_{cr} <50 mL/minute: Avoid use.

Monitoring and Teaching Issues

Physical Assessment: See Warnings/Precautions, Contraindications, and Dosing for use cautions. Assess therapeutic effectiveness according to rational for use. Instruct patients with diabetes to use serum glucose monitoring (phenazopyridine may interfere with certain urine testing reagents - see Effects on Lab Values). Teach patient appropriate use, side effects and interventions, and adverse symptoms to report (see Patient Education). Note breast-feeding caution.

Patient Education: Take exactly as directed. May discolor urine (orange/yellow); this is normal, but will also stain fabric. If diabetic, use serum glucose tests; this medication may interfere with accuracy of urine testing. Report persistent headache, dizziness, or stomach cramping. **Breast-feeding precaution:** Consult prescriber if breast-feeding.

Dietary Issues: Should be taken after meals.

Geriatric Considerations: Use of this agent in the elderly is limited since accumulation of phenazopyridine can occur in patients with renal insufficiency. It should not be used in patients with a Cl_{cr} <50 mL/minute.

Phenazopyridine Hydrochloride *see* Phenazopyridine *on page 1065*

Phencyclidine *see page 1568*

Phenelzine (FEN el zeen)

U.S. Brand Names Nardil®

Synonyms Phenelzine Sulfate

Generic Available No

Pharmacologic Category Antidepressant, Monoamine Oxidase Inhibitor

Pregnancy Risk Factor C

Lactation Excretion in breast milk unknown/not recommended

Use Symptomatic treatment of atypical, nonendogenous, or neurotic depression

Use - Unlabeled/Investigational Selective mutism

Mechanism of Action/Effect Thought to act by increasing endogenous concentrations of norepinephrine, dopamine, and serotonin through inhibition of the enzyme (monoamine oxidase) responsible for the breakdown of these neurotransmitters

Contraindications Hypersensitivity to phenelzine or any component of the formulation; uncontrolled hypertension; pheochromocytoma; hepatic disease; congestive heart failure; concurrent use of sympathomimetics (and related compounds), CNS depressants, ethanol, meperidine, bupropion, buspirone, guanethidine, serotonergic drugs (including SSRIs) - do not use within 5 weeks of fluoxetine discontinuation or 2 weeks of other antidepressant discontinuation; general anesthesia, local vasoconstrictors; spinal anesthesia (hypotension

(Continued)

Phenelzine *(Continued)*

may be exaggerated); foods with a high content of tyramine, tryptophan, or dopamine, chocolate, or caffeine (may cause hypertensive crisis)

Warnings/Precautions Safety in children <16 years of age has not been established; use with caution in patients who are hyperactive, hyperexcitable, or who have glaucoma, suicidal tendencies, hyperthyroidism, or diabetes; avoid use of meperidine within 2 weeks of phenelzine use. Hypertensive crisis may occur with tyramine, tryptophan, or dopamine-containing foods. Should not be used in combination with other antidepressants. Use with caution in depressed patients at risk of suicide. May cause orthostatic hypotension (especially at dosages >30 mg/day) - use with caution in patients with hypotension or patients who would not tolerate transient hypotensive episodes - effects may be additive when used with other agents known to cause orthostasis (phenothiazines). Has been associated with activation of hypomania and/or mania in bipolar patients. May worsen psychotic symptoms in some patients. Use with caution in patients at risk of seizures, or in patients receiving other drugs which may lower seizure threshold. Discontinue at least 48 hours prior to myelography. Use with caution in patients with renal impairment.

The MAO inhibitors are effective and generally well tolerated by older patients. It is the potential interactions with tyramine- or tryptophan-containing foods and other drugs, and their effects on blood pressure that have limited their use.

Pregnancy risk C.

Drug Interactions

Decreased Effect: Phenelzine (and other MAO inhibitors) inhibits the antihypertensive response to guanadrel or guanethidine.

Increased Effect/Toxicity: In general, the combined use of phenelzine with TCAs, venlafaxine, trazodone, dexfenfluramine, sibutramine, lithium, meperidine, fenfluramine, dextromethorphan, and SSRIs should be avoided due to the potential for severe adverse reactions (serotonin syndrome, death). MAO inhibitors (including phenelzine) may inhibit the metabolism of barbiturates and prolong their effect. Phenelzine in combination with amphetamines, other stimulants (methylphenidate), levodopa, metaraminol, reserpine, and decongestants (pseudoephedrine) may result in severe hypertensive reactions. Foods (eg, cheese) and beverages (eg, ethanol) containing tyramine should be avoided; hypertensive crisis may result. Phenelzine may increase the pressor response of norepinephrine and may prolong neuromuscular blockade produced by succinylcholine. Tramadol may increase the risk of seizures and serotonin syndrome in patients receiving an MAO inhibitor. Phenelzine may produce additive hypoglycemic effect in patients receiving hypoglycemic agents and may produce delirium in patients receiving disulfiram.

Nutritional/Ethanol Interactions

Ethanol: Avoid ethanol (alcoholic beverages containing tyramine may induce a severe hypertensive response).

Food: Clinically-severe elevated blood pressure may occur if phenelzine is taken with tyramine-containing foods. Avoid foods containing tryptophan, dopamine, chocolate, or caffeine.

Effects on Lab Values ↓ glucose

Adverse Reactions Frequency not defined.

Cardiovascular: Orthostatic hypotension, edema

Central nervous system: Dizziness, headache, drowsiness, sleep disturbances, fatigue, hyper-reflexia, twitching, ataxia, mania

Dermatologic: Rash, pruritus

Endocrine & metabolic: Decreased sexual ability (anorgasmia, ejaculatory disturbances, impotence), hypernatremia, hypermetabolic syndrome

Gastrointestinal: Xerostomia, constipation, weight gain

Genitourinary: Urinary retention

Hematologic: Leukopenia

Hepatic: Hepatitis

Neuromuscular & skeletal: Weakness, tremor, myoclonus

Ocular: Blurred vision, glaucoma

Miscellaneous: Diaphoresis

Overdosage/Toxicology Symptoms of overdose include tachycardia, palpitations, muscle twitching, seizures, insomnia, restlessness, transient hypertension, hypotension, drowsiness, hyperpyrexia, and coma. Treatment is symptom-directed and supportive.

Pharmacodynamics/Kinetics

Absorption: Well absorbed

Onset: Therapeutic: 2-4 weeks

Duration: May continue to have a therapeutic effect and interactions 2 weeks after discontinuing therapy

Formulations Tablet, as sulfate: 15 mg

Dosing

Adults: Depression: Oral: 15 mg 3 times/day; may increase to 60-90 mg/day during early phase of treatment, then reduce dose for maintenance therapy slowly after maximum benefit is obtained. Takes 2-4 weeks for a significant response to occur.

Elderly: Oral: Initial: 7.5 mg/day; increase by 7.5-15 mg/day every 3-4 days as tolerated; usual therapeutic dose: 15-60 mg/day in 3-4 divided doses.

Pediatrics: Selective mutism (unlabeled use): Oral: 30-60 mg/day

Stability

Storage: Protect from light

Monitoring and Teaching Issues

Physical Assessment: Assess other medications patient may be taking for effectiveness and interactions (see Drug Interactions). See Contraindications and Warnings/Precautions for use cautions. Monitor therapeutic response and adverse reactions at beginning of therapy and periodically with long-term use (see Adverse Reactions and Overdose/Toxicology). Taper dosage slowly when discontinuing; allow 3-4 weeks between discontinuing phenelzine and starting another antidepressant. Advise diabetics to monitor serum glucose closely (phenelzine may lower glucose level). Assess knowledge/teach patient appropriate use, interventions to reduce side effects (including tyramine-free diet - see Tyramine Foods List *on page 1601*), and adverse symptoms to report (see Patient Education). **Pregnancy risk factor C** - benefits of use should outweigh possible risks. Breast-feeding is not recommended.

Patient Education: Take exactly as directed; do not increase dose or frequency. It may take 2-3 weeks to achieve desired results. Avoid alcohol, caffeine, and other prescription or OTC medications not approved by prescriber. Avoid tyramine-containing foods (eg, pickles, aged cheese, wine). Maintain adequate hydration (2-3 L/day of fluids) unless advised by prescriber to restrict fluids. You may experience postural hypotension (use caution when climbing stairs or changing position from lying or sitting to standing); drowsiness, lightheadedness, dizziness (use caution when driving or engaging in tasks requiring alertness until response to drug is known); anorexia, dry mouth (small, frequent meals, frequent mouth care, chewing gum, or sucking lozenges may help); constipation (increased exercise, fluids, fruit, or fiber may help); or diarrhea (buttermilk, yogurt, or boiled milk may help). Diabetic patients should monitor serum glucose closely (Nardil® may effect glucose levels). Report persistent insomnia; chest pain, palpitations, irregular or rapid heartbeat, or swelling of extremities; muscle cramping, tremors, or altered gait; blurred vision or eye pain; yellowing of eyes or skin; pale stools/dark urine; or worsening of condition. **Pregnancy/breast-feeding precautions:** Inform prescriber if you are or intend to become pregnant. Breast-feeding is not recommended.

Geriatric Considerations: MAO inhibitors are effective and generally well tolerated by older patients. Potential interactions with tyramine- or tryptophan-containing foods (see Warnings/Precautions) and other drugs, and adverse effects on blood pressure have limited the use of MAO inhibitors. They are usually reserved for patients who do not tolerate or respond to traditional "cyclic" or "second generation" antidepressants. Brain activity due to monoamine oxidase increases with age and even more so in patients with Alzheimer's disease. Therefore, MAO inhibitors may have an increased role in treating depressed patients with Alzheimer's disease. Phenelzine is less stimulating than tranylcypromine.

Additional Information Pyridoxine deficiency has occurred; symptoms include numbness and edema of hands; may respond to supplementation.

The MAO inhibitors are usually reserved for patients who do not tolerate or respond to other antidepressants. The brain activity of monoamine oxidase increases with age and even more so in patients with Alzheimer's disease. Therefore, the MAO inhibitors may have an increased role in patients with Alzheimer's disease who are depressed. Phenelzine is less stimulating than tranylcypromine.

Related Information

Antidepressant Agents *on page 1553*
Antidepressant Medication Guidelines *on page 1613*
Tyramine Foods List *on page 1601*

Phenelzine Sulfate *see* Phenelzine *on page 1065*

Phenergan® *see* Promethazine *on page 1133*

Phenergan® VC *see* Promethazine and Phenylephrine *on page 1135*

Phenergan® VC With Codeine *see* Promethazine, Phenylephrine, and Codeine *on page 1136*

Phenergan® With Codeine *see* Promethazine and Codeine *on page 1135*

Phenergan® With Dextromethorphan *see* Promethazine and Dextromethorphan *on page 1135*

Pheniramine and Naphazoline *see page 1509*

Phenobarbital (fee noe BAR bi tal)

U.S. Brand Names Luminal® Sodium

Synonyms Phenobarbital Sodium; Phenobarbitone; Phenylethylmalonylurea

Restrictions C-IV

Generic Available Yes

Pharmacologic Category Anticonvulsant, Barbiturate; Barbiturate

Pregnancy Risk Factor D

Lactation Enters breast milk/not recommended (AAP recommends use "with caution")

Use Management of generalized tonic-clonic (grand mal) and partial seizures; sedative

Use - Unlabeled/Investigational Febrile seizures in children; may also be used for prevention and treatment of neonatal hyperbilirubinemia and lowering of bilirubin in chronic cholestasis; neonatal seizures; management of sedative/hypnotic withdrawal

Mechanism of Action/Effect Short-acting barbiturate with sedative, hypnotic, and anticonvulsant properties. Barbiturates depress the sensory cortex, decrease motor activity, alter cerebellar function, and produce drowsiness, sedation, and hypnosis. In high doses, barbiturates exhibit anticonvulsant activity; barbiturates produce dose-dependent respiratory depression.

Contraindications Hypersensitivity to barbiturates or any component of the formulation; marked hepatic impairment; dyspnea or airway obstruction; porphyria; pregnancy

Warnings/Precautions Potential for drug dependency exists, abrupt cessation may precipitate withdrawal, including status epilepticus in epileptic patients. Do not administer to patients in acute pain. Use caution in elderly, debilitated, renally or hepatic dysfunction, and pediatric patients. May cause paradoxical responses, including agitation and hyperactivity, particularly in acute pain and pediatric patients. Use with caution in patients with depression or suicidal tendencies, or in patients with a history of drug abuse. Tolerance, psychological and physical dependence may occur with prolonged use. May cause CNS depression, which may impair physical or mental abilities. Effects with other sedative drugs or ethanol may be potentiated. May cause respiratory depression or hypotension, particularly when administered intravenously. Use with caution in hemodynamically unstable patients (hypovolemic shock, CHF) or patients with respiratory disease. Due to its long half-life and risk of dependence, phenobarbital is not recommended as a sedative in the elderly. Use has been associated with cognitive deficits in children. Use with caution in patients with hypoadrenalism.

(Continued)

Phenobarbital *(Continued)*

Drug Interactions

Cytochrome P450 Effect: Substrate of CYP2C8/9, **2C19**, 2E1; Induces **CYP1A2, 2A6, 2B6, 2C8/9, 3A4**

Decreased Effect: Barbiturates are hepatic enzyme inducers, and may increase the metabolism of antipsychotics, some beta-blockers (unlikely with atenolol and nadolol), calcium channel blockers, chloramphenicol, cimetidine, corticosteroids, cyclosporine, disopyramide, doxycycline, ethosuximide, felbamate, furosemide, griseofulvin, lamotrigine, phenytoin, propafenone, quinidine, tacrolimus, TCAs, and theophylline. Barbiturates may increase the metabolism of estrogens and reduce the efficacy of oral contraceptives; an alternative method of contraception should be considered. Barbiturates inhibit the hypoprothrombinemic effects of oral anticoagulants via increased metabolism. Barbiturates may enhance the metabolism of methadone resulting in methadone withdrawal.

Increased Effect/Toxicity: When combined with other CNS depressants, ethanol, narcotic analgesics, antidepressants, or benzodiazepines, additive respiratory and CNS depression may occur. Barbiturates may enhance the hepatotoxic potential of acetaminophen overdoses. Chloramphenicol, MAO inhibitors, valproic acid, and felbamate may inhibit barbiturate metabolism. Barbiturates may impair the absorption of griseofulvin, and may enhance the nephrotoxic effects of methoxyflurane. Concurrent use of phenobarbital with meperidine may result in increased CNS depression. Concurrent use of phenobarbital with primidone may result in elevated phenobarbital serum concentrations.

Nutritional/Ethanol Interactions

Ethanol: Avoid ethanol (may increase CNS depression).

Food: May cause decrease in vitamin D and calcium.

Herb/Nutraceutical: Avoid evening primrose (seizure threshold decreased). Avoid valerian, St John's wort, kava kava, gotu kola (may increase CNS depression).

Effects on Lab Values ↑ ammonia (B), LFTs, copper (serum); ↓ bilirubin (S); assay interference of LDH

Adverse Reactions Frequency not defined.

Cardiovascular: Bradycardia, hypotension, syncope

Central nervous system: Drowsiness, lethargy, CNS excitation or depression, impaired judgment, "hangover" effect, confusion, somnolence, agitation, hyperkinesia, ataxia, nervousness, headache, insomnia, nightmares, hallucinations, anxiety, dizziness

Dermatologic: Rash, exfoliative dermatitis, Stevens-Johnson syndrome

Gastrointestinal: Nausea, vomiting, constipation

Hematologic: Agranulocytosis, thrombocytopenia, megaloblastic anemia

Local: Pain at injection site, thrombophlebitis with I.V. use

Renal: Oliguria

Respiratory: Laryngospasm, respiratory depression, apnea (especially with rapid I.V. use), hypoventilation, apnea

Miscellaneous: Gangrene with inadvertent intra-arterial injection

Overdosage/Toxicology Symptoms of overdose include unsteady gait, slurred speech, confusion, jaundice, hypothermia, hypotension, respiratory depression, and coma. In severe overdose, charcoal hemoperfusion may accelerate removal. Treatment is symptom-directed and supportive.

Pharmacodynamics/Kinetics

Absorption: Oral: 70% to 90%

Half-Life Elimination: Neonates: 45-500 hours; Infants: 20-133 hours; Children: 37-73 hours; Adults: 53-140 hours

Time to Peak: Serum: Oral: 1-6 hours

Metabolism: Hepatic via hydroxylation and glucuronide conjugation

Onset: Oral: Hypnosis: 20-60 minutes; I.V.: ~5 minutes; Peak effect: I.V.: ~30 minutes

Duration: Oral: 6-10 hours; I.V.: 4-10 hours

Formulations

Elixir: 20 mg/5 mL (5 mL, 7.5 mL, 15 mL, 120 mL, 473 mL, 946 mL, 4000 mL)

Injection, as sodium: 30 mg/mL (1 mL); 60 mg/mL (1 mL); 65 mg/mL (1 mL); 130 mg/mL (1 mL)

Luminal®: 60 mg/mL (1 mL); 130 mg/mL (1 mL)

Tablet: 15 mg, 16 mg, 30 mg, 32 mg, 60 mg, 65 mg, 100 mg

Dosing

Adults:

Sedation: Oral, I.M.: 30-120 mg/day in 2-3 divided doses

Hypnotic: Oral, I.M., I.V., S.C.: 100-320 mg at bedtime

Preoperative sedation: I.M.: 100-200 mg 1-1.5 hours before procedure

Anticonvulsant: Status epilepticus: **Loading dose:** I.V.: 300-800 mg initially followed by 120-240 mg/dose at 20-minute intervals until seizures are controlled or a total dose of 1-2 g

Anticonvulsant maintenance dose: Oral, I.V.: 1-3 mg/kg/day in divided doses or 50-100 mg 2-3 times/day

Sedative/hypnotic withdrawal (unlabeled use): Initial daily requirement is determined by substituting phenobarbital 30 mg for every 100 mg pentobarbital used during tolerance testing; then daily requirement is decreased by 10% of initial dose.

Elderly: Not recommended for use in the elderly.

Pediatrics:

Children:

Sedation: Oral: 2 mg/kg 3 times/day

Hypnotic: I.M., I.V., S.C.: 3-5 mg/kg at bedtime

Preoperative sedation: Oral, I.M., I.V.: 1-3 mg/kg 1-1.5 hours before procedure

Anticonvulsant: Status epilepticus: **Loading dose:** I.V.: Infants and Children: 10-20 mg/kg in a single or divided dose; in select patients may administer additional 5 mg/kg/dose every 15-30 minutes until seizure is controlled or a total dose of 40 mg/kg is reached

Anticonvulsant maintenance dose: Oral, I.V.:

Infants: 5-8 mg/kg/day in 1-2 divided doses

Children:

1-5 years: 6-8 mg/kg/day in 1-2 divided doses

5-12 years: 4-6 mg/kg/day in 1-2 divided doses

>12 years: 1-3 mg/kg/day in divided doses or 50-100 mg 2-3 times/day

Renal Impairment:

Cl_{cr} <10 mL/minute: Administer every 12-16 hours.

Moderately dialyzable (20% to 50%)

Hepatic Impairment: Increased side effects may occur in severe liver disease. Monitor plasma levels and adjust dose accordingly.

Administration

I.V.: Avoid rapid I.V. administration >50 mg/minute. Avoid intra-arterial injection.

Stability

Storage: Protect elixir from light. Not stable in aqueous solutions. Use only clear solutions. Do not add to acidic solutions; precipitation may occur.

Compatibility: Stable in dextran 6% in dextrose, dextran 6% in NS, D_5LR, $D_5{}^1/_4NS$, $D_5{}^1/_2NS$, D_5NS, D_5W, $D_{10}W$, LR, $^1/_2NS$, NS

Y-site administration: Incompatible with amphotericin B cholesteryl sulfate complex, hydromorphone

Compatibility in syringe: Incompatible with hydromorphone, pentazocine, ranitidine, sufentanil

Compatibility when admixed: Incompatible with chlorpromazine, cimetidine, clindamycin, dimenhydrinate, diphenhydramine, droperidol, ephedrine, hydralazine, hydrocortisone sodium succinate, hydroxyzine, insulin (regular), kanamycin, levorphanol, meperidine, morphine, norepinephrine, pancuronium, penicillin G, pentazocine, phenytoin, procaine, prochlorperazine edisylate, prochlorperazine mesylate, promazine, promethazine, streptomycin, succinylcholine, vancomycin

Monitoring Laboratory Tests Phenobarbital serum concentrations, CBC, LFTs

Monitoring and Teaching Issues

Physical Assessment: Assess effectiveness and interactions of other medications patient may be taking (see Contraindications, Warnings/Precautions, and Drug Interactions). Assess for history of addiction; long-term use can result in dependence, abuse, or tolerance; periodically evaluate need for continued use. Monitor cardio/respiratory and CNS status; use safety precautions. Monitor effectiveness of therapy and adverse reactions (see above). **Oral:** Monitor therapeutic response and adverse reactions (see Adverse Reactions) at beginning of therapy and periodically with long-term use. Assess knowledge/teach patient appropriate use, possible side effects, and symptoms to report (see Patient Education). **Pregnancy risk factor D** - determine that patient is not pregnant before beginning treatment. Instruct patients of childbearing age about appropriate barrier contraceptive measures. Breast-feeding is not recommended.

Patient Education: I.M./I.V.: Patient instructions and information are determined by patient condition and therapeutic purpose. If self-administered, use exactly as directed; do not increase dose or frequency. Drug may cause physical and/or psychological dependence. While using this medication, do not use alcohol and other prescription or OTC medications (especially pain medications, sedatives, antihistamines, or hypnotics) without consulting prescriber. Maintain adequate hydration (2-3 L/day of fluids) unless advised by prescriber to restrict fluids. You may experience drowsiness, dizziness, or blurred vision (use caution when driving or engaging in tasks requiring alertness until response to drug is known); nausea, vomiting, or loss of appetite (small, frequent meals, frequent mouth care, chewing gum, or sucking lozenges may help); or constipation (increased exercise, fluids, fruit, or fiber may help). Report skin rash or irritation; CNS changes (confusion, depression, increased sedation, excitation, headache, insomnia, or nightmares); difficulty breathing or shortness of breath; changes in urinary pattern or menstrual pattern; muscle weakness or tremors; or difficulty swallowing or feeling of tightness in throat. **Pregnancy/breast-feeding precautions:** Do not get pregnant while taking this medication; use appropriate barrier contraceptive measures. Breast-feeding is not recommended.

Dietary Issues: Vitamin D: Loss in vitamin D due to malabsorption; increase intake of foods rich in vitamin D. Supplementation of vitamin D and/or calcium may be necessary. Sodium content of injection (65 mg, 1 mL): 6 mg (0.3 mEq).

Geriatric Considerations: Due to its long half-life and risk of dependence, phenobarbital is not recommended as a sedative or hypnotic in the elderly. Interpretive guidelines from the Health Care Financing Administration discourage the use of this agent as a sedative/hypnotic in long-term care residents.

Breast-feeding Issues: Sedation has been reported in nursing infants; infantile spasms may occur after weaning from breast milk. AAP recommends USE WITH CAUTION.

Pregnancy Issues: Crosses the placenta. Cardiac defect reported; hemorrhagic disease of newborn due to fetal vitamin K depletion may occur; may induce maternal folic acid deficiency; withdrawal symptoms observed in infant following delivery. Epilepsy itself, number of medications, genetic factors, or a combination of these probably influence the teratogenicity of anticonvulsant therapy. Benefit:risk ratio usually favors continued use during pregnancy.

Additional Information Injectable solutions contain propylene glycol.

Related Information

Compatibility of Drugs *on page 1564*

Peak and Trough Guidelines *on page 1544*

Seizure Treatment *on page 1700*

Phenobarbital, Belladonna, and Ergotamine Tartrate *see* Belladonna, Phenobarbital, and Ergotamine *on page 152*

Phenobarbital, Hyoscyamine, Atropine, and Scopolamine *see* Hyoscyamine, Atropine, Scopolamine, and Phenobarbital *on page 687*

Phenobarbital Sodium *see* Phenobarbital *on page 1067*

Phenobarbitone *see* Phenobarbital *on page 1067*

Phenolsulfonphthalein *see page 1461*

Phenoxymethyl Penicillin *see* Penicillin V Potassium *on page 1048*

Phentermine *see page 1693*

Phentolamine (fen TOLE a meen)

U.S. Brand Names Regitine®

Synonyms Phentolamine Mesylate

Generic Available Yes

Pharmacologic Category Alpha$_1$ Blocker

Pregnancy Risk Factor C

Lactation Excretion in breast milk unknown

Use Diagnosis of pheochromocytoma and treatment of hypertension associated with pheochromocytoma or other caused by excess sympathomimetic amines; as treatment of dermal necrosis after extravasation of drugs with alpha-adrenergic effects (norepinephrine, dopamine, epinephrine, dobutamine)

Mechanism of Action/Effect Competitively blocks alpha-adrenergic receptors to produce brief antagonism of circulating epinephrine and norepinephrine to reduce hypertension caused by alpha effects of these catecholamines; also has a positive inotropic and chronotropic effect on the heart

Contraindications Hypersensitivity to phentolamine or any component of the formulation; renal impairment; coronary or cerebral arteriosclerosis

Warnings/Precautions Myocardial infarction, cerebrovascular spasm and cerebrovascular occlusion have occurred following administration. Use with caution in patients with gastritis or peptic ulcer, tachycardia, or a history of cardiac arrhythmias. Pregnancy risk C.

Drug Interactions

Decreased Effect: Decreased effect of phentolamine with epinephrine and ephedrine.

Increased Effect/Toxicity: Phentolamine's toxicity is increased with ethanol (disulfiram reaction).

Effects on Lab Values ↑ LFTs rarely

Adverse Reactions Frequency not defined.

Cardiovascular: Hypotension, tachycardia, arrhythmia, flushing, orthostatic hypotension
Central nervous system: Weakness, dizziness
Gastrointestinal: Nausea, vomiting, diarrhea
Respiratory: Nasal congestion
Postmarketing and/or case reports: Pulmonary hypertension

Overdosage/Toxicology Symptoms of overdose include tachycardia, shock, vomiting, and dizziness. If fluid replacement is inadequate to treat hypotension, only alpha-adrenergic vasopressors such as norepinephrine should be used. Mixed agents such as epinephrine may cause more hypotension.

Pharmacodynamics/Kinetics

Half-Life Elimination: 19 minutes

Metabolism: Hepatic

Onset: I.M.: 15-20 minutes; I.V.: Immediate

Duration: I.M.: 30-45 minutes; I.V.: 15-30 minutes

Formulations Injection, as mesylate: 5 mg/mL (1 mL)

Dosing

Adults & Elderly:

Treatment of alpha-adrenergic drug extravasation: S.C.:
Infiltrate area with a small amount (eg, 1 mL) of solution (made by diluting 5-10 mg in 10 mL of NS) within 12 hours of extravasation; do not exceed 0.1-0.2 mg/kg or 5 mg total
If dose is effective, normal skin color should return to the blanched area within 1 hour.
Diagnosis of pheochromocytoma: I.M., I.V.: 5 mg
Surgery for pheochromocytoma: Hypertension: I.M., I.V.: 5 mg given 1-2 hours before procedure and repeated as needed every 2-4 hours
Hypertensive crisis: I.V.: 5-20 mg

Pediatrics:

Treatment of alpha-adrenergic drug extravasation: S.C.: Children: Infiltrate area with a small amount (eg, 1 mL) of solution (made by diluting 5-10 mg in 10 mL of NS) within 12 hours of extravasation; do not exceed 0.1-0.2 mg/kg or 5 mg total
Diagnosis of pheochromocytoma: I.M., I.V.: Children: 0.05-0.1 mg/kg/dose, maximum single dose: 5 mg
Surgery for pheochromocytoma: Hypertension: I.M., I.V.: Children: 0.05-0.1 mg/kg/dose given 1-2 hours before procedure; repeat as needed every 2-4 hours until hypertension is controlled; maximum single dose: 5 mg.

Administration

I.V.:

Vasoconstrictor (alpha-adrenergic agonist) extravasation: Infiltrate the area of extravasation with multiple small injections using only 27- or 30-gauge needles and changing the needle between each skin entry. Be careful not to cause so much swelling of the extremity or digit that a compartment syndrome occurs.
Pheochromocytoma: Inject each 5 mg over 1 minute.

Stability

Reconstitution: Reconstituted solution is stable for 48 hours at room temperature and 1 week when refrigerated.

Compatibility: Stable in NS

Monitoring and Teaching Issues

Physical Assessment: See Contraindications, Warnings/Precautions, and Drug Interactions for use cautions. See Dosing and Administration for specifics according to purpose for use. When used to treat dermal necrosis after extravasation of drugs with alpha-adrenergic effects, monitor effectiveness of treatment closely. Assess patient response (eg, Cardiac status - Adverse Reactions and Overdose/Toxicology). Teach patient adverse symptoms to report (see Patient Education). **Pregnancy risk factor C** - benefits of use should outweigh possible risks. Note breast-feeding caution.

Patient Education: This medication can only be administered by infusion or injection. Report immediately any pain at infusion/injection site. May cause orthostatic hypotension (use caution when changing position or call for assistance). Report dizziness, rapid heartbeat, feelings of weakness, or nausea/vomiting. **Pregnancy/breast-feeding precautions:** Inform prescriber if you are or intend to become pregnant. Consult prescriber if breast-feeding.

Phentolamine Mesylate *see* Phentolamine *on page 1070*

Phenylalanine Mustard *see* Melphalan *on page 848*

Phenylazo Diamino Pyridine Hydrochloride *see* Phenazopyridine *on page 1065*

Phenylephrine (fen il EF rin)

U.S. Brand Names AK-Dilate® Ophthalmic; AK-Nefrin® Ophthalmic; Alconefrin® Nasal [OTC]; Children's Nostril®; Mydfrin® Ophthalmic; Neo-Synephrine® Injection; Neo-Synephrine® Nasal [OTC]; Neo-Synephrine® Ophthalmic; Nostril® Nasal [OTC]; Prefrin™ Ophthalmic; Relief® Ophthalmic; Rhinall® Nasal [OTC]; Vicks Sinex® Nasal [OTC]

Synonyms Phenylephrine Hydrochloride

Generic Available Yes

Pharmacologic Category Alpha/Beta Agonist; Ophthalmic Agent, Antiglaucoma; Ophthalmic Agent, Mydriatic

Pregnancy Risk Factor C

Lactation Excretion in breast milk unknown

Use Treatment of hypotension, vascular failure in shock; as a vasoconstrictor in regional analgesia; symptomatic relief of nasal and nasopharyngeal mucosal congestion; as a mydriatic in ophthalmic procedures and treatment of wide-angle glaucoma; supraventricular tachycardia

Mechanism of Action/Effect Potent, direct-acting alpha-adrenergic stimulator with weak beta-adrenergic activity; causes vasoconstriction of the arterioles of the nasal mucosa and conjunctiva; activates the dilator muscle of the pupil to cause contraction; produces vasoconstriction of arterioles in the body; produces systemic arterial vasoconstriction

Contraindications Hypersensitivity to phenylephrine, bisulfite (some products contain metabisulfite), or any component of the formulation; hypertension; ventricular tachycardia

Warnings/Precautions Use with caution in the elderly, patients with hyperthyroidism, bradycardia, partial heart block, myocardial disease, or severe CAD. Not a substitute for volume replacement. Avoid hypertension; monitor blood pressure closely and adjust infusion rate. Infuse into a large vein if possible. Watch I.V. site closely. Avoid extravasation. The elderly can be more sensitive to side effects from the nasal decongestant form. Rebound congestion can occur when the drug is discontinued after chronic use. Pregnancy risk C.

Drug Interactions

Decreased Effect: Alpha- and beta-adrenergic blocking agents may have a decreased effect if taken with phenylephrine.

Increased Effect/Toxicity: Phenylephrine, taken with sympathomimetics, may induce tachycardia or arrhythmias. If taken with MAO inhibitors or oxytocic agents, actions may be potentiated.

Nutritional/Ethanol Interactions Herb/Nutraceutical: Avoid ephedra, yohimbe (may cause CNS stimulation).

Adverse Reactions Frequency not defined.

Cardiovascular: Reflex bradycardia, excitability, restlessness, arrhythmias (rare), precordial pain or discomfort, pallor, hypertension, severe peripheral and visceral vasoconstriction, decreased cardiac output

Central nervous system: Headache, anxiety, weakness, dizziness, tremor, paresthesia, restlessness

Endocrine & metabolic: Metabolic acidosis

Local: Extravasation which may lead to necrosis and sloughing of surrounding tissue, blanching of skin

Neuromuscular & skeletal: Pilomotor response, weakness

Renal: Decreased renal perfusion, reduced urine output, reduced urine output

Respiratory: Respiratory distress

Overdosage/Toxicology Symptoms of overdose include vomiting, hypertension, palpitations, paresthesia, and ventricular extrasystoles. Treatment is supportive. In extreme cases, I.V. phentolamine may be used.

Pharmacodynamics/Kinetics

Half-Life Elimination: 2.5 hours; prolonged after long-term infusion

Metabolism: Hepatically and via intestinal monoamine oxidase to phenolic conjugates

Onset: I.M., S.C.: 10-15 minutes; I.V.: Immediate

Duration: I.M.: 0.5-2 hours; I.V.: 15-30 minutes; S.C.: 1 hour

Formulations

Injection, as hydrochloride (Neo-Synephrine®): 1% [10 mg/mL] (1 mL)

Solution, intranasal drops, as hydrochloride:

Alconefrin®, Neo-Synephrine®: 0.5% (15 mL, 30 mL)

Alconefrin® 12: 0.16% (30 mL)

Alconefrin® 25, Neo-Synephrine®, Children's Nostril®, Rhinall®: 0.25% (15 mL, 30 mL, 40 mL)

Neo-Synephrine®: 0.125% (15 mL)

Solution, intranasal spray, as hydrochloride:

Alconefrin® 25, Neo-Synephrine®, Rhinall®: 0.25% (15 mL, 30 mL, 40 mL)

Neo-Synephrine®: 1% (15 mL)

Neo-Synephrine®, Nostril®, Vicks Sinex®: 0.5% (15 mL, 30 mL)

Solution, ophthalmic, as hydrochloride:

AK-Dilate®, Mydfrin®, Neo-Synephrine®, Phenoptic®: 2.5% (2 mL, 3 mL, 5 mL, 15 mL)

AK-Dilate®, Neo-Synephrine®, Neo-Synephrine® Viscous: 10% (1 mL, 2 mL, 5 mL, 15 mL)

AK-Nefrin®, Prefrin™ Liquifilm®, Relief®: 0.12% (0.3 mL, 15 mL, 20 mL)

(Continued)

Phenylephrine *(Continued)*

Dosing

Adults:

Nasal decongestant (therapy should not exceed 5 continuous days): Nasal: Instill 1-2 sprays or instill 1-2 drops every 4 hours of 0.25% to 0.5% solution as needed; 1% solution may be used in adults in cases of extreme nasal congestion. Do not use nasal solutions more than 3 days.

Hypotension/shock:

I.M., S.C.: 2-5 mg/dose every 1-2 hours as needed (initial dose should not exceed 5 mg)

I.V. bolus: 0.1-0.5 mg/dose every 10-15 minutes as needed (initial dose should not exceed 0.5 mg)

I.V. infusion: 10 mg in 250 mL D_5W or NS (1:25,000 dilution) (40 mcg/mL); start at 100-180 mcg/minute (2-5 mL/minute; 50-90 drops/minute) initially; when blood pressure is stabilized, maintenance rate: 40-60 mcg/minute (20-30 drops/minute); rates up to 360 mcg/minute have been reported; dosing range: 0.4-9.1 mcg/kg/minute

Note: Concentrations up to 100-500 mg in 250 mL have been used.

Paroxysmal supraventricular tachycardia: I.V.: 0.25-0.5 mg/dose over 20-30 seconds

Ocular procedures: Ophthalmic: Instill 1 drop of 2.5% or 10% solution, may repeat in 10-60 minutes as needed.

Elderly:

Nasal decongestant: Administer 2-3 drops or 1-2 sprays every 4 hours of 0.125% to 0.25% solution as needed; do not use more than 3 days.

Ophthalmic preparations for pupil dilation: Instill 1 drop of 2.5% solution, may repeat in 1 hour if necessary.

Refer to adult dosing for other uses and Geriatric Considerations for cautions on I.V. use.

Pediatrics:

Ocular procedures: Ophthalmic:

Infants <1 year: Instill 1 drop of 2.5% 15-30 minutes before procedures

Children: Refer to adult dosing.

Nasal decongestant (therapy should not exceed 5 continuous days): Nasal:

2-6 years: Instill 1 drop every 2-4 hours of 0.125% solution as needed

6-12 years: Instill 1-2 sprays or instill 1-2 drops every 4 hours of 0.25% solution as needed

>12 years: Refer to adult dosing.

Hypotension/shock: Children:

I.M., S.C.: 0.1 mg/kg/dose every 1-2 hours as needed (maximum: 5 mg)

I.V. bolus: 5-20 mcg/kg/dose every 10-15 minutes as needed

I.V. infusion: 0.1-0.5 mcg/kg/minute

Paroxysmal supraventricular tachycardia: I.V.: Children: 5-10 mcg/kg/dose over 20-30 seconds

Administration

I.V.: Concentration and rate of infusion can be calculated using the following formulas: Dilute 0.6 mg x weight (kg) to 100 mL; then the dose in mcg/kg/minute = 0.1 x the infusion rate in mL/hour.

Stability

Storage: Stable for 48 hours in 5% dextrose in water at pH 3.5-7.5; do not use brown colored solutions

Reconstitution: Stable for 48 hours in 5% dextrose in water at pH 3.5-7.5. Do not use brown colored solutions.

Compatibility: Stable in dextran 6% in dextrose, dextran 6% in NS, D_5LR, $D_5{}^1/_4NS$, $D_5{}^1/_2NS$, D_5NS, D_5W, $D_{10}W$, LR, $^1/_2NS$, NS, sodium bicarbonate 5%

Y-site administration: Incompatible with thiopental

Monitoring Laboratory Tests Parenteral use: Monitor arterial blood gases

Monitoring and Teaching Issues

Physical Assessment: Assess other medications patient may be taking for effectiveness and interactions (see Warnings/Precautions and Drug Interactions). Monitor therapeutic response and adverse reactions according to use (see Contraindications, Adverse Reactions, and Overdose/Toxicology). **Parenteral:** Monitor arterial blood gases, adverse reactions, and infusion site (see Adverse Reactions, Overdose/Toxicology, and Administration). **Nasal/ophthalmic:** Assess knowledge/teach patient appropriate use, interventions to reduce side effects, and adverse symptoms to report (see Patient Education). **Pregnancy risk factor C** - benefits of use should outweigh possible risks. Note breast-feeding caution. Systemic absorption from ophthalmic instillation is minimal.

Patient Education: Nasal decongestant: Do not use for more than 3 days in a row. Clear nose as much as possible before use. Tilt head back and instill recommended dose of drops or spray. Do not blow nose for 5-10 minutes. You may experience transient stinging or burning.

Ophthalmic: Do not let tip of applicator touch eye; do not contaminate tip of applicator (may cause eye infection, eye damage, or vision loss). Open eye, look at ceiling, and instill prescribed amount of solution. Close eye and roll eye in all directions, and apply gentle pressure to inner corner of eye for 1-2 minutes after instillation. Temporary stinging or blurred vision may occur. Report persistent pain, burning, double vision, severe headache, or if condition worsens.

Pregnancy/breast-feeding precautions: Inform prescriber if you are pregnant. Consult prescriber if breast-feeding.

Geriatric Considerations: Phenylephrine I.V. should be used with extreme caution in the elderly. The 10% ophthalmic solution has caused increased blood pressure in elderly patients and its use should, therefore, be avoided. Since topical decongestants can be obtained OTC, elderly patients should be counseled about their proper use and in what disease states they should be avoided (see Warnings/Precautions).

Additional Information Phenylephrine allows for close titration of blood pressure and should be used in patients with hypotension or shock due to peripheral vasodilation. Phenylephrine should not constitute sole therapy in patients with hypotension due to aortic dysfunction or hypovolemia. An important benefit of this drug is the short half-life, allowing rapid changes in dosage with prompt appropriate blood pressure responses. When administered intravenously, it should be used in intensive care settings or under very close monitoring.

Related Information

Inotropic and Vasoconstrictor Comparison *on page 1580*

Ophthalmic Agents *on page 1509*

Phenylephrine and Promethazine *see* Promethazine and Phenylephrine *on page 1135*

Phenylephrine Hydrochloride *see* Phenylephrine *on page 1071*

Phenylephrine, Promethazine, and Codeine *see* Promethazine, Phenylephrine, and Codeine *on page 1136*

Phenylethylmalonylurea *see* Phenobarbital *on page 1067*

Phenylisohydantoin *see* Pemoline *on page 1042*

Phenytek™ *see* Phenytoin *on page 1073*

Phenytoin (FEN i toyn)

U.S. Brand Names Dilantin®; Phenytek™

Synonyms Diphenylhydantoin; DPH; Phenytoin Sodium; Phenytoin Sodium, Extended; Phenytoin Sodium, Prompt

Generic Available Yes: Excludes chewable tablet, extended release capsule

Pharmacologic Category Antiarrhythmic Agent, Class Ib; Anticonvulsant, Hydantoin

Pregnancy Risk Factor D

Lactation Enters breast milk/use caution (AAP rates "compatible")

Use Management of generalized tonic-clonic (grand mal), complex partial seizures; prevention of seizures following head trauma/neurosurgery

Use - Unlabeled/Investigational Ventricular arrhythmias, including those associated with digitalis intoxication, prolonged QT interval and surgical repair of congenital heart diseases in children; epidermolysis bullosa

Mechanism of Action/Effect Stabilizes neuronal membranes and decreases seizure activity by increasing efflux or decreasing influx of sodium ions across cell membranes in the motor cortex during generation of nerve impulses; prolongs effective refractory period and suppresses ventricular pacemaker automaticity, shortens action potential in the heart

Contraindications Hypersensitivity to phenytoin, other hydantoins, or any component of the formulation; pregnancy

Warnings/Precautions May increase frequency of petit mal seizures; I.V. form may cause hypotension, skin necrosis at I.V. site; avoid I.V. administration in small veins; use with caution in patients with porphyria; discontinue if rash or lymphadenopathy occurs; use with caution in patients with hepatic dysfunction, sinus bradycardia, SA block, or AV block; use with caution in elderly or debilitated patients, or in any condition associated with low serum albumin levels, which will increase the free fraction of phenytoin in the serum and, therefore, the pharmacologic response. Sedation, confusional states, or cerebellar dysfunction (loss of motor coordination) may occur at higher total serum concentrations, or at lower total serum concentrations when the free fraction of phenytoin is increased. Abrupt withdrawal may precipitate status epilepticus.

Drug Interactions

Cytochrome P450 Effect: Substrate of **CYP2C8/9, 2C19**, 3A4; Induces **CYP2B6, 2C8/9, 2C19, 3A4**

Decreased Effect: The blood levels of phenytoin may be decreased by carbamazepine, rifampin, amiodarone, cisplatin, disulfiram, vinblastine, bleomycin, folic acid, phenobarbital, ethanol (chronic), pyridoxine, vigabatrin, and theophylline. Sucralfate and continuous NG feedings may decrease absorption of phenytoin. Phenytoin induces hepatic enzymes, and may decrease the effect of oral contraceptives, itraconazole, mebendazole, methadone, oral midazolam, valproic acid, cyclosporine, theophylline, doxycycline, quinidine, mexiletine, disopyramide. Phenytoin also may increase the metabolism of alprazolam, amiodarone, bromfenac, carbamazepine, clozapine, cyclosporine, diazepam, disopyramide, doxycycline, felbamate, furosemide, itraconazole, lamotrigine, mebendazole, meperidine, methadone, metyrapone, mexiletine, midazolam, oral contraceptives, quetiapine, quinidine, tacrolimus, teniposide, theophylline, thyroid hormones, triazolam, and valproic acid resulting in decreased levels/effect. Phenytoin may inhibit the anti-Parkinson effect of levodopa. Long-term concurrent use of phenytoin may inhibit hypoprothrombinemic response to warfarin. Phenytoin may reduce the effectiveness of some nondepolarizing neuromuscular blocking agents.

Increased Effect/Toxicity: Phenytoin serum concentrations may be increased by isoniazid, chloramphenicol, ticlopidine, or fluconazole. In addition, trimethoprim, sulfamethoxazole, valproic acid, sulfamethizole, sulfaphenazole, nifedipine, omeprazole, phenylbutazone, phenobarbital, amiodarone, chloramphenicol, cimetidine, ciprofloxacin, disulfiram, enoxacin, norfloxacin, felbamate, fluconazole, fluoxetine, influenza vaccine, isoniazid, and metronidazole inhibit the metabolism of phenytoin resulting in increased serum phenytoin concentrations. Valproic acid may increase, decrease, or have no effect on phenytoin serum concentrations. Phenytoin may increase the effect of dopamine (enhanced hypotension), warfarin (transiently enhanced anticoagulation), or increase the rate of conversion of primidone to phenobarbital resulting in increased phenobarbital serum concentrations. Phenytoin may enhance the hepatotoxic potential of acetaminophen. Concurrent use of acetazolamide and phenytoin may result in an increased risk of osteomalacia. Concurrent use of phenytoin and lithium has resulted in lithium intoxication. Phenytoin enhances the conversion of primidone to phenobarbital resulting in elevated phenobarbital serum concentrations. Valproic acid and sulfisoxazole may displace phenytoin from binding sites, transiently increasing phenytoin free levels.

Nutritional/Ethanol Interactions

Ethanol:

Acute use: Avoid or limit ethanol (inhibits metabolism of phenytoin). Watch for sedation.

Chronic use: Avoid or limit ethanol (stimulates metabolism of phenytoin).

(Continued)

Phenytoin *(Continued)*

Food: Phenytoin serum concentrations may be altered if taken with food. If taken with enteral nutrition, phenytoin serum concentrations may be decreased. Tube feedings decrease bioavailability; hold tube feedings 2 hours before and 2 hours after phenytoin administration. May decrease calcium, folic acid, and vitamin D levels.

Herb/Nutraceutical: Avoid evening primrose (seizure threshold decreased). Avoid valerian, St John's wort, kava kava, gotu kola (may increase CNS depression).

Effects on Lab Values ↑ glucose, alkaline phosphatase (S); ↓ thyroxine (S), calcium (S)

Adverse Reactions I.V. effects: Hypotension, bradycardia, cardiac arrhythmias, cardiovascular collapse (especially with rapid I.V. use), venous irritation and pain, thrombophlebitis

Effects not related to plasma phenytoin concentrations: Hypertrichosis, gingival hypertrophy, thickening of facial features, carbohydrate intolerance, folic acid deficiency, peripheral neuropathy, vitamin D deficiency, osteomalacia, systemic lupus erythematosus

Concentration-related effects: Nystagmus, blurred vision, diplopia, ataxia, slurred speech, dizziness, drowsiness, lethargy, coma, rash, fever, nausea, vomiting, gum tenderness, confusion, mood changes, folic acid depletion, osteomalacia, hyperglycemia

Related to elevated concentrations:

>20 mcg/mL: Far lateral nystagmus

>30 mcg/mL: 45° lateral gaze nystagmus and ataxia

>40 mcg/mL: Decreased mentation

>100 mcg/mL: Death

Cardiovascular: Hypotension, bradycardia, cardiac arrhythmias, cardiovascular collapse

Central nervous system: Psychiatric changes, slurred speech, dizziness, drowsiness, headache, insomnia

Dermatologic: Rash

Gastrointestinal: Constipation, nausea, vomiting, gingival hyperplasia, enlargement of lips

Hematologic: Leukopenia, thrombocytopenia, agranulocytosis

Hepatic: Hepatitis

Local: Thrombophlebitis

Neuromuscular & skeletal: Tremor, peripheral neuropathy, paresthesia

Ocular: Diplopia, nystagmus, blurred vision

Rarely seen effects: Blood dyscrasias, coarsening of facial features, dyskinesias, hepatitis, hypertrichosis, lymphadenopathy, lymphoma, pseudolymphoma, SLE-like syndrome, Stevens-Johnson syndrome, venous irritation and pain

Overdosage/Toxicology Symptoms of overdose include unsteady gait, slurred speech, confusion, nausea, hypothermia, fever, hypotension, respiratory depression, coma. Treatment is symptomatic.

Pharmacodynamics/Kinetics

Absorption: Oral: Slow

Bioavailability: Form dependent

Half-Life Elimination: Oral: 22 hours (range: 7-42 hours)

Time to Peak: Serum (form dependent): Oral: Extended-release capsule: 4-12 hours; Immediate release preparation: 2-3 hours

Metabolism: Follows dose-dependent capacity-limited (Michaelis-Menten) pharmacokinetics with increased V_{max} in infants >6 months of age and children versus adults; major metabolite (via oxidation), HPPA, undergoes enterohepatic recirculation

Onset: I.V.: ~0.5-1 hour

Formulations

Capsule, extended release, as sodium:

Dilantin®: 30 mg [contains sodium benzoate], 100 mg

Phenytek™: 200 mg, 300 mg

Capsule, prompt release, as sodium: 100 mg

Injection, solution, as sodium: 50 mg/mL (2 mL, 5 mL) [contains alcohol]

Suspension, oral (Dilantin®): 125 mg/5 mL (240 mL) [contains alcohol <0.6%, sodium benzoate; orange-vanilla flavor]

Tablet, chewable (Dilantin®): 50 mg

Dosing

Adults & Elderly:

Status epilepticus: I.V.: Loading dose: Manufacturer recommends 10-15 mg/kg, however, 15-25 mg/kg has been used clinically; maintenance dose: 300 mg/day or 5-6 mg/kg/day in 3 divided doses or 1-2 divided doses using extended release

Anticonvulsant: Oral: Loading dose: 15-20 mg/kg; based on phenytoin serum concentrations and recent dosing history; administer oral loading dose in 3 divided doses given every 2-4 hours to decrease GI adverse effects and to ensure complete oral absorption; maintenance dose: 300 mg/day or 5-6 mg/kg/day in 3 divided doses or 1-2 divided doses using extended release (range 200-1200 mg/day)

Pediatrics:

Status epilepticus: I.V.:

Infants and Children: Loading dose: 15-20 mg/kg in a single or divided dose; maintenance dose: Initial: 5 mg/kg/day in 2 divided doses, usual doses:

6 months to 3 years: 8-10 mg/kg/day

4-6 years: 7.5-9 mg/kg/day

7-9 years: 7-8 mg/kg/day

10-16 years: 6-7 mg/kg/day, some patients may require every 8 hours dosing

Anticonvulsant: Children: Oral: Refer to adult dosing.

Renal Impairment: Phenytoin level in serum may be difficult to interpret in renal failure. Monitoring of free (unbound) concentrations or adjustment to allow interpretation is recommended.

Hepatic Impairment: Safe in usual doses in mild liver disease; clearance may be substantially reduced in cirrhosis and plasma level monitoring with dose adjustment advisable. Free phenytoin levels should be monitored closely.

Administration

Oral: Suspension: Shake well prior to use. Absorption is impaired when phenytoin suspension is given concurrently to patients who are receiving continuous nasogastric feedings. A method to resolve this interaction is to divide the daily dose of phenytoin and withhold the administration of nutritional supplements for 1-2 hours before and after each phenytoin dose.

I.M.: Although approved for I.M. use, I.M. administration is not recommended due to erratic absorption and pain on injection. Fosphenytoin may be considered.

I.V.: Vesicant. Fosphenytoin may be considered for loading in patients who are in status epilepticus, hemodynamically unstable or develop hypotension/bradycardia with I.V. administration of phenytoin. Phenytoin may be administered by IVP or IVPB administration. The maximum rate of I.V. administration is 50 mg/minute. Highly sensitive patients (eg, elderly, patients with pre-existing cardiovascular conditions) should receive phenytoin more slowly (eg, 20 mg/minute).

Other: S.C. administration is not recommended because of the possibility of local tissue damage.

Stability

Storage:

Capsule, tablet: Store below 30°C (86°F); protect from light and moisture

Oral suspension: Store at room temperature of 20°C to 25°C (68°F to 77°F); protect from freezing and light.

Solution for injection: Store at room temperature of 15°C to 30°C (59°F to 86°F); use only clear solutions free of precipitate and haziness, slightly yellow solutions may be used. Precipitation may occur if solution is refrigerated and may dissolve at room temperature.

Reconstitution: I.V.: Further dilution of the solution for I.V. infusion is controversial and no consensus exists as to the optimal concentration and length of stability. Stability is concentration and pH dependent. Based on limited clinical consensus, NS or LR are recommended diluents; dilutions of 1-10 mg/mL have been used and should be administered as soon as possible after preparation (some recommend to discard if not used within 4 hours). Do not refrigerate.

Compatibility: Incompatible with D_5NS, D_5W, fat emulsion 10%, LR, ½NS

Compatibility in syringe: Incompatible with hydromorphone, sufentanil

Compatibility when admixed: Incompatible with amikacin, aminophylline, bretylium, chloramphenicol, dimenhydrinate, diphenhydramine, dobutamine, hydroxyzine, insulin (regular), kanamycin, levorphanol, lidocaine, lincomycin, meperidine, metaraminol, morphine, nitroglycerin, norepinephrine, penicillin G potassium, pentobarbital, phenobarbital, phenylephrine, phytonadione, procainamide, procaine, prochlorperazine edisylate, promazine, promethazine, streptomycin, vancomycin, vitamin B complex with C

Monitoring Laboratory Tests Plasma phenytoin level, CBC, liver function. **Note:** Serum phenytoin concentrations should be interpreted in terms of the unbound concentration. Adjustment should be made in patients with renal impairment and/or hypoalbuminemia.

Monitoring and Teaching Issues

Physical Assessment: See Warnings/Precautions and Dosing for use cautions. Assess potential for interactions with other prescriptions, OTC medications, or herbal products patient may be taking (see extensive list of Drug Interactions). Assess results of laboratory tests (see above), therapeutic effectiveness, and adverse response - when beginning therapy and at regular intervals during treatment (see Warnings/Precautions, Adverse Reactions, and Overdose/Toxicology). When discontinuing oral formulation, taper dose gradually; abrupt discontinuance can cause status epilepticus. **I.V.:** See I.V. Administration specifics. Infusion site should be monitored closely (vesicant). Patient should be monitored closely for adverse/toxic results (see Adverse Reactions). Teach patient proper use (oral), side effects and interventions, and adverse symptoms to report (see Patient Education). **Pregnancy risk factor D** - determine that patient is not pregnant before beginning treatment. Instruct patients of childbearing age about appropriate barrier contraceptive measures (phenytoin may interfere with effectiveness of oral contraceptives). Note breast-feeding caution.

Patient Education: Inform prescriber of all prescriptions, OTC medications, or herbal products you are taking, and any allergies you have. Do not take anything new during treatment without consulting prescriber. Take exactly as directed, preferably on an empty stomach. Do not alter dose or discontinue without consulting prescriber. Do not crush, break, or chew extended release capsules. Shake liquid suspension well before using. Follow recommended diet, avoid alcohol, and maintain adequate hydration (2-3 L/day of fluids) unless advised to restrict fluids. May cause gum or mouth soreness (use good oral hygiene and have frequent dental exams); drowsiness, dizziness, nervousness, or headache (use caution when driving or engaging in tasks that require alertness until response to drug is known); or nausea or vomiting (small, frequent meals, frequent mouth care, chewing gum, or sucking lozenges may help). Report chest pain, irregular heartbeat, or palpitations; slurred speech, unsteady gait, coordination difficulties, or change in mentation; skin rash; unresolved nausea, vomiting, or constipation; swollen glands; swollen, sore, or bleeding gums; unusual bruising or bleeding; acute persistent fatigue; vision changes; or other persistent adverse effects. **Pregnancy/breast-feeding precautions:** Do not get pregnant; use contraceptive measures to prevent possible harm to the fetus (effectiveness of oral contraceptives may be affected by phenytoin). Consult prescriber if breast-feeding.

Dietary Issues:

Folic acid: Phenytoin may decrease mucosal uptake of folic acid; to avoid folic acid deficiency and megaloblastic anemia, some clinicians recommend giving patients on anticonvulsants prophylactic doses of folic acid and cyanocobalamin. However, folate supplementation may increase seizures in some patients (dose dependent). Discuss with healthcare provider prior to using any supplements.

Calcium: Hypocalcemia has been reported in patients taking prolonged high-dose therapy with an anticonvulsant. Some clinicians have given an additional 4000 units/week of vitamin D (especially in those receiving poor nutrition and getting no sun exposure) to prevent hypocalcemia.

(Continued)

Phenytoin *(Continued)*

Vitamin D: Phenytoin interferes with vitamin D metabolism and osteomalacia may result; may need to supplement with vitamin D

Tube feedings: Tube feedings decrease phenytoin absorption. To avoid decreased serum levels with continuous NG feeds, hold feedings for 2 hours prior to and 2 hours after phenytoin administration, if possible. There is a variety of opinions on how to administer phenytoin with enteral feedings. Be **consistent** throughout therapy.

Sodium content of 1 g injection: 88 mg (3.8 mEq)

Geriatric Considerations: Elderly may have low albumin which will increase free fraction and increase drug response. Monitor closely in those who are hypoalbuminemic. Free fraction measurements advised, also elderly may display a higher incidence of adverse effects (cardiovascular) when using the I.V. loading regimen; therefore, recommended to decrease loading I.V. dose to 25 mg/minute (see Warnings/Precautions).

Breast-feeding Issues: Clinical effects on the infant: Methemoglobinemia, drowsiness and decreased sucking reported in 1 case. Benefit:risk ratio usually favors continued use breast-feeding. AAP considers **compatible** with breast-feeding.

Pregnancy Issues: Crosses the placenta. Cardiac defects and multiple other malformations reported; characteristic pattern of malformations called "fetal hydantoin syndrome"; hemorrhagic disease of newborn due to fetal vitamin K depletion, maternal folic acid deficiency may occur. Epilepsy itself, number of medications, genetic factors, or a combination of these probably influence the teratogenicity of anticonvulsant therapy. Benefit:risk ratio usually favors continued use during pregnancy.

Related Information

Peak and Trough Guidelines *on page 1544*
Seizure Treatment *on page 1700*

Phenytoin Sodium *see* Phenytoin *on page 1073*
Phenytoin Sodium, Extended *see* Phenytoin *on page 1073*
Phenytoin Sodium, Prompt *see* Phenytoin *on page 1073*
Phillips'® Milk of Magnesia [OTC] *see* Magnesium Supplements *on page 831*
Phillips'® Stool Softener Laxative [OTC] *see* Docusate *on page 432*
PhosLo® *see* Calcium Supplements *on page 202*

Phosphate Supplements (FOS fate SUP la ments)

U.S. Brand Names Fleet® Enema [OTC]; Fleet® Phospho®-Soda [OTC]; K-Phos® M.F.; K-Phos® Neutral; K-Phos® No. 2; K-Phos® Original; Neutra-Phos® [OTC]; Neutra-Phos®-K [OTC]; Uro-KP-Neutral®

Synonyms Potassium Acid Phosphate; Potassium Phosphate; Potassium Phosphate and Sodium Phosphate; Sodium Phosphate

Generic Available Yes

Pharmacologic Category Cathartic; Electrolyte Supplement, Oral; Electrolyte Supplement, Parenteral; Laxative, Bowel Evacuant

Pregnancy Risk Factor C

Lactation Use caution

Use Treatment and prevention of hypophosphatemia; short-term treatment of constipation (oral/rectal); evacuation of the colon for rectal and bowel exams; source of phosphate in large volume I.V. fluids and parenteral nutrition; urinary acidifier (potassium acid phosphate) for reduction in formation of calcium stones

Mechanism of Action/Effect Phosphorus participates in bone deposition, calcium metabolism, utilization of B complex vitamins, and as a buffer in acid-base equilibrium; as a laxative, exerts osmotic effect in the small intestine by drawing water into the lumen of the gut, producing distension, promoting peristalsis, and evacuation of the bowel

Contraindications Hypersensitivity to sodium phosphate salts or any component of the formulation; hyperphosphatemia, hyperkalemia (potassium salt form), hypocalcemia, hypomagnesemia, hypernatremia (sodium salt form), severe renal impairment, severe tissue trauma, heat cramps, CHF, abdominal pain (rectal forms), fecal impaction (rectal forms); patients with infected phosphate kidney stones; congenital megacolon, toxic megacolon, bowel obstruction, bowel perforation, imperforate anus (enema); CHF; ascites

I.V.: Should not be used in diseases with high phosphate levels, low calcium levels or hypernatremia.

Oral solution: Should not be used in patients with kidney disease or on a sodium-restricted diet.

Tablet: Should not be used in patients with unstable angina pectoris, gastric retention, ileus, acute obstruction or pseudo-obstruction, severe chronic constipation, acute colitis, or hypomotility syndrome (ie, hypothyroidism, scleroderma).

Warnings/Precautions Use with caution in patients with impaired renal function (oral solution contraindicated) or pre-existing electrolyte imbalances (including patients on diuretics which may effect electrolyte levels or dehydration); and those at risk of hypocalcemia, hyperphosphatemia, hypernatremia, and acidosis.

Intravenous preparation: Must be diluted before use; infuse slowly.

Tablet preparation: Prolongation of the QT interval has been reported with use of the tablet formulation; use with caution with other medication known to cause this effect; use caution within 3 months of acute myocardial infarction or cardiac surgery. Do not use with other phosphate-containing products, fatalities have been reported. Not for use in patients <18 years of age.

If using as a bowel evacuant, correct electrolyte abnormalities before treatment; inadequate fluid intake may lead to excessive fluid loss and hypovolemia. May cause colonic mucosal aphthous ulcerations; use with caution in patients with an acute exacerbation of chronic inflammatory bowel disease (absorption may be enhanced) and in debilitated patients. Enemas and oral solution are available in pediatric and adult sizes; prescribe by "volume" not "by bottle".

Enema preparation: Use caution in patients with a colostomy; not for use in children <2 years of age. Enema tips are latex free.

Drug Interactions

Decreased Effect: Oral phosphate preparations may reduce absorption of some medications due to rapid intestinal peristalsis; do not administer with sucralfate, iron supplements, or antacids which contain aluminum, calcium, or magnesium (may result in binding of the phosphate and reduced absorption).

Increased Effect/Toxicity: Potassium-containing preparations should be used with caution in patients receiving ACE-inhibitors, salt substitutes, or potassium-sparing diuretics.

Adverse Reactions Frequency not defined.

Cardiovascular: Hypotension, edema; **potassium salt form:** arrhythmias, heart block, cardiac arrest

Central nervous system: Tetany, mental confusion, seizures, dizziness, headache, calcium phosphate precipitation

Endocrine & metabolic: Hyperphosphatemia, hyperkalemia **(potassium salt form)**, hypocalcemia, hypernatremia **(sodium salt form)**

Gastrointestinal: Nausea, vomiting, diarrhea, flatulence (oral use), abdominal bloating, abdominal pain, mucosal bleeding, superficial mucosal ulcerations

Local: Phlebitis (parenteral forms)

Neuromuscular & skeletal: Paresthesia, bone and joint pain, arthralgia, weakness, muscle cramps

Renal: Acute renal failure

Case reports: Tablet: Atrial fibrillation following severe vomiting

Pharmacodynamics/Kinetics

Absorption: Oral: 1% to 20%

Half-Life Elimination: Oral forms excreted in feces; I.V. forms are excreted in the urine with over 80% of dose reabsorbed by the kidney

Onset: Catharsis: Oral: 3-6 hours; Rectal: 2-5 minutes

Formulations

Enema: Monobasic sodium phosphate 19 g and dibasic sodium phosphate 7 g per 118 mL delivered dose (133 mL)

- Fleet® Enema: Monobasic sodium phosphate 19 g and dibasic sodium phosphate 7 g per 118 mL delivered dose (133 mL)
- Fleet® Enema for Children: Monobasic sodium phosphate 9.5 g and dibasic sodium phosphate 3.5 g per 59 mL delivered dose (66 mL)

Injection: solution, as potassium phosphate: Phosphate 3 mmol and potassium 4.4 mEq per mL (5 mL, 15 mL, 50 mL)

Injection, solution, as sodium phosphate: Phosphate 3 mmol and sodium 4 mEq per mL (5 mL, 15 mL, 50 mL)

Powder:

- Neutra-Phos®: Phosphorus 250 mg [8 mmol], potassium 278 mg [7.125 mEq], and sodium 164 mg [7.125 mEq] per packet (100s)
- Neutra-Phos®-K: Elemental phosphorus 250 mg [8 mmol] and potassium 556 mg [14.25 mEq] per packet (100s) [sodium free]

Solution, oral (Fleet® Phospho®-Soda): Phosphate 4 mmol and sodium 4.82 mEq per mL (45 mL, 90 mL) [equivalent to monobasic sodium phosphate monohydrate 2.4 g and dibasic sodium phosphate heptahydrate 0.9 g per 5 mL; ginger-lemon flavor or unflavored]

Tablet:

- K-Phos® M.F.: Phosphorus 125.6 mg [4 mmol], potassium 44.5 mg [1.1 mEq], and sodium 67 mg [2.9 mEq]
- K-Phos® Neutral: Phosphorus 250 mg [8 mmol], potassium 45 mg [1.1 mEq], and sodium 298 mg [13 mEq] per tablet
- K-Phos® No. 2: Phosphorus 250 mg [8 mmol], potassium 88 mg [2.3 mEq], and sodium 134 mg [5.8 mEq]
- K-Phos® Original: Phosphorus 114 mg [3.7 mmol] and potassium 144 mg [3.7 mEq] per tablet [sodium free]
- Uro-KP-Neutral®: Phosphorus 258 mg [8 mmol], potassium 49.4 mg [1.27 mEq], and sodium 262.4 mg [10.9 mEq]

Dosing

Adults: Phosphate supplements are either sodium or potassium salt forms. Consider the contribution of these electrolytes also when determining appropriate phosphate replacement.

I.V. doses should be incorporated into the patient's maintenance I.V. fluids; intermittent I.V. infusion should be reserved for severe depletion situations; requires continuous cardiac monitoring (for potassium salts). It is difficult to determine total body phosphorus deficit, the following dosages are empiric guidelines: **Note:** Doses listed as mmol of **phosphate**:

Hypophosphatemia: Intermittent I.V. infusion: Varying dosages: 0.15-0.3 mmol/kg/dose over 12 hours; may repeat as needed to achieve desired serum level **or**

- 15 mmol/dose over 2 hours; use if serum phosphorus <2 mg/dL **or**
- Low dose: 0.16 mmol/kg over 4-6 hours; use if serum phosphorus level 2.3-3 mg/dL
- Intermediate dose: 0.32 mmol/kg over 4-6 hours; use if serum phosphorus level 1.6-2.2 mg/dL
- High dose: 0.64 mmol/kg over 8-12 hours; use if serum phosphorus <1.5 mg/dL

Maintenance:

- I.V.: 50-70 mmol/day
- Oral: 50-150 mmol/day in divided doses

Laxative:

- Oral:
  - 1-2 capsules or packets (250-500 mg phosphorus/8-16 mmol) 4 times/day; dilute as instructed
  - Fleet® Phospho®-Soda:® 20-45 mL as a single dose
- Rectal: Enema: Contents of one 4.5 oz enema as a single dose, may repeat

Urinary acidification: Oral (K-Phos® Original): 2 tablets 4 times/day

(Continued)

Phosphate Supplements *(Continued)*

Bowel cleansing prior to colonoscopy (Visicol™): Oral: A total of 40 tablets divided as follows:

Evening before colonoscopy: 3 tablets every 15 minutes for 6 doses, then 2 additional tablets in 15 minutes (total of 20 tablets)

3-5 hours prior to colonoscopy: 3 tablets every 15 minutes for 6 doses, then 2 additional tablets in 15 minutes (total of 20 tablets)

Note: Each dose should be taken with a minimum of 8 oz. of clear liquids. Do not repeat treatment within 7 days. Do not use additional agents, especially sodium phosphate products.

Elderly: Use with caution due to increased risk of renal impairment in the elderly.

Pediatrics: Phosphate supplements are either sodium or potassium salt forms. Consider the contribution of these electrolytes also when determining appropriate phosphate replacement.

I.V. doses should be incorporated into the patient's maintenance I.V. fluids; intermittent I.V. infusion should be reserved for severe depletion situations; requires continuous cardiac monitoring (for potassium salts). It is difficult to determine total body phosphorus deficit, the following dosages are empiric guidelines: **Note:** Doses listed as mmol of **phosphate**:

Hypophosphatemia: Intermittent I.V. infusion:

Children:

Low dose: 0.08 mmol/kg over 6 hours; use if recent losses and uncomplicated

Intermediate dose: 0.16-0.24 mmol/kg over 4-6 hours; use if serum phosphorus level 0.5-1 mg/dL

High dose: 0.36 mmol/kg over 6 hours; use if serum phosphorus <0.5 mg/dL

Maintenance:

Children:

I.V.: 0.5-1.5 mmol/kg/day

Oral: 2-3 mmol/kg/day in divided doses

Laxative: Oral

Neutra-Phos®, Neutra-Phos®-K, or Uro-KP-Neutral®:

Children <4 years: 1 capsule or packet (250 mg phosphorus/8 mmol) 4 times/day; dilute as instructed

Children >4 years: 1-2 capsules or packets (250-500 mg phosphorus/8-16 mmol) 4 times/day; dilute as instructed

Fleet® Phospho®-Soda:® Oral:

Children 5-9 years: 5-10 mL as a single dose

Children 10-12 years: 10-20 mL as a single dose

Children ≥12 years: 20-45 mL as a single dose

Laxative: Rectal:

Fleet® Enema:

Children 2-4 years: One-half contents of one 2.25 oz pediatric enema

Children 5-12 years: Contents of one 2.25 oz pediatric enema, may repeat

Children ≥12 years: Contents of one 4.5 oz enema as a single dose, may repeat

Renal Impairment: Use with caution; ionized inorganic phosphate is excreted by the kidneys; oral solution is contraindicated in patients with kidney disease.

Hepatic Impairment: Not expected to be metabolized in the liver.

Administration

Oral: Administer with food to reduce the risk of diarrhea. Do not swallow the capsule. Contents of 1 capsule or packet should be diluted in 75 mL water before administration. Administer tablets with a full glass of water. Maintain adequate fluid intake. Dilute oral solution with an equal volume of cool water. K-Phos® Original tablets (urinary acidifier) should be dissolved in 6-8 ounces of water before administration.

I.V.: For intermittent infusion, if peripheral line, dilute to a maximum concentration of 0.05 mmol/mL. If central line, dilute to a maximum concentration of 0.12 mmol/mL; maximum rate of infusion: 0.06 mmol/kg/hour; do **not** infuse with calcium containing I.V. fluids.

Stability

Storage: Phosphate salts may precipitate when mixed with calcium salts. Solubility is improved in amino acid parenteral nutrition solutions.

Compatibility: Check with a pharmacist to determine compatibility.

Monitoring Laboratory Tests Serum potassium (potassium salt forms), sodium (sodium salt forms), calcium, phosphorus, magnesium, renal function, reflexes; cardiac monitor (when intermittent infusion or high-dose I.V. replacement of potassium salts needed)

Monitoring and Teaching Issues

Physical Assessment: Assess other medications patient may be taking for effectiveness and interactions (see Drug Interactions). See Contraindications and Warnings/Precautions for use cautions. Monitor laboratory tests (serum Ca, K, Na, phosphate levels), therapeutic response, and adverse reactions at beginning of therapy and periodically throughout therapy (see Adverse Reactions and Overdose/Toxicology). Assess knowledge/teach patient appropriate use according to product and purpose, interventions to reduce side effects, and adverse symptoms to report (see Patient Education). **Pregnancy risk factor C** - benefits of use should outweigh possible risk. Note breast-feeding caution.

I.V.: Monitor infusion site on a regular basis.

Supplements: Monitor cardiac status on a regular basis (continuous EKG during highly concentrated infusions). Note Dosing information. Instruct patient about adverse reactions to report.

Patient Education: Supplements: Take as directed; do not take more than directed. Swallow tablet whole with full glass of water or juice. Take with or after meals (do not take on an empty stomach). If taking potassium salt, take any antacids 2 hours before or after potassium. For capsules or packets, dissolve effervescent tablet or contents of packet or capsule in 4-6 ounces of water or juice and stir. Consult prescriber about advisability of increasing amount or about taking dietary supplements. Report tingling of hands or feet;

unresolved nausea or vomiting or diarrhea; chest pain or palpitations; persistent abdominal pain; feelings of weakness, dizziness, listlessness, confusion, acute muscle weakness, or cramping; blood in stool or tarry stools; or easy bruising or unusual bleeding.

Enema: Use as directed - no more than once in 24 hours and no longer than 1 week unless advised by healthcare provider. Prolonged use of any laxative may cause dependence. Do not use if you are nauseated, vomiting, or have abdominal pain unless direct by healthcare provider. Do not use with any other laxative products. Consult healthcare provider prior to using, if you are pregnant or breast-feeding. Not for oral use. Insert bottle gently into rectum with tip of bottle pointed towards naval. Do not force insertion. Squeeze bottle gently and steadily to expel liquid; stop if resistance is felt. Contact healthcare provider immediately if no liquid/stool is returned, or if rectal bleeding occurs.

Pregnancy/breast-feeding precautions: Consult prescriber if pregnant, anticipating being pregnant, or breast-feeding.

Dietary Issues: Avoid giving with oxalate (ie, berries, nuts, chocolate, beans, celery, tomato) or phytate-containing (ie, bran, whole wheat) foods.

Phospholine Iodide® *see* Ophthalmic Agents, Glaucoma *on page 1002*

Phosphonoformate *see* Foscarnet *on page 603*

Phosphonoformic Acid *see* Foscarnet *on page 603*

Photofrin® *see* Porfimer *on page 1101*

p-Hydroxyampicillin *see* Amoxicillin *on page 88*

Phylloquinone *see* Phytonadione *on page 1080*

Physostigmine *see* Ophthalmic Agents, Glaucoma *on page 1002*

Physostigmine (fye zoe STIG meen)

U.S. Brand Names Antilirium®

Synonyms Eserine Salicylate; Physostigmine Salicylate; Physostigmine Sulfate

Generic Available Yes: Ophthalmic

Pharmacologic Category Acetylcholinesterase Inhibitor; Ophthalmic Agent, Antiglaucoma

Pregnancy Risk Factor C

Lactation Excretion in breast milk unknown

Use Reverse toxic CNS effects caused by anticholinergic drugs; used as miotic in treatment of glaucoma

Mechanism of Action/Effect Inhibits destruction of acetylcholine by acetylcholinesterase which facilitates transmission of impulses across myoneural junction and prolongs the central and peripheral effects of acetylcholine

Contraindications Hypersensitivity to physostigmine or any component of the formulation; GI or GU obstruction; physostigmine therapy of drug intoxications should be used with extreme caution in patients with asthma, gangrene, severe cardiovascular disease, or mechanical obstruction of the GI tract or urogenital tract. In these patients, physostigmine should be used only to treat life-threatening conditions.

Warnings/Precautions Use with caution in patients with epilepsy, asthma, diabetes, gangrene, cardiovascular disease, bradycardia. Discontinue if excessive salivation or emesis, frequent urination or diarrhea occur. Reduce dosage if excessive sweating or nausea occurs. Administer I.V. slowly or at a controlled rate not faster than 1 mg/minute. Due to the possibility of hypersensitivity or overdose/cholinergic crisis, atropine should be readily available; ointment may delay corneal healing, may cause loss of dark adaptation; not intended as a first-line agent for anticholinergic toxicity or Parkinson's disease. Pregnancy risk C.

Drug Interactions

Increased Effect/Toxicity: Increased toxicity with bethanechol, methacholine. Succinylcholine may increase neuromuscular blockade with systemic administration.

Effects on Lab Values ↑ aminotransferase [ALT (SGPT)/AST (SGOT)] (S), amylase (S)

Adverse Reactions Frequency not defined.

Ophthalmic:

Central nervous system: Headache, browache
Dermatologic: Burning, redness
Ocular: Lacrimation, marked miosis, blurred vision, eye pain
Miscellaneous: Diaphoresis

Systemic:

Cardiovascular: Palpitations, bradycardia
Central nervous system: Restlessness, nervousness, hallucinations, seizures
Gastrointestinal: Nausea, salivation, diarrhea, stomach pains
Genitourinary: Frequent urge to urinate
Neuromuscular & skeletal: Muscle twitching
Ocular: Lacrimation, miosis
Respiratory: Dyspnea, bronchospasm, respiratory paralysis, pulmonary edema
Miscellaneous: Diaphoresis

Overdosage/Toxicology Symptoms of overdose include muscle weakness, blurred vision, excessive sweating, tearing and salivation, nausea, vomiting, bronchospasm, and seizures. If physostigmine is used in excess or in the absence of an anticholinergic overdose, patients may manifest signs of cholinergic toxicity. At this point a cholinergic agent (eg, atropine 0.015-0.05 mg/kg) may be necessary.

Pharmacodynamics/Kinetics

Absorption: I.M., ophthalmic, S.C.: Readily absorbed

Half-Life Elimination: 15-40 minutes

Metabolism: Hepatic and via hydrolysis by cholinesterases

Onset: Ophthalmic: ~2 minutes; Parenteral: ~5 minutes

Duration: Ophthalmic: 12-48 hours; Parenteral: 0.5-5 hours

Formulations

Injection, as salicylate: 1 mg/mL (2 mL)
Ointment, ophthalmic, as sulfate: 0.25% (3.5 g, 3.75 g)

(Continued)

Physostigmine *(Continued)*

Dosing

Adults & Elderly:

Anticholinergic drug overdose:

I.M., I.V., S.C.: 0.5-2 mg to start; repeat every 20 minutes until response occurs or adverse effect occurs.

Repeat 1-4 mg every 30-60 minutes as life-threatening signs (arrhythmias, seizures, deep coma) recur; maximum I.V. rate: 1 mg/minute.

Glaucoma: Ophthalmic: Ointment: Instill a small quantity to lower fornix up to 3 times/day.

Pediatrics: Children: Anticholinergic drug overdose: Reserve for life-threatening situations only: I.V.: 0.01-0.03 mg/kg/dose (maximum: 0.5 mg/minute). May repeat after 5-10 minutes to a maximum total dose of 2 mg or until response occurs or adverse cholinergic effects occur,

Administration

I.V.: Infuse slowly I.V. at a maximum rate of 0.5 mg/minute in children or 1 mg/minute in adults

Topical: Ophthalmic: Apply thin ribbon of ointment inside lower eyelid. Close eye and roll eyeball in all directions. Do not blink for $^1/_2$ minute. Do not use any other eye preparation for at least 10 minutes.

Other: Ophthalmic: Apply thin ribbon of ointment inside lower eyelid. Close eye and roll eyeball in all directions. Do not blink for $^1/_2$ minute. Do not use any other eye preparation for at least 10 minutes.

Stability

Storage: Do not use solution if cloudy or dark brown.

Compatibility: Stable in dextran 6% in dextrose, dextran 6% in NS, D_5W, $D_{10}W$, D_5LR, $D_5{}^1/_4NS$, $D_5{}^1/_2NS$, D_5NS, fat emulsion 10%, LR, $^1/_2NS$, NS

Y-site administration: Incompatible with dobutamine

Compatibility when admixed: Incompatible Phenytoin, ranitidine

Monitoring and Teaching Issues

Physical Assessment: When used to reverse neuromuscular block, patient must be monitored closely until full return of neuromuscular functioning. Assess bladder and sphincter adequacy prior to administering medication. Assess other medications patient may be taking for effectiveness and interactions (see Drug Interactions). See Contraindications and Warnings/Precautions for use cautions. Monitor therapeutic effects and adverse reactions (cholinergic crisis - see Warnings/Precautions, Adverse Reactions, and Overdose/Toxicology). Assess knowledge/teach patient appropriate use of ophthalmic forms, interventions to reduce side effects, and adverse symptoms to report (see Patient Education). **Pregnancy risk factor C** - benefits of use should outweigh possible risks. Note breast-feeding caution.

Patient Education: Systemic: Maintain adequate hydration (2-3 L/day of fluids) unless advised by prescriber to restrict fluids. May cause dizziness, drowsiness, or hypotension (rise slowly from sitting or lying position and use caution when driving or climbing stairs); vomiting or loss of appetite (small, frequent meals, frequent mouth care, chewing gum, or sucking lozenges may help); or diarrhea (boiled milk, yogurt, or buttermilk may help). Report persistent abdominal discomfort; significantly increased salivation, sweating, tearing, or urination; flushed skin; chest pain or palpitations; acute headache; unresolved diarrhea; excessive fatigue, insomnia, dizziness, or depression; increased muscle, joint, or body pain; vision changes or blurred vision; or shortness of breath or wheezing. **Pregnancy/breast-feeding precautions:** Inform prescriber if you are or intend to become pregnant. Consult prescriber if breast-feeding.

Ophthalmic: For ophthalmic use only. Wash hands before using. Do not let tip of applicator touch eye; do not contaminate tip of applicator (may cause eye infection, eye damage, or vision loss). Tilt head back and look upward. Apply thin ribbon of ointment inside lower eyelid. Close eye and roll eyeball in all directions. Do not blink for $^1/_2$ minute. Do not use any other eye preparation for at least 10 minutes. Do not share medication with anyone else. Wear sunglasses when in sunlight; you may be more sensitive to bright light. Inform prescriber if condition worsens or fails to improve or if you experience eye pain, vision changes, or other adverse eye response; excess sweating; urinary frequency; severe headache; or skin rash, redness, or burning.

Geriatric Considerations: Studies on the use of physostigmine in Alzheimer's disease have reported variable results. Doses generally were in the range of 2-4 mg 4 times/day. Limitations to the use of physostigmine include a short half-life requiring frequent dosing, variable absorption from the GI tract, and no commercially available oral product; therefore, not recommended for treatment of Alzheimer's disease.

Related Information

Glaucoma Drug Comparison *on page 1575*

Physostigmine Salicylate *see* Physostigmine *on page 1079*

Physostigmine Sulfate *see* Physostigmine *on page 1079*

Phytomenadione *see* Phytonadione *on page 1080*

Phytonadione (fye toe na DYE one)

U.S. Brand Names AquaMEPHYTON®; Mephyton®

Synonyms Methylphytyl Napthoquinone; Phylloquinone; Phytomenadione; Vitamin K_1

Generic Available Yes: Injection

Pharmacologic Category Vitamin, Fat Soluble

Pregnancy Risk Factor C

Lactation Enters breast milk/compatible

Use Prevention and treatment of hypoprothrombinemia caused by drug-induced or anticoagulant-induced vitamin K deficiency, hemorrhagic disease of the newborn; phytonadione is more effective and is preferred to other vitamin K preparations in the presence of impending hemorrhage; oral absorption depends on the presence of bile salts

Mechanism of Action/Effect Promotes liver synthesis of clotting factors (II, VII, IX, X); however, the exact mechanism as to this stimulation is unknown. Menadiol is a water soluble form of vitamin K; phytonadione has a more rapid and prolonged effect than menadione; menadiol sodium diphosphate (K_4) is half as potent as menadione (K_3).

Contraindications Hypersensitivity to phytonadione or any component of the formulation

Warnings/Precautions Severe reactions resembling anaphylaxis or hypersensitivity have occurred rarely during or immediately after I.V. administration (even with proper dilution and rate of administration), as well as I.M. administration. Restrict I.V. administration for emergency use only. Allergic reactions have also occurred with I.M. and S.C. injection. Ineffective in hereditary hypoprothrombinemia, hypoprothrombinemia caused by severe liver disease. Severe hemolytic anemia has been reported rarely in neonates following large doses (10-20 mg) of phytonadione. Pregnancy risk C.

Drug Interactions

Decreased Effect: The anticoagulant effects of warfarin, dicumarol, anisindione are reversed by phytonadione.

Adverse Reactions <1% (Limited to important or life-threatening): Anaphylaxis, cyanosis, diaphoresis, dizziness (rarely), dyspnea, hemolysis in neonates and in patients with G6PD deficiency, hypersensitivity reactions, hypotension (rare)

Pharmacodynamics/Kinetics

Absorption: Oral: From intestines in presence of bile

Metabolism: Rapidly hepatic

Onset: Increased coagulation factors: Oral: 6-12 hours; Parenteral: 1-2 hours; prothrombin may become normal after 12-14 hours

Formulations

Injection, aqueous, colloidal: 2 mg/mL (0.5 mL)

Injection, aqueous: 10 mg/mL (1 mL)

Tablet: 5 mg

Dosing

Adults & Elderly: S.C. is the preferred (per manufacturer) parenteral route; I.V. route should be restricted for emergency use only

Minimum daily requirement (not well established): 0.03 mcg/kg/day

Oral anticoagulant overdose: Oral, I.V., S.C.: 1-10 mg/dose depending on degree of INR elevation

Serious bleeding or major overdose: I.V. (slow infusion): 10 mg; may repeat every 12 hours (have required doses up to 25 mg)

Vitamin K deficiency (due to drugs, malabsorption or decreased synthesis of vitamin K):

Oral: 5-25 mg/24 hours

I.M., I.V., S.C.: 10 mg

Pediatrics: S.C. is the preferred (per manufacturer) parenteral route; I.V. route should be restricted for emergency use only.

Minimum daily requirement: Not well established

Infants: 1-5 mcg/kg/day

Hemorrhagic disease of the newborn:

Prophylaxis: I.M.: 0.5-1 mg within 1 hour of birth

Treatment: I.M., S.C.: 1-2 mg/dose/day

Oral anticoagulant overdose: Infants and Children:

No bleeding, rapid reversal needed, patient **will require** further oral anticoagulant therapy: S.C., I.V.: 0.5-2 mg

No bleeding, rapid reversal needed, patient **will not require** further oral anticoagulant therapy: S.C., I.V.: 2-5 mg

Significant bleeding, not life-threatening: S.C., I.V.: 0.5-2 mg

Significant bleeding, life-threatening: I.V.: 5 mg over 10-20 minutes

Vitamin K deficiency (due to drugs, malabsorption or decreased synthesis of vitamin K):

Infants and Children:

Oral: 2.5-5 mg/24 hours

I.M., I.V., S.C.: 1-2 mg/dose as a single dose

Administration

I.V.: Dilute in normal saline, D_5W or D_5NS and infuse slowly; rate of infusion should not exceed 1 mg/minute. **This route should be used only if administration by another route is not feasible.** I.V. administration should not exceed 1 mg/minute; for I.V. infusion, dilute in PF (preservative free) D_5W or normal saline.

Stability

Storage: Protect injection from light at all times; may be autoclaved.

Monitoring Laboratory Tests PT

Monitoring and Teaching Issues

Physical Assessment: See Contraindications, Warnings/Precautions (eg, infusion cautions), Drug Interactions and Adverse Reactions for use cautions. Note dosing specifics according to purpose for use. Assess results of laboratory tests (see above) and patient response (degree of bleeding). Teach patient proper use, possible side effects and interventions, and adverse symptoms to report (see Patient Education). **Pregnancy risk factor C** - benefits of use should outweigh possible risks.

Patient Education: Inform prescriber of all prescriptions, OTC medications, or herbal products you are taking, and any allergies you have. Do not take anything new during treatment (especially any aspirin-containing products or NSAIDs) without consulting prescriber. Oral: Take only as directed; do not take more or more often than prescribed. Consult prescriber for recommended diet. Report bleeding gums; blood in urine, stool, or vomitus; unusual bruising of bleeding; or abdominal cramping. **Pregnancy precaution:** Inform prescriber if you are or intend to become pregnant.

Additional Information Injection contains benzyl alcohol 0.9% as preservative

Pilocar® *see* Ophthalmic Agents, Glaucoma *on page 1002*

Pilocar® *see* Pilocarpine *on page 1082*

Pilocarpine *see* Ophthalmic Agents, Glaucoma *on page 1002*

Pilocarpine (pye loe KAR peen)

U.S. Brand Names Isopto® Carpine; Ocusert Pilo-20® [DSC]; Ocusert Pilo-40® [DSC]; Pilocar®; Pilopine HS®; Piloptic®; Salagen®

Synonyms Pilocarpine Hydrochloride

Generic Available Yes: Solution

Pharmacologic Category Cholinergic Agonist; Ophthalmic Agent, Antiglaucoma; Ophthalmic Agent, Miotic

Pregnancy Risk Factor C

Lactation Excretion in breast milk unknown/not recommended

Use

Ophthalmic: Management of chronic simple glaucoma, chronic and acute angle-closure glaucoma

Oral: Symptomatic treatment of xerostomia caused by salivary gland hypofunction resulting from radiotherapy for cancer of the head and neck or Sjögren's syndrome

Use - Unlabeled/Investigational Counter effects of cycloplegics

Mechanism of Action/Effect Directly stimulates cholinergic receptors in the eye causing miosis (by contraction of the iris sphincter), loss of accommodation (by constriction of ciliary muscle), and lowering of intraocular pressure (with decreased resistance to aqueous humor outflow)

Contraindications Hypersensitivity to pilocarpine or any component of the formulation; acute inflammatory disease of the anterior chamber of the eye; in addition, tablets are also contraindicated in patients with uncontrolled asthma, angle-closure glaucoma, severe hepatic impairment

Warnings/Precautions Use caution with cardiovascular disease; patients may have difficulty compensating for transient changes in hemodynamics or rhythm induced by pilocarpine.

Ophthalmic products: May cause decreased visual acuity, especially at night or with reduced lighting.

Oral tablets: Use caution with controlled asthma, chronic bronchitis or COPD; may increase airway resistance, bronchial smooth muscle tone, and bronchial secretions. Use caution with cholelithiasis, biliary tract disease, nephrolithiasis; adjust dose with moderate hepatic impairment.

Pregnancy risk C.

Drug Interactions

Cytochrome P450 Effect: Inhibits CYP2A6, 2E1, 3A4

Decreased Effect: May decrease effects of anticholinergic drugs (atropine, ipratropium).

Increased Effect/Toxicity: Concurrent use with beta-blockers may cause conduction disturbances.

Nutritional/Ethanol Interactions Food: Avoid administering oral formulation with high-fat meal; fat decreases the rate of absorption, maximum concentration and increases the time it takes to reach maximum concentration.

Adverse Reactions

Ophthalmic: Frequency not defined:

- Cardiovascular: Hypertension, tachycardia
- Dermatologic: Diaphoresis
- Gastrointestinal: Diarrhea, nausea, salivation, vomiting
- Ocular: Burning, ciliary spasm, conjunctival vascular congestion, corneal granularity (gel 10%), lacrimation, lens opacity, myopia, retinal detachment, supraorbital or temporal headache, visual acuity decreased
- Respiratory: Bronchial spasm, pulmonary edema

Oral (frequency varies by indication and dose):

>10%:

- Cardiovascular: Flushing (8% to 13%)
- Central nervous system: Chills (3% to 15%), dizziness (5% to 12%), headache (11%)
- Dermatologic: Diaphoresis (29% to 68%)
- Gastrointestinal: Nausea (6% to 15%)
- Genitourinary: Urinary frequency (9% to 12%)
- Neuromuscular & skeletal: Weakness (2% to 12%)
- Respiratory: Rhinitis (5% to 14%)

1% to 10%:

- Cardiovascular: Edema (<1% to 5%), facial edema, hypertension (3%), palpitation, tachycardia
- Central nervous system: Pain (4%), fever, somnolence
- Dermatologic: Pruritus, rash
- Gastrointestinal: Diarrhea (4% to 7%), dyspepsia (7%), vomiting (3% to 4%), constipation, flatulence, glossitis, salivation increased, stomatitis, taste perversion
- Genitourinary: Vaginitis, urinary incontinence
- Neuromuscular & skeletal: Myalgias, tremor
- Ocular: Lacrimation (6%), amblyopia (4%), abnormal vision, blurred vision, conjunctivitis,
- Otic: Tinnitus
- Respiratory: Cough increased, dysphagia, epistaxis, sinusitis
- Miscellaneous: Allergic reaction, voice alteration

<1% (Limited to important or life-threatening): Abnormal dreams, alopecia, angina pectoris, anorexia, anxiety, arrhythmia, body odor, bone disorder, cholelithiasis, colitis, confusion, dry eyes, dry mouth, EKG abnormality, myasthenia, photosensitivity reaction, nervousness, pancreatitis, paresthesias, salivary gland enlargement, sputum increased, taste loss, tongue disorder, urinary impairment, urinary urgency, yawning

Overdosage/Toxicology Symptoms of overdose include bronchospasm, bradycardia, involuntary urination, vomiting, hypotension, and tremor. Atropine is the treatment of choice for intoxications manifesting with significant muscarinic symptoms. Atropine I.V. 2-4 mg every 3-60 minutes should be repeated to control symptoms and then continued as needed for 1-2 days following acute ingestion. Epinephrine 0.1-1 mg S.C. may be useful for reversing severe cardiovascular or pulmonary sequelae.

Pharmacodynamics/Kinetics

Half-Life Elimination: Oral: 0.76-1.35 hours; increased with hepatic impairment

Onset:

Ophthalmic: Miosis: 10-30 minutes; Intraocular pressure reduction: 1 hour
Oral: 20 minutes

Duration:

Ophthalmic: Miosis: 4-8 hours; Intraocular pressure reduction: 4-12 hours
Oral: 3-5 hours

Formulations

Gel, ophthalmic, as hydrochloride (Pilopine HS®): 4% (3.5 g) [contains benzalkonium chloride]

Ocular therapeutic system:

Ocusert Pilo-20® [DSC]: Releases 20 mcg/hour for 1 week (8s)
Ocusert Pilo-40® [DSC]: Releases 40 mcg/hour for 1 week (8s)

Solution, ophthalmic, as hydrochloride: 1% (15 mL), 2% (15 mL), 4% (15 mL), 6% (15 mL) [may contain benzalkonium chloride]

Isopto® Carpine: 1% (15 mL); 2% (15 mL, 30 mL); 4% (15 mL, 30 mL); 6% (15 mL); 8% (15 mL) [contains benzalkonium chloride]

Pilocar®: 0.5% (15 mL); 1% (1 mL, 15 mL); 2% (1 mL, 15 mL); 3% (15 mL); 4% (1 mL, 15 mL); 6% (15 mL) [contains benzalkonium chloride]

Piloptic®: 0.5% (15 mL); 1% (15 mL); 2% (15 mL); 3% (15 mL); 4% (15 mL); 6% (15 mL) [contains benzalkonium chloride]

Tablet, as hydrochloride (Salagen®): 5 mg

Dosing

Adults & Elderly:

Glaucoma: Ophthalmic

Solution: Instill 1-2 drops up to 6 times/day; adjust the concentration and frequency as required to control elevated intraocular pressure.

Gel: Instill 0.5" ribbon into lower conjunctival sac once daily at bedtime.

Ocular systems: Systems are labeled in terms of mean rate of release of pilocarpine over 7 days; begin with 20 mcg/hour at night and adjust based on response.

To counteract the mydriatic effects of sympathomimetic agents (unlabeled use): Ophthalmic solution: Instill 1 drop of a 1% solution in the affected eye.

Xerostomia: Oral:

Following head and neck cancer: 5 mg 3 times/day, titration up to 10 mg 3 times/day may be considered for patients who have not responded adequately; do not exceed 2 tablets/dose

Sjögren's syndrome: 5 mg 4 times/day

Hepatic Impairment: Oral: Patients with moderate impairment: 5 mg 2 times/day regardless of indication; adjust dose based on response and tolerability. Do not use with severe impairment (Child-Pugh score 10-15)

Administration

Oral: Avoid administering with high fat meal. Fat decreases the rate of absorption, maximum concentration, and increases the time it takes to reach maximum concentration.

Other: Ophthalmic: If both solution and gel are used, the solution should be applied first, then the gel at least 5 minutes later. Following administration of the solution, finger pressure should be applied on the lacrimal sac for 1-2 minutes.

Stability

Storage:

Gel: Store at room temperature of 2°C to 27°C (36°F to 80°F). Do not freeze; avoid excessive heat.

Tablets: Store at controlled room temperature of 15°C to 30°C (59°F to to 86°F).

Monitoring Laboratory Tests Intraocular pressure, fundoscopic exam, visual field testing

Monitoring and Teaching Issues

Physical Assessment: Monitor for adverse effects and response to treatment. Monitor results of intraocular pressure testing and visual field testing on a periodic basis. Teach patient appropriate administration of ophthalmic solution. **Pregnancy risk factor C.** Breast-feeding is not recommended.

Patient Education: Use as often as recommended. Avoid taking oral medication with a high fat meal.

Ophthalmic: Wash hands before using. Do not let tip of applicator touch eye; do not contaminate tip of applicator (may cause eye infection, eye damage, or vision loss). Sit or lie down. Open eye, look at ceiling, and instill prescribed amount of solution. Do not blink for 30 seconds, close eye and roll eye in all directions, and apply gentle pressure to inner corner of eye for 1-2 minutes. Temporary stinging or blurred vision may occur. You may experience altered dark adaptation; use caution when driving at night or in poorly lit environments. Report persistent pain, redness, burning, double vision, or severe headache. **Breast-feeding precaution:** Breast-feeding is not recommended.

Geriatric Considerations: Assure the patient or a caregiver can adequately administer ophthalmic medication dosage form.

Related Information

Glaucoma Drug Comparison *on page 1575*

Pilocarpine and Epinephrine (pye loe KAR peen & ep i NEF rin)

U.S. Brand Names E-Pilo-x®; P_xE_x®

Synonyms Epinephrine and Pilocarpine

Generic Available No

Pharmacologic Category Ophthalmic Agent, Antiglaucoma; Ophthalmic Agent, Miotic

Pregnancy Risk Factor C

Lactation Excretion in breast milk unknown

Use Treatment of glaucoma; counter effect of cycloplegics

(Continued)

Pilocarpine and Epinephrine *(Continued)*

Formulations Solution, ophthalmic: Epinephrine bitartrate 1% and pilocarpine hydrochloride 1%, 2%, 3%, 4%, 6% (10 mL, 15 mL)

Dosing

Adults & Elderly:

Glaucoma: Ophthalmic: Instill 1-2 drops up to 6 times/day.

Counteract mydriatics: Ophthalmic: Instill 1-2 drops.

Monitoring and Teaching Issues

Physical Assessment: See individual components listed in Related Information. **Pregnancy risk factor C** - benefits of use should outweigh possible risks. Note breast-feeding caution.

Patient Education: See individual components listed in Related Information. **Pregnancy/ breast-feeding precautions:** Inform prescriber if you are or intend to become pregnant. Consult prescriber if breast-feeding.

Related Information

Epinephrine *on page 470*
Pilocarpine *on page 1082*

Pilocarpine Hydrochloride *see* Pilocarpine *on page 1082*

Pilopine HS® *see* Ophthalmic Agents, Glaucoma *on page 1002*

Pilopine HS® *see* Pilocarpine *on page 1082*

Piloptic® *see* Ophthalmic Agents, Glaucoma *on page 1002*

Piloptic® *see* Pilocarpine *on page 1082*

Pima® *see* Potassium Iodide *on page 1105*

Pimecrolimus (pim e KROE li mus)

U.S. Brand Names Elidel®

Generic Available No

Pharmacologic Category Immunosuppressant Agent; Topical Skin Product

Pregnancy Risk Factor C

Lactation Excretion in breast milk unknown/not recommended

Use Short-term and intermittent long-term treatment of mild to moderate atopic dermatitis in patients not responsive to conventional therapy or when conventional therapy is not appropriate

Mechanism of Action/Effect Inhibits T cell activation by blocking proinflammatory cytokine secretion.

Contraindications Hypersensitivity to pimecrolimus or any component of the formulation; Netherton's syndrome

Warnings/Precautions Do not apply to areas of active cutaneous viral infections. May increased risk of varicella zoster, herpes simplex viral infections, or eczema herpeticum. Consider discontinuation if lymphadenopathy or worsening of skin papillomas occur. Minimize or avoid natural/artificial sunlight exposure. No data to support use in immunocompromised patients. Not recommended in children <2 years of age. Pregnancy risk C.

Drug Interactions

Cytochrome P450 Effect: Substrate of CYP3A4

Increased Effect/Toxicity: CYP3A inhibitors may increase pimecrolimus levels in patients where increased absorption expected.

Adverse Reactions

>10% :

Central nervous system: Headache (7% to 25%), pyrexia (1% to 13%)

Local: Burning at application site (2% to 26%)

Respiratory: Nasopharyngitis (8% to 27%), cough (2% to 16%), upper respiratory tract infection (4% to 19%), bronchitis (0.4% to 11%)

Miscellaneous: Influenza (3% to 13%)

1% to 10%:

Dermatologic: Skin papilloma (warts) (up to 3%), molluscum contagiosum (0.7% to 2%), herpes simplex dermatitis (up to 2%)

Gastrointestinal: Diarrhea (0.6% to 8%), constipation (up to 4%)

Local: Irritation at application site (0.4% to 6%), erythema at application site (0.4% to 2%), pruritus at application site (0.6% to 6%)

Ocular: Eye infection (up to 1%)

Otic: Ear infection (0.6% to 6%), nasal congestion (0.6% to 3%)

Respiratory: Pharyngitis (0.7% to 8%), sinusitis (0.6% to 3%)

Miscellaneous: Viral infection (up to 7%), herpes simplex infections (0.4% to 4%), tonsillitis (0.4% to 6%)

Overdosage/Toxicology No experience with overdose reported.

Pharmacodynamics/Kinetics

Absorption: Poor when applied to 13% to 62% body surface area for up to a year

Formulations Cream, topical: 1% (15 g, 30 g, 100 g)

Dosing

Adults & Elderly: Mild to moderate atopic dermatitis: Topical: Apply thin layer to affected area twice daily; rub in gently and completely. **Note:** Continue as long as signs and symptoms persist; discontinue if resolution occurs; re-evaluate if symptoms persist >6 weeks.

Pediatrics: Children ≥2 years: Topical: Refer to adult dosing.

Administration

Topical: Do not use with occlusive dressings. Continue as long as signs and symptoms persist; discontinue if resolution occurs; re-evaluate if symptoms persist >6 weeks.

Stability

Storage: Store at 15°C to 30°C (59°F to 86°F). Do not freeze.

Monitoring and Teaching Issues

Physical Assessment: See Use, Contraindications, Warnings/Precautions, and Drug Interactions for use cautions. See Administration directions. Assess knowledge/teach patient appropriate use, interventions to reduce side effects, and adverse symptoms to report (see Patient Education). **Pregnancy risk factor C** - benefits of use should outweigh possible risks. Breast-feeding is not recommended.

Patient Education: This medication is for external use only. Do not use for any skin disorder except that for which it was prescribed. Avoid getting any medication in or close to eyes. Apply as often as directed by prescriber, in thin film to affected area. Do not cover with bandages or occlusive dressings. Wash and dry hands thoroughly before applying. Wash hands thoroughly after applying (if affected area is not on hands). Protect affected skin area from direct sunlight or UV light. Discontinue therapy after signs and symptoms have disappeared; restart treatment at first sign of recurrence. You may experience burning at sight of application, this will usually last less than 5 days, and go away as skin condition improves. You may experience headache, fever, cough, nasal or throat irritation, flu-like symptoms, diarrhea, or constipation; contact prescriber if these persist. Contact prescriber if skin condition worsens or if symptoms persist longer than 6 weeks. **Pregnancy/breast-feeding precautions:** Inform prescriber if you are or intend to become pregnant. Breast-feeding is not recommended.

Pimozide (PI moe zide)

U.S. Brand Names Orap™

Generic Available No

Pharmacologic Category Antipsychotic Agent, Diphenylbutylperidine

Pregnancy Risk Factor C

Lactation Excretion in breast milk unknown

Use Suppression of severe motor and phonic tics in patients with Tourette's disorder who have failed to respond satisfactorily to standard treatment

Use - Unlabeled/Investigational Psychosis; reported use in individuals with delusions focused on physical symptoms (ie, preoccupation with parasitic infestation); Huntington's chorea

Mechanism of Action/Effect A potent centrally-acting dopamine-receptor antagonist resulting in its characteristic neuroleptic effects

Contraindications Hypersensitivity to pimozide or any component of the formulation; severe CNS depression; coma; history of dysrhythmia; prolonged QT syndrome; concurrent use of drugs that are inhibitors of CYP3A4, including concurrent use of azole antifungals, macrolide antibiotics (such as clarithromycin or erythromycin), mesoridazine, nefazodone, protease inhibitors (ie, indinavir, nelfinavir, ritonavir, saquinavir), thioridazine, zileuton, and ziprasidone; simple tics other than Tourette's

Warnings/Precautions May cause hypotension, use with caution in patients with autonomic instability. Moderately sedating, use with caution in disorders where CNS depression is a feature. Use with caution in Parkinson's disease. Caution in patients with hemodynamic instability; bone marrow suppression; predisposition to seizures; subcortical brain damage; severe cardiac, hepatic, renal, or respiratory disease. Esophageal dysmotility and aspiration have been associated with antipsychotic use - use with caution in patients at risk of pneumonia (ie, Alzheimer's disease). Caution in breast cancer or other prolactin-dependent tumors (may elevate prolactin levels). May alter temperature regulation or mask toxicity of other drugs due to antiemetic effects. May alter cardiac conduction - life-threatening arrhythmias have occurred with high doses (>10 mg). May prolong QT interval predisposing patients to ventricular arrhythmias. May cause orthostatic hypotension - use with caution in patients at risk of this effect or those who would tolerate transient hypotensive episodes (cerebrovascular disease, cardiovascular disease, or other medications which may predispose).

May cause anticholinergic effects (confusion, agitation, constipation, xerostomia, blurred vision, urinary retention); therefore, they should be used with caution in patients with decreased gastrointestinal motility, urinary retention, BPH, xerostomia, or visual problems. Conditions which also may be exacerbated by cholinergic blockade include narrow-angle glaucoma (screening is recommended) and worsening of myasthenia gravis. Relative to neuroleptics, pimozide has a moderate potency of cholinergic blockade.

May cause extrapyramidal symptoms, including pseudoparkinsonism, acute dystonic reactions, akathisia, and tardive dyskinesia (risk of these reactions is high relative to other neuroleptics). May be associated with neuroleptic malignant syndrome (NMS) or pigmentary retinopathy.

Avoid grapefruit juice due to potential inhibition of pimozide metabolism.

Pregnancy risk C.

Drug Interactions

Cytochrome P450 Effect: Substrate of **CYP1A2, 3A4**; Inhibits **CYP2D6**, 3A4

Decreased Effect: Barbiturates and carbamazepine may increase the metabolism of pimozide, lowering its serum levels. Benztropine (and other anticholinergics) may inhibit the therapeutic response to pimozide. Antipsychotics such as pimozide inhibit the ability of bromocriptine to lower serum prolactin concentrations. The antihypertensive effects of guanethidine and guanadrel may be inhibited by pimozide. Pimozide may inhibit the antiparkinsonian effect of levodopa. Pimozide (and possibly other low potency antipsychotics) may reverse the pressor effects of epinephrine.

Increased Effect/Toxicity: Pimozide levels/toxicity may be increased by macrolide antibiotics (clarithromycin, erythromycin, dirithromycin, troleandomycin), azole antifungals (fluconazole, itraconazole), protease inhibitors (amprenavir, nelfinavir, ritonavir), nefazodone, ziprasidone, mesoridazine, thioridazine, and zileuton; may predispose to life-threatening arrhythmias. Chloroquine, propranolol, and sulfadoxine-pyrimethamine also may increase pimozide concentrations. Concurrent use with TCA may produce increased toxicity or altered therapeutic response. Pimozide plus lithium may (rarely)

(Continued)

Pimozide *(Continued)*

produce neurotoxicity. Pimozide and CNS depressants (ethanol, narcotics) may produce additive CNS depressant effects. Pimozide with fluoxetine has been associated with the development of bradycardia (case report). Metoclopramide may increase risk of extrapyramidal symptoms (EPS).

Nutritional/Ethanol Interactions

Food: Pimozide serum concentration may be increased when taken with grapefruit juice; avoid concurrent use.

Ethanol: Avoid ethanol (may increase CNS depression).

Herb/Nutraceutical: St John's wort may decrease pimozide levels. Avoid kava kava, gotu kola, valerian, St John's wort (may increase CNS depression).

Effects on Lab Values ↑ prolactin (S)

Adverse Reactions Frequency not defined.

Cardiovascular: Facial edema, tachycardia, orthostatic hypotension, chest pain, hypertension, palpitations, ventricular arrhythmias, QT prolongation

Central nervous system: Extrapyramidal symptoms (akathisia, akinesia, dystonia, pseudoparkinsonism, tardive dyskinesia), drowsiness, NMS, headache, dizziness, excitement

Dermatologic: Rash

Endocrine & metabolic: Edema of breasts, decreased libido

Gastrointestinal: Constipation, xerostomia, weight gain/loss, nausea, salivation, vomiting, anorexia

Genitourinary: Impotence

Hematologic: Blood dyscrasias

Hepatic: Jaundice

Neuromuscular & skeletal: Weakness, tremor

Ocular: Visual disturbance, decreased accommodation, blurred vision

Miscellaneous: Diaphoresis

Overdosage/Toxicology Symptoms of overdose include hypotension, respiratory depression, EKG abnormalities, extrapyramidal symptoms. Treatment is supportive and symptomatic.

Pharmacodynamics/Kinetics

Absorption: 50%

Half-Life Elimination: 50 hours

Time to Peak: Serum: 6-8 hours

Metabolism: Hepatic; significant first-pass effect

Formulations Tablet: 1 mg, 2 mg

Dosing

Adults: Tourette's disorder: Oral: Initial: 1-2 mg/day, then increase dosage as needed every other day; range is usually 7-16 mg/day; maximum: 20 mg/day or 0.3 mg/kg/day should not be exceeded. **Note:** Sudden unexpected deaths have occurred in patients taking doses >10 mg.

Elderly: Recommend initial dose of 1 mg/day; periodically attempt gradual reduction of dose to determine if tic persists; follow up for 1-2 weeks before concluding the tic is a persistent disease phenomenon and not a manifestation of drug withdrawal. **Note:** Recommend obtaining a baseline EKG and done periodically, especially with dose increases or addition of drugs which may interact.

Pediatrics:

Children ≤12 years: Tourette's disorder: Oral: Initial: 1-2 mg/day in divided doses; usual range: 2-4 mg/day; do not exceed 10 mg/day (0.2 mg/kg/day)

Children >12 years: Tourette's disorder: Oral: Refer to adult dosing.

Hepatic Impairment: Reduced dose is necessary.

Monitoring Laboratory Tests Baseline EKG and periodically during therapy, ophthalmic exam

Monitoring and Teaching Issues

Physical Assessment: Assess other medications patient is taking for effectiveness and interactions (see Drug Interactions). See Contraindications and Warnings/Precautions for use cautions. Assess patient/caregiver knowledge of rationale for therapy and risks involved. Monitor ophthalmic exam and laboratory tests, therapeutic response, and adverse reactions at beginning of therapy and periodically with long-term use (see Adverse Reactions and Overdose/Toxicology). Initiate at lower doses (see Dosing) and decrease dosage slowly when discontinuing. Assess knowledge/teach patient appropriate use, interventions to reduce side effects, and adverse symptoms to report (see Patient Education). **Pregnancy risk factor C** - benefits of use should outweigh possible risks. Note breast-feeding caution.

Patient Education: Use exactly as directed; do not increase dose or frequency. It may take 2-3 weeks to achieve desired results; do not discontinue without consulting prescriber. Avoid alcohol or caffeine and other prescription or OTC medications not approved by prescriber. Avoid grapefruit juice. Maintain adequate hydration (2-3 L/day of fluids) unless advised by prescriber to restrict fluids. You may experience excess drowsiness, restlessness, dizziness, or blurred vision (use caution driving or when engaging in tasks requiring alertness until response to drug is known); or constipation, dry mouth, anorexia (increased exercise, fluids, fruit, or fiber may help). Report persistent CNS effects (eg, trembling fingers, altered gait or balance, excessive sedation, seizures, unusual muscle or facial movements, anxiety, abnormal thoughts, confusion, personality changes); unresolved constipation or GI effects; breast swelling (male and female) or decreased sexual ability; vision changes; difficulty breathing; unusual cough or flu-like symptoms; or worsening of condition. **Pregnancy/breast-feeding precautions:** Inform prescriber if you are or intend to become pregnant. Consult prescriber if breast-feeding.

Geriatric Considerations: (See Warnings/Precautions, Adverse Reactions, and Overdose/Toxicology.) Elderly patients have an increased risk of adverse response to side effects or adverse reactions to antipsychotics.

Additional Information Less sedation but pimozide is more likely to cause acute extrapyramidal symptoms than chlorpromazine.

Related Information

Antipsychotic Agents *on page 1558*

Antipsychotic Medication Guidelines *on page 1614*

Pindolol (PIN doe lole)

U.S. Brand Names Visken®

Generic Available Yes

Pharmacologic Category Beta Blocker With Intrinsic Sympathomimetic Activity

Pregnancy Risk Factor B

Lactation Enters breast milk/use caution

Use Management of hypertension

Use - Unlabeled/Investigational Potential augmenting agent for antidepressants; ventricular arrhythmias/tachycardia, antipsychotic-induced akathisia, situational anxiety; aggressive behavior associated with dementia

Mechanism of Action/Effect Blocks both $beta_1$- and $beta_2$-receptors and has mild intrinsic sympathomimetic activity; pindolol has negative inotropic and chronotropic effects and can significantly slow AV nodal conduction. Augmentive action of antidepressants thought to be mediated via a serotonin 1A autoreceptor antagonism.

Contraindications Hypersensitivity to pindolol, beta-blockers, or any component of the formulation; uncompensated congestive heart failure; cardiogenic shock; bradycardia, sinus node dysfunction, or heart block (2nd or 3rd degree) except in patients with a functioning artificial pacemaker; pulmonary edema; severe hyperactive airway disease (asthma or COPD); Raynaud's disease

Warnings/Precautions Administer very cautiously to patients with CHF, asthma, diabetes mellitus, hyperthyroidism. May mask signs and symptoms of thyrotoxicosis. Abrupt withdrawal of the drug should be avoided, drug should be discontinued over 1-2 weeks. Do not use in pregnant or nursing women. May potentiate hypoglycemia in a diabetic patient and mask signs and symptoms. Use with caution in patients with myasthenia gravis or peripheral vascular disease. May cause CNS depression; use caution in patients with a history of psychiatric illness. May potentiate anaphylactic reactions and/or blunt response to epinephrine treatment. Beta-blockers with intrinsic sympathomimetic activity (including pindolol) do not appear to be of benefit in CHF.

Drug Interactions

Cytochrome P450 Effect: Substrate of **CYP2D6**; Inhibits CYP2D6

Decreased Effect: Decreased levels/effect of pindolol with aluminum salts, barbiturates, calcium salts, cholestyramine, colestipol, NSAIDs, penicillins (ampicillin), rifampin, salicylates, and sulfinpyrazone due to decreased bioavailability and plasma levels. Beta-blockers may decrease the effect of sulfonylureas (possibly hyperglycemia). Nonselective beta-blockers blunt the effect of beta-2 adrenergic agonists (albuterol).

Increased Effect/Toxicity: Pindolol may increase the effects of other drugs which slow AV conduction (digoxin, verapamil, diltiazem), alpha-blockers (prazosin, terazosin), and alpha-adrenergic stimulants (epinephrine, phenylephrine). Pindolol may mask the tachycardia from hypoglycemia caused by insulin and oral hypoglycemics. In patients receiving concurrent therapy, the risk of hypertensive crisis is increased when either clonidine or the beta-blocker is withdrawn. Reserpine has been shown to enhance the effect of beta-blockers. Beta-blockers may increase the action or levels of ethanol, disopyramide, nondepolarizing muscle relaxants, and theophylline although the effects are difficult to predict.

Nutritional/Ethanol Interactions Herb/Nutraceutical: Avoid dong quai if using for hypertension (has estrogenic activity). Avoid ephedra, yohimbe, ginseng (may worsen hypertension).

Adverse Reactions

1% to 10%:

Cardiovascular: Chest pain (3%), edema (6%)

Central nervous system: Nightmares/vivid dreams (5%), dizziness (9%), insomnia (10%), fatigue (8%), nervousness (7%), anxiety (<2%)

Dermatologic: Rash, itching (4%)

Gastrointestinal: Nausea (5%), abdominal discomfort (4%)

Neuromuscular & skeletal: Weakness (4%), paresthesia (3%), arthralgia (7%), muscle pain (10%)

Respiratory: Dyspnea (5%)

<1% (Limited to important or life-threatening): Bradycardia, CHF, confusion, hallucinations, hypotension, mental depression, thrombocytopenia

Overdosage/Toxicology Symptoms of intoxication include cardiac disturbances, CNS toxicity, bronchospasm, hypoglycemia, and hyperkalemia. The most common cardiac symptoms include hypotension and bradycardia. Atrioventricular block, intraventricular conduction disturbances, cardiogenic shock, and asystole may occur with severe overdose, especially with membrane-depressant drugs (eg, propranolol). CNS effects include convulsions, and coma. Respiratory arrest is commonly seen with propranolol and other membrane-depressant and lipid-soluble drugs. Treatment includes symptomatic treatment of seizures, hypotension, hyperkalemia, and hypoglycemia.

Pharmacodynamics/Kinetics

Absorption: Rapid, 50% to 95%

Half-Life Elimination: 2.5-4 hours; prolonged with renal impairment, age, and cirrhosis

Time to Peak: Serum: 1-2 hours

Metabolism: Hepatic (60% to 65%) to conjugates

Formulations Tablet: 5 mg, 10 mg

Dosing

Adults:

Hypertension: Oral: Initial: 5 mg twice daily, increase as necessary by 10 mg/day every 3-4 weeks; maximum daily dose: 60 mg.

Antidepressant augmentation: Oral: 2.5 mg 3 times/day

(Continued)

Pindolol *(Continued)*

Elderly: Oral: Initial: 5 mg once daily; increase as necessary by 5 mg/day every 3-4 weeks.

Renal Impairment: Reduction is necessary in severe impairment.

Hepatic Impairment: Reduce dose in severely impaired.

Monitoring and Teaching Issues

Physical Assessment: See Contraindications, Warnings/Precautions, and Dosing for use cautions. Assess potential for interactions with other prescriptions, OTC medications, or herbal products patient may be taking (eg, anything that affects blood pressure or cardiac status - see Drug Interactions). Assess patient response at beginning of therapy, when adjusting dosage, and periodically with long-term therapy (eg, cardiac, respiratory, hemodynamic status - see Adverse Reactions and Overdose/Toxicology). Caution patient to monitor serum glucose levels closely (may alter glucose tolerance, potentiate hypoglycemia, or mask symptoms of hypoglycemia). Teach patient appropriate use, possible side effects and interventions, and adverse symptoms to report (see Patient Education). Note breast-feeding caution.

Patient Education: Inform prescriber of all prescriptions, OTC medications, or herbal products you are taking, and any allergies you have. Do not take anything new during treatment unless approved by prescriber. Take exactly as directed. Do not alter dose or discontinue without consulting prescriber. If diabetic, monitor serum glucose closely (drug may alter glucose tolerance or mask signs of hypoglycemia). May cause nervousness, fatigue, dizziness, insomnia, or postural hypotension (use caution when changing position from lying or sitting to standing, when driving, or climbing stairs until response to medication is known); or nausea or abdominal discomfort (small, frequent meals, frequent mouth care, chewing gum, or sucking lozenges may help). Report chest pain or swelling of extremities or unusual weight gain (>5 lb/week), unusual muscle weakness or pain; or other persistent adverse effects. Consult prescriber if breast-feeding.

Dietary Issues: May be taken without regard to meals.

Geriatric Considerations: Due to alterations in the beta-adrenergic autonomic nervous system, beta-adrenergic blockade may result in less hemodynamic response than seen in younger adults. Studies indicate that despite decreased sensitivity to the chronotropic effects of beta blockade with age, there appears to be an increased myocardial sensitivity to the negative inotropic effect during stress (eg, exercise). Controlled trials have shown the overall response rate for propranolol to be only 20% to 50% in elderly populations. Therefore, all beta-adrenergic blocking drugs may result in a decreased response as compared to younger adults (see Pharmacodynamics and Pharmacokinetics).

Breast-feeding Issues: There is limited experience with pindolol; however, other beta-blockers like metoprolol are considered compatible by the AAP. Monitor the infant for signs of beta-blockade (hypotension, bradycardia, etc) with long-term use.

Related Information

Beta-Blockers *on page 1561*

Pink Bismuth *see* Bismuth *on page 169*

PIO *see* Pemoline *on page 1042*

Pioglitazone (pye oh GLI ta zone)

U.S. Brand Names Actos®

Generic Available No

Pharmacologic Category Antidiabetic Agent, Thiazolidinedione

Pregnancy Risk Factor C

Lactation Excretion in breast milk unknown/not recommended

Use

Type 2 diabetes mellitus (noninsulin dependent, NIDDM), monotherapy: Adjunct to diet and exercise, to improve glycemic control

Type 2 diabetes mellitus (noninsulin dependent, NIDDM), combination therapy with sulfonylurea, metformin, or insulin: When diet, exercise, and a single agent alone does not result in adequate glycemic control

Mechanism of Action/Effect Thiazolidinedione antidiabetic agent that lowers blood glucose by improving target cell response to insulin, without increasing pancreatic insulin secretion. It has a mechanism of action that is dependent on the presence of insulin for activity. Pioglitazone is a potent and selective agonist for peroxisome proliferator-activated receptor-gamma (PPARgamma). Activation of nuclear PPARgamma receptors influences the production of a number of gene products involved in glucose and lipid metabolism.

Contraindications Hypersensitivity to pioglitazone or any component of the formulation; active liver disease (transaminases >2.5 times the upper limit of normal at baseline); patients who have experienced jaundice during troglitazone therapy

Warnings/Precautions Should not be used in diabetic ketoacidosis. Mechanism requires the presence of insulin, therefore use in type 1 diabetes (insulin dependent, IDDM) is not recommended. May potentiate hypoglycemia when used in combination with sulfonylureas or insulin. Use with caution in premenopausal, anovulatory women - may result in a resumption of ovulation, increasing the risk of pregnancy. Use with caution in patients with anemia (may reduce hemoglobin and hematocrit). May increase plasma volume and/or increase cardiac hypertrophy. Use with caution in patients with edema. Monitor closely for signs and symptoms of heart failure. Avoid use in patients with NYHA Class III or IV heart failure. Discontinue if heart failure develops. Use with caution in patients with minor elevations in transaminases (AST or ALT). Idiosyncratic hepatotoxicity has been reported with another thiazolidinedione agent (troglitazone) and postmarketing case reports of hepatitis (with rare hepatic failure) have been received for pioglitazone. Monitoring should include periodic determinations of liver function. Pregnancy risk C.

Drug Interactions

Cytochrome P450 Effect: Substrate of **CYP2C8/9, 3A4**; Inhibits CYP2C8/9, 2C19; Induces CYP3A4

Decreased Effect: Effects of oral contraceptives may be decreased, based on data from a related compound. This has not been specifically evaluated for pioglitazone. CYP3A4 inducers may decrease the therapeutic effect of pioglitazone.

Increased Effect/Toxicity: Ketoconazole (*in vitro*) inhibits metabolism of pioglitazone. Other inhibitors of CYP3A4, including itraconazole, are likely to decrease pioglitazone metabolism. Patients receiving inhibitors of CYP3A4 should have their glycemic control evaluated more frequently.

Nutritional/Ethanol Interactions

Ethanol: Caution with ethanol (may cause hypoglycemia).

Food: Peak concentrations are delayed when administered with food, but the extent of absorption is not affected. Pioglitazone may be taken without regard to meals.

Herb/Nutraceutical: St John's wort may decrease levels. Caution with chromium, garlic, gymnema (may cause hypoglycemia).

Adverse Reactions

>10%:

- Endocrine & metabolic: Decreased serum triglycerides, increased HDL-cholesterol
- Gastrointestinal: Weight gain
- Respiratory: Upper respiratory tract infection (13%)

1% to 10%:

- Cardiovascular: Edema (5%) (in combination trials with sulfonylureas or insulin, the incidence of edema was as high as 15%)
- Central nervous system: Headache (9%), fatigue (4%)
- Endocrine & metabolic: Aggravation of diabetes mellitus (5%), hypoglycemia (range 2% to 15% when used in combination with sulfonylureas or insulin)
- Hematologic; Anemia (1%)
- Neuromuscular & skeletal: Myalgia (5%)
- Respiratory: Sinusitis (6%), pharyngitis (5%)

<1% (Limited to important or life-threatening): Congestive heart failure, elevated CPK, elevated transaminases, hepatic failure (very rare), hepatitis

Overdosage/Toxicology Experience in overdose is limited. Symptoms may include hypoglycemia. Treatment is supportive.

Pharmacodynamics/Kinetics

Half-Life Elimination: Parent drug: 3-7 hours; Total: 16-24 hours

Time to Peak: ~2 hours

Metabolism: Hepatic (99%) via CYP2C8/9 and 3A4 to both active and inactive metabolites

Onset: Delayed; Peak effect: Glucose control: Several weeks

Formulations Tablet: 15 mg, 30 mg, 45 mg

Dosing

Adults & Elderly: Type 2 Diabetes: Oral:

Monotherapy: Initial: 15-30 mg once daily; if response is inadequate, the dosage may be increased in increments up to 45 mg once daily; maximum recommended dose: 45 mg once daily

Combination therapy:

- With sulfonylureas: Initial: 15-30 mg once daily; dose of sulfonylurea should be reduced if the patient reports hypoglycemia
- With metformin: Initial: 15-30 mg once daily; it is unlikely that the dose of metformin will need to be reduced due to hypoglycemia
- With insulin: Initial: 15-30 mg once daily; dose of insulin should be reduced by 10% to 25% if the patient reports hypoglycemia or if the plasma glucose falls to below 100 mg/dL. Doses greater than 30 mg/day have not been evaluated in combination regimens.

A 1-week washout period is recommended in patients with normal liver enzymes who are changed from troglitazone to pioglitazone therapy.

Renal Impairment: No adjustment is necessary.

Hepatic Impairment: Clearance is significantly lower in hepatic impairment. Therapy should not be initiated if the patient exhibits active liver disease or increased transaminases (>2.5 times the upper limit of normal) at baseline.

Administration

Oral: May be administered without regard to meals.

Monitoring Laboratory Tests Hemoglobin A_{1c}, liver enzymes (prior to initiation and every 2 months for the first year of treatment, then periodically). If the ALT is increased to >2.5 times the upper limit of normal, liver function testing should be performed more frequently until the levels return to normal or pretreatment values. Patients with an elevation in ALT >3 times the upper limit of normal should be rechecked as soon as possible. If the ALT levels remain >3 times the upper limit of normal, therapy with pioglitazone should be discontinued.

Monitoring and Teaching Issues

Physical Assessment: Assess other medications patient may be taking (see Warnings/Precautions and Drug Interactions). Monitor laboratory results (see Adverse Reactions and Monitoring Laboratory Tests) and response to therapy frequently until patient is stable. Monitor for adverse response (see Adverse Reactions). Assess knowledge/teach risks of hyper-/hypoglycemia, symptoms, and treatment. Refer patient to a diabetic educator, if available. **Pregnancy risk factor C** - benefits of use should outweigh possible risks. **Note:** Advise women using oral contraceptives about need for alternative method of contraception. Breast-feeding is not recommended.

Patient Education: Use exactly as directed; do not increase dose or frequency or discontinue without consulting prescriber. May be taken without regard to meals. Avoid or use caution with alcohol while taking this medication. If dose is missed, take as soon as possible. If dose is missed completely one day, do not double dose the next day. Follow dietary, exercise, and glucose monitoring instructions of prescriber (more frequent monitoring may be advised in periods of stress, trauma, surgery, increased exercise etc). Report respiratory infection, unusual weight gain, aggravation of hyper-/hypoglycemic condition, unusual swelling of extremities, shortness of breath, fatigue, yellowing of skin or eyes, dark urine, pale stool, nausea/vomiting, or muscle pain. **Pregnancy/breast-feeding precautions:** Inform prescriber if you are or intend to become pregnant. Use alternate means of contraception if using oral contraceptives. Breast-feeding is not recommended.

(Continued)

Pioglitazone *(Continued)*

Dietary Issues: Management of type 2 diabetes mellitus (noninsulin dependent, NIDDM) should include diet control. May be taken without regard to meals.

Breast-feeding Issues: In animal studies, pioglitazone has been found to be excreted in milk. It is not known whether pioglitazone is excreted in human milk. Should not be administered to a nursing woman.

Pregnancy Issues: Treatment during mid-late gestation was associated with delayed parturition, embryotoxicity and postnatal growth retardation in animal models. Abnormal blood glucose levels are associated with a higher incidence of congenital abnormalities. Insulin is the drug of choice for the control of diabetes mellitus during pregnancy.

Related Information

Antidiabetic Oral Agents Comparison *on page 1556*
Diabetes Mellitus Management *on page 1661*

Piperacillin (pi PER a sil in)

U.S. Brand Names Pipracil®

Synonyms Piperacillin Sodium

Generic Available No

Pharmacologic Category Antibiotic, Penicillin

Pregnancy Risk Factor B

Lactation Enters breast milk (small amounts - other penicillins are compatible with breast-feeding)

Use Treatment of susceptible infections such as septicemia, acute and chronic respiratory tract infections, skin and soft tissue infections, and urinary tract infections due to susceptible strains of *Pseudomonas*, *Proteus*, and *Escherichia coli* and *Enterobacter*; active against some streptococci and some anaerobic bacteria; febrile neutropenia (as part of combination regimen)

Mechanism of Action/Effect Inhibits bacterial cell wall synthesis by binding to one or more of the penicillin binding proteins (PBPs); which in turn inhibits the final transpeptidation step of peptidoglycan synthesis in bacterial cell walls, thus inhibiting cell wall biosynthesis. Bacteria eventually lyse due to ongoing activity of cell wall autolytic enzymes (autolysins and murein hydrolases) while cell wall assembly is arrested.

Contraindications Hypersensitivity to piperacillin, other penicillins, or any component of the formulation

Warnings/Precautions Dosage modification required in patients with impaired renal function; history of seizure activity; use with caution in patients with a history of beta-lactam allergy

Drug Interactions

Decreased Effect: Tetracyclines may decrease penicillin effectiveness. High concentrations of piperacillin may cause physical inactivation of aminoglycosides and lead to potential toxicity in patients with mild-moderate renal dysfunction. Although anecdotal reports suggest oral contraceptive efficacy could be reduced by penicillins, this has been refuted by more rigorous scientific and clinical data.

Increased Effect/Toxicity: Probenecid may increase penicillin levels. Neuromuscular blockers may increase duration of blockade.

Effects on Lab Values May interfere with urinary glucose tests using cupric sulfate (Benedict's solution, Clinitest®); may inactivate aminoglycosides *in vitro*; false-positive urinary and serum proteins, positive Coombs' test [direct]

Adverse Reactions Frequency not defined.

Central nervous system: Confusion, convulsions, drowsiness, fever, Jarisch-Herxheimer reaction
Dermatologic: Rash
Endocrine & metabolic: Electrolyte imbalance
Hematologic: Abnormal platelet aggregation and prolonged PT (high doses), hemolytic anemia, Coombs' reaction (positive)
Local: Thrombophlebitis
Neuromuscular & skeletal: Myoclonus
Renal: Acute interstitial nephritis
Miscellaneous: Anaphylaxis, hypersensitivity reactions

Overdosage/Toxicology Symptoms of penicillin overdose include neuromuscular hypersensitivity (eg, agitation, hallucinations, asterixis, encephalopathy, confusion, and seizures). Electrolyte imbalance may occur if the preparation contains potassium or sodium salts, especially in renal failure. Hemodialysis may be helpful to aid in removal of the drug from blood; otherwise, treatment is supportive or symptom-directed.

Pharmacodynamics/Kinetics

Absorption: I.M.: 70% to 80%

Half-Life Elimination: Dose dependent; prolonged with moderately severe renal or hepatic impairment:

Neonates: 1-5 days old: 3.6 hours; >6 days old: 2.1-2.7 hours
Children: 1-6 months: 0.79 hour; 6 months to 12 years: 0.39-0.5 hour
Adults: 36-80 minutes

Time to Peak: Serum: I.M.: 30-50 minutes

Formulations Injection, powder for reconstitution, as sodium: 2 g, 3 g, 4 g, 40 g

Dosing

Adults: Susceptible infections:
I.M.: 2-3 g/dose every 6-12 hours; maximum: 24 g/24 hours
I.V.: 3-4 g/dose every 4-6 hours; maximum: 24 g/24 hours

Elderly: Adjust dose for renal impairment:
I.M.: 1-2 g every 8-12 hours
I.V.: 2-4 g every 6-8 hours

Pediatrics: Susceptible infections:
Neonates: I.M., I.V.: 100 mg/kg every 12 hours

Infants and Children: I.M., I.V.: 200-300 mg/kg/day in divided doses every 4-6 hours
Higher doses have been used in cystic fibrosis: 350-500 mg/kg/day in divided doses every 4-6 hours

Renal Impairment:

Cl_{cr} 10-50 mL/minute: Administer every 6-8 hours.
Cl_{cr} <10 mL/minute: Administer every 8 hours.
Moderately dialyzable (20% to 50%)
Continuous arteriovenous or venovenous hemofiltration: Dose as for Cl_{cr} 10-50 mL/minute.

Administration

I.M.: Do not administer more than 2 g per injection site.

I.V.: Administer around-the-clock to promote less variation in peak and trough serum levels. Give at least 1 hour apart from aminoglycosides. Rapid administration can lead to seizures. Administer direct I.V. over 3-5 minutes. Intermittently infusion over 30 minutes.

Stability

Storage: Reconstituted solution is stable (I.V. infusion) in NS or D_5W for 24 hours at room temperature, 7 days when refrigerated, or 4 weeks when frozen. After freezing, thawed solution is stable for 24 hours at room temperature or 48 hours when refrigerated. 40 g bulk vial should **not** be frozen after reconstitution.

Compatibility: Stable in dextran 6% in NS, D_5NS, D_5W, LR, NS, sterile water for injection, bacteriostatic water

Y-site administration: Incompatible with amphotericin B cholesteryl sulfate complex, filgrastim, fluconazole, gatifloxacin, gemcitabine, ondansetron, sargramostim, vinorelbine

Compatibility when admixed: Incompatible with aminoglycosides

Monitoring Laboratory Tests Perform culture and sensitivity before administering first dose.

Monitoring and Teaching Issues

Physical Assessment: Assess for allergy history prior to starting therapy. See Contraindications and Warnings/Precautions for use cautions. Assess potential for interactions with other prescriptions, OTC medications, or herbal products patient may be taking (see Drug Interactions). Assess for therapeutic effectiveness and adverse reactions (eg, hypersensitivity reactions, opportunistic infection - see Adverse Reactions and Overdose/Toxicology). Caution diabetic patients about altered response to Clinitest®. Teach patient possible side effects and interventions, and adverse symptoms to report (see Patient Education).

Patient Education: Inform prescriber of all prescriptions, OTC medications, or herbal products you are taking, and any allergies you have. Do not take anything new during treatment unless approved by prescriber. This drug can only be given by injection or infusion. Report immediately any redness, swelling, burning, or pain at infusion site or any signs of allergic reaction (eg, difficulty breathing or swallowing, chest tightness, rash, hives, swelling of lips or mouth). Maintain adequate hydration (2-3 L/day of fluids) unless advised by prescriber to restrict fluids. If diabetic, drug may cause false test results with Clinitest®, consult prescriber for alternative method of glucose monitoring. May cause confusion or drowsiness (use caution when driving or engaging in tasks that require alertness until response to drug is known). Report chest pain, palpitations, or irregular heartbeat; persistent adverse effects.

Dietary Issues: Sodium content of 1 g: 1.85 mEq

Geriatric Considerations: Antipseudomonal penicillins should not be used alone and are often combined with an aminoglycoside as empiric therapy for lower respiratory infection and sepsis in which gram-negative (including *Pseudomonas*) and/or anaerobes are of a high probability. Because of piperacillin's lower sodium content, it is preferred over ticarcillin in patients with a history of heart failure and/or renal or hepatic disease. Adjust dose for renal function.

Additional Information As of September 2002, piperacillin is not available from the manufacturer. This product is anticipated to return to the market in 2003.

Piperacillin and Tazobactam Sodium

(pi PER a sil in & ta zoe BAK tam SOW dee um)

U.S. Brand Names Zosyn®

Synonyms Piperacillin Sodium and Tazobactam Sodium

Generic Available No

Pharmacologic Category Antibiotic, Penicillin

Pregnancy Risk Factor B

Lactation Enters breast milk/use caution (other penicillins are compatible)

Use Treatment of infections of lower respiratory tract, urinary tract, skin and skin structures, gynecologic, bone and joint infections, and septicemia caused by susceptible organisms. Tazobactam expands activity of piperacillin to include beta-lactamase producing strains of *S. aureus*, *H. influenzae*, *Bacteroides*, and other gram-negative bacteria.

Mechanism of Action/Effect Piperacillin interferes with bacterial cell wall synthesis during active multiplication, causing cell wall death and resultant bactericidal activity against susceptible bacteria; tazobactam prevents degradation of piperacillin by binding to the active side on beta-lactamase; tazobactam inhibits many beta-lactamases, including staphylococcal penicillinase and Richmond and Sykes Types II, III, IV, and V, including extended spectrum enzymes; it has only limited activity against Class I beta-lactamases other than Class 1C

Contraindications Hypersensitivity to penicillins, beta-lactamase inhibitors, or any component of the formulation

Warnings/Precautions Due to sodium load and to the adverse effects of high serum concentrations of penicillins, dosage modification is required in patients with impaired or underdeveloped renal function; use with caution in patients with seizures or in patients with history of beta-lactam allergy; safety and efficacy have not been established in children <12 years of age

Drug Interactions

Decreased Effect: Tetracyclines may decrease penicillin effectiveness. Aminoglycosides may cause physical inactivation of aminoglycosides in the presence of high concentrations

(Continued)

Piperacillin and Tazobactam Sodium *(Continued)*

of piperacillin and potential toxicity in patients with mild-moderate renal dysfunction. Although anecdotal reports suggest oral contraceptive efficacy could be reduced by penicillins, this has been refuted by more rigorous scientific and clinical data.

Increased Effect/Toxicity: Probenecid may increase penicillin levels. Neuromuscular blockers may increase duration of blockade.

Effects on Lab Values Positive Coombs' [direct] test 3.8%, ALT, AST, bilirubin, and LDH

Adverse Reactions

>10%: Gastrointestinal: Diarrhea (11%)

1% to 10%:

Cardiovascular: Hypertension (2%)

Central nervous system: Insomnia (7%), headache (7% to 8%), agitation (2%), fever (2%), dizziness (1%)

Dermatologic: Rash (4%), pruritus (3%)

Gastrointestinal: Constipation (7% to 8%), nausea (7%), vomiting/dyspepsia (3%)

Respiratory: Rhinitis/dyspnea (~1%)

Miscellaneous: Serum sickness-like reaction

<1% (Limited to important or life-threatening): Cholestatic jaundice, *Clostridium difficile* colitis, eosinophilia, erythema multiforme, hemolytic anemia, hepatitis, hepatotoxicity, interstitial nephritis, leukopenia, neutropenia, positive direct Coombs' test, prolonged PT and PTT, seizures, Stevens-Johnson syndrome, thrombocytopenia

Overdosage/Toxicology Symptoms of penicillin overdose include neuromuscular hypersensitivity (eg, agitation, hallucinations, asterixis, encephalopathy, confusion, and seizures). Electrolyte imbalance may occur if the preparation contains potassium or sodium salts, especially in renal dysfunction. Hemodialysis may be helpful to aid in removal of the drug from blood; otherwise, treatment is supportive or symptom-directed.

Pharmacokinetic Note Both AUC and peak concentrations are dose proportional. Hepatic impairment does not affect the kinetics of piperacillin or tazobactam significantly.

Pharmacodynamics/Kinetics

Half-Life Elimination: Piperacillin: 1 hour; Metabolite: 1-1.5 hours; Tazobactam: 0.7-0.9 hour

Metabolism: Piperacillin: 6% to 9%; Tazobactam: ~26%

Formulations Vials at an 8:1 ratio of piperacillin sodium/tazobactam sodium:

Injection:

Piperacillin sodium 2 g and tazobactam sodium 0.25 g

Piperacillin sodium 3 g and tazobactam sodium 0.375 g

Piperacillin sodium 4 g and tazobactam sodium 0.5 g

Dosing

Adults & Elderly:

Severe infections: I.V.: Piperacillin/tazobactam 4/0.5 g every 8 hours or 3/0.375 g every 6 hours

Moderate infections: I.M., I.V.: Piperacillin/tazobactam 2/0.25 g every 6-8 hours; treatment should be continued for ≥7-10 days depending on severity of disease. (**Note:** I.M. route not FDA-approved.)

Pediatrics: Not FDA-approved for children <12 years of age.

Infants <6 months: I.V.: 150-300 mg of piperacillin component/kg/day in divided doses every 6-8 hours

Infants and Children ≥6 months: I.V.: 240 mg of piperacillin component/kg/day in divided doses every 8 hours; higher doses have been used for serious pseudomonal infections: 300-400 mg of piperacillin component/kg/day in divided doses every 6 hours.

Renal Impairment:

Cl_{cr} >40 mL/minute: No change

Cl_{cr} 20-40 mL/minute: Administer 2/0.25 g every 6 hours.

Cl_{cr} <20 mL/minute: Administer 2/0.25 g every 8 hours.

Hemodialysis: Administer 2/0.25 g every 8 hours with an additional dose of 0.75 g after each dialysis.

Hemodialysis removes 30% to 40% of piperacillin and tazobactam. Peritoneal dialysis removes 11% to 21% of tazobactam and 6% of piperacillin.

Continuous arteriovenous or venovenous hemofiltration: Dose as for Cl_{cr} 10-50 mL/minute.

Hepatic Impairment: Hepatic impairment does not affect the kinetics of piperacillin or tazobactam significantly.

Administration

I.V.: Administer by I.V. infusion over 30 minutes. Discontinue primary infusion, if possible, during infusion and administer aminoglycosides separately from Zosyn®.

Stability

Storage: Store at controlled room temperature. After reconstitution, solution is stable in NS or D_5W for 24 hours at room temperature and 7 days when refrigerated.

Reconstitution: Use single-dose vials immediately after reconstitution (discard unused portions after 24 hours at room temperature and 48 hours if refrigerated). Reconstitute with 5 mL of diluent per 1 g of piperacillin and then further dilute. Compatible diluents include NS, SW, dextran 6%, D_5W, D_5W with potassium chloride 40 mEq, bacteriostatic saline and water.

Compatibility: Stable in dextran 6% in NS, D_5W, NS, sterile water for injection, bacteriostatic water; **incompatible** with LR

Y-site administration: Incompatible with acyclovir, alatrofloxacin, amphotericin B, amphotericin B cholesteryl sulfate complex, chlorpromazine, cisplatin, dacarbazine, daunorubicin, dobutamine, doxorubicin, doxorubicin liposome, doxycycline, droperidol, famotidine, ganciclovir, gatifloxacin, gemcitabine, haloperidol, hydroxyzine, idarubicin, minocycline, mitomycin, mitoxantrone, nalbuphine, prochlorperazine edisylate, promethazine, streptozocin

Monitoring Laboratory Tests LFTs, creatinine, BUN, CBC with differential, serum electrolytes, urinalysis, PT, PTT; perform culture and sensitivity before administering first dose.

Monitoring and Teaching Issues

Physical Assessment: Assess for allergy history prior to starting therapy. See Contraindications, Warnings/Precautions, and Dosing for use cautions. Assess potential for interactions with other prescriptions, OTC medications, or herbal products patient may be taking (see Drug Interactions). Assess results of laboratory tests (see above), therapeutic effectiveness, and adverse reactions (eg, hypersensitivity reactions, opportunistic infection - see Adverse Reactions and Overdose/Toxicology). Caution diabetic patients about altered response to Clinitest®. Teach patient possible side effects and interventions, and adverse symptoms to report (see Patient Education). Note breast-feeding caution.

Patient Education: Inform prescriber of all prescriptions, OTC medications, or herbal products you are taking, and any allergies you have. Do not take anything new during treatment unless approved by prescriber. This drug can only be given by injection or infusion; report immediately any redness, swelling, burning, or pain at infusion site or any signs of allergic reaction (eg, difficulty breathing or swallowing, chest tightness, rash, hives, swelling of lips or mouth). Maintain adequate hydration (2-3 L/day of fluids) unless advised by prescriber to restrict fluids. If diabetic, drug may cause false test results with Clinitest®; consult prescriber for alternative method of glucose monitoring. May cause diarrhea (consult prescriber for approved medication); nausea or vomiting (small, frequent meals, frequent mouth care, chewing gum or sucking lozenges may help); or constipation (increased exercise, fluids, fruit, or fiber may help). Report acute or persistent headache; rash; CNS changes (eg, agitation, confusion, hallucinations, or seizures); persistent abdominal pain, cramping or diarrhea; unusual fever; or other persistent adverse effects. **Breast-feeding precaution:** Consult prescriber if breast-feeding.

Dietary Issues: Sodium content of 1 g injection: 54 mg (2.35 mEq)

Geriatric Considerations: Has not been studied exclusively in the elderly.

Breast-feeding Issues: Use by the breast-feeding mother may result in bowel flora change, diarrhea, candidiasis, allergic response, or antibiotic effect on the infant. Use caution.

Related Information

Piperacillin *on page 1090*

Piperacillin Sodium *see* Piperacillin *on page 1090*

Piperacillin Sodium and Tazobactam Sodium *see* Piperacillin and Tazobactam Sodium *on page 1091*

Pipracil® *see* Piperacillin *on page 1090*

Pirbuterol (peer BYOO ter ole)

U.S. Brand Names Maxair™; Maxair™ Autohaler™

Synonyms Pirbuterol Acetate

Generic Available No

Pharmacologic Category $Beta_2$ Agonist

Pregnancy Risk Factor C

Lactation Excretion in breast milk unknown

Use Prevention and treatment of reversible bronchospasm including asthma

Mechanism of Action/Effect Pirbuterol is a $beta_2$-adrenergic agonist with a similar structure to albuterol, specifically a pyridine ring has been substituted for the benzene ring in albuterol. The increased $beta_2$ selectivity of pirbuterol results from the substitution of a tertiary butyl group on the nitrogen of the side chain, which additionally imparts resistance of pirbuterol to degradation by monoamine oxidase and provides a lengthened duration of action in comparison to the less selective previous beta-agonist agents.

Contraindications Hypersensitivity to pirbuterol, albuterol, or any component of the formulation

Warnings/Precautions Excessive use may result in tolerance. Use with caution in patients with hyperthyroidism, diabetes mellitus. Cardiovascular disorders including coronary insufficiency or hypertension or sensitivity to sympathomimetic amines. Pregnancy risk C.

Drug Interactions

Decreased Effect: Decreased effect with beta-blockers.

Increased Effect/Toxicity: Increased toxicity with other beta agonists, MAO inhibitors, tricyclic antidepressants.

Adverse Reactions

>10%:

Central nervous system: Nervousness, restlessness

Neuromuscular & skeletal: Trembling

1% to 10%:

Cardiovascular: Tachycardia, pounding heartbeat

Central nervous system: Headache, dizziness, lightheadedness

Gastrointestinal: Taste changes, vomiting, nausea

<1% (Limited to important or life-threatening): Arrhythmias, chest pain, hypertension, insomnia, paradoxical bronchospasm

Overdosage/Toxicology Symptoms of overdose include hypertension, tachycardia, angina, and hypokalemia. In cases of overdose, supportive therapy should be instituted, and prudent use of a cardioselective beta-adrenergic blocker (eg, atenolol or metoprolol) should be considered, keeping in mind the potential for induction of bronchoconstriction in an asthmatic individual. Dialysis has not been shown to be of value in the treatment of overdose with pirbuterol.

Pharmacodynamics/Kinetics

Half-Life Elimination: 2-3 hours

Metabolism: Hepatic

Onset: Peak effect: Therapeutic: Oral: 2-3 hours with peak serum concentration of 6.2-9.8 mcg/L; Inhalation: 0.5-1 hour

Formulations Aerosol for oral inhalation, as acetate:

Maxair™ Autohaler™: 0.2 mg per actuation (2.8 g - 80 inhalations, 14 g - 400 inhalations)

Maxair™: 0.2 mg per actuation (25.6 g - 300 inhalations)

(Continued)

Pirbuterol *(Continued)*

Dosing

Adults & Elderly: Bronchospasm: Inhalation: 2 inhalations every 4-6 hours for prevention; 2 inhalations at an interval of at least 1-3 minutes, followed by a third inhalation in treatment of bronchospasm, not to exceed 12 inhalations/day

Pediatrics: Children ≥12 years: Refer to adult dosing.

Administration

Inhalation: Shake inhaler well before use.

Stability

Storage: Store between 15°C and 30°C (59°F and 86°F).

Monitoring and Teaching Issues

Physical Assessment: Assess effectiveness and interactions of other medications patient may be taking (see Drug Interactions). See Contraindications and Warnings/Precautions for use cautions. Monitor effectiveness of therapy and adverse reactions (see Adverse Reactions) at beginning of therapy and periodically with long-term use. For inpatient care, monitor vital signs and lung sounds prior to and periodically during therapy. Assess knowledge/teach patient appropriate use, interventions to reduce side effects, and adverse symptoms to report (see Patient Education). **Pregnancy risk factor C** - benefits of use should outweigh possible risks. Note breast-feeding caution.

Patient Education: Use exactly as directed (see Administration below). Do not use more often than recommended. Maintain adequate hydration (2-3 L/day of fluids) unless advised by prescriber to restrict fluids. You may experience nervousness, dizziness, or fatigue (use caution when driving or engaging in tasks requiring alertness until response to drug is known); or dry mouth or stomach upset (small, frequent meals, frequent mouth care, chewing gum, or sucking hard candy may help). Report unresolved GI upset; dizziness or fatigue; vision changes; chest pain, rapid heartbeat, or palpitations; nervousness or insomnia; muscle cramping or tremor; or unusual cough. **Pregnancy/breast-feeding precautions:** Inform prescriber if you are or intend to become pregnant. Consult prescriber if breast-feeding.

Aerosol: Store canister upside down; do not freeze. Shake canister before using. Sit when using medication. Close eyes when administering pirbuterol to avoid spray getting into eyes. Exhale slowly and completely through nose; inhale deeply through mouth while administering aerosol. Hold breath for 5-10 seconds after inhalation. Wait at least 1 full minute between inhalations. Wash mouthpiece between use. If more than one inhalation medication is used, use bronchodilator first and wait 5 minutes between medications.

Maxair™ Autohaler™: Hold upright. Raise lever so that it stays up and snaps into place. Shake well. Exhale. Seal lips tightly around mouthpiece, inhale deeply. A "click" will be heard and you will feel a soft puff when the medication has been triggered. Continue to take a full, deep breath. Remove inhaler from mouth, hold breath for 10 seconds, then exhale slowly. **Note:** A test-fire slide has been added to the bottom of the Autohaler™ actuator/mouthpiece. The inhaler should be primed prior to using for the first time or if it has not been used in 48 hours. To prime, remove mouthpiece; point mouthpiece away from yourself or others, and push the lever so that it stays up. Push the white test-fire slide located on the bottom of the mouthpiece to release the priming spray. In order to release a second priming spray, push lever to "down" position, then repeat steps. When two priming sprays have been done, return lever to "down" position.

Geriatric Considerations: Elderly patients may find it beneficial to utilize a spacer device when using a metered dose inhaler. Difficulty in using the inhaler often limits its effectiveness. The Maxair™ Autohaler™ may be easier for the elderly to use.

Related Information

Inhalant (Asthma, Bronchospasm) Agents Comparison *on page 1577*

Pirbuterol Acetate *see* Pirbuterol *on page 1093*

Piroxicam (peer OKS i kam)

U.S. Brand Names Feldene®

Generic Available Yes

Pharmacologic Category Nonsteroidal Anti-inflammatory Drug (NSAID)

Pregnancy Risk Factor B/D (3rd trimester or near term)

Lactation Enters breast milk (small amounts)/compatible

Use Management of inflammatory disorders; symptomatic treatment of acute and chronic rheumatoid arthritis, osteoarthritis, and ankylosing spondylitis; also used to treat sunburn

Mechanism of Action/Effect Inhibits prostaglandin synthesis, acts on the hypothalamus heat-regulating center to reduce fever, blocks prostaglandin synthetase action which prevents formation of the platelet-aggregating substance thromboxane A_2; decreases pain receptor sensitivity. Other proposed mechanisms of action for salicylate anti-inflammatory action are lysosomal stabilization, kinin and leukotriene production, alteration of chemotactic factors, and inhibition of neutrophil activation. This latter mechanism may be the most significant pharmacologic action to reduce inflammation.

Contraindications Hypersensitivity to piroxicam, aspirin, other NSAIDs or any component of the formulation; active GI bleeding; pregnancy (3rd trimester or near term)

Warnings/Precautions Use with caution in patients with CHF, hypertension, dehydration, decreased renal or hepatic function, history of GI disease (bleeding or ulcers), or those receiving anticoagulants. Elderly are at a high risk for CNS and gastrointestinal adverse effects from NSAIDs. As many as 60% of elderly can develop peptic ulceration and/or hemorrhage asymptomatically.

Use lowest effective dose for shortest period possible. Use of NSAIDs can compromise existing renal function especially when Cl_{cr} is <30 mL/minute. Withhold for at least 4-6 half-lives prior to surgical or dental procedures. May have adverse effects on fetus. Use with caution with dehydration. Use in children is not recommended.

Pregnancy risk B/D (3rd trimester or near term).

Drug Interactions

Cytochrome P450 Effect: Substrate of CYP2C8/9

Decreased Effect: Decreased effect of diuretics, beta-blockers. Decreased effect with aspirin, antacids, and cholestyramine.

Increased Effect/Toxicity: Increased effect/toxicity of lithium, warfarin, and methotrexate (controversial).

Nutritional/Ethanol Interactions

Ethanol: Avoid ethanol (may enhance gastric mucosal irritation).

Food: Onset of effect may be delayed if piroxicam is taken with food.

Herb/Nutraceutical: Avoid cat's claw, dong quai, evening primrose, feverfew, garlic, red clover, horse chestnut, green tea, ginseng, ginkgo (all have additional antiplatelet activity).

Effects on Lab Values ↑ chloride (S), sodium (S), bleeding time

Adverse Reactions

1% to 10%:

Cardiovascular: Edema

Central nervous system: Headache, dizziness, somnolence, vertigo

Dermatologic: Pruritus, rash

Gastrointestinal: Stomatitis, anorexia, epigastric distress, nausea, constipation, abdominal discomfort, flatulence, diarrhea, indigestion

Hematologic: Decreases in hemoglobin and hematocrit, anemia, leukopenia, eosinophilia

Renal: Elevated BUN, elevated serum creatinine, Polyuria, acute renal failure

Otic: Tinnitus

<1% (Limited to important or life-threatening): Abnormal LFTs, aplastic anemia, bone marrow depression, bronchospasm, chest pain, CHF, dyspnea, erythema multiforme, hemolytic anemia, hepatitis, hyperglycemia, hypertension, hypoglycemia, jaundice, Stevens-Johnson syndrome, thrombocytopenia, toxic epidermal necrolysis

Overdosage/Toxicology Symptoms of overdose include nausea, epigastric distress, CNS depression, leukocytosis, and renal failure. Management of NSAID intoxication is supportive and symptomatic. Multiple doses of activated charcoal may interrupt enterohepatic recycling of some NSAIDs.

Pharmacodynamics/Kinetics

Half-Life Elimination: 45-50 hours

Metabolism: Hepatic

Onset: Analgesic: ~1 hour; Peak effect: 3-5 hours

Formulations Capsule: 10 mg, 20 mg

Dosing

Adults: Inflammation, rheumatoid arthritis: Oral: 10-20 mg/day once daily; although associated with increase in GI adverse effects, doses >20 mg/day have been used (ie, 30-40 mg/day)

Elderly: Refer to adult dosing. **Note:** Some clinicians have used 10 mg every other day to initiate therapy in the elderly to help avoid side effects and produce therapeutic effect at minimal dose.

Pediatrics: Oral: Children: 0.2-0.3 mg/kg/day once daily; maximum dose: 15 mg/day

Hepatic Impairment: Reduced dose is necessary.

Monitoring Laboratory Tests Occult blood loss, hemoglobin, hematocrit, and periodic renal and hepatic function tests

Monitoring and Teaching Issues

Physical Assessment: Assess effectiveness and interactions of other medications patient may be taking (see Contraindications and Drug Interactions). Monitor laboratory tests (see above) and therapeutic and adverse reactions (eg, GI effects, hepatotoxicity, ototoxicity) at beginning of therapy and periodically throughout therapy (see Warnings/Precautions, Adverse Reactions, and Overdose/Toxicology). Schedule ophthalmic evaluations for patients who develop eye complaints during long-term NSAID therapy. Advise diabetic patients to use serum glucose testing (see Effects on Lab Values). Assess knowledge/teach patient appropriate use, interventions to reduce side effects, and adverse symptoms to report (see Patient Education). **Pregnancy risk factor B/D** - see Pregnancy Risk Factor for use cautions.

Patient Education: Take this medication exactly as directed; do not increase dose without consulting prescriber. Do not break capsules. Take with food or milk to reduce GI distress. Maintain adequate hydration (2-3 L/day of fluids) unless advised by prescriber to restrict fluids. Do not use alcohol, aspirin or aspirin-containing medication, or any other anti-inflammatory medications without consulting prescriber. You may experience drowsiness, dizziness, or nervousness (use caution when driving or engaging in tasks requiring alertness until response to drug is known); anorexia, nausea, vomiting, flatulence, or heartburn (small, frequent meals, frequent mouth care, sucking lozenges, or chewing gum may help); or fluid retention (weigh yourself weekly and report unusual weight gain [3-5 lb/wk]). GI bleeding, ulceration, or perforation can occur with or without pain; discontinue medication and contact prescriber if persistent abdominal pain or cramping, or blood in stool occurs. Report unusual swelling of extremities or unusual weight gain; breathlessness, difficulty breathing, or unusual cough; chest pain, rapid heartbeat, palpitations; unusual bruising/bleeding; blood in urine, stool, mouth, or vomitus; unusual fatigue; changes in urinary pattern (polyuria or anuria); skin rash or itching; or change in hearing or ringing in ears. **Pregnancy precaution:** Inform prescriber if you are or intend to become pregnant. This drug should not be used in the 3rd trimester of pregnancy.

Dietary Issues: May be taken with food to decrease GI adverse effect.

Geriatric Considerations: Elderly are at high risk for adverse effects from NSAIDs. As much as 60% of elderly can develop peptic ulceration and/or hemorrhage asymptomatically. The concomitant use of H_2 blockers, omeprazole, and sucralfate is not generally effective as prophylaxis with the exception of NSAID-induced duodenal ulcers which may be prevented by the use of ranitidine. Misoprostol is the only prophylactic agent proven effective. Also, concomitant disease and drug use contribute to the risk for GI adverse effects. Use lowest effective dose for shortest period possible. Consider renal function decline with age. Use of NSAIDs can compromise existing renal function especially when

(Continued)

Piroxicam *(Continued)*

Cl_{cr} is ≤30 mL/minute. Tinnitus may be a difficult and unreliable indication of toxicity due to age-related hearing loss or eighth cranial nerve damage. CNS adverse effects such as confusion, agitation, and hallucination are generally seen in overdose or high-dose situations, but elderly may demonstrate these adverse effects at lower doses than younger adults.

Related Information

Nonsalicylate/Nonsteroidal Anti-inflammatory Comparison *on page 1587*

p-Isobutylhydratropic Acid *see* Ibuprofen *on page 688*

Pit *see* Oxytocin *on page 1024*

Pitocin® *see* Oxytocin *on page 1024*

Pitressin® *see* Vasopressin *on page 1391*

Plan B® *see* Levonorgestrel *on page 793*

Plantago Seed *see* Psyllium *on page 1152*

Plantain Seed *see* Psyllium *on page 1152*

Plaquenil® *see* Hydroxychloroquine *on page 681*

Plaque Vaccine *see page 1498*

Plasbumin® *see* Albumin *on page 50*

Platinol® *see* Cisplatin *on page 298*

Platinol®-AQ *see* Cisplatin *on page 298*

Plavix® *see* Clopidogrel *on page 319*

Plendil® *see* Felodipine *on page 548*

Pletal® *see* Cilostazol *on page 288*

Plicamycin (plye kay MYE sin)

U.S. Brand Names Mithracin®

Synonyms Mithramycin

Generic Available No

Pharmacologic Category Antidote; Antineoplastic Agent, Antibiotic

Pregnancy Risk Factor X

Lactation Excretion in breast milk unknown/not recommended

Use Malignant testicular tumors, in the treatment of hypercalcemia and hypercalciuria of malignancy unresponsive to conventional treatment; Paget's disease; blast crisis of chronic granulocytic leukemia

Mechanism of Action/Effect Forms a complex with DNA in the presence of magnesium or other divalent cations inhibiting DNA-directed RNA synthesis

Contraindications Hypersensitivity to plicamycin or any component of the formulation; thrombocytopenia; thrombocytopathy; coagulation disorders or any other condition where a bleeding tendency is increased; bone marrow function impaired; pregnancy

Warnings/Precautions The U.S. Food and Drug Administration (FDA) currently recommends that procedures for proper handling and disposal of antineoplastic agents be considered. Use with caution in patients with hepatic or renal impairment. Reduce dosage in patients with renal impairment. Discontinue if bleeding or epistaxis occurs. **Note:** Dosing of plicamycin is in **micrograms**.

Drug Interactions

Increased Effect/Toxicity: Calcitonin, etidronate, or glucagon taken with plicamycin may result in additive hypoglycemic effects.

Nutritional/Ethanol Interactions Ethanol: Avoid ethanol (due to GI irritation).

Adverse Reactions Note: Adverse reactions appear to be dose-related and less common at the lower doses used to treat hypercalcemia.

>10%: Gastrointestinal: Anorexia, stomatitis, nausea, vomiting, diarrhea

Nausea and vomiting occur in almost 100% of patients within the first 6 hours after treatment; incidence increases with rapid injection; stomatitis has also occurred

Time course for nausea/vomiting: Onset 4-6 hours; Duration: 4-24 hours

1% to 10%:

Cardiovascular: Facial flushing

Central nervous system: Fever, headache, depression, drowsiness

Endocrine & metabolic: Hypocalcemia

Hematologic: Myelosuppressive: Mild leukopenia and thrombocytopenia

WBC: Moderate, but uncommon

Platelets: Moderate, rapid onset

Onset: 7-10 days

Nadir: 14 days

Recovery: 21 days

Clotting disorders: May also depress hepatic synthesis of clotting factors, leading to a form of coagulopathy; petechiae, increased prothrombin time, epistaxis, and thrombocytopenia may be seen and may require discontinuation of the drug. Epistaxis is frequently the first sign of this bleeding disorder.

Hepatic: Hepatotoxicity

Local: Pain at injection site

Irritant chemotherapy

Renal: Azotemia, nephrotoxicity

Miscellaneous: Hemorrhagic diathesis

Overdosage/Toxicology Symptoms of overdose include bone marrow suppression, bleeding syndrome, and thrombocytopenia. Treatment is symptom-directed and supportive.

Pharmacodynamics/Kinetics

Half-Life Elimination: Plasma: 1 hour

Onset: Decreasing calcium levels: ~24 hours; Peak effect: Decreasing calcium levels: 48-72 hours

Duration: Decreasing calcium levels: 5-15 days

Formulations Injection, powder for reconstitution: 2.5 mg

Dosing

Adults & Elderly: Refer to individual protocols. Dose should be diluted in 1 L of D_5W or NS and administered over 4-6 hours.

Note: Dosage should be based on the patient's body weight. If a patient has abnormal fluid retention (eg, edema, hydrothorax, or ascites), the patient's ideal weight rather than actual body weight should be used to calculate the dose.

Testicular cancer: I.V.: 25-30 mcg/kg/day for 8-10 days

Blastic chronic granulocytic leukemia: I.V.: 25 mcg/kg over 2-4 hours every other day for 3 weeks

Paget's disease: I.V.: 15 mcg/kg/day once daily for 10 days

Hypercalcemia: I.V.: 25 mcg/kg single dose which may be repeated in 48 hours if no response occurs

or 25 mcg/kg for 3-4 days

or 25-50 mcg/kg every other day for 3-8 doses

Renal Impairment:

Cl_{cr} 10-50 mL/minute: Decrease dosage to 75% of normal dose.

Cl_{cr} <10 mL/minute: Decrease dosage to 50% of normal dose.

Hemodialysis effects: Unknown

CAPD effects: Unknown

CAVH effects: Unknown

Hepatic Impairment: Treatment of hypercalcemia in patients with hepatic dysfunction: Reduce dose to 12.5 mcg/kg/day.

Administration

I.V.: Irritant. Rapid I.V. infusion has been associated with an increased incidence of nausea and vomiting; an antiemetic given prior to and during plicamycin infusion may be helpful. Administer I.V. infusion over 4-6 hours.

Stability

Storage: Store intact vials under refrigeration (2°C to 8°C). Vials are stable at room temperature (<25°C) for up to 3 months.

Reconstitution: Dilute powder in 4.9 mL SWI to result in a concentration of 500 mcg/mL which is stable for 24 hours at room temperature (25°C) and 48 hours under refrigeration (4°C). Further dilution in 1000 mL D_5W or NS is stable for 24 hours at room temperature.

Standard I.V. dilution: Dose/1000 mL D_5W or NS; solution is stable for 24 hours at room temperature (25°C).

Compatibility: Stable in D_5W, NS, sterile water for injection

Y-site administration: Incompatible with cefepime

Monitoring Laboratory Tests Hepatic and renal function, CBC, platelet count, prothrombin time, serum electrolytes

Monitoring and Teaching Issues

Physical Assessment: Assess effectiveness and interactions of other medications patient may be taking (see Drug Interactions). See Warnings/Precautions, Contraindications, and Administration for use cautions. Monitor effectiveness of therapy and monitor laboratory tests frequently during therapy (see above). Monitor closely for adverse response (see Adverse Reactions and Overdose/Toxicology). Assess knowledge/teach patient possible side effects and appropriate interventions and adverse symptoms to report (see Patient Education). **Pregnancy risk factor X** - determine that patient is not pregnant before beginning treatment. Instruct patients of childbearing age about appropriate contraceptive measures. Breast-feeding is not recommended.

Patient Education: This medication can only be administered I.V. and frequent blood tests will be necessary to monitor effects of the drug. Report pain, swelling, or irritation at infusion site. Do not take alcohol, and prescription or OTC medications containing aspirin or ibuprofen without consulting prescriber. Maintain adequate hydration (2-3 L/day of fluids) unless advised by prescriber to restrict fluids. Maintain good oral hygiene (use soft toothbrush or cotton applicators several times a day and rinse mouth frequently). You will be susceptible to infection (avoid crowds and exposure to infection and do not receive any vaccinations unless approved by prescriber). Report persistent fever or chills, unhealed sores, oral or vaginal sores, foul-smelling urine, easy bruising or bleeding, yellowing of eyes or skin, or change in color of urine or stool. **Pregnancy/breast-feeding precautions:** Do not get pregnant while taking this medication - use appropriate contraceptive measures. Breast-feeding is not recommended.

PMPA *see* Tenofovir *on page 1287*

Pneumococcal 7 Valent Conjugate Vaccine *see page 1498*

Pneumococcal Vaccine *see page 1498*

Pneumovax® 23 *see page 1498*

Pnu-Imune® 23 *see page 1498*

Podocon-25™ *see* Podophyllum Resin *on page 1097*

Podofin® *see* Podophyllum Resin *on page 1097*

Podophyllin *see* Podophyllum Resin *on page 1097*

Podophyllum Resin (po DOF fil um REZ in)

U.S. Brand Names Podocon-25™; Podofin®

Synonyms Mandrake; May Apple; Podophyllin

Generic Available No

Pharmacologic Category Keratolytic Agent

Pregnancy Risk Factor X

Lactation Enters breast milk/contraindicated

Use Topical treatment of benign growths including external genital and perianal warts, papillomas, fibroids; compound benzoin tincture generally is used as the medium for topical application

(Continued)

Podophyllum Resin *(Continued)*

Mechanism of Action/Effect Directly affects epithelial cell metabolism by arresting mitosis through binding to a protein subunit of spindle microtubules (tubulin)

Contraindications Not to be used on birthmarks, moles, or warts with hair growth; cervical, urethral, oral warts; not to be used by diabetic patient or patient with poor circulation; pregnancy

Warnings/Precautions Use of large amounts of drug should be avoided. Avoid contact with the eyes as it can cause severe corneal damage; do not apply to moles, birthmarks, or unusual warts. To be applied by prescriber only. For external use only; 25% solution should not be applied to or near mucous membranes.

Adverse Reactions

1% to 10%:

Dermatologic: Pruritus

Gastrointestinal: Nausea, vomiting, abdominal pain, diarrhea

<1% (Limited to important or life-threatening): Hepatotoxicity, leukopenia, peripheral neuropathy, renal failure, thrombocytopenia

Formulations Liquid, topical: 25% (15 mL) [in benzoin tincture]

Dosing

Adults & Elderly: Treatment of benign growths (warts, papillomas, fibroids): Topical: 10% to 25% solution in compound benzoin tincture; apply drug to dry surface, use 1 drop at a time allowing drying between drops until area is covered. Total volume should be limited to <0.5 mL per treatment session.

Condylomata acuminatum: 25% solution is applied daily. Use a 10% solution when applied to or near mucous membranes.

Verrucae: 25% solution is applied 3-5 times/day directly to the wart.

Pediatrics: Refer to adult dosing.

Administration

Topical: Shake well before using. **Only to be applied by physician.** Solution should be washed off within 1-4 hours for genital and perianal warts and within 1-2 hours for accessible meatal warts. Use protective occlusive dressing around warts to prevent contact with unaffected skin. For external use only.

Monitoring and Teaching Issues

Physical Assessment: See Contraindications, Warnings/Precautions, and Administration. **Pregnancy risk factor X** - determine that patient is not pregnant before starting therapy. Do not give to sexually-active female patients unless capable of complying with barrier contraceptive use. Breast-feeding is contraindicated.

Patient Education: Cover with occlusive dressing to prevent contact with unaffected skin. Wash off medication as instructed by professional who applied the treatment. **Pregnancy/breast-feeding precautions:** Inform prescriber if you are pregnant. Do not get pregnant during or for 1 month following therapy. Consult prescriber for instruction on appropriate barrier contraceptive measures. This drug may cause severe fetal defects. Do not breast-feed.

Polaramine® [DSC] *see* Dexchlorpheniramine *on page 385*

Poliovirus Vaccine, Inactivated *see page 1498*

Polycitra®-K *see* Potassium Citrate and Citric Acid *on page 1104*

Polycitra® Syrup *see page 1522*

Polyethylene Glycol-Electrolyte Solution

(pol i ETH i leen GLY kol ee LEK troe lite soe LOO shun)

U.S. Brand Names Colyte®; GoLYTELY®; MiraLax™; NuLytely®; OCL®

Synonyms Electrolyte Lavage Solution

Generic Available No

Pharmacologic Category Cathartic; Laxative, Bowel Evacuant

Pregnancy Risk Factor C

Lactation Excretion in breast milk unknown/use caution

Use Bowel cleansing prior to GI examination or following toxic ingestion (electrolyte containing solutions only); treatment of occasional constipation (MiraLax™)

Mechanism of Action/Effect Induces catharsis by strong electrolyte and osmotic effects

Contraindications Hypersensitivity to polyethylene glycol or any component of the formulation; gastrointestinal obstruction, gastric retention, bowel perforation, toxic colitis, megacolon

Warnings/Precautions Do not add flavorings as additional ingredients before use. Observe unconscious or semiconscious patients with impaired gag reflex or those who are otherwise prone to regurgitation or aspiration during administration. Use with caution in ulcerative colitis. Caution against the use of hot loop polypectomy. Do not use MiraLax™ for longer than 2 weeks. Pregnancy risk C.

Drug Interactions

Decreased Effect: Oral medications should not be administered within 1 hour of start of therapy.

Adverse Reactions Frequency not defined.

Dermatologic: Dermatitis, rash, urticaria

Gastrointestinal: Nausea, abdominal fullness, bloating, abdominal cramps, vomiting, anal irritation, diarrhea, flatulence

Postmarketing and/or case reports: Anaphylaxis, asystole, dehydration and hypokalemia (reported in children), dyspnea (acute), esophageal perforation, Mallory-Weiss tear, pulmonary edema, upper GI bleeding, vomiting with aspiration of PEG

Pharmacodynamics/Kinetics

Onset: Oral: Bowel cleansing: ~1-2 hours; Constipation: 48-96 hours

Formulations

Powder for oral solution:

Colyte®:

PEG 3350 240 g, sodium sulfate 22.72 g, sodium bicarbonate 6.72 g, sodium chloride 5.84 g, and potassium chloride 2.98 g (to make 4000 mL) [cherry, citrus berry, lemon-lime, and pineapple flavors]

PEG 3350 227.1 g, sodium sulfate 21.5 g, sodium bicarbonate 6.36 g, sodium chloride 5.53 g, and potassium chloride 2.82 g (to make 4000 mL) [pineapple and regular flavors]

GoLYTELY®:

Disposable jug: PEG 3350 236 g, sodium sulfate 22.74 g, sodium bicarbonate 6.74 g, sodium chloride 5.86 g, and potassium chloride 2.97 g (to make 4000 mL) [pineapple and regular flavors]

Packets: PEG 3350 227.1 g, sodium sulfate 21.5 g, sodium bicarbonate 6.36 g, sodium chloride 5.53 g, and potassium chloride 2.82 g (to make 4000 mL) [regular flavor]

MiraLax™: PEG 3350 255 g (to make 14 oz); PEG 3350 527 g (to make 26 oz)

NuLytely®: PEG 3350 420 g, sodium bicarbonate 5.72 g, sodium chloride 11.2 g, and potassium chloride 1.48 (to make 4000 mL) [cherry, lemon-lime, and orange flavors]

Solution, oral (OCL®): PEG 3350 6 g, sodium sulfate decahydrate 1.29 g, sodium bicarbonate 168 mg, potassium chloride 75 mg, and polysorbate 80 30 mg per 100 mL (1500 mL)

Dosing

Adults & Elderly:

Bowel cleansing prior to GI exam (solutions with electrolytes only):

Oral: 240 mL (8 oz) every 10 minutes, until 4 L are consumed or the rectal effluent is clear; rapid drinking of each portion is preferred to drinking small amounts continuously. Ideally, patients should fast for ~3-4 hours prior to administration; absolutely no solid food for at least 2 hours before the solution is given. The solution may be given via nasogastric tube to patients who are unwilling or unable to drink the solution.

Nasogastric tube: 20-30 mL/minute (1.2-1.8 L/hour); the first bowel movement should occur ~1 hour after the start of administration. Ideally, patients should fast for ~3-4 hours prior to administration; absolutely no solid food for at least 2 hours before the solution is given.

Occasional constipation (MiraLax™): Oral: 17 g of powder (~1 heaping tablespoon) dissolved in 8 oz of water; once daily; do not use for >2 weeks.

Pediatrics: Children ≥6 months: Bowel cleansing (solutions with electrolytes only): Ideally, patients should fast for ~3-4 hours prior to administration; absolutely no solid food for at least 2 hours before the solution is given.

Oral: 25-40 mL/kg/hour for 4-10 hours until rectal effluent is clear

Nasogastric tube: 25 mL/kg/hour until rectal effluent is clear

Administration

Oral: Bowel cleansing prior to GI exam (solutions with electrolytes only): Oral: Rapid drinking of each portion is preferred to drinking small amounts continuously. Do not add flavorings as additional ingredients before use. Chilled solution often more palatable.

Stability

Storage: Store at 15°C to 30°C (59°F to 86°F) before reconstitution.

Reconstitution:

Powder for solution (with electrolytes): Use within 48 hours of preparation; refrigerate reconstituted solution; tap water may be used for preparation of the solution; shake container vigorously several times to ensure dissolution of powder. Do not add additional flavorings to solution.

MiraLax™: Dissolve powder in 8 ounces of water, juice, cola, or tea

Monitoring Laboratory Tests Electrolytes, serum glucose, BUN, urine osmolality

Monitoring and Teaching Issues

Physical Assessment: See Contraindications, Warnings/Precautions, Drug Interactions, and Adverse Reactions for use cautions. Instruct patient in appropriate use (see above for specific instructions according to formulation and purpose). **Pregnancy risk factor C** - benefits of use should outweigh possible risks. Note breast-feeding caution.

Patient Education: Follow instructions exactly; directions will differ according to the formulation and the purpose for which this medication is taken. Do not eat any solid foods for at least 2 -3 hours before taking and do not take any other oral medication for 1 hour before taking. For bowel cleansing prior to GI exam, take 240 mL (8 oz) every 10 minutes, until 4 L is consumed or the rectal effluent is clear. Rapid drinking of each portion is preferred to drinking small amounts continuously. The first bowel movement should occur approximately 1 hour after the start of administration. May cause abdominal bloating and distention before bowel starts to move. If severe discomfort or distention occurs, stop drinking temporarily or drink each portion at longer intervals until these symptoms disappear. Continue drinking until the watery stool is clear and free of solid matter. This usually requires at least 3 L. It is best to drink all of the solutions. Discard any unused portion. **Pregnancy/breast-feeding precautions:** Inform prescriber if you are or intend to become pregnant. Consult prescriber if breast-feeding.

Dietary Issues: Bowel cleansing prior to GI exam: Ideally, the patient should fast for ~3-4 hours prior to administration, but in no case should solid food be given for at least 2 hours before the solution is given.

Breast-feeding Issues: Significant changes in the mother's fluid or electrolyte balance would not be expected.

Related Information

Laxatives: Classification and Properties *on page 1581*

Polygam® S/D *see* Immune Globulin (Intravenous) *on page 703*

Polymyxin B (pol i MIX in bee)

Synonyms Polymyxin B Sulfate

Generic Available Yes

Pharmacologic Category Antibiotic, Irrigation; Antibiotic, Miscellaneous

Pregnancy Risk Factor B (per expert opinion)

Lactation Excretion in breast milk unknown/use caution

Use Treatment of acute infections caused by susceptible strains of *Pseudomonas aeruginosa*; used occasionally for gut decontamination; parenteral use of polymyxin B has mainly been replaced by less toxic antibiotics, reserved for life-threatening infections caused by organisms resistant to the preferred drugs (eg, pseudomonal meningitis - intrathecal administration)

Mechanism of Action/Effect Binds to phospholipids, alters permeability, and damages the bacterial cytoplasmic membrane permitting leakage of intracellular constituents

Contraindications Hypersensitivity to polymyxin B or any component of the formulation; concurrent use of neuromuscular blockers

Warnings/Precautions Use with caution in patients with impaired renal function (modify dosage) neurotoxic reactions are usually associated with high serum levels, found in patients with impaired renal function. Avoid concurrent or sequential use of other nephrotoxic and neurotoxic drugs, particularly bacitracin, colistin, and the aminoglycosides. The drug's neurotoxicity can result in respiratory paralysis from neuromuscular blockade, especially when the drug is given soon after anesthesia or muscle relaxants. Polymyxin B sulfate is toxic when given parenterally; avoid parenteral use whenever possible.

Drug Interactions

Increased Effect/Toxicity: Increased/prolonged effect of neuromuscular blocking agents.

Adverse Reactions Frequency not defined (limited to important or life-threatening):

Central nervous system: Neurotoxicity (irritability, drowsiness, ataxia, perioral paresthesia, numbness of the extremities, and blurring of vision); dizziness

Neuromuscular & skeletal: Neuromuscular blockade

Renal: Nephrotoxicity

Respiratory: Respiratory arrest

Overdosage/Toxicology Symptoms of overdose include respiratory paralysis, ototoxicity, and nephrotoxicity. Supportive care is indicated as treatment.

Pharmacodynamics/Kinetics

Absorption: Well absorbed from peritoneum; minimal from GI tract (except in neonates) from mucous membranes or intact skin

Half-Life Elimination: 4.5-6 hours; prolonged with renal impairment

Time to Peak: Serum: I.M.: ~2 hours

Formulations Powder: 500,000 units/vial

Dosing

Adults & Elderly:

Ear canal infections (external): Otic (in combination with other drugs): Instill 1-2 drops, 3-4 times/day; should be used sparingly to avoid accumulation of excess debris.

Systemic infections:

I.M.: 25,000-30,000 units/kg/day divided every 4-6 hours

I.V.: 15,000-25,000 units/kg/day divided every 12 hours

Intrathecal: 50,000 units/day for 3-4 days, then every other day for at least 2 weeks

Note: Total daily dose should not exceed 2,000,000 units/day.

Bladder irrigation (in combination with 57 mg neomycin sulfate): Continuous irrigant or rinse in the urinary bladder for up to 10 days using 20 mg (equal to 200,000 units) added to 1 L of normal saline; usually no more than 1 L of irrigant is used per day unless urine flow rate is high; administration rate is adjusted to patient's urine output.

Topical irrigation or topical solution: 500,000 units/L of normal saline; topical irrigation should not exceed 2 million units/day in adults.

Ocular infections: Ophthalmic: A concentration of 0.1% to 0.25% is administered as 1-3 drops every hour, then increasing the interval as response indicates to 1-2 drops 4-6 times/day.

Pediatrics:

Ear canal infections (external): Otic (in combination with other drugs): 1-2 drops, 3-4 times/day; should be used sparingly to avoid accumulation of excess debris

Systemic infections: Infants <2 years:

I.M.: Up to 40,000 units/kg/day divided every 6 hours (not routinely recommended due to pain at injection sites)

I.V.: Up to 40,000 units/kg/day divided every 12 hours

Intrathecal: 20,000 units/day for 3-4 days, then 25,000 units every other day for at least 2 weeks after CSF cultures are negative and CSF (glucose) has returned to within normal limits

Children ≥2 years: Refer to adult dosing.

Renal Impairment:

Cl_{cr} 20-50 mL/minute: Administer 75% to 100% of normal dose every 12 hours.

Cl_{cr} 5-20 mL/minute: Administer 50% of normal dose every 12 hours.

Cl_{cr} <5 mL/minute: Administer 15% of normal dose every 12 hours.

Administration

I.M.: Administer into upper outer quadrant of gluteal muscle; however, I.M. route is not recommended due to severe pain at injection site.

I.V.: Infuse over 60-90 minutes.

Stability

Storage: Prior to reconstitution, store at room temperature of 15°C to 30°C (59°F to 86°F) and protect from light. After reconstitution, store under refrigeration at 2°C to 8°C (36°F to 46°F). Discard any unused solution after 72 hours. **Incompatible** with strong acids/alkalies, calcium, magnesium, cephalothin, cefazolin, chloramphenicol, heparin, penicillins.

Compatibility: when admixed: Incompatible with amphotericin B, calcium chloride, calcium gluconate, cefazolin, chloramphenicol, chlorothiazide, heparin, magnesium sulfate

Monitoring Laboratory Tests Perform culture and sensitivity prior to beginning therapy. Establish baseline renal function prior to initiating therapy. Monitor renal function closely.

Monitoring and Teaching Issues

Physical Assessment: Assess for allergy history prior to starting therapy. See Contraindications, Warnings/Precautions, and Dosing for use cautions. Assess potential for interactions with other prescriptions, OTC medications, or herbal products patient may be taking (eg, other nephrotoxic and neurotoxic drugs - see Drug Interactions). See Administration specifics; infusion site must be monitored closely to prevent extravasation. Assess results of laboratory tests (see above), therapeutic effectiveness, and adverse reactions (eg, neurotoxicity - irritability, drowsiness, ataxia, perioral paresthesia, numbness of the extremities, and blurring of vision; neuromuscular blockade - see Adverse Reactions and Overdose/Toxicology). Teach patient possible side effects and interventions and adverse symptoms to report (see Patient Education). Note breast-feeding caution.

Patient Education: Wound irrigation/bladder irrigation/gut sterilization/I.V.: Immediately report numbness or tingling of mouth, tongue, or extremities; constant blurring of vision; increased nervousness or irritability; excessive drowsiness; or difficulty breathing. For I.V. immediately report swelling, redness, burning, or pain at infusion site.

Ophthalmic: Tilt head back, place medication into eyes (as frequently as prescribed), close eyes, apply light pressure over inside corner of the eye for 1 minute. Do not let tip of applicator touch eye; do not contaminate tip of applicator (may cause eye infection, eye damage, or vision loss). You may experience some stinging or burning or temporary blurring of vision; use caution driving or when engaging in hazardous tasks until vision clears. Report any adverse effects including difficulty breathing or unusual numbness or tingling of mouth or tongue, increased nervousness or irritability, or excessive drowsiness.

Breast-feeding precaution: Consult prescriber if breast-feeding.

Additional Information 1 mg = 10,000 units

Polymyxin B and Bacitracin *see* Bacitracin and Polymyxin B *on page 144*

Polymyxin B and Hydrocortisone *see page 1519*

Polymyxin B and Neomycin *see* Neomycin and Polymyxin B *on page 960*

Polymyxin B, Bacitracin, and Neomycin *see* Bacitracin, Neomycin, and Polymyxin B *on page 144*

Polymyxin B, Bacitracin, Neomycin, and Hydrocortisone *see* Bacitracin, Neomycin, Polymyxin B, and Hydrocortisone *on page 145*

Polymyxin B Sulfate *see* Polymyxin B *on page 1100*

Poly-Pred® *see page 1509*

Polysporin® *see page 1509*

Polysporin® Ophthalmic *see* Bacitracin and Polymyxin B *on page 144*

Polysporin® Topical [OTC] *see* Bacitracin and Polymyxin B *on page 144*

Polythiazide and Prazosin *see* Prazosin and Polythiazide *on page 1113*

Polytrim® *see page 1509*

Porfimer (POR fi mer)

U.S. Brand Names Photofrin®

Synonyms CL184116; Dihematoporphyrin Ether; Porfimer Sodium

Generic Available No

Pharmacologic Category Antineoplastic Agent, Miscellaneous

Pregnancy Risk Factor C

Lactation Enters breast milk/contraindicated

Use Orphan drug: Photodynamic therapy (PDT) with porfimer for palliation of patients with completely obstructing esophageal cancer, or of patients with partially obstructing esophageal cancer who cannot be satisfactorily treated with Nd:YAG laser therapy; completely- or partially-obstructing endobronchial nonsmall cell lung cancer; microinvasive endobronchial nonsmall cell lung cancer

Mechanism of Action/Effect Photosensitizing agent used in the photodynamic therapy (PDT) of tumors: cytotoxic and antitumor actions of porfimer are light and oxygen dependent. Cellular damage caused by porfimer PDT is a consequence of the propagation of radical reactions.

Contraindications Hypersensitivity to porfimer, porphyrins, or any component of the formulation; porphyria; tracheoesophageal or bronchoesophageal fistula; tumors eroding into a major blood vessel

Warnings/Precautions The U.S. Food and Drug Administration (FDA) currently recommends that procedures for proper handling and disposal of antineoplastic agents be considered. Appropriate safety equipment is recommended for preparation, administration, and disposal of antineoplastics. If porfimer contacts the skin, wash and flush thoroughly with water.

If the esophageal tumor is eroding into the trachea or bronchial tree, the likelihood of tracheoesophageal or bronchoesophageal fistula resulting from treatment is sufficiently high that PDT is not recommended. All patients who receive porfimer sodium will be photosensitive and must observe precautions to avoid exposure of skin and eyes to direct sunlight or bright indoor light for 30 days. The photosensitivity is due to residual drug which will be present in all parts of the skin. Exposure of the skin to ambient indoor light is, however, beneficial because the remaining drug will be inactivated gradually and safely through a photobleaching reaction. Patients should not stay in a darkened room during this period and should be encouraged to expose their skin to ambient indoor light. Ocular discomfort has been reported; for 30 days, when outdoors, patients should wear dark sunglasses which have an average white light transmittance <4%.

Pregnancy risk C.

Drug Interactions

Decreased Effect: Compounds that quench active oxygen species or scavenge radicals (eg, dimethyl sulfoxide, beta-carotene, ethanol, mannitol) would be expected to decrease

(Continued)

Porfimer *(Continued)*

photodynamic therapy (PDT) activity. Allopurinol, calcium channel blockers, and some prostaglandin synthesis inhibitors could interfere with porfimer. Drugs that decrease clotting, vasoconstriction, or platelet aggregation could decrease the efficacy of PDT. Glucocorticoid hormones may decrease the efficacy of the treatment.

Increased Effect/Toxicity: Concomitant administration of other photosensitizing agents (eg, tetracyclines, sulfonamides, phenothiazines, sulfonylureas, thiazide diuretics, griseofulvin) could increase the photosensitivity reaction.

Adverse Reactions

>10%:

Cardiovascular: Atrial fibrillation, chest pain
Central nervous system: Fever, pain, insomnia
Dermatologic: Photosensitivity reaction
Gastrointestinal: abdominal pain, constipation, dysphagia, nausea, vomiting
Emetic potential: Low (10% to 30%)
Hematologic: Anemia
Neuromuscular & skeletal: Back pain
Respiratory: Dyspnea, pharyngitis, pleural effusion, pneumonia, respiratory insufficiency

1% to 10%:

Cardiovascular: Hypertension, hypotension, edema, cardiac failure, tachycardia, chest pain (substernal)
Central nervous system: Anxiety, confusion
Endocrine & metabolic: Dehydration
Gastrointestinal: Diarrhea, heartburn, eructation, esophageal edema, esophageal tumor bleeding, esophageal stricture, esophagitis, hematemesis, melena, weight loss, anorexia
Genitourinary: Urinary tract infection
Neuromuscular & skeletal: Weakness
Respiratory: Coughing, tracheoesophageal fistula
Miscellaneous: Moniliasis, surgical complication

Overdosage/Toxicology Increased symptoms and damage to normal tissue might be expected with overdose of laser light following porfimer injection. Effects of overdose on the duration of photosensitivity are unknown. Laser treatment should not be given if an overdose of porfimer is administered. In the event of overdose, patients should protect their eyes and skin from direct sunlight or bright indoor lights for 30 days. At this time, patients should be tested for residual photosensitivity. Porfimer is not dialyzable.

Pharmacodynamics/Kinetics

Half-Life Elimination: 250 hours

Time to Peak: Serum: ~2 hours

Formulations Injection, powder for reconstitution, as sodium: 75 mg

Dosing

Adults & Elderly:

Cancer photodynamic therapy: I.V.: 2 mg/kg over 3-5 minutes

Photodynamic therapy (PDT) is a two-stage process requiring administration of both drug and light. The first stage of PDT is the I.V. injection of porfimer. Illumination with laser light 40-50 hours following the injection with porfimer constitutes the second stage of therapy. A second laser light application may be given 90-120 hours after injection, preceded by gentle debridement of residual tumor.

Patients may receive a second course of PDT a minimum of 30 days after the initial therapy; up to three courses of PDT (each separated by a minimum of 30 days) can be given. Before each course of treatment, evaluate patients for the presence of a tracheoesophageal or bronchoesophageal fistula.

Pediatrics: I.V. (refer to individual protocols): Children: Safety and efficacy have not been established.

Administration

I.V.: Administer slow I.V. injection over 3-5 minutes.

Stability

Storage: Store intact vials at controlled room temperature of 20°C to 25°C/68°F to 77°F.

Reconstitution: Reconstitute each vial of porfimer with 31.8 mL of either 5% dextrose injection or 0.9% sodium chloride injection resulting in a final concentration of 2.5 mg/mL and a pH of 7-8. Shake well until dissolved. Protect the reconstituted product from bright light and use immediately. Reconstituted porfimer is an opaque solution in which detection of particulate matter by visual inspection is extremely difficult.

Compatibility: Do not mix porfimer with other drugs in the same solution.

Monitoring and Teaching Issues

Physical Assessment: See Contraindications, Warnings/Precautions, and Dosing for use cautions. Assess potential for interactions with other prescriptions, OTC medications, or herbal products patient may be taking (eg, other nephrotoxic and neurotoxic drugs - see Drug Interactions). See Administration specifics; infusion site must be monitored closely to prevent extravasation. Patients will be photosensitive and must be protected from direct sunlight or bright indoor light for 30 days after treatment. Ambient indoor light is, however, beneficial (should not stay in dark rooms). Assess patient response (see Adverse Reactions and Overdose/Toxicology). Teach patient (caregiver) possible side effects and interventions and adverse symptoms to report (see Patient Education). **Pregnancy risk factor C** - benefits of use should outweigh possible risks. Breast-feeding is contraindicated

Patient Education: Inform prescriber of all prescriptions, OTC medications, or herbal products you are taking, and any allergies you have. Do not take anything new during treatment unless approved by prescriber. This drug can only be given by injection or infusion. Report immediately any redness, swelling, burning, or pain at infusion site. The infusion will be followed by laser light therapy. Maintain adequate hydration (2-3 L/day of fluids) unless advised by prescriber to restrict fluids. You will be highly sensitive to bright light. Avoid exposure to sunlight or bright indoor light for at least 30 days following treatment (cover skin with protective clothing and wear dark sunglasses with light transmittance

<4% when outdoors - severe blistering, burning, and skin/eye damage can result). Conventional sunscreens do not protect against photosensitization. After 30 days, test small area of skin (not face) for remaining sensitivity. Retest sensitivity if traveling to a different geographic area with greater sunshine. Exposure to indoor normal light is beneficial since it will help dissipate photosensitivity gradually. May cause nausea or vomiting (small, frequent meals, frequent mouth care, sucking lozenges, or chewing gum may help); or constipation (increased exercise, fluids, fruit, or fiber may help). Report rapid heart rate, chest pain or palpitations, difficulty breathing or air hunger, persistent fever or chills, foul-smelling urine or burning on urination, swelling of extremities, increased anxiety, confusion, or hallucination. **Pregnancy/breast-feeding precautions:** Inform prescriber if you are pregnant. Do not breast-feed.

Porfimer Sodium *see* Porfimer *on page 1101*

Portia™ *see* Ethinyl Estradiol and Levonorgestrel *on page 523*

Post Peel Healing Balm [OTC] *see* Hydrocortisone *on page 673*

Posture® [OTC] *see* Calcium Supplements *on page 202*

Potasalan® *see* Potassium Supplements *on page 1106*

Potassium Acetate *see* Potassium Supplements *on page 1106*

Potassium Acetate, Potassium Bicarbonate, and Potassium Citrate *see* Potassium Supplements *on page 1106*

Potassium Acid Phosphate *see* Phosphate Supplements *on page 1076*

Potassium Acid Phosphate *see* Potassium Supplements *on page 1106*

Potassium Bicarbonate *see* Potassium Supplements *on page 1106*

Potassium Bicarbonate and Potassium Chloride *see* Potassium Supplements *on page 1106*

Potassium Bicarbonate and Potassium Chloride (Effervescent)

(poe TASS ee um bye KAR bun ate & poe TASS ee um KLOR ide, ef er VES ent)

U.S. Brand Names Klorvess® Effervescent; K-Lyte/Cl®

Synonyms Potassium Bicarbonate and Potassium Chloride (Effervescent)

Generic Available No

Pharmacologic Category Electrolyte Supplement, Oral

Pregnancy Risk Factor C

Lactation Enters breast milk/compatible

Use Treatment or prevention of hypokalemia

Warnings/Precautions Use with caution in patients with renal disease, cardiac disease.

Drug Interactions

Increased Effect/Toxicity: Potassium-sparing diuretics, salt substitutes, ACE inhibitors

Formulations

Tablet for oral solution, effervescent:

Klorvess®: 20 mEq per packet

K-Lyte/Cl®: 25 mEq, 50 mEq per packet

Dosing

Adults & Elderly: Hypokalemia: Oral:

Prevention: 16-24 mEq/day in 2-4 divided doses

Treatment: 40-100 mEq/day in 2-4 divided doses

Monitoring and Teaching Issues

Physical Assessment: Assess for adequate kidney function, use of ACE inhibitors, or potassium-sparing diuretics prior to starting therapy. Monitor cardiac status and serum potassium levels on a regular basis with long-term therapy. Instruct patient on appropriate diet and administration. **Pregnancy risk factor C.**

Patient Education: Take as directed; do not take more than directed. Dissolve granules, powder, or tablets in 4-6 oz of water or juice and stir before drinking. Do not take on an empty stomach; take with or after meals. Consult prescriber about increasing dietary potassium intake (eg, salt substitutes, orange juice, bananas, etc). Report tingling of hands or feet, unresolved nausea or vomiting, chest pain, palpitations, persistent abdominal pain, muscle cramping or weakness, tarry stools, easy bruising, or unusual bleeding. **Pregnancy precaution:** Inform prescriber if you are pregnant.

Potassium Bicarbonate and Potassium Citrate *see* Potassium Supplements *on page 1106*

Potassium Chloride *see* Potassium Supplements *on page 1106*

Potassium Chloride and Potassium Gluconate *see* Potassium Supplements *on page 1106*

Potassium Citrate (poe TASS ee um SIT rate)

U.S. Brand Names Urocit®-K

Generic Available No

Pharmacologic Category Alkalinizing Agent

Pregnancy Risk Factor Not available

Lactation Enters breast milk/compatible

Use Prevention of uric acid nephrolithiasis; prevention of calcium renal stones in patients with hypocitraturia; urinary alkalinizer when sodium citrate is contraindicated

Contraindications Severe renal insufficiency; sodium-restricted diet (sodium citrate); untreated Addison's disease; severe myocardial damage; acute dehydration; patients with hyperkalemia; patients with delayed gastric emptying, esophageal compression, intestinal obstruction or stricture, or those taking anticholinergic medication; patients with active urinary tract infection

Warnings/Precautions Use caution in patients with CHF, hypertension, edema, or any condition sensitive to sodium or potassium intake. Citrate is converted to bicarbonate in the liver. This conversion may be blocked in patients who are severely ill, in shock, or in hepatic failure. Use caution with potassium-sparing diuretics and drugs that slow GI transit time.

(Continued)

Potassium Citrate *(Continued)*

Drug Interactions

Increased Effect/Toxicity: Concurrent administration with potassium-containing medications, potassium-sparing diuretics, ACE inhibitors, or cardiac glycosides could lead to toxicity.

Adverse Reactions

>10%: Gastrointestinal: Diarrhea, nausea, stomach pain, flatulence, vomiting (oral)

1% to 10%:

Cardiovascular: Bradycardia

Endocrine & metabolic: Hyperkalemia, metabolic alkalosis in patients with severe renal failure

Neuromuscular & skeletal: Weakness

Respiratory: Dyspnea

<1% (Limited to important or life-threatening): Arrhythmias, chest pain, heart block, hypotension

Pharmacodynamics/Kinetics

Metabolism: Hepatic to bicarbonate

Formulations Tablet: 540 mg [5 mEq]; 1080 mg [10 mEq]

Dosing

Adults & Elderly: Alkalinizer, bicarbonate precursor: Oral: 10-20 mEq 3 times/day with meals up to 100 mEq/day

Administration

Oral: Swallow tablets whole with a full glass of water.

Stability

Storage: Store in a cool, dry place.

Monitoring and Teaching Issues

Physical Assessment: See Contraindications and Warnings/Precautions for use cautions. Assess effectiveness and interactions of other medications patient may be taking (see Drug Interactions). Assess kidney function prior to starting therapy. Monitor cardiac status and serum potassium at beginning of therapy and at regular intervals with long-term therapy. Assess knowledge/teach patient appropriate use, recommended diet, and adverse symptoms to report (see Patient Education).

Patient Education: Take as directed; do not take more than directed. Swallow tablet whole with full glass of water or juice and stir before sipping slowly, with or after meals (do not take on an empty stomach). Take any antacids 2 hours before or after potassium. Consult prescriber about advisability of increasing dietary potassium. Report tingling of hands or feet; unresolved nausea or vomiting; chest pain or palpitations; persistent abdominal pain; feelings of weakness, dizziness, listlessness, confusion; acute muscle weakness or cramping; blood in stool or tarry stools; or easy bruising or unusual bleeding.

Dietary Issues: May be taken with meals.

Potassium Citrate *see* Potassium Supplements *on page 1106*

Potassium Citrate and Citric Acid (poe TASS ee um SIT rate & SI trik AS id)

U.S. Brand Names Polycitra®-K

Synonyms Citric Acid and Potassium Citrate

Generic Available No

Pharmacologic Category Alkalinizing Agent

Pregnancy Risk Factor A

Lactation Excretion in breast milk unknown/compatible

Use Treatment of metabolic acidosis; alkalinizing agent in conditions where long-term maintenance of an alkaline urine is desirable

Contraindications Severe renal insufficiency, oliguria, or azotemia; potassium-restricted diet; untreated Addison's disease; adynamia episodica hereditaria; acute dehydration; heat cramps; anuria; severe myocardial damage; hyperkalemia from any cause

Warnings/Precautions Use with caution in patients with CHF, hypertension, pulmonary edema, or severe renal impairment. Large doses may cause hyperkalemia and alkalosis.

Drug Interactions

Increased Effect/Toxicity: Concurrent administration with potassium-containing medications, potassium-sparing diuretics, ACE inhibitors, or cardiac glycosides could lead to toxicity.

Adverse Reactions

>10%: Gastrointestinal: Diarrhea, nausea, stomach pain, flatulence, vomiting (oral)

1% to 10%:

Cardiovascular: Bradycardia

Endocrine & metabolic: Hyperkalemia, metabolic alkalosis in patients with severe renal failure

Neuromuscular & skeletal: Weakness

Respiratory: Dyspnea

<1% (Limited to important or life-threatening): Arrhythmias, chest pain, heart block, hypotension

Pharmacodynamics/Kinetics

Metabolism: To potassium bicarbonate; citric acid is metabolized to CO_2 and H_2O

Formulations

Crystals for reconstitution: Potassium citrate 3300 mg and citric acid 1002 mg per packet

Solution, oral: Potassium citrate 1100 mg and citric acid 334 mg per 5 mL

Dosing

Adults & Elderly: Alkalinizer: Oral:

Mild to moderate hypocitraturia: 10 mEq 3 times/day with meals

Severe hypocitraturia: Initial: 20 mEq 3 times/day or 15 mEq 4 times/day with meals or within 30 minutes after meals; do not exceed 100 mEq/day

Stability

Storage: Protect from excessive heat or freezing.

Monitoring and Teaching Issues

Physical Assessment: See Contraindications and Warnings/Precautions for use cautions. Assess kidney function prior to starting therapy. Monitor cardiac status and serum potassium at beginning of therapy and at regular intervals with long-term therapy. Assess knowledge/teach patient appropriate use, recommended diet, and adverse symptoms to report (see Patient Education).

Patient Education: Take as directed; do not take more than directed. Dilute crystals or solution in at least 6 oz of juice or water; stir and drink. May drink additional water or juice after dose. Take with or after meals (do not take on an empty stomach). Take any antacids 2 hours before or after potassium. Consult prescriber about advisability of increasing dietary potassium. Report tingling of hands or feet; unresolved nausea or vomiting; chest pain or palpitations; persistent abdominal pain; feelings of weakness, dizziness, listlessness, or confusion; acute muscle weakness or cramping; blood in stool or tarry stools; or easy bruising or unusual bleeding.

Related Information

Potassium Citrate *on page 1103*

Sodium Citrate and Citric Acid *on page 1236*

Potassium Citrate and Potassium Gluconate *see* Potassium Supplements *on page 1106*

Potassium Gluconate *see* Potassium Supplements *on page 1106*

Potassium Iodide (poe TASS ee um EYE oh dide)

U.S. Brand Names Pima®; SSKI®

Synonyms KI; Lugol's Solution; Strong Iodine Solution

Generic Available Yes

Pharmacologic Category Antithyroid Agent; Expectorant

Pregnancy Risk Factor D

Lactation Enters breast milk/use caution (AAP rates "compatible")

Use Expectorant for the symptomatic treatment of chronic pulmonary diseases complicated by mucous; reduce thyroid vascularity prior to thyroidectomy and management of thyrotoxic crisis; block thyroidal uptake of radioactive isotopes of iodine in a radiation emergency or other exposure to radioactive iodine

Use - Unlabeled/Investigational Lymphocutaneous and cutaneous sporotrichosis

Mechanism of Action/Effect Reduces viscosity of mucus by increasing respiratory tract secretions; inhibits secretion of thyroid hormone, fosters colloid accumulation in thyroid follicles

Contraindications Hypersensitivity to iodine or any component of the formulation; hyperkalemia; pulmonary edema; impaired renal function; hyperthyroidism; iodine-induced goiter; pregnancy

Warnings/Precautions Prolonged use can lead to hypothyroidism; cystic fibrosis patients have an exaggerated response; can cause acne flare-ups, can cause dermatitis; use with caution in patients with a history of thyroid disease, Addison's disease, cardiac disease, myotonia congenita, tuberculosis, acute bronchitis

Drug Interactions

Increased Effect/Toxicity: Lithium may cause additive hypothyroid effects; ACE-inhibitors, potassium-sparing diuretics, and potassium/potassium-containing products may lead to hyperkalemia, cardiac arrhythmias, or cardiac arrest

Adverse Reactions Frequency not defined.

Cardiovascular: Irregular heart beat

Central nervous system: Confusion, tiredness, fever

Dermatologic: Skin rash

Endocrine & metabolic: Goiter, salivary gland swelling/tenderness, thyroid adenoma, swelling of neck/throat, myxedema, lymph node swelling

Gastrointestinal: Diarrhea, gastrointestinal bleeding, metallic taste, nausea, stomach pain, stomach upset, vomiting

Neuromuscular & skeletal: Numbness, tingling, weakness

Miscellaneous: Chronic iodine poisoning (with prolonged treatment/high doses); iodism, hypersensitivity reactions (angioedema, cutaneous and mucosal hemorrhage, serum sickness-like symptoms)

Overdosage/Toxicology Symptoms of overdose include angioedema, laryngeal edema or cutaneous hemorrhages, muscle weakness, paralysis, peaked T waves, flattened P waves, prolongation of QRS complex, and ventricular arrhythmias.

Symptoms of iodism or chronic iodine poisoning may manifest as burning of mouth or throat, severe headache, metallic taste, sore teeth and gums, head cold symptoms, eye irritation including eyelid swelling, unusual increase in salivation, acneform skin lesions in seborrheic areas, or severe skin eruption (rare).

Removal of potassium can be accomplished by various means: Removal through the GI tract with Kayexalate® administration; by way of the kidney through diuresis, mineralocorticoid administration, or increased sodium intake; by hemodialysis or peritoneal dialysis; or by shifting potassium back into the cells by insulin and glucose infusion or by administration of sodium bicarbonate. Calcium chloride reverses cardiac effects.

Pharmacodynamics/Kinetics

Onset: 24-48 hours; Peak effect: 10-15 days after continuous therapy

Duration: May persist for up to 6 weeks

Formulations

Solution, oral:

SSKI®: 1 g/mL (30 mL, 240 mL) [contains sodium thiosulfate]

Lugol's solution, strong iodine: Potassium iodide 100 mg/mL with iodine 50 mg/mL

Syrup (Pima®): 325 mg/5 mL [equivalent to iodide 249 mg/5 mL] (473 mL) [black raspberry flavor]

(Continued)

Potassium Iodide *(Continued)*

Dosing

Adults & Elderly: RDA: 150 mcg (iodide)

Expectorant: Oral:

Pima®: 325-650 mg 3 times/day

SSKI®: 300-600 mg 3-4 times/day

Preoperative thyroidectomy: Oral: 50-250 mg (1-5 drops SSKI®) 3 times/day **or** 0.1-0.3 mL (3-5 drops) of strong iodine (Lugol's solution) 3 times/day; administer for 10 days before surgery

Radiation protectant to radioactive isotopes of iodine (Pima®): Oral: 195 mg once daily for 10 days; start 24 hours prior to exposure

To reduce risk of thyroid cancer following nuclear accident (dosing should continue until risk of exposure has passed or other measures are implemented): Children >68 kg and Adults (including pregnant/lactating women): Oral: 130 mg once daily

Thyrotoxic crisis: Oral: 300-500 mg (6-10 drops SSKI®) 3 times/day or 1 mL strong iodine (Lugol's solution) 3 times/day

Sporotrichosis (cutaneous, lymphocutaneous): Oral: Initial: 5 drops (SSKI®) 3 times/day; increase to 40-50 drops (SSKI®) 3 times/day as tolerated for 3-6 months

Pediatrics:

Expectorant: Oral: Children:

<3 years: Pima®: 162 mg 3 times day

>3 years: Pima®: 325 mg 3 times/day

Preoperative thyroidectomy: Refer to adult dosing.

Radiation protectant to radioactive isotopes of iodine (Pima®): Oral:

Infants up to 1 year: 65 mg once daily for 10 days; start 24 hours prior to exposure

>1 year: 130 mg once daily for 10 days; start 24 hours prior to exposure

To reduce risk of thyroid cancer following nuclear accident (dosing should continue until risk of exposure has passed or other measures are implemented): Oral (children >68 kg: Refer to adult dosing):

Infants <1 month: 16 mg once daily

1 month to 3 years: 32 mg once daily

3-18 years: 65 mg once daily

Thyrotoxic crisis: Oral:

Infants <1 year: 150-250 mg (3-5 drops SSKI®) 3 times/day

Children: Refer to adult dosing.

Administration

Oral:

Pima®: When used as an expectorant, take each dose with at least 4-6 ounces of water

SSKI®: Dilute in a glassful of water, fruit juice or milk. Take with food to decrease gastric irritation

Stability

Storage: Store at controlled room temperature of 25°C (77°F) excursions permitted to 15°C to 30°C (59°F to 86°F). Protect from light. Keep tightly closed.

SSKI®: If exposed to cold, crystallization may occur. Warm and shake to redissolve. If solution becomes brown/yellow, it should be discarded.

Compatibility: SSKI®: May be mixed in water, fruit juice, or milk.

Monitoring Laboratory Tests Thyroid function

Monitoring and Teaching Issues

Physical Assessment: See Contraindications, Warnings/Precautions, Drug Interactions, and Dosing for use cautions. Assess results of laboratory tests (see above), therapeutic effectiveness (according to purpose for use), and adverse reactions (see Adverse Reactions and Overdose/Toxicology). Teach patient proper use, possible side effects and interventions, and adverse symptoms to report (see Patient Education). **Pregnancy risk factor D** - determine that patient is not pregnant before beginning treatment. Instruct patients of childbearing age about appropriate barrier contraceptive measures. Note breast-feeding caution.

Patient Education: Inform prescriber of all prescriptions, OTC medications, or herbal products you are taking, and any allergies you have. Do not take anything new during treatment unless approved by prescriber. Take after meals. Dilute in 6 oz of water, fruit juice, milk, or broth. Do not exceed recommended dosage. May cause metallic taste, nausea, or vomiting (small, frequent meals, frequent mouth care, chewing gum, or sucking lozenges may help); soreness of teeth or gums (use soft toothbrush and frequent mouth rinses); fever, headache, or sore joints (consult prescriber for approved medication); or acne or skin irritation. Discontinue and report any swelling of lips, mouth, or tongue; difficulty swallowing; chest pain or irregular heartbeat; unusual muscle weakness; or other persistent adverse effects. **Pregnancy/breast-feeding precautions:** Do not get pregnant while taking this medication. Consult prescriber for appropriate barrier contraceptive measures. Consult prescriber if breast-feeding.

Dietary Issues: SSKI®: Take with food to decrease gastric irritation.

Breast-feeding Issues: AAP considers this drug compatible, but iodine in breast milk may affect thyroid function. May cause skin rash in nursing infant.

Pregnancy Issues: Iodide crosses the placenta (may cause hypothyroidism and goiter in fetus/newborn). Use as an expectorant during pregnancy is contraindicated by the AAP. Use for protection against thyroid cancer secondary to radioactive iodine exposure is considered acceptable based upon risk/benefit, keeping in mind the dose and duration.

Additional Information 10 drops of SSKI® = potassium iodide 500 mg

Potassium Phosphate *see* Phosphate Supplements *on page 1076*

Potassium Phosphate and Sodium Phosphate *see* Phosphate Supplements *on page 1076*

Potassium Supplements (poe TASS ee um SUP la ments)

U.S. Brand Names Cena-K®; Effer-K™; Gen-K®; Glu-K® [OTC]; K+® 10; Kaochlor®; Kaochlor® SF; Kaon®; Kaon-Cl®; Kaon-Cl-10®; Kay Ciel®; K+ Care®; K+ Care® ET; K-Dur-10®; K-Dur-20®; K-G®; K-Lease®; K-Lor™; Klor-Con® 8; Klor-Con® 10; Klor-Con/25®;

Klor-Con®/EF; Klorvess®; Klorvess® Effervescent; Klotrix®; K-Lyte®; K-Lyte/Cl®; K-Norm®; Kolyum®; K-Phos® Original; K-Tab®; Micro-K® 10 Entencaps; Micro-K® Entencaps; Micro-K® LS; Potasalan®; Rum-K®; Slow-K®; Ten-K®; Tri-K®; Twin-K®; Urocit®-K

Synonyms KCl (Potassium Chloride); Potassium Acetate; Potassium Acetate, Potassium Bicarbonate, and Potassium Citrate; Potassium Acid Phosphate; Potassium Bicarbonate; Potassium Bicarbonate and Potassium Chloride; Potassium Bicarbonate and Potassium Citrate; Potassium Chloride; Potassium Chloride and Potassium Gluconate; Potassium Citrate; Potassium Citrate and Potassium Gluconate; Potassium Gluconate

Generic Available Yes

Pharmacologic Category Electrolyte Supplement; Electrolyte Supplement, Oral; Electrolyte Supplement, Parenteral

Pregnancy Risk Factor C

Lactation Enters breast milk/compatible

Use Potassium deficiency; treatment or prevention of hypokalemia

Mechanism of Action/Effect Potassium is the major cation of intracellular fluid and is essential for the conduction of nerve impulses in heart, brain, and skeletal muscle; contraction of cardiac, skeletal, and smooth muscles; and maintenance of normal renal function, acid-base balance (acetate form), carbohydrate metabolism, and gastric secretion.

Contraindications Hypersensitivity to formulation; severe renal impairment; untreated Addison's disease; heat cramps; hyperkalemia; severe tissue trauma; solid oral dosage forms are contraindicated in patients in whom there is a structural, pathological, and/or pharmacologic cause for delay or arrest in passage through the GI tract; oral liquid preparation should be used in patients with esophageal compression or delayed gastric emptying time

Warnings/Precautions Use with caution in patients with cardiac disease, patients receiving potassium-sparing drugs. Patients must be on a cardiac monitor during intermittent infusions. Potassium injections should be administered only in patients with adequate urine flow. Injection must be diluted before I.V. use and infused slowly (see Administration). Some oral products contain tartrazine which may cause allergic reactions in susceptible individuals.

Drug Interactions

Increased Effect/Toxicity: Potassium-sparing diuretics, salt substitutes, ACE inhibitors such as captopril and enalapril may result in increased serum potassium.

Adverse Reactions Adverse reactions are usually dependent on rate of elimination or serum concentration. Frequency not defined:

Cardiovascular (with rapid I.V. administration or at high serum concentrations): Arrhythmias and cardiac arrest, heart block, hypotension, bradycardia, chest pain

Central nervous system: Mental confusion

Endocrine & metabolic: Hyperkalemia, metabolic alkalosis (acetate salt)

Gastrointestinal (with oral administration): Nausea, vomiting, diarrhea, abdominal pain, GI lesions, flatulence

Local: Pain at the site of injection, phlebitis, tissue necrosis with extravasation

Neuromuscular & skeletal: Muscle weakness, paresthesia, flaccid paralysis

Respiratory: Dyspnea

Pharmacodynamics/Kinetics

Absorption: Well from upper GI tract; enters cells via active transport from extracellular fluid

Half-Life Elimination: Largely by the kidneys

Formulations

Potassium acetate: Injection: 2 mEq/mL (20 mL, 50 mL, 100 mL); 4 mEq/mL (50 mL)

Potassium acetate, potassium bicarbonate, and potassium citrate: Solution, oral (Tri-K®): 45 mEq/15 mL from potassium acetate 1500 mg, potassium bicarbonate 1500 mg, and potassium citrate 1500 mg per 15 mL

Potassium acid phosphate (K-Phos® Original): 500 mg [potassium 3.67 mEq; sodium free]

Potassium bicarbonate: Tablet for oral solution, effervescent: 6.5 mEq, 20 mEq, 25 mq; K+ Care® ET: 25 mEq

Potassium bicarbonate and potassium chloride: Tablet for oral solution, effervescent: Klorvess®: 20 mEq per packet; K-Lyte/Cl®: 25 mEq, 50 mEq per packet

Potassium bicarbonate and potassium citrate: Tablet, effervescent: 25 mEq; Effer-K™, Klor-Con®/EF, K-Lyte®: 25 mEq

Potassium chloride:

Capsule, controlled release, microencapsulated: 600 mg [8 mEq]; 750 mg [10 mEq]

K-Lease®, K-Norm®, Micro-K® 10 Extencaps®: 750 mg [10 mEq]

Micro-K® Extencaps®: 600 mg [8 mEq]

Crystals for oral suspension, extended release (Micro-K® LS®): 20 mEq per packet

Liquid: 10% [20 mEq/15 mL] (480 mL, 4000 mL); 20% [40 mEq/15 mL] (480 mL, 4000 mL)

Cena-K®, Kaochlor®, Kaochlor® SF, Kay Ciel®, Klorvess®, Potasalan®: 10% [20 mEq/15 mL] (480 mL, 4000 mL)

Cena-K®, Kaon-Cl® 20%: 20% [40 mEq/15 mL] (480 mL, 4000 mL)

Rum-K®: 15% [30 mEq/15 mL] (480 mL, 4000 mL)

Infusion: 0.1 mEq/mL (100 mL); 0.2 mEq/mL (50 mL, 100 mL); 0.3 mEq/mL (100 mL); 0.4 mEq/mL (50 mL, 100 mL); 0.6 mEq/mL (50 mL); 0.8 mEq/mL (50 mL)

Injection, concentrate: 2 mEq/mL

Powder:

Gen-K®, K+ Care®, Kay Ciel®, K-Lor™, Klor-Con®: 20 mEq per packet (30s, 100s)

K+ Care®: 15 mEq per packet (30s, 100s)

K+ Care®, Klor-Con®/25: 25 mEq per packet (30s, 100s)

Tablet, controlled release, microencapsulated:

K-Dur® 10, Ten-K®: 750 mg [10 mEq]

K-Dur® 20: 1500 mg [20 mEq]

Tablet, controlled release, wax matrix: 600 mg [8 mEq]; 750 mg [10 mEq]

K+ 10®, Kaon-Cl-10®, Klor-Con® 10, Klotrix®, K-Tab®: 750 mg [10 mEq]

Kaon-Cl®: 500 mg [6.7 mEq]

Klor-Con® 8, Slow-K®: 600 mg [8 mEq]

(Continued)

Potassium Supplements *(Continued)*

Potassium chloride and potassium gluconate: Solution, oral (Kolyum®): Potassium 20 mEq/15 mL

Potassium citrate: Tablet (Urocit®-K): 540 mg [5 mEq]; 1080 mg [10 mEq]

Potassium citrate and potassium gluconate: Solution, oral (Twin-K®): 20 mEq/5 mL from potassium citrate 170 mg and potassium gluconate 170 mg per 5 mL

Potassium gluconate:
- Elixir (K-G®, Kaon®): 20 mEq/15 mL
- Tablet (Glu-K®): 2 mEq

Dosing

Adults: I.V. doses should be incorporated into the patient's maintenance I.V. fluids; intermittent I.V. potassium administration should be reserved for severe depletion situations and requires EKG monitoring. Doses listed as mEq of **potassium**. When using microencapsulated or wax matrix formulations, use no more than 20 mEq as a single dose.

Normal daily requirement: Oral, I.V.: 40-80 mEq/day

Prevention of hypokalemia during diuretic therapy: Oral: 20-40 mEq/day in 1-2 divided doses

Treatment of hypokalemia: Oral, I.V.: 40-100 mEq/day in divided doses

Treatment of hypokalemia: I.V. intermittent infusion (must be diluted prior to administration): 10-20 mEq/dose (maximum dose: 40 mEq/dose) to infuse over 2-3 hours (maximum dose: 40 mEq over 1 hour)

Elderly: Refer to adult dosing and Special Geriatric Considerations.

Pediatrics: I.V. doses should be incorporated into the patient's maintenance I.V. fluids; intermittent I.V. potassium administration should be reserved for severe depletion situations and requires EKG monitoring. Doses listed as mEq of **potassium**. When using microencapsulated or wax matrix formulations, use no more than 20 mEq as a single dose.

Normal daily requirement: Oral, I.V.:
- Neonates and Infants: 2-6 mEq/kg/day
- Children: 2-3 mEq/kg/day

Prevention of hypokalemia during diuretic therapy: Oral:
- Neonates, Infants, and Children: 1-2 mEq/kg/day in 1-2 divided doses

Treatment of hypokalemia: Oral, I.V.: Neonates, Infants, and Children: 2-5 mEq/kg/day in divided doses

Treatment of hypokalemia: I.V. intermittent infusion (must be diluted prior to administration): Neonates, Infants, and Children: 0.5-1 mEq/kg/dose (maximum dose: 30 mEq) to infuse at 0.3-0.5 mEq/kg/hour (maximum dose: 1 mEq/kg/hour)

Administration

Oral: Sustained release and wax matrix tablets should be swallowed whole; do not crush or chew. Effervescent tablets must be dissolved in water before use. Administer with food. Granules can be diluted or dissolved in water or juice. Do not administer liquid full strength, must be diluted in 2-6 parts of water or juice.

I.V.: Potassium must be diluted prior to parenteral administration. Maximum recommended concentration (peripheral line): 80 mEq/L; maximum recommended concentration (central line): 150 mEq/L or 15 mEq/100 mL. In severely fluid-restricted patients (with central lines): 200 mEq/L or 20 mEq/100 mL has been used. Maximum rate of infusion, see Dosage, I.V. intermittent infusion.

Monitoring Laboratory Tests Serum potassium, glucose, chloride, pH, urine output (if indicated), cardiac monitor (if intermittent I.V. infusion or potassium I.V. infusion rates >0.25 mEq/kg/hour)

Monitoring and Teaching Issues

Physical Assessment: Assess other medications patient may be taking for effectiveness and interactions (see Drug Interactions). See Contraindications and Warnings/Precautions for use cautions. Monitor serum K, therapeutic response, and adverse reactions at beginning of therapy and periodically throughout therapy (see Adverse Reactions). Assess knowledge/teach patient appropriate use, interventions to reduce side effects, and adverse symptoms to report (see Patient Education).

I.V.: Requires frequent monitoring of the infusion site and cardiac status on a regular basis (continuous EKG during highly concentrated infusions). Instruct patient about adverse reactions to report.

Patient Education: Oral: Take as directed; do not take more than directed. Dissolve tablet or powder in 4-6 ounces of water or juice and stir drinking. Do not chew or crush extended release capsules. Take potassium with or after meals (do not take on an empty stomach). Take any antacids 2 hours before or after potassium. Consult prescriber about advisability of increasing dietary potassium. Report tingling of hands or feet; unresolved nausea or vomiting; chest pain or palpitations; persistent abdominal pain; feelings of weakness, dizziness, listlessness, confusion, acute muscle weakness or cramping; blood in stool or black or tarry stools; or easy bruising or unusual bleeding.

Geriatric Considerations: Elderly may require less potassium than younger adults due to decreased renal function. For elderly who do not respond to replacement therapy, check serum magnesium. Due to long-term diuretic use, elderly may be hypomagnesemic.

Pounds/Kilograms Conversion *see page 1534*

Pramipexole (pra mi PEX ole)

U.S. Brand Names Mirapex®

Generic Available No

Pharmacologic Category Anti-Parkinson's Agent, Dopamine Agonist

Pregnancy Risk Factor C

Lactation Excretion in breast milk unknown/not recommended

Use Treatment of the signs and symptoms of idiopathic Parkinson's disease

Use - Unlabeled/Investigational Treatment of depression

Mechanism of Action/Effect Pramipexole is a nonergot dopamine agonist with specificity for the D_2 subfamily dopamine receptor, and has also been shown to bind to D_3 and D_4 receptors. By binding to these receptors, it is thought that pramipexole can stimulate dopamine activity on the nerves of the striatum and substantia nigra.

Contraindications Hypersensitivity to pramipexole or any component of the formulation

Warnings/Precautions Caution should be taken in patients with renal insufficiency and in patients with pre-existing dyskinesias. May cause orthostatic hypotension; Parkinson's disease patients appear to have an impaired capacity to respond to a postural challenge. Use with caution in patients at risk of hypotension (such as those receiving antihypertensive drugs) or where transient hypotensive episodes would be poorly tolerated (cardiovascular disease or cerebrovascular disease). May cause hallucinations, particularly in older patients.

Although not reported for pramipexole, other dopaminergic agents have been associated with a syndrome resembling neuroleptic malignant syndrome on withdrawal or significant dosage reduction after long-term use. Dopaminergic agents from the ergot class have also been associated with fibrotic complications, such as retroperitoneum, lungs, and pleura.

Pramipexole has been associated with somnolence, particularly at higher dosages (>1.5 mg/day). In addition, patients have been reported to fall asleep during activities of daily living, including driving, while taking this medication. Patients should be advised of this issue, cautioned against driving or performing activities requiring alertness, and advised of factors which may increase risk (sleep disorders, other sedating medications, or concomitant medications which increase pramipexole concentrations). Patients should be instructed to report daytime somnolence or sleepiness to the prescriber.

Pregnancy risk C.

Drug Interactions

Decreased Effect: Dopamine antagonists (antipsychotics, metoclopramide) may decrease the efficiency of pramipexole.

Increased Effect/Toxicity: Cimetidine in combination with pramipexole produced a 50% increase in AUC and a 40% increase in half-life. Drugs secreted by the cationic transport system (diltiazem, triamterene, verapamil, quinidine, quinine, ranitidine) decrease the clearance of pramipexole by ~20%.

Nutritional/Ethanol Interactions

Ethanol: Avoid ethanol (may increase CNS depression).

Food: Food intake does not affect the extent of drug absorption, although the time to maximal plasma concentration is delayed by 60 minutes when taken with a meal.

Herb/Nutraceutical: Avoid valerian, St John's wort, SAMe, kava kava (may increase risk of serotonin syndrome and/or excessive sedation).

Adverse Reactions

Frequency not defined, dose-related: Falling asleep during activities of daily living

>10%:

Cardiovascular: Postural hypotension

Central nervous system: Asthenia, dizziness, somnolence, insomnia, hallucinations, abnormal dreams

Gastrointestinal: Nausea, constipation

Neuromuscular & skeletal: Weakness, dyskinesia, EPS

1% to 10%:

Cardiovascular: Edema, postural hypotension, syncope, tachycardia, chest pain

Central nervous system: Malaise, confusion, amnesia, dystonias, akathisia, thinking abnormalities, myoclonus, hyperesthesia, gait abnormalities, hypertonia, paranoia

Endocrine & metabolic: Decreased libido

Gastrointestinal: Anorexia, weight loss, xerostomia

Genitourinary: Urinary frequency (up to 6%), impotence

Neuromuscular & skeletal: Muscle twitching, leg cramps, arthritis, bursitis

Ocular: Vision abnormalities (3%)

Respiratory: Dyspnea, rhinitis

<1% (Limited to important or life-threatening): Liver transaminases increased

Pharmacodynamics/Kinetics

Bioavailability: 90%

Half-Life Elimination: ~8 hours; Elderly: 12-14 hours

Time to Peak: Serum: ~2 hours

Formulations Tablet: 0.125 mg, 0.25 mg, 0.5 mg, 1 mg, 1.5 mg

Dosing

Adults & Elderly: Parkinson's disease: Oral: Initial: 0.375 mg/day given in 3 divided doses; increase gradually by 0.125 mg/dose every 5-7 days; range: 1.5-4.5 mg/day.

Administration

Oral: Doses should be titrated gradually in all patients to avoid the onset of intolerable side effects. The dosage should be increased to achieve a maximum therapeutic effect, balanced against the side effects of dyskinesia, hallucinations, somnolence, and dry mouth.

Monitoring and Teaching Issues

Physical Assessment: See Contraindications, Warnings/Precautions, and Dosing for use cautions. Assess potential for interactions with other prescriptions, OTC medications, or herbal products patient may be taking (see extensive list of Drug Interactions). Assess for therapeutic effectiveness (improvement of symptoms) and adverse response (see Adverse Reactions and Overdose/Toxicology). Teach patient appropriate use, interventions to reduce side effects, and adverse symptoms to report (see Patient Education). **Pregnancy risk factor C** - benefits of use should outweigh possible risks. Breast-feeding is not recommended.

Patient Education: Inform prescriber of all prescriptions, OTC medications, or herbal products you are taking, and any allergies you have. Do not take anything new during treatment unless approved by prescriber. Take exactly as directed. Avoid alcohol. May cause drowsiness and extreme sedation or somnolence (use caution when driving or engaging in hazardous activities until response to drug is known); postural hypotension

(Continued)

Pramipexole *(Continued)*

(use caution when changing position - rise slowly from sitting or lying position to standing and use caution when climbing stairs); constipation (increased exercise, fluids, fruit, or fiber may help); or urinary frequency. Consult prescriber about persistent adverse effects. **Pregnancy/breast-feeding precautions:** Inform prescriber if you are or intend to become pregnant. Breast-feeding is not recommended.

Prandin® *see* Repaglinide *on page 1176*

Pravachol® *see* Pravastatin *on page 1110*

Pravastatin (PRA va stat in)

U.S. Brand Names Pravachol®

Synonyms Pravastatin Sodium

Generic Available No

Pharmacologic Category Antilipemic Agent, HMG-CoA Reductase Inhibitor

Pregnancy Risk Factor X

Lactation Enters breast milk/contraindicated

Use

Primary prevention of coronary events: In combination with dietary therapy in hypercholesterolemic patients without established coronary heart disease, to reduce cardiovascular morbidity (myocardial infarction, coronary revascularization procedures) and mortality.

Secondary prevention of coronary events:

In combination with dietary therapy in hypercholesterolemic patients with established coronary heart disease, to slow the progression of coronary atherosclerosis, to reduce cardiovascular morbidity (myocardial infarction, coronary vascular procedures) and to reduce mortality; to reduce the risk of stroke and transient ischemic attacks

In combination with dietary therapy in patients with a history of prior myocardial infarction or unstable angina and "normal" cholesterol concentrations (total cholesterol ~219 mg/dL, LDL-C ~150 mg/dL); pravastatin may reduce cardiovascular mortality, the risk for recurrent myocardial infarction, stroke, and TIA, and the risk for undergoing coronary revascularization procedures.

Hyperlipidemias: As an adjunct to diet to reduce elevations in total cholesterol, LDL-C, apolipoprotein B, and triglycerides (elevations of one or more components are present in Fredrickson type IIa, IIb, III, and IV hyperlipidemias).

Mechanism of Action/Effect Pravastatin is a competitive inhibitor of 3-hydroxy-3-methylglutaryl coenzyme A (HMG-CoA) reductase, which is the rate-limiting enzyme involved in *de novo* cholesterol synthesis.

Contraindications Hypersensitivity to pravastatin or any component of the formulation; active liver disease; unexplained persistent elevations of serum transaminases; pregnancy; breast-feeding

Warnings/Precautions Secondary causes of hyperlipidemia should be ruled out prior to therapy. Liver function must be monitored by periodic laboratory assessment. Rhabdomyolysis with acute renal failure has occurred with fluvastatin and other HMG-CoA reductase inhibitors. Risk may be increased with concurrent use of other drugs which may cause rhabdomyolysis (including gemfibrozil, fibric acid derivatives, or niacin at doses ≥1 g/day). Temporarily discontinue in any patient experiencing an acute or serious condition predisposing to renal failure secondary to rhabdomyolysis. Use caution in patients with previous liver disease or heavy ethanol use. Treatment in patients <18 years of age is not recommended.

Drug Interactions

Cytochrome P450 Effect: Substrate of CYP3A4; Inhibits CYP2C8/9, 2D6, 3A4

Decreased Effect: Concurrent administration of cholestyramine or colestipol can decrease pravastatin absorption.

Increased Effect/Toxicity: Clofibrate, fenofibrate, gemfibrozil, and niacin may increase the risk of myopathy and rhabdomyolysis. Imidazole antifungals (itraconazole, ketoconazole), P-glycoprotein inhibitors may increase pravastatin concentrations.

Nutritional/Ethanol Interactions

Ethanol: Consumption of large amounts of ethanol may increase the risk of liver damage with HMG-CoA reductase inhibitors.

Herb/Nutraceutical: St John's wort may decrease pravastatin levels.

Adverse Reactions As reported in short-term trials; safety and tolerability with long-term use were similar to placebo

1% to 10%:

Cardiovascular: Chest pain (4%)

Central nervous system: Headache (2% to 6%), fatigue (4%), dizziness (1% to 3%)

Dermatologic: Rash (4%)

Gastrointestinal: Nausea/vomiting (7%), diarrhea (6%), heartburn (3%)

Hepatic: Increased transaminases (>3x normal on two occasions - 1%)

Neuromuscular & skeletal: Myalgia (2%)

Respiratory: Cough (3%)

Miscellaneous: Influenza (2%)

<1% (Limited to important or life-threatening): Allergy, lens opacity, libido change, memory impairment, muscle weakness, neuropathy, paresthesia, taste disturbance, tremor, vertigo

Postmarketing and/or case reports: Anaphylaxis, cholestatic jaundice, cirrhosis, cranial nerve dysfunction, dermatomyositis, erythema multiforme, ESR increase, fulminant hepatic necrosis, gynecomastia, hemolytic anemia, hepatitis, hepatoma, lupus erythematosus-like syndrome, myopathy, pancreatitis, peripheral nerve palsy, polymyalgia rheumatica, positive ANA, purpura, rhabdomyolysis, Stevens-Johnson syndrome, vasculitis

Additional class-related events or case reports (not necessarily reported with pravastatin therapy): Angioedema, cataracts, depression, dyspnea, eosinophilia, erectile dysfunction, facial paresis, hypersensitivity reaction, impaired extraocular muscle movement, impotence, leukopenia, malaise, memory loss, ophthalmoplegia, paresthesia, peripheral neuropathy, photosensitivity, psychic disturbance, skin discoloration, thrombocytopenia, thyroid dysfunction, toxic epidermal necrolysis, transaminases increased, vomiting

Overdosage/Toxicology Very little adverse events. Treatment is symptomatic.

Pharmacodynamics/Kinetics

Absorption: Poor

Bioavailability: 17%

Half-Life Elimination: ~2-3 hours

Time to Peak: Serum: 1-1.5 hours

Metabolism: Hepatic to at least two metabolites

Onset: Several days; Peak effect: 4 weeks

Formulations Tablet, as sodium: 10 mg, 20 mg, 40 mg, 80 mg

Dosing

Adults: Oral:

Dyslipidemia: 10-40 mg once daily.

Initial: 40 mg once daily (10 mg in patients with renal/hepatic dysfunction or receiving immunosuppressants, such as cyclosporine); titrate dosage to response (usual range: 10-80 mg); maximum dose: 80 mg once daily (maximum dose of 20 mg once daily recommended in patients receiving immunosuppressants, such as cyclosporine)

Elderly: No specific dosage recommendations. Clearance is reduced in the elderly, resulting in an increase in AUC between 25% to 50%. However, substantial accumulation is not expected.

Renal Impairment: Initial: 10 mg/day

Hepatic Impairment: Initial: 10 mg/day

Administration

Oral: May be taken without regard to meals.

Stability

Storage: Store at 25°C (77°F); excursions permitted to 15°C to 30°C (59°F to 86°F). Protect from moisture and light.

Monitoring Laboratory Tests Obtain baseline LFTs and total cholesterol profile; creatine phosphokinase due to possibility of myopathy. Repeat LFTs prior to elevation of dose. May be measured when clinically indicated and/or periodically thereafter.

Monitoring and Teaching Issues

Physical Assessment: See Contraindications, Warnings/Precautions, and Dosing for use cautions. Assess potential for interactions with other prescriptions, OTC medications, or herbal products patient may be taking (see Drug Interactions). Assess results of laboratory tests (see above) and patient response at beginning of therapy, when increasing dose, and periodically thereafter (see Adverse Reactions and Overdose/Toxicology). Teach patient proper use, possible side effects and interventions, and adverse symptoms to report (see Patient Education). **Pregnancy risk factor X** - determine that patient is not pregnant before starting therapy. Do not give to females of childbearing age unless capable of complying with barrier contraceptive use. Breast-feeding is contraindicated.

Patient Education: Inform prescriber of all prescriptions, OTC medications, or herbal products you are taking, and any allergies you have. Do not take anything new during treatment unless approved by prescriber. Take at same time each day. Follow diet and exercise regimen as prescribed. Avoid excess alcohol. You will have periodic blood tests to assess effectiveness. May cause mild nausea or vomiting (small, frequent meals, frequent mouth care, chewing gum, or sucking lozenges may help); diarrhea (buttermilk, boiled milk, or yogurt may help); or headache (see prescriber for analgesic). Report chest pain; CNS changes (memory loss, depression, personality changes); numbness, weakness, tingling, pain, or cramping in extremities or muscles; vision changes; rash; or other persistent adverse reactions. **Pregnancy/breast-feeding precautions:** Inform prescriber if you are pregnant. Consult prescriber for appropriate barrier contraceptive measures to use during and for 1 month following therapy. This drug may cause severe fetal defects. Do not donate blood during or for 1 month following therapy. Do not breast-feed.

Dietary Issues: May be taken without regard to meals. Before initiation of therapy, patients should be placed on a standard cholesterol-lowering diet for 6 weeks and the diet should be continued during drug therapy.

Geriatric Considerations: Effective and well tolerated in the elderly. The definition of and, therefore, when to treat hyperlipidemia in the elderly is a controversial issue. The National Cholesterol Education Program recommends that all adults 20 years of age and older maintain a plasma cholesterol <200 mg/dL. By this definition, 60% of all elderly would be considered to have a borderline high (200-239 mg/dL) or high (≥240 mg/dL) plasma cholesterol. However, plasma cholesterol has been shown to be a less reliable predictor of coronary heart disease in the elderly. Therefore, it is the authors' belief that pharmacologic treatment be reserved for those who are unable to obtain a desirable plasma cholesterol level by diet alone and for whom the benefits of treatment are believed to outweigh the potential adverse effects, drug interactions, and cost of treatment.

Related Information

Hyperlipidemia Management *on page 1682*
Lipid-Lowering Agents *on page 1582*

Pravastatin Sodium *see* Pravastatin *on page 1110*
Prazepam *see page 1560*

Prazosin (PRA zoe sin)

U.S. Brand Names Minipress®

Synonyms Furazosin; Prazosin Hydrochloride

Generic Available Yes

Pharmacologic Category Alpha$_1$ Blocker

Pregnancy Risk Factor C

Lactation Excretion in breast milk unknown/use caution

Use Treatment of hypertension

Use - Unlabeled/Investigational Benign prostatic hyperplasia; Raynaud's syndrome

(Continued)

Prazosin *(Continued)*

Mechanism of Action/Effect Competitively inhibits postsynaptic alpha-adrenergic receptors which results in vasodilation of veins and arterioles and a decrease in total peripheral resistance and blood pressure

Contraindications Hypersensitivity to quinazolines (doxazosin, prazosin, terazosin) or any component of the formulation

Warnings/Precautions May cause significant orthostatic hypotension and syncope, especially with first dose. Risk is increased at doses >1 mg, hypovolemia, or in patients receiving concurrent beta-blocker therapy. Anticipate a similar effect if therapy is interrupted for a few days, if dosage is rapidly increased, or if another antihypertensive drug is introduced. Pregnancy risk C.

Drug Interactions

Decreased Effect: Decreased antihypertensive effect if taken with NSAIDs.

Increased Effect/Toxicity: Prazosin's hypotensive effect may be increased with beta-blockers, diuretics, ACE inhibitors, calcium channel blockers, and other antihypertensive medications. Concurrent use with tricyclic antidepressants (TCAs) and low-potency antipsychotics may increase risk of orthostasis.

Nutritional/Ethanol Interactions

Ethanol: Avoid ethanol (may increase vasodilation).

Food: Food has variable effects on absorption.

Herb/Nutraceutical: Avoid dong quai if using for hypertension (has estrogenic activity). Avoid ephedra, yohimbe, ginseng (may worsen hypertension). Avoid saw palmetto (due to limited experience with this combination). Avoid garlic (may have increased antihypertensive effect).

Effects on Lab Values Increased urinary UMA 17%, norepinephrine metabolite 42%

Adverse Reactions

>10%: Central nervous system: Dizziness (10%)

1% to 10%:

Cardiovascular: Palpitations (5%), edema, orthostatic hypotension, syncope (1%)

Central nervous system: Headache (8%), drowsiness (8%), weakness (7%), vertigo, depression, nervousness

Dermatologic: Rash (1% to 4%)

Endocrine & metabolic: Decreased energy (7%)

Gastrointestinal: Nausea (5%), vomiting, diarrhea, constipation

Genitourinary: Urinary frequency (1% to 5%)

Ocular: Blurred vision, reddened sclera, xerostomia

Respiratory: Dyspnea, epistaxis, nasal congestion

<1% (Limited to important or life-threatening): Allergic reaction, alopecia, angina, cataplexy, cataracts (both development and disappearance have been reported), hallucinations, impotence, leukopenia, lichen planus, myocardial infarction, narcolepsy (worsened), pancreatitis, paresthesia, pigmentary mottling and serous retinopathy, priapism, pruritus, systemic lupus erythematosus, tinnitus, urticaria, vasculitis

Overdosage/Toxicology Symptoms of overdose include hypotension and drowsiness. Treatment is otherwise supportive and symptomatic.

Pharmacodynamics/Kinetics

Bioavailability: 43% to 82%

Half-Life Elimination: 2-4 hours; prolonged with congestive heart failure

Metabolism: Extensively hepatic

Onset: BP reduction: ~2 hours; Maximum decrease: 2-4 hours

Duration: 10-24 hours

Formulations Capsule, as hydrochloride: 1 mg, 2 mg, 5 mg

Dosing

Adults:

Hypertension: Oral: Initial: 1 mg/dose 2-3 times/day; usual maintenance dose: 3-15 mg/day in divided doses 2-4 times/day; maximum daily dose: 20 mg

Hypertensive urgency: Oral: 10-20 mg once, may repeat in 30 minutes

Raynaud's (unlabeled use): Oral: 0.5-3 mg twice daily

Benign prostatic hyperplasia (unlabeled use): Oral: 2 mg twice daily

Elderly: Oral (first dose given at bedtime): Initial: 1 mg 1-2 times/day

Pediatrics: Oral: Children: Initial: 5 mcg/kg/dose (to assess hypotensive effects); usual dosing interval: every 6 hours; increase dosage gradually up to maximum of 25 mcg/kg/dose every 6 hours.

Stability

Storage: Store in airtight container. Protect from light.

Monitoring and Teaching Issues

Physical Assessment: See Contraindications, Warnings/Precautions, and Dosing for use cautions. Assess potential for interactions with other prescriptions, OTC medications, or herbal products patient may be taking (see Drug Interactions). Assess therapeutic effectiveness and adverse reactions at beginning of therapy and on a regular basis with long-term therapy (see Adverse Reactions and Overdose/Toxicology). When discontinuing, monitor blood pressure and taper dose slowly over 1 week or more. Teach patient proper use, possible side effects and interventions, and adverse symptoms to report (see Patient Education). **Pregnancy risk factor C** - benefits of use should outweigh possible risks. Note breast-feeding caution.

Patient Education: Inform prescriber of all prescriptions, OTC medications, or herbal products you are taking, and any allergies you have. Do not take anything new during treatment unless approved by prescriber. Take as directed with or without meals; do not skip dose or discontinue without consulting prescriber. Avoid alcohol. Follow recommended diet and exercise program. May cause drowsiness, dizziness, or impaired judgment (use caution when driving or engaging in tasks that require alertness until response to drug is known); postural hypotension (use caution when rising from sitting or lying position or when climbing stairs); or dry mouth or nausea (frequent mouth care or sucking lozenges may help). Report increased nervousness or depression; sudden weight gain (weigh yourself in the same clothes at the same time of day once a week); palpitations or rapid heartbeat; difficulty breathing; muscle weakness, fatigue, or pain; vision changes or hearing; rash; changes in urinary pattern (void before taking medications); or other persistent side effects. **Pregnancy/breast-feeding precautions:** Inform prescriber if you are or intend to become pregnant. Consult prescriber if breast-feeding.

Geriatric Considerations: See Warnings/Precautions and Pharmacokinetics. Adverse effects such as dry mouth and urinary problems can be particularly bothersome in the elderly.

Prazosin and Polythiazide (PRA zoe sin & pol i THYE a zide)

U.S. Brand Names Minizide®

Synonyms Polythiazide and Prazosin

Generic Available No

Pharmacologic Category Antihypertensive Agent Combination

Pregnancy Risk Factor C

Lactation Excretion in breast milk unknown

Use Management of mild to moderate hypertension

Formulations Capsule:

1: Prazosin 1 mg and polythiazide 0.5 mg
2: Prazosin 2 mg and polythiazide 0.5 mg
5: Prazosin 5 mg and polythiazide 0.5 mg

Dosing

Adults & Elderly: Hypertension: Oral: Initial: 1 capsule 2-3 times/day; maintenance: May be slowly increased to a total daily dose of 20 mg. Therapeutic dosages often used range from 6-15 mg in divided doses.

Monitoring and Teaching Issues

Physical Assessment: See individual components listed in Related Information. **Pregnancy risk factor C** - benefits of use should outweigh possible risks. Note breast-feeding caution.

Patient Education: Also see Prazosin.

Based on Polythiazide component: A few people who take this medication become more sensitive to sunlight and may experience skin rash, redness, itching, or severe sunburn, especially if sunblock SPF ≥15 is not used on exposed skin areas.

Pregnancy/breast-feeding precautions: Inform prescriber if you are or intend to become pregnant. Consult prescriber if breast-feeding.

Related Information

Prazosin *on page 1111*

Prazosin Hydrochloride *see* Prazosin *on page 1111*

Precedex™ *see* Dexmedetomidine *on page 386*

Precose® *see* Acarbose *on page 33*

Pred Forte® *see page 1509*

Pred Forte® *see* PrednisoLONE *on page 1113*

Pred-G® *see page 1509*

Pred Mild® *see page 1509*

Pred Mild® *see* PrednisoLONE *on page 1113*

Prednicarbate *see* Topical Corticosteroids *on page 1334*

PrednisoLONE (pred NIS oh lone)

U.S. Brand Names AK-Pred®; Econopred®; Econopred® Plus; Inflamase® Forte; Inflamase® Mild; Orapred®; Pediapred®; Pred Forte®; Pred Mild®; Prelone®

Synonyms Deltahydrocortisone; Metacortandralone; Prednisolone Acetate; Prednisolone Acetate, Ophthalmic; Prednisolone Sodium Phosphate; Prednisolone Sodium Phosphate, Ophthalmic; Prednisolone Tebutate

Generic Available Yes

Pharmacologic Category Corticosteroid, Ophthalmic; Corticosteroid, Systemic

Pregnancy Risk Factor C

Lactation Enters breast milk/compatible

Use Treatment of palpebral and bulbar conjunctivitis; corneal injury from chemical, radiation, thermal burns, or foreign body penetration; endocrine disorders, rheumatic disorders, collagen diseases, dermatologic diseases, allergic states, ophthalmic diseases, respiratory diseases, hematologic disorders, neoplastic diseases, edematous states, and gastrointestinal diseases; useful in patients with inability to activate prednisone (liver disease)

Mechanism of Action/Effect Decreases inflammation by suppression of migration of polymorphonuclear leukocytes and reversal of increased capillary permeability; suppresses the immune system by reducing activity and volume of the lymphatic system

Contraindications Hypersensitivity to prednisolone or any component of the formulation; acute superficial herpes simplex keratitis; systemic fungal infections; varicella

Warnings/Precautions Use with caution in patients with hyperthyroidism, cirrhosis, nonspecific ulcerative colitis, hypertension, osteoporosis, thromboembolic tendencies, CHF, convulsive disorders, myasthenia gravis, thrombophlebitis, peptic ulcer, and diabetes. Acute adrenal insufficiency may occur with abrupt withdrawal after long-term therapy or with stress. Because of the risk of adverse effects, systemic corticosteroids should be used cautiously in the elderly, in the smallest possible dose, and for the shortest possible time. Pregnancy risk C.

Drug Interactions

Cytochrome P450 Effect: Substrate of CYP3A4; Inhibits CYP3A4

Decreased Effect: Systemic: Decreased effect or corticosteroids with barbiturates, aminoglutethimide, phenytoin, and rifampin. Decreased effect of salicylates, vaccines, and

(Continued)

PrednisoLONE *(Continued)*

toxoids. Prednisolone may decrease the effect of isoniazid. Corticosteroids may decrease the effect of warfarin or IUD contraceptives.

Increased Effect/Toxicity: Systemic: The combined use of cyclosporine and prednisolone may result in elevated levels of both agents. Oral contraceptives may enhance the effect of prednisolone.

Nutritional/Ethanol Interactions

Ethanol: Avoid ethanol (may increase gastric mucosal irritation).

Food: Prednisolone interferes with calcium absorption. Limit caffeine.

Herb/Nutraceutical: St John's wort may decrease prednisolone levels. Avoid cat's claw, echinacea (have immunostimulant properties).

Effects on Lab Values Response to skin tests

Adverse Reactions Systemic:

>10%:

Central nervous system: Insomnia, nervousness
Gastrointestinal: Increased appetite, indigestion

1% to 10%:

Central nervous system: Dizziness or lightheadedness, headache
Dermatologic: Hirsutism, hypopigmentation
Endocrine & metabolic: Diabetes mellitus
Neuromuscular & skeletal: Arthralgia
Ocular: Cataracts, glaucoma
Respiratory: Epistaxis
Miscellaneous: Diaphoresis

<1% (Limited to important or life-threatening): Cushing's syndrome, edema, fractures, hallucinations, hypersensitivity reactions, hypertension, muscle wasting, osteoporosis, pancreatitis, pituitary-adrenal axis suppression, pseudotumor cerebri, seizures

Overdosage/Toxicology When consumed in high doses for prolonged periods, systemic hypercorticism and adrenal suppression may occur, in those cases discontinuation of the corticosteroid should be done judiciously.

Pharmacodynamics/Kinetics

Half-Life Elimination: 3.6 hours; Biological: 18-36 hours; End-stage renal disease: 3-5 hours

Metabolism: Primarily hepatic, but also metabolized in most tissues, to inactive compounds

Duration: 18-36 hours

Formulations

Solution, ophthalmic, as sodium phosphate: 1% (5 mL, 10 mL, 15 mL) [contains benzalkonium chloride]

AK-Pred®: 1% (5 mL, 15 mL) [contains benzalkonium chloride]
Inflamase® Forte: 1% (5 mL, 10 mL, 15 mL) [contains benzalkonium chloride]
Inflamase® Mild: 0.125% (5 mL, 10 mL) [contains benzalkonium chloride]

Suspension, ophthalmic, as acetate: 1% (5 mL, 10 mL, 15 mL) [contains benzalkonium chloride]

Econopred®: 0.125% (5 mL, 10 mL) [contains benzalkonium chloride]
Econopred® Plus: 1% (5 mL, 10 mL) [contains benzalkonium chloride]
Pred Forte®: 1% (1 mL, 5 mL, 10 mL, 15 mL) [contains benzalkonium chloride and sodium bisulfite]
Pred Mild®: 0.12% (5 mL, 10 mL) [contains benzalkonium chloride and sodium bisulfite]

Solution, oral, as sodium phosphate: Prednisolone base 5 mg/5 mL (120 mL)

Orapred®: 20 mg/5 mL (240 mL) [equivalent to prednisolone base 15 mg/5 mL; dye free; contains alcohol 2%, sodium benzoate; grape flavor]
Pediapred®: 6.7 mg/5 mL (120 mL) [equivalent to prednisolone base 5 mg/5 mL; dye free; raspberry flavor]

Syrup, as base: 5 mg/5 mL (120 mL); 15 mg/5 mL (240 mL, 480 mL)

Prelone®: 5 mg/5 mL (120 mL) [dye free, sugar free; contains alcohol ≤0.4%, benzoic acid; wild cherry flavor]; 15 mg/5 mL (240 mL, 480 mL) [contains alcohol 5%, benzoic acid; wild cherry flavor]

Tablet, as base: 5 mg [contains sodium benzoate]

Dosing

Adults: Dose depends upon condition being treated and response of patient. Consider alternate day therapy for long-term therapy. Discontinuation of long-term therapy requires gradual withdrawal by tapering the dose.

Usual dose (range):

Oral, I.V., I.M. (sodium phosphate salt): 5-60 mg/day
I.M. (acetate salt): 4-60 mg/day

Rheumatoid arthritis: Oral: Initial: 5-7.5 mg/day, adjust dose as necessary

Multiple sclerosis (sodium phosphate): Oral: 200 mg/day for 1 week followed by 80 mg every other day for 1 month

Multiple sclerosis (acetate salt): I.M.: 200 mg/day for 1 week followed by 80 mg every other day for 1 month

Intra-articular, intralesional, soft-tissue administration:

Tebutate salt: 4-40 mg/dose
Acetate salt: 4-100 mg/dose
Sodium phosphate salt: 2-30 mg/dose

Conjunctivitis: Ophthalmic (suspension/solution): Instill 1-2 drops into conjunctival sac every hour during day, every 2 hours at night until favorable response is obtained, then use 1 drop every 4 hours.

Elderly: Use lowest effective adult dose. Dose depends upon condition being treated and response of patient; alternate day dosing may be attempted in some disease states.

Pediatrics: Dose depends upon condition being treated and response of patient; dosage for infants and children should be based on severity of the disease and response of the patient rather than on strict adherence to dosage indicated by age, weight, or body surface area.

Consider alternate day therapy for long-term therapy. Discontinuation of long-term therapy requires gradual withdrawal by tapering the dose.

Acute asthma:

Oral: 1-2 mg/kg/day in divided doses 1-2 times/day for 3-5 days

I.V. (sodium phosphate salt): 2-4 mg/kg/day divided 3-4 times/day

Anti-inflammatory or immunosuppressive dose: Oral, I.V., I.M. (sodium phosphate salt): 0.1-2 mg/kg/day in divided doses 1-4 times/day

Nephrotic syndrome: Oral:

Initial (first 3 episodes): 2 mg/kg/day **or** 60 mg/m^2/day (maximum: 80 mg/day) in divided doses 3-4 times/day until urine is protein free for 3 consecutive days (maximum: 28 days); followed by 1-1.5 mg/kg/dose **or** 40 mg/m^2/dose given every other day for 4 weeks

Maintenance (long-term maintenance dose for frequent relapses): 0.5-1 mg/kg/dose given every other day for 3-6 months

Conjunctivitis: Ophthalmic (suspension/solution): Children: Refer to adult dosing.

Renal Impairment: Slightly dialyzable (5% to 20%)

Administration

Oral: Give oral formulation with food or milk to decrease GI effects.

I.V.: Do **not** give acetate or tebutate salt I.V.

Monitoring Laboratory Tests Blood glucose, electrolytes

Monitoring and Teaching Issues

Physical Assessment: Assess other medications patient may be taking for effectiveness and interactions (see Drug Interactions). See Contraindications and Warnings/Precautions for use cautions. Monitor laboratory tests, therapeutic response, and adverse effects according to indications for therapy, dose, route, and duration of therapy (see Dosing, Warnings/Precautions, Adverse Reactions). With systemic administration, diabetics should monitor glucose levels closely. Assess knowledge/teach patient appropriate use, interventions to reduce side effects, and adverse symptoms to report (see Patient Education). When used for long-term therapy (>10-14 days), do not discontinue abruptly; decrease dosage incrementally. **Pregnancy risk factor C** - benefits of use should outweigh possible risks.

Patient Education: Take exactly as directed; do not increase dose or discontinue abruptly without consulting prescriber. Take oral medication with or after meals. Avoid alcohol. Limit intake of caffeine or stimulants. Prescriber may recommend increased dietary vitamins, minerals, or iron. If diabetic, monitor glucose levels closely (antidiabetic medication may need to be adjusted). Inform prescriber if you are experiencing greater than normal levels of stress (medication may need adjustment). Some forms of this medication may cause GI upset (oral medication may be taken with meals to reduce GI upset; small, frequent meals and frequent mouth care may reduce GI upset). You may be more susceptible to infection (avoid crowds and exposure to infection). Report promptly excessive nervousness or sleep disturbances; any signs of infection (sore throat, unhealed injuries); excessive growth of body hair or loss of skin color; vision changes; excessive or sudden weight gain (>3 lb/week); swelling of face or extremities; difficulty breathing; muscle weakness; change in color of stools (black or tarry) or persistent abdominal pain; or worsening of condition or failure to improve. **Pregnancy precaution:** Inform prescriber if you are or intend to become pregnant.

Ophthalmic: For ophthalmic use only. Wash hands before using. Tilt head back and look upward. Put drops of suspension inside lower eyelid. Close eye and roll eyeball in all directions. Do not blink for ½ minute. Apply gentle pressure to inner corner of eye for 30 seconds. Do not use any other eye preparation for at least 10 minutes. Do not let tip of applicator touch eye; do not contaminate tip of applicator (may cause eye infection, eye damage, or vision loss). Do not share medication with anyone else. Wear sunglasses when in sunlight; you may be more sensitive to bright light. Inform prescriber if condition worsens or fails to improve or if you experience eye pain, disturbances of vision, or other adverse eye response.

Dietary Issues: Should be taken after meals or with food or milk to decrease GI effects; increase dietary intake of pyridoxine, vitamin C, vitamin D, folate, calcium, and phosphorus.

Geriatric Considerations: Useful in patients with inability to activate prednisone (liver disease). Because of the risk of adverse effects, systemic corticosteroids should be used cautiously in the elderly, in the smallest possible dose, and for the shortest possible time.

Additional Information

Sodium phosphate injection: For I.V., I.M., intra-articular, intralesional, or soft tissue administration

Tebutate injection: For intra-articular, intralesional, or soft tissue administration only

Related Information

Corticosteroids Comparison, Systemic Equivalencies *on page 1572*
FDA Name Differentiation Project: The Use of Tall-man Letters *on page 12*
Ophthalmic Agents *on page 1509*

Prednisolone Acetate *see* PrednisoLONE *on page 1113*

Prednisolone Acetate, Ophthalmic *see* PrednisoLONE *on page 1113*

Prednisolone and Gentamicin *see page 1509*

Prednisolone Sodium Phosphate *see* PrednisoLONE *on page 1113*

Prednisolone Sodium Phosphate, Ophthalmic *see* PrednisoLONE *on page 1113*

Prednisolone Tebutate *see* PrednisoLONE *on page 1113*

PredniSONE (PRED ni sone)

U.S. Brand Names Deltasone®; Liquid Pred®; Meticorten®; Orasone®

Synonyms Deltacortisone; Deltadehydrocortisone

Generic Available Yes

Pharmacologic Category Corticosteroid, Systemic

Pregnancy Risk Factor B

(Continued)

PredniSONE *(Continued)*

Lactation Enters breast milk/compatible

Use Treatment of a variety of diseases including adrenocortical insufficiency, hypercalcemia, rheumatic, and collagen disorders; dermatologic, ocular, respiratory, gastrointestinal, and neoplastic diseases; organ transplantation and a variety of diseases including those of hematologic, allergic, inflammatory, and autoimmune in origin; not available in injectable form, prednisolone must be used

Use - Unlabeled/Investigational Investigational: Prevention of postherpetic neuralgia and relief of acute pain in the early stages

Mechanism of Action/Effect Decreases inflammation by suppression of migration of polymorphonuclear leukocytes and reversal of increased capillary permeability; suppresses the immune system by reducing activity and volume of the lymphatic system; suppresses adrenal function at high doses

Contraindications Hypersensitivity to prednisone or any component of the formulation; serious infections, except tuberculous meningitis; systemic fungal infections; varicella

Warnings/Precautions Use with caution in patients with hypothyroidism, cirrhosis, CHF, ulcerative colitis, thromboembolic disorders, and patients with an increased risk for peptic ulcer disease. Corticosteroids should be used with caution in patients with diabetes, hypertension, osteoporosis, glaucoma, cataracts, or tuberculosis. Use caution in hepatic impairment. May retard bone growth. Gradually taper dose to withdraw therapy. Because of the risk of adverse effects, systemic corticosteroids should be used cautiously in the elderly, in the smallest possible dose, and for the shortest possible time.

Drug Interactions

Cytochrome P450 Effect: Substrate of CYP3A4; Induces CYP2C19, 3A4

Decreased Effect: Decreased effect with barbiturates, phenytoin, rifampin; decreased effect of salicylates, vaccines, and toxoids.

Increased Effect/Toxicity: Concurrent use with NSAIDs may increase the risk of GI ulceration.

Nutritional/Ethanol Interactions

Ethanol: Avoid ethanol (may increase gastric mucosal irritation)

Food: Prednisone interferes with calcium absorption, Limit caffeine.

Herb/Nutraceutical: St John's wort may decrease prednisone levels. Avoid cat's claw, echinacea (have immunostimulant properties).

Effects on Lab Values Response to skin tests

Adverse Reactions

>10%:

Central nervous system: Insomnia, nervousness

Gastrointestinal: Increased appetite, indigestion

1% to 10%:

Central nervous system: Dizziness or lightheadedness, headache

Dermatologic: Hirsutism, hypopigmentation

Endocrine & metabolic: Diabetes mellitus, glucose intolerance, hyperglycemia

Neuromuscular & skeletal: Arthralgia

Ocular: Cataracts, glaucoma

Respiratory: Epistaxis

Miscellaneous: Diaphoresis

<1% (Limited to important or life-threatening): Cushing's syndrome, edema, fractures, hallucinations, hypertension, muscle-wasting, osteoporosis, pancreatitis, pituitary-adrenal axis suppression, seizures

Overdosage/Toxicology When consumed in high doses for prolonged periods, systemic hypercorticism and adrenal suppression may occur. In those cases, discontinuation of the corticosteroid should be done judiciously.

Pharmacokinetic Note See Prednisolone monograph for complete information.

Pharmacodynamics/Kinetics

Half-Life Elimination: Normal renal function: 2.5-3.5 hours

Metabolism: Hepatically converted from prednisone (inactive) to prednisolone (active); may be impaired with hepatic dysfunction

Formulations

Solution, oral: 1 mg/mL (5 mL, 120 mL, 500 mL) [contains alcohol 5%]

Solution, oral concentrate: 5 mg/mL (30 mL) [contains alcohol 30%]

Syrup: 1 mg/mL (120 mL, 240 mL)

Tablet: 1 mg, 2.5 mg, 5 mg, 10 mg, 20 mg, 50 mg

Dosing

Adults: Dose depends upon condition being treated and response of patient; consider alternate day therapy for long-term therapy. Discontinuation of long-term therapy requires gradual withdrawal by tapering the dose.

Physiologic replacement: Oral: 4-5 mg/m^2/day

Immunosuppression/chemotherapy adjunct: Oral: Range: 5-60 mg/day in divided doses 1-4 times/day

Allergic reaction (contact dermatitis): Oral:

Day 1: 30 mg divided as 10 mg before breakfast, 5 mg at lunch, 5 mg at dinner, 10 mg at bedtime

Day 2: 5 mg at breakfast, 5 mg at lunch, 5 mg at dinner, 10 mg at bedtime

Day 3: 5 mg 4 times/day (with meals and at bedtime)

Day 4: 5 mg 3 times/day (breakfast, lunch, bedtime)

Day 5: 5 mg 2 times/day (breakfast, bedtime)

Day 6: 5 mg before breakfast

Acute asthma: 1-2 mg/kg/day in divided doses 1-2 times/day for 3-5 days

Asthma maintenance:

Moderate persistent: Inhaled corticosteroid (medium dose) or inhaled corticosteroid (low-medium dose) with a long-acting bronchodilator

Severe persistent: Inhaled corticosteroid (high dose) and corticosteroid tablets or syrup long term: 2 mg/kg/day, generally not to exceed 60 mg/day

Pneumocystis carinii pneumonia (PCP): Oral:

40 mg twice daily for 5 days **followed by**

40 mg once daily for 5 days **followed by**

20 mg once daily for 11 days or until antimicrobial regimen is completed

Thyrotoxicosis: Oral: 60 mg/day

Note: Dosing adjustment in hyperthyroidism: Prednisone dose may need to be increased to achieve adequate therapeutic effects

Chemotherapy (refer to individual protocols): Oral: Range: 20 mg/day to 100 mg/m²/day

Rheumatoid arthritis: Oral: Use lowest possible daily dose (often ≤7.5 mg/day)

Idiopathic thrombocytopenia purpura (ITP): Oral: 60 mg daily for 4-6 weeks, gradually tapered over several weeks

Systemic lupus erythematosus (SLE): Oral:

Acute: 1-2 mg/kg/day in 2-3 divided doses

Maintenance: Reduce to lowest possible dose, usually <1 mg/kg/day as single dose (morning)

Elderly: Refer to adult dosing; use the lowest effective dose. Oral dose depends upon condition being treated and response of patient. Alternate day dosing may be attempted.

Pediatrics: Note: Dose depends upon condition being treated and response of patient; dosage for infants and children should be based on severity of the disease and response of the patient rather than on strict adherence to dosage indicated by age, weight, or body surface area. Consider alternate day therapy for long-term therapy. Discontinuation of long-term therapy requires gradual withdrawal by tapering the dose.

Physiologic replacement: Oral: Children: 4-5 mg/m²/day

Anti-inflammatory or immunosuppressive dose: Oral: 0.05-2 mg/kg/day divided 1-4 times/day

Acute asthma: Oral: 1-2 mg/kg/day in divided doses 1-2 times/day for 3-5 days

Alternatively (for 3- to 5-day "burst"):

<1 year: 10 mg every 12 hours

1-4 years: 20 mg every 12 hours

5-13 years: 30 mg every 12 hours

>13 years: 40 mg every 12 hours

Asthma long-term therapy (alternative dosing by age): Oral:

<1 year: 10 mg every other day

1-4 years: 20 mg every other day

5-13 years: 30 mg every other day

>13 years: 40 mg every other day

Asthma maintenance: Children ≥5 years: Refer to adult dosing.

Nephrotic syndrome: Oral:

Initial (first 3 episodes): 2 mg/kg/day **or** 60 mg/m²/day (maximum: 80 mg/day) in divided doses 3-4 times/day until urine is protein free for 3 consecutive days (maximum: 28 days); followed by 1-1.5 mg/kg/dose **or** 40 mg/m²/dose given every other day for 4 weeks

Maintenance dose (long-term maintenance dose for frequent relapses): 0.5-1 mg/kg/dose given every other day for 3-6 months

Renal Impairment: Hemodialysis effects: Supplemental dose is not necessary.

Administration

Oral: Take with food to decrease GI upset.

Monitoring Laboratory Tests Blood glucose, electrolytes

Monitoring and Teaching Issues

Physical Assessment: Assess effectiveness and interactions of other medications patient may be taking (see Drug Interactions). See Contraindications and Warnings/Precautions for use cautions. Monitor for effectiveness of therapy and adverse reactions according to dose and length of therapy. Assess knowledge/teach patient appropriate use, possible side effects/interventions, and adverse symptoms to report (ie, opportunistic infection, adrenal suppression - see Adverse Reactions, Overdose/Toxicology, and Patient Education). Instruct diabetics to monitor serum glucose levels closely; corticosteroids can alter glucose tolerance. Dose may need to be increased if patient is experiencing higher than normal levels of stress. When discontinuing, taper dose and frequency slowly.

Patient Education: Take exactly as directed. Do not take more than prescribed dose and do not discontinue abruptly; consult prescriber. Take with or after meals. Take once-a-day dose with food in the morning. Avoid alcohol. Limit intake of caffeine or stimulants. Maintain adequate nutrition; consult prescriber for possibility of special dietary recommendations. If diabetic, monitor serum glucose closely and notify prescriber of changes; this medication can alter hypoglycemic requirements. Notify prescriber if you are experiencing higher than normal levels of stress; medication may need adjustment. Periodic ophthalmic examinations will be necessary with long-term use. You will be susceptible to infection (avoid crowds and exposure to infection). You may experience insomnia or nervousness; use caution when driving or engaging in tasks requiring alertness until response to drug is known. Report weakness, change in menstrual pattern, vision changes, signs of hyperglycemia, signs of infection (eg, fever, chills, mouth sores, perianal itching, vaginal discharge), other persistent side effects, or worsening of condition.

Dietary Issues: Should be taken after meals or with food or milk; increase dietary intake of pyridoxine, vitamin C, vitamin D, folate, calcium, and phosphorus.

Geriatric Considerations: Because of the risk of adverse effects, systemic corticosteroids should be used cautiously in the elderly, in the smallest possible dose, and for the shortest possible time.

Breast-feeding Issues: Crosses into breast milk. No data on clinical effects on the infant. AAP considers **compatible** with breast-feeding.

Pregnancy Issues: Crosses the placenta. Immunosuppression reported in 1 infant exposed to high-dose prednisone plus azathioprine throughout gestation. One report of congenital cataracts. Available evidence suggests safe use during pregnancy.

(Continued)

PredniSONE *(Continued)*

Additional Information Tapering of corticosteroids after a short course of therapy (<7-10 days) is generally not required unless the disease/inflammatory process is slow to respond. Tapering after prolonged exposure is dependent upon the individual patient, duration of corticosteroid treatments, and size of steroid dose, Recovery of the HPA axis may require several months. Subtle but important HPA axis suppression may be present for as long as several months after a course of as few as 10-14 days duration. Testing of HPA axis (cosyntropin) may be required, and signs/symptoms of adrenal insufficiency should be monitored in patients with a history of use.

Related Information

Corticosteroids Comparison, Systemic Equivalencies *on page 1572*
FDA Name Differentiation Project: The Use of Tall-man Letters *on page 12*

Prefrin™ *see page 1509*
Prefrin™ Ophthalmic *see* Phenylephrine *on page 1071*
Pregnenedione *see* Progesterone *on page 1130*
Pregnyl® *see* Chorionic Gonadotropin (Human) *on page 284*
Prelone® *see* PrednisoLONE *on page 1113*
Premarin® *see* Estrogens (Conjugated/Equine) *on page 503*
Premjact® [OTC] *see* Lidocaine *on page 800*
Premphase® *see* Estrogens (Conjugated/Equine) and Medroxyprogesterone *on page 505*
Prempro™ *see* Estrogens (Conjugated/Equine) and Medroxyprogesterone *on page 505*
Preparation H® Hydrocortisone [OTC] *see* Hydrocortisone *on page 673*
Pre-Pen® *see page 1461*
Prepidil® *see* Dinoprostone *on page 421*
Prevacid® *see* Lansoprazole *on page 772*
Prevalite® *see* Cholestyramine Resin *on page 282*
PREVEN™ *see* Ethinyl Estradiol and Levonorgestrel *on page 523*
Prevnar™ *see page 1498*
Prevpac® *see* Lansoprazole, Amoxicillin, and Clarithromycin *on page 774*
Priftin® *see* Rifapentine *on page 1188*
Prilocaine and Lidocaine *see* Lidocaine and Prilocaine *on page 803*
Prilosec® *see* Omeprazole *on page 999*
Primaclone *see* Primidone *on page 1119*
Primacor® *see* Milrinone *on page 908*

Primaquine (PRIM a kween)

Synonyms Primaquine Phosphate; Prymaccone

Generic Available No

Pharmacologic Category Aminoquinoline (Antimalarial)

Pregnancy Risk Factor C

Lactation Excretion in breast milk unknown

Use Provides radical cure of *P. vivax* or *P. ovale* malaria after a clinical attack has been confirmed by blood smear or serologic titer and postexposure prophylaxis

Mechanism of Action/Effect Eliminates the primary tissue exoerythrocytic forms of *P. falciparum*; disrupts mitochondria and binds to DNA

Contraindications Hypersensitivity to primaquine, similar alkaloids, or any component of the formulation; acutely ill patients who have a tendency to develop granulocytopenia (rheumatoid arthritis, SLE); patients receiving other drugs capable of depressing the bone marrow (eg, quinacrine and primaquine)

Warnings/Precautions Use with caution in patients with G6PD deficiency, NADH methemoglobin reductase deficiency. Do not exceed recommended dosage. Pregnancy risk C.

Drug Interactions

Cytochrome P450 Effect: Substrate of **CYP3A4**; Inhibits CYP2D6, 3A4; Induces CYP1A2

Increased Effect/Toxicity: Increased toxicity/levels with quinacrine.

Nutritional/Ethanol Interactions Ethanol: Avoid ethanol (due to GI irritation).

Adverse Reactions

>10%:

- Gastrointestinal: Abdominal pain, nausea, vomiting
- Hematologic: Hemolytic anemia

1% to 10%: Hematologic: Methemoglobinemia

<1% (Limited to important or life-threatening): Agranulocytosis, arrhythmias, leukocytosis, leukopenia

Overdosage/Toxicology Symptoms of acute overdose include abdominal cramps, vomiting, cyanosis, methemoglobinemia (possibly severe), leukopenia, acute hemolytic anemia (often significant), and granulocytopenia. With chronic overdose, symptoms include ototoxicity and retinopathy. Treatment is supportive.

Pharmacodynamics/Kinetics

Absorption: Well absorbed

Half-Life Elimination: 3.7-9.6 hours

Time to Peak: Serum: 1-2 hours

Metabolism: Hepatic to carboxyprimaquine (active)

Formulations Tablet, as phosphate: 26.3 mg [15 mg base]

Dosing

Adults & Elderly: Malaria: Oral: 15 mg/day (base) once daily for 14 days or 45 mg base once weekly for 8 weeks

Pediatrics: Malaria: Oral: Children: 0.3 mg base/kg/day once daily for 14 days (not to exceed 15 mg/day) or 0.9 mg base/kg once weekly for 8 weeks not to exceed 45 mg base/week

Administration

Oral: Take with meals to decrease adverse GI effects. Drug has a bitter taste.

Monitoring Laboratory Tests Periodic CBC, visual color check of urine, glucose, electrolytes; if hemolysis suspected - CBC, haptoglobin, peripheral smear, urinalysis dipstick for occult blood

Monitoring and Teaching Issues

Physical Assessment: See Contraindications and Warnings/Precautions for use cautions. Assess potential for interactions with other prescriptions, OTC medications, or herbal products patient may be taking (see Drug Interactions). Assess results of laboratory tests (see above), therapeutic effectiveness, and adverse reactions (see Adverse Reactions and Overdose/Toxicology). Teach patient appropriate use, possible side effects/interventions, and adverse symptoms to report (see Patient Education). **Pregnancy risk factor C** - benefits of use should outweigh possible risks. Note breast-feeding caution.

Patient Education: Inform prescriber of all prescriptions, OTC medications, or herbal products you are taking, and any allergies you have. Do not take anything new during treatment unless approved by prescriber. It is important to complete full course of therapy for full effect. May be taken with meals to decrease GI upset and bitter aftertaste. Avoid alcohol. You should have regular ophthalmic exams (every 4-6 months) if using this medication over extended periods. May cause nausea, vomiting, or loss of appetite (small, frequent meals, frequent mouth care, sucking lozenges, or chewing gum may help). Report persistent GI disturbance, chest pain or palpitation, unusual fatigue, easy bruising or bleeding, visual or hearing disturbances, changes in urine (darkening, tinged with red, decreased volume), or any other persistent adverse reactions. **Pregnancy/breast-feeding precautions:** Inform prescriber if you are or intend to become pregnant. Consult prescriber if breast-feeding.

Primaquine Phosphate *see* Primaquine *on page 1118*

Primatene® Mist [OTC] *see* Epinephrine *on page 470*

Primaxin® *see* Imipenem and Cilastatin *on page 698*

Primidone (PRI mi done)

U.S. Brand Names Mysoline®

Synonyms Desoxyphenobarbital; Primaclone

Generic Available Yes: Tablet

Pharmacologic Category Anticonvulsant, Miscellaneous; Barbiturate

Pregnancy Risk Factor D

Lactation Enters breast milk/not recommended (AAP recommends use "with caution")

Use Management of grand mal, psychomotor, and focal seizures

Use - Unlabeled/Investigational Benign familial tremor (essential tremor)

Mechanism of Action/Effect Decreases neuron excitability, raises seizure threshold similar to phenobarbital; primidone has two active metabolites, phenobarbital and phenylethylmalonamide (PEMA); PEMA may enhance the activity of phenobarbital

Contraindications Hypersensitivity to primidone, phenobarbital, or any component of the formulation; porphyria; pregnancy

Warnings/Precautions Use with caution in patients with renal or hepatic impairment, pulmonary insufficiency; abrupt withdrawal may precipitate status epilepticus. Potential for drug dependency exists. Do not administer to patients in acute pain. Use caution in elderly, debilitated, or pediatric patients - may cause paradoxical responses. May cause CNS depression, which may impair physical or mental abilities. Patients must cautioned about performing tasks which require mental alertness (ie, operating machinery or driving). Effects with other sedative drugs or ethanol may be potentiated. Use with caution in patients with depression or suicidal tendencies, or in patients with a history of drug abuse. Tolerance or psychological and physical dependence may occur with prolonged use. Primidone's metabolite, phenobarbital, has been associated with cognitive deficits in children. Use with caution in patients with hypoadrenalism.

Drug Interactions

Cytochrome P450 Effect: Metabolized to phenobarbital; Induces **CYP1A2, 2B6, 2C8/9, 3A4**

Decreased Effect: Primidone may induce the hepatic metabolism of many drugs due to enzyme induction, and may reduce the efficacy of beta-blockers, chloramphenicol, cimetidine, clozapine, corticosteroids, cyclosporine, disopyramide, doxycycline, ethosuximide, furosemide, griseofulvin, haloperidol, lamotrigine, methadone, nifedipine, oral contraceptives, phenothiazine, phenytoin, propafenone, quinidine, tacrolimus, TCAs, theophylline, warfarin, and verapamil.

Increased Effect/Toxicity: Central nervous system depression (and possible respiratory depression) may be increased when combined with other CNS depressants, benzodiazepines, valproic acid, chloramphenicol, or antidepressants. MAO inhibitors may prolong the effect of primidone.

Nutritional/Ethanol Interactions

Ethanol: Avoid ethanol (may increase CNS depression).

Food: Protein-deficient diets increase duration of action of primidone.

Herb/Nutraceutical: Avoid valerian, St John's wort, kava kava, gotu kola (may increase CNS depression).

Effects on Lab Values ↑ alkaline phosphatase (S); ↓ calcium (S)

Adverse Reactions Frequency not defined.

Central nervous system: Drowsiness, vertigo, ataxia, lethargy, behavior change, fatigue, hyperirritability

Dermatologic: Rash

Gastrointestinal: Nausea, vomiting, anorexia

Genitourinary: Impotence

Hematologic: Agranulocytopenia, agranulocytosis, anemia

Ocular: Diplopia, nystagmus

Overdosage/Toxicology Symptoms of overdose include unsteady gait, slurred speech, confusion, jaundice, hypothermia, fever, hypotension, coma, and respiratory arrest. Assure

(Continued)

Primidone *(Continued)*

adequate hydration and renal function. Urinary alkalinization with I.V. sodium bicarbonate also helps to enhance elimination. Repeat oral doses of activated charcoal significantly reduce the half-life of primidone through nonrenal elimination. Hemodialysis or hemoperfusion is of uncertain value. Patients in stage IV coma due to high serum drug levels may require charcoal hemoperfusion.

Pharmacodynamics/Kinetics

Bioavailability: 60% to 80%

Half-Life Elimination: Age dependent: Primidone: 10-12 hours; PEMA: 16 hours; Phenobarbital: 52-118 hours

Time to Peak: Serum: ~4 hours

Metabolism: Hepatic to phenobarbital (active) and phenylethylmalonamide (PEMA)

Formulations

Suspension, oral: 250 mg/5 mL (240 mL)

Tablet: 50 mg, 250 mg

Dosing

Adults & Elderly: Seizure disorders (grand mal, psychomotor, and focal): Oral: Initial: 125-250 mg/day at bedtime; increase by 125-250 mg/day every 3-7 days; usual dose: 750-1500 mg/day in divided doses 3-4 times/day with maximum dosage of 2 g/day.

Pediatrics: Seizure disorders (grand mal, psychomotor, and focal): Oral: Children:

<8 years: Initial: 50-125 mg/day given at bedtime; increase by 50-125 mg/day increments every 3-7 days; usual dose: 10-25 mg/kg/day in divided doses 3-4 times/day.

≥8 years: Refer to adult dosing.

Renal Impairment:

Cl_{cr} 50-80 mL/minute: Administer every 8 hours.

Cl_{cr} 10-50 mL/minute: Administer every 8-12 hours.

Cl_{cr} <10 mL/minute: Administer every 12-24 hours.

Moderately dialyzable (20% to 50%)

Administer dose postdialysis or administer supplemental 30% dose.

Hepatic Impairment: Increased side effects may occur in severe liver disease. Monitor plasma levels and adjust dose accordingly.

Stability

Storage: Protect from light.

Monitoring Laboratory Tests Serum primidone and phenobarbital concentration, CBC. Monitor CBC at 6-month intervals to compare with baseline obtained at start of therapy. Since elderly patients metabolize phenobarbital at a slower rate than younger adults, it is suggested to measure both primidone and phenobarbital levels together.

Monitoring and Teaching Issues

Physical Assessment: Assess effectiveness and interactions of other medications patient may be taking (see Contraindications and Drug Interactions). Monitor therapeutic response, laboratory values, and adverse reactions (see Adverse Reactions) at beginning of therapy and periodically with long-term use. Taper dosage slowly when discontinuing. Assess knowledge/teach patient appropriate use and seizure precautions, interventions to reduce side effects, and adverse symptoms to report (see Patient Education). **Pregnancy risk factor D** - determine that patient is not pregnant before beginning treatment. Instruct patients of childbearing age about appropriate barrier contraceptive measures. Breast-feeding is not recommended.

Patient Education: Take exactly as directed; do not increase dose or frequency or discontinue without consulting prescriber. Drug may cause physical and/or psychological dependence. While using this medication, do not use alcohol and other prescription or OTC medications (especially pain medications, sedatives, antihistamines, or hypnotics) without consulting prescriber. Maintain adequate hydration (2-3 L/day of fluids) unless advised by prescriber to restrict fluids. You may experience drowsiness, dizziness, or blurred vision (use caution when driving or engaging in tasks requiring alertness until response to drug is known); nausea, vomiting, or loss of appetite (small, frequent meals, frequent mouth care, chewing gum, or sucking lozenges may help); or impotence (reversible). Wear identification of epileptic status and medications. Report behavioral or CNS changes (confusion, depression, increased sedation, excitation, headache, insomnia, or lethargy); muscle weakness, or tremors; unusual bruising or bleeding (mouth, urine, stool); or worsening of seizure activity or loss of seizure control. **Pregnancy/breast-feeding precautions:** Do not get pregnant while taking this drug; use appropriate contraceptive measures. Breast-feeding is not recommended.

Dietary Issues: Folic acid: Low erythrocyte and CSF folate concentrations. Megaloblastic anemia has been reported. To avoid folic acid deficiency and megaloblastic anemia, some clinicians recommend giving patients on anticonvulsants prophylactic doses of folic acid and cyanocobalamin.

Geriatric Considerations: Due to CNS effects, monitor closely when initiating drug in the elderly. Since elderly metabolize phenobarbital at a slower rate than younger adults, it is suggested to measure both primidone and phenobarbital levels together. Adjust dose for renal function in the elderly when initiating or changing dose.

Breast-feeding Issues: Sedation and feeding problems may occur in nursing infants. AAP recommends USE WITH CAUTION.

Pregnancy Issues: Crosses the placenta. Dysmorphic facial features; hemorrhagic disease of newborn due to fetal vitamin K depletion, maternal folic acid deficiency may occur. Epilepsy itself, number of medications, genetic factors, or a combination of these probably influence the teratogenicity of anticonvulsant therapy. Benefit:risk ratio usually favors continued use during pregnancy.

Related Information

Peak and Trough Guidelines *on page 1544*

Phenobarbital *on page 1067*

Primsol® *see* Trimethoprim *on page 1366*

Principen® *see* Ampicillin *on page 101*

Prinivil® *see* Lisinopril *on page 808*
Prinzide® *see* Lisinopril and Hydrochlorothiazide *on page 810*
Pristinamycin *see* Quinupristin and Dalfopristin *on page 1166*
ProAmatine® *see* Midodrine *on page 903*

Probenecid (proe BEN e sid)

Synonyms Benemid [DSC]
Generic Available Yes
Pharmacologic Category Uricosuric Agent
Pregnancy Risk Factor B
Lactation Excretion in breast milk unknown
Use Prevention of gouty arthritis; hyperuricemia; prolongation of beta-lactam effect (ie, serum levels)
Mechanism of Action/Effect Competitively inhibits the reabsorption of uric acid at the proximal convoluted tubule, thereby promoting its excretion and reducing serum uric acid levels; increases plasma levels of weak organic acids (penicillins, cephalosporins, or other beta-lactam antibiotics) by competitively inhibiting their renal tubular secretion
Contraindications Hypersensitivity to probenecid or any component of the formulation; high-dose aspirin therapy; moderate to severe renal impairment; children <2 years of age
Warnings/Precautions Use with caution in patients with peptic ulcer. Use extreme caution in the use of probenecid with penicillin in patients with renal insufficiency. Probenecid may not be effective in patients with a creatinine clearance <30-50 mL/minute. May cause exacerbation of acute gouty attack.
Drug Interactions
Cytochrome P450 Effect: Inhibits CYP2C19
Decreased Effect: Salicylates (high-dose) may decrease uricosuria. Decreased urinary levels of nitrofurantoin may decrease efficacy.
Increased Effect/Toxicity: Increases methotrexate toxic potential. Probenecid increases the serum concentrations of quinolones and beta-lactams such as penicillins and cephalosporins. Also increases levels/toxicity of acyclovir, diflunisal, ketorolac, thiopental, benzodiazepines, dapsone, fluoroquinolones, methotrexate, NSAIDs, sulfonylureas, zidovudine.
Effects on Lab Values False-positive glucosuria with Clinitest®
Adverse Reactions Frequency not defined.
Cardiovascular: Flushing of face
Central nervous system: Headache, dizziness
Dermatologic: Rash, itching
Gastrointestinal: Anorexia, nausea, vomiting, sore gums
Genitourinary: Painful urination
Hematologic: Aplastic anemia, hemolytic anemia, leukopenia
Hepatic: Hepatic necrosis
Neuromuscular & skeletal: Gouty arthritis (acute)
Renal: Renal calculi, nephrotic syndrome, urate nephropathy
Miscellaneous: Anaphylaxis
Overdosage/Toxicology Symptoms of overdose include nausea, vomiting, tonic-clonic seizures, and coma. Activated charcoal is especially effective at binding probenecid, for GI decontamination.
Pharmacodynamics/Kinetics
Absorption: Rapid and complete
Half-Life Elimination: Dose dependent: Normal renal function: 6-12 hours
Time to Peak: Serum: 2-4 hours
Metabolism: Hepatic
Onset: Effect on penicillin levels: 2 hours
Formulations Tablet: 500 mg
Dosing
Adults & Elderly:
Hyperuricemia with gout: Oral: 250 mg twice daily for 1 week; increase to 250-500 mg/day; may increase by 500 mg/month, if needed, to maximum of 2-3 g/day (dosages may be increased by 500 mg every 6 months if serum urate concentrations are controlled)
Prolong penicillin serum levels: Oral: 500 mg 4 times/day
Gonorrhea: Oral: 1 g 30 minutes before penicillin, ampicillin, or amoxicillin
Neurosyphilis: Oral: Aqueous procaine penicillin 2.4 million units/day I.M. plus probenecid 500 mg 4 times/day for 10-14 days
Pediatrics:
Note: Note recommended in children <2 years of age.
Prolong penicillin serum levels: Oral: Children 2-14 years: 25 mg/kg starting dose, then 40 mg/kg/day given 4 times/day
Treatment of gonorrhea: Oral: Children <45 kg: 25 mg/kg x 1 (maximum: 1 g/dose) 30 minutes before penicillin, ampicillin, or amoxicillin
Renal Impairment: Cl_{cr} <50 mL/minute: Avoid use.
Monitoring Laboratory Tests Uric acid, renal function, CBC
Monitoring and Teaching Issues
Physical Assessment: Assess effectiveness and interactions of other medications patient may be taking (see Contraindications and Drug Interactions). Monitor therapeutic response, laboratory values, and adverse reactions (see Adverse Reactions and Overdose/Toxicology) at beginning of therapy and periodically with long-term use. Assess knowledge/teach patient appropriate use, interventions to reduce side effects, and adverse symptoms to report (see Patient Education). Note breast-feeding caution.
Patient Education: Take as directed; do not discontinue without consulting prescriber. May take 6-12 months to reduce gouty attacks (attacks may increase in frequency and severity for first few months of therapy). Take with food or antacids or alkaline ash foods (milk, nuts, beets, spinach, turnip greens). Maintain adequate hydration (2-3 L/day of fluids) unless
(Continued)

Probenecid *(Continued)*

advised by prescriber to restrict fluids. Avoid aspirin or aspirin-containing substances. If diabetic, use serum glucose monitoring. If you experience severe headache, contact prescriber for medication. You may experience dizziness or lightheadedness (use caution when driving, changing position, or engaging in tasks requiring alertness until response to drug is known); or nausea, vomiting, indigestion, or loss of appetite (small, frequent meals, frequent mouth care, chewing gum, or sucking lozenges may help). Report skin rash or itching, persistent headache, blood in urine or painful urination, excessive tiredness or easy bruising or bleeding, or sore gums. **Breast-feeding precaution:** Consult prescriber if breast-feeding.

Dietary Issues: Drug may cause GI upset; take with food if GI upset. Drink plenty of fluids.

Geriatric Considerations: Since probenecid loses its effectiveness when the Cl_{cr} is <30 mL/minute, its usefulness in the elderly is limited.

Additional Information Avoid fluctuation in uric acid (increase or decrease); may precipitate gout attack.

Probenecid and Colchicine *see* Colchicine and Probenecid *on page 330*

Probiotica® [OTC] *see Lactobacillus on page 766*

Procainamide (proe kane A mide)

U.S. Brand Names Procanbid®; Pronestyl®; Pronestyl-SR®

Synonyms PCA; Procainamide Hydrochloride; Procaine Amide Hydrochloride

Generic Available Yes

Pharmacologic Category Antiarrhythmic Agent, Class Ia

Pregnancy Risk Factor C

Lactation Enters breast milk/use caution (AAP rates "compatible")

Use Treatment of ventricular tachycardia (VT), premature ventricular contractions, paroxysmal atrial tachycardia (PSVT), and atrial fibrillation (AF); prevent recurrence of ventricular tachycardia, paroxysmal supraventricular tachycardia, atrial fibrillation or flutter

Use - Unlabeled/Investigational ACLS guidelines:

Intermittent/recurrent VF or pulseless VT not responsive to earlier interventions
Monomorphic VT (EF >40%, no CHF)
Polymorphic VT with normal baseline QT interval
Wide complex tachycardia of unknown type (EF >40%, no CHF, patient stable)
Refractory paroxysmal SVT
Atrial fibrillation or flutter (EF >40%, no CHF) including pre-excitation syndrome

Mechanism of Action/Effect Decreases myocardial excitability and conduction velocity and may depress myocardial contractility, by increasing the electrical stimulation threshold of ventricle, His-Purkinje system and through direct cardiac effects

Contraindications Hypersensitivity to procaine, other ester-type local anesthetics, or any component of the formulation; complete heart block (except in patients with a functioning artificial pacemaker); second-degree AV block (without a functional pacemaker); various types of hemiblock (without a functional pacemaker); SLE; torsade de pointes; concurrent cisapride use; QT prolongation

Warnings/Precautions Monitor and adjust dose to prevent QT_c prolongation. Watch for proarrhythmic effects. May precipitate or exacerbate CHF. Reduce dosage in renal impairment. May increase ventricular response rate in patients with atrial fibrillation or flutter; control AV conduction before initiating. Correct hypokalemia before initiating therapy; hypokalemia may worsen toxicity. Use caution in digoxin-induced toxicity (can further depress AV conduction). Reduce dose if first-degree heart block occurs. Use caution with concurrent use of other antiarrhythmics. Avoid use in myasthenia gravis (may worsen condition). Hypersensitivity reactions can occur.

Potentially fatal blood dyscrasias have occurred with therapeutic doses; close monitoring is recommended during the first 3 months of therapy.

Long-term administration leads to the development of a positive antinuclear antibody (ANA) test in 50% of patients which may result in a drug-induced lupus erythematosus-like syndrome (in 20% to 30% of patients); discontinue procainamide with SLE symptoms and choose an alternative agent

Pregnancy risk C.

Drug Interactions

Cytochrome P450 Effect: Substrate of **CYP2D6**

Increased Effect/Toxicity: Amiodarone, cimetidine, ofloxacin (and potentially other renally eliminated quinolones), ranitidine, and trimethoprim increase procainamide and NAPA blood levels; consider reducing procainamide dosage by 25% with concurrent use. Cisapride and procainamide may increase the risk of malignant arrhythmia; concurrent use is contraindicated. Neuromuscular blocking agents: Procainamide may potentiate neuromuscular blockade.

Drugs which may prolong the QT interval include amiodarone, amitriptyline, astemizole, bepridil, cisapride, disopyramide, erythromycin, haloperidol, imipramine, pimozide, quinidine, sotalol, mesoridazine, thioridazine, and some quinolone antibiotics (sparfloxacin, gatifloxacin, moxifloxacin); concurrent use may result in additional prolongation of the QT interval.

Nutritional/Ethanol Interactions

Ethanol: Avoid ethanol (acute ethanol administration reduces procainamide serum concentrations).

Herb/Nutraceutical: Avoid ephedra (may worsen arrhythmia).

Adverse Reactions

>1%:

Cardiovascular: Hypotension (I.V., up to 5%)
Dermatologic: Rash

Gastrointestinal: Diarrhea (3% to 4%), nausea, vomiting, taste disorder, GI complaints (3% to 4%)

<1% (Limited to important or life-threatening): Agranulocytosis, angioneurotic edema, aplastic anemia, arrhythmia (proarrhythmic effect, new or worsened), bone marrow suppression, cerebellar ataxia, cholestasis, demyelinating polyradiculoneuropathy, depressed myocardial contractility, depression, disorientation, drug fever, granulomatous hepatitis, hallucinations, hemolytic anemia, hepatic failure, hypoplastic anemia, leukopenia, mania, myasthenia gravis (worsened), myocarditis, myopathy, neuromuscular blockade, neutropenia, pancreatitis, pancytopenia, paradoxical increase in ventricular rate in atrial fibrillation/flutter, pericarditis, peripheral neuropathy, pleural effusion, positive ANA, positive Coombs' test, pruritus, pseudo-obstruction, psychosis, pulmonary embolism, QT prolongation (excessive), rash, respiratory failure due to myopathy, second-degree heart block, SLE-like syndrome, thrombocytopenia (0.5%), torsade de pointes, tremor, urticaria, vasculitis, ventricular arrhythmias

Overdosage/Toxicology Procainamide has a low toxic:therapeutic ratio and may easily produce fatal intoxication (acute toxic dose: 5 g in adults). Symptoms of overdose include sinus bradycardia, sinus node arrest or asystole, P-R, QRS, or QT interval prolongation, torsade de pointes (polymorphous ventricular tachycardia), and depressed myocardial contractility, which along with alpha-adrenergic or ganglionic blockade, may result in hypotension and pulmonary edema. Other effects are seizures, coma, and respiratory arrest. Treatment is symptomatic and effects usually respond to conventional therapies. **Note:** Do not use other Type 1A or 1C antiarrhythmic agents to treat ventricular tachycardia. Sodium bicarbonate may treat wide QRS intervals or hypotension. Markedly impaired conduction or high degree AV block, unresponsive to bicarbonate, indicates consideration of a pacemaker.

Pharmacodynamics/Kinetics

Bioavailability: Oral: 75% to 95%

Half-Life Elimination:

Procainamide (hepatic acetylator, phenotype, cardiac and renal function dependent):
Children: 1.7 hours; Adults: 2.5-4.7 hours; Anephric: 11 hours

NAPA (renal function dependent):
Children: 6 hours; Adults: 6-8 hours; Anephric: 42 hours

Time to Peak: Serum: Capsule: 45 minutes to 2.5 hours; I.M.: 15-60 minutes

Metabolism: Hepatic via acetylation to produce N-acetyl procainamide (NAPA) (active metabolite)

Onset: I.M. 10-30 minutes

Formulations

Capsule, as hydrochloride: 250 mg, 375 mg, 500 mg
Injection, as hydrochloride: 100 mg/mL (10 mL); 500 mg/mL (2 mL)
Tablet, as hydrochloride: 250 mg, 375 mg, 500 mg
Tablet, sustained release, as hydrochloride: 250 mg, 500 mg, 750 mg, 1000 mg
Procanbid®: 500 mg, 1000 mg

Dosing

Adults & Elderly: Dose must be titrated to patient's response.

Antiarrhythmic:

Oral: 250-500 mg/dose every 3-6 hours or 500 mg to 1 g every 6 hours sustained release; usual dose: 50 mg/kg/24 hours; maximum: 4 g/24 hours

I.M.: 0.5-1 g every 4-8 hours until oral therapy is possible

I.V. (infusion requires use of an infusion pump): Loading dose: 15-18 mg/kg administered as slow infusion over 25-30 minutes or 100-200 mg/dose repeated every 5 minutes as needed to a total dose of 1 g; maintenance dose: 1-4 mg/minute by continuous infusion.

Infusion rate: **2 g/250 mL** D_5W/NS (I.V. infusion requires use of an infusion pump):
1 mg/minute: 7.5 mL/hour
2 mg/minute: 15 mL/hour
3 mg/minute: 22.5 mL/hour
4 mg/minute: 30 mL/hour
5 mg/minute: 37.5 mL/hour
6 mg/minute: 45 mL/hour

Intermittent/recurrent VF or pulseless VT:

Initial: 20-30 mg/minute (maximum: 50 mg/minute if necessary), up to a total of 17 mg/kg. ACLS guidelines: I.V.: Infuse 20 mg/minute until arrhythmia is controlled, hypotension occurs, QRS complex widens by 50% of its original width, or total of 17 mg/kg is given.

Note: Reduce to 12 mg/kg in setting of cardiac or renal dysfunction

I.V. maintenance infusion: 1-4 mg/minute; monitor levels and do not exceed 3 mg/minute for >24 hours in adults with renal failure.

Pediatrics: Must be titrated to patient's response:

Arrhythmias:

Oral: 15-50 mg/kg/24 hours divided every 3-6 hours

I.M.: 50 mg/kg/24 hours divided into doses of $^1/_8$ to $^1/_4$ every 3-6 hours in divided doses until oral therapy is possible

I.V. (infusion requires use of an infusion pump):

Load: 3-6 mg/kg/dose over 5 minutes not to exceed 100 mg/dose; may repeat every 5-10 minutes to maximum of 15 mg/kg/load

Maintenance as continuous I.V. infusion: 20-80 mcg/kg/minute; maximum: 2 g/24 hours

Renal Impairment:

Cl_{cr} 10-50 mL/minute: Administer every 6-12 hours.

Cl_{cr} <10 mL/minute: Administer every 8-24 hours.

Dialysis:

Procainamide: Moderately hemodialyzable (20% to 50%): 200 mg supplemental dose posthemodialysis is recommended.

N-acetylprocainamide: Not dialyzable (0% to 5%)

Procainamide/N-acetylprocainamide: Peritoneal dialysis: Not dialyzable (0% to 5%)

(Continued)

Procainamide *(Continued)*

Procainamide/N-acetylprocainamide: Replace by blood level during continuous arteriovenous or venovenous hemofiltration.

Hepatic Impairment: Reduce dose by 50%.

Administration

Oral: Do **not** crush or chew sustained release drug product.

I.V.: Maximum rate: 50 mg/minute; give around-the-clock to promote less variation in peak and trough serum levels.

Stability

Storage: Procainamide may be stored at room temperature up to 27°C; however, refrigeration retards oxidation, which causes color formation. The solution is initially colorless but may turn slightly yellow on standing. Injection of air into the vial causes the solution to darken. Solutions darker than a light amber should be discarded.

Reconstitution: Minimum volume: 1 g/250 mL NS/D_5W

Stability of admixture at room temperature in D_5W or NS is 24 hours. Some information indicates that procainamide may be subject to greater decomposition in D_5W unless the admixture is refrigerated or the pH is adjusted. Procainamide is believed to form an association complex with dextrose - the bioavailability of procainamide in this complex is not known and the complex formation is reversible.

Compatibility: Stable in $^1/_2$NS, NS, sterile water for injection

Y-site administration: Incompatible with milrinone

Compatibility when admixed: Incompatible with esmolol, ethacrynate, milrinone, phenytoin

Monitoring Laboratory Tests CBC with differential, platelet count

Monitoring and Teaching Issues

Physical Assessment: Assess other medications patient may be taking for effectiveness and interactions (see Drug Interactions). See Warnings/Precautions for use cautions. I.V. requires use of infusion pump and continuous cardiac and hemodynamic monitoring. Monitor laboratory tests, therapeutic response, and adverse reactions (see Warnings/Precautions and Adverse Reactions) at beginning of therapy, when titrating dosage, and on a regular basis with long-term therapy. **Note:** Procainamide has a low TI and overdose may easily produce severe and life-threatening reactions (see Overdose/Toxicology). Assess knowledge/teach patient appropriate use, interventions to reduce side effects, and adverse symptoms to report (see Patient Education). **Pregnancy risk factor C** - benefits of use should outweigh possible risks. Note breast-feeding caution.

Patient Education: Oral: Take exactly as directed; do not take additional doses or discontinue without consulting prescriber. Avoid alcohol. You will need regular cardiac checkups and blood tests while taking this medication. You may experience dizziness, lightheadedness, or visual changes (use caution when driving or engaging in tasks requiring alertness until response to drug is known); loss of appetite (small, frequent meals, frequent mouth care, chewing gum, or sucking lozenges may help); headaches (prescriber may recommend mild analgesic); or diarrhea (yogurt, or boiled milk may help - if persistent consult prescriber). Report chest pain, palpitation, or erratic heartbeat; increased weight or swelling of hands or feet; acute diarrhea; or unusual fatigue and tiredness. **Pregnancy/breast-feeding precautions:** Inform prescriber if you are or intend to become pregnant. Consult prescriber if breast-feeding.

Dietary Issues: Should be taken with water on an empty stomach.

Geriatric Considerations: Monitor closely since clearance is reduced in those >60 years of age. If clinically possible, start doses at lowest recommended dose. Also, elderly frequently have drug therapy which may interfere with the use of procainamide. Adjust dose for renal function in the elderly.

Breast-feeding Issues: Considered compatible by the AAP. However, the AAP stated concern regarding long-term effects and potential for infant toxicity. Use caution and monitor closely if continuing to breast-feed while taking procainamide.

Related Information

Antiarrhythmic Drugs *on page 1551*
Peak and Trough Guidelines *on page 1544*

Procainamide Hydrochloride *see* Procainamide *on page 1122*

Procaine (PROE kane)

U.S. Brand Names Novocain®

Synonyms Procaine Hydrochloride

Generic Available Yes

Pharmacologic Category Local Anesthetic

Pregnancy Risk Factor C

Lactation Excretion in breast milk unknown

Use Produces spinal anesthesia and epidural and peripheral nerve block by injection and infiltration methods

Mechanism of Action/Effect Blocks both the initiation and conduction of nerve impulses by decreasing the neuronal membrane's permeability to sodium ions, which results in inhibition of depolarization with resultant blockade of conduction

Contraindications Hypersensitivity to procaine, PABA, parabens, other ester local anesthetics, or any component of the formulation

Warnings/Precautions Patients with cardiac diseases, hyperthyroidism, or other endocrine diseases may be more susceptible to toxic effects of local anesthetics. Some preparations contain metabisulfite. Pregnancy risk C.

Drug Interactions

Decreased Effect: Decreased effect of sulfonamides with the PABA metabolite of procaine, chloroprocaine, and tetracaine. Decreased/increased effect of vasopressors, ergot alkaloids, and MAO inhibitors on blood pressure when using anesthetic solutions with a vasoconstrictor.

Adverse Reactions

1% to 10%: Local: Burning sensation at site of injection, tissue irritation, pain at injection site

<1% (Limited to important or life-threatening): Aseptic meningitis resulting in paralysis, chills, CNS stimulation followed by CNS depression

Overdosage/Toxicology Treatment is symptomatic and supportive. Termination of anesthesia by pneumatic tourniquet inflation should be attempted when procaine is administered by infiltration or regional injection.

Pharmacodynamics/Kinetics

Half-Life Elimination: 7.7 minutes

Metabolism: Rapidly hydrolyzed by plasma enzymes to para-aminobenzoic acid and diethylaminoethanol (80% conjugated before elimination)

Onset: 2-5 minutes

Duration: Patient, type of block, concentration, and method of anesthesia dependent: 0.5-1.5 hours

Formulations Injection, as hydrochloride: 1% [10 mg/mL] (2 mL, 6 mL, 30 mL, 100 mL); 2% [20 mg/mL] (30 mL, 100 mL); 10% (2 mL)

Dosing

Adults & Elderly: Spinal anesthesia, epidural and peripheral nerve block: Injection and infiltration methods: Dose varies with procedure, desired depth, and duration of anesthesia, desired muscle relaxation, vascularity of tissues, physical condition, and age of patient.

Pediatrics: Dose varies with procedure, desired depth, and duration of anesthesia, desired muscle relaxation, vascularity of tissues, physical condition, and age of patient.

Stability

Compatibility: Stable in dextran 6% in dextrose, dextran 6% in NS, D_5LR, $D_5{}^1/_4NS$, $D_5{}^1/_2NS$, D_5NS, D_5W, $D_{10}W$, LR, $^1/_2NS$, NS

Compatibility when admixed: Incompatible with amobarbital, amphotericin B, chlorothiazide, magnesium sulfate, phenobarbital, phenytoin, sodium bicarbonate

Monitoring and Teaching Issues

Physical Assessment: Monitor response, degree of pain sensation, and injection site. **Epidural:** Monitor CNS status (see Adverse Reactions). **Pregnancy risk factor C.** Note breast-feeding caution.

Patient Education: The purpose of this medication is to reduce pain sensation. Report local burning or pain at injection site. **Pregnancy/breast-feeding precautions:** Inform prescriber if you are or intend to become pregnant. Consult prescriber if breast-feeding.

Procaine Amide Hydrochloride *see* Procainamide *on page 1122*

Procaine Benzylpenicillin *see* Penicillin G Procaine *on page 1047*

Procaine Hydrochloride *see* Procaine *on page 1124*

Procaine Penicillin G *see* Penicillin G Procaine *on page 1047*

Procanbid® *see* Procainamide *on page 1122*

Procarbazine (proe KAR ba zeen)

U.S. Brand Names Matulane®

Synonyms Benzmethyzin; N-Methylhydrazine; Procarbazine Hydrochloride

Generic Available No

Pharmacologic Category Antineoplastic Agent, Alkylating Agent

Pregnancy Risk Factor D

Lactation Excretion in breast milk unknown/not recommended

Use Treatment of Hodgkin's disease; other uses include non-Hodgkin's lymphoma, brain tumors, melanoma, lung cancer, multiple myeloma

Mechanism of Action/Effect Mechanism of action is not clear, methylating of nucleic acids; inhibits DNA, RNA, and protein synthesis; may damage DNA directly and suppresses mitosis; metabolic activation required by host

Contraindications Hypersensitivity to procarbazine or any component of the formulation; pre-existing bone marrow aplasia; ethanol ingestion; pregnancy

Warnings/Precautions The U.S. Food and Drug Administration (FDA) currently recommends that procedures for proper handling and disposal of antineoplastic agents be considered. Appropriate safety equipment is recommended for preparation, administration, and disposal of antineoplastics. If procarbazine contacts the skin, wash and flush thoroughly with water. Use with caution in patients with pre-existing renal or hepatic impairment. Modify dosage in patients with renal or hepatic impairment or marrow disorders. Reduce dosage with serum creatinine >2 mg/dL or total bilirubin >3 mg/dL. Procarbazine possesses MAO inhibitor activity. Procarbazine is a carcinogen which may cause acute leukemia. Procarbazine may cause infertility.

Drug Interactions

Increased Effect/Toxicity: Procarbazine exhibits weak MAO inhibitor activity. Foods containing high amounts of tyramine should, therefore, be avoided. When an MAO inhibitor is given with food high in tyramine, hypertensive crisis, intracranial bleeding, and headache have been reported.

Sympathomimetic amines (epinephrine and amphetamines) and antidepressants (tricyclics) should be used cautiously with procarbazine. Barbiturates, narcotics, phenothiazines, and other CNS depressants can cause somnolence, ataxia, and other symptoms of CNS depression. Ethanol has caused a disulfiram-like reaction with procarbazine. May result in headache, respiratory difficulties, nausea, vomiting, sweating, thirst, hypotension, and flushing.

Nutritional/Ethanol Interactions

Ethanol: Avoid ethanol and ethanol-containing products.

Food: Clinically severe and possibly life-threatening elevations in blood pressure may occur if procarbazine is taken with tyramine-containing foods.

(Continued)

Procarbazine *(Continued)*

Adverse Reactions

>10%:

Central nervous system: Mental depression, manic reactions, hallucinations, dizziness, headache, nervousness, insomnia, nightmares, ataxia, disorientation, confusion, seizure, CNS stimulation

Endocrine & metabolic: Amenorrhea

Gastrointestinal: Severe nausea and vomiting occur frequently and may be dose-limiting; anorexia, abdominal pain, stomatitis, dysphagia, diarrhea, and constipation; use a nonphenothiazine antiemetic, when possible

Emetic potential: Moderately high (60% to 90%)

Time course of nausea/vomiting: Onset: 24-27 hours; Duration: variable

Hematologic: Thrombocytopenia, hemolytic anemia, anemia

Myelosuppressive: May be dose-limiting toxicity; procarbazine should be discontinued if leukocyte count is <4000/mm^3 or platelet count <100,000/mm^3

WBC: Moderate

Platelets: Moderate

Onset (days): 14

Nadir (days): 21

Recovery (days): 28

Neuromuscular & skeletal: Weakness, paresthesia, neuropathies, decreased reflexes, foot drop, tremors

Ocular: Nystagmus

Respiratory: Pleural effusion, cough

1% to 10%:

Dermatologic: Alopecia, hyperpigmentation

Gastrointestinal: Diarrhea, stomatitis, constipation

Hepatic: Hepatotoxicity

Neuromuscular & skeletal: Peripheral neuropathy

<1% (Limited to important or life-threatening): Disulfiram-like reactions, hypertensive crisis, orthostatic hypotension, pneumonitis

Overdosage/Toxicology Symptoms of overdose include arthralgia, alopecia, paresthesia, bone marrow suppression, hallucinations, nausea, vomiting, diarrhea, seizures, and coma. Treatment is supportive. Adverse effects such as marrow toxicity may begin as late as 2 weeks after exposure.

Pharmacodynamics/Kinetics

Absorption: Rapid and complete

Half-Life Elimination: 1 hour

Metabolism: Hepatic and renal

Formulations Capsule, as hydrochloride: 50 mg

Dosing

Adults: Refer to individual protocols.

Chemotherapy: Oral: Initial: 2-4 mg/kg/day in single or divided doses for 7 days then increase dose to 4-6 mg/kg/day until response is obtained or leukocyte count decreased <4000/mm^3 or the platelet count decreased <100,000/mm^3; maintenance: 1-2 mg/kg/day

Commonly used doses in combination chemotherapy regimens are in the range of 60-100 mg/m^2/day for 10-14 days. Doses are commonly rounded to the nearest 50 mg. Alternating daily doses may be utilized to achieve an "average" (eg, 150 mg alternating with 200 mg in a 1.7 m^2 patient).

In MOPP, 100 mg/m^2/day on days 1-14 of a 28-day cycle

Elderly: Refer to adult dosing; use with caution. Adjust for renal impairment.

Pediatrics: Refer to individual protocols. Dose based on patient's ideal weight if the patient is obese or has abnormal fluid retention. Oral: Children:

BMT aplastic anemia conditioning regimen: 12.5 mg/kg/dose every other day for 4 doses

Hodgkin's disease: MOPP/IC-MOPP regimens: 100 mg/m^2/day for 14 days and repeated every 4 weeks

Neuroblastoma and medulloblastoma: Doses as high as 100-200 mg/m^2/day once daily have been used.

Renal Impairment: Use with caution, may result in increased toxicity.

Hepatic Impairment: Use with caution; may result in increased toxicity.

Stability

Storage: Protect from light

Monitoring Laboratory Tests CBC with differential, platelet and reticulocyte count, urinalysis, liver and renal function

Monitoring and Teaching Issues

Physical Assessment: See Contraindications and Warnings/Precautions for use cautions. Assess potential for interactions with other prescriptions, OTC medications, or herbal products patient may be taking (see Drug Interactions). Emetic potential is high; antiemetic is generally required. Assess results of laboratory tests (see above) and patient response frequently (see Adverse Reactions and Overdose/Toxicology). Instruct patient about dietary cautions (procarbazine has some MAO inhibitory effects - see Tyramine Foods List). Teach patient proper use, possible side effects and interventions, and adverse symptoms to report (see Patient Education). **Pregnancy risk factor D** - determine that patient is not pregnant before beginning treatment. Instruct patients of childbearing age about necessity for barrier contraceptive measures during and for one month following therapy. Breast-feeding is not recommended.

Patient Education: Inform prescriber of all prescriptions, OTC medications, or herbal products you are taking, and any allergies you have. Do not take anything new during treatment unless approved by prescriber. Take as directed. Maintain adequate hydration (2-3 L/day of fluids) unless advised by prescriber to restrict fluids. Avoid alcohol; may cause acute disulfiram reaction (headache, respiratory difficulties, nausea, vomiting, sweating, thirst, hypotension, and flushing). Avoid tyramine-containing foods (aged cheese, chocolate, pickles, aged meat, wine, etc) - could cause serious hypertensive effects. You will be more sensitive to infection (avoid crowds and exposure to infection and do not have any vaccinations without consulting prescriber). May cause considerable nausea or vomiting (consult prescriber for approved antiemetic); mental depression, nervousness, insomnia, nightmares, dizziness, confusion, or lethargy (use caution when driving or engaging in tasks that require alertness until response to drug is known); rash, hair loss, or hyperpigmentation (reversible), loss of libido, sterility, or amenorrhea. Report persistent fever, chills, sore throat; unusual bleeding; blood in urine, stool (black stool), or vomitus; unresolved depression; mania; hallucinations; nightmares; disorientation; seizures; chest pain or palpitations; difficulty breathing; or vision changes. **Pregnancy/breast-feeding precautions:** Inform prescriber if you are pregnant. Do not get pregnant during or for 1 month following therapy. Male: Do not cause a female to become pregnant. Male/female: Consult prescriber for instruction on appropriate contraceptive measures. This drug may cause severe fetal defects. Breast-feeding is not recommended.

Related Information

Tyramine Foods List *on page 1601*

Procarbazine Hydrochloride *see* Procarbazine *on page 1125*

Procardia® *see* NIFEdipine *on page 970*

Procardia XL® *see* NIFEdipine *on page 970*

Procetofene *see* Fenofibrate *on page 549*

Prochlorperazine (proe klor PER a zeen)

U.S. Brand Names Compazine®; Compro™

Synonyms Prochlorperazine Edisylate; Prochlorperazine Maleate

Generic Available Yes: Injection and tablet

Pharmacologic Category Antipsychotic Agent, Phenothiazine, Piperazine

Pregnancy Risk Factor C

Lactation Enters breast milk/not recommended

Use Management of nausea and vomiting; psychosis; anxiety

Use - Unlabeled/Investigational Dementia behavior

Mechanism of Action/Effect Blocks postsynaptic mesolimbic dopaminergic D_1 and D_2 receptors in the brain, including the medullary chemoreceptor trigger zone; exhibits a strong alpha-adrenergic and anticholinergic blocking effect and depresses the release of hypothalamic and hypophyseal hormones; believed to depress the reticular activating system, thus affecting basal metabolism, body temperature, wakefulness, vasomotor tone and emesis

Contraindications Hypersensitivity to prochlorperazine or any component of the formulation (cross-reactivity between phenothiazines may occur); severe CNS depression; coma; bone marrow suppression; should not be used in children <2 years of age or <10 kg

Warnings/Precautions May be sedating; use with caution in disorders where CNS depression is a feature. May impair physical or mental abilities; patients must cautioned about performing tasks which require mental alertness (ie, operating machinery or driving). Effects with other sedative drugs or ethanol may be potentiated. Avoid use in Reye's syndrome. Use with caution in Parkinson's disease; hemodynamic instability; bone marrow suppression; predisposition to seizures; subcortical brain damage; and in severe cardiac, hepatic, renal or respiratory disease. Caution in breast cancer or other prolactin-dependent tumors (may elevate prolactin levels). May alter temperature regulation or mask toxicity of other drugs due to antiemetic effects. May alter cardiac conduction - life threatening arrhythmias have occurred with therapeutic doses of phenothiazines. May cause orthostatic hypotension; use with caution in patients at risk of hypotension or where transient hypotensive episodes would be poorly tolerated (cardiovascular disease or cerebrovascular disease). Hypotension may occur following administration, particularly when parenteral form is used or in high dosages.

Due to anticholinergic effects, use with caution in patients with decreased gastrointestinal motility, urinary retention, BPH, xerostomia, visual problems, narrow-angle glaucoma (screening is recommended) and myasthenia gravis. May cause extrapyramidal symptoms, including pseudoparkinsonism, acute dystonic reactions, akathisia and tardive dyskinesia. May be associated with neuroleptic malignant syndrome (NMS).

Pregnancy risk C.

Drug Interactions

Decreased Effect: Barbiturates and carbamazepine may increase the metabolism of prochlorperazine, lowering its serum levels. Benztropine (and other anticholinergics) may inhibit the therapeutic response to prochlorperazine. Antipsychotics such as prochlorperazine inhibit the ability of bromocriptine to lower serum prolactin concentrations. The antihypertensive effects of guanethidine and guanadrel may be inhibited by prochlorperazine. Prochlorperazine may inhibit the antiparkinsonian effect of levodopa. Prochlorperazine (and possibly other low potency antipsychotics) may reverse the pressor effects of epinephrine.

Increased Effect/Toxicity: Chloroquine, propranolol, and sulfadoxine-pyrimethamine may increase prochlorperazine concentrations. Concurrent use with TCA may produce increased toxicity or altered therapeutic response. Prochlorperazine plus lithium may rarely produce neurotoxicity. Prochlorperazine may produce additive CNS depressant effects with CNS depressants (ethanol, narcotics). Metoclopramide may increase risk of extrapyramidal symptoms (EPS).

Nutritional/Ethanol Interactions

Ethanol: Avoid ethanol (may increase CNS depression).

Food: Limit caffeine.

Herb/Nutraceutical: Avoid dong quai, St John's wort (may also cause photosensitization). Avoid kava kava, gotu kola, valerian, St John's wort (may increase CNS depression).

Effects on Lab Values False-positives for phenylketonuria, urinary amylase, uroporphyrins, urobilinogen

Adverse Reactions Frequency not defined.

Cardiovascular: Hypotension, orthostatic hypotension, hypertension, tachycardia, bradycardia, dizziness, cardiac arrest

(Continued)

Prochlorperazine *(Continued)*

Central nervous system: Extrapyramidal symptoms (pseudoparkinsonism, akathisia, dystonias, tardive dyskinesia), dizziness, cerebral edema, seizures, headache, drowsiness, paradoxical excitement, restlessness, hyperactivity, insomnia, neuroleptic malignant syndrome (NMS), impairment of temperature regulation

Dermatologic: Increased sensitivity to sun, rash, discoloration of skin (blue-gray)

Endocrine & metabolic: Hypoglycemia, hyperglycemia, galactorrhea, lactation, breast enlargement, gynecomastia, menstrual irregularity, amenorrhea, SIADH, changes in libido

Gastrointestinal: Constipation, weight gain, vomiting, stomach pain, nausea, xerostomia, salivation, diarrhea, anorexia, ileus

Genitourinary: Difficulty in urination, ejaculatory disturbances, incontinence, polyuria, ejaculating dysfunction, priapism

Hematologic: Agranulocytosis, leukopenia, eosinophilia, hemolytic anemia, thrombocytopenic purpura, pancytopenia

Hepatic: Cholestatic jaundice, hepatotoxicity

Neuromuscular & skeletal: Tremor

Ocular: Pigmentary retinopathy, blurred vision, cornea and lens changes

Respiratory: Nasal congestion

Miscellaneous: Diaphoresis

Overdosage/Toxicology Symptoms of overdose include deep sleep, coma, extrapyramidal symptoms, abnormal involuntary muscle movements, and hypotension. Treatment is symptom-directed and supportive.

Pharmacodynamics/Kinetics

Half-Life Elimination: 23 hours

Metabolism: Primarily hepatic

Onset: Oral: 30-40 minutes; I.M.: 10-20 minutes; Rectal: ~60 minutes

Duration: I.M., oral extended-release: 12 hours; Rectal, immediate release: 3-4 hours

Formulations

Capsule, sustained action, as maleate: 10 mg, 15 mg, 30 mg

Injection, as edisylate: 5 mg/mL (2 mL, 10 mL)

Suppository, rectal: 2.5 mg, 5 mg, 25 mg (12/box)

Syrup, as edisylate: 5 mg/5 mL (120 mL)

Tablet, as maleate: 5 mg, 10 mg, 25 mg

Dosing

Adults:

Antiemetic:

Oral:

Tablet: 5-10 mg 3-4 times/day; usual maximum: 40 mg/day

Capsule, sustained action: 15 mg on arising or 10 mg every 12 hours

I.M.: 5-10 mg every 3-4 hours; usual maximum: 40 mg/day

I.V.: 2.5-10 mg; maximum 10 mg/dose or 40 mg/day; may repeat dose every 3-4 hours as needed

Rectal: 25 mg twice daily

Surgical nausea/vomiting: Adults:

I.M.: 5-10 mg 1-2 hours before induction; may repeat once if necessary

I.V.: 5-10 mg 15-30 minutes before induction; may repeat once if necessary

Antipsychotic:

Oral: Tablet: 5-10 mg 3-4 times/day; doses up to 150 mg/day may be required in some patients for treatment of severe disturbances.

I.M.: 10-20 mg every 4-6 hours may be required in some patients for treatment of severe disturbances; change to oral as soon as possible.

Nonpsychotic anxiety: Oral: Usual dose: 15-20 mg/day in divided doses; do not give doses >20 mg/day or for longer than 12 weeks

Elderly: Dementia behavior (nonpsychotic): Initial: 2.5-5 mg 1-2 times/day; increase dose at 4- to 7-day intervals by 2.5-5 mg/day. Increase dosing intervals (twice daily, 3 times/day, etc) as necessary to control response or side effects. Maximum daily dose should probably not exceed 75 mg in the elderly. Gradual increases (titration) may prevent some side effects or decrease their severity. See Geriatric Considerations.

Pediatrics: Not recommended in children <10 kg or <2 years.

Antiemetic:

Oral, rectal:

>10 kg: 0.4 mg/kg/24 hours in 3-4 divided doses; **or**

9-14 kg: 2.5 mg every 12-24 hours as needed; maximum: 7.5 mg/day

14-18 kg: 2.5 mg every 8-12 hours as needed; maximum: 10 mg/day

18-39 kg: 2.5 mg every 8 hours or 5 mg every 12 hours as needed; maximum: 15 mg/day

I.M.: 0.1-0.15 mg/kg/dose; usual: 0.13 mg/kg/dose; change to oral as soon as possible.

Antipsychotic: Children 2-12 years:

Oral, rectal: 2.5 mg 2-3 times/day; increase dosage as needed to maximum daily dose of 20 mg for 2-5 years and 25 mg for 6-12 years.

I.M.: 0.13 mg/kg/dose; change to oral as soon as possible.

Renal Impairment: Not dialyzable (0% to 5%)

Administration

Oral: Avoid skin contact with oral solution contact dermatitis has occurred.

I.M.: I.M. should be administered into the upper outer quadrant of the buttock. Avoid skin contact with injection solution, contact dermatitis has occurred.

I.V.: IVP should be administered at a concentration of 5 mg/mL at a rate not to exceed 5 mg/minute. Avoid skin contact with injection solution; contact dermatitis has occurred.

Stability

Storage: Protect from light. Clear or slightly yellow solutions may be used.

Compatibility: Stable in dextran 6% in dextrose, dextran 6% in NS, D_5W, $D_{10}W$, D_5LR, $D_5{}^1/_4NS$, $D_5{}^1/_2NS$, D_5NS, LR, $^1/_2NS$, NS

Y-site administration: Incompatible with aldesleukin, allopurinol, amifostine, amphotericin B cholesteryl sulfate complex, aztreonam, cefepime, etoposide phosphate, fludarabine, foscarnet, filgrastim, gemcitabine, piperacillin/tazobactam

Compatibility in syringe: Incompatible with dimenhydrinate, ketorolac, midazolam, morphine tartrate, pentobarbital, thiopental

Compatibility when admixed: Incompatible with aminophylline, amphotericin B, ampicillin, calcium salts, cephalothin, foscarnet, chloramphenicol, chlorothiazide, floxacillin, furosemide, heparin, hydrocortisone sodium succinate, methohexital, midazolam, penicillin G sodium, phenobarbital, phenytoin, thiopental

Monitoring Laboratory Tests Baseline liver and kidney function, CBC prior to and periodically during therapy

Monitoring and Teaching Issues

Physical Assessment: Assess all other medications patient may be taking (see Drug Interactions and Warnings/Precautions). For I.V., continuously monitor blood pressure and heart rate during administration. Monitor blood pressure and heart rate, fluid balance, and dehydration. Monitor for seizures, especially with known seizure disorder. Monitor for excessive sedation, neuromuscular malignant syndrome, autonomic instability (eg, anticholinergic effects), and extrapyramidal symptoms. **Pregnancy risk factor C** - benefits of use should outweigh possible risks. Breast-feeding is not recommended.

Patient Education: Take exact amount as prescribed. Do not change brand names. Do not crush or chew tablets or capsules. Do not discontinue without consulting prescriber. Avoid alcohol or other sedatives or sleep-inducing drugs. Avoid skin contact with drug; wash immediately with warm soapy water. You may experience appetite changes; small, frequent meals may help. Maintain adequate hydration (2-3 L/day of fluids) unless advised by prescriber to restrict fluids. May cause dizziness, tremors, or visual disturbance (especially during early therapy); use caution when driving or engaging in tasks that require alertness until response to drug is known. Do not change position rapidly (rise slowly). May cause photosensitivity reaction; use sunscreen, wear protective clothing and eyewear, and avoid direct sunlight. Report immediately any changes in gait or muscular tremors. Report unresolved changes in voiding or elimination (constipation or diarrhea), acute dizziness or unresolved sedation, vision changes, palpitations, yellowing of skin or eyes, or changes in color of urine or stool (pink or red brown urine is expected). **Pregnancy/breast-feeding precautions:** Inform prescriber if you are or intend to become pregnant. Breast-feeding is not recommended.

Dietary Issues: Increase dietary intake of riboflavin; should be administered with food or water.

Geriatric Considerations: Due to side effect profile (dystonias, EPS) this is not a preferred drug in the elderly for antiemetic therapy.

Pregnancy Issues: Crosses the placenta. Isolated reports of congenital anomalies, however, some included exposures to other drugs. Available evidence with use of occasional low doses suggests safe use during pregnancy.

Additional Information Not recommended as an antipsychotic due to inferior efficacy compared to other phenothiazines.

Related Information

Antiemetics for Chemotherapy-Induced Nausea and Vomiting *on page 1639*
Antipsychotic Medication Guidelines *on page 1614*
Compatibility of Drugs in Syringe *on page 1566*

Prochlorperazine Edisylate *see* Prochlorperazine *on page 1127*
Prochlorperazine Maleate *see* Prochlorperazine *on page 1127*
Procort® [OTC] *see* Topical Corticosteroids *on page 1334*
Procrit® *see* Epoetin Alfa *on page 476*
Proctocort® *see* Hydrocortisone *on page 673*
Proctocort™ *see* Topical Corticosteroids *on page 1334*
ProctoCream® HC *see* Hydrocortisone *on page 673*
Proctofene *see* Fenofibrate *on page 549*
Proctosol-HC® *see* Hydrocortisone *on page 673*

Procyclidine (proe SYE kli deen)

U.S. Brand Names Kemadrin®

Synonyms Procyclidine Hydrochloride

Generic Available No

Pharmacologic Category Anticholinergic Agent; Anti-Parkinson's Agent, Anticholinergic

Pregnancy Risk Factor C

Lactation Excretion in breast milk unknown/not recommended

Use Relieves symptoms of parkinsonian syndrome and drug-induced extrapyramidal symptoms

Mechanism of Action/Effect Thought to act by blocking excess acetylcholine at cerebral synapses; many of its effects are due to its pharmacologic similarities with atropine; it exerts an antispasmodic effect on smooth muscle, is a potent mydriatic; inhibits salivation

Contraindications Angle-closure glaucoma; safe use in children not established

Warnings/Precautions Use with caution in hot weather or during exercise. Elderly patients frequently develop increased sensitivity and require strict dosage regulation - side effects may be more severe in elderly patients with atherosclerotic changes. Use with caution in patients with tachycardia, cardiac arrhythmias, hypertension, hypotension, prostatic hyperplasia (especially in the elderly) or any tendency toward urinary retention, liver or kidney disorders and obstructive disease of the GI or GU tract. When given in large doses or to susceptible patients, may cause weakness and inability to move particular muscle groups. Pregnancy risk C.

Drug Interactions

Decreased Effect: May increase gastric degradation of levodopa and decrease the amount of levodopa absorbed by delaying gastric emptying; the opposite may be true for digoxin.

(Continued)

Procyclidine *(Continued)*

Therapeutic effects of cholinergic agents (tacrine, donepezil) and neuroleptics may be antagonized.

Increased Effect/Toxicity: Central and/or peripheral anticholinergic syndrome can occur when administered with amantadine, rimantadine, narcotic analgesics, phenothiazines and other antipsychotics (especially with high anticholinergic activity), tricyclic antidepressants, quinidine and some other antiarrhythmics, and antihistamines.

Nutritional/Ethanol Interactions Ethanol: Avoid ethanol.

Adverse Reactions Frequency not defined.

Cardiovascular: Tachycardia, palpitations

Central nervous system: Confusion, drowsiness, headache, loss of memory, fatigue, ataxia, giddiness, lightheadedness

Dermatologic: Dry skin, increased sensitivity to light, rash

Gastrointestinal: Constipation, xerostomia, dry throat, nausea, vomiting, epigastric distress

Genitourinary: Difficult urination

Neuromuscular & skeletal: Weakness

Ocular: Increased intraocular pain, blurred vision, mydriasis

Respiratory: Dry nose

Miscellaneous: Diaphoresis (decreased)

Overdosage/Toxicology Symptoms of overdose include disorientation, hallucinations, delusions, blurred vision, dysphagia, absent bowel sounds, hyperthermia, hypertension, and urinary retention. For anticholinergic overdose with severe life-threatening symptoms, physostigmine 1-2 mg S.C. or I.V. slowly, may be given to reverse these effects.

Pharmacodynamics/Kinetics

Onset: 30-40 minutes

Duration: 4-6 hours

Formulations Tablet, as hydrochloride: 5 mg

Dosing

Adults: Parkinson's disease or treatment of EPS: Oral: 2.5 mg 3 times/day after meals; if tolerated, gradually increase dose, to a maximum of 20 mg/day if necessary.

Elderly: Oral: Initial: 2.5 mg once or twice daily, gradually increasing as necessary. Avoid use if possible (see Geriatric Considerations).

Hepatic Impairment: Decrease dose to a twice daily dosing regimen.

Administration

Oral: Should be administered after meals to minimize stomach upset.

Monitoring and Teaching Issues

Physical Assessment: Assess effectiveness and interactions of other medications patient may be taking (see Contraindications and Drug Interactions). Monitor therapeutic response, renal function, and adverse reactions (eg, anticholinergic syndrome - see Adverse Reactions) at beginning of therapy and periodically throughout therapy (see Warnings/Precautions, Adverse Reactions, and Overdose/Toxicology). Assess knowledge/teach patient appropriate use, interventions to reduce side effects, and adverse symptoms to report (see Patient Education). **Pregnancy risk factor C** - benefits of use should outweigh possible risks. Breast-feeding is not recommended.

Patient Education: Take exactly as directed (after meals); do not increase, decrease, or discontinue without consulting prescriber. Take at the same time each day. Do not use alcohol and all prescription or OTC sedatives or CNS depressants without consulting prescriber. You may experience drowsiness, dizziness, confusion, and blurred vision (use caution when driving, climbing stairs, or engaging in tasks requiring alertness until response to drug is known); increased susceptibility to heat stroke, decreased perspiration (use caution in hot weather - maintain adequate fluids and reduce exercise activity); constipation (increased exercise, fluids, fruit, or fiber may help); or dry skin or nasal passages (consult prescriber for appropriate relief). Report unresolved constipation, chest pain or palpitations, difficulty breathing, CNS changes (hallucination, loss of memory, nervousness, etc), painful or difficult urination, increased muscle spasticity or rigidity, skin rash, or significant worsening of condition. **Pregnancy/breast-feeding precautions:** Inform prescriber if you are or intend to become pregnant. Breast-feeding is not recommended.

Dietary Issues: Should be taken after meals to minimize stomach upset.

Geriatric Considerations: Anticholinergic agents are generally not well tolerated in the elderly and their use should be avoided when possible (see Warnings/Precautions, Adverse Reactions). In the elderly, anticholinergic agents should not be used as prophylaxis against extrapyramidal symptoms. Elderly patients frequently develop increased sensitivity and require strict dosage regulation - side effects may be more severe in elderly patients with atherosclerotic changes.

Procyclidine Hydrochloride *see* Procyclidine *on page 1129*

Prodium™ [OTC] *see* Phenazopyridine *on page 1065*

Profasi® *see* Chorionic Gonadotropin (Human) *on page 284*

Profenal® Ophthalmic *see page 1461*

Progestasert® *see* Progesterone *on page 1130*

Progesterone (proe JES ter one)

U.S. Brand Names Crinone®; Progestasert®; Prometrium®

Synonyms Pregnenedione; Progestin

Generic Available Yes: Injection

Pharmacologic Category Progestin

Pregnancy Risk Factor B (Prometrium®, per manufacturer); none established for gel (Crinone®), injection (contraindicated), or intrauterine device (contraindicated)

Lactation Excreted in breast milk/use caution (AAP rates "compatible")

Use

Oral: Prevention of endometrial hyperplasia in nonhysterectomized, postmenopausal women who are receiving conjugated estrogen tablets; secondary amenorrhea

I.M.: Amenorrhea; abnormal uterine bleeding due to hormonal imbalance

Intrauterine device (IUD): Contraception in women who have had at least one child, are in a stable and mutually-monogamous relationship, and have no history of pelvic inflammatory disease; amenorrhea; functional uterine bleeding

Intravaginal gel: Part of assisted reproductive technology (ART) for infertile women with progesterone deficiency; secondary amenorrhea

Mechanism of Action/Effect Natural steroid hormone that induces secretory changes in the endometrium, promotes mammary gland development, relaxes uterine smooth muscle, blocks follicular maturation and ovulation, and maintains pregnancy

Contraindications Hypersensitivity to progesterone or any component of the formulation; thrombophlebitis; undiagnosed vaginal bleeding; carcinoma of the breast; cerebral apoplexy; severe liver dysfunction; missed abortion; diagnostic test for pregnancy; pregnancy (see Pregnancy Risk Factor)

Capsule: Contains peanut oil; contraindicated in patients with allergy to peanuts

IUD: Should also not be used in patients with current or history of ectopic pregnancy, pelvic inflammatory disease, sexually-transmitted disease, postpartum endometritis, incomplete involution of uterus; vaginitis or cervicitis, genital actinomycosis, uterus <6 cm or >10 cm, cervical cancer, or conditions associated with increased susceptibility to infection.

Warnings/Precautions Use with caution in patients with impaired liver function, depression, diabetes, and epilepsy. Except when used as indicated in ART, use of any progestin during the first 4 months of pregnancy is not recommended. Monitor closely for loss of vision, proptosis, diplopia, migraine, and signs or symptoms of embolic disorders. Not a progestin of choice in the elderly for hormonal cycling. May cause some degree of fluid retention, use with caution in conditions which may be aggravated by this factor, including CHF, renal dysfunction, epilepsy, migraine, or asthma. Patients should be warned that progesterone may cause transient dizziness or drowsiness during initial therapy. Use of progestin treatment may adversely effect carbohydrate and lipid metabolism

Use of the IUD is associated with increased risk of ectopic pregnancy if pregnancy occurs. In addition, women should be informed that the IUD does not protect against HIV infection, pelvic inflammatory disease, or other sexually-transmitted diseases.

Drug Interactions

Cytochrome P450 Effect: Substrate of CYP1A2, 2A6, 2C8/9, **2C19**, 2D6, **3A4**; Inhibits CYP2C8/9, 2C19

Decreased Effect: Aminoglutethimide may decrease effect by increasing hepatic metabolism.

Increased Effect/Toxicity: Ketoconazole may increase the bioavailability of progesterone. Progesterone may increase concentrations of estrogenic compounds during concurrent therapy with conjugated estrogens.

Nutritional/Ethanol Interactions

Food: Food increases oral bioavailability.

Herb/Nutraceutical: St John's wort may decrease progesterone levels.

Effects on Lab Values Thyroid function, metyrapone, liver function, coagulation tests, endocrine function tests

Adverse Reactions

Oral capsule:

>10%:

Central nervous system: Dizziness (16%)

Endocrine & metabolic: Breast pain (11%)

5% to 10%:

Central nervous system: Headache (10%), fatigue (7%), emotional lability (6%), irritability (5%)

Gastrointestinal: Abdominal pain (10%), abdominal distention (6%)

Neuromuscular & skeletal: Musculoskeletal pain (6%)

Respiratory: Upper respiratory tract infection (5%)

Miscellaneous: Viral infection (7%)

<5% (Limited to important or life-threatening): Angina pectoris, anxiety, arthritis, bronchitis, chest pain, depression, edema, fever, gastroenteritis, hemorrhagic rectum, hepatitis (reversible), hypertension, hypertonia, hypotension, insomnia, leukorrhea, lymphadenopathy, myalgia, pneumonitis, somnolence, syncope, uterine fibroid, vaginal dryness, vaginitis, verruca, vomiting

Additional adverse reactions seen with **intrauterine device:** Abdominal adhesions, abscess formation, amenorrhea, bradycardia and syncope (secondary to insertion), cervical erosion, complete or partial IUD expulsion, delayed menses, dysmenorrhea, dyspareunia, ectopic pregnancy, embedment or fragmentation of the IUD, endometritis, fetal damage, leukorrhea, local inflammatory reaction, pelvic infection, perforation of uterus and cervix, peritonitis, pregnancy, prolonged menstrual flow, septic abortion, septicemia, spontaneous abortion, spotting, tubo-ovarian abscess

Additional adverse reactions seen with **injection (I.M.):** Acne, alopecia, amenorrhea, anaphylactoid reactions, breakthrough bleeding, breast tenderness, cervical erosion changes, cervical secretion changes, depression, fever, galactorrhea, hirsutism, insomnia, menstrual flow changes, pain at the injection site, pruritus, rash, somnolence, spotting, urticaria

Overdosage/Toxicology Toxicity is unlikely following single exposure of excessive doses. Supportive treatment is adequate in most cases.

(Continued)

Progesterone *(Continued)*

Pharmacodynamics/Kinetics

Half-Life Elimination: 5 minutes

Time to Peak: Oral: 1.5-2.3 hours

Metabolism: Hepatic

Duration: 24 hours

Formulations

Capsule (Prometrium®): 100 mg, 200 mg [contains peanut oil]

Gel, vaginal (Crinone®): 4% (45 mg); 8% (90 mg)

Injection [in oil]: 50 mg/mL (10 mL) [may contain benzyl alcohol, sesame oil]

Intrauterine system, reservoir [in silicone fluid] (Progestasert®): 38 mg [delivers progesterone 65 mcg/day over 1 year]

Dosing

Adults & Elderly: Female:

Amenorrhea: I.M.: 5-10 mg/day for 6-8 consecutive days

Amenorrhea, secondary:

Intravaginal gel: 45 mg (4% gel) every other day for 6 doses; if response is inadequate, may increase to 90 mg (8% gel) at same schedule

Oral: 400 mg every evening for 10 days

ART in patients who require progesterone supplementation: Intravaginal gel: 90 mg (8% gel) once daily. If pregnancy occurs, may continue treatment for 10-12 weeks.

ART in patients with partial or complete ovarian failure: Intravaginal gel: 90 mg (8% gel) twice daily. If pregnancy occurs, continue treatment for 10-12 weeks.

Contraception: Intrauterine device: Insert a single system into the uterine cavity; contraceptive effectiveness is retained for 1 year and system must be replaced 1 year after insertion

Endometrial hyperplasia prevention (in postmenopausal women with a uterus who are receiving daily conjugated estrogen tablets): Oral: 200 mg as a single daily dose every evening for 12 days sequentially per 28-day cycle

Functional uterine bleeding: I.M.: 5-10 mg/day for 6 doses

Administration

I.M.: Administer deep I.M. only

Other: Vaginal gel: (A small amount of gel will remain in the applicator following insertion): Administer into the vagina directly from sealed applicator. Remove applicator from wrapper; holding applicator by thickest end, shake down to move contents to thin end; while holding applicator by flat section of thick end, twist off tab; gently insert into vagina and squeeze thick end of applicator.

For use at altitudes above 2500 feet: Remove applicator from wrapper; hold applicator on both sides of bubble in the thick end; using a lancet, make a single puncture in the bubble to relieve air pressure; holding applicator by thickest end, shake down to move contents to thin end; while holding applicator by flat section of thick end, twist off tab; gently insert into vagina and squeeze thick end of applicator.

Stability

Storage: Store at controlled room temperature.

Monitoring and Teaching Issues

Physical Assessment: See Contraindications, Warnings/Precautions, and Dosing for use cautions. Assess potential for interactions with other prescriptions, OTC medications, or herbal products patient may be taking (see Drug Interactions). Assess therapeutic effectiveness and patient response (eg, blood pressure, mammogram, and results of Pap smears and pregnancy tests before beginning treatment and at least annually with vaginal insert - see Adverse Reactions and Overdose/Toxicology). Teach patient proper use according to formulation, possible side effects and interventions (eg, annual physicals, Pap smears, and vision assessment), and adverse symptoms to report (see Patient Education). **Pregnancy risk factor B** - see Pregnancy Risk Factor for use cautions.

Patient Education: Inform prescriber of all prescriptions, OTC medications, or herbal products you are taking, and any allergies you have. Do not take anything new during treatment unless approved by prescriber. Use exactly as directed. It is important that you you have an annual physical assessment, Pap smear, and vision assessment while taking this medication. May cause temporary dizziness or drowsiness (use caution when driving or engaging in tasks that are potentially hazardous until response to drug is known). Report immediately muscle pain or soreness; warmth, swelling, or redness in calves; shortness of breath; sudden loss or change in vision; change in menstrual pattern (unusual bleeding, amenorrhea, breakthrough spotting); breast tenderness that does not go away; acute abdominal cramping; signs of vaginal infection (drainage, pain, itching); or CNS changes (eg, blurred vision, confusion, acute anxiety, or unresolved depression). **Pregnancy/breast-feeding precautions:** If you suspect you may be pregnant contact prescriber immediately. Consult prescriber if breast-feeding.

Vaginal gel: A small amount of gel will remain in the applicator following insertion. Administer into the vagina directly from sealed applicator. Remove applicator from wrapper; holding applicator by thickest end, shake down to move contents to thin end; while holding applicator by flat section of thick end, twist off tab; gently insert into vagina and squeeze thick end of applicator.

Geriatric Considerations: Not a progestin of choice in the elderly for hormonal cycling.

Pregnancy Issues: There is an increased risk of minor birth defects in children whose mothers take progesterones during the first 4 months of pregnancy. Hypospadias has been reported in male and mild masculinization of the external genitalia has been reported in female babies exposed during the first trimester. Crinone® is indicated for use in ART.

Progestin *see* Progesterone *on page 1130*

Prograf® *see* Tacrolimus *on page 1271*

Proguanil and Atovaquone *see* Atovaquone and Proguanil *on page 131*

Proleukin® *see* Aldesleukin *on page 54*

Prolixin® *see* Fluphenazine *on page 581*
Prolixin Decanoate® *see* Fluphenazine *on page 581*
Prolixin Enanthate® [DSC] *see* Fluphenazine *on page 581*
Proloprim® *see* Trimethoprim *on page 1366*
Promazine *see page 1558*
Promazine *see page 1614*

Promethazine (proe METH a zeen)

U.S. Brand Names Anergan®; Phenergan®

Synonyms Promethazine Hydrochloride

Generic Available Yes

Pharmacologic Category Antiemetic

Pregnancy Risk Factor C

Lactation Enters breast milk/not recommended

Use Symptomatic treatment of various allergic conditions; antiemetic; motion sickness; sedative; analgesic adjunct for control of postoperative pain; anesthetic adjunct

Mechanism of Action/Effect Blocks postsynaptic mesolimbic dopaminergic receptors in the brain; exhibits a strong alpha-adrenergic blocking effect and depresses the release of hypothalamic and hypophyseal hormones; competes with histamine for the H_1-receptor; reduces stimuli to the brainstem reticular system

Contraindications Hypersensitivity to promethazine or any component of the formulation (cross-reactivity between phenothiazines may occur); severe CNS depression; coma; intra-arterial or subcutaneous injection

Warnings/Precautions Do not give S.C. or intra-arterially, necrotic lesions may occur. Injection may contain sulfites which may cause allergic reactions in some patients. Rapid I.V. administration may produce a transient fall in blood pressure; rate of administration should not exceed 25 mg/minute. Slow I.V. administration may produce a slightly elevated blood pressure. Not considered an antihistamine of choice in the elderly.

May be sedating and may impair physical or mental abilities. Effects with other sedative drugs or ethanol may be potentiated. Use with caution in Parkinson's disease, hemodynamic instability, bone marrow suppression, predisposition to seizures, subcortical brain damage, and in severe cardiac, hepatic, renal, or respiratory disease. Caution in breast cancer or other prolactin-dependent tumors (may elevate prolactin levels). May alter temperature regulation or mask toxicity of other drugs due to antiemetic effects. May alter cardiac conduction (life-threatening arrhythmias have occurred with therapeutic doses of phenothiazines). May cause orthostatic hypotension. Use caution in cardiovascular or cerebrovascular disease.

Due to anticholinergic effects, use caution in patients with decreased gastrointestinal motility, urinary retention, BPH, xerostomia, visual problems, narrow-angle glaucoma, and myasthenia gravis. May cause extrapyramidal symptoms, including pseudoparkinsonism, acute dystonic reactions, akathisia, and tardive dyskinesia. May be associated with neuroleptic malignant syndrome (NMS). Ampuls contain sodium metabisulfite.

Pregnancy risk C.

Drug Interactions

Cytochrome P450 Effect: Substrate of **CYP2B6, 2D6**; Inhibits CYP2D6

Decreased Effect: Barbiturates and carbamazepine may increase the metabolism of promethazine, lowering its serum levels. Benztropine (and other anticholinergics) may inhibit the therapeutic response to promethazine. Promethazine may inhibit the ability of bromocriptine to lower serum prolactin concentrations. The antihypertensive effects of guanethidine and guanadrel may be inhibited by promethazine. Promethazine may inhibit the antiparkinsonian effect of levodopa. Promethazine (and possibly other low potency antipsychotics) may reverse the pressor effects of epinephrine.

Increased Effect/Toxicity: Chloroquine, propranolol, and sulfadoxine-pyrimethamine also may increase promethazine concentrations. Concurrent use with TCA may produce increased toxicity or altered therapeutic response. Promethazine plus lithium may rarely produce neurotoxicity. Concurrent use of promethazine and CNS depressants (ethanol, narcotics) may produce additive depressant effects.

Nutritional/Ethanol Interactions

Ethanol: Avoid ethanol (may increase CNS depression).

Herb/Nutraceutical: Avoid valerian, St John's wort, kava kava, gotu kola (may increase CNS depression).

Effects on Lab Values Alters the flare response in intradermal allergen tests

Adverse Reactions Frequency not defined.

Cardiovascular: Postural hypotension, tachycardia, dizziness, nonspecific QT changes

Central nervous system: Drowsiness, dystonias, akathisia, pseudoparkinsonism, tardive dyskinesia, neuroleptic malignant syndrome, seizures

Dermatologic: Photosensitivity, dermatitis, skin pigmentation (slate gray)

Endocrine & metabolic: Lactation, breast engorgement, false-positive pregnancy test, amenorrhea, gynecomastia, hyper- or hypoglycemia

Gastrointestinal: Xerostomia, constipation, nausea

Genitourinary: Urinary retention, ejaculatory disorder, impotence

Hematologic: Agranulocytosis, eosinophilia, leukopenia, hemolytic anemia, aplastic anemia, thrombocytopenic purpura

Hepatic: Jaundice

Ocular: Blurred vision, corneal and lenticular changes, epithelial keratopathy, pigmentary retinopathy

Overdosage/Toxicology Symptoms of overdose include CNS depression, respiratory depression, possible CNS stimulation, dry mouth, fixed and dilated pupils, and hypotension. Treatment is symptom-directed and supportive.

Pharmacodynamics/Kinetics

Time to Peak: Maximum serum concentration: 4.4 hours (syrup); 6.7-8.6 hours (suppositories)

(Continued)

Promethazine *(Continued)*

Metabolism: Hepatic

Onset: I.M.: ~20 minutes; I.V.: 3-5 minutes

Peak effect: C_{max}: 9.04 mg/mL (suppository); 19.3 mg/mL (syrup)

Duration: 2-6 hours

Formulations

Injection, as hydrochloride: 25 mg/mL (1 mL, 10 mL); 50 mg/mL (1 mL, 10 mL)

Suppository, rectal, as hydrochloride: 12.5 mg, 25 mg, 50 mg

Syrup, as hydrochloride: 6.25 mg/5 mL (5 mL, 120 mL, 480 mL, 4000 mL); 25 mg/5 mL (120 mL, 480 mL, 4000 mL)

Tablet, as hydrochloride: 12.5 mg, 25 mg, 50 mg

Dosing

Adults:

Antihistamine (including allergic reactions to blood or plasma):

Oral, rectal: 12.5 mg 3 times/day and 25 mg at bedtime

I.M., I.V.: 25 mg, may repeat in 2 hours when necessary; switch to oral route as soon as feasible

Antiemetic: Oral, I.M., I.V., rectal: 12.5-25 mg every 4 hours as needed

Motion sickness: Oral, rectal: 25 mg 30-60 minutes before departure, then every 12 hours as needed

Sedation: Oral, I.M., I.V., rectal: 25-50 mg/dose

Elderly: Refer to adult dosing and Geriatric Considerations.

Pediatrics:

Antihistamine: Oral, Rectal: Children: 0.1 mg/kg/dose every 6 hours during the day and 0.5 mg/kg/dose at bedtime as needed

Antiemetic: Oral, I.M., I.V., Rectal: Children: 0.25-1 mg/kg 4-6 times/day as needed

Motion sickness: Oral, Rectal: Children: 0.5 mg/kg/dose 30 minutes to 1 hour before departure, then every 12 hours as needed

Sedation: Oral, I.M., I.V., Rectal: Children: 0.5-1 mg/kg/dose every 6 hours as needed

Renal Impairment: Not dialyzable (0% to 5%)

Administration

I.M.: Administer into deep muscle.

I.V.: Avoid I.V. use. If necessary, may dilute to a maximum concentration of 25 mg/mL and infuse at a maximum rate of 25 mg/minute.

Stability

Storage: Protect from light and from freezing.

Compatibility: Stable in dextran 6% in dextrose, dextran 6% in NS, D_5W, $D_{10}W$, D_5LR, $D_5{}^1/_4NS$, $D_5{}^1/_2NS$, D_5NS, LR, $^1/_2NS$, NS

Y-site administration: Incompatible with aldesleukin, allopurinol, amphotericin B cholesteryl sulfate complex, cefazolin, cefepime, cefoperazone, cefotetan, doxorubicin liposome, foscarnet, methotrexate, piperacillin/tazobactam

Compatibility in syringe: Incompatible with cefotetan, chloroquine, diatrizoate sodium 75%, diatrizoate meglumine 52% with diatrizoate sodium 8%, diatrizoate meglumine 34.3% with diatrizoate sodium 35%, dimenhydrinate, heparin, iodipamide meglumine 52%, iothalamate meglumine 60%, iothalamate sodium 80%, ketorolac, pentobarbital, thiopental

Compatibility when admixed: Incompatible with aminophylline, chloramphenicol, chlorothiazide, dimenhydrinate, floxacillin, furosemide, heparin, hydrocortisone sodium succinate, methohexital, penicillin G sodium, pentobarbital, phenobarbital, phenytoin, thiopental

Monitoring and Teaching Issues

Physical Assessment: See Contraindications, Warnings/Precautions, and Dosing for use cautions. Assess potential for interactions with other prescriptions, OTC medications, or herbal products patient may be taking (see extensive list of Drug Interactions). See Administration for I.V. and I.M. use. Assess for therapeutic effectiveness and adverse response (see Adverse Reactions and Overdose/Toxicology). Use and teach sedation safety measures (side rails up, call light within reach, etc). Teach patient appropriate use (oral), interventions to reduce side effects, and adverse symptoms to report (see Patient Education). **Pregnancy risk factor C** - benefits of use should outweigh possible risks. Breast-feeding is not recommended.

Patient Education: Inform prescriber of all prescriptions, OTC medications, or herbal products you are taking, and any allergies you have. Do not take anything new during treatment unless approved by prescriber (especially anything that may cause CNS depression). Take this drug as prescribed; do not increase dosage. Avoid alcohol. May cause dizziness, drowsiness, or blurred vision (use caution when driving or engaging in tasks requiring alertness until response to drug is known); or nausea, dry mouth, appetite disturbances (small, frequent meals, frequent mouth care, chewing gum, or sucking lozenges may help). Report unusual weight gain, unresolved nausea or diarrhea, chest pain or palpitations, excess sedation or stimulation, or sore throat or difficulty breathing. **Pregnancy/breast-feeding precautions:** Inform prescriber if you are or intend to become pregnant. Breast-feeding is not recommended.

Dietary Issues: Increase dietary intake of riboflavin; should be administered with food or water.

Geriatric Considerations: Because promethazine is a phenothiazine (and can, therefore, cause side effects such as extrapyramidal symptoms), it is not considered an antihistamine of choice in the elderly.

Pregnancy Issues: Crosses the placenta. Possible respiratory depression if drug is administered near time of delivery; behavioral changes, EEG alterations, impaired platelet aggregation reported with use during labor. Available evidence with use of occasional low doses suggests safe use during pregnancy.

Related Information

Antiemetics for Chemotherapy-Induced Nausea and Vomiting *on page 1639*

Compatibility of Drugs in Syringe *on page 1566*

Promethazine and Codeine (proe METH a zeen & KOE deen)

U.S. Brand Names Phenergan® With Codeine; Prothazine-DC®

Synonyms Codeine and Promethazine

Restrictions C-V

Generic Available Yes

Pharmacologic Category Antihistamine/Antitussive

Pregnancy Risk Factor C

Lactation Enters breast milk (codeine)/not recommended

Use Temporary relief of coughs and upper respiratory symptoms associated with allergy or the common cold

Formulations Syrup: Promethazine hydrochloride 6.25 mg and codeine phosphate 10 mg per 5 mL (120 mL, 180 mL, 473 mL)

Dosing

Adults: Upper respiratory symptoms: Oral: 10-20 mg/dose every 4-6 hours as needed; maximum: 120 mg codeine/day; or 5-10 mL every 4-6 hours as needed

Elderly: Refer to dosing in individual monographs.

Pediatrics: Upper respiratory symptoms: Oral (in terms of codeine):

Children: 1-1.5 mg/kg/day every 4 hours as needed; maximum: 30 mg/day **or**

2-6 years: 1.25-2.5 mL every 4-6 hours or 2.5-5 mg/dose every 4-6 hours as needed; maximum: 30 mg codeine/day

6-12 years: 2.5-5 mL every 4-6 hours as needed or 5-10 mg/dose every 4-6 hours as needed; maximum: 60 mg codeine/day

Monitoring and Teaching Issues

Physical Assessment: See individual components listed in Related Information. **Pregnancy risk factor C** - benefits of use should outweigh possible risks. Breast-feeding is not recommended.

Patient Education: See individual components listed in Related Information. **Pregnancy/breast-feeding precautions:** Inform prescriber if you are or intend to become pregnant. Breast-feeding is not recommended.

Related Information

Codeine *on page 327*
Promethazine *on page 1133*

Promethazine and Dextromethorphan

(proe METH a zeen & deks troe meth OR fan)

U.S. Brand Names Phenameth® DM; Phenergan® With Dextromethorphan

Synonyms Dextromethorphan and Promethazine

Generic Available Yes

Pharmacologic Category Antihistamine/Antitussive

Pregnancy Risk Factor C

Lactation Excretion in breast milk unknown/not recommended

Use Temporary relief of coughs and upper respiratory symptoms associated with allergy or the common cold

Formulations Syrup: Promethazine hydrochloride 6.25 mg and dextromethorphan hydrobromide 15 mg per 5 mL (120 mL, 480 mL, 4000 mL) [contains alcohol 7%]

Dosing

Adults: Cough and upper respiratory symptoms: Oral: 5 mL every 4-6 hours, up to 30 mL in 24 hours

Elderly: Refer to dosing in individual monographs.

Pediatrics: Cough and upper respiratory symptoms: Oral: Children:

2-6 years: 1.25-2.5 mL every 4-6 hours up to 10 mL in 24 hours

6-12 years: 2.5-5 mL every 4-6 hours up to 20 mL in 24 hours

Monitoring and Teaching Issues

Physical Assessment: See individual components listed in Related Information. **Pregnancy risk factor C** - benefits of use should outweigh possible risks. Breast-feeding is not recommended.

Patient Education: See also Promethazine.

Based on Dextromethorphan component: Shake well; do not exceed recommended dosage; take with a large glass of water; if cough lasts more than 1 week or is accompanied by a rash, fever, or headache, notify physician.

Pregnancy/breast-feeding precautions: Inform prescriber if you are or intend to become pregnant. Breast-feeding is not recommended.

Related Information

Promethazine *on page 1133*

Promethazine and Phenylephrine (proe METH a zeen & fen il EF rin)

U.S. Brand Names Phenergan® VC; Promethazine VC; Promethazine VC Plain; Prometh VC Plain

Synonyms Phenylephrine and Promethazine

Generic Available Yes

Pharmacologic Category Antihistamine/Decongestant Combination

Pregnancy Risk Factor C

Lactation Excretion in breast milk unknown/not recommended

Use Temporary relief of upper respiratory symptoms associated with allergy or the common cold

Formulations Liquid: Promethazine hydrochloride 6.25 mg and phenylephrine hydrochloride 5 mg per 5 mL (120 mL, 240 mL, 473 mL)

Dosing

Adults: Upper respiratory symptoms: Oral: 5 mL every 4-6 hours, not to exceed 30 mL in 24 hours

(Continued)

Promethazine and Phenylephrine *(Continued)*

Elderly: Refer to dosing in individual monographs.

Pediatrics: Upper respiratory symptoms: Oral: Children:

2-6 years: 1.25 mL every 4-6 hours, not to exceed 7.5 mL in 24 hours

6-12 years: 2.5 mL every 4-6 hours, not to exceed 15 mL in 24 hours

>12 years: Refer to adult dosing.

Monitoring and Teaching Issues

Physical Assessment: See individual components listed in Related Information. **Pregnancy risk factor C** - benefits of use should outweigh possible risks. Breast-feeding is not recommended.

Patient Education: See individual components listed in Related Information. **Pregnancy/breast-feeding precautions:** Inform prescriber if you are or intend to become pregnant. Breast-feeding is not recommended.

Related Information

Phenylephrine *on page 1071*
Promethazine *on page 1133*

Promethazine Hydrochloride *see* Promethazine *on page 1133*

Promethazine, Phenylephrine, and Codeine

(proe METH a zeen, fen il EF rin, & KOE deen)

U.S. Brand Names Phenergan® VC With Codeine; Promethist® With Codeine; Prometh® VC With Codeine

Synonyms Codeine, Promethazine, and Phenylephrine; Phenylephrine, Promethazine, and Codeine

Restrictions C-V

Generic Available Yes

Pharmacologic Category Antihistamine/Decongestant/Antitussive

Pregnancy Risk Factor C

Lactation Enters breast milk/not recommended

Use Temporary relief of coughs and upper respiratory symptoms including nasal congestion

Formulations Liquid: Promethazine hydrochloride 6.25 mg, phenylephrine hydrochloride 5 mg, and codeine phosphate 10 mg per 5 mL (120 mL, 240 mL, 480 mL, 4000 mL) [contains alcohol 7%]

Dosing

Adults: Cough and upper respiratory symptoms: Oral: 5 mL every 4-6 hours, not to exceed 30 mL/24 hours

Elderly: Refer to dosing in individual monographs.

Pediatrics: Cough and upper respiratory symptoms: Oral:

Children (expressed in terms of codeine dosage): 1-1.5 mg/kg/day every 4 hours, maximum: 30 mg/day **or**

<2 years: Not recommended

2-6 years:

Weight 25 lb: 1.25-2.5 mL every 4-6 hours, not >6 mL/24 hours

Weight 30 lb: 1.25-2.5 mL every 4-6 hours, not >7 mL/24 hours

Weight 35 lb: 1.25-2.5 mL every 4-6 hours, not >8 mL/24 hours

Weight 40 lb: 1.25-2.5 mL every 4-6 hours, not >9 mL/24 hours

6 to <12 years: 2.5-5 mL every 4-6 hours, not >15 mL/24 hours

Monitoring and Teaching Issues

Physical Assessment: See individual components listed in Related Information. **Pregnancy risk factor C** - benefits of use should outweigh possible risks. Breast-feeding is not recommended.

Patient Education: See individual components listed in Related Information. **Pregnancy/breast-feeding precautions:** Inform prescriber if you are or intend to become pregnant. Breast-feeding is not recommended.

Related Information

Codeine *on page 327*
Phenylephrine *on page 1071*
Promethazine *on page 1133*

Promethazine VC *see* Promethazine and Phenylephrine *on page 1135*
Promethazine VC Plain *see* Promethazine and Phenylephrine *on page 1135*
Promethist® With Codeine *see* Promethazine, Phenylephrine, and Codeine *on page 1136*
Prometh VC Plain *see* Promethazine and Phenylephrine *on page 1135*
Prometh® VC With Codeine *see* Promethazine, Phenylephrine, and Codeine *on page 1136*
Prometrium® *see* Progesterone *on page 1130*
Promit® *see* Dextran 1 *on page 391*
Pronap-100® *see* Propoxyphene and Acetaminophen *on page 1142*
Pronestyl® *see* Procainamide *on page 1122*
Pronestyl-SR® *see* Procainamide *on page 1122*

Propafenone (proe pa FEEN one)

U.S. Brand Names Rythmol®

Synonyms Propafenone Hydrochloride

Generic Available Yes

Pharmacologic Category Antiarrhythmic Agent, Class Ic

Pregnancy Risk Factor C

Lactation Excretion in breast milk unknown

Use Life-threatening ventricular arrhythmias

Use - Unlabeled/Investigational Supraventricular tachycardias, including those patients with Wolff-Parkinson-White syndrome

Mechanism of Action/Effect Propafenone is a class 1c antiarrhythmic agent which possesses local anesthetic properties, blocks the fast inward sodium current, and slows the rate of increase of the action potential. Prolongs conduction and refractoriness in all areas of the myocardium, with a slightly more pronounced effect on intraventricular conduction; it prolongs effective refractory period, reduces spontaneous automaticity and exhibits some beta-blockade activity.

Contraindications Hypersensitivity to propafenone or any component of the formulation; sinoatrial, AV, and intraventricular disorders of impulse generation and/or conduction (except in patients with a functioning artificial pacemaker); sinus bradycardia; cardiogenic shock; uncompensated cardiac failure; hypotension; bronchospastic disorders; uncorrected electrolyte abnormalities; concurrent use of amprenavir, cimetidine, metoprolol, propranolol quinidine, and ritonavir (see Drug Interactions)

Warnings/Precautions Patients with bronchospastic disease should generally not receive this drug. May worsen CHF in some patients. May cause or unmask a variety of conduction disturbances, or lead to the development of new arrhythmias (proarrhythmic events). May alter pacing and sensing thresholds of artificial pacemakers. Administer cautiously in significant hepatic dysfunction. Pregnancy risk C.

Drug Interactions

Cytochrome P450 Effect: Substrate of CYP1A2, **2D6**, 3A4; Inhibits CYP1A2, 2D6

Decreased Effect: Enzyme inducers (phenobarbital, phenytoin, rifabutin, rifampin) may decrease propafenone blood levels.

Increased Effect/Toxicity: Amprenavir, cimetidine, metoprolol, propranolol, quinidine, and ritonavir may increase propafenone levels; concurrent use is contraindicated. Digoxin (reduce dose by 25%), cyclosporine, local anesthetics, theophylline, and warfarin blood levels are increased by propafenone.

Nutritional/Ethanol Interactions

Food: Propafenone serum concentrations may be increased if taken with food.

Herb/Nutraceutical: St John's wort may decrease propafenone levels. Avoid ephedra (may worsen arrhythmia).

Adverse Reactions

1% to 10%:

Cardiovascular: New or worsened arrhythmias (proarrhythmic effect) (2% to 10%), angina (2% to 5%), CHF (1% to 4%), ventricular tachycardia (1% to 3%), palpitations (1% to 3%), AV block (first-degree) (1% to 3%), syncope (1% to 2%), increased QRS interval (1% to 2%), chest pain (1% to 2%), PVCs (1% to 2%), bradycardia (1% to 2%), edema (0% to 1%), bundle branch block (0% to 1%), atrial fibrillation (1%), hypotension (0% to 1%), intraventricular conduction delay (0% to 1%)

Central nervous system: Dizziness (4% to 15%), fatigue (2% to 6%), headache (2% to 5%), weakness (1% to 2%), ataxia (0% to 2%), insomnia (0% to 2%), anxiety (1% to 2%), drowsiness (1%)

Dermatologic: Rash (1% to 3%)

Gastrointestinal: Nausea/vomiting (2% to 11%), unusual taste (3% to 23%), constipation (2% to 7%), dyspepsia (1% to 3%), diarrhea (1% to 3%), xerostomia (1% to 2%), anorexia (1% to 2%), abdominal pain (1% to 2%), flatulence (0% to 1%)

Neuromuscular & skeletal: Tremor (0% to 1%), arthralgia (0% to 1%)

Ocular: Blurred vision (1% to 6%)

Respiratory: Dyspnea (2% to 5%)

Miscellaneous: Diaphoresis (1%)

<1% (Limited to important or life-threatening): Agranulocytosis, alopecia, amnesia, anemia, apnea, AV block (second or third degree), AV dissociation, cardiac arrest, cholestasis (0.1%), coma, confusion, CHF, depression, granulocytopenia, hepatitis (0.03%), hyperglycemia, impotence, increased bleeding time, leukopenia, lupus erythematosus, mania, memory loss, nephrotic syndrome, paresthesia, peripheral neuropathy, pruritus, psychosis, purpura, renal failure, seizures (0.3%), SIADH, sinus node dysfunction, thrombocytopenia, tinnitus, vertigo

Overdosage/Toxicology Propafenone has a narrow therapeutic index and severe toxicity may occur slightly above the therapeutic range, especially if combined with other antiarrhythmic drugs. Acute single ingestion of twice the daily therapeutic dose is life-threatening. Symptoms of overdose include increased P-R, QRS, or QT intervals and amplitude of the T wave, AV block, bradycardia, hypotension, ventricular arrhythmias (monomorphic or polymorphic ventricular tachycardia), and asystole. Other symptoms include dizziness, blurred vision, headache, and GI upset. Treatment is supportive. **Note:** Class 1A antiarrhythmic agents should not be used to treat cardiotoxicity caused by Class 1C drugs. Sodium bicarbonate may reverse QRS prolongation, bradycardia, and hypotension. Ventricular pacing may be needed.

Pharmacodynamics/Kinetics

Absorption: Well absorbed

Bioavailability: 150 mg: 3.4%; 300 mg: 10.6%

Half-Life Elimination: Single dose (100-300 mg): 2-8 hours; Chronic dosing: 10-32 hours

Time to Peak: 150 mg dose: 2 hours; 300 mg dose: 3 hours

Metabolism: Hepatic; two genetically determined metabolism groups exist: fast or slow metabolizers; 10% of Caucasians are slow metabolizers; exhibits nonlinear pharmacokinetics; when dose is increased from 300-900 mg/day, serum concentrations increase tenfold; this nonlinearity is thought to be due to saturable first-pass effect

Formulations Tablet, as hydrochloride: 150 mg, 225 mg, 300 mg

Dosing

Adults & Elderly: Ventricular arrhythmias: Oral: 150 mg every 8 hours, increase at 3- to 4-day intervals up to 300 mg every 8 hours. **Note:** Patients who exhibit significant widening of QRS complex or second- or third-degree AV block may need dose reduction.

Hepatic Impairment: Reduced dose is necessary.

Monitoring and Teaching Issues

Physical Assessment: Assess other medications patient may be taking for effectiveness and interactions (see Drug Interactions). See Warnings/Precautions and Contraindications

(Continued)

Propafenone *(Continued)*

for use cautions. Monitor laboratory tests, therapeutic response, and adverse reactions (see Warnings/Precautions and Adverse Reactions) at beginning of therapy, when titrating dosage, and on a regular basis with long-term therapy. **Note:** Propafenone has a low TI and overdose may easily produce severe and life-threatening reactions (see Overdose/Toxicology). Assess knowledge/teach patient appropriate use, interventions to reduce side effects, and adverse symptoms to report (see Patient Education). **Pregnancy risk factor C** - benefits of use should outweigh possible risks. Note breast-feeding caution.

Patient Education: Take exactly as directed; do not take additional doses or discontinue without consulting prescriber. You will need regular cardiac checkups. You may experience dizziness, drowsiness, or visual changes (use caution when driving or engaging in tasks requiring alertness until response to drug is known); abnormal taste, nausea or vomiting, or loss of appetite (small, frequent meals, frequent mouth care, chewing gum, or sucking lozenges may help); headaches (prescriber may recommend mild analgesic); or diarrhea (yogurt, or boiled milk may help - if persistent consult prescriber). Report chest pain, palpitation, or erratic heartbeat; difficulty breathing, increased weight or swelling of hands or feet; acute persistent diarrhea or constipation; or vision changes. **Pregnancy/breast-feeding precautions:** Inform prescriber if you are or intend to become pregnant. Consult prescriber if breast-feeding.

Dietary Issues: Administer at the same time in relation to meals each day, either always with meals or always between meals.

Geriatric Considerations: Elderly may have age-related decreases in hepatic Phase I metabolism. Propafenone is dependent upon liver metabolism, therefore, monitor closely in the elderly and adjust dose more gradually during initial treatment (see Warnings/Precautions). No differences in clearance noted with impaired renal function and, therefore, no adjustment for renal function in the elderly is necessary.

Related Information

Antiarrhythmic Drugs *on page 1551*

Propafenone Hydrochloride *see* Propafenone *on page 1136*

Proparacaine *see page 1461*

Proparacaine and Fluorescein *see page 1461*

Propecia® *see* Finasteride *on page 560*

Prophylaxis for Exposure to Common Communicable Diseases *see page 1651*

Propine® *see* Ophthalmic Agents, Glaucoma *on page 1002*

Propofol (PROE po fole)

U.S. Brand Names Diprivan®

Generic Available Yes

Pharmacologic Category General Anesthetic

Pregnancy Risk Factor B

Lactation Excreted in breast milk/contraindicated

Use Induction of anesthesia for inpatient or outpatient surgery in patients ≥3 years of age; maintenance of anesthesia for inpatient or outpatient surgery in patients >2 months of age; in adults, for the induction and maintenance of monitored anesthesia care sedation during diagnostic procedures; may be used (for patients >18 years of age who are intubated and mechanically ventilated) as an alternative to benzodiazepines for the treatment of agitation in the intensive care unit

Use - Unlabeled/Investigational Postoperative antiemetic; refractory delirium tremens (case reports)

Mechanism of Action/Effect Propofol is a hindered phenolic compound with intravenous general anesthetic properties. The drug is unrelated to any of the currently used barbiturate, opioid, benzodiazepine, arylcyclohexylamine, or imidazole intravenous anesthetic agents.

Contraindications

Absolute contraindications:

Patients with a hypersensitivity to propofol or any component of the formulation

Patients who are not intubated or mechanically ventilated

Patients who are pregnant

When general anesthesia or sedation is contraindicated

Relative contraindications:

Pediatric intensive care unit patients: Safety and efficacy of propofol are not established

Patients with severe cardiac disease (ejection fraction <50%) or respiratory disease - propofol may have more profound adverse cardiovascular responses

Patients with a history of epilepsy or seizures; risk of seizure during recovery phase

Patients with increased intracranial pressure or impaired cerebral circulation - substantial decreases in mean arterial pressure and subsequent decreases in cerebral perfusion pressure may occur

Patients with hyperlipidemia as evidenced by increased serum triglyceride levels or serum turbidity

Patients who are hypotensive, hypovolemic, hemodynamically unstable, or abnormally low vascular tone (eg, sepsis)

Warnings/Precautions Use slower rate of induction in the elderly; transient local pain may occur during I.V. injection; perioperative myoclonia has occurred; do not administer with blood or blood products through the same I.V. catheter; not for obstetrics, including cesarean section deliveries. Abrupt discontinuation prior to weaning or daily wake up assessments should be avoided. Abrupt discontinuation can result in rapid awakening, anxiety, agitation, and resistance to mechanical ventilation. Several deaths associated with severe metabolic acidosis have been reported in pediatric ICU patients on long-term propofol infusion. Propofol emulsion contains soybean oil, egg phosphatide, and glycerol.

Drug Interactions

Cytochrome P450 Effect: Substrate of CYP1A2, 2A6, **2B6, 2C8/9**, 2C19, 2D6, 2E1, 3A4; Inhibits CYP1A2, 2C8/9, 2D6, 2E1, 3A4

Decreased Effect: Theophylline may antagonize the effect of propofol, requiring dosage increases.

Increased Effect/Toxicity: Increased toxicity:

Neuromuscular blockers:

Atracurium: Anaphylactoid reactions (including bronchospasm) have been reported in patients who have received concomitant atracurium and propofol.

Vecuronium: Propofol may potentiate the neuromuscular blockade of vecuronium.

Central nervous system depressants: Additive CNS depression and respiratory depression may necessitate dosage reduction when used with anesthetics, benzodiazepines, opiates, ethanol, narcotics, phenothiazines.

Nutritional/Ethanol Interactions Food: EDTA, an ingredient of propofol emulsion, may lead to decreased zinc levels in patients on prolonged therapy (>5 days) or those predisposed to deficiency (burns, diarrhea, and/or major sepsis).

Effects on Lab Values ↑ porphyrin (U); ↓ cortisol (S), but does not appear to inhibit adrenal responsiveness to ACTH; ↓ cholesterol (S)

Adverse Reactions

>10%:

Cardiovascular: Hypotension (3% to 26% adults, 17% children)

Central nervous system: Movement (17% children)

Local: Injection site burning, stinging, or pain (adults 18%, children 10%)

Respiratory: Apnea, lasting 30-60 seconds (24% adults, 10% children); Apnea, lasting >60 seconds (12% adults, 5% children)

3% to 10%:

Cardiovascular: Hypertension (8% children)

Central nervous system: Movement (adults)

Dermatologic: Pruritus (adults), rash

Endocrine & metabolic: Hyperlipidemia

Respiratory: Respiratory acidosis during weaning

1% to 3%:

Cardiovascular: Arrhythmia, bradycardia, decreased cardiac output, tachycardia

Dermatologic: Pruritus (children)

<1% (Limited to important or life-threatening): Anaphylaxis, anaphylactoid reaction, anticholinergic syndrome, bigeminy, cardiac arrest, delirium; discoloration (green) of urine, hair, or nailbed; dystonia, EKG abnormal, hemorrhage, hypoxia, infusion site reactions, laryngospasm, pancreatitis, perioperative myoclonia (rarely including convulsions and opisthotonos), premature atrial contractions, premature pulmonary edema, rhabdomyolysis, syncope, thrombosis, increased serum triglycerides, tissue necrosis following accidental extravasation

Overdosage/Toxicology

Symptoms of overdose include hypotension, bradycardia, and cardiovascular collapse.

Treatment is symptomatic and supportive. Hypotension usually responds to I.V. fluids and/or Trendelenburg positioning. Parenteral inotropes may be needed. Bradycardia may respond to atropine.

Pharmacodynamics/Kinetics

Half-Life Elimination: Biphasic: Initial: 40 minutes; Terminal: 4-7 hours (up to 1-3 days)

Metabolism: Hepatic to water-soluble sulfate and glucuronide conjugates

Onset: Anesthetic: Bolus infusion (dose dependent): 9-51 seconds (average: 30 seconds)

Duration: Dose and rate dependent: 3-10 minutes

Formulations Injection [with EDTA preservative]: 10 mg/mL (20 mL, 50 mL, 100 mL)

Dosing

Adults: Dosage must be individualized based on total body weight and titrated to the desired clinical effect. Wait at least 3-5 minutes between dosage adjustments to clinically assess drug effects. Smaller doses are required when used with narcotics. The following are general dosing guidelines (see "Symbols and Abbreviations Used in This Handbook" in front section of this book for explanation of ASA classes):

Induction:

General anesthesia:

ASA I or II, <55 years: I.V.: 2-2.5 mg/kg (~40 mg every 10 seconds until onset of induction)

Debilitated, ASA III or IV, hypovolemic: Refer to elderly dosing.

Cardiac anesthesia: I.V.: 0.5-1.5 mg/kg (~20 mg every 10 seconds until onset of induction)

Neurosurgical patients: I.V.: 1-2 mg/kg (~20 mg every 10 seconds until onset of induction)

Maintenance:

ASA I or II, <55 years:

I.V. infusion: Initial: 150-200 mcg/kg/minute for 10-15 minutes; decrease by 30% to 50% during first 30 minutes of maintenance; usual infusion rate: 100-200 mcg/kg/minute (6-12 mg/kg/hour)

I.V. intermittent bolus: 20-50 mg increments as needed

Debilitated, ASA III or IV, hypovolemic: I.V. Infusion: Refer to elderly dosing.

Cardiac anesthesia: I.V. infusion:

Low-dose propofol with primary opioid: 50-100 mcg/kg/minute (see manufacturer's labeling)

Primary propofol with secondary opioid: 100-150 mcg/kg/minute

Neurosurgical patients: I.V. infusion: 100-200 mcg/kg/minute (6-12 mg/kg/hour)

Monitored anesthesia care sedation:

Initiation:

ASA I or II, <55 years: Slow I.V. infusion: 100-150 mcg/kg/minute for 3-5 minutes **or** slow injection: 0.5 mg/kg over 3-5 minutes

Debilitated, neurosurgical, or ASA III or IV patients: Use similar doses to healthy adults; avoid rapid I.V. boluses

(Continued)

Propofol *(Continued)*

Maintenance:

ASA I or II, <55 years: I.V. infusion using variable rates (preferred over intermittent boluses): 25-75 mcg/kg/minute **or** incremental bolus doses: 10 mg or 20 mg

Debilitated, neurosurgical, or ASA III or IV patients: Use 80% of healthy adult dose; **do not** use rapid bolus doses (single or repeated)

ICU sedation in intubated mechanically-ventilated patients: Avoid rapid bolus injection; individualize dose and titrate to response

Continuous infusion: Initial: 0.3 mg/kg/hour; increase by 0.3-0.6 mg/kg/hour every 5-10 minutes until desired sedation level is achieved; usual maintenance: 0.3-3 mg/kg/hour or higher. Reduce dose by 80% in debilitated, and ASA III or IV patients. Reduce dose after adequate sedation established and adjust to response (ie, evaluate frequently to use minimum dose for sedation). Some clinicians recommend daily interruption of infusion to perform clinical evaluation.

Elderly:

General anesthesia:

Induction: Elderly, debilitated, ASA III or IV, hypovolemic: I.V.: 1-1.5 mg/kg (~20 mg every 10 seconds until onset of induction)

Maintenance: Elderly, debilitated, ASA III or IV, hypovolemic: I.V. infusion: 50-100 mcg/kg/minute (3-6 mg/kg/hour)

Monitored anesthesia care sedation:

Initiation: Elderly, debilitated, ASA III or IV, neurosurgical: I.V.: Use doses similar to healthy adults; avoid rapid I.V. boluses

Maintenance: Elderly, debilitated, ASA III or IV, neurosurgical: I.V.: Use 80% of healthy adult dose; **do not** use rapid bolus doses (single or repeated)

Pediatrics: Dosage must be individualized based on total body weight and titrated to the desired clinical effect; wait at least 3-5 minutes between dosage adjustments to clinically assess drug effects; smaller doses are required when used with narcotics; the following are general dosing guidelines (see "Symbols and Abbreviations Used in This Handbook" in front section of this book for explanation of ASA classes):

General anesthesia:

Induction: I.V.: Children 3-16 years, ASA I or II: 2.5-3.5 mg/kg over 20-30 seconds; use a lower dose for children ASA III or IV

Maintenance: I.V. infusion: Children 2 months to 16 years, ASA I or II: Initial: 200-300 mcg/kg/minute; decrease dose after 30 minutes if clinical signs of light anesthesia are absent; usual infusion rate: 125-150 mcg/kg/minute (range: 125-300 mcg/kg/minute; 7.5-18 mg/kg/hour); children ≤5 years may require larger infusion rates compared to older children.

Administration

I.V.: To reduce pain associated with injection, use larger veins of forearm or antecubital fossa; lidocaine I.V. (1 mL of a 1% solution) may also be used prior to administration. Do not use filter with <5 micron for administration. Soybean fat emulsion is used as a vehicle for propofol. Strict aseptic technique must be maintained in handling although a preservative has been added. Do not administer through the same I.V. catheter with blood or plasma. The American College of Critical Care Medicine recommends the use of a central vein for administration in an ICU setting.

Stability

Storage: Store at room temperature 4°C to 22°C (40°F to 72°F); refrigeration is not recommended. Protect from light. If transferred to a syringe or other container prior to administration, use within 6 hours. If used directly from vial/prefilled syringe, use within 12 hours. Shake well before use. Do not use if there is evidence of separation of phases of emulsion.

Reconstitution: Does not need to be diluted; however, propofol may be further diluted in 5% dextrose in water to a concentration of 2 mg/mL and is stable for 8 hours at room temperature.

Compatibility: Do not mix with other therapeutic agents.

Stable in D_5LR, $D_5{}^1/_4NS$, $D_5{}^1/_2NS$, D_5W, LR

Y-site administration: Incompatible with amikacin, amphotericin B, atracurium, bretylium, calcium chloride, ciprofloxacin, diazepam, digoxin, doxorubicin, gentamicin, methotrexate, methylprednisolone sodium succinate, metoclopramide, minocycline, mitoxantrone, phenytoin, tobramycin, verapamil

Monitoring Laboratory Tests Monitor zinc levels in patients predisposed to deficiency (burns, diarrhea, major sepsis). In patients at risk for renal impairment, urinalysis and urine sediment should be monitored prior to treatment and every other day of sedation. Serum triglyceride levels should be obtained prior to initiation of therapy (ICU setting) and every 3-7 days thereafter.

Monitoring and Teaching Issues

Physical Assessment: Dosage and rate of administration should be individualized and titrated to the desired effect, according to relevant clinical factors, premedication, concomitant medications, age, and general condition of patient. See Use, Contraindications, and Warnings/Precautions for appropriate use cautions. Assess other medications for effectiveness and safety. Other drugs that cause CNS depression may increase CNS depression induced by propofol (monitor and adjust dosage as necessary). Continuous monitoring of vital signs, cardiac and respiratory status, and level of sedation is mandatory during infusion and until full consciousness is regained (see Adverse Reactions). Safety precautions must be maintained until patient is fully alert. Propofol is an anesthetic; pain must be treated with appropriate analgesic agents. Do not discontinue abruptly (may result in rapid awakening associated with anxiety, agitation, and resistance to mechanical ventilation). Titrate infusion rate so patient awakes slowly. **Note:** After long-term administration, it will take longer for reduction of propofol levels than if propofol is used for short-term anesthesia. For long-term use, monitor fluid levels (intake and output) during and following infusion (urine will be green). Reposition patient and provide appropriate skin care, mouth care, and care of patient's eyes every 2-3 hours while sedated. Provide appropriate emotional and sensory support (auditory and environmental). Breast-feeding is contraindicated.

Patient Education: This is an anesthetic. Patient education should be appropriate to individual situation. With long-term use appropriate emotional and sensory support is strongly recommended. Following return of consciousness, do not attempt to change position or rise from bed without assistance. Report immediately any pounding or unusual heartbeat, difficulty breathing, or acute dizziness. **Breast-feeding precaution:** Do not breast-feed.

Dietary Issues: Propofol is formulated in an oil-in-water emulsion. If on parenteral nutrition, may need to adjust the amount of lipid infused. Propofol emulsion contains 1.1 kcal/mL.

Pregnancy Issues: Propofol is not recommended for obstetrics, including cesarean section deliveries. Propofol crosses the placenta and may be associated with neonatal depression.

Additional Information On March 26, 2001, a specific warning was issued concerning the use of propofol in pediatric ICU patients. In the opinion of the FDA, a clinical trial evaluating the use of propofol as a sedative agent in this population was associated with a higher number of deaths as compared to standard sedative agents. The warning reminded health-care professionals that propofol is not approved in the U.S. for sedation in pediatric ICU patients. A new clinical trial is planned to evaluate differences in safety within this population.

Propoxyphene (proe POKS i feen)

U.S. Brand Names Darvon®; Darvon-N®

Synonyms Dextropropoxyphene; Propoxyphene Hydrochloride; Propoxyphene Napsylate

Restrictions C-IV

Generic Available Yes: Capsule

Pharmacologic Category Analgesic, Narcotic

Pregnancy Risk Factor C/D (prolonged use)

Lactation Enters breast milk/use caution (AAP rates "compatible")

Use Management of mild to moderate pain

Mechanism of Action/Effect Binds to opiate receptors in the CNS, causing inhibition of ascending pain pathways, altering the perception of and response to pain; produces generalized CNS depression

Contraindications Hypersensitivity to propoxyphene or any component of the formulation; pregnancy (prolonged use)

Warnings/Precautions Give with caution in patients dependent on opiates. Substitution may result in acute opiate withdrawal symptoms. Use with caution in patients with severe renal or hepatic dysfunction. When given in excessive doses, either alone or in combination with other CNS depressants or propoxyphene products, propoxyphene is a major cause of drug-related deaths. Avoid use in severely depressed or suicidal patients. **Do not exceed recommended dosage.** Pregnancy risk C/D (prolonged use).

Drug Interactions

Cytochrome P450 Effect: Inhibits CYP2C8/9, 2D6, 3A4

Decreased Effect: Decreased effect with cigarette smoking.

Increased Effect/Toxicity: CNS depressants (phenothiazines, tranquilizers, anxiolytics, sedatives, hypnotics, or alcohol) may potentiate pharmacologic effects. Propoxyphene may inhibit the metabolism and increase the serum concentrations of carbamazepine, phenobarbital, MAO inhibitors, tricyclic antidepressants, and warfarin.

Nutritional/Ethanol Interactions

Ethanol: Avoid or limit ethanol (may increase CNS depression). Watch for sedation.

Food: May decrease rate of absorption, but may slightly increase bioavailability. Glucose may cause hyperglycemia; monitor blood glucose concentrations.

Effects on Lab Values False-positive methadone test; ↑ LFTs; ↓ glucose (S), 17-OHCS (U)

Adverse Reactions Frequency not defined.

Cardiovascular: Hypotension, bundle branch block

Central nervous system: Dizziness, lightheadedness, sedation, paradoxical excitement and insomnia, fatigue, drowsiness, mental depression, hallucinations, paradoxical CNS stimulation, increased intracranial pressure, nervousness, headache, restlessness, malaise, confusion

Dermatologic: Rash, urticaria

Endocrine & metabolic: May decrease glucose, urinary 17-OHCS

Gastrointestinal: Anorexia, stomach cramps, xerostomia, biliary spasm, nausea, vomiting, constipation, paralytic ileus

Genitourinary: Decreased urination, ureteral spasms

Neuromuscular & skeletal: Weakness

Hepatic: Increased liver enzymes (may increase LFTs)

Respiratory: Dyspnea

Miscellaneous: Psychologic and physical dependence with prolonged use, histamine release

Overdosage/Toxicology Symptoms of overdose include CNS disturbances, respiratory depression, hypotension, pulmonary edema, and seizures. Naloxone, 2 mg I.V. with repeat administration as necessary up to a total of 10 mg, can also be used to reverse toxic effects of the opiate. Charcoal is very effective (>95%) at binding propoxyphene.

Pharmacodynamics/Kinetics

Bioavailability: 30% to 70%

Half-Life Elimination: Adults: Parent drug: 8-24 hours (mean: ~15 hours); Norpropoxyphene: 34 hours

Metabolism: Hepatic to active metabolite (norpropoxyphene) and inactive metabolites; first-pass effect

Onset: 0.5-1 hour

Duration: 4-6 hours

Formulations

Capsule, as hydrochloride: 65 mg

Tablet, as napsylate: 100 mg

Dosing

Adults: Pain management: Oral:

Hydrochloride: 65 mg every 3-4 hours as needed for pain; maximum: 390 mg/day

Napsylate: 100 mg every 4 hours as needed for pain; maximum: 600 mg/day

(Continued)

Propoxyphene *(Continued)*

Elderly: Oral:
Hydrochloride: 65 mg every 4-6 hours as needed for pain
Napsylate: 100 mg every 4-6 hours as needed for pain

Pediatrics: Pain management: Oral: Children: Doses for children are not well established; doses of the hydrochloride of 2-3 mg/kg/d divided every 6 hours have been used.

Renal Impairment:
Cl_{cr} <10 mL/minute: Avoid use.
Not dialyzable (0% to 5%)

Hepatic Impairment: Reduced doses should be used.

Administration

Oral: Should be administered with glass of water on an empty stomach. Food may decrease rate of absorption, but may slightly increase bioavailability.

Monitoring and Teaching Issues

Physical Assessment: Assess other medications patient may be taking for effectiveness and interactions (see Drug Interactions). Monitor therapeutic effectiveness, cardio/respiratory and CNS status, adverse reactions and signs of overdose (see Overdose/Toxicology) at beginning of therapy and periodically with long-term use. Assess knowledge/teach patient appropriate use, interventions to reduce side effects, and adverse symptoms to report (see Patient Education). **Pregnancy risk factor C/D** - see Pregnancy Risk Factor for use cautions. Assess knowledge/instruct patient on use of barrier contraceptive measures; danger of use during pregnancy must outweigh risk to fetus. Note breast-feeding caution.

Patient Education: Take as directed; do not take a larger dose or more often than prescribed. Do not use alcohol, other prescription or OTC sedatives, tranquilizers, antihistamines, or pain medications without consulting prescriber. May cause dizziness, drowsiness, or impaired judgment; avoid driving or engaging in tasks requiring alertness until response to drug is known. If you experience vomiting or loss of appetite, frequent mouth care, small, frequent meals, chewing gum, or sucking lozenges may help. Increased fluid intake, exercise, fiber in diet may help with constipation (if unresolved consult prescriber). Report unresolved nausea or vomiting, difficulty breathing or shortness of breath, or unusual weakness. **Pregnancy/breast-feeding precautions:** Inform prescriber if you are or intend to become pregnant. Nursing women should take this drug 4-5 hours before breast-feeding.

Dietary Issues: May administer with food if gastrointestinal distress occurs.

Geriatric Considerations: The elderly may be particularly susceptible to the CNS depressant effects of narcotics.

Additional Information 100 mg of napsylate = 65 mg of hydrochloride
Propoxyphene hydrochloride: Darvon®
Propoxyphene napsylate: Darvon-N®

Related Information
Narcotic/Opioid Analgesic Comparison *on page 1583*

Propoxyphene and Acetaminophen
(proe POKS i feen & a seet a MIN oh fen)

U.S. Brand Names Darvocet-N® 50; Darvocet-N® 100; Pronap-100®; Wygesic®

Synonyms Propoxyphene Hydrochloride and Acetaminophen; Propoxyphene Napsylate and Acetaminophen

Restrictions C-IV

Generic Available Yes

Pharmacologic Category Analgesic Combination (Narcotic)

Pregnancy Risk Factor C

Lactation Enters breast milk/compatible

Use Management of mild to moderate pain

Formulations
Tablet:
Darvocet-N® 50: Propoxyphene napsylate 50 mg and acetaminophen 325 mg
Darvocet-N® 100, Pronap-100®: Propoxyphene napsylate 100 mg and acetaminophen 650 mg
Wygesic®: Propoxyphene hydrochloride 65 mg and acetaminophen 650 mg

Dosing

Adults & Elderly: Pain management: Oral:
Darvocet-N®: 1-2 tablets every 4 hours as needed; maximum: 600 mg propoxyphene napsylate/day
Darvocet-N® 100: 1 tablet every 4 hours as needed; maximum: 600 mg propoxyphene napsylate/day
Note: Formulations contain significant amounts of acetaminophen; intake should be limited to <4 g acetaminophen/day (less in patients with hepatic impairment/ethanol abuse)

Hepatic Impairment: Limit acetaminophen intake; refer to adult dosing.

Monitoring and Teaching Issues

Physical Assessment: See individual components listed in Related Information. **Pregnancy risk factor C** - benefits of use should outweigh possible risks.

Patient Education: See individual components listed in Related Information. **Pregnancy precaution:** Inform prescriber if you are or intend to become pregnant.

Related Information
Acetaminophen *on page 35*
Propoxyphene *on page 1141*

Propoxyphene and Aspirin (proe POKS i feen & AS pir in)

U.S. Brand Names Darvon® Compound-65 Pulvules®; PC-Cap®

Synonyms Propoxyphene Hydrochloride and Aspirin; Propoxyphene Napsylate and Aspirin

Restrictions C-IV

Generic Available Yes

Pharmacologic Category Analgesic Combination (Narcotic)

Pregnancy Risk Factor D

Lactation Enters breast milk/use caution due to aspirin content

Use Management of mild to moderate pain

Formulations Capsule (Darvon® Compound-65, PC-Cap®): Propoxyphene hydrochloride 65 mg and aspirin 389 mg with caffeine 32.4 mg

Dosing

Adults: Pain management: Oral: 1-2 capsules every 4 hours as needed

Elderly: Refer to dosing in individual monographs.

Renal Impairment: Dose reduction is recommended.

Hepatic Impairment: Use with caution. Limited, low-dose therapy is usually well tolerated in hepatic disease/cirrhosis; however, cases of hepatotoxicity at daily acetaminophen dosages <4 g/day have been reported. Avoid chronic use in hepatic impairment.

Monitoring and Teaching Issues

Physical Assessment: See individual components listed in Related Information. **Pregnancy risk factor D** - determine that patient is not pregnant before beginning treatment. Instruct patients of childbearing age about appropriate barrier contraceptive measures. Note breast-feeding caution.

Patient Education: See individual components listed in Related Information. **Pregnancy/breast-feeding precautions:** Inform prescriber if you are or intend to become pregnant. Consult prescriber if breast-feeding.

Related Information

Aspirin *on page 121*
Propoxyphene *on page 1141*

Propoxyphene Hydrochloride *see* Propoxyphene *on page 1141*

Propoxyphene Hydrochloride and Acetaminophen *see* Propoxyphene and Acetaminophen *on page 1142*

Propoxyphene Hydrochloride and Aspirin *see* Propoxyphene and Aspirin *on page 1142*

Propoxyphene Napsylate *see* Propoxyphene *on page 1141*

Propoxyphene Napsylate and Acetaminophen *see* Propoxyphene and Acetaminophen *on page 1142*

Propoxyphene Napsylate and Aspirin *see* Propoxyphene and Aspirin *on page 1142*

Propranolol (proe PRAN oh lole)

U.S. Brand Names Inderal®; Inderal® LA

Synonyms Propranolol Hydrochloride

Generic Available Yes

Pharmacologic Category Antiarrhythmic Agent, Class II; Beta Blocker, Nonselective

Pregnancy Risk Factor C (manufacturer); D (2nd and 3rd trimesters - expert analysis)

Lactation Enters breast milk/use caution (AAP rates "compatible")

Use Management of hypertension; angina pectoris; pheochromocytoma; essential tremor; tetralogy of Fallot cyanotic spells; arrhythmias (such as atrial fibrillation and flutter, AV nodal re-entrant tachycardias, and catecholamine-induced arrhythmias); prevention of myocardial infarction; migraine headache; symptomatic treatment of hypertrophic subaortic stenosis

Use - Unlabeled/Investigational Tremor due to Parkinson's disease; ethanol withdrawal; aggressive behavior; antipsychotic-induced akathisia; prevention of bleeding esophageal varices; anxiety; schizophrenia; acute panic; gastric bleeding in portal hypertension

Mechanism of Action/Effect Nonselective beta-adrenergic blocker (class II antiarrhythmic); competitively blocks response to $beta_1$- and $beta_2$-adrenergic stimulation which results in decreases in heart rate, myocardial contractility, blood pressure, and myocardial oxygen demand

Contraindications Hypersensitivity to propranolol, beta-blockers, or any component of the formulation; uncompensated congestive heart failure (unless the failure is due to tachyarrhythmias being treated with propranolol), cardiogenic shock, bradycardia or heart block (2nd or 3rd degree), pulmonary edema, severe hyperactive airway disease (asthma or COPD), Raynaud's disease; pregnancy (2nd and 3rd trimesters)

Warnings/Precautions Administer cautiously in compensated heart failure and monitor for a worsening of the condition (efficacy of propranolol in CHF has not been demonstrated). Beta-blocker therapy should not be withdrawn abruptly (particularly in patients with CAD), but gradually tapered to avoid acute tachycardia, hypertension, and/or ischemia. Use caution in patient with peripheral vascular disease. Use caution with concurrent use of beta-blockers and either verapamil or diltiazem; bradycardia or heart block can occur. Avoid concurrent I.V. use of both agents. Use cautiously in patients with diabetes; may mask prominent hypoglycemic symptoms. May mask signs of thyrotoxicosis. Can cause fetal harm when administered in pregnancy. Use cautiously in hepatic dysfunction (dosage adjustment required). Use care with anesthetic agents which decrease myocardial function. Pregnancy risk C.

Drug Interactions

Cytochrome P450 Effect: Substrate of **CYP1A2, 2C19, 2D6**, 3A4; Inhibits CYP1A2, 2D6

Decreased Effect: Aluminum salts, barbiturates, calcium salts, cholestyramine, colestipol, NSAIDs, penicillins (ampicillin), rifampin, salicylates, and sulfinpyrazone decrease effect of beta-blockers due to decreased bioavailability and plasma levels. Beta-blockers may decrease the effect of sulfonylureas. Ascorbic acid decreases propranolol Cp_{max} and AUC and increases the T_{max} significantly resulting in a greater decrease in the reduction of heart rate, possibly due to decreased absorption and first pass metabolism (n=5). Nefazodone decreased peak plasma levels and AUC of propranolol and increases time to reach steady-state; monitoring of clinical response is recommended. Nonselective beta-blockers blunt the response to beta-2 adrenergic agonists (albuterol).

Increased Effect/Toxicity: The heart rate lowering effects of propranolol are additive with other drugs which slow AV conduction (digoxin, verapamil, diltiazem). Reserpine increases the effects of propranolol. Concurrent use of propranolol may increase the effects of

(Continued)

Propranolol *(Continued)*

alpha-blockers (prazosin, terazosin), alpha-adrenergic stimulants (epinephrine, phenylephrine), and the vasoconstrictive effects of ergot alkaloids. Propranolol may mask the tachycardia from hypoglycemia caused by insulin and oral hypoglycemics. In patients receiving concurrent therapy, the risk of hypertensive crisis is increased when either clonidine or the beta-blocker is withdrawn. Beta-blockers may increase the action or levels of ethanol, disopyramide, nondepolarizing muscle relaxants, and theophylline although the effects are difficult to predict.

Beta-blocker effects may be enhanced by oral contraceptives, flecainide, haloperidol (hypotensive effects), H_2-antagonists (cimetidine, possibly ranitidine), hydralazine, loop diuretics, possibly MAO inhibitors, phenothiazines, propafenone, quinidine (in extensive metabolizers), ciprofloxacin, thyroid hormones (when hypothyroid patient is converted to euthyroid state). Beta-blockers may increase the effect/toxicity of flecainide, haloperidol (hypotensive effects), hydralazine, phenothiazines, acetaminophen, anticoagulants (warfarin), and benzodiazepines.

Nutritional/Ethanol Interactions

Food: Propranolol serum levels may be increased if taken with food. Protein-rich foods may increase bioavailability; a change in diet from high carbohydrate/low protein to low carbohydrate/high protein may result in increased oral clearance.

Herb/Nutraceutical: Avoid dong quai if using for hypertension (has estrogenic activity). Avoid ephedra, yohimbe, ginseng (may worsen hypertension or arrhythmia). Avoid natural licorice (causes sodium and water retention and increases potassium loss). Avoid garlic (may have increased antihypertensive effect).

Effects on Lab Values ↑ thyroxine (S)

Adverse Reactions Frequency not defined.

Cardiovascular: Bradycardia, CHF, reduced peripheral circulation, chest pain, hypotension, impaired myocardial contractility, worsening of AV conduction disturbance, cardiogenic shock, Raynaud's syndrome, mesenteric thrombosis (rare)

Central nervous system: Mental depression, lightheadedness, amnesia, emotional lability, confusion, hallucinations, dizziness, insomnia, fatigue, vivid dreams, lethargy, cold extremities, vertigo, syncope, cognitive dysfunction, psychosis, hypersomnolence

Dermatologic: Rash, alopecia, exfoliative dermatitis, psoriasiform eruptions, eczematous eruptions, hyperkeratosis, nail changes, pruritus, urticaria, ulcerative lichenoid, contact dermatitis

Endocrine & metabolic: Hypoglycemia, hyperglycemia, hyperlipidemia, hyperkalemia

Gastrointestinal: Diarrhea, nausea, vomiting, stomach discomfort, constipation, anorexia

Genitourinary: Impotence, proteinuria (rare), oliguria (rare), interstitial nephritis (rare), Peyronie's disease

Hematologic: Agranulocytosis, thrombocytopenia, thrombocytopenic purpura

Neuromuscular & skeletal: Weakness, carpal tunnel syndrome (rare), paresthesias, myotonus, polyarthritis, arthropathy

Respiratory: Wheezing, pharyngitis, bronchospasm, pulmonary edema

Ocular: Hyperemia of the conjunctiva, decreased tear production, decreased visual acuity, mydriasis

Miscellaneous: Lupus-like syndrome (rare)

Overdosage/Toxicology Symptoms of intoxication include cardiac disturbances, CNS toxicity, bronchospasm, hypoglycemia, and hyperkalemia. The most common cardiac symptoms include hypotension and bradycardia. Atrioventricular block, intraventricular conduction disturbances, cardiogenic shock, and asystole may occur with severe overdose, especially with membrane-depressant drugs (eg, propranolol). CNS effects include convulsions and coma. Respiratory arrest is commonly seen with propranolol and other membrane-depressant and lipid-soluble drugs. Treatment is symptom-directed and supportive.

Pharmacodynamics/Kinetics

Bioavailability: 30% to 40%; may be increased with Down syndrome

Half-Life Elimination: Neonates and Infants: Possible increased half-life; Children: 3.9-6.4 hours; Adults: 4-6 hours

Metabolism: Hepatic to active and inactive compounds; extensive first-pass effect

Onset: Beta-blockade: Oral: 1-2 hours

Duration: ~6 hours

Formulations

Capsule, long-acting, as hydrochloride: 60 mg, 80 mg, 120 mg, 160 mg

Injection, as hydrochloride: 1 mg/mL (1 mL)

Solution, oral, as hydrochloride: 4 mg/mL (5 mL, 500 mL); 8 mg/mL (5 mL, 500 mL) [strawberry-mint flavor]

Solution, oral concentrate, as hydrochloride: 80 mg/mL (30 mL)

Tablet, as hydrochloride: 10 mg, 20 mg, 40 mg, 60 mg, 80 mg, 90 mg

Dosing

Adults:

Angina: Oral: 80-320 mg/day in doses divided 2-4 times/day

Long-acting formulation: Initial: 80 mg once daily; maximum dose: 320 mg once daily.

Myocardial infarction prophylaxis: Oral: 180-240 mg/day in 3-4 divided doses

Hypertension: Oral: Initial: 40 mg twice daily; increase dosage every 3-7 days; usual dose: ≤320 mg divided in 2-3 doses/day; maximum daily dose: 640 mg.

Long-acting formulation: Initial: 80 mg once daily; usual maintenance: 120-160 mg once daily; maximum daily dose: 640 mg.

Tachyarrhythmias:

Oral: 10-30 mg/dose every 6-8 hours

I.V.: 1 mg/dose slow IVP; repeat every 5 minutes up to a total of 5 mg.

Migraine headache prophylaxis: Oral: Initial: 80 mg/day divided every 6-8 hours; increase by 20-40 mg/dose every 3-4 weeks to a maximum of 160-240 mg/day given in divided doses every 6-8 hours. If satisfactory response not achieved within 6 weeks of starting therapy, drug should be withdrawn gradually over several weeks.

Long-acting formulation: Initial: 80 mg once daily; effective dose range: 160-240 mg once daily

Thyrotoxicosis:

Oral: 10-40 mg/dose every 6 hours

I.V.: 1-3 mg/dose slow IVP as a single dose

Pheochromocytoma: Oral: 30-60 mg/day in divided doses

Hypertrophic subaortic stenosis: Oral: 20-40 mg 3-4 times/day; long-acting formulation: 80-160 mg once daily.

Essential tremor: Oral: 20-40 mg twice daily initially; maintenance doses: usually 120-320 mg/day

Akathisia: Oral: 30-120 mg/day in 2-3 divided doses

Elderly: Tachyarrhythmias: Initial: 10 mg twice daily; increase dosage every 3-7 days; usual dose range: 10-320 mg given 1-2 times/day. Refer to adult dosing for additional uses.

Pediatrics:

Tachyarrhythmias:

Oral: Children: Initial: 0.5-1 mg/kg/day in divided doses every 6-8 hours; titrate dosage upward every 3-7 days; usual dose: 2-4 mg/kg/day; higher doses may be needed; do not exceed 16 mg/kg/day or 60 mg/day.

I.V.: Children: 0.01-0.1 mg/kg slow IVP over 10 minutes; maximum dose: 1 mg

Hypertension: Oral: Children: Initial: 0.5-1 mg/kg/day in divided doses every 6-12 hours; increase gradually every 3-7 days; maximum: 2 mg/kg/24 hours

Migraine headache prophylaxis: Oral: Children: 0.6-1.5 mg/kg/day **or**

≤35 kg: 10-20 mg 3 times/day

>35 kg: 20-40 mg 3 times/day

Tetralogy spells: Children:

Oral: 1-2 mg/kg/day every 6 hours as needed, may increase by 1 mg/kg/day to a maximum of 5 mg/kg/day, or if refractory may increase slowly to a maximum of 10-15 mg/kg/day.

I.V.: 0.15-0.25 mg/kg/dose slow IVP; may repeat in 15 minutes.

Thyrotoxicosis: Adolescents: Oral: 10-40 mg/dose every 6 hours

Renal Impairment:

Cl_{cr} 31-40 mL/minute: Administer every 24-36 hours or administer 50% of normal dose.

Cl_{cr} 10-30 mL/minute: Administer every 24-48 hours or administer 50% of normal dose.

Cl_{cr} <10 mL/minute: Administer every 40-60 hours or administer 25% of normal dose.

Not dialyzable (0% to 5%); supplemental dose is not necessary.

Peritoneal dialysis effects: Supplemental dose is not necessary.

Hepatic Impairment: Marked slowing of heart rate may occur in cirrhosis with conventional doses; low initial dose and regular heart rate monitoring.

Administration

I.V.: I.V. administration should not exceed 1 mg/minute. I.V. dose is much smaller than oral dose.

Stability

Storage: Protect injection from light. Solutions have maximum stability at pH of 3 and decompose rapidly in alkaline pH. Propranolol is stable for 24 hours at room temperature in D_5W or NS.

Compatibility: Stable in D_5½NS, D_5NS, D_5W, LR, ½NS, NS

Y-site administration: Incompatible with amphotericin B cholesteryl sulfate complex, diazoxide

Compatibility in syringe: Incompatible with HCO_3

Compatibility when admixed: Incompatible with HCO_3

Monitoring and Teaching Issues

Physical Assessment: Assess effectiveness and interactions of other medications patient may be taking (see Drug Interactions). Monitor therapeutic response and adverse reactions when starting or adjusting dosage (see Warnings/Precautions and Adverse Reactions). I.V. infusion requires hemodynamic monitoring. Monitor serum glucose closely in diabetic patients. Beta-blockers may alter serum glucose levels. Assess knowledge/teach patient appropriate use, orthostatic precautions, interventions to reduce side effects, and adverse symptoms to report (see Patient Education). **Pregnancy risk factor C/D** - benefits of use should outweigh possible risks. Note breast-feeding caution.

Patient Education: Take exactly as directed; do not increase, decrease, or discontinue without consulting prescriber. Tablets may be crushed and taken with liquids. Do not chew or crush long-acting forms; take whole. Take at the same time each day. Do not alter dietary intake of protein or carbohydrates without consulting prescriber. You may experience orthostatic hypotension, dizziness, drowsiness, or blurred vision (use caution when driving, climbing stairs, or changing position - rising from sitting or lying to standing - or engaging in tasks requiring alertness until response to drug is known); nausea, vomiting, or stomach discomfort (small, frequent meals, frequent mouth care, chewing gum, or sucking lozenges may help); or decreased sexual ability (reversible). If diabetic, monitor serum glucose closely. Report unusual swelling of extremities, difficulty breathing, unresolved cough, or unusual weight gain, cold extremities, persistent diarrhea, confusion, hallucinations, headache, nervousness, lack of improvement, or worsening of condition. **Pregnancy/breast-feeding precautions:** Inform prescriber if you are or intend to become pregnant. Consult prescriber if breast-feeding.

Dietary Issues: Administer with food.

Geriatric Considerations: Since bioavailability increased in the elderly, about twofold geriatric patients may require lower maintenance doses, therefore, as serum and tissue concentrations increase $beta_1$ selectivity diminishes; due to alterations in the beta-adrenergic autonomic nervous system, beta-adrenergic blockade may result in less hemodynamic response than seen in younger adults.

Breast-feeding Issues: Propranolol is excreted in breast milk and is considered compatible by the AAP. It is recommended that the infant be monitored for signs or symptoms of beta-blockade (hypotension, bradycardia, etc) with long-term use.

Pregnancy Issues: Crosses the placenta. IUGR, hypoglycemia, bradycardia, respiratory depression, hyperbilirubinemia, polycythemia, polydactyly reported. IUGR probably related

(Continued)

Propranolol *(Continued)*

to maternal hypertension. Preterm labor has been reported. Available evidence suggests safe use during pregnancy.

Additional Information Not indicated for hypertensive emergencies. Do not abruptly discontinue therapy, taper dosage gradually over 2 weeks.

Related Information

Antiarrhythmic Drugs *on page 1551*
Beta-Blockers *on page 1561*

Propranolol and Hydrochlorothiazide

(proe PRAN oh lole & hye droe klor oh THYE a zide)

U.S. Brand Names Inderide®; Inderide® LA

Synonyms Hydrochlorothiazide and Propranolol

Generic Available Yes: Immediate release

Pharmacologic Category Antihypertensive Agent Combination

Pregnancy Risk Factor C

Lactation Enters breast milk/compatible

Use Management of hypertension

Formulations

Capsule, long-acting (Inderide® LA):
- 80/50: Propranolol hydrochloride 80 mg and hydrochlorothiazide 50 mg
- 120/50: Propranolol hydrochloride 120 mg and hydrochlorothiazide 50 mg
- 160/50: Propranolol hydrochloride 160 mg and hydrochlorothiazide 50 mg

Tablet (Inderide®):
- 40/25: Propranolol hydrochloride 40 mg and hydrochlorothiazide 25 mg
- 80/25: Propranolol hydrochloride 80 mg and hydrochlorothiazide 25 mg

Dosing

Adults: Hypertension: Oral: Dose is individualized; typical dosages of **hydrochlorothiazide**: 12.5-50 mg/day; initial dose of **propranolol** 80 mg/day

Daily dose of tablet form should be divided into 2 daily doses; may be used to maximum dosage of up to 160 mg of propranolol; higher dosages would result in higher than optimal thiazide dosages.

Long acting capsules may be given once daily.

Elderly: Refer to dosing in individual monographs.

Monitoring and Teaching Issues

Physical Assessment: See individual components listed in Related Information. **Pregnancy risk factor C** - benefits of use should outweigh possible risks.

Patient Education: See individual components listed in Related Information. **Pregnancy precaution:** Inform prescriber if you are or intend to become pregnant.

Related Information

Hydrochlorothiazide *on page 664*
Propranolol *on page 1143*

Propranolol Hydrochloride *see* Propranolol *on page 1143*
Propulsid® *see* Cisapride *on page 294*
2-Propylpentanoic Acid *see* Valproic Acid and Derivatives *on page 1382*

Propylthiouracil

(proe pil thye oh YOOR a sil)

Synonyms PTU

Generic Available Yes

Pharmacologic Category Antithyroid Agent

Pregnancy Risk Factor D

Lactation Enters breast milk/use caution (AAP rates "compatible")

Use Palliative treatment of hyperthyroidism as an adjunct to ameliorate hyperthyroidism in preparation for surgical treatment or radioactive iodine therapy; management of thyrotoxic crisis

Mechanism of Action/Effect Inhibits the synthesis of thyroid hormones by blocking the oxidation of iodine in the thyroid gland; blocks synthesis of thyroxine and triiodothyronine

Contraindications Hypersensitivity to propylthiouracil or any component of the formulation; pregnancy

Warnings/Precautions Use with caution in patients >40 years of age because PTU may cause hypoprothrombinemia and bleeding. Use with extreme caution in patients receiving other drugs known to cause agranulocytosis; may cause agranulocytosis, thyroid hyperplasia, thyroid carcinoma (usage >1 year). Discontinue in the presence of agranulocytosis, aplastic anemia, ANCA-positive vasculitis, hepatitis, unexplained fever, or exfoliative dermatitis. Safety and efficacy have not been established in children <6 years of age.

Drug Interactions

Decreased Effect: Oral anticoagulant activity is increased only until metabolic effect stabilizes. Anticoagulants may be potentiated by anti-vitamin K effect of propylthiouracil. Correction of hyperthyroidism may alter disposition of beta-blockers, digoxin, and theophylline, necessitating a dose reduction of these agents.

Increased Effect/Toxicity: Propylthiouracil may increase the anticoagulant activity of warfarin.

Nutritional/Ethanol Interactions Food: Propylthiouracil serum levels may be altered if taken with food.

Adverse Reactions Frequency not defined.

Cardiovascular: Edema, cutaneous vasculitis, leukocytoclastic vasculitis, ANCA-positive vasculitis

Central nervous system: Fever, drowsiness, vertigo, headache, drug fever, dizziness, neuritis

Dermatologic: Skin rash, urticaria, pruritus, exfoliative dermatitis, alopecia, erythema nodosum

Endocrine & metabolic: Goiter, weight gain, swollen salivary glands

Gastrointestinal: Nausea, vomiting, loss of taste perception, stomach pain, constipation
Hematologic: Leukopenia, agranulocytosis, thrombocytopenia, bleeding, aplastic anemia
Hepatic: Cholestatic jaundice, hepatitis
Neuromuscular & skeletal: Arthralgia, paresthesia
Renal: Nephritis, glomerulonephritis, acute renal failure
Respiratory: Interstitial pneumonitis, alveolar hemorrhage
Miscellaneous: SLE-like syndrome

Overdosage/Toxicology Symptoms of overdose include nausea, vomiting, epigastric pain, headache, fever, arthralgia, pruritus, edema, pancytopenia, epigastric distress, headache, fever, CNS stimulation, or depression. Treatment is supportive. Monitor bone marrow response. Forced diuresis, dialysis, and charcoal hemoperfusion have been used to enhance elimination.

Pharmacodynamics/Kinetics

Bioavailability: 80% to 95%

Half-Life Elimination: 1.5-5 hours; End-stage renal disease: 8.5 hours

Time to Peak: Serum: ~1 hour

Metabolism: Hepatic

Onset: Therapeutic: 24-36 hours; Peak effect: Remission: 4 months of continued therapy

Duration: 2-3 hours

Formulations Tablet: 50 mg

Dosing

Adults:

Hyperthyroidism: Oral: Initial: 300-450 mg/day in divided doses every 8 hours (severe hyperthyroidism may require 600-1200 mg/day); maintenance: 100-150 mg/day in divided doses every 8-12 hours

Note: Administer in 3 equally divided doses at approximately 8-hour intervals. Adjust dosage to maintain T_3, T_4, and TSH levels in normal range; elevated T_3 may be sole indicator of inadequate treatment. Elevated TSH indicates excessive antithyroid treatment.

Elderly: Use lower dose recommendations; adjust for renal impairment.
Initial: 150-300 mg/day in divided doses every 8 hours
Maintenance: 100-150 mg/day in divided doses every 8-12 hours

Pediatrics:

Hyperthyroidism: Oral: Children: Initial: 5-7 mg/kg/day **or** 150-200 mg/m^2/day in divided doses every 8 hours **or**
6-10 years: 50-150 mg/day
>10 years: 150-300 mg/day
Maintenance: Determined by patient response **or** $^1/_3$ to $^2/_3$ of the initial dose in divided doses every 8-12 hours. This usually begins after 2 months on an effective initial dose.

Note: Administer in 3 equally divided doses at approximately 8-hour intervals. Adjust dosage to maintain T_3, T_4, and TSH levels in normal range; elevated T_3 may be sole indicator of inadequate treatment. Elevated TSH indicates excessive antithyroid treatment.

Renal Impairment:
Cl_{cr} 10-50 mL/minute: Administer 75% of normal dose.
Cl_{cr} <10 mL/minute: Administer 50% of normal dose.

Monitoring Laboratory Tests CBC with differential, prothrombin time, liver and thyroid function (T_4, T_3, TSH); periodic blood counts are recommended for chronic therapy.

Monitoring and Teaching Issues

Physical Assessment: See Contraindications, Warnings/Precautions, Drug Interactions, and Dosing for use cautions. Assess results of laboratory tests (see above) and patient response according to purpose for use (eg, hyper/hypothyroidism and bleeding tendency - see Adverse Reactions and Overdose/Toxicology). Teach patient proper use, possible side effects and interventions, and adverse symptoms to report (see Patient Education). **Pregnancy risk factor D** - determine that patient is not pregnant before beginning treatment. Instruct patients of childbearing age about necessity for barrier contraceptive measures during and for one month following therapy. Note breast-feeding caution.

Patient Education: Take as directed, at the same time each day at around-the-clock intervals; at the same time in relation to meals, either always with meals or always between meals. Do not miss doses or make up missed doses. This drug may need to be taken for an extended period of time to achieve appropriate results and you may need periodic blood tests to assess effectiveness of therapy. May cause nausea or vomiting (small, frequent meals may help); constipation (increased exercise, fluids, fruit, or fiber may help); or dizziness or drowsiness (use caution when driving or engaging in tasks that require alertness until response to drug is known). Report rash, skin eruptions, or loss of hair; fever; unusual bleeding or bruising; unusual weight gain (>5 lb/week); unresolved headache or fever; yellowing of eyes or skin; changes in color of urine or feces; or joint or muscle pain or weakness. **Pregnancy/breast-feeding precautions:** Inform prescriber if you are pregnant. Do not get pregnant while taking this medication. Consult prescriber for appropriate contraceptive measures. Consult prescriber if breast-feeding.

Dietary Issues: Administer at the same time in relation to meals each day, either always with meals or always between meals.

Geriatric Considerations: The use of antithyroid thioamides is as effective in the elderly as they are in younger adults; however, the expense, potential adverse effects, and inconvenience (compliance, monitoring) make them undesirable. The use of radioiodine, due to ease of administration and less concern for long-term side effects and reproduction problems, makes it a more appropriate therapy.

Pregnancy Issues: Crosses the placenta and may induce goiter and hypothyroidism in the developing fetus (cretinism). May need to monitor infant's thyroid function periodically.

Additional Information Preferred over methimazole in thyroid storm due to inhibition of peripheral conversion as well as synthesis of thyroid hormone.

2-Propylvaleric Acid *see* Valproic Acid and Derivatives *on page 1382*
Proscar® *see* Finasteride *on page 560*

Prostacyclin *see* Epoprostenol *on page 479*
Prostaglandin E_1 *see* Alprostadil *on page 65*
Prostaglandin E_2 *see* Dinoprostone *on page 421*
Prostigmin® *see* Neostigmine *on page 960*
Prostin E_2® *see* Dinoprostone *on page 421*
Prostin F_2 Alpha® *see page 1461*
Prostin VR Pediatric® *see* Alprostadil *on page 65*

Protamine Sulfate (PROE ta meen SUL fate)

Generic Available Yes

Pharmacologic Category Antidote

Pregnancy Risk Factor C

Lactation Excretion in breast milk unknown

Use Treatment of heparin overdosage; neutralize heparin during surgery or dialysis procedures

Mechanism of Action/Effect Combines with strongly acidic heparin to form a stable complex (salt) neutralizing the anticoagulant activity of both drugs

Contraindications Hypersensitivity to protamine or any component of the formulation

Warnings/Precautions For I.V. use only. May not be totally effective in some patients following cardiac surgery despite adequate doses. May cause hypersensitivity reaction in patients with a history of allergy to fish (have epinephrine 1:1000 available) and in patients sensitized to protamine (via protamine zinc insulin). Rapid administration can cause severe hypotensive and anaphylactoid-like reactions. Heparin rebound associated with anticoagulation and bleeding has been reported to occur occasionally. Symptoms typically occur 8-9 hours after protamine administration, but may occur as long as 18 hours later. Pregnancy risk C.

Adverse Reactions Frequency not defined.

Cardiovascular: Sudden fall in blood pressure, bradycardia, flushing, hypotension
Central nervous system: Lassitude
Gastrointestinal: Nausea, vomiting
Hematologic: Hemorrhage
Respiratory: Dyspnea, pulmonary hypertension
Miscellaneous: Hypersensitivity reactions

Overdosage/Toxicology Symptoms of overdose include hypertension. May cause hemorrhage. Doses exceeding 100 mg may cause paradoxical anticoagulation.

Pharmacodynamics/Kinetics

Duration: Onset of action: I.V.: Heparin neutralization: ~5 minutes

Formulations Injection: 10 mg/mL (5 mL, 25 mL)

Dosing

Adults & Elderly:

Heparin neutralization: I.V.: Protamine dosage is determined by the dosage of heparin; 1 mg of protamine neutralizes 90 USP units of heparin (lung) and 115 USP units of heparin (intestinal); maximum dose: 50 mg

Heparin overdosage, following intravenous administration: I.V.: Since blood heparin concentrations decrease rapidly **after** administration, adjust the protamine dosage depending upon the duration of time since heparin administration as follows: See table.

Time Elapsed	Dose of Protamine (mg) to Neutralize 100 units of Heparin
Immediate	1-1.5
30-60 min	0.5-0.75
>2 h	0.25-0.375

Heparin overdosage, following S.C. injection: I.V.: 1-1.5 mg protamine per 100 units heparin; this may be done by a portion of the dose (eg, 25-50 mg) given slowly I.V. followed by the remaining portion as a continuous infusion over 8-16 hours (the expected absorption time of the S.C. heparin dose)

Pediatrics: Refer to adult dosing.

Administration

I.V.: For I.V. use only. Administer slow IVP (50 mg over 10 minutes). Rapid I.V. infusion causes hypotension. Reconstitute vial with 5 mL sterile water. Resulting solution equals 10 mg/mL. Inject without further dilution over 1-3 minutes; maximum of 50 mg in any 10-minute period.

Stability

Storage: Refrigerate; avoid freezing. Remains stable for at least 2 weeks at room temperature; preservative-free formulation does not require refrigeration.

Compatibility: Stable in D_5W, NS

Compatibility in syringe: Incompatible with diatrizoate meglumine 52%, diatrizoate sodium 8%, diatrizoate sodium 60%, ioxaglate meglumine 39.3%, ioxaglate sodium 19.6%

Compatibility when admixed: Incompatible with cephalosporins, penicillins

Monitoring Laboratory Tests Coagulation test, APTT or ACT

Monitoring and Teaching Issues

Physical Assessment: See Warnings/Precautions and Contraindications for use cautions. Monitor effectiveness of therapy by monitoring laboratory tests frequently during therapy (see above). Monitor closely for adverse response (see Adverse Reactions and Overdose/Toxicology). Assess knowledge/teach patient possible side effects and adverse symptoms to report (see Patient Education). **Pregnancy risk factor C.** Note breast-feeding caution.

Patient Education: Report any difficulty breathing, rash or flushing, feeling of warmth, tingling or numbness, dizziness, or disorientation. **Pregnancy/breast-feeding precautions:** Inform prescriber if you are pregnant. Consult prescriber if breast-feeding.

Related Information

Antidotes, Antivenins, and Antitoxins *on page 1460*

Heparin *on page 653*

Protein C (Activated), Human, Recombinant *see* Drotrecogin Alfa *on page 455*

Prothazine-DC® *see* Promethazine and Codeine *on page 1135*

Protirelin *see page 1461*

Protonix® *see* Pantoprazole *on page 1033*

Protopam® *see page 1460*

Protopic® *see* Tacrolimus *on page 1271*

Protostat® Oral *see* Metronidazole *on page 895*

Protriptyline (proe TRIP ti leen)

U.S. Brand Names Vivactil®

Synonyms Protriptyline Hydrochloride

Generic Available Yes

Pharmacologic Category Antidepressant, Tricyclic (Secondary Amine)

Pregnancy Risk Factor C

Lactation Excretion in breast milk unknown/not recommended

Use Treatment of depression

Mechanism of Action/Effect Increases the synaptic concentration of serotonin and/or norepinephrine in the central nervous system by inhibition of their reuptake by the presynaptic neuronal membrane

Contraindications Hypersensitivity to protriptyline (cross-reactivity to other cyclic antidepressants may occur) or any component of the formulation; use of MAO inhibitors within 14 days; use of cisapride; use in a patient during the acute recovery phase of MI

Warnings/Precautions May cause drowsiness/sedation, resulting in impaired performance of tasks requiring alertness (ie, operating machinery or driving). Sedative effects may be additive with other CNS depressants and/or ethanol. May worsen psychosis in some patients or precipitate a shift to mania or hypomania in patients with bipolar disease. May cause hyponatremia/SIADH. May increase the risks associated with electroconvulsive therapy. Discontinue, when possible, prior to elective surgery. Therapy should not be abruptly discontinued in patients receiving high doses for prolonged periods.

Use with caution in patients at risk of hypotension (orthostasis) or in patients where transient hypotensive episodes would be poorly tolerated (cardiovascular disease or cerebrovascular disease). Use with caution in elderly patients, patients with diabetes, thyroid disease (or patients receiving thyroid supplements), hepatic dysfunction, renal dysfunction, urinary retention, benign prostatic hyperplasia, narrow-angle glaucoma, xerostomia, visual problems, constipation, or a history of bowel obstruction.

Use caution in patients with depression, particularly if suicidal risk may be present. Use with caution in patients with a history of cardiovascular disease, previous seizure disorder or condition/drug therapy predisposing to seizures.

Pregnancy risk C.

Drug Interactions

Decreased Effect: Carbamazepine, phenobarbital, and rifampin may increase the metabolism of protriptyline, decreasing its effects. Protriptyline inhibits the antihypertensive response to bethanidine, clonidine, debrisoquin, guanadrel, guanethidine, guanabenz, guanfacine. Cimetidine and methylphenidate may decrease the metabolism of protriptyline. Cholestyramine and colestipol may bind TCAs and reduce their absorption.

Increased Effect/Toxicity: Protriptyline increases the effects of amphetamines, anticholinergics, other CNS depressants (sedatives, hypnotics, or ethanol), chlorpropamide, tolazamide, and warfarin. When used with MAO inhibitors, hyperpyrexia, hypertension, tachycardia, confusion, seizures, and **deaths have been reported** (serotonin syndrome). The SSRIs (to varying degrees), cimetidine, grapefruit juice, indinavir, methylphenidate, ritonavir, quinidine, diltiazem, and verapamil inhibit the metabolism of TCAs and clinical toxicity may result. Use of lithium with a TCA may increase the risk for neurotoxicity. Phenothiazines may increase concentration of some TCAs and TCAs may increase concentration of phenothiazines. Pressor response to I.V. epinephrine, norepinephrine, and phenylephrine may be enhanced in patients receiving TCAs (**Note:** Effect is unlikely with epinephrine or levonordefrin dosages typically administered as infiltration in combination with local anesthetics). Combined use of beta-agonists or drugs which prolong QT_c (including quinidine, procainamide, disopyramide, cisapride, sparfloxacin, gatifloxacin, moxifloxacin) with TCAs may predispose patients to cardiac arrhythmias.

Nutritional/Ethanol Interactions

Ethanol: Avoid ethanol (may increase CNS depression).

Food: Grapefruit juice may inhibit the metabolism of some TCAs and clinical toxicity may result.

Herb/Nutraceutical: Avoid valerian, St John's wort, SAMe, kava kava (may increase risk of serotonin syndrome and/or excessive sedation).

Effects on Lab Values ↑ glucose

Adverse Reactions Frequency not defined.

Cardiovascular: Arrhythmias, hypotension, myocardial infarction, stroke, heart block, hypertension, tachycardia, palpitations

Central nervous system: Dizziness, drowsiness, headache, confusion, delirium, hallucinations, restlessness, insomnia, nightmares, fatigue, delusions, anxiety, agitation, hypomania, exacerbation of psychosis, panic, seizures, incoordination, ataxia, EPS

Dermatologic: Alopecia, photosensitivity, rash, petechiae, urticaria, itching

Endocrine & metabolic: Breast enlargement, galactorrhea, SIADH, gynecomastia, increased or decreased libido

Gastrointestinal: Xerostomia, constipation, unpleasant taste, weight gain, increased appetite, nausea, diarrhea, heartburn, vomiting, anorexia, weight loss, trouble with gums, decreased lower esophageal sphincter tone may cause GE reflux

(Continued)

Protriptyline *(Continued)*

Genitourinary: Difficult urination, impotence, testicular edema
Hematologic: Agranulocytosis, leukopenia, eosinophilia, thrombocytopenia, purpura
Hepatic: Cholestatic jaundice, increased liver enzymes
Neuromuscular & skeletal: Fine muscle tremors, weakness, tremor, numbness, tingling
Ocular: Blurred vision, eye pain, increased intraocular pressure
Otic: Tinnitus
Miscellaneous: Diaphoresis (excessive), allergic reactions

Overdosage/Toxicology Symptoms of overdose include confusion, hallucinations, urinary retention, hypotension, tachycardia, seizures, and hyperthermia. Following initiation of essential overdose management, toxic symptoms should be treated. Ventricular arrhythmias often respond to systemic alkalinization (sodium bicarbonate 0.5-2 mEq/kg I.V.) Physostigmine (1-2 mg I.V. slowly for adults) may be indicated for reversing life-threatening cardiac arrhythmias.

Pharmacodynamics/Kinetics

Half-Life Elimination: 54-92 hours (average: 74 hours)

Time to Peak: Serum: 24-30 hours

Metabolism: Extensively hepatic via N-oxidation, hydroxylation, and glucuronidation; first-pass effect (10% to 25%)

Formulations Tablet, as hydrochloride: 5 mg, 10 mg

Dosing

Adults: Depression: Oral: 15-60 mg in 3-4 divided doses

Elderly: Oral: Initial: 5-10 mg/day

Pediatrics: Depression: Oral: Adolescents: 15-20 mg/day

Monitoring and Teaching Issues

Physical Assessment: See Contraindications, Warnings/Precautions, and Dosing for use cautions. Assess potential for interactions with other prescriptions, OTC medications, or herbal products patient may be taking (see extensive list of Drug Interactions). Assess for suicidal tendencies before beginning therapy. May cause physiological or psychological dependence, tolerance, or abuse; periodically evaluate need for continued use. Assess therapeutic response (mental status, mood, affect) and adverse reactions (eg, suicidal ideation - see Adverse Reactions and Overdose/Toxicology) at beginning of therapy and periodically with long-term use. Taper dosage slowly when discontinuing (allow 3-4 weeks between discontinuing this medication and starting another antidepressant). Caution diabetic patients to monitor glucose levels closely; may increase or decrease serum glucose levels. Teach patient appropriate use, interventions to reduce side effects, and adverse symptoms to report (see Patient Education). **Pregnancy risk factor C** - benefits of use should outweigh possible risks. Breast-feeding is not recommended.

Patient Education: Inform prescriber of all prescriptions, OTC medications, or herbal products you are taking, and any allergies you have. Do not take anything new during treatment unless approved by prescriber. Take exactly as directed; take once-a-day dose at bedtime. Do not increase dose or frequency; may take 2-3 weeks to achieve desired results. This drug may cause physical and/or psychological dependence. Avoid alcohol and grapefruit juice. Maintain adequate hydration (2-3 L/day of fluids) unless advised by prescriber to restrict fluids. May cause drowsiness, lightheadedness, impaired coordination, dizziness, or blurred vision (use caution when driving or engaging in tasks requiring alertness until response to drug is known); nausea, vomiting, loss of appetite, or disturbed taste (small, frequent meals, good mouth care, chewing gum, or sucking lozenges may help); constipation (increased exercise, fluids, fruit, or fiber may help); urinary retention (void before taking medication); postural hypotension (use caution climbing stairs or when changing position from lying or sitting to standing); altered sexual drive or ability (reversible); or photosensitivity (use sunscreen, wear protective clothing and eyewear, and avoid direct sunlight). Report chest pain, palpitations, or rapid heartbeat; persistent CNS effects (eg, nervousness, restlessness, insomnia, anxiety, excitation, headache, agitation, impaired coordination, changes in cognition); muscle cramping, weakness, tremors, or rigidity; blurred vision or eye pain; breast enlargement or swelling; yellowing of skin or eyes; or worsening of condition. **Pregnancy/breast-feeding precautions:** Inform prescriber if you are or intend to become pregnant. Breast-feeding is not recommended.

Dietary Issues: May be taken with food to decrease GI distress.

Geriatric Considerations: Little data on use in the elderly. Strong anticholinergic properties which may limit protriptyline's use; more often stimulating rather than sedating effects.

Related Information

Antidepressant Agents *on page 1553*
Antidepressant Medication Guidelines *on page 1613*

Protriptyline Hydrochloride *see* Protriptyline *on page 1149*
Protropin® *see* Human Growth Hormone *on page 658*
Proventil® *see* Albuterol *on page 52*
Proventil® HFA *see* Albuterol *on page 52*
Proventil® Repetabs® *see* Albuterol *on page 52*
Provera® *see* MedroxyPROGESTERone *on page 842*
Provigil® *see* Modafinil *on page 920*
Provocholine® *see page 1461*
Prozac® *see* Fluoxetine *on page 578*
Prozac® Weekly™ *see* Fluoxetine *on page 578*
Prudoxin™ *see* Doxepin *on page 443*
Prymaccone *see* Primaquine *on page 1118*

Pseudoephedrine (soo doe e FED rin)

U.S. Brand Names Cenafed® [OTC]; Children's Silfedrine® [OTC]; Children's Sudafed® Nasal Decongestant [OTC]; Decofed® [OTC]; Dimetapp® Decongestant Liqui-Gels® [OTC]; Efidac/24® [OTC]; Genaphed® [OTC]; PediaCare® Decongestant Infants [OTC]; Sudafed® [OTC];

Sudafed® 12 Hour [OTC]; Triaminic® AM Decongestant Formula [OTC]; Triaminic® Infant Decongestant [OTC]

Synonyms *d*-Isoephedrine Hydrochloride; Pseudoephedrine Hydrochloride; Pseudoephedrine Sulfate

Generic Available Yes

Pharmacologic Category Alpha/Beta Agonist

Pregnancy Risk Factor C

Lactation Enters breast milk/use caution (AAP rates "compatible")

Use Temporary symptomatic relief of nasal congestion due to common cold, upper respiratory allergies, and sinusitis; also promotes nasal or sinus drainage

Mechanism of Action/Effect Directly stimulates alpha-adrenergic receptors of respiratory mucosa causing vasoconstriction; directly stimulates beta-adrenergic receptors causing bronchial relaxation, increased heart rate and contractility

Contraindications Hypersensitivity to pseudoephedrine or any component of the formulation; MAO inhibitor therapy

Warnings/Precautions Use with caution in patients >60 years of age. Administer with caution to patients with hypertension, hyperthyroidism, diabetes mellitus, cardiovascular disease, ischemic heart disease, increased intraocular pressure, or prostatic hyperplasia. Elderly patients are more likely to experience adverse reactions to sympathomimetics. Overdosage may cause hallucinations, seizures, CNS depression, and death. Avoid prolonged use; generally limited to not more than 5 days. Pregnancy risk C.

Drug Interactions

Decreased Effect: Decreased effect of methyldopa, reserpine.

Increased Effect/Toxicity: MAO inhibitors may increase blood pressure effects of pseudoephedrine. Sympathomimetic agents may increase toxicity.

Nutritional/Ethanol Interactions

Food: Onset of effect may be delayed if pseudoephedrine is taken with food.

Herb/Nutraceutical: Avoid ephedra, yohimbe (may cause hypertension).

Effects on Lab Values Interferes with urine detection of amphetamine (false-positive)

Adverse Reactions Frequency not defined.

Cardiovascular: Tachycardia, palpitations, arrhythmias

Central nervous system: Nervousness, transient stimulation, insomnia, excitability, dizziness, drowsiness, convulsions, hallucinations, headache

Gastrointestinal: Nausea, vomiting

Genitourinary: Dysuria

Neuromuscular & skeletal: Weakness, tremor

Respiratory: Dyspnea

Miscellaneous: Diaphoresis

Overdosage/Toxicology Symptoms of overdose include seizures, nausea, vomiting, cardiac arrhythmias, hypertension, agitation, hallucinations, and death. There is no specific antidote for pseudoephedrine intoxication. Treatment is primarily supportive.

Pharmacodynamics/Kinetics

Absorption: Rapid

Half-Life Elimination: 9-16 hours

Metabolism: Partially hepatic

Onset: Decongestant: Oral: 15-30 minutes

Duration: Immediate release tablet: 4-6 hours; Extended release: ≤12 hours

Formulations

Gelcap, as hydrochloride: 30 mg

Liquid, as hydrochloride: 15 mg/5 mL (120 mL); 30 mg/5 mL (120 mL, 240 mL, 473 mL)

Solution, oral drops, as hydrochloride: 7.5 mg/0.8 mL (15 mL)

Syrup, as hydrochloride: 15 mg/5 mL (118 mL); 30 mg/mL (480 mL, 4000 mL)

Tablet, as hydrochloride: 30 mg, 60 mg

Tablet, chewable: 15 mg

Tablet, extended release, as sulfate: 120 mg, 240 mg

Dosing

Adults: Nasal congestion: Oral: 30-60 mg every 4-6 hours, sustained release: 120 mg every 12 hours; maximum: 240 mg/24 hours

Elderly: Nasal congestion: 30-60 mg every 6 hours as needed

Pediatrics: Nasal congestion: Oral:

<2 years: 4 mg/kg/day in divided doses every 6 hours

2-5 years: 15 mg every 6 hours; maximum: 60 mg/24 hours

6-12 years: 30 mg every 6 hours; maximum: 120 mg/24 hours

Renal Impairment: Reduce dose.

Administration

Oral: Do not crush extended release drug product, swallow whole.

Monitoring and Teaching Issues

Physical Assessment: Assess effectiveness and interactions of other medications patient may be taking (see Drug Interactions). See Contraindications and Warnings/Precautions for use cautions. Monitor effectiveness of therapy and adverse reactions (see Adverse Reactions) at beginning of therapy and periodically with long-term use. Assess knowledge/teach patient appropriate use, interventions to reduce side effects, and adverse symptoms to report (see Patient Education). **Pregnancy risk factor C** - benefits of use should outweigh possible risks. Note breast-feeding caution.

Patient Education: Take only as prescribed; do not exceed prescribed dose or frequency. Do not chew or crush timed release forms. Maintain adequate hydration (2-3 L/day of fluids) unless advised by prescriber to restrict fluids. You may experience nervousness, insomnia, dizziness, or drowsiness (use caution when driving or engaging in tasks requiring alertness until response to drug is known). Report persistent CNS changes (dizziness, tremor, agitation, or convulsions); difficulty breathing; chest pain, palpitations, or rapid heartbeat; muscle tremor; or lack of improvement or worsening or condition. **Pregnancy/breast-feeding precautions:** Inform prescriber if you are or intend to become pregnant. Consult prescriber if breast-feeding.

(Continued)

Pseudoephedrine *(Continued)*

Dietary Issues: Should be taken with water or milk to decrease GI distress.

Geriatric Considerations: Elderly patients should be counseled about the proper use of over-the-counter cough and cold preparations. Elderly are more predisposed to adverse effects of sympathomimetics since they frequently have cardiovascular diseases and diabetes mellitus as well as multiple drug therapies. It may be advisable to treat with a short-acting/immediate-release formulation before initiating sustained-release/long-acting formulations.

Related Information

Pharmacotherapy of Urinary Incontinence *on page 1699*

Pseudoephedrine and Acrivastine *see* Acrivastine and Pseudoephedrine *on page 42*

Pseudoephedrine and Azatadine *see* Azatadine and Pseudoephedrine *on page 137*

Pseudoephedrine and Carbinoxamine *see* Carbinoxamine and Pseudoephedrine *on page 217*

Pseudoephedrine and Fexofenadine *see* Fexofenadine and Pseudoephedrine *on page 557*

Pseudoephedrine and Guaifenesin *see* Guaifenesin and Pseudoephedrine *on page 648*

Pseudoephedrine and Loratadine *see* Loratadine and Pseudoephedrine *on page 821*

Pseudoephedrine, Guaifenesin, and Codeine *see* Guaifenesin, Pseudoephedrine, and Codeine *on page 649*

Pseudoephedrine Hydrochloride *see* Pseudoephedrine *on page 1150*

Pseudoephedrine Sulfate *see* Pseudoephedrine *on page 1150*

Pseudo GG TR *see* Guaifenesin and Pseudoephedrine *on page 648*

Pseudomonic Acid A *see* Mupirocin *on page 931*

Pseudovent™, Pseudovent™-Ped *see* Guaifenesin and Pseudoephedrine *on page 648*

Psorcon™ *see* Topical Corticosteroids *on page 1334*

Psorcon™ E *see* Topical Corticosteroids *on page 1334*

Psyllium (SIL i yum)

U.S. Brand Names Fiberall® Powder [OTC]; Fiberall® Wafer [OTC]; Hydrocil® [OTC]; Konsyl® [OTC]; Konsyl-D® [OTC]; Metamucil® [OTC]; Metamucil® Smooth Texture [OTC]; Modane® Bulk [OTC]; Perdiem® Plain [OTC]; Reguloid® [OTC]; Serutan® [OTC]; Syllact® [OTC]

Synonyms Plantago Seed; Plantain Seed; Psyllium Hydrophilic Mucilloid

Generic Available Yes

Pharmacologic Category Antidiarrheal; Laxative, Bulk-Producing

Pregnancy Risk Factor B

Lactation Excretion in breast milk unknown/compatible

Use Treatment of chronic atonic or spastic constipation and in constipation associated with rectal disorders; management of irritable bowel syndrome

Mechanism of Action/Effect Adsorbs water in the intestine to form a viscous liquid which promotes peristalsis and reduces transit time

Contraindications Hypersensitivity to psyllium or any component of the formulation; fecal impaction; GI obstruction

Warnings/Precautions May contain aspartame which is metabolized in the GI tract to phenylalanine which is contraindicated in individuals with phenylketonuria. Use with caution in patients with esophageal strictures, ulcers, stenosis, or intestinal adhesions. Elderly may have insufficient fluid intake which may predispose them to fecal impaction and bowel obstruction.

Drug Interactions

Decreased Effect: Decreased effect of warfarin, digitalis, potassium-sparing diuretics, salicylates, tetracyclines, nitrofurantoin when taken together. Separate administration times to reduce potential for drug-drug interaction.

Adverse Reactions Frequency not defined.

Gastrointestinal: Esophageal or bowel obstruction, diarrhea, constipation, abdominal cramps

Respiratory: Bronchospasm

Miscellaneous: Anaphylaxis upon inhalation in susceptible individuals, rhinoconjunctivitis

Overdosage/Toxicology Symptoms of overdose include abdominal pain, diarrhea, and constipation.

Pharmacodynamics/Kinetics

Absorption: None; small amounts of grain extracts present in the preparation have been reportedly absorbed following colonic hydrolysis

Onset: 12-24 hours; Peak effect: 2-3 days

Formulations

Granules for oral solution: 4.03 g per rounded teaspoon (100 g, 250 g); 2.5 g per rounded teaspoon

Powder for oral solution, psyllium hydrophilic: 3.4 g per rounded teaspoon (210 g, 300 g, 420 g, 630 g)

Wafers: 3.4 g

Dosing

Adults & Elderly: Constipation, IBS: Oral (administer at least 3 hours before or after other drugs): 1-2 rounded teaspoonfuls or 1-2 packets or 1-2 wafers in 8 oz glass of liquid 1-3 times/day.

Pediatrics: Constipation: Oral (administer at least 3 hours before or after other drugs): Children 6-11 years (approximately 1/2 adult dosage): 1/2 to 1 rounded teaspoonful in 4 oz glass of liquid 1-3 times/day

Administration

Oral: Inhalation of psyllium dust may cause sensitivity to psyllium (eg, runny nose, watery eyes, wheezing). Must be mixed in a glass of water or juice. Drink a full glass of liquid with each dose. Separate dose from other drug therapies.

Monitoring and Teaching Issues

Physical Assessment: See Contraindications, Warnings/Precautions, Drug Interactions, and Dosing for use cautions. Teach patient proper use (according to formulation), possible side effects and interventions, and adverse symptoms to report (see Patient Education).

Patient Education: Take as directed. Granules/powder: Mix in large glass of water or juice (8 oz or more) and drink immediately. Maintain adequate hydration (2-3 L/day of fluids), unless advised to restrict fluids. Mix carefully; do not inhale powder. Separate this medication from other medications by at least 1 hour. Results may begin in 12 hours; full results may take 2-3 days. Do not increase dose. Report persistent constipation; watery diarrhea; difficulty, pain, or choking with swallowing; difficulty breathing; or unusual coughing.

Dietary Issues: Should be taken with large amount of fluids. Some products contain aspartame, dextrose, or sucrose, as well as additional ingredients. Check individual product information for caloric and nutritional value.

Geriatric Considerations: Elderly may have insufficient fluid intake which may predispose them to fecal impaction and bowel obstruction. Patients should have a 1 month trial, with at least 14 g/day, before effects in bowel function are determined. Bloating and flatulence are mostly a problem in first 4 weeks of therapy.

Additional Information 3.4 g psyllium hydrophilic mucilloid per 7 g powder is equivalent to a rounded teaspoonful or one packet.

Related Information

Laxatives: Classification and Properties *on page 1581*

Psyllium Hydrophilic Mucilloid *see* Psyllium *on page 1152*

Pteroylglutamic Acid *see* Folic Acid *on page 596*

PTU *see* Propylthiouracil *on page 1146*

Pulmicort Respules™ *see* Budesonide *on page 179*

Pulmicort Turbuhaler® *see* Budesonide *on page 179*

Pulmozyme® *see* Dornase Alfa *on page 439*

Purinethol® *see* Mercaptopurine *on page 855*

P_xE_x® *see* Pilocarpine and Epinephrine *on page 1083*

Pyrazinamide (peer a ZIN a mide)

Synonyms Pyrazinoic Acid Amide

Generic Available Yes

Pharmacologic Category Antitubercular Agent

Pregnancy Risk Factor C

Lactation Enters breast milk

Use Adjunctive treatment of tuberculosis in combination with other antituberculosis agents in combination with rifampin or rifabutin for prevention of tuberculosis (as an alternative to isoniazid monotherapy)

Mechanism of Action/Effect Converted to pyrazinoic acid in susceptible strains of *Mycobacterium* which lowers the pH of the environment; bacteriostatic or bactericidal depending on the drug's concentration at the site of infection

Contraindications Hypersensitivity to pyrazinamide or any component of the formulation; acute gout; severe hepatic damage

Warnings/Precautions Administer with at least one other effective agent for tuberculosis; use with caution in patients with renal failure, chronic gout, diabetes mellitus, or porphyria. Use with caution in patients receiving concurrent medications associated with hepatotoxicity (particularly with rifampin), or in patients with a history of alcoholism (even if ethanol consumption is discontinued during therapy). Pregnancy risk C.

Drug Interactions

Increased Effect/Toxicity: Combination therapy with rifampin and pyrazinamide has been associated with severe and fatal hepatotoxic reactions.

Effects on Lab Values Reacts with Acetest® and Ketostix® to produce pinkish-brown color.

Adverse Reactions

1% to 10%:

Central nervous system: Malaise

Gastrointestinal: Nausea, vomiting, anorexia

Neuromuscular & skeletal: Arthralgia, myalgia

<1% (Limited to important or life-threatening): Hepatotoxicity, interstitial nephritis, porphyria, thrombocytopenia

Overdosage/Toxicology Symptoms of overdose include gout, gastric upset, and hepatic damage (mild). Treatment is supportive.

Pharmacokinetic Note Bacteriostatic or bactericidal depending on drug's concentration at infection site.

Pharmacodynamics/Kinetics

Absorption: Well absorbed

Half-Life Elimination: 9-10 hours

Time to Peak: Serum: Within 2 hours

Metabolism: Hepatic

Formulations Tablet: 500 mg

Dosing

Adults: Note: A four-drug regimen (isoniazid, rifampin, pyrazinamide, and either streptomycin or ethambutol) is preferred for the initial, empiric treatment of TB. When the drug susceptibility results are available, the regimen should be altered as appropriate.

Tuberculosis: Oral:

Daily therapy: 15-30 mg/kg/day (maximum: 2 g/day)

Directly observed therapy (DOT):

Twice weekly: 50-70 mg/kg (maximum: 4 g)

Three times/week: 50-70 mg/kg (maximum: 3 g)

Prevention of tuberculosis (in combination with rifampin or rifabutin): Oral: 30 mg/kg/day for 2 months

(Continued)

Pyrazinamide *(Continued)*

Note: Calculate dose on ideal body weight rather than total body weight.

Elderly: Start with a lower daily dose (15 mg/kg) and increase as tolerated.

Pediatrics: Tuberculosis: Children: Refer to adult dosing.

Renal Impairment:

Cl_{cr} <50 mL/minute: Avoid use or reduce dose to 12-20 mg/kg/day.

Avoid use in hemo- and peritoneal dialysis as well as continuous arteriovenous or venovenous hemofiltration.

Hepatic Impairment: Reduce dose.

Monitoring Laboratory Tests Periodic liver function, serum uric acid, sputum culture, chest x-ray 2-3 months into treatment and at completion

Monitoring and Teaching Issues

Physical Assessment: See Contraindications, Warnings/Precautions, Drug Interactions, and Dosing for use cautions. Schedule and assess results of laboratory tests regularly (see above). Teach patient proper use and necessity scheduled laboratory tests, possible side effects and interventions, and adverse symptoms to report (see Patient Education). **Pregnancy risk factor C** - benefits of use should outweigh possible risks.

Patient Education: Take as directed, with food. It is imperative to take for full length of therapy; do not miss doses and do not discontinue without consulting prescriber. You will need regular medical follow-up and laboratory tests while taking this medication. May cause nausea or loss of appetite (small, frequent meals, frequent mouth care, sucking lozenges, or chewing gum may help). Report change in color of urine, pale stools, easy bruising or bleeding, blood in urine or difficulty urinating, yellowing of skin or eyes, extreme joint pain, unusual fever, or unresolved nausea or vomiting, **Pregnancy precaution:** Inform prescriber if you are or intend to become pregnant.

Geriatric Considerations: Pyrazinamide is used in the 2-month intensive treatment phase of a 6-month treatment plan. Most elderly acquired their *Mycobacterium tuberculosis* infection before effective chemotherapy was available; however, older persons with new infections (not reactivation), or who are from areas where drug-resistant *M. tuberculosis* is endemic, or who are HIV-infected should receive 3-4 drug therapies including pyrazinamide.

Related Information

Tuberculosis *on page 1705*

Pyrazinamide, Rifampin, and Isoniazid *see* Rifampin, Isoniazid, and Pyrazinamide *on page 1188*

Pyrazinoic Acid Amide *see* Pyrazinamide *on page 1153*

Pyridiate® *see* Phenazopyridine *on page 1065*

Pyridium® *see* Phenazopyridine *on page 1065*

Pyridostigmine (peer id oh STIG meen)

U.S. Brand Names Mestinon®; Mestinon® Timespan®; Regonol® [DSC]

Synonyms Pyridostigmine Bromide

Generic Available No

Pharmacologic Category Acetylcholinesterase Inhibitor

Pregnancy Risk Factor C

Lactation Enters breast milk/compatible

Use Symptomatic treatment of myasthenia gravis; also used as an antidote for nondepolarizing neuromuscular blockers

Mechanism of Action/Effect Inhibits destruction of acetylcholine by acetylcholinesterase which facilitates transmission of impulses across myoneural junction

Contraindications Hypersensitivity to pyridostigmine, bromides, or any component of the formulation; GI or GU obstruction

Warnings/Precautions Use with caution in patients with epilepsy, asthma, bradycardia, hyperthyroidism, cardiac arrhythmias, or peptic ulcer. Use with caution in renal impairment (lower dosages may be required). Adequate facilities should be available for cardiopulmonary resuscitation when testing and adjusting dose for myasthenia gravis. Have atropine and epinephrine ready to treat hypersensitivity reactions. Overdosage may result in cholinergic crisis, this must be distinguished from myasthenic crisis. Anticholinesterase insensitivity can develop for brief or prolonged periods. Safety and efficacy in pediatric patients have not been established. Regonol® injection contains 1% benzyl alcohol as the preservative (not intended for use in newborns). Pregnancy risk C.

Drug Interactions

Decreased Effect: Neuromuscular blockade reversal effect of pyridostigmine may be decreased by aminoglycosides, quinolones, tetracyclines, bacitracin, colistin, polymyxin B, sodium colistimethate, quinidine, elevated serum magnesium concentrations.

Increased Effect/Toxicity: Increased effect of depolarizing neuromuscular blockers (succinylcholine). Increased toxicity with edrophonium. Increased bradycardia/hypotension with beta-blockers.

Effects on Lab Values ↑ aminotransferase [ALT (SGPT)/AST (SGOT)] (S), amylase (S)

Adverse Reactions Frequency not defined.

Cardiovascular: Arrhythmias (especially bradycardia), hypotension, decreased carbon monoxide, tachycardia, AV block, nodal rhythm, nonspecific EKG changes, cardiac arrest, syncope, flushing

Central nervous system: Convulsions, dysarthria, dysphonia, dizziness, loss of consciousness, drowsiness, headache

Dermatologic: Skin rash, thrombophlebitis (I.V.), urticaria

Gastrointestinal: Hyperperistalsis, nausea, vomiting, salivation, diarrhea, stomach cramps, dysphagia, flatulence

Genitourinary: Urinary urgency

Neuromuscular & skeletal: Weakness, fasciculations, muscle cramps, spasms, arthralgias

Ocular: Small pupils, lacrimation

Respiratory: Increased bronchial secretions, laryngospasm, bronchiolar constriction, respiratory muscle paralysis, dyspnea, respiratory depression, respiratory arrest, bronchospasm

Miscellaneous: Diaphoresis (increased), anaphylaxis, allergic reactions

Overdosage/Toxicology Symptoms of overdose include muscle weakness, blurred vision, excessive sweating, tearing and salivation, nausea, vomiting, diarrhea, hypertension, bradycardia, and paralysis. Atropine is the treatment of choice for intoxications manifesting significant muscarinic symptoms. Atropine I.V. 2-4 mg every 3-60 minutes should be repeated to control symptoms and then continued as needed for 1-2 days following acute ingestion. Monitor cardiac function and support ventilation.

Pharmacodynamics/Kinetics

Absorption: Oral: Very poor (10% to 20%)

Half-Life Elimination: 1-2 hours; Renal failure: ≤6 hours

Metabolism: Hepatic

Onset: Oral, I.M.: 15-30 minutes; I.V. injection: 2-5 minutes

Duration: Oral: Up to 6-8 hours (due to slow absorption); I.V.: 2-3 hours

Formulations

Injection, solution, as bromide:

Mestinon®: 5 mg/mL (2 mL)

Regonol®: 5 mg/mL (2 mL, 5 mL) [contains benzyl alcohol 1%] [DSC]

Syrup, as bromide (Mestinon®): 60 mg/5 mL (480 mL) [contains alcohol 5%; raspberry flavor]

Tablet, as bromide (Mestinon®): 60 mg

Tablet, sustained release, as bromide (Mestinon® Timespan®): 180 mg

Dosing

Adults & Elderly:

Myasthenia gravis:

Oral: Highly individualized dosing ranges: 60-1500 mg/day, usually 600 mg/day divided into 5-6 doses, spaced to provide maximum relief

Sustained release formulation: Highly individualized dosing ranges: 180-540 mg once or twice daily (doses separated by at least 6 hours); **Note:** Most clinicians reserve sustained release dosage form for bedtime dose only.

I.M. or slow I.V. Push (To supplement oral dosage pre- and postoperatively during labor and postpartum, during myasthenic crisis, or when oral therapy is impractical): ~1/30th of oral dose; observe patient closely for cholinergic reactions

I.V. infusion (To supplement oral dosage pre- and postoperatively, during labor and postpartum, during myasthenic crisis, or when oral therapy is impractical): Initial: 2 mg/hour with gradual titration in increments of 0.5-1 mg/hour, up to a maximum rate of 4 mg/hour

Reversal of nondepolarizing muscle relaxants: **Note:** Atropine sulfate (0.6-1.2 mg) I.V. immediately prior to pyridostigmine to minimize side effects: I.V.: 0.1-0.25 mg/kg/dose; 10-20 mg is usually sufficient*

*Full recovery usually occurs ≤15 minutes, but ≥30 minutes may be required

Pediatrics:

Myasthenia gravis:

Oral: Children: 7 mg/kg/24 hours divided into 5-6 doses. Most clinicians reserve sustained release dosage form for bedtime dose only.

I.M., slow I.V. push: Children: 0.05-0.15 mg/kg/dose

Reversal of nondepolarizing muscle relaxants: **Note:** Atropine sulfate (0.6-1.2 mg) I.V. immediately prior to pyridostigmine to minimize side effects: I.V.: Children: Dosing range: 0.1-0.25 mg/kg/dose*

Renal Impairment: Lower dosages may be required due to prolonged elimination; no specific recommendations have been published.

Administration

Oral: Do **not** crush sustained release drug product.

Stability

Storage: Protect from light.

Monitoring and Teaching Issues

Physical Assessment: When used to reverse neuromuscular block (anesthesia or excessive acetylcholine), monitor patient safety until full return of neuromuscular functioning. Assess bladder and sphincter adequacy prior to administering medication. See Contraindications and Warnings/Precautions for use cautions. Monitor therapeutic effects and adverse reactions (eg, cholinergic crisis - see Warnings/Precautions, Adverse Reactions, and Overdose/Toxicology). Assess knowledge/teach patient appropriate use (self-injections, oral), interventions to reduce side effects, and adverse symptoms to report (see Patient Education). **Pregnancy risk factor C** - benefits of use should outweigh possible risks.

Patient Education: This drug will not cure myasthenia gravis, but may help reduce symptoms. Use as directed; do not increase dose or discontinue without consulting prescriber. Take extended release tablets at bedtime; do not chew or crush extended release tablets. Maintain adequate hydration (2-3 L/day of fluids) unless advised by prescriber to restrict fluids. May cause dizziness, drowsiness, or hypotension (rise slowly from sitting or lying position and use caution when driving or climbing stairs); vomiting or loss of appetite (small, frequent meals, frequent mouth care, chewing gum, or sucking lozenges may help); or diarrhea (boiled milk, yogurt, or buttermilk may help). Report persistent abdominal discomfort; significantly increased salivation, sweating, tearing, or urination; flushed skin; chest pain or palpitations; acute headache; unresolved diarrhea; excessive fatigue, insomnia, dizziness, or depression; increased muscle, joint, or body pain; vision changes or blurred vision; or shortness of breath or wheezing. **Pregnancy precaution:** Inform prescriber if you are or intend to become pregnant.

Geriatric Considerations: See Warnings/Precautions and Adverse Reactions.

Breast-feeding Issues: Neonates of myasthenia gravis mothers may have difficulty in sucking and swallowing (as well as breathing). Neonatal pyridostigmine may be indicated by symptoms (confirmed by edrophonium test).

(Continued)

Pyridostigmine *(Continued)*

Pregnancy Issues: Safety has not been established for use during pregnancy. The potential benefit to the mother should outweigh the potential risk to the fetus. When pyridostigmine is needed in myasthenic mothers, giving dose parenterally 1 hour before completion of the second stage of labor may facilitate delivery and protect the neonate during the immediate postnatal state.

Pyridostigmine Bromide *see* Pyridostigmine *on page 1154*

Pyridoxine (peer i DOKS een)

U.S. Brand Names Aminoxin® [OTC]; Nestrex® [OTC]

Synonyms Pyridoxine Hydrochloride; Vitamin B_6

Generic Available Yes

Pharmacologic Category Vitamin, Water Soluble

Pregnancy Risk Factor A/C (dose exceeding RDA recommendation)

Lactation Enters breast milk/compatible

Use Prevention and treatment of vitamin B_6 deficiency, pyridoxine-dependent seizures in infants; adjunct to treatment of acute toxicity from isoniazid, cycloserine, or hydralazine overdose

Mechanism of Action/Effect Precursor to pyridoxal, which functions in the metabolism of proteins, carbohydrates, and fats; pyridoxal also aids in the release of liver and muscle-stored glycogen and in the synthesis of GABA (within the central nervous system) and heme

Contraindications Hypersensitivity to pyridoxine or any component of the formulation

Warnings/Precautions Dependence and withdrawal may occur with doses >200 mg/day. Pregnancy risk A/C (dose exceeding RDA).

Drug Interactions

Decreased Effect: Pyridoxine may decrease serum levels of levodopa, phenobarbital, and phenytoin (patients taking levodopa without carbidopa should avoid supplemental vitamin B_6 >5 mg per day, which includes multivitamin preparations).

Effects on Lab Values Urobilinogen

Adverse Reactions Frequency not defined.

Central nervous system: Headache, seizures (following very large I.V. doses), sensory neuropathy

Endocrine & metabolic: Decreased serum folic acid secretions

Gastrointestinal: Nausea

Hepatic: Increased AST

Neuromuscular & skeletal: Paresthesia

Miscellaneous: Allergic reactions

Overdosage/Toxicology Symptoms of overdose include ataxia and sensory neuropathy with doses of 50 mg to 2 g daily over prolonged periods.

Pharmacodynamics/Kinetics

Absorption: Enteral, parenteral: Well absorbed

Half-Life Elimination: 15-20 days

Metabolism: Via 4-pyridoxic acid (active form) and other metabolites

Formulations

Injection, as hydrochloride: 100 mg/mL (10 mL, 30 mL)

Tablet, as hydrochloride: 25 mg, 50 mg, 100 mg, 250 mg, 500 mg

Tablet, enteric coated, as hydrochloride: 20 mg

Dosing

Adults & Elderly:

Recommended daily allowance (RDA):

Male: 1.7-2.0 mg

Female: 1.4-1.6 mg

Dietary deficiency: Oral: 10-20 mg/day for 3 weeks

Drug-induced neuritis (eg, isoniazid, hydralazine, penicillamine, cycloserine): Oral:

Treatment: 100-200 mg/24 hours

Prophylaxis: 25-100 mg/24 hours

Treatment of seizures and/or coma from acute isoniazid toxicity: A dose of pyridoxine hydrochloride equal to the amount of INH ingested can be given I.M./I.V. in divided doses together with other anticonvulsants; if the amount INH ingested is not known, administer 5 g I.V. pyridoxine.

Treatment of acute hydralazine toxicity: A pyridoxine dose of 25 mg/kg in divided doses I.M./I.V. has been used.

Pediatrics:

Recommended daily allowance (RDA):

1-3 years: 0.9 mg

4-6 years: 1.3 mg

7-10 years: 1.6 mg

Pyridoxine-dependent Infants:

Oral: 2-100 mg/day

I.M., I.V., S.C.: 10-100 mg

Dietary deficiency: Oral: Children: 5-25 mg/24 hours for 3 weeks, then 1.5-2.5 mg/day in multiple vitamin product

Drug-induced neuritis (eg, isoniazid, hydralazine, penicillamine, cycloserine): Oral: Children:

Treatment: 10-50 mg/24 hours

Prophylaxis: 1-2 mg/kg/24 hours

Treatment of seizures and/or coma from acute isoniazid toxicity: A dose of pyridoxine hydrochloride equal to the amount of INH ingested can be given I.M./I.V. in divided doses together with other anticonvulsants. If the amount INH ingested is not known, administer 5 g I.V. pyridoxine.

Treatment of acute hydralazine toxicity; A pyridoxine dose of 25 mg/kg in divided doses I.M./I.V. has been used.

Administration

I.M.: Burning may occur at the injection site after I.M. or S.C. administration.

I.V.: Seizures have occurred following I.V. administration of very large doses.

Stability

Storage: Protect from light.

Compatibility: Stable in fat emulsion 10%

Monitoring and Teaching Issues

Physical Assessment: See Contraindications and Warnings/Precautions for use cautions. Assess effectiveness and interactions of other medications patient may be taking (see Drug Interactions). Monitor effectiveness of therapy and adverse effects at beginning of therapy and regularly with long-term use (see Adverse Reactions). Assess knowledge/teach patient appropriate use, dietary instructions, interventions to reduce side effects, and adverse symptoms to report (see Patient Education). **Pregnancy risk factor A/C** - see Pregnancy Risk Factor for use cautions.

Patient Education: Take exactly as directed. Do not take more than recommended. Do not chew or crush extended release tablets. Do not exceed recommended intake of dietary B_6 (eg, red meat, bananas, potatoes, yeast, lima beans, and whole grain cereals). You may experience burning or pain at injection site; notify prescriber if this persists. **Pregnancy precaution:** Inform prescriber if you are pregnant.

Geriatric Considerations: Use with caution in patients with Parkinson's disease treated with levodopa.

Breast-feeding Issues: Crosses into breast milk; possible inhibition of lactation at doses >600 mg/day. AAP considers **compatible** with breast-feeding.

Pyridoxine Hydrochloride *see* Pyridoxine *on page 1156*

Pyrimethamine (peer i METH a meen)

U.S. Brand Names Daraprim®

Generic Available No

Pharmacologic Category Antimalarial Agent

Pregnancy Risk Factor C

Lactation Enters breast milk/contraindicated (AAP rates "compatible")

Use Prophylaxis of malaria due to susceptible strains of plasmodia; used in conjunction with quinine and sulfadiazine for the treatment of uncomplicated attacks of chloroquine-resistant *P. falciparum* malaria; used in conjunction with fast-acting schizonticide to initiate transmission control and suppression cure; synergistic combination with sulfonamide in treatment of toxoplasmosis

Mechanism of Action/Effect Inhibits parasitic dihydrofolate reductase, resulting in inhibition of vital tetrahydrofolic acid synthesis

Contraindications Hypersensitivity to pyrimethamine or any component of the formulation; chloroguanide; resistant malaria; megaloblastic anemia secondary to folate deficiency

Warnings/Precautions When used for more than 3-4 days, it may be advisable to give leucovorin to prevent hematologic complications. Use with caution in patients with impaired renal or hepatic function or with possible G6PD. Pregnancy risk C (may be carcinogenic).

Drug Interactions

Cytochrome P450 Effect: Inhibits CYP2D6

Decreased Effect: Pyrimethamine effectiveness is decreased by acid.

Increased Effect/Toxicity: Increased effect with sulfonamides (synergy), methotrexate, and TMP/SMZ.

Adverse Reactions Frequency not defined.

Cardiovascular: Arrhythmias (large doses)

Central nervous system: Depression, fever, insomnia, lightheadedness, malaise, seizures

Dermatologic: Abnormal skin pigmentation, dermatitis, erythema multiforme, rash, Stevens-Johnson syndrome

Gastrointestinal: Anorexia, abdominal cramps, vomiting, diarrhea, xerostomia, atrophic glossitis

Hematologic: Megaloblastic anemia, leukopenia, pancytopenia, thrombocytopenia, pulmonary eosinophilia

Miscellaneous: Anaphylaxis

Overdosage/Toxicology Symptoms of overdose include megaloblastic anemia, leukopenia, thrombocytopenia, anorexia, CNS stimulation, seizures, nausea, vomiting, and hematemesis. Following GI decontamination, leucovorin should be administered in an I.M. or I.V. dosage of 5-15 mg/day or orally for 5-7 days, or as required to reverse symptoms of folic acid deficiency. Provide other supportive treatment as required.

Pharmacodynamics/Kinetics

Absorption: Well absorbed

Half-Life Elimination: 80-95 hours

Time to Peak: Serum: 1.5-8 hours

Metabolism: Hepatic

Onset: ~1 hour

Formulations Tablet: 25 mg

Dosing

Adults & Elderly:

Malaria chemoprophylaxis (for areas where chloroquine-resistant *P. falciparum* exists): Oral: 25 mg once weekly

Note: Begin prophylaxis 2 weeks before entering endemic area. Dosage should be continued for all age groups for at least 6-10 weeks after leaving endemic areas.

Chloroquine-resistant *P. falciparum* malaria (when used in conjunction with quinine and sulfadiazine): Oral: 25 mg twice daily for 3 days.

Toxoplasmosis: Oral: 50-75 mg/day together with 1-4 g of a sulfonamide for 1-3 weeks depending on patient's tolerance and response, then reduce dose by 50% and continue for 4-5 weeks **or** 25-50 mg/day for 3-4 weeks.

(Continued)

Pyrimethamine *(Continued)*

Pediatrics:

Malaria chemoprophylaxis (for areas where chloroquine-resistant *P. falciparum* exists):
Oral:
Children: 0.5 mg/kg once weekly; not to exceed 25 mg/dose **or**
<4 years: 6.25 mg once weekly
4-10 years: 12.5 mg once weekly
Children >10 years: 25 mg once weekly
Note: Begin prophylaxis 2 weeks before entering endemic area. Dosage should be continued for all age groups for at least 6-10 weeks after leaving endemic areas.

Chloroquine-resistant *P. falciparum* malaria (when used in conjunction with quinine and sulfadiazine): Oral: Children:
<10 kg: 6.25 mg/day once daily for 3 days
10-20 kg: 12.5 mg/day once daily for 3 days
20-40 kg: 25 mg/day once daily for 3 days

Congenital toxoplasmosis: Oral: Infants; 1 mg/kg once daily for 6 months with sulfadiazine then every other month with sulfa, alternating with spiramycin.

Toxoplasmosis: Oral: Children: Loading dose: 2 mg/kg/day divided into 2 equal daily doses for 1-3 days (maximum: 100 mg/day) followed by 1 mg/kg/day divided into 2 doses for 4 weeks; maximum: 25 mg/day
With sulfadiazine or trisulfapyrimidines: 2 mg/kg/day divided every 12 hours for 3 days followed by 1 mg/kg/day once daily or divided twice daily for 4 weeks given with trisulfapyrimidines or sulfadiazine.

Note: In HIV, life-long suppression is necessary to prevent relapse; leucovorin (5-10 mg/day) is given concurrently.

Administration

Oral: Take with meals to minimize GI distress.

Stability

Storage: Pyrimethamine tablets may be crushed to prepare oral suspensions of the drug in water, cherry syrup, or sucrose-containing solutions at a concentration of 1 mg/mL; stable at room temperature for 5-7 days.

Monitoring Laboratory Tests CBC, including platelet counts twice weekly; liver and renal function

Monitoring and Teaching Issues

Physical Assessment: See Contraindications, Warnings/Precautions, Drug Interactions, and Dosing for use cautions. Assess results of regularly scheduled laboratory tests (see above), therapeutic effectiveness (according to purpose for therapy), and adverse reactions (see Adverse Reactions and Overdose/Toxicology - eg, folic acid deficiency and renal function). Teach patient appropriate use, possible side effects and interventions, and adverse symptoms to report (see Patient Education). **Pregnancy risk factor C** - benefits of use should outweigh possible risks (may be carcinogenic). Breast-feeding is contraindicated.

Patient Education: Inform prescriber of all prescriptions, OTC medications, or herbal products you are taking, and any allergies you have. Do not take anything new during treatment unless approved by prescriber. Take with meals. Tablets may be crushed to prepare oral suspensions of the drug in water, cherry syrup, or sucrose-containing solutions at a concentration of 1 mg drug/mL of liquid. It is important to complete full course of therapy for full effect. Regular blood tests will be necessary during therapy. If used for prophylaxis, consult with prescriber in order to begin 2 weeks before traveling to endemic areas, continue during travel period, and for 6-10 weeks following return. May cause GI distress or loss of appetite (small, frequent meals, frequent mouth care, sucking lozenges, or chewing gum may help); dizziness, lightheadedness, insomnia, or changes in mentation (use caution when driving or with tasks that require alertness until response to drug is known); or changes in skin pigmentation or rash. Report persistent GI disturbance (nausea, vomiting, diarrhea, cramping); chest pain or palpitation; unusual fatigue, easy bruising, bleeding, or bloody emesis; or other adverse reactions. **Pregnancy/breast-feeding precautions:** Inform prescriber if you are or intend to become pregnant. Do not breast-feed.

Quazepam *see page 1608*
Quelicin® *see* Succinylcholine *on page 1252*
Quelicin® Injection *see page 1461*
Questran® *see* Cholestyramine Resin *on page 282*
Questran® Light *see* Cholestyramine Resin *on page 282*

Quetiapine (kwe TYE a peen)

U.S. Brand Names Seroquel®

Synonyms Quetiapine Fumarate

Generic Available No

Pharmacologic Category Antipsychotic Agent, Dibenzothiazepine

Pregnancy Risk Factor C

Lactation Excretion in breast milk unknown/not recommended

Use Treatment of schizophrenia

Use - Unlabeled/Investigational Treatment of mania, bipolar disorder (children and adults); autism, psychosis (children)

Mechanism of Action/Effect Mechanism of action of quetiapine, as with other antipsychotic drugs, is unknown. However, it has been proposed that this drug's antipsychotic activity is mediated through a combination of dopamine type 2 (D_2) and serotonin type 2 ($5\text{-}HT_2$) antagonism. However, it is an antagonist at multiple neurotransmitter receptors in the brain: serotonin $5\text{-}HT_{1A}$ and $5\text{-}HT_2$, dopamine D_1 and D_2, histamine H_1, and adrenergic $alpha_1$- and $alpha_2$-receptors; but appears to have no appreciable affinity at cholinergic muscarinic and benzodiazepine receptors.

Antagonism at receptors other than dopamine and 5-HT_2 with similar receptor affinities may explain some of the other effects of quetiapine. The drug's antagonism of histamine H_1 receptors may explain the somnolence observed with it. The drug's antagonism of adrenergic alpha$_1$-receptors may explain the orthostatic hypotension observed with it.

Contraindications Hypersensitivity to quetiapine or any component of the formulation; severe CNS depression; bone marrow suppression; blood dyscrasias; severe hepatic disease, coma

Warnings/Precautions May be sedating, use with caution in disorders where CNS depression is a feature. Use with caution in Parkinson's disease. May cause orthostatic hypotension; use caution in patients predisposed to hypotension or with hemodynamic instability; prior myocardial infarction, cerebrovascular disease or ischemic heart disease. Caution in patients with hypercholesterolemia; thyroid disease; predisposition to seizures; subcortical brain damage; hepatic impairment; or severe cardiac, renal, or respiratory disease. May alter temperature regulation or mask toxicity of other drugs due to antiemetic effects. May alter cardiac conduction - life-threatening arrhythmias have occurred with therapeutic doses of neuroleptics.

Due to anticholinergic effects, use with caution in patients with decreased gastrointestinal motility, urinary retention, BPH, xerostomia, visual problems, narrow-angle glaucoma (screening is recommended), and myasthenia gravis. Relative to other antipsychotics, quetiapine has a moderate potency of cholinergic blockade. Risk of neuroleptic malignant syndrome, extrapyramidal symptoms or tardive dyskinesias appears to be very low relative to other antipsychotics. May cause hyperglycemia - use with caution in patients with diabetes or other disorders of glucose regulation.

Has been noted to cause cataracts in animals, lens examination on initiation of therapy and every 6 months is recommended.

Pregnancy risk C.

Drug Interactions

Cytochrome P450 Effect: Substrate of CYP2D6, **3A4**

Decreased Effect: The metabolism of quetiapine may be increased when administered with enzyme-inducing drugs (phenytoin, rifampin, barbiturates, carbamazepine). Thioridazine increases quetiapine's clearance (by 65%).

Increased Effect/Toxicity: Quetiapine reduces the metabolism of lorazepam (by 20%). The effects of other centrally-acting drugs, sedatives, or ethanol may be potentiated by quetiapine. Quetiapine may enhance the effects of antihypertensive agents. Although data is not yet available, caution is advised with inhibitors of CYP3A4 (eg, ketoconazole, erythromycin), which may increase levels of quetiapine. Cimetidine increases blood levels of quetiapine (quetiapine's clearance is reduced by by 20%). Metoclopramide may increase risk of extrapyramidal symptoms (EPS).

Nutritional/Ethanol Interactions

Ethanol: Avoid ethanol (may cause excessive impairment in cognition/motor function).

Food: In healthy volunteers, administration of quetiapine with food resulted in an increase in the peak serum concentration and AUC (each by ~15%) compared to the fasting state.

Herb/Nutraceutical: St John's wort may decrease quetiapine levels. Avoid valerian, St John's wort, kava kava, gotu kola (may increase CNS depression).

Adverse Reactions

>10%:

Central nervous system: Headache, somnolence

Gastrointestinal: Weight gain

1% to 10%:

Cardiovascular: Postural hypotension, tachycardia, palpitations

Central nervous system: Dizziness

Dermatologic: Rash

Gastrointestinal: Abdominal pain, constipation, xerostomia, dyspepsia, anorexia

Hematologic: Leukopenia

Neuromuscular & skeletal: Dysarthria, back pain, weakness

Respiratory: Rhinitis, pharyngitis, cough, dyspnea

Miscellaneous: Diaphoresis

<1% (Limited to important or life-threatening): Diabetes mellitus, hyperglycemia, hyperlipidemia, hypothyroidism, increased appetite, increased salivation, involuntary movements, leukocytosis, QT prolongation, rash, tardive dyskinesia, vertigo

Pharmacodynamics/Kinetics

Absorption: Accumulation is predictable upon multiple dosing

Bioavailability: 100%

Half-Life Elimination: Mean: Terminal: ~6 hours

Time to Peak: Plasma: 1.5 hours

Metabolism: Primarily hepatic; both metabolites are pharmacologically inactive

Formulations Tablet, as fumarate: 25 mg, 100 mg, 200 mg, 300 mg

Dosing

Adults: Schizophrenia/psychosis: Oral: 25-100 mg 2-3 times/day; usual starting dose 25 mg twice daily, increased in increments of 25-50 mg 2-3 times/day on the second or third day. By the fourth day, the dose should be in the range of 300-400 mg/day in 2-3 divided doses. Further adjustments may be made, as needed, at intervals of at least 2 days in adjustments of 25-50 mg twice daily. Usual maintenance range: 150-750 mg/day.

Elderly: Lower clearance in elderly patients (40%), resulting in higher concentrations. Dosage adjustment may be required.

Pediatrics: Children and Adolescents:

Autism (unlabeled use): Oral: 100-350 mg/day (1.6-5.2 mg/kg/day)

Psychosis and mania (unlabeled use): Oral: Initial: 25 mg twice daily; titrate as necessary to 450 mg/day

Hepatic Impairment: Lower clearance in hepatic impairment (30%), may result in higher concentrations. Dosage adjustment may be required.

Monitoring Laboratory Tests Eye examination every 6 months while on this medication

(Continued)

Quetiapine *(Continued)*

Monitoring and Teaching Issues

Physical Assessment: Assess other medications patient is taking for effectiveness and interactions (especially drugs affected by P450 enzymes - see Drug Interactions). See Contraindications and Warnings/Precautions for use cautions. Monitor results of ophthalmic exam and laboratory tests (see above), therapeutic response, and adverse reactions at beginning of therapy and periodically with long-term use (see Adverse Reactions and Overdose/Toxicology). Initiate at lower doses (see Dosing) and taper dosage slowly when discontinuing. Assess knowledge/teach patient appropriate use, interventions to reduce side effects, and adverse symptoms to report (see Patient Education). **Pregnancy risk factor C** - benefits of use should outweigh possible risks. Breast-feeding is not recommended.

Patient Education: Use exactly as directed; do not increase dose or frequency. It may take 2-3 weeks to achieve desired results; do not discontinue without consulting prescriber. Avoid alcohol or caffeine and other prescription or OTC medications not approved by prescriber. Maintain adequate hydration (2-3 L/day of fluids) unless advised by prescriber to restrict fluids. You may experience excess drowsiness, restlessness, dizziness, or blurred vision (use caution driving or when engaging in tasks requiring alertness until response to drug is known); mouth sores or GI upset (small, frequent meals, frequent mouth care, chewing gum, or sucking lozenges may help); constipation (increased exercise, fluids, fruit, or fiber may help); or postural hypotension (use caution climbing stairs or when changing position from lying or sitting to standing). Report persistent CNS effects (eg, somnolence, agitation, insomnia); severe dizziness; vision changes; difficulty breathing; or worsening of condition. **Pregnancy/breast-feeding precautions:** Inform prescriber if you are or intend to become pregnant. Breast-feeding is not recommended.

Dietary Issues: May be taken with or without food.

Geriatric Considerations: (See Warnings/Precautions, Adverse Reactions, and Overdose/Toxicology.) Elderly patients have an increased risk of adverse response to side effects or adverse reactions to antipsychotics.

Additional Information Quetiapine has a very low incidence of extrapyramidal symptoms such as restlessness and abnormal movement, and is at least as effective as conventional antipsychotics.

Related Information

Antipsychotic Agents *on page 1558*
Antipsychotic Medication Guidelines *on page 1614*

Quetiapine Fumarate *see* Quetiapine *on page 1158*
Quibron® *see* Theophylline and Guaifenesin *on page 1303*
Quibron®-T *see* Theophylline *on page 1300*
Quibron®-T/SR *see* Theophylline *on page 1300*
Quinaglute® Dura-Tabs® *see* Quinidine *on page 1163*
Quinalbarbitone Sodium *see* Secobarbital *on page 1220*

Quinapril (KWIN a pril)

U.S. Brand Names Accupril®

Synonyms Quinapril Hydrochloride

Generic Available No

Pharmacologic Category Angiotensin-Converting Enzyme (ACE) Inhibitor

Pregnancy Risk Factor C/D (2nd and 3rd trimesters)

Lactation Excretion in breast milk unknown

Use Management of hypertension; treatment of congestive heart failure

Use - Unlabeled/Investigational Treatment of left ventricular dysfunction after myocardial infarction

Mechanism of Action/Effect Competitive inhibitor of angiotensin-converting enzyme (ACE); prevents conversion of angiotensin I to angiotensin II, a potent vasoconstrictor; results in lower levels of angiotensin II which causes an increase in plasma renin activity and a reduction in aldosterone secretion

Contraindications Hypersensitivity to quinapril or any component of the formulation; angioedema related to previous treatment with an ACE inhibitor; bilateral renal artery stenosis; primary hyperaldosteronism; patients with idiopathic or hereditary angioedema; pregnancy (2nd and 3rd trimesters)

Warnings/Precautions Anaphylactic reactions can occur. Angioedema can occur at any time during treatment (especially following first dose). Careful blood pressure monitoring with first dose (hypotension can occur especially in volume depleted patients). Dosage adjustment needed in renal impairment. Use with caution in hypovolemia; collagen vascular diseases; valvular stenosis (particularly aortic stenosis); hyperkalemia; or before, during, or immediately after anesthesia. Avoid rapid dosage escalation, which may lead to renal insufficiency. Neutropenia/agranulocytosis with myeloid hyperplasia can rarely occur. Hypersensitivity reactions may be seen during hemodialysis with high-flux dialysis membranes (eg, AN69). Use with caution in unilateral renal artery stenosis and pre-existing renal insufficiency. Deterioration in renal function can occur with initiation. Due to rare hepatotoxic reactions, discontinue if jaundice or marked elevation of transaminases occurs. Pregnancy risk C/D (2nd and 3rd trimesters).

Drug Interactions

Decreased Effect: Quinapril may reduce the absorption of quinolones and tetracycline antibiotics. Aspirin (high dose) may reduce the therapeutic effects of ACE inhibitors; at low dosages this does not appear to be significant. Rifampin may decrease the effect of ACE inhibitors. Antacids may decrease the bioavailability of ACE inhibitors (may be more likely to occur with captopril); separate administration times by 1-2 hours. NSAIDs, specifically indomethacin, may reduce the hypotensive effects of ACE inhibitors.

Increased Effect/Toxicity: Potassium supplements, co-trimoxazole (high dose), angiotensin II receptor antagonists (candesartan, losartan, irbesartan, etc), or potassium-sparing diuretics (amiloride, spironolactone, triamterene) may result in elevated serum potassium levels when combined with quinapril. ACE inhibitor effects may be increased by phenothiazines or probenecid (increases levels of captopril). ACE inhibitors may increase serum concentrations/effects of digoxin, lithium, and sulfonlyureas.

Diuretics have additive hypotensive effects with ACE inhibitors, and hypovolemia increases the potential for adverse renal effects of ACE inhibitors. In patients with compromised renal function, coadministration with NSAIDs may result in further deterioration of renal function. Allopurinol and ACE inhibitors may cause a higher risk of hypersensitivity reaction when taken concurrently.

Nutritional/Ethanol Interactions Herb/Nutraceutical: Avoid dong quai if using for hypertension (has estrogenic activity). Avoid ephedra, yohimbe, ginseng (may worsen hypertension). Avoid garlic (may have increased antihypertensive effect).

Adverse Reactions Note: Frequency ranges include data from hypertension and heart failure trials. Higher rates of adverse reactions have generally been noted in patients with CHF. However, the frequency of adverse effects associated with placebo is also increased in this population.

1% to 10%:

- Cardiovascular: Hypotension (3%), chest pain (2%), first-dose hypotension (up to 3%)
- Central nervous system: Dizziness (4% to 8%), headache (2% to 6%), fatigue (3%)
- Dermatologic: Rash (1%)
- Endocrine & metabolic: Hyperkalemia (2%)
- Gastrointestinal: Vomiting/nausea (1% to 2%), diarrhea (1.7%)
- Neuromuscular & skeletal: Myalgias (2% to 5%), back pain (1%)
- Renal: Increased BUN/serum creatinine (2%, transient elevations may occur with a higher frequency), worsening of renal function (in patients with bilateral renal artery stenosis or hypovolemia)
- Respiratory: Upper respiratory symptoms, cough (2% to 4%; up to 13% in some studies), dyspnea (2%)

<1% (Limited to important or life-threatening): Acute renal failure, agranulocytosis, alopecia, amblyopia, angina, angioedema, arrhythmia, arthralgia, depression, dermatopolymyositis, edema, eosinophilic pneumonitis, exfoliative dermatitis, hemolytic anemia, hepatitis, hyperkalemia, hypertensive crisis, impotence, insomnia, myocardial infarction, orthostatic hypotension, pancreatitis, paresthesia, pemphigus, photosensitivity, pruritus, shock, somnolence, stroke, syncope, thrombocytopenia, vertigo

A syndrome which may include fever, myalgia, arthralgia, interstitial nephritis, vasculitis, rash, eosinophilia and positive ANA, and elevated ESR has been reported with ACE inhibitors. In addition, pancreatitis, hepatic necrosis, neutropenia, and/or agranulocytosis (particularly in patients with collagen-vascular disease or renal impairment) have been associated with many ACE inhibitors.

Overdosage/Toxicology Mild hypotension has been the primary toxic effect seen with acute overdose. Bradycardia may also occur. Hyperkalemia occurs even with therapeutic doses, especially in patients with renal insufficiency and those taking NSAIDs. Treatment is symptom-directed and supportive.

Pharmacodynamics/Kinetics

Absorption: Quinapril: ≥60%

Half-Life Elimination: Quinapril: 0.8 hours; Quinaprilat: 3 hours; increases as Cl_{cr} decreases

Time to Peak: Serum: Quinapril: 1 hour; Quinaprilat: ~2 hours

Metabolism: Rapidly hydrolyzed to quinaprilat, the active metabolite

Onset: 1 hour

Duration: 24 hours

Formulations Tablet, as hydrochloride: 5 mg, 10 mg, 20 mg, 40 mg

Dosing

Adults:

Hypertension: Oral: Initial: 10-20 mg once daily, adjust according to blood pressure response at peak and trough blood levels; initial dose may be reduced to 5 mg in patients receiving diuretic therapy if the diuretic is continued (normal dosage range is 20-80 mg/day for hypertension)

Congestive heart failure or post-MI: Oral: Initial: 5 mg once daily, titrated at weekly intervals to 20-40 mg daily in 2 divided doses

Elderly: Oral: Initial: 2.5-5 mg/day; increase dosage at increments of 2.5-5 mg at 1- to 2-week intervals; adjust for renal impairment.

Renal Impairment: Lower initial doses should be used; after initial dose (if tolerated), administer initial dose twice daily; may be increased at weekly intervals to optimal response:

Hypertension: Oral: Initial:

- Cl_{cr} >60 mL/minute: Administer 10 mg/day
- Cl_{cr} 30-60 mL/minute: Administer 5 mg/day
- Cl_{cr} 10-30 mL/minute: Administer 2.5 mg/day

Congestive heart failure: Oral: Initial:

- Cl_{cr} >30 mL/minute: Administer 5 mg/day
- Cl_{cr} 10-30 mL/minute: Administer 2.5 mg/day

Hepatic Impairment: In patients with alcoholic cirrhosis, hydrolysis of quinapril to quinaprilat is impaired; however, the subsequent elimination of quinaprilat is unaltered.

Stability

Storage: Store at room temperature.

Reconstitution: Unstable in aqueous solutions. To prepare solution for oral administration, mix prior to administration and use within 10 minutes.

Monitoring Laboratory Tests CBC, renal function tests, electrolytes If patient has renal impairment, a baseline WBC with differential and serum creatinine should be evaluated and monitored closely during the first 3 months of therapy.

(Continued)

Quinapril *(Continued)*

Monitoring and Teaching Issues

Physical Assessment: See Contraindications, Warnings/Precautions, and Dosing for use cautions. Assess potential for interactions with other prescriptions, OTC medications, or herbal products patient may be taking (see Drug Interactions). May be advisable to administer first dose in prescriber's office with careful blood pressure monitoring (hypotension angioedema can occur at any time during treatment, especially following first dose). Assess results of laboratory tests (see above) and patient response at beginning of therapy, when adjusting dose, and periodically with long-term therapy (eg, BP, cardiac status and fluid balance - see Adverse Reactions and Overdose/Toxicology). Teach patient appropriate use, possible side effects and interventions, and adverse symptoms to report (see Patient Education). **Pregnancy risk factor C/D** - determine that patient is not pregnant prior to beginning therapy. Instruct patient in appropriate use of barrier contraceptives (see Pregnancy Issues). Note breast-feeding caution.

Patient Education: Inform prescriber of all prescriptions, OTC medications, or herbal products you are taking, and any allergies you have. Do not take anything new during treatment unless approved by prescriber. Take as directed; do not alter dose or discontinue without consulting prescriber. Take first dose at bedtime or when sitting down (hypotension may occur). This drug does not eliminate need for diet or exercise regimen as recommended by prescriber. May cause increased cough (if persistent or bothersome, contact prescriber); postural hypotension (use caution when rising from lying or sitting position or climbing stairs); headache (consult prescriber for approved analgesic); dizziness (use caution when driving or engaging in tasks that require alertness until response to drug is known); nausea or vomiting (small, frequent meals, frequent mouth care, sucking lozenges, or chewing gum may help); or muscle or back pain (consult prescriber for approved analgesic). Immediately report swelling of face, mouth, lips, tongue or throat; chest pain or difficulty breathing. Report persistent cough; persistent pain in muscles, joints, or back; skin rash; or other persistent adverse reactions. **Pregnancy/breast-feeding precautions:** Inform prescriber if you are or intend to become pregnant. This drug should not be used in the 2nd or 3rd trimester of pregnancy. Consult prescriber for appropriate contraceptive measures if necessary. Consult prescriber if breast-feeding.

Geriatric Considerations: Due to frequent decreases in glomerular filtration (also creatinine clearance) with aging, elderly patients may have exaggerated responses to ACE inhibitors. Differences in clinical response due to hepatic changes are not observed.

Pregnancy Issues: ACE inhibitors can cause fetal injury or death if taken during the 2nd or 3rd trimester. Discontinue ACE inhibitors as soon as pregnancy is detected.

Related Information

Angiotensin Agents *on page 1547*
Heart Failure *on page 1670*

Quinapril and Hydrochlorothiazide

(KWIN a pril & hye droe klor oh THYE a zide)

U.S. Brand Names Accuretic™

Synonyms Hydrochlorothiazide and Quinapril

Generic Available No

Pharmacologic Category Angiotensin-Converting Enzyme (ACE) Inhibitor; Antihypertensive; Diuretic, Thiazide

Pregnancy Risk Factor C (1st trimester)/D (2nd and 3rd trimesters)

Lactation Enters breast milk/use caution

Use Treatment of hypertension (not for initial therapy)

Formulations Tablet:

10/25: Quinapril hydrochloride 10 mg and hydrochlorothiazide 12.5 mg
20/12.5: Quinapril hydrochloride 20 mg and hydrochlorothiazide 12.5 mg
20/25: Quinapril hydrochloride 20 mg and hydrochlorothiazide 25 mg

Dosing

Adults:

Hypertension: Oral:

Patients who have failed quinapril monotherapy: Quinapril 10 mg/ hydrochlorothiazide 12.5 mg **or** quinapril 20 mg/hydrochlorothiazide 12.5 mg once daily

Patients with adequate blood pressure control on hydrochlorothiazide 25 mg/day, but significant potassium loss: Quinapril 10 mg/hydrochlorothiazide 12.5 mg **or** quinapril 20 mg/hydrochlorothiazide 12.5 mg once daily

Note: Clinical trials of quinapril/hydrochlorothiazide combinations used quinapril doses of 2.5-40 mg/day and hydrochlorothiazide doses of 6.25-25 mg/day .

Pediatrics: Safety and efficacy have not been established.

Renal Impairment: Cl_{cr} <30 mL/minute/1.73 m^2 or serum creatinine ≤3 mg/dL: Use is not recommended.

Monitoring and Teaching Issues

Physical Assessment: See individual components listed in Related Information. **Pregnancy risk factor C/D** - determine that patient is not pregnant prior to beginning therapy. Instruct patient in appropriate use of barrier contraceptives (see Pregnancy Issues). Note breast-feeding caution.

Patient Education: See individual components listed in Related Information. **Pregnancy/breast-feeding precautions:** Do not get pregnant while taking this medication. Consult prescriber for appropriate contraceptive measures. Consult prescriber if breast-feeding.

Related Information

Hydrochlorothiazide *on page 664*
Quinapril *on page 1160*

Quinapril Hydrochloride *see* Quinapril *on page 1160*
Quinidex® Extentabs® *see* Quinidine *on page 1163*

Quinidine (KWIN i deen)

U.S. Brand Names Quinaglute® Dura-Tabs®; Quinidex® Extentabs®

Synonyms Quinidine Gluconate; Quinidine Polygalacturonate; Quinidine Sulfate

Generic Available Yes

Pharmacologic Category Antiarrhythmic Agent, Class Ia

Pregnancy Risk Factor C

Lactation Enters breast milk/compatible

Use Prophylaxis after cardioversion of atrial fibrillation and/or flutter to maintain normal sinus rhythm; prevent recurrence of paroxysmal supraventricular tachycardia, paroxysmal AV junctional rhythm, paroxysmal ventricular tachycardia, paroxysmal atrial fibrillation, and atrial or ventricular premature contractions; has activity against *Plasmodium falciparum* malaria

Mechanism of Action/Effect Class 1a antiarrhythmic agent; depresses phase O of the action potential; decreases myocardial excitability and conduction velocity, and myocardial contractility by decreasing sodium influx during depolarization and potassium efflux in repolarization; also reduces calcium transport across cell membrane

Contraindications Hypersensitivity to quinidine or any component of the formulation; thrombocytopenia; thrombocytopenic purpura; myasthenia gravis; heart block greater than first degree; idioventricular conduction delays (except in patients with a functioning artificial pacemaker); those adversely affected by anticholinergic activity; concurrent use of quinolone antibiotics which prolong QT interval, cisapride, amprenavir, or ritonavir

Warnings/Precautions Monitor and adjust dose to prevent excessive QT_c prolongation. May cause new or worsened arrhythmia (proarrhythmic effect). May precipitate or exacerbate CHF. Reduce dosage in hepatic impairment. In patients with atrial fibrillation or flutter, block the AV node before initiating. Correct hypokalemia before initiating therapy; hypokalemia may worsen toxicity. Use may cause digoxin-induced toxicity (adjust digoxin's dose). Use caution with concurrent use of other antiarrhythmics. Hypersensitivity reactions can occur. Can unmask sick sinus syndrome (causes bradycardia). Has been associated with severe hepatotoxic reactions, including granulomatous hepatitis. Hemolysis may occur in patients with G6PD (glucose-6-phosphate dehydrogenase) deficiency. Pregnancy risk C.

Drug Interactions

Cytochrome P450 Effect: Substrate of CYP2C8/9, 2E1, **3A4**; Inhibits CYP2C8/9, **2D6**, 3A4

Decreased Effect: Analgesic efficacy of codeine may be reduced. Enzyme inducers (aminoglutethimide, carbamazepine, phenobarbital, phenytoin, primidone, rifabutin, rifampin) may decrease quinidine blood levels.

Increased Effect/Toxicity: Quinidine potentiates nondepolarizing and depolarizing muscle relaxants. Quinidine may increase plasma concentration of digoxin; closely monitor digoxin concentrations. Digoxin dosage may need to be reduced (by 50%) when quinidine is initiated; new steady-state digoxin plasma concentrations occur in 5-7 days. When combined with quinidine, amiloride may cause prolonged ventricular conduction leading to arrhythmias. Urinary alkalinizers (antacids, sodium bicarbonate, acetazolamide) increase quinidine blood levels. Warfarin effects may be increased by quinidine.

Amprenavir, amiodarone, cimetidine, clarithromycin, diltiazem, erythromycin, itraconazole, ketoconazole, nelfinavir, ritonavir, troleandomycin, and verapamil (as well as other inhibitors of cytochrome P450 isoenzyme 3A4 may increase quinidine blood levels). Quinidine may increase blood levels of metoprolol mexiletine, nifedipine, propafenone, propranolol, and timolol.

Effects may be additive with drugs which prolong the QT interval, including amiodarone, amitriptyline, astemizole, bepridil, cisapride (use is contraindicated), disopyramide, erythromycin, haloperidol, imipramine, pimozide, procainamide, sotalol, thioridazine, and some quinolones (sparfloxacin, gatifloxacin, moxifloxacin - concurrent use is contraindicated).

Nutritional/Ethanol Interactions

Food: Dietary salt intake may alter the rate and extent of quinidine absorption. A decrease in dietary salt may lead to an increase in quinidine serum concentrations. Avoid changes in dietary salt intake. Quinidine serum levels may be increased if taken with food. Food has a variable effect on absorption of sustained release formulation. The rate of absorption of quinidine may be decreased following the ingestion of grapefruit juice. In addition, CYP3A4 metabolism of quinidine may be reduced by grapefruit juice. Grapefruit juice should be avoided. Excessive intake of fruit juices or vitamin C may decrease urine pH and result in increased clearance of quinidine with decreased serum concentration. Alkaline foods may result in increased quinidine serum concentrations.

Herb/Nutraceutical: St John's wort may decrease quinidine levels. Avoid ephedra (may worsen arrhythmia).

Adverse Reactions

Frequency not defined: Hypotension, syncope

>10%:

Cardiovascular: QT_c prolongation (modest prolongation is common, however, excessive prolongation is rare and indicates toxicity)

Central nervous system: Lightheadedness (15%)

Gastrointestinal: Diarrhea (35%), upper GI distress, bitter taste, diarrhea, anorexia, nausea, vomiting, stomach cramping (22%)

1% to 10%:

Cardiovascular: Angina (6%), palpitation (7%), new or worsened arrhythmias (proarrhythmic effect)

Central nervous system: Syncope (1% to 8%), headache (7%), fatigue (7%), weakness (5%), sleep disturbance (3%), tremor (2%), nervousness (2%), incoordination (1%)

Dermatologic: Rash (5%)

Ocular: Blurred vision

Otic: Tinnitus

Respiratory: Wheezing

<1% (Limited to important or life-threatening): Abnormal pigmentation, acute psychotic reactions, agranulocytosis, angioedema, arthralgia, bronchospasm, cerebral hypoperfusion

(Continued)

Quinidine *(Continued)*

(possibly resulting in ataxia, apprehension, and seizures), cholestasis, confusion, delirium, depression, drug-induced lupus-like syndrome, eczematous dermatitis, esophagitis, exacerbated bradycardia (in sick sinus syndrome), exfoliative rash, fever, flushing, granulomatous hepatitis, hallucinations, heart block, hemolytic anemia, hepatotoxic reaction (rare), impaired hearing, increased CPK, lichen planus, livedo reticularis, lymphadenopathy, melanin pigmentation of the hard palate, myalgia, mydriasis, nephropathy, optic neuritis, pancytopenia, paradoxical increase in ventricular rate during atrial fibrillation/flutter, photosensitivity, pneumonitis, pruritus, psoriaform rash, QT_c prolongation (excessive), respiratory depression, sicca syndrome, tachycardia, thrombocytopenia, thrombocytopenic purpura, torsade de pointes, urticaria, uveitis, vascular collapse, vasculitis, ventricular fibrillation, ventricular tachycardia, vertigo, visual field loss

Note: Cinchonism, a syndrome which may include tinnitus, high-frequency hearing loss, deafness, vertigo, blurred vision, diplopia, photophobia, headache, confusion, and delirium has been associated with quinidine use. Usually associated with chronic toxicity, this syndrome has also been described after brief exposure to a moderate dose in sensitive patients. Vomiting and diarrhea may also occur as isolated reactions to therapeutic quinidine levels.

Overdosage/Toxicology Has a low toxic:therapeutic ratio and may easily produce fatal intoxication (acute toxic dose: 1 g in adults). Symptoms of overdose include sinus bradycardia, sinus node arrest or asystole, P-R, QRS, or QT interval prolongation, torsade de pointes (polymorphous ventricular tachycardia), and depressed myocardial contractility, which along with alpha-adrenergic or ganglionic blockade, may result in hypotension and pulmonary edema. Other effects are anticholinergic (dry mouth, dilated pupils, and delirium) as well as seizures, coma, and respiratory arrest. Treatment is symptomatic and effects usually respond to conventional therapies. **Note:** Do not use other Class 1A or 1C antiarrhythmic agents to treat ventricular tachycardia. Sodium bicarbonate may treat wide QRS intervals or hypotension. Markedly impaired conduction or high degree AV block, unresponsive to bicarbonate, indicates consideration of a pacemaker.

Pharmacodynamics/Kinetics

Bioavailability: Sulfate: 80%; Gluconate: 70%

Half-Life Elimination: Plasma: Children: 2.5-6.7 hours; Adults: 6-8 hours; prolonged with elderly, cirrhosis, and congestive heart failure

Metabolism: Extensively hepatic (50% to 90%) to inactive compounds

Formulations

Injection, solution, as gluconate: 80 mg/mL (10 mL) [equivalent to quinidine base 50 mg]

Tablet, as sulfate: 200 mg, 300 mg

Tablet, extended release, as gluconate (Quinaglute® Dura-Tabs®): 324 mg [equivalent to quinidine base 202 mg]

Tablet, extended release, as sulfate (Quinidex® Extentabs®): 300 mg [equivalent to quinidine base 249 mg]

Dosing

Adults:

Note: Dosage expressed in terms of the salt: 267 mg of quinidine gluconate = 275 mg of quinidine polygalacturonate = 200 mg of quinidine sulfate.

Test dose: Oral, I.M.: 200 mg administered several hours before full dosage (to determine possibility of idiosyncratic reaction)

Antiarrhythmic:

Oral:

Sulfate: 100-600 mg/dose every 4-6 hours; begin at 200 mg/dose and titrate to desired effect (maximum daily dose: 3-4 g)

Gluconate: 324-972 mg every 8-12 hours

I.M.: 400 mg/dose every 4-6 hours

I.V.: 200-400 mg/dose diluted and given at a rate ≤10 mg/minute

Elderly: In general, elderly patient should be cautious, usually beginning on the low end of the dosing range, due to the potential for altered response due to decreased hepatic, cardiac, or renal function.

Pediatrics:

Note: Dosage expressed in terms of the salt: 267 mg of quinidine gluconate = 200 mg of quinidine sulfate.

Test dose for idiosyncratic reaction (sulfate, oral or gluconate, I.M.): Children: 2 mg/kg or 60 mg/m^2

Antiarrhythmic: Oral (quinidine sulfate): Children: 15-60 mg/kg/day in 4-5 divided doses or 6 mg/kg every 4-6 hours; usual 30 mg/kg/day or 900 mg/m^2/day given in 5 daily doses

I.V. **not** recommended (quinidine gluconate): Children: 2-10 mg/kg/dose given at a rate ≤10 mg/minute every 3-6 hours as needed

Renal Impairment:

Cl_{cr} <10 mL/minute: Administer 75% of normal dose.

Hemodialysis effects: Slightly hemodialyzable (5% to 20%); 200 mg supplemental dose posthemodialysis is recommended; not dialyzable (0% to 5%) by peritoneal dialysis.

Hepatic Impairment: Larger loading dose may be indicated; reduce maintenance doses by 50% and monitor serum levels closely.

Administration

Oral: Do not crush, chew, or break sustained release dosage forms. Give around-the-clock to promote less variation in peak and trough serum levels.

I.V.: Give around-the-clock to promote less variation in peak and trough serum levels. Maximum I.V. infusion rate: 10 mg/minute. Minimize use of PVC tubing to enhance bioavailability.

Stability

Storage: Do not use discolored parenteral solution.

Compatibility: Stable in D_5W, NS

Y-site administration: Incompatible with furosemide

Compatibility when admixed: Incompatible with atracurium

Monitoring Laboratory Tests Routine CBC, liver and renal function during long-term administration

Monitoring and Teaching Issues

Physical Assessment: Assess other medications patient may be taking for effectiveness and interactions (see Drug Interactions and Contraindications). See Warnings/Precautions and Contraindications for use cautions. I.V. requires use of infusion pump and continuous cardiac and hemodynamic monitoring. Monitor laboratory tests (see above), therapeutic response, and adverse reactions (see Warnings/Precautions and Adverse Reactions) at beginning of therapy, when titrating dosage, and on a regular basis with long-term therapy. **Note:** Quinidine has a low TI and overdose may easily produce severe and life-threatening reactions (see Overdose/Toxicology). Assess knowledge/teach patient appropriate use, interventions to reduce side effects, and adverse symptoms to report (see Patient Education). **Pregnancy risk factor C** - benefits of use should outweigh possible risks.

Patient Education: Take exactly as directed, around-the-clock; do not take additional doses or discontinue without consulting prescriber. Do not crush, chew, or break sustained release dosage forms. Do not take with grapefruit juice. You will need regular cardiac checkups and blood tests while taking this medication. You may experience dizziness, drowsiness, or visual changes (use caution when driving or engaging in tasks requiring alertness until response to drug is known); abnormal taste, nausea or vomiting, or loss of appetite (small, frequent meals, frequent mouth care, chewing gum, or sucking lozenges may help); headaches (prescriber may recommend mild analgesic); or diarrhea (yogurt or boiled milk may help - if persistent consult prescriber). Report chest pain, palpitation, or erratic heartbeat; difficulty breathing or wheezing; CNS changes (confusion, delirium, fever, consistent dizziness); skin rash; sense of fullness or ringing in ears; or vision changes. **Pregnancy precaution:** Inform prescriber if you are or intend to become pregnant.

Dietary Issues: Administer with food or milk to decrease gastrointestinal irritation. Avoid changes in dietary salt intake.

Geriatric Considerations: Clearance may be decreased with a resultant increased half-life. Must individualize dose. Bioavailability and half-life are increased in the elderly due to decreases in both renal and hepatic function with age.

Related Information

Antiarrhythmic Drugs *on page 1551*
Peak and Trough Guidelines *on page 1544*

Quinidine Gluconate *see* Quinidine *on page 1163*

Quinidine Polygalacturonate *see* Quinidine *on page 1163*

Quinidine Sulfate *see* Quinidine *on page 1163*

Quinine (KWYE nine)

Synonyms Quinine Sulfate

Generic Available Yes

Pharmacologic Category Antimalarial Agent

Pregnancy Risk Factor X

Lactation Enters breast milk/compatible

Use In conjunction with other antimalarial agents, suppression or treatment of chloroquine-resistant *P. falciparum* malaria; treatment of *Babesia microti* infection in conjunction with clindamycin

Use - Unlabeled/Investigational Prevention and treatment of nocturnal recumbency leg muscle cramps

Mechanism of Action/Effect Depresses oxygen uptake and carbohydrate metabolism; intercalates into DNA, disrupting the parasite's replication and transcription; affects calcium distribution within muscle fibers and decreases the excitability of the motor end-plate region; cardiovascular effects similar to quinidine

Contraindications Hypersensitivity to quinine or any component of the formulation; tinnitus, optic neuritis, G6PD deficiency; history of black water fever; thrombocytopenia with quinine or quinidine; pregnancy

Warnings/Precautions Use with caution in patients with cardiac arrhythmias (quinine has quinidine-like activity) and in patients with myasthenia gravis.

Drug Interactions

Cytochrome P450 Effect: Substrate of CYP1A2, 2C19, 3A4; Inhibits CYP2C8/9, **2D6**, 3A4

Decreased Effect: Phenobarbital, phenytoin, and rifampin may decrease quinine serum concentrations.

Increased Effect/Toxicity: Beta-blockers + quinine may increase bradycardia. Quinine may enhance warfarin anticoagulant effect. Quinine potentiates nondepolarizing and depolarizing muscle relaxants. Quinine may increase plasma concentration of digoxin. Closely monitor digoxin concentrations. Digoxin dosage may need to be reduced (by one-half) when quinine is initiated. New steady-state digoxin plasma concentrations occur in 5-7 days. Verapamil, amiodarone, alkalinizing agents, and cimetidine may increase quinine serum concentrations.

Nutritional/Ethanol Interactions Herb/Nutraceutical: St John's wort may decrease quinine levels.

Effects on Lab Values Positive Coombs' [direct]

Adverse Reactions

Frequency not defined:

- Central nervous system: Severe headache
- Gastrointestinal: Nausea, vomiting, diarrhea
- Ocular: Blurred vision
- Otic: Tinnitus
- Miscellaneous: Cinchonism (risk of cinchonism is directly related to dose and duration of therapy)

(Continued)

Quinine *(Continued)*

<1% (Limited to important or life-threatening): Anginal symptoms, diplopia, epigastric pain, fever, flushing of the skin, hemolysis in G6PD deficiency, hepatitis, hypersensitivity reactions, hypoglycemia, impaired hearing, nightblindness, optic atrophy, pruritus, rash, thrombocytopenia

Overdosage/Toxicology Symptoms of mild toxicity include nausea, vomiting, and cinchonism. Severe intoxication may cause ataxia, obtundation, convulsions, coma, and respiratory arrest. With massive intoxication quinidine-like cardiotoxicity (hypotension, QRS and QT interval prolongation, AV block, and ventricular arrhythmias) may be fatal. Retinal toxicity occurs 9-10 hours after ingestion (blurred vision, impaired color perception, constriction of visual fields and blindness). Other toxic effects include hypokalemia, hypoglycemia, hemolysis, and congenital malformations when taken during pregnancy. Treatment includes symptomatic therapy with conventional agents. **Note:** Avoid Type 1A and 1C antiarrhythmic drugs. Treat cardiotoxicity with sodium bicarbonate. Dialysis and hemoperfusion procedures are ineffective in enhancing elimination.

Pharmacodynamics/Kinetics

Absorption: Readily, mainly from upper small intestine

Half-Life Elimination: Children: 6-12 hours; Adults: 8-14 hours

Time to Peak: Serum: 1-3 hours

Metabolism: Primarily hepatic

Formulations

Capsule, as sulfate: 200 mg, 325 mg

Tablet, as sulfate: 260 mg

Dosing

Adults & Elderly:

Treatment of chloroquine-resistant malaria: Oral: 650 mg every 8 hours for 3-7 days with tetracycline

Suppression of malaria: Oral: 325 mg twice daily and continued for 6 weeks after exposure

Babesiosis: Oral: 650 mg every 6-8 hours for 7 days

Leg cramps: Oral: 200-300 mg at bedtime

Pediatrics:

Treatment of chloroquine-resistant malaria: Oral: Children: 25-30 mg/kg/day in divided doses every 8 hours for 3-7 days with tetracycline (consider risk versus benefit in children <8 years of age)

Babesiosis: Oral: Children: 25 mg/kg/day divided every 8 hours for 7 days

Renal Impairment:

Cl_{cr} 10-50 mL/minute: Administer every 8-12 hours or 75% of normal dose.

Cl_{cr} <10 mL/minute: Administer every 24 hours or 30% to 50% of normal dose.

Not removed by hemo- or peritoneal dialysis; dose for Cl_{cr} <10 mL/minute.

Continuous arteriovenous or venovenous hemofiltration: Dose as for Cl_{cr} 10-50 mL/minute.

Administration

Oral: Do not crush sustained release preparations. Avoid use of aluminum-containing antacids because of drug absorption problems. Swallow dose whole to avoid bitter taste. May be administered with food.

Stability

Storage: Protect from light.

Monitoring and Teaching Issues

Physical Assessment: Assess allergy history prior to beginning therapy. See Contraindications, Warnings/Precautions, and Dosing for use cautions. Assess potential for interactions with other prescriptions, OTC medications, or herbal products patient may be taking (especially digoxin - see Drug Interactions). Assess therapeutic effectiveness (according to purpose for therapy) and adverse reactions (see Adverse Reactions and Overdose/Toxicology). Teach patient appropriate use, possible side effects/interventions, and adverse symptoms to report (see Patient Education). **Pregnancy risk factor X** - determine that patient is not pregnant before starting therapy. Do not give to females of childbearing age unless patient is capable of complying with barrier contraceptive use during and for 2 months following therapy.

Patient Education: Inform prescriber of all prescriptions, OTC medications, or herbal products you are taking, and any allergies you have. Do not take anything new during treatment unless approved by prescriber (avoid use of any aluminum-containing antacids). Take on schedule as directed, with full 8 oz of water. May take with food. Do not crush sustained release preparations. Do not increase dose without consulting prescriber - overdose can cause severe systemic effects. You will need to return for follow-up blood tests. May cause severe headache (consult prescriber for approved analgesic); nausea or vomiting (small, frequent meals, frequent mouth care, chewing gum, or sucking lozenges may help); or diarrhea (buttermilk, boiled milk, or yogurt may help). Report any vision changes (blurring, nightblindness, double vision, etc); ringing in ears; or other persistent side effects. Seek emergency help for chest pain, difficulty breathing, or seizures. **Pregnancy precautions:** Inform prescriber if you are pregnant. Consult prescriber for appropriate barrier contraceptive measures to use during and for 2 months following therapy. This drug may cause fetal defects. Do not donate blood during or for 1 month following therapy.

Dietary Issues: May be taken with food.

Geriatric Considerations: Efficacy in nocturnal leg cramps is not well supported in the medical and pharmacy literature, however, some patients do respond. Nonresponders should be evaluated for other possible etiologies.

Quinine Sulfate *see* Quinine *on page 1165*

Quinol *see* Hydroquinone *on page 679*

Quinupristin and Dalfopristin (kwi NYOO pris tin & dal FOE pris tin)

U.S. Brand Names Synercid®

Synonyms Pristinamycin; RP59500

Generic Available No

Pharmacologic Category Antibiotic, Streptogramin

Pregnancy Risk Factor B

Lactation Excretion in breast milk unknown/use caution

Use Treatment of serious or life-threatening infections associated with vancomycin-resistant *Enterococcus faecium* bacteremia; treatment of complicated skin and skin structure infections caused by methcillin-susceptible *Staphylococcus aureus* or *Streptococcus pyogenes*

Has been studied in the treatment of a variety of infections caused by *Enterococcus faecium* (not *E. fecalis*) including vancomycin-resistant strains. May also be effective in the treatment of serious infections caused by *Staphylococcus* species including those resistant to methicillin.

Mechanism of Action/Effect Quinupristin/dalfopristin inhibits bacterial protein synthesis by binding to different sites on the 50S bacterial ribosomal subunit thereby inhibiting protein synthesis.

Contraindications Hypersensitivity to quinupristin, dalfopristin, pristinamycin, or virginiamycin, or any component of the formulation

Warnings/Precautions Use with caution in patients with hepatic or renal dysfunction. May cause pain and phlebitis when infused through a peripheral line (not relieved by hydrocortisone or diphenhydramine). May inhibit the metabolism of many drugs metabolized by CYP3A4. Concurrent therapy with astemizole and cisapride (which may prolong QT_c interval and lead to arrhythmias) should be avoided. Superinfection may occur. As with many antibiotics, antibiotic-associated colitis and pseudomembranous colitis may occur. May cause arthralgias, myalgias, and hyperbilirubinemia.

Drug Interactions

Cytochrome P450 Effect: Quinupristin: Inhibits CYP3A4

Increased Effect/Toxicity: Astemizole and cisapride (which may prolong QT_c interval and lead to arrhythmias) should be avoided. The metabolism of midazolam and nifedipine have been demonstrated to be inhibited *in vitro.* An increase in cyclosporine levels has been documented in patients receiving concomitant therapy. Other medications metabolized by CYP3A4, including protease inhibitors, non-nucleoside reverse transcriptase inhibitors, benzodiazepines, calcium channel blockers, some HMG-CoA reductase inhibitors, immunosuppressive agents, corticosteroids, carbamazepine, quinidine, lidocaine, and disopyramide are predicted to have increased plasma concentrations during concurrent dosing.

Adverse Reactions

>10%:

Hepatic: Hyperbilirubinemia (3% to 35%)

Local: Inflammation at infusion site (38% to 42%), local pain (40% to 44%), local edema (17% to 18%), infusion site reaction (12% to 13%)

1% to 10%:

Central nervous system: Pain (2% to 3%), headache (2%)

Dermatologic: Pruritus (2%), rash (3%)

Endocrine & metabolic: Hyperglycemia (1%)

Gastrointestinal: Nausea (3% to 5%), diarrhea (3%), vomiting (3% to 4%)

Hematologic: Anemia (3%)

Hepatic: Increased LDH (3%), increased GGT (2%)

Local: Thrombophlebitis (2%)

Neuromuscular & skeletal: Arthralgia (<1% to 8%), myalgia (<1% to 5%), Increased CPK (2%)

<1% (Limited to important or life-threatening): Allergic reaction, anaphylactoid reaction, angina, apnea, arrhythmia, cardiac arrest, coagulation disorder, dysautonomia, dyspnea, encephalopathy, gout, hematuria, hemolytic anemia, hepatitis, hyperkalemia, hypotension, maculopapular rash, mesenteric artery occlusion, myasthenia, neuropathy, pancreatitis, pancytopenia, paraplegia, paresthesia, pericarditis, pleural effusion, pseudomembranous colitis, respiratory distress, seizures, shock, stomatitis, syncope, thrombocytopenia, urticaria

Overdosage/Toxicology Symptoms may include dyspnea, emesis, tremors and ataxia. Treatment is supportive. Not removed by hemodialysis or peritoneal dialysis.

Pharmacodynamics/Kinetics

Half-Life Elimination: Quinupristin: 0.85 hour; Dalfopristin: 0.7 hour (mean elimination half-lives, including metabolites: 3 and 1 hours, respectively)

Metabolism: To active metabolites via nonenzymatic reactions

Formulations Injection, powder for reconstitution: 500 mg (dalfopristin 350 mg and quinupristin 150 mg)

Dosing

Adults & Elderly:

Vancomycin-resistant *Enterococcus faecium:* I.V.: 7.5 mg/kg every 8 hours

Complicated skin and skin structure infection: I.V.: 7.5 mg/kg every 12 hours

Pediatrics: Limited information: Dosages similar to adult dosing have been used in the treatment of complicated skin/soft tissue infections and infections caused by vancomycin-resistant *Enterococcus faecium*

CNS shunt infection due to vancomycin-resistant *Enterococcus faecium*: I.V.: 7.5 mg/kg/dose every 8 hours. Concurrent intrathecal doses of 1-2 mg/day have been administered for up to 68 days.

Renal Impairment: No adjustment is necessary in renal failure, hemodialysis, or peritoneal dialysis.

Hepatic Impairment: Pharmacokinetic data suggest dosage adjustment may be necessary; however, specific recommendations have not been proposed.

Administration

I.V.: Line should be flushed with 5% dextrose in water prior to and following administration. Incompatible with saline. Infusion should be completed over 60 minutes (toxicity may be increased with shorter infusion). Compatible (Y-site injection) with aztreonam, ciprofloxacin, haloperidol, metoclopramide or potassium chloride when admixed in 5% dextrose in water. Also compatible (Y-site injection) with fluconazole (used as undiluted solution). If

(Continued)

Quinupristin and Dalfopristin *(Continued)*

severe venous irritation occurs following peripheral administration of quinupristin/dalfopristin diluted in 250 mL 5% dextrose in water, consideration should be given to increasing the infusion volume to 500 mL or 750 mL, changing the infusion site, or infusing by a peripherally inserted central catheter (PICC) or a central venous catheter.

Stability

Storage: Store unopened vials under refrigeration (2°C to 8°C/36°F to 46°F).

Reconstitution: Reconstitute single dose vial with 5 mL of 5% dextrose in water or sterile water for injection. Swirl gentle to dissolve - do not shake (to limit foam formation). The reconstituted solution should be diluted within 30 minutes. Stability of the diluted solution prior to the infusion is established as 5 hours at room temperature or 54 hours if refrigerated at 2°C to 8°C. Reconstituted solution should be added to at least 250 mL of 5% dextrose in water for peripheral administration (increase to 500 mL or 750 mL if necessary to limit venous irritation). An infusion volume of 100 mL may be used for central line infusions. Do not freeze solution.

Monitoring and Teaching Issues

Physical Assessment: Assess effectiveness and interactions of other medications (see Drug Interactions). See Warnings/Precautions and Contraindications for use cautions. See Administration for exact infusion protocols to prevent (or treat) severe venous irritation. Monitor infusion site closely. Monitor therapeutic effectiveness (reduction of infection) and adverse reactions and toxicity (see Adverse Reactions, and Overdose/Toxicology). Assess knowledge/teach patient adverse reactions to report (see Patient Education). Note breast-feeding caution.

Patient Education: This drug can only be administered by intravenous infusion. Report immediately any pain, irritation, redness, burning, swelling at infusion site. You may experience other side effects. Report headache, rash, nausea, vomiting, diarrhea, pain, heat or swelling in muscle areas, especially in lower extremities; difficulty breathing, tremors, or difficulty speaking. Consult prescriber if breast-feeding.

Quixin™ *see* Levofloxacin *on page 790*

QVAR™ *see* Beclomethasone *on page 149*

Rabeprazole (ra BE pray zole)

U.S. Brand Names Aciphex®

Synonyms Pariprazole

Generic Available No

Pharmacologic Category Proton Pump Inhibitor

Pregnancy Risk Factor B

Lactation Excretion in breast milk unknown/not recommended

Use Short-term (4-8 weeks) treatment and maintenance of erosive or ulcerative gastroesophageal reflux disease (GERD); symptomatic GERD; short-term (up to 4 weeks) treatment of duodenal ulcers; long-term treatment of pathological hypersecretory conditions, including Zollinger-Ellison syndrome

Use - Unlabeled/Investigational *H. pylori* eradication; maintenance of duodenal ulcer

Mechanism of Action/Effect Suppresses gastric acid secretion by inhibiting the parietal cell H^+/K^+ ATP pump

Contraindications Hypersensitivity to rabeprazole, substituted benzimidazoles, or any component of the formulation

Warnings/Precautions Use caution in severe hepatic impairment. Relief of symptoms with rabeprazole does not preclude the presence of a gastric malignancy

Drug Interactions

Cytochrome P450 Effect: Substrate of **CYP2C19, 3A4**; Inhibits CYP2C19, 3A4

Decreased Effect: Rabeprazole may decrease bioavailability of ketoconazole or itraconazole.

Increased Effect/Toxicity: Rabeprazole (in extremely high concentrations) may increase serum levels of digoxin and cyclosporine.

Nutritional/Ethanol Interactions Ethanol: Avoid ethanol (may cause gastric mucosal irritation).

Adverse Reactions

1% to 10%: Central nervous system: Headache (2.4%)

<1% (Limited to important or life-threatening): Anaphylaxis, agranulocytosis, allergic reactions, alopecia, amnesia, angina, angioedema, apnea, asthma, bradycardia, bundle branch block, cholecystitis, coma, delirium, depression, dysphagia, dyspnea, extrapyramidal reaction, gout, hemolytic anemia, interstitial pneumonia, jaundice, leukopenia, myocardial infarction, neuralgia, neuropathy, pancreatitis, pancytopenia, paresthesia, photosensitivity, pulmonary embolus, QT prolongation, rash, renal calculus, retinal degeneration, rhabdomyolysis, seizures, strabismus, syncope, tachycardia, thrombocytopenia, ventricular tachycardia, vertigo

Overdosage/Toxicology No experience with large overdose; rabeprazole is not dialyzable. Treatment of overdosage should be symptomatic and supportive.

Pharmacodynamics/Kinetics

Absorption: Oral: Well absorbed within 1 hour

Bioavailability: Oral: 52%

Half-Life Elimination: Dose dependent: 0.85-2 hours

Time to Peak: Serum: 2-5 hours

Metabolism: Hepatic via CYP3A and 2C19 to inactive metabolites

Onset: 1 hour; Peak effect, plasma: ~2-5 hours

Duration: 24 hours

Formulations Tablet, delayed release, enteric coated: 20 mg

Dosing

Adults & Elderly:

GERD: Oral: 20 mg once daily for 4-8 weeks; maintenance: 20 mg once daily

Duodenal ulcer: Oral: 20 mg/day after breakfast for 4 weeks

Hypersecretory conditions: Oral: 60 mg once daily; dose may need to be adjusted as necessary. Doses as high as 100 mg and 60 mg twice daily have been used.

Stability

Storage: Rapidly degraded in acid conditions; may give antacid with rabeprazole

Monitoring and Teaching Issues

Physical Assessment: Assess other medications, especially those dependent on cytochrome P450 metabolism (eg, digoxin) and those requiring acid environment for absorption (eg, ketoconazole, ampicillin) (see Drug Interactions). Monitor therapeutic effectiveness (reduction in symptoms) and adverse reactions and toxicity (see Adverse Reactions, and Overdose/Toxicology). Assess knowledge/teach patient appropriate use, interventions to reduce side effects, and adverse reactions to report (see Patient Education). Breast-feeding is not recommended.

Patient Education: Take as directed. Swallow whole, do not crush or chew. Follow recommended diet and activity instructions. Avoid alcohol. You may experience headache (use of mild analgesic may help) or other side effects. Report these to prescriber if they persist. **Breast-feeding precaution:** Breast-feeding is not recommended.

Geriatric Considerations: No difference in efficacy or safety was noted in elderly subjects as compared to younger subjects. No dosage adjustment is necessary in the elderly.

Rabies (Immune Globulin Human) *see page 1498*

Rabies Virus Vaccine *see page 1498*

rAHF *see* Antihemophilic Factor (Recombinant) *on page 112*

R-albuterol *see* Levalbuterol *on page 783*

Raloxifene (ral OX i feen)

U.S. Brand Names Evista®

Synonyms Keoxifene Hydrochloride; Raloxifene Hydrochloride

Generic Available No

Pharmacologic Category Selective Estrogen Receptor Modulator (SERM)

Pregnancy Risk Factor X

Lactation Contraindicated

Use Prevention and treatment of osteoporosis in postmenopausal women

Mechanism of Action/Effect A selective estrogen receptor modulator, meaning that it affects some of the same receptors that estrogen does, but not all, and in some instances, it antagonizes or blocks estrogen; it acts like estrogen to prevent bone loss and improve lipid profiles (decreases total and LDL-cholesterol but does not raise triglycerides), but it has the potential to block some estrogen effects such as those that lead to breast cancer and uterine cancer

Contraindications Hypersensitivity to raloxifene or any component of the formulation; active thromboembolic disorder; pregnancy (not intended for use in premenopausal women)

Warnings/Precautions Use caution in patients with history of or at high risk for venous thromboembolism/pulmonary embolism; patients with cardiovascular disease; history of cervical/uterine carcinoma; renal/hepatic insufficiency (however, pharmacokinetic data are lacking); concurrent use of estrogens; women with a history of elevated triglycerides in response to treatment with oral estrogens (or estrogen/progestin). Discontinue at least 72 hours prior to and during prolonged immobilization (postoperative recovery or prolonged bedrest).

Drug Interactions

Decreased Effect: Ampicillin and cholestyramine reduce raloxifene absorption/blood levels.

Increased Effect/Toxicity: Raloxifene has the potential to interact with highly protein-bound drugs (increase effects of either agent). Use caution with highly protein-bound drugs, warfarin, clofibrate, indomethacin, naproxen, ibuprofen, diazepam, phenytoin, or tamoxifen.

Adverse Reactions Note: Has been associated with increased risk of thromboembolism (DVT, PE) and superficial thrombophlebitis; risk is similar to reported risk of HRT

>10%:

Cardiovascular: Hot flashes

Neuromuscular & skeletal: Arthralgia

Respiratory: Sinusitis

Miscellaneous: Flu syndrome, infection

1% to 10%:

Cardiovascular: Chest pain

Central nervous system: Fever, migraine, depression, insomnia

Dermatologic: Rash, diaphoresis

Endocrine & metabolic: Peripheral edema

Gastrointestinal: Nausea, dyspepsia, vomiting, flatulence, GI disorder, gastroenteritis, weight gain

Genitourinary: Urinary tract infection, vaginitis, cystitis, leukorrhea, endometrial disorder

Neuromuscular & skeletal: Myalgia, leg cramps, arthritis

Respiratory: Pharyngitis, cough, pneumonia, laryngitis

<1% (Limited to important or life-threatening): Hypertriglyceridemia, retinal vein occlusion (very rare)

Overdosage/Toxicology Incidence of overdose in humans has not been reported. In an 8-week study of postmenopausal women, a dose of raloxifene 600 mg/day was safely tolerated. No mortality was seen after a single oral dose in rats or mice at 810 times the human dose for rats and 405 times the human dose for mice. There is no specific antidote for raloxifene.

(Continued)

Raloxifene *(Continued)*

Pharmacodynamics/Kinetics

Absorption: ~60%

Bioavailability: ~2%

Half-Life Elimination: 27.7-32.5 hours

Metabolism: Extensive first-pass effect

Onset: 8 weeks

Formulations Tablet, as hydrochloride: 60 mg

Dosing

Adults & Elderly: Osteoporosis prevention or treatment (postmenopausal women): Oral: 1 tablet (60 mg) daily; may be administered any time of the day without regard to meals.

Hepatic Impairment: Avoid use; safety has not been established.

Administration

Oral: Raloxifene should be stopped 72 hours prior to or during prolonged immobilization due to risk of thromboembolic events.

Monitoring Laboratory Tests Monitor lipid profile, bone mineral density

Monitoring and Teaching Issues

Physical Assessment: See Contraindications and Warnings/Precautions for use cautions. Assess potential for interactions with other prescriptions, OTC medications, or herbal products patient may be taking (see Drug Interactions). Assess results of laboratory work (see above) and patient response (eg, DVT or PE - see Adverse Reactions and Overdose/Toxicology). Teach patient appropriate use, possible side effects and interventions, and adverse symptoms to report (eg, thromboembolism - see Patient Education). **Pregnancy risk factor X** - determine that patient is not pregnant before starting therapy. For use in postmenopausal women only. Breast-feeding is contraindicated.

Patient Education: Inform prescriber of all prescriptions, OTC medications, or herbal products you are taking, and any allergies you have. Do not take anything new during treatment unless approved by prescriber. May be taken at any time of day without regard to meals. This medication is given to reduce incidence of osteoporosis; it will not reduce menopausal hot flashes or flushing (cool environment may reduce hot flashes). May cause flu-like symptoms at beginning of therapy (these will resolve with use); GI disturbances (eg, nausea, vomiting, dyspepsia - small, frequent meals, frequent mouth care, chewing gum, or sucking lozenges may help); or joint pain (consult prescriber for approved analgesic). Report immediately any pain, redness, warmth, or cramping in leg muscles; sudden chest pain; or difficulty breathing. Report fever, acute migraine, insomnia or emotional depression, unusual weight gain (>5 lb/week), unresolved gastric distress, urinary infection or vaginal burning or itching, or unusual cough. **Pregnancy/breast-feeding precautions:** Inform prescriber if you are pregnant. For use in postmenopausal women only. Breast-feeding is contraindicated.

Geriatric Considerations: No need to cycle with progesterone.

Additional Information The decrease in estrogen-related adverse effects with the selective estrogen-receptor modulators in general and raloxifene in particular should improve compliance and decrease the incidence of cardiovascular events and fractures while not increasing breast cancer.

Related Information

Estrogen Replacement Therapy *on page 1666*
Osteoporosis Management *on page 1696*

Raloxifene Hydrochloride *see* Raloxifene *on page 1169*

Ramipril (ra MI pril)

U.S. Brand Names Altace®

Generic Available No

Pharmacologic Category Angiotensin-Converting Enzyme (ACE) Inhibitor

Pregnancy Risk Factor C/D (2nd and 3rd trimesters)

Lactation Enters breast milk/not recommended

Use Treatment of hypertension, alone or in combination with thiazide diuretics; treatment of congestive heart failure; treatment of left ventricular dysfunction after myocardial infarction; to reduce risk of heart attack, stroke, and death in patients at increased risk for these problems

Mechanism of Action/Effect Ramipril is an ACE inhibitor which prevents the formation of angiotensin II from angiotensin I and exhibits pharmacologic effects that are similar to captopril. Ramipril must undergo conversion in the liver to its biologically active metabolite, ramiprilat. The pharmacodynamic effects of ramipril result from the high-affinity, competitive, reversible binding of ramiprilat to angiotensin-converting enzyme thus preventing the formation of the potent vasoconstrictor angiotensin II.

Contraindications Hypersensitivity to ramipril or any component of the formulation; prior hypersensitivity (including angioedema) to ACE inhibitors; bilateral renal artery stenosis; primary hyperaldosteronism; pregnancy (2nd and 3rd trimesters)

Warnings/Precautions Angioedema can occur at any time during treatment (especially following first dose). Careful blood pressure monitoring with first dose (hypotension can occur especially in volume depleted patients). Dosage adjustment needed in renal impairment. Use with caution in hypovolemia; collagen vascular diseases; valvular stenosis (particularly aortic stenosis); hyperkalemia; or before, during, or immediately after anesthesia. Avoid rapid dosage escalation, which may lead to renal insufficiency. Neutropenia/agranulocytosis with myeloid hyperplasia can rarely occur. Hypersensitivity reactions may be seen during hemodialysis with high-flux dialysis membranes (eg, AN69). Use with caution in unilateral renal artery stenosis and pre-existing renal insufficiency. Pregnancy risk C/D (2nd and 3rd trimesters).

Drug Interactions

Decreased Effect: Aspirin (high dose) may reduce the therapeutic effects of ACE inhibitors; at low dosages this does not appear to be significant. Rifampin may decrease the effect of ACE inhibitors. Antacids may decrease the bioavailability of ACE inhibitors (may be more likely to occur with captopril); separate administration times by 1-2 hours. NSAIDs, specifically indomethacin, may reduce the hypotensive effects of ACE inhibitors. More likely to occur in low renin or volume dependent hypertensive patients.

Increased Effect/Toxicity: Potassium supplements, co-trimoxazole (high dose), angiotensin II receptor antagonists (candesartan, losartan, irbesartan, etc), or potassium-sparing diuretics (amiloride, spironolactone, triamterene) may result in elevated serum potassium levels when combined with ramipril. ACE inhibitor effects may be increased by phenothiazines or probenecid (increases levels of captopril). ACE inhibitors may increase serum concentrations/effects of digoxin, lithium, and sulfonlyureas.

Diuretics have additive hypotensive effects with ACE inhibitors, and hypovolemia increases the potential for adverse renal effects of ACE inhibitors. In patients with compromised renal function, coadministration with NSAIDs may result in further deterioration of renal function. Allopurinol and ACE inhibitors may cause a higher risk of hypersensitivity reaction when taken concurrently.

Nutritional/Ethanol Interactions Herb/Nutraceutical: Avoid dong quai if using for hypertension (has estrogenic activity). Avoid ephedra, yohimbe, ginseng (may worsen hypertension). Avoid garlic (may have increased antihypertensive effect).

Effects on Lab Values Increases BUN, creatinine, potassium, positive Coombs' [direct]; decreases cholesterol (S); may cause false-positive results in urine acetone determinations using sodium nitroprusside reagent

Adverse Reactions Note: Frequency ranges include data from hypertension and heart failure trials. Higher rates of adverse reactions have generally been noted in patients with CHF. However, the frequency of adverse effects associated with placebo is also increased in this population.

>10%: Respiratory: Cough (increased) (7% to 12%)

1% to 10%:

Cardiovascular: Hypotension (11%), angina (3%), postural hypotension (2%), syncope (2%)

Central nervous system: Headache (1% to 5%), dizziness (2% to 4%), fatigue (2%), vertigo (2%)

Endocrine & metabolic: Hyperkalemia (1% to 10%)

Gastrointestinal: Nausea/vomiting (1% to 2%)

Neuromuscular & skeletal: Chest pain (noncardiac) (1%)

Renal: Renal dysfunction (1%), elevation in serum creatinine (1% to 2%), increased BUN (<1% to 3%); transient elevations of creatinine and/or BUN may occur more frequently

Respiratory: Cough (estimated 1% to 10%)

<1% (Limited to important or life-threatening): Agitation, agranulocytosis, amnesia, anaphylactoid reaction, angina, angioedema, arrhythmia, bone marrow depression, convulsions, depression, dysphagia, dyspnea, edema, eosinophilia, erythema multiforme, hearing loss, hemolytic anemia, hepatitis, hypersensitivity reactions (urticaria, rash, fever), impotence, insomnia, myalgia, myocardial infarction, neuropathy, onycholysis, pancreatitis, pancytopenia, paresthesia, pemphigoid, pemphigus, photosensitivity, proteinuria, somnolence, Stevens-Johnson syndrome, symptomatic hypotension, syncope, thrombocytopenia, toxic epidermal necrolysis, vertigo

Worsening of renal function may occur in patients with bilateral renal artery stenosis or in hypovolemia. In addition, a syndrome which may include fever, myalgia, arthralgia, interstitial nephritis, vasculitis, rash, eosinophilia and positive ANA, and elevated ESR has been reported with ACE inhibitors. Risk of pancreatitis and/or agranulocytosis may be increased in patients with collagen vascular disease or renal impairment.

Overdosage/Toxicology Mild hypotension has been the primary toxic effect seen with acute overdose. Bradycardia may also occur. Hyperkalemia occurs even with therapeutic doses, especially in patients with renal insufficiency and those taking NSAIDs. Treatment is symptom-directed and supportive.

Pharmacodynamics/Kinetics

Absorption: Well absorbed (50% to 60%)

Half-Life Elimination: Ramiprilat: Effective: 13-17 hours; Terminal: >50 hours

Time to Peak: Serum: ~1 hour

Metabolism: Hepatic to the active form, ramiprilat

Onset: 1-2 hours

Duration: 24 hours

Formulations Capsule: 1.25 mg, 2.5 mg, 5 mg, 10 mg

Dosing

Adults:

Hypertension: Oral: 2.5-5 mg once daily, maximum: 20 mg/day

Reduction in risk of MI, stroke, and death from cardiovascular causes: Oral: Initial: 2.5 mg once daily for 1 week, then 5 mg once daily for the next 3 weeks, then increase as tolerated to 10 mg once daily (may be given as divided dose)

Heart failure postmyocardial infarction: Oral: Initial: 2.5 mg twice daily titrated upward, if possible, to 5 mg twice daily.

Note: The dose of any concomitant diuretic should be reduced. If the diuretic cannot be discontinued, initiate therapy with 1.25 mg. After the initial dose, the patient should be monitored carefully until blood pressure has stabilized.

Elderly: Refer to adult dosing (see Geriatric Considerations). Adjust for renal function for elderly since glomerular filtration rates are decreased; may see exaggerated hypotensive effects if renal clearance is not considered.

Renal Impairment:

Cl_{cr} <40 mL/minute: Administer 25% of normal dose.

Renal failure and hypertension: Administer 1.25 mg once daily, titrated upward as possible.

Renal failure and heart failure: Administer 1.25 mg once daily, increasing to 1.25 mg twice daily up to 2.5 mg twice daily as tolerated.

Administration

Oral: Capsule is usually swallowed whole, but may be may be mixed in water, apple juice, or applesauce.

(Continued)

Ramipril *(Continued)*

Stability

Storage: Stable for 24 hours at room temperature or 48 hours under refrigeration.

Monitoring Laboratory Tests CBC, renal function tests, electrolytes; If patient has renal impairment then a baseline WBC with differential and serum creatinine should be evaluated and monitored closely during the first 3 months of therapy.

Monitoring and Teaching Issues

Physical Assessment: See Contraindications, Warnings/Precautions, and Dosing for use cautions. Assess potential for interactions with other prescriptions, OTC medications, or herbal products patient may be taking (see Drug Interactions). May be advisable to administer first dose in prescriber's office with careful blood pressure monitoring (hypotension and angioedema can occur at any time during treatment, especially following first dose). Assess results of laboratory tests (see above) and patient response at beginning of therapy, when adjusting dose, and periodically with long-term therapy (eg, blood pressure, cardiac status and fluid balance - see Adverse Reactions and Overdose/Toxicology). Teach patient appropriate use, possible side effects and interventions, and adverse symptoms to report (see Patient Education). **Pregnancy risk factor C/D** - determine that patient is not pregnant prior to beginning therapy. Instruct patient in appropriate use of barrier contraceptives (see Pregnancy Issues). Breast-feeding is not recommended.

Patient Education: Inform prescriber of all prescriptions, OTC medications, or herbal products you are taking, and any allergies you have. Do not take anything new without consulting prescriber. Take as directed; do not alter dose or discontinue without consulting prescriber. Take first dose at bedtime or when sitting down (hypotension may occur). This drug does not eliminate need for diet or exercise regimen as recommended by prescriber. May cause increased cough (if persistent or bothersome, contact prescriber); headache (consult prescriber for approved analgesic); postural hypotension (use caution when rising from lying or sitting position or climbing stairs); dizziness (use caution when driving or engaging in tasks that require alertness until response to drug is known); or nausea or vomiting (small, frequent meals, frequent mouth care, sucking lozenges, or chewing gum may help). Immediately report swelling of face, mouth, lips, tongue or throat; chest pain or irregular heartbeat. Report difficulty breathing or persistent cough; persistent pain in muscles, joints, or back; or other persistent adverse reactions. **Pregnancy/breast-feeding precautions:** Inform prescriber if you are or intend to become pregnant. This drug should not be used in the 2nd or 3rd trimester of pregnancy. Consult prescriber for appropriate contraceptive measures if necessary. Consult prescriber if breast-feeding.

Geriatric Considerations: Due to frequent decreases in glomerular filtration (also creatinine clearance) with aging, elderly patients may have exaggerated responses to ACE inhibitors. Differences in clinical response due to hepatic changes are not observed.

Breast-feeding Issues: The manufacturer states that after single dose studies, ramipril was not excreted in breast milk; however, since the amount excreted with daily dosing is unknown, nursing while taking ramipril is not recommended.

Pregnancy Issues: ACE inhibitors can cause fetal injury or death if taken during the 2nd or 3rd trimester. Discontinue ACE inhibitors as soon as pregnancy is detected.

Related Information

Angiotensin Agents *on page 1547*
Heart Failure *on page 1670*

Ranitidine (ra NI ti deen)

U.S. Brand Names Zantac®; Zantac® 75 [OTC]

Synonyms Ranitidine Hydrochloride

Generic Available Yes: Except effervescent granules and tablets, injection

Pharmacologic Category Histamine H_2 Antagonist

Pregnancy Risk Factor B

Lactation Enters breast milk/use caution

Use

Zantac®: Short-term and maintenance therapy of duodenal ulcer, gastric ulcer, gastroesophageal reflux, active benign ulcer, erosive esophagitis, and pathological hypersecretory conditions; as part of a multidrug regimen for *H. pylori* eradication to reduce the risk of duodenal ulcer recurrence

Zantac® 75 [OTC]: Relief of heartburn, acid indigestion, and sour stomach

Use - Unlabeled/Investigational Recurrent postoperative ulcer, upper GI bleeding, prevention of acid-aspiration pneumonitis during surgery, and prevention of stress-induced ulcers

Mechanism of Action/Effect Competitive inhibition of histamine at H_2-receptors, gastric acid secretion, gastric volume and hydrogen ion concentration are reduced

Contraindications Hypersensitivity to ranitidine or any component of the formulation

Warnings/Precautions Use with caution in patients with hepatic impairment; dosage modification required in patients with renal impairment; long-term therapy may be associated with vitamin B_{12} deficiency

Drug Interactions

Cytochrome P450 Effect: Substrate of CYP1A2, 2C19, 2D6; Inhibits CYP1A2, 2D6

Decreased Effect:

Decreased effect: Variable effects on warfarin; antacids may decrease absorption of ranitidine; ketoconazole and itraconazole absorptions are decreased; may produce altered serum levels of procainamide and ferrous sulfate; decreased effect of nondepolarizing muscle relaxants, cefpodoxime, cyanocobalamin (decreased absorption), diazepam, oxaprozin

Decreased toxicity of atropine

Increased Effect/Toxicity: Increased the effect/toxicity of cyclosporine (increased serum creatinine), gentamicin (neuromuscular blockade), glipizide, glyburide, midazolam (increased concentrations), metoprolol, pentoxifylline, phenytoin, quinidine, and triazolam.

Nutritional/Ethanol Interactions

Ethanol: Avoid ethanol (may cause gastric mucosal irritation).

Food: Does not interfere with absorption of ranitidine.

Effects on Lab Values False-positive urine protein using Multistix®, gastric acid secretion test, skin test allergen extracts, serum creatinine and serum transaminase concentrations, urine protein test

Adverse Reactions Frequency not defined (limited to important or life-threatening):

Cardiovascular: Arrhythmias, vasculitis

Central nervous system: Dizziness, hallucinations, headache, mental confusion, somnolence, vertigo

Dermatologic: Erythema multiforme, rash

Gastrointestinal: Pancreatitis

Hematologic: Acquired hemolytic anemia, agranulocytosis, aplastic anemia, granulocytopenia, leukopenia, pancytopenia, thrombocytopenia

Hepatic: Hepatic failure

Miscellaneous: Anaphylaxis, hypersensitivity reactions

Overdosage/Toxicology Symptoms of overdose include abnormal gait, hypotension, and adverse effects seen with normal use. Treatment is primarily symptomatic and supportive.

Pharmacodynamics/Kinetics

Absorption: Oral: 50%

Bioavailability: Oral: 48%

Half-Life Elimination:

Oral: Normal renal function: 2.5-3 hours; Cl_{cr} 25-35 mL/minute: 4.8 hours

I.V.: Normal renal function: 2-2.5 hours

Time to Peak: Serum: Oral: 2-3 hours; I.M.: ≤15 minutes

Metabolism: Hepatic to N-oxide, S-oxide, and N-desmethyl metabolites

Formulations

Capsule, as hydrochloride: 150 mg, 300 mg

Granules, effervescent, as hydrochloride (Zantac® EFFERdose®): 150 mg (60s) [contains sodium 7.55 mEq/packet, phenylalanine 16.84 mg/packet, and sodium benzoate]

Infusion, as hydrochloride [premixed in NaCl 0.45%; preservative free] (Zantac®): 50 mg (50 mL)

Injection, solution, as hydrochloride (Zantac®): 25 mg/mL (2 mL, 6 mL, 40 mL) [contains phenol 0.5% as preservative]

Syrup, as hydrochloride: 15 mg/mL (10 mL) [contains alcohol 7.5%; peppermint flavor]

Zantac®: 15 mg/mL (473 mL) [contains alcohol 7.5%; peppermint flavor]

Tablet, as hydrochloride: 75 mg [OTC], 150 mg, 300 mg

Zantac®: 150 mg, 300 mg

Zantac® 75: 75 mg

Tablet, effervescent, as hydrochloride (Zantac® EFFERdose®): 150 mg [contains sodium 7.96 mEq/tablet, phenylalanine 16.84 mg/tablet, and sodium benzoate]

Dosing

Adults:

Duodenal ulcer: Oral: Treatment: 150 mg twice daily, or 300 mg once daily after the evening meal or at bedtime; maintenance: 150 mg once daily at bedtime

Helicobacter pylori eradication: Oral: 150 mg twice daily; requires combination therapy

Pathological hypersecretory conditions:

Oral: 150 mg twice daily; adjust dose or frequency as clinically indicated; doses of up to 6 g/day have been used

I.V.: Continuous infusion for Zollinger-Ellison: 1 mg/kg/hour; measure gastric acid output at 4 hours, if >10 mEq or if patient is symptomatic, increase dose in increments of 0.5 mg/kg/hour; doses of up to 2.5 mg/kg/hour have been used

Gastric ulcer, benign: Oral: 150 mg twice daily; maintenance: 150 mg once daily at bedtime

Erosive esophagitis: Oral: Treatment: 150 mg 4 times/day; maintenance: 150 mg twice daily

Prevention of heartburn: Oral: Zantac®75 [OTC]: 75 mg 30-60 minutes before eating food or drinking beverages which cause heartburn; maximum: 150 mg in 24 hours; do not use for more than 14 days

Patients not able to take oral medication:

I.M.: 50 mg every 6-8 hours

I.V.: Intermittent bolus or infusion: 50 mg every 6-8 hours

Continuous I.V. infusion: 6.25 mg/hour

Elderly: Ulcer healing rates and incidence of adverse effects are similar in the elderly, when compared to younger patients; dosing adjustments not necessary based on age alone

Pediatrics:

Duodenal and gastric ulcer

Oral: Children 1 month to 16 years:

Treatment: 2-4 mg/kg/day divided twice daily; maximum treatment dose: 300 mg/day

Maintenance: 2-4 mg/kg once daily; maximum maintenance dose: 150 mg/day

I.V.: 2-4 mg/kg/day divided every 6-8 hours; maximum: 150 mg/day

GERD and erosive esophagitis: Children 1 month to 16 years:

Oral: 5-10 mg/kg/day divided twice daily; maximum: GERD: 300 mg/day, erosive esophagitis: 600 mg/day

I.V.: 2-4 mg/kg/day divided every 6-8 hours; maximum: 150 mg/day **or as an alternative**

Continuous infusion: Initial: 1 mg/kg/dose for one dose followed by infusion of 0.08-0.17 mg/kg/hour or 2-4 mg/kg/day

Prevention of heartburn: Oral: Children ≥12 years: Zantac® 75 [OTC]: 75 mg 30-60 minutes before eating food or drinking beverages which cause heartburn; maximum: 150 mg/24 hours; do not use for more than 14 days

Renal Impairment: Adults: Cl_{cr} <50 mL/minute: Administer 150 mg every 24 hours; adjust dose cautiously if needed.

Hemodialysis: Adjust dosing schedule so that dose coincides with the end of hemodialysis.

(Continued)

Ranitidine *(Continued)*

Hepatic Impairment: Patients with hepatic impairment may have minor changes in ranitidine half-life, distribution, clearance, and bioavailability; dosing adjustments are not necessary; monitor patient.

Administration

Oral: Efferdose® formulations: Dissolve each dose in 6-8 ounces of water before drinking

I.M.: No dilution is needed

I.V.:

Intermittent bolus: Dilute vials to 2.5 mg/mL; infuse at 4 mL/minute (5 minutes)

Intermittent infusion: Dilute vials to 0.5 mg/mL; infuse at 5-7 mL/minute (15-20 minutes)

Continuous I.V. infusion: Administer at 6.25 mg/hour and titrate dosage based on gastric pH by continuous infusion over 24 hours

Stability

Storage:

Injection: Vials; Store between 4°C to 30°C (39°F to 86°F); protect from light. Solution is a clear, colorless to yellow solution; slight darkening does not affect potency.

Premixed bag: Store between 2°C to 25°C (36°F to 77°F); protect from light.

Efferdose® formulations: Store between 2°C to 30°C (36°F to 86°F).

Syrup; Store between 4°C to 25°C (39°F to 77°F); protect from light.

Tablets; Store in dry place, between 15°C to 30°C (59°F to 86°F); protect from light.

Reconstitution: Vials can be mixed with NS or D_5W; solutions are stable for 48 hours at room temperature

Intermittent bolus injection: Dilute to maximum of 2.5 mg/mL

Intermittent infusion: Dilute to maximum of 0.5 mg/mL

Compatibility: Injection: Do not add other medications to premixed bag.

Stable in $D_5{}^1/_2NS$, D_5W, $D_{10}W$, fat emulsion 10%, LR, NS, sodium bicarbonate 5%

Y-site administration: Incompatible with amphotericin B cholesteryl sulfate complex, hetastarch, insulin (regular)

Compatibility in syringe: Incompatible with hydroxyzine, methotrimeprazine, midazolam, pentobarbital, phenobarbital

Compatibility when admixed: Incompatible with amphotericin B, atracurium, cefamandole, cefazolin, cefoxitin, ceftazidime, cefuroxime, ethacrynate, metaraminol, phytonadione

Monitoring Laboratory Tests AST, ALT, serum creatinine; when used to prevent stress-related GI bleeding, measure the intragastric pH and try to maintain pH >4; occult blood with GI bleeding; monitor renal function and adjust dosage as indicated.

Monitoring and Teaching Issues

Physical Assessment: See Contraindications, Warnings/Precautions, and Dosing for use cautions. Assess potential for interactions with other prescriptions, OTC medications, or herbal products patient may be taking (see Drug Interactions). Assess results of laboratory tests (see above) and patient response (see Adverse Reactions and Overdose/Toxicology). Teach patient appropriate use, possible side effects and interventions, and adverse symptoms to report (see Patient Education). Note breast-feeding caution.

Patient Education: Inform prescriber of all prescriptions, OTC medications, or herbal products you are taking, and any allergies you have. Do not take anything new without consulting prescriber. Take exactly as directed; do not increase dose - may take several days before you notice relief. Allow 1 hour between any other antacids (if approved by prescriber) and ranitidine. Avoid alcohol. Follow diet as prescriber recommends. May cause drowsiness, dizziness, or fatigue (use caution when driving or engaging in tasks requiring alertness until response to drug is known). Report chest pain or irregular heartbeat; skin rash; CNS changes (mental confusion, hallucinations, somnolence); unusual persistent weakness or lethargy; yellowing of skin or eyes; or change in color of urine or stool. Consult prescriber if breast-feeding.

Dietary Issues: Oral dosage forms may be taken with or without food.

Geriatric Considerations: H_2 blockers are the preferred drugs for treating PUD in elderly due to cost and ease of administration. These agents are no less or more effective than any other therapy. The preferred agents, due to side effects and drug interaction profile and pharmacokinetics are ranitidine, famotidine, and nizatidine. Treatment for PUD in elderly is recommended for 12 weeks since their lesions are larger; therefore, take longer to heal. Always adjust dose based upon creatinine clearance. Serum half-life is increased to 3-4 hours in elderly patients.

Related Information

Compatibility of Drugs in Syringe *on page 1566*

Ranitidine Hydrochloride *see* Ranitidine *on page 1172*

Rapamune® *see* Sirolimus *on page 1232*

Rasburicase (ras BYOOR i kayse)

U.S. Brand Names Elitek™

Generic Available No

Pharmacologic Category Enzyme; Enzyme, Urate-Oxidase (Recombinant)

Pregnancy Risk Factor C

Lactation Excretion in breast milk unknown/not recommended

Use Initial management of uric acid levels in pediatric patients with leukemia, lymphoma, and solid tumor malignancies receiving anticancer therapy expected to result in tumor lysis and elevation of plasma uric acid

Mechanism of Action/Effect Converts uric acid to allantoin (an inactive and soluble metabolite of uric acid); it does not inhibit the formation of uric acid.

Contraindications Hypersensitivity, hemolytic or methemoglobinemia reactions to rasburicase or any component of the formulation; glucose-6-phosphatase dehydrogenase (G6PD) deficiency

Warnings/Precautions Hypersensitivity reactions (including anaphylaxis), methemoglobinemia, and severe hemolysis have been reported; discontinue **immediately and permanently** in patients developing any of these reactions. Hemolysis may be associated with G6PD deficiency; patients at higher risk for G6PD deficiency should be screened prior to therapy. Enzymatic degradation of uric acid in blood samples will occur if left at room temperature; specific guidelines for the collection of plasma uric acid samples must be followed. Rasburicase is immunogenic and can elicit an antibody response; studies in healthy volunteers detected neutralizing antibodies from 1-6 weeks after exposure and lasted for up to 494 days. Safety and efficacy have been established for a single treatment course; administration of more than one course is not recommended. Administer concurrently with standard intravenous hydration therapy. Efficacy in adults has not been established. Pregnancy risk C.

Adverse Reactions As reported in patients receiving rasburicase with antitumor therapy versus active-control:

>10%:
- Central nervous system: Fever (5% to 46%), headache (26%)
- Dermatologic: Rash (13%)
- Gastrointestinal: Vomiting (50%), nausea (27%), abdominal pain (20%), constipation (20%), mucositis (2% to 15%), diarrhea (≤1% to 20%)

1% to 10%:
- Hematologic: Neutropenia with fever (4%), neutropenia (2%)
- Respiratory: Respiratory distress (3%)
- Miscellaneous: Sepsis (3%)

<1% (Limited to important or life-threatening): Anaphylaxis, convulsions, hemolysis, methemoglobinemia, pulmonary edema

Overdosage/Toxicology No cases of overdose have been reported; low or undetectable serum levels of uric acid would be expected. Treatment should be symptom-directed and supportive.

Pharmacodynamics/Kinetics

Half-Life Elimination: Elimination: Pediatric patients: 18 hours

Formulations Injection, powder for reconstitution: 1.5 mg [packaged with three 1 mL ampules of diluent]

Dosing

Adults: Refer to pediatric dosing. Insufficient data collected in adult patients to determine response to treatment.

Elderly: Refer to pediatric dosing. Insufficient data collected in geriatric patients to determine response to treatment.

Pediatrics: Management of uric acid levels: I.V.: 0.15 mg/kg or 0.2 mg/kg once daily for 5 days; begin chemotherapy 4-24 hours after the first dose

Administration

I.V.: To be given as an I.V. infusion over 30 minutes; do **not** administer as a bolus infusion. Do **not** filter during infusion. If not possible to administer through a separate line, I.V. line should be flushed with at least 15 mL saline prior to and following rasburicase infusion.

Stability

Storage: Prior to reconstitution, store with diluent at 2°C to 8°C (36°F to 46°F). Do not freeze; protect from light.

Reconstitution: Reconstitute each vial with 1 mL of the provided diluent. Mix by gently swirling; do **not** shake or vortex. Discard if discolored or containing particulate matter. Total dose should be further diluted in NS to a final volume of 50 mL. Both the reconstituted and final solution may be stored up to 24 hours at 2°C to 8°C (36°F to 46°F). Discard unused product.

Monitoring and Teaching Issues

Physical Assessment: See Contraindications, Warnings/Precautions (eg, severe hypersensitivity reactions), and Dosing for use cautions. See I.V. Administration for specifics. Patient must be observed closely for hypersensitivity reaction (which can occur within minutes of administration). Assess results of laboratory tests, therapeutic effectiveness, and adverse reactions (see Adverse Reactions and Overdose/Toxicology) prior to initiating therapy and on a regular basis throughout therapy. Teach patient possible side effects and interventions and adverse symptoms to report (see Patient Education).

Patient Education: This medication can only be administered by infusion; you will be monitored closely during and following infusion. Report immediately any pain, burning, swelling at infusion site, or any signs of allergic reaction (eg.,difficulty breathing or swallowing, back pain, chest tightness, rash, hives, swelling of lips or mouth). Report headache, nausea, or difficulty breathing.

R&C® Lice [DSC] *see* Permethrin *on page 1061*

Rebetol® *see* Ribavirin *on page 1181*

Rebetron® *see* Interferon Alfa-2b and Ribavirin *on page 722*

Rebif® *see* Interferon Beta-1a *on page 727*

Recombinant Hirudin *see* Lepirudin *on page 776*

Recombinant Human Deoxyribonuclease *see* Dornase Alfa *on page 439*

Recombinant Human Follicle Stimulating Hormone *see* Follitropins *on page 597*

Recombinant Plasminogen Activator *see* Reteplase *on page 1179*

Recombinate™ *see* Antihemophilic Factor (Recombinant) *on page 112*

Recombivax HB® *see page 1498*

Redutemp® [OTC] *see* Acetaminophen *on page 35*

ReFacto® *see* Antihemophilic Factor (Recombinant) *on page 112*

Refludan® *see* Lepirudin *on page 776*

Regitine® *see* Phentolamine *on page 1070*

Reglan® *see* Metoclopramide *on page 889*

Regonol® [DSC] *see* Pyridostigmine *on page 1154*

Regular Iletin® II *see* Insulin Preparations *on page 714*

Reguloid® [OTC] *see* Psyllium *on page 1152*

Relafen® *see* Nabumetone *on page 937*

Relefact® TRH Injection *see page 1461*

Relenza® *see* Zanamivir *on page 1418*

Relief® *see page 1509*

Relief® Ophthalmic *see* Phenylephrine *on page 1071*

Remeron® *see* Mirtazapine *on page 910*

Remeron® SolTab™ *see* Mirtazapine *on page 910*

Remicade® *see* Infliximab *on page 712*

Remifentanil *see page 1583*

Reminyl® *see* Galantamine *on page 616*

Renagel® *see* Sevelamer *on page 1225*

Renova® *see* Tretinoin (Topical) *on page 1355*

ReoPro® *see* Abciximab *on page 31*

Repaglinide (re PAG li nide)

U.S. Brand Names Prandin®

Generic Available No

Pharmacologic Category Antidiabetic Agent, Miscellaneous

Pregnancy Risk Factor C

Lactation Excretion in breast milk unknown/not recommended

Use Management of type 2 diabetes mellitus (noninsulin dependent, NIDDM)

An adjunct to diet and exercise to lower the blood glucose in patients with type 2 diabetes mellitus whose hyperglycemia cannot be controlled satisfactorily by diet and exercise alone

In combination with metformin or thiazolidinediones to lower blood glucose in patients whose hyperglycemia cannot be controlled by exercise, diet and either agent alone

Mechanism of Action/Effect Nonsulfonylurea hypoglycemic agent which blocks ATP-dependent potassium channels, depolarizing the membrane and facilitating calcium entry through calcium channels. Increased intracellular calcium stimulates insulin release from the pancreatic beta cells.

Contraindications Hypersensitivity to repaglinide or any component of the formulation; diabetic ketoacidosis, with or without coma (treat with insulin); type 1 diabetes (insulin dependent, IDDM)

Warnings/Precautions Use with caution in patients with hepatic or renal impairment. All oral hypoglycemic agents are capable of producing hypoglycemia. Proper patient selection, dosage, and instructions to the patients are important to avoid hypoglycemic episodes. It may be necessary to discontinue repaglinide and administer insulin if the patient is exposed to stress (fever, trauma, infection, surgery). Safety and efficacy have not been established in pediatric patients. Pregnancy risk C.

Drug Interactions

Cytochrome P450 Effect: Substrate of CYP2C8/9, **3A4**

Decreased Effect: Drugs which induce cytochrome P450 isoenzyme 3A4 may increase metabolism of repaglinide (phenytoin, rifampin, barbiturates, carbamazepine). Certain drugs (thiazides, diuretics, corticosteroids, phenothiazines, thyroid products, estrogens, oral contraceptives, phenytoin, nicotinic acid, sympathomimetics, calcium channel blockers, isoniazid) tend to produce hyperglycemia and may lead to loss of glycemic control.

Increased Effect/Toxicity: Agents that inhibit CYP3A4 (eg, ketoconazole, miconazole, erythromycin) may increase repaglinide concentrations. The effect of repaglinide may be potentiated when given concomitantly with other highly protein-bound drugs (ie, phenylbutazone, oral anticoagulants, hydantoins, salicylates, NSAIDs, sulfonamides). Concurrent use of other hypoglycemic agents may increase risk of hypoglycemia.

Nutritional/Ethanol Interactions

Ethanol: Avoid ethanol (may cause hypoglycemia).

Food: When given with food, the AUC of repaglinide is decreased.

Herb/Nutraceutical: St John's wort may decrease repaglinide levels. Avoid gymnema, garlic (may cause hypoglycemia).

Adverse Reactions

>10%:

Central nervous system: Headache (9% to 11%)

Endocrine & metabolic: Hypoglycemia (16% to 31%)

Respiratory: Upper respiratory tract infection (10% to 16%)

1% to 10%:

Cardiovascular: Chest pain (2% to 3%)

Gastrointestinal: Nausea (3% to 5%), heartburn (2% to 4%), vomiting (2% to 3%) constipation (2% to 3%), diarrhea (4% to 5%), tooth disorder (<1% to 2%)

Genitourinary: Urinary tract infection (2% to 3%)

Neuromuscular & skeletal: Arthralgia (3% to 6%), back pain (5% to 6%), paresthesia (2% to 3%)

Respiratory: Sinusitis (3% to 6%), rhinitis (3% to 7%), bronchitis (2% to 6%)

Miscellaneous: Allergy (1% to 2%)

<1% (Limited to important or life-threatening): Alopecia, anaphylactoid reaction, hemolytic anemia, hepatic dysfunction (severe), leukopenia, liver function tests increased, pancreatitis, Stevens-Johnson syndrome, thrombocytopenia

Overdosage/Toxicology Symptoms of severe hypoglycemia include seizures, cerebral damage, tingling of lips and tongue, nausea, yawning, confusion, agitation, tachycardia, sweating, convulsions, stupor, and coma. Management includes glucose administration (oral for milder hypoglycemia or by injection in more severe forms) and symptomatic treatment.

Pharmacodynamics/Kinetics

Absorption: Rapid and complete

Bioavailability: Mean absolute: ~56%

Half-Life Elimination: 1 hour

Time to Peak: Plasma: ~1 hour

Metabolism: Hepatic via CYP3A4 isoenzyme and glucuronidation to inactive metabolites

Onset: Single dose: Increased insulin levels: ~15-60 minutes

Duration: 4-6 hours

Formulations Tablet: 0.5 mg, 1 mg, 2 mg

Dosing

Adults & Elderly: Type 2 diabetes: Oral:

Note: Doses should be taken within 15 minutes of the meal, but time may vary from immediately preceding the meal to as long as 30 minutes before the meal

Patients not previously treated or whose Hb A_{1c} is <8%: Initial: 0.5 mg before each meal

Patients previously treated with blood glucose-lowering agents whose Hb A_{1c} is ≥8%: Initial: 1 or 2 mg before each meal.

Dose adjustment: Determine dosing adjustments by blood glucose response, usually fasting blood glucose. Double the preprandial dose up to 4 mg until satisfactory blood glucose response is achieved. At least 1 week should elapse to assess response after each dose adjustment.

Dose range: 0.5-4 mg taken with meals. Repaglinide may be dosed preprandial 2, 3 or 4 times/day in response to changes in the patient's meal pattern. Maximum recommended daily dose: 16 mg.

Note: Patients receiving other oral hypoglycemic agents: When repaglinide is used to replace therapy with other oral hypoglycemic agents, it may be started the day after the final dose is given. Observe patients carefully for hypoglycemia because of potential overlapping of drug effects. When transferred from longer half-life sulfonylureas (eg, chlorpropamide), close monitoring may be indicated for up to ≥1 week.

Note: Combination therapy: If repaglinide monotherapy does not result in adequate glycemic control, metformin or a thiazolidinedione may be added. Or, if metformin or thiazolidinedione therapy does not provide adequate control, repaglinide may be added. The starting dose and dose adjustments for combination therapy are the same as repaglinide monotherapy. Carefully adjust the dose of each drug to determine the minimal dose required to achieve the desired pharmacologic effect. Failure to do so could result in an increase in the incidence of hypoglycemic episodes. Use appropriate monitoring of FPG and Hb A_{1c} measurements to ensure that the patient is not subjected to excessive drug exposure or increased probability of secondary drug failure. If glucose is not achieved after a suitable trial of combination therapy, consider discontinuing these drugs and using insulin.

Renal Impairment:

Cl_{cr} 40-80 mL/minute (mild to moderate renal dysfunction): Initial dosage adjustment does not appear to be necessary.

Cl_{cr} 20-40 mL/minute: Initiate 0.5 mg with meals; titrate carefully.

Hepatic Impairment: Use conservative initial and maintenance doses. Use longer intervals between dosage adjustments.

Administration

Oral: Administer repaglinide 15-30 minutes before meals.

Stability

Storage: Do not store above 25°C (77°F). Protect from moisture.

Monitoring Laboratory Tests Fasting blood glucose and glycosylated hemoglobin (Hb A_{1c}) levels

Monitoring and Teaching Issues

Physical Assessment: See Contraindications, Warnings/Precautions, and Dosing for use cautions. Assess potential for interactions with other prescriptions, OTC medications, or herbal products patient may be taking (especially anything that is metabolized via the cytochrome P450 isoenzyme 3A4 route - see Drug Interactions). Assess results of laboratory tests (see above) and patient response on a regular basis throughout therapy (see Adverse Reactions and Overdose/Toxicology). Teach patient proper use (or refer patient to diabetic educator), possible side effects and appropriate interventions, and adverse symptoms to report (eg, signs of hypoglycemia - see Patient Education). **Pregnancy risk factor C** - benefits of use should outweigh possible risks (see Pregnancy Issues). Breast-feeding is not recommended.

Patient Education: Inform prescriber of all prescriptions, OTC medications, or herbal products you are taking, and any allergies you have. Do not take anything new without consulting prescriber. Take this medication exactly as directed (3-4 times a day) 15-30 minutes prior to a meal. If you skip a meal (or add an extra meal) skip (or add) a dose for that meal. Do not change dosage or discontinue without consulting prescriber. Follow dietary and lifestyle directions of prescriber or diabetic educator. Avoid alcohol. You will be instructed in signs of hypo- or hyperglycemia by prescriber or diabetic educator; be alert for adverse hypoglycemia (lightheadedness, tachycardia or palpitations, sweaty palms or profuse perspiration, yawning, tingling of lips and tongue, seizures, or change in sensorium) and follow prescriber's instructions for intervention. May cause headache or mild GI effects during first weeks of therapy (nausea, vomiting, diarrhea, constipation, heartburn), if these do not diminish, consult prescriber for approved medication. Report chest pain; difficulty breathing or symptoms of upper respiratory infection; urinary tract infection (burning or itching on urination); muscle pain or back pain; or other adverse effects. **Pregnancy/breast-feeding precautions:** Inform prescriber if you are or intend to become pregnant. Do not breast-feed.

Dietary Issues: Administer repaglinide 15-30 minutes before meals. Dietary modification based on ADA recommendations is a part of therapy. May cause hypoglycemia. Must be able to recognize symptoms of hypoglycemia (palpitations, tachycardia, sweaty palms, diaphoresis, lightheadedness).

(Continued)

Repaglinide *(Continued)*

Geriatric Considerations: Repaglinide has not been studied exclusively in the elderly; information from the manufacturer states that no differences in its effectiveness or adverse effects had been identified between persons younger than and older than 65 years of age. How "tightly" a geriatric patient's blood glucose should be controlled is controversial; however, a fasting blood glucose <150 mg/dL is now an acceptable end-point. Such a decision should be based on the patient's functional status, how well he/she recognizes hypoglycemic or hyperglycemic symptoms, and how to respond to them and their other disease states.

Breast-feeding Issues: It is not known whether repaglinide is excreted in breast milk. Because the potential for hypoglycemia in nursing infants may exist, decide whether to discontinue repaglinide or discontinue breast-feeding. If repaglinide is discontinued and if diet alone is inadequate for controlling blood glucose, consider insulin therapy.

Pregnancy Issues: Safety in pregnant women has not been established. Use during pregnancy only if clearly needed. Insulin is the drug of choice for the control of diabetes mellitus during pregnancy.

Related Information

Antidiabetic Oral Agents Comparison *on page 1556*
Diabetes Mellitus Management *on page 1661*

Repan® *see* Butalbital, Acetaminophen, and Caffeine *on page 192*

Repronex® *see* Menotropins *on page 850*

Requip® *see* Ropinirole *on page 1206*

Rescriptor® *see* Delavirdine *on page 372*

Resectisol® Irrigation Solution *see* Mannitol *on page 835*

Reserpine (re SER peen)

Generic Available Yes

Pharmacologic Category Rauwolfia Alkaloid

Pregnancy Risk Factor C

Lactation Enters breast milk/use caution

Use Management of mild to moderate hypertension

Use - Unlabeled/Investigational Management of tardive dyskinesia, schizophrenia

Mechanism of Action/Effect Reduces blood pressure via depletion of sympathetic biogenic amines (norepinephrine and dopamine); this also commonly results in sedative effects

Contraindications Hypersensitivity to reserpine or any component of the formulation; active peptic ulcer disease; ulcerative colitis; history of mental depression (especially with suicidal tendencies); MAO inhibitors

Warnings/Precautions Use extreme caution in treating patients with a history of depression; watch for signs and symptoms of depression. Discontinue at the first sign of depression. Use cautiously in patients with a history of PUD (increases GI motility and secretion) or gallstones (biliary colic may be precipitated). Preoperative withdrawal does not ensure circulatory stability. Make anesthesiologist aware of medical regimen. Avoid in severe renal impairment. Avoid use with MAO inhibitors. Pregnancy risk C.

Drug Interactions

Decreased Effect: Tricyclic antidepressants may increase antihypertensive effect.

Increased Effect/Toxicity: Reserpine may cause hypertensive reactions in patients receiving an MAO inhibitor; use an alternative antihypertensive. Reserpine may increase the effect of beta-blockers. May increase effects of CNS depressants and/or ethanol. May increase the effects/toxicity of levodopa, quinidine, procainamide, and digitalis glycosides.

Nutritional/Ethanol Interactions

Ethanol: Avoid ethanol (may increase CNS depression).

Herb/Nutraceutical: Avoid dong quai if using for hypertension (has estrogenic activity). Avoid ephedra, yohimbe (may worsen hypertension). Avoid valerian, St John's wort, kava kava, gotu kola (may increase CNS depression). Avoid garlic (may have increased antihypertensive effect).

Effects on Lab Values ↓ catecholamines (U)

Adverse Reactions Frequency not defined.

Cardiovascular: Peripheral edema, arrhythmias, bradycardia, chest pain, PVC, hypotension

Central nervous system: Dizziness, headache, nightmares, nervousness, drowsiness, fatigue, mental depression, parkinsonism, dull sensorium, syncope, paradoxical anxiety

Dermatologic: Rash, pruritus, flushing of skin

Gastrointestinal: Anorexia, diarrhea, dry mouth, nausea, vomiting, increased salivation, weight gain, increased gastric acid secretion

Genitourinary: Impotence, decreased libido

Hematologic: Thrombocytopenia purpura

Ocular: Blurred vision

Respiratory: Nasal congestion, dyspnea, epistaxis

Overdosage/Toxicology Symptoms of overdose include hypotension, bradycardia, CNS depression, sedation, coma, hypothermia, miosis, tremor, diarrhea, and vomiting. Treatment is symptom-directed and supportive. Anticholinergic agents may be useful in reducing parkinsonian effects and bradycardia.

Pharmacodynamics/Kinetics

Absorption: ~40%

Half-Life Elimination: 50-100 hours

Metabolism: Extensively hepatic (>90%)

Onset: Antihypertensive: 3-6 days

Duration: 2-6 weeks

Formulations Tablet: 0.1 mg, 0.25 mg

Dosing

Adults:

Hypertension: Oral: 0.1-0.25 mg/day in 1-2 doses; initial: 0.5 mg/day for 1-2 weeks; maintenance: reduce to 0.1-0.25 mg/day (full antihypertensive effects may take as long as 3 weeks)

Tardive dyskinesia/schizophrenia: Oral: Initial: 0.5 mg/day; usual range: 0.1-1 mg

Elderly: Oral: Initial: 0.05 mg once daily increasing by 0.05 mg every week as necessary (full antihypertensive effects may take as long as 3 weeks).

Pediatrics: Children: Hypertension: 0.01-0.02 mg/kg/24 hours divided every 12 hours; maximum dose: 0.25 mg/day (not recommended in children)

Renal Impairment:

Cl_{cr} <10 mL/minute: Avoid use.

Not removed by hemo- or peritoneal dialysis; supplemental dose is not necessary.

Stability

Storage: Protect oral dosage forms from light.

Monitoring and Teaching Issues

Physical Assessment: See Contraindications, Warnings/Precautions, and Dosing for use cautions. Assess potential for interactions with other prescriptions, OTC medications, or herbal products patient may be taking (see Drug Interactions). Assess blood pressure and cardiac status prior to starting therapy, during first doses, when changing dose, and regularly thereafter (see Adverse Reactions and Overdose/Toxicology). Teach patient proper use, possible side effects and appropriate interventions, and adverse symptoms to report (eg, signs of hypoglycemia - see Patient Education). **Pregnancy risk factor C** - benefits of use should outweigh possible risks (see Pregnancy Issues). Note breast-feeding caution.

Patient Education: Inform prescriber of all prescriptions, OTC medications, or herbal products you are taking, and any allergies you have. Do not take anything new without consulting prescriber. Take as directed; do not alter dose or discontinue without consulting prescriber. May take up to 2 weeks to see effects of therapy. Avoid alcohol and maintain recommended diet. May cause mild nervousness, dizziness, or fatigue (use caution when driving or engaging in hazardous activities until response to drug is known); orthostatic hypotension (use caution when rising from sitting or lying position or when climbing stairs until response to therapy is known): nausea or loss of appetite (small, frequent meals or sucking lozenges may help); constipation (increased exercise, fluids, fruit, or fiber, may help); nasal stuffiness (avoid OTC medications, and consult prescriber for approved medication); or impotence (will resolve when medication is discontinued). Report chest pain, rapid heartbeat, or palpitations; difficulty breathing; sudden increase in weight; swelling in ankles or hands; black tarry stools; or unusual feelings of depression. **Pregnancy/breast-feeding precautions:** Inform prescriber if you are or intend to become pregnant. Consult prescriber if breast-feeding.

Geriatric Considerations: Some studies advocate the use of reserpine because of its low cost, long half-life, and efficacy, but it is generally not considered a first-line drug. If it is to be used, doses should not exceed 0.25 mg and the patient should be monitored for depressed mood.

Additional Information Adverse effects are usually dose related, mild, and infrequent when administered for the management of hypertension.

Reserpine and Hydrochlorothiazide *see* Hydrochlorothiazide and Reserpine *on page 666*

Respa-1st® *see* Guaifenesin and Pseudoephedrine *on page 648*

Respa® DM *see* Guaifenesin and Dextromethorphan *on page 647*

Respa-GF® *see* Guaifenesin *on page 646*

Respaire®-60 SR *see* Guaifenesin and Pseudoephedrine *on page 648*

Respaire®-120 SR *see* Guaifenesin and Pseudoephedrine *on page 648*

Respbid® *see* Theophylline *on page 1300*

Restoril® *see* Temazepam *on page 1281*

Retavase® *see* Reteplase *on page 1179*

Reteplase (RE ta plase)

U.S. Brand Names Retavase®

Synonyms Recombinant Plasminogen Activator; r-PA

Generic Available No

Pharmacologic Category Thrombolytic Agent

Pregnancy Risk Factor C

Lactation Excretion in breast milk unknown/use caution

Use Management of acute myocardial infarction (AMI); improvement of ventricular function; reduction of the incidence of CHF and the reduction of mortality following AMI

Mechanism of Action/Effect Reteplase initiates local fibrinolysis by binding to fibrin in a thrombus (clot) and converting entrapped plasminogen to plasmin. Dissolution of thrombus occluding a coronary artery restores perfusion to ischemic myocardium. Reteplase is manufactured by recombinant DNA technology using *E. coli.*

Contraindications Hypersensitivity to reteplase or any component of the formulation; active internal bleeding; history of cerebrovascular accident; recent intracranial or intraspinal surgery or trauma; intracranial neoplasm, arteriovenous malformations, or aneurysm; known bleeding diathesis; severe uncontrolled hypertension

Warnings/Precautions Concurrent heparin anticoagulation can contribute to bleeding; careful attention to all potential bleeding sites. I.M. injections and nonessential handling of the patient should be avoided. Venipunctures should be performed carefully and only when necessary. If arterial puncture is necessary, use an upper extremity vessel that can be manually compressed. If serious bleeding occurs then the infusion of anistreplase and heparin should be stopped.

For the following conditions the risk of bleeding is higher with use of reteplase and should be weighed against the benefits of therapy: recent major surgery (eg, CABG, obstetrical

(Continued)

Reteplase *(Continued)*

delivery, organ biopsy, previous puncture of noncompressible vessels), cerebrovascular disease, recent gastrointestinal or genitourinary bleeding, recent trauma including CPR, hypertension (systolic BP >180 mm Hg and/or diastolic BP >110 mm Hg), high likelihood of left heart thrombus (eg, mitral stenosis with atrial fibrillation), acute pericarditis, subacute bacterial endocarditis, hemostatic defects including ones caused by severe renal or hepatic dysfunction, significant hepatic dysfunction, pregnancy, diabetic hemorrhagic retinopathy or other hemorrhagic ophthalmic conditions, septic thrombophlebitis or occluded AV cannula at seriously infected site, advanced age (eg, >75 years), patients receiving oral anticoagulants, any other condition in which bleeding constitutes a significant hazard or would be particularly difficult to manage because of location.

Coronary thrombolysis may result in reperfusion arrhythmias. Follow standard MI management. Rare anaphylactic reactions can occur. Safety and efficacy in pediatric patients have not been established.

Pregnancy risk C.

Drug Interactions

Decreased Effect: Aminocaproic acid (antifibrinolytic agent) may decrease effectiveness of thrombolytic agents.

Increased Effect/Toxicity: The risk of bleeding associated with reteplase may be increased by oral anticoagulants (warfarin), heparin, low molecular weight heparins, and drugs which affect platelet function (eg, NSAIDs, dipyridamole, ticlopidine, clopidogrel, IIb/IIIa antagonists). Concurrent use with aspirin and heparin may increase the risk of bleeding; however, aspirin and heparin were used concomitantly with reteplase in the majority of patients in clinical studies.

Adverse Reactions Bleeding is the most frequent adverse effect associated with reteplase. Heparin and aspirin have been administered concurrently with reteplase in clinical trials. The incidence of adverse events is a reflection of these combined therapies, and are comparable with comparison thrombolytics.

>10%: Local: Injection site bleeding (4.6% to 48.6%)

1% to 10%:

Gastrointestinal: Bleeding (1.8% to 9.0%)

Genitourinary: Bleeding (0.9% to 9.5%)

Hematologic: Anemia (0.9% to 2.6%)

<1% (Limited to important or life-threatening): Allergic/anaphylactoid reactions, cholesterol embolization, intracranial hemorrhage (0.8%)

Other adverse effects noted are frequently associated with myocardial infarction (and therefore may or may not be attributable to Retavase®) and include arrhythmias, arrest, cardiac reinfarction, cardiogenic shock, embolism, hypotension, pericarditis, pulmonary edema, tamponade, thrombosis

Overdosage/Toxicology Symptoms of overdose include increased incidence of intracranial bleeding. Treatment is supportive.

Pharmacodynamics/Kinetics

Half-Life Elimination: 13-16 minutes

Onset: Thrombolysis: 30-90 minutes

Formulations Injection, powder for reconstitution [preservative free]: 10.4 units [equivalent to reteplase 18.1 mg; packaged with sterile water for injection]

Dosing

Adults & Elderly: 10 units I.V. over 2 minutes, followed by a second dose 30 minutes later of 10 units I.V. over 2 minutes; withhold second dose if serious bleeding or anaphylaxis occurs.

Pediatrics: Not recommended

Administration

I.V.: Infuse over 2 minutes.

Stability

Storage: Dosage kits should be stored at 2°C to 25°C (36°F to 77°F) and remain sealed until use in order to protect from light.

Reconstitution: Reteplase should be reconstituted using the diluent, syringe, needle, and dispensing pin provided with each kit.

Monitoring and Teaching Issues

Physical Assessment: See Contraindications, Warnings/Precautions, and Dosing for use cautions. Assess potential for interactions with other prescriptions, OTC medications, or herbal products patient may be taking (especially those medications that may affect coagulation or platelet function - see Drug Interactions). See Administration specifics for infusion. Neurological status (eg, intracranial hemorrhage), vital signs, and EKG should be monitored prior to, during, and after therapy. Assess infusion site and monitor for hemorrhage during and following therapy (see Adverse Reactions and Overdose/Toxicology). Bedrest and bleeding precautions should be maintained. Avoid I.M. injections and nonessential handling of the patient. Venipunctures should be performed carefully and only when necessary. If arterial puncture is necessary, use an upper extremity vessel that can be manually compressed. Patient instructions determined by patient condition (see Patient Education). **Pregnancy risk factor C** - benefits of use should outweigh possible risks. Note breast-feeding caution.

Patient Education: Inform prescriber of all prescriptions, OTC medications, or herbal products you are taking, and any allergies you have. This medication can only be administered by infusion; you will be monitored closely during and after treatment. You will have a tendency to bleed easily; use caution to prevent injury (use electric razor, soft toothbrush, and caution with knives, needles, or anything sharp). Follow instructions for strict bedrest to reduce the risk of injury. If bleeding occurs, report immediately and apply pressure to bleeding spot until bleeding stops completely. Report unusual pain (acute headache, joint pain, chest pain); unusual bruising or bleeding; blood in urine, stool, or vomitus; bleeding gums; vision changes; or difficulty breathing. **Pregnancy/breast-feeding precautions:**

Inform prescriber if you are or intend to become pregnant. Consult prescriber if breast-feeding.

Retin-A® *see* Tretinoin (Topical) *on page 1355*
Retin-A® Micro *see* Tretinoin (Topical) *on page 1355*
Retinoic Acid *see* Tretinoin (Topical) *on page 1355*
Retrovir® *see* Zidovudine *on page 1419*
Reversol® *see* Edrophonium *on page 458*
Revex® *see* Nalmefene *on page 943*
Rēv-Eyes™ *see page 1461*
ReVia® *see* Naltrexone *on page 946*
rFSH-alpha *see* Follitropins *on page 597*
rFSH-beta *see* Follitropins *on page 597*
rFVIIa *see* Factor VIIa (Recombinant) *on page 541*
rGM-CSF *see* Sargramostim *on page 1215*
r-hCG *see* Chorionic Gonadotropin (Recombinant) *on page 285*
Rheumatrex® *see* Methotrexate *on page 874*
rhFSH-alpha *see* Follitropins *on page 597*
rhFSH-beta *see* Follitropins *on page 597*
Rhinall® Nasal [OTC] *see* Phenylephrine *on page 1071*
Rhinatate® Tablet *see page 1522*
Rhinocort® *see* Budesonide *on page 179*
Rhinocort® Aqua™ *see* Budesonide *on page 179*
Rh_o(D) Immune Globulin *see page 1498*
Rh_o(D) Immune Globulin (Intravenous-Human) *see page 1498*
RhoGAM™ *see page 1498*
***r*HuEPO-α** *see* Epoetin Alfa *on page 476*

Ribavirin (rye ba VYE rin)

U.S. Brand Names Rebetol®; Virazole®

Synonyms RTCA; Tribavirin

Generic Available No

Pharmacologic Category Antiviral Agent

Pregnancy Risk Factor X

Lactation Excretion in breast milk unknown/not recommended

Use

Inhalation: Treatment of patients with respiratory syncytial virus (RSV) infections; may also be used in other viral infections including influenza A and B and adenovirus; specially indicated for treatment of severe lower respiratory tract RSV infections in patients with an underlying compromising condition (prematurity, bronchopulmonary dysplasia and other chronic lung conditions, congenital heart disease, immunodeficiency, immunosuppression), and recent transplant recipients

Oral capsules: The combination therapy of oral ribavirin with interferon alfa-2b, recombinant (Intron® A) injection is indicated for the treatment of chronic hepatitis C in patients with compensated liver disease who have relapsed after alpha interferon therapy or were previously untreated with alpha interferons

Use - Unlabeled/Investigational Treatment of West Nile virus; hemorrhagic fever virus infections with renal syndrome (Lassa, Venezuelan, Korean hemorrhagic fever, Sabia, Argentian hemorrhagic fever, Bolivian hemorrhagic fever, Junin, Machupa)

Mechanism of Action/Effect Inhibits viral protein synthesis

Contraindications Hypersensitivity to ribavirin or any component of the formulation; women of childbearing age who will not use contraception reliably; pregnancy

Additional contraindications for oral formulation: Male partners of pregnant women; Cl_{cr}< 50 mL/minute; hemoglobinopathies (eg, thalassemia major, sickle cell anemia); as monotherapy for treatment of chronic hepatitis C; patients with autoimmune hepatitis, anemia, severe heart disease

Warnings/Precautions

Inhalation: Use with caution in patients requiring assisted ventilation because precipitation of the drug in the respiratory equipment may interfere with safe and effective patient ventilation; monitor carefully in patients with COPD and asthma for deterioration of respiratory function. Ribavirin is potentially mutagenic, tumor-promoting, and gonadotoxic. Although not reported with inhalation therapy, consider monitoring for anemia 1-2 weeks post-treatment. Pregnant healthcare workers may consider unnecessary occupational exposure; ribavirin has been detected in healthcare workers' urine. Healthcare professionals or family members who are pregnant (or may become pregnant) should be counseled about potential risks of exposure and counseled about risk reduction strategies.

Oral: Anemia has been observed in patients receiving the interferon/ribavirin combination. Severe psychiatric events have also occurred including depression and suicidal behavior during combination therapy; avoid use in patients with a psychiatric history. Hemolytic anemia is a significant toxicity; usually occurring within 1-2 weeks. Assess cardiac disease before initiation. Anemia may worsen underlying cardiac disease; use caution. If any deterioration in cardiovascular status occurs, discontinue therapy. Negative pregnancy test required before initiation and monthly thereafter. Avoid pregnancy in female patients and female partners of patients during therapy by using two effective forms of contraception; continue contraceptive measures for at least 6 months after completion of therapy. If patient or female partner becomes pregnant during treatment, she should be counseled about potential risks of exposure. Discontinue therapy in suspected/confirmed pancreatitis. Use caution in elderly patients; higher frequency of anemia; take renal function into consideration before initiating. Safety and efficacy have not been established in organ transplant patients, decompensated liver disease, concurrent hepatitis B virus or HIV exposure, or pediatric patients.

(Continued)

Ribavirin *(Continued)*

Drug Interactions

Decreased Effect: Decreased effect of zidovudine.

Increased Effect/Toxicity: Concomitant use of ribavirin and nucleoside analogues may increase the risk of developing lactic acidosis (includes adefovir, didanosine, lamivudine, stavudine, zalcitabine, zidovudine). Concurrent use with didanosine has been noted to increase the risk of pancreatitis and/or peripheral neuropathy in addition to lactic acidosis. Suspend therapy of signs/symptoms of toxicity are present.

Nutritional/Ethanol Interactions Food: Oral formulation: High-fat meal (54 g fat) increases the AUC and C_{max} by 70%.

Adverse Reactions

Inhalation:

1% to 10%:

Central nervous system: Fatigue, headache, insomnia

Gastrointestinal: Nausea, anorexia

Hematologic: Anemia

<1%: Apnea, bronchospasm, cardiac arrest, conjunctivitis, digitalis toxicity, hypotension, mild worsening of respiratory function

Note: Incidence of adverse effects (approximate) in healthcare workers: Headache (51%); conjunctivitis (32%); rhinitis, nausea, rash, dizziness, pharyngitis, and lacrimation (10% to 20%)

Oral (all adverse reactions are documented while receiving combination therapy with interferon alpha-2b):

>10%:

Central nervous system: Dizziness (17% to 26%), headache (63% to 66%)*, fatigue (60% to 70%)*, fever (32% to 41%)*, insomnia (26% to 39%), irritability (23% to 32%), depression (23% to 36%)*, emotional lability (7% to 12%)*, impaired concentration (10% to 14%)*

Dermatologic: Alopecia (27% to 32%), rash (20% to 28%), pruritus (13% to 21%)

Gastrointestinal: Nausea (38% to 47%), anorexia (21% to 27%), dyspepsia (14% to 16%), vomiting (9% to 12%)*

Hematologic: Decreased hemoglobin (25% to 36%), decreased WBC, absolute neutrophil count <0.5 x 10^9/L (5% to 11%), thrombocytopenia (6% to 14%), hyperbilirubinemia (24% to 34%), hemolysis

Neuromuscular & skeletal: Myalgia (61% to 64%)*, arthralgia (29% to 33%)*, musculoskeletal pain (20% to 28%), rigors (40% to 43%)

Respiratory: Dyspnea (17% to 19%), sinusitis (9% to 12%)*, nasal congestion

Miscellaneous: Flu-like syndrome (13% to 18%)*

*Similar to interferon alone

1% to 10%:

Cardiovascular: Chest pain (5% to 9%)*

Central nervous system: Nervousness (~5%)*

Gastrointestinal: Taste perversion (6% to 8%)

Hematologic: Hemolytic anemia (~10%)

Neuromuscular & skeletal: Weakness (9% to 10%)

*Similar to interferon alone

<1% (Limited to important or life-threatening): Diabetes mellitus, gout, hearing disorder, pancreatitis, pulmonary dysfunction, suicidal ideation, thyroid function test abnormalities, vertigo

Overdosage/Toxicology Treatment is symptom-directed and supportive. Not effectively removed by hemodialysis.

Pharmacodynamics/Kinetics

Absorption: Systemic from respiratory tract following nasal and oral inhalation; dependent upon respiratory factors and method of drug delivery; maximal absorption occurs with the use of aerosol generator via endotracheal tube; highest concentrations in respiratory tract and erythrocytes

Bioavailability: Oral: 64%

Half-Life Elimination: Plasma:

Children: 6.5-11 hours

Adults: 24 hours, significantly prolonged in the erythrocyte (16-40 days), which can be used as a marker for intracellular metabolism

Time to Peak: Serum: Inhalation: At end of inhalation period; Oral: Multiple doses: 3 hours

Metabolism: Hepatically and intracellularly; may be necessary for drug action

Formulations

Capsule (Rebetol®): 200 mg

Powder for aerosol (Virazole®): 6 g

Dosing

Adults & Elderly:

Chronic hepatitis C (in combination with interferon alfa-2b): Oral:

≤75 kg: 400 mg in the morning, then 600 mg in the evening

>75 kg: 600 mg in the morning, then 600 mg in the evening

Note: If HCV-RNA is undetectable at 24 weeks, duration of therapy is 48 weeks. In patients who relapse following interferon therapy, duration of dual therapy is 24 weeks.

Note: Also refer to Interferon Alfa-2B and Ribavirin Combination Pack monograph.

Chronic hepatitis C (in combination with peginterferon alfa-2b): Oral: 400 mg twice daily; duration of therapy is 1 year; after 24 weeks of treatment, if serum HCV-RNA is not below the limit of detection of the assay, consider discontinuation.

Pediatrics:

Infants and Children: RSV infection:

Aerosol inhalation: Use with Viratek® small particle aerosol generator (SPAG-2) at a concentration of 20 mg/mL (6 g reconstituted with 300 mL of sterile water without preservatives)

Aerosol only: 12-18 hours/day for 3 days, up to 7 days in length

Children: Chronic hepatitis C (in combination with interferon alfa-2b): Oral: **Note:** Safety and efficacy have not been established; dosing based on pharmacokinetic profile:
25-36 kg: 400 mg/day; 200 mg twice daily
37-49 kg: 600 mg/day; 200 mg in morning and 400 mg in evening
50-61 kg: 800 mg/day; 400 mg twice daily
>61 kg: Refer to adult dosing.
Note: Also refer to Interferon Alfa-2B and Ribavirin Combination Pack monograph.

Renal Impairment: Cl_{cr} <50 mL/minute: Oral is route contraindicated.

Administration

Oral: Administer concurrently with interferon alfa-2b.

Inhalation: Ribavirin should be administered in well-ventilated rooms (at least 6 air changes/hour). In mechanically-ventilated patients, ribavirin can potentially be deposited in the ventilator delivery system depending on temperature, humidity, and electrostatic forces; this deposition can lead to malfunction or obstruction of the expiratory valve, resulting in inadvertently high positive end-expiratory pressures. The use of one-way valves in the inspiratory lines, a breathing circuit filter in the expiratory line, and frequent monitoring and filter replacement have been effective in preventing these problems. Solutions in SPAG-2 unit should be discarded at least every 24 hours and when the liquid level is low before adding newly reconstituted solution. Should not be mixed with other aerosolized medication.

Stability

Storage:
Inhalation: Store vials in a dry place at 15°C to 25°C (59°F to 78°F).
Oral: Store at 15°C to 30°C (59°F to 86°F).

Reconstitution: Inhalation: Do not use any water containing an antimicrobial agent to reconstitute drug. Reconstituted solution is stable for 24 hours at room temperature.

Compatibility: Inhalation: Should not be mixed with other aerosolized medication

Monitoring Laboratory Tests

Inhalation: Respiratory function, CBC

Oral: CBC with differential (pretreatment, 2- and 4 weeks after initiation); pretreatment and monthly pregnancy test for women of childbearing age; LFTs, TSH, HCV-RNA after 24 weeks of therapy

Monitoring and Teaching Issues

Physical Assessment: See Contraindications and extensive Warnings/Precautions for use cautions. Handle with care (see Warnings/Precautions and Adverse Effects for healthcare professional's exposure risks). See Administration - Inhalation and Warnings/Precautions for use with mechanically ventilated patients. Assess results of laboratory tests (see above), respiratory status, and adverse reactions (see Adverse Reactions and Overdose/Toxicology). Teach patient proper use (according to formulation), possible side effects and appropriate interventions, and adverse symptoms to report (see Patient Education). **Pregnancy risk factor X** - determine that patient is not pregnant before beginning treatment. Do not give to women of childbearing age or males who may have intercourse with childbearing women unless both male and female are capable of complying with using two effective forms of contraception during therapy and 6 months following therapy. Breast-feeding is not recommended.

Patient Education: For oral administration, take as directed. For aerosol use, follow directions for use of aerosol device. Do not allow pregnant women or women of childbearing age to handle medication. Maintain adequate hydration (2-3 L/day of fluids) unless advised by prescriber to restrict fluids. You will need regular blood tests while taking this drug. You may experience increased susceptibility to infection (avoid crowds and exposure to infection and do not have any vaccinations without consulting prescriber). May cause confusion, impaired concentration, or headache (use cautions when driving or engaging in potentially hazardous tasks until response to drug is known); nausea, vomiting, or anorexia (small, frequent meals, frequent mouth care, chewing gum, or sucking lozenges may help); diarrhea (buttermilk, boiled milk, or yogurt may relieve diarrhea); or loss of hair (reversible). Report rash, infection (fever, chills, unusual bleeding or bruising, infection, or unhealed sores or white plaques in mouth); tingling, weakness, or pain in extremities; or other persistent adverse effects. **Pregnancy/breast-feeding precautions:** Inform prescriber if you are pregnant. Both males and females should use appropriate barrier contraceptive measures during and for 60-90 days following end of therapy. Do not allow family members or friends who are pregnant (or may become pregnant) to handle inhalation powder. This drug may cause serious fetal defects. Consult prescriber for appropriate barrier contraceptive measures. Do not donate blood during or for 6 months following therapy. Breast-feeding is not recommended.

Dietary Issues: Take oral formulation without regard to food, but always in a consistent manner with respect to food intake (ie, always take with food or always take on an empty stomach).

Pregnancy Issues: Produced significant embryocidal and/or teratogenic effects in all animal studies at ~0.01 times the maximum recommended daily human dose. Use is contraindicated in pregnancy. May cause birth defects and/or death of the exposed fetus. Avoid pregnancy during therapy and for 6 months after completion of therapy in female patients and in female partners of male patients. If pregnancy occurs during use or within 6 months after treatment, report to company (800-727-7064).

Ribavirin and Interferon Alfa-2b Combination Pack *see* Interferon Alfa-2b and Ribavirin *on page 722*

Riboflavin (RYE boe flay vin)

Synonyms Lactoflavin; Vitamin B_2; Vitamin G

Generic Available Yes

Pharmacologic Category Vitamin, Water Soluble

Pregnancy Risk Factor A/C (dose exceeding RDA recommendation)

Lactation Enters breast milk/compatible

Use Prevention of riboflavin deficiency and treatment of ariboflavinosis

(Continued)

Riboflavin *(Continued)*

Mechanism of Action/Effect Component of flavoprotein enzymes that work together, which are necessary for normal tissue respiration; also needed for activation of pyridoxine and conversion of tryptophan to niacin

Warnings/Precautions Riboflavin deficiency often occurs in the presence of other B vitamin deficiencies. Pregnancy risk A/C (dose exceeding RDA).

Drug Interactions

Decreased Effect: Decreased absorption with probenecid.

Effects on Lab Values Large doses may interfere with urinalysis based on spectrometry. May cause false elevations in fluorometric determinations of catecholamines and urobilinogen.

Adverse Reactions Frequency not defined: Genitourinary: Discoloration of urine (yellow-orange)

Pharmacodynamics/Kinetics

Absorption: Readily via GI tract, however, food increases extent; decreased with hepatitis, cirrhosis, or biliary obstruction

Half-Life Elimination: Biologic: 66-84 minutes

Metabolism: None

Formulations

Capsule: 100 mg

Tablet: 25 mg, 50 mg, 100 mg

Dosing

Adults & Elderly:

Riboflavin deficiency: Oral: 5-30 mg/day in divided doses

Recommended daily allowance: Oral: 1.2-1.7 mg

Pediatrics:

Riboflavin deficiency: Oral: Children: 2.5-10 mg/day in divided doses

Recommended daily allowance: Oral: Children: 0.4-1.8 mg

Monitoring and Teaching Issues

Physical Assessment: Assess knowledge/teach patient appropriate use, dietary instruction, possible side effects, and adverse symptoms to report (see Patient Education). **Pregnancy risk factor A/C** - see Pregnancy Risk Factor for use cautions.

Patient Education: Take with food. Large doses may cause bright yellow or orange urine.

Additional Information Dietary sources of riboflavin include liver, kidney, dairy products, green vegetables, eggs, whole grain cereals, yeast, and mushroom.

RID® Spray [OTC] *see* Permethrin *on page 1061*

Rifabutin (rif a BYOO tin)

U.S. Brand Names Mycobutin®

Synonyms Ansamycin

Generic Available No

Pharmacologic Category Antibiotic, Miscellaneous; Antitubercular Agent

Pregnancy Risk Factor B

Lactation Excretion in breast milk unknown

Use Prevention of disseminated *Mycobacterium avium* complex (MAC) in patients with advanced HIV infection; also utilized in multiple drug regimens for treatment of MAC

Mechanism of Action/Effect Inhibits DNA-dependent RNA polymerase at the beta subunit which prevents chain initiation

Contraindications Hypersensitivity to rifabutin, any other rifamycins, or any component of the formulation; rifabutin is contraindicated in patients with a WBC $<1000/mm^3$ or a platelet count $<50,000/mm^3$

Warnings/Precautions Rifabutin as a single agent must not be administered to patients with active tuberculosis since its use may lead to the development of tuberculosis that is resistant to both rifabutin and rifampin. Rifabutin should be discontinued in patients with AST >500 units/L or if total bilirubin is >3 mg/dL. Use with caution in patients with liver impairment. Modification of dosage should be considered in patients with renal impairment.

Drug Interactions

Cytochrome P450 Effect: Substrate of **CYP1A2, 3A4**; Induces **CYP3A4**

Decreased Effect: Rifabutin may decreased plasma concentrations (due to induction of liver enzymes) of verapamil, methadone, digoxin, cyclosporine, corticosteroids, oral anticoagulants, theophylline, barbiturates, chloramphenicol, itraconazole, ketoconazole, oral contraceptives, quinidine, protease inhibitors (indinavir, nelfinavir, ritonavir, saquinavir), non-nucleoside reverse transcriptase inhibitors, halothane, and clarithromycin.

Increased Effect/Toxicity: Concentrations of rifabutin are increased by indinavir (reduce rifabutin to 50% of standard dose) and ritonavir (reduce rifabutin dose to 150 mg every other day). Fluconazole increases rifabutin concentrations.

Nutritional/Ethanol Interactions Food: High-fat meal may decrease the rate but not the extent of absorption.

Adverse Reactions

>10%:

Dermatologic: Rash

Gastrointestinal: Vomiting, nausea; discoloration of feces, saliva (reddish orange)

Genitourinary: Discoloration of urine (reddish orange)

Miscellaneous: Discoloration of sputum, sweat, and/or tears (reddish orange)

1% to 10%:

Central nervous system: Headache

Gastrointestinal: Abdominal pain, diarrhea, anorexia, flatulence, eructation

Hematologic: Anemia, thrombocytopenia

<1% (Limited to important or life-threatening): Chest pain, dyspnea, leukopenia, neutropenia, uveitis

Overdosage/Toxicology Symptoms of overdose include nausea, vomiting, hepatotoxicity, lethargy, CNS disturbances, and depression. Treatment is supportive. Hemodialysis will remove rifabutin; however, its effect on outcome is unknown.

Pharmacodynamics/Kinetics

Absorption: Readily, 53%

Bioavailability: Absolute: HIV: 20%

Half-Life Elimination: Terminal: 45 hours (range: 16-69 hours)

Time to Peak: Serum: 2-4 hours

Metabolism: To active and inactive metabolites

Formulations Capsule: 150 mg

Dosing

Adults & Elderly: Disseminated MAC in advanced HIV infection:

Treatment: Oral:

Patients not receiving NNRTIs or protease inhibitors:

Initial phase: 5 mg/kg daily (maximum: 300 mg)

Second phase: 5 mg/kg daily or twice weekly

Patients receiving nelfinavir, amprenavir, indinavir: Reduce dose to 150 mg/day; no change in dose if administered twice weekly

Prophylaxis: Oral: 300 mg once daily (alone or in combination with azithromycin)

Pediatrics: Disseminated MAC in advanced HIV infection: Children >1 year:

Treatment: Oral: Patients not receiving NNRTIs or protease inhibitors:

Initial phase (2 weeks to 2 months): 10-20 mg/kg daily (maximum: 300 mg).

Second phase: 10-20 mg/kg daily (maximum: 300 mg) or twice weekly

Prophylaxis: Oral: 5 mg/kg daily; higher dosages have been used in limited trials

Renal Impairment: Cl_{cr} <30 mL/minute: Reduce dose by 50%

Administration

Oral: Rifabutin is best taken on an empty stomach but may be taken with meals to minimize nausea or vomiting.

Monitoring Laboratory Tests Periodic liver function, CBC with differential, platelet count

Monitoring and Teaching Issues

Physical Assessment: See Contraindications, Warnings/Precautions, and Dosing for use cautions. Assess potential for interactions with other prescriptions, OTC medications, or herbal products patient may be taking (see Drug Interactions). Assess results of laboratory tests (see above) and patient response (see Adverse Reactions and Overdose/Toxicology). Teach patient proper use, possible side effects and appropriate interventions, and adverse symptoms to report (see Patient Education). **Pregnancy risk factor B** - may interfere with effectiveness of oral contraceptives. Advise patient about alternative contraceptive methods. Note breast-feeding caution.

Patient Education: Inform prescriber of all prescriptions, OTC medications, or herbal products you are taking, and any allergies you have. Do not take anything new without consulting prescriber. Take as directed, with or without food. Complete full course of therapy; do not skip doses. Will discolor urine, stool, saliva, tears, sweat, and other body fluid a red-brown color. Stains on clothing or contact lenses are permanent. Report skin rash; persistent vomiting or diarrhea; fever, chills, or flu-like symptoms; dark urine or pale stools; unusual bleeding or bruising; or unusual confusion, depression, or fatigue. **Pregnancy/breast-feeding precautions:** This drug may interfere with effectiveness of oral contraceptives; consult prescriber for alternative contraceptive measures. Consult prescriber if breast-feeding.

Dietary Issues: May be taken with meals or without food or mix with applesauce.

Rifadin® *see* Rifampin *on page 1185*

Rifamate® *see* Rifampin and Isoniazid *on page 1187*

Rifampicin *see* Rifampin *on page 1185*

Rifampin (RIF am pin)

U.S. Brand Names Rifadin®; Rimactane®

Synonyms Rifampicin

Generic Available Yes

Pharmacologic Category Antibiotic, Miscellaneous; Antitubercular Agent

Pregnancy Risk Factor C

Lactation Enters breast milk/compatible

Use Management of active tuberculosis in combination with other agents; eliminate meningococci from asymptomatic carriers; prophylaxis of *Haemophilus influenzae* type b infection; used in combination with other anti-infectives in the treatment of staphylococcal infections; *Legionella* pneumonia

Mechanism of Action/Effect Inhibits bacterial RNA synthesis by binding to the beta subunit of DNA-dependent RNA polymerase, blocking RNA transcription

Contraindications Hypersensitivity to rifampin, any rifamycins, or any component of the formulation; concurrent use of amprenavir (possibly other protease inhibitors)

Warnings/Precautions Use with caution and modify dosage in patients with liver impairment. Discontinue therapy if clinical symptoms or any signs of significant hepatocellular damage develop. Use with caution in patients with porphyria. Not for use in meningococcal disease, only for short-term treatment of asymptomatic carrier states. Use with caution in patients receiving concurrent medications associated with hepatotoxicity (particularly with pyrazinamide), or in patients with a history of alcoholism (even if ethanol consumption is discontinued during therapy).

Monitor for compliance and effects including hypersensitivity, thrombocytopenia in patients on intermittent therapy. May discolor urine, feces, saliva, sweat, tears, and CSF (red/orange); remove soft contact lenses during therapy. Regimens of 600 mg once or twice weekly have been associated with a high incidence of adverse reactions including a flu-like syndrome. I.V. formulation is not intended for I.M. or S.C. administration.

Pregnancy risk C.

(Continued)

Rifampin *(Continued)*

Drug Interactions

Cytochrome P450 Effect: Substrate of **CYP2A6, 2C8/9, 3A4**; Induces **CYP1A2, 2A6, 2B6, 2C8/9, 2C19, 3A4**

Decreased Effect: Rifampin induces liver enzymes which may decrease the plasma concentration of calcium channel blockers (verapamil, diltiazem, nifedipine), methadone, digoxin, cyclosporine, corticosteroids, haloperidol, oral anticoagulants, theophylline, barbiturates, chloramphenicol, imidazole antifungals (ketoconazole), oral contraceptives, acetaminophen, benzodiazepines, hydantoins, sulfa drugs, enalapril, beta-blockers, clofibrate, dapsone, antiarrhythmics (disopyramide, mexiletine, quinidine, tocainide), doxycycline, fluoroquinolones, levothyroxine, nortriptyline, tacrolimus, zidovudine, protease inhibitors (ie, amprenavir), and non-nucleoside reverse transcriptase inhibitors.

Increased Effect/Toxicity: Rifampin levels may be increased when given with co-trimoxazole, probenecid, or ritonavir. Rifampin given with halothane or isoniazid increases the potential for hepatotoxicity. Combination therapy with rifampin and pyrazinamide has been associated with severe and fatal hepatotoxic reactions.

Nutritional/Ethanol Interactions

Ethanol: Avoid ethanol (may increase risk of hepatotoxicity).

Food: Food decreases the extent of absorption; rifampin concentrations may be decreased if taken with food.

Herb/Nutraceutical: St John's wort may decrease rifampin levels.

Effects on Lab Values Positive Coombs' reaction [direct], inhibit standard assay's ability to measure serum folate and B_{12}

Adverse Reactions

Frequency not defined:

- Cardiovascular: Flushing, edema
- Central nervous system: Headache, drowsiness, dizziness, confusion, numbness, behavioral changes, ataxia
- Dermatologic: Pruritus, urticaria, pemphigoid reaction
- Hematologic: Eosinophilia, leukopenia, hemolysis, hemolytic anemia, thrombocytopenia (especially with high-dose therapy)
- Hepatic: Hepatitis (rare)
- Neuromuscular & skeletal: Myalgia, weakness, osteomalacia
- Ocular: Visual changes, exudative conjunctivitis

1% to 10%:

- Dermatologic: Rash (1% to 5%)
- Gastrointestinal (1% to 2%): Epigastric distress, anorexia, nausea, vomiting, diarrhea, cramps, pseudomembranous colitis, pancreatitis
- Hepatic: Increased LFTs (up to 14%)

Overdosage/Toxicology Symptoms of overdose include nausea, vomiting, hepatotoxicity, lethargy, and CNS depression. Treatment is supportive. Plasma rifampin concentrations are not significantly affected by hemodialysis or peritoneal dialysis.

Pharmacodynamics/Kinetics

Absorption: Oral: Well absorbed; food may delay or slightly reduce peak

Half-Life Elimination: 3-4 hours, prolonged with hepatic impairment; End-stage renal disease: 1.8-11 hours

Time to Peak: Serum: Oral: 2-4 hours

Metabolism: Hepatic; undergoes enterohepatic recirculation

Duration: ≤24 hours

Formulations

Capsule: 150 mg, 300 mg

- Rifadin®: 150 mg, 300 mg
- Rimactane®: 300 mg

Injection, powder for reconstitution (Rifadin®): 600 mg

Dosing

Adults & Elderly:

Tuberculosis therapy: Oral, I.V.: **Note:** A four-drug regimen (isoniazid, rifampin, pyrazinamide, and either streptomycin or ethambutol) is preferred for the initial, empiric treatment of TB. When the drug susceptibility results are available, the regimen should be altered as appropriate.

- Daily therapy: 10 mg/kg/day (maximum: 600 mg/day)
- Directly observed therapy (DOT): Twice weekly: 10 mg/kg (maximum: 600 mg); 3 times/week: 10 mg/kg (maximum: 600 mg)

Tuberculosis prevention: As an alternative to isoniazid: Oral, I.V.: 10 mg/kg/day (maximum: 600 mg/day) for 2 months in combination with pyrazinamide

H. influenzae **prophylaxis:** Oral, I.V.: 600 mg every 24 hours for 4 days

Leprosy: Oral, I.V.:

- Multibacillary: 600 mg once monthly for 24 months in combination with ofloxacin and minocycline
- Paucibacillary: 600 mg once monthly for 6 months in combination with dapsone
- Single lesion: 600 mg as a single dose in combination with ofloxacin 400 mg and minocycline 100 mg

Meningococcal meningitis prophylaxis: Oral, I.V.: 600 mg every 12 hours for 2 days

Nasal carriers of *Staphylococcus aureus*: Oral, I.V.: 600 mg/day for 5-10 days in combination with other antibiotics

Synergy for *Staphylococcus aureus* infections: Oral, I.V.: 300-600 mg twice daily with other antibiotics

Pediatrics:

Tuberculosis therapy: Oral, I.V.:

Note: A four-drug regimen (isoniazid, rifampin, pyrazinamide, and either streptomycin or ethambutol) is preferred for the initial, empiric treatment of TB. When the drug susceptibility results are available, the regimen should be altered as appropriate.

Infants and Children <12 years:

Daily therapy: 10-20 mg/kg/day usually as a single dose (maximum: 600 mg/day)

Directly observed therapy (DOT): Twice weekly: 10-20 mg/kg (maximum: 600 mg); 3 times/week: 10-20 mg/kg (maximum: 600 mg)

H. influenzae **prophylaxis:** Oral, I.V.: Infants and Children: 20 mg/kg/day every 24 hours for 4 days, not to exceed 600 mg/dose

Meningococcal prophylaxis: Oral:

<1 month: 10 mg/kg/day in divided doses every 12 hours for 2 days

Infants and Children: 20 mg/kg/day in divided doses every 12 hours for 2 days

Nasal carriers of *Staphylococcus aureus*: Oral, I.V.: 15 mg/kg/day divided every 12 hours for 5-10 days in combination with other antibiotics

Renal Impairment: Plasma rifampin concentrations are not significantly affected by hemodialysis or peritoneal dialysis.

Hepatic Impairment: Dose reductions are necessary to reduce hepatotoxicity.

Administration

Oral: Should be administered 1 hour before or 2 hours after a meal on an empty stomach with a glass of water. Food may delay and reduce the amount of rifampin absorbed.

I.M.: Do not administer I.M. or S.C.

I.V.: Preferable administered at 500 mL over 3 hours. In selected situations, can be administered at 100 mL over 30 minutes.

Stability

Storage: Rifampin powder is reddish brown. Intact vials should be stored at room temperature and protected from excessive heat and light.

Reconstitution: Reconstituted vials are stable for 24 hours at room temperature. Stability of parenteral admixture at room temperature (25°C) is 4 hours in D_5W, 24 hours in NS.

Compatibility:

Y-site administration: Incompatible with diltiazem

Compatibility when admixed: Incompatible with minocycline

Monitoring Laboratory Tests Periodic monitoring of liver function (AST, ALT), CBC; sputum culture, chest x-ray 2-3 months into treatment

Monitoring and Teaching Issues

Physical Assessment: See Contraindications, Warnings/Precautions, and Dosing for use cautions. Assess potential for interactions with other prescriptions, OTC medications, or herbal products patient may be taking (see Drug Interactions). Assess results of laboratory tests (see above) and patient response (see Adverse Reactions and Overdose/Toxicology). Teach patient proper use, possible side effects and appropriate interventions, and adverse symptoms to report (see Patient Education). **Pregnancy risk factor C** - benefits of use should outweigh possible risks. **Note:** May interfere with effectiveness of oral contraceptives. Advise patient about alternative contraceptive methods while taking rifampin.

Patient Education: Inform prescriber of all prescriptions, OTC medications, or herbal products you are taking, and any allergies you have. Do not take anything new without consulting prescriber. Take as per recommended schedule; on an empty stomach, 1 hour before or 2 hours after meals. Complete full course of therapy; do not skip doses. Will discolor urine, stool, saliva, tears, sweat, and other body fluid a red-brown color. Stains on clothing or contact lenses are permanent. Report persistent vomiting or diarrhea; rash; fever, chills, or flu-like symptoms; unusual bruising or bleeding; or other persistent adverse effects. **Pregnancy/breast-feeding precautions:** Inform prescriber is you are or intend to become pregnant. This drug may interfere with effectiveness of oral contraceptives; consult prescriber for alternative contraceptive measures.

Dietary Issues: Rifampin is best taken on an empty stomach.

Geriatric Considerations: Rifampin, in combination with isoniazid, is the foundation of tuberculosis treatment. Since most older patients acquired their *Mycobacterium tuberculosis* infection before effective chemotherapy was available, either a 9-month regimen of isoniazid and rifampin or a 6-month regimen of isoniazid and rifampin with pyrazinamide (the first 2 months) should be effective.

Related Information

Tuberculosis *on page 1705*

Rifampin and Isoniazid (RIF am pin & eye soe NYE a zid)

U.S. Brand Names Rifamate®

Synonyms Isoniazid and Rifampin

Generic Available No

Pharmacologic Category Antibiotic, Miscellaneous

Pregnancy Risk Factor C

Lactation Enters breast milk/compatible

Use Management of active tuberculosis; see individual agents for additional information

Formulations Capsule: Rifampin 300 mg and isoniazid 150 mg

Dosing

Adults: Tuberculosis: Oral: 2 capsules/day

Elderly: Refer to dosing in individual monographs.

Monitoring and Teaching Issues

Physical Assessment: See individual components listed in Related Information. **Pregnancy risk factor C** - benefits of use should outweigh possible risks.

Patient Education: See individual components listed in Related Information. **Pregnancy precaution:** Inform prescriber if you are or intend to become pregnant.

Related Information

Isoniazid *on page 746*

Rifampin *on page 1185*

Rifampin, Isoniazid, and Pyrazinamide

(RIF am pin, eye soe NYE a zid, & peer a ZIN a mide)

U.S. Brand Names Rifater®

Synonyms Isoniazid, Rifampin, and Pyrazinamide; Pyrazinamide, Rifampin, and Isoniazid

Generic Available No

Pharmacologic Category Antibiotic, Miscellaneous

Pregnancy Risk Factor C

Lactation Excretion in breast milk unknown

Use Management of active tuberculosis; see individual agents for additional information

Formulations Tablet: Rifampin 120 mg, isoniazid 50 mg, and pyrazinamide 300 mg

Dosing

Adults: Tuberculosis: Oral: Patients weighing:

≤44 kg: 4 tablets

45-54 kg: 5 tablets

≥55 kg: 6 tablets

Doses should be administered in a single daily dose.

Elderly: Refer to dosing in individual monographs.

Monitoring and Teaching Issues

Physical Assessment: See individual components listed in Related Information. **Pregnancy risk factor C** - benefits of use should outweigh possible risks. Note breast-feeding caution.

Patient Education: See individual components listed in Related Information. **Pregnancy/breast-feeding precautions:** Inform prescriber if you are or intend to become pregnant. Consult prescriber if breast-feeding.

Related Information

Isoniazid *on page 746*

Pyrazinamide *on page 1153*

Rifampin *on page 1185*

Rifapentine (RIF a pen teen)

U.S. Brand Names Priftin®

Generic Available No

Pharmacologic Category Antitubercular Agent

Pregnancy Risk Factor C

Lactation Excretion in breast milk unknown/contraindicated

Use Treatment of pulmonary tuberculosis; rifapentine must always be used in conjunction with at least one other antituberculosis drug to which the isolate is susceptible; it may also be necessary to add a third agent (either streptomycin or ethambutol) until susceptibility is known.

Mechanism of Action/Effect Inhibits DNA-dependent RNA polymerase in susceptible strains of *Mycobacterium tuberculosis* (but not in mammalian cells). Rifapentine is bactericidal against both intracellular and extracellular MTB organisms. Strains which are resistant to other rifamycins including rifampin are likely to be resistant to rifapentine. Cross-resistance does not appear between rifapentine and other nonrifamycin antimycobacterial agents.

Contraindications Hypersensitivity to rifapentine, rifampin, rifabutin, any rifamycin analog, or any component of the formulation

Warnings/Precautions Compliance with dosing regimen is absolutely necessary for successful drug therapy. Patients with abnormal liver tests and/or liver disease should only be given rifapentine when absolutely necessary and under strict medical supervision. Monitoring of liver function tests should be carried out prior to therapy and then every 2-4 weeks during therapy if signs of liver disease occur or worsen, rifapentine should be discontinued. Pseudomembranous colitis has been reported to occur with various antibiotics including other rifamycins. If this is suspected, rifapentine should be stopped and the patient treated with specific and supportive treatment. Experience in treating TB in HIV-infected patients is limited.

Rifapentine may produce a red-orange discoloration of body tissues/fluids including skin, teeth, tongue, urine, feces, saliva, sputum, tears, sweat, and cerebral spinal fluid. Contact lenses may become permanently stained.

Pregnancy risk C.

Drug Interactions

Cytochrome P450 Effect: Induces **CYP2C8/9, 3A4**

Decreased Effect: Rifapentine may increase the metabolism of coadministered drugs that are metabolized by these enzymes. Enzymes are induced within 4 days after the first dose and returned to baseline 14 days after discontinuation of rifapentine. The magnitude of enzyme induction is dose and frequency dependent.

Rifampin has been shown to accelerate the metabolism and may reduce activity of the following drugs (therefore, rifapentine may also do the same): Phenytoin, disopyramide, mexiletine, quinidine, tocainide, chloramphenicol, clarithromycin, dapsone, doxycycline, fluoroquinolones, warfarin, fluconazole, itraconazole, ketoconazole, barbiturates, benzodiazepines, beta-blockers, diltiazem, nifedipine, verapamil, corticosteroids, cardiac glycoside preparations, clofibrate, oral or other systemic hormonal contraceptives, haloperidol, HIV protease inhibitors, sulfonylureas, cyclosporine, tacrolimus, levothyroxine, methadone, progestins, quinine, delavirdine, zidovudine, sildenafil, theophylline, amitriptyline, and nortriptyline.

Rifapentine should be used with extreme caution, if at all, in patients who are also taking protease inhibitors.

Patients using oral or other systemic hormonal contraceptives should be advised to change to nonhormonal methods of birth control when receiving concomitant rifapentine.

Increased Effect/Toxicity: Rifapentine metabolism is mediated by esterase activity, therefore, there is minimal potential for rifapentine metabolism to be affected by other drug therapy.

Nutritional/Ethanol Interactions Food: Food increases AUC and maximum serum concentration by 43% and 44% respectively as compared to fasting conditions.

Effects on Lab Values Rifampin has been shown to inhibit standard microbiological assays for serum folate and vitamin B_{12}. This should be considered for rifapentine; therefore, alternative assay methods should be considered.

Adverse Reactions

>10%: Endocrine & metabolic: Hyperuricemia (most likely due to pyrazinamide from initiation phase combination therapy)

1% to 10%:

Cardiovascular: Hypertension

Central nervous system: Headache, dizziness

Dermatologic: Rash, pruritus, acne

Gastrointestinal: Anorexia, nausea, vomiting, dyspepsia, diarrhea

Genitourinary: Pyuria, proteinuria, hematuria, urinary casts

Hematologic: Neutropenia, lymphopenia, anemia, leukopenia, thrombocytosis

Hepatic: Increased ALT, AST

Neuromuscular & skeletal: Arthralgia, pain

Respiratory: Hemoptysis

<1% (Limited to important or life-threatening): Aggressive reaction, arthrosis, gout, hepatitis, hyperkalemia, pancreatitis, purpura, thrombocytopenia

Overdosage/Toxicology There is no experience with treatment of acute overdose with rifapentine; experience with other rifamycins suggests that gastric lavage followed by activated charcoal may help adsorb any remaining drug from the GI tract. Hemodialysis or forced diuresis is not expected to enhance elimination of unchanged rifapentine in an overdose.

Pharmacodynamics/Kinetics

Absorption: Food increases AUC and C_{max} by 43% and 44% respectively.

Bioavailability: ~70%

Half-Life Elimination: Rifapentine: 14-17 hours; 25-desacetyl rifapentine: 13 hours

Time to Peak: Serum: 5-6 hours

Metabolism: Hepatic; hydrolyzed by an esterase and esterase enzyme to form the active metabolite 25-desacetyl rifapentine

Formulations Tablet, film coated: 150 mg

Dosing

Adults & Elderly: Note: Rifapentine should not be used alone; initial phase should include a 3- to 4-drug regimen.

Tuberculosis, intensive phase of short-term therapy: 600 mg (four 150 mg tablets) given twice weekly (at intervals not less than 72 hours); following the intensive phase, treatment should continue with rifapentine 600 mg once weekly for 4 months in combination with INH or appropriate agent for susceptible organisms.

Stability

Storage: Store at room temperature (15°C to 30°C; 59°F to 86°F). Protect from excessive heat and humidity.

Monitoring Laboratory Tests Perform baseline liver function tests at beginning of therapy. Patients with pre-existing hepatic problems should have liver function tests monitored every 2-4 weeks during therapy. Perform CBC monthly.

Monitoring and Teaching Issues

Physical Assessment: Assess for allergy history related to other antitubercular medications before beginning therapy. See Contraindications, Warnings/Precautions, and Dosing for use cautions. Assess potential for interactions with other prescriptions, OTC medications, or herbal products patient may be taking (see Drug Interactions). Assess results of laboratory tests (see above) and patient response (see Adverse Reactions and Overdose/Toxicology) periodically throughout therapy. Teach patient proper use, possible side effects and appropriate interventions, and adverse symptoms to report (see Patient Education). **Pregnancy risk factor C** - benefits of use should outweigh possible risks (see Pregnancy Issues). **Note:** May interfere with effectiveness of oral contraceptives. Advise patient about alternative contraceptive methods. Breast-feeding is contraindicated.

Patient Education: Inform prescriber of all prescriptions, OTC medications, or herbal products you are taking, and any allergies you have. Do not take anything new without consulting prescriber. Take as per recommended schedule; preferably on an empty stomach, 1 hour before or 2 hours after meals. Complete full course of therapy; do not skip doses. Will discolor urine, stool, saliva, tears, sweat, and other body fluid a red-brown color. Stains on clothing or contact lenses are permanent. Report changes in urinary pattern or pain on urination; vomiting; fever, chills, or flu-like symptoms; muscle weakness or unusual fatigue; dark urine, pale stools, or unusual bleeding or bruising; yellowing skin or eyes; skin rash; swelling of extremities; chest pain or palpitations; or persistent GI upset. **Pregnancy/breast-feeding precautions:** Inform prescriber is you are or intend to become pregnant. This drug may interfere with effectiveness of oral contraceptives; consult prescriber for alternative contraceptive measures. Do not breast-feed.

Breast-feeding Issues: May discolor breast milk

Pregnancy Issues: Has been shown to be teratogenic in rats and rabbits. Rat offspring showed cleft palates, right aortic arch, and delayed ossification and increased number of ribs. Rabbits displayed ovarian agenesis, pes varus, arhinia, microphthalmia, and irregularities of the ossified facial tissues. Rat studies also show decreased fetal weight, increased number of stillborns, and decreased gestational survival. No adequate well-controlled studies in pregnant women are available. Rifapentine should be used during pregnancy only if the potential benefit justifies the potential risk to the fetus.

Additional Information Rifapentine has only been studied in patients with tuberculosis receiving a 6-month short-course intensive regimen approval. Outcomes have been based on 6-month follow-up treatment observed in clinical trial 008 as a surrogate for the 2-year

(Continued)

Rifapentine *(Continued)*

follow-up generally accepted as evidence for efficacy in the treatment of pulmonary tuberculosis.

Rifater® *see* Rifampin, Isoniazid, and Pyrazinamide *on page 1188*

rIFN-A *see* Interferon Alfa-2a *on page 717*

rIFN beta-1a *see* Interferon Beta-1a *on page 727*

rIFN beta-1b *see* Interferon Beta-1b *on page 729*

Rilutek® *see* Riluzole *on page 1190*

Riluzole (RIL yoo zole)

U.S. Brand Names Rilutek®

Synonyms 2-Amino-6-Trifluoromethoxy-benzothiazole; RP54274

Generic Available No

Pharmacologic Category Glutamate Inhibitor

Pregnancy Risk Factor C

Lactation Excretion in breast milk unknown

Use Orphan drug: Treatment of amyotrophic lateral sclerosis (ALS); riluzole can extend survival or time to tracheostomy

Mechanism of Action/Effect Inhibitory effect on glutamate release, inactivation of voltage-dependent sodium channels; and ability to interfere with intracellular events that follow transmitter binding at excitatory amino acid receptors

Contraindications Severe hypersensitivity reactions to riluzole or any component of the formulation

Warnings/Precautions Among 4000 patients given riluzole for ALS, there were 3 cases of marked neutropenia (ANC <500/mm^3), all seen within the first 2 months of treatment. Use with caution in patients with concomitant renal insufficiency. Use with caution in patients with current evidence or history of abnormal liver function. Monitor liver chemistries. Pregnancy risk C.

Drug Interactions

Cytochrome P450 Effect: Substrate of **CYP1A2**

Decreased Effect: Drugs that induce CYP1A2 (eg, cigarette smoke, charbroiled food, rifampin, omeprazole) could increase the rate of riluzole elimination.

Increased Effect/Toxicity: Inhibitors of CYP1A2 (eg, caffeine, theophylline, amitriptyline, quinolones) could decrease the rate of riluzole elimination resulting in accumulation of riluzole.

Nutritional/Ethanol Interactions

Ethanol: Avoid ethanol (due to CNS depression).

Food: A high-fat meal decreases absorption of riluzole (decreasing AUC by 20% and peak blood levels by 45%).

Adverse Reactions

>10%:

Gastrointestinal: Nausea (10% to 21%)

Neuromuscular & skeletal: Weakness (15% to 20%)

Respiratory: Decreased lung function (10% to 16%)

1% to 10%:

Cardiovascular: Hypertension, tachycardia, postural hypotension, edema

Central nervous system: headache, dizziness, somnolence, insomnia, malaise, depression, vertigo, agitation, tremor, circumoral paresthesia

Dermatologic: Pruritus, eczema, alopecia

Gastrointestinal: Abdominal pain, diarrhea, anorexia, dyspepsia, vomiting, stomatitis

Neuromuscular & skeletal: Arthralgia, back pain

Respiratory: Rhinitis, increased cough

Miscellaneous: Aggravation reaction

<1% (Limited to important or life-threatening): Exfoliative dermatitis, neutropenia, seizures

Overdosage/Toxicology No specific antidote or treatment information is available. Treatment should be supportive and directed toward alleviating symptoms.

Pharmacodynamics/Kinetics

Absorption: 90%; high fat meal decreases AUC by 20%, peak blood levels by 45%

Bioavailability: Oral: Absolute: 50%

Half-Life Elimination: 12 hours

Metabolism: Extensively hepatic to six major and a number of minor metabolites via CYP1A2 dependent hydroxylation and glucuronidation

Formulations Tablet: 50 mg

Dosing

Adults & Elderly:

ALS treatment: Oral: 50 mg every 12 hours; no increased benefit can be expected from higher daily doses, but adverse events are increased.

Dosage adjustment in smoking: Cigarette smoking is known to induce CYP1A2; patients who smoke cigarettes would be expected to eliminate riluzole faster. There is no information, however, on the effect of, or need for, dosage adjustment in these patients.

Dosage adjustment in special populations: Females and Japanese patients may possess a lower metabolic capacity to eliminate riluzole compared with male and Caucasian subjects, respectively.

Renal Impairment: Use with caution in patients with concomitant renal insufficiency.

Hepatic Impairment: Use with caution in patients with current evidence or history of abnormal liver function indicated by significant abnormalities in serum transaminase, bilirubin or GGT levels. Baseline elevations of several LFTs (especially elevated bilirubin) should preclude use of riluzole.

Stability

Storage: Protect from bright light.

Monitoring Laboratory Tests Monitor serum aminotransferases including ALT levels before and during therapy. Evaluate serum ALT levels every month during the first 3 months of therapy, every 3 months during the remainder of the first year and periodically thereafter. Evaluate ALT levels more frequently in patients who develop elevations. Maximum increases in serum ALT usually occurred within 3 months after the start of therapy and were usually transient when <5 x ULN.

In trials, if ALT levels were <5 x ULN, treatment continued and ALT levels usually returned to below 2 x ULN within 2-6 months. Treatment in studies was discontinued, however, if ALT levels exceed 5 x ULN, so that there is no experience with continued treatment of ALS patients once ALT values exceed 5 x ULN.

If a decision is made to continue treatment in patients when the ALT exceeds 5 x ULN, frequent monitoring (at least weekly) of complete liver function is recommended. Discontinue treatment if ALT exceeds 10 x ULN or if clinical jaundice develops.

Monitoring and Teaching Issues

Physical Assessment: Assess effectiveness and interactions of other medications patient may be taking (see Drug Interactions and Dosing). Monitor laboratory tests (see above), therapeutic response, and adverse reactions at beginning of therapy and periodically throughout therapy (see Warnings/Precautions, Adverse Reactions, and Overdose/Toxicology). Assess knowledge/teach patient appropriate use, interventions to reduce side effects, and adverse symptoms to report (see Patient Education). **Pregnancy risk factor C** - benefits of use should outweigh possible risks. Note breast-feeding caution.

Patient Education: This drug will not cure or stop disease but it may slow progression. Take as directed, at the same time each day, preferably on an empty stomach, 1 hour before or 2 hours after meals. Avoid alcohol. You may experience increased spasticity, dizziness or sleepiness; use caution when driving or engaging in tasks requiring alertness until response to drug is known. Small frequent meals, frequent mouth care, chewing gum, or sucking lozenges may reduce nausea, vomiting, or anorexia. Report fever; severe vomiting, diarrhea, or constipation; change in color of urine or stool; yellowing of skin or eyes; acute back pain or muscle pain; or worsening of condition. **Pregnancy/breast-feeding precautions:** Inform prescriber if you are or intend to become pregnant. Consult prescriber if breast-feeding.

Geriatric Considerations: In clinical trials, no difference was demonstrated between elderly and younger adults. However, renal changes with age can be expected to result in higher serum concentrations of the parent drug and its metabolites.

Additional Information May be obtained through Rhone-Poulenc Rorer Inc (Collegeville, PA) for compassionate use (through treatment IND process) by calling 800-727-6737 for treatment of amyotrophic lateral sclerosis. May be more effective for amyotrophic lateral sclerosis of bulbar onset. In animal models, riluzole was a potent inhibitor of seizures induced by ouabain.

Rimactane® *see* Rifampin *on page 1185*

Rimantadine (ri MAN ta deen)

U.S. Brand Names Flumadine®

Synonyms Rimantadine Hydrochloride

Generic Available Yes: Tablet

Pharmacologic Category Antiviral Agent

Pregnancy Risk Factor C

Lactation Enters breast milk/contraindicated

Use Prophylaxis (adults and children >1 year of age) and treatment (adults) of influenza A viral infection

Mechanism of Action/Effect Exerts its inhibitory effect on three antigenic subtypes of influenza A virus (H1N1, H2N2, H3N2) early in the viral replicative cycle, possibly inhibiting the uncoating process; it has no activity against influenza B virus and is two- to eightfold more active than amantadine

Contraindications Hypersensitivity to drugs of the adamantine class, including rimantadine and amantadine, or any component of the formulation

Warnings/Precautions Use with caution in patients with renal and hepatic dysfunction. Avoid use, if possible, in patients with recurrent and eczematoid dermatitis, uncontrolled psychosis, or severe psychoneurosis. An increase in seizure incidence may occur in patients with seizure disorders. Discontinue drug if seizures occur. Consider the development of resistance during rimantadine treatment of the index case as likely if failure of rimantadine prophylaxis among family contact occurs and if index case is a child. Viruses exhibit cross-resistance between amantadine and rimantadine. Pregnancy risk C.

Drug Interactions

Decreased Effect: Acetaminophen may cause a small reduction in AUC and peak concentration of rimantadine. Peak plasma and AUC concentrations of rimantadine are slightly reduced by aspirin.

Increased Effect/Toxicity: Cimetidine increases blood levels/toxicity of rimantadine.

Nutritional/Ethanol Interactions Food: Food does not affect rate or extent of absorption

Adverse Reactions 1% to 10%:

Cardiovascular: Orthostatic hypotension, edema

Central nervous system: Dizziness (2%), confusion, headache (1%), insomnia (2%), difficulty in concentrating, anxiety (1%), restlessness, irritability, hallucinations; incidence of CNS side effects may be less than that associated with amantadine

Gastrointestinal: Nausea (3%), vomiting (2%), xerostomia (2%), abdominal pain (1%), anorexia (2%)

Genitourinary: Urinary retention

Overdosage/Toxicology Agitation, hallucinations, ventricular cardiac arrhythmias (torsade de pointes and PVCs), slurred speech, anticholinergic effects (dry mouth, urinary retention and mydriasis), ataxia, tremor, myoclonus, seizures, and death have been reported with

(Continued)

Rimantadine *(Continued)*

amantadine, a related drug. Treatment is symptomatic (do not use physostigmine). Tachyarrhythmias may be treated with beta-blockers such as propranolol. Dialysis is not recommended except possibly in renal failure.

Pharmacodynamics/Kinetics

Absorption: Tablets and syrup formulations are equally absorbed

Half-Life Elimination: 25.4 hours; prolonged with elderly

Time to Peak: 6 hours

Metabolism: Extensively hepatic

Onset: Antiviral activity: No data exist establishing a correlation between plasma concentration and antiviral effect

Formulations

Syrup, as hydrochloride: 50 mg/5 mL (240 mL) [raspberry flavor]
Tablet, as hydrochloride: 100 mg

Dosing

Adults:

Prophylaxis of influenza A: Oral: 100 mg twice daily
Treatment of influenza A: Oral: 100 mg twice daily

Elderly: Prophylaxis and treatment: Oral: Decrease to 100 mg/day in elderly patients (see Geriatric Considerations).

Pediatrics:

Prophylaxis of influenza A: Oral:
Children <10 years: 5 mg/kg once daily; maximum: 150 mg
Children >10 years: Refer to adult dosing.

Renal Impairment: Cl_{cr} ≤10 mL/minute: Administer 50% of normal dose.

Hepatic Impairment: Administer 50% normal dose with severe hepatic impairment.

Administration

Oral: Initiation of rimantadine within 48 hours of the onset of influenza A illness halves the duration of illness and significantly reduces the duration of viral shedding and increased peripheral airways resistance. Continue therapy for 5-7 days after symptoms begin.

Monitoring and Teaching Issues

Physical Assessment: See Contraindications, Warnings/Precautions, and Drug Interactions for use cautions. Assess therapeutic effectiveness and adverse reactions (see Adverse Reactions and Overdose/Toxicology). Teach patient appropriate use, possible side effects/interventions (eg, postural hypotension), and adverse symptoms to report (see Patient Education). **Pregnancy risk factor C** - benefits of use should outweigh possible risks. Breast-feeding is contraindicated.

Patient Education: Inform prescriber of all prescriptions, OTC medications, or herbal products you are taking, and any allergies you have. Do not take anything new during treatment unless approved by prescriber. Take as directed. Complete full course of therapy even if feeling better. Take a missed dose as soon as possible. If almost time for next dose, skip the missed dose and return to your regular schedule. Do not take a double dose. May cause orthostatic hypotension (use caution when changing position (rising from sitting or lying) or climbing stairs until response is known). Report CNS changes (eg, confusion, insomnia, anxiety, restlessness, irritability, hallucinations); difficulty urinating; or severe nausea or vomiting. **Pregnancy/breast-feeding precautions:** Inform prescriber if you are or intend to become pregnant. Do not breast-feed.

Geriatric Considerations: Adverse CNS and GI effects occur frequently if dosage is not adjusted. Monitor GI effects in the elderly or patients with renal or hepatic impairment. Dosing must be individualized (100 mg 1-2 times/day). It is recommended that nursing home patients receive 100 mg/day (see Pharmacodynamics/Kinetics).

Breast-feeding Issues: Use in nursing mothers due to potential adverse effect in infants; rimantadine is concentrated in milk.

Pregnancy Issues: Embryotoxic in high dose rat studies.

Rimantadine Hydrochloride *see* Rimantadine *on page 1191*
Rimexolone *see page 1509*
Rimso®-50 *see* Dimethyl Sulfoxide *on page 420*
Riopan® [OTC] *see* Magaldrate *on page 830*
Riopan Plus® [OTC] *see* Magaldrate and Simethicone *on page 831*
Riopan Plus® Double Strength [OTC] *see* Magaldrate and Simethicone *on page 831*

Risedronate (ris ED roe nate)

U.S. Brand Names Actonel®

Synonyms Risedronate Sodium

Generic Available No

Pharmacologic Category Bisphosphonate Derivative

Pregnancy Risk Factor C

Lactation Excretion in breast milk unknown/not recommended

Use Paget's disease of the bone; treatment and prevention of glucocorticoid-induced osteoporosis; treatment and prevention of osteoporosis in postmenopausal women

Mechanism of Action/Effect A bisphosphonate which inhibits bone resorption via actions on osteoclasts or on osteoclast precursors; decreases the rate of bone resorption direction, leading to an indirect decrease in bone formation

Contraindications Hypersensitivity to risedronate, bisphosphonates, or any component of the formulation; hypocalcemia; abnormalities of the esophagus which delay esophageal emptying such as stricture or achalasia; inability to stand or sit upright for at least 30 minutes; severe renal impairment (Cl_{cr} <30 mL/minute)

Warnings/Precautions Bisphosphonates may cause upper gastrointestinal disorders such as dysphagia, esophageal ulcer, and gastric ulcer. Use caution in patients with renal impairment; hypocalcemia must be corrected before therapy initiation with alendronate; ensure adequate calcium and vitamin D intake, especially for patients with Paget's disease in whom the pretreatment rate of bone turnover may be greatly elevated. Pregnancy risk C.

Drug Interactions

Decreased Effect: Calcium supplements and antacids interfere with absorption of risedronate (take at a different time of the day than risedronate).

Nutritional/Ethanol Interactions Food: Food may reduce absorption (similar to other bisphosphonates); mean oral bioavailability is decreased when given with food.

Adverse Reactions

Seen in patients taking 30 mg/day for Paget's disease:

>10%:

- Central nervous system: Headache (18%)
- Dermatologic: Rash (11%)
- Gastrointestinal: Diarrhea (20%), abdominal pain (11%)
- Neuromuscular & skeletal: Arthralgia (33%)
- Miscellaneous: Flu-like syndrome (10%)

1% to 10%:

- Cardiovascular: Peripheral edema (8%)
- Central nervous system: Chest pain (7%), dizziness (7%)
- Gastrointestinal: Nausea (10%), constipation (7%), belching (3%), colitis (3%, placebo 3%)
- Neuromuscular & skeletal: Weakness (5%), bone pain (5%, placebo 5%), leg cramps (3%, placebo 3%), myasthenia (3%)
- Ocular: Amblyopia (3%, placebo 3%), dry eye (3%)
- Otic: Tinnitus (3%, placebo 3%)
- Respiratory: Sinusitis (5%), bronchitis (3%, placebo 5%) <1%: Acute iritis
- Miscellaneous: Neoplasm (3%)

Events observed in patients taking 5 mg/day for osteoporosis were similar to those seen with placebo

Overdosage/Toxicology Symptoms of overdose include hypocalcemia, hypophosphatemia, and upper GI adverse events (upset stomach, heartburn, esophagitis, gastritis, or ulcer). Gastric lavage may remove unabsorbed drug. Treat with milk or antacids to bind risedronate; dialysis would not be beneficial.

Pharmacodynamics/Kinetics

Absorption: Rapid

Bioavailability: Poor, ~0.54% to 0.75%

Half-Life Elimination: Terminal: 480 hours

Metabolism: None

Onset: May require weeks

Formulations Tablet, as sodium: 5 mg, 30 mg, 35 mg

Dosing

Adults:

Paget's disease of bone: Oral: 30 mg once daily for 2 months

Retreatment may be considered (following post-treatment observation of at least 2 months) if relapse occurs, or if treatment fails to normalize serum alkaline phosphatase. For retreatment, the dose and duration of therapy are the same as for initial treatment. No data are available on more than one course of retreatment.

Osteoporosis (postmenopausal) prevention and treatment: Oral: 5 mg once daily; efficacy for use longer than 1 year has not been established; **alternatively,** a dose of 35 mg once weekly has been demonstrated to be effective

Osteoporosis (glucocorticoid-induced) prevention and treatment: Oral: 5 mg once daily

Note: Risedronate should be taken at least 30 minutes before the first food or drink of the day other than water. Patients should receive supplemental calcium and vitamin D if dietary intake is inadequate.

Elderly: Dosage adjustment is not necessary in patients with Cl_{cr} ≥30 mL/minute.

Renal Impairment: Cl_{cr} <30 mL/minute: Not recommended

Administration

Oral: Risedronate should be administered 30 or more minutes before the first food or drink of the day other than water. Risedronate should be taken in an upright position with a full glass (6-8 oz) of plain water and the patient should avoid lying down for 30 minutes to minimize the possibility of GI side effects.

Stability

Storage: Store at room temperature of 20°C to 25°C (68°F to 77°F).

Monitoring Laboratory Tests Alkaline phosphatase should be periodically measured; serum calcium, phosphorus, and possibly potassium due to its drug class. Use of absorptiometry may assist in noting benefit in osteoporosis.

Monitoring and Teaching Issues

Physical Assessment: See Contraindications and Warnings/Precautions for use cautions. Assess results of laboratory tests (see above), effectiveness of treatment, and development of adverse reactions. Teach appropriate use and administration of medication (see Administration), lifestyle and dietary changes that will have a beneficial impact on Paget's disease or osteoporosis, possible side effects and interventions, and adverse reactions to report. **Pregnancy risk factor C** - benefits of use should outweigh risks. Breast-feeding is not recommended.

Patient Education: Inform prescriber of all prescriptions, OTC medications, or herbal products you are taking, and any allergies you have. Do not take anything new during treatment unless approved by prescriber. In order to be effective, this medication must be taken exactly as directed, with a full glass of water first thing in the morning, at least 30 minutes before the first food or beverage of the day. Wait at least 30 minutes after taking this medication before taking anything else. Stay in sitting or standing position for 30 minutes following administration and until after the first food of the day to reduce potential for esophageal irritation. Consult prescriber to determine necessity of lifestyle changes (eg, decreased smoking, decreased alcohol intake, dietary supplements of calcium, or increased dietary vitamin D). May cause GI upset (eg, flatulence, bloating, nausea, acid

(Continued)

Risedronate *(Continued)*

regurgitation); small, frequent meals may help. Report unresolved muscle or bone pain or leg cramps; acute abdominal pain; chest pain, palpitations, or swollen extremities; disturbed vision or excessively dry eyes; ringing in the ears; or persistent flu-like symptoms. Also notify prescriber at once if experiencing difficulty swallowing, pain when swallowing, or severe or persistent heartburn. **Pregnancy/breast-feeding precautions:** Inform prescriber if you are or intend to become pregnant. Breast-feeding is recommended.

Dietary Issues: Take ≥30 minutes before the first food or drink of the day other than water.

Risedronate Sodium *see* Risedronate *on page 1192*

Risperdal® *see* Risperidone *on page 1194*

Risperdal Consta™ [Investigational] *see* Risperidone *on page 1194*

Risperidone (ris PER i done)

U.S. Brand Names Risperdal®; Risperdal Consta™ [Investigational]

Generic Available No

Pharmacologic Category Antipsychotic Agent, Benzisoxazole

Pregnancy Risk Factor C

Lactation Enters breast milk/contraindicated

Use Management of psychotic disorders (eg, schizophrenia)

Use - Unlabeled/Investigational Behavioral symptoms associated with dementia in elderly; treatment of bipolar disorder, mania, Tourette's disorder; treatment of pervasive developmental disorder and autism in children and adolescents

Mechanism of Action/Effect Risperidone is a benzisoxazole derivative, mixed serotonin-dopamine antagonist; binds to 5-HT_2-receptors in the CNS and in the periphery with a very high affinity; binds to dopamine-D_2 receptors with less affinity. The binding affinity to the dopamine-D_2 receptor is 20 times lower than the 5-HT_2 affinity. The addition of serotonin antagonism to dopamine antagonism (classic neuroleptic mechanism) is thought to improve negative symptoms of psychoses and reduce the incidence of extrapyramidal side effects. Alpha$_1$, alpha$_2$ adrenergic, and histaminergic receptors are also antagonized with high affinity. Risperidone has low to moderate affinity for 5-HT_{1C}, 5-HT_{1D}, and 5-HT_{1A} receptors, weak affinity for D_1 and no affinity for muscarinics or beta$_1$ and beta$_2$ receptors

Contraindications Hypersensitivity to risperidone or any component of the formulation

Warnings/Precautions Low to moderately sedating, use with caution in disorders where CNS depression is a feature. Use with caution in Parkinson's disease. Use with caution in patients with hemodynamic instability; bone marrow suppression; predisposition to seizures; subcortical brain damage; or severe cardiac, hepatic, renal, or respiratory disease. Neuroleptics may cause swallowing difficulties, caution in patients predisposed to aspiration. Use with caution in breast cancer or other prolactin-dependent tumors (may elevate prolactin levels). May alter temperature regulation or mask toxicity of other drugs due to antiemetic effects. May alter cardiac conduction (low risk relative to other neuroleptics) - life-threatening arrhythmias have occurred with therapeutic doses of neuroleptics.

Risperidone has a low potential for anticholinergic effects, but should be used with caution in patients with decreased gastrointestinal motility, urinary retention, BPH, xerostomia, visual problems, narrow-angle glaucoma (screening is recommended), and myasthenia gravis.

May cause extrapyramidal symptoms including pseudoparkinsonism, acute dystonic reactions, akathisia, and tardive dyskinesia (risk of these reactions is dose dependent and low relative to other neuroleptics). May be associated with neuroleptic malignant syndrome (NMS). May rarely cause hyperglycemia - use with caution in patients with diabetes or other disorders of glucose regulation.

Pregnancy risk C.

Drug Interactions

Cytochrome P450 Effect: Substrate of **CYP2D6**, 3A4; Inhibits CYP2D6, 3A4

Decreased Effect: Risperidone may antagonize effects of levodopa. Carbamazepine decreases risperidone serum concentrations.

Increased Effect/Toxicity: Risperidone may enhance the hypotensive effects of antihypertensive agents. Clozapine decreases clearance of risperidone. Metoclopramide may increase risk of extrapyramidal symptoms (EPS).

Nutritional/Ethanol Interactions

Ethanol: Avoid ethanol (may increase CNS depression).

Food: Risperidone serum concentration may be increased if taken with grapefruit juice.

Herb/Nutraceutical: Avoid kava kava, gotu kola, valerian, St John's wort (may increase CNS depression).

Adverse Reactions

Frequency not defined: Gastrointestinal: Dysphagia, esophageal dysmotility

>10%: Central nervous system: Insomnia, agitation, anxiety, headache

1% to 10%:

Cardiovascular: Hypotension (especially orthostatic), tachycardia

Central nervous system: Sedation, dizziness, restlessness, extrapyramidal reactions (dose dependent), dystonic reactions, pseudoparkinson, tardive dyskinesia, neuroleptic malignant syndrome, altered central temperature regulation

Dermatologic: Photosensitivity (rare), rash, dry skin

Endocrine & metabolic: Amenorrhea, galactorrhea, gynecomastia, sexual dysfunction

Gastrointestinal: Constipation, GI upset, xerostomia, dyspepsia, vomiting, abdominal pain, nausea, anorexia, weight gain

Genitourinary: Polyuria

Ocular: Abnormal vision

Respiratory: Rhinitis, coughing, sinusitis, pharyngitis, dyspnea

<1% (Limited to important or life-threatening): Diabetes mellitus, hyperglycemia

Pharmacodynamics/Kinetics

Absorption: Rapid and well absorbed; food does not affect either rate or extent

Bioavailability: Tablet: 70%; Solution: 74.5%

Half-Life Elimination: 20 hours (risperidone and its active metabolite 9-hydroxyrisperidone)

Time to Peak: Plasma:

Risperidone: Within 1 hour

9-hydroxyrisperidone: Extensive metabolizers: 3 hours; Poor metabolizers: 17 hours

Metabolism: Extensively hepatic via CYP2D6 to 9-hydroxyrisperidone (equi-effective with risperidone); *N*-dealkylation is a second minor pathway

Formulations

Injection, microspheres for reconstitution, extended release (Risperdal Consta™): 25 mg, 37.5 mg, 50 mg [currently investigational, not commercially available]

Solution, oral: 1 mg/mL (30 mL) [contains benzoic acid]

Tablet: 0.25 mg, 0.5 mg, 1 mg, 2 mg, 3 mg, 4 mg

Dosing

Adults: Psychosis: Recommended starting dose: 0.5-1 mg twice daily; slowly increase to the optimum range of 3-6 mg/day; may be given as a single daily dose once maintenance dose is achieved; daily dosages >10 mg does not appear to confer any additional benefit, and the incidence of extrapyramidal symptoms is higher than with lower doses

Elderly: In elderly patients, a starting dose of 0.5 mg twice daily is recommended, and titration should progress slowly. Additional monitoring of renal function and orthostatic blood pressure may be warranted. If once-a-day dosing in the elderly or debilitated patient is considered, a twice daily regimen should be used to titrate to the target dose, and this dose should be maintained for 2-3 days prior to attempts to switch to a once-daily regimen.

Pediatrics: Children and Adolescents:

Autism (unlabeled use): Oral: Initial: 0.25 mg at bedtime; titrate to 1 mg/day (0.1 mg/kg/day)

Bipolar disorder (unlabeled use): Oral: Initial: 0.5 mg; titrate to 0.5-3 mg/day

Pervasive developmental disorder (unlabeled use): Oral: Initial: 0.25 mg twice daily; titrate up 0.25 mg/day every 5-7 days; optimal dose range: 0.75-3 mg/day

Schizophrenia: Oral: Initial: 0.5 mg twice daily; titrate as necessary up to 2-6 mg/day

Tourette's disorder (unlabeled use): Oral: Initial: 0.5 mg; titrate to 2-4 mg/day

Renal Impairment: Starting dose of 0.25-0.5 mg twice daily is advisable.

Hepatic Impairment: Starting dose of 0.25-0.5 mg twice daily is advisable.

Administration

Oral: Oral solution can be mixed with water, coffee, orange juice, or low-fat milk, but is **not compatible** with cola, grapefruit juice, or tea. May be administered with or without food.

Monitoring Laboratory Tests Ophthalmic exam

Monitoring and Teaching Issues

Physical Assessment: Assess other medications patient is taking for effectiveness and interactions (see Drug Interactions). See Contraindications and Warnings/Precautions for use cautions. Monitor therapeutic response, results of ophthalmic exam, and adverse reactions at beginning of therapy and periodically with long-term use (see Adverse Reactions and Overdose/Toxicology). Initiate at lower doses (see Dosing) and taper dosage slowly when discontinuing. Assess knowledge/teach patient appropriate use, interventions to reduce side effects, and adverse symptoms to report (see Patient Education). **Pregnancy risk factor C** - benefits of use should outweigh possible risks. Breast-feeding is contraindicated.

Patient Education: Use exactly as directed; do not increase dose or frequency. It may take several weeks to achieve desired results; do not discontinue without consulting prescriber. Dilute solution with water, milk, or orange juice; do not dilute with grapefruit juice or beverages containing tannin or pectinate (eg, colas, tea). Avoid concurrent grapefruit juice. Avoid alcohol or caffeine and other prescription or OTC medications not approved by prescriber. Maintain adequate hydration (2-3 L/day of fluids) unless advised by prescriber to restrict fluids. You may experience excess sedation, drowsiness, restlessness, dizziness, or blurred vision (use caution driving or when engaging in tasks requiring alertness until response to drug is known); dry mouth, nausea, or GI upset (small, frequent meals, frequent mouth care, chewing gum, or sucking lozenges may help); postural hypotension (use caution climbing stairs or when changing position from lying or sitting to standing); or urinary retention (void before taking medication). Report persistent CNS effects (eg, trembling fingers, altered gait or balance, excessive sedation, seizures, unusual muscle or skeletal movements, anxiety, abnormal thoughts, confusion, personality changes); chest pain, palpitations, rapid heartbeat, severe dizziness; swelling or pain in breasts (male and female), altered menstrual pattern, sexual dysfunction; pain or difficulty on urination; vision changes; skin rash or yellowing of skin; difficulty breathing; or worsening of condition. **Pregnancy/breast-feeding precautions:** Inform prescriber if you are or intend to become pregnant. Do not breast-feed.

Dietary Issues: May be taken with or without food.

Geriatric Considerations: (See Warnings/Precautions, Adverse Reactions, Elderly Dosing, and Overdose/Toxicology.) Elderly patients have an increased risk of adverse response to side effects or adverse reactions to antipsychotics.

Additional Information Risperdal Consta™ is an currently an investigational dosage form and not commercially available. It is an injectable formulation of risperidone using the extended release Medisorb® drug-delivery system; small polymeric microspheres degrade slowly, releasing the medication at a controlled rate. If FDA approved, Risperdal Consta™ will be manufactured by Alkermes and marketed in the U.S. by Janssen Pharmaceutica Products. It is expected to be supplied in a dose-pack, including vial with active ingredient in microsphere formulation, syringe with diluent, needle-free vial access device, and safety needle.

Related Information

Antipsychotic Agents *on page 1558*

Antipsychotic Medication Guidelines *on page 1614*

Ritalin® *see* Methylphenidate *on page 882*
Ritalin® LA *see* Methylphenidate *on page 882*
Ritalin-SR® *see* Methylphenidate *on page 882*

Ritonavir (rye TON a veer)

U.S. Brand Names Norvir®

Generic Available No

Pharmacologic Category Antiretroviral Agent, Protease Inhibitor

Pregnancy Risk Factor B

Lactation Excretion in breast milk unknown/contraindicated

Use Treatment of HIV infection; should always be used as part of a multidrug regimen (at least 3 antiretroviral agents)

Mechanism of Action/Effect Ritonavir prevents cleavage of protein precursors essential for HIV infection of new cells and viral replication. Saquinavir- and zidovudine-resistant HIV isolates are generally susceptible to ritonavir. Used in combination therapy, resistance to ritonavir develops slowly; strains resistant to ritonavir are cross-resistant to indinavir and saquinavir.

Contraindications Hypersensitivity to ritonavir or any component of the formulation; concurrent amiodarone, astemizole, bepridil, cisapride, dihydroergotamine, ergonovine, ergotamine, flecainide, lovastatin, methylergonovine, midazolam, pimozide, propafenone, quinidine, simvastatin, St John's wort, triazolam

Warnings/Precautions Use caution in patients with hepatic insufficiency. Safety and efficacy have not been established in children <2 years of age. Use caution with benzodiazepines, rifabutin, sildenafil, and certain analgesics (meperidine, piroxicam, propoxyphene). Selected HMG-CoA reductase inhibitors are contraindicated (see Contraindications); atorvastatin should be used at the lowest possible dose, while fluvastatin or pravastatin may be safer alternatives. Avoid concurrent use of St John's wort. Warn patients that redistribution of fat may occur.

Drug Interactions

Cytochrome P450 Effect: Substrate of CYP1A2, 2B6, **2D6, 3A4**; Inhibits CYP2C8/9, 2C19, **2D6**, 2E1, **3A4**; Induces CYP1A2, 2C8/9, 3A4

Decreased Effect: The administration of didanosine (buffered formulation) should be separated from ritonavir by 2.5 hours to limit interaction with ritonavir. Concurrent use of rifampin, rifabutin, dexamethasone, and many anticonvulsants may lower serum concentration of ritonavir. Ritonavir may reduce the concentration of ethinyl estradiol which may result in loss of contraception (including combination products). Theophylline concentrations may be reduced in concurrent therapy. Levels of didanosine and zidovudine may be decreased by ritonavir, however, no dosage adjustment is necessary. In addition, ritonavir may decrease the serum concentrations of the following drugs: Atovaquone, divalproex, lamotrigine, methadone, phenytoin, warfarin.

Increased Effect/Toxicity: Concurrent use of amiodarone, bepridil, cisapride, flecainide, pimozide, propafenone, and quinidine is contraindicated. Serum concentrations/toxicity of many benzodiazepines may be increased; midazolam and triazolam are contraindicated. Concurrent use of ergot alkaloids (dihydroergotamine, ergotamine, ergonovine, methylergonovine) with ritonavir is also contraindicated (may cause vasospasm and peripheral ischemia). HMG-CoA reductase inhibitors serum concentrations may be increased by ritonavir, increasing the risk of myopathy/rhabdomyolysis; lovastatin and simvastatin are contraindicated; fluvastatin and pravastatin may be safer alternatives. Serum concentrations of meperidine's neuroexcitatory metabolite (normeperidine) are increased by ritonavir, which may increase the risk of CNS toxicity/seizures. Rifabutin and rifabutin metabolite serum concentrations may be increased by ritonavir; reduce rifabutin dose to 150 mg every other day. Sildenafil serum concentrations may be increased by ritonavir; when used concurrently, do not exceed a maximum sildenafil dose of 25 mg in a 48-hour period. Saquinavir's serum concentrations are increased by ritonavir; the dosage of both agents should be reduced to 400 mg twice daily. Concurrent therapy with amprenavir may result in increased serum concentrations: dosage adjustment is recommended. Metronidazole or disulfiram may cause disulfiram reaction (oral solution contains 43% ethanol).

Ritonavir may also increase the serum concentrations of the following drugs (dose decrease may be needed): Benzodiazepines, beta-blockers (metoprolol, timolol), bupropion, calcium channel blockers (diltiazem, nifedipine, verapamil), carbamazepine, clarithromycin, clonazepam, clorazepate, clozapine, cyclosporin, dexamethasone, disopyramide, dronabinol, ethosuximide, fluoxetine (and other SSRIs), indinavir, ketoconazole, lidocaine, methamphetamine, mexiletine, nefazodone, perphenazine, prednisone, propoxyphene, piroxicam, quinine, risperidone, tacrolimus, tramadol, thioridazine, tricyclic antidepressants (including desipramine), and zolpidem. Serum concentrations of rifabutin may be increased by ritonavir; dosage adjustment required.

Nutritional/Ethanol Interactions

Food: Food enhances absorption.

Herb/Nutraceutical: St John's wort may decrease ritonavir serum levels. Avoid use.

Adverse Reactions

Protease inhibitors cause hyperglycemia and dyslipidemia (elevated cholesterol/triglycerides) and a redistribution of fat (protease paunch, buffalo hump, facial atrophy and breast engorgement).

>10%:

Endocrine & metabolic: Increased GGT, increased triglycerides
Gastrointestinal: Diarrhea, nausea, vomiting, taste perversion
Hematologic: Anemia, decreased WBCs
Neuromuscular & skeletal: Weakness

1% to 10%:

Cardiovascular: Vasodilation
Central nervous system: Headache, fever, malaise, paresthesia, dizziness, insomnia, somnolence, thinking abnormally
Dermatologic: Rash

Endocrine & metabolic: Hyperlipidemia, increased glucose, increased uric acid, increased potassium, increased calcium
Gastrointestinal: Abdominal pain, anorexia, constipation, heartburn, flatulence, local throat irritation
Hematologic: Decreased neutrophils, increased eosinophils, increased, neutrophils, increased prothrombin time, increased WBC
Hepatic: Increased LFTs
Neuromuscular & skeletal: Myalgia, increased CPK
Respiratory: Pharyngitis
Miscellaneous: Diaphoresis

Overdosage/Toxicology Human experience is limited; there is no specific antidote for overdose with ritonavir. Oral solution contains 43% ethanol by volume, potentially causing significant ethanol-related toxicity in younger patients. Dialysis is unlikely to be beneficial in significant removal of the drug. Charcoal or gastric lavage may be useful to remove unabsorbed drug.

Pharmacodynamics/Kinetics

Absorption: Variable, with or without food

Half-Life Elimination: 3-5 hours

Metabolism: Hepatic; five metabolites, low concentration of an active metabolite achieved in plasma (oxidative); see Drug Interactions

Formulations

Capsule: 100 mg [contains ethanol and polyoxyl 35 castor oil]
Solution: 80 mg/mL (240 mL) [contains ethanol and polyoxyl 35 castor oil]

Dosing

Adults & Elderly: HIV infection: Oral: 600 mg twice daily; dose escalation tends to avoid nausea that many patients experience upon initiation of full dosing. Escalate the dose as follows: 300 mg twice daily for 1 day, 400 mg twice daily for 2 days, 500 mg twice daily for 1 day, then 600 mg twice daily. Ritonavir may be better tolerated when used in combination with other antiretrovirals by initiating the drug alone and subsequently adding the second agent within 2 weeks.

Note: Dosage adjustments for ritonavir when administered in combination therapy:
Amprenavir: Adjustments necessary for each agent:
Amprenavir 1200 mg with ritonavir 200 mg once daily **or**
Amprenavir 600 mg with ritonavir 100 mg twice daily
Amprenavir plus efavirenz (3-drug regimen): Amprenavir 1200 mg twice daily plus ritonavir 200 mg twice daily plus efavirenz at standard dose
Indinavir: Adjustments necessary for agent:
Indinavir 800 mg twice daily plus ritonavir 100-200 mg twice daily **or**
Indinavir 400 mg twice daily plus ritonavir 400 mg twice daily
Nelfinavir or saquinavir: Ritonavir 400 mg twice daily

Pediatrics: HIV infection: Oral: Children ≥2 years: 250 mg/m^2 twice daily; titrate dose upward to 400 mg/m^2 twice daily (maximum: 600 mg twice daily)

Hepatic Impairment: No adjustment required in mild impairment; insufficient data in moderate-severe impairment; caution advised with severe impairment

Administration

Oral: Administer with food. Liquid formulations usually have an unpleasant taste. Consider mixing it with chocolate milk or a liquid nutritional supplement.

Stability

Storage:

Capsule: Store under refrigeration at 2°C to 80°C (36°F to 46°F); may be left out at room temperature of <25°C (<77°F) if used within 30 days. Protect from light. Avoid exposure to excessive heat.
Solution: Store at room temperature at 20°C to 25°C (68°F to 77°F). Do not refrigerate.

Monitoring Laboratory Tests Triglycerides, cholesterol, LFTs, CBC, CPK, uric acid, basic HIV monitoring, viral load, and CD4 count, glucose

Monitoring and Teaching Issues

Physical Assessment: See Contraindications, Warnings/Precautions, and Dosing for use cautions. Assess potential for interactions with other prescriptions, OTC medications, or herbal products patient may be taking (see extensive list of Drug Interactions). Assess result of laboratory tests (see above) and patient response at regular intervals during therapy (see Adverse Reactions and Overdose/Toxicology). Teach patient proper use, possible side effects and appropriate interventions (eg, glucose testing; protease inhibitors may cause hyperglycemia - exacerbation or new-onset diabetes), and adverse symptoms to report - see Patient Education. **Pregnancy risk factor B** - may decrease effects of ethinyl estradiol containing contraceptives. Advise patient about alternative contraceptive measures. Breast-feeding is contraindicated.

Patient Education: Inform prescriber of all prescriptions, OTC medications, or herbal products you are taking, and any allergies you have. Do not take anything new during treatment unless approved by prescriber. Ritonavir is not a cure for HIV, nor has it been shown to reduce transmission of HIV. Take as often directed, with meals. Mix liquid formulation with chocolate milk or liquid nutritional supplement. Capsules may be stored in refrigerator (do not freeze) or stored at room temperature (<77°F) if used within 30 days. Protect from light. Avoid exposure to excessive heat. Solution should be stored at room temperature (68°F to 77°F). Do not refrigerate. Maintain adequate hydration (2-3 L/day of fluids) unless advised by prescriber to restrict fluids. Ritonavir may be prescribed with a combination of other medications; time these medications as directed by prescriber. You may be advised to check your glucose levels (this drug can cause exacerbation or new-onset diabetes). May cause body changes due to redistribution of body fat, facial atrophy, or breast enlargement (normal effects of drug); dizziness, insomnia, abnormal thinking (use caution when driving or engaging in potentially hazardous tasks until response to drug is known); nausea, vomiting, or taste perversion (small, frequent meals, frequent mouth care, chewing gum, or sucking lozenges may help); muscle weakness (consult prescriber for approved analgesic); or headache or insomnia (consult prescriber

(Continued)

Ritonavir *(Continued)*

for medication). Report any persistent adverse effect. **Pregnancy/breast-feeding precautions:** May reduce effectiveness of some contraceptives. Consult prescriber for appropriate contraceptive measures. Do not breast-feed.

Dietary Issues: Should be taken with food. Oral solution contains 43% ethanol by volume.

Breast-feeding Issues: HIV-infected mothers are discouraged from breast-feeding to decrease potential transmission of HIV.

Pregnancy Issues: According to preliminary data, placental passage of ritonavir is minimal. Pregnancy and protease inhibitors are both associated with an increased risk of hyperglycemia. Glucose levels should be closely monitored. Healthcare professionals are encouraged to contact the antiretroviral pregnancy registry to monitor outcomes of pregnant women exposed to antiretroviral medications (1-800-258-4263).

Additional Information Potential compliance problems, frequency of administration and adverse effects should be discussed with patients before initiating therapy to help prevent the emergence of resistance.

Related Information

Tuberculosis *on page 1705*

Rituxan® *see* Rituximab *on page 1198*

Rituximab (ri TUK si mab)

U.S. Brand Names Rituxan®

Synonyms C2B8

Generic Available No

Pharmacologic Category Antineoplastic Agent, Monoclonal Antibody

Pregnancy Risk Factor C

Lactation Excretion in breast milk unknown/contraindicated

Use Treatment of patients with relapsed or refractory low-grade or follicular, CD20 positive, B-cell non-Hodgkin's lymphoma; treatment (as part of combination therapy with radiolabeled ibritumomab) of patients with relapsed or refractory low-grade, follicular, or transformed B-cell non-Hodgkin's lymphoma (including rituximab refractory follicular non-Hodgkin's lymphoma)

Mechanism of Action/Effect Binds to the CD20 antigen on B-lymphocytes and recruits immune effector functions to mediate B-cell lysis *in vitro*. The antibody induces cell death in the DHL-4 human B-cell lymphoma line.

Contraindications Type I hypersensitivity or anaphylactic reactions to murine proteins or any component of the formulation

Warnings/Precautions Rituximab is associated with hypersensitivity reactions which may respond to adjustments in the infusion rate. Hypotension, bronchospasm, and angioedema have occurred as part of an infusion-related symptom complex (see Administration). In most cases, patients who have experienced nonlife-threatening reactions have been able to complete the full course of therapy. Medications for the treatment of hypersensitivity reactions (eg, epinephrine, antihistamines, corticosteroids) should be available for immediate use in the event of such a reaction during administration.

Discontinue infusions in the event of serious or life-threatening cardiac arrhythmias. Patients who develop clinically significant arrhythmias should undergo cardiac monitoring during and after subsequent infusions of rituximab. Patients with pre-existing cardiac conditions including arrhythmias and angina have had recurrences of these events during rituximab therapy; monitor these patients throughout the infusion and immediate postinfusion periods.

Pregnancy risk C.

Adverse Reactions Infusion-related symptoms are common. The incidence of infusion-related events decreased from 80% during the first infusion to ~40% with subsequent infusions. Fever, chills/rigors, and other infusion-related events occurred in the majority of patients during the first rituximab infusion. Angioedema may occur in up to 13% of patients. These reactions generally occurred within 30 minutes to 2 hours of beginning the first infusion, and resolved with slowing or interruption of the infusion and with supportive care.

>10%:

- Central nervous system: Headache (14%)
- Gastrointestinal: Nausea (18%)
- Hematologic: Leukopenia (11%)
- Miscellaneous: Fever (49%), chills (32%), asthenia (16%), angioedema (13%)
- Immunologic: Rituximab-induced B-cell depletion (70% to 80%)

1% to 10%:

- Cardiovascular: Hypotension (10%)
- Central nervous system: Myalgia (7%), dizziness (7%)
- Dermatologic: Pruritus (10%), rash (10%), urticaria (8%)
- Gastrointestinal: Vomiting (7%), abdominal pain (6%)
- Hematologic: During the treatment period (up to 30 days following the last dose), the following occurred: Severe thrombocytopenia, severe neutropenia, and severe anemia
- Respiratory: Bronchospasm occurred in 8%; 25% of these patients were treated with bronchodilators; rhinitis (8%)
- Miscellaneous: Throat irritation (6%)

<1% (Limited to important or life-threatening): Angina, aplastic anemia (pure red-cell aplasia), arrhythmia (ventricular and supraventricular), hemolytic anemia, myocardial infarction

Note: The following adverse events were reported more frequently in retreated patients: Anemia, anorexia, asthenia, depression, dizziness, flushing, leukopenia, night sweats, peripheral edema, pruritus, respiratory symptoms, tachycardia, throat irritation, thrombocytopenia

Overdosage/Toxicology There has been no experience with overdosage in human clinical trials; single doses higher than 500 mg/m^2 have not been tested

Pharmacodynamics/Kinetics

Absorption: I.V.: Immediate and results in a rapid and sustained depletion of circulating and tissue-based B cells

Half-Life Elimination:
>100 mg/m^2: 4.4 days (range 1.6-10.5 days)
375 mg/m^2: 50 hours (following first dose) to 174 hours (following fourth dose)

Duration: Detectable in serum 3-6 months after completion of treatment; B-cell recovery begins ~6 months following completion of treatment; median B-cell levels return to normal by 12 months following completion of treatment

Formulations Injection, solution [preservative free]: 10 mg/mL (10 mL, 50 mL)

Dosing

Adults & Elderly: Refer to individual protocols. **Note:** Do not administer I.V. push or bolus (hypersensitivity reactions may occur). Consider premedication (consisting of acetaminophen and diphenhydramine) before each infusion of rituximab. Premedication may attenuate infusion-related events. Because transient hypotension may occur during infusion, give consideration to withholding antihypertensive medications 12 hours prior to rituximab infusion.

Non-Hodgkin's lymphoma: I.V.: 375 mg/m^2 once weekly for 4 doses (days 1, 8, 15, and 22).

As part of combination therapy with ibritumomab (Zevalin™ therapeutic regimen): Two infusions of rituximab are completed, separated by 7-9 days (corresponding to two infusions of ibritumomab with differing radiolabels).

Rituximab dose (also see Ibritumomab monograph):

Step 1: 250 mg/m^2 at an initial rate of 50 mg/hour. If hypersensitivity or infusion-related events do not occur, increase infusion in increments of 50 mg/hour every 30 minutes, to a maximum of 400 mg/hour. Infusions should be temporarily slowed or interrupted if hypersensitivity or infusion related events occur. The infusion may be resumed at ½ the previous rate upon improvement of symptoms.

Step 2: 250 mg/m^2 at an initial rate of 100 mg/hour (50 mg/hour if infusion-related events occurred with the first infusion). If hypersensitivity or infusion-related events do not occur, increase infusion in increments of 100 mg/hour every 30 minutes, to a maximum of 400 mg/hour, as tolerated.

Administration

I.V.: Consider premedication (consisting of acetaminophen and diphenhydramine) before each infusion of rituximab. Premedication may attenuate infusion-related events. Because transient hypotension may occur during infusion, give consideration to withholding antihypertensive medications 12 hours prior to rituximab infusion.

Do **not** administer as an I.V. push or bolus. Rituximab is associated with hypersensitivity reactions which may respond to adjustments in the infusion rate. Hypotension, bronchospasm, and angioedema have occurred as part of an infusion-related symptom complex. Interrupt rituximab infusion for severe reactions and resume at a 50% reduction in rate (eg, from 100 to 50 mg/hour) when symptoms have completely resolved. Treatment of these symptoms with diphenhydramine and acetaminophen is recommended; additional treatment with bronchodilators or I.V. saline may be indicated. In most cases, patients who have experienced nonlife-threatening reactions have been able to complete the full course of therapy.

Stability

Storage: Store under refrigeration; protect vials from direct sunlight. Solutions for infusion are stable at 2°C to 8°C/36°F to 46°F for 24 hours and at room temperature for an additional 12 hours.

Reconstitution: Withdraw necessary amount of rituximab and dilute to a final concentration of 1-4 mg/mL into an infusion bag containing either 0.9% sodium chloride or 5% dextrose in water.

Monitoring Laboratory Tests CBC w/differential, peripheral CD20+ cells. Patients with elevated HAMA/HACA titers may have an allergic reaction when treated with rituximab or other antibodies from a mouse genetic source.

Monitoring and Teaching Issues

Physical Assessment: Prior to therapy, assess patient history to mouse antibodies (see Monitoring Laboratory Tests). See Contraindications, Warnings/Precautions, and Dosing for use cautions. See Administration for premedication considerations. Assess results of laboratory tests prior to, during, and following therapy (see Monitoring Laboratory Tests). Assess therapeutic response and adverse reactions (especially infusion-related reactions - see Warnings/Precautions, Adverse Reactions, and Dosing). Teach patient appropriate interventions to reduce side effects and adverse reactions to report. **Pregnancy risk factor C** - benefits of use should outweigh possible risks. Breast-feeding is contraindicated.

Patient Education: Inform prescriber of all prescriptions, OTC medications, or herbal products you are taking, and any allergies you have. Do not take anything new during treatment unless approved by prescriber. This medication can only be administered by infusion. You may experience a reaction during the infusion of this medication including high fever, chills, difficulty breathing, or congestion. You will be closely monitored and comfort measures provided. Maintain adequate hydration (2-3 L/day of fluids) during entire course of therapy unless advised by prescriber to restrict fluids. You will be susceptible to infection and people may wear masks and gloves while caring for you to protect you as much as possible (avoid crowds and exposure to infection and do not have any vaccinations without consulting prescriber). May cause dizziness or trembling (use caution until response to medication is known); or nausea or vomiting (small, frequent meals, frequent mouth care may help). Report persistent dizziness, swelling of extremities, unusual weight gain, difficulty breathing, chest pain or tightness; symptoms of respiratory infection, wheezing or bronchospasms, or difficulty breathing; unresolved GI effects; skin rash or redness; sore or irritated throat; fatigue, chills, fever, unhealed sores, white plaques in mouth or genital area; unusual bruising or bleeding; or other unusual effects related to this medication. **Pregnancy/breast-feeding precautions:** Inform prescriber if you are or intend to become pregnant. Do not breast-feed.

Additional Information Rapid infusion or bolus administration are associated with a high incidence of infusion-related reactions.

Rivastigmine (ri va STIG meen)

U.S. Brand Names Exelon®

Synonyms ENA 713; SDZ ENA 713

Generic Available No

Pharmacologic Category Acetylcholinesterase Inhibitor (Central)

Pregnancy Risk Factor B

Lactation Excretion in breast milk unknown/use caution

Use Mild to moderate dementia from Alzheimer's disease

Mechanism of Action/Effect A deficiency of cortical acetylcholine is thought to account for some of the symptoms of Alzheimer's disease; rivastigmine increases acetylcholine in the central nervous system through reversible inhibition of its hydrolysis by cholinesterase

Contraindications Hypersensitivity to rivastigmine, other carbamate derivatives, or any component of the formulation

Warnings/Precautions Significant nausea, vomiting, anorexia, and weight loss are associated with use, occurring more frequently in women and during the titration phase. Use caution in patients with a history of peptic ulcer disease or concurrent NSAID use. Caution in patients undergoing anesthesia who will receive succinylcholine-type muscle relaxation, patients with sick sinus syndrome, bradycardia or supraventricular conduction conditions, urinary obstruction, seizure disorders, or pulmonary conditions such as asthma or COPD. There are no trials evaluating the safety and efficacy in children.

Drug Interactions

Decreased Effect: Anticholinergic agents effects may be reduced with rivastigmine.

Increased Effect/Toxicity:

Beta-blockers without ISA activity may increase risk of bradycardia.

Calcium channel blockers (diltiazem or verapamil) may increase risk of bradycardia.

Cholinergic agonists effects may be increased with rivastigmine.

Cigarette use increases the clearance of rivastigmine by 23%.

Depolarizing neuromuscular blocking agents effects may be increased with rivastigmine.

Digoxin may increase risk of bradycardia.

Nutritional/Ethanol Interactions

Cigarette use: Increases the clearance of rivastigmine by 23%.

Ethanol: Avoid ethanol (due to risk of sedation; may increase GI irritation).

Food: Food delays absorption by 90 minutes, lowers C_{max} by 30% and increases AUC by 30%.

Adverse Reactions

>10%:

Central nervous system: Dizziness (21%), headache(17%)

Gastrointestinal: Nausea (47%), vomiting (31%), diarrhea (19%), anorexia (17%), abdominal pain (13%)

2% to 10%:

Central nervous system: Fatigue (9%), insomnia (9%), confusion (8%), depression (6%), anxiety (5%), malaise (5%), somnolence (5%), hallucinations (4%), aggressiveness (3%)

Cardiovascular: Syncope (3%), hypertension (3%)

Gastrointestinal: Dyspepsia (9%), constipation (5%), flatulence (4%), weight loss (3%), eructation (2%)

Genitourinary: Urinary tract infection (7%)

Neuromuscular & skeletal: Weakness (6%), tremor (4%)

Respiratory: Rhinitis (4%)

Miscellaneous: Increased diaphoresis (4%), flu-like syndrome (3%)

<2% (Limited to important or life-threatening; reactions may be at a similar frequency to placebo): Acute renal failure, allergic reaction, angina pectoris, aphasia, apnea, apraxia, ataxia, atrial fibrillation, AV block, bradycardia, bronchospasm, bundle branch block, cardiac arrest, cardiac failure, cholecystitis, convulsions, delirium, dysphonia, GI hemorrhage, intestinal obstruction, intracranial hemorrhage, migraine, myocardial infarction, pancreatitis, peripheral ischemia, peripheral neuropathy, postural hypotension, psychosis, pulmonary embolism, rash, sick sinus syndrome, Stevens-Johnson syndrome, supraventricular tachycardia, thrombocytopenia, thrombophlebitis, thrombosis, urticaria, vomiting (severe) with esophageal rupture (following inappropriate reinitiation of dose)

Overdosage/Toxicology In cases of asymptomatic overdoses, rivastigmine should be held for 24 hours. Cholinergic crisis, caused by significant acetylcholinesterase inhibition, is characterized by severe nausea, vomiting, salivation, sweating, bradycardia, hypotension, respiratory depression, collapse, and convulsions. Treatment is supportive and symptomatic. Dialysis would not be helpful.

Pharmacodynamics/Kinetics

Absorption: Fasting: Rapid and complete within 1 hour

Bioavailability: 40%

Half-Life Elimination: 1.5 hours

Time to Peak: 1 hour

Metabolism: Extensively via cholinesterase-mediated hydrolysis in the brain; metabolite undergoes N-demethylation and/or sulfate conjugation hepatically; minimal CYP involvement; linear kinetics at 3 mg twice daily, but nonlinear at higher doses

Formulations

Capsule, as tartrate: 1.5 mg, 3 mg, 4.5 mg, 6 mg

Solution, oral, as tartrate: 2 mg/mL (120 mL) [contains sodium benzoate]

Dosing

Adults: Alzheimer's dementia: Oral: Initial: 1.5 mg twice daily for 2 weeks; if tolerated, may be increased to 3 mg twice daily; further increases may be attempted no more frequently than every 2 weeks, to 4.5 mg twice daily and then to 6 mg twice daily; maximum dose: 6 mg twice daily. If gastrointestinal adverse events occur, the patient should be instructed to discontinue treatment for several doses then restart at the same or next lower dosage level; antiemetics have been used to control GI symptoms. If treatment is interrupted for longer than several days, restart the treatment at the lowest dose and titrate as previously described.

Elderly: Refer to adult dosing. Clearance is significantly lower in patients older than 60 years of age, but dosage adjustments are not recommended. Titrate dose to individual's tolerance.

Renal Impairment: Dosage adjustments are not recommended, however, titrate the dose to the individual's tolerance.

Hepatic Impairment: Clearance is significantly reduced in mild to moderately impaired patients. Although dosage adjustments are not recommended, use lowest possible dose and titrate according to individual's tolerance. May consider waiting >2 weeks between dosage adjustments.

Administration

Oral: Should be administered with meals (breakfast or dinner). Capsule should be swallowed whole. Liquid form is available for patients who cannot swallow capsules (can be swallowed directly from syringe or mixed with water, milk, or juice). Stir well and drink within 4 hours of mixing.

Stability

Storage: Store below 77°F (25°C). Store solution in an upright position and protect from freezing.

Monitoring Laboratory Tests Cognitive function at periodic intervals

Monitoring and Teaching Issues

Physical Assessment: See Warnings/Precautions for use cautions. Assess bladder and sphincter adequacy prior to administering medication. Assess other medications for effectiveness and interactions (see Contraindications and Drug Interactions). Monitor therapeutic effects and adverse reactions at beginning of therapy and regularly with long-term use (see Adverse Reactions and Overdose/Toxicology). Assess knowledge/teach patient appropriate use, possible side effects and interventions, and adverse symptoms to report. Note breast-feeding caution.

Patient Education: This drug is not a cure for Alzheimer's disease, but it may reduce the symptoms. Use as directed; do not increase dose or discontinue without consulting prescriber. Swallow capsule whole with meals (do not crush or chew). Liquid can be swallowed directly from syringe or mixed with water, milk, or juice; stir well and drink within 4 hours of mixing. Maintain adequate hydration (2-3 L/day of fluids) unless advised by prescriber to restrict fluids. Avoid alcohol. May cause dizziness, drowsiness, or postural hypotension (rise slowly from sitting or lying position and use caution when driving or climbing stairs); vomiting or loss of appetite (small, frequent meals, frequent mouth care, sucking lozenges, or chewing gum may help); diarrhea (buttermilk, boiled milk, or yogurt may help); or constipation (increased exercise, fluids, fruit, or fiber may help); or urinary frequency. Report persistent abdominal discomfort, diarrhea, or constipation; significantly increased salivation, sweating, tearing, or urination; chest pain, palpitations, acute headache; CNS changes (eg, excessive fatigue, agitation, insomnia, dizziness, confusion, aggressiveness, depression); increased muscle, joint, or body pain; vision changes or blurred vision; shortness of breath, coughing, or wheezing; skin rash; or other persistent adverse reactions. **Breast-feeding precaution:** Consult prescriber if breast-feeding.

Dietary Issues: Should be taken with meals.

Rizatriptan (rye za TRIP tan)

U.S. Brand Names Maxalt®; Maxalt-MLT®

Synonyms MK462

Generic Available No

Pharmacologic Category Serotonin 5-HT_{1D} Receptor Agonist

Pregnancy Risk Factor C

Lactation Excretion in breast milk unknown/not recommended

Use Acute treatment of migraine with or without aura

Mechanism of Action/Effect Selective agonist for serotonin (5-HT-$_{1D}$ receptor) in cranial arteries to cause vasoconstriction and reduce sterile inflammation associated with antidromic neuronal transmission correlating with relief of migraine

Contraindications Hypersensitivity to rizatriptan or any component of the formulation; documented ischemic heart disease or Prinzmetal's angina; uncontrolled hypertension; basilar or hemiplegic migraine; during or within 2 weeks of MAO inhibitors; during or within 24 hours of treatment with another 5-HT_1 agonist, or an ergot-containing or ergot-type medication (eg, methysergide, dihydroergotamine)

Warnings/Precautions Use only in patients with a clear diagnosis of migraine; use with caution in elderly or patients with hepatic or renal impairment, history of hypersensitivity to sumatriptan or adverse effects from sumatriptan, and in patients at risk of coronary artery disease. (as predicted by presence of risk factors); establish absence of cardiovascular disease and administer initial dose in appropriately staffed setting (physician's office) Do not use with ergotamines. May increase blood pressure transiently; may cause coronary vasospasm (less than sumatriptan); avoid in patients with signs/symptoms suggestive of reduced arterial flow (ischemic bowel, Raynaud's) which could be exacerbated by vasospasm. Phenylketonurics (tablets contain phenylalanine).

Patients who experience sensations of chest pain/pressure/tightness or symptoms suggestive of angina following dosing should be evaluated for coronary artery disease or Prinzmetal's angina before receiving additional doses.

Caution in dialysis patients or hepatically impaired. Reconsider diagnosis of migraine if no response to initial dose. Long-term effects on vision have not been evaluated.

Pregnancy risk C.

Drug Interactions

Increased Effect/Toxicity: Use within 24 hours of another selective 5-HT_1 antagonist or ergot-containing drug should be avoided due to possible additive vasoconstriction. Use with propranolol increased plasma concentration of rizatriptan by 70%. Rarely, concurrent use with SSRIs results in weakness and incoordination; monitor closely. MAO inhibitors and nonselective MAO inhibitors increase concentration of rizatriptan.

Nutritional/Ethanol Interactions Food: Food delays absorption.

(Continued)

Rizatriptan *(Continued)*

Adverse Reactions

1% to 10%:

Cardiovascular: Systolic/diastolic blood pressure increases (5-10 mm Hg), chest pain (5%), palpitation

Central nervous system: Dizziness, drowsiness, fatigue (13% to 30%, dose related)

Dermatologic: Skin flushing

Endocrine & metabolic: Mild increase in growth hormone, hot flashes

Gastrointestinal: Nausea, abdominal pain, dry mouth (<5%)

Respiratory: Dyspnea

<1% (Limited to important or life-threatening): Akinesia, angina, angioedema, arrhythmia, bradycardia, bradykinesia, decreased mental activity, myalgia, myocardial ischemia, myocardial infarction, neck pain/stiffness, neurological/psychiatric abnormalities, pruritus, stroke, syncope, tachycardia, tinnitus, toxic epidermal necrolysis, wheezing

Pharmacodynamics/Kinetics

Bioavailability: 40% to 50%

Half-Life Elimination: 2-3 hours

Time to Peak: 1-1.5 hours

Metabolism: Via monoamine oxidase-A; first-pass effect

Onset: ~30 minutes

Duration: 14-16 hours

Formulations

Tablet, as benzoate (Maxalt®): 5 mg, 10 mg

Tablet, orally-disintegrating, as benzoate (Maxalt-MLT®): 5 mg [contains phenylalanine 1.05 mg/tablet; peppermint flavor]; 10 mg [contains phenylalanine 2.1 mg/tablet; peppermint flavor]

Dosing

Adults & Elderly: Note: In patients with risk factors for coronary artery disease, following adequate evaluation to establish the absence of coronary artery disease, the initial dose should be administered in a setting where response may be evaluated (physician's office or similarly staffed setting). EKG monitoring may be considered.

Migraine: Oral: 5-10 mg, repeat after 2 hours if significant relief is not attained; maximum: 30 mg in a 24-hour period (use 5 mg dose in patients receiving propranolol with a maximum of 15 mg in 24 hours)

Note: For orally-disintegrating tablets (Maxalt-MLT™): Patient should be instructed to place tablet on tongue and allow to dissolve. Dissolved tablet will be swallowed with saliva.

Stability

Storage: Store in blister pack until administration.

Monitoring Laboratory Tests Consider monitoring vital signs and EKG with first dose in patients with unrecognized coronary disease, such as patients with significant hypertension, hypercholesterolemia, obese patients, diabetics, smokers with other risk factors or strong family history of coronary artery disease

Monitoring and Teaching Issues

Physical Assessment: See Contraindications and Warnings/Precautions (clear diagnosis of migraine) for use cautions. Assess potential for interactions with other prescriptions, OTC medications, or herbal products patient may be taking (eg, ergot-containing drugs - see Drug Interactions). See Monitoring Laboratory Tests. Assess effectiveness and adverse response (see Adverse Reactions and Overdose/Toxicology). Teach patient proper use, possible side effects and appropriate interventions, and adverse symptoms to report (see Patient Education). **Pregnancy risk factor C** - benefits of use should outweigh possible risks. Breast-feeding is not recommended.

Patient Education: Inform prescriber of all prescription (including oral contraceptives) and OTC medications or herbal products you are taking, and any allergies you have. This drug is to be used to reduce your migraine, not to prevent or reduce the number of attacks. Follow exact instructions for use. For orally-disintegrating tablets (Maxalt-MLT®), do not open blister pack before using. Open with dry hands, place on tongue, and allow to dissolve (dissolved tablet will be swallowed with saliva). Do not crush, break, or chew. Do not take within 24 hours of any other migraine medication without first consulting prescriber. If first dose brings relief, second dose may be taken anytime after 2 hours if migraine returns. Do not take more than two doses without consulting prescriber. May cause dizziness or drowsiness (use caution when driving or engaging in tasks requiring alertness until response to drug is known); dry mouth (frequent mouth care and sucking on lozenges may help); skin flushing or hot flashes (cool clothes or a cool environment may help); or mild abdominal discomfort or nausea or vomiting. Report immediately any chest pain, palpitations, or irregular heartbeat; severe dizziness, acute headache, stiff or painful neck or facial swelling; muscle weakness or pain; changes in mental acuity; blurred vision or eye pain; or excessive perspiration or urination. **Pregnancy/breast-feeding precautions:** Inform prescriber if you are or intend to become pregnant. Breast-feeding is not recommended.

Dietary Issues: Orally-disintegrating tablet contains phenylalanine (1.05 mg per 5 mg tablet, 2.10 mg per 10 mg tablet).

Related Information

Antimigraine Drugs *on page 1557*

rLFN-α2 *see* Interferon Alfa-2b *on page 719*

RMS® *see* Morphine Sulfate *on page 926*

Robafen® AC *see* Guaifenesin and Codeine *on page 647*

Robaxin® *see* Methocarbamol *on page 873*

Robaxisal® *see* Methocarbamol and Aspirin *on page 874*

Robinul® *see* Glycopyrrolate *on page 638*

Robinul® Forte *see* Glycopyrrolate *on page 638*

Robitussin® [OTC] *see* Guaifenesin *on page 646*

Rocuronium (roe kyoor OH nee um)

U.S. Brand Names Zemuron®

Synonyms ORG 946; Rocuronium Bromide

Generic Available No

Pharmacologic Category Neuromuscular Blocker Agent, Nondepolarizing

Pregnancy Risk Factor C

Lactation Excretion in breast milk unknown/use caution

Use Adjunct to general anesthesia to facilitate both rapid sequence and routine endotracheal intubation and to relax skeletal muscles during surgery; to facilitate mechanical ventilation in ICU patients; does not relieve pain or produce sedation

Contraindications Hypersensitivity to rocuronium or any component of the formulation

Warnings/Precautions Use with caution in patients with valvular heart disease, pulmonary disease, hepatic impairment; ventilation must be supported during neuromuscular blockade; certain clinical conditions may result in potentiation or antagonism of neuromuscular blockade:

Potentiation: Electrolyte abnormalities, severe hyponatremia, severe hypocalcemia, severe hypokalemia, hypermagnesemia, neuromuscular diseases, acidosis, acute intermittent porphyria, renal failure, hepatic failure

Antagonism: Alkalosis, hypercalcemia, demyelinating lesions, peripheral neuropathies, diabetes mellitus

Increased sensitivity in patients with myasthenia gravis, Eaton-Lambert syndrome; resistance in burn patients (>30% of body) for period of 5-70 days postinjury; resistance in patients with muscle trauma, denervation, immobilization, infection

Pregnancy risk C.

Drug Interactions

Decreased Effect: Effect of nondepolarizing neuromuscular blockers may be reduced by carbamazepine (chronic use), corticosteroids (also associated with myopathy - see increased effect), phenytoin (chronic use), sympathomimetics, and theophylline.

Increased Effect/Toxicity: Increased effects are possible with aminoglycosides, beta-blockers, clindamycin, calcium channel blockers, halogenated anesthetics, imipenem, ketamine, lidocaine, loop diuretics (furosemide), macrolides (case reports), magnesium sulfate, procainamide, quinidine, quinolones, tetracyclines, and vancomycin. May increase risk of myopathy when used with high- dose corticosteroids for extended periods.

Adverse Reactions

>1%: Cardiovascular: Transient hypotension and hypertension

<1% (Limited to important or life-threatening): Abnormal EKG, anaphylaxis, arrhythmia, bronchospasm, edema, hiccups, injection site pruritus, nausea, rash, rhonchi, shock, tachycardia, vomiting, wheezing

Overdosage/Toxicology

Symptoms of overdose include prolonged skeletal muscle block, muscle weakness and apnea

Treatment is maintenance of a patent airway and controlled ventilation until recovery of normal neuromuscular block is observed, further recovery may be facilitated by administering an anticholinesterase agent (eg, neostigmine, edrophonium, or pyridostigmine) with atropine, to antagonize the skeletal muscle relaxation; support of the cardiovascular system with fluids and pressors may be necessary

Pharmacodynamics/Kinetics

Metabolism: Minimally hepatic

Onset: Good intubation conditions in 1-2 minutes; maximum neuromuscular blockade within 4 minutes

Duration: ~30 minutes (with standard doses, increases with higher doses)

Formulations Injection, solution, as bromide: 10 mg/mL (5 mL, 10 mL)

Dosing

Adults & Elderly: Administer I.V.; dose to effect; doses will vary due to interpatient variability; use ideal body weight for obese patients

Tracheal intubation: I.V.:

Initial: 0.6 mg/kg is expected to provide approximately 31 minutes of clinical relaxation under opioid/nitrous oxide/oxygen anesthesia with neuromuscular block sufficient for intubation attained in 1-2 minutes; lower doses (0.45 mg/kg) may be used to provide 22 minutes of clinical relaxation with median time to neuromuscular block of 1-3 minutes; maximum blockade is achieved in <4 minutes

Maximum: 0.9-1.2 mg/kg may be given during surgery under opioid/nitrous oxide/oxygen anesthesia without adverse cardiovascular effects and is expected to provide 58-67 minutes of clinical relaxation; neuromuscular blockade sufficient for intubation is achieved in <2 minutes with maximum blockade in <3 minutes

Maintenance: 0.1, 0.15, and 0.2 mg/kg administered at 25% recovery of control T_1 (defined as 3 twitches of train-of-four) provides a median of 12, 17, and 24 minutes of clinical duration under anesthesia

Rapid sequence intubation: 0.6-1.2 mg/kg in appropriately premedicated and anesthetized patients with excellent or good intubating conditions within 2 minutes

Continuous infusion: Initial: 0.01-0.012 mg/kg/minute only after early evidence of spontaneous recovery of neuromuscular function is evident; infusion rates have ranged from 0.004-0.016 mg/kg/minute.

(Continued)

Rocuronium *(Continued)*

ICU: 10 mcg/kg/minute; adjust dose to maintain appropriate degree of neuromuscular blockade (eg, 1 or 2 twitches on train-of-four)

Pediatrics: Administer I.V.; dose to effect; doses will vary due to interpatient variability; use ideal body weight for obese patients

Tracheal intubation: I.V.: Children:

Initial: 0.6 mg/kg under halothane anesthesia produce excellent to good intubating conditions within 1 minute and will provide a median time of 41 minutes of clinical relaxation in children 3 months to 1 year of age, and 27 minutes in children 1-12 years

Maintenance: 0.075-0.125 mg/kg administered upon return of T_1 to 25% of control provides clinical relaxation for 7-10 minutes

Administration

I.V.: Administer I.V. only; may be given undiluted as a bolus injection or via a continuous infusion using an infusion pump

Stability

Storage: Store under refrigeration (2°C to 8°C), do not freeze; when stored at room temperature, it is stable for 30 days; unlike vecuronium, it is stable in 0.9% sodium chloride and 5% dextrose in water, this mixture should be used within 24 hours of preparation

Monitoring and Teaching Issues

Physical Assessment: Only clinicians experienced in the use of neuromuscular blocking agents should administer and/or manage the use of mivacurium. See Contraindications, Warnings/Precautions, and Dosing for use cautions. Assess potential for interactions with other prescription or OTC medications or herbal products patient may be taking (eg, other drugs that affect neuromuscular activity may increase/decrease neuromuscular block induced by rocuronium - see Drug Interactions). Dosage and rate of administration should be individualized and titrated to the desired effect, according to relevant clinical factors, premedication, concomitant medication, age, and general condition of the patient. Ventilatory support must be instituted and maintained until adequate respiratory muscle function and/or airway protection are assured. This drug does not cause anesthesia or analgesia; pain must be treated with appropriate agents. Continuous monitoring of vital signs, cardiac and respiratory status, and neuromuscular block (objective assessment with peripheral external nerve stimulator) are mandatory until full muscle tone has returned (see Adverse Reactions). Safety precautions must be maintained until full muscle tone has returned. Muscle tone returns in a predictable pattern; starting with diaphragm, abdomen, chest, limbs, and finally muscles of the neck, face, and eyes. **Note:** It may take longer for return of muscle tone in obese or elderly persons or patients with renal or hepatic disease, myasthenia gravis, myopathy, other neuromuscular diseases, dehydration, electrolyte imbalance, or severe acid/base imbalance. Provide appropriate teaching/support prior to, during, and following administration.

Long-term use: Vital signs and fluid levels should be monitored regularly during treatment. Every 2- to 3-hour repositioning, and skin, mouth, and eye care is necessary while patient is sedated. Emotional and sensory support (auditory and environmental) should be provided. **Pregnancy risk factor C** - benefits of use should outweigh possible risks. Note breast-feeding caution.

Patient Education: Patient education should be appropriate for patient condition. Reassurance of constant monitoring and emotional support should precede and follow administration. Patients should be reminded as muscle tone returns not to attempt to change position or rise from bed without assistance and to report and skin rash, hives, pounding heartbeat, difficulty breathing, or muscle tremors. **Pregnancy/breast-feeding precautions:** Inform prescriber if you are pregnant. Consult prescriber if breast-feeding.

Additional Information Rocuronium is classified as an intermediate-duration neuromuscular-blocking agent. Do not mix in the same syringe with barbiturates. Rocuronium does not relieve pain or produce sedation.

Rocuronium Bromide *see* Rocuronium *on page 1203*

Rofecoxib (roe fe COX ib)

U.S. Brand Names Vioxx®

Generic Available No

Pharmacologic Category Nonsteroidal Anti-inflammatory Drug (NSAID), COX-2 Selective

Pregnancy Risk Factor C/D (3rd trimester)

Lactation Excretion in breast milk unknown/not recommended

Use Relief of the signs and symptoms of osteoarthritis; management of acute pain in adults; treatment of primary dysmenorrhea; relief of signs and symptoms of rheumatoid arthritis in adults

Mechanism of Action/Effect Inhibits prostaglandin synthesis by decreasing the activity of the enzyme, cyclooxygenase-2 (COX-2), which results in decreased formation of prostaglandin precursors. Rofecoxib does not inhibit cyclooxygenase-1 (COX-1) at therapeutic concentrations.

Contraindications Hypersensitivity to rofecoxib or any component of the formulation, aspirin, or other NSAIDs; pregnancy (3rd trimester)

Warnings/Precautions Gastrointestinal irritation, ulceration, bleeding, and perforation may occur with NSAIDs (rofecoxib has been associated with rates of these events which are lower than naproxen, a nonselective NSAID). Use with caution in patients with a history of GI disease (bleeding or ulcers), decreased renal function, hepatic disease, CHF, hypertension, or asthma. Edema, GI irritation, and/or hypertension occur at an increased frequency with chronic use of 50 mg/day. Use with caution in patients with ischemic heart disease; antiplatelet therapies should be considered (rofecoxib is not a substitute for antiplatelet agents). Anaphylactoid reactions may occur, even with no prior exposure to rofecoxib. Pregnancy risk C/D (3rd trimester).

Drug Interactions

Cytochrome P450 Effect: Substrate of CYP2C8/9; Inhibits **CYP1A2**; Induces CYP3A4

Decreased Effect: Efficacy of thiazide diuretics, loop diuretics (furosemide), or ACE-inhibitors may be diminished by rofecoxib. Rifampin reduces the serum concentration of rofecoxib by ~50%.

Increased Effect/Toxicity: Cimetidine increases AUC of rofecoxib by 23%. Rofecoxib may increase plasma concentrations of methotrexate, lithium, and theophylline. Rofecoxib may be used with low-dose aspirin, however, rates of gastrointestinal bleeding may be increased with coadministration. Rofecoxib may increase the INR in patients receiving warfarin and may increase the risk of bleeding complications.

Nutritional/Ethanol Interactions

Ethanol: Avoid ethanol (may increase gastric mucosal irritation)

Food: Time to peak concentrations are delayed when taken with a high-fat meal, however, peak concentration and AUC are unchanged.

Adverse Reactions

2% to 10%:

Cardiovascular: Peripheral edema (4%), hypertension (up to 10%)

Central nervous system: Headache (5%), dizziness (3%), weakness (2%)

Gastrointestinal: Diarrhea (7%), nausea (5%), heartburn (4%), epigastric discomfort (4%), dyspepsia (4%), abdominal pain (3%), dry socket (post-dental extraction alveolitis 2%)

Genitourinary: Urinary tract infection (3%)

Neuromuscular & skeletal: Back pain (3%)

Respiratory: Upper respiratory infection (9%), bronchitis (2%), sinusitis (3%)

Miscellaneous: Flu-like syndrome (3%)

<2% (Limited to important or life-threatening): Allergy, alopecia, angina, arrhythmia, asthma, atopic dermatitis, atrial fibrillation, blurred vision, decreased mental acuity, depression, dyspnea, esophageal reflux, esophagitis, fluid retention, gastritis, hematochezia, hematoma, hemorrhoids, muscle cramps, neuropathy, paresthesia, pruritus, rash, somnolence, syncope, tendonitis, tinnitus, urinary retention, urticaria, venous insufficiency, vertigo

<0.1% (Limited to important or life-threatening): Breast cancer, cholecystitis, colitis, colonic neoplasm, CHF, deep vein thrombosis, duodenal ulcer, gastrointestinal bleeding, intestinal obstruction, lymphoma, myocardial infarction, pancreatitis, prostatic cancer, stroke, transient ischemic attack, unstable angina, urolithiasis

Overdosage/Toxicology Symptoms may include epigastric pain, drowsiness, lethargy, nausea, and vomiting. Gastrointestinal bleeding may occur. Rare manifestations include hypertension, respiratory depression, coma, and acute renal failure. Treatment is symptomatic and supportive. Hemodialysis does not remove rofecoxib.

Pharmacodynamics/Kinetics

Half-Life Elimination: 17 hours

Time to Peak: 2-3 hours

Metabolism: Hepatic (99%); minor metabolism via CYP2C8/9 isoenzyme

Onset: 45 minutes

Duration: Up to >24 hours

Formulations

Suspension, oral: 12.5 mg/5 mL (150 mL); 25 mg/5 mL (150 mL) [strawberry flavor]

Tablet: 12.5 mg, 25 mg, 50 mg

Dosing

Adults:

Osteoarthritis: Oral: 12.5 mg once daily; may be increased to a maximum of 25 mg once daily

Acute pain or dysmenorrhea: Oral: 50 mg once daily as needed (use for longer than 5 days has not been studied)

Rheumatoid arthritis: Oral: 25 mg once daily

Elderly: No specific adjustment is recommended; however, the AUC in elderly patients may be increased by 34% as compared to younger subjects. Use the lowest recommended dose. Refer to adult dosing.

Renal Impairment: Use in advanced renal disease is not recommended.

Hepatic Impairment: No specific dosage adjustment is recommended (AUC may be increased by 69%).

Monitoring and Teaching Issues

Physical Assessment: Assess allergy history (salicylates) prior to beginning therapy. See Contraindications and Warnings/Precautions for use cautions. Assess effectiveness and interactions of other medications patient may be taking (see Drug Interactions, ie, lithium). Monitor effectiveness of therapy and adverse reactions (see Adverse Reactions and Overdose/Toxicology). Assess knowledge/teach patient appropriate use, interventions to reduce side effects, and adverse symptoms to report (see Patient Education). **Pregnancy risk factor C/D** - see Pregnancy Risk Factor for use cautions. Breast-feeding is not recommended.

Patient Education: Do not take more than recommended dose. May be taken with food to reduce GI upset. Do not take with antacids. Avoid alcohol, aspirin, and OTC medication unless approved by prescriber. You may experience dizziness, confusion, or blurred vision (avoid driving or engaging in tasks requiring alertness until response to drug is known); or anorexia, nausea, vomiting, taste disturbance, gastric distress (small, frequent meals, frequent mouth care, sucking lozenges, or chewing gum may help). GI bleeding, ulceration, or perforation can occur with or without pain; rofecoxib has rates of these events which are lower than nonselective NSAIDs. Stop taking medication and report stomach pain or cramping, unusual bleeding or bruising, or blood in vomitus, stool, or urine immediately. Report persistent insomnia; skin rash; unusual fatigue or easy bruising or bleeding; muscle pain, tremors, or weakness; sudden weight gain; chest pain; changes in hearing (ringing in ears); vision changes; changes in urination pattern; or difficulty breathing. **Pregnancy/breast-feeding precautions:** Inform prescriber if you are or intend to become pregnant. This drug should not be used in the 3rd trimester of pregnancy. Breast-feeding is not recommended.

(Continued)

Rofecoxib *(Continued)*

Dietary Issues: May be taken without regard to meals.

Breast-feeding Issues: In animal studies, rofecoxib has been found to be excreted in milk. It is not known whether rofecoxib is excreted in human milk. Because many drugs are excreted in milk, and the potential for serious adverse reactions exists, a decision should be made whether to discontinue nursing or discontinue the drug, taking into account the importance of the drug to the mother.

Pregnancy Issues: In late pregnancy may cause premature closure of the ductus arteriosus.

Related Information

Nonsalicylate/Nonsteroidal Anti-inflammatory Comparison *on page 1587*

Roferon-A® *see* Interferon Alfa-2a *on page 717*

Rolaids® Calcium Rich [OTC] *see* Calcium Supplements *on page 202*

Romazicon™ *see page 1460*

Romazicon® *see* Flumazenil *on page 570*

Romilar® AC *see* Guaifenesin and Codeine *on page 647*

Romycin® *see* Erythromycin (Systemic) *on page 486*

Rondec® Drops *see* Carbinoxamine and Pseudoephedrine *on page 217*

Rondec® Tablets *see* Carbinoxamine and Pseudoephedrine *on page 217*

Rondec-TR® *see* Carbinoxamine and Pseudoephedrine *on page 217*

Ropinirole (roe PIN i role)

U.S. Brand Names Requip®

Synonyms Ropinirole Hydrochloride

Generic Available No

Pharmacologic Category Anti-Parkinson's Agent, Dopamine Agonist

Pregnancy Risk Factor C

Lactation Excretion in breast milk unknown/not recommended

Use Treatment of idiopathic Parkinson's disease; in patients with early Parkinson's disease who were not receiving concomitant levodopa therapy as well as in patients with advanced disease on concomitant levodopa

Contraindications Hypersensitivity to ropinirole or any component of the formulation

Warnings/Precautions Syncope, sometimes associated with bradycardia, was observed in association with ropinirole in both early Parkinson's disease (without levodopa) patients and advanced Parkinson's disease (with levodopa) patients. Use with caution in patients at risk of hypotension (ie, those receiving antihypertensive drugs) or where transient hypotensive episodes would be poorly tolerated (cardiovascular disease or cerebrovascular disease). Parkinson's patients being treated with dopaminergic agonists ordinarily require careful monitoring for signs and symptoms of postural hypotension, especially during dose escalation, and should be informed of this risk. May cause hallucinations. Use with caution in patients with pre-existing dyskinesia, severe hepatic or renal dysfunction.

Patients treated with ropinirole have reported falling asleep while engaging in activities of daily living. Discontinue if significant daytime sleepiness or episodes of falling asleep occur. The significance of data concerning retinal changes observed in animal studies remains uncertain.

Other dopaminergic agents have been associated with a syndrome resembling neuroleptic malignant syndrome on withdrawal or significant dosage reduction after long-term use.

Pregnancy risk C.

Drug Interactions

Cytochrome P450 Effect: Substrate of **CYP1A2**, 3A4; Inhibits CYP1A2, **2D6**

Decreased Effect: Antipsychotics, enzyme inducers (barbiturates, carbamazepine, phenytoin, rifampin, rifabutin), cigarette smoking, and metoclopramide may reduce the effect or serum concentrations of ropinirole.

Increased Effect/Toxicity: Inhibitors of CYP1A2 inhibitors may increase serum concentrations of ropinirole; inhibitors include cimetidine, ciprofloxacin, erythromycin, fluvoxamine, isoniazid, ritonavir, and zileuton. Estrogens may also reduce the metabolism of ropinirole; dosage adjustments may be needed.

Nutritional/Ethanol Interactions

Ethanol: Avoid ethanol (may increase CNS depression).

Herb/Nutraceutical: Avoid kava kava, gotu kola, valerian, St John's wort (may increase CNS depression).

Adverse Reactions

Early Parkinson's disease (without levodopa):

>10%:

Cardiovascular: Syncope (12%)

Central nervous system: Dizziness (40%), somnolence (40%), fatigue (11%)

Gastrointestinal: Nausea (60%), vomiting (12%)

Miscellaneous: Viral infection (11%)

1% to 10%:

Cardiovascular: Dependent/leg edema (6% to 7%), orthostasis (6%), hypertension (5%), chest pain (4%), flushing (3%), palpitations (3%), peripheral ischemia (3%), hypotension (2%), tachycardia (2%),

Central nervous system: Pain (8%), confusion (5%), hallucinations (5%, dose related), hypoesthesia (4%), amnesia (3%), malaise (3%), vertigo (2%), yawning (3%)

Gastrointestinal: Constipation (>5%), dyspepsia (10%), abdominal pain (6%), xerostomia (5%), anorexia (4%), flatulence (3%)

Genitourinary: Urinary tract infection (5%), impotence (3%)

Hepatic: Elevated alkaline phosphatase (3%)

Neuromuscular & skeletal: Weakness (6%)

Ocular: Abnormal vision (6%), xerophthalmia (2%)

Respiratory: Pharyngitis (6%), rhinitis (4%), sinusitis (4%), dyspnea (3%)
Miscellaneous: Diaphoresis (increased) (6%)

Advanced Parkinson's disease (with levodopa):

>10%:

Central nervous system: Dizziness (26%), somnolence (20%), headache (17%)
Gastrointestinal: Nausea (30%)
Neuromuscular & skeletal: Dyskinesias (34%)

1% to 10%:

Cardiovascular: Syncope (3%), hypotension (2%)
Central nervous system: Hallucinations (10%, dose related), aggravated parkinsonism, confusion (9%), pain (5%), paresis (3%), amnesia (5%), anxiety (6%), abnormal dreaming (3%), insomnia
Gastrointestinal: Abdominal pain (9%), vomiting (7%), constipation (6%), diarrhea (5%), dysphagia (2%), flatulence (2%), increased salivation (2%), xerostomia, weight loss (2%)
Genitourinary: Urinary tract infections
Hematologic: Anemia (2%)
Neuromuscular & skeletal: Falls (10%), arthralgia (7%), tremor (6%), hypokinesia (5%), paresthesia (5%), arthritis (3%)
Respiratory: Upper respiratory tract infection (9%), dyspnea (3%)
Miscellaneous: Injury, increased diaphoresis (7%), viral infection, increased drug level (7%)

Other adverse effects (all phase 2/3 trials):

<1% (Limited to important or life-threatening): Acute renal failure, aphasia, asthma, bradycardia, bundle branch block, cardiac arrest, cardiac failure, cholecystitis, coma, delirium, dementia, eosinophilia, extrapyramidal symptoms, gangrene, gastrointestinal hemorrhage, gastrointestinal ulceration, leukopenia, lymphopenia, manic reaction, pancreatitis, paralysis, paranoid reaction, peripheral neuropathy, photosensitivity, pleural effusion, pulmonary edema, pulmonary embolism, rash, renal calculus, renal failure (acute), seizures, SIADH, stupor, suicide attempt, thrombocytopenia, thrombosis, torticollis, urticaria, ventricular tachycardia

Overdosage/Toxicology No reports of intentional overdose; symptoms reported with accidental overdosage were agitation, increased dyskinesia, sedation, orthostatic hypotension, chest pain, confusion, nausea, and vomiting. It is anticipated that the symptoms of overdose will be related to its dopaminergic activity. General supportive measures are recommended. Vital signs should be maintained, if necessary. Removal of any unabsorbed material (eg, by gastric lavage) should be considered. Removal by hemodialysis is unlikely.

Pharmacodynamics/Kinetics

Absorption: Not affected by food

Bioavailability: Absolute: 55%

Half-Life Elimination: ~6 hours

Time to Peak: ~1-2 hours; T_{max} increased by 2.5 hours when taken with food

Metabolism: Extensively hepatic via CYP1A2 to inactive metabolites; first-pass effect

Formulations Tablet, as hydrochloride: 0.25 mg, 0.5 mg, 1 mg, 2 mg, 4 mg, 5 mg

Dosing

Adults & Elderly:

Parkinson's disease: Oral:

Initial: Recommended starting dose is 0.25 mg 3 times/day;

Adjustment: **Note:** The dosage should be increased to achieve a maximum therapeutic effect, balanced against the principal side effects of nausea, dizziness, somnolence and dyskinesia. Based on individual patient response, the dosage should be titrated with weekly increments as described below:

- Week 1: 0.25 mg 3 times/day; total daily dose: 0.75 mg
- Week 2: 0.5 mg 3 times/day; total daily dose: 1.5 mg
- Week 3: 0.75 mg 3 times/day; total daily dose: 2.25 mg
- Week 4: 1 mg 3 times/day; total daily dose: 3 mg

After week 4, if necessary, daily dosage may be increased by 1.5 mg per day on a weekly basis up to a dose of 9 mg/day, and then by up to 3 mg/day weekly to a total of 24 mg/day

Renal Impairment: Removal by hemodialysis is unlikely.

Monitoring and Teaching Issues

Physical Assessment: See Contraindications, Warnings/Precautions, and Dosing for use cautions. Assess potential for interactions with other prescriptions, OTC medications, or herbal products patient may be taking (see Drug Interactions). Assess therapeutic effectiveness and adverse responses on a regular basis during therapy (see Adverse Reactions and Overdose/Toxicology). Teach patient proper use, side effects and appropriate interventions, and adverse reactions to report (see Patient Education). **Pregnancy risk factor C** - benefits of use should outweigh possible risks. Breast-feeding is not recommended.

Patient Education: Inform prescriber of all prescriptions, OTC medications, or herbal products you are taking (especially anything that may cause drowsiness), and any allergies you have. Take exactly as directed, without regard to food. May cause dizziness, postural hypotension, or sudden, overwhelming sleepiness (use caution when driving or engaging in tasks that require alertness until response to drug is known); dizziness or postural hypotension (use caution and avoid quick moves when rising from sitting or lying position, when climbing stairs, or engaging in activities that require quick movements); or nausea, vomiting, lack of appetite, or mouth sores (small, frequent meals, frequent mouth care, chewing gum, or sucking lozenges may help). Report unusual and persistent sleepiness; chest pain or palpitations; CNS changes (confusion, hallucinations, amnesia, abnormal dreaming, insomnia); skeletal weakness or increased random tremors or movements, gait changes, or difficulty walking; signs of urinary tract or respiratory infection (pain or burning on urination, pus or blood in urine, or unusual cough and chest tightness); or unusual persistent adverse reactions. **Pregnancy/breast-feeding precautions:** Inform prescriber if you are or intend to become pregnant. Breast-feeding is not recommended.

(Continued)

Ropinirole *(Continued)*

Dietary Issues: May be taken with or without food.

Additional Information If therapy with a drug known to be a potent inhibitor of CYP1A2 is stopped or started during treatment with ropinirole, adjustment of ropinirole dose may be required. Ropinirole binds to melanin-containing tissues (ie, eyes, skin) in pigmented rats. After a single dose, long-term retention of drug was demonstrated, with a half-life in the eye of 20 days; not known if ropinirole accumulates in these tissues over time.

Ropinirole Hydrochloride *see* Ropinirole *on page 1206*

Rosiglitazone (ROSE i gli ta zone)

U.S. Brand Names Avandia®

Generic Available No

Pharmacologic Category Antidiabetic Agent, Thiazolidinedione

Pregnancy Risk Factor C

Lactation Excretion in breast milk unknown/not recommended

Use Type 2 diabetes mellitus (noninsulin dependent, NIDDM):

Monotherapy: Improve glycemic control as an adjunct to diet and exercise

Combination therapy: In combination with metformin or a sulfonylurea when diet, exercise, and metformin or a sulfonylurea alone do not result in adequate glycemic control; **or** when diet, exercise, and rosiglitazone alone do not result in adequate glycemic control

Mechanism of Action/Effect Thiazolidinedione antidiabetic agent that lowers blood glucose by improving target cell response to insulin, without increasing pancreatic insulin secretion. It has a mechanism of action that is dependent on the presence of insulin for activity.

Contraindications Hypersensitivity to rosiglitazone or any component of the formulation; active liver disease (transaminases >2.5 times the upper limit of normal at baseline); contraindicated in patients who previously experienced jaundice during troglitazone therapy

Warnings/Precautions Should not be used in diabetic ketoacidosis. Mechanism requires the presence of insulin, therefore use in type 1 diabetes (insulin dependent, IDDM) is not recommended. Use with caution in premenopausal, anovulatory women; may result in resumption of ovulation, increasing the risk of pregnancy. May result in hormonal imbalance; development of menstrual irregularities should prompt reconsideration of therapy. Use with caution in patients with anemia or depressed leukocyte counts (may reduce hemoglobin, hematocrit, and/or WBC). May increase plasma volume and/or increase cardiac hypertrophy. Use with caution in patients with edema. Monitor closely for signs and symptoms of heart failure. Avoid use in patients with NYHA Class III or IV heart failure. Discontinue if heart failure develops. Use with caution in patients with elevated transaminases (AST or ALT). Idiosyncratic hepatotoxicity has been reported with another thiazolidinedione agent (troglitazone) and (rarely) with rosiglitazone; discontinue if jaundice occurs. Monitoring should include periodic determinations of liver function. Pregnancy risk C.

Drug Interactions

Cytochrome P450 Effect: Substrate of **CYP2C8/9**; Inhibits CYP2C8/9

Increased Effect/Toxicity: When rosiglitazone was coadministered with glyburide, metformin, digoxin, warfarin, ethanol, or ranitidine, no significant pharmacokinetic alterations were observed.

Nutritional/Ethanol Interactions

Ethanol: Avoid ethanol (may cause hypoglycemia).

Food: Peak concentrations are lower by 28% and delayed when administered with food, but these effects are not believed to be clinically significant.

Herb/Nutraceutical: Avoid garlic, gymnema (may cause hypoglycemia).

Adverse Reactions

>10%:

Endocrine & metabolic: Increased total cholesterol, increased LDL-cholesterol, increased HDL-cholesterol

Gastrointestinal: Weight gain

1% to 10%:

Cardiovascular: Edema (5%)

Central nervous system: Headache (6%), fatigue (4%)

Endocrine & metabolic: Hyperglycemia (4%), hypoglycemia (<1% to 2%)

Gastrointestinal: Diarrhea (2%)

Hematologic: Anemia (2%)

Neuromuscular & skeletal: Back pain (4%)

Respiratory: Upper respiratory tract infection (10%), sinusitis (3%)

Miscellaneous: Injury (8%)

<1% (Limited to important or life-threatening): Congestive heart failure or exacerbation of CHF, elevated transaminases, increased bilirubin, pulmonary edema

Isolated case reports of hepatotoxic reactions have been reported in patients receiving rosiglitazone; causality not established

Overdosage/Toxicology Experience in overdose is limited. Symptoms may include hypoglycemia. Treatment is supportive.

Pharmacodynamics/Kinetics

Bioavailability: 99%

Half-Life Elimination: 3.15-3.59 hours

Time to Peak: 1 hour

Metabolism: Hepatic (99%) via CYP2C8; minor metabolism via CYP2C9

Onset: Delayed; Maximum effect: Up to 12 weeks

Formulations Tablet: 2 mg, 4 mg, 8 mg

Dosing

Adults & Elderly: Type 2 diabetes: Oral: Initial: 4 mg daily as a single daily dose or in divided doses twice daily. If response is inadequate after 12 weeks of treatment, the dosage may be increased to 8 mg daily as a single daily dose or in divided doses twice daily.

Renal Impairment: No adjustment is necessary.

Hepatic Impairment: Clearance is significantly lower in hepatic impairment. Therapy should not be initiated if the patient exhibits active liver disease of increased transaminases (>2.5 times the upper limit of normal) at baseline. For patients with normal hepatic enzymes who are switched from troglitazone to rosiglitazone, a 1-week washout is recommended before initiating therapy with rosiglitazone.

Monitoring Laboratory Tests Hemoglobin A_{1c}, liver enzymes (prior to initiation of therapy, every 2 months for the first year of therapy, then periodically thereafter). Patients with an elevation in ALT >3 times the upper limit of normal should be rechecked as soon as possible. If the ALT levels remain >3 times the upper limit of normal, therapy with rosiglitazone should be discontinued. Monitor serum glucose as recommended by prescriber.

Monitoring and Teaching Issues

Physical Assessment: Monitor laboratory results closely. Assess other medications patient may be taking (see Warnings/Precautions and Drug Interactions). Monitor response to therapy closely until response is stable. Advise women using oral contraceptives about need for alternative method of contraception. Assess knowledge/teach risks of hyper-/hypoglycemia, its symptoms, treatment, and predisposing conditions. Refer patient to a diabetic educator, if possible. Teach appropriate use of medication, interventions to reduce side effects, and adverse reactions to report (see Patient Education). **Pregnancy risk factor C** - benefits of use should outweigh possible risks. Breast-feeding is not recommended.

Patient Education: May be taken without regard to meals. Follow directions of prescriber. If dose is missed at the usual meal, take it with next meal. Do not double dose if daily dose is missed completely. Monitor urine or serum glucose as recommended by prescriber. More frequent monitoring is required during periods of stress, trauma, surgery, pregnancy, increased activity or exercise. Avoid alcohol. Report chest pain, rapid heartbeat or palpitations, abdominal pain, fever, rash, hypoglycemia reactions, yellowing of skin or eyes, dark urine or light stool, or unusual fatigue or nausea/vomiting. Report unusually rapid weight gain; swelling of ankles, legs, or abdomen; or weakness or shortness of breath. **Pregnancy/breast-feeding precautions:** In anovulatory, premenopausal women, ovulation may occur, increasing the risk of pregnancy. Adequate contraception is recommended. Use alternate means of contraception if using oral contraceptives. Breast-feeding is not recommended.

Dietary Issues: Management of type 2 diabetes mellitus (noninsulin dependent, NIDDM) should include diet control. May be taken without regard to meals.

Breast-feeding Issues: In animal studies, rosiglitazone has been found to be excreted in milk. It is not known whether rosiglitazone is excreted in human milk. Should not be administered to a nursing woman.

Pregnancy Issues: Treatment during mid to late gestation was associated with fetal death and growth retardation in animal models. Abnormal blood glucose levels are associated with a higher incidence of congenital abnormalities. Insulin is the drug of choice for the control of diabetes mellitus during pregnancy.

Related Information

Antidiabetic Oral Agents Comparison *on page 1556*
Diabetes Mellitus Management *on page 1661*

Rowasa® *see* Mesalamine *on page 858*
Roxanol® *see* Morphine Sulfate *on page 926*
Roxanol 100® *see* Morphine Sulfate *on page 926*
Roxanol®-T *see* Morphine Sulfate *on page 926*
Roxicet® *see* Oxycodone and Acetaminophen *on page 1022*
Roxicet® 5/500 *see* Oxycodone and Acetaminophen *on page 1022*
Roxicodone™ *see* Oxycodone *on page 1020*
Roxicodone™ Intensol™ *see* Oxycodone *on page 1020*
RP54274 *see* Riluzole *on page 1190*
RP59500 *see* Quinupristin and Dalfopristin *on page 1166*
r-PA *see* Reteplase *on page 1179*
R-Tannamine® Tablet *see page 1522*
R-Tannate® Tablet *see page 1522*
RTCA *see* Ribavirin *on page 1181*
RU-486 *see* Mifepristone *on page 905*
RU-38486 *see* Mifepristone *on page 905*
Rubella and Mumps Vaccines, Combined *see page 1498*
Rubella Virus Vaccine, Live *see page 1498*
Rubex® *see* DOXOrubicin *on page 446*
Rubidomycin Hydrochloride *see* DAUNOrubicin Hydrochloride *on page 369*
Rum-K® *see* Potassium Supplements *on page 1106*
Ryna-C® Liquid *see page 1522*
Rynatan® Pediatric Suspension *see page 1522*
Rynatan® Tablet *see page 1522*
Rynatan® Tablet *see* Azatadine and Pseudoephedrine *on page 137*
Rythmol® *see* Propafenone *on page 1136*

Sacrosidase (sak RO se dase)

U.S. Brand Names Sucraid®

Generic Available No

Pharmacologic Category Enzyme, Gastrointestinal

Pregnancy Risk Factor C

Lactation Enters breast milk/compatible

Use Orphan drug: Oral replacement therapy in sucrase deficiency, as seen in congenital sucrase-isomaltase deficiency (CSID)

(Continued)

Sacrosidase *(Continued)*

Mechanism of Action/Effect Sacrosidase is a naturally-occurring gastrointestinal enzyme which breaks down the disaccharide sucrose to its monosaccharide components. Hydrolysis is necessary to allow absorption of these nutrients.

Contraindications Hypersensitivity to yeast, yeast products, or glycerin

Warnings/Precautions Hypersensitivity reactions to sacrosidase, including bronchospasm, have been reported. Administer initial doses in a setting where acute hypersensitivity reactions may be treated within a few minutes. Skin testing for hypersensitivity may be performed prior to administration to identify patients at risk. Pregnancy risk C.

Drug Interactions

Increased Effect/Toxicity: Drug-drug interactions have not been evaluated.

Nutritional/Ethanol Interactions Food: May be inactivated or denatured if administered with fruit juice, warm or hot food or liquids. Since isomaltase deficiency is not addressed by supplementation of sacrosidase, adherence to a low-starch diet may be required.

Adverse Reactions

1% to 10%: Gastrointestinal: Abdominal pain, vomiting, nausea, diarrhea, constipation

<1% (Limited to important or life-threatening symptoms): Bronchospasm, dehydration, headache, hypersensitivity reaction, insomnia, nervousness

Overdosage/Toxicology Symptoms may include epigastric pain, drowsiness, lethargy, nausea, and vomiting. Gastrointestinal bleeding may occur. Rare manifestations include hypertension, respiratory depression, coma, and acute renal failure. Treatment is symptomatic and supportive. Forced diuresis, hemodialysis and/or urinary alkalinization are not likely to be useful.

Pharmacodynamics/Kinetics

Absorption: Amino acids

Metabolism: GI tract to individual amino acids

Formulations Solution, oral: 8500 int. units per mL (118 mL)

Dosing

Adults & Elderly: Sucrase deficiency: Oral: 17,000 int. units (2 mL) per meal or snack. Doses should be diluted with 2-4 ounces of water, milk or formula with each meal or snack. Approximately one-half of the dose may be taken before, and the remainder of a dose taken at the completion of each meal or snack.

Pediatrics: Children >15 kg: Refer to adult dosing.

Stability

Storage: Store under refrigeration at 4°C to 8°C (36°F to 46°F). Protect from heat or light.

Monitoring and Teaching Issues

Physical Assessment: See Contraindications and Warnings/Precautions for use cautions (eg, hypersensitivity testing). Monitor effectiveness of therapy and adverse reactions at beginning of therapy and periodically with long-term use (see Adverse Reactions). Assess knowledge/teach patient appropriate use, interventions to reduce side effects, and adverse symptoms to report (see Patient Education). **Pregnancy risk factor C** - benefits of use should outweigh possible risks.

Patient Education: Use exactly as directed. Dilute dose in 2-4 oz of water, milk, or formula; do not dilute with fruit juice or warm or cold liquids. Take half the dose at beginning of meal and half the dose at end of meal. Maintain adequate hydration (2-3 L/day of fluids) unless advised by prescriber to restrict fluids. Follow prescribers recommended diet exactly. You may experience headache or nervousness (use caution when driving or engaging in tasks requiring alertness until response to drug is known); or nausea, vomiting, or GI disturbance (frequent mouth care, chewing gum, or sucking hard candy may help). Report immediately skin rash or difficulty breathing; persistent vomiting, abdominal pain, or blood in stools; change in CNS status (depression, agitation, lethargy); or other adverse response. **Pregnancy precaution:** Inform prescriber if you are or intend to become pregnant.

Additional Information Oral solution contains 50% glycerol.

Safe Prescription Writing *see page 17*

Safe Tussin® 30 [OTC] *see* Guaifenesin and Dextromethorphan *on page 647*

Saizen® *see* Human Growth Hormone *on page 658*

Salagen® *see* Pilocarpine *on page 1082*

Salbutamol *see* Albuterol *on page 52*

Salflex® *see* Salsalate *on page 1212*

Salicylazosulfapyridine *see* Sulfasalazine *on page 1262*

Salicylsalicylic Acid *see* Salsalate *on page 1212*

Salmeterol (sal ME te role)

U.S. Brand Names Serevent®; Serevent® Diskus®

Synonyms Salmeterol Xinafoate

Generic Available No

Pharmacologic Category $Beta_2$ Agonist

Pregnancy Risk Factor C

Lactation Enters breast milk/use caution

Use Maintenance treatment of asthma and in prevention of bronchospasm (inhalation aerosol in patients >12 years of age; inhalation powder in patients ≥4 years of age) with reversible obstructive airway disease, including patients with symptoms of nocturnal asthma, who require regular treatment with inhaled, short-acting $beta_2$ agonists; prevention of exercise-induced bronchospasm; maintenance treatment of bronchospasm associated with COPD

Mechanism of Action/Effect Relaxes bronchial smooth muscle by selective action on $beta_2$-receptors with little effect on heart rate; because salmeterol acts locally in the lung, therapeutic effect is not predicted by plasma levels

Contraindications Hypersensitivity to salmeterol, adrenergic amines, or any component of the formulation; need for acute bronchodilation; within 2 weeks of MAO inhibitor use

Warnings/Precautions Salmeterol is not meant to relieve acute asthmatic symptoms. **Acute episodes should be treated with short-acting $beta_2$ agonist.** Do not increase the frequency of salmeterol. Patients receiving maintenance dosages should not use additional salmeterol for exercise-induced asthma prevention. Cardiovascular effects are not common with salmeterol when used in recommended doses. All beta agonists may cause elevation in blood pressure, heart rate, and result in excitement (CNS). Use with caution in patients with prostatic hyperplasia, diabetes, cardiovascular disorders, convulsive disorders, thyrotoxicosis, or others who are sensitive to the effects of sympathomimetic amines. Paroxysmal bronchospasm (which can be fatal) has been reported with this and other inhaled agents. If this occurs, discontinue treatment. The elderly may be at greater risk of cardiovascular side effects; safety and efficacy have not been established in children <4 years of age. Pregnancy risk C.

Drug Interactions

Decreased Effect: Beta-adrenergic blockers (eg, propranolol)

Increased Effect/Toxicity:

Increased toxicity (cardiovascular): MAO inhibitors, tricyclic antidepressants

Increased effect: Inhaled corticosteroids: The addition of salmeterol has been demonstrated to improve response to inhaled corticosteroids (as compared to increasing steroid dosage).

Adverse Reactions

>10%:

Central nervous system: Headache

Respiratory: Pharyngitis

1% to 10%:

Cardiovascular: Tachycardia, palpitations, elevation or depression of blood pressure, cardiac arrhythmias

Central nervous system: Nervousness, CNS stimulation, hyperactivity, insomnia, malaise, dizziness

Gastrointestinal: GI upset, diarrhea, nausea

Neuromuscular & skeletal: Tremors (may be more common in the elderly), myalgias, back pain, arthralgia

Respiratory: Upper respiratory infection, cough, bronchitis

<1% (Limited to important or life-threatening): Arrhythmias, atrial fibrillation, hypertension, immediate hypersensitivity reactions (rash, urticaria, bronchospasm), laryngeal spasm, paradoxical bronchospasms

Overdosage/Toxicology Decontamination: Lavage/activated charcoal. Prudent use of a cardioselective beta-adrenergic blocker (eg, atenolol or metoprolol). Keep in mind the potential for induction of bronchoconstriction in an asthmatic. Dialysis has not been shown to be of value in treatment of overdose with salmeterol.

Pharmacodynamics/Kinetics

Half-Life Elimination: 3-4 hours

Metabolism: Hepatically hydroxylated

Onset: 5-20 minutes (average 10 minutes); Peak effect: 2-4 hours

Duration: 12 hours

Formulations

Aerosol for oral inhalation, as xinafoate (Serevent®): 21 mcg/spray [60 inhalations] (6.5 g), [120 inhalations] (13 g)

Powder for oral inhalation (Serevent® Diskus®): 50 mcg [46 mcg/inhalation] (60 doses)

Dosing

Adults:

Note: Do **not** use spacer with inhalation powder.

Asthma, maintenance and prevention:

Inhalation, aerosol: 42 mcg (2 puffs) twice daily (12 hours apart)

Inhalation, powder (Serevent® Diskus®): One inhalation (50 mcg) twice daily

Exercise-induced asthma, prevention:

Inhalation, aerosol: 42 mcg (2 puffs) 30-60 minutes prior to exercise; additional doses should not be used for 12 hours.

Inhalation, powder (Serevent® Diskus®): One inhalation (50 mcg) at least 30 minutes prior to exercise; additional doses should not be used for 12 hours.

COPD (maintenance treatment of associated bronchospasm):

Inhalation, aerosol: 42 micrograms (2 puffs) twice daily (morning and evening, 12 hours apart)

Inhalation, powder (Serevent® Diskus®): One inhalation (50 mcg) twice daily, ~12 hours apart

Elderly: Refer to adult dosing and Geriatric Considerations.

Pediatrics:

Note: Do **not** use spacer with inhalation powder.

Asthma, maintenance and prevention:

Inhalation, aerosol: Children ≥12 years: 42 mcg (2 puffs) twice daily (12 hours apart)

Inhalation, powder (Serevent® Diskus®): Children ≥4 years: One inhalation (50 mcg) twice daily

Exercise-induced asthma, prevention:

Inhalation, aerosol: Children ≥12 years: 42 mcg (2 puffs) 30-60 minutes prior to exercise; additional doses should not be used for 12 hours.

Inhalation, powder (Serevent® Diskus®): Children ≥4 years: One inhalation (50 mcg) at least 30 minutes prior to exercise; additional doses should not be used for 12 hours.

Administration

Inhalation: Inhalation: Shake well before use. **Not** to be used for the relief of acute attacks.

Stability

Storage:

Aerosol: Store at 15°C to 30°C (59°F to 86°F). Protect from freezing temperature. The therapeutic effect may decrease when the canister is cold therefore the canister should

(Continued)

Salmeterol *(Continued)*

remain at room temperature. Store canister with nozzle end down. Do not store at temperatures >120°F.

Inhalation powder (Serevent® Diskus®): Store at controlled room temperature 20°C to 25°C (68°F to 77°F) in a dry place away from direct heat or sunlight. Stable for 6 weeks after removal from foil pouch.

Monitoring Laboratory Tests Pulmonary function

Monitoring and Teaching Issues

Physical Assessment: Not for use to relieve acute asthmatic attacks. Assess effectiveness and interactions of other medications patient may be taking (see Drug Interactions). See Contraindications and Warnings/Precautions for use cautions. Monitor effectiveness of therapy and adverse reactions at beginning of therapy and periodically with long-term use (see Adverse Reactions and Overdose/Toxicology). For inpatient care, monitor vital signs and lung sounds prior to and periodically during therapy. Assess knowledge/teach patient appropriate use, interventions to reduce side effects, and adverse symptoms to report (see Patient Education). **Pregnancy risk factor C** - benefits of use should outweigh possible risks. Note breast-feeding caution.

Patient Education: Use exactly as directed (see Administration below). Do not use more often than recommended (excessive use may result in tolerance, overdose may result in serious adverse effects) and do not discontinue without consulting prescriber. Do not use for acute attacks. Maintain adequate hydration (2-3 L/day of fluids) unless advised by prescriber to restrict fluids. You may experience nervousness, dizziness, or fatigue (use caution when driving or engaging in tasks requiring alertness until response to drug is known); or dry mouth, stomach upset (small, frequent meals, frequent mouth care, chewing gum, or sucking hard candy may help). Report unresolved GI upset; dizziness or fatigue; vision changes; chest pain, rapid heartbeat, or palpitations; insomnia; nervousness or hyperactivity; muscle cramping, tremors, or pain; unusual cough; or skin rash. **Pregnancy/breast-feeding precautions:** Inform prescriber if you are or intend to become pregnant. Consult prescriber if breast-feeding.

Inhalation: Store canister upside down; do not freeze. Shake canister before using. Sit when using medication. Close eyes when administering salmeterol to avoid spray getting into eyes. Exhale slowly and completely through nose; inhale deeply through mouth while administering aerosol. Hold breath for 5-10 seconds after inhalation. Wait at least 1 full minute between inhalations. Wash mouthpiece between use. If more than one inhalation medication is used, use bronchodilator first and wait 5 minutes between medications.

Geriatric Considerations: Geriatric patients were included in four clinical studies of salmeterol; no apparent differences in efficacy and safety were noted in geriatric patients compared to younger adults. Because salmeterol is only to be used for prevention of bronchospasm, patients also need a short-acting beta-agonist to treat acute attacks. Elderly patients should be carefully counseled about which inhaler to use and the proper scheduling of doses; a spacer device may be utilized to maximize effectiveness.

Related Information

Inhalant (Asthma, Bronchospasm) Agents Comparison *on page 1577*

Salmeterol and Fluticasone *see* Fluticasone and Salmeterol *on page 591*

Salmeterol Xinafoate *see* Salmeterol *on page 1210*

Salsalate (SAL sa late)

U.S. Brand Names Amigesic®; Argesic®-SA; Disalcid®; Mono-Gesic®; Salflex®

Synonyms Disalicylic Acid; Salicylsalicylic Acid

Generic Available Yes

Pharmacologic Category Salicylate

Pregnancy Risk Factor C/D (3rd trimester)

Lactation Enters breast milk/contraindicated

Use Treatment of minor pain or fever; arthritis

Mechanism of Action/Effect Inhibits prostaglandin synthesis, acts on the hypothalamus heat-regulating center to reduce fever, blocks prostaglandin synthetase action which prevents formation of the platelet-aggregating substance thromboxane A_2

Contraindications Hypersensitivity to salsalate or any component of the formulation; GI ulcer or bleeding; pregnancy (3rd trimester)

Warnings/Precautions Use with caution in patients with platelet and bleeding disorders, renal dysfunction, erosive gastritis, or peptic ulcer disease, dehydration, previous nonreaction does not guarantee future safe taking of medication. Pregnancy risk C/D (3rd trimester).

Drug Interactions

Decreased Effect: Decreased effect with urinary alkalinizers, antacids, and corticosteroids. Decreased effect of uricosurics and spironolactone.

Increased Effect/Toxicity: Increased effect/toxicity of oral anticoagulants, hypoglycemics, and methotrexate.

Nutritional/Ethanol Interactions

Ethanol: Avoid ethanol (may enhance gastric mucosal irritation).

Food: Salsalate peak serum levels may be delayed if taken with food.

Herb/Nutraceutical: Avoid cat's claw, dong quai, evening primrose, feverfew, garlic, ginger, ginkgo, red clover, horse chestnut, green tea, ginseng (all have additional antiplatelet activity).

Effects on Lab Values False-negative results for glucose oxidase urinary glucose tests (Clinistix®); false-positives using the cupric sulfate method (Clinitest®); also, interferes with Gerhardt test, VMA determination; 5-HIAA, xylose tolerance test and T_3 and T_4

Adverse Reactions

>10%: Gastrointestinal: Nausea, heartburn, stomach pains, dyspepsia

1% to 10%:

- Central nervous system: Drowsiness
- Dermatologic: Rash
- Gastrointestinal: Gastrointestinal ulceration

Hematologic: Hemolytic anemia
Neuromuscular & skeletal: Weakness
Respiratory: Dyspnea
Miscellaneous: Anaphylactic shock

<1% (Limited to important or life-threatening): Bronchospasm, does not appear to inhibit platelet aggregation, hepatotoxicity, impaired renal function, iron-deficiency anemia, leukopenia, occult bleeding, thrombocytopenia

Overdosage/Toxicology Symptoms of overdose include respiratory alkalosis, hyperpnea, tachypnea, tinnitus, headache, hyperpyrexia, metabolic acidosis, hypoglycemia, and coma. Nomograms, such as the "Done" nomogram, can be very helpful for estimating the severity of aspirin poisoning and for directing treatment using serum salicylate levels. Treatment can also be based upon symptomatology.

Pharmacodynamics/Kinetics

Absorption: Complete, from small intestine

Half-Life Elimination: 7-8 hours

Metabolism: Hepatically hydrolyzed to two moles of salicylic acid (active)

Onset: Therapeutic: 3-4 days of continuous dosing

Formulations

Capsule: 500 mg
Tablet: 500 mg, 750 mg

Dosing

Adults & Elderly: Pain, inflammation (arthritis): Oral: 3 g/day in 2-3 divided doses

Renal Impairment: Patients with end-stage renal disease undergoing hemodialysis: Administer 750 mg twice daily with an additional 500 mg after dialysis.

Monitoring and Teaching Issues

Physical Assessment: Assess effectiveness and interactions of other medications patient may be taking (see Contraindications and Drug Interactions). Monitor laboratory tests (see above) and therapeutic response and adverse reactions (eg, GI effects, hepatotoxicity) at beginning of therapy and periodically throughout therapy (see Warnings/Precautions, Adverse Reactions, and Overdose/Toxicology). Schedule ophthalmic evaluations for patients who are on long-term NSAID therapy. Assess knowledge/teach patient appropriate use, interventions to reduce side effects, and adverse symptoms to report (see Patient Education). **Pregnancy risk factor C/D** - see Pregnancy Risk Factor for use cautions; benefits of use should outweigh possible risks. Breast-feeding is contraindicated.

Patient Education: Take this medication exactly as directed; do not increase dose without consulting prescriber. Do not crush tablets or break capsules. Take with food or milk to reduce GI distress. Maintain adequate hydration (2-3 L/day of fluids) unless advised by prescriber to restrict fluids. Do not use alcohol, aspirin or aspirin-containing medication, or any other anti-inflammatory medications without consulting prescriber. You may experience drowsiness (use caution when driving or engaging in tasks requiring alertness until response to drug is known); or nausea or heartburn (small, frequent meals, frequent mouth care, sucking lozenges, or chewing gum may help). GI bleeding, ulceration, or perforation can occur with or without pain; discontinue medication and contact prescriber if persistent abdominal pain or cramping, or blood in stool occurs. Report breathlessness or difficulty breathing; unusual bruising or bleeding; blood in urine, stool, mouth, or vomitus; unusual fatigue; skin rash or itching; change in urinary pattern; or change in hearing or ringing in ears. **Pregnancy/breast-feeding precautions:** Inform prescriber if you are or intend to become pregnant. This drug should not be used in the 3rd trimester of pregnancy. Do not breast-feed.

Dietary Issues: May be taken with food to decrease GI distress.

Geriatric Considerations: Elderly are at high risk for adverse effects from NSAIDs. As much as 60% of elderly can develop peptic ulceration and/or hemorrhage asymptomatically. The concomitant use of H_2 blockers, omeprazole, and sucralfate is not effective as prophylaxis with the exception of NSAID-induced duodenal ulcers which may be prevented by the use of ranitidine. Misoprostol is the only prophylactic agent proven effective. Also, concomitant disease and drug use contribute to the risk for GI adverse effects. Use lowest effective dose for shortest period possible. Consider renal function decline with age. Use of NSAIDs can compromise existing renal function especially when Cl_{cr} is ≤30 mL/minute. Tinnitus may be a difficult and unreliable indication of toxicity due to age-related hearing loss or eighth cranial nerve damage. CNS adverse effects such as confusion, agitation, and hallucinations are generally seen in overdose or high-dose situations, but elderly may demonstrate these adverse effects at lower doses than younger adults.

Breast-feeding Issues: Salsalate is metabolized to salicylate which is contraindicated while breast-feeding.

Related Information

Nonsalicylate/Nonsteroidal Anti-inflammatory Comparison *on page 1587*

Salt Poor Albumin *see* Albumin *on page 50*

Sal-Tropine® *see page 1509*

Sal-Tropine™ *see* Atropine *on page 134*

Sandimmune® *see* CycloSPORINE *on page 343*

Sandostatin® *see* Octreotide *on page 991*

Sandostatin LAR® *see* Octreotide *on page 991*

Sanorex® *see* Mazindol *on page 837*

Sansert® *see* Methysergide *on page 888*

Santyl® *see* Collagenase *on page 332*

Saquinavir (sa KWIN a veer)

U.S. Brand Names Fortovase®; Invirase®

Synonyms Saquinavir Mesylate

Generic Available No

Pharmacologic Category Antiretroviral Agent, Protease Inhibitor

Pregnancy Risk Factor B

(Continued)

Saquinavir *(Continued)*

Lactation Excretion in breast milk unknown/contraindicated

Use Treatment of HIV infection in selected patients; used in combination with at least two other antiretroviral agents

Mechanism of Action/Effect As an inhibitor of HIV protease, saquinavir prevents the cleavage of viral polyprotein precursors which are needed to generate functional proteins in and maturation of HIV-infected cells

Contraindications Hypersensitivity to saquinavir or any component of the formulation; exposure to direct sunlight without sunscreen or protective clothing; coadministration with cisapride, astemizole, triazolam, midazolam, or ergot derivatives

Warnings/Precautions The indication for saquinavir for the treatment of HIV infection is based on changes in surrogate markers. At present, there are no results from controlled clinical trials evaluating its effect on patient survival or the clinical progression of HIV infection (ie, occurrence of opportunistic infections or malignancies); use caution in patients with hepatic insufficiency; safety and efficacy have not been established in children <16 years of age. May exacerbate pre-existing hepatic dysfunction; use with caution in patients with hepatitis B or C and in cirrhosis. Not recommended for use in patients receiving lovastatin or simvastatin; use caution with atorvastatin or cerivastatin. May be associated with fat redistribution (buffalo hump, protease paunch, breast engorgement, facial atrophy). Avoid concurrent use of St John's wort (may lead to loss of virologic response and/or resistance).

Drug Interactions

Cytochrome P450 Effect: Substrate of CYP2D6, **3A4**; Inhibits CYP2C8/9, 2C19, 2D6, **3A4**

Decreased Effect: Nevirapine, rifabutin, rifampin, phenobarbital, phenytoin, dexamethasone, and carbamazepine may decrease saquinavir concentrations. Saquinavir may decrease delavirdine concentrations.

Increased Effect/Toxicity:

Decreased effect: Rifampin may decrease saquinavir's plasma levels and AUC by 40% to 80%; other enzyme inducers may induce saquinavir's metabolism (eg, phenobarbital, phenytoin, dexamethasone, carbamazepine); may decrease delavirdine concentrations

Increased effect: Ketoconazole significantly increases plasma levels and AUC of saquinavir; as a known, although not potent inhibitor of the cytochrome P450 system, saquinavir may decrease the metabolism of astemizole, as well as cisapride and ergot derivatives (and result in rare but serious effects including cardiac arrhythmias); other drugs which may have increased adverse effects if coadministered with saquinavir include benzodiazepines (midazolam and triazolam), calcium channel blockers, clindamycin, dapsone, ergot alkaloids, and quinidine. Both clarithromycin and saquinavir levels/effects may be increased with coadministration. Delavirdine may increase concentration; ritonavir may increase AUC >17-fold; concurrent administration of nelfinavir results in increase in nelfinavir (18%) and saquinavir (mean: 392%).

Saquinavir increased serum concentrations of simvastatin, lovastatin, and atorvastatin; risk of myopathy/rhabdomyolysis may be increased. Use cautiously with HMG-CoA reductase inhibitors. Avoid use with simvastatin and lovastatin. Use caution with atorvastatin and cerivastatin (fluvastatin and pravastatin are not metabolized by CYP3A4).

Sildenafil serum concentrations are increased in concurrent therapy (limit sildenafil dosage to 25 mg).

Nutritional/Ethanol Interactions

Food: A high-fat meal maximizes bioavailability. Saquinavir levels may increase if taken with grapefruit juice.

Herb/Nutraceutical: Saquinavir serum concentrations may be decreased by St John's wort; avoid concurrent use.

Adverse Reactions Protease inhibitors cause dyslipidemia which includes elevated cholesterol and triglycerides and a redistribution of body fat centrally to cause "protease paunch", buffalo hump, facial atrophy, and breast enlargement. These agents also cause hyperglycemia.

1% to 10%:

Dermatologic: Rash

Endocrine & metabolic: Hyperglycemia

Gastrointestinal: Diarrhea, abdominal discomfort, nausea, abdominal pain, buccal mucosa ulceration

Neuromuscular & skeletal: Paresthesia, weakness, increased CPK

<1% (Limited to important or life-threatening): Acute myeloblastic leukemia, ascites, ataxia, bullous skin eruption, exacerbation of chronic liver disease, hemolytic anemia, jaundice, polyarthritis, portal hypertension, seizures, Stevens-Johnson syndrome, thrombocytopenia, thrombophlebitis

Pharmacodynamics/Kinetics

Absorption: Poor; increased with high fat meal; Fortovase® has improved absorption over Invirase®

Bioavailability: Invirase®: ~4%; Fortovase®: 12% to 15%

Metabolism: Extensively hepatic via CYP3A4; extensive first-pass effect

Formulations

Capsule, as mesylate (Invirase®): 200 mg

Capsule, soft gelatin (Fortovase®): 200 mg

Dosing

Adults: HIV infection: Oral: **Note:** Fortovase® and Invirase® are not bioequivalent and should not be used interchangeably; only Fortovase® should be used to initiate therapy:

Fortovase®: Six 200 mg capsules (1200 mg) 3 times/day within 2 hours after a meal in combination with a nucleoside analog

Invirase®: Three 200 mg capsules (600 mg) 3 times/day within 2 hours after a full meal in combination with a nucleoside analog

Note: Dosage adjustment of either Fortovase® or Invirase® in combination with ritonavir: 400 mg twice daily

Note: Dosage adjustments of Fortovase® when administered in combination therapy:

Delavirdine: Fortovase® 800 mg 3 times/day

Lopinavir and ritonavir (Kaletra™): Fortovase® 800 mg twice daily

Nelfinavir: Fortovase® 800 mg 3 times/day or 1200 mg twice daily

Elderly: Clinical studies did not include sufficient numbers of patients ≥65 years of age. Use caution due to increased frequency of organ dysfunction.

Pediatrics: Children and Adolescents <16 years: Safety and efficacy have not been established; dosages of 33-50 mg/kg/dose 3 times/day are under study

Administration

Oral: Take saquinavir within 2 hours after a full meal. Avoid direct sunlight when taking saquinavir.

Stability

Storage:

Fortovase®: Store in refrigerator. Storage at room temperature is stable for 3 months.

Invirase®: Store at room temperature.

Monitoring Laboratory Tests CBC, renal and liver function, electrolytes, triglycerides, cholesterol, glucose, CD4 cell count, plasma levels of HIV RNA

Monitoring and Teaching Issues

Physical Assessment: See Contraindications, Warnings/Precautions, and Dosing for use cautions. Assess potential for interactions with other prescriptions, OTC medications, or herbal products patient may be taking (see Drug Interactions). Assess result of laboratory tests (see above) and patient response at regular intervals during therapy (see Adverse Reactions and Overdose/Toxicology). Teach patient proper use, possible side effects and appropriate interventions (eg, glucose testing; protease inhibitors may cause hyperglycemia [exacerbation or new-onset diabetes], and adverse symptoms to report - see Patient Education). Breast-feeding is contraindicated.

Patient Education: Inform prescriber of all prescriptions, OTC medications, or herbal products you are taking, and any allergies you have. Do not take anything new during treatment unless approved by prescriber. Ritonavir is not a cure for HIV, nor has it been found to reduce transmission of HIV. Take as directed, with meals. Avoid grapefruit juice. Maintain adequate hydration (2-3 L/day of fluids) unless advised by prescriber to restrict fluids. Saquinavir may be prescribed with a combination of other medications; time these medications as directed by prescriber. You may be advised to check your glucose levels (this drug can cause exacerbation or new-onset diabetes). Avoid exposure to direct sunlight (wear protective clothing, use sunblock, and avoid direct sunlight). May cause body changes due to redistribution of body fat, facial atrophy, or breast enlargement (normal effects of drug); dizziness, insomnia, abnormal thinking (use caution when driving or engaging in potentially hazardous tasks until response to drug is known); nausea, vomiting, or taste perversion (small, frequent meals, frequent mouth care, chewing gum, or sucking lozenges may help); mouth sores (frequent oral care is necessary); muscle weakness (consult prescriber for approved analgesic); headache; or insomnia (consult prescriber for medication). Report any persistent adverse effects. **Breast-feeding precaution:** Do not breast-feed.

Dietary Issues: Administer within 2 hours of a meal.

Breast-feeding Issues: HIV-infected mothers are discouraged from breast-feeding to decrease postnatal transmission of HIV.

Pregnancy Issues: Preliminary data show that saquinavir pharmacokinetics may be affected by pregnancy; studies are not yet complete. Pregnancy and protease inhibitors are both associated with an increased risk of hyperglycemia. Glucose levels should be closely monitored. Health professionals are encouraged to contact the antiretroviral pregnancy registry to monitor outcomes of pregnant women exposed to antiretroviral medications (1-800-258-4263).

Additional Information The indication for saquinavir for the treatment of HIV infection is based on changes in surrogate markers. At present, there are no results from controlled clinical trials evaluating the effect of regimens containing saquinavir on patient survival or the clinical progression of HIV infection, such as the occurrence of opportunistic infections or malignancies; in cell culture, saquinavir is additive to synergistic with AZT, ddC, and DDI without enhanced toxicity. According to the manufacturer, Invirase® will be phased out over time and completely replaced by Fortovase®. Potential compliance problems, frequency of administration and adverse effects should be discussed with patients before initiating therapy to help prevent the emergence of resistance.

Related Information

Tuberculosis *on page 1705*

Saquinavir Mesylate *see* Saquinavir *on page 1213*

Sarafem™ *see* Fluoxetine *on page 578*

Sargramostim (sar GRAM oh stim)

U.S. Brand Names Leukine™

Synonyms GM-CSF; Granulocyte-Macrophage Colony Stimulating Factor; rGM-CSF

Generic Available No

Pharmacologic Category Colony Stimulating Factor

Pregnancy Risk Factor C

Lactation Excretion in breast milk unknown

Use

Myeloid reconstitution after autologous bone marrow transplantation: Non-Hodgkin's lymphoma (NHL), acute lymphoblastic leukemia (ALL), Hodgkin's lymphoma, metastatic breast cancer

Myeloid reconstitution after allogeneic bone marrow transplantation

Peripheral stem cell transplantation: Metastatic breast cancer, non-Hodgkin's lymphoma, Hodgkin's lymphoma, multiple myeloma

(Continued)

Sargramostim *(Continued)*

Orphan drug:

Acute myelogenous leukemia (AML) following induction chemotherapy in older adults to shorten time to neutrophil recovery and to reduce the incidence of severe and life-threatening infections and infections resulting in death

Bone marrow transplant (allogeneic or autologous) failure or engraftment delay

Safety and efficacy of GM-CSF given simultaneously with cytotoxic chemotherapy have not been established. Concurrent treatment may increase myelosuppression.

Mechanism of Action/Effect Stimulates proliferation, differentiation and functional activity of neutrophils, eosinophils, monocytes, and macrophages; see table.

Comparative Effects — G-CSF vs. GM-CSF

Proliferation/Differentiation	G-CSF (Filgrastim)	GM-CSF (Sargramostim)
Neutrophils	Yes	Yes
Eosinophils	No	Yes
Macrophages	No	Yes
Neutrophil migration	Enhanced	Inhibited

Contraindications Hypersensitivity to sargramostim, yeast-derived products, or any component of the formulation; concurrent myelosuppressive chemotherapy or radiation therapy. The solution for injection contains benzyl alcohol and should not be used in neonates.

Warnings/Precautions Simultaneous administration, or administration 24 hours preceding/following cytotoxic chemotherapy or radiotherapy is not recommended. Use with caution in patients with pre-existing cardiac problems, hypoxia, fluid retention, pulmonary infiltrates or CHF, renal or hepatic impairment. rapid increase in peripheral blood counts. If ANC is >20,000/mm^3, or platelets >500,000/mm^3 decrease dose by 50% or discontinue drug (counts will fall to normal within 3-7 days after discontinuing drug). Growth factor potential: caution with myeloid malignancies. Precaution should be exercised in the usage of GM-CSF in any malignancy with myeloid characteristics. GM-CSF can potentially act as a growth factor for any tumor type, particularly myeloid malignancies. Tumors of nonhematopoietic origin may have surface receptors for GM-CSF. Pregnancy risk C.

Drug Interactions

Increased Effect/Toxicity: Lithium, corticosteroids may potentiate myeloproliferative effects.

Adverse Reactions

>10%:

Cardiovascular: Hypotension, tachycardia, flushing, and syncope may occur with the first dose of a cycle ("first-dose effect"); peripheral edema (11%)
Central nervous system: Headache (26%)
Dermatologic: Rash, alopecia
Endocrine & metabolic: Polydypsia
Gastrointestinal: Diarrhea (52% to 89%), stomatitis, mucositis
Local: Local reactions at the injection site (~50%)
Neuromuscular & skeletal: Myalgia (18%), arthralgia (21%), bone pain
Renal: Increased serum creatinine (14%)
Respiratory: Dyspnea (28%)

1% to 10%:

Cardiovascular: Transient supraventricular arrhythmias; chest pain; capillary leak syndrome; pericardial effusion (4%)
Central nervous system: Headache
Gastrointestinal: Nausea, vomiting
Hematologic: Leukocytosis, thrombocytopenia
Neuromuscular & skeletal: Weakness
Respiratory: Cough; pleural effusion (1%)

<1% (Limited to important or life-threatening): Anaphylaxis, anorexia, arrhythmia, constipation, eosinophilia, fever, lethargy, malaise, pericarditis, rigors, sore throat, thrombophlebitis, thrombosis

Overdosage/Toxicology Symptoms of overdose include dyspnea, malaise, nausea, fever, headache, and chills. Discontinue drug and wait for levels to fall. Treatment is supportive. Monitor CBC, respiratory symptoms, and fluid status. Discontinue drug and wait for levels to fall, monitor for pulmonary edema. Toxicity of GM-CSF is dose dependent. Severe reactions such as capillary leak syndrome are seen at higher doses (>15 mcg/kg/day).

Pharmacodynamics/Kinetics

Half-Life Elimination: 2 hours

Time to Peak: Serum: S.C.: 1-2 hours

Onset: Increase in WBC: 7-14 days

Duration: WBCs return to baseline within 1 week of discontinuing drug

Formulations Injection: 250 mcg, 500 mcg

Dosing

Adults & Elderly:

Existing clinical data suggest that starting GM-CSF between 24 and 72 hours subsequent to chemotherapy may provide optimal neutrophil recover. Continue therapy until the occurrence of an absolute neutrophil count of 10,000/µL after the neutrophil nadir.

The available data suggest that rounding the dose to the nearest vial size may enhance patient convenience and reduce costs without clinical detrement.

Myeloid reconstitution after peripheral stem cell, allogeneic or autologous bone marrow transplant: I.V.: 250 mcg/m^2/day for 21 days to begin 2-4 hours after the marrow infusion on day 0 of autologous bone marrow transplant or ≥24 hours after chemotherapy or 12 hours after last dose of radiotherapy.

If a severe adverse reaction occurs, reduce or temporarily discontinue the dose until the reaction abates.

If blast cells appear or progression of the underlying disease occurs, disrupt treatment.

Interrupt or reduce the dose by half if ANC is >20,000 cells/mm^3

Patients should not receive sargramostim until the postmarrow infusion ANC is <500 cells/mm^3.

Neutrophil recovery following chemotherapy in AML: I.V.: 250 mcg/m^2/day over a 4-hour period starting approximately day 11 or 4 days following the completion of induction chemotherapy, if day 10 bone marrow is hypoblastic with <5% blasts.

If a second cycle of chemotherapy is necessary, administer ~4 days after the completion of chemotherapy if the bone marrow is hypoblastic with <5% blasts.

Continue sargramostim until ANC is >1500 cells/mm^3 for consecutive days or a maximum of 42 days.

Discontinue sargramostim immediately if leukemic regrowth occurs.

If a severe adverse reaction occurs, reduce the dose by 50% or temporarily discontinue the dose until the reaction abates.

Mobilization of peripheral blood progenitor cells: I.V.: 250 mcg/m^2/day over 24 hours or S.C. once daily.

Continue the same dose through the period of PBPC collection.

The optimal schedule for PBPC collection has not been established (usually begun by day 5 and performed daily until protocol specified targets are achieved).

If WBC >50,000 cells/mm^3, reduce the dose by 50%.

If adequate numbers of progenitor cells are not collected, consider other mobilization therapy.

Postperipheral blood progenitor cell transplantation: I.V.: 250 mcg/m^2/day over 24 hours or S.C. once daily beginning immediately following infusion of progenitor cells and continuing until ANC is >1500 for 3 consecutive days is attained.

BMT failure or engraftment delay: I.V.: 250 mcg/m^2/day for 14 days as a 2-hour infusion.

The dose can be repeated after 7 days off therapy if engraftment has not occurred.

If engraftment still has not occurred, a third course of 500 mcg/m^2/day for 14 days may be tried after another 7 days off therapy; if there is still no improvement, it is unlikely that further dose escalation will be beneficial.

If a severe adverse reaction occurs, reduce or temporarily discontinue the dose until the reaction abates.

If blast cells appear or disease progression occurs, discontinue treatment.

Note: Doses may be given via I.V. infusion over ≥2 hours or S.C.

Pediatrics: Refer to adult dosing.

Administration

I.V.: I.V. infusion should be over at least 2 hours; incompatible with dextrose-containing solutions.

Other: Administer by S.C. (undiluted). Do not shake solution. When administering GM-CSF subcutaneously, rotate injection sites.

Stability

Storage: Sargramostim is available as a sterile, white, preservative-free, lyophilized powder. Sargramostim should be stored at 2°C to 8°C (36°F to 46°F). Vials should not be frozen or shaken.

Reconstitution: Sargramostim is stable after dilution in 1 mL of bacteriostatic or nonbacteriostatic sterile water for injection for 30 days at 2°C to 8°C or 25°C. Sargramostim may also be further diluted in 0.9% sodium chloride to a concentration ≥10 mcg/mL for I.V. infusion administration. This diluted solution is stable for 48 hours at room temperature and refrigeration. If the final concentration of sargramostim is <10 mcg/mL, human albumin should be added to the saline prior to the addition of sargramostim to prevent absorption of the components to the delivery system. It is recommended that 1 mg of human albumin per 1 mL of 0.9% sodium chloride (eg, 1 mL of 5% human albumin per 50 mL of 0.9% sodium chloride) be added.

Standard diluent: Dose ≥250 mcg/25 mL NS

Compatibility: Stable in NS, sterile water for injection, bacteriostatic water; **incompatible** with dextrose-containing solutions

Y-site administration: Incompatible with acyclovir, ampicillin, ampicillin/sulbactam, cefoperazone, chlorpromazine, ganciclovir, haloperidol, hydrocortisone sodium phosphate, hydrocortisone sodium succinate, hydromorphone, hydroxyzine, imipenem/cilastatin, lorazepam, methylprednisolone sodium succinate, mitomycin, morphine, nalbuphine, ondansetron, piperacillin, sodium bicarbonate, tobramycin

Monitoring Laboratory Tests To avoid potential complications of excessive leukocytosis (WBC >50,000 cells/mm^3, ANC >20,000 cells/mm^3) a CBC with differential is recommended twice per week during therapy. Sargramostim therapy should be interrupted or the dose reduced by half if the ANC is >20,000 cells/mm^3. Monitoring of renal and hepatic function in patients displaying renal or hepatic dysfunction prior to initiation of treatment is recommended and at least biweekly during sargramostim administration.

Monitoring and Teaching Issues

Physical Assessment: See Contraindications, Warnings/Precautions, and Dosing for use cautions. See specific I.V. directions above. Patient must be monitored closely for "first dose effects" (see Adverse Reactions). Assess results of laboratory tests (see above) closely. Assess patient response (eg, fluid balance, CNS response, and GI effects - see Adverse Reactions and Overdose/Toxicology) on a frequent basis. Teach patient use if self-administered (eg, appropriate injection technique and syringe/needle disposal), possible side effects and appropriate interventions, and adverse symptoms to report (see Patient Education). **Pregnancy risk factor C** - benefits of use should outweigh possible risks (see Pregnancy Issues). Note breast-feeding caution.

Patient Education: I.V.: Immediately report any redness, swelling, pain, or burning at infusion site. You will require frequent blood tests during treatment. May cause bone pain (request analgesic); or nausea and vomiting (small, frequent meals may help); or hair loss (reversible). Report signs or symptoms of edema (eg, swollen extremities, difficulty breathing, rapid weight gain); onset of severe headache; acute back or chest pain;

(Continued)

Sargramostim *(Continued)*

muscular tremors or seizure activity. **Pregnancy/breast-feeding precautions:** Inform prescriber if you are or intend to become pregnant. Consult prescriber if breast-feeding.

Pregnancy Issues: Animal reproduction studies have not been conducted. It is not known whether sargramostim can cause fetal harm when administered to a pregnant woman or can affect reproductive capability. Sargramostim should be given to a pregnant woman only if clearly needed.

Additional Information

Reimbursement Hotline (Leukine™): 1-800-321-4669
Professional Services (Immunex): 1-800-334-6273

Sarnol®-HC [OTC] *see* Hydrocortisone *on page 673*
Scalpicin® *see* Topical Corticosteroids *on page 1334*
S-Citalopram *see* Escitalopram *on page 489*
Scopace® *see* Scopolamine *on page 1218*

Scopolamine (skoe POL a meen)

U.S. Brand Names Isopto® Hyoscine; Scopace®; Transderm Scōp®

Synonyms Hyoscine; Scopolamine Hydrobromide

Generic Available Yes

Pharmacologic Category Anticholinergic Agent

Pregnancy Risk Factor C

Lactation Enters breast milk/compatible

Use Preoperative medication to produce amnesia and decrease salivary and respiratory secretions; to produce cycloplegia and mydriasis; treatment of iridocyclitis; prevention of motion sickness; prevention of nausea/vomiting associated with anesthesia or opiate analgesia (patch); symptomatic treatment of postencephalitic parkinsonism and paralysis agitans (oral); inhibits excessive motility and hypertonus of the gastrointestinal tract in such conditions as the irritable colon syndrome, mild dysentery, diverticulitis, pylorospasm, and cardiospasm

Mechanism of Action/Effect Blocks the action of acetylcholine at parasympathetic sites in smooth muscle, secretory glands and the CNS; increases cardiac output, dries secretions, antagonizes histamine and serotonin

Contraindications Hypersensitivity to scopolamine or any component of the formulation; narrow-angle glaucoma; acute hemorrhage, gastrointestinal or genitourinary obstruction, thyrotoxicosis, tachycardia secondary to cardiac insufficiency, paralytic ileus

Warnings/Precautions Use with caution with hepatic or renal impairment since adverse CNS effects occur more often in these patients. Anticholinergic agents are not well tolerated in the elderly and their use should be avoided when possible. Pregnancy risk C.

Drug Interactions

Decreased Effect: Decreased effect of acetaminophen, levodopa, ketoconazole, digoxin, riboflavin, and potassium chloride in wax matrix preparations.

Increased Effect/Toxicity: Additive adverse effects with other anticholinergic agents.

Nutritional/Ethanol Interactions Ethanol: Avoid ethanol (may increase CNS depression).

Adverse Reactions Frequency not defined.

Ophthalmic: Note: Systemic adverse effects have been reported following ophthalmic administration.

Cardiovascular: Vascular congestion, edema
Central nervous system: Drowsiness
Dermatologic: Eczematoid dermatitis
Ocular: Blurred vision, photophobia, local irritation, increased intraocular pressure, follicular conjunctivitis, exudate
Respiratory: Congestion

Systemic:

Cardiovascular: Orthostatic hypotension, ventricular fibrillation, tachycardia, palpitations
Central nervous system: Confusion, drowsiness, headache, loss of memory, ataxia, fatigue
Dermatologic: Dry skin, increased sensitivity to light, rash
Endocrine & metabolic: Decreased flow of breast milk
Gastrointestinal: Constipation, xerostomia, dry throat, dysphagia, bloated feeling, nausea, vomiting
Genitourinary: Dysuria
Local: Irritation at injection site
Neuromuscular & skeletal: Weakness
Ocular: Increased intraocular pain, blurred vision
Respiratory: Dry nose, diaphoresis (decreased)
Postmarketing and/or case reports (Limited to important or life-threatening): Hallucinations, restlessness

Overdosage/Toxicology Symptoms of overdose include dilated pupils, flushed skin, tachycardia, hypertension, and EKG abnormalities. CNS manifestations resemble acute psychosis. CNS depression, circulatory collapse, respiratory failure, and death can occur. For a scopolamine overdose with severe life-threatening symptoms, physostigmine 1-2 mg S.C. or I.V. slowly should be given to reverse toxic effects.

Pharmacodynamics/Kinetics

Absorption: Well absorbed from all routes

Metabolism: Hepatic

Onset: Oral, I.M.: 0.5-1 hour; I.V.: 10 minutes

Peak effect: 20-60 minutes; may take 3-7 days for full recovery; transdermal: 24 hours

Duration: Oral, I.M.: 4-6 hours; I.V.: 2 hours

Formulations

Injection, as hydrobromide: 0.4 mg/mL (0.5 mL, 1 mL)
Solution, ophthalmic, as hydrobromide (Isopto® Hyoscine, Scopace®): 0.25% (5 mL, 15 mL)
Tablet, as hydrobromide: 0.4 mg
Transdermal system (Transderm Scōp®): 0.33 mg/24 hours [2.5 cm^2] total scopolamine 1.5 mg per patch [releases ~1 mg over 72 hours]

Dosing

Adults:

Preoperatively:

I.M., I.V., S.C.: 0.3-0.65 mg; may be repeated every 4-6 hours

Transdermal patch: Apply 2.5 cm^2 patch to hairless area behind ear the night before surgery or 1 hour prior to cesarean section (the patch should be applied no sooner than 1 hour before surgery for best results, and removed 24 hours after surgery)

Motion sickness:

Transdermal patch: Apply 1 disc behind the ear at least 4 hours prior to exposure and every 3 days as needed; effective if applied as soon as 2-3 hours before anticipated need, best if 12 hours before.

Oral: 0.4-0.8 mg prior to exposure

Parkinsonism, spasticity: Oral: 0.4-0.8 mg as a range; the dosage may be cautiously increased in parkinsonism and spastic states.

Ophthalmic refraction: Ophthalmic: Instill 1-2 drops of 0.25% to eye(s) 1 hour before procedure.

Iridocyclitis: Ophthalmic: Instill 1-2 drops of 0.25% to eye(s) up to 4 times/day.

Elderly: Avoid use; see Geriatric Considerations.

Pediatrics:

Preoperatively: I.M., S.C.: Children: 6 mcg/kg/dose (maximum: 0.3 mg/dose) or 0.2 mg/m^2 may be repeated every 6-8 hours **or** alternatively:

4-7 months: 0.1 mg

7 months to 3 years: 0.15 mg

3-8 years: 0.2 mg

8-12 years: 0.3 mg

Motion sickness: Transdermal: Children >12 years: Refer to adult dosing.

Ophthalmic refraction: Ophthalmic: Children: Instill 1 drop of 0.25% to eye(s) twice daily for 2 days before procedure.

Iridocyclitis: Ophthalmic: Children: Instill 1 drop of 0.25% to eye(s) up to 3 times/day.

Administration

I.V.: Inject over 2-3 minutes.

Topical: Topical disc is programmed to deliver *in vivo* 1 mg over 3 days. Once applied, do not remove the patch for 3 full days. Apply to hairless area of skin behind the ear.

Stability

Reconstitution: Avoid acid solutions, because hydrolysis occurs at pH <3.

Compatibility: Physically compatible when mixed in the same syringe with atropine, butorphanol, chlorpromazine, dimenhydrinate, diphenhydramine, droperidol, fentanyl, glycopyrrolate, hydromorphone, hydroxyzine, meperidine, metoclopramide, morphine, pentazocine, pentobarbital, perphenazine, prochlorperazine, promazine, promethazine, or thiopental.

Monitoring and Teaching Issues

Physical Assessment: See Contraindications, Warnings/Precautions, and Dosing for use cautions. Assess potential for interactions with other prescriptions, OTC medications, or herbal products patient may be taking (eg, ergot-containing drugs - see Drug Interactions). When used preoperatively, safety precautions should be observed and patient should be advised about blurred vision. For all uses, assess therapeutic effectiveness and adverse reactions (see Adverse Reactions and Overdose/Toxicology). Teach patient appropriate use (according to formulation and purpose), interventions to reduce side effects, and adverse symptoms to report (see Patient Education). **Pregnancy risk factor C** - benefits of use should outweigh possible risks. (Systemic effects have been reported following ophthalmic administration.)

Patient Education: Inform prescriber of all prescription (including oral contraceptives) and OTC medications or herbal products you are taking, and any allergies you have. Use as directed. May cause drowsiness, confusion, impaired judgment, or vision changes (use caution when driving or engaging in tasks requiring alertness until response to drug is known); dry mouth, nausea, or vomiting (small, frequent meals, frequent mouth care, chewing gum, or sucking lozenges may help); orthostatic hypotension (use caution when climbing stairs and when rising from lying or sitting position); constipation (increased exercise, fluids, fruit, or fiber may help; if not effective consult prescriber); increased sensitivity to heat and decreased perspiration (avoid extremes of heat, reduce exercise in hot weather); or decreased milk if breast-feeding. Report hot, dry, flushed skin; blurred vision or vision changes; difficulty swallowing; chest pain, palpitations, or rapid heartbeat; painful or difficult urination; increased confusion, depression, or loss of memory; rapid or difficult respirations; muscle weakness or tremors; or eye pain.

Pregnancy precaution: Inform prescriber if you are or intend to become pregnant.

Transdermal: Apply patch behind ear the day before traveling. Wash hands before and after applying, and avoid contact with the eyes. Do not remove for 3 days.

Ophthalmic: Instill as often as recommended. Wash hands before using. Do not let tip of applicator touch eye; do not contaminate tip of applicator (may cause eye infection, eye damage, or vision loss). Sit or lie down, open eye, look at ceiling, and instill prescribed amount of solution. Do not blink for 30 seconds, close eye and roll eye in all directions, and apply gentle pressure to inner corner of eye for 1-2 minutes. Temporary stinging or blurred vision may occur.

Geriatric Considerations: Because of its long duration of action as a mydriatic agent, it should be avoided in elderly patients. Anticholinergic agents are not well tolerated in the elderly and their use should be avoided when possible.

Related Information

Antiemetics for Chemotherapy-Induced Nausea and Vomiting *on page 1639*

Ophthalmic Agents *on page 1509*

Scopolamine Hydrobromide *see* Scopolamine *on page 1218*

Scopolamine, Hyoscyamine, Atropine, and Phenobarbital *see* Hyoscyamine, Atropine, Scopolamine, and Phenobarbital *on page 687*

Scot-Tussin® Sugar Free Expectorant [OTC] *see* Guaifenesin *on page 646*

SDZ ENA 713 *see* Rivastigmine *on page 1200*

Sebizon® *see* Sulfacetamide *on page 1256*

Secobarbital (see koe BAR bi tal)

U.S. Brand Names Seconal™

Synonyms Quinalbarbitone Sodium; Secobarbital Sodium

Restrictions C-II

Generic Available Yes

Pharmacologic Category Barbiturate

Pregnancy Risk Factor D

Lactation Enters breast milk/use caution (AAP rates "compatible")

Use Preanesthetic agent; short-term treatment of insomnia

Mechanism of Action/Effect Interferes with transmission of impulses from the thalamus to the cortex of the brain resulting in an imbalance in central inhibitory and facilitatory mechanisms

Contraindications Hypersensitivity to barbiturates or any component of the formulation; marked hepatic impairment; dyspnea or airway obstruction; porphyria; pregnancy

Warnings/Precautions Should be used only after evaluation of potential causes of sleep disturbance. Failure of sleep disturbance to resolve after 7-10 days may indicate psychiatric or medical illness. Do not administer to patients in acute pain. Use caution in elderly patients, debilitated patients, hepatic impairment, renally impairment, or pediatric patients. May cause paradoxical responses, including agitation and hyperactivity, particularly in acute pain and pediatric patients. Use with caution in patients with depression or suicidal tendencies, or in patients with a history of drug abuse. Tolerance, psychological and physical dependence may occur with prolonged use. May cause CNS depression, which may impair physical or mental abilities. Effects with other sedative drugs or ethanol may be potentiated. May cause respiratory depression or hypotension, Use with caution in hemodynamically unstable patients or patients with respiratory disease.

Drug Interactions

Cytochrome P450 Effect: Induces **CYP2A6, 2C8/9**

Decreased Effect: Barbiturates, such as secobarbital, are hepatic enzyme inducers, and may increase the metabolism of antipsychotics, some beta-blockers (unlikely with atenolol and nadolol), calcium channel blockers, chloramphenicol, cimetidine, corticosteroids, cyclosporine, disopyramide, doxycycline, ethosuximide, felbamate, furosemide, griseofulvin, lamotrigine, phenytoin, propafenone, quinidine, tacrolimus, TCAs, and theophylline. Barbiturates may increase the metabolism of estrogens and reduce the efficacy of oral contraceptives; an alternative method of contraception should be considered. Barbiturates inhibit the hypoprothrombinemic effects of oral anticoagulants via increased metabolism. Barbiturates may enhance the metabolism of methadone resulting in methadone withdrawal.

Increased Effect/Toxicity: Increased toxicity when combined with other CNS depressants, antidepressants, benzodiazepines, chloramphenicol, or valproic acid; respiratory and CNS depression may be additive. MAO inhibitors may prolong the effect of secobarbital. Barbiturates may enhance the hepatotoxic potential of acetaminophen (due to an increased formation of toxic metabolites). Chloramphenicol may inhibit the metabolism of barbiturates.

Nutritional/Ethanol Interactions

Ethanol: Avoid ethanol (may increase CNS depression).

Herb/Nutraceutical: Avoid valerian, St John's wort, kava kava, gotu kola (may increase CNS depression).

Adverse Reactions Frequency not defined.

Cardiovascular: Hypotension

Central nervous system: Dizziness, lightheadedness, "hangover" effect, drowsiness, CNS depression, fever, confusion, mental depression, unusual excitement, nervousness, faint feeling, headache, insomnia, nightmares, hallucinations

Dermatologic: Exfoliative dermatitis, rash, Stevens-Johnson syndrome

Gastrointestinal: Nausea, vomiting, constipation

Hematologic: Agranulocytosis, megaloblastic anemia, thrombocytopenia, thrombophlebitis, urticaria apnea

Local: Pain at injection site

Respiratory: Respiratory depression, laryngospasm

Overdosage/Toxicology Symptoms of overdose include unsteady gait, slurred speech, confusion, jaundice, hypothermia, fever, hypotension, respiratory depression, and coma. Charcoal hemoperfusion or hemodialysis may be useful, especially in the presence of very high serum barbiturate levels when the patient is in shock, coma, or renal failure. Forced alkaline diuresis is of no value in the treatment of intoxications with short-acting barbiturates.

Pharmacodynamics/Kinetics

Half-Life Elimination: 15-40 hours, mean: 28 hours

Time to Peak: Serum: Within 2-4 hours

Metabolism: Hepatic, by microsomal enzyme system

Onset: Onset of hypnosis: 15-30 minutes

Duration: 3-4 hours with 100 mg dose

Formulations Capsule, as sodium: 100 mg

Dosing

Adults: Insomnia (hypnotic): Oral: 100 mg/dose at bedtime; range: 100-200 mg/dose

Elderly: Not recommended for use in the elderly (see Geriatric Considerations).

Pediatrics:

Preoperative sedation: Oral: Children: 2-6 mg/kg (maximum dose: 100 mg/dose) 1-2 hours before procedure

Sedation: Oral: Children: 6 mg/kg/day divided every 8 hours

Renal Impairment: Slightly dialyzable (5% to 20%)

Administration

I.V.: Maximum infusion rate: 50 mg/15 seconds; avoid intra-arterial injection.

Stability

Reconstitution: Do not shake vial during reconstitution, rotate ampul. Aqueous solutions are not stable, reconstitute with aqueous polyethylene glycol. Aqueous (sterile water) solutions should be used within 30 minutes. Do not use bacteriostatic water for injection or lactated Ringer's.

Compatibility: I.V. formulation: **Incompatible** with benzquinamide (in syringe), cimetidine (same syringe), codeine, erythromycin, glycopyrrolate (same syringe), hydrocortisone, insulin, levorphanol, methadone, norepinephrine, pentazocine, phenytoin, sodium bicarbonate, tetracycline, and vancomycin

Monitoring and Teaching Issues

Physical Assessment: Assess effectiveness and interactions of other medications patient may be taking (see Drug Interactions). See Contraindications and Warnings/Precautions for use cautions. Assess patient for history of addiction; long-term use can result in dependence, abuse, or tolerance and evaluate periodically for need for continued use. After long-term use, taper dosage slowly when discontinuing. **I.V.** (see Administration): Monitor infusion site frequently; patient should be carefully monitored and safety/seizure precautions observed. **Oral:** For inpatient use, institute safety measures. For outpatient use, monitor effectiveness and adverse reactions (see Adverse Reactions) at beginning of therapy and periodically with long-term use. Assess knowledge/teach patient appropriate use, interventions to reduce side effects, and adverse symptoms to report (see Patient Education). **Pregnancy risk factor D** - determine that patient is not pregnant before beginning treatment. Instruct both male and female patients about appropriate barrier contraceptive measures. Note breast-feeding caution.

Patient Education: Use exactly as directed; do not increase dose or frequency or discontinue without consulting prescriber. Drug may cause physical and/or psychological dependence. While using this medication, do not use alcohol or other prescription or OTC medications (especially, pain medications, sedatives, antihistamines, or hypnotics) without consulting prescriber. Maintain adequate hydration (2-3 L/day of fluids) unless advised by prescriber to restrict fluids. You may experience drowsiness, dizziness, or blurred vision (use caution when driving or engaging in tasks requiring alertness until response to drug is known); nausea or vomiting (small, frequent meals, frequent mouth care, chewing gum, or sucking lozenges may help); or constipation (increased exercise, fluids, fruit, or fiber may help). Report skin rash or irritation; CNS changes (confusion, depression, increased sedation, excitation, headache, insomnia, or nightmares); difficulty breathing or shortness of breath; difficulty swallowing or feeling of tightness in throat; unusual weakness or unusual bleeding in mouth, urine, or stool; or other unanticipated adverse effects. **Pregnancy/breast-feeding precautions:** Do not get pregnant while taking this medication. Use appropriate barrier contraceptive measures. Consult prescriber if breast-feeding.

Geriatric Considerations: Use of this agent in the elderly is not recommended due to its long half-life and addiction potential.

Related Information

Antipsychotic Medication Guidelines *on page 1614*
Compatibility of Drugs in Syringe *on page 1566*

Secobarbital Sodium *see* Secobarbital *on page 1220*

Seconal™ *see* Secobarbital *on page 1220*

Secretin *see page 1461*

Secretin Ferring Powder *see page 1461*

Seizure Treatment *see page 1700*

Selected Adverse Effects *see page 1523*

Selected Prescription Combination Products *see page 1522*

Selegiline (seh LEDGE ah leen)

U.S. Brand Names Atapryl®; Eldepryl®; Selpak®

Synonyms Deprenyl; L-Deprenyl; Selegiline Hydrochloride

Generic Available Yes

Pharmacologic Category Antidepressant, Monoamine Oxidase Inhibitor; Anti-Parkinson's Agent, MAO Type B Inhibitor

Pregnancy Risk Factor C

Lactation Excretion in breast milk unknown

Use Adjunct in the management of parkinsonian patients in which levodopa/carbidopa therapy is deteriorating

Use - Unlabeled/Investigational Early Parkinson's disease; attention-deficit/hyperactivity disorder (ADHD); negative symptoms of schizophrenia; extrapyramidal symptoms; depression; Alzheimer's disease (studies have shown some improvement in behavioral and cognitive performance)

Mechanism of Action/Effect Potent monoamine oxidase (MAO) type B inhibitor; MAO type B plays a major role in the metabolism of dopamine; selegiline may also increase dopaminergic activity by interfering with dopamine reuptake at the synapse

Contraindications Hypersensitivity to selegiline or any component of the formulation; concomitant use of meperidine

Warnings/Precautions Increased risk of nonselective MAO inhibition occurs with doses >10 mg/day. A MAO inhibitor type "B", there should **not** be a problem with tyramine-containing products as long as the typical doses are employed, however, rare reactions have been reported. Pregnancy risk C.

Drug Interactions

Cytochrome P450 Effect: Substrate of CYP1A2, 2A6, **2B6, 2C8/9**, 2D6, 3A4; Inhibits CYP1A2, 2A6, 2C8/9, 2C19, 2D6, 2E1, 3A4

Increased Effect/Toxicity: Concurrent use of selegiline (high dose) in combination with amphetamines, methylphenidate, dextromethorphan, fenfluramine, meperidine,
(Continued)

Selegiline *(Continued)*

nefazodone, sibutramine, tramadol, trazodone, tricyclic antidepressants, and venlafaxine may result in serotonin syndrome; these combinations are best avoided. Concurrent use of selegiline with an SSRI may result in mania or hypertension; it is generally best to avoid these combinations. Selegiline (>10 mg/day) in combination with tyramine (cheese, ethanol) may increase the pressor response; avoid high tyramine-containing foods in patients receiving >10 mg/day of selegiline. The toxicity of levodopa (hypertension), lithium (hyperpyrexia), and reserpine may be increased by MAO inhibitors.

Nutritional/Ethanol Interactions

Ethanol: Avoid ethanol. Avoid beverages containing tyramine (wine [Chianti and hearty red] and beer).

Food: Selegiline may cause sudden and severe high blood pressure when taken with food high in tyramine (cheeses, sour cream, yogurt, pickled herring, chicken liver, canned figs, raisins, bananas, avocados, soy sauce, broad bean pods, yeast extracts, meats prepared with tenderizers, and many foods aged to improve flavor). Small amounts of caffeine may produce irregular heartbeat or high blood pressure and can interact with this medication for up to 2 weeks after stopping its use.

Herb/Nutraceutical: Avoid valerian, St John's wort, SAMe, kava kava (may increase risk of serotonin syndrome and/or excessive sedation).

Adverse Reactions Frequency not defined.

Cardiovascular: Orthostatic hypotension, hypertension, arrhythmias, palpitations, angina, tachycardia, peripheral edema, bradycardia, syncope

Central nervous system: Hallucinations, dizziness, confusion, anxiety, depression, drowsiness, behavior/mood changes, dreams/nightmares, fatigue, delusions

Dermatologic: Rash, photosensitivity

Gastrointestinal: Xerostomia, nausea, vomiting, constipation, weight loss, anorexia, diarrhea, heartburn

Genitourinary: Nocturia, prostatic hyperplasia, urinary retention, sexual dysfunction

Neuromuscular & skeletal: Tremor, chorea, loss of balance, restlessness, bradykinesia

Ocular: Blepharospasm, blurred vision

Miscellaneous: Diaphoresis (increased)

Overdosage/Toxicology Symptoms of overdose include tachycardia, palpitations, muscle twitching, and seizures. Both hypertension or hypotension can occur with intoxication. While treating hypertension, care is warranted to avoid sudden drops in blood pressure, since this may worsen MAO inhibitor toxicity. Cardiac arrhythmias are best treated with phenytoin or procainamide. Treatment is generally symptom-directed and supportive.

Pharmacodynamics/Kinetics

Half-Life Elimination: Steady state: 10 hours

Metabolism: Hepatic to amphetamine and methamphetamine

Onset: Therapeutic: Within 1 hour

Duration: 24-72 hours

Formulations

Capsule, as hydrochloride (Eldepryl®): 5 mg

Tablet, as hydrochloride: 5 mg

Dosing

Adults: Parkinson's disease: Oral: 5 mg twice daily with breakfast and lunch or 10 mg in the morning

Elderly: Oral: Initial: 5 mg in the morning; may increase to a total of 10 mg/day.

Pediatrics: Children and Adolescents: ADHD (unlabeled use): Oral: 5-15 mg/day

Monitoring and Teaching Issues

Physical Assessment: Assess effectiveness and interactions of other medications patient may be taking (see Warnings/Precautions and Drug Interactions). Monitor therapeutic response according to rationale for therapy and adverse reactions at beginning of therapy and periodically throughout therapy (see Warnings/Precautions, Adverse Reactions, and Overdose/Toxicology). Patient should be cautioned against eating foods high in tyramine (see Tyramine Foods List *on page 1601*). Assess knowledge/teach patient appropriate use, interventions to reduce side effects, and adverse symptoms to report (see Patient Education). **Pregnancy risk factor C** - benefits of use should outweigh possible risks. Note breast-feeding caution.

Patient Education: Take exactly as directed (may be prescribed in conjunction with levodopa/carbidopa); do not change dosage or discontinue without consulting prescriber. Therapeutic effects may take several weeks or months to achieve and you may need frequent monitoring during first weeks of therapy. Take with meals if GI upset occurs, before meals if dry mouth occurs, after eating if drooling or if nausea occurs. Take at the same time each day. Avoid tyramine-containing foods (low potential for reaction). Maintain adequate hydration (2-3 L/day of fluids) unless advised by prescriber to restrict fluids; void before taking medication. Do not use alcohol and prescription or OTC sedatives or CNS depressants without consulting prescriber. You may experience drowsiness, dizziness, confusion, or vision changes (use caution when driving, climbing stairs, or engaging in tasks requiring alertness until response to drug is known); orthostatic hypotension (use caution when changing position - rising to standing from sitting or lying); constipation (increased exercise, fluids, fruit, or fiber may help); runny nose or flu-like symptoms (consult prescriber for appropriate relief); or nausea, vomiting, loss of appetite, or stomach discomfort (small, frequent meals, frequent mouth care, chewing gum, or sucking lozenges may help). Report unresolved constipation or vomiting; chest pain, palpitations, irregular heartbeat; CNS changes (hallucination, loss of memory, seizures, acute headache, nervousness, etc); painful or difficult urination; increased muscle spasticity, rigidity, or involuntary movements; skin rash; or significant worsening of condition. **Pregnancy/breast-feeding precautions:** Inform prescriber if you are or intend to become pregnant. Consult prescriber if breast-feeding.

Geriatric Considerations: Selegiline is also being studied in Alzheimer's disease, but further studies are needed to assess its usefulness. Do not use at daily doses exceeding 10 mg/day because of the risks associated with nonselective inhibition of MAO.

Additional Information When adding selegiline to levodopa/carbidopa, the dose of the latter can usually be decreased. Studies are investigating the use of selegiline in early Parkinson's disease to slow the progression of the disease.

Related Information

Tyramine Foods List *on page 1601*

Selegiline Hydrochloride *see* Selegiline *on page 1221*

Selpak® *see* Selegiline *on page 1221*

Semprex®-D *see* Acrivastine and Pseudoephedrine *on page 42*

Senna *see page 1581*

Septra® *see* Sulfamethoxazole and Trimethoprim *on page 1259*

Septra® DS *see* Sulfamethoxazole and Trimethoprim *on page 1259*

Serax® *see* Oxazepam *on page 1015*

Serentil® *see* Mesoridazine *on page 861*

Serevent® *see* Salmeterol *on page 1210*

Serevent® Diskus® *see* Salmeterol *on page 1210*

Sermorelin Acetate *see page 1461*

Seromycin® Pulvules® *see* CycloSERINE *on page 342*

Serophene® *see* ClomiPHENE *on page 312*

Seroquel® *see* Quetiapine *on page 1158*

Serostim® *see* Human Growth Hormone *on page 658*

Serotonin Syndrome *see page 1527*

Sertraline (SER tra leen)

U.S. Brand Names Zoloft®

Synonyms Sertraline Hydrochloride

Generic Available No

Pharmacologic Category Antidepressant, Selective Serotonin Reuptake Inhibitor

Pregnancy Risk Factor C

Lactation Enters breast milk/not recommended (AAP rates "of concern")

Use Treatment of major depression; obsessive-compulsive disorder (OCD); panic disorder; post-traumatic stress disorder (PTSD); premenstrual dysphoric disorder (PMDD)

Use - Unlabeled/Investigational Eating disorders; anxiety disorders; impulse control disorders

Mechanism of Action/Effect Antidepressant with selective inhibitory effects on presynaptic serotonin (5-HT) reuptake and only very weak effects on norepinephrine and dopamine neuronal uptake

Contraindications Hypersensitivity to sertraline or any component of the formulation; use of MAO inhibitors within 14 days; concurrent use of pimozide; concurrent use of sertraline oral concentrate with disulfiram is contraindicated

Warnings/Precautions Potential for severe reaction when used with MAO inhibitors - serotonin syndrome may occur. May precipitate a shift to mania or hypomania in patients with bipolar disease. Has a very low potential to impair cognitive or motor performance. Does not appear to potentiate the effects of alcohol, however, ethanol use is not advised. Use caution if suicidal risk may be present. Use caution in patients with a previous seizure disorder, predisposing condition, or concurrent current drug therapy predisposing to seizures. Use with caution in patients with hepatic or renal dysfunction and in elderly patients. May cause hyponatremia/SIADH. Sertraline acts as a mild uricosuric - use with caution in patients at risk of uric acid nephropathy. Use with caution in patients at risk of bleeding or receiving anticoagulant therapy - may cause impairment in platelet aggregation. Use with caution in patients where weight loss is undesirable. May cause or exacerbate sexual dysfunction. Use oral concentrate formulation with caution in patients with latex sensitivity; dropper dispenser contains dry natural rubber. Pregnancy risk C.

Drug Interactions

Cytochrome P450 Effect: Substrate of **CYP2B6, 2C8/9, 2C19**, 2D6, **3A4**; Inhibits CYP1A2, **2B6**, 2C8/9, **2C19**, 2D6, 3A4

Decreased Effect: Sertraline may decrease the metabolism of tolbutamide; monitor for changes in glucose control.

Increased Effect/Toxicity:

MAO inhibitors: Sertraline should not be used with nonselective MAO inhibitors (phenelzine, isocarboxazid) or other drugs with MAO inhibition (linezolid); fatal reactions have been reported. Wait 5 weeks after stopping sertraline before starting a nonselective MAO inhibitor and 2 weeks after stopping an MAO inhibitor before starting sertraline. Concurrent selegiline has been associated with mania, hypertension, or serotonin syndrome (risk may be reduced relative to nonselective MAO inhibitors). Sertraline may increase serum concentrations of pimozide; concurrent use is contraindicated.

Combined used of SSRIs and amphetamines, buspirone, meperidine, nefazodone, serotonin agonists (such as sumatriptan), sibutramine, other SSRIs, sympathomimetics, ritonavir, tramadol, and venlafaxine may increase the risk of serotonin syndrome. Sertraline may increase serum levels/effects of benzodiazepines (alprazolam and diazepam), carbamazepine, carvedilol, clozapine, cyclosporine (and possibly tacrolimus), dextromethorphan, digoxin, haloperidol, HMG-CoA reductase inhibitors (lovastatin and simvastatin - increasing the risk of rhabdomyolysis, despite sertraline's weak inhibition), phenytoin, propafenone, trazodone, tricyclic antidepressants, and valproic acid. Concurrent lithium may increase risk of nephrotoxicity. Risk of hyponatremia may increase with concurrent use of loop diuretics (bumetanide, furosemide, torsemide). Sertraline may increase the hypoprothrombinemic response to warfarin.

Combined use of sumatriptan (and other serotonin agonists) may result in toxicity; weakness, hyper-reflexia, and incoordination have been observed with sumatriptan and SSRIs. In addition, concurrent use may theoretically increase the risk of serotonin syndrome; includes sumatriptan, naratriptan, rizatriptan, and zolmitriptan.

(Continued)

Sertraline *(Continued)*

Phenothiazines: CYP3A4 inhibitors (including sertraline) may inhibit the metabolism of thioridazine or mesoridazine, resulting in increased plasma levels and increasing the risk of QT_c interval prolongation. This may lead to serious ventricular arrhythmias, such as torsade de pointes-type arrhythmias and sudden death. Do not use together. Wait at least 5 weeks after discontinuing sertraline prior to starting thioridazine.

Nutritional/Ethanol Interactions

Ethanol: Avoid ethanol (may increase CNS depression).

Food: Sertraline average peak serum levels may be increased if taken with food.

Herb/Nutraceutical: Avoid valerian, St John's wort, kava kava, gotu kola (may increase CNS depression).

Effects on Lab Values Minor ↑ triglycerides (S), LFTs; ↓ uric acid (S)

Adverse Reactions

>10%:

Central nervous system: Insomnia, somnolence, dizziness, headache, fatigue
Gastrointestinal: Xerostomia, diarrhea, nausea
Genitourinary: Ejaculatory disturbances

1% to 10%:

Cardiovascular: Palpitations
Central nervous system: Agitation, anxiety, nervousness
Dermatologic: Rash
Endocrine & metabolic: Decreased libido
Gastrointestinal: Constipation, anorexia, dyspepsia, flatulence, vomiting, weight gain
Genitourinary: Micturition disorders
Neuromuscular & skeletal: Tremors, paresthesia
Ocular: Visual difficulty, abnormal vision
Otic: Tinnitus
Miscellaneous: Diaphoresis (increased)

<1% (Limited to important or life-threatening): Acute renal failure, agranulocytosis, angioedema, aplastic anemia, atrial arrhythmias, AV block, blindness, extrapyramidal symptoms, hepatic failure, hypothyroidism, jaundice, lupus-like syndrome, neuroleptic malignant syndrome, oculogyric crisis, optic neuritis, pancreatitis (rare), photosensitivity, psychosis, pulmonary hypertension, QT_c prolongation, serotonin syndrome, serum sickness, SIADH, Stevens-Johnson syndrome (and other severe dermatologic reactions), thrombocytopenia, vasculitis, ventricular tachycardia (including torsade de pointes)

Overdosage/Toxicology Among 634 patients who overdosed on sertraline alone, 8 resulted in a fatal outcome. Symptoms of overdose include somnolence, vomiting, tachycardia, nausea, dizziness, agitation, and tremor. Treatment is symptomatic and supportive.

Pharmacodynamics/Kinetics

Absorption: Slow

Bioavailability: 88%

Half-Life Elimination: Parent drug: 26 hours; Metabolite N-desmethylsertraline: 66 hours (range: 62-104 hours)

Time to Peak: Plasma: 4.5-8.4 hours

Metabolism: Hepatic; extensive first-pass metabolism

Formulations

Solution, oral concentrate: 20 mg/mL (60 mL)
Tablet, as hydrochloride: 25 mg, 50 mg, 100 mg

Dosing

Adults:

Depression and obsessive-compulsive disorder: Oral: Initial: 50 mg/day

Note: May increase by 50 mg/day increments at intervals of not less than 1 week if tolerated to 100 mg/day; additional increases may be necessary; maximum: 200 mg/day. If somnolence is noted, give at bedtime.

Panic disorder and post-traumatic stress disorder: Oral: Initial 25 mg once daily; increased after 1 week to 50 mg once daily (see "Note" above)

PMDD: 50 mg/day either daily throughout menstrual cycle **or** limited to the luteal phase of menstrual cycle, depending on physician assessment. Patients not responding to 50 mg/day may benefit from dose increases (50 mg increments per menstrual cycle) up to 150 mg/day when dosing throughout menstrual cycle **or** up to 100 mg day when dosing during luteal phase only. If a 100 mg/day dose has been established with luteal phase dosing, a 50 mg/day titration step for 3 days should be utilized at the beginning of each luteal phase dosing period.

Elderly: Oral: Initial: 25 mg/day in the morning; increase by 25 mg/day increments every 2-3 days if tolerated to 50-100 mg/day; additional increases may be necessary; maximum: 200 mg/day.

Pediatrics:

Depression/obsessive-compulsive disorder: Oral: Children:

6-12 years: Initial: 25 mg once daily
13-17 years: Initial: 50 mg once daily
May increase by 50 mg/day increments at intervals of not less than 1 week if tolerated to 100 mg/day; additional increases may be necessary; maximum: 200 mg/day. If somnolence is noted, give at bedtime.

Renal Impairment: Multiple-dose pharmacokinetics are unaffected by renal impairment.

Hemodialysis effect: Not removed by hemodialysis

Hepatic Impairment: Sertraline is extensively metabolized by the liver. Caution should be used in patients with hepatic impairment. A lower dose or less frequent dosing should be used.

Administration

Oral: Oral concentrate: Must be diluted before use. Immediately before administration, use the dropper provided to measure the required amount of concentrate; mix with 4 ounces (1/2 cup) of water, ginger ale, lemon/lime soda, lemonade, or orange juice **only**. Do not mix with any other liquids than these. The dose should be taken immediately after mixing; do not mix in advance. A slight haze may appear after mixing; this is normal. **Note:** Use with caution in patients with latex sensitivity; dropper dispenser contains dry natural rubber.

Stability

Storage: Tablets should be stored at controlled room temperature of 15°C to 30°C (59°F to 86°F).

Monitoring and Teaching Issues

Physical Assessment: Assess other medications patient may be taking for effectiveness and interactions (see Drug Interactions). See Warnings/Precautions for use cautions. Monitor therapeutic response (ie, mental status, mood, affect, suicidal ideation) and adverse reactions at beginning of therapy and periodically with long-term use (see Adverse Reactions and Overdose/Toxicology). Taper dosage slowly when discontinuing. Assess knowledge/teach patient appropriate use, interventions to reduce side effects, and adverse symptoms to report (see Patient Education). **Pregnancy risk factor C** - benefits of use should outweigh possible risks. Breast-feeding is not recommended.

Patient Education: Take exactly as directed; do not increase dose or frequency. It may take 2-3 weeks to achieve desired results. Take in the morning to reduce the incidence of insomnia. Avoid alcohol, caffeine, and other prescription or OTC medications not approved by prescriber. Maintain adequate hydration (2-3 L/day of fluids) unless advised by prescriber to restrict fluids. You may experience drowsiness, dizziness, or lightheadedness (use caution when driving or engaging in tasks requiring alertness until response to drug is known); nausea, vomiting, anorexia, or dry mouth (small, frequent meals, frequent mouth care, chewing gum, or sucking lozenges may help); postural hypotension (use caution when climbing stairs or changing position from sitting or lying to standing); urinary pattern changes (void before taking medication); or male sexual dysfunction (reversible). Report persistent insomnia or daytime sedation, agitation, nervousness, fatigue; muscle cramping, tremors, weakness, or change in gait; chest pain, palpitations, or swelling of extremities; vision changes or eye pain; hearing changes (ringing in ears); difficulty breathing or breathlessness; skin rash or irritation; or worsening of condition. **Pregnancy/ breast-feeding precautions:** Inform prescriber if you are or intend to become pregnant. Breast-feeding is not recommended.

Geriatric Considerations: Sertraline's favorable side effect profile makes it a useful alternative to the traditional tricyclic antidepressants. Its potential stimulation effect and anorexia may be bothersome.

Additional Information Buspirone (15-60 mg/day) may be useful in treatment of sexual dysfunction during treatment with a selective serotonin reuptake inhibitor. May exacerbate tics in Tourette's syndrome.

Related Information

Antidepressant Agents *on page 1553*
Antidepressant Medication Guidelines *on page 1613*

Sertraline Hydrochloride *see* Sertraline *on page 1223*

Serutan® [OTC] *see* Psyllium *on page 1152*

Serzone® *see* Nefazodone *on page 954*

Sevelamer (se VEL a mer)

U.S. Brand Names Renagel®

Synonyms Sevelamer Hydrochloride

Generic Available No

Pharmacologic Category Phosphate Binder

Pregnancy Risk Factor C

Lactation Excretion in breast milk unknown/use caution (not absorbed systemically but may alter maternal nutrition)

Use Reduction of serum phosphorous in patients with end-stage renal disease

Mechanism of Action/Effect Sevelamer (a polymeric compound) binds phosphate within the intestinal lumen, limiting absorption and decreasing serum phosphate concentrations without altering calcium, aluminum, or bicarbonate concentrations.

Contraindications Hypersensitivity to sevelamer or any component of the formulation; hypophosphatemia; bowel obstruction

Warnings/Precautions Use with caution in patients with gastrointestinal disorders including dysphagia, swallowing disorders, severe gastrointestinal motility disorders, or major gastrointestinal surgery. May cause reductions in vitamin D, E, K, and folic acid absorption. Long-term studies of carcinogenic potential have not been completed. Capsules should not be taken apart or chewed. Pregnancy risk C.

Drug Interactions

Decreased Effect: Sevelamer may bind to some drugs in the gastrointestinal tract and decrease their absorption. When changes in absorption of oral medications may have significant clinical consequences (such as antiarrhythmic and antiseizure medications), these medications should be taken at least 1 hour before or 3 hours after a dose of sevelamer.

Adverse Reactions

>10%:

Cardiovascular: Hypotension (11%), thrombosis (10%)
Central nervous system: Headache (10%)
Endocrine & metabolic: Decreased absorption of vitamins D, E, K and folic acid
Gastrointestinal: Diarrhea (16%), dyspepsia (5% to 11%), vomiting (12%)
Neuromuscular & skeletal: Pain (13%)
Miscellaneous: Infection (15%)

1% to 10%:

Cardiovascular: Hypertension (9%)
Gastrointestinal: Nausea (7%), flatulence (4%), diarrhea (4%), constipation (2%)
Respiratory: Cough (4%)

Overdosage/Toxicology Sevelamer is not absorbed systemically. There are no reports of overdosage in patients.

(Continued)

Sevelamer *(Continued)*

Pharmacodynamics/Kinetics

Absorption: None

Formulations

Capsule: 403 mg

Tablet: 400 mg, 800 mg

Dosing

Adults & Elderly: Reduction of serum phosphorous (ESRD): Oral:

Patients not taking a phosphate binder: 800-1600 mg 3 times/day with meals; the initial dose may be based on serum phosphorous.

Phosphorous: Initial:

>6.0 mg/dL and <7.5 mg/dL: 800 mg 3 times/day

≥7.5 mg/dL and <9.0 mg/dL: 1200-1600 mg 3 times/day

≥9.0 mg/dL: 1600 mg 3 times/day

Dosage should be adjusted based on serum phosphorous concentration, with a goal of lowering to <6.0 mg/dL; maximum daily dose studied was equivalent to 30 capsules/day.

Stability

Storage: Store at controlled room temperature.

Monitoring Laboratory Tests Serum phosphorus

Monitoring and Teaching Issues

Physical Assessment: See Contraindications and Warnings/Precautions for use cautions. Assess knowledge/teach patient appropriate use, possible side effects/interventions, and adverse symptoms to report (see Patient Education). **Pregnancy risk factor C** - benefits of use should outweigh possible risks. Note breast-feeding caution.

Patient Education: Take as directed, with meals. Do not break or chew capsules or tablets (contents will expand in water). You may experience headache or dizziness (use caution when driving or engaging in tasks requiring alertness until response to drug is known); nausea or vomiting (small, frequent meals, frequent mouth care, or sucking hard candy may help); diarrhea (yogurt or buttermilk may help); hypotension (use caution when rising from sitting or lying position or when climbing stairs or bending over); or mild neuromuscular pain or stiffness (mild analgesic may help). Report persistent adverse reactions. **Pregnancy/breast-feeding precautions:** Inform prescriber if you are or intend to become pregnant. Consult prescriber if breast-feeding.

Breast-feeding Issues: It is not known whether sevelamer is excreted in human milk. Because sevelamer may cause a reduction in the absorption of some vitamins, it should be used with caution in nursing women.

Additional Information Switching patients from calcium acetate to sevelamer: 667 mg of calcium acetate is equivalent to 800 mg sevelamer

Sevelamer Hydrochloride *see* Sevelamer *on page 1225*

Sibutramine (si BYOO tra meen)

U.S. Brand Names Meridia®

Synonyms Sibutramine Hydrochloride Monohydrate

Restrictions C-IV; recommended only for obese patients with a body mass index ≥30 kg/m^2 or ≥27 kg/m^2 in the presence of other risk factors such as hypertension, diabetes, and/or dyslipidemia

Generic Available No

Pharmacologic Category Anorexiant

Pregnancy Risk Factor C

Lactation Excretion in breast milk unknown/not recommended

Use Management of obesity, including weight loss and maintenance of weight loss, and should be used in conjunction with a reduced calorie diet

Mechanism of Action/Effect Sibutramine blocks the neuronal uptake of norepinephrine and, to a lesser extent, serotonin and dopamine

Contraindications Hypersensitivity to sibutramine or any component of the formulation; during or within 2 weeks of MAO inhibitors (eg, phenelzine, selegiline) or concomitant centrally-acting appetite suppressants; anorexia nervosa; uncontrolled or poorly controlled hypertension; congestive heart failure; coronary heart disease; conduction disorders (arrhythmias); stroke; concurrent use of serotonergic agents (eg, SSRIs sumatriptan, dihydroergotamine, dextromethorphan, meperidine, pentazocine, fentanyl, lithium)

Warnings/Precautions Use with caution in severe renal impairment or severe hepatic dysfunction, seizure disorder, hypertension, gallstones, narrow-angle glaucoma, nursing mothers, elderly patients. Primary pulmonary hypertension (PPH), a rare and frequently fatal pulmonary disease, has been reported to occur in patients receiving other agents with serotonergic activity which have been used as anorexiants. Although not reported in clinical trials, it is possible that sibutramine may share this potential, and patients should be monitored closely. Stimulants may unmask tics in individuals with coexisting Tourette's syndrome.

Serious, potentially life-threatening toxicities may occur when thyroid hormones (at dosages above usual daily hormonal requirements) are used in combination with sympathomimetic amines to induce weight loss. Treatment of obesity is not an approved use for thyroid hormone.

Pregnancy risk C.

Drug Interactions

Cytochrome P450 Effect: Substrate of **CYP3A4**

Decreased Effect: Inducers of CYP3A4 (including phenytoin, phenobarbital, carbamazepine, and rifampin) theoretically may reduce sibutramine serum concentrations.

Increased Effect/Toxicity: Serotonergic agents such as buspirone, selective serotonin reuptake inhibitors (eg, citalopram, fluoxetine, fluvoxamine, paroxetine, sertraline), sumatriptan (and similar serotonin agonists), dihydroergotamine, lithium, tryptophan, some opioid/analgesics (eg, meperidine, tramadol), and venlafaxine, when combined with sibutramine may result in serotonin syndrome. Dextromethorphan, MAO inhibitors and other drugs that can raise the blood pressure (eg decongestants, centrally-acting weight loss products, amphetamines, and amphetamine-like compounds) can increase the possibility of sibutramine-associated cardiovascular complications. Sibutramine may increase serum levels of tricyclic antidepressants. Theoretically, inhibitors of CYP3A4 (including ketoconazole, itraconazole, erythromycin) may increase sibutramine levels.

Nutritional/Ethanol Interactions

Ethanol: Avoid excess ethanol ingestion.

Herb/Nutraceutical: St John's wort may decrease sibutramine levels.

Adverse Reactions

>10%

Central nervous system: Headache, insomnia

Gastrointestinal: Anorexia, xerostomia, constipation

Respiratory: Rhinitis

1% to 10%

Cardiovascular: Tachycardia, vasodilation, hypertension, palpitations, chest pain, edema

Central nervous system: Migraine, dizziness, nervousness, anxiety, depression, somnolence, CNS stimulation, emotional liability

Dermatologic: Rash

Endocrine & metabolic: Dysmenorrhea

Gastrointestinal: Increased appetite, nausea, dyspepsia, gastritis, vomiting, taste perversion, abdominal pain

Neuromuscular & skeletal: Weakness, arthralgia, back pain

Respiratory: Pharyngitis, sinusitis, cough, laryngitis

Miscellaneous: Diaphoresis, flu-like syndrome, allergic reactions, thirst

Postmarketing and/or reports (frequency not defined; limited to important or life-threatening): Alopecia, anaphylactic shock, anaphylactoid reaction, angina, arrhythmia, atrial fibrillation, cardiac arrest, cholecystitis, cholelithiasis, CHF, GI hemorrhage, goiter, hyperthyroidism, hypothyroidism, impotence, increased intraocular pressure, intestinal obstruction, mania, photosensitivity, serotonin syndrome, stroke, syncope, torsade de pointes, transient ischemic attack, vascular headache, ventricular dysrhythmias

Overdosage/Toxicology Symptoms of overdose include hypertension, tachycardia, headache, and palpitations. Treatment is supportive.

Pharmacodynamics/Kinetics

Absorption: Rapid

Time to Peak: Within 3-4 hours

Metabolism: Hepatic; undergoes first-pass metabolism via CYP3A4

Formulations Capsule, as hydrochloride: 5 mg, 10 mg, 15 mg

Dosing

Adults: Obesity: Oral: Initial: 10 mg once daily; after 4 weeks may titrate up to 15 mg once daily as needed and tolerated (may be used for up to 2 years, per manufacturer labeling).

Elderly: Use with caution; adjust dose based on renal or hepatic function.

Hepatic Impairment: No adjustment necessary for mild to moderate liver failure. Sibutramine is contraindicated in patients with severe liver failure.

Administration

Oral: May take with or without food.

Monitoring and Teaching Issues

Physical Assessment: Assess effectiveness and interactions of other medications patient may be taking (see Contraindications, Warnings/Precautions, and Drug Interactions). Monitor blood pressure, vital signs, and adverse reactions at start of therapy, when changing dosage, and at regular intervals during therapy (see Adverse Reactions). Assess knowledge/teach patient appropriate use, possible side effects, and symptoms to report (see Patient Education). **Pregnancy risk factor C** - use only if benefits outweigh possible risks. Breast-feeding is not recommended.

Patient Education: Take exactly as directed; do not increase dose or frequency without consulting prescriber. May be taken with meals (do not take at bedtime). Avoid alcohol, caffeine, or OTC medications that act as stimulants. You may experience restlessness, dizziness, sleepiness (use caution when driving or engaging in tasks requiring alertness until response to drug is known); insomnia (taking medication early in morning may help, warm milk, and quiet environment at bedtime may help); increased appetite, nausea or vomiting (small, frequent meals, frequent mouth care may help); constipation (increased exercise, fluids, fruit, or fiber may help); diarrhea (buttermilk, boiled milk, or yogurt may help); or altered menstrual periods (reversible when drug is discontinued). Report chest pain, palpitations, or irregular heartbeat; excessive nervousness, excitation, or sleepiness; back pain, muscle weakness, or tremors; CNS changes (acute headache, aggressiveness, restlessness, excitation, sleep disturbances); menstrual pattern changes; rash; blurred vision; runny nose, sinusitis, cough, or difficulty breathing. **Pregnancy/breast-feeding precautions:** Inform prescriber if you are or intend to become pregnant. Breast-feeding is not recommended.

Dietary Issues: Sibutramine, as an appetite suppressant, is the most effective when combined with a low calorie diet and behavior modification counseling.

Additional Information Physicians should carefully evaluate patients for history of drug abuse and follow such patients closely, observing them for signs of misuse or abuse (eg, development of tolerance, excessive increases of doses, drug seeking behavior).

Unlike dexfenfluramine and fenfluramine, the medication does not cause the release of serotonin from neurons. Tests done on humans show no evidence of valvular heart disease and experiments done on animals show no evidence of the neurotoxicity which was found in similar testing using animals treated with fenfluramine and dexfenfluramine; has minimal potential for abuse.

Related Information

Obesity Treatment Guidelines for Adults *on page 1693*

Sibutramine Hydrochloride Monohydrate *see* Sibutramine *on page 1226*

Siladryl® Allergy [OTC] *see* DiphenhydrAMINE *on page 422*
Silapap® Children's [OTC] *see* Acetaminophen *on page 35*
Silapap® Infants [OTC] *see* Acetaminophen *on page 35*

Sildenafil (sil DEN a fil)

U.S. Brand Names Viagra®

Synonyms UK 92480

Generic Available No

Pharmacologic Category Phosphodiesterase Enzyme Inhibitor

Pregnancy Risk Factor B

Use Treatment of erectile dysfunction

Use - Unlabeled/Investigational Psychotropic-induced sexual dysfunction

Mechanism of Action/Effect Sildenafil enhances the effect of nitric oxide by inhibiting phosphodiesterase type 5 (PDE5), resulting in smooth muscle relaxation and inflow of blood into the corpus cavernosum with sexual stimulation.

Contraindications Hypersensitivity to sildenafil or any component of the formulation; concurrent use of organic nitrates (nitroglycerin) in any form (potentiates the hypotensive effects)

Warnings/Precautions A thorough medical history and physical examination to diagnose erectile dysfunction should be undertaken to determine potential underlying causes and appropriate treatment. There is a potential cardiac risk associated with sexual activity which may need to be considered in patients with cardiovascular disease before starting sildenafil therapy. Use with caution in patients predisposed to priapism (ie, sickle cell anemia, multiple myeloma or leukemia). Use with caution in patients with anatomical deformation of the penis (ie, angulation, cavernosal fibrosis, or Peyronie's disease). Use of sildenafil with other approaches to treat erectile dysfunction is **not** recommended. May cause hypotension; use caution in patients with MI, stroke, or life-threatening arrhythmia (within last 6 months); resting hypotension or hypertension; history of unstable angina or cardiac failure; and retinitis pigmentosa.

Drug Interactions

Cytochrome P450 Effect: Substrate of CYP2C8/9, **3A4**; Inhibits CYP1A2, 2C8/9, 2C19, 2D6, 2E1, 3A4

Decreased Effect: Enzyme inducers (including phenytoin, carbamazepine, phenobarbital, rifampin) may decrease the serum concentration and efficacy of sildenafil.

Increased Effect/Toxicity: Sildenafil potentiates the hypotensive effects of nitrates (amyl nitrate, isosorbide dinitrate, isosorbide mononitrate, nitroglycerin); severe reactions have occurred and concurrent use is contraindicated. Sildenafil may potentiate the effect of other antihypertensives. Serum concentrations/toxicity of sildenafil may be increased by inhibitors of CYP3A4, including amprenavir, cimetidine, ciprofloxacin, clarithromycin, clozapine, diltiazem, disulfiram, digoxin, erythromycin, ethanol, fluconazole, fluoxetine, fluvoxamine, grapefruit juice, ritonavir, isoniazid, itraconazole, ketoconazole, labetalol, levodopa, loxapine, metoprolol, metronidazole, miconazole, nefazodone, nelfinavir, omeprazole, phenytoin, rifabutin, rifampin, ritonavir, troleandomycin, valproic acid, and verapamil. Sildenafil may potentiate bleeding in patients receiving heparin. A reduction in sildenafil's dose is recommended when used with ritonavir or indinavir (no more than 25 mg/dose; no more than 25 mg in 48 hours).

Nutritional/Ethanol Interactions

Food: Amount and rate of absorption of sildenafil is reduced when taken with a high-fat meal. Serum concentrations/toxicity may be increased with grapefruit juice; avoid concurrent use.

Herb/Nutraceutical: St John's wort may decrease sildenafil levels.

Adverse Reactions

>10%: Central nervous system: Headache

Note: Dyspepsia and abnormal vision (color changes, blurred or increased sensitivity to light) occurred at an incidence of >10% with doses of 100 mg.

1% to 10%:

Cardiovascular: Flushing
Central nervous system: Dizziness
Dermatologic: Rash
Genitourinary: Urinary tract infection
Ophthalmic: Abnormal vision (color changes, blurred or increased sensitivity to light)
Respiratory: Nasal congestion

<2% (Limited to important of life-threatening): Allergic reaction, angina pectoris, anorgasmia, asthma, AV block, cardiac arrest, cardiomyopathy, cataract, cerebral thrombosis, colitis, dyspnea, edema, exfoliative dermatitis, eye hemorrhage, gout, heart failure, hyperglycemia, hypotension, migraine, myocardial ischemia, neuralgia, photosensitivity, postural hypotension, priapism, rectal hemorrhage, seizures, shock, syncope, vertigo

Overdosage/Toxicology In studies with healthy volunteers of single doses up to 800 mg, adverse events were similar to those seen at lower doses but incidence rates were increased

Pharmacodynamics/Kinetics

Absorption: Rapid
Bioavailability: 40%
Half-Life Elimination: 4 hours
Time to Peak: 30-120 minutes
Metabolism: Hepatic via CYP3A4 (major) and CYP2C9 (minor route)
Onset: ~60 minutes
Duration: 2-4 hours

Formulations Tablet, as citrate: 25 mg, 50 mg, 100 mg

Dosing

Adults: Erectile dysfunction: Oral: 50 mg tablet, approximately 1 hour before sexual activity (30 minutes - 4 hours). An initial and maximum dose of 25 mg is recommended in patients with factors which may increase sildenafil levels (age >65, hepatic impairment, severe renal impairment, and concomitant use of inhibitors of CYP3A4 such as erythromycin, ketoconazole, and itraconazole). Adjust dose in other patients based on effectiveness or tolerance, decrease to 25 mg or increase to the maximum daily dose of 100 mg. Do not take more than once daily.

Elderly: Initial: 25 mg, 1 hour before sexual activity. Age >65 years was associated with increased serum sildenafil concentrations which may increase side effects and efficacy.

Renal Impairment: Cl_{cr} <30 mL/minute: Initial: 25 mg, 1 hour before sexual activity.

Hepatic Impairment: Hepatic impairment; cirrhosis: Initial: 25 mg, 1 hour before sexual activity.

Administration

Oral: Administer orally ~1 hour before sexual activity (may be used anytime from 4 hours to 30 minutes before).

Stability

Storage: Store tablets at controlled room temperature of 15°C to 30°C (59°F to 86°F).

Monitoring and Teaching Issues

Physical Assessment: Monitor other medications patient may be taking for effectiveness and interactions (see Drug Interactions and Contraindications). Instruct patient on appropriate use and cautions, possible side effects (see Adverse Reactions), and symptoms to report (see Patient Education).

Patient Education: Inform prescriber of all other medications you are taking; serious side effects can result when sildenafil is used with nitrates and some other medications. Do not combine sildenafil with other approaches to treating erectile dysfunction without consulting prescriber. **Note:** Sildenafil provides no protection against sexually-transmitted diseases, including HIV. You may experience headache, flushing, or abnormal vision (color changes, blurred or increased sensitivity to light); use caution when driving at night or in poorly lit environments. Report immediately acute allergic reactions; chest pain or palpitations; persistent dizziness; sign of urinary tract infection; skin rash; difficulty breathing; genital swelling; or other adverse reactions.

Breast-feeding Issues: Sildenafil is not indicated for use in women.

Pregnancy Issues: Sildenafil is not indicated for use in women.

Additional Information Sildenafil is ~10 times more selective for PDE5 as compared to PDE6. This enzyme is found in the retina and is involved in phototransduction. At higher plasma levels, interference with PDE6 is believed to be the basis for changes in color vision noted in some patients.

Silexin® [OTC] *see* Guaifenesin and Dextromethorphan *on page 647*

Silphen® [OTC] *see* DiphenhydrAMINE *on page 422*

Silvadene® *see* Silver SulfaDIAZINE *on page 1229*

Silver SulfaDIAZINE (SIL ver sul fa DYE a zeen)

U.S. Brand Names Silvadene®; SSD® AF; SSD® Cream; Thermazene®

Generic Available No

Pharmacologic Category Antibiotic, Topical

Pregnancy Risk Factor B

Lactation For external use

Use Prevention and treatment of infection in second and third degree burns

Mechanism of Action/Effect Acts upon the bacterial cell wall and cell membrane. Bactericidal for many gram-negative and gram-positive bacteria and is effective against yeast. Active against *Pseudomonas aeruginosa*, *Pseudomonas maltophilia*, *Enterobacter* species, *Klebsiella* species, *Serratia* species, *Escherichia coli*, *Proteus mirabilis*, *Morganella morganii*, *Providencia rettgeri*, *Proteus vulgaris*, *Providencia* species, *Citrobacter* species, *Acinetobacter calcoaceticus*, *Staphylococcus aureus*, *Staphylococcus epidermidis*, *Enterococcus* species, *Candida albicans*, *Corynebacterium diphtheriae*, and *Clostridium perfringens*

Contraindications Hypersensitivity to silver sulfadiazine or any component of the formulation; premature infants or neonates <2 months of age (sulfonamides may displace bilirubin and cause kernicterus); pregnancy (approaching or at term)

Warnings/Precautions Use with caution in patients with G6PD deficiency, renal impairment, or history of allergy to other sulfonamides. Sulfadiazine may accumulate in patients with impaired hepatic or renal function. Use of analgesic might be needed before application. Systemic absorption is significant and adverse reactions may be due to sulfa component.

Drug Interactions

Decreased Effect: Topical proteolytic enzymes are inactivated by silver sulfadiazine.

Adverse Reactions Frequency not defined.

Dermatologic: Itching, rash, erythema multiforme, discoloration of skin, photosensitivity

Hematologic: Hemolytic anemia, leukopenia, agranulocytosis, aplastic anemia

Hepatic: Hepatitis

Renal: Interstitial nephritis

Miscellaneous: Allergic reactions may be related to sulfa component

Pharmacodynamics/Kinetics

Absorption: Significant percutaneous absorption of silver sulfadiazine can occur especially when applied to extensive burns

Half-Life Elimination: 10 hours; prolonged with renal impairment

Time to Peak: Serum: 3-11 days of continuous therapy

Formulations Cream: 1% [10 mg/g] (20 g, 50 g, 85 g, 100 g, 400 g, 1000 g)

Dosing

Adults & Elderly: Antiseptic, burns: Topical: Apply once or twice daily

Pediatrics: Refer to adult dosing.

Administration

Topical: Apply with a sterile-gloved hand. Apply to a thickness $^1/_{16}$". Burned area should be covered with cream at all times.

Stability

Storage: Discard if cream is darkened (reacts with heavy metals resulting in release of silver).

(Continued)

Silver SulfaDIAZINE *(Continued)*

Monitoring Laboratory Tests Serum electrolytes, urinalysis, renal function, CBC in patients with extensive burns on long-term treatment

Monitoring and Teaching Issues

Physical Assessment: Monitor development of granulation. Observe for hypersensitivity reactions in unburned areas. Long-term use over large areas - monitor kidney function, and serum sulfa levels (significant absorption can occur).

Patient Education: Usually applied by professional in burn care setting. Patient instruction should be appropriate to extent of burn, patient understanding, etc.

Additional Information Contains methylparaben and propylene glycol

Simethicone and Magaldrate *see* Magaldrate and Simethicone *on page 831*

Simulect® *see* Basiliximab *on page 147*

Simvastatin (SIM va stat in)

U.S. Brand Names Zocor®

Generic Available No

Pharmacologic Category Antilipemic Agent, HMG-CoA Reductase Inhibitor

Pregnancy Risk Factor X

Lactation Enters breast milk/contraindicated

Use Adjunct to dietary therapy to decrease elevated serum total and LDL-cholesterol, apolipoprotein B (apo-B), and triglyceride levels, and to increase HDL-cholesterol in patients with primary hypercholesterolemia (heterozygous, familial and nonfamilial) and mixed dyslipidemia (Fredrickson types IIa and IIb); treatment of homozygous familial hypercholesterolemia; treatment of isolated hypertriglyceridemia (Fredrickson type IV) and type III hyperlipoproteinemia

"Secondary prevention" in patients with coronary heart disease and hypercholesterolemia to reduce the risk of total mortality by reducing coronary death; reduce the risk of nonfatal myocardial infarction; reduce the risk of undergoing myocardial revascularization procedures; and reduce the risk of stroke or transient ischemic attack

Mechanism of Action/Effect Simvastatin is a derivative of lovastatin that acts by competitively inhibiting 3-hydroxy-3-methylglutaryl-coenzyme A (HMG-CoA) reductase, the enzyme that catalyzes the rate-limiting step in cholesterol biosynthesis; lowers total and LDL-cholesterol with increase in HDL

Contraindications Hypersensitivity to simvastatin or any component of the formulation; acute liver disease; unexplained persistent elevations of serum transaminases; pregnancy; breast-feeding

Warnings/Precautions Liver function must be monitored by periodic laboratory assessment. Rhabdomyolysis with acute renal failure has occurred. Risk is dose-related and is increased with concurrent use of lipid-lowering agents which may cause rhabdomyolysis (gemfibrozil, fibric acid derivatives, or niacin at doses ≥1 g/day) or during concurrent use with potent CYP3A4 inhibitors (including amiodarone, clarithromycin, cyclosporine, erythromycin, itraconazole, ketoconazole, nefazodone, grapefruit juice in large quantities, verapamil, or protease inhibitors such as indinavir, nelfinavir, or ritonavir). Weigh the risk versus benefit when combining any of these drugs with simvastatin. Temporarily discontinue in any patient experiencing an acute or serious condition predisposing to renal failure secondary to rhabdomyolysis.

Drug Interactions

Cytochrome P450 Effect: Substrate of **CYP3A4**; Inhibits CYP2C8/9, 2D6

Decreased Effect: When taken within 1 before or up to 2 hours after cholestyramine, a decrease in absorption of simvastatin can occur.

Increased Effect/Toxicity: Risk of myopathy/rhabdomyolysis may be increased by concurrent use of lipid-lowering agents which may cause rhabdomyolysis (gemfibrozil, fibric acid derivatives, or niacin at doses ≥1 g/day), or during concurrent use of potent CYP3A4 inhibitors (including amiodarone, clarithromycin, cyclosporine, danazol, diltiazem, erythromycin, fluconazole, itraconazole, ketoconazole, nefazodone, verapamil or protease inhibitors such as indinavir, nelfinavir, ritonavir or saquinavir). In large quantities (ie, >1 quart/day), grapefruit juice may also increase simvastatin serum concentrations, increasing the risk of rhabdomyolysis. In general, concurrent use with CYP3A4 inhibitors is not recommended; manufacturer recommends limiting simvastatin dose to 20 mg/day when used with amiodarone or verapamil, and 10 mg/day when used with cyclosporine, gemfibrozil, or fibric acid derivatives. The anticoagulant effect of warfarin may be increased by simvastatin. Cholesterol-lowering effects are additive with bile-acid sequestrants (colestipol and cholestyramine).

Nutritional/Ethanol Interactions

Food: Simvastatin serum concentration may be increased when taken with grapefruit juice; avoid concurrent intake of large quantities (>1 quart/day).

Herb/Nutraceutical: St John's wort may decrease simvastatin levels.

Adverse Reactions

1% to 10%:

Gastrointestinal: Constipation (2%), dyspepsia (1%), flatulence (2%)

Neuromuscular & skeletal: CPK elevation (>3x normal on one or more occasions - 5%)

Respiratory: Upper respiratory infection (2%)

<1% (Limited to important or life-threatening): Depression, lichen planus, photosensitivity, thrombocytopenia, vertigo

Additional class-related events: Alopecia, anaphylaxis, angioedema, anxiety, cataracts, cholestatic jaundice, depression, dermatomyositis, dyspnea, eosinophilia, erythema multiforme, facial paresis, fulminant hepatic necrosis, gynecomastia, hemolytic anemia, hepatitis, hypersensitivity reaction, impotence, leukopenia, myopathy, ophthalmoplegia, pancreatitis, paresthesia, peripheral nerve palsy, peripheral neuropathy, photosensitivity, polymyalgia rheumatica, psychic disturbance, rash, renal failure (secondary to rhabdomyolysis), rhabdomyolysis, Stevens-Johnson syndrome, systemic lupus erythematosus-like syndrome, thrombocytopenia, thyroid dysfunction, toxic epidermal necrolysis, urticaria, vasculitis, vertigo

Overdosage/Toxicology Very few adverse events. Treatment is symptomatic.

Pharmacodynamics/Kinetics

Absorption: 85%

Bioavailability: <5%

Half-Life Elimination: Unknown

Time to Peak: 1.3-2.4 hours

Metabolism: Hepatic via CYP3A4; extensive first-pass effect

Onset: >3 days; Peak effect: 2 weeks

Formulations Tablet: 5 mg, 10 mg, 20 mg, 40 mg, 80 mg

Dosing

Adults:

Dyslipidemia: Oral: Initial: 20 mg once daily in the evening

Patients who require only a moderate reduction of LDL-cholesterol may be started at 10 mg

Patients who require a reduction of >45% in low-density lipoprotein (LDL) cholesterol: 40 mg once daily in the evening

Maintenance: Recommended dosage range: 5-80 mg/day as a single dose in the evening; doses should be individualized according to the baseline LDL-cholesterol levels, the recommended goal of therapy, and the patient's response.

Adjustments: Should be made at intervals of 4 weeks or more.

Familial hypercholesteremia: Oral: 40 mg in the evening or 80 mg/day in 3 divided doses of 20 mg, 20 mg, and an evening dose of 40 mg.

Note: Patients who are concomitantly receiving cyclosporine: Initial: 5 mg, should not exceed 10 mg/day.

Note: Patients receiving concomitant fibrates or niacin: Dose should **not** exceed 10 mg/day.

Note: Patients receiving concomitant amiodarone or verapamil: Dose should **not** exceed 20 mg/day.

Elderly: Oral: Initial: Maximum reductions in LDL-cholesterol may be achieved with daily dose ≤20 mg.

Renal Impairment: Because simvastatin does not undergo significant renal excretion, modification of dose should not be necessary in patients with mild to moderate renal insufficiency.

Severe renal impairment: Cl_{cr} <10 mL/minute: Initial: 5 mg/day with close monitoring.

Administration

Oral: May be taken without regard to meals.

Stability

Storage: Tablets should be stored in tightly-closed containers at temperatures between 5°C to 30°C (41°F to 86°F).

Monitoring Laboratory Tests Creatine phosphokinase levels due to possibility of myopathy; serum cholesterol (total and fractionated); obtain liver function tests prior to initiation, 6 and 12 weeks after initiation or first dose, and periodically thereafter (semiannually).

Monitoring and Teaching Issues

Physical Assessment: See Contraindications, Warnings/Precautions, and Dosing for use cautions. Assess potential for interactions with other prescriptions, OTC medications, or herbal products patient may be taking (see Drug Interactions). Assess results of laboratory tests (see above) and patient response at beginning of therapy, when increasing dose and periodically during long-term therapy (see Adverse Reactions and Overdose/Toxicology). Teach patient use, possible side effects and interventions, and adverse symptoms to report (see Patient Education). **Pregnancy risk factor X** - determine that patient is not pregnant before starting therapy. Do not give to females of childbearing age unless patient is capable of complying with barrier contraceptive use. Breast-feeding is contraindicated.

Patient Education: Inform prescriber of all prescriptions, OTC medications, or herbal products you are taking, and any allergies you have. Do not take anything new during treatment unless approved by prescriber. Take as directed, same time each day without regard to meals, and 1 hour prior to of 2 hours after any other medication. Avoid grapefruit juice while taking this medication. Follow diet and exercise regimen as prescribed. You will have periodic blood tests while taking this medication. May cause mild GI upset (should diminish with use). Report chest pain; CNS changes (dizziness, memory loss, depression, personality changes); numbness, weakness, tingling, pain or cramping in extremities or muscles; vision changes; rash; or other persistent adverse reactions. **Pregnancy/breast-feeding precautions:** Inform prescriber if you are pregnant. Consult prescriber for appropriate barrier contraceptive measures to use during and for 1 month following therapy. This drug may cause severe fetal defects. Do not donate blood during or for 1 month following therapy. Do not breast-feed.

Geriatric Considerations: Effective and well tolerated in the elderly. The definition of and, therefore, when to treat hyperlipidemia in the elderly is a controversial issue. The National Cholesterol Education Program recommends that all adults 20 years of age and older maintain a plasma cholesterol <200 mg/dL. By this definition, 60% of all elderly would be considered to have a borderline high (200-239 mg/dL) or high (≥240 mg/dL) plasma cholesterol. However, plasma cholesterol has been shown to be a less reliable predictor of coronary heart disease in the elderly. Therefore, it is the authors' belief that pharmacologic treatment be reserved for those who are unable to obtain a desirable plasma cholesterol level by diet alone and for whom the benefits of treatment are believed to outweigh the potential adverse effects, drug interactions, and cost of treatment. HMG-CoA reductase inhibitory activity is increased by ~45% in elderly patients; efficacy and toxicity were not different as compared to younger patients.

Related Information

Hyperlipidemia Management *on page 1682*
Lipid-Lowering Agents *on page 1582*

Sincalide *see page 1461*
Sinemet® *see* Levodopa and Carbidopa *on page 789*
Sinemet® CR *see* Levodopa and Carbidopa *on page 789*
Sinequan® *see* Doxepin *on page 443*
Singulair® *see* Montelukast *on page 923*
Sirdalud® *see* Tizanidine *on page 1328*

Sirolimus (sir OH li mus)

U.S. Brand Names Rapamune®

Generic Available No

Pharmacologic Category Immunosuppressant Agent

Pregnancy Risk Factor C

Lactation Excretion in breast milk unknown/not recommended

Use Prophylaxis of organ rejection in patients receiving renal transplants, in combination with cyclosporine and corticosteroids

Mechanism of Action/Effect Sirolimus inhibits T-lymphocyte activation and proliferation in response to antigenic and cytokine stimulation. Its mechanism differs from other immunosuppressants. It inhibits acute rejection of allografts and prolongs graft survival.

Contraindications Hypersensitivity to sirolimus or any component of the formulation

Warnings/Precautions Immunosuppressive agents, including sirolimus, increase the risk of infection and may be associated with the development of lymphoma. Only physicians experienced in the management of organ transplant patients should prescribe sirolimus. May increase serum lipids (cholesterol and triglycerides). Use with caution in patients with hyperlipidemia. May decrease GFR and increase serum creatinine. Use caution in patients with renal impairment, or when used concurrently with medications which may alter renal function. Has been associated with an increased risk of lymphocele. Avoid concurrent use of ketoconazole. Sirolimus is neither approved nor recommended for use in liver transplant patients; studies indicate an association with an increase risk of hepatic artery thrombosis and graft failure in these patients. Pregnancy risk C.

Drug Interactions

Cytochrome P450 Effect: Substrate of **CYP3A4**; Inhibits CYP3A4

Decreased Effect: Inducers of CYP3A4 (eg, rifampin, phenobarbital, carbamazepine, rifabutin, phenytoin) are likely to decrease serum concentrations of sirolimus.

Increased Effect/Toxicity: Cyclosporine increases sirolimus concentrations during concurrent therapy, and cyclosporine levels may be increased. Diltiazem, ketoconazole, and rifampin increase serum concentrations of sirolimus. Other inhibitors of CYP3A4 (eg, calcium channel blockers, antifungal agents, macrolide antibiotics, gastrointestinal prokinetic agents, HIV-protease inhibitors) are likely to increase sirolimus concentrations. Voriconazole may increase serum concentration of sirolimus (concurrent use is contraindicated).

Nutritional/Ethanol Interactions

Food: Do not administer with grapefruit juice; may decrease clearance of sirolimus. Ingestion with high-fat meals decreases peak concentrations but increases AUC by 35%. Sirolimus should be taken consistently either with or without food to minimize variability.

Herb/Nutraceutical: St John's wort may decrease sirolimus levels; avoid concurrent use. Avoid cat's claw, echinacea (have immunostimulant properties).

Adverse Reactions Incidence of many adverse effects are dose related

>20%:

Cardiovascular: Hypertension (39% to 49%), peripheral edema (54% to 64%), edema (16% to 24%), chest pain (16% to 24%)

Central nervous system: Fever (23% to 34%), headache (23% to 34%), pain (24% to 33%), insomnia (13% to 22%)

Dermatologic: Acne (20% to 31%)

Endocrine & metabolic: Hypercholesterolemia (38% to 46%), hypophosphatemia (15% to 23%), hyperlipidemia (38% to 57%), hypokalemia (11% to 21%)

Gastrointestinal: Abdominal pain (28% to 36%), nausea (25% to 36%), vomiting (19% to 25%), diarrhea (25% to 42%), constipation (28% to 38%), dyspepsia (17% to 25%), weight gain (8% to 21%)

Genitourinary: Urinary tract infection (20% to 33%)

Hematologic: Anemia (23% to 37%), thrombocytopenia (13% to 40%)

Neuromuscular & skeletal: Arthralgia (25% to 31%), weakness (22% to 40%), back pain (16% to 26%), tremor (21% to 31%)

Renal: Increased serum creatinine (35% to 40%)

Respiratory: Dyspnea (22% to 30%), upper respiratory infection (20% to 26%), pharyngitis (16% to 21%)

3% to 20% (Limited to important or life-threatening):

Cardiovascular: Atrial fibrillation, CHF, postural hypotension, syncope, thrombosis

Central nervous system: Anxiety, confusion, depression, emotional lability, neuropathy, somnolence

Dermatologic: Hirsutism, pruritus, skin hypertrophy, rash (10% to 20%)

Endocrine & metabolic: Cushing's syndrome, diabetes mellitus, hypercalcemia, hyperglycemia, hyperphosphatemia, hypocalcemia, hypoglycemia, hypomagnesemia, hyponatremia, hyperkalemia (12% to 17%)

Gastrointestinal: Esophagitis, gastritis, gingival hyperplasia, ileus

Genitourinary: Impotence

Hematologic: TTP, hemolytic-uremic syndrome, hemorrhage, leukopenia (9% to 15%)

Hepatic: Increased transaminases, ascites

Neuromuscular & skeletal: Increased CPK, bone necrosis, tetany, paresthesia

Otic: Deafness

Renal: Acute tubular necrosis, nephropathy (toxic), urinary retention

Respiratory: Asthma, pulmonary edema, pleural effusion

Miscellaneous: Flu-like syndrome, infection, peritonitis, sepsis

<1% (Limited to important or life-threatening): Pneumonitis with no identified infectious etiology (sometimes with an interstitial pattern), fascial dehiscence, anastomotic disruption; in liver transplant patients, an increase in hepatic artery thrombosis and graft failure were noted in clinical trials (not an approved use)

Overdosage/Toxicology Experience with overdosage has been limited. Dose-limiting toxicities include immune suppression. Reported symptoms of overdose include atrial fibrillation. Treatment is supportive, dialysis is not likely to facilitate removal.

Pharmacodynamics/Kinetics

Absorption: Rapid

Bioavailability: 14%

Half-Life Elimination: Mean: 62 hours

Time to Peak: 1-3 hours

Metabolism: Extensively hepatic via CYP3A4 and P-glycoprotein

Formulations

Solution, oral: 1 mg/mL (1 mL, 2 mL, 5 mL, 60 mL, 150 mL)

Tablet: 1 mg

Dosing

Adults & Elderly: Immunosuppression: Oral:

<40 kg: Loading dose: 3 mg/m^2 (day 1); followed by a maintenance of 1 mg/m^2/day.

≥40 kg: Loading dose: For *de novo* transplant recipients, a loading dose of 3 times the daily maintenance dose should be administered on day 1 of dosing. Maintenance dose: 2 mg/day. Doses should be taken 4 hours after cyclosporine, and should be taken consistently either with or without food.

Pediatrics: Immunosuppression: Oral: Children ≥13 years: Loading dose: 3 mg/m^2 (day 1); followed by a maintenance of 1 mg/m^2/day.

Renal Impairment: No adjustment is necessary.

Hepatic Impairment: Reduce maintenance dose by approximately 33% in hepatic impairment. Loading dose is unchanged.

Administration

Oral: Amber oral dose syringe should be used to withdraw solution from the bottle. Syringe should then be emptied, or, if a pouch is used, the entire contents should be squeezed out into a glass or plastic cup. The solution in the cup should be mixed with at least 2 ounces of water or orange juice. No other liquids should be used for dilution. Patient should drink diluted solution immediately. The cup should then be refilled with an additional 4 ounces of water or orange juice, stirred vigorously, and the patient should drink the contents at once.

Stability

Storage: Protect from light and store under refrigeration (2°C to 8°C/36°F to 46°F). (Stable for 24 months under these conditions). A slight haze may develop in refrigerated solutions, but the quality of the product is not affected. After opening, solution should be used in 1 month. If necessary, may be stored at temperatures up to 25°C (77°F) for several days after opening (not longer than 30 days). Product may be stored in amber syringe for a maximum of 24 hours (at room temperature or refrigerated). Discard syringe after use. Solution should be used immediately following dilution.

Monitoring Laboratory Tests Monitor sirolimus levels in pediatric patients, patients with hepatic impairment, or on concurrent inhibitors or inducers of CYP3A4, and/or if cyclosporine dosing is markedly reduced or discontinued. Also monitor serum cholesterol and triglycerides, blood pressure, and serum creatinine. Routine therapeutic drug level monitoring is not required in most patients.

Monitoring and Teaching Issues

Physical Assessment: Assess effectiveness and interactions of other medications (see Drug Interactions). See Warnings/Precautions and Contraindications for use cautions. Monitor laboratory tests at beginning and periodically during therapy. Monitor therapeutic response and adverse reactions and toxicity (see Adverse Reactions, and Overdose/Toxicology). Assess knowledge/teach patient appropriate use (see Administration), interventions to reduce side effects, and adverse reactions to report (see Patient Education). **Pregnancy risk factor C** - benefits of use should outweigh possible risks. Breast-feeding is not recommended.

Patient Education: Take as directed; do not alter dose or discontinue without consulting prescriber. Do not ever mix sirolimus solution with anything other than water or orange juice. May be taken with or without food, but should be taken consistently with regard to food (always on an empty stomach or always with food). Consult prescriber about timing of any other prescribed or OTC medications. Maintain adequate hydration (2-3 L/day of fluids) during entire course of therapy unless advised by prescriber to restrict fluids. You will be susceptible to infection (avoid crowds and exposure to infection). If you are diabetic, monitor glucose levels closely (drug may alter glucose levels). You may experience nausea, vomiting, loss of appetite (small, frequent meals, good mouth care, chewing gum, or sucking hard candy may help); constipation (increase exercise, fluids, fruit, or fiber may help); or diarrhea (yogurt or buttermilk); or muscle or back pain (mild analgesic). Inform prescriber of any adverse effects including, but not limited to, unresolved GI problems; difficulty breathing, cough, infection; skin rash or irritation; headache, insomnia, anxiety, confusion, emotional lability; changes in voiding pattern, burning, itching, or pain on urination; persistent bone, joint, or muscle cramping, pain or weakness; chest pain, palpitations, swelling of extremities; vision changes or hearing; or any other adverse reactions. **Pregnancy/breast-feeding precautions:** Inform prescriber if you are or intend to become pregnant. Breast-feeding is not recommended.

Dietary Issues: Take consistently, with or without food, to minimize variability.

Pregnancy Issues: Embryotoxicity and fetotoxicity may occur, as evidenced by increased mortality, reduced fetal weights and delayed ossification. Effective contraception must be initiated before therapy with sirolimus and continued for 12 weeks after discontinuation.

SK *see* Streptokinase *on page 1247*

SK and F 104864 *see* Topotecan *on page 1339*

Skelid® *see* Tiludronate *on page 1321*

SKF 104864 *see* Topotecan *on page 1339*
SKF 104864-A *see* Topotecan *on page 1339*
Skin Test Antigens, Multiple *see page 1461*
Sleepinal® [OTC] *see* DiphenhydrAMINE *on page 422*
Slo-bid™ *see* Theophylline *on page 1300*
Slo-Niacin® [OTC] *see* Niacin *on page 965*
Slo-Phyllin® *see* Theophylline *on page 1300*
Slo-Phyllin® GG *see* Theophylline and Guaifenesin *on page 1303*
Slow FE® [OTC] *see* Iron Supplements *on page 744*
Slow-K® *see* Potassium Supplements *on page 1106*
Slow-Mag® [OTC] *see* Magnesium Supplements *on page 831*
SMZ-TMP *see* Sulfamethoxazole and Trimethoprim *on page 1259*
Sodium 2-Mercaptoethane Sulfonate *see* Mesna *on page 860*
Sodium Acid Carbonate *see* Sodium Bicarbonate *on page 1234*
Sodium Benzoate and Caffeine *see* Caffeine and Sodium Benzoate *on page 198*

Sodium Bicarbonate (SOW dee um bye KAR bun ate)

U.S. Brand Names Neut®

Synonyms Baking Soda; $NaHCO_3$; Sodium Acid Carbonate; Sodium Hydrogen Carbonate

Generic Available Yes

Pharmacologic Category Alkalinizing Agent; Antacid; Electrolyte Supplement, Oral; Electrolyte Supplement, Parenteral

Pregnancy Risk Factor C

Lactation Enters breast milk/compatible

Use Management of metabolic acidosis; gastric hyperacidity; as an alkalinization agent for the urine; treatment of hyperkalemia; management of overdose of certain drugs, including tricyclic antidepressants and aspirin

Mechanism of Action/Effect Dissociates to provide bicarbonate ion which neutralizes hydrogen ion concentration and raises blood and urinary pH

Contraindications Alkalosis, hypernatremia, severe pulmonary edema, hypocalcemia, unknown abdominal pain

Warnings/Precautions **Use of I.V. $NaHCO_3$ should be reserved for documented metabolic acidosis and for hyperkalemia-induced cardiac arrest.** Routine use in cardiac arrest is not recommended. Avoid extravasation, tissue necrosis can occur due to the hypertonicity of $NaHCO_3$. May cause sodium retention especially if renal function is impaired; not to be used in treatment of peptic ulcer; use with caution in patients with CHF, edema, cirrhosis, or renal failure. Not the antacid of choice for the elderly because of sodium content and potential for systemic alkalosis. Pregnancy risk C.

Drug Interactions

Decreased Effect: Decreased effect/levels of lithium, chlorpropamide, and salicylates due to urinary alkalinization.

Increased Effect/Toxicity: Increased toxicity/levels of amphetamines, ephedrine, pseudoephedrine, flecainide, quinidine, and quinine due to urinary alkalinization.

Nutritional/Ethanol Interactions Herb/Nutraceutical: Concurrent doses with iron may decrease iron absorption.

Adverse Reactions Frequency not defined.

Cardiovascular: Cerebral hemorrhage, CHF (aggravated), edema
Central nervous system: Tetany
Gastrointestinal: Belching
Endocrine & metabolic: Hypernatremia, hyperosmolality, hypocalcemia, hypokalemia, increased affinity of hemoglobin for oxygen-reduced pH in myocardial tissue necrosis when extravasated, intracranial acidosis, metabolic alkalosis, milk-alkali syndrome (especially with renal dysfunction)
Gastrointestinal: Flatulence (with oral), gastric distension
Respiratory: Pulmonary edema

Overdosage/Toxicology Symptoms of overdose include hypocalcemia, hypokalemia, hypernatremia, and seizures. Treatment is symptom-directed and supportive.

Pharmacodynamics/Kinetics

Absorption: Oral: Well absorbed

Onset: Oral: Rapid; I.V.: 15 minutes

Duration: Oral: 8-10 minutes; I.V.: 1-2 hours

Formulations

Injection:
- 4% [40 mg/mL = 2.4 mEq/5 mL] (5 mL)
- 4.2% [42 mg/mL = 5 mEq/10 mL] (10 mL)
- 5% [50 mg/mL = 5.95 mEq/10 mL] (500 mL)
- 7.5% [75 mg/mL = 8.92 mEq/10 mL] (10 mL, 50 mL)
- 8.4% [84 mg/mL = 10 mEq/10 mL] (10 mL, 50 mL)

Powder: 120 g, 480 g

Tablet: 325 mg [3.8 mEq]; 520 mg [6.3 mEq]; 650 mg [7.6 mEq]

Dosing

Adults:

Cardiac arrest: I.V.: Initial: 1 mEq/kg/dose one time; maintenance: 0.5 mEq/kg/dose every 10 minutes or as indicated by arterial blood gases

Routine use of $NaHCO_3$ is not recommended and should be given only after adequate alveolar ventilation has been established and effective cardiac compressions are provided

Metabolic acidosis: I.V.: Dosage should be based on the following formula if blood gases and pH measurements are available:

HCO_3^-(mEq) = 0.2 x weight (kg) x base deficit (mEq/L) **or**

HCO_3^-(mEq) = 0.5 x weight (kg) x [24 - serum HCO_3^- (mEq/L)]

If acid-base status is not available: Dose for older Children and Adults: 2-5 mEq/kg I.V. infusion over 4-8 hours; subsequent doses should be based on patient's acid-base status

Hyperkalemia: I.V.: 1 mEq/kg over 5 minutes

Chronic renal failure: Oral: Initiate when plasma HCO_3^- <15 mEq/L Start with 20-36 mEq/day in divided doses, titrate to bicarbonate level of 18-20 mEq/L

Renal tubular acidosis: Oral:

Distal: 0.5-2 mEq/kg/day in 4-5 divided doses

Urine alkalinization: Oral: Initial: 48 mEq (4 g), then 12-24 mEq (1-2 g) every 4 hours; dose should be titrated to desired urinary pH; doses up to 16 g/day (200 mEq) in patients <60 years and 8 g (100 mEq) in patients >60 years

Antacid: Oral: 325 mg to 2 g 1-4 times/day

Elderly: Not recommended for use in the elderly (see Geriatric Considerations).

Pediatrics:

Cardiac arrest: I.V.: Infants and Children: I.V.: 0.5-1 mEq/kg/dose repeated every 10 minutes or as indicated by arterial blood gases; rate of infusion should not exceed 10 mEq/minute; neonates and children <2 years of age should receive 4.2% (0.5 mEq/mL) solution.

Note: Routine use of $NaHCO_3$ is not recommended and should be given only after adequate alveolar ventilation has been established and effective cardiac compressions are provided

Metabolic acidosis: I.V.; Infants and Children: Dosage should be based on the following formula if blood gases and pH measurements are available:

HCO_3^-(mEq) = 0.3 x weight (kg) x base deficit (mEq/L) **or**

HCO_3^-(mEq) = 0.5 x weight (kg) x [24 - serum HCO_3^- (mEq/L)]

If acid-base status is not available: Dose for older Children: 2-5 mEq/kg I.V. infusion over 4-8 hours; subsequent doses should be based on patient's acid-base status.

Chronic renal failure: Oral: Children: Initiate when plasma HCO_3^- <15 mEq/L: 1-3 mEq/kg/day

Renal tubular acidosis, distal: Oral: Children: 2-3 mEq/kg/day

Renal tubular acidosis, proximal: Children: Initial: 5-10 mEq/kg/day; maintenance: Increase as required to maintain serum bicarbonate in the normal range

Urine alkalinization: Oral: Children: 1-10 mEq (84-840 mg)/kg/day in divided doses every 4-6 hours; dose should be titrated to desired urinary pH.

Administration

I.V.: Vesicant. Advise patient of milk-alkali syndrome if use is long-term.

Stability

Storage: Store injection at room temperature. Protect from heat and from freezing. Use only clear solutions.

Compatibility: Stable in dextran 6% in dextrose, dextran 6% in NS, $D_5{}^1/_4$NS, $D_5{}^1/_2$NS, D_5NS, D_5W, D_{10}W, $^1/_2$NS, NS; incompatible with acids, acidic salts, alkaloid salts, calcium salts, catecholamines, and atropine

Y-site administration: Incompatible with allopurinol, amiodarone, amphotericin B cholesteryl sulfate complex, calcium chloride, doxorubicin liposome, idarubicin, imipenem/cilastatin inamrinone, leucovorin, midazolam, nalbuphine, ondansetron, oxacillin, sargramostim, verapamil, vincristine, vindesine, vinorelbine

Compatibility in syringe: Incompatible with etidocaine, glycopyrrolate, mepivacaine, metoclopramide, thiopental

Compatibility when admixed: Incompatible with amiodarone, ascorbic acid injection, carboplatin, carmustine, cefotaxime, ciprofloxacin, cisplatin, dobutamine, dopamine, epinephrine, hydromorphone, imipenem/cilastatin, isoproterenol, labetalol, levorphanol, magnesium sulfate, meropenem, morphine, norepinephrine, pentazocine, procaine, streptomycin, succinylcholine, ticarcillin/clavulanate potassium, vitamin B complex with C

Monitoring and Teaching Issues

Physical Assessment: Assess other medications patient may be taking for effectiveness and interactions (see Warnings/Precautions and Drug Interactions). **I.V.:** Monitor therapeutic response and adverse reactions (see Adverse Reactions and Overdose/Toxicology) and infusion site (if extravasation occurs, elevate extravasation site and apply warm compresses). Teach patient adverse symptoms to report (see Patient Education). **Oral:** Monitor effectiveness of treatment and adverse response (see Adverse Reactions). Assess knowledge/teach patient appropriate use, interventions to reduce side effects, and adverse symptoms to report (see Patient Education). **Pregnancy risk factor C** - benefits of use should outweigh possible risks.

Patient Education: Do not use for chronic gastric acidity. Take as directed. Chew tablets thoroughly and follow with a full glass of water, preferably on an empty stomach (2 hours before or after food). Take at least 2 hours before or after any other medications. Report CNS effects (eg, irritability, confusion); muscle rigidity or tremors; swelling of feet or ankles; difficulty breathing; chest pain or palpitations; respiratory changes; or tarry stools. **Pregnancy precaution:** Inform prescriber if you are or intend to become pregnant.

Dietary Issues: Oral product should be administered 1-3 hours after meals.

Sodium content of injection 50 mL, 8.4% = 1150 mg = 50 mEq; each 6 mg of $NaHCO_3$ contains 12 mEq sodium; 1 mEq $NaHCO_3$ = 84 mg

Geriatric Considerations: Not the antacid of choice for the elderly because of sodium content and potential for systemic alkalosis (see maximum daily dose under Usual Dosage).

Additional Information Each 84 mg of sodium bicarbonate provides 1 mEq of sodium and bicarbonate ions; each gram of sodium bicarbonate provides 12 mEq of sodium and bicarbonate ions.

Related Information

Compatibility of Drugs *on page 1564*

Sodium Citrate and Citric Acid (SOW dee um SIT rate & SI trik AS id)

U.S. Brand Names Bicitra®; Oracit®

Synonyms Modified Shohl's Solution

Generic Available No

Pharmacologic Category Alkalinizing Agent

Pregnancy Risk Factor Not established

Lactation Excretion in breast milk unknown/compatible

Use Treatment of metabolic acidosis; alkalinizing agent in conditions where long-term maintenance of an alkaline urine is desirable

Contraindications Severe renal insufficiency, sodium-restricted diet

Warnings/Precautions Conversion to bicarbonate may be impaired in patients with hepatic failure, in shock, or who are severely ill.

Drug Interactions

Decreased Effect: Decreased effect/levels of lithium, chlorpropamide, and salicylates due to urinary alkalinization.

Increased Effect/Toxicity: Increased toxicity/levels of amphetamines, ephedrine, pseudoephedrine, flecainide, quinidine, and quinine due to urinary alkalinization.

Adverse Reactions Frequency not defined.

Central nervous system: Tetany

Endocrine & metabolic: Metabolic alkalosis, hyperkalemia

Gastrointestinal: Diarrhea, nausea, vomiting

Overdosage/Toxicology Symptoms of overdose include hypokalemia, hypernatremia, tetany, and seizures. Treatment is symptom-directed and supportive.

Formulations

Solution, oral:

Bicitra®: Sodium citrate 500 mg and citric acid 334 mg per 5 mL (15 mL unit dose, 480 mL)

Oracit®: Sodium citrate 490 mg and citric acid 640 mg per 5 mL

Dosing

Adults & Elderly: Alkalinizing agent/bicarbonate precursor: Oral: 15-30 mL with water after meals and at bedtime

Pediatrics: Alkalinizing agent/bicarbonate precursor: Oral: Infants and Children: 2-3 mEq/kg/day in divided doses 3-4 times/day **or** 5-15 mL with water after meals and at bedtime

Administration

Oral: Dilute with 30-90 mL of chilled water to enhance taste. Give after meals.

Monitoring and Teaching Issues

Physical Assessment: See Contraindications and Warnings/Precautions for use cautions. Assess kidney function prior to starting therapy. Monitor cardiac status and serum potassium at beginning of therapy and at regular intervals with long-term therapy. Assess knowledge/teach patient appropriate use, possible side effects, and adverse symptoms to report (see Patient Education).

Patient Education: Take as often as directed, preferably on an empty stomach, 1 hour before or 2 hours after meals, and at least 2 hours before or after any other medications. Dilute with 4-6 oz of chilled water. You may experience diarrhea or nausea and vomiting; if severe, contact prescriber. Report CNS changes status (eg, irritability, tremors, confusion); swelling of feet or ankles; difficulty breathing or palpitations; abdominal pain or tarry stools.

Dietary Issues: Should be taken after meals to avoid laxative effect.

Additional Information 1 mL of Bicitra® contains 1 mEq of sodium and the equivalent of 1 mEq of bicarbonate.

Related Information

Potassium Citrate and Citric Acid *on page 1104*

Sodium Citrate and Potassium Citrate Mixture *see page 1522*

Sodium Ferric Gluconate *see* Ferric Gluconate *on page 555*

Sodium Hyaluronate *see page 1509*

Sodium Hyaluronate *see page 1461*

Sodium Hydrogen Carbonate *see* Sodium Bicarbonate *on page 1234*

Sodium Nafcillin *see* Nafcillin *on page 941*

Sodium Nitroferricyanide *see* Nitroprusside *on page 980*

Sodium Nitroprusside *see* Nitroprusside *on page 980*

Sodium Phosphate *see* Phosphate Supplements *on page 1076*

Sodium Phosphate/Biphosphate Enema *see page 1581*

Sodium Polystyrene Sulfonate (SOW dee um pol ee STYE reen SUL fon ate)

U.S. Brand Names Kayexalate®; Kionex™; SPS®

Generic Available Yes

Pharmacologic Category Antidote

Pregnancy Risk Factor C

Lactation Excretion in breast milk unknown/use caution

Use Treatment of hyperkalemia

Mechanism of Action/Effect Removes potassium by exchanging sodium ions for potassium ions in the intestine before the resin is passed from the body; exchange capacity is 1 mEq/g *in vivo*, and *in vitro* capacity is 3.1 mEq/g, therefore, a wide range of exchange capacity exists such that close monitoring of serum electrolytes is necessary

Contraindications Hypersensitivity to sodium polystyrene sulfonate or any component of the formulation; hypernatremia

Warnings/Precautions Use with caution in patients with severe CHF, hypertension, edema, or renal failure. Large oral doses may cause fecal impaction (especially in the elderly). Enema will reduce the serum potassium faster than oral administration, but the oral route will result in a greater reduction over several hours. Pregnancy risk C.

Drug Interactions

Increased Effect/Toxicity: Systemic alkalosis and seizure has occurred after cation-exchange resins were administered with nonabsorbable cation-donating antacids and laxatives (eg, magnesium hydroxide, aluminum carbonate).

Adverse Reactions Frequency not defined.

Endocrine & metabolic: Hypokalemia, hypocalcemia, hypomagnesemia, sodium retention

Gastrointestinal: Fecal impaction, constipation, loss of appetite, nausea, vomiting

Overdosage/Toxicology Symptoms of overdose include hypokalemia including cardiac dysrhythmias, confusion, irritability, EKG changes, muscle weakness, and GI effects. Treatment is supportive, limited to management of fluid and electrolytes.

Pharmacodynamics/Kinetics

Absorption: None

Onset: 2-24 hours

Formulations

Powder for suspension, oral/rectal: 454 g

Suspension, oral/rectal: 1.25 g/5 mL (60 mL, 120 mL, 200 mL, 500 mL) [contains alcohol 0.3% and sorbitol 33%]

Dosing

Adults: Hyperkalemia:

Oral: 15 g (60 mL) 1-4 times/day

Rectal: 30-50 g every 6 hours

Elderly: Refer to adult dosing and Geriatric Considerations.

Pediatrics: Hyperkalemia:

Oral: Children: 1 g/kg/dose every 6 hours

Rectal: Children: 1 g/kg/dose every 2-6 hours (in small children and infants, employ lower doses by using the practical exchange ratio of 1 mEq K^+/g of resin as the basis for calculation)

Administration

Oral: Administer oral (or NG) as ~25% sorbitol solution; never mix in orange juice. Chilling the oral mixture will increase palatability.

Other: Rectal: Enema route is less effective than oral administration. Administer cleansing enema first. Retain enema in colon for at least 30-60 minutes and for several hours, if possible. Enema should be followed by irrigation with normal saline to prevent necrosis.

Monitoring Laboratory Tests Serum electrolytes (potassium, sodium, calcium, magnesium), EKG

Monitoring and Teaching Issues

Physical Assessment: Monitor laboratory tests (see Monitoring Laboratory Tests). Monitor EKG until potassium levels are normal. Monitor for adverse reactions (see Adverse Reactions) and teach patient interventions and importance of reporting adverse symptoms promptly (see Patient Education). **Pregnancy risk factor C** - benefits of use should outweigh possible risks. Note breast-feeding caution.

Patient Education: Emergency instructions depend on patient's condition. You will be monitored for effects of this medication and frequent blood tests may be necessary. Oral: Take as directed. Mix well with a full glass of liquid (not orange juice). You may experience nausea or vomiting (small, frequent meals, frequent mouth care, chewing gum, or sucking lozenges may help); or constipation or fecal impaction (increased dietary fluids and exercise may help). Report persistent constipation or GI distress; chest pain or rapid heartbeat; or mental confusion or muscle weakness. **Pregnancy/breast-feeding precautions:** Inform prescriber if you are pregnant. Consult prescriber if breast-feeding.

Dietary Issues: Do **not** mix in orange juice.

Geriatric Considerations: Large doses in the elderly may cause fecal impaction and intestinal obstruction. Best to administer using sorbitol 70% as vehicle.

Additional Information 1 g of resin binds approximately 1 mEq of potassium; sodium content of 1 g: 31 mg (1.3 mEq)

Sodium Sulamyd® *see page 1509*

Sodium Sulamyd® *see* Sulfacetamide *on page 1256*

Sodium Sulfacetamide *see* Sulfacetamide *on page 1256*

Sodium Thiosulfate *see page 1460*

Solagé™ *see* Mequinol and Tretinoin *on page 854*

Solagé™ Topical Solution *see page 1522*

Solaquin® [OTC] *see* Hydroquinone *on page 679*

Solaquin Forte® *see* Hydroquinone *on page 679*

Solaraze™ *see* Diclofenac *on page 400*

Solarcaine® [OTC] *see* Benzocaine *on page 156*

Solarcaine® Aloe Extra Burn Relief [OTC] *see* Lidocaine *on page 800*

Solu-Cortef® *see* Hydrocortisone *on page 673*

Solu-Cortef® *see* Topical Corticosteroids *on page 1334*

Solu-Medrol® *see* MethylPREDNISolone *on page 885*

Solurex® *see* Dexamethasone *on page 382*

Solurex L.A.® *see* Dexamethasone *on page 382*

Soma® *see* Carisoprodol *on page 221*

Soma® Compound *see* Carisoprodol and Aspirin *on page 222*

Soma® Compound w/Codeine *see* Carisoprodol, Aspirin, and Codeine *on page 223*

Somatrem *see* Human Growth Hormone *on page 658*

Somatropin *see* Human Growth Hormone *on page 658*

Sominex® [OTC] *see* DiphenhydrAMINE *on page 422*

Sominex® Maximum Strength [OTC] *see* DiphenhydrAMINE *on page 422*

Sonata® *see* Zaleplon *on page 1416*

Sorbitol (SOR bi tole)

Generic Available Yes

Pharmacologic Category Genitourinary Irrigant; Laxative, Miscellaneous

Lactation Excretion in breast milk unknown

Use Genitourinary irrigant in transurethral prostatic resection or other transurethral resection or other transurethral surgical procedures; diuretic; humectant; sweetening agent; hyperosmotic laxative; facilitate the passage of sodium polystyrene sulfonate through the intestinal tract

Mechanism of Action/Effect A polyalcoholic sugar with osmotic cathartic actions

Contraindications Anuria

Warnings/Precautions Use with caution in patients with severe cardiopulmonary or renal impairment and in patients unable to metabolize sorbitol; large volumes may result in fluid overload and/or electrolyte changes

Adverse Reactions Frequency not defined.

Cardiovascular: Edema

Endocrine & metabolic: Fluid and electrolyte losses, lactic acidosis

Gastrointestinal: Diarrhea, nausea, vomiting, abdominal discomfort, dry mouth

Overdosage/Toxicology Symptoms of overdose include nausea, diarrhea, fluid and electrolyte loss. Treatment is supportive to ensure fluid and electrolyte balance.

Pharmacodynamics/Kinetics

Absorption: Oral, rectal: Poor

Metabolism: Primarily hepatic to fructose

Onset: 0.25-1 hour

Formulations

Solution: 70% (480 mL, 3840 mL)

Solution, genitourinary irrigation: 3% (1500 mL, 3000 mL); 3.3% (2000 mL)

Dosing

Adults & Elderly:

Hyperosmotic laxative (as single dose, at infrequent intervals):

Oral: 30-150 mL (as 70% solution)

Rectal enema: 120 mL as 25% to 30% solution

Adjunct to sodium polystyrene sulfonate: 15 mL as 70% solution orally until diarrhea occurs (10-20 mL/2 hours) or 20-100 mL as an oral vehicle for the sodium polystyrene sulfonate resin

When administered with charcoal:

Oral: 4.3 mL/kg of 70% sorbitol with 1 g/kg of activated charcoal every 4 hours until first stool containing charcoal is passed

Transurethral surgical procedures: Irrigation: Topical: 3% to 3.3% as transurethral surgical procedure irrigation

Pediatrics: Hyperosmotic laxative (as single dose, at infrequent intervals):

Children 2-11 years:

Oral: 2 mL/kg (as 70% solution)

Rectal enema: 30-60 mL as 25% to 30% solution

Children >12 years: Oral, Rectal enema: Refer to adult dosing.

When administered with charcoal: Oral: Children: 4.3 mL/kg of 35% sorbitol with 1 g/kg of activated charcoal

Stability

Storage: Protect from freezing. Avoid storage in temperatures >150°F.

Monitoring Laboratory Tests Electrolytes

Monitoring and Teaching Issues

Physical Assessment: When used as cathartic, determine cause of constipation before use. Assess knowledge/teach patient about use of nonpharmacological interventions to prevent constipation. Note breast-feeding caution.

Patient Education: Cathartic: Use of cathartics on a regular basis will have adverse effects. Increased exercise, increased fluid intake, or increased dietary fruit and fiber may be effective in preventing and resolving constipation. **Breast-feeding precaution:** Consult prescriber if breast-feeding.

Geriatric Considerations: Causes for constipation must be evaluated prior to initiating treatment. Nonpharmacological dietary treatment should be initiated before laxative use. Sorbitol is as effective as lactulose but is much less expensive.

Related Information

Laxatives: Classification and Properties *on page 1581*

Sorine™ *see* Sotalol *on page 1238*

Sotalol (SOE ta lole)

U.S. Brand Names Betapace®; Betapace AF™; Sorine™

Synonyms Sotalol Hydrochloride

Generic Available Yes: Betapace®

Pharmacologic Category Antiarrhythmic Agent, Class II; Antiarrhythmic Agent, Class III; Beta Blocker, Nonselective

Pregnancy Risk Factor B

Lactation Enters breast milk/use caution (AAP rates "compatible")

Use Treatment of documented ventricular arrhythmias (ie, sustained ventricular tachycardia), that in the judgment of the physician are life-threatening; maintenance of normal sinus rhythm in patients with symptomatic atrial fibrillation and atrial flutter who are currently in sinus rhythm. Manufacturer states substitutions should not be made for Betapace AF™ since Betapace AF™ is distributed with a patient package insert specific for atrial fibrillation/flutter.

Mechanism of Action/Effect

Beta-blocker which contains both beta-adrenoreceptor-blocking (Vaughan Williams Class II) and cardiac action potential duration prolongation (Vaughan Williams Class III) properties

Class II effects: Increased sinus cycle length, slowed heart rate, decreased AV nodal conduction, and increased AV nodal refractoriness

Class III effects: Prolongation of the atrial and ventricular monophasic action potentials, and effective refractory prolongation of atrial muscle, ventricular muscle, and atrioventricular accessory pathways in both the antegrade and retrograde directions

Sotalol is a racemic mixture of *d*- and *l*-sotalol; both isomers have similar Class III antiarrhythmic effects while the *l*-isomer is responsible for virtually all of the beta-blocking activity

Sotalol has both $beta_1$- and $beta_2$-receptor blocking activity

The beta-blocking effect of sotalol is a noncardioselective [half maximal at about 80 mg/day and maximal at doses of 320-640 mg/day]. Significant beta blockade occurs at oral doses as low as 25 mg/day.

Significant Class III effects are seen only at oral doses ≥160 mg/day.

Contraindications Hypersensitivity to sotalol or any component of the formulation; bronchial asthma; sinus bradycardia; second- and third-degree AV block (unless a functioning pacemaker is present); congenital or acquired long QT syndromes; cardiogenic shock; uncontrolled congestive heart failure; concurrent use with cisapride, gatifloxacin, moxifloxacin, or sparfloxacin. Betapace AF® is contraindicated in patients with significantly reduced renal filtration (Cl_{cr} <40 mL/minute).

Warnings/Precautions Must be initiated (or reinitiated) in a setting with continuous monitoring and staff familiar with the recognition and treatment of life-threatening arrhythmias. Patients must be monitored with continuous EKG for a minimum of 3 days (on their maintenance dose). Use cautiously in the renally-impaired (dosage adjustment required). Creatinine clearance must be calculated prior to dosing.

Monitor and adjust dose to prevent QT_c prolongation. Watch for proarrhythmic effects. Correct electrolyte imbalances before initiating (especially hypokalemia and hyperkalemia). Consider pre-existing conditions such as sick sinus syndrome before initiating. Conduction abnormalities can occur particularly sinus bradycardia. Use cautiously within the first 2 weeks post-MI (experience limited), in compensated heart failure, diabetes, or in patients with PVD. Beta-blocker therapy should not be withdrawn abruptly (particularly in patients with CAD), but gradually tapered to avoid acute tachycardia, hypertension, and/or ischemia. Use caution with concurrent use of beta-blockers and either verapamil or diltiazem; bradycardia or heart block can occur. Can mask signs of thyrotoxicosis. Use care with anesthetic agents which decrease myocardial function.

Drug Interactions

Decreased Effect: Decreased effect of sotalol may occur with aluminum-magnesium antacids (if taken within 2 hours), aluminum salts, barbiturates, calcium salts, cholestyramine, colestipol, NSAIDs, penicillins (ampicillin), rifampin, salicylates, and sulfinpyrazone due to decreased bioavailability and plasma levels. Beta-blockers may decrease the effect of sulfonylureas. Beta-agonists such as albuterol, terbutaline may have less of a therapeutic effect when administered concomitantly.

Increased Effect/Toxicity: Increased effect/toxicity of beta-blockers with calcium blockers since there may be additive effects on AV conduction or ventricular function. Sotalol in combination with amiodarone. Other agents which prolong QT interval, including Class I antiarrhythmic agents, bepridil, cisapride (use is contraindicated), erythromycin, haloperidol, pimozide, phenothiazines, tricyclic antidepressants, specific quinolones (sparfloxacin, gatifloxacin, moxifloxacin), or astemizole may increase the effect of sotalol on the prolongation of QT interval. When used concurrently with clonidine, sotalol may increase the risk of rebound hypertension after or during withdrawal of either agent. Beta-blocker and catecholamine depleting agents (reserpine or guanethidine) may result in additive hypotension or bradycardia. Beta-blockers may increase the action or levels of ethanol, nondepolarizing muscle relaxants, and theophylline although the effects are difficult to predict.

Nutritional/Ethanol Interactions

Food: Sotalol peak serum concentrations may be decreased if taken with food.

Herb/Nutraceutical: Avoid ephedra (may worsen arrhythmia).

Adverse Reactions

>10%:

- Cardiovascular: Bradycardia (16%), chest pain (16%), palpitations (14%)
- Central nervous system: Fatigue (20%), dizziness (20%), lightheadedness (12%)
- Neuromuscular & skeletal: Weakness (13%)
- Respiratory: Dyspnea (21%)

1% to 10%:

- Cardiovascular: Congestive heart failure (5%), peripheral vascular disorders (3%), edema (8%), abnormal EKG (7%), hypotension (6%), proarrhythmia (5% in ventricular arrhythmia patients; less than 1% in atrial fibrillation/flutter), syncope (5%)
- Central nervous system: Mental confusion (6%), anxiety (4%), headache (8%), sleep problems (8%), depression (4%)
- Dermatologic: Itching/rash (5%)
- Endocrine & metabolic: Decreased sexual ability (3%)
- Gastrointestinal: Diarrhea (7%), nausea/vomiting (10%), stomach discomfort (3% to 6%), flatulence (2%)
- Genitourinary: Impotence (2%)
- Hematologic: Bleeding (2%)
- Neuromuscular & skeletal: Paresthesia (4%), extremity pain (7%), back pain (3%)
- Ocular: Visual problems (5%)
- Respiratory: Upper respiratory problems (5% to 8%), asthma (2%)

<1% (Limited to important or life-threatening): Alopecia, bronchiolitis obliterans with organized pneumonia (BOOP), cold extremities, diaphoresis, eosinophilia, leukocytoclastic vasculitis, leukopenia, paralysis, phlebitis, photosensitivity reaction, pruritus, pulmonary edema, Raynaud's phenomenon, red crusted skin, retroperitoneal fibrosis, serum transaminases increased, skin necrosis after extravasation, thrombocytopenia, vertigo

Overdosage/Toxicology Symptoms of intoxication include cardiac disturbances, CNS toxicity, bronchospasm, hypoglycemia and hyperkalemia. The most common cardiac symptoms include hypotension and bradycardia; atrioventricular block, intraventricular conduction disturbances, cardiogenic shock, and asystole may occur with severe overdose, especially with membrane-depressant drugs (eg, propranolol); CNS effects include convulsions, coma,

(Continued)

Sotalol *(Continued)*

and respiratory arrest is commonly seen with propranolol and other membrane-depressant and lipid-soluble drugs.

Treatment includes symptomatic treatment of seizures, hypotension, hyperkalemia and hypoglycemia. Bradycardia and hypotension resistant to atropine, isoproterenol or pacing may respond to glucagon. Wide QRS defects caused by the membrane-depressant poisoning may respond to hypertonic sodium bicarbonate. Repeat-dose charcoal, hemoperfusion, or hemodialysis may be helpful in removal of only those beta-blockers with a small V_d, long half-life, or low intrinsic clearance (acebutolol, atenolol, nadolol, sotalol).

Pharmacodynamics/Kinetics

Absorption: Decreased 20% to 30% by meals compared to fasting

Bioavailability: 90% to 100%

Half-Life Elimination: 12 hours; Children: 9.5 hours; terminal half-life decreases with age <2 years (may by ≥1 week in neonates)

Metabolism: None

Onset: Rapid, 1-2 hours; Peak effect: 2.5-4 hours

Duration: 8-16 hours

Formulations Tablet, as hydrochloride:

Betapace® [light blue]: 80 mg, 120 mg, 160 mg, 240 mg
Betapace AF™ [white]: 80 mg, 120 mg, 160 mg
Sorine™ [white]: 80 mg, 120 mg, 160 mg, 240 mg

Dosing

Adults: Sotalol should be initiated and doses increased in a hospital with facilities for cardiac rhythm monitoring and assessment. Proarrhythmic events can occur after initiation of therapy and with each upward dosage adjustment.

Ventricular arrhythmias (Betapace®, Sorine™): Oral:

Initial: 80 mg twice daily; dose may be increased gradually to 240-320 mg/day; allow 3 days between dosing increments (to attain steady-state plasma concentrations and to allow monitoring of QT intervals).

Most patients respond to 160-320 mg/day in 2-3 divided doses.

Some patients, with life-threatening refractory ventricular arrhythmias, may require doses as high as 480-640 mg/day; prescribed ONLY when the potential benefit outweighs the increased of adverse events.

Atrial fibrillation or atrial flutter (Betapace AF™): Oral: Initial: 80 mg twice daily

If the initial dose does not reduce the frequency of relapses of atrial fibrillation/flutter and is tolerated without excessive QT prolongation (not >520 msec) after 3 days, the dose may be increased to 120 mg twice daily. This may be further increased to 160 mg twice daily if response is inadequate and QT prolongation is not excessive.

Elderly: Age does not significantly alter the pharmacokinetics of sotalol, but impaired renal function in elderly patients can increase the terminal half-life, resulting in increased drug accumulation.

Pediatrics: Sotalol should be initiated and doses increased in a hospital with facilities for cardiac rhythm monitoring and assessment. Proarrhythmic events can occur after initiation of therapy and with each upward dosage adjustment.

Note: The safety and efficacy of sotalol in children have not been established

Supraventricular arrhythmias: Oral: **Note:** Dosing per manufacturer, based on pediatric pharmacokinetic data; wait at least 36 hours between dosage adjustments to allow monitoring of QT intervals

≤2 years: Dosage should be adjusted (decreased) by plotting of the child's age on a logarithmic scale; see graph or refer to manufacturer's package labeling.

>2 years: Initial: 90 mg/m²/day in 3 divided doses; may be incrementally increased to a maximum of 180 mg/m²/day

Age Factor Nomogram

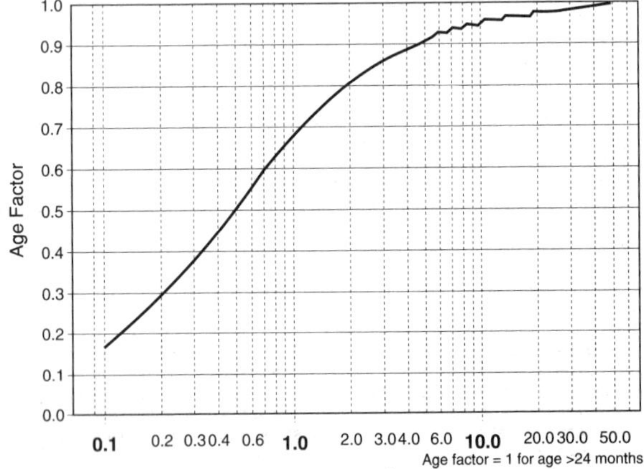

Adapted from U.S. Food and Drug Administration.
http://www.fda.gov/cder/foi/label/2001/2115s3lbl.PDF

Renal Impairment:

Children: Safety and efficacy in children with renal impairment have not been established.

Adults: Impaired renal function can increase the terminal half-life, resulting in increased drug accumulation. Sotalol (Betapace AF™) is contraindicated per the manufacturer for treatment of atrial fibrillation/flutter in patients with a Cl_{cr} <40 mL/minute.

Ventricular arrhythmias (Betapace®, Sorine™):

Cl_{cr} >60 mL/minute: Administer every 12 hours.
Cl_{cr} 30-60 mL/minute: Administer every 24 hours.
Cl_{cr} 10-30 mL/minute: Administer every 36-48 hours.
Cl_{cr} <10 mL/minute: Individualize dose.

Atrial fibrillation/flutter (Betapace AF™):

Cl_{cr} >60 mL/minute: Administer every 12 hours.
Cl_{cr} 40-60 mL/minute: Administer every 24 hours.
Cl_{cr} <40 mL/minute: Use is contraindicated.

Dialysis: Hemodialysis would be expected to reduce sotalol plasma concentrations because sotalol is not bound to plasma proteins and does not undergo extensive metabolism. Administer dose postdialysis or administer supplemental 80 mg dose. Peritoneal dialysis does not remove sotalol; supplemental dose is not necessary.

Stability

Storage: Store at 25°C (77°F). Excursions permitted to 15°C to 30°C (59°F to 86°F).

Monitoring Laboratory Tests Serum magnesium, potassium

Monitoring and Teaching Issues

Physical Assessment: See Contraindications, Warnings/Precautions, and Dosing for use cautions. Assess potential for interactions with other prescriptions, OTC medications, or herbal products patient may be taking (see Drug Interactions). Assess blood pressure and heart rate prior to and following first dose and with any change in dosage. Assess results of laboratory tests (see above), therapeutic effectiveness, and adverse effects (eg, cardiac and pulmonary status - see Adverse Reactions and Overdose /Toxicology). Advise diabetic patients to monitor glucose levels closely (beta-blockers may alter glucose tolerance). Do not discontinue abruptly; dose should be tapered gradually. Teach patient appropriate use, possible side effects/interventions (hypotension precautions), and adverse symptoms to report (see Patient Education). Note breast-feeding caution.

Patient Education: Inform prescriber of all prescriptions, OTC medications, or herbal products you are taking, and any allergies you have. Do not take any new medications without consulting prescriber. Take exactly as directed; do not adjust dosage or discontinue without consulting prescriber. Take pulse daily (prior to medication) and follow prescriber's instruction about holding of medication. If diabetic, monitor serum sugar closely (drug may alter glucose tolerance or mask signs of hypoglycemia). May cause fatigue, dizziness, lightheadedness, or postural hypotension (use caution when changing position from lying or sitting to standing, when driving, or climbing stairs until response to medication is known); alteration in sexual performance (reversible); nausea or vomiting (small, frequent meals, frequent mouth care, sucking lozenges, or chewing gum may help); or diarrhea (boiled milk, buttermilk, or yogurt may help). Report immediately any chest pain, palpitations, irregular heartbeat; swelling of extremities, difficulty breathing, new cough, or unusual fatigue; persistent nausea, vomiting, or diarrhea; or unusual muscle weakness. **Breast-feeding precaution:** Consult prescriber if breast-feeding.

Dietary Issues: Administer on an empty stomach.

Geriatric Considerations: Since elderly frequently have Cl_{cr} <60 mL/minute, attention to dose, creatinine clearance, and monitoring is important. Make dosage adjustments at 3-day intervals or after 5-6 doses at any dosage.

Breast-feeding Issues: Sotalol is considered compatible by the AAP. It is recommended that the infant be monitored for signs or symptoms of beta-blockade (hypotension, bradycardia, etc) with long-term use.

Pregnancy Issues: Although there are no adequate and well controlled studies in pregnant women, sotalol has been shown to cross the placenta, and is found in amniotic fluid. There has been a report of subnormal birth weight with sotalol, therefore, sotalol should be used during pregnancy only if the potential benefit outweighs the potential risk.

Additional Information Pharmacokinetics in children are more relevant for BSA than age.

Related Information

Antiarrhythmic Drugs *on page 1551*
Beta-Blockers *on page 1561*

Sotalol Hydrochloride *see* Sotalol *on page 1238*

SPA *see* Albumin *on page 50*

Spacol *see* Hyoscyamine *on page 685*

Spacol T/S *see* Hyoscyamine *on page 685*

Sparfloxacin (spar FLOKS a sin)

U.S. Brand Names Zagam®

Generic Available No

Pharmacologic Category Antibiotic, Quinolone

Pregnancy Risk Factor C

Lactation Enters breast milk/contraindicated

Use Treatment of adults with community-acquired pneumonia caused by *C. pneumoniae, H. influenzae, H. parainfluenzae, M. catarrhalis, M. pneumoniae* or *S. pneumoniae*; treatment of acute bacterial exacerbations of chronic bronchitis caused by *C. pneumoniae, E. cloacae, H. influenzae, H. parainfluenzae, K. pneumoniae, M. catarrhalis, S. aureus* or *S. pneumoniae*

Mechanism of Action/Effect Inhibits DNA-gyrase in susceptible organisms; inhibits relaxation of supercoiled DNA and promotes breakage of double-stranded DNA

(Continued)

Sparfloxacin *(Continued)*

Contraindications Hypersensitivity to sparfloxacin, any component of the formulation, or other quinolones; a concurrent administration with drugs which increase the QT interval including: amiodarone, bepridil, bretylium, cisapride, disopyramide, furosemide, procainamide, quinidine, sotalol, albuterol, astemizole, chloroquine, halofantrine, phenothiazines, prednisone, and tricyclic antidepressants

Warnings/Precautions Not recommended in children <18 years of age, other quinolones have caused transient arthropathy in children. CNS stimulation may occur (tremor, restlessness, confusion, rarely hallucinations or seizures). Use with caution in patients with known or suspected CNS disorder or renal dysfunction. Although quinolones may exacerbate myasthenia gravis, sparfloxacin appears to be an exception; caution is still warranted.

Prolonged use may result in superinfection. May cause photosensitivity; severe reactions have been reported rarely (avoid exposure during and for several days following fluoroquinolone therapy). Superinfection may occur; pseudomembranous colitis should be considered in patients who present with diarrhea. Tendon inflammation and/or rupture have been reported with other quinolone antibiotics. Risk may be increased with concurrent corticosteroids, particularly in the elderly. Discontinue at first sign of tendon inflammation or pain. Severe hypersensitivity reactions, including anaphylaxis, have occurred with quinolone therapy. Discontinue immediately if an allergic reaction occurs.

Pregnancy risk C.

Drug Interactions

Cytochrome P450 Effect: Inhibits **CYP1A2**

Decreased Effect: Decreased absorption with antacids containing aluminum, didanosine (chewable/buffered tablets or pediatric powder for oral solution), magnesium, zinc, iron and/or calcium (by up to 98% if given at the same time). Phenytoin serum levels may be reduced by quinolones. Antineoplastic agents may also decrease serum levels of fluoroquinolones.

Increased Effect/Toxicity: Quinolones cause increased levels of caffeine, warfarin, cyclosporine, and theophylline (although one study indicates that sparfloxacin may not affect theophylline metabolism). Cimetidine, and probenecid increase quinolone levels. An increased incidence of seizures may occur with foscarnet and NSAIDs. Sparfloxacin does not appear to alter warfarin levels, but warfarin effect may be increased due possible effects on gastrointestinal flora. Concurrent use of corticosteroids may increase risk of tendon rupture.

Nutritional/Ethanol Interactions Herb/Nutraceutical: Avoid dong quai, St John's wort (may also cause photosensitization).

Adverse Reactions

1% to 10%:

- Cardiovascular: QT_c interval prolongation (1.3%)
- Central nervous system: Insomnia, dizziness, headache, agitation, sleep disorders, anxiety, delirium
- Dermatologic: Photosensitivity reaction, pruritus, vasodilatation
- Gastrointestinal: Diarrhea, dyspepsia, nausea, abdominal pain, vomiting, flatulence, taste perversion, dry mouth
- Hematologic: Leukopenia, eosinophilia, anemia
- Hepatic: Increased LFTs

<1% (Limited to important or life-threatening): Angina pectoris, angioedema, arrhythmia, asthma, atrial fibrillation, atrial flutter, complete AV block, dyspnea, ecchymosis, exfoliative dermatitis, migraine, postural hypotension; quinolones have been associated with tendonitis and tendon rupture

Overdosage/Toxicology

Symptoms of overdose include acute renal failure, seizures

GI decontamination and supportive care; not removed by peritoneal or hemodialysis

Pharmacodynamics/Kinetics

Absorption: Unaffected by food or milk; reduced ~50% by concurrent administration of aluminum- and magnesium-containing antacids

Half-Life Elimination: Mean terminal: 20 hours (range: 16-30 hours)

Time to Peak: 3-5 hours

Metabolism: Hepatic, but does not utilize CYP

Formulations Tablet: 200 mg

Dosing

Adults & Elderly: Susceptible infections: Oral: Loading dose: 2 tablets (400 mg) on day 1; maintenance dose: 1 tablet (200 mg) daily for 9 additional days (completes 10 days therapy with a total of 11 tablets)

Renal Impairment: Cl_{cr} <50 mL/minute: Administer 400 mg on day 1 as a loading dose, then 200 mg every 48 hours for a total of 8 additional days of therapy (total 6 tablets).

Administration

Oral: May be taken without regard to meals, however, should be administered at the same time each day. Antacids containing magnesium and aluminum or sucralfate, didanosine (chewable/buffered tablets or pediatric oral solution) should be taken 4 hours after sparfloxacin.

Monitoring Laboratory Tests Perform culture and sensitivity prior to beginning therapy. Monitor CBC, renal and hepatic function periodically if therapy is prolonged.

Monitoring and Teaching Issues

Physical Assessment: Assess allergy history before initiating therapy. See Contraindications and Warnings/Precautions for use cautions. Assess potential for interactions with other prescriptions, OTC medications, or herbal products patient may be taking (see Drug Interactions). Assess results of laboratory tests (see above) and patient response (see Adverse Reactions and Overdose/Toxicology). Teach patient appropriate use (according to formulation), possible side effects and interventions (eg, photosensitivity), and adverse symptoms to report (eg, opportunistic infection - see Patient Education). **Pregnancy risk**

factor C - benefits of use should outweigh possible risks. Breast-feeding is contraindicated.

Patient Education: Inform prescriber of all prescriptions, OTC medications, or herbal products you are taking, and any allergies you have. Do not take anything new during treatment unless approved by prescriber. Take as directed, at the same time each day - do not take with antacids. Take entire prescription even if feeling better, if dose is missed take as soon as possible, do not double doses. Maintain adequate hydration (2-3 L/day of fluids) unless advised by prescriber to restrict fluids. May cause dizziness, lightheadedness, or anxiety (use caution when driving or engaging in tasks that require alertness until response to drug is known); nausea, vomiting, or dry mouth (small, frequent meals, frequent mouth care, sucking lozenges, or chewing gum may help); photosensitivity (use sunscreen, wear protective clothing and eyewear, and avoid direct sunlight during and for several days following therapy). If inflammation or tendon pain occurs, discontinue use immediately and report to prescriber. If allergic reaction occurs (itching urticaria, difficulty breathing, facial edema or difficulty swallowing, loss of consciousness, tingling, chest pain, palpitations), discontinue use immediately and report to prescriber. Report palpitations or chest pain; persistent diarrhea or constipation; or signs of superinfection (unusual fever or chills; vaginal itching or foul-smelling vaginal discharge; easy bruising or bleeding). **Pregnancy/ breast-feeding precautions:** Inform prescriber if you are or intend to become pregnant. Do not breast-feed.

Dietary Issues: May be taken without regard to meals; should be taken at the same time each day.

Geriatric Considerations: Elderly patients may be more susceptible to the cardiac adverse effects of sparfloxacin. Adjust dose based on renal function; evaluate patient's drug regimen prior to initiating therapy to avoid or make allowances for possible drug interactions since elderly frequently have diseases requiring medications that can interact with quinolones.

Breast-feeding Issues: Quinolones are known to distribute well into breast milk; consequently use during lactation should be avoided if possible.

Additional Information As of September 2002, sparfloxacin is not available from the manufacturer. This product is anticipated to return to the market in 2003.

Spectinomycin (spek ti noe MYE sin)

U.S. Brand Names Trobicin®

Synonyms Spectinomycin Hydrochloride

Generic Available No

Pharmacologic Category Antibiotic, Miscellaneous

Pregnancy Risk Factor B

Lactation Enters breast milk/effect on infant unknown

Use Treatment of uncomplicated gonorrhea

Mechanism of Action/Effect A bacteriostatic antibiotic that selectively binds to the 30s subunits of ribosomes, and thereby inhibiting bacterial protein synthesis

Contraindications Hypersensitivity to spectinomycin or any component of the formulation

Warnings/Precautions Since spectinomycin is ineffective in the treatment of syphilis and may mask symptoms, all patients should be tested for syphilis at the time of diagnosis and 3 months later.

Adverse Reactions <1% (Limited to important or life-threatening): Abdominal cramps, chills, dizziness, headache, nausea, vomiting

Overdosage/Toxicology Symptoms of overdose include paresthesia, dizziness, blurring of vision, ototoxicity, renal damage, nausea, sleeplessness, decrease in hemoglobin

Pharmacodynamics/Kinetics

Absorption: I.M.: Rapid and almost complete

Half-Life Elimination: 1.7 hours

Time to Peak: ~1 hour

Duration: Up to 8 hours

Formulations Injection, powder for reconstitution, as hydrochloride: 2 g

Dosing

Adults & Elderly:

Uncomplicated urethral, cervical, pharyngeal, or rectal gonorrhea: I.M.: 2 g deep I.M. or 4 g where antibiotic resistance is prevalent 1 time; 4 g (10 mL) dose should be given as two 5 mL injections, followed by adequate chlamydial treatment (doxycycline 100 mg twice daily for 7 days)

Disseminated gonococcal infection: I.M.: 2 g every 12 hours

Pediatrics: Gonorrhea: I.M.: Children:

<45 kg: 40 mg/kg/dose 1 time (ceftriaxone preferred)

≥45 kg: Refer to adult dosing.

Children >8 years who are allergic to PCNS/cephalosporins may be treated with oral tetracycline.

Renal Impairment: Hemodialysis effects: 50% removed by hemodialysis

Administration

I.M.: For I.M. use only.

Stability

Reconstitution: Use reconstituted solutions within 24 hours; reconstitute with supplied diluent only.

Monitoring Laboratory Tests Test for syphilis before treatment and 3 months later (see Warnings/Precautions).

Monitoring and Teaching Issues

Physical Assessment: Assess knowledge/teach patient sexually transmitted diseases precautions. Monitor effectiveness and evaluate laboratory results (see above). Note breast-feeding caution.

Patient Education: This medication can only be administered I.M. You will need to return for follow-up blood tests. **Breast-feeding precaution:** Consult prescriber if breast-feeding.

Spectinomycin Hydrochloride *see* Spectinomycin *on page 1243*
Spectracef™ *see* Cefditoren *on page 236*
Spherulin® *see page 1461*

Spironolactone (speer on oh LAK tone)

U.S. Brand Names Aldactone®

Generic Available Yes

Pharmacologic Category Diuretic, Potassium Sparing

Pregnancy Risk Factor C/D in pregnancy-induced hypertension (per expert analysis)

Lactation Enters breast milk/compatible

Use Management of edema associated with excessive aldosterone excretion; hypertension; primary hyperaldosteronism; hypokalemia; treatment of hirsutism; cirrhosis of liver accompanied by edema or ascites. The benefits of spironolactone were additive to the benefits of ACE inhibition in patients with severe CHF (further reducing mortality by 30% over 2 years) in RALES - a large controlled clinical trial.

Mechanism of Action/Effect Competes with aldosterone for receptor sites in the distal renal tubules, increasing sodium chloride and water excretion while conserving potassium and hydrogen ions; may block the effect of aldosterone on arteriolar smooth muscle as well

Contraindications Hypersensitivity to spironolactone or any component of the formulation; anuria; acute renal insufficiency; significant impairment of renal excretory function; hyperkalemia; pregnancy

Warnings/Precautions Avoid potassium supplements, potassium-containing salt substitutes, a diet rich in potassium, or other drugs that can cause hyperkalemia. Monitor for fluid and electrolyte imbalances. Gynecomastia is related to dose and duration of therapy. Diuretic therapy should be carefully used in severe hepatic dysfunction; electrolyte and fluid shifts can cause or exacerbate encephalopathy. Discontinue use prior to adrenal vein catheterization. C/D in pregnancy-induced hypertension (per expert analysis)

Drug Interactions

Decreased Effect: The effects of digoxin (loss of positive inotropic effect) and mitotane may be reduced by spironolactone. Salicylates and NSAIDs (indomethacin) may decrease the natriuretic effect of spironolactone.

Increased Effect/Toxicity: Concurrent use of spironolactone with other potassium-sparing diuretics, potassium supplements, angiotensin-receptor antagonists, co-trimoxazole (high dose), and ACE inhibitors can increase the risk of hyperkalemia, especially in patients with renal impairment. Cholestyramine can cause hyperchloremic acidosis in cirrhotic patients; avoid concurrent use.

Nutritional/Ethanol Interactions

Food: Food increases absorption.

Herb/Nutraceutical: Avoid natural licorice (due to mineralocorticoid activity)

Effects on Lab Values May cause false elevation in serum digoxin concentrations measured by RIA.

Adverse Reactions Incidence of adverse events is not always reported (mean daily dose 26 mg).

Cardiovascular: Edema (2%, placebo 2%)

Central nervous system: Disorders (23%, placebo 21%) which may include drowsiness, lethargy, headache, mental confusion, drug fever, ataxia, fatigue

Dermatologic: Maculopapular, erythematous cutaneous eruptions, urticaria, hirsutism, eosinophilia

Endocrine & metabolic: Gynecomastia (men 9%; placebo 1%), breast pain (men 2%; placebo 0.1%), serious hyperkalemia (2%, placebo 1%), hyponatremia, dehydration, hyperchloremic metabolic acidosis (in decompensated hepatic cirrhosis), impotence, menstrual irregularities, amenorrhea, postmenopausal bleeding

Gastrointestinal: Disorders (29%, placebo 29%) which may include anorexia, nausea, cramping, diarrhea, gastric bleeding, ulceration, gastritis, vomiting

Hematologic: Agranulocytosis

Hepatic: Cholestatic/hepatocellular toxicity

Renal: Increased BUN concentration

Miscellaneous: Deepening of the voice, anaphylactic reaction, breast cancer

Overdosage/Toxicology Symptoms of overdose include drowsiness, confusion, clinical signs of dehydration and electrolyte imbalance, and hyperkalemia. Ingestion of large amounts of potassium-sparing diuretics may result in life-threatening hyperkalemia. This can be treated with I.V. glucose, with concurrent regular insulin. Sodium bicarbonate may also be used as a temporary measure. If needed, Kayexalate® oral or rectal solutions in sorbitol may also be used.

Pharmacodynamics/Kinetics

Half-Life Elimination: 78-84 minutes

Time to Peak: Serum: 1-3 hours (primarily as the active metabolite)

Metabolism: Hepatic to multiple metabolites, including canrenone (active)

Formulations Tablet: 25 mg, 50 mg, 100 mg

Dosing

Adults: To reduce delay in onset of effect, a loading dose of 2 or 3 times the daily dose may be administered on the first day of therapy. Oral:

Edema, hypertension, hypokalemia: 25-200 mg/day in 1-2 divided doses

Diagnosis of primary aldosteronism: 100-400 mg/day in 1-2 divided doses

Hirsutism in women: 50-200 mg/day in 1-2 divided doses

CHF, severe (with ACE inhibitor and a loop diuretic ± digoxin): 25 mg/day, increased or reduced depending on individual response and evidence of hyperkalemia

Elderly: Oral: Initial: 25-50 mg/day in 1-2 divided doses; increase by 25-50 mg every 5 days as needed. Adjust for renal impairment.

Pediatrics: Administration with food increases absorption. To reduce delay in onset of effect, a loading dose of 2 or 3 times the daily dose may be administered on the first day of therapy.

Edema, hypertension: Oral:
Neonates: 1-3 mg/kg/day divided every 12-24 hours
Children: 1.5-3.5 mg/kg/day **or** 60 mg/m²/day in divided doses every 6-24 hours
Diagnosis of primary aldosteronism: 125-375 mg/m²/day in divided doses
Vaso-occlusive disease: Children: 7.5 mg/kg/day in divided doses twice daily (not FDA approved)

Renal Impairment:
Cl_{cr} 10-50 mL/minute: Administer every 12-24 hours.
Cl_{cr} <10 mL/minute: Avoid use.

Stability
Storage: Protect from light.

Monitoring Laboratory Tests Serum electrolytes (potassium, sodium), renal function

Monitoring and Teaching Issues

Physical Assessment: See Contraindications and Warnings/Precautions for use cautions. Diuretic effect may be delayed 2-3 days and antihypertensive effect may be delayed 2-3 weeks (see Dosing to reduce delayed effect). Assess potential for interactions with other prescriptions, OTC medications, or herbal products patient may be taking (see Drug Interactions). Assess results of laboratory tests (see above) and patient response (eg, fluid status and electrolytes - see Adverse Reactions and Overdose/Toxicology). Teach patient appropriate use, possible side effects and interventions (eg, photosensitivity), and adverse symptoms to report (eg, opportunistic infection - see Patient Education). **Pregnancy risk factor C/D** - see Pregnancy Risk Factor for use cautions; determine that patient is not pregnant before beginning treatment. Instruct patients of childbearing age about necessity for barrier contraceptive measures.

Patient Education: Inform prescriber of all prescriptions, OTC medications, or herbal products you are taking, and any allergies you have. Do not take anything new during treatment unless approved by prescriber. Take as directed, with meals. Do not increase dietary potassium. Avoid natural licorice. Weigh yourself weekly at the same time, in the same clothes, and report weight loss >5 lb/week. May cause dizziness, drowsiness, confusion, or headache (use caution when driving or engaging in tasks requiring alertness until response to drug is known); nausea, vomiting, or dry mouth (small, frequent meals, frequent mouth care, sucking lozenges, or chewing gum may help); or decreased sexual ability, gynecomastia, impotence, menstrual irregularities (reversible with discontinuing of medication). Report mental confusion; clumsiness; persistent fatigue, chills, numbness, or muscle weakness in hands, feet, or face; acute persistent diarrhea; breast tenderness or increased body hair in females; breast enlargement or inability to achieve erection in males; chest pain, rapid heartbeat, or palpitations; excessive thirst; or difficulty breathing. **Pregnancy precaution:** Do not get pregnant while taking this medication. Consult prescriber for appropriate barrier contraceptive measures.

Dietary Issues: Should be taken with food to decrease gastrointestinal irritation and to increase absorption. Excessive potassium intake (eg, salt substitutes, low-salt foods, bananas, nuts) should be avoided.

Geriatric Considerations: See Warnings/Precautions; monitor serum potassium.

Breast-feeding Issues: Crosses into breast milk; AAP considers **compatible** with breast-feeding.

Pregnancy Issues: One report of oral cleft. Generally, use of diuretics during pregnancy is avoided due to risk of decreased placental perfusion.

Related Information
Heart Failure *on page 1670*

Spironolactone and Hydrochlorothiazide *see* Hydrochlorothiazide and Spironolactone *on page 666*

Sporanox® *see* Itraconazole *on page 755*

SPS® *see* Sodium Polystyrene Sulfonate *on page 1236*

SSD® AF *see* Silver SulfaDIAZINE *on page 1229*

SSD® Cream *see* Silver SulfaDIAZINE *on page 1229*

SSKI® *see* Potassium Iodide *on page 1105*

Stadol® *see* Butorphanol *on page 196*

Stadol® NS *see* Butorphanol *on page 196*

Stagesic® *see* Hydrocodone and Acetaminophen *on page 667*

Starlix® *see* Nateglinide *on page 951*

Staticin® *see* Erythromycin (Systemic) *on page 486*

Stavudine (STAV yoo deen)

U.S. Brand Names Zerit®

Synonyms d4T

Generic Available No

Pharmacologic Category Antiretroviral Agent, Reverse Transcriptase Inhibitor (Nucleoside)

Pregnancy Risk Factor C

Lactation Excretion in breast milk unknown/contraindicated

Use Treatment of adults with HIV infection in combination with other antiretroviral agents

Mechanism of Action/Effect Inhibits reverse transcriptase of the human immunodeficiency virus (HIV)

Contraindications Hypersensitivity to stavudine or any component of the formulation

Warnings/Precautions Use with caution in patients who demonstrate previous hypersensitivity to zidovudine, didanosine, zalcitabine, pre-existing bone marrow suppression, renal insufficiency, or peripheral neuropathy. Peripheral neuropathy may be the dose-limiting side effect. Zidovudine should not be used in combination with stavudine. Lactic acidosis and severe hepatomegaly with steatosis have been reported with stavudine use, including fatal cases. Risk may be increased in obesity, prolonged nucleoside exposure, or in female patients. Suspend therapy in patients with suspected lactic acidosis; consider discontinuation of stavudine if lactic acidosis is confirmed. Pregnant women may be at increased risk of lactic acidosis and liver damage. Severe motor weakness (resembling Guillain-Barré syndrome)
(Continued)

Stavudine *(Continued)*

has also been reported (including fatal cases, usually in association with lactic acidosis); manufacturer recommends discontinuation if motor weakness develops (with or without lactic acidosis). Pancreatitis (including some fatal cases) has occurred during combination therapy (didanosine with or without hydroxyurea). Risk increased when used in combination regimen with didanosine and hydroxyurea. Suspend therapy with agents toxic to the pancreas (including stavudine, didanosine, or hydroxyurea) in patients with suspected pancreatitis. Pregnancy risk C.

Drug Interactions

Decreased Effect: Stavudine may decrease the activity of zidovudine (based on *in vitro* data).

Increased Effect/Toxicity: Drugs associated with peripheral neuropathy (chloramphenicol, cisplatin, dapsone, ethionamide, gold, hydralazine, iodoquinol, isoniazid, lithium, metronidazole, nitrofurantoin, pentamidine, phenytoin, ribavirin, vincristine) may increase risk for stavudine peripheral neuropathy. Risk of neuropathy, pancreatitis, or lactic acidosis and severe hepatomegaly is increased with concurrent use of didanosine and hydroxyurea. Concomitant use of ribavirin and nucleoside analogues may increase the risk of developing lactic acidosis (includes adefovir, didanosine, lamivudine, stavudine, zalcitabine, zidovudine).

Adverse Reactions All adverse reactions reported below were similar to comparative agent (zidovudine), except for peripheral neuropathy, which was greater with stavudine

>10%:
- Neuromuscular & skeletal: Peripheral neuropathy (dose related)
- Central nervous system: Headache, chills/fever, malaise, insomnia, anxiety, depression, pain
- Gastrointestinal: Nausea, vomiting, anorexia, diarrhea, abdominal pain

1% to 10%
- Hematologic: Neutropenia, thrombocytopenia
- Hepatic: increased bilirubin
- Neuromuscular & skeletal: Myalgia, arthralgia, back pain, weakness

Postmarketing and/or case reports (limited to important or life-threatening): Allergic reaction, anemia, anorexia, hepatomegaly, hepatic failure, hepatic steatosis, insomnia, lactic acidosis, leukopenia, motor weakness (severe), pancreatitis, redistribution/accumulation of body fat

Pharmacodynamics/Kinetics

Bioavailability: 86.4%

Half-Life Elimination: 1-1.6 hours

Time to Peak: Serum: 1 hour

Formulations

Capsule: 15 mg, 20 mg, 30 mg, 40 mg

Powder, oral solution: 1 mg/mL (200 mL)

Dosing

Adults: HIV infection (in combination with other antiretrovirals): Oral (Dose may be cut in half if symptoms of peripheral neuropathy occur):
- ≥60 kg: 40 mg every 12 hours
- <60 kg: 30 mg every 12 hours

Elderly: Older patients should be closely monitored for signs and symptoms of peripheral neuropathy. Dosage should be carefully adjusted to renal function.

Pediatrics: HIV infection: Oral:
- Newborns (Birth to 13 days): 0.5 mg/kg every 12 hours
- Children:
  - >14 days and <30 kg: 1 mg/kg every 12 hours
  - ≥30 kg: 30 mg every 12 hours

Renal Impairment:
- Cl_{cr} >50 mL/minute:
  - ≥60 kg: Administer 40 mg every 12 hours.
  - <60 kg: Administer 30 mg every 12 hours.
- Cl_{cr} 26-50 mL/minute:
  - ≥60 kg: Administer 20 mg every 12 hours.
  - <60 kg: Administer 15 mg every 12 hours.
- Cl_{cr} 10-25 mL/minute:
  - ≥60 kg: Administer 20 mg every 24 hours.
  - <60 kg: Administer 15 mg every 24 hours.
- Hemodialysis:
  - ≥60 kg: Administer 20 mg every 24 hours.
  - <60 kg: Administer 15 mg every 24 hours.

Administration

Oral: May be taken without regard to meals.

Stability

Reconstitution: Reconstituted oral solution should be refrigerated and is stable for 30 days.

Monitoring Laboratory Tests Liver function

Monitoring and Teaching Issues

Physical Assessment: See Contraindications, and Warnings/Precautions, and Dosing for use cautions. Assess potential for interactions with other prescriptions, OTC medications, or herbal products patient may be taking (see Drug Interactions). Assess results of laboratory tests (see above) and patient response (eg, peripheral neuropathy, CNS changes, hematological changes, and opportunistic infection - see Adverse Reactions and Overdose/Toxicology) on a regular basis throughout therapy. Teach patient proper use (see Administration, Storage, and Reconstitution), possible side effects and interventions, and adverse symptoms to report (see Patient Education). **Pregnancy risk factor C** - benefits of use should outweigh possible risks. Breast-feeding is contraindicated.

Patient Education: Inform prescriber of all prescriptions, OTC medications, or herbal products you are taking, and any allergies you have. Do not take anything new during treatment unless approved by prescriber. This drug will not cure HIV; use appropriate precautions to prevent spread of HIV to other persons. Take as directed, with or without food. Powder: Pour powder into 4 oz of water, stir, and drink immediately (do not mix with fruit juice or other acid-containing liquids). Maintain adequate hydration (2-3 L/day of fluids) unless advised by prescriber to restrict fluids. You may be more susceptible to infection (avoid crowds and exposure to infection and do not have any vaccinations without consulting prescriber). May cause nausea or vomiting (small, frequent meals, frequent mouth care, chewing gum, or sucking lozenges may help); diarrhea (boiled milk, yogurt, or buttermilk may help); or headache, back, muscle, or joint pain (consult prescriber for approved analgesic). Report immediately any loss of sensation, numbness, or tingling in fingers, toes, or feet. Report persistent unresolved abdominal distress (nausea, vomiting, diarrhea); or signs of infection (burning on urination, perineal itching, white plaques in mouth, unhealed sores, persistent sore throat or cough). **Pregnancy/breast-feeding precautions:** Inform prescriber if you are pregnant. Do not breast-feed.

Dietary Issues: May be taken without regard to meals.

Breast-feeding Issues: HIV-infected mothers are discouraged from breast-feeding to decrease potential transmission of HIV.

Pregnancy Issues: Cases of fatal and nonfatal lactic acidosis, with or without pancreatitis, have been reported in pregnant women. It is not known if pregnancy itself potentiates this known side effect; however, pregnant women may be at increased risk of lactic acidosis and liver damage. Hepatic enzymes and electrolytes should be monitored frequently during the 3rd trimester of pregnancy. Use during pregnancy only if the potential benefit to the mother outweighs the potential risk of this complication. Stavudine crosses the placenta *ex vivo*. Health professionals are encouraged to contact the antiretroviral pregnancy registry to monitor outcomes of pregnant women exposed to antiretroviral medications (1-800-258-4263).

Additional Information Potential compliance problems, frequency of administration and adverse effects should be discussed with patients before initiating therapy to help prevent the emergence of resistance.

S-T Cort® *see* Topical Corticosteroids *on page 1334*

Stelazine® *see* Trifluoperazine *on page 1361*

STI571 *see* Imatinib *on page 695*

Stilbestrol *see* Diethylstilbestrol *on page 407*

Stilphostrol® *see* Diethylstilbestrol *on page 407*

Stimate™ *see* Desmopressin *on page 380*

St. Joseph® Pain Reliever [OTC] *see* Aspirin *on page 121*

Streptase® *see* Streptokinase *on page 1247*

Streptokinase (strep toe KYE nase)

U.S. Brand Names Streptase®

Synonyms SK

Generic Available No

Pharmacologic Category Thrombolytic Agent

Pregnancy Risk Factor C

Lactation Excretion in breast milk unknown

Use Thrombolytic agent used in treatment of recent severe or massive deep vein thrombosis, pulmonary emboli, myocardial infarction, and occluded arteriovenous cannulas

Mechanism of Action/Effect Activates the conversion of plasminogen to plasmin by forming a complex, exposing plasminogen-activating site, and cleaving a peptide bond that converts plasminogen to plasmin; plasmin degrades fibrin, fibrinogen and other procoagulant proteins into soluble fragments; effective both outside and within the formed thrombus/embolus

Contraindications Hypersensitivity to anistreplase, streptokinase, or any component of the formulation; active internal bleeding; history of CVA; recent (within 2 months) intracranial or intraspinal surgery or trauma; intracranial neoplasm, arteriovenous malformation, or aneurysm; known bleeding diathesis; severe uncontrolled hypertension

Warnings/Precautions Concurrent heparin anticoagulation can contribute to bleeding; careful attention to all potential bleeding sites. I.M. injections and nonessential handling of the patient should be avoided. Venipunctures should be performed carefully and only when necessary. If arterial puncture is necessary, use an upper extremity vessel that can be manually compressed. If serious bleeding occurs then the infusion of streptokinase and heparin should be stopped.

For the following conditions the risk of bleeding is higher with use of thrombolytics and should be weighed against the benefits of therapy: recent (within 10 days) major surgery (eg, CABG, obstetrical delivery, organ biopsy, previous puncture of noncompressible vessels), cerebrovascular disease, recent (within 10 days) gastrointestinal or genitourinary bleeding, recent trauma (within 10 days) including CPR, hypertension (systolic BP >180 mm Hg and/or diastolic BP >110 mm Hg), high likelihood of left heart thrombus (eg, mitral stenosis with atrial fibrillation), acute pericarditis, subacute bacterial endocarditis, hemostatic defects including ones caused by severe renal or hepatic dysfunction, significant hepatic dysfunction, pregnancy, diabetic hemorrhagic retinopathy or other hemorrhagic ophthalmic conditions, septic thrombophlebitis or occluded AV cannula at seriously infected site, advanced age (eg, >75 years), patients receiving oral anticoagulants, any other condition in which bleeding constitutes a significant hazard or would be particularly difficult to manage because of location.

Coronary thrombolysis may result in reperfusion arrhythmias. Hypotension, occasionally severe, can occur (not from bleeding or anaphylaxis). Follow standard MI management. Rare anaphylactic reactions can occur. Cautious repeat administration in patients who have received anistreplase or streptokinase within 1 year (streptokinase antibody may decrease effectiveness or risk of allergic reactions). Safety and efficacy in pediatric patients have not been established.

(Continued)

Streptokinase *(Continued)*

Streptokinase is not indicated for restoration of patency of intravenous catheters. Serious adverse events relating to the use of streptokinase in the restoration of patency of occluded intravenous catheters have involved the use of high doses of streptokinase in small volumes (250,000 international units in 2 mL). Uses of lower doses of streptokinase in infusions over several hours, generally into partially occluded catheters, or local instillation into the catheter lumen and subsequent aspiration, have been described in the medical literature. Healthcare providers should consider the risk for potentially life-threatening reactions (hypersensitivity, apnea, bleeding) associated with the use of streptokinase in the management of occluded intravenous catheters.

Pregnancy risk C.

Drug Interactions

Decreased Effect: Antifibrinolytic agents (aminocaproic acid) may decrease effectiveness to thrombolytic agents.

Increased Effect/Toxicity: The risk of bleeding with streptokinase is increased by oral anticoagulants (warfarin), heparin, low molecular weight heparins, and drugs which affect platelet function (eg, NSAIDs, dipyridamole, ticlopidine, clopidogrel, IIb/IIIa antagonists). Although concurrent use with aspirin and heparin may increase the risk of bleeding. Aspirin and heparin were used concomitantly with streptokinase in the majority of patients in clinical studies of MI.

Nutritional/Ethanol Interactions Herb/Nutraceutical: Avoid cat's claw, dong quai, evening primrose, feverfew, red clover, horse chestnut, garlic, green tea, ginseng, ginkgo (all have additional antiplatelet activity).

Adverse Reactions As with all drugs which may affect hemostasis, bleeding is the major adverse effect associated with streptokinase. Hemorrhage may occur at virtually any site. Risk is dependent on multiple variables, including the dosage administered, concurrent use of multiple agents which alter hemostasis, and patient predisposition (including hypertension). Rapid lysis of coronary artery thrombi by thrombolytic agents may be associated with reperfusion-related atrial and/or ventricular arrhythmias.

>10%:
- Cardiovascular: Hypotension
- Local: Injection site bleeding

1% to 10%:
- Central nervous system: Fever (1% to 4%)
- Dermatologic: Bruising, rash, pruritus
- Gastrointestinal: Gastrointestinal hemorrhage, nausea, vomiting
- Genitourinary: Genitourinary hemorrhage
- Hematologic: Anemia
- Neuromuscular & skeletal: Muscle pain
- Ocular: Eye hemorrhage, periorbital edema
- Respiratory: Bronchospasm, epistaxis
- Miscellaneous: Diaphoresis

<1% (Limited to important or life-threatening): Acute tubular necrosis, allergic reactions, anaphylactic shock, anaphylactoid reactions, anaphylaxis, angioneurotic edema, ARDS, back pain (during infusion), cholesterol embolization, elevated transaminases, erysipelas-like rash, Guillain-Barré syndrome, hemarthrosis, intracranial hemorrhage, laryngeal edema, morbilliform, Parsonage-Turner syndrome, pericardial hemorrhage, respiratory depression, retroperitoneal hemorrhage, splenic rupture, urticaria

Additional cardiovascular events associated with use in myocardial infarction: Asystole, AV block, cardiac arrest, cardiac tamponade, cardiogenic shock, electromechanical dissociation, heart failure, mitral regurgitation, myocardial rupture, pericardial effusion, pericarditis, pulmonary edema, recurrent ischemia/infarction, thromboembolism, ventricular tachycardia

Overdosage/Toxicology Symptoms of overdose include epistaxis, bleeding gums, hematoma, spontaneous ecchymoses, and oozing at the catheter site. If uncontrollable bleeding occurs, discontinue infusion. Whole blood or blood products may be used to reverse bleeding.

Pharmacodynamics/Kinetics

Half-Life Elimination: 83 minutes

Onset: Activation of plasminogen occurs almost immediately

Duration: Fibrinolytic effect: Several hours; Anticoagulant effect: 12-24 hours

Formulations Injection, powder for reconstitution: 250,000 units, 750,000 units, 1,500,000 units

Dosing

Adults & Elderly: I.V.:

Antibodies to streptokinase remain for at least 3-6 months after initial dose: See Warnings/Precautions.

An intradermal skin test of 100 units has been suggested to predict allergic response to streptokinase. If a positive reaction is not seen after 15-20 minutes, a therapeutic dose may be administered.

Guidelines for acute myocardial infarction (AMI): I.V.: 1.5 million units over 60 minutes

Administration:

Dilute two 750,000 unit vials of streptokinase with 5 mL dextrose 5% in water (D_5W) each, gently swirl to dissolve.

Add this dose of the 1.5 million units to 150 mL D_5W.

This should be infused over 60 minutes; an in-line filter ≥0.45 micron should be used.

Monitor for the first few hours for signs of anaphylaxis or allergic reaction. **Infusion should be slowed if lowering of 25 mm Hg in blood pressure or terminated if asthmatic symptoms appear.**

If heparin is administered, start when aPTT is less than 2 times the upper limit of control; do not use a bolus, but initiate infusion adjusted to a target a PTT of 1.5-2 times the upper limit of control. If heparin is not administered by infusion, initiate 7500-12,500 units S.C. every 12 hours.

Guidelines for acute pulmonary embolism (APE): I.V.: 3 million unit dose over 24 hours

Administration:

Dilute four 750,000 unit vials of streptokinase with 5 mL dextrose 5% in water (D_5W) each, gently swirl to dissolve.

Add this dose of 3 million units to 250 mL D_5W, an in-line filter ≥0.45 micron should be used.

Administer 250,000 units (23 mL) over 30 minutes followed by 100,000 units/hour (9 mL/hour) for 24 hours.

Monitor for the first few hours for signs of anaphylaxis or allergic reaction. **Infusion should be slowed if blood pressure is lowered by 25 mm Hg or if asthmatic symptoms appear.**

Begin heparin 1000 units/hour about 3-4 hours after completion of streptokinase infusion or when PTT is <100 seconds.

Guidelines for thromboses: I.V.: Administer 250,000 units to start, then 100,000 units/hour for 24-72 hours depending on location.

Cannula occlusion: 250,000 units into cannula, clamp for 2 hours, then aspirate contents and flush with normal saline; **Not recommended; see Warnings/Precautions**

Pediatrics: Children: Safety and efficacy not established; limited studies have used the following doses.

Thromboses: I.V.: *Chest,* 1998 recommendations: Initial (loading dose): 2000 units/kg followed by 2000 units/kg/hour for 6-12 hours **or** initial (loading dose): 3500-4000 units/kg over 30 minutes followed by I.V. continuous infusion: 1000-1500 units/kg/hour; dose should be individualized based on response.

Clotted catheter: I.V.: **Note:** Not recommended due to possibility of allergic reactions with repeated doses: 10,000-25,000 units diluted in NS to a final volume equivalent to catheter volume; instill into catheter and leave in place for 1 hour, then aspirate contents out of catheter and flush catheter with normal saline.

Administration

I.M.: Do **not** administer by intramuscular injection.

I.V.: For I.V. or intracoronary use only. Infusion pump is required. Use in-line filter >0.8 micron.

Stability

Storage: Streptokinase, a white lyophilized powder, may have a slight yellow color in solution due to the presence of albumin. Intact vials should be stored at room temperature. Stability of parenteral admixture at room temperature (25°C) is 8 hours and at refrigeration (4°C) is 24 hours.

Reconstitution: Reconstituted solutions should be refrigerated and are stable for 24 hours.

Compatibility: Stable in D_5W, NS; **incompatible** with dextrans

Monitoring Laboratory Tests PT, APTT, platelet count, hematocrit, fibrinogen concentration

Monitoring and Teaching Issues

Physical Assessment: See Contraindications, Warnings/Precautions, and Dosing for use cautions. **Note:** Streptokinase is not indicated for restoration of patency of intravenous catheters; potentially life-threatening reactions (eg, hypersensitivity, apnea, bleeding) are associated with the use of streptokinase in the management of occluded intravenous catheters. Assess potential for interactions with other prescriptions, OTC medications, or herbal products patient may be taking (especially those medications that may affect coagulation or platelet function - see Drug Interactions). Assess results of laboratory results (see above). See Administration infusion specifics; assess infusion site and monitor for systemic hemorrhage during and following therapy (see Adverse Reactions and Overdose/Toxicology). Neurological status (eg, intracranial hemorrhage), vital signs, and EKG (reperfusion arrhythmias) should be monitored prior to, during, and after therapy. Bedrest and bleeding precautions should be maintained. Avoid I.M. injections and nonessential handling of the patient; venipunctures should be performed carefully and only when necessary. If arterial puncture is necessary, use an upper extremity vessel that can be manually compressed. Patient instructions determined by patient condition (see Patient Education). **Pregnancy risk factor C** - benefits of use should outweigh possible risks. Note breast-feeding caution.

Patient Education: Inform prescriber of all prescriptions, OTC medications, or herbal products you are taking, and any allergies you have. This medication can only be administered by infusion; you will be monitored closely during and after treatment: immediately report burning, pain, redness, swelling, or oozing at infusion site, acute headache, joint pain, chest pain, or altered vision, You will have a tendency to bleed easily; use caution to prevent injury (use electric razor, soft toothbrush, and caution with knives, needles, or anything sharp). Follow instructions for strict bedrest to reduce the risk of injury. If bleeding occurs, report immediately and apply pressure to bleeding spot until bleeding stops completely. Report unusual bruising or bleeding; blood in urine, stool, or vomitus; bleeding gums; vision changes; or difficulty breathing. **Pregnancy/breast-feeding precautions:** Inform prescriber if you are or intend to become pregnant. Consult prescriber if breast-feeding.

Geriatric Considerations: Investigators applied analysis to data for patients ≥75 years of age from two large trials studying the impact of streptokinase on patient outcome after acute myocardial infarction. Their conclusion was that age alone is not a contraindication to the use of streptokinase and that thrombolytic therapy is cost-effective and is beneficial toward the survival of elderly patients. Additional studies are needed to determine if a weight-adjusted dose will maintain efficacy but decrease adverse events such as stroke.

Streptomycin (strep toe MYE sin)

Synonyms Streptomycin Sulfate

Generic Available Yes

Pharmacologic Category Antibiotic, Aminoglycoside; Antitubercular Agent

Pregnancy Risk Factor D

Lactation Enters breast milk/compatible

(Continued)

Streptomycin *(Continued)*

Use Part of combination therapy of active tuberculosis; used in combination with other agents for treatment of streptococcal or enterococcal endocarditis, mycobacterial infections, plague, tularemia, and brucellosis

Mechanism of Action/Effect Inhibits bacterial protein synthesis by binding directly to the 30S ribosomal subunits causing faulty peptide sequence to form in the protein chain

Contraindications Hypersensitivity to streptomycin or any component of the formulation; pregnancy

Warnings/Precautions Use with caution in patients with pre-existing vertigo, tinnitus, hearing loss, neuromuscular disorders, or renal impairment. Modify dosage in patients with renal impairment. Aminoglycosides are associated with nephrotoxicity or ototoxicity. The ototoxicity may be proportional to the amount of drug given and the duration of treatment. Tinnitus or vertigo are indications of vestibular injury and impending hearing damage. Renal damage is usually reversible.

Drug Interactions

Increased Effect/Toxicity: Increased/prolonged effect with depolarizing and nondepolarizing neuromuscular blocking agents. Concurrent use with amphotericin or loop diuretics may increase nephrotoxicity.

Effects on Lab Values False-positive urine glucose with Benedict's solution

Adverse Reactions Frequency not defined.

Cardiovascular: Hypotension
Central nervous system: Neurotoxicity, drowsiness, headache, drug fever, paresthesia
Dermatologic: Skin rash
Gastrointestinal: Nausea, vomiting
Hematologic: Eosinophilia, anemia
Neuromuscular & skeletal: Arthralgia, weakness, tremor
Otic: Ototoxicity (auditory), ototoxicity (vestibular)
Renal: Nephrotoxicity
Respiratory: Difficulty in breathing

Overdosage/Toxicology Symptoms of overdose include ototoxicity, nephrotoxicity, and neuromuscular toxicity. The treatment of choice following a single acute overdose appears to be maintenance of urine output of at least 3 mL/kg/hour during the acute treatment phase. Dialysis is of questionable value in enhancing aminoglycoside elimination. If required, hemodialysis is preferred over peritoneal dialysis in patients with normal renal function. Chelation with penicillins is experimental.

Pharmacodynamics/Kinetics

Absorption: I.M.: Well absorbed

Half-Life Elimination: Newborns: 4-10 hours; Adults: 2-4.7 hours, prolonged with renal impairment

Time to Peak: I.M.: Within 1 hour

Formulations Injection, as sulfate: 400 mg/mL (2.5 mL) [1 g vial]

Dosing

Adults:

Tuberculosis: I.M.:
Daily therapy: I.M.: 15 mg/kg/day (maximum: 1 g)
Directly observed therapy (DOT), twice weekly: I.M.: 25-30 mg/kg (maximum: 1.5 g)
DOT, 3 times/week: I.M.: 25-30 mg/kg (maximum: 1 g)
Enterococcal endocarditis: I.M.: 1 g every 12 hours for 2 weeks, 500 mg every 12 hours for 4 weeks in combination with penicillin
Streptococcal endocarditis: I.M., I.V.: 1 g every 12 hours for 1 week, 500 mg every 12 hours for 1 week
Tularemia: I.M., I.V.: 1-2 g/day in divided doses for 7-10 days or until patient is afebrile for 5-7 days
Plague: I.M., I.V.: 2-4 g/day in divided doses until the patient is afebrile for at least 3 days

Elderly: Intramuscular: 10 mg/kg/day, not to exceed 750 mg/day; dosing interval should be adjusted for renal function. Some authors suggest not to give more than 5 days/week or give as 20-25 mg/kg/dose twice weekly.

Pediatrics: Tuberculosis: I.M., I.V.: Children:
Daily therapy: 20-40 mg/kg/day (maximum: 1 g/day)
Directly observed therapy (DOT): Twice weekly: 20-40 mg/kg (maximum: 1 g)
DOT: 3 times/week: 25-30 mg/kg (maximum: 1 g)

Renal Impairment:
Cl_{cr} 10-50 mL/minute: Administer every 24-72 hours.
Cl_{cr} <10 mL/minute: Administer every 72-96 hours.
Removed by hemo- and peritoneal dialysis: Administer dose postdialysis.

Administration

I.M.: Inject deep I.M. into large muscle mass.

I.V.: I.V. administration is not recommended. Has been administered intravenously over 30-60 minutes.

Stability

Storage: Depending upon manufacturer, reconstituted solution remains stable for 2-4 weeks when refrigerated and 24 hours at room temperature. Exposure to light causes darkening of solution without apparent loss of potency.

Compatibility:

Compatibility in syringe: Incompatible with heparin

Compatibility when admixed: Incompatible with amobarbital, amphotericin B, chlorothiazide, heparin, methohexital, norepinephrine, pentobarbital, phenobarbital, phenytoin, sodium bicarbonate

Monitoring Laboratory Tests Hearing (audiogram), BUN, creatinine; serum concentration of the drug should be monitored. Perform culture and sensitivity prior to initiating therapy.

Monitoring and Teaching Issues

Physical Assessment: Assess for allergy history prior to starting therapy. See Contraindications, Warnings/Precautions, and Dosing for use cautions. Assess potential for interactions with other prescriptions, OTC medications, or herbal products patient may be taking (eg, nephrotoxic or ototoxic drugs - see Drug Interactions). Assess results of laboratory tests (see above) and patient response (eg, ototoxicity, neurotoxicity, nephrotoxicity - see Adverse Reactions and Overdose/Toxicology) on a regular basis during therapy. Teach patient possible side effects and interventions and adverse symptoms to report (see Patient Education). **Pregnancy risk factor D** - determine that patient is not pregnant before beginning treatment. Instruct patients of childbearing age about necessity for barrier contraceptive measures.

Patient Education: Inform prescriber of all prescriptions, OTC medications, or herbal products you are taking, and any allergies you have. This medication can only be given by intramuscular injection. Therapy for TB may last several months. Do not discontinue even if you are feeling better. Maintain adequate hydration (2-3 L/day of fluids) unless advised by prescriber to restrict fluids. May cause headache or dizziness (use caution when driving or engaging in tasks requiring alertness until response to drug is known); or nausea, vomiting, or loss of appetite (small, frequent meals, frequent mouth care, sucking lozenges, or chewing gum may help). Report immediately change in hearing or sense of fullness in ears; pain, weakness, tremors, or numbness in muscles; unusual clumsiness or change in strength or altered gait; change in urinary pattern or back pain; or difficulty breathing or chest pain. **Pregnancy precaution:** Do not get pregnant while taking this medication. Consult prescriber for appropriate barrier contraceptive measures.

Geriatric Considerations: Streptomycin is indicated for persons from endemic areas of drug-resistant *Mycobacterium tuberculosis* or who are HIV infected. Since most older patients acquired the *M. tuberculosis* infection prior to the availability of effective chemotherapy, isoniazid and rifampin are usually effective unless resistant organisms are suspected or the patient is HIV infected. Adjust dose interval for renal function.

Related Information

Tuberculosis *on page 1705*

Streptomycin Sulfate *see* Streptomycin *on page 1249*

Streptozocin (strep toe ZOE sin)

U.S. Brand Names Zanosar®

Generic Available No

Pharmacologic Category Antineoplastic Agent, Alkylating Agent

Pregnancy Risk Factor C

Lactation Enters breast milk/contraindicated

Use Treatment of metastatic islet cell carcinoma of the pancreas, carcinoid tumor and syndrome, Hodgkin's disease, palliative treatment of colorectal cancer

Mechanism of Action/Effect Interferes with the normal function of DNA by alkylation and cross-linking the strands of DNA, and by possible protein modification

Warnings/Precautions The U.S. Food and Drug Administration (FDA) currently recommends that procedures for proper handling and disposal of antineoplastic agents be considered. Appropriate safety equipment is recommended for preparation, administration, and disposal of antineoplastics. If streptozocin contacts the skin, wash and flush thoroughly with water.

Renal toxicity is dose-related and cumulative and may be severe or fatal. Discontinue treatment in the presence of significant renal toxicity. Do not use in combination with other nephrotoxic drugs.

Pregnancy risk C.

Drug Interactions

Decreased Effect: Phenytoin results in negation of streptozocin cytotoxicity.

Increased Effect/Toxicity: Doxorubicin prolongs half-life and thus prolonged leukopenia and thrombocytopenia.

Adverse Reactions

>10%:

Gastrointestinal: Nausea and vomiting in all patients usually 1-4 hours after infusion; diarrhea in 10% of patients

Emetic potential: High (>90%)

Time course of nausea/vomiting: Onset 1-3 hours; Duration: 1-12 hours

Hepatic: Increased LFTs and hypoalbuminemia

Renal: Nephrotoxicity (25% to 75%), proteinuria, decreased Cl_{cr}, increased BUN, hypophosphatemia, renal tubular acidosis

1% to 10%:

Endocrine & metabolic: Hypoglycemia: Seen in 6% of patients; may be prevented with the administration of nicotinamide

Local: Pain at injection site

Vesicant chemotherapy

<1% (Limited to important or life-threatening): Leukopenia, liver dysfunction, secondary malignancy, thrombocytopenia

Myelosuppressive:

WBC: Mild

Platelets: Mild

Onset: 7 days

Nadir: 14 days

Recovery: 21 days

Overdosage/Toxicology Symptoms of overdose include bone marrow suppression, nausea, and vomiting. Treatment of bone marrow suppression is supportive.

(Continued)

Streptozocin *(Continued)*

Pharmacodynamics/Kinetics

Half-Life Elimination: 35-40 minutes

Metabolism: Rapidly hepatic

Duration: Disappears from serum in 4 hours

Formulations Injection: 1 g

Dosing

Adults & Elderly: Refer to individual protocols.

Single agent therapy: I.V.: 1-1.5 g/m^2 weekly for 6 weeks followed by a 4-week observation period

Combination therapy: I.V.: 0.5-1 g/m^2 for 5 consecutive days followed by a 4- to 6-week observation period

Pediatrics: Refer to adult dosing.

Renal Impairment:

Cl_{cr} 10-50 mL/minute: Administer 75% of dose.

Cl_{cr} <10 mL/minute: Administer 50% of dose.

Hepatic Impairment: Dose should be reduced in patients with severe liver disease.

Administration

I.V.: Vesicant. Slow I.V. infusion in ≥100 mL D_5W or NS over 30-60 minutes; may be administered by rapid I.V. push.

Stability

Storage: Refrigerate vials. Protect from light.

Reconstitution: Solution is stable 48 hours at room temperature and 96 hours with refrigeration. May be diluted in D_5W or sodium chloride.

Compatibility: Stable in D_5W, NS

Y-site administration: Incompatible with allopurinol, aztreonam, cefepime, piperacillin/tazobactam

Monitoring Laboratory Tests Liver function tests, CBC, renal function tests (BUN, serum creatinine) at baseline and weekly during therapy

Monitoring and Teaching Issues

Physical Assessment: See Contraindications, Warnings/Precautions, and Dosing for use cautions. See Drug Interactions. Administer antiemetic prior to therapy (emetic potential >90%). See Administration, Compatibility, and Reconstitution. Infusion site should be monitored closely to prevent extravasation. Assess results of laboratory tests (see above) and patient response (see Adverse Reactions and Overdose/Toxicology) regularly during therapy. Diabetic patients should monitor glucose levels closely (may precipitate hypoglycemia - see Adverse Reactions). Teach patient (or caregiver) possible side effects and interventions, and adverse symptoms to report (see Patient Education). **Pregnancy risk factor C** - determine that patient is not pregnant before beginning treatment and do not give to women of childbearing age or to males who may have intercourse with women of childbearing age unless both male and female are capable of complying with barrier contraceptive measures during therapy and for 1 month following therapy. Breast-feeding is contraindicated.

Patient Education: Inform prescriber of all prescriptions, OTC medications, or herbal products you are taking, and any allergies you have. Do not take anything new during treatment unless approved by prescriber. This drug can only be given I.V.; report immediately any redness, swelling, pain, or burning at infusion site. Maintain adequate hydration (2-3 L/day of fluids) unless advised by prescriber to restrict fluids. You will be more sensitive to infection (avoid crowds and exposure to infection and do not have any vaccinations without consulting prescriber). If diabetic, monitor glucose levels closely; may cause hypoglycemia. May cause nausea and vomiting (consult prescriber for antiemetic); nervousness, dizziness, confusion, or lethargy (use caution when driving or engaging in tasks requiring alertness until response to drug is known); or loss of body hair (reversible when treatment is finished). Report unusual back pain, change in urinary pattern; persistent fever, chills, or sore throat; unusual bleeding; blood in urine, vomitus, or stool; chest pain, palpitations, or difficulty breathing; or swelling of feet or lower legs. **Pregnancy/breast-feeding precautions:** Inform prescriber if you are pregnant. Do not get pregnant during or for 1 month following therapy. Male: Do not cause a female to become pregnant. Male/female: Consult prescriber for instruction on appropriate barrier contraceptive measures. This drug may cause severe fetal damage.

Strong Iodine Solution *see* Potassium Iodide *on page 1105*

Sublimaze® *see* Fentanyl *on page 552*

Suboxone® *see* Buprenorphine and Naloxone *on page 186*

Subutex® *see* Buprenorphine *on page 184*

Succimer *see page 1460*

Succinylcholine (suks in il KOE leen)

U.S. Brand Names Anectine® Chloride; Anectine® Flo-Pack®; Quelicin®

Synonyms Succinylcholine Chloride; Suxamethonium Chloride

Generic Available Yes

Pharmacologic Category Neuromuscular Blocker Agent, Depolarizing

Pregnancy Risk Factor C

Lactation Excretion in breast milk unknown/use caution

Use Adjunct to general anesthesia to facilitate both rapid sequence and routine endotracheal intubation and to relax skeletal muscles during surgery; to reduce the intensity of muscle contractions of pharmacologically- or electrically-induced convulsions; does not relieve pain or produce sedation

Mechanism of Action/Effect Acts similar to acetylcholine, produces depolarization of the motor endplate at the myoneural junction which causes sustained flaccid skeletal muscle paralysis produced by state of accommodation that developes in adjacent excitable muscle membranes

Contraindications Hypersensitivity to succinylcholine or any component of the formulation; personal or familial history of malignant hyperthermia; myopathies associated with elevated serum creatine phosphokinase (CPK) values; narrow-angle glaucoma, penetrating eye injuries; disorders of plasma pseudocholinesterase

Warnings/Precautions **Use with caution in pediatrics and adolescents** secondary to undiagnosed skeletal muscle myopathy and potential for ventricular dysrhythmias and cardiac arrest resulting from hyperkalemia; use with caution in patients with pre-existing hyperkalemia, paraplegia, extensive or severe burns, extensive denervation of skeletal muscle because of disease or injury to the CNS or with degenerative or dystrophic neuromuscular disease; may increase vagal tone Pregnancy risk C.

Drug Interactions

Increased Effect/Toxicity:

Increased toxicity: Anticholinesterase drugs (neostigmine, physostigmine, or pyridostigmine) in combination with succinylcholine can cause cardiorespiratory collapse; cyclophosphamide, oral contraceptives, lidocaine, thiotepa, pancuronium, lithium, magnesium salts, aprotinin, chloroquine, metoclopramide, terbutaline, and procaine enhance and prolong the effects of succinylcholine

Prolonged neuromuscular blockade: Inhaled anesthetics, local anesthetics, calcium channel blockers, antiarrhythmics (eg, quinidine or procainamide), antibiotics (eg, aminoglycosides, tetracyclines, vancomycin, clindamycin), immunosuppressants (eg, cyclosporine)

Effects on Lab Values ↑ potassium (S)

Adverse Reactions

>10%:

- Ocular: Increased intraocular pressure
- Miscellaneous: Postoperative stiffness

1% to 10%:

- Cardiovascular: Bradycardia, hypotension, cardiac arrhythmias, tachycardia
- Gastrointestinal: Intragastric pressure, salivation

<1% (Limited to important or life-threatening): Apnea, bronchospasm, circulatory collapse, erythema, hyperkalemia, hypertension, itching, malignant hyperthermia, myalgia, myoglobinuria, rash

Overdosage/Toxicology

Symptoms of overdose include respiratory paralysis and cardiac arrest.

Bradyarrhythmias can often be treated with atropine 0.1 mg (infants). Do not treat with anticholinesterase drugs (eg, neostigmine, physostigmine) since this may worsen its toxicity by interfering with its metabolism.

Pharmacodynamics/Kinetics

Metabolism: Rapidly hydrolyzed by plasma pseudocholinesterase

Onset: I.M.: 2-3 minutes; I.V.: Complete muscular relaxation: 30-60 seconds

Duration: I.M.: 10-30 minutes; I.V.: 4-6 minutes with single administration

Formulations

Injection, as chloride: 20 mg/mL (10 mL); 50 mg/mL (10 mL); 100 mg/mL (5 mL, 10 mL, 20 mL)

Injection, powder for reconstitution, as chloride: 500 mg, 1 g

Dosing

Adults & Elderly: Neuromuscular blockade: Dose to effect; doses will vary due to interpatient variability; use ideal body weight for obese patients

I.M.: 2.5-4 mg/kg, total dose should not exceed 150 mg

I.V.: 1-1.5 mg/kg, up to 150 mg total dose

Maintenance: 0.04-0.07 mg/kg every 5-10 minutes as needed

Continuous infusion: 10-100 mcg/kg/minute (or 0.5-10 mg/minute); dilute to concentration of 1-2 mg/mL in D_5W or NS

Note: Initial dose of succinylcholine must be increased when nondepolarizing agent pretreatment used because of the antagonism between succinylcholine and nondepolarizing neuromuscular blocking agents

Pediatrics: Neuromuscular blockade: Because of the risk of malignant hyperthermia, use of continuous infusions is not recommended in infants and children:

Small Children: Intermittent: Initial: 2 mg/kg/dose one time; maintenance: 0.3-0.6 mg/kg/dose at intervals of 5-10 minutes as necessary

Older Children and Adolescents: Intermittent: Initial: 1 mg/kg/dose one time; maintenance: 0.3-0.6 mg/kg every 5-10 minutes as needed

Hepatic Impairment: Dose should be reduced in patients with severe liver disease.

Administration

I.M.: I.M. injections should be made deeply, preferably high into deltoid muscle.

I.V.: May be given by rapid I.V. injection without further dilution.

Stability

Storage: Refrigerate at 2°C to 8°C (36°F to 46°F); however, remains stable for 14 days unrefrigerated; powder form does not require refrigeration. Stability of parenteral admixture at refrigeration temperature (4°C) is 24 hours in D_5W or NS.

Compatibility:

Stable in dextran 6% in dextrose, dextran 6% in NS, D_5LR, $D_5{}^1/_4NS$, $D_5{}^1/_2NS$, D_5NS, D_5W, $D_{10}W$, LR, $^1/_2NS$, NS

Y-site administration: Incompatible with thiopental

Compatibility when admixed: Incompatible with methohexital, nafcillin, sodium bicarbonate, thiopental

Monitoring Laboratory Tests Serum potassium and calcium

Monitoring and Teaching Issues

Physical Assessment: Only clinicians experienced in the use of neuromuscular-blocking drugs should administer and/or manage the use of succinylcholine. Dosage and rate of administration should be individualized and titrated to the desired effect, according to

(Continued)

Succinylcholine *(Continued)*

relevant clinical factors, premedication, concomitant medications, age, and general condition of patient. See Use, Contraindications, and Warnings/Precautions for appropriate use cautions. Ventilatory support must be instituted and maintained until adequate respiratory muscle function and/or airway protection are assured. Assess other medications for effectiveness and safety. Other drugs that affect neuromuscular activity may increase/decrease neuromuscular block induced by succinylcholine. This drug does not cause anesthesia or analgesia; pain must be treated with appropriate analgesic agents. Continuous monitoring of vital signs, cardiac status, respiratory status, and degree of neuromuscular block (objective assessment with external nerve stimulator) is mandatory during infusion and until full muscle tone has returned (see Adverse Reactions). Muscle tone returns in a predictable pattern, starting with limbs, abdomen, chest diaphragm, intercostals, and finally muscles of the neck, face, and eyes. Safety precautions must be maintained until full muscle tone has returned. Provide appropriate patient teaching/support prior to and following administration. **Pregnancy risk factor C.** Note breast-feeding caution.

Patient Education: Patient will usually be unconscious prior to administration. Education should be appropriate to individual situation. Reassurance of constant monitoring and emotional support to reduce fear and anxiety should precede and follow administration. Following return of muscle tone, do not attempt to change position or rise from bed without assistance. Report immediately any skin rash or hives, pounding heartbeat, difficulty breathing, or muscle tremors. **Pregnancy/breast-feeding precautions:** Inform prescriber if you are pregnant. Consult prescriber if breast-feeding.

Related Information

Diagnostics and Surgical Aids *on page 1461*

Succinylcholine Chloride *see* Succinylcholine *on page 1252*

Sucraid® *see* Sacrosidase *on page 1209*

Sucralfate (soo KRAL fate)

U.S. Brand Names Carafate®

Synonyms Aluminum Sucrose Sulfate, Basic

Generic Available Yes

Pharmacologic Category Gastrointestinal Agent, Miscellaneous

Pregnancy Risk Factor B

Lactation Enters breast milk/compatible

Use Short-term management of duodenal ulcers; maintenance of duodenal ulcers

Use - Unlabeled/Investigational Gastric ulcers; suspension may be used topically for treatment of stomatitis due to cancer chemotherapy and other causes of esophageal and gastric erosions; GERD, esophagitis; treatment of NSAID mucosal damage; prevention of stress ulcers; postsclerotherapy for esophageal variceal bleeding

Mechanism of Action/Effect Forms a complex by binding with positively charged proteins in exudates, forming a viscous paste-like, adhesive substance, when combined with gastric acid adheres to the damaged mucosal area. This selectively forms a protective coating that protects the lining against peptic acid, pepsin, and bile salts.

Contraindications Hypersensitivity to sucralfate or any component of the formulation

Warnings/Precautions Successful therapy with sucralfate should not be expected to alter the posthealing frequency of recurrence or the severity of duodenal ulceration. Use with caution in patients with chronic renal failure who have an impaired excretion of absorbed aluminum. Because of the potential for sucralfate to alter the absorption of some drugs, take other medications 2 hours before sucralfate when alterations in bioavailability are believed to be critical. Do not give antacids within 30 minutes of administration.

Drug Interactions

Decreased Effect: Sucralfate may alter the absorption of digoxin, phenytoin (hydantoins), warfarin, ketoconazole, quinidine, quinolones, tetracycline, theophylline. Because of the potential for sucralfate to alter the absorption of some drugs; separate administration (take other medications at least 2 hours before sucralfate). The potential for decreased absorption should be considered when alterations in bioavailability are believed to be critical.

Nutritional/Ethanol Interactions Food: Sucralfate may interfere with absorption of vitamin A, vitamin D, vitamin E, and vitamin K.

Adverse Reactions

1% to 10%: Gastrointestinal: Constipation

<1% (Limited to important or life-threatening): Bezoar formation, hypersensitivity (pruritus, urticaria, angioedema), rash

Overdosage/Toxicology Toxicity is minimal, may cause constipation

Pharmacodynamics/Kinetics

Absorption: Oral: <5%

Metabolism: None

Onset: Paste formation and ulcer adhesion: 1-2 hours

Duration: Up to 6 hours

Formulations

Suspension, oral: 1 g/10 mL (10 mL, 420 mL)

Tablet: 1 g

Dosing

Adults & Elderly:

Stress ulcer prophylaxis: Oral: 1 g 4 times/day

Stress ulcer treatment: Oral: 1 g every 4 hours

Duodenal ulcer: Oral:

Treatment: 1 g 4 times/day, 1 hour before meals or food and at bedtime for 4-8 weeks, or alternatively 2 g twice daily; treatment is recommended for 4-8 weeks in adults, the elderly will require 12 weeks.

Maintenance: Prophylaxis: 1 g twice daily

Stomatitis (unlabeled use): Oral: 1 g/10 mL suspension; swish and spit or swish and swallow 4 times/day.

Pediatrics: Dose not established, doses of 40-80 mg/kg/day divided every 6 hours have been used

Stomatitis (unlabeled use): Oral: Children: 2.5-5 mL (1 g/10 mL suspension), swish and spit or swish and swallow 4 times/day

Renal Impairment: Aluminum salt is minimally absorbed (<5%), however, may accumulate in renal failure.

Administration

Oral: Tablet may be broken or dissolved in water before ingestion. Administer with water on an empty stomach.

Stability

Storage: Suspension: Shake well. Refrigeration is **not** necessary; do **not** freeze.

Monitoring and Teaching Issues

Physical Assessment: See Contraindications and Warnings/Precautions for use cautions. Assess potential for interactions with other prescriptions, OTC medications, or herbal products patient may be taking (see Drug Interactions). Monitor patient response (see Adverse Reactions and Overdose/Toxicology). Teach patient proper use (eg, timing of other medications), possible side effects (eg, constipation) and interventions, and adverse symptoms to report (see Patient Education) on a regular basis during therapy.

Patient Education: Take recommended dose with water on an empty stomach, 1 hour before or 2 hours after meals. Take any other medications at least 2 hours before taking sucralfate. Do not take antacids (if prescribed) within 30 minutes of taking sucralfate. May cause constipation (increased exercise, fluids, fruit, or fiber may help). If constipation persists, consult prescriber for approved stool softener.

Dietary Issues: Administer with water on an empty stomach.

Geriatric Considerations: Caution should be used in the elderly due to reduced renal function. Patients with Cl_{cr} <30 mL/minute may be at risk for aluminum intoxication. Due to low side effect profile, this may be an agent of choice in the elderly with PUD.

Sucrets® [OTC] *see* Dyclonine *on page 457*

Sudafed® [OTC] *see* Pseudoephedrine *on page 1150*

Sudafed® 12 Hour [OTC] *see* Pseudoephedrine *on page 1150*

Sufentanil *see page 1583*

Sular® *see* Nisoldipine *on page 975*

Sulbactam and Ampicillin *see* Ampicillin and Sulbactam *on page 103*

Sulf-10® *see page 1509*

Sulf-10® *see* Sulfacetamide *on page 1256*

Sulfabenzamide, Sulfacetamide, and Sulfathiazole

(sul fa BENZ a mide, sul fa SEE ta mide, & sul fa THYE a zole)

U.S. Brand Names V.V.S.®

Synonyms Triple Sulfa

Generic Available Yes

Pharmacologic Category Antibiotic, Vaginal

Pregnancy Risk Factor C (avoid if near term)

Lactation Excretion in breast milk unknown

Use Treatment of *Haemophilus vaginalis* vaginitis

Mechanism of Action/Effect Interferes with microbial folic acid synthesis and growth via inhibition of para-aminobenzoic acid metabolism

Contraindications Hypersensitivity to sulfabenzamide, sulfacetamide, sulfathiazole, or any component of the formulation; renal dysfunction; pregnancy (if near term)

Warnings/Precautions Associated with Stevens-Johnson syndrome; if local irritation or systemic toxicity develops, discontinue therapy. Pregnancy risk C (avoid if near term).

Adverse Reactions Frequency not defined.

Dermatologic: Pruritus, urticaria, Stevens-Johnson syndrome

Local: Local irritation

Miscellaneous: Allergic reactions

Pharmacodynamics/Kinetics

Absorption: Absorption from vagina is variable and unreliable

Metabolism: Primarily via acetylation

Formulations

Cream, vaginal: Sulfabenzamide 3.7%, sulfacetamide 2.86%, and sulfathiazole 3.42% (78 g [with applicator], 90 g, 120 g)

Tablet, vaginal: Sulfabenzamide 184 mg, sulfacetamide 143.75 mg, and sulfathiazole 172.5 mg [with applicator] (20 tablets/box)

Dosing

Adults & Elderly: *Haemophilus vaginalis* vaginitis: Intravaginal:

Cream: Insert 1 applicatorful in vagina twice daily for 4-6 days. Dosage may then be decreased to $^1/_2$ to $^1/_4$ of an applicatorful twice daily.

Tablet: Insert 1 tablet intravaginally twice daily for 10 days.

Monitoring and Teaching Issues

Physical Assessment: Assess patient knowledge/teach appropriate administration and adverse symptoms to report (see Patient Education). **Pregnancy risk factor C.** Note breast-feeding caution.

Patient Education: This medication is to be inserted into vagina; do not ingest tablets. Complete full course of therapy. Wash hands before inserting applicator gently into vagina and releasing cream or tablet. Wash hands and applicator with soap and water following each application. Discontinue and notify prescriber immediately if burning, irritation, or allergic reaction occurs. **Pregnancy/breast-feeding precautions:** Inform prescriber if you are pregnant before use. Consult prescriber if breast-feeding.

Related Information

Sulfacetamide *on page 1256*

Sulfacetamide (sul fa SEE ta mide)

U.S. Brand Names AK-Sulf®; Bleph®-10; Carmol® Scalp; Cetamide®; Klaron®; Ocu-Sul®; Sebizon®; Sodium Sulamyd®; Sulf-10®

Synonyms Sodium Sulfacetamide; Sulfacetamide Sodium

Generic Available Yes

Pharmacologic Category Antibiotic, Ophthalmic; Antibiotic, Sulfonamide Derivative

Pregnancy Risk Factor C

Lactation Excretion in breast milk unknown

Use Treatment and prophylaxis of conjunctivitis due to susceptible organisms; corneal ulcers; adjunctive treatment with systemic sulfonamides for therapy of trachoma; topical application in scaling dermatosis (seborrheic); bacterial infections of the skin

Mechanism of Action/Effect Interferes with bacterial growth by inhibiting bacterial folic acid synthesis through competitive antagonism of PABA

Contraindications Hypersensitivity to sulfacetamide or any component of the formulation, sulfonamides; infants <2 months of age

Warnings/Precautions Inactivated by purulent exudates containing PABA; use with caution in severe dry eye; ointment may retard corneal epithelial healing; sulfite in some products may cause hypersensitivity reactions. Chemical similarities are present among sulfonamides, sulfonylureas, carbonic anhydrase inhibitors, thiazides, and loop diuretics (except ethacrynic acid). Use in patients with sulfonamide allergy is specifically contraindicated in product labeling, however, a risk of cross-reaction exists in patients with allergy to any of these compounds; avoid use when previous reaction has been severe. Pregnancy risk C.

Drug Interactions

Decreased Effect: Silver containing products are incompatible with sulfacetamide solutions.

Adverse Reactions

1% to 10%: Local: Irritation, stinging, burning

<1% (Limited to important or life-threatening): Exfoliative dermatitis, Stevens-Johnson syndrome, toxic epidermal necrolysis

Pharmacodynamics/Kinetics

Half-Life Elimination: 7-13 hours

Formulations

Lotion, as sodium: 10% (59 mL, 85 g)

Ointment, ophthalmic, as sodium: 10% (3.5 g)

Solution, ophthalmic, as sodium: 10% (1 mL, 2 mL, 2.5 mL, 5 mL, 15 mL); 15% (5 mL, 15 mL); 30% (15 mL)

Dosing

Adults & Elderly:

Conjunctivitis: Ophthalmic:

Ointment: Apply to lower conjunctival sac 1-4 times/day and at bedtime.

Solution: Instill 1-3 drops several times daily up to every 2-3 hours in lower conjunctival sac during waking hours and less frequently at night.

Seborrheic dermatitis: Topical: Apply at bedtime and allow to remain overnight. In severe cases, may apply twice daily.

Secondary cutaneous bacterial infections: Topical: Apply 2-4 times/day until infection clears.

Pediatrics:

Conjunctivitis: Ophthalmic: Children >2 months: Refer to adult dosing.

Dermatologic: Topical: Children >12 years: Refer to adult dosing.

Stability

Storage: Protect from light. Discolored solution should not be used.

Compatibility: Incompatible with silver and zinc sulfate. Sulfacetamide is inactivated by blood or purulent exudates.

Monitoring and Teaching Issues

Physical Assessment: Assess for previous sulfonamide allergic reactions (see Warnings/Precautions). Monitor effectiveness of therapy. Assess knowledge/teach patient appropriate use (ophthalmic/topical), interventions to reduce side effects, and adverse symptoms to report (see Patient Education). **Pregnancy risk factor C** - benefits of use should outweigh possible risks. Note breast-feeding caution.

Patient Education: Use as directed. Complete full course of therapy even if condition appears improved.

Ophthalmic: Store at room temperature. Shake solution before using. Apply prescribed amount as often as directed. Wash hands before using. Do not let tip of applicator touch eye; do not contaminate tip of applicator (may cause eye infection, eye damage, or vision loss). When using solution, tilt head back and look upward. Gently pull down lower lid and put drop(s) in inner corner of eye. When using ointment, place medicine inside the lower lid, close eye, and roll eyeball in all directions. Do not blink for ½ minute. Apply gentle pressure to inner corner of eye for 30 seconds. Wipe away excess from skin around eye. Do not use any other eye preparation for at least 10 minutes. Do not share medication with anyone else. May cause sensitivity to bright light (dark glasses may help); temporary stinging or blurred vision may occur. Inform prescriber if you experience eye pain, redness, burning, watering, dryness, double vision, puffiness around eye, vision changes, or other adverse eye response; worsening of condition or lack of improvement within 3-4 days.

Topical: For external use only. Apply a thin film of lotion to affected area as often as directed. Do not cover with occlusive dressing. Report increased skin redness, irritation, or development of open sores; or if condition worsens or does not improve.

Pregnancy/breast-feeding precautions: Inform prescriber if you are pregnant. Consult prescriber if breast-feeding.

Geriatric Considerations: Assess whether patient can adequately instill drops or ointment.

Breast-feeding Issues: Systemic sulfonamides are excreted in breast milk. Sodium sulfacetamide is an eye drop and the extent of absorption is unknown.

Related Information

Ophthalmic Agents *on page 1509*

Sulfacetamide and Fluorometholone *see page 1509*

Sulfacetamide and Prednisolone *see page 1509*

Sulfacetamide Sodium *see* Sulfacetamide *on page 1256*

Sulfacet-R® Topical *see page 1522*

SulfaDIAZINE (sul fa DYE a zeen)

Generic Available Yes

Pharmacologic Category Antibiotic, Sulfonamide Derivative

Pregnancy Risk Factor B/D (at term)

Lactation Enters breast milk/contraindicated

Use Treatment of urinary tract infections and nocardiosis, rheumatic fever prophylaxis; adjunctive treatment in toxoplasmosis; uncomplicated attack of malaria

Mechanism of Action/Effect Interferes with bacterial growth by inhibiting bacterial folic acid synthesis through competitive antagonism of PABA

Contraindications Hypersensitivity to any sulfa drug or any component of the formulation; porphyria; children <2 months of age unless indicated for the treatment of congenital toxoplasmosis; sunscreens containing PABA; pregnancy (at term)

Warnings/Precautions Use with caution in patients with impaired hepatic function or impaired renal function, G6PD deficiency; dosage modification required in patients with renal impairment; fluid intake should be maintained ≥1500 mL/day, or administer sodium bicarbonate to keep urine alkaline; more likely to cause crystalluria because it is less soluble than other sulfonamides. Chemical similarities are present among sulfonamides, sulfonylureas, carbonic anhydrase inhibitors, thiazides, and loop diuretics (except ethacrynic acid). Use in patients with sulfonamide allergy is specifically contraindicated in product labeling, however, a risk of cross-reaction exists in patients with allergy to any of these compounds; avoid use when previous reaction has been severe.

Drug Interactions

Cytochrome P450 Effect: Substrate of **CYP2C8/9**, 2E1, 3A4; Inhibits CYP2C8/9

Decreased Effect: Decreased effect with PABA or PABA metabolites of drugs (eg, procaine, proparacaine, tetracaine, sunblock).

Increased Effect/Toxicity: Increased effect of oral anticoagulants and oral hypoglycemic agents.

Nutritional/Ethanol Interactions

Food: Avoid large quantities of vitamin C or acidifying agents (cranberry juice) to prevent crystalluria.

Herb/Nutraceutical: Avoid dong quai, St John's wort (may also cause photosensitization).

Adverse Reactions Frequency not defined.

Central nervous system: Fever, dizziness, headache

Dermatologic: Lyell's syndrome, Stevens-Johnson syndrome, itching, rash, photosensitivity

Endocrine & metabolic: Thyroid function disturbance

Gastrointestinal: Anorexia, nausea, vomiting, diarrhea

Genitourinary: Crystalluria

Hematologic: Granulocytopenia, leukopenia, thrombocytopenia, aplastic anemia, hemolytic anemia

Hepatic: Hepatitis, jaundice

Renal: Hematuria, acute nephropathy, interstitial nephritis

Miscellaneous: Serum sickness-like reactions

Overdosage/Toxicology Symptoms of overdose include drowsiness, dizziness, anorexia, abdominal pain, nausea, vomiting, hemolytic anemia, acidosis, jaundice, fever, and agranulocytosis. Doses as little as 2-5 g/day may produce toxicity. The aniline radical is responsible for hematologic toxicity. High volume diuresis may aid in elimination and prevention of renal failure. Leucovorin 5-15 mg/day has been used to speed recovery of bone marrow.

Pharmacodynamics/Kinetics

Absorption: Well absorbed

Half-Life Elimination: 10 hours

Time to Peak: Within 3-6 hours

Metabolism: Via N-acetylation

Formulations Tablet: 500 mg

Dosing

Adults & Elderly:

Toxoplasmosis: Oral: 2-6 g/day divided every 6 hours in conjunction with pyrimethamine 50-75 mg/day and with supplemental folinic acid

Asymptomatic meningococcal carriers: 1 g twice daily for 2 days

Nocardiosis: 4-8 g/day for a minimum of 6 weeks

Prevention of recurrent attacks of rheumatic fever: 1 g/day

Pediatrics:

Asymptomatic meningococcal carriers: Oral:

Infants 1-12 months: 500 mg once daily for 2 days

Children 1-12 years: 500 mg twice daily for 2 days

Congenital toxoplasmosis: Oral:

Newborns and Children <2 months: 100 mg/kg/day divided every 6 hours in conjunction with pyrimethamine 1 mg/kg/day once daily and supplemental folinic acid 5 mg every 3 days for 6 months

Children >2 months: 25-50 mg/kg/dose 4 times/day

Toxoplasmosis: Oral:

Children >2 months: Loading dose: 75 mg/kg; maintenance dose: 120-150 mg/kg/day, maximum dose: 6 g/day; divided every 4-6 hours in conjunction with pyrimethamine 2

(Continued)

SulfaDIAZINE *(Continued)*

mg/kg/day divided every 12 hours for 3 days followed by 1 mg/kg/day once daily with supplemental folinic acid

Prevention of recurrent attacks of rheumatic fever: Oral:

>30 kg: 1 g/day; <30 kg: 0.5 g/day

Administration

Oral: Tablets may be crushed to prepare oral suspension of the drug in water or with a sucrose-containing solution. Aqueous suspension with concentrations of 100 mg/mL should be stored in the refrigerator and used within 7 days. Administer around-the-clock to promote less variation in peak and trough serum levels.

Monitoring Laboratory Tests Perform culture and sensitivity prior to initiating therapy.

Monitoring and Teaching Issues

Physical Assessment: Assess for allergy history prior to starting therapy. See Contraindications, Warnings/Precautions, and Dosing for use cautions. Assess potential for interactions with other prescriptions, OTC medications, or herbal products patient may be taking (see Drug Interactions). Monitor patient response (see Adverse Reactions and Overdose/Toxicology). Teach patient proper use, possible side effects and interventions, and adverse symptoms to report (see Patient Education) on a regular basis during therapy. **Pregnancy risk factor B/D** - see Pregnancy Risk Factor for use cautions. Breast-feeding is contraindicated.

Patient Education: Inform prescriber of all prescriptions, OTC medications, or herbal products you are taking, and any allergies you have. Take as directed, at regular intervals around-the-clock. Take on an empty stomach, 1 hour before or 2 hours after meals with full glass of water. Complete full course of therapy even if you are feeling better. Take a missed dose as soon as possible. If almost time for next dose, skip the missed dose and return to your regular schedule. Do not take a double dose. Avoid large quantities of vitamin C. Maintain adequate hydration (2-3 L/day of fluids) to prevent kidney damage unless advised by prescriber to restrict fluids. May cause dizziness or headache (use caution when driving or engaging in tasks requiring alertness until response to drug is known); photosensitivity (use sunblock, wear protective clothing and eyewear, and avoid direct sunlight); nausea, vomiting, or loss of appetite (small, frequent meals, frequent mouth care, sucking lozenges, or chewing gum may help). Report skin rash, persistent nausea, vomiting, or diarrhea; opportunistic infection (sore throat, fever, vaginal itching or discharge, unusual bruising or bleeding, fatigue); blood in urine or change in urinary pattern; persistent headache; abdominal pain; or difficulty breathing. **Pregnancy/breast-feeding precautions:** Inform prescriber if you are or intend to become pregnant. Do not breast-feed.

Dietary Issues: Supplemental folinic acid should be administered to reverse symptoms or prevent problems due to folic acid deficiency.

Related Information

FDA Name Differentiation Project: The Use of Tall-man Letters *on page 12*

Sulfamethoxazole (sul fa meth OKS a zole)

U.S. Brand Names Gantanol®

Generic Available Yes

Pharmacologic Category Antibiotic, Sulfonamide Derivative

Pregnancy Risk Factor B/D (at term)

Lactation Enters breast milk/compatible

Use Treatment of urinary tract infections, nocardiosis, toxoplasmosis, acute otitis media, and acute exacerbations of chronic bronchitis due to susceptible organisms

Mechanism of Action/Effect Interferes with bacterial growth by inhibiting bacterial folic acid synthesis through competitive antagonism of PABA

Contraindications Hypersensitivity to any sulfa drug or any component of the formulation; porphyria; children <2 months of age unless indicated for the treatment of congenital toxoplasmosis; sunscreens containing PABA; pregnancy (at term)

Warnings/Precautions Maintain adequate fluid intake to prevent crystalluria; use with caution in patients with renal or hepatic impairment, and patients with G6PD deficiency; should not be used for group A beta-hemolytic streptococcal infections. Chemical similarities are present among sulfonamides, sulfonylureas, carbonic anhydrase inhibitors, thiazides, and loop diuretics (except ethacrynic acid). Use in patients with sulfonamide allergy is specifically contraindicated in product labeling, however, a risk of cross-reaction exists in patients with allergy to any of these compounds; avoid use when previous reaction has been severe.

Drug Interactions

Cytochrome P450 Effect: Substrate of **CYP2C8/9**, 3A4; Inhibits CYP2C8/9

Decreased Effect: Decreased effect with PABA or PABA metabolites of drugs (eg, procaine, proparacaine, tetracaine).

Increased Effect/Toxicity: Increased effect of oral anticoagulants, oral hypoglycemic agents, and methotrexate.

Nutritional/Ethanol Interactions Food: The presence of food delays but does not reduce absorption. Avoid large quantities of vitamin C or acidifying agents (cranberry juice) to prevent crystalluria.

Effects on Lab Values May interfere with Jaffé alkaline picrate reaction assay for creatinine resulting in overestimations of ∼10% in the range of normal values. Decreased effect with PABA or PABA metabolites of drugs (ie, procaine, proparacaine, tetracaine).

Adverse Reactions

>10%:

Central nervous system: Fever, dizziness, headache

Dermatologic: Itching, rash, photosensitivity

Gastrointestinal: Anorexia, nausea, vomiting, diarrhea

1% to 10%:

Dermatologic: Lyell's syndrome, Stevens-Johnson syndrome

Hematologic: Granulocytopenia, leukopenia, thrombocytopenia, aplastic anemia, hemolytic anemia

Hepatic: Hepatitis

<1% (Limited to important or life-threatening): Acute nephropathy, hematuria, interstitial nephritis, vasculitis

Overdosage/Toxicology Symptoms of overdose include drowsiness, dizziness, anorexia, abdominal pain, nausea, vomiting, hemolytic anemia, acidosis, jaundice, fever, and agranulocytosis. The aniline radical is responsible for hematologic toxicity. High volume diuresis may aid in elimination and prevention of renal failure. Leucovorin 5-15 mg/day has been used to speed recovery of bone marrow.

Pharmacodynamics/Kinetics

Absorption: 90%

Half-Life Elimination: 9-12 hours; prolonged with renal impairment

Time to Peak: Serum: 1-4 hours

Metabolism: Primarily hepatic via N-acetylation and glucuronidation with 10% to 20% as the N-acetylated form in plasma

Formulations Tablet: 500 mg

Dosing

Adults: Susceptible infections: Oral: 2 g stat, 1 g 2-3 times/day; maximum: 3 g/24 hours

Elderly: Oral: Same as adults unless Cl_{cr} <30 mL/minute; see Renal Impairment. Single dose or 3-day dosing has not been shown to be reliable for treating urinary tract infections in the elderly.

Pediatrics: Susceptible infections: Oral: Children >2 months: 50-60 mg/kg as single dose followed by 50-60 mg/kg/day divided every 12 hours; maximum: 3 g/24 hours or 75 mg/kg/day

Renal Impairment:

Cl_{cr} 10-50 mL/minute: Administer every 18 hours.

Cl_{cr} <10 mL/minute: Administer every 24 hours.

Moderately dialyzable (20% to 50%)

Administration

Oral: Administer around-the-clock to promote less variation in peak and trough serum levels.

Stability

Storage: Protect from light

Monitoring Laboratory Tests Perform culture and sensitivity prior to initiating therapy.

Monitoring and Teaching Issues

Physical Assessment: Assess for allergy history prior to starting therapy. See Contraindications, Warnings/Precautions, and Dosing for use cautions. Assess potential for interactions with other prescriptions, OTC medications, or herbal products patient may be taking (see Drug Interactions). Monitor patient response (see Adverse Reactions and Overdose/Toxicology). Caution diabetic patients using oral hypoglycemics to monitor glucose levels closely (may increase effect of oral hypoglycemics). Teach patient proper use, possible side effects and interventions, and adverse symptoms to report (see Patient Education) on a regular basis during therapy. **Pregnancy risk factor B/D** - see Pregnancy Risk Factor for use cautions.

Patient Education: Inform prescriber of all prescriptions, OTC medications, or herbal products you are taking, and any allergies you have. Take as directed, at regular intervals around-the-clock. Take on an empty stomach, 1 hour before or 2 hours after meals with full glass of water. Complete full course of therapy even if you are feeling better. Take a missed dose as soon as possible. If almost time for next dose, skip the missed dose and return to your regular schedule. Do not take a double dose. Avoid large quantities of vitamin C or acidifying agents (cranberry juice). Maintain adequate hydration (2-3 L/day of fluids) to prevent kidney damage unless advised by prescriber to restrict fluids. Diabetics taking oral hypoglycemics should monitor glucose levels closely (may increase effect of oral hypoglycemics). May cause dizziness or headache (use caution when driving or engaging in tasks requiring alertness until response to drug is known); photosensitivity (use sunblock, wear protective clothing and eyewear, and avoid direct sunlight); or nausea, vomiting, or loss of appetite (small, frequent meals, frequent mouth care, sucking lozenges, or chewing gum may help). Report skin rash; persistent nausea, vomiting, or diarrhea; opportunistic infection (sore throat, fever, vaginal itching or discharge, unusual bruising or bleeding, fatigue); or blood in urine or change in urinary pattern. **Pregnancy/breast-feeding precautions:** Inform prescriber if you are or intend to become pregnant

Dietary Issues: Should be taken 1 hour before or 2 hours after a meal on an empty stomach.

Geriatric Considerations: Sulfamethoxazole is an effective anti-infective agent. Most prescribers prefer the combination of sulfamethoxazole and trimethoprim for its dual mechanism of action. Trimethoprim penetrates the prostate. Adjust dose for renal function.

Sulfamethoxazole and Trimethoprim

(sul fa meth OKS a zole & trye METH oh prim)

U.S. Brand Names Bactrim™; Bactrim™ DS; Septra®; Septra® DS; Sulfatrim®; Sulfatrim® DS

Synonyms Co-Trimoxazole; SMZ-TMP; TMP-SMZ; Trimethoprim and Sulfamethoxazole

Generic Available Yes

Pharmacologic Category Antibiotic, Sulfonamide Derivative; Antibiotic, Miscellaneous

Pregnancy Risk Factor C/D (at term - expert analysis)

Lactation Enters breast milk/compatible

Use

Oral treatment of urinary tract infections due to *E. coli*, *Klebsiella* and *Enterobacter* sp, *M. morganii*, *P. mirabilis* and *P. vulgaris*; acute otitis media in children and acute exacerbations of chronic bronchitis in adults due to susceptible strains of *H. influenzae* or *S. pneumoniae*; prophylaxis of *Pneumocystis carinii* pneumonitis (PCP), traveler's diarrhea due to enterotoxigenic *E. coli* or *Cyclospora*

I.V. treatment or severe·or complicated infections when oral therapy is not feasible, for documented PCP, empiric treatment of PCP in immune compromised patients; treatment

(Continued)

Sulfamethoxazole and Trimethoprim *(Continued)*

of documented or suspected shigellosis, typhoid fever, *Nocardia asteroides* infection, or other infections caused by susceptible bacteria

Use - Unlabeled/Investigational Cholera and salmonella-type infections and nocardiosis; chronic prostatitis; as prophylaxis in neutropenic patients with *P. carinii* infections, in leukemics, and in patients following renal transplantation, to decrease incidence of gram-negative rod infections

Mechanism of Action/Effect Sulfamethoxazole interferes with bacterial folic acid synthesis; trimethoprim inhibits enzymes of the folic acid pathway

Contraindications Hypersensitivity to any sulfa drug, trimethoprim, or any component of the formulation; porphyria; megaloblastic anemia due to folate deficiency; infants <2 months of age; marked hepatic damage; severe renal disease; pregnancy (at term)

Warnings/Precautions Use with caution in patients with G6PD deficiency, impaired renal or hepatic function. Adjust dosage in patients with renal impairment. Injection vehicle contains benzyl alcohol and sodium metabisulfite. Fatalities associated with severe reactions including Stevens-Johnson syndrome, toxic epidermal necrolysis, hepatic necrosis, agranulocytosis, aplastic anemia, and other blood dyscrasias. Discontinue use at first sign of rash. Elderly patients and patients with HIV appear at greater risk for more severe adverse reactions. May cause hypoglycemia (particularly in malnourished, renal, or hepatic impairment). Use caution in patients with porphyria or thyroid dysfunction. May cause hyperkalemia. Slow acetylators may be more prone to adverse reactions.

Chemical similarities are present among sulfonamides, sulfonylureas, carbonic anhydrase inhibitors, thiazides, and loop diuretics (except ethacrynic acid). Use in patients with sulfonamide allergy is specifically contraindicated in product labeling, however, a risk of cross-reaction exists in patients with allergy to any of these compounds; avoid use when previous reaction has been severe.

Pregnancy risk C/D (near term).

Drug Interactions

Cytochrome P450 Effect:

Sulfamethoxazole: Substrate of **CYP2C8/9**, 3A4; Inhibits CYP2C8/9

Trimethoprim: Substrate of **CYP2C8/9, 3A4**; Inhibits CYP2C8/9

Decreased Effect: Co-trimoxazole causes decreased effect of cyclosporines and tricyclic antidepressants. Procaine and indomethacin may cause decreased effect of co-trimoxazole.

Increased Effect/Toxicity: Co-trimoxazole may cause an increased effect of sulfonylureas and oral anticoagulants (warfarin). Co-trimoxazole may displace highly protein-bound drugs like methotrexate, phenytoin, or cyclosporine causing increased free serum concentrations, leading to increased toxicity of these agents. May also compete for renal excretion of methotrexate. Co-trimoxazole may enhance the nephrotoxicity of cyclosporine and may increase digoxin concentrations.

Nutritional/Ethanol Interactions Herb/Nutraceutical: Avoid dong quai, St John's wort (may also cause photosensitization).

Effects on Lab Values ↑ creatinine (Jaffé alkaline picrate reaction); increased serum methotrexate by dihydrofolate reductase method; does not interfere with RAI method

Adverse Reactions The most common adverse reactions include gastrointestinal upset (nausea, vomiting, anorexia) and dermatologic reactions (rash or urticaria). Rare, life-threatening reactions have been associated with co-trimoxazole, including severe dermatologic reactions and hepatotoxic reactions. Most other reactions listed are rare, however, frequency cannot be accurately estimated.

Cardiovascular: Allergic myocarditis

Central nervous system: Confusion, depression, hallucinations, seizures, aseptic meningitis, peripheral neuritis, fever, ataxia, kernicterus in neonates

Dermatologic: Rashes, pruritus, urticaria, photosensitivity; rare reactions include erythema multiforme, Stevens-Johnson syndrome, toxic epidermal necrolysis, exfoliative dermatitis, and Henoch-Schönlein purpura

Endocrine & metabolic: Hyperkalemia (generally at high dosages), hyperglycemia

Gastrointestinal: Nausea, vomiting, anorexia, stomatitis, diarrhea, pseudomembranous colitis, pancreatitis

Hematologic: Thrombocytopenia, megaloblastic anemia, granulocytopenia, eosinophilia, pancytopenia, aplastic anemia, methemoglobinemia, hemolysis (with G6PD deficiency), agranulocytosis

Hepatic: Elevated serum transaminases, hepatotoxicity (including hepatitis, cholestasis, and hepatic necrosis), hyperbilirubinemia

Neuromuscular & skeletal: Arthralgia, myalgia, rhabdomyolysis

Renal: Interstitial nephritis, crystalluria, renal failure, nephrotoxicity (in association with cyclosporine), diuresis

Respiratory: Cough, dyspnea, pulmonary infiltrates

Miscellaneous: Serum sickness, angioedema, periarteritis nodosa (rare), systemic lupus erythematosus (rare)

Overdosage/Toxicology Symptoms of overdose include nausea, vomiting, GI distress, hematuria, and crystalluria. Bone marrow suppression may occur. Treatment is supportive. Adequate fluid intake is essential. Peritoneal dialysis is not effective and hemodialysis is only moderately effective in removing co-trimoxazole. Leucovorin 5-15 mg/day may accelerate hematologic recovery.

Pharmacokinetic Note See individual agents.

Formulations The 5:1 ratio (SMX:TMP) remains constant in all dosage forms:

Injection: Sulfamethoxazole 80 mg and trimethoprim 16 mg per mL (5 mL, 10 mL, 20 mL, 30 mL, 50 mL)

Suspension, oral: Sulfamethoxazole 200 mg and trimethoprim 40 mg per 5 mL (20 mL, 100 mL, 150 mL, 200 mL, 480 mL)

Tablet: Sulfamethoxazole 400 mg and trimethoprim 80 mg

Tablet, double strength: Sulfamethoxazole 800 mg and trimethoprim 160 mg

Dosing

Adults & Elderly: Dosage recommendations are based on the trimethoprim component.

Urinary tract infection/chronic bronchitis: Oral: 1 double strength tablet every 12 hours for 10-14 days

Sepsis: I.V.: 20 TMP/kg/day divided every 6 hours

Pneumocystis carinii:

Prophylaxis: Oral: 1 double strength tablet daily or 3 times weekly

Treatment: Oral, I.V.: 15-20 mg TMP/kg/day divided in 3-4 doses daily

Cholera: Oral, I.V.: 160 mg TMP twice daily for 3 days

Cyclospora: Oral, I.V.: 160 mg TMP twice daily for 7 days

Nocardia: Oral, I.V.: 640 mg TMP/day in divided doses for several months (duration is controversial; an average of 7 months has been reported)

Pediatrics: Recommendations are based on the trimethoprim component. Children >2 months:

Mild to moderate infections: Oral, I.V.: 8 mg TMP/kg/day in divided doses every 12 hours

Serious infection/*Pneumocystis*: I.V.: 20 mg TMP/kg/day in divided doses every 6 hours

Urinary tract infection prophylaxis: Oral: 2 mg TMP/kg/dose daily

Prophylaxis of *Pneumocystis*: Oral, I.V.: 10 mg TMP/kg/day or 150 mg TMP/m^2/day in divided doses every 12 hours for 3 days/week; dose should not exceed 320 mg trimethoprim and 1600 mg sulfamethoxazole 3 days/week.

Cholera: Oral, I.V.: 5 mg TMP/kg twice daily for 3 days

Cyclospora: Oral, I.V.: 5 mg TMP/kg twice daily for 7 days

Renal Impairment:

Cl_{cr} 15-30 mL/minute: Reduce dose by 50%.

Cl_{cr} <15 mL/minute: Not recommended

Administration

I.V.: Infuse over 60-90 minutes, must dilute well before giving.

Stability

Storage: Do not refrigerate injection. Less soluble in more alkaline pH. Protect from light.

Reconstitution: Do not refrigerate injection. Do not use NS as a diluent. Injection vehicle contains benzyl alcohol and sodium metabisulfite.

Stability of parenteral admixture at room temperature (25°C):

5 mL/125 mL D_5W = 6 hours

5 mL/100 mL D_5W = 4 hours

5 mL/75 mL D_5W = 2 hours

Compatibility: Stable in D_5½NS, LR, ½NS

Y-site administration: Incompatible with fluconazole, midazolam, vinorelbine

Compatibility when admixed: Incompatible with fluconazole, verapamil

Monitoring Laboratory Tests Perform culture and sensitivity testing prior to initiating therapy.

Monitoring and Teaching Issues

Physical Assessment: Assess for previous allergy history prior to therapy. See Contraindications, Warnings/Precautions, and Dosing for use cautions. Assess potential for interactions with other prescriptions, OTC medications, or herbal products patient may be taking (see Drug Interactions). **I.V.:** See Administration and Reconstitution. Assess results of laboratory tests, therapeutic response (according to purpose for use), and adverse reactions (see Adverse Reactions and Overdose/Toxicology). Instruct diabetic patients regarding Clinitest®. Teach patient possible side effects and interventions and adverse symptoms to report (see Patient Education). **Pregnancy risk factor C/D** - benefits of use should outweigh possible risks.

Patient Education: Inform prescriber of all prescriptions, OTC medications, or herbal products you are taking, and any allergies you have. Do not take anything new during treatment unless approved by prescriber. Take oral medication with 8 oz of water on an empty stomach, 1 hour before or 2 hours after meals, for best absorption. Finish all medication; do not skip doses. May cause false test results with Clinitest®; use of another type of glucose testing is preferable. May cause increased sensitivity to sunlight (use sunblock, wear protective clothing and dark glasses, and avoid direct exposure to sunlight); or nausea or vomiting (small, frequent meals, frequent mouth care, sucking lozenges, or chewing gum may help). Report immediately rash; palpitations or chest pain; CNS changes (eg, hallucinations, abnormal anxiety, seizures); sore throat, unusual coughing, or shortness of breath; blackened stool; or unusual bruising or bleeding. **Pregnancy precaution:** Inform prescriber if you are or intend to become pregnant.

Dietary Issues: Should be taken with a glass of water on empty stomach.

Geriatric Considerations: Elderly patients appear at greater risk for more severe adverse reactions. Adjust dose based on renal function.

Pregnancy Issues: Do not use at term to avoid kernicterus in the newborn and use during pregnancy only if risks outweigh the benefits since folic acid metabolism may be affected.

Related Information

Sulfamethoxazole *on page 1258*

Trimethoprim *on page 1366*

Sulfanilamide (sul fa NIL a mide)

U.S. Brand Names AVC™

Generic Available Yes

Pharmacologic Category Antifungal Agent, Vaginal

Pregnancy Risk Factor C (avoid use after 7th month)

Lactation Contraindicated

Use Treatment of vulvovaginitis caused by *Candida albicans*

Mechanism of Action/Effect Interferes with microbial folic acid synthesis and growth via inhibition of para-aminiobenzoic acid metabolism

Contraindications Hypersensitivity to sulfanilamide or any component of the formulation; pregnancy (near term)

(Continued)

Sulfanilamide *(Continued)*

Warnings/Precautions Since sulfonamides may be absorbed from vaginal mucosa, the same precaution for oral sulfonamides apply (eg, blood dyscrasias); if a rash develops, terminate therapy immediately. Use vaginal applicators very cautiously after the 7th month of pregnancy. Pregnancy risk C (avoid after 7th month).

Adverse Reactions Frequency not defined.

Dermatologic: Stevens-Johnson syndrome (infrequent)

Genitourinary: Burning, increased discomfort, irritation of penis of sexual partner

Miscellaneous: Allergic reactions, systemic reactions (rare)

Pharmacodynamics/Kinetics

Absorption: Not absorbed

Formulations

Cream, vaginal [with applicator]: 15% [150 mg/g] (120 g)

Suppository, vaginal: 1.05 g (16s)

Dosing

Adults & Elderly: Vulvovaginal candidiasis: Intravaginal: Insert 1 applicatorful once or twice daily through one complete menstrual cycle or insert 1 suppository intravaginally once or twice daily for 30 days.

Administration

Other: For vaginal use only.

Monitoring and Teaching Issues

Physical Assessment: See Contraindications and Warnings/Precautions for use cautions. Assess knowledge/teach patient appropriate administration, possible side effects/interventions, and adverse symptoms to report (see Patient Education). **Pregnancy risk factor C** - see Pregnancy Risk Factor for use cautions. Breast-feeding is contraindicated.

Patient Education: Complete full course of therapy as directed. Insert vaginally as directed by prescriber or see package insert. You may be sensitive to direct sunlight (wear protective clothing, use sunblock, and avoid excessive exposure to direct sunlight). Sexual partner may experience irritation of penis; best to refrain from intercourse during period of treatment. Report persistent vaginal burning, itching, or irritation; rash; yellowing of eyes or skin; dark urine or pale stool; unresolved nausea or vomiting; or painful urination. **Pregnancy/breast-feeding precautions:** Inform prescriber if you are or intend to become pregnant. Do not breast-feed.

Sulfasalazine (sul fa SAL a zeen)

U.S. Brand Names Azulfidine®; Azulfidine® EN-tabs®

Synonyms Salicylazosulfapyridine

Generic Available Yes

Pharmacologic Category 5-Aminosalicylic Acid Derivative

Pregnancy Risk Factor B/D (at term)

Lactation Enters breast milk/use caution (AAP recommends use "with caution")

Use Management of ulcerative colitis; enteric coated tablets are also used for rheumatoid arthritis (including juvenile rheumatoid arthritis) in patients who inadequately respond to analgesics and NSAIDs

Use - Unlabeled/Investigational Ankylosing spondylitis, collagenous colitis, Crohn's disease, psoriasis, psoriatic arthritis, juvenile chronic arthritis

Mechanism of Action/Effect Acts locally in the colon to decrease the inflammatory response and systemically interferes with secretion by inhibiting prostaglandin synthesis

Contraindications Hypersensitivity to sulfasalazine, sulfa drugs, salicylates, or any component of the formulation; porphyria; GI or GU obstruction; pregnancy (at term)

Warnings/Precautions Use with caution in patients with renal impairment; impaired hepatic function or urinary obstruction, blood dyscrasias, severe allergies or asthma, or G6PD deficiency; may cause folate deficiency (consider providing 1 mg/day folate supplement). Chemical similarities are present among sulfonamides, sulfonylureas, carbonic anhydrase inhibitors, thiazides, and loop diuretics (except ethacrynic acid). Use in patients with sulfonamide allergy is specifically contraindicated in product labeling, however, a risk of cross-reaction exists in patients with allergy to any of these compounds; avoid use when previous reaction has been severe. Safety and efficacy have not been established in children <2 years of age.

Drug Interactions

Decreased Effect: Decreased effect with iron, digoxin and PABA or PABA metabolites of drugs (eg, procaine, proparacaine, tetracaine).

Increased Effect/Toxicity: Sulfasalazine may increase hydantoin levels. Effects of thiopental, oral hypoglycemics, and oral anticoagulants may be increased. Sulfasalazine may increase the risk of myelosuppression with azathioprine, mercaptopurine, or thioguanine (due to TPMT inhibition); may also increase the toxicity of methotrexate. Risk of thrombocytopenia may be increased with thiazide diuretics. Concurrent methenamine may increase risk of crystalluria.

Nutritional/Ethanol Interactions

Food: May impair folate absorption.

Herb/Nutraceutical: Avoid dong quai, St John's wort (may also cause photosensitization)

Adverse Reactions

>10%:

Central nervous system: Headache (33%)

Dermatologic: Photosensitivity

Gastrointestinal: Anorexia, nausea, vomiting, diarrhea (33%), gastric distress

Genitourinary: Reversible oligospermia (33%)

<3% (Limited to important or life-threatening): Alopecia, anaphylaxis, aplastic anemia, ataxia, crystalluria, depression, epidermal necrolysis, exfoliative dermatitis, granulocytopenia, hallucinations, Heinz body anemia, hemolytic anemia, hepatitis, interstitial nephritis, jaundice, leukopenia, Lyell's syndrome, myelodysplastic syndrome, nephropathy (acute), neutropenic enterocolitis, pancreatitis, peripheral neuropathy, photosensitization, pruritus,

rhabdomyolysis, seizures, serum sickness-like reactions, skin discoloration, Stevens-Johnson syndrome, thrombocytopenia, thyroid function disturbance, urine discoloration, urticaria, vasculitis, vertigo

Additional events reported with sulfonamides and/or 5-ASA derivatives: Cholestatic jaundice, eosinophilia pneumonitis, erythema multiforme, fibrosing alveolitis, hepatic necrosis, Kawasaki-like syndrome, SLE-like syndrome, pericarditis, seizures, transverse myelitis

Overdosage/Toxicology Symptoms of overdose include drowsiness, dizziness, anorexia, abdominal pain, nausea, vomiting, hemolytic anemia, acidosis, jaundice, fever, and agranulocytosis. The aniline radical is responsible for hematologic toxicity. High volume diuresis may aid in elimination and prevention of renal failure. Leucovorin 5-15 mg/day has been used to speed recovery of bone marrow.

Pharmacodynamics/Kinetics

Absorption: 10% to 15% as unchanged drug from small intestine

Half-Life Elimination: 5.7-10 hours

Metabolism: Via colonic intestinal flora to sulfapyridine and 5-aminosalicylic acid (5-ASA); following absorption, sulfapyridine undergoes N-acetylation and ring hydroxylation while 5-ASA undergoes N-acetylation

Formulations

Tablet: 500 mg

Tablet, enteric coated: 500 mg

Dosing

Adults & Elderly:

Ulcerative colitis: Oral (enteric coated tablet): Initial: 1 g 3-4 times/day, 2 g/day maintenance in divided doses; may initiate therapy with 0.5-1 g/day

Rheumatoid arthritis: Oral (enteric coated tablet): Initial: 0.5-1 g/day; increase weekly to maintenance dose of 2 g/day in 2 divided doses; maximum: 3 g/day (if response to 2 g/day is inadequate after 12 weeks of treatment)

Pediatrics:

Ulcerative colitis: Oral: Children ≥2 years: Initial: 40-60 mg/kg/day in 3-6 divided doses; maintenance dose: 20-30 mg/kg/day in 4 divided doses

Juvenile rheumatoid arthritis: Oral: Children ≥6 years: 30-50 mg/kg/day in 2 divided doses; Initial: Begin with $^1/_4$ to $^1/_3$ of expected maintenance dose; increase weekly; maximum: 2 g/day typically

Renal Impairment:

Cl_{cr} 10-30 mL/minute: Administer twice daily.

Cl_{cr} <10 mL/minute: Administer once daily.

Hepatic Impairment: Avoid use.

Administration

Oral: GI intolerance is common during the first few days of therapy (give with meals).

Stability

Storage: Protect from light.

Monitoring and Teaching Issues

Physical Assessment: Assess for allergy history prior to starting therapy. See Contraindications, Warnings/Precautions, and Dosing for use cautions. Assess potential for interactions with other prescriptions, OTC medications, or herbal products patient may be taking (see Drug Interactions). Monitor patient response (see Adverse Reactions and Overdose/Toxicology). Caution diabetic patient to monitor glucose levels closely (decreased effect of oral hypoglycemic agents). Teach patient proper use, possible side effects and interventions, and adverse symptoms to report (see Patient Education) on a regular basis during therapy. **Pregnancy risk factor B/D** - see Pregnancy Risk Factor for use cautions. Note breast-feeding caution.

Patient Education: Inform prescriber of all prescriptions, OTC medications, or herbal products you are taking, and any allergies you have. Take as directed, at regular intervals around-the-clock with food. Do not crush, chew, or dissolve coated tablets. Complete full course of therapy even if you are feeling better. Take a missed dose as soon as possible. If almost time for next dose, skip the missed dose and return to your regular schedule. Do not take a double dose. Maintain adequate hydration (2-3 L/day of fluids) to prevent kidney damage unless advised by prescriber to restrict fluids. If diabetic, monitor glucose levels closely (may cause decreased effect of oral hypoglycemic agents). Orange-yellow color of urine is normal. May cause dizziness or headache (use caution when driving or engaging in tasks requiring alertness until response to drug is known); photosensitivity (use sunblock, wear protective clothing and eyewear, and avoid direct sunlight); or nausea, vomiting, or loss of appetite (small, frequent meals, frequent mouth care, sucking lozenges, or chewing gum may help). Report rash; persistent nausea, vomiting, or diarrhea; opportunistic infection (sore throat, fever, vaginal itching or discharge, unusual bruising or bleeding, fatigue); blood in urine or change in urinary pattern; swelling of face, lips, or tongue, tightness in chest, bad cough, blue skin color, or other persistent adverse effects. **Pregnancy/breast-feeding precautions:** Inform prescriber if you are or intend to become pregnant. Consult prescriber if breast-feeding.

Dietary Issues: Since sulfasalazine impairs folate absorption, consider providing 1 mg/day folate supplement.

Geriatric Considerations: Adjust dose for renal function (see Additional Information).

Breast-feeding Issues: Sulfonamides are excreted in human breast milk and may cause kernicterus in the newborn. Although sulfapyridine has poor bilirubin-displacing ability, use with caution in women who are breast-feeding. The AAP classifies this agent to be used with caution since adverse effects have been reported in nursing infants.

Sulfatrim® *see* Sulfamethoxazole and Trimethoprim *on page 1259*

Sulfatrim® DS *see* Sulfamethoxazole and Trimethoprim *on page 1259*

Sulfinpyrazone (sul fin PEER a zone)

U.S. Brand Names Anturane®

Generic Available Yes

Pharmacologic Category Uricosuric Agent

(Continued)

Sulfinpyrazone *(Continued)*

Pregnancy Risk Factor C/D (near term - expert analysis)

Lactation Excretion in breast milk unknown

Use Treatment of chronic gouty arthritis and intermittent gouty arthritis

Use - Unlabeled/Investigational To decrease the incidence of sudden death postmyocardial infarction

Mechanism of Action/Effect Acts by increasing the urinary excretion of uric acid, thereby decreasing blood urate levels; this effect is therapeutically useful in treating patients with acute intermittent gout, chronic tophaceous gout, and acts to promote resorption of tophi; also has antithrombic and platelet inhibitory effects

Contraindications Hypersensitivity to sulfinpyrazone, phenylbutazone, other pyrazoles, or any component of the formulation; active peptic ulcer; GI inflammation; blood dyscrasias; pregnancy (near term)

Warnings/Precautions Safety and efficacy are not established in children <18 years of age. Use with caution in patients with impaired renal function and urolithiasis. Pregnancy risk C/D (near term).

Drug Interactions

Cytochrome P450 Effect: Substrate of **CYP2C8/9**, 3A4; Inhibits CYP2C8/9; Induces CYP3A4

Decreased Effect: Decreased effect/levels of theophylline, verapamil. Decreased uricosuric activity with salicylates, niacins.

Increased Effect/Toxicity: Increased effect of oral hypoglycemics and anticoagulants. Risk of acetaminophen hepatotoxicity is increased, while therapeutic effects may be reduced.

Nutritional/Ethanol Interactions Herb/Nutraceutical: Avoid dong quai, St John's wort (may also cause photosensitization).

Effects on Lab Values ↓ uric acid (S)

Adverse Reactions Frequency not defined.

Cardiovascular: Flushing
Central nervous system: Dizziness, headache
Dermatologic: Dermatitis, rash
Gastrointestinal (most frequent adverse effects): Nausea, vomiting, stomach pain
Genitourinary: Polyuria
Hematologic: Anemia, leukopenia, increased bleeding time (decreased platelet aggregation)
Hepatic: Hepatic necrosis
Renal: Nephrotic syndrome, uric acid stones

Overdosage/Toxicology Symptoms of overdose include drowsiness, dizziness, anorexia, abdominal pain, nausea, vomiting, hemolytic anemia, acidosis, jaundice, fever, and agranulocytosis. The aniline radical is responsible for hematologic toxicity. High volume diuresis may aid in elimination and prevention of renal failure. Leucovorin 5-15 mg/day has been used to speed recovery of bone marrow.

Pharmacodynamics/Kinetics

Absorption: Rapid and complete
Half-Life Elimination: 2.7-6 hours
Time to Peak: Serum: 1.6 hours
Metabolism: Hepatic to two active metabolites

Formulations

Capsule: 200 mg
Tablet: 100 mg

Dosing

Adults: Gouty arthritis: Oral: 100-200 mg twice daily; maximum daily dose: 800 mg
Elderly: Refer to adult dosing (see Geriatric Considerations).
Renal Impairment: Cl_{cr} <50 mL/minute: Avoid use.

Monitoring Laboratory Tests Serum and urinary uric acid, CBC

Monitoring and Teaching Issues

Physical Assessment: Assess effectiveness and interactions of other medications patient may be taking (see Contraindications and Drug Interactions). Monitor therapeutic response (eg, frequency and severity of gouty attacks), laboratory values, and adverse reactions (see Adverse Reactions and Overdose/Toxicology) at beginning of therapy and periodically with long-term use. Assess knowledge/teach patient appropriate use, interventions to reduce side effects, and adverse symptoms to report (see Patient Education). **Pregnancy risk factor C/D** - benefits of use should outweigh possible risks. Note breast-feeding caution.

Patient Education: Take as directed, with meals or antacids and a full glass of water. Avoid aspirin, aspirin-containing medications, or acetaminophen products and avoid large quantities of vitamin C. It is very important to maintain adequate hydration (2-3 L/day of fluids) to prevent kidney damage unless advised by prescriber to restrict fluids. You may experience nausea or vomiting (small, frequent meals, frequent mouth care, chewing gum, or sucking lozenges may help). Report skin rash, persistent stomach pain, painful urination or bloody urine, unusual bruising or bleeding, fatigue, or yellowing of eyes or skin. **Pregnancy/breast-feeding precautions:** Inform prescriber if you are or intend to become pregnant. Consult prescriber if breast-feeding.

Dietary Issues: Should be taken with food or milk.

Geriatric Considerations: Since sulfinpyrazone loses its effectiveness when the Cl_{cr} is <50 mL/minute, its usefulness in the elderly is limited.

SulfiSOXAZOLE (sul fi SOKS a zole)

U.S. Brand Names Gantrisin®; Truxazole®

Synonyms Sulfisoxazole Acetyl; Sulphafurazole

Generic Available Yes

Pharmacologic Category Antibiotic, Sulfonamide Derivative

Pregnancy Risk Factor B/D (near term)

Lactation Enters breast milk/compatible

Use Treatment of urinary tract infections, otitis media, *Chlamydia*; nocardiosis; treatment of acute pelvic inflammatory disease in prepubertal children; often used in combination with trimethoprim

Mechanism of Action/Effect Interferes with bacterial growth by inhibiting bacterial folic acid synthesis through competitive antagonism of PABA

Contraindications Hypersensitivity to sulfisoxazole, any sulfa drug, or any component of the formulation; porphyria; infants <2 months of age (sulfas compete with bilirubin for protein binding sites); patients with urinary obstruction; sunscreens containing PABA; pregnancy (at term)

Warnings/Precautions Use with caution in patients with G6PD deficiency (hemolysis may occur), hepatic or renal impairment; dosage modification required in patients with renal impairment; risk of crystalluria should be considered in patients with impaired renal function. Chemical similarities are present among sulfonamides, sulfonylureas, carbonic anhydrase inhibitors, thiazides, and loop diuretics (except ethacrynic acid). Use in patients with sulfonamide allergy is specifically contraindicated in product labeling, however, a risk of cross-reaction exists in patients with allergy to any of these compounds; avoid use when previous reaction has been severe.

Drug Interactions

Cytochrome P450 Effect: Substrate of **CYP2C8/9**; Inhibits CYP2C8/9

Decreased Effect: Decreased effect with PABA or PABA metabolites of drugs (eg, procaine, proparacaine, tetracaine), thiopental. May decrease cyclosporine levels.

Increased Effect/Toxicity: Increased effect of oral anticoagulants, methotrexate, and oral hypoglycemic agents. May increase phenytoin levels. Risk of adverse reactions (thrombocytopenia purpura) may be increased by thiazide.

Nutritional/Ethanol Interactions

Food: Interferes with folate absorption.

Herb/Nutraceutical: Avoid dong quai, St John's wort (may also cause photosensitization).

Effects on Lab Values False-positive protein in urine; false-positive urine glucose with Clinitest®

Adverse Reactions Frequency not defined.

Cardiovascular: Vasculitis

Central nervous system: Fever, dizziness, headache

Dermatologic: Itching, rash, photosensitivity, Lyell's syndrome, Stevens-Johnson syndrome

Endocrine & metabolic: Thyroid function disturbance

Gastrointestinal: Anorexia, nausea, vomiting, diarrhea

Genitourinary: Crystalluria, hematuria,

Hematologic: Granulocytopenia, leukopenia, thrombocytopenia, aplastic anemia, hemolytic anemia

Hepatic: Jaundice, hepatitis

Renal: Interstitial nephritis

Miscellaneous: Serum sickness-like reactions

Overdosage/Toxicology Symptoms of overdose include drowsiness, dizziness, anorexia, abdominal pain, nausea, vomiting, hemolytic anemia, acidosis, jaundice, fever, and agranulocytosis. Doses as little as 2-5 g/day may produce toxicity. The aniline radical is responsible for hematologic toxicity. High volume diuresis may aid in elimination and prevention of renal failure. Leucovorin 5-15 mg/day has been used to speed recovery of bone marrow.

Pharmacodynamics/Kinetics

Absorption: Sulfisoxazole acetyl is hydrolyzed in GI tract to sulfisoxazole which is readily absorbed

Half-Life Elimination: 4-7 hours; prolonged with renal impairment

Time to Peak: Serum: 2-3 hours

Metabolism: Hepatic via acetylation and glucuronide conjugation to inactive compounds

Formulations

Suspension, oral, pediatric, as acetyl: 500 mg/5 mL (480 mL) [raspberry flavor]

Tablet: 500 mg

Dosing

Adults: Susceptible infections: Oral: 2-4 g stat, 4-8 g/day in divided doses every 4-6 hours

Elderly: Oral: Urinary tract infections: 2 g stat, 2-8 g/day every 6 hours; adjust dose for Cl_{cr}. Single and 3-day dosing for urinary tract infections in the elderly are not reliable.

Pediatrics: Not for use in patients <2 months of age:

Children >2 months: Oral: Initial: 75 mg/kg, followed by 120-150 mg/kg/day in divided doses every 4-6 hours; not to exceed 6 g/day

Renal Impairment:

Cl_{cr} 10-50 mL/minutes: Administer every 8-12 hours.

Cl_{cr} <10 mL/minute: Administer every 12-24 hours.

Hemodialysis effects: >50% is removed by hemodialysis.

Administration

Oral: Administer around-the-clock to promote less variation in peak and trough serum levels.

Stability

Storage: Protect from light.

Monitoring Laboratory Tests CBC, urinalysis, renal function. Obtain specimen for culture prior to first dose.

Monitoring and Teaching Issues

Physical Assessment: Assess for allergy history prior to starting therapy. See Contraindications, Warnings/Precautions, and Dosing for use cautions. Assess potential for interactions with other prescriptions, OTC medications, or herbal products patient may be taking (see Drug Interactions). Monitor patient response (see Adverse Reactions and Overdose/Toxicology). Caution diabetic patients; may cause increased effect of oral hypoglycemics and may alter Clinitest® response (use another form of glucose testing). Teach patient proper use, possible side effects and interventions, and adverse symptoms to report (see Patient Education) on a regular basis during therapy. **Pregnancy risk factor B/D** - see Pregnancy Risk Factor for use cautions.

(Continued)

SulfiSOXAZOLE *(Continued)*

Patient Education: Inform prescriber of all prescriptions, OTC medications, or herbal products you are taking, and any allergies you have. Take as directed with a full glass of water, at regular intervals around-the-clock, on an empty stomach (1 hour before or 2 hours after a meal). Complete full course of therapy even if you are feeling better. Take a missed dose as soon as possible. If almost time for next dose, skip the missed dose and return to your regular schedule. Do not take a double dose. Maintain adequate hydration (2-3 L/day of fluids) to prevent kidney damage unless advised by prescriber to restrict fluids. If diabetic, this medication may cause increased effect of oral hypoglycemics - monitor glucose levels closely; may alter Clinitest® response; use of alternative method of glucose monitoring is preferable. May cause dizziness or headache (use caution when driving or engaging in tasks requiring alertness until response to drug is known); photosensitivity (use sunblock, wear protective clothing and eyewear, and avoid direct sunlight); or nausea, vomiting, or loss of appetite (small, frequent meals, frequent mouth care, sucking lozenges, or chewing gum may help). Report persistent nausea, vomiting, or diarrhea; opportunistic infection (sore throat, fever, vaginal itching or discharge, unusual bruising or bleeding, fatigue); blood in urine or change in urinary pattern; swelling of face, lips, or tongue; tightness in chest; bad cough; or other persistent adverse effects. **Pregnancy/breast-feeding precautions:** Inform prescriber if you are or intend to become pregnant.

Dietary Issues: Should be taken with a glass of water on an empty stomach.

Geriatric Considerations: Sulfisoxazole is an effective anti-infective agent. Most prescribers prefer the combination of sulfamethoxazole and trimethoprim for its dual mechanism of action. Trimethoprim penetrates the prostate. Adjust dose for renal function.

Related Information

FDA Name Differentiation Project: The Use of Tall-man Letters *on page 12*

Sulfisoxazole Acetyl *see* SulfiSOXAZOLE *on page 1264*

Sulfisoxazole and Erythromycin *see* Erythromycin and Sulfisoxazole *on page 486*

Sulfur and Sodium Sulfacetamide *see page 1522*

Sulindac (sul IN dak)

U.S. Brand Names Clinoril®

Generic Available Yes

Pharmacologic Category Nonsteroidal Anti-inflammatory Drug (NSAID)

Pregnancy Risk Factor B/D (3rd trimester)

Lactation Excretion in breast milk unknown

Use Management of inflammatory disease, rheumatoid disorders, acute gouty arthritis; structurally similar to indomethacin but acts like aspirin; safest NSAID for use in mild renal impairment

Mechanism of Action/Effect Inhibits prostaglandin synthesis by decreasing the activity of the enzyme, cyclooxygenase, which results in decreased formation of prostaglandin precursors

Contraindications Hypersensitivity to sulindac, any component of the formulation, aspirin or other NSAIDs; pregnancy (3rd trimester)

Warnings/Precautions Use with caution in patients with CHF, hypertension, dehydration, decreased renal or hepatic function, history of peptic ulcer disease or GI disease (bleeding or ulcers), or those receiving anticoagulants. Elderly are at a high risk for CNS and gastrointestinal adverse effects from NSAIDs. As many as 60% of elderly can develop peptic ulceration and/or hemorrhage asymptomatically.

Use lowest effective dose for shortest period possible. Use of NSAIDs can compromise existing renal function especially when Cl_{cr} is <30 mL/minute. Withhold for at least 4-6 half-lives prior to surgical or dental procedures. May have adverse effects on fetus. Use with caution with dehydration. Use in children is not recommended.

Drug Interactions

Decreased Effect: Decreased effect of diuretics, beta-blockers, hydralazine, and captopril.

Increased Effect/Toxicity: Increased toxicity with probenecid, NSAIDs. Increased toxicity of digoxin, anticoagulants, methotrexate, lithium, aminoglycosides antibiotics (reported in neonates), cyclosporine (increased nephrotoxicity), and potassium-sparing diuretics (hyperkalemia).

Nutritional/Ethanol Interactions

Ethanol: Avoid ethanol (may enhance gastric mucosal irritation).

Food: Food may decrease the rate but not the extent of oral absorption. The therapeutic effect of sulindac may be decreased if taken with food.

Herb/Nutraceutical: Avoid cat's claw, dong quai, evening primrose, feverfew, garlic, ginger, ginkgo, red clover, horse chestnut, green tea, ginseng (all have additional antiplatelet activity).

Effects on Lab Values ↑ chloride (S), sodium (S), bleeding time

Adverse Reactions

1% to 10%:

Cardiovascular: Edema

Central nervous system: Dizziness, headache, nervousness

Dermatologic: Pruritus, rash

Gastrointestinal: GI pain, heartburn, nausea, vomiting, diarrhea, constipation, flatulence, anorexia, abdominal cramps

Otic: Tinnitus

<1% (Limited to important or life-threatening): Agranulocytosis, anaphylaxis, angioneurotic edema, aplastic anemia, arrhythmia, aseptic meningitis, bone marrow depression, bronchial spasm, CHF, crystalluria, depression, dyspnea, erythema multiforme, exfoliative dermatitis, GI bleeding, GI perforation, hemolytic anemia, hepatic failure, hepatitis, hypersensitivity reaction, hypertension, increased prothrombin time, interstitial nephritis, jaundice, leukopenia, nephrotic syndrome, neutropenia, pancreatitis, peptic ulcer, proteinuria, psychosis, renal failure, renal impairment, seizures, Stevens-Johnson syndrome, thrombocytopenia, toxic epidermal necrolysis

Overdosage/Toxicology Symptoms of overdose include dizziness, vomiting, nausea, abdominal pain, hypotension, coma, stupor, metabolic acidosis, leukocytosis, and renal failure. Management of NSAID intoxication is supportive and symptomatic. Seizures tend to be short-lived and often do not require drug treatment.

Pharmacodynamics/Kinetics

Absorption: 90%

Half-Life Elimination: Parent drug: 7 hours; Active metabolite: 18 hours

Metabolism: Hepatic; prodrug requiring metabolic activation to sulfide metabolite (active) for therapeutic effects and to sulfone metabolites (inactive)

Onset: Analgesic: ~1 hour

Duration: 12-24 hours

Formulations Tablet: 150 mg, 200 mg

Dosing

Adults & Elderly: Maximum therapeutic response may not be realized for up to 3 weeks.

Pain, inflammation: Oral: 150-200 mg twice daily or 300-400 mg once daily; not to exceed 400 mg/day.

Pediatrics: Dose not established

Hepatic Impairment: Dose reduction is necessary.

Administration

Oral: Should be administered with food or milk.

Monitoring Laboratory Tests Liver enzymes, BUN, serum creatinine, CBC, platelets

Monitoring and Teaching Issues

Physical Assessment: Assess effectiveness and interactions of other medications patient may be taking (see Contraindications and Drug Interactions). Monitor laboratory tests (see Monitoring Laboratory Tests), therapeutic response according to purpose for therapy, and adverse reactions (eg, GI bleeding, hepatotoxicity, ototoxicity) at beginning of therapy and periodically throughout therapy (see Warnings/Precautions, Adverse Reactions, and Overdose/Toxicology). Schedule ophthalmic evaluations for patients who are taking NSAIDs for long periods of time. Assess knowledge/teach patient appropriate use, interventions to reduce side effects, and adverse symptoms to report (see Patient Education). **Pregnancy risk factor B/D** - see Pregnancy Risk Factor for use cautions. Note breast-feeding caution.

Patient Education: Take this medication exactly as directed; do not increase dose without consulting prescriber. Take with food or milk to reduce GI distress. Maintain adequate hydration (2-3 L/day of fluids) unless advised by prescriber to restrict fluids. Do not use alcohol, aspirin or aspirin-containing medication, or any other anti-inflammatory medications without consulting prescriber. Regularly scheduled ophthalmic exams are advised with long-term use of NSAIDs. You may experience dizziness, nervousness, or headache (use caution when driving or engaging in tasks requiring alertness until response to drug is known); nausea, vomiting, or heartburn (small, frequent meals, frequent mouth care, sucking lozenges, or chewing gum may help); or constipation (increased exercise, fluids, fruit, or fiber may help). GI bleeding, ulceration, or perforation can occur with or without pain; discontinue medication and contact prescriber if persistent abdominal pain, cramping, or blood in stool occurs. Report breathlessness or difficulty breathing; unusual bruising or bleeding; blood in urine, stool, mouth, or vomitus; unusual fatigue; skin rash or itching; change in urinary pattern; or change in hearing or ringing in ears. **Pregnancy/breast-feeding precautions:** Inform prescriber if you are or intend to become pregnant. This drug should not be used in the 3rd trimester of pregnancy. Consult prescriber if breast-feeding.

Dietary Issues: Drug may cause GI upset, bleeding, ulceration, perforation; take with food or milk to minimize GI upset.

Geriatric Considerations: Elderly are at high risk for adverse effects from NSAIDs. As much as 60% of elderly who develop GI complications can develop peptic ulceration and/or hemorrhage asymptomatically. The concomitant use of H_2 blockers, omeprazole, and sucralfate is not effective as prophylaxis with the exception of NSAID-induced duodenal ulcers which may be prevented by the use of ranitidine. Misoprostol is the only prophylactic agent proven effective. Also, concomitant disease and drug use contribute to the risk for GI adverse effects. Use lowest effective dose for shortest period possible. Consider renal function decline with age. Use of NSAIDs can compromise existing renal function especially when Cl_{cr} is ≤30 mL/minute. Tinnitus may be a difficult and unreliable indication of toxicity due to age-related hearing loss or eighth cranial nerve damage. CNS adverse effects such as confusion, agitation, and hallucination are generally seen in overdose or high-dose situations, but elderly may demonstrate these adverse effects at lower doses than younger adults.

Related Information

Nonsalicylate/Nonsteroidal Anti-inflammatory Comparison *on page 1587*

Sulphafurazole *see* SulfiSOXAZOLE *on page 1264*

Sumatriptan Succinate (SOO ma trip tan SUKS i nate)

U.S. Brand Names Imitrex®

Generic Available No

Pharmacologic Category Serotonin 5-HT_{1D} Receptor Agonist

Pregnancy Risk Factor C

Lactation Enters breast milk/use caution (AAP rates "compatible")

Use Acute treatment of migraine with or without aura

Sumatriptan injection: Acute treatment of cluster headache episodes

Mechanism of Action/Effect Selective agonist for serotonin (5-HT_{1D} receptor) in cranial arteries to cause vasoconstriction and reduces sterile inflammation associated with antidromic neuronal transmission correlating with relief of migraine

Contraindications Hypersensitivity to sumatriptan or any component of the formulation; patients with ischemic heart disease or signs or symptoms of ischemic heart disease (including Prinzmetal's angina, angina pectoris, myocardial infarction, silent myocardial

(Continued)

Sumatriptan Succinate *(Continued)*

ischemia); cerebrovascular syndromes (including strokes, transient ischemic attacks); peripheral vascular syndromes (including ischemic bowel disease); uncontrolled hypertension; use within 24 hours of ergotamine derivatives; use with in 24 hours of another 5-HT_1 agonist; concurrent administration or within 2 weeks of discontinuing an MAO inhibitor, specifically MAO type A inhibitors; management of hemiplegic or basilar migraine; prophylactic treatment of migraine; severe hepatic impairment; not for I.V. administration

Warnings/Precautions Sumatriptan is indicated only in patients ≥18 years of age with a clear diagnosis of migraine or cluster headache. Cardiac events, cerebral/subarachnoid hemorrhage, and stroke have been reported with 5-HT_1 agonist administration. Do not give to patients with risk factors for CAD until a cardiovascular evaluation has been performed. If the evaluation is satisfactory, the healthcare provider should administer the first dose and cardiovascular status should be periodically evaluated.

Significant elevation in blood pressure, including hypertensive crisis, has also been reported on rare occasions in patients with and without a history of hypertension. Vasospasm-related reactions have been reported other than coronary artery vasospasm. Peripheral vascular ischemia and colonic ischemia with abdominal pain and bloody diarrhea have occurred.

Use with caution in patients with history of seizure disorder. Safety and efficacy in pediatric patients have not been established.

Pregnancy risk C.

Drug Interactions

Increased Effect/Toxicity: Increased toxicity with ergot-containing drugs, avoid use, wait 24 hours from last ergot containing drug (dihydroergotamine, or methysergide) before administering sumatriptan. MAO inhibitors decrease clearance of sumatriptan increasing the risk of systemic sumatriptan toxic effects. Sumatriptan may enhance CNS toxic effects when taken with selective serotonin reuptake inhibitors (SSRIs) like fluoxetine, fluvoxamine, paroxetine, or sertraline.

Adverse Reactions

>10%:

Central nervous system: Dizziness (injection 12%), warm/hot sensation (injection 11%)

Gastrointestinal: Bad taste (nasal spray 13% to 24%), nausea (nasal spray 11% to 13%), vomiting (nasal spray 11% to 13%)

Local: Injection: Pain at the injection site (59%)

Neuromuscular & skeletal: Tingling (injection 13%)

1% to 10%:

Cardiovascular: Chest pain/tightness/heaviness/pressure (injection 2% to 3%, tablet 1% to 2%)

Central nervous system: Burning (injection 7%), dizziness (nasal spray 1% to 2%, tablet >1%), feeling of heaviness (injection 7%), flushing (injection 7%), pressure sensation (injection 7%), feeling of tightness (injection 5%), numbness (injection 5%), drowsiness (injection 3%, tablet >1%), malaise/fatigue (tablet 2% to 3%, injection 1%), feeling strange (injection 2%), headache (injection 2%, tablet >1%), tight feeling in head (injection 2%), nonspecified pain (tablet 1% to 2%, placebo 1%), vertigo (tablet <1% to 2%, nasal spray 1% to 2%), migraine (tablet >1%), sleepiness (tablet >1%), cold sensation (injection 1%), anxiety (injection 1%)

Gastrointestinal: Nausea (tablet >1%), vomiting (tablet >1%), hyposalivation (tablet >1%), abdominal discomfort (injection 1%), dysphagia (injection 1%)

Neuromuscular & skeletal: Neck, throat, and jaw pain/tightness/pressure (injection 2% to 5%, tablet 2% to 3%), mouth/tongue discomfort (injection 5%), paresthesia (tablet 3% to 5%), weakness (injection 5%), myalgia (injection 2%), muscle cramps (injection 1%)

Ocular: Vision alterations (injection 1%)

Respiratory: Nasal disorder/discomfort (nasal spray 2% to 4%, injection 2%), throat discomfort (injection 3%, nasal spray 1% to 2%)

Miscellaneous: Warm/cold sensation (tablet 2% to 3%, placebo 2%), nonspecified pressure/tightness/heaviness (tablet 1% to 3%, placebo 2%), diaphoresis (injection 2%)

<1% (Limited to important or life-threatening): Abdominal aortic aneurysm, acute renal failure, agitation, anaphylactoid reactions, anaphylaxis, angioneurotic edema, arrhythmia, atrial fibrillation, bronchospasm, cerebral ischemia, deafness, diarrhea, dysphagia, dystonic reaction, ECG changes, hallucinations, heart block, hematuria, hemolytic anemia, hypersensitivity reactions increased ICP, intestinal obstruction, ischemic colitis, nose/throat hemorrhage, numbness of tongue, optic neuropathy (ischemic), pancytopenia, paresthesia, photosensitivity, Prinzmetal's angina, pruritus, psychomotor disorders, pulmonary embolism, rash, Raynaud syndrome, seizures, shock, stroke, subarachnoid hemorrhage, swallowing disorders, syncope, thrombocytopenia, transient myocardial ischemia, vasculitis, vision loss, visual disturbance (accommodation disorder), xerostomia

Overdosage/Toxicology Single oral doses ≤400 mg, injectable doses ≤16 mg, and nasal doses of 40 mg have been reported without adverse effects. Treatment of overdose should be supportive and symptomatic. Monitor for at least 12 hours or until signs and symptoms subside. It is not known if hemodialysis or peritoneal dialysis is effective.

Pharmacodynamics/Kinetics

Bioavailability: S.C.: 97% ± 16% of that following I.V. injection

Half-Life Elimination: Injection, tablet: 2.5 hours; Nasal spray: 2 hours

Time to Peak: Serum: 5-20 minutes

Onset: ~30 minutes

Formulations

Injection: 12 mg/mL (0.5 mL, 2 mL)

Solution, intranasal spray [100 μL unit dose spray device]: 5 mg, 20 mg

Tablet: 25 mg, 50 mg, 100 mg

Dosing

Adults: Migraine, cluster headache (injection):

Oral: 25 mg (taken with fluids); maximum recommended dose is 100 mg. If a satisfactory response has not been obtained at 2 hours, a second dose of up to 100 mg may be given. Efficacy of this second dose has not been examined. If a headache returns, additional doses may be taken at intervals of at least 2 hours up to a daily maximum of 300 mg. There is no evidence that an initial dose of 100 mg provides substantially greater relief than 25 mg.

Intranasal: Single dose of 5, 10, or 20 mg administered in one nostril; a 10 mg dose may be achieved by administration of a single 5 mg dose in each nostril; if headache returns, the dose may be repeated once after 2 hours, not to exceed a total daily dose of 40 mg

S.C.: 6 mg; a second injection may be administered at least 1 hour after the initial dose, but not more than two injections in a 24-hour period

Elderly: Due to increased risk of CAD, decreased hepatic function, and more pronounced blood pressure increases, use of the tablet dosage form in elderly patients is not recommended. Use of the nasal spray has not been studied in the elderly. Pharmacokinetics of injectable sumatriptan in the elderly are similar to healthy patients.

Renal Impairment: Dosage adjustment is not necessary.

Hepatic Impairment: Bioavailability of oral sumatriptan is increased with liver disease. If treatment is needed, do not exceed single doses of 50 mg. The nasal spray has not been studied in patients with hepatic impairment, however, because the spray does not undergo first-pass metabolism, levels would not be expected to alter. Use of all dosage forms is contraindicated with severe hepatic impairment.

Administration

Oral: Oral: Should be taken with fluids as soon as symptoms to appear.

I.V.: Do **not** administer I.V.; may cause coronary vasospasm.

Other: Administer subcutaneously.

Stability

Storage: Store at 2°C to 20°C (36°F to 86°F). Protect from light.

Monitoring and Teaching Issues

Physical Assessment: See Contraindications, Warnings/Precautions (clear diagnosis of migraine), and Dosing for use cautions. Assess potential for interactions with other prescriptions, OTC medications, or herbal products patient may be taking (eg, ergot-containing drugs - see Drug Interactions). Assess therapeutic effectiveness and adverse response (see Adverse Reactions and Overdose/Toxicology). Teach patient proper use according to formulation (eg, appropriate injection technique and syringe/needle disposal), possible side effects and appropriate interventions, and adverse symptoms to report (see Patient Education). **Pregnancy risk factor C** - benefits of use should outweigh possible risks. Note breast-feeding caution.

Patient Education: Inform prescriber of all prescription (including oral contraceptives) and OTC medications or herbal products you are taking, and any allergies you have. Take at first sign of migraine attack. This drug is to be used to reduce your migraine, not to prevent or reduce the number of attacks. Follow exact instructions for use.

Nasal spray: Administer dose into one nostril. If headache returns or is not fully resolved after the first dose, the dose may be repeated after 2 hours. **Do not exceed 40 mg in 24 hours.**

Oral: If headache returns or is not fully resolved after first dose, the dose may be repeated after 2 hours. **Do not exceed 200 mg in 24 hours.** Take whole with fluids.

S.C.: If headache returns or is not fully resolved after first dose, the dose may be repeated after 1 hour. **Do not exceed two injections in 24 hours.**

All forms: Do not take any form of this drug within 24 hours of any other migraine medication without consulting prescriber. May cause dizziness, fatigue, or drowsiness (use caution when driving or engaging in tasks that require alertness until response to drug is known); or nausea or vomiting (small, frequent meals, frequent mouth care, chewing gum, or sucking on lozenges may help). Report chest tightness or pain; excessive drowsiness; acute abdominal pain; skin rash or burning sensation; muscle weakness, soreness, or numbness; difficulty breathing; or any other persistent adverse reactions. **Pregnancy/breast-feeding precautions:** Inform prescriber if you are or intend to become pregnant. Consult prescriber if breast-feeding.

Geriatric Considerations: Use cautiously in the elderly, particularly since many elderly have cardiovascular disease which would put them at risk for cardiovascular adverse effects. Safety and efficacy in the elderly (>65 years) have not been established. Pharmacokinetic disposition is, however, similar to that in young adults.

Related Information

Antimigraine Drugs *on page 1557*

Summer's Eve® SpecialCare™ Medicated Anti-Itch Cream [OTC] *see* Hydrocortisone *on page 673*

Sumycin® *see* Tetracycline *on page 1296*

Superdophilus® [OTC] *see Lactobacillus on page 766*

Suprax® *see* Cefixime *on page 239*

Suprofen *see page 1461*

Sureprin 81™ [OTC] *see* Aspirin *on page 121*

Surfak® [OTC] *see* Docusate *on page 432*

Surgicel® *see page 1461*

Surmontil® *see* Trimipramine *on page 1368*

Suspen® *see* Penicillin V Potassium *on page 1048*

Sustiva® *see* Efavirenz *on page 459*

Suxamethonium Chloride *see* Succinylcholine *on page 1252*

Swim-Ear® *see page 1519*

Syllact® [OTC] *see* Psyllium *on page 1152*

Symax SL *see* Hyoscyamine *on page 685*

Symax SR *see* Hyoscyamine *on page 685*

Symbols & Abbreviations Used in This Handbook *see page 13*

Symmetrel® *see* Amantadine *on page 72*
Synacort® *see* Topical Corticosteroids *on page 1334*
Synalar® *see* Topical Corticosteroids *on page 1334*
Synalar-HP® *see* Topical Corticosteroids *on page 1334*
Synalgos®-DC *see* Dihydrocodeine Compound *on page 415*
Synarel® *see* Nafarelin *on page 940*
Synemol® *see* Topical Corticosteroids *on page 1334*
Synercid® *see* Quinupristin and Dalfopristin *on page 1166*
Synthroid® *see* Levothyroxine *on page 797*
Syprine® *see page 1460*
T_4 *see* Levothyroxine *on page 797*
Tac™-3 *see* Triamcinolone *on page 1356*
Tac™-40 *see* Triamcinolone *on page 1356*

Tacrine (TAK reen)

U.S. Brand Names Cognex®

Synonyms Tacrine Hydrochloride; Tetrahydroaminoacrine; THA

Generic Available No

Pharmacologic Category Acetylcholinesterase Inhibitor (Central)

Pregnancy Risk Factor C

Lactation Excretion in breast milk unknown/not recommended

Use Treatment of mild to moderate dementia of the Alzheimer's type

Mechanism of Action/Effect Centrally-acting cholinesterase inhibitor. It elevates acetylcholine in cerebral cortex by slowing the degradation of acetylcholine.

Contraindications Hypersensitivity to tacrine, acridine derivatives, or any component of the formulation; patients previously treated with tacrine who developed jaundice

Warnings/Precautions The use of tacrine has been associated with elevations in serum transaminases; serum transaminases (specifically ALT) must be monitored throughout therapy; use extreme caution in patients with current evidence of a history of abnormal liver function tests; use caution in patients with urinary tract obstruction (bladder outlet obstruction or prostatic hyperplasia), asthma, and sick-sinus syndrome (tacrine may cause bradycardia). Also, patients with cardiovascular disease, asthma, or peptic ulcer should use cautiously. Use with caution in patients with a history of seizures. May cause nausea, vomiting, or loose stools. Abrupt discontinuation or dosage decrease may worsen cognitive function. May be associated with neutropenia. Pregnancy risk C.

Drug Interactions

Cytochrome P450 Effect: Substrate of **CYP1A2**; Inhibits CYP1A2

Decreased Effect: Enzyme inducers and cigarette smoking may reduce tacrine plasma levels via enzyme induction (CYP1A2). Tacrine may worsen Parkinson's disease and inhibit the effects of levodopa. Tacrine may antagonize the therapeutic effect of anticholinergic agents (benztropine, trihexphenidyl).

Increased Effect/Toxicity: Tacrine in combination with other cholinergic agents (eg, ambenonium, edrophonium, neostigmine, pyridostigmine, bethanechol), will likely produce additive cholinergic effects. Tacrine in combination with beta-blockers may produce additive bradycardia. Tacrine may increase the levels/effect of succinylcholine and theophylline. in elevated plasma levels. Fluvoxamine, enoxacin, and cimetidine increase tacrine concentrations via enzyme inhibition (CYP1A2).

Nutritional/Ethanol Interactions Food: Food decreases bioavailability.

Adverse Reactions

>10%:
- Central nervous system: Headache, dizziness
- Gastrointestinal: Nausea, vomiting, diarrhea
- Miscellaneous: Elevated transaminases

1% to 10%:
- Cardiovascular: Flushing
- Central nervous system: Confusion, ataxia, insomnia, somnolence, depression, anxiety, fatigue
- Dermatologic: Rash
- Gastrointestinal: Dyspepsia, anorexia, abdominal pain, flatulence, constipation, weight loss
- Neuromuscular & skeletal: Myalgia, tremor
- Respiratory: Rhinitis

Overdosage/Toxicology Provide general supportive measures. Can cause cholinergic crisis characterized by severe nausea, vomiting, salivation, sweating, bradycardia, hypotension, collapse, and convulsions. Increased muscle weakness is a possibility and may result in death if respiratory muscles are involved.

Tertiary anticholinergics, such as atropine, may be used as an antidote for overdose. I.V. atropine sulfate titrated to effect is recommended at an initial dose of 1-2 mg I.V. with subsequent doses based upon clinical response. Atypical increases in blood pressure and heart rate have been reported with other cholinomimetics when coadministered with quaternary anticholinergics such as glycopyrrolate.

Pharmacodynamics/Kinetics

Absorption: Oral: Rapid

Bioavailability: Absolute: 17%

Half-Life Elimination: Serum: 2-4 hours; Steady-state: 24-36 hours

Time to Peak: Plasma: 1-2 hours

Metabolism: Extensively by CYP450 to multiple metabolites; first pass effect

Formulations Capsule, as hydrochloride: 10 mg, 20 mg, 30 mg, 40 mg

Dosing

Adults & Elderly: Alzheimer's disease: Oral: Initial: 10 mg 4 times/day; may increase by 40 mg/day adjusted every 6 weeks; maximum: 160 mg/day; best administered separate from meal times.

Dose adjustment based upon transaminase elevations:

ALT ≤3 x ULN*: Continue titration

ALT >3 to ≤5 x ULN*: Decrease dose by 40 mg/day, resume when ALT returns to normal

ALT >5 x ULN*: Stop treatment, may rechallenge upon return of ALT to normal

*ULN = upper limit of normal

Patients with clinical jaundice confirmed by elevated total bilirubin (>3 mg/dL) should not be rechallenged with tacrine

Hepatic Impairment: Patients with clinical jaundice confirmed by elevated total bilirubin (>3 mg/dL) should not be rechallenged with tacrine.

Monitoring Laboratory Tests ALT (SGPT) levels and other liver enzymes at least every other week from weeks 4-16 weeks, then monitor once every 3 months

Monitoring and Teaching Issues

Physical Assessment: Assess bladder and sphincter adequacy prior to administering medication. Assess other medications patient may be taking for effectiveness and interactions (see Drug Interactions). Monitor laboratory tests throughout therapy (see above), therapeutic effect, and adverse reactions (eg, cholinergic crisis - see Warnings/Precautions, Adverse Reactions, and Overdose/Toxicology). Assess knowledge/teach patient appropriate use, interventions to reduce side effects, and adverse symptoms to report (see Patient Education). **Pregnancy risk factor C** - benefits of use should outweigh possible risks. Breast-feeding is not recommended.

Patient Education: This medication will not cure the disease, but may help reduce symptoms. Use as directed; do not increase dose or discontinue without consulting prescriber. Maintain adequate hydration (2-3 L/day of fluids) unless advised by prescriber to restrict fluids. May cause dizziness, sedation, or hypotension (rise slowly from sitting or lying position and use caution when driving or climbing stairs); vomiting or loss of appetite (small, frequent meals, frequent mouth care, or chewing gum, or sucking lozenges may help); or diarrhea (boiled milk, yogurt, or buttermilk may help). Report persistent abdominal discomfort; significantly increased salivation, sweating, tearing, or urination; flushed skin; chest pain or palpitations; acute headache; unresolved diarrhea; excessive fatigue, insomnia, dizziness, or depression; increased muscle, joint, or body pain; vision changes or blurred vision; shortness of breath or wheezing; or signs of jaundice (yellowing of eyes or skin, dark colored urine or light colored stool, abdominal pain, or easy fatigue). **Pregnancy/breast-feeding precautions:** Inform prescriber if you are or intend to become pregnant. Breast-feeding is not recommended.

Dietary Issues: Give with food if GI side effects are intolerable.

Geriatric Considerations: Tacrine is currently FDA-approved for the treatment of Alzheimer's disease, it is clearly not a cure. At least 25% of patients may not tolerate the drug and only 50% of patients demonstrate some improvement in symptoms or a slowing of deterioration. While worth a trial in mild to moderate dementia of the Alzheimer's type, patients and their families must be counseled about the limitations of the drug and the importance of regular monitoring of liver function tests. No specific dosage adjustments are necessary due to age.

Tacrine Hydrochloride *see* Tacrine *on page 1270*

Tacrolimus (ta KROE li mus)

U.S. Brand Names Prograf®; Protopic®

Synonyms FK506

Generic Available No

Pharmacologic Category Immunosuppressant Agent; Topical Skin Product

Pregnancy Risk Factor C

Lactation Enters breast milk/contraindicated

Use

Oral/injection: Potent immunosuppressive drug used in liver or kidney transplant recipients

Topical: Moderate to severe atopic dermatitis in patients not responsive to conventional therapy or when conventional therapy is not appropriate

Use - Unlabeled/Investigational Potent immunosuppressive drug used in heart, lung, small bowel transplant recipients; immunosuppressive drug for peripheral stem cell/bone marrow transplantation

Mechanism of Action/Effect Suppresses cellular immunity (inhibits T-lymphocyte activation)

Contraindications Hypersensitivity to tacrolimus or any component of the formulation

Warnings/Precautions

Oral/injection: Insulin-dependent post-transplant diabetes mellitus (PTDM) has been reported (1% to 20%); risk increases in African-American and Hispanic kidney transplant patients. Increased susceptibility to infection and the possible development of lymphoma may occur. Nephrotoxicity and neurotoxicity have been reported, especially with higher doses; avoid concurrent use with cyclosporine. May cause seizures. Use caution in renal or hepatic dysfunction, dosing adjustments may be required. Delay initiation if postoperative oliguria occurs. Use may be associated with the development of hypertension (common). Myocardial hypertrophy has been reported (rare). Each mL of injection contains polyoxyl 60 hydrogenated castor oil (HCO-60) (200 mg) and dehydrated alcohol USP 80% v/v. Anaphylaxis has been reported with the injection, use should be reserved for those patients not able to take oral medications.

Topical: Infections at the treatment site should be cleared prior to therapy. Patients with atopic dermatitis are predisposed to skin infections, including eczema herpeticum, varicella zoster, and herpes simplex. Discontinue use in patients with unknown cause of lymphadenopathy or acute infectious mononucleosis. Not recommended for use in patients with Netherton's syndrome. Safety not established in patients with generalized erythroderma.

Pregnancy risk C.

(Continued)

Tacrolimus *(Continued)*

Drug Interactions

Cytochrome P450 Effect: Substrate of **CYP3A4**; Inhibits CYP3A4

Decreased Effect:

Antacids: Impaired tacrolimus absorption (separate administration by at least 2 hours).

Agents which may decrease tacrolimus plasma concentrations and reduce the therapeutic effect include rifampin, rifabutin, phenytoin, phenobarbital, and carbamazepine.

St John's wort may reduce tacrolimus serum concentrations (avoid concurrent use).

Increased Effect/Toxicity: Amphotericin B and other nephrotoxic antibiotics have the potential to increase tacrolimus-associated nephrotoxicity. Agents which may increase tacrolimus plasma concentrations resulting in toxicity are erythromycin, clarithromycin, clotrimazole, fluconazole, itraconazole, ketoconazole, diltiazem, nicardipine, verapamil, bromocriptine, cimetidine, cisapride, danazol, metoclopramide, methylprednisolone, and cyclosporine (synergistic immunosuppression). Voriconazole may increase tacrolimus serum concentrations; decrease tacrolimus dosage by 66% when initiating voriconazole.

Nutritional/Ethanol Interactions

Food: Decreases rate and extent of absorption. High-fat meals have most pronounced effect (35% decrease in AUC, 77% decrease in C_{max}). Grapefruit juice, CYP3A4 inhibitor, may increase serum level and/or toxicity of tacrolimus; avoid concurrent use.

Herb/Nutraceutical: St John's wort: May reduce tacrolimus serum concentrations (avoid concurrent use).

Adverse Reactions

Oral, I.V.:

≥15%:

Cardiovascular: Chest pain, hypertension

Central nervous system: Dizziness, headache, insomnia, tremor (headache and tremor are associated with high whole blood concentrations and may respond to decreased dosage)

Dermatologic: Pruritus, rash

Endocrine & metabolic: Diabetes mellitus, hyperglycemia, hyperkalemia, hyperlipemia, hypomagnesemia, hypophosphatemia

Gastrointestinal: Abdominal pain, constipation, diarrhea, dyspepsia, nausea, vomiting

Genitourinary: Urinary tract infection

Hematologic: Anemia, leukocytosis, thrombocytopenia

Hepatic: Ascites

Neuromuscular & skeletal: Arthralgia, back pain, weakness, paresthesia

Renal: Abnormal kidney function, increased creatinine, oliguria, urinary tract infection, increased BUN

Respiratory: Atelectasis, dyspnea, increased cough

3% to 15% (Limited to important or life-threatening):

Cardiovascular: Abnormal EKG, angina pectoris, deep thrombophlebitis, hemorrhage, hypotension, postural hypotension, thrombosis

Central nervous system: Agitation, amnesia, anxiety, confusion, depression, encephalopathy, hallucinations, psychosis, somnolence

Dermatologic: Acne, alopecia, exfoliative dermatitis, hirsutism, photosensitivity reaction, skin discoloration

Endocrine & metabolic: Cushing's syndrome, decreased bicarbonate, decreased serum iron, diabetes mellitus, hypercalcemia, hypercholesterolemia, hyperphosphatemia

Gastrointestinal: Dysphagia, esophagitis, GI perforation/hemorrhage, ileus

Hematologic: Coagulation disorder, decreased prothrombin, leukopenia

Hepatic: Cholangitis, jaundice, hepatitis

Neuromuscular & skeletal: Incoordination, myasthenia, neuropathy, osteoporosis

Respiratory: Asthma, pneumothorax, pulmonary edema

Miscellaneous: Abscess, allergic reaction, flu-like syndrome, peritonitis, sepsis

Postmarketing and/or case reports (Limited to important or life-threatening): Acute renal failure, anaphylaxis, coma, deafness, delirium, hearing loss, hemolytic-uremic syndrome, leukoencephalopathy, lymphoproliferative disorder (related to EBV), myocardial hypertrophy (associated with ventricular dysfunction), pancreatitis, seizures, Stevens-Johnson syndrome, thrombocytopenic purpura, torsade de pointes

Topical:

>10%:

Central nervous system: Headache (5% to 20%), fever (1% to 21%)

Dermatologic: Skin burning (43% to 58%), pruritus (41% to 46%), erythema (12% to 28%)

Respiratory: Increased cough (18% children)

Miscellaneous: Flu-like syndrome (23% to 28%), allergic reaction (4% to 12%)

Overdosage/Toxicology Symptoms are extensions of immunosuppressive activity and adverse effects. Symptomatic and supportive treatment is required. Hemodialysis is not effective.

Pharmacodynamics/Kinetics

Absorption: Better in resected patients with a closed stoma; unlike cyclosporine, clamping of the T-tube in liver transplant patients does not alter trough concentrations or AUC

Oral: Incomplete and variable; food within 15 minutes of administration decreases absorption (27%)

Topical: Serum concentrations range from undetectable to 20 ng/mL (<5 ng/mL in majority of adult patients studied)

Bioavailability: Oral: Adults: 7% to 28%, Children: 10% to 52%; Topical: <0.5%; Absolute: Unknown

Half-Life Elimination: Variable, 21-61 hours in healthy volunteers

Time to Peak: 0.5-4 hours

Metabolism: Extensively hepatic via CYP3A4 to eight possible metabolites (major metabolite, 31-demethyl tacrolimus, shows same activity as tacrolimus *in vitro*)

Formulations

Capsule: 0.5 mg, 1 mg, 5 mg

Injection: 5 mg/mL (1 mL) [contains alcohol and surfactant]
Ointment, topical: 0.03% (30 g, 60 g); 0.1% (30 g, 60g)

Dosing

Adults & Elderly:

Kidney transplant:

Oral: Initial dose: 0.2 mg/kg/day in 2 divided doses, given every 12 hours; initial dose may be given within 24 hours of transplant, but should be delayed until renal function has recovered; African-American patients may require larger doses to maintain trough concentration

Typical whole blood trough concentrations: Months 1-3: 7- 20 ng/mL; months 4-12: 5-15 ng/mL

I.V.: **Note:** I.V. route should only be used in patients not able to take oral medications, anaphylaxis has been reported. Initial dose: 0.03-0.05 mg/kg/day as a continuous infusion; begin no sooner than 6 hours post-transplant, starting at lower end of the dosage range; adjunctive therapy with corticosteroids is recommended; continue only until oral medication can be tolerated

Liver transplant:

Oral: Initial dose: 0.1-0.15 mg/kg/day in 2 divided doses, given every 12 hours; begin oral dose no sooner than 6 hours post-transplant; adjunctive therapy with corticosteroids is recommended; if switching from I.V. to oral, the oral dose should be started 8-12 hours after stopping the infusion

Typical whole blood trough concentrations: Months 1-12: 5-20 ng/mL

I.V.: **Note:** I.V. route should only be used in patients not able to take oral medications, anaphylaxis has been reported. Initial dose: 0.03-0.05 mg/kg/day as a continuous infusion; begin no sooner than 6 hours post-transplant starting at lower end of the dosage range; adjunctive therapy with corticosteroids is recommended; continue only until oral medication can be tolerated

Prevention of graft-vs-host disease: I.V.: 0.03 mg/kg/day as continuous infusion

Atopic dermatitis (moderate to severe): Topical: Apply 0.03% or 0.1% ointment to affected area twice daily; rub in gently and completely; continue applications for 1 week after symptoms have cleared

Pediatrics:

Liver transplant: Patients without pre-existing renal or hepatic dysfunction have required and tolerated higher doses than adults to achieve similar blood concentrations. It is recommended that therapy be initiated at high end of the recommended adult I.V. and oral dosing ranges; dosage adjustments may be required.

Oral: Initial dose: 0.15-0.20 mg/kg/day in 2 divided doses, given every 12 hours; begin oral dose no sooner than 6 hours post-transplant; adjunctive therapy with corticosteroids is recommended; if switching from I.V. to oral, the oral dose should be started 8-12 hours after stopping the infusion

Typical whole blood trough concentrations: Months 1-12: 5-20 ng/mL

I.V.: **Note:** I.V. route should only be used in patients not able to take oral medications, anaphylaxis has been reported. Initial dose: 0.03-0.05 mg/kg/day as a continuous infusion; begin no sooner than 6 hours post-transplant; adjunctive therapy with corticosteroids is recommended; continue only until oral medication can be tolerated

Moderate to severe atopic dermatitis: Topical: Children ≥2 years: Apply 0.03% ointment to affected area twice daily; rub in gently and completely; continue applications for 1 week after symptoms have cleared

Renal Impairment: Evidence suggests that lower doses should be used. Patients should receive doses at the lowest value of the recommended I.V. and oral dosing ranges. Further reductions in dose below these ranges may be required. Tacrolimus therapy should usually be delayed up to 48 hours or longer in patients with postoperative oliguria.

Hemodialysis: Not removed by hemodialysis; supplemental dose is not necessary.

Peritoneal dialysis: Significant drug removal is unlikely based on physiochemical characteristics.

Hepatic Impairment: Use of tacrolimus in liver transplant recipients experiencing post-transplant hepatic impairment may be associated with increased risk of developing renal insufficiency related to high whole blood levels of tacrolimus. The presence of moderate-to-severe hepatic dysfunction (serum bilirubin >2 mg/dL) appears to affect the metabolism of FK506. The half-life of the drug was prolonged and the clearance reduced after I.V. administration. The bioavailability of FK506 was also increased after oral administration. The higher plasma concentrations as determined by ELISA, in patients with severe hepatic dysfunction are probably due to the accumulation of FK506 metabolites of lower activity. These patients should be monitored closely and dosage adjustments should be considered. Some evidence indicates that lower doses could be used in these patients.

Administration

I.V.: Administer by I.V. continuous infusion only (use infusion pump). Tacrolimus is dispensed in a 50 mL glass container with no overfill. It is intended to be infused over 12 hours. Polyolefin administration sets should be used. Dilute with 0.9% sodium chloride or D_5W to a concentration of 0.004-0.02 mg/mL prior to administration.

Stability

Storage:

Injection: Prior to dilution, store at 5°C to 25°C (41°F to 77°F). Polyvinyl-containing sets (eg, Venoset®, Accuset®) adsorb significant amounts of the drug, and their use may lead to a lower dose being delivered to the patient. FK506 admixtures prepared in 5% dextrose injection or 0.9% sodium chloride injection should be stored in polyolefin containers or glass bottles. Infusion of FK506 through PVC tubings did not result in decreased concentration of the drug, however, loss by absorption may be more important when lower concentrations of FK506 are used. Stable for 24 hours in D_5W or NS in glass or polyolefin containers.

Capsules and ointment: Store at room temperature 25°C (77°F).

Monitoring Laboratory Tests Renal function, hepatic function, serum electrolytes, glucose. Since pharmacokinetics show great inter- and intrapatient variability over time, monitoring of serum concentrations (trough for oral therapy) has proven helpful to prevent organ rejection

(Continued)

Tacrolimus *(Continued)*

and reduce drug-related toxicity. Measure 3 times/week for first few weeks, then gradually decrease frequency as patient stabilizes.

Monitoring and Teaching Issues

Physical Assessment: Assess other medications patient may be taking for effectiveness and interactions (see Warnings/Precautions and Drug Interactions). See Warnings/Precautions for use cautions. Monitor blood pressure frequently. Monitor laboratory tests prior to, during, and following therapy (see Monitoring Laboratory Tests). Monitor response to therapy and adverse reactions (see Warnings/Precautions, Adverse Reactions, and Dosing). Diabetic patients should be advised to monitor glucose levels closely (this medication may alter glucose levels). Monitor/instruct patient on appropriate use, interventions to reduce side effects, to monitor for signs of opportunistic infection, and adverse reactions to report (see Patient Education). **Pregnancy risk factor C.** Breast-feeding is contraindicated.

Patient Education: Take as directed, on an empty stomach. Be consistent with timing and consistency of meals if GI intolerance occurs (per manufacturer). Do not take within 2 hours before or after antacids. Do not alter dose and do not discontinue without consulting prescriber. Maintain adequate hydration (2-3 L/day of fluids) during entire course of therapy unless advised by prescriber to restrict fluids. You will be susceptible to infection (avoid crowds and exposure to infection). If you are diabetic, monitor glucose levels closely (drug may alter glucose levels). You may experience nausea, vomiting, loss of appetite (small, frequent meals, frequent mouth care may help); diarrhea (boiled milk, yogurt, or buttermilk may help); constipation (increased exercise, fluids, fruit, fluid, or fiber may help; if unresolved, consult prescriber); or muscle or back pain (mild analgesics may be recommended). Report chest pain; acute headache or dizziness; symptoms of respiratory infection, cough, or difficulty breathing; unresolved GI effects; fatigue, chills, fever, unhealed sores, white plaques in mouth, irritation in genital area; unusual bruising or bleeding; pain or irritation on urination or change in urinary patterns; rash or skin irritation; or other unusual effects.

Topical: Before applying, wash area gently and thoroughly. Apply in thin film to affected area. Do not cover skin with bandages. Wash hands only if not treating skin on the hands. Protect skin from sunlight or exposure to UV light. Consult prescriber if breast-feeding.

Pregnancy/breast-feeding precautions: Inform prescriber if you are or intend to become pregnant. Do not breast-feed.

Dietary Issues: Capsule: Take on an empty stomach; be consistent with timing and composition of meals if GI intolerance occurs (per manufacturer).

Breast-feeding Issues: Concentrations in breast milk are equivalent to plasma concentrations; breast-feeding is not advised.

Pregnancy Issues: Tacrolimus crosses the placenta and reaches concentrations four times greater than maternal plasma concentrations. Neonatal hyperkalemia and renal dysfunction have been reported.

Additional Information Additional dosing considerations:

Switch from I.V. to oral therapy: Threefold increase in dose

Pediatric patients: About 2 times higher dose compared to adults

Liver dysfunction: Decrease I.V. dose; decrease oral dose

Renal dysfunction: Does not affect kinetics; decrease dose to decrease levels if renal dysfunction is related to the drug

Tagamet® *see* Cimetidine *on page 289*

Tagamet® HB [OTC] *see* Cimetidine *on page 289*

Talacen® *see* Pentazocine Compound *on page 1052*

Talwin® *see* Pentazocine *on page 1051*

Talwin® Compound *see* Pentazocine Compound *on page 1052*

Talwin® NX *see* Pentazocine *on page 1051*

Tambocor™ *see* Flecainide *on page 562*

Tamiflu® *see* Oseltamivir *on page 1010*

Tamoxifen (ta MOKS i fen)

U.S. Brand Names Nolvadex®

Synonyms Tamoxifen Citrate

Generic Available Yes

Pharmacologic Category Antineoplastic Agent, Estrogen Receptor Antagonist

Pregnancy Risk Factor D

Lactation Enters breast milk/contraindicated

Use Palliative or adjunctive treatment of advanced breast cancer; reduce the incidence of breast cancer in women at high risk (at least 35 years of age with 5-year predicted risk ≥1.67% calculated by Gail Model); reduce risk of invasive breast cancer in women with ductal carcinoma *in situ* (DCIS); metastatic male breast cancer

Use - Unlabeled/Investigational Treatment of mastalgia, gynecomastia, pancreatic carcinoma; induction of ovulation; treatment of precocious puberty in females, secondary to McCune-Albright syndrome

Mechanism of Action/Effect Competitively binds to estrogen receptors on tumors and other tissue targets, producing a nuclear complex that decreases DNA synthesis and inhibits estrogen effects; nonsteroidal agent with potent antiestrogenic properties which compete with estrogen for binding sites in breast and other tissues; cells accumulate in the G_0 and G_1 phases; therefore, tamoxifen is cytostatic rather than cytocidal.

Contraindications Hypersensitivity to tamoxifen or any component of the formulation; concurrent warfarin therapy (when used for cancer risk reduction); pregnancy

Warnings/Precautions Serious and life-threatening events (including stroke, pulmonary emboli, and uterine malignancy) have occurred at an incidence greater than placebo during use for cancer risk reduction; these events are rare, but require consideration in risk:benefit evaluation. Use with caution in patients with leukopenia, thrombocytopenia, or hyperlipidemias; ovulation may be induced; decreased visual acuity, retinopathy, corneal changes, and increased incidence of cataracts have been reported; hypercalcemia in patients with bone metastasis; hepatocellular carcinomas have been reported in some studies, relationship to treatment is unclear. Endometrial hyperplasia and polyps have occurred. Increased risk of uterine or endometrial cancer; monitor.

Drug Interactions

Cytochrome P450 Effect: Substrate of CYP2A6, 2B6, **2C8/9, 2D6**, 2E1, **3A4**; Inhibits CYP2B6, 2C8/9, 3A4

Decreased Effect: CYP3A4 inducers may decrease serum levels of tamoxifen. Letrozole serum levels may be reduced by tamoxifen.

Increased Effect/Toxicity: Allopurinol and tamoxifen results in exacerbation of allopurinol-induced hepatotoxicity. Cyclosporine serum levels may be increased when taken with tamoxifen. Bromocriptine may increase serum levels of tamoxifen. Concomitant use of warfarin is contraindicated when used for risk reduction; results in significant enhancement of the anticoagulant effects of warfarin.

Nutritional/Ethanol Interactions Herb/Nutraceutical: Avoid black cohosh, dong quai in estrogen-dependent tumors.

Effects on Lab Values T_4 elevations (which may be explained by increases in thyroid-binding globulin) have been reported; not accompanied by clinical hyperthyroidism

Adverse Reactions Note: Differences in the frequency of some adverse events may be related to use for a specific indication.

Frequency not defined: Depression, dizziness, headache, hypercalcemia, lightheadedness, peripheral edema, pruritus vulvae, taste disturbance, vaginal dryness

>10%:

- Cardiovascular: Fluid retention (32%)
- Central nervous system: Mood changes (up to 12%; may include depression)
- Dermatologic: Skin changes (19%)
- Endocrine & metabolic: Hot flashes (64% to 80%), weight loss (23%)
- Gastrointestinal: Nausea (26%)
- Genitourinary: Vaginal bleeding (up to 23%), vaginal discharge (30% to 55%), menstrual irregularities (25%)
- Neuromuscular & skeletal: Bone pain, tumor pain, and local disease flare (including increase in lesion size and erythema) during treatment of metastatic breast cancer (generally resolves with continuation)

1% to 10%:

- Dermatologic: Alopecia (<1% to 5%)
- Gastrointestinal: Constipation (up to 4%)
- Hematologic: Thrombocytopenia (<1% to 2%)
- Hepatic: SGOT increased (2%), serum bilirubin increased (2%)
- Renal: Serum creatinine increased (up to 2%)
- Miscellaneous: Infection/sepsis (up to 6%), allergic reaction (up to 3%)

<1% (Limited to important or life-threatening): Angioedema, bullous pemphigoid, deep vein thrombosis, erythema multiforme, hypersensitivity reactions, hypertriglyceridemia, interstitial pneumonitis, pancreatitis, phlebitis, pulmonary embolism, rash, retinopathy (optic disc swelling, retinal hemorrhage, visual impairment associated with doses >200 mg/day), Stevens-Johnson syndrome

Overdosage/Toxicology Symptoms of overdose include hypercalcemia and edema. Provide general supportive care.

Pharmacodynamics/Kinetics

Absorption: Well absorbed

Half-Life Elimination: Distribution: 7-14 hours; Elimination: 5-7 days; Metabolites: 14 days

Time to Peak: Serum: 5 hours

Metabolism: Hepatic (via CYP3A4) to major metabolites, desmethyltamoxifen and 4-hydroxytamoxifen; undergoes enterohepatic recirculation

Formulations Tablet, as citrate: 10 mg, 20 mg

Dosing

Adults & Elderly: Refer to individual protocols.

Breast cancer:

- Metastatic (males and females) or adjuvant therapy (females): Oral: 20-40 mg/day; dosages >20 mg/day in divided doses; 20 mg/day is most common
- DCIS (females): Oral: 20 mg once daily for 5 years
- Prevention (high-risk females): Oral: 20 mg/day for 5 years
- **Note:** Higher dosages (up to 700 mg/day) have been investigated for use in modulation of multidrug resistance (MDR), but are not routinely used in clinical practice.

Induction of ovulation (unlabeled use): Oral: 5-40 mg twice daily for 4 days

Pediatrics: Female: Precocious puberty and McCune-Albright syndrome (unlabeled use): Oral: A dose of 20 mg/day has been reported in patients 2-10 years of age; safety and efficacy have not been established for treatment of longer than 1 year duration

Stability

Storage: Store at room temperature of 20°C to 25°C (68°F to 77°F).

Monitoring Laboratory Tests WBC and platelet counts

Monitoring and Teaching Issues

Physical Assessment: See Contraindications, Warnings/Precautions, and Dosing for use cautions. Assess potential for interactions with other prescriptions, OTC medications, or herbal products patient may be taking (see Drug Interactions). Assess results of laboratory tests (see above), therapeutic response (eg, complaints of bone pain is usually an indication of a good therapeutic response and will usually subside as treatment continues), and adverse reactions (see Adverse Reactions and Overdose/Toxicology). Teach patient proper use, possible side effects and interventions (eg, periodic ophthalmic evaluations with long-term use), and adverse symptoms to report (see Patient Education). **Pregnancy risk factor D** - determine that patient is not pregnant before beginning treatment. Instruct

(Continued)

Tamoxifen *(Continued)*

patients of childbearing age on appropriate barrier contraceptive measures. Breast-feeding is contraindicated.

Patient Education: Inform prescriber of all prescriptions, OTC medications, or herbal products you are taking, and any allergies you have. Do not take anything new during treatment unless approved by prescriber. Take exactly as directed. It is important to maintain adequate hydration (2-3 L/day of fluids) unless advised by prescriber to restrict fluids, and adequate nutrition (small, frequent meals may help) during therapy. You should schedule an annual ophthalmic examination is this medication is used long-term. You may experience hot flashes, hair loss, loss of libido (these will subside when treatment is completed). Bone pain may indicate a good therapeutic responses (consult prescriber for mild analgesics). May cause nausea or vomiting (small, frequent meals, frequent mouth care, sucking lozenges, or chewing gum may help); or photosensitivity (use sunscreen, wear protective clothing and eyewear, and avoid direct sunlight). Notify prescriber if menstrual irregularities or vaginal bleeding occur. Report unusual bleeding or bruising, severe weakness, sedation, mental changes, swelling or pain in calves, difficulty breathing, or any vision changes. **Pregnancy/breast-feeding precautions:** Do not get pregnant while taking this medication. Consult prescriber for appropriate contraceptive measures. Do not breast-feed.

Geriatric Considerations: Studies have shown tamoxifen to be effective in the treatment of primary breast cancer in elderly women. Comparative studies with other antineoplastic agents in elderly women with breast cancer had more favorable survival rates with tamoxifen. Initiation of hormone therapy rather than chemotherapy is justified for elderly patients with metastatic breast cancer who are responsive.

Pregnancy Issues: No adequate or well-controlled studies in pregnant women. For sexually-active women of childbearing age, initiate during menstruation (negative β-hCG immediately prior to initiation in women with irregular cycles). Pregnancy should be avoided for 2 months after treatment has been discontinued.

Additional Information Oral clonidine is being studied for the treatment of tamoxifen-induced "hot flashes." The tumor flare reaction may indicate a good therapeutic response, and is often considered a good prognostic factor.

Related Information

Estrogen Replacement Therapy *on page 1666*

Tamoxifen Citrate *see* Tamoxifen *on page 1274*

Tanoral® Tablet *see page 1522*

Tapazole® *see* Methimazole *on page 871*

Targretin® *see* Bexarotene *on page 165*

Tarka® *see* Trandolapril and Verapamil *on page 1347*

Tasmar® *see* Tolcapone *on page 1331*

TAT *see page 1498*

Taxol® *see* Paclitaxel *on page 1025*

Taxotere® *see* Docetaxel *on page 430*

Tazarotene (taz AR oh teen)

U.S. Brand Names Avage™; Tazorac®

Generic Available No

Pharmacologic Category Keratolytic Agent

Pregnancy Risk Factor X

Lactation Excretion in breast milk unknown/use caution

Use Topical treatment of facial acne vulgaris; topical treatment of stable plaque psoriasis of up to 20% body surface area involvement; mitigation (palliation) of facial skin wrinkling, facial mottled hyper/hypopigmentation, and benign facial lentigines

Contraindications Hypersensitivity to tazarotene, other retinoids or vitamin A derivatives (isotretinoin, tretinoin, etretinate), or any component of the formulation; use in women of childbearing potential who are unable to comply with birth control requirements; pregnancy (negative pregnancy test required)

Warnings/Precautions Women of childbearing potential must use adequate contraceptive measures because of potential teratogenicity. May cause photosensitivity; exposure to sunlight should be avoided unless deemed medically necessary, and in such cases, exposure should be minimized (including use of sunscreens/protective clothing) during use of tazarotene. Risk may be increased by concurrent therapy with known photosensitizers (thiazides, tetracyclines, fluoroquinolones, phenothiazines, sulfonamides). For external use only; avoid contact with eyes, eyelids, and mouth. Not for use on eczematous, broken, or sunburned skin; not for treatment of lentigo maligna. Avoid application over extensive areas; specifically, safety and efficacy of gel applied over >20% of BSA have not been established. Safety and efficacy in children <12 years of age have not been established.

Drug Interactions

Increased Effect/Toxicity: Increased toxicity may occur with sulfur, benzoyl peroxide, salicylic acid, resorcinol, or any product with strong drying effects (including alcohol-containing compounds) due to increased drying actions. May augment phototoxicity of sensitizing medications (thiazides, tetracyclines, fluoroquinolones, phenothiazines, sulfonamides).

Adverse Reactions Percentage of incidence varies with formulation and/or strength:

>10%: Dermatologic: Burning/stinging, desquamation, dry skin, erythema, pruritus, skin pain, worsening of psoriasis

1% to 10%: Dermatologic: Contact dermatitis, discoloration, fissuring, hypertriglyceridemia, inflammation, irritation, localized bleeding, rash

Frequency not defined:

Dermatologic: Photosensitization

Neuromuscular & skeletal: Peripheral neuropathy

Overdosage/Toxicology

Excessive topical use may lead to marked redness, peeling, or discomfort. Oral ingestion may lead to the same adverse effects as those associated with excessive oral intake of Vitamin A (hypervitaminosis A) or other retinoids.

Treatment: If oral ingestion occurs, monitor the patient and administer appropriate supportive measures as necessary

Pharmacodynamics/Kinetics

Absorption: Minimal following cutaneous application (≤6% of dose)

Half-Life Elimination: 18 hours

Metabolism: Prodrug, rapidly metabolized via esterases to an active metabolite (tazarotenic acid) following topical application and systemic absorption; tazarotenic acid undergoes further hepatic metabolism

Duration: Therapeutic: Psoriasis: Effects have been observed for up to 3 months after a 3-month course of topical treatment

Formulations

Cream:

Avage™: 0.1% (15 g, 30 g) [contains benzyl alcohol]

Tazorac® 0.05% (15 g, 30 g, 60 g); 0.1% (15 g, 30 g, 60 g) [contains benzyl alcohol]

Gel (Tazorac®): 0.05% (30 g, 100 g); 0.1% (30 g, 100 g) [contains benzyl alcohol]

Dosing

Adults & Elderly: Note: In patients experiencing excessive pruritus, burning, skin redness, or peeling, discontinue until integrity of the skin is restored, or reduce dosing to an interval the patient is able to tolerate.

Acne: Topical: Tazorac® cream/gel 0.1%: Cleanse the face gently. After the skin is dry, apply a thin film of tazarotene (2 mg/cm^2) once daily, in the evening, to the skin where the acne lesions appear; use enough to cover the entire affected area

Palliation of fine facial wrinkles, facial mottled hyper/hypopigmentation, benign facial lentigines: Topical: Avage™: Apply a pea-sized amount once daily to clean dry face at bedtime; lightly cover entire face including eyelids if desired. Emollients or moisturizers may be applied before or after; if applied before tazarotene, ensure cream or lotion has absorbed into the skin and has dried completely.

Psoriasis: Topical:

Tazorac® gel 0.05% or 0.1%: Apply once daily, in the evening, to psoriatic lesions using enough (2 mg/cm^2) to cover only the lesion with a thin film to no more than 20% of body surface area. If a bath or shower is taken prior to application, dry the skin before applying. Unaffected skin may be more susceptible to irritation, avoid application to these areas. **Note:** In patients experiencing excessive pruritus, burning, skin redness, or peeling, discontinue until integrity of the skin is restored, or reduce dosing to an interval the patient is able to tolerate.

Tazorac® cream 0.05% or 0.1%: Apply once daily, in the evening, to psoriatic lesions using enough (2 mg/cm^2) to cover only the lesion with a thin film to no more than 20% of body surface area. If a bath or shower is taken prior to application, dry the skin before applying. Unaffected skin may be more susceptible to irritation, avoid application to these areas. **Note:** In patients experiencing excessive pruritus, burning, skin redness, or peeling, discontinue until integrity of the skin is restored, or reduce dosing to an interval the patient is able to tolerate.

Pediatrics: Topical: **Note:** In patients experiencing excessive pruritus, burning, skin redness, or peeling, discontinue until integrity of the skin is restored, or reduce dosing to an interval the patient is able to tolerate.

Children ≥12 years:

Acne: Topical: Tazorac® cream/gel 0.1%: Cleanse the face gently. After the skin is dry, apply a thin film of tazarotene (2 mg/cm^2) once daily, in the evening, to the skin where the acne lesions appear; use enough to cover the entire affected area

Psoriasis: Topical: Tazorac® gel 0.05% or 0.1%: Apply once daily, in the evening, to psoriatic lesions using enough (2 mg/cm^2) to cover only the lesion with a thin film to no more than 20% of body surface area. If a bath or shower is taken prior to application, dry the skin before applying. Unaffected skin may be more susceptible to irritation, avoid application to these areas.

Children ≥17 years: Palliation of fine facial wrinkles, facial mottled hyper/hypopigmentation, benign facial lentigines: Topical: Avage™: Refer to adult dosing.

Administration

Topical: Do not apply to eczematous or sunburned skin; apply thin film to affected areas; avoid eyes and mouth

Stability

Storage: Store at room temperature of 25°C (77°F), away from heat and direct light; do not freeze.

Monitoring and Teaching Issues

Physical Assessment: See Contraindications, Warnings/Precautions, and Dosing for use cautions. Assess potential for interactions with other prescriptions, OTC medications, or herbal products patient may be taking (eg, accumulated photosensitivity - see Drug Interactions). Assess therapeutic effectiveness and adverse response on a regular basis during therapy (see Adverse Reactions and Overdose/Toxicology). Teach patient proper use, side effects and appropriate interventions, and adverse reactions to report (see Patient Education). **Pregnancy risk factor X** - determine that patient is not pregnant before beginning treatment. Do not give to women of childbearing age unless they are capable of complying with barrier contraceptive use. Instruct patients of childbearing age about appropriate barrier contraceptive measures. Note breast-feeding caution.

Patient Education: Inform prescriber of all prescriptions, OTC medications, or herbal products you are taking, and any allergies you have. This medication is for external use only; avoid using near eyes or mouth. Use exactly as directed; do not use more than recommended (severe skin reactions may occur). Avoid any other skin products (including cosmetics or personal products that may contain medications, spices, alcohols, or irritants) that are not approved by your prescriber. May cause photosensitivity, which will cause severe rash or burning (use sunblock SPF 15 or higher, wear protective clothing and

(Continued)

Tazarotene *(Continued)*

eyewear, and avoid direct sunlight, sunlamps, or tanning beds). Report redness or discoloration, irritation, open sores, bleeding, burning, stinging, excessive dryness, or swelling of skin; or worsening of condition. **Pregnancy/breast-feeding precautions:** Inform prescriber if you are pregnant. Do not get pregnant during treatment. Consult prescriber for instruction on appropriate contraceptive measures. This drug may cause severe fetal defects. Do not allow anyone who may be or become pregnant to touch this medication. Consult prescriber if breast-feeding.

Application: Wash affected area gently and completely dry before applying medication. Apply a thin layer to cover affected area. Wash off any medication that gets on unaffected skin areas and wash hands thoroughly after application.

Pregnancy Issues: May cause fetal harm if administered to a pregnant woman. A negative pregnancy test should be obtained 2 weeks prior to treatment; treatment should begin during a normal menstrual period.

Tazicef® *see* Ceftazidime *on page 249*

Tazidime® *see* Ceftazidime *on page 249*

Tazorac® *see* Tazarotene *on page 1276*

3TC *see* Lamivudine *on page 768*

3TC, Abacavir, and Zidovudine *see* Abacavir, Lamivudine, and Zidovudine *on page 31*

T-Cell Growth Factor *see* Aldesleukin *on page 54*

TCGF *see* Aldesleukin *on page 54*

TCN *see* Tetracycline *on page 1296*

TDF *see* Tenofovir *on page 1287*

Tegaserod (teg a SER od)

U.S. Brand Names Zelnorm™

Synonyms HTF919; Tegaserod Maleate

Generic Available No

Pharmacologic Category Serotonin 5-HT_4 Receptor Agonist

Pregnancy Risk Factor B

Lactation Excretion in breast milk unknown/not recommended

Use Short-term treatment of constipation-predominate irritable bowel syndrome (IBS) in women

Mechanism of Action/Effect Normalizes impaired motility by stimulating peristalsis and decreasing transit time in the gastrointestinal tract.

Contraindications Hypersensitivity to tegaserod or any component of the formulation; severe renal impairment; moderate or severe hepatic impairment; history of bowel obstruction, symptomatic gallbladder disease, suspected sphincter of Oddi dysfunction, or abdominal adhesions. Treatment should **not** be started in patients with diarrhea or in those who experience diarrhea frequently.

Warnings/Precautions Discontinue immediately with new or sudden worsening abdominal pain. Diarrhea may occur after the start of treatment, most cases reported as a single episode within the first week of therapy, and may resolve with continued dosing. Patients who develop severe diarrhea, or diarrhea with severe cramping, abdominal pain, or dizziness should consult healthcare provider. Use caution with mild hepatic impairment. Safety and efficacy have not been established in males or patients <18 years of age.

Nutritional/Ethanol Interactions Food: Bioavailability is decreased by 40% to 65% and C_{max} is decreased by 20% to 40% when taken with food. T_{max} is prolonged from 1 hour up to 2 hours when taken following a meal, but decreased to 0.7 hours when taken 30 minutes before a meal.

Adverse Reactions

>10%:

Central nervous system: Headache (15%)

Gastrointestinal: Abdominal pain (12%)

1% to 10%:

Central nervous system: Dizziness (4%), migraine (2%)

Gastrointestinal: Diarrhea (9%), nausea (8%), flatulence (6%)

Neuromuscular & skeletal: Back pain (5%), arthropathy (2%), leg pain (1%)

<1% (Limited to important or life-threatening): Albuminuria, angina pectoris, arrhythmia, bile duct stone, cramps, cholecystitis with elevated transaminases, hypotension, pruritus, renal pain, SGOT increased, SGPT increased, sphincter of Oddi spasm (suspected), syncope, tenesmus, vertigo

Overdosage/Toxicology Treatment should be symptom-directed and supportive. Diarrhea, headache, abdominal pain, orthostatic hypotension, flatulence, nausea, and vomiting were reported in healthy volunteers with doses of 90-180 mg. Unlikely to be removed by dialysis.

Pharmacodynamics/Kinetics

Bioavailability: Fasting: 10%

Half-Life Elimination: I.V.: 11 ± 5 hours

Time to Peak: 1 hour

Metabolism: GI: Hydrolysis in the stomach; Hepatic: oxidation, conjugation, and glucuronidation; metabolite (negligible activity); significant first-pass effect

Formulations Tablet, as maleate: 2 mg, 6 mg

Dosing

Adults: IBS with constipation: Female: Oral: 6 mg twice daily, before meals, for 4-6 weeks; may consider continuing treatment for an additional 4-6 weeks in patients who respond initially.

Renal Impairment: C_{max} and AUC of the inactive metabolite are increased with renal impairment.

Mild to moderate impairment: No dosage adjustment recommended

Severe impairment: Use is contraindicated

Hepatic Impairment: C_{max} and AUC of tegaserod are increased with hepatic impairment.
Mild impairment: No dosage adjustment recommended; however, user caution
Moderate to severe impairment: Use is contraindicated

Administration

Oral: Administer 30 minutes before meals.

Stability

Storage: Store at controlled room temperature of 15°C to 30°C (59°F to 86°F). Protect from moisture.

Monitoring and Teaching Issues

Physical Assessment: See Contraindications, Warnings/Precautions, and Drug Interactions for use cautions. Assess therapeutic effectiveness and adverse response when beginning therapy and at regular intervals during treatment (see Adverse Reactions and Overdose/Toxicology). Teach patient appropriate use, side effects and interventions, and adverse symptoms to report (see Patient Education). Breast-feeding is not recommended.

Patient Education: Inform prescriber of all prescriptions, OTC medications, or herbal products you are taking, and any allergies you have. Do not take anything new during treatment without consulting prescriber. Take exactly as directed, on an empty stomach, at least 30 minutes before meals. If you miss a dose, skip that dose and continue with regular schedule; do not double doses. May cause headache or dizziness (use caution when driving or engaging in tasks requiring alertness until response to drug is known); nausea or vomiting (small, frequent meals, frequent mouth care, chewing gum, or sucking lozenges may help); or diarrhea (should resolve within a week). Report immediately if you experience severe diarrhea, abdominal cramping, or increased abdominal pain. **Breast-feeding precaution:** Breast-feeding is not recommended.

Dietary Issues: Take on an empty stomach, 30 minutes before meals.

Additional Information In clinical trials, constipation was defined as <3 bowel movements per week, hard or lumpy stools, or straining with a bowel movement.

Tegaserod Maleate *see* Tegaserod *on page 1278*

Tegretol® *see* Carbamazepine *on page 213*

Tegretol®-XR *see* Carbamazepine *on page 213*

Tegrin®-HC [OTC] *see* Topical Corticosteroids *on page 1334*

Teladar® *see* Topical Corticosteroids *on page 1334*

Telmisartan (tel mi SAR tan)

U.S. Brand Names Micardis®

Generic Available No

Pharmacologic Category Angiotensin II Receptor Blocker

Pregnancy Risk Factor C (1st trimester); D (2nd and 3rd trimesters)

Lactation Enters breast milk/not recommended

Use Treatment of hypertension; may be used alone or in combination with other antihypertensive agents

Mechanism of Action/Effect Telmisartan is a nonpeptide angiotensin receptor antagonist. Angiotensin II acts as a vasoconstrictor. In addition to causing direct vasoconstriction, angiotensin II also stimulates the release of aldosterone. Once aldosterone is released, sodium as well as water are reabsorbed. The end result is an elevation in blood pressure. Telmisartan binds to the AT1 angiotensin II receptor. This binding prevents angiotensin II from binding to the receptor thereby blocking the vasoconstriction and the aldosterone secreting effects of angiotensin II.

Contraindications Hypersensitivity to telmisartan or any component of the formulation; hypersensitivity to other A-II receptor antagonists; primary hyperaldosteronism; bilateral renal artery stenosis; pregnancy (2nd and 3rd trimesters)

Warnings/Precautions Avoid use or use a smaller dose in patients who are volume depleted; correct depletion first. Deterioration in renal function can occur with initiation. Use with caution in unilateral renal artery stenosis and pre-existing renal insufficiency; significant aortic/mitral stenosis. Use with caution in patients who have biliary obstructive disorders or hepatic dysfunction. Pregnancy risk C (1st trimester)/D (2nd and 3rd trimesters).

Drug Interactions

Cytochrome P450 Effect: Inhibits CYP2C19

Decreased Effect: Telmisartan decreased the trough concentrations of warfarin during concurrent therapy, however, INR was not changed.

Increased Effect/Toxicity: Telmisartan may increase serum digoxin concentrations. Potassium salts/supplements, co-trimoxazole (high dose), ACE inhibitors, and potassium-sparing diuretics (amiloride, spironolactone, triamterene) may increase the risk of hyperkalemia with telmisartan.

Nutritional/Ethanol Interactions Herb/Nutraceutical: Avoid dong quai if using for hypertension (has estrogenic activity). Avoid ephedra, yohimbe, ginseng (may worsen hypertension). Avoid garlic (may have increased antihypertensive effect).

Adverse Reactions May be associated with worsening of renal function in patients dependent on renin-angiotensin-aldosterone system.

1% to 10%:
- Cardiovascular: Hypertension (1%), chest pain (1%), peripheral edema (1%)
- Central nervous system: Headache (1%), dizziness (1%), pain (1%), fatigue (1%)
- Gastrointestinal: Diarrhea (3%), dyspepsia (1%), nausea (1%), abdominal pain (1%)
- Genitourinary: Urinary tract infection (1%)
- Neuromuscular & skeletal: Back pain (3%), myalgia (1%)
- Respiratory: Upper respiratory infection (7%), sinusitis (3%), pharyngitis (1%), cough (2%)
- Miscellaneous: Flu-like syndrome (1%)

<1% (Limited to important or life-threatening): Abnormal vision, allergic reaction, angina, angioedema, depression, dyspnea, epistaxis, gout, impotence, increased serum creatinine and BUN, insomnia, involuntary muscle contractions, migraine, paresthesia, pruritus, rash, somnolence, tinnitus, vertigo

(Continued)

Telmisartan *(Continued)*

Overdosage/Toxicology Symptoms of overdose may include hypotension, dizziness, and tachycardia. Vagal stimulation may result in bradycardia. Treatment is supportive.

Pharmacokinetic Note Orally active, not a prodrug.

Pharmacodynamics/Kinetics

Bioavailability: Dose dependent: 42% to 58%

Half-Life Elimination: Terminal: 24 hours

Metabolism: Hepatic via conjugation to inactive metabolites; not metabolized via CYP

Onset: 1-2 hours; Peak effect: 0.5-1 hours

Duration: Up to 24 hours

Formulations Tablet: 20 mg, 40 mg, 80 mg

Dosing

Adults & Elderly: Hypertension: Oral: Initial: 40 mg once daily; usual maintenance dose range: 20-80 mg/day. Patients with volume depletion should be initiated on the lower dosage with close supervision.

Hepatic Impairment: Supervise patients closely.

Monitoring Laboratory Tests Monitor electrolytes, serum creatinine, BUN, urinalysis, symptomatic hypotension, and tachycardia

Monitoring and Teaching Issues

Physical Assessment: See Contraindications, Warnings/Precautions, and Dosing for use cautions. Assess potential for interactions with other prescriptions, OTC medications, or herbal products patient may be taking (see Drug Interactions). Assess results of laboratory tests (see above), therapeutic effectiveness, and adverse response on a regular basis during therapy (eg, hypotension - see Adverse Reactions and Overdose/Toxicology). Teach patient proper use, need for regular blood pressure monitoring, possible side effects and appropriate interventions, and adverse symptoms to report (see Patient Education). **Pregnancy risk factor C/D** - see Pregnancy Risk Factor for use cautions. Instruct patient of childbearing age about appropriate use of barrier contraceptives. Breast-feeding is not recommended.

Patient Education: Inform prescriber of all prescriptions, OTC medications, or herbal products you are taking, and any allergies you have. Do not take anything new during treatment unless approved by prescriber. Take exactly as directed and do not alter dose or discontinue without consulting prescriber. Monitor blood pressure on a regular basis at same time of day - as advised by prescriber. This drug does not eliminate need for diet or exercise regimen as recommended by prescriber. May cause dizziness, fainting, or light-headedness (use caution when driving or engaging in tasks that require alertness until response to drug is known); or postural hypotension (use caution when rising from lying or sitting position or climbing stairs). Report unusual weight gain and swelling of ankles, hands, face, lips, throat, or tongue; persistent fatigue; dry cough or difficulty breathing; palpitations or chest pain; CNS changes; GI disturbances; muscle or bone pain, cramping, or tremors; change in urinary pattern; changes in hearing or vision; or other adverse response. **Pregnancy/breast-feeding precautions:** Inform prescriber if you are or intend to become pregnant. This drug should not be used in the 2nd or 3rd trimester of pregnancy. Consult prescriber for appropriate contraceptive measures if necessary. Consult prescriber if breast-feeding.

Dietary Issues: May be taken without regard to food.

Related Information

Angiotensin Agents *on page 1547*

Telmisartan and HCTZ *see* Telmisartan and Hydrochlorothiazide *on page 1280*

Telmisartan and Hydrochlorothiazide

(tel mi SAR tan & hye droe klor oh THYE a zide)

U.S. Brand Names Micardis® HCT

Synonyms HCTZ and Telmisartan; Hydrochlorothiazide and Telmisartan; Telmisartan and HCTZ

Pharmacologic Category Angiotensin II Receptor Blocker Combination; Antihypertensive Agent Combination

Pregnancy Risk Factor C (1st trimester); D (2nd and 3rd trimesters)

Lactation Enters breast milk/not recommended

Use Treatment of hypertension; combination product should not be used for initial therapy

Formulations

Tablet:

Telmisartan 40 mg and hydrochlorothiazide 12.5 mg

Telmisartan 80 mg and hydrochlorothiazide 12.5 mg

Dosing

Adults: Hypertension: Oral: Replacement therapy: Combination product can be substituted for individual titrated agents. Initiation of combination therapy when monotherapy has failed to achieve desired effects:

Patients currently on telmisartan: Initial dose if blood pressure is not currently controlled on monotherapy of 80 mg telmisartan: Telmisartan 80 mg/hydrochlorothiazide 12.5 mg once daily; may titrate up to telmisartan 160 mg/hydrochlorothiazide 25 mg if needed.

Patients currently on HCTZ: Initial dose if blood pressure is not currently controlled on monotherapy of 25 mg once daily, or is controlled and experiencing hypokalemia: Telmisartan 80 mg/hydrochlorothiazide 12.5 mg once daily; may titrate up to telmisartan 160 mg/hydrochlorothiazide 25 mg if blood pressure remains uncontrolled after 2-4 weeks of therapy.

Elderly: Refer to adult dosing. Monitor renal function.

Renal Impairment:

Cl_{cr} >30 mL/minute: Usual recommended dose

Cl_{cr} <30 mL/minute: Not recommended

Hepatic Impairment: Dosing should be started at telmisartan 40 mg/hydrochlorothiazide 12.5 mg. Do **not** use in patients with severe hepatic impairment.

Monitoring and Teaching Issues

Physical Assessment: See individual components listed in Related Information. **Pregnancy risk factor C/D** - see Pregnancy Risk Factor for use cautions; benefits of use should outweigh possible risks. Breast-feeding is not recommended.

Patient Education: See individual components listed in Related Information. **Pregnancy/breast-feeding precautions:** Use appropriate contraceptive measures; do not get pregnant while taking this drug. Inform prescriber if you are or intend to become pregnant. Breast-feeding is not recommended.

Related Information

Hydrochlorothiazide *on page 664*
Telmisartan *on page 1279*

Temazepam (te MAZ e pam)

U.S. Brand Names Restoril®

Restrictions C-IV

Generic Available Yes

Pharmacologic Category Benzodiazepine

Pregnancy Risk Factor X

Lactation Enters breast milk/not recommended (AAP rates "of concern")

Use Short-term treatment of insomnia

Use - Unlabeled/Investigational Treatment of anxiety; adjunct in the treatment of depression; management of panic attacks

Mechanism of Action/Effect Binds to stereospecific benzodiazepine receptors on the postsynaptic GABA neuron at several sites within the central nervous system, including the limbic system, reticular formation. Enhancement of the inhibitory effect of GABA on neuronal excitability results by increased neuronal membrane permeability to chloride ions. This shift in chloride ions results in hyperpolarization (a less excitable state) and stabilization.

Contraindications Hypersensitivity to temazepam or any component of the formulation (cross-sensitivity with other benzodiazepines may exist); narrow-angle glaucoma (not in product labeling, however, benzodiazepines are contraindicated); pregnancy

Warnings/Precautions As a hypnotic, should be used only after evaluation of potential causes of sleep disturbance. Failure of sleep disturbance to resolve after 7-10 days may indicate psychiatric or medical illness. Use is not recommended in patients with depressive disorders or psychoses. Avoid use in patients with sleep apnea. Use with caution in patients receiving concurrent CYP3A4 inhibitors, particularly when these agents are added to therapy. Use with caution in elderly or debilitated patients, patients with hepatic disease (including alcoholics), renal impairment, respiratory disease, impaired gag reflex, or obese patients.

Causes CNS depression (dose-related) which may impair physical and mental capabilities. Use with caution in patients receiving other CNS depressants or psychoactive agents. Benzodiazepines have been associated with falls and traumatic injury and should be used with extreme caution in patients who are at risk of these events (especially the elderly). May cause physical or psychological dependence - use with caution in patients with a history of drug dependence.

Benzodiazepines have been associated with anterograde amnesia. Paradoxical reactions, including hyperactive or aggressive behavior, have been reported with benzodiazepines, particularly in adolescent/pediatric or psychiatric patients. Does not have analgesic, antidepressant, or antipsychotic properties.

Drug Interactions

Cytochrome P450 Effect: Substrate of CYP2B6, 2C8/9, 2C19, 3A4

Decreased Effect: Oral contraceptives may increase the clearance of temazepam. Temazepam may decrease the antiparkinsonian efficacy of levodopa. Theophylline and other CNS stimulants may antagonize the sedative effects of temazepam. Carbamazepine, rifampin, rifabutin may enhance the metabolism of temazepam and decrease its therapeutic effect.

Increased Effect/Toxicity: Temazepam potentiates the CNS depressant effects of narcotic analgesics, barbiturates, phenothiazines, ethanol, antihistamines, MAO inhibitors, sedative-hypnotics, and cyclic antidepressants. Serum levels of temazepam may be increased by inhibitors of CYP3A4, including cimetidine, ciprofloxacin, clarithromycin, clozapine, diltiazem, disulfiram, digoxin, erythromycin, ethanol, fluconazole, fluoxetine, fluvoxamine, grapefruit juice, isoniazid, itraconazole, ketoconazole, labetalol, levodopa, loxapine, metoprolol, metronidazole, miconazole, nefazodone, omeprazole, phenytoin, rifabutin, rifampin, troleandomycin, valproic acid, and verapamil.

Nutritional/Ethanol Interactions

Ethanol: Avoid ethanol (may increase CNS depression).

Food: Serum levels may be increased by grapefruit juice.

Herb/Nutraceutical: St John's wort may decrease temazepam levels. Avoid valerian, St John's wort, kava kava, gotu kola (may increase CNS depression).

Adverse Reactions

1% to 10%:

- Central nervous system: Confusion, dizziness, drowsiness, fatigue, anxiety, headache, lethargy, hangover, euphoria, vertigo
- Dermatologic: Rash
- Endocrine & metabolic: Decreased libido
- Gastrointestinal: Diarrhea
- Neuromuscular & skeletal: Dysarthria, weakness
- Otic: Blurred vision
- Miscellaneous: Diaphoresis

<1% (Limited to important or life-threatening): Amnesia, ataxia, blood dyscrasias, drug dependence, paradoxical reactions, vomiting

Overdosage/Toxicology Symptoms of overdose include somnolence, confusion, coma, hypoactive reflexes, dyspnea, hypotension, slurred speech, and impaired coordination. Treatment for benzodiazepine overdose is supportive. Flumazenil has been shown to selectively

(Continued)

Temazepam *(Continued)*

block the binding of benzodiazepines to CNS receptors, resulting in a reversal of benzodiazepine-induced CNS depression but not always respiratory depression due to toxicity.

Pharmacodynamics/Kinetics

Half-Life Elimination: 9.5-12.4 hours

Time to Peak: Serum: 2-3 hours

Metabolism: Hepatic

Formulations Capsule: 7.5 mg, 15 mg, 30 mg

Dosing

Adults: Insomnia: Oral: 15-30 mg at bedtime

Elderly: 15 mg in elderly or debilitated patients

Monitoring and Teaching Issues

Physical Assessment: For short-term use. Assess effectiveness and interactions of other medications patient may be taking (see Drug Interactions). See Contraindications and Warnings/Precautions for use cautions. Assess for history of addiction (long-term use can result in dependence, abuse, or tolerance) and periodically evaluate need for continued use. After long-term use, taper dosage slowly when discontinuing. For inpatient use, institute safety measures and monitor effectiveness and adverse reactions. For outpatients, monitor therapeutic effectiveness and adverse reactions (see Adverse Reactions) at beginning of therapy and periodically with long-term use. Assess knowledge/teach patient appropriate use, interventions to reduce side effects, and adverse symptoms to report (see Patient Education). **Pregnancy risk factor X** - determine that patient is not pregnant before starting therapy. Do not give to sexually-active female patients unless capable of complying with barrier contraceptive use. Breast-feeding is not recommended.

Patient Education: Use exactly as directed; do not increase dose or frequency or discontinue without consulting prescriber. Drug may cause physical and/or psychological dependence. May take with food to decrease GI upset. While using this medication, do not use alcohol or other prescription or OTC medications (especially, pain medications, sedatives, antihistamines, or hypnotics) without consulting prescriber. Maintain adequate hydration (2-3 L/day of fluids) unless advised by prescriber to restrict fluids. You may experience drowsiness, dizziness, lightheadedness, or blurred vision (use caution when driving or engaging in tasks requiring alertness until response to drug is known); or dry mouth or GI discomfort (small, frequent meals, frequent mouth care, chewing gum, or sucking lozenges may help). Report CNS changes (confusion, depression, increased sedation, excitation, headache, abnormal thinking, insomnia, or nightmares, memory impairment, impaired coordination); muscle pain or weakness; difficulty breathing; persistent dizziness, chest pain, or palpitations; alterations in normal gait; vision changes; or ineffectiveness of medication. **Pregnancy/breast-feeding precautions:** Inform prescriber if you are pregnant. Do not get pregnant during or for 1 month following therapy. Consult prescriber for instruction on appropriate barrier contraceptive measures. This drug may cause severe fetal defects. Breast-feeding is not recommended.

Geriatric Considerations: Because of its lack of active metabolites, temazepam is recommended in the elderly when a benzodiazepine hypnotic is indicated. Hypnotic use should be limited to 10-14 days. If insomnia persists, the patient should be evaluated for etiology.

Other Issues: Taper dosage gradually after long-term therapy. Abrupt withdrawal may cause tremors, nausea, vomiting, abdominal and/or muscle cramps.

Additional Information Abrupt discontinuation after sustained use (generally >10 days) may cause withdrawal symptoms.

Related Information

Anxiolytic/Hypnotic Use in Long-Term Care Facilities *on page 1608*
Benzodiazepines *on page 1560*

Temodar® *see* Temozolomide *on page 1282*
Temovate® *see* Topical Corticosteroids *on page 1334*

Temozolomide (te mo ZOLE oh mide)

U.S. Brand Names Temodar®

Generic Available No

Pharmacologic Category Antineoplastic Agent, Alkylating Agent

Pregnancy Risk Factor D

Lactation Excretion in breast milk unknown/not recommended

Use Treatment of adult patients with refractory (first relapse) anaplastic astrocytoma who have experienced disease progression on nitrosourea and procarbazine

Use - Unlabeled/Investigational Glioma, first relapse/advanced metastatic malignant melanoma

Mechanism of Action/Effect Prodrug, hydrolyzed to MTIC (active form). The cytotoxic effects of MTIC is through alkylation of DNA (O^6, N^7 of guanine).

Contraindications Hypersensitivity to temozolomide or any component of the formulation; hypersensitivity to DTIC (since both drugs are metabolized to MTIC); pregnancy

Warnings/Precautions Must have ANC >1500/µL, platelet count >100,000/µL before starting each cycle. Geriatric patients and women have a higher incidence of myelosuppression. Safety/efficacy in pediatrics not established. Use caution in patients with severe hepatic or renal impairment. The U.S. Food and Drug Administration (FDA) currently recommends that procedures for proper handling and disposal of antineoplastic agents be considered.

Drug Interactions

Decreased Effect: Although valproic acid reduces the clearance of temozolomide by 5%, the clinical significance of this is unknown.

Nutritional/Ethanol Interactions Food: Food reduces rate and extent of absorption.

Adverse Reactions

>10%:

Cardiovascular: Peripheral edema (11%)

Central nervous system: Headache (41%), fatigue (34%), convulsions (23%), hemiparesis (29%), dizziness (19%), fever (11%), coordination abnormality (11%), amnesia (10%), insomnia (10%), somnolence. In the case of CNS malignancies, it is difficult to distinguish the relative contributions of temozolomide and progressive disease to CNS symptoms.

Gastrointestinal: Nausea (53%), vomiting (42%), constipation (33%), diarrhea (16%)
Hematologic: Neutropenia (grade 3-4, 14%), thrombocytopenia (grade 3-4 19%)
Neuromuscular & skeletal: Weakness (13%)

1% to 10%:

Central nervous system: Ataxia (8%), confusion (5%), anxiety (7%), depression (6%)
Dermatologic: Rash (8%), pruritus (8%)
Endocrine & metabolic: Hypercorticism (8%), breast pain (6%), weight gain (5%)
Gastrointestinal: Dysphagia (7%), abdominal pain (9%), anorexia (9%)
Genitourinary: Increased micturition frequency (6%)
Hematologic: Anemia (8%; grade 3-4, 4%)
Neuromuscular & skeletal: Paresthesia (9%), back pain (8%), myalgia (5%)
Ocular: Diplopia (5%), vision abnormality (5%)
Respiratory: Pharyngitis (8%), sinusitis (6%), cough (5%)

<1% (Limited to important or life-threatening): Allergic reactions, anaphylaxis, erythema multiforme

Overdosage/Toxicology Dose-limiting toxicity is hematological. In the event of an overdose, hematological evaluation is necessary. Treatment is supportive.

Pharmacodynamics/Kinetics

Bioavailability: 100%

Half-Life Elimination: Mean: Parent drug: 1.8 hours

Time to Peak: Empty stomach: 1 hour

Metabolism: Prodrug, hydrolyzed to the active form, MTIC; MTIC is eventually eliminated as CO_2 and 5-aminoimidazole-4-carboxamide (AIC), a natural constituent in urine

Formulations Capsule: 5 mg, 20 mg, 100 mg, 250 mg

Dosing

Adults: Refer to individual protocols.

Antineoplastic: Oral: Usual dose: 150-200 mg/m^2/day for 5 days; repeat every 28 days.

Dosage is adjusted according to nadir neutrophil and platelet counts of previous cycle and counts at the time of the next cycle

Measure day 22 ANC and platelets. Measure day 29 ANC and platelets. Based on lowest counts at either day 22 or day 29:

On day 22 or day 29, if ANC <1000/µL or the platelet count is <50,000/µL, postpone therapy until ANC >1500/µL and platelet count >100,000/µL. Reduce dose by 50 mg/m^2 for subsequent cycle.

If ANC 1000-1500/µL or platelets 50,000-100,000/µL, postpone therapy until ANC >1500/µL and platelet count >100,000/µL; maintain initial dose.

If ANC >1500/µL (on day 22 and day 29) and platelet count >100,000/µL, increase dose to, or maintain dose at 200 mg/m^2/day for 5 for subsequent cycle.

Temozolomide therapy can be continued until disease progression. Treatment could be continued for a maximum of 2 years in the clinical trial, but the optimum duration of therapy is not known.

Elderly: Dosage is adjusted according to nadir neutrophil and platelet counts of previous cycle and counts at the time of the next cycle. Patients ≥70 years of age had a higher incidence of grade 4 neutropenia and thrombocytopenia in the first cycle of therapy than patients <70 years of age.

Renal Impairment: Caution should be used when administered to patients with severe renal impairment (Cl_{cr} <39 mL/minute).

Hepatic Impairment: Caution should be used when administering to patients with severe hepatic impairment.

Administration

Oral: Capsules should not be opened or chewed but swallowed whole with a glass of water. May be administered on an empty stomach to reduce nausea and vomiting. Bedtime administration may be advised.

Stability

Storage: Store at controlled room temperature (15°C to 10°C/59°F to 86°F).

Monitoring Laboratory Tests A complete blood count on day 22 of cycle or within 48 hours of that day and weekly until the ANC >1500 µL, platelet count >100,000/µL

Monitoring and Teaching Issues

Physical Assessment: See Contraindications, Warnings/Precautions, Drug Interactions, and Dosing for use cautions. Assess results of laboratory tests (see above) and patient response (see Adverse Reactions and Overdose/Toxicology). Teach patient proper use, possible side effects, and appropriate interventions (see Patient Education). **Pregnancy risk factor D** - determine that patient is not pregnant before beginning treatment. Instruct patients of childbearing age on appropriate barrier contraceptive measures. Breast-feeding is not recommended.

Patient Education: Take exactly as directed. Take on an empty stomach (1 hour before or 2 hours after meals or at bedtime) to reduce GI upset. Do not open, crush, or chew capsules; swallow whole with full 8 oz of water. May cause headache, dizziness, confusion, fatigue, anxiety, insomnia, or impaired coordination (use caution when driving or engaging in tasks requiring alertness until response to medication is known); nausea, vomiting, or loss of appetite (small, frequent meals, good mouth care, chewing gum, or sucking hard candy may help); or hot flashes (cool dark room or cold compresses may help). Report chest pain, palpitations, acute headache, visual disturbances; unresolved GI problems; itching or burning on urination or vaginal discharge; acute joint, back, bone, or muscle pain; difficulty breathing, unusual cough, or respiratory infection; or other adverse reactions. **Pregnancy/breast-feeding precautions:** Inform prescriber if you pregnant. Do not get pregnant while taking this medication. Consult prescriber for appropriate contraceptive measures. Breast-feeding is not recommended.

Dietary Issues: The incidence of nausea/vomiting is decreased when the drug is taken on an empty stomach.

(Continued)

Temozolomide *(Continued)*

Pregnancy Issues: May cause fetal harm when administered to pregnant women. Animal studies, at doses less than used in humans, resulted in numerous birth defects. Testicular toxicity was demonstrated in animal studies using smaller doses than recommended for cancer treatment. Male and female patients should avoid pregnancy while receiving drug.

Tenecteplase (ten EK te plase)

U.S. Brand Names TNKase™

Generic Available No

Pharmacologic Category Thrombolytic Agent

Pregnancy Risk Factor C

Lactation Use caution

Use Thrombolytic agent used in the management of acute myocardial infarction for the lysis of thrombi in the coronary vasculature to restore perfusion and reduce mortality.

Mechanism of Action/Effect Initiates fibrinolysis by binding to fibrin and converting plasminogen to plasmin.

Contraindications Hypersensitivity to tenecteplase or any component of the formulation; active internal bleeding; history of stroke; intracranial/intraspinal surgery or trauma within 2 months; intracranial neoplasm; arteriovenous malformation or aneurysm; bleeding diathesis; severe uncontrolled hypertension

Warnings/Precautions Stop antiplatelet agents and heparin if serious bleeding occurs. Avoid I.M. injections and nonessential handling of the patient for a few hours after administration. Monitor for bleeding complications. Venipunctures should be performed carefully and only when necessary. If arterial puncture is necessary then use an upper extremity that can be compressed manually. For the following conditions the risk of bleeding is higher with use of tenecteplase and should be weighed against the benefits: recent major surgery, cerebrovascular disease, recent GI or GU bleed, recent trauma, uncontrolled HTN (systolic BP ≥180 mm Hg and/or diastolic BP ≥110 mm Hg), suspected left heart thrombus, acute pericarditis, subacute bacterial endocarditis, hemostatic defects, severe hepatic dysfunction, pregnancy, hemorrhagic diabetic retinopathy or other hemorrhagic ophthalmic conditions, septic thrombophlebitis or occluded AV cannula at seriously infected site, advanced age (>75 years of age), anticoagulants, recent administration of GP IIb/IIIa inhibitors. Coronary thrombolysis may result in reperfusion arrhythmias. Caution should be used with readministration of tenecteplase. Safety and efficacy has not been established in pediatric patients. Cholesterol embolism has rarely been reported. Pregnancy risk C.

Drug Interactions

Decreased Effect: Aminocaproic acid (antifibrinolytic agent) may decrease effectiveness.

Increased Effect/Toxicity: Drugs which affect platelet function (eg, NSAIDs, dipyridamole, ticlopidine, clopidogrel, IIb/IIIa antagonists) may potentiate the risk of hemorrhage; use with caution.

Heparin and aspirin: Use with aspirin and heparin may increase bleeding. However, aspirin and heparin were used concomitantly with tenecteplase in the majority of patients in clinical studies.

Warfarin or oral anticoagulants: Risk of bleeding may be increased during concurrent therapy.

Adverse Reactions As with all drugs which may affect hemostasis, bleeding is the major adverse effect associated with tenecteplase. Hemorrhage may occur at virtually any site. Risk is dependent on multiple variables, including the dosage administered, concurrent use of multiple agents which alter hemostasis, and patient predisposition. Rapid lysis of coronary artery thrombi by thrombolytic agents may be associated with reperfusion-related arterial and/or ventricular arrhythmias.

>10%:

- Local: Hematoma (12% minor)
- Hematologic: Bleeding (22% minor: ASSENT-2 trial)

1% to 10%:

- Central nervous system: Stroke (2%)
- Gastrointestinal: GI hemorrhage (1% major, 2% minor), epistaxis (2% minor)
- Genitourinary: GU bleeding (4% minor)
- Hematologic: Bleeding (5% major; ASSENT-2 trial)
- Local: Bleeding at catheter puncture site (4% minor), hematoma (2% major)
- Respiratory: Pharyngeal (3% minor)

The incidence of stroke and bleeding increase with age above 65 years.

<1% (Limited to important or life-threatening): Anaphylaxis, angioedema, bleeding at catheter puncture site (<1% major), cholesterol embolism (clinical features may include livedo reticularis, "purple toe" syndrome, acute renal failure, gangrenous digits, hypertension, pancreatitis, myocardial infarction, cerebral infarction, spinal cord infarction, retinal artery occlusion, bowel infarction, rhabdomyolysis), GU bleeding (<1% major), intracranial hemorrhage (0.9%), laryngeal edema, rash, respiratory tract bleeding, retroperitoneal bleeding, urticaria

Additional cardiovascular events associated with use in myocardial infarction: Arrhythmias, AV block, cardiac arrest, cardiac tamponade, cardiogenic shock, electromechanical dissociation, embolism, fever, heart failure, hypotension, mitral regurgitation, myocardial reinfarction, myocardial rupture, nausea, pericardial effusion, pericarditis, pulmonary edema, recurrent myocardial ischemia, thrombosis, vomiting

Overdosage/Toxicology Increased incidence of bleeding

Pharmacodynamics/Kinetics

Half-Life Elimination: 90-130 minutes

Metabolism: Primarily hepatic

Formulations Injection, powder for reconstitution, recombinant: 50 mg

Dosing

Adults: Coronary thrombosis/AMI: I.V.: The recommended total dose should not exceed 50 mg and is based on weight. Administer as a bolus over 5 seconds:

<60 kg: 30 mg dose
≥60 to <70 kg: 35 mg
≥70 to <80 kg: 40 mg
≥80 to <90 kg: 45 mg
≥90 kg: 50 mg

All patients received 150-325 mg of aspirin as soon as possible and then daily. Intravenous heparin was initiated as soon as possible and PTT was maintained between 50-70 seconds.

Elderly: Refer to adult dosing. Although dosage adjustments are not recommended, the elderly have a higher incidence of morbidity and mortality with the use of tenecteplase. The 30-day mortality in the ASSENT-2 trial was 2.5% for patients younger than 65 years, 8.5% for patients between 65 and 74 years, and 16.2% for patients 75 years and older. The intracranial hemorrhage rate was 0.4% for patient younger than 65 years, 1.6% for patients between 65 and 74 years, and 1.7% for patients 75 years and older. The risks and benefits of use should be weighted carefully in the elderly.

Renal Impairment: No adjustment is necessary.

Hepatic Impairment: Severe hepatic failure is a relative contraindication. Recommendations were not made for mild to moderate hepatic impairment.

Administration

I.V.: Tenecteplase should be reconstituted using the supplied 10 mL syringe with TwinPak™ Dual Cannula Device and 10 mL SWFI. Do not shake when reconstituting. Slight foaming is normal; will dissipate if left standing for several minutes. Any unused solution should be discarded. The reconstituted solution is 5 mg/mL. Dextrose-containing lines must be flushed with a saline solution before and after administration. Check frequently for signs of bleeding. Avoid I.M. injections and unessential handling of patient.

Stability

Storage: Store at room temperature not to exceed 30°C (86°F) or under refrigeration 2°C to 8°C (36°F to 46°F).

Reconstitution: Tenecteplase should be reconstituted using the supplied 10 cc syringe with TwinPak™ Dual Cannula Device and 10 mL sterile water for injection. Tenecteplase is incompatible with dextrose solutions. Dextrose-containing lines must be flushed with a saline solution before and after administration. Administer as a single I.V. bolus over 5 seconds. If reconstituted and not used immediately, store in refrigerator and use within 8 hours.

Monitoring Laboratory Tests CBC, PTT, signs and symptoms of bleeding, EKG monitoring

Monitoring and Teaching Issues

Physical Assessment: See Contraindications, Warnings/Precautions, and Dosing for use cautions. Assess potential for interactions with other prescriptions, OTC medications, or herbal products patient may be taking - especially those medications that may affect coagulation or platelet function (see Drug Interactions). Note infusion specifics above. Vital signs, laboratory results (see above), and EKG should be monitored prior to, during, and after therapy. Arrhythmias may occur; antiarrhythmic drugs should be immediately available. Assess infusion site and monitor for hemorrhage every 10 minutes (or according to institutional policy) during therapy and for 1 hour following therapy (see Adverse Reactions and Overdose/Toxicology). Strict bedrest should be maintained and bleeding precautions should be instituted (avoid invasive procedures and activities that could cause trauma). Patient instruction is determined by patient condition (see Patient Education). **Pregnancy risk factor C** - benefits of use should outweigh possible risks. Note breast-feeding caution.

Patient Education: Inform prescriber of all prescriptions, OTC medications, or herbal products you are taking, and any allergies you have. This medication can only be administered by infusion; you will be monitored closely during and after treatment. You will have a tendency to bleed easily; use caution to prevent injury (use electric razor, soft toothbrush, and use caution with knives, needles, or anything sharp). Follow instructions for strict bedrest to reduce the risk of injury. If bleeding occurs, report immediately and apply pressure to bleeding spot until bleeding stops completely. Report immediately any unusual pain (acute headache, joint pain, chest pain); unusual bruising or bleeding; blood in urine, stool, or vomitus; bleeding gums; vision changes; or difficulty breathing. **Pregnancy/breast-feeding precautions:** Inform prescriber if you are or intend to become pregnant. Consult prescriber if breast-feeding.

Teniposide (ten i POE side)

U.S. Brand Names Vumon

Synonyms EPT; VM-26

Generic Available No

Pharmacologic Category Antineoplastic Agent, Miscellaneous

Pregnancy Risk Factor D

Lactation Not recommended

Use Treatment of acute lymphocytic leukemia, small cell lung cancer

Mechanism of Action/Effect Inhibits mitotic activity; inhibits cells from entering mitosis

Contraindications Hypersensitivity to teniposide, Cremophor® EL (polyoxyethylated castor oil), or any component of the formulation; pregnancy

Warnings/Precautions The U.S. Food and Drug Administration (FDA) currently recommends that procedures for proper handling and disposal of antineoplastic agents be considered. Teniposide injection contains benzyl alcohol and should be avoided in neonates. The injection contains about 43% alcohol; the possible CNS depressant effect, especially with higher doses of teniposide, should be considered.

Drug Interactions

Cytochrome P450 Effect: Substrate of **CYP3A4**; Inhibits CYP2C8/9, 3A4

Decreased Effect: Barbiturates, phenytoin (and other CYP3A4 inducers) may decrease teniposide efficacy.

Increased Effect/Toxicity: Alteration of methotrexate (MTX) transport has been found as a slow efflux of MTX and its polyglutamated form out of the cell, leading to intercellular

(Continued)

Teniposide *(Continued)*

accumulation of MTX. Sodium salicylate, sulfamethizole, and tolbutamide displace teniposide from protein-binding sites which could cause substantial increases in free drug levels, resulting in potentiation of toxicity. Concurrent use of vincristine may increase the incidence of peripheral neuropathy.

Nutritional/Ethanol Interactions Herb/Nutraceutical: St John's wort may decrease teniposide levels.

Adverse Reactions

>10%:

Gastrointestinal: Mucositis (75%); diarrhea, nausea, vomiting (20% to 30%); anorexia

Hematologic: Myelosuppression, leukopenia, neutropenia (95%), thrombocytopenia (65% to 80%), anemia

Onset: 5-7 days

Nadir: 7-10 days

Recovery: 21-28 days

1% to 10%:

Cardiovascular: Hypotension (2%), associated with rapid (<30 minutes) infusions

Dermatologic: Alopecia (9%), rash (3%)

Miscellaneous: Anaphylactoid reactions (5%) (fever, rash, hypertension, hypotension, dyspnea, bronchospasm), usually seen with rapid (<30 minutes) infusions

<1% (Limited to important or life-threatening): Lethargy, peripheral neuropathies, somnolence

Overdosage/Toxicology Symptoms of overdose include bone marrow suppression, leukopenia, thrombocytopenia, nausea, and vomiting. Treatment is supportive.

Pharmacodynamics/Kinetics

Half-Life Elimination: 5 hours

Metabolism: Extensively hepatic

Formulations Injection: 10 mg/mL (5 mL)

Dosing

Adults & Elderly:

Antineoplastic: I.V. (refer to individual protocols): 50-180 mg/m^2 once or twice weekly for 4-6 weeks or 20-60 mg/m^2/day for 5 days

Small cell lung cancer: I.V.: 80-90 mg/m^2/day for 5 days every 4-6 weeks

Dosage adjustment in Down syndrome patient: Reduce initial dosing give the first course at half the usual dose. Patients with both Down syndrome and leukemia may be especially sensitive to myelosuppressive chemotherapy.

Pediatrics:

Antineoplastic: I.V. (refer to individual protocols): 130 mg/m^2/week, increasing to 150 mg/m^2 after 3 weeks and up to 180 mg/m^2 after 6 weeks

Acute lymphoblastic leukemia (ALL): I.V.: 165 mg/m^2 twice weekly for 8-9 doses **or** 250 mg/m^2 weekly for 4-8 weeks

Renal Impairment: Data is insufficient, but dose adjustments may be necessary in patient with significant renal impairment.

Hepatic Impairment: Data is insufficient, but dose adjustments may be necessary in patient with significant hepatic impairment.

Administration

I.V.: Irritant. Slow I.V. infusion over ≥30 minutes.

Stability

Storage: Store ampuls in refrigerator at 2°C to 8°C (36°F to 46°F).

Reconstitution: Reconstituted solutions are stable at room temperature for up to 24 hours after preparation. Teniposide must be diluted with either D_5W or 0.9% sodium chloride solutions to a final concentration of 0.1, 0.2, 0.4, or 1 mg/mL. In order to prevent extraction of the plasticizer DEHP, **solutions should be prepared in non-DEHP-containing containers such as glass or polyolefin containers**. The use of polyvinyl chloride (PVC) containers is not recommended. Administer 1 mg/mL solutions within 4 hours of preparation to reduce the potential for precipitation. Precipitation may occur at any concentration.

Compatibility: Stable in D_5W, LR, NS

Y-site administration: Incompatible with Idarubicin, heparin

Monitoring Laboratory Tests CBC, platelet count

Monitoring and Teaching Issues

Physical Assessment: See Contraindications, Warnings/Precautions, and Dosing for use cautions. Assess potential for interactions with other prescriptions, OTC medications, or herbal products patient may be taking (see Drug Interactions). Premedication with antiemetic may be beneficial. See specific infusion directions above. Infusion site should be closely monitored to prevent extravasation. Patient should be monitored closely during infusion for possible hypotension (may require discontinuing infusion and administering supportive therapy) or hypersensitivity reactions (chills, fever, tachycardia, dyspnea, hypotension). Assess results of laboratory tests, therapeutic effectiveness, and adverse reactions prior to each infusion and throughout therapy (see Adverse Reactions and Overdose/Toxicology). Teach patient possible side effects and interventions and adverse symptoms to report (see Patient Education). **Pregnancy risk factor D** - determine that patient is not pregnant before beginning treatment. Instruct patients of childbearing age on appropriate barrier contraceptive measures. Breast-feeding is not recommended.

Patient Education: Inform prescriber of all prescriptions, OTC medications, or herbal products you are taking, and any allergies you have. Do not take anything new during treatment unless approved by prescriber. This medication can only be administered by infusion. Report immediately any swelling, pain, burning, or redness at infusion site. It is important to maintain adequate hydration (2-3 L/day of fluids) unless advised by prescriber to restrict fluids, and adequate nutrition (small, frequent meals may help). You will be more susceptible to infection (avoid crowds and exposure to infection and do not have any vaccinations without consulting prescriber). May cause nausea or vomiting (small, frequent meals, frequent mouth care, sucking lozenges, or chewing gum may help); diarrhea (buttermilk, boiled milk, or yogurt may help); or loss of hair (reversible). Report unusual bleeding or bruising, persistent fever or chills, sore throat, sores in mouth or vagina, or difficulty breathing. **Pregnancy/breast-feeding precautions:** Do not get pregnant while taking this medication. Consult prescriber for appropriate barrier contraceptive measures. Breast-feeding is not recommended.

Related Information

Antiemetics for Chemotherapy-Induced Nausea and Vomiting *on page 1639*

Ten-K® *see* Potassium Supplements *on page 1106*

Tenofovir (te NOE fo veer)

U.S. Brand Names Viread™

Synonyms PMPA; TDF; Tenofovir Disoproxil Fumarate

Generic Available No

Pharmacologic Category Antiretroviral Agent, Reverse Transcriptase Inhibitor (Nucleotide)

Pregnancy Risk Factor B

Lactation Excretion in breast milk unknown/contraindicated

Use Management of HIV infections in combination with at least two other antiretroviral agents

Mechanism of Action/Effect Tenofovir blocks replication of HIV virus by inhibiting the reverse transcriptase enzyme. It is chemically similar to adenosine 5'-monophosphate (a nucleotide), which is required to form DNA.

Contraindications Hypersensitivity to tenofovir or any component of the formulation

Warnings/Precautions Lactic acidosis and severe hepatomegaly with steatosis have been reported with nucleoside analogues, including fatal cases; use with caution in patients with risk factors for liver disease (risk may be increased in obese patients or prolonged exposure) and suspend treatment in any patient who develops clinical or laboratory findings suggestive of lactic acidosis (transaminase elevation may/may not accompany hepatomegaly and steatosis).

Avoid use in patients with renal impairment (Cl_{cr} <60 mL/minute); data to support dosage adjustment not yet available. May have potential to cause osteomalacia and/or renal toxicity (based on preclinical animal studies); monitor renal function and possible bone abnormalities during therapy. Use caution in hepatic impairment. Safety and effectiveness not established in pediatric patients.

Drug Interactions

Cytochrome P450 Effect: Inhibits CYP1A2

Decreased Effect: Serum levels of lopinavir and/or ritonavir may be decreased by tenofovir.

Increased Effect/Toxicity: Concurrent use has been noted to increase serum concentrations/exposure to didanosine and its metabolites, potentially increasing the risk of didanosine toxicity (pancreatitis, peripheral neuropathy, or lactic acidosis); suspend therapy of signs/symptoms of toxicity are present. Drugs which may compete for renal tubule secretion (including acyclovir, cidofovir, ganciclovir, valacyclovir, valganciclovir) may increase the serum concentrations of tenofovir. Drugs causing nephrotoxicity may also reduce elimination of tenofovir.

Nutritional/Ethanol Interactions Food: Fatty meals may increase the bioavailability of tenofovir. Tenofovir should be taken with food.

Adverse Reactions Clinical trials involved addition to prior antiretroviral therapy. Frequencies listed are treatment-emergent adverse effects noted at higher frequency than in the placebo group.

>10%: Gastrointestinal: Nausea (11%)

1% to 10%:

- Endocrine & metabolic: Glycosuria (3%, frequency equal to placebo); other metabolic effects (hyperglycemia, hypertriglyceridemia) noted at frequencies less than placebo
- Gastrointestinal: Diarrhea (9%), vomiting (5%), flatulence (4%), abdominal pain (3%, frequency equal to placebo), anorexia (3%)
- Hematologic: Neutropenia (1%, frequency equal to placebo)
- Hepatic: Increased transaminases (2% to 4%)
- Neuromuscular & skeletal: Weakness (8%, frequency equal to placebo)

Note: Uncommon, but significant adverse reactions reported with other reverse transcriptase inhibitors include pancreatitis, peripheral neuropathy, and myopathy. These have not been reported in clinical trials with tenofovir prior to marketing approval.

Overdosage/Toxicology Limited experience with overdose. Treatment is supportive.

Pharmacodynamics/Kinetics

Bioavailability: Fasting: 25%; increases ~40% with high-fat meal

Time to Peak: Fasting: 1 hour; With food: 2 hours

Metabolism: Not by CYP; converted intracellularly by hydrolysis to tenofovir, then phosphorylated to the active tenofovir diphosphate

Formulations Tablet, as disoproxil fumarate: 300 mg [equivalent to 245 mg tenofovir disoproxil]

Dosing

Adults: HIV infection: Oral: 300 mg once daily

Note: When used concurrently with didanosine, tenofovir should be administered at least 2 hours before or 1 hour after didanosine.

Renal Impairment: Avoid use in renal impairment (Cl_{cr} <60 mL/minute). No dosage guidelines available.

Stability

Storage: Store at 25°C (77°F); excursions permitted to 15°C to 30°C (59°F to 86°F).

Monitoring Laboratory Tests CBC with differential, reticulocyte count, serum creatine kinase, CD4 cell count, HIV RNA plasma levels, renal and hepatic function tests, bone density (long-term), serum phosphorus

Monitoring and Teaching Issues

Physical Assessment: See Contraindications, Warnings/Precautions, and Dosing for use cautions. Assess potential for interactions with other prescriptions, OTC medications, or

(Continued)

Tenofovir *(Continued)*

herbal products patient may be taking (see Drug Interactions). Assess results of laboratory tests (see above), therapeutic response, and adverse reactions (see Adverse Reactions and Overdose/Toxicology) on a regular basis throughout therapy. Teach patient proper use, possible side effects and interventions, and adverse symptoms to report (see Patient Education). **Pregnancy risk factor B** - benefits of use should outweigh possible risks. Breast-feeding is contraindicated.

Patient Education: Inform prescriber of all prescriptions, OTC medications, or herbal products you are taking (especially anything that may cause drowsiness), and any allergies you have. Take exactly as directed with food (space other medications as instructed). This drug will not cure HIV; use appropriate precautions to prevent spread to other persons. Maintain adequate hydration (2-3 L/day of fluids) unless advised by prescriber to restrict fluids. You may be susceptible to infection (avoid crowds and exposure to infection and do not have any vaccinations without consulting prescriber). May cause nausea, vomiting, loss of appetite (small, frequent meals, frequent mouth care, chewing gum, or sucking lozenges may help); or diarrhea (boiled milk, yogurt, or buttermilk may help). Report immediately any loss of sensation, numbness, or tingling in fingers, toes, or feet; persistent unresolved abdominal distress (nausea, vomiting, diarrhea); signs of opportunistic infection (burning on urination, perineal itching, white plaques in mouth, unhealed sores, persistent sore throat or cough) **Pregnancy/breast-feeding precautions:** Inform prescriber if you are pregnant and do not get pregnant while taking this medicine. Breast-feeding is not recommended. HIV-infected mothers are discouraged from breast-feeding to decrease potential transmission of HIV.

Dietary Issues: Take with food to increase absorption.

Breast-feeding Issues: HIV-infected mothers are discouraged from breast-feeding to decrease potential transmission of HIV.

Pregnancy Issues: No adequate or well-controlled studies in pregnant women. Use in pregnancy only if clearly needed. Cases of lactic acidosis/hepatic steatosis syndrome have been reported in pregnant women receiving nucleoside analogues. It is not known if pregnancy itself potentiates this known side effect; however, pregnant women may be at increased risk of lactic acidosis and liver damage. Hepatic enzymes and electrolytes should be monitored frequently during the 3rd trimester of pregnancy in women receiving nucleoside analogues. Health professionals are encouraged to contact the Antiretroviral Pregnancy Registry to monitor outcomes of pregnant women exposed to antiretroviral medications (1-800-258-4263).

Additional Information Approval was based on two clinical trials involving patients who were previously treated with antiretrovirals with continued evidence of HIV replication despite therapy. The risk:benefit ratio for untreated patients has not been established (studies currently ongoing), however, patients who received tenofovir showed significant decreases in HIV replication as compared to continuation of standard therapy. At the time of approval, there are no long-term trials to demonstrate inhibition of clinical HIV progression by tenofovir.

Tenofovir Disoproxil Fumarate *see* Tenofovir *on page 1287*

Tenoretic® *see* Atenolol and Chlorthalidone *on page 128*

Tenormin® *see* Atenolol *on page 126*

Tenuate® *see* Diethylpropion *on page 406*

Tenuate® Dospan® *see* Diethylpropion *on page 406*

Tequin® *see* Gatifloxacin *on page 621*

Tera-Cortril® *see page 1509*

Terazol® 3 *see* Terconazole *on page 1292*

Terazol® 7 *see* Terconazole *on page 1292*

Terazosin (ter AY zoe sin)

U.S. Brand Names Hytrin®

Generic Available Yes

Pharmacologic Category Alpha$_1$ Blocker

Pregnancy Risk Factor C

Lactation Excretion in breast milk unknown

Use Management of mild to moderate hypertension; alone or in combination with other agents such as diuretics or beta-blockers; benign prostate hyperplasia (BPH)

Mechanism of Action/Effect Alpha$_1$-specific blocking agent with minimal alpha$_2$ effects; this allows peripheral postsynaptic blockade, with the resultant decrease in arterial tone, while preserving the negative feedback loop which is mediated by the peripheral presynaptic alpha$_2$-receptors; terazosin relaxes the smooth muscle of the bladder neck, thus reducing bladder outlet obstruction

Contraindications Hypersensitivity to quinazolines (doxazosin, prazosin, terazosin) or any component of the formulation

Warnings/Precautions Can cause significant orthostatic hypotension and syncope, especially with first dose. Prostate cancer should be ruled out before starting for BPH. Anticipate a similar effect if therapy is interrupted for a few days, if dosage is rapidly increased, or if another antihypertensive drug is introduced. Pregnancy risk C.

Drug Interactions

Decreased Effect: Decreased antihypertensive response with NSAIDs. Alpha-blockers reduce the response to pressor agents (norepinephrine).

Increased Effect/Toxicity: Terazosin's hypotensive effect is increased with beta-blockers, diuretics, ACE inhibitors, calcium channel blockers, and other antihypertensive medications.

Nutritional/Ethanol Interactions Herb/Nutraceutical: Avoid dong quai if using for hypertension (has estrogenic activity). Avoid ephedra, yohimbe, ginseng (may worsen hypertension). Avoid saw palmetto. Avoid garlic (may have increased antihypertensive effect).

Adverse Reactions Asthenia, postural hypotension, dizziness, somnolence, nasal congestion/rhinitis, and impotence were the only events noted in clinical trials to occur at a frequency significantly greater than placebo ($p<0.05$).

>10%: Central nervous system: Dizziness, headache, muscle weakness

1% to 10%:

Cardiovascular: Edema, palpitations, chest pain, peripheral edema (3%), orthostatic hypotension (2.7% to 3.9%), tachycardia

Central nervous system: Fatigue, nervousness, drowsiness

Gastrointestinal: Dry mouth

Genitourinary: Urinary incontinence

Ocular: Blurred vision

Respiratory: Dyspnea, nasal congestion

<1% (Limited to important or life-threatening): Allergic reactions, anaphylaxis, atrial fibrillation, priapism, sexual dysfunction, syncope (0.8%), thrombocytopenia

Overdosage/Toxicology Symptoms of overdose include hypotension, drowsiness, and shock. Treatment is supportive and symptomatic.

Pharmacodynamics/Kinetics

Absorption: Rapid

Half-Life Elimination: 9.2-12 hours

Time to Peak: Serum: ~1 hour

Metabolism: Extensively hepatic

Onset: 1-2 hours

Formulations

Capsule: 1 mg, 2 mg, 5 mg, 10 mg

Tablet: 1 mg, 2 mg, 5 mg, 10 mg

Dosing

Adults & Elderly:

Hypertension: Oral: Initial: 1 mg at bedtime; slowly increase dose to achieve desired blood pressure, up to 20 mg/day; usual dose: 1-5 mg/day.

Benign prostatic hyperplasia: Oral: Initial: 1 mg at bedtime, increasing as needed; most patients require 10 mg day. If no response after 4-6 weeks of 10 mg/day, may increase to 20 mg/day.

Monitoring and Teaching Issues

Physical Assessment: See Contraindications, Warnings/Precautions, and Dosing for use cautions. Assess potential for interactions with other prescriptions, OTC medications, or herbal products patient may be taking (see Drug Interactions). Assess therapeutic effectiveness (blood pressure) and adverse reactions at beginning of therapy and on a regular basis with long-term therapy (see Adverse Reactions and Overdose/Toxicology). When discontinuing, dose should be tapered and blood pressure monitored closely. Teach patient proper use, possible side effects and interventions, and adverse symptoms to report (see Patient Education). **Pregnancy risk factor C** - benefits of use should outweigh possible risks. Note breast-feeding caution.

Patient Education: Inform prescriber of all prescriptions, OTC medications, or herbal products you are taking, and any allergies you have. Do not take anything new during treatment unless approved by prescriber. Take as directed; at bedtime. Do not skip dose or discontinue without consulting prescriber. Follow recommended diet and exercise program. May cause drowsiness, dizziness, or impaired judgment (use caution when driving or engaging in tasks that require alertness until response to drug is known); postural hypotension (use caution when rising from sitting or lying position or when climbing stairs); dry mouth or nausea (frequent mouth care or sucking lozenges may help); urinary incontinence (void before taking medication); or sexual dysfunction (reversible, may resolve with continued use). Report altered CNS status (eg, fatigue, lethargy, confusion, nervousness); sudden weight gain (weigh yourself in the same clothes at the same time of day once a week); unusual or persistent swelling of ankles, feet, or extremities; palpitations or rapid heartbeat; difficulty breathing; muscle weakness; or other persistent side effects. **Pregnancy/breast-feeding precautions:** Inform prescriber if you are or intend to become pregnant. Consult prescriber if breast-feeding.

Dietary Issues: May be taken without regard to meals at the same time each day.

Geriatric Considerations: Adverse reactions such as dry mouth and urinary problems can be particularly bothersome in the elderly.

Related Information

Pharmacotherapy of Urinary Incontinence *on page 1699*

Terbinafine (TER bin a feen)

U.S. Brand Names Lamisil®; Lamisil® AT™; Lamisil® Dermgel; Lamisil® Solution

Synonyms Terbinafine Hydrochloride

Generic Available No

Pharmacologic Category Antifungal Agent, Oral; Antifungal Agent, Topical

Pregnancy Risk Factor B

Lactation Excreted in breast milk/not recommended

Use Active against most strains of *Trichophyton mentagrophytes*, *Trichophyton rubrum*; may be effective for infections of *Microsporum gypseum* and *M. nanum*, *Trichophyton verrucosum*, *Epidermophyton floccosum*, *Candida albicans*, and *Scopulariopsis brevicaulis*

Oral: Onychomycosis of the toenail or fingernail due to susceptible dermatophytes

Topical: Antifungal for the treatment of tinea pedis (athlete's foot), tinea cruris (jock itch), and tinea corporis (ringworm)

Use - Unlabeled/Investigational Topical: Cutaneous candidiasis and pityriasis versicolor

Contraindications Hypersensitivity to terbinafine, naftifine, or any component of the formulation; pre-existing liver or renal disease (≤50 mL/minute GFR)

Warnings/Precautions While rare, the following complications have been reported and may require discontinuation of therapy: Changes in the ocular lens and retina, pancytopenia, neutropenia, Stevens-Johnson syndrome, toxic epidermal necrolysis. Rare cases of hepatic failure, including fatal cases, have been reported following oral treatment of onychomycosis.

(Continued)

Terbinafine *(Continued)*

Not recommended for use in patients with active or chronic liver disease. Discontinue if symptoms or signs of hepatobiliary dysfunction or cholestatic hepatitis develop. If irritation/sensitivity develop with topical use, discontinue therapy. **Use caution in writing and/or filling prescription/orders. Confusion between Lamictal® (lamotrigine) and Lamisil® (terbinafine) has occurred.**

Drug Interactions

Cytochrome P450 Effect: Substrate of **CYP3A4**; Inhibits CYP2D6; Induces CYP3A4

Decreased Effect: Cyclosporine clearance is increased (~15%) with concomitant terbinafine; rifampin increases terbinafine clearance (100%); rifampin increases the metabolism of terbinafine (decreases serum concentration)

Increased Effect/Toxicity: Terbinafine clearance is decreased by cimetidine (33%); caffeine clearance is decreased by terbinafine (19%); effects of drugs metabolized by CYP2D6 (including beta-blockers, SSRIs, MAO inhibitors, tricyclic antidepressants) may be increased; warfarin effects may be increased

Adverse Reactions

Oral:

1% to 10%:

Central nervous system: Headache, dizziness, vertigo

Dermatologic: Rash, pruritus, and alopecia with oral therapy

Gastrointestinal: Nausea, diarrhea, dyspepsia, abdominal pain, appetite decrease, taste disturbance

Hematologic: Lymphocytopenia

Hepatic: Liver enzyme elevations

Ocular: Visual disturbance

Miscellaneous: Allergic reaction

<1% (Limited to important or life-threatening): Agranulocytosis, allergic reactions, anaphylaxis, hepatic failure, neutropenia, Stevens-Johnson syndrome, taste disturbance (with prolonged recovery and weight loss), thrombocytopenia, toxic epidermal necrolysis; changes in ocular lens and retina have been reported (clinical significance unknown)

Topical: 1% to 10%:

Dermatologic: Pruritus, contact dermatitis, irritation, burning, dryness

Local: Irritation, stinging

Pharmacodynamics/Kinetics

Absorption: Topical: Limited (<5%); Oral: >70%

Bioavailability: Oral: 80%

Half-Life Elimination: 22-26 hours; very slow release of drug from skin and adipose tissues occurs

Time to Peak: Plasma: 1-2 hours

Metabolism: Hepatic; no active metabolites; first-pass effect (40%); little effect on CYP

Formulations

Cream: 1% (15 g, 30 g)

Gel: 1% (5 g, 15 g, 30 g)

Solution, topical spray: 1%

Tablet: 250 mg

Dosing

Adults & Elderly:

Superficial mycoses (onychomycosis): Oral:

Fingernail: 250 mg/day for up to 6 weeks; may be given in two divided doses

Toenail: 250 mg/day for 12 weeks; may be given in two divided doses

Systemic mycosis: Oral: 250-500 mg/day for up to 16 months

Athlete's foot (tinea pedis): Topical:

Cream: Apply to affected area twice daily for at least 1 week, not to exceed 4 weeks

Gel: Apply to affected area once daily for 7 days

Solution: Apply to affected area twice daily for 7 days

Ringworm and jock itch (tinea versicolor, tinea corporis, tinea cruris): Topical:

Cream: Apply to affected area once or twice daily for at least 1 week, not to exceed 4 weeks

Gel: Apply to affected area once daily for 7 days

Solution: Apply to affected area once daily for 7 days in tinea corporis and tinea cruris; apply to affected area twice daily for 7 days in tinea versicolor

Renal Impairment: Oral administration: Although specific guidelines are not available, dose reduction in significant renal insufficiency (GFR <50 mL/minute) is recommended.

Stability

Storage:

Cream: Store at 5°C to 30°C (41°F to 86°F).

Solution: Store at 8°C to 25°C (46°F to 77°F).

Monitoring and Teaching Issues

Patient Education: Topical: Avoid contact with eyes, nose, or mouth. Advise physician if eyes or skin becomes yellow or if irritation, itching, or burning develops. Do not use occlusive dressings concurrent with therapy. Full clinical effect may require several months due to the time required for a new nail to grow. **Breast-feeding precaution:** Nursing women should not use on breast tissue.

Breast-feeding Issues: Although minimal concentrations of terbinafine cross into breast milk after topical use, oral or topical treatment during lactation should be avoided.

Pregnancy Issues: Avoid use in pregnancy since treatment of onychomycosis is postponable.

Additional Information Due to potential toxicity, the manufacturer recommends confirmation of diagnosis testing of nail specimens prior to treatment of onychomycosis.

A meta-analysis of efficacy studies for toenail infections revealed that weighted average mycological cure rates for continuous therapy were 36.7% (griseofulvin), 54.7% (itraconazole), and 77% (terbinafine). Cure rate for 4-month pulse therapy for itraconazole and terbinafine were 73.3% and 80%. Additionally, the final outcome measure of final costs per cured infections for continuous therapy was significantly lower for terbinafine.

Terbinafine Hydrochloride *see* Terbinafine *on page 1289*

Terbutaline (ter BYOO ta leen)

U.S. Brand Names Brethine®

Synonyms Brethaire [DSC]; Bricanyl [DSC]

Generic Available No

Pharmacologic Category $Beta_2$ Agonist

Pregnancy Risk Factor B

Lactation Enters breast milk/compatible

Use Bronchodilator in reversible airway obstruction and bronchial asthma; tocolytic agent

Use - Unlabeled/Investigational Tocolytic agent (management of preterm labor)

Mechanism of Action/Effect Relaxes bronchial smooth muscle by action on $beta_2$-receptors with less effect on heart rate

Contraindications Hypersensitivity to terbutaline or any component of the formulation; cardiac arrhythmias associated with tachycardia; tachycardia caused by digitalis intoxication

Warnings/Precautions Excessive or prolonged use may lead to tolerance. Paradoxical bronchoconstriction may occur with excessive use. If it occurs, discontinue terbutaline immediately. When used for tocolysis, there is some risk of maternal pulmonary edema, which has been associated with the following risk factors, excessive hydration, multiple gestation, occult sepsis and underlying cardiac disease. To reduce risk, limit fluid intake to 2.5-3 L/day, limit sodium intake, maintain maternal pulse to <130 beats/minute.

Drug Interactions

Decreased Effect: Decreased effect with beta-blockers.

Increased Effect/Toxicity: Increased toxicity with MAO inhibitors, tricyclic antidepressants.

Nutritional/Ethanol Interactions Herb/Nutraceutical: Avoid ephedra, yohimbe (may cause CNS stimulation).

Adverse Reactions

>10%:

Central nervous system: Nervousness, restlessness

Neuromuscular & skeletal: Trembling

1% to 10%:

Cardiovascular: Tachycardia, hypertension, pounding heartbeat

Central nervous system: Dizziness, lightheadedness, drowsiness, headache, insomnia

Gastrointestinal: Dry mouth, nausea, vomiting, bad taste in mouth

Neuromuscular & skeletal: Muscle cramps, weakness

Miscellaneous: Diaphoresis

<1% (Limited to important or life-threatening): Arrhythmia, chest pain, paradoxical bronchospasm

Overdosage/Toxicology Symptoms of overdose include seizures, nausea, vomiting, tachycardia, cardiac dysrhythmias, and hypokalemia. In cases of overdose, supportive therapy should be instituted. Prudent use of a cardioselective beta-adrenergic blocker (eg, atenolol or metoprolol) should be considered, keeping in mind the potential for induction of bronchoconstriction in an asthmatic. Dialysis has not been shown to be of value in the treatment of overdose with terbutaline.

Pharmacodynamics/Kinetics

Bioavailability: S.C. doses are more bioavailable than oral

Half-Life Elimination: 11-16 hours

Metabolism: Hepatic to inactive sulfate conjugates

Onset: Oral: 30-45 minutes; S.C.: 6-15 minutes

Formulations

Injection, as sulfate: 1 mg/mL (1 mL)

Tablet, as sulfate: 2.5 mg, 5 mg

Dosing

Adults:

Bronchoconstriction:

Oral: 5 mg/dose every 6 hours 3 times/day; if side effects occur, reduce dose to 2.5 mg every 6 hours; not to exceed 15 mg in 24 hours.

S.C.: 0.25 mg/dose repeated in 15-30 minutes for one time only; a total dose of 0.5 mg should not be exceeded within a 4-hour period.

Premature labor (tocolysis):

Acute: I.V. 2.5-10 mcg/minute; increased gradually every 10-20 minutes. Effective maximum dosages from 17.5-30 mcg/minute have been use with caution. Duration of infusion is at least 12 hours.

Maintenance: Oral: 2.5-10 mg every 4-6 hours for as long as necessary to prolong pregnancy depending on patient tolerance

Elderly: Not recommended for use in the elderly (see Geriatric Considerations).

Pediatrics: Bronchoconstriction:

Oral: Children:

<12 years: Initial: 0.05 mg/kg/dose 3 times/day, increased gradually as required; maximum: 0.15 mg/kg/dose 3-4 times/day or a total of 5 mg/24 hours

12-15 years: 2.5 mg every 6 hours 3 times/day; not to exceed 7.5 mg in 24 hours

>15 years: 5 mg/dose every 6 hours 3 times/day; if side effects occur, reduce dose to 2.5 mg every 6 hours; not to exceed 15 mg in 24 hours

S.C.: Children:

<12 years: 0.005-0.01 mg/kg/dose to a maximum of 0.3 mg/dose every 15-20 minutes for 3 doses

≥12 years: Refer to adult dosing.

Renal Impairment:

Cl_{cr} 10-50 mL/minute: Administer 50% of normal dose.

(Continued)

Terbutaline *(Continued)*

Cl_{cr} <10 mL/minute: Avoid use.

Administration

Oral: Administer around-the-clock to promote less variation in peak and trough serum levels.

I.V.: Use infusion pump.

Stability

Storage: Store injection at room temperature. Protect from heat, light, and from freezing. Use only clear solutions.

Compatibility: Stable in D_5W, ½NS, NS

Compatibility when admixed: Incompatible with bleomycin

Monitoring Laboratory Tests Serum potassium

Tocolysis: If patient receives therapy for more than 1 week, monitor serum glucose.

Monitoring and Teaching Issues

Physical Assessment: Respiratory use: Assess effectiveness and interactions of other medications patient may be taking (see Drug Interactions). See Contraindications and Warnings/Precautions for use cautions. Monitor therapeutic effectiveness and adverse reactions (see Adverse Reactions) at beginning of therapy and periodically with long-term use. For inpatient care, monitor vital signs and lung sounds prior to and periodically during therapy. Assess knowledge/teach patient appropriate use, interventions to reduce side effects, and adverse symptoms to report (see Patient Education). **Preterm labor use: Inpatient:** Monitor maternal vital signs; respiratory, cardiac, and electrolyte status; frequency, duration, and intensity of contractions; and fetal heart rate. For outpatients, assess knowledge/teach patient appropriate use, interventions to reduce side effects, and adverse symptoms to report (see Patient Education).

Patient Education: Use exactly as directed (see following administration information). Do not use more often than recommended (excessive use may result in tolerance, overdose may result in serious adverse effects) and do not discontinue without consulting prescriber. Maintain adequate hydration (2-3 L/day of fluids) unless advised by prescriber to restrict fluids. You may experience nervousness, dizziness, or fatigue (use caution when driving or engaging in tasks requiring alertness until response to drug is known); or dry mouth, stomach upset (small, frequent meals, frequent mouth care, chewing gum, or sucking hard candy may help). Report unresolved GI upset; dizziness or fatigue; vision changes; chest pain, rapid heartbeat, or palpitations; insomnia, nervousness, or hyperactivity; muscle cramping, tremors, or pain; unusual cough; or rash (hypersensitivity).

Preterm labor: Notify prescriber immediately if labor resumes or adverse side effects are noted.

Related Information

Inhalant (Asthma, Bronchospasm) Agents Comparison *on page 1577*

Terconazole (ter KONE a zole)

U.S. Brand Names Terazol® 3; Terazol® 7

Synonyms Triaconazole

Generic Available No

Pharmacologic Category Antifungal Agent, Vaginal

Pregnancy Risk Factor C

Lactation Excretion in breast milk unknown

Use Local treatment of vulvovaginal candidiasis

Mechanism of Action/Effect Triazole ketal antifungal agent; involves inhibition of fungal cytochrome P450

Contraindications Hypersensitivity to terconazole or any component of the formulation

Warnings/Precautions Should be discontinued if sensitization or irritation occurs. Microbiological studies (KOH smear and/or cultures) should be repeated in patients not responding to terconazole in order to confirm the diagnosis and rule out other pathogens. Pregnancy risk C.

Adverse Reactions

1% to 10%:

Central nervous system; Fever, chills

Gastrointestinal: Abdominal pain

Genitourinary: Vulvar/vaginal burning, dysmenorrhea

<1% (Limited to important or life-threatening): Burning or itching of penis of sexual partner, flu-like syndrome, polyuria; vulvar itching, soreness, edema, or discharge

Pharmacodynamics/Kinetics

Absorption: Extent of systemic absorption after vaginal administration may be dependent on presence of a uterus; 5% to 8% in women who had a hysterectomy versus 12% to 16% in nonhysterectomy women

Formulations

Cream, vaginal:

Terazol® 7: 0.4% (45 g)

Terazol® 3: 0.8% (20 g)

Suppository, vaginal (Terazol® 3): 80 mg (3s)

Dosing

Adults & Elderly: Vulvovaginal candidiasis: Intravaginal:

Terazol® 3 vaginal cream: Insert 1 applicatorful intravaginally at bedtime for 3 consecutive days.

Terazol® 7 vaginal cream: Insert 1 applicatorful intravaginally at bedtime for 7 consecutive days.

Terazol® 3 vaginal suppository: Insert 1 suppository intravaginally at bedtime for 3 consecutive days.

Stability

Storage: Store at room temperature of 13°C to 30°C (59°F to 86°F).

Monitoring and Teaching Issues

Physical Assessment: See Contraindications and Warnings/Precautions for use cautions. Assess knowledge/teach patient appropriate administration, possible side effects/interventions, and adverse symptoms to report (see Patient Education). **Pregnancy risk factor C** - benefits of use should outweigh possible risks. Note breast-feeding caution.

Patient Education: Complete full course of therapy as directed. Insert vaginally as directed by prescriber or see package insert. Sexual partner may experience irritation of penis; best to refrain from intercourse during period of treatment. Suppositories may cause breakdown of rubber/latex products such as diaphragms; avoid concurrent use. Report persistent vaginal burning, itching, irritation, or discharge. **Pregnancy/breast-feeding precautions:** Inform prescriber if you are or intend to become pregnant. Consult prescriber if breast-feeding.

Geriatric Considerations: Assess patient's ability to self-administer; may be difficult in patients with arthritis or limited range of motion.

Teriparatide *see page 1461*

Teslac® *see* Testolactone *on page 1293*

TESPA *see* Thiotepa *on page 1309*

Tessalon® *see* Benzonatate *on page 157*

Testim™ *see* Testosterone *on page 1294*

Testoderm® *see* Testosterone *on page 1294*

Testoderm® TTS [DSC] *see* Testosterone *on page 1294*

Testoderm® with Adhesive *see* Testosterone *on page 1294*

Testolactone (tes toe LAK tone)

U.S. Brand Names Teslac®

Restrictions C-III

Generic Available No

Pharmacologic Category Androgen

Pregnancy Risk Factor C

Lactation Excretion in breast milk unknown

Use Palliative treatment of advanced disseminated breast carcinoma

Mechanism of Action/Effect Testolactone is a synthetic testosterone derivative without significant androgen activity. The drug inhibits steroid aromatase activity, thereby blocking the production of estradiol and estrone from androgen precursors such as testosterone and androstenedione. Unfortunately, the enzymatic block provided by testolactone is transient and is usually limited to a period of 3 months.

Contraindications Hypersensitivity to testolactone or any component of the formulation; in men for the treatment of breast cancer

Warnings/Precautions The U.S. Food and Drug Administration (FDA) currently recommends that procedures for proper handling and disposal of antineoplastic agents be considered. Use with caution in hepatic, renal, or cardiac disease; prolonged use may cause drug-induced hepatic disease; or history of porphyria. Pregnancy risk C.

Drug Interactions

Increased Effect/Toxicity: Increased effects of oral anticoagulants.

Effects on Lab Values Plasma estradiol concentrations by RIA

Adverse Reactions 1% to 10%:

Cardiovascular: Edema

Central nervous system: Malaise

Dermatologic: Maculopapular rash

Endocrine & metabolic: Hypercalcemia,

Gastrointestinal: Anorexia, diarrhea, nausea, edema of the tongue

Neuromuscular & skeletal: Paresthesias, peripheral neuropathies

Overdosage/Toxicology Increased toxicity: Increased effects of oral anticoagulants

Pharmacodynamics/Kinetics

Absorption: Well absorbed

Metabolism: Hepatic

Formulations Tablet: 50 mg

Dosing

Adults & Elderly: Breast carcinoma (palliative): Female: Oral: 250 mg 4 times/day for at least 3 months; desired response may take as long as 3 months.

Monitoring Laboratory Tests Plasma calcium levels

Monitoring and Teaching Issues

Physical Assessment: Assess effectiveness and interactions of other medications patient may be taking (see Drug Interactions, eg, anticoagulants). See Warnings/Precautions and Contraindications for use cautions. Monitor effectiveness of therapy, laboratory tests, and adverse response (see Adverse Reactions and Overdose/Toxicology). Assess knowledge/teach patient appropriate use, possible side effects and appropriate interventions, and adverse symptoms to report (see Patient Education). **Pregnancy risk factor C.** Note breast-feeding caution.

Patient Education: Take as directed; do not discontinue without consulting prescriber. Effectiveness of therapy may take several months. Maintain adequate hydration (2-3 L/day of fluids) unless advised by prescriber to restrict fluids, and diet and exercise program recommended by prescriber. You may experience nausea or vomiting (small, frequent meals, frequent mouth care, sucking lozenges, or chewing gum may help). Report fluid retention (swelling of ankles, feet, or hands; difficulty breathing or sudden weight gain); numbness, tingling, or swelling of fingers, toes, or face; skin rash, redness, or irritation; or other adverse reactions. **Pregnancy/breast-feeding precautions:** Inform prescriber if you are pregnant or intend to become pregnant. Consult prescriber if breast-feeding.

Testopel® *see* Testosterone *on page 1294*

Testosterone (tes TOS ter one)

U.S. Brand Names Androderm®; AndroGel®; Delatestryl®; Depo®-Testosterone; Testim™; Testoderm®; Testoderm® TTS [DSC]; Testoderm® with Adhesive; Testopel®

Synonyms Testosterone Cypionate; Testosterone Enanthate

Restrictions C-III

Generic Available No

Pharmacologic Category Androgen

Pregnancy Risk Factor X

Lactation Enters breast milk/contraindicated

Use

Injection: Androgen replacement therapy in the treatment of delayed male puberty; male hypogonadism (primary or hypogonadotropic); inoperable female breast cancer (enanthate only)

Pellet: Androgen replacement therapy in the treatment of delayed male puberty; male hypogonadism (primary or hypogonadotropic)

Topical: Male hypogonadism (primary or hypogonadotropic)

Mechanism of Action/Effect Principal endogenous androgen responsible for promoting the growth and development of the male sex organs and maintaining secondary sex characteristics in androgen-deficient males

Contraindications Hypersensitivity to testosterone or any component of the formulation (including soy); severe renal or cardiac disease; benign prostatic hyperplasia with obstruction; undiagnosed genital bleeding; males with carcinoma of the breast or prostate; pregnancy

Warnings/Precautions When used to treat delayed male puberty, perform radiographic examination of the hand and wrist every 6 months to determine the rate of bone maturation. May accelerate bone maturation without producing compensating gain in linear growth. Has both androgenic and anabolic activity, the anabolic action may enhance hypoglycemia. Use caution in elderly patients or patients with other demographic factors which may increase the risk of prostatic carcinoma; careful monitoring is required. May cause fluid retention; use caution in patients with cardiovascular disease or other edematous conditions. Prolonged use has been associated with serious hepatic effects (hepatitis, hepatic neoplasms, cholestatic hepatitis, jaundice). May potentiate sleep apnea in some male patients (obesity or chronic lung disease). Gels have not been evaluated in males <18 years of age; safety and efficacy of injection have not been established in males <12 years of age.

Drug Interactions

Cytochrome P450 Effect: Substrate of CYP2B6, 2C8/9, 2C19, 3A4; Inhibits CYP3A4

Increased Effect/Toxicity: Warfarin and testosterone: Effects of oral anticoagulants may be enhanced. Testosterone may increase levels of oxyphenbutazone. May enhance fluid retention from corticosteroids.

Nutritional/Ethanol Interactions Herb/Nutraceutical: St John's wort may decrease testosterone levels.

Effects on Lab Values May cause a decrease in creatinine and creatine excretion and an increase in the excretion of 17-ketosteroids, thyroid function tests.

Adverse Reactions Frequency not defined.

Cardiovascular: Flushing, edema

Central nervous system: Excitation, aggressive behavior, sleeplessness, anxiety, mental depression, headache

Dermatologic: Hirsutism (increase in pubic hair growth), acne

Endocrine & metabolic: Menstrual problems (amenorrhea), virilism, breast soreness, gynecomastia, hypercalcemia, hypoglycemia

Gastrointestinal: Nausea, vomiting, GI irritation

Genitourinary: Prostatic hyperplasia, prostatic carcinoma, impotence, testicular atrophy, epididymitis, priapism, bladder irritability

Hepatic: Hepatic dysfunction, cholestatic hepatitis, hepatic necrosis

Hematologic: Leukopenia, polycythemia, suppression of clotting factors

Miscellaneous: Hypersensitivity reactions

Pharmacodynamics/Kinetics

Absorption: Transdermal gel: ~10% of dose

Half-Life Elimination: 10-100 minutes

Metabolism: Hepatic; forms metabolites

Duration: Route and ester dependent; I.M.: Cypionate and enanthate esters have longest duration, ≤2-4 weeks

Formulations

Gel, topical

AndroGel®: 25 mg/2.5 g (30s); 50 mg/5 g (30s) [1% unit-dose packet]

Testim™: 50 mg/5 g (30s) [1% unit-dose tube]

Injection, in oil, as cypionate (Depo® Testosterone): 100 mg/mL (10 mL); 200 mg/mL (1 mL, 10 mL) [contains benzyl alcohol, benzyl benzoate, and cottonseed oil]

Injection, in oil, as enanthate (Delatestryl®): 200 mg/mL (1 mL) [prefilled syringe; contains sesame oil]; (5 mL) [multidose vial; contains sesame oil]

Pellet, for subcutaneous implantation (Testopel®): 75 mg (1 pellet/vial)

Transdermal system:

Androderm®: 2.5 mg/day (60s); 5 mg/day (30s)

Testoderm®: 4 mg/day (30s); 6 mg/day (30s)

Testoderm® TTS [DSC]: 5 mg/day (30s) [contains alcohol]

Testoderm® with Adhesive: 6 mg/day (30s)

Dosing

Adults & Elderly:

Female: Inoperable breast cancer: I.M.: Testosterone enanthate: 200-400 mg every 2-4 weeks

Male:

I.M.: Long-acting formulations: Testosterone enanthate (in oil)/testosterone cypionate (in oil):

Hypogonadism: 50-400 mg every 2-4 weeks

Delayed puberty: 50-200 mg every 2-4 weeks for a limited duration

Pellet (for subcutaneous implantation): Hypogonadism, delayed puberty: 150-450 mg every 3-6 months

Transdermal: Primary male hypogonadism **or** hypogonadotropic hypogonadism:

Testoderm®: Apply 6 mg patch daily to scrotum (if scrotum is inadequate, use a 4 mg daily system)

Androderm®: Apply two systems nightly to clean, dry area on the back, abdomen, upper arms, or thighs for 24 hours for a total of 5 mg day

AndroGel®, Testim™: 5 g (to deliver 50 mg of testosterone with 5 mg systemically absorbed) applied once daily (preferably in the morning) to clean, dry, intact skin of the shoulder and upper arms. AndroGel® may also be applied to the abdomen. Dosage may be increased to a maximum of 10 g (100 mg). Upon opening the packet(s), the entire contents should be squeezed into the palm of the hand and immediately applied to the application site(s). Application sites should be allowed to dry for a few minutes prior to dressing. Hands should be washed with soap and water after application. **Do not apply testosterone gel to the genitals**.

Pediatrics: Adolescents:

Male hypogonadism:

I.M.:

Initiation of pubertal growth: 40-50 mg/m^2/dose (cypionate or enanthate ester) monthly until the growth rate falls to prepubertal levels

Terminal growth phase: 100 mg/m^2/dose (cypionate or enanthate ester) monthly until growth ceases

Maintenance virilizing dose: 100 mg/m^2/dose (cypionate or enanthate ester) twice monthly

Pellet (for subcutaneous implantation): Refer to adult dosing.

Delayed puberty (male):

I.M.: 40-50 mg/m^2/dose monthly (cypionate or enanthate ester) for 6 months

Pellet (for subcutaneous implantation): Refer to adult dosing.

Hepatic Impairment: Reduce dose.

Administration

I.M.: Warm injection to room temperature and shaking vial will help redissolve crystals that have formed after storage. Administer by deep I.M. injection into the upper outer quadrant of the gluteus maximus.

Topical: Transdermal:

Androderm®: Apply patch to clean, dry area of skin on the arm, back, or upper buttocks.

Testoderm®: Apply patch to clean, dry scrotal skin. Dry shave scrotal hair for optimal skin contact. Do not use chemical depilatories.

AndroGel®, Testim™: Apply gel (preferably in the morning) to clean, dry, intact skin of the shoulder and upper arms (AndroGel® may also be applied to the abdomen). Upon opening the packet(s), the entire contents should be squeezed into the palm of the hand and immediately applied to the application site(s). Application sites should be allowed to dry for a few minutes prior to dressing. Hands should be washed with soap and water after application. **Do not apply testosterone gel to the genitals**.

Monitoring Laboratory Tests Periodic liver function tests, PSA, cholesterol, hemoglobin and hematocrit; radiologic examination of wrist and hand every 6 months (when using in prepubertal children)

Gel: Morning serum testosterone levels 14 days after start of therapy

Monitoring and Teaching Issues

Physical Assessment: (For use in children see pediatric reference). See Contraindications, Warnings/Precautions, and Dosing for use cautions. Assess potential for interactions with other prescriptions, OTC medications, or herbal products patient may be taking (see Drug Interactions). Assess results of laboratory tests (see above), therapeutic effects (according to purpose for use), and adverse reactions (see Adverse Reactions and Overdose/Toxicology) regularly during therapy. Caution diabetic patients - may cause hypoglycemic reaction. Teach patient proper use (according to formulation), possible side effects and appropriate interventions, and adverse symptoms to report (see Patient Education). **Pregnancy risk factor X** - determine that patient is not pregnant before beginning treatment. Instruct patients of childbearing age or males who may have intercourse with women of childbearing age on appropriate barrier contraceptive measures. Breast-feeding is contraindicated.

Patient Education: Diabetics should monitor serum glucose closely and notify prescriber of changes; this medication may alter hypoglycemic requirements. You may experience acne, growth of body hair, loss of libido, impotence, or menstrual irregularity (usually reversible); nausea or vomiting (small frequent meals, frequent mouth care, sucking lozenges, or chewing gum may help). Report changes in menstrual pattern; enlarged or painful breasts; deepening of voice or unusual growth of body hair; persistent penile erection; fluid retention (swelling of ankles, feet, or hands, difficulty breathing or sudden weight gain); unresolved changes in CNS (nervousness, chills, insomnia, depression, aggressiveness); altered urinary patterns; change in color of urine or stool; yellowing of eyes or skin; unusual bruising or bleeding; or other persistent adverse reactions.

Transdermal:

Androderm®: Apply patch to clean, dry area of skin on the arm, back, or upper buttocks.

Testoderm®: Apply patch to clean, dry scrotal skin. Dry shave scrotal hair for optimal skin contact. Do not use chemical depilatories.

AndroGel®, Testim™: Apply gel (preferably in the morning) to clean, dry, intact skin of the shoulder and upper arms (AndroGel® may also be applied to the abdomen). Upon opening the packet(s), the entire contents should be squeezed into the palm of the hand and immediately applied to the application site(s). Application sites should be

(Continued)

Testosterone *(Continued)*

allowed to dry for a few minutes prior to dressing. Hands should be washed with soap and water after application. **Do not apply testosterone gel to the genitals.**

Pregnancy/breast-feeding precautions: Inform prescriber if you are pregnant. Do not get pregnant during or for 1 month following therapy. Male: Do not cause a female to become pregnant. Male/female: Consult prescriber for instruction on appropriate contraceptive measures. This drug may cause severe fetal defects. Do not breast-feed.

Geriatric Considerations: Geriatric patients may have an increased risk of prostatic hyperplasia or prostatic carcinoma.

Related Information

Controlled Substances Comparison *on page 1568*

Testosterone Cypionate *see* Testosterone *on page 1294*

Testosterone Enanthate *see* Testosterone *on page 1294*

Testred® *see* MethylTESTOSTERone *on page 887*

Tetanus Antitoxin *see page 1498*

Tetanus Immune Globulin, Human *see page 1498*

Tetanus Toxoid, Adsorbed *see page 1498*

Tetanus Toxoid, Fluid *see page 1498*

TetraCap® *see* Tetracycline *on page 1296*

Tetracycline (tet ra SYE kleen)

U.S. Brand Names Brodspec®; EmTet®; Sumycin®; TetraCap®; Topicycline®; Wesmycin®

Synonyms Achromycin [DSC]; TCN; Tetracycline Hydrochloride

Generic Available Yes

Pharmacologic Category Antibiotic, Ophthalmic; Antibiotic, Tetracycline Derivative; Antibiotic, Topical

Pregnancy Risk Factor D (systemic)/B (topical)

Lactation Enters breast milk/not recommended (AAP rates "compatible")

Use Treatment of susceptible bacterial infections of both gram-positive and gram-negative organisms; also infections due to *Mycoplasma*, *Chlamydia*, and *Rickettsia*; indicated for acne, exacerbations of chronic bronchitis, and treatment of gonorrhea and syphilis in patients that are allergic to penicillin; as part of a multidrug regimen for *H. pylori* eradication to reduce the risk of duodenal ulcer recurrence

Mechanism of Action/Effect Inhibits protein synthesis of susceptible bacteria; bacteriostatic - causes call death.

Contraindications Hypersensitivity to tetracycline or any component of the formulation; do not administer to children ≤8 years of age; pregnancy (systemic use)

Warnings/Precautions Use of tetracyclines during tooth development may cause permanent discoloration of the teeth and enamel, hypoplasia and retardation of skeletal development and bone growth with risk being the greatest for children <4 years and those receiving high doses; use with caution in patients with renal or hepatic impairment (eg, elderly) and in pregnancy; dosage modification required in patients with renal impairment since it may increase BUN as an antianabolic agent; pseudotumor cerebri has been reported with tetracycline use (usually resolves with discontinuation); outdated drug can cause nephropathy; superinfection possible; use protective measure to avoid photosensitivity

Drug Interactions

Cytochrome P450 Effect: Substrate of **CYP3A4**; Inhibits CYP3A4

Decreased Effect: Calcium, magnesium- or aluminum-containing antacids, iron, zinc, sodium bicarbonate, sucralfate, didanosine, or quinapril may decrease tetracycline absorption. Therapeutic effect of penicillins may be reduced with coadministration of tetracycline. Although anecdotal reports suggest oral contraceptive efficacy could be reduced by tetracyclines, this has been refuted by more rigorous scientific and clinical data.

Increased Effect/Toxicity: Methoxyflurane anesthesia when concurrent with tetracycline may cause fatal nephrotoxicity. Warfarin with tetracyclines may cause increased anticoagulation.

Nutritional/Ethanol Interactions

Food: Tetracycline serum concentrations may be decreased if taken with dairy products.

Herb/Nutraceutical: Avoid dong quai, St John's wort (may also cause photosensitization)

Effects on Lab Values False-negative urine glucose with Clinistix®

Adverse Reactions

>10%: Gastrointestinal: Discoloration of teeth and enamel hypoplasia (young children)

1% to 10%:

Dermatologic: Photosensitivity

Gastrointestinal: Nausea, diarrhea

<1% (Limited to important or life-threatening): Acute renal failure, anaphylaxis, bulging fontanels in infants, diabetes insipidus, esophagitis, exfoliative dermatitis, hepatotoxicity, hypersensitivity reactions, increased intracranial pressure, pancreatitis, paresthesia, pericarditis, pigmentation of nails, pruritus, pseudomembranous colitis, pseudotumor cerebri, staphylococcal enterocolitis, superinfection, thrombophlebitis, vomiting

Overdosage/Toxicology Symptoms of overdose include nausea, anorexia, and diarrhea. Treatment is supportive.

Pharmacodynamics/Kinetics

Absorption: Oral: 75%

Half-Life Elimination: Normal renal function: 8-11 hours; End-stage renal disease: 57-108 hours

Time to Peak: Serum: Oral: 2-4 hours

Formulations

Capsule, as hydrochloride: 250 mg, 500 mg

Ointment, as hydrochloride: 3% [30 mg/mL] (14.2 g, 30 g)

Ointment, ophthalmic: 1% [10 mg/mL] (3.5 g)

Solution, topical: 2.2 mg/mL (70 mL)
Suspension, ophthalmic: 1% [10 mg/mL] (0.5 mL, 1 mL, 4 mL)
Suspension, oral, as hydrochloride: 125 mg/5 mL (60 mL, 480 mL)
Tablet, as hydrochloride: 250 mg, 500 mg

Dosing

Adults & Elderly:

Antibacterial:

Ophthalmic:

Ointment: Instill every 2-12 hours.

Suspension: Instill 1-2 drops 2-4 times/day or more often as needed.

Topical: Apply to affected areas 1-4 times/day.

Oral:

Systemic infection: 250-500 mg/dose every 6 hours

Helicobacter pylori eradication: 500 mg 2-4 times/day depending on regimen; requires combination therapy with at least one other antibiotic and an acid-suppressing agent (proton pump inhibitor or H_2 blocker)

Periodontitis: 250 mg every 6 hours until improvement (usually 10 days)

Pediatrics:

Antibacterial, systemic: Children >8 years: Oral: 25-50 mg/kg/day in divided doses every 6 hours

Children >8 years: Ophthalmic and Topical: Refer to adult dosing.

Renal Impairment:

Cl_{cr} 50-80 mL/minute: Administer every 8-12 hours.

Cl_{cr} 10-50 mL/minute: Administer every 12-24 hours.

Cl_{cr} <10 mL/minute: Administer every 24 hours.

Slightly dialyzable (5% to 20%) via hemo- and peritoneal dialysis or via continuous arterio-venous or venovenous hemofiltration; supplemental dose is not necessary.

Hepatic Impairment: Avoid use or maximum dose is 1 g/day.

Administration

Oral: Oral should be given on an empty stomach (ie, 1 hour prior to, or 2 hours after meals) to increase total absorption. Administer at least 1-2 hours prior to, or 4 hours after antacid because aluminum and magnesium cations may chelate with tetracycline and reduce its total absorption. Administer around-the-clock to promote less variation in peak and trough serum levels.

Stability

Storage: Outdated tetracyclines have caused a Fanconi-like syndrome (nausea, vomiting, acidosis, proteinuria, glycosuria, aminoaciduria, polydipsia, polyuria, hypokalemia). Protect oral dosage forms from light.

Compatibility: in solution: Incompatible with aminophylline, amphotericin B, ampicillin, calcium gluconate, carbenicillin, cefazolin, erythromycin, furosemide, heparin sodium, hydrocortisone, pentobarbital, sodium bicarbonate

Monitoring Laboratory Tests Renal, hepatic, and hematologic function; WBC. Perform culture and sensitivity studies prior to initiating therapy to determine the causative organism and its susceptibility to tetracycline.

Monitoring and Teaching Issues

Physical Assessment: Assess effectiveness and interactions of other medications patient may be taking (see Drug Interactions). Monitor laboratory tests, therapeutic response, and adverse reactions (see Adverse Reactions) at beginning of therapy and periodically throughout therapy. Assess knowledge/teach patient appropriate use, interventions to reduce side effects, and adverse symptoms to report (see Patient Education). **Pregnancy risk factor B/D** - see Pregnancy Risk Factor - assess knowledge/instruct patient on need to use appropriate barrier contraceptive measures and the need to avoid pregnancy. Breast-feeding is not recommended; may cause discoloration of infant's teeth.

Patient Education: Take this medication exactly as directed. Take all of the prescription even if you see an improvement in your condition. Do not use more or more often than recommended.

Oral: Preferable to take on an empty stomach, 1 hour before or 2 hours after meals. Take at regularly scheduled times, around-the-clock. Avoid antacids, iron, or dairy products within 2 hours of taking tetracycline. You may experience photosensitivity (use sunscreen, wear protective clothing and eyewear, and avoid direct sunlight); dizziness or lightheadedness (use caution when driving or engaging in tasks requiring alertness until response to drug is known); or nausea/vomiting (small, frequent meals, frequent mouth care, chewing gum, or sucking lozenges may help). Report rash or intense itching, yellowing of skin or eyes, fever or chills, blackened stool, vaginal itching or discharge, foul-smelling stools, excessive thirst or urination, acute headache, unresolved diarrhea, difficulty breathing, condition does not improve, or worsening of condition.

Pregnancy/breast-feeding precautions: Do not get pregnant while taking this medication. Use appropriate barrier contraceptive measures. Breast-feeding is not recommended.

Ophthalmic: Do not let tip of applicator touch eye; do not contaminate tip of applicator (may cause eye infection, eye damage, or vision loss). Sit down, tilt head back, instill solution or drops inside lower eyelid, and roll eyeball in all directions. Close eye and apply gentle pressure to inner corner of eye for 30 seconds. May experience temporary stinging or blurred vision. Inform prescriber if condition worsens or does not improve in 3-4 days.

Topical: Wash area and pat dry (unless contraindicated). Avoid getting in mouth or eyes. You may experience temporary stinging or burning which will resolve quickly. Treated skin may turn yellow; this will wash off. May stain clothing (permanent). Report rash. Inform prescriber if condition worsens or does not improve in a few days.

Geriatric Considerations: The role of tetracycline has decreased because of the emergence of resistant organisms. Doxycycline is the tetracycline of choice when one is indicated because of its better GI absorption, less interactions with divalent cations, longer half-life, and the fact that the majority is cleared by nonrenal mechanisms.

(Continued)

Tetracycline *(Continued)*

Breast-feeding Issues: Negligible absorption by infant; potential to stain infants' unerupted teeth

Related Information

Compatibility of Drugs *on page 1564*
Helicobacter pylori Treatment *on page 1676*
Ophthalmic Agents *on page 1509*

Tetracycline, Bismuth Subsalicylate, and Metronidazole *see* Bismuth Subsalicylate, Metronidazole, and Tetracycline *on page 170*

Tetracycline Hydrochloride *see* Tetracycline *on page 1296*

Tetracycline, Metronidazole, and Bismuth Subsalicylate *see* Bismuth Subsalicylate, Metronidazole, and Tetracycline *on page 170*

Tetrahydroaminoacrine *see* Tacrine *on page 1270*

Tetrahydrocannabinol *see page 1568*

Tetrahydrocannabinol *see* Dronabinol *on page 452*

Tetrahydrozoline *see page 1509*

Tetramune® *see page 1498*

Tetrasine® *see page 1509*

Teveten® *see* Eprosartan *on page 480*

Texacort® *see* Hydrocortisone *on page 673*

Texacort® *see* Topical Corticosteroids *on page 1334*

TG *see* Thioguanine *on page 1305*

6-TG *see* Thioguanine *on page 1305*

THA *see* Tacrine *on page 1270*

Thalidomide (tha LI doe mide)

U.S. Brand Names Thalomid®

Restrictions Thalidomide is approved for marketing only under a special distribution program. This program, called the "System for Thalidomide Education and Prescribing Safety" (STEPS™), has been approved by the FDA. Prescribing and dispensing of thalidomide is restricted to prescribers and pharmacists registered with the program. Prior to dispensing, an authorization number must be obtained (1-888-423-5436) from Celgene (write authorization number on prescription). No more than a 4-week supply should be dispensed. Blister packs should be dispensed intact (do not repackage capsules). Prescriptions must be filled within 7 days.

Generic Available No

Pharmacologic Category Immunosuppressant Agent

Pregnancy Risk Factor X

Lactation Excretion in breast milk unknown/contraindicated

Use Treatment and maintenance of cutaneous manifestations of erythema nodosum leprosum

Orphan status: Treatment of Crohn's disease

Use - Unlabeled/Investigational Treatment or prevention of graft-versus-host reactions after bone marrow transplantation; AIDS-related aphthous stomatitis; Langerhans cell histiocytosis, Behçet's syndrome; hypnotic agent; also may be effective in rheumatoid arthritis, discoid lupus erythematosus, and erythema multiforme; useful in type 2 lepra reactions, but not type 1; renal cell carcinoma, multiple myeloma, myeloma, Waldenström's macroglobulinemia

Mechanism of Action/Effect A derivative of glutethimide; mode of action for immunosuppression is unclear; inhibition of neutrophil chemotaxis and decreased monocyte phagocytosis may occur; may cause 50% to 80% reduction of tumor necrosis factor - alpha.

Contraindications Hypersensitivity to thalidomide or any component of the formulation; neuropathy (peripheral); pregnancy or women in childbearing years unless alternative therapies are inappropriate and adequate precautions are taken to avoid pregnancy; patient unable to comply with STEPS™ program.

Warnings/Precautions Liver, hepatic, neurological disorders, constipation, CHF, hypertension; safety and efficacy have not been established in children <12 years of age. Use caution in patients with a history of seizures, receiving concurrent therapy with drugs which alter seizure threshold, or conditions which predispose to seizures.

Drug Interactions

Increased Effect/Toxicity: Other medications known to cause peripheral neuropathy should be used with caution in patients receiving thalidomide; thalidomide may enhance the sedative activity of other drugs such as ethanol, barbiturates, reserpine, and chlorpromazine

Nutritional/Ethanol Interactions

Ethanol: Avoid ethanol (may increase sedation).
Herb/Nutraceutical: Avoid cat's claw (has immunostimulant properties).

Adverse Reactions

Controlled clinical trials: ENL:

- >10%:
  - Central nervous system: Somnolence (37.5%), headache (12.5%)
  - Dermatologic: Rash (20.8%)
- 1% to 10% (Limited to important or life-threatening):
  - Dermatologic: Rash (maculopapular) (4.2%)
  - Genitourinary: Impotence (8.2%)

HIV-seropositive:

- General: An increased viral load has been noted in patients treated with thalidomide. This is of uncertain clinical significance - see monitoring
- >10%:
  - Central nervous system: Somnolence (36% to 37%), dizziness (18.7% to 19.4%), fever (19.4% to 21.9%), headache (16.7% to 18.7%)

Dermatologic: Rash (25%), maculopapular rash (16.7% to 18.7%), acne (3.1% to 11.1%)

Gastrointestinal: AST increase (2.8% to 12.5%), diarrhea (11.1% to 18.7%), nausea (≤12.5%), oral moniliasis (6.3% to 11.1%)

Hematologic: Leukopenia (16.7% to 25%), anemia (5.6% to 12.5%)

Neuromuscular & skeletal: Paresthesia (5.6% to 15.6%), weakness (5.6% to 21.9%)

Miscellaneous: Diaphoresis (≤12.5%), lymphadenopathy (5.6% to 12.5%)

1% to 10% (Limited to important or life-threatening): Central nervous system: Agitation (≤9.4%)

Literature reports of other adverse reactions (limited to important or life-threatening): Acute renal failure, bradycardia, chronic myelogenous leukemia (CML), dyspnea, erythema nodosum, Hodgkin's disease, hypersensitivity, hyperthyroidism, lymphopenia, myxedema, orthostatic hypotension, pancytopenia, photosensitivity, Raynaud's syndrome, seizures, Stevens-Johnson syndrome, suicide attempt, toxic epidermal necrolysis

Pharmacodynamics/Kinetics

Half-Life Elimination: 8.7 hours

Time to Peak: Plasma: 2-6 hours

Metabolism: Hepatic

Formulations Capsule: 50 mg

Dosing

Adults & Elderly:

Cutaneous ENL: Oral:

Initiate dosing at 100-300 mg/day taken once daily at bedtime with water (at least 1 hour after evening meal)

Patients weighing <50 kg: Initiate at lower end of the dosing range

Severe cutaneous reaction or previously requiring high dose may be initiated at 400 mg/day; doses may be divided, but taken 1 hour after meals

Dosing should continue until active reaction subsides (usually at least 2 weeks), then tapered in 50 mg decrements every 2-4 weeks

Patients who flare during tapering or with a history or requiring prolonged maintenance should be maintained on the minimum dosage necessary to control the reaction. Efforts to taper should be repeated every 3-6 months, in increments of 50 mg every 2-4 weeks.

Behçet's syndrome (unlabeled use): Oral: 100-400 mg/day

Graft-vs-host reactions (unlabeled use): Oral: 100-1600 mg/day; usual initial dose: 200 mg 4 times/day for use up to 700 days

AIDS-related aphthous stomatitis (unlabeled use): Oral: 200 mg twice daily for 5 days, then 200 mg/day for up to 8 weeks

Discoid lupus erythematosus (unlabeled use): Oral: 100-400 mg/day; maintenance dose: 25-50 mg

Pediatrics: Graft-vs-host reactions (unlabeled use): Oral: Children: 3 mg/kg 4 times/day

Stability

Storage: Store at 15°C to 30°C (50°F to 86°F). Protect from light. Keep in original package.

Monitoring Laboratory Tests Required pregnancy testing, WBC with differential. In HIV-seropositive patients: viral load after 1 and 3 months, then every 3 months. Pregnancy testing is required within 24 hours of initiation of therapy.

Monitoring and Teaching Issues

Physical Assessment: Patient must be capable of complying with STEPS™ program (see Use). Instruct patient on risks of pregnancy, appropriate contraceptive measures (see Patient Education), and necessity for frequent pregnancy testing (schedule pregnancy testing at time of dispensing and give patient schedule in writing). Assess other medications patient may be taking for possible interactions (see Drug Interactions). Monitor closely for adverse reactions (see Adverse Reactions). Instruct patient on signs and symptoms to report (see Patient Education), and appropriate interventions for adverse reactions.

Pregnancy risk factor X - pregnancy test is required within 24 hours prior to beginning therapy, weekly during first month of therapy, and monthly thereafter for all women of childbearing age. Effective contraception with at least two reliable forms of contraception must be used for 1 month prior to beginning therapy, during therapy, and for 1 month following discontinuance of therapy. (Women who have undergone a hysterectomy or have been postmenopausal for at least 24 consecutive months are the only exception.) Do not prescribe, administer, or dispense to women of childbearing age or males who may have intercourse with women of childbearing age unless both female and male are capable of complying with contraceptive measures. (Even males who have undergone vasectomy must acknowledge these risks in writing, and must use a latex condom during any sexual contact with women of childbearing age.) Oral and written warnings concerning contraception and the hazards of thalidomide must be conveyed to females and males and they must acknowledge their understanding in writing. Parents or guardians must consent and sign acknowledgment for patients between 12 and 18 years of age following therapy. Breast-feeding is contraindicated.

Patient Education: You will be given oral and written instructions about the necessity of using two methods of contraception and and the necessity of keeping return visits for pregnancy testing. Do not donate blood while taking this medicine. Male patients should not donate sperm. You may experience sleepiness, dizziness, lack of concentration (use caution when driving, climbing stairs, or engaging in tasks requiring alertness until response to drug is known); nausea or vomiting or loss of appetite (small, frequent meals, frequent mouth care, chewing gum, or sucking lozenges may help); constipation or diarrhea; oral thrush (frequent mouth care is necessary); or sexual dysfunction (reversible). Report any of the above if persistent or severe. Report chest pain or palpitations or swelling of extremities; back, neck, or muscle pain or stiffness; skin rash or eruptions; increased nervousness, anxiety, or insomnia; or any other symptom of adverse reactions. **Pregnancy/breast-feeding precautions:** Do not get pregnant (females) or cause pregnancy (males) during treatment. The use of two forms of contraception are required for 1 month prior to therapy, during therapy, and for 1 month following discontinuation of therapy.

(Continued)

Thalidomide *(Continued)*

Pregnancy tests will be routinely conducted during therapy. Do not breast-feed while taking this medication or for 1 month following discontinuation.

Dietary Issues: Should be taken at least 1 hour after the evening meal.

Pregnancy Issues: Embryotoxic with limb defects noted from the 27th to 40th gestational day of exposure; all cases of phocomelia occur from the 27th to 42nd gestational day; fetal cardiac, gastrointestinal, and genitourinary tract abnormalities have also been described. Effective contraception must be used for at least 4 weeks before initiating therapy, during therapy, and for 4 weeks following discontinuation of thalidomide. Males (even those vasectomized) must use a latex condom during any sexual contact with women of child-bearing age.

Thalitone® *see* Chlorthalidone *on page 279*

Thalomid® *see* Thalidomide *on page 1298*

THC *see* Dronabinol *on page 452*

Theo-24® *see* Theophylline *on page 1300*

Theochron® *see* Theophylline *on page 1300*

Theo-Dur® *see* Theophylline *on page 1300*

Theolair™ *see* Theophylline *on page 1300*

Theophylline (thee OF i lin)

U.S. Brand Names Aerolate III®; Aerolate JR®; Aerolate SR®; Elixophyllin®; Quibron®-T; Quibron®-T/SR; Respbid®; Slo-bid™; Slo-Phyllin®; Theo-24®; Theochron®; Theo-Dur®; Theolair™; T-Phyl®; Uni-Dur®; Uniphyl®

Synonyms Theophylline Anhydrous

Generic Available Yes

Pharmacologic Category Theophylline Derivative

Pregnancy Risk Factor C

Lactation Enters breast milk/compatible

Use Treatment of symptoms and reversible airway obstruction due to chronic asthma, chronic bronchitis, or COPD

Mechanism of Action/Effect Causes bronchodilatation, diuresis, CNS and cardiac stimulation, and gastric acid secretion by blocking phosphodiesterase which increases tissue concentrations of cyclic adenine monophosphate (cAMP) which in turn promotes catecholamine stimulation of lipolysis, glycogenolysis, and gluconeogenesis and induces release of epinephrine from adrenal medulla cells.

Contraindications Hypersensitivity to theophylline or any component of the formulation

Warnings/Precautions If a patient develops signs and symptoms of theophylline toxicity (eg, persistent, repetitive vomiting), a serum theophylline level should be measured and subsequent doses held. Due to potential saturation of theophylline clearance at serum levels in or (in some patients) less than the therapeutic range, dosage adjustment should be made in small increments (maximum: 25%). Due to wider interpatient variability, theophylline serum level measurements must be used to optimize therapy and prevent serious toxicity. Use with caution in patients with peptic ulcer, hyperthyroidism, seizure disorders, hypertension, and patients with cardiac arrhythmias (excluding bradyarrhythmias). Pregnancy risk C.

Drug Interactions

Cytochrome P450 Effect: Substrate of **CYP1A2**, 2C8/9, 2D6, **2E1, 3A4**; Inhibits CYP1A2

Decreased Effect: Changes in diet may affect the elimination of theophylline. Charcoal-broiled foods may increase elimination, reducing half-life by 50%. The following factors decrease theophylline serum levels: Smoking (cigarettes, marijuana), high protein/low carbohydrate diet, charcoal, phenytoin, phenobarbital, carbamazepine, rifampin, ritonavir, I.V. isoproterenol, aminoglutethimide, barbiturates, hydantoins, ketoconazole, sulfinpyrazone, isoniazid, loop diuretics, and sympathomimetics.

Increased Effect/Toxicity: Changes in diet may affect the elimination of theophylline. The following may increase serum theophylline levels: propranolol, allopurinol (>600 mg/day), erythromycin, cimetidine, troleandomycin, ciprofloxacin (other quinolone antibiotics), oral contraceptives, beta-blockers, calcium channel blockers, corticosteroids, disulfiram, ephedrine, influenza virus vaccine, interferon, macrolides, mexiletine, thiabendazole, thyroid hormones, carbamazepine, isoniazid, and loop diuretics. Other inhibitors of cytochrome P450 1A2 may increase theophylline levels.

Nutritional/Ethanol Interactions Food: Food does not appreciably affect the absorption of liquid, fast-release products, and most sustained release products; however, food may induce a sudden release (dose-dumping) of once-daily sustained release products resulting in an increase in serum drug levels and potential toxicity. Avoid excessive amounts of caffeine. Avoid extremes of dietary protein and carbohydrate intake. Limit charcoal-broiled foods.

Adverse Reactions

Adverse reactions/theophylline serum level: (Adverse effects do not necessarily occur according to serum levels. Arrhythmia and seizure can occur without seeing the other adverse effects).

15-25 mcg/mL: GI upset, diarrhea, nausea/vomiting, abdominal pain, nervousness, headache, insomnia, agitation, dizziness, muscle cramp, tremor

25-35 mcg/mL: Tachycardia, occasional PVC

>35 mcg/mL: Ventricular tachycardia, frequent PVC, seizure

Uncommon at serum theophylline concentrations ≤20 mcg/mL

1% to 10%:

Cardiovascular: Tachycardia

Central nervous system: Nervousness, restlessness

Gastrointestinal: Nausea, vomiting

<1% (Limited to important or life-threatening): Insomnia, irritability, seizures, tremor

Overdosage/Toxicology Symptoms of overdose include nausea, vomiting, insomnia, irritability, tachycardia, seizures, tonic-clonic seizures, insomnia, and circulatory failure. If seizures have not occurred, induce vomiting; ipecac syrup is preferred. Do not induce emesis in the presence of impaired consciousness. Repeated doses of charcoal have been shown to be effective in enhancing the total body clearance of theophylline. Do not repeat charcoal doses if an ileus is present. Charcoal hemoperfusion may be considered if serum theophylline levels exceed 40 mcg/mL, the patient is unable to tolerate repeat oral charcoal administrations, or if severe toxic symptoms are present. Clearance with hemoperfusion is better than clearance from hemodialysis. Administer a cathartic, especially if sustained release agents were used. Phenobarbital administered prophylactically may prevent seizures.

Pharmacodynamics/Kinetics

Absorption: Oral (formulation dependent): ≤100%

Half-Life Elimination: Highly variable and age, liver and cardiac function, lung disease, and smoking history dependent

Metabolism: Hepatic

Onset: I.V.: <30 minutes

Formulations

Capsule, immediate release: 100 mg, 200 mg

Capsule, timed release:
- 8-12 hours (Aerolate®): 65 mg [III], 130 mg [JR], 260 mg [SR]
- 8-12 hours (Slo-bid™): 50 mg, 75 mg, 100 mg, 125 mg, 200 mg, 300 mg
- 8-12 hours (Slo-Phyllin® Gyrocaps®): 60 mg, 125 mg, 250 mg
- 24 hours (Theo-24®): 100 mg, 200 mg, 300 mg

Elixir (Elixophyllin®): 80 mg/15 mL (15 mL, 30 mL, 480 mL, 4000 mL)

Infusion [in D_5W]: 0.4 mg/mL (1000 mL); 0.8 mg/mL (500 mL, 1000 mL); 1.6 mg/mL (250 mL, 500 mL); 2 mg/mL (100 mL); 3.2 mg/mL (250 mL); 4 mg/mL (50 mL, 100 mL);

Solution, oral (Theolair™): 80 mg/15 mL (15 mL, 18.75 mL, 30 mL, 480 mL)

Syrup (Slo-Phyllin®): 80 mg/15 mL (15 mL, 30 mL, 500 mL)

Tablet, immediate release:
- Quibron®-T: 300 mg
- Slo-Phyllin®: 100 mg, 200 mg
- Theolair™: 125 mg, 250 mg

Tablet, controlled release (Theo-X®): 100 mg, 200 mg, 300 mg

Tablet, timed release:
- 8-12 hours (Quibron®-T/SR): 300 mg
- 8-12 hours (Respbid®): 250 mg, 500 mg
- 8-12 hours (T-Phyl®): 200 mg
- 8-24 hours (Theo-Dur®): 100 mg, 200 mg, 300 mg, 450 mg
- 12-24 hours: 100 mg, 200 mg, 300 mg, 450 mg
- 12-24 hours (Theochron®): 100 mg, 200 mg, 300 mg
- 24 hours (Theolair™-SR): 200 mg, 300 mg, 500 mg
- 24 hours (Uni-Dur®, Uniphyl®): 400 mg, 600 mg

Dosing

Adults:

Initial dosage recommendation: Loading dose (to achieve a serum concentration of about 10 mcg/mL; loading doses should be given using a rapidly absorbed oral product **not** a sustained release product):

If no theophylline has been administered in the previous 24 hours: 4-6 mg/kg theophylline

If theophylline has been administered in the previous 24 hours: Administer ½ loading dose; 2-3 mg/kg theophylline can be given in emergencies when serum concentrations are not available

On the average, for every 1 mg/kg theophylline given, blood concentrations will rise 2 mcg/mL

Maintenance dose: See table.

Maintenance Dose for Acute Symptoms

Population Group	Oral Theophylline (mg/kg/day)	I.V. Aminophylline
Otherwise healthy nonsmoking adults (including elderly patients)	10 (not to exceed 900 mg/day)	0.5 mg/kg/h
Cardiac decompensation, cor pulmonale and/or liver dysfunction	5 (not to exceed 400 mg/day)	0.25 mg/kg/h

*For continuous I.V. infusion divide total daily dose by 24 = mg/kg/h.

Bronchodilation: Oral:

Nonsustained release: 16-20 mg/kg/day divided into 4 doses/day

Sustained release: 9-13 mg/kg/day divided into 2-3 doses/day

These recommendations, based on mean clearance rates for age or risk factors, were calculated to achieve a serum concentration of 10 mcg/mL. In healthy adults, a slow-release product can be used (9-13 mg/kg in divided dose). The total daily dose can be divided every 8-12 hours.

Use ideal body weight for obese patients. Dose should be adjusted further based on serum concentrations. Guidelines for obtaining theophylline serum concentrations are shown in the table under Monitoring Laboratory Tests.

Elderly: Elderly patients should be started with a 25% reduction in the adult dose.

Pediatrics:

Loading dose:

Apnea of prematurity: Neonates: Oral: 4 mg/kg/dose

Treatment of acute bronchospasm: Infants and Children: Oral (to achieve a serum level of about 10 mcg/mL; loading doses should be given using a rapidly absorbed oral product **not** a sustained release product):

If no theophylline has been administered in the previous 24 hours: 5 mg/kg theophylline

If theophylline has been administered in the previous 24 hours: 2.5 mg/kg theophylline may be given in emergencies when serum levels are not available

(Continued)

Theophylline *(Continued)*

A modified loading dose (mg/kg) may be calculated (when the serum level is known) by: [Blood level desired - blood level measured] divided by 2 (for every 1 mg/kg theophylline given, the blood level will rise by approximately 2 mcg/mL)

Maintenance dose: See table.

Maintenance Dose for Acute Symptoms

Population Group	Oral Theophylline (mg/kg/day)
Premature infant or newborn - 6 wk (for apnea/bradycardia)	4*
6 wk to 6 mo	10*
Infants 6 mo to 1 y	12-18*
Children 1-9 y	20-24
Children 9-12 y, adolescent daily smokers of cigarettes or marijuana, and otherwise healthy adult smokers <50 y	16
Adolescents 12-16 y (nonsmokers)	13
Otherwise healthy nonsmoking adults (including elderly patients)	10 (not to exceed 900 mg/day)
Cardiac decompensation, cor pulmonale, and/or liver dysfunction	5 (not to exceed 400 mg/day)
***Alternative dosing regimen for full-term infants <1 year of age:** Total daily dose (mg) = [(0.2 x age in weeks) + 5] x weight (kg) Postnatal Age <26 weeks: Total daily dose divided every 8 hours Postnatal Age >26 weeks: Total daily dose divided every 6 hours	

These recommendations, based on mean clearance rates for age or risk factors, were calculated to achieve a serum level of 10 mcg/mL (5 mcg/mL for newborns with apnea/bradycardia). In newborns and infants, a fast-release oral product can be used. The total daily dose can be divided every 12 hours in newborns and every 6-8 hours in infants. In children and healthy adults, a slow-release product can be used. The total daily dose can be divided every 8-12 hours.

Use ideal body weight for obese patients

Dose should be further adjusted based on serum levels. Guidelines for drawing theophylline serum levels are shown in the table.

Administration

Oral: Sustained release preparations should be taken with a full glass of water, swallowed whole, or cut in half if scored. Do **not** crush. Sustained release capsule forms may be opened and the contents sprinkled on soft foods; do **not** chew beads.

Stability

Compatibility: Stable in D_5W

Y-site administration: Incompatible with hetastarch, phenytoin

Compatibility when admixed: Incompatible with ascorbic acid injection, ceftriaxone, cimetidine

Monitoring Laboratory Tests Therapeutic levels:

Asthma: 10-15 mg/mL (peak level)

Toxic concentration: >20 mg/mL; see table.

Guidelines for Drawing Theophylline Serum Levels

Dosage Form	Time to Draw Level
I.V. bolus	30 min after end of 30 min infusion
I.V. continuous infusion	12-24 h after initiation of infusion
P.O. liquid, fast-release tab	Peak: 1 h postdose after at least 1 day of therapy Trough: Just before a dose after at least one day of therapy
P.O. slow-release product	Peak: 4 h postdose after at least 1 day of therapy Trough: Just before a dose after at least one day of therapy

Monitoring and Teaching Issues

Physical Assessment: Assess effectiveness and interactions of other medications patient may be taking (see Drug Interactions). See Contraindications and Warnings/Precautions for use cautions. Monitor effectiveness of therapy (respiratory rate, lung sounds, characteristics of cough and sputum) and adverse reactions (see Adverse Reactions) at beginning of therapy and periodically with long-term use. For inpatient care, monitor vital signs and lung sounds prior to and periodically during therapy. Assess knowledge/teach patient appropriate use, interventions to reduce side effects, and adverse symptoms to report (see Patient Education). **Pregnancy risk factor C** - benefits of use should outweigh possible risks.

Patient Education: Take exactly as directed; do not exceed recommended dosage. Avoid smoking (smoking may interfere with drug absorption as well as exacerbate condition for which medication is prescribed). If you are smoking when dosage is prescribed; inform prescriber if you stop smoking (dosage may need to be adjusted to prevent toxicity). Preferable to take on empty stomach, 1 hour before or 2 hours after meals, with a full glass of water. Do not chew of crush sustained release forms; capsules may be opened and contents sprinkled on soft food (do not chew beads). Avoid dietary stimulants (eg, caffeine, tea, colas, or chocolate - may increase adverse side effects). Maintain adequate hydration (2-3 L/day of fluids) unless advised by prescriber to restrict fluids. You may experience nausea, vomiting, or lose of appetite (small, frequent meals, frequent mouth care, chewing gum, or sucking lozenges may help). Report acute insomnia or restlessness, chest pain or rapid heartbeat, emotional lability or agitation, muscle tremors or cramping, acute headache, abdominal pain and cramping, blackened stool, or worsening of respiratory condition. **Pregnancy precaution:** Inform prescriber if you are or intend to become pregnant.

Dietary Issues: Should be taken with water 1 hour before or 2 hours after meals.

Geriatric Considerations: Although there is a great intersubject variability for half-lives of methylxanthines (2-10 hours), elderly as a group have slower hepatic clearance. Therefore, use lower initial doses and monitor closely for response and adverse reactions. Additionally, elderly are at greater risk for toxicity due to concomitant disease (eg, CHF, arrhythmias), and drug use (eg, cimetidine, ciprofloxacin, etc) (see Warnings/Precautions and Drug Interactions).

Additional Information Theophylline salt / theophylline content (percent)

Theophylline anhydrous (eg, most oral solids): 100% theophylline
Theophylline monohydrate (eg, oral solutions): 91% theophylline
Aminophylline (theophylline) (eg, injection): 80% (79% to 86%) theophylline
Oxtriphylline (choline theophylline) (eg, Choledyl®): 64% theophylline

Related Information

Compatibility of Drugs *on page 1564*
Peak and Trough Guidelines *on page 1544*

Theophylline and Guaifenesin (thee OF i lin & gwye FEN e sin)

U.S. Brand Names Bronchial®; Glycerol-T®; Quibron®; Slo-Phyllin® GG

Synonyms Guaifenesin and Theophylline

Generic Available Yes

Pharmacologic Category Theophylline Derivative

Pregnancy Risk Factor C

Lactation Enters breast milk/compatible

Use Symptomatic treatment of bronchospasm associated with bronchial asthma, chronic bronchitis, and pulmonary emphysema

Formulations

Capsule:
Theophylline 150 mg and guaifenesin 90 mg
Theophylline 300 mg and guaifenesin 180 mg
Elixir: Theophylline 150 mg and guaifenesin 90 mg per 15 mL (480 mL)

Dosing

Adults: Bronchospasm: Oral: 16 mg/kg/day or 400 mg theophylline/day in divided doses every 6-8 hours

Elderly: Refer to dosing in individual monographs.

Monitoring and Teaching Issues

Physical Assessment: See individual components listed in Related Information. **Pregnancy risk factor C** - benefits of use should outweigh possible risks.

Patient Education: See individual components listed in Related Information. **Pregnancy precaution:** Inform prescriber if you are or intend to become pregnant.

Related Information

Guaifenesin *on page 646*
Theophylline *on page 1300*

Theophylline Anhydrous *see* Theophylline *on page 1300*
Theracort® [OTC] *see* Hydrocortisone *on page 673*
Theramycin Z® *see* Erythromycin (Systemic) *on page 486*
Thermazene® *see* Silver SulfaDIAZINE *on page 1229*

Thiabendazole (thye a BEN da zole)

U.S. Brand Names Mintezol®

Synonyms Tiabendazole

Generic Available No

Pharmacologic Category Anthelmintic

Pregnancy Risk Factor C

Lactation Excretion in breast milk unknown

Use Treatment of strongyloidiasis, cutaneous larva migrans, visceral larva migrans, dracunculiasis, trichinosis, and mixed helminthic infections

Mechanism of Action/Effect Inhibits helminth-specific mitochondrial fumarate reductase

Contraindications Hypersensitivity to thiabendazole or any component of the formulation

Warnings/Precautions Use with caution in patients with renal or hepatic impairment, malnutrition or anemia, or dehydration. Pregnancy risk C.

Drug Interactions

Cytochrome P450 Effect: Substrate of CYP1A2

Increased Effect/Toxicity: Increased levels of theophylline and other xanthines.

Effects on Lab Values ↑ glucose

Adverse Reactions Frequency not defined.

Central nervous system: Seizures, hallucinations, delirium, dizziness, drowsiness, headache, chills
Dermatologic: Rash, Stevens-Johnson syndrome, pruritus, angioedema
Endocrine & metabolic: Hyperglycemia
Gastrointestinal: Anorexia, diarrhea, nausea, vomiting, drying of mucous membranes, abdominal pain
Genitourinary: Malodor of urine, hematuria, crystalluria, enuresis
Hematologic: Leukopenia
Hepatic: Jaundice, cholestasis, hepatic failure, hepatotoxicity
Neuromuscular & skeletal: Numbness, incoordination
Ocular: Visual changes, dry eyes, sicca syndrome
Otic: Tinnitus
(Continued)

Thiabendazole *(Continued)*

Renal: Nephrotoxicity
Miscellaneous: Anaphylaxis, hypersensitivity reactions, lymphadenopathy

Overdosage/Toxicology Symptoms of overdose include altered mental status and visual problems. Treatment is supportive.

Pharmacodynamics/Kinetics

Absorption: Rapid and well absorbed
Half-Life Elimination: 1.2 hours
Time to Peak: Oral suspension: Within 1-2 hours
Metabolism: Rapidly hepatic

Formulations

Suspension, oral: 500 mg/5 mL (120 mL)
Tablet, chewable: 500 mg [orange flavor]

Dosing

Adults & Elderly: Purgation is not required prior to use; drinking of fruit juice aids in expulsion of worms by removing the mucous to which the intestinal tapeworms attach themselves.

Parasitic infections: Oral: 50 mg/kg/day divided every 12 hours; maximum: 3 g/day
Treatment duration:
Strongyloidiasis: For 2 consecutive days
Cutaneous larva migrans: For 2-5 consecutive days
Visceral larva migrans: For 5-7 consecutive days
Trichinosis: For 2-4 consecutive days
Dracunculosis: 50-75 mg/kg/day divided every 12 hours for 3 days

Pediatrics: Parasitic infections: Children: Refer to adult dosing.
Renal Impairment: Use with caution.
Hepatic Impairment: Use with caution.

Monitoring and Teaching Issues

Physical Assessment: Assess effectiveness and interactions of other medications patient may be taking (see Drug Interactions). See Warnings/Precautions and Contraindications for use cautions. Worm infestations are easily transmitted, all close family members should be treated. Instruct patient/caregiver on appropriate use, transmission prevention, possible side effects and appropriate interventions, and adverse symptoms to report (see Patient Education). **Pregnancy risk factor C** - benefits of use should outweigh possible risks. Note breast-feeding caution.

Patient Education: Take exactly as directed for full course of medication. Tablets may be chewed, swallowed whole, or crushed and mixed with food. Increase dietary intake of fruit juices. All family members and close friends should also be treated. To reduce possibility of reinfection, wash hands and scrub nails carefully with soap and hot water before handling food, before eating, and before and after toileting. Keep hands out of mouth. Disinfect toilet daily and launder bed lines, undergarments, and nightclothes daily with hot water and soap. Do not go barefoot and do not sit directly on grass or ground. May cause dizziness, fainting, or lightheadedness (use caution when driving or engaging in tasks requiring alertness until response to drug is known); or abdominal pain, nausea, dry mouth, or vomiting (small, frequent meals, frequent mouth care, sucking lozenges, or chewing gum may help). Report skin rash or itching, unresolved diarrhea or vomiting, CNS changes (hallucinations, delirium, acute headache), change in color of urine or stool, or easy bruising or unusual bleeding. **Pregnancy/breast-feeding precautions:** Inform prescriber if you are pregnant. Consult prescriber if breast-feeding.

Thiamazole *see* Methimazole *on page 871*
Thiamilate® *see* Thiamine *on page 1304*

Thiamine (THYE a min)

U.S. Brand Names Thiamilate®

Synonyms Aneurine Hydrochloride; Thiamine Hydrochloride; Thiaminium Chloride Hydrochloride; Vitamin B_1

Generic Available Yes

Pharmacologic Category Vitamin, Water Soluble

Pregnancy Risk Factor A/C (dose exceeding RDA recommendation)

Lactation Enters breast milk/compatible

Use Treatment of thiamine deficiency including beriberi, Wernicke's encephalopathy syndrome, and peripheral neuritis associated with pellagra, alcoholic patients with altered sensorium; various genetic metabolic disorders

Mechanism of Action/Effect An essential coenzyme in carbohydrate metabolism by combining with adenosine triphosphate to form thiamine pyrophosphate

Contraindications Hypersensitivity to thiamine or any component of the formulation

Warnings/Precautions Use with caution with parenteral route (especially I.V.) of administration. Pregnancy risk C (dose exceeding RDA).

Nutritional/Ethanol Interactions Food: High carbohydrate diets may increase thiamine requirement.

Effects on Lab Values False-positive for uric acid using the phosphotungstate method and for urobilinogen using the Ehrlich's reagent; large doses may interfere with the spectrophotometric determination of serum theophylline concentration

Adverse Reactions <1% (Limited to important or life-threatening): Cardiovascular collapse and death, paresthesia

Pharmacodynamics/Kinetics

Absorption: Oral: Adequate; I.M.: Rapid and complete

Formulations

Injection, as hydrochloride: 100 mg/mL (1 mL, 2 mL, 10 mL, 30 mL); 200 mg/mL (30 mL)
Tablet, as hydrochloride: 50 mg, 100 mg, 250 mg, 500 mg
Tablet, enteric coated, as hydrochloride (Thiamilate®): 20 mg

Dosing

Adults & Elderly:

Recommended daily allowance: >14 years: 1-1.5 mg

Thiamine deficiency (beriberi): I.M. or I.V. 5-30 mg/dose 3 times/day (if critically ill); then orally 5-30 mg/day in single or divided doses 3 times/day for 1 month

Wernicke's encephalopathy: I.V., I.M.: Initial: 100 mg I.V., then 50-100 mg/day I.M. or I.V. until consuming a regular, balanced diet

Dietary supplement (depends on caloric or carbohydrate content of the diet): Oral: 1-2 mg/day

Note: The above doses can be found in multivitamin preparations.

Metabolic disorders: Oral: 10-20 mg/day (dosages up to 4 g/day in divided doses have been used)

Pediatrics:

Recommended daily allowance:
- <6 months: 0.3 mg
- 6 months to 1 year: 0.4 mg
- 1-3 years: 0.7 mg
- 4-6 years: 0.9 mg
- 7-10 years: 1 mg
- 11-14 years: 1.1-1.3 mg
- >14 years: 1-1.5 mg

Thiamine deficiency (beriberi):

Children: I.M., I.V.: 10-25 mg/dose daily (if critically ill), or 10-50 mg/dose orally every day for 2 weeks, then 5-10 mg/dose orally daily for 1 month

Dietary supplement (depends on caloric or carbohydrate content of the diet): Oral:

Infants: 0.3-0.5 mg/day

Children: 0.5-1 mg/day

Note: The above doses can be found in multivitamin preparations

Administration

I.M.: Parenteral form may be administered by I.M. or slow I.V. injection.

I.V.: Doses are usually administered over 1-2 minutes.

Stability

Storage: Protect oral dosage forms from light.

Compatibility: Stable in dextran 6% in dextrose, dextran 6% in NS, D_5LR, $D_5{}^1/_4NS$, $D_5{}^1/_2NS$, D_5NS, D_5W, $D_{10}W$, fat emulsion 10%, LR, $^1/_2NS$, NS

Monitoring and Teaching Issues

Physical Assessment: Assess knowledge/teach patient appropriate administration (injection technique and needle disposal if I.M. self-administered) and dietary instruction. **Pregnancy risk factor A/C** - see Pregnancy Risk Factor for use cautions.

Patient Education: Take exactly as directed; do not discontinue without consulting prescriber (deficiency state can occur in as little as 3 weeks). Follow dietary instructions (dietary sources include legumes, pork, beef, whole grains, yeast, fresh vegetables). **Pregnancy precaution:** Inform prescriber if you are or intend to become pregnant.

Dietary Issues: Dietary sources include legumes, pork, beef, whole grains, yeast, and fresh vegetables. A deficiency state can occur in as little as 3 weeks following total dietary absence.

Thiamine Hydrochloride *see* Thiamine *on page 1304*

Thiaminium Chloride Hydrochloride *see* Thiamine *on page 1304*

Thiethylperazine *see page 1639*

Thioguanine (thye oh GWAH neen)

Synonyms 2-Amino-6-Mercaptopurine; TG; 6-TG; 6-Thioguanine; Tioguanine

Generic Available No

Pharmacologic Category Antineoplastic Agent, Antimetabolite

Pregnancy Risk Factor D

Lactation Excretion in breast milk unknown

Use Remission induction, consolidation, and maintenance therapy of acute myelogenous (nonlymphocytic) leukemia; treatment of chronic myelogenous leukemia and granulocytic leukemia

Mechanism of Action/Effect Purine analog that is incorporated into DNA and RNA resulting in the blockage of synthesis and metabolism of purine nucleotides

Contraindications Hypersensitivity to thioguanine or any component of the formulation; history of previous therapy resistance with either thioguanine or mercaptopurine (there is usually complete cross resistance between these two); pregnancy

Warnings/Precautions The U.S. Food and Drug Administration (FDA) currently recommends that procedures for proper handling and disposal of antineoplastic agents be considered. Use with caution and reduce dose of thioguanine in patients with renal or hepatic impairment. Thioguanine is potentially carcinogenic and teratogenic. Myelosuppression may be delayed. Patients with genetic deficiency of thiopurine methyltransferase (TPMT) or who are receiving drugs which inhibit this enzyme (olsalazine) may be highly sensitive to myelosuppressive effects.

Drug Interactions

Increased Effect/Toxicity: Allopurinol can be used in full doses with 6-TG unlike 6-MP. Use with busulfan may cause hepatotoxicity and esophageal varices. Aminosalicylates (olsalazine, mesalamine, sulfasalazine) may inhibit TPMT, increasing toxicity/myelosuppression of thioguanine.

Nutritional/Ethanol Interactions Food: Enhanced absorption if administered between meals.

Adverse Reactions

>10%:

Hematologic: Leukopenia; Thrombocytopenia; Myelosuppressive:

WBC: Moderate

(Continued)

Thioguanine *(Continued)*

Platelets: Moderate
Onset: 7-10 days
Nadir: 14 days
Recovery: 21 days

1% to 10%:
Dermatologic: Skin rash
Endocrine & metabolic: Hyperuricemia
Gastrointestinal: Mild nausea or vomiting, anorexia, stomatitis, diarrhea
Emetic potential: Low (<10%)
Neuromuscular & skeletal: Unsteady gait

<1% (Limited to important or life-threatening): Hepatitis, jaundice, neurotoxicity, veno-occlusive hepatic disease

Overdosage/Toxicology Symptoms of overdose include bone marrow suppression, nausea, vomiting, malaise, hypertension, and sweating. Treatment is supportive. Dialysis is not useful.

Pharmacodynamics/Kinetics

Absorption: 30%

Half-Life Elimination: Terminal: 11 hours

Time to Peak: Serum: Within 8 hours

Metabolism: Rapidly and extensively hepatic to 2-amino-6-methylthioguanine (active) and inactive compounds

Formulations Tablet, scored: 40 mg

Dosing

Adults & Elderly: Total daily dose can be given at one time; offers little advantage over mercaptopurine; is sometimes ordered as 6-thioguanine, with 6 being part of the drug name and not some kind of unit or strength.

Antineoplastic: Oral (**refer to individual protocols**): 2-3 mg/kg/day calculated to nearest 20 mg or 75-200 mg/m²/day in 1-2 divided doses for 5-7 days or until remission is attained

Pediatrics: Total daily dose can be given at one time; offers little advantage over mercaptopurine; is sometimes ordered as 6-thioguanine, with 6 being part of the drug name and not a unit or strength.

Antineoplastic: Oral (refer to individual protocols):
Infants and Children <3 years: Combination drug therapy for acute nonlymphocytic leukemia: 3.3 mg/kg/day in divided doses twice daily for 4 days
Children >3 years: Refer to adult dosing.

Renal Impairment: Reduce dose.

Hepatic Impairment: Reduce dose.

Monitoring Laboratory Tests CBC with differential and platelet count, liver function, serum uric acid, renal function

Monitoring and Teaching Issues

Physical Assessment: See Contraindications, Warnings/Precautions, and Dosing for use cautions (eg, antiemetic, steroid eye drops). Assess potential for interactions with other prescriptions, OTC medications, or herbal products patient may be taking (see Drug Interactions). Assess results of laboratory tests (see above) and monitor adverse response (see Adverse Reactions and Overdose/Toxicology). Teach patient appropriate use, possible side effects and interventions (eg, importance of adequate hydration), and adverse symptoms to report (see Patient Education). **Pregnancy risk factor D** - determine that patient is not pregnant before beginning treatment. Instruct patients of childbearing age about appropriate barrier contraceptive measures. Note breast-feeding caution.

Patient Education: Inform prescriber of all prescriptions, OTC medications, or herbal products you are taking, and any allergies you have. Do not take anything new during treatment unless approved by prescriber. Take exactly as directed. Maintain adequate hydration (2-3 L/day of fluids) unless advised by prescriber to restrict fluids. May cause nausea and vomiting, diarrhea, or loss of appetite (small, frequent meals may help/request medication); weakness or lethargy (use caution when driving or engaging in tasks requiring alertness until response to drug is known); mouth sores (use good oral care); or headache (request medication). You will be susceptible to infection (avoid crowds and exposure to infection). Report signs or symptoms of infection (eg, fever, chills, sore throat, burning urination, fatigue); bleeding (eg, tarry stools, easy bruising); vision changes; unresolved mouth sores, nausea, or vomiting; CNS changes (hallucinations); or difficulty breathing. **Pregnancy/breast-feeding precautions:** Do not get pregnant. Consult prescriber for appropriate contraceptive measures. The drug may cause permanent sterility and may cause birth defects. Consult prescriber if breast-feeding.

6-Thioguanine *see* Thioguanine *on page 1305*
Thiophosphoramide *see* Thiotepa *on page 1309*
Thioplex® *see* Thiotepa *on page 1309*

Thioridazine (thye oh RID a zeen)

U.S. Brand Names Mellaril®

Synonyms Thioridazine Hydrochloride

Generic Available Yes

Pharmacologic Category Antipsychotic Agent, Phenothiazine, Piperidine

Pregnancy Risk Factor C

Lactation Excretion in breast milk unknown/not recommended

Use Management of schizophrenic patients who fail to respond adequately to treatment with other antipsychotic drugs, either because of insufficient effectiveness or the inability to achieve an effective dose due to intolerable adverse effects from those medications

Use - Unlabeled/Investigational Psychosis

Mechanism of Action/Effect Blocks postsynaptic mesolimbic dopaminergic receptors in the brain; exhibits a strong alpha-adrenergic blocking effect and depresses the release of hypothalamic and hypophyseal hormones

Contraindications Hypersensitivity to thioridazine or any component of the formulation (cross-reactivity between phenothiazines may occur); severe CNS depression; circulatory collapse; severe hypotension; bone marrow suppression; blood dyscrasias; coma; in combination with other drugs that are known to prolong the QT_c interval; in patients with congenital long QT syndrome or a history of cardiac arrhythmias; concurrent use with medications that inhibit the metabolism of thioridazine (fluoxetine, paroxetine, fluvoxamine, propranolol, pindolol); patients known to have genetic defect leading to reduced levels of activity of CYP2D6

Warnings/Precautions Thioridazine has dose-related effects on ventricular repolarization leading to QT_c prolongation, a potentially life-threatening effect. Therefore, it should be reserved for patients with schizophrenia who have failed to respond to adequate levels of other antipsychotic drugs. May cause orthostatic hypotension - use with caution in patients at risk of this effect or those who would tolerate transient hypotensive episodes (cerebrovascular disease, cardiovascular disease, or other medications which may predispose).

Highly sedating, use with caution in disorders where CNS depression is a feature. Use with caution in Parkinson's disease. Caution in patients with hemodynamic instability; bone marrow suppression; predisposition to seizures; subcortical brain damage; severe cardiac, hepatic, renal, or respiratory disease. Esophageal dysmotility and aspiration have been associated with antipsychotic use - use with caution in patients at risk of pneumonia (ie, Alzheimer's disease). Caution in breast cancer or other prolactin-dependent tumors (may elevate prolactin levels). May alter temperature regulation or mask toxicity of other drugs due to antiemetic effects.

Due to anticholinergic effects, use caution in patients with decreased gastrointestinal motility, urinary retention, BPH, xerostomia, visual problems, narrow-angle glaucoma (screening is recommended) and myasthenia gravis. Relative to other neuroleptics, thioridazine has a high potency of cholinergic blockade.

May cause extrapyramidal symptoms, including pseudoparkinsonism, acute dystonic reactions, akathisia, and tardive dyskinesia (risk of these reactions is low relative to other neuroleptics). May be associated with neuroleptic malignant syndrome (NMS). Doses exceeding recommended doses may cause pigmentary retinopathy.

Pregnancy risk C.

Drug Interactions

Cytochrome P450 Effect: Substrate of CYP2C19, **2D6**; Inhibits CYP1A2, **2D6**, 2E1

Decreased Effect: Aluminum salts may decrease the absorption of phenothiazines. The efficacy of amphetamines may be diminished by antipsychotics; in addition, amphetamines may increase psychotic symptoms; avoid concurrent use. Anticholinergics may inhibit the therapeutic response to phenothiazines and excess anticholinergic effects may occur (includes benztropine, trihexyphenidyl, biperiden, and drugs with significant anticholinergic activity). Chlorpromazine (and possibly other low potency antipsychotics) may diminish the pressor effects of epinephrine. The antihypertensive effects of guanethidine or guanadrel may be inhibited by phenothiazines. Phenothiazines may inhibit the antiparkinsonian effect of levodopa. Enzyme inducers may enhance the hepatic metabolism of phenothiazines; larger doses may be required; includes rifampin, rifabutin, barbiturates, phenytoin, and cigarette smoking.

Increased Effect/Toxicity: Concurrent use of phenothiazines with an antihypertensive may produce additive hypotensive effects (particularly orthostasis). Concurrent use of beta-blockers may increase the risk of arrhythmia; propranolol and pindolol are **contraindicated**. Phenothiazines inhibit the ability of bromocriptine to lower serum prolactin concentrations. Serum concentrations of carvedilol or valproic acid may be increased by phenothiazines. The sedative effects of CNS depressants or ethanol may be additive with phenothiazines. Phenothiazines and trazodone may produce additive hypotensive effects Concurrent use of phenothiazines and tricyclic antidepressants may produce increased toxicity or altered therapeutic response. Metoclopramide may increase risk of extrapyramidal symptoms (EPS).

QT_c-prolonging agents: Effects on QT_c interval may be additive with phenothiazines, increasing the risk of malignant arrhythmias; includes type Ia antiarrhythmics, TCAs, and some quinolone antibiotics (sparfloxacin, moxifloxacin and gatifloxacin). **These agents are contraindicated with thioridazine.** Potassium depleting agents may increase the risk of serious arrhythmias with thioridazine (includes many diuretics, aminoglycosides, and amphotericin).

CYP2D6 inhibitors: Metabolism of phenothiazines may be decreased; increasing clinical effect or toxicity. Inhibitors include amiodarone, cimetidine, delavirdine, fluoxetine, paroxetine, propafenone, quinidine, and ritonavir; monitor for increased effect/toxicity. **Thioridazine is contraindicated with inhibitors of this enzyme, including fluoxetine and paroxetine.** Inhibitors of CYP1A2, including cimetidine, ciprofloxacin, fluvoxamine, isoniazid, ritonavir, and zileuton may also decrease thioridazine metabolism. **Concurrent use with fluvoxamine is contraindicated.**

Phenothiazines may produce neurotoxicity with lithium; this is a rare effect. Rare cases of respiratory paralysis have been reported with concurrent use of phenothiazines and polypeptide antibiotics. Naltrexone in combination with thioridazine has been reported to cause lethargy and somnolence. Phenylpropanolamine has been reported to result in cardiac arrhythmias when combined with thioridazine.

Nutritional/Ethanol Interactions

Ethanol: Avoid ethanol (may increase CNS depression).

Herb/Nutraceutical: Avoid kava kava, valerian, St John's wort, gotu kola (may increase CNS depression). Avoid dong quai, St John's wort (may also cause photosensitization).

Effects on Lab Values False-positives for phenylketonuria, urinary amylase, uroporphyrins, urobilinogen

Adverse Reactions Frequency not defined.

Cardiovascular: Hypotension, orthostatic hypotension, peripheral edema, EKG changes

(Continued)

Thioridazine *(Continued)*

Central nervous system: EPS (pseudoparkinsonism, akathisia, dystonias, tardive dyskinesia), dizziness, drowsiness, neuroleptic malignant syndrome (NMS), impairment of temperature regulation, lowering of seizures threshold

Dermatologic: Increased sensitivity to sun, rash, discoloration of skin (blue-gray)

Endocrine & metabolic: Changes in menstrual cycle, changes in libido, breast pain, galactorrhea, amenorrhea

Gastrointestinal: Constipation, weight gain, nausea, vomiting, stomach pain, xerostomia, nausea, vomiting, diarrhea

Genitourinary: Difficulty in urination, ejaculatory disturbances, urinary retention, priapism

Hematologic: Agranulocytosis, leukopenia

Hepatic: Cholestatic jaundice, hepatotoxicity

Neuromuscular & skeletal: Tremor, seizure

Ocular: Pigmentary retinopathy, blurred vision, cornea and lens changes

Respiratory: Nasal congestion

Overdosage/Toxicology Symptoms of overdose include deep sleep, coma, extrapyramidal symptoms, abnormal involuntary muscle movements, hypotension, and arrhythmias.

Immediate cardiac monitoring, including continuous electrocardiographic monitoring, to detect arrhythmias. Avoid use of medications that also prolong the QT_c interval, such as disopyramide, procainamide, and quinidine. Following initiation of essential overdose management, toxic symptom treatment and supportive treatment should be initiated. Hypotension usually responds to I.V. fluids or Trendelenburg positioning. If unresponsive to these measures, the use of a parenteral inotrope may be required (eg, norepinephrine 0.1-0.2 mcg/kg/minute titrated to response); do not use epinephrine or dopamine. Seizures commonly respond to diazepam (I.V. 5-10 mg bolus in adults every 15 minutes if needed up to a total of 30 mg; I.V. 0.25-0.4 mg/kg/dose up to a total of 10 mg in children) or to phenytoin. Avoid barbiturates (may potentiate respiratory depression). Neuroleptics often cause extrapyramidal symptoms (eg, dystonic reactions) requiring management with diphenhydramine 1-2 mg/kg (adults) up to a maximum of 50 mg I.M. or I.V. slow push followed by a maintenance dose for 48-72 hours. When these reactions are unresponsive to diphenhydramine, benztropine mesylate I.V. 1-2 mg (adults) may be effective. These agents are generally effective within 2-5 minutes.

Pharmacodynamics/Kinetics

Half-Life Elimination: 21-25 hours

Time to Peak: Serum: ~1 hour

Duration: 4-5 days

Formulations

Solution, oral concentrate, as hydrochloride: 30 mg/mL (120 mL); 100 mg/mL (3.4 mL, 120 mL)

Tablet, as hydrochloride: 10 mg, 15 mg, 25 mg, 50 mg, 100 mg, 150 mg, 200 mg

Dosing

Adults:

Schizophrenia/psychosis: Oral: Initial: 50-100 mg 3 times/day with gradual increments as needed and tolerated; maximum: 800 mg/day in 2-4 divided doses; if >65 years, initial dose: 10 mg 3 times/day

Depressive disorders, dementia: Oral: Initial: 25 mg 3 times/day; maintenance dose: 20-200 mg/day

Elderly: Behavioral symptoms associated with dementia: Oral: Initial: 10-25 mg 1-2 times/day; increase at 4- to 7-day intervals by 10-25 mg/day; increase dose intervals (qd, bid, etc) as necessary to control response or side effects. Maximum daily dose: 400 mg; gradual increases (titration) may prevent some side effects or decrease their severity.

Pediatrics:

Schizophrenia/psychosis: Oral:

Children >2-12 years: Range: 0.5-3 mg/kg/day in 2-3 divided doses; usual: 1 mg/kg/day; maximum: 3 mg/kg/day

Children >12 years: Refer to adult dosing.

Behavior problems: Oral:

Children >2-12 years: Initial: 10 mg 2-3 times/day, increase gradually.

Children >12 years: Refer to adult dosing.

Severe psychoses: Oral:

Children >2-12 years: Initial: 25 mg 2-3 times/day, increase gradually.

Children >12 years: Refer to adult dosing.

Renal Impairment: Not dialyzable (0% to 5%)

Administration

Oral: Oral concentrate must be diluted in 2-4 oz of liquid (eg, water, fruit juice, carbonated drinks, milk, or pudding) before administration. Do not take antacid within 2 hours of taking drug. Thioridazine concentrate is not compatible with carbamazepine suspension; schedule dosing at least 1-2 hours apart from each other. **Note:** Avoid skin contact with oral suspension or solution; may cause contact dermatitis.

Stability

Storage: Protect all dosage forms from light.

Monitoring Laboratory Tests Baseline EKG, serum potassium; do not initiate if QT_c >450 msec

Monitoring and Teaching Issues

Physical Assessment: Assess other medications patient is taking for effectiveness and interactions (see Drug Interactions). See Contraindications and Warnings/Precautions for use cautions. Review ophthalmic exam and monitor laboratory results (see above), therapeutic response (mental status, mood, affect, gait), and adverse reactions at beginning of therapy and periodically with long-term use (see Adverse Reactions and Overdose/Toxicology). Avoid skin contact with liquid medication; may cause contact dermatitis (wash immediately with warm, soapy water). Initiate at lower doses (see Dosing) and taper dosage slowly when discontinuing. Assess knowledge/teach patient appropriate use, interventions to reduce side effects, and adverse symptoms to report (see Patient Education). **Pregnancy risk factor C** - benefits of use should outweigh possible risks. Breast-feeding is not recommended.

Patient Education: Use exactly as directed; do not increase dose or frequency. Do not discontinue without consulting prescriber. Tablets/capsules may be taken with food. Mix oral solution with 2-4 oz of liquid (eg, juice, milk, water, pudding). Do not take within 2 hours of any antacid. Store away from light. Avoid alcohol or caffeine and other prescription or OTC medications not approved by prescriber. Maintain adequate hydration (2-3 L/day of fluids) unless advised by prescriber to restrict fluids. Avoid skin contact with liquid medication; may cause contact dermatitis (wash immediately with warm, soapy water). May turn urine red-brown (normal). You may experience excess drowsiness, lightheadedness, dizziness, or blurred vision (use caution driving or when engaging in tasks requiring alertness until response to drug is known); nausea, vomiting, or dry mouth (small, frequent meals, frequent mouth care, chewing gum, or sucking lozenges may help); constipation (increased exercise, fluids, fruit, or fiber may help); postural hypotension (use caution climbing stairs or when changing position from lying or sitting to standing); urinary retention (void before taking medication); ejaculatory dysfunction (reversible); decreased perspiration (avoid strenuous exercise in hot environments); or photosensitivity (use sunscreen, wear protective clothing and eyewear, and avoid direct sunlight). Report persistent CNS effects (eg, trembling fingers, altered gait or balance, excessive sedation, seizures, unusual movements, anxiety, abnormal thoughts, confusion, personality changes); chest pain, palpitations, rapid heartbeat, severe dizziness; unresolved urinary retention or changes in urinary pattern; altered menstrual pattern, change in libido, swelling or pain in breasts (male or female); vision changes; skin rash, irritation, or changes in color of skin (gray-blue); or worsening of condition. **Pregnancy/breast-feeding precautions:** Inform prescriber if you are or intend to become pregnant. Breast-feeding is not recommended.

Geriatric Considerations: (See Warnings/Precautions, Adverse Reactions, and Overdose/Toxicology.) Elderly patients have an increased risk of adverse response to side effects or adverse reactions to antipsychotics.

Related Information

Antipsychotic Agents *on page 1558*
Antipsychotic Medication Guidelines *on page 1614*

Thioridazine Hydrochloride *see* Thioridazine *on page 1306*

Thiotepa (thye oh TEP a)

U.S. Brand Names Thioplex®

Synonyms TESPA; Thiophosphoramide; Triethylenethiophosphoramide; TSPA

Generic Available Yes

Pharmacologic Category Antineoplastic Agent, Alkylating Agent

Pregnancy Risk Factor D

Lactation Enters breast milk/not recommended

Use Treatment of superficial tumors of the bladder; palliative treatment of adenocarcinoma of breast or ovary; lymphomas and sarcomas; controlling intracavitary effusions caused by metastatic tumors; I.T. use: CNS leukemia/lymphoma, CNS metastases

Mechanism of Action/Effect Alkylating agent that reacts with DNA phosphate groups to produce cross-linking of DNA strands leading to inhibition of DNA, RNA, and protein synthesis; mechanism of action has not been explored as thoroughly as the other alkylating agents, it is presumed that the aziridine rings open and react as nitrogen mustard; reactivity is enhanced at a lower pH

Contraindications Hypersensitivity to thiotepa or any component of the formulation; severe myelosuppression with leukocyte count <3000/mm^3 or platelet count <150,000 mm^3, except in stem cell transplant; pregnancy

Warnings/Precautions The U.S. Food and Drug Administration (FDA) currently recommends that procedures for proper handling and disposal of antineoplastic agents be considered. Appropriate safety equipment is recommended for preparation, administration, and disposal of antineoplastics. If thiotepa contacts the skin, wash and flush thoroughly with water. Potentially mutagenic, carcinogenic, and teratogenic. Reduce dosage in patients with hepatic, renal, or bone marrow damage.

Drug Interactions

Cytochrome P450 Effect: Inhibits CYP2B6

Increased Effect/Toxicity: Other alkylating agents or irradiation used concomitantly with thiotepa intensifies toxicity rather than enhancing therapeutic response. Prolonged muscular paralysis and respiratory depression may occur when neuromuscular blocking agents are administered. Succinylcholine and other neuromuscular blocking agents' action can be prolonged due to thiotepa inhibiting plasma pseudocholinesterase.

Nutritional/Ethanol Interactions

Ethanol: Avoid ethanol (due to GI irritation).

Herb/Nutraceutical: Avoid black cohosh, dong quai in estrogen-dependent tumors.

Adverse Reactions

>10%:

Hematopoietic: Myelosuppression (dose-related and cumulative): Anemia and pancytopenia may become fatal; careful hematologic monitoring is required; intravesical administration may cause bone marrow suppression as well.

Hematologic: Myelosuppressive:
WBC: Moderate
Platelets: Severe
Onset: 7-10 days
Nadir: 14 days
Recovery: 28 days

1% to 10%:

Central nervous system: Dizziness, fever, headache

Dermatologic: Alopecia, rash, pruritus, hyperpigmentation with high-dose therapy

(Continued)

Thiotepa *(Continued)*

Endocrine & metabolic: Hyperuricemia
Gastrointestinal: Anorexia, nausea and vomiting rarely occur
Emetic potential: Low (<10%)
Genitourinary: Hemorrhagic cystitis
Local: Pain at injection site
Renal: Hematuria
Miscellaneous: Tightness of the throat, allergic reactions

<1% (Limited to important or life-threatening): Carcinogenesis: Like other alkylating agents, this drug is carcinogenic.

BMT:

Central nervous system: Confusion, inappropriate behavior, somnolence
Dermatologic: Hyperpigmentation
Gastrointestinal: Mucositis, mild nausea and vomiting
Hepatic: Serum transaminitis, hyperbilirubinemia

Overdosage/Toxicology Symptoms of overdose include nausea, vomiting, precipitation of uric acid in kidney tubules, bone marrow suppression, and bleeding. Therapy is supportive only. Thiotepa is dialyzable. Transfusions of whole blood or platelets have been proven beneficial.

Pharmacodynamics/Kinetics

Absorption: Intracavitary instillation: Unreliable (10% to 100%) through bladder mucosa; I.M.: variable

Half-Life Elimination: Terminal: Dose-dependent clearance: 109 minutes

Metabolism: Extensively hepatic

Formulations Injection, powder for reconstitution: 15 mg

Dosing

Adults & Elderly: Refer to individual protocols. Dosing must be based on the clinical and hematologic response of the patient.

Usual dose (range):
I.M., I.V., S.C.: 30-60 mg/m^2 once per week
I.V. doses of 0.3-0.4 mg/kg by rapid I.V. administration every 1-4 weeks, or 0.2 mg/kg or 6-8 mg/m^2/day for 4-5 days every 2-4 weeks
I.M. doses of 15-30 mg in various schedules have been given
Intracavitary: 0.6-0.8 mg/kg
Intrapericardial dose: Usually 15-30 mg
Intravesical: Used for treatment of carcinoma of the bladder; patients should be dehydrated for 8-12 hours prior to treatment; instill 60 mg (in 30-60 mL of sterile water) into the bladder and retain for a minimum of 2 hours. Patient should be positioned every 15 minutes for maximal area exposure. Instillations usually once a week for 4 weeks.
Intratumor: Use a 22-gauge needle to inject thiotepa directly into the tumor. Initial: 0.6-0.8 mg/kg (diluted to 10 mg/mL) are used every 1-4 weeks; maintenance dose: 0.07-0.8 mg/kg are administered at 1- to 4-week intervals
Ophthalmic: 0.05% solution in LR has been instilled into the eye every 3 hours for 6-8 weeks for the prevention of pterygium recurrence

BMT high dose: I.V.: 360-1125 mg/m^2 as a single dose or divided into 2 daily doses; generally combined with other high-dose chemotherapeutic drugs.

Pediatrics: Refer to individual protocols; dosing must be based on the clinical and hematologic response of the patient. Children: Sarcomas: I.V.: 25-65 mg/m^2 as a single dose every 21 days.

Administration

I.V.: Administer I.V., intracavitary, and intrathecally. Administer over 1 minute.

Other: Thiotepa is usually administered intravenously, either as a short bolus or push, or a 1-hour infusion; or as an intravesical infusion. The drug is occasionally administered as intracavitary, intramuscular, or intrathecal injections. Intrathecal doses are usually diluted to a concentration of 1 mg/mL in preservative-free sterile water or normal saline. Bladder irrigations should be diluted in 50-100 mL of sterile water or normal saline, and retained for at least 2 hours. The patient should be repositioned every 15 minutes for maximal exposure.

Stability

Storage: Store intact vials under refrigeration (2°C to 8°C) and protect from light.

Reconstitution: Dilute powder 1.5 mL SWI to a concentration of 10 mg/mL which is stable for 8 hours at refrigeration. Further dilution in NS, D_5W, or lactated Ringer's should be used immediately (within 1 hour of preparation). Thiotepa is stable for 24 hours at a concentration of 5 mg/mL in NS at 8°C and 23°C; however, stability decreases significantly at concentrations <5 mg/mL (1 hour).

Standard I.V. dilution:
I.V. push: Dose/syringe (concentration = 10 mg/mL)
IVPB: Dose/250 mL D_5W
Further dilution in NS, D_5W, or lactated Ringer's should be used immediately (within one hour of preparation)
Continuous 24-hour I.V. infusion:
Dose ≥250 mg: qs to 50 mL (total volume) in NS
Dose 230-250 mg: qs to 45 mL (total volume) in NS
Dose 200-230 mg: qs to 40 mL (total volume) in NS
Thiotepa is stable for 24 hours at a concentration of 5 mg/mL in NS at 8°C and 23°C; however, stability decreases significantly at concentrations <5 mg/mL (1 hour).

Standard intravesicular dilution: 60 mg/30-60 mL SWI
Intravesicular doses should be prepared with 60 mg of drug diluted into 30-60 mL SWI. Solution is placed via catheter and retained for 2 hours for maximum effect.

Standard intrathecal dilution: 10-15 mg/3-5 mL lactated Ringer's
Intrathecal doses of 1-10 mg/m^2 should be diluted to 1-5 mg in lactated Ringer's.
All solutions should be **prepared fresh** and administered within 1 hour of preparation.

Compatibility:

Y-site administration: Incompatible with cisplatin, filgrastim, minocycline, vinorelbine

Compatibility when admixed: Incompatible with cisplatin

Monitoring Laboratory Tests CBC with differential, platelet count, uric acid, urinalysis

Monitoring and Teaching Issues

Physical Assessment: See Contraindications, Warnings/Precautions, and Dosing specifics for use cautions (eg, intravesical, intratumor, ophthalmic). Assess potential for interactions with other prescriptions, OTC medications, or herbal products patient may be taking (see Drug Interactions). See I.V. specifics above, Closely assess results of laboratory tests (eg, anemia and pancytopenia can become fatal - see Monitoring Laboratory Tests above) and monitor adverse response (see Adverse Reactions and Overdose/Toxicology). Teach patient possible side effects and interventions (eg, importance of adequate hydration) and adverse symptoms to report (see Patient Education). **Pregnancy risk factor D** - determine that patient is not pregnant before beginning treatment. Do not give to women of childbearing age or to males who may have intercourse with women of childbearing age unless both male and female are capable of complying with barrier contraceptive measures during therapy and for 1 month following therapy. Breast-feeding is not recommended.

Patient Education: Inform prescriber of all prescriptions, OTC medications, or herbal products you are taking, and any allergies you have. Do not take anything new during treatment unless approved by prescriber (especially aspirin or aspirin-containing products). This drug can only be administered I.V. Report immediately any redness, pain, swelling, or burning at infusion site. You will require regular blood tests to assess response to therapy. Maintain adequate hydration (2-3 L/day of fluids) to prevent kidney damage unless advised by prescriber to restrict fluids. You may have increased sensitivity to infection (avoid crowds and exposure to infection and do not have any vaccinations unless approved by prescriber). May cause nausea, vomiting, or loss of appetite (small, frequent meals, chewing gum, or sucking lozenges may help; antiemetic may be prescribed); amenorrhea or changed sperm production; rash; or hair loss. Report unusual bleeding or bruising; persistent fever or chills; sore throat; sores in mouth or vagina; blackened stool; or difficulty breathing. **Pregnancy/breast-feeding precautions:** Inform prescriber if you are pregnant. Do not get pregnant (females) or cause a pregnancy (males) during therapy and for 1 month following completion of therapy. Consult prescriber for instruction on appropriate barrier contraceptive measures. This drug may cause severe fetal defects. Breast-feeding is not recommended.

Additional Information A 1 mg/mL solution is considered isotonic.

Thiothixene (thye oh THIKS een)

U.S. Brand Names Navane®

Synonyms Tiotixene

Generic Available Yes

Pharmacologic Category Antipsychotic Agent, Thioxanthene Derivative

Pregnancy Risk Factor C

Lactation Excretion in breast milk unknown/not recommended

Use Management of schizophrenia

Use - Unlabeled/Investigational Psychotic disorders

Mechanism of Action/Effect Elicits antipsychotic activity by postsynaptic blockade of CNS dopamine receptors resulting in inhibition of dopamine-mediated effects; also has alpha-adrenergic blocking activity

Contraindications Hypersensitivity to thiothixene or any component of the formulation; severe CNS depression; circulatory collapse; blood dyscrasias; coma

Warnings/Precautions May be sedating, use with caution in disorders where CNS depression is a feature. Use with caution in Parkinson's disease. Caution in patients with hemodynamic instability; predisposition to seizures; subcortical brain damage; bone marrow suppression; severe cardiac, hepatic, renal, or respiratory disease. Esophageal dysmotility and aspiration have been associated with antipsychotic use - use with caution in patients at risk of pneumonia (ie, Alzheimer's disease). Caution in breast cancer or other prolactin-dependent tumors (may elevate prolactin levels). May alter temperature regulation or mask toxicity of other drugs due to antiemetic effects. May alter cardiac conduction - life-threatening arrhythmias have occurred with therapeutic doses of neuroleptics. May cause orthostatic hypotension - use with caution in patients at risk of this effect or those who would tolerate transient hypotensive episodes (cerebrovascular disease, cardiovascular disease, or other medications which may predispose). Safety and efficacy in children <12 years of age have not been established.

May cause anticholinergic effects, use caution in patients with decreased gastrointestinal motility, urinary retention, BPH, xerostomia, visual problems, narrow-angle glaucoma (screening is recommended), and myasthenia gravis. Relative to other neuroleptics, thiothixene has a low potency of cholinergic blockade.

May cause extrapyramidal symptoms, including pseudoparkinsonism, acute dystonic reactions, akathisia, and tardive dyskinesia (risk of these reactions is high relative to other neuroleptics). May be associated with neuroleptic malignant syndrome (NMS) or pigmentary retinopathy.

Pregnancy risk C.

Drug Interactions

Cytochrome P450 Effect: Substrate of **CYP1A2**; Inhibits CYP2D6

Decreased Effect: Thiothixene inhibits the activity of guanadrel, guanethidine, levodopa, and bromocriptine. Benztropine (and other anticholinergics) may inhibit the therapeutic response to thiothixene. Barbiturates and cigarette smoking may enhance the hepatic metabolism of thiothixene. Thiothixene and low potency antipsychotics may reverse the pressor effects of epinephrine.

Increased Effect/Toxicity: Thiothixene and CNS depressants (ethanol, narcotics) may produce additive CNS depressant effects. Thiothixene may increase the effect/toxicity of

(Continued)

Thiothixene *(Continued)*

antihypertensives, benztropine (and other anticholinergic agents), lithium, trazodone, and TCAs. Thiothixene's concentrations may be increased by chloroquine, sulfadoxine-pyrimethamine, and propranolol. Metoclopramide may increase risk of extrapyramidal symptoms (EPS).

Nutritional/Ethanol Interactions

Ethanol: Avoid ethanol (may increase CNS depression).

Herb/Nutraceutical: Avoid kava kava, valerian, St John's wort, gotu kola (may increase CNS depression).

Effects on Lab Values ↑ cholesterol (S), glucose; ↓ uric acid (S); may cause false-positive pregnancy test

Adverse Reactions Frequency not defined:

Cardiovascular: Hypotension, tachycardia, syncope, nonspecific EKG changes

Central nervous system: Extrapyramidal symptoms (pseudoparkinsonism, akathisia, dystonias, lightheadedness, tardive dyskinesia), dizziness, drowsiness, restlessness, agitation, insomnia

Dermatologic: Discoloration of skin (blue-gray), rash, pruritus, urticaria, photosensitivity

Endocrine & metabolic: Changes in menstrual cycle, changes in libido, breast pain, galactorrhea, lactation, amenorrhea, gynecomastia, hyperglycemia, hypoglycemia

Gastrointestinal: Weight gain, nausea, vomiting, stomach pain, constipation, xerostomia, increased salivation

Genitourinary: Difficulty in urination, ejaculatory disturbances, impotence

Hematologic: Leukopenia, leukocytes

Neuromuscular & skeletal: Tremors

Ocular: Pigmentary retinopathy, blurred vision

Respiratory: Nasal congestion

Miscellaneous: Diaphoresis

Overdosage/Toxicology Symptoms of overdose include muscle twitching, drowsiness, dizziness, rigidity, tremor, hypotension, and cardiac arrhythmias. Treatment is symptom-directed and supportive.

Pharmacodynamics/Kinetics

Half-Life Elimination: >24 hours with chronic use

Metabolism: Extensively hepatic

Formulations

Capsule: 1 mg, 2 mg, 5 mg, 10 mg, 20 mg

Injection, powder for reconstitution, as hydrochloride: 5 mg/mL (2 mL)

Solution, oral concentrate, as hydrochloride: 5 mg/mL (30 mL, 120 mL)

Dosing

Adults:

Mild to moderate psychosis:

Oral: 2 mg 3 times/day, up to 20-30 mg/day; more severe psychosis: Initial: 5 mg 2 times/day, may increase gradually, if necessary; maximum: 60 mg/day

I.M.: 4 mg 2-4 times/day, increase dose gradually; usual: 16-20 mg/day; maximum: 30 mg/day; change to oral dose as soon as able

Rapid tranquilization of the agitated patient (administered every 30-60 minutes):

Oral: 5-10 mg; I.M.: 10-20 mg

Average total dose for tranquilization: 15-30 mg

Elderly: Nonpsychotic patients, dementia behavior: Initial: 1-2 mg 1-2 times/day; increase dose at 4- to 7-day intervals by 1-2 mg/day. Increase dosing intervals (bid, tid, etc) as necessary to control response or side effects; maximum daily dose: 30 mg. Gradual increases in dose may prevent some side effects or decrease their severity.

Pediatrics:

Children <12 years (unlabeled): Oral: 0.25 mg/kg/24 hours in divided doses (dose not well established; use not recommended)

Children >12 years: Mild to moderate psychosis: Refer to adult dosing.

Renal Impairment: Not dialyzable (0% to 5%)

Administration

Oral: Oral concentration contains 7% alcohol. Dilute immediately before administration with water, fruit juice, milk, etc. **Note:** Avoid skin contact with oral medication; may cause contact dermatitis.

Stability

Storage: Refrigerate powder for injection.

Reconstitution: Reconstituted powder for injection is stable at room temperature for 48 hours.

Monitoring Laboratory Tests Baseline liver and kidney function, CBC prior to and periodically during therapy, ophthalmic exam

Monitoring and Teaching Issues

Physical Assessment: Assess other medications patient is taking for effectiveness and interactions (see Drug Interactions). See Contraindications and Warnings/Precautions for use cautions. Review ophthalmic exam and monitor laboratory results (see above), therapeutic response, and adverse reactions at beginning of therapy and periodically with long-term use (see Adverse Reactions and Overdose/Toxicology). With I.M. use, monitor closely for hypotension. Avoid skin contact with liquid medication; may cause contact dermatitis (wash immediately with warm, soapy water). Initiate at lower doses (see Dosing) and taper dosage slowly when discontinuing. Assess knowledge/teach patient appropriate use, interventions to reduce side effects, and adverse symptoms to report (see Patient Education). **Note:** Thiothixene may cause false-positive pregnancy test (see Effects on Lab Values). **Pregnancy risk factor C** - benefits of use should outweigh possible risks. Breast-feeding is not recommended.

Patient Education: Use exactly as directed; do not increase dose or frequency. Do not discontinue without consulting prescriber. Tablets/capsules may be taken with food. Mix oral solution with 2-4 oz of liquid (eg, juice, milk, water, pudding). Do not take within 2 hours of any antacid. Avoid alcohol or caffeine and other prescription or OTC medications not approved by prescriber. Maintain adequate hydration (2-3 L/day of fluids) unless advised by prescriber to restrict fluids. May turn urine red-brown (normal). You may experience excess drowsiness, lightheadedness, dizziness, or blurred vision (use caution driving or when engaging in tasks requiring alertness until response to drug is known); nausea or vomiting (small, frequent meals, frequent mouth care, chewing gum, or sucking lozenges may help); constipation (increased exercise, fluids, fruit, or fiber may help); postural hypotension (use caution climbing stairs or when changing position from lying or sitting to standing); urinary retention (void before taking medication); ejaculatory dysfunction (reversible); decreased perspiration (avoid strenuous exercise in hot environments); or photosensitivity (use sunscreen, wear protective clothing and eyewear, and avoid direct sunlight). Report persistent CNS effects (eg, trembling fingers, altered gait or balance, excessive sedation, seizures, unusual movements, anxiety, abnormal thoughts, confusion, personality changes); chest pain, palpitations, rapid heartbeat, severe dizziness; unresolved urinary retention or changes in urinary pattern; altered menstrual pattern, change in libido, swelling or pain in breasts (male or female); vision changes; skin rash, irritation, or changes in color of skin (gray-blue); or worsening of condition. **Pregnancy/breast-feeding precautions:** Inform prescriber if you are or intend to become pregnant. Breast-feeding is not recommended.

Geriatric Considerations: (See Warnings/Precautions, Adverse Reactions, and Overdose/Toxicology.) Elderly patients have an increased risk of adverse response to side effects or adverse reactions to antipsychotics.

Additional Information Coadministration of two or more antipsychotics does not improve clinical response and may increase the potential for adverse effects.

Related Information

Antipsychotic Agents *on page 1558*
Antipsychotic Medication Guidelines *on page 1614*

Thorazine® *see* ChlorproMAZINE *on page 277*

Thrombinar® *see page 1461*

Thrombin, Topical *see page 1461*

Thrombogen® *see page 1461*

Thrombostat® *see page 1461*

Thymocyte Stimulating Factor *see* Aldesleukin *on page 54*

Thypinone® Injection *see page 1461*

Thyrogen® *see page 1461*

Thyroid (THYE royd)

U.S. Brand Names Armour® Thyroid; Nature-Throid® NT; Westhroid®

Synonyms Desiccated Thyroid; Thyroid Extract; Thyroid USP

Generic Available Yes

Pharmacologic Category Thyroid Product

Pregnancy Risk Factor A

Lactation Enters breast milk/compatible

Use Replacement or supplemental therapy in hypothyroidism; pituitary TSH suppressants (thyroid nodules, thyroiditis, multinodular goiter, thyroid cancer), thyrotoxicosis, diagnostic suppression tests

Mechanism of Action/Effect The primary active compound is T_3 (triiodothyronine), which may be converted from T_4 (thyroxine) and then circulates throughout the body to influence growth and maturation of various tissues

Contraindications Hypersensitivity to beef or pork or any component of the formulation; recent myocardial infarction; thyrotoxicosis uncomplicated by hypothyroidism; uncorrected adrenal insufficiency

Warnings/Precautions Ineffective for weight reduction. High doses may produce serious or even life-threatening toxic effects particularly when used with some anorectic drugs. Use cautiously in patients with pre-existing cardiovascular disease (angina, CHD), elderly since they may be more likely to have compromised cardiovascular function. Chronic hypothyroidism predisposes patients to coronary artery disease. Desiccated thyroid contains variable amounts of T_3, T_4, and other triiodothyronine compounds which are more likely to cause cardiac signs or symptoms due to fluctuating levels. Should avoid use in the elderly for this reason. Many clinicians consider levothyroxine to be the drug of choice for thyroid replacement.

Drug Interactions

Decreased Effect: Thyroid hormones increase the therapeutic need for oral hypoglycemics or insulin. Cholestyramine can bind thyroid and reduce its absorption. Phenytoin may decrease thyroxine serum levels. Thyroid hormone may decrease effect of oral sulfonylureas.

Increased Effect/Toxicity: Thyroid may potentiate the hypoprothrombinemic effect of oral anticoagulants. Tricyclic antidepressants (TAD) coadministered with thyroid hormone may increase potential for toxicity of both drugs.

Effects on Lab Values Many drugs may have effects on thyroid function tests: para-aminosalicylic acid, aminoglutethimide, amiodarone, barbiturates, carbamazepine, chloral hydrate, clofibrate, colestipol, corticosteroids, danazol, diazepam, estrogens, ethionamide, fluorouracil, I.V. heparin, insulin, lithium, methadone, methimazole, mitotane, nitroprusside, oxyphenbutazone, phenylbutazone, PTU, perphenazine, phenytoin, propranolol, salicylates, sulfonylureas, and thiazides.

Adverse Reactions <1% (Limited to important or life-threatening): Alopecia, cardiac arrhythmia, chest pain, dyspnea, excessive bone loss with overtreatment (excess thyroid replacement), hand tremors, myalgia, palpitations, tachycardia, tremor

Overdosage/Toxicology Chronic excessive use results in signs and symptoms of hyperthyroidism, weight loss, nervousness, sweating, tachycardia, insomnia, heat intolerance, palpitations, vomiting, psychosis, fever, seizures, angina, arrhythmias, and CHF in those predisposed.

(Continued)

Thyroid *(Continued)*

Reduce dose or temporarily discontinue therapy. Hypothalamic-pituitary-thyroid axis will return to normal in 6-8 weeks. Serum T_4 levels do not correlate well with toxicity. In massive acute ingestion, reduce GI absorption and give general supportive care.

Pharmacodynamics/Kinetics

Absorption: T_4: 48% to 79%; T_3: 95%; desiccated thyroid contains thyroxine, liothyronine, and iodine (primarily bound)

Half-Life Elimination: Serum: Liothyronine: 1-2 days; Thyroxine: 6-7 days

Metabolism: Thyroxine: Largely converted to liothyronine

Formulations

Capsule, pork source in soybean oil (S-P-T): 60 mg, 120 mg, 180 mg, 300 mg

Tablet:

Armour® Thyroid: 15 mg, 30 mg, 60 mg, 90 mg, 120 mg, 180 mg, 240 mg, 300 mg

Thyroid USP: 15 mg, 30 mg, 60 mg, 120 mg, 180 mg, 300 mg

Dosing

Adults: Hypothyroidism: Oral: Initial: 15-30 mg; increase with 15 mg increments every 2-4 weeks; use 15 mg in patients with cardiovascular disease or myxedema. Maintenance dose: Usually 60-120 mg/day; monitor TSH and clinical symptoms.

Note: Thyroid cancer requires larger amounts than replacement therapy.

Elderly: Not recommended for use in the elderly (see Geriatric Considerations).

Pediatrics: Hypothyroidism: Oral: See table.

Recommended Pediatric Dosage for Congenital Hypothyroidism

Age	Daily Dose (mg)	Daily Dose/kg (mg)
0-6 mo	15-30	4.8-6
6-12 mo	30-45	3.6-4.8
1-5 y	45-60	3-3.6
6-12 y	60-90	2.4-3
>12 y	>90	1.2-1.8

Monitoring Laboratory Tests Monitor T_4 and TSH. TSH is the most reliable guide for evaluating adequacy of thyroid replacement dosage. TSH may be elevated during the first few months of thyroid replacement despite patients being clinically euthyroid. In cases where T_4 remains low and TSH is within normal limits, an evaluation of "free" (unbound) T_4 is needed to evaluate further increase in dosage.

Monitoring and Teaching Issues

Physical Assessment: See Contraindications, Warnings/Precautions, and Dosing for use cautions. Assess potential for interactions with other prescriptions, OTC medications, or herbal products patient may be taking (eg, high doses may produce serious or even life-threatening toxic effects particularly when used with some anorectic drugs - see extensive list of Drug Interactions). Assess results of laboratory tests (see above), therapeutic effects, and adverse response (eg, hypo-/hyperthyroidism - see Adverse Reactions and Overdose/Toxicology) regularly during therapy. **Important:** Many drugs may have effects on thyroid function tests (see Effects on Lab Values) when assessing results of thyroid function tests. Caution patients with diabetes to monitor glucose levels closely (may increase need for oral hypoglycemics or insulin). Teach patient appropriate use, possible side effects and interventions, and adverse symptoms to report (see Patient Education).

Patient Education: Inform prescriber of all prescriptions, OTC medications, or herbal products you are taking, and any allergies you have. Do not take anything new during treatment unless approved by prescriber. Thyroid replacement therapy is generally for life. Take as directed, in the morning before breakfast. Do not take antacids or iron preparations within 8 hours of thyroid medication. Do not change brands and do not discontinue without consulting prescriber. Consult prescriber if drastically increasing or decreasing intake of goitrogenic food (eg, asparagus, cabbage, peas, turnip greens, broccoli, spinach, Brussels sprouts, lettuce, soybeans). If diabetic, monitor glucose levels closely (may increase need for oral hypoglycemics or insulin). Report chest pain, rapid heart rate, palpitations, heat intolerance, excessive sweating, increased nervousness, agitation, or lethargy.

Dietary Issues: Should be taken on an empty stomach.

Geriatric Considerations: Desiccated thyroid contains variable amounts of T_3, T_4, and other triiodothyronine compounds which are more likely to cause cardiac signs or symptoms due to fluctuating levels. Should avoid use in the elderly for this reason. Many clinicians consider levothyroxine to be the drug of choice.

Related Information

Levothyroxine *on page 797*

Thyroid Extract *see* Thyroid *on page 1313*

Thyroid Stimulating Hormone *see* Thyrotropin *on page 1314*

Thyroid USP *see* Thyroid *on page 1313*

Thyrotropic Hormone *see* Thyrotropin *on page 1314*

Thyrotropin (thye roe TROE pin)

U.S. Brand Names Thytropar®

Synonyms Thyroid Stimulating Hormone; Thyrotropic Hormone; TSH

Generic Available No

Pharmacologic Category Diagnostic Agent

Pregnancy Risk Factor C

Lactation Enters breast milk/compatible

Use Diagnostic aid to differentiate thyroid failure; diagnosis of decreased thyroid reserve, to differentiate between primary and secondary hypothyroidism and between primary hypothyroidism and euthyroidism in patients receiving thyroid replacement

Mechanism of Action/Effect Stimulates formation and secretion of thyroid hormone, increases uptake of iodine by thyroid gland

Contraindications Hypersensitivity to thyrotropin or any component of the formulation; coronary thrombosis, untreated Addison's disease

Warnings/Precautions Use with caution in patients with angina pectoris or cardiac failure, patients with hypopituitarism, or adrenal cortical suppression as may be seen with corticosteroid therapy. May cause thyroid hyperplasia. Pregnancy risk C.

Adverse Reactions <1% (Limited to important or life-threatening): Anaphylaxis with repeated administration, fever, tachycardia

Overdosage/Toxicology Symptoms of overdose include weight loss, nervousness, sweating, tachycardia, insomnia, heat intolerance, menstrual irregularities, headache, angina pectoris, and CHF. Acute massive overdose may require cardiac glycosides for CHF. Fever should be controlled with the help of acetaminophen. Antiadrenergic agents, particularly propranolol 1-3 mg I.V. every 6 hours or 80-160 mg/day, can be used to treat increased sympathetic activity.

Pharmacodynamics/Kinetics

Half-Life Elimination: Thyroid state dependent: 35 minutes

Formulations Injection: 10 units

Dosing

Adults & Elderly: Diagnostic aid: I.M., S.C.: 10 units/day for 1-3 days; follow by a radioiodine study 24 hours past last injection, no response in thyroid failure, substantial response in pituitary failure

Stability

Reconstitution: Refrigerate at 2°C to 8°C (36°F to 46°F) after reconstitution. Use within 2 weeks.

Monitoring and Teaching Issues

Physical Assessment: Monitor for adverse reactions or overdose response (see Adverse Reactions and Overdose/Toxicology). **Pregnancy risk factor C** - benefits of use should outweigh possible risks.

Patient Education: You will receive this medication for 3 days prior to the radiologic studies. You may experience some nausea or vomiting. Report dizziness, faintness, palpitations, or any respiratory difficulties. **Pregnancy precaution:** Inform prescriber if you are or intend to become pregnant.

Thyrotropin Alpha *see page 1461*

Thytropar® *see* Thyrotropin *on page 1314*

Tiabendazole *see* Thiabendazole *on page 1303*

Tiagabine (tye AG a bene)

U.S. Brand Names Gabitril®

Synonyms Tiagabine Hydrochloride

Generic Available No

Pharmacologic Category Anticonvulsant, Miscellaneous

Pregnancy Risk Factor C

Lactation Enters breast milk/not recommended

Use Adjunctive therapy in adults and children ≥12 years of age in the treatment of partial seizures

Use - Unlabeled/Investigational Bipolar disorder

Mechanism of Action/Effect The exact mechanism by which tiagabine exerts antiseizure activity is not definitively known; however, *in vitro* experiments demonstrate that it enhances the activity of gamma aminobutyric acid (GABA), the major neuroinhibitory transmitter in the nervous system; it is thought that binding to the GABA uptake carrier inhibits the uptake of GABA into presynaptic neurons, allowing an increased amount of GABA to be available to postsynaptic neurons; based on *in vitro* studies, tiagabine does not inhibit the uptake of dopamine, norepinephrine, serotonin, glutamate, or choline

Contraindications Hypersensitivity to tiagabine or any component of the formulation

Warnings/Precautions Anticonvulsants should not be discontinued abruptly because of the possibility of increasing seizure frequency; tiagabine should be withdrawn gradually to minimize the potential of increased seizure frequency, unless safety concerns require a more rapid withdrawal. Rarely, nonconvulsive status epilepticus has been reported following abrupt discontinuation or dosage reduction.

Use with caution in patients with hepatic impairment. Experience in patients not receiving enzyme-inducing drugs has been limited - caution should be used in treating any patient who is not receiving one of these medications. Weakness, sedation, and confusion may occur with tiagabine use. Patients must cautioned about performing tasks which require mental alertness (ie, operating machinery or driving). Effects with other sedative drugs or ethanol may be potentiated. May cause potentially serious rash, including Stevens-Johnson syndrome.

Pregnancy risk C.

Drug Interactions

Cytochrome P450 Effect: Substrate of **3A4**

Decreased Effect: Primidone, phenobarbital, phenytoin, and carbamazepine increase tiagabine clearance by 60%.

Increased Effect/Toxicity: Valproate increased free tiagabine concentrations by 40%.

Nutritional/Ethanol Interactions

Ethanol: Avoid ethanol (may increase CNS depression).

Food: Food reduces the rate but not the extent of absorption.

Herb/Nutraceutical: St John's wort may decrease tiagabine levels. Avoid valerian, St John's wort, kava kava, gotu kola (may increase CNS depression).

(Continued)

Tiagabine *(Continued)*

Adverse Reactions

>10%:

Central nervous system: Dizziness, somnolence
Gastrointestinal: Nausea
Neuromuscular & skeletal: Weakness

1% to 10%:

Central nervous system: Nervousness, difficulty with concentration, insomnia, ataxia, confusion, speech disorder, depression, emotional lability, abnormal gait, hostility
Dermatologic: Rash, pruritus
Gastrointestinal: Diarrhea, vomiting, increased appetite
Neuromuscular & skeletal: Tremor, paresthesia
Ocular: Nystagmus
Otic: Hearing impairment
Respiratory: Pharyngitis, cough

Overdosage/Toxicology Somnolence, impaired consciousness, agitation, confusion, speech difficulty, hostility, depression, weakness, myoclonus, and seizures may occur. Treatment is supportive.

Pharmacodynamics/Kinetics

Absorption: Rapid (within 1 hour); prolonged with food

Bioavailability: Oral: Absolute: 90%

Half-Life Elimination: 6.7 hours

Time to Peak: Plasma: 45 minutes

Metabolism: Hepatic via CYP (primarily 3A4)

Formulations Tablet: 2 mg, 4 mg, 12 mg, 16 mg, 20 mg

Dosing

Adults & Elderly: Partial seizures (adjunct): Oral: Initial: 4 mg once daily for 1 week; may increase by 4-8 mg weekly to response or up to 56 mg daily in 2-4 divided doses

Pediatrics: Partial seizures: Oral: Children 12-18 years: 4 mg once daily for 1 week; may increase to 8 mg daily in 2 divided doses for 1 week; then may increase by 4-8 mg weekly to response or up to 32 mg daily in 2-4 divided doses

Monitoring Laboratory Tests A therapeutic range for tiagabine has not been established. Monitor complete blood counts, renal function tests, liver function tests, and routine blood chemistry.

Monitoring and Teaching Issues

Physical Assessment: Assess effectiveness and interactions of other medications patient may be taking (see Contraindications, Warnings/Precautions, and Drug Interactions). Monitor therapeutic response (seizure activity, force, type, duration), laboratory values, and adverse reactions (see Adverse Reactions) at beginning of therapy and periodically with long-term use. Taper dosage slowly when discontinuing. Assess knowledge/teach patient appropriate use, seizure safety precautions, interventions to reduce side effects, and adverse symptoms to report (see Patient Education). **Pregnancy risk factor C** - benefits of use should outweigh possible risks. Breast-feeding is not recommended.

Patient Education: Take exactly as directed; do not increase dose or frequency or discontinue without consulting prescriber. While using this medication, do not use alcohol and other prescription or OTC medications (especially pain medications, sedatives, antihistamines, or hypnotics) without consulting prescriber. Maintain adequate hydration (2-3 L/day of fluids) unless advised by prescriber to restrict fluids. You may experience drowsiness, dizziness, disturbed concentration, or blurred vision (use caution when driving or engaging in tasks requiring alertness until response to drug is known); or nausea, vomiting, or loss of appetite (small, frequent meals, frequent mouth care, chewing gum, or sucking lozenges may help). Wear identification of epileptic status and medications. Report behavioral or CNS changes; skin rash; muscle cramping, weakness, tremors, changes in gait; vision difficulties; persistent GI distress (cramping, pain, vomiting); chest pain, irregular heartbeat, or palpitations; cough or difficulty breathing; or worsening of seizure activity or loss of seizure control. **Pregnancy/breast-feeding precautions:** Inform prescriber if you are or intend to become pregnant. Breast-feeding is not recommended.

Dietary Issues: Take with food.

Geriatric Considerations: There has been limited clinical experience with geriatric patients during clinical evaluation - use with caution.

Tiagabine Hydrochloride *see* Tiagabine *on page 1315*
Tiazac® *see* Diltiazem *on page 418*
Ticar® *see* Ticarcillin *on page 1316*

Ticarcillin (tye kar SIL in)

U.S. Brand Names Ticar®

Synonyms Ticarcillin Disodium

Generic Available No

Pharmacologic Category Antibiotic, Penicillin

Pregnancy Risk Factor B

Lactation Enters breast milk/compatible

Use Treatment of susceptible infections such as septicemia, acute and chronic respiratory tract infections, skin and soft tissue infections, and urinary tract infections due to susceptible strains of *Pseudomonas*, and other gram-negative bacteria

Mechanism of Action/Effect Interferes with bacterial cell wall synthesis during active multiplication, causing cell wall death and resultant bactericidal activity against susceptible bacteria

Contraindications Hypersensitivity to ticarcillin, any component of the formulation, or penicillins

Warnings/Precautions Due to sodium load and adverse effects (anemia, neuropsychological changes), use with caution and modify dosage in patients with renal impairment. Serious and occasionally severe or fatal hypersensitivity (anaphylactoid) reactions have been reported in patients on penicillin therapy (especially with a history of beta-lactam hypersensitivity and/or a history of sensitivity to multiple allergens). Use with caution in patients with seizures.

Drug Interactions

Decreased Effect: Tetracyclines may decrease penicillin effectiveness. Aminoglycosides may cause physical inactivation of aminoglycosides in the presence of high concentrations of ticarcillin and potential toxicity in patients with mild-moderate renal dysfunction. Although anecdotal reports suggest oral contraceptive efficacy could be reduced by penicillins, this has been refuted by more rigorous scientific and clinical data.

Increased Effect/Toxicity: Probenecid may increase penicillin levels. Neuromuscular blockers may have an increased duration of action (neuromuscular blockade).

Effects on Lab Values False-positive urinary or serum protein, positive Coombs' test

Adverse Reactions Frequency not defined.

Central nervous system: Confusion, convulsions, drowsiness, fever, Jarisch-Herxheimer reaction

Dermatologic: Rash

Endocrine & metabolic: Electrolyte imbalance

Gastrointestinal: *Clostridium difficile* colitis

Hematologic: Bleeding, eosinophilia, hemolytic anemia, leukopenia, neutropenia, positive Coombs' reaction, thrombocytopenia

Hepatic: Hepatotoxicity, jaundice

Local: Thrombophlebitis

Neuromuscular & skeletal: Myoclonus

Renal: Interstitial nephritis (acute)

Miscellaneous: Anaphylaxis, hypersensitivity reactions

Overdosage/Toxicology Symptoms of penicillin overdose include neuromuscular hypersensitivity (eg, agitation, hallucinations, asterixis, encephalopathy, confusion, and seizures). Electrolyte imbalance may occur if the preparation contains potassium or sodium salts, especially in renal failure. Hemodialysis may be helpful to aid in removal of the drug from blood; otherwise, treatment is supportive or symptom-directed.

Pharmacodynamics/Kinetics

Absorption: I.M.: 86%

Half-Life Elimination:

Neonates: <1 week old: 3.5-5.6 hours; 1-8 weeks old: 1.3-2.2 hours

Children 5-13 years: 0.9 hour

Adults: 66-72 minutes; prolonged with renal and/or hepatic impairment

Time to Peak: Serum: I.M.: 30-75 minutes

Formulations Injection, powder for reconstitution, as disodium: 3 g, 20 g

Dosing

Adults:

Susceptible infections: I.M., I.V.: 1-4 g every 4-6 hours, usual dose: 3 g I.V. every 4-6 hours

Note: Ticarcillin is generally given I.V., I.M. injection is only for the treatment of uncomplicated urinary tract infections and dose should not exceed 2 g/injection when administered I.M.

Elderly: Ticarcillin is generally given I.M. only for the treatment of uncomplicated urinary tract infections.

I.V.: 3 g every 4-6 hours; adjust dosing interval for renal impairment.

Pediatrics:

Susceptible infections: I.M., I.V.:

Infants and Children:

Systemic infections: I.V.: 200-300 mg/kg/day in divided doses every 4-6 hours

Urinary tract infections: I.M., I.V.: 50-100 mg/kg/day in divided doses every 6-8 hours

Maximum dose: 24 g/day

Note: Ticarcillin is generally given I.V., I.M. injection is only for the treatment of uncomplicated urinary tract infections and dose should not exceed 2 g/injection when administered I.M.

Renal Impairment:

Cl_{cr} 30-60 mL/minute: 2 g every 4 hours or 3 g every 8 hours

Cl_{cr} 10-30 mL/minute: 2 g every 8 hours or 3 g every 12 hours

Cl_{cr} <10 mL/minute: 2 g every 12 hours

Moderately dialyzable (20% to 50%)

Continuous arteriovenous or venovenous hemodiafiltration effects: Dose as for Cl_{cr} 10-50 mL/minute

Administration

I.M.: Do not give more than 2 g per injection.

I.V.: Administer around-the-clock. Administer 1 hour apart from aminoglycosides. Intermittently infusion over 30 minutes to 2 hours.

Stability

Storage: Reconstituted solution is stable for 72 hours at room temperature and 14 days when refrigerated or 30 days when frozen. For I.V. infusion in NS or D_5W.

Compatibility: Stable in D_5W, LR, NS, sterile water for injection

Y-site administration: Incompatible with amphotericin B cholesteryl sulfate complex, fluconazole

Compatibility in syringe: Incompatible with doxapram

Compatibility when admixed: Incompatible with gentamicin, aminoglycosides

Monitoring Laboratory Tests Serum electrolytes, bleeding time, and periodic tests of renal, hepatic, and hematologic function; perform culture and sensitivity before administering first dose.

Monitoring and Teaching Issues

Physical Assessment: Assess for allergy history prior to starting therapy. See Contraindications and Warnings/Precautions for use cautions. Assess potential for interactions with other prescriptions, OTC medications, or herbal products patient may be taking (see Drug Interactions). Caution diabetic patients about altered response to Clinitest®. Assess results

(Continued)

Ticarcillin *(Continued)*

of laboratory tests (see above), therapeutic effectiveness, and adverse reactions (eg, hypersensitivity reactions, opportunistic infection - see Adverse Reactions and Overdose/Toxicology). Teach patient possible side effects and interventions, and adverse symptoms to report (see Patient Education).

Patient Education: Inform prescriber of all prescriptions, OTC medications, or herbal products you are taking, and any allergies you have. Do not take anything new during treatment unless approved by prescriber. This drug can only be given by injection or infusion. Report immediately any redness, swelling, burning, or pain at infusion site or any signs of allergic reaction (eg, difficulty breathing or swallowing, chest tightness, rash, hives, swelling of lips or mouth). Maintain adequate hydration (2-3 L/day of fluids) unless advised by prescriber to restrict fluids. If diabetic, drug may cause false test results with Clinitest®, consult prescriber for alternative method of glucose monitoring. May cause confusion or drowsiness (use caution when driving or engaging in tasks that require alertness until response to drug is known). Report persistent diarrhea or abdominal pain (do not use antidiarrheal medication without consulting prescriber); bloody urine or stool; muscle pain; mouth sores; difficulty breathing; skin rash; or signs of opportunistic infection (eg, fever, chills, unhealed sores, white plaques in mouth or vagina, purulent vaginal discharge, fatigue).

Dietary Issues: Sodium content of 1 g: 119.6-149.5 mg (5.2-6.5 mEq)

Geriatric Considerations: When used as empiric therapy or for documented pseudomonal pneumonia, it is best to combine with an aminoglycoside such as gentamicin or tobramycin. High sodium may limit use in patients with congestive heart failure. Adjust dose for renal function.

Ticarcillin and Clavulanate Potassium

(tye kar SIL in & klav yoo LAN ate poe TASS ee um)

U.S. Brand Names Timentin®

Synonyms Ticarcillin and Clavulanic Acid

Generic Available No

Pharmacologic Category Antibiotic, Penicillin

Pregnancy Risk Factor B

Lactation Enters breast milk (other penicillins are compatible with breast-feeding)

Use Treatment of infections of lower respiratory tract, urinary tract, skin and skin structures, bone and joint, and septicemia caused by susceptible organisms. Clavulanate expands activity of ticarcillin to include beta-lactamase producing strains of *S. aureus*, *H. influenzae*, *Bacteroides* species, and some other gram-negative bacilli

Mechanism of Action/Effect Ticarcillin interferes with bacterial cell wall synthesis during active multiplication, causing cell wall death and resultant bactericidal activity against susceptible bacteria; clavulanic acid prevents degradation of ticarcillin by binding to the active site on beta-lactamase

Contraindications Hypersensitivity to ticarcillin, clavulanate, any penicillin, or any component of the formulation

Warnings/Precautions Use with caution and modify dosage in patients with renal impairment. Serious and occasionally fatal hypersensitivity (anaphylactoid) reactions have been reported in patients on penicillin therapy. These reactions are more likely to occur in individuals with a history of cephalosporin hypersensitivity and/or a history of sensitivity to multiple allergens.

Drug Interactions

Decreased Effect: Tetracyclines may decrease penicillin effectiveness. Aminoglycosides may cause physical inactivation of aminoglycosides in the presence of high concentrations of ticarcillin and potential toxicity in patients with mild-moderate renal dysfunction. Although anecdotal reports suggest oral contraceptive efficacy could be reduced by penicillins, this has been refuted by more rigorous scientific and clinical data.

Increased Effect/Toxicity: Probenecid may increase penicillin levels. Neuromuscular blockers may have an increased duration of action (neuromuscular blockade).

Effects on Lab Values Positive Coombs' test, false-positive urinary proteins

Adverse Reactions Frequency not defined.

Central nervous system: Confusion, convulsions, drowsiness, fever, Jarisch-Herxheimer reaction

Dermatologic: Rash, erythema multiforme, toxic epidermal necrolysis, Stevens-Johnson syndrome

Endocrine & metabolic: Electrolyte imbalance

Gastrointestinal: *Clostridium difficile* colitis

Hematologic: Bleeding, hemolytic anemia, leukopenia, neutropenia, positive Coombs' reaction, thrombocytopenia

Hepatic: Hepatotoxicity, jaundice

Local: Thrombophlebitis

Neuromuscular & skeletal: Myoclonus

Renal: Interstitial nephritis (acute)

Miscellaneous: Anaphylaxis, hypersensitivity reactions

Overdosage/Toxicology Symptoms of overdose include neuromuscular hypersensitivity and seizures. Hemodialysis may be helpful to aid in removal of the drug from blood; otherwise, treatment is supportive or symptom-directed.

Pharmacokinetic Note See Ticarcillin monograph.

Pharmacodynamics/Kinetics

Half-Life Elimination:

Clavulanic acid: 66-90 minutes

Metabolism:

Clavulanic acid: Hepatic

Formulations

Infusion [premixed, frozen]: Ticarcillin disodium 3 g and clavulanate potassium 0.1 g (100 mL)

Injection, powder for reconstitution: Ticarcillin disodium 3 g and clavulanate potassium 0.1 g (3.1 g, 31 g)

Dosing

Adults:

Systemic infections: I.V.: 3.1 g (ticarcillin 3 g plus clavulanic acid 0.1 g) every 4-6 hours; maximum: 18-24 g/day

Urinary tract infections: I.V.: 3.1 g every 6-8 hours

Elderly: I.V. (based on ticarcillin): 3 g every 4-6 hours; adjust for renal function.

Pediatrics:

Systemic infections: Children <60 kg: 200-300 mg of ticarcillin component/kg/day in divided doses every 4-6 hours

Children >60 kg: 3.1 g (ticarcillin 3 g plus clavulanic acid 0.1 g) every 4-6 hours; maximum: 24 g/day

Renal Impairment:

Cl_{cr} 30-60 mL/minute: Administer 2 g every 4 hours or 3.1 g every 8 hours.

Cl_{cr} 10-30 mL/minute: Administer 2 g every 8 hours or 3.1 g every 12 hours.

Cl_{cr} <10 mL/minute: Administer 2 g every 12 hours.

Cl_{cr} <10 mL/minute with hepatic dysfunction: 2 g every 24 hours.

Moderately dialyzable (20% to 50%)

Continuous arteriovenous or venovenous hemodiafiltration effects: Dose as for Cl_{cr} 10-50 mL/minute.

Peritoneal dialysis: Administer 3.1 g every 12 hours.

Hemodialysis: Administer 2 g every 12 hours; supplemented with 3.1 g after each dialysis.

Hepatic Impairment: Cl_{cr} <10 mL/minute with hepatic dysfunction: Administer 2 g every 24 hours.

Administration

I.V.: Infuse over 30 minutes. Administer 1 hour apart from aminoglycosides. Give around-the-clock.

Stability

Storage: Reconstituted solution is stable for 6 hours at room temperature and 72 hours when refrigerated. I.V. infusion in NS is stable for 24 hours at room temperature, 7 days when refrigerated, or 30 days when frozen. Darkening of solution indicates loss of potency of clavulanate potassium.

Compatibility: Stable in D_5W, LR, NS, sterile water for injection

Y-site administration: Incompatible with alatrofloxacin, amphotericin B cholesteryl sulfate complex

Compatibility when admixed: Incompatible with sodium bicarbonate, aminoglycosides

Monitoring Laboratory Tests Serum electrolytes, bleeding time, and periodic tests of renal, hepatic, and hematologic function; perform culture and sensitivity before administering first dose.

Monitoring and Teaching Issues

Physical Assessment: Assess for allergy history prior to starting therapy. See Contraindications and Warnings/Precautions for use cautions. Assess potential for interactions with other prescriptions, OTC medications, or herbal products patient may be taking (see Drug Interactions). Caution diabetic patients about altered response to Clinitest®. Assess results of laboratory tests (see above), therapeutic effectiveness, and adverse reactions (eg, hypersensitivity reactions, opportunistic infection - see Adverse Reactions and Overdose/Toxicology). Teach patient possible side effects and interventions and adverse symptoms to report (see Patient Education).

Patient Education: Inform prescriber of all prescriptions, OTC medications, or herbal products you are taking, and any allergies you have. Do not take anything new during treatment unless approved by prescriber. This drug can only be given by injection or infusion. Report immediately any redness, swelling, burning, or pain at infusion site or any signs of allergic reaction (eg, difficulty breathing or swallowing, chest tightness, rash, hives, swelling of lips or mouth). Maintain adequate hydration (2-3 L/day of fluids) unless advised by prescriber to restrict fluids. If diabetic, drug may cause false test results with Clinitest®, consult prescriber for alternative method of glucose monitoring. May cause confusion or drowsiness (use caution when driving or engaging in tasks that require alertness until response to drug is known). Report persistent diarrhea or abdominal pain (do not use antidiarrheal medication without consulting prescriber), fever, chills, unhealed sores, bloody urine or stool, muscle pain, mouth sores, difficulty breathing, or skin rash; or signs of opportunistic infection (eg, fever, chills, unhealed sores, white plaques in mouth or vagina, purulent vaginal discharge, fatigue).

Dietary Issues: Sodium content of 1 g: 4.75 mEq; potassium content of 1 g: 0.15 mEq

Geriatric Considerations: When used as empiric therapy or for a documented pseudomonal pneumonia, it is best to combine with an aminoglycoside such as gentamicin or tobramycin. High sodium content may limit use in patients with congestive heart failure. Adjust dose for renal function.

Related Information

Ticarcillin *on page 1316*

Ticarcillin and Clavulanic Acid *see* Ticarcillin and Clavulanate Potassium *on page 1318*

Ticarcillin Disodium *see* Ticarcillin *on page 1316*

Ticlid® *see* Ticlopidine *on page 1319*

Ticlopidine (tye KLOE pi deen)

U.S. Brand Names Ticlid®

Synonyms Ticlopidine Hydrochloride

Generic Available Yes

Pharmacologic Category Antiplatelet Agent

Pregnancy Risk Factor B

Lactation Excretion in breast milk unknown

(Continued)

Ticlopidine *(Continued)*

Use Platelet aggregation inhibitor that reduces the risk of thrombotic stroke in patients who have had a stroke or stroke precursors. **Note:** Due to its association with life-threatening hematologic disorders, ticlopidine should be reserved for patients who are intolerant to aspirin, or who have failed aspirin therapy. Adjunctive therapy (with aspirin) following successful coronary stent implantation to reduce the incidence of subacute stent thrombosis.

Use - Unlabeled/Investigational Protection of aortocoronary bypass grafts, diabetic microangiopathy, ischemic heart disease, prevention of postoperative DVT, reduction of graft loss following renal transplant

Mechanism of Action/Effect Ticlopidine is an inhibitor of platelet function with a mechanism which is different from other antiplatelet drugs. The drug significantly increases bleeding time. This effect may not be solely related to ticlopidine's effect on platelets. The prolongation of the bleeding time caused by ticlopidine is further increased by the addition of aspirin in *ex vivo* experiments. Although many metabolites of ticlopidine have been found, none have been shown to account for *in vivo* activity.

Contraindications Hypersensitivity to ticlopidine or any component of the formulation; active pathological bleeding such as PUD or intracranial hemorrhage; severe liver dysfunction; hematopoietic disorders (neutropenia, thrombocytopenia, a past history of TTP)

Warnings/Precautions Use with caution in patients who may have an increased risk of bleeding (such as, ulcers). Consider discontinuing 10-14 days before elective surgery. Use caution in mixing with other antiplatelet drugs. Use with caution in patients with severe liver disease or severe renal impairment (experience is limited). May cause life-threatening hematologic reactions, including neutropenia, agranulocytosis, thrombotic thrombocytopenia purpura (TTP), and aplastic anemia. Routine monitoring is required. Monitor for signs and symptoms of neutropenia including WBC count. Discontinue if the absolute neutrophil count falls to <1200/mm^3 or if the platelet count falls to <80,000/mm^3.

Drug Interactions

Cytochrome P450 Effect: Substrate of **CYP3A4**; Inhibits **CYP1A2, 2C8/9, 2C19**, 2D6

Decreased Effect: Decreased effect of ticlopidine with antacids (decreased absorption). Ticlopidine may decrease the effect of digoxin, cyclosporine.

Increased Effect/Toxicity: Ticlopidine may increase effect/toxicity of aspirin, anticoagulants, theophylline, and NSAIDs. Cimetidine may increase ticlopidine blood levels. Phenytoin blood levels may be increased by ticlopidine (case reports).

Nutritional/Ethanol Interactions

Food: Ticlopidine bioavailability may be increased (20%) if taken with food. High-fat meals increase absorption, antacids decrease absorption.

Herb/Nutraceutical: Avoid cat's claw, dong quai, evening primrose, feverfew, garlic, ginkgo, ginger, red clover, horse chestnut, green tea, ginseng (all have additional antiplatelet activity).

Effects on Lab Values ↑ cholesterol (S), alkaline phosphatase, transaminases (S)

Adverse Reactions As with all drugs which may affect hemostasis, bleeding is associated with ticlopidine. Hemorrhage may occur at virtually any site. Risk is dependent on multiple variables, including the use of multiple agents which alter hemostasis and patient susceptibility.

>10%:

Endocrine & metabolic: Increased total cholesterol (increases of ~8% to 10% within 1 month of therapy)

Gastrointestinal: Diarrhea (13%)

1% to 10%: Central nervous system: Dizziness (1%)

Dermatologic: Rash (5%), purpura (2%), pruritus (1%)

Gastrointestinal: Nausea (7%), dyspepsia (7%), gastrointestinal pain (4%), vomiting (2%), flatulence (2%), anorexia (1%)

Hematologic: Neutropenia (2%)

Hepatic: Abnormal liver function test (1%)

<1% (Limited to important or life-threatening): Agranulocytosis, anaphylaxis, angioedema, aplastic anemia, arthropathy, bone marrow suppression, bronchiolitis obliterans-organized pneumonia, chronic diarrhea, conjunctival bleeding, eosinophilia, erythema multiforme, erythema nodosum, exfoliative dermatitis, gastrointestinal bleeding, hematuria, hemolytic anemia, hepatic necrosis, hepatitis, hyponatremia, intracranial bleeding (rare), jaundice, maculopapular rash, menorrhagia, myositis, nephrotic syndrome, pancytopenia, peptic ulcer, peripheral neuropathy, pneumonitis (allergic), positive ANA, renal failure, sepsis, serum creatinine increased, serum sickness, Stevens-Johnson syndrome, systemic lupus erythematosus, thrombocytopenia (immune), thrombocytosis, thrombotic thrombocytopenic purpura, urticaria, vasculitis

Overdosage/Toxicology Symptoms of overdose include ataxia, seizures, vomiting, abdominal pain, and hematologic abnormalities. Specific treatments are lacking. Treatment is symptomatic and supportive.

Pharmacodynamics/Kinetics

Half-Life Elimination: 24 hours

Metabolism: Extensively hepatic; has at least one active metabolite

Onset: ~6 hours; Peak effect: 3-5 days; serum levels do not correlate with clinical antiplatelet activity

Formulations Tablet, as hydrochloride: 250 mg

Dosing

Adults:

Stroke prevention: Oral: 250 mg twice daily with food

Coronary artery stenting (initiate after successful implantation): Oral: 250 mg twice daily with food (in combination with antiplatelet doses of aspirin) for up to 30 days

Elderly: Dosage in the elderly has not been determined; however, in two large clinical trials, the average age of subjects was 63 and 66 years.

Administration

Oral: Administer with food.

Monitoring Laboratory Tests CBC with differential and platelet counts every 2 weeks starting the second week through the third month of treatment; more frequent monitoring is recommended for patients whose absolute neutrophil counts have been consistently declining or are 30% less than baseline values. Liver function tests (alkaline phosphatase and transaminases) should be performed in the first 4 months of therapy if liver dysfunction is suspected.

Monitoring and Teaching Issues

Physical Assessment: Monitor effectiveness of therapy (laboratory results) frequently at beginning of treatment and regularly thereafter (see Monitoring Laboratory Tests). Monitor and teach patient bleeding precautions, possible side effects, and adverse symptoms to report (see Patient Education). Note breast-feeding caution.

Patient Education: Take exact dosage prescribed, with food. Do not use aspirin or aspirin-containing medications and OTC medications without consulting prescriber. You may experience easy bleeding or bruising (use soft toothbrush or cotton swabs and frequent mouth care, use electric razor, avoid sharp knives or scissors). Report unusual bleeding or bruising, persistent fever, sore throat, weakness, paleness, changes in neurological status; blood in urine, stool, or vomitus; delayed healing of any wounds; skin rash; yellowing of skin or eyes; changes in color of urine or stool; pain or burning on urination; difficulty breathing; or skin rash. **Breast-feeding precaution:** Consult prescriber if breast-feeding.

Dietary Issues: Should be taken with food to reduce stomach upset.

Geriatric Considerations: Because of the risk of neutropenia and its relative expense as compared with aspirin, ticlopidine should only be used in patients with a documented intolerance to aspirin.

Ticlopidine Hydrochloride *see* Ticlopidine *on page 1319*

Tigan® *see* Trimethobenzamide *on page 1365*

Tikosyn™ *see* Dofetilide *on page 433*

Tilade® *see* Nedocromil *on page 953*

Tiludronate (tye LOO droe nate)

U.S. Brand Names Skelid®

Synonyms Tiludronate Disodium

Generic Available No

Pharmacologic Category Bisphosphonate Derivative

Pregnancy Risk Factor C

Lactation Excretion in breast milk unknown

Use Treatment of Paget's disease of the bone in patients who have a level of serum alkaline phosphatase (SAP) at least twice the upper limit of normal, or who are symptomatic, or who are at risk for future complications of their disease

Mechanism of Action/Effect A biphosphonate which inhibits osteoclast activity, reducing enzymatic and transport processes that lead to resorption of bone. At least two possible mechanisms may be involved: detachment of osteoclasts from the bone surface (due to inhibition of protein-tyrosine-phosphatase) and inhibition of the osteoclastic proton pump, required to alter local pH to solubilize ions and bone matrix during resorption.

Contraindications Hypersensitivity to biphosphonates or any component of the formulation

Warnings/Precautions Not recommended in severe renal impairment (Cl_{cr} <30 mL/minute). May cause upper gastrointestinal problems (eg, dysphagia, esophageal diseases, gastritis, duodenitis, ulcers). Pregnancy risk C.

Drug Interactions

Decreased Effect: Concurrent administration of calcium salts, aluminum- or magnesium-containing antacids, and aspirin markedly decrease absorption/bioavailability (by 50% to 60%) of tiludronate if given within 2 hours of a dose.

Increased Effect/Toxicity: Administration of indomethacin increases bioavailability of tiludronate two- to fourfold.

Nutritional/Ethanol Interactions Food: In single-dose studies, the bioavailability of tiludronate was reduced by 90% when an oral dose was administered with, or 2 hours after, a standard breakfast compared to the same dose administered after an overnight fast and 4 hours before a standard breakfast.

Adverse Reactions The following events occurred >2% and at a frequency > placebo:

1% to 10%:

Cardiovascular: Chest pain (3%), edema (3%)

Central nervous system: Dizziness (4%), paresthesia (4%)

Dermatologic: Rash (3%), skin disorder (3%)

Gastrointestinal: Nausea (9%), diarrhea (9%), heartburn (5%), vomiting (4%), flatulence (3%)

Neuromuscular & skeletal: Arthrosis (3%)

Ocular: cataract (3%), conjunctivitis (3%), glaucoma (3%)

Respiratory: Rhinitis (5%), sinusitis (5%), coughing (3%), pharyngitis (3%)

<1% (Limited to important or life-threatening): Stevens-Johnson syndrome

Overdosage/Toxicology Hypocalcemia is a potential consequence of overdose. Treatment is supportive.

(Continued)

Tiludronate *(Continued)*

Pharmacodynamics/Kinetics

Absorption: Rapid

Bioavailability: 6%; reduced by food

Half-Life Elimination: Healthy volunteers: 50 hours; Pagetic patients: 150 hours

Time to Peak: Plasma: ~2 hours

Metabolism: Little, if any

Onset: Delayed, may require several weeks

Formulations Dosage expressed in terms of tiludronic acid:

Tablet, as disodium: 240 mg [tiludronic acid 200 mg]

Dosing

Adults: Paget's disease: Oral: 400 mg (2 tablets of tiludronic acid) daily for a period of 3 months

Elderly: Plasma concentrations of tiludronic acid are higher in elderly patients, but no dosage reduction is recommended. Refer to adult dosing.

Renal Impairment: Tiludronate is excreted renally. It is not recommended for use in patients with severe renal impairment (Cl_{cr} <30 mL/minute) and is not removed by dialysis.

Administration

Oral: Take with 6-8 oz of plain water. Do not take within 2 hours of food, aspirin, indomethacin, or calcium-, magnesium-, or aluminum-containing medications.

Stability

Storage: Do not remove tablet from foil strips until they are to be used.

Monitoring Laboratory Tests Serum calcium, alkaline phosphatase

Monitoring and Teaching Issues

Physical Assessment: See Contraindications and Warnings/Precautions for use cautions. Assess results of laboratory tests (see above), effectiveness of treatment, and development of adverse reactions (see Adverse Reactions and Overdose/Toxicology). Teach appropriate use and administration of medication (see Administration), lifestyle and dietary changes that will have a beneficial impact on Paget's disease, possible side effects and interventions, and adverse reactions to report. **Pregnancy risk factor C** - benefits of use should outweigh possible risks. Note breast-feeding caution.

Patient Education: Inform prescriber of all prescriptions, OTC medications, or herbal products you are taking, and any allergies you have. Do not take anything new during treatment unless approved by prescriber. Do not remove medication from foil strip until ready to be used. Take as directed, on an empty stomach with a full glass of water. Do not take within 2 hours of food, aspirin, indomethacin, or calcium-, magnesium-, or aluminum-containing medications. Stay in sitting or standing position for 30 minutes following administration. Consult prescriber to determine possibility of lifestyle changes (eg, decreased smoking, decreased alcohol intake, dietary supplements of calcium, or increased dietary vitamin D). May cause mild skin rash; or abdominal pain, diarrhea, or constipation (report if persistent). Report unresolved muscle or bone pain or leg cramps; acute abdominal pain; chest pain, palpitations, or swollen extremities; disturbed vision or excessively dry eyes; ringing in the ears; persistent rash or skin disorder; or unusual weakness or increased perspiration. **Pregnancy/breast-feeding precautions:** Inform prescriber if you are or intend to become pregnant. Consult prescriber if breast-feeding.

Dietary Issues: Do not take within 2 hours of food.

Tiludronate Disodium *see* Tiludronate *on page 1321*

Timentin® *see* Ticarcillin and Clavulanate Potassium *on page 1318*

Timolol *see* Ophthalmic Agents, Glaucoma *on page 1002*

Timolol (TYE moe lole)

U.S. Brand Names Betimol®; Blocadren®; Timoptic®; Timoptic® OcuDose®; Timoptic-XE®

Synonyms Timolol Hemihydrate; Timolol Maleate

Generic Available Yes: Except hemihydrate and preservative free maleate ophthalmic solutions

Pharmacologic Category Beta Blocker, Nonselective; Ophthalmic Agent, Antiglaucoma

Pregnancy Risk Factor C (manufacturer); D (2nd and 3rd trimesters - expert analysis)

Lactation Enters breast milk/use caution (AAP rates "compatible")

Use Ophthalmic dosage form used in treatment of elevated intraocular pressure such as glaucoma or ocular hypertension; oral dosage form used for treatment of hypertension and angina, to reduce mortality following myocardial infarction, and for prophylaxis of migraine

Mechanism of Action/Effect Blocks both $beta_1$- and $beta_2$-adrenergic receptors, reduces intraocular pressure by reducing aqueous humor production or possibly outflow; reduces blood pressure by blocking adrenergic receptors and decreasing sympathetic outflow, produces a negative chronotropic and inotropic activity through an unknown mechanism

Contraindications Hypersensitivity to timolol or any component of the formulation; sinus bradycardia; sinus node dysfunction; heart block greater than first degree (except in patients with a functioning artificial pacemaker); cardiogenic shock; uncompensated cardiac failure; bronchospastic disease; pregnancy (2nd and 3rd trimesters)

Warnings/Precautions Administer cautiously in compensated heart failure and monitor for a worsening of the condition. Beta-blocker therapy should not be withdrawn abruptly (particularly in patients with CAD), but gradually tapered to avoid acute tachycardia, hypertension, and/or ischemia. Use caution with concurrent use of beta-blockers and either verapamil or diltiazem; bradycardia or heart block can occur. Beta-blockers can aggravate symptoms in patients with peripheral vascular disease. Patients with bronchospastic disease should generally not receive beta-blockers - monitor closely if used in patients at risk of bronchospasm. Use cautiously in patients with diabetes; may mask prominent hypoglycemic symptoms. May mask signs of thyrotoxicosis. Use cautiously in severe renal impairment: marked hypotension can occur in patients maintained on hemodialysis. Use care with anesthetic agents which decrease myocardial function. Can worsen myasthenia gravis. Similar reactions found with systemic administration may occur with topical (ophthalmic) administration. Pregnancy risk C/D (2nd and 3rd trimesters).

Drug Interactions

Cytochrome P450 Effect: Substrate of **CYP2D6**; Inhibits CYP2D6

Decreased Effect: Decreased effect of timolol with aluminum salts, barbiturates, calcium salts, cholestyramine, colestipol, NSAIDs, penicillins (ampicillin), rifampin, salicylates, and sulfinpyrazone due to decreased bioavailability and plasma levels. Beta-blockers may decrease the effect of sulfonylureas. Beta-blockers may affect the action or levels of ethanol, disopyramide, nondepolarizing muscle relaxants, and theophylline, although the effects are difficult to predict.

Increased Effect/Toxicity: The heart rate lowering effects of timolol are additive with other drugs which slow AV conduction (digoxin, verapamil, diltiazem). Reserpine increases the effects of timolol. Concurrent use of timolol may increase the effects of alpha-blockers (prazosin, terazosin), alpha-adrenergic stimulants (epinephrine, phenylephrine), and the vasoconstrictive effects of ergot alkaloids. Timolol may mask the tachycardia from hypoglycemia caused by insulin and oral hypoglycemics. In patients receiving concurrent therapy, the risk of hypertensive crisis is increased when either clonidine or the beta-blocker is withdrawn. Beta-blockers may increase the action or levels of ethanol, disopyramide, nondepolarizing muscle relaxants, and theophylline although the effects are difficult to predict.

Adverse Reactions

Ophthalmic:

>10%: Ocular: Conjunctival hyperemia

1% to 10%: Ocular: Anisocoria, corneal punctate keratitis, keratitis, corneal staining, decreased corneal sensitivity, eye pain, vision disturbances

<1% (Limited to important or life-threatening): Systemic allergic reaction (anaphylaxis, angioedema, rash, urticaria)

Systemic:

>10%:
- Central nervous system: Drowsiness, insomnia
- Endocrine & metabolic: Decreased sexual ability

1% to 10%:
- Cardiovascular: Bradycardia, palpitations, edema, CHF, reduced peripheral circulation
- Central nervous system: Mental depression
- Gastrointestinal: Diarrhea or constipation, nausea, vomiting, stomach discomfort
- Respiratory: Bronchospasm
- Miscellaneous: Cold extremities

<1% (Limited to important or life-threatening): Anaphylaxis, angina, arrhythmias, confusion, depression, dyspnea, hallucinations, leukopenia, memory loss, nightmares, orthostatic hypotension, psoriasis, rash, Raynaud's phenomenon, retroperitoneal fibrosis, thrombocytopenia

Overdosage/Toxicology Symptoms of intoxication include cardiac disturbances, CNS toxicity, bronchospasm, hypoglycemia and hyperkalemia. The most common cardiac symptoms include hypotension and bradycardia. Atrioventricular block, intraventricular conduction disturbances, cardiogenic shock, and asystole may occur with severe overdose, especially with membrane-depressant drugs (eg, propranolol). CNS effects including convulsions, coma, and respiratory arrest are commonly seen with propranolol and other membrane-depressant and lipid-soluble drugs. Treatment is symptom-directed and supportive.

Pharmacodynamics/Kinetics

Half-Life Elimination: 2-2.7 hours; prolonged with renal impairment

Metabolism: Extensively hepatic; extensive first-pass effect

Onset: Hypotensive: Oral: 15-45 minutes; Peak effect: 0.5-2.5 hours

Duration: ~4 hours; Ophthalmic: Intraocular: 24 hours

Formulations

Gel-forming solution, ophthalmic, as maleate (Timoptic-XE®): 0.25% (2.5 mL, 5 mL); 0.5% (2.5 mL, 5 mL)

Solution, ophthalmic, as hemihydrate (Betimol®): 0.25% (5 mL, 10 mL, 15 mL); 0.5% (5 mL, 10 mL, 15 mL) [contains benzalkonium chloride]

Solution, ophthalmic, as maleate: 0.25% (5 mL, 10 mL, 15 mL); 0.5% (5 mL, 10 mL, 15 mL) [contains benzalkonium chloride]

Timoptic®: 0.25% (5 mL, 10 mL); 0.5% (5 mL, 10 mL) [contains benzalkonium chloride]

Solution, ophthalmic, as maleate [preservative free] (Timoptic® OcuDose®): 0.25% (0.2 mL);0.5% (0.2 mL) [single use]

Tablet, as maleate (Blocadren®): 5 mg, 10 mg, 20 mg

Dosing

Adults & Elderly:

Glaucoma: Ophthalmic:

Solution: Initial: 0.25% solution, instill 1 drop twice daily; increase to 0.5% solution if response not adequate; decrease to 1 drop/day if controlled; do not exceed 1 drop twice daily of 0.5% solution.

Gel-forming solution (Timoptic-XE®): Instill 1 drop (either 0.25% or 0.5%) once daily

Hypertension: Oral: Initial: 10 mg twice daily, increase gradually every 7 days, usual dosage: 20-40 mg/day in 2 divided doses; maximum: 60 mg/day.

Prevention of myocardial infarction: Oral: 10 mg twice daily initiated within 1-4 weeks after infarction.

Migraine prophylaxis: Oral: Initial: 10 mg twice daily, increase to maximum of 30 mg/day.

Pediatrics: Children: Ophthalmic: Refer to adult dosing.

Administration

Other: Administer other topically-applied ophthalmic medications at least 10 minutes before Timoptic-XE®; wash hands before use; invert closed bottle and shake once before use; remove cap carefully so that tip does not touch anything; hold bottle between thumb and index finger; use index finger of other hand to pull down the lower eyelid to form a pocket

(Continued)

Timolol *(Continued)*

for the eye drop and tilt head back; place the dispenser tip close to the eye and gently squeeze the bottle to administer 1 drop; remove pressure after a single drop has been released; **do not allow the dispenser tip to touch the eye**; replace cap and store bottle in an upright position in a clean area; do **not** enlarge hole of dispenser; do **not** wash tip with water, soap, or any other cleaner

Monitoring and Teaching Issues

Physical Assessment: See Contraindications and Warnings/Precautions for use cautions. Assess other medications patient may be taking for effectiveness and interactions (see Drug Interactions). Monitor therapeutic effectiveness (according to purpose of therapy) and adverse reactions (see Warnings/Precautions, Adverse Reactions, and Overdose/Toxicology) at beginning of therapy and regularly with long-term therapy. Assess knowledge/ teach patient appropriate use, interventions to reduce side effects, and adverse symptoms to report (see Patient Education). **Pregnancy risk factor C/D** - benefits of use should outweigh possible risks. Note breast-feeding caution.

Patient Education: Oral: Take exact dose prescribed; do not increase, decrease, or discontinue dosage without consulting prescriber. Take at the same time each day. Does not replace recommended diet or exercise program. If diabetic, monitor serum glucose closely. May cause postural hypotension (use caution when rising from sitting or lying position or climbing stairs); dizziness, drowsiness, or blurred vision (use caution when driving or engaging in tasks requiring alertness until response to drug is known); decreased sexual ability (reversible); or nausea or vomiting (small, frequent meals or frequent mouth care may help). Report swelling of extremities, difficulty breathing, or new cough; weight gain (>3 lb/week); unresolved diarrhea or vomiting; or cold blue extremities. **Pregnancy/ breast-feeding precautions:** Inform prescriber if you are or intend to become pregnant. Consult prescriber if breast-feeding.

Ophthalmic: For ophthalmic use only. Apply prescribed amount as often as directed. Wash hands before using. Do not let tip of applicator touch eye; do not contaminate tip of applicator (may cause eye infection, eye damage, or vision loss). Tilt head back and look upward. Gently pull down lower lid and put drop(s) inside lower eyelid at inner corner. Close eye and roll eyeball in all directions. Do not blink for $^1/_2$ minute. Apply gentle pressure to inner corner of eye for 30 seconds. Wipe away excess from skin around eye. Do not use any other eye preparation for at least 10 minutes. Do not share medication with anyone else. Temporary stinging or blurred vision may occur. Immediately report any adverse cardiac or CNS effects (usually signifies overdose). Report persistent eye pain, redness, burning, watering, dryness, double vision, puffiness around eye, vision changes, other adverse eye response, worsening of condition or lack of improvement.

Dietary Issues: Oral product should be administered with food at the same time each day.

Geriatric Considerations: Due to alterations in the beta-adrenergic autonomic nervous system, beta-adrenergic blockade may result in less hemodynamic response than seen in younger adults.

Breast-feeding Issues: Timolol is excreted in breast milk and is considered compatible by the AAP. It is recommended that the infant be monitored for signs or symptoms of beta-blockade (hypotension, bradycardia, etc) with long-term use.

Related Information

Beta-Blockers *on page 1561*
Glaucoma Drug Comparison *on page 1575*

Timolol Hemihydrate *see* Timolol *on page 1322*
Timolol Maleate *see* Timolol *on page 1322*
Timoptic® *see* Ophthalmic Agents, Glaucoma *on page 1002*
Timoptic® *see* Timolol *on page 1322*
Timoptic® OcuDose® *see* Ophthalmic Agents, Glaucoma *on page 1002*
Timoptic® OcuDose® *see* Timolol *on page 1322*
Timoptic-XE® *see* Ophthalmic Agents, Glaucoma *on page 1002*
Timoptic-XE® *see* Timolol *on page 1322*

Tinzaparin (tin ZA pa rin)

U.S. Brand Names Innohep®

Synonyms Tinzaparin Sodium

Generic Available No

Pharmacologic Category Low Molecular Weight Heparin

Pregnancy Risk Factor B

Lactation Excretion in breast milk unknown/use caution

Use Treatment of acute symptomatic deep vein thrombosis, with or without pulmonary embolism, in conjunction with warfarin sodium

Mechanism of Action/Effect Standard heparin consists of components with molecular weights ranging from 4000-30,000 daltons with a mean of 16,000 daltons. Heparin acts as an anticoagulant by enhancing the inhibition rate of clotting proteases by antithrombin III, impairing normal hemostasis and inhibition of factor Xa. Low molecular weight heparins have a small effect on the activated partial thromboplastin time and strongly inhibit factor Xa. The primary inhibitory activity of tinzaparin is through antithrombin. Tinzaparin is derived from porcine heparin that undergoes controlled enzymatic depolymerization. The average molecular weight of tinzaparin ranges between 5500 and 7500 daltons which is distributed as (<10%) 2000 daltons (60% to 72%) 2000-8000 daltons, and (22% to 36%) >8000 daltons. The antifactor Xa activity is approximately 100 int. units/mg.

Contraindications Hypersensitivity to tinzaparin sodium, heparin, sulfites, benzyl alcohol, pork products, or any component of the formulation; active major bleeding; heparin-induced thrombocytopenia (current or history of)

Warnings/Precautions **Patients with recent or anticipated neuraxial anesthesia (epidural or spinal anesthesia) are at risk of spinal or epidural hematoma and subsequent paralysis.** Consider risk versus benefit prior to neuraxial anesthesia; risk is increased by concomitant agents which may alter hemostasis, as well as traumatic or repeated epidural or spinal puncture, and indwelling epidural catheters. Patient should be observed closely for signs and symptoms of neurological impairment. Not to be used interchangeably (unit for unit) with heparin or any other low molecular weight heparins. Monitor patient closely for signs or symptoms of bleeding. Certain patients are at increased risk of bleeding. Risk factors include bacterial endocarditis; congenital or acquired bleeding disorders; active ulcerative or angiodysplastic GI diseases; severe uncontrolled hypertension; hemorrhagic stroke; use shortly after brain, spinal, or ophthalmologic surgery; patients treated concomitantly with platelet inhibitors; recent GI bleeding; thrombocytopenia or platelet defects; severe liver disease; hypertensive or diabetic retinopathy; or in patients undergoing invasive procedures. Safety and efficacy in pediatric patients has not been established. Use with caution in the elderly (delayed elimination may occur). Heparin can cause hyperkalemia by affecting aldosterone; similar reactions could occur with LMWHs. Monitor for hyperkalemia. Discontinue therapy if platelets are <100,000/mm^3. For subcutaneous injection only, do not mix with other injections or infusions. Clinical experience is limited in patients with BMI >40 kg.

Drug Interactions

Increased Effect/Toxicity: Drugs which affect platelet function (eg, aspirin, NSAIDs, dipyridamole, ticlopidine, clopidogrel, sulfinpyrazone, dextran) may potentiate the risk of hemorrhage. Thrombolytic agents increase the risk of hemorrhage.

Warfarin: Risk of bleeding may be increased during concurrent therapy. Tinzaparin is commonly continued during the initiation of warfarin therapy to assure anticoagulation and to protect against possible transient hypercoagulability

Effects on Lab Values Asymptomatic increases in AST (SGOT) (8.8%) and ALT (SGPT) (13%) have been reported. Elevations were >3 times the upper limit of normal and were reversible and rarely associated with increases in bilirubin.

Adverse Reactions As with all anticoagulants, bleeding is the major adverse effect of tinzaparin. Hemorrhage may occur at virtually any site. Risk is dependent on multiple variables.

>10%:
- Hepatic: Increased ALT (13%)
- Local: Injection site hematoma (16%)

1% to 10%:
- Cardiovascular: Angina pectoris, chest pain (2%), hypertension, hypotension, tachycardia
- Central nervous system: Confusion, dizziness, fever (2%), headache (2%), insomnia, pain (2%)
- Dermatologic: Bullous eruption, pruritus, rash (1%), skin disorder
- Gastrointestinal: Constipation (1%), dyspepsia, flatulence, nausea (2%), nonspecified gastrointestinal disorder, vomiting (1%)
- Genitourinary: Dysuria, urinary retention, urinary tract infection (4%)
- Hematologic: Anemia, hematoma, hemorrhage (2%), thrombocytopenia (1%)
- Hepatic: Increased AST (9%)
- Local: Deep vein thrombosis, injection site hematoma
- Neuromuscular & skeletal: Back pain (2%)
- Renal: Hematuria (1%)
- Respiratory: Dyspnea (1%), epistaxis (2%), pneumonia, pulmonary embolism (2%), respiratory disorder
- Miscellaneous: Impaired healing, infection, unclassified reactions

<1% (Limited to important or life-threatening): Agranulocytosis, allergic purpura, allergic reaction, angioedema, arrhythmia, cholestatic hepatitis, epidermal necrolysis, gastrointestinal hemorrhage, granulocytopenia, hemarthrosis, hematoma, hemoptysis, intracranial hemorrhage, ischemic necrosis, major bleeding, myocardial infarction, ocular hemorrhage, pancytopenia, priapism, purpura, rash, retroperitoneal/intra-abdominal bleeding, severe thrombocytopenia, skin necrosis, spinal epidural hematoma, Stevens-Johnson syndrome, urticaria, vaginal hemorrhage

Postmarketing and/or case reports: The following adverse effects have been reported in infants of women receiving tinzaparin during pregnancy (relationship has not been established): Cleft palate (one report), optic nerve hypoplasia (one report), trisomy 21 (one report), fetal death/miscarriage, fetal distress, neonatal hypotonia, cutis aplasia of the scalp

Overdosage/Toxicology Overdose may lead to bleeding; bleeding may occur at any site. In case of overdose, discontinue medication, apply pressure to bleeding site if possible, and replace volume and hemostatic blood elements as required. If these measures are ineffective, or if bleeding is severe, protamine sulfate may be administered at 1 mg per every 100 anti-Xa int. units of tinzaparin.

Pharmacodynamics/Kinetics

Bioavailability: 87%

Half-Life Elimination: 3-4 hours

Time to Peak: 4-5 hours

Metabolism: Partially metabolized by desulphation and depolymerization

Onset: 2-3 hours

Formulations Injection: 20,000 anti-Xa int. units/mL (2 mL vial)

Dosing

Adults: Treatment of DVT: S.C.: 175 anti-Xa int. units/kg of body weight once daily. Warfarin sodium should be started when appropriate. Administer tinzaparin for at least 6 days and until patient is adequately anticoagulated with warfarin.

Note: To calculate the volume of solution to administer per dose: Volume to be administered (mL) = patient weight (kg) x 0.00875 mL/kg (may be rounded off to the nearest 0.05 mL)

Elderly: Refer to adult dosing. No significant differences in safety or response were seen when used in patients ≥65 years of age. However, increased sensitivity to tinzaparin in elderly patients may be possible due to a decline in renal function.

Renal Impairment: Patients with severe renal impairment had a 24% decrease in clearance, use with caution.

(Continued)

Tinzaparin *(Continued)*

Hepatic Impairment: No adjustment necessary.

Administration

I.V.: Patient should be lying down or sitting. Administer by deep S.C. injection, alternating between the left and right anterolateral and left and right posterolateral abdominal wall. Vary site daily. The entire needle should be introduced into the skin fold formed by the thumb and forefinger. Hold the skin fold until injection is complete. To minimize bruising, do not rub the injection site.

Stability

Storage: Store at 25°C (77°F). Excursions permitted to 15°C to 30°C (59°F to 86°F).

Monitoring Laboratory Tests CBC including platelet count and hematocrit or hemoglobin, and stool for occult blood; the monitoring of PT and/or PTT is not necessary. Patients receiving both warfarin and tinzaparin should have their INR drawn just prior to the next scheduled dose of tinzaparin.

Monitoring and Teaching Issues

Physical Assessment: See Contraindications, Warnings/Precautions, and Dosing for use cautions. Assess potential for interactions with other prescription and OTC medications or herbal products patient may be taking (especially anything that will impact coagulation or platelet aggregation - see Drug Interactions). Assess laboratory tests (see above), therapeutic effectiveness, and adverse response (eg, thrombolytic reactions - see Adverse Reactions and Overdose/Toxicology). Teach patient appropriate use (if self-administered, appropriate injection technique and syringe disposal), possible side effects and interventions (eg, bleeding precautions), and adverse symptoms to report (see Patient Education). Note breast-feeding caution.

Patient Education: Inform prescriber of all prescriptions, OTC medications, or herbal products you are taking, and any allergies you have. Do not take anything new during treatment unless approved by prescriber. This drug can only be administered by injection. Use exactly as directed (if self-administered, follow exact instructions for injection and syringe disposal). Do not alter dosage or discontinue without consulting prescriber. You may have a tendency to bleed easily while taking this drug (brush teeth with soft brush, use waxed dental floss, use electric razor, avoid scissors or sharp knives, and avoid potentially harmful activities). Report immediately any unusual bleeding or bruising (eg, mouth, nose, blood in urine or stool); chest pain or palpitations; confusion, dizziness, or headache; skin rash or itching; GI upset (eg, nausea, vomiting, abdominal pain, acute constipation); warmth, swelling, pain, or redness in calves or other areas; back or muscle pain; respiratory difficulties; or other persistent adverse reactions. **Breast-feeding precaution:** Consult prescriber if breast-feeding.

Pregnancy Issues: There are no adequate, well-controlled studies in pregnant women. Cases of teratogenic effects and/or fetal death have been reported (relationship to tinzaparin not established). Use during pregnancy only if clearly needed. Pregnant women, or those who become pregnant while receiving tinzaparin, should be informed of the potential risks to the fetus.

Additional Information Contains sodium metabisulfite and benzyl alcohol, 10 mg/mL

Related Information

Heparins *on page 1576*

Tinzaparin Sodium *see* Tinzaparin *on page 1324*

Tioconazole (tye oh KONE a zole)

U.S. Brand Names 1-Day™ [OTC]; Vagistat®-1 [OTC]

Generic Available No

Pharmacologic Category Antifungal Agent, Vaginal

Pregnancy Risk Factor C

Lactation Excretion in breast milk unknown/not recommended

Use Local treatment of vulvovaginal candidiasis

Mechanism of Action/Effect A 1-substituted imidazole derivative with a broad antifungal spectrum against a wide variety of dermatophytes and yeasts

Contraindications Hypersensitivity to tioconazole or any component of the formulation

Warnings/Precautions For vaginal use only. Petrolatum-based vaginal products may damage rubber or latex condoms or diaphragms. Separate use by 3 days. Pregnancy risk C.

Adverse Reactions Frequency not defined.

Central nervous system: Headache

Gastrointestinal: Abdominal pain

Dermatologic: Burning, desquamation

Genitourinary: Discharge, dyspareunia, dysuria, irritation, itching, nocturia, vaginal pain, vaginitis, vulvar swelling

Pharmacodynamics/Kinetics

Absorption: Intravaginal: Systemic (small amounts)

Onset: Some improvement: Within 24 hours; Complete relief: Within 7 days

Formulations Ointment, vaginal: 6.5% (4.6 g) [with applicator]

Dosing

Adults & Elderly: Vulvovaginal candidiasis: Vaginal: Insert 1 applicatorful in vagina, just prior to bedtime, as a single dose

Stability

Storage: Store at room temperature.

Monitoring and Teaching Issues

Physical Assessment: Assess knowledge/teach patient appropriate administration, possible side effects/interventions, and adverse symptoms to report (see Patient Education). **Pregnancy risk factor C** - 25% systemically absorbed. Breast-feeding is not recommended.

Patient Education: Consult with healthcare provider if treating a vaginal yeast infection for the first time. Insert high into the vagina. Refrain from intercourse during treatment. May interact with condoms and vaginal contraceptive diaphragms (ie, weaken latex); do not rely on these products for 3 days following treatment. Do not use tampons, douches, spermicides, or other vaginal products during treatment. Although product is used for a single day, relief from symptoms usually takes longer than 1 day. Report persistent (>3 days) vaginal burning, irritation, or discharge. **Breast-feeding precaution:** Breast-feeding is not recommended.

Tioguanine *see* Thioguanine *on page 1305*

Tiotixene *see* Thiothixene *on page 1311*

Tirofiban (tye roe FYE ban)

U.S. Brand Names Aggrastat®

Synonyms MK383; Tirofiban Hydrochloride

Generic Available No

Pharmacologic Category Antiplatelet Agent, Glycoprotein IIb/IIIa Inhibitor

Pregnancy Risk Factor B

Lactation Excretion in breast milk unknown/contraindicated

Use In combination with heparin, is indicated for the treatment of acute coronary syndrome, including patients who are to be managed medically and those undergoing PTCA or atherectomy. In this setting, it has been shown to decrease the rate of a combined endpoint of death, new myocardial infarction or refractory ischemia/repeat cardiac procedure.

Mechanism of Action/Effect A reversible antagonist of fibrinogen binding to the GP IIb/IIIa receptor, the major platelet surface receptor involved in platelet aggregation. Platelet aggregation inhibition is reversible following cessation of the infusion.

Contraindications Hypersensitivity to tirofiban or any component of the formulation; active internal bleeding or a history of bleeding diathesis within the previous 30 days; history of intracranial hemorrhage, intracranial neoplasm, arteriovenous malformation, or aneurysm; history of thrombocytopenia following prior exposure; history of CVA within 30 days or any history of hemorrhagic stroke; major surgical procedure or severe physical trauma within the previous month; history, symptoms, or findings suggestive of aortic dissection; severe hypertension (systolic BP >180 mm Hg and/or diastolic BP >110 mm Hg); concomitant use of another parenteral GP IIb/IIIa inhibitor; acute pericarditis

Warnings/Precautions Bleeding is the most common complication. Watch closely for bleeding, especially the arterial access site for the cardiac catheterization. Prior to pulling the sheath, heparin should be discontinued for 3-4 hours and ACT <180 seconds or APTT <45 seconds. Use standard compression techniques after sheath removal. Watch the site closely afterwards for further bleeding. Use with extreme caution in patients with platelet counts <150,000/mm^3, patients with hemorrhagic retinopathy, and chronic dialysis patients. Use caution with administration of other drugs affecting hemostasis. Adjust the dose with severe renal dysfunction (Cl_{cr} <30 mL/minute). The use of tirofiban, aspirin and heparin together causes more bleeding than aspirin and heparin alone.

Drug Interactions

Decreased Effect: Levothyroxine and omeprazole decrease tirofiban levels; however, the clinical significance of this interaction remains to be demonstrated.

Increased Effect/Toxicity: Use of tirofiban with aspirin and heparin is associated with an increase in bleeding over aspirin and heparin alone; however, efficacy of tirofiban is improved. Risk of bleeding is increased when used with thrombolytics, oral anticoagulants, NSAIDs, dipyridamole, ticlopidine, and clopidogrel. Avoid concomitant use of other IIb/IIIa antagonists. Cephalosporins which contain the MTT side chain may theoretically increase the risk of hemorrhage.

Adverse Reactions Bleeding is the major drug-related adverse effect. Patients received background treatment with aspirin and heparin. Major bleeding was reported in 1.4% to 2.2%; minor bleeding in 10.5% to 12%; transfusion was required in 4% to 4.3%.

>1% (nonbleeding adverse events):

Cardiovascular: Bradycardia (4%), coronary artery dissection (5%), edema (2%)

Central nervous system: Dizziness (3%), fever (>1%), headache (>1%), vasovagal reaction (2%)

Gastrointestinal: Nausea (>1%)

Genitourinary: Pelvic pain (6%)

Hematologic: Thrombocytopenia: <90,000/mm^3 (1.5%), <50,000/mm^3 (0.3%)

Neuromuscular & skeletal: Leg pain (3%)

Miscellaneous: Diaphoresis (2%)

<1% (Limited to important or life-threatening): Acutely decreased platelets in association with fever, anaphylaxis, GI bleeding (0.1% to 0.2%), GU bleeding (up to 0.1%), hemopericardium, intracranial bleeding (up to 0.1%), pulmonary alveolar hemorrhage, rash, retroperitoneal bleeding (up to 0.6%), severe (<10,000/mm^3) thrombocytopenia (rare), spinal-epidural hematoma

Overdosage/Toxicology The most frequent manifestation of overdose is bleeding. Treatment is cessation of therapy and assessment of transfusion. Tirofiban is dialyzable.

Pharmacodynamics/Kinetics

Half-Life Elimination: 2 hours

Metabolism: Minimally hepatic

Formulations

Injection [premixed] 50 mcg/mL (500 mL)

Injection, solution: 250 mcg/mL (50 mL)

Dosing

Adults & Elderly: Acute coronary syndromes: I.V.: Initial rate of 0.4 mcg/kg/minute for 30 minutes and then continued at 0.1 mcg/kg/minute. Dosing should be continued through angiography and for 12-24 hours after angioplasty or atherectomy.

(Continued)

Tirofiban *(Continued)*

Renal Impairment: Cl_{cr} <30 mL/minute: Reduce dose to 50% of normal rate.

Administration

I.V.: Infuse over 30 minutes. Tirofiban injection must be diluted to a concentration of 50 mcg/mL (premixed solution does not require dilution). Unused solution should be discarded. Do not administer via the same IV line as diazepam.

Stability

Storage: Store at 25°C (77°F); do not freeze. Protect from light during storage.

Compatibility: Stable in $D_5{}^1/_2NS$, D_5W, NS

Y-site administration: Incompatible with diazepam

Monitoring Laboratory Tests Platelet count, persistent reductions <90,000/mm^3 may require interruption or discontinuation of infusion. Hemoglobin and hematocrit should be monitored prior to treatment, within 6 hours following loading infusion, and at least daily thereafter during therapy. Platelet count may need to be monitored earlier in patients who received prior glycoprotein IIb/IIa antagonists. Because tirofiban requires concurrent heparin therapy, aPTT levels should also be followed.

Monitoring and Teaching Issues

Physical Assessment: Monitor vital signs and laboratory results prior to, during, and after therapy. Assess infusion insertion site during and after therapy. Observe and teach bleeding precautions. Monitor closely for signs of unusual or excessive bleeding. Breast-feeding is contraindicated.

Patient Education: Emergency use may dictate depth of patient education. This medication can only be administered I.V. You will have a tendency to bleed easily following this medication. Use caution to prevent injury (use electric razor, use soft toothbrush, use caution with sharps). If bleeding occurs, apply pressure to bleeding spot until bleeding stops completely. Report unusual bruising or bleeding (eg, blood in urine, stool, or vomitus, bleeding gums, vaginal bleeding, nosebleeds); unusual and persistent fever; dizziness or vision changes; back, leg, or pelvic pain; or persistent nausea or vomiting. **Breast-feeding precaution:** Do not breast-feed.

Tirofiban Hydrochloride *see* Tirofiban *on page 1327*

Tizanidine (tye ZAN i deen)

U.S. Brand Names Zanaflex®

Synonyms Sirdalud®

Generic Available Yes

Pharmacologic Category Alpha$_2$-Adrenergic Agonist

Pregnancy Risk Factor C

Lactation Excretion in breast milk unknown/not recommended

Use Skeletal muscle relaxant used for treatment of muscle spasticity

Use - Unlabeled/Investigational Tension headaches, low back pain, and trigeminal neuralgia

Contraindications Hypersensitivity to tizanidine or any component of the formulation

Warnings/Precautions Reduce dose in patients with liver or renal disease; use with caution in patients with hypotension or cardiac disease. Tizanidine clearance is reduced by more than 50% in elderly patients with renal insufficiency (Cl_{cr} <25 mL/minute) compared to healthy elderly subjects; this may lead to a longer duration of effects and, therefore, should be used with caution in renally impaired patients. Pregnancy risk C.

Drug Interactions

Increased Effect/Toxicity:

Increased effect: Oral contraceptives

Increased toxicity: Additive hypotensive effects may be seen with diuretics, other alpha adrenergic agonists, or antihypertensives; CNS depression with alcohol, baclofen or other CNS depressants

Nutritional/Ethanol Interactions

Ethanol: Avoid ethanol (may increase CNS depression).

Food: Increases maximum concentration of tizanidine by 33% and reduces the time to peak by 40 minutes; extent of absorption is unchanged.

Herb/Nutraceutical: Avoid valerian, St John's wort, kava kava, gotu kola (may increase CNS depression).

Adverse Reactions

>10%:

Cardiovascular: Hypotension

Central nervous system: Sedation, daytime drowsiness, somnolence

Gastrointestinal: Xerostomia

1% to 10%:

Cardiovascular: Bradycardia, syncope

Central nervous system: Fatigue, dizziness, anxiety, nervousness, insomnia

Dermatologic: Pruritus, skin rash

Gastrointestinal: Nausea, vomiting, dyspepsia, constipation, diarrhea

Hepatic: Elevation of liver enzymes

Neuromuscular & skeletal: Muscle weakness, tremor

<1% (Limited to important or life-threatening): Delusions, hepatic failure, palpitations, psychotic-like symptoms, ventricular extrasystoles, visual hallucinations

Overdosage/Toxicology

Symptoms of overdose include dry mouth, bradycardia, hypotension

Treatment: Lavage (within 2 hours of ingestion) with activated charcoal; benzodiazepines for seizure control; atropine can be given for treatment of bradycardia; flumazenil has been used to reverse coma successfully; forced diuresis is not helpful; multiple dosing of activated charcoal may be helpful. Following attempts to enhance drug elimination, hypotension should be treated with I.V. fluids and/or Trendelenburg positioning.

Pharmacodynamics/Kinetics

Bioavailability: 40%

Half-Life Elimination: 2.5 hours

Time to Peak: Serum: 1-5 hours

Duration: 3-6 hours

Formulations Tablet: 2 mg, 4 mg

Dosing

Adults & Elderly:

Spasticity: Usual initial dose: 4 mg, may increase by 2-4 mg as needed for satisfactory reduction of muscle tone every 6-8 hours to a maximum of three doses in any 24 hour period

Range: 2-4 mg 3 times/day

Maximum dose: 36 mg/day

Renal Impairment: May require dose reductions or less frequent dosing

Hepatic Impairment: May require dose reductions or less frequent dosing.

Monitoring and Teaching Issues

Physical Assessment: See Contraindications, Warnings/Precautions, and Dosing for use cautions. Assess potential for interactions with other prescriptions, OTC medications, or herbal products patient may be taking (see Drug Interactions). Assess results of laboratory tests (see above), therapeutic response, and adverse reactions (see Adverse Reactions and Overdose/Toxicology) on a regular basis throughout therapy. Teach patient proper use, possible side effects and interventions, and adverse symptoms to report (see Patient Education). **Pregnancy risk factor C** - benefits of use should outweigh possible risks. Breast-feeding is not recommended.

Patient Education: Inform prescriber of all prescriptions, OTC medications, or herbal products you are taking (especially anything that may cause drowsiness), and any allergies you have. Take exactly as directed; do not change dosage or discontinue without consulting prescriber. If you miss a dose, take the missed dose as soon as possible if it is within an hour or so of the regular time. If not within an hour or so, skip the missed dose and go back to your regular dosing schedule. Do not double doses. Avoid alcohol. May cause dizziness, nervousness, insomnia, or daytime drowsiness (use caution when driving or engaging in tasks that require alertness until response to drug is known); postural hypotension (use caution and avoid quick moves when rising from sitting or lying position, climbing stairs, or engaging in activities that require quick movements); or nausea, vomiting, dry mouth, mouth sores, or upset stomach (small, frequent meals, frequent mouth care, chewing gum, or sucking lozenges may help). Report persistent dizziness or GI symptoms; chest pain or palpitations; CNS disturbances (delusions, confusion); muscle weakness or tremors; rash; difficulty breathing; or other persistent adverse effects. **Pregnancy/breast-feeding precautions:** Inform prescriber if you are or intend to become pregnant. Breast-feeding is not recommended.

TMP *see* Trimethoprim *on page 1366*

TMP-SMZ *see* Sulfamethoxazole and Trimethoprim *on page 1259*

TNKase™ *see* Tenecteplase *on page 1284*

TOBI™ *see* Tobramycin *on page 1329*

TobraDex® *see page 1509*

Tobramycin (toe bra MYE sin)

U.S. Brand Names AKTob®; Nebcin®; TOBI™; Tobrex®

Synonyms Tobramycin Sulfate

Generic Available Yes

Pharmacologic Category Antibiotic, Aminoglycoside; Antibiotic, Ophthalmic

Pregnancy Risk Factor C

Lactation Enters breast milk/compatible

Use Treatment of documented or suspected infections caused by susceptible gram-negative bacilli including *Pseudomonas aeruginosa*; topically used to treat superficial ophthalmic infections caused by susceptible bacteria. Tobramycin solution for inhalation is indicated for the management of cystic fibrosis patients (>6 years of age) with *Pseudomonas aeruginosa*.

Mechanism of Action/Effect Interferes with bacterial protein synthesis by binding to 30S and 50S ribosomal subunits resulting in a defective bacterial cell membrane

Contraindications Hypersensitivity to tobramycin, other aminoglycosides, or any component of the formulation

Warnings/Precautions Use with caution in patients with renal impairment, pre-existing auditory or vestibular impairment, and in patients with neuromuscular disorders. Dosage modification required in patients with impaired renal function (I.M. & I.V.). Aminoglycosides are associated with significant nephrotoxicity or ototoxicity; the ototoxicity is directly proportional to the amount of drug given and the duration of treatment. Tinnitus or vertigo are indications of vestibular injury. Ototoxicity is often irreversible, while renal damage is usually reversible. Pregnancy risk C.

Drug Interactions

Increased Effect/Toxicity: Increased antimicrobial effect of tobramycin with extended spectrum penicillins (synergistic). Neuromuscular blockers may have an increased duration of action (neuromuscular blockade). Amphotericin B, cephalosporins, and loop diuretics may increase the risk of nephrotoxicity.

Effects on Lab Values ↑ protein, BUN, aminotransferase [AST (SGOT)/ALT (SGPT)] (S), alkaline phosphatase, creatinine; ↓ magnesium, potassium, sodium, calcium (S)

Adverse Reactions

1% to 10%:

Neuromuscular & skeletal: Neurotoxicity (neuromuscular blockade)

Otic: Ototoxicity (auditory), ototoxicity (vestibular)

Renal: Nephrotoxicity

<1% (Limited to important or life-threatening): Anemia, dyspnea, eosinophilia

(Continued)

Tobramycin *(Continued)*

Overdosage/Toxicology Symptoms of overdose include ototoxicity, nephrotoxicity, and neuromuscular toxicity. Treatment of choice following a single acute overdose appears to be maintenance of urine output of at least 3 mL/kg/hour during the acute treatment phase. Dialysis is of questionable value in enhancing aminoglycoside elimination. If required, hemodialysis is preferred over peritoneal dialysis in patients with normal renal function. Chelation with penicillins is investigational.

Pharmacodynamics/Kinetics

Absorption: I.M.: Rapid and complete

Half-Life Elimination:

Neonates: ≤1200 g: 11 hours; >1200 g: 2-9 hours

Adults: 2-3 hours; directly dependent upon glomerular filtration rate

Adults with impaired renal function: 5-70 hours

Time to Peak: Serum: I.M.: 30-60 minutes; I.V.: ~30 minutes

Formulations

Injection, as sulfate (Nebcin®): 10 mg/mL (2 mL, 6 mL, 8 mL); 40 mg/mL (1 mL, 2 mL, 30 mL, 50 mL)

Injection, powder for reconstitution (Nebcin®): 40 mg/mL (1.2 g vials)

Ointment, ophthalmic (Tobrex®): 0.3% (3.5 g)

Solution for nebulization (TOBI™): 60 mg/mL (5 mL)

Solution, ophthalmic: 0.3% (5 mL)

AKTob®, Tobrex®: 0.3% (5 mL)

Dosing

Adults: Note: Individualization is critical because of the low therapeutic index.

Use of ideal body weight (IBW) for determining the mg/kg/dose appears to be more accurate than dosing on the basis of total body weight (TBW)

In morbid obesity, dosage requirement may best be estimated using a dosing weight of IBW + 0.4 (TBW - IBW)

Initial and periodic peak and trough plasma drug levels should be determined, particularly in critically ill patients with serious infections or in disease states known to significantly alter aminoglycoside pharmacokinetics (eg, cystic fibrosis, burns, or major surgery). Two to three serum level measurements should be obtained after the initial dose to measure the half-life in order to determine the frequency of subsequent doses.

Severe life-threatening infections: I.M., I.V.: 2-2.5 mg/kg/dose

Urinary tract infection: I.M., I.V.: 1.5 mg/kg/dose

Synergy (for gram-positive infections): I.M., I.V.: 1 mg/kg/dose

Ocular infection: Ophthalmic: Instill 1-2 drops of solution every 4 hours; apply ointment 2-3 times/day; for severe infections apply ointment every 3-4 hours, or solution 2 drops every 30-60 minutes initially, then reduce to less frequent intervals

Inhalation: Aerosol:

Standard aerosolized tobramycin: 60-80 mg 3 times/day

High-dose regimen (TOBI™): Adults with cystic fibrosis and *Pseudomonas aeruginosa*: 300 mg every 12 hours (do not administer doses <6 hours apart); administer in repeated cycles of 28 days on drug followed by 28 days off drug

Some clinicians suggest a daily dose of 4-7 mg/kg for all patients with normal renal function. This dose is at least as efficacious with similar, if not less, toxicity than conventional dosing

Elderly: Dosage should be based on an estimate of ideal body weight.

I.M., I.V.: 1.5-5 mg/kg/day in 1-2 divided doses

I.V.: Once daily or extended interval: 5-7 mg/kg/dose given every 24, 36, or 48 hours based on Cl_{cr} (see Renal Impairment and Geriatric Considerations).

Pediatrics: Individualization is critical because of the low therapeutic index

Susceptible infections:

Infants and Children <5 years: I.M., I.V.: 2.5 mg/kg/dose every 8 hours

Children >5 years: 1.5-2.5 mg/kg/dose every 8 hours

Note: Some patients may require larger or more frequent doses if serum levels document the need (ie, cystic fibrosis or febrile granulocytopenic patients).

Ocular infection: Ophthalmic: Children: Refer to adult dosing.

Inhalation: Aerosol:

Standard aerosolized tobramycin: Children: 40-80 mg 2-3 times/day

High-dose regimen (TOBI™): Children ≥6 years with cystic fibrosis and *Pseudomonas aeruginosa* infection: 300 mg every 12 hours (do not administer doses less than 6 hours apart); administer in repeated cycles of 28 days on drug followed by 28 days off drug.

Renal Impairment:

Cl_{cr} ≥60 mL/minute: Administer every 8 hours.

Cl_{cr} 40-60 mL/minute: Administer every 12 hours.

Cl_{cr} 20-40 mL/minute: Administer every 24 hours.

Cl_{cr} 10-20 mL/minute: Administer every 48 hours.

Cl_{cr} <10 mL/minute: Administer every 72 hours.

Dialyzable; 30% removal of aminoglycosides occurs during 4 hours of HD - administer dose after dialysis and follow levels.

Continuous arteriovenous or venovenous hemofiltration: Dose as for Cl_{cr} of 10-40 mL/minute and follow levels.

Administration via CAPD fluid:

Gram-negative infection: 4-8 mg/L (4-8 mcg/mL) of CAPD fluid

Gram-positive infection (ie, synergy): 3-4 mg/L (3-4 mcg/mL) of CAPD fluid

Administration IVPB/I.M.: Dose as for Cl_{cr} <10 mL/minute and follow levels.

Hepatic Impairment: Monitor plasma concentrations.

Administration

I.V.: Infuse over 30-60 minutes. Give penicillins or cephalosporins at least 1 hour apart from tobramycin.

Topical: Eye solutions: Allow 5 minutes between application of "multiple-drop" therapy.

Stability

Storage: Tobramycin is stable at room temperature both as the clear, colorless solution and as the dry powder. Reconstituted solutions remain stable for 24 hours at room temperature and 96 hours when refrigerated.

Reconstitution: Stability of parenteral admixture at room temperature (25°C) and at refrigeration temperature (4°C) is 48 hours.

Standard diluent: Dose/100 mL NS
Minimum volume: 50 mL NS

Compatibility: Stable in dextran 40 10% in dextrose, D_5NS, D_5W, $D_{10}W$, mannitol 20%, LR, NS

Y-site administration: Incompatible with allopurinol, amphotericin B cholesteryl sulfate complex, cefoperazone, heparin, hetastarch, indomethacin, propofol, sargramostim

Compatibility in syringe: Incompatible with cefamandole, clindamycin, heparin

Compatibility when admixed: Incompatible with cefamandole, cefepime, cefotaxime, cefotetan, floxacillin, heparin, penicillins

Monitoring Laboratory Tests Urinalysis, BUN, serum creatinine, peak and trough plasma tobramycin levels. Obtain drug levels after the third dose. Peak levels are drawn 30 minutes after the end of a 30-minute infusion or 1 hour after initiation of infusion or I.M. injection. The trough is drawn just before the next dose. Perform culture and sensitivity studies prior to initiating therapy to determine the causative organism and its susceptibility to tobramycin.

Monitoring and Teaching Issues

Physical Assessment: Assess effectiveness and interactions of other medications patient may be taking (see Contraindications and Drug Interactions). Assess patient's hearing level before, during, and following therapy. Monitor therapeutic response, laboratory values (see above), and adverse reactions (see Warnings/Precautions, Adverse Reactions, and Overdose/Toxicology) at beginning of therapy and periodically throughout therapy. Assess knowledge/ teach patient appropriate use, interventions to reduce side effects, and adverse symptoms to report (see Patient Education). **Pregnancy risk factor C** - benefits of use should outweigh possible risks.

Patient Education: Systemic: Maintain adequate hydration (2-3 L/day of fluids) unless advised by prescriber to restrict fluids. Report decreased urine output, swelling of extremities, difficulty breathing, vaginal itching or discharge, rash, diarrhea, oral thrush, unhealed wounds, dizziness, change in hearing acuity or ringing in ears, or worsening of condition. **Pregnancy precaution:** Inform prescriber if you are pregnant.

Ophthalmic: Use as frequently as recommended; do not overuse. Do not let tip of applicator touch eye; do not contaminate tip of applicator (may cause eye infection, eye damage, or vision loss). Sit down, tilt head back, instill solution or drops inside lower eyelid, and roll eyeball in all directions. Close eye and apply gentle pressure to inner corner of eye for 30 seconds. May experience temporary stinging or blurred vision. Do not use any other eye preparation for 10 minutes. Inform prescriber if condition worsens or does not improve in 3-4 days.

Dietary Issues: May require supplementation of calcium, magnesium, potassium.

Geriatric Considerations: Aminoglycosides are important therapeutic interventions for susceptible organisms and as empiric therapy in seriously ill patients. Their use is not without risk of toxicity; however, these risks can be minimized if initial dosing is adjusted for estimated renal function and appropriate monitoring is performed. High-dose, once-daily aminoglycosides have been advocated as an alternative to traditional dosing regimens. To date, there is little information on the safety and efficacy of these regimens in persons with a creatinine clearance <60 mL/minute/70 kg. A dosing nomogram based upon creatinine clearance has been proposed. Additional studies comparing high-dose, once-daily aminoglycosides to traditional dosing regimens in the elderly are needed before once-daily aminoglycoside dosing can be routinely adopted to this patient population.

Breast-feeding Issues: Tobramycin is not absorbed orally, so any drug in breast milk is not available to the infant.

Related Information

Ophthalmic Agents *on page 1509*
Peak and Trough Guidelines *on page 1544*

Tobramycin and Dexamethasone *see page 1509*

Tobramycin Sulfate *see* Tobramycin *on page 1329*

Tobrex® *see page 1509*

Tobrex® *see* Tobramycin *on page 1329*

Tofranil® *see* Imipramine *on page 700*

Tofranil-PM® *see* Imipramine *on page 700*

Tolazamide *see page 1661*

Tolcapone (TOLE ka pone)

U.S. Brand Names Tasmar®

Generic Available No

Pharmacologic Category Anti-Parkinson's Agent, COMT Inhibitor

Pregnancy Risk Factor C

Lactation Excretion in breast milk unknown/contraindicated

Use Adjunct to levodopa and carbidopa for the treatment of signs and symptoms of idiopathic Parkinson's disease

Mechanism of Action/Effect Tolcapone is a selective and reversible inhibitor of catechol-o-methyltransferase (COMT)

Contraindications Hypersensitivity to tolcapone or any component of the formulation

(Continued)

Tolcapone *(Continued)*

Warnings/Precautions Due to reports of fatal liver injury, reserve for use only in patients who do not have severe movement abnormalities and who do not respond to or who are not appropriate candidates for other available treatments. Use with caution in patients with pre-existing dyskinesias, hepatic impairment, or severe renal impairment. May cause/exacerbate orthostatic hypotension (common in Parkinson's disease) use caution in patients at risk or where transient hypotensive episodes would be poorly tolerated. Monitor carefully for signs and symptoms of postural hypotension, especially during dose escalation, and inform patient of this risk. May cause hallucinations, which may improve with reduction in levodopa therapy. Use with caution in patients with lower gastrointestinal disease or an increased risk of dehydration - tolcapone has been associated with delayed development of diarrhea (onset after 2-12 weeks).

It is not recommended that patients receive tolcapone concomitantly with nonselective MAO inhibitors (see Drug Interactions). Selegiline is a selective MAO type B inhibitor and can be taken with tolcapone.

Although not reported for tolcapone, other dopaminergic agents have been associated with a syndrome resembling neuroleptic malignant syndrome on withdrawal or significant dosage reduction after long-term use. Dopaminergic agents from the ergot class have also been associated with fibrotic complications, such as retroperitoneum, lungs, and pleura.

Pregnancy risk C.

Drug Interactions

Cytochrome P450 Effect: Inhibits CYP2C8/9

Increased Effect/Toxicity: Tolcapone may increase the effect/levels of methyldopa, dobutamine, apomorphine, and isoproterenol due to inhibition of catechol-O-methyl transferase enzymes (COMT).

Nutritional/Ethanol Interactions

Ethanol: Avoid ethanol (may increase CNS depression).

Food: Tolcapone, taken with food within 1 hour before or 2 hours after the dose, decreases bioavailability by 10% to 20%.

Avoid valerian, St John's wort, kava kava, gotu kola (may increase CNS depression).

Adverse Reactions

>10%:

Cardiovascular: Orthostatic hypotension
Central nervous system: Sleep disorder, excessive dreaming, somnolence, headache
Gastrointestinal: Nausea, diarrhea, anorexia
Neuromuscular & skeletal: Dyskinesia, dystonia, muscle cramps

1% to 10%:

Central nervous system: Hallucinations, fatigue, loss of balance, hyperkinesia
Gastrointestinal: Vomiting, constipation, xerostomia, abdominal pain, flatulence, dyspepsia
Genitourinary: Urine discoloration
Neuromuscular & skeletal: Paresthesia, stiffness
Miscellaneous: Diaphoresis (increased)

Pharmacodynamics/Kinetics

Absorption: Rapid

Bioavailability: 65%

Half-Life Elimination: 2-3 hours

Time to Peak: ~2 hours

Metabolism: Glucuronidation

Formulations Tablet: 100 mg, 200 mg

Dosing

Adults & Elderly: Parkinson's disease: Oral: Initial: 100-200 mg 3 times/day; levodopa therapy may need to be decreased upon initiation of tolcapone.

Monitoring and Teaching Issues

Physical Assessment: Assess effectiveness and interactions of other medications patient may be taking (see Contraindications and Drug Interactions). Monitor therapeutic response (eg, mental status, involuntary movements) and adverse reactions at beginning of therapy and periodically throughout therapy (see Warnings/Precautions, Adverse Reactions, and Overdose/Toxicology). Assess knowledge/teach patient appropriate use, interventions to reduce side effects, and adverse symptoms to report (see Patient Education). **Pregnancy risk factor C** - benefits of use should outweigh possible risks. Breast-feeding is contraindicated.

Patient Education: Take exactly as directed (may be prescribed in conjunction with levodopa/carbidopa); do not change dosage or discontinue without consulting prescriber. Therapeutic effects may take several weeks or months to achieve and you may need frequent monitoring during first weeks of therapy. Best to take 2 hours before or after a meal; however, may be taken with meals if GI upset occurs. Take at the same time each day. Maintain adequate hydration (2-3 L/day of fluids) unless advised by prescriber to restrict fluids. Do not use alcohol and prescription or OTC sedatives or CNS depressants without consulting prescriber. Urine or perspiration may appear darker. You may experience drowsiness, dizziness, confusion, or vision changes (use caution when driving, climbing stairs, or engaging in tasks requiring alertness until response to drug is known); orthostatic hypotension (use caution when changing position - rising to standing from sitting or lying); increased susceptibility to heat stroke, decreased perspiration (use caution in hot weather - maintain adequate fluids and reduce exercise activity); constipation (increased exercise, fluids, or fruit, or fiber may help); dry skin or nasal passages (consult prescriber for appropriate relief); or nausea, vomiting, loss of appetite, or stomach discomfort (small, frequent meals, frequent mouth care, chewing gum, or sucking lozenges may help). Report unresolved constipation or vomiting; chest pain or irregular heartbeat; difficulty breathing; acute headache or dizziness; CNS changes (hallucination, loss of memory, nervousness, etc); painful or difficult urination; abdominal pain or blood in stool; increased muscle spasticity, rigidity, or involuntary movements; skin rash; or significant worsening of condition. **Pregnancy/breast-feeding precautions:** Inform prescriber if you are or intend to become pregnant. Do not breast-feed.

Tolterodine (tole TER oh dine)

U.S. Brand Names Detrol™; Detrol® LA

Synonyms Tolterodine Tartrate

Generic Available No

Pharmacologic Category Anticholinergic Agent

Pregnancy Risk Factor C

Lactation Excretion in breast milk unknown/not recommended

Use Treatment of patients with an overactive bladder with symptoms of urinary frequency, urgency, or urge incontinence

Mechanism of Action/Effect Tolterodine is a competitive antagonist of muscarinic receptors. In animal models, tolterodine demonstrates selectivity for urinary bladder receptors over salivary receptors. Urinary bladder contraction is mediated by muscarinic receptors. Tolterodine increases residual urine volume and decreases detrusor muscle pressure.

Contraindications Hypersensitivity to tolterodine or any component of the formulation; urinary retention, gastric retention, or uncontrolled narrow-angle glaucoma

Warnings/Precautions Use with caution in patients with bladder flow obstruction, may increase the risk of urinary retention. Use with caution in patients with gastrointestinal obstructive disorders (ie pyloric stenosis), may increase the risk of gastric retention. Use with caution in patients with controlled (treated) narrow-angle glaucoma; metabolized in the liver and excreted in the urine and feces, dosage adjustment is required for patients with renal or hepatic impairment. Patients on CYP3A4 inhibitors require lower dose. Safety and efficacy in pediatric patients have not been established. Pregnancy risk C.

Drug Interactions

Cytochrome P450 Effect: Substrate of CYP2C8/9, 2C19, **2D6, 3A4**

Increased Effect/Toxicity:

Serum levels and/or toxicity of tolterodine may be increased by drugs which inhibit CYP2D6; effect was seen with fluoxetine. Inhibitors include amiodarone, cimetidine, delavirdine, paroxetine, propafenone, quinidine, and ritonavir. No dosage adjustment was needed in patients coadministered tolterodine and fluoxetine.

Serum level and/or toxicity of tolterodine may be increased by drugs which inhibit CYP3A4, particularly in patients who are poor metabolizers via CYP2D6; effect was seen with ketoconazole. Other inhibitors include amiodarone, cimetidine, clarithromycin, cyclosporine, erythromycin, delavirdine, diltiazem, dirithromycin, disulfiram, fluoxetine, fluvoxamine, grapefruit juice, indinavir, itraconazole, nefazodone, nevirapine, propoxyphene, quinupristin-dalfopristin, ritonavir, saquinavir, verapamil, vinblastine, zafirlukast, zileuton.

Nutritional/Ethanol Interactions

Food: Increases bioavailability (~53% increase) of tolterodine tablets, but does not affect the pharmacokinetics of tolterodine extended release capsules; adjustment of dose is not needed. As a CYP3A4 inhibitor, grapefruit juice may increase the serum level and/or toxicity of tolterodine, but unlikely secondary to high oral bioavailability.

Herb/Nutraceutical: St John's wort (*Hypericum*) appears to induce CYP3A enzymes.

Adverse Reactions As reported with immediate release tablet, unless otherwise specified

>10%: Gastrointestinal: Dry mouth (35%; extended release capsules 23%)

1% to 10%:

Cardiovascular: Chest pain (2%)

Central nervous system: Headache (7%; extended release capsules 6%), somnolence (3%; extended release capsules 3%), fatigue (4%; extended release capsules 2%), dizziness (5%; extended release capsules 2%), anxiety (extended release capsules 1%)

Dermatologic: Dry skin (1%)

Gastrointestinal: Abdominal pain (5%; extended release capsules 4%), constipation (7%; extended release capsules 6%), dyspepsia (4%; extended release capsules 3%), diarrhea (4%), weight gain (1%)

Genitourinary: Dysuria (2%; extended release capsules 1%)

Neuromuscular & skeletal: Arthralgia (2%)

Ocular: Abnormal vision (2%; extended release capsules 1%), dry eyes (3%; extended release capsules 3%)

Respiratory: Bronchitis (2%), sinusitis (extended release capsules 2%)

<1% (Limited to important or life-threatening): Anaphylactoid reactions, peripheral edema, tachycardia

Overdosage/Toxicology Overdosage with tolterodine can potentially result in severe central anticholinergic effects and should be treated accordingly. EKG monitoring is recommended in the event of overdosage.

Pharmacodynamics/Kinetics

Absorption: Immediate release tablet: Rapid

Bioavailability: Immediate release tablet: 77%; increased with food

Half-Life Elimination:

Immediate release tablet: Extensive metabolizers: ~2 hours; Poor metabolizers: ~10 hours

Extended release capsule: Extensive metabolizers: ~7 hours; Poor metabolizers: ~18 hours

Time to Peak: Immediate release tablet: 1-2 hours; Extended release tablet: 2-6 hours

Metabolism: Extensively hepatic, primarily via CYP2D6 (some metabolites share activity) and 3A4 usually (minor pathway). In patients with a genetic deficiency of CYP2D6, metabolism via 3A4 predominates. Forms three active metabolites.

Formulations

Capsule, extended release, as tartrate: 2 mg, 4 mg

Tablet, as tartrate: 1 mg, 2 mg

(Continued)

Tolterodine *(Continued)*

Dosing

Adults & Elderly: Treatment of overactive bladder: Oral:

Immediate release tablet: 2 mg twice daily; the dose may be lowered to 1 mg twice daily based on individual response and tolerability

Dosing adjustment in patients concurrently taking CYP3A4 inhibitors: 1 mg twice daily

Extended release capsule: 4 mg once a day; dose may be lowered to 2 mg daily based on individual response and tolerability

Dosing adjustment in patients concurrently taking CYP3A4 inhibitors: 2 mg daily

Pediatrics: Safety and efficacy in pediatric patients have not been established

Renal Impairment: Use with caution (studies conducted in patients with Cl_{cr} 10-30 mL/minute):

Immediate release tablet: 1 mg twice daily

Extended release capsule: 2 mg daily

Hepatic Impairment:

Immediate release tablet: 1 mg twice daily

Extended release capsule: 2 mg daily

Stability

Storage: Store at room temperature, protect from light

Monitoring and Teaching Issues

Physical Assessment: See Contraindications (eg, patient's ability to void), Warnings/Precautions, and Dosing for use cautions. Assess potential for interactions with other prescriptions, OTC medications, or herbal products patient may be taking (eg, ergot-containing drugs - see Drug Interactions). Assess therapeutic effectiveness and adverse reactions (see Adverse Reactions and Overdose/Toxicology). Teach patient appropriate use (according to formulation and purpose), interventions to reduce side effects, and adverse symptoms to report (see Patient Education). **Pregnancy risk factor C** - benefits of use should outweigh risks. Breast-feeding is not recommended.

Patient Education: Inform prescriber of all prescription (including oral contraceptives) and OTC medications or herbal products you are taking, and any allergies you have. Take as directed, preferably with food. Do not break, crush, or chew extended release medication. May cause headache (consult prescriber for a mild analgesic); dizziness, nervousness, or sleepiness (use caution when driving, climbing stairs, or engaging in tasks requiring alertness until response to drug is known); or abdominal discomfort, diarrhea, constipation, nausea, or vomiting (small, frequent meals, increased exercise, adequate hydration may help). Report back pain, muscle spasms, alteration in gait, or numbness of extremities; unresolved or persistent constipation, diarrhea, or vomiting; or symptoms of upper respiratory infection or flu. Report immediately any chest pain or palpitations, difficulty urinating, or pain on urination. **Pregnancy/breast-feeding precautions:** Inform prescriber if you are or intend to become pregnant. Breast-feeding is not recommended.

Related Information

Pharmacotherapy of Urinary Incontinence *on page 1699*

Tolterodine Tartrate *see* Tolterodine *on page 1333*

Tolu-Sed® DM [OTC] *see* Guaifenesin and Dextromethorphan *on page 647*

Topamax® *see* Topiramate *on page 1337*

Topicaine® [OTC] *see* Lidocaine *on page 800*

Topical Corticosteroids (TOP i kal kor ti koe STER oyds)

U.S. Brand Names Aclovate®; A-hydroCort®; AK-Dex®; Ala-Cort®; Ala-Scalp®; Alphatrex®; Anucort-HC® Suppository; Anusol® HC-1 [OTC]; Anusol® HC-2.5% [OTC]; Anusol-HC® Suppository; Aristocort®; Baldex®; Betatrex®; Beta-Val®; Capex™; Cetacort®; Clocort® Maximum Strength; Cloderm®; Cordran®; Cordran® SP; Cormax®; Cortaid® Maximum Strength [OTC]; Cortaid® With Aloe [OTC]; Cort-Dome®; Cortef® Feminine Itch; Cortenema®; Corticaine®; Cortifoam®; Cortizone®-5 [OTC]; Cortizone®-10 [OTC]; Cutivate™; Dalalone®; Dalalone L.A.®; Decaspray®; Delcort®; Delta-Tritex®; Dermacort®; Derma-Smoothe/FS®; Dermatop®; DermiCort®; Dermolate® [OTC]; Dermtex® HC With Aloe; DesOwen®; Dexasone®; Dexasone® L.A.; Dexone®; Dexone® LA; Diprolene®; Diprolene® AF; Diprosone®; Eldecort®; Elocon®; Florone®; Flutex®; FS Shampoo® [DSC]; Gynecort® [OTC]; Halog®; Halog®-E; Hemril-HC® Uniserts®; Hexadrol®; Hexadrol® Phosphate; Hi-Cor 1.0®; Hi-Cor 2.5®; Hycort®; Hydrocort®; HydroTex® [OTC]; Hytone®; Kenalog®; Kenalog® H; Kenalog® in Orabase®; Kenonel®; LactiCare-HC®; Lanacort® [OTC]; Lidex®; Lidex-E®; Locoid®; Luxiq™; Maxiflor®; Maxivate®; Nasonex®; Nutracort®; Olux™; Orabase® HCA; Pandel®; Penecort®; Procort® [OTC]; Proctocort™; Psorcon™; Psorcon™ E; Scalpicin®; Solu-Cortef®; S-T Cort®; Synacort®; Synalar®; Synalar-HP®; Synemol®; Tegrin®-HC [OTC]; Teladar®; Temovate®; Texacort®; Topicort®; Topicort®-LP; Triacet™; Triderm®; Tridesilon®; Ultravate™; Valisone® [DSC]; Westcort®

Synonyms Alclometasone; Betamethasone; Clobetasol; Clocortolone; Corticosteroids, Topical; Desonide; Desoximetasone; Dexamethasone; Diflorasone; Fluocinolone; Fluocinonide; Flurandrenolide; Fluticasone; Halcinonide; Halobetasol; Hydrocortisone; Mometasone; Prednicarbate; Triamcinolone

Pharmacologic Category Corticosteroid, Topical

Pregnancy Risk Factor C

Lactation Excretion in breast milk unknown/use caution

Use

Topical corticosteroids: Relief of inflammatory and pruritic manifestations of corticosteroid-responsive dermatologic conditions. Significant differences in potency are present within this class. The following list is designed to facilitate comparison.

Lowest potency:

Alclometasone 0.05% cream, ointment (Aclovate®)

Betamethasone 0.1% cream

Betamethasone 0.2% cream

Desonide 0.05% cream, ointment, lotion (DesOwen®, Tridesilon®)

Dexamethasone 0.04% aerosol (Decaspray®)
Hydrocortisone 1% cream, ointment, lotion
Hydrocortisone 2.5% cream, ointment
Methylprednisolone acetate 0.25% ointment (Medrol®)
Methylprednisolone acetate 1% ointment (Medrol®)

Low potency:
Betamethasone valerate 0.025% cream (Valisone® reduced strength)
Clocortolone 0.1% cream (Cloderm®)
Fluocinolone acetonide 0.01% cream, solution (Synalar®)
Flurandrenolide 0.025% cream, ointment (Cordran®, Cordran® SP)
Hydrocortisone valerate 0.2% cream (Westcort®)
Triamcinolone acetonide 0.025% cream, ointment (Kenalog®)

Intermediate potency:
Betamethasone benzoate 0.025% cream, gel, lotion
Betamethasone valerate 0.1% cream, ointment, lotion (Valisone®)
Desoximetasone 0.05% cream, ointment (Topicort® LP)
Fluocinolone acetonide 0.025% cream
Flurandrenolide 0.05% cream, ointment, lotion (Cordran®, Cordran® SP)
Fluticasone propionate 0.05% cream (Cutivate™)
Halcinonide 0.025% cream, ointment (Halog®)
Mometasone furoate 0.1% cream, ointment, lotion
Triamcinolone acetonide 0.1% cream, ointment (Kenalog®)

High potency:
Amcinonide 0.1% cream, ointment (Cyclocort®)
Betamethasone dipropionate 0.05% cream, ointment, lotion (Diprosone®)
Desoximetasone 0.25% cream, ointment (Topicort®)
Fluocinolone 0.2% cream (Synalar® HP)
Fluocinonide 0.05% cream, ointment (Lidex®)
Halcinonide 0.1% cream, ointment, solution (Halog®)
Triamcinolone acetonide 0.5% cream, ointment (Kenalog®)

Very high potency:
Augmented betamethasone dipropionate 0.05% ointment (Diprolene®)
Clobetasol propionate 0.05% cream, ointment (Temovate®)
Diflorasone 0.05% gel, ointment (Florone®, Maxiflor®, Psorcon™)
Halobetasol propionate 0.05% cream, ointment (Ultravate™)

Nasal corticosteroids: Treatment of the symptoms of perennial and seasonal allergic disorders (also see individual monographs for beclomethasone, flunisolide)
Age restrictions:
Mometasone: Children age 3 and older
Fluticasone: Children age 4 and older

Mechanism of Action/Effect Reverses capillary permeability and release of inflammatory mediators (leukotrienes and prostaglandins); suppresses migration of polymorphonuclear leukocytes; agents may be grouped by potency (see Use)

Contraindications Hypersensitivity to any specific agent or component; viral, fungal, or tubercular skin infection

Warnings/Precautions May cause adrenal suppression or insufficiency, application to abraded or inflamed skin or large areas of the body may increase the risk of systemic absorption and adrenal suppression. Use only low-potency agents on or near the face. Use of fluticasone topical in pediatric patients for more than 4 weeks of use has not been established. Pregnancy factor C (however, exposure to fetus after topical application may be minimal due to low absorption).

Adverse Reactions When systemic absorption occurs, adrenocortical suppression may occur, as well as other systemic effects of steroids, including Cushing's syndrome, hypokalemia, glaucoma, and cataracts.

1% to 10%:
Dermatologic: Secondary infection, allergic contact dermatitis, dryness, rash, folliculitis, furunculosis, pustules, pyoderma, hyperesthesia
Local: Burning, itching

<1% (Limited to important or life-threatening symptoms): Hypertrichosis, acneform eruptions, hypopigmentation, perioral dermatitis, bruising, maceration of skin, hirsutism, skin atrophy, striae, telangiectasia

Pharmacodynamics/Kinetics

Absorption: Negligible, under normal circumstances, approximately 1% reaches systemic circulation; occlusive dressings may dramatically increase absorption

Metabolism: Hepatic

Formulations

Alclometasone:
Cream, as dipropionate (Aclovate®): 0.05% (15 g, 45 g, 60 g)
Ointment, as dipropionate (Aclovate®): 0.05% (15 g, 45 g, 60 g)

Betamethasone:
Cream, as dipropionate: 0.05% (15 g, 45 g, 60 g)
Alphatrex®, Diprosone®: 0.05% (15 g, 45 g)
Maxivate®: 0.05% (45 g)
Cream, as dipropionate augmented (Diprolene® AF): 0.05% (15 g, 50 g)
Cream, as valerate: 0.1% (15 g, 45 g)
Betatrex®, Valisone® [DSC]: 0.1% (15 g, 45 g)
Beta-Val®: 0.1% (15 g, 45 g)
Foam, as valerate (Luxiq™): 0.12% (50 g, 100 g) [contains alcohol 60.4%]
Gel, topical, as dipropionate augmented (Diprolene®): 0.05% (15 g, 50 g)
Lotion, as dipropionate: 0.05% (20 mL, 60 mL)
Alphatrex®, Maxivate®: 0.05% (60 mL)
Diprosone®: 0.05% (20 mL, 60 mL)
Lotion, as dipropionate augmented (Diprolene®): 0.05% (30 mL, 60 mL)
Lotion, as valerate (Beta-Val®, Betatrex®, Valisone® [DSC]): 0.1% (60 mL)

(Continued)

Topical Corticosteroids *(Continued)*

Ointment, as dipropionate: 0.05% (15 g, 45 g)
Alphatrex®, Maxivate®: 0.05% (45 g)
Diprosone®: 0.05% (15 g, 45 g)
Ointment, as dipropionate augmented: 0.05% (15 g, 45 g, 50 g); Diprolene®: 0.05% (15 g, 50 g)
Ointment, as valerate (Betatrex®, Valisone® [DSC]): 0.1% (15 g, 45 g)

Clobetasol propionate:
Cream, as propionate: 0.05% (15 g, 30 g, 45 g)
Cream, as propionate [in emollient base]: 0.05% (15 g, 30 g, 60 g)
Foam, scalp, as propionate (Olux™): 0.05% (100 g)
Gel, as propionate: 0.05% (15 g, 30 g, 45 g)
Ointment, as propionate: 0.05% (15 g, 30 g, 45 g)
Solution, scalp, as propionate: 0.05% (25 mL, 50 mL)

Clocortolone (Cloderm®): Cream, as pivalate: 0.1% (15 g, 45 g)

Desonide:
Cream: 0.05% (15 g, 60 g)
Lotion: 0.05% (60 mL, 120 mL)
Ointment: 0.05% (15 g, 60 g)

Desoximetasone:
Cream:
Topicort®: 0.25% (15 g, 60 g, 120 g)
Topicort®-LP: 0.05% (15 g, 60 g)
Gel (Topicort®): 0.05% (15 g, 60 g)
Ointment (Topicort®): 0.25% (15 g, 60 g)

Dexamethasone:
Aerosol, topical: 0.04% (25 g)
Cream, as sodium phosphate: 0.1% (15 g, 30 g)
Ointment, ophthalmic, as sodium phosphate: 0.05% (3.5 g)

Diflorasone:
Cream, as diacetate: 0.05% (15 g, 30 g, 60 g)
Ointment, as diacetate: 0.05% (15 g, 30 g, 60 g)

Fluocinolone:
Cream, as acetonide: 0.01% (15 g, 60 g); 0.025% (15 g, 60 g); Synalar®: 0.025% (15 g, 60 g)
Oil, topical, as acetonide (Derma-Smoothe/FS®): 0.01% (120 mL) [contains peanut oil]
Ointment, as acetonide: 0.025% (15 g, 60 g); Synalar®: 0.025% (15 g, 30 g, 60 g)
Shampoo, as acetonide (Capex™): 0.01% (120 mL)
Solution, topical, as acetonide: 0.01% (20 mL, 60 mL); Synalar®: 0.01% (20 mL, 60 mL)

Fluocinonide:
Cream: 0.05% (15 g, 30 g, 60 g, 120 g)
Cream, anhydrous, emollient (Lidex®): 0.05% (15 g, 30 g, 60 g, 120 g)
Cream, aqueous, emollient (Lidex-E®): 0.05% (15 g, 30 g, 60 g, 120 g)
Gel: 0.05% (15 g, 60 g); Lidex®: 0.05% (15 g, 30 g, 60 g, 120 g)
Ointment: 0.05% (15 g, 30 g, 60 g); Lidex®: 0.05% (15 g, 30 g, 60 g, 120 g)
Solution, topical: 0.05% (20 mL, 60 mL); Lidex®: 0.05% (20 mL, 60 mL)

Flurandrenolide:
Cream, emulsified, as base (Cordran® SP): 0.025% (30 g, 60 g); 0.05% (15 g, 30 g, 60 g)
Lotion (Cordran®): 0.05% (15 mL, 60 mL)
Ointment (Cordran®): 0.025% (30 g, 60 g); 0.05% (15 g, 30 g, 60 g)
Tape, topical (Cordran®): 4 mcg/cm2 (7.5 cm x 60 cm, 7.5 cm x 200 cm rolls)

Fluticasone:
Cream, as propionate (Cutivate™): 0.05% (15 g, 30 g, 60 g)
Ointment, as propionate (Cutivate™): 0.005% (15 g, 30 g, 60 g)

Halcinonide:
Cream (Halog®): 0.1% (15 g, 30 g, 60 g, 240 g)
Cream, emollient base (Halog®-E): 0.1% (30 g, 60 g)
Ointment (Halog®): 0.1% (15 g, 30 g, 60 g, 240 g)
Solution, topical (Halog®): 0.1% (20 mL, 60 mL)

Halobetasol:
Cream, as propionate (Ultravate™): 0.05% (15 g, 45 g)
Ointment, as propionate (Ultravate™): 0.05% (15 g, 45 g)

Hydrocortisone:
Aerosol, rectal, as acetate: 10% (20 g)
Aerosol, topical, as base: 0.5% (45 g, 58 g); 1% (45 mL)
Cream, as acetate: 0.5% (15 g, 22.5 g, 30 g); 1% (15 g, 30 g, 120 g)
Cream, as base: 0.2% (15 g, 30 g, 60 g, 120 g, 454 g); 0.5% (15 g, 30 g, 60 g, 120 g, 454 g); 1% (15 g, 20 g, 30 g, 60 g, 90 g, 120 g, 240 g, 454 g); 2.5% (15 g, 20 g, 30 g, 60 g, 120 g, 240 g, 454 g)
Cream, as buteprate: 0.1%, 1% (15 g, 45 g)
Cream, as butyrate: 0.1% (15 g, 45 g)
Cream, rectal, as base: 1% (30 g); 2.5% (30 g)
Cream, as valerate: 0.2% (15 g, 45 g, 60 g)
Gel, as base: 0.5% (15 g, 30 g); 1% (15 g, 30 g)
Lotion, as acetate: 0.5%
Lotion, as base: 0.25% (120 mL); 0.5% (30 mL, 60 mL, 120 mL); 1% (60 mL, 118 mL, 120 mL); 2% (30 mL); 2.5% (60 mL, 120 mL)
Ointment, as acetate: 0.5% (15 g, 30 g); 1% (15 g, 21 g, 30 g)
Ointment, as base: 0.2% (15 g, 30 g); 0.5% (30 g); 1% (15 g, 20 g, 28 g, 30 g, 60 g, 120 g, 240 g, 454 g); 2.5% (20 g, 30 g)
Ointment, as butyrate: 0.1% (15 g, 45 g)
Ointment, as valerate: 0.2% (15 g, 45 g, 60 g, 120 g)
Ointment, ophthalmic, as acetate: 0.5%
Ointment, rectal, as base: 1% (30 g)

Solution, topical, as base: 1% (45 mL, 75 mL, 120 mL)
Solution, topical, as butyrate: 0.1% (20 mL, 50 mL)
Suppositories, rectal, as acetate: 10 mg, 25 mg
Suspension, rectal, as base: 100 mg/60 mL (7s)

Mometasone:
Cream, (Elocon®): 0.1% (15 g, 45 g)
Lotion, (Elocon®): 0.1% (30 mL, 60 mL)
Ointment, (Elocon®): 0.1% (15 g, 45 g)

Prednicarbate:
Cream (Dermatop®): 0.1% (15 g, 60 g)
Ointment (Dermatop®): 0.1% (15 g, 60 g)

Triamcinolone:
Aerosol, topical, as acetonide: 0.2 mg/2 second spray (23 g, 63 g)
Cream, as acetonide: 0.025% (15 g, 60 g, 80 g, 240 g, 454 g); 0.1% (15 g, 30 g, 60 g, 80 g, 90 g, 120 g, 240 g); 0.5% (15 g, 20 g, 30 g, 240 g)
Lotion, as acetonide: 0.025% (60 mL); 0.1% (15 mL, 60 mL)
Ointment, as acetonide: 0.025% (15 g, 30 g, 60 g, 80 g, 120 g, 454 g); 0.1% (15 g, 30 g, 60 g, 80 g, 120 g, 240 g, 454 g); 0.5% (15 g, 20 g, 30 g, 240 g)
Paste, oral, topical, as acetonide (Kenalog® in Orabase®): 0.1% (5 g)

Dosing

Adults & Elderly: Therapy should be discontinued when control is achieved. If no improvement is seen, reassessment of diagnosis may be necessary.

Alclometasone: Apply a thin film to the affected area 2-3 times/day.
Betamethasone: Apply thin film 2-4 times/day.
Clobetasol: Apply twice daily for up to 2 weeks with no more than 50 g/week.
Clocortolone: Apply sparingly and gently; rub into affected area from 1-4 times/day.
Desonide: Apply 2-4 times/day sparingly.
Desoximetasone: Apply sparingly in a thin film twice daily.
Dexamethasone: Apply 1-4 times/day.
Diflorasone: Apply ointment sparingly 1-3 times/day; apply cream sparingly 2-4 times/day.
Fluocinolone: Apply a thin layer to affected area 2-4 times/day.
Flurandrenolide:
Ointment, cream: Apply sparingly 1-2 times/day.
Tape: Apply once daily.
Cream, lotion, ointment: Apply sparingly 2-3 times/day.
Fluticasone:
Topical (approved for use in pediatric patients ≥3 months): Apply sparingly in a thin film twice daily.
Nasal spray (approved for use in children 4 years of age or older): 1 spray into each nostril daily
Halcinonide: Apply sparingly 1-3 times/day, occlusive dressing may be used for severe or resistant dermatoses. A thin film of cream or ointment is effective; do not overuse.
Halobetasol: Apply sparingly to skin twice daily, rub in gently and completely. Treatment should not exceed 2 consecutive weeks and total dosage should not exceed 50 g/week.
Hydrocortisone: Apply to affected area 3-4 times/day.
Mometasone:
Topical: Apply sparingly to area once daily. Do not use occlusive dressings.
Nasal spray: One spray into each nostril daily.
Prednicarbate: Apply a thin film to affected area twice daily.
Triamcinolone: Apply a thin film 2-3 times/day.

Administration

Topical: For external use only. Do not use on open wounds, weeping lesions, or burns. Do not use occlusive dressings. Use only low-potency agents on or near the face.

Stability

Storage: Store at room temperature.

Monitoring and Teaching Issues

Physical Assessment: See Contraindications and Warnings/Precautions for use cautions. When applied to large areas of skin or for extensive periods of time, monitor for adverse skin or systemic reactions. Assess knowledge/teach patient appropriate application and use and adverse symptoms (see Adverse Reactions) to report (see Patient Education). **Pregnancy risk factor C** - systemic absorption may be minimal with appropriate use. Note breast-feeding caution.

Patient Education: For external use only. Use exactly as directed; do not overuse. Do not apply to open wounds or weeping areas. Before using, wash and dry area gently. Apply a thin film to affected area and rub in gently. If dressing is necessary, use a porous dressing. Avoid contact with eyes. Avoid exposing treated area to direct sunlight; sunburn can occur. Report increased swelling, redness, rash, itching, signs of infection, worsening of condition, or lack of healing. **Pregnancy/breast-feeding precautions:** Inform prescriber if you are or intend to become pregnant. Consult prescriber if breast-feeding.

Additional Information Hydrocortisone base topical cream, lotion, and ointments in concentrations of 0.25%, 0.5%, and 1% may be OTC or prescriptive depending on the product labeling.

Topicort® *see* Topical Corticosteroids *on page 1334*
Topicort®-LP *see* Topical Corticosteroids *on page 1334*
Topicycline® *see* Tetracycline *on page 1296*

Topiramate (toe PYE ra mate)

U.S. Brand Names Topamax®
Generic Available No
Pharmacologic Category Anticonvulsant, Miscellaneous
Pregnancy Risk Factor C
Lactation Excretion in breast milk unknown/not recommended

(Continued)

Topiramate *(Continued)*

Use In adults and pediatric patients (ages 2-16 years), adjunctive therapy for partial onset seizures and adjunctive therapy of primary generalized tonic-clonic seizures; treatment of seizures associated with Lennox-Gastaut syndrome in patients ≥2 years of age

Use - Unlabeled/Investigational Bipolar disorder, infantile spasms, neuropathic pain, migraine, cluster headache

Mechanism of Action/Effect Mechanism is not fully understood, it is thought to decrease seizure frequency by blocking sodium channels in neurons, enhancing GABA activity and by blocking glutamate activity

Contraindications Hypersensitivity to topiramate or any component of the formulation

Warnings/Precautions Avoid abrupt withdrawal of topiramate therapy, it should be withdrawn slowly to minimize the potential of increased seizure frequency. The risk of kidney stones is about 2-4 times that of the untreated population, the risk of this event may be reduced by increasing fluid intake. Use cautiously in patients with hepatic or renal impairment and during pregnancy. May cause paresthesias. Sedation, psychomotor slowing, confusion, and mood disturbances may occur with topiramate use. Has been associated with secondary angle-closure glaucoma in adults and children, typically within 1 month of initiation. Safety and efficacy have not been established in children <2 years of age. Pregnancy risk C.

Drug Interactions

Cytochrome P450 Effect: Inhibits CYP2C19; Induces CYP3A4

Decreased Effect: Phenytoin can decrease topiramate levels by as much as 48%, carbamazepine reduces it by 40%, and valproic acid reduces topiramate by 14%. Digoxin levels and ethinyl estradiol blood levels are decreased when coadministered with topiramate. Topiramate may decrease valproic acid concentration by 11%.

Increased Effect/Toxicity: Concomitant administration with other CNS depressants will increase its sedative effects. Coadministration with other carbonic anhydrase inhibitors may increase the chance of nephrolithiasis. Topiramate may increase phenytoin concentration by 25%.

Nutritional/Ethanol Interactions

Ethanol: Avoid ethanol (may increase CNS depression).

Herb/Nutraceutical: Avoid evening primrose (seizure threshold decreased).

Adverse Reactions

>10%:

Central nervous system: Dizziness, ataxia, somnolence, psychomotor slowing, nervousness, memory difficulties, speech problems, fatigue

Gastrointestinal: Nausea

Neuromuscular & skeletal: Paresthesia, tremor

Ocular: Nystagmus, diplopia, abnormal vision

Respiratory: Upper respiratory infections

1% to 10%:

Cardiovascular: Chest pain, edema

Central nervous system: Language problems, abnormal coordination, confusion, depression, difficulty concentrating, hypoesthesia

Endocrine & metabolic: Hot flashes

Gastrointestinal: Dyspepsia, abdominal pain, anorexia, constipation, xerostomia, gingivitis, weight loss

Neuromuscular & skeletal: Myalgia, weakness, back pain, leg pain, rigors

Otic: Decreased hearing

Renal: Nephrolithiasis

Respiratory: Pharyngitis, sinusitis, epistaxis

Miscellaneous: Flu-like symptoms

<1% (Limited to important or life-threatening): Apraxia, AV block, bone marrow depression, delirium, dyskinesia, encephalopathy, eosinophilia, granulocytopenia, hepatic failure, hepatitis, manic reaction, neuropathy, pancreatitis, pancytopenia, paranoid reaction, photosensitivity, psychosis, renal calculus, renal tubular acidosis, suicidal behavior, syndrome of acute myopia/secondary angle-closure glaucoma, tinnitus

Overdosage/Toxicology Activated charcoal has not been shown to adsorb topiramate and is therefore not recommended. Hemodialysis can remove the drug; however, most cases do not require removal and instead are best treated with supportive measures.

Pharmacodynamics/Kinetics

Absorption: Good; unaffected by food

Bioavailability: 80%

Half-Life Elimination: Mean: Adults: 21 hours; shorter in pediatric patients; clearance is 50% higher in pediatric patients

Time to Peak: Serum: ~2-4 hours

Metabolism: Minimally hepatic via hydroxylation, hydrolysis, glucuronidation

Formulations

Capsule, sprinkle (Topamax®): 15 mg, 25 mg

Tablet (Topamax®): 25 mg, 100 mg, 200 mg

Dosing

Adults & Elderly:

Partial onset seizures (adjunctive therapy), primary generalized tonic-clonic seizures (adjunctive therapy): Oral: Initial: 25-50 mg/day; titrate in increments of 25-50 mg per week until an effective daily dose is reached; the daily dose may be increased by 25 mg at weekly intervals for the first 4 weeks; thereafter, the daily dose may be increased by 25-50 mg weekly to an effective daily dose (usually at least 400 mg); usual maximum dose: 1600 mg/day

Note: A more rapid titration schedule has been previously recommended (ie, 50 mg/week), and may be attempted in some clinical situations; however, this may reduce the patient's ability to tolerate topiramate.

Migraine, cluster headache (unlabeled uses): Oral: Initial: 25 mg/day, titrated at weekly intervals in 25 mg increments, up to 200 mg/day

Pediatrics: Children 2-16 years: Partial onset seizures (adjunctive therapy), primary generalized tonic-clonic seizures (adjunctive therapy), and seizures associated with Lennox-Gastaut syndrome: Oral: Initial dose titration should begin at 25 mg (or less, based on a range of 1-3 mg/kg/day) nightly for the first week. Dosage may be increased in increments of 1-3 mg/kg/day (administered in two divided doses) at 1- or 2-week intervals to a total daily dose of 5-9 mg/kg/day.

Renal Impairment: Cl_{cr} <70 mL/minute: Administer 50% dose and titrate more slowly.

Hemodialysis: Supplemental dose may be needed during hemodialysis

Dialyzable: ~30%

Hepatic Impairment: Clearance may be reduced.

Administration

Oral: May be administered without regard to meals

Capsule sprinkles: May be swallowed whole or opened to sprinkle the contents on soft food (drug/food mixture should not be chewed).

Tablet: Because of bitter taste, tablets should not be broken.

Stability

Storage: Store at room temperature; protect capsules from moisture.

Monitoring and Teaching Issues

Physical Assessment: Assess effectiveness and interactions of other medications patient may be taking (see Drug Interactions). Monitor therapeutic response (seizure activity, force, type, duration), laboratory values, and adverse reactions (see Adverse Reactions) at beginning of therapy and periodically with long-term use. Taper dosage slowly when discontinuing. Assess knowledge/teach patient appropriate use, seizure safety precautions, interventions to reduce side effects, and adverse symptoms to report (see Patient Education). **Pregnancy risk factor C** - benefits of use should outweigh possible risks. Breast-feeding is not recommended.

Patient Education: Take exactly as directed; do not increase dose or frequency or discontinue without consulting prescriber. While using this medication, do not use alcohol and other prescription or OTC medications (especially pain medications, sedatives, antihistamines, or hypnotics) without consulting prescriber. Maintain adequate hydration (2-3 L/day of fluids) unless advised by prescriber to restrict fluids. You may experience drowsiness, dizziness, disturbed concentration, memory changes, or blurred vision (use caution when driving or engaging in tasks requiring alertness until response to drug is known); or mouth sores, nausea, vomiting, or loss of appetite (small, frequent meals, frequent mouth care, chewing gum, or sucking lozenges may help). Wear identification of epileptic status and medications. Adults should be aware of and follow state laws about driving with a seizure disorder. Report behavioral or CNS changes; skin rash; muscle cramping, weakness, tremors, changes in gait; chest pain, irregular heartbeat, or palpitations; hearing loss; cough or difficulty breathing; or worsening of seizure activity or loss of seizure control. Seek immediate medical evaluation if you experience sudden vision changes and/or periorbital pain. **Pregnancy/breast-feeding precautions:** Inform prescriber if you are pregnant or intend to become pregnant. Breast-feeding is not recommended.

Geriatric Considerations: Since drug is renally excreted and most elderly will have creatinine clearance <70 mL/minute, doses must be reduced 50% and titrated more slowly. Obtain a serum creatinine and calculate creatinine clearance prior to starting therapy. Follow the recommended titration schedule and adjust time intervals to meet patient's needs.

Breast-feeding Issues: Topiramate has been shown to be secreted in the milk of lactating rats. Excretion in human milk is unknown, but would be expected based upon topiramate's low molecular weight and low protein binding.

Pregnancy Issues: No studies in pregnant women; use only if benefit to the mother outweighs the risk to the fetus. Postmarketing experience includes reports of hypospadias following *in vitro* exposure to topiramate.

Additional Information May be associated with weight loss in some patients

TOPO *see* Topotecan *on page 1339*

Toposar® *see* Etoposide *on page 536*

Topotecan (toe poe TEE kan)

U.S. Brand Names Hycamtin™

Synonyms Hycamptamine; SK and F 104864; SKF 104864; SKF 104864-A; TOPO; Topotecan Hydrochloride; TPT

Generic Available No

Pharmacologic Category Antineoplastic Agent, Natural Source (Plant) Derivative

Pregnancy Risk Factor D

Lactation Enters breast milk/contraindicated

Use Treatment of metastatic carcinoma of the ovary after failure of initial or subsequent chemotherapy; second-line treatment of small cell lung cancer

Use - Unlabeled/Investigational Investigational: Treatment of nonsmall cell lung cancer, sarcoma (pediatrics)

Mechanism of Action/Effect Inhibits topoisomerase I (an enzyme which relaxes torsionally strained-coiled duplex DNA) to prevent DNA replication and translocation; topotecan acts in S phase

Contraindications Hypersensitivity to topotecan or any component of the formulation; pregnancy

Warnings/Precautions The U.S. Food and Drug Administration (FDA) currently recommends that procedures for proper handling and disposal of antineoplastic agents be considered. Appropriate safety equipment is recommended for preparation, administration, and disposal of antineoplastics. If paclitaxel contacts the skin, wash and flush thoroughly with water. Monitor bone marrow function. Should only administer to patients with adequate bone marrow reserves, baseline neutrophils at least 1500 cells/mm^3 and platelet counts at least 100,000/mm^3.

(Continued)

Topotecan *(Continued)*

Drug Interactions

Increased Effect/Toxicity: Concurrent administration of TPT and G-CSF in clinical trials results in severe myelosuppression. Concurrent *in vitro* exposure to TPT and the topoisomerase II inhibitor etoposide results in no altered effect; sequential exposure results in potentiation. Concurrent exposure to TPT and 5-azacytidine results in potentiation both *in vitro* and *in vivo*. Myelosuppression was more severe when given in combination with cisplatin.

Nutritional/Ethanol Interactions Ethanol: Avoid ethanol (due to GI irritation).

Adverse Reactions

>10%:

Central nervous system: Headache
Dermatologic: Alopecia (reversible)
Gastrointestinal: Nausea, vomiting, diarrhea
Emetic potential: Moderately low (10% to 30%)
Hematologic: Myelosuppressive: Principle dose-limiting toxicity; white blood cell count nadir is 8-11 days after administration and is more frequent than thrombocytopenia (at lower doses); recover is usually within 21 days and cumulative toxicity has not been noted.
WBC: Mild to severe
Platelets: Mild (at low doses)
Nadir: 8-11 days
Recovery: 14-21 days

1% to 10%:

Neuromuscular & skeletal: Paresthesia
Respiratory: Dyspnea

Pharmacodynamics/Kinetics

Absorption: Oral: ~30%

Half-Life Elimination: 3 hours

Metabolism: Undergoes a rapid, pH-dependent opening of the lactone ring to yield a relatively inactive hydroxy acid in plasma

Formulations Injection, powder for reconstitution, as hydrochloride: 4 mg (base)

Dosing

Adults & Elderly: Refer to individual protocols.

Metastatic ovarian cancer and small cell lung cancer: IVPB: 1.5 mg/m^2/day for 5 days; repeated every 21 days (neutrophil count should be >1500/mm^3 and platelet count should be >100,000/mm^3)

Dosage adjustment for hematological effects: If neutrophil count <1500/mm^3, reduce dose by 0.25 mg/m^2/day for 5 days for next cycle

Renal Impairment:

Cl_{cr} 20-39 mL/minute: Administer 50% of normal dose.
Cl_{cr} <20 mL/minute: Do not use, insufficient data available.
Hemodialysis: Supplemental dose is not necessary.
CAPD effects: Unknown
CAVH effects: Unknown

Hepatic Impairment: Bilirubin 1.5-10 mg/dL: No adjustment necessary.

Administration

I.V.: Administer lower doses IVPB over 30 minutes.

Stability

Storage: Store intact vials of lyophilized powder for injection at room temperature and protected from light. Topotecan should be initially reconstituted with 4 mL SWI. This solution is stable for 24 hours at room temperature. Topotecan should be further diluted in 100 mL D_5W. This solution is stable for 24 hours at room temperature.

Reconstitution: Standard I.V. dilution: Dose/100 mL D_5W; stability is pH dependent; although topotecan may be further diluted in 0.9% NaCl, stability is longer in D_5W

Compatibility: Stable in D_5W, NS

Y-site administration: Incompatible with dexamethasone sodium phosphate, fluorouracil, mitomycin

Monitoring Laboratory Tests CBC with differential and platelet count, renal function tests

Monitoring and Teaching Issues

Physical Assessment: See Contraindications, Warnings/Precautions, Drug Interactions, and Dosing for use cautions. Infusion site should be monitored closely to prevent extravasation. Assess results of laboratory tests, therapeutic effectiveness, and adverse reactions prior to each infusion and throughout therapy (eg, signs of myelosuppression - see Adverse Reactions and Overdose/Toxicology). Teach patient possible side effects and interventions and adverse symptoms to report (see Patient Education). **Pregnancy risk factor D** - determine that patient is not pregnant before beginning treatment. Instruct patients of childbearing age on appropriate barrier contraceptive measures. Breast-feeding is contraindicated.

Patient Education: Inform prescriber of all prescriptions, OTC medications, or herbal products you are taking, and any allergies you have. Do not take anything new during treatment unless approved by prescriber. This medication can only be administered I.V. Report immediately any redness, pain, swelling, or burning at infusion site. Maintain adequate hydration (2-3 L/day of fluids) unless advised by prescriber to restrict fluids. Maintain good oral hygiene (use soft toothbrush or cotton applicators several times a day and rinse mouth frequently). You will be susceptible to infection (avoid crowds and exposure to infection do not have any vaccinations unless approved by prescriber). May cause nausea, vomiting, or loss of appetite (small, frequent meals, frequent mouth care, sucking lozenges, or chewing gum may help, or consult prescriber); or hair loss (reversible). Report signs of opportunistic infection (eg, persistent fever or chills, unhealed sores, oral or vaginal sores, foul-smelling urine, painful urination, easy bruising or bleeding); unusual or persistent weakness or lethargy; numbness or tingling in extremities; or difficulty breathing. **Pregnancy/breast-feeding precautions:** Inform prescriber if you are pregnant. Do not get pregnant while taking this medication. Consult prescriber for appropriate contraceptive measures. This medication may cause severe fetal harm. Do not breast-feed.

Pregnancy Issues: Animal studies found reduced fetal body weight, eye, brain, skull, and vertebrae malformations. May cause fetal harm in pregnant women.

Additional Information Manufacturer reports that reconstituted solutions of topotecan diluted in D_5W or 0.9% NaCl are stable for 24 hours at room temperature and under ambient lighting. It has been suggested that topotecan be mixed in dextrose solutions (pH 4.5) rather than saline solutions with a relatively higher pH which would further the conversion of lactone to the hydroxy acid form; however, topotecan solutions in 0.9% NaCl of various concentrations in a final volume of 21 mL have been reported to remain >90% stable in the lactone form over 7 days at room temperature. Further, topotecan was reported to be stable in the lactone form for up to 24 hours at room temperature and up to 7 days refrigerated in solutions of D_5W or 0.9% NaCl in PVC infusion bags, polyolefin infusion bags, and glass bottles.

Topotecan Hydrochloride *see* Topotecan *on page 1339*

Toprol-XL® *see* Metoprolol *on page 893*

Toradol® *see* Ketorolac *on page 761*

Toremifene (TORE em i feen)

U.S. Brand Names Fareston®

Synonyms FC1157a; Toremifene Citrate

Generic Available No

Pharmacologic Category Antineoplastic Agent, Estrogen Receptor Antagonist

Pregnancy Risk Factor D

Lactation Excretion in breast milk unknown/contraindicated

Use Treatment of metastatic breast cancer in postmenopausal women with estrogen-receptor (ER) positive or ER unknown tumors

Mechanism of Action/Effect Nonsteroidal agent that competitively binds to estrogen receptors on tumors and other tissue targets (including breast and other tissues), producing a nuclear complex that decreases DNA synthesis and inhibits estrogen effects. Cells accumulate in the G_0 and G_1 phases; therefore, toremifene is cytostatic rather than cytocidal.

Contraindications Hypersensitivity to toremifene or any component of the formulation; pregnancy

Warnings/Precautions Hypercalcemia and tumor flare have been reported in some breast cancer patients with bone metastases during the first weeks of treatment. Tumor flare is a syndrome of diffuse musculoskeletal pain and erythema with increased size of tumor lesions that later regress. It is often accompanied by hypercalcemia. Tumor flare does not imply treatment failure or represent tumor progression. Institute appropriate measures if hypercalcemia occurs, and if severe, discontinue treatment. Drugs that decrease renal calcium excretion (eg, thiazide diuretics) may increase the risk of hypercalcemia in patients receiving toremifene. Leukopenia and thrombocytopenia have been reported rarely.

Patients with a history of thromboembolic disease should generally not be treated with toremifene.

Drug Interactions

Cytochrome P450 Effect: Substrate of CYP1A2, **3A4**

Decreased Effect: Phenobarbital, phenytoin, and carbamazepine increase the rate of toremifene metabolism and lower blood levels.

Increased Effect/Toxicity: Enzyme inhibitors (such as ketoconazole or erythromycin) may increase blood levels of toremifene. Concurrent therapy with warfarin results in significant enhancement of anticoagulant effects; has been speculated that a ↓ in antitumor effect of tamoxifen may also occur due to alterations in the percentage of active tamoxifen metabolites.

Adverse Reactions

>10%:

- Endocrine & metabolic: Hot flashes (35%), vaginal discharge (13%)
- Gastrointestinal: Nausea, vomiting
  - Emetic potential: Moderate (30% to 40%)
- Miscellaneous: Diaphoresis (20%)

1% to 10%:

- Cardiovascular: Thromboembolism (venous thrombosis, pulmonary embolism, arterial thrombosis), cardiac failure, myocardial infarction, angina, edema
- Central nervous system: Dizziness
- Endocrine & metabolic: Hypercalcemia (patients with bone metastases), galactorrhea, vitamin deficiency, menstrual irregularities
- Gastrointestinal: Elevated transaminase levels
- Genitourinary: Vaginal bleeding or discharge, endometriosis, priapism, possible endometrial cancer
- Ocular: Ophthalmologic effects (visual acuity changes, cataracts, or retinopathy), corneal opacities, dry eyes, blurred vision

Other events observed with unclear association with toremifene: Alopecia, anorexia, asthenia, dermatitis, dyspnea, jaundice, paresis, pruritus, rigors, skin discoloration, tremor

Overdosage/Toxicology Theoretically, overdose may manifest as an increase of antiestrogenic effects such as hot flashes; estrogenic effects such as vaginal bleeding; or nervous system disorders such as vertigo, dizziness, ataxia, and nausea. No specific antidote exists and treatment is symptomatic.

Pharmacodynamics/Kinetics

Absorption: Well absorbed

Half-Life Elimination: ~5 days

Time to Peak: Serum: ~3 hours

Metabolism: Extensively hepatic, principally by CYP3A4 to N-demethyltoremifene, which is also antiestrogenic but with weak *in vivo* antitumor potency

Formulations Tablet, as citrate: 60 mg

(Continued)

Toremifene *(Continued)*

Dosing

Adults & Elderly: Refer to individual protocols.

Metastatic breast carcinoma: Oral: 60 mg once daily, generally continued until disease progression is observed

Renal Impairment: No adjustment is necessary.

Hepatic Impairment: Toremifene is extensively metabolized in the liver and dosage adjustments may be indicated in patients with liver disease; however, no specific guidelines have been developed.

Monitoring Laboratory Tests Obtain periodic complete blood counts, calcium levels, and liver function tests. Closely monitor patients with bone metastases for hypercalcemia during the first few weeks of treatment. Leukopenia and thrombocytopenia have been reported rarely; monitor leukocyte and platelet counts during treatment.

Monitoring and Teaching Issues

Physical Assessment: See Contraindications, Warnings/Precautions, and Dosing for use cautions. Infusion site should be monitored closely to prevent extravasation. Assess potential for interactions with other prescriptions, OTC medications, or herbal products patient may be taking (see Drug Interactions). Assess results of laboratory tests (see above), therapeutic effectiveness, and adverse reactions throughout therapy (see Adverse Reactions and Overdose/Toxicology). Teach patient proper use, possible side effects and interventions and adverse symptoms to report (see Patient Education). **Pregnancy risk factor D** - determine that patient is not pregnant before beginning treatment. Instruct patients of childbearing age on appropriate barrier contraceptive measures. Breast-feeding is contraindicated.

Patient Education: Inform prescriber of all prescriptions, OTC medications, or herbal products you are taking, and any allergies you have. Do not take anything new during treatment unless approved by prescriber. Take as directed, without regard to food. You may experience an initial "flare" of this disease (eg, increased bone pain and hot flashes), which will subside with continued use. May cause nausea, vomiting, or loss of appetite (frequent mouth care, small, frequent meals, chewing gum, or sucking lozenges may help); dizziness (use caution when driving, climbing stairs, or engaging in tasks requiring alertness until response to drug is known); or loss of hair (reversible). Report vomiting that occurs immediately after taking medication; chest pain, palpitations, or swollen extremities; vaginal bleeding, hot flashes, or excessive perspiration; chest pain, unusual coughing, or difficulty breathing; or any vision changes or dry eyes. **Pregnancy/breast-feeding precautions:** Do not get pregnant while taking this medication. Consult prescriber for appropriate contraceptive measures. Do not breast-feed.

Related Information

Estrogen Replacement Therapy *on page 1666*

Toremifene Citrate *see* Toremifene *on page 1341*

Tornalate [DSC] *see* Bitolterol *on page 173*

Torsemide (TOR se mide)

U.S. Brand Names Demadex®

Generic Available Yes: Tablet

Pharmacologic Category Diuretic, Loop

Pregnancy Risk Factor B

Lactation Excretion in breast milk unknown/use caution

Use Management of edema associated with congestive heart failure and hepatic or renal disease; used alone or in combination with antihypertensives in treatment of hypertension; I.V. form is indicated when rapid onset is desired

Mechanism of Action/Effect Inhibits reabsorption of sodium and chloride in the ascending loop of Henle and distal renal tubule, interfering with the chloride-binding cotransport system, thus causing increased excretion of water, sodium, chloride, magnesium, and calcium; does not alter GFR, renal plasma flow, or acid-base balance

Contraindications Hypersensitivity to torsemide, any component of the formulation, or any sulfonylureas; anuria

Warnings/Precautions Ototoxicity has been associated with loop diuretics and has been seen with oral torsemide. Do not administer intravenously in less than 2 minutes; single doses should not exceed 200 mg. Avoid electrolyte imbalances in cirrhosis that might lead to hepatic encephalopathy. Monitor fluid status and renal function in an attempt to prevent dehydration, oliguria, azotemia, and reversible increases in BUN and creatinine. Monitor closely for electrolyte imbalances particularly hypokalemia and correct when necessary. Coadministration with antihypertensives may increase the risk of hypotension.

Chemical similarities are present among sulfonamides, sulfonylureas, carbonic anhydrase inhibitors, thiazides, and loop diuretics (except ethacrynic acid). Use in patients with sulfonylurea allergy is specifically contraindicated in product labeling, however, a risk of cross-reaction exists in patients with allergy to any of these compounds; avoid use when previous reaction has been severe.

Drug Interactions

Cytochrome P450 Effect: Substrate of **CYP2C8/9**; Inhibits CYP2C19

Decreased Effect: Torsemide efficacy may be decreased with NSAIDs. Torsemide action may be reduced with probenecid. Diuretic action may be impaired in patients with cirrhosis and ascites if used with salicylates. Glucose tolerance may be decreased when used with sulfonylureas.

Increased Effect/Toxicity: Torsemide-induced hypokalemia may predispose to digoxin toxicity and may increase the risk of arrhythmia with drugs which may prolong QT interval, including type Ia and type III antiarrhythmic agents, cisapride, and some quinolones (sparfloxacin, gatifloxacin, and moxifloxacin). The risk of toxicity from lithium and salicylates (high dose) may be increased by loop diuretics. Hypotensive effects and/or adverse renal effects of ACE inhibitors and NSAIDs are potentiated by bumetanide-induced hypovolemia.

The effects of peripheral adrenergic-blocking drugs or ganglionic blockers may be increased by bumetanide.

Torsemide may increase the risk of ototoxicity with other ototoxic agents (aminoglycosides, cis-platinum), especially in patients with renal dysfunction. Synergistic diuretic effects occur with thiazide-type diuretics. Diuretics tend to be synergistic with other antihypertensive agents, and hypotension may occur.

Nutritional/Ethanol Interactions Herb/Nutraceutical: Avoid dong quai if using for hypertension (has estrogenic activity). Avoid ephedra, yohimbe, ginseng (may worsen hypertension). Avoid garlic (may have increased antihypertensive effect).

Adverse Reactions

1% to 10%:

Cardiovascular: Edema (1.1%), EKG abnormality (2%), chest pain (1.2%)

Central nervous system: Headache (7.3%), dizziness (3.2%), insomnia (1.2%), nervousness (1%)

Endocrine & metabolic: Hyperglycemia, hyperuricemia, hypokalemia

Gastrointestinal: Diarrhea (2%), constipation (1.8%), nausea (1.8%), dyspepsia (1.6%), sore throat (1.6%)

Genitourinary: Excessive urination (6.7%)

Neuromuscular & skeletal: Weakness (2%), arthralgia (1.8%), myalgia (1.6%)

Respiratory: Rhinitis (2.8%), cough increase (2%)

<1% (Limited to important or life-threatening): Angioedema, atrial fibrillation, GI hemorrhage, hypernatremia hypotension, hypovolemia, rash, rectal bleeding, shunt thrombosis, syncope, ventricular tachycardia

Overdosage/Toxicology Symptoms include electrolyte depletion, volume depletion, hypotension, dehydration, and circulatory collapse. Electrolyte depletion may manifest as weakness, dizziness, mental confusion, anorexia, lethargy, vomiting, and cramps. Treatment is supportive.

Pharmacodynamics/Kinetics

Absorption: Oral: Rapid

Bioavailability: 80% to 90%

Half-Life Elimination: 2-4; Cirrhosis: 7-8 hours

Metabolism: Hepatic (80%) via CYP

Onset: Diuresis: 30-60 minutes; Peak effect: 1-4 hours

Duration: ~6 hours

Formulations

Injection: 10 mg/mL (2 mL, 5 mL)

Tablet: 5 mg, 10 mg, 20 mg, 100 mg

Dosing

Adults:

Note: The oral form may be given regardless of meal times. Patients may be switched from the I.V. form to the oral and vice-versa with no change in dose.

Congestive heart failure: Oral, I.V.: 10-20 mg once daily; may increase gradually for chronic treatment by doubling dose until the diuretic response is apparent (for acute treatment. I.V. dose may be repeated every 2 hours with double the dose as needed).

Chronic renal failure: Oral, I.V.: 20 mg once daily; increase as above.

Hepatic cirrhosis: Oral, I.V.: 5-10 mg once daily with an aldosterone antagonist or a potassium-sparing diuretic; increase as above.

Hypertension: Oral, I.V.: 5 mg once daily; increase to 10 mg after 4-6 weeks if an adequate hypotensive response is not apparent. If still not effective, an additional antihypertensive agent may be added.

Elderly: Usual starting dose should be 5 mg; refer to adult dosing.

Administration

I.V.: I.V. injections should be given over ≥2 minutes.

Stability

Compatibility: Stable in D_5W, NS, ½NS

Monitoring Laboratory Tests Renal function, electrolytes

Monitoring and Teaching Issues

Physical Assessment: Assess for allergy to sulfonylurea before beginning therapy. See Contraindications, Warnings/Precautions, and Dosing for use cautions. Assess potential for interactions with other prescriptions, OTC medications, or herbal products patient may be taking (especially anything that may impact fluid balance or increase potential for ototoxicity or hypotension - see Drug Interactions). See Administration for I.V. specifics. Assess results of laboratory tests, therapeutic effectiveness, and adverse response on a regular basis during therapy (eg, dehydration, electrolyte imbalance, postural hypotension - see Adverse Reactions and Overdose/Toxicology). Caution diabetics about closely monitoring glucose levels (glucose tolerance may be decreased). Teach patient appropriate use, possible side effects and appropriate interventions, and adverse symptoms to report (see Patient Education). Note breast-feeding caution.

Patient Education: Inform prescriber of all prescriptions, OTC medications, or herbal products you are taking, and any allergies you have. Do not take anything new during treatment unless approved by prescriber. Take as directed, with food or milk (to reduce GI distress), early in the day, or if twice daily, take last dose in late afternoon in order to avoid sleep disturbance and achieve maximum therapeutic effect. Include orange juice or bananas (or other potassium-rich foods) in daily diet. Do not take potassium supplements without consulting prescriber. Weigh yourself each day, at the same time, in the same clothes when beginning therapy, and weekly on long-term therapy; report unusual or unanticipated weight gain or loss. May cause postural hypotension (change position slowly when rising from sitting or lying); transient drowsiness, blurred vision, or dizziness (avoid driving or engaging in tasks that require alertness until response to drug is known); reduced tolerance to heat (avoid strenuous activity in hot weather or excessively hot showers); or constipation (increased exercise and increased dietary fiber, fruit, or fluids may help). Report unusual weight gain or loss (>5 lb/week), swelling of ankles and hands;

(Continued)

Torsemide *(Continued)*

persistent fatigue; unresolved constipation or diarrhea; weakness, fatigue, or dizziness; vomiting; cramps; change in hearing; or chest pain or palpitations. **Breast-feeding precaution:** Consult prescriber if breast-feeding.

Pregnancy Issues: A decrease in fetal weight, an increase in fetal resorption, and delayed fetal ossification has occurred in animal studies.

Additional Information 10-20 mg torsemide is approximately equivalent to furosemide 40 mg or bumetanide 1 mg.

Touro® DM *see* Guaifenesin and Dextromethorphan *on page 647*

Touro Ex® *see* Guaifenesin *on page 646*

Touro LA® *see* Guaifenesin and Pseudoephedrine *on page 648*

tPA *see* Alteplase *on page 67*

T-Phyl® *see* Theophylline *on page 1300*

TPT *see* Topotecan *on page 1339*

Tracrium® *see* Atracurium *on page 132*

Tramadol (TRA ma dole)

U.S. Brand Names Ultram®

Synonyms Tramadol Hydrochloride

Generic Available Yes

Pharmacologic Category Analgesic, Non-narcotic

Pregnancy Risk Factor C

Lactation Excreted in breast milk/contraindicated

Use Relief of moderate to moderately-severe pain

Mechanism of Action/Effect Binds to μ-opiate receptors in the CNS causing inhibition of ascending pain pathways, altering the perception of and response to pain; also inhibits the reuptake of norepinephrine and serotonin, which also modifies the ascending pain pathway

Contraindications Hypersensitivity to tramadol, opioids, or any component of the formulation; opioid-dependent patients; acute intoxication with alcohol, hypnotics, centrally-acting analgesics, opioids, or psychotropic drugs

Warnings/Precautions Should be used only with extreme caution in patients receiving MAO inhibitors. May cause CNS depression and/or respiratory depression, particularly when combined with other CNS depressants. Use with caution and reduce dosage when administered to patients receiving other CNS depressants. An increased risk of seizures may occur in patients receiving serotonin reuptake inhibitors (SSRIs or anorectics), tricyclic antidepressants, other cyclic compounds (including cyclobenzaprine, promethazine), neuroleptics, MAO inhibitors, or drugs which may lower seizure threshold. Patients with a history of seizures, or with a risk of seizures (head trauma, metabolic disorders, CNS infection, or malignancy, or during ethanol/drug withdrawal) are also at increased risk.

Elderly patients and patients with chronic respiratory disorders may be at greater risk of adverse events. Use with caution in patients with increased intracranial pressure or head injury. Use tramadol with caution and reduce dosage in patients with liver disease or renal dysfunction and in patients with myxedema, hypothyroidism, or hypoadrenalism. Not recommended during pregnancy or in nursing mothers. Tolerance or drug dependence may result from extended use; abrupt discontinuation should be avoided. Safety and efficacy in pediatric patients have not been established.

Pregnancy risk C.

Drug Interactions

Cytochrome P450 Effect: Substrate of **CYP2D6**, 3A4

Decreased Effect: Carbamazepine may decrease analgesic efficacy of tramadol (half-life decreases 33% to 50%) and may increase the risk of seizures in patients requiring anticonvulsants.

Increased Effect/Toxicity: Amphetamines may increase the risk of seizures with tramadol. Cimetidine increases the half-life of tramadol by 20% to 25%. SSRIs may increase the risk of seizures with tramadol. Tricyclic antidepressants may increase the risk of seizures. Linezolid may be associated with increased risk of seizures (due to MAO inhibition). MAO inhibitors may increases the risk of seizures. It is not clear if drugs with selective MAO type B inhibition are safer than nonselective agents. Avoid drugs with MAO activity (ie, linezolid). Naloxone may increase the risk of seizures in tramadol overdose. Neuroleptic agents may increase the risk of tramadol-associated seizures and may have additive CNS depressant effects. Opioids may increase the risk of seizures, and may have additive CNS depressant effects. Quinidine (and other inhibitors of CYP2D6) may increase the tramadol serum concentrations.

Nutritional/Ethanol Interactions

Ethanol: Avoid ethanol (may increase CNS depression).

Food: Does not affect the rate or extent of absorption.

Herb/Nutraceutical: Avoid valerian, St John's wort, kava kava, gotu kola (may increase CNS depression).

Adverse Reactions Incidence of some adverse effects may increase over time

>10%:

Central nervous system: Dizziness, headache, somnolence, vertigo

Gastrointestinal: Constipation, nausea

1% to 10%:

Cardiovascular: Vasodilation

Central nervous system: Agitation, anxiety, confusion, coordination impaired, emotional lability, euphoria, hallucinations, malaise, nervousness, sleep disorder, tremor

Dermatologic: Pruritus, rash

Endocrine & metabolic: Menopausal symptoms

Gastrointestinal: Abdominal pain, anorexia, diarrhea, dry mouth, dyspepsia, flatulence, vomiting

Genitourinary: Urinary frequency, urinary retention
Neuromuscular & skeletal: Hypertonia, spasticity, weakness
Ocular: Miosis, visual disturbance
Miscellaneous: Diaphoresis

<1% (Limited to important or life-threatening): Allergic reaction, amnesia, anaphylaxis, angioedema, bronchospasm, cognitive dysfunction, creatinine increased, death, depression, dyspnea, gastrointestinal bleeding, liver failure, seizure, serotonin syndrome, Stevens-Johnson syndrome, suicidal tendency, syncope, toxic epidermal necrolysis, vesicles

Overdosage/Toxicology Symptoms of overdose include CNS and respiratory depression, lethargy, coma, seizure, cardiac arrest, and death. Treatment may include naloxone 2 mg I.V. (0.01 mg/kg children) with repeat administration as needed up to 18 mg. Naloxone may increase the risk of seizures in tramadol overdose.

Pharmacodynamics/Kinetics

Absorption: Rapid and complete

Bioavailability: 75%

Half-Life Elimination: Tramadol: ~6 hours; Active metabolite: 7 hours; prolonged in elderly, hepatic or renal impairment

Time to Peak: 2 hours

Metabolism: Extensively hepatic via demethylation, glucuronidation, and sulfation; has pharmacologically active metabolite formed by CYP2D6

Onset: ~1 hour

Duration: 9 hours

Formulations Tablet, as hydrochloride: 50 mg

Dosing

Adults: Moderate to severe chronic pain: Oral: 50-100 mg every 4-6 hours, not to exceed 400 mg/day

For patients not requiring rapid onset of effect, tolerability may be improved by starting dose at 25 mg/day and titrating dose by 25 mg every 3 days, until reaching 25 mg 4 times/day. Dose may then be increased by 50 mg every 3 days as tolerated, to reach dose of 50 mg 4 times/day.

Elderly: Oral: >75 years: 50-100 mg every 4-6 hours not to exceed 300 mg/day; see renal or hepatic dosing.

Renal Impairment: Cl_{cr} <30 mL/minute: Administer 50-100 mg dose every 12 hours; maximum: 200 mg/day.

Hepatic Impairment: Cirrhosis: Recommended dose is 50 mg every 12 hours.

Stability

Storage: Store at controlled room temperature of 25°C (77°F).

Monitoring and Teaching Issues

Physical Assessment: Assess other medications patient may be taking for additive or adverse interactions (see Warnings/Precautions, Contraindications, and Drug Interactions). Monitor therapeutic effectiveness and adverse reactions or overdose (see Adverse Reactions) at beginning of therapy and periodically during therapy. May cause physical and/or psychological dependence. Assess knowledge/teach patient appropriate use, interventions to reduce side effects, and adverse symptoms to report (see Patient Education). **Pregnancy risk factor C** - benefits of use should outweigh possible risks. Breast-feeding is contraindicated.

Patient Education: If self-administered, use exactly as directed; do not increase dose or frequency. Drug may cause physical and/or psychological dependence. While using this medication, do not use alcohol and other prescription or OTC medications (especially pain medications, sedatives, antihistamines, or cough preparations) without consulting prescriber. Maintain adequate hydration (2-3 L/day of fluids) unless advised by prescriber to restrict fluids. You may experience drowsiness, dizziness, or blurred vision (use caution when driving or engaging in tasks requiring alertness until response to drug is known); nausea, vomiting, or loss of appetite (small, frequent meals, frequent mouth care, chewing gum, or sucking lozenges may help); or constipation (increased exercise, fluids, fruit, or fiber may help). Report severe unresolved constipation, difficulty breathing or shortness of breath, excessive sedation or increased insomnia and restlessness, changes in urinary pattern or menstrual pattern, seizures, muscle weakness or tremors, or chest pain or palpitations. **Pregnancy/breast-feeding precautions:** Inform prescriber if you are or intend to become pregnant. Do not breast-feed.

Dietary Issues: May be taken with or without food.

Geriatric Considerations: One study in the elderly found that tramadol 50 mg was similar in efficacy as acetaminophen 300 mg with codeine 30 mg.

Breast-feeding Issues: Not recommended for post-delivery analgesia in nursing mothers.

Pregnancy Issues: Tramadol has been shown to cross the placenta. Postmarketing reports following tramadol use during pregnancy include neonatal seizures, withdrawal syndrome, fetal death and stillbirth. Not recommended for use during labor and delivery.

Tramadol Hydrochloride *see* Tramadol *on page 1344*
Trandate® *see* Labetalol *on page 764*

Trandolapril (tran DOE la pril)

U.S. Brand Names Mavik®

Generic Available No

Pharmacologic Category Angiotensin-Converting Enzyme (ACE) Inhibitor

Pregnancy Risk Factor C/D (2nd and 3rd trimesters)

Lactation Enters breast milk/contraindicated

Use Management of hypertension alone or in combination with other antihypertensive agents; treatment of left ventricular dysfunction after myocardial infarction

Use - Unlabeled/Investigational As a class, ACE inhibitors are recommended in the treatment of systolic congestive heart failure

(Continued)

Trandolapril *(Continued)*

Mechanism of Action/Effect Competitive inhibitor of angiotensin-converting enzyme (ACE); prevents conversion of angiotensin I to angiotensin II, a potent vasoconstrictor; results in lower levels of angiotensin II which causes an increase in plasma renin activity and a reduction in aldosterone secretion

Contraindications Hypersensitivity to trandolapril or any component of the formulation; history of angioedema-related to previous treatment with an ACE inhibitor; bilateral renal artery stenosis; primary hyperaldosteronism; pregnancy (2nd and 3rd trimesters)

Warnings/Precautions Angioedema can occur at any time during treatment (especially following first dose). Careful blood pressure monitoring with first dose (hypotension can occur especially in volume depleted patients). Dosage adjustment needed in severe renal dysfunction (Cl_{cr} <30 mL/minute) or in hepatic cirrhosis. Use with caution in hypovolemia; collagen vascular diseases; valvular stenosis (particularly aortic stenosis); hyperkalemia; or before, during, or immediately after anesthesia. Avoid rapid dosage escalation, which may lead to renal insufficiency. Neutropenia/agranulocytosis with myeloid hyperplasia can rarely occur with captopril (another ACE inhibitor). Use with caution in unilateral renal artery stenosis and pre-existing renal insufficiency. Pregnancy risk C/D (2nd and 3rd trimesters).

Drug Interactions

Decreased Effect: Aspirin (high dose) may reduce the therapeutic effects of ACE inhibitors; at low dosages this does not appear to be significant. Rifampin may decrease the effect of ACE inhibitors. Antacids may decrease the bioavailability of ACE inhibitors (may be more likely to occur with captopril); separate administration times by 1-2 hours. NSAIDs, specifically indomethacin, may reduce the hypotensive effects of ACE inhibitors. More likely to occur in low renin or volume dependent hypertensive patients.

Increased Effect/Toxicity: Potassium supplements, co-trimoxazole (high dose), angiotensin II receptor antagonists (candesartan, losartan, irbesartan, etc), or potassium-sparing diuretics (amiloride, spironolactone, triamterene) may result in elevated serum potassium levels when combined with trandolapril. ACE inhibitor effects may be increased by phenothiazines or probenecid (increases levels of captopril). ACE inhibitors may increase serum concentrations/effects of digoxin, lithium, and sulfonlyureas.

Diuretics have additive hypotensive effects with ACE inhibitors, and hypovolemia increases the potential for adverse renal effects of ACE inhibitors. In patients with compromised renal function, coadministration with NSAIDs may result in further deterioration of renal function. Allopurinol and ACE inhibitors may cause a higher risk of hypersensitivity reaction when taken concurrently.

Nutritional/Ethanol Interactions Herb/Nutraceutical: Avoid dong quai if using for hypertension (has estrogenic activity). Avoid ephedra, yohimbe, ginseng (may worsen hypertension). Avoid garlic (may have increased antihypertensive effect).

Adverse Reactions Note: Frequency ranges include data from hypertension and heart failure trials. Higher rates of adverse reactions have generally been noted in patients with CHF. However, the frequency of adverse effects associated with placebo is also increased in this population.

>1%:

Cardiovascular: Hypotension (<1% to 11%), bradycardia (<1% to 4.7%), intermittent claudication (3.8%), stroke (3.3%)

Central nervous system: Dizziness (1.3% to 23%), syncope (5.9%), asthenia (3.3%)

Endocrine & metabolic: Elevated uric acid (15%), hyperkalemia (5.3%), hypocalcemia (4.7%)

Gastrointestinal: Dyspepsia (6.4%), gastritis (4.2%)

Neuromuscular & skeletal: Myalgia (4.7%)

Renal: Elevated BUN (9%), elevated serum creatinine (1.1% to 4.7%) Respiratory: Cough (1.9% to 35%)

<1% (Limited to important or life-threatening): Angina, angioedema, anxiety, AV block (first-degree), dyspnea, gout, impotence, increased ALT, increased serum creatinine, insomnia, laryngeal edema, muscle pain, neutropenia, pancreatitis, paresthesia, pruritus, rash, symptomatic hypotension, thrombocytopenia, vertigo. Worsening of renal function may occur in patients with bilateral renal artery stenosis or in hypovolemic patients. In addition, a syndrome which may include fever, myalgia, arthralgia, interstitial nephritis, vasculitis, rash, eosinophilia and positive ANA, and elevated ESR has been reported with ACE inhibitors.

Overdosage/Toxicology Mild hypotension has been the primary toxic effect seen with acute overdose. Bradycardia may also occur. Hyperkalemia occurs even with therapeutic doses, especially in patients with renal insufficiency and those taking NSAIDs. Treatment is symptom-directed and supportive.

Pharmacodynamics/Kinetics

Absorption: Rapid

Half-Life Elimination:

Trandolapril: 6 hours; Trandolaprilat: Effective: 10 hours, Terminal: 24 hours

Time to Peak: Parent: 1 hour; Active metabolite trandolaprilat: 4-10 hours

Metabolism: Hepatically hydrolyzed to active metabolite, trandolaprilat

Onset: 1-2 hours; Peak effect: Reduction in blood pressure: 6 hours

Duration: Prolonged; 72 hours after single dose

Formulations Tablet: 1 mg, 2 mg, 4 mg

Dosing

Adults & Elderly:

Hypertension: Oral; Initial dose in patients not receiving a diuretic: 1 mg/day (2 mg/day in black patients). Adjust dosage according to the blood pressure response. Make dosage adjustments at intervals of ≥1 week. Most patients have required dosages of 2-4 mg/day. There is a little experience with doses >8 mg/day. Patients inadequately treated with once daily dosing at 4 mg may be treated with twice daily dosing. If blood pressure is not adequately controlled with trandolapril monotherapy, a diuretic may be added.

Heart failure postmyocardial infarction or left ventricular dysfunction postmyocardial infarction: Oral: Initial: 1 mg/day; titrate patients (as tolerated) towards the target dose of 4 mg/day. If a 4 mg dose is not tolerated, patients can continue therapy with the greatest tolerated dose.

Renal Impairment: Cl_{cr} ≤30 mL/minute: Administer lowest doses, starting at 0.5 mg/day.

Hepatic Impairment: Patients with hepatic cirrhosis: Start dose at 0.5 mg.

Monitoring Laboratory Tests CBC, electrolytes, renal function, serum calcium; if patient has renal impairment then a baseline WBC with differential and serum creatinine should be evaluated and monitored closely during the first 3 months of therapy.

Monitoring and Teaching Issues

Physical Assessment: See Warnings/Precautions, Contraindications, and Dosing for use cautions. Assess potential for interactions with other prescriptions, OTC medications, or herbal products patient may be taking (especially anything that may impact fluid balance or cardiac status - see Drug Interactions). Assess results of laboratory tests (see above), therapeutic effectiveness, and adverse reactions with first dose and on a regular basis during therapy (eg, hypovolemia, angioedema, postural hypotension - see Adverse Reactions and Overdose/Toxicology). Teach patient appropriate use (according to purpose for use), possible side effects/interventions, and adverse symptoms to report (see Patient Education). **Pregnancy risk factor C/D** - see Pregnancy Risk Factor for use cautions. Instruct patient is use of appropriate barrier contraceptives (see Pregnancy Issues). Breast feeding is contraindicated.

Patient Education: Inform prescriber of all prescriptions, OTC medications, or herbal products you are taking, and any allergies you have. Do not take anything new during treatment unless approved by prescriber. Take exactly as directed; do not discontinue without consulting prescriber. Do not take antacids within 2 hours of this medication. Take first dose at bedtime. This drug does not eliminate need for diet or exercise regimen as recommended by prescriber. May cause dizziness, fainting, or lightheadedness (use caution when driving or engaging in tasks that require alertness until response to drug is known); postural hypotension (use caution when rising from lying or sitting position or climbing stairs); or diarrhea (buttermilk, boiled milk, yogurt may help). Report immediately any swelling of face, mouth, lips, tongue or throat. Report chest pain or palpitations; swelling of extremities, mouth, or tongue; skin rash; difficulty breathing or unusual cough; or other persistent adverse reactions. **Pregnancy/breast-feeding precautions:** Inform prescriber if you are or intend to become pregnant. This drug should not be used in the 2nd or 3rd trimester of pregnancy. Consult prescriber for appropriate contraceptive measures if necessary. Consult prescriber if breast-feeding.

Geriatric Considerations: Due to frequent decreases in glomerular filtration (also creatinine clearance) with aging, elderly patients may have exaggerated responses to ACE inhibitors. Differences in clinical response due to hepatic changes are not observed.

Pregnancy Issues: ACE inhibitors can cause fetal injury or death if taken during the 2nd or 3rd trimester. Discontinue ACE inhibitors as soon as pregnancy is detected.

Related Information

Angiotensin Agents *on page 1547*
Heart Failure *on page 1670*

Trandolapril and Verapamil (tran DOE la pril & ver AP a mil)

U.S. Brand Names Tarka®

Synonyms Verapamil and Trandolapril

Generic Available No

Pharmacologic Category Antihypertensive Agent Combination

Pregnancy Risk Factor C/D (2nd and 3rd trimesters)

Lactation Enters breast milk/contraindicated

Use Combination drug for the treatment of hypertension, however, not indicated for initial treatment of hypertension; replacement therapy in patients receiving separate dosage forms (for patient convenience); when monotherapy with one component fails to achieve desired antihypertensive effect, or when dose-limiting adverse effects limit upward titration of monotherapy

Formulations

Tablet, combination [trandolapril component is immediate release, verapamil component is sustained release]:

Trandolapril 1 mg and verapamil hydrochloride 240 mg
Trandolapril 2 mg and verapamil hydrochloride 180 mg
Trandolapril 2 mg and verapamil hydrochloride 240 mg
Trandolapril 4 mg and verapamil hydrochloride 240 mg

Dosing

Adults: Hypertension: Oral: Individualize dose. Patients receiving trandolapril (up to 8 mg) and verapamil (up to 240 mg) in separate tablets may wish to receive Tarka® at equivalent dosages once daily.

Elderly: Refer to dosing in individual monographs.

Renal Impairment: Usual regimen need not be adjusted unless patient's creatinine clearance is <30 mL/minute. Titration of individual components must be done prior to switching to combination product

Hepatic Impairment: Has not been evaluated in hepatic impairment. Verapamil is hepatically metabolized, adjustment of dosage in hepatic impairment is recommended.

Monitoring and Teaching Issues

Physical Assessment: See individual components listed in Related Information. **Pregnancy risk factor C/D** - see Pregnancy Risk Factor for use cautions. Assess knowledge/instruct patient on need to use appropriate contraceptive measures and the need to avoid pregnancy. Breast-feeding is contraindicated.

Patient Education: See individual components listed in Related Information. **Pregnancy/breast-feeding precautions:** Inform prescriber if you are or intend to become pregnant. Do not breast-feed.

(Continued)

Trandolapril and Verapamil *(Continued)*

Related Information

Trandolapril *on page 1345*
Verapamil *on page 1396*

Transamine Sulphate *see* Tranylcypromine *on page 1348*
Transderm Scōp® *see* Scopolamine *on page 1218*
***trans*-Retinoic Acid** *see* Tretinoin (Topical) *on page 1355*
Tranxene® *see* Clorazepate *on page 320*

Tranylcypromine (tran il SIP roe meen)

U.S. Brand Names Parnate®

Synonyms Transamine Sulphate; Tranylcypromine Sulfate

Generic Available No

Pharmacologic Category Antidepressant, Monoamine Oxidase Inhibitor

Pregnancy Risk Factor C

Lactation Excretion in breast milk unknown/not recommended

Use Treatment of major depressive episode without melancholia

Use - Unlabeled/Investigational Post-traumatic stress disorder

Mechanism of Action/Effect Thought to act by increasing endogenous concentrations of epinephrine, norepinephrine, dopamine, and serotonin through inhibition of the enzyme (monoamine oxidase) responsible for the breakdown of these neurotransmitters

Contraindications Hypersensitivity to tranylcypromine or any component of the formulation; uncontrolled hypertension; pheochromocytoma; hepatic or renal disease; cerebrovascular defect; cardiovascular disease (CHF); concurrent use of sympathomimetics (and related compounds), CNS depressants, ethanol, meperidine, bupropion, buspirone, dexfenfluramine, dextromethorphan, guanethidine, and serotonergic drugs (including SSRIs) - do not use within 5 weeks of fluoxetine discontinuation or 2 weeks of other antidepressant discontinuation; general anesthesia (discontinue 10 days prior to elective surgery); local vasoconstrictors; spinal anesthesia (hypotension may be exaggerated); foods which are high in tyramine, tryptophan, or dopamine, chocolate, or caffeine.

Warnings/Precautions Safety in children <16 years of age has not been established; use with caution in patients who are hyperactive, hyperexcitable, or who have glaucoma, suicidal tendencies, hyperthyroidism, or diabetes; avoid use of meperidine within 2 weeks of tranylcypromine use. Toxic reactions have occurred with dextromethorphan. Hypertensive crisis may occur with tyramine, tryptophan, or dopamine-containing foods. Should not be used in combination with other antidepressants. Hypotensive effects of antihypertensives (beta-blockers, thiazides) may be exaggerated. Use with caution in depressed patients at risk of suicide. May cause orthostatic hypotension (especially at dosages >30 mg/day) - use with caution in patients with hypotension or patients who would not tolerate transient hypotensive episodes - effects may be additive when used with other agents known to cause orthostasis (phenothiazines). Has been associated with activation of hypomania and/or mania in bipolar patients. May worsen psychotic symptoms in some patients. Use with caution in patients at risk of seizures, or in patients receiving other drugs which may lower seizure threshold. Discontinue at least 48 hours prior to myelography. Use with caution in patients receiving disulfiram. Use with caution in patients with renal impairment.

The MAO inhibitors are effective and generally well tolerated by older patients. It is the potential interactions with tyramine or tryptophan-containing foods and other drugs, and their effects on blood pressure that have limited their use.

Pregnancy risk C.

Drug Interactions

Cytochrome P450 Effect: Inhibits CYP1A2, **2A6**, 2C8/9, 2C19, 2D6, 2E1, 3A4

Decreased Effect: Tranylcypromine inhibits the antihypertensive response to guanadrel or guanethidine.

Increased Effect/Toxicity: In general, the combined use of tranylcypromine with TCAs, venlafaxine, trazodone, dexfenfluramine, sibutramine, lithium, meperidine, fenfluramine, dextromethorphan, and SSRIs should be avoided due to the potential for severe adverse reactions (serotonin syndrome, death). Tranylcypromine in combination with amphetamines, other stimulants (methylphenidate), levodopa, metaraminol, buspirone, bupropion, reserpine, and decongestants (pseudoephedrine) may result in severe hypertensive reactions. MAO inhibitors (including tranylcypromine) may inhibit the metabolism of barbiturates and prolong their effect. Foods (eg, cheese) and beverages (eg, ethanol) containing tyramine should be avoided; hypertensive crisis may result. Tranylcypromine may increase the pressor response of norepinephrine and may prolong neuromuscular blockade produced by succinylcholine. Tramadol may increase the risk of seizures and serotonin syndrome in patients receiving an MAO inhibitor. Tranylcypromine may produce additive hypoglycemic effect in patients receiving hypoglycemic agents and may produce delirium in patients receiving disulfiram. Tryptophan combined use with an MAO inhibitor has been reported to cause disorientation, confusion, anxiety, delirium, agitation, hypomanic signs, ataxia, and myoclonus; concurrent use is contraindicated.

Nutritional/Ethanol Interactions

Ethanol: Avoid ethanol (many contain tyramine).

Food: Clinically-severe elevated blood pressure may occur if tranylcypromine is taken with tyramine-containing food. Avoid foods containing tryptophan or dopamine, chocolate or caffeine.

Herb/Nutraceutical: Avoid valerian, St John's wort, SAMe, ginseng. Avoid ginkgo (may lead to MAO inhibitor toxicity). Avoid ephedra, yohimbe (can cause hypertension).

Effects on Lab Values ↓ glucose

Adverse Reactions Frequency not defined.

Cardiovascular: Orthostatic hypotension, edema

Central nervous system: Dizziness, headache, drowsiness, sleep disturbances, fatigue, hyper-reflexia, twitching, ataxia, mania, akinesia, confusion, disorientation, memory loss

Dermatologic: Rash, pruritus, urticaria, localized scleroderma, cystic acne (flare), alopecia
Endocrine & metabolic: Sexual dysfunction (anorgasmia, ejaculatory disturbances, impotence), hypernatremia, hypermetabolic syndrome, SIADH
Gastrointestinal: Xerostomia, constipation, weight gain
Genitourinary: Urinary retention, incontinence
Hematologic: Leukopenia, agranulocytosis
Hepatic: Hepatitis
Neuromuscular & skeletal: Weakness, tremor, myoclonus
Ocular: Blurred vision, glaucoma
Miscellaneous: Diaphoresis

Overdosage/Toxicology Symptoms of overdose include tachycardia, palpitations, muscle twitching, seizures, insomnia, transient hypotension, hypertension, hyperpyrexia, and coma. Treatment is symptom-directed and supportive.

Pharmacodynamics/Kinetics

Half-Life Elimination: 90-190 minutes

Time to Peak: Serum: ~2 hours

Onset: Therapeutic: 2-3 weeks continued dosing

Formulations Tablet, as sulfate: 10 mg

Dosing

Adults: Depression: Oral: 10 mg twice daily for 2 weeks, increase by 10 mg increments at 1- to 3-week intervals; maximum: 60 mg/day

Elderly: Refer to adult dosing and Geriatric Considerations.

Hepatic Impairment: Use with care and monitor plasma levels and patient response closely.

Monitoring Laboratory Tests Blood glucose

Monitoring and Teaching Issues

Physical Assessment: Assess other medications patient may be taking for effectiveness and interactions (see Drug Interactions). See Warnings/Precautions for use cautions. Evaluate need for continued therapy on a regular basis. Monitor laboratory tests, therapeutic response according to rationale for therapy, and adverse reactions at beginning of therapy and periodically with long-term use (see Adverse Reactions and Overdose/Toxicology). Taper dosage slowly when discontinuing. Assess knowledge/teach patient appropriate use, interventions to reduce side effects, and adverse symptoms to report (see Patient Education). See Tyramine Foods List *on page 1601*. **Pregnancy risk factor C** - benefits of use should outweigh possible risks. Breast-feeding is not recommended.

Patient Education: Take exactly as directed; do not increase dose or frequency. It may take 2-3 weeks to achieve desired results. Take in the morning to reduce the incidence of insomnia. Avoid alcohol, caffeine, and other prescription or OTC medications not approved by prescriber. Avoid tyramine-containing foods (eg, pickles, aged cheese, wine); see prescriber for complete list of foods to be avoided. Maintain adequate hydration (2-3 L/day of fluids) unless advised by prescriber to restrict fluids. You may experience drowsiness, dizziness, or blurred vision (use caution when driving or engaging in tasks requiring alertness until response to drug is known); anorexia or dry mouth (small, frequent meals, frequent mouth care, chewing gum, or sucking lozenges may help); constipation (increased exercise, fluids, fruit, or fiber may help); diarrhea (buttermilk, yogurt, or boiled milk may help); or orthostatic hypotension (use caution when climbing stairs or changing position from lying or sitting to standing); or altered sexual ability (reversible). Report persistent excessive sedation; muscle cramping, tremors, weakness, or change in gait; chest pain, palpitations, rapid heartbeat, or swelling of extremities; vision changes; or worsening of condition. **Pregnancy/breast-feeding precautions:** Inform prescriber if you are or intend to become pregnant. Breast-feeding is not recommended.

Dietary Issues: Avoid food which contains high amounts of tyramine. Avoid foods containing tryptophan or dopamine, including chocolate and caffeine.

Geriatric Considerations: MAO inhibitors are effective and generally well tolerated by older patients. Potential interactions with tyramine- or tryptophan-containing foods (see Warnings/Precautions), other drugs, and adverse effects on blood pressure have limited use of MAO inhibitors. They are usually reserved for patients who do not tolerate or respond to traditional "cyclic" or "second generation" antidepressants. Tranylcypromine is the preferred MAO inhibitor because its enzymatic-blocking effects are more rapidly reversed. The brain activity of monoamine oxidase increases with age and even more so in patients with Alzheimer's disease. Therefore, MAO inhibitors may have an increased role in treating depressed patients with Alzheimer's disease.

Additional Information Tranylcypromine has a more rapid onset of therapeutic effect than other MAO inhibitors, but causes more severe hypertensive reactions.

Related Information

Antidepressant Agents *on page 1553*
Antidepressant Medication Guidelines *on page 1613*
Tyramine Foods List *on page 1601*

Tranylcypromine Sulfate *see* Tranylcypromine *on page 1348*

Trastuzumab (tras TU zoo mab)

U.S. Brand Names Herceptin®

Generic Available No

Pharmacologic Category Monoclonal Antibody

Pregnancy Risk Factor B

Lactation Excretion in breast milk unknown/not recommended

Use

Single agent for the treatment of patients with metastatic breast cancer whose tumors overexpress the HER-2/*neu* protein and who have received one or more chemotherapy regimens for their metastatic disease

Combination therapy with paclitaxel for the treatment of patients with metastatic breast cancer whose tumors overexpress the HER-2/*neu* protein and who have not received chemotherapy for their metastatic disease

(Continued)

Trastuzumab *(Continued)*

Note: HER-2/*neu* protein overexpression or amplification has been noted in ovarian, gastric, colorectal, endometrial, lung, bladder, prostate, and salivary gland tumors. It is not yet known whether trastuzumab may be effective in these other carcinomas which overexpress HER-2/*neu* protein.

Mechanism of Action/Effect Trastuzumab is a monoclonal antibody which binds to the extracellular domain of the human epidermal growth factor receptor 2 protein (HER-2). It mediates antibody-dependent cellular cytotoxicity against cells which overproduce HER-2.

Contraindications No specific contraindications noted in product labeling. However, patients experiencing severe hypersensitivity reactions have been reported to have repeat episodes despite pretreatment with antihistamines and corticosteroids.

Warnings/Precautions Congestive heart failure associated with trastuzumab may be severe and has been associated with disabling cardiac failure, death, mural thrombus, and stroke. Left ventricular function should be evaluated in all patients prior to and during treatment with trastuzumab. Discontinuation should be strongly considered in patients who develop a clinically significant decrease in ejection fraction during therapy. Combination therapy which includes anthracyclines and cyclophosphamide increases the incidence and severity of cardiac dysfunction. Extreme caution should be used when treating patients with pre-existing cardiac disease or dysfunction, and in patients with previous exposure to anthracyclines. Advanced age may also predispose to cardiac toxicity. Use with caution in patients with known hypersensitivity to trastuzumab, Chinese hamster ovary cell preparations or any component of this product.

Serious adverse events, including hypersensitivity reaction (anaphylaxis), infusion reactions (including fatalities), and pulmonary events (including adult respiratory distress syndrome) have been associated with trastuzumab. Most of these events occur within 24 hours of infusion, however, delayed reactions have occurred. Use with caution in pre-existing pulmonary disease. Discontinuation of trastuzumab should be strongly considered in any patient who develops anaphylaxis, angioedema, or acute respiratory distress syndrome. Retreatment of patients who experienced severe hypersensitivity reactions has been attempted (with premedication). Some patients tolerated retreatment, while others experienced a second severe reaction.

Drug Interactions

Increased Effect/Toxicity: Paclitaxel may result in a decrease in clearance of trastuzumab, increasing serum concentrations.

Adverse Reactions

>10%:

- Central nervous system: Pain (47%), fever (36%), chills (32%), headache (26%)
- Dermatologic: Rash (18%)
- Gastrointestinal: Nausea (33%), diarrhea (25%), vomiting (23%), abdominal pain (22%), anorexia (14%)
- Neuromuscular & skeletal: Weakness (42%), back pain (22%)
- Respiratory: Cough (26%), dyspnea (22%), rhinitis (14%), pharyngitis (12%)
- Miscellaneous: Infection (20%)

1% to 10%:

- Cardiovascular: Peripheral edema (10%), CHF (7%), tachycardia (5%)
- Central nervous system: Insomnia (14%), dizziness (13%), paresthesia (9%), depression (6%), peripheral neuritis (2%), neuropathy (1%)
- Dermatologic: Herpes simplex (2%), acne (2%)
- Gastrointestinal: Nausea and vomiting (8%)
- Genitourinary: Urinary tract infection (5%)
- Hematologic: Anemia (4%), leukopenia (3%)
- Neuromuscular & skeletal: Bone pain (7%), arthralgia (6%)
- Respiratory: Sinusitis (9%)
- Miscellaneous: Flu syndrome (10%), accidental injury (6%), allergic reaction (3%)

<1% (Limited to important or life-threatening): Amblyopia, anaphylactoid reaction, arrhythmia, ascites, cardiac arrest, cellulitis, coagulopathy, deafness, esophageal ulcer, hematemesis, hemorrhage, hepatic failure, hepatitis, hydrocephalus, hypotension, hypothyroidism, ileus, intestinal obstruction, pancreatitis, pancytopenia, pericardial effusion, radiation injury, shock, stomatitis, syncope, vascular thrombosis

Overdosage/Toxicology There is no experience with overdose in human clinical trials. Treatment is supportive.

Pharmacodynamics/Kinetics

Half-Life Elimination: Mean: 5.8 days (range: 1-32 days)

Formulations Injection [vial; with vial of bacteriostatic water]: 440 mg

Dosing

Adults & Elderly: Metastatic breast carcinoma: I.V.:

Loading dose: 4 mg/kg over 90 minutes; do not administer as an I.V. bolus or I.V. push.

Maintenance dose: 2 mg/kg once weekly (may be infused over 30 minutes if prior infusions are well tolerated).

Renal Impairment: No adjustment is necessary.

Hepatic Impairment: No adjustment necessary.

Administration

I.V.: Administer initial infusion over 90 minutes. Subsequent weekly infusions may be administered over 30 minutes if prior infusions are well tolerated. During the first infusion with trastuzumab, a complex of symptoms most commonly consisting of chills, and/or fever were observed in ~40% of patients. These symptoms were usually mild to moderate in severity and were treated with acetaminophen, diphenhydramine and meperidine (with or without reduction in the rate of trastuzumab infusion). These symptoms occurred infrequently with subsequent trastuzumab infusions.

Stability

Storage: Store under refrigeration at 2°C to 8°C (36°F to 46°F) prior to reconstitution.

Reconstitution: Prepare each vial by reconstituting with 20 mL of bacteriostatic water for injection (supplied in carton). If patient has a known hypersensitivity to benzyl alcohol, it may be reconstituted with sterile water for injection. Stable for 28 days after reconstitution if refrigerated; do not freeze. If sterile water for injection without preservative is used for reconstitution, it must be used immediately. After dilution in 0.9% sodium chloride for injection in polyethylene bags, solution is stable for 24 hours.

Monitoring and Teaching Issues

Physical Assessment: Monitor therapeutic response and adverse reactions (see Warnings/Precautions and Adverse Reactions). Monitor vital signs during transfusion. Assess knowledge/teach patient interventions to reduce side effects and adverse symptoms to report (see Patient Education). Breast-feeding is not recommended.

Patient Education: This medication can only be administered by infusion. Report immediately any adverse reactions during infusion (eg, difficulty breathing, chills, fever, headache, backache, or nausea/vomiting) so appropriate medication can be administered. You will be susceptible to infection (avoid crowds and exposure to infection). You may experience dizziness or weakness (use caution when driving or engaging in tasks requiring alertness until response to drug is known); nausea or vomiting (small, frequent meals, frequent mouth care, chewing gum, or sucking lozenges may help); diarrhea (boiled milk, yogurt, or buttermilk may help); or headache, back or joint pain (mild analgesics may offer relief). Report persistent GI effects; sore throat, runny nose, or difficulty breathing; chest pain, irregular heartbeat, palpitations, swelling of extremities, or unusual weight gain; muscle or joint weakness, numbness, or pain; skin rash or irritation; itching or pain on urination; unhealed sores, white plaques in mouth or genital area, unusual bruising or bleeding; or other unusual adverse effects. **Breast-feeding precaution:** Breast-feeding is not recommended.

Breast-feeding Issues: It is not known whether trastuzumab is secreted in human milk. Because many immunoglobulins are secreted in milk, and the potential for serious adverse reactions exists, patients should discontinue nursing during treatment and for 6 months after the last dose.

Travatan™ Trusopt® *see* Ophthalmic Agents, Glaucoma *on page 1002*

Travoprost *see page 1575*

Travoprost *see* Ophthalmic Agents, Glaucoma *on page 1002*

Trazodone (TRAZ oh done)

U.S. Brand Names Desyrel®

Synonyms Trazodone Hydrochloride

Generic Available Yes

Pharmacologic Category Antidepressant, Serotonin Reuptake Inhibitor/Antagonist

Pregnancy Risk Factor C

Lactation Enters breast milk/contraindicated (AAP rates "of concern")

Use Treatment of depression

Use - Unlabeled/Investigational Potential augmenting agent for antidepressants, hypnotic

Mechanism of Action/Effect Inhibits reuptake of serotonin, causes adrenoreceptor subsensitivity, and induces significant changes in 5HT presynaptic receptor adrenoreceptors. Trazodone also significantly blocks histamine (H1) and alpha$_1$ adrenergic receptors.

Contraindications Hypersensitivity to trazodone or any component of the formulation

Warnings/Precautions Priapism, including cases resulting in permanent dysfunction, has occurred with the use of trazodone. Not recommended for use in a patient during the acute recovery phase of MI. Trazodone should be initiated with extreme caution in patients who are receiving concurrent or recent therapy with a MAO inhibitor. May cause sedation, resulting in impaired performance of tasks requiring alertness (ie, operating machinery or driving). Sedative effects may be additive with other CNS depressants and ethanol. The degree of sedation is very high relative to other antidepressants. May worsen psychosis in some patients or precipitate a shift to mania or hypomania in patients with bipolar disease. May increase the risks associated with electroconvulsive therapy. This agent should be discontinued, when possible, prior to elective surgery. Therapy should not be abruptly discontinued in patients receiving high doses for prolonged periods.

Use with caution in patients at risk of hypotension or in patients where transient hypotensive episodes would be poorly tolerated (cardiovascular or cerebrovascular disease). The risk of postural hypotension is high relative to other antidepressants. Use caution in patients with depression, particularly if suicidal risk may be present. Use caution in patients with a previous seizure disorder or condition predisposing to seizures such as brain damage, alcoholism, or concurrent therapy with other drugs which lower the seizure threshold. Use with caution in patients with hepatic or renal dysfunction and in elderly patients. Use with caution in patients with a history of cardiovascular disease (including previous MI, stroke, tachycardia, or conduction abnormalities). However, the risk of conduction abnormalities with this agent is low relative to other antidepressants.

Pregnancy risk C.

Drug Interactions

Cytochrome P450 Effect: Substrate of CYP2D6, **3A4**; Inhibits CYP2D6

Decreased Effect: Trazodone inhibits the hypotensive response to clonidine.

Increased Effect/Toxicity: Trazodone, in combination with other serotonergic agents (buspirone, MAO inhibitors), may produce additive serotonergic effects, including serotonin syndrome. Trazodone, in combination with other psychotropics (low potency antipsychotics), may result in additional hypotension. Trazodone, in combination with ethanol, may result in additive sedation and impairment of motor skills. Fluoxetine may inhibit the metabolism of trazodone resulting in elevated plasma levels.

Nutritional/Ethanol Interactions

Ethanol: Avoid ethanol (may increase CNS depression).

Food: Time to peak serum levels may be increased if trazodone is taken with food.

(Continued)

Trazodone *(Continued)*

Herb/Nutraceutical: Avoid valerian, St John's wort, SAMe, kava kava (may increase risk of serotonin syndrome and/or excessive sedation).

Adverse Reactions

>10%:

Central nervous system: Dizziness, headache, sedation

Gastrointestinal: Nausea, xerostomia

1% to 10%:

Cardiovascular: Syncope, hypertension, hypotension, edema

Central nervous system: Confusion, decreased concentration, fatigue, incoordination

Gastrointestinal: Diarrhea, constipation, weight gain/loss

Neuromuscular & skeletal: Tremor, myalgia

Ocular: Blurred vision

Respiratory: Nasal congestion

<1% (Limited to important or life-threatening): Agitation, bradycardia, extrapyramidal reactions, hepatitis, priapism, rash, seizures, tachycardia, urinary retention

Overdosage/Toxicology Symptoms of overdose include drowsiness, vomiting, hypotension, tachycardia, incontinence, coma, and priapism. Treatment is symptom-directed and supportive.

Pharmacodynamics/Kinetics

Half-Life Elimination: 7-8 hours, two compartment kinetics

Time to Peak: Serum: 30-100 minutes; delayed with food (up to 2.5 hours)

Metabolism: Hepatic

Onset: Therapeutic: 1-3 weeks

Formulations Tablet, as hydrochloride: 50 mg, 100 mg, 150 mg, 300 mg

Dosing

Adults:

Depression: Oral: Initial: 150 mg/day in 3 divided doses (may increase by 50 mg/day every 3-7 days); maximum: 600 mg/day

Note: Therapeutic effects may take up to 6 weeks. Therapy is normally maintained for 6-12 months after optimum response is reached to prevent recurrence of depression.

Sedation/hypnotic (unlabeled use): Oral: 25-50 mg at bedtime (often in combination with daytime SSRIs). May increase up to 200 mg at bedtime.

Elderly: Therapeutic effects may take up to 4 weeks. Therapy is normally maintained for several months after optimum response is reached to prevent recurrence of depression.

Oral: 25-50 mg at bedtime with 25-50 mg/day dose increase every 3 days for inpatients and weekly for outpatients, if tolerated; usual dose: 75-150 mg/day

Pediatrics:

Children 6-12 years: Depression: Initial: 1.5-2 mg/kg/day in divided doses; increase gradually every 3-4 days as needed; maximum: 6 mg/kg/day in 3 divided doses

Adolescents: Depression: Initial: 25-50 mg/day; increase to 100-150 mg/day in divided doses

Administration

Oral: Dosing after meals may decrease lightheadedness and postural hypotension.

Monitoring Laboratory Tests Baseline liver function prior to and periodically during therapy

Monitoring and Teaching Issues

Physical Assessment: Assess other medications patient may be taking for effectiveness and interactions (see Drug Interactions). See Contraindications and Warnings/Precautions for use cautions. Periodically review need for continued therapy. Monitor laboratory tests, therapeutic response according to rationale for therapy, and adverse reactions at beginning of therapy and periodically with long-term use (see Adverse Reactions and Overdose/Toxicology). Taper dosage slowly when discontinuing (allow 3-4 weeks between discontinuing Desyrel® and starting another antidepressant). Assess knowledge/teach patient appropriate use, interventions to reduce side effects, and adverse symptoms to report (see Patient Education). **Pregnancy risk factor C** - benefits of use should outweigh possible risks. Breast-feeding is contraindicated.

Patient Education: Take exactly as directed; do not increase dose or frequency. It may take 2-4 weeks to achieve desired results. Take after meals. Avoid alcohol, caffeine, and other prescription or OTC medications not approved by prescriber. Maintain adequate hydration (2-3 L/day of fluids) unless advised by prescriber to restrict fluids. You may experience drowsiness, lightheadedness, dizziness (use caution when driving or engaging in tasks requiring alertness until response to drug is known); postural hypotension (use caution when climbing stairs or changing position from lying or sitting to standing); nausea, dry mouth (small, frequent meals, frequent mouth care, chewing gum, or sucking lozenges may help); constipation (increased exercise, fluids, fruit, or fiber may help); or diarrhea (buttermilk, yogurt, or boiled milk may help). Report persistent dizziness or headache; muscle cramping, tremors, or altered gait; blurred vision or eye pain; chest pain or irregular heartbeat; or worsening of condition. **Pregnancy/breast-feeding precautions:** Inform prescriber if you are or intend to become pregnant. Do not breast-feed.

Geriatric Considerations: Very sedating, but little anticholinergic effects.

Additional Information Therapeutic effect for sleep occurs in 1-3 hours

Related Information

Antidepressant Agents *on page 1553*

Trazodone Hydrochloride *see* Trazodone *on page 1351*

Treatment of Sexually Transmitted Diseases *see page 1701*

Trelstar™ Depot *see* Triptorelin *on page 1371*

Trelstar™ LA *see* Triptorelin *on page 1371*

Trental® *see* Pentoxifylline *on page 1057*

Tretinoin and Mequinol *see* Mequinol and Tretinoin *on page 854*

Tretinoin, Fluocinolone Acetonide, and Hydroquinone *see* Fluocinolone, Hydroquinone, and Tretinoin *on page 574*

Tretinoin (Oral) (TRET i noyn OR al)

U.S. Brand Names Vesanoid®

Synonyms All-*trans*-Retinoic Acid

Generic Available No

Pharmacologic Category Antineoplastic Agent, Miscellaneous

Pregnancy Risk Factor D

Lactation Enters breast milk/not recommended

Use Acute promyelocytic leukemia (APL): Induction of remission in patients with APL, French American British (FAB) classification M3 (including the M3 variant), characterized by the presence of the t(15;17) translocation or the presence of the PML/RARα gene who are refractory to or who have relapsed from anthracycline chemotherapy, or for whom anthracycline-based chemotherapy is contraindicated. Tretinoin is for the induction of remission only. All patients should receive an accepted form of remission consolidation or maintenance therapy for APL after completion of induction therapy with tretinoin.

Mechanism of Action/Effect Retinoid that induces maturation of acute promyelocytic leukemia (APL) cells in cultures; induces cytodifferentiation and decreased proliferation of APL cells

Contraindications Sensitivity to parabens, vitamin A, other retinoids, or any component of the formulation; pregnancy

Warnings/Precautions Patients with acute promyelocytic leukemia (APL) are at high risk and can have severe adverse reactions to tretinoin. Administer under the supervision of a physician who is experienced in the management of patients with acute leukemia and in a facility with laboratory and supportive services sufficient to monitor drug tolerance and to protect and maintain a patient compromised by drug toxicity, including respiratory compromise.

May cause retinoic acid-APL (RA-APL) syndrome (fever, dyspnea, pulmonary infiltrates, pleural/pericardial effusions, cardiac dysfunction). May be treated with high-dose steroids. The majority of patients do not require termination of tretinoin therapy. During treatment, rapidly evolving leukocytosis is associated with a higher risk of life-threatening complications.

Not to be used in women of childbearing potential unless the woman is capable of complying with effective contraceptive measures; therapy is normally begun on the second or third day of next normal menstrual period; two reliable methods of effective contraception must be used during therapy and for 1 month after discontinuation of therapy, unless abstinence is the chosen method. Within one week prior to the institution of tretinoin therapy, the patient should have blood or urine collected for a serum or urine pregnancy test with a sensitivity of at least 50 mIU/L. When possible, delay tretinoin therapy until a negative result from this test is obtained. When a delay is not possible, place the patient on two reliable forms of contraception. Repeat pregnancy testing and contraception counseling monthly throughout the period of treatment.

Initiation of therapy with tretinoin may be based on the morphological diagnosis of APL. Confirm the diagnosis of APL by detection of the t(15;17) genetic marker by cytogenetic studies. If these are negative, PML/RARα fusion should be sought using molecular diagnostic techniques. The response rate of other AML subtypes to tretinoin has not been demonstrated.

Retinoids have been associated with pseudotumor cerebri (benign intracranial hypertension), especially in children. Up to 60% of patients experienced reversible hypercholesterolemia or hypertriglyceridemia. Monitor liver function during treatment.

Drug Interactions

Cytochrome P450 Effect: Substrate of CYP2A6, 2B6, 2C8/9; Inhibits CYP2C8/9; Induces CYP2E1

Increased Effect/Toxicity: Ketoconazole increases the mean plasma AUC of tretinoin. Other drugs which inhibit CYP3A4 would be expected to increase tretinoin concentrations, potentially increasing toxicity.

Nutritional/Ethanol Interactions

Ethanol: Avoid ethanol (may increase CNS depression).

Food: Absorption of retinoids has been shown to be enhanced when taken with food.

Herb/Nutraceutical: St John's wort may decrease tretinoin levels. Avoid dong quai, St John's wort (may also cause photosensitization). Avoid additional vitamin A supplementation. May lead to vitamin A toxicity.

Adverse Reactions Virtually all patients experience some drug-related toxicity, especially headache, fever, weakness and fatigue. These adverse effects are seldom permanent or irreversible nor do they usually require therapy interruption

About 25% of patients with APL, who have been treated with tretinoin, have experienced a syndrome called the retinoic acid-APL (RA-APL) syndrome (fever, dyspnea, weight gain, pulmonary infiltrates and pleural or pericardial effusions). Occasionally accompanied by impaired myocardial contractility and episodic hypotension, with or without concomitant leukocytosis. High-dose steroids given at the first suspicion of RA-APL syndrome appear to reduce morbidity and mortality (dexamethasone 10 mg I.V. every 12 hours for 3 days or until resolution of symptoms). Many patients do not require termination of tretinoin therapy during treatment of the RA-APL syndrome.

>10%:

- Cardiovascular: Arrhythmias, flushing, hypotension, hypertension, peripheral edema, chest discomfort, edema
- Central nervous system: Dizziness, anxiety, insomnia, depression, confusion, malaise, pain
- Dermatologic: Burning, redness, cheilitis, inflammation of lips, dry skin, pruritus, photosensitivity
- Endocrine & metabolic: Increased triglycerides, increased cholesterol (up to 60%)
- Gastrointestinal: GI hemorrhage, abdominal pain, other GI disorders, diarrhea, constipation, heartburn, abdominal distention, weight gain/loss, anorexia, dry mouth

(Continued)

Tretinoin (Oral) *(Continued)*

Hematologic: Hemorrhage, disseminated intravascular coagulation Hepatic: Increased transaminases (50% to 60%)
Local: Phlebitis, injection site reactions
Neuromuscular & skeletal: Bone pain, arthralgia, myalgia, paresthesia
Ocular: Itching of eye
Renal: Renal insufficiency
Respiratory: Upper respiratory tract disorders, dyspnea, respiratory insufficiency, pleural effusion, pneumonia, rales, expiratory wheezing, dry nose
Miscellaneous: Infections, shivering

1% to 10% (Limited to important or life-threatening):
Cardiovascular: Cardiac failure, cardiac arrest, myocardial infarction, stroke, myocarditis, pericarditis, pulmonary hypertension, cardiomyopathy, cerebral hemorrhage
Central nervous system: Intracranial hypertension, agitation, hallucination, aphasia, cerebellar edema, convulsions, coma, CNS depression, encephalopathy, hypotaxia, no light reflex, neurologic reaction, spinal cord disorder, dementia, somnolence, hypothermia
Dermatologic: Skin peeling on hands or soles of feet, rash, cellulitis
Hepatic: Ascites, hepatitis
Neuromuscular & skeletal: Tremor, hyporeflexia, dysarthria, facial paralysis, hemiplegia, asterixis, abnormal gait
Ocular: Dry eyes, photophobia
Renal: Acute renal failure, renal tubular necrosis
Respiratory: Asthma, pulmonary/laryngeal edema

<1% (Limited to important or life-threatening): Alopecia, hepatitis, pseudomotor cerebri

Overdosage/Toxicology Symptoms of overdose include transient headache, facial flushing, cheilosis, abdominal pain, dizziness, and ataxia. All signs or symptoms have been transient and have resolved without apparent residual effects.

Pharmacodynamics/Kinetics

Half-Life Elimination: Terminal: Parent drug: 0.5-2 hours

Time to Peak: Serum: 1-2 hours

Metabolism: Hepatic via CYP

Formulations Capsule: 10 mg

Dosing

Adults & Elderly: Induction of remission in patients with APL: Oral: 45 mg/m^2/day administered as two evenly divided doses until complete remission is documented. Discontinue therapy 30 days after achievement of complete remission or after 90 days of treatment, whichever occurs first. If after initiation of treatment the presence of the t(15;17) translocation is not confirmed by cytogenetics or by polymerase chain reaction studies and the patient has not responded to tretinoin, consider alternative therapy.

Note: Tretinoin is for the induction of remission only. Optimal consolidation or maintenance regimens have not been determined. All patients should therefore receive a standard consolidation or maintenance chemotherapy regimen for APL after induction therapy with tretinoin unless otherwise contraindicated.

Pediatrics: Oral: Children: There are limited clinical data on the pediatric use of tretinoin. Of 15 pediatric patients (age range: 1-16 years) treated with tretinoin, the incidence of complete remission was 67%. Safety and efficacy in pediatric patients <1 year of age have not been established. Some pediatric patients experience severe headache and pseudotumor cerebri, requiring analgesic treatment and lumbar puncture for relief. Increased caution is recommended. Consider dose reduction in children experiencing serious or intolerable toxicity; however, the efficacy and safety of tretinoin at doses <45 mg/m^2/day have not been evaluated.
Also see Note in adult dosing.

Administration

Oral: Administer with meals. Do not crush capsules.

Monitoring Laboratory Tests Monitor the patient's hematologic profile, coagulation profile, liver function results and triglyceride and cholesterol levels frequently. Consider temporary discontinuation if LFTs are >5 times the upper limit of normal.

Monitoring and Teaching Issues

Physical Assessment: See extensive and specific Warnings/Precautions, and Contraindications for use cautions. Assess potential for interactions with other prescriptions, OTC medications, or herbal products patient may be taking (see Drug Interactions). Assess results of laboratory tests closely. Patient will require close monitoring (eg, cardiac, CNS, and respiratory status) on a regular (frequent) basis during therapy. Teach patient appropriate use, possible side effects/ interventions, and adverse symptoms to report (see Patient Education). **Pregnancy risk factor D** - determine that patient is not pregnant before beginning treatment. Instruct patients of childbearing age or males who may have intercourse with women of childbearing age on use of appropriate barrier contraceptive measures during and for 1 month following therapy (see Warnings Precautions). Breast-feeding is not recommended.

Patient Education: Inform prescriber of all prescriptions, OTC medications, or herbal products you are taking, and any allergies you have. Do not take anything new during treatment unless approved by prescriber. Take with food. Do not crush, chew, or dissolve capsules. Maintain adequate hydration (2-3 L/day of fluids) unless advised by prescriber to restrict fluids. Avoid alcohol and foods containing vitamin A, and foods with high fat content. May cause lethargy, dizziness, visual changes, confusion, anxiety (avoid driving or engaging in tasks requiring alertness until response to drug is known); nausea, vomiting, loss of appetite, or dry mouth (small, frequent meals, chewing gum, or sucking lozenges may help); photosensitivity (use sunscreen, wear protective clothing and eyewear, and avoid direct sunlight); dry, itchy skin; or dry or irritated eyes (avoid contact lenses). Report persistent vomiting or diarrhea, difficulty breathing, unusual bleeding or bruising, acute GI pain, bone pain, swelling of extremities, unusual weight gain, or vision changes immediately. **Pregnancy/breast-feeding precautions:** Do not get pregnant (females) or cause a pregnancy (males) while taking this medication and for 1 month following completion of therapy. Consult prescriber for appropriate barrier contraceptive measures. Breast-feeding is not recommended.

Tretinoin (Topical) (TRET i noyn TOP i kal)

U.S. Brand Names Altinac™; Avita®; Renova®; Retin-A®; Retin-A® Micro

Synonyms Retinoic Acid; *trans*-Retinoic Acid; Vitamin A Acid

Generic Available Yes

Pharmacologic Category Retinoic Acid Derivative

Pregnancy Risk Factor C

Lactation Enters breast milk/compatible

Use Treatment of acne vulgaris; photodamaged skin; palliation of fine wrinkles, mottled hyperpigmentation, and tactile roughness of facial skin as part of a comprehensive skin care and sun avoidance program

Use - Unlabeled/Investigational Some skin cancers

Mechanism of Action/Effect Keratinocytes in the sebaceous follicle become less adherent which allows for easy removal; decreases microcomedone formation

Contraindications Hypersensitivity to tretinoin or any component of the formulation; sunburn

Warnings/Precautions Use with caution in patients with eczema; avoid excessive exposure to sunlight and sunlamps; avoid contact with abraded skin, mucous membranes, eyes, mouth, angles of the nose. Palliation of fine wrinkles, mottled hyperpigmentation, and tactile roughness of facial skin: Do not use the 0.05% cream for longer than 48 weeks or the 0.02% cream for longer than 52 weeks. Not for use on moderate- to heavily-pigmented skin. Gel is flammable; do not expose to high temperatures or flame. Pregnancy risk C.

Drug Interactions

Cytochrome P450 Effect: Substrate of CYP2A6, 2B6, 2C8/9; Inhibits CYP2C8/9; Induces CYP2E1

Increased Effect/Toxicity: Topical application of sulfur, benzoyl peroxide, salicylic acid, resorcinol, or any product with strong drying effects potentiates adverse reactions with tretinoin.

Photosensitizing medications (thiazides, tetracyclines, fluoroquinolones, phenothiazines, sulfonamides) augment phototoxicity and should not be used when treating palliation of fine wrinkles, mottled hyperpigmentation, and tactile roughness of facial skin.

Nutritional/Ethanol Interactions

Food: Avoid excessive intake of vitamin A (cod liver oil, halibut fish oil).

Herb/Nutraceutical: Avoid dong quai, St John's wort (may also cause photosensitization). Avoid excessive amounts of vitamin A supplements.

Adverse Reactions

>10%: Dermatologic: Excessive dryness, erythema, scaling of the skin, pruritus

1% to 10%:

Dermatologic: Hyperpigmentation or hypopigmentation, photosensitivity, initial acne flare-up

Local: Edema, blistering, stinging

Overdosage/Toxicology

Excessive application may lead to marked redness, peeling or discomfort. Oral ingestion of the topical product may lead to the same adverse reactions seen with excessive vitamin A intake (increased intracranial pressure, jaundice, ascites, cutaneous desquamation; symptoms of acute overdose [12,000 units/kg] include nausea, vomiting, and diarrhea); toxic signs of an overdose commonly respond to drug discontinuation, and generally return to normal spontaneously within a few days to weeks. Toxic signs of a topical overdose commonly respond to drug discontinuation, and generally resolve spontaneously within a few days to weeks.

When confronted with signs of increased intracranial pressure, treatment with mannitol (0.25 g/kg I.V. up to 1 g/kg/dose repeated every 5 minutes as needed), dexamethasone (1.5 mg/kg I.V. load followed with 0.375 mg/kg every 6 hours for 5 days), and/or hyperventilation should be employed.

Pharmacodynamics/Kinetics

Absorption: Minimal

Metabolism: Hepatic for the small amount absorbed

Formulations

Cream, topical:

Altinac™: 0.025% (20 g, 45 g); 0.05% (20 g, 45 g); 0.1% (20 g, 45 g)

Avita®: 0.025% (20 g, 45 g)

Retin-A®: 0.025% (20 g, 45 g); 0.05% (20 g, 45 g); 0.1% (20 g, 45 g)

Cream, emollient, topical (Renova®): 0.02% (40 g); 0.05% (20 g, 40 g, 60 g)

Gel, topical:

Retin-A®: 0.01% (15 g, 45 g); 0.025% (15 g, 45 g)

Retin-A® Micro [microsphere]: 0.04% (20 g, 45 g); 0.1% (20 g, 45 g)

Liquid, topical (Retin-A®): 0.05% (28 mL)

Dosing

Adults:

Acne vulgaris: Topical: Begin therapy with a weaker formulation of tretinoin (0.025% cream, 0.04% microsphere gel, or 0.01% gel) and increase the concentration as tolerated; apply once daily to acne lesions before retiring or on alternate days; if stinging or irritation develop, decrease frequency of application

Palliation of fine wrinkles, mottled hyperpigmentation, and tactile roughness of facial skin: Topical: Pea-sized amount of the 0.02% or 0.05% emollient cream applied to entire face once daily in the evening

Elderly: Use of the 0.02% emollient cream in patients 65-71 years of age showed similar improvement in fine wrinkles as seen in patients <65 years. Safety and efficacy of the 0.02% cream have not been established in patients >71 years of age. Safety and efficacy of the 0.05% cream have not been established in patients >50 years of age.

(Continued)

Tretinoin (Topical) *(Continued)*

Pediatrics: Children >12 years: Acne vulgaris: Topical: Refer to adult dosing.

Stability

Storage: Store at 25°C (77°F); gel is flammable, keep away from heat and flame

Monitoring and Teaching Issues

Physical Assessment: Assess knowledge/instruct patient on appropriate application, possible adverse effects, and symptoms to report (see Patient Education). **Pregnancy risk factor C.**

Patient Education: For once-daily use, do not overuse. Avoid increased intake of vitamin A. Thoroughly wash hands before applying. Wash area to be treated at least 30 minutes before applying. Do not wash face more frequently than 2-3 times a day. Do not apply to areas near your mouth, eyes, corners of your nose, or open sores. Avoid using topical preparations that contain alcohol or harsh chemicals during treatment. It may take several weeks before the full benefit of the medication is seen. You may experience increased sensitivity to sunlight; protect skin with sunblock (minimum SPF 15), wear protective clothing, and avoid direct sunlight. Stop treatment and inform prescriber if rash, skin irritation, redness, scaling, or excessive dryness occurs. When used for hyperpigmentation and tactile redness of facial skin, wrinkles will not be eliminated. Must be used in combination with a comprehensive skin care program. **Pregnancy precaution:** Inform prescriber if you are pregnant.

Gel: Flammable; do not expose to flame and do not smoke during use.

Pregnancy Issues: Clinical effects on the fetus: Oral tretinoin is teratogenic and fetotoxic in rats at doses 1000 and 500 times the topical human dose, respectively. Tretinoin does not appear to be teratogenic when used topically since it is rapidly metabolized by the skin; however, there are rare reports of fetal defects. Use for acne only if benefit to mother outweighs potential risk to fetus. During pregnancy, do not use for palliation of fine wrinkles, mottled hyperpigmentation, and tactile roughness of facial skin.

Trexall™ *see* Methotrexate *on page 874*

Triacet™ *see* Topical Corticosteroids *on page 1334*

Triacet™ *see* Triamcinolone *on page 1356*

Triaconazole *see* Terconazole *on page 1292*

Triam-A® *see* Triamcinolone *on page 1356*

Triamcinolone *see* Topical Corticosteroids *on page 1334*

Triamcinolone (trye am SIN oh lone)

U.S. Brand Names Amcort®; Aristocort®; Aristocort® A; Aristocort® Forte; Aristocort® Intralesional; Aristospan® Intra-Articular; Aristospan® Intralesional; Atolone®; Azmacort®; Delta-Tritex®; Flutex®; Kenacort®; Kenaject-40®; Kenalog®; Kenalog-10®; Kenalog-40®; Kenalog® H; Kenalog® in Orabase®; Kenonel®; Nasacort®; Nasacort® AQ; Tac™-3; Tac™-40; Triacet™; Triam-A®; Triam Forte®; Triderm®; Tri-Kort®; Trilog®; Trilone®; Tri-Nasal®; Tristoject®

Synonyms Triamcinolone Acetonide, Aerosol; Triamcinolone Acetonide, Parenteral; Triamcinolone Diacetate, Oral; Triamcinolone Diacetate, Parenteral; Triamcinolone Hexacetonide; Triamcinolone, Oral

Generic Available Yes

Pharmacologic Category Corticosteroid, Adrenal; Corticosteroid, Inhalant (Oral); Corticosteroid, Nasal; Corticosteroid, Systemic; Corticosteroid, Topical

Pregnancy Risk Factor C

Lactation Excretion in breast milk unknown

Use

Inhalation: Control of bronchial asthma and related bronchospastic conditions.

Intranasal: Management of seasonal and perennial allergic rhinitis in patients ≥12 years of age

Systemic: Adrenocortical insufficiency, rheumatic disorders, allergic states, respiratory diseases, systemic lupus erythematosus, and other diseases requiring anti-inflammatory or immunosuppressive effects

Topical: Inflammatory dermatoses responsive to steroids

Mechanism of Action/Effect Decreases inflammation by suppression of migration of polymorphonuclear leukocytes and reversal of increased capillary permeability; suppresses the immune system by reducing activity and volume of the lymphatic system; suppresses adrenal function at high doses

Contraindications Hypersensitivity to triamcinolone or any component of the formulation; systemic fungal infections; serious infections (except septic shock or tuberculous meningitis); primary treatment of status asthmaticus

Warnings/Precautions Not to be used in status asthmaticus or for the relief of acute bronchospasm. May cause suppression of hypothalamic-pituitary-adrenal (HPA) axis, particularly in younger children or in patients receiving high doses for prolonged periods. Fatalities have occurred due to adrenal insufficiency in asthmatic patients during and after transfer from systemic corticosteroids to aerosol steroids; aerosol steroids do **not** provide the systemic steroid needed to treat patients having trauma, surgery, or infections. Withdrawal and discontinuation of the corticosteroid should be done slowly and carefully

Controlled clinical studies have shown that orally-inhaled and intranasal corticosteroids may cause a reduction in growth velocity in pediatric patients, which appears to be related to dose and duration of exposure.

May suppress the immune system, patients may be more susceptible to infection. Use with caution in patients with systemic infections or ocular herpes simplex. Avoid exposure to chickenpox and measles. Corticosteroids should be used with caution in patients with diabetes, hypertension, osteoporosis, peptic ulcer, glaucoma, cataracts, or tuberculosis. Use caution in hepatic impairment.

Pregnancy risk C.

Drug Interactions

Decreased Effect: Decreased effect with barbiturates and phenytoin. Rifampin increased metabolism of triamcinolone. Vaccine and toxoid effects may be reduced.

Increased Effect/Toxicity: Salicylates or NSAIDs coadministered oral corticosteroids may increase risk of GI ulceration.

Nutritional/Ethanol Interactions

Ethanol: Avoid ethanol (may enhance gastric mucosal irritation).

Food: Triamcinolone interferes with calcium absorption.

Herb/Nutraceutical: Avoid cat's claw, echinacea (have immunostimulant properties).

Adverse Reactions

Systemic:

>10%:

- Central nervous system: Insomnia, nervousness
- Gastrointestinal: Increased appetite, indigestion

1% to 10%:

- Central nervous system: Dizziness or lightheadedness, headache
- Dermatologic: Hirsutism, hypopigmentation
- Endocrine & metabolic: Diabetes mellitus
- Neuromuscular & skeletal: Arthralgia
- Ocular: Cataracts, glaucoma
- Respiratory: Epistaxis
- Miscellaneous: Diaphoresis

<1% (Limited to important or life-threatening): Cushing's syndrome, edema, hypertension, pituitary-adrenal axis suppression, seizures

Topical:

1% to 10%:

- Dermatologic: Itching, allergic contact dermatitis, erythema, dryness papular rashes, folliculitis, furunculosis, pustules, pyoderma, vesiculation, hyperesthesia, skin infection (secondary)
- Local: Burning, irritation

<1% (Limited to important or life-threatening): Cataracts (posterior subcapsular), gastric ulcer, glaucoma

Overdosage/Toxicology When consumed in high doses for prolonged periods, systemic hypercorticism and adrenal suppression may occur. In those cases, discontinuation of the corticosteroid should be done judiciously.

Pharmacodynamics/Kinetics

Absorption: Topical: Systemic

Half-Life Elimination: Biologic: 18-36 hours

Time to Peak: I.M.: 8-10 hours

Duration: Oral: 8-12 hours

Formulations

Aerosol for oral inhalation (Azmacort®): 100 mcg/metered spray (20 g)

Aerosol, topical, as acetonide: 0.2 mg/2 second spray (23 g, 63 g)

Cream, as acetonide: 0.025% (15 g, 60 g, 80 g, 240 g, 454 g); 0.1% (15 g, 30 g, 60 g, 80 g, 90 g, 120 g, 240 g); 0.5% (15 g, 20 g, 30 g, 240 g)

Injection, as acetonide: 10 mg/mL (5 mL); 40 mg/mL (1 mL, 5 mL, 10 mL)

Injection, as diacetate: 25 mg/mL (5 mL); 40 mg/mL (1 mL, 5 mL, 10 mL)

Injection, as hexacetonide: 5 mg/mL (5 mL); 20 mg/mL (1 mL, 5 mL)

Lotion, as acetonide: 0.025% (60 mL); 0.1% (15 mL, 60 mL)

Ointment, as acetonide: 0.025% (15 g, 30 g, 60 g, 80 g, 120 g, 454 g); 0.1% (15 g, 30 g, 60 g, 80 g, 120 g, 240 g, 454 g); 0.5% (15 g, 20 g, 30 g, 240 g)

Paste, oral, topical, as acetonide (Kenalog® in Orabase®): 0.1% (5 g)

Suspension, intranasal spray:

- Nasacort®, Nasacort® AQ™: 55 mcg per actuation (15 mL)
- Tri-Nasal®: 50 mcg per actuation (15 mL)

Syrup: 2 mg/5 mL (120 mL); 4 mg/5 mL (120 mL)

Tablet: 1 mg, 2 mg, 4 mg, 8 mg

Dosing

Adults:

Allergic rhinitis: Intranasal: 2 sprays in each nostril once daily; may increase after 4-7 days up to 4 sprays once daily or 1 spray 4 times/day in each nostril.

Steroid-responsive dermatoses: Topical: Apply a thin film 2-3 times/day.

Systemic anti-inflammatory/immunosuppressant:

- Oral: 4-48 mg/day
- I.M.: Acetonide or hexacetonide: 60 mg (of 40 mg/mL), additional 20-100 mg doses (usual: 40-80 mg) may be given when signs or symptoms recur, best at 6-week intervals to minimize HPA suppression
  - **Note:** In general, single I.M. dose of 4-7 times oral dose will control patient from 4-7 days up to 3-4 weeks.

Pulmonary inflammation/asthma: Oral inhalation: 2 inhalations 3-4 times/day, not to exceed 16 inhalations/day

Arthritis: Intra-articular (hexacetonide): 2-20 mg every 3-4 weeks as hexacetonide salt

- Soft-tissue: Intralesional (use 10 mg/mL) (diacetate or acetonide): 1 mg/injection site, may be repeated one or more times/week depending upon patients response; maximum; 30 mg at any one time; may use multiple injections if they are more than 1 cm apart
- Intra-articular, intrasynovial, and soft-tissue injection (use 10 mg/mL or 40 mg/mL) (diacetate or acetonide): 2.5-40 mg depending upon location, size of joints, and degree of inflammation; repeat when signs or symptoms recur.
- Sublesional (as acetonide): Up to 1 mg per injection site and may be repeated one or more times weekly; multiple sites may be injected if they are 1 cm or more apart, not to exceed 30 mg

See table on following page.

(Continued)

Triamcinolone *(Continued)*

Triamcinolone Dosing

	Acetonide	Diacetate	Hexacetonide
Intrasynovial	2.5-40 mg	5-40 mg	
Intralesional	1-30 mg	5-40 mg (not >25 mg per lesion)	Up to 0.5 mg/sq inch affected area
Sublesional	1-30 mg		
Systemic I.M.	2.5-60 mg/dose (usual adult dose: 60 mg)	~40 mg/wk	
Intra-articular	2.5-40 mg	2-40 mg	2-20 mg average
large joints	15-40 mg		10-20 mg
small joints	2.5-10 mg		2-6 mg
Tendon sheaths	2.5-10 mg		
Intradermal	1 mg/site		

Elderly: Refer to adult dosing; use with caution (see Geriatric Considerations).

Pediatrics: In general, single I.M. dose of 4-7 times oral dose will control patient from 4-7 days up to 3-4 weeks

Children >12 years: Refer to adult dosing.

Children 6-12 years:

Asthma: Oral inhalation: 1-2 inhalations 3-4 times/day, not to exceed 12 inhalations/day

Allergic rhinitis: Nasal spray: Initial 1 spray in each nostril once daily (maximum 2 sprays in each nostril once daily)

Anti-inflammatory, systemic: I.M. (acetonide or hexacetonide): 0.03-0.2 mg/kg at 1- to 7-day intervals

Joint/tendon inflammation: Intra-articular, intrabursal, or tendon-sheath injection: 2.5-15 mg, repeated as needed

Administration

Oral: Once daily doses should be given in the morning.

I.M.: Inject I.M. dose deep in large muscle mass, avoid deltoid.

Inhalation: Inhaler: Rinse mouth and throat after use to prevent candidiasis. Use spacer device provided with Azmacort®.

Topical: Apply a thin film sparingly and avoid topical application on the face. Do not use on open skin or wounds. Do not occlude area unless directed.

Other: Avoid subcutaneous administration.

Monitoring and Teaching Issues

Physical Assessment: Assess other medications patient may be taking for effectiveness and interactions (see Drug Interactions). See Contraindications and Warnings/Precautions for use cautions. Monitor laboratory tests, therapeutic response, and adverse effects according to indications for therapy, dose, route (systemic or topical), and duration of therapy (see Dosing, Warnings/Precautions, Adverse Reactions). With systemic administration, diabetics should monitor glucose levels closely (corticosteroids may alter glucose levels). Assess knowledge/teach patient appropriate use, interventions to reduce side effects, and adverse symptoms to report (see Patient Education). When used for long-term therapy (longer than 10-14 days) do not discontinue abruptly; decrease dosage incrementally. **Pregnancy risk factor C** - benefits of use should outweigh possible risks. Note breast-feeding caution.

Patient Education: Take exactly as directed; do not increase dose or discontinue abruptly without consulting prescriber. Take oral medication with or after meals. Avoid alcohol. Limit intake of caffeine or stimulants. Prescriber may recommend increased dietary vitamins, minerals, or iron. If diabetic, monitor glucose levels closely (antidiabetic medication may need to be adjusted). Inform prescriber if you are experiencing greater than normal levels of stress (medication may need adjustment). Some forms of this medication may cause GI upset (oral medication may be taken with meals to reduce GI upset; or small, frequent meals and frequent mouth care may reduce GI upset). You may be more susceptible to infection (avoid crowds and exposure to infection). Report promptly excessive nervousness or sleep disturbances; any signs of infection (sore throat, unhealed injuries); excessive growth of body hair or loss of skin color; vision changes; excessive or sudden weight gain (>3 lb/week); swelling of face or extremities; difficulty breathing; muscle weakness; change in color of stools (black or tarry) or persistent abdominal pain; or worsening of condition or failure to improve. **Pregnancy/breast-feeding precautions:** Inform prescriber if you are or intend to become pregnant. Consult prescriber if breast-feeding.

Aerosol: Shake gently before use. Use at regular intervals, no more frequently than directed. Not for use during acute asthmatic attack. Follow directions that accompany product. Rinse mouth and throat after use to prevent candidiasis. Do not use intranasal product if you have a nasal infection, nasal injury, or recent nasal surgery. If using two products, consult prescriber in which order to use the two products. Report unusual cough or spasm; persistent nasal bleeding, burning, or irritation; or worsening of condition.

Inhalation: Sit when using. Take deep breaths for 3-5 minutes, and clear nasal passages before administration (use decongestant as needed). Hold breath for 5-10 seconds after use, and wait 1-3 minutes between inhalations. Follow package insert instructions for use. Do not exceed maximum dosage. If also using inhaled bronchodilator, use before triamcinolone. Rinse mouth and throat after use to reduce aftertaste and prevent candidiasis.

Topical: For external use only. Not for eyes or mucous membranes or open wounds. Apply in very thin layer to occlusive dressing. Apply dressing to area being treated. Avoid prolonged or excessive use around sensitive tissues, genital, or rectal areas. Inform prescriber if condition worsens (swelling, redness, irritation, pain, open sores) or fails to improve.

Dietary Issues: May be taken with food to decrease GI distress.

Geriatric Considerations: Because of the risk of adverse effects, systemic corticosteroids should be used cautiously in the elderly, in the smallest possible dose, and for the shortest possible time. Azmacort® (metered dose inhaler) comes with its own spacer device attached and may be easier to use in older patients.

Breast-feeding Issues: No data on crossing into breast milk or clinical effects on the infant.

Additional Information 16 mg triamcinolone is equivalent to 100 mg cortisone (no mineralocorticoid activity).

Effects of inhaled/intranasal steroids on growth have been observed in the absence of laboratory evidence of HPA axis suppression, suggesting that growth velocity is a more sensitive indicator of systemic corticosteroid exposure in pediatric patients than some commonly used tests of HPA axis function. The long-term effects of this reduction in growth velocity associated with orally-inhaled and intranasal corticosteroids, including the impact on final adult height, are unknown. The potential for "catch up" growth following discontinuation of treatment with inhaled corticosteroids has not been adequately studied.

Related Information

Corticosteroids Comparison, Systemic Equivalencies *on page 1572*

Inhalant (Asthma, Bronchospasm) Agents Comparison *on page 1577*

Triamcinolone Acetonide, Aerosol *see* Triamcinolone *on page 1356*

Triamcinolone Acetonide, Parenteral *see* Triamcinolone *on page 1356*

Triamcinolone and Nystatin *see* Nystatin and Triamcinolone *on page 990*

Triamcinolone Diacetate, Oral *see* Triamcinolone *on page 1356*

Triamcinolone Diacetate, Parenteral *see* Triamcinolone *on page 1356*

Triamcinolone Hexacetonide *see* Triamcinolone *on page 1356*

Triamcinolone, Oral *see* Triamcinolone *on page 1356*

Triam Forte® *see* Triamcinolone *on page 1356*

Triaminic® AM Decongestant Formula [OTC] *see* Pseudoephedrine *on page 1150*

Triaminic® Infant Decongestant [OTC] *see* Pseudoephedrine *on page 1150*

Triamterene and Hydrochlorothiazide *see* Hydrochlorothiazide and Triamterene *on page 667*

Triazolam (trye AY zoe lam)

U.S. Brand Names Halcion®

Restrictions C-IV

Generic Available Yes

Pharmacologic Category Benzodiazepine

Pregnancy Risk Factor X

Lactation Enters breast milk/not recommended

Use Short-term treatment of insomnia

Mechanism of Action/Effect Binds to stereospecific benzodiazepine receptors on the postsynaptic GABA neuron at several sites within the central nervous system, including the limbic system, reticular formation. Enhancement of the inhibitory effect of GABA on neuronal excitability results by increased neuronal membrane permeability to chloride ions. This shift in chloride ions results in hyperpolarization (a less excitable state) and stabilization.

Contraindications Hypersensitivity to triazolam or any component of the formulation (cross-sensitivity with other benzodiazepines may exist); concurrent therapy with CYP3A4 inhibitors (including ketoconazole, itraconazole, and nefazodone); pregnancy

Warnings/Precautions As a hypnotic, should be used only after evaluation of potential causes of sleep disturbance. Failure of sleep disturbance to resolve after 7-10 days may indicate psychiatric or medical illness. Use is not recommended in patients with depressive disorders or psychoses. Avoid use in patients with sleep apnea. Use with caution in patients receiving concurrent CYP3A4 inhibitors, particularly when these agents are added to therapy. Use with caution in elderly or debilitated patients, patients with hepatic disease (including alcoholics), renal impairment, respiratory disease, impaired gag reflex, or obese patients.

Causes CNS depression (dose-related) which may impair physical and mental capabilities. Use with caution in patients receiving other CNS depressants or psychoactive agents. Benzodiazepines have been associated with falls and traumatic injury and should be used with extreme caution in patients who are at risk of these events (especially the elderly). May cause physical or psychological dependence - use with caution in patients with a history of drug dependence.

Benzodiazepines have been associated with anterograde amnesia. Paradoxical reactions, including hyperactive or aggressive behavior, have been reported with benzodiazepines, particularly in adolescent/pediatric or psychiatric patients. Does not have analgesic, antidepressant, or antipsychotic properties.

Drug Interactions

Cytochrome P450 Effect: Substrate of **CYP3A4**; Inhibits CYP2C8/9

Decreased Effect: Carbamazepine, rifampin, and rifabutin may enhance the metabolism of triazolam and decrease its therapeutic effect.

Increased Effect/Toxicity: Triazolam levels may be increased by cimetidine, ciprofloxacin, clarithromycin, clozapine, CNS depressants, diltiazem, disulfiram, digoxin, erythromycin, ethanol, fluconazole, fluoxetine, fluvoxamine, grapefruit juice, isoniazid, itraconazole, ketoconazole, labetalol, levodopa, loxapine, metoprolol, metronidazole, miconazole, nefazodone, omeprazole, phenytoin, rifabutin, rifampin, troleandomycin, valproic acid, and verapamil. Concurrent use of some protease inhibitors (including ritonavir and amprenavir) is contraindicated.

Nutritional/Ethanol Interactions

Ethanol: Avoid ethanol (may increase CNS depression).

Food: Food may decrease the rate of absorption. Triazolam serum concentration may be increased by grapefruit juice; avoid concurrent use.

(Continued)

Triazolam *(Continued)*

Herb/Nutraceutical: St John's wort may decrease levels. Avoid valerian, St John's wort, kava kava, gotu kola (may increase CNS depression).

Adverse Reactions

>10%: Central nervous system: Drowsiness, anteriograde amnesia

1% to 10%:

Central nervous system: Headache, dizziness, nervousness, lightheadedness, ataxia

Gastrointestinal: Nausea, vomiting

<1% (Limited to important or life-threatening): Confusion, depression, euphoria, memory impairment

Overdosage/Toxicology Symptoms of overdose include somnolence, confusion, coma, diminished reflexes, dyspnea, and hypotension. Treatment for benzodiazepine overdose is supportive. Flumazenil has been shown to selectively block the binding of benzodiazepines to CNS receptors, resulting in reversal of benzodiazepine-induced CNS depression but not always respiratory depression.

Pharmacodynamics/Kinetics

Half-Life Elimination: 1.7-5 hours

Metabolism: Extensively hepatic

Onset: Hypnotic: 15-30 minutes

Duration: 6-7 hours

Formulations Tablet: 0.125 mg, 0.25 mg

Dosing

Adults: Note: Onset of action is rapid, patient should be in bed when taking medication.

Insomnia (short-term): Oral: 0.125-0.25 mg at bedtime

Dental (preprocedure): Oral: 0.25 mg taken the evening before oral surgery; or 0.25 mg 1 hour before procedure

Elderly: Oral: Insomnia (short-term use): 0.0625-0.125 mg at bedtime (see Geriatric Considerations).

Hepatic Impairment: Reduce dose or avoid use in cirrhosis.

Administration

Oral: May take with food. Tablet may be crushed or swallowed whole. Onset of action is rapid, patient should be in bed when taking medication.

Monitoring and Teaching Issues

Physical Assessment: Assess other medications patient may be taking for effectiveness and interactions (see Drug Interactions). See Contraindications and Warnings/Precautions for use cautions. Assess for history of addiction; long-term use can result in dependence, abuse, or tolerance; periodically evaluate need for continued use. Monitor therapeutic response according to rationale for therapy and adverse reactions at beginning of therapy and periodically with long-term use (see Adverse Reactions and Overdose/Toxicology). Taper dosage slowly when discontinuing. Assess knowledge/teach patient appropriate use, interventions to reduce side effects, and adverse symptoms to report (see Patient Education). **Pregnancy risk factor X** - determine that patient is not pregnant before starting therapy. Do not give to sexually-active female patients unless capable of complying with barrier contraceptive use. Breast-feeding is not recommended.

Patient Education: Take exactly as directed; do not increase dose or frequency. It may take 2-3 weeks to achieve desired results. Drug may cause physical and/or psychological dependence. Do not use alcohol or other prescription or OTC medications (especially pain medications, sedatives, antihistamines, or hypnotics) without consulting prescriber. Maintain adequate hydration (2-3 L/day of fluids) unless advised by prescriber to restrict fluids. You may experience drowsiness, lightheadedness, impaired coordination, dizziness, or blurred vision (use caution when driving or engaging in tasks requiring alertness until response to drug is known); nausea, vomiting, or dry mouth (small, frequent meals, frequent mouth care, chewing gum, or sucking lozenges may help); constipation (increased exercise, fluids, fruit, or fiber may help); altered sexual drive or ability (reversible); or photosensitivity (use sunscreen, wear protective clothing and eyewear, and avoid direct sunlight). Report persistent CNS effects (eg, memory impairment, confusion, depression, increased sedation, excitation, headache, agitation, insomnia or nightmares, dizziness, fatigue, impaired coordination, changes in personality, or changes in cognition); changes in urinary pattern; muscle cramping, weakness, tremors, or rigidity; ringing in ears or visual disturbances; chest pain, palpitations, or rapid heartbeat; excessive perspiration; excessive GI symptoms (cramping, constipation, vomiting, anorexia); or worsening of condition. **Pregnancy/breast-feeding precautions:** Inform prescriber if you are pregnant. Do not get pregnant during or for 1 month following therapy. Consult prescriber for instruction on appropriate contraceptive measures. This drug may cause severe fetal defects. Breast-feeding is not recommended.

Geriatric Considerations: Due to the higher incidence of CNS adverse reactions and its short half-life, this benzodiazepine is not a drug of first choice. For short-term only.

Additional Information Onset of action is rapid, patient should be in bed when taking medication. Prescription should be written for 7-10 days and should not be prescribed in quantities exceeding a 1-month supply. Abrupt discontinuation after sustained use (generally >10 days) may cause withdrawal symptoms.

Related Information

Anxiolytic/Hypnotic Use in Long-Term Care Facilities *on page 1608*
Benzodiazepines *on page 1560*

Tribavirin *see* Ribavirin *on page 1181*
Trichloroacetaldehyde Monohydrate *see* Chloral Hydrate *on page 268*
***Trichophyton* Skin Test** *see page 1461*
TriCor® *see* Fenofibrate *on page 549*
Tricosal® *see* Choline Magnesium Trisalicylate *on page 283*
Triderm® *see* Topical Corticosteroids *on page 1334*
Triderm® *see* Triamcinolone *on page 1356*

Tridesilon® *see* Topical Corticosteroids *on page 1334*
Trientine *see page 1460*
Triethanolamine Polypeptide Oleate Condensate *see page 1519*
Triethylenethiophosphoramide *see* Thiotepa *on page 1309*

Trifluoperazine (trye floo oh PER a zeen)

U.S. Brand Names Stelazine®

Synonyms Trifluoperazine Hydrochloride

Generic Available Yes

Pharmacologic Category Antipsychotic Agent, Phenothiazine, Piperazine

Pregnancy Risk Factor C

Lactation Enters breast milk/not recommended (AAP rates "of concern")

Use Treatment of schizophrenia

Use - Unlabeled/Investigational Management of psychotic disorders

Mechanism of Action/Effect Blocks postsynaptic mesolimbic dopaminergic receptors in the brain; exhibits alpha-adrenergic blocking effect and depresses the release of hypothalamic and hypophyseal hormones

Contraindications Hypersensitivity to trifluoperazine or any component of the formulation (cross-reactivity between phenothiazines may occur); severe CNS depression; bone marrow suppression; blood dyscrasias; severe hepatic disease; coma

Warnings/Precautions May result in hypotension, particularly after I.M. administration. May be sedating, use with caution in disorders where CNS depression is a feature. Use with caution in Parkinson's disease. Caution in patients with hemodynamic instability; predisposition to seizures; subcortical brain damage; hepatic impairment; severe cardiac, renal, or respiratory disease. Esophageal dysmotility and aspiration have been associated with antipsychotic use - use with caution in patients at risk of pneumonia (ie, Alzheimer's disease). Caution in breast cancer or other prolactin-dependent tumors (may elevate prolactin levels). May alter temperature regulation or mask toxicity of other drugs due to antiemetic effects. May alter cardiac conduction - life-threatening arrhythmias have occurred with therapeutic doses of phenothiazines. May cause orthostatic hypotension - use with caution in patients at risk of this effect or those who would tolerate transient hypotensive episodes (cerebrovascular disease, cardiovascular disease or other medications which may predispose). Safety in children <6 months of age has not been established.

Due to anticholinergic effects, should be used with caution in patients with decreased gastrointestinal motility, urinary retention, BPH, xerostomia, visual problems, narrow-angle glaucoma (screening is recommended) and myasthenia gravis. Relative to other antipsychotics, trifluoperazine has a low potency of cholinergic blockade.

May cause extrapyramidal symptoms, including pseudoparkinsonism, acute dystonic reactions, akathisia, and tardive dyskinesia (risk of these reactions is high relative to other neuroleptics). May be associated with neuroleptic malignant syndrome (NMS) or pigmentary retinopathy.

Pregnancy risk C.

Drug Interactions

Cytochrome P450 Effect: Substrate of **CYP1A2**

Decreased Effect: Phenothiazines inhibit the effects of levodopa, guanadrel, guanethidine, and bromocriptine. Benztropine (and other anticholinergics) may inhibit the therapeutic response to trifluoperazine and excess anticholinergic effects may occur. Cigarette smoking and barbiturates may enhance the hepatic metabolism of trifluoperazine. Trifluoperazine and possibly other low potency antipsychotics may reverse the pressor effects of epinephrine.

Increased Effect/Toxicity: Trifluoperazine's effects on CNS depression may be additive when trifluoperazine is combined with CNS depressants (narcotic analgesics, ethanol, barbiturates, cyclic antidepressants, antihistamines, or sedative-hypnotics). Trifluoperazine may increase the effects/toxicity of anticholinergics, antihypertensives, lithium (rare neurotoxicity), trazodone, or valproic acid. Concurrent use with TCA may produce increased toxicity or altered therapeutic response. Chloroquine and propranolol may increase trifluoperazine concentrations. Hypotension may occur when trifluoperazine is combined with epinephrine. May increase the risk of arrhythmia when combined with antiarrhythmics, cisapride, pimozide, sparfloxacin, or other drugs which prolong QT interval. Metoclopramide may increase risk of extrapyramidal symptoms (EPS).

Nutritional/Ethanol Interactions

Ethanol: Avoid ethanol (may increase CNS depression).

Herb/Nutraceutical: Avoid kava kava, gotu kola, valerian, St John's wort (may increase CNS depression). Avoid dong quai, St John's wort (may also cause photosensitization).

Effects on Lab Values False-positive for phenylketonuria; ↑ cholesterol (S), glucose; ↓ uric acid (S)

Adverse Reactions Frequency not defined.

Cardiovascular: Hypotension, orthostatic hypotension, cardiac arrest

Central nervous system: Extrapyramidal symptoms (pseudoparkinsonism, akathisia, dystonias, tardive dyskinesia), dizziness, headache, neuroleptic malignant syndrome (NMS), impairment of temperature regulation, lowering of seizures threshold

Dermatologic: Increased sensitivity to sun, rash, discoloration of skin (blue-gray)

Endocrine & metabolic: Changes in menstrual cycle, changes in libido, breast pain, hyperglycemia, hypoglycemia, gynecomastia, lactation, galactorrhea

Gastrointestinal: Constipation, weight gain, nausea, vomiting, stomach pain, xerostomia

Genitourinary: Difficulty in urination, ejaculatory disturbances, urinary retention, priapism

Hematologic: Agranulocytosis, leukopenia, pancytopenia, thrombocytopenic purpura, eosinophilia, hemolytic anemia, aplastic anemia

Hepatic: Cholestatic jaundice, hepatotoxicity

Neuromuscular & skeletal: Tremor

Ocular: Pigmentary retinopathy, cornea and lens changes

Respiratory: Nasal congestion

(Continued)

Trifluoperazine *(Continued)*

Overdosage/Toxicology Symptoms of overdose include deep sleep, coma, extrapyramidal symptoms, abnormal involuntary muscle movements, hypo- or hypertension, and cardiac arrhythmias. Treatment is symptom-directed and supportive.

Pharmacodynamics/Kinetics

Half-Life Elimination: >24 hours with chronic use

Metabolism: Extensively hepatic

Formulations

Injection, as hydrochloride: 2 mg/mL (10 mL)

Solution, oral concentrate, as hydrochloride: 10 mg/mL (60 mL)

Tablet, as hydrochloride: 1 mg, 2 mg, 5 mg, 10 mg

Dosing

Adults:

Schizophrenia/psychoses:

Outpatients: Oral: 1-2 mg twice daily

Hospitalized or well supervised patient: Initial: 2-5 mg twice daily with optimum response in the 15-20 mg/day range; do not exceed 40 mg/day.

I.M.: 1-2 mg every 4-6 hours as needed up to 10 mg/24 hours maximum

Nonpsychotic anxiety: Oral: 1-2 mg twice daily; maximum: 6 mg/day; therapy for anxiety should not exceed 12 weeks; do not exceed 6 mg/day for longer than 12 weeks when treating anxiety; agitation, jitteriness, or insomnia may be confused with original neurotic or psychotic symptoms.

Elderly:

Schizophrenia/psychoses:

Oral: Refer to adult dosing. Dose selection should start at the low end of the dosage range and titration must be gradual.

I.M.: Initial: 1 mg every 4-6 hours; increase at 1 mg increments; do not exceed 6 mg/day

Behavioral symptoms associated with dementia behavior: Oral: Initial: 0.5-1 mg 1-2 times/day; increase dose at 4- to 7-day intervals by 0.5-1 mg/day; increase dosing intervals (bid, tid, etc) as necessary to control response or side effects. Maximum daily dose: 40 mg. Gradual increases (titration) may prevent some side effects or decrease their severity.

Pediatrics: Children 6-12 years: Schizophrenia/psychoses:

Oral: Hospitalized or well supervised patients: Initial: 1 mg 1-2 times/day, gradually increase until symptoms are controlled or adverse effects become troublesome; maximum: 15 mg/day.

I.M.: 1 mg twice daily

Renal Impairment: Not dialyzable (0% to 5%)

Administration

Oral: Oral concentrate must be diluted in 2-4 oz of liquid (water, carbonated drinks, fruit juices, tomato juice, milk, or pudding). Wash hands if undiluted concentrate is spilled on skin to prevent contact dermatosis. **Note:** Avoid skin contact with oral medication; may cause contact dermatitis.

I.M.: Give I.M. injection deep in upper outer quadrant of buttock.

Stability

Storage: Store injection at room temperature. Protect from heat and from freezing. Use only clear or slightly yellow solutions.

Monitoring Laboratory Tests Baseline liver and kidney function, CBC prior to and periodically during therapy, ophthalmic exam

Monitoring and Teaching Issues

Physical Assessment: Assess other medications patient is taking for effectiveness and interactions (see Drug Interactions). See Contraindications and Warnings/Precautions for use cautions. Review ophthalmic exam and monitor laboratory results (see above), therapeutic response according to rationale for therapy, and adverse reactions at beginning of therapy and periodically with long-term use (see Adverse Reactions and Overdose/Toxicology). With I.M. use, monitor closely for hypotension. **Note:** Avoid skin contact with liquid medication; may cause contact dermatitis (wash immediately with warm, soapy water). Initiate at lower doses (see Dosing) and taper dosage slowly when discontinuing. Assess knowledge/teach patient appropriate use, interventions to reduce side effects, and adverse symptoms to report (see Patient Education). **Pregnancy risk factor C** - benefits of use should outweigh possible risks. Breast-feeding is not recommended.

Patient Education: Use exactly as directed; do not increase dose or frequency. Do not discontinue without consulting prescriber. Tablets/capsules may be taken with food. Mix oral solution with 2-4 oz of liquid (eg, juice, milk, water, pudding). Do not take within 2 hours of any antacid. Avoid alcohol or caffeine and other prescription or OTC medications not approved by prescriber. Maintain adequate hydration (2-3 L/day of fluids) unless advised by prescriber to restrict fluids. Avoid skin contact with liquid medication; may cause contact dermatitis (wash immediately with warm, soapy water). You may experience excess drowsiness, lightheadedness, dizziness, or blurred vision (use caution driving or when engaging in tasks requiring alertness until response to drug is known); nausea or vomiting (small, frequent meals, frequent mouth care, chewing gum, or sucking lozenges may help); constipation (increased exercise, fluids, fruit, or fiber may help); postural hypotension (use caution climbing stairs or when changing position from lying or sitting to standing); urinary retention (void before taking medication); ejaculatory dysfunction (reversible); decreased perspiration (avoid strenuous exercise in hot environments); or photosensitivity (use sunscreen, wear protective clothing and eyewear, and avoid direct sunlight). Report persistent CNS effects (eg, trembling fingers, altered gait or balance, excessive sedation, seizures, unusual movements, anxiety, abnormal thoughts, confusion, personality changes); chest pain, palpitations, rapid heartbeat, severe dizziness; unresolved urinary retention or changes in urinary pattern; altered menstrual pattern, changes in libido, swelling or pain in breasts (male or female); vision changes; skin rash, irritation, or changes in color of skin (gray-blue); or worsening of condition. **Pregnancy/breast-feeding**

precautions: Inform prescriber if you are or intend to become pregnant. Breast-feeding is not recommended.

Dietary Issues: May be taken with food to decrease GI distress.

Geriatric Considerations: (See Warnings/Precautions, Adverse Reactions, and Overdose/Toxicology.) Elderly patients have an increased risk of adverse response to side effects or adverse reactions to antipsychotics.

Additional Information Do not exceed 6 mg/day for longer than 12 weeks when treating anxiety. Agitation, jitteriness, or insomnia may be confused with original neurotic or psychotic symptoms.

Related Information

Antipsychotic Agents *on page 1558*
Antipsychotic Medication Guidelines *on page 1614*

Trifluoperazine Hydrochloride *see* Trifluoperazine *on page 1361*

Trifluorothymidine *see* Trifluridine *on page 1363*

Trifluridine (trye FLURE i deen)

U.S. Brand Names Viroptic®

Synonyms F_3T; Trifluorothymidine

Generic Available No

Pharmacologic Category Antiviral Agent, Ophthalmic

Pregnancy Risk Factor C

Lactation Excretion in breast milk unknown

Use Treatment of primary keratoconjunctivitis and recurrent epithelial keratitis caused by herpes simplex virus types I and II

Mechanism of Action/Effect Interferes with viral replication by incorporating into viral DNA in place of thymidine, inhibiting thymidylate synthetase resulting in the formation of defective proteins

Contraindications Hypersensitivity to trifluridine or any component of the formulation

Warnings/Precautions Mild local irritation of conjunctiva and cornea may occur when instilled but usually is a transient effect. Pregnancy risk C.

Adverse Reactions

>10%: Local: Burning, stinging

<1% (Limited to important or life-threatening): Epithelial keratopathy, increased intraocular pressure, keratitis, palpebral edema, stromal edema

Pharmacodynamics/Kinetics

Absorption: Ophthalmic: Systemic absorption negligible, corneal penetration adequate

Formulations Solution, ophthalmic: 1% (7.5 mL)

Dosing

Adults & Elderly: Herpes keratoconjunctivitis, keratitis: Ophthalmic: Instill 1 drop into affected eye every 2 hours while awake, to a maximum of 9 drops/day, until re-epithelialization of corneal ulcer occurs. Then use 1 drop every 4 hours for another 7 days. Do **not** exceed 21 days of treatment. If improvement has not taken place in 7-14 days, consider another form of therapy.

Stability

Storage: Refrigerate at 2°C to 8°C (36°F to 46°F). Storage at room temperature may result in a solution altered pH which could result in ocular discomfort upon administration and/or decreased potency.

Monitoring and Teaching Issues

Physical Assessment: Monitor effectiveness of therapy, not for long-term use (see Dosing). Assess knowledge/teach patient appropriate use, interventions to reduce side effects, and adverse symptoms to report (see Patient Education). **Pregnancy risk factor C** - systemic absorption minimal or unlikely. Note breast-feeding caution.

Patient Education: For ophthalmic use only. Store in refrigerator; do not use discolored solution. Apply prescribed amount as often as directed. Wash hands before using. Do not let tip of applicator touch eye; do not contaminate tip of applicator (may cause eye infection, eye damage, or vision loss). Tilt head back and look upward. Gently pull down lower lid and put drop(s) in inner corner of eye. Close eye and roll eyeball in all directions. Do not blink for 1/2 minute. Apply gentle pressure to inner corner of eye for 30 seconds. Wipe away excess from skin around eye. Do not use any other eye preparation for at least 10 minutes. Do not touch tip of applicator to eye or contaminate tip of applicator. Do not share medication with anyone else. May cause sensitivity to bright light (dark glasses may help); or temporary stinging or blurred vision may occur. Inform prescriber if you experience eye pain, redness, burning, watering, dryness, double vision, puffiness around eye, vision changes, or other adverse eye response; or worsening of condition or lack of improvement within 7-14 days. **Pregnancy/breast-feeding precautions:** Inform prescriber if you are pregnant. Consult prescriber if breast-feeding.

Geriatric Considerations: Assess ability to self-administer.

Trihexyphenidyl (trye heks ee FEN i dil)

U.S. Brand Names Artane®

Synonyms Benzhexol Hydrochloride; Trihexyphenidyl Hydrochloride

Generic Available Yes

Pharmacologic Category Anticholinergic Agent; Anti-Parkinson's Agent, Anticholinergic

Pregnancy Risk Factor C

Lactation Excretion in breast milk unknown

Use Adjunctive treatment of Parkinson's disease; treatment of drug-induced extrapyramidal symptoms

Mechanism of Action/Effect Exerts a direct inhibitory effect on the parasympathetic nervous system. It also has a relaxing effect on smooth musculature; exerted both directly on the muscle itself and indirectly through parasympathetic nervous system (inhibitory effect)

(Continued)

Trihexyphenidyl *(Continued)*

Contraindications Hypersensitivity to trihexyphenidyl or any component of the formulation; narrow-angle glaucoma; pyloric or duodenal obstruction; stenosing peptic ulcers; bladder neck obstructions; achalasia; myasthenia gravis

Warnings/Precautions Use with caution in hot weather or during exercise. Elderly patients require strict dosage regulation. Use with caution in patients with tachycardia, cardiac arrhythmias, hypertension, hypotension, prostatic hyperplasia or any tendency toward urinary retention, liver or kidney disorders, and obstructive disease of the GI or GU tract. May exacerbate mental symptoms when used to treat extrapyramidal symptoms. When given in large doses or to susceptible patients, may cause weakness. Does not improve symptoms of tardive dyskinesias. Pregnancy risk C.

Drug Interactions

Decreased Effect: May increase gastric degradation of levodopa and decrease the amount of levodopa absorbed by delaying gastric emptying; the opposite may be true for digoxin. Therapeutic effects of cholinergic agents (tacrine, donepezil) and neuroleptics may be antagonized.

Increased Effect/Toxicity: Central and/or peripheral anticholinergic syndrome can occur when administered with amantadine, rimantadine, narcotic analgesics, phenothiazines and other antipsychotics (especially with high anticholinergic activity), tricyclic antidepressants, quinidine and some other antiarrhythmics, and antihistamines.

Nutritional/Ethanol Interactions Ethanol: Avoid ethanol (may increase CNS depression).

Adverse Reactions Frequency not defined.

Cardiovascular: Tachycardia

Central nervous system: Confusion, agitation, euphoria, drowsiness, headache, dizziness, nervousness, delusions, hallucinations, paranoia

Dermatologic: Dry skin, increased sensitivity to light, rash

Gastrointestinal: Constipation, xerostomia, dry throat, ileus, nausea, vomiting, parotitis

Genitourinary: Urinary retention

Neuromuscular & skeletal: Weakness

Ocular: Blurred vision, mydriasis, increase in intraocular pressure, glaucoma

Respiratory: Dry nose

Miscellaneous: Diaphoresis (decreased)

Overdosage/Toxicology Symptoms of overdose include blurred vision, urinary retention, and tachycardia. For anticholinergic overdose with severe life-threatening symptoms, physostigmine 1-2 mg S.C. or I.V. slowly, may be given to reverse these effects.

Pharmacodynamics/Kinetics

Half-Life Elimination: 3.3-4.1 hours

Time to Peak: Serum: 1-1.5 hours

Onset: Peak effect: Within 1 hour

Formulations

Elixir, as hydrochloride: 2 mg/5 mL (480 mL)

Tablet, as hydrochloride: 2 mg, 5 mg

Dosing

Adults: Parkinson's disease or drug-induced EPS: Oral: Initial: 1-2 mg/day, increase by 2 mg increments at intervals of 3-5 days; usual dose: 5-15 mg/day in 3-4 divided doses

Elderly: Parkinsonism: Oral: 1 mg on first day, increase by 2 mg every 3-5 days as needed until a total of 6-10 mg/day (in 3-4 divided doses) is reached. If the patient is on concomitant levodopa therapy, the daily dose is reduced to 1-2 mg 3 times/day. Avoid use if possible (see Geriatric Considerations).

Administration

Oral: Tolerated best if given in 3 daily doses and with food. High doses may be divided into 4 doses, at meal times and at bedtime. Patients may be switched to sustained-action capsules when stabilized on conventional dosage forms.

Monitoring Laboratory Tests Intraocular pressure monitoring and gonioscopic evaluations should be performed periodically.

Monitoring and Teaching Issues

Physical Assessment: Assess effectiveness and interactions of other medications patient may be taking (see Contraindications and Drug Interactions). Monitor renal function, therapeutic response, and adverse reactions (eg, anticholinergic syndrome) at beginning of therapy and periodically throughout therapy (see Warnings/Precautions, Adverse Reactions, and Overdose/Toxicology). Assess knowledge/teach patient appropriate use, interventions to reduce side effects, and adverse symptoms to report (see Patient Education). **Pregnancy risk factor C** - benefits of use should outweigh possible risks. Note breast-feeding caution.

Patient Education: Take exactly as directed; with meals if GI upset occurs, before meals if dry mouth occurs, after eating if drooling or if nausea occurs. Take at the same time each day. Maintain adequate hydration (2-3 L/day of fluids) unless advised by prescriber to restrict fluids; void before taking medication. Do not use alcohol and all prescription or OTC sedatives or CNS depressants without consulting prescriber. You may experience drowsiness, confusion, or vision changes (use caution when driving, climbing stairs, or engaging in tasks requiring alertness until response to drug is known); increased susceptibility to heat stroke, decreased perspiration (use caution in hot weather - maintain adequate fluids and reduce exercise activity); constipation (increased exercise, fluids, fruit, or fiber may help); or dry skin or nasal passages (consult prescriber for appropriate relief). Report unresolved constipation; chest pain or palpitations; difficulty breathing; CNS changes (hallucination, loss of memory, nervousness, etc); painful or difficult urination; increased muscle spasticity or rigidity; skin rash; or significant worsening of condition. **Pregnancy/breast-feeding precautions:** Inform prescriber if you are or intend to become pregnant. Consult prescriber if breast-feeding.

Geriatric Considerations: Anticholinergic agents are generally not well tolerated in the elderly and their use should be avoided when possible. Elderly patients require strict dosage regulation. In the elderly, anticholinergic agents should not be used as prophylaxis against extrapyramidal symptoms.

Additional Information Incidence and severity of side effects are dose related. Patients may be switched to sustained-action capsules when stabilized on conventional dosage forms.

Trihexyphenidyl Hydrochloride *see* Trihexyphenidyl *on page 1363*

Tri-Immunol® *see page 1498*

Tri-K® *see* Potassium Supplements *on page 1106*

Tri-Kort® *see* Triamcinolone *on page 1356*

Trilafon® *see* Perphenazine *on page 1062*

Trileptal® *see* Oxcarbazepine *on page 1017*

Tri-Levlen® *see* Ethinyl Estradiol and Levonorgestrel *on page 523*

Trilisate® *see* Choline Magnesium Trisalicylate *on page 283*

Trilog® *see* Triamcinolone *on page 1356*

Trilone® *see* Triamcinolone *on page 1356*

Tri-Luma™ *see* Fluocinolone, Hydroquinone, and Tretinoin *on page 574*

Trimethaphan Camsylate *see page 1461*

Trimethobenzamide (trye meth oh BEN za mide)

U.S. Brand Names Benzacot®; Tigan®

Synonyms Trimethobenzamide Hydrochloride

Generic Available Yes

Pharmacologic Category Anticholinergic Agent; Antiemetic

Pregnancy Risk Factor C

Lactation Excretion in breast milk unknown

Use Treatment of postoperative nausea and vomiting; nausea associated with gastroenteritis

Mechanism of Action/Effect Acts centrally to inhibit the medullary chemoreceptor trigger zone

Contraindications Hypersensitivity to trimethobenzamide, benzocaine (or similar local anesthetics), or any component of the formulation; injection contraindicated in children; suppositories contraindicated in premature infants or neonates

Warnings/Precautions May mask emesis due to Reye's syndrome or mimic CNS effects of Reye's syndrome in patients with emesis of other etiologies. Use in patients with acute vomiting should be avoided. May cause drowsiness; patient should avoid tasks requiring alertness (eg, driving, operating machinery). May cause extrapyramidal symptoms (EPS) which may be confused with CNS symptoms of primary disease responsible for emesis. Pregnancy risk C.

Nutritional/Ethanol Interactions Ethanol: Concomitant use should be avoided.

Adverse Reactions Frequency not defined.

Cardiovascular: Hypotension

Central nervous system: Coma, depression, disorientation, dizziness, drowsiness, EPS, headache, opisthotonos, Parkinson-like syndrome, seizures

Hematologic: Blood dyscrasias

Hepatic: Jaundice

Neuromuscular & skeletal: Muscle cramps

Ocular: Blurred vision

Miscellaneous: Hypersensitivity reactions

Overdosage/Toxicology Symptoms of overdose include hypotension, seizures, CNS depression, cardiac arrhythmias, disorientation, and confusion. Treatment is symptom-directed and supportive.

Pharmacodynamics/Kinetics

Absorption: Rectal: ~60%

Bioavailability: Oral: 100%

Half-Life Elimination: 7-9 hours

Time to Peak: Oral: 45 minutes; I.M.: 30 minutes

Onset: Antiemetic: Oral: 10-40 minutes; I.M.: 15-35 minutes

Duration: 3-4 hours

Formulations

Capsule, as hydrochloride: 250 mg, 300 mg

Injection, solution, as hydrochloride: 100 mg/mL (2 mL, 20 mL)

Suppository, rectal, as hydrochloride: 100 mg, 200 mg [contains benzocaine]

Dosing

Adults & Elderly: Nausea, vomiting:

Oral: 250-300 mg 3-4 times/day

I.M., rectal: 200 mg 3-4 times/day

Pediatrics: Rectal use is contraindicated in neonates and premature infants.

Nausea, vomiting:

Rectal: Children <14 kg: 100 mg 3-4 times/day

Oral, rectal: Children 14-40 kg: 100-200 mg 3-4 times/day

Administration

I.M.: Administer I.M. only. Inject deep into upper outer quadrant of gluteal muscle.

Stability

Storage: Store at room temperature. Protect from heat and from freezing. Use only clear solutions.

Monitoring and Teaching Issues

Physical Assessment: See Warnings/Precautions, Contraindications (eg, GI or GU obstruction), and Dosing for use cautions. Assess potential for interactions with other prescriptions, OTC medications, or herbal products patient may be taking (see Drug Interactions). Assess results of laboratory tests (see above), therapeutic effectiveness, and adverse reactions with first dose and on a regular basis during therapy (eg, hypovolemia, angioedema, postural hypotension - see Adverse Reactions and Overdose/Toxicology). Teach patient appropriate use (according to purpose for use), possible side effects/interventions, and adverse symptoms to report (see Patient Education). **Pregnancy risk factor C** - benefits of use should outweigh possible risks. Note breast-feeding caution.

(Continued)

Trimethobenzamide *(Continued)*

Patient Education: Inform prescriber of all prescriptions, OTC medications, or herbal products you are taking, and any allergies you have. Do not take anything new during treatment unless approved by prescriber. Take as directed before meals; do not increase dose and do not discontinue without consulting prescriber. May cause drowsiness or blurred vision (use caution when driving or engaging in tasks that require alertness until response to drug is known) or diarrhea (buttermilk or yogurt may help). Report chest pain or palpitations, persistent dizziness or blurred vision, or CNS changes (disorientation, depression, confusion). **Pregnancy/breast-feeding precautions:** Inform prescriber if you are or intend to become pregnant. Consult prescriber if breast-feeding.

Related Information

Antiemetics for Chemotherapy-Induced Nausea and Vomiting *on page 1639*

Trimethobenzamide Hydrochloride *see* Trimethobenzamide *on page 1365*

Trimethoprim (trye METH oh prim)

U.S. Brand Names Primsol®; Proloprim®

Synonyms TMP

Generic Available Yes

Pharmacologic Category Antibiotic, Miscellaneous

Pregnancy Risk Factor C

Lactation Enters breast milk/use caution (AAP rates "compatible")

Use Treatment of urinary tract infections due to susceptible strains of *E. coli*, *P. mirabilis*, *K. pneumoniae*, *Enterobacter* sp and coagulase-negative *Staphylococcus* including *S. saprophyticus*; acute otitis media in children; acute exacerbations of chronic bronchitis in adults; in combination with other agents for treatment of toxoplasmosis, *Pneumocystis carinii*; treatment of superficial ocular infections involving the conjunctiva and cornea

Mechanism of Action/Effect Inhibits folic acid reduction to tetrahydrofolate, and thereby inhibits microbial growth

Contraindications Hypersensitivity to trimethoprim or any component of the formulation; megaloblastic anemia due to folate deficiency

Warnings/Precautions Use with caution in patients with impaired renal or hepatic function or with possible folate deficiency. Pregnancy risk C.

Drug Interactions

Cytochrome P450 Effect: Substrate of **CYP2C8/9, 3A4**; Inhibits CYP2C8/9

Increased Effect/Toxicity: Increased effect/toxicity/levels of phenytoin. Concurrent use with ACE inhibitors increases risk of hyperkalemia. Increased myelosuppression with methotrexate. May increase levels of digoxin. Concurrent use with dapsone may increase levels of dapsone and trimethoprim. Concurrent use with procainamide may increase levels of procainamide and trimethoprim.

Adverse Reactions Frequency not defined.

Central nervous system: Aseptic meningitis (rare), fever

Dermatologic: Maculopapular rash (3% to 7% at 200 mg/day; incidence higher with larger daily doses), erythema multiforme (rare), exfoliative dermatitis (rare), pruritus (common), phototoxic skin eruptions, Stevens-Johnson syndrome (rare), toxic epidermal necrolysis (rare)

Endocrine & metabolic: Hyperkalemia, hyponatremia

Gastrointestinal: Epigastric distress, glossitis, nausea, vomiting

Hematologic: Leukopenia, megaloblastic anemia, methemoglobinemia, neutropenia, thrombocytopenia

Hepatic: Liver enzyme elevation, cholestatic jaundice (rare)

Renal: BUN and creatinine increased

Miscellaneous: Anaphylaxis, hypersensitivity reactions

Overdosage/Toxicology Symptoms of acute toxicity include nausea, vomiting, confusion, and dizziness. Chronic overdose results in bone marrow suppression. Treatment of acute overdose is supportive following GI decontamination. Use oral leucovorin 5-15 mg/day for treatment of chronic overdose. Hemodialysis is only moderately effective in eliminating drug.

Pharmacodynamics/Kinetics

Absorption: Readily and extensive

Half-Life Elimination: 8-14 hours; prolonged with renal impairment

Time to Peak: Serum: 1-4 hours

Metabolism: Partially hepatic

Formulations

Solution, oral (Primsol®): 50 mg (base)/5 mL (480 mL) [contains sodium benzoate; bubblegum flavor]

Tablet: 100 mg

Proloprim®: 100 mg, 200 mg

Dosing

Adults & Elderly: Susceptible infections: Oral: 100 mg every 12 hours or 200 mg every 24 hours

Pediatrics: Oral: Children (>2 months or age): 4 mg/kg/day in divided doses every 12 hours

Renal Impairment:

Cl_{cr} 15-30 mL/minute: Administer 100 mg every 18 hours or 50 mg every 12 hours.

Cl_{cr} <15 mL/minute: Administer 100 mg every 24 hours or avoid use.

Moderately dialyzable (20% to 50%)

Administration

Oral: Administer with milk or food.

Stability

Storage: Protect the 200 mg tablet from light.

Monitoring Laboratory Tests Periodic CBC during long-term therapy. Perform culture and sensitivity prior to initiating therapy.

Monitoring and Teaching Issues

Physical Assessment: See Contraindications and Warnings/Precautions for use cautions. Assess potential for interactions with other prescriptions, OTC medications, or herbal products patient may be taking (see Drug Interactions). Assess results of laboratory tests (see above), therapeutic effectiveness and adverse reactions (see Adverse Reactions and Overdose/Toxicology). Teach patient possible side effects and interventions and adverse symptoms to report (see Patient Education). **Pregnancy risk factor C** - benefits of use should outweigh possible risks. Note breast-feeding caution.

Patient Education: Inform prescriber of all prescriptions, OTC medications, or herbal products you are taking, and any allergies you have. Do not take anything new during treatment unless approved by prescriber. Take per recommended schedule. Complete full course of therapy even if feeling better; do not skip doses. Maintain adequate hydration (2-3 L/day of fluids) unless advised by prescriber to restrict fluids. May cause nausea, vomiting, or GI upset (small, frequent meals, frequent mouth care, sucking lozenges, or chewing gum may help). Report skin rash, redness, or irritation; feelings of acute fatigue or weakness; unusual bleeding or bruising; or other persistent adverse effects. **Pregnancy precaution:** Inform prescriber if you are or intend to become pregnant. Consult prescriber if breast-feeding.

Dietary Issues: May cause folic acid deficiency, supplements may be needed. Should be taken with milk or food.

Geriatric Considerations: Trimethoprim is often used in combination with sulfamethoxazole; it can be used alone in patients who are allergic to sulfonamides; adjust dose for renal function (see Pharmacokinetics and Usual Dosage).

Trimethoprim and Polymyxin B *see page 1509*

Trimethoprim and Sulfamethoxazole *see* Sulfamethoxazole and Trimethoprim *on page 1259*

Trimethylpsoralen *see* Trioxsalen *on page 1370*

Trimetrexate Glucuronate (tri me TREKS ate gloo KYOOR oh nate)

U.S. Brand Names Neutrexin®

Generic Available No

Pharmacologic Category Antineoplastic Agent, Miscellaneous

Pregnancy Risk Factor D

Lactation Excretion in breast milk unknown/contraindicated

Use Alternative therapy for the treatment of moderate-to-severe *Pneumocystis carinii* pneumonia (PCP) in immunocompromised patients, including patients with acquired immunodeficiency syndrome (AIDS), who are intolerant of, or are refractory to, co-trimoxazole therapy or for whom co-trimoxazole and pentamidine are contraindicated. **Concurrent folinic acid (leucovorin) must always be administered.**

Mechanism of Action/Effect Exerts an antimicrobial effect through potent inhibition of the enzyme dihydrofolate reductase (DHFR)

Contraindications Hypersensitivity to trimetrexate, methotrexate, leucovorin, or any component of the formulation; severe existing myelosuppression; pregnancy

Warnings/Precautions The U.S. Food and Drug Administration (FDA) currently recommends that procedures for proper handling and disposal of antineoplastic agents be considered. Appropriate safety equipment is recommended for preparation, administration, and disposal of antineoplastics. If trimetrexate contacts the skin, immediately wash with soap and water. **Must be administered with concurrent leucovorin to avoid potentially serious or life-threatening toxicities**. Leucovorin therapy must extend for 72 hours past the last dose of trimetrexate. Hypersensitivity/allergic-type reactions have been reported, primarily when given as a bolus infusion, at higher than recommended doses for PCP, or in combination with 5-FU or leucovorin. Use with caution in patients with mild myelosuppression, severe hepatic or renal dysfunction, hypoproteinemia, hypoalbuminemia, or previous extensive myelosuppressive therapies.

Drug Interactions

Increased Effect/Toxicity: Cimetidine, clotrimazole, and ketoconazole may decrease trimetrexate metabolism, resulting in increased serum levels. Trimetrexate may increase toxicity (infections) of live virus vaccines.

Adverse Reactions

>10%:

Hematologic: Neutropenia

Hepatic: LFTs increased

1% to 10%:

Central nervous system: Seizures, fever

Dermatologic: Rash

Gastrointestinal: Stomatitis, nausea, vomiting

Hematologic: Thrombocytopenia, anemia

Neuromuscular & skeletal: Peripheral neuropathy

Renal: Increased serum creatinine

Miscellaneous: Flu-like illness, hypersensitivity reactions, anaphylactoid reactions

Pharmacodynamics/Kinetics

Half-Life Elimination: 15-17 hours

Metabolism: Extensively hepatic

Formulations Injection, powder for reconstitution: 25 mg, 200 mg

Dosing

Adults & Elderly: *Pneumocystis carinii* pneumonia (PCP): I.V.: 45 mg/m^2 once daily for 21 days; concurrent leucovorin 20 mg/m^2 every 6 hours must be administered daily (oral or I.V.) during treatment and for 72 hours past the last dose of trimetrexate glucuronate (for a total of 24 days).

Alternative dosing based on weight: See table on following page.

Hepatic Impairment: Although it may be necessary to reduce the dose in patients with liver dysfunction, no specific recommendations exist.

(Continued)

Trimetrexate Glucuronate *(Continued)*

Trimetrexate Weight-Based Dosing

Body Weight (kg)	Trimetrexate Glucuronate (mg/kg/day)	Leucovorin[1] (mg/kg/qid)
<50	1.5	0.6
50-80	1.2	0.5
>50	1	0.5

[1]Oral doses of leucovorin should be rounded to the next higher 25 mg increment.

Administration

I.V.: Infuse over 60 minutes.

Stability

Storage: Prior to reconstitution, vials should stored at controlled room temperature of 20°C to 25°C (68°F to 77°F). Protect from light.

Reconstitution: Reconstitute with D_5W or SWFI to a concentration of 12.5 mg/mL. Do not use if cloudy or if precipitate forms. Following reconstitution, the solution should be used immediately, but is stable for 6 hours at room temperature or 24 hours under refrigeration. Prior to administration, solution should be further diluted with D_5W to a concentration of 0.25 mg/mL to 2 mg/mL. This final diluted solution is stable under refrigeration or at room temperature for 24 hours.

Compatibility: Stable in D_5W, sterile water for injection

Precipitate occurs with leucovorin or any solution containing chloride ion.

Y-site administration: Incompatible with foscarnet, indomethacin

Compatibility when admixed: Incompatible with chloride-containing solutions, leucovorin

Monitoring Laboratory Tests Absolute neutrophil counts (ANC), platelet count, renal function tests (serum creatinine, BUN), hepatic function (ALT, AST, alkaline phosphatase)

Monitoring and Teaching Issues

Physical Assessment: See Contraindications and Warnings/Precautions for use cautions. Assess potential for interactions with other prescriptions, OTC medications, or herbal products patient may be taking (see Drug Interactions). Assess results of laboratory tests (see above), therapeutic effectiveness and adverse reactions (see Adverse Reactions and Overdose/Toxicology). Teach patient possible side effects and interventions, and adverse symptoms to report (see Patient Education). **Pregnancy risk factor D** - determine that patient is not pregnant before beginning treatment. Instruct patients of childbearing age on appropriate barrier contraceptive measures. Breast-feeding is contraindicated.

Patient Education: Inform prescriber of all prescriptions, OTC medications, or herbal products you are taking, and any allergies you have. Do not take anything new during treatment unless approved by prescriber (especially aspirin or aspirin-containing products.). This medication can only be administered I.V. Report immediately any redness, swelling, or pain at infusion site. Maintain adequate hydration (2-3 L/day of fluids) unless advised by prescriber to restrict fluids. You may be more susceptible to infection (avoid crowds and exposure to infection and do not have any vaccinations unless approved by prescriber). Report persistent fever, chills, or joint pain; numbness or tingling of extremities; vomiting, nausea, or acute abdominal pain; mouth sores; increased bruising or bleeding; blood in urine or stool; changes in sensorium (eg, confusion, hallucinations, seizures); increased difficulty breathing; or acute persistent malaise or weakness. **Pregnancy/ breast-feeding precautions:** Inform prescriber if you are pregnant. Do not get pregnant while taking this medication or for one month after completing therapy. Consult prescriber for appropriate contraceptive measures. Do not breast-feed.

Geriatric Considerations: No specific recommendations are available for the elderly. Use with caution in patients with liver dysfunction (see Usual Dosage).

Additional Information Not a vesicant; methotrexate derivative

Trimipramine (trye MI pra meen)

U.S. Brand Names Surmontil®

Synonyms Trimipramine Maleate

Generic Available No

Pharmacologic Category Antidepressant, Tricyclic (Tertiary Amine)

Pregnancy Risk Factor C

Lactation Enters breast milk/contraindicated

Use Treatment of depression

Mechanism of Action/Effect Increases the synaptic concentration of serotonin and/or norepinephrine in the central nervous system by inhibition of their reuptake by the presynaptic neuronal membrane

Contraindications Hypersensitivity to trimipramine, any component of the formulation, or other dibenzodiazepines; use of MAO inhibitors within 14 days; use in a patient during the acute recovery phase of MI

Warnings/Precautions May cause drowsiness/sedation, resulting in impaired performance of tasks requiring alertness (ie, operating machinery or driving). Sedative effects may be additive with other CNS depressants and/or ethanol. May worsen psychosis in some patients or precipitate a shift to mania or hypomania in patients with bipolar disease. May cause hyponatremia/SIADH. May increase the risks associated with electroconvulsive therapy. Discontinue, when possible, prior to elective surgery. Therapy should not be abruptly discontinued in patients receiving high doses for prolonged periods.

Use with caution in patients at risk of hypotension (orthostasis) or in patients where transient hypotensive episodes would be poorly tolerated (cardiovascular disease or cerebrovascular disease). Use with caution in elderly patients, patients with diabetes, thyroid disease (or patients receiving thyroid supplements), hepatic dysfunction, renal dysfunction, urinary retention, benign prostatic hyperplasia, narrow-angle glaucoma, xerostomia, visual problems, constipation, or a history of bowel obstruction.

Use caution in patients with depression, particularly if suicidal risk may be present. Use with caution in patients with a history of cardiovascular disease, previous seizure disorder, or condition/drug therapy predisposing to seizures. Not for use in patients <12 years of age.

Pregnancy risk C.

Drug Interactions

Cytochrome P450 Effect: Substrate of **CYP2C19, 2D6, 3A4**

Decreased Effect: Carbamazepine, phenobarbital, and rifampin may increase the metabolism of trimipramine resulting in decreased effect of trimipramine. Trimipramine inhibits the antihypertensive response to bethanidine, clonidine, debrisoquin, guanadrel, guanethidine, guanabenz, and guanfacine. Cholestyramine and colestipol may bind TCAs and reduce their absorption; monitor for altered response.

Increased Effect/Toxicity: Trimipramine increases the effects of amphetamines, anticholinergics, other CNS depressants (sedatives, hypnotics, or ethanol), chlorpropamide, tolazamide, and warfarin. When used with MAO inhibitors, hyperpyrexia, hypertension, tachycardia, confusion, seizures, and **deaths have been reported** (serotonin syndrome). Serotonin syndrome has also been reported with ritonavir (rare). The SSRIs (to varying degrees), cimetidine, grapefruit juice, indinavir, methylphenidate, ritonavir, quinidine, diltiazem, and verapamil inhibit the metabolism of TCAs and clinical toxicity may result. Use of lithium with a TCA may increase the risk for neurotoxicity. Phenothiazines may increase concentration of some TCAs and TCAs may increase concentration of phenothiazines. Pressor response to I.V. epinephrine, norepinephrine, and phenylephrine may be enhanced in patients receiving TCAs (**Note:** Effect is unlikely with epinephrine or levonordefrin dosages typically administered as infiltration in combination with local anesthetics). Combined use of beta-agonists or drugs which prolong QT_c (including quinidine, procainamide, disopyramide, cisapride, sparfloxacin, gatifloxacin, moxifloxacin) with TCAs may predispose patients to cardiac arrhythmias.

Nutritional/Ethanol Interactions

Ethanol: Avoid ethanol (may increase CNS depression).

Food: Grapefruit juice may inhibit the metabolism of some TCAs and clinical toxicity may result.

Herb/Nutraceutical: Avoid valerian, St John's wort, SAMe, kava kava (may increase risk of serotonin syndrome and/or excessive sedation).

Effects on Lab Values ↑ glucose

Adverse Reactions Frequency not defined.

Cardiovascular: Arrhythmias, hypotension, hypertension, tachycardia, palpitations, heart block, stroke, myocardial infarction

Central nervous system: Headache, exacerbation of psychosis, confusion, delirium, hallucinations, nervousness, restlessness, delusions, agitation, insomnia, nightmares, anxiety, seizures, drowsiness

Dermatologic: Photosensitivity, rash, petechiae, itching

Endocrine & metabolic: Sexual dysfunction, breast enlargement, galactorrhea, SIADH

Gastrointestinal: Xerostomia, constipation, increased appetite, nausea, unpleasant taste, weight gain, diarrhea, heartburn, vomiting, anorexia, trouble with gums, decreased lower esophageal sphincter tone may cause GE reflux

Genitourinary: Difficult urination, urinary retention, testicular edema

Hematologic: Agranulocytosis, eosinophilia, purpura, thrombocytopenia

Hepatic: Cholestatic jaundice, increased liver enzymes

Neuromuscular & skeletal: Tremors, numbness, tingling, paresthesia, incoordination, ataxia, peripheral neuropathy, extrapyramidal symptoms

Ocular: Blurred vision, eye pain, disturbances in accommodation, mydriasis, increased intraocular pressure

Otic: Tinnitus

Miscellaneous: Allergic reactions

Overdosage/Toxicology Symptoms of overdose include agitation, confusion, hallucinations, urinary retention, hypothermia, hypotension, tachycardia, and cardiac arrhythmias. Following initiation of essential overdose management, toxic symptoms should be treated.

Ventricular arrhythmias and EKG changes (QRS widening) often respond to systemic alkalinization (sodium bicarbonate 0.5-2 mEq/kg I.V.). Physostigmine (1-2 mg I.V. slowly for adults) may be indicated for reversing life-threatening cardiac arrhythmias. Treatment is symptomatic and supportive.

Pharmacodynamics/Kinetics

Bioavailability: 18% to 63%

Half-Life Elimination: 16-40 hours

Metabolism: Hepatic; significant first-pass effect

Formulations Capsule, as maleate: 25 mg, 50 mg, 100 mg

Dosing

Adults: Depression: Oral: 50-150 mg/day as a single bedtime dose up to a maximum of 200 mg/day for outpatients and 300 mg/day for inpatients

Elderly: Oral: Initial: 25 mg at bedtime; increase by 25 mg/day every 3 days for inpatients and weekly for outpatients, as tolerated, to a maximum of 100 mg/day (see Geriatric Considerations).

Stability

Storage: Solutions stable at a pH of 4-5; turns yellowish or reddish on exposure to light. Slight discoloration does not affect potency; marked discoloration is associated with loss of potency. Capsules stable for 3 years following date of manufacture.

Monitoring and Teaching Issues

Physical Assessment: Assess other medications patient may be taking for effectiveness and interactions (see Drug Interactions). See Contraindications and Warnings/Precautions for use cautions. Monitor therapeutic response according to rationale for therapy, and

(Continued)

Trimipramine *(Continued)*

adverse reactions at beginning of therapy and periodically with long-term use (see Adverse Reactions and Overdose/Toxicology). Taper dosage slowly when discontinuing (allow 3-4 weeks between discontinuing Surmontil® and starting another antidepressant). Assess knowledge/teach patient appropriate use, interventions to reduce side effects, and adverse symptoms to report (see Patient Education). **Pregnancy risk factor C** - benefits of use should outweigh possible risks. Breast-feeding is contraindicated.

Patient Education: Take exactly as directed; do not increase dose or frequency. It may take 2-3 weeks to achieve desired results. Take at bedtime. Avoid alcohol, caffeine, and other prescription or OTC medications not approved by prescriber. Maintain adequate hydration (2-3 L/day of fluids) unless advised by prescriber to restrict fluids. You may experience drowsiness, lightheadedness, dizziness, or blurred vision (use caution when driving or engaging in tasks requiring alertness until response to drug is known); nausea, altered taste, dry mouth (small, frequent meals, frequent mouth care, chewing gum, or sucking lozenges may help); constipation (increased exercise, fluids, fruit, or fiber may help); diarrhea (buttermilk, yogurt, or boiled milk may help); increased appetite (monitor dietary intake to avoid excess weight gain); postural hypotension (use caution when climbing stairs or changing position from lying or sitting to standing); urinary retention (void before taking medication); or sexual dysfunction (reversible). Report persistent CNS effects (eg, insomnia, restlessness, fatigue, anxiety, impaired cognitive function, seizures); muscle cramping or tremors; chest pain, palpitations, rapid heartbeat, swelling of extremities, or severe dizziness; unresolved urinary retention; vision changes or eye pain; yellowing of eyes or skin; pale stools/dark urine; or worsening of condition. **Pregnancy/breast-feeding precautions:** Inform prescriber if you are or intend to become pregnant. Do not breast-feed.

Geriatric Considerations: Similar to doxepin in its side effect profile. Has not been well studied in the elderly. Very anticholinergic and, therefore, not considered a drug of first choice in the elderly when selecting an antidepressant.

Additional Information May cause alterations in bleeding time.

Related Information

Antidepressant Agents *on page 1553*
Antidepressant Medication Guidelines *on page 1613*

Trimipramine Maleate *see* Trimipramine *on page 1368*

Trimox® *see* Amoxicillin *on page 88*

Trinalin® *see* Azatadine and Pseudoephedrine *on page 137*

Tri-Nasal® *see* Triamcinolone *on page 1356*

Tri-Norinyl® *see* Ethinyl Estradiol and Norethindrone *on page 527*

Triotann® Tablet *see page 1522*

Trioxsalen (trye OKS a len)

U.S. Brand Names Trisoralen®

Synonyms Trimethylpsoralen

Generic Available No

Pharmacologic Category Psoralen

Pregnancy Risk Factor C

Lactation Excretion in breast milk unknown

Use In conjunction with controlled exposure to ultraviolet light or sunlight for repigmentation of idiopathic vitiligo; increasing tolerance to sunlight with albinism; enhance pigmentation

Mechanism of Action/Effect Psoralens are thought to form covalent bonds with pyrimidine bases in DNA which inhibit the synthesis of DNA. This reaction involves excitation of the trioxsalen molecule by radiation in the long-wave ultraviolet light (UVA) resulting in transference of energy to the trioxsalen molecule producing an excited state. Binding of trioxsalen to DNA occurs only in the presence of ultraviolet light. The increase in skin pigmentation produced by trioxsalen and UVA radiation involves multiple changes in melanocytes and interaction between melanocytes and keratinocytes. In general, melanogenesis is stimulated but the size and distribution of melanocytes is unchanged.

Contraindications Hypersensitivity to psoralens, melanoma, a history of melanoma, or other diseases associated with photosensitivity; porphyria; acute lupus erythematosus; patients <12 years of age

Warnings/Precautions Serious burns from UVA or sunlight can occur if dosage or exposure schedules are exceeded. Patients must wear protective eyewear to prevent cataracts. Use with caution in patients with severe hepatic or cardiovascular disease. Pregnancy risk C.

Adverse Reactions

>10%:

Dermatologic: Itching
Gastrointestinal: Nausea

1% to 10%:

Central nervous system: Dizziness, headache, mental depression, insomnia, nervousness
Dermatologic: Severe burns from excessive sunlight or ultraviolet exposure
Gastrointestinal: Gastric discomfort

Pharmacodynamics/Kinetics

Absorption: Rapid

Half-Life Elimination: ~2 hours

Onset: Peak effect: Photosensitivity: 2 hours

Duration: Skin sensitivity to light: 8-12 hours

Formulations Tablet: 5 mg

Dosing

Adults & Elderly: Repigmentation of idiopathic vitiligo, albinism, enhance pigmentation: Oral: 10 mg/day as a single dose, 2-4 hours before controlled exposure to UVA (for 15-35 minutes) or sunlight. Do not continue for longer than 14 days.

Pediatrics: Children >12 years: Oral: Refer to adult dosing.

Administration

Oral: To minimize gastric discomfort, tablets may be taken with milk or after a meal.

Monitoring and Teaching Issues

Physical Assessment: See Contraindications and Warnings/Precautions for use cautions. This medication will be administered in conjunction with ultraviolet light of ultraviolet radiation therapy. Teach patient appropriate use, safety measures, and sunlight precautions. **Pregnancy risk factor C** - benefits of use should outweigh possible risks. Note breast-feeding caution.

Patient Education: This medication is used in conjunction with specific ultraviolet treatment. Follow prescriber's directions exactly for oral medication which can be taken with food or milk to reduce nausea. Avoid use of any other skin treatments unless approved by prescriber. You must wear protective eyewear during treatments. Avoid use of any other skin treatments unless approved by prescriber. Control exposure to direct sunlight as per prescriber's instructions for 8-12 hours following treatment. If sunlight cannot be avoided, use sunblock (consult prescriber for specific SPF level), wear protective clothing, and wrap-around protective eyewear. Consult prescriber immediately if burning, blistering, or skin irritation occur. **Pregnancy/breast-feeding precautions:** Inform prescriber if you are or intend to become pregnant. Consult prescriber if breast-feeding.

Tripedia® *see page 1498*

Triphasil® *see* Ethinyl Estradiol and Levonorgestrel *on page 523*

Triple Antibiotic® *see* Bacitracin, Neomycin, and Polymyxin B *on page 144*

Triple Care® Antifungal [OTC] *see* Miconazole *on page 899*

Triple Sulfa *see* Sulfabenzamide, Sulfacetamide, and Sulfathiazole *on page 1255*

Triptorelin (trip toe REL in)

U.S. Brand Names Trelstar™ Depot; Trelstar™ LA

Synonyms Triptorelin Pamoate

Generic Available No

Pharmacologic Category Luteinizing Hormone-Releasing Hormone Analog

Pregnancy Risk Factor X

Lactation Excretion in breast milk unknown/contraindicated

Use Palliative treatment of advanced prostate cancer as an alternative to orchiectomy or estrogen administration

Mechanism of Action/Effect Causes suppression of ovarian and testicular steroidogenesis due to decreased levels of LH and FSH with subsequent decrease in testosterone (male) and estrogen (female) levels. After chronic and continuous administration, usually 2-4 weeks after initiation, a sustained decrease in LH and FSH secretion occurs.

Contraindications Hypersensitivity to triptorelin or any component of the formulation, other LHRH agonists or LHRH; pregnancy

Warnings/Precautions Transient increases in testosterone can lead to worsening symptoms (bone pain, hematuria, bladder outlet obstruction) of prostate cancer during the first few weeks of therapy. Cases of spinal cord compression have been reported with LHRH agonists. Hypersensitivity reactions including angioedema and anaphylaxis have rarely occurred. Safety and efficacy has not established in pediatric population.

Drug Interactions

Decreased Effect: Not studied. Hyperprolactinemic drugs (dopamine antagonists such as antipsychotics, and metoclopramide) are contraindicated.

Increased Effect/Toxicity: Not studied. Hyperprolactinemic drugs (dopamine antagonists such as antipsychotics, and metoclopramide) are contraindicated.

Effects on Lab Values Pituitary-gonadal function may be suppressed with chronic administration and for up to 8 weeks after triptorelin therapy has been discontinued.

Adverse Reactions As reported with Trelstar™ Depot and Trelstar™ LA; frequency of effect may vary by product:

>10%:

Endocrine & metabolic: Hot flashes (59% to 73%), glucose increased, hemoglobin decreased, RBC count decreased

Hepatic: Alkaline phosphatase increased, ALT increased, AST increased

Neuromuscular & skeletal: Skeletal pain (12% to 13%)

Renal: BUN increased

1% to 10%:

Cardiovascular: Leg edema (6%), hypertension (4%), chest pain (2%), peripheral edema (1%)

Central nervous system: Headache (5% to 7%), dizziness (1% to 3%), pain (2% to 3%), emotional lability (1%), fatigue (2%), insomnia (2%)

Dermatologic: Rash (2%), pruritus (1%)

Endocrine & metabolic: Alkaline phosphatase increased (2%), breast pain (2%), gynocomastia (2%), libido decreased (2%)

Gastrointestinal: Nausea (3%), anorexia (2%), constipation (2%), dyspepsia (2%), vomiting (2%), abdominal pain (1%), diarrhea (1%)

Genitourinary: Dysuria (5%), impotence (2% to 7%), urinary retention (1%), urinary tract infection (1%)

Hematologic: Anemia (1%)

Local: Injection site pain (4%)

Neuromuscular & skeletal: Leg pain (2% to 5%), back pain (3%), arthralgia (2%), leg cramps (2%), myalgia (1%), weakness (1%)

Ocular: Conjunctivitis (1%), eye pain (1%)

Respiratory: Cough (2%), dyspnea (1%), pharyngitis (1%)

Postmarketing and/or case reports (Limited to important or life-threatening): Anaphylaxis, angioedema, hypersensitivity reactions, renal dysfunction, spinal cord compression

Overdosage/Toxicology Accidental or intentional overdose unlikely. If it were to occur, supportive and symptomatic treatment would be indicated.

(Continued)

Triptorelin *(Continued)*

Pharmacodynamics/Kinetics

Absorption: Oral: Not active

Half-Life Elimination: 2.8 ± 1.2 hours

Moderate to severe renal impairment: 6.5-7.7 hours

Hepatic impairment: 7.6 hours

Time to Peak: 1-3 hours

Metabolism: Unknown; unlikely to involve CYP; no known metabolites

Formulations Injection, powder for reconstitution, as pamoate [also available packaged with Debioclip™ (prefilled syringe containing sterile water)]:

Trelstar™ Depot: 3.75 mg

Trelstar™ LA: 11.25 mg

Dosing

Adults & Elderly: Advanced prostate carcinoma: I.M.: 3.75 mg once monthly

Renal Impairment: Specific guidelines are not available.

Hepatic Impairment: Specific guidelines are not available.

Administration

I.M.: Must be administered under the supervision of a physician. Administer by I.M. injection into the buttock; alternate injection sites.

Debioclip™: Follow manufacturer's instructions for mixing prior to use.

Stability

Storage:

Trelstar™ Depot: Store at 15°C to 30°C (59°F to 86°F)

Trelstar™ LA: Store at 20°C to 25°C (68°F to 77°F)

Reconstitution: Reconstitute with 2 mL sterile water for injection. Shake well to obtain a uniform suspension. Withdraw the entire contents into the syringe and inject immediately.

Monitoring Laboratory Tests Serum testosterone levels, prostate-specific antigen

Monitoring and Teaching Issues

Physical Assessment: See Contraindications, Warnings/Precautions, and Dosing for use cautions. Assess results of laboratory tests (see above), therapeutic effectiveness, and adverse response (see Adverse Reactions and Overdose/Toxicology). See Administration details. Teach patient possible side effects and appropriate interventions and adverse symptoms to report (see Patient Education). **Pregnancy risk factor X** - used to treat advanced prostate cancer. Breast-feeding is contraindicated.

Patient Education: This medication can only be administered by injection. Report swelling, pain, or burning at injection site. May cause disease flare (increased bone pain), blood in urine, or urinary retention during early treatment (usually resolves within 1 week); impotence; or hot flashes (cool cloth on forehead, cool environment, and light clothing may help - contact prescriber if these become intolerable). Report any persistent adverse GI upset; chest pain, rapid heartbeat, or palpations; numbness in extremities; acute headache; alterations in urinary pattern; or other persistent adverse effects. **Pregnancy/breast-feeding precautions:** This drug will cause severe fetal defects. Do not breast-feed.

Triptorelin Pamoate *see* Triptorelin *on page 1371*

Trisenox™ *see* Arsenic Trioxide *on page 117*

Trisoralen® *see* Trioxsalen *on page 1370*

Tristoject® *see* Triamcinolone *on page 1356*

Tri-Tannate® Tablet *see page 1522*

Trivagizole 3™ *see* Clotrimazole *on page 322*

Trivora® *see* Ethinyl Estradiol and Levonorgestrel *on page 523*

Trizivir® *see* Abacavir, Lamivudine, and Zidovudine *on page 31*

Trobicin® *see* Spectinomycin *on page 1243*

Trocaine® [OTC] *see* Benzocaine *on page 156*

Tropicacyl® *see page 1509*

Tropicacyl® *see page 1461*

Tropicamide *see page 1509*

Tropicamide *see page 1461*

Trovafloxacin (TROE va flox a sin)

U.S. Brand Names Trovan®

Synonyms Alatrofloxacin Mesylate; CP-99,219-27

Generic Available No

Pharmacologic Category Antibiotic, Quinolone

Pregnancy Risk Factor C

Lactation Enters breast milk/contraindicated

Use Should be used only in life- or limb-threatening infections

Treatment of nosocomial pneumonia, community-acquired pneumonia, complicated intra-abdominal infections, gynecologic/pelvic infections, complicated skin and skin structure infections

Mechanism of Action/Effect Inhibits DNA gyrase and topoisomerase IV in susceptible organisms; blocks relaxation of supercoiled DNA and promoted breakage of double-stranded DNA. Activity *in vitro* includes atypical, gram-negative, gram-positive (including penicillin-resistant pneumococci), intra- and extracellular aerobic organisms.

Contraindications History of hypersensitivity to trovafloxacin, alatrofloxacin, quinolone antimicrobial agents, or any component of the formulation

Warnings/Precautions For use only in serious life- or limb-threatening infections. Initiation of therapy must occur in an inpatient healthcare facility. May alter GI flora resulting in pseudomembranous colitis due to *Clostridium difficile*. Use with caution in patients with seizure disorders or severe cerebral atherosclerosis. May cause photosensitivity. CNS stimulation may occur which may lead to tremor, restlessness, confusion, hallucinations, paranoia, depression, nightmares, insomnia, or lightheadedness. Hepatic reactions have resulted in death. Risk of hepatotoxicity is increased if therapy exceeds 14 days. Tendon inflammation and/or rupture have been reported with other quinolone antibiotics. Risk may be increased with concurrent corticosteroids, particularly in the elderly. Discontinue at first sign of tendon inflammation or pain. Quinolones may exacerbate myasthenia gravis.

Severe hypersensitivity reactions, including anaphylaxis, have occurred with quinolone therapy. If an allergic reaction occurs (itching, urticaria, dyspnea, facial edema, loss of consciousness, tingling, cardiovascular collapse), discontinue drug immediately. Prolonged use may result in superinfection; pseudomembranous colitis may occur and should be considered in all patients who present with diarrhea.

Pregnancy risk C.

Drug Interactions

Decreased Effect: Coadministration with antacids containing aluminum or magnesium, citric acid/sodium citrate, sucralfate, and iron markedly reduces absorption of trovafloxacin. Separate oral administration by at least 2 hours. Coadministration of intravenous morphine also reduces absorption. Separate I.V. morphine by 2 hours (when trovafloxacin is taken in fasting state) or 4 hours (when taken with food). Do not administer multivalent cations (eg, calcium, magnesium) through the same intravenous line.

Increased Effect/Toxicity: Concurrent use of corticosteroids may increase risk of tendon rupture.

Nutritional/Ethanol Interactions

Food: Dairy products such as milk or yogurt may reduce absorption of oral trovafloxacin; avoid concurrent use. Enteral feedings may also limit absorption.

Herb/Nutraceutical: Avoid dong quai, St John's wort (may also cause photosensitization).

Adverse Reactions Note: Fatalities have occurred in patients developing hepatic necrosis.

1% to 10% (range reported in clinical trials):
- Central nervous system: Dizziness (2% to 11%), lightheadedness (<1% to 4%), headache (1% to 5%)
- Dermatologic: Rash (<1% to 2%), pruritus (<1% to 2%)
- Gastrointestinal: Nausea (4% to 8%), abdominal pain (<1% to 1%), vomiting, diarrhea
- Genitourinary: Vaginitis (<1% to 1%)
- Hepatic: Increased LFTs
- Local: Injection site reaction, pain, or inflammation

<1% (Limited to important or life-threatening): Allergic/anaphylactoid reaction, anaphylaxis, bronchospasm, convulsions, dyskinesia, hepatic necrosis, interstitial nephritis, pancreatitis, phototoxicity, pseudomembranous colitis, Stevens-Johnson syndrome, tendonitis; quinolones have been associated with tendon rupture,

Overdosage/Toxicology Empty the stomach by vomiting or gastric lavage. Observe carefully and give symptomatic and supportive treatment; maintain adequate hydration.

Pharmacodynamics/Kinetics

Bioavailability: 88%

Half-Life Elimination: 9-12 hours

Time to Peak: Oral: Within 2 hours

Metabolism: Hepatic conjugation; glucuronidation 13%, acetylation 9%

Formulations

Injection, as mesylate (alatrofloxacin): 5 mg/mL (40 mL, 60 mL)

Tablet, as mesylate (trovafloxacin): 100 mg, 200 mg

Dosing

Adults & Elderly:
- Nosocomial pneumonia: I.V.: 300 mg single dose followed by 200 mg/day orally for a total duration of 10-14 days
- Community-acquired pneumonia: Oral, I.V.: 200 mg/day for 7-14 days
- Complicated intra-abdominal infections, including postsurgical infections/gynecologic and pelvic infections: I.V.: 300 mg as a single dose followed by 200 mg/day orally for a total duration of 7-14 days
- Skin and skin structure infections, complicated, including diabetic foot infections: Oral, I.V.: 200 mg/day for 10-14 days

Renal Impairment: No adjustment is necessary. Trovafloxacin is not sufficiently removed by hemodialysis.

Hepatic Impairment:
- Mild to moderate cirrhosis:
  - Initial dose for normal hepatic function: 300 mg I.V.; 200 mg I.V. or oral; 100 mg oral
  - Reduced dose: 200 mg I.V.; 100 mg I.V. or oral; 100 mg oral
- Severe cirrhosis: No data available

Administration

Oral: Take without regard to meals.

I.V.: Not for I.M. or S.C. Administer over 60 minutes.

Stability

Storage: Store undiluted vials of solution at 15°C to 30°C (50°F to 86°F).

Reconstitution: Diluted solutions are stable for up to 7 days when refrigerated and up to 3 days at room temperature. Dilute to a concentration of 0.5-2 mg/mL in dextrose 5% in water, 0.45% sodium chloride, dextrose 5% in water and 0.45% sodium chloride, dextrose 5% in water and 0.2% sodium chloride, or lactated Ringer's in dextrose 5% in water; should not be diluted with 0.9% sodium chloride or lactated Ringer's.

Compatibility: Stable in D_5W, D_5LR, $D_5\frac{1}{4}NS$, $D_5\frac{1}{2}NS$, $\frac{1}{2}NS$; **incompatible** with 0.9% NS, NS, LR; dilute to a concentration of 0.5-2 mg/mL in D_5W, 0.45% NS, D_5W and 0.45% NS, D_5W and 0.2% NS, or LR in D_5W

Y-site administration: Incompatible with aztreonam, ceftazidime, ceftriaxone, dobutamine, famotidine, furosemide, heparin, insulin (regular), magnesium sulfate, morphine, piperacillin/tazobactam, ticarcillin/clavulanate

Monitoring Laboratory Tests Perform culture and sensitivity testing prior to initiating therapy. Monitor CBC, liver function tests if therapy is longer than 21 days.

(Continued)

Trovafloxacin *(Continued)*

Monitoring and Teaching Issues

Physical Assessment: Assess allergy history before initiating therapy. See Contraindications, Warnings/Precautions, and Dosing for use cautions. Assess potential for interactions with other prescriptions, OTC medications, or herbal products patient may be taking (see extensive list of Drug Interactions). **I.V.:** See specifics above and monitor closely for severe hypersensitivity reactions, including anaphylaxis. If an allergic reaction occurs, drug should be discontinued immediately. Assess results of laboratory tests (see above), therapeutic effectiveness, and adverse effects (eg, hypersensitivity reactions can occur days after therapy has started), (see Adverse Reactions and Overdose/Toxicology) regularly during therapy. Teach patient appropriate use (according to formulation), possible side effects and interventions, and adverse symptoms to report (see Patient Education). **Pregnancy risk factor C** - benefits of use should outweigh possible risks. Breast-feeding is contraindicated.

Patient Education: Inform prescriber of all prescriptions, OTC medications, or herbal products you are taking, and any allergies you have. Do not take anything new during treatment unless approved by prescriber. Take exactly as directed: at least 2 hours before or 2 hours after antacids or other drug products containing calcium, iron, or zinc. Take entire prescription even if feeling better. Maintain adequate hydration (2-3 L/day of fluids) unless advised by prescriber to restrict fluids. May cause dizziness, lightheadedness, or confusion (use caution when driving or engaging in tasks that require alertness until response to drug is known); nausea or vomiting (small, frequent meals, frequent mouth care, sucking lozenges, or chewing gum may help); or photosensitivity (use sunscreen, wear protective clothing and eyewear, and avoid direct sunlight). If inflammation or tendon pain occurs, discontinue use immediately and report to prescriber. If signs of allergic reaction (eg, itching urticaria, difficulty breathing, facial edema or difficulty swallowing, loss of consciousness, tingling, chest pain, palpitations) occurs, discontinue use immediately and report to prescriber. Report CNS disturbances (eg, hallucinations, gait disturbances); palpitations or chest pain; persistent diarrhea or constipation; signs of infection (eg, sore throat, chills, unusual fever, burning, itching on urination, vaginal discharge, white plaques in mouth); easy bruising or bleeding; difficulty breathing; or worsening of condition. Report immediately any pain, inflammation, or rupture of tendon. **Pregnancy/breast-feeding precautions:** Inform prescriber if you are or intend to become pregnant. Do not breast-feed.

Pregnancy Issues: Quinolones have been associated with an increase in skeletal malformations in animal models. Use during pregnancy only if potential benefit outweighs possible risks.

Trovan® *see* Trovafloxacin *on page 1372*

Truxazole® *see* SulfiSOXAZOLE *on page 1264*

Truxcillin® *see* Penicillin V Potassium *on page 1048*

TSH *see* Thyrotropin *on page 1314*

TSPA *see* Thiotepa *on page 1309*

T-Stat® *see* Erythromycin (Systemic) *on page 486*

Tuberculosis *see page 1705*

Tums® [OTC] *see* Calcium Supplements *on page 202*

Tums® E-X Extra Strength Tablet [OTC] *see* Calcium Supplements *on page 202*

Tums® Ultra® [OTC] *see* Calcium Supplements *on page 202*

Tussi-Organidin® DM NR *see* Guaifenesin and Dextromethorphan *on page 647*

Tussi-Organidin® NR *see* Guaifenesin and Codeine *on page 647*

Tussi-Organidin® S-NR *see* Guaifenesin and Codeine *on page 647*

Tusstat® *see* DiphenhydrAMINE *on page 422*

Twilite® [OTC] *see* DiphenhydrAMINE *on page 422*

Twin-K® *see* Potassium Supplements *on page 1106*

Tylenol® [OTC] *see* Acetaminophen *on page 35*

Tylenol® Arthritis Pain [OTC] *see* Acetaminophen *on page 35*

Tylenol® Children's [OTC] *see* Acetaminophen *on page 35*

Tylenol® Extra Strength [OTC] *see* Acetaminophen *on page 35*

Tylenol® Infants [OTC] *see* Acetaminophen *on page 35*

Tylenol® Junior Strength [OTC] *see* Acetaminophen *on page 35*

Tylenol® Sore Throat [OTC] *see* Acetaminophen *on page 35*

Tylenol® With Codeine *see* Acetaminophen and Codeine *on page 37*

Tylox® *see* Oxycodone and Acetaminophen *on page 1022*

Tympangesic® *see page 1519*

TyphimV® *see page 1498*

Typhoid Vaccine *see page 1498*

Tyramine Foods List *see page 1601*

U-90152S *see* Delavirdine *on page 372*

UAD Otic® *see page 1519*

UCB-P071 *see* Cetirizine *on page 263*

UK *see* Urokinase *on page 1375*

UK 92480 *see* Sildenafil *on page 1228*

UK109496 *see* Voriconazole *on page 1407*

Ultram® *see* Tramadol *on page 1344*

Ultrase® *see* Pancrelipase *on page 1029*

Ultrase® MT *see* Pancrelipase *on page 1029*

Ultravate™ *see* Topical Corticosteroids *on page 1334*

Unasyn® *see* Ampicillin and Sulbactam *on page 103*

Uni-Dur® *see* Theophylline *on page 1300*

Urokinase (yoor oh KIN ase)

U.S. Brand Names Abbokinase®

Synonyms UK

Generic Available No

Pharmacologic Category Thrombolytic Agent

Pregnancy Risk Factor B

Lactation Excretion in breast milk unknown/use caution

Use Thrombolytic agent for the lysis of acute massive pulmonary emboli or pulmonary emboli with unstable hemodynamics

Use - Unlabeled/Investigational Thrombolytic agent used in treatment of recent severe or massive deep vein thrombosis, myocardial infarction, and occluded I.V. or dialysis cannulas

Mechanism of Action/Effect Promotes thrombolysis by directly activating plasminogen to plasmin, which degrades fibrin, fibrinogen, and other procoagulant plasma proteins

Contraindications Hypersensitivity to urokinase or any component of the formulation; active internal bleeding; history of CVA; recent (within 2 months) intracranial or intraspinal surgery or trauma; intracranial neoplasm, arteriovenous malformation, or aneurysm; known bleeding diathesis; severe uncontrolled hypertension

Warnings/Precautions Concurrent heparin anticoagulation can contribute to bleeding; careful attention to all potential bleeding sites. I.M. injections and nonessential handling of the patient should be avoided. Venipunctures should be performed carefully and only when necessary. If arterial puncture is necessary, use an upper extremity vessel that can be manually compressed. If serious bleeding occurs, then the infusion of urokinase and heparin should be stopped.

For the following conditions the risk of bleeding is higher with use of anistreplase and should be weighed against the benefits of therapy: recent (within 10 days) major surgery (eg, CABG, obstetrical delivery, organ biopsy, previous puncture of noncompressible vessels), cerebrovascular disease, recent (within 10 days) gastrointestinal or genitourinary bleeding, recent trauma (within 10 days) including CPR, hypertension (systolic BP >180 mm Hg and/or diastolic BP >110 mm Hg), high likelihood of left heart thrombus (eg, mitral stenosis with atrial fibrillation), acute pericarditis, subacute bacterial endocarditis, hemostatic defects including ones caused by severe renal or hepatic dysfunction, significant hepatic dysfunction, pregnancy, diabetic hemorrhagic retinopathy or other hemorrhagic ophthalmic conditions, septic thrombophlebitis or occluded AV cannula at seriously infected site, advanced age (eg, >75 years), patients receiving oral anticoagulants, any other condition in which bleeding constitutes a significant hazard or would be particularly difficult to manage because of location.

Coronary thrombolysis may result in reperfusion arrhythmias. Follow standard MI management. Rare anaphylactoid reactions can occur. Safety and efficacy in pediatric patients have not been established.

Drug Interactions

Decreased Effect: Aminocaproic acid (an antifibrinolytic agent) may decrease the effectiveness of thrombolytic therapy.

Increased Effect/Toxicity: Oral anticoagulants (warfarin), heparin, low molecular weight heparins, and drugs which affect platelet function (eg, NSAIDs, dipyridamole, ticlopidine, clopidogrel, IIb/IIIa antagonists) may potentiate the risk of hemorrhage.

Adverse Reactions As with all drugs which may affect hemostasis, bleeding is the major adverse effect associated with urokinase. Hemorrhage may occur at virtually any site. Risk is dependent on multiple variables, including the dosage administered, concurrent use of multiple agents which alter hemostasis, and patient predisposition.

>10%: Local: Injection site: Bleeding (5% decrease in hematocrit reported in 37% patients; most bleeding occurring at external incisions or injection sites, but also reported in other areas)

<1% (Limited to important or life-threatening): Allergic reaction (includes bronchospasm, orolingual edema, urticaria, skin rash, pruritus); cardiac arrest, cerebral vascular accident, chest pain, cholesterol embolism, diaphoresis, hemiplegia, intracranial hemorrhage, retroperitoneal hemorrhage, myocardial infarction, pulmonary edema, recurrent pulmonary embolism, reperfusion ventricular arrhythmias, stroke, substernal pain, thrombocytopenia, vascular embolization (cerebral and distal); infusion reactions (most occurring within 1 hour) including acidosis, back pain, chills, cyanosis, dyspnea, fever, hypertension, hypotension, hypoxia, nausea, rigors, tachycardia, vomiting

Overdosage/Toxicology Symptoms of overdose include epistaxis, bleeding gums, hematoma, spontaneous ecchymoses, and oozing at the catheter site. In the event of overdose, stop the infusion and reverse bleeding with blood products that contain clotting factors.

(Continued)

Urokinase *(Continued)*

Pharmacodynamics/Kinetics

Half-Life Elimination: 6.4-18.8 minutes

Onset: I.V.: Fibrinolysis occurs rapidly

Duration: ≥4 hours

Formulations Injection, powder for reconstitution: 250,000 int. units [contains human albumin 250 mg and mannitol 25 mg]

Dosing

Adults & Elderly:

Deep vein thrombosis (unlabeled use): I.V.: Loading: 4400 units/kg over 10 minutes, then 4400 units/kg/hour for 12 hours

Myocardial infarction (unlabeled use): Intracoronary: 750,000 units over 2 hours (6000 units/minute over up to 2 hours)

Occluded I.V. catheters (unlabeled use):

5000 units in each lumen over 1-2 minutes, leave in lumen for 1-4 hours, then aspirate. May repeat with 10,000 units in each lumen if 5000 units fails to clear the catheter. **Do not infuse into the patient**. Volume to instill into catheter is equal to the volume of the catheter. Will not dissolve drug precipitate or anything other than blood products.

I.V. infusion: 200 units/kg/hour in each lumen for 12-48 hours at a rate of at least 20 mL/hour

Dialysis patient: 5000 units is administered in each lumen over 1-2 minutes; leave urokinase in lumen for 1-2 days, then aspirate.

Acute pulmonary embolism: I.V.: Loading: 4400 int. units/kg over 10 minutes; maintenance: 4400 int. units/kg/hour for 12 hours. Following infusion, anticoagulation treatment is recommended to prevent recurrent thrombosis. Do not start anticoagulation until aPTT has decreased to less than twice the normal control value. If heparin is used, do not administer loading dose. Treatment should be followed with oral anticoagulants.

Pediatrics: Children: Deep vein thrombosis, pulmonary embolus, or occluded catheter: I.V.: Refer to adult dosing.

Administration

I.V.: Solution may be filtered using a 0.22 or 0.45 micron filter during I.V. therapy. Administer using a pump which can deliver a total volume of 195 mL. The loading dose should be administered at 90 mL/hour over 10 minutes. The maintenance dose should be administered at 15 mL/hour over 12 hours. I.V. tubing should be flushed with NS or D_5W to ensure total dose is administered.

Stability

Storage: Prior to reconstitution, store in refrigerator at 2°C to 8°C (36°F to 46°F). Prior to infusion, solution should be further diluted in D_5W or NS.

Reconstitution: Reconstitute vial with 5 mL sterile water for injection (preservative free) by gently rolling and tilting; do not shake. Contains no preservatives; should not be reconstituted until immediately before using; discard unused portion. Solution will look pale and straw colored. May filter through ≤0.45 micron filter.

Compatibility: Stable in NS

Monitoring Laboratory Tests CBC, platelet count, aPTT, urinalysis

Monitoring and Teaching Issues

Physical Assessment: See Contraindications, Warnings/Precautions, and Dosing for use cautions. Assess potential for interactions with other prescriptions, OTC medications, or herbal products patient may be taking (especially those medications that may affect coagulation or platelet function - see Drug Interactions). Note infusion specifics above; assess infusion site and monitor for systemic hemorrhage during and following therapy (see Adverse Reactions and Overdose/Toxicology). Assess results of laboratory results (see above). Patient should be monitored closely prior to, during, and after therapy (eg, neurological status - intracranial hemorrhage; vital signs; and EKG - reperfusion arrhythmias). Bedrest and bleeding precautions should be maintained. Avoid I.M. injections and nonessential handling of the patient. Venipunctures should be performed carefully and only when necessary. If arterial puncture is necessary, use an upper extremity vessel that can be manually compressed. Patient instructions are determined by patient condition (see Patient Education). Note breast-feeding caution.

Patient Education: Inform prescriber of all prescriptions, OTC medications, or herbal products you are taking, and any allergies you have. This medication can only be administered by infusion; you will be monitored closely during and after treatment; immediately report burning, pain, redness, swelling, or oozing at infusion site, acute headache, joint pain, chest pain, or altered vision. You will have a tendency to bleed easily; use caution to prevent injury (use electric razor, soft toothbrush, and caution with knives, needles, or anything sharp). Follow instructions for strict bedrest to reduce the risk of injury. If bleeding occurs, report immediately and apply pressure to bleeding spot until bleeding stops completely. Report chest pain, palpitations, irregular heartbeat; unusual bruising or bleeding; blood in urine, stool, or vomiting; bleeding gums; muscle pain; or difficulty breathing. **Breast-feeding precaution:** Consult prescriber if breast-feeding.

Uro-KP-Neutral® *see* Phosphate Supplements *on page 1076*
Urolene Blue® *see page 1461*
Uro-Mag® [OTC] *see* Magnesium Supplements *on page 831*
Urso® *see* Ursodiol *on page 1376*
Ursodeoxycholic Acid *see* Ursodiol *on page 1376*

Ursodiol (ER soe dye ole)

U.S. Brand Names Actigall®; Urso®

Synonyms Ursodeoxycholic Acid

Generic Available Yes: Capsule

Pharmacologic Category Gallstone Dissolution Agent

Pregnancy Risk Factor B

Lactation Excretion in breast milk unknown

Use Actigall®: Gallbladder stone dissolution; prevention of gallstones in obese patients experiencing rapid weight loss; Urso®: Primary biliary cirrhosis

Use - Unlabeled/Investigational Liver transplantation

Mechanism of Action/Effect Decreases the cholesterol content of bile and bile stones by reducing the secretion of cholesterol from the liver and the fractional reabsorption of cholesterol by the intestines. Mechanism of action in primary biliary cirrhosis is not clearly defined.

Contraindications Hypersensitivity to ursodiol, bile acids, or any component of the formulation; not to be used with cholesterol, radiopaque, bile pigment stones, or stones >20 mm in diameter; allergy to bile acids

Warnings/Precautions Gallbladder stone dissolution may take several months of therapy. Complete dissolution may not occur and recurrence of stones within 5 years has been observed in 50% of patients. Use with caution in patients with a nonvisualizing gallbladder and those with chronic liver disease.

Drug Interactions

Decreased Effect: Decreased effect with aluminum-containing antacids, cholestyramine, colestipol, clofibrate, and oral contraceptives (estrogens).

Adverse Reactions

>10%:

Central nervous system: Headache (up to 25%), dizziness (up to 17%)

Gastrointestinal: In treatment of primary biliary cirrhosis: Constipation (up to 26%)

1% to 10%:

Dermatologic: Rash (<1% to 3%), alopecia (<1% to 5%)

Gastrointestinal:

In gallstone dissolution: Most GI events (diarrhea, nausea, vomiting) are similar to placebo and attributable to gallstone disease.

In treatment of primary biliary cirrhosis: Diarrhea (1%)

Hematologic: Leukopenia (3%)

Miscellaneous: Allergy (5%)

<1% (Limited to important or life-threatening): Abdominal pain, biliary pain, fatigue, metallic taste, nausea, pruritus, vomiting

In treatment of primary biliary cirrhosis: Constipation, dyspepsia, headache

Overdosage/Toxicology Symptoms of overdose include diarrhea. No specific therapy for diarrhea or overdose.

Pharmacodynamics/Kinetics

Half-Life Elimination: 100 hours

Metabolism: Undergoes extensive enterohepatic recycling; following hepatic conjugation and biliary secretion, the drug is hydrolyzed to active ursodiol, where it is recycled or transformed to lithocholic acid by colonic microbial flora

Formulations

Capsule (Actigall®): 300 mg

Tablet, film coated (Urso®): 250 mg

Dosing

Adults & Elderly:

Gallstone:

Dissolution: Oral: 8-10 mg/kg/day in 2-3 divided doses; use beyond 24 months is not established; obtain ultrasound images at 6-month intervals for the first year of therapy; 30% of patients have stone recurrence after dissolution

Prevention: Oral: 300 mg twice daily

Primary biliary cirrhosis: Oral: 13-15 mg/kg/day in 4 divided doses (with food)

Administration

Oral: Do not administer with aluminum-based antacids. If aluminum based antacids are needed, administer 2 hours after ursodiol. Urso® should be taken with food.

Stability

Storage: Do not store above 30°C (86°F)

Monitoring Laboratory Tests

Gallstone disease: ALT, AST, ALP; sonogram may be required

Hepatic disease: Monitor hepatic function tests frequently

Monitoring and Teaching Issues

Physical Assessment: See Contraindications, Warnings/Precautions, Drug Interactions, and Dosing for use cautions. Assess results of laboratory tests (see above), therapeutic effectiveness, and adverse reactions (see Adverse Reactions and Overdose/Toxicology). Teach patient proper use, possible side effects signs to report (see Patient Education). Note breast-feeding caution.

Patient Education: Take medication as directed with food. Drug will need to be taken for 1-3 months after stone is dissolved and stones may recur. Report any persistent nausea, vomiting, abdominal pain, or yellowing of skin or eyes. **Breast-feeding precaution:** Consult prescriber if breast-feeding.

Dietary Issues: Urso® should be taken with food.

Geriatric Considerations: No specific clinical studies in the elderly. Would recommend starting at lowest recommended dose with scheduled monitoring.

Uvadex® *see* Methoxsalen *on page 878*

Vagifem® *see* Estradiol *on page 494*

Vagistat®-1 [OTC] *see* Tioconazole *on page 1326*

Valacyclovir (val ay SYE kloe veer)

U.S. Brand Names Valtrex®

Synonyms Valacyclovir Hydrochloride

Generic Available No

Pharmacologic Category Antiviral Agent, Oral

Pregnancy Risk Factor B

Lactation Enters breast milk/use caution

(Continued)

Valacyclovir *(Continued)*

Use Treatment of herpes zoster (shingles) in immunocompetent patients; episodic treatment or prophylaxis of recurrent genital herpes in immunocompetent patients; for first episode genital herpes; treatment of herpes labialis (cold sores)

Mechanism of Action/Effect Valacyclovir is rapidly converted to acyclovir before it exerts its antiviral activity against HSV-1, HSV-2, or VZV. Inhibits viral DNA synthesis and replication.

Contraindications Hypersensitivity to valacyclovir, acyclovir, or any component of the formulation

Warnings/Precautions Thrombotic thrombocytopenic purpura/hemolytic uremic syndrome has occurred in immunocompromised patients (at doses of 8 g/day); use caution and adjust the dose in elderly patients or those with renal insufficiency and in patients receiving concurrent nephrotoxic agents; treatment should begin as soon as possible after the first signs and symptoms (within 72 hours of onset of first diagnosis or within 24 hours of onset of recurrent episodes); safety and efficacy in children have not been established, except in adolescents for the treatment of herpes labialis

Drug Interactions

Decreased Effect: Cimetidine and/or probenecid has decreased the rate but not the extent of valacyclovir conversion to acyclovir leading to decreased effectiveness of valacyclovir.

Increased Effect/Toxicity: Valacyclovir and acyclovir have increased CNS side effects with zidovudine and probenecid.

Adverse Reactions

>10%: Central nervous system: Headache (14% to 35%)

1% to 10%:

Central nervous system: Dizziness (2% to 4%), depression (0% to 7%)

Endocrine: Dysmenorrhea (≤1% to 8%)

Gastrointestinal: Abdominal pain (2% to 11%), vomiting (<1% to 6%), nausea (6% to 15%)

Hematologic: Leukopenia (≤1%), thrombocytopenia (≤1%)

Hepatic: AST increased (1% to 4%)

Neuromuscular & skeletal: Arthralgia (≤1 to 6%)

<1% (Limited to important or life-threatening): Acute hypersensitivity reactions, agitation, anaphylaxis, aplastic anemia, auditory hallucinations, coma, confusion, encephalopathy, erythema multiforme, hepatitis, mania, photosensitivity reaction, psychosis, rash, renal failure, thrombotic thrombocytopenic purpura/hemolytic uremic syndrome, visual hallucinations

Overdosage/Toxicology Precipitation in renal tubules may occur. Treatment is symptomatic and includes hemodialysis, especially if compromised renal function develops.

Pharmacodynamics/Kinetics

Absorption: Rapid

Bioavailability: ~55% once converted to acyclovir

Half-Life Elimination: Normal renal function: Adults: 2.5-3.3 hours (acyclovir), ~30 minutes (valacyclovir); End-stage renal disease: 14-20 hours (acyclovir)

Metabolism: Hepatic; valacyclovir is rapidly and nearly completely converted to acyclovir and L-valine by first-pass effect; acyclovir is hepatically metabolized to a very small extent by aldehyde oxidase and by alcohol and aldehyde dehydrogenase (inactive metabolites)

Formulations Caplet, as hydrochloride: 500 mg, 1000 mg

Dosing

Adults & Elderly:

Herpes zoster (shingles): Oral: 1 g 3 times/day for 7 days

Genital herpes: Oral:

Initial episode: 1 g 2 times/day for 10 days

Episodic treatment: 500 mg twice daily for 3 days

Prophylaxis: 500-1000 mg once daily

Herpes labialis (cold sores): Oral: 2 g twice daily for 1 day (separate doses by ~12 hours)

Pediatrics: Herpes labialis (cold sores): Adolescents ≥12 years: Refer to adult dosing.

Renal Impairment:

Herpes zoster: Adults:

Cl_{cr} 30-49 mL/minute: 1 g every 12 hours

Cl_{cr} 10-29 mL/minute: 1 g every 24 hours

Cl_{cr} <10 mL/minute: 500 mg every 24 hours

Genital herpes: Adults:

Initial episode:

Cl_{cr} 10-29 mL/minute: 1 g every 24 hours

Cl_{cr} <10 mL/minute: 500 mg every 24 hours

Episodic treatment: Cl_{cr} <10-29 mL/minute: 500 mg every 24 hours

Prophylaxis: Cl_{cr} <10-29 mL/minute:

For usual dose of 1 g every 24 hours, decrease dose to 500 mg every 24 hours

For usual dose of 500 mg every 24 hours, decrease dose to 500 mg every 48 hours

Herpes labialis: Adolescents ≥12 years and Adults:

Cl_{cr} 30-49 mL/minute: 1 g every 12 hours for 2 doses

Cl_{cr} 10-29 mL/minute: 500 mg every 12 hours for 2 doses

Cl_{cr} <10 mL/minute: 500 mg as a single dose

Hemodialysis: Dialyzable (~33% removed during 4-hour session); administer dose postdialysis

Chronic ambulatory peritoneal dialysis/continuous arteriovenous hemofiltration dialysis: Pharmacokinetic parameters are similar to those in patients with ESRD; supplemental dose not needed following dialysis

Administration

Oral: If GI upset occurs, administer with meals.

Stability

Storage: Store at 15°C to 25°C (59°F to 77°F).

Monitoring and Teaching Issues

Physical Assessment: See Warnings/Precautions, Contraindications, and Drug Interactions for use cautions. Assess therapeutic effects and adverse responses (eg, CNS changes - see Adverse Reactions and Overdose/Toxicology). Teach patient appropriate use, possible side effects and appropriate interventions, and adverse symptoms to report (see Patient Education). Note breast-feeding caution.

Patient Education: This medication is not a cure for genital herpes; it is not known if it will prevent transmission to others. Take as directed, with or without food. Begin use at first sign of herpes. Maintain adequate hydration (2-3 L/day of fluids) unless advised by prescriber to restrict fluids. May cause headache, dizziness (use caution when driving or engaging in potentially hazardous tasks until response to drug is known); or nausea, vomiting, abdominal pain (small, frequent meals, frequent mouth care, chewing gum, or sucking lozenges may help). Immediately report difficulty breathing difficulty swallowing, rash, or hives. Consult prescriber if breast-feeding.

Dietary Issues: May be taken with or without food.

Geriatric Considerations: More convenient dosing and increased bioavailability, without increasing side effects, make valacyclovir a favorable choice compared to acyclovir. Has been shown to accelerate resolution of postherpetic pain. Adjust dose for renal impairment.

Breast-feeding Issues: Avoid use in breast-feeding, if possible, since the drug distributes in high concentrations in breast milk.

Valacyclovir Hydrochloride *see* Valacyclovir *on page 1377*

Valcyte™ *see* Valganciclovir *on page 1380*

Valdecoxib (val de KOKS ib)

U.S. Brand Names Bextra®

Generic Available No

Pharmacologic Category Nonsteroidal Anti-inflammatory Drug (NSAID), COX-2 Selective

Pregnancy Risk Factor C/D (3rd trimester)

Lactation Excretion in breast milk unknown/not recommended

Use Relief of signs and symptoms of osteoarthritis and adult rheumatoid arthritis; treatment of primary dysmenorrhea

Mechanism of Action/Effect Inhibits cyclooxygenase-2 (COX-2) and as a result, prostaglandin synthesis resulting in decreased pain.

Contraindications Hypersensitivity to valdecoxib, sulfonamides, or any component of the formulation; patients who have experienced asthma, urticaria, or allergic-type reactions to aspirin or NSAIDs; pregnancy (3rd trimester)

Warnings/Precautions Gastrointestinal irritation, ulceration, bleeding, and perforation may occur with NSAIDs. Use with caution in patients with a history of GI bleeding, ulcers, or risk factor for GI bleeding. Anaphylactic/anaphylactoid reactions may occur, even with no prior exposure to valdecoxib. Serious dermatologic reactions have been reported; discontinue in any patients who develop rash or any signs of hypersensitivity. Use with caution in patients with decreased renal function, hepatic disease, CHF, hypertension, dehydration, or asthma. Use caution in patients with known or suspected deficiency of cytochrome P450 isoenzyme 2C9. Use in patients with severe hepatic impairment (Child-Pugh Class C) is not recommended. Safety and efficacy have not been established for patients <18 years of age. Pregnancy risk C/D (3rd trimester).

Drug Interactions

Cytochrome P450 Effect: Substrate of CYP2C8/9, 3A4; Inhibits CYP2C8/9, 2C19

Decreased Effect: ACE inhibitors, angiotensin II antagonists, hydralazine, loop and thiazide diuretics effects reduced.

Increased Effect/Toxicity: Anticoagulants and antiplatelet drugs may increase risk of bleeding. Warfarin efficacy may increase. Corticosteroids may increase risk of GI ulceration. CYP2C8/9 and 3A4 inhibitors may increase valdecoxib levels. Cyclosporine, dextromethorphan, lithium levels increased. Serum concentrations/toxicity of methotrexate may be increased.

Nutritional/Ethanol Interactions

Ethanol: Avoid ethanol (may enhance gastric mucosal irritation).

Food: Time to peak level is delayed by 1-2 hours when taken with high-fat meal, but other parameters are unaffected.

Herb/Nutraceutical: Avoid cat's claw, dong quai, evening primrose, feverfew, garlic, ginger, ginkgo, red clover, horse chestnut, green tea, ginseng (may cause increased risk of bleeding).

Adverse Reactions

2% to 10%:

Cardiovascular: Peripheral edema (2% to 3%), hypertension (2%)

Central nervous system: Headache (5% to 9%), dizziness (3%)

Dermatologic: Rash (1% to 2%)

Gastrointestinal: Dyspepsia (8% to 9%), abdominal pain (7% to 8%), nausea (6% to 7%), diarrhea (5% to 6%), flatulence (3% to 4%), abdominal fullness (2%)

Neuromuscular & skeletal: Back pain (2% to 3%), myalgia (2%)

Otic: Earache, tinnitus

Respiratory: Upper respiratory tract infection (6% to 7%), sinusitis (2% to 3%)

Miscellaneous: Influenza-like symptoms (2%)

<2% (Limited to important or life threatening): Allergy, anaphylaxis, aneurysm, angina, angioedema, aortic stenosis, arrhythmia, atrial fibrillation, bradycardia, breast neoplasm, cardiomyopathy, carotid stenosis, colitis, CHF, convulsion, coronary thrombosis, depression exacerbation, diabetes mellitus, diverticulosis, duodenal ulcer, emphysema, erythema multiforme, esophageal perforation, exfoliative dermatitis, facial edema, gastric ulcer, gastroesophageal reflux, gastrointestinal bleeding, gout, heart block, hepatitis, hiatal

(Continued)

Valdecoxib *(Continued)*

hernia, hyperlipemia, hyperparathyroidism, hypertension exacerbation, hypertensive encephalopathy, hypotension, impotence, intermittent claudication, liver function tests increased, lymphadenopathy, lymphangitis, lymphopenia, migraine, mitral insufficiency, myocardial infarction, myocardial ischemia, neuropathy, osteoporosis, ovarian cyst (malignant), pericarditis, periorbital swelling, photosensitivity, pneumonia, rash (erythematous, maculopapular, psoriaform), Stevens-Johnson syndrome, syncope, tachycardia, thrombocytopenia, thrombophlebitis, toxic epidermal necrolysis, unstable angina, urinary tract infection, vaginal hemorrhage, ventricular fibrillation, vertigo

Overdosage/Toxicology Symptoms of overdose may include epigastric pain, drowsiness, lethargy, nausea, and vomiting; gastrointestinal bleeding may occur. Rare manifestations include hypertension, respiratory depression, coma, and acute renal failure. Treatment is symptomatic and supportive. Forced diuresis, hemodialysis, hemoperfusion, and/or urinary alkalinization may not be useful.

Pharmacodynamics/Kinetics

Bioavailability: 83%

Half-Life Elimination: 8-11 hours

Time to Peak: 2.25-3 hours

Metabolism: Extensively hepatic via CYP3A4 and 2C9; glucuronidation

Onset: Dysmenorrhea: 60 minutes

Formulations Tablet: 10 mg, 20 mg

Dosing

Adults & Elderly:

Osteoarthritis and rheumatoid arthritis: Oral: 10 mg once daily; **Note:** No additional benefits seen with 20 mg/day

Primary dysmenorrhea: Oral: 20 mg twice daily as needed

Pediatrics: Not indicated for pediatric patients.

Renal Impairment: Not recommended for use in advanced disease.

Hepatic Impairment: Not recommended for use in advanced liver dysfunction (Child-Pugh Class C).

Administration

Oral: Avoid dehydration. Encourage patient to drink plenty of fluids.

Stability

Storage: Store at 15°C to 30°C (59°F to 86°F).

Monitoring and Teaching Issues

Physical Assessment: See Contraindications and Warnings/Precautions for use cautions. Assess effectiveness and interactions of other prescription, OTC, or herbal medication patient may be taking (see Drug Interactions). Assess allergy history (salicylates, NSAIDs). Monitor for effectiveness of therapy and adverse reactions. Assess knowledge/teach patient appropriate use, interventions to reduce possible side effects, and adverse symptoms to report (see Adverse Reactions, Overdose/Toxicology, and Patient Education). **Pregnancy risk factor C/D** - see Pregnancy Risk Factor for use cautions; benefits of use should outweigh possible risks. Breast-feeding is not recommended.

Patient Education: Use exactly as directed. May be taken with food to reduce GI upset. Do not take with antacids. Avoid alcohol, aspirin, or other medication unless approved by prescriber. Maintain adequate hydration (2-3 L/day of fluids) unless advised by prescriber to restrict fluids. GI bleeding, ulceration, or perforation can occur with or without pain. Stop taking medication and report immediately abdominal tenderness, stomach pain or cramping; unusual bleeding or bruising; or blood in vomitus, stool, or urine. You may experience dizziness, confusion, or blurred vision (avoid driving or engaging in tasks requiring alertness until response to drug is known); or anorexia, nausea, vomiting (small, frequent meals, frequent mouth care, chewing gum or sucking lozenges may help). Report any skin rash, muscle aches, unusual fatigue, lethargy, yellowing of skin or eyes, flu-like symptoms, easy bruising or bleeding, sudden weight gain, changes in urinary pattern, difficulty breathing, or signs of upper respiratory infection. **Pregnancy/breast-feeding precautions:** Inform prescriber if you are or intend to become pregnant. This drug should not be used in the 3rd trimester of pregnancy. Breast-feeding is not recommended.

Dietary Issues: May be taken with or without food.

Pregnancy Issues: Use should be avoided in late pregnancy because it may cause premature closure of the ductus arteriosus.

Valganciclovir (val gan SYE kloh veer)

U.S. Brand Names Valcyte™

Synonyms Valganciclovir Hydrochloride

Generic Available No

Pharmacologic Category Antiviral Agent

Pregnancy Risk Factor C

Lactation Excretion in breast milk unknown/contraindicated

Use Treatment of cytomegalovirus (CMV) retinitis in patients with acquired immunodeficiency syndrome (AIDS)

Mechanism of Action/Effect Valganciclovir is a prodrug of ganciclovir, and is rapidly metabolized in the body to form ganciclovir. Ganciclovir inhibits the formation of viral DNA within infected cells, blocking reproduction of the virus.

Contraindications Hypersensitivity to valganciclovir, ganciclovir, acyclovir, or any component of the formulation; absolute neutrophil count <500/mm^3; platelet count <25,000/mm^3; hemoglobin <8 g/dL

Warnings/Precautions Dosage adjustment or interruption of valganciclovir therapy may be necessary in patients with neutropenia and/or thrombocytopenia and patients with impaired renal function. Not approved for use in children. Due to differences in bioavailability, valganciclovir tablets cannot be substituted for ganciclovir capsules on a one-to-one basis. Safety and efficacy not established in pediatric patients. Pregnancy risk C.

Drug Interactions

Decreased Effect: Reported for ganciclovir: A decrease in blood levels of ganciclovir AUC may occur when used with didanosine.

Increased Effect/Toxicity: Reported for ganciclovir: Immunosuppressive agents may increase hematologic toxicity of ganciclovir. Imipenem/cilastatin may increase seizure potential. Oral ganciclovir increases blood levels of zidovudine, although zidovudine decreases steady-state levels of ganciclovir. Since both drugs have the potential to cause neutropenia and anemia, some patients may not tolerate concomitant therapy with these drugs at full dosage. Didanosine levels are increased with concurrent ganciclovir. Other nephrotoxic drugs (eg, amphotericin and cyclosporine) may have additive nephrotoxicity with ganciclovir.

Nutritional/Ethanol Interactions Food: Coadministration with a high-fat meal increased AUC by 30%.

Adverse Reactions

>10%:

Central nervous system: Fever (31%), headache (9% to 22%), insomnia (16%)

Gastrointestinal: Diarrhea (16% to 41%), nausea (8% to 30%), vomiting (21%), abdominal pain (15%)

Hematologic: Granulocytopenia (11% to 27%), anemia (8% to 26%)

Ocular: Retinal detachment (15%)

1% to 10%:

Central nervous system: Peripheral neuropathy (9%), paresthesia (8%), seizures (<5%), psychosis, hallucinations (<5%), confusion (<5%), agitation (<5%)

Hematologic: Thrombocytopenia (8%), pancytopenia (<5%), bone marrow depression (<5%), aplastic anemia (<5%), bleeding (potentially life-threatening due to thrombocytopenia <5%)

Renal: Decreased renal function (<5%)

Miscellaneous: Local and systemic infections, including sepsis (<5%); allergic reaction (<5%)

<1% (Limited to important or life-threatening): Valganciclovir is expected to share the toxicities which may occur at a low incidence or due to idiosyncratic reactions which have been associated with ganciclovir

Overdosage/Toxicology Symptoms of overdose with ganciclovir include neutropenia, vomiting, hypersalivation, bloody diarrhea, cytopenia, and testicular atrophy. Treatment is supportive. Hemodialysis removes 50% of the drug. Hydration may be of some benefit.

Pharmacodynamics/Kinetics

Absorption: Well absorbed; high-fat meal increases AUC by 30%

Bioavailability: With food: 60%

Half-Life Elimination: Ganciclovir: 4.08 hours, prolonged with renal impairment; Severe renal impairment: Up to 68 hours

Metabolism: Converted to ganciclovir by intestinal mucosal cells and hepatocytes

Formulations Tablet, as hydrochloride: 450 mg [valganciclovir hydrochloride 496.3 mg equivalent to valganciclovir 450 mg]

Dosing

Adults & Elderly: CMV retinitis: Oral:

Induction (active retinitis): 900 mg twice daily for 21 days (with food)

Maintenance: Following induction treatment, or for patients with inactive CMV retinitis who require maintenance therapy: Recommended dose: 900 mg once daily (with food)

Renal Impairment:

Induction dose (for 21 days):

Cl_{cr} 40-59 mL/minute: 450 mg twice daily

Cl_{cr} 25-39 mL/minute: 450 mg once daily

Cl_{cr} 10-24 mL/minute: 450 mg every 2 days

Maintenance dose:

Cl_{cr} 40-59 mL/minute: 450 mg once daily

Cl_{cr} 25-39 mL/minute: 450 mg every 2 days

Cl_{cr} 10-24 mL/minute: 450 mg twice weekly

Note: Valganciclovir is not recommended in patients receiving hemodialysis. For patients on hemodialysis (Cl_{cr} <10 mL/minute), it is recommended that ganciclovir be used (dose adjusted as specified for ganciclovir).

Administration

Oral: Avoid direct contact with broken or crushed tablets. Consideration should be given to handling and disposal according to guidelines issued for antineoplastic drugs. However, there is no consensus on the need for these precautions.

Stability

Storage: Store at 25°C (77°F), excursions permitted to 15°C to 30°C (59°F to 86°F).

Monitoring Laboratory Tests Retinal exam (at least every 4-6 weeks), CBC, platelet counts, serum creatinine

Monitoring and Teaching Issues

Physical Assessment: See Contraindications, Warnings/Precautions, and Dosing for use cautions. Assess potential for interactions with other prescriptions, OTC medications, or herbal products patient may be taking (see Drug Interactions). Assess results of laboratory tests (see Monitoring Lab Tests), therapeutic effects, and adverse response (eg, peripheral neuropathy, neutropenia, anemia, nephrotoxicity, retinal detachment - see Adverse Reactions and Overdose/Toxicology) on a regular basis during therapy. Teach proper use, possible side effects and appropriate interventions, and adverse symptoms to report (see Patient Education). **Pregnancy risk factor C** - determine appropriateness of use. Barrier contraceptive use is appropriate during therapy and for 60-90 days after therapy for both males and females. Breast-feeding is contraindicated.

Patient Education: Inform prescriber of all prescriptions, OTC medications, or herbal products you are taking, and any allergies you have. Do not take anything new during treatment unless approved by prescriber. This medication is not a cure for CMV retinitis. Take exactly as directed; do not alter dosage or discontinue without consulting prescriber.

(Continued)

Valganciclovir *(Continued)*

You will need frequent and regular laboratory tests and ophthalmic exams while taking this medication. Maintain adequate hydration (2-3 L/day of fluids) unless advised by prescriber to restrict fluids. You may be more susceptible to infection (avoid crowds or exposure to infection and do not have any vaccinations unless approved by prescriber). May cause headache or insomnia (use caution when driving or engaging in hazardous tasks until response to drug is known); nausea or vomiting (small, frequent meals, good mouth care, sucking lozenges, or chewing gum may help); diarrhea (boiled milk, yogurt, or buttermilk may help); or photosensitivity (use sunscreen, wear protective clothing and eyewear, and avoid direct sunlight). Report fever; chills; unusual bleeding or bruising; infection or unhealed sores; white plaques in mouth or vaginal discharge; CNS disturbances (eg, hallucinations, confusion, nightmares); or weakness or loss of feeling in nerves or muscles.

Pregnancy/breast-feeding precautions: Inform prescriber if you are pregnant. Males and females should use appropriate barrier contraceptive measures during and for 90 days following end of therapy. Do not breast-feed.

Dietary Issues: Should be taken with meals.

Breast-feeding Issues: HIV-infected mothers are discouraged from breast-feeding to decrease the potential transmission of HIV.

Pregnancy Issues: Valganciclovir is converted to ganciclovir and shares its reproductive toxicity. Ganciclovir may adversely affect spermatogenesis and fertility; due to its mutagenic potential, contraceptive precautions for female and male patients need to be followed during and for at least 90 days after therapy with this drug.

Valganciclovir Hydrochloride *see* Valganciclovir *on page 1380*

Valisone® [DSC] *see* Betamethasone *on page 160*

Valisone® [DSC] *see* Topical Corticosteroids *on page 1334*

Valium® *see* Diazepam *on page 397*

Valorin [OTC] *see* Acetaminophen *on page 35*

Valorin Extra [OTC] *see* Acetaminophen *on page 35*

Valproate Semisodium *see* Valproic Acid and Derivatives *on page 1382*

Valproate Sodium *see* Valproic Acid and Derivatives *on page 1382*

Valproic Acid *see* Valproic Acid and Derivatives *on page 1382*

Valproic Acid and Derivatives (val PROE ik AS id & dah RIV ah tives)

U.S. Brand Names Depacon®; Depakene®; Depakote® Delayed Release; Depakote® ER; Depakote® Sprinkle®

Synonyms Dipropylacetic Acid; Divalproex Sodium; DPA; 2-Propylpentanoic Acid; 2-Propylvaleric Acid; Valproate Semisodium; Valproate Sodium; Valproic Acid

Generic Available Yes (valproic acid)

Pharmacologic Category Anticonvulsant, Miscellaneous

Pregnancy Risk Factor D

Lactation Enters breast milk/compatible

Use

Mania associated with bipolar disorder (Depakote®)

Migraine prophylaxis (Depakote®, Depakote® ER)

Monotherapy and adjunctive therapy in the treatment of patients with complex partial seizures that occur either in isolation or in association with other types of seizures (Depacon™, Depakote®)

Sole and adjunctive therapy of simple and complex absence seizures (Depacon™, Depakene®, Depakote®)

Adjunctively in patients with multiple seizure types that include absence seizures (Depacon™, Depakene®)

Use - Unlabeled/Investigational Behavior disorders in Alzheimer's disease

Mechanism of Action/Effect Causes increased availability of gamma-aminobutyric acid (GABA), an inhibitory neurotransmitter, to brain neurons or may enhance the action of GABA or mimic its action at postsynaptic receptor sites

Contraindications Hypersensitivity to valproic acid, derivatives, or any component of the formulation; hepatic dysfunction; urea cycle disorders; pregnancy

Warnings/Precautions Hepatic failure resulting in fatalities has occurred in patients; children <2 years of age are at considerable risk; other risk factors include organic brain disease, mental retardation with severe seizure disorders, congenital metabolic disorders, and patients on multiple anticonvulsants. Hepatotoxicity has been reported after 3 days to 6 months of therapy. Monitor patients closely for appearance of malaise, weakness, facial edema, anorexia, jaundice, and vomiting; may cause severe thrombocytopenia, inhibition of platelet aggregation and bleeding; tremors may indicate overdosage; use with caution in patients receiving other anticonvulsants.

Cases of life-threatening pancreatitis, occurring at the start of therapy or following years of use, have been reported in adults and children. Some cases have been hemorrhagic with rapid progression of initial symptoms to death.

May cause teratogenic effects such as neural tube defects (eg, spina bifida). Use in women of childbearing potential requires that benefits of use in mother be weighed against the potential risk to fetus, especially when used for conditions not associated with permanent injury or risk of death (eg, migraine).

Hyperammonemic encephalopathy, sometimes fatal, has been reported following the initiation of valproate therapy in patients with known or suspected urea cycle disorders (UCD), particularly those with ornithine transcarbamylase deficiency. Although a rare genetic disorder, UCD evaluation should be considered for the following patients, prior to the start of therapy: History of unexplained encephalopathy or coma; encephalopathy associated with protein load; pregnancy or postpartum encephalopathy; unexplained mental retardation; history of elevated plasma ammonia or glutamine; history of cyclical vomiting and lethargy; episodic extreme irritability, ataxia; low BUN or protein avoidance; family history of UCD or unexplained infant deaths (particularly male); signs or symptoms of UCD (hyperammonemia, encephalopathy, respiratory alkalosis). Patients who develop symptoms of hyperammonemic encephalopathy during therapy with valproate should receive prompt evaluation for UCD and valproate should be discontinued.

Hyperammonemia may occur with therapy and may be present with normal liver function tests. Ammonia levels should be measured in patients who develop unexplained lethargy and vomiting, or changes in mental status. Discontinue therapy if ammonia levels are increased and evaluate for possible UCD.

In vitro studies have suggested valproate stimulates the replication of HIV and CMV viruses under experimental conditions. The clinical consequence of this is unknown, but should be considered when monitoring affected patients.

Anticonvulsants should not be discontinued abruptly because of the possibility of increasing seizure frequency; valproate should be withdrawn gradually to minimize the potential of increased seizure frequency, unless safety concerns require a more rapid withdrawal. Concomitant use with clonazepam may induce absence status.

CNS depression may occur with valproate use. Patients must be cautioned about performing tasks which require mental alertness (operating machinery or driving). Effects with other sedative drugs or ethanol may be potentiated.

Drug Interactions

Cytochrome P450 Effect: For valproic acid: Substrate of CYP2A6, 2B6, 2C8/9, 2C19, 2E1; Inhibits CYP2C8/9, 2C19, 2D6, 3A4; Induces CYP2A6

Decreased Effect: Valproic acid may displace clozapine from protein binding site resulting in decreased clozapine serum concentrations. Carbamazepine, lamotrigine, and phenytoin may induce the metabolism of valproic acid. Cholestyramine (and possibly colestipol) may bind valproic acid in GI tract, decreasing absorption. Acyclovir may reduce valproic acid levels.

Increased Effect/Toxicity: Absence seizures have been reported in patients receiving VPA and clonazepam. Valproic acid may increase, decrease, or have no effect on carbamazepine and phenytoin levels. Valproic acid may increase serum concentrations of carbamazepine - epoxide (active metabolite). Valproic acid may increase serum concentrations of diazepam, lamotrigine, nimodipine, and phenobarbital, and tricyclic antidepressants. Chlorpromazine (and possibly other phenothiazines), macrolide antibiotics (clarithromycin, erythromycin, troleandomycin), felbamate, and isoniazid may inhibit the metabolism of valproic acid. Aspirin or other salicylates may displace valproic acid from protein-binding sites, leading to acute toxicity.

CYP2C18/19 inhibitors: May increase serum concentrations of valproic acid; inhibitors include cimetidine, felbamate, fluoxetine, and fluvoxamine

Nutritional/Ethanol Interactions

Ethanol: Avoid ethanol (may increase CNS depression).

Food: Food may delay but does not affect the extent of absorption. Valproic acid serum concentrations may be decreased if taken with food. Milk has no effect on absorption.

Herb/Nutraceutical: Avoid evening primrose (seizure threshold decreased)

Effects on Lab Values Valproic acid may cause abnormalities in liver function tests; false-positive result for urine ketones; accuracy of thyroid function tests

Adverse Reactions

Adverse reactions reported when used as monotherapy for complex partial seizures:

>10%:

Central nervous system: Somnolence (18% to 30%), dizziness (13% to 18%), insomnia (9% to 15%), nervousness (7% to 11%)

Dermatologic: Alopecia (13% to 24%)

Gastrointestinal: Nausea (26% to 34%), diarrhea (19% to 23%), vomiting (15% to 23%), abdominal pain (9% to 12%), dyspepsia (10% to 11%), anorexia (4% to 11%)

Hematologic: Thrombocytopenia (1% to 24%)

Neuromuscular & skeletal: Tremor (19% to 57%), weakness (10% to 21%)

Respiratory: Respiratory tract infection (13% to 20%), pharyngitis (2% to 8%), dyspnea (1% to 5%)

1% to 10%

Cardiovascular: Hypertension, palpitation, peripheral edema (3% to 8%), tachycardia, chest pain

Central nervous system: Amnesia (4% to 7%), abnormal dreams, anxiety, confusion, depression (4% to 5%), malaise, personality disorder

Dermatologic: Bruising (4% to 5%), dry skin, petechia, pruritus, rash

Endocrine & metabolic: Amenorrhea, dysmenorrhea

Gastrointestinal: Eructation, flatulence, hematemesis, increased appetite, pancreatitis, periodontal abscess, taste perversion, weight gain (4% to 9%)

Genitourinary: Urinary frequency, urinary incontinence, vaginitis

Hepatic: Increased AST and ALT

Neuromuscular & skeletal: Abnormal gait, arthralgia, back pain, hypertonia, incoordination, leg cramps, myalgia, myasthenia, paresthesia, twitching

Ocular: Amblyopia/blurred vision (4% to 8%), abnormal vision, nystagmus (1% to 7%)

Otic: Deafness, otitis media, tinnitus (1% to 7%)

Respiratory: Epistaxis, increased cough, pneumonia, sinusitis

Additional adverse effects (Limited to important or life-threatening): Anaphylaxis, aplastic anemia, asterixis, ataxia, bone marrow suppression, cerebral atrophy (reversible), cutaneous vasculitis, decreased carnitine, dementia, encephalopathy (rare), eosinophilia, erythema multiforme, Fanconi-like syndrome (rare, in children), hallucinations, hemorrhage, hyperammonemia, hyperglycinemia, hypofibrinogenemia, hyponatremia, inappropriate ADH secretion, incoordination, intermittent porphyria, lupus erythematosus, pancreatitis (rare, may be hemorrhagic/life-threatening), pancytopenia, Parkinsonism, photosensitivity, psychosis, Stevens-Johnson syndrome, toxic epidermal necrolysis (rare), vertigo

(Continued)

Valproic Acid and Derivatives *(Continued)*

Overdosage/Toxicology Symptoms of overdose include coma, deep sleep, motor restlessness, and visual hallucinations. Supportive treatment is necessary. Naloxone has been used to reverse CNS depressant effects, but may block the action of other anticonvulsants.

Pharmacodynamics/Kinetics

Bioavailability: Extended release: 90% of I.V. dose and 81% to 90% of delayed release dose

Half-Life Elimination: Increased in neonates and with liver disease; Children: 4-14 hours; Adults: 9-16 hours

Time to Peak: Serum: 1-4 hours; Divalproex (enteric coated): 3-5 hours

Metabolism: Extensively hepatic via glucuronide conjugation and mitochondrial beta-oxidation. The relationship between dose and total valproate concentration is nonlinear; concentration does not increase proportionally with the dose, but increases to a lesser extent due to saturable plasma protein binding. The kinetics of unbound drug are linear.

Formulations

Capsule, as valproic acid (Depakene®): 250 mg

Capsule, sprinkles, as divalproex sodium (Depakote® Sprinkle®): 125 mg

Injection, solution, as sodium valproate (Depacon®): 100 mg/mL (5 mL)

Syrup, as sodium valproate: 250 mg/5 mL (5 mL, 480 mL)

Depakene®: 250 mg/mL (480 mL)

Tablet, delayed release, as divalproex sodium (Depakote®): 125 mg, 250 mg, 500 mg

Tablet, extended release, as divalproex sodium (Depakote® ER): 500 mg

Dosing

Adults & Elderly:

Seizures:

Oral: Initial: 10-15 mg/kg/day in 1-3 divided doses; increase by 5-10 mg/kg/day at weekly intervals until therapeutic levels are achieved; maintenance: 30-60 mg/kg/day in 2-3 divided doses. Adult usual dose: 1000-2500 mg/day

I.V.: Administer as a 60-minute infusion (≤20 mg/minute) with the same frequency as oral products; switch patient to oral products as soon as possible. Rapid infusions have been given: ≤15 mg/kg over 5-10 minutes (1.5-3 mg/kg/minute).

Rectal: Dilute syrup 1:1 with water for use as a retention enema; loading dose: 17-20 mg/kg one time; maintenance: 10-15 mg/kg/dose every 8 hours

Mania: Oral: 750 mg/day in divided doses; dose should be adjusted as rapidly as possible to desired clinical effect; a loading dose of 20 mg/kg may be used; maximum recommended dosage: 60 mg/kg/day

Migraine prophylaxis: Oral:

Extended release tablets: 500 mg once daily for 7 days, then increase to 1000 mg once daily; adjust dose based on patient response; usual dosage range 500-1000 mg/day

Delayed release tablets: 250 mg twice daily; adjust dose based on patient response, up to 1000 mg/day

Pediatrics: Seizures: Oral, I.V., Rectal: Children >10 years: Refer to adult dosing.

Renal Impairment: A 27% reduction in clearance of unbound valproate is seen in patients with Cl_{cr} <10 mL/minute. Hemodialysis reduces valproate concentrations by 20%, therefore no dose adjustment is needed in patients with renal failure. Protein binding is reduced, monitoring only total valproate concentrations may be misleading.

Hepatic Impairment: Dosage reduction is required. Clearance is decreased with liver impairment. Hepatic disease is also associated with increased albumin concentrations and 2- to 2.6-fold increase in the unbound fraction. Free concentrations of valproate may be elevated while total concentrations appear normal.

Administration

Oral: Do not crush enteric coated drug product or capsules.

I.V.: Depacon®: Final concentration: ≤20 mg/minute over 60 minutes; use for longer than 14 days has not been studied. Alternatively, may be administered as a rapid infusion over 5-10 minutes (1.5-3 mg/kg/minute).

Stability

Storage: Store vials at room temperature 15°C to 30°C (59°F to 86°F).

Reconstitution: Injection is physically compatible and chemically stable in D_5W, NS, and LR for at least 24 hours when stored in glass or PVC.

Monitoring Laboratory Tests Liver enzymes, CBC with platelets, ammonium levels

Monitoring and Teaching Issues

Physical Assessment: Assess effectiveness and interactions of other medications patient may be taking (see Drug Interactions). **I.V.:** Keep patient under observation, observe safety/seizure precautions, and monitor therapeutic response (type of seizure activity, force, and duration). For outpatients, monitor therapeutic effect, laboratory values, and adverse reactions (see Adverse Reactions) at beginning of therapy and periodically with long-term use. Taper dosage slowly when discontinuing. Assess knowledge/teach patient seizure safety precautions, appropriate use, interventions to reduce side effects, and adverse symptoms to report (see Patient Education). **Note:** Valproic acid will alter results of urine ketones (use serum glucose testing) and reduce effectiveness of oral contraceptives (use alternative form of contraception to prevent pregnancy). Some adverse reactions including hepatic failure and thrombocytopenia can occur 3 days to 6 months after beginning therapy. **Pregnancy risk factor D** - determine that patient is not pregnant before beginning treatment. Instruct patients of childbearing age about appropriate barrier contraceptive measures.

Patient Education: When used to treat generalized seizures, patient instructions are determined by patient's condition and ability to understand. Oral: Take as directed; do not alter dose or timing of medication. Do not increase dose or take more than recommended. Do not crush or chew capsule or enteric-coated pill. While using this medication, do not use alcohol and other prescription or OTC medications (especially pain medications, sedatives, antihistamines, or hypnotics) without consulting prescriber. Maintain adequate hydration (2-3 L/day of fluids) unless advised by prescriber to restrict fluids. If diabetic, monitor serum glucose closely (valproic acid will alter results of urine ketones). Report alterations in menstrual cycle; abdominal cramps, unresolved diarrhea, vomiting, or constipation; skin rash; unusual bruising or bleeding; blood in urine, stool, or vomitus; malaise; weakness; facial swelling; yellowing of skin or eyes; persistent abdominal pain; excessive sedation; or restlessness. **Pregnancy precaution:** Do not get pregnant while taking this medication; use appropriate contraceptive measures.

Dietary Issues: Valproic acid may cause GI upset; take with large amount of water or food to decrease GI upset. May need to split doses to avoid GI upset.

Coated particles of divalproex sodium may be mixed with semisolid food (eg, applesauce or pudding) in patients having difficulty swallowing; particles should be swallowed and not chewed

Valproate sodium oral solution will generate valproic acid in carbonated beverages and may cause mouth and throat irritation; do not mix valproate sodium oral solution with carbonated beverages; sodium content of valproate sodium syrup (5 mL): 23 mg (1 mEq)

Breast-feeding Issues: Crosses into breast milk. AAP considers **compatible** with breast-feeding.

Pregnancy Issues: Crosses the placenta. Neural tube, cardiac, facial (characteristic pattern of dysmorphic facial features), skeletal, multiple other defects reported. Epilepsy itself, number of medications, genetic factors, or a combination of these probably influence the teratogenicity of anticonvulsant therapy. Risk of neural tube defects with use during first 30 days of pregnancy warrants discontinuation prior to pregnancy and through this period of possible. Use in women of childbearing potential requires that benefits of use in mother be weighed against the potential risk to fetus, especially when used for conditions not associated with permanent injury or risk of death (eg, migraine).

Additional Information

Extended release tablets have 10% to 20% less fluctuation in serum concentration than delayed release tablets. Extended release tablets are not bioequivalent to delayed release tablets.

Related Information

Peak and Trough Guidelines *on page 1544*

Valrubicin (val ru BYE cin)

U.S. Brand Names Valstar®

Generic Available No

Pharmacologic Category Antineoplastic Agent, Anthracycline

Pregnancy Risk Factor C

Lactation Excretion in breast milk unknown/not recommended

Use Intravesical therapy of BCG-refractory carcinoma *in situ* of the urinary bladder

Mechanism of Action/Effect Blocks function of DNA topoisomerase II; inhibits DNA synthesis, causes extensive chromosomal damage, and arrests cell development

Contraindications Hypersensitivity to anthracyclines, Cremophor® EL, or any component of the formulation; concurrent urinary tract infection or small bladder capacity (unable to tolerate a 75 mL instillation)

Warnings/Precautions The U.S. Food and Drug Administration (FDA) currently recommends that procedures for proper handling and disposal of antineoplastic agents be considered. Appropriate safety equipment is recommended for preparation, administration, and disposal of antineoplastics. If valrubicin contacts the skin, wash and flush thoroughly with water. Complete response observed in only 1 of 5 patients, delay of cystectomy may lead to development of metastatic bladder cancer, which is lethal. If complete response is not observed after 3 months or disease recurs, cystectomy must be reconsidered. Do not administer if mucosal integrity of bladder has been compromised or bladder perforation is present. Following TURP, status of bladder mucosa should be evaluated prior to initiation of therapy. Administer under the supervision of a physician experienced in the use of intravesical chemotherapy. Aseptic technique must be used during administration. All patients of reproductive age should use an effective method of contraception during the treatment period. Irritable bladder symptoms may occur during instillation and retention. Caution in patients with severe irritable bladder symptoms. Do not clamp urinary catheter. Red-tinged urine is typical for the first 24 hours after instillation. Prolonged symptoms or discoloration should prompt contact with the physician. Pregnancy risk C.

Drug Interactions

Decreased Effect: No specific drug interactions studies have been performed. Systemic exposure to valrubicin is negligible, and interactions are unlikely.

Increased Effect/Toxicity: No specific drug interactions studies have been performed. Systemic exposure to valrubicin is negligible, and interactions are unlikely.

Adverse Reactions

>10%: Genitourinary: Frequency (61%), dysuria (56%), urgency (57%), bladder spasm (31%), hematuria (29%), bladder pain (28%), urinary incontinence (22%), cystitis (15%), urinary tract infection (15%)

1% to 10%:

Cardiovascular: Chest pain (2%), vasodilation (2%), peripheral edema (1%)

Central nervous system: Headache (4%), malaise (4%), dizziness (3%), fever (2%)

Dermatologic: Rash (3%)

Endocrine & metabolic: Hyperglycemia (1%)

Gastrointestinal: Abdominal pain (5%), nausea (5%), diarrhea (3%), vomiting (2%), flatulence (1%)

Genitourinary: Nocturia (7%), burning symptoms (5%), urinary retention (4%), urethral pain (3%), pelvic pain (1%), hematuria (microscopic) (3%)

Hematologic: Anemia (2%)

Neuromuscular & skeletal: Weakness (4%), back pain (3%), myalgia (1%)

Respiratory: Pneumonia (1%)

<1% (Limited to important or life-threatening): Decreased urine flow, pruritus, skin irritation, taste disturbance, tenesmus, urethritis

(Continued)

Valrubicin *(Continued)*

Overdosage/Toxicology Inadvertent paravenous extravasation has not been associated with skin ulceration or necrosis. Myelosuppression is possible following inadvertent systemic administration, or following significant systemic absorption from intravesical instillation.

Pharmacodynamics/Kinetics

Absorption: Well absorbed into bladder tissue, negligible systemic absorption. Trauma to mucosa may increase absorption, and perforation greatly increases absorption with significant systemic myelotoxicity.

Metabolism: Negligible after intravesical instillation and 2 hour retention

Formulations Injection, solution: 40 mg/mL (5 mL) [contains Cremophor® EL 50% (polyoxyethyleneglycol triricinoleate) and dehydrated alcohol 50%]

Dosing

Adults & Elderly: Urinary carcinoma *in situ*: Intravesical: 800 mg once weekly for 6 weeks

Renal Impairment: No adjustment is necessary.

Hepatic Impairment: No adjustment necessary.

Administration

I.V.: Instill slowly via gravity flow through a urinary catheter (following sterile insertion). Withdraw the catheter and allow patient to retain solution for 2 hours. After 2 hours, the patient should void.

Stability

Storage: Store unopened vials under refrigeration at 2°C to 8°C (36°F to 48°F). Stable for 12 hours when diluted in 0.9% sodium chloride.

Reconstitution: Withdraw contents of four vials, each containing 200 mg in 5 mL (allowed to warm to room temperature without heating), and dilute with 55 mL of 0.9% sodium chloride injection, USP.

Monitoring Laboratory Tests Cystoscopy, biopsy, and urine cytology every 3 months for recurrence or progression

Monitoring and Teaching Issues

Physical Assessment: This medication is administered by a physician through a urinary bladder catheter, using aseptic technique. **Note:** Caution must be used to prevent exposure to this mediation (see Warnings/Precautions). Monitor patient response during and following instillation. Instruct patient on appropriate interventions to reduce side effects and adverse symptoms to report (see Patient Education). **Pregnancy risk factor C** - determine that patient is not pregnant before beginning treatment. Instruct patients of childbearing age on appropriate barrier contraceptive measures. Breast-feeding is not recommended.

Patient Education: This medication will be instilled into your bladder through a catheter to be retained for as long as possible. Your urine will be red tinged for the next 24 hours; report promptly if this continues for a longer period. May cause altered urination patterns (frequency, dysuria, or incontinence), some bladder pain, pain on urination, or pelvic pain; report if these persist. If diabetic, monitor glucose levels closely (may cause hyperglycemia). It is important that you maintain adequate hydration (2-3 L/day of fluids) unless advised by prescriber to restrict fluids. May cause dizziness or fatigue (use caution when driving or engaging in tasks requiring alertness until response to drug is known); or nausea, vomiting, or taste disturbance (small, frequent meals, frequent mouth care, chewing gum, or sucking lozenges may help). Report chest pain or palpitations; persistent dizziness; swelling of extremities; persistent nausea, vomiting, diarrhea, or abdominal pain; muscle weakness, pain, or tremors; unusual cough or difficulty breathing; or other adverse effects. **Pregnancy/breast-feeding precautions:** Inform prescriber if you are pregnant. Do not get pregnant while taking this medication and for 1 month following therapy; consult prescriber for appropriate barrier contraceptives. Breast-feeding is not recommended.

Breast-feeding Issues: It is not known whether valrubicin is secreted in human milk. Because many immunoglobulins are secreted in milk, and the potential for serious adverse reactions exists, a decision should be made whether to discontinue nursing or discontinue the drug, taking into account the importance of the drug to the mother.

Valsartan (val SAR tan)

U.S. Brand Names Diovan®

Generic Available No

Pharmacologic Category Angiotensin II Receptor Blocker

Pregnancy Risk Factor C/D (2nd and 3rd trimesters)

Lactation Excretion in breast milk unknown/contraindicated

Use Alone or in combination with other antihypertensive agents in treating essential hypertension; treatment of heart failure (NYHA Class II-IV) in patients intolerant to angiotensin converting enzyme (ACE) inhibitors

Mechanism of Action/Effect As a prodrug, valsartan produces direct antagonism of the angiotensin II (AT2) receptors. Valsartan blocks the vasoconstrictor and aldosterone-secreting effects of angiotensin II. It displaces angiotensin II from the AT1 receptor and produces its blood pressure lowering effects by antagonizing AT1-induced vasoconstriction, aldosterone release, catecholamine release, arginine vasopressin release, water intake, and hypertrophic responses. This action results in more efficient blockade of the cardiovascular effects of angiotensin II and fewer side effects than the ACE inhibitors.

Contraindications Hypersensitivity to valsartan or any component of the formulation; hypersensitivity to other A-II receptor antagonists; primary hyperaldosteronism; bilateral renal artery stenosis; pregnancy (2nd and 3rd trimesters)

Warnings/Precautions Avoid use or use a smaller dose in patients who are volume depleted; correct depletion first. Deterioration in renal function can occur with initiation. Use with caution in unilateral renal artery stenosis and pre-existing renal insufficiency; significant aortic/mitral stenosis. Use caution in patients with severe renal impairment or significant hepatic dysfunction.

Heart failure: Concomitant use of valsartan, an ACE inhibitor, and a beta-blocker is not recommended; this combination has been associated with unfavorable outcomes in clinical trials. Monitor renal function closely in patients with severe heart failure; changes in renal function should be anticipated and dosage adjustments of valsartan or concomitant medications may be needed.

Pregnancy risk C/D (2nd and 3rd trimesters).

Drug Interactions

Cytochrome P450 Effect: Inhibits CYP2C8/9

Decreased Effect: Phenobarbital, ketoconazole, troleandomycin, sulfaphenazole

Increased Effect/Toxicity: Valsartan blood levels may be increased by cimetidine and monoxidine; clinical effect is unknown. Concurrent use of potassium salts/supplements, co-trimoxazole (high dose), ACE inhibitors, and potassium-sparing diuretics (amiloride, spironolactone, triamterene) may increase the risk of hyperkalemia.

Nutritional/Ethanol Interactions

Food: Decreases rate and extent of absorption by 50% and 40%, respectively.

Herb/Nutraceutical: Avoid dong quai if using for hypertension (has estrogenic activity). Avoid ephedra, yohimbe, ginseng (may worsen hypertension). Avoid garlic (may have increased antihypertensive effect).

Adverse Reactions

Hypertension: Similar incidence to placebo; independent of race, age, and gender.

>1%:

Central nervous system: Dizziness (2% to 8%), fatigue (2%)
Endocrine & metabolic: Serum potassium increased (4.4%)
Gastrointestinal: Abdominal pain (2%)
Hematologic: Neutropenia (1.9%)
Respiratory: Cough (2.6% versus 1.5% in placebo)
Miscellaneous: Viral infection (3%)

>1% but frequency ≤ placebo: Headache, upper respiratory infection, cough, diarrhea, rhinitis, sinusitis, nausea, pharyngitis, edema, arthralgia

Heart failure:

>10%: Central nervous system: Dizziness (17%)

1% to 10%:

Cardiovascular: Hypotension (7%), postural hypotension (2%)
Central nervous system: Fatigue (3%)
Endocrine & metabolic: Hyperkalemia (2%)
Gastrointestinal: Diarrhea (5%)
Neuromuscular & skeletal: Arthralgia (3%), back pain (3%)
Renal: Creatinine elevated >50% (4%)

All indications:

<1%: Allergic reactions, anemia, angioedema, anorexia, anxiety, asthenia, back pain, chest pain, constipation, creatinine increased (0.8% in hypertensive patients), dyspepsia, dyspnea, flatulence, hematocrit/hemoglobin decreased, impotence, insomnia, muscle cramps, myalgia, orthostatic effects, palpitations, paresthesia, pruritus, rash, serum transaminases increased, somnolence, syncope, vertigo, vomiting, xerostomia. May be associated with worsening of renal function in patients dependent on renin-angiotensin-aldosterone system.

Postmarketing and/or case reports: Angioedema, hepatitis, impaired renal function, hyperkalemia (hypertensive patients), alopecia

Overdosage/Toxicology Only mild toxicity (hypotension, bradycardia, hyperkalemia) has been reported with large overdoses (up to 5 g of captopril and 300 mg of enalapril). No fatalities have been reported. Treatment is symptomatic. Not removed by hemodialysis.

Pharmacodynamics/Kinetics

Bioavailability: 25% (range 10% to 35%)

Half-Life Elimination: 6 hours

Time to Peak: 2-4 hours

Metabolism: To inactive metabolite

Onset: Peak antihypertensive effect: 2-4 weeks

Formulations

Capsule: 80 mg, 160 mg, 320 mg [DSC]
Tablet: 40 mg, 80 mg, 160 mg, 320 mg

Dosing

Adults & Elderly:

Hypertension: Oral: Initial: 80 mg or 160 mg once daily (in patients who are not volume depleted); majority of effect within 2 weeks, maximal effects in 4-6 weeks; dose may be increased to achieve desired effect; maximum recommended dose: 320 mg/day

Heart failure: Oral: Initial: 40 mg twice daily; titrate dose to 80-160 mg twice daily, as tolerated; maximum daily dose: 320 mg. **Note:** Do not use with ACE inhibitors and beta blockers.

Renal Impairment:

Cl_{cr} >10 mL/minute: No dosage adjustment necessary.
Dialysis: Not significantly removed.

Hepatic Impairment: Mild to moderate liver disease: ≤80 mg/day

Administration

Oral: Administer with or without food.

Stability

Storage: Store at controlled room temperature of 15°C to 30°C (59°F to 86°F). Protect from moisture.

Monitoring Laboratory Tests Baseline and periodic electrolyte panels, renal and liver function, urinalysis

Monitoring and Teaching Issues

Physical Assessment: See Warnings/Precautions, Contraindications, and Dosing for use cautions. Assess effectiveness and interactions of other medications patient may be taking (see Drug Interactions). Assess results of laboratory tests (see above), effectiveness of therapy, and adverse response on a regular basis during therapy (see Adverse Reactions and Overdose/Toxicology). Teach patient appropriate use according to drug form and

(Continued)

Valsartan *(Continued)*

purpose of therapy, possible side effects and appropriate interventions, and adverse symptoms to report (see Patient Education). **Pregnancy risk factor C/D** - see Pregnancy Risk Factor for use cautions. Teach appropriate use of barrier contraceptives. Breast-feeding is contraindicated.

Patient Education: Inform prescriber of all prescriptions, OTC medications, or herbal products you are taking, and any allergies you have. Do not take anything new during treatment unless approved by prescriber. Take exactly as directed and do not discontinue without consulting prescriber. This drug does not eliminate need for diet or exercise regimen as recommended by prescriber. May cause dizziness, fainting, or lightheadedness (use caution when driving or engaging in tasks that require alertness until response to drug is known); postural hypotension (use caution when rising from lying or sitting position or climbing stairs); diarrhea (boiled milk, buttermilk, or yogurt may help); or decreased libido (will resolve). Report chest pain or palpitations; unrelenting headache; swelling of extremities, face, or tongue; muscle weakness or pain; difficulty breathing or unusual cough; flu-like symptoms; or other persistent adverse reactions. **Pregnancy/breast-feeding precautions:** Inform prescriber if you are or intend to become pregnant. This drug should not be used in the 2nd or 3rd trimester of pregnancy. Consult prescriber for appropriate contraceptive measures if necessary. Do not breast-feed.

Dietary Issues: Avoid salt substitutes which contain potassium. May be taken with or without food.

Pregnancy Issues: Medications which act on the renin-angiotensin system are reported to have the following fetal/neonatal effects: Hypotension, neonatal skull hypoplasia, anuria, renal failure, and death; oligohydramnios is also reported. These effects are reported to occur with exposure during the 2nd and 3rd trimesters. Valsartan should be discontinued as soon as possible after pregnancy is detected.

Additional Information Valsartan may have an advantage over losartan due to minimal metabolism requirements and consequent use in mild to moderate hepatic impairment.

Related Information

Angiotensin Agents *on page 1547*

Valsartan and Hydrochlorothiazide

(val SAR tan & hye droe klor oh THYE a zide)

U.S. Brand Names Diovan HCT®

Synonyms Hydrochlorothiazide and Valsartan

Generic Available No

Pharmacologic Category Antihypertensive Agent Combination

Pregnancy Risk Factor C (1st trimester); D (2nd and 3rd trimester)

Lactation Excretion in breast milk unknown/not recommended

Use Treatment of hypertension (not indicated for initial therapy)

Formulations Tablet:

80 mg/12.5 mg: Valsartan 80 mg and hydrochlorothiazide 12.5 mg
160 mg/12.5 mg: Valsartan 160 mg and hydrochlorothiazide 12.5 mg
160 mg/25 mg: Valsartan 160 mg and hydrochlorothiazide 25 mg

Dosing

Adults & Elderly: Hypertension: Oral: Dose is individualized.

Monitoring and Teaching Issues

Physical Assessment: See individual components listed in Related Information. **Pregnancy risk factor C/D** - see Pregnancy Risk Factor for use cautions. Assess knowledge/instruct patient on need to use appropriate contraceptive measures and the need to avoid pregnancy. Breast-feeding is not recommended.

Patient Education: See individual components listed in Related Information. **Pregnancy/breast-feeding precautions:** Inform prescriber if you are or intend to become pregnant. Breast-feeding is not recommended.

Related Information

Hydrochlorothiazide *on page 664*
Valsartan *on page 1386*

Valstar® *see* Valrubicin *on page 1385*
Valtrex® *see* Valacyclovir *on page 1377*
Vanatrip® *see* Amitriptyline *on page 84*
Vancenase® AQ 84 mcg *see* Beclomethasone *on page 149*
Vancenase® Pockethaler® *see* Beclomethasone *on page 149*
Vanceril® *see* Beclomethasone *on page 149*
Vancocin® *see* Vancomycin *on page 1388*

Vancomycin (van koe MYE sin)

U.S. Brand Names Vancocin®

Synonyms Vancomycin Hydrochloride

Generic Available Yes

Pharmacologic Category Antibiotic, Miscellaneous

Pregnancy Risk Factor C

Lactation Enters breast milk/use caution

Use Treatment of patients with infections caused by staphylococcal species and streptococcal species; used orally for staphylococcal enterocolitis or for antibiotic-associated pseudomembranous colitis produced by *C. difficile*

Mechanism of Action/Effect Inhibits bacterial cell wall synthesis

Contraindications Hypersensitivity to vancomycin or any component of the formulation; avoid in patients with previous severe hearing loss

Warnings/Precautions Use with caution in patients with renal impairment or those receiving other nephrotoxic or ototoxic drugs. Dosage modification is required in patients with impaired renal function (especially elderly). Pregnancy risk C.

Drug Interactions

Increased Effect/Toxicity: Increased toxicity with other ototoxic or nephrotoxic drugs. Increased neuromuscular blockade with most neuromuscular blocking agents.

Adverse Reactions

Oral:

>10%: Gastrointestinal: Bitter taste, nausea, vomiting, stomatitis

1% to 10%:

Central nervous system: Chills, drug fever

Hematologic: Eosinophilia

<1% (Limited to important or life-threatening): Interstitial nephritis, ototoxicity, renal failure, skin rash, thrombocytopenia, vasculitis

Parenteral:

>10%:

Cardiovascular: Hypotension accompanied by flushing

Dermatologic: Erythematous rash on face and upper body (red neck or red man syndrome)

1% to 10%:

Central nervous system: Chills, drug fever

Hematologic: Eosinophilia

<1% (Limited to important or life-threatening): Ototoxicity, renal failure, thrombocytopenia, vasculitis

Overdosage/Toxicology Symptoms of overdose include ototoxicity and nephrotoxicity. There is no specific therapy for overdose with vancomycin. Care is symptomatic and supportive. Peritoneal filtration and hemofiltration (not dialysis) have been shown to reduce the serum concentration of vancomycin. High flux dialysis may remove up to 25% of the drug.

Pharmacodynamics/Kinetics

Absorption: Oral: Poor; I.M.: Erratic; Intraperitoneal: ~38%

Half-Life Elimination: Biphasic: Terminal:

Newborns: 6-10 hours

Infants and Children 3 months to 4 years: 4 hours

Children >3 years: 2.2-3 hours

Adults: 5-11 hours; significantly prolonged with renal impairment

End-stage renal disease: 200-250 hours

Time to Peak: Serum: I.V.: 45-65 minutes

Formulations

Capsule, as hydrochloride: 125 mg, 250 mg

Infusion [premixed in iso-osmotic dextrose]: 500 mg (100 mL); 1 g (200 mL)

Injection, powder for reconstitution, as hydrochloride: 500 mg, 1 g, 5 g, 10 g

Vancocin®: 500 mg, 1 g, 10 g

Powder for oral solution, as hydrochloride (Vancocin®): 1 g [provides 250 mg/5 mL when mixed]; 10 g [provides 500 mg/6 mL when mixed]

Dosing

Adults:

Systemic infections: I.V.: Initial dosage recommendation: Normal renal function: 1 g every 12 hours **or** select individualized dosage based on weight (10-15 mg/kg)

Note: Select interval based on estimated Cl_{cr} >60 mL/minute every 12 hours, 40-60 mL/minute every 24 hours, <40 mL/minute every 24 hours; monitor levels.

Prophylaxis for bacterial endocarditis: I.V.:

Dental, oral, or upper respiratory tract surgery: 1 g 1 hour before surgery

GI/GU procedure: 1 g plus 1.5 mg/kg gentamicin 1 hour prior to surgery

CNS infections: **Intrathecal:** Vancomycin is available as a powder for injection and may be diluted to 1-5 mg/mL concentration in preservative-free 0.9% sodium chloride for administration into the CSF Up to 20 mg/day

Antibiotic lock technique (for catheter infections): 2 mg/mL in SWI/NS or D_5W; instill 3-5 mL into catheter port as a flush solution instead of heparin lock. (**Note:** Do not mix with any other solutions.)

Intrathecal: 20 mg/day; vancomycin is available as a powder for injection and may be diluted to 1-5 mg/mL concentration in preservative free 0.9% sodium chloride for administration into the CSF.

Pseudomembranous colitis produced by *C. difficile*: Oral: 125 mg 4 times/day for 10 days. **Note:** Due to the emergence of resistant enterococci, the use of vancomycin is limited in most settings

Elderly: Refer to adult dosing. Elderly may require greater dosage reduction than expected.

Pediatrics: Initial dosage recommendation: I.V.:

Neonates:

Postnatal age ≤7 days:

<1200 g: 15 mg/kg/dose every 24 hours

1200-2000 g: 10 mg/kg/dose every 12 hours

>2000 g: 15 mg/kg/dose every 12 hours

Postnatal age >7 days:

<1200 g: 15 mg/kg/dose every 24 hours

≥1200 g: 10 mg/kg/dose divided every 8 hours

Infants >1 month and Children:

40 mg/kg/day in divided doses every 6 hours

Prophylaxis for bacterial endocarditis: I.V.:

Dental, oral, or upper respiratory tract surgery: 20 mg/kg 1 hour prior to the procedure

GI/GU procedure: 20 mg/kg plus gentamicin 2 mg/kg 1 hour prior to surgery

CNS infections:

Intrathecal: Vancomycin is available as a powder for injection and may be diluted to 1-5 mg/mL concentration in preservative-free 0.9% sodium chloride for administration into the CSF

Neonates: 5-10 mg/day

Children: 5-20 mg/day

I.V.: Infants >1 month and Children with staphylococcal central nervous system infection: 60 mg/kg/day in divided doses every 6 hours

(Continued)

Vancomycin *(Continued)*

Antibiotic lock technique (for catheter infections): 2 mg/mL in SWI/NS or D_5W; instill 3-5 mL into catheter port as a flush solution instead of heparin lock (**Note:** Do not mix with any other solutions)

Pseudomembranous colitis produced by *C. difficile*: Oral:

Neonates: 10 mg/kg/day in divided doses

Children: 40 mg/kg/day in divided doses, added to fluids

Note: Use is restricted in most settings

Renal Impairment: Vancomycin levels should be monitored in patients with any renal impairment.

Cl_{cr} >60 mL/minute: Start with 1 g or 10-15 mg/kg/dose every 12 hours.

Cl_{cr} 40-60 mL/minute: Start with 1 g or 10-15 mg/kg/dose every 24 hours.

Cl_{cr} <40 mL/minute: Will need longer intervals; determine by serum concentration monitoring.

Hemodialysis: Not dialyzable (0% to 5%); generally not removed; exception minimal-moderate removal by some of the newer high-flux filters. Dose may need to be administered more frequently. Monitor serum concentrations.

Continuous ambulatory peritoneal dialysis (CAPD): Not significantly removed; administration via CAPD fluid: 15-30 mg/L (15-30 mcg/mL) of CAPD fluid.

Continuous arteriovenous hemofiltration: Dose as for Cl_{cr} 10-40 mL/minute.

Antibiotic lock technique (for catheter infections): 2 mg/mL in SWI/NS or D_5W; instill 3-5 mL into catheter port as a flush solution instead of heparin lock (**Note:** Do not mix with any other solutions).

Hepatic Impairment: Reduce dose by 60%.

Administration

Oral: May be administered with food. Shake well before administration.

I.M.: Do not administer I.M.

I.V.: Administer vancomycin by I.V. intermittent infusion over at least 60 minutes at a final concentration not to exceed 5 mg/mL. Administration of antihistamines just before the infusion may also prevent or minimize Red man syndrome.

Stability

Storage: Refrigerate oral solution.

Reconstitution: Vancomycin reconstituted intravenous solutions are stable for 14 days at room temperature or refrigeration. Stability of parenteral admixture at room temperature (25°C) or refrigeration temperature (4°C) is 7 days.

Standard diluent: 500 mg/150 mL D_5W; 750 mg/250 mL D_5W; 1 g/250 mL D_5W

Minimum volume: Maximum concentration is 5 mg/mL to minimize thrombophlebitis.

After the oral solution is reconstituted, it should be refrigerated and used within 2 weeks.

Compatibility: Stable in dextran 6% in NS, D_5LR, D_5NS, D_5W, $D_{10}W$, LR, NS

Y-site administration: Incompatible with albumin, amphotericin B cholesteryl sulfate complex, cefepime, gatifloxacin, heparin, idarubicin, omeprazole

Compatibility in syringe: Incompatible with heparin

Compatibility when admixed: Incompatible with amobarbital, chloramphenicol, chlorothiazide, dexamethasone sodium phosphate, penicillin G potassium, pentobarbital, phenobarbital, phenytoin

Monitoring Laboratory Tests Perform culture and sensitivity studies prior to first dose. Periodic renal function, urinalysis, serum vancomycin concentrations, WBC, audiogram with prolonged use. Obtain drug levels after the third dose unless otherwise directed. Peaks are drawn 1 hour after the completion of a 1- to 2-hour infusion. Troughs are obtained just before the next dose.

Monitoring and Teaching Issues

Physical Assessment: See Warnings/Precautions and Contraindications for use cautions. Assess effectiveness and interactions of other medications patient may be taking (eg, anything that is ototoxic or nephrotoxic - see Drug Interactions). See specifics above for I.V. administration (eg, premedication and Red Man syndrome). Infusion site must be monitored closely to prevent extravasation. Assess results of laboratory tests (see above), effectiveness of therapy, and adverse response on a regular basis during therapy (see Adverse Reactions and Overdose/Toxicology). Teach patient appropriate use (oral), possible side effects and appropriate interventions, and adverse symptoms to report (see Patient Education). **Pregnancy risk C** - benefits of use should outweigh possible risks. Note breast-feeding caution.

Patient Education: Inform prescriber of all prescriptions, OTC medications, or herbal products you are taking, and any allergies you have. Do not take anything new during treatment unless approved by prescriber. I.V. report immediately and chills or pain at infusion site, skin rash or redness, or difficulty breathing. Take as directed with food, for as long as prescribed. Maintain adequate hydration (2-3 L/day of fluids) unless advised by prescriber to restrict fluids.

Oral/I.V.: May cause nausea, vomiting, or GI upset (small, frequent meals, frequent mouth care, sucking lozenges, or chewing gum may help). Report rash or hives; chills or fever; persistent GI disturbances; opportunistic infection (sore throat, chills, fever, burning, itching on urination, vaginal discharge, white plaques in mouth); difficulty breathing; decreased urine output; chest pain or palpitations; changes in hearing or fullness in ears; or worsening of condition.

Pregnancy/breast-feeding precautions: Inform prescriber if you are or intend to become pregnant. Consult prescriber if breast-feeding.

Dietary Issues: May be taken with food.

Geriatric Considerations: As a result of age-related changes in renal function and volume of distribution, accumulation and toxicity are a risk in the elderly. Careful monitoring and dosing adjustment is necessary.

Breast-feeding Issues: Vancomycin is excreted in breast milk but is poorly absorbed from the gastrointestinal tract. Therefore, systemic absorption would not be expected. Theoretically, vancomycin in the GI tract may affect the normal bowel flora in the infant, resulting in diarrhea.

Additional Information Because of its long half-life, vancomycin should be dosed on an every 12 hour basis; monitoring of peak and trough serum levels is advisable. The "red man syndrome" characterized by skin rash and hypotension is not an allergic reaction but rather is associated with too rapid infusion of the drug. To alleviate or prevent the reaction, infuse vancomycin at a rate of ≥30 minutes for each 500 mg of drug being administered (eg, 1 g over ≥60 minutes); 1.5 g over ≥90 minutes.

Related Information

Compatibility of Drugs *on page 1564*
Peak and Trough Guidelines *on page 1544*

Vancomycin Hydrochloride *see* Vancomycin *on page 1388*

Vaniqa™ *see* Eflornithine *on page 461*

Vanoxide-HC® *see* Benzoyl Peroxide and Hydrocortisone *on page 158*

Vantin® *see* Cefpodoxime *on page 246*

VAQTA® *see page 1498*

Varicella Virus Vaccine *see page 1498*

Varicella-Zoster Immune Globulin (Human) *see page 1498*

Varivax® *see page 1498*

Vaseretic® *see* Enalapril and Hydrochlorothiazide *on page 466*

Vasocidin® *see page 1509*

VasoClear® [OTC] *see page 1509*

Vasocon-A® [OTC] *see page 1509*

Vasocon Regular® *see page 1509*

Vasopressin (vay soe PRES in)

U.S. Brand Names Pitressin®

Synonyms ADH; Antidiuretic Hormone; 8-Arginine Vasopressin; Vasopressin Tannate

Generic Available No

Pharmacologic Category Antidiuretic Hormone Analog; Hormone, Posterior Pituitary

Pregnancy Risk Factor C

Lactation Enters breast milk/use caution

Use Treatment of diabetes insipidus; prevention and treatment of postoperative abdominal distention; differential diagnosis of diabetes insipidus

Use - Unlabeled/Investigational Adjunct in the treatment of GI hemorrhage and esophageal varices; pulseless ventricular tachycardia (VT)/ventricular fibrillation (VF); vasodilatory shock (septic shock)

Mechanism of Action/Effect Increases cyclic adenosine monophosphate (cAMP) which increases water permeability at the renal tubule resulting in decreased urine volume and increased osmolality. Causes peristalsis by directly stimulating the smooth muscle in the GI tract.

Contraindications Hypersensitivity to vasopressin or any component of the formulation

Warnings/Precautions Use with caution in patients with seizure disorders, migraine, asthma, vascular disease, renal disease, cardiac disease, chronic nephritis with nitrogen retention, goiter with cardiac complications, arteriosclerosis. I.V. infiltration may lead to severe vasoconstriction and localized tissue necrosis, gangrene of extremities or tongue, and ischemic colitis.

Pregnancy risk C.

Drug Interactions

Decreased Effect: Lithium, epinephrine, demeclocycline, heparin, and ethanol block antidiuretic activity to varying degrees.

Increased Effect/Toxicity: Chlorpropamide, urea, clofibrate, carbamazepine, and fludrocortisone potentiate antidiuretic response.

Nutritional/Ethanol Interactions Ethanol: Avoid ethanol (due to effects on ADH).

Adverse Reactions Frequency not defined.

Cardiovascular: Increased blood pressure, arrhythmias, venous thrombosis, vasoconstriction (with higher doses), chest pain, myocardial infarction
Central nervous system: Pounding in the head, fever, vertigo
Dermatologic: Urticaria, circumoral pallor
Gastrointestinal: Flatulence, abdominal cramps, nausea, vomiting
Genitourinary: Uterine contraction
Neuromuscular & skeletal: Tremor
Respiratory: Bronchial constriction
Miscellaneous: Diaphoresis

Overdosage/Toxicology Symptoms of overdose include drowsiness, weight gain, confusion, listlessness, and water intoxication. Water intoxication requires withdrawal of the drug. Severe intoxication may require osmotic diuresis and loop diuretics.

Pharmacodynamics/Kinetics

Half-Life Elimination: Nasal: 15 minutes; Parenteral: 10-20 minutes

Metabolism: Nasal/Parenteral: Hepatic, renal

Onset: Nasal: 1 hour

Duration: Nasal: 3-8 hours; I.M., S.C.: 2-8 hours

Formulations Injection, solution, aqueous: 20 pressor units/mL (0.5 mL, 1 mL, 10 mL)

Pitressin®: 20 pressor units/mL (1 mL)

(Continued)

Vasopressin *(Continued)*

Dosing

Adults & Elderly:

Diabetes insipidus (highly variable dosage; titrated based on serum and urine sodium and osmolality in addition to fluid balance and urine output):

I.M., S.C.: 5-10 units 2-4 times/day as needed (dosage range 5-60 units/day)

Continuous I.V. infusion: 0.5 milliunit/kg/hour (0.0005 unit/kg/hour); double dosage as needed every 30 minutes to a maximum of 0.01 unit/kg/hour

Intranasal: Administer on cotton pledget, as nasal spray, or by dropper

Abdominal distention: I.M.: 5 mg stat, 10 mg every 3-4 hours

GI hemorrhage (unlabeled use):

Continuous I.V. infusion: 0.5 milliunits/kg/hour (0.0005 unit/kg/hour); double dosage as needed every 30 minutes to a maximum of 10 milliunits/kg/hour

I.V.: Initial: 0.2-0.4 unit/minute, then titrate dose as needed; if bleeding stops, continue at same dose for 12 hours, taper off over 24-48 hours.

Pulseless VT/VF (ACLS protocol): I.V.: 40 int. units (as a single dose only); if no I.V. access, administer 40 int. units diluted with NS (to a total volume of 10 mL) endotracheally

Vasodilatory shock/septic shock (unlabeled use): I.V.: 0.04 units/minute continuous infusion, usually not titrated

Pediatrics:

Diabetes insipidus (highly variable dosage; titrated based on serum and urine sodium and osmolality in addition to fluid balance and urine output):

I.M., S.C.:

Children: 2.5-10 units 2-4 times/day as needed

Continuous I.V. infusion: Children: 0.5 milliunit/kg/hour (0.0005 unit/kg/hour); double dosage as needed every 30 minutes to a maximum of 0.01 unit/kg/hour

Intranasal: Administer on cotton pledget, as nasal spray, or by dropper

GI hemorrhage (unlabeled use): I.V. infusion: Dilute in NS or D_5W to 0.1-1 unit/mL

Children: Initial: 0.002-0.005 units/kg/minute; titrate dose as needed; maximum: 0.01 unit/kg/minute; continue at same dosage (if bleeding stops) for 12 hours, then taper off over 24-48 hours

Hepatic Impairment: Some patients respond to much lower doses with cirrhosis.

Administration

I.V.: I.V. infusion administration requires the use of an infusion pump and should be administered in a peripheral line. Dilute in NS or D_5W to 0.1-1 unit/mL.

Infusion rates:

100 units in 500 mL D_5W rate

0.1 unit/minute: 30 mL/hour

0.2 units/minute: 60 mL/hour

0.3 units/minute: 90 mL/hour

0.4 units/minute: 120 mL/hour

0.5 units/minute: 150 mL/hour

0.6 units/minute: 180 mL/hour

Topical: Topical administration on nasal mucosa: Administer injectable vasopressin on cotton plugs, as nasal spray, or by dropper. Should not be inhaled.

Stability

Storage: Store injection at room temperature. Protect from heat and from freezing. Use only clear solutions.

Compatibility: Stable in D_5W, NS

Monitoring Laboratory Tests Serum and urine sodium, urine specific gravity, urine and serum osmolality

Monitoring and Teaching Issues

Physical Assessment: See Warnings/Precautions, Contraindications, and Drug Interactions for use cautions. See specifics above for I.V. or intranasal administration. Infusion site must be monitored closely to prevent extravasation (see Administration). Assess results of laboratory tests (see above), effectiveness of therapy, and adverse response on a regular basis during therapy (eg, cardiac status, blood pressure, CNS status, fluid balance, signs or symptoms of water intoxication, or intranasal irritation - see Adverse Reactions and Overdose/Toxicology). Teach patient possible side effects and appropriate interventions and adverse symptoms to report (see Patient Education).

Patient Education: Inform prescriber of all prescriptions, OTC medications, or herbal products you are taking, and any allergies you have. Do not take anything new during treatment unless approved by prescriber. Avoid alcohol. This drug will usually be administered by infusion or injection. Report immediately any redness, swelling, pain, or burning at infusion/injection site. When self-administered follow directions exactly. May cause dizziness, drowsiness (use caution when driving or engaging in potentially hazardous tasks until response to drug is known); nausea, vomiting, cramping (small, frequent meals, frequent mouth care, chewing gum, or sucking lozenges may help), Report persistent nausea, vomiting, abdominal cramps; tremor, acute headache, or dizziness; chest pain or irregular heartbeat; difficulty breathing or excess perspiration; CNS changes (confusion, drowsiness); or runny nose or painful nasal membranes (intranasal).

Geriatric Considerations: Elderly patients should be cautioned not to increase their fluid intake beyond that sufficient to satisfy their thirst in order to avoid water intoxication and hyponatremia. Under experimental conditions, the elderly have shown to have a decreased responsiveness to vasopressin with respect to its effects on water homeostasis.

Breast-feeding Issues: Based on case reports, vasopressin and desmopressin have been used safely during nursing.

Additional Information Vasopressin increases factor VIII levels and may be useful in hemophiliacs.

Vasopressin Tannate *see* Vasopressin *on page 1391*

Vasotec® *see* Enalapril *on page 463*

Vasotec® I.V. *see* Enalapril *on page 463*
VCR *see* VinCRIStine *on page 1401*
V-Dec-M® *see* Guaifenesin and Pseudoephedrine *on page 648*
Vectrin® [DSC] *see* Minocycline *on page 909*

Vecuronium (ve KYOO roe nee um)

U.S. Brand Names Norcuron®

Synonyms ORG NC 45

Generic Available Yes

Pharmacologic Category Neuromuscular Blocker Agent, Nondepolarizing

Pregnancy Risk Factor C

Lactation Excretion in breast milk unknown/use caution

Use Adjunct to general anesthesia to facilitate endotracheal intubation and to relax skeletal muscles during surgery; to facilitate mechanical ventilation in ICU patients; does not relieve pain or produce sedation

Mechanism of Action/Effect Blocks acetylcholine from binding to receptors on motor endplate inhibiting depolarization

Contraindications Hypersensitivity to vecuronium or any component of the formulation

Warnings/Precautions Ventilation must be supported during neuromuscular blockade; certain clinical conditions may result in potentiation or antagonism of neuromuscular blockade:

Potentiation: Electrolyte abnormalities, severe hyponatremia, severe hypocalcemia, severe hypokalemia, hypermagnesemia, neuromuscular diseases, acidosis, acute intermittent porphyria, renal failure, hepatic failure

Antagonism: Alkalosis, hypercalcemia, demyelinating lesions, peripheral neuropathies, diabetes mellitus

Increased sensitivity in patients with myasthenia gravis, Eaton-Lambert syndrome; resistance in burn patients (>30% of body) for period of 5-70 days postinjury; resistance in patients with muscle trauma, denervation, immobilization, infection; use with caution in patients with hepatic or renal impairment; does not counteract bradycardia produced by anesthetics/vagal stimulation.

Pregnancy risk C.

Drug Interactions

Increased Effect/Toxicity: Increased effects are possible with aminoglycosides, beta-blockers, clindamycin, calcium channel blockers, halogenated anesthetics, imipenem, ketamine, lidocaine, loop diuretics (furosemide), macrolides (case reports), magnesium sulfate, procainamide, quinidine, quinolones, tetracyclines, and vancomycin. May increase risk of myopathy when used with high- dose corticosteroids for extended periods.

Adverse Reactions <1% (Limited to important or life-threatening): Bradycardia, circulatory collapse, edema, flushing, hypersensitivity reaction, hypotension, itching, rash, tachycardia

Overdosage/Toxicology

Symptoms of overdose include prolonged skeletal muscle weakness and apnea cardiovascular collapse.

Use neostigmine, edrophonium, or pyridostigmine with atropine to antagonize skeletal muscle relaxation; support of ventilation and the cardiovascular system through mechanical means, fluids, and pressors may be necessary.

Pharmacodynamics/Kinetics

Onset: Good intubation conditions: Within 2.5-3 minutes

Duration: Maximum neuromuscular blockade: Within 3-5 minutes

Formulations Injection, powder for reconstitution, as bromide: 10 mg, 20 mg [may be supplied with diluent containing benzyl alcohol]

Dosing

Adults & Elderly: Neuromuscular blockade: I.V. (do not administer I.M.):

Initial: 0.08-0.1 mg/kg or 0.04-0.06 mg/kg after initial dose of succinylcholine for intubation; maintenance: 0.01-0.015 mg/kg 25-40 minutes after initial dose, then 0.01-0.015 mg/kg every 12-15 minutes (higher doses will allow less frequent maintenance doses); may be administered as a continuous infusion at 0.8-2 mcg/kg/minute

Pretreatment/priming: Adults: 10% of intubating dose given 3-5 minutes before initial dose

ICU: Adults: 0.05-0.1 mg/kg bolus followed by 0.8-1.7 mcg/kg/minute once initial recovery from bolus observed or 0.1-0.2 mg/kg/dose every 1 hour

Pediatrics: Neuromuscular blockade: I.V. (do not administer I.M.):

Infants >7 weeks to 1 year: Initial: 0.08-0.1 mg/kg/dose; maintenance: 0.05-0.1 mg/kg/ every 60 minutes as needed

Children >1 year: Refer to adult dosing.

Hepatic Impairment: Dose reductions are necessary in patients with liver disease.

Administration

I.V.: Dilute vial to a maximum concentration of 2 mg/mL and give by rapid direct injection. For continuous infusion, dilute to a maximum concentration of 1 mg/mL.

Stability

Storage: Stable for 5 days at room temperature when reconstituted with bacteriostatic water. Stable for 24 hours at room temperature when reconstituted with preservative-free sterile water (avoid preservatives in neonates). Do not mix with alkaline drugs.

Monitoring and Teaching Issues

Physical Assessment: Only clinicians experienced in the use of neuromuscular blocking drugs should administer and/or manage the use of vecuronium. Dosage and rate of administration should be individualized and titrated to the desired effect, according to relevant clinical factors, premedication, concomitant medications, age, and general condition of patient. See Use, Contraindications, and Warnings/Precautions for appropriate use cautions. Ventilatory support must be instituted and maintained until adequate respiratory muscle function and/or airway protection are assured. Assess other medications for effectiveness and safety. Other drugs that affect neuromuscular activity may increase/decrease

(Continued)

Vecuronium *(Continued)*

neuromuscular block induced by vecuronium; monitor and adjust dosage as necessary. This drug does not cause anesthesia or analgesia; pain must be treated with appropriate analgesic agents. Continuous monitoring of vital signs, cardiac status, respiratory status, and degree of neuromuscular block (objective assessment with peripheral external nerve stimulator) is mandatory during infusion and until full muscle tone has returned (see Adverse Reactions). Muscle tone returns in a predictable pattern, starting with diaphragm, abdomen, chest, limbs, and finally muscles of the neck, face, and eyes. Safety precautions must be maintained until full muscle tone has returned. **Note:** It may take longer for return of muscle tone in obese or elderly patients or patients with renal or hepatic disease, myasthenia gravis, myopathy, other neuromuscular disease, dehydration, electrolyte imbalance, or severe acid/base imbalance. Provide appropriate patient teaching /support prior to and following administration.

Long-term use: Monitor fluid levels (intake and output) during and following infusion. Reposition patient and provide appropriate skin care, mouth care, and care of patient's eyes every 2-3 hours while sedated. Provide appropriate emotional and sensory support (auditory and environmental).

Pregnancy risk factor C. Note breast-feeding caution.

Patient Education: Patient will usually be unconscious prior to administration. Patient education should be appropriate to individual situation. Reassurance of constant monitoring and emotional support to reduce fear and anxiety should precede and follow administration. Following return of muscle tone, do not attempt to change position or rise from bed without assistance. Report immediately any skin rash or hives, pounding heartbeat, difficulty breathing, or muscle tremors. **Pregnancy/breast-feeding precautions:** Inform prescriber if you are pregnant or breast-feeding.

Pregnancy Issues: Use in cesarean section has been reported. Umbilical venous concentrations were 11% of maternal.

Additional Information Vecuronium is classified as an intermediate-duration neuromuscular-blocking agent. It produces minimal, if any, histamine release; does not relieve pain or produce sedation. It may produce cumulative effect on duration of blockade.

Veetids® *see* Penicillin V Potassium *on page 1048*

Velban® [DSC] *see* VinBLAStine *on page 1399*

Velosef® *see* Cephradine *on page 261*

Velosulin® BR (Buffered) *see* Insulin Preparations *on page 714*

Venlafaxine (VEN la faks een)

U.S. Brand Names Effexor®; Effexor® XR

Generic Available No

Pharmacologic Category Antidepressant, Serotonin/Norepinephrine Reuptake Inhibitor

Pregnancy Risk Factor C

Lactation Enters breast milk/contraindicated

Use Treatment of depression, generalized anxiety disorder (GAD)

Use - Unlabeled/Investigational Obsessive-compulsive disorder (OCD), chronic fatigue syndrome; hot flashes; neuropathic pain; attention-deficit/hyperactivity disorder (ADHD) and autism in children

Mechanism of Action/Effect Venlafaxine and its active metabolite o-desmethylvenlafaxine (ODV) are potent inhibitors of neuronal serotonin and norepinephrine reuptake and weak inhibitors of dopamine reuptake

Contraindications Hypersensitivity to venlafaxine or any component of the formulation; use of MAO inhibitors within 14 days; should not initiate MAO inhibitor within 7 days of discontinuing venlafaxine

Warnings/Precautions May cause sustained increase in blood pressure; may cause increase in anxiety, nervousness, insomnia; may cause weight loss (use with caution in patients where weight loss is undesirable). May worsen psychosis in some patients or precipitate a shift to mania or hypomania in patients with bipolar disease. May increase the risks associated with electroconvulsive therapy. Use caution in patients with depression, particularly if suicidal risk may be present. The risks of cognitive or motor impairment, as well as the potential for anticholinergic effects are very low. May cause or exacerbate sexual dysfunction. Abrupt discontinuation or dosage reduction after extended (≥6 weeks) therapy may lead to agitation, dysphoria, nervousness, anxiety, and other symptoms. When discontinuing therapy, dosage should be tapered gradually over at least a 2-week period. Use caution in patients with increased intraocular pressure or at risk of acute narrow-angle glaucoma. Pregnancy risk C.

Drug Interactions

Cytochrome P450 Effect: Substrate of CYP2C8/9, 2C19, **2D6, 3A4**; Inhibits CYP2B6, 2D6, 3A4

Decreased Effect: Serum levels of indinavir may be reduced be venlafaxine (AUC reduced by 28%) - clinical significance not determined. Enzyme inducers (carbamazepine, phenytoin, phenobarbital) may reduce the serum concentrations of venlafaxine.

Increased Effect/Toxicity: Concurrent use of MAO inhibitors (phenelzine, isocarboxazid), or drugs with MAO inhibitor activity (linezolid) may result in serotonin syndrome; should not be used within 2 weeks of each other. Selegiline may have a lower risk of this effect, particularly at low dosages, due to selectivity for MAO type B. In addition, concurrent use of buspirone, lithium, meperidine, nefazodone, selegiline, serotonin agonists (sumatriptan, naratriptan), sibutramine, SSRIs, trazodone, or tricyclic antidepressants may increase the risk of serotonin syndrome. Serum levels of haloperidol may be increased by venlafaxine. Inhibitors of CYP2D6 or CYP3A4 may increase the serum levels and/or toxicity of venlafaxine.

Nutritional/Ethanol Interactions

Ethanol: Avoid ethanol (may increase CNS effects).

Herb/Nutraceutical: Avoid valerian, St John's wort, SAMe, kava kava, tryptophan (may increase risk of serotonin syndrome and/or excessive sedation).

Effects on Lab Values ↑ thyroid, uric acid, glucose, potassium, AST, cholesterol (S)

Adverse Reactions

≥10%:

Central nervous system: Headache (25%), somnolence (23%), dizziness (19%), insomnia (18%), nervousness (13%)

Gastrointestinal: Nausea (37%), xerostomia (22%), constipation (15%), anorexia (11%)

Genitourinary: Abnormal ejaculation/orgasm (12%)

Neuromuscular & skeletal: Weakness (12%)

Miscellaneous: Diaphoresis (12%)

1% to 10%:

Cardiovascular: Vasodilation (4%), hypertension (dose-related; 3% in patients receiving <100 mg/day, up to 13% in patients receiving >300 mg/day), tachycardia (2%), chest pain (2%), postural hypotension (1%)

Central nervous system: Anxiety (6%), abnormal dreams (4%), yawning (3%), agitation (2%), confusion (2%), abnormal thinking (2%), depersonalization (1%), depression (1%)

Dermatologic: Rash (3%), pruritus (1%)

Endocrine & metabolic: Decreased libido

Gastrointestinal: Diarrhea (8%), vomiting (6%), dyspepsia (5%), flatulence (3%), taste perversion (2%), weight loss (1%)

Genitourinary: Impotence (6%), urinary frequency (3%), impaired urination (2%), orgasm disturbance (2%), urinary retention (1%)

Neuromuscular & skeletal: Tremor (5%), hypertonia (3%), paresthesia (3%), twitching (1%)

Ocular: Blurred vision (6%), mydriasis (2%)

Otic: Tinnitus (2%)

Miscellaneous: Infection (6%), chills (3%), trauma (2%)

<1% (Limited to important or life-threatening): Agranulocytosis, akathisia, anaphylaxis, aplastic anemia, asthma, catatonia, delirium, dyspnea, epidermal necrolysis, erythema multiforme, erythema nodosum, exfoliative dermatitis, extrapyramidal symptoms, hallucinations, hemorrhage (including ophthalmic and gastrointestinal), hepatic failure, hepatic necrosis, hirsutism, manic reaction (0.5%), pancreatitis, psychosis, rash (maculopapular, pustular, or vesiculobullous), seizures, serotonin syndrome, SIADH, Stevens-Johnson syndrome, tardive dyskinesia, torticollis, vertigo

Overdosage/Toxicology Symptoms of overdose include somnolence and occasionally tachycardia. Most overdoses resolve with only supportive treatment. Use of activated charcoal, inductions of emesis, or gastric lavage should be considered for acute ingestion. Forced diuresis, dialysis, and hemoperfusion not effective due to large volume of distribution.

Pharmacodynamics/Kinetics

Absorption: Oral: 92% to 100%; food has no significant effect on absorption of venlafaxine or formation of the active metabolite O-desmethylvenlafaxine (ODV)

Bioavailability: Absolute: ~45%

Half-Life Elimination: Venlafaxine: 3-7 hours; ODV: 9-13 hours; Steady-state plasma: Venlafaxine/ODV: Within 3 days of multiple dose therapy

Prolonged with cirrhosis and dialysis:

Adults: Cirrhosis: Venlafaxine: ~30%, ODV: ~60%

Adults: Dialysis: Venlafaxine: ~180%, ODV: ~142%

Time to Peak:

Immediate release: Venlafaxine: 2 hours, ODV: 3 hours

Extended release: Venlafaxine: 5.5 hours, ODV: 9 hours

Metabolism: Hepatic via CYP2D6 to active metabolite, O-desmethylvenlafaxine (ODV); other metabolites include N-desmethylvenlafaxine and N,O-didesmethylvenlafaxine

Formulations

Capsule, extended release, as hydrochloride (Effexor® XR): 37.5 mg, 75 mg, 150 mg

Tablet, as hydrochloride (Effexor®): 25 mg, 37.5 mg, 50 mg, 75 mg, 100 mg

Dosing

Adults: Depression or generalized anxiety (GAD): Oral:

Immediate-release tablets: 75 mg/day, administered in 2 or 3 divided doses, taken with food; dose may be increased in 75 mg/day increments at intervals of at least 4 days, up to 225-375 mg/day.

Extended-release capsules: 75 mg once daily taken with food; for some new patients, it may be desirable to start at 37.5 mg/day for 4-7 days before increasing to 75 mg once daily. Dose may be increased by up to 75 mg/day increments every 4 days as tolerated, up to a maximum of 225 mg/day.

Note: When discontinuing this medication after more than 1 week of treatment, it is generally recommended that the dose be tapered. If venlafaxine is used for 6 weeks or more, the dose should be tapered over 2 weeks when discontinuing its use.

Elderly: No specific recommendations for elderly, but may be best to start lower at 25-50 mg twice daily and increase as tolerated by 25 mg/dose. Adjust dose for renal impairment (see Renal Impairment). Hold dose until dialysis in dialysis patients.

Pediatrics: Children and Adolescents:

ADHD (unlabeled use): Initial: 12.5 mg/day

Children <40 kg: Increase by 12.5 mg/week to maximum of 50 mg/day in 2 divided doses

Children ≥40 kg: Increase by 25 mg/week to maximum of 75 mg/day in 3 divided doses.

Mean dose: 60 mg or 1.4 mg/kg administered in 2-3 divided doses

Autism (unlabeled use): Oral: Initial: 12.5 mg/day; adjust to 6.25-50 mg/day

Renal Impairment:

Cl_{cr} 10-70 mL/minute: Decrease dose by 25%.

Hemodialysis: Decrease total daily dose by 50% given after completion of dialysis.

(Continued)

Venlafaxine *(Continued)*

Hepatic Impairment: Reduce total dosage by 50%.

Administration

Oral: Administer with food.

Monitoring and Teaching Issues

Physical Assessment: Assess other medications patient may be taking for effectiveness and interactions (see Drug Interactions). See Contraindications and Warnings/Precautions for use cautions. Monitor therapeutic response according to rationale for therapy and adverse reactions at beginning of therapy and periodically with long-term use (see Adverse Reactions and Overdose/Toxicology). Taper dosage slowly when discontinuing. Assess knowledge/teach patient appropriate use, interventions to reduce side effects, and adverse symptoms to report (see Patient Education). **Pregnancy risk factor C** - benefits of use should outweigh possible risks. Breast-feeding is contraindicated.

Patient Education: Take exactly as directed; do not increase dose or frequency. It may take 2-3 weeks to achieve desired results. Take with food. Avoid alcohol, caffeine, and other prescription or OTC medications not approved by prescriber. Maintain adequate hydration (2-3 L/day of fluids) unless advised by prescriber to restrict fluids. You may experience excess drowsiness, lightheadedness, dizziness, or blurred vision (use caution when driving or engaging in tasks requiring alertness until response to drug is known); nausea, vomiting, anorexia, altered taste, dry mouth (small, frequent meals, frequent mouth care, chewing gum, or sucking lozenges may help); constipation (increased exercise, fluids, fruit, or fiber may help); diarrhea (buttermilk, yogurt, or boiled milk may help); postural hypotension (use caution when climbing stairs or changing position from lying or sitting to standing); urinary retention (void before taking medication); or sexual dysfunction (reversible). Report persistent CNS effects (eg, insomnia, restlessness, fatigue, anxiety, abnormal thoughts, confusion, personality changes, impaired cognitive function); muscle cramping or tremors; chest pain, palpitations, rapid heartbeat, swelling of extremities, or severe dizziness; unresolved urinary retention; vision changes or eye pain; hearing changes or ringing in ears; skin rash or irritation; or worsening of condition. **Pregnancy/ breast-feeding precautions:** Inform prescriber if you are or intend to become pregnant. Do not breast-feed.

Dietary Issues: Should be taken with food.

Geriatric Considerations: Has not been studied exclusively in the elderly, however, its low anticholinergic activity, minimal sedation, and hypotension makes this a potentially valuable antidepressant in treating elderly with depression. No dose adjustment is necessary for age alone, additional studies are necessary; adjust dose for renal function in the elderly.

Related Information

Antidepressant Agents *on page 1553*
Antidepressant Medication Guidelines *on page 1613*

Venofer® *see* Iron Sucrose *on page 742*
Venoglobulin®-S *see* Immune Globulin (Intravenous) *on page 703*
Ventolin® *see* Albuterol *on page 52*
Ventolin® HFA *see* Albuterol *on page 52*
VePesid® *see* Etoposide *on page 536*

Verapamil (ver AP a mil)

U.S. Brand Names Calan®; Calan® SR; Covera-HS®; Isoptin® SR; Verelan®; Verelan® PM

Synonyms Iproveratril Hydrochloride; Verapamil Hydrochloride

Generic Available Yes

Pharmacologic Category Antiarrhythmic Agent, Class IV; Calcium Channel Blocker

Pregnancy Risk Factor C

Lactation Enters breast milk (small amounts)/compatible

Use Orally for treatment of angina pectoris (vasospastic, chronic stable, unstable) and hypertension; I.V. for supraventricular tachyarrhythmias (PSVT, atrial fibrillation, atrial flutter)

Use - Unlabeled/Investigational Migraine; hypertrophic cardiomyopathy; bipolar disorder (manic manifestations)

Mechanism of Action/Effect Inhibits calcium ion from entering the "slow channels" or select voltage-sensitive areas of vascular smooth muscle and myocardium during depolarization. Produces a relaxation of coronary vascular smooth muscle and coronary vasodilation. Increases myocardial oxygen delivery in patients with vasospastic (Prinzmetal's) angina. Slows automaticity and conduction of AV node.

Contraindications Hypersensitivity to verapamil or any component of the formulation; severe left ventricular dysfunction; hypotension (systolic pressure <90 mm Hg) or cardiogenic shock; sick sinus syndrome (except in patients with a functioning artificial pacemaker); second- or third-degree AV block (except in patients with a functioning artificial pacemaker); atrial flutter or fibrillation and an accessory bypass tract (WPW, Lown-Ganong-Levine syndrome)

Warnings/Precautions Avoid use in heart failure; can exacerbate condition. Can cause hypotension. Rare increases in liver function tests can be observed. Can cause first-degree AV block or sinus bradycardia. Other conduction abnormalities are rare. Use caution when using verapamil together with a beta-blocker. Avoid use of I.V. verapamil with an I.V. beta-blocker; can result in asystole. Use caution in patients with hypertrophic cardiomyopathy (IHSS). Use with caution in patients with attenuated neuromuscular transmission (Duchenne's muscular dystrophy, myasthenia gravis). Adjust the dose in severe renal dysfunction and hepatic dysfunction. Verapamil significantly increases digoxin serum concentrations (adjust digoxin's dose). Pregnancy risk C.

Drug Interactions

Cytochrome P450 Effect: Substrate of CYP1A2, 2B6, 2C8/9, 2C18, 2E1, **3A4**; Inhibits CYP1A2, 2C8/9, 2D6, **3A4**

Decreased Effect: Rifampin or phenobarbital may decrease verapamil serum concentrations by increased hepatic metabolism. Lithium levels may be decreased by verapamil. Nafcillin decreases plasma concentration of verapamil.

Increased Effect/Toxicity: Use of verapamil with amiodarone, beta-blockers, or flecainide may lead to bradycardia and decreased cardiac output. Aspirin and concurrent verapamil use may increase bleeding times. Azole antifungals, cimetidine, erythromycin may inhibit verapamil metabolism, increasing serum concentrations/effect of verapamil. Lithium neurotoxicity may result when verapamil is added. Effect of nondepolarizing neuromuscular blocker is prolonged by verapamil. Grapefruit juice may increase verapamil serum concentrations.

Cisapride and astemizole levels may be increased by verapamil, potentially resulting in life-threatening arrhythmias; avoid concurrent use. Serum concentrations of the following drugs may be increased by verapamil: Alfentanil, buspirone, carbamazepine, cyclosporine, digoxin, doxorubicin, ethanol, HMG-CoA reductase inhibitors (atorvastatin, cerivastatin, lovastatin, simvastatin), midazolam, prazosin, quinidine, tacrolimus, and theophylline.

Nutritional/Ethanol Interactions

Ethanol: Avoid or limit ethanol (may increase ethanol levels).

Food: Grapefruit juice may increase the serum concentration of verapamil; avoid concurrent use.

Herb/Nutraceutical: St John's wort may decrease levels. Avoid dong quai if using for hypertension (has estrogenic activity). Avoid ephedra, yohimbe, ginseng (may worsen arrhythmia or hypertension). Avoid garlic (may have increased antihypertensive effect).

Effects on Lab Values ↑ alkaline phosphatase, CPK, LDH, aminotransferase [AST (SGOT)/ ALT (SGPT)] (S)

Adverse Reactions

>10%: Gastrointestinal: Gingival hyperplasia (up to 19%), constipation (12% up to 42% in clinical trials)

1% to 10%:

Cardiovascular: Bradycardia (1.2 to 1.4%), first-, second-, or third-degree AV block (1.2%), CHF (1.8%), hypotension (2.5% to 3%), peripheral edema (1.9%), symptomatic hypotension (1.5% I.V.), severe tachycardia (1%)

Central nervous system: Dizziness (1.2% to 3.3%), fatigue (1.7%), headache (1.2% to 2.2%)

Dermatologic: Rash (1.2%)

Gastrointestinal: Nausea (0.9% to 2.7%)

Respiratory: Dyspnea (1.4%)

<1% (Limited to important or life-threatening): Alopecia, angina, arthralgia, asystole, atrioventricular dissociation, bronchial/laryngeal spasm, cerebrovascular accident, chest pain, claudication, confusion, diarrhea, dry mouth, ecchymosis, electrical mechanical dissociation (EMD), emotional depression, eosinophilia, equilibrium disorders, erythema multiforme, exanthema, exfoliative dermatitis, galactorrhea/hyperprolactinemia, GI obstruction, gingival hyperplasia, gynecomastia, hair color change, impotence, muscle cramps, myocardial infarction, myoclonus, paresthesia, Parkinsonian syndrome, psychotic symptoms, purpura (vasculitis), rash, respiratory failure, rotary nystagmus, shakiness, shock, somnolence, Stevens-Johnson syndrome, syncope, urticaria, ventricular fibrillation, vertigo

Overdosage/Toxicology Primary cardiac symptoms of calcium blocker overdose include hypotension and bradycardia (second- or third-degree atrioventricular block, or sinus arrest with junctional rhythm). Intraventricular conduction is usually not affected so QRS duration is normal (verapamil does prolong the PR interval).

Noncardiac symptoms include confusion, stupor, nausea, vomiting, metabolic acidosis and hyperglycemia. Following initial gastric decontamination, if possible, repeated calcium administration may promptly reverse depressed cardiac contractility (but not sinus node depression or peripheral vasodilation). Large doses of calcium chloride (up to 1 g/hour for 24 hours) have been used in refractory cases. Glucagon, epinephrine, and amrinone may treat refractory hypotension. Glucagon and epinephrine also increase heart rate (outside the U.S., 4-aminopyridine may be available as an antidote). Dialysis and hemoperfusion are not effective in enhancing elimination although repeat-dose activated charcoal may serve as an adjunct with sustained-release preparations.

Pharmacodynamics/Kinetics

Bioavailability: Oral: 20% to 30%

Half-Life Elimination: Infants: 4.4-6.9 hours; Adults: Single dose: 2-8 hours, Multiple doses: Up to 12 hours; prolonged with hepatic cirrhosis

Metabolism: Hepatic via multiple CYP isoenzymes; extensive first-pass effect

Onset: Oral (immediate release tablets): Peak effect: 2 hours; I.V.: Peak effect: 1-5 minutes

Duration: Oral: Immediate release tablets: 6-8 hours; I.V.: 10-20 minutes

Formulations

Caplet, sustained release (Calan® SR): 120 mg, 180 mg, 240 mg

Capsule, extended release: 120 mg, 180 mg, 240 mg

Verelan® PM: 100 mg, 200 mg, 300 mg

Capsule, sustained release, as hydrochloride (Verelan®): 120 mg, 180 mg, 240 mg, 360 mg

Injection, solution, as hydrochloride: 2.5 mg/mL (2 mL, 4 mL)

Tablet, as hydrochloride (Calan®): 40 mg, 80 mg, 120 mg

Tablet, extended release: 120 mg, 180 mg, 240 mg

Covera HS®: 180 mg, 240 mg

Tablet, sustained release, as hydrochloride (Isoptin® SR): 120 mg, 180 mg, 240 mg

Dosing

Adults:

Angina: Oral: Initial: 80-120 mg twice daily (elderly or small stature: 40 mg twice daily); range: 240-480 mg/day in 3-4 divided doses

Hypertension: Oral: Usual dose is 80 mg 3 times/day or 240 mg/day (sustained release); range 240-480 mg/day (no evidence of additional benefit in doses >360 mg/day)

Arrhythmia (SVT): I.V.: 2.5-5 mg (over 2 minutes); second dose of 5-10 mg (~0.15 mg/kg) may be given 15-30 minutes after the initial dose if patient tolerates, but does not respond to initial dose; maximum total dose: 20 mg

Elderly:

Oral: 120-480 mg/24 hours divided 3-4 times/day

(Continued)

Verapamil *(Continued)*

Sustained release: 120 mg/day; adjust dose after 24 hours by increases of 120 mg/day. When switching from immediate release forms, total daily dose may remain the same.

Controlled onset: initiate therapy with 180 mg in the evening; titrate upward as needed to obtain desired response and avoiding adverse effects.

Pediatrics: Children: SVT:

I.V.:

<1 year: 0.1-0.2 mg/kg over 2 minutes; repeat every 30 minutes as needed

1-15 years: 0.1-0.3 mg/kg over 2 minutes; maximum: 5 mg/dose, may repeat dose in 15 minutes if adequate response not achieved; maximum for second dose: 10 mg/dose

Oral (dose not well established):

1-5 years: 4-8 mg/kg/day in 3 divided doses **or** 40-80 mg every 8 hours

>5 years: 80 mg every 6-8 hours

Renal Impairment: Cl_{cr} <10 mL/minute: Administer 50% to 75% of normal dose.

Hepatic Impairment: In cirrhosis, reduce dose to 20% to 50% of normal and monitor EKG.

Administration

Oral: Administer sustained release product with food or milk; sprinkling contents of capsules onto food does not affect absorption; should be dosed 1-2 times/day; **do not crush sustained release drug product.** Other oral formulations may be given with or without food.

Stability

Storage: Store injection at room temperature. Protect from heat and from freezing. Use only clear solutions. Protect I.V. solution from light.

Compatibility: Stable in dextran 40 10% in NS, dextran 75 6% in NS, D_5LR, $D_5{}^1/_2NS$, D_5NS, D_5W, LR, $^1/_2NS$, NS

Y-site administration: Incompatible with albumin, amphotericin B cholesteryl sulfate complex, ampicillin, nafcillin, oxacillin, propofol, sodium bicarbonate

Compatibility when admixed: Incompatible with albumin, amphotericin B, floxacillin, hydralazine, trimethoprim/sulfamethoxazole

Monitoring and Teaching Issues

Physical Assessment: Assess other medications patient may be taking for effectiveness and interactions (see Drug Interactions). I.V. requires use of infusion pump and continuous cardiac and hemodynamic monitoring. Monitor laboratory tests (see above), therapeutic response, and adverse reactions (see Warnings/Precautions, Adverse Reactions, and Overdose/Toxicology) when beginning therapy, when titrating dosage, and periodically during long-term oral therapy. Assess knowledge/teach patient appropriate use (oral), interventions to reduce side effects, and adverse symptoms to report (see Patient Education). **Pregnancy risk factor C** - benefits of use should outweigh possible risks.

Patient Education: Oral: Take as directed. Do not alter dosage or discontinue therapy without consulting prescriber. Do not crush or chew extended release form. Avoid grapefruit juice; avoid (or limit) alcohol and caffeine. You may experience dizziness or lightheadedness (use caution when driving or engaging in tasks requiring alertness until response to drug is known); nausea or vomiting (small, frequent meals, frequent mouth care, chewing gum, or sucking lozenges may help); constipation (increased exercise, fluids, fruit, or fiber may help); or diarrhea (buttermilk, boiled milk, or yogurt may help). Report chest pain, palpitations, or irregular heartbeat; unusual cough, difficulty breathing, or swelling of extremities (feet/ankles); muscle tremors or weakness; confusion or acute lethargy; or skin irritation or rash. **Pregnancy precaution:** Inform prescriber if you are or intend to become pregnant.

Dietary Issues: Sustained release product should be administered with food or milk, other formulations may be administered without regard to meals; sprinkling contents of capsule onto food does not affect oral absorption.

Geriatric Considerations: Elderly may experience a greater hypotensive response. Theoretically, constipation may be more of a problem in the elderly. Calcium channel blockers are no more effective in the elderly than other therapies, however, they do not cause significant CNS effects, which is an advantage over some antihypertensive agents. Generic verapamil products which are bioequivalent in young adults may not be bioequivalent in the elderly. Use generics cautiously.

Breast-feeding Issues: Crosses into breast milk. AAP considers **compatible** with breast-feeding.

Pregnancy Issues: Crosses the placenta. One report of suspected heart block when used to control fetal supraventricular tachycardia. May exhibit tocolytic effects.

Related Information

Antiarrhythmic Drugs *on page 1551*
Calcium Channel Blockers *on page 1563*
Compatibility of Drugs *on page 1564*

Verapamil and Trandolapril *see* Trandolapril and Verapamil *on page 1347*
Verapamil Hydrochloride *see* Verapamil *on page 1396*
Verazinc® [OTC] *see* Zinc Supplements *on page 1423*
Verelan® *see* Verapamil *on page 1396*
Verelan® PM *see* Verapamil *on page 1396*
Vergon® [OTC] *see* Meclizine *on page 840*
Vermox® *see* Mebendazole *on page 838*
Versacaps® *see* Guaifenesin and Pseudoephedrine *on page 648*
Versed® [DSC] *see* Midazolam *on page 900*
Vesanoid® *see* Tretinoin (Oral) *on page 1353*
Vexol® *see page 1509*
VFEND® *see* Voriconazole *on page 1407*
Viadur® *see* Leuprolide *on page 781*
Viagra® *see* Sildenafil *on page 1228*
Vibramycin® *see* Doxycycline *on page 450*

Vibra-Tabs® *see* Doxycycline *on page 450*

Vicks® 44E [OTC] *see* Guaifenesin and Dextromethorphan *on page 647*

Vicks® Pediatric Formula 44E [OTC] *see* Guaifenesin and Dextromethorphan *on page 647*

Vicks Sinex® Nasal [OTC] *see* Phenylephrine *on page 1071*

Vicodin® *see* Hydrocodone and Acetaminophen *on page 667*

Vicodin® ES *see* Hydrocodone and Acetaminophen *on page 667*

Vicodin® HP *see* Hydrocodone and Acetaminophen *on page 667*

Vicoprofen® *see* Hydrocodone and Ibuprofen *on page 671*

Vidarabine (vye DARE a been)

U.S. Brand Names Vira-A® [DSC]

Synonyms Adenine Arabinoside; Ara-A; Arabinofuranosyladenine; Vidarabine Monohydrate

Generic Available No

Pharmacologic Category Antiviral Agent, Ophthalmic

Pregnancy Risk Factor C

Lactation Excretion in breast milk unknown

Use Treatment of acute keratoconjunctivitis and epithelial keratitis due to herpes simplex virus type 1 and 2; superficial keratitis caused by herpes simplex virus

Mechanism of Action/Effect Inhibits viral DNA synthesis by blocking DNA polymerase

Contraindications Hypersensitivity to vidarabine or any component of the formulation; sterile trophic ulcers

Warnings/Precautions Not effective against RNA virus, adenoviral ocular infections, bacterial fungal or chlamydial infections of the cornea, or trophic ulcers; temporary visual haze may be produced; neoplasia has occurred with I.M. vidarabine-treated animals; although *in vitro* studies have been inconclusive, they have shown mutagenesis Pregnancy risk C.

Drug Interactions

Increased Effect/Toxicity: Allopurinol (may increase vidarabine levels).

Adverse Reactions Frequency not defined: Ocular: Burning eyes, foreign body sensation, keratitis, lacrimation, photophobia, uveitis

Overdosage/Toxicology No untoward effects anticipated with ingestion

Formulations Ointment, ophthalmic, as monohydrate: 3% [30 mg/mL = 28 mg/mL base] (3.5 g) [DSC]

Dosing

Adults & Elderly: Keratoconjunctivitis: Ophthalmic: Instill 1/2" of ointment in lower conjunctival sac every 3 hours up to 5 times/day while awake until complete re-epithelialization has occurred, then twice daily for an additional 7 days.

Pediatrics: Refer to adult dosing.

Monitoring and Teaching Issues

Physical Assessment: Monitor effectiveness of therapy (for length of therapy see Dosing). Assess knowledge/teach patient appropriate use, interventions to reduce side effects, and adverse symptoms to report (see Patient Education). **Pregnancy risk factor C** - benefits of use should outweigh possible risks. Note breast-feeding caution.

Patient Education: For ophthalmic use only. Store in refrigerator. Apply prescribed amount as often as directed. Wash hands before using. Do not let tip of applicator touch eye; do not contaminate tip of applicator (may cause eye infection, eye damage, or vision loss). Tilt head back and look upward. Gently pull down lower lid and put drop(s) in inner corner of eye. Close eye and roll eyeball in all directions. Do not blink for 1/2 minute. Apply gentle pressure to inner corner of eye for 30 seconds. Wipe away excess from skin around eye. Do not use any other eye preparation for at least 10 minutes. Do not touch tip of applicator to eye or contaminate tip of applicator. Do not share medication with anyone else. May cause sensitivity to bright light (dark glasses may help); temporary stinging or blurred vision may occur. Inform prescriber if you experience eye pain, redness, burning, watering, dryness, double vision, puffiness around eye, vision changes, or other adverse eye response; or worsening of condition or lack of improvement within 7-14 days. **Pregnancy/breast-feeding precautions:** Inform prescriber if you are pregnant. Consult prescriber if breast-feeding.

Geriatric Considerations: Assess ability to self-administer ophthalmic ointment.

Vidarabine Monohydrate *see* Vidarabine *on page 1399*

Videx® *see* Didanosine *on page 403*

Videx® EC *see* Didanosine *on page 403*

VinBLAStine (vin BLAS teen)

U.S. Brand Names Velban® [DSC]

Synonyms Vinblastine Sulfate; Vincaleukoblastine; VLB

Generic Available Yes

Pharmacologic Category Antineoplastic Agent, Natural Source (Plant) Derivative

Pregnancy Risk Factor D

Lactation Enters breast milk/not recommended

Use Treatment of Hodgkin's and non-Hodgkin's lymphoma, testicular, lung, head and neck, breast, and renal carcinomas, Mycosis fungoides, Kaposi's sarcoma, histiocytosis, choriocarcinoma, and idiopathic thrombocytopenic purpura

Mechanism of Action/Effect VLB arrests cell cycle growth in metaphase. Also inhibits RNA synthesis and amino acid metabolism resulting in inhibition of metabolic pathways and cell growth.

Contraindications For I.V. use only; **I.T. use may result in death**; hypersensitivity to vinblastine or any component of the formulation; severe bone marrow suppression or presence of bacterial infection not under control prior to initiation of therapy; pregnancy

Warnings/Precautions The U.S. Food and Drug Administration (FDA) currently recommends that procedures for proper handling and disposal of antineoplastic agents be considered. Appropriate safety equipment is recommended for preparation, administration, and

(Continued)

VinBLAStine *(Continued)*

disposal of antineoplastics. If vinblastine contacts the skin, wash and flush thoroughly with water.

Drug is a vesicant. Avoid extravasation. Dosage modification required in patients with impaired liver function and neurotoxicity. Using small amounts of drug daily for long periods may increase neurotoxicity and is therefore not advised. For I.V. use only. **Intrathecal administration results in death**. Use with caution in patients with cachexia or ulcerated skin. Monitor closely for shortness of breath or bronchospasm in patients receiving mitomycin C.

Drug Interactions

Cytochrome P450 Effect: Substrate of CYP2D6, **3A4**; Inhibits CYP2D6, 3A4

Decreased Effect: Phenytoin plasma levels may be reduced with concomitant combination chemotherapy with vinblastine. Alpha-interferon enhances interferon toxicity; phenytoin may ↓ plasma levels.

Increased Effect/Toxicity: Vinblastine levels may be increased when given with drugs that inhibit cytochrome P450 3A enzyme substrate. Previous or simultaneous use with mitomycin-C has resulted in acute shortness of breath and severe bronchospasm within minutes or several hours after *Vinca* alkaloid injection and may occur up to 2 weeks after the dose of mitomycin. Mitomycin-C in combination with administration of VLB may cause acute shortness of breath and severe bronchospasm, onset may be within minutes or several hours after VLB injection.

Nutritional/Ethanol Interactions Herb/Nutraceutical: St John's wort may decrease vinblastine levels. Avoid black cohosh, dong quai in estrogen-dependent tumors.

Adverse Reactions

>10%:

Dermatologic: Alopecia

Gastrointestinal: Nausea, vomiting, constipation, diarrhea (less common), stomatitis, abdominal cramps, anorexia, metallic taste

Emetic potential: Moderate (30% to 60%)

Hematologic: Leukopenia, severe bone marrow suppression (dose-limiting toxicity - unlike vincristine)

Myelosuppressive:

WBC: Moderate - severe

Platelets: Moderate - severe

Onset: 4-7 days

Nadir: 4-10 days

Recovery: 17 days

1% to 10%:

Cardiovascular: Hypertension, Raynaud's phenomenon

Central nervous system: Depression, malaise, headache, seizures

Dermatologic: Rash, photosensitivity, dermatitis

Endocrine & metabolic: Hyperuricemia

Gastrointestinal: Paralytic ileus, stomatitis

Genitourinary: Urinary retention

Local: **Vesicant chemotherapy**

Neuromuscular & skeletal: Jaw pain, myalgia, paresthesia

Respiratory: Bronchospasm

<1% (Limited to important or life-threatening): Hemorrhagic colitis, neurotoxicity (rare; symptoms may include peripheral neuropathy, loss of deep tendon reflexes, headache, weakness, urinary retention, GI symptoms, tachycardia, orthostatic hypotension, convulsions), rectal bleeding

Overdosage/Toxicology Symptoms of overdose include bone marrow suppression, mental depression, paresthesia, loss of deep tendon reflexes, and neurotoxicity. There are no antidotes for vinblastine. Treatment is supportive and symptomatic, including fluid restriction or hypertonic saline (3% sodium chloride) for drug-induced secretion of inappropriate antidiuretic hormone (SIADH).

Pharmacodynamics/Kinetics

Half-Life Elimination: Biphasic: Initial: 0.164 hours; Terminal: 25 hours

Metabolism: Hepatic to active metabolite

Formulations

Injection, solution, as sulfate: 1 mg/mL (10 mL) [contains benzyl alcohol]

Injection, powder for reconstitution, as sulfate: 10 mg

Dosing

Adults & Elderly: Refer to individual protocols. Varies depending upon clinical and hematological response. Give at intervals of at least 14 days and only after leukocyte count has returned to at least 4000/mm^3; maintenance therapy should be titrated according to leukocyte count. Dosage should be reduced in patients with recent exposure to radiation therapy or chemotherapy; single doses in these patients should not exceed 5.5 mg/m^2.

Antineoplastic (typical dosages): I.V.: 4-20 mg/m^2 (0.1-0.5 mg/kg) every 7-10 days **or** 5-day continuous infusion of 1.5-2 mg/m^2/day **or** 0.1-0.5 mg/kg/week

Pediatrics: Refer to adult dosing.

Renal Impairment: Not removed by hemodialysis

Hepatic Impairment:

Serum bilirubin 1.5-3.0 mg/dL or AST 60-180 units: Administer 50% of normal dose.

Serum bilirubin 3.0-5.0 mg/dL: Administer 25% of dose.

Serum bilirubin >5.0 mg/dL or AST >180 units: Omit dose.

Administration

I.V.: Vesicant. Drug is for I.V. administration only. **Fatal if given intrathecally.** May be administered by I.V. push or into a free flowing I.V. IVP over at least 1 minute is the desired route of administration because of potential for extravasation. However, has also been administered by continuous intravenous infusion - **central line only for continuous intravenous infusion administration**.

Stability

Storage: Store intact vials under refrigeration (2°C to 8°C) and protect from light.

Reconstitution: Standard I.V. dilution:

I.V. push: Dose/syringe (concentration = 1 mg/mL)

Maximum syringe size for IVP is a 30 mL syringe and syringe should be ≤75% full.

Continuous intravenous infusion: Dose = 250-1000 mL D_5W or NS

Solutions are stable for 21 days at room temperature (25°C) and refrigeration (4°C). Protect from light.

Compatibility: Stable in D_5W, LR, NS, bacteriostatic water

Y-site administration: Incompatible with cefepime, furosemide

Compatibility in syringe: Incompatible with furosemide

Monitoring Laboratory Tests CBC with differential and platelet count, serum uric acid, hepatic function

Monitoring and Teaching Issues

Physical Assessment: See Contraindications, Warnings/Precautions, and Dosing for use cautions. Assess potential for interactions with other prescriptions, OTC medications, or herbal products patient may be taking (especially mitomycin - see Drug Interactions). Premedication with antiemetic is advisable. Infusion site must be monitored closely to prevent extravasation (see Administration). Assess results of laboratory tests (see above), therapeutic effectiveness, and adverse reactions prior to each infusion and throughout therapy (see Adverse Reactions and Overdose/Toxicology). Teach patient possible side effects and interventions and adverse symptoms to report (see Patient Education). **Pregnancy risk factor D** - determine that patient is not pregnant before beginning treatment. Teach patients of childbearing age, and males who may have intercourse with females of childbearing age, appropriate use of barrier contraceptives. Breast-feeding is not recommended.

Patient Education: Inform prescriber of all prescriptions, OTC medications, or herbal products you are taking, and any allergies you have. Do not take anything new during treatment unless approved by prescriber. This medication can only be administered by infusion; report immediately any redness, swelling, burning, or pain at infusion site. Maintain adequate hydration (2-3 L/day of fluids) unless advised by prescriber to restrict fluids, and nutrition (small, frequent meals will help). You will be more susceptible to infection (avoid crowds and exposure to infection and do not have any vaccinations unless approved by prescriber). May cause hair loss (will grow back after therapy); nausea or vomiting (request antiemetic); photosensitivity (use sunscreen, wear protective clothing and eyewear, and avoid direct sunlight); feelings of extreme weakness or lethargy (use caution when driving or engaging in tasks requiring alertness until response to drug is known); or mouth sores (use soft toothbrush, waxed dental floss, and frequent oral care). Report numbness or tingling in fingers or toes (use care to prevent injury); weakness or pain in muscles or jaw; signs of infection (eg, fever, chills, sore throat, burning urination, fatigue); unusual bleeding (eg, tarry stools, easy bruising, blood in stool, urine, or mouth); unresolved mouth sores; skin rash or itching; or difficulty breathing. **Pregnancy/breast-feeding precautions:** Do not get pregnant (females) or cause a pregnancy (males) during this therapy. Consult prescriber for appropriate contraceptive measures. Breast-feeding is not recommended.

Related Information

FDA Name Differentiation Project: The Use of Tall-man Letters *on page 12*

Vinblastine Sulfate *see* VinBLAStine *on page 1399*

Vincaleukoblastine *see* VinBLAStine *on page 1399*

Vincasar PFS® *see* VinCRIStine *on page 1401*

VinCRIStine (vin KRIS teen)

U.S. Brand Names Oncovin® [DSC]; Vincasar PFS®

Synonyms LCR; Leurocristine; VCR; Vincristine Sulfate

Generic Available Yes

Pharmacologic Category Antineoplastic Agent, Natural Source (Plant) Derivative

Pregnancy Risk Factor D

Lactation Enters breast milk/not recommended

Use Treatment of leukemias, Hodgkin's disease, non-Hodgkin's lymphomas, Wilms' tumor, neuroblastoma, rhabdomyosarcoma

Mechanism of Action/Effect Binds to microtubular protein of the mitotic spindle causing metaphase arrest; cell-cycle phase specific in the M and S phases

Contraindications Hypersensitivity to vincristine or any component of the formulation; **for I.V. use only, fatal if given intrathecally**; patients with demyelinating form of Charcot-Marie-Tooth syndrome; pregnancy

Warnings/Precautions For I.V. use only. The U.S. Food and Drug Administration (FDA) currently recommends that procedures for proper handling and disposal of antineoplastic agents be considered. Appropriate safety equipment is recommended for preparation, administration, and disposal of antineoplastics. If vincristine contacts the skin, wash and flush thoroughly with water.

Dosage modification required in patients with impaired hepatic function or who have pre-existing neuromuscular disease. Drug is a vesicant. Avoid extravasation. Use with caution in the elderly. Avoid eye contamination. Observe closely for shortness of breath, bronchospasm, especially in patients treated with mitomycin C. Alterations in mental status such as depression, confusion, or insomnia; constipation, paralytic ileus, and urinary tract disturbances may occur. All patients should be on a prophylactic bowel management regimen. Administer allopurinol to prevent uric acid nephropathy.

Intrathecal administration of VCR has uniformly caused death; VCR should never be administered by this route. Neurologic effects of VCR may be additive with those of other neurotoxic agents and spinal cord irradiation.

(Continued)

VinCRIStine *(Continued)*

Drug Interactions

Cytochrome P450 Effect: Substrate of **CYP3A4**; Inhibits CYP3A4

Decreased Effect: Digoxin and phenytoin levels may decrease with combination chemotherapy.

Increased Effect/Toxicity: Vincristine levels may be increased when given with drugs that inhibit cytochrome P450 3A enzyme (itraconazole has been shown to increase onset and severity of neuromuscular adverse effects of vincristine). Digoxin plasma levels and renal excretion may decrease with combination chemotherapy including vincristine. Vincristine should be given 12-24 hours before asparaginase to minimize toxicity (may decrease the hepatic clearance of vincristine). Acute pulmonary reactions may occur with mitomycin-C. Previous or simultaneous use with mitomycin-C has resulted in acute shortness of breath and severe bronchospasm within minutes or several hours after *Vinca* alkaloid injection and may occur up to 2 weeks after the dose of mitomycin.

Nutritional/Ethanol Interactions Herb/Nutraceutical: St John's wort may decrease vincristine levels.

Adverse Reactions

>10%: Dermatologic: Alopecia occurs in 20% to 70% of patients

1% to 10%:

Cardiovascular: Orthostatic hypotension or hypertension, hypertension, hypotension

Central nervous system: Motor difficulties, seizures, headache, CNS depression, cranial nerve paralysis, fever

Dermatologic: Rash

Endocrine & metabolic: Hyperuricemia

Gastrointestinal: Constipation and possible paralytic ileus secondary to neurologic toxicity; oral ulceration, abdominal cramps, anorexia, metallic taste, bloating, nausea, vomiting, weight loss, diarrhea

Genitourinary: Bladder atony (related to neurotoxicity)

Emetic potential: Low (<10%)

Local: Phlebitis

Vesicant chemotherapy

Neuromuscular & skeletal: Jaw pain, leg pain, myalgia, cramping, numbness, weakness

Peripheral neuropathy: Frequently the dose-limiting toxicity of VCR. Most frequent in patients >40 years of age; occurs usually after an average of 3 weekly doses, but may occur after just one dose. Manifested as loss of the deep tendon reflexes in the lower extremities, numbness, tingling, pain, paresthesias of the fingers and toes (stocking glove sensation), and "foot drop" or "wrist drop"

Ocular: Photophobia

<1% (Limited to important or life-threatening): Mild leukopenia and thrombocytopenia, SIADH (rare, may be related to neurologic toxicity; symptomatic hyponatremia may cause seizures)

Overdosage/Toxicology Symptoms of overdose include bone marrow suppression, mental depression, paresthesia, loss of deep tendon reflexes, alopecia, and nausea. Severe symptoms may occur with 3-4 mg/m^2.

There are no antidotes for vincristine. Treatment is supportive and symptomatic, including fluid restriction or hypertonic saline (3% sodium chloride) for drug-induced secretion of inappropriate antidiuretic hormone (SIADH). Case reports suggest that folinic acid may be helpful in treating vincristine overdose. It is suggested that 100 mg folinic acid be given I.V. every 3 hours for 24 hours, then every 6 hours for 48 hours. This is in addition to supportive care. The use of pyridoxine, leucovorin factor, cyanocobalamin, or thiamine has been used with little success for drug-induced peripheral neuropathy.

Pharmacodynamics/Kinetics

Absorption: Oral: Poor

Half-Life Elimination: Terminal: 24 hours

Metabolism: Extensively hepatic

Formulations Injection, solution, as sulfate: 1 mg/mL (1 mL, 2 mL)

Dosing

Adults & Elderly: Refer to individual protocols as dosages vary with protocol used. Adjustments are made depending upon clinical and hematological response and upon adverse reactions.

Antineoplastic (typical dosages): I.V.: 0.4-1.4 mg/m^2 (up to 2 mg maximum); may repeat every week. The average total dose per course of treatment should be around 2-2.5 mg. Some recommend capping the dose at 2 mg maximum to reduce toxicity; however, it is felt that this measure can reduce the efficacy of the drug.

Pediatrics: Refer to individual protocols as dosages vary with protocol used; adjustments are made depending upon clinical and hematological response and upon adverse reaction.

Chemotherapy:

Children ≤10 kg or BSA <1 m^2: Initial therapy: 0.05 mg/kg once weekly then titrate dose; maximum single dose: 2 mg

Children >10 kg or BSA ≥1 m^2: 1-2 mg/m^2, may repeat once weekly for 3-6 weeks; maximum single dose: 2 mg

Neuroblastoma: I.V. continuous infusion with doxorubicin: 1 mg/m^2/day for 72 hours

Hepatic Impairment:

Serum bilirubin 1.5-3.0 mg/dL or AST 60-180 units: Administer 50% of normal dose.

Serum bilirubin 3.0-5.0 mg/dL: Administer 25% of dose.

Serum bilirubin >5.0 mg/dL or AST >180 units: Omit dose.

Administration

I.V.: Vesicant. For I.V. use only. **Fatal if given intrathecally.** IVP over at least 1 minute is the desired route of administration because of potential for extravasation. However, has also been administered IVPB over 15 minutes - **central line only for IVPB administration.**

Stability

Storage: Store intact vials at refrigeration (2°C to 8°C) and protect from light.

Reconstitution: Further dilution in NS or D_5W is stable for 21 days at room temperature (25°C) and refrigeration (4°C).

Standard I.V. dilution:

I.V. push: Dose/syringe (concentration = 1 mg/mL)

Maximum syringe size for IVP is 30 mL syringe and syringe should be ≤75% full

IVPB: Dose/50 mL D_5W

Compatibility: Stable in D_5W, LR, NS

Y-site administration: Incompatible with cefepime, furosemide, idarubicin, sodium bicarbonate

Compatibility in syringe: Incompatible with furosemide

Monitoring Laboratory Tests Serum electrolytes (sodium), hepatic function, CBC, serum uric acid

Monitoring and Teaching Issues

Physical Assessment: See Contraindications, Warnings/Precautions, and Dosing for use cautions. Assess potential for interactions with other prescriptions, OTC medications, or herbal products patient may be taking (especially mitomycin - see Drug Interactions). Premedication with antiemetic is advisable. Constipation may result in upper colon impaction; all patients should be on prophylactic bowel management regimen. Infusion site must be monitored closely to prevent extravasation (see Administration). Assess results of laboratory tests (see above), therapeutic effectiveness and adverse reactions prior to each infusion and throughout therapy (eg, CNS, neuromuscular, urological, and neurological reactions - see Adverse Reactions and Overdose/Toxicology). Teach patient possible side effects and interventions and adverse symptoms to report (see Patient Education). **Pregnancy risk factor D** - determine that patient is not pregnant before beginning treatment. Teach patients of childbearing age and males who may have intercourse with females of childbearing age appropriate use of barrier contraceptives. Breast-feeding is not recommended.

Patient Education: Inform prescriber of all prescriptions, OTC medications, or herbal products you are taking, and any allergies you have. Do not take anything new during treatment unless approved by prescriber. This medication can only be administered by infusion; report immediately any redness, swelling, burning, or pain at infusion site. Maintain adequate hydration (2-3 L/day of fluids) unless advised by prescriber to restrict fluids, and nutrition (small, frequent meals will help). You will be more susceptible to infection (avoid crowds and exposure to infection and do not have any vaccinations unless approved by prescriber). May cause hair loss (will grow back after therapy); nausea or vomiting (request antiemetic); photosensitivity (use sunscreen, wear protective clothing and eyewear, and avoid direct sunlight); feelings of extreme weakness or lethargy (use caution when driving or engaging in tasks requiring alertness until response to drug is known); or mouth sores (use soft toothbrush, waxed dental floss, and frequent oral care). Report numbness or tingling in fingers or toes (use care to prevent injury); weakness, numbness, or pain in muscles or extremities; signs of infection (eg, fever, chills, sore throat, burning urination, fatigue); unusual bleeding (eg, tarry stools, easy bruising, blood in stool, urine, or mouth); unresolved mouth sores; skin rash or itching; or difficulty breathing. **Pregnancy/breast-feeding precautions:** Do not get pregnant (females) or cause a pregnancy (males) during this therapy. Consult prescriber for appropriate contraceptive measures. Breast-feeding is not recommended.

Related Information

FDA Name Differentiation Project: The Use of Tall-man Letters *on page 12*

Vincristine Sulfate *see* VinCRIStine *on page 1401*

Vinorelbine (vi NOR el been)

U.S. Brand Names Navelbine®

Synonyms Vinorelbine Tartrate

Generic Available No

Pharmacologic Category Antineoplastic Agent, Natural Source (Plant) Derivative

Pregnancy Risk Factor D

Lactation Enters breast milk/contraindicated

Use Treatment of nonsmall cell lung cancer (as a single agent or in combination with cisplatin)

Use - Unlabeled/Investigational Breast cancer, ovarian carcinoma (cisplatin-resistant), Hodgkin's disease

Mechanism of Action/Effect Mitotic inhibition that causes metaphase arrest in neoplastic cells

Contraindications For I.V. use only; **I.T. use may result in death**; hypersensitivity to vinorelbine or any component of the formulation; severe bone marrow suppression (granulocyte counts <1000 cells/mm^3) or presence of bacterial infection not under control prior to initiation of therapy; pregnancy

Warnings/Precautions The U.S. Food and Drug Administration (FDA) currently recommends that procedures for proper handling and disposal of antineoplastic agents be considered. Avoid extravasation; dosage modification required in patients with impaired liver function and neurotoxicity. Frequently monitor patients for myelosuppression both during and after therapy. Granulocytopenia is dose-limiting. **Intrathecal administration may result in death**. Use with caution in patients with cachexia or ulcerated skin.

Acute shortness of breath and severe bronchospasm have been reported, most commonly when administered with mitomycin. Fatal cases of interstitial pulmonary changes and ARDS have also been reported. May cause severe constipation (grade 3-4), paralytic ileus, intestinal obstruction, necrosis, and/or perforation.

(Continued)

Vinorelbine *(Continued)*

Drug Interactions

Cytochrome P450 Effect: Substrate of CYP2D6, **3A4**; Inhibits CYP2D6, 3A4

Increased Effect/Toxicity: Previous or simultaneous use with mitomycin-C has resulted in acute shortness of breath and severe bronchospasm within minutes or several hours after *Vinca* alkaloid injection and may occur up to 2 weeks after the dose of mitomycin.

Cisplatin: Incidence of granulocytopenia is significantly higher than with single-agent vinorelbine.

Nutritional/Ethanol Interactions Herb/Nutraceutical: St John's wort may decrease vinorelbine levels.

Adverse Reactions

>10%:

Central nervous system: Fatigue (27%)

Dermatologic: Alopecia (12%)

Gastrointestinal: Nausea (44%, severe <2%), constipation (35%), vomiting (20%), diarrhea (17%)

Emetic potential: Moderate (30% to 60%)

Hematologic: May cause severe bone marrow suppression and is the dose-limiting toxicity of vinorelbine; severe granulocytopenia (90%) may occur following the administration of vinorelbine; leukopenia (92%), anemia (83%)

Myelosuppressive:

WBC: Moderate - severe

Onset: 4-7d days

Nadir: 7-10 days

Recovery: 14-21 days

Hepatic: Elevated SGOT (67%), elevated total bilirubin (13%)

Local: Injection site reaction (28%), injection site pain (16%)

Neuromuscular & skeletal: Weakness (36%), peripheral neuropathy (20% to 25%)

1% to 10%:

Cardiovascular: Chest pain (5%)

Gastrointestinal: Paralytic ileus (1%)

Hematologic: Thrombocytopenia (5%)

Local: Extravasation: Vesicant and can cause tissue irritation and necrosis if infiltrated; if extravasation occurs, follow institutional policy, which may include hyaluronidase and hot compresses; phlebitis (7%)

Vesicant chemotherapy

Neuromuscular & skeletal: Mild to moderate peripheral neuropathy manifested by paresthesia and hyperesthesia, loss of deep tendon reflexes (<5%); myalgia (<5%), arthralgia (<5%), jaw pain (<5%)

Respiratory: Dyspnea (3% to 7%)

<1% (Limited to important or life-threatening): Anaphylaxis, angioedema, deep vein thrombosis, dysphagia, esophagitis, gait instability, hemorrhagic cystitis, pancreatitis, pulmonary edema, pulmonary embolus, radiation recall (dermatitis, esophagitis), severe peripheral neuropathy (generally reversible), SIADH

Overdosage/Toxicology Symptoms of overdose include bone marrow suppression, mental depression, paresthesia, loss of deep tendon reflexes, and neurotoxicity. There are no antidotes for vinorelbine. Treatment is supportive and symptomatic, including fluid restriction or hypertonic saline (3% sodium chloride) for drug-induced secretion of inappropriate antidiuretic hormone (SIADH).

Pharmacodynamics/Kinetics

Absorption: Unreliable; must be given I.V.

Half-Life Elimination: Triphasic: Terminal: 27.7-43.6 hours

Metabolism: Extensively hepatic to two metabolites, deacetylvinorelbine (active) and vinorelbine N-oxide

Formulations Injection, solution, as tartrate [preservative free]: 10 mg/mL (1 mL, 5 mL)

Dosing

Adults & Elderly: Varies depending upon clinical and hematological response (refer to individual protocols).

Nonsmall cell lung cancer: I.V.:

Single-agent therapy: 30 mg/m^2 every 7 days

Combination therapy with cisplatin: 25 mg/m^2 every 7 days (with cisplatin 100 mg/m^2 every 4 weeks)

Dosage adjustment in hematological toxicity (based on granulocyte counts):

Granulocytes ≥1500 cells/mm^3 on day of treatment: Administer 30 mg/m^2.

Granulocytes 1000-1499 cells/mm^3 on day of treatment: Administer 15 mg/m^2.

Granulocytes <1000 cells/mm^3 on day of treatment: Do not administer. Repeat granulocyte count in 1 week. If 3 consecutive doses are held because granulocyte count is <1000 cells/mm^3, discontinue vinorelbine.

For patients who, during treatment, have experienced fever or sepsis while granulocytopenic or had 2 consecutive weekly doses held due to granulocytopenia, subsequent doses of vinorelbine should be:

22.5 mg/m^2 for granulocytes ≥1500 cells/mm^3

11.25 mg/m^2 for granulocytes 1000-1499 cells/mm^3

Renal Impairment: If moderate or severe neurotoxicity develops, discontinue vinorelbine.

Hepatic Impairment:

Serum bilirubin ≤2 mg/dL: Administer 30 mg/m^2.

Serum bilirubin 2.1-3 mg/dL: Administer 15 mg/m^2.

Serum bilirubin >3 mg/dL: Administer 7.5 mg/m^2.

In patients with concurrent hematologic toxicity and hepatic impairment, administer the lower doses determined from the above recommendations under Adult Dosing.

Administration

I.V.: Vesicant. For I.V. use only. **Fatal if given intrathecally.** Administer I.V. over 20-30 minutes; central line only for IVPB administration. Avoid extravasation.

Stability

Storage: Store intact vials under refrigeration (2°C to 8°C). Vials are stable at room temperature for up to 72 hours.

Reconstitution: Further dilution in D_5W or NS is stable for 24 hours at room temperature.

Standard I.V. dilution:

I.V. push: Dose/syringe (concentration = 1.5-3 mg/mL)

Maximum syringe size for IVP is a 30 mL syringe and syringe should be ≤75% full.

IVPB: Dose/50-250 mL D_5W or NS (concentration = 0.5-2 mg/mL)

Solutions are stable for 24 hours at room temperature.

Compatibility: Stable in $D_5{}^1/_2NS$, D_5W, LR, NS, $^1/_2NS$

Y-site administration: Incompatible with acyclovir, allopurinol, aminophylline, amphotericin B, amphotericin B cholesteryl sulfate complex, ampicillin, cefazolin, cefoperazone, cefotetan, ceftriaxone, cefuroxime, co-trimoxazole, fluorouracil, furosemide, ganciclovir, methylprednisolone sodium succinate, mitomycin, piperacillin, sodium bicarbonate, thiotepa

Monitoring Laboratory Tests CBC with differential and platelet count, serum uric acid, hepatic function

Monitoring and Teaching Issues

Physical Assessment: See Contraindications, Warnings/Precautions, and Dosing for use cautions. Assess potential for interactions with other prescriptions, OTC medications, or herbal products patient may be taking (see Drug Interactions). Premedication with antiemetic is advisable. May cause severe constipation, paralytic ileus, intestinal obstruction, necrosis, and/or perforation; prophylactic bowel management regimen may be advisable. Infusion site must be monitored closely to prevent extravasation (see Administration). Assess results of laboratory tests (see above) and monitor for adverse reactions prior to each infusion and throughout therapy (see Adverse Reactions and Overdose/Toxicology). Teach patient possible side effects and interventions and adverse symptoms to report (see Patient Education). **Pregnancy risk factor D** - determine that patient is not pregnant before beginning treatment. Teach patients of childbearing age, and males who may have intercourse with females of childbearing age, appropriate use of barrier contraceptives. Breast-feeding is contraindicated.

Patient Education: Inform prescriber of all prescriptions, OTC medications, or herbal products you are taking, and any allergies you have. Do not take anything new during treatment unless approved by prescriber. This medication can only be administered by infusion; report immediately any redness, swelling, burning, or pain at infusion site. Maintain adequate hydration (2-3 L/day of fluids) unless advised by prescriber to restrict fluids, and nutrition (small, frequent meals will help). You will be more susceptible to infection (avoid crowds and exposure to infection and do not have any vaccinations unless approved by prescriber). May cause hair loss (will grow back after therapy); nausea or vomiting (request antiemetic); photosensitivity (use sunscreen, wear protective clothing and eyewear, and avoid direct sunlight); feelings of weakness or lethargy (use caution when driving or engaging in tasks requiring alertness until response to drug is known); or mouth sores (use soft toothbrush, waxed dental floss and frequent oral care). Report numbness or tingling in fingers or toes (use care to prevent injury); weakness, numbness, or pain in muscles or extremities; signs of infection (eg, fever, chills, sore throat, burning urination, fatigue); unusual bleeding (eg, tarry stools, easy bruising, blood in stool, urine, or mouth); unresolved mouth sores; skin rash or itching; or difficulty breathing. **Pregnancy/breast-feeding precautions:** Do not get pregnant (females) or cause a pregnancy (males) during this therapy. Consult prescriber for appropriate contraceptive measures. Do not breast-feed.

Vinorelbine Tartrate *see* Vinorelbine *on page 1403*

Viokase® *see* Pancrelipase *on page 1029*

Viosterol *see* Ergocalciferol *on page 483*

Vioxx® *see* Rofecoxib *on page 1204*

Vira-A® [DSC] *see* Vidarabine *on page 1399*

Viracept® *see* Nelfinavir *on page 956*

Viramune® *see* Nevirapine *on page 963*

Virazole® *see* Ribavirin *on page 1181*

Viread™ *see* Tenofovir *on page 1287*

Virilon® *see* MethylTESTOSTERone *on page 887*

Viroptic® *see* Trifluridine *on page 1363*

Viscoat® *see page 1509*

Viscoat® *see page 1461*

Visine® Extra *see page 1509*

Visken® *see* Pindolol *on page 1087*

Vistaril® *see* HydrOXYzine *on page 684*

Vistide® *see* Cidofovir *on page 286*

Vitamin A Acid *see* Tretinoin (Topical) *on page 1355*

Vitamin B_1 *see* Thiamine *on page 1304*

Vitamin B_2 *see* Riboflavin *on page 1183*

Vitamin B_3 *see* Niacin *on page 965*

Vitamin B_6 *see* Pyridoxine *on page 1156*

Vitamin B_{12} *see* Cyanocobalamin *on page 337*

Vitamin B_{12} *see* Hydroxocobalamin *on page 680*

Vitamin D_2 *see* Ergocalciferol *on page 483*

Vitamin E (VYE ta min ee)

U.S. Brand Names Aqua Gem E® [OTC]; Aquasol E® [OTC]; E-Gems® [OTC]; Key-E® [OTC]; Key- E® Kaps [OTC]

Synonyms *d*-Alpha Tocopherol; *dl*-Alpha Tocopherol

Generic Available Yes

Pharmacologic Category Vitamin, Fat Soluble

Pregnancy Risk Factor A/C (dose exceeding RDA recommendation)

Lactation Excretion in breast milk unknown/compatible

Use Prevention and treatment hemolytic anemia secondary to vitamin E deficiency, dietary supplement

Use - Unlabeled/Investigational To reduce the risk of bronchopulmonary dysplasia or retrolental fibroplasia in infants exposed to high concentrations of oxygen; prevention and treatment of tardive dyskinesia and Alzheimer's disease

Mechanism of Action/Effect Prevents oxidation of vitamin A and C; protects polyunsaturated fatty acids in membranes from attack by free radicals and protects red blood cells against hemolysis

Contraindications Hypersensitivity to vitamin E or any component of the formulation; I.V. route

Warnings/Precautions May induce vitamin K deficiency. Necrotizing enterocolitis has been associated with oral administration of large dosages (eg, >200 units/day) of a hyperosmolar vitamin E preparation in low birth weight infants. Pregnancy risk C (dose exceeding RDA).

Drug Interactions

Decreased Effect: Vitamin E may impair the hematologic response to iron in children with iron-deficiency anemia; monitor.

Increased Effect/Toxicity: Vitamin E may alter the effect of vitamin K actions on clotting factors resulting in an increase hypoprothrombinemic response to warfarin; monitor.

Adverse Reactions <1% (Limited to important or life-threatening): Blurred vision, contact dermatitis with topical preparation, gonadal dysfunction

Pharmacodynamics/Kinetics

Absorption: Oral: Depends on presence of bile; reduced in conditions of malabsorption, in low birth weight premature infants, and as dosage increases; water miscible preparations are better absorbed than oil preparations

Metabolism: Hepatic to glucuronides

Formulations

Capsule: 100 units, 200 units, 400 units, 500 units, 600 units, 1000 units
- Aqua Gem E®: 200 units, 400 units
- E-Gems®: 30 units, 100 units, 600 units, 800 units, 1000 units, 1200 units
- Key-E Kaps®: 200 units, 400 units

Cream: 100 units/g (60 g)
- Key-E®: 30 units/g (60 g, 120 g, 480 g)

Oil: 100 units/0.25 mL (60 mL); 1150 units/0.25 mL (30 mL, 60 mL, 120 mL)
- E-Gem®: 100 units/10 drops (15 mL, 60 mL)

Ointment, topical (Key-E®): 30 units/g (60 g, 120 g, 480 g)

Powder (Key-E®): 700 units/dose (15 g, 75 g, 1000 g)

Solution, oral drops (Aquasol E®): 15 units/0.3 mL (12 mL, 30 mL)

Suppository (Key-E®): 30 units (12s, 24s)

Spray (Key-E®): 30 units/3 seconds (105 g)

Tablet: 100 units, 200 units, 400 units, 500 units, 800 units
- Key-E®: 100 units, 200 units, 400 units

Dosing

Adults & Elderly: One unit of vitamin E = 1 mg *dl*-alpha-tocopherol acetate. Oral:

Recommended daily allowance (RDA): 15 mg (22.5 units); upper limit of intake should not exceed 1000 mg/day
- Pregnant female:
  - ≤18 years: 15 mg (22.5 units); upper level of intake should not exceed 800 mg/day
  - 19-50 years: 15 mg (22.5 units); upper level of intake should not exceed 1000 mg/day
- Lactating female:
  - ≤18 years: 19 mg (28.5 units); upper level of intake should not exceed 800 mg/day
  - 19-50 years: 19 mg (28.5 units); upper level of intake should not exceed 1000 mg/day

Vitamin E deficiency: 60-75 units/day

Prevention of vitamin E deficiency: Oral: 30 units/day
- Cystic fibrosis: Oral: 100-400 units/day
- Beta-thalassemia: Oral: 750 units/day

Sickle cell: Oral: 450 units/day

Alzheimer's disease: Oral; 1000 units twice daily

Tardive dyskinesia: Oral: 1600 units/day

Superficial dermatologic irritation: Topical: Apply a thin layer over affected area.

Pediatrics: One unit of vitamin E = 1 mg *dl*-alpha-tocopherol acetate. Oral:

Recommended daily allowance (RDA):
- Premature infants ≤3 months: 17 mg (25 units)
- Infants:
  - ≤6 months: 3 mg (4.5 units)
  - 7-12 months: 4 mg (6 units)
- Children:
  - 1-3 years: 6 mg (9 units); upper limit of intake should not exceed 200 mg/day
  - 4-8 years: 7 mg (10.5 units); upper limit of intake should not exceed 300 mg/day
  - 9-13 years: 11 mg (16.5 units); upper limit of intake should not exceed 600 mg/day
  - 14-18 years: 15 mg (22.5 units); upper limit of intake should not exceed 800 mg/day

Vitamin E deficiency:
- Children (with malabsorption syndrome): 1 unit/kg/day of water miscible vitamin E (to raise plasma tocopherol concentrations to the normal range within 2 months and to maintain normal plasma concentrations)

Prevention of vitamin E deficiency: Adults: 30 units/day

Prevention of retinopathy of prematurity or BPD secondary to O_2 therapy (AAP considers this use investigational and routine use is not recommended):

Retinopathy prophylaxis: 15-30 units/kg/day to maintain plasma levels between 1.5-2 µg/mL (may need as high as 100 units/kg/day)

Cystic fibrosis, beta-thalassemia, sickle cell anemia may require higher daily maintenance doses:

Cystic fibrosis: Oral: 100-400 units/day

Beta-thalassemia: Oral: 750 units/day

Administration

Oral: Swallow capsules whole, do not crush or chew.

Stability

Storage: Protect from light.

Monitoring and Teaching Issues

Physical Assessment: Assess effectiveness and interactions of other medications patient may be taking (see Drug Interactions). Assess knowledge/teach patient appropriate use (according to formulation prescribed) and adverse symptoms to report (see Patient Education). **Pregnancy risk factor A/C** - see Pregnancy Risk Factor for use cautions.

Patient Education: Take exactly as directed; do not take more than the recommended dose. Do not use mineral oil or other vitamin E supplements without consulting prescriber. Report persistent nausea, vomiting, or cramping; or gonadal dysfunction. **Pregnancy precaution:** Inform prescriber if you are pregnant.

Additional Information 1 mg *dl*-alpha tocopheryl acetate = 1 int. unit

Vitamin G *see* Riboflavin *on page 1183*

Vitamin K_1 *see* Phytonadione *on page 1080*

Vitrasert® *see* Ganciclovir *on page 618*

Vivactil® *see* Protriptyline *on page 1149*

Vivelle® *see* Estradiol *on page 494*

Vivelle-Dot® *see* Estradiol *on page 494*

Vivotif Berna™ *see page 1498*

VLB *see* VinBLAStine *on page 1399*

VM-26 *see* Teniposide *on page 1285*

Volmax® *see* Albuterol *on page 52*

Voltaren® *see page 1509*

Voltaren® *see* Diclofenac *on page 400*

Voltaren Ophthalmic® *see* Diclofenac *on page 400*

Voltaren®-XR *see* Diclofenac *on page 400*

Voriconazole (vor i KOE na zole)

U.S. Brand Names VFEND®

Synonyms UK109496

Generic Available No

Pharmacologic Category Antifungal Agent, Oral; Antifungal Agent, Parenteral

Pregnancy Risk Factor D

Lactation Excretion in breast milk unknown/not recommended

Use Treatment of invasive aspergillosis; treatment of serious fungal infections caused by *Scedosporium apiospermum* and *Fusarium* spp (including *Fusarium solani*) in patients intolerant of, or refractory to, other therapy

Mechanism of Action/Effect Interferes with fungal cytochrome P450 activity, decreasing ergosterol synthesis (principal sterol in fungal cell membrane) and inhibiting fungal cell membrane formation.

Contraindications Hypersensitivity to voriconazole or any component of the formulation (cross-reaction with other azole antifungal agents may occur but has not been established, use caution); coadministration of CYP3A4 substrates which may lead to QT_c prolongation (astemizole, cisapride, pimozide, or quinidine); coadministration with barbiturates (long acting), carbamazepine, ergot alkaloids, rifampin, rifabutin, and sirolimus; pregnancy (unless risk:benefit justifies use)

Warnings/Precautions Visual changes are commonly associated with treatment. Patients should be warned to avoid tasks which depend on vision, including operating machinery or driving. Changes are reversible on discontinuation following brief exposure/treatment regimens (≤28 days).

Serious hepatic reactions (including hepatitis, cholestasis, and fulminant hepatic failure) have occurred during treatment, primarily in patients with serious concomitant medical conditions. However, hepatotoxicity has occurred in patients with no identifiable risk factors. Use caution in patients with pre-existing hepatic impairment (dose adjustment required).

Voriconazole tablets contain lactose; avoid administration in hereditary galactose intolerance, Lapp lactase deficiency, or glucose-galactose malabsorption. Avoid/limit use of intravenous formulation in patients with renal impairment (intravenous formulation contains SBECD). Infusion-related reactions may occur with intravenous dosing. Consider discontinuation of infusion if reaction is severe.

Avoid use in pregnancy, unless an evaluation of the potential benefit justifies possible risk to the fetus. Safety and efficacy have not been established in children <12 years of age.

Drug Interactions

Cytochrome P450 Effect: Substrate of **CYP2C8/9, 2C19**, 3A4; Inhibits CYP2C8/9, 2C19, 3A4

Decreased Effect: Rifampin decreases voriconazole's serum concentration to levels which are no longer effective; avoid concurrent use. Other inducers (barbiturates, carbamazepine, rifabutin) may share this effect (rifabutin is contraindicated due to increased serum

(Continued)

Voriconazole *(Continued)*

concentrations). Phenytoin may decrease serum concentrations of voriconazole; prospective adjustment of voriconazole dosage is recommended. Serum levels of voriconazole may be decreased by efavirenz or nevirapine.

Increased Effect/Toxicity: Voriconazole may increase the serum concentrations of cisapride, pimozide leading to malignant arrhythmias; use in contraindicated. Serum levels of ergot alkaloids may be increased by voriconazole, leading to ergot toxicity; concurrent use is contraindicated. Rifabutin serum levels are increased by voriconazole; concurrent use is contraindicated. Serum concentrations of busulfan, docetaxel, and dofetilide; avoid concurrent use.

Serum concentrations of immunosuppressants (cyclosporine, sirolimus, and tacrolimus) may be increased; concurrent use of sirolimus is contraindicated. Decrease cyclosporine dosage by 50% when initiating voriconazole, decreased tacrolimus dosage by 66% when initiating voriconazole.

Serum levels of voriconazole may be increased by efavirenz or delavirdine. Indinavir did not appear to alter voriconazole serum concentrations during concurrent treatment; other protease inhibitors may result in increased voriconazole concentrations.

Voriconazole may increase the serum concentrations of benzodiazepines (oxidatively metabolized), buspirone, calcium channel blockers, methylprednisolone, quinidine, sulfonylureas, trimetrexate, vinca alkaloids, or zolpidem. In addition, the anticoagulant effect of warfarin may be increased. Serum concentrations of HMG-CoA reductase inhibitors may be increased (except pravastatin and fluvastatin); increasing the risk of myopathy/rhabdomyolysis. Changes in gastric acidity (due to H_2 antagonists or proton pump inhibitors) do not appear to significantly affect voriconazole absorption. However, voriconazole may significantly increase serum levels of omeprazole. For omeprazole dosages >40 mg/day, reduce omeprazole dosage by 50%. Serum levels of other proton pump inhibitors may also be increased.

Nutritional/Ethanol Interactions

Food: May decrease voriconazole absorption. Voriconazole should be taken 1 hour before or 1 hour after a meal. Avoid grapefruit juice (may increase voriconazole serum levels).

Herb/Nutraceutical: St John's wort may decrease voriconazole levels.

Adverse Reactions Note: Includes adverse reactions reported from all trials, including trials conducted in immunocompromised patients; cause:effect relationship not established for many reactions

>10%: Ocular: Visual changes (photophobia, color changes, increased or decreased visual acuity, or blurred vision occur in ~30%)

1% to 10%:

- Cardiovascular: Tachycardia (3%), hypertension (2%), hypotension (2%), vasodilation (2%), peripheral edema (1%)
- Central nervous system: Fever (6%), chills (4%), headache (3%), hallucinations (3%), dizziness (1%)
- Dermatologic: Rash (6%), pruritus (1%)
- Endocrine & metabolic: Hypokalemia (2%), hypomagnesemia (1%)
- Gastrointestinal: Nausea (6%), vomiting (5%), abdominal pain (2%), diarrhea (1%), xerostomia (1%)
- Hematologic: Thrombocytopenia (1%)
- Hepatic: Alkaline phosphatase increased (4%), serum transaminases increased (2%), AST increased (2%), ALT increased (2%), cholestatic jaundice (1%)
- Renal: Acute renal failure (1%)

<1% (Limited to important or life-threatening): Acute tubular necrosis, adrenal cortical insufficiency, agranulocytosis, allergic reaction, anaphylactoid reaction, anemia (aplastic), anemia (macrocytic, megaloblastic, or microcytic), angioedema, aplastic anemia, ataxia, atrial arrhythmia, atrial fibrillation, AV block, bigeminy, bone marrow depression, bone necrosis, bradycardia, brain edema, bundle branch block, cardiac arrest, cerebral hemorrhage, cholecystitis, cholelithiasis, color blindness, coma, congestive heart failure, convulsion, delirium, dementia, depersonalization, depression, DIC, discoid lupus erythematosus, duodenal ulcer perforation, dyspnea, encephalopathy, enlarged liver, enlarged spleen, eosinophilia, erythema multiforme, exfoliative dermatitis, extrapyramidal symptoms, fixed drug eruption, gastrointestinal hemorrhage, grand mal seizure, Guillain-Barré syndrome, hematemesis, hemolytic anemia, hepatic coma, hepatic failure, hepatitis, intestinal perforation, intracranial hypertension, leukopenia, lung edema, myasthenia, myocardial infarction, neuropathy, night blindness, optic atrophy, optic neuritis, pancreatitis, pancytopenia, papilledema, paresthesia, photosensitivity, psychosis, pulmonary embolus, QT interval prolongation, respiratory distress syndrome, sepsis, Stevens-Johnson syndrome, suicidal ideation, supraventricular tachycardia, syncope, thrombotic thrombocytopenic purpura, toxic epidermal necrolysis, ventricular arrhythmia, ventricular fibrillation, ventricular tachycardia (including possible torsade de pointes), vertigo, visual field defect

Overdosage/Toxicology Limited experience in overdose. Symptoms may include changes in vision, cholinergic symptoms (salivation, mydriasis), and CNS depression. Following intravenous overdose, toxicity from the vehicle, SBECD, may also occur. Both voriconazole and the intravenous vehicle may be eliminated via hemodialysis.

Pharmacodynamics/Kinetics

Absorption: Well absorbed after oral administration

Bioavailability: 96%

Half-Life Elimination: Variable, dose dependent

Time to Peak: 1-2 hours

Metabolism: Hepatic, nonlinear (via CYP isoenzymes)

Formulations

Injection, powder for reconstitution: 200 mg [contains SBECD 3200 mg]

Tablet: 50 mg, 200 mg [contains lactose]

Dosing

Adults & Elderly: Fungal infections: I.V.: Initial: Loading dose: 6 mg/kg every 12 hours for 2 doses; followed by maintenance dose of 4 mg/kg every 12 hours

Conversion to oral dosing:

Patients >40 kg: 200 mg every 12 hours

Patients ≤40 kg: 100 mg every 12 hours

Note: Dosage may be increased by 100 mg/dose in patients who fail to respond adequately (50 mg/dose in patients ≤ 40 kg)

Dosage adjustment in patients unable to tolerate treatment:

I.V.: Dose may be reduced to 3 mg/kg every 12 hours

Oral: Dose may be reduced in 50 mg increments to a minimum dosage of 200 mg every 12 hours in patients weighing >40 kg (100 mg every 12 hours in patients ≤40 kg)

Dosage adjustment in patients receiving concomitant phenytoin:

I.V.: Increase maintenance dosage to 5 mg/kg every 12 hours

Oral: Increase dose from 200 mg to 400 mg every 12 hours in patients >40 kg (100 mg to 200 mg every 12 hours in patients ≤40 kg)

Pediatrics: Children ≥12 years: Refer to adult dosing.

Renal Impairment: In patients with Cl_{cr} <50 mL/minute, accumulation of the intravenous vehicle (SBECD) occurs. After initial loading dose, oral voriconazole should be administered to these patients, unless an assessment of the benefit:risk to the patient justifies the use of I.V. voriconazole. Monitor serum creatinine and change to oral voriconazole therapy when possible.

Hepatic Impairment:

Mild to moderate hepatic dysfunction (Child-Pugh class A and B): Following standard loading dose, reduce maintenance dosage by 50%

Severe hepatic impairment: Should only be used if benefit outweighs risk; monitor closely for toxicity

Administration

Oral: Administer 1 hour before or 1 hour after a meal.

I.V.: Infuse over 1-2 hours (rate not to exceed 3 mg/kg/hour)

Stability

Storage: Store tablets and unreconstituted powder for injection at 15°C to 30°C (59°F to 86°F).

Reconstitution: Reconstitute 200 mg vial with 19 mL of sterile water for injection (use of automated syringe is not recommended). Resultant solution (20 mL) has a concentration of 10 mg/mL. Must dilute to 0.5-5 mg/mL prior to infusion. Reconstituted solutions should be used as soon as possible. Diluted solutions are stable for up to 24 hours under refrigeration at 2°C to 8°C (37°F to 46°F).

Compatibility: Stable in LR, ½NS, NS, D_5W, D_5LR, D_5NS, D_5½NS; **incompatible** with alkaline solutions, bicarbonate, aminofusin 10%, electrolyte solutions.

Monitoring and Teaching Issues

Physical Assessment: Assess allergy history prior to beginning therapy. See Contraindications, Warnings/Precautions, and Dosing for use cautions. Assess potential for interactions with other prescriptions, OTC medications, or herbal products patient may be taking (see Drug Interactions). See specific Administration and Compatibility directions. Assess results of laboratory tests (see Monitoring Laboratory Tests), therapeutic effects, and adverse response (see Adverse Reactions and Overdose/Toxicology) on a regular basis. Teach patient use, possible side effects (eg, vision changes) and interventions, and adverse symptoms to report (see Patient Education). **Pregnancy risk factor D** - determine that patient is not pregnant before beginning treatment. Do not give to women of childbearing age unless patient is capable of complying with barrier contraceptive measures during therapy. Instruct patient in appropriate contraceptive measures. Breast-feeding is not recommended.

Patient Education: Inform prescriber of all prescriptions, OTC medications, or herbal products you are taking, and any allergies you have. Do not take anything new during treatment unless approved by prescriber. Take full course of medication as ordered. Preferable to take on empty stomach (1 hour before or 2 hours after a meal). Maintain adequate hydration (2-3 L/day of fluids) unless advised by prescriber to restrict fluids. You may experience headache, dizziness, blurred vision, photophobia, or changes in visual acuity (use caution when driving or engaging in tasks that require alertness until response to drug is known - vision changes are reversible on discontinuation following brief treatment); or nausea or vomiting (small, frequent meals, frequent mouth care, sucking lozenges, or chewing gum may help). Report immediately any change in vision. Report skin rash; chest pain, palpitations, or rapid heartbeat; fever, chills, or hallucinations; persistent GI upset; urinary pattern changes; yellowing of skin or eyes; changes in color of stool or urine; or any other persistent side effects. **Pregnancy/breast-feeding precautions:** Inform prescriber if you are pregnant. Do not get pregnant while taking this drug. Fetal harm can occur. Consult prescriber for appropriate contraceptive measures. Breast-feeding is not recommended.

Dietary Issues: Oral: Should be taken 1 hour before or 1 hour after a meal.

Breast-feeding Issues: Excretion in breast milk has not been investigated; avoid breast-feeding until additional data are available.

Pregnancy Issues: Voriconazole can cause fetal harm when administered to a pregnant woman. Voriconazole was teratogenic in animal studies, and lowered plasma estradiol in animal models. Should be used in pregnant woman only if benefit to mother justifies potential risk to the fetus.

VoSol HC® *see page 1519*

VoSol® Otic *see page 1519*

VP-16 *see* Etoposide *on page 536*

VP-16-213 *see* Etoposide *on page 536*

Vumon *see* Teniposide *on page 1285*

V.V.S.® *see* Sulfabenzamide, Sulfacetamide, and Sulfathiazole *on page 1255*

Vytone® *see* Iodoquinol and Hydrocortisone *on page 732*

Warfarin (WAR far in)

U.S. Brand Names Coumadin®

Synonyms Warfarin Sodium

Generic Available Yes: Tablet

Pharmacologic Category Anticoagulant, Coumarin Derivative

Pregnancy Risk Factor D

Lactation Does not enter breast milk, only metabolites are excreted (AAP rates "compatible")

Use Prophylaxis and treatment of venous thrombosis, pulmonary embolism and thromboembolic disorders; atrial fibrillation with risk of embolism and as an adjunct in the prophylaxis of systemic embolism after myocardial infarction

Use - Unlabeled/Investigational Prevention of recurrent transient ischemic attacks and to reduce risk of recurrent myocardial infarction

Mechanism of Action/Effect Interferes with hepatic synthesis of vitamin K-dependent coagulation factors (II, VII, IX, X)

Contraindications Hypersensitivity to warfarin or any component of the formulation; hemorrhagic tendencies; hemophilia; thrombocytopenia purpura; leukemia; recent or potential surgery of the eye or CNS; major regional lumbar block anesthesia or surgery resulting in large, open surfaces; patients bleeding from the GI, respiratory, or GU tract; threatened abortion; aneurysm; ascorbic acid deficiency; history of bleeding diathesis; prostatectomy; continuous tube drainage of the small intestine; polyarthritis; diverticulitis; emaciation; malnutrition; cerebrovascular hemorrhage; eclampsia/pre-eclampsia; blood dyscrasias; severe uncontrolled or malignant hypertension; severe hepatic disease; pericarditis or pericardial effusion; subacute bacterial endocarditis; visceral carcinoma; following spinal puncture and other diagnostic or therapeutic procedures with potential for significant bleeding; history of warfarin-induced necrosis; an unreliable, noncompliant patient; alcoholism; patient who has a history of falls or is a significant fall risk; pregnancy

Warnings/Precautions Use care in the selection of patients appropriate for this treatment. Ensure patient cooperation especially from the alcoholic, illicit drug user, demented, or psychotic patient. Use with caution in trauma, acute infection (antibiotics and fever may alter affects), renal insufficiency, prolonged dietary insufficiencies (vitamin K deficiency), moderate-severe hypertension, polycythemia vera, vasculitis, open wound, active TB, history of PUD, anaphylactic disorders, indwelling catheters, severe diabetes, thyroid disease, severe renal disease, and menstruating and postpartum women. Use with caution in protein C deficiency.

Hemorrhage is the most serious risk of therapy. Patient must be instructed to report bleeding, accidents, or falls. Patient must also report any new or discontinued medications, herbal or alternative products used, significant changes in smoking or dietary habits. Necrosis or gangrene of the skin and other tissues can occur (rarely) due to early hypercoagulability. "Purple toes syndrome," due to cholesterol microembolization, may rarely occur (often after several weeks of therapy). Women may be at risk of developing ovarian hemorrhage at the time of ovulation. The elderly may be more sensitive to anticoagulant therapy.

Drug Interactions

Cytochrome P450 Effect: Substrate of CYP1A2, **2C8/9**, 2C19, 3A4; Inhibits CYP2C8/9, 2C19

Decreased Effect: See table.

Decreased Anticoagulant Effects

Induction of Enzymes		Increased Procoagulant Factors	Decreased Drug Absorption	Other
Barbiturates Carbamazepine Glutethimide Griseofulvin	Nafcillin Phenytoin Rifampin	Estrogens Oral contraceptives Vitamin K (including nutritional supplements)	Aluminum hydroxide Cholestyramine* Colestipol*	Ethchlorvynol Griseofulvin Spironolactone† Sucralfate

Decreased anticoagulant effect may occur when these drugs are administered with oral anticoagulants.

*Cholestyramine and colestipol may increase the anticoagulant effect by binding vitamin K in the gut; yet, the decreased drug absorption appears to be of more concern.

†Diuretic-induced hemoconcentration with subsequent concentration of clotting factors has been reported to decrease the effects of oral anticoagulants.

Increased Effect/Toxicity:
See tables.

Increased Bleeding Tendency

Inhibit Platelet Aggregation	Inhibit Procoagulant Factors	Ulcerogenic Drugs
Cephalosporins Dipyridamole Indomethacin Oxyphenbutazone Penicillin, parenteral Phenylbutazone Salicylates Sulfinpyrazone	Antimetabolites Quinidine Quinine Salicylates	Adrenal corticosteroids Indomethacin Oxyphenbutazone Phenylbutazone Potassium products Salicylates

Use of these agents with oral anticoagulants may increase the chances of hemorrhage.

Enhanced Anticoagulant Effects

Decrease Vitamin K	Displace Anticoagulant	Inhibit Metabolism	Other
Oral antibiotics: Can ↑/↓ INR Check INR 3 days after a patient begins antibiotics to see the INR value and adjust the warfarin dose accordingly	Chloral hydrate Clofibrate Diazoxide Ethacrynic acid Miconazole (including intravaginal use) Nalidixic acid Phenylbutazone Salicylates Sulfonamides Sulfonylureas	Allopurinol Amiodarone Azole antifungals Capecitabine Chloramphenicol Chlorpropamide Cimetidine Ciprofloxacin Co-trimoxazole Disulfiram Ethanol (acute ingestion)[1] Flutamide Isoniazid Metronidazole Norfloxacin Ofloxacin Omperazole Phenylbutazone Phenytoin Propafenone Propoxyphene Protease inhibitors Quinidine "Statins"[2] Sulfinpyrazone Sulfonamides Tamoxifen Tolbutamide Zafirlukast Zileuton	Acetaminophen Anabolic steroids Clarithromycin Clofibrate Danazol Erythromycin Gemfibrozil Glucagon Influenza vaccine Propranolol Propylthiouracil Ranitidine SSRIs Sulindac Tetracycline Thyroid drugs Vitamin E (≥400 int. units)

[1] The hypoprothrombinemic effect of oral anticoagulants has been reported to be both increased and decreased during chronic and excessive alcohol ingestion. Data are insufficient to predict the direction of this interaction in alcoholic patients.

[2] Particularly lovastatin and fluvastatin; others (atorvastatin, pravastatin) rarely associated with increased PT.

Nutritional/Ethanol Interactions

Ethanol: Avoid ethanol. Acute ethanol ingestion (binge drinking) decreases the metabolism of warfarin and increases PT/INR. Chronic daily ethanol use increases the metabolism of warfarin and decreases PT/INR.

Food: The anticoagulant effects of warfarin may be decreased if taken with foods rich in vitamin K. Vitamin E may increase warfarin effect.

Herb/Nutraceutical: St John's wort may decrease warfarin levels. Alfalfa contains large amounts of vitamin K as do many enteral products. Coenzyme Q_{10} may decrease response to warfarin. Avoid cat's claw, dong quai, bromelains, evening primrose, feverfew, red clover, horse chestnut, garlic, green tea, ginseng, ginkgo (all have additional antiplatelet activity).

Effects on Lab Values Warfarin ↑ PTT

Adverse Reactions As with all anticoagulants, bleeding is the major adverse effect of warfarin. Hemorrhage may occur at virtually any site. Risk is dependent on multiple variables, including the intensity of anticoagulation and patient susceptibility.

Additional adverse effects are often related to idiosyncratic reactions, and the frequency cannot be accurately estimated.

Cardiovascular: Vasculitis, edema, hemorrhagic shock

Central nervous system: Fever, lethargy, malaise, asthenia, pain, headache, dizziness, stroke

Dermatologic: Rash, dermatitis, bullous eruptions, urticaria, pruritus, alopecia

Gastrointestinal: Anorexia, nausea, vomiting, stomach cramps, abdominal pain, diarrhea, flatulence, gastrointestinal bleeding, taste disturbance, mouth ulcers

Genitourinary: Priapism, hematuria

Hematologic: Hemorrhage, leukopenia, unrecognized bleeding sites (eg, colon cancer) may be uncovered by anticoagulation, retroperitoneal hematoma, agranulocytosis

Hepatic: Increased transaminases, hepatic injury, jaundice,

Neuromuscular & skeletal: Paresthesia, osteoporosis

Respiratory: Hemoptysis, epistaxis, pulmonary hemorrhage, tracheobronchial calcification

Miscellaneous: Hypersensitivity/allergic reactions

Skin necrosis/gangrene, due to paradoxical local thrombosis, is a known but rare risk of warfarin therapy. Its onset is usually within the first few days of therapy and is frequently localized to the limbs, breast or penis. The risk of this effect is increased in patients with protein C or S deficiency.

"Purple toes syndrome," caused by cholesterol microembolization, also occurs rarely. Typically, this occurs after several weeks of therapy, and may present as a dark, purplish, mottled discoloration of the plantar and lateral surfaces. Other manifestations of cholesterol microembolization may include rash, livedo reticularis, rash, gangrene, abrupt and intense pain in lower extremities, abdominal, flank, or back pain, hematuria, renal insufficiency, hypertension, cerebral ischemia, spinal cord infarction, or other symptom of vascular compromise.

Overdosage/Toxicology Symptoms of overdose include internal or external hemorrhage and hematuria. Avoid emesis and lavage to avoid possible trauma and incidental bleeding. When an overdose occurs, the drug should be immediately discontinued and vitamin K_1 (phytonadione) may be administered, up to 25 mg I.V. for adults. When hemorrhage occurs, fresh frozen plasma transfusions can help control bleeding by replacing clotting factors. In urgent bleeding, prothrombin complex concentrates may be needed.

(Continued)

Warfarin *(Continued)*

Management of elevated INR: See table.

Management of Elevated INR

INR	Patient Situation	Action
>3 and <5	No bleeding or need for rapid reversal (ie, no need for surgery)	Omit next few warfarin dose and/or restart at lower dose when INR approaches desired range. If only minimally above range, then no dosage reduction may be required.
>5 and <9.0	No bleeding or need for rapid reversal	Omit next 1-2 doses, monitor INR more frequently, and restart at lower dose when INR approaches target range **or** omit dose and give 1-2.5 mg vitamin K orally (use this if patient has risk factors for bleeding).
	No bleeding but reversal needed for surgery or dental extraction within 24 hours	Vitamin K 2-4 mg orally (expected reversal within 24 hours); give additional 1-2 mg if INR remains high at 24 hours.
>9.0 and <20.0	No bleeding	Stop warfarin, give vitamin K 3-5 mg orally; follow INR closely; repeat vitamin K if needed. Reassess need and dose of warfarin when INR approaches desirable range.
Rapid reversal required (ie, INR >20)	Serious bleeding or major warfarin overdose	Stop warfarin, give vitamin K 10 mg by slow I.V. infusion. May repeat vitamin K every 12 hours and give fresh plasma transfusion or prothrombin complex concentrate as needed. When appropriate, heparin can be given until the patient becomes responsive to warfarin.

Pharmacodynamics/Kinetics

Absorption: Oral: Rapid

Half-Life Elimination: 20-60 hours; Mean: 40 hours; highly variable among individuals

Metabolism: Hepatic

Onset: Anticoagulation: Oral: 36-72 hours; Peak effect: Full therapeutic effect: 5-7 days; INR may increase in 36-72 hours

Duration: 2-5 days

Formulations

Injection, powder for reconstitution, as sodium: 5 mg

Tablet, as sodium: 1 mg, 2 mg, 2.5 mg, 3 mg, 4 mg, 5 mg, 6 mg, 7.5 mg, 10 mg

Dosing

Adults: Prevention/treatment of thrombosis/embolism:

Oral: Initial dosing must be individualized based upon patient's end organ function, concurrent therapy, and risk of bleeding; ACCP recommendation: 5 mg/day for 2-5 days, then adjust dose according to results of prothrombin time; usual maintenance dose ranges from 2-10 mg/day (selected sensitive patients may require less; resistant patients may require higher dosages).

Note: Lower starting doses may be required for patients with hepatic impairment, poor nutrition, CHF, elderly, or a high risk of bleeding. Higher initial doses may be reasonable in selected patients (ie, receiving enzyme-inducing agents and with low risk of bleeding).

I.V. (administer as a slow bolus injection): 2-5 mg/day

Elderly: Oral: Initial dose ≤5 mg. Usual maintenance dose: 2-5 mg/day. The elderly tend to require lower dosages to produce a therapeutic level of anticoagulation (due to changes in the pattern of warfarin metabolism).

Pediatrics: Prevention/treatment of thrombosis: Oral: Infants and Children: 0.05-0.34 mg/kg/day; infants <12 months of age may require doses at or near the high end of this range; consistent anticoagulation may be difficult to maintain in children <5 years of age.

Hepatic Impairment: Monitor effect at usual doses. The response to oral anticoagulants may be markedly enhanced in obstructive jaundice, hepatitis, and cirrhosis. Prothrombin index should be closely monitored.

Administration

Oral: Do not take with food. Take at the same time each day.

I.V.: Administer as a slow bolus injection over 1-2 minutes. Avoid all I.M. injections.

Stability

Storage: Protect from light.

Reconstitution: Injection is stable for 4 hours at room temperature after reconstitution with 2.7 mL of sterile water (yields 2 mg/mL solution).

Compatibility: Stable in D_5LR, $D_5\frac{1}{2}NS$, D_5NS, D_5W, $D_{10}W$

Y-site administration: Incompatible with aminophylline, bretylium, ceftazidime, cimetidine, ciprofloxacin, dobutamine, esmolol, gentamicin, labetalol, metronidazole, promazine, lactated Ringer's

Compatibility in syringe: Incompatible with heparin

Monitoring Laboratory Tests Prothrombin time (desirable range usually 1.5-2 times the control), hematocrit, INR (desirable range usually 2.0-3.0 with standard therapy, 2.5-3.5 with high-dose therapy)

Monitoring and Teaching Issues

Physical Assessment: See Contraindications and Warnings/Precautions for use cautions. Assess potential for interactions with other prescriptions, OTC medications, or herbal products patient may be taking (see Drug Interactions). Assess results of laboratory tests closely (see above). Patient should be monitored closely for therapeutic effectiveness and adverse reactions (eg, thrombolytic reactions - see Adverse Reactions and Overdose/Toxicology). Teach patient possible side effects and interventions (eg, safety precautions) and adverse symptoms to report (see Patient Education). **Pregnancy risk factor D** - determine that patient is not pregnant before beginning treatment. Teach patients of childbearing age appropriate use of barrier contraceptives.

Patient Education: It is imperative that you inform prescriber of all prescriptions, OTC medications, or herbal products you are taking, and any allergies you have. Do not take anything new during treatment unless approved by prescriber. Take exactly as directed; if dose is missed, take as soon as possible. Do not double dose. Follow diet and activity as recommended by prescriber; check with prescriber before changing diet. Avoid alcohol. You will have a tendency to bleed easily while taking this drug (use soft toothbrush, waxed dental floss, electric razor, and avoid scissors or sharp knives and potentially harmful activities). May cause nausea, vomiting, disturbed taste (small, frequent meals, frequent mouth care, sucking lozenges, or chewing gum may help). Report any unusual bleeding or bruising (eg, bleeding gums, nosebleed, blood in urine, dark stool, bloody emesis); skin rash or irritation; unusual fever; persistent nausea or GI upset; pain in joints or back; or swelling or pain at injection site. **Pregnancy precautions:** Do not get pregnant while taking this medication. Consult prescriber for appropriate barrier contraceptive measures.

Dietary Issues: Foods high in vitamin K (eg, beef liver, pork liver, green tea and leafy green vegetables) inhibit anticoagulant effect. Do not change dietary habits once stabilized on warfarin therapy; a balanced diet with a consistent intake of vitamin K is essential; avoid large amounts of alfalfa, asparagus, broccoli, Brussels sprouts, cabbage, cauliflower, green teas, kale, lettuce, spinach, turnip greens, watercress decrease efficacy of warfarin. It is recommended that the diet contain a CONSISTENT vitamin K content of 70-140 mcg/day. Check with healthcare provider before changing diet.

Geriatric Considerations: Before committing an elderly patient to long-term anticoagulation therapy, their risk for bleeding complications secondary to falls, drug interactions, living situation, and cognitive status should be considered. A risk of bleeding complications has been associated with increased age.

Breast-feeding Issues: Warfarin does not pass into breast milk and can be given to nursing mothers (AAP rates "compatible"). However, limited data suggests prolonged PT may occur in some infants. Women who are breast-feeding should be carefully monitored to avoid excessive anticoagulation. Evaluation of coagulation tests and vitamin K status of breast-feeding infant is considered prudent.

Pregnancy Issues: Oral anticoagulants cross the placenta and produce fetal abnormalities. Warfarin should not be used during pregnancy because of significant risks. Adjusted-dose heparin can be given safely throughout pregnancy in patients with venous thromboembolism.

Related Information

Anticoagulant Therapy Guidelines *on page 1635*
Peak and Trough Guidelines *on page 1544*

Warfarin Sodium *see* Warfarin *on page 1410*
WelChol™ *see* Colesevelam *on page 331*
Wellbutrin® *see* BuPROPion *on page 186*
Wellbutrin SR® *see* BuPROPion *on page 186*
Wesmycin® *see* Tetracycline *on page 1296*
Westcort® *see* Hydrocortisone *on page 673*
Westcort® *see* Topical Corticosteroids *on page 1334*
Westhroid® *see* Thyroid *on page 1313*
WinRho SD® *see page 1498*
WinRho SDF® *see page 1498*
Wyamine® Sulfate Injection *see page 1461*
Wycillin® *see* Penicillin G Procaine *on page 1047*
Wygesic® *see* Propoxyphene and Acetaminophen *on page 1142*
Wymox® *see* Amoxicillin *on page 88*
Xalatan® *see* Ophthalmic Agents, Glaucoma *on page 1002*
Xanax® *see* Alprazolam *on page 63*
Xeloda® *see* Capecitabine *on page 207*
Xenical® *see* Orlistat *on page 1008*
Xigris® *see* Drotrecogin Alfa *on page 455*
Xopenex® *see* Levalbuterol *on page 783*
Xylocaine® *see* Lidocaine *on page 800*
Xylocaine® MPF *see* Lidocaine *on page 800*
Xylocaine® MPF With Epinephrine *see* Lidocaine and Epinephrine *on page 803*
Xylocaine® Viscous *see* Lidocaine *on page 800*
Xylocaine® With Epinephrine *see* Lidocaine and Epinephrine *on page 803*
Xylo-Pfan® [OTC] *see page 1461*
Yasmin® *see* Ethinyl Estradiol and Drospirenone *on page 519*
Yellow Fever Vaccine *see page 1498*
YF-VAX® *see page 1498*
Yodoxin® *see* Iodoquinol *on page 731*
Zaditor™ *see page 1509*
Zaditor™ *see* Ophthalmic Agents, Glaucoma *on page 1002*

Zafirlukast (za FIR loo kast)

U.S. Brand Names Accolate®
Synonyms ICI 204, 219
Generic Available No
Pharmacologic Category Leukotriene Receptor Antagonist
Pregnancy Risk Factor B
Lactation Enters breast milk/contraindicated

(Continued)

Zafirlukast *(Continued)*

Use Prophylaxis and chronic treatment of asthma in adults and children ≥5 years of age

Mechanism of Action/Effect Leukotrienes are inflammatory mediators of asthma. Zafirlukast blocks leukotriene receptors and is able to reduce bronchoconstriction and inflammatory cell infiltration.

Contraindications Hypersensitivity to zafirlukast or any component of the formulation

Warnings/Precautions The clearance of zafirlukast is reduced in patients with stable alcoholic cirrhosis such that the C_{max} and AUC are approximately 50% to 60% greater than those of normal adults.

Zafirlukast is not indicated for use in the reversal of bronchospasm in acute asthma attacks, including status asthmaticus. Therapy with zafirlukast can be continued during acute exacerbations of asthma.

An increased proportion of zafirlukast patients >55 years of age reported infections as compared to placebo-treated patients. These infections were mostly mild or moderate in intensity and predominantly affected the respiratory tract. Infections occurred equally in both sexes, were dose-proportional to total milligrams of zafirlukast exposure and were associated with coadministration of inhaled corticosteroids.

Rare hepatic events have been reported, including hepatitis, hyperbilirubinemia, and hepatic failure. Female patients may be at greater risk. Discontinue **immediately** if liver dysfunction is suspected. If hepatic dysfunction is suspected (due to clinical signs/symptoms) liver function tests should be measured immediately. Do not resume or restart if hepatic function tests are consistent with dysfunction.

Rare cases of eosinophilic vasculitis (Churg-Strauss) have been reported in patients receiving zafirlukast (usually, but not always, associated with reduction in concurrent steroid dosage). No causal relationship established.

Drug Interactions

Cytochrome P450 Effect: Substrate of **CYP2C8/9**; Inhibits CYP1A2, 2C8/9, 2C19, 2D6, 3A4

Decreased Effect: Zafirlukast concentrations may be reduced by erythromycin.

Increased Effect/Toxicity: Zafirlukast concentrations are increased by aspirin. Warfarin effect may be increased with zafirlukast. Zafirlukast may increase theophylline levels.

Nutritional/Ethanol Interactions Food: Decreases bioavailability of zafirlukast by 40%.

Adverse Reactions

>10%: Central nervous system: Headache (12.9%)

1% to 10%:

Central nervous system: Dizziness, pain, fever

Gastrointestinal: Nausea, diarrhea, abdominal pain, vomiting, dyspepsia

Hepatic: SGPT elevation

Neuromuscular & skeletal: Back pain, myalgia, weakness

<1% (Limited to important or life-threatening): Agranulocytosis, arthralgia, bleeding, edema, hepatic failure, hepatitis, hyperbilirubinemia, hypersensitivity reactions (urticaria, angioedema, rash), systemic eosinophilia with clinical features of Churg-Strauss syndrome (rare)

Overdosage/Toxicology There is no experience with overdose in humans to date. Treatment is supportive.

Pharmacodynamics/Kinetics

Bioavailability: Reduced 40% with food

Half-Life Elimination: 10 hours

Time to Peak: Serum: 3 hours

Metabolism: Extensively hepatic via CYP2C9

Formulations Tablet: 10 mg, 20 mg

Dosing

Adults & Elderly: Children ≥12 years and Adults: Asthma: Oral: 20 mg twice daily

Pediatrics: Asthma: Oral:

Children 5-11 years: 10 mg twice daily. Safety and effectiveness have not been established in children <5 years of age.

Children ≥12 years: Refer to adult dosing.

Hepatic Impairment: Clearance of zafirlukast is reduced with a greater C_{max} and AUC of 50% to 60% in patients with alcoholic cirrhosis.

Administration

Oral: Administer 1 hour before or 2 hours after meals.

Stability

Storage: Store tablets at controlled room temperature (20°C to 25°C; 68°F to 77°F); protect from light and moisture; dispense in original airtight container

Monitoring and Teaching Issues

Physical Assessment: Not for use in acute asthma attack. Assess effectiveness and interactions of other medications patient may be taking (see Drug Interactions). See Contraindications and Warnings/Precautions for use cautions. Monitor effectiveness of therapy and adverse reactions (see Adverse Reactions) at beginning of therapy and periodically with long-term use. Assess knowledge/teach patient appropriate use, interventions to reduce side effects, and adverse symptoms to report (see Patient Education). Breast-feeding is contraindicated.

Patient Education: Do not use during acute bronchospasm. Take regularly as prescribed, even during symptom-free periods. This medication should be taken on an empty stomach, 1 hour before or 2 hours after meals. Do not take more than recommended or discontinue use without consulting prescriber. Do not stop taking other antiasthmatic medications unless instructed by prescriber. Avoid aspirin or aspirin-containing medications unless approved by prescriber. You may experience headache, drowsiness, dizziness, or blurred vision (use caution when driving or engaging in tasks requiring alertness until response to drug is known); or gastric upset, nausea, or vomiting (small, frequent meals, frequent mouth care, chewing gum, or sucking lozenges may help). Report persistent CNS or GI symptoms; muscle or back pain; weakness, fever, chills; yellowing of skin or eyes; dark urine or pale stool; or skin rash. Contact prescriber immediately if experiencing right upper abdominal pain, nausea, fatigue, itching, flu-like symptoms; swelling of the eyes, face, neck, or throat; anorexia; or worsening of condition. **Breast-feeding precaution:** Do not breast-feed.

Dietary Issues: Should be taken on an empty stomach (1 hour before or 2 hours after meals).

Geriatric Considerations: The mean dose (mg/kg) normalized AUC and C_{max} increase and plasma clearance decreases with increasing age. In patients >65 years of age, there is a two- to threefold greater C_{max} and AUC compared to younger adults.

Pregnancy Issues: At 2000 mg/kg/day in rats, maternal toxicity and deaths were seen with increased incidence of early fetal resorption. Spontaneous abortions occurred in cynomolgus monkeys at a maternally toxic dose of 2000 mg/kg/day orally. There are no adequate and well controlled trials in pregnant women.

Zagam® *see* Sparfloxacin *on page 1241*

Zalcitabine (zal SITE a been)

U.S. Brand Names Hivid®

Synonyms ddC; Dideoxycytidine

Generic Available No

Pharmacologic Category Antiretroviral Agent, Reverse Transcriptase Inhibitor (Nucleoside)

Pregnancy Risk Factor C

Lactation Excretion in breast milk unknown/contraindicated

Use In combination with at least two other antiretrovirals in the treatment of patients with HIV infection; it is not recommended that zalcitabine be given in combination with didanosine, stavudine, or lamivudine due to overlapping toxicities, virologic interactions, or lack of clinical data

Mechanism of Action/Effect Inhibits cell protein synthesis leading to cell death with viral replication.

Contraindications Hypersensitivity to zalcitabine or any component of the formulation

Warnings/Precautions Careful monitoring of pancreatic enzymes and liver function tests in patients with a history of pancreatitis, increased amylase, those on parenteral nutrition or with a history of ethanol abuse; discontinue use immediately if pancreatitis is suspected; lactic acidosis and severe hepatomegaly and failure have rarely occurred with zalcitabine resulting in fatality (stop treatment if lactic acidosis or hepatotoxicity occur); some cases may possibly be related to underlying hepatitis B; use with caution in patients on digitalis, or with CHF, renal failure, or hyperphosphatemia; zalcitabine can cause severe peripheral neuropathy; avoid use, if possible, in patients with pre-existing neuropathy or at risk of developing neuropathy. Risk factors include CD4 counts <50 cells/mm^3, diabetes mellitus, weight loss, other drugs known to cause peripheral neuropathy. Pregnancy risk C.

Drug Interactions

Decreased Effect: It is not recommended that zalcitabine be given in combination with didanosine, stavudine, or lamivudine due to overlapping toxicities, virologic interactions, or lack of clinical data. Doxorubicin and lamivudine have been shown *in vitro* to decrease zalcitabine phosphorylation. Magnesium/aluminum-containing antacids and metoclopramide may decrease the absorption of zalcitabine.

Increased Effect/Toxicity: Amphotericin, foscarnet, and aminoglycosides may potentiate the risk of developing peripheral neuropathy or other toxicities associated with zalcitabine by interfering with the renal elimination of zalcitabine. Other drugs associated with peripheral neuropathy include chloramphenicol, cisplatin, dapsone, disulfiram, ethionamide, glutethimide, gold, hydralazine, iodoquinol, isoniazid, metronidazole, nitrofurantoin, phenytoin, ribavirin, and vincristine. Concomitant use with zalcitabine may increase risk of peripheral neuropathy. Concomitant use of zalcitabine with didanosine is not recommended. Concomitant use of ribavirin and nucleoside analogues may increase the risk of developing lactic acidosis (includes adefovir, didanosine, lamivudine, stavudine, zalcitabine, zidovudine).

Nutritional/Ethanol Interactions Food: Food decreases peak plasma concentrations by 39%. Extent and rate of absorption may be decreased with food.

Effects on Lab Values May cause abnormalities in CBC, WBC, hemoglobin, platelet count, AST, ALT, or alkaline phosphatase.

Adverse Reactions

>10%:

Central nervous system: Fever (5% to 17%), malaise (2% to 13%)

Neuromuscular & skeletal: Peripheral neuropathy (28%)

1% to 10%:

Central nervous system: Headache (2%), dizziness (1%), fatigue (4%), seizures (1.3%)

Dermatologic: Rash (2% to 11%), pruritus (3% to 5%)

Endocrine & metabolic: Hypoglycemia (2% to 6%), hyponatremia (4%), hyperglycemia (1% to 6%)

Gastrointestinal: Nausea (3%), dysphagia (1% to 4%), anorexia (4%), abdominal pain (3% to 8%), vomiting (1% to 3%), diarrhea (<1% to 10%), weight loss, oral ulcers (3% to 7%), increased amylase (3% to 8%)

Hematologic: Anemia (occurs as early as 2-4 weeks), granulocytopenia (usually after 6-8 weeks)

Hepatic: Abnormal hepatic function (9%), hyperbilirubinemia (2% to 5%)

Neuromuscular & skeletal: Myalgia (1% to 6%), foot pain

Respiratory: Pharyngitis (2%), cough (6%), nasal discharge (4%)

<1% (Limited to important or life-threatening): Anaphylaxis, atrial fibrillation, constipation, hepatic failure, hepatitis, hypocalcemia, jaundice, lactic acidosis, night sweats, pancreatitis, redistribution/accumulation of body fat, syncope

Overdosage/Toxicology Symptoms of overdose include delayed peripheral neurotoxicity. Treatment is supportive.

(Continued)

Zalcitabine *(Continued)*

Pharmacodynamics/Kinetics

Absorption: Well, but variable; decreased 39% with food

Bioavailability: >80%

Half-Life Elimination: 2.9 hours; Renal impairment: ≤8.5 hours

Metabolism: Intracellularly to active triphosphorylated agent

Formulations Tablet: 0.375 mg, 0.75 mg

Dosing

Adults & Elderly: HIV infection (component of combination therapy): Oral: Daily dose: 0.75 mg every 8 hours

Pediatrics: HIV infection: Oral:

Children <13 years: Safety and efficacy have not been established.

Adolescents: Refer to adult dosing.

Renal Impairment:

Cl_{cr} 10-40 mL/minute: Administer 0.75 mg every 12 hours.

Cl_{cr} <10 mL/minute: Administer 0.75 mg every 24 hours.

Moderately dialyzable (20% to 50%)

Administration

Oral: Food decreases absorption; take on an empty stomach. Administer around-the-clock. Do not take at the same time with dapsone.

Stability

Storage: Tablets should be stored in tightly closed bottles at room temperature (59°F to 86°F)

Monitoring Laboratory Tests CBC and serum chemistry (prior to initiation and appropriate intervals), renal function, CD4 counts, serum amylase, triglyceride, calcium (see Zidovudine monograph)

Monitoring and Teaching Issues

Physical Assessment: See Contraindications, Warnings/Precautions and Dosing for use cautions. Assess potential for interactions with other prescriptions, OTC medications, or herbal products patient may be taking (eg, especially those that are related to neuropathy - see Drug Interactions). Assess results of laboratory tests (see above), therapeutic response, and adverse reactions (see Adverse Reactions and Overdose/Toxicology) on a regular basis throughout therapy. Teach patient proper use (see Administration and Storage), possible side effects and interventions, and adverse symptoms to report (see Patient Education). **Pregnancy Risk Factor C** - benefits of use should outweigh possible risks. Breast-feeding is contraindicated - CDC recommends that women with HIV not breast-feed in order to prevent transmission of HIV.

Patient Education: Inform prescriber of all prescriptions, OTC medications, or herbal products you are taking, and any allergies you have. Do not take anything new during treatment unless approved by prescriber. This is not a cure for HIV nor has it been found to reduce transmission of HIV. Take as directed, around-the-clock, preferably on an empty stomach, 1 hour before or 2 hours after meals. Do not take antacids or other medication within 1 hour of taking this medication. May cause headache, dizziness, fatigue (use caution when driving or engaging in potentially hazardous tasks until response to drug is known); nausea, vomiting, lack of appetite, mouth sores (small, frequent meals, frequent mouth care, chewing gum, or sucking lozenges may help). Report muscle weakness or pain; tingling, numbness, or pain in toes or fingers; weakness of extremities; chest pain, palpitations, or rapid heartbeat; swelling of extremities; weight gain or loss >5 lb/week; signs of infection (eg, fever, chills, sore throat, burning urination, fatigue); unusual bleeding (eg, tarry stools, easy bruising, or blood in stool, urine, or mouth); skin rash or irritation. **Pregnancy/breast-feeding precautions:** Inform prescriber if you are or intend to become pregnant. Do not breast-feed.

Breast-feeding Issues: HIV-infected mothers are discouraged from breast-feeding to decrease potential transmission of HIV.

Pregnancy Issues: It is not known if zalcitabine crosses the human placenta. Cases of lactic acidosis/hepatic steatosis syndrome have been reported in pregnant women receiving nucleoside analogue drugs. It is not known if pregnancy itself potentiates this known side effect; however, pregnant women may be at increased risk of lactic acidosis and liver damage. Hepatic enzymes and electrolytes should be monitored frequently during the 3rd trimester of pregnancy in women receiving nucleoside analogues. Health professionals are encouraged to contact the antiretroviral pregnancy registry to monitor outcomes of pregnant women exposed to antiretroviral medications (1-800-258-4263).

Additional Information Potential compliance problems, frequency of administration and adverse effects should be discussed with patients before initiating therapy to help prevent the emergence of resistance.

Zaleplon (ZAL e plon)

U.S. Brand Names Sonata®

Restrictions C-IV

Generic Available No

Pharmacologic Category Hypnotic, Nonbenzodiazepine

Pregnancy Risk Factor C

Lactation Enters breast milk/not recommended

Use Short-term (7-10 days) treatment of insomnia (has been demonstrated to be effective for up to 5 weeks in controlled trial)

Mechanism of Action/Effect Zaleplon is unrelated to benzodiazepines, barbiturates, or other hypnotics. However, it interacts with the benzodiazepine GABA receptor complex. Nonclinical studies have shown that it binds selectively to the brain omega-1 receptor situated on the alpha subunit of the GABA-A receptor complex.

Contraindications Hypersensitivity to zaleplon or any component of the formulation

Warnings/Precautions Failure of sleep disturbance to resolve after 7-10 days may indicate psychiatric and/or medical illness. Use with caution in patients with depression, particularly if suicidal risk may be present. Use with caution in patients with a history of drug dependence. Abrupt discontinuance may lead to withdrawal symptoms. May impair physical and mental capabilities; caution in patients receiving other CNS depressants or psychoactive medications. Effects with other sedative drugs or ethanol may be potentiated. Use with caution in the elderly, those with compromised respiratory function, or renal and hepatic impairment. Because of the rapid onset of action, zaleplon should be administered immediately prior to bedtime or after the patient has gone to bed and is having difficulty falling asleep. Capsules contain tartrazine (FD&C yellow #5); avoid in patients with sensitivity (caution in patients with asthma). Pregnancy risk C.

Drug Interactions

Cytochrome P450 Effect: Substrate of CYP3A4

Decreased Effect: CYP3A4 inducers (eg, phenytoin, carbamazepine, phenobarbital) could lead to ineffectiveness of zaleplon.

Increased Effect/Toxicity: Zaleplon potentiates the CNS effects of CNS depressants, including alcohol, imipramine, and thioridazine. Cimetidine increases concentrations of zaleplon. Avoid concurrent use or use 5 mg zaleplon as starting dose in patient receiving cimetidine.

Nutritional/Ethanol Interactions

Ethanol: Avoid ethanol (may increase CNS depression).

Food: High fat meal prolonged absorption; delayed t_{max} by 2 hours, and reduced C_{max} by 35%.

Herb/Nutraceutical: St John's wort may decrease zaleplon levels. Avoid valerian, St John's wort, kava kava, gotu kola (may increase CNS depression).

Adverse Reactions

1% to 10%:

Cardiovascular: Peripheral edema, chest pain

Central nervous system: Amnesia, anxiety, depersonalization, dizziness, hallucinations, hypesthesia, somnolence, vertigo, malaise, depression, lightheadedness, impaired coordination, fever, migraine

Dermatologic: Photosensitivity reaction, rash, pruritus

Gastrointestinal: Abdominal pain, anorexia, colitis, dyspepsia, nausea, constipation, xerostomia

Genitourinary: Dysmenorrhea

Neuromuscular & skeletal: Paresthesia, tremor, myalgia, weakness, back pain, arthralgia

Ocular: Abnormal vision, eye pain

Otic: Hyperacusis

Miscellaneous: Parosmia

1% (Limited to important or life-threatening): Alopecia, angina, ataxia, bundle branch block, dysarthria, dystonia, eosinophilia, facial paralysis, glaucoma, intestinal obstruction, paresthesia, pericardial effusion, ptosis, pulmonary embolus, syncope, urinary retention, ventricular tachycardia

Overdosage/Toxicology Symptoms include CNS depression, ranging from drowsiness to coma. Mild overdose is associated with drowsiness, confusion, and lethargy. Serious case may result in ataxia, respiratory depression, hypotension, hypotonia, coma, and rarely death. Treatment is supportive.

Pharmacodynamics/Kinetics

Absorption: Rapid and almost complete

Bioavailability: 30%

Half-Life Elimination: 1 hour

Time to Peak: Serum: 1 hour

Metabolism: Extensive, primarily via aldehyde oxidase to form 5-oxo-zaleplon and to a lesser extent by CYP3A4 to desethylzaleplon; all metabolites are pharmacologically inactive

Onset: Rapid; Peak effect: ~1 hour

Duration: 6-8 hours

Formulations Capsule: 5 mg, 10 mg [contains tartrazine]

Dosing

Adults: Insomnia (short-term use): Oral: 10 mg at bedtime (range: 5-20 mg); has been used for up to 5 weeks of treatment in controlled trial setting

Elderly: Reduce dose to 5 mg at bedtime

Renal Impairment: No adjustment for mild to moderate renal impairment; use in severe renal impairment has not been adequately studied.

Hepatic Impairment: Mild to moderate impairment: 5 mg; not recommended for use in patients with severe hepatic impairment.

Administration

Oral: Administer immediately before bedtime or when the patient is in bed and cannot fall asleep.

Stability

Storage: Store at controlled room temperature of 20°C to 25°C (68°F to 77°F); protect from light

Monitoring and Teaching Issues

Physical Assessment: Evaluate etiology of insomnia; failure of sleep disturbance after 7-10 days may indicate psychiatric and/or medical illness. Assess effectiveness and interactions of other medications (see Drug Interactions). See Warnings/Precautions for use cautions. Evaluate risk for suicide, and assess for history of addiction (long-term use may result in dependence, abuse, or tolerance). Prescription quantities should not exceed a 1 month supply; monitor therapeutic response and periodically evaluate need for continued use. Assess knowledge/teach patient appropriate use, interventions to reduce side effects, and adverse reactions to report (see Patient Education). **Pregnancy risk factor C** - benefits of use should outweigh possible risks. Breast-feeding is not recommended.

Patient Education: Take exactly as directed; immediately before bedtime, or when you cannot fall asleep. Do not alter dosage or frequency, may be habit forming. Avoid alcohol and other prescription or OTC medications (especially medications to relieve pain, induce sleep, reduce anxiety, treat or prevent cold, coughs, or allergies) unless approved by

(Continued)

Zaleplon *(Continued)*

prescriber. You may experience drowsiness, dizziness, somnolence, vertigo, lightheadedness, blurred vision (avoid driving or engaging in activities that require alertness until response to drug is known); photosensitivity (avoid exposure to direct sunlight, wear protective clothing, and sunscreen); nausea or GI discomfort (small, frequent meals, good mouth care, chewing gum, or sucking hard candy may help); constipation (increase exercise, fluids, fruit, or fiber may help); or menstrual disturbances (reversible when drug is discontinued). Discontinue drug and report any severe CNS disturbances (hallucinations, acute nervousness or anxiety, persistent sleepiness or lethargy, impaired coordination, amnesia, or impaired thought processes); skin rash or irritation; eye pain or major vision changes; difficulty breathing; chest pain; ear pain; or muscle weakness or pain. **Pregnancy/breast-feeding precautions:** Inform prescriber if you are or intend to become pregnant. Breast-feeding is not recommended.

Additional Information Prescription quantities should not exceed a 1-month supply.

Zanaflex® *see* Tizanidine *on page 1328*

Zanamivir (za NA mi veer)

U.S. Brand Names Relenza®

Generic Available No

Pharmacologic Category Antiviral Agent; Neuraminidase Inhibitor

Pregnancy Risk Factor C

Lactation Excretion in breast milk unknown/use caution

Use Treatment of uncomplicated acute illness due to influenza virus in adults and children ≥7 years of age. Treatment should only be initiated in patients who have been symptomatic for no more than 2 days.

Use - Unlabeled/Investigational Investigational: Prophylaxis against influenza A/B infections

Mechanism of Action/Effect Zanamivir inhibits influenza virus neuraminidase enzymes, potentially altering virus particle aggregation and release.

Contraindications Hypersensitivity to zanamivir or any component of the formulation

Warnings/Precautions Patients must be instructed in the use of the delivery system. No data are available to support the use of this drug in patients who begin treatment after 48 hours of symptoms, as a prophylactic treatment for influenza, or in patients with significant underlying medical conditions. Bronchospasm, decreased lung function, and other serious adverse reactions, including those with fatal outcomes, have been reported. Not recommended for use in patients with underlying chronic airway disease, such as asthma or COPD, due to lack of efficacy and risk of serious adverse effects. For a patient with an underlying airway disease where a medical decision has been made to use zanamivir, a fast-acting bronchodilator should be made available, and used prior to each dose. Discontinue if bronchospasm occur or if there is a decline in respiratory function. Consider primary or concomitant bacterial infections. Not a substitute for influenza vaccine. Pregnancy risk C.

Drug Interactions

Decreased Effect: No clinically significant pharmacokinetic interactions are predicted.

Increased Effect/Toxicity: No clinically significant pharmacokinetic interactions are predicted.

Adverse Reactions Most adverse reactions occurred at a frequency which was equal to the control (lactose vehicle).

>1.5%:

- Central nervous system: Headache (2%), dizziness (2%)
- Gastrointestinal: Nausea (3%), diarrhea (3% adults, 2% children), vomiting (1% adults, 2% children)
- Respiratory: Sinusitis (3%), bronchitis (2%), cough (2%), other nasal signs and symptoms (2%), infection (ear, nose, and throat; 2% adults, 5% children)

<1.5% (Limited to important or life-threatening): Allergic or allergic-like reaction (including oropharyngeal edema), arrhythmias, bronchospasm, dyspnea, facial edema, rash (including serious cutaneous reactions), seizures, syncope, urticaria

Overdosage/Toxicology Information is limited, and symptoms appear similar to reported adverse events from clinical studies.

Pharmacodynamics/Kinetics

Absorption: Inhalation: 4% to 17%

Half-Life Elimination: Serum: 2.5-5.1 hours

Metabolism: None

Formulations Powder for oral inhalation: 5 mg/blister (20s) [4 blisters per Rotadisk®, 5 Rotadisk® per package]

Dosing

Adults & Elderly:

Influenza treatment: 2 inhalations (10 mg total) twice daily for 5 days. Two doses should be taken on the first day of dosing, regardless of interval, while doses should be spaced by approximately 12 hours on subsequent days.

Prophylaxis of influenza (investigational use): 2 inhalations (10 mg) once daily for duration of exposure period (6 weeks has been used in clinical trial)

Pediatrics: Influenza treatment: Children ≥7 years: Refer to adult dosing.

Administration

Inhalation: Must be used with Diskhaler® delivery device. Patients who are scheduled to use an inhaled bronchodilator should use their bronchodilator prior to zanamivir.

Stability

Storage: Store at room temperature (25°C) 77°F. Do not puncture blister until taking a dose using the Diskhaler®.

Monitoring and Teaching Issues

Physical Assessment: This is **not** a substitute for the influenza vaccine. Therapy must be started within 48 hours of first influenza symptoms. Teach patient appropriate use (inhalation device), interventions to reduce side effects, and adverse reactions to report (see Adverse Reactions and Patient Education). **Pregnancy risk factor C** - benefits of use should outweigh possible risks. Note breast-feeding caution.

Patient Education: Use delivery device exactly as directed; complete full 5-day regimen, even if symptoms improve sooner. If you have asthma or COPD you may be at risk for bronchospasm; see prescriber for appropriate bronchodilator before using zanamivir. Stop using this medication and contact your physician if you experience shortness of breath, increased wheezing, or other signs of bronchospasm. You may experience dizziness or headache (use caution when driving or engaging in hazardous tasks until response to drug is known). Report unresolved diarrhea, vomiting, or nausea; acute fever or muscle pain; or other acute and persistent adverse effects. **Pregnancy/breast-feeding precautions:** Inform prescriber if you are or intend to become pregnant. Consult prescriber if breast-feeding.

Breast-feeding Issues: Zanamivir has been shown to be excreted in the milk of animals, but its excretion in human milk is unknown. Caution should be used when zanamivir is administered to a nursing mother.

Additional Information Majority of patients included in clinical trials were infected with influenza A, however, a number of patients with influenza B infections were also enrolled. Patients with lower temperature or less severe symptoms appeared to derive less benefit from therapy. No consistent treatment benefit was demonstrated in patients with chronic underlying medical conditions.

Zanosar® *see* Streptozocin *on page 1251*

Zantac® *see* Ranitidine *on page 1172*

Zantac® 75 [OTC] *see* Ranitidine *on page 1172*

Zarontin® *see* Ethosuximide *on page 533*

Zaroxolyn® *see* Metolazone *on page 891*

ZDV *see* Zidovudine *on page 1419*

ZDV, Abacavir, and Lamivudine *see* Abacavir, Lamivudine, and Zidovudine *on page 31*

Zeasorb®-AF [OTC] *see* Miconazole *on page 899*

Zebeta® *see* Bisoprolol *on page 171*

Zeldox *see* Ziprasidone *on page 1424*

Zelnorm™ *see* Tegaserod *on page 1278*

Zemplar™ *see* Paricalcitol *on page 1036*

Zemuron® *see* Rocuronium *on page 1203*

Zenapax® *see* Daclizumab *on page 354*

Zephrex® *see* Guaifenesin and Pseudoephedrine *on page 648*

Zephrex LA® *see* Guaifenesin and Pseudoephedrine *on page 648*

Zerit® *see* Stavudine *on page 1245*

Zestoretic® *see* Lisinopril and Hydrochlorothiazide *on page 810*

Zestril® *see* Lisinopril *on page 808*

Ziac® *see* Bisoprolol and Hydrochlorothiazide *on page 172*

Ziagen® *see* Abacavir *on page 30*

Zidovudine (zye DOE vyoo deen)

U.S. Brand Names Retrovir®

Synonyms Azidothymidine; AZT; Compound S; ZDV

Generic Available No

Pharmacologic Category Antiretroviral Agent, Reverse Transcriptase Inhibitor (Nucleoside)

Pregnancy Risk Factor C

Lactation Enters breast milk/not recommended

Use Management of patients with HIV infections in combination with at least two other antiretroviral agents; for prevention of maternal/fetal HIV transmission as monotherapy

Mechanism of Action/Effect Zidovudine is a thymidine analog which interferes with the HIV virus that results in inhibition of viral replication.

Contraindications Life-threatening hypersensitivity to zidovudine or any component of the formulation

Warnings/Precautions Often associated with hematologic toxicity including granulocytopenia, severe anemia requiring transfusions, or (rarely) pancytopenia. Use with caution in patients with bone marrow compromise (granulocytes <1000 cells/mm^3 or hemoglobin <9.5 mg/dL); dosage adjustment may be required in patients who develop anemia or neutropenia. Lactic acidosis and severe hepatomegaly with steatosis have been reported, including fatal cases; use with caution in patients with risk factors for liver disease (risk may be increased in obese patients or prolonged exposure) and suspend treatment with zidovudine in any patient who develops clinical or laboratory findings suggestive of lactic acidosis (transaminase elevation may/may not accompany hepatomegaly and steatosis). Prolonged use has been associated with symptomatic myopathy. Reduce dose in patients with renal impairment. Pregnancy risk C.

Drug Interactions

Cytochrome P450 Effect: Substrate of CYP2A6, 2C8/9, 2C19, 3A4

Decreased Effect: *In vitro* evidence suggests zidovudine's antiretroviral activity may be antagonized by doxorubicin, ribavirin, and/or stavudine; avoid concurrent use.

Increased Effect/Toxicity: Coadministration of zidovudine with drugs that are nephrotoxic (amphotericin B), cytotoxic (flucytosine, vincristine, vinblastine, doxorubicin, interferon), inhibit glucuronidation or excretion (acetaminophen, cimetidine, indomethacin, lorazepam, probenecid, aspirin), or interfere with RBC/WBC number or function (acyclovir, ganciclovir, pentamidine, dapsone). Clarithromycin may increase blood levels of zidovudine (although total body exposure was unaffected, peak plasma concentrations were increased).

(Continued)

Zidovudine *(Continued)*

Valproic acid significantly increases zidovudine's blood levels (believed due to inhibition first pass metabolism). Concomitant use of ribavirin and nucleoside analogues may increase the risk of developing lactic acidosis (includes adefovir, didanosine, lamivudine, stavudine, zalcitabine, zidovudine).

Adverse Reactions

>10%:

Central nervous system: Severe headache (42%), fever (16%)

Dermatologic: Rash (17%)

Gastrointestinal: Nausea (46% to 61%), anorexia (11%), diarrhea (17%), pain (20%), vomiting (6% to 25%)

Hematologic: Anemia (23% in children), leukopenia, granulocytopenia (39% in children)

Neuromuscular & skeletal: Weakness (19%)

1% to 10%:

Central nervous system: Malaise (8%), dizziness (6%), insomnia (5%), somnolence (8%)

Dermatologic: Hyperpigmentation of nails (bluish-brown)

Gastrointestinal: Dyspepsia (5%)

Hematologic: Changes in platelet count

Neuromuscular & skeletal: Paresthesia (6%)

<1% (Limited to important or life-threatening): Bone marrow suppression, cholestatic jaundice, confusion, granulocytopenia, gynecomastia, hepatotoxicity, mania, myopathy, neurotoxicity, oral pigmentation changes, pancytopenia, seizures, tenderness, thrombocytopenia

Overdosage/Toxicology Symptoms of overdose include nausea, vomiting, ataxia, and granulocytopenia. Erythropoietin, thymidine, and cyanocobalamin have been used experimentally to treat zidovudine-induced hematopoietic toxicity, yet none are presently specified as the agent of choice. Treatment is supportive.

Pharmacodynamics/Kinetics

Absorption: Oral: 66% to 70%

Half-Life Elimination: Terminal: 60 minutes

Time to Peak: Serum: 30-90 minutes

Metabolism: Hepatic via glucuronidation to inactive metabolites; extensive first-pass effect

Formulations

Capsule: 100 mg

Injection, solution: 10 mg/mL (20 mL)

Syrup: 50 mg/5 mL (240 mL) [contains sodium benzoate; strawberry flavor]

Tablet: 300 mg

Dosing

Adults & Elderly:

Prevention of maternal-fetal HIV transmission: Maternal (may delay treatment until after 10-12 weeks gestation): Oral (per HIV/ATIS 2001 guidelines): 200 mg 3 times/day or 300 mg twice daily until the start of labor

During labor and delivery, administer zidovudine I.V. at 2 mg/kg over 1 hour followed by a continuous I.V. infusion of 1 mg/kg/hour until the umbilical cord is clamped

HIV infection:

Oral: 300 mg twice daily or 200 mg 3 times/day

I.V.: 1-2 mg/kg/dose (infused over 1 hour) administered every 4 hours around-the-clock (6 doses/day)

Prevention of HIV following needlesticks: Oral: 200 mg 3 times/day plus lamivudine 150 mg twice daily; a protease inhibitor (eg, indinavir) may be added for high risk exposures; begin therapy within 2 hours of exposure if possible

Note: Patients should receive I.V. therapy only until oral therapy can be administered

Pediatrics:

Prevention of maternal-fetal HIV transmission:

Neonatal: Oral: 2 mg/kg/dose every 6 hours for 6 weeks beginning 6-12 hours after birth; infants unable to receive oral dosing may receive 1.5 mg/kg I.V. infused over 30 minutes every 6 hours

Maternal (may delay treatment until after 10-12 weeks gestation): Oral (per HIV/ATIS 2001 guidelines): 200 mg 3 times/day or 300 mg twice daily until start of labor

During labor and delivery, administer zidovudine I.V. at 2 mg/kg over 1 hour followed by a continuous I.V. infusion of 1 mg/kg/hour until the umbilical cord is clamped

Treatment of HIV infection:

Oral: Children 3 months to 12 years:

160 mg/m^2/dose every 8 hours; dosage range: 90 mg/m^2/dose to 180 mg/m^2/dose every 6-8 hours; some Working Group members use a dose of 180 mg/m^2 every 12 hours when using in drug combinations with other antiretroviral compounds, but data on this dosing in children is limited

I.V. continuous infusion: 20 mg/m^2/hour

I.V. intermittent infusion: 120 mg/m^2/dose every 6 hours

Renal Impairment: Cl_{cr} <10 mL/minute: May require minor dose adjustment.

Hemodialysis: At least partially removed by hemo- and peritoneal dialysis. Administer dose after hemodialysis or administer 100 mg supplemental dose. During CAPD, dose as for Cl_{cr} <10 mL/minute.

Continuous arteriovenous or venovenous hemodiafiltration effects: Administer 100 mg every 8 hours.

Hepatic Impairment: Reduce dose by 50% or double dosing interval in patients with cirrhosis.

Administration

Oral: Administer around-the-clock to promote less variation in peak and trough serum levels. Oral zidovudine may be administered without regard to food.

I.M.: Do not give I.M.

I.V.: Infuse over 1 hour. Avoid rapid infusion or bolus injection.

Stability

Storage: Store undiluted vials at room temperature and protect from light.

Reconstitution: After dilution to ≤4 mg/mL, the solution is physically and chemically stable for 24 hours at room temperature and 48 hours if refrigerated. Attempt to administer diluted solution within 8 hours, if stored at room temperature or 24 hours if refrigerated to minimize potential for microbially contaminated solutions.

Compatibility: Stable in D_5W, NS; incompatible with blood products and protein solutions

Monitoring Laboratory Tests Monitor CBC and platelet count at least every 2 weeks, MCV, serum creatinine kinase, CD4 cell count

Monitoring and Teaching Issues

Physical Assessment: See Warnings/Precautions and Dosing for use cautions. Assess potential for interactions with other prescriptions, OTC medications, or herbal products patient may be taking (see Drug Interactions). Assess results of laboratory tests (see above) and patient response (eg, CNS changes, hematological changes, and gastrointestinal disturbances - see Adverse Reactions and Overdose/Toxicology) on a regular basis throughout therapy. Teach patient proper use (see Administration, Storage, and Reconstitution), possible side effects and interventions, and adverse symptoms to report (see Patient Education). **Pregnancy risk factor C** - benefits of use should outweigh possible risks. Breast-feeding is not recommended.

Patient Education: Inform prescriber of all prescriptions, OTC medications, or herbal products you are taking, and any allergies you have. Do not take anything new during treatment unless approved by prescriber. This drug will not cure HIV; use appropriate precautions to prevent spread of HIV to other persons. Take as directed; may be taken without regard to food. Take around-the-clock. Maintain adequate hydration (2-3 L/day of fluids) unless advised by prescriber to restrict fluids. You may be more susceptible to infection (avoid crowds and exposure to infection and do not have any vaccinations unless approved by prescriber). May cause headache or insomnia; if these persist notify prescriber. Report unresolved nausea or vomiting; signs of infection (eg, fever, chills, sore throat, burning urination, flu-like symptoms, fatigue); unusual bleeding (eg, tarry stools, easy bruising, or blood in stool, urine, or mouth); pain, tingling, or numbness of toes or fingers; skin rash or irritation; or muscle weakness or tremors. **Pregnancy/breast-feeding precautions:** Inform prescriber if you are or intend to become pregnant. Breast-feeding is not recommended.

Dietary Issues: May be taken without regard to food.

Breast-feeding Issues: HIV-infected mothers are discouraged from breast-feeding to decrease potential transmission of HIV.

Pregnancy Issues: Zidovudine crosses the placenta. The use of zidovudine reduces the maternal-fetal transmission of HIV by ~70% and should be considered for antenatal and intrapartum therapy whenever possible. In HIV infected mothers not previously on antiretroviral therapy, treatment may be delayed until after 10-12 weeks gestation. Cases of lactic acidosis/hepatic steatosis syndrome have been reported in pregnant women receiving nucleoside analogues. It is not known if pregnancy itself potentiates this known side effect; however, pregnant women may be at increased risk of lactic acidosis and liver damage. Hepatic enzymes and electrolytes should be monitored frequently during the 3rd trimester of pregnancy in women receiving nucleoside analogues. Health professionals are encouraged to contact the antiretroviral pregnancy registry to monitor outcomes of pregnant women exposed to antiretroviral medications (1-800-258-4263).

Other Issues: Anemia occurs usually after 4-6 weeks of therapy. Dose adjustments and/or transfusions may be required.

Additional Information Potential compliance problems, frequency of administration and adverse effects should be discussed with patients before initiating therapy to help prevent the emergence of resistance.

Zidovudine, Abacavir, and Lamivudine *see* Abacavir, Lamivudine, and Zidovudine *on page 31*

Zidovudine and Lamivudine (zye DOE vyoo deen & la MI vyoo deen)

U.S. Brand Names Combivir®

Synonyms AZT + 3TC; Lamivudine and Zidovudine

Generic Available No

Pharmacologic Category Antiretroviral Agent, Reverse Transcriptase Inhibitor (Nucleoside)

Pregnancy Risk Factor C

Lactation Enters breast milk/contraindicated

Use Treatment of HIV infection when therapy is warranted based on clinical and/or immunological evidence of disease progression. Combivir® given twice daily, provides an alternative regimen to lamivudine 150 mg twice daily plus zidovudine 600 mg/day in divided doses; this drug form reduces capsule/tablet intake for these two drugs to 2 per day instead of up to 8.

Formulations Tablet: Zidovudine 300 mg and lamivudine 150 mg

Dosing

Adults: Treatment of HIV infection: Oral: 1 tablet twice daily. Because this is a fixed-dose combination product, avoid use in patients requiring dosage reduction including children <12 years of age, renally impaired patients with a creatinine clearance ≤50 mL/minute, patients with low body weight (<50 kg or 1110 pounds), or those experiencing dose-limiting adverse effects.

Elderly: Refer to Special Geriatric Considerations.

Pediatrics: Children >12 years: Refer to adult dosing.

Monitoring and Teaching Issues

Physical Assessment: See individual components listed in Related Information. **Pregnancy risk factor C** - benefits of use should outweigh possible risks. Breast-feeding is contraindicated.

Patient Education: Combivir® is not a cure for HIV and you may continue to experience HIV-associated illness. Major toxicities are neutropenia and/or anemia; have blood counts

(Continued)

Zidovudine and Lamivudine *(Continued)*

checked regularly while on therapy. **Pregnancy/breast-feeding precautions:** Inform prescriber if you are or intend to become pregnant. Do not breast-feed.

Related Information

Lamivudine *on page 768*
Zidovudine *on page 1419*

Zilactin®-B [OTC] *see* Benzocaine *on page 156*
Zilactin® Baby [OTC] *see* Benzocaine *on page 156*
Zilactin-L® [OTC] *see* Lidocaine *on page 800*

Zileuton (zye LOO ton)

U.S. Brand Names Zyflo™

Generic Available No

Pharmacologic Category 5-Lipoxygenase Inhibitor

Pregnancy Risk Factor C

Lactation Excretion in breast milk unknown

Use Prophylaxis and chronic treatment of asthma in children ≥12 years of age and adults

Mechanism of Action/Effect Specific inhibitor of 5-lipoxygenase and thus inhibits leukotriene (LTB1, LTC1, LTD1 and LTE1) formation. Leukotrienes are substances that induce numerous biological effects including augmentation of neutrophil and eosinophil migration, neutrophil and monocyte aggregation, leukocyte adhesion, increased capillary permeability and smooth muscle contraction.

Contraindications Hypersensitivity to zileuton or any component of the formulation; active liver disease or transaminase elevations greater than or equal to three times the upper limit of normal (≥3 x ULN)

Warnings/Precautions Elevations of one or more liver function tests may occur during therapy. These laboratory abnormalities may progress, remain unchanged or resolve with continued therapy. Use with caution in patients who consume substantial quantities of ethanol or have a past history of liver disease. Zileuton is not indicated for use in the reversal of bronchospasm in acute asthma attacks, including status asthmaticus. Zileuton can be continued during acute exacerbations of asthma. Pregnancy risk C.

Drug Interactions

Cytochrome P450 Effect: Substrate of CYP1A2, 2C8/9, 3A4; Inhibits CYP1A2

Increased Effect/Toxicity: Zileuton increases concentrations/effects of of beta-blockers (propranolol), theophylline, and warfarin. Potentially, it may increase levels of many drugs, including cisapride, due to inhibition of CYP3A4.

Nutritional/Ethanol Interactions

Ethanol: Avoid ethanol (may increase CNS depression).

Herb/Nutraceutical: St John's wort may decrease zileuton levels.

Adverse Reactions

>10%:
- Central nervous system: Headache (24.6%)
- Hepatic: ALT elevation (12%)

1% to 10%:
- Cardiovascular: Chest pain
- Central nervous system: Pain, dizziness, fever, insomnia, malaise, nervousness, somnolence
- Gastrointestinal: Dyspepsia, nausea, abdominal pain, constipation, flatulence
- Hematologic: Low white blood cell count
- Neuromuscular & skeletal: Myalgia, arthralgia, weakness
- Ocular: Conjunctivitis

<1% (Limited to important or life-threatening): Rash, urticaria

Overdosage/Toxicology Symptoms of overdose: Human experience is limited. Oral minimum lethal doses in mice and rats were 500-1000 mg/kg and 300-1000 mg/kg, respectively (providing >3 and 9 times the systemic exposure achieved at the maximum recommended human daily oral dose, respectively). No deaths occurred, but nephritis was reported in dogs at an oral dose of 1000 mg/kg. Treat symptomatically; institute supportive measures as required.

Pharmacodynamics/Kinetics

Absorption: Rapid

Bioavailability: Unknown

Half-Life Elimination: 2.5 hours

Time to Peak: Serum: 1.7 hours

Metabolism: Several metabolites in plasma and urine; metabolized via CYP1A2, 2C9, and 3A4

Formulations Tablet: 600 mg

Dosing

Adults & Elderly: Asthma: Oral: 600 mg 4 times/day with meals and at bedtime

Pediatrics: Asthma: Oral: Children ≥12 years: Refer to adult dosing.

Renal Impairment: Dosing adjustment is **not** necessary in renal impairment or renal failure (even during dialysis).

Hepatic Impairment: Contraindicated in patients with active liver disease.

Administration

Oral: Can be administered without regard to meals (ie, with or without food).

Monitoring Laboratory Tests Liver function tests

Monitoring and Teaching Issues

Physical Assessment: Not for use to relieve acute asthmatic attacks. Assess effectiveness and interactions of other medications patient may be taking (see Drug Interactions). See Contraindications and Warnings/Precautions for use cautions. Monitor results of laboratory tests, effectiveness of therapy, and adverse reactions (see Adverse Reactions) at beginning of therapy and periodically with long-term use. For inpatient care, monitor vital signs and lung sounds prior to and periodically during therapy. Assess knowledge/teach patient appropriate use, interventions to reduce side effects, and adverse symptoms to report (see Patient Education). **Pregnancy risk factor C** - benefits of use should outweigh possible risks. Note breast-feeding caution.

Patient Education: This medication is not for an acute asthmatic attack; in acute attack, follow instructions of prescriber. Do not stop other asthma medication unless advised by prescriber. Take with meals and at bedtime on a continuous bases; do not discontinue even if feeling better (this medication may help reduce incidence of acute attacks). Avoid alcohol and other medications unless approved by your prescriber. You may experience mild headache (mild analgesic may help); fatigue or dizziness (use caution when driving); or nausea or heartburn (small, frequent meals, frequent mouth care, sucking lozenges, or chewing gum may help). Report persistent headache, chest pain, rapid heartbeat, or palpitations; skin rash or itching; unusual bleeding (eg, tarry stools, easy bruising, or blood in stool, urine, or mouth); skin rash or irritation; muscle weakness or tremors; redness, irritation, or infections of the eye; or worsening of asthmatic condition. **Pregnancy/breast-feeding precautions:** Inform prescriber if you are or intend to become pregnant. Consult prescriber if breast-feeding.

Geriatric Considerations: No differences in the pharmacokinetics found between younger adults and elderly; no dosage adjustments necessary. However, monitor liver effects closely as with any patient regardless of age.

Breast-feeding Issues: Zileuton and its metabolites are excreted in rat milk; it is not known if zileuton is excreted in breast milk.

Pregnancy Issues: Developmental studies indicated adverse effects (reduced body weight and increased skeletal variations) in rats at an oral dose of 300 mg/kg/day. There are no adequate and well controlled studies in pregnant women.

Zinacef® *see* Cefuroxime *on page 255*

Zinc Acetate *see* Zinc Supplements *on page 1423*

Zinca-Pak® Zincate® *see* Zinc Supplements *on page 1423*

Zinc Carbonate *see* Zinc Supplements *on page 1423*

Zinc Chloride *see* Zinc Supplements *on page 1423*

Zinc Gluconate *see* Zinc Supplements *on page 1423*

Zinc Sulfate *see* Zinc Supplements *on page 1423*

Zinc Supplements (zink SUP la ments)

U.S. Brand Names Cold-eze® [OTC]; Eye-Sed® [OTC]; Orazinc® [OTC]; Verazinc® [OTC]; Zinca-Pak® Zincate®

Synonyms Zinc Acetate; Zinc Carbonate; Zinc Chloride; Zinc Gluconate; Zinc Sulfate

Generic Available Yes

Pharmacologic Category Mineral, Oral; Mineral, Parenteral; Trace Element

Pregnancy Risk Factor C (A for zinc acetate)

Lactation Excretion in breast milk unknown/compatible

Use Cofactor for replacement therapy to different enzymes helps maintain normal growth rates, normal skin hydration and senses of taste and smell; zinc supplement (oral and parenteral) for treatment and prevention of zinc deficiency states; may improve wound healing in those who are deficient; promote wound healing in patients with pressure sores; lozenges are used to diminish symptoms and duration of the common cold; maintenance treatment of Wilson's disease (zinc acetate)

Mechanism of Action/Effect Provides for normal growth and tissue repair; cofactor for more than 70 enzymes which are important to carbohydrate and protein metabolism; helps to maintain normal growth and tissue repair, normal skin hydration, and senses of taste and smell; in Wilson's disease, zinc cation inhibits the absorption of dietary copper by inducing the synthesis of metallothionein, a metal-binding protein present in the intestinal mucosa, which binds metals, including copper, forming a nontoxic complex that is not absorbed systematically but excreted in the stool; ophthalmic astringent and weak antiseptic due to precipitation of protein and clearing mucus from outer surface of the eye

Contraindications Hypersensitivity to zinc salts or any component

Warnings/Precautions Do not administer undiluted by direct injection into a peripheral vein because of potential for phlebitis, tissue irritation, and potential to increase renal loss of minerals from a bolus injection. Administration of zinc in absence of copper may decrease plasma copper levels. Excessive dose may increase HDL and impair immune system function.

Drug Interactions

Decreased Effect: Decreased penicillamine and tetracycline effect. Iron may decrease the uptake of zinc. Bran products, dairy products reduce absorption of zinc.

Nutritional/Ethanol Interactions Zinc serum concentration may be decreased if taken with food, dairy products, or caffeine.

Adverse Reactions

Frequency not defined:

- Cardiovascular: Tachycardia (excessive doses)
- Central nervous system: Hypothermia (excessive doses)
- Ocular: Blurred vision (excessive doses)
- Miscellaneous: Profuse diaphoresis

<1% (Limited to important or life-threatening symptoms): Hypotension, indigestion, nausea, vomiting, neutropenia, leukopenia, jaundice, pulmonary edema

Overdosage/Toxicology Symptoms of overdose include hypotension, pulmonary edema, diarrhea, vomiting, oliguria, nausea, gastric ulcers, restlessness, dizziness, profuse sweating, decreased consciousness, blurred vision, tachycardia, hypothermia, hyperamylasemia, and jaundice.

This agent is corrosive and emesis or gastric lavage should be avoided, instead dilute rapidly with milk or water. Calcium disodium edetate or dimercaprol can be very effective at binding zinc. Supportive care should always be instituted.

(Continued)

Zinc Supplements *(Continued)*

Pharmacodynamics/Kinetics

Absorption: Poor from GI tract (20% to 30%)

Formulations

Zinc acetate: Zinc acetate: Capsule (Galzin™): 25 mg elemental zinc, 50 mg elemental zinc

Zinc carbonate, complex: Liquid: 15 mg/mL (30 mL)

Zinc chloride: Injection: 1 mg/mL (10 mL)

Zinc gluconate (14.3% zinc): Tablet: 10 mg (elemental zinc 1.4 mg), 15 mg (elemental zinc 2 mg), 50 mg (elemental zinc 7 mg), 78 mg (elemental zinc 11 mg)

Zinc sulfate (23% zinc):

Capsule: 110 mg (elemental zinc 25 mg), 220 mg (elemental zinc 50 mg)

Injection: 1 mg/mL (10 mL, 30 mL); 4 mg/mL (10 mL); 5 mg/mL (5 mL, 10 mL)

Tablet: 66 mg (elemental zinc 15 mg), 110 mg (elemental zinc 25 mg), 200 mg (elemental zinc 45 mg)

Dosing

Adults & Elderly: Clinical response may not occur for up to 6-8 weeks.

RDA: Oral: Male: 15 mg **elemental** zinc/day; Female: 12 mg **elemental** zinc/day

Zinc deficiency: Oral: 25-50 mg **elemental** zinc/dose (110-220 mg zinc sulfate) 3 times/day

Supplement to parenteral nutrition solutions (clinical response may not occur for up to 6-8 weeks): I.V. (all doses are mcg of **elemental** zinc):

Stable metabolically: 2.5-4 mg **elemental** zinc/day; catabolic state: Increase by an additional 2 mg/day (eg, 4.5-6 mg **elemental** zinc/day)

Stable with fluid loss from small bowel: Additional 12.2 mg **elemental** zinc/L parenteral nutrition or 17.1 mg **elemental** zinc/kg of stool or ileostomy output

Wound healing: Oral: 50 mg **elemental** zinc (220 mg zinc sulfate) 3 times daily in patients with low serum zinc levels (<110 mcg/dL)

Pediatrics: Clinical response may not occur for up to 6-8 weeks.

RDA: Oral:

Neonates and Infants <12 months: 5 mg **elemental** zinc/day

Children 1-10 years: 10 mg **elemental** zinc/day

Children ≥11 years: Male: 15 mg **elemental** zinc/day; Female: 12 mg **elemental** zinc/day

Zinc deficiency: Oral: Infants and Children: 0.5-1 mg **elemental** zinc/kg/day divided 1-3 times/day; larger doses may be needed if impaired intestinal absorption or an excessive loss of zinc (eg, excessive, prolonged diarrhea)

Supplement to parenteral nutrition solutions (clinical response may not occur for up to 6-8 weeks): I.V. (all doses are mcg of **elemental** zinc):

Premature Infants: 400 mcg/kg/day

Term Infants <3 months: 300 mcg/kg/day

Infants ≥3 months and Children ≤5 years: 100 mcg/kg/day (maximum: 5 mg/day)

Children >5 years and Adolescents: 2-5 mg/day

Administration

Oral: Administer oral formulation with food if GI upset occurs; in patients with Wilson's disease, administer zinc acetate 1 hour before or after meals or beverage (except water); zinc acetate capsules should be swallowed whole; do not open or chew

I.V.: Dilute as component of daily parenteral nutrition or maintenance fluids. Do not give undiluted by direct injection into a peripheral vein due to potential for phlebitis and tissue irritation, and potential to increase renal losses of minerals from a bolus injection.

Monitoring Laboratory Tests Patients on TPN therapy should have periodic serum copper and serum zinc levels; alkaline phosphatase, taste acuity, mental depression, wound healing (if indicated), growth (if indicated), skin integrity; Wilson's disease: 24-hour urinary copper excretion, neuropsychiatric evaluations, LFTs

Monitoring and Teaching Issues

Physical Assessment: See Contraindications and Warnings/Precautions for use cautions. Assess effectiveness and interactions of other medications patient may be taking (see Drug Interactions). Assess knowledge/teach patient appropriate use and adverse symptoms to report (see Patient Education).

Patient Education: Take as directed; do not take more than recommended. Take with food; however, avoid foods high in calcium, phosphorous, or phytate. Stop medication and contact prescriber if you develop severe nausea or vomiting or acute indigestion; easy bruising or bleeding; persistent dizziness; or unusual respiratory difficulty. Lozenges are to be dissolved slowly in mouth.

Dietary Issues: Coffee, foods high in phytate (eg, whole grain cereals & legumes), bran, and dairy products reduce zinc absorption; avoid foods high in calcium or phosphorus.

Zinecard® *see* Dexrazoxane *on page 389*

Ziprasidone (zi PRAY si done)

U.S. Brand Names Geodon®

Synonyms Zeldox; Ziprasidone Hydrochloride; Ziprasidone Mesylate

Generic Available No

Pharmacologic Category Antipsychotic Agent, Benzylisothiazolylpiperazine

Pregnancy Risk Factor C

Lactation Excretion in breast milk unknown/not recommended

Use Treatment of schizophrenia

Use - Unlabeled/Investigational Tourette's syndrome

Mechanism of Action/Effect Blocks a number of CNS receptors, including dopamine, serotonin, alpha$_1$ adrenergic, and histamine receptors. Also inhibits reuptake of serotonin and epinephrine. Results in improvement in positive and negative symptoms of schizophrenia.

Contraindications Hypersensitivity to ziprasidone or any component of the formulation; history (or current) prolonged QT; congenital long QT syndrome; recent myocardial infarction; history of arrhythmias; uncompensated heart failure; concurrent use of other QT_c-prolonging agents including amiodarone, arsenic trioxide, chlorpromazine, cisapride, class Ia antiarrhythmics (quinidine, procainamide), dofetilide, dolasetron, droperidol, halofantrine, levomethadyl, mefloquine, mesoridazine, pentamidine, pimozide, some quinolone antibiotics (moxifloxacin, sparfloxacin, gatifloxacin), sotalol, tacrolimus, and thioridazine

Warnings/Precautions May result in QT_c prolongation (dose-related), which has been associated with the development of malignant ventricular arrhythmias (torsade de pointes) and sudden death. Observed prolongation was greater than with other atypical antipsychotic agents (risperidone, olanzapine, quetiapine), but less than with thioridazine. Avoid hypokalemia, hypomagnesemia. Use caution in patients with bradycardia. Discontinue in patients found to have persistent QT_c intervals >500 msec. Patients with symptoms of dizziness, palpitations, or syncope should receive further cardiac evaluation.

May cause extrapyramidal symptoms, including pseudoparkinsonism, acute dystonic reactions, akathisia, and tardive dyskinesia. Disturbances of temperature regulation have been reported with antipsychotics (not reported in premarketing trials of ziprasidone). Antipsychotic use may also be associated with neuroleptic malignant syndrome (NMS). Use with caution in patients at risk of seizures, including those with a history of seizures (head trauma, brain damage, alcoholism, or concurrent medications which may lower seizure threshold). Elderly patients may be at increased risk of seizures due to an increased prevalence of predisposing factors.

May cause orthostatic hypotension; use with caution in patients with cerebrovascular disease, cardiovascular disease, hypovolemia, or other medications which may predispose to orthostasis.

Cognitive and/or motor impairment (sedation) is common with ziprasidone, resulting in impaired performance of tasks requiring alertness (ie, operating machinery or driving). Use with caution in disorders where CNS depression is a feature. Use with caution in Parkinson's disease. Esophageal dysmotility and aspiration have been associated with antipsychotic use; use with caution in patients at risk of aspiration pneumonia (ie, Alzheimer's disease). Caution in breast cancer or other prolactin-dependent tumors (may elevate prolactin levels). Ziprasidone has been associated with a fairly high incidence of rash (5%); discontinue if alternative etiology is not identified. Safety and efficacy have not been established in pediatric patients.

I.M. administration: Use caution in patients with renal impairment.

Pregnancy risk C.

Drug Interactions

Cytochrome P450 Effect: Substrate of CYP1A2, 3A4; Inhibits CYP2D6, 3A4

Decreased Effect: Carbamazepine may decrease serum concentrations of ziprasidone. Other enzyme-inducing agents may share this potential. Amphetamines may decrease the efficacy of ziprasidone. Ziprasidone may inhibit the efficacy of levodopa.

Increased Effect/Toxicity:

Ketoconazole may increase serum concentrations of ziprasidone. Other CYP3A4 inhibitors may share this potential. Inhibitors include amiodarone, clarithromycin, erythromycin, delavirdine, diltiazem, dirithromycin, disulfiram, fluoxetine, fluvoxamine, grapefruit juice, indinavir, itraconazole, ketoconazole, nefazodone, nevirapine, propoxyphene, quinupristin-dalfopristin, ritonavir, saquinavir, verapamil, zafirlukast, zileuton

Concurrent use with QT_c-prolonging agents may result in additive effects on cardiac conduction, potentially resulting in malignant or lethal arrhythmias. Concurrent use is contraindicated. Includes amiodarone, arsenic trioxide, chlorpromazine, cisapride; class Ia antiarrhythmics (quinidine, procainamide); dofetilide, dolasetron, droperidol, halofantrine, levomethadyl, mefloquine, mesoridazine, pentamidine, pimozide; some quinolone antibiotics (moxifloxacin, sparfloxacin, gatifloxacin); sotalol, tacrolimus, and thioridazine. Potassium- or magnesium-depleting agents (diuretics, aminoglycosides, cyclosporine, and amphotericin B) may increase the risk of QT_c prolongation. Antihypertensive agents may increase the risk of orthostatic hypotension. CNS depressants may increase the degree of sedation caused by ziprasidone. Metoclopramide may increase risk of extrapyramidal symptoms (EPS).

Nutritional/Ethanol Interactions

Ethanol: Avoid ethanol (may increase CNS depression).

Food: Administration with food increases serum levels twofold. Grapefruit juice may increase serum concentration of ziprasidone.

Herb/Nutraceutical: St John's wort may decrease serum levels of ziprasidone, due to a potential effect on CYP3A4. This has not been specifically studied. Avoid kava kava, chamomile (may increase CNS depression).

Effects on Lab Values ↑ cholesterol, triglycerides, eosinophils

Adverse Reactions Note: Although minor QT_c prolongation (mean 10 msec at 160 mg/day) may occur more frequently (incidence not specified), clinically relevant prolongation (>500 msec) was rare (0.06%).

>10%:

Central nervous system: Somnolence (8% to 20%), headache (3% to 13%)

Gastrointestinal: Nausea (4% to 12%)

1% to 10%:

Cardiovascular: Bradycardia (2%), hypertension (2%), tachycardia (2%), postural hypotension (1% to 5%), vasodilation (1%)

Central nervous system: Akathisia (2% to 8%), dizziness (3% to 10%), extrapyramidal symptoms (2% to 5%), dystonia (4%), hypertonia (3%), insomnia (3%), agitation (2%), anxiety (2%), speech disorder (2%), psychosis (1%)

Dermatologic: Rash (with urticaria, 4% to 5%), fungal dermatitis (2%), furunculosis (2%)

Endocrine & metabolic: Dysmenorrhea (2%)

Gastrointestinal: Constipation (2% to 9%), dyspepsia (1% to 8%), diarrhea (3% to 5%), xerostomia (1% to 4%), vomiting (3%), abdominal pain (2%), anorexia (2%), weight gain (10%), rectal hemorrhage (2%)

Genitourinary: Priapism (1%)

Local: Pain at injection site (7% to 9%)

(Continued)

Ziprasidone *(Continued)*

Neuromuscular & skeletal: Weakness (2% to 5%), paresthesia (2%), cogwheel rigidity (1%), hypertonia (1%), myalgia (1%)

Ocular: Abnormal vision (3%)

Respiratory: Respiratory disorder (8%, primarily cold symptoms, upper respiratory infection), rhinitis (1% to 4%), cough increased (3%)

Miscellaneous: Accidental injury (4%), diaphoresis (2%)

<1% (Limited to important or life-threatening): Akinesia, angina, atrial fibrillation, ataxia, AV block (first degree), bundle branch block, cerebral infarction, cholestatic jaundice, choreoathetosis, delirium, dysarthria, dyskinesia, dysphagia, dyspnea, eosinophilia, exfoliative dermatitis, gout, gynecomastia, hemorrhage, hepatitis, jaundice, myocarditis, neuropathy, oculogyric crisis, opisthotonos, photophobia, photosensitivity reaction, pneumonia, pulmonary embolism, QT_c prolongation >500 msec (0.06%), seizure (0.4%), sexual dysfunction (male and female), stroke, syncope (0.6%), tenosynovitis, thrombocytopenia, thyroiditis, torticollis, urinary retention, withdrawal syndrome

Overdosage/Toxicology Reported symptoms include somnolence, slurring of speech, and hypertension. Acute extrapyramidal symptoms may also occur. Treatment is symptom-directed and supportive. Not removed by dialysis.

Pharmacodynamics/Kinetics

Absorption: Well absorbed

Bioavailability: Oral (with food): 60% (up to twofold increase with food); I.M.: 100%

Half-Life Elimination: Oral: 7 hours; I.M.: 2-5 hours

Time to Peak: Oral: 6-8 hours; I.M.: ≤60 minutes

Metabolism: Extensively hepatic, primarily via aldehyde oxidase; less than 1/3 of total metabolism via CYP3A4 and CYP1A2 (minor)

Formulations

Capsule, as hydrochloride: 20 mg, 40 mg, 60 mg, 80 mg

Injection, powder for reconstitution, as mesylate: 20 mg

Dosing

Adults: Psychosis:

Oral: Initial: 20 mg twice daily (with food)

Adjustment: Increases (if indicated) should be made no more frequently than every 2 days; ordinarily patients should be observed for improvement over several weeks before adjusting the dose.

Maintenance: Range 20-100 mg twice daily; however, dosages >80 mg twice daily are generally not recommended.

I.M.: 10 mg every 2 hours **or** 20 mg every 4 hours; maximum: 40 mg/day; oral therapy should replace I.M. administration as soon as possible

Elderly: No dosage adjustment is recommended; consider initiating at a low end of the dosage range, with slower titration.

Pediatrics: Children and adolescents: Tourette's syndrome (unlabeled use): Oral: 5-40 mg/day

Renal Impairment:

Oral: No dosage adjustment is recommended

I.M.: Cyclodextrin, an excipient in the I.M. formulation, is cleared by renal filtration; use with caution.

Hepatic Impairment: No adjustment necessary.

Administration

Oral: Administer with food.

Stability

Storage:

Capsule: Store at controlled room temperature of 15°C to 30°C (59°F to 86°F).

Vials for injection: Prior to reconstitution, store at controlled room temperature of 15°C to 30°C (59°F to 86°F); protect from light. Following reconstitution, injection may be stored at room temperature up to 24 hours, or up to 7 days if refrigerated; protect from light.

Reconstitution: Each vial should be reconstituted with 1.2 mL SWI; shake vigorously; will form a pale, pink solution containing 20 mg/mL ziprasidone.

Monitoring Laboratory Tests Serum potassium, magnesium, improvements in symptomatology. The value of routine ECG screening or monitoring has not been established. Potential for extrapyramidal symptoms. Fever, confusion, and/or stiffness should prompt evaluation of possible NMS.

Monitoring and Teaching Issues

Physical Assessment: Assess seizure risk (seizure history, ethanol use, head trauma, brain damage, or current therapy with medications that reduce seizure threshold) and cardiac status (bradycardia, QT prolongation) before starting therapy. Assess other medications patient may be taking for effectiveness and interactions (especially those dependent on cytochrome P450 metabolism - see Drug Interactions). See Contraindications, Warnings/Precautions, and Dosing for extensive use cautions. Monitor closely for therapeutic response and adverse reactions at beginning and at regular periods throughout therapy (see Adverse Reactions and Overdose/Toxicology). Assess knowledge/teach appropriate use of this medication, interventions to reduce side effects, and adverse symptoms to report (see Patient Education). **Pregnancy risk factor C** - benefits of use should outweigh possible risks. Breast-feeding is not recommended.

Patient Education: Use this mediation exactly as directed; do not alter dosage or discontinue without consulting prescriber - may take 2-3 weeks to achieve desired results. Do not share this medication with anyone else. Avoid alcohol, caffeine, grapefruit or grapefruit juice, other prescription or OTC medication unless approved by prescriber. Maintain adequate hydration (2-3 L/day of fluids) unless advised by prescriber to restrict fluids. You may experience drowsiness, lightheadedness, impaired coordination, dizziness, or blurred vision (use caution when driving or engaging in tasks hazardous tasks until response to drug is known); dry mouth, nausea, or GI upset (small, frequent meals, good mouth care, sucking lozenges or chewing gum may help); postural hypotension (rise slowly when changing position from lying or sitting to standing or when climbing stairs); urinary retention (void before taking medication); or constipation (increased exercise, fluids, fruit, or fiber may help). Report immediately persistent CNS effects (eg, trembling, altered gait or balance, excessive sedation, seizures, unusual muscle or skeletal movements, excessive anxiety, hallucinations, nightmares, suicidal thoughts, or confusion); swelling or pain in breasts (male or female); altered menstrual pattern; sexual dysfunction; alteration in urinary pattern; vision changes; rash; difficulty breathing; or chest pain or palpitations. **Pregnancy/breast-feeding precautions:** Inform prescriber if you are or intend to become pregnant. Do not breast-feed.

Pregnancy Issues: Developmental toxicity demonstrated in animals. There are no adequate and well-controlled studies in pregnant women. Use only if potential benefit justifies risk to the fetus.

Additional Information The increased potential to prolong QT_c, as compared to other available antipsychotic agents, should be considered in the evaluation of available alternatives.

Related Information

Antipsychotic Agents *on page 1558*

Ziprasidone Hydrochloride *see* Ziprasidone *on page 1424*
Ziprasidone Mesylate *see* Ziprasidone *on page 1424*
Zithromax® *see* Azithromycin *on page 139*
Zithromax® TRI-PAK™ *see* Azithromycin *on page 139*
Zithromax® Z-PAK® *see* Azithromycin *on page 139*
Zocor® *see* Simvastatin *on page 1230*
Zofran® *see* Ondansetron *on page 1000*
Zofran® ODT *see* Ondansetron *on page 1000*
Zoladex® *see* Goserelin *on page 641*
Zoledronate *see* Zoledronic Acid *on page 1427*

Zoledronic Acid (ZOE le dron ik AS id)

U.S. Brand Names Zometa®

Synonyms CGP-42446; Zoledronate

Generic Available No

Pharmacologic Category Bisphosphonate Derivative

Pregnancy Risk Factor D

Lactation Excretion in breast milk unknown/not recommended

Use Treatment of hypercalcemia of malignancy, multiple myeloma, and bone metastases of solid tumors in conjunction with standard antineoplastic therapy

Mechanism of Action/Effect A bisphosphonate which inhibits bone resorption via actions on osteoclasts or on osteoclast precursors; inhibits osteoclastic activity and skeletal calcium release induced by tumors.

Contraindications Hypersensitivity to zoledronic acid, other bisphosphonates, or any component of the formulation; pregnancy

Warnings/Precautions Renal toxicity has been reported with doses >4 mg or infusions administered over <15 minutes. Renal function should be assessed prior to and after treatment; if decreased after treatment, additional treatments should be withheld until renal function returns to within 10% of baseline. Use caution in patients with previous renal impairment; adverse reactions may be greater in patients with impaired renal function. Use is not recommended in patients with severe renal impairment (serum creatinine >3 mg/dL) and bone metastases (limited data). Adequate hydration is required during treatment (urine output ~2 L/day); avoid overhydration, especially in patients with heart failure; diuretics should not be used before correcting hypovolemia. Use caution in patients with aspirin-sensitive asthma (may cause bronchoconstriction), hepatic dysfunction, and the elderly. Safety and efficacy have not been established in pediatric patients. Pregnancy risk C.

Drug Interactions

Increased Effect/Toxicity: Aminoglycosides may also lower serum calcium levels; loop diuretics increase risk of hypocalcemia; thalidomide increases renal toxicity

Adverse Reactions

>10%:

Cardiovascular: Leg edema (up to 19%)

Central nervous system: Fever (30% to 44%), headache (18%), insomnia (15%), anxiety (9% to 14%), dizziness (14%), agitation (13%)

Dermatologic: Alopecia (11%)

Endocrine & metabolic: Hypophosphatemia (13%), hypokalemia (12%), dehydration (up to 12%)

Gastrointestinal: Diarrhea (17% to 22%), abdominal pain (12% to 16%)

Genitourinary: Urinary tract infection (11% to 14%)

Hematologic: Anemia (22% to 29%), neutropenia (11%)

Neuromuscular & skeletal: Myalgia (21%), paresthesias (18%), arthralgia (18%) skeletal pain (12%)

Respiratory: Dyspnea (22%), coughing (12% to 19%)

1% to 10%:

Cardiovascular: Hypotension (10%), chest pain

Central nervous system: Hypoesthesia (10%)

Dermatologic: Dermatitis (10%)

Endocrine & metabolic: Hypomagnesemia (up to 10%), hypocalcemia, hypophosphatemia (9%), hypermagnesemia (Grade 3: 2%)

Gastrointestinal: Anorexia (9%), mucositis, dysphagia

Genitourinary: Urinary tract infection (14%)

Hematologic: Thrombocytopenia, pancytopenia

Neuromuscular & skeletal: Arthralgia, rigors (10%)

Renal: Serum creatinine increased

Respiratory: Pleural effusion , upper respiratory tract infection (8%)

(Continued)

Zoledronic Acid *(Continued)*

<1% (Limited to important or life-threatening): Conjunctivitis, flu-like symptoms, injection site reactions, pruritus, rash

Symptoms of hypercalcemia include polyuria, nephrolithiasis, anorexia, nausea, vomiting, constipation, weakness, fatigue, confusion, stupor, and coma. These may not be drug-related adverse events, but related to the underlying metabolic condition.

Overdosage/Toxicology Clinically significant hypocalcemia, hypophosphatemia, and hypomagnesemia may occur.

Pharmacodynamics/Kinetics

Half-Life Elimination: Triphasic; Terminal: 167 hours

Onset: Maximum effect may not been seen for 7 days.

Formulations Injection, powder for reconstitution: 4 mg [as monohydrate 4.264 mg]

Dosing

Adults & Elderly:

Hypercalcemia of malignancy (albumin-corrected serum calcium ≥12 mg/dL): I.V.: 4 mg (maximum) given as a single dose infused over **no less than 15 minutes**; patients should be adequately hydrated prior to treatment (restoring urine output to ~2 L/day). Monitor serum calcium and wait at least 7 days before considering retreatment. Dosage adjustment may be needed in patients with decreased renal function following treatment.

Multiple myeloma or metastatic bone lesions from solid tumors: I.V.: 4 mg given over 15 minutes every 3-4 weeks; duration of treatment ranges from 9-15 months

Note: Patients should receive a daily calcium supplement and multivitamin containing vitamin D

Renal Impairment: Specific dosing guidelines are not available.

Hypercalcemia of malignancy: Patients with serum creatinine ≥4.5 mg/dL were excluded from clinical trials.

Bone metastases: Patients with serum creatinine >3 mg/dL were excluded from clinical trials.

Hepatic Impairment: Specific guidelines are not available.

Administration

I.V.: In order to prevent renal toxicity, infuse solution over at least 15 minutes.

Stability

Storage: Prior to dilution, vials should be stored at 25°C (77°F). Following final dilution, solution should be used immediately or stored under at 2°C to 8°C (36°F to 46°F).

Reconstitution: Reconstitute powder with 5 mL sterile water for injection. Once fully dissolved, further dilute in 100 mL NS or D_5W prior to administration. Infusion of solution must be completed within 24 hours of initial reconstitution of powder.

Compatibility: Incompatible with calcium-containing solutions (eg, LR)

Monitoring Laboratory Tests Monitor serum creatinine prior to each dose. Serum electrolytes, phosphate, magnesium, and hemoglobin/hematocrit should be evaluated regularly. Monitor serum calcium to assess response and avoid over-treatment.

Monitoring and Teaching Issues

Physical Assessment: See Contraindications, Warnings/Precautions, and Dosing for use cautions. Assess potential for interactions with other prescriptions, OTC medications, and herbal products patient may be taking (see Drug Interactions). See I.V. Administration instructions. Note recommendations for daily calcium and vitamin D supplements. Assess results of laboratory tests (see above) and patient response to therapy (see Adverse Reactions and Overdose/Toxicology). Teach patient possible side effects and interventions (eg, need for adequate hydration) and adverse symptoms to report (see Patient Education). **Pregnancy risk factor D** - determine that patient is not pregnant before beginning treatment. Instruct patients of childbearing age about appropriate barrier contraceptive measures during therapy. Breast-feeding is not recommended.

Patient Education: This medication can only be administered intravenously. Avoid vitamins during infusion or for 2-3 hours after completion. You may experience some nausea or vomiting (small, frequent meals, good mouth care, sucking lozenges, or chewing gum may help) or recurrent bone pain (consult prescriber for analgesic). Report unusual muscle twitching or spasms, severe diarrhea/constipation, acute bone pain, or other persistent adverse effects. **Pregnancy/breast-feeding precautions:** Inform prescriber if you are or intend to become pregnant. Do not get pregnant during therapy. Consult prescriber for instructions on appropriate contraceptive measures. This drug may cause fetal defects. Breast-feeding is not recommended.

Dietary Issues: Multiple myeloma or metastatic bone lesions from solid tumors: Take daily calcium supplement (500 mg) and daily multivitamin (with 400 int. units vitamin D).

Pregnancy Issues: Animal studies resulted in embryotoxicity and losses. May cause fetal harm when administered to a pregnant woman. Use only if the benefit to the mother outweighs the potential risk to the fetus.

Zolmitriptan (zohl mi TRIP tan)

U.S. Brand Names Zomig®; Zomig-ZMT™

Synonyms 311C90

Generic Available No

Pharmacologic Category Serotonin $5\text{-}HT_{1D}$ Receptor Agonist

Pregnancy Risk Factor C

Lactation Excretion in breast milk unknown/use caution

Use Acute treatment of migraine with or without auras

Mechanism of Action/Effect Zolmitriptan is a selective $5\text{-}HT_{1B/1D}$ agonist

Contraindications Hypersensitivity to zolmitriptan or any component of the formulation; ischemic heart disease or Prinzmetal's angina; signs or symptoms of ischemic heart disease; uncontrolled hypertension; symptomatic Wolff-Parkinson-White syndrome or arrhythmias associated with other cardiac accessory conduction pathway disorders; use with ergotamine derivatives (within 24 hours of); use within 24 hours of another $5\text{-}HT_1$ agonist; concurrent administration or within 2 weeks of discontinuing an MAO inhibitor; management of hemiplegic or basilar migraine

Warnings/Precautions Zolmitriptan is indicated only in patient populations with a clear diagnosis of migraine. Not for prophylactic treatment of migraine headaches. Cardiac events (including myocardial infarction, ventricular arrhythmia, cardiac arrest, and death) have been reported with 5-HT_1 agonist administration. Should not be given to patients who have risk factors for CAD without adequate cardiac evaluation. Patients with suspected CAD should have cardiovascular evaluation to rule out CAD before considering zolmitriptan's use; if cardiovascular evaluation negative, first dose would be safest if given in the healthcare provider's office. Periodic evaluation of those without cardiovascular disease, but with continued risk factors should be done. Significant elevation in blood pressure, including hypertensive crisis, has also been reported. Vasospasm-related reactions have been reported other than coronary artery vasospasm. Peripheral vascular ischemia and colonic ischemia with abdominal pain and bloody diarrhea have occurred. Use with caution in patients with hepatic impairment. Zomig-ZMT™ tablets contain phenylalanine. Safety and efficacy not established in patients <18 years of age. Pregnancy risk C.

Drug Interactions

Cytochrome P450 Effect: Substrate of CYP1A2

Increased Effect/Toxicity: Ergot-containing drugs may lead to vasospasm; cimetidine, MAO inhibitors, oral contraceptives, propranolol increase levels of zolmitriptan; concurrent use with SSRIs and sibutramine may lead to serotonin syndrome.

Nutritional/Ethanol Interactions Ethanol: Limit use (may have additive CNS toxicity).

Effects on Lab Values No interferences have been identified

Adverse Reactions

1% to 10%:

Cardiovascular: Chest pain (2% to 4%), palpitations (up to 2%)

Central nervous system: Dizziness (6% to 10%), somnolence (5% to 8%), pain (2% to 3%), vertigo (≤2%)

Gastrointestinal: Nausea (4% to 9%), xerostomia (3% to 5%), dyspepsia (1% to 3%), dysphagia (≤2%)

Neuromuscular & skeletal: Paresthesia (5% to 9%), weakness (3% to 9%), warm/cold sensation (5% to 7%), hypesthesia (1% to 2%), myalgia (1% to 2%), myasthenia (up to 2%)

Miscellaneous: Neck/throat/jaw pain (4% to 10%), diaphoresis (up to 3%), allergic reaction (up to 1%)

<1% (Limited to important or life-threatening): Angina, apnea, arrhythmia, ataxia, bronchospasm, cerebral ischemia, coronary artery vasospasm, cyanosis, eosinophilia, esophagitis, hallucinations, hematemesis, hypertension, hypertensive crisis, melena, miscarriage, myocardial infarction, myocardial ischemia, pancreatitis, photosensitivity, QT prolongation, rash, syncope, tetany, thrombocytopenia, tinnitus, ulcer, urticaria

Events related to other serotonin 5-HT_{1D} receptor agonists: Cardiac arrest, cerebral hemorrhage, colonic ischemia, peripheral vascular ischemia, stroke, subarachnoid hemorrhage, ventricular fibrillation

Overdosage/Toxicology Treatment is symptom-directed and supportive. It is not known if hemodialysis or peritoneal dialysis is effective.

Pharmacodynamics/Kinetics

Absorption: Well absorbed

Bioavailability: 40%

Half-Life Elimination: 2.8-3.7 hours

Time to Peak: Serum: Tablet: 1.5 hours; Orally-disintegrating: 3 hours

Metabolism: Converted to an active N-desmethyl metabolite (2-6 times more potent than zolmitriptan)

Onset: 0.5-1 hour

Formulations

Tablet (Zomig®): 2.5 mg, 5 mg

Tablet, orally-disintegrating (Zomig-ZMT™): 2.5 mg [contains phenylalanine 2.81 mg/tablet; orange flavor]; 5 mg [contains phenylalanine 5.62 mg/tablet; orange flavor]

Dosing

Adults: Migraine headache: Oral:

Tablet: Initial: ≤2.5 mg at the onset of migraine headache; may break 2.5 mg tablet in half

Orally-disintegrating tablet: Initial: 2.5 mg at the onset of migraine headache

Note: Use the lowest possible dose to minimize adverse events. If the headache returns, the dose may be repeated after 2 hours; do not exceed 10 mg within a 24-hour period. Controlled trials have not established the effectiveness of a second dose if the initial one was ineffective

Elderly: No dosage adjustment needed, but elderly patients are more likely to have underlying cardiovascular disease and should have careful evaluation of cardiovascular system before prescribing.

Renal Impairment: No dosage adjustment recommended. There is a 25% reduction in zolmitriptan's clearance in patients with severe renal impairment (Cl_{cr} 5-25 mL/minute)

Hepatic Impairment: Administer with caution in patients with liver disease, generally using doses <2.5 mg. Patients with moderate-to-severe hepatic impairment may have decreased clearance of zolmitriptan, and significant elevation in blood pressure was observed in some patients.

Administration

Oral: Administer as soon as migraine headache starts. Tablets may be broken. Orally-disintegrating tablets: Must be taken whole; do not break, crush or chew; place on tongue and allow to dissolve; administration with liquid is not required

Stability

Storage: Store at 20°C to 25°C (68°F to 77°F); protect from light and moisture

Monitoring and Teaching Issues

Physical Assessment: See Contraindications, Warnings/Precautions (clear diagnosis of migraine) for use cautions. Assess potential for interactions with other prescriptions, OTC

(Continued)

Zolmitriptan *(Continued)*

medications, or herbal products patient may be taking (eg, ergot-containing drugs - see Drug Interactions). Assess effectiveness and adverse response (see Adverse Reactions and Overdose/Toxicology). Teach patient proper use, possible side effects and appropriate interventions, and adverse symptoms to report (see Patient Education). **Pregnancy risk factor C** - benefits of use should outweigh possible risks. Note breast-feeding caution.

Patient Education: Inform prescriber of all prescriptions (including oral contraceptives), OTC medications, or herbal products you are taking, and any allergies you have. This drug is to be used to reduce your migraine, not to prevent or reduce the number of attacks. Follow exact instructions for use. Remove orally-disintegrating tablet from blister package just before using, place on tongue, and allow to dissolve. Do not crush, break, or chew. Regular tablet may be broken in half for use. Do not take within 24 hours of any other migraine medication without first consulting prescriber. If first dose brings relief, second dose may be taken anytime after 2 hours if migraine returns. If you have no relief with first dose, do not take a second dose without consulting prescriber. Do not exceed 10 mg in 24 hours. May cause dizziness or drowsiness (use caution when driving or engaging in tasks requiring alertness until response to drug is known); or dry mouth (frequent mouth care and sucking on lozenges may help). Report immediately any chest pain, heart throbbing, or tightness in throat; swelling of eyelids, face, or lips; skin rash or hives; easy bruising; blood in urine, stool, or vomitus; pain or itching with urination; or pain, warmth, or numbness in extremities. **Pregnancy/breast-feeding precautions:** Inform prescriber if you are or intend to become pregnant. Consult prescriber if breast-feeding.

Geriatric Considerations: Zolmitriptan use in the elderly patient has not been studied.

Pregnancy Issues: In pregnant animals, zolmitriptan caused embryolethality and fetal abnormalities at doses ≥11 times the equivalent human dose.

Additional Information Not recommended if the patient has risk factors for heart disease (high blood pressure, high cholesterol, obesity, diabetes, smoking, strong family history of heart disease, postmenopausal woman, or a male >40 years of age).

This agent is intended to relieve migraine, but not to prevent or reduce the number of attacks. Use only to treat an actual migraine attack.

Related Information

Antimigraine Drugs *on page 1557*

Zoloft® *see* Sertraline *on page 1223*

Zolpidem (zole PI dem)

U.S. Brand Names Ambien®

Synonyms Zolpidem Tartrate

Restrictions C-IV

Generic Available No

Pharmacologic Category Hypnotic, Nonbenzodiazepine

Pregnancy Risk Factor B

Lactation Enters breast milk/use caution (AAP rates "compatible")

Use Short-term treatment of insomnia

Mechanism of Action/Effect Structurally dissimilar to benzodiazepine, however, has much or all of its actions explained by its effects on benzodiazepine (BZD) receptors, especially the omega-1 receptor; retains hypnotic and much of the anxiolytic properties of the BZD, but has reduced effects on skeletal muscle and seizure threshold.

Contraindications Hypersensitivity to zolpidem or any component of the formulation

Warnings/Precautions Should be used only after evaluation of potential causes of sleep disturbance. Failure of sleep disturbance to resolve after 7-10 days may indicate psychiatric or medical illness. Use with caution in patients with decreased respiratory function or or depression. Behavioral changes have been associated with sedative-hypnotics. Causes CNS depression, which may impair physical and mental capabilities. Effects with other sedative drugs or ethanol may be potentiated. Closely monitor elderly or debilitated patients for impaired cognitive or motor performance; not recommended for use in children <18 years of age. Avoid use in patients with sleep apnea or a history of sedative-hypnotic abuse.

Drug Interactions

Cytochrome P450 Effect: Substrate of CYP1A2, 2C8/9, 2C19, 2D6, **3A4**

Decreased Effect: Rifampin may reduce levels and effect of zolpidem. Other enzyme inducers may have a similar effect.

Increased Effect/Toxicity: Use of zolpidem in combination with other centrally-acting drugs may produce additive CNS depression. Concurrent use of drugs which inhibit cytochrome P450 3A4 (including erythromycin, clarithromycin, diltiazem, itraconazole, ketoconazole, nefazodone, and verapamil) may increase the levels of zolpidem.

Nutritional/Ethanol Interactions

Ethanol: Avoid ethanol (may increase CNS depression).

Herb/Nutraceutical: St John's wort may decrease zolpidem levels. Avoid valerian, St John's wort, kava kava, gotu kola (may increase CNS depression).

Effects on Lab Values ↑ aminotransferase [ALT (SGPT)/AST (SGOT)], bilirubin (S); ↓ RAI uptake

Adverse Reactions

1% to 10%:

- Cardiovascular: Palpitations
- Central nervous system: Headache, drowsiness, dizziness, lethargy, lightheadedness, depression, abnormal dreams, amnesia
- Dermatologic: Rash
- Gastrointestinal: Nausea, diarrhea, xerostomia, constipation
- Respiratory: Sinusitis, pharyngitis

<1% (Limited to important or life-threatening): Confusion, depression, falls, impaired concentration, manic reaction, tremor, vomiting

Overdosage/Toxicology Symptoms of overdose include coma and hypotension. Treatment for overdose is supportive. Rarely is mechanical ventilation required. Flumazenil has been shown to selectively block binding to CNS receptors, resulting in a reversal of CNS depression, but not always respiratory depression.

Pharmacodynamics/Kinetics

Absorption: Rapid

Half-Life Elimination: 2-2.6 hours; Cirrhosis: Up to 9.9 hours

Metabolism: Hepatic to inactive metabolites

Onset: 30 minutes

Duration: 6-8 hours

Formulations Tablet, as tartrate: 5 mg, 10 mg

Dosing

Adults: Insomnia (Duration of therapy should be limited to 7-10 days): Oral: 10 mg immediately before bedtime; maximum: 10 mg

Elderly: 5 mg immediately before bedtime

Renal Impairment: Not dialyzable

Hepatic Impairment: Decrease dose to 5 mg.

Monitoring and Teaching Issues

Physical Assessment: For short-term use. Assess effectiveness and interactions of other medications patient may be taking (see Drug Interactions). See Contraindications and Warnings/Precautions for use cautions. Assess for history of addiction; long-term use can result in dependence, abuse, or tolerance; periodically evaluate need for continued use. After long-term use, taper dosage slowly when discontinuing. For inpatient use, institute safety measures and monitor effectiveness and adverse reactions. For outpatients, monitor for effectiveness of therapy and adverse reactions (see Adverse Reactions) at beginning of therapy and periodically with long-term use. Assess knowledge/teach patient appropriate use, interventions to reduce side effects, and adverse symptoms to report (see Patient Education). Note breast-feeding caution.

Patient Education: Use exactly as directed; do not increase dose or frequency or discontinue without consulting prescriber. Drug may cause physical and/or psychological dependence. While using this medication, do not use alcohol or other prescription or OTC medications (especially, pain medications, sedatives, antihistamines, or hypnotics) without consulting prescriber. Maintain adequate hydration (2-3 L/day of fluids) unless advised by prescriber to restrict fluids. You may experience drowsiness, dizziness, or blurred vision (use caution when driving or engaging in tasks requiring alertness until response to drug is known); nausea (small, frequent meals, frequent mouth care, chewing gum, or sucking lozenges may help); or diarrhea (buttermilk, boiled milk, yogurt may help). Report CNS changes (confusion, depression, increased sedation, excitation, headache, abnormal thinking, insomnia, or nightmares); muscle pain or weakness; difficulty breathing; chest pain or palpitations; or ineffectiveness of medication. **Breast-feeding precaution:** Consult prescriber if breast-feeding.

Geriatric Considerations: In doses >5 mg, there was subjective evidence of impaired sleep on the first post-treatment night. There have been few reports of increased hypotension and/or falls in the elderly with this drug. Can be considered a drug of choice in the elderly when a hypnotic is indicated.

Additional Information Causes less disturbances in sleep stages as compared to benzodiazepines. Time spent in sleep stages 3 and 4 are maintained; decreases sleep latency. Should not be prescribed in quantities exceeding a 1-month supply.

Related Information

Anxiolytic/Hypnotic Use in Long-Term Care Facilities *on page 1608*

Zolpidem Tartrate *see* Zolpidem *on page 1430*

Zometa® *see* Zoledronic Acid *on page 1427*

Zomig® *see* Zolmitriptan *on page 1428*

Zomig-ZMT™ *see* Zolmitriptan *on page 1428*

Zonalon® *see* Doxepin *on page 443*

Zonegran® *see* Zonisamide *on page 1431*

Zonisamide (zoe NIS a mide)

U.S. Brand Names Zonegran®

Generic Available No

Pharmacologic Category Anticonvulsant, Miscellaneous

Pregnancy Risk Factor C

Lactation Excretion in breast milk unknown/contraindicated

Use Adjunct treatment of partial seizures in children >16 years of age and adults with epilepsy

Mechanism of Action/Effect The exact mechanism of action is not known. May stabilize neuronal membranes and suppress neuronal hypersynchronization through action at sodium and calcium channels. Does not affect GABA activity.

Contraindications Hypersensitivity to zonisamide, sulfonamides, or any component of the formulation

Warnings/Precautions Rare, but potentially fatal sulfonamide reactions have occurred following the use of zonisamide. These reactions include Stevens-Johnson syndrome and toxic epidermal necrolysis, usually appearing within 2-16 weeks of drug initiation. Discontinue zonisamide if rash develops. Chemical similarities are present among sulfonamides, sulfonylureas, carbonic anhydrase inhibitors, thiazides, and loop diuretics (except ethacrynic acid). Use in patients with sulfonamide allergy is specifically contraindicated in product labeling, however, a risk of cross-reaction exists in patients with allergy to any of these compounds; avoid use when previous reaction has been severe.

Decreased sweating (oligohydrosis) and hyperthermia requiring hospitalization have been reported in children. Discontinue zonisamide in patients who develop acute renal failure or a significant sustained increase in creatinine/BUN concentration. Kidney stones have been reported. Use cautiously in patients with renal or hepatic dysfunction. Do not use if estimated Cl_{cr} <50 mL/minute. Significant CNS effects include psychiatric symptoms, psychomotor slowing, and fatigue or somnolence. Fatigue and somnolence occur within the first month of

(Continued)

Zonisamide *(Continued)*

treatment, most commonly at doses of 300-500 mg/day. Abrupt withdrawal may precipitate seizures; discontinue or reduce doses gradually. Safety and efficacy in children <16 years of age has not been established.

Pregnancy risk C.

Drug Interactions

Cytochrome P450 Effect: Substrate of CYP2C19, **3A4**

Decreased Effect:

Note: Zonisamide did NOT affect steady state levels of carbamazepine, phenytoin, or valproate; zonisamide half-life is decreased by carbamazepine, phenytoin, phenobarbital, and valproate

Enzyme inducers: May increase the metabolism of zonisamide, reducing its effectiveness; inducers include phenytoin, carbamazepine, phenobarbital, and rifampin

Increased Effect/Toxicity: Sedative effects may be additive with other CNS depressants; monitor for increased effect; includes barbiturates, benzodiazepines, narcotic analgesics, ethanol, and other sedative agents. Serum level and/or toxicity of zonisamide may be increased by CYP3A4 inhibitors; inhibitors include amiodarone, cimetidine, clarithromycin, erythromycin, delavirdine, diltiazem, dirithromycin, disulfiram, fluoxetine, fluvoxamine, grapefruit juice, indinavir, itraconazole, ketoconazole, metronidazole, nefazodone, nevirapine, propoxyphene, quinupristin-dalfopristin, ritonavir, saquinavir, verapamil, zafirlukast, zileuton; monitor for increased response.

Nutritional/Ethanol Interactions

Ethanol: Avoid ethanol (may increase CNS depression).

Food: Food delays time to maximum concentration, but does not affect bioavailability.

Adverse Reactions Adjunctive Therapy: Frequencies noted in patients receiving other anticonvulsants:

>10%:

Central nervous system: Somnolence (17%), dizziness (13%)

Gastrointestinal: Anorexia (13%)

1% to 10%:

Central nervous system: Headache (10%), agitation/irritability (9%), fatigue (8%), tiredness (7%), ataxia (6%), confusion (6%), decreased concentration (6%), memory impairment (6%), depression (6%), insomnia (6%), speech disorders (5%), mental slowing (4%), anxiety (3%), nervousness (2%), schizophrenic/schizophreniform behavior (2%), difficulty in verbal expression (2%), status epilepticus (1%), tremor (1%), convulsion (1%), hyperesthesia (1%), incoordination (1%)

Dermatologic: Rash (3%), bruising (2%), pruritus (1%)

Gastrointestinal: Nausea (9%), abdominal pain (6%), diarrhea (5%), dyspepsia (3%), weight loss (3%), constipation (2%), dry mouth (2%), taste perversion (2%), vomiting (1%)

Neuromuscular & skeletal: Paresthesia (4%), weakness (1%), abnormal gait (1%)

Ocular: Diplopia (6%), nystagmus (4%), amblyopia (1%)

Otic: Tinnitus (1%)

Respiratory: Rhinitis (2%), pharyngitis (1%), increased cough (1%)

Miscellaneous: Flu-like syndrome (4%) accidental injury (1%)

<1% (Limited to important and/or life threatening symptoms): Agranulocytosis, allergic reaction, alopecia, aplastic anemia, apnea, atrial fibrillation, bladder calculus, cholangitis, cholecystitis, cholestatic jaundice, colitis, deafness, duodenitis, dysarthria, dyskinesia, dyspnea, dystonia, encephalopathy, esophagitis, facial paralysis, gingival hyperplasia, glaucoma, gum hemorrhage, gynecomastia, heart failure, hematemesis, hemoptysis, hirsutism, hyperthermia, impotence, leukopenia, lupus erythematosus, menorrhagia, movement disorder, myoclonus, nephrolithiasis, neuropathy, oculogyric crisis, oligohydrosis, paresthesia, peripheral neuritis, pulmonary embolus, rash, rectal hemorrhage, Stevens-Johnson syndrome, stroke, syncope, thrombocytopenia, toxic epidermal necrolysis, urinary retention, urticaria

Overdosage/Toxicology No specific antidotes are available; experience with doses >800 mg/day is limited. Emesis or gastric lavage, with airway protection, should be done following a recent overdose. General supportive care and close observation are indicated. Renal dialysis may not be effective due to low protein binding (40%).

Pharmacodynamics/Kinetics

Half-Life Elimination: 63 hours

Time to Peak: 2-6 hours

Metabolism: Hepatic via CYP3A4; forms N-acetyl zonisamide and 2-sulfamoylacetyl phenol (SMAP)

Formulations Capsule: 100 mg

Dosing

Adults: Adjunctive treatment of partial seizures: Oral: Initial: 100 mg/day. Dose may be increased to 200 mg/day after 2 weeks. Further dosage increases to 300 mg and 400 mg/day can then be made with a minimum of 2 weeks between adjustments, in order to reach steady state at each dosage level. Doses of up to 600 mg/day have been studied, however, there is no evidence of increased response with doses >400 mg/day.

Elderly: Data from clinical trials is insufficient for patients older than 65. Begin dosing at the low end of the dosing range.

Pediatrics: Children >16 years: Refer to adult dosing.

Renal Impairment: Slower titration and frequent monitoring are indicated. Do not use if Cl_{cr} is <50 mL/minute.

Hepatic Impairment: Slower titration and frequent monitoring are indicated.

Stability

Storage: Store at controlled room temperature 25°C (77°F). Protect from moisture and light.

Monitoring and Teaching Issues

Physical Assessment: Assess other medications patient may be taking for increased risk of drug/drug interactions (see Drug Interactions). See Warnings/Precautions and Adverse

Reactions for use cautions. Monitor therapeutic response, laboratory results, and adverse reactions (see Adverse Reactions) at beginning of therapy and periodically with long-term use. Observe and teach seizure precautions. Assess knowledge/teach patient appropriate use, interventions to reduce side effects, and adverse symptoms to report (see Patient Education). **Pregnancy risk factor C** - benefits of use should outweigh possible risks. Breast-feeding is contraindicated.

Patient Education: Take exactly as directed, as the same time each day, with or without food. Do not increase frequency, alter dose, or discontinue without consulting prescriber. If you miss a dose, take as soon as possible. If it is almost time for your next dose, skip the missed dose. Do not chew, crush, or open capsules; swallow whole. Maintain adequate hydration (2-3 L/day of fluids) unless advised by prescriber to restrict fluids. Avoid grapefruit juice while on this medication. While using this medication, avoid alcohol, herbal remedies, OTC or prescriptions drugs (especially pain medication, antihistamines, psychiatric medications, sedatives, or hypnotics) unless approved by your prescriber. Wear/carry identification of epileptic status and medications. You may experience drowsiness, dizziness, or blurred vision (use caution when driving or engaging in tasks requiring alertness until response to drug is known); or nausea, vomiting, constipation, dry mouth, or loss of appetite (small, frequent meals, frequent mouth care, chewing gum, or sucking hard candy may help). Report CNS changes (changes in speech patterns, mentation changes, changes in cognition or memory, unusual thought patterns, coordination difficulties, or excessive drowsiness); difficulty breathing or tightening of the throat; swelling of mouth, lips, or tongue; muscle cramping, weakness, or pain; rash or skin irritations; unusual bruising or bleeding (mouth, urine, stool); fever, sore throat, sores in your mouth; swelling of extremities; sudden back pain, pain on urination, or dark/bloody urine (signs of kidney stones); or other adverse response including change in seizure type or frequency. **Pregnancy/breast-feeding precautions:** Inform prescriber if you are or intend to become pregnant. Do not breast-feed.

Dietary Issues: May be taken with or without food.

Breast-feeding Issues: Use during lactation only if the potential benefits outweigh the potential risks.

Pregnancy Issues: Fetal abnormalities and death have been reported in animals, however, there are no studies in pregnant women.

ZORprin® *see* Aspirin *on page 121*

Zosyn® *see* Piperacillin and Tazobactam Sodium *on page 1091*

Zovia™ *see* Ethinyl Estradiol and Ethynodiol Diacetate *on page 521*

Zovirax® *see* Acyclovir *on page 43*

Zyban® *see* BuPROPion *on page 186*

Zydone® *see* Hydrocodone and Acetaminophen *on page 667*

Zyflo™ *see* Zileuton *on page 1422*

Zyloprim® *see* Allopurinol *on page 60*

Zymase® [DSC] *see* Pancrelipase *on page 1029*

Zyprexa® *see* Olanzapine *on page 995*

Zyprexa® Zydis® *see* Olanzapine *on page 995*

Zyrtec® *see* Cetirizine *on page 263*

Zyvox™ *see* Linezolid *on page 806*

CONTROLLED SUBSTANCE INDEX

CONTROLLED SUBSTANCE II

CONTROLLED SUBSTANCE III

CONTROLLED SUBSTANCE IV

CONTROLLED SUBSTANCE V

PHARMACOLOGIC CATEGORY INDEX

(Continued)

APPENDIX TABLE OF CONTENTS

Additional Medicines

Adverse Reactions Information

Calculations/Conversions/Laboratory Values

APPENDIX TABLE OF CONTENTS *(Continued)*

Overdose and Toxicology

Treatment/Prophylaxis Guidelines

ANTIDOTES, ANTIVENINS, AND ANTITOXINS

Agent	Use
Alcohol, ethyl (Lavacol®)	Antidote for ethylene glycol overdose; antidote for methanol overdose
Antivenin (*Crotalidae* polyvalent)	Neutralization of the venoms of North and South America crotalids: rattlesnakes, copperheads, cottonmouth, tropical moccasins, fer-de-lance, bushmaster
Antivenin (*Latrodectus mactans*)	Treatment of patients with symptoms of black widow spider bites
Antivenin (*Micrurus fluvius*)	Neutralization of the venom of Eastern coral snakes and Texas coral snakes but does not neutralize the venom of Arizona or Sonoran coral snakes
Cyanide antidote kit	Treatment of cyanide poisoning
Dimecaprol (BAL in Oil®)	Antidote to gold, arsenic (except arsine), and mercury poisoning (except nonalkyl mercury); adjunct to edetate calcium disodium in lead poisoning; possibly effective for antimony, bismuth, chromium, copper, nickel, tungsten, or zinc
Diphtheria antitoxin	Treatment of diphtheria (neutralizes unbound toxin, available from CDC)
Flumazenil (Romazicon™)	Benzodiazepine antagonist - reverses sedative effects of benzodiazepines used in general anesthesia; for management of benzodiazepine overdose; flumazenil **does not** antagonize the CNS effects of other GABA agonists (such as ethanol, barbiturates, or general anesthetics), **does not** reverse narcotics
Fomepizole (Antizol®)	Known or suspected ethylene glycol (antifreeze) and methanol toxicity, alone or in combination with dialysis. **Unlabeled use**: Known or suspected propylene glycol toxicity
Insect sting kit (Ana-Kit®)	Anaphylaxis emergency treatment of insect bites or stings by the sensitive patient that may occur within minutes of insect sting or exposure to an allergic substance
Pralidoxime (Protopam®)	Reverse muscle paralysis with toxic exposure to organophosphate anticholinesterase pesticides and chemicals; control of overdose of drugs used to treat myasthenia gravis (ambenonium, neostigmine, pyridostigmine)
Protamine	Treatment of heparin overdosage; neutralize heparin during surgery or dialysis procedures
Sodium thiosulfate	Parenteral: Used alone or with sodium nitrite or amyl nitrite in cyanide poisoning or arsenic poisoning; reduce the risk of nephrotoxicity associated with cisplatin therapy
Succimer (Chemet®)	Treatment of lead poisoning in children with blood levels higher than 45 μg/dL. Not indicated for prophylaxis of lead poisoning in a lead-containing environment.
Trientine (Syprine®)	Treatment of Wilson's disease in patients intolerant to penicillamine

DIAGNOSTICS AND SURGICAL AIDS

Agent	Use
Apraclonidine (Iopidine®)	Prevention and treatment of postsurgical intraocular pressure elevation
Benzylpenicilloyl-Polylysine (Pre-Pen®)	Adjunct in assessing the risk of administering penicillin (penicillin or benzylpenicillin) in adults with a history of clinical penicillin hypersensitivity
Candida albicans (Monilia) (Dermatophytin-O)	Screen for the detection of nonresponsiveness to antigens in immunocompromised individuals
Cellulose, oxidized (Oxycel®; Surgicel®)	Temporary packing for the control of capillary, venous, or small arterial hemorrhage
Chondroitin sulfate - sodium hyaluronate (Viscoat®)	Surgical aid in anterior segment procedures, protects corneal endothelium and coats intraocular lens thus protecting it
Chymopapain (Chymodiactin®)	Alternative to surgery in patients with herniated lumbar intervertebral disks
Coccidioidin skin test (Spherulin®; BioCox®)	Intradermal skin test in diagnosis of coccidioidomycosis; differential diagnosis of this disease from histoplasmosis, sarcoidosis, and other mycotic and bacterial infections. The skin test may be negative in severe forms of disease (anergy) or when prolonged periods of time have passed since infection.
Corticotropin (Acthar®; H.P. Acthar® Gel)	Diagnostic aid in adrenocortical insufficiency; repository dosage form is used for acute exacerbations of multiple sclerosis or severe muscle weakness in myasthenia gravis; cosyntropin is preferred
Cosyntropin (Cortrosyn® Injection)	Diagnostic test to differentiate primary adrenal from secondary (pituitary) adrenocortical insufficiency
Cyclopentolate (AK-Pentolate®; Cyclogyl®; I-Pentolate®)	Diagnostic procedures requiring mydriasis and cycloplegia
Cyclopentolate and phenylephrine (Cyclomydril® Ophthalmic)	Induce mydriasis greater than that produced with cyclopentolate alone
Dapiprazole (Rēv-Eyes™)	Reverse dilation due to drugs (adrenergic or parasympathomimetic) after eye exams
Dimercaprol (BAL in Oil®)	Antidote to gold, arsenic (except arsine), and mercury poisoning (except nonalkyl mercury); adjunct to edetate calcium disodium in lead poisoning; possibly effective for antimony, bismuth, chromium, copper, nickel, tungsten, or zinc
Dinoprost (Prostin F_2 Alpha®)	Abort 2nd trimester pregnancy
d-Xylose (Xylo-Pfan® [OTC])	Also referred to as wood sugar; used in evaluating intestinal absorption and diagnosing malabsorptive states
Fluorescein sodium (AK-Fluor® Injection; Fluorescite® Injection; Fluorets® Ophthalmic Strips; Fluor-I-Strip®; Fluor-I-Strip-AT®; Fluress® Ophthalmic Solution; Ful-Glo® Ophthalmic Strips)	Demonstrates defects of corneal epithelium; diagnostic aid in ophthalmic angiography
Gelatin, absorbable (Gelfilm® Ophthalmic; Gelfoam® Topical)	Adjunct to provide hemostasis in surgery; used in open prostatic surgery
Histoplasmin (Histolyn-CYL® Injection)	Diagnose histoplasmosis; assess cell-mediated immunity
Hydroxyamphetamine and tropicamide (Paremyd® Ophthalmic)	Diagnostic mydriasis with cycloplegia
Hydroxypropyl methylcellulose (Gonak™; Goniosol®)	Ophthalmic surgical aid in cataract extraction and intraocular implantation; gonioscopic examination
Indocyanine green (Cardio-Green®)	Determine hepatic function, cardiac output, and liver blood flow and for ophthalmic angiography
Mephentermine (Wyamine® Sulfate Injection)	Treatment of hypotension secondary to ganglionic blockade or spinal anesthesia; may be used as an emergency measure to maintain blood pressure until whole blood replacement becomes available
Methacholine (Provocholine®)	Diagnosis of bronchial airway hyperactivity
Methylene blue (Urolene Blue®)	Antidote for cyanide poisoning and drug-induced methemoglobinemia, indicator dye, chronic urolithiasis. **Unlabeled use:** Has been used topically (0.1% solutions) in conjunction with polychromatic light to photoinactivate viruses such as herpes simplex; has been used alone or in combination with vitamin C for the management of chronic urolithiasis.
Metocurine iodide (Metubine® Iodide)	Adjunct to anesthesia to induce skeletal muscle relaxation
Microfibrillar collagen hemostat (Avitene®; Helistat®; Hemotene®)	Adjunct to hemostasis when control of bleeding by ligature is ineffective or impractical
Mumps skin test antigen	Assess the status of cell-mediated immunity
Pentagastrin (Peptavlon®)	Evaluate gastric acid secretory function in pernicious anemia, gastric carcinoma; used with suspected duodenal ulcer or Zollinger-Ellison tumor
Phenolsulfonphthalein	Evaluation of renal blood flow to aid in the determination of renal function

DIAGNOSTICS AND SURGICAL AIDS *(Continued)*

Agent	Use
Proparacaine (AK-Taine®; Alcaine®; I-Paracaine®; Ophthetic®)	Anesthesia for tonometry, gonioscopy; suture removal from cornea; removal of corneal foreign body; cataract extraction, glaucoma surgery; short operative procedure involving the cornea and conjunctiva
Proparacaine and fluorescein (Fluoracaine® Ophthalmic)	Anesthesia for tonometry, gonioscopy; suture removal from cornea; removal of corneal foreign body; cataract extraction, glaucoma surgery
Protirelin (Relefact® TRH Injection; Thypinone® Injection)	Adjunct in the diagnostic assessment of thyroid function, and an adjunct to other diagnostic procedures in assessment of patients with pituitary or hypothalamic dysfunction; causes release of prolactin from the pituitary and is used to detect defective control of prolactin secretion
Secretin (Secretin Ferring Powder)	Diagnose Zollinger-Ellison syndrome, chronic pancreatic dysfunction, and some hepatobiliary diseases such as obstructive jaundice resulting from cancer or stones in the biliary tract
Sermorelin acetate (Geref® Injection; Geref® Diagnostic)	Geref® Diagnostic: For the evaluation of short children whose height is at least 2 standard deviations below the mean height for their chronological age and sex, presenting with low basal serum levels of IGF-1 and IGF-1-BP3. A single intravenous injection of sermorelin is indicated for evaluating the ability of the somatotroph of the pituitary gland to secrete growth hormone (GH). A normal plasma GH response demonstrates that the somatotroph is intact. Geref® injection: Treatment of idiopathic growth hormone deficiency
Sincalide (Kinevac®)	Postevacuation cholecystography; gallbladder bile sampling; stimulate pancreatic secretion for analysis
Skin test antigens, multiple (Multitest CMI®)	Detection of nonresponsiveness to antigens by means of delayed hypersensitivity skin testing
Sodium hyaluronate (AMO Vitrax®; Amvisc®; Amvisc® Plus; Healon®; Healon® GV)	Surgical aid in cataract extraction, intraocular implantation, corneal transplant, glaucoma filtration, and retinal attachment surgery
Succinylcholine (Anectine® Chloride Injection; Anectine® Flo-Pack®; Quelicin® Injection)	Produces skeletal muscle relaxation in procedures of short duration such as endotracheal intubation or endoscopic exams
Suprofen (Profenal® Ophthalmic)	Inhibition of intraoperative miosis
Thrombin, topical (Thrombinar®; Thrombogen®; Thrombostat®)	Hemostasis whenever minor bleeding from capillaries and small venules is accessible
Thyrotropin Alpha (Thyrogen®)	As an adjunctive diagnostic tool for serum thyroglobulin (Tg) testing with or without radioiodine imaging in the follow-up of patients with well-differentiated thyroid cancer
Trichophyton skin test (Dermatophytin® Injection)	Assess cell-mediated immunity
Tropicamide (Mydriacyl®; Opticyl®; Tropicacyl®)	Short-acting mydriatic used in diagnostic procedures, as well as preoperatively and postoperatively; treatment of some cases of acute itis, iridocyclitis, and keratitis

HERBAL AND NUTRITIONAL PRODUCTS

TOP HERBAL PRODUCTS

This section contains general information on commonly encountered herbal or nutritional products. A more complete listing of products follows.

Alpha-lipoic Acid

Synonyms: Alpha-lipoate; Lipoic Acid; Thioctic acid
Use: Treatment of glaucoma and neuropathies
Mechanism of Action/Effect: Sulfur-containing cofactor normally synthesized in humans; potent antioxidant
Warnings: Use with caution in individuals who may be predisposed to hypoglycemia (including individuals receiving antidiabetic agents).
Drug Interactions: Oral hypoglycemics or insulin
Adverse Reactions: Rash
Dosing: Oral: 20-600 mg/day (common dose: 25-50 mg twice daily)

Androstenedione

Use: Increase strength and muscle mass
Mechanism of Action/Effect: Weak androgenic steroid hormone believed to facilitate faster recovery from exercise and to promote muscle development in response to training
Contraindication: Hypertension
Warnings: Use with caution in individuals with CHF, prostate conditions, and hormone-sensitive tumors. The FDA requires specific labeling on this supplement, noting that these supplements "contain steroid hormones that may cause breast enlargement, testicular shrinkage, and infertility in males, and increased facial and body hair, voice deepening and clitoral enlargement in females."
Drug Interactions: Estrogens and androgenic drugs
Dosing: Oral: 50-100 mg/day (usually about 1 hour before exercising)

Arginine

Synonyms: L-Arginine
Use: Treatment of high cholesterol, poor circulation,inflammatory bowel disease, immunity enhancement, male infertility; promotes lean body mass, surgery and wound healing, sexual vitality and enhancement
Mechanism of Action/Effect: Precursor to nitric oxide; plays a key role in the urea cycle, which is the biochemical pathway that metabolized protein and other nitrogen-containing compounds
Warnings: Use caution in individuals with herpes simplex; may stimulate growth of virus.
Drug Interactions: Nitroglycerin and sildenafil
Dosing: Oral: 3-6 g/day

Bifidobacterium bifidum/Lactobacillus acidophilus

Use:

B. bifidum: Treatment of Crohn's disease, diarrhea, ulcerative colitis; maintenance of anaerobic microflora in the colon

L. acidophilus: Treatment of constipation, infant diarrhea, lactose intolerance; recolonization of the GI tract with beneficial bacteria during and after antibiotic use

Mechanism of Action/Effect: Natural components of colonic flora, used to facilitate recolonization with benign symbiotic organisms; promote vitamin K synthesis and absorption
Drug Interactions: Antibiotics eliminate *B. bifidum* and *L. acidophilus*
Adverse Reactions: No known toxicity or serious side effect
Dosing: Oral: 5-10 billion colony forming units (CFU) per day (dairy free); refrigerate to maintain optimum potency

Bilberry

Synonym: *Vaccinium myrtillus*
Use: Treatment of ophthalmologic disorders (eg, macular degeneration, diabetic retinopathy, cataracts) and vascular disorders (eg, varicose veins, phlebitis)
Mechanism of Action/Effect: Reportedly inhibits a variety of inflammatory mediators, including histamine, proteases, leukotrienes, and prostaglandins; may decrease capillary permeability and inhibit platelet aggregation
Contraindication: Active bleeding (eg, peptic ulcer, intracranial bleeding)
Warnings: Use with caution in individuals with a history of bleeding, hemostatic disorders, or drug-related hemostatic problems. Use with caution in individuals taking anticoagulants (eg, warfarin, aspirin, aspirin-containing products, NSAIDs) or antiplatelet agents (eg, ticlopidine, clopidogrel, dipyridamole). Discontinue use prior to dental or surgical procedures (generally at least 14 days before).
Drug Interactions: Oral hypoglycemics or insulin (effects may be altered)
Dosing: Oral: 80 mg 2-3 times/day

HERBAL AND NUTRITIONAL PRODUCTS *(Continued)*

Black Cohosh

Synonym: *Cimicifuga racemosa*
Use: Treatment of vasomotor symptoms of menopause, premenstrual syndrome (PMS), mild depression, arthritis
Mechanism of Action/Effect: Contains multiple phytoestrogens and salicylic acid (small amounts)
Contraindications: Pregnancy (may stimulate uterine contractions) and lactation; history of estrogen-dependent tumors or endometrial cancer
Warnings: Use with caution in individuals allergic to salicylates (unknown whether the amount of salicylic acid is likely to affect platelet aggregation or have other effects associated with salicylates); those receiving hormone replacement therapy, taking oral contraceptives, or with a history of thromboembolic disease or stroke
Drug Interactions: Oral contraceptives, hormonal replacement therapy
Adverse Reactions: High doses: Nausea, vomiting, headache, hypotension
Dosing: Oral: 20-40 mg twice daily

Chamomile

Synonyms: *Matricaria chamomilla*; *Matricaria recutita*
Use: Topical anti-inflammatory with hypnotic properties; treatment of hemorrhoids, irritable bowel, eczema, mastitis and leg ulcers; cigarette tobacco flavoring
Mechanism of Action/Effect: Antispasmodic; anti-inflammatory; antiulcer; antibacterial and sedative effects also documented
Contraindications: Hypersensitivity to *Asteraceae/Compositae* family or ragweed pollens
Warnings: Use with caution in asthmatics; cross sensitivity may occur in individuals allergic to ragweed pollens, asters, or chrysanthemums.
Drug Interactions: May increase effect of coumarin-type anticoagulants at high doses; may potentiate sedatives (benzodiazepines, barbiturates)
Adverse Reactions: Contact dermatitis, emesis (from dried flowering heads), anaphylaxis, hypersensitivity reactions (especially in atopic individuals)
Dosing:

Tea: ±150 mL H_2O poured over heaping tablespoon (±3 g) of chamomile, covered and steeped 5-10 minutes; tea is used 3-4 times/day for GI upset

Liquid extract: 1-4 mL 3 times/day

Pregnancy Implications: Excessive use should be avoided due to potential teratogenicity.

Chasteberry

Synonyms: Chastetree; *Vitex agnus-castus*
Use: Treatment of acne vulgaris, corpus luteum insufficiency, hyperprolactinemia, insufficient lactation, menopause, menstrual disorders (eg, amenorrhea, endometriosis, premenstrual syndrome)
Mechanism of Action/Effect: Noted to possess significant effect on pituitary function; demonstrated to have progesterone-like effects (may stimulate luteinizing hormone [LH] and inhibit follicle-stimulating hormone [FSH]
Contraindications: Pregnancy and lactation (based on case reports of uterine stimulation and emmenagogue effects)
Warnings: Use with caution in individuals receiving hormonal therapy.
Drug Interactions: Hormonal replacement therapy, oral contraceptives, dopamine antagonists (eg, metoclopramide and antipsychotics)
Dosing: Oral: 400 mg/day in the morning (preferably on an empty stomach)

Chondroitin Sulfate

Use: Treatment of osteoarthritis
Mechanism of Action/Effect: Reported to act synergistically with glucosamine to support the maintenance of strong, healthy cartilage and maintain joint function; inhibits synovial enzymes (elastase, hyaluronidase) which may contribute to cartilage destruction and loss of joint function (studies inconclusive)
Adverse Reactions: No known toxicity or serious side effects.
Dosing: Oral: 300-1500 mg/day

Chromium

Use: Improves glycemic control; increases lean body mass; reduces obesity; improves lipid profile by decreasing total cholesterol and triglycerides, increasing HDL (dosages in excess of >300 mg/day reported to benefit breast cancer, diabetes, and cardiovascular diseases)
Mechanism of Action/Effect: Chromium picolinate is the only active form of chromium. It appears that chromium, in its trivalent form, increases insulin sensitivity and improves glucose transport into cells. The mechanism by which this happens could include one or more of the following: Increase the number of insulin receptors, enhance

insulin binding to target tissues, promote activation of insulin-receptor tyrosine dinase activity, enhance beta-cell sensitivity in the pancreas.
Drug Interactions: Any medications that may also affect blood sugars (eg, beta-blockers, thiazides, oral hypoglycemics, and insulin); discuss chromium use prior to initiating
Adverse Reactions: Nausea, loose stools, flatulence, changes in appetite; isolated reports of anemia, cognitive impairment, renal failure
Dosing: 50-600 mcg/day

Coenzyme Q_{10}

Synonym: Ubiquinone
Use: Treatment of angina, chronic fatigue syndrome, CHF, hypertension, muscular dystrophy, obesity, periodontal disease
Mechanism of Action/Effect: Functions as a lipid-soluble antioxidant, providing protection against free radical damage; involved in ATP generation, the primary source of energy in human physiology
Drug Interactions: Drugs which can cause depletion of CoQ_{10}: Hydralazine, thiazide diuretics, HMG-CoA reductase inhibitors, sulfonylureas, beta blockers, tricyclic antidepressants, chlorpromazine, clonidine, methyldopa, diazoxide, biguanides, haloperidol; CoQ_{10} may decrease response to warfarin
Warnings: Controlled trials have not demonstrated benefit in heart failure.
Dosing: Oral: 30-200 mg/day

Cranberry

Synonym: *Vaccinium macrocarpon*
Use: Prevention of nephrolithiasis, urinary tract infection
Mechanism of Action/Effect: Although early research indicated that cranberry worked through urinary acidification, current research indicates that a cranberry-derived glycoprotein inhibits *E. coli* adherence to the epithelial cells of the urinary tract.
Dosing: Oral: 300-400 mg twice daily or 8-16 oz/day of 100% cranberry juice

Dehydroepiandosterone

Synonym: DHEA
Use: Treatment of depression, diabetes, fatigue, aging, lupus
Mechanism of Action/Effect: Precursor for the synthesis of over 50 hormones (including estrogen and testosterone); secreted by the adrenal glands, DHEA has been shown to stimulate production of insulin growth factor-1 (IGF-1) and change the response to insulin, decreasing the insulin requirement in individuals with diabetes. Supplementation may also increase circulating testosterone levels.
Contraindications: History of prostate or breast cancer
Warnings: Use with caution in individuals with hepatic dysfunction, diabetes, or those predisposed to hypoglycemia. Blood glucose should be closely monitored in diabetics and the dosage of antidiabetic agents should be closely monitored among health care providers.
Drug Interactions: May interact with androgens, estrogens, corticosteroids, insulin, oral hypoglycemic agents
Adverse Reactions: No known toxicity or serious side effects; long-term human studies have not been conducted
Dosing: Oral: 5-50 mg/day; 100 mg/day has been used in elderly individuals

Dong Quai

Synonyms: *Angelica sinensis*; Chinese angelica
Use: Treatment of anemia, hypertension, menopause, dysmenorrhea, PMS, amenorrhea; improves energy (particularly in females)
Mechanism of Action/Effect: Reported to cause vasodilation and may have hematopoietic properties; rich in phytoestrogens which may demonstrate similar pharmacological effects, but are less potent than pure estrogenic compounds
Contraindications: Active bleeding (eg, peptic ulcer, intracranial bleeding); may alter hemostasis, based on potential interference with platelet aggregation (observed with related species)
Warnings: Use with caution in individuals at risk of hypotension and those who would tolerate hypotension poorly (eg, cerebrovascular or cardiovascular disease); individuals taking antihypertensive medications, hormone replacement therapy, oral contraceptives, or with a history of estrogen-dependent tumors, endometrial cancer, thromboembolic disease, or stroke; individuals with a history of bleeding, hemostatic disorders, or drug-related hemostatic problems; those taking anticoagulants (may potentiate effects of warfarin) or antiplatelet agents (eg, ticlopidine, clopidogrel, dipyridamole); and in pregnant and lactating women. May cause photosensitization; avoid prolonged exposure to sunlight or other sources of ultraviolet radiation (ie, tanning booths). Discontinue use prior to dental or surgical procedures (generally at least 14 days before).
Drug Interactions: Antihypertensives, anticoagulants, antiplatelet drugs, hormonal replacement therapy, oral contraceptives, photosensitizing medications
Dosing: Oral: 200 mg twice daily

HERBAL AND NUTRITIONAL PRODUCTS *(Continued)*

Echinacea

Synonyms: American Coneflower; Black Susans; Comb Flower; *Echinacea angustifolia*; Indian Head; Purple Coneflower; Scury Root; Snakeroot

Use: Treatment of cold and flu, minor upper respiratory tract infections, urinary tract infections

Mechanism of Action/Effect: Has antihyaluronidase and anti-inflammatory activity; caffeic acid glycosides and isolutylamides associated with the plant can cause immune stimulation (leukocyte phagocytosis and T-cell activation)

Contraindications: Allergy to sunflowers, daisies, ragweed; autoimmune diseases (eg, collagen vascular disease [lupus, RA], HIV/AIDS), multiple sclerosis, tuberculosis, pregnancy; per Commission E: Parenteral administration is contraindicated, but oral use is not contraindicated during pregnancy

Warnings: May alter immunosuppression; long-term use may cause immunosuppression. Persons allergic to sunflowers may display cross-allergy potential. Use as a preventative treatment should be discouraged.

Drug Interactions: May alter response to immunosuppressive therapy

Adverse Reactions: Tingling sensation of tongue, allergic reactions (rare); may become immunosuppressive with continuous use over 6-8 weeks

Per Commission E: None known for oral and external use

Dosing: Continuous use should not exceed 8 weeks; may be applied topically.

Per Commission E: Expressed juice (of fresh herb): 6-9 mL/day

Capsule/tablet or tea form: 500 mg to 2 g 3 times/day

Liquid extract: 0.25-1 mL 3 times/day

Tincture: 1-2 mL 3 times/day

Evening Primrose

Synonyms: Evening Primrose Oil; *Oenothera biennis*

Use: Treatment of diabetic neuropathy, endometriosis, hyperglycemia, irritable bowel syndrome, multiple sclerosis, omega-6-fatty acid supplementation, PMS, menopause, rheumatoid arthritis

Mechanism of Action/Effect: Contains high amounts of gamma-linolenic acid, or GLA, an essential omega-6 fatty acid which reportedly reduces generation of arachidonic acid metabolites in short-term use, improving symptoms of various inflammatory and immune conditions; reported to stimulate hormone synthesis

Contraindications: Seizure disorders (may lower seizure threshold, based on animal studies), schizophrenia, active bleeding (may inhibit platelet aggregation), individuals receiving anticonvulsant or antipsychotic medications

Warnings: Use with caution in individuals with a history of bleeding, hemostatic disorders, or drug-related hemostatic problems; individuals taking anticoagulants (eg, warfarin, aspirin, aspirin-containing products, NSAIDs) or antiplatelet agents (eg, ticlopidine, clopidogrel, dipyridamole). Discontinue use prior to dental or surgical procedures (generally at least 14 days before).

Drug Interactions: Anticonvulsants (seizure threshold decreased), anticoagulants, antiplatelet agents

Dosing: Oral: 500 mg to 8 g/day

Feverfew

Synonyms: Altamisa; Bachelor's Buttons; Featherfew; Featherfoil; Nosebleed; *Tanacetum parthenium*; Wild Quinine

Use: Prophylaxis and treatment of migraine headaches; treatment of menstrual complaints and fever

Mechanism of Action/Effect: Active ingredient is parthenolide (~0.2% concentration), which is a serotonin antagonist; also, the plant may be an inhibitor of prostaglandin synthesis and platelet aggregation; may have spasmolytic activity

Contraindications: Pregnancy and lactation; children <2 years of age; allergies to feverfew and other members of Asteraceae, daisy, ragweed, chamomile

Warning: Use with caution in patients taking medications with serotonergic properties.

Drug Interactions: Anticoagulants (eg, aspirin, aspirin-containing products, NSAIDs)

Adverse Reactions: Mouth ulcerations, contact dermatitis, abdominal pain, nausea, vomiting, loss of taste; postfeverfew syndrome on discontinuation (nervousness, insomnia, still joints, headache)

Dosing: 125 mg 1-2 times/day

Garlic

Synonyms: *Allium savitum*; Comphor of the Poor; Nectar of the Gods; Poor Mans Treacle; Rustic Treacle; Stinking Rose

Use: Treatment of hypertension; lowers LDL cholesterol and triglycerides and raises HDL cholesterol; may lower blood glucose and decrease thrombosis; potential anti-inflammatory and antitumor effects

Mechanism of Action/Effect: Allinin garlic is converted to allicin (after the bulb is ground), which is odoriferous and may have some antioxidant activity; ajoene (a byproduct of allicin) has potent platelet inhibition effects; garlic can also decrease LDL cholesterol levels and increase fibrinolytic activity

Contraindication: Pregnancy

Warnings: Onset of cholesterol-lowering and hypotensive effects may require months. Use with caution in patients receiving treatment for hyperglycemia or hypertension.

Drug Interactions: Iodine uptake may be reduced with garlic ingestion; can exacerbate bleeding in patients taking aspirin or anticoagulant agents; may increase the risk of hypoglycemia; may increase response to antihypertensives

Adverse Reactions: Skin blistering, eczema, systemic contact dermatitis, immunologic contact urticaria, GI upset and changes in intestinal flora (rare) per Commission E, lacrimation, asthma (upon inhalation of garlic dust), allergic reactions (rare), change in odor of skin and breath (per Commission E)

Half-Life Elimination: N-acetyl-S-allyl-L-cysteine: 6 hours

Excretion: Pulmonary and renal

Dosing: Adults: 4-12 mg allicin/day

Average daily dose for cardiovascular benefit: 0.25-1 g/kg or 1-4 cloves daily in an 80 kg individual in divided doses

Toxic dose: >5 cloves or >25 mL of extract can cause GI symptoms

Additional Information: 1% as active as penicillin as an antibiotic; number one over-the-counter medication in Germany; enteric-coated products may demonstrate best results.

Ginger

Synonym: *Zingiber officinale*

Pregnancy Risk Factor: Per Commission E, not to be used for morning sickness during pregnancy (some contradictory recommendations exist); high doses may be abortifacient

Use: Antiemetic; digestive aid; treatment of nausea and motion sickness, headaches, colds and flu, arthritis; flavoring agent in beverages and mouthwashes

Mechanism of Action/Effect: Unknown; appears to decrease prostaglandin synthesismay increase GI motility; may have cardiotonic activity and inhibit platelet aggregation (very high doses)

Contraindication: Gallstones (per Commission E)

Warnings: Use with caution in diabetics, patients on cardiac glycosides, and those receiving anticoagulants.

Drug Interactions: May alter response to cardiotonic, hypoglycemic, anticoagulant, and antiplatelet agents

Dosing:

Prevention of motion sickness or digestive aid: 1-4 g/day (250 mg of ginger root powder 3-4 times/day)

Per Commission E: 2-4 g/day or equivalent preparations

Ginkgo Biloba

Synonyms: Kew Tree; Maidenhair Tree

Use: Treatment of tinnitus, visual disorders, traumatic brain injury, vertigo of vascular origin

Europe: Treatment of intermittent claudication, arterial insufficiency, and cerebral vascular disease (dementia)

Per Commission E: Demential syndromes including memory deficits, etc (tinnitus, headache); depressive emotional conditions, primary degenerative dementia, vascular dementia, or both

Investigational: Treatment of asthma, impotence (male)

Mechanism of Action/Effect: Dilates blood vessels and inhibits platelet aggregation; leaf extract contain terpenoids and flavonoids which can allegedly inactivate oxygen-free radicals causing vasodilatation and antagonize effects of platelet activating factor (PAF); fruit pulp contains ginkolic acids which are allergens (seeds are not sensitizing)

Contraindications: Pregnancy, clotting disorders, hypersensitivity to ginkgo biloba preparations (per Commission E)

Warnings: Use with caution following recent surgery or trauma. Effects may require 1-2 months. Controlled studies have not demonstrated consistent efficacy in dementia.

Drug Interactions: Due to effects on PAF, use with caution in patients receiving anticoagulants or platelet inhibitors.

Adverse Reactions: Palpitations, bilateral subdural hematomas, dizziness, seizures (in children), restlessness, urticaria, cheilitis, nausea, diarrhea, vomiting, stomatitis, proctitis, stomach or intestinal upsets, hyphema

Rare (per Commission E): Headache, allergic skin reactions, stomach or GI upset

Onset of Effect: 1 hour

Peak Absorption: 2-3 hours

Duration of Action: 7 hours

Bioavailability: 70% to 100%

Half-life: Ginkgolide A: 4 hours; ginkgolide B: 10.6 hours; bilobalide: 3.2 hours

Dosing: ~40 mg 3 times/day with meals; 60-80 mg twice daily to 3 times/day (depending on indication); maximum dose: 360 mg/day

HERBAL AND NUTRITIONAL PRODUCTS *(Continued)*

Cerebral ischemia: 120 mg/day in 2-3 divided doses (24% flavonoid-glycoside extract, 6% terpene glycosides); beneficial effects for cerebral ischemia in the elderly occur after 1 month of use

Ginseng, Panax

Synonyms: Asian Ginseng; *Panax ginseng*

Use: Adrenal tonic; immunosupportive; enhances physical/mental performance and energy levels; adjunct support for chemotherapy/radiation

Mechanism of Action/Effect: Ginsenosides are believed to act via hormone receptors in the hypothalamus, pituitary glands, and other tissues. Ginsenosides stimulate secretion of adrenocorticotropic hormone (ACTH), leading to production of increased release of adrenal hormones, including cortisol. Specific triterpenoid saponins (diols) are claimed to be mediate improvements in endurance and learning. These compounds are also believed to contribute to sedative and antihypertensive properties. A second group (triols) reportedly increase blood pressure and function as central nervous system stimulants. *Panax ginseng* is reported to have immunostimulating effects. *Panax ginseng* has been claimed to facilitate adaptation to stress caused by chemotherapy and radiation.

Contraindications: Renal failure, acute infection, active bleeding (may alter hemostasis), pregnancy and lactation

Adverse Reactions: Mastalgia, vaginal breakthrough bleeding **Note:** Prolonged use or high dosages may cause Ginseng Abuse Syndrome (diarrhea, hypertension, nervousness, dermatologic eruptions, insomnia) and/or palpitations and tachycardia in sensitive individuals

Warnings: Use with caution in individuals with hyper- or hypotension; those with a history of bleeding, hemostatic disorders, or drug-related hemostatic problems; those receiving MAO inhibitors or stimulants (eg, decongestants, caffeine). Discontinue use prior to dental or surgical procedures (generally at least 14 days before).

Drug Interactions: Antihypertensives, MAO inhibitors, central nervous stimulants (caffeine), sympathomimetics, and hormonal therapies; anticoagulant medications, including warfarin, aspirin, aspirin-containing products, NSAIDs, or antiplatelet agents (eg, ticlopidine, clopidogrel, dipyridamole).

Dosing: Oral: 100-600 mg/day in divided doses

Ginseng, Siberian

Synonyms: *Eleutherococcus senticosus;* Siberian Ginseng

Use: Believed to facilitate adaptation to stress and to act as an immune stimulant.; reported to enhance athletic performance and physical endurance, increase mental alertness and amount of quality work performed, and decrease sick days

Contraindication: Active bleeding; hemostasis may be affected

Warnings: Use with caution in individuals with hypertension or those receiving antihypertensive medications (may potentiate effects); individuals at risk of hypotension, elderly , or those who would not tolerate transient hyper- or hypotensive episodes (ie, cerebrovascular or cardiovascular disease); diabetics; those with a history of bleeding, hemostatic disorders, or drug-related hemostatic problems. Discontinue use prior to dental or surgical procedures (generally at least 14 days before). Extensive or prolonged use may heighten estrogenic activity (based on pharmacological activity).

Drug Interactions: Barbiturates, antihypertensives, insulin, oral hypoglycemics, digoxin, stimulants (including OTC); anticoagulants (eg, warfarin, aspirin, aspirin-containing products, NSAIDs) or antiplatelet agents (eg, ticlopidine, clopidogrel, dipyridamole)

Dosing: Oral: 100-200 mg twice daily

Glucosamine

Use: Treatment of osteoarthritis, rheumatoid arthritis, tendonitis, gout, bursitis

Mechanism of Action/Effect: An amino sugar, which is a key component in the synthesis of proteoglycans, a group of proteins found in cartilage which are negatively charged, and attract water so they can produce synovial fluid in the joints; the theory is that supplying the body with these precursors will replenish important synovial fluid, and lead to production of new cartilage. Glucosamine also appears to inhibit cartilage-destroying enzymes (eg, collagenase and phospholipase A2), thus stopping the degenerative processes of osteoarthritis. A third mechanism may be glucosamine's ability to prevent production of damaging superoxide radicals, which may lead to cartilage destruction.

Adverse Reactions: Flatulence, nausea

Warnings: Use caution in patients with diabetes; may cause insulin resistance

Drug Interactions: May increase effect of oral anticoagulants and alter response to insulin or oral hypoglycemics

Dosing: 500 mg 3 times/day (sulfate form)

Golden Seal

Synonyms: Eye Balm; Eye Root; *Hydrastis canadensis*; Indian Eye; Jaundice Root; Orange Root; Turmeric Root; Yellow Indian Paint; Yellow Root
Use: Treatment of hemorrhoids, postpartum hemorrhage, mucosal inflammation/ gastritis (efficacy not established in clinical studies); produces GI and peripheral vascular activity; used in sterile eyewashes; used as a mouthwash and laxative
Mechanism of Action/Effect: Contains the alkaloids hydrastine (4%) and berberine (6%), which at higher doses can cause vasoconstriction, hypertension, and mucosal irritation. Berberine can produce hypotension.
Contraindications: Pregnancy and lactation
Warnings: Should not be used in patients with hypertension, glaucoma, diabetes, history of stroke, or heart disease.
Drug Interaction: May interfere with vitamin B absorption
Adverse Reactions: High doses: Stimulation/agitation, nausea, vomiting, diarrhea, mouth and throat irritation, extremity numbness, respiratory failure
Dosing:
Root: 0.5-1 g 3 times/day
Solid form: Usual dose: 5-10 grains

Green Tea

Synonym: *Camellia sinensis*
Use: Platelet-aggregation inhibitor; antioxidant with anticarcinogenic activity; supportive in cancer prevention and cardiovascular disease; may lower cholesterol
Mechanism of Action/Effect: Reportedly has antioxidant properties and protects against oxidative damage to cells and tissues. Demonstrated to increase HDL cholesterol, decrease LDL cholesterol, and decrease triglycerides. Green tea has also been reported to block the peroxidation of LDL, inhibit formation of thromboxane formation, and block platelet aggregation. Human studies have noted a correlation between consumption of green tea and improvement in prognosis in some forms of breast cancer.
Contraindications: Active bleeding (eg, peptic ulcer, intracerebral bleeding)
Warnings: Nondecaffeinated products should be used with caution in individuals with peptic ulcer disease or cardiovascular disease. Use with caution in individuals with a history of bleeding, hemostatic disorders, or drug-related hemostatic problems; those receiving anticoagulants (reported to antagonize the effects of warfarin) or antiplatelet agents (eg, ticlopidine, clopidogrel, dipyridamole). Discontinue use prior to dental or surgical procedures (generally at least 14 days before). Use with caution when taking other stimulants (caffeine, decongestants), unless a caffeine-free product is used. **Note:** Addition of milk to tea may significantly lower the antioxidant potential of this agent.
Drug Interactions: Anticoagulants (eg, warfarin, aspirin, aspirin-containing products, NSAIDs), antiplatelet agents (eg, ticlopidine, clopidogrel, dipyridamole), stimulants (including OTC decongestants)
Adverse Reactions: If product is not decaffeinated, caffeine may cause gastric irritation, decreased appetite, insomnia, tachycardia, palpitations, and nervousness in sensitive individuals.
Dosing: Oral: 250-500 mg/day

Hawthorn

Synonyms: *Crataegus laevigata; Crataegus monogyna; Crataegus oxyacantha; Crataegus pinnatifida*; English Hawthorn; Haw; Maybush; Whitehorn
Use: Sedative; treatment of cardiovascular abnormalities (eg, arrhythmia, angina), increased cardiac output, increased contractility of heart muscle
Mechanism of Action/Effect: Contains flavonoids, catechin, and epicatechin which may be cardioprotective and have vasodilatory properties; shown to dilate coronary vessels
Contraindications: Pregnancy and lactation
Drug Interactions: Antihypertensives (effect enhanced), ACE inhibitors, digoxin; effects with Viagra® are unknown
Adverse Reactions: Hypotension, bradycardia, hypertension, depression, fatigue, rash, nausea
Dosing: Daily dose of total flavonoids: 10 mg
Per Commission E: 160-900 mg native water-ethanol extract (ethanol 45% v/v or methanol 70% v/v, drug-extract ratio: 4-7:1, with defined flavonoid or procyanidin content), corresponding to 30-168.7 mg procyanidins, calculated as epicatechin, or 3.5-19.8 mg flavonoids, calculated as hyperoside in accordance with DAB 10 (German pharmacopoeia #10) in 2 or 3 individual doses; duration of administration: 6 weeks minimum

Horse Chestnut

Synonym: *Aesculus hippocastanum*
Use: Treatment of varicose veins, hemorrhoids, other venous insufficiencies, deep venous thrombosis, lower extremity edema

HERBAL AND NUTRITIONAL PRODUCTS *(Continued)*

Mechanism of Action/Effect: Reportedly functions as an anti-inflammatory, which may be related to quercetin's reported ability to inhibit cyclo-oxygenase and lipoxygenase, the enzymes which form inflammatory prostaglandins and leukotrienes; quercetin is also an inhibitor of phosphodiesterase, which has been correlated to cardiotonic, hypotensive, spasmolytic, antiplatelet, and sedative actions; inhibits platelet aggregation and supports collagen structures
Contraindications: Active bleeding (eg, peptic ulcer, intracranial bleeding)
Warnings: Use with caution in individuals with hepatic or renal impairment, a history of bleeding, hemostatic disorders, or drug-related hemostatic problems. Discontinue use prior to dental or surgical procedures (generally at least 14 days before).
Drug Interactions: Anticoagulants (eg, warfarin, aspirin, aspirin-containing products, NSAIDs) and antiplatelet agents (eg, ticlopidine, clopidogrel, dipyridamole)
Adverse Reaction: GI upset
Dosing:
 Oral: 300 mg 1-2 times/day, standardized to 50 mg escin per dose
 Topical: Apply 2% escin gel 1-2 times/day to affected area

Kava

Synonyms: Awa; Kew; *Piper methysticum*; Tonga
Use: Treatment of anxiety, stress, and restlessness (per Commission E); sleep inducement
Mechanism of Action/Effect: Contains alpha-pyrones in root extracts; may possess central dopaminergic antagonistic properties
Contraindications: Per Commission E: Pregnancy, endogenous depression
Warnings: Extended continuous intake can cause a temporary yellow discoloration of skin, hair, and nails. In this case, further application must be discontinued. In rare cases, allergic skin reactions occur. Also, accommodative disturbances (eg, enlargement of the pupils and disturbances of the oculomotor equilibrium) have been described.
Drug Interactions: Coma can occur from concomitant administration of alprazolam; may potentiate alcohol or CNS depressants, barbiturates, psychopharmacological agents
Adverse Reactions: Euphoria, depression, somnolence, skin discoloration (prolonged use), muscle weakness, eye disturbances, hepatotoxicity
Dosing: Per Commission E: Do not use for >3 months without medical advice. Herb and preparations equivalent to 60-120 mg kavalactones

Melaleuca Oil

Use: Dermal agent for burns; marketed as fungicidal, bactericidal
Mechanism of Action/Effect: Consists of plant terpenes, pinenes, and cineole, derived from the *Melaleuca alternifolia* tree, the colorless or pale yellow oil can cause CNS depression; may be bacteriostatic
Adverse Reactions: Allergic reactions or dermatitis (rare)
Dosing: Topical: Minimal toxic dose: Infant: <10 mL

Melatonin

Use: Treatment of sleep disorders (eg, jet lag, insomnia, neurologic problems, shift work), aging, cancer, immune system support
Mechanism of Action/Effect: Hormone responsible for regulating the body's circadian rhythm and sleep patterns; release is prompted by darkness and inhibited by light. Secretion appears to peak during childhood, and declines gradually through adolescence and adulthood. Melatonin receptors have been found in blood cells, the brain, gut, and ovaries; may also have a role in regulating cardiovascular and reproductive function through its antioxidant properties.
Contraindications: Immune disorders; pregnancy and lactation
Drug Interactions: Medications commonly used as sedatives or hypnotics, or those that induce sedation, drowsiness (eg, benzodiazepines, narcotics); CNS depressants (prescription, supplements such as 5-HTP); other herbs known to cause sedation include kava, valerian
Adverse Reactions: Reduced alertness, headache, irritability, increased fatigue, drowsiness, sedation
Dosing: Sleep disturbances: 0.3-5 mg/day

Red Yeast Rice

Synonym: *Monascus purpureus*
Use: Hypercholesterolemic agent; may lower triglycerides and LDL cholesterol and raise HDL cholesterol
Mechanism of Action/Effect: Eight compounds with HMG-CoA reductase inhibitory activity have been identified, including lovastatin and its active hydroxy acid metabolite.
Contraindications: Pregnancy, or if trying to become pregnant, and lactation (based on pharmacological activity); known hypersensitivity to rice or yeast; children and adults <20 years of age; hepatic disease, history of liver disease, or those who may be at risk

of liver disease; serious infection, recent major surgery, other serious disease, or organ transplant individuals; any individual who consumes more than 1-2 alcohol-containing drinks per day
Warnings: Use with caution in individuals currently receiving other cholesterol-lowering medications. HMG-CoA reductase inhibitors have been associated with rare (less than 1% to 2% incidence) but serious adverse effects, including hepatic and skeletal muscle disorders (myopathy, rhabdomyolysis). The risk of these disorders may be increased by concomitant therapy with specific medications. Discontinue use at the first sign of hepatic dysfunction.
Drug Interactions: HMG-CoA reductase inhibitors, other cholesterol-lowering agents, anticoagulants, gemfibrozil, erythromycin, itraconazole, ketoconazole, cyclosporine, niacin, clofibrate, fenofibrate
Adverse Reaction: GI upset
Dosing: Oral: 1200 mg twice daily

SAMe

Synonym: S-adenosylmethionine
Use: Treatment of depression
Mechanism of Action/Effect: Not defined; functions as a cofactor in many synthetic pathways
Contraindication: Active bleeding (eg, peptic ulcer, intracranial bleeding)
Warnings: Use caution when combining with other antidepressants, tryptophan, or 5-HTP. SAMe is not effective in the treatment of depressive symptoms associated with bipolar disorder.
Drug Interactions: May potentiate activity and/or toxicities of MAO inhibitors, tricyclic antidepressants, or SSRIs; may potentiate the antidepressant effects of 5-HTP, tryptophan, and St John's wort
Adverse Reactions: Dry mouth, nausea, restlessness
Dosing: Oral: 400-1600 mg/day

Sassafras Oil

Synonym: *Sassafras albidum*
Use: Mild counterirritant on the skin (ie, lice or insect bites)
Mechanism of Action/Effect: Contains safrole (up to 80%) which inhibits liver microsomal enzymes; its metabolite may cause hepatic tumors
Adverse Reactions: Primarily related to sassafras oil and safrole: Tachycardia, flushing, hypotension, sinus tachycardia, anxiety, hallucinations, vertigo, aphasia, contact dermatitis, vomiting, fatty changes of liver, hepatic necrosis, mydriasis, diaphoresis; little documentation of adverse effects due to ingestion of herbal tea
Absorption: Orally
Metabolism: Hepatic
Excretion: Renal primarily
Warnings: Considered unsafe by the FDA; should not be ingested (banned in food by FDA since 1960)
Dosing: Tea can contain as much as 200 mg (3 mg/kg) of safrole.
Toxic: 0.66 mg/kg (based on rodent studies); Lethal: ~5 mL

Saw Palmetto

Synonyms: Palmetto Scrub; *Sabal serrulata; Sabasilis serrulatae; Serenoa repens*
Use: Treatment of benign prostatic hyperplasia
Mechanism of Action/Effect: Liposterolic extract of the berries may inhibit the enzymes 5α-reductase, along with cyclo-oxygenase and 5-lipoxygenase, thus exhibiting antiandrogen and anti-inflammatory effects; does not reduce prostatic enlargement but may help increase urinary flow (not FDA approved)
Contraindications: Pregnancy and lactation
Adverse Reactions: Headache, gynecomastia, stomach problems (rare, per Commission E)
Absorption: Oral: Low
Dosing: Adults: Dried fruit: 0.5-1 g 3 times/day

Schisandra

Synonym: *Schizandra chinensis*
Use: Promoted as an adaptogen/health tonic; hepatic protection and detoxification; increased endurance, stamina, and work performance
Mechanism of Action/Effect: Stimulates hepatic glycogen synthesis, protein synthesis, and increases microsomal enzyme activity; functions as an antioxidant
Contraindication: Pregnancy (based on uterine stimulation in animal studies)
Drug Interactions: Cytochrome P450 enzyme induction may alter the metabolism of many drugs (calcium channel blockers noted to be decreased)
Dosing: Oral: 100 mg twice daily

Senna

Synonyms: *C. angustifolia; Cassia acutifolia*; Senna Alexandria
Use: Catharsis

HERBAL AND NUTRITIONAL PRODUCTS *(Continued)*

Mechanism of Action/Effect: Contains up to 3% anthraquinone glycosides which can cause colonic stimulation

Contraindications: Per Commission E: Intestinal obstruction, acute intestinal inflammation (eg, Crohn's disease), colitis ulcerosa, appendicitis, abdominal pain of unknown origin, children <12 years, pregnancy

Drug Interactions: Per Commission E: Potentiation of cardiac glycosides (with long-term use) is possible due to loss in potassium; effect on antiarrhythmics is possible; potassium deficiency can be increased by simultaneous application of thiazide diuretics, corticosteroids, and licorice root.

Adverse Reactions: Palpitations, tetany, dizziness, finger clubbing (reversible), hypokalemia, vomiting (with fresh plant leaves or pods), diarrhea, abdominal cramping, nausea, melanosis coli (reversible), cachexia, red discoloration in alkaline urine (yellow-brown in acidic urine), hepatitis, oliguria, proteinuria, dyspnea

Per Commission E: Long-term use/abuse can cause electrolyte imbalance; in single incidents, cramp-like discomforts of GI tract requiring a reduction in dosage.

Metabolism: Hydrolyzed by bacteria in the colon thus releasing active sennosides

Excretion: Urine and feces

Onset of Action: Oral: 6-8 hours; Suppository: 0.5-2 hours

Dosing:

- Sennosides:
  - Children >6 years: 20 mg at bedtime
  - Adults: 20-40 mg with water at bedtime
- Senna granules: 2.5-5 mL (163-326 mg) at bedtime; maximum dose: 10 mL (652 mg)/day
- Senna tablets:
  - Children >60 pounds: 1 tablet (187 mg) at bedtime; maximum daily dose: 2 tablets
  - Adults: 1-2 tablets (187-374 mg) at bedtime; maximum daily dose: 4 tablets (**Note:** Extra strength senna tablets contain 374 mg each.)
- Senna syrup:
  - 1 month to 1 year: 1.25-2.5 mL (55-109 mg) at bedtime, up to 5 mL/day
  - 1-5 years: 2.5-5 mL (109-218 mg) at bedtime, up to 10 mL/day
  - 5-15 years: 5-10 mL (218-436 mg) at bedtime, up to 20 mL/day
  - Adults: 10-15 mL (436-654 mg); maximum daily dose: 30 mL (1308 mg)
- Senna suppositories:
  - Children >60 pounds: $^1/_2$ suppository (326 mg)
  - Adults: 1 suppository (652 mg) at bedtime; can repeat in 2 hours
- Tea: $^1/_2$ to 2 teaspoons of leaves (0.5-4 g of the herb)

Soy Isoflavones

Synonym: Isoflavones

Use: Treatment of decreased bone loss, hypercholesterolemia, menopausal symptoms

Mechanism of Action/Effect: Contains plant-derived estrogenic compounds, however, the estrogenic potency has been estimated to be only 1/1000 to 1/100,000 that of estradiol; reported to inhibit bone reabsorption in postmenopausal women and lower serum lipids, including LDL cholesterol and triglycerides, along with increases in HDL cholesterol

Contraindication: History of estrogenic tumors (endometrial or breast cancer)

Warnings: May alter response to hormonal therapy; use with caution in individuals with history of thromboembolism or stroke

Drug Interactions: Weak estrogenic effect; may interact with estrogen-containing medications (close monitoring is recommended)

Dosing: Oral: 500-1000 mg/day soy extract

St Johns Wort

Synonyms: Amber Touch-and-Feel; Goatweed; *Hypercium perforatum*; Klamath Weed; Rosin Rose

Use: Treatment of mild-moderate depression, stress, anxiety, insomnia, vitiligo (topical); popular drug for AIDS patients due to possible antiretroviral activity; topically for wound healing

Per Commission E: Psychovegetative disorders, depressive moods, anxiety and/or nervous unrest; oily preparations for dyspeptic complaints; oily preparations externally for treatment of post-therapy of acute and contused injuries, myalgia, first degree burns

Mechanism of Action/Effect: Active ingredients are xanthones, flavonoids (hypericin) which can act as monoamine oxidase inhibitors, although *in vitro* activity is minimal; majority of activity appears to be related to GABA modulation; may be related to dopamine, serotonin, norepinephrine modulation also

Contraindications: Endogenous depression, pregnancy, children <<2 years of age; concurrent use of indinavir or therapeutic immunosuppressants (cyclosporine)

Warnings: May be photosensitizing; use caution with tyramine-containing foods; appears to induce hepatic cytochrome P450 3A3/4 enzymes, potentially reducing effect of many medications.
Drug Interactions: Avoid amphetamines or other stimulants and concurrent use with SSRI or other antidepressants. Use caution with MAO inhibitors, levodopa, 5-hydroxytryptophan, and drugs metabolized by CYP3A3/4. Treatment failure with HIV medications and immunosuppressants has been associated with use.
Adverse Reactions: Sinus tachycardia, photosensitization (especially in fair-skinned person, per Commission E), stomach pains, abdominal pain
Dosing: Based on hypericin extract content: Oral: 300 mg 3 times/day

Valerian

Synonyms: Radix; Red Valerian; *Valeriana edulis; Valeriana wallichi*
Use: Sleep-promoting agent and minor tranquilizer; treatment of anxiety, panic attacks, intestinal cramps, headache

Per Commission E: Restlessness, sleep disorders based on nervous conditions
Mechanism of Action/Effect: May affect neurotransmitter levels (serotonin, GABA, and norepinephrine); also has antispasmodic properties
Drug Interactions: Not synergistic with alcohol; potentiation of other CNS depressants is possible
Adverse Reactions: Cardiac disturbances (unspecified), lightheadedness, restlessness, fatigue, nausea, tremor, blurred vision
Dosing:

Sedative: 1-3 g (1-3 mL of tincture)
Sleep aid: 1-3 mL of tincture at bedtime
Dried root: 0.3-1 g

Vanadium

Use: Treatment of type 1 and type 2 diabetes
Mechanism of Action/Effect: Reported to be a cofactor in nicotinamide adenine dinucleotide phosphate (NADPH) oxidation reactions, lipoprotein lipase activity, amino acid transport, and hematopoiesis; may improve/augment glucose regulation
Warning: Use with caution in diabetics or in those predisposed to hypoglycemia; may alter glucose regulation. Effects of drugs with hypoglycemic activity may be potentiated (including insulin and oral hypoglycemics). Closely monitor blood sugar, dosage of these agents (including insulin) may require adjustment. This should be carefully coordinated among the individual's healthcare providers.
Drug Interactions: Oral hypoglycemics or insulin
Adverse Reactions: No dietary toxicity or serious side effects reported, however industrial exposure has resulted in toxicity.
Dosing: Oral: RDI: 250 mcg 1-3 times/day

HERBS AND COMMON NATURAL AGENTS

The authors have chosen to include this list of natural products and proposed medical claims. However, due to limited scientific investigation to support these claims, this list is not intended to imply that these claims have been scientifically proven.

Proposed Medicinal Claims

Herb	Medicinal Claim
Agrimony	Digestive disorders
Alfalfa	Source of carotene (vitamin A); contains natural fluoride
Allspice	General health
Aloe	Healing agent
Anise seed	Prevent gas
Astragalus	Enhance energy reserves; immune system modulation; adaptogen
Barberry bark	Treat halitosis
Bayberry bark	Relieve and prevent varicose veins
Bay leaf	Relieves cramps
Bee pollen	Renewal of enzymes, hormones, vitamins, amino acids, and others
Bergamot herb	Calming effect
Bilberry leaf	Increases night vision; reduces eye fatigue; antioxidant; circulation
Birch bark	Treat urinary problems; used for rheumatism
Blackberry leaf	Treat diarrhea

HERBAL AND NUTRITIONAL PRODUCTS *(Continued)*

Proposed Medicinal Claims *(continued)*

Herb	Medicinal Claim
Black cohosh	Relieves menstrual cramps; phytoestrogen
Blueberry leaf	Diarrhea
Blue Cohosh	Regulate menstrual flow
Blue flag	Treatment of skin diseases and constipation
Boldo leaf	Stimulates digestion; treatment of gallstones
Boneset	Treatment of colds and flu
Bromelain	Digestive enzyme
Buchu leaf	Diuretic
Buckthorn bark	Expels worms; laxative
Burdock leaf and root	Treatment of severe skin problems; cases of arthritis
Butternut bark	Works well for constipation
Calendula flower	Mending and healing of cuts or wounds topically
Capsicum (Cayenne)	Normalizes blood pressure; circulation
Caraway seed	Aids digestion
Cascara sagrada bark	Remedies for chronic constipation
Catnip	Calming effect in children
Celery leaf and seed	Blood pressure; diuretic
Centaury	Stimulates the salivary gland
Chamomile flower	Excellent for a nervous stomach; relieves cramping associated with the menstrual cycle
Chickweed	Rich in vitamin C and minerals (calcium, magnesium, and potassium); diuretic; thyroid stimulant
Chicory root	Effective in disorders of the kidneys, liver, and urinary canal
Cinnamon bark	Prevents infection and indigestion; helps break down fats during digestion
Cleavers	Treatment of kidney and bladder disorders; useful in obstructions of the urinary organ
Cloves	General medicinal
Coriander seed	Stomach tonic
Cornsilk	Diuretic
Cranberry	Urinary tract health
Cubeb berry	Chronic bladder trouble; increases flow of urine
Damiana leaf	Sexual impotency
Dandelion leaf	Diuretic
Dandelion root	Detoxify poisons in the liver; beneficial in lowering blood pressure
Dill weed	Digestive health
Dong Quai root	Female troubles; menopause and PMS symptoms; anemia; blood pressure
Echinacea root	Treat strep throat, lymph glands; immune modulating
Eucalyptus leaf	Mucolytic
Elder	Antiviral
Elecampane root	Cough with mucus
Eyebright herb	Eyesight
Fennel seed	Remedies for gas and acid stomach
Fenugreek seed	Allergies, coughs, digestion, emphysema, headaches, migraines, intestinal inflammation, ulcers, lungs, mucous membranes, and sore throat
Feverfew herb	Migraines; helps reduce inflammation in arthritis joints
Garlic capsules	Lowers blood cholesterol; anti-infective
Gentian	Digestive health
Ginger root	Antiemetic

Proposed Medicinal Claims *(continued)*

Herb	Medicinal Claim
Ginkgo biloba	Improves blood circulation to the brain; asthma; vertigo; tinnitus; impotence
Ginseng root, Siberian	Resistance against stress; slows the aging process; adaptogen
Goldenseal	Treatment of bladder infections, cankers, mouth sores, mucous membranes, and ulcers
Gota kola	"Memory herb"; nerve tonic; wound healing
Gravelroot (Queen of the Meadow)	Remedy for stones in the kidney and bladder
Green barley	Antioxidant
Hawthorn	Antioxidant; cardiotonic
Henna	External use only
Hibiscus flower	Diuretic
Hops flower	Insomnia; used to decrease the desire for alcohol
Horehound	Acute or chronic sore throat and coughs
Horsetail (Shavegrass)	Rich in minerals, especially silica; used to develop strong fingernails and hair, good for split ends; diuretic
Ho shou wu	Rejuvenator
Hydrangea root	Backaches
Juniper berry	Diuretic
Kava kava root	Calm nervousness; anxiety; pain
Kelp	High contents of natural plant iodine, for proper function of the thyroid; high levels of natural calcium, potassium, and magnesium
Lavender oil	Wound healing; decrease scarring (topical)
Lecithin	Break up cholesterol; prevent arteriosclerosis
Licorice root	Expectorant; used in peptic ulceration; adrenal exhaustion
Malva flower	Soothes inflammation in the mouth and throat; helpful for earaches
Marjoram	Beneficial for a sour stomach or loss of appetite
Marshmallow leaf	Demulcent
Milk thistle herb	Liver detoxifier; antioxidant
Motherwort	Nervousness
Mugwort	Used for rheumatism and gout
Mullein leaf	High in iron, magnesium, and potassium; sinuses; relieves swollen joints; soothing bronchial tissue
Mustard seed	General medicinal
Myrrh gum	Removes bad breath; sinus problems
Nettle leaf	Remedy for dandruff; antihistiminic qualities
Nettle root	Used in benign prostatic hyperplasia (BPH)
Nutmeg	Gas
Oregano leaf	Settles the stomach after meals; helps treat colds
Oregon grape root	Gallbladder problems
Papaya leaf	Digestive stimulant; contains the enzyme papain
Paprika (sweet)	Stimulates the appetite and gastric secretions
Passion flower	Mild sedative
Pau d'arco	Protects immune system; antifungal
Peppermint leaf	Excellent for headaches; digestive stimulation
Pleurisy root	Mucolytic
Poppy seed blue	Excellent in the making of breads and desserts
Prickly ash bark	Increases circulation
Psyllium seed	Lubricant to the intestinal tract
Red clover	Phytoestrogenic properties
Red raspberry leaf	Decreases menstrual bleeding
Rhubarb root	Powerful laxative

HERBAL AND NUTRITIONAL PRODUCTS *(Continued)*

Proposed Medicinal Claims *(continued)*

Herb	Medicinal Claim
Rose hips	High content of vitamin C
Saw palmetto berry	Used in benign prostatic hyperplasia (BPH)
Scullcap	Nerve sedative
Seawrack (Bladderwrack)	Combat obesity; contains iodine
Senna leaf	Laxative
Shepherd's purse	Female reproductive health
Sheep sorrel	Diuretic
Slippery elm bark	Normalize bowel movement; beneficial for hemorrhoids and constipation
Solomon's seal root	Poultice for bruises
Spikenard	Skin ailments such as acne, pimples, blackheads, rashes, and general skin problems
Star anise	Promotes appetite and relieves flatulence
St John's wort	Mild to moderate depression
Summer savory leaf	Treats diarrhea, upset stomach, and sore throat
Thyme leaf	Ulcers (peptic)
Uva-ursi leaf	Diuretic; used in urinary tract health
Valerian root	Promotes sleep
Vervain	Remedy for fevers
White oak bark	Strong astringent
White willow bark	Used for minor aches and pains in the body; aspirin content
Wild alum root	Powerful astringent; used as rinse for sores in mouth and bleeding gums
Wild cherry	Cough suppressant
Wild Oregon grape root	Chronic skin disease
Wild yam root	Used in female reproductive health
Wintergreen leaf	Valuable for colic and gas in the bowels
Witch hazel bark and leaf	Hemorrhoids
Wormwood	Antiparasitic
Yarrow root	Fevers
Yellow dock root	Good in all skin problems
Yerba santa	Bronchial congestion
Yohimbe	Natural aphrodisiac
Yucca root	Reduces inflammation of the joints

HERB-DRUG INTERACTIONS / CAUTIONS

Herb	Drug Interaction/Caution
Acidophilus/bifidobacterium	Antibiotics (oral)
Activated charcoal	Vitamins or oral medications may be adsorbed
Alfalfa	Do not use with lupus due to amino acid L-canavanine; causes pancytopenia at high doses; warfarin (alfalfa contains a large amount of vitamin K)
Aloe vera	Caution in pregnancy, may cause uterine contractions; digoxin, diuretics (hypokalemia)
Ashwagandha	May cause sedation and other CNS effects
Asparagus root	Causes diuresis
Barberry	Normal metabolism of vitamin B may be altered with high doses
Birch	If taking a diuretic, drink plenty of fluids
Black cohosh	Estrogen-like component; pregnant and nursing women should probably avoid this herb; also women with estrogen-dependent cancer and women who are taking birth control pills or estrogen supplements after menopause; caution also in people taking sedatives or blood pressure medications
Black haw	Do not give to children <6 years of age (salicin content) with flu or chickenpox due to potential Reye's syndrome; do not take if allergic to aspirin
Black pepper (*Piper nigrum*)	Antiasthmatic drugs (decreases metabolism)
Black tea	May inhibit body's utilization of thiamine
Blessed thistle	Do not use with gastritis, ulcers, or hyperacidity since herb stimulates gastric juices
Blood root	Large doses can cause nausea, vomiting, CNS sedation, low BP, shock, coma, and death
Broom (*Cytisus scoparius*)	MAO inhibitors lead to sudden blood pressure changes
Bugleweed (*Lycopus virginicus*)	May interfere with nuclear imaging studies of the thyroid gland (thyroid uptake scan)
Cat's claw (*Uncaria tomentosa*)	Avoid in organ transplant patients or patients on ulcer medications, antiplatelet drugs, NSAIDs, anticoagulants, immunosuppressive therapy, intravenous immunoglobulin therapy
Chaste tree berry (*Vitex agnus-castus*)	Interferes with actions of oral contraceptives, HRT, and other endocrine therapies; may interfere with metabolism of dopamine-receptor antagonists
Chicory (*Cichorium intybus*)	Avoid with gallstones due to bile-stimulating properties
Chlorella (*Chlorella vulgaris*)	Contains significant amounts of vitamin K
Chromium picolinate	Picolinic acid causes notable changes in brain chemicals (serotonin, dopamine, norepinephrine); do not use if patient has behavioral disorders or diabetes
Cinnabar root (*Salviae multorrhizae*)	Warfarin (increases INR)
Deadly nightshade (*Atropa belladonna*)	Contains atropine
Dong quai	Warfarin (increases INR), estrogens, oral contraceptives, photosensitizing drugs, histamine replacement therapy, anticoagulants, antiplatelet drugs, antihypertensives
Echinacea	Caution with other immunosuppressive therapies; stimulates TNF and interferons
Ephedra	Avoid with blood pressure medications, antidepressants, and MAOIs
Evening primrose oil	May lower seizure threshold; do not combine with anticonvulsants or phenothiazines
Fennel	Do not use in women who have had breast cancer or who have been told not to take birth control pills
Fenugreek	Practice moderation in patients on diabetes drugs, MAO inhibitors, cardiovascular agents, hormonal medicines, or warfarin due to the many components of fenugreek

HERBAL AND NUTRITIONAL PRODUCTS *(Continued)*

Herb	Drug Interaction/Caution
Feverfew	Antiplatelets, anticoagulants, NSAIDs
Forskolin, coleonol	This herb lowers blood pressure (vasodilator) and is a bronchodilator and increases the contractility of the heart, inhibits platelet aggregation, and increases gastric acid secretion
Foxglove	Digitalis-containing herb
Garlic	Blood sugar-lowering medications, warfarin, and aspirin at medicinal doses of garlic
Ginger	May inhibit platelet aggregation by inhibiting thromboxane synthetase at large doses; *in vitro* and animal studies indicate that ginger may interfere with diabetics; has anticoagulant effect, so avoid in medicinal amounts in patients on warfarin or heart medicines
Ginkgo biloba	Warfarin (ginkgo decreases blood clotting rate); NSAIDs, MAO inhibitors
Ginseng	Blood sugar-lowering medications (additive effects) and other stimulants
Ginseng (American, Korean)	Furosemide (decreases efficacy)
Ginseng (Siberian)	Digoxin (increases digoxin level)
Glucomannan	Diabetics (herb delays absorption of glucose from intestines, decreasing mean fasting sugar levels)
Goldenrod	Diuretics (additive properties)
Gymnema	Blood sugar-lowering medications (additive effects)
Hawthorn	Digoxin or other heart medications (herb dilates coronary vessels and other blood vessels, also inotropic)
Hibiscus	Chloroquine (reduced effectiveness of chloroquine)
Hops	Those with estrogen-dependent breast cancer should not take hops (contains estrogen-like chemicals); patients with depression (accentuate symptoms); alcohol or sedative (additive effects)
Horehound	May cause arrhythmias at high doses
Horseradish	In medicinal amounts with thyroid medications
Kava	CNS depressants (additive effects, eg, alcohol, barbiturates, etc); benzodiazepines
Kelp	Thyroid medications (additive effects or opposite effects by negative feedback); kelp contains a high amount of sodium
Labrador tea	Plant has narcotic properties, possible additive effects with other CNS depressants
Lemon balm	Do not use with Graves disease since it inhibits certain thyroid hormones
Licorice	Acts as a corticosteroid at high doses (about 1.5 lbs candy in 9 days) which can lead to hypertension, edema, hypernatremia, and hypokalemia (pseudoaldosteronism); do not use in persons with hypertension, glaucoma, diabetes, kidney or liver disease, or those on hormonal therapy; may interact with digitalis (due to hypokalemia)
Lobelia	Contains lobeline which has nicotinic activity; may mask withdrawal symptoms from nicotine; it can act as a polarizing neuromuscular blocker
Lovage	Is a diuretic
Ma huang	MAO inhibitors, digoxin, beta-blockers, methyldopa, caffeine, theophylline, decongestants (increases toxicity)
Marshmallow	May delay absorption of other drugs taken at the same time; may interfere with treatments of lowering blood sugar
Meadowsweet	Contains salicylates
Melatonin	Acts as contraceptive at high doses; antidepressants (decreases efficacy)
Mistletoe	May interfere with medications for blood pressure, depression, and heart disease

Herb	Drug Interaction/Caution
L-phenylalanine	MAO inhibitors
Pleurisy root	Digoxin (plant contains cardiac glycosides); also contains estrogen-like compounds; may alter amine concentrations in the brain and interact with antidepressants
Prickly ash (Northern)	Contains coumarin-like compounds
Prickly ash (Southern)	Contains neuromuscular blockers
Psyllium	Digoxin (decreases absorption)
Quassia	High doses may complicate heart or blood-thinning treatments (quassia may be inotropic)
Red clover	May have estrogen-like actions; avoid when taking birth control pills, HRT, people with heart disease or at risk for blood clots, patients who suffer from estrogen-dependent cancer; do not take with warfarin
Red pepper	May increase liver metabolism of other medications and may interfere with high blood pressure medications or MAO inhibitors
Rhubarb, Chinese	Do not use with digoxin (enhanced effects)
St John's wort	Indinavir, cyclosporine, SSRIs or any antidepressants, tetracycline (increases sun sensitivity); digoxin (decreases digoxin concentration); may also interact with diltiazem, nicardipine, verapamil, etoposide, paclitaxel, vinblastine, vincristine, glucocorticoids, cyclosporine, dextromethorphan, ephedrine, lithium, meperidine, pseudoephedrine, selegiline, yohimbine, ACE inhibitors (serotonin syndrome, hypertension, possible exacerbation of allergic reaction)
Saw palmetto	Acts an antiandrogen; do not take with prostate medicines or HRT
Squill	Digoxin or persons with potassium deficiency; also not with quinidine, calcium, laxatives, saluretics, prednisone (long-term)
Tonka bean	Contains coumarin, interacts with warfarin
Vervain	Avoid large amounts of herb with blood pressure medications or HRT
Wild Oregon grape	High doses may alter metabolism of vitamin B
Wild yam	May interfere with hormone precursors
Wintergreen	Warfarin, increased bleeding
Sweet woodruff	Contains coumarin
Yarrow	Interferes with anticoagulants and blood pressure medications
Yohimbe	Do not consume tyramine-rich foods; do not take with nasal decongestants, PPA-containing diet aids, antidepressants, or mood-altering drugs

HERBAL AND NUTRITIONAL PRODUCTS *(Continued)*

Herbs Contraindicated During Lactation According to German Commission E

- Aloe (*Aloe vera*)
- Basil (*Ocimum basillcum*)
- Buckthorn bark and berry (*Rhamnus frangula, R. cathartica*)
- Cascara sagrada (*Rhamnus purshiana*)
- Coltsfoot leaf (*Tussilago farfara*)
- Combinations of senna, peppermint oil and caraway oil
- Kava kava root (*Piper methysticum*)
- Petasite root (*Pefasites* spp)
- Indian snakeroot (*Rauwolfia serpentina*)
- Rhubarb root (*Rheum palmatum*)
- Senna (*Cassia senna*)

Herbs Contraindicated During Pregnancy According to German Commission E

- Aloe (*Aloe vera*)
- Autumn crocus (*Colchicum autumnale*)
- Black cohosh root (*Cimicifuga racemosa*)
- Buckthorn bark and berry (*Rhamnus frangula, R. cathartica*)
- Cascara sagrada bark (*Rhamnus purshiana*)
- Chaste tree fruit (*Vitex agnus-castus*)
- Cinchona bark (*Cinchona* spp)
- Cinnamon bark (*Cinnamomum zeylanicum*)
- Coltsfoot leaf (*Tussliago farfara*)
- *Echinacea purpurea* herb (*Echinacea purpurea*)
- Fennel oil (*Foeniculum vulgare*)
- Combination of licorice, peppermint, and chamomile
- Combination of licorice, primrose, marshmallow, and anise
- Combination of senna, peppermint oil, and caraway oil
- Ginger root (*Zingiber officinale*)*
- Indian snakeroot (*Rauwolfia serpentina*)
- Juniper berry (*Juniperus comunis*)
- Kava kava root (*Piper methysticum*)
- Licorice root (*Glycyrrhiza glabra*)
- Marsh tea (*Ledum palustre*)
- Mayapple root (*Podophyllum peltatum*)
- Petasite root (*Petasites* spp)
- Rhubarb root (*Rheum palmatum*)
- Sage leaf (*Salvia officinalis*)
- Senna (*Cassia senna*)

*A subsequent review of the clinical literature could find no basis for the contraindication of ginger, a common spice, during pregnancy (Fulder and Tenne, 1996).

IMMUNIZATION RECOMMENDATIONS

Standards for Pediatric Immunization Practices

Standard 1.	Immunization services are readily available.
Standard 2.	There are no barriers or unnecessary prerequisites to the receipt of vaccines.
Standard 3.	Immunization services are available free or for a minimal fee.
Standard 4.	Providers utilize all clinical encounters to screen and, when indicated, immunize children.
Standard 5.	Providers educate parents and guardians about immunizations in general terms.
Standard 6.	Providers question parents or guardians about contraindications and, before immunizing a child, inform them in specific terms about the risks and benefits of the immunizations their child is to receive.
Standard 7.	Providers follow only true contraindications.
Standard 8.	Providers administer simultaneously all vaccine doses for which a child is eligible at the time of each visit.
Standard 9.	Providers use accurate and complete recording procedures.
Standard 10.	Providers co-schedule immunization appointments in conjunction with appointments for other child health services.
Standard 11.	Providers report adverse events following immunization promptly, accurately, and completely.
Standard 12.	Providers operate a tracking system.
Standard 13.	Providers adhere to appropriate procedures for vaccine management.
Standard 14.	Providers conduct semiannual audits to assess immunization coverage levels and to review immunization records in the patient populations they serve.
Standard 15.	Providers maintain up-to-date, easily retrievable medical protocols at all locations where vaccines are administered.
Standard 16.	Providers operate with patient-oriented and community-based approaches.
Standard 17.	Vaccines are administered by properly trained individuals.
Standard 18.	Providers receive ongoing education and training on current immunization recommendations.

Recommended by the National Vaccine Advisory Committee, April 1992.
Approved by the United States Public Health Service, May 1992.
Endorsed by the American Academy of Pediatrics, May 1992.

The Standards represent the consensus of the National Vaccine Advisory Committee (NVAC) and of a broad group of medical and public health experts about what constitutes the most desirable immunization practices. It is recognized by the NVAC that not all of the current immunization practices of public and private providers are in compliance with the Standards. Nevertheless, the Standards are expected to be useful as a means of helping providers to identify needed changes, to obtain resources if necessary, and to actually implement the desirable immunization practices in the future.

IMMUNIZATION RECOMMENDATIONS *(Continued)*

Recommended Childhood Immunization Schedule United States, 2002

Range of Recommended Ages | Catch-up Vaccination | Preadolescent Assessment

Age ► / Vaccine ▼	Birth	1 mo	2 mo	4 mo	6 mo	12 mo	15 mo	18 mo	24 mo	4-6 y	11-12 y	13-18 y
Hepatitis B[1]	Hep B #1	only if mother $HB_sAg(-)$							Hep B series			
		Hep B #2			Hep B #3							
Diphtheria, tetanus, pertussis[2]			DTaP	DTaP	DTaP		DTaP			DTaP	Td	
H. influenzae type b[3]			Hib	Hib	Hib	Hib						
Inactivated polio[4]			IPV	IPV	IPV					IPV		
Measles, mumps, rubella[5]						MMR #1				MMR #2	MMR #2	
Varicella[6]						Varicella			Varicella			
Pneumococcal[7]			PCV	PCV	PCV	PCV			PCV	PPV		
Vaccines below this line are for selected populations												
Hepatitis A[8]									Hepatitis A series			
Influenza[9]					Influenza (yearly)							

This schedule indicates the recommended ages for routine administration of currently licensed childhood vaccines, as of December 1, 2001, for children through 18 years of age. Any dose not given at the recommended age should be given at any subsequent visit when indicated and feasible. ▭ Indicates age groups that warrant special effort to administer those vaccines not previously given. Additional vaccines may be licensed and recommended during the year. Licensed combination vaccines may be used whenever any components of the combination are indicated and the vaccine's other components are not contraindicated. Providers should consult the manufacturers' package inserts for detailed recommendations.

1 All infants should receive the first dose of **hepatitis B vaccine (Hep B)** soon after birth and before hospital discharge; the 1st dose may also be given by 2 months of age if the infant's mother is HB_sAg-negative. Only monovalent hepatitis B vaccine can be used for the birth dose. Monovalent or combination vaccine containing Hep B may be used to complete the series; four doses of vaccine may be administered if combination vaccine is used. The 2nd dose should be given at least 4 weeks after the 1st dose, except for Hib-containing vaccine which cannot be administered before 6 weeks of age. The 3rd dose should be given at least 16 weeks after the 1st dose and at least 8 weeks after the 2nd dose. The last dose in the vaccination series (3rd or 4th dose) should not be administered before 6 months of age.

Infants born to HB_sAg-positive mothers should receive hepatitis B vaccine and 0.5 mL hepatitis B immune globulin (HBIG) within 12 hours of birth at separate sites. The 2nd dose is recommended at 1-2 months of age and the vaccination series should be completed (3rd or 4th dose) at 6 months of age.

Infants born to mothers whose HB_sAg status is unknown should receive the 1st dose of the hepatitis B vaccine series within 12 hours of birth. Maternal blood should be drawn at the time of delivery to determine the mother's HB_sAg status; if the HB_sAg test is positive, the infant should receive HBIG as soon as possible (no later than 1 week of age).

2 **Diphtheria and tetanus toxoids and acellular pertussis vaccine (DTaP).** The 4th dose of DTaP may be administered as early as 12 months of age, provided 6 months have elapsed since the 3rd dose and the child is unlikely to return at 15-18 months of age. **Tetanus and diphtheria toxoids (Td)** is recommended at 11-12 years of age if at least 5 years have elapsed since the last dose of tetanus and diphtheria toxoid-containing vaccine. Subsequent routine Td boosters are recommended every 10 years.

3 ***Haemophilus influenzae* type b (Hib) conjugate vaccines.** Three Hib conjugate vaccines are licensed for infant use. If PRP-OMP (PedvaxHIB® or ComVax® [Merck]) is administered at 2 and 4 months of age, a dose at 6 months of age is not required. DTaP/Hib combination products should not be used for primary immunization in infants at 2, 4, or 6 months of age, but can be used as boosters following any Hib vaccine.

4 **Inactivated polio vaccine (IPV).** An all-IPV schedule is recommended for routine childhood polio vaccination in the United States. All children should receive four doses of IPV at 2 months, 4 months, 6-18 months, and 4-6 years of age.

5 **Measles, mumps, and rubella vaccine (MMR).** The 2nd dose of MMR is recommended routinely at 4-6 years of age but may be administered during any visit, provided at least 4 weeks have elapsed since the 1st dose and that both doses are administered beginning at or after 12 months of age. Those who have not previously received the 2nd dose should complete the schedule by the 11- to 12-year old visit.

6 **Varicella vaccine** is recommended at any visit at or after 12 months of age for susceptible children (ie, those who lack a reliable history of chickenpox). Susceptible persons >13 years of age should receive 2 doses, given at least 4 weeks apart.

7 The heptavalent **pneumococcal conjugate vaccine (PCV)** is recommended for all children 2-23 months of age. It is also recommended for certain children 24-59 months of age. **Pneumococcal polysaccharide vaccine (PPV)** is recommended in addition to PCV for certain high-risk groups. See *MMWR Morb Mortal Wkly Rep*, 2000, 49(RR-9),1-35.

8 **Hepatitis A vaccine** is recommended for use in selected states and regions, and for certain high-risk groups; consult your local public health authority. See *MMWR Morb Mortal Wkly Rep*, 1999, 48(RR-12): 1-37.

9 **Influenza vaccine** is recommended annually for children >6 months of age with certain risk factors (including but not limited to asthma, cardiac disease, sickle cell disease, HIV, diabetes (see *MMWR Morb Mortal Wkly Rep*, 2001, 50(RR-4):1-44), and can be administered to all others wishing to obtain immunity. Children ≤12 years of age should receive vaccine in a dosage appropriate for their age (0.25 mL if 6-35 months of age or 0.5 mL if ≥3 years of age). Children ≤8 years of age who are receiving influenza vaccine for the first time should receive two doses separated by at least 4 weeks.

Approved by the Advisory Committee on Immunization Practices (*www.cdc.gov/nip/acip*), the American Academy of Pediatrics (*www.aap.org*), and the American Academy of Family Physicians (www.aafp.org).

For additional information about the vaccines, vaccine supply, and contraindications for immunization, please visit the National Immunization Program web site at *www.cdc.gov/nip* or call the National Immunization Hotline at (800) 232-2522 (English) or (800) 232-0233 (Spanish).

RECOMMENDATIONS OF THE ADVISORY COMMITTEE ON IMMUNIZATION PRACTICES (ACIP)

Recommended Poliovirus Vaccination Schedules for Children

Vaccine	Child's Age			
	2 mo	4 mo	12-18 mo	4-6 y
Sequential IPV [1]/OPV[1]/OPV[2]	IPV	IPV	OPV	OPV
OPV[1]	OPV	OPV	OPV[3]	OPV
IPV[2]	IPV	IPV	IPV	OPV

[1]Inactivated poliovirus vaccine.

[2]Live, oral poliovirus vaccine.

[3]For children who receive only OPV, the third dose of OPV may be administered as early as 6 months of age.

Adapted from "Poliomyelitis Prevention in the United States: Introduction of a Sequential Vaccination Schedule of Inactivated Poliovirus Vaccine Followed by Oral Poliovirus Vaccine" *MMWR Morb Mortal Wkly Rep*, 1997, 46(RR-3).

Recommendations for Measles Immunization[1]

Category	Recommendations
Unvaccinated, no history of measles (12-15 mo)	A 2-dose schedule (with MMR) is recommended if born after 1956. The first dose is recommended at 12-15 mo; the second is recommended at 4-6 y
Children 6-11 mo in epidemic situations	Immunize (with monovalent measles vaccine or, if not available, MMR); reimmunization (with MMR) at 12-15 mo is necessary, and a third dose is indicated at 4-6 y
Children 4-12 y who have received 1 dose of measles vaccine at ≥12 mo	Reimmunize (1 dose)
Students in college and other post-high school institutions who have received 1 dose of measles vaccine at ≥12 mo	Reimmunize (1 dose)
History of vaccination before the first birthday	Consider susceptible and immunize (2 doses)
Unknown vaccine, 1963-1967	Consider susceptible and immunize (2 doses)
Further attenuated or unknown vaccine given with IG	Consider susceptible and immunize (2 doses)
Egg allergy	Immunize; no reactions likely
Neomycin allergy, nonanaphylactic	Immunize; no reactions likely
Tuberculosis	Immunize; vaccine does not exacerbate infection
Measles exposure	Immunize and/or give IG, depending on circumstances
HIV-infected	Immunize (2 doses) unless severely immunocompromised
Immunoglobulin or blood	Immunize at the appropriate interval

[1] MMR = measles-mumps-rubella vaccine; IG = immune globulin; HIV = human immunodeficiency virus.

Adapted from "Report of the Committee on Infectious Diseases," *2000 Red Book®*, 25th ed, 391.

IMMUNIZATION RECOMMENDATIONS *(Continued)*

Recommended Immunization Schedules for Children Not Immunized in the First Year of Life*

Recommended Time/Age	Immunization(s)[1,2,3]	Comments
	Younger Than 7 Years	
First visit	DTaP (or DTP), Hib, HBV, MMR, OPV[3]	If indicated, tuberculin testing may be done at same visit. If child is ≥5 y of age, Hib is not indicated in most circumstances.
Interval after first visit		
1 mo (4 wk)	DTaP (or DTP), HBV, Var[4]	The second dose of OPV may be given if accelerated poliomyelitis vaccination is necessary, such as for travelers to areas where polio is endemic.
2 mo	DTaP (or DTP), Hib, OPV[3]	Second dose of Hib is indicated only if the first dose was received when <15 mo.
≥8 mo	DTaP (or DTP), HBV, OPV[3]	OPV and HBV are not given if the third doses were given earlier.
Age 4-6 y (at or before school entry)	DTaP (or DTP), OPV,[3] MMR[5]	DTaP (or DTP) is not necessary if the fourth dose was given after the fourth birthday; OPV is not necessary if the third dose was given after the fourth birthday.
Age 11-12 y	See Childhood Immunization Schedule	
	7-12 Years	
First visit	HBV, MMR, Td, OPV[3]	
Interval after first visit		
2 mo (8 wk)	HBV, MMR,[5] Var,[4] Td, OPV[3]	OPV also may be given 1 mo after the first visit if accelerated poliomyelitis vaccination is necessary.
8-14 mo	HBV,[6] Td, OPV[3]	OPV is not given if the third dose was given earlier.
Age 11-12 y	See Childhood Immunization Schedule	

*Table is not completely consistent with all package inserts. For products used, also consult manufacturer's package insert for instructions on storage, handling, dosage, and administration. Biologics prepared by different manufacturers may vary, and package inserts of the same manufacturer may change from time to time. Therefore, the physician should be aware of the contents of the current package insert.

Vaccine abbreviations: HBV indicates hepatitis B virus vaccine; Var, varicella vaccine; DTP, diphtheria and tetanus toxoids and pertussis vaccine; DTaP, diphtheria and tetanus toxoids and acellular pertussis vaccine; Hib, *Haemophilus influenzae* type b conjugate vaccine; OPV, oral poliovirus vaccine; IPV, inactivated poliovirus vaccine; MMR, live measles-mumps-rubella vaccine; Td, adult tetanus toxoid (full dose) and diphtheria toxoid (reduced dose), for children ≥7 years and adults.

[1]If all needed vaccines cannot be administered simultaneously, priority should be given to protecting the child against those diseases that pose the greatest immediate risk. In the United States, these diseases for children <2 years usually are measles and *Haemophilus influenzae* type b infection; for children >7 years, they are measles, mumps, and rubella. Before 13 years of age, immunity against hepatitis B and varicella should be ensured.

[2]DTaP, HBV, Hib, MMR, and Var can be given simultaneously at separate sites if failure of the patient to return for future immunizations is a concern.

[3]IPV is also acceptable. However, for infants and children starting vaccination late (ie, after 6 months of age), OPV is preferred in order to complete an accelerated schedule with a minimum number of injections.

[4]Varicella vaccine can be administered to susceptible children any time after 12 months of age. Unvaccinated children who lack a reliable history of chickenpox should be vaccinated before their 13th birthday.

[5]Minimal interval between doses of MMR is 1 month (4 weeks).

[6]HBV may be given earlier in a 0-, 2-, and 4-month schedule.

Adapted from "Report of the Committee on Infectious Diseases," *1997 Red Book®*, 24th ed.

Minimum Age for Initial Vaccination and Minimum Interval Between Vaccine Doses, by Type of Vaccine

Vaccine	Minimum[1] *Age* for First Dose	Minimum[1] *Interval* From Dose 1 to 2	Minimum[1] *Interval* From Dose 2 to 3	Minimum[1] *Interval* From Dose 3 to 4
DTP (DT)[2]	6 wk[3]	4 wk	4 wk	6 mo
Combined DTP-Hib	6 wk	1 mo	1 mo	6 mo
DTaP[1]	6 wk			6 mo
Hib (primary series)				
HbOC	6 wk	1 mo	1 mo	[4]
PRP-T	6 wk	1 mo	1 mo	[4]
PRP-OMP	6 wk	1 mo	[4]	
OPV			6 wk	
IPV[5]	6 wk	4 wk	6 mo[6]	
MMR	12 mo[7]	1 mo		
Hepatitis B	Birth	1 mo	2 mo[8]	
Varicella-zoster	12 mo	4 wk		

DTP = diphtheria-tetanus-pertussis.

DTaP = diphtheria-tetanus-acellular pertussis.

Hib = *Haemophilus influenzae* type b conjugate.

IPV = inactivated poliovirus vaccine.

MMR = measles-mumps-rubella.

OPV = poliovirus vaccine, live oral, trivalent.

[1]These minimum acceptable ages and intervals may not correspond with the optimal recommended ages and intervals for vaccination. See tables for the current recommended routine and accelerated vaccination schedules.

[2]DTaP can be used in place of the fourth (and fifth) dose of DTP for children who are at least 15 months of age. Children who have received all four primary vaccination doses before their fourth birthday should receive a fifth dose of DTP (DT) or DTaP at 4-6 years of age before entering kindergarten or elementary school **and** at least 6 months after the fourth dose. The total number of doses of diphtheria and tetanus toxoids should not exceed six each before the seventh birthday.

[3]The American Academy of Pediatrics permits DTP to be administered as early as 4 weeks of age in areas with high endemicity and during outbreaks.

[4]The booster dose of Hib vaccine which is recommended following the primary vaccination series should be administered no earlier than 12 months of age **and** at least 2 months after the previous dose of Hib vaccine.

[5]See text to differentiate conventional inactivated poliovirus vaccine from enhanced-potency IPV.

[6]For unvaccinated adults at increased risk of exposure to poliovirus with <3 months but >2 months available before protection is needed, three doses of IPV should be administered at least 1 month apart.

[7]Although the age for measles vaccination may be as young as 6 months in outbreak areas where cases are occurring in children <1 year of age, children initially vaccinated before the first birthday should be revaccinated at 12-15 months of age and an additional dose of vaccine should be administered at the time of school entry or according to local policy. Doses of MMR or other measles-containing vaccines should be separated by at least 1 month.

[8]This final dose is recommended no earlier than 4 months of age.

Modified from *MMWR Morb Mortal Wkly Rep*, 1994, 43(RR-1).

IMMUNIZATION RECOMMENDATIONS *(Continued)*

Recommended Immunization Schedule For HIV-Infected Children[1]

Age ▶ / Vaccine ▼	Birth	1 mo	2 mos	4 mos	6 mos	12 mos	15 mos	18 mos	24 mos	4-6 yrs	11-12 yrs	14-16 yrs
Recommendations for these vaccines are the same as those for immunocompetent children												
Hepatitis B[2]	Hep B-1											
		Hep B-2			Hep B-3						Hep B[3]	
Diphtheria, Tetanus, Pertussis[4]			DTaP	DTaP	DTaP		DTaP			DTaP	Td	
Haemophilus influenzae type b[5]			Hib	Hib	Hib	Hib						
Recommendations for these vaccines differ from those for immunocompetent children												
Polio[6]			IPV	IPV	IPV					IPV		
Measles, Mumps, Rubella[7]	Do not give to severely immunosuppressed (Category 3) children.					MMR	MMR					
Influenza[8]					Influenza (a dose is required every year)							
Streptococcus pneumoniae[9]									*pneumococcal*			
Varicella[10]	Give only to asymptomatic nonimmunosuppressed (Category 1) children. CONTRAINDICATED in all other HIV-infected children.					Varicella						

Note: Modified from the immunization schedule for immunocompetent children. This schedule also applies to children born to HIV-infected mothers whose HIV infection status has not been determined. Once a child is known not to be HIV-infected, the schedule for immunocompetent children applies. This schedule indicates the recommended age for routine administration of currently licensed childhood vaccines. Some combination vaccines are available and may be used whenever administration of all componenets of the vaccine is indicated. Providers should consult the manufacturers' package inserts for detailed recommendations.

1 Vaccines are listed under the routinely recommended ages. Bars indicate range of acceptable ages for vaccination. Shaded bars indicate catch-up vaccination: at 11-12 years of age, hepatitis B vaccine should be administered to children not previously vaccinated.

2 ***Infants born to HBsAg-negative mothers*** should receive 2.5 mcg of Merch vaccine (Recombivax HB®) or 10 mcg of Smith Kline Beecham (SB) vaccine (Engerix-B®). The 2nd dose should be administered >1 mo after the 1st dose.

Infants born to HBsAg-positive mothers should receive 0.5 mL of hepatitis B immune globulin (HBIG) within 12 h of birth and either 5 mcg of Merck vaccine (Recombivax HB®) or 10 mcg of SB vaccine (Engerix-B®) at a separate site. The 2nd dose is recommended at 1-2 months of age and the 3rd dose at 6 months of age.

Infants born to mothers whose HBsAg status is unknown should receive either 5 mcg of Merck vaccine (Recombivax HB®) or 10 mcg of SB vaccine (Engerix-B®) within 12 h of birth. The 2nd dose of vaccine is recommended at 1 month of age and the 3rd dose at 6 of age. Blood should be drawn at the time of delivery to determine the mother's HBsAg status; if it is positive, the infant should receive HBIG as soon as possible (no later than 1 week of age). The dosage and timing of subsequent vaccine doses should be based upon the mother's HBsAg status.

3 Children and adolescents who have not been vaccinated against hepatitis B in infancy can begin the series during any childhood visit. Those who have not previously received 3 doses of hepatitis B vaccine should initiate or complete the series during the 11 to 12 year old visit. The 2nd dose should be administered at least 1 month after the 1st dose, and the 3rd dose should be administered at least 4 mos after the 1st dose and at 2 mos after 2nd dose.

4 DTaP (diphtheria and tetanus toxoids and acellular pertusssis vaccine) is the preferred vaccine for all doses in the vaccination series, including copletion of the series in children who have received >1 dose of whole-cell DtP vaccine. The 4th dose of DTaP may be administered as early as 12 months of age, provided 6 months have elapsed since the 3rd dose, and if the child is considered unlikely to return at 15-18 months of age. Td (tetanus and diphtheria toxoids, absorbed for adult use) is recommended at 11-12 years of age if at least 5 years have elapsed since the last dose of DTaP or DT. Subsequent routine Td boosters are recommended every 10 years.

5 Three H. influenzae type b (Hib) conjugate vaccines are licensed for infant use. If PRP-OMP (PedvaxHIB® [Merck]) is administered at 2 and 4 months of age, a dose at 6 months is not required. After the primary series has been completed, any Hib conjugate vaccine may be used as a booster.

6 Inactivated poliovirus vaccine (IPV) is the only polio vaccine recommended for HIV-infected persons and their household contacts. Although the third dose fo IPV is generally administered at 12-18 months, the 3rd dose of IPV has been approved to be administered as early as 6 months of age. Oral poliovirus vaccine (OPV) should NOT be administered to HIV-infected persons or their household contacts.

7 MMR should not be administered to severely immunocompromised children. HIV-infected children without severe immunosuppression should routinely receive their first dose of MMR as soon as possible upon reaching the first birthday. Consideration should be given to administering the 2nd dose of MMR vaccine as soon as one month (ie, minimum 28 days) after the first dose, rather than waiting until school entry.

8 Influenza virus vaccine should be administered to all HIV-infected children >6 months of age each year. Children aged 6 months to 8 years who are receiving influenza vaccine for the first time should receive two doses of split virus vaccine separated by at least one month. In subsequent years, a single dose of vaccine (split virus for persons ≥12 y of age, whole or split virus for persons >12 y of age) should be administered each year. The dose of vaccine for children aged 6-35 months is 0.25 mL: the dose for children aged ≥3 years is 0.5 mL.

9 The 23-valent pneumococcal vaccine should be administered to HIV-infected children at 24 months of age. Revaccination should generally be offered to HIV-infected children vaccinated 3-5 years (children aged ≤10 years) or >5 years (children aged >10 years) earlier.

10 Varicella zoster virus vaccine, 0.5 mL, is given as a subcutaneous dose between 12 mos and 12 y of age; a second dose should be given 3 mos later. The vaccine should be given only to asymptomatic, nonimmunosuppressed children.

Adapted from the American Academy of Pediatrics and American Academy of Family Practice Physicians, Advisory Committee on Immunization Practices and the Centers for Disease Control.

Vaccines Licensed in the U.S. and Administration

Vaccine[1]	Type	Route
Adenovirus[2]	Live virus	Oral
Anthrax[3]	Inactivated bacteria	S.C.
BCG	Live bacteria	I.D. (preferred) or S.C.
Cholera	Inactivated bacteria	S.C., I.M., or I.D.
Diphtheria-tetanus (dT, DT)	Toxoids	I.M.
DTP	Toxoids and inactivated bacteria	I.M.
DTaP	Toxoids and inactivated bacterial components	I.M.
Hepatitis A	Inactivated viral antigen	I.M.
Hepatitis B	Inactivated viral antigen	I.M.
Hib conjugates	Polysaccharide-protein conjugate	I.M.
Hib conjugate-DTP (HbOC-DTP and PRP-T reconstituted with DTP)	Polysaccharide-protein conjugate with toxoids and inactivated bacteria	I.M.
Hib conjugate-DTaP (PRP-T reconstituted with DTaP)	Polysaccharide-protein conjugate with toxoids and inactivated bacterial components	I.M.
Hib conjugate (PRP-OMP)-hepatitis B	Polysaccharide-protein conjugate with inactivated virus	I.M.
Influenza	Inactivated virus (whole virus), viral components	I.M.
Japanese encephalitis	Inactivated virus	S.C.
Lyme disease[4]	Inactivated protein	I.M.
Measles	Live virus	S.C.
MMR	Live viruses	S.C.
Measles-rubella	Live viruses	S.C.
Meningococcal	Polysaccharide	S.C.
Mumps	Live virus	S.C.
Pertussis[5]	Inactivated bacteria	I.M.
Plague	Inactivated bacteria	I.M.
Pneumococcal	Polysaccharide	I.M. or S.C.
Poliovirus		
IPV	Inactivated virus	S.C.
OPV	Live virus	Oral
Rabies	Inactivated virus	I.M. or I.D.[6]
Rubella	Live virus	S.C.
Tetanus	Toxoid	I.M.
Typhoid		
Parenteral	Inactivated bacteria	S.C.
Parenteral	Capsular polysaccharide	S.C. (boosters may be I.D.)
Oral	Live bacteria	Oral
Varicella	Live virus	S.C.
Yellow fever	Live virus	S.C.

[1]BCG = bacillus Calmette-Guérin; DTP = diphtheria and tetanus toxoids and pertussis, adsorbed; DTaP = diphtheria and tetanus toxoids and acellular pertussis, adsorbed; Hib = *Haemophilus influenzae* type b; MMR = live measles-mumps-rubella viruses; OPV = oral poliovirus; IPV = inactivated poliovirus; dT = diphtheria and tetanus toxoids (for children ≥7 years of age and adults); DT = diphtheria and tetanus toxoids (for children <7 years of age).

[2]Available only to the U.S. Armed Forces; no longer being manufactured but existing supplies continue to be used

[3]Not commercially available in the U.S.; presently, all anthrax vaccine lots are owned by the U.S. Department of Defense. The Centers for Disease Control (CDC) does not currently recommend routine vaccination of the general public.

[4]Withdrawn from the market

[5]Distributed by Bio Port Corporation in Lansing, Michigan

[6]Human diploid cell rabies vaccine for intradermal use is different in constitution and potency from the I.M. vaccine; it should be used for pre-exposure immunization only. Rabies vaccine adsorbed and RabAvert should not be given intradermally.

Adapted from "Report of the Committee on Infectious Diseases," *2000 Red Book®*, 25th ed, 7-8

IMMUNIZATION RECOMMENDATIONS *(Continued)*

Recommendations for Pneumococcal Conjugate Vaccine Use Among Healthy Children During Moderate and Severe Shortages

Age at First Vaccination (mo)	No Shortage[1]	Moderate Shortage	Severe Shortage
<6	2, 4, 6, and 12-15 mo	2, 4, and 6 mo (defer fourth dose)	2 doses at 2-mo interval in first 6 months of life (defer third and fourth doses)
7-11	2 doses at 2-mo interval; 12-15 mo dose	2 doses at 2-mo interval; 12-15-mo dose	2 doses at 2-mo interval (defer third dose)
12-23	2 doses at 2-mo interval	2 doses at 2-mo interval	1 dose (defer second dose)
>24	1 dose should be considered	No vaccination	No vaccination
Reduction in vaccine doses used[2]		21%	46%

[1]The vaccine schedule for no shortage is included as a reference. Providers should not use the" no shortage schedule", regardless of their vaccine supply, until the national shortage is resolved.

[2]Assumes that ~ 85% of vaccine is administered to healthy infants beginning at age <7 months; ~5% is administered to high-risk infants beginning at age <7 months; and ~10% is administered to healthy children beginning at age 7-24 months. Actual vaccine savings will depend on a provider's vaccine use.

Adapted from the Advisory Committee on Immunization Practices, "Updated Recommendations on Use of Pneumococcal Conjugate Vaccine in a Setting of Vaccine Shortage," *MMWR Morb Mortal Wkly Rep*, 2001, 50(50):1140-2.

Immune Globulins and Antitoxins[1] Available in the United States, by Type of Antibodies and Indications for Use

Immunobiologic	Type	Indication(s)
C. botulinum antitoxin	Specific equine antibodies	Treatment of botulism
Cytomegalovirus immune globulin, intravenous (CMV-IGIV)	Specific human antibodies	Prophylaxis for bone marrow and kidney transplant recipients
Diphtheria antitoxin	Specific equine antibodies	Treatment of respiratory diphtheria
Immune globulin (IG)	Pooled human antibodies	Hepatitis A pre- and postexposure prophylaxis; measles postexposure prophylaxis
Immune globulin, intravenous (IGIV)	Pooled human antibodies	Replacement therapy for antibody deficiency disorders; immune thrombocytopenic purpura (ITP); hypogammaglobulinemia in chronic lymphocytic leukemia; Kawasaki disease
Hepatitis B immune globulin (HBIG)	Specific human antibodies	Hepatitis B postexposure prophylaxis
Rabies immune globulin (HRIG)[2]	Specific human antibodies	Rabies postexposure management of persons not previously immunized with rabies vaccine
Tetanus immune globulin (TIG)	Specific human antibodies	Tetanus treatment; postexposure prophylaxis of persons not adequately immunized with tetanus toxoid
Vaccinia immune globulin (VIG)	Specific human antibodies	Treatment of eczema vaccinatum, vaccinia necrosum, and ocular vaccinia
Varicella-zoster immune globulin (VZIG)	Specific human antibodies	Postexposure prophylaxis of susceptible immunocompromised persons, certain susceptible pregnant women, and perinatally exposed newborn infants

[1]Immune globulin preparations and antitoxins are administered intramuscularly unless otherwise indicated.

[2]HRIG is administered around the wounds in addition to the intramuscular injection.

Modified from *MMWR Morb Mortal Wkly Rep*, 1994, 43(RR-1).

Suggested Intervals Between Immunoglobulin Administration and Measles Immunization (MMR or Monovalent Measles Vaccine)[1]

Indication for Immunoglobulin	Dose	(mg IgG/kg)	Interval (mo)[2]
Tetanus (TIG)	I.M.: 250 units	~10	3
Hepatitis A prophylaxis (IG)			
Contact prophylaxis	I.M.: 0.02 mL/kg	3.3	3
International travel	I.M.: 0.06 mL/kg	10	3
Hepatitis B prophylaxis (HBIG)	I.M.: 0.06 mL/kg	10	3
Rabies prophylaxis (RIG)	I.M.: 20 IU/kg	22	4
Measles prophylaxis (IG)			
Standard	I.M.: 0.25 mL/kg	40	5
Immunocompromised host	I.M.: 0.50 mL/kg	80	6
Varicella prophylaxis (VZIG)	I.M.: 125 units/10 kg (max: 625 units)	20-39	5
Blood transfusion			
Washed RBCs	I.V.: 10 mL/kg	Negligible	0
RBCs, adenine-saline added	I.V.: 10 mL/kg	10	3
Packed RBCs	I.V.: 10 mL/kg	20-60	5
Whole blood cells	I.V.: 10 mL/kg	80-100	6
Plasma or platelet products	I.V.: 10 mL/kg	160	7
Replacement (or therapy) of immune deficiencies	I.V.	300-400	8
ITP (IGIV)	I.V.	400	8
IRSV-IGIV	I.V.	750	9
ITP	I.V.	1000	10
ITP or Kawasaki disease	I.V.	1600-2000	11

[1]MMR = measles-mumps-rubella; IgG = immunoglobulin G; IG = immune globulin; TIG = tetanus IG; HBIG = hepatitis B IG; RIG = rabies IG; VZIG = varicella-zoster IG; RBC = red blood cell; IGIV = IG intravenous; ITP = immune (formerly termed "idiopathic") thrombocytopenic purpura; RSV-IGIV = respiratory syncytial virus IGIV.

[2]These intervals should provide sufficient time for decreases in passive antibodies in all children to allow for an adequate response to measles vaccine. Physicians should not assume that children are fully protected against measles during these intervals. Additional doses of IG or measles vaccine may be indicated after exposure to measles.

Adapted from "Report of the Committee on Infectious Diseases," *2000 Red Book®*, 25th ed, 390.

IMMUNIZATION RECOMMENDATIONS *(Continued)*

HAEMOPHILUS INFLUENZAE VACCINATION

Currently Recommended Regimens for Routine *Haemophilus influenzae* Type b Conjugate Immunization for Children Immunized Beginning at 2-6 Months of Age[1]

Vaccine Product at Initiation	Total No. of Doses to Be Administered	Recommended Regimens
HbOC or PRP-T	4	3 doses at 2-month intervals initially; fourth dose at 12-15 months of age; any conjugate vaccine for dose 4[2]
PRP-OMP	3	2 doses at 2-month intervals initially; when feasible, same vaccine for doses 1 and 2; third dose at 12-15 months of age; any conjugate vaccine for dose 3[2]

[1]These vaccines may be given in combination products or as reconstituted products with DTaP or DTP, provided the combination or reconstituted vaccine is approved by the U.S. Food and Drug Administration for the child's age and the administration of the other vaccine component(s) also is justified.

[2]The safety and efficacy of PRP-OMP, PRP-T, HbOC, and PRP-D are likely to be equivalent for children ≥12 months of age. If a different product is given for dose 2, then the recommendations for that product (eg, HbOC or PRP-T) apply.

Adapted from "Report of the Committee on Infectious Diseases," *2000 Red Book®*, 25th ed, 268.

Recommendations for *Haemophilus influenzae* Type b Conjugate Immunization for Children in Whom Initial Immunization Is Delayed Until 7 Months of Age or Older[1]

Age at Initiation of Immunization (mo)	Vaccine Product at Initiation	Total No. of Doses to Be Administered	Recommended Vaccine Regimens
7-11	HbOC, PRP-T, or PRP-OMP	3	2 doses at 2-month intervals; third dose at 12-15 months, given at 2 months after dose 2; any conjugate vaccine for dose 3[2]
12-14	HbOC, PRP-T, PRP-OMP, or PRP-D	2	2-month interval between doses
15-59	HbOC, PRP-T, PRP-OMP, or PRP-D	1[3]	Any conjugate vaccine
60 and older[4]	HbOC, PRP-T, PRP-OMP, or PRP-D	1 or 2[3]	Any conjugate vaccine

[1]These vaccines may be given in combination products or as reconstituted products with DTaP or DTP, provided the combination or reconstituted vaccine is approved by the U.S. Food and Drug Administration for the child's age and administration of the other vaccine component(s) also is justified.

[2]The safety and efficacy of PRP-OMP, PRP-T, HbOC, or PRP-D are likely to be equivalent for use as a booster dose for children 12 months or older.

[3]Two doses separated by 2 months are recommended by some experts for children with certain underlying diseases associated with increased risk of disease and impaired antibody responses to *H. influenzae* type conjugate vaccination.

[4]Only for children with chronic illness known to be associated with an increased risk for *H. influenzae* type b disease.

Adapted from "Report of the Committee on Infectious Diseases," *2000 Red Book®*, 25th ed, 269.

Recommendations for *Haemophilus influenzae* Type b Conjugate Immunization in Children With a Lapse in Vaccination[1]

Age at Presentation (mo)	Previous Immunization History	Recommended Regimen
7-11	1 dose of HbOC or PRP-T	1 or 2 doses of conjugate vaccine at 7-11 months of age (depending on age), with a booster dose given at least 2 months later, at 12-15 months of age
	2 doses of HbOC or PRP-T or 1 dose of PRP-OMP	1 dose of conjugate vaccine at 7-11 months of age with a booster dose given at least 2 months later at 12-15 month of age
12-14	2 doses before 12 months[2]	A single dose of any licensed conjugate vaccine[3]
	1 dose before 12 months[2]	2 additional doses of any licensed conjugate vaccine, separated by 2 months[3]
15-59	Any incomplete schedule	A single dose of any licensed conjugate[3]

[1]These vaccines may be given in combination products or as reconstituted products with DTaP or DTP, provided the combination or reconstituted vaccine is approved by the U.S. Food and Drug Administration for the child's age and the administration of the other vaccine component(s) also is justified.

[2]PRP-OMP, PRP-T, or HbOC.

[3]The safety and efficacy of PRP-OMP, PRP-T, HbOC, or PRP-D are likely to be equivalent for children ≥12 months of age.

Adapted from "Report of the Committee on Infectious Diseases," *2000 Red Book*®, 25th ed, 271.

IMMUNIZATION RECOMMENDATIONS *(Continued)*

POSTEXPOSURE PROPHYLAXIS FOR HEPATITIS B[1]

Exposure	Hepatitis B Immune Globulin	Hepatitis B Vaccine
Perinatal	0.5 mL I.M. within 12 h of birth	0.5 mL[2] I.M. within 12 h of birth (no later than 7 d), and at 1 and 6 mo[3]; test for HB_sAg and anti-HB_s at 12-15 mo
Sexual	0.06 mL/kg I.M. within 14 d of sexual contact; a second dose should be given if the index patient remains HB_sAg-positive after 3 mo and hepatitis B vaccine was not given initially	1 mL I.M. at 0, 1, and 6 mo for homosexual and bisexual men and regular sexual contacts of persons with acute and chronic hepatitis B
Percutaneous; exposed person unvaccinated		
Source known HB_sAg-positive	0.06 mL/kg I.M. within 24 h	1 mL I.M. within 7 d, and at 1 and 6 mo[4]
Source known, HB_sAg status not known	Test source for HB_sAg; if source is positive, give exposed person 0.06 mL/kg I.M. once within 7 d	1 mL I.M. within 7 d, and at 1 and 6 mo[4]
Source not tested or unknown	Nothing required	1 mL I.M. within 7 d, and at 1 and 6 mo
Percutaneous; exposed person vaccinated		
Source known HB_sAg-positive	Test exposed person for anti-HB_s.[5] If titer is protective, nothing is required; if titer is not protective, give 0.06 mL/kg within 24 h.	Review vaccination status[6]
Source known, HB_sAg status not known	Test source for HB_sAg and exposed person for anti-HB_s. If source is HB_sAg-negative, or if source is HB_sAg-positive but anti-HB_s titer is protective, nothing is required. If source is HB_sAg-positive and anti-HB_s titer is not protective or if exposed person is a known nonresponder, give 0.06 mL/kg I.M. within 24 h. A second dose of hepatitis B immune globulin can be given 1 mo later if a booster dose of hepatitis B vaccine is not given.	Review vaccination status[6]
Source not tested or unknown	Test exposed person for anti-HB_s. If anti-HB_s titer is protective, nothing is required. If anti-HB_s titer is not protective, 0.06 mL/kg may be given along with a booster dose of hepatitis B vaccine.	Review vaccination status[6]

[1]HB_sAg = hepatitis B surface antigen; anti-HB_s = antibody to hepatitis B surface antigen; I.M. = intramuscularly; SRU = standard ratio units.

[2]Each 0.5 mL dose of plasma-derived hepatitis B vaccine contains 10 mcg of HB_sAg; each 0.5 mL dose of recombinant hepatitis B vaccine contains 5 mcg (Merck Sharp & Dohme) or 10 mcg (SmithKline Beecham) of HB_sAg.

[3]If hepatitis B immune globulin and hepatitis B vaccine are given simultaneously, they should be given at separate sites.

[4]If hepatitis B vaccine is not given, a second dose of hepatitis B immune globulin should be given 1 month later.

[5]Anti-HB_s titers <10 SRU by radioimmunoassay or negative by enzyme immunoassay indicate lack of protection. Testing the exposed person for anti-HB_s is not necessary if a protective level of antibody has been shown within the previous 24 months.

[6]If the exposed person has not completed a three-dose series of hepatitis B vaccine, the series should be completed. Test the exposed person for anti-HB_s. If the antibody level is protective, nothing is required. If an adequate antibody response in the past is shown on retesting to have declined to an inadequate level, a booster dose (1 mL) of hepatitis B vaccine should be given. If the exposed person has inadequate antibody or is a known nonresponder to vaccination, a booster dose can be given along with one dose of hepatitis B immune globulin.

PREVENTION OF HEPATITIS A THROUGH ACTIVE OR PASSIVE IMMUNIZATION

Recommendations of the Advisory Committee on Immunization Practices (ACIP)

PROPHYLAXIS AGAINST HEPATITIS A VIRUS INFECTION

Recommended Doses of Immune Globulin (IG) for Hepatitis A Pre-exposure and Postexposure Prophylaxis

Setting	Duration of Coverage	IG Dose[1]
Pre-exposure	Short-term (1-2 months)	0.02 mL/kg
	Long-term (3-5 months)	0.06 mL/kg[2]
Postexposure	—	0.02 mL/kg

[1]IG should be administered by intramuscular injection into either the deltoid or gluteal muscle. For children <24 months of age, IG can be administered in the anterolateral thigh muscle.

[2]Repeat every 5 months if continued exposure to HAV occurs.

Recommended Dosages of Havrix®[1]

Vaccinee's Age (y)	Dose (EL.U.)[2]	Volume (mL)	No. Doses	Schedule (mo)[3]
2-18	720	0.5	2	0, 6-12
>18	1440	1.0	2	0, 6-12

[1]Hepatitis A vaccine, inactivated, SmithKline Beecham Biologicals.

[2]ELISA units.

[3]0 months represents timing of the initial dose; subsequent numbers represent months after the initial dose.

Recommended Dosages of VAQTA®[1]

Vaccinee's Age (y)	Dose (units)	Volume (mL)	No. Doses	Schedule (mo)[2]
2-17	25	0.5	2	0, 6-18
>17	50	1.0	2	0, 6

[1]Hepatitis A vaccine, inactivated, Merck & Company, Inc.

[2]0 months represents timing of the initial dose; subsequent numbers represent months after the initial dose.

From *MMWR Morb Mortal Wkly Rep*, 1996, 45(RR-15).

IMMUNIZATION RECOMMENDATIONS *(Continued)*

RECOMMENDATIONS FOR TRAVELERS

Recommended Immunizations for Travelers to Developing Countries[1]

Immunizations	Length of Travel		
	Brief, <2 wk	**Intermediate, 2 wk - 3 mo**	**Long-term Residential, >3 mo**
Review and complete age-appropriate childhood schedule • DTaP; poliovirus vaccine, and *H. influenzae* type b vaccine may be given at 4 wk intervals if necessary to complete the recommended schedule before departure • Measles: 2 additional doses given if younger than 12 mo of age at first dose • Varicella • Hepatitis B[2]	+	+	+
Yellow fever[3]	+	+	+
Hepatitis A[4]	+	+	+
Typhoid fever[4]	±	+	+
Meningococcal disease[5]	±	±	±
Rabies[6]	±	+	+
Japanese encephalitis[3]	±	±	+

[1]+ = recommended; ± = consider.

[2]If insufficient time to complete 6-month primary series, accelerated series can be given.

[3]For endemic regions, see *Health Information for International Travel* in *Red Book®*. For high-risk activities in areas experiencing outbreaks, vaccine is recommended even for brief travel.

[4]Indicated for travelers who will consume food and liquids in areas of poor sanitation.

[5]For endemic regions of Africa, during local epidemics, and travel to Saudi Arabia for the Hajj.

[6]Indicated for person with high risk of animal exposure, and for travelers to endemic countries.

Adapted from "Report of the Committee on Infectious Diseases," *2000 Red Book®*, 25th ed, 78.

Recommendations for Pre-exposure Immunoprophylaxis of Hepatitis A Virus Infection for Travelers[1]

Age (y)	Likely Exposure (mo)	Recommended Prophylaxis
<2	<3	IG 0.02 mL/kg[2]
	3-5	IG 0.06 mL/kg[2]
	Long-term	IG 0.06 mL/kg at departure and every 5 mo if exposure to HAV continues[2]
≥2	<3[3]	HAV vaccine[4,5] or
	3-5[3]	HAV vaccine[4,5] or IG 0.06 mL/kg[2]
	Long-term	HAV vaccine[4,5]

[1] IG = immune globulin; HAV= hepatitis A virus.

[2]IG should be administered deep into a large muscle mass. Ordinarily, no more than 5 mL should be administered in one site in an adult or large child; lesser amounts (maximum 3 mL) should be given to small children and infants.

[3]Vaccine is preferable, but IG is an acceptable alternative.

[4]To ensure protection in travelers whose departure is imminent, IG also may be given.

[5]Dose and schedule of hepatitis A vaccine as recommended according to age.

Adapted from "Report of the Committee on Infectious Diseases," *2000 Red Book®*, 25th ed, 282.

Prevention of Malaria[1]

Drug	Adult Dosage	Pediatric Dosage
	Chloroquine-Sensitive Areas	
Chloroquine phosphate[2,3]	500 mg (300 mg base), once/week[4]	5 mg/kg base once/week, up to adult dose of 300 mg base[4]
	Chloroquine-Resistant Areas	
Mefloquine[3,5]	250 mg once/week[4]	<15 kg: 5 mg/kg[4] 15-19 kg: 1/4 tablet[4] 20-30 kg: 1/2 tablet[4] 31-45 kg: 3/4 tablet[4] >45 kg: 1 tablet[4]
Doxycycline[3]	100 mg/d[6]	2 mg/kg/d, up to 100 mg/d[6]
Atovaquone/Proguanil	250 mg/100 mg (1 tablet) daily[7]	11-20 kg: 62.5 mg/25 mg[7] 21-30 kg: 125 mg/50 mg[7] 31-40 kg: 187.5 mg/75 mg[7]
Alternative:		
Primaquine[8]	30 mg base daily	0.5 mg/kg base daily
Chloroquine phosphate[3]	Same as above	Same as above
plus		
pyrimethamine-sulfadoxine for presumptive treatment[9]	Carry a single dose (3 tablets) for self-treatment of febrile illness when medical care is not immediately available	<1 y: 1/4 tablet 1-3 y: 1/2 tablet 4-8 y: 1 tablet 9-14 y: 2 tablets
or plus		
proguanil[10]	200 mg daily	<2 y: 50 mg daily 2-6 y: 100 mg 7-10 y: 150 mg >10 y: 200 mg

[1]No drug regimen guarantees protection against malaria. If fever develops within a year (particularly within the first 2 months) after travel to malarious areas, travelers should be advised to seek medical attention. Insect repellents, insecticide-impregnated bed nets, and proper clothing are important adjuncts for malaria prophylaxis.

[2]In pregnancy, chloroquine prophylaxis has been used extensively and safely.

[3]For prevention of attack after departure from areas where *P. vivax* and *P. ovale* are endemic, which includes almost all areas where malaria is found (except Haiti), some experts prescribe in addition primaquine phosphate 15 mg base (26.3 mg)/d or, for children, 0.3 mg base/kg/d during the last 2 weeks of prophylaxis. Others prefer to avoid the toxicity of primaquine and rely on surveillance to detect cases when they occur; particularly when exposure was limited or doubtful.

[4]Beginning 1-2 weeks before travel and continuing weekly for the duration of stay and for 4 weeks after leaving.

[5]The drug has not been approved for use during pregnancy; however, it has been reported to be safe for prophylactic use during the second or third trimester of pregnancy and possibly during early pregnancy as well (CDC Health Information for International Travel, 1999-2000, page 120; Smoak BL, et al, *J Infect Dis*, 1997, 176:831). Mefloquine is not recommended for patients with cardiac conduction abnormalities. Patients with a history of seizures or psychiatric disorders should avoid mefloquine (*Medical Letter*, 1990, 32:13). Resistance to mefloquine has been reported in some areas, such as Thailand; in these areas, doxycycline should be used for prophylaxis. In children <8 years of age, proguanil plus sulfisoxazole has been used (Suh KN and Keystone JS, *Infect Dis Clin Pract*, 1996, 5:541).

[6]Beginning 1-2 days before travel and continuing for the duration of stay and for 4 weeks after leaving. Use of tetracyclines is contraindicated in pregnancy and in children <8 years old. Doxycycline can cause gastrointestinal disturbances, vaginal moniliasis, and photosensitivity reactions.

[7]Shanks GE et al, *Clin Infect Dis*, 1998, 27:494; Lell B et al, *Lancet*, 1998, 351:709. Beginning 1-2 days before travel and continuing for the duration of stay and for 1 week after leaving.

[8]Several studies have shown that daily primaquine, beginning 1 day before departure and continued until 2 days after leaving the malaria area, provides effective prophylaxis against chloroquine-resistant *P. falciparum* (Schwartz E and Regev-Yochay G, *Clin Infect Dis*, 1999, 29:1502). Some studies have shown less efficacy against *P. vivax*.

[9]In areas with strains resistant to pyrimethamine-sulfadoxine, atovaquone/proguanil or atovaquone plus doxycycline can also be used for presumptive treatment.

[10]Proguanil (Paludrine – Wyeth Ayerst, Canada; Zeneca, United Kingdom), which is not available alone in the U.S.A. but is widely available in Canada and overseas, is recommended mainly for use in Africa south of the Sahara. Prophylaxis is recommended during exposure and for 4 weeks afterwards. Proguanil has been used in pregnancy without evidence of toxicity (Phillips-Howard PA and Wood D, *Drug Saf*, 1996, 14:131).

Adapted from "Report of the Committee on Infectious Diseases," *2000 Red Book®*, 25th ed, 709-10.

IMMUNIZATION RECOMMENDATIONS *(Continued)*

ADVERSE EVENTS AND VACCINATION

Reportable Events Following Vaccination[1]

These events are reportable by law to the Vaccine Adverse Event Reporting System (VAERS) (1-800-822-7967). In addition, individuals are encouraged to report any clinically significant or unexpected events (even if uncertain whether the vaccine caused the event) for any vaccine, whether or not it is listed in the table. Manufacturers also are required to report to the VAERS program all adverse events made known to them for any vaccine.

Vaccine		Adverse Event	Interval From Vaccination to Onset of Event for Reporting[2]
Tetanus toxoid-containing vaccines (eg, DTaP, DTP, DTP-Hib; DT; dT or TT)	A.	Anaphylaxis or anaphylactic shock	0-7 d
	B.	Brachial neuritis	0-28 d
	C.	Any acute complication or sequela (including death) of above events	No limit
	D.	Events described in manufacturer's package insert as contraindications to additional doses of vaccine	No limit
Pertussis antigen-containing vaccines (eg, DTaP, DTP, P, DTP-Hib)	A.	Anaphylaxis or anaphylactic shock	0-7 d
	B.	Encephalopathy (or encephalitis)	0-7 d
	C.	Any acute complication or sequela (including death) of above events	No limit
	D.	Events described in manufacturer's package insert as contraindications to additional doses of vaccine	No limit
Measles, mumps, and rubella virus-containing vaccines in any combination (eg, MMR, MR, M, R)	A.	Anaphylaxis or anaphylactic shock	0-7 d
	B.	Encephalopathy (or encephalitis)	0-15 d
	C.	Any acute complication or sequela (including death) of above events	No limit
	D.	Events described in manufacturer's package insert as contraindications to additional doses of vaccine	No limit
Rubella virus-containing vaccines (eg, MMR, MR, R)	A.	Chronic arthritis	0-42 d
	B.	Any acute complication or sequela (including death) of above events	No limit
	C.	Events described in manufacturer's package insert as contraindications to additional doses of vaccine	No limit
Measles virus-containing vaccines (eg, MMR, MR, M)	A.	Thrombocytopenic purpura	0-30 d
	B.	Vaccine-strain measles viral infection in an immunodeficient recipient	0-6 mo
	C.	Any acute complication or sequela (including death) of above events	No limit
	D.	Events described in manufacturer's package insert as contraindications to additional doses of vaccine	No limit
Live poliovirus-containing vaccines (OPV)	A.	Paralytic polio	
		• in a nonimmunodeficient recipient	0-30 d
		• in an immunodeficient recipient	0-6 mo
		• in a vaccine-associated community case	No limit
	B.	Vaccine-strain polio viral infection	
		• in a nonimmunodeficient recipient	0-30 d
		• in an immunodeficient recipient	0-6 mo
		• in a vaccine-associated community case	No limit
	C.	Any acute complication or sequela (including death) of above events	No limit
	D.	Events described in manufacturer's package insert as contraindications to additional doses of vaccine	No limit
Polio inactivated	A.	Anaphylaxis or anaphylactic shock	0-7 d
	B.	Any acute complication or sequela (including death) of above events	No limit
	C.	Events described in manufacturer's package insert as contraindications to additional doses of vaccine	No limit
Hepatitis B	A.	Anaphylaxis or anaphylactic shock	0-7 d
	B.	Any acute complication or sequela (including death) of above events	No limit
	C.	Events described in manufacturer's package insert as contraindications to additional doses of vaccine	No limit
Haemophilus influenzae type b polysaccharide vaccines (unconjugated, PRP vaccines)	A.	Early onset Hib disease	0-7 d
	B.	Any acute complication or sequela (including death) of above events	No limit
	C.	Events described in manufacturer's package insert as contraindications to additional doses of vaccine	No limit
Haemophilus influenzae type b polysaccharide conjugate vaccines	A.	No condition specified for compensation	Not applicable
	B.	Events described in manufacturer's package insert as contraindications to additional doses of vaccine	No limit
Varicella virus-containing vaccine	A.	No condition specified for compensation	Not applicable
	B.	Events described in manufacturer's package insert as contraindications to additional doses of vaccine	No limit

Vaccine	Adverse Event	Interval From Vaccination to Onset of Event for Reporting[2]
Any new vaccine recommended by the CDC for routine administration to children, after publication by Secretary, HHS of a notice of coverage	A. No condition specified for compensation B. Events described in manufacturer's package insert as contraindications to additional doses of vaccine	

[1]Effective October 22, 1998.

[2]Taken from the Reportable Events Table (RET), which lists conditions reportable by law (42 USC §300aa-25) to the Vaccine Adverse Event Reporting System (VAERS), including conditions found in the manufacturer's package insert. In addition, physicians are encouraged to report **ANY** clinically significant or unexpected events (even if you are not certain the vaccine caused the event) for **ANY** vaccine, whether or not it is listed on the RET. Manufacturers also are required by regulation (21 CFR§600.80) to report to the VAERS program all adverse events made known to them for any vaccine. VAERS reporting forms and information can be obtained by calling 1-800-822-7967 or from the Web site (http://www.fda.gov/cber/vaers/report.htm).

Adapted from "Report of the Committee on Infectious Diseases," *2000 Red Book®*, 25th ed, 760-2.

IMMUNIZATIONS[1] (VACCINES)

Drug	Use	Stability	Administration/ Patient Information
Anthrax vaccine adsorbed[2]	Used for individuals who may come in contact with animal products which come from anthrax endemic areas and may be contaminated with *Bacillus anthracis* spores and for high-risk persons such as veterinarians and other handling potentially infected animals; Department of Defense is implementing an anthrax vaccination program for active duty and reserve personnel against the biological warfare agent anthrax	Refrigerate; do not freeze.	Injection may be deferred in patients with acute respiratory disease or other active infection. Persons receiving immunosuppressive agents may not have adequate response to immunization. If immunosuppression therapy is short-term, immunization should be delayed. If immunosuppression therapy is long-term, an extra dose of vaccine should be given a month or more after immunosuppressive therapy is discontinued.
BCG vaccine	Bladder instillation of vaccine as immunotherapy for treatment of bladder cancer (TheraCys®; TICE® BCG). BCG vaccine is not routinely recommended for use in the U.S. for prevention of tuberculosis. BCG should be administered with caution to persons in groups at high risk for HIV infection or persons know to be severely immunocompromised. Although limited data suggests that the vaccine may be safe for use in asymptomatic children infected with HIV, BCG vaccination is not recommended for HIV infected adults or for persons with symptomatic disease. Vaccination should be restricted to persons at exceptionally high risk for tuberculosis infection. HIV infected persons thought to be infected with *Mycobacterium tuberculosis* should be strongly recommended for tuberculosis preventive therapy.	Refrigerate between 2°C and 8°C (35°F to 46°F) and protect from light. Use within 2 hours of mixing (TICE® BCG; TheraCys®).	**Immunization against tuberculosis:** 0.2-0.3 mL percutaneous; initial lesion usually appears after 10-14 days consisting of small red papule at injection site and reaches maximum diameter of 3 mm in 4-6 weeks. Conduct postvaccinal tuberculin test in 2-3 months. If test is negative, repeat vaccination. **Immunotherapy for bladder cancer:** TICE® BCG vaccine 6 x 10^8 viable organisms in 50 mL NS (preservative free) instilled into bladder and retained for 2 hours weekly for 6 weeks; refer to individual protocols.
Cholera vaccine	Primary immunization for cholera prophylaxis. The World Health Organization no longer recommends cholera vaccination for travel to or from cholera-endemic areas. Some countries may still require evidence of a complete primary series or a booster dose given within 6 months of arrival. Vaccination should not be considered as an alternative to continued careful selection of foods and water. Ideally, cholera and yellow fever vaccines should be administered at least 3 weeks apart.	Refrigerate; avoid freezing.	0.5 mL in two doses 1 week to 1 month or more apart. There is no data on the safety of cholera vaccination during pregnancy. Use in pregnancy should reflect actual increased risk. Persons who have had severe local or systemic reactions to a previous dose should not be revaccinated. Have epinephrine (1:1000) available for immediate use. Defer immunization in individuals with moderate or severe febrile illness. May cause malaise, fever, headache, pain, swelling, tenderness, erythema, and induration at the injection site. Local reaction can occur up to 7 days after injection. Review history of elderly to assure no drug or disease is contraindicated with use of this vaccine.
Diphtheria and tetanus toxoid	Active immunity against diphtheria and tetanus when pertussis vaccine is contraindicated	Refrigerate.	**Children:** 6 weeks to 1 year of age: Three 0.5 mL doses at least 4 weeks apart; administer a reinforcing dose 6-12 months after the third injection. **Children 1-6 years:** Two 0.5 mL doses at least 4 weeks apart; reinforcing dose 6-12 months after second injection. If final dose is given after seventh birthday, use adult preparation. **Children 4-6 years**(booster immunization): 0.5 mL; not necessary if all 4 doses were given after fourth birthday - routinely administer booster doses at 10-year intervals with the adult preparation.
Diphtheria, tetanus toxoids, and acellular pertussis vaccine (Acel-Imune®; Certiva®; Infanrix™; Tripedia®)	Active immunization against diphtheria, tetanus, and pertussis from age 6 weeks through seventh birthday	Refrigerate at 2°C to 8°C (35°F to 46°F); do not freeze.	I.M.: After at least three doses of whole-cell DTP, administer 0.5 mL at 18 months (at least 6 months after third DTwP dose), then another dose at 4-5 years of age. DTaP should not be used in children <15 months of age and should not be used in children who have received fewer than 3 doses of DTP.

Drug	Use	Stability	Administration/ Patient Information
Diphtheria, tetanus toxoids, and whole-cell pertussis vaccine (Tri-Immunol®)	Active immunization of infants and children through 6 years of age (between 2 months and the seventh birthday) against diphtheria, tetanus, and pertussis. Recommended for both primary immunization and routine recall. Start immunization at once if whooping cough or diphtheria is present in the community.		The primary immunization for children 2 months to 6 years of age, ideally beginning at the age of 2-3 months or at 6-week check-up. Administer 0.5 mL I.M. on three occasions at 4- to 8-week intervals with a re-enforcing dose administered 1 year after the third injection. The booster doses (0.5 mL I.M.) are administered when the child is 4-6 years of age.
Diphtheria, tetanus toxoids, whole-cell pertussis vaccine, and *Haemophilus* b conjugate vaccine (Tetramune®)	Active immunization of infants and children through 5 years of age (between 2 months and the sixth birthday) against diphtheria, tetanus, pertussis, and *Haemophilus* b disease when indications for immunization with DTP vaccine and HIB vaccine coincide.	Refrigerate. May be frozen (not diluent) without affecting potency.	The primary immunization for children 2 months to 5 years of age, ideally beginning at the age of 2-3 months or at 6-week checkup. Administer 0.5 mL I.M. on three occasions at 2-month intervals, followed by a fourth 0.5 mL dose at 15 months of age. If adverse reactions occurred with previous doses, immunization should be completed with diphtheria and tetanus toxoid absorbed (pediatric). Any febrile illness or active infection is reason for delaying use of *Haemophilus* b conjugate vaccine.
Haemophilus b conjugate vaccine (ActHIB®; HibTITER®; PedvaxHIB™)	Routine immunization of children 2 months to 5 years of age against invasive disease caused by *H. influenzae* type b. Nonimmunized children ≥5 years of age with a chronic illness known to be associated with increased risk of *Haemophilus influenzae* type b disease, specifically, persons with anatomic or functional asplenia or sickle cell anemia or those who have undergone splenectomy, should receive Hib vaccine, as well as adults with specific dysfunction or certain complement deficiencies who are at especially high risk of *H. influenzae* type b infection (HIV-infected adults); patients with Hodgkin's disease or other hematologic neoplasms and immunosuppression (vaccinated at least 2 weeks before the initiation of chemotherapy or 3 months after the end of chemotherapy). *Haemophilus* b conjugate vaccines are not indicated for prevention of bronchitis or other infections due to *H. influenzae* in adults.	Store in refrigerator, may be frozen (not diluent) without affecting potency). Reconstituted Hib-Imune® remains stable for only 8 hours, whereas HibVAX® remains stable for 30 days when refrigerated.	**I.M. injection:** 0.5 mL according to "brand-specific" schedules; do not inject I.V. The same brand should be used throughout the entire vaccination series. If the healthcare provider does not know which vaccine was previously used, an infant (2-6 months of age) should be given a primary series of three doses. Have epinephrine 1:1000 available. **HibTITER®:** Age at 1st dose: 2-6 months: Primary series: 3 doses, 2 months apart; booster: 15 months (at least 2 months after previous dose). Age at 1st dose: 7-11 months: Primary series: 2 doses, 2 months apart; booster: 15 months (at least 2 months after previous dose). Age at 1st dose: 12-14 months: Primary series: 1 dose; booster: 15 months (at least 2 months after previous dose). Age at 1st dose: 15-60 months: Primary series: 1 dose; no booster. **PedvaxHIB®:** Age at 1st dose: 2-6 months: Primary series: 2 doses, 2 months apart; booster: 12 months (at least 2 months after previous dose). Age at 1st dose: 7-11 months: Primary series: 2 doses, 2 months apart; booster: 15 months (at least 2 months after previous dose). Age at 1st dose: 12-14 months: Primary series: 1 dose; booster: 15 months (at least 2 months after previous dose). Age at 1st dose: 15-60 months: Primary series: 1 dose; no booster. **ProHIBIT®:** Age at 1st dose: 15-60 months: Primary series: 1 dose; no booster .
Hepatitis A vaccine (Havrix®; VAQTA®)	For populations desiring protection against hepatitis A or for populations at high risk of exposure to hepatitis A virus (travelers to developing countries, household and sexual contacts of persons infected with hepatitis A), child day care employees, illicit drug users, patients with chronic liver disease, male homosexuals, institutional workers (eg, institutions for the mentally and physically handicapped persons, prisons, etc), and healthcare workers who may be exposed to hepatitis A virus (eg, laboratory employees); protection lasts for approximately 15 years		**I.M.injection** (do not administer I.V.): Use caution in patients with serious active infection, cardiovascular disease, or pulmonary disorders; treatment for anaphylactic reactions should be immediately available. **Havrix®:** Children 2-18 years: 720 ELISA units (administered as 2 injections of 360 ELISA units [0.5 mL]) 15-30 days prior to travel with a booster 6-12 months following primary immunization. The deltoid muscle should be used for I.M. injection. Adults: 1440 ELISA units (1 mL) 15-30 days prior to travel with a booster 6-12 months following primary immunization. Injection should be in the deltoid. **VAQTA®:** Children 2-17 years: 25 units (0.5 mL) with 25 units (0.5 mL) booster to be given 6-18 months after primary immunization. Adults: 50 units (1 mL) with 50 units (1 mL) booster to be given 6 months after primary immunization.

IMMUNIZATIONS[1] (VACCINES) *(Continued)*

Drug	Use	Stability	Administration/ Patient Information
Hepatitis B immune globulin (BayHepB™; Nabi-HB®)	Provide prophylactic passive immunity to hepatitis B infection to those individuals exposed; newborns of mothers known to be hepatitis B surface antigen positive; hepatitis B immune globulin is not indicated for treatment of active hepatitis B infections and is ineffective in the treatment of chronic active hepatitis B infection	Refrigerate at 2°C to 8°C (36°F to 46°F); do not freeze.	For I.M. injection (do not administer I.V.) only in gluteal or deltoid region. To prevent injury from injection, care should be taken when given to patients with thrombocytopenia or bleeding disorders. **I.M.:** Postexposure prophylaxis: 0.06 mL/kg; usual dose: 3-5 mL; repeat at 28-30 days after exposure. **Newborns:** Hepatitis B: 0.5 mL as soon after birth as possible (within 12 hours); may repeat at 3 months in order for a higher rate of prevention of the carrier state to be achieved. At this time, an active vaccination program with the vaccine may begin.
Hepatitis B vaccine (Engerix-B®; Recombivax HB®)	Immunization against infection caused by all known subtypes of hepatitis B virus, in individuals considered at high risk of potential exposure to hepatitis B virus or HB_sAg-positive materials.	Refrigerate; do not freeze.	For I.M. injection (do not administer I.V.). The deltoid muscle is the preferred site (adults). Administer with caution in patients receiving anticoagulant therapy. S.C. injection may be administered in patients at risk of hemorrhage which may result in an increased incidence of local reactions and a reduced therapeutic effect. Patient will receive three doses of hepatitis B vaccine; immunity will last approximately 5-7 years. Refer to specific product labeling for dosing.
Immune globulin, intramuscular (BayGam™)	Household and sexual contacts of persons with hepatitis A, measles, varicella, and possibly rubella; travelers to high-risk areas outside tourist routes; staff, attendees, and parents of diapered attendees in day-care center outbreaks. For travelers, IG is not an alternative to careful selection of foods and water; immune globulin can interfere with the antibody response to parenterally administered live virus vaccines. Frequent travelers should be tested for hepatitis A antibody, immune hemolytic anemia, and neutropenia (with TTP, I.V. route is usually used).	Refrigerate; do not freeze.	For I.M. injection only (do not administer I.V.); do not mix with other medications. Skin testing should not be performed as local irritation can occur and be misinterpreted as a positive reaction. **Hepatitis A:** Pre-exposure prophylaxis upon travel into endemic areas (hepatitis A vaccine preferred); postexposure prophylaxis: 0.02 mL/kg given within 2 weeks of exposure. **Measles: Prophylaxis:** 0.25 mL/kg/dose (max: 15 mL) given within 6 days of exposure followed by live attenuated measles vaccine in 3 months or at 15 months of age (whichever is later). **Leukemia, lymphoma, immunodeficiency disorders, generalized malignancy, or receiving immunosuppressive therapy:** 0.5 mL/kg (max: 15 mL). **Poliomyelitis: Prophylaxis:** 0.3 mL/kg/dose as a single dose **Rubella: Prophylaxis:** 0.55 mL/kg/dose within 72 hours of exposure **Varicella: Prophylaxis:** 0.6-1.2 mL/kg (varicella-zoster immune globulin preferred) within 72 hours of exposure **IgG deficiency:** 1.3 mL/kg, then 0.66 mL/kg in 3-4 weeks **Hepatitis B: Prophylaxis:** 0.06 mL/kg/dose (HBIG preferred)

Drug	Use	Stability	Administration/ Patient Information
Influenza virus vaccine (Fluogen®; FluShield®; Fluvirin®; Fluzone®)	Provide active immunity to influenza virus strains contained in the vaccine; for high-risk persons, previous year vaccines do not prevent present year influenza. Those at risk for influenza injection include persons ≥65 years of age; institutionalized patients; persons of any age with chronic disorders of pulmonary and/or cardiovascular system; persons who have required medical follow-up following hospitalization for other chronic diseases such as diabetes, renal disease, immunodepressive disorders, etc; and travelers, especially those at risk. Children and teenagers (6 months to 18 years) who are receiving long-term aspirin therapy and, therefore, may be at risk for developing Reye's syndrome after influenza.	Refrigerate	For I.M. administration only **Children:** 6-35 mo: 1-2 doses of 0.25 mL with ≥4 weeks between doses and the last dose administered before December **3-8 years:** 1-2 doses of 0.5 mL (in anterolateral aspect of thigh) with≥4 weeks between doses and the last dose administered before December **Children ≥9 years and Adults:** 0.5 mL each year of appropriate vaccine for the year, one dose is all that is necessary. Administer late in the fall to allow maximum titers to develop by peak epidemic periods usually occurring in early December. Waiting until the second or third trimester to vaccinate pregnant women with a high-risk condition may be reasonable. Antigenic response may not be as great as expected in patients requiring immunosuppressive drug. Hypersensitivity reactions may occur. Because of potential for febrile reactions, risks and benefits must carefully be considered in patients with a history of febrile convulsions. Influenza vaccines from previous seasons must not be used. Patients with sulfite sensitivity may be affected by this product.
Japanese encephalitis virus vaccine, inactivated (JE-VAX®)	Active immunization against Japanese encephalitis for persons 1 year of age and older who plan to spend 1 month or more in endemic areas in Asia, especially persons traveling during the transmission season or visiting rural areas. Consider vaccination for shorter trips to epidemic areas or extensive outdoor activities in rural endemic areas. Elderly (>55 years of age) individuals should be considered for vaccination, since they have increased risk of developing symptomatic illness after infection. Those planning travel to or residence in endemic areas should consult the Travel Advisory Service (Central Campus) for specific advice.	Refrigerate at 2°C to 8°C. Do not freeze. Discard 8 hours after reconstitution.	For S.C. injection (do not administer I.V.): U.S. recommended primary immunization schedule: **Children >3 years and Adults:** Three 1 mL doses given on days 0, 7, and 30. Give third dose on day 14 when time does not permit waiting; 2 doses a week apart produce immunity in about 80% of recipients. The longest regimen yields highest titers after 6 months. **Children 1-3 years:** Three 0.5 mL doses given on days 0, 7, and 30; abbreviated schedules should be used only when necessary due to time constraints. Booster dose: Give after 2 years, or according to current recommendation. Epinephrine should be immediately available. Severe adverse reactions may occur within minutes following vaccination, or up to 17 days later; most reactions occur within 10 days, with the majority within 48 hours. Observe vaccinees for 30 minutes after vaccination. Warn them of the possibility of delayed generalized urticaria and to remain where medical care is readily available for 10 days following any dose of the vaccine. Because of the potential for severe adverse reactions, Japanese encephalitis vaccine is **not** recommended for all persons traveling to or residing in Asia. Immunization of infants should be deferred whenever possible. **Note**: Travel should not commence for at least 10 days after the last dose of vaccine to allow adequate antibody formation and recognition of any delayed adverse reaction. Advise concurrent use of other means to reduce the risk of mosquito exposure when possible, including bed nets, insect repellents, protective clothing, avoidance of travel in endemic areas, and avoidance of outdoor activity during twilight and evening periods.
Lyme disease vaccine (LYMErix™) [3]	Active immunization against Lyme disease in individuals between 15-70 years of age. Individuals most at risk are those who live, work, or travel to *B. burgdorferi*-infected, tick-infected, grassy/wooded areas.	Store between 2°C and 8°C (36°F and 46°F).	I.M.: Vaccination with three doses of 30 mcg (0.5 mL), administered at 0, 1, and 12 months, is recommended for optimal protection.

IMMUNIZATIONS[1] (VACCINES) *(Continued)*

Drug	Use	Stability	Administration/ Patient Information
Measles and rubella vaccines, combined (M-R-VAX® II)	Simultaneous immunization against measles and rubella; **Note:** Trivalent measles-mumps-rubella (M-M-R® II) vaccine is the preferred agent for most children and many adults. Persons born prior to 1957 are generally considered immune and need not be vaccinated.	Refrigerate prior to use. Use as soon as possible. Discard if not used within 8 hours of reconstitution.	S.C.: Children ≥15 months and Adults: Inject 0.5 mL into outer aspect of upper arm; no routine booster for rubella.
Measles, mumps, and rubella vaccines, combined (M-M-R® II)	Measles, mumps, and rubella prophylaxis	Refrigerate and protect from light prior to reconstitution. Use as soon as possible. Discard 8 hours after reconstitution.	Administer 0.5 mL S.C. in outer aspect of the upper arm to children 12 months of age, then repeat at 4-6 years of age. If the second dose was not received, the schedule should be completed by the 11- to 12-year old visit. Females should not become pregnant within 3 months of vaccination. MMR vaccine should not be given within 3 months of immune globulin or whole blood. Have epinephrine available during and after administration. Should not be administered to severely immunocompromised persons with the exception of asymptomatic children with HIV (ACIP and AAP recommendation). Severely immunocompromised patients and symptomatic HIV-infected patients who are exposed to measles should receive immune globulin, regardless of prior vaccination status. Defer immunization during any acute illness.
Measles virus vaccine, live (Attenuvax®)	Immunization for adults born after 1957 without documentation of live vaccine on or after first birthday, physician-diagnosed measles, or laboratory evidence of immunity should be vaccinated, ideally with two doses of vaccine separated by no less than 1 month. For those previously vaccinated with one dose of measles vaccine, revaccination is recommended for students entering colleges and other institutions of higher education, for healthcare workers at the time of employment, and for international travelers who visit endemic areas.	Refrigerate at 2°C to 8°C. Discard if left at room temperature for over 8 hours. Protect from light.	S.C.: Children ≥15 months and Adults: Inject 0.5 mL into outer aspect of upper arm; no routine booster.
Meningococcal polysaccharide vaccine, groups A, C, Y, and W-135 (Menomune®-A/C/Y/W-135)	Immunization of persons 2 years of age and older in epidemic or endemic areas as might be determined in a population delineated by neighborhood, school, dormitory, or other reasonable boundary. The prevalent serogroup in such a situation should match a serogroup in the vaccine. Individuals at particular high-risk include persons with terminal component complement deficiencies and those with anatomic or function asplenia. For use with travelers visiting areas of a country that are recognized as having hyperendemic or epidemic meningococcal disease. Vaccinations should be considered for household or institutional contacts of persons with meningococcal disease as an adjunct to appropriate antibiotic chemoprophylaxis as well as medical and laboratory personnel at risk of exposure to meningococcal disease.	Discard remainder of vaccine within 5 days after reconstitution. Store reconstituted vaccine in refrigerator.	S.C.: 0.5 mL; do not inject intradermally or I.V. Have epinephrine 1:1000 available to control allergic reaction. Patients who undergo splenectomy secondary to trauma or nonlymphoid tumors respond well, however, those asplenic patients with lymphoid tumors who receive either chemotherapy or irradiation respond poorly. Avoid in pregnancy unless there is a substantial risk of infection.
Mumps virus vaccine (live/attenuated) (Mumpsvax®)	Mumps prophylaxis by promoting active immunity **Note:** Trivalent measles-mumps-rubella (M-M-R® II) vaccine is the preferred agent for most children and many adults. Persons born prior to 1957 are generally considered immune and need not be vaccinated.	Refrigerate; protect from light. Discard within 8 hours after reconstitution.	Children ≥15 months and Adults: 0.5 mL S.C. in outer aspect of upper arm; no booster

Drug	Use	Stability	Administration/ Patient Information
Plague vaccine	Vaccinate selected travelers to countries where avoidance of rodents and fleas is impossible; laboratory and field personnel working with *Yersinia pestis* organisms possibly resistant to antimicrobials; those engaged in *Yersinia pestis* aerosol experiments or in field operations in areas with enzootic plague where regular exposure to potentially infected wild rodents, rabbits, or their fleas cannot be prevented. Prophylactic antibiotics may be indicated following definite exposure, whether or not the exposed persons have been vaccinated.		Three I.M. doses: First dose 1 mL, second dose (0.2 mL) 1 month later, third dose (0.2 mL) 5 months after the second dose; booster doses (0.2 mL) at 1-to 2-year intervals if exposure continues. Do not use in pregnant females unless there is substantial and unavoidable risk of exposure.
Pneumococcal 7 valent conjugate vaccine (Diphtheria CRM_{197} Protein; Prevnar™)	Immunization of infants and toddlers against active disease caused by *Streptococcus pneumoniae* due to serotypes included in the vaccine		Infants: I.M.: 0.5 mL at approximately 2 month-interval for 3 consecutive doses, followed by a fourth dose of 0.5 mL at 12-15 months of age. The first dose may be given as young as 2 months of age, but is typically given at 2 months of age. **Previously Unvaccinated Infants and Children:** 7-11 months: 0.5 mL for a total of 3 doses; 2 doses at least 4 weeks apart, followed by a third dose after the 1-year birthday, separated from the second dose by at least 2 months. 12-23 months: 0.5 mL for a total of two doses, separated by at least 2 months. 24-59 months: Healthy Children: 0.5 mL as a single dose. Children with sickle cell disease, asplenia, HIV infection, chronic illness, or immunocompromising conditions (not including bone marrow transplants ~ results pending; use PPV23 (pneumococcal polysaccharide vaccine, polyvalent) at 12- and 24-months until studies are complete): 0.5 mL for a total of 2 doses, separated by 2 months **Previously Vaccinated Children with a lapse in vaccination administration:** 7-11 months: Previously received 1 or 2 doses PCV7: 0.5 mL dose at 7-11 months of age, followed by a second dose ≥2 months later at 12-15 months of age. 12-23 months: Previously received 1 dose before 12 months of age: 0.5 mL dose, followed by a second dose ≥2 months later. Use is contraindicated if hypersensitivity to the vaccine, including diphtheria toxoid, and with current or recent severe or moderate febrile illness. Use caution with thrombocytopenia, latex sensitivity. Not for I.V. use. Use of the pneumococcal conjugate vaccine does not replace the use of the 23-valent vaccine in children >24 months of age with sickle cell disease, asplenia, HIV infection, chronic illness, or if immunocompromised. Injection contains 2 mcg of each saccharide for each of 6 serotypes and 4 mcg of a 7th serotype; also 20 mcg of CRM_{197} carrier protein and 0.125 mg of aluminum phosphate adjuvant/0.5 mL per dose.

IMMUNIZATIONS[1] (VACCINES) *(Continued)*

Drug	Use	Stability	Administration/ Patient Information
Pneumococcal vaccine (Pneumovax® 23; Pnu-Imune®23)	For children >2 years of age and adults who are at increased risk of pneumococcal disease and its complications because of underlying health conditions; older adults, including all those ≥65 years of age	Refrigerate	Administer S.C. or I.M. (deltoid muscle or lateral migthigh). Do not inject I.V. Have epinephrine injection (1:1000) available. I.M., S.C.: 0.5 mL. Revaccination should be considered if ≥6 years have elapsed since initial vaccination, for patients who received 14-valent pneumococcal vaccine and are at highest risk (asplenic) for fatal infection, or at ≥6 years in patients with nephrotic syndrome, renal failure, or transplant recipients. Use with caution in individuals who have had episodes of pneumococcal infection within the preceeding 3 years (pre-existing pneumococcal antibodies may result in increased reactions to vaccine). May cause relapse in patients with stable idiopathic thrombocytopenia purpura. Federal law requires that the date of administration, the vaccine manufacturer, lot number of vaccine, and the administering person's name, title, and address be entered into the patient's permanent medical record.
Poliovirus vaccine, inactivated (IPOL™)	AAP recommends three poliomyelitis vaccines schedules: OPV-only, IPV-only and sequential IPV-OPV. Inactivated poliovirus vaccine contains three types of poliovirus grown either in monkey kidney or human diploid cells and inactivated with formaldehyde. IPV is of enhanced potency and is highly immunogenic. OPV schedule ONLY is recommended when parents or providers who prefer not to have the child receive the additional injections needed if IPV were to be used, for infants and children starting vaccination regimens after 6 months of age in whom an accelerated schedule is necessary to complete immunizations, an OPV-only regimen will minimize the number of injections required at each visit. In populations with low vaccination rates, OPV may be preferred in order to expedite implementation of the routine childhood immunization schedule. IPV schedule ONLY is recommended for immunocompromised persons and their household contacts (OPV would be contraindicated); for infants and children in which an adult household member is know to be inadequately vaccinated against poliomyelitis, because unimmunized adults are at increased risk of vaccine-associated paralytic poliomyelitis (VAPP); when the number of injections is not likely to decrease compliance and when IPV is preferred by healthcare providers or parents or other caregivers. IPV Primary immunization is also recommended for unvaccinated adults because the risk of VAPP after OPV is slightly higher in adults than in children. Sequential IPV/OPV schedule is recommended to reduce the total number of injections required to reduce the risk of VAPP while maintaining optimal intestinal immunity, especially for travelers to areas where poliovirus is still endemic. The rationale of sequential use of IPV and OPV is that two doses of IPV induce sufficient humoral immunity to prevent VAPP in recipients from subsequent administration of OPV, given to induce optimal intestinal immunity as well as to sustain humoral immunity.		Oral: **Infants:** Primary series: 0.5 mL at 6-12 weeks of age, second dose 6-8 weeks after first dose (commonly at 4 months), and third dose 8-12 months after second dose (commonly at 18 months) Booster: All children who have received primary immunization series, should receive a single follow-up dose and all children who have not should complete primary series. **Children (older) and Adults** (adolescents through 18 years of age): Two 0.5 mL doses 6-8 weeks apart and a third dose of 0.5 mL 8-12 months after second dose. S.C.: Enhanced-potency inactivated poliovirus vaccine (E-IPV) is preferred for primary vaccination of adults, two doses 4-8 weeks apart, a third dose 6-12 months after the second. For adults with a completed primary series and for whom a booster is indicated, either OPV or E-IPV can be given. If immediate protection is needed, either OPV or E-IPV is recommended.

Drug	Use	Stability	Administration/ Patient Information
Rabies immune globulin (human) (BayRab™; Imogam®)	Part of postexposure prophylaxis of persons with rabies exposure who lack a history of pre-exposure or postexposure prophylaxis with rabies vaccine or a recently documented neutralizing antibody response to previous rabies vaccination. It is preferable to give RIG with the first dose of vaccine, but it can be given up to 8 days after vaccination.	Refrigerate	I.M.: 20 units/kg in a single dose (RIG should always be administered in conjunction with rabies vaccine (HDCV)). Infiltrate half of the dose locally around the wound; administer the remainder I.M. Use with caution in individuals with thrombocytopenia, bleeding disorders, or prior allergic reactions to immune globulins. Severe adverse reactions can occur if the patient receives RIG I.V.
Rabies virus vaccine (Imovax® Rabies ID Vaccine; Imovax® Rabies Vaccine)	Pre-exposure rabies immunization for high-risk persons; postexposure antirabies immunization along with local treatment and immune globulin	Refrigerate. Reconstituted vaccine should be used immediately.	**Pre-exposure prophylaxis:** 1 mL I.M. or 0.1 mL I.D. on days 0, 7, and 21-28. **Note**: Prolonging the interval between doses does not interfere with immunity achieved after concluding dose of the basic series. **Postexposure prophylaxis:** All postexposure treatment should begin with immediate cleansing of the wound with soap and water. Persons not previously immunized should be given rabies immune globulin 20 units/kg body weight, half infiltrated at bite site if possible, remainder I.M. and 5 doses of rabies vaccine, 1 mL I.M. one each on days 0, 3, 7, 14, and 28. Persons who have previously received postexposure prophylaxis with rabies vaccine, received a recommended I.M. or I.D. pre-exposure series of rabies vaccine, or have a previously documented rabies antibody titer considered adequate should receive 2 doses of rabies vaccine, 1 mL I.M. one each on days 0 and 3. Complete pre-exposure prophylaxis does not eliminate the need for additional therapy with rabies vaccine after a rabies exposure. The FDA has not approved the I.D. use of rabies vaccine for postexposure prophylaxis. Recommendations for I.D. use of HDCV are currently being discussed. The decision for postexposure rabies vaccination depends on the species of biting animal, the circumstances of biting incident, and the type of exposure (bite, saliva contamination of wound, etc). The type of and schedule for postexposure prophylaxis depends upon the person's previous rabies vaccination status or the result of a previous or current serologic test for rabies antibody. Rabies vaccine is available only in I.M. form; it cannot be given intradermally.
Rh_o(D) immune globulin (BayRho®-D; BayRho®-D Mini-Dose; Gamulin® Rh; MICRhoGAM™; Mini-Gamulin® Rh; RhoGAM™)	Prevention of isoimmunization in Rh-negative individuals exposed to Rh-positive blood during delivery of an Rh-positive infant, as a result of an abortion, following amniocentesis or abdominal trauma, or following a transfusion accident; prevention of hemolytic disease of the newborn if there is a subsequent pregnancy with an Rh-positive fetus	Reconstituted solution should be refrigerated and will remain stable for 30 days. Solutions that have been frozen should be discarded.	I.M. (administered I.M. to mothers not to infant): **Obstetrical use:** 1 vial (300 mcg) prevents maternal sensitization if fetal packed red blood cell volume that has entered the circulation is ≤15 mL; it if is more, give additional vials. The number of vials = RBC volume of the calculated fetomaternal hemorrhage divided by 15 mL. **Postpartum prophylaxis:** 300 mcg within 72 hours of delivery. **Antepartum prophylaxis:** 300 mcg at approximately 26-28 weeks gestation; followed by 300 mcg within 72 hours of delivery if infant is Rh-positive. **Following miscarriage, abortion, or termination of ectopic pregnancy at up to 13 weeks gestation:** 50 mcg ideally within 3 hours, but may be given up to 72 hours after. If pregnancy has been terminated at 13 or more weeks of gestation, administer 300 mcg.

IMMUNIZATIONS[1] (VACCINES) *(Continued)*

Drug	Use	Stability	Administration/ Patient Information
$Rh_o(D)$ immune globulin (intravenous-human) (WinRho SD®; WinRho SDF®)	Prevention of Rh isoimmunization in nonsensitized $Rh_o(D)$ antigen-negative women within 7 hours after spontaneous or induced abortion, amniocentesis, chorionic villus sampling, ruptured tubal pregnancy, abdominal trauma, transplacental hemorrhage, or in the normal course of pregnancy unless the blood type of the fetus or father is known to be $Rh_o(D)$ antigen-negative; suppression of Rh isoimmunization in $Rh_o(D)$ antigen-negative female children and female adults in their childbearing years transfused with $Rh_o(D)$ antigen-positive RBCs or blood components containing $Rh_o(D)$ antigen-positive RBCs; treatment of immune thrombocytopenia purpura in nonsplenectomized $Rh_o(D)$ antigen-positive patients	Store at 2°C to 8°C. Do not freeze. If not used immediately, store the product at room temperature for 4 hours. Discard unused portions.	**Prevention of Rh isoimmunization:** I.V.: 1500 units (300 mcg) at 28 weeks gestation or immediately after amniocentesis if before 34 weeks gestation or after chorionic villus sampling; repeat this dose every 12 weeks during the pregnancy, 600 units (120 mcg) at delivery (within 72 hours) and after invasive intrauterine procedures such as abortion, amniocentesis, or any other manipulation if at >34 weeks gestation. If the Rh status of the baby is not known at 72 hours, administer $Rh_o(D)$ immune globulin to the mother at 72 hours after delivery. If >72 hours have elapsed, do not withhold $Rh_o(D)$ immune globulin, but administer as soon as possible, up to 28 days after delivery. I.M.: reconstitute vial with 1.25 mL and administer as above. **Transfusion:** Administer within 72 hours after exposure for treatment of incompatible blood transfusions or massive fetal hemorrhage as follows: I.V.: 3000 units (600 mcg) every 8 hours until the total dose is administered (45 units [9 mcg] of Rh-positive blood/mL blood; 90 units [18 mcg] Rh positive red cells/mL cells). I.M.: 6000 units (1200 mcg) every 12 hours until the total dose is administered (60 units [12 mcg] of Rh-positive blood/mL blood; 120 units [24 mcg] Rh-positive red cells/mL cells). **Treatment of ITP:** I.V.: Initial: 25-50 mcg/kg depending on the patient's Hg concentration; maintenance: 25-60 mcg/kg depending on the clinical response.
Rubella virus vaccine, live (Meruvax® II)	Selective active immunization against rubella; vaccination is routinely recommended for persons from 12 months of age to puberty. All adults, both male and female, lacking documentation of live vaccine on or after first birthday, or laboratory evidence of immunity (particularly women of childbearing age and young adults who work in or congregate in hospitals, colleges, and on military bases) should be vaccinated. Susceptible travelers should be vaccinated. **Note:** Trivalent measles-mumps-rubella (M-M-R® II) vaccine is the preferred agent for most children and many adults. Persons born prior to 1957 are generally considered immune and need not be vaccinated.	Refrigerate, discard reconstituted vaccine after 8 hours.	Children ≥12 months and Adults: S.C.: 0.5 mL in outer aspect of upper arm. Children vaccinated before 12 months of age should be revaccinated. Federal law requires that the date of administration, the vaccine manufacturer, lot number of vaccine, and the administering person's name, title, and address be entered into the patient's permanent medical record.
Tetanus antitoxin	Tetanus prophylaxis or treatment of active tetanus only when tetanus immune globulin (TIG) is not available. Tetanus immune globulin (Hyper-Tet®) is the preferred tetanus immunoglobulin for the treatment of active tetanus. May be given concomitantly with tetanus toxoid adsorbed when immediate treatment is required, but active immunization is desirable.	Refrigerate; do not freeze.	**Prophylaxis:** I.M., S.C.: Children <30 kg: 1500 units Children and Adults ≥30 kg: 3000-5000 units **Treatment:** Children and Adults: Inject 10,000-40,000 units into wound; administer 40,000-100,000 units I.V. Tetanus antitoxin is not the same as tetanus immune globulin. Sensitivity testing should be conducted in all individuals regardless of clinical history. Have epinephrine 1:1000 available.
Tetanus immune globulin (human) (BayTet™)	Passive immunization against tetanus; tetanus immune globulin is preferred over tetanus antitoxin for treatment of active tetanus; part of the management of an unclean wound in a person whose history of previous receipt of tetanus toxoid is unknown or who has received less than three doses of tetanus toxoid; elderly may require TIG more often than younger patients with tetanus infection due to declining antibody titers with age	Refrigerate at 2°C to 8°C (36°F to 46°F).	Administer I.M. **Prophylaxis:** Children: 4 units/kg; some recommend administering 250 units to small children; Adults: 250 units **Treatment:** Children: 500-3000 units, some should infiltrate locally around the wound; Adults: 3000-6000 units Do not give I.V. Never administer tetanus toxoid (Td) and TIG in the same syringe (toxoid will be neutralized). Toxoid may be given at a separate site. Have epinephrine 1:1000 available. Boosters will be necessary.

Drug	Use	Stability	Administration/ Patient Information
Tetanus toxoid (adsorbed)	Selective induction of active immunity against tetanus in selected patients. **Note:** Tetanus and diphtheria toxoids for adult use (Td) is the preferred immunizing agent for most adults and for children after 7 years of age. Young children should receive trivalent DTwP or DTaP (diphtheria/tetanus/pertussis – whole cell or acellular), as part of their childhood immunization program, unless pertussis is contraindicated, then TD is warranted.	Refrigerate; do not freeze.	Administer I.M. in the area of the vastus lateralis (midthigh laterally) or deltoid. Primary immunization: 0.5 mL; repeat 0.5 mL at 4-8 weeks after the first dose and at 6-12 months after the second dose. Routine booster doses are recommended only every 5-10 years. Have epinephrine 1:1000 available. Not equivalent to tetanus toxoid fluid. Tetanus toxoid adsorbed is the preferred toxoid for immunization and Td, TD, or DTaP/DTwP are the preferred adsorbed forms. Avoid injection into a blood vessel.
Tetanus toxoid (fluid)	Detection of delayed hypersensitivity and assessment of cell-mediated immunity; active immunization against tetanus in the rare adult or child who is allergic to the aluminum adjuvant (a product containing adsorbed tetanus toxoid is preferred)	Refrigerate	Do not administer I.V. Anergy testing: Intradermal: 0.1 mL. Primary immunization (**Note:** Td, TD, DTaP/DTwP are recommended): Inject three doses of 0.5 mL I.M. or S.C. at 4- to 8-week intervals. Give fourth dose 6-12 months after third dose. Booster doses: I.M., S.C.: 0.5 mL every 10 years. Have epinephrine 1:1000 available.
Typhoid vaccine (Typhim®; Vivotif Berna™)	**Parenteral:** Promotes active immunity to typhoid fever for patients intimately exposed to a typhoid carrier or foreign travel to a typhoid fever endemic area. **Oral:** Immunize children older than 6 years and adults who expect intimate exposure of or household contact with typhoid fever, travelers to areas of the world with a risk of exposure to typhoid fever, and workers in microbiology laboratories with expected frequent contact with *S. typhi*. **Typhoid vaccine:** Live, attenuated TY21a typhoid vaccine should not be administered to immunocompromised persons, including those known to be infected with HIV. Parenteral inactivated vaccine is a theoretically safer alternative for this group.	Refrigerate. Do not freeze. Potency is not harmed if mistakenly placed in a freezer; however, remove from the freezer as soon as possible and place in refrigerator. Can be used if exposed to temperature ≤80°F.	**S.C. (AKD and H-P):** Children 6 months to 10 years: 0.25 mL; repeat in ≥4 weeks (total immunization is 2 doses). Children >10 years and Adults: 0.5 mL; repeat dose in ≥4 weeks (total immunization is 2 doses). Booster: 0.25 mL every 3 years for children 6 months to 10 years and 0.5 mL every 3 years for children >10 years and adults. **Oral:** Adults: Primary immunization: 1 capsule on alternate days (day 1, 3, 5, and 7); booster: Repeat full course of primary immunization every 5 years. Postpone use in the presence of acute infection. Use during pregnancy only when clearly needed. Not all recipients of typhoid vaccine will be fully protected against typhoid fever. Travelers should take all necessary precautions to avoid contact or ingestion of potentially contaminated food or water sources. Unless a complete immunization schedule is followed, an optimum immune response may not be achieved. Doses of vaccine are different between S.C. and intradermal; only S.C. injection should be used. Oral capsule should be taken 1 hour before a meal with cold or lukewarm drink. Do not chew or swallow whole. Systemic adverse effects may persist for 1-2 days. Take all 4 doses exactly as directed on alternate days to obtain a maximal response. Vaccinating the elderly is often overlooked. If no record of immunization can be recalled, repeat primary series.
Varicella virus vaccine (Varivax®)	The American Association of Pediatrics recommends that the chickenpox vaccine should be given to all healthy children between 12 months and 18 years. children between 12 months and 13 years who have not been immunized or who have not had chickenpox should receive 1 vaccination while children 13-18 years of age require 2 vaccinations 4-8 weeks apart. The vaccine has been added to the childhood immunization schedule for infants 12-28 months of age and children 11-12 years of age who have not been vaccinated previously or who have not had the disease. It is recommended to be given with the measles, mumps, and rubella (MMR) vaccine.	Freeze (-157°C). Store diluent separately at room temperature or in refrigerator. Discard if reconstituted vaccine is not used within 30 minutes.	Children 12 months to 12 years: S.C.: 0.5 mL. Children 12 years to Adults: S.C.: 2 doses of 0.5 mL separated by 4-8 weeks.

IMMUNIZATIONS[1] (VACCINES) *(Continued)*

Drug	Use	Stability	Administration/ Patient Information
Varicella-zoster immune globulin (human)	Passive immunization of susceptible immunodeficient patients after exposure to varicella. Most effective if begun within 72 hours of exposure. There is no evidence that VZIG modifies established varicella-zoster infections. **Restrict administration to:** Patients with neoplastic disease (leukemia, lymphoma); congenital or acquired immunodeficiency; immunosuppressive therapy with steroids, antimetabolites, or other immunosuppressive treatment regimens; newborns or mothers who had onset of chickenpox within 5 days before delivery or within 48 hours after delivery; premature infant (≥28 weeks gestation) whose mother has no history of chickenpox; premature infants (<28 weeks gestation or ≤1000 g VZIG) regardless of maternal history. **One of the following types of exposure to chickenpox or zoster patients may warrant administration**: Continuous household contact; playmate contact (>1 hour play indoors); hospital contact (in same 2-4 bedroom or adjacent beds in a large ward or prolonged face-to-face contact with an infectious staff member of patient); susceptible to varicella-zoster; age <15 years (administer to immunocompromised adolescents and adults and to other older patients on an individual basis). An acceptable alternative to VZIG prophylaxis is to treat varicella, if it occurs, with high-dose I.V. acyclovir.	Refrigerate at 2°C to 8°C.	High-risk susceptible patients who are exposed again more than 3 weeks after a prior dose of VZIG should receive another full dose; there is no evidence VZIG modifies established varicella-zoster infections. I.M.: Administer by deep injection in the gluteal muscle or in another large muscle mass. Inject 125 units/10 kg (22 lb); maximum dose: 625 units (5 vials); minimum dose: 125 units; do not administer fractional doses. Do not inject I.V. VZIG is not indicated for prophylaxis or therapy of normal adults who are exposed to or who develop varicella. It is not indicated for treatment of herpes zoster. VZIG provides passive immunity for those susceptible to varicella, with neoplastic disease, in immunosuppressed elderly, or those institutionalized who are exposed to other patients with varicella. CDC provides specific guidelines for use. Age is the most important risk factor for reactivation of varicella-zoster.
Yellow fever vaccine (YF-VAX®)	Vaccinate selected persons traveling or living in areas where yellow fever infection exists.	Ship vaccine on dry ice. Do not use vaccine unless shipping case contains some dry ice on arrival. Maintain vaccine continuously at a temperature between 0°C to 5°C. Sterilize and discard all unused rehydrated vaccine and containers after 1 hour. Avoid vigorous shaking.	Single dose S.C.: 0.5 mL 10 days to 10 years before travel; booster every 10 years. If a pregnant woman is to be vaccinated only to satisfy an international requirement, efforts should be made to obtain a waiver letter.

[1]Contact Poison Control Center.

[2]Not commercially available in the U.S.; presently, all anthrax vaccine lots are owned by the U.S. Department of Defense. The Centers for Disease Control (CDC) does not currently recommend routine vaccination of the general public.

[3]Withdrawn from market

OPHTHALMIC AGENTS

Note: Consult product literature for full prescribing information. See also, Ophthalmic Agents, Glaucoma in the Alphabetical Listing of Drugs section.

Patient Instructions: Wash hands before instilling. Sit or lie down to instill. Open eye, look at ceiling, and instill prescribed amount of medication. Close eye and apply gentle pressure to inner corner of eye. Do not let tip of applicator touch eye or contaminate tip of applicator. Temporary stinging or burning may occur. Report persistent pain, burning, vision disturbances, swelling, itching, rash, or worsening of condition.

ANTIBIOTIC / ANTIBACTERIAL

Bacitracin

Brand Names: AK-Tracin®
Use: Treatment of susceptible bacterial infections against gram-positive bacilli
Dose: Children and Adults: Instill 1/4" to 1/2" ribbon every 3-4 hours into conjunctival sac for acute infections or 2-3 times/day for mild-moderate infections for 7-10 days.
Strength: Ointment, ophthalmic (AK-Tracin®): 500 units/g (3.5 g)

Bacitracin and Polymyxin B

Brand Names: AK-Poly-Bac®; Polysporin®
Use: Treatment of superficial infections caused by susceptible organisms
Dose: Children and Adults: Instill 1/2" ribbon every 3-4 hours for acute infections or 2-3 times/day for mild-moderate infections for 7-10 days.
Strength: Ointment, ophthalmic (AK-Poly-Bac®; Polysporin®): Bacitracin 500 units and polymyxin B sulfate 10,000 units per g (3.5 g)

Bacitracin, Neomycin, and Polymyxin B

Brand Names: Neosporin® Ophthalmic Ointment
Use: Short-term treatment of superficial external ocular infections caused by susceptible organisms
Dose: Children and Adults: Instill 1/2" ribbon into the conjunctival sac every 3-4 hours for acute infections or 2-3 times/day for mild-moderate infections for 7-10 days.
Strength: Ointment, ophthalmic (Neosporin® Ophthalmic Ointment): Bacitracin 400 units, neomycin sulfate 3.5 mg, and polymyxin B sulfate 10,000 units per g (3.5 g)

Chloramphenicol

Brand Names: Chloromycetin®; Chloroptic® S.O.P.; Ocu-Chlor®
Use: Treatment of infection caused by susceptible organisms
Dose: Children and Adults: Instill 1-2 drops 4-6 times/day or 1/2"of ointment every 3-4 hours. Increase interval between applications after 72 hours to 2-3 times/day. Continue treatment for ~7 days.
Strength:
- Ointment, ophthalmic; 1% [10 mg/g] (3.5 g); Chloromycetin®; Chloroptic® S.O.P.; Ocu-Chlor®: 1% [10 mg/g]
- Powder for ophthalmic solution (Chloromycetin®): 25 mg/vial (15 mL)
- Solution, ophthalmic (Chloroptic®, Ocu-Chlor®): 0.5% [5 mg/mL] (2.5 mL, 7.5 mL, 15 mL)

Ciprofloxacin

Brand Names: Ciloxan®
Use: Treatment for superficial ocular infections (eg, corneal ulcers, conjunctivitis) due to susceptible strains
Dose:
- Solution: Children >1 year and Adults: Instill 1-2 drops every 2 hours while awake for 2 days then 1-2 drops every 4 hours while awake for the next 5 days.
- Ointment: Children>2 years and Adults: Instill 1/2" ribbon into the lower conjunctival sac 3 times/day for the first 2 days then twice daily for the next 5 days.

Strength:
- Ointment, ophthalmic, as hydrochloride (Ciloxan®): 3.33 mg/g [0.3% base] (3.5 g)
- Solution, ophthalmic, as hydrochloride (Ciloxan®): 3.33 mg/g [0.3% base] (2.5 mL, 5 mL, 10 mL)

Erythromycin

Brand Names: Romycin®
Use: Treatment of superficial eye infections involving the conjunctiva or cornea; neonatal ophthalmia

OPHTHALMIC AGENTS *(Continued)*

Dose:

Neonates: Prophylaxis of neonatal gonococcal or chlamydial conjunctivitis: Instill 0.5-1 cm ribbon into each conjunctival sac

Children and Adults: Instill one or more times daily, depending on severity of infection.

Strength: Ointment, ophthalmic: 0.5% [5 mg/g] (1 g, 3.5 g); Romycin®: 0.5% [5 mg/g] (3.5 g)

Gentamicin

Brand Names: Garamycin®; Genoptic®; Genoptic® S.O.P; Gentacidin®; Gentak®
Use: Treatment of ophthalmic infections caused by susceptible bacteria
Dose: Children and Adults:

Ointment: Instill ½" 2-3 times/day to every 3-4 hours.

Solution: Instill 1-2 drops every 2-4 hours; up to 2 drops every hour for severe infections.

Strength:

Ointment, ophthalmic, as sulfate: 0.3% [3 mg/g] (3.5 g)

Solution, ophthalmic, as sulfate: 0.3% (5 mL, 15 mL) [contains benzalkonium chloride]; Garamycin®, Gentacidin®: 0.3% (5 mL) [contains benzalkonium chloride[; Genoptic®: 0.3% (1 mL, 5 mL) [contains benzalkonium chloride[; Gentak®: 0.3% (5 mL, 15 mL) [contains benzalkonium chloride]

Neomycin, Polymyxin B, and Gramicidin

Brand Names: Neosporin® Ophthalmic Solution
Use: Treatment of superficial ocular infections
Dose: Children and Adults: Instill 1-2 drops 4-6 times/day or more frequently as required for severe infections.
Strength: Solution, ophthalmic: Neomycin sulfate 1.75 mg, polymyxin B sulfate 10,000 units, and gramicidin 0.025 mg per mL (2 mL, 10 mL); Neosporin® Ophthalmic Solution: Neomycin sulfate 1.75 mg, polymyxin B sulfate 10,000 units, and gramicidin 0.025 mg per mL (2 mL, 10 mL)

Ofloxacin

Brand Names: Ocuflox®
Use: Treatment of superficial ocular infections involving conjunctiva or cornea due to strains of susceptible organisms
Dose: Children and Adults: Instill 1-2 drops every 2-4 hours for the first 2 days, then use 4 times/day for the next 5 days.
Strength: Solution, ophthalmic (Ocuflox®): 0.3% (5 mL, 10 mL) [contains benzalkonium chloride]

Sulfacetamide

Brand Names: AK-Sulf®; Bleph®-10; Cetamide®; Sodium Sulamyd®; Sulf-10®
Use: Treatment and prophylaxis of conjunctivitis due to susceptible organisms; corneal ulcers; adjunctive treatment with systemic sulfonamides for therapy of trachoma **Note:** Do not use in patients with sulfonamide allergy.
Dose: Children and Adults:

Ointment: Apply to lower conjunctival sac 1-4 times/day and at bedtime.

Solution: Instill 1-3 drops several times daily up to every 2-3 hours in lower conjunctival sac during waking hours and less frequently at night.

Strength:

Ointment, ophthalmic: 10% (3.5 g)

Solution, ophthalmic: 10% (1 mL, 2 mL, 2.5 mL, 5 mL, 15 mL); 15% (5 mL, 15 mL); 30% (15 mL)

Tetracycline

Brand Names: Achromycin®
Use: Treatment of susceptible bacterial infections of both gram-positive and gram-negative organisms
Dose: Children >8 years and Adults:

Ointment, ophthalmic (Achromycin®): Instill every 2-12 hours.

Suspension, ophthalmic (Achromycin®): Instill 1-2 drops 2-4 times/day or more often as needed.

Strength:

Ointment, ophthalmic: 1% [10 mg/mL] (3.5 g)

Suspension, ophthalmic: 1% [10 mg/mL] (0.5 mL, 1 mL, 4 mL)

Tobramycin

Brand Names: AKTob®; Tobrex®
Use: Treatment of superficial ophthalmic infections caused by susceptible bacteria
Dose: Children and Adults:

Ointment: Apply 2-3 times/day. For severe infections, apply every 3-4 hours then reduce to less frequent intervals.

Solution: Instill 1-2 drops every 4 hours. For severe infections, instill 2 drops every 30-60 minutes initially then reduce to less frequent intervals.

Strength:

Ointment, ophthalmic (Tobrex®): 0.3% (3.5 g)

Solution, ophthalmic: 0.3% (5 mL); AKTob®, Tobrex®: 0.3% (5 mL)

Trimethoprim and Polymyxin B

Brand Names: Polytrim®
Use: Treatment of surface ocular bacterial conjunctivitis and blepharoconjunctivitis
Dose: Children and Adults: Instill 1-2 drops every 4-6 hours.
Strength: Solution, ophthalmic (Polytrim®): Trimethoprim sulfate 1 mg and polymyxin B sulfate 10,000 units per mL (10 mL)

ANTIBIOTIC / ANTI-INFLAMMATORY

Bacitracin, Neomycin, Polymyxin B, and Hydrocortisone

Brand Names: Cortisporin® Ophthalmic Ointment
Use: Prevention and treatment of susceptible superficial topical infections
Dose: Children and Adults: Instill ½" ribbon to inside of lower lid every 3-4 hours until improvement occurs.
Strength: Ointment, ophthalmic: Bacitracin 400 units, neomycin sulfate 3.5 mg, polymyxin B sulfate 10,000 units, and hydrocortisone 10 mg per g (3.5 g); Cortisporin® Ophthalmic Ointment: Bacitracin 400 units, neomycin sulfate 3.5 mg, polymyxin B sulfate 10,000 units, and hydrocortisone 10 mg per g (3.5 g)

Chloramphenicol and Prednisolone

Brand Names: Chloroptic-P®
Use: Topical anti-infective and corticosteroid for treatment of ocular infections
Dose: Children and Adults: Instill 1-2 drops 2-4 times/day.
Strength: Ointment, ophthalmic (Chloroptic-P®): Chloramphenicol 1% and prednisolone 0.5% (3.5 g)

Neomycin and Dexamethasone

Brand Names: NeoDexadron®
Use: Treatment of steroid responsive inflammatory conditions of the palpebral and bulbar conjunctiva, lid, cornea, and anterior segment of the globe
Dose: Children and Adults: Instill 1-2 drops every 3-4 hours.
Strength: Solution, ophthalmic (NeoDexadron®): Neomycin sulfate 0.35% [3.5 mg/mL] and dexamethasone sodium phosphate 0.1% [1 mg/mL] (5 mL) [contains benzalkonium chloride and sodium bisulfite]

Neomycin, Polymyxin B, and Dexamethasone

Brand Names: AK-Trol®; Dexacidin®; Dexacine™; Maxitrol®
Use: Treatment of steroid-responsive inflammatory ocular conditions where bacterial infection or risk of bacterial infection exists in which a corticosteroid is indicated
Dose: Children and Adults:

Ointment: Instill ~½" ribbon 3-4 times/day or apply at bedtime as an adjunct with drops.

Suspension: Instill 1-2 drops every 3-4 hours. In severe disease, drops may be used hourly and tapered to discontinuation.

Strength:

Ointment, ophthalmic: Neomycin sulfate 3.5 mg, polymyxin B sulfate 10,000 units, and and dexamethasone 0.1% per g (3.5 g, 5 g); Dexacine™, Maxitrol®: Neomycin sulfate 3.5 mg, polymyxin B sulfate 10,000 units, and and dexamethasone 0.1% per g (3.5 g, 5 g)

Suspension, ophthalmic: Neomycin sulfate 3.5 mg, polymyxin B sulfate 10,000 units, and dexamethasone 0.1% per mL (5 mL, 10 mL); AK-Trol®, Dexacidin®, Maxitrol®: Neomycin sulfate 3.5 mg, polymyxin B sulfate 10,000 units, and dexamethasone 0.1% per mL (5 mL, 10 mL)

Neomycin, Polymyxin B, and Hydrocortisone

Brand Names: Cortisporin® Ophthalmic
Use: Treatment of steroid-responsive inflammatory conditions where bacterial infection or risk of bacterial infection exists and in which a corticosteroid is indicated
Dose: Children and Adults: Instill 1-2 drops 2-4 times/day or more frequently as required for severe infections. In acute infections, instill 1-2 drops every 15-30 minutes, gradually reducing the frequency of administration as the infection is controlled.

OPHTHALMIC AGENTS *(Continued)*

Strength: Suspension, ophthalmic (Cortisporin®): Neomycin sulfate 5 mg [equivalent to 3.5 mg base], polymyxin B sulfate 10,000 units, and hydrocortisone 10 mg per mL (7.5 mL) [contains thimerosal]

Neomycin, Polymyxin B, and Prednisolone

Brand Names: Poly-Pred®
Use: Treatment of steroid-responsive inflammatory ocular conditions where bacterial infection or risk of bacterial infection exists
Dose: Children and Adults: Instill 1-2 drops every 3-4 hours. Acute infections may require every 30-minute instillation initially with frequency of administration reduced as the infection is brought under control. To treat the lids: Instill 1-2 drops every 3-4 hours, close the eye, and rub the excess on the lids and lid margins.
Strength: Suspension, ophthalmic (Poly-Pred®): Neomycin sulfate 0.35%, polymyxin B sulfate 10,000 units, and prednisolone acetate 0.5% per mL (5 mL, 10 mL)

Prednisolone and Gentamicin

Brand Names: Pred-G®
Use: Treatment of steroid-responsive inflammatory conditions and superficial ocular infections
Dose: Children and Adults:
Ointment: Instill 1/4"- 1/3" 2-4 times/day.
Suspension: Instill 1 drop 2-4 times/day. During the initial 24-48 hours, the dosing frequency may be increased if necessary.
Strength:
Ointment, ophthalmic (Pred-G®): Prednisolone acetate 0.6% and gentamicin sulfate 0.3% (3.5 g)
Suspension, ophthalmic (Pred-G®): Prednisolone acetate 1% and gentamicin sulfate 0.3% (2 mL, 5 mL, 10 mL)

Sulfacetamide and Fluorumetholone

Brand Names: FML-S®
Use: Treatment of steroid-responsive inflammatory ocular conditions where infection is present or there is risk of infection **Note:** Do not use in sulfa-allergic patients.
Dose: Children >2 months and Adults: Instill 1-3 drops every 2-3 hours while awake.
Strength: Suspension, ophthalmic: Sulfacetamide sodium 10% and fluorumetholone 0.1% (5 mL, 10 mL)

Sulfacetamide and Prednisolone

Brand Names: AK-Cide®; Blephamide®; Cetapred®; Isopto® Cetapred®; Metimyd®; Vasocidin®
Use: Treatment of steroid-responsive inflammatory ocular conditions where infection is present or there is a risk of infection
Dose: Children >2 months and Adults:
Ointment: Apply to lower conjunctival sac 1-4 times/day.
Suspension: Instill 1-3 drops every 2-3 hours while awake.
Strength:
Ointment, ophthalmic:
AK-Cide®, Metimyd®, Vasocidin®: Sulfacetamide sodium 10% and prednisolone acetate 0.5% (3.5 g)
Blephamide®: Sulfacetamide sodium 10% and prednisolone acetate 0.2% (3.5 g)
Cetapred®: Sulfacetamide sodium 10% and prednisolone acetate 0.25% (3.5 g)
Suspension, ophthalmic: Sulfacetamide sodium 10% and prednisolone sodium phosphate 0.25% (5 mL);
AK-Cide®, Metimyd®: Sulfacetamide sodium 10% and prednisolone acetate 0.5% (5 mL);
Blephamide®: Sulfacetamide sodium 10% and prednisolone acetate 0.2% (2.5 mL, 5 mL, 10 mL);
Isopto® Cetapred®: Sulfacetamide sodium 10% and prednisolone acetate 0.25% (5 mL, 15 mL);
Vasocidin®: Sulfacetamide sodium 10% and prednisolone sodium phosphate 0.25% (5 mL, 10 mL)

Tobramycin and Dexamethasone

Brand Names: TobraDex®
Use: Treatment of external ocular infections caused by susceptible bacteria and steroid responsive inflammatory conditions of the palpebral and bulbar conjunctiva, lid, cornea, and anterior segment of the globe
Dose: Children and Adults:

Ointment: Instill 2-3 times/day; every 3-4 hours for severe infections, then reduce to less frequent intervals..

Suspension: Instill 1-2 drops every 4 hours. For severe infections, instill 2 drops every 30-60 minutes initially, then reduce to less frequent intervals.

Strength:

Ointment, ophthalmic: Tobramycin 0.3%, dexamethasone 0.1% (3.5 g); TobraDex®: Tobramycin 0.3%, dexamethasone 0.1% (3.5 g)

Suspension, ophthalmic: Tobramycin 0.3%, dexamethasone 0.1% (2.5 mL, 5 mL); TobraDex®: Tobramycin 0.3%, dexamethasone 0.1% (2.5 mL, 5 mL)

ANTIHISTAMINE AND ANTIHISTAMINE/DECONGESTANT

Ketotifen

Brand Names: Zaditor™

Use: Temporary prevention of eye itching due to allergic conjunctivitis

Dose: Children ≤3 years and Adults: Instill 1 drop twice daily every 8-12 hours.

Strength: Solution, ophthalmic, as fumarate (Zaditor™): 0.025% (5 mL) [contains benzalkonium chloride]

Levocabastine

Brand Names: Liovistin®

Use: Temporary relief of allergic conjunctivitis

Dose: Children ≤12 years and Adults: Instill 1 drop 4 times/day for up to 2 weeks.

Strength: Suspension, ophthalmic, as hydrochloride (Liovistin®): 0.05% (2.5 mL, 5 mL, 10 mL)

Olopatadine

Brand Names: Patanol®

Use: Treatment of the signs and symptoms of allergic conjunctivitis

Dose: Adults: Instill 1-2 drops twice daily every 6-8 hours.

Strength: Solution, ophthalmic (Patanol®): 0.1% (5 mL) [contains benzalkonium chloride]

Naphazoline and Antazoline Phosphate

Brand Names: Vasocon®-A [OTC]

Use: Treatment of topical ocular congestion, irritation, and itching

Dose: Children and Adults: Instill 1-2 drops every 3-4 hours.

Strength: Solution, ophthalmic (Vasocon®-A [OTC]): Naphazoline hydrochloride 0.05% and antazoline phosphate 0.5% (15 mL) [contains benzalkonium chloride]

Naphazoline and Pheniramine

Brand Names: Naphcon-A® [OTC]; Opcon-A® [OTC]; Visine-A™ [OTC]

Use: Topical ocular vasoconstrictor

Dose: Children and Adults: Instill 1-2 drops every 3-4 hours.

Strength: Solution, ophthalmic: Naphazoline hydrochloride 0.025% and pheniramine 0.3% (15 mL) [contains benzalkonium chloride]; Naphcon-A® [OTC], Opcon-A® [OTC], Visine-A™ [OTC]: Naphazoline hydrochloride 0.025% and pheniramine 0.3% (15 mL) [contains benzalkonium chloride]

ANTI-INFLAMMATORY, STEROID

Loteprednol

Brand Names: Alrex™; Lotemax™

Use:

Suspension, 0.2% (Alrex™): Temporary relief of signs and symptoms of seasonal allergic conjunctivitis

Suspension, 0.5% (Lotemax™): Treatment of steroid-responsive inflammatory conditions of the palpebral and bulbar conjunctiva, cornea, and anterior segment of the globe such as allergic conjunctivitis, acne rosacea, superficial punctate keratitis, herpes zoster keratitis, iritis, cyclitis, selected infective conjunctivitis, when the inherent hazard of steroid use is accepted to obtain an advisable diminution in edema and inflammation; treatment of postoperative inflammation following ocular surgery

Dose: Adults:

Alrex™: Instill 1 drop 4 times/day.

Lotemax™: Inflammatory conditions: Apply 1-2 drops into the conjunctival sac 4 times/day. During the initial treatment within the first week, the dosing may be increased up to 1 drop every hour. Advise patients not to discontinue therapy prematurely. If signs and symptoms fail to improve after 2 days, re-evaluate

OPHTHALMIC AGENTS *(Continued)*

the patient. Postoperative inflammation: Apply 1-2 drops into the conjunctival sac 4 times/day beginning 24 hours after surgery and continuing throughout the first 2 weeks of the postoperative period.

Strength: Suspension, ophthalmic, as etabonate: 0.2% (Alrex™): 5 mL, 10 mL; 0.5% (Lotemax™): 2.5 mL, 5 mL, 10 mL, 15 mL

Prednisolone

Brand Names: Inflamase® Mild; Pred Forte®; Pred Mild®

Use: Treatment of ophthalmic diseases, palpebral and bulbar conjunctivitis, and corneal injury from chemical, radiation, thermal burns, or foreign body penetration

Dose: Children and Adults: Instill 1-2 drops into conjunctival sac every hour during day; every 2 hours at night until favorable response, then use 1 drop every 4 hours.

Strength:

Solution, ophthalmic, as sodium phosphate: 0.125% (5 mL, 10 mL); 1% (5 mL, 10 mL, 15 mL)

Suspension, ophthalmic, as acetate: 0.12% (5 mL, 10 mL); 0.125% (5 mL, 10 mL, 15 mL); 1% (1 mL, 5 mL, 10 mL, 15 mL)

Rimexolone

Brand Names: Vexol®

Use: Treatment of postoperative inflammation following ocular surgery; treatment of anterior uveitis

Dose: Adults: Instill 1 drop in conjunctival sac 2-4 times/day up to every 4 hours; may be used every 1-2 hours during first 1-2 days.

Strength: Suspension, ophthalmic (Vexol®): 1% (5 mL, 10 mL) [contains benzalkonium chloride]

ANTI-INFLAMMATORY, NONSTEROIDAL

Diclofenac

Brand Names: Voltaren®

Use: Treatment of postoperative inflammation following cataract surgery; temporary relief of pain and photophobia in patients undergoing corneal refractive surgery

Dose: Adults:

Cataract surgery: Instill 1 drop 4 times/day beginning 24 hours after surgery and continuing for 2 weeks.

Corneal refractive surgery: Instill 1-2 drops within the hour prior to surgery, within 15 minutes following surgery, and then continue for 4 times/day, up to 3 days.

Strength: Solution, ophthalmic, as sodium (Voltaren®): 0.1% (2.5 mL, 5 mL)

Flurbiprofen

Brand Names: Ocufen®

Use: Inhibition of intraoperative miosis; prevention and management of postoperative ocular inflammation and postoperative cystoid macular edema remains to be determined

Dose: Children and Adults: Instill 1 drop every 30 minutes for 2 hours prior to surgery (total of 4 drops).

Strength: Solution, ophthalmic, as sodium: 0.03% (2.5 mL, 5 mL, 10 mL) [contains thimerosal 0.005% as preservative]; Ocufen®: 0.03% (2.5 mL, 5 mL, 10 mL) [contains thimerosal 0.005% as preservative]

Ketorolac Tromethamine

Brand Names: Acular®; Acular® PF

Use: Temporary relief of ocular itching due to seasonal allergic conjunctivitis; postoperative inflammation following cataract surgery; reduction of ocular pain and photophobia following incisional refractive surgery

Dose: Children ≥3 years and Adults:

Allergic conjunctivitis (relief of ocular itching): Instill 1 drop 4 times/day.

Inflammation following cataract surgery: Instill 1 drop (0.25 mg) 4 times/day beginning 24 hours after surgery; continue for 2 weeks.

Pain and photophobia following incisional refractive surgery: Instill 1 drop (0.25 mg) 4 times/day for up to 3 days.

Strength: Solution, ophthalmic, as tromethamine: Acular®: 0.5% (3 mL, 5 mL, 10 mL) [contains benzalkonium chloride]; Acular® P.F. [preservative free]: 0.5% (0.4 mL)

ANTI-INFLAMMATORY, MAST CELL STABILIZER

Cromolyn Sodium

Brand Names: Crolom®; Opticrom®
Use: Treatment of vernal keratoconjunctivitis, vernal conjunctivitis, and vernal keratitis
Dose: Children >4 years and Adults: Instill 1-2 drops 4-6 times/day.
Strength: Solution, ophthalmic, as sodium: 4% (2.5 mL, 10 mL) [contains benzalkonium chloride]; Crolom®, Opticrom®: 4% (2.5 mL, 10 mL) [contains benzalkonium chloride]

Ketotifen

Brand Names: Zaditor™
Use: Temporary prevention of itching due to allergic conjunctivitis
Dose: Children ≥3 years and Adults: Instill 1 drop twice daily every 8-12 hours.
Strength: Solution, ophthalmic, as fumarate (Zaditor™): 0.025% (5 mL) [contains benzalkonium chloride]

Lodoxamide Tromethamine

Brand Names: Alomide®
Use: Treatment of vernal keratoconjunctivitis, vernal conjunctivitis, and vernal keratitis
Dose: Children ≥3 years and Adults: Instill 1-2 drops up to 4 times/day for up to 3 months.
Strength: Solution, ophthalmic (Alomide®): 0.1% (10 mL)

Nedocromil

Brand Names: Alocril™
Use: Treatment of itching associated with allergic conjunctivitis
Dose: Children and Adults: Instill 1-2 drops in each eye twice daily.
Strength: Solution, ophthalmic, as sodium (Alocril™): 2% (5 mL) [contains benzalkonium chloride]

MIOTIC

Acetylcholine

Brand Names: Miochol-E®
Use: Produce complete miosis in cataract surgery, keratoplasty, iridectomy, and other anterior segment surgery where rapid miosis is required
Dose: Adults: Instill 0.5-2 mL of 1% injection (5-20 mg) into anterior chamber before or after securing one or more sutures.
Strength: Powder for suspension, intraocular, as chloride (Miochol-E®): 1:100 [10 mg/mL] (2 mL)

Echothiophate Iodide

Brand Names: Phospholine Iodide®
Use: Treatment of open-angle glaucoma; may be useful in specific cases of narrow-angle glaucoma; accommodative esotropia
Dose: Adults:

- Glaucoma: Instill 1 drop twice daily into eyes with 1 dose just prior to bedtime; some patients have been treated with 1 dose daily or every other day.
- Accommodative esotropia:
  - Diagnosis: Instill 1 drop of 0.125% once daily into both eyes at bedtime for 2-3 weeks.
  - Treatment: Use lowest concentration and frequency which gives satisfactory response, with a maximum dose of 0.125% once daily, although more intensive therapy may be used for short period of time.

Strength: Powder, ophthalmic (Phospholine Iodide®): 1.5 mg [0.03%] (5 mL); 3 mg [0.06%] (5 mL); 6.25 mg [0.125%] (5 mL); 12.5 mg [0.25%] (5 mL)

MYDRIATIC

Atropine

Brand Names: Atropine-Care®; Atropisol®; Isopto® Atropine; Sal-Tropine®
Use: Produce mydriasis and cycloplegia for examination of the retina and optic disc and accurate measurement of refractile errors; uveitis
Dose:

Children:

OPHTHALMIC AGENTS *(Continued)*

Mydriasis, cycloplegia (preprocedure): Solution (0.5%): Instill 1-2 drops twice daily for 1-3 days before the procedure.
Uveitis: Solution (0.5%): Instill 1-2 drops up to 3 times/day.

Adults:

Mydriasis, cycloplegia (preprocedure): Solution (1%): Instill 1-2 drops 1 hour before the procedure.
Uveitis: Instill 1-2 drops solution (1%) 4 times/day or a small amount of ointment in the conjunctival sac up to 3 times/day. Compress the lacrimal sac by digital pressure for 1-3 minutes after instillation.

Strength:

Ointment, ophthalmic, as sulfate: 1% (3.5 g)
Solution, ophthalmic, as sulfate: 1% (5 mL, 15 mL); Atropine-Care®: 1% (2 mL); Atropisol®: 1% (1 mL); Isopto® Atropine: 1% (5 mL, 15 mL)

Cyclopentolate

Brand Names: Cyclogyl®; Diopentolate®
Use: Produces mydriasis and cycloplegia in diagnostic procedures
Dose:

Neonates and Infants: Cyclopentolate and phenylephrine combination formulation is the preferred agent for use in neonates and infants due to lower cyclopentolate concentration and reduced risk for systemic reactions.
Children: Instill 1 drop of 0.5%, 1%, or 2% solution followed by 1 drop of 0.5% or 1% solution in 5 minutes, if necessary.
Adults: Instill 1 drop of 1% solution followed by another drop in 5 minutes; use 2% solution in heavily pigmented iris.

Strength: Solution, ophthalmic, as hydrochloride: 0.5% (2 mL, 5 mL, 15 mL); 1% (2 mL, 5 mL, 15 mL); 2% (2 mL, 5 mL, 15 mL); Cyclogyl®, Diopentolate®: 0.5% (2 mL, 5 mL, 15 mL); 1% (2 mL, 5 mL, 15 mL); 2% (2 mL, 5 mL, 15 mL)

Homatropine

Brand Names: Isopto® Homatropine
Use: Produce cycloplegia and mydriasis for refraction; treatment of acute inflammatory conditions of the uveal tract
Dose:

Children:

Mydriasis and cycloplegia for refraction: Instill 1 drop immediately before the procedure. Repeat at 10-minute intervals as needed.
Uveitis: Instill 1 drop 2-3 times/day.

Adults:

Mydriasis and cycloplegia for refraction: Instill 1-2 drops of 2% solution or 1 drop of 5% solution before the procedure. Repeat at 5- to 10-minute intervals as needed; maximum of 3 doses for refraction.
Uveitis: Instill 1-2 drops of 2% or 5% solution 2-3 times/day up to every 3-4 hours as needed.

Strength: Solution, ophthalmic, as hydrobromide: 2% (1 mL, 5 mL); 5% (1 mL, 2 mL, 5 mL); Isopto® Homatropine: 2% (5 mL, 15 mL); 5% (5 mL, 15 mL)

Phenylephrine

Brand Names: AK-Dilate®; AK-Nefrin®; Mydfrin®; Neo-Synephrine®; Neo-Synephrine® Viscous; Phenoptic®; Prefrin™ Liquifilm; Relief®
Use: Produce mydriasis in ophthalmic procedures; treatment of wide-angle glaucoma
Dose: Ophthalmic procedures:

Infants <1 year: Instill 1 drop of 2.5% solution 15-30 minutes before procedure.
Children and Adults: Instill 1 drop of 2.5% or 10% solution; repeat in 10-60 minutes, as needed.

Strength: Solution, ophthalmic, as hydrochloride: AK-Dilate®, Mydfrin®, Neo-Synephrine®, Phenoptic®: 2.5% (2 mL, 3 mL, 5 mL, 15 mL); AK-Dilate®, Neo-Synephrine®, Neo-Synephrine® Viscous: 10% (1 mL, 2 mL, 5 mL, 15 mL); AK-Nefrin®, Prefrin™ Liquifilm®, Relief®: 0.12% (0.3 mL, 15 mL, 20 mL)

Scopolamine

Brand Names: Isopto® Hyoscine; Scopace®
Use: Produce cycloplegia and mydriasis; treatment of iridocyclitis
Dose:

Children:

Iridocyclitis: Instill 1drop up to 3 times/day.
Refraction: Instill 1 drop twice daily for 2 days before procedure.

Adults:

Iridocyclitis: Instill 1-2 drops up to 4 times/day.
Refraction: Instill 1-2 drops 1 hour before procedure.

Strength: Solution, ophthalmic, as hydrobromide (Isopto® Hyoscine, Scopace®): 0.25% (5 mL, 15 mL)

Tropicamide

Brand Names: Mydriacyl®
Use: Short-acting mydriatic used in diagnostic procedures; as well as preoperatively and postoperatively; treatment of some cases of acute iritis, iridocyclitis, and keratitis
Dose: Children and Adults (individuals with heavily pigmented eyes may require larger doses):

Cycloplegia: Instill 1-2 drops (1%). May repeat in 5 minutes. Exam must be performed within 30 minutes after the repeat dose. If the patient is not examined within 20-30 minutes, instill an additional drop.

Mydriasis: Instill 1-2 drops (0.5%) 15-20 minutes before exam; may repeat every 30 minutes as needed.

Strength: Solution, ophthalmic: 0.5% (2 mL, 15 mL); 1% (2 mL, 3 mL, 15 mL); Mydriacyl®: 0.5% (2 mL, 15 mL); 1% (2 mL, 3 mL, 15 mL)

SURGICAL AID

Chondroitin Sulfate - Sodium Hyaluronate

Brand Names: Viscoat®
Use: Surgical aid in anterior segment procedures; protects corneal endothelium and coats intraocular lens thus protecting it
Dose: Children and Adults: Carefully introduce (using a 27-gauge needle or cannula) into anterior chamber after thoroughly cleaning the chamber with a balanced salt solution
Strength: Solution, ophthalmic (Viscoat®): Sodium chondroitin 40 mg and sodium hyaluronate 30 mg (0.25 mL, 0.5 mL)

Sodium Hyaluronate

Brand Names: AMO Vitrax®; Amvisc®; Amvisc® Plus; Healon®; Healon® GV
Use: Surgical aid in cataract extraction, intraocular implantation, corneal transplant, glaucoma filtration, and retinal attachment surgery
Dose: Children and Adults: Depends upon procedure; slowly introduce a sufficient quantity into eye.
Strength: Injection, intraocular: AMO Vitrax®: 30 mg/mL (0.65 mL); Amvisc®: 12 mg/mL (0.5 mL, 0.8 mL); Amvisc® Plus: 16 mg/mL (0.5 mL, 8 mL); Healon®: 10 mg/mL (0.4 mL, 0.55 mL, 0.85 mL, 2 mL); Healon® GV: 14 mg/mL (0.55 mL, 0.85 mL)

TOXIN

Botulinum Toxin Type A

Brand Names: Botox®, Botox® Cosmetic
Use: Treatment of strabismus and blepharospasm associated with dystonia (including benign essential blepharospasm or VII nerve disorders in patients 12 years of age); cervical dystonia (spasmodic torticollis) in patients 16 years of age; temporary improvement in the appearance of lines/wrinkles of the face (moderate to severe glabellar lines associated with corrugator and/or procerus muscle activity) in adult patients 65 years of age.
Dose: I.M.:

Children 16 years and Adults: Cervical dystonia: For dosing guidance, the mean dose is 236 units (25th to 75th percentile range 198-300 units) divided among the affected muscles in patients previously treated with botulinum toxin. Initial dose in previously untreated patients should be lower. Sequential dosing should be based on the patient's head and neck position, localization of pain, muscle hypertrophy, patient response, and previous adverse reactions. The total dose injected into the sternocleidomastoid muscles should be 100 units to decrease the occurrence of dysphagia.

Children ≥12 years and Adults:

Blepharospasm: Initial dose: 1.25-2.5 units injected into the medial and lateral pretarsal orbicularis oculi of the upper and lower lid; dose may be increased up to twice the previous dose if the response from the initial dose lasted 2 months; maximum dose per site: 5 units; cumulative dose in a 30-day period: 200 units. Tolerance may occur if treatments are given more often than every 3 months, but the effect is not usually permanent.

Strabismus: Initial dose: Vertical muscles and for horizontal strabismus <20 prism diopters: 1.25-2.5 units in any one muscle; horizontal strabismus of 20-50 prism diopters: 2.5-5 units in any one muscle; persistent VI nerve palsy >1 month: 1.5-2.5 units in the medial rectus muscle. Re-examine patients 7-14 days after each injection to assess the effect of that dose. Subsequent doses

OPHTHALMIC AGENTS *(Continued)*

for patients experiencing incomplete paralysis of the target may be increased up to twice the previous administered dose. The maximum recommended dose as a single injection for any one muscle is 25 units. Do not administer subsequent injections until the effects of the previous dose are gone.

Adults ≤65 years: Reduction of glabellar lines: An effective dose is determined by gross observation of the patient's ability to activate the superficial muscles injected. The location, size and use of muscles may vary markedly among individuals. Inject 0.1 mL dose into each of five sites, two in each corrugator muscle and one in the procerus muscle (total dose 0.5 mL).

Strength: Injection, powder for reconstitution (Botox®, Botox® Cosmetic): 100 units Clostridium botulinum toxin type A

VASOCONSTRICTOR

Naphazoline

Brand Names: AK-Con™; Albalon®; Allersol®; Clear Eyes® [OTC]; Clear Eyes® ACR [OTC]; Naphcon® [OTC]; VasoClear® [OTC]
Use: Topical ocular vasoconstrictor; temporary relief of congestion, itching, and minor irritations; control hyperemia in patients with superficial corneal vascularity
Dose:

Children <6 years: Not recommended for use due to CNS depression (especially in infants).

Children >6 years and Adults: Instill 1-2 drops into conjunctival sac every 3-4 hours; therapy generally should not exceed 3-4 days.

Strength:

Solution, ophthalmic, as hydrochloride: 0.1% (15 mL);

AK-Con™, Albalon®, Allersol®: 0.1% (15 mL) [contains benzalkonium chloride];

Clear Eyes®: 0.012% (6 mL, 15 mL, 30 mL) [contains glycerin 0.2% and benzalkonium chloride];

Clear Eyes® ACR: 0.012% (15 mL, 30 mL) [contains glycerin 0.2%, zinc sulfate 0.25%, and benzalkonium chloride] ;

Naphcon®: 0.012% (15 mL) [contains benzalkonium chloride];

VasoClear®: 0.02% (15 mL) [contains benzalkonium chloride]

Naphazoline and Antazoline

Brand Names: Vasocon-A® [OTC]
Use: Symptomatic relief of topical ocular congestion, irritation, and itching
Dose: Children and Adults: Instill 1-2 drops every 3-4 hours.
Strength: Solution, ophthalmic (Vasocon-A®): Naphazoline hydrochloride 0.05% and antazoline phosphate 0.5% (15 mL) [contains benzalkonium chloride]

Naphazoline and Pheniramine

Brand Names: Naphcon-A® [OTC]; Opcon-A® [OTC]; Visine-A™ [OTC]
Use: Topical ocular vasoconstrictor
Dose: Instill 1-2 drops every 3-4 hours.
Strength: Solution, ophthalmic: Naphazoline hydrochloride 0.025% and pheniramine 0.3% (15 mL) [contains benzalkonium chloride]; Naphcon-A®, Opcon-A®, Visine-A™: Naphazoline hydrochloride 0.025% and pheniramine 0.3% (15 mL) [contains benzalkonium chloride]

Tetrahydrozoline

Brand Names: Collyrium Fresh® [OTC]; Eyesine® [OTC]; Geneye® [OTC]; Mallazine® Eye Drops [OTC]; Murine® Plus Ophthalmic [OTC]; Optigene® [OTC]; Tetrasine® [OTC]; Tetrasine® Extra Ophthalmic [OTC]; Tyzine®; Visine® Extra [OTC]
Use: Symptomatic relief of nasal congestion and conjunctival congestion
Dose: Adults: Conjunctival congestion: Instill 1-2 drops 2-4 times/day.
Strength: Solution, ophthalmic, as hydrochloride: 0.05% (15 mL); Collyrium Fresh®, Eyesine®, Geneye®, Mallazine® Eye Drops, Murine® Plus Ophthalmic, Optigene®, Tetrasine®, Tetrasine® Extra Ophthalmic, Tyzine®, Visine® Extra: 0.05% (15 mL)

OTIC AGENTS

Consult product literature for full prescribing information.

Patient Instructions: Wash hands before instilling. Tilt head with affected ear upward. Gently grasp ear lobe and lift back and upward. Instill prescribed drops into ear canal. Do not push dropper into ear. Remain with head tilted for 2 minutes. Report ringing in ears, discharge, or worsening of condition.

CERUMENOLYTICS

Carbamide Peroxide [OTC]

Brand Names: Auro® Ear Drops; Debrox® Otic; E•R•O Ear; Mollifene® Ear Wax Removing Formula; Murine® Ear Drops

Use: Emulsify and disperse ear wax

Dose: Individualize dose according to patient size. Tip of applicator should not enter ear canal. Keep drops in ear for several minutes by keeping head tilted and placing cotton in ear.

Children <12 years: Tilt head sideways and individualize the dose according to patient size; 3 drops (range: 1-5 drops) twice daily for up to 4 days. Tip of applicator should not enter ear canal. Keep drops in ear for several minutes by keeping head tilted and placing cotton in ear.

Children ≥12 years and Adults: Tilt head sideways and instill 5-10 drops twice daily up to 4 days. Tip of applicator should not enter ear canal. Keep drops in ear for several minutes by keeping head tilted and placing cotton in ear.

Strengths: Solution, otic: 6.5% [in glycerin] (15 mL, 30 mL)

Triethanolamine Polypeptide Oleate Condensate [OTC]

Brand Names: Cerumenex®

Use: Emulsify/disperse ear wax

Dose: Children and Adults: Fill ear canal and insert cotton plug. Allow to remain 15-30 minutes. Flush ear with lukewarm water as a single treatment. If a second application is needed for unusually hard impactions, repeat the procedure.

Strengths: Solution, otic (Cerumenex®): 10% triethanolamine oleate (6 mL, 12 mL)

ANTIBIOTICS

Chloramphenicol [Rx]

Brand Names: Chloromycetin®

Use: Treatment of infections

Dose: Children and Adults: Instill 2-3 drops 3 times/day.

Strengths: Solution, otic (Chloromycetin®): 0.5% (15 mL)

Ofloxacin [Rx]

Brand Names: Floxin®

Use: Treatment of otitis externa, otitis media with tympanostomy tubes, chronic suppurative otitis media (>12 years); acute otitis media

Dose:

Children 1-12 years: Otitis externa or acute otitis media with tympanostomy tubes: Instill 5 drops twice daily for 10 days.

Children ≥12 years and Adults:

Otitis externa: Instill 10 drops twice daily for 10 days.

Chronic otitis media with perforated tympanic membranes or chronic suppurative otitis media: Instill 10 drops twice daily for 14 days.

Strengths: Solution, otic (Floxin®): 0.3% (5 mL, 10 mL)

OTIC AGENTS *(Continued)*

ANTI-INFECTIVE/ANTI-INFLAMMATORY

Acetic Acid and Hydrocortisone [Rx]

Brand Names: Acetasol HC®; VoSol HC®
Use: Anti-inflammatory; drying agent
Dose: Children and Adults: Insert saturated wick into ear. Leave in 24 hours, keeping moist with 3-5 drops every 4-6 hours. Keep moist for 24 hours. Remove wick and instill 5 drops 3 or 4 times/day.
Strengths: 1% hydrocortisone, 2% acetic acid, 3% propylene glycol diacetate

Ciprofloxacin and Hydrocortisone [Rx]

Brand Names: Cipro® HC Otic
Use: Treatment of acute otitis externa (swimmer's ear)
Dose: Children >1 year and Adults: The recommended dosage for all patients is three drops of the suspension in the affected ear twice daily for seven day; twice-daily dosing schedule is more convenient for patients than that of existing treatments with hydrocortisone, which are typically administered three or four times a day; a twice-daily dosage schedule may be especially helpful for parents and caregivers of young children.
Strengths: Suspension, otic (Cipro® HC Otic): Ciprofloxacin hydrochloride 0.2% and hydrocortisone 1% (10 mL)

Colistin, Neomycin, and Hydrocortisone [Rx]

Brand Names: Coly-Mycin® S Otic; Cortisporin-TC® Otic
Use: Treatment of superficial and susceptible bacterial infections of the external auditory canal; susceptible bacterial infections of mastoidectomy and fenestration cavities
Dose:
- Children: 3 drops 3-4 times/day
- Adults: Instill 4 drops 3-4 times/day

Strengths: Suspension, otic:
- Coly-Mycin® S: Colistin sulfate 0.3%, neomycin sulfate 0.47%, and hydrocortisone acetate 1% (5 mL, 10 mL);
- Cortisporin-TC®: Colistin 0.3%, neomycin 0.33%, and hydrocortisone 1% (5 mL, 10 mL)

m-Cresyl Acetate [Rx]

Brand Names: Cresylate®
Use: Treatment of external otitis infections caused by susceptible bacteria or fungus; acts as an acidifier, anti-infective, and antifungal
Dose: Children and Adults: Instill 2-4 drops as required.
Strengths: Solution, otic (Cresylate®): 25% with isopropanol 25%, chlorobutanol 1%, benzyl alcohol 1%, and castor oil 5% in propylene glycol (15 mL dropper bottle)

Neomycin, Polymyxin B, and Hydrocortisone [Rx]

Brand Names: AntibiOtic® Ear; Cortisporin® Otic; PediOtic®
Use: Treatment of acute otitis externa (swimmer's ear)
Dose: Duration of use should be limited to 10 days unless otherwise directed by the physician.
- Children: Instill 3 drops 3-4 times/day
- Adults: Instill 4 drops 3-4 times/day

Strengths:
- Solution, otic (AntibiOtic® Ear, Cortisporin® Otic): Neomycin sulfate 5 mg [equivalent to 3.5 mg base], polymyxin B sulfate 10,000 units, and hydrocortisone 10 mg per mL (10 mL) [contains potassium metabisulfite]
- Suspension, otic: Neomycin sulfate 5 mg [equivalent to 3.5 mg base], polymyxin B sulfate 10,000 units, and hydrocortisone 10 mg per mL (10 mL);
  - AntibiOtic® Ear, Cortisporin® Otic: Neomycin sulfate 5 mg [equivalent to 3.5 mg base], polymyxin B sulfate 10,000 units, and hydrocortisone 10 mg per mL (10 mL);
  - PediOtic®: Neomycin sulfate 5 mg [equivalent to 3.5 mg base], polymyxin B sulfate 10,000 units, and hydrocortisone 10 mg per mL (7.5 mL)

Polymyxin B and Hydrocortisone [Rx]

Brand Names: Otobiotic®
Use: Treatment of superficial bacterial infections of the external ear canal
Dose: Children and Adults: Instill 4 drops 3-4 times/day
Strengths: Solution, otic (Otobiotic®): Polymyxin B sulfate 10,000 units and hydrocortisone 0.5% [5 mg/mL] per mL (15 mL)

MISCELLANEOUS OTIC PREPARATIONS

Aluminum Acetate and Acetic Acid [Rx]

Brand Names: Otic Domeboro®
Use: Treatment of superficial infections of external auditory canal
Dose: Children and Adults: Insert saturated wick and keep moist for 24 hours by instilling 4-6 drops every 2-3 hours.
Strengths: Solution, otic: Acetic acid 2% in aluminum acetate 0.8% (60 mL); Otic Domeboro®: Acetic acid 2% in aluminum acetate 0.8% (60 mL)

Acetic Acid, Propylene Glycol Diacetate, and Hydrocortisone [Rx]

Brand Names: Acetasol® HC; VoSol®
Use: Treatment of superficial infections of external auditory canal caused by organisms susceptible to the action of the antimicrobial complicated by swelling
Dose: Adults: Instill 4 drops 3-4 times/day
Strengths: Solution, otic: 2% acetic acid with 3% propylene glycol diacetate, and 1% hydrocortisone (10 mL); Acetasol® HC, VoSol®: 2% acetic acid with 3% propylene glycol diacetate, and 1% hydrocortisone (10 mL)

Antipyrine and Benzocaine [Rx]

Brand Names: Allergan®; Auralgan®; Auroto®
Use: Temporary relief of pain and reduction of swelling associated with acute congestive and serous otitis media, otitis externa (swimmer's ear); facilitates ear wax removal
Dose: Children and Adults: Fill ear canal. Moisten cotton pledget, place in ear canal, and repeat every 1-2 hours until pain and congestion are relieved. For ear wax removal, instill drops 3-4 times/day for 2-3 days.
Strengths: Solution, otic: Antipyrine 5.4% and benzocaine 1.4% (10 mL, 15 mL);
Allergen®, Auroto®: Antipyrine 5.4% and benzocaine 1.4% (15 mL);
Auralgan®: Antipyrine 5.4% and benzocaine 1.4% (10 mL)

Boric Acid [OTC]

Use: Prophylaxis of otitis externa (swimmer's ear)
Dose: Children and Adults: Instill 3-8 drops.
Strengths: Ointment, otic, topical: 10% (30 g)

Isopropyl Alcohol [OTC]

Brand Names: Swim-Ear®
Use: Drying agent
Dose: Children and Adults: Instill 4-5 drops after exposure to water.
Strengths: Solution: Isopropyl alcohol 95%, glycerin 5%

SELECTED PRESCRIPTION COMBINATION PRODUCTS*

Brand Name	Generic Name
Allergan® Ear Drops	Antipyrine and benzocaine
Auralgan®	Antipyrine and benzocaine
Auroto®	Antipyrine and benzocaine
Carmol-HC® Topical	Urea and hydrocortisone
Codehist® DH Liquid	Chlorpheniramine, pseudoephedrine, and codeine
D.A.II™ Tablet	Chlorpheniramine, phenylephrine, and methscopolamine
Dallergy®	Chlorpheniramine, phenylephrine, and methscopolamine
Decohistine® DH Liquid	Chlorpheniramine, pseudoephedrine, and codeine
Dihistine® DH Liquid	Chlorpheniramine, pseudoephedrine, and codeine
Dura-Vent®/DA	Chlorpheniramine, phenylephrine, and methscopolamine
Extendryl®, Extendryl® SR, Extendryl® Jr	Chlorpheniramine, phenylephrine, and methscopolamine
Polycitra® Syrup	Sodium citrate and potassium citrate mixture
Rhinatate® Tablet	Chlorpheniramine, pyrilamine, and phenylephrine
R-Tannamine® Tablet	Chlorpheniramine, pyrilamine, and phenylephrine
R-Tannate® Tablet	Chlorpheniramine, pyrilamine, and phenylephrine
Ryna-C® Liquid	Chlorpheniramine, pseudoephedrine, and codeine
Rynatan® Pediatric Suspension	Chlorpheniramine, pyrilamine, and phenylephrine
Solagé™ Topical Solution	Mequinol and tretinoin
Tanoral® Tablet	Chlorpheniramine, pyrilamine, and phenylephrine
Triotann® Tablet	Chlorpheniramine, pyrilamine, and phenylephrine
Tri-Tannate® Tablet	Chlorpheniramine, pyrilamine, and phenylephrine

*See individual monographs for detailed information.

SELECTED ADVERSE EFFECTS

Adverse drug reactions can range from inconvenient to life-threatening. The type of effects, the severity, and frequency of occurrence is dependent on the medication and dosage of the medication being used, as well as the individual's response to the therapy. Early recognition by healthcare providers or patients of these adverse side effects is a major factor if appropriate intervention is to implemented. The following are definitions of selected adverse effects, and examples of some (by no means all) medications associated with these adverse effects.

Name	Description
Acute tubular necrosis	Acute renal failure characterized by direct toxicity to tubular cells. Cellular debris (casts) are a prominent feature of urinary sediment. Usually requires several days of treatment. **Examples of associated drugs:** Aminoglycosides
Ageusia	Loss of sense of taste **Examples of associated drugs:** Bleomycin, cisplatin, diltiazem
Akathisia	Evidenced by an uncontrollable constant need for motion, pacing, and squirming or restlessness; usually develops within first 2 months of antipsychotic treatment **Examples of associated drugs:** Phenergan, haldo
Alopecia	Loss of body hair **Examples of associated drugs:** Chemotherapeutic agents, beta-blockers
Anemia	A condition in which the number of red blood cells, the amount of hemoglobin, and the volume of packed red blood cells of blood is less than normal; manifested by pallor of the skin and mucus membranes, shortness of breath, palpitation of the heart, soft systolic murmurs, lethargy, fatigability, nose bleeds, bleeding gums, easy bruising, hematuria or blood in stool **Examples of associated drugs:** Amoxicillin, warfarin
Angioedema	Localized swelling of the subcutaneous tissue of face, hands, feet, and genitalia **Examples of associated drugs:** ACE inhibitors
Anhidrosis	Deficiency of or absence of sweat; since sweating is necessary for cooling, persons with anhidrosis are at increased risk for hyperthermia
Anorexia	Loss of desire for food **Examples of associated drugs:** CNS stimulants
Anticholinergic effects	Usually used to describe blockade of muscarinic receptors. Symptoms include blurred vision, mydriasis, increased intraocular pressure, headache, flushing, tachycardia, nervousness, constipation, dizziness, insomnia, mental confusion or excitement, dry mouth, altered taste perception, dysphagia, constipation, palpitations, bradycardia, urinary hesitancy or retention, impotence, decreased sweating, susceptibility to heat prostration, thickening or drying of bronchial secretions. **Examples of associated drugs:** Tricyclic antidepressants, antihistamines
Anticoagulant skin necrosis	Occurs early in therapy (3-5) days with oral anticoagulants (eg, warfarin). A paradoxical effect of oral anticoagulant therapy which involves microembolization and necrosis of skin often localized to the abdomen, breast, buttock, and thigh regions. Genetic deficiency of protein C appears to be a risk factor. **Examples of associated drugs:** Oral anticoagulants (eg, warfarin)
Cushing's syndrome	Usually a response to excess levels of circulating glucocorticoids; resembles Cushing's disease (pituitary tumor); characterized by obesity, hyperglycemia, glycosuria, muscle weakness, menstrual irregularities, fluid and electrolyte disturbances, hirsutism, myopathy, and decreased resistance to infection **Examples of associated drugs:** Prednisone
Disulfiram reaction	Many drugs will produce a disulfiram-type reaction when the patient ingests alcohol. Symptoms includes nausea and/or vomiting, pounding or throbbing headache, systemic flushing, respiratory difficulties (dyspnea, hyperventilation), sweating, excessive thirst, cardiac disturbances (chest pain, palpitations), vertigo, visual disturbances (blurred or double vision), and CNS disturbances (confusion, convulsions). **Examples of associated drugs:** Metronidazole, cephalosporins with MTT side chains
Drug fever	Persistent fever which may be associated with low-grade allergic reaction to a drug entity. Often develops several days after initial defervescence from antibiotics. Other causes of fever related to drugs may be due to dopamine inhibition (see neuroleptic malignant syndrome). **Examples of associated drugs:** Beta-lactams, macrolides
Dysgeusia	Impairment of or perversion of sense of taste
Dystonia	Develops early in therapy – sometimes within hours of first dose. Typically, appears as severe spasms of the muscles of face, neck, tongue, and back. Oculogyric crisis (upward deviation of the eyes) and opisthotonus (tetanic spasm of back muscles cause trunk to arch forward, with head and lower extremities thrown backward. Acute cramping can cause dislocation of joints and laryngeal dystonia can impair respiration (can be fatal, requires emergency treatment). **Examples of associated drugs:** Haldol, phenothiazines
Eosinophilic pneumonitis	Development of interstitial pneumonitis due to eosinophilic infiltrates. Shortness of breath and inflammation are prominent features. **Examples of associated drugs:** Mesalamine
Erythema multiforme	Cutaneous eruption of macules, papules, and/or subdermal vesicles (multiform appearance), including characteristic "target" or "iris" lesions over the dorsal aspect of the hands and forearms. Self-limiting eruptions are termed "minor", while major erruptions may be referred to as Stevens-Johnson syndrome. **Examples of associated drugs:** Phenytoin, sulfonamides

SELECTED ADVERSE EFFECTS *(Continued)*

Name	Description
Extrapyramidal movement disorders	Movement disorders associated with antipsychotic effects: Dystonia, pseudoparkinsonism, akathisia, tardive dyskinesia **Examples of associated drugs:** Metoclopramide, haldol, phenothiazines
Hallucinations	**Examples of associated drugs:** Opiates
Hepatotoxicity	Hepatocellular damage or multilobular hepatic necrosis can result in liver dysfunction manifested as jaundice or hepatitis; yellowing of skin or eyes is usually a later manifestation; anorexia, fatigue or malaise, nausea, darkening in color of urine or light colored stool may occur first **Examples of associated drugs:** Troglitazone
Interstitial nephritis	Acute renal failure characterized by localized inflammatory/allergic reaction, pronounced eosinophilic collection in interstitial cells of kidney. Eosinophils may appear in urine. Usually develops after several days of therapy. **Examples of associated drugs:** Beta-lactams, NSAIDs
Leukopenia/ neutropenia	**Examples of associated drugs:** Beta-lactams, procainamide
Methemoglobinemia	Rare reaction in which the hemoglobin molecule is altered, rendering it unable to effectively carry oxygen after exposure to a chemical initiator. Cyanosis, respiratory distress, lactic acidosis, and shock may progress rapidly after exposure. May occur with any route of administration, including topical. **Examples of associated drugs:** Nitrates, local anesthetics
Myositis/ rhabdomyolysis	Inflammation/toxicity to muscle cells characterized by muscle pain/stiffness. Pronounced lysis of muscle cells leads to dramatic increase in serum CPK and possible precipitation of myoglobin in urine. **Examples of associated drugs:** HMG CoA reductase inhibitors (particularly when combined with drugs like erythromycin or cyclosporin)
Neuroleptic malignant syndrome	Rare, but may cause 30% to 50% fatality, response to antipsychotic therapy – usually with high-potency drugs. Manifests as extremely rigid musculoskeletal posturing, extremely high fevers, sweating, dysrhythmias, and acute fluctuations of blood pressure and consciousness, respiratory failure and/or cardiac collapse (requires immediate supportive care and withdrawal of antipsychotic medication). **Examples of associated drugs:** Haldol, phenothiazines
Neuromuscular blockade	Weakness, respiratory failure as neuromuscular transmission may be interrupted. Patients with decreased neuromuscular transmission (ie, myasthenia gravis) are at particular risk. **Examples of associated drugs:** Aminoglycosides, macrolides
Neutropenia	Usually associated with antineoplastic medications. A reduction in circulating neutrophils (white blood cells that are essential in fighting infection) means that both severity and incidence of infections are significantly increased. Usually, benign infections such as candidiasis can become systemically life-threatening. **Examples of associated drugs:** Beta-lactams, procainamide, carbamazepine
Opportunistic infection	Many medications reduce the natural resistance to infection and/or mask the more obvious indications of an infection when persons are receiving antineoplastics, antivirals, antibiotics, and glucocorticoids. Symptoms include sore throat, fever, chills, unhealed sores, purulent vaginal discharge, white plaques in mouth, fatigue, and joint pain. **Examples of associated drugs:** Chemotherapeutic agents, broad-spectrum antibiotics, immunosuppressants
Optic neuritis	Blurred vision, altered color discrimination, and constriction of visual fields **Examples of associated drugs:** Quinidine, cisplatin
Orthostatic hypotension	Reduced muscle tone in the venous wall which causes blood to pool in lower extremity veins when the person assumes an erect position from lying or sitting; blood return to the heart is decreased because of this pooling, resulting in decreased cardiac output, and abrupt fall in blood pressure **Examples of associated drugs:** Tricyclic antidepressants, beta-blockers
Paradoxical response	A response to a medication that is opposite of the anticipated response or side effects (eg, a paradoxical response to CNS depressants may be CNS excitation such as hyperactivity, aggression, decreased ability to concentrate, etc) **Examples of associated drugs:** Benzodiazepines, phenobarbital
Photophobia	Blocking muscarinic receptors on the sphincter of the iris decreases ability to adapt to bright light with intolerance for any bright light; both artificial lighting and outside sunlight **Examples of associated drugs:** Anticholinergics
Photosensitization/ phototoxicity	Phototoxic and photoallergic reactions result from a combination of a sensitizing agent and ultraviolet light. The sensitizing agent in phototoxic reactions may be systemically ingested or locally applied. The reaction occurs within hours of exposure. Photoallergy results from chemical change to the structure of a sensitizing agent, and may require several days before symptoms appear. **Examples of associated drugs:** Fluoroquinolones, tetracyclines
Postural hypotension	See orthostatic hypotension.
Pseudoparkinsonism	Blocking of dopamine receptors produces symptoms that resemble Parkinson's disease: Bradycardia, facies, drooling, tremors, rigidity, gait disturbance, and stooped posture (usually develops within first month of therapy) **Examples of associated drugs:** Antipsychotic medications, haldol
Pulmonary fibrosis	Restrictive airway disease due to fibrous changes in the lungs, often manifest only after long-term drug administration. **Examples of associated drugs:** Nitrofurantoin, melphalan, amiodarone

Name	Description
Purple toes syndrome	Peripheral ischemia and cyanosis generally localized to the plantar surfaces and sides of the toes which may occasionally progress to necrosis or gangrene. The effect is believed to be caused by cholesterol microemboli. Effects are noted after weeks to months of therapy. **Examples of associated drugs:** Oral anticoagulants
QTc prolongation	Lengthening of the corrected Q-T interval (on ECG) which may predispose to the development of polymorphic ventricular tachycardia (Torsade de pointes). **Examples of associated drugs:** Type Ia and III antiarrhythmics, selected fluoroquinolones, erythromycin, thioridazine, mesoridazine
Seizures (drug-induced)	An infrequent, nonspecific effect of a variety of medications, particularly at high concentrations. Drug-induced seizures may occur due to lowering of seizure threshold, blockade of inhibitory neurotransmitters (GABA) or direct neuroexcitatory effects. **Examples of associated drugs:** Tricyclic antidepressants (lower seizure threshold), high-dose beta-lactam or fluoroquinolone antibiotics (GABA blockade); theophylline or accumulation of normeperidine (neuroexcitation)
Serotonin syndrome	Presence of three or more of the following: Altered mental status (40% – primarily confusion or hypomania), agitation, tremor (50%), shivering, diarrhea, hyperreflexia (pronounced) in lower extremities, myoclonus (50%), ataxia or incoordination, fever (50% incidence; temperature >105°F associated with grave prognosis), diaphoresis **Examples of associated drugs:** Serotonin reuptake inhibitors, MOMA (ecstasy), clomipramine, combinations of many drugs
Stevens-Johnson syndrome (SJS)	Rare reaction; symptoms include widespread lesions of the skin and mucous membranes, fever, malaise, and toxemia; reducing or discontinuing the sulfonamide at the first sign of skin rash may reduce the incidence of SJS **Examples of associated drugs:** Associated primarily with sulfonamides and associated compounds such as sulfonylureas, thiazide diuretics, and loop diuretics; anticonvulsants
Stomatitis	**Examples of associated drugs:** Chemotherapeutic agents
Sulfite hypersensitivity	Reactions occur within 2-15 minutes after ingestion of inhalation and include nasal pruritus, rhinorrhea, conjunctivitis, generalized urticaria, dyspnea, wheezing, angioedema, flushing, weakness, and anaphylaxis; patients frequently have underlying allergies or asthmatic disease. **Examples of associated drugs:** Sulfite derivatives are common antioxidant preservatives used in foods and medications. Sulfite derivatives include sodium bisulfite, potassium bisulfite, sodium metabisulfite, sodium sulfites, potassium metabisulfite, and sulfur dioxide. Most common food sources are fresh fruits and vegetables, shellfish, soft drinks, beer, wine, dried foods, and fruit drinks. Sympathomimetic medications are very susceptible to oxidation and frequently contain bisulfites in concentrations of 0.3% to 0.75%.
Tardive dyskinesia	Usually develops with long-term therapy – symptoms may be irreversible. Characterized by wormlike, writhing movements of tongue and facial muscles, lip-smacking, or flicking tongue movements; can progress to involuntary movements of digits or limbs. **Examples of associated drugs:** Haldol, phenothiazines
Tendonitis/Achilles' tendon rupture	Pain associated with tendon area, most commonly in the Achilles' region, which may progress to tendon rupture, particularly if the effect is not recognized and therapy is continued. **Examples of associated drugs:** Fluoroquinolone antibiotics
Teratogenic effects	Neonatal abnormalities (physical and mental) that result from impaired development at some stage in the fetal development; specificity of defects depends on several factors, including the period of fetal development when the medication was used (eg, some drugs are teratogenic during the early period of fetal development, some are teratogenic during later periods of development, and some have negative impact on fetal development during any period of the pregnancy) **Examples of associated drugs:** Phenytoin, metronidazole
Thrombocytopenia	**Examples of associated drugs:** H_2 antagonists, beta-lactams
Tyramine reaction	Specific foods in the presence of MAO inhibitors; see Food/Drug Interactions for a list of tyramine-containing foods which the patient taking MAO inhibitors should be advised to avoid. Normally, dietary tyramine is inactivated by MAO (monamine oxidase) in the intestinal wall and by hepatic MAO. In the presence of MAO inhibitors, dietary tyramine is not inactivated, passes without metabolism into the circulation to promote the release of accumulated norepinephrine stores in the sympathetic nerve terminals, thereby causing massive vasoconstriction and acute stimulation of the heart. Reactions can be severe and usually require emergency treatment. **Examples of associated drugs:** MAO inhibitors
Vestibulotoxicity	Form of ototoxicity which affects vestibular function, as opposed to hearing. Primary symptom is ataxia or difficulty maintaining balance. **Examples of associated drugs:** Aminoglycosides
Virilization	Acne, deepening of voice, increased body and facial hair, baldness, clitoral enlargement, increased libido, menstrual irregularities (Hair loss, voice changes, and enlargement of clitoris may be irreversible.) **Examples of associated drugs:** Minoxidil, phenytoin
Xerostomia	Dry mouth results from blockade of muscarinic receptors on salivary glands. Decreased salivation and excessively dry mouth are extremely uncomfortable but also interfere with mastication and swallowing, resulting in poor nutrition. **Examples of associated drugs:** Clonidine, anticholinergics

DISCOLORATION OF FECES DUE TO DRUGS

Black
Acetazolamide
Aluminum hydroxide
Aminophylline
Amphetamine
Amphotericin B
Bismuth salts
Chlorpropamide
Clindamycin
Corticosteroids
Cyclophosphamide
Cytarabine
Digitalis
Ethacrynic acid
Ferrous salts
Fluorouracil
Hydralazine
Hydrocortisone
Iodide-containing drugs
Melphalan
Methotrexate
Methylprednisolone
Phenylephrine
Potassium salts
Prednisolone
Procarbazine
Sulfonamides
Tetracycline
Theophylline
Thiotepa
Triamcinolone
Warfarin

Blue
Chloramphenicol
Methylene blue

Green
Indomethacin
Medroxyprogesterone

Yellow/Yellow-Green
Senna

Orange-Red
Phenazopyridine
Rifampin

Pink/Red
Anticoagulants
Aspirin
Barium
Heparin
Oxyphenbutazone
Phenylbutazone
Tetracycline syrup

White/Speckling
Antibiotics (oral)
Barium

DISCOLORATION OF URINE DUE TO DRUGS

Black/Brown/Dark
Cascara
Chloroquine
Ferrous salts
Metronidazole
Nitrofurantoin
Quinine
Senna

Blue
Triamterene

Blue-Green
Amitriptyline
Methylene blue
Propofol

Orange/Yellow
Heparin
Phenazopyridine
Rifampin
Sulfasalazine
Warfarin

Red/Pink
Daunorubicin
Doxorubicin
Heparin
Ibuprofen
Oxyphenbutazone
Phenylbutazone
Phenytoin
Rifampin
Senna

FEVER DUE TO DRUGS

Most Common	Less Common	
Cephalosporins	Allopurinol	Hydralazine
Iodides	Antihistamines	Hydroxyurea
Isoniazid	Azathioprine	Ibuprofen
Methyldopa	Barbiturates	Mercaptopurine
Penicillins	Bleomycin	Nitrofurantoin
Phenytoin	Carbamazepine	Para-aminosalicylic acid
Procainamide	Cimetidine	Pentazocine
Quinidine	Cisplatin	Procarbazine
Streptomycin	Clofibrate	Propylthiouracil
Sulfas	Colistimethate	Sulindac
Vancomycin	Diazoxide	Streptozocin
	Folic acid	Triamterene

Drug Intell Clin Pharm, Table 2, "Drugs Implicated in Causing a Fever," 1986, 20:416.

SEROTONIN SYNDROME

DIAGNOSTIC CRITERIA

- Recent addition or dosage increase of any agent increasing serotonin activity or availability (usually within 1 day)
- Absence of abused substances, metabolic infectious etiology, or withdrawal
- No recent addition or dosage increase of a neuroleptic agent prior to onset of signs and symptoms
- Presence of three or more of the following: (% incidence)

Agitation (34%)
Abdominal pain (4%)
Ataxia/incoordination (40%)
Diaphoresis (45%)
Diarrhea (8%)
Hyperpyrexia (45%)
Hypertension/hypotension (35%)
Hyperthermia
Hyperreflexia (52%)
Mental status change – cognitive behavioral changes:
- Anxiety (15%)
- Euphoria/hypomania (21%)
- Confusion (51%)
- Agitation (34%)
- Disorientation
- Coma/unresponsiveness (29%)

Muscle rigidity (51%)
Mydriasis
Myoclonus (58%)
Nausea (23%)
Nystagmus (15%)
Restlessness/hyperactivity (48%)
Salivation (2%)
Seizures (12%)
Shivering (26%)
Sinus tachycardia (36%)
Tachypnea (26%)
Tremor (43%)
Unreactive pupils (20%)

DRUG INTERACTIONS

Drugs (as Single Causative Agent) Which Can Induce Serotonin Syndrome

Specific serotonin reuptake inhibitors (SSRI)
MDMA (Ecstasy)
Clomipramine

Drug Combinations Which Can Induce Serotonin Syndrome[1]

Alprazolam – Clomipramine
Amphetamines – MAO inhibitors
Amphetamines – SSRIs (Citalopram, Fluoxetine, Fluvoxamine, Paroxetine, Sertraline)
Amphetamines – Tricyclic antidepressants
Amitriptyline – Dihydroergotamine
Amitriptyline – Lithium – Trazodone
Amitriptyline – Sertraline
Anorexiants – MAO inhibitors
Bromocriptine – Levodopa/Carbidopa
Buspirone – Nefazodone
Buspirone – SSRIs (Citalopram, Fluoxetine, Fluvoxamine, Paroxetine, Sertraline)
Buspirone – Trazodone
Buspirone – Tricyclic antidepressants
Carbamazepine – Fluoxetine
Citalopram – Moclobemide
Clomipramine – Alprazolam
Clomipramine – Clorgiline
Clomipramine – Lithium
Clomipramine – MAO inhibitors
Clomipramine – Moclobemide
Clomipramine – S-adenosylmethionine
Clomipramine – Tranylcypromine
Clorgiline – Clomipramine
Dextromethorphan – MAO inhibitors
Dextromethorphan – SSRIs (Citalopram, Fluoxetine, Fluvoxamine, Paroxetine, Sertraline)
Dextropropoxyphene – Phenelzine – Trazodone
Dihydroergotamine – Amitriptyline
Dihydroergotamine – Paroxetine
Dihydroergotamine – SSRIs (Citalopram, Fluoxetine, Fluvoxamine, Paroxetine, Sertraline)
Dihydroergotamine – Tricyclic antidepressants
Fentanyl – SSRIs (Citalopram, Fluoxetine, Fluvoxamine, Paroxetine, Sertraline)
Fluoxetine – Carbamazepine
Fluoxetine – Remoxipride
Fluoxetine – Tryptophan
Levodopa/Carbidopa – Bromocriptine
Linezolid - SSRIs (Citalopram, Fluoxetine, Fluvoxamine, Paroxetine, Sertraline)
Linezolid – Tramadol
Linezolid – Tricyclic antidepressants
Lithium – Amitriptyline – Trazodone
Lithium – Clomipramine
Lithium – SSRIs (Citalopram, Fluoxetine, Fluvoxamine, Paroxetine, Sertraline)
Lithium – Tricyclic antidepressants
Lithium – Venlafaxine
Lysergic acid diethylamide (LSD) – SSRIs (Citalopram, Fluoxetine, Fluvoxamine, Paroxetine, Sertraline)
Metoclopramide – Sertraline

SEROTONIN SYNDROME *(Continued)*

Metoclopramide – Venlafaxine
MAO inhibitors – Amphetamines
MAO inhibitors – Anorexiants
MAO inhibitors – Clomipramine
MAO inhibitors – Dextromethorphan
MAO inhibitors – Meperidine
MAO inhibitors – Nefazodone
MAO inhibitors – Serotonin agonists
MAO inhibitors – S-adenosylmethionine
MAO inhibitors – SSRIs (Citalopram, Fluoxetine, Fluvoxamine, Paroxetine, Sertraline)
MAO inhibitors – St John's Wort
MAO inhibitors – Tramadol
MAO inhibitors – Trazodone
MAO inhibitors – Tricyclic antidepressants
MAO inhibitors – Tryptophan
MAO inhibitors – Venlafaxine
Meperidine – MAO inhibitors
Meperidine – Moclobemide
Meperidine – Nefazodone
Meperidine – SSRIs (Citalopram, Fluoxetine, Fluvoxamine, Paroxetine, Sertraline)
Moclobemide – Citalopram
Moclobemide – Clomipramine
Moclobemide – Meperidine
Moclobemide – Pethidine
Moclobemide – SSRIs (Citalopram, Fluoxetine, Fluvoxamine, Paroxetine, Sertraline)
Moclobemide – Tricyclic antidepressants
Nefazodone – Buspirone
Nefazodone – MAO inhibitors
Nefazodone – Meperidine
Nefazodone – Serotonin agonists
Nefazodone – SSRIs (Citalopram, Fluoxetine, Fluvoxamine, Paroxetine, Sertraline)
Nefazodone – Trazodone
Nefazodone – Tramadol
Nefazodone – Valproic Acid
Nortriptyline – Trazodone
Paroxetine – Dihydroergotamine
Paroxetine – Trazodone
Pethidine – Moclobemide
Phenelzine – Trazodone – Dextropropoxyphene
Remoxipride – Fluoxetine
S-adenosylmethionine – Clomipramine
S-adenosylmethionine – MAO inhibitors
S-adenosylmethionine – SSRIs (Citalopram, Fluoxetine, Fluvoxamine, Paroxetine, Sertraline)
S-adenosylmethionine – Tricyclic antidepressants
Selegiline (high-dose) – SSRIs (Citalopram, Fluoxetine, Fluvoxamine, Paroxetine, Sertraline)
Selegiline (high-dose) – Tricyclic antidepressants
Selegiline (high-dose) – Venlafaxine
Serotonin agonists (Sumatriptan, others) – MAO inhibitors
Serotonin agonists (Sumatriptan, others) – Nefazodone
Serotonin agonists (Sumatriptan, others) – SSRIs (Citalopram, Fluoxetine, Fluvoxamine, Paroxetine, Sertraline)
Serotonin agonists (Sumatriptan, others) – TCAs
Serotonin agonists (Sumatriptan, others) – Tramadol
Sertraline – Amitriptyline
Sibutramine – SSRIs (Citalopram, Fluoxetine, Fluvoxamine, Paroxetine, Sertraline)
SSRIs – Amphetamines
SSRIs – Buspirone
SSRIs – Dextromethorphan
SSRIs – Dihydroergotamine
SSRIs – Fentanyl
SSRIs – Linezolid
SSRIs – Lithium
SSRIs – Lysergic acid diethylamide (LSD)
SSRIs – MAO inhibitors
SSRIs – Meperidine
SSRIs – Moclobemide
SSRIs – Nefazodone
SSRIs – S-adenosylmethionine
SSRIs – Selegiline (high-dose)
SSRIs – Serotonin agonists
SSRIs – Sibutramine
SSRIs – St John's Wort
SSRIs – Tramadol
SSRIs – Trazodone
SSRIs – Tricyclic antidepressants
SSRIs – Tryptophan
St John's Wort – MAO inhibitors
St John's Wort – SSRIs (Citalopram, Fluoxetine, Fluvoxamine, Paroxetine, Sertraline)
St John's Wort – Tricyclic antidepressants
Sympathomimetics – Tricyclic antidepressants
Tramadol – Linezolid
Tramadol – MAO inhibitors
Tramadol – Nefazodone
Tramadol – Serotonin agonists
Tramadol – SSRIs (Citalopram, Fluoxetine, Fluvoxamine, Paroxetine, Sertraline)
Tramadol – TCAs
Tranylcypromine – Clomipramine
Trazodone – Buspirone
Trazodone – Lithium – Amitriptyline
Trazodone – MAO inhibitors
Trazodone – Nefazodone
Trazodone – Nortriptyline
Trazodone – Paroxetine
Trazodone – SSRIs (Citalopram, Fluoxetine, Fluvoxamine, Paroxetine, Sertraline) (theoretical)
Tricyclic antidepressants – Amphetamines
Tricyclic antidepressants – Buspirone
Tricyclic antidepressants – Dihydroergotamine
Tricyclic antidepressants – Linezolid
Tricyclic antidepressants – Lithium
Tricyclic antidepressants – MAO inhibitors
Tricyclic antidepressants – Moclobemide
Tricyclic antidepressants – S-adenosylmethionine
Tricyclic antidepressants – Serotonin agonists
Tricyclic antidepressants – SSRIs (Citalopram, Fluoxetine,

Fluvoxamine, Paroxetine, Sertraline)
Tricyclic antidepressants – St John's Wort
Tricyclic antidepressants – Sympathomimetics
Tricyclic antidepressants – Tramadol
Tryptophan – Fluoxetine
Tryptophan – MAO inhibitors
Tryptophan – SSRIs (Citalopram, Fluoxetine, Fluvoxamine, Paroxetine, Sertraline)
Valproic acid – Nefazodone
Venlafaxine – Lithium
Venlafaxine – MAO inhibitors
Venlafaxine – Selegiline (high-dose)

[1]When administered within 2 weeks of each other.

TREATMENT GUIDELINES

Therapy is primarily supportive with I.V. crystalloid solutions utilized for hypotension and cooling blankets for mild hyperthermia. Endotracheal intubation and paralysis may be required to treat refractory muscular contractions. Recovery is seen within 1 day in 70% of cases; mortality rate is about 11%.

- Norepinephrine is the preferred vasopressor.
- Chlorpromazine (25 mg I.M.) or dantrolene sodium (1 mg/kg I.V. – maximum dose 10 mg/kg) may have a role in controlling fevers, although there is no proven benefit.
- Benzodiazepines are the first-line treatment in controlling rigors and thus, limiting fever and rhabdomyolysis, while clonazepam may be specifically useful in treating myoclonus.
- Tachycardia or tremor can be treated with beta-blocking agents; although due to its blockade of 5-HTIA receptors, the syndrome may worsen.
- Serotonin blockers such as diphenhydramine (50 mg I.M.), cyproheptadine (adults: 4-8 mg every 2-4 hours up to 0.5 mg/kg/day; children: up to 0.25 mg/kg/day), or chlorpromazine (25 mg I.M.) have been used with variable efficacy.
- Methysergide (2-6 mg/day) and nitroglycerin (I.V. infusion of 2 mg/kg/minute with lorazepam) also has been utilized with variable efficacy in case reports.
- It appears that cyproheptadine is most consistently beneficial.

Pharmacokinetics of Selective Serotonin-Reuptake Inhibitors (SSRIs)

SSRI	Half-life (h)	Metabolite Half-life	Peak Plasma Level (h)	% Protein Bound	Bioavailability (%)
Citalopram	35	N/A	4	80	80
Fluoxetine	Initial: 24-72 Chronic: 96-144	Norfluoxetine 4-16 days	6-8	95	72
Fluvoxamine	16	N/A	3	80	53
Paroxetine	21	N/A	5	95	>90
Sertraline	26	N-desmethyl-sertraline 2-4 days	5-8	98	—

References

Gardner DM and Lynd LD, "Sumatriptan Contraindications and the Serotonin Syndrome," *Ann Pharmacother*, 1998, 32(1):33-8

Gitlin MJ, "Venlafaxine, Monoamine Oxidase Inhibitors, and the Serotonin Syndrome," *J Clin Psychopharmacol*, 1997, 17:66-7.

Heisler MA, Guidery JR, and Arnecke B, "Serotonin Syndrome Induced by Administration of Venlafaxine and Phenelzine," *Ann Pharmacother*, 1996, 30:84.

Hodgman MJ, Martin TG, and Krenzelok EP, "Serotonin Syndrome Due to Venlafaxine and Maintenance Tranylcypromine Therapy," *Hum Exp Toxicol*, 1997, 16:14-7.

John L, Perreault MM, Tao T, et al, "Serotonin Syndrome Associated With Nefazodone and Paroxetine," *Ann Emerg Med*, 1997, 29:287-9.

LoCurto MJ, "The Serotonin Syndrome," *Emerg Clin North Am*, 1997, 15(3):665-75.

Martin TG, "Serotonin Syndrome," *Ann Emerg Med*, 1996, 28:520-6.

Mills K, "Serotonin Toxicity: A Comprehensive Review for Emergency Medicine," *Top Emerg Med*, 1993, 15:54-73.

Mills KC, "Serotonin Syndrome: A Clinical Update," *Crit Care Clin*, 1997, 13(4):763-83.

Nisijima K, Shimizu M, Abe T, et al, "A Case of Serotonin Syndrome Induced by Concomitant Treatment With Low-Dose Trazodone, and Amitriptyline and Lithium," *Int Clin Psychopharmacol*, 1996, 11:289-90.

Sobanski T, Bagli M, Laux G, et al, "Serotonin Syndrome After Lithium Add-On Medication to Paroxetine," *Pharmacopsychiatry*, 1997, 30:106-7.

Sporer, "The Serotonin Syndrome: Implicated Drugs, Pathophysiology and Management," *Drug Safety*, 1995, 13(2):94-104.

Sternbach H, "The Serotonin Syndrome," *Am J Psychiatry*, 1991, 146:705-7.

Van Berkum MM, Thiel J, Leikin JB, et al, "A Fatality Due to Serotonin Syndrome," *Medical Update for Psychiatrists*, 1997, 2:55-7.

CALCULATIONS/CONVERSIONS/ LABORATORY VALUES

APOTHECARY/METRIC CONVERSIONS

Approximate Liquid Measures

Basic equivalent: 1 fluid ounce = 30 mL

Examples:

1 gallon	3800 mL	15 minims	1 mL
1 quart	960 mL	10 minims	0.6 mL
1 pint	480 mL	1 gallon	128 fluid ounces
8 fluid ounces	240 mL	1 quart	32 fluid ounces
4 fluid ounces	120 mL	1 pint	16 fluid ounces

Approximate Household Equivalents

1 teaspoonful	5 mL	1 tablespoonful	15 mL

Weights

Basic equivalents:

1 ounce = 30 g   15 grains = 1 g

Examples:

4 ounces	120 g	1/100 grain	600 mcg
2 ounces	60 g	1/150 grain	400 mcg
10 grains	600 mg	1/200 grain	300 mcg
7 1/2 grains	500 mg	16 ounces	1 pound
1 grain	60 mg		

Metric Conversions

Basic equivalents:

1 g	1000 mg	1 mg	1000 mcg

Examples:

5 g	5000 mg	5 mg	5000 mcg
0.5 g	500 mg	0.5 mg	500 mcg
0.05 g	50 mg	0.05 mg	50 mcg

Exact Equivalents

1 g	=	15.43 grains (gr)	0.1 mg	=	1/600 gr
1 mL	=	16.23 minims	0.12 mg	=	1/500 gr
1 minim	=	0.06 mL	0.15 mg	=	1/400 gr
1 gr	=	64.8 mg	0.2 mg	=	1/300 gr
1 pint (pt)	=	473.2 mL	0.3 mg	=	1/200 gr
1 oz	=	28.35 g	0.4 mg	=	1/150 gr
1 lb	=	453.6 g	0.5 mg	=	1/120 gr
1 kg	=	2.2 lbs	0.6 mg	=	1/100 gr
1 qt	=	946.4 mL	0.8 mg	=	1/80 gr
			1 mg	=	1/65 gr

Solids*

1/4 grain	=	15 mg
1/2 grain	=	30 mg
1 grain	=	60 mg
1 1/2 grains	=	90 mg
5 grains	=	300 mg
10 grains	=	600 mg

*Use exact equivalents for compounding and calculations requiring a high degree of accuracy.

BODY SURFACE AREA OF ADULTS AND CHILDREN

Calculating Body Surface Area in Children

In a child of average size, find weight and corresponding surface area on the boxed scale to the left; or, use the nomogram to the right. Lay a straightedge on the correct height and weight points for the child, then read the intersecting point on the surface area scale.

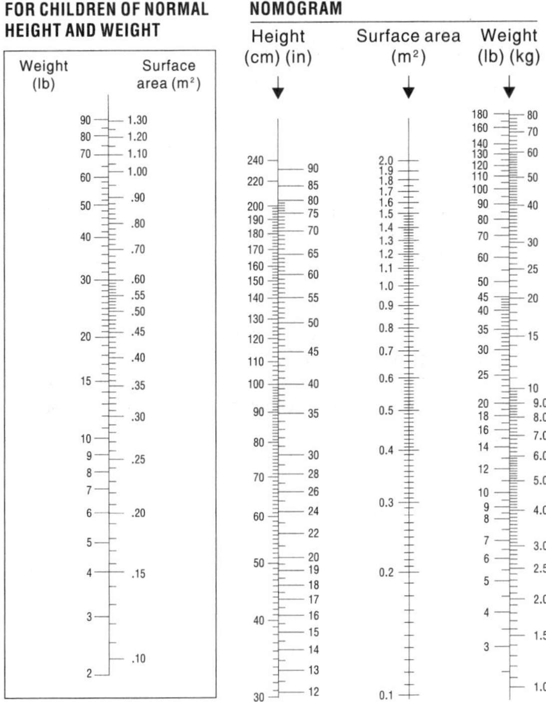

BODY SURFACE AREA FORMULA (Adult and Pediatric)

$$BSA\ (m^2) = \sqrt{\frac{Ht\ (in) \times Wt\ (lb)}{3131}} \quad \text{or, in metric: } BSA\ (m^2) = \sqrt{\frac{Ht\ (cm) \times Wt\ (kg)}{3600}}$$

References

Lam TK and Leung DT, "More on Simplified Calculation of Body Surface Area," *N Engl J Med*, 1988, 318(17):1130 (Letter).

Mosteller RD, "Simplified Calculation of Body Surface Area", *N Engl J Med*, 1987, 317(17):1098 (Letter).

IDEAL BODY WEIGHT CALCULATION (IBW is in kg)

Adults (18 years and older)

IBW (male) = 50 + (2.3 x height in inches over 5 feet)

IBW (female) = 45.5 + (2.3 x height in inches over 5 feet)

Children (height is in cm)

a. 1-18 years

$$IBW = \frac{(height^2 \times 1.65)}{1000}$$

b. 5 feet and taller

IBW (male) = 39 + (2.27 x height in inches over 5 feet)

IBW (female) = 42.2 + (2.27 x height in inches over 5 feet)

CALCULATIONS/CONVERSIONS/LABORATORY VALUES *(Continued)*

CREATININE CLEARANCE ESTIMATING METHODS IN PATIENTS WITH STABLE RENAL FUNCTION

These formulas provide an acceptable estimate of the patient's creatinine clearance **except** in the following instances.

- Patient's serum creatinine is changing rapidly (either up or down).
- Patients are markedly emaciated.

In above situations, certain assumptions have to be made.

- In patients with rapidly rising serum creatinines (ie, >0.5-0.7 mg/dL/day), it is best to assume that the patient's creatinine clearance is probably <10 mL/minute.
- In emaciated patients, although their actual creatinine clearance is less than their calculated creatinine clearance (because of decreased creatinine production), it is not possible to easily predict how much less.

Infants

Estimation of creatinine clearance using serum creatinine and body length (to be used when an adequate timed specimen cannot be obtained). **Note:** This formula may not provide an accurate estimation of creatinine clearance for infants younger than 6 months of age and for patients with severe starvation or muscle wasting.

$Cl_{cr} = K \times L/S_{cr}$

where:

Cl_{cr} = creatinine clearance in mL/minute/1.73 m^2
K = constant of proportionality that is age specific

Age	K
Low birth weight ≤1 y	0.33
Full-term ≤1 y	0.45
2-12 y	0.55
13-21 y female	0.55
13-21 y male	0.70

L = length in cm
S_{cr} = serum creatinine concentration in mg/dL

Reference

Schwartz GJ, Brion LP, and Spitzer A, "The Use of Plasma Creatinine Concentration for Estimating Glomerular Filtration Rate in Infants, Children, and Adolescents," *Pediatr Clin North Amer*, 1987, 34(3):571-90.

Children (1-18 years)

Method 1: (Traub SL and Johnson CE, "Comparison of Methods of Estimating Creatinine Clearance in Children," *Am J Hosp Pharm*, 1980, 37(2):195-201)

$$Cl_{cr} = \frac{0.48 \times (\text{height}) \times BSA}{S_{cr} \times 1.73}$$

where

BSA = body surface area in m^2
Cl_{cr} = creatinine clearance in mL/min
S_{cr} = serum creatinine in mg/dL
Height = in cm

Method 2: Nomogram (Traub SL and Johnson CE, "Comparison of Methods of Estimating Creatinine Clearance in Children," *Am J Hosp Pharm*, 1980, 37(2):195-201)

Children 1-18 Years

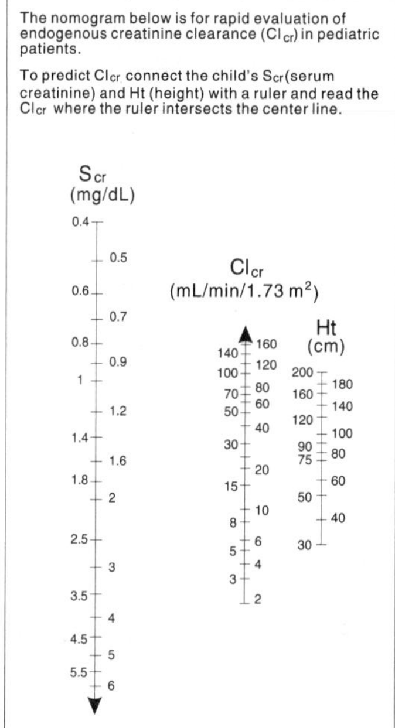

Adults (18 years and older)

Method 1: (Cockroft DW and Gault MH, *Nephron*, 1976, 16:31-41)

Estimated creatinine clearance (Cl_{cr}) (mL/min):

$$\text{Male} = \frac{(140 - \text{age})\ \text{IBW (kg)}}{72 \times S_{cr}}$$

$$\text{Female} = \text{estimated } Cl_{cr} \text{ male} \times 0.85$$

Note: The use of the patient's ideal body weight (IBW) is recommended for the above formula except when the patient's actual body weight is less than ideal. Use of the IBW is especially important in obese patients.

Method 2: (Jelliffe RW, *Ann Intern Med*, 1973, 79:604)

Estimated creatinine clearance (Cl_{cr}) (mL/min/1.73 m^2):

$$\text{Male} = \frac{98\text{-}0.8\ (\text{age} - 20)}{\text{serum creatinine}}$$

$$\text{Female} = \text{estimated } Cl_{cr} \text{ male} \times 0.90$$

CALCULATIONS/CONVERSIONS/LABORATORY VALUES *(Continued)*

Pounds/Kilograms Conversion

1 pound = 0.45359 kilograms
1 kilogram = 2.2 pounds

lb	kg	lb	kg	lb	kg
1	0.45	70	31.75	140	63.50
5	2.27	75	34.02	145	65.77
10	4.54	80	36.29	150	68.04
15	6.80	85	38.56	155	70.31
20	9.07	90	40.82	160	72.58
25	11.34	95	43.09	165	74.84
30	13.61	100	45.36	170	77.11
35	15.88	105	47.63	175	79.38
40	18.14	110	49.90	180	81.65
45	20.41	115	52.16	185	83.92
50	22.68	120	54.43	190	86.18
55	24.95	125	56.70	195	88.45
60	27.22	130	58.91	200	90.72
65	29.48	135	61.24		

FAHRENHEIT/CENTIGRADE CONVERSIONS

Celsius to Fahrenheit = (°C x 9/5) + 32 = °F
Fahrenheit to Celsius = (°F – 32) x 5/9 = °C

°C	°F	°C	°F	°C	°F
100.0	212.0	39.0	102.2	36.8	98.2
50.0	122.0	38.8	101.8	36.6	97.9
41.0	105.8	38.6	101.5	36.4	97.5
40.8	105.4	38.4	101.1	36.2	97.2
40.6	105.1	38.2	100.8	36.0	96.8
40.4	104.7	38.0	100.4	35.8	96.4
40.2	104.4	37.8	100.1	35.6	96.1
40.0	104.0	37.6	99.7	35.4	95.7
39.8	103.6	37.4	99.3	35.2	95.4
39.6	103.3	37.2	99.0	35.0	95.0
39.4	102.9	37.0	98.6	0	32.0
39.2	102.6				

LABORATORY REFERENCE VALUES FOR ADULTS

Automated Chemistry (CHEMISTRY A)

Test	Values	Remarks
Serum/Plasma		
Acetone	Negative	
Albumin	3.2-5 g/dL	
Alcohol, ethyl	Negative	
Aldolase	1.2-7.6 IU/L	
Ammonia	20-70 mcg/dL	Specimen to be placed on ice as soon as collected
Amylase	30-110 units/L	
Bilirubin, direct	0-0.3 mg/dL	
Bilirubin, total	0.1-1.2 mg/dL	
Calcium	8.6-10.3 mg/dL	
Calcium, ionized	2.24-2.46 mEq/L	
Chloride	95-108 mEq/L	
Cholesterol, total	≤220 mg/dL	Fasted blood required – normal value affected by dietary habits This reference range is for a general adult population
HDL cholesterol	40-60 mg/dL	Fasted blood required – normal value affected by dietary habits
LDL cholesterol	65-170 mg/dL	LDLC calculated by Friewald formula... which has certain inaccuracies and is invalid at trig levels >300 mg/dL
CO_2	23-30 mEq/L	
Creatine kinase (CK) isoenzymes		
CK-BB	0%	
CK-MB (cardiac)	0%-3.9%	
CK-MM (muscle)	96%-100%	
CK-MB levels must be both ≥4% and 10 IU/L to meet diagnostic criteria for CK-MB positive result consistent with myocardial injury.		
Creatine phosphokinase (CPK)	8-150 IU/L	
Creatinine	0.5-1.4 mg/dL	
Ferritin	13-300 ng/mL	
Folate	3.6-20 ng/dL	
GGT (gamma-glutamyltranspeptidase)		
male	11-63 IU/L	
female	8-35 IU/L	
GLDH	To be determined	
Glucose (2-h postprandial)	Up to 140 mg/dL	
Glucose, fasting	60-110 mg/dL	
Glucose, nonfasting (2-h postprandial)	60-140 mg/dL	
Hemoglobin A_{1c}	8	
Hemoglobin, plasma free	<2.5 mg/100 mL	
Hemoglobin, total glycosolated (Hb A_1)	4%-8%	
Iron	65-150 mcg/dL	
Iron binding capacity, total (TIBC)	250-420 mcg/dL	
Lactic acid	0.7-2.1 mEq/L	Specimen to be kept on ice and sent to lab as soon as possible
Lactate dehydrogenase (LDH)	56-194 IU/L	
Lactate dehydrogenase (LDH) isoenzymes		
LD_1	20%-34%	
LD_2	29%-41%	
LD_3	15%-25%	
LD_4	1%-12%	
LD_5	1%-15%	
Flipped LD_1/LD_2 ratios (>1 may be consistent with myocardial injury) particularly when considered in combination with a recent CK-MB positive result		
Lipase	23-208 units/L	
Magnesium	1.6-2.5 mg/dL	Increased by slight hemolysis
Osmolality	289-308 mOsm/kg	
Phosphatase, alkaline		
adults 25-60 y	33-131 IU/L	

CALCULATIONS/CONVERSIONS/LABORATORY VALUES *(Continued)*

Automated Chemistry (CHEMISTRY A) *(continued)*

Test	Values	Remarks
adults 61 y or older	51-153 IU/L	
infancy-adolescence	Values range up to 3-5 times higher than adults	
Phosphate, inorganic	2.8-4.2 mg/dL	
Potassium	3.5-5.2 mEq/L	Increased by slight hemolysis
Prealbumin	>15 mg/dL	
Protein, total	6.5-7.9 g/dL	
SGOT (AST)	<35 IU/L (20-48)	
SGPT (ALT) (10-35)	<35 IU/L	
Sodium	134-149 mEq/L	
Transferrin	>200 mg/dL	
Triglycerides	45-155 mg/dL	Fasted blood required
Urea nitrogen (BUN)	7-20 mg/dL	
Uric acid		
male	2.0-8.0 mg/dL	
female	2.0-7.5 mg/dL	
Cerebrospinal Fluid		
Glucose	50-70 mg/dL	
Protein		
adults and children	15-45 mg/dL	CSF obtained by lumbar puncture
newborn infants	60-90 mg/dL	

On CSF obtained by cisternal puncture: About 25 mg/dL

On CSF obtained by ventricular puncture: About 10 mg/dL

Note: Bloody specimen gives erroneously high value due to contamination with blood proteins

Urine

(24-hour specimen is required for all these tests unless specified)

Test	Values	Remarks
Amylase	32-641 units/L	The value is in units/L and **not** calculated for total volume
Amylase, fluid (random samples)		Interpretation of value left for physician, depends on the nature of fluid
Calcium	Depends upon dietary intake	
Creatine		
male	150 mg/24 h	Higher value on children and during pregnancy
female	250 mg/24 h	
Creatinine	1000-2000 mg/24 h	
Creatinine clearance (endogenous)		
male	85-125 mL/min	A blood sample must accompany urine specimen
female	75-115 mL/min	
Glucose	1 g/24 h	
5-hydroxyindoleacetic acid	2-8 mg/24 h	
Iron	0.15 mg/24 h	Acid washed container required
Magnesium	146-209 mg/24 h	
Osmolality	500-800 mOsm/kg	With normal fluid intake
Oxalate	10-40 mg/24 h	
Phosphate	400-1300 mg/24 h	
Potassium	25-120 mEq/24 h	Varies with diet; the interpretation of urine electrolytes and osmolality should be left for the physician
Sodium	40-220 mEq/24 h	
Porphobilinogen, qualitative	Negative	
Porphyrins, qualitative	Negative	
Proteins	0.05-0.1 g/24 h	
Salicylate	Negative	
Urea clearance	60-95 mL/min	A blood sample must accompany specimen
Urea N	10-40 g/24 h	Dependent on protein intake
Uric acid	250-750 mg/24 h	Dependent on diet and therapy

Automated Chemistry (CHEMISTRY A) *(continued)*

Test	Values	Remarks
Urobilinogen	0.5-3.5 mg/24 h	For qualitative determination on random urine, send sample to urinalysis section in Hematology Lab
Xylose absorption test		
children	16%-33% of ingested xylose	
adults	>4 g in 5 h	
Feces		
Fat, 3-day collection	<5 g/d	Value depends on fat intake of 100 g/d for 3 days preceding and during collection
Gastric Acidity		
Acidity, total, 12 h	10-60 mEq/L	Titrated at pH 7

Blood Gases

	Arterial	Capillary	Venous
pH	7.35-7.45	7.35-7.45	7.32-7.42
pCO_2 (mm Hg)	35-45	35-45	38-52
pO_2 (mm Hg)	70-100	60-80	24-48
HCO_3 (mEq/L)	19-25	19-25	19-25
TCO_2 (mEq/L)	19-29	19-29	23-33
O_2 saturation (%)	90-95	90-95	40-70
Base excess (mEq/L)	-5 to +5	-5 to +5	-5 to +5

HEMATOLOGY

Complete Blood Count

Age	Hgb (g/dL)	Hct (%)	RBC (mill/mm^3)	RDW
0-3 d	15.0-20.0	45-61	4.0-5.9	<18
1-2 wk	12.5-18.5	39-57	3.6-5.5	<17
1-6 mo	10.0-13.0	29-42	3.1-4.3	<16.5
7 mo to 2 y	10.5-13.0	33-38	3.7-4.9	<16
2-5 y	11.5-13.0	34-39	3.9-5.0	<15
5-8 y	11.5-14.5	35-42	4.0-4.9	<15
13-18 y	12.0-15.2	36-47	4.5-5.1	<14.5
Adult male	13.5-16.5	41-50	4.5-5.5	<14.5
Adult female	12.0-15.0	36-44	4.0-4.9	<14.5

Age	MCV (fL)	MCH (pg)	MCHC (%)	Plts (x 10^3/mm^3)
0-3 d	95-115	31-37	29-37	250-450
1-2 wk	86-110	28-36	28-38	250-450
1-6 mo	74-96	25-35	30-36	300-700
7 mo to 2 y	70-84	23-30	31-37	250-600
2-5 y	75-87	24-30	31-37	250-550
5-8 y	77-95	25-33	31-37	250-550
13-18 y	78-96	25-35	31-37	150-450
Adult male	80-100	26-34	31-37	150-450
Adult female	80-100	26-34	31-37	150-450

CALCULATIONS/CONVERSIONS/LABORATORY VALUES *(Continued)*

WBC and Diff

Age	WBC (x $10^3/mm^3$)	Segs	Bands	Lymphs	Monos
0-3 d	9.0-35.0	32-62	10-18	19-29	5-7
1-2 wk	5.0-20.0	14-34	6-14	36-45	6-10
1-6 mo	6.0-17.5	13-33	4-12	41-71	4-7
7 mo to 2 y	6.0-17.0	15-35	5-11	45-76	3-6
2-5 y	5.5-15.5	23-45	5-11	35-65	3-6
5-8 y	5.0-14.5	32-54	5-11	28-48	3-6
13-18 y	4.5-13.0	34-64	5-11	25-45	3-6
Adults	4.5-11.0	35-66	5-11	24-44	3-6

Segs = segmented neutrophils
Bands = band neutrophils
Lymphs = lymphocytes
Monos = monocytes

Age	Eosinophils	Basophils	Atypical Lymphs	No. of NRBCs
0-3 d	0-2	0-1	0-8	0-2
1-2 wk	0-2	0-1	0-8	0
1-6 mo	0-3	0-1	0-8	0
7 mo to 2 y	0-3	0-1	0-8	0
2-5 y	0-3	0-1	0-8	0
5-8 y	0-3	0-1	0-8	0
13-18 y	0-3	0-1	0-8	0
Adults	0-3	0-1	0-8	0

Erythrocyte Sedimentation Rates and Reticulocyte Counts

Sedimentation rate, Westergren	Children	0-20 mm/hour
	Adult male	0-15 mm/hour
	Adult female	0-20 mm/hour
Sedimentation rate, Wintrobe	Children	0-13 mm/hour
	Adult male	0-10 mm/hour
	Adult female	0-15 mm/hour
Reticulocyte count	Newborns	2%-6%
	1-6 mo	0%-2.8%
	Adults	0.5%-1.5%

LABORATORY REFERENCE VALUES FOR CHILDREN

Chemistry

Albumin	0-1 y	2-4 g/dL
	1 y to adult	3.5-5.5 g/dL
Ammonia	Newborns	90-150 μg/dL
	Children	40-120 μg/dL
	Adults	18-54 μg/dL
Amylase	Newborns	0-60 units/L
	Adults	30-110 units/L
Bilirubin, conjugated, direct	Newborns	<1.5 mg/dL
	1 mo to adult	0-0.5 mg/dL
Bilirubin, total	0-3 d	2-10 mg/dL
	1 mo to adult	0-1.5 mg/dL
Bilirubin, unconjugated, indirect		0.6-10.5 mg/dL
Calcium	Newborns	7-12 mg/dL
	0-2 y	8.8-11.2 mg/dL
	2 y to adult	9-11 mg/dL
Calcium, ionized, whole blood		4.4-5.4 mg/dL
Carbon dioxide, total		23-33 mEq/L
Chloride		95-105 mEq/L
Cholesterol	Newborns	45-170 mg/dL
	0-1 y	65-175 mg/dL
	1-20 y	120-230 mg/dL
Creatinine	0-1 y	≤0.6 mg/dL
	1 y to adult	0.5-1.5 mg/dL
Glucose	Newborns	30-90 mg/dL
	0-2 y	60-105 mg/dL
	Children to adults	70-110 mg/dL
Iron	Newborns	110-270 μg/dL
	Infants	30-70 μg/dL
	Children	55-120 μg/dL
	Adults	70-180 μg/dL
Iron binding	Newborns	59-175 μg/dL
	Infants	100-400 μg/dL
	Adults	250-400 μg/dL
Lactic acid, lactate		2-20 mg/dL
Lead, whole blood		<30 μg/dL
Lipase	Children	20-140 units/L
	Adults	0-190 units/L
Magnesium		1.5-2.5 mEq/L
Osmolality, serum		275-296 mOsm/kg
Osmolality, urine		50-1400 mOsm/kg
Phosphorus	Newborns	4.2-9 mg/dL
	6 wk to ≤18 mo	3.8-6.7 mg/dL
	18 mo to 3 y	2.9-5.9 mg/dL
	3-15 y	3.6-5.6 mg/dL
	>15 y	2.5-5 mg/dL
Potassium, plasma	Newborns	4.5-7.2 mEq/L
	2 d to 3 mo	4-6.2 mEq/L
	3 mo to 1 y	3.7-5.6 mEq/L
	1-16 y	3.5-5 mEq/L
Protein, total	0-2 y	4.2-7.4 g/dL
	>2 y	6-8 g/dL
Sodium		136-145 mEq/L
Triglycerides	Infants	0-171 mg/dL
	Children	20-130 mg/dL
	Adults	30-200 mg/dL
Urea nitrogen, blood	0-2 y	4-15 mg/dL
	2 y to adult	5-20 mg/dL
Uric acid	Male	3-7 mg/dL
	Female	2-6 mg/dL

CALCULATIONS/CONVERSIONS/LABORATORY VALUES *(Continued)*

Chemistry *(continued)*

Enzymes

Alanine aminotransferase (ALT)	0-2 mo	8-78 units/L
(SGPT)	>2 mo	8-36 units/L
Alkaline phosphatase (ALKP)	Newborns	60-130 units/L
	0-16 y	85-400 units/L
	>16 y	30-115 units/L
Aspartate aminotransferase (AST)	Infants	18-74 units/L
(SGOT)	Children	15-46 units/L
	Adults	5-35 units/L
Creatine kinase (CK)	Infants	20-200 units/L
	Children	10-90 units/L
	Adult male	0-206 units/L
	Adult female	0-175 units/L
Lactate dehydrogenase (LDH)	Newborns	290-501 units/L
	1 mo to 2 y	110-144 units/L
	>16 y	60-170 units/L

Blood Gases

	Arterial	Capillary	Venous
pH	7.35-7.45	7.35-7.45	7.32-7.42
pCO_2 (mm Hg)	35-45	35-45	38-52
pO_2 (mm Hg)	70-100	60-80	24-48
HCO_3 (mEq/L)	19-25	19-25	19-25
TCO_2 (mEq/L)	19-29	19-29	23-33
O_2 saturation (%)	90-95	90-95	40-70
Base excess (mEq/L)	-5 to +5	-5 to +5	-5 to +5

Thyroid Function Tests

T_4 (thyroxine)	1-7 d	10.1-20.9 μg/dL
	8-14 d	9.8-16.6 μg/dL
	1 mo to 1 y	5.5-16 μg/dL
	>1 y	4-12 μg/dL
FTI	1-3 d	9.3-26.6
	1-4 wk	7.6-20.8
	1-4 mo	7.4-17.9
	4-12 mo	5.1-14.5
	1-6 y	5.7-13.3
	>6 y	4.8-14
T_3 by RIA	Newborns	100-470 ng/dL
	1-5 y	100-260 ng/dL
	5-10 y	90-240 ng/dL
	10 y to adult	70-210 ng/dL
T_3 uptake		35%-45%
TSH	Cord	3-22 μU/mL
	1-3 d	<40 μU/mL
	3-7 d	<25 μU/mL
	>7 d	0-10 μU/mL

MILLIEQUIVALENT AND MILLIMOLE CALCULATIONS & CONVERSIONS

DEFINITIONS & CALCULATIONS

Definitions

mole	=	gram molecular weight of a substance (aka molar weight)
millimole (mM)	=	milligram molecular weight of a substance (a millimole is 1/1000 of a mole)
equivalent weight	=	gram weight of a substance which will combine with or replace one gram (one mole) of hydrogen; an equivalent weight can be determined by dividing the molar weight of a substance by its ionic valence
milliequivalent (mEq)	=	milligram weight of a substance which will combine with or replace one milligram (one millimole) of hydrogen (a milliequivalent is 1/1000 of an equivalent)

Calculations

$$\text{moles} = \frac{\text{weight of a substance (grams)}}{\text{molecular weight of that substance (grams)}}$$

$$\text{millimoles} = \frac{\text{weight of a substance (milligrams)}}{\text{molecular weight of that substance (milligrams)}}$$

$$\text{equivalents} = \text{moles x valence of ion}$$

$$\text{milliequivalents} = \text{millimoles x valence of ion}$$

$$\text{moles} = \frac{\text{equivalents}}{\text{valence of ion}}$$

$$\text{millimoles} = \frac{\text{milliequivalents}}{\text{valence of ion}}$$

$$\text{millimoles} = \text{moles x 1000}$$

$$\text{milliequivalents} = \text{equivalents x 1000}$$

Note: Use of equivalents and milliequivalents is valid only for those substances which have fixed ionic valences (eg, sodium, potassium, calcium, chlorine, magnesium bromine, etc). For substances with variable ionic valences (eg, phosphorous), a reliable equivalent value cannot be determined. In these instances, one should calculate millimoles (which are fixed and reliable) rather than milliequivalents.

MILLIEQUIVALENT CONVERSIONS

To convert mg/100 mL to mEq/L the following formula may be used:

$$\frac{\text{(mg/100 mL) x 10 x valence}}{\text{atomic weight}} = \text{mEq/L}$$

To convert mEq/L to mg/100 mL the following formula may be used:

$$\frac{\text{(mEq/L) x atomic weight}}{\text{10 x valence}} = \text{mg/100 mL}$$

To convert mEq/L to volume of percent of a gas the following formula may be used:

$$\frac{\text{(mEq/L) x 22.4}}{10} = \text{volume percent}$$

Valences and Atomic Weights of Selected Ions

Substance	Electrolyte	Valence	Molecular Wt
Calcium	Ca^{++}	2	40
Chloride	Cl^{-}	1	35.5
Magnesium	Mg^{++}	2	24
Phosphate	HPO_4^{--} (80%)	1.8	96*
pH = 7.4	$H_2PO_4^{-}$ (20%)	1.8	96*
Potassium	K^{+}	1	39
Sodium	Na^{+}	1	23
Sulfate	SO_4^{--}	2	96*

*The molecular weight of phosphorus only is 31, and sulfur only is 32.

CALCULATIONS/CONVERSIONS/LABORATORY VALUES *(Continued)*

Approximate Milliequivalents — Weights of Selected Ions

Salt	mEq/g Salt	Mg Salt/mEq
Calcium carbonate [$CaCO_3$]	20	50
Calcium chloride [$CaCl_2 \bullet 2H_2O$]	14	74
Calcium gluceptate [$Ca(C_7H_{13}O_8)_2$]	4	245
Calcium gluconate [$Ca(C_6H_{11}O_7)_2 \bullet H_2O$]	5	224
Calcium lactate [$Ca(C_3H_5O_3)_2 \bullet 5H_2O$]	7	154
Magnesium gluconate [$Mg(C_6H_{11}O_7)_2 \bullet H_2O$]	5	216
Magnesium oxide [MgO]	50	20
Magnesium sulfate [$MgSO_4$]	17	60
Magnesium sulfate [$MgSO_4 \bullet 7H_2O$]	8	123
Potassium acetate [$K(C_2H_3O_2)$]	10	98
Potassium chloride [KCl]	13	75
Potassium citrate [$K_3(C_6H_5O_7) \bullet H_2O$]	9	108
Potassium iodide [KI]	6	166
Sodium acetate [$Na(C_2H_3O_2)$]	12	82
Sodium acetate [$Na(C_2H_3O_2) \bullet 3H_2O$]	7	136
Sodium bicarbonate [$NaHCO_3$]	12	84
Sodium chloride [NaCl]	17	58
Sodium citrate [$Na_3(C_6H_5O_7) \bullet 2H_2O$]	10	98
Sodium iodine [NaI]	7	150
Sodium lactate [$Na(C_3H_5O_3)$]	9	112
Zinc sulfate [$ZnSO_4 \bullet 7H_2O$]	7	144

CORRECTED SODIUM

Corrected Na^+ = measured Na^+ + [1.5 x (glucose – 150 divided by 100)]

Note: Do not correct for glucose <150.

WATER DEFICIT

Water deficit = 0.6 x body weight [1 – (140 divided by Na^+)]

Note: Body weight is estimated weight in kg when fully hydrated; **Na^+** is serum or plasma sodium. Use corrected Na^+ if necessary. Consult medical references for recommendations for replacement of deficit.

TOTAL SERUM CALCIUM CORRECTED FOR ALBUMIN LEVEL

[(Normal albumin – patient's albumin) x 0.8] + patient's measured total calcium

ACID-BASE ASSESSMENT

Henderson-Hasselbalch Equation

$$pH = 6.1 + \log (HCO_3^- / (0.03)(pCO_2))$$

Alveolar Gas Equation

PIO_2 = FiO_2 x (total atmospheric pressure – vapor pressure of H_2O at 37°C)

= FiO_2 x (760 mm Hg – 47 mm Hg)

PAO_2 = $PIO_2 - PACO_2 / R$

Alveolar/arterial oxygen gradient = $PAO_2 - PaO_2$

Normal ranges:

Children	15-20 mm Hg
Adults	20-25 mm Hg

where:

PIO_2 = Oxygen partial pressure of inspired gas (mm Hg) (150 mm Hg in room air at sea level)

FiO_2	=	Fractional pressure of oxygen in inspired gas (0.21 in room air)
PAO_2	=	Alveolar oxygen partial pressure
$PACO_2$	=	Alveolar carbon dioxide partial pressure
PaO_2	=	Arterial oxygen partial pressure
R	=	Respiratory exchange quotient (typically 0.8, increases with high carbohydrate diet, decreases with high fat diet)

Acid-Base Disorders

Acute metabolic acidosis (<12 h duration):

$$PaCO_2 \text{ expected} = 1.5\ (HCO_3^-) + 8 \pm 2$$

or

$$\text{expected change in pCO} = (1\text{-}1.5) \times \text{change in } HCO_3^-$$

Acute metabolic alkalosis (<12 h duration):

$$\text{expected change in } pCO_2 = (0.5\text{-}1) \times \text{change in } HCO_3^-$$

Acute respiratory acidosis (<6 h duration):

$$\text{expected change in } HCO_3^- = 0.1 \times pCO_2$$

Acute respiratory acidosis (>6 h duration):

$$\text{expected change in } HCO_3^- = 0.4 \times \text{change in } pCO_2$$

Acute respiratory alkalosis (<6 h duration):

$$\text{expected change in } HCO_3^- = 0.2 \times \text{change in } pCO_2$$

Acute respiratory alkalosis (>6 h duration):

$$\text{expected change in } HCO_3^- = 0.5 \times \text{change in } pCO_2$$

ACID-BASE EQUATION

H^+ (in mEq/L) = (24 x $PaCO_2$) divided by HCO_3^-

Aa GRADIENT

Aa gradient [(713)(FiO_2 – ($PaCO_2$ divided by 0.8))] – PaO_2

Aa gradient	=	alveolar-arterial oxygen gradient
FiO_2	=	inspired oxygen (expressed as a fraction)
$PaCO_2$	=	arterial partial pressure carbon dioxide (mm Hg)
PaO_2	=	arterial partial pressure oxygen (mm Hg)

BICARBONATE DEFICIT

HCO_3^- deficit = (0.4 x wt in kg) x (HCO_3^- desired – HCO_3^- measured)

Note: In clinical practice, the calculated quantity may differ markedly from the actual amount of bicarbonate needed or that which may be safely administered.

RETICULOCYTE INDEX

(% retic divided by 2) x (patient's Hct divided by normal Hct) or (% retic divided by 2) x (patient's Hgb divided by normal Hgb)

Normal index: 1.0

Good marrow response: 2.0-6.0

CALCULATIONS/CONVERSIONS/LABORATORY VALUES *(Continued)*

Peak and Trough Guidelines

Drug	When to Sample	Therapeutic Levels*	Usual Half-Life	Steady State (Ideal Sampling Time)	Potentially Toxic Levels*
Antibiotics					
Gentamicin Tobramycin	30 min after 30 min infusion Trough: <0.5 h before next dose	Peak: 4-10 mcg/mL Trough: <2.0 mcg/mL	2 h	15 h	Peak: >12 mcg/mL Trough: >2 mcg/mL
Amikacin		Peak: 20-35 mcg/mL Trough: <8 mcg/mL	2 h	15 h	Peak: >35 mcg/mL Trough: >8 mcg/mL
Vancomycin	Peak: 1 h after 1 h infusion Trough: <0.5 h before next dose	Peak: 30-40 mcg/mL Trough: 5-10 mcg/mL	6-8 h	24 h	Peak: >80 mcg/mL Trough: >13 mcg/mL
Anticonvulsants					
Carbamazepine	Trough: Just before next oral dose In combination with other anticonvulsants	4-12 mcg/mL 4-8 mcg/mL	15-20 h	7-12 d	>12 mcg/mL
Ethosuximide	Trough: Just before next oral dose	40-100 mcg/mL	30-60 h	10-13 d	>100 mcg/mL
Phenobarbital	Trough: Just before next dose	15-40 mcg/mL	40-120 h	20 d	>40 mcg/mL
Phenytoin Free phenytoin	Trough: Just before next dose Draw at same time as total level	10-20 mcg/mL 1-2 mcg/mL	Concentration dependent	5-14 d	>20 mcg/mL
Primidone	Trough: Just before next dose (**Note:** Primidone is metabolized to phenobarb, order levels separately)	5-12 mcg/mL	10-12 h	5 d	>12 mcg/mL
Valproic acid	Trough: Just before next dose	50-100 mcg/mL	5-20 h	4 d	>150 mcg/mL
Bronchodilators					
Aminophylline (I.V.)	18-24 h after starting or changing a maintenance dose given as a constant infusion	10-20 mcg/mL	Nonsmoking adult: 8 h Children and smoking adults: 4 h	2 d	>20 mcg/mL
Theophylline (P.O.)	Peak levels: Not recommended Trough level: Just before next dose	10-20 mcg/mL		2 d	
Cardiovascular Agents					
Digoxin	Trough: Just before next dose (levels drawn earlier than 6 h after a dose will be artificially elevated)	0.5-2 ng/mL	36 h	5 d	>2 ng/mL

Peak and Trough Guidelines *(continued)*

Drug	When to Sample	Therapeutic Levels*	Usual Half-Life	Steady State (Ideal Sampling Time)	Potentially Toxic Levels*
Lidocaine	Steady-state levels are usually achieved after 6-12 h	1.2-5.0 mcg/mL	1.5 h	5-10 h	>6 mcg/mL
Procainamide	Trough: Just before next oral dose I.V.: 6-12 h after infusion started Combined procainamide plus NAPA	4-10 mcg/mL NAPA: 6-10 h 5-30 mcg/mL	Procain: 2.7-5 h >30 (NAPA + procain)	20 h	>10 mcg/mL
Quinidine	Trough: Just before next oral dose	2-5 mcg/mL	6 h	24 h	>10 mcg/mL
Warfarin	Same time of day each draw	See Warfarin monograph	42 h	5-7 d	See Warfarin monograph
Other Agents					
Amitriptyline plus nortriptyline	Trough: Just before next dose	120-250 ng/mL		4-80 d	
Cyclosporine	Trough: Just before next dose	Months post-transplant: Plasma: 50-150 ng/mL Whole blood: 150-450 ng/mL		Variable	
Desipramine	Trough: Just before next dose	50-300 ng/mL	12-54 h	3-11 d	
Imipramine plus desipramine	Trough: Just before next dose	150-300 ng/mL	9-24 h	2-5 d	
Lithium	Trough: Just before next dose	0.6-1.2 mEq/mL (acute)	18-20 h	2-7 d	>3 mEq/mL
Nortriptyline	Trough: Just before next dose	50-140 ng/mL		4-19 d	

*Due to methodology differences, reference ranges may vary from laboratory to laboratory; check with the laboratory service used for their appropriate levels.

CALCULATIONS/CONVERSIONS/LABORATORY VALUES *(Continued)*

PEDIATRIC DOSAGE ESTIMATIONS

Dosage Estimations Based on Weight:

Augsberger's rule:

(1.5 x weight in kg + 10) % of adult dose = child's approximate dose

Clark's rule:

$$\frac{\text{weight (in pounds)}}{150} \times \text{adult dose} = \text{child's approximate dose}$$

Dosage Estimations Based on Age:

Augsberger's rule:

(4 x age in years + 20) % of adult dose = child's approximate dose

Bastedo's rule:

$$\frac{\text{age in years} + 3}{30} \times \text{adult dose} = \text{child's approximate dose}$$

Cowling's rule:

$$\frac{\text{age at next birthday (in years)}}{24} \times \text{adult dose} = \text{child's approximate dose}$$

Dilling's rule:

$$\frac{\text{age (in years)}}{20} \times \text{adult dose} = \text{child's approximate dose}$$

Fried's rule for infants (younger than 1 year):

$$\frac{\text{age (in months)}}{150} \times \text{adult dose} = \text{infant's approximate dose}$$

Young's rule:

$$\frac{\text{age (in years)}}{\text{age} + 12} \times \text{adult dose} = \text{child's approximate dose}$$

ANGIOTENSIN AGENTS

Comparisons of Indications and Adult Dosages

Drug	Hypertension	CHF	Renal Dysfunction	Dialyzable	Strengths (mg)
Benazepril (Lotensin®)	20-80 mg per day qd-bid Maximum: 80 mg qd	Not FDA approved LV dysfunction (post-MI): 20-40 mg/day in 1-2 divided doses	Cl_{cr} <30 mL/min: 5 mg/day initially Maximum: 40 mg qd	Yes	Tablets 5, 10, 20, 40
Candesartan[1] (Atacand®)	8-32 mg qd qd-bid Maximum: 32 mg qd	Not FDA approved	No adjustment necessary	No	Tablets 4, 8, 16, 32
Captopril (Capoten®)	25-150 mg qd bid-tid Maximum: 450 mg qd	6.25-100 mg tid Maximum: 450 mg qd	Cl_{cr} 10-50 mL/min: 75% of usual dose Cl_{cr} <10 mL/min: 50% of usual dose	Yes	Tablets 12.5, 25, 50, 100
Enalapril (Vasotec®)	5-40 mg qd qd-bid Maximum: 40 mg qd	2.5-20 mg bid Maximum: 20 mg bid	Cl_{cr} 30-80 mL/min: 5 mg/day initially Cl_{cr} <30 mL/min: 2.5 mg/day initially	Yes	Tablets 2.5, 5, 10, 20
Enalaprilat[2]	0.625 mg, 1.25 mg, 2.5 mg q6h Maximum: 5 mg q6h	Not FDA approved	Cl_{cr} <30 mL/min: 0.625 mg	Yes	2.5 mg/2 mL vial
Eprosartan[1] (Teveten®)	400-800 mg qd qd-bid	Not FDA approved	No dosage adjustment necessary	Unknown	Tablets 400, 600
Fosinopril (Monopril®)	10-40 mg qd Maximum: 80 mg qd	10-40 mg qd	No dosage reduction necessary	Not well dialyzed	Tablets 10, 20, 40
Irbesartan[1] (Avapro®)	150 mg qd Maximum: 300 mg qd	Not FDA approved	No dosage reduction necessary	No	Tablets 75, 150, 300
Lisinopril (Prinivil®, Zestril®)	10-40 mg qd Maximum: 80 mg qd	5-20 mg qd	Cl_{cr} 10-30 mL/min: 5 mg/day initially Cl_{cr} <10 mL/min: 2.5 mg/day initially	Yes	Tablets 5, 10, 20, 40
Losartan[1] (Cozaar®)	25-100 mg qd or bid	Not FDA approved	No adjustment necessary	No	Tablets 25, 50
Moexipril (Univasc®)	7.5-30 mg qd qd-bid Maximum: 30 mg qd	Not FDA approved	Cl_{cr} <30 mL/min: 3.75 mg/day initially Maximum: 15 mg/day	Unknown	Tablets 7.5, 15
Olmesartan (Benicar™)	5-40 mg qd	Not FDA approved	No adjustment necessary	Unknown	Tablets 5, 20, 40
Perindopril (Aceon®)	4-16 mg qd	4 mg qd (Not FDA approved)	Cl_{cr} 30-60 mL/min: 2 mg qd Cl_{cr} 15-29 mL/min: 2 mg qod Cl_{cr} <15 mL/min: 2 mg on dialysis days	Yes	Tablets 2, 4, 8
Quinapril (Accupril®)	10-80 mg qd qd-bid	5-20 mg bid	Cl_{cr} 30-60 mL/min: 5 mg/day initially Cl_{cr} <10 mL/min: 2.5 mg qd initially	Not well dialyzed	Tablets 5, 10, 20, 40

ANGIOTENSIN AGENTS *(Continued)*

Comparisons of Indications and Adult Dosages *(continued)*

Drug	Hypertension	CHF	Renal Dysfunction	Dialyzable	Strengths (mg)
Ramipril (Altace™)	2.5-20 mg qd qd-bid	2.5-20 mg qd	Cl_{cr} <40 mL/min: 1.25 mg/day Maximum: 5 mg qd	Unknown	Capsules 1.25, 2.5, 5
Telmisartan[1] (Micardis®)	20-80 mg qd	Not FDA approved	No dosage reduction necessary	No	Tablets 20, 40, 80
Trandolapril (Mavik®)	2-4 mg qd maximum: 8 mg/d qd-bid	Not FDA approved	Cl_{cr} <30 mL/min: 0.5 mg/day initially	No	Tablets 1 mg, 2 mg, 4 mg
Valsartan[1] (Diovan®)	80-160 mg qd	Not FDA approved	Decrease dose only if Cl_{cr} <10 mL/minute	No	Tablets 80, 160, 320

Dosage is based on 70 kg adult with normal hepatic and renal function.

[1]Angiotensin II antagonist.

[2]Enalaprilat is the only available ACE inhibitor in a parenteral formulation.

Comparative Pharmacokinetics

Drug	Prodrug	Absorption (%)	Serum $t_{1/2}$ (h) Normal Renal Function	Serum Protein Binding (%)	Elimination	Onset of BP Lowering Action (h)	Peak BP Lowering Effects (h)	Duration of BP Lowering Effects (h)
Benazepril	Yes	37		~97	Renal (32%), biliary (~12%)	1	2-4	24
Benazeprilat			10-11 (effective)	~95%				
Captopril	No	60-75 (fasting)	1.9 (elimination)	25-30	Renal	0.25-0.5	1-1.5	~6
Enalapril	Yes	55-75	2	50-60	Renal (60%-80%), fecal	1	4-6	12-24
Enalaprilat			11 (effective)					
Fosinopril		36			Renal (~50%), biliary (~50%)	1		24
Fosinoprilat			12 (effective)	>99				
Moexipril	Yes		1	90	Fecal (53%), renal (8%)		1-2	>24
Moexiprilat			2-10	50				
Perindopril	Yes		1.5-3	60	Renal		3-7	
Perindoprilat			3-10 (effective)	10-20				
Quinapril	Yes	>60	0.8	97	Renal (~60%) as metabolite, fecal	1	2-4	24
Quinaprilat			2					
Ramipril	Yes	50-60	1-2	73	Renal (60%), fecal (40%)	1-2	3-6	24
Ramiprilat			13-17 (effective)	56				
Trandolapril	Yes		6	80	Renal (33%), fecal (66%)	1-2	6	≥24
Trandolaprilat			10	65-94				

ANGIOTENSIN AGENTS *(Continued)*

Comparative Pharmacokinetics of Angiotensin II Receptor Antagonists

	Candesartan (Atacand®)	Eprosartan (Teveten®)	Irbesartan (Avapro®)	Losartan (Cozaar®)	Telmisartan (Micardis®)	Valsartan (Diovan™)
Prodrug	Yes[1]	No	No	Yes[2]	No	No
Time to peak	3-4 h	1-2 h	1.5-2	1 h / 3-4 h[2]	0.5-1 h	2-4 h
Bioavailability	15%	13%	60%-80%	33%	42%-58%	25%
Food – area-under-the-curve	No effect	No effect	No effect	9%-10%	9.6%-20%	9%-40%
Elimination half-life	9 h	5-9 h	11-15 h	1.5-2 h / 6-9 h[2]	24 h	6 h
Elimination altered in renal dysfunction	Yes[3]	No	No	No	No	No
Precautions in severe renal dysfunction	Yes	Yes	Yes	Yes	Yes	Yes
Elimination altered in hepatic dysfunction	No	No	No	Yes	Yes	Yes
Precautions in hepatic dysfunction	No	Yes	No	No	Yes	No
Protein binding	>99%	98%	90%	~99%	>99.5%	95%

[1]Candesartan cilexetil: Active metabolite candesartan.

[2]Losartan: Active metabolite E-3174.

[3]Dosage adjustments are not necessary.

ANTIARRHYTHMIC DRUGS

Antiarrhythmic Agents and Their Indications/Adverse Effects

Drug(s)	Indication	Route of Administration	Adverse Effects
Acebutolol	VT, VF	P.O.	Bradycardia, hypotension, fatigue
Adenosine	SVT, PSVT	I.V.	Flushing, dizziness, bradycardia, syncope
Amiodarone	VT	P.O.	CNS, GI, thyroid, pulmonary fibrosis, liver, corneal deposits
Bretylium	VT, VF	I.V.	GI, orthostatic hypotension, CNS
Digoxin	AF, PSVT	P.O./I.V.	GI, CNS, arrhythmias
Diltiazem	AF, PSVT	P.O./I.V.	Hypotension, GI, liver
Disopyramide	AF, VT	P.O.	Anticholinergic effects, CHF
Dofetilide	SVT	P.O.	CNS, arrhythmias (torsade de pointes)
Esmolol	VT, SVT	I.V.	CHF, CNS, lupus-like syndrome, hypotension, bradycardia, bronchospasm
Flecainide	VT	P.O.	CHF, GI, CNS, blurred vision
Ibutilide	AF, VT, VF	I.V.	Torsade de pointes, hypotension, branch bundle block, AV block, nausea, headache
Lidocaine	VT, VF, PVC	I.V.	CNS, GI
Magnesium	VT, VF	I.V.	Hypotension, CNS, hypothermia, myocardial depression
Mexiletine	VT	P.O.	GI, CNS
Moricizine	VT	P.O.	Dizziness, nausea, rash, seizures
Procainamide	AF, VT, WPW	P.O./I.V.	GI, CNS, lupus, fever, hematological, anticholinergic effects
Propafenone	VT	P.O.	GI, blurred vision, dizziness
Propranolol	SVT, VT, PVC, digoxin toxicity	P.O./I.V.	CHF, bradycardia, hypotension, CNS, fatigue
Quinidine	AF, PSVT, VT, WPW	P.O./I.V.	Hypotension, GI, thrombocytopenia, cinchonism
Sotalol	AF, VT	P.O.	Bradycardia, hypotension, CHF, CNS, fatigue
Tocainide	VT	P.O.	GI, CNS, pulmonary, agranulocytosis
Verapamil	AF, PSVT	P.O./I.V.	Hypotension, CHF, bradycardia, vertigo, constipation

AF = atrial fibrillation; PSVT = paroxysmal supraventricular tachycardia; VT = ventricular tachycardia; WPW = Wolf-Parkinson-White arrhythmias; VF = ventricular fibrillation; SVT = supraventricular tachycardia.

ANTIARRHYTHMIC DRUGS *(Continued)*

Vaughan Williams Classification of Antiarrhythmic Drugs Based on Cardiac Effects

Type	Drug(s)	Conduction Velocity*	Refractory Period	Automaticity
I	Moricizine†	0/↓	↓	↓
Ia	Disopyramide Procainamide Quinidine	↓	↑	↓
Ib	Lidocaine Mexiletine Tocainide	0/↓	↓	↓
Ic	Flecainide Indecainide Propafenone‡	↓↓	0	↓
II	Beta-blockers	0	0	↓
III	Amiodarone Bretylium Dofetilide Ibutilide Sotalol‡	0	↑↑	0
IV	Diltiazem Verapamil§	↓	↑	↓

*Variables for normal tissue models in ventricular tissue.

†Also has type Ia action to decrease conduction velocity more than most type Ib.

‡Also has type II, beta-blocking action.

§Variables for SA and AV nodal tissue only.

ANTIDEPRESSANT AGENTS

Comparison of Usual Dosage, Mechanism of Action, and Adverse Effects

Drug	Initial Dose	Usual Dosage (mg/d)	Dosage Forms	Adverse Effects						Comments
				ACH	Drowsiness	Orthostatic Hypotension	Cardiac Arrhythmias	GI Distress	Weight Gain	
Tricyclic Antidepressants & Related Compounds[1]										
Amitriptyline (Elavil®, Vanatrip®)	25-75 mg qhs	100-300	T, I	4+	4+	4+	3+	1	4+	Also used in chronic pain, migraine, and as a hypnotic; contraindicated with cisapride
Amoxapine	50 mg bid	100-400	T	2+	2+	2+	2+	0	2+	May cause extrapyramidal symptom (EPS)
Clomipramine[2] (Anafranil®)	25-75 mg qhs	100-250	C	4+	4+	2+	3+	1+	4+	Approved for OCD
Desipramine (Norpramin®)	25-75 mg qhs	100-300	T	1+	2+	2+	2+	0	1+	Blood levels useful for therapeutic monitoring
Doxepin (Sinequan®, Zonalon®)	25-75 mg qhs	100-300	C, L	3+	4+	2+	2+	0	4+	
Imipramine (Tofranil®, Tofranil-PM®)	25-75 mg qhs	100-300	T, C	3+	3+	4+	3+	1+	4+	Blood levels useful for therapeutic monitoring
Maprotiline (Ludiomil®)	25-75 mg qhs	100-225	T	2+	3+	2+	2+	0	2+	
Nortriptyline (Aventyl®, Pamelor®)	25-50 mg qhs	50-150	C, L	2+	2+	1+	2+	0	1+	Blood levels useful for therapeutic monitoring
Protriptyline (Vivactil®)	15 mg qAM	15-60	T	2+	1+	2+	3+	1+	1+	
Trimipramine (Surmontil®)	25-75 mg qhs	100-300	C	4+	4+	3+	3+	0	4+	
Selective Serotonin Reuptake Inhibitors[3]										
Citalopram (Celexa™)	20 mg qAM	20-60	T	0	0	0	0	3+[4]	1+	
Escitalopram (Lexpro™)	10 mg qAM	10-20	T	0	0	0	0	3+	1+	
Fluoxetine (Prozac®, Prozac® Weekly™, Sarafem™)	10-20 mg qAM	20-80	C, L, T	0	0	0	0	3+[4]	1+	CYP2B6 and 2D6 inhibitor

ANTIDEPRESSANT AGENTS *(Continued)*

Comparison of Usual Dosage, Mechanism of Action, and Adverse Effects *(continued)*

Drug	Initial Dose	Usual Dosage (mg/d)	Dosage Forms	Adverse Effects						Comments
				ACH	Drowsiness	Orthostatic Hypotension	Cardiac Arrhythmias	GI Distress	Weight Gain	
Fluvoxamine (Luvox®)[1]	50 mg qhs	100-300	T	0	0	0	0	3+[4]	1+	Contraindicated with pimozide, thioridazine, mesoridazine, CYP1A2, 2B6, and 2C19 inhibitors
Paroxetine (Paxil®, Paxil® CR™)	10-20 mg qAM	20-50	T, L	1+	1+	0	0	3+[4]	2+	CYP2D6 and 2B6 inhibitor
Sertraline (Zoloft®)	25-50 mg qAM	50-200	T	0	0	0	0	3+[4]	1+	CYP2B6 and 2C19 inhibitor
Dopamine-Reuptake Blocking Compounds										
Bupropion (Wellbutrin®, Wellbutrin SR®, Zyban®)	100 mg bid-tid IR[5] 150 mg qAM-bid SR[6]	300-450[7]	T	0	0	0	1+	1+	0	Contraindicated with seizures, bulimia, and anorexia; low incidence of sexual dysfunction
Serotonin/Norepinephrine Reuptake Inhibitors[8]										
Venlafaxine (Effexor®, Effexor® XR)	25 mg bid-tid IR 37.5 mg qd XR	75-375	T	1+	1+	0	1+	3+[4]	0	High-dose is useful to treat refractory depression
5HT2 Receptor Antagonist Properties										
Nefazodone (Serzone®)	100 mg bid	300-600	T	1+	1+	0	0	1+	0	Contraindicated with carbamazepine, pimozide, astemizole, cisapride, and terfenadine; caution with triazolam and alprazolam; low incidence of sexual dysfunction
Trazodone (Desyrel®)	50 mg tid	150-600	T	0	4+	3+	1+	1+	2+	
Noradrenergic Antagonist										
Mirtazapine (Remeron®, Remeron® SolTab™)	15 mg qhs	15-45	T	1+	3+	0	0	0	3+	Dose >15 mg/d less sedating, low incidence of sexual dysfunction

Comparison of Usual Dosage, Mechanism of Action, and Adverse Effects *(continued)*

Drug	Initial Dose	Usual Dosage (mg/d)	Dosage Forms	Adverse Effects						Comments
				ACH	Drowsiness	Orthostatic Hypotension	Cardiac Arrhythmias	GI Distress	Weight Gain	
Monoamine Oxidase Inhibitors										
Phenelzine (Nardil®)	15 mg tid	15-90	T	2+	2+	2+	1+	1+	3+	Diet must be low in tyramine; contraindicated with sympathomimetics and other antidepressants
Tranylcypromine (Parnate®)	10 mg bid	10-60	T	2+	1+	2+	1+	1+	2+	

Key: ACH = anticholinergic effects (dry mouth, blurred vision, urinary retention, constipation); 0 - 4+ = absent or rare - relatively common. T = tablet, L = liquid, I = injectable, C = capsule; IR = immediate release, SR = sustained release.

[1]**Important note:** A 1-week supply taken all at once in a patient receiving the maximum dose can be fatal.

[2]Not approved by FDA for depression. Approved for OCD.

[3]Flat dose response curve, headache, nausea, and sexual dysfunction are common side effects for SSRIs.

[4]Nausea is usually mild and transient.

[5]IR: 100 mg bid, may be increased to 100 mg tid no sooner than 3 days after beginning therapy.

[6]SR: 150 mg qAM, may be increased to 150 mg bid as early as day 4 of dosing.

[7]To minimize seizure risk, do not exceed IR 150 mg/dose or SR 200 mg/dose.

[8]Do not use with sibutramine; relatively safe in overdose.

ANTIDIABETIC ORAL AGENTS COMPARISON

Contraindications to Therapy and Potential Adverse Effects of Oral Antidiabetic Agents

	Sulfonylureas/ Insulin Secretagogues	Metformin	Acarbose/ Miglitol	Pioglitazone/ Rosiglitazone
Contraindications				
Insulin dependency	A	A	A*	
Pregnancy/lactation	A	A	A	
Hypersensitivity to the agent	A	A	A	A
Hepatic impairment	R	A	R	A
Renal impairment	R	A	R	
Congestive heart failure		A		R
Chronic lung disease		A		
Peripheral vascular disease		A		
Steroid-induced diabetes	R	R		
Inflammatory bowel disease		A	A	
Major recurrent illness	R	A		
Surgery	R	A		
Alcoholism	R	A		A
Adverse Effects				
Hypoglycemia	Yes	No	No	No
Body weight gain	Yes	No	No	Yes
Hypersensitivity	Yes	No	No	No
Drug interactions	Yes	No	No	Yes/No
Lactic acidosis	No	Yes	No	No
Gastrointestinal disturbances	No	Yes	Yes	No

*Can be used in conjunction with insulin. A = absolute; R = relative.

Approved Indications for Thiazolidinedione Derivatives

Indication	Pioglitazone (Actos®)	Rosiglitazone (Avandia®)
Monotherapy		
	X	X
Combination Therapy - Dual Therapy		
Combination with sulfonylureas	X	X
Combination therapy with Glucophage® (metformin)	X	X
Combination therapy with insulin	X	–
Combination Therapy - Triple Therapy		
Combination therapy with sulfonylureas and Glucophage® (metformin)	–	–

Comparative Lipid Effects

Parameter	Pioglitazone (Actos®)	Rosiglitazone (Avandia®)
LDL	No significant change	↑ up to 12.1%
HDL	↑ up to 13%	↑ up to 18.5%
Total Cholesterol	No significant change	↑
Total Cholesterol/HDL Ratio	–	–
LDL/HDL Ratio	–	No change
Triglycerides	↓ up to 28%	Variable effects

ANTIMIGRAINE DRUGS

5-HT_1 Receptor Agonists: Pharmacokinetic Differences

Pharmacokinetic Parameter	Almotriptan (Axert™)	Frovatriptan (Frova™)	Naratriptan (Amerge®)	Rizatriptan (Maxalt®, Maxalt-MLT™)		Sumatriptan (Imitrex®)			Zolmitriptan (Zomig®, Zomig-ZMT™)	
	Oral (6.25 mg)	Oral	Oral	Tablets	Disintegrating Tablets	S.C. (6 mg)	Oral (100 mg)	Nasal (20 mg)	Oral (5 mg)	Oral (10 mg)
Onset	<60 min	<2 h	1-3 h	30-120 min	30-120 min	10 min	30-60 min	<60 min	45 min	
Duration	Short	Long	Long	Short	Short	Short	Short	Short	Short	
Time to peak serum concentration (h)	1-3	2-4	2-4	1-1.5	1.6-2.5	5-20	1.5-2.5	1	1.5	2-3.5
Average bioavailability (%)	70	20-30	70	45	—	96	14	17	40-46	46-49
Volume of distribution (L)	180-200	210-280	170	110-140	110-140	170	170	NA	—	402
Half-life (h)	3-4	26	6	2-3	2-3	2	2-2.5[1]	2	2.8-3.4	2.5-3.7
Fraction excreted unchanged in urine (%)	40	32	50	14	14	22	22	—	8	8

[1]With extended dosing the half-life extends to 7 hours.

ANTIPSYCHOTIC AGENTS

Antipsychotic Agent	Dosage Forms	I.M./P.O. Potency	Equiv. Dosages (approx) (mg)	Usual Adult Daily Maint. Dose (mg)	Sedation (Incidence)	Extrapyramidal Side Effects	Anticholinergic Side Effects	Cardiovascular Side Effects	Comments
Chlorpromazine (Thorazine®)	Cap, Conc, Inj, Supp, Syr, Tab	4:1	100	200-1000	High	Moderate	Moderate	Moderate/high	
Clozapine (Clozaril®)	Tab		50	75-900	High	Very Low	High	High	~1% incidence of agranulocytosis; weekly-biweekly CBC required; potential for weight gain, lipid abnormalities, and diabetes
Fluphenazine (Permitil®, Prolixin®, Prolixin Decanoate®, Prolixin Enanthate®)	Conc, Elix, Inj, Tab	2:1	2	0.5-20	Low	High	Low	Low	
Haloperidol (Haldol®, Haldol® Decanoate)	Conc, Inj, Tab	2:1	2	0.5-20	Low	High	Low	Low	
Loxapine (Loxitane®, Loxitane® C, Loxitane® I.M.)	Cap, Conc, Inj		10	25-250	Moderate	Moderate	Low	Low	
Mesoridazine (Serentil®)	Inj, Liq, Tab	3:1	50	30-400	High	Low	High	Moderate	Prolongs QTc; use only in treatment of refractory illness
Molindone (Moban®)	Conc, Tab		15	15-225	Low	Moderate	Low	Low	May cause less weight gain
Olanzapine (Zyprexa®, Zyprexa® Zydis®)	Tab		4	5-20	Moderate/High	Low	Moderate	Moderate	Potential for weight gain, lipid abnormalities, diabetes
Perphenazine (Trilafon®)	Conc, Inj, Tab		10	16-64	Low	Moderate	Low	Low	
Pimozide (Orap™)	Tab		2	1-20	Moderate	High	Moderate	Low	Contraindicated with CYP3A inhibitors
Promazine (Sparine®)	Inj, Tab		200	40-1000	Moderate	Moderate	High	Moderate	

Antipsychotic Agent	Dosage Forms	I.M./P.O. Potency	Equiv. Dosages (approx) (mg)	Usual Adult Daily Maint. Dose (mg)	Sedation (Incidence)	Extrapyramidal Side Effects	Anticholinergic Side Effects	Cardiovascular Side Effects	Comments
Quetiapine (Seroquel®)	Tab		80	50-800	Moderate	Very Low	Moderate	Moderate	Moderate weight gain; potential for lipid abnormalities
Risperidone (Risperdal®)	Sol, Tab		1	0.5-6	Low/Moderate	Low	Low	Low/Moderate	Moderate weight gain
Thioridazine (Mellaril®)	Conc, Tab		100	200-800	High	Low	High	Moderate/high	May cause irreversible retinitis pigmentosa at doses >800 mg/d; prolongs QTc; use only in treatment of refractory illness
Thiothixene (Navane®)	Cap, Conc, Powder for inj	4:1	4	5-40	Low	High	Low	Low/moderate	
Trifluoperazine (Stelazine®)	Conc, Inj, Tab		5	2-40	Low	High	Low	Low	
Ziprasidone (Geodon®)	Cap, Powder for inj	2:1	40	40-160	Low/Moderate	Low	Low	Low/Moderate	Low weight gain; contraindicated with QTc-prolonging agents

BENZODIAZEPINES

Agent	Dosage Forms	Relative Potency	Peak Blood Levels (oral) (h)	Protein Binding (%)	Volume of Distribution (L/kg)	Major Active Metabolite	Half-Life (parent) (h)	Half-Life[1] (metabolite) (h)	Usual Initial Dose	Adult Oral Dosage Range
Anxiolytic										
Alprazolam (Alprazolam Intensol®, Xanax®)	Sol, Tab	0.5	1-2	80	0.9-1.2	No	12-15	—	0.25-0.5 tid	0.75-4 mg/d
Chlordiazepoxide (Librium®)	Cap, Powd for inj	10	2-4	90-98	0.3	Yes	5-30	24-96	5-25 mg tid-qid	15-100 mg/d
Diazepam (Diastat® Rectal Delivery System, Diazepam Intensol®, Valium®)	Gel, Inj, Sol, Tab	5	0.5-2	98	1.1	Yes	20-80	50-100	2-10 mg bid-qid	4-40 mg/d
Lorazepam (Ativan®)[2]	Inj, Sol, Tab	1	1-6	88-92	1.3	No	10-20	—	0.5-2 mg tid-qid	2-4 mg/d
Oxazepam (Serax®)	Cap, Tab	15-30	2-4	86-99	0.6-2	No	5-20	—	10-30 mg tid-qid	30-120 mg/d
Sedative/Hypnotic										
Estazolam (ProSom™)	Tab	0.3	2	93	—	No	10-24	—	1 mg qhs	1-2 mg
Flurazepam (Dalmane®)	Cap	5	0.5-2	97	—	Yes	Not significant	40-114	15 mg qhs	15-60 mg
Quazepam (Doral®)	Tab	5	2	95	5	Yes	25-41	28-114	15 mg qhs	7.5-15 mg
Temazepam (Restoril®)	Cap	5	2-3	96	1.4	No	10-40	—	15-30 mg qhs	15-30 mg
Triazolam (Halcion®)	Tab	0.1	1	89-94	0.8-1.3	No	2.3	—	0.125-0.25 qhs	0.125-0.25 mg
Miscellaneous										
Clonazepam (Klonopin™)	Tab	0.25-0.5	1-2	86	1.8-4	No	18-50 h	—	0.5 mg tid	1.5-20 mg/d
Clorazepate (Tranxene®)	Cap, Tab	7.5	1-2	80-95	—	Yes	Not significant	50-100 h	7.5-15 mg bid-qid	15-60 mg
Midazolam (Versed®)	Inj, Syr		0.4-0.7[3]	95	0.8-6.6	No	2-5 h	—	NA	

[1]Significant metabolite.

[2]Reliable bioavailability when given I.M.

[3]I.V. only.

NA = not available.

BETA-BLOCKERS

Agent	Adrenergic Receptor Blocking Activity	Lipid Solubility	Protein Bound (%)	Half-Life (h)	Bioavail-ability (%)	Primary (Secondary) Route of Elimination	Indications	Usual Dosage
Acebutolol (Sectral®)	beta$_1$	Low	15-25	3-4	40 7-fold[1]	Hepatic (renal)	Hypertension, arrhythmias	P.O.: 400-1200 mg/d
Atenolol (Tenormin®)	beta$_1$	Low	<5-10	6-9[2]	50-60 4-fold[1]	Renal (hepatic)	Hypertension, angina pectoris, acute MI	P.O.: 50-200 mg/d I.V.: 5 mg x 2 doses
Betaxolol (Kerlone®)	beta$_1$	Low	50-55	14-22	84-94	Hepatic (renal)	Hypertension	P.O.: 10-20 mg/d
Bisoprolol (Zebeta™)	beta$_1$	Low	26-33	9-12	80	Renal (hepatic)	Hypertension, heart failure	P.O.: 2.5-5 mg
Carteolol (Cartrol®)	beta$_1$ beta$_2$	Low	20-30	6	80-85	Renal	Hypertension	P.O.: 2.5-10 mg/d
Carvedilol (Coreg™)				7-10	25-35	Bile into feces	Hypertension, heart failure (mild to severe)	P.O.: 6.25 mg twice daily
Esmolol (Brevibloc®)	beta$_1$	Low	55	0.15	NA 5-fold[1]	Red blood cell	Supraventricular tachycardia, sinus tachycardia	I.V. infusion: 25-300 mcg/kg/min
Labetalol (Normodyne®, Trandate®)	alpha$_1$ beta$_1$ beta$_2$	Moderate	50	5.5-8	18-30 10-fold[1]	Renal (hepatic)	Hypertension	P.O.: 200-2400 mg/d I.V.: 20-80 mg at 10-min intervals up to a maximum of 300 mg **or** continuous infusion of 2 mg/min
Metoprolol (Lopressor®, Toprol XL®)	beta$_1$	Moderate	10-12	3-7	50 10-fold[1] (Toprol XL®: 77)	Hepatic/renal	Hypertension, angina pectoris, acute MI, heart failure (mild to moderate; XL formulation only)	P.O.: 100-450 mg/d I.V.: Post-MI 15 mg Angina: 15 mg then 2-5 mg/hour Arrhythmias: 0.2 mg/kg
Nadolol (Corgard®)	beta$_1$ beta$_2$	Low	25-30	20-24	30 5-8 fold[1]	Renal	Hypertension, angina pectoris	P.O.: 40-320 mg/d
Penbutolol (Levatol™)	beta$_1$ beta$_2$	High	80-98	5	≅100	Hepatic (renal)	Hypertension	P.O.: 20-80 mg/d
Pindolol (Visken®)	beta$_1$ beta$_2$	Moderate	57	3-4[2]	90 4-fold[1]	Hepatic (renal)	Hypertension	P.O.: 20-60 mg/d
Propranolol (Inderal®, various)	beta$_1$ beta$_2$	High	90	3-5[2]	30 20-fold[1]	Hepatic	Hypertension, angina pectoris, arrhythmias	P.O.: 40-480 mg/d I.V.: Reflex tachycardia 1-10 mg
Propranolol long-acting (Inderal-LA®)	beta$_1$ beta$_2$	High	90	9-18	20-30 fold[1]	Hepatic	Hypertrophic subaortic stenosis, prophylaxis (post-MI)	P.O.: 180-240 mg/d

BETA-BLOCKERS *(Continued)*

Agent	Adrenergic Receptor Blocking Activity	Lipid Solubility	Protein Bound (%)	Half-Life (h)	Bioavail-ability (%)	Primary (Secondary) Route of Elimination	Indications	Usual Dosage
Sotalol (Betapace®, Betapace AF™, Sorine®)	$beta_1$ $beta_2$	Low	0	12	90-100	Renal	Ventricular arrhythmias/ tachyarrhythmias	P.O. 160-320 mg/d
Timolol (Blocadren®)	$beta_1$ $beta_2$	Low to moderate	<10	4	75 7-fold[1]	Hepatic (renal)	Hypertension, prophylaxis (post-MI)	P.O.: 20-60 mg/d P.O.: 20 mg/d

Dosage is based on 70 kg adult with normal hepatic and renal function.

Note: All $beta_1$-selective agents will inhibit $beta_2$ receptors at higher doses.

[1]Interpatient variations in plasma levels.

[2]Half-life increased to 16-27 h in creatinine clearance of 15-35 mL/min and >27 h in creatinine clearance <15 mL/min.

CALCIUM CHANNEL BLOCKERS

Comparative Pharmacokinetics

Agent	Bioavailability (%)	Protein Binding (%)	Onset (min)	Peak (h)	Half-Life (h)	Volume of Distribution	Route of Metabolism	Route of Excretion
Dihydropyridines								
Nifedipine (prototype) (Adalat® CC, Procardia®/Procardia XL®)	Immediate/sustained release 45-70/86	92-98	20	Immediate/ sustained release 0.5/6	2-5	ND	Liver, inactive metabolites	60%-80% urine, feces, bile
Amlodipine (Norvasc®)	52-88	97	6 h	6-9	33.8	21 L/kg	Liver, inactive metabolites, not a significant first-pass metabolism/presystemic metabolism	Bile, gut wall
Felodipine (Plendil®)	10-25	>99	3-5 h	2.5-5	10-36	10.3 L/kg	Liver, inactive metabolites, extensive metabolism by several pathways including cytochrome P-450, extensive first-pass metabolism/presystemic metabolism	70% urine, 10% feces
Isradipine (DynaCirc®)	15-24	97	120	0.5-2.5	8	2.9 L/kg	Liver, inactive metabolites, extensive first-pass metabolism	90% urine, 10% feces
Nicardipine (Cardene®)	35	>95	20	0.5-2	2-4	ND	Liver, saturable first-pass metabolism	60% urine, 35% feces
Nimodipine (Nimotop®)	13	>95	ND	≤1	1-2	0.43 L/kg	Liver, inactive metabolites, high first-pass metabolism	Urine
Nisoldipine (Sular®)	4-8	>99	ND	6-12	7-12	4-5 L/kg	Liver, 1 active metabolite (10%), presystemic metabolism	70%-75% kidney, 6%-12% feces
Phenylalkylamines								
Verapamil (prototype) (Calan®, Isoptin®)	20-35	83-92	30	1-2.2	3-7	4.5-7 L/kg	Liver	70% urine, 16% feces
Benzothiazepines								
Diltiazem (prototype) (Cardizem®/Cardizem® CD, Dilacor® XR)	40-67	70-80	30-60	Immediate/ sustained release 2-3/6-11	Immediate/ sustained release 3.5-6/5-7	ND	Liver; drugs which inhibit/induce hepatic microsomal enzymes may alter disposition	Urine
Miscellaneous								
Bepridil (Vascor®)	59	>99	60	2-3	24	ND	Liver	70% urine, 22% feces

COMPATIBILITY OF DRUGS

Drug Compatibility Guide

KEY

Y = Compatible
N = Incompatible
Blank = Information about compatibility was not available

	aminophylline	amphotericin B	ampicillin	atropine	calcium gluconate	carbenicillin	cefazolin	cimetidine	clindamycin	diazepam	dopamine	epinephrine	erythromycin	fentanyl	furosemide	gentamicin
aminophylline	■		Y		Y	N	N		N	Y	Y	N	N			
amphotericin B		■	N		N	N		N			N					N
ampicillin	Y	N	■	N	N	Y	Y		N		N		N			N
atropine			N	■				Y		N		N		Y		
calcium gluconate	Y	N	N		■		N		N		Y	N	Y			
carbenicillin	N	N	Y			■		Y	Y		Y	N	N			N
cefazolin	N		Y		N		■	N		Y			N			N
cimetidine		N		Y		Y	N	■	Y			Y	Y		Y	Y
clindamycin	N		N		N	Y		Y	■							Y
diazepam	Y			N			Y			■		N			N	
dopamine	Y	N	N		Y	Y					■					N
epinephrine	N			N	N	N		Y		N		■	N		N	
erythromycin	N		N		Y	N	N	Y				N	■			
fentanyl				Y										■		
furosemide								Y		N		N			■	N
gentamicin		N	N			N	N		Y		Y				N	■
glycopyrrolate				Y						N						
heparin sodium	Y	Y	Y	N	Y			Y	Y	N	Y	Y	N		Y	N
hydrocortisone	Y	Y	N		Y	Y	Y		Y		Y		Y			
hydroxyzine	N			Y						N				Y		
levarterenol	N			N	Y	N	N	Y		N		N			N	
lidocaine	Y	N	Y		Y	Y	N	Y		N	Y	N	Y			
meperidine	N			Y						N		Y		Y		
morphine	N			Y						N				Y		
nitroglycerin	Y										Y				Y	
pentobarbital	Y			N			N	N	N	N			N	N		
potassium chloride	Y	N	Y	Y	Y	Y	Y	Y	Y	N	Y	N	Y		Y	
sodium bicarbonate	Y	Y		N	N				Y	N		N	Y			
tetracycline	N	N	N		N	N	N	Y			Y		N		N	
vancomycin	N				Y			Y					Y			
verapamil	Y	N	Y	Y	Y	Y	Y	Y	Y	Y	Y	Y	Y		Y	Y
vitamin B & C complex	N		Y	Y	Y	N	Y	Y	Y	N	Y	Y	N		Y	Y

NOTE: Because the compatibility of two or more drugs in solution depends on several variables such as the solution itself, drug concentration and the method of mixing (bottle, syringe, or Y-site), this table is intended to be used solely as a guide to general drug compatibilities. Before mixing any drugs, the healthcare professional should ascertain if a potential incompatibility exists by referring to an appropriate information source.

(continued)

KEY

Y = Compatible
N = Incompatible
Blank = Information about compatibility was not available

	glycopyrrolate	heparin sodium	hydrocortisone	hydroxyzine	levarterenol	lidocaine	meperidine	morphine	nitroglycerin	pentobarbital	potassium chloride	sodium bicarbonate	tetracycline	vancomycin	verapamil	vitamin B & C complex
aminophylline		Y	Y	N	N	Y	N	N	Y	Y	Y	Y	N	N	Y	N
amphotericin B		Y	Y			N					N	Y	N		N	
ampicillin		Y	N			Y					Y		N		Y	Y
atropine	Y	N		Y	N		Y	Y		N	Y	N			Y	Y
calcium gluconate		Y	Y		Y	Y					Y	N	N	Y	Y	Y
carbenicillin			Y		N	Y					Y		N		Y	N
cefazolin			Y		N	N				N	Y		N		Y	Y
cimetidine		Y			Y	Y				N	Y		Y	Y	Y	Y
clindamycin		Y	Y							N	Y	Y			Y	Y
diazepam	N	N		N	N	N	N	N		N	N	N			Y	N
dopamine		Y	Y			Y			Y		Y		Y		Y	Y
epinephrine		Y			N	N	Y				N	N			Y	Y
erythromycin		N	Y			Y				N	Y	Y	N	Y	Y	N
fentanyl				Y			Y	Y		N						
furosemide		Y			N				Y		Y		N		Y	Y
gentamicin		N													Y	Y
glycopyrrolate	■			Y		Y	Y	Y		N		N				
heparin sodium		■	N	N	Y	Y	N	N			Y	Y	N	N	Y	Y
hydrocortisone		N	■		Y	Y				N	Y	Y	N	Y	Y	Y
hydroxyzine	Y	N		■		Y	Y	Y		N						N
levarterenol		Y	Y		■					N	Y		Y		Y	Y
lidocaine	Y	Y	Y	Y		■			Y	Y	Y	Y	Y		Y	Y
meperidine	Y	N		Y			■	N		N		N			Y	
morphine	Y	N		Y			N	■		N	Y	N			Y	Y
nitroglycerin						Y			■						Y	
pentobarbital	N		N	N	N	Y	N	N		■		N	N	N	Y	
potassium chloride		Y	Y		Y	Y		Y			■	Y	Y	Y	Y	
sodium bicarbonate	N	Y	Y			Y	N	N		N	Y	■	N	N	Y	N
tetracycline		N	N		Y	Y				N	Y	N	■			Y
vancomycin		N	Y							N	Y	N		■	Y	Y
verapamil		Y	Y		Y	Y	Y	Y	Y	Y	Y	Y		Y	■	Y
vitamin B & C complex		Y	Y	N	Y	Y		Y				N	Y	Y	Y	■

Reprinted from Malseed RT, Goldstein FJ, & Balkon N, *Pharmacology: Drug Therapy and Nursing Management* (4th ed), Philadelphia: JB Lippincott Co (1995). Used with permission.

COMPATIBILITY OF DRUGS IN SYRINGE

Compatibility of Drugs in Syringe

	atropine	butorphanol	chlorpromazine	cimetidine	dimenhydrinate	diphenhydramine	fentanyl	glycopyrrolate	heparin	hydroxyzine	meperidine
atropine	■	Y	Y	Y	M	M	M	Y	M	Y	Y
butorphanol	Y	■	Y	Y	N	Y	Y			Y	M
chlorpromazine	Y	Y	■	N	N	M	M	Y	N	M	M
cimetidine	Y	Y	N	■		Y	Y	Y	Y	Y	Y
dimenhydrinate	M	N	N		■	M	M	N	M	N	M
diphenhydramine	M	Y		Y	M	■		Y		M	M
fentanyl	M	Y	M		M	M	■		M	Y	M
glycopyrrolate	Y		Y	Y	N	Y		■		Y	Y
heparin	M		N		M		M		■		N
hydroxyzine	Y	Y	M	Y	N	M	Y	Y		■	M
meperidine	Y	M	M	Y	M	M	M	Y	N	M	■
metoclopramide	M		M		M	Y	M		M	M	M
midazolam	Y	Y	Y	Y	N	Y	Y	Y		Y	Y
morphine	M	Y	M	Y	M	M	M	Y	N	Y	N
nalbuphine	Y			Y						Y	
pentazocine	M	Y	M	Y	M	M	M	N	N	Y	M
pentobarbital	M	N	N	N	N	N	N	N		N	N
prochlorperazine	M	Y	Y	Y	N	M	M	Y		M	M
promethazine	M	Y	M	Y	N	M	M	Y	N	M	Y
ranitidine	Y		Y		Y	Y	Y	Y		N	Y
secobarbital				N				N			
thiopental			N		N	N		N			N

KEY

Y = Compatible in a syringe
M = Moderately compatible, inject immediately after combining
N = Incompatible, do not mix in syringe
Blank = Information about compatibility is not currently available

(continued)

	metoclopramide	midazolam	morphine	nalbuphine	pentazocine	pentobarbital	prochlorperazine	promethazine	ranitidine	secobarbital	thiopental
atropine	M	Y	M	Y	M	M	M	M	Y		
butorphanol		Y	Y		Y	N	Y	Y			
chlorpromazine	M	Y	M		M	N	Y	M	Y		N
cimetidine		Y	Y	Y	Y	N	Y	Y		N	
dimenhydrinate	M	N	M		M	N	N	N	Y		N
diphenhydramine	Y	Y	M		M	N	M	M	Y		N
fentanyl	M	Y	M		M	N	M	M	Y		
glycopyrrolate		Y	Y		N	N	Y	Y	Y	N	N
heparin	M		N		N			N			
hydroxyzine	M	Y	Y	Y	Y	N	M	M	N		
meperidine	M	Y	N		M	N	M	Y	Y		N
metoclopramide	■	Y	M		M		M	M	Y		
midazolam	Y	■	Y	Y		N	N	Y	N		
morphine	M	Y	■		M	N	M	M	Y		N
nalbuphine		Y		■		N	Y	Y	Y		
pentazocine	M		M		■	N	M	Y	Y		
pentobarbital	N	N	N	N	N	■	N	N			Y
prochlorperazine	M	N	M	Y	M	N	■	M	Y		N
promethazine	M	Y	M	Y	Y	N	M	■	Y		N
ranitidine	Y	N	Y	Y	Y		Y	Y	■		
secobarbital										■	
thiopental			N			Y	N	N			■

Reprinted from Malseed RT, Goldstein FJ, & Balkon N, *Pharmacology: Drug Therapy and Nursing Management* (4th ed), Philadelphia: JB Lippincott Co (1995). Used with permission.

CONTROLLED SUBSTANCES COMPARISON

Drugs	CSA Schedules	Trade or Other Names	Medical Uses	Physical Dependence	Psychological Dependence	Tolerance	Duration (h)	Usual Method	Possible Effects	Effects of Overdose	Withdrawal Syndrome
					Narcotics						
Heroin	I	Diacetylmorphine, horse, smack	None in U.S; analgesic, antitussive	High	High	Yes	3-6	Injected, sniffed, smoked	Euphoria, drowsiness, respiratory depression, constricted pupils, nausea	Slow and shallow breathing, clammy skin, convulsions, coma, possible death	Watery eyes, runny nose, yawning, lose of appetite, irritability, tremors, panic, cramps, nausea, chills and sweating
Morphine	II	Duramorph, MS-Contin, Roxanol, Oramorph SR	Analgesic	High	High	Yes	3-6	Oral, smoked, injected			
Codeine	II, III, V	Tylenol w/codeine, Empirin w/codeine, Robitussin A-C, Fiorinal w/codeine, APAP w/codeine	Analgesic, antitussive	Moderate	Moderate	Yes	3-6	Oral, injected			
Hydrocodone	II, III	Tussionex, Vicodin, Hycodan, Lorcet	Analgesic, antitussive	High	High	Yes	3-6	Oral			
Hydromorphone	II	Dilaudid	Analgesic	High	High	Yes	3-6	Oral, injected			
Oxycodone	II	Percodan, Percocet, Tylox, Roxicet, Roxicodone	Analgesic	High	High	Yes	4-5	Oral			
Methadone and LAAM	I, II	Dolophine, methadone, levo-alpha-acetylmethadol, levomethadyl acetate	Analgesic, treatment of dependence	High	High	Yes	12-72	Oral, injected			
Fentanyl and analogs	I, II	Innovar, Sublimaze, Alfenta, Sufenta, Duragesic	Analgesic, adjunct to anesthesia, anesthetic	High	High	Yes	0.1-72	Injected, transdermal patch			
Other narcotics	II, III, IV, V	Percodan, Percocet, Tylox, opium, Darvon, Talwin,* buprenorphine, meperidine (pethidine), Demerol	Analgesic, antidiarrheal	High-low	High-low	Yes	Variable	Oral, injected			

Drugs	CSA Schedules	Trade or Other Names	Medical Uses	Physical Dependence	Psychological Dependence	Tolerance	Duration (h)	Usual Method	Possible Effects	Effects of Overdose	Withdrawal Syndrome
Depressants											
Acetaminophen, Isometheptene, and Dichloralphenazone	IV	Isocom, Isopap, Midchlor, Midrin, Migratine	Hypnotic	Moderate	Moderate	Yes	5-8	Oral	Slurred speech, disorientation, drunken behavior without odor of alcohol	Shallow respiration, clammy skin, dilated pupils, weak and rapid pulse, coma, possible death	Anxiety, insomnia, tremors, delirium, convulsions, possible death
Chloral hydrate	IV	Noctec Somnos, Felsules	Hypnotic	Moderate	Moderate	Yes	5-8	Oral			
Barbiturates	II, III, IV	Amytal, Fiorinal, Nembutal, Seconal, Tuinal, phenobarbital, pentobarbital	Anesthetic, anticonvulsant, sedative, hypnotic, veterinary euthanasia agent	High-moderate	High-moderate	Yes	1-16	Oral, injected			
Benzodiazepines	IV	Ativan, Dalmane, Diazepam, Librium, Xanax, Serax, Valium, Tranxene, Verstran, Versed, Halcion, Paxipam, Restoril	Antianxiety, sedative, anticonvulsant, hypnotic	Low	Low	Yes	4-8	Oral, injected			
Glutethimide	II	Doriden	Sedative, hypnotic	High	Moderate	Yes	4-8	Oral			
Other depressants	I, II, III, IV	Equanil, Miltown, Noludar, Placidyl, Valmid, methaqualone	Antianxiety, sedative, hypnotic	Moderate	Moderate	Yes	4-8	Oral			

CONTROLLED SUBSTANCES COMPARISON *(Continued)*

Drugs	CSA Schedules	Trade or Other Names	Medical Uses	Physical Dependence	Psychological Dependence	Tolerance	Duration (h)	Usual Method	Possible Effects	Effects of Overdose	Withdrawal Syndrome
Stimulants											
Cocaine†	II	Coke, flake, snow, crack	Local anesthetic	Possible	High	Yes	1-2	Sniffed, smoked, injected	Increased alertness, excitation, euphoria, increased pulse rate and blood pressure, insomnia, loss of appetite	Agitation, increased body temperature, hallucinations, convulsions, possible death	Apathy, long periods of sleep, irritability, depression, disorientation
Amphetamine/ methamphetamine	II	Biphetamine, Desoxyn, Dexedrine, Obetrol, ice	Attention deficit disorder, narcolepsy, weight control	Possible	High	Yes	2-4	Oral, injected, smoked			
Methylphenidate	II	Ritalin	Attention deficit disorder, narcolepsy	Possible	High	Yes	2-4	Oral, injected			
Other stimulants	I, II, III, IV	Adipex, Didrex, Ionamin, Melfiat, Plegine, Captagon, Sanorex, Tenuate, Tepanil, Prelu-2, Preludin	Weight control	Possible	High	Yes	2-4	Oral, injected			
Cannabis											
Marijuana	I	Pot, Acapulco gold, grass, Reefer, Sinsemilla, Thai sticks	None	Unknown	Moderate	Yes	2-4	Smoked, oral	Euphoria, relaxed inhibitions, increased appetite, disorientation	Fatigue, paranoia, possible psychosis	Occasional reports of insomnia, hyperactivity, decreased appetite
Tetrahydro-cannabinol	I, II	THC, Marinol	Antinauseant	Unknown	Moderate	Yes	2-4	Smoked, oral			
Hashish and hashish oil	I	Hash, hash oil	None	Unknown	Moderate	Yes	2-4	Smoked, oral			

Drugs	CSA Schedules	Trade or Other Names	Medical Uses	Physical Dependence	Psychological Dependence	Tolerance	Duration (h)	Usual Method	Possible Effects	Effects of Overdose	Withdrawal Syndrome
Hallucinogens											
LSD	I	Acid, Microdot	None	None	Unknown	Yes	8-12	Oral	Illusions and hallucinations, altered perception of time and distance	Longer, more intense "trip" episodes, psychosis, possible death	Unknown
Mescaline and peyote	I	Mescal, buttons, cactus	None	None	Unknown	Yes	8-12	Oral			
Amphetamine variants	I	2,5-DMA, STP, MDA, MDMA, ecstasy, DOM, DOB	None	Unknown	Unknown	Yes	Variable	Oral, injected			
Phencyclidine and analogs	I, II	PCE, PCPy, TCP, PCP, hog, loveboat, angel dust	None	Unknown	High	Yes	Days	Oral, smoked			
Other hallucinogens	I	Bufotenine, Ibogaine, DMT, DET, Psilocybin, Psilocyn	None	None	Unknown	Possible	Variable	Smoked, oral, injected, sniffed			
Anabolic Steroids											
Testosterone (Cypionate, Enanthate)	III	Depo-testosterone, Delatestryl	Hypogonadism	Unknown	Unknown	Unknown	14-28 days	Injected	Virilization, acne, testicular atrophy, gynecomastia, aggressive behavior, edema	Unknown	Possible depression
Nandrolone (Decanoate, Phenpropionate)	III	Nortestosterone, Durabolin, Deca-durabolin, Deca	Anemia, breast cancer	Unknown	Unknown	Unknown	14-21 days	Injected			
Oxymetholone	III	Anadrol-50	Anemia	Unknown	Unknown	Unknown	24	Oral			

*Not designated a narcotic under the CSA.

†Designated a narcotic under the CSA.

From U.S. Department of Justice Drug Enforcement Administration, *Drugs of Abuse*, 1996, with permission.

CORTICOSTEROIDS

Corticosteroids, Systemic Equivalencies

Glucocorticoid	Pregnancy Category	Approximate Equivalent Dose (mg)	Routes of Administration	Relative Anti-inflammatory Potency	Relative Mineralocorticoid Potency	Protein Binding (%)	Half-life	
							Plasma (min)	Biologic (h)
Short-Acting								
Cortisone	D	25	P.O., I.M.	0.8	2	90	30	8-12
Hydrocortisone	C	20	I.M., I.V.	1	2	90	80-118	8-12
Intermediate-Acting								
Methylprednisolone[1]	—	4	P.O., I.M., I.V.	5	0	—	78-188	18-36
Prednisolone	B	5	P.O., I.M., I.V., intra-articular, intradermal, soft tissue injection	4	1	90-95	115-212	18-36
Prednisone	B	5	P.O.	4	1	70	60	18-36
Triamcinolone[1]	C	4	P.O., I.M., intra-articular, intradermal, intrasynovial, soft tissue injection	5	0	—	200+	18-36
Long-Acting								
Betamethasone	C	0.6-0.75	P.O., I.M., intra-articular, intradermal, intrasynovial, soft tissue injection	25	0	64	300+	36-54
Dexamethasone	C	0.75	P.O., I.M., I.V., intra-articular, intradermal, soft tissue injection	25-30	0	—	110-210	36-54
Mineralocorticoids								
Fludrocortisone	C	—	P.O.	10	125	42	210+	18-36

[1]May contain propylene glycol as an excipient in injectable forms.

GUIDELINES FOR SELECTION AND USE OF TOPICAL CORTICOSTEROIDS

The quantity prescribed and the frequency of refills should be monitored to reduce the risk of adrenal suppression. In general, short courses of high-potency agents are preferable to prolonged use of low potency. After control is achieved, control should be maintained with a low potency preparation.

1. Low-to-medium potency agents are usually effective for treating thin, acute, inflammatory skin lesions; whereas, high or super-potent agents are often required for treating chronic, hyperkeratotic, or lichenified lesions.
2. Since the stratum corneum is thin on the face and intertriginous areas, low-potency agents are preferred but a higher potency agent may be used for 2 weeks.
3. Because the palms and sole shave a thick stratum corneum, high or super-potent agents are frequently required.
4. Low potency agents are preferred for infants and the elderly. Infants have a high body surface area to weight ratio; elderly patients have thin, fragile skin.
5. The vehicle in which the topical corticosteroid is formulated influences the absorption and potency of the drug. Ointment bases are preferred for thick, lichenified lesions; they enhance penetration of the drug. Creams are preferred for acute and subacute dermatoses; they may be used on moist skin areas or intertriginous areas. Solutions, gels, and sprays are preferred for the scalp or for areas where a non-oil-based vehicle is needed.
6. In general, super-potent agents should not be used for longer than 3 weeks unless the lesion is limited to a small body area. Medium-to-high potency agents usually cause only rare adverse effects when treatment is limited to 3 months or less, and use on the face and intertriginous areas are avoided. If long-term treatment is needed, intermittent vs continued treatment is recommended.
7. Most preparations are applied once or twice daily. More frequent application may be necessary for the palms or soles because the preparation is easily removed by normal activity and penetration is poor due to a thick stratum corneum. Every-other-day or weekend-only application may be effective for treating some chronic conditions.

Corticosteroids, Topical

Steroid		Vehicle
Very High Potency		
0.05%	Augmented betamethasone dipropionate	Ointment
0.05%	Clobetasol propionate	Cream, ointment
0.05%	Diflorasone diacetate	Ointment
0.05%	Halobetasol propionate	Cream, ointment
High Potency		
0.1%	Amcinonide	Cream, ointment, lotion
0.05%	Betamethasone dipropionate, augmented	Cream
0.05%	Betamethasone dipropionate	Cream, ointment
0.1%	Betamethasone valerate	Ointment
0.05%	Desoximetasone	Gel
0.25%	Desoximetasone	Cream, ointment
0.05%	Diflorasone diacetate	Cream, ointment
0.2%	Fluocinolone acetonide	Cream
0.05%	Fluocinonide	Cream, ointment, gel
0.1%	Halcinonide	Cream, ointment
0.5%	Triamcinolone acetonide	Cream, ointment
Intermediate Potency		
0.025%	Betamethasone benzoate	Cream, gel, lotion
0.05%	Betamethasone dipropionate	Lotion
0.1%	Betamethasone valerate	Cream
0.1%	Clocortolone pivalate	Cream
0.05%	Desoximetasone	Cream
0.025%	Fluocinolone acetonide	Cream, ointment
0.05%	Flurandrenolide	Cream, ointment, lotion, tape
0.005%	Fluticasone propionate	Ointment
0.05%	Fluticasone propionate	Cream
0.1%	Hydrocortisone butyrate[1]	Ointment, solution
0.2%	Hydrocortisone valerate[1]	Cream, ointment
0.1%	Mometasone furoate[1]	Cream, ointment, lotion
0.1%	Prednicarbate	Cream, ointment
0.025%	Triamcinolone acetonide	Cream, ointment, lotion
0.1%	Triamcinolone acetonide	Cream, ointment, lotion

CORTICOSTEROIDS *(Continued)*

Corticosteroids, Topical *(continued)*

Steroid		Vehicle
Low Potency		
0.05%	Alclometasone dipropionate[1]	Cream, ointment
0.05%	Desonide	Cream
0.01%	Dexamethasone	Aerosol
0.04%	Dexamethasone	Aerosol
0.1%	Dexamethasone sodium phosphate	Cream
0.01%	Fluocinolone acetonide	Cream, solution
0.25%	Hydrocortisone[1]	Lotion
0.5%	Hydrocortisone[1]	Cream, ointment, lotion, aerosol
0.5%	Hydrocortisone acetate[1]	Cream, ointment
1%	Hydrocortisone acetate[1]	Cream, ointment
1%	Hydrocortisone	Cream, ointment, lotion, solution
2.5%	Hydrocortisone	Cream, ointment, lotion

[1]Not fluorinated.

GLAUCOMA DRUG COMPARISON

Ophthalmic Agent	Reduces Aqueous Humor Production	Increases Aqueous Humor Outflow	Average Duration of Action	Strengths Available
Cholinesterase Inhibitors*				
Demecarium	No data	Significant	7 d	0.125%, 0.25%
Echothiophate	No data	Significant	2 wk	0.06%, 0.125%
Physostigmine	No data	Significant	24 h	0.25%
Direct-Acting Cholinergic Agents				
Carbachol	Some activity	Significant	8 h	1.5%, 2.25%
Pilocarpine	Some activity	Significant	5 h	0.25%, 0.5%, 1%, 2%, 3%, 4%, 8%, 10%
Sympathomimetics				
Dipivefrin	Some activity	Moderate	12 h	0.1%
Epinephrine	Some activity	Moderate	18 h	0.1%, 0.5%, 1%, 2%
Beta-Blockers				
Betaxolol	Significant	Some activity	12 h	0.25%, 0.5%
Carteolol	Yes	No	12 h	1%
Levobetaxolol	Significant	No data	12 h	0.5%
Levobunolol	Significant	Some activity	18 h	0.25%, 0.5%
Metipranolol	Significant	Some activity	18 h	0.3%
Timolol	Significant	Some activity	18 h	0.25%, 0.5%
Carbonic Anhydrase Inhibitors				
Acetazolamide	Significant	No data	10 h	125 mg, 250 mg tabs, 500 mg cap
Brinzolamide	Yes	No data	8 h	1%
Dorzolamide	Yes	No	8 h	2%
Methazolamide	Significant	No data	14 h	25 mg, 50 mg
Prostaglandin Agonist				
Bimatoprost			>24h	0.03%
Latanoprost		Yes	8-12 h	0.005%
Travoprost			>24 h	0.004%
Alpha-2 Agonists				
Apraclonidine	Yes	Yes	8 h	0.5%, 1%
Brimonidine	Yes	Yes	8 h	0.2%

*All miotic drugs significantly affect accommodation.

Also see Ophthalmic Agents, Glaucoma in the Alphabetical Listing of Drugs section.

HEPARINS

Name	Type	Limitation	Dose (S.C. unless otherwise noted)	Average MW (in daltons)
Low Molecular Weight Heparins				
Dalteparin (Fragmin®)	Prophylaxis	Abdominal surgery[1] Abdominal surgery[2]	2500 units/d 5000 units/d	4000-6000
		Hip surgery[1]	5000 units/d postoperatively	
	Treatment	DVT[3]	100 units/kg bid 200 units/kg qd	4000-6000
		Unstable[4] angina Non-Q-wave MI	120 units/kg (max: 10,000 units) q12h for 5-8 d	
Enoxaparin (Lovenox®)	Prophylaxis	Hip or knee replacement	30 mg twice daily[5]	3500-5500
		High-risk hip replacement or abdominal surgery	40 mg once daily	
	Treatment	DVT or PE	1 mg/kg q12h	
		Acute coronary	1 mg/kg q12h	
Tinzaparin (Innohep®)	Treatment	DVT or PE	175 anti-Xa int. units/ kg/day	5500-7500
Heparin				
Heparin (Hep-Lock®)	Prophylaxis	Risk of thromboembolic disease	5000 units q8-12h	3000-30,000
	Treatment	Thrombosis or embolization	80 units/kg IVP then 20,000-40,000 units daily as continuous I.V. infusion	
	Treatment[3]	Unstable angina[3]	80 units/kg IVP then 20,000-40,000 units daily as continuous I.V. infusion	
Heparinoid				
Danaparoid (Orgaran®)	Prophylaxis	Hip replacement	750 units bid	6500
	Treatment[3]		2000 units q12h	

[1]Patients with low risk of DVT.

[2]Patients with high risk of DVT.

[3]Not FDA approved.

[4]Patients >60 years of age may require a lower dose of heparin.

[5]Patients weighing <100 lb or ≥65 years of age may receive 0.5 mg/kg/dose every 12 hours.

INHALANT (ASTHMA, BRONCHOSPASM) AGENTS COMPARISON

Medications Commonly Used for Asthma, Bronchospasm, and COPD

Agent	Indications	Onset	Duration	Frequency	Comments
		Anticholinergics			
Ipratropium bromide (Atrovent®)	Bronchospasm associated with COPD		6 h	2 puffs qid	Additive bronchodilating effects used with α-, β_2-adrenergic agonists
		Bronchodilators			
Albuterol (Proventil®, Proventil® HFA, Ventolin®)	Prevent exercise-induced bronchospasm; relief and prevention of bronchospasm	5 min	6-8 h	2 puffs q4-6h	
Bitolterol mesylate (Tornalate®)	Prevent and treat bronchial asthma and reversible bronchospasm	5 min	8 h	2 puffs q8h	Contains a high alcohol content that may irritate the airway
Epinephrine (Bronkaid® Mist, Primatene® Mist)	Acute paroxysms of bronchial asthma; treatment of postintubation and infectious croup	1-5 min	Individualize dosing		OTC; shorter-acting and less effective than prescription β-agonists
Formoterol (Foradil® Aerolizer™)	Long-term maintenance of asthma, prevention of bronchospasm in patients ≥5 y; prevention of exercise-induced bronchospasm in patients ≥12 y		12 h	q12h	Not meant to relieve acute asthmatic symptoms
Ipratropium bromide and albuterol sulfate (Combivent®)	Patients with chronic obstructive pulmonary disease (COPD) on a regular aerosol bronchodilator who continue to have evidence of bronchospasm and who require a second bronchodilator			2 puffs qid	Additional doses may be administered; however, total doses should not exceed 12 in 24 hours
Isoetharine HCl (Bronkometer)	Bronchial asthma and reversible bronchospasm with bronchitis and emphysema	5 min	1-3 h	1-2 puffs q4h	May cause cardiac stimulation
Levalbuterol (Xopenex™)	Bronchospasm in adults and adolescents ≥12 years of age with reversible obstructive airway disease	10-17 min	5-6 h	0.63 mg tid at 6-8 h intervals	
Metaproterenol sulfate (Alupent®, Metaprel®)	Bronchial asthma and reversible bronchospasm; acute asthmatic attacks in children ≥6 years of age	5-30 min	4-6 h	2-3 puffs q3-4h (max 12 puffs/d)	Contraindicated in patients with arrhythmias; should not be used with other β-adrenergic aerosol inhalers because of additive effects
Pirbuterol acetate (Maxair™)	Prevent and reverse bronchospasm with reversible bronchospasm	Within 5 min	4-6 h	2 puffs q4-6h	
Salmeterol (Serevent®)	Long-term maintenance treatment of asthma and prevention of bronchospasm in patients >12 years of age	20 min	12 h	2 puffs q12h	Not meant to relieve acute asthmatic symptoms
Terbutaline sulfate (Brethaire®)	Bronchial asthma and reversible bronchospasm with bronchitis or emphysema	5-30 min	6-8 h	2 puffs q4-6h	

INHALANT (ASTHMA, BRONCHOSPASM) AGENTS COMPARISON *(Continued)*

Medications Commonly Used for Asthma, Bronchospasm, and COPD *(continued)*

Agent	Indications	Onset	Duration	Frequency	Comments
		Corticosteroids*			
Beclomethasone dipropionate (Beclovent®, Vanceril®)	Bronchial asthma		6-8 h	2 puffs q6-8h	Coughing and wheezing are more common
Dexamethasone Na phosphate (Decadron® phosphate respihaler)	Bronchial asthma		6-8 h	3 puffs q6-8h (max 12 puffs/d)	
Flunisolide (AeroBid®)	Bronchial asthma		12 h	2 puffs bid (max 4 puffs bid)	
Fluticasone (Flonase®, Flovent®)	Maintenance treatment of asthma as prophylactic therapy; also indicated for patients requiring oral corticosteroid therapy for asthma to assist in total discontinuation or reduction of total oral dose; NOT indicated for the relief of acute bronchospasm		—	2-4 puffs qd (44-220 mcg)	May allow weaning from oral steroids in selected patients
Triamcinolone acetonide (Azmacort™)	Bronchial asthma		6-8 h	2 puffs q6-8h (max 16 puffs/d)	Asthma should be reasonably stable before Azmacort™ treatment
		Miscellaneous			
Cromolyn (Intal®)	Severe bronchial asthma; prevent exercise-induced bronchospasm		6 h	2 puffs qid	Only useful in prophylaxis; has low toxicity and is as effective as theophylline in many patients
Nedocromil sodium (Tilade®)	Mild to moderate bronchial asthma		6 h	2 puffs qid	Must be taken regularly for benefit — even during symptom-free periods

*Not indicated for rapid relief of bronchospasm. Dysphonia and oral candidiasis can occur. Long-term use is associated with cataract formation.

ESTIMATED COMPARATIVE DAILY DOSAGES FOR INHALED CORTICOSTEROIDS

Adults

Drug	Low Dose	Medium Dose	High Dose
Beclomethasone dipropionate	168-504 mcg	504-840 mcg	>840 mcg
42 mcg/puff	4-12 puffs	12-20 puffs	>20 puffs
84 mcg/puff	2-6 puffs	6-10 puffs	>10 puffs
Beclomethasone dipropionate HFA	80-240 mcg	240-640 mcg	>640 mcg
40 mcg/puff	2-6 puffs	6-16 puffs	>16 puffs
80 mcg/puff	1-3 puffs	3-8 puffs	>8 puffs
Budesonide Turbuhaler	200-600 mcg	600-1200 mcg	>1200 mcg
200 mcg/inhalation	1-3 inhalations	3-6 inhalations	>6 inhalations
Flunisolide	500-1000 mcg	1000-2000 mcg	>2000 mcg
250 mcg/puff	2-4 puffs	4-8 puffs	>8 puffs
Fluticasone	88-264 mcg	264-660 mcg	>660 mcg
MDI: 44, 110, 220 mcg/puff			
DPI: 50, 100, 250 mcg/dose			
Triamcinolone acetonide	400-1000 mcg	1000-2000 mcg	>2000 mcg
100 mcg/puff	4-10 puffs	10-20 puffs	>20 puffs

Children

Drug	Low Dose	Medium Dose	High Dose
Beclomethasone dipropionate	84-336 mcg	336-672 mcg	>672 mcg
42 mcg/puff	2-8 puffs	8-16 puffs	>16 puffs
84 mcg/puff	1-4 puffs	4-8 puffs	>8 puffs
Beclomethasone dipropionate HFA	80-160 mcg	160-320 mcg	>320 mcg
40 mcg/puff	2-4 puffs	4-8 puffs	>8 puffs
80 mcg/puff	1-2 puffs	2-4 puffs	>4 puffs
Budesonide Turbuhaler	200-400 mcg	400-800 mcg	>800 mcg
200 mcg/inhalation	1-2 inhalations	2-4 inhalations	>4 inhalations
Inhalation suspension for nebulization	0.5 mg	1 mg	2 mg
Flunisolide	500-750 mcg	1000-1250 mcg	>1250 mcg
250 mcg/puff	2-3 puffs	4-5 puffs	>5 puffs
Fluticasone	88-176 mcg	176-440 mcg	>440 mcg
MDI: 44, 110, 220 mcg/puff			
DPI: 50, 100, 250 mcg/dose			
Triamcinolone acetonide	400-800 mcg	800-1200 mcg	>1200 mcg
100 mcg/puff	4-8 puffs	8-12 puffs	>12 puffs

INOTROPIC AND VASOCONSTRICTOR COMPARISON

Cardiovascular Comparison

Drug	Hemodynamic Effects			
	CO	TPR	Mean BP	Renal Perfusion
Dobutamine (Dobutrex®)	↑	↓	↑	—
Dopamine (Intropin®)	↑	+/—*	—/↑*	↑*
Epinephrine (Adrenalin®)	↑	↓	↑	↓
Inamrinone (Inocor®)	↑	↓	—	↑
Isoproterenol (Isuprel®)	↑	↓	↓	+/—†
Mephentermine (Wyamine®)	↑	—/↑	↑	+/—
Metaraminol (Aramine®)	↓	↑	↑	↓
Methoxamine	—/↓	↑	↑	↓
Milrinone (Primacor®)	↑	↓	—	↑
Norepinephrine (Levophed®)	—/↓	↑	↑	↓
Phenylephrine (Neo-Synephrine®)	↓	↑	↑	↓

↑ = increase ↓ = decrease, — = no change, * = dose dependent

†In patients with cardiogenic or septic shock, renal perfusion commonly increases, however, in the normal patient, renal perfusion may be reduced with isoproterenol.

LAXATIVES: CLASSIFICATION AND PROPERTIES

Laxative	Onset of Action	Site of Action	Mechanism of Action
Saline			
Magnesium citrate (Citroma®) Magnesium hydroxide (Milk of Magnesia)	30 min to 3 h	Small and large intestine	Attract/retain water in intestinal lumen increasing intraluminal pressure; cholecystokinin release
Sodium phosphate/ biphosphate enema (Fleet® Enema)	2-15 min	Colon	
Irritant/Stimulant			
Cascara Casanthranol Senna (Senokot®)	6-10 h	Colon	Direct action on intestinal mucosa; stimulate myenteric plexus; alter water and electrolyte secretion
Bisacodyl (Dulcolax®) tablets, suppositories	15 min to 1 h	Colon	
Castor oil	2-6 h	Small intestine	
Cascara aromatic fluid extract	6-10 h	Colon	
Bulk-Producing			
Methylcellulose Psyllium (Metamucil®) Malt soup extract (Maltsupex®) Calcium polycarbophil (Mitrolan®, FiberCon®)	12-24 h (up to 72 h)	Small and large intestine	Holds water in stool; mechanical distention; malt soup extract reduces fecal pH
Lubricant			
Mineral oil	6-8 h	Colon	Lubricates intestine; retards colonic absorption of fecal water; softens stool
Surfactants/Stool Softener			
Docusate sodium (Colace®) Docusate calcium (Surfak®) Docusate potassium (Dialose®)	24-72 h	Small and large intestine	Detergent activity; facilitates admixture of fat and water to soften stool
Miscellaneous and Combination Laxatives			
Glycerin suppository	15-30 min	Colon	Local irritation; hyperosmotic action
Lactulose (Cephulac®)	24-48 h	Colon	Delivers osmotically active molecules to colon
Docusate/casanthranol (Peri-Colace®)	8-12 h	Small and large intestine	Casanthranol – mild stimulant; docusate – stool softener
Polyethylene glycol-electrolyte solution (GoLYTELY®)	30-60 min	Small and large intestine	Nonabsorbable solution which acts as an osmotic agent
Sorbitol 70%	24-48 h	Colon	Delivers osmotically active molecules to colon

LIPID-LOWERING AGENTS

Effects on Lipoproteins

Drug	Total Cholesterol (%)	LDLC (%)	HDLC (%)	TG (%)
Bile-acid resins	↓20-25	↓20-35	→	↑5-20
Fibric acid derivatives	↓10	↓10 (↑)	↑10-25	↓40-55
HMG-CoA RI (statins)	↓15-35	↓20-40	↑2-15	↓7-25
Nicotinic acid	↓25	↓20	↑20	↓40
Probucol	↓10-15	↓<10	↓30	→

Lipid-Lowering Agents

Drug	Dose/Day	Effect on LDL (%)	Effect on HDL (%)	Effect on TG (%)
HMG-CoA Reductase Inhibitors				
Atorvastatin	10 mg	-39	+6	-13
	20 mg	-43	+5	-20
	40 mg	-50	+5	-32
	80 mg	-60	+5	-37
Fluvastatin	20 mg	-22	+2	-5
	40 mg	-25	+3	-12
	80 mg	-36	+4	-12
Lovastatin	20 mg	-27	+7	-8
	40 mg	-32	+5	-2
	80 mg	-42	+8	-13
Pravastatin	10 mg	-22	+5	-3
	20 mg	-32	+3	-15
	40 mg	-34	+6	-10
Simvastatin	5 mg	-26	+7	-12
	10 mg	-30	+5	-17
	20 mg	-38	+10	-15
	40 mg	-41	+8	-24
	80 mg	-47		
Bile Acid Sequestrants				
Cholestyramine	4-24 g/day	-15 to -30	+3 to +5	+0 to +20
Colestipol	7-30 g/day	-15 to -30	+3 to +5	+0 to +20
Colesevelam	6 tab/day	-10	+10 to +25	-40 to -55
Fibric Acid Derivative				
Clofibrate	500 mg 4 times/day	-10	+10 to +25	-40 to -55
Fenofibrate	67-200 mg/day	-20 to -25	+1 to -34	-30 to -50
Gemfibrozil	600 mg bid	-5 to -10*	+10 to +20	-40 to -60
Niacin	1.5-6 g/day	-21 to -27	+10 to +35	-10 to -50

*May increase LDL in some patients.

Recommended Liver Function Monitoring for HMG-CoA Reductase Inhibitors

Agent	Initial and After Elevation in Dose	6 Weeks*	12 Weeks*	Periodically
Atorvastatin (Lipitor®)	x		x	x
Fluvastatin (Lescol®)	x		x	x
Lovastatin (Mevacor®)	x	x	x	x
Pravastatin (Pravachol®)	x			x
Simvastatin (Zocor®)	x			x

*After initiation of therapy or any elevation in dose.

NARCOTIC / OPIOID ANALGESIC COMPARISON

I.V. administration is most reliable and rapid; I.M. or S.C. use may cause delayed absorption and peak effect, especially with impaired tissue perfusion. Many agents undergo a significant first-pass effect. All are metabolized by the liver and excreted primarily in urine.

Dose Equivalents for Opioid Analgesics in Opioid-Naive Adults ≥50 kg*

Drug	Approximate Equianalgesic Dose		Usual Starting Dose for Moderate to Severe Pain	
	Oral	Parenteral	Oral	Parenteral
Opioid Agonist				
Morphine†	30 mg q3-4h (repeat around-the-clock dosing) 60 mg q3-4h (single dose or intermittent dosing)	10 mg q3-4h	30 mg q3-4h	10 mg q3-4h
Codeine	130 mg q3-4h	75 mg q3-4h	60 mg q3-4h	60 mg q2h (I.M./S.C.)
Hydromorphone† (Dilaudid®)	7.5 mg q3-4h	1.5 mg q3-4h	6 mg q3-4h	1.5 mg q3-4h
Levorphanol (Levo-Dromoran®)	4 mg q6-8h	2 mg q6-8h	4 mg q6-8h	2 mg q6-8h (S.C.)
Meperidine (Demerol®; Meperitab®)	300 mg q2-3h	100 mg q3h	NR	100 mg q3h
Methadone (Dolophine®, others)	20 mg q6-8h	10 mg q6-8h	20 mg q6-8h	10 mg q6-8h
Oxymorphone† (Numorphan®)	NA	1 mg q3-4h	NA	1 mg q3-4h
Combination Opioid/NSAID Preparations#				
Hydrocodone (in Lorcet®, Lortab®, Vicodin®, others)	30 mg q3-4h	NA	10 mg q3-4h	NA
Oxycodone (Roxicodone®, also in Percocet®, Percodan®, Tylox®, others)	30 mg q3-4h	NA	10 mg q3-4h	NA
Opioid Agonist-Antagonist and Partial Agonist				
Buprenorphine (Buprenex®)	NA	0.3-0.4 mg q6-8h	NA	0.4 q6-8h
Butorphanol (Stadol®)	NA	2 mg q3-4h	NA	2 mg q3-4h
Nalbuphine (Nubain®)	NA	10 mg q3-4h	NA	10 mg q3-4h
Pentazocine (Talwin®, others)	150 mg q3-4h	60 mg q3-4h	50 mg q4-6h	NR

Note: Tables vary in the suggested doses that are equianalgesic to morphine. Clinical response is the criterion that must be applied for each patient; titration to clinical response is necessary. Because there is not complete cross tolerance among these drugs, it is usually necessary to use a lower than equianalgesic dose when changing drugs and to retitrate to response.

Caution: Recommended doses do not apply to patients with renal or hepatic insufficiency or other conditions affecting drug metabolism and kinetics.

***Caution:** Recommended doses do not apply for adult patients with body weight <50 kg. For recommended starting doses for adults <50 kg body weight, see following table.

†**Caution:** For morphine, hydromorphone, and oxymorphone, rectal administration is an alternate route for patients unable to take oral medications. Equianalgesic doses may differ from oral and parenteral doses because of pharmacokinetic differences. **Note:** A short-acting opioid should normally be used for initial therapy of moderate to severe pain.

‡**Caution:** Codeine doses >65 mg often are not appropriate because of diminishing incremental analgesia with increasing doses but continually increasing nausea, constipation, and other side effects.

NA = not available; NR = not recommended.

NARCOTIC / OPIOID ANALGESIC COMPARISON *(Continued)*

Dose Equivalents for Opioid Analgesics in Opioid-Naive Adults <50 kg*

Drug	Approximate Equianalgesic Dose		Usual Starting Dose for Moderate to Severe Pain	
	Oral	Parenteral	Oral	Parenteral
Opioid Agonist				
Morphine†	30 mg q3-4h (repeat around-the-clock dosing) 60 mg q3-4h (single dose or intermittent dosing)	10 mg q3-4h	0.3 mg/kg q3-4h	0.1 mg/kg q3-4h
Codeine‡	130 mg q3-4h	75 mg q3-4h	1 mg/kg q3-4h#	NR
Hydromorphone† (Dilaudid®)	7.5 mg q3-4h	1.5 mg q3-4h	0.06 mg/kg q3-4h	0.015 mg/kg q3-4h
Levorphanol (Levo-Dromoran®)	4 mg q6-8h	2 mg q6-8h	0.04 mg/kg q6-8h	0.02 mg/kg q6-8h
Meperidine (Demerol®; Meperitab®)	300 mg q2-3h	100 mg q3h	NR	0.75 mg/kg q2-3h
Methadone (Dolophine®, others)	20 mg q6-8h	10 mg q6-8h	0.2 mg/kg q6-8h	0.1 mg/kg q6-8h
Oxymorphone† (Numorphan®)	NA	1 mg q3-4h	NR	NR
Combination Opioid/NSAID Preparations				
Hydrocodone (in Lorcet®, Lortab®, Vicodin®, others)	30 mg q3-4h	NA	0.2 mg/kg q3-4h#	NA
Oxycodone (Roxicodone®, also in Percocet®, Percodan®, Tylox®, others)	30 mg q3-4h	NA	0.2 mg/kg q3-4h#	NA
Opioid Agonist-Antagonist and Partial Agonist				
Buprenorphine (Buprenex®)	NA	0.3-0.4 mg q6-8h	NA	0.4 q6-8h
Butorphanol (Stadol®)	NA	2 mg q3-4h	NA	2 mg q3-4h
Nalbuphine (Nubain®)	NA	10 mg q3-4h	NA	10 mg q3-4h
Pentazocine (Talwin®, others)	150 mg q3-4h	60 mg q3-4h	50 mg q4-6h	NR

Note: Tables vary in the suggested doses that are equianalgesic to morphine. Clinical response is the criterion that must be applied for each patient; titration to clinical response is necessary. Because there is not complete cross tolerance among these drugs, it is usually necessary to use a lower than equianalgesic dose when changing drugs and to retitrate to response.

Caution: Recommended doses do not apply to patients with renal or hepatic insufficiency or other conditions affecting drug metabolism and kinetics.

***Caution:** Doses listed for patients with body weight <50 kg cannot be used as initial starting doses in babies younger than 6 months of age.

†**Caution:** For morphine, hydromorphone, and oxymorphone, rectal administration is an alternate route for patients unable to take oral medications. Equianalgesic doses may differ from oral and parenteral doses because of pharmacokinetic differences. **Note:** A short-acting opioid should normally be used for initial therapy of moderate to severe pain.

‡**Caution:** Codeine doses >65 mg often are not appropriate because of diminishing incremental analgesia with increasing doses but continually increasing nausea, constipation, and other side effects.

#**Caution:** Doses of aspirin and acetaminophen in combination opioid/NSAID preparations must also be adjusted to the patient's body weight.

NA = not available; NR = not recommended.

Comparative Pharmacokinetics

Drug	Onset (min)	Peak (h)	Duration (h)	Half-Life (h)	Average Dosing Interval (h)		Equianalgesic Doses* (mg)	
							I.M.	Oral
Alfentanil	Immediate	ND	ND	1-2	—	—	ND	NA
Buprenorphine	15	1	4-8	2-3			0.4	—
Butorphanol	I.M.: 30-60; I.V.: 4-5	0.5-1	3-5	2.5-3.5	3	(3-6)	2	—
Codeine	P.O.: 30-60; I.M.: 10-30	0.5-1	4-6	3-4	3	(3-6)	120	200
Fentanyl	I.M.: 7-15; I.V.: Immediate	ND	1-2	1.5-6	1	(0.5-2)	0.1	NA
Hydrocodone	ND	ND	4-8	3.3-4.4	6	(4-8)	ND	ND
Hydromorphone	P.O.: 15-30	0.5-1	4-6	2-4	4	(3-6)	1.5	7.5
Levorphanol	P.O.: 10-60	0.5-1	4-8	12-16	6	(6-24)	2 (A); 1 (C)	4 (A); 1 (C)
Meperidine	P.O./I.M./S.C.: 10-15; I.V.: ≤5	0.5-1	2-4	3-4	3	(2-4)	75	300
Methadone	P.O.: 30-60; I.V.: 10-20	0.5-1	4-6 (acute); >8 (chronic)	15-30	8	(6-12)	10 (A); 2-4 (C)	20 (A); 2-4 (C)
Morphine	P.O.: 15-60 I.V.: ≤5	P.O./I.M./S.C.: 0.5-1; I.V.: 0.3	3-6	2-4	4	(3-6)	10	60# (A); 30 (C)
Nalbuphine	I.M.: 30; I.V.: 1-3	1	3-6	5		—	10	—
Oxycodone	P.O.: 10-15	0.5-1	4-6	3-4	4	(3-6)	NA	20
Oxymorphone	5-15	0.5-1	3-6				1	10†
Pentazocine	15-20	0.25-1	3-4	2-3	3	(3-6)		
Propoxyphene	P.O.: 30-60	2-2.5	4-6	3.5-15	6	(4-8)	ND	130‡-200§
Remifentanil	1-3	<0.3	0.1-0.2	0.15-0.3	—	—	ND	ND
Sufentanil	1.3-3	ND	ND	2.5-3	—	—	0.02	NA

Adapted from The American Pain Society, *Principles of Analgesic Use in the Treatment of Acute Pain and Cancer Pain,* 4th ed, Skokie, IL, The American Pain Society, 1999.

ND = no data available. NA = not applicable. (A) = acute. (C) = chronic

*Based on acute, short-term use. Chronic administration may alter pharmacokinetics and decrease the oral parenteral dose ratio. The morphine oral-parenteral ratio decreases to ~1.5-2.5:1 upon chronic dosing.

#Extensive survey data suggest that the relative potency of I.M.:P.O. morphine of 1:6 changes to 1:2-3 with chronic dosing.

†Rectal

‡HCl salt

§Napsylate salt

NARCOTIC / OPIOID ANALGESIC COMPARISON *(Continued)*

Comparative Pharmacology

Drug	Analgesic	Antitussive	Constipation	Respiratory Depression	Sedation	Emesis
Phenanthrenes						
Codeine	+	+++	+	+	+	+
Hydrocodone	+	+++		+		
Hydromorphone	++	+++	+	++	+	+
Levorphanol	++	++	++	++	++	+
Morphine	++	+++	++	++	++	++
Oxycodone	++	+++	++	++	++	++
Oxymorphone	++	+	++	+++		+++
Phenylpiperidines						
Alfentanil	++					
Fentanyl	++			+		+
Meperidine	++	+	+	++	+	
Sufentanil	+++					
Diphenylheptanes						
Methadone	++	++	++	++	+	+
Propoxyphene	+			+	+	+
Agonist/Antagonist						
Buprenorphine	++	N/A	+++	+++	++	++
Butorphanol	++	N/A	+++	+++	++	+
Dezocine	++		+	++	+	++
Nalbuphine	++	N/A	+++	+++	++	++
Pentazocine	++	N/A	+	++	++ or stimulation	++

NONSALICYLATE/NONSTEROIDAL ANTI-INFLAMMATORY AGENTS

Name	Plasma Half-Life (h)	Time to Peak (h)[1]	Usual Duration (h)	Maximum Recommended Daily Dose (mg)	Considerations
Celecoxib (Celebrex®)	11	2-3	12	400	Selective COX-2 inhibitor
Choline magnesium salicylate (Trilisate®, Tricosal®)	2-30	2	8-24	4500	Nonacetylated salicylates: limited antiplatelet effects
Diclofenac potassium immediate release (Cataflam®)	1-2	1	8	200	Less GI distress, less CNS depression
Diclofenac sodium delayed release (Voltaren®)	1-2	2-3	8-12	200	Less GI distress, less CNS depression
Diflunisal (Dolobid®)	8-12	2-3	8-12	1500	
Etodolac (Lodine®)	7	1-2	6-8	1200	Less GI distress
Fenoprofen (Nalfon®)	2-3	1-2	4-6	3200	Increased nephrotoxicity, increased antiplatelet activity
Flurbiprofen (Ansaid®)	3-6	1.5-2	6-12	300	Increased GI distress
Ibuprofen (Motrin®, Advil®)	2	1-2	4-6	3200	Less GI distress, moderately increased nephrotoxicity
Indomethacin (Indocin®)	4.5	3-4	4-6	200	Increased nephrotoxicity, GI distress, and CNS depression
Indomethacin SR, (Indocin® SR)	4.5-6	2-4	6-12	150	
Ketoprofen (Orudis®, Oruvail®)	1-4	0.5-2	4-6	300	
Ketorolac (Toradol®)	5-6	1	6-8	P.O.: 40[2] I.M.: 120	Increased nephrotoxicity and GI distress
Meclofenamate (Meclomen®)	2-3	0.5-1.5	2-4	400	Less hepatic injury, increased GI distress
Mefenamic acid (Ponstel®)	3.5	2-4	2-6	1000	
Meloxicam (Mobic®)	15-20	5-10	>24	15	
Nabumetone (Relafen®)	24	3-6	>24	2000	Less GI distress
Naproxen (Naprosyn®)	9-20	1-2	2-7	1500	Less GI distress
Naproxen sodium (Anaprox®)	12-13	1-2	8-12	1375	
Oxaprozin (Daypro™)	42-50	3-5	>24	1800	Less GI distress
Piroxicam (Feldene®)	30-86	P.O.: 3-5	24	40	Less hepatic injury
Rofecoxib (Vioxx®)	17	2-3	>24	50	Selective COX-2 inhibitor
Salsalate (Disalcid®)	7-8	2	8-24	3 g	Nonacetylated salicylates: limited antiplatelet effects
Sulindac (Clinoril®)	7 (16)[3]	2-4	12	400	
Tolmetin (Tolectin®)	5	0.5-1	6-8	2000	
Valdecoxib (Bextra®)	8-11	2.25-3	12-24	40	Selective COX-2 inhibitor

Dosage is based on a 70 kg adult with normal hepatic and renal function.

[1]Food decreases the rate of absorption and may delay the time to peak levels.

[2]150 mg on the first day.

[3]Half-life of active sulfide metabolite.

CYTOCHROME P450 ENZYMES: SUBSTRATES, INHIBITORS, AND INDUCERS

INTRODUCTION

Most drugs are eliminated from the body, at least in part, by being chemically altered to less lipid-soluble products (ie, metabolized), and thus more likely to be excreted via the kidneys or the bile. Phase I metabolism includes drug hydrolysis, oxidation, and reduction, and results in drugs that are more polar in their chemical structure, while Phase II metabolism involves the attachment of an additional molecule onto the drug (or partially metabolized drug) in order to create an inactive and/or more water soluble compound. Phase II processes include (primarily) glucuronidation, sulfation, glutathione conjugation, acetylation, and methylation.

Virtually any of the Phase I and II enzymes can be inhibited by some xenobiotic or drug. Some of the Phase I and II enzymes can be induced. Inhibition of the activity of metabolic enzymes will result in increased concentrations of the substrate (drug), whereas induction of the activity of metabolic enzymes will result in decreased concentrations of the substrate. For example, the well-documented enzyme-inducing effects of phenobarbital may include a combination of Phase I and II enzymes. Phase II glucuronidation may be increased via induced UDP-glucuronosyltransferase (UGT) activity, whereas Phase I oxidation may be increased via induced cytochrome P450 (CYP) activity. However, for most drugs, the primary route of metabolism (and the primary focus of drug-drug interaction) is Phase I oxidation, and specifically, metabolism.

CYP enzymes may be responsible for the metabolism (at least partial metabolism) of approximately 75% of all drugs, with the CYP3A subfamily responsible for nearly half of this activity. Found throughout plant, animal, and bacterial species, CYP enzymes represent a superfamily of xenobiotic metabolizing proteins. There have been several hundred CYP enzymes identified in nature, each of which has been assigned to a family (1, 2, 3, etc), subfamily (A, B, C, etc) and given a specific enzyme number (1, 2, 3, etc) according to the similarity in amino acid sequence that it shares with other enzymes. Of these many enzymes, only a few are found in humans, and even fewer appear to be involved in the metabolism of xenobiotics (eg, drugs). The key human enzyme subfamilies include CYP1A, CYP2A, CYP2B, CYP2C, CYP2D, CYP2E, and CYP3A.

CYP enzymes are found in the endoplasmic reticulum of cells in a variety of human tissues (eg, skin, kidneys, brain, lungs), but their predominant sites of concentration and activity are the liver and intestine. Though the abundance of CYP enzymes throughout the body is relatively equally distributed among the various subfamilies, the relative contribution to drug metabolism is (in decreasing order of magnitude) CYP3A4 (nearly 50%), CYP2D6 (nearly 25%), CYP2C8/9 (nearly 15%), then CYP1A2, CYP2C19, CYP2A6, and CYP2E1. Owing to their potential for numerous drug-drug interactions, those drugs that are identified early in their preclinical as substrates of CYP3A enzymes are often given a lower priority for continued research and development in favor of drugs that appear to be less affected by (or less likely to affect) this enzyme subfamily.

Each enzyme subfamily possesses unique selectivity toward potential substrates. For example, CYP1A2 preferentially binds medium-sized, planar, lipophilic molecules, while CYP2D6 preferentially binds molecules that possess a basic nitrogen atom. Some CYP subfamilies exhibit polymorphism (ie, multiple allelic variants that manifest differing catalytic properties). The best described polymorphisms involve CYP2C9, CYP2C19, and CYP2D6. Individuals possessing "wild type" gene alleles exhibit normal functioning CYP capacity. Others, however, possess allelic variants that leave the person with a subnormal level of catalytic potential (so called "poor metabolizers"). Poor metabolizers would be more likely to experience toxicity from drugs metabolized by the affected enzymes (or less effects if the enzyme is responsible for converting a prodrug to it's active form as in the case of codeine). The percentage of people classified as poor metabolizers varies by enzyme and population group. As an example, approximately 7% of Caucasians and only about 1% of Orientals appear to be CYP2D6 poor metabolizers.

CYP enzymes can be both inhibited and induced by other drugs, leading to increased or decreased serum concentrations (along with the associated effects), respectively. Induction occurs when a drug causes an increase in the amount of smooth endoplasmic reticulum, secondary to increasing the amount of the affected CYP enzymes in the tissues. This "revving up" of the CYP enzyme system may take several days to reach peak activity, and likewise, may take several days, even months, to return to normal following discontinuation of the inducing agent.

CYP inhibition occurs via several potential mechanisms. Most commonly, a CYP inhibitor competitively (and reversibly) binds to the active site on the enzyme, thus preventing the substrate from binding to the same site, and preventing the substrate from being metabolized. The affinity of an inhibitor for an enzyme may be expressed by an inhibition constant (Ki) or IC50 (defined as the concentration of the inhibitor required to cause 50% inhibition under a given set of conditions). In addition to reversible competition for an enzyme site, drugs may inhibit enzyme activity by binding to sites on the enzyme other than that to which the substrate would bind, and thereby cause a change in the functionality or physical structure of the enzyme. A drug may also bind to the enzyme in an irreversible (ie, "suicide") fashion. In such a case, it is not the concentration of drug at the enzyme site that is important (constantly binding and releasing), but the shear number of molecules available for binding (once bound, always bound).

Although an inhibitor or inducer may be known to affect a variety of CYP subfamilies, it may only inhibit one or two in a clinically important fashion. Likewise, although a substrate is known to be at least partially metabolized by a variety of CYP enzymes, only one or two enzymes may contribute significantly enough to its overall metabolism to warrant concern when used with potential inducers or inhibitors. Therefore, when attempting to predict the level of risk of using two drugs that may affect each other via altered CYP function, it is important to identify the relative effectiveness of the inhibiting/inducing drug on the CYP subfamilies that significantly contribute to the metabolism of the substrate. The contribution of a specific CYP pathway to substrate metabolism should be considered not only in light of other known CYP pathways, but also other nonoxidative pathways for substrate metabolism (eg, glucuronidation) and transporter proteins (eg, P-glycoprotein) that may affect the presentation of a substrate to a metabolic pathway.

HOW TO USE THE TABLES

The following CYP SUBSTRATES, INHIBITORS, and INDUCERS tables provide a comprehensive perspective on drugs that are affected by, or affect, cytochrome P450 (CYP) enzymes.

The CYP Substrates table contains a list of drugs reported to be metabolized, at least in part, by one or more CYP enzymes. An enzyme that appears to play a clinically significant role in a drug's metabolism is marked with a solid dot "•", and an enzyme whose role does not appear to be clinically significant is marked with an open dot "o". The designation of clinically significant is the result of a two-phase review. The first phase considered the clinical relevance of a substrate's concentration being increased twofold, or decreased by one-half. If either of these changes (which might occur in the presence of an effective enzyme inhibitor or inducer) was considered to present a clinically significant concern, the drug was subjected to a second phase. The second phase considered the contribution of each CYP enzyme to the overall metabolism of the drug. The enzyme pathway was considered clinically relevant if it was responsible for at least 30% of the metabolism of the drug.

The CYP Inhibitors table contains a list of drugs that are reported to inhibit one or more CYP enzymes. Enzymes that appear to be effectively inhibited by a drug are marked with a solid dot "•", and enzymes that do not appear to be effectively inhibited are marked with an open dot "o". The designation of "effectively inhibited" is the compiled result of the authors' review of published clinical reports, available Ki data, and assessments published by other experts in the field.

The CYP Inducers table contains a list of drugs that are reported to induce one or more CYP enzymes. Enzymes that appear to be effectively induced by a drug are marked with a solid dot "•", and enzymes that do not appear to be effectively induced are marked with an open dot "o". The designation of "effectively induced" is the compiled result of the authors' review of published clinical reports and assessments published by other experts in the field.

In all cases, only those enzymes marked with either a solid or open dot should be considered relevant to the drug identified at the beginning of the row. In general, clinically significant interactions are more likely to occur between substrates and either inhibitors or inducers of the same enzyme(s), all of which have been marked with a solid dot "•". However, these assessments possess a degree of subjectivity on behalf of the authors, at times based on limited indications regarding the significance of CYP effects of particular agents. The authors have attempted to balance a conservative, clinically-sensitive presentation of the data with a desire to avoid the numbing effect of a "beware of everything" approach. Even so, other potential interactions (ie, those involving enzymes marked with an open dot "o") may warrant consideration in some cases. It is important to note that information related to CYP metabolism of drugs is expanding at a rapid pace, and thus, the contents of this table should only be considered to represent a "snapshot" of the information available at the time of publication.

Selected Readings

Drug-Drug Interactions, Rodrigues AD, ed, New York, NY: Marcel Dekker, Inc, 2002.

Metabolic Drug Interactions, Levy R, Thummel K, Trager W, et al, eds, Philadephia, PA: Lippincott Williams & Wilkins, 2000.

Michalets EL, "Update: Clinically Significant Cytochrome P-450 Drug Interactions," *Pharmacotherapy*, 1998, 18(1):84-112.

Thummel KE and Wilkinson GR, "*In vitro* and *in vivo* Drug Interactions Involving Human CYP3A," *Annu Rev Pharmacol Toxicol*, 1998, 38:389-430.

Zhang Y and Benet LZ, "The Gut as a Barrier to Drug Absorption: Combined Role of Cytochrome P450 3A and P-Glycoprotein," *Clin Pharmacokinet*, 2001, 40(3):159-68.

Selected Websites

http://www.gentest.com

http://www.imm.ki.se/CYPalleles

http://medicine.iupui.edu/flockhart

http://www.mhc.com/Cytochromes

CYTOCHROME P450 ENZYMES: SUBSTRATES, INHIBITORS, AND INDUCERS *(Continued)*

CYP Substrates

Drug	1A2	2A6	2B6	2C8/9	2C19	2D6	2E1	3A4
Acetaminophen	o	o		o		o	o	o
Albendazole	o							o
Albuterol								•
Alfentanil								•
Almotriptan						o		o
Alosetron	o			•				o
Alprazolam								•
Aminophylline	•						o	o
Amiodarone	o			•	o	o		o
Amitriptyline	o		o	o	o	•		o
Amlodipine								•
Amoxapine						•		
Amphetamine						o		
Amprenavir				o				•
Argatroban								o
Aspirin				o				
Atorvastatin								•
Azelastine	o				o	o		o
Azithromycin								o
Benzphetamine			o					•
Benztropine						o		
Betaxolol	•					•		
Bexarotene								o
Bezafibrate								o
Bisoprolol						o		•
Bosentan				•				•
Brinzolamide								o
Bromazepam								•
Bromocriptine								•
Budesonide								o
Bupivacaine	o				o	o		o
Buprenorphine								•
BuPROPion	o	o	•	o		o	o	o
BusPIRone						o		•
Busulfan								•
Caffeine	•			o		o	o	o
Candesartan				o				
Capsaicin							o	
Captopril						•		
Carbamazepine				o				•
Carisoprodol					•			
Carteolol						o		
Carvedilol	o			•		•	o	o
Celecoxib				o				o
Cerivastatin								•
Cetirizine								o
Cevimeline						o		o
Chlordiazepoxide								•
Chloroquine						•		•
Chlorpheniramine						o		•
ChlorproMAZINE	o					•		o
ChlorproPAMIDE				o				
Chlorzoxazone	o	o				o	•	o
Cilostazol	o				o	o		o
Cisapride	o	o	o	o	o			•
Citalopram					•	o		•
Clarithromycin								•
Clobazam								•
Clofibrate								o
ClomiPRAMINE	•				•	•		o
Clonazepam								•
Clopidogrel	o							o

CYP Substrates *(continued)*

Drug	1A2	2A6	2B6	2C8/9	2C19	2D6	2E1	3A4
Clorazepate								•
Clozapine	•	o		o	o	o		o
Cocaine								•
Codeine						•		o
Colchicine								•
Cyclobenzaprine	•					o		o
Cyclophosphamide		o	•	o	•			o
CycloSPORINE								•
Dacarbazine	•						•	
Dantrolene								•
Dapsone				o	o		o	•
Delavirdine						o		•
Desipramine	o					•		
Desogestrel					•			
Dexamethasone								o
Dexmedetomidine		•						
Dextroamphetamine						•		
Dextromethorphan		o		o	o	•	o	o
Diazepam	o		o	o	•			•
Diclofenac	o		o	o	o	o		o
Dicumarol				•				
Digitoxin								•
Digoxin								o
Dihydrocodeine compound						•		
Dihydroergotamine								•
Diltiazem				o		o		•
Dirithromycin								o
Disopyramide								•
Disulfiram	o	o	o			o	o	o
Docetaxel								•
Dofetilide								o
Dolasetron				o				o
Domperidone								o
Donepezil						o		o
Dorzolamide				o				o
Doxepin	•					•		•
DOXOrubicin						•		•
Doxycycline								•
Drospirenone								o
Dutasteride								o
Efavirenz			•					•
Enalapril								•
Enflurane							•	
Ergoloid mesylates								•
Ergonovine								•
Ergotamine								•
Erythromycin			o					•
Escitalopram					•			•
Esomeprazole					•			o
Estazolam								o
Estradiol	•	o	o	o	o	o	o	•
Estrogens, conjugated A/synthetic	•	o	o	o	o	o	o	•
Estrogens, conjugated equine	•	o	o	o	o	o	o	•
Estrogens, conjugated esterified	•		o	o			o	•
Estrone	•		o	o			o	•
Estropipate	•		o	o			o	•
Ethinyl estradiol								•
Ethosuximide								•
Etonogestrel								o
Etoposide	o						o	•
Exemestane								o
Felbamate							o	•
Felodipine								•

CYTOCHROME P450 ENZYMES: SUBSTRATES, INHIBITORS, AND INDUCERS *(Continued)*

CYP Substrates *(continued)*

Drug	1A2	2A6	2B6	2C8/9	2C19	2D6	2E1	3A4
Fenofibrate								o
Fentanyl								•
Fexofenadine								o
Finasteride								o
Flecainide	o					•		
Fluoxetine	o		o	•	o	•	o	o
Fluphenazine						•		
Flurazepam								•
Flurbiprofen				o				
Flutamide	•							•
Fluticasone								o
Fluvastatin				o		o		o
Fluvoxamine	•					•		
Formoterol		o		o	o	o		
Fosphenytoin (as phenytoin)				•	•			o
Frovatriptan	o							
Fulvestrant								•
Galantamine						o		o
Gemfibrozil								o
Glimepiride				•				
GlipiZIDE				•				
Granisetron								o
Guanabenz	•							
Halazepam								o
Halofantrine				o		o		•
Haloperidol	o					•		•
Halothane		o	o	o		o	•	o
Hydrocodone						•		
Hydrocortisone								o
Ibuprofen				o	o			
Ifosfamide		•	o	•	•			•
Imatinib	o			o	o	o		•
Imipramine	o		o		•	•		o
Imiquimod	o							o
Indinavir						o		•
Indomethacin				o	o			
Irbesartan				o				
Irinotecan			•					•
Isoflurane							•	
Isoniazid							•	
Isosorbide								•
Isosorbide dinitrate								•
Isosorbide mononitrate								•
Isradipine								•
Itraconazole								•
Ivermectin								o
Ketamine			•	•				•
Ketoconazole								•
Labetalol						•		
Lansoprazole				o	•			•
Letrozole		o						•
Levobupivacaine	o							o
Levomethadyl acetate hydrochloride			o					•
Levonorgestrel								•
Lidocaine	o	o	o	o		•		•
Lomustine						•		
Lopinavir								o
Loratadine						o		o
Losartan				•				•
Lovastatin								•
Maprotiline						•		

CYP Substrates *(continued)*

Drug	1A2	2A6	2B6	2C8/9	2C19	2D6	2E1	3A4
MedroxyPROGESTERone								•
Mefenamic acid				o				
Mefloquine								•
Meloxicam				o				o
Mephenytoin			o	•	•			
Mephobarbital			o	o	•			
Mestranol				•				•
Methadone				o	o	o		•
Methamphetamine						•		
Methoxsalen		o						
Methoxyflurane		o	o				•	o
Methsuximide					•			
Methylergonovine								•
Methylphenidate						•		
MethylPREDNISolone								o
Methysergide								•
Metoclopramide	o					o		
Metoprolol					o	•		
Mexiletine	•					•		
Miconazole								•
Midazolam			o					•
Mifepristone								o
Mirtazapine	•			o		•		•
Moclobemide					•	•		
Modafinil								•
Mometasone furoate								o
Montelukast				•				•
Moricizine								•
Morphine sulfate						o		
Naproxen	o			o				
Nateglinide				•				•
Nefazodone						•		•
Nelfinavir				o	•	o		•
Nevirapine			o			o		•
NiCARdipine	o			o		o	o	•
Nicotine	o	o	o	o	o	o	o	o
NIFEdipine						o		•
Nilutamide					•			
Nimodipine								•
Nisoldipine								•
Nitrendipine								•
Norelgestromin								o
Norethindrone								•
Norgestrel								•
Nortriptyline	o				o	•		o
Olanzapine	o					o		
Omeprazole		o		o	•	o		o
Ondansetron	o			o		o	o	•
Orphenadrine	o		o			o		o
Oxybutynin								o
Oxycodone						•		
Paclitaxel				•				•
Pantoprazole					•			o
Paroxetine						•		
Pentamidine					•			
Perphenazine	o			o	o	•		o
Phencyclidine								•
Phenobarbital				o	•		o	
Phenytoin				•	•			o
Pimecrolimus								o
Pimozide	•							•
Pindolol						•		
Pioglitazone				•				•
Pipecuronium				o				
Piroxicam				o				

CYTOCHROME P450 ENZYMES: SUBSTRATES, INHIBITORS, AND INDUCERS *(Continued)*

CYP Substrates *(continued)*

Drug	1A2	2A6	2B6	2C8/9	2C19	2D6	2E1	3A4
Pravastatin								o
Prazepam								o
PrednisoLONE								o
PredniSONE								o
Primaquine								•
Procainamide						•		
Progesterone	o	o		o	•	o		•
Proguanil	o				o			o
Promethazine			•			•		
Propafenone	o					•		o
Propofol	o	o	•	•	o	o	o	o
Propranolol	•				•	•		o
Quazepam								o
Quetiapine						o		•
Quinidine				o			o	•
Quinine	o				o			o
Rabeprazole					•			•
Ranitidine	o				o	o		
Repaglinide				o				•
Rifabutin	•							•
Rifampin		•		•				•
Riluzole	•							
Risperidone						•		o
Ritonavir	o		o			•		•
Rofecoxib				o				
Ropinirole	•							o
Ropivacaine	o		o			o		o
Rosiglitazone				•				
Saquinavir						o		•
Selegiline	o	o	•	•		o		o
Sertraline			•	•	•	o		•
Sevoflurane		o	o				•	o
Sibutramine								•
Sildenafil				o				•
Simvastatin								•
Sirolimus								•
Spiramycin								•
Sufentanil								•
SulfaDIAZINE				•			o	o
Sulfamethoxazole				•				o
Sulfinpyrazone				•				o
SulfiSOXAZOLE				•				
Suprofen				o				
Tacrine	•							
Tacrolimus								•
Tamoxifen		o	o	•		•	o	•
Tamsulosin						•		•
Temazepam			o	o	o			o
Teniposide								•
Terbinafine								•
Testosterone			o	o	o			o
Tetracycline								•
Theophylline	•			o		o	•	•
Thiabendazole	o							
Thioridazine					o	•		
Thiothixene	•							
Tiagabine								•
Ticlopidine								•
Timolol						•		
TOLBUTamide				•	o			
Tolcapone (metabolites)		o						o
Tolterodine				o	o	•		•

CYP Substrates *(continued)*

Drug	1A2	2A6	2B6	2C8/9	2C19	2D6	2E1	3A4
Toremifene	o							•
Torsemide				•				
Tramadol						•		o
Trazodone						o		•
Tretinoin		o	o	o				
Triazolam								•
Trifluoperazine	•							
Trimethadione				o	o		•	o
Trimethoprim				•				•
Trimipramine					•	•		•
Troleandomycin								•
Valdecoxib				o				o
Valproic acid		o	o	o	o		o	
Venlafaxine				o	o	•		•
Verapamil	o		o	o			o	•
VinBLAStine						o		•
VinCRIStine								•
Vinorelbine						o		•
Voriconazole				•	•			o
Warfarin	o			•	o			o
Yohimbine						o		
Zafirlukast				•				
Zaleplon								o
Zidovudine		o		o	o			o
Zileuton	o			o				o
Ziprasidone	o							o
Zolmitriptan	o							
Zolpidem	o			o	o	o		•
Zonisamide					o			•
Zopiclone				•				•
Zuclopenthixol						•		

CYTOCHROME P450 ENZYMES: SUBSTRATES, INHIBITORS, AND INDUCERS *(Continued)*

CYP Inhibitors

Drug	1A2	2A6	2B6	2C8/9	2C19	2D6	2E1	3A4
Acebutolol						o		
AcetaZOLAMIDE								o
Albendazole	o							
Alosetron	o						o	
Amiodarone	o	o	o	•	o	•		•
Amitriptyline	o			o	o	o	o	
Amlodipine			o	o		o		o
Amphetamine						o		
Amprenavir					o			•
Anastrozole	o			o				o
Atorvastatin								o
Azelastine			o	o	o	•		o
Azithromycin								o
Bepridil						o		
Betamethasone								o
Betaxolol						o		
Biperiden						o		
Bromazepam							o	
Bromocriptine								•
BuPROPion						•		
Caffeine	•							
Candesartan				o				
Celecoxib						o		
Cerivastatin								o
Chloramphenicol				o				o
Chloroquine						o		
Chlorpheniramine						•		
ChlorproMAZINE						o	o	
Chlorzoxazone							o	o
Cholecalciferol				o	o	o		
Cimetidine	•			o	o	•	o	•
Ciprofloxacin	•							•
Cisapride						o		
Citalopram	o		o		o	o		
Clarithromycin	o							•
Clemastine						•		o
Clofazimine								o
Clofibrate		o						
ClomiPRAMINE						•		
Clopidogrel				o				
Clotrimazole		o		o			o	o
Clozapine				o		o		o
Cocaine						•		o
Codeine						o		
CycloSPORINE				o				o
Danazol								o
Delavirdine	o			o	o	o		o
Desipramine						o	o	
Dexmedetomidine	o			o		•		o
Dextromethorphan						o		
Diazepam					o			o
Diclofenac				o			o	
Dihydroergotamine								o
Diltiazem				o		o		•
Dimethyl sulfoxide				o	o			
DiphenhydrAMINE						o		
Disulfiram	o	o	o	o		o	•	o
Dolasetron						o		
DOXOrubicin						o		o
Doxycycline								o
Drospirenone	o			o	o			o
Econazole							o	

CYP Inhibitors *(continued)*

Drug	1A2	2A6	2B6	2C8/9	2C19	2D6	2E1	3A4
Efavirenz				o	o			o
Enoxacin	•							•
Entacapone	o	o		o	o	o	o	o
Eprosartan				o				
Ergotamine								o
Erythromycin	o							•
Escitalopram						o		
Estradiol	o							
Estrogens, conjugated A/synthetic	o							
Estrogens, conjugated equine	o							
Ethinyl estradiol	o		o		o			o
Ethotoin					o			
Etoposide				o				o
Felbamate					o			
Felodipine				o		o		o
Fentanyl								o
Fexofenadine						o		
Flecainide						o		
Fluconazole	o			•	•			•
Fluoxetine	o		•	o	o	•		o
Fluphenazine	o					o	o	
Flurazepam							o	
Flurbiprofen				o				
Flutamide	o							
Fluvastatin	o			•		o		o
Fluvoxamine	•		•	o	•	o		•
Fomepizole		•						
Grapefruit juice								•
Halofantrine						o		
Haloperidol						•		
HydrALAZINE								o
HydrOXYzine						o		
Ibuprofen				o				
Imatinib				o		o		•
Imipramine	o				o	o	o	
Indinavir				o	o	o		•
Indomethacin				o	o			
Interferon gamma-1b							o	
Irbesartan				o				o
Isoflurane			o					
Isoniazid	o			o	o	o	o	o
Itraconazole								•
Ketoconazole	o	o	o	o	o	o		•
Ketoprofen				o				
Labetalol						o		
Lansoprazole				o	•	o		o
Leflunomide				o				
Letrozole		o			o			
Levofloxacin	•							
Lidocaine	o					o		
Lomefloxacin	•							
Lomustine						o		o
Losartan	o			o	o			o
Lovastatin				o		o		
Mefenamic acid				o				
Mefloquine								o
Meloxicam				o				
Mephobarbital					o			
Mestranol	o		o		o			o
Methadone						•		o
Methimazole	o	o	o	o	o	o	o	o
Methoxsalen	•	•		o	o	o	o	o
Methsuximide					o			

CYTOCHROME P450 ENZYMES: SUBSTRATES, INHIBITORS, AND INDUCERS *(Continued)*

CYP Inhibitors *(continued)*

Drug	1A2	2A6	2B6	2C8/9	2C19	2D6	2E1	3A4
Methylphenidate						o		
MethylPREDNISolone								o
Metoclopramide						o		
Metoprolol						o		
Metronidazole				o				o
Metyrapone		o						
Mexiletine	o							
Miconazole		o		o			o	o
Midazolam				o				o
Mifepristone						o		o
Mirtazapine	o							o
Mitoxantrone								o
Moclobemide	o				o	o		
Modafinil				o	o			
Montelukast				o				
Nalidixic acid	•							
Nateglinide				o				
Nefazodone	o		o			o		•
Nelfinavir	o		o	o	o	o		•
Nevirapine	o					o		o
NiCARdipine				o	o	o		o
Nicotine		o						
NIFEdipine	o			o		o		o
Nilutamide					o			
Nisoldipine	o							o
Nitrendipine								o
Norfloxacin	•							o
Nortriptyline						o	o	
Ofloxacin	o							
Olanzapine	o			o	o	o		o
Omeprazole				o	•	o		•
Ondansetron	o			o		o		
Orphenadrine	o	o	o	o	o	o	o	•
Oxcarbazepine					o			
Oxprenolol						o		
Oxybutynin						o		o
Paroxetine	o		•	o	o	•		o
Pentamidine						o		
Pentoxifylline	o							
Pergolide						•		o
Perphenazine	o					•		
Phencyclidine								o
Pilocarpine		o					o	o
Pimozide						•		o
Pindolol						o		
Pioglitazone				o	o			
Pipecuronium				o				
Pravastatin				o		o		o
Praziquantel						o		
PrednisoLONE								o
Primaquine						o		o
Probenecid					o			
Progesterone				o	o			
Promethazine						o		
Propafenone	o					o		
Propofol	o			o		o	o	o
Propoxyphene				o		o		o
Propranolol	o					o		
Pyrimethamine						o		
Quinidine				o		•		o
Quinine				o		•		o
Quinupristin								o

CYP Inhibitors *(continued)*

Drug	1A2	2A6	2B6	2C8/9	2C19	2D6	2E1	3A4
Rabeprazole					o			o
Ranitidine	o					o		
Risperidone						o		o
Ritonavir				o	o	•	o	•
Rofecoxib	•							
Ropinirole	o					•		
Rosiglitazone				o				
Saquinavir				o	o	o		•
Selegiline	o	o		o	o	o	o	o
Sertraline	o		•	o	•	o		o
Sildenafil	o			o	o	o	o	o
Simvastatin				o		o		
Sirolimus								o
Sparfloxacin	•							
SulfaDIAZINE				o				
Sulfamethoxazole				o				
Sulfinpyrazone				o				
SulfiSOXAZOLE				o				
Tacrine	o							
Tacrolimus								o
Tamoxifen			o	o				o
Telmisartan					o			
Teniposide				o				o
Tenofovir	o							
Terbinafine						o		
Testosterone								o
Tetracycline								o
Theophylline	o							
Thioridazine	o					•	o	
Thiotepa			o					
Thiothixene						o		
Ticlopidine	•			•	•	o		
Timolol						o		
Tocainide	o							
TOLBUTamide				o				
Tolcapone				o				
Topiramate					o			
Torsemide					o			
Tranylcypromine	o	•		o	o	o	o	o
Trazodone						o		
Tretinoin				o				
Triazolam				o				
Trimethoprim				o				
Tripelennamine						o		
Triprolidine						o		
Troleandomycin								•
Valdecoxib				o	o			
Valproic acid				o	o	o		o
Valsartan				o				
Venlafaxine			o			o		o
Verapamil	o			o		o		•
VinBLAStine						o		o
VinCRIStine								o
Vinorelbine						o		o
Voriconazole				o	o			o
Warfarin				o	o			
Yohimbine						o		
Zafirlukast	o			o	o	o		o
Zileuton	o							
Ziprasidone						o		o

CYTOCHROME P450 ENZYMES: SUBSTRATES, INHIBITORS, AND INDUCERS *(Continued)*

CYP Inducers

Drug	1A2	2A6	2B6	2C8/9	2C19	2D6	2E1	3A4
Aminoglutethimide	•				•			•
Amobarbital		•						
Azatadine								o
Bosentan				o				o
Calcitriol								o
Carbamazepine	•		•	•	•			•
Clofibrate			o				o	o
Colchicine				o			o	o
Cyclophosphamide			o	o				
Dexamethasone		o	o	o				o
Dicloxacillin								o
Efavirenz (in liver only)			o					o
Estradiol								o
Estrogens, conjugated A/synthetic								o
Estrogens, conjugated equine								o
Felbamate								o
Fosphenytoin (as phenytoin)			•	•	•			•
Griseofulvin	o			o				o
Hydrocortisone								o
Ifosfamide				o				
Insulin preparations	o							
interferon alfa-2a	o							
Interferon alfa-2b	o							
Isoniazid (after D/C)							o	
Lansoprazole	o							
MedroxyPROGESTERone								o
Mephobarbital		o						
Metyrapone								o
Modafinil	o		o					o
Moricizine	o							o
Nafcillin								•
Nevirapine			•					•
Norethindrone					o			
Omeprazole	o							
Oxcarbazepine								•
Paclitaxel								o
Pantoprazole	o							o
Pentobarbital		•						•
Phenobarbital	•	•	•	•				•
Phenytoin			•	•	•			•
Pioglitazone								o
PredniSONE					o			o
Primaquine	o							
Primidone	•		•	•				•
Rifabutin								•
Rifampin	•	•	•	•	•			•
Rifapentine				•				•
Ritonavir (long-term)	o			o				o
Rofecoxib								o
Secobarbital		•		•				
Sulfinpyrazone								o
Terbinafine								o
Topiramate								o
Tretinoin							o	
Troglitazone								o
Valproic acid		o						

TYRAMINE FOODS LIST

Food Types*	Allowed	Minimize Intake	Not Allowed
Beverages	Milk, decaffeinated coffee, tea, soda	Chocolate beverage, caffeine-containing drinks, clear spirits	Acidophilus milk, beer, ale, wine, malted beverages, alcohol-free and reduced alcohol beer and wine products
Breads/cereals	All except those containing cheese	None	Cheese bread and crackers
Dairy products	Cottage cheese, farmers or pot cheese, cream cheese, ricotta cheese, all milk, eggs, ice cream, pudding (except chocolate)	Yogurt (limit to 4 oz per day)	All other cheeses (aged cheese, American, Camembert, cheddar, Gouda, gruyere, mozzarella, parmesan, provolone, romano, Roquefort, stilton
Meat, fish, and poultry	All fresh or frozen	Aged meats, hot dogs, canned fish and meat	Chicken and beef liver, dried and pickled fish, pickled herring, summer or dry sausage, pepperoni, dried meats (ie, Genoa salami, hard salami, pepperoni, Lebanon bologna), meat extracts, bologna, liverwurst
Starches — potatoes/rice	All	None	Soybean (including paste)
Vegetables	All fresh, frozen, canned, or dried vegetable juices except those not allowed	Chili peppers, Chinese pea pods	Fava beans, sauerkraut, pickles, olives, Italian broad beans
Fruit	Fresh, frozen, or canned fruits and fruit juices	Avocado, banana, raspberries, figs	Banana peel extract
Soups	All soups not listed to limit or avoid	Commercially canned soups	Soups which contain broad beans, fava beans, cheese, beer, wine, any made with flavor cubes or meat extract, miso soup
Fats	All except fermented	Sour cream	Packaged gravy
Sweets	Sugar, hard candy, honey, molasses, syrups	Chocolate candies	None
Desserts	Cakes, cookies, gelatin, pastries, sherbets, sorbets	Chocolate desserts	Cheese-filled desserts
Miscellaneous	Salt, nuts, spices, herbs, flavorings, Worcestershire sauce	Soy sauce, peanuts	Brewer's yeast, yeast concentrates, all aged and fermented products, monosodium glutamate, vitamins with Brewer's yeast

*Foods high in tyramine.

MATERNAL/FETAL MEDICATIONS

Adapted from Briggs GG, "Medication Use During the Perinatal Period," *J Am Pharm Assoc*, 1998, 38:717-27.

Antibiotics in Pregnancy

Antibiotics Which Are Generally Regarded as Safe	
Antibiotic	**Comments**
Aminoglycosides (limited use)	
Penicillins	
Cephalosporins	
Clindamycin	
Erythromycin	
Antibiotics to Be Avoided	
Tetracyclines	Staining of deciduous teeth (4th month through term)
Aminoglycosides (prolonged use)	Eighth cranial nerve damage (hearing loss, vestibulotoxicity)
Fluoroquinolones	Potentially mutagenic, cartilage damage, arthropathy, and teratogenicity
Erythromycin estolate	Hepatotoxic in mother
Ribavirin	Possibly fetotoxic

Treatment and Prevention of Infection

Prophylaxis	
Preterm premature rupture of membranes	Ampicillin, amoxicillin, cefazolin, amoxicillin/clavulanate, ampicillin/sulbactam, erythromycin
Prevention of bacterial endocarditis	Ampicillin 2 g and gentamicin 1.5 mg/kg (max 120 mg) within 30 min of delivery, followed by 1 g ampicillin (I.V.) or amoxicillin (oral) 6 hours later
Cesarean section	Cefazolin (I.V. or uterine irrigation) or clindamycin/ gentamicin
Treatment	
Bacterial vaginosis	Clindamycin (oral or gel) in first trimester (gel has been associated with higher rate of preterm deliveries) Metronidazole (oral) for 7 days or gel for 5 days (after first trimester)
Chorioamnionitis	Ampicillin plus gentamicin (clindamycin, erythromycin, or vancomycin if PCN allergic)
Genital herpes	First episode: Oral acyclovir Near term treatment may reduce Cesarian sections I.V. therapy for disseminated infection
Group B streptococci	Penicillin G 5 million units once, then 2.5 million units q4h Ampicillin 2 g once, then 1 g q4h Clindamycin or erythromycin if PCN allergic
HIV*	***Note:** Always consult HIV guidelines (www.hivatis.org) Zidovudine (limits maternal-fetal transmission) Oral dosing during pregnancy/I.V. prior to delivery Other antiretroviral agents - effects unknown Lamivudine during labor used in combination with zidovudine in women who have not received prior antiretroviral therapy
Postpartum endometritis	Ampicillin (vancomycin if PCN allergic) plus clindamycin (or metronidazole) plus gentamicin until afebrile
Pyelonephritis	Ampicillin-gentamicin Cefazolin Co-trimoxazole
Urinary tract infection	Amoxicillin/ampicillin (resistance has increased) Co-trimoxazole Nitrofurantoin Cephalexin
Vaginal candidiasis	Buconizole for 7 days Clotrimazole for 7 days Miconazole for 7 days Terconazole for 7 days

Preterm Labor: Tocolytic Agents

Drug Class	Route	Fetal/Neonatal Toxicities	Maternal Toxicities
Beta-adrenergic agonists			
Ritodrine, terbutaline	Oral, I.V., S.C.	Fetal tachycardia, intraventricular septal hypertrophy, neonatal hyperinsulinemia/ hypoglycemia	Pulmonary, edema, myocardial infarction, hypokalemia, hypotension, hyperglycemia, tachycardia
Magnesium	I.V.	Neurologic depression in newborn (loss of reflexes, hypotonia, respiratory depression); fetal hypocalcemia and hypercalcuria; abnormal fetal bone mineralization and enamel hypoplasia	Hypotension, respiratory depression, ileus/ constipation, hypocalcemia, pulmonary edema, hypotension, headache/dizziness
NSAIDs			
Indomethacin	Oral, P.R.	Ductus arteriosis: premature closure, ricuspid regurgitation, primary pulmonary hypertension of the newborn, PDA; intraventricular hemorrhage, necrotizing enterocolitis, renal failure	GI bleeding, oligohydramnios, pulmonary edema, acute renal failure
Calcium channel blockers			
Nifedipine	Oral	Hypoxia secondary to maternal hypotension	Hypotension, flushing, tachycardia, headache
Nitrates			
Nitroglycerin	I.V./ S.L.	Hypoxia secondary to maternal hypotension	Hypotension, headache, dizziness

Pregnancy-Induced Hypertension*

Drug Class	Maternal/Fetal Effects
Antihypertensives Contraindicated in PIH	
Diuretics	Reduction of maternal plasma volume exacerbates disease; use in chronic hypertension acceptable (if no superimposed pregnancy-induced hypertension)
ACE-inhibitors	Teratogenic in second and third trimester; fetal/newborn anuria and hypotension, fetal oligohydramnios; neonatal death (congenital abnormalities of skull and renal failure)
Hypertension Treatment†	
Central-acting	
Methyldopa	Relatively safe in second/third trimester
Beta-blockers	
Acebutolol, atenolol, metoprolol, pindolol, propranolol	Increased risk of IUGR
Alpha-/beta-blocking	
Labetolol	See beta-blockers
Vasodilators	
Hydralazine	Relatively safe in second/third trimester
Nitrates	
Nitroglycerin	Relatively safe in second/third trimester
Calcium channel blockers	
Nifedipine	Relatively safe in second/third trimester

*Includes management of pre-eclampsia/eclampsia and HELLP syndrome. **Note:** Prevention may include low-dose aspirin (81 mg/day) or calcium supplementation (2 g/day).

†All agents must be carefully titrated to avoid fetal hypoxia.

MATERNAL/FETAL MEDICATIONS *(Continued)*

Other Maternal-Fetal Drug Therapy

Drug	Dose/Route
Fetal Lung Maturation	
Betamethasone	Two 12 mg doses I.M. at a 24-hour interval
Dexamethasone	Four 6 mg doses I.M. at 12-hour intervals
Doses repeated weekly up to 34 weeks gestation	
Cervical Ripening	
Oxytocin	I.V. dosing - often ineffective
Hygroscopic cervical dilators	
Dinoprostone (prostaglandin E2)	Gel (0.5 mg) or vaginal insert (10 mg, releasing 0.3 mg/h)
Misoprostol (prostaglandin E1)	Oral tablets inserted intravaginally 25-50 mcg q3-4h for up to 24 hours; oral dosing is investigational. **Note:** Manufacturer warnings issued in 2000 emphasize the risk of this off-label use.
Analgesia During Labor	
Meperidine	25-50 mg I.V. q1-2h or 50-100 mg I.M. q2-4h
Fentanyl	50-100 mcg q1h
Butorphanol	No advantage over other agents
Nalbuphine	No advantage over other agents
Tramadol	No advantage over other agents
Postpartum Hemorrhage	
Oxytocin	I.V. usually; also I.M. or intramyometrially (IMM)
Methylergonovine	I.M. or I.M.M.; contraindicated in hypertension
Carboprost (PG F2 alpha)	Pyrexia is common; contraindicated in cardiac, pulmonary, renal, or hepatic disease
Misoprostil	Rectal administration has been investigated

MATERNAL/FETAL TOXICOLOGY

Drugs and Chemicals Proven to Be Teratogenic in Humans

Drug/ Chemical	Fetal Adverse Effects	Relative Risk for Teratogenicity	Clinical Intervention
Alcohol	**Fetal alcohol syndrome:** Mental retardation, microcephaly, poor coordination, hypotonia, hyperactivity, short upturned nose, micrognathia or retrognathia (infancy) or prognathia (adolescence), short palpebral fissures, hypoplastic philtrum, thinned upper lips, microphthalmia, antenatal/postnatal growth retardation, occasional pathologies of eyes, mouth, heart, kidneys, gonads, skin, muscle, and skeleton	In alcoholic women consuming >2 g/kg/d ethanol over first trimester: 2- to 3-fold higher risk for congenital malformations (about 10%)	To calculate accurate dose of alcohol: **Prospective:** To discontinue exposure; if woman is alcoholic, refer to addiction center **During pregnancy:** To alleviate fears in mild or occasional drinkers who may terminate pregnancy based on unrealistic perception of risk, level 2 ultrasound to rule out visible malformation
Alkylating agents (busulfan, chlorambucil, cyclophosphamide, mechlorethamine)	Growth retardation, cleft palate, microphthalmia hypoplastic ovaries, cloudy corneas, agenesis of kidney, malformations of digits, cardiac defects, multiple other anomalies	Based on case reports, between 10% and 50% of cases were malformed for different drugs. It is possible that adverse outcome was over-represented.	Level 2 ultrasound to rule out visible malformations. Supplement folic acid to women receiving antifolates (eg, methotrexate).
Antimetabolite agents (aminopterin azauridine, cytarabine, 5-FU, 6-MP, methotrexate)	Hydrocephalus, meningoencephalocele, anencephaly, malformed skull, cerebral hypoplasia, growth retardation, eye and ear malformations, malformed nose and cleft palate, malformed extremities and fingers **Aminopterin syndrome:** Cranial dysostosis, hydrocephalus, hypertelorism, anomalies of external ear, micrognathia, posterior cleft palate	Based on case reports 7%-75% of cases were malformed. It is possible that adverse outcome was over-represented.	Level 2 ultrasound to rule out visible malformations.
Carbamazepine	Increased risk for neural tube defects (NTDs)	NTDs estimated at 1% with carbamazepine	Periconceptional folate; maternal and/ or amniotic α-fetoprotein; ultrasound to rule out NTD.
Carbon monoxide	Cerebral atrophy, mental retardation, microcephaly, convulsions, spastic disorders, intrauterine or postnatal death	Based on case reports, when mother is severely poisoned, high risk for neurological sequelae; no increased risk in mild accidental exposures	Measure maternal carboxyhemoglobin levels. Treat with 100% oxygen for 5 hours after maternal carboxyhemoglobin returns to normal because fetal equilibration takes longer. If hyperbaric chamber available, should be used, as elimination half-life of CO is more rapid. Fetal monitoring by an obstetrician; sonographic follow-up.

MATERNAL/FETAL TOXICOLOGY *(Continued)*

Drugs and Chemicals Proven to Be Teratogenic in Humans *(continued)*

Drug/ Chemical	Fetal Adverse Effects	Relative Risk for Teratogenicity	Clinical Intervention
Diethylstilbestrol (DES)	**Female offspring:** Clear cell vaginal or cervical adenocarcinoma in young female adults exposed in utero (before 18th week); irregular menses (oligomenorrhea), reduced pregnancy rates, increased rate of preterm deliveries, increased perinatal mortality and spontaneous abortion **Male offspring:** Cysts of epididymis, cryptorchidism, hypogonadism, diminished spermatogenesis	Exposure before 18 weeks of gestation: ≤1.4/1000 of exposed female with carcinoma. Congenital morphological changes in vaginal epithelium in 39% of exposures.	**Diagnosis:** Direct observation of mucosa and Shiller's test. **Treatment:** Mechanical excision or destruction in relatively confined area. Surgery and radiotherapy for diffused tumor.
Lead	Lower scores in developmental tests	Higher risk when maternal lead is >10 µg/dL	**Maternal lead levels >10 µg/dL:** Investigate for possible source of contamination. **Levels >25 µg/dL:** Consider chelation
Lithium carbonate	Possibly higher risk for Ebstein's anomaly; no detectable higher risk for other malformations		Women who need lithium should continue therapy, with sonographic follow-up. Patients may need higher doses because of increased clearance rate.
Methyl mercury, mercuric sulfide	Microcephaly, eye malformations, cerebral palsy, mental retardation, malocclusion of teeth	Women of affected babies consumed 9-27 ppm mercury; greater risk when ingested at 6-8 gestational months. Relative risk was not elucidated, but 13/220 babies born in Minamata, Japan, at time of contamination had severe disease.	Good correlation between mercury concentrations in maternal hair follicles and neurological outcome of the fetus. Hair mercury content >50 ppm was used successfully as a cut point for termination. In acute poisoning, the fetus is 4-10 times more sensitive than the adult to methylmercury toxicity.
PCBs	**Stillbirth** **Signs at birth:** White eye discharge, 30% (32/108); teeth present, 8.7% (11/127); irritated/swollen gums, 11% (11/99); hyperpigmentation ("cola" staining), 42.5% (54/127); deformed/small nails, 24.6% (30/122); acne, 12.8% (16/125) **Subsequent history:** Bronchitis or pneumonia, 27.2% (30/124); chipped or broken teeth, 35.5% (38/107); hair loss, 12.2% (14/115); acne scars, 9.6% (11/115); generalized itching, 27.8% (32/1150) **Developmental:** Do not meet milestones; lower scores than unexposed controls; evidence of CNS damage	4%-20% (6/159-8/39)	These figures, which are from cases poisoned by high consumption of PCB-contaminated rice oil, cannot be extrapolated to cases in which maternal poisoning has not been verified. Women working near PCBs (eg, hydroelectric facilities) should use effective protection.
Penicillamine	Skin hyperelastosis	Few case reports; risk unknown	

Drugs and Chemicals Proven to Be Teratogenic in Humans *(continued)*

Drug/ Chemical	Fetal Adverse Effects	Relative Risk for Teratogenicity	Clinical Intervention
Phenytoin	**Fetal hydantoin syndrome:** Low nasal bridge, inner epicanthal folds, ptosis, strabismus, hypertelorism, low set or abnormal ears, wide mouth, large fontanels, anomalies and hypoplasia of distal phalanges and nails, skeletal abnormalities, microcephaly and mental retardation, growth deficiency, neuroblastoma, cardiac defects, cleft palate/lip	5%-10% of typical syndrome; about 30% of partial picture. Relative risk of 7 for offspring IQ ≤84.	Neurologist should consider changing to other medications. Keep phenytoin concentrations at lower effective levels. Level 2 ultrasound to rule out visible malformations, vitamin K to neonate. Epilepsy itself increases teratogenic risk.
Systemic retinoids (isotretinoin, etretinate)	Spontaneous abortions; deformities of cranium, ears, face, heart, limbs, liver; hydrocephalus, microcephalus, heart defects. Cognitive defects even without dysmorphology	For isotretinoin: 38% risk. 80% of malformation are CNS.	Treated women should have an effective method of contraception. Pregnancy termination. If diagnosed too late, sonographic follow-up to rule out confirmed malformations.
Tetracycline	Yellow, gray-brown, or brown staining of deciduous teeth, destruction of enamel	From 4 months of gestation and on, occurs in 50% of fetuses exposed to tetracycline; 12.5% to oxytetracycline	If exposure before 14-16 weeks of gestation, no known risk
Thalidomide	Limb phocomelia, amelia, hypoplasia, congenital heart defects, renal malformations, cryptorchidism, abducens paralysis, deafness, microtia, anotia	About 20% risk when exposure to drug occurs in days 34-50 of gestation.	Thalidomide is an effective drug for some forms of leprosy. Treated women should have an effective mode of contraception.
Trimethadione	**Fetal trimethadione syndrome:** Intrauterine growth retardation, cardiac anomalies, microcephaly, cleft palate and lip, abnormal ears, dysmorphic face, mental retardation, tracheoesophageal fistula, postnatal death	Based on case reports: 83% risk; 32% infantile or neonatal death	No need for this antiepileptic to date
Valproic acid	Lumbosacral spina bifida with meningomyelocele; CNS defects, microcephaly, cardiac defects	1.2% risk of neural tube defects	Level 2 ultrasound and maternal α-fetoproteins or amniocentesis to rule out neural tube defects. Epilepsy itself increases teratogenic risk.
Warfarin	**Fetal warfarin syndrome:** Nasal hypoplasia, chondrodysplasia punctata, branchydactyly, skull defects, abnormal ears, malformed eyes, CNS malformations, microcephaly, hydrocephalus, skeletal deformities, mental retardation, optic atrophy, spasticity, Dandy Walker malformations	16% of exposed fetuses have malformation; another 3% hemorrhages; 8% stillbirths	**Prospective:** Switch to heparin for the first trimester. Deliver by a cesarean section. Women should be followed up in a high-risk perinatal unit.

Reprinted with permission from "Drugs and Chemicals Proven to Be Teratogenic in Humans," *Maternal-Fetal Toxicology: A Clinician's Guide*, 2nd ed, Koren G, ed, New York, NY: Marcel Dekker, Inc, 1994, 37-43.

ANXIOLYTIC/HYPNOTIC USE IN LONG-TERM CARE FACILITIES

One of the regulations regarding medication use in long-term care facilities concerns "unnecessary drugs." The regulation states, "Each resident's drug regimen must be free from unnecessary drugs." Recently, the Health Care Financing Administration (HCFA) issued the final interpretive guidelines on this regulation. The following is a summary of these guidelines as they pertain to anxiolytic/hypnotic agents.

A. **Long-Acting Benzodiazepines**

Long-acting benzodiazepine drugs should not be used in residents unless an attempt with a shorter-acting drug has failed. If they are used, the doses must be no higher than the listed dose, unless higher doses are necessary for maintenance or improvement in the resident's functional status. Daily use should be less than 4 continuous months unless an attempt at a gradual dose reduction is unsuccessful. Residents on diazepam for seizure disorders or for the treatment of tardive dyskinesia are exempt from this restriction. Residents on clonazepam for bipolar disorder, tardive dyskinesia, nocturnal myoclonus, or seizure disorder are also exempt. Residents on long-acting benzodiazepines should have a gradual dose reduction at least twice within 1 year before it can be concluded that the gradual dose reduction is "clinically contraindicated."

Generic	Brand	Maximum Daily Geriatric Dose (mg)
Chlordiazepoxide	Librium®	20
Clonazepam	Klonopin™	1.5
Clorazepate	Tranxene®	15
Diazepam	Valium®	5
Flurazepam	Dalmane®	15
Halazepam	Paxipam®	40
Quazepam	Doral®	7.5

B. **Benzodiazepine or Other Anxiolytic/Sedative Drugs**

Anxiolytic/sedative drugs should be used for purposes other than sleep induction only when other possible causes of the resident's distress have been ruled out and the use results in maintenance or improvement in the resident's functional status. Daily use should not exceed 4 continuous months unless an attempt at gradual dose reduction has failed. Anxiolytics should only be used for generalized anxiety disorder, dementia with agitated states that either endangers the resident or others, or is a source of distress or dysfunction; panic disorder or symptomatic anxiety associated with other psychiatric disorders. The dose should not exceed those listed below unless a higher dose is needed as evidenced by the resident's response. Gradual dosage reductions should be attempted at least twice within 1 year before it can be concluded that a gradual dose reduction is "clinically contraindicated."

Short-Acting Benzodiazepines

Generic	Brand	Maximum Daily Geriatric Dose (mg)
Alprazolam	Xanax®	0.75
Estazolam[1]	ProSom®	0.5
Lorazepam	Ativan®	2
Oxazepam	Serax®	30

[1]Primarily used as a hypnotic agent.

Other Anxiolytic and Sedative Drugs

Generic	Brand	Maximum Daily Geriatric Dose (mg)
Chloral hydrate	Noctec®, etc	750
Diphenhydramine	Benadryl®	50
Hydroxyzine	Atarax®, Vistaril®	50

Note: Chloral hydrate, diphenhydramine, and hydroxyzine are not necessarily drugs of choice for treatment of anxiety disorders. HCFA lists them only in the event of their possible use.

C. Drugs Used for Sleep Induction

Drugs for sleep induction should only be used when all possible reasons for insomnia have been ruled out (ie, pain, noise, caffeine). The use of the drug must result in the maintenance or improvement of the resident's functional status. Daily use of a hypnotic should not exceed 10 consecutive days unless an attempt at a gradual dose reduction is unsuccessful. The dose should not exceed those listed below unless a higher dose has been deemed necessary. Gradual dose reductions should be attempted at least three times within 6 months before it can be concluded that a gradual dose reduction is "clinically contraindicated."

Hypnotic Drugs

Generic	Brand	Daily Geriatric Dose (mg)
Alprazolam[1]	Xanax®	0.25
Chloral hydrate	Noctec®	500
Diphenhydramine	Benadryl®	25
Estazolam	ProSom™	0.5
Hydroxyzine	Atarax®, Vistaril®	50
Lorazepam[1]	Ativan®	1
Oxazepam[1]	Serax®	15
Temazepam	Restoril®	7.5
Triazolam	Halcion®	0.125
Zaleplon	Sonata®	5
Zolpidem	Ambien®	5

[1]Not officially indicated as a hypnotic agent.

Note: Chloral hydrate, diphenhydramine, and hydroxyzine are not necessarily drugs of choice for sleep disorders. HCFA lists them only in the event of their possible use.

D. Miscellaneous Hypnotic/Sedative/Anxiolytic Drugs

The initiation of the following medications should not occur in any dose in any resident. Residents currently using these drugs or residents admitted to the facility while using these drugs should receive gradual dose reductions. Newly admitted residents should have a period of adjustment before attempting reduction. Dose reductions should be attempted at least twice within 1 year before it can be concluded that it is "clinically contraindicated."

Examples of Barbiturates

Generic	Brand
Amobarbital	Amytal®
Amobarbital/Secobarbital	Tuinal®
Butabarbital	Butisol Sodium®
Combinations	Fiorinal®, etc
Pentobarbital	Nembutal®
Secobarbital	Seconal™

Miscellaneous Hypnotic/Sedative/Anxiolytic Agents

Generic	Brand
Ethchlorvynol	Placidyl®
Glutethimide	Doriden®
Meprobamate	Equanil®, Miltown®
Methyprylon	Noludar®
Paraldehyde	Paral®

FEDERAL OBRA REGULATIONS RECOMMENDED MAXIMUM DOSES

Antidepressants

Drug	Brand Name	Usual Max Daily Dose for Age ≥65	Usual Max Daily Dose
Amitriptyline	Elavil®	150 mg	300 mg
Amoxapine	Asendin®	200 mg	400 mg
Desipramine	Norpramin®	150 mg	300 mg
Doxepin	Adapin®, Sinequan®	150 mg	300 mg
Imipramine	Tofranil®	150 mg	300 mg
Maprotiline	Ludiomil®	150 mg	300 mg
Nortriptyline	Aventyl®, Pamelor®	75 mg	150 mg
Protriptyline	Vivactil®	30 mg	60 mg
Trazodone	Desyrel®	300 mg	600 mg
Trimipramine	Surmontil®	150 mg	300 mg

Antipsychotics

Drug	Brand Name	Usual Max Daily Dose for Age ≥65	Usual Max Daily Dose	Daily Oral Dose for Residents With Organic Mental Syndromes
Acetophenazine	Tindal®	150 mg	300 mg	20 mg
Chlorpromazine	Thorazine®	800 mg	1600 mg	75 mg
Chlorprothixene	Taractan®	800 mg	1600 mg	75 mg
Clozapine	Clozaril®	25 mg	450 mg	50 mg
Fluphenazine	Prolixin®	20 mg	40 mg	4 mg
Haloperidol	Haldol®	50 mg	100 mg	4 mg
Loxapine	Loxitane®	125 mg	250 mg	10 mg
Mesoridazine	Serentil®	250 mg	500 mg	25 mg
Molindone	Moban®	112 mg	225 mg	10 mg
Perphenazine	Trilafon®	32 mg	64 mg	8 mg
Promazine	Sparine®	50 mg	500 mg	150 mg
Risperidone	Risperdal®	1 mg	16 mg	2 mg
Thioridazine	Mellaril®	400 mg	800 mg	75 mg
Thiothixene	Navane®	30 mg	60 mg	7 mg
Trifluoperazine	Stelazine®	40 mg	80 mg	8 mg
Trifluopromazine	Vesprin®	100 mg	20 mg	–
Quetiapine	Seroquel®		800 mg	200 mg

Anxiolytics*

Drug	Brand Name	Usual Daily Dose for Age ≥65	Usual Daily Dose for Age ≤65
Alprazolam	Xanax®	2 mg	4 mg
Chlordiazepoxide	Librium®	40 mg	100 mg
Clorazepate	Tranxene®	30 mg	60 mg
Diazepam	Valium®	20 mg	60 mg
Halazepam	Paxipam®	80 mg	160 mg
Lorazepam	Ativan®	3 mg	6 mg
Meprobamate	Miltown®	600 mg	1600 mg
Oxazepam	Serax®	60 mg	90 mg
Prazepam	Centrax®	30 mg	60 mg

***Note:** HCFA-OBRA guidelines strongly urge clinicians not to use barbiturates, glutethimide, and ethchlorvynol due to their side effects, pharmacokinetics, and addiction potential in the elderly. Also, HCFA discourages use of long-acting benzodiazepines in the elderly.

Hypnotics*

Drug	Brand Name	Usual Max Single Dose for Age ≥65	Usual Max Single Dose
Alprazolam	Xanax®	0.25 mg	1.5 mg
Amobarbital	Amytal®	105 mg	300 mg
Butabarbital	Butisol®	100 mg	200 mg
Chloral hydrate	Noctec®	750 mg	1500 mg
Chloral hydrate	Various	500 mg	1000 mg
Diphenhydramine	Benadryl®	25 mg	50 mg
Ethchlorvynol	Placidyl®	500 mg	1000 mg
Flurazepam	Dalmane®	15 mg	30 mg
Glutethimide	Doriden®	500 mg	1000 mg
Halazepam	Paxipam®	20 mg	40 mg
Hydroxyzine	Atarax®	50 mg	100 mg
Lorazepam	Ativan®	1 mg	2 mg
Oxazepam	Serax®	15 mg	30 mg
Pentobarbital	Nembutal®	100 mg	200 mg
Secobarbital	Seconal®	100 mg	200 mg
Temazepam	Restoril®	15 mg	30 mg
Triazolam	Halcion®	0.125 mg	0.5 mg

***Should not be used for more than 10 continuous days Note:** HCFA-OBRA guidelines strongly urge clinicians not to use the following drugs in the elderly due to their side effects, pharmacokinetics, and addiction potential: barbiturates, glutethimide, and ethchlorvynol. Also, HCFA discourages use of long-acting benzodiazepines, diphenhydramine, and hydroxyzine in the elderly.

HCFA GUIDELINES FOR UNNECESSARY DRUGS IN LONG-TERM CARE FACILITIES

Procedures: §483.25(1)(1)

Consider drug therapy "unnecessary" only after determining that the facility's use of the drug is:

- in excessive dose (including duplicate drug therapy)
- for excessive duration
- without adequate monitoring
- without adequate indications of use
- in the presence of adverse consequences which indicate the dose should be reduced or discontinued, or
- any combination of the reasons above

Allow the facility the opportunity to provide a rationale for the use of drugs prescribed outside the preceding guidelines. The facility may not justify the use of a drug prescribed outside the proceeding guidelines solely on the basis of "the doctor ordered it." This justification would render the regulation meaningless. The rationale must be based on sound risk-benefit analysis of the resident's symptoms and potential adverse effects of the drug.

Examples of evidence that would support a justification of why a drug is being used outside these guidelines but in the best interests of the resident may include, but are not limited to:

- a physician's note indicating for example, that the dosage, duration, indication, and monitoring are clinically appropriate, **and the reasons why they are clinically appropriate**; this note should demonstrate that the physician has carefully considered the risk/benefit to the resident in using drugs outside the guidelines
- a medical or psychiatric consultation or evaluation (eg, geriatric depression scale) that confirms the physician's judgment that use of a drug outside the guidelines is in the best interest of the resident
- physician, nursing, or other health professional documentation indicating that the resident is being monitored for adverse consequences or complications of the drug therapy
- documentation confirming that previous attempts at dosage reduction have been unsuccessful
- documentation (including MDS documentation) showing resident's subjective or objective improvement, or maintenance of function while taking the medication
- documentation showing that a resident's decline or deterioration is evaluated by the interdisciplinary team to determine whether a particular drug, or a particular dose, or duration of therapy, may be the cause
- documentation showing why the resident's age, weight, or other factors would require a unique drug dose or drug duration, indication, monitoring, and
- other evidence the survey team may deem appropriate

If the survey team determines that there is a deficiency in the use of antipsychotics, cite the facility under either the "unnecessary drug" regulation or the "antipsychotic drug" regulation, but not both.

Note: The unnecessary drug criterion of "adequate indications for use" does not simply mean that the **physician's order** must include a reason for using the drug (although such order writing is encouraged). It means that the **resident** lacks a valid clinical reason for use of the drug as evidenced by the survey team's evaluation of some, but not necessarily all, of the following: resident assessment, plan of care, reports of significant change, progress notes, laboratory reports, professional consults, drug orders, observation and interview of the resident, and other information.

ANTIDEPRESSANT MEDICATION GUIDELINES

The under diagnosis and under treatment of depression in nursing homes has been documented in a *Journal of the American Medical Association* paper entitled "Depression and Mortality in the Nursing home" (*JAMA*, February 27, 1991, 265(8)). HCFA continues to support the accurate identification and treatment of depression in nursing homes.

The surveyor should not urge a facility to use behavioral monitoring charts (documenting quantitatively [number of episodes] and objectively [withdrawn behavior, such as, staying in their room, refusal to speak, etc]) when antidepressant drugs are used in nursing homes. Such charts are promoted in the interpretative guidelines for antipsychotic and benzodiazepine and other anxiolytic/sedative drugs, but **not** for antidepressant drugs. These charts may be helpful for monitoring the effects of antidepressant drugs in nursing homes, but they may place additional paperwork burden on the facility and thus act as a deterrent to the appropriate diagnosis and treatment of this condition.

The following is a list of commonly used antidepressant drugs, those marked with an asterisk are not necessarily drugs of choice for the elderly but are listed here in the event of their potential use.

Generic Name	Brand Name
Amitriptyline*	Elavil®
Amoxapine	Asendin®
Bupropion	Wellbutrin®
Citalopram*	Celexa®
Clomipramine*	Anafranil®
Desipramine	Norpramin®
Doxepin*	Sinequan®
Fluoxetine	Prozac®
Fluvoxamine	Luvox®
Imipramine*	Tofranil
Isocarboxazid*	Marplan®
Maprotiline	Ludiomil®
Mirtazapine	Remeron®
Nefazodone	Serzone®
Nortriptyline	Aventyl®, Pamelor®
Paroxetine	Paxil™
Phenelzine*	Nardil®
Protriptyline	Vivactil®
Sertraline	Zoloft™
Tranylcypromine*	Parnate®
Trazodone	Desyrel®
Trimipramine*	Surmontil®
Venlafaxine	Effexor®

ANTIPSYCHOTIC MEDICATION GUIDELINES

Appropriate indications for use of antipsychotic medications are outlined in the Health Care Finance Administration's Omnibus Reconciliation Act (OBRA) of 1987. These regulations require that antipsychotics be used to treat specific conditions (listed below) and not solely for behavior control.

Approved indications include:

- acute psychotic episode
- atypical psychosis
- brief reactive psychosis
- delusional disorder
- Huntington's disease
- psychotic mood disorder (including manic depression and depression with psychotic features)
- schizo-affective disorder
- schizophrenia
- schizophrenic form disorder
- Tourette's disease
- short-term (7 days) for hiccups, nausea, vomiting, or pruritus
- organic mental syndrome with psychotic or agitated features:
  - behaviors are quantitatively and objectively documented
  - behaviors must be **persistent**
  - behaviors are not caused by preventable reasons
  - patient presents a danger to self or others
  - continuous crying or screaming if this impairs functional status
  - psychotic symptoms (hallucinations, paranoia, delusions) which cause resident distress or impaired functional capacity

"Clinically contraindicated" means that a resident with a "specific condition" who has had a history of recurrence of psychotic symptoms (eg, delusions, hallucinations) which have been stabilized with a maintenance dose of an antipsychotic drug without incurring significant side effects (eg, tardive dyskinesia) **should not receive gradual dose reductions**. In residents with organic mental syndromes (eg, dementia, delirium), "clinically contraindicated" means that a gradual dose reduction has been attempted **twice** in 1 year and that attempt resulted in the return of symptoms for which the drug was prescribed to a degree that a cessation in the gradual dose reduction, or a return to previous dose levels was necessary.

If the medication is being used outside the guidelines, the physician must provide justification why the continued use of the drug and the dose of the drug is clinically appropriate.

Antipsychotics should not be used if one or more of the following is/are the **only** indication:

- wandering
- poor self care
- restlessness
- impaired memory
- anxiety
- depression (without psychotic features)
- insomnia
- unsociability
- indifference to surroundings
- fidgeting
- nervousness
- uncooperativeness
- agitated behaviors which do **not** represent danger to the resident or others

Selection of an antipsychotic agent should be based on the side effect profile since all antipsychotic agents are equally effective at equivalent doses. Coadministration of two or more antipsychotics does not have any pharmacological basis or clinical advantage and increases the potential for side effects. See Antipsychotic Agents table in Comparison Charts.

DOSING GUIDELINES

1. Daily dosages should be equal to or less than those listed below, unless documentation exists to support the need for higher doses to maintain or improve functional status.

Generic	Brand	Daily Dose for Patients With Organic Mental Syndrome
Acetophenazine	Tindal®	20 mg
Chlorpromazine	Thorazine®	75 mg
Clozapine	Clozaril®	50 mg
Fluphenazine	Prolixin®	4 mg
Haloperidol	Haldol®	4 mg
Loxapine	Loxitane®	10 mg
Mesoridazine	Serentil®	25 mg
Molindone	Moban®	10 mg
Olanzapine	Zyprexa®	5 mg
Perphenazine	Trilafon®	8 mg
Pimozide	Orap™	4 mg
Prochlorperazine	Compazine®	10 mg
Promazine	Sparine®	150 mg
Quetiapine	Seroquel®	100 mg
Risperidone	Risperdal®	2 mg
Thioridazine	Mellaril®	75 mg
Thiothixene	Navane®	7 mg
Trifluoperazine	Stelazine®	8 mg

2. The dose of prochlorperazine may be exceeded for short-term (up to 7 days) for treatment of nausea and vomiting. Residents with nausea and vomiting secondary to cancer or cancer chemotherapy can also be treated with higher doses for longer periods of time.
3. The residents must receive adequate monitoring for significant side effects such as tardive dyskinesia, postural hypotension, cognitive-behavioral impairment, akathisia, and parkinsonism.
4. Gradual dosage reductions are to be attempted twice in 1 year if prescribed for OMS. If symptoms for which the drug has been prescribed return and both reduction attempts have proven unsuccessful, the physician may indicate further reductions are clinically contraindicated.
5. "Clinically contraindicated" means that a resident **need not undergo** a "gradual dose reduction" or "behavioral interventions" if:
   - The resident has a "specific condition" and has a history of recurrence of psychotic symptoms (eg, delusions, hallucinations), which have been stabilized with a maintenance dose of an antipsychotic drug without incurring significant side effects.
   - The resident has organic mental syndrome (now called "delirium, dementia, and amnestic and other cognitive disorders" by DSM IV) and has had a gradual dose reduction attempted **twice** in 1 year and that attempt resulted in the return of symptoms for which the drug was prescribed to a degree that a cessation in the gradual dose reduction, or a return to previous dose reduction was necessary.
   - The resident's physician provides a justification why the continued use of the drug and the dose of the drug is clinically appropriate. This justification should include: a) a diagnosis, but not simply a diagnostic label or code, but the description of symptoms, b) a discussion of the differential psychiatric and medical diagnosis (eg, why the resident's behavioral symptom is thought to be a result of a dementia with associated psychosis and/or agitated behaviors, and not the result of an unrecognized painful medical condition or a psychosocial or environmental stressor), c) a description of the justification for the choice of a particular treatment, or treatments, and d) a discussion of why the present dose is necessary to manage the symptoms of the resident. This information need not necessarily be in the physician's progress notes, but must be a part of the resident's clinical record.

Examples of evidence that would support a justification of why a drug is being used outside these guidelines but in the best interests of the resident may include, but are not limited to the following.

ANTIPSYCHOTIC MEDICATION GUIDELINES *(Continued)*

1. A physician's note indicating for example, that the dosage, duration, indication, and monitoring are clinically appropriate, **and the reasons why they are clinically appropriate**; this note should demonstrate that the physician has carefully considered the risk/benefit to the resident in using drugs outside the guidelines.
2. A medical or psychiatric consultation or evaluation (eg, Geriatric Depression Scale) that confirms the physician's judgment that use of a drug outside the guidelines is in the best interest of the resident.
3. Physician, nursing, or other health professional documentation indicating that the resident is being monitored for adverse consequences or complications of the drug therapy.
4. Documentation confirming that previous attempts at dosage reduction have been unsuccessful.
5. Documentation (including MDS documentation) showing resident's subjective or objective improvement, or maintenance of function while taking the medication.
6. Documentation showing that a resident's decline or deterioration is evaluated by the interdisciplinary team to determine whether a particular drug, or a particular dose, or duration of therapy, may be the cause.
7. Documentation showing why the resident's age, weight, or other factors would require a unique drug dose or drug duration, indication, or monitoring.
8. Other evidence you may deem appropriate.

OVERDOSE AND TOXICOLOGY

GENERAL STABILIZATION OF THE PATIENT

The recommended treatment plan for the poisoned patient is not unlike general treatment plans taught in advanced cardiac life support (ACLS) or advanced trauma life support (ATLS) courses. In this manner, the initial approach to the poisoned patient should be essentially similar in every case, irrespective of the toxin ingested, just as the initial approach to the trauma patient is the same, irrespective of the mechanism of injury. This approach, which can be termed as routine poison management, essentially includes the following aspects.

- Stabilization: ABCs (airway, breathing, circulation; administration of glucose, thiamine, oxygen, and naloxone)
- History, physical examination leading toward the identification of class of toxin (toxidrome recognition)
- Prevention of absorption (decontamination)
- Specific antidote, if available
- Removal of absorbed toxin (enhancing excretion)
- Support and monitoring for adverse effects

Drug	Effect	Comment
25-50 g **dextrose** ($D_{50}W$) intravenously to reverse the effects of drug-induced hypoglycemia (adult) 1 mL/kg $D_{50}W$ diluted 1:1 (child)	This can be especially effective in patients with limited glycogen stores (ie, neonates and patients with cirrhosis)	Extravasation into the extremity of this hyperosmolar solution can cause Volkmann's contractures
50-100 mg intravenous **thiamine**	Prevent Wernicke's encephalopathy	A water-soluble vitamin with low toxicity; rare anaphylactoid reactions have been reported
Initial dosage of **naloxone** should be 2 mg in adult patients preferably by the intravenous route, although intramuscular, subcutaneous, intralingual, and endotracheal routes may also be utilized. Pediatric dose is 0.1 mg/kg from birth until 5 years of age	Specific opioid antagonist without any agent properties	It should be noted that some semisynthetic opiates (such as meperidine or propoxyphene) may require higher initial doses for reversal, so that a total dose of 6-10 mg is not unusual for the adults. If the patient responds to a bolus dose and then relapses to a lethargic or comatose state, a naloxone drip can be considered. This can be accomplished by administering two-thirds of the bolus dose that revives the patient per hour or injecting 4 mg naloxone in 1 L crystalloid solution and administering at a rate of 100 mL/hour 0.4 mg/hour)
Oxygen, utilized in 100% concentration	Useful for carbon monoxide, hydrogen, sulfide, and asphyxiants	While oxygen is antidotal for carbon monoxide intoxication, the only relative toxic contraindication is in paraquat intoxication (in that it can promote pulmonary fibrosis)
Flumazenil	Benzodiazepine antagonist	Not routinely recommended due to increased risk of seizures

OVERDOSE AND TOXICOLOGY *(Continued)*

LABORATORY EVALUATION OF OVERDOSE

Unknown ingestion: Electrolytes, anion gap, serum osmolality, arterial blood gases, serum drug concentration

Known ingestion: Labs tailored to agent

ANION GAP

Definition: The difference in concentration between unmeasured cation and anion equivalents in serum

Anion gap = $Na^+ - Cl^- + HCO_3^-$

(The normal anion gap is 10-14 mEq/L)

DIFFERENTIAL DIAGNOSIS

Increased Anion Gap Acidosis

Organic anions:

- Lactate (sepsis, hypovolemia, seizures, large tumor burden)
- Pyruvate
- Uremia
- Ketoacidosis (β-hydroxybutyrate and acetoacetate)
- Amino acids and their metabolites
- Other organic acids

Inorganic anions:

- Hyperphosphatemia
- Sulfates
- Nitrates

Decreased Anion Gap

Organic cations:

- Hypergammaglobulinemia

Inorganic cations:

- Hyperkalemia
- Hypercalcemia
- Hypermagnesemia

Medications and toxins:

- Lithium

Hypoalbuminemia

TOXINS AFFECTING THE ANION GAP

Drugs Causing Increased Anion Gap (>12 mEq/L)

Nonacidotic

- Carbenicillin
- Sodium salts

Metabolic Acidosis

- Acetaminophen (ingestion >75-100 g)
- Acetazolamide
- Amiloride
- Ascorbic acid
- Benzalkonium chloride
- Benzyl alcohol
- Beta-adrenergic drugs
- Bialaphos
- 2-butanone
- Carbon monoxide
- Centrimonium bromide
- Chloramphenicol
- Colchicine
- Cyanide
- Dapsone
- Dimethyl sulfate
- Dinitrophenol
- Endosulfan
- Epinephrine (I.V. overdose)
- Ethanol
- Ethylene dibromide
- Ethylene glycol
- Fenoprofen
- Fluoroacetate
- Formaldehyde
- Fructose (I.V.)
- Glycol ethers
- Hydrogen sulfide
- Ibuprofen (ingestion >300 mg/kg)
- Inorganic acid
- Iodine
- Iron
- Isoniazid
- Ketamine
- Ketoprofen
- Metaldehyde
- Metformin
- Methanol
- Methenamine mandelate
- Monochloracetic acid
- Nalidixic acid

Naproxen
Niacin
Papaverine
Paraldehyde
Pennyroyal oil
Pentachlorophenol
Phenelzine
Phenformin (off the market)
Phenol
Phenylbutazone
Phosphoric acid
Potassium chloroplatinite
Propylene glycol
Salicylates
Sorbitol (I.V.)
Strychnine
Surfactant herbicide
Tetracycline (outdated)
Theophylline
Tienilic acid
Toluene
Tranylcypromine
Vacor
Verapamil

Drugs Causing Decreased Anion Gap (<6 mEq/L)

Acidosis

Ammonium chloride
Bromide
Iodide
Lithium
Polymyxin B
Tromethamine

OSMOLALITY

Definition: The summed concentrations of all osmotically active solute particles

Predicted serum osmolality =

2 Na^+ + glucose (mg/dL) / 18 + BUN (mg/dL) / 2.8

The normal range of serum osmolality is 285-295 mOsm/L.

Differential diagnosis of increased serum osmolal gap (>10 mOsm/L)

Medications and toxins

- Alcohols (ethanol, methanol, isopropanol, glycerol, ethylene glycol)
- Mannitol
- Paraldehyde

Calculated Osm

Osmolal gap = measured Osm – calculated Osm

0 to +10: Normal

>10: Abnormal

<0: Probable lab or calculation error

Drugs Causing Increased Osmolar Gap

(by freezing-point depression, gap is >10 mOsm)

Ethanol*
Ethylene glycol*
Glycerol
Hypermagnesemia (>9.5 mEq/L)
Isopropanol* (acetone)
Iodine (questionable)
Mannitol
Methanol*
Propylene glycol
Severe alcoholic ketoacidosis or lactic acidosis
Sorbitol*

*Toxins increasing both anion and osmolar gap.

Toxins Associated With Oxygen Saturation Gap

(>5% difference between measured and calculated value)

Carbon monoxide
Cyanide (questionable)
Hydrogen sulfide (possible)
Methemoglobin

OVERDOSE AND TOXICOLOGY *(Continued)*

Toxins Eliminated by Multiple Dosing of Activated Charcoal

Acetaminophen
Amitriptyline
Atrazine (?)
Baclofen (?)
Bupropion (?)
Carbamazepine
Chlordecone
Cyclosporine
Dapsone
Dextropropoxyphene
Diazepam (desmethyldiazepam)
Digitoxin
Digoxin (with renal impairment)
Disopyramide
Glutethimide
Maprotiline
Meprobamate
Methotrexate
Methyprylon
Nadolol
Nortriptyline
Phencyclidine (?)
Phenobarbital
Phenylbutazone
Phenytoin (?)
Piroxicam
Propoxyphene
Propranolol (?)
Salicylates (?)
Theophylline
Valproic acid
Vancomycin (?)

The following agents have been studied and have not been demonstrated to result in enhanced elimination:

Amiodarone
Chlopropamide
Imipramine
Tobramycin

Toxins Eliminated by Forced Saline Diuresis

Barium
Bromides
Chromium
Cimetidine (?)
Cis-platinum
Cyclophosphamide
Hydrazine
Iodide
Iodine
Isoniazid (?)
Meprobamate
Methyl iodide
Mushrooms (Group I)
Nickel
Potassium chloroplatinite
Thallium
Valproic acid (?)

Toxins Eliminated by Alkaline Diuresis

2,4-D-chlorophenoxyacetic acid
Barbital (serum levels >10 mg/dL)
Chlorpropamide
Fluoride
Iopanoic Acid (?)
Isoniazid (?)
Mephobarbital
Methotrexate
2-Methyl-4-chlorophenoxyacetic acid (MCPA)
Orellanine (?)
Phenobarbital
Primidone
Quinolones antibiotic
Salicylates
Sulfisoxazole
Uranium

A urine flow of 3-5 mL/kg/hour should be achieved with a combination of isotonic fluids or diuretics. Alkalinization can be achieved by administration of 44-88 mEq of sodium bicarbonate per liter to titrate a urine pH of 7.5; 20-40 mEq/L of potassium chloride may also be required (potassium should not be administered in patients with renal insufficiency). It should be noted that the efficacy of forced diuresis has only been studied for salicylates and phenobarbital. Although several drugs can exhibit enhanced elimination through an acidic urine (tranylcypromine, quinine, chlorpheniramine, fenfluramine, strychnine, cathinone or khat, amphetamines, phencyclidine, nicotine, bismuth, diethylcarbamazine citrate, ephedrine, flecainide, local anesthetics), the practice of acidifying the urine should be discouraged in that it can produce metabolic acidosis and promote renal failure in the presence of rhabdomyolysis.

Drugs and Toxins Removed by Hemoperfusion (Charcoal)

Amanita phalloides (?)
Atenolol (?)
Bromisoval
Bromoethylbutyramide
Caffeine
Carbamazepine
Carbon tetrachloride (?)
Carbromal
Chloral hydrate (trichloroethanol)
Chloramphenicol
Chlorfenvinfos (?)
Chlorpropamide
Clonidine
Colchicine (?)
Creosote (?)
Dapsone
Demeton-S-methyl sulfoxide
Diltiazem (?)
Dimethoate
Disopyramide
Ethchlorvynol
Ethylene oxide
Glutethimide
Levothyroxine (?)
Lindane
Liotrix
Meprobamate
Methaqualone
Methotrexate
Methsuximide
Methyprylon (?)
Metoprolol (?)
Nadolol (?)
Orellanine (?)
Oxalic acid (?)
Paraquat
Parathion (?)
Pentamidine
Phenelzine (?)
Phenobarbital
Phenol
Phenytoin
Podophyllin (?)
Procainamide (?)
Quinidine (?)
Rifabutin (?)
Sotalol (?)
Thallium
Thyroglobulin/thyroid hormone
Theophylline
Valproic acid
Verapamil (?)

Continuous arteriovenous hemofiltration has been used to treat lithium, paraquat, N-acetyl-procainamide and vancomycin ingestions with varying results. It is capable of filtering molecules with a molecular weight up to 50,000 but some substances such as thallium and formaldehyde cannot be removed by this method despite their low molecular weight.

Exchange transfusion is a useful modality to enhance drug elimination in neonatal or infant drug toxicity. Usually double or triple volume exchanges are performed. It has been utilized to treat barbiturate, acetaminophen, iron, caffeine, methyl salicylate, propafenone, ganciclovir, sodium nitrite, lead, phenazopyridine hydrochloride, pine oil, theophylline overdose, and nitrate exposure in pediatric patients. Exchange transfusions (500-2000 mL) volume replacement have also been used to treat adults with 80-150 g ingestions of parathion.

OVERDOSE AND TOXICOLOGY *(Continued)*

TREATMENTS

Drug or Drug Class	Signs/Symptoms	Treatment/Comments
Acetaminophen	Generally asymptomatic	Assess severity of ingestion; adult doses ≥140 mg/kg are thought to be toxic. Obtain serum concentration ≥4 hours postingestion and use acetaminophen nomogram to evaluate need for acetylcysteine. Gastric decontamination within 2-4 hours after ingestion. May administer activated charcoal for one dose, this may decrease absorption of acetylcysteine if given within 1 hour of acetylcysteine. For unknown ingested quantities and for significant ingestion give acetylcysteine orally (diluted 1:4 with juice or carbonated beverage); initial: 140 mg/kg then give 70 mg/kg every 4 hours for 17 doses. I.V. protocols are used in some institutions.
Alpha-adrenergic blocking agents	Hypotension, drowsiness	Give activated charcoal, additional treatment if symptomatic; use I.V. fluids, dopamine, or norepinephrine to treat hypotension. Epinephrine may worsen hypotension due to beta effects.
Aminoglycosides	Ototoxicity, nephrotoxicity, neuromuscular toxicity	Hemodialysis or peritoneal dialysis may be useful in patients with decreased renal function; calcium may reverse the neuromuscular toxicity.
Anticholinergics, antihistamines	Coma, hallucinations, delirium, tachycardia, dry skin, urinary retention, dilated pupils	For life-threatening arrhythmias or seizures. Adults: 2 mg/dose physostigmine, may repeat 1-2 mg in 20 minutes and give 1-4 mg slow I.V. over 5-10 minutes if signs and symptoms recur (relatively contraindicated if QRS >0.1 msec).
Barbiturates	Respiratory depression, circulatory collapse, bradycardia, hypotension, hypothermia, slurred speech, confusion, coma	Repeated oral doses of activated charcoal given every 3-6 hours will increase clearance. Adults: 30-60 g. Assure GI motility, adequate hydration, and renal function. Urinary alkalinization with I.V. sodium bicarbonate will increase renal elimination of longer-acting barbiturates (eg, phenobarbital). Charcoal hemoperfusion may be required in severe overdose.

TREATMENTS *(continued)*

Drug or Drug Class	Signs/Symptoms	Treatment/Comments
Benzodiazepines	Respiratory depression, apnea (after rapid I.V.), hypoactive reflexes, hypotension, slurred speech, unsteady gait, coma	Dialysis is of limited value; support blood pressure and respiration until symptoms subside. Flumazenil: Initial dose: 0.2 mg given I.V. over 30 seconds. If further response is desired after 30 seconds, give 0.3 mg over another 30 seconds. Further doses of 0.5 mg can be given over 30 seconds at 1-minute intervals up to a total of 3 mg. Continuous infusions may be used in rare instances since duration of benzodiazepines is longer than flumazenil.
Beta-adrenergic blockers	Hypotension, bronchospasm, bradycardia, hypoglycemia, seizures	Activated charcoal; treat symptomatically; glucagon, atropine, isoproterenol, dobutamine, or cardiac pacing may be needed to treat bradycardia, conduction defects, or hypotension.
Carbamazepine	Dizziness, drowsiness, ataxia, involuntary movements, opisthotonos, seizures, nausea, vomiting, agitation, nystagmus, coma, urinary retention, respiratory depression, tachycardia, arrhythmias	Use supportive therapy, general poisoning management as needed. Use repeated oral doses of activated charcoal given every 3-6 hours to decrease serum concentrations. Charcoal hemoperfusion may be needed. Treat hypotension with I.V. fluids, dopamine, or norepinephrine. Monitor EKG. Diazepam may control convulsions but may exacerbate respiratory depression.
Cardiac glycosides	Hyperkalemia may develop rapidly and result in life-threatening cardiac arrhythmias, progressive bradyarrhythmias, second or third degree heart block unresponsive to atropine, ventricular fibrillation, asystole	Obtain serum drug level, induce emesis or perform gastric lavage. Give activated charcoal to reduce further absorption. Atropine may reverse heart block. Digoxin immune Fab (digoxin specific antibody fragments) is used in serious cases. Each 40 mg of digoxin immune Fab binds with 0.6 mg of digoxin.
Cholinergic	Nausea, vomiting, diarrhea, miosis, CNS depression, excessive salivation, excessive sweating, muscle weakness	Suction oral secretions, decontaminate skin, atropinize patient. Atropine dose must be individualized. Adults: Initial atropine dose: 1 mg; titrate dose upward. Pralidoxime (2-PAM) may need to be added for moderate to severe intoxications.
Cyanide	Myocardial depression, lactic acidosis, hypotension, respiratory depression, shock and cyanosis despite high oxygen saturation	Cyanide antidote kit: 1) Inhale vapor from 0.3 mL amyl nitrate ampul until I.V. sodium nitrite available; 2) sodium nitrite 300 mg I.V. then 3) sodium thiosulfate 12.5 g I.V. over 10 minutes
Heparin	Severe hemorrhage	1 mg of protamine sulfate will neutralize approximately 90 units of heparin sodium (bovine) or 115 units of heparin sodium (porcine) or 100 units of heparin calcium (porcine).

OVERDOSE AND TOXICOLOGY *(Continued)*

TREATMENTS *(continued)*

Drug or Drug Class	Signs/Symptoms	Treatment/Comments
Hydantoin derivatives	Nausea, vomiting, nystagmus, slurred speech, ataxia, coma	Gastric lavage or emesis; repeated oral doses of activated charcoal may increase clearance of phenytoin. Use 0.5-1 g/kg (30-60 g/dose) activated charcoal every 3-6 hours until nontoxic serum concentration is obtained. Assure adequate GI motility, supportive therapy.
Iron	Lethargy, nausea, vomiting, green or tarry stools, hypotension, weak rapid pulse, metabolic acidosis, shock, coma, hepatic necrosis, renal failure, local GI erosions	If immediately after ingestion and not already vomiting, give ipecac or lavage with saline solution. Give deferoxamine mesylate I.V. at 15 mg/kg/hour in cases of severe poisoning (serum iron >350 µg/mL) until the urine color is normal, the patient is asymptomatic, or a maximum daily dose of 8 g is reached. Urine output should be maintained >2 mL/kg/hour to avoid hypovolemic shock.
Isoniazid	Nausea, vomiting, blurred vision, CNS depression, intractable seizures, coma, metabolic acidosis	Control seizures with diazepam. Give pyridoxine I.V. equal dose to the suspected overdose of isoniazid or up to 5 g empirically. Give activated charcoal.
Nonsteroidal anti-inflammatory drugs	Dizziness, abdominal pain, sweating, apnea, nystagmus, cyanosis, hypotension, coma, seizures (rarely)	Induce emesis. Give activated charcoal via NG tube. Fluid therapy is commonly effective in managing the hypotension that may occur following an acute NSAIDs overdose, except when this is due to an acute blood loss. Seizures tend to be very short-lived and often do not require drug treatment; although, recurrent seizures should be treated with I.V. diazepam. Since many of the NSAIDs undergo enterohepatic cycling, multiple doses of charcoal may be needed to reduce the potential for delayed toxicities. Provide symptomatic and supportive care.
Opioids and morphine analogs	Respiratory depression, miosis, hypothermia, bradycardia, circulatory collapse, pulmonary edema, apnea	Establish airway and adequate ventilation. Give naloxone 0.4 mg and titrate to a maximum of 10 mg. Additional doses may be needed every 20-60 minutes. May need to institute continuous infusion, as duration of action of opiates can be longer than duration of action of naloxone.
Organophosphates (insecticides, pyridostigmine, neostigmine)	Bronchospasm, diarrhea, diaphoresis, ventricular dysrhythmia, fasiculations, flacid paralysis, lethargy, coma	Atropine 2-5 mg every 15 minutes until symptoms abate (0.05 mg/kg children). If severe, may add pralidoxime 1-2 g over 15-30 minutes (20-50 mg/kg children); may repeat every 8-12 hours or continuous infusion 0.5 g/hour (10-20 mg/kg/hour children).

TREATMENTS *(continued)*

Drug or Drug Class	Signs/Symptoms	Treatment/Comments
Phenothiazines	Deep, unarousable sleep, anticholinergic symptoms, extrapyramidal signs, diaphoresis, rigidity, tachycardia, cardiac dysrhythmias, hypotension	Activated charcoal; do **not** dialyze. Use I.V. benztropine mesylate 1-2 mg/dose slowly over 3-6 minutes for extrapyramidal signs. Use I.V. fluids and norepinephrine to treat hypotension. Avoid epinephrine which may cause hypotension due to phenothiazine-induced alpha-adrenergic blockade and unopposed epinephrine B_2 action. Use benzodiazepines for seizure management and to decrease rigidity.
Salicylates	Nausea, vomiting, respiratory alkalosis, hyperthermia, dehydration, hyperapnea, tinnitus, headache, dizziness, metabolic acidosis, coma, hypoglycemia, seizures	Induce emesis or gastric lavage immediately. Give several doses of activated charcoal, rehydrate, and use sodium bicarbonate to correct metabolic acidosis and enhance renal elimination by alkalinizing the urine. Control hyperthermia by cooling blankets or sponge baths. Correct coagulopathy with vitamin K I.V. and platelet transfusions as necessary. Hypoglycemia may be treated with I.V. dextrose. Seizures should be treated with I.V. benzodiazepines (diazepam 5-10 mg I.V.). Give supplemental potassium after renal function has been determined to be adequate. Monitor electrolytes; obtain stat serum salicylate level and follow.
Tricyclic antidepressants	Agitation, confusion, hallucinations, urinary retention, hypothermia, hypotension, tachycardia, arrhythmias, seizures	Give activated charcoal ± lavage. Use sodium bicarbonate for QRS >0.1 msec; alkalinization by hyperventilation has been used in patients on mechanical ventilation; I.V. fluids and norepinephrine may be used for hypotension; benzodiazepines may be used for seizure management.
Warfarin	Internal or external hemorrhage, hematuria	For moderate overdoses, give oral, S.C., or I.D., or slow I.V. (I.V. associated with anaphylactoid reactions) phytonadione; usual dose: 2.5-10 mg, adjust per prothrombin time. For severe hemorrhage, give fresh frozen plasma or whole blood. See Warfarin monograph.
Xanthine derivatives	Vomiting, abdominal pain, bloody diarrhea, tachycardia, extrasystoles, tachypnea, tonic/clonic seizures	Give activated charcoal orally. Repeated oral doses of activated charcoal increase clearance. Use 0.5-1 g/kg (30-60 g/dose) of activated charcoal every 1-4 hours (depending on the severity of ingestion) until nontoxic serum concentrations are obtained. Assure adequate GI motility, supportive therapy. Charcoal hemoperfusion or hemodialysis can also be effective in decreasing serum concentrations and should be used if the serum concentration approaches 90-100 mcg/mL in acute overdoses.

ANIMAL AND HUMAN BITES GUIDELINES

WOUND MANAGEMENT

Irrigation: Critically important; irrigate all penetration wounds using 20 mL syringe, 19 gauge needle and >250 mL 1% povidone iodine solution. This method will reduce wound infection by a factor of 20. When there is high risk of rabies, use viricidal 1% benzalkonium chloride in addition to the 1% povidone iodine. Irrigate wound with normal saline after antiseptic irrigation.

Debridement: Remove all crushed or devitalized tissue remaining after irrigation. Minimize removal on face, over thin skin areas, or anywhere you would create a worse situation than the bite itself already has. Do not extend puncture wounds surgically, rather, manage them with irrigation and antibiotics.

Suturing: Close most dog bites if <8 hours (<12 hours on face); do not routinely close puncture wounds, or deep or severe bites on the hands or feet, as these are at highest risk for infection. Cat and human bites should not be sutured unless cosmetically important. Wound edge freshening, where feasible, reduces infection; minimize sutures in the wound and use monofilament on the surface.

Immobilization: Critical in hand wounds; important for infected extremities.

Hospitalization/I.V. Antibiotics: Admit for I.V. antibiotics all significant human bites to the hand, especially closed fist injuries, and bites involving penetration of the bone or joint (a high index of suspicion is needed). Consider I.V. antibiotics for significant established wound infections with cellulitis or lymphangitis, any infected bite on the hand, any infected cat bite, and any infection in an immunocompromised or asplenic patient. Outpatient treatment with I.V. antibiotics may be possible in selected cases by consulting with infectious disease.

LABORATORY ASSESSMENT

Gram's Stain: Not useful prior to onset of clinically apparent infection; examination of purulent material may show a predominant organism in established infection, aiding antibiotic selection; not warranted unless results will change your treatment.

Culture: Not useful or cost effective prior to onset of clinically apparent infection.

X-ray: Whenever you suspect bony involvement, especially in craniofacial dog bites in very small children or severe bite/crush in an extremity; cat bites with their long needle like teeth may cause osteomyelitis or a septic joint, especially in the hand or wrist.

IMMUNIZATIONS

Tetanus: All bite wounds are contaminated. If not immunized in last 5 years, or if not current in a child, give DPT, DT, Td, or TT as indicated. For absent or incomplete primary immunization, give 250 units tetanus immune globulin (TIG) in addition.

Rabies: In the U.S. 30,000 persons are treated each year in an attempt to prevent 1-5 cases. Domestic animals should be quarantined for 10 days to prove need for prophylaxis. High risk animal bites (85% of cases = bat, skunk, raccoon) usually receive treatment consisting of:

- human rabies immune globulin (HRIG): 20 units/kg I.M. (unless previously immunized with HDCV)
- human diploid cell vaccine (HDCV): 1 mL I.M. on days 0, 3, 7, 14, and 28 (unless previously immunized with HDCV - then give only first 2 doses)

Consult with Infectious Disease before ordering rabies prophylaxis.

BITE WOUNDS AND PROPHYLACTIC ANTIBIOTICS

Parenteral vs Oral: If warranted, consider an initial I.V. dose to rapidly establish effective serum levels, especially if high risk, delayed treatment, or if patient reliability is poor.

Dog Bite:

1. Rarely get infected (~5%)
2. Infecting organisms: Coagulase-negative staph, coagulase-positive staph, alpha strep, diphtheroids, beta strep, *Pseudomonas aeruginosa*, gamma strep, *Pasteurella multocida*
3. Prophylactic antibiotics are seldom indicated. Consider for high risk wounds such as distal extremity puncture wounds, severe crush injury, bites occurring in cosmetically sensitive areas (eg, face), or in immunocompromised or asplenic patients.

Cat Bite:

1. Often get infected (~25% to 50%)
2. Infecting organisms: *Pasteurella multocida* (first 24 hours), coagulase-positive staph, anaerobic cocci (after first 24 hours)
3. Prophylactic antibiotics are indicated in all cases.

Human Bite:

1. Intermediate infection rate (~15% to 20%)
2. Infecting organisms: Coagulase-positive staph, alpha, beta, gamma strep, *Haemophilus*, *Eikenella corrodens*, anaerobic streptococci, *Fusobacterium*, *Veillonella*, bacteroides.
3. Prophylactic antibiotics are indicated in almost all cases except superficial injuries.

See the following table for prophylactic antibiotic summary.

Bite Wound Antibiotic Regimens

	Dog Bite	Cat Bite	Human Bite
Prophylactic Antibiotics			
Prophylaxis	No routine prophylaxis, consider if involves face or hand, or immunosuppressed or asplenic patients	Routine prophylaxis	Routine prophylaxis
Prophylactic antibiotic	Amoxicillin	Amoxicillin	Amoxicillin
Penicillin allergy	Doxycycline if >10 y or co-trimoxazole	Doxycycline if >10 y or co-trimoxazole	Doxycycline if >10 y or erythromycin and cephalexin*
Outpatient Oral Antibiotic Treatment (mild to moderate infection)			
Established infection	Amoxicillin and clavulanic acid	Amoxicillin and clavulanic acid	Amoxicillin and clavulanic acid
Penicillin allergy (mild infection only)	Doxycycline if >10 y	Doxycycline if >10 y	Cephalexin* or clindamycin
Outpatient Parenteral Antibiotic Treatment (moderate infections – single drug regimens)			
	Ceftriaxone	Ceftriaxone	Cefotetan
Inpatient Parenteral Antibiotic Treatment			
Established infection	Ampicillin + cefazolin	Ampicillin + cefazolin	Ampicillin + clindamycin
Penicillin allergy	Cefazolin*	Ceftriaxone*	Cefotetan* or imipenem
Duration of Prophylactic and Treatment Regimens			
Prophylaxis: 5 days			
Treatment: 10-14 days			

*Contraindicated if history of immediate hypersensitivity reaction (anaphylaxis) to penicillin.

ANTIMICROBIAL DRUGS OF CHOICE

The following table lists the antibacterial drugs of choice for various infecting organisms. This table is reprinted with permission from *The Medical Letter*, 2001, 43(1111-1112):69-78. Users should not assume that all antibiotics which are appropriate for a given organism are listed or that those not listed are inappropriate. The infection caused by the organism may encompass varying degrees of severity, and since the antibiotics listed may not be appropriate for the differing degrees of severity, or because of other patient-related factors, it cannot be assumed that the antibiotics listed for any specific organism are interchangeable. This table should not be used by itself without first referring to *The Medical Letter*, an infectious disease manual, or the infectious disease department. Therefore, only use this table as a tool for obtaining more information about the therapies available.

Infecting Organism	Drug of First Choice	Alternative Drugs
GRAM-POSITIVE COCCI		
**Enterococcus*[1]		
endocarditis or other severe infection	Penicillin G or ampicillin + gentamicin or streptomycin[2]	Vancomycin + gentamicin or streptomycin[2]; linezolid; quinupristin/dalfopristin
uncomplicated urinary tract infection	Ampicillin or amoxicillin	Nitrofurantoin; a fluoroquinolone[3]; fosfomycin
**Staphylococcus aureus* or *epidermidis*		
methicillin-sensitive	A penicillinase-resistant penicillin[4]	A cephalosporin[5,6]; vancomycin; amoxicillin/clavulanic acid; ticarcillin/clavulanic acid; piperacillin/tazobactam; ampicillin/sulbactam; imipenem or meropenem; clindamycin; a fluoroquinolone[3]
methicillin-resistant[7]	Vancomycin ± gentamicin ± rifampin	Linezolid; quinupristin/dalfopristin; a fluoroquinolone[3]; a tetracycline[8]; trimethoprim-sulfamethoxazole
Streptococcus pyogenes (group A[9]) and groups C and G	Penicillin G or V[10]	Clindamycin; erythromycin; a cephalosporin[5,6]; vancomycin; clarithromycin[11]; azithromycin
Streptococcus, group B	Penicillin G or ampicillin	A cephalosporin[5,6]; vancomycin; erythromycin
**Streptococcus*, viridans group[1]	Penicillin G ± gentamicin	A cephalosporin[5,6]; vancomycin
Streptococcus bovis	Penicillin G	A cephalosporin[5,6]; vancomycin
Streptococcus, anaerobic or *Peptostreptococcus*	Penicillin G	Clindamycin; a cephalosporin[5,6]; vancomycin
**Streptococcus pneumoniae*[12] (pneumococcus), penicillin-susceptible (MIC <0.1 mcg/mL)	Penicillin G or V[10]; amoxicillin	A cephalosporin[5,6]; erythromycin; azithromycin; clarithromycin[11]; levofloxacin[13]; gatifloxacin[13] or moxifloxacin[13]; meropenem; imipenem; trimethoprim-sulfamethoxazole; clindamycin; a tetracycline[8]
penicillin-intermediate resistance (MIC 0.1-≤2 mcg/mL)	Penicillin G I.V. (12 million units/day for adults); ceftriaxone or cefotaxime	Levofloxacin[13]; gatifloxacin[13] or moxifloxacin[13]; vancomycin; clindamycin
penicillin-high level resistance (MIC ≥2 mcg/mL)	**Meningitis:** Vancomycin + ceftriaxone or cefotaxime ± rifampin	Meropenem; imipenem
	Other Infections: Vancomycin + ceftriaxone or cefotaxime; or levofloxacin,[13] gatifloxacin[13] or moxifloxacin[13]	Linezolid; quinupristin/dalfopristin
GRAM-NEGATIVE COCCI		
Moraxella (Branhamella) catarrhalis	Cefuroxime[5]; a fluoroquinolone[3]	Trimethoprim-sulfamethoxazole; amoxicillin/clavulanic acid; erythromycin; a tetracycline[8]; cefotaxime[5]; ceftizoxime[5]; ceftriaxone[5]; cefuroxime axetil[5]; cefixime[5]; cefpodoxime[5]; clarithromycin[11]; azithromycin

Infecting Organism	Drug of First Choice	Alternative Drugs
**Neisseria gonorrhoeae* (gonococcus)[14]	Ceftriaxone[5] or cefixime[5]; or ciprofloxacin,[13] gatifloxacin[13] or ofloxacin[13]	Cefotaxime[5]; penicillin G
Neisseria meningitidis[15] (meningococcus)	Penicillin G	Cefotaxime[5]; ceftizoxime[5]; ceftriaxone[5]; chloramphenicol[16]; a sulfonamide[17]; a fluoroquinolone[3]
GRAM-POSITIVE BACILLI		
Bacillus anthracis (anthrax)	Penicillin G	Ciprofloxacin[13]; erythromycin; a tetracycline[8]
Bacillus cereus, subtilis	Vancomycin	Imipenem or meropenem; clindamycin
Clostridium perfringens[18]	Penicillin G; clindamycin	Metronidazole; imipenem or meropenem; chloramphenicol[16]
Clostridium tetani[19]	Metronidazole	Penicillin G; a tetracycline[8]
Clostridium difficile[20]	Metronidazole	Vancomycin (oral)
Corynebacterium diphtheriae[21]	Erythromycin	Penicillin G
Corynebacterium, JK group	Vancomycin	Penicillin G + gentamicin; erythromycin
**Erysipelothrix rhusiopathiae*	Penicillin G	Erythromycin, a cephalosporin[5,6]; a fluoroquinolone[3]
Listeria monocytogenes	Ampicillin ± gentamicin	Trimethoprim-sulfamethoxazole
ENTERIC GRAM-NEGATIVE BACILLI		
**Bacteroides*	Metronidazole or clindamycin	Imipenem or meropenem; amoxicillin/clavulanic acid; ticarcillin/ clavulanic acid; piperacillin/ tazobactam; ampicillin/sulbactam; cefoxitin[5]; cefotetan[5]; chloramphenicol[16]; cefmetazole[5]; penicillin G; gatifloxacin[13] or moxifloxacin[13]
**Campylobacter fetus*	Imipenem or meropenem	Gentamicin
**Campylobacter jejuni*	Erythromycin or azithromycin	A fluoroquinolone[2]; a tetracycline[8]; gentamicin
**Citrobacter freundii*	Imipenem or meropenem[22]	A fluoroquinolone[3]; amikacin; a tetracycline[8]; trimethoprim-sulfamethoxazole; cefotaxime[5,22]; ceftizoxime[5,22]; ceftriaxone[5,22]; cefepime[5,22] or ceftazidime[5,22]
**Enterobacter*	Imipenem or meropenem[22]	Gentamicin, tobramycin or amikacin; trimethoprim-sulfamethoxazole; ciprofloxacin[13]; ticarcillin[23]; mezlocillin[23] or piperacillin[23]; aztreonam[22]; cefotaxime[5,22]; ceftizoxime[5,22]; ceftriaxone[5,22]; cefepime[5,22] or ceftazidime[5,22]
**Escherichia coli*[24]	Cefotaxime, ceftizoxime, ceftriaxone, cefepime or ceftazidime[5,22]	Ampicillin ± gentamicin, tobramycin or amikacin; carbenicillin[23]; ticarcillin[23]; mezlocillin[23] or piperacillin[23]; gentamicin, tobramycin or amikacin; amoxicillin/clavulanic acid[22]; ticarcillin/clavulanic acid[23]; piperacillin/tazobactam[23]; ampicillin/ sulbactam[22]; trimethoprim/ sulfamethoxazole; imipenem or meropenem[22]; aztreonam[22]; a fluoroquinolone[3]; another cephalosporin[5,6]
**Helicobacter pylori*[25]	Omeprazole + amoxicillin + clarithromycin; or tetracycline HCl[8] + metronidazole + bismuth subsalicylate	Tetracycline HCl[8] + clarithromycin[11] + bismuth subsalicylate; amoxicillin + metronidazole + bismuth subsalicylate; amoxicillin + clarithromycin[11]

ANTIMICROBIAL DRUGS OF CHOICE *(Continued)*

Infecting Organism	Drug of First Choice	Alternative Drugs
**Klebsiella pneumoniae*[24]	Cefotaxime, ceftizoxime, ceftriaxone, cefepime or ceftazidime[5,22]	Imipenem or meropenem[22]; gentamicin, tobramycin or amikacin; amoxicillin/clavulanic acid[22]; ticarcillin/clavulanic acid[23]; piperacillin/tazobactam[23]; ampicillin/sulbactam[22]; trimethoprim-sulfamethoxazole; aztreonam[22]; a fluoroquinolone[3]; mezlocillin[23] or piperacillin[23]; another cephalosporin[5,6]
**Proteus mirabilis*[24]	Ampicillin[26]	A cephalosporin[5,6,22]; ticarcillin[23]; mezlocillin[23] or piperacillin[23]; gentamicin, tobramycin, or amikacin; trimethoprim-sulfamethoxazole; imipenem or meropenem[22]; aztreonam[23]; a fluoroquinolone[3]; chloramphenicol[16]
Proteus, indole-positive (including *Providencia rettgeri, Morganella morganii*, and *Proteus vulgaris*)	Cefotaxime, ceftizoxime, ceftriaxone, cefepime, or ceftazidime[5,22]	Imipenem or meropenem[22]; gentamicin, tobramycin, or amikacin; carbenicillin[23]; ticarcillin[23]; mezlocillin[23] or piperacillin[23]; amoxicillin/clavulanic acid[22]; ticarcillin/clavulanic acid[23]; piperacillin/tazobactam[23]; ampicillin/sulbactam[22]; aztreonam[22]; trimethoprim-sulfamethoxazole; a fluoroquinolone[3]
**Providencia stuartii*	Cefotaxime, ceftizoxime, ceftriaxone, cefepime, or ceftazidime[5,22]	Imipenem or meropenem[22]; ticarcillin/clavulanic acid[23]; piperacillin/tazobactam[23]; gentamicin, tobramycin, or amikacin; carbenicillin[23]; ticarcillin,[23] mezlocillin,[23] or piperacillin[23]; aztreonam[22]; trimethoprim-sulfamethoxazole; a fluoroquinolone[3]
**Salmonella typhi*[27] (typhoid fever)	A fluoroquinolone[3] or ceftriaxone[5]	Chloramphenicol[16]; trimethoprim-sulfamethoxazole; ampicillin; amoxicillin; azithromycin[28]
*other *Salmonella*[29]	Cefotaxime[5] or ceftriaxone[5] or a fluoroquinolone[3]	Ampicillin or amoxicillin; trimethoprim-sulfamethoxazole; chloramphenicol[16]
**Serratia*	Imipenem or meropenem[22]	Gentamicin or amikacin; cefotaxime, ceftizoxime, ceftriaxone, cefepime, or ceftazidime[5,22]; aztreonam[22]; trimethoprim-sulfamethoxazole; carbenicillin[30], ticarcillin[30], mezlocillin[30] or piperacillin[30]; a fluoroquinolone[3]
**Shigella*	A fluoroquinolone[3]	Azithromycin; trimethoprim-sulfamethoxazole; ampicillin; ceftriaxone[5]
**Yersinia enterocolitica*	Trimethoprim-sulfamethoxazole	A fluoroquinolone[3]; gentamicin, tobramycin, or amikacin; cefotaxime or ceftizoxime[5]
OTHER GRAM-NEGATIVE BACILLI		
**Acinetobacter*	Imipenem or meropenem[22]	An aminoglycoside; ciprofloxacin[13]; trimethoprim-sulfamethoxazole; ticarcillin,[23] mezlocillin[23], or piperacillin[23]; ceftazidime[22]; minocycline[8]; doxycycline[8]; sulbactam[31]; polymyxin
**Aeromonas*	Trimethoprim-sulfamethoxazole	Gentamicin or tobramycin; imipenem; a fluoroquinolone[3]
Bartonella henselae or *quintana* (bacillary angiomatosis)	Erythromycin	Doxycycline[8]; azithromycin
Bartonella henselae[32] (cat scratch bacillus)	Azithromycin	Ciprofloxacin[13]; erythromycin; trimethoprim-sulfamethoxazole; gentamicin; rifampin
Bordetella pertussis (whooping cough)	Erythromycin	Azithromycin or clarithromycin[11]; trimethoprim-sulfamethoxazole
**Brucella*	A tetracycline[8] + rifampin	A tetracycline[8] + streptomycin or gentamicin; chloramphenicol[16] ± streptomycin; trimethoprim-sulfamethoxazole ± gentamicin; ciprofloxacin[13] + rifampin

Infecting Organism	Drug of First Choice	Alternative Drugs
**Burkholderia cepacia*	Trimethoprim-sulfamethoxazole	Ceftazidime[5]; chloramphenicol[16]; imipenem
Burkholderia (Pseudomonas) mallei (glanders)	Streptomycin + a tetracycline[8]	Streptomycin + chloramphenicol[16]; imipenem
**Burkholderia (Pseudomonas) pseudomallei* (melioidosis)	Imipenem; ceftazidime[5]	Meropenem; chloramphenicol[16] + doxycycline[8] + trimethoprim-sulfamethoxazole; amoxicillin/clavulanic acid
Calymmatobacterium granulomatis (granuloma inguinale)	Trimethoprim-sulfamethoxazole	Doxycycline[8] or ciprofloxacin[13] ± gentamicin
Capnocytophaga canimorsus[33]	Penicillin G	Cefotaxime[5]; ceftizoxime[5]; ceftriaxone[5]; imipenem or meropenem; vancomycin; a fluoroquinolone[3]; clindamycin
**Eikenella corrodens*	Ampicillin	An erythromycin; a tetracycline[8]; amoxicillin/clavulanic acid; ampicillin/sulbactam; ceftriaxone[5]
**Francisella tularensis* (tularemia)	Streptomycin	Gentamicin; a tetracycline[8]; chloramphenicol[16]; ciprofloxacin[13]
**Fusobacterium*	Penicillin G	Metronidazole; clindamycin; cefoxitin[5]; chloramphenicol[16]
Gardnerella vaginalis (bacterial vaginosis)	Oral metronidazole[34]	Topical clindamycin or metronidazole; oral clindamycin
**Haemophilus ducreyi* (chancroid)	Azithromycin or ceftriaxone	Ciprofloxacin[13] or erythromycin
**Haemophilus influenzae*		
meningitis, epiglottitis, arthritis, and other serious infections	Cefotaxime or ceftriaxone[5]	Cefuroxime[5] (not for meningitis); chloramphenicol[16]; meropenem
upper respiratory infections and bronchitis	Trimethoprim-sulfamethoxazole	Cefuroxime[5]; amoxicillin/clavulanic acid; cefuroxime axetil[5]; cefpodoxime[5]; cefaclor[5]; cefotaxime[5]; ceftizoxime[5]; ceftriaxone[5]; cefixime[5]; a tetracycline[8]; clarithromycin[11]; azithromycin; a fluoroquinolone[3]; ampicillin or amoxicillin
Legionella species	Azithromycin or a fluoroquinolone[3] ± rifampin	Doxycycline[8] ± rifampin; trimethoprim-sulfamethoxazole; erythromycin
Leptotrichia buccalis	Penicillin G	A tetracycline[8]; clindamycin; erythromycin
Pasteurella multocida	Penicillin G	A tetracycline[8]; a cephalosporin[5,6]; amoxicillin/clavulanic acid; ampicillin/sulbactam
**Pseudomonas aeruginosa*		
urinary tract infection	Ciprofloxacin[13]	Levofloxacin[13]; carbenicillin, ticarcillin, piperacillin, or mezlocillin; ceftazidime[5]; cefepime[5]; imipenem or meropenem; aztreonam; tobramycin; gentamicin; amikacin
other infections	Ticarcillin, mezlocillin, or piperacillin + tobramycin, gentamicin, or amikacin[35]	Ceftazidime[5], imipenem, meropenem, aztreonam, cefepime[5] + tobramycin, gentamicin, or amikacin; ciprofloxacin[13]
Spirillum minus (rat bite fever)	Penicillin G	A tetracycline[8]; streptomycin
**Stenotrophomonas maltophilia*	Trimethoprim-sulfamethoxazole	Minocycline[8]; a fluoroquinolone[3]
Streptobacillus moniliformis (rat bite fever, Haverhill fever)	Penicillin G	A tetracycline[8]; streptomycin
Vibrio cholerae (cholera)[36]	A tetracycline[8]	A fluoroquinolone[3]; trimethoprim-sulfamethoxazole
Vibrio vulnificus	A tetracycline[8]	Cefotaxime[5]
Yersinia pestis (plague)	Streptomycin ± a tetracycline[8]	Chloramphenicol[16]; gentamicin; trimethoprim-sulfamethoxazole
ACID-FAST BACILLI		
**Mycobacterium tuberculosis*	Isoniazid + rifampin + pyrazinamide ± ethambutol or streptomycin[16]	A fluoroquinolone[3]; cycloserine[16]; capreomycin[16] or kanamycin[16] or amikacin[16]; ethionamide[16]; para-aminosalicylic acid[16]; ± clofazimine[16]

ANTIMICROBIAL DRUGS OF CHOICE *(Continued)*

Infecting Organism	Drug of First Choice	Alternative Drugs
**Mycobacterium kansasii*	Isoniazid + rifampin ± ethambutol or streptomycin[16]	Clarithromycin[11] or azithromycin; ethionamide[16]; cycloserine[16]
**Mycobacterium avium* complex	Clarithromycin[11] or azithromycin + ethambutol ± rifabutin	Ciprofloxacin[13]; amikacin[16]
prophylaxis	Clarithromycin[11] or azithromycin ± rifabutin	
**Mycobacterium fortuitum/ chelonae* complex	Amikacin + clarithromycin[11]	Cefoxitin[5]; rifampin; a sulfonamide; doxycycline[8]; ethambutol; linezolid
Mycobacterium marinum (balnei)[37]	Minocycline[8]	Trimethoprim-sulfamethoxazole; rifampin; clarithromycin[11]; doxycycline[8]
Mycobacterium leprae (leprosy)	Dapsone + rifampin ± clofazimine	Minocycline[8]; ofloxacin[13]; sparfloxacin[13]; clarithromycin[11]
ACTINOMYCETES		
Actinomyces israelii (actinomycosis)	Penicillin G	A tetracycline[8]; erythromycin; clindamycin
Nocardia	Trimethoprim-sulfamethoxazole	Sulfisoxazole; amikacin[16]; a tetracycline[8]; imipenem or meropenem; cycloserine[16]; linezolid
**Rhodococcus equi*	Vancomycin ± a fluoroquinolone[3], rifampin, imipenem or meropenem; amikacin	Erythromycin
Tropheryma whippelii (agent of Whipple's disease)	Trimethoprim-sulfamethoxazole	Penicillin G; a tetracycline[8]
CHLAMYDIAE		
Chlamydia psittaci (psittacosis, ornithosis)	A tetracycline[8]	Chloramphenicol[16]
Chlamydia trachomatis		
(trachoma)	Azithromycin	A tetracycline[8] (topical plus oral); a sulfonamide (topical plus oral)
(inclusion conjunctivitis)	Erythromycin (oral or I.V.)	A sulfonamide
(pneumonia)	Erythromycin	A sulfonamide
(urethritis, cervicitis)	Azithromycin or doxycycline[8]	Erythromycin; ofloxacin[13]; amoxicillin
(lymphogranuloma venereum)	A tetracycline[8]	Erythromycin
Chlamydia pneumoniae (TWAR strain)	Erythromycin; a tetracycline[8]; clarithromycin[11] or azithromycin	A fluoroquinolone[3]
EHRLICHIA		
Ehrlichia chaffeensis	Doxycycline[8]	Chloramphenicol[16]
Ehrlichia ewingii	Doxycycline[8]	
Ehrlichia phagocytophila	Doxycycline[8]	Rifampin
MYCOPLASMA		
Mycoplasma pneumoniae	Erythromycin; a tetracycline[8]; clarithromycin[11] or azithromycin	A fluoroquinolone[3]
Ureaplasma urealyticum	Erythromycin	A tetracycline[8]; clarithromycin[11]; azithromycin; ofloxacin[13]
RICKETTSIA – Rocky Mountain spotted fever, endemic typhus (murine), epidemic typhus (louse-borne), scrub typhus (*Orientia tsutsugamushi*), trench fever, Q fever	Doxycycline[8]	Chloramphenicol[16]; a fluoroquinolone[3]; rifampin

Infecting Organism	Drug of First Choice	Alternative Drugs
SPIROCHETES		
Borrelia burgdorferi (Lyme disease)[38]	Doxycycline[8]; amoxicillin; cefuroxime axetil[5]	Ceftriaxone[5]; cefotaxime[5]; penicillin G; azithromycin; clarithromycin[11]
Borrelia recurrentis (relapsing fever)	A tetracycline[8]	Penicillin G
Leptospira	Penicillin G	A tetracycline[8]
Treponema pallidum (syphilis)	Penicillin G[10]	A tetracycline[8]; ceftriaxone[5]
Treponema pertenue (yaws)	Penicillin G	A tetracycline[8]

***Resistance may be a problem; susceptibility tests should be used to guide therapy.**

[1]Disk sensitivity testing may not provide adequate information; beta-lactamase assays, "E" tests, and dilution tests for susceptibility should be used in serious infections.

[2]Aminoglycoside resistance is increasingly common among enterococci; treatment options include ampicillin 2 g I.V. q4h, continuous infusion of ampicillin, a combination of ampicillin plus a fluoroquinolone, or a combination of ampicillin, imipenem, and vancomycin.

[3]Among the fluoroquinolones, levofloxacin, gatifloxacin, and moxifloxacin have excellent *in vitro* activity against *S. pneumoniae*, including penicillin- and cephalosporin-resistant strains. Levofloxacin, gatifloxacin, and moxifloxacin also have good activity against many strains of *S. aureus*, but resistance has become frequent among methicillin-resistant strains. Ciprofloxacin has the greatest activity against *Pseudomonas aeruginosa*. For urinary tract infections, norfloxacin, lomefloxacin, or enoxacin can be used. For tuberculosis, levofloxacin, ofloxacin, ciprofloxacin, gatifloxacin, or moxifloxacin could be used. Ciprofloxacin, ofloxacin, levofloxacin, and gatifloxacin are available for intravenous use. None of these agents are recommended for children or pregnant women.

[4]For oral use against staphylococci, cloxacillin or dicloxacillin is preferred; for severe infections, a parenteral formulation of nafcillin or oxacillin should be used. Ampicillin, amoxicillin, carbenicillin, ticarcillin, and piperacillin are not effective against penicillinase-producing staphylococci. The combinations of clavulanic acid with amoxicillin or ticarcillin, sulbactam with ampicillin, and tazobactam with piperacillin may be active against these organisms.

[5]The cephalosporins have been used as alternatives to penicillins in patients allergic to penicillins, but such patients may also have allergic reactions to cephalosporins.

[6]For parenteral treatment of staphylococcal or nonenterococcal streptococcal infections, a first-generation cephalosporin such as cefazolin can be used. For oral therapy, cephalexin or cephradine can be used. The second-generation cephalosporins cefamandole, cefprozil, cefuroxime, cefonicid, cefotetan, cefmetazole, cefoxitin, and loracarbef are more active than the first-generation drugs against gram-negative bacteria. Cefuroxime is active against ampicillin-resistant strains of *H. influenzae*. Cefoxitin, cefotetan, and cefmetazole are the most active of the cephalosporins against *B. fragilis*, but cefotetan and cefmetazole have been associated with prothrombin deficiency. The third-generation cephalosporins cefotaxime, cefoperazone, ceftizoxime, ceftriaxone, and ceftazidime, and the fourth-generation cefepime have greater activity than the second-generation drugs against enteric gram-negative bacilli. Ceftazidime has poor activity against many gram-positive cocci and anaerobes, and ceftizoxime has poor activity against penicillin-resistant *S. pneumoniae*. Cefepime has *in vitro* activity against gram-positive cocci similar to cefotaxime and ceftriaxone and somewhat greater activity against enteric gram-negative bacilli. The activity of cefepime against *Pseudomonas aeruginosa* is similar to that of ceftazidime. Cefixime, cefpodoxime, cefdinir, and ceftibuten are oral cephalosporins with more activity than second-generation cephalosporins against facultative gram-negative bacilli; they have no useful activity against anaerobes or *P. aeruginosa*, and cefixime and ceftibuten have no useful activity against staphylococci. With the exception of cefoperazone (which, like cefamandole, can cause bleeding), ceftazidime and cefepime, the activity of all currently available cephalosporins against *P. aeruginosa* is poor or inconsistent.

[7]Many strains of coagulase-positive staphylococci and coagulase-negative staphylococci are resistant to penicillinase-resistant penicillins; these strains are also resistant to cephalosporins, imipenem, and meropenem, and are often resistant to fluoroquinolones, trimethoprim/sulfamethoxazole, and clindamycin.

[8]Tetracyclines are generally not recommended for pregnant women or children younger than 8 years old.

[9]For serious soft-tissue infection due to group A streptococci, clindamycin may be more effective than penicillin. Group A streptococci may, however, be resistant to clindamycin; therefore, some *Medical Letter* consultants suggest using both clindamycin and penicillin, with or without I.V. immune globulin, to treat serious soft-tissue infections. Group A streptococci may also be resistant to erythromycin, azithromycin, and clarithromycin.

[10]Penicillin V (or amoxicillin) is preferred for oral treatment of infections caused by nonpenicillinase-producing streptococci. For initial therapy of severe infections, penicillin G, administered parenterally, is first choice. For somewhat longer action in less severe infections due to group A streptococci, pneumococci or *Treponema pallidum*, procaine penicillin G, an intramuscular formulation, can be given once or twice daily, but is seldom used now. Benzathine penicillin G, a slowly absorbed preparation, is usually given in a single monthly injection for prophylaxis of rheumatic fever, once for treatment of group A streptococcal pharyngitis and once or more for treatment of syphilis.

[11]Not recommended for use in pregnancy.

[12]Some strains of *S. pneumoniae* are resistant to erythromycin, clindamycin, trimethoprim-sulfamethoxazole, clarithromycin, azithromycin and chloramphenicol, and resistance to the newer fluoroquinolones is increasing. Nearly all strains tested so far are susceptible to linezolid and quinupristin/dalfopristin *in vitro* (Patel R, Rouse MS, Piper KE, et al, "*In Vitro* Activity of Linezolid Against Vancomycin-Resistant Enterococci, Methicillin-Resistant *Staphylococcus aureus* and Penicillin-Resistant *Streptococcus pneumoniae*," *Diagn Microbiol Infect Dis*, 1999, 34(2):119-22; Verhaegen J and Verbist L, "*In Vitro* Activities of 16 Non-beta-lactam Antibiotics Against Penicillin-

ANTIMICROBIAL DRUGS OF CHOICE *(Continued)*

Susceptible and Penicillin-Resistant *Streptococcus pneumoniae*," *J Antimicrob Chemother*, 1999, 43(4):563-7.

[13]Usually not recommended for use in children or pregnant women.

[14]Patients with gonorrhea should be treated presumptively for coinfection with *C. trachomatis* with azithromycin or doxycycline.

[15]Rare strains of *N. meningitidis* are resistant or relatively resistant to penicillin. A fluoroquinolone or rifampin is recommended for prophylaxis after close contact with infected patients.

[16]Because of the possibility of serious adverse effects, this drug should be used only for severe infections when less hazardous drugs are ineffective.

[17]Sulfonamide-resistant strains are frequent in the U.S.A; sulfonamides should be used only when susceptibility is established by susceptibility tests.

[18]Debridement is primary. Large doses of penicillin G are required. Hyperbaric oxygen therapy may be a useful adjunct to surgical debridement in management of the spreading, necrotizing type of infection.

[19]For prophylaxis, a tetanus toxoid booster and, for some patients, tetanus immune globulin (human) are required.

[20]In order to decrease the emergence of vancomycin-resistant enterococci in hospitals and to reduce costs, most clinicians now recommend use of metronidazole first in treatment of patients with *C. difficile* colitis, with oral vancomycin used only for seriously ill patients or those who do not respond to metronidazole.

[21]Antitoxin is primary; antimicrobials are used only to halt further toxin production and to prevent the carrier state.

[22]In severely ill patients, most *Medical Letter* consultants would add gentamicin, tobramycin, or amikacin.

[23]In severely ill patients, most *Medical Letter* consultants would add gentamicin, tobramycin, or amikacin (but see footnote 35).

[24]For an acute, uncomplicated urinary tract infection, before the infecting organism is known, the drug of first choice is trimethoprim-sulfamethoxazole.

[25]Eradication of *H. pylori* with various antibacterial combinations, given concurrently with an H_2-receptor blocker or proton pump inhibitor, has led to rapid healing of active peptic ulcers and low recurrence rates (Mégraud F and Marshall BJ, "How to Treat *Helicobacter pylori*. First-line, Second-line, and Future Therapies," *Gastroenterol Clin North Am*, 2000, 29(4):759-73.

[26]Large doses (6 g or more daily) are usually necessary for systemic infections. In severely ill patients, some *Medical Letter* consultants would add gentamicin, tobramycin, or amikacin.

[27]A fluoroquinolone or amoxicillin is the drug of choice for *S. typhi* carriers.

[28]Frenck RW Jr, Nakhla I, Sultan Y, et al, "Azithromycin Versus Ceftriaxone for the Treatment of Uncomplicated Typhoid Fever in Children," *Clin Infect Dis*, 2000, 31(5):1134-8.

[29]Most cases of *Salmonella* gastroenteritis subside spontaneously without antimicrobial therapy. Immunosuppressed patients, young children, and the elderly may benefit the most from antibacterials.

[30]In severely ill patients, most *Medical Letter* consultants would add gentamicin or amikacin (but see footnote 35).

[31]Sulbactam may be useful to treat multidrug resistant *Acinetobacter*. It is only available in combination with ampicillin as Unasyn®. *Medical Letter* consultants recommend 3 g I.V. q4h.

[32]Role of antibiotics is not clear (Conrad DA, "Treatment of Cat-Scratch Disease," *Curr Opin Pediatr*, 2001, 13(1):56-9.

[33]Pers C, Gahrn-Hansen B, Frederiksen W, et al, "*Capnocytophaga canimorsus* Septicemia in Denmark, 1982-1995: Review of 39 Cases," *Clin Infect Dis*, 1996, 23(1):71-5.

[34]Metronidazole is effective for bacterial vaginosis even though it is not usually active *in vitro* against *Gardnerella*.

[35]Neither gentamicin, tobramycin, netilmicin, or amikacin should be mixed in the same bottle with carbenicillin, ticarcillin, mezlocillin, or piperacillin for intravenous administration. When used in high doses or in patients with renal impairment, these penicillins may inactivate the aminoglycosides.

[36]Antibiotic therapy is an adjunct to and not a substitute for prompt fluid and electrolyte replacement.

[37]Most infections are self-limited without drug treatment.

[38]For treatment of erythema migrans, facial nerve palsy, mild cardiac disease, and some cases of arthritis, oral therapy is satisfactory; for more serious neurologic or cardiac disease or arthritis, parenteral therapy with ceftriaxone, cefotaxime, or penicillin G is recommended (*Medical Letter*, 2000, 42:37).

ANTICOAGULANT THERAPY GUIDELINES

This section focuses on treatment of atrial fibrillation and management of patients with prosthetic valves.

ATRIAL FIBRILLATION (AF)

The goal of anticoagulation in patients with AF is to prevent stroke and thromboembolic events and to promote thrombus dissolution, if present, prior to elective cardioversion. Anticoagulation in patients with atrial fibrillation is required prior to cardioversion if the patient has been in AF for more than 48 hours or if a thrombus is observed by echocardiography. Patients with a longer or unknown duration of AF may undergo transesophageal echocardiography (TEE) to aid in the assessment for anticoagulation therapy. Anticoagulation therapy is maintained for 3-4 weeks prior to cardioversion and continued for 4 weeks after successful cardioversion. It is important that anticoagulation be maintained after cardioversion because even though the atrium is electrically in sinus rhythm, the mechanical force is diminished and the likelihood of clotting is still high. Obviously, if there are other indications for anticoagulation, it should be continued. In the absence of contraindications, daily aspirin should be started after warfarin therapy is completed.

The need for chronic antithrombotic therapy in AF depends on patient risk factors. The risk of stroke in AF is approximately 6 times that of patients without AF. The risk for stroke increases with age (>60 years); if the patient has had a previous transient ischemic attack, stroke, or systemic embolus; if the patient has hypertension (treated or untreated); or with poor ventricular function, rheumatic mitral valve disease, or a prosthetic heart valve. These risk factors should be considered when deciding on the intensity of oral anticoagulation or when prescribing chronic antithrombotic therapy (see table). Patients with diabetes, coronary artery disease, or thyrotoxicosis are at a high risk for stroke. Patients with chronic or paroxysmal AF should be on chronic antithrombotic therapy. Warfarin (INR 2.0-3.0) and aspirin (325 mg daily) are considered first-line therapies for the prophylaxis of thromboembolic events in AF.

Recommendations for Atrial Fibrillation

Risk Factors*	Age	Recommended Therapy
None	<65 y	Aspirin
None	65-75 y	Aspirin or warfarin
≥1	<65 to 75 y	Warfarin
None or ≥1	>75 y	Warfarin

*Risk factors: Prior TIA or stroke, systemic embolus, hypertension (treated or untreated), poor left ventricular function, rheumatic mitral valve disease, or prosthetic heart valve.

HEPARIN THERAPY

Heparin therapy may be initially started to anticoagulate patients with AF. Therapy may be switched to warfarin therapy on the first day if a therapeutic aPTT can be achieved. The aPTT should be evaluated at baseline and every 6 hours following the start of heparin therapy or if dosage adjustments are made. The optimal dose of heparin is achieved when aPTT is maintained between 1.5-2.5 times the patient's baseline aPPT. Please refer to Heparin *on page 653*, which includes dosing information.

WARFARIN THERAPY

The target INR range for warfarin therapy in AF is 2.0-3.0. Patients with mechanical heart valves may require a higher range (see below). Patients should **not** receive loading doses of warfarin (ie, 10 mg daily for 3 days then 5 mg daily) as the steady-state INR is not achieved more quickly. The intensity of anticoagulation therapy should be monitored closely until the patient has reached a stable PT/INR. Once the patient is stabilized on a fixed dose of warfarin, the PT/INR can be monitored on a monthly basis if the patient demonstrates a stable PT/INR on chronic therapy. If dosage adjustments are made, PT/INR should be evaluated in approximately 2 weeks. Supratherapeutic INR values are managed based on the presence and severity of bleeding (see table). Patients on warfarin should be warned to seek medical evaluation if they develop a very severe headache, abdominal pain, unusual bleeding, backache, or if they experience significant trauma, particularly head injuries. Please refer to Warfarin *on page 1409* for complete drug information.

ANTICOAGULANT THERAPY GUIDELINES *(Continued)*

Initiation of Oral Anticoagulation Therapy with Warfarin

The dosing of warfarin must be individualized according to the patient's response to the drug as indicated by the PT/INR. Use of a large loading dose may increase the incidence of hemorrhagic and other complications, does not offer more rapid protection against thrombus formation, and is not recommended. Low initiation doses (eg, 2-5 mg/day) are recommended for elderly and/or debilitated patients and patients with potential for increased responsiveness to warfarin.

Step 1: Obtain baseline PT/INR

Begin therapy with warfarin with a dose of 2-5 mg per day with dosage adjustment based on the results of PT/INR determinations. **Note:** Consider lower dosages (<5 mg) for elderly, malnourished, hepatic impairment, or when high risk of bleeding.

For patients on heparin: Since the anticoagulant effect of warfarin is delayed, heparin is preferred initially for rapid anticoagulation. Conversion to warfarin may begin concomitantly with heparin therapy or may be delayed 3-6 days. When warfarin has produced the desired therapeutic range, INR, or prothrombin time, heparin may be discontinued.

Step 2: Day that the PT/INR is stabilized in the therapeutic range: Check PT/INR daily. Adjust warfarin dose based on the results of PT/INR determinations.

Patients stabilized in the therapeutic range: Intervals between subsequent PT/INR determinations should be based upon the physician's judgment of the patient's reliability and response to warfarin in order to maintain the individual within the therapeutic range. Acceptable intervals for PT/INR determinations are normally with the range of 1-4 weeks after a stable dosage has been determined. Most patients are satisfactorily maintained on warfarin at a dose of 2-10 mg daily.

Monitoring — The International Normalized Ratio (INR)

Because PT results are very dependent on the thromboplastin reagent used, a system of standardizing the prothrombin time in oral anticoagulant therapy was introduced by the World Health Organization in 1983. It is based upon determination of an INR, which is equivalent to the PT ratio one would obtain if a sensitive reference thromboplastin were used for the PT.

- Thromboplastin sensitivity is determined by the manufacturer and is expressed as an International Sensitivity Index (ISI)
- The INR can be calculated as **INR = (observed PT ratio)**^{ISI}
- The calculation of the INR from the PT ratio is usually performed by the laboratory

Reminder

- Be aware of potential drug interactions and other factors that may affect INR (refer to prescribing information for warfarin)
- Patient/staff education about warfarin is an important part of therapy. Effective therapeutic levels with minimal complications are in part dependent upon cooperative and well-instructed patients who communicate effectively with their physician. Various warfarin patient educational guides are available to health professionals on request.

Management of Supratherapeutic INR

INR	Patient Situation	Action
>3 and ≤5	No bleeding or need for rapid reversal (ie, no need for surgery)	Omit next few warfarin dose and/or restart at lower dose when INR approaches desired range. If only minimally above range, then no dosage reduction may be required.
>5 and <9.0	No bleeding or need for rapid reversal	Omit next 1-2 doses, monitor INR more frequently, and restart at lower dose when INR approaches target range **or** omit dose and give 1-2.5 mg vitamin K orally (use this if patient has risk factors for bleeding).
	No bleeding but reversal needed for surgery or dental extraction within 24 hours	Vitamin K 2-4 mg orally (expected reversal within 24 hours); give additional 1-2 mg if INR remains high at 24 hours.
>9.0 and <20.0	No bleeding	Stop warfarin, give vitamin K 3-5 mg orally; follow INR closely; repeat vitamin K if needed. Reassess need and dose of warfarin when INR approaches desirable range.
Rapid reversal required (ie, INR >20)	Serious bleeding or major warfarin overdose	Stop warfarin, give vitamin K 10 mg by slow I.V. infusion. May repeat vitamin K every 12 hours and give fresh plasma transfusion or prothrombin complex concentrate as needed. When appropriate, heparin can be given until the patient becomes responsive to warfarin.

WARFARIN INTERACTIONS

Numerous factors, alone or in combination, including travel, changes in diet, environment, physical state, and medication may influence response of the patient to anticoagulants. It is generally good practice to monitor the patient's response with additional PT/INR determinations in the period immediately after discharge from the hospital, and whenever other medications are initiated, discontinued, or taken irregularly. The following factors are listed for reference; however, other factors may also affect the anticoagulant response.

Intensity of warfarin anticoagulation is affected by foods high in vitamin K, alcohol, diseases such as congestive heart failure, and by concomitant drug therapy. Drugs that inhibit or induce P450 2C9 isoenzyme will have the greatest effect on INR (see following table). It is important to note that just as the therapeutic effect of warfarin requires several days to become apparent, treatment with vitamin K may also inhibit the effects of warfarin for several days. Foods high in vitamin K decrease PT/INR and include green leafy vegetables (eg, kale, broccoli, spinach, parsley, collard greens). Acute alcohol consumption can increase PT/INR while chronic ingestion can decrease PT/INR. Drug interactions with warfarin may occur by several mechanisms, including impairment of absorption, induction or inhibition of metabolism, competition for protein-binding sites, and platelet inhibition. Drugs that inhibit or induce P450 2C9 (responsible for metabolism of S-warfarin) may have the greatest effect on INR. Select and important drug-drug interactions are depicted in the following table.

Selected Warfarin Drug Interactions

Drug	Effect on P450	Isoenzyme		
		1A2	2C9	3A4
Amiodarone	Inhibit		X	X
Carbamazepine	Induce		X	X
Ciprofloxacin	Inhibit	X		
Cimetidine	Inhibit	X		
Dicloxacillin	Induce			
Erythromycin	Inhibit	X		X
Fluconazole	Inhibit		X	X
Metronidazole	Inhibit		X	
Nafcillin	Induce			
Omeprazole	Inhibit			X
Phenobarbital	Induce	X	X	X
Phenytoin	Induce	X	X	X
Rifampin	Induce	X	X	X
SSRI	Inhibit	X		
TMP/SMX (Bactrim®)	Inhibit		X	
Zileuton	Inhibit	X		
Zafirlukast	Inhibit		X	

ANTICOAGULANT THERAPY GUIDELINES *(Continued)*

PROSTHETIC HEART VALVES

Patients with mechanical prosthetic valves require life-long anticoagulation therapy. The optimal intensity of anticoagulation is not established. The risk of thromboembolism is greater in valve patients who have atrial fibrillation (AF); have an enlarged left atrium (>5.5 cm); have a history of systemic embolism, left ventricular systolic dysfunction, coronary artery disease, left atrial thrombus; have ball valve; or have more than one mechanical valve. The risk for thromboembolism is also higher for mechanical valves in the mitral position compared to aortic. These factors should be weighed in each patient before deciding the desired level of anticoagulation to prevent thromboembolism and to avoid bleeding complications. Ranges for anticoagulation intensity in patients with prosthetic valves are described in the following table.

Prosthetic Valves

Valve Location	Type	Recommended INR / Therapy
Mechanical	Mitral - bileaflet or tilting disk	2.5-3.5 or 2.0-3.0 plus aspirin 80-100 mg daily
	Mitral - cage disk or ball	2.5-3.5 plus aspirin (80-100 mg daily)
	Aortic - bileaflet (eg, St Jude, CarboMedics)	2.0-3.0 if normal left ventricular function, left atrial size, and sinus rhythm 2.5-3.5 or 2.0-3.0 plus aspirin (80-100 mg daily) if AF and high-risk patients
	Mitral or aortic valve and history of systemic embolism despite adequate warfarin therapy	2.5-3.5 plus aspirin 80-100 mg daily
Bioprosthetic	Mitral or aortic	2.0-3.0 for 3 months after insertion or indefinitely if patient has AF; left atrial thrombus or permanent pacemaker, duration uncertain; prior systemic embolism, duration of therapy should be increased to 3-12 months; chronic low-dose aspirin therapy (≤160 mg daily) after warfarin therapy

As a general rule, concomitant warfarin and aspirin therapy should be avoided, except in special situations. For patients with mechanical prosthetic valves who suffer a systemic thromboembolism despite adequate anticoagulation therapy, low-dose aspirin should be added and the INR should be maintained between 2.5 and 3.5. The combination of warfarin and low-dose aspirin in all mechanical valve patients is uncertain; patients at the highest risk for thromboembolism should be considered. For patients who cannot tolerate aspirin, dypyridamole 150 mg daily may be combined with warfarin therapy.

REFERENCES

Guidelines

Proceedings of the American College of Chest Physicians – 6th Consensus Conference on Antithrombotic Therapy, *Chest*, 2001, 119(1 Suppl):1S-370S.

Drug Therapy

Crowther MA, Ginsberg JB, Kearon C, et al, "A Randomized Trial Comparing 5 mg and 10 mg Warfarin Loading Doses," *Arch Intern Med*, 1999, 159:46-8.

ANTIEMETICS FOR CHEMOTHERAPY-INDUCED NAUSEA AND VOMITING

GENERAL PRINCIPLES FOR MANAGING NAUSEA AND VOMITING

1. Prophylaxis is **much** better than treatment of actual vomiting. For agents with a moderate-to-high (30% to 100%) incidence of nausea, patients should be pretreated with an antiemetic. Depending on the antiemetic agent(s) and route(s) of administration, pretreatment may range from 1 hour to 5 minutes prior to administration of the antineoplastic agent(s).
2. Doses and intervals of the antiemetic regimen need to be individualized for each patient. "PRN" regimens should **not** be used. A fixed schedule of drug administration is preferable.
3. If a patient has had no nausea for 24 hours while on their scheduled antiemetic regimen, it is usually possible to switch to a "PRN" regimen. The patient should be advised to resume the fixed schedule at the **first** sign of recurrent nausea, and continue it until they have had at least 24 hours without nausea.
4. Titrate antiemetic dose to patient tolerance.
5. In most cases, combination regimens are required for optimum control of nausea. Do not be afraid to use two or more agents, from different pharmacologic categories, to achieve optimal results.
6. To the extent possible, avoid duplication of agents from the same pharmacologic category.
7. Anticipatory nausea and vomiting can often be minimized if the patient receives effective prophylaxis against nausea from the first cycle of therapy.
8. If anticipatory nausea does develop, an anxiolytic agent is usually the drug of choice.
9. "If it's not broken - **don't** fix it!" Regardless of your own preferences, if the patient's current antiemetic regimen is working, don't change it.
10. For moderately emetogenic regimens, a steroid and dopamine blocker (eg, metoclopramide, prochlorperazine, thiethylperazine) may be the most cost-effective regimen.
11. For highly emetogenic regimens, a steroid and serotonin receptor blocker (eg, dolasetron, granisetron, ondansetron) combination is the preferred regimen.
12. A dopamine blocker (eg, metoclopramide, prochlorperazine, thiethylperazine) is a good first alternative if the serotonin blocker fails.
13. Although most nausea or vomiting develops within the first 24 hours after treatment, delayed reactions (1-7 days after chemotherapy) are not uncommon.
14. Other antiemetics (eg, cannabinoids, antihistamines, or anticholinergics) have limited use as initial therapy. They are best used in combination with more effective agents (steroids, dopamine, or serotonin blockers); or, as second- or third-line therapy.
15. Serotonin blockers are most effective in scheduled prophylactic regimens; rather than in "PRN" regimens to chase existing vomiting.
16. The serotonin blockers appear to have a "ceiling" dose, above which there is little or no added antiemetic effect.

ANTIEMETICS FOR CHEMOTHERAPY-INDUCED NAUSEA AND VOMITING *(Continued)*

Time Course of Nausea and Vomiting

Drug	Onset (h)	Duration (h)
Azacitidine	1-3	3-4
Carboplatin	2-6	1-48
Carmustine	2-6	4-6
Cisplatin	1-4	12-96
Cyclophosphamide	6-8	8-24
Cytarabine	1-3	3-8
Dacarbazine	1-2	2-4
Dactinomycin	2-5	4-24
Daunorubicin	1-3	4-24
Doxorubicin	1-3	4-24
Ifosfamide	2-3	12-72
Lomustine	2-6	4-6
Mechlorethamine	1-3	2-8
Mitomycin	1-2	48-72
Plicamycin	4-6	4-24
Procarbazine	24-27	Variable
Streptozocin	1-3	1-12

Emetogenic Potential of Single Chemotherapeutic Agents

Very High (>90%)

Cisplatin
Cytarabine (>2 g)
Dacarbazine
Didemnin-B
JM-216
Mechlorethamine
Melphalan (I.V.)
Streptozocin

High (60% to 90%)

Aldesleukin
Amifostine
Carmustine
Cyclophosphamide (>1 g)
Cytarabine (<2 g)
Dactinomycin
Elsamitrucin
Estramustine
Etoposide
Hydroxyurea
Idarubicin
Irinotecan
Lomustine
Mitotane
Mitomycin
Mitoxantrone
Semustine
Toremifene
Tretinoin

Moderate (30% to 60%)

Altretamine
Amonafide
Amsacrine
Asparaginase
Azacytidine
Carboplatin
Cladribine
Cyclophosphamide (<1 g)
Daunorubicin
Dexrazocane
Diazequone
Docetaxel
Doxorubicin
Epirubicin
Ifosfamide
Interferons
Interleukin-6
Mitoguazone
PALA
Pegaspergase
Pentostatin
Plicamycin
Procarbazine
Teniposide
Tomudex
Topotecan
Trimetrexate
Vinblastine
Vinorelbine

Low (10% to 30%)

Floxuridine
Fluorouracil
Flutamide
Gemcitabine
Levamisole
Melphalan (oral)
Methotrexate (high dose)
Steroids
Suramin
Tamoxifen
Thioguanine
Vindesine

Very Low (<10%)

Androgens
Aminoglutethimide
Anastrozole
Bicalutamide
Bleomycin
Busulfan
Chlorambucil
Estrogens
Fludarabine
Goserelin
Homoharringtonine
Leucovorin
Leuprolide
Megestrol
Mercaptopurine
Mesna
Methotrexate (low dose)
Paclitaxel
Thiotepa
Vincristine

Drugs With a High Incidence but Low Severity of Nausea/Vomiting

Amonafide
Carboplatin
Cyclophosphamide (<1 g)
Dexrazoxane
Docetaxel
Gemcitabine
Hydroxyurea
Interferons
Mitoguazone
Mitoxantrone
Tretinoin
Vinblastine

Drugs With a Low Incidence but High Severity of Nausea/Vomiting

Lomustine
Methotrexate (high dose)
Semustine

Potency of Antiemetic Drugs

Potency	Type of Antiemetic Drug
Active against highly emetogenic chemotherapy	Serotonin antagonist Substituted benzamide (high dose)
Active against mildly or moderately emetogenic chemotherapy	Butyrophenone Cannabinoid Corticosteroid Phenothiazine
Minimally active	Anticholinergic agent Antihistamine Benzodiazepine

REPRESENTATIVE ANTIEMETIC REGIMENS

Highly emetogenic chemotherapy:

Dexamethasone 10-20 mg P.O. or I.V. + a serotonin antagonist daily 15-30 minutes before treatment on each day of chemotherapy

Recommended serotonin antagonist regimens:
- Dolasetron 100 mg P.O. once daily
- Granisetron 2 mg P.O. once daily
- Granisetron 1 mg P.O. every 12 hours
- Granisetron 10 mcg/kg I.V. once daily
- Granisetron 1 mg I.V. once daily
- Ondansetron 0.45 mg/kg I.V. once daily
- Ondansetron 24-32 mg I.V. once daily
- Ondansetron 0.15 mg/kg I.V. every 8 hours
- Ondansetron 8-10 mg I.V. every 8 hours

For continuous infusion therapy, carboplatin, and high-dose (>1 g/m^2) cyclophosphamide regimens, the following regimen may be preferred:

Dexamethasone 10 mg P.O. or I.V. + a serotonin antagonist every 12 hours

Recommended serotonin antagonist regimens:
- Granisetron 1 mg P.O.
- Granisetron 10 mcg/kg I.V.
- Ondansetron 10-16 mg I.V.
- Ondansetron 16-24 mg P.O.

Moderately emetogenic chemotherapy:

Dexamethasone 10 mg P.O. or I.V. + a serotonin antagonist daily 15-30 minutes before treatment on each day of chemotherapy

Recommended serotonin antagonist regimens:
- Granisetron 1 mg P.O. once daily
- Ondansetron 16 mg P.O. once daily
- Ondansetron 8-10 mg I.V. once daily

For continuous infusion therapy, the following regimen may be preferred:

Dexamethasone 4 mg P.O. or I.V. + ondansetron 8 mg P.O. or I.V. every 12 hours on each day of chemotherapy

Mildly emetogenic chemotherapy (all agents are given 15-30 minutes before treatment, and may be repeated every 4-6 hours if necessary. With the exceptions of dexamethasone (given over 5-15 minutes) and droperidol (given by I.V. push), intravenous doses should be given over 30 minutes.):

ANTIEMETICS FOR CHEMOTHERAPY-INDUCED NAUSEA AND VOMITING *(Continued)*

Dexamethasone 4 mg P.O./I.V./I.M.
Droperidol 1.25-5 mg I.M./I.V. push
Haloperidol 2 mg P.O./I.V./I.M.
Metoclopramide 30 mg P.O./I.V./I.M.
Prochlorperazine 10-20 mg P.O./I.V./I.M.
Thiethylperazine 10-20 mg P.O./I.V./I.M.

Delayed nausea and vomiting:

Dexamethasone + a dopamine or serotonin antagonist. Therapy should start within 12-24 hours of administration of the emetogenic chemotherapy.

Recommended regimens:

Dexamethasone

8 mg P.O. every 12 hours for 2 days, then 4 mg P.O. every 12 hours for 2 days **or**

20 mg P.O. 1 hour before chemotherapy; 10 mg P.O. 12 hours after chemotherapy, then 8 mg P.O. every 12 hours for 4 doses, then 4 mg P.O. every 12 hours for 4 doses

Recommended dopamine/serotonin antagonist regimens:

Droperidol 1.25-2.5 mg I.V./I.M. every 4 hours for 4 days
Metoclopramide 0.5 mg/kg P.O. every 6 hours for 4 days
Ondansetron 8 mg P.O. every 8 hours for 4 days
Prochlorperazine 10 mg P.O. every 6 hours for 4 days
Prochlorperazine 15 mg (sustained release) P.O. 1 hour before chemotherapy, then every 12 hours for 5 doses
Thiethylperazine 10 mg P.O. every 6 hours for 4 days

Recommended Doses of Serotonin ($5HT_3$) Antiemetics Prophylaxis of Acute Highly Emetogenic Chemotherapy-Induced Nausea/Vomiting

ASCO	ASHP	NCCN	MASCC
Dolasetron			
100 mg P.O.	100-200 mg P.O.	100 mg P.O.	100-200 mg P.O.
1.8 mg/kg* I.V.	1.8 mg/kg* I.V.	1.8 mg/kg* I.V.	1.8 mg/kg I.V.
Granisetron			
2 mg P.O.	2 mg P.O.	2 mg P.O.†	2 mg P.O.
10 mcg/kg‡ I.V	10 mcg/kg I.V.	10 mcg/kg§ I.V.	10 mcg/kg I.V.
Ondansetron			
12-24 mg P.O.	24 mg P.O.	8 mg P.O. bid	12-16 mg P.O.
8 mg I.V.¶	8 mg I.V.	8 mg I.V.#	8 mg I.V.

*Or 100 mg
†Or 100 mg
‡Or 1 mg
§Maximum: 1 mg
¶Or 0.15 mg/kg
#Maximum: 32 mg/24 hours

ASTHMA

Adapted from National Asthma Education and Prevention Program (NAEPP) Expert Panel Report, "Guidelines for the Diagnosis and Management of Asthma – Update on Selected Topics 2002," NIH Publication No. 02-5075 (www.nhlbi.nih.gov/guidelines/asthma/index.html)

MANAGEMENT OF ASTHMA IN ADULTS AND CHILDREN >5 YEARS OF AGE

Goals of Asthma Treatment

- Minimal or no chronic symptoms day or night
- Minimal or no exacerbations
- No limitations on activities; no school/work missed
- Minimal use of inhaled short-acting beta$_2$-agonist (<1 time/day, <1 canister/month)
- Minimal or no adverse effects from medications
- Children >5 years of age and adults only: PEF >80% of personal best

All Patients

- Short-acting bronchodilator: **Inhaled beta$_2$-agonists** as needed for symptoms.
- Intensity of treatment will depend on severity of exacerbation; see "Management of Asthma Exacerbations".
- Use of short-acting inhaled beta$_2$-agonists on a daily basis, or increasing use, indicates the need to initiate or titrate long-term control therapy.

Education

- Teach self-management.
- Teach about controlling environmental factors (avoidance of allergens or other factors that contribute to asthma severity).
- Review administration technique and compliance with patient.
- May use a written action plan to help educate.

ASTHMA *(Continued)*

Stepwise Approach for Managing Asthma in Adults and Children >5 Years of Age: Treatment[1]

Symptoms[2]	Lung Function[3]	Long-Term Control (Daily Medications)
STEP 4: Severe Persistent		
Day: Continual Night: Frequent	PEF/FEV_1 ≤60% PEF variability >30%	**• Preferred treatment:** **– High dose inhaled corticosteroid** **AND** **– Long-acting inhaled $beta_2$-agonist** AND, if needed – Long-term oral corticosteroids (2 mg/kg/day, generally do not exceed 60 mg/day). (Make repeated attempts to reduce systemic corticosteroids and maintain control with high-dose inhaled corticosteroids.)
STEP 3: Moderate Persistent		
Day: Every day Night: >1 night/week	PEF/FEV_1 >60% - <80% PEF variability >30%	**• Preferred treatment:** **– Low-medium dose inhaled corticosteroid** **AND** **– Long-acting inhaled $beta_2$-agonist** • Alternatives: – Increase inhaled corticosteroids within medium-dose range **OR** – Low-medium dose inhaled corticosteroids and either leukotriene receptor antagonist or theophylline
		If needed (especially with recurring severe exacerbations): **• Preferred treatment:** – Increase inhaled corticosteroids within medium-dose range, and add long-acting inhaled $beta_2$-agonist • Alternatives: – Increase inhaled corticosteroids in medium-dose range, and add either leukotriene receptor antagonist or theophylline
STEP 2: Mild Persistent		
Day: >2 days/week but <1 time/day Night: >2 nights/month	PEF/FEV_1 ≥80% PEF variability 20%-30%	**• Preferred treatment:** **– Low-dose inhaled corticosteroid** • Alternatives: Cromolyn, leukotriene receptor antagonist, nedocromil, or sustained release theophylline (serum concentration 5-15 mcg/mL)
STEP 1: Mild Intermittent		
Day: ≤2 days/week Night: ≤2 nights/month	PEF/FEV_1 ≥80% PEF variability <20%	No daily medication needed. A course of systemic corticosteroids is recommended for severe exacerbations.

[1]Classify severity. The presence of one of the features of severity is sufficient to place a patient in that category. An individual should be assigned to the most severe grade in which any feature occurs. The characteristics noted are general and may overlap because asthma is highly variable. Furthermore, an individual's classification may change over time.

[2]Patients at any level of severity can have mild, moderate, or severe exacerbations. Some patients with intermittent asthma experience severe and life-threatening exacerbations separated by long periods of normal lung function and no symptoms.

[3]PEF is % of personal best and FEV_1 is % predicted.

↓ Step down
Review treatment every 1-6 months; a gradual stepwise reduction in treatment may be possible.

↑Step up
If control is not maintained, consider step up. First, review patient medication technique, adherence, and environmental control.

Notes:

- **The stepwise approach presents general guidelines to assist clinical decision making; it is not intended to be a specific prescription. Asthma is highly**

variable; clinicians should tailor specific medication plans to the needs and circumstances of individual patients.

- Gain control as quickly as possible; then decrease treatment to the least medication necessary to maintain control.
- A rescue course of systemic corticosteroids may be needed at any time and at any step.
- Some patients with intermittent asthma experience severe and life-threatening exacerbations separated by long periods of normal lung function and no symptoms. This may be especially common with exacerbations provoked by respiratory infections. A short course of systemic corticosteroids is recommended.
- At each step, patients should control their environment to avoid or control factors that make their asthma worse.
- Antibiotics are not recommended for treatment of acute asthma exacerbations except where there is evidence or suspicion of bacterial infection.
- Consultation with an asthma specialist is recommended for moderate or severe persistent asthma.
- Peak flow monitoring for patients with moderate-severe asthma should be considered.

MANAGEMENT OF ASTHMA IN INFANTS AND YOUNG CHILDREN

All Patients

- Bronchodilator as needed for symptoms ≤2 times/week. Intensity of treatment will depend upon severity of exacerbation (see "Management of Asthma Exacerbations"). Either:
  - Preferred treatment: Inhaled short-acting beta$_2$-agonist by nebulizer or face mask and spacer/holding chamber

    or
  - Alternative treatment: Oral beta$_2$-agonist
- With viral respiratory infection:
  - Bronchodilator q4-6h up to 24 hours (longer with physician consult) but, in general, repeat no more than once every 6 weeks.
  - Consider systemic corticosteroid if current exacerbation is severe or patient has history of severe exacerbations.
- Use of short-acting inhaled beta$_2$-agonist on a daily basis, or increasing use, indicates the need to initiate or titrate long-term control therapy.

Education

- Teach self-management or caregiver management.
- Teach about controlling environmental factors.
- Review administration technique and compliance with patient.
- May use a written action plan to help educate.

ASTHMA *(Continued)*

Stepwise Approach for Managing Infants and Young Children (≤5 Years of Age) With Acute or Chronic Asthma[1]

Symptoms[2]	Long-Term Control (Daily Medications)
STEP 4: Severe Persistent	
Day: Continual Night: Frequent	**• Preferred treatment:** **– High dose inhaled corticosteroid** **AND** **– Long-acting inhaled $beta_2$-agonist** AND, if needed – Long-term oral corticosteroids (2 mg/kg/day, generally do not exceed 60 mg/day). (Make repeated attempts to reduce systemic corticosteroids and maintain control with high-dose inhaled corticosteroids.)
STEP 3: Moderate Persistent	
Day: Every day Night: >1 night/week	**• Preferred treatment:** **– Low-dose inhaled corticosteroid** **AND** **Long-acting inhaled $beta_2$-agonist** **OR** **Medium-dose inhaled corticosteroid** • Alternatives: – Low-dose inhaled corticosteroid and either leukotriene receptor antagonist or theophylline
	If needed (especially with recurring severe exacerbations): **• Preferred treatment:** **– Medium-dose inhaled corticosteroid and long-acting inhaled $beta_2$-agonist** • Alternatives: – Medium-dose inhaled corticosteroid and either leukotriene receptor antagonist or theophylline
STEP 2: Mild Persistent	
Day: >2 days/week but <1 time/day Night: >2 nights/month	**• Preferred treatment:** **– Low-dose inhaled corticosteroid (with nebulizer or MDI with holding chamber with or without face mask or DPI)** • Alternatives: – Cromolyn (nebulizer is preferred or MDI with holding chamber) **OR** – Leukotriene receptor antagonist
STEP 1: Mild Intermittent	
Day: ≤2 days/week Night: ≤2 nights/month	No daily medication needed

[1]Classify severity. The presence of one of the features of severity is sufficient to place a patient in that category. An individual should be assigned to the most severe grade in which any feature occurs. The characteristics noted in this figure are general and may overlap because asthma is highly variable. Furthermore, an individual's classification may change over time.

[2]Patients at any level of severity can have mild, moderate, or severe exacerbations. Some patients with intermittent asthma experience severe and life-threatening exacerbations separated by long periods of normal lung function and no symptoms.

↓ Step Down
Review treatment every 1-6 month; a gradual stepwise reduction in treatment may be possible.

↑ Step Up
If control is not achieved, consider step up. But first: review patient medication technique, adherence, and environmental control (avoidance of allergens or other precipitant factors)

Notes:

- **The stepwise approach presents guidelines to assist clinical decision making. Asthma is highly variable; clinicians should tailor specific medication plans to the needs and circumstances of individual patients.**
- Gain control as quickly as possible; then decrease treatment to the least medication necessary to maintain control.
- A rescue course of systemic corticosteroid may be needed at any time and step.
- In general, use of short-acting $beta_2$-agonist on a daily basis indicates the need for additional long-term control therapy.
- There are very few studies on asthma therapy for infants.
- Studies comparing medications in children <5 years of age are not available.
- Consultation with an asthma specialist is recommended for moderate or severe persistent asthma. Consider consultation for patient with mild persistent asthma.
- Initiation of long-term control therapy should be considered in infants and young children who have had >3 episodes of wheezing in the past year that lasted >1 day and affected sleep and who have risk factors for asthma.
- Inhaled corticosteroids improve health outcomes for children with mild-moderate persistent asthma. Monitor growth of children taking corticosteroids by any route. If growth appears slowed, weigh the benefits against the risks.
- Antibiotics are not recommended for treatment of acute asthma exacerbations except where there is evidence or suspicion of bacterial infection.

Management of Asthma Exacerbations: Home Treatment*

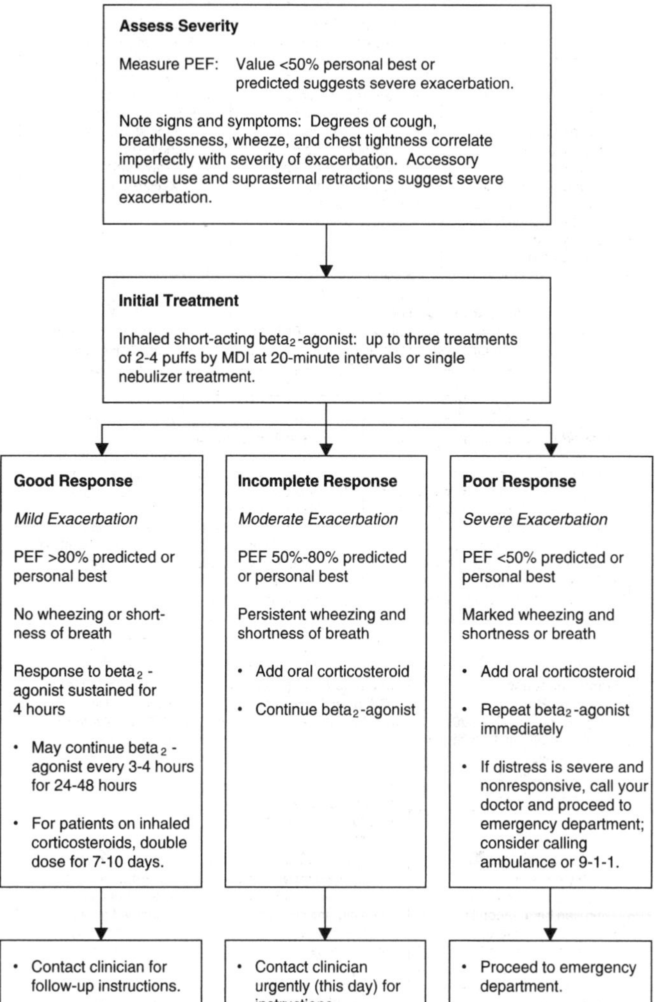

*Patients at high risk of asthma-related death should receive immediate clinical attention after initial treatment. Additional therapy may be required.

ASTHMA *(Continued)*

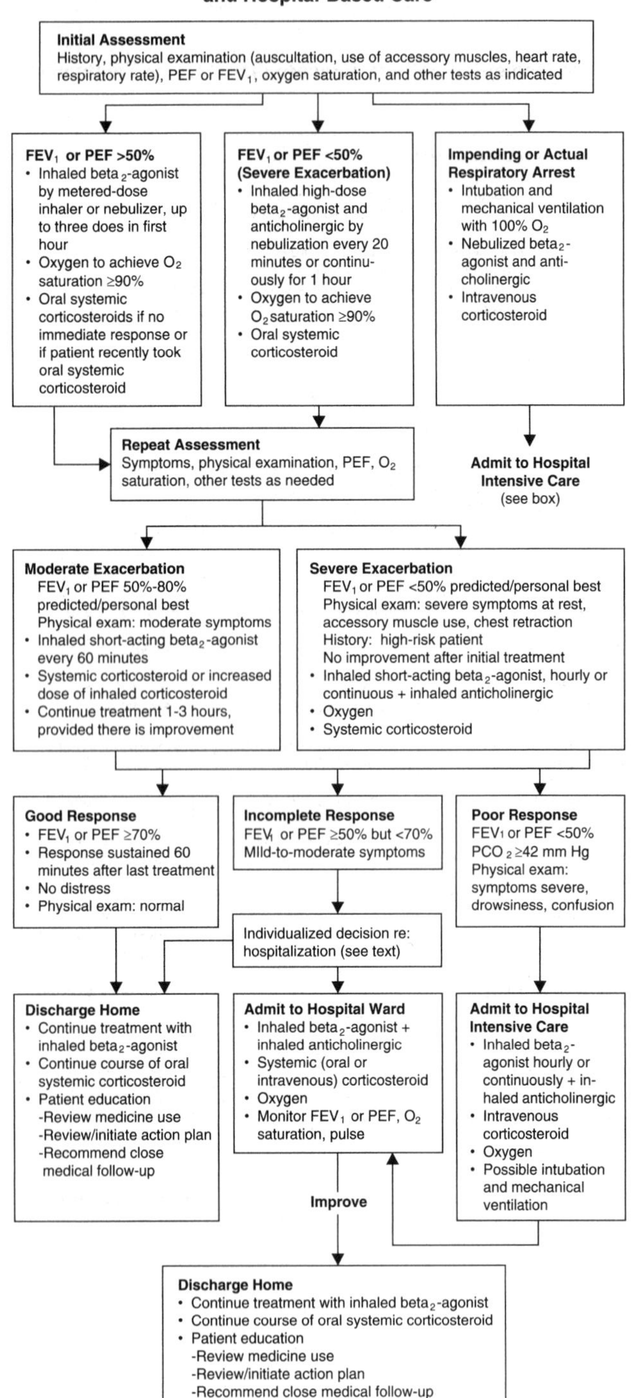

ESTIMATED COMPARATIVE DAILY DOSAGES FOR INHALED CORTICOSTEROIDS

Adults

Drug	Low Dose	Medium Dose	High Dose
Beclomethasone dipropionate	168-504 mcg	504-840 mcg	>840 mcg
42 mcg/puff	4-12 puffs	12-20 puffs	>20 puffs
84 mcg/puff	2-6 puffs	6-10 puffs	>10 puffs
Beclomethasone dipropionate HFA	80-240 mcg	240-640 mcg	>640 mcg
40 mcg/puff	2-6 puffs	6-16 puffs	>16 puffs
80 mcg/puff	1-3 puffs	3-8 puffs	>8 puffs
Budesonide Turbuhaler	200-600 mcg	600-1200 mcg	>1200 mcg
200 mcg/inhalation	1-3 inhalations	3-6 inhalations	>6 inhalations
Flunisolide	500-1000 mcg	1000-2000 mcg	>2000 mcg
250 mcg/puff	2-4 puffs	4-8 puffs	>8 puffs
Fluticasone MDI: 44, 110, 220 mcg/puff DPI: 50, 100, 250 mcg/dose	88-264 mcg	264-660 mcg	>660 mcg
Triamcinolone acetonide	400-1000 mcg	1000-2000 mcg	>2000 mcg
100 mcg/puff	4-10 puffs	10-20 puffs	>20 puffs

Children

Drug	Low Dose	Medium Dose	High Dose
Beclomethasone dipropionate	84-336 mcg	336-672 mcg	>672 mcg
42 mcg/puff	2-8 puffs	8-16 puffs	>16 puffs
84 mcg/puff	1-4 puffs	4-8 puffs	>8 puffs
Beclomethasone dipropionate HFA	80-160 mcg	160-320 mcg	>320 mcg
40 mcg/puff	2-4 puffs	4-8 puffs	>8 puffs
80 mcg/puff	1-2 puffs	2-4 puffs	>4 puffs
Budesonide Turbuhaler	200-400 mcg	400-800 mcg	>800 mcg
200 mcg/inhalation	1-2 inhalations	2-4 inhalations	>4 inhalations
Inhalation suspension for nebulization	0.5 mg	1 mg	2 mg
Flunisolide	500-750 mcg	1000-1250 mcg	>1250 mcg
250 mcg/puff	2-3 puffs	4-5 puffs	>5 puffs
Fluticasone MDI: 44, 110, 220 mcg/puff DPI: 50, 100, 250 mcg/dose	88-176 mcg	176-440 mcg	>440 mcg
Triamcinolone acetonide	400-800 mcg	800-1200 mcg	>1200 mcg
100 mcg/puff	4-8 puffs	8-12 puffs	>12 puffs

Notes:

- **The most important determinant of appropriate dosing is the clinician's judgment of the patient's response to therapy.** The clinician must monitor the patient's response on several clinical parameters and adjust the dose accordingly. The stepwise approach to therapy emphasizes that once control of asthma is achieved, the dose of mediation should be carefully titrated to the minimum dose required to maintain control, thus reducing the potential for adverse effect.
- The reference point for the range in the dosages for children is data on the safety on inhaled corticosteroids in children, which, in general, suggest that the dose ranges are equivalent to beclomethasone dipropionate 200-400 mcg/day (low dose), 400-800 mcg/day (medium dose), and >800 mcg/day (high dose).
- Some dosages may be outside package labeling.
- Metered-dose inhaler (MDI) dosages are expressed as the actuator dose (the amount of drug leaving the actuator and delivered to the patient), which is the labeling required in the United States. This is different from the dosage expressed as the valve dose (the amount of drug leaving the valve, all of which is not available to the patient), which is used in many European countries and in some of the scientific literature. Dry powder inhaler (DPI) doses (eg, Turbuhaler) are expressed as the amount of drug in the inhaler following activation.

ASTHMA *(Continued)*

ESTIMATED CLINICAL COMPARABILITY OF DOSES FOR INHALED CORTICOSTEROIDS

Data from *in vitro* and in clinical trials suggest that the different inhaled corticosteroid preparations are not equivalent on a per puff or microgram basis. However, it is not entirely clear what implications these differences have for dosing recommendations in clinical practice because there are few data directly comparing the preparations. Relative dosing for clinical comparability is affected by differences in topical potency, clinical effects at different doses, delivery device, and bioavailability. The Expert Panel developed recommended dose ranges for different preparations based on available data and the following assumptions and cautions about estimating relative doses needed to achieve comparable clinical effect.

Relative Topical Potency Using Human Skin Blanching

- The standard test for determining relative topical anti-inflammatory potency is the topical vasoconstriction (MacKenzie skin blanching) test.
- The MacKenzie topical skin blanching test correlates with binding affinities and binding half-lives for human lung corticosteroid receptors (see following table) (Dahlberg, et al, 1984; Hogger and Rohdewald 1994).
- The relationship between relative topical anti-inflammatory effect and clinical comparability in asthma management is not certain. However, recent clinical trials suggest that different in vitro measures of anti-inflammatory effect is not certain. However, recent clinical trials suggest that different in vitro measures of anti-inflammatory effect correlate with clinical efficacy (Barnes and Pedersen 1993; Johnson 1996; Kamada, et al, 1996; Ebden, et al, 1986; Leblanc, et al, 1994; Gustaffson, et al, 1993; Lundback, et al, 1993; Barnes, et al, 1993; Fabbri, et al, 1993; Langdon and Capsey, 1994; Ayres, et al, 1995; Rafferty, et al, 1985; Bjorkander, et al, 1982, Stiksa, et al, 1982; Willey, et al, 1982.)

Medication	Topical Potency (Skin Blanching)[1]	Corticosteroid Receptor Binding Half-Life	Receptor Binding Affinity
Beclomethasone dipropionate (BDP)	600	7.5 hours	13.5
Budesonide (BUD)	980	5.1 hours	9.4
Flunisolide (FLU)	330	3.5 hours	1.8
Fluticasone propionate (FP)	1200	10.5 hours	18.0
Triamcinolone acetonide (TAA)	330	3.9 hours	3.6

[1]Numbers are assigned in reference to dexamethasone, which has a value of "1" in the MacKenzie test.

Relative Doses to Achieve Similar Clinical Effects

- Clinical effects are evaluated by a number of outcome parameters (eg, changes in spirometry, peak flow rates, symptom scores, quick-relief beta$_2$-agonist use, frequency of exacerbations, airway responsiveness).
- The daily dose and duration of treatment may affect these outcome parameters differently (eg, symptoms and peak flow may improve at lower doses and over a shorter treatment time than bronchial reactivity) (van Essen-Zandvliet, et al, 1992; Haahtela, et al, 1991)
- Delivery systems influence comparability. For example, the delivery device for budesonide (Turbuhaler) delivers approximately twice the amount of drug to the airway as the MDI, thus enhancing the clinical effect (Thorsson, et al, 1994; Agertoft and Pedersen, 1993).
- Individual patients may respond differently to different preparations, as noted by clinical experience.
- Clinical trials comparing effects in reducing symptoms and improving peak expiratory flow demonstrate:
  - BDP and BUD achieved comparable effects at similar microgram doses by MDI (Bjorkander, et al, 1982; Ebden, et al, 1986; Rafferty, et al, 1985).
  - BDP achieved effects similar to twice the dose of TAA on a microgram basis.

Reference

National Asthma Education and Prevention Program (NAEPP), Clinical Practice Guidelines, Expert Panel Report 2, "Guidelines for the Diagnosis and Management of Asthma," NIH Publication No. 97-4051, July 1997.

PROPHYLAXIS FOR EXPOSURE TO COMMUNICABLE DISEASES

Disease	Exposure	Prophylaxis/Management
Anthrax	Postexposure inhalational	Doxycycline and ciprofloxacin; 60-day (oral and intravenous) regimens have been recommended.
Invasive *Haemophilus influenzae* disease	Close contact with an infected child for more than 4 hours	Give rifampin 20 mg/kg orally once daily for 4 days (600 mg maximum daily dose) to entire family with at least one household contact <48 months old. Contraindication: Pregnant contacts.
Hepatitis A	Direct contact with an infected child, or sharing of food or utensils	Give 0.02 mL/kg immune globulin (IG) within 7 days of exposure.
Hepatitis B	Needlestick (used needle); mucous membrane exposure with blood or body fluid; direct inoculation of blood or body fluid into open cut, lesion, or laceration	**Known source and employee status unknown: Test patient for HB_sAg and employee for anti-HB_s.** If patient is HB_sAg negative and the patient does not have non-A, non-B hepatitis, do nothing. If patient is HB_sAg negative and has non-A, non-B hepatitis, **offer** ISG (optional). If patient is HB_sAg positive, give HBIG and hepatitis B vaccine within 48 hours of exposure. Employee antibody status may not be available for up to a week, so the above should be given as soon as patient's antigen status is known. Occasionally, the patient's antigen status will be unavailable for more than 24 hours. In these cases, HBIG should be given if the patient is high risk (ie, Asian immigrants, institutionalized patients, homosexuals, intravenous drug abusers, hemodialysis patients, patients with a history of hepatitis). If the employee is anti-HB_s negative, give the second and third doses of hepatitis B vaccine. **Known source and employee documented anti-HB_s positive:** If source has non-A, non-B hepatitis, offer ISG (optional). If employee is believed to be anti-HB_s positive due to vaccination, has received 3 doses of vaccine, and has not had an anti-HB_s test done, draw serum for anti-HB_s
Measles	15 minutes or more in the same room with a child with measles from 2 days before the onset of symptoms to 4 days after the appearance of the rash	Children who have not been vaccinated and have not had natural infection should be isolated from the 7th through the 18th day after exposure and/or for 4 days after the rash appears. Those who have not been vaccinated should be vaccinated within 72 hours of exposure if no contraindication exists, or receive immune globulin (IG) 0.25 mL/kg I.M. for immunocompetent individuals and 0.5 mL/kg (maximum: 15 mL) for immunosuppressed individuals. Children who are younger than 15 months of age should be revaccinated at 15 months of age but at least 3 months after receipt of vaccine or IG. Older individuals who have received IG should be vaccinated 3 months later.
Meningococcal disease	Household contact or direct contact with secretions	Household, day care center, and nursery school children should receive rifampin prophylaxis for 2 days. Dosages are given every 12 hours for a total of 4 doses. Dosage is 10 mg/kg/dose for children ages 1 month to 12 years (maximum: 600 mg/dose), 5 mg/kg/dose for infants <1 month of age, and 600 mg/dose for adults. Alternatively, ciprofloxacin 750 mg as a single dose may be used. Contraindication: Pregnant contacts **Because prophylaxis is not always effective, exposed children should be monitored for symptoms.** **Employee exposure: Anyone who develops a febrile illness should receive prompt medical evaluation. If indicated, antimicrobial therapy should be administered.**

PROPHYLAXIS FOR EXPOSURE TO COMMUNICABLE DISEASES *(Continued)*

Disease	Exposure	Prophylaxis/Management
Pertussis	Housed in the same room with an infected child or spent 15 minutes in the playroom with the infected child	**Prophylaxis:** Contacts <7 years old who have had at least 4 doses of pertussis vaccine should receive a booster dose of DTP, unless a dose has been given within the past 3 years, and should receive erythromycin 40-50 mg/kg/day orally for 14 days. Contacts <7 years old who are not immunized or who have received less than 4 doses of DTP should have DTP immunization initiated or continued according to the recommended schedule. Children who have received their third dose 6 months or more before exposure should be given their fourth dose at this time. Erythromycin should also be given for 14 days. Contacts ≥7 years of age and above should receive prophylactic erythromycin (maximum: 1 g/day) for 10-14 days. All exposed patients should be watched closely for respiratory symptoms for 14 days after exposure has stopped because immunity conferred by the vaccine is not absolute and the efficacy of erythromycin in prophylaxis has not been established.
Tuberculosis	Housed in the same room with a child with contagious tuberculosis (tuberculosis is contagious if the child has a cough plus AFB seen on smear plus cavitation on CXR)	Place PPD immediately and 10 weeks after exposure. Start on INH. Consult Infectious Diseases if seroconversion occurs.
Varicella-zoster	1 hour or more in the same room with a contagious child from 24 hours before vesicles appear to when all vesicles are crusted, which is usually 5-7 days after vesicles appear. In household exposure, communicability is 48 hours before vesicles appear.	**Immunocompetent** children who have not been vaccinated or had natural infection, should have titers drawn only if they will still be hospitalized for more than 10 days after exposure. If titers are negative, they should be isolated from 10 to 21 days after exposure and/or until all lesions are crusted and dry. If VZIG was given the child should be isolated from 10 to 28 days after exposure. **Immunocompromised** children who have not been vaccinated or had natural infection should first have titers drawn, and then receive VZIG (varicella-zoster immune globulin) **1 vial/10 kg I.M.** up to a maximum of 5 vials as soon as possible but at most 96 hours after exposure. Fractional doses are not recommended. If titers are positive, nothing further need be done. If titers are negative, the child should be isolated from 10 to 28 days after exposure and should be monitored very carefully for the appearance of vesicles so that treatment can be initiated. VZIG is available from the Blood Bank.

COMMUNITY-ACQUIRED PNEUMONIA IN ADULTS

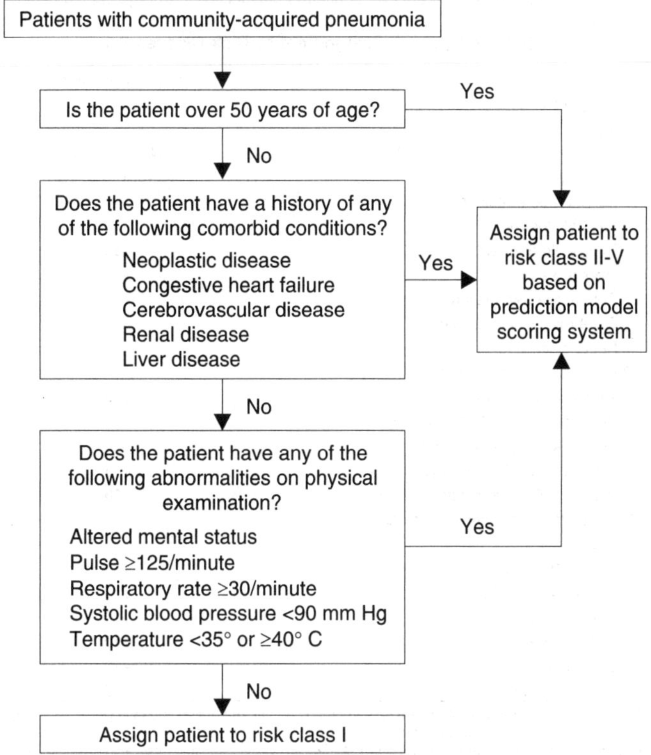

Stratification of Risk Score

Risk	Risk class	Based on
Low	I	Algorithm
	II	≤ 70 total points
	III	71-90 total points
Moderate	IV	91-130 total points
High	V	> 130 total points

COMMUNITY-ACQUIRED PNEUMONIA IN ADULTS *(Continued)*

The table below is the prediction model for identification of patient risk for persons with community-acquired pneumonia. This model may be used to help guide the initial decision on site of care; however, its use may not be appropriate for all patients with this illness and, therefore, should be applied in conjunction with physician judgment.

Scoring System: Assignment to Risk Classes II-V

Patient Characteristic	Points Assigned[1]
Demographic factors	
Age	
Male	No. of years
Female	No. of years -10
Nursing home resident	+10
Comorbid illnesses	
Neoplastic disease[2]	+30
Liver disease[3]	+20
Congestive heart failure[4]	+10
Cerebrovascular disease[5]	+10
Renal disease[6]	+10
Physical examination findings	
Altered mental status[7]	+20
Respiratory rate >30 breaths/minute	+20
Systolic blood pressure <90 mm Hg	+20
Temperature <35°C or >40°C	+15
Pulse >125 beats/minute	+10
Laboratory or radiographic findings	
Arterial pH <7.35	+30
BUN >30 mg/dL	+20
Sodium <130 mEq/L	+20
Glucose >250 mg/dL	+10
Hematocrit <30%	+10
pO_2 <60 mm Hg[8]	+10
Pleural effusion	+10

[1]A total point score for a given patient is obtained by adding the patient's age in years (age -10, for females) and the points for each applicable patient characteristic.
[2]Any cancer except basal or squamous cell cancer of the skin that was active at the time of presentation or diagnosed within 1 year of presentation.
[3]A clinical or histologic diagnosis of cirrhosis or other form of chronic liver disease such as chronic active hepatitis.
[4]Systolic or diastolic ventricular dysfunction documented by history and physical examination, as well as chest radiography, echocardiography, Muga scanning, or left ventriculography.
[5]A clinical diagnosis of stroke, transient ischemic attack, or stroke documented by MRI or computed axial tomography.
[6]A history of chronic renal disease or abnormal blood urea nitrogen (BUN) and creatinine values documented in the medical record.
[7]Disorientation (to person, place, or time, not known to be chronic), stupor, or coma.
[8]In the Pneumonia Patient Outcome Research Team cohort study, an oxygen saturation value <90% on pulse oximetry or intubation before admission was also considered abnormal.

Risk-Class Mortality Rates for Patients With Pneumonia

		Validation Cohort		
Risk Class	No. of Points	No. of Patients	Mortality (%)	Recommended Site of Care
I	No predictors	3034	0.1	Outpatient
II	≤70	5778	0.6	Outpatient
III	71-90	6790	2.8	Outpatient or brief inpatient
IV	91-130	13,104	8.2	Inpatient
V	>130	9333	29.2	Inpatient

Epidemiological Conditions Related to Specific Pathogens in Patients With Selected Community-Acquired Pneumonia

Condition	Commonly Encountered Pathogens
Alcoholism	*Streptococcus pneumoniae*, anaerobes
COPD and/or smoker	*S. pneumoniae, Haemophilus influenzae, Moraxella catarrhalis, Legionella* species
Nursing home residency	*S. pneumoniae*, gram-negative bacilli, *H. influenzae, Staphylococcus aureus*, anaerobes, *Chlamydia pneumoniae*
Poor dental hygiene	Anaerobes
Epidemic Legionnaires' disease	*Legionella* species
Exposure to bats or soil enriched with bird droppings	*Histoplasma capsulatum*
Exposure to birds	*Chlamydia psittaci*
Exposure to rabbits	*Francisella tularensis*
HIV infection (early stage)	*S. pneumoniae, H. influenzae, Mycobacterium tuberculosis*
HIV infection (late stage)	Above plus *P. carinii, Cryptococcus, Histoplasma* species
Travel to southwestern United States	*Coccidioides* species
Exposure to farm animals or parturient cats	*Coxiella burnetii* (Q fever)
Influenza active in community	Influenza, *S. pneumoniae, S. aureus, Streptococcus pyogenes, H. influenzae*
Suspected large-volume aspiration	Anaerobes (chemical pneumonitis, obstruction)
Structural disease of the lung (bronchiectasis, cystic fibrosis, etc)	*Pseudomonas aeruginosa, Burkholderia (Pseudomonas) cepacia, S. aureus*
Injection drug use	*S. aureus*, anaerobes, *M. tuberculosis, S. pneumoniae*
Airway obstruction	Anaerobes, *S. pneumoniae, H. influenzae, S. aureus*

COPD = chronic obstructive pulmonary disease.

COMMUNITY-ACQUIRED PNEUMONIA IN ADULTS *(Continued)*

Flow Chart Approach to Treating Outpatients and Inpatients with Community-Acquired Pneumonia

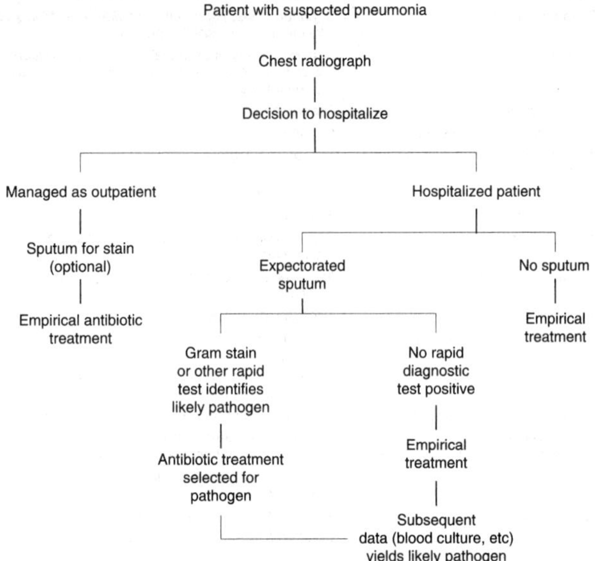

Community-Acquired Pneumonia

Possible reasons for failure of empirical treatment in patients with community-acquired pneumonia.

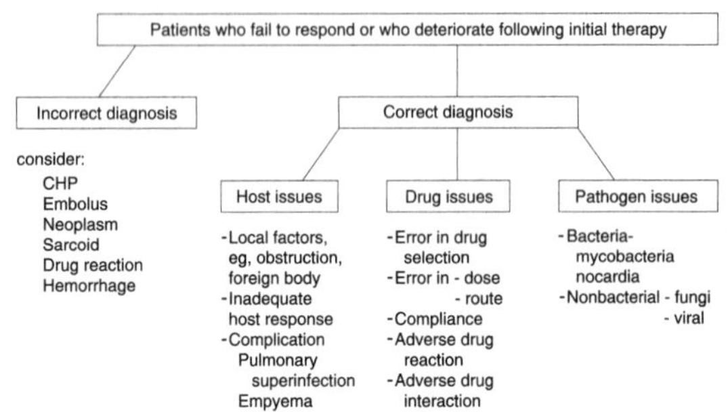

Pathogen-Directed Antimicrobial Therapy for Community-Acquired Pneumonia

Organism	Preferred Antimicrobial	Alternative Antimicrobial
Streptococcus pneumoniae		
Penicillin susceptible (MIC, <2 mcg/mL)	Penicillin G, amoxicillin	Cephalosporins (cefazolin, cefuroxime, cefotaxime, ceftriaxone, or cefepime), oral cephalosporins (cefpodoxime, cefprozil, or cefuroxime), imipenem or meropenem, macrolides,[1] clindamycin, fluoroquinolone,[2] doxycycline, ampicillin ± sulbactam or piperacillin ± tazobactam
Penicillin resistant (MIC, ≥2 mcg/mL)	Agents based on *in vitro* susceptibility tests, including cefotaxime and ceftriaxone, fluoroquinolone,[2] vancomycin	—
Haemophilus influenzae	Cephalosporins (2nd or 3rd generation), doxycycline, beta-lactam/beta-lactamase inhibitor, azithromycin, TMP-SMZ	Fluoroquinolone,[2] clarithromycin
Moraxella catarrhalis	Cephalosporin (2nd or 3rd generation), TMP-SMZ, macrolide, beta-lactam/beta-lactamase inhibitor	Fluoroquinolone[2]
Anaerobe	Beta-lactam/beta-lactamase inhibitor, clindamycin	Imipenem
Staphylococcus aureus[3]		
Methicillin-susceptible	Nafcillin/oxacillin ± rifampin or gentamicin[3]	Cefazolin or cefuroxime, vancomycin, clindamycin, TMP-SMZ
Methicillin-resistant	Vancomycin ± rifampin or gentamicin	Linezolid
Enterobacteriaceae (coliforms: *Escherichia coli, Klebsiella, Proteus, Enterobacter*)	Cephalosporin (3rd generation) ± aminoglycoside, carbapenem	Aztreonam, beta-lactam/beta-lactamase inhibitor, fluoroquinolone[2]
Pseudomonas aeruginosa[3]	Aminoglycoside + antipseudomonal beta-lactam: ticarcillin, piperacillin, mezlocillin, ceftazidime, cefepime, aztreonam, or carbapenem	Aminoglycoside + ciprofloxacin, ciprofloxacin + antipseudomonal beta-lactam
Legionella	Macrolide[1] ± rifampin, fluoroquinolone[2] (including ciprofloxacin)	Doxycycline ± rifampin
Mycoplasma pneumoniae	Doxycycline, macrolide[1]	Fluoroquinolone[2]
Chlamydia pneumoniae	Doxycycline, macrolide[1]	Fluoroquinolone[2]
Chlamydia psittaci	Doxycycline	Erythromycin, chloramphenicol
Nocardia	TMP-SMZ, sulfonamide ± minocycline or amikacin	Imipenem ± amikacin, doxycycline or minocycline
Coxiella burnetii (Q fever)	Tetracycline	Chloramphenicol
Influenza virus	Amantadine or rimantadine (influenza A), zanamivir or oseltamivir (influenza A or B)	—
Hantavirus	Supportive care	—

Note: TMP-SMZ = trimethoprim-sulfamethoxazole.

[1]Erythromycin, clarithromycin, azithromycin, or dirithromycin; *S. pneumoniae*, especially strains with reduced susceptibility to penicillin, should have verified *in vitro* susceptibility.

[2]Levofloxacin, gatifloxacin, moxifloxacin, trovafloxacin, or other fluoroquinolone with enhanced activity against *S. pneumoniae*; ciprofloxacin is appropriate for *Legionella*, *C. pneumoniae*, fluoroquinolone-susceptible *S. aureus*, and most gram-negative bacilli; ciprofloxacin may not be as effective as other quinolones against *S. pneumoniae*.

[3]*In vitro* susceptibility tests are required for optimal treatment; against *Enterobacter* species, the preferred antibiotics are fluoroquinolones and carbapenems.

COMMUNITY-ACQUIRED PNEUMONIA IN ADULTS *(Continued)*

Empirical Selection of Antimicrobial Agents for Treating Patients With Community-Acquired Pneumonia

Outpatients

Generally preferred (not in any particular order): Doxycycline, a macrolide, or a fluoroquinolone

Selection considerations

These agents have activity against the most likely pathogens in this setting, which include *Streptococcus pneumoniae, Mycoplasma pneumoniae*, and *Chlamydia pneumoniae*

Selection should be influenced by regional antibiotic susceptibility patterns for *S. pneumoniae* and the presence of other risk factors for drug-resistant *S. pneumoniae*

Penicillin-resistant pneumococci may be resistant to macrolides and/or doxycycline

For older patients or those with underlying disease, a fluoroquinolone may be a preferred choice; some authorities prefer to reserve fluoroquinolones for such patients

Hospitalized Patients

General medical ward

Generally preferred: An extended-spectrum cephalosporin combined with a macrolide or a beta-lactam/beta-lactamase inhibitor combined with a macrolide or a fluoroquinolone (alone)

Intensive care unit

Generally preferred: An extended-spectrum cephalosporin or beta-lactam/beta-lactamase inhibitor plus either fluoroquinolone or macrolide

Alternatives or modifying factors

Structural lung disease: Antipseudomonal agents (piperacillin, piperacillin-tazobactam, carbapenem, or cefepime) plus a fluoroquinolone (including high-dose ciprofloxacin)

Beta-lactam allergy: Fluoroquinolone ± clindamycin

Suspected aspiration: Fluoroquinolone ± clindamycin, metronidazole, or a beta-lactam/beta-lactamase inhibitor

Note:

Beta-lactam/beta-lactamase inhibitor: Ampicillin-sulbactam or piperacillin-tazobactam.

Extended-spectrum cephalosporin: Cefotaxime or ceftriaxone.

Fluoroquinolone: Gatifloxacin, levofloxacin, moxifloxacin, or other fluoroquinolone with enhanced activity against *S. pneumoniae* (for aspiration pneumonia, some fluoroquinolones show *in vitro* activity against anaerobic pulmonary pathogens, although there are no clinical studies to verify activity *in vivo*).

Macrolide: Azithromycin, clarithromycin, or erythromycin.

References

Bartlett JG, Breiman RF, Mandell LA, et al, "Community-Acquired Pneumonia in Adults: Guidelines for Management. The Infectious Diseases Society of America," *Clin Infect Dis*, 1998, 26(4):811-38.

Bartlett JG, Dowell SF, Mandell LA, et al, "Practice Guidelines for the Management of Community-Acquired Pneumonia in Adults. The Infectious Diseases Society of America," *Clin Infect Dis*, 2000, 31(2):347-82.

DEPRESSION

For depression in the elderly see OBRA Guidelines *on page 1613*.

Criteria for Major Depressive Episode

A. Five (or more) of the following symptoms have been present during the same 2-week period and represent a change from previous functioning; at least one of the symptoms is either (1) depressed mood or (2) loss of interest or pleasure.

1. Depressed mood most of the day, nearly every day
2. Marked diminished interest or pleasure in all, or almost all, activities
3. Significant weight loss (not dieting) or weight gain, or decrease or increase in appetite nearly every day
4. Insomnia or hypersomnia nearly every day
5. Psychomotor agitation or retardation nearly every day
6. Fatigue or loss of energy nearly every day
7. Feelings of worthlessness or excessive or inappropriate guilt (may be delusional) nearly every day
8. Diminished ability to think or concentrate, or indecisiveness
9. Recurrent thoughts of death, recurrent suicidal ideation without a specific plan, or a suicide attempt or a specific suicide plan

B. The symptoms cause clinically significant distress or impairment in social, occupational or other important areas of functioning.

C. The symptoms are not due to the direct physiologic effects of a substance or a general medical condition (eg, hypothyroidism).

Medications That May Precipitate Depression

Anti-inflammatory & analgesic agents	Indomethacin, pentazocine, phenacetin, phenylbutazone
Antimicrobial agents	Cycloserine, ethambutol, sulfonamides, select gram-negative antibiotics
Cardiovascular/antihypertensive agents	Clonidine, digitalis, diuretics, guanethidine, hydralazine, indapamide, methyldopa, prazosin, procainamide, propranolol, reserpine
CNS-agents	Alcohol, amantadine, amphetamine & derivatives, barbiturates, benzodiazepines, chloral hydrate, carbamazepine, cocaine, haloperidol, L-dopa, phenothiazines, succinimide derivatives
Hormonal agents	ACTH, corticosteroids, estrogen, melatonin, oral contraceptives, progesterone
Miscellaneous	Antineoplastic agents, cimetidine, disulfiram, organic pesticides, physostigmine

Medical Disorders and Psychiatric Disorders Associated With Depression

Endocrine diseases	Acromegaly, Addison's disease, Cushing's disease, diabetes mellitus, hyperparathyroidism, hypoparathyroidism, hyperthyroidism, hypothyroidism, insulinoma, pheochromocytoma, pituitary dysfunction
Deficiency states	Pernicious anemia, severe anemia, Wernicke's encephalopathy
Infections	Encephalitis, fungal infections, meningitis, neurosyphilis, influenza, mononucleosis, tuberculosis, AIDS
Collagen disorders	Rheumatoid arthritis
Systemic lupus erythematosus	
Metabolic disorders	Electrolyte imbalance, hypokalemia, hyponatremia, hepatic encephalopathy, Pick's disease, uremia, Wilson's disease
Cardiovascular disease	Cerebral arteriosclerosis, chronic bronchitis, congestive heart failure, emphysema, myocardial infarction, paroxysmal dysrhythmias, pneumonia
Neurologic disorders	Alzheimer's disease, amyotrophic lateral sclerosis, brain tumors, chronic pain syndrome, Cruetzfeld-Jakob disease, Huntington's disease, multiple sclerosis, myasthenia gravis, Parkinson's disease, poststroke, trauma (postconcussion)
Malignant disease	Breast, gastrointestinal, lung, pancreas, prostate
Psychiatric disorders	Alcoholism, anxiety disorders, eating disorders, schizophrenia

DEPRESSION *(Continued)*

Somatic Treatments of Depression in the Patient With Medical Illness

Condition	First Choice	Second-Line Options	Alternatives
Thyroid			
Hypothyroid	Thyroid (T)	T_4 or T_3 + antidepressant (SSRIs , TCAs, new generation agents)	ECT, other antidepressants psychostimulants
Hyperthyroid	Antidepressant and antihyperthyroid medications	Select a different group of antidepressants	
Diabetes mellitus	SSRIs, other new generation antidepressants	TCAs (second amine or low-dose tertiary amine) MAOIs	ECT, buspirone, psychostimulants, thyroid supplements, mood stabilizers
Cardiovascular disorders	SSRIs, bupropion	ECT, psychostimulants β-blockers, buspirone	ECT, TCAs, MAOIs, mood stabilizers
Renal disease	Fluoxetine, sertraline	TCAs, other new generation antidepressants, psychostimulants	ECT, anticonvulsants, lithium (if dialysis or CLOSELY monitored)
Hepatic disease (reduced dose ALL)	Sertraline	Other new generation antidepressants, TCAs-secondary amines	TCAs-tertiary amines
HIV	Bupropion, SSRIs, psychostimulants	TCAs	ECT
Transplant	**Closely monitor.** See cardiovascular, renal, liver, pulmonary, new antidepressant agents, TCAs-secondary amines		
Neurologic	Newer generation antidepressants, TCAs - secondary amines	Selegiline, anticonvulsants	Bromocriptine
Malignancy	Newer generation antidepressants, TCAs - secondary amines, psychostimulants	TCAs - tertiary amines of pain, MAOIs	ECT
Respiratory	Activating antidepressants, buspirone		More sedating antidepressants, ECT
Gastrointestinal	TCAs - secondary amines, new generation antidepressants	TCAs - tertiary amines	ECT

DIABETES MELLITUS MANAGEMENT

OVERVIEW

Diabetes represents a significant health care problem in the United States and worldwide. Of the nearly 16 million Americans with diabetes, the majority (90% to 95%) have type 2 diabetes. Of this number, roughly one-third are undiagnosed. The incidence of type 2 diabetes is increasing around the world. There is strong evidence to support an interaction between a genetic predisposition and behavioral or environmental factors, such as obesity and physical inactivity, in the development of this disease. In individuals at high risk of developing type 2 diabetes, it has been shown that the development of diabetes may be prevented by changes in lifestyle (*N Engl J Med*, 2001, 344:1343-50).

Within the United States, type 1 diabetes is estimated to affect 500,000 to 1 million people, and therefore represents the minority of individuals with diabetes. In addition to type 1 and type 2 diabetes, approximately 2% to 5% of pregnancies are complicated by the development of gestational diabetes, which usually remits following delivery. This occurs in women with no previous history of type 1 or type 2 diabetes. However, women who have had gestational diabetes are at an increased risk for later development of type 2 diabetes. In addition to the causes noted above, diabetes may result from genetic syndromes, surgery (pancreatectomy), chemicals and/or drugs, recurrent pancreatitis, malnutrition, and viral infections.

COMPLICATIONS OF DIABETES

Complications due to diabetes comprise the seventh leading cause of death in the United States. The greatest number of these deaths are related to cardiovascular complications (myocardial infarction, CHF, and stroke), which have been estimated to result in more than 77,000 deaths annually.

In addition to cardiovascular effects, diabetes is the leading cause of new blindness in people 20-74 years of age, and diabetic nephropathy is the most common cause of end-stage renal disease. Mild to severe forms of diabetic neuropathy are common. Neuropathy and circulatory insufficiency combine to make diabetes the most frequent cause of nontraumatic lower-limb amputations. The rate of impotence in diabetic males over 50 years of age has been estimated to be as high as 50% to 60%. Control of hyperglycemia may significantly decrease the rate at which diabetic complications develop, and provides compelling justification for early diagnosis and management of this disorder.

DIAGNOSIS

Diabetes

Diagnosis of diabetes is made by any of the three criteria described below. In the absence of unequivocal hyperglycemia with acute metabolic decompensation, these criteria should be confirmed by repeat testing on a different day. The third method (OGGT) is not recommended for routine clinical use.

1. Symptoms of diabetes (polydipsia, polyuria, unexplained weight loss) plus casual plasma glucose concentration ≥200 mg/dL (11.1 mmol/L). Casual plasma glucose is defined as any time of day without regard to time of last meal.

OR

2. Fasting plasma glucose (no caloric intake for at least 8 hours) ≥126 mg/dL (7 mmol/L)

OR

3. A 2-hour plasma glucose ≥200 mg/dL (11.1 mmol/L) during an oral glucose tolerance test (OGTT).

DIABETES MELLITUS MANAGEMENT *(Continued)*

Intermediate Disorders of Glucose Homeostasis

1. Impaired fasting glucose:

   FPG ≥110 mg/dL (6.1 mmol/L) and <126 mg/dL (7 mmol/L)

2. Impaired fasting glucose

   Two-hour plasma glucose ≥140 mg/dL (7.8 mmol/L) and <200 mg/dL (11.1 mmol/L)

Gestation Diabetes Mellitus (GDM)

Low risk: Routine screening not recommended; must fulfill **all** criteria

- <25 years of age
- Normal body weight
- No family history of diabetes (ie, first-degree relatives)
- No history of abnormal glucose metabolism
- No history of poor obstetric outcome
- Not a member of an ethnic/racial group with a high prevalence of diabetes (Hispanic, Native American, Asian, African, Pacific Islander)

Average risk: Testing at 24-28 weeks gestation is recommended (oral glucose tolerance test - OGTT)

High risk: Initial screening (OGTT) as soon as feasible; repeat at 24-28 weeks gestation

- Marked obesity
- Personal history of GDM
- Glycosuria
- Strong family history

GOALS

The goals of diabetes treatment include normalization of hyperglycemia, avoidance of hypoglycemia, and slowing the development of diabetic complications. The following table lists guidelines for the evaluation of glucose control and parameters for addressing hyperglycemia.

	Normal	Goal	Action Suggested
Plasma (mg/dL)			
Average preprandial glucose	<110	90-130	<90 or >150
Average bedtime glucose	<120	110-150	<110 or >180
Whole Blood (mg/dL)			
Average preprandial glucose	<100	80-120	<80 or >140
Average bedtime glucose	<110	100-140	<100 or >160
Hb A_{1C} (%)	<6	<7	>8

Consult website (http://diabetes.org) for frequently updated guidelines

MANAGEMENT

Current American Diabetes Association (ADA) recommendations emphasize a multidisciplinary approach to the management of diabetes, with an emphasis on the participation of the patient and/or caregivers in the monitoring and management of the disease. Consultation with a diabetes educator and dietitian may help to prepare the patient to manage his/her disease and adjust to the necessary changes in diet and lifestyle. Patients must be educated about disease monitoring procedures, including blood glucose self-monitoring equipment and tests. Patients should be encouraged to wear or carry appropriate identification to inform health care providers of the disease in the event of an emergency. Foot care and other issues related to possible complications should be addressed. It is extremely important to educate patients concerning the recognition and management of hypoglycemic symptoms. The management of diabetes is constantly adapting to new information, techniques, and technologies. For the most current information on diabetes diagnosis and management, visit the ADA website (www.diabetes.org).

Pharmacological Algorithm for Treatment of Type 2 Diabetes (Patients inadequately controlled with diet and exercise)

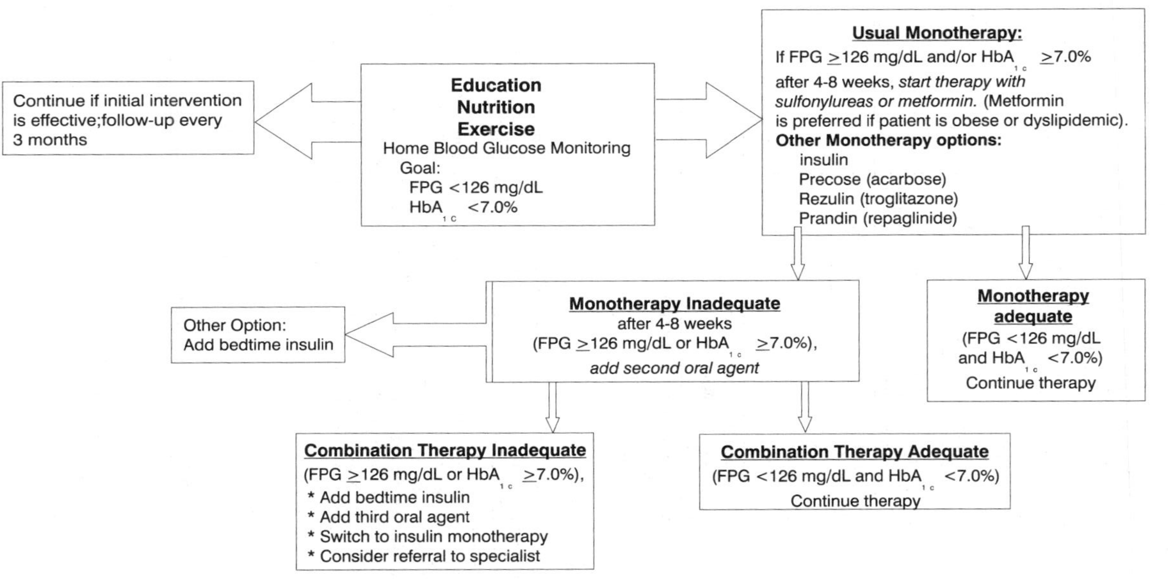

Modified from DeFronzo RA, "Pharmacological Treatment for Type 2 Diabetes Mellitus," *Ann Intern Med*, 1999, 131:281-303.

DIABETES MELLITUS MANAGEMENT *(Continued)*

DRUG TREATMENT

Insulin

Insulin therapy is required in type 1 diabetes, and may be necessary in some individuals with type 2 diabetes. Product selection and combination is designed to limit fluctuations in blood glucose values. There is solid scientific documentation of the benefit of tight glucose control, either by insulin pump or multiple daily injections (4-6 times daily). However, the benefits must be balanced against the risk of hypoglycemia, the patient's ability to adhere to the regimen, and other issues regarding the complexity of management. In addition to the educational issues outlined above, patients should be instructed in administration techniques, timing of administration, and sick-day management.

Types of Insulin	Onset (h)	Peak (h)	Duration (h)
Lispro (Humalog®)	0.25	0.5-1.5	6-8
Insulin aspart injection (NovoLog®)	0.5	1-3	3-5
Insulin, regular (Novolin® R)	0.5-1	2-3	8-12
Isophane insulin suspension (NPH) (Novolin® N)	1-1.5	4-12	24
Insulin zinc suspension (Lente®)	1-2.5	8-12	18-24
Isophane insulin suspension and regular insulin injection (Novolin® 70/30)	0.5	2-12	24
Extended insulin zinc suspension (Ultralente®)	4-8	16-18	>36
Insulin glargine (Lantus®)	—	—	24

Oral Agents

A large number of drugs for oral administration have become available for diabetic management. The drug classes vary in terms of their magnitude of effect on glycemic control, mechanism of action, and adverse effect profiles. In many cases, the adverse effect profile may influence the selection of a particular drug. The risk of hypoglycemia is higher for drugs which prompt insulin secretion (particularly sulfonylureas or insulin secretagogues). At least two drugs have been withdrawn from the U.S. market due to toxicities. Phenformin was removed many years ago after a number of cases of fatal lactic acidosis were reported. Metformin (a drug similar to phenformin) carries some risk of this reaction, but it is tremendously lower than the risk associated with phenformin. Troglitazone, a prototye thiazolidinedione, was associated with hepatic failure and several deaths, and it was withdrawn shortly after introduction. Currently, marketed drugs from this class appear to have a lower risk of these reactions. See Contraindications to Therapy and Potential Adverse Effects of Oral Antidiabetic Agents *on page 1556*.

Effect on Glycemic Control of Oral Hypoglycemic Agents as Monotherapy

Agent	Fasting Blood Glucose	Postprandial Blood Glucose	Hb A_{1c}
Precose® (acarbose) 25-100 mg 3 times/day	-25 mg/dL	-49 mg/dL	-0.44% to -0.74%
Glucophage® (metformin) Up to 2500 mg/day	-52 mg/dL	–	-1.4%
Amaryl® (glimepiride) 1-8 mg/day	-60 mg/dL	–	-1.5% to 2%
Diaβeta®/Micronase® (glyburide) 1.25-20 mg/day			
Glynase™ PresTab™ (glyburide) 0.75-12 mg/day			
Prandin® (repaglinide) 0.25-4 mg 3 times/day	-31 to -82 mg/dL	-48 mg/dL	-0.6% to -1.9%
Avandia® (rosiglitazone) 4-8 mg/day	-25 to -55 mg/dL	–	-0.1% to 0.7%*
Actos® (pioglitazone) 15-45 mg/day	-27 to -55 mg/dL	–	-0.1% to 0.6%*
Glyset™ (miglitol) 25-50 mg 3 times/day	–	-35 to -60 mg/dL	-0.3% to -0.82%
Starlix® (nateglinide) 60-120 mg 3 times/day	–	–	-0.3% to -0.5%

*Previously treated subjects

Class	Key Adverse Effects
Alpha-glucosidase inhibitors:	
Acarbose, Miglitol	GI distress, bloating, flatulence
Sulfonylureas:	
Glimepiride, Glyburide, Glipizide	Hypoglycemia, allergic reactions, resistance
Older Agents:	
Acetohexamide, Chlorpropamide, Tolazamide	SIADH (with chlorpropamide)
Biguanide:	
Metformin	GI distress (common), lactic acidosis (rare)
Thiazolidinediones:	
Rosiglitazone, Pioglitazone	Hepatic dysfunction, hepatic failure
Secretagogues:	
Repaglinide, Natagrelide	Hypoglycemia

References

The Expert Committee on the Diagnosis and Classification of Diabetes Mellitus, "Report of the Expert Committee on the Diagnosis and Classification of Diabetes Mellitus," *Diabetes Care*, 2002, 25 (Suppl 1).

The Diabetes Control and Complications Trial Research Group, "The Effect of Intensive Treatment of Diabetes on the Development and Progression of Long-Term Complications in Insulin-dependent Diabetes Mellitus," *N Engl J Med*, 1993, 329(14):977-86.

UK Prospective Diabetes Study Group, " Intensive Blood Glucose Control With Sulphonylureas or Insulin Compared With Conventional Treatment and Risk of Complications in Patients With Type 2 Diabetes (UKPDS 33)," *Lancet*, 1998, 352(9131):837-53.

Tuomilehto J, Lindstrom J, Eriksson JG, et al, "Prevention of Type 2 Diabetes Mellitus by Changes in Lifestyle Among Subjects With Impaired Glucose Tolerance," *N Engl J Med*, 2001, 344(18):1343-50.

ESTROGEN REPLACEMENT THERAPY

HORMONAL REPLACEMENT WITH ESTROGEN

Estrogen replacement therapy continues to be a controversial topic. Several benefits have been demonstrated, primarily for the reduction of menopausal symptoms and improvements in bone mineral density. However, this therapy does carry a number of associated risks. In recent years, a number of proposed benefits have been refuted, particularly with respect to estrogen use and cardiovascular disease. It should be noted that treatment or primary prevention of coronary heart disease has never been an approved indication for estrogen therapy. The decision to use estrogen therapy for one of its approved uses must be made on an individualized basis, taking into account the individual's risk of breast cancer, venous thromboembolism, and coronary heart disease.

Controversial or Recently Refuted Proposed Benefits

Central nervous system: Estrogen replacement was believed to improve memory in patients with Alzheimer's disease. Clinical trials have not supported this claim (*JAMA*, 2000, 283:1007-15; *Neurology*, 2000, 54:295-301).

Cardiovascular: Treatment or prevention of coronary heart disease has never been an approved indication for estrogen therapy. Estrogen replacement was believed to have a potential benefit on the development and/or progression of coronary heart disease. Unopposed estrogen therapy has been associated with increases in HDL cholesterol and decreases in LDL cholesterol, but elevations in triglycerides were also observed (*JAMA*, 1995, 273:199-203). However, investigators in three key clinical trials which evaluated the relationship between combination therapy (conjugated equine estrogen, or CEE, with medroxyprogesterone, or MPA) and the occurrence of coronary heart events have concluded that CEE/MPA therapy should not be used for either the prevention or treatment of coronary heart disease in postmenopausal women (*JAMA*, 1998, 280:605-13; *JAMA*, 2002, 288:49-57, 321-33). It should be noted that investigations of estrogen therapy alone (without progestin in women without an intact uterus) have not been completed.

SUMMARY OF ESTROGEN EFFECTS

The following list summarizes the benefits and risks of hormonal replacement therapy. Many controversies remain to be resolved. The scientific literature concerning these agents continues to develop, and the benefits and risks of therapy will, no doubt, continue to evolve. Current medical literature, individual monographs, and product literature should also be consulted to guide prescribing.

Proposed Beneficial Effects of Estrogen Replacement

- Endocrine/metabolic:
  - Blocks menopausal vasomotor symptoms (hot flashes)
  - Relief of other menopausal symptoms (vaginal atrophy/dryness)
  - Beneficial effects on serum lipids: increased HDL, decreased LDL
- Musculoskeletal:
  - Decreases bone resorption
  - Increases bone mineral density (in both cortical and trabecular bone)
- Genitourinary:
  - May improve symptoms in some patients with stress incontinence
  - Decreases incidence of urinary tract infection
- Dermatologic:
  - Maintains skin thickness and elasticity

Selected Adverse Effects

- Neoplastic:
  - Increased risk of breast cancer[1]
  - Increased risk of endometrial cancer[2]
- Cardiovascular:
  - Hypertension
- Endocrine/metabolic:
  - May increase serum glucose
  - May increase serum triglycerides[2]
- Hematologic:
  - Increased risk of thromboembolism[3] - DVT, stroke, pulmonary embolism
- Gastrointestinal:
  - Increased risk of gallbladder disease

[1]Risk may be increased in combination with progestin.

[2]Risk is attenuated by progestin.

[3]Although baseline risk may be low, increased by estrogen therapy

ESTROGEN PRODUCTS

Estrogen is available in a variety of products. These products are differentiated based on their source (natural versus synthetic), number of estrogen compounds contained in the product, and the route of administration. The majority of beneficial effects have been demonstrated with conjugated estrogens from an equine source. Due to its chemical complexity (over 10 active estrogenic compounds have been identified), it is difficult to say whether all of the effects attributed to this product may be generalized to other estrogens. In addition, the route of administration may influence the systemic response. Finally, some of the physiologic changes correlated to menopause may result from cellular changes which are not reversed by exogenous hormonal replacement. The following table lists the available compounds, representative brand names, and notes concerning key clinical issues.

ESTROGEN REPLACEMENT THERAPY *(Continued)*

Estrogen Replacement Products

Agent/Source	Representative Brand Names	Form	Use	Notes
Multiple Component Products				
Conjugated estrogens (equine)	Premarin®	Tab Vaginal I.V.	Menopausal symptoms, vulvar/ vaginal atrophy, and prevention of osteoporosis	Contains at least 10 active estrogenic compounds
Conjugated estrogens with medroxyprogesterone	Prempro™ Premphase®	Tab	Menopausal symptoms, atrophic vaginitis, and prevention of osteoporosis	Combination without cyclic effects
Conjugated estrogens (synthetic)	Cenestin™	Tab	Menopausal symptoms and vulvar/vaginal atrophy	Not biologically equivalent to Premarin®; consists of 9 active estrogenic compounds
Esterified estrogens	Estratab® Menest®	Tab	Menopausal symptoms, vulvar/ vaginal atrophy, and prevention of osteoporosis	
Estradiol with norethindrone	Activelle™ CombiPatch™	Tab TD	Menopausal symptoms	
Ethinyl estradiol with norethindrone	Femhrt™	Tab	Menopausal symptoms, prevention of osteoporosis, acne, and contraception	
Estradiol and norgestimate	Ortho-Prefest®	Tab	Menopausal symptoms, vulvar/ vaginal atrophy, and prevention of osteoporosis	
Estradiol and testosterone	Depo-Testadiol® Depotestogen® Duo-Cyp® Valertest No. 1®	Injection (I.M.)	Menopausal symptoms	
Estrogens (esterified) and methyltestosterone	Estratest® Estratest® H.S.	Tab	Menopausal symptoms	
Single Component Products				
Estradiol	Alora® Esclim® Estrace® Climara® Estraderm® Vivelle®	TD Tab Vaginal	Menopausal symptoms, vulvar/ vaginal atrophy, urogenital symptoms (postmenopausal), and prevention of osteoporosis	
Estropipate (piprazine estrone sulfate)	Ogen® Ortho-Est®	Tab Vaginal	Menopausal symptoms, vulvar/ vaginal atrophy, and prevention of osteoporosis	
Selective Estrogen Receptor Modulator (SERM)				
Raloxifene	Evista®	Tab	Prevention and treatment of osteoporosis	

*Relative to menopausal management.

TD = transdermal.

SELECTIVE ESTROGEN RECEPTOR MODULATORS

Selective estrogen receptor modulators (SERMs) are nonsteroidal modulators of estrogen-receptor mediated reactions. The key difference between these agents and estrogen replacement therapies is the potential to exert tissue-specific effects. Due to their chemical differences, these agents retain some of estrogen's beneficial effects on bone metabolism and lipid levels, but differ in their actions on breast and endometrial tissues, potentially limiting adverse effects related to nonspecific hormone stimulation. Among the SERMs, tamoxifen and toremifene retain stimulatory effects in endometrial tissue, while raloxifene does not stimulate endometrial or breast tissue, limiting the potential for endometrial or breast cancer related to this agent. Presumably, because of this activity, tamoxifen is approved for breast cancer prevention in high-risk women, as well as, for adjuvant treatment of breast cancer. Toremifene is also indicated for the treatment of breast cancer. Raloxifene is the only SERM which has been approved by the FDA for osteoporosis prevention. Its role in breast cancer management or prevention continues to be defined. As with estrogen replacement, each of these therapies has been associated with an increased risk of thromboembolism, and is contraindicated in patients with a history of thromboembolic disease.

The following table briefly summarizes the comparative effects of agents used in hormonal replacement therapy.

Receptor Interactions/Effects

Agent	Endometrial	Breast	Bone	Lipids
Estrogens	Agonist	Agonist	Highest Increase*	↓ LDL ↑LDL
Tamoxifen	Agonist	Antagonist	Increased†	↓ LDL‡
Toremifene	Agonist	Antagonist	Increased	↓ LDL‡ Increased HDL
Raloxifene	Antagonist	Antagonist	Increased	↓ LDL‡

*In a comparative trial, conjugated estrogens increased hip mineral density by approximately two times that observed with raloxifene.

†May effect specific skeletal areas preferentially (lumbar versus radial).

‡Effects are less than with conjugated estrogens.

Note: Effects on HDL may vary based on product and/or route of administration.

It should be noted that the effects on bone observed with SERMs appear to be less than those observed with estrogen replacement. In one study, the effect of raloxifene on hip bone mineral density was approximately half of that observed with conjugated estrogens. In addition, the effects on lipid profiles are less than with estrogen replacement. Tamoxifen's effects on bone may be inconsistent, with one study noting some effect on lumbar density while radial bone mineral density was not preserved. Some authors recommend the use of raloxifene in patients where carcinoma of the breast or endometrium is of concern. However, it has been noted that the limited ability to block some of the vasomotor symptoms of menopause may limit compliance.

OTHER HORMONAL THERAPY

Methyltestosterone has been used either as a sole agent or in combination with estrogen. Its primary effects are to block vasomotor symptoms and increase libido in postmenopausal women. When used in combination with estrogen, the beneficial effect on lipids is less than with estrogen alone. Increases in bone mineral density are observed with combination treatment.

HEART FAILURE

This section outlines a general approach to treatment of chronic systolic heart failure and highlights various aspects of drug therapy. Patient assessment, management, and select drug therapies for heart failure are listed in the following table, followed by general considerations for each class of drugs. Detailed consensus recommendations for the management of chronic heart failure are found at http://www.acc.org/clinical/guidelines/failure/hf_index.htm.

DRUG THERAPY

Drug Therapy for Systolic Heart Failure

Drug Therapy*	Role	Benefit	Comment
		Routine Use	
ACEI	Standard therapy for patients with asymptomatic and symptomatic heart failure (NYHA class I-IV)	Improves morbidity and mortality	– Achieve target or maximum tolerated dose – Optimize diuretic therapy, if needed, prior to initiating ACEI therapy – Ramipril may improve cardiovascular morbidity and mortality in high-risk patients without heart failure
Beta-blockers	Standard therapy for patients with **stable** NYHA class II-III heart failure	Improves morbidity and mortality	– Beneficial effects specific to individual agents – Need close patient contact / follow-up
Diuretics	Standard therapy for the treatment of symptoms of heart failure	Improves symptoms; spironolactone improves mortality in severe (NYHA class IV) heart failure	– Achieve and maintain euvolemia – Combine with standard therapy – Consider spironolactone in severe heart failure
Digoxin	Patients with symptoms despite optimal standard therapy	Improves symptoms and frequency of hospitalizations for heart failure	– No beneficial impact on mortality – No therapeutic range for efficacy (toxicity >2 ng/mL) – Potential for drug interactions
		Selected Patients	
Aldosterone antagonist	Recent or current symptoms at rest despite digoxin, diuretics, ACEI and (usually) a beta-blocker	May reduce morbidity and mortality	– Initiate only in patients with S_{cr} <2.5 mg/dL and serum potassium <5.0 mmol/L
Angiotensin-II receptor blockers	Patients intolerant to ACEI	Very limited data showing similar improvements in morbidity and mortality compared to ACEI	– Mechanistically similar to ACEI – Should not be considered equivalent or superior to ACEI
Beta-type natriuretic peptide	Patients with acutely decompensated NYHA Class IV	Short-term symptomatic improvement	Hemodynamic effects/ symptomatic improvement not sustained
Hydralazine/ISDN	Patients intolerant to ACEI	Improves mortality	– Requires frequent daily dosing – No outcome data for combined therapy with standard therapy
Treprostinil	Patients with NYHA Class II-IV pulmonary artery hypertension	Decreases exercise-associated symptoms	Dosage must be carefully and individually titrated

*See following information and also individual monographs.

Angiotensin-Converting Enzyme Inhibitors (ACEI)

ACEIs improve morbidity and mortality and are "standard therapy" for treatment of symptomatic or asymptomatic systolic heart failure (NYHA class I-IV) unless contraindicated. Therapy should be initiated and titrated to the established target or maximum tolerated dose (see following table) and continued long-term unless the patient cannot tolerate or develops a contraindication. Contraindications include hypotension (systolic pressure <90 mm Hg; diastolic pressure <60 mm Hg), shock, angioedema, anuric renal failure, pregnancy, significant hyperkalemia, and bilateral renal artery stenosis. Patients on diuretic therapy or those with asymptomatic low blood pressure should be monitored more closely for signs of symptomatic hypotension with initiation of therapy. ACEIs should not be used to treat hemodynamically unstable heart failure. See specific ACEI monographs.

ACEI	Initial Dose	Maximum Dose
Captopril	6.25-12.5 mg tid	50 mg tid
Enalapril	2.5 mg bid	10-20 mg bid
Fosinopril	5-10 mg daily	40 mg daily
Lisinopril	2.5-5 mg daily	20-40 mg daily
Quinapril	10 mg bid	40 mg bid
Ramipril	1.25-2.5 mg bid	10 mg daily
Trandolapril	1 mg daily	4 mg daily

*Doses are based on clinical trials and national guidelines.

Beta-Blockers

Carvedilol, sustained release metoprolol (CR/XL), and bisoprolol have demonstrated in clinical trials to decrease morbidity and mortality in patients with mild to moderate heart failure (NYHA class II-III) when combined with standard therapy (target doses of ACEI, diuretics, ± digoxin). Other beta-blockers (eg, bucindolol and celiprolol) have no benefit or may tend to increase mortality. Only carvedilol is FDA approved for the treatment of heart failure. (See individual drug monographs for carvedilol, metoprolol, and bisoprolol.)

All patients on standard therapy with **stable** NYHA class II-III systolic heart failure should be on beta-blocker therapy. Beta-blocker therapy may be considered for patients on standard therapy with mild systolic heart failure (NYHA class I). Patients with sympathetic nervous system activation (eg, heart rate >85 beats/minute) may derive greatest benefit. Beta-blocker therapy is not recommended for patients with unstable heart failure and in those that cannot tolerate therapy or where therapy is contraindicated.

Contraindications to beta blockade include bradycardia, 2nd or 3rd degree AV block, hypotension (systolic pressure <90 mm Hg/diastolic pressure <60 mm Hg), decompensated heart failure, and noncompliance. Special consideration should be given in evaluating the risk versus benefit for beta blockade in patients with coexisting conditions, including poorly controlled diabetes, severe COPD, and severe reactive airway disease. These patients should be followed more frequently if beta-blocker therapy is prescribed.

In general, therapy should be initiated at low dose and titrated slowly, no faster than doubling the dose at weekly intervals to tolerated or target doses (see following table). This should be done by practitioners or clinics with experience and capabilities for close patient contact and follow-up. During initiation and titration of therapy, it is imperative that patients be frequently monitored for signs of worsening heart failure. Significant weight gain, increasing shortness of breath, edema, paroxysmal nocturnal dyspnea, and dyspnea on exertion may necessitate slowing or decreasing the dose of beta-blocker with dose adjustment of ACEI and diuretic therapies. Patients should be well educated on potential signs of worsening heart failure, importance of diet and drug compliance, and the need to notify the practitioner or clinic immediately if symptoms of worsening heart failure occur.

HEART FAILURE *(Continued)*

Initial and Target Doses for Beta-Blocker Therapy in Heart Failure*

Beta-Blocker	Starting Dose	Target Dose	Comment
Bisoprolol	1.25 mg/day	10 mg/day	– β_1-selective: possible benefit in patients with reactive airway disease – Inconvenient dosage forms for initial dose titration
Carvedilol	3.125 mg twice daily	25-50 mg twice daily	– FDA approved for heart failure – Nonselective beta-blocker/ α_1-blocker – Possible greater reduction in blood pressure (α-blocking effects) – Convenient dosages
Metoprolol XL/CR	12.5-25 mg/day	200 mg/day	– Compelling data for mortality benefit – β_1-selective: possible benefit in patients with reactive airway disease – Inconvenient dosage forms for initial dose titration – Less potential to decrease blood pressure (no α-blocking properties)

*Doses are those used in clinical trials.

Digoxin

Digoxin improves symptoms of heart failure and decreases hospitalizations for heart failure, but does not improve mortality. Digoxin should be used in patients who have symptoms despite optimal standard therapy (ACEIs, diuretics, beta-blocker). There is no compelling evidence for a target therapeutic serum level for digoxin in the treatment of heart failure. Digoxin should be avoided in patients with sinus and AV block. Caution should be used with digoxin in patients with potential drug interactions, unstable renal function, hypokalemia, and hypomagnesemia.

Diuretics

Diuretic therapy should be initiated immediately in patients with heart failure who have signs of volume overload. Patients with mild volume overload can be managed adequately on thiazide diuretics. Patients with more severe volume overload, particularly in patients with a creatinine clearance <30 mL/minute should be started on a loop diuretic. Therapy should eliminate symptoms of heart failure (eg, edema) and may be monitored and dosed by changes in body weight. Resistance to therapy, as is seen in severe heart failure, may necessitate intravenous diuretic therapy or the use of more than one diuretic. See monographs for individual diuretics.

Diuretic Therapy for Heart Failure

Diuretic	Initial Dose (mg)	Target Dose (mg)	Recommended Maximal Dose (mg)	Comment
Thiazide Diuretics				
Chlorthalidone Hydrochlorothiazide	25 qd	As needed	50 qd	– Postural hypotension, hypokalemia, hyperglycemia, hyperuricemia, rash; rare severe reaction includes pancreatitis, bone marrow suppression, and anaphylaxis
Loop Diuretics				
Bumetanide Furosemide Torsemide	0.5-1 qd-bid 10-40 qd-bid 10-20 mg qd-bid	As needed	10 qd 240 bid 200 mg qd	– Same as thiazide diuretics
Thiazide-Related Diuretic				
Metolazone	2.5*	As needed	10 qd	– Same as thiazide diuretics
Potassium-Sparing Diuretics				
Amiloride Triamterene	5 qd 50 qd	As needed	40 qd 100 bid	– Hyperkalemia (especially if administered with ACEI), rash
Aldosterone Antagonist				
Spironolactone	25 qd	As needed	50 qd	– Hyperkalemia (especially if administered with ACEI), gynecomastia – Decreases mortality in severe heart failure (initiate only in patients with S_{cr} <2.5 mg/dL and serum potassium <5.0 mmol/L)

*Given as a single test dose initially.

Adapted from U.S. Department of Health & Human Services, the Agency for Healthcare Policy and Research (ACHPR) Publication No. 94-0613, June, 1994.

HEART FAILURE *(Continued)*

Hydralazine/Isosorbide Dinitrate (ISDN)

The combination of hydralazine (initial dose 10 mg qid up to 75 mg qid) and isosorbide dinitrate (initial dose 5 mg tid up to 40 mg tid), may be considered in patients intolerant to ACEI therapy. It has been shown to improve mortality in patients with heart failure not on ACEI therapy. The combination is sometimes added to standard therapy if symptoms or fatigue persist. However, there is little data to suggest that the addition of hydralazine/ISDN to standard therapy further improves morbidity and mortality. ACEI therapy is superior compared to hydralazine/ISDN in improving mortality. The chronic use of other direct vasodilators may increase morbidity and mortality in this population.

Angiotensin II Receptor Blockers (ARBs)

The renin-angiotensin-aldosterone system plays a key role in the progression of heart failure. For this reason, the role of ARBs in this patient population is being extensively evaluated. Mechanistically, angiotensin II is also produced through non-ACE systems and heart failure patients have "escape" of angiotensin II levels with chronic ACEI therapy. For these reasons, ARB therapy may confer a positive impact on morbidity and mortality by directly blocking the detrimental affects of angiotensin II. It is not established if ARB therapy provides similar mortality benefits as ACEIs or if there is an added benefit in combining an ABR to standard (ACEI) therapy.

In the Evaluation of Losartan in the Elderly (ELITE) trial, losartan and captopril therapy produced similar effects on renal function (primary study endpoint). The risk for cardiovascular events (secondary study endpoint) were significantly decreased in those treated with losartan. A follow-up study (ELITE-II) showed similar cardiovascular events and no differences in hospitalization rates between patients randomized to captopril or losartan. In another ARB trial (RESOLVD), candesartan and enalapril therapy alone and the combination of these two agents were evaluated. The findings of this trial showed no difference in clinical effects overall and a trend for improved left ventricular structure with ARB and ACEI combination therapy. The addition of ARBs to ACEI therapy (as well as other heart failure treatment) did not result in a decrease in mortality, although hospitalization was significantly reduced (ValHeFT) and the combined endpoint of mortality and morbidity was reduced. In a subgroup analysis, patients taking both an ACEI and a beta-blocker at baseline had a higher mortality after valsartan was added. Ongoing studies will give more data on the potential role of ARBs in the treatment of heart failure.

Current recommendations for ARB therapy is in those heart failure patients who are intolerant of ACEI therapy (see drug monographs).

Aldosterone Antagonists

In the RALES study, a large, long-term trial (*N Engl J Med*, 1999, 341:709-17), low-dose spironolactone, when added to prior ACEI therapy in patients with recent or current Class IV symptoms, resulted in a reduced risk of hospitalization and death. Patients who were also receiving digitalis and beta-blockers appeared to demonstrate the most marked effect. Therapy should only be initiated in patients with a serum potassium <5.0 mmol/L and a serum creatinine <2.5 mg/dL. Close monitoring of serum potassium is required.

B-type Natriuretic Peptide

Infusions of nesiritide have been shown to result in improvement of symptoms in acutely decompensated patients with CHF. Careful monitoring and titration is required and duration of the symptomatic response following infusion has been limited, in most cases, to a few days.

PHARMACOLOGICAL MANAGEMENT OF PATIENTS WITH HEART FAILURE

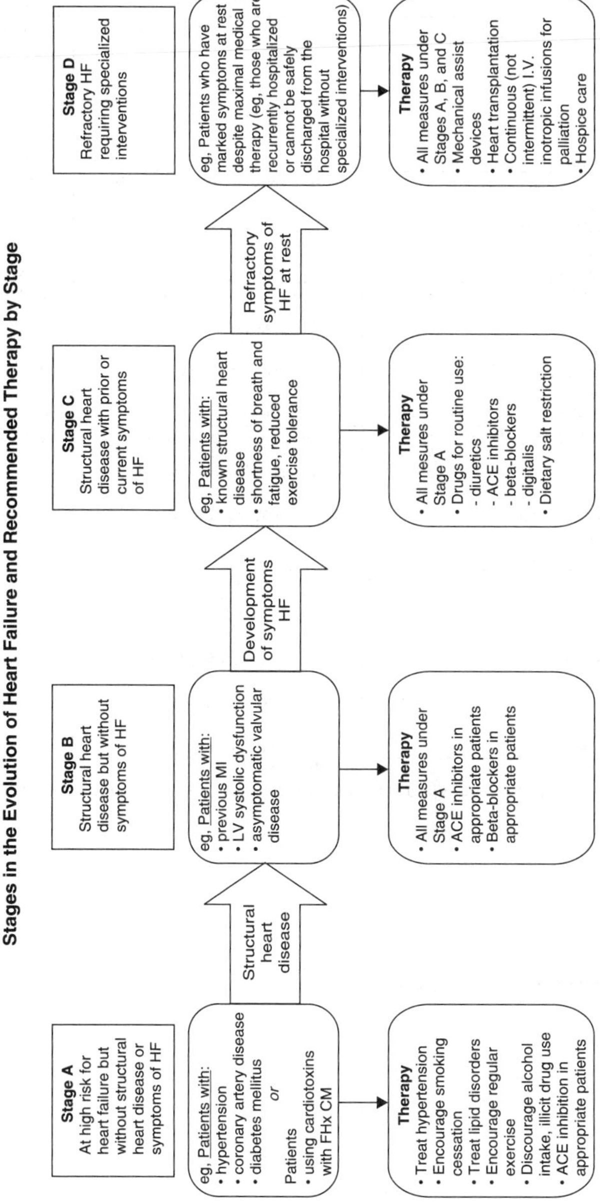

Adapted from Hunt SA, Barker DW, and Chin MJ, "ACC/AHA Guidelines for the Evaluation and Management of Chronic Heart Failure in the Adult," *J Heart Lung Transplant*, 2002,21(2):189-203.

HELICOBACTER PYLORI TREATMENT

Multiple Drug Regimens for the Treatment of *H. pylori* Infection

Drug	Dosages	Duration of Therapy
H_2-receptor antagonist[1]	Any one given at appropriate dose	4 weeks
plus		
Bismuth subsalicylate	525 mg 4 times/day	2 weeks
plus		
Metronidazole	250 mg 4 times/day	2 weeks
plus		
Tetracycline	500 mg 4 times/day	2 weeks
Proton pump inhibitor[1]	Esomeprazole 40 mg once daily	10 days
plus		
Clarithromycin	500 mg twice daily	10 days
plus		
Amoxicillin	1000 mg twice daily	10 days
Proton pump inhibitor[1]	Lansoprazole 30 mg twice daily or Omeprazole 20 mg twice daily	10-14 days
plus		
Clarithromycin	500 mg twice daily	10-14 days
plus		
Amoxicillin	1000 mg twice daily	10-14 days
Proton pump inhibitor	Lansoprazole 30 mg twice daily or Omeprazole 20 mg twice daily	2 weeks
plus		
Clarithromycin	500 mg twice daily	2 weeks
plus		
Metronidazole	500 mg twice daily	2 weeks
Proton pump inhibitor	Lansoprazole 30 mg once daily or Omeprazole 20 mg once daily	2 weeks
plus		
Bismuth	525 mg 4 times/day	2 weeks
plus		
Metronidazole	500 mg 3 times/day	2 weeks
plus		
Tetracycline	500 mg 4 times/day	2 weeks

[1]FDA-approved regimen

Modified from Howden CS and Hunt RH, "Guidelines for the Management of *Helicobacter pylori* Infection," *AJG*, 1998, 93:2336.

HYPERLIPIDEMIA MANAGEMENT

MORTALITY

There is a strong link between serum cholesterol and cardiovascular mortality. This association becomes stronger in patients with established coronary artery disease. Lipid-lowering trials show that reductions in LDL cholesterol are followed by reductions in mortality. In general, each 1% fall in LDL cholesterol confers a 2% reduction in cardiovascular events. The aim of therapy for hyperlipidemia is to decrease cardiovascular morbidity and mortality by lowering cholesterol to a target level using safe and cost-effective treatment modalities. The target LDL cholesterol is determined by the number of patient risk factors (see the following Risk Factors and Goal LDL Cholesterol tables). The goal is achieved through diet, lifestyle modification, and drug therapy. The basis for these recommendations is provided by longitudinal interventional studies, demonstrating that lipid-lowering in patients with prior cardiovascular events (secondary prevention) and in patients with hyperlipidemia but no prior cardiac event (primary prevention) lowers the occurrence of future cardiovascular events, including stroke. In a recent randomized study of relatively low-risk patients with LDLs ≥115 mg/dL, who were referred for revascularization (angioplasty), those assigned to aggressive lipid-lowering therapy were at the same or lower risk for subsequent ischemic events than those who underwent angioplasty (*N Engl J Med*, 1999, 341:170-6).

Major Risk Factors That Modify LDL Goals

Positive risk factors	Male ≥45 years
	Female ≥55 years
	Family history of premature coronary heart disease, defined as CHD in male first-degree relative <55 years; CHD in female first-degree relative <65 years
	Cigarette smoking
	Hypertension (blood pressure ≥140/90 mm Hg) or taking antihypertensive medication
	Low HDL (<40 mg/dL/1.03 mmol/L)
Negative risk factors	High HDL (≥60 mg/dL/1.6 mmol/L)[1]

[1]If HDL is ≥60 mg/dL, may subtract one positive risk factor.

Treatment Goals for LDL Cholesterol

Risk Factors	Target LDL Cholesterol	Target Non-HDL Cholesterol[1]
0-1 risk factor	<160 mg/dL	<190 mg/dL
Multiple (2+) risk factors	<130 mg/dL	<160 mg/dL
CHD or CHD risk equivalents[2]	<100 mg/dL	<130 mg/dL
Diabetes (with or without established coronary artery disease)	<100 mg/dL	<130 mg/dL

[1]Non-HDL cholesterol = total cholesterol minus HDL; for use in patients with serum triglyceride ≥200 mg/dL

[2]CHD risk equivalent: Other form of atherosclerotic disease (peripheral arterial disease, abdominal aortic aneurysm, and symptomatic carotid artery disease).

Any person with elevated LDL cholesterol or other form of hyperlipidemia should undergo evaluation to rule out secondary dyslipidemia. Causes of secondary dyslipidemia include diabetes, hypothyroidism, obstructive liver disease, chronic renal failure, and drugs that increase LDL and decrease HDL (progestins, anabolic steroids, corticosteroids).

Elevated Serum Triglyceride Levels

Elevated serum triglyceride levels may be an independent risk factor for coronary heart disease. Factors that contribute to hypertriglyceridemia include obesity, inactivity, cigarette smoking, excess alcohol intake, high carbohydrate diets (>60% of energy intake), type 2 diabetes, chronic renal failure, nephrotic syndrome, certain medications (corticosteroids, estrogens, retinoids, higher doses of beta-blockers), and genetic disorders. Non-HDL cholesterol (total cholesterol minus HDL cholesterol) is a secondary focus for clinicians treating patients with high serum triglyceride levels (≥200 mg/dL). The goal for non-HDL cholesterol in patients with high serum triglyceride levels can be set 30 mg/dL higher than usual LDL cholesterol goals. Patients with serum triglyceride levels <200 mg/dL should aim for the target LDL cholesterol goal.

HYPERLIPIDEMIA MANAGEMENT *(Continued)*

ATP classification of serum triglyceride levels:

- Normal triglycerides: <150 mg/dL
- Borderline-high: 150-199 mg/dL
- High: 200-499 mg/dL
- Very high: ≥500 mg/dL

NONDRUG THERAPY

Dietary therapy and lifestyle modifications should be individualized for each patient. A total lifestyle change is recommended for all patients. Dietary and lifestyle modifications should be tried for 3 months, if deemed appropriate. Nondrug and drug therapy should be initiated simultaneously in patients with highly elevated cholesterol (see LDL Cholesterol Goals and Cutpoints for Therapeutic Lifestyle Changes and Drug Therapy in Different Risk Categories table). Increasing physical activity and smoking cessation will aid in the treatment of hyperlipidemia and improve cardiovascular health.

Note: Refer to the National Cholesterol Education Program reference for details concerning the calculation of 10-year risk of CHD using Framingham risk scoring. Risk assessment tool is available online at http://hin.nhlbi.nih.gov/atpiii/calculator.asp?usertype=prof, last accessed March 14, 2002.

Total Lifestyle Change (TLC) Diet

	Recommended Intake
Total fat	25%-35% of total calories
Saturated fat[1]	<7% of total calories
Polyunsaturated fat	≤10% of total calories
Monounsaturated fat	≤20% of total calories
Carbohydrates[2]	50%-60% of total calories
Fiber	20-30 g/day
Protein	~15% of total calories
Cholesterol	<200 mg/day
Total calories[3]	Balance energy intake and expenditure to maintain desirable body weight/prevent weight gain

[1]*Trans* fatty acids (partially hydrogenated oils) intake should be kept low. These are found in potato chips, other snack foods, margarines and shortenings, and fast-foods.

[2]Complex carbohydrates including grains (especially whole grains, fruits, and vegetables).

[3]Daily energy expenditure should include at least moderate physical activity.

LDL Cholesterol Goals and Cutpoints for Therapeutic Lifestyle Changes (TLC) and Drug Therapy in Different Risk Categories

Risk Category	LDL-C Goal	LDL Level at Which to Initiate TLC	LDL Level at Which to Consider Drug Therapy
CHD or CHD risk equivalents (10-year risk >20%)	<100 mg/dL	≥100 mg/dL	≥130 mg/dL (100-129 mg/dL: drug optional)[1]
2+ risk factors (10-year risk ≤20%)	<130 mg/dL	≥130 mg/dL	10-year risk 10%-20%: ≥130 mg/dL
			10-year risk <10%: ≥160 mg/dL
0-1 risk factor[2]	<160 mg/dL	≥160 mg/dL	≥190 mg/dL (160-189 mg/dL: drug optional)

[1]Some authorities recommend use of LDL-lowering drugs in this category if an LDL cholesterol <100 mg/dL cannot be achieved by therapeutic lifestyle changes. Others prefer use of drugs that primarily modify triglycerides and HDL (eg, nicotinic acid or fibrate). Clinical judgment also may call for deferring drug therapy in this subcategory.

[2]Almost all people with 0-1 risk factor have a 10-year risk <10%, thus 10-year risk assessment in people with 0-1 risk factor is not necessary.

DRUG THERAPY

Drug therapy should be selected based on the patient's lipid profile, concomitant disease states, and the cost of therapy. The following table lists specific advantages and disadvantages for various classes of lipid-lowering medications. The cost and expected reduction in lipids with therapy are listed in the Lipid-Lowering Agents table. Refer to individual drug monographs for detailed information.

Advantages and Disadvantages of Specific Lipid-Lowering Therapies

	Advantages	Disadvantages
Bile acid sequestrants	Good choice for ↑ LDL, especially when combined with a statin (↓ LDL ≤50%); low potential for systemic side effects; good choice for younger patients	May increase triglycerides; higher incidence of adverse effects; moderately expensive; drug interactions; inconvenient dosing
Niacin	Good choice for almost any lipid abnormality; inexpensive; greatest increase in HDL	High incidence of adverse effects; may adversely affect NIDDM and gout; sustained release niacin may decrease the incidence of flushing and circumvent the need for multiple daily dosing; sustained release niacin may not increase HDL cholesterol or decrease triglycerides as well as immediate release niacin
HMG-CoA reductase inhibitors	Produces greatest ↓ in LDL; generally well-tolerated; convenient once-daily dosing; proven decrease in mortality	Expensive
Gemfibrozil	Good choice in patients with ↑ triglycerides where niacin is contraindicated or not well-tolerated; gemfibrozil is well tolerated	Variable effects on LDL

Lipid-Lowering Agents

Drug	Dose/Day	Effect on LDL (%)	Effect on HDL (%)	Effect on TG (%)
HMG-CoA Reductase Inhibitors				
Atorvastatin	10 mg 20 mg 40 mg 80 mg	-39 -43 -50 -60	+6 +5 +5 +5	-13 -20 -32 -37
Fluvastatin	20 mg 40 mg 80 mg	-22 -25 -36	+2 +3 +4	-5 -12 -12
Lovastatin	20 mg 40 mg 80 mg	-27 -32 -42	+7 +5 +8	-8 -2 -13
Pravastatin	10 mg 20 mg 40 mg	-22 -32 -34	+5 +3 +6	-3 -15 -10
Simvastatin	5 mg 10 mg 20 mg 40 mg 80 mg	-26 -30 -38 -41 -47	+7 +5 +10 +8	-12 -17 -15 -24
Bile Acid Sequestrants				
Cholestyramine	4-24 g/day	-15 to -30	+3 to +5	+0 to +20
Colestipol	7-30 g/day	-15 to -30	+3 to +5	+0 to +20
Colesevelam	6 tab/day	-10	+10 to +25	-40 to -55
Fibric Acid Derivative				
Clofibrate	500 mg 4 times/day	-10	+10 to +25	-40 to -55
Fenofibrate	67-200 mg/day	-20 to -25	+1 to -34	-30 to -50
Gemfibrozil	600 mg bid	-5 to -10*	+10 to +20	-40 to -60
Niacin	1.5-6 g/day	-21 to -27	+10 to +35	-10 to -50

*May increase LDL in some patients.

Recommended Liver Function Monitoring for HMG-CoA Reductase Inhibitors

Agent	Initial and After Elevation in Dose	6 Weeks*	12 Weeks*	Periodically
Atorvastatin (Lipitor®)	x		x	x
Fluvastatin (Lescol®)	x		x	x
Lovastatin (Mevacor®)	x	x	x	x
Pravastatin (Pravachol®)	x			x
Simvastatin (Zocor®)	x			x

*After initiation of therapy or any elevation in dose.

HYPERLIPIDEMIA MANAGEMENT *(Continued)*

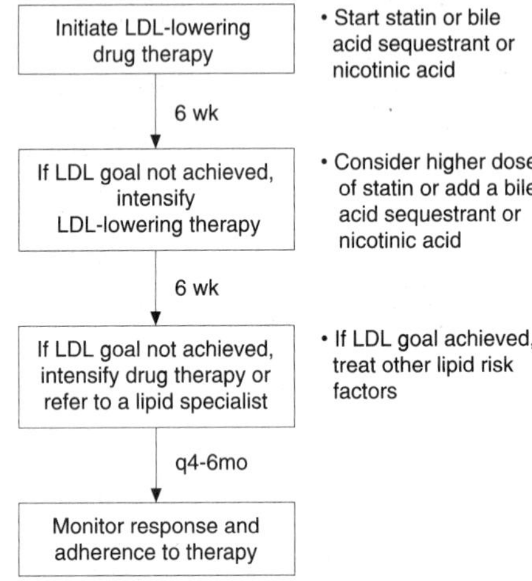

DRUG SELECTION

Lipid Profile	Monotherapy	Combination Therapies
Increased LDL with normal HDL and triglycerides (TG)	Resin Niacin[1] Statin	Resin plus niacin[1] or statin Statin plus niacin[1,2]
Increased LDL and increased TG (200-499 mg/dL)[2]	Intensify LDL-lowering therapy	Statin plus niacin[1,3] Statin plus fibrate[3]
Increased LDL and increased TG (≥500 mg/dL)[2]	Consider combination therapy (niacin,[1] fibrates, statin)	
Increased TG	Niacin[1] Fibrates	Niacin[1] plus fibrates
Increased LDL and low HDL	Niacin[1] Statin	Statin plus niacin[1,2]

[1]Avoid in diabetics.

[2]Emphasize weight reduction and increased physical activity.

[3]Risk of myopathy with combination.

Resins = bile acid sequestrants; statins = HMG-CoA reductase inhibitors; fibrates = fibric acid derivatives (eg, gemfibrozil, fenofibrate).

COMBINATION DRUG THERAPY

If after at least 6 weeks of therapy at the maximum recommended or tolerated dose, the patient's LDL cholesterol is not at target, consider optimizing nondrug measures, prescribing a higher dose of current lipid-lowering drug, or adding another lipid-lowering medication to the current therapy. Successful drug combinations include statin and niacin, statin and bile acid sequestrant, or niacin and bile acid sequestrant. At maximum recommended doses, LDL cholesterol may be decreased by 50% to 60% with combination therapy. This is the same reduction achieved by atorvastatin 40 mg twice daily. If a bile acid sequestrant is used with other lipid-lowering agents, space doses 1 hour before or 4 hours after the bile acid sequestrant administration. Statins combined with either fenofibrate, clofibrate, gemfibrozil, or niacin increase the risk of rhabdomyolysis. In this situation, patient education (muscle pain/weakness) and careful follow-up are warranted.

References

Guidelines

Gavin JR, Alberti KGMM, Davidson MB, et al, for the Members of the Expert Committee on the Diagnosis and Classification of Diabetes Mellitus, "American Diabetes Association: Clinical Practice Recommendations," *Diabetes Care*, 1999, 22(Suppl 1):S1-S114.

National Cholesterol Education Program, "Third Report of the Expert Panel on Detection, Evaluation, and Treatment of High Blood Cholesterol in Adults (Adult Treatment Panel III)," *JAMA*, 2001, 285:2486-97.

Others

Berthold HK, Sudhop T, and von Bergmann K, "Effect of a Garlic Oil Preparation on Serum Lipoproteins and Cholesterol Metabolism: A Randomized Controlled Trial," *JAMA*, 1998, 279:1900-2.

Bertolini S, Bon GB, Campbell LM, et al, "Efficacy and Safety of Atorvastatin Compared to Pravastatin in Patients With Hypercholesterolemia," *Atherosclerosis*, 1997, 130:191-7.

Blankenhorn DH, Nessim SA, Johnson RL, et al, "Beneficial Effects of Combined Colestipol-Niacin Therapy on Coronary Atherosclerosis and Venous Bypass Grafts," *JAMA*, 1987, 257:3233-40.

Brown G, Albers JJ, Fisher LD, et al, "Regression of Coronary Artery Disease as a Result of Intensive Lipid-Lowering Therapy in Men With High Levels of Apolipoprotein B," *N Engl J Med*, 1990, 323:1289-98.

Capuzzi DM, Guyton JR, Morgan JM, et al, "Efficacy and Safety of an Extended-Release Niacin (Niaspan®): A Long-Term Study," *Am J Cardiol*, 1998, 82:74U-81U.

Coronary Drug Project Research Program, "Clofibrate and Niacin in Coronary Heart Disease," *JAMA*, 1975, 231:360-81.

Dart A, Jerums G, Nicholson G, et al, "A Multicenter, Double-Blind, One-Year Study Comparing Safety and Efficacy of Atorvastatin Versus Simvastatin in Patients With Hypercholesterolemia," *Am J Cardiol*, 1997, 80:39-44.

Davidson MH, Dillon MA, Gordon B, et al, "Colesevelam Hydrochloride (Cholestagel): A New Potent Bile Acid Sequestrant Associated With a Low Incidence of Gastrointestinal Side Effects," *Arch Intern Med*, 1999, 159(16):1893-900.

Davidson M, McKenney J, Stein E, et al, "Comparison of One-Year Efficacy and Safety of Atorvastatin Versus Lovastatin in Primary Hypercholesterolemia," *Am J Cardiol*, 1997, 79:1475-81.

Frick MH, Heinonen OP, Huttunen JK, et al, "Helsinki Heart Study: Primary-Prevention Trial With Gemfibrozil in Middle-Aged Men With Dyslipidemia," *N Engl J Med*, 1987, 317:1237-45.

Garber AM, Browner WS, and Hulley SB, "Clinical Guideline, Part 2: Cholesterol Screening in Asymptomatic Adults, Revisited," *Ann Intern Med*, 1995, 124:518-31.

Johannesson M, Jonsson B, Kjekshus J, et al, "Cost-Effectiveness of Simvastatin Treatment to Lower Cholesterol Levels in Patients With Coronary Heart Disease. Scandinavian Simvastatin Survival Study Group," *N Engl N Med*, 1997, 336:332-6.

Jones P, Kafonek S, Laurora I, et al, "Comparative Dose Efficacy Study of Atorvastatin Versus Simvastatin, Pravastatin, Lovastatin, and Fluvastatin in Patients With Hypercholesterolemia," *Am J Cardiol*, 1998, 81:582-7.

Kasiske BL, Ma JZ, Kalil RS, et al, "Effects of Antihypertensive Therapy on Serum Lipids," *Ann Intern Med*, 1995, 133-41.

Lipid Research Clinics Program, "The Lipid Research Clinics Coronary Primary Prevention Trial Results: I. Reduction in Incidence of Coronary Heart Disease," *JAMA*, 1984, 251:351-64.

Multiple Risk Factor Intervention Trial Research Group, "Multiple Risk Factor Intervention Trial: Risk Factor Changes and Mortality Results," *JAMA*, 1982, 248:1465-77.

Pitt B, Waters D, Brown WV, et al, "Aggressive Lipid-Lowering Therapy Compared With Angioplasty in Stable Coronary Artery Disease. Atorvastatin Versus Revascularization Treatment Investigators," *N Engl J Med*, 1999, 341(2):70-6.

Ross SD, Allen IE, Connelly JE, et al, "Clinical Outcomes in Statin Treatment Trials: A Meta-Analysis," *Arch Intern Med*, 1999, 159:1793-802.

Sacks FM, Pfeffer MA, Moye LA, et al, "The Effect of Pravastatin on Coronary Events After Myocardial Infarction in Patients With Average Cholesterol Levels," *N Engl J Med*, 1996, 335:1001-9.

Scandinavian Simvastatin Survival Study, "Randomized Trial of Cholesterol Lowering in 4444 Patients With Coronary Heart Disease: The Scandinavian Simvastatin Survival Study (4S)," *Lancet*, 1994, 344:1383-9.

Schrott HG, Bittner V, Vittinghoff E, et al, "Adherence to National Cholesterol Education Program Treatment Goals in Postmenopausal Women With Heart Disease. The Heart and Estrogen/Progestin Replacement Study (HERS)," *JAMA*, 1997, 277:1281-6.

Shepherd J, Cobbe SM, Ford I, et al, "Prevention of Coronary Heart Disease With Pravastatin in Men With Hypercholesterolemia, The West of Scotland Coronary Prevention Study Group," *N Engl J Med*, 1995, 333:1301-7.

Stein EA, Davidson MH, Dobs AS, et al, "Efficacy and Safety of Simvastatin 80 mg/day in Hypercholesterolemic Patients. The Expanded Dose Simvastatin U.S. Study Group," *Am J Cardiol*, 1998, 82:311-6.

HYPERTENSION

The optimal blood pressure for adults is <120/80 mm Hg. Consistent systolic pressure ≥140 mm Hg or a diastolic pressure ≥90 mm Hg, in the absence of a secondary cause, define hypertension. Hypertension affects approximately 25% (50 million people) of the United States population. Of those patients on antihypertensive medication, only one in four patients have their blood pressure controlled (<140/90 mm Hg). Recent mortality rates for stroke and heart disease, in which hypertension is an antecedent, remain unchanged. The prevention, detection, evaluation, and treatment of high blood pressure is therefore paramount for each person and for all healthcare providers.

The Sixth Report of the Joint National Committee (JNC VI) is an excellent reference and guide for the treatment of hypertension (*Arch Intern Med*, 1997, 157:2413-46). For adults, hypertension is classified in stages (see Table 1). Initial follow up of adult patients is based on office blood pressure recordings (see Table 3). Based on these initial assessments, treatment strategies for patients with hypertension are stratified based on their blood pressure and their risk group classification (see Table 4). Patients in Risk **Group A** have no risk factors; **Group B**, at least one risk factor (other than diabetes), and no cardiovascular disease or target-organ disease (see Table 5); **Group C**, have cardiovascular disease or diabetes or target-organ disease (see Table 5). Risk factors include smoking, dyslipidemia, diabetes, age >60 years, male gender, postmenopausal women, and family history of cardiovascular disease (cardiovascular event in first degree female relatives <65 years and in first degree male relatives <55 years).

Table 1. Adult Classification of Blood Pressure

Category	Systolic (mm Hg)		Diastolic (mm Hg)
Optimal	<120	and	<80
Normal	<130	and	<85
High normal	130-139	or	85-89
Hypertension			
Stage 1	140-159	or	90-99
Stage 2	160-179	or	100-109
Stage 3	≥180	or	≥110
Isolated systolic	≥140	and	<90

Adapted from the Sixth Report of the Joint National Committee on Prevention, Detection, Evaluation, and Treatment of High Blood Pressure, NIH Publication No. 98-4080, November 1997.

Table 2. Normal Blood Pressure in Children

Age (y)	Girls' SBP/DBP (mm Hg)		Boys' SBP/DBP (mm Hg)	
	50th Percentile for Height	75th Percentile for Height	50th Percentile for Height	75th Percentile for Height
1	104/58	105/59	102/57	104/58
6	111/73	112/73	114/74	115/75
12	123/80	124/81	123/81	125/82
17	129/84	130/85	136/87	138/88

SBP = systolic blood pressure.

DBP = diastolic blood pressure.

Adapted from the report by the NHBPEP Working Group on Hypertension Control in Children and Adolescents, *Pediatrics*, 1996, 98(4 Pt 1):649-58.

Table 3. Blood Pressure Screening and Follow-up

Initial Screening BP (mm Hg)		Follow-up Recommended
Systolic	Diastolic	
<130	<85	Recheck in 2 years
130-139	85-89	Recheck in 1 year
140-159	90-99	Confirm within 2 months
160-179	100-109	Evaluate/treatment within 1 month
≥180	≥110	Evaluate/treatment immediately or within 1 week

Adapted from the Sixth Report of the Joint National Committee on Prevention, Detection, Evaluation, and Treatment of High Blood Pressure, NIH Publication No. 98-4080, November 1997.

Table 4. Blood Pressure and Risk Stratification

Blood Pressure Stages	Risk Group A (no RF or TOD)	Risk Group B (≥1 RF, not including diabetes, no TOD)	Risk Group C (TOD and/or diabetes regardless of RF)
High normal (130-139/85-89 mm Hg)	Lifestyle modification	Lifestyle modification	Drug therapy[1] and lifestyle modification
Stage 1 (140-159/90-99 mm Hg)	Lifestyle modification (up to 12 mo)	Lifestyle modification (up to 6 mo)[2]	Drug therapy and lifestyle modification
Stages 2 and 3 (≥160/≥100 mm Hg)	Drug therapy and lifestyle modification	Drug therapy and lifestyle modification	Drug therapy and lifestyle modification

[1]For those with heart failure, renal insufficiency, or diabetes.

[2]For patients with multiple risk factors, consider starting both drug and lifestyle modification together.

RF = risk factor.

TOD = target-organ disease.

Adapted from the Sixth Report of the Joint National Committee on Prevention, Detection, Evaluation, and Treatment of High Blood Pressure, NIH Publication No. 98-4080, November 1997.

Table 5. Target-Organ Disease

Organ System	Manifestation
Cardiac	Clinical, EKG, or radiologic evidence of coronary artery disease; prior MI, angina, post-CABG; left ventricular hypertrophy (LVH); left ventricular dysfunction or cardiac failure
Cerebrovascular	Transient ischemic attack or stroke
Peripheral vascular	Absence of pulses in extremities (except dorsalis pedis), claudication, aneurysm
Renal	Serum creatinine ≥130 μmol/L (1.5 mg/dL); proteinuria (≥1+); microalbuminuria
Retinopathy	Hemorrhages or exudates, with or without papilledema

Adapted from the Sixth Report of the Joint National Committee on Prevention, Detection, Evaluation, and Treatment of High Blood Pressure, NIH Publication No. 98-4080, November 1997.

Treatment of hypertension should be individualized. Lower blood pressures should be achieved in patients with diabetes or renal disease. The Hypertension Treatment Algorithm on the following page may be used to select specific antihypertensives based on specific or compelling indications. Special consideration for starting combination therapy should be made in each patient. Starting drug therapy at a low dose and titrating upward if blood pressure is not controlled is recommended. The benefit of these strategies is to minimize the occurrence of adverse effects while achieving optimal blood pressure control. One caveat for starting at a low dose and then titrating upward is that patients and clinicians must commit to well-timed follow-up so that blood pressure is controlled in a timely manner. Lifestyle modification and risk reduction should be initiated and continued throughout treatment.

COMBINATION THERAPY IN THE TREATMENT OF HYPERTENSION

Important concerns in treating hypertension are the efficacy and side effects of therapy. In the past, progressive increases in dosage of a single drug were used to improve blood pressure control. Historically (based on the Joint National Committee [JNC] recommendations), the maximum doses of recommended drugs have decreased from those proposed in earlier JNC reports.

More recently, the concept of combination therapy has begun to gain increasing favor. This is reflected most clearly in the report of the Sixth Joint National Committee on Detection, Evaluation, and Treatment of High Blood Pressure (JNC VI). Specifically, JNC VI endorses the use of low doses of two antihypertensive drugs in fixed-dose combinations as a possible route for initial treatment of hypertension. This recommendation extends earlier JNC V recognition that combining drugs with different modes of action may allow smaller doses of drugs to be used to achieve control, and minimize the potential for dose-dependent side effects.

Combination therapy thus constitutes the use of an additional antihypertensive medication before the first therapeutic agent is necessarily at maximum dose, or the use of two agents in low doses at the onset of antihypertensive treatment. The rationale, background, and experience with combination therapy are nicely reviewed in Kaplan NM and Sever PS, "Combination Therapy: A Key to Comprehensive Patient Care," *Am J Hyperten*, 1997, 10(7 part 2):127S and by Moser M and Black HR, "The Role of Combination Therapy in the Treatment of Hypertension," *Am J Hyperten*, 11:73S-8S).

HYPERTENSION *(Continued)*

Fundamental to the combination therapy approach are the following considerations.

- Drugs with different and complementary mechanisms of action may often produce synergistic reductions in blood pressure, classically evident in the use of diuretics and ACE inhibitors.
- Low doses of a single drug are less likely to induce side effects.
- More than 50% of all hypertensive patients will need more than one drug to achieve blood pressure control.

In effect, this therapeutic strategy allows exploitation of the steepest part of the antihypertensive dose response curve, achieving synergistic or additive therapeutic benefit while limiting potential for side effects. Disadvantages include first, the need to take two drugs, often resulting in taking two separate tablets. It is important to ensure that both therapeutic preparations have equivalent durations of action. Second, the cost of separate products may exceed that of increased doses of a single medication.

In mitigation, fixed-dose combinations of antihypertensive preparations are available with recent options, including Lexxel™ (calcium channel blocker and ACE inhibitor), Hyzaar® (angiotensin receptor blocker and hydrochlorothiazide), Capozide® (ACE inhibitor and hydrochlorothiazide), and Ziac™ (beta-blocker and hydrochlorothiazide). These combinations help address cost and convenience issues in combination therapy.

HYPERTENSION TREATMENT ALGORITHM

Begin or continue lifestyle modifications

↓

Not at goal blood pressure (<140/90 mm Hg)
Lower BP goals for patients with diabetes or renal disease

↓

Initial Drug Choices (<140/90 mm Hg)
Uncomplicated Hypertension
(Based on Randomized Controlled Trials)

Diuretics, beta-blockers

Compelling Indications
(Based on Randomized Controlled Trials)

Diabetes Mellitus (Type I) with Proteinuria
ACE inhibitors

Isolated Systolic Hypertension
(Older Persons)
Diuretics preferred
Long-acting dihydropyridines
Calcium antagonists

Heart Failure
ACE inhibitors
Beta-blockers (non-ISA)
Diuretics

Myocardial Infarction
Beta-blockers (non-ISA)
ACE inhibitors (with systolic dysfunction)

Start with a low dose of a long-acting once-daily drug and titrate dose. Low-dose combinations may be appropriate.

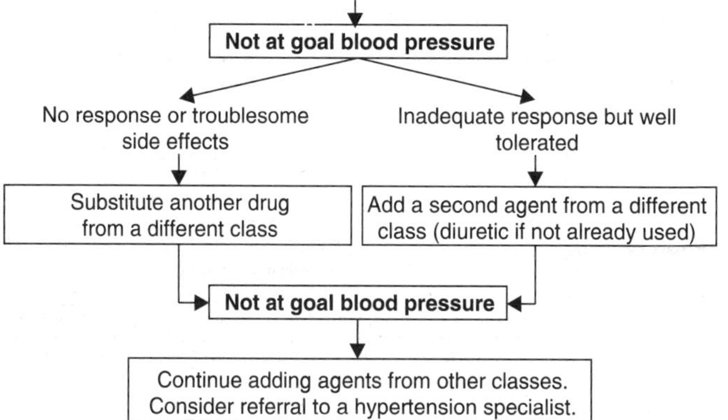

Adapted from *Arch Intern Med*, 1998, 157:2450.

HYPERTENSION *(Continued)*

COMPELLING INDICATIONS FOR SPECIFIC THERAPIES

Indication	Drug Therapy
COMPELLING INDICATIONS UNLESS CONTRAINDICATED	
Diabetes mellitus (type I) with proteinuria	ACEI
Heart failure	ACEI, diuretics, beta-blockers (carvedilol, metoprolol XL/CR, bisoprolol, hydralazine + isosorbide dinitrate)
Isolated systolic hypertension (older patients)	Diuretics (preferred), CCB (long-acting)
Myocardial infarction	Beta-blockers (non-ISA), ACEI (with systolic dysfunction)
High-risk patients (CVD plus risk factors)	ACEI (ramipril)
MAY HAVE FAVORABLE EFFECTS ON COMORBID CONDITIONS	
Angina	Beta-blockers, CCB (long-acting)
Atrial tachycardia and fibrillation	Beta-blockers, CCB (non-DHP)
Cyclosporine-induced hypertension (caution with the dose of cyclosporine)	CCB
Diabetes mellitus (types I and II) with proteinuria	ACEI (preferred), CCB
Diabetes mellitus (type II)	Low-dose diuretics (≤25 mg HCTZ)
Dyslipidemia	Alpha-blockers
Essential tremor	Beta-blockers (noncardioselective)
Heart failure	Losartan, candesartan
Hyperthyroidism	Beta-blockers
Migraine	Beta-blockers (noncardioselective), CCB (long-acting) (non-DHP)
Myocardial infarction (non-Q-wave with normal systolic function and no edema)	Diltiazem, verapamil (long-acting)
Osteoporosis	Thiazides
Preoperative hypertension	Beta-blockers
Prostatism (BPH)	Alpha-blockers
Renal insufficiency (caution in renovascular hypertension and creatinine ≥265.2 mmol/L [3 mg/dL])	ACEI
MAY HAVE UNFAVORABLE EFFECTS ON COMORBID CONDITIONS[1]	
Bronchospastic disease	Beta-blockers[2]
Depression	Beta-blockers, central alpha-agonists, reserpine[2]
Diabetes mellitus (types I and II)	Beta-blockers, high-dose diuretics
Dyslipidemia	Beta-blockers (non-ISA), diuretics (high-dose)
Gout	Diuretics
Second or third degree heart block	Beta-blockers,[2] CCB (non-DHP)[2]
Heart failure	Beta-blockers (with high ISA), CCB (except amlodipine, felodipine)
Liver disease	Labetalol hydrochloride, methyldopa[2]
Peripheral vascular disease	Beta-blockers
Pregnancy	ACEI,[2] angiotensin II receptor blockers[2]
Renal insufficiency	Potassium-sparing agents
Renovascular disease	ACEI, angiotensin II receptor blockers

ACEI = angiotensin-converting enzyme inhibitors; BPH = benign prostatic hyperplasia; CCB = calcium antagonists; CVD = cardiovascular disease; DHP = dihydropyridine; HCTZ = hydrochlorothiazide; ISA = intrinsic sympathomimetic activity; MI = myocardial infarction; and non-CS = noncardioselective.

Conditions and drugs are listed in alphabetical order.

[1]These drugs may be used with special monitoring unless contraindicated.

[2]Contraindicated.

HYPERTENSION AND PREGNANCY

The report of the NHBPEP Working Group on High Blood Pressure in Pregnancy permits continuation of drug therapy in women with chronic hypertension (**except for ACE inhibitors**). In addition, angiotensin II receptor blockers should not be used during pregnancy. In women with chronic hypertension with diastolic levels ≥100 mm Hg (lower when end organ damage or underlying renal disease is present) and in women with acute hypertension when levels are ≥105 mm Hg, the following agents are suggested (see table).

Suggested Drug	Comments
Central alpha-agonists	Methyldopa (C) is the drug of choice recommended by the NHBPEP Working Group.
Beta-blockers	Atenolol (C) and metoprolol (C) appear to be safe and effective in late pregnancy. Labetalol (C) also appears to be effective (alpha- and beta-blockers).
Calcium antagonists	Potential synergism with magnesium sulfate may lead to precipitous hypotension. (C)
ACE inhibitors, angiotensin II receptor blockers	Fetal abnormalities, including death, can be caused, and these drugs **should not** be used in pregnancy. (D)
Diuretics	Diuretics (C) are recommended for chronic hypertension if prescribed before gestation or if patients appear to be salt-sensitive. They are not recommended in pre-eclampsia.
Direct vasodilators	Hydralazine (C) is the parenteral drug of choice based on its long history of safety and efficacy. (C)

Adapted from Sibai and Lindheimer. There are several other antihypertensive drugs for which there are very limited data. The U.S. Food and Drug Administration classifies pregnancy risk as follows: C = adverse effects in animals; no controlled trials in humans; use if risk appears justified; D = positive evidence of fetal risk. ACE = angiotensin-converting enzyme.

HYPERTENSIVE EMERGENCIES AND URGENCIES

General Treatment Principles in the Treatment of Hypertensive Emergencies

Principle	Considerations
Admit the patient to the hospital, preferably in the ICU. Monitor vital signs appropriately.	Establish I.V. access and place patient on a cardiac monitor. Place a femoral intra-arterial line and pulmonary arterial catheter, if indicated, to assess cardiopulmonary function and intravascular volume status.
Perform rapid but thorough history and physical examination.	Determine cause of, or precipitating factors to, hypertensive crisis if possible (remember to obtain a medication history including Rx, OTC, and illicit drugs). Obtain details regarding any prior history of hypertension (severity, duration, treatment), as well as other coexisting illnesses. Assess the extent of hypertensive end organ damage. Determine if a hypertensive urgency or emergency exists.
Determine goal blood pressure based on premorbid level, duration, severity and rapidity of increase of blood pressure, concomitant medical conditions, race, and age.	Acute decreases in blood pressure to normal or subnormal levels during the initial treatment period may reduce perfusion to the brain, heart, and kidneys, and must be avoided except in specific instances (ie, dissecting aortic aneurysm). Gradually establish a normal (or reasonable) blood pressure over the next 1-2 weeks.
Select an appropriate antihypertensive regimen depending on the individual patient and clinical setting.	Initiate a controlled decrease in blood pressure. Avoid concomitant administration of multiple agents that may cause precipitous falls in blood pressure. Select the agent with the best hemodynamic profile based on the primary treatment goal. Avoid diuretics and sodium restriction during the initial treatment period unless there is a clear clinical indication (ie, CHF, pulmonary edema). Avoid sedating antihypertensives in patients with hypertensive encephalopathy, CVA, or other CNS disorders in whom mental status must be monitored. Use caution with direct vasodilating agents that induce reflex tachycardia or increase cardiac output in patients with coronary heart disease, history of angina or myocardial infarction, or dissecting aortic aneurysm. Preferably choose an agent that does not adversely affect glomerular filtration rate or renal blood flow and also agents that have favorable effects on cerebral blood flow and its autoregulation, especially for patients with hypertensive encephalopathy or CVAs. Select the most efficacious agent with the fewest adverse effects based on the underlying cause of the hypertensive crisis and other individual patient factors.
Initiate a chronic antihypertensive regimen after the patient's blood pressure is stabilized	Begin oral antihypertensive therapy once goal blood pressure is achieved before gradually tapering parenteral medications. Select the best oral regimen based on cost, ease of administration, adverse effect profile, and concomitant medical conditions.

HYPERTENSION *(Continued)*

Oral Agents Used in the Treatment of Hypertensive Urgencies and Emergencies

Drug	Dose	Onset	Cautions
Captopril[1]	P.O.: 25 mg, repeat as required	15-30 min	Hypotension, renal failure in bilateral renal artery stenosis
Clonidine	P.O.: 0.1-0.2 mg, repeated every hour as needed to a total dose of 0.6 mg	30-60 min	Hypotension, drowsiness, dry mouth
Labetalol	P.O.: 200-400 mg, repeat every 2-3 h	30 min to 2 h	Bronchoconstriction, heart block, orthostatic hypotension

[1]There is no clearly defined clinical advantage in the use of sublingual over oral routes of administration with these agents.

Recommendations for the Use of Intravenous Antihypertensive Drugs in Selected Hypertensive Emergencies

Condition	Agent(s) of Choice	Agent(s) to Avoid or Use With Caution	General Treatment Principles
Hypertensive encephalopathy	Nitroprusside, labetalol, diazoxide	Methyldopa, reserpine	Avoid drugs with CNS-sedating effects
Acute intracranial or subarachnoid hemorrhage	Nicardipine,[1] nitroprusside, trimethaphan	Beta-blockers	Careful titration with a short-acting agent
Cerebral infarction	Nicardipine,[1] nitroprusside, labetalol, trimethaphan	Beta-blockers, minoxidil, diazoxide	Careful titration with a short-acting agent. Avoid agents that may decrease cerebral blood flow.
Head trauma	Esmolol, labetalol	Methyldopa, reserpine, nitroprusside, nitroglycerin, hydralazine	Avoid drugs with CNS-sedating effects, or those that may increase intracranial pressure
Acute myocardial infarction, myocardial ischemia	Nitroglycerin, nicardipine[1] (calcium channel blockers), labetalol	Hydralazine, diazoxide, minoxidil	Avoid drugs which cause reflex tachycardia and increased myocardial oxygen consumption
Acute pulmonary edema	Nitroprusside, nitroglycerin, loop diuretics	Beta-blockers (labetalol), minoxidil, methyldopa	Avoid drugs which may cause sodium and water retention and edema exacerbation
Renal dysfunction	Hydralazine, calcium channel blockers	Nitroprusside, ACE inhibitors, beta-blockers (labetalol)	Avoid drugs with increased toxicity in renal failure and those that may cause decreased renal blood flow.
Eclampsia	Hydralazine, labetalol, nitroprusside[2]	Trimethaphan, diuretics, diazoxide (diazoxide may cause cessation of labor)	Avoid drugs that may cause adverse fetal effects, compromise placental circulation, or decrease cardiac output.
Pheochromocytoma	Phentolamine, nitroprusside, beta-blockers (eg, esmolol) only after alpha blockade (phentolamine)	Beta-blockers in the absence of alpha blockade, methyldopa, minoxidil	Use drugs of proven efficacy and specificity. Unopposed beta blockade may exacerbate hypertension.
Dissecting aortic aneurysm	Nitroprusside and beta blockade, trimethaphan	Hydralazine, diazoxide, minoxidil	Avoid drugs which may increase cardiac output.
Postoperative hypertension	Nitroprusside, nicardipine,[1] labetalol	Trimethaphan	Avoid drugs which may exacerbate postoperative ileus.

[1]The use of nicardipine in these situations is by the recommendation of the author based on a review of the literature.

[2]Reserve nitroprusside for eclamptic patients with life-threatening hypertension unresponsive to other agents due to the potential risk to the fetus (cyanide and thiocyanate metabolites may cross the placenta).

Selected Intravenous Agents for Hypertensive Emergencies

Drug	Dose[1]	Onset of Action	Duration of Action	Adverse Effects[2]	Special Indications
Vasodilators					
Sodium nitroprusside	0.25-10 mcg/kg/min as I.V. infusion[3] (max: 10 min only)	Immediate	1-2 min	Nausea, vomiting, muscle twitching, sweating, thiocyanate and cyanide intoxication	Most hypertensive emergencies; caution with high intracranial pressure or azotemia
Nicardipine hydrochloride	5-15 mg/h I.V.	5-10 min	1-4 h	Tachycardia, headache, flushing, local phlebitis	Most hypertensive emergencies except acute heart failure; caution with coronary ischemia
Fenoldopam mesylate	0.1-0.3 mcg/kg/min I.V. infusion	<5 min	30 min	Tachycardia, headache, nausea, flushing	Most hypertensive emergencies; caution with glaucoma
Nitroglycerin	5-100 mcg/min as I.V. infusion[3]	2-5 min	3-5 min	Headache, vomiting, methemoglobinemia, tolerance with prolonged use	Coronary ischemia
Enalaprilat	1.25-5 mg every 6 hours I.V.	15-30 min	6 h	Precipitous fall in pressure in high-renin states; response variable	Acute left ventricular failure; avoid in acute myocardial infarction
Hydralazine hydrochloride	10-20 mg I.V. 10-50 mg I.M.	10-20 min 20-30 min	3-8 h	Tachycardia, flushing, headache, vomiting, aggravation of angina	Eclampsia
Diazoxide	50-100 mg I.V. bolus repeated, or 15-30 mg/min infusion	2-4 min	6-12 h	Nausea, flushing, tachycardia, chest pain	Now obsolete; when no intensive monitoring available
Adrenergic Inhibitors					
Labetalol hydrochloride	20-80 mg I.V. bolus every 10 min; 0.5-2 mg/min I.V. infusion	5-10 min	3-6 h	Vomiting, scalp tingling, burning in throat, dizziness, nausea, heart block, orthostatic hypotension	Most hypertensive emergencies except acute heart failure
Esmolol hydrochloride	250-500 mcg/kg/min for 1 min, then 50-100 mcg/kg/min for 4 min; may repeat	1-2 min	10-20 min	Hypotension, nausea	Aortic dissection, perioperative
Phentolamine	5-15 mg I.V.	1-2 min	3-10 min	Tachycardia, flushing, headache	Catecholamine excess

[1]These doses may vary from those in the *Physicians' Desk Reference* (51st edition).

[2]Hypotension may occur with all agents.

[3]Require special delivery system.

HYPERTENSION *(Continued)*

Resources

Guidelines

1999 World Health Organization-International Society of Hypertension Guidelines for the Management of Hypertension. Guidelines Subcommittee, *J Hypertens*, 1999, 17:151-83.

National High Blood Pressure Education Program Working Group on Hypertension Control in Children and Adolescents. Update on the 1987 Task Force Report on High Blood Pressure in Children and Adolescents: A Working Group Report From the National High Blood Pressure Education Program, *Pediatrics*, 1996, 98(4 Pt 1):649-58.

National High Blood Pressure Education Program Working Group. 1995 Update of the Working Group Reports on Chronic Renal Failure and Renovascular Hypertension, *Arch Intern Med*, 1996, 156:1938-47.

"The Sixth Report of the National Committee on Detection, Evaluation, and Treatment of High Blood Pressure (JNC-VI)," *Arch Intern Med*, 1997, 157:2413-46.

I.V. TO ORAL CONVERSION

1. **Consider drug class and indication. Conversion is acceptable only if the risk and benefit evaluation justifies conversion. Conversion should never be made only because of drug costs. The cost of failed therapy is much higher.**

   Assuming access is available, intravenous dosing rapidly produces effective serum concentrations, suitable when this benefit outweighs the risk of venous irritation/trauma, infection, and cost. Conversion from I.V. to oral is often dependent on the patient's specific clinical situation. As the clinical situation improves, oral administration may be acceptable. In general, changing the route of administration for a drug treating the patient's primary problem is to be approached with more caution than a drug which is a continuation of prior therapy.

2. **Consider pharmaceutical and pharmacokinetic issues.**

   Specifically, adjustments for bioavailability or to standard oral dosing must be made. It should be recognized that standard oral dosing is often a much lower total daily dose as compared to oral dosing (this is particularly true for some antibiotics. In addition, the patient must be able to ingest or receive the drug in the dosage form available. Drugs not available in a liquid dosage form may be difficult to convert.

3. **Consider the patient's ability to absorb drug.**

   The reliability of swallowing or enteral access should be considered. If the patient is receiving medications by an enteral access device such as an enteral feeding tube (eg, PEG, PEJ, or nasogastric), the function of these tubes should be assured. In addition, the functional status of the gastrointestinal tract must be evaluated. Obviously, NPO status normally precludes conversion to oral therapy. However, gastrointestinal motility should be assessed in all patients when a conversion is planned. The presence or suspicion of obstruction, use of multiple promotility agents, or problems with nausea/emesis should be assessed. Agents with complete absorption in ambulatory patients may not be well absorbed in acute illness. For patients receiving continuous enteral feedings, conversion should not be attempted until the patient has demonstrated an ability to tolerate feedings up to their goal rate. In addition, the presence or absence of diarrhea should be assessed as indicators of the patient's potential to absorb medications.

4. **Prospectively identify potential interferences with absorption.**

   Absorption of some medications may be dramatically altered in the presence of enteral feedings or specific electrolytes in the gastrointestinal tract. For example, sucralfate may reduce the absorption of fluoroquinolones to ineffective levels. In this instance, one may consider the replacement with an H_2 antagonist to eliminate potential interferences or selection of comparable nonquinolone antibiotic coverage. Other drug binding agents include bile acid sequestrants and activated charcoal.

5. **Monitoring**

   With any change in the route of administration, consider that a recurrence may require reconsideration of the route.

SPECIFIC MEDICATION GROUPS

Antibiotics

May be readily converted to oral therapy in most situations. Most institutions encourage evaluation of an initial response (3- to 5-day period) prior to oral therapy. In most cases, a lack of clinical improvement over the evaluation period or a recent change in the status should delay prompting to oral therapy.

I.V. TO ORAL CONVERSION *(Continued)*

I.V. Agent	Usual I.V. Dose	Oral Agent	Common Oral Dose
Ampicillin	1 g q6h	Amoxicillin	500 mg q6h†
Ampicillin/ Sulbactam	1.5-3 g q6h	Amoxicillin/ clavulanate	500 mg q8h or 875 mg q12h
Azithromycin	500 mg qd		250 mg qd
Cefazolin	1 g q8h	Cephalexin	500 mg q6h
Cefuroxime	750 mg q8h	Cefuroxime axetil	250-500 mg q12h*†
Ciprofloxacin	400-600 mg q12h		500-750 mg q12h
Clindamycin	300-600 mg q8h		300-450 mg orally q6h
Co-trimoxazole	7.5-20 mg/kg		Equivalent # tablets (divide q6h or q12h)
Doxycycline	100 mg q12h		100 mg q12h
Erythromycin	500-1000 mg q6h		500 mg q6h
Fluconazole	100 mg qd		100 mg qd
Gatifloxacin	200-400 mg q24h		200-400 mg q24h
Levofloxacin	500 mg q24h		500 mg q24h
Metronidazole	500 mg q8-12h		500 mg q8h or 250 mg q6h
Ofloxacin	200-400 mg q12h		200-400 mg q12h
Trovafloxacin	100-200 mg qd		100-200 mg qd

*Poor oral absorption.

†Oral dose represents dose reduction.

Others

- H_2 antagonists – generally converted 1:1 to equivalent dose and scheduled orally.
- Methylprednisolone – may be converted to oral prednisone (each 4 mg methylprednisolone = 5 mg prednisone).
- Aminophylline – must be calculated based on infusion rate. However, a simple conversion calculation is possible: dose in mg/h x 10 = dose of sustained release product to be given every 12 hours (ie, a typical infusion of 30 mg/h = 300 mg of sustained release theophylline q12h or 150 mg q6h of nonsustained release product.

OBESITY TREATMENT GUIDELINES FOR ADULTS

Summary of Clinical Practice Guidelines

National Heart, Lung, and Blood Institute, June 1998

Note: Weight loss treatment for children and adolescents are not covered by these guidelines.

ASSESSMENT

Assessment of weight involves evaluating body mass index, waist circumference, and the patient's risk factors

A. Body mass Index (BMI)

1. BMI should be calculated for all adults (see table). Those with normal BMI should be reassessed in 2 years. A very muscular person may have a high BMI without the additional health risks.
2. Overweight is defined as a BMI of 25-29.9 kg/m^2.
3. Obesity is defined as a BMI of ≥30 kg/m^2

B. Abdominal Fat

1. Excess abdominal fat, not proportional to total body fat, is an independent predictor for risk and morbidity.
2. Waist circumference for men >40 inches or women >35 inches is an increased risk for those with a BMI of 25-34.9.

C. Risk Factors

1. Coronary heart disease or other atherosclerotic diseases, type 2 diabetes, and sleep apnea are factors associated with a very high risk of developing disease complications and mortality.
2. Other obesity-associated diseases: Gynecological abnormalities, osteoarthritis, gallstones, stress incontinence
3. Cardiovascular risk factors: Cigarette smoking, hypertension, high-risk LDL-cholesterol, low HDL-cholesterol, impaired fasting glucose, family history of premature CHD
4. Other risk factors: Physical inactivity, high serum triglycerides

   Weight loss is recommended for those who are obese and for those who are classified as overweight or have a high waist circumference and two or more risk factors.

Body Mass Index (BMI), kg/m^2
Height (feet, inches)

Weight (lb)	5'0"	5'3"	5'6"	5'9"	6'0"	6'3"
140	27	25	23	21	19	18
150	29	27	24	22	20	19
160	31	28	26	24	22	20
170	33	30	28	25	23	21
180	35	32	29	27	25	23
190	37	34	31	28	26	24
200	39	36	32	30	27	25
210	41	37	34	31	29	26
220	43	39	36	33	30	28
230	45	41	37	34	31	29
240	47	43	39	36	33	30
250	49	44	40	37	34	31

OBESITY TREATMENT GUIDELINES FOR ADULTS *(Continued)*

TREATMENT

Patients who are overweight or obese, but are not candidates for weight loss or do not wish to lose weight, should be counseled to avoid further weight gain.

A. Goals of Treatment

1. Prevent further weight gain.
2. Reduce body weight. The initial goal is to reduce body weight by 10% from baseline over the suggested time period of 6 months.
3. Maintain a lower body weight, long term.

B. Nonpharmacologic treatment should include:

1. An individually-planned diet which includes a decrease in fat as well as total calories.
2. An increase in physical activity. Physical activity should be gradually increased to a goal of 30 minutes per day of moderate-intensity activity.
3. Behavior therapy, which should include tools to help overcome individual barriers to weight loss.

Nonpharmacologic treatment should be tried for 6 months before starting physician-prescribed drug therapy.

C. Drug Therapy

In select patients with BMI ≥30, or BMI ≥27 with 2 or more risk factors, who did not lose weight or maintain weight loss, drug therapy can be started along with dietary therapy and physical activity.

D. Surgery

Patients with severe clinical obesity, BMI ≥40 or BMI ≥35 with coexisting conditions, can be considered for weight loss surgery when other methods have failed. Lifelong surveillance after surgery is necessary.

Medications for the Treatment of Obesity

Generic (Trade) Name	Therapeutic Category / Mechanism of Action	Usual Adult Dosage
Orlistat (Xenical®)	Lipase inhibitor; a reversible inhibitor of gastric and pancreatic lipases thus inhibiting absorption of dietary fats by 30% (at doses of 120 mg 3 times/day)	120 mg 3 times/day with each main meal containing fat (during or up to 1 hour after the meal); omit dose if meal is occasionally missed or contains no fat.
Amphetamine	The amphetamines are noncatecholamine sympathomimetic amines with CNS stimulant activity. The anorexigenic effect is probably secondary to the CNS-stimulating effect; the site of action is probably the hypothalamic feeding center.	Long-acting capsule: 10 or 15 mg/day, up to 30 mg/day; Immediate release tablets: 5-30 mg/day in divided doses
Benzphetamine (Didrex®)	Anorexiant; noncatechol sympathomimetic amines with pharmacologic actions similar to ephedrine; anorexigenic effect is probably secondary to the CNS-stimulating effect; the site of action is probably the hypothalamic feeding center	25-50 mg 2-3 times/day, preferably twice daily (midmorning and midafternoon); maximum dose: 50 mg 3 times/day
Diethylpropion (Tenuate®; Tenuate® Dospan®)	Anorexiant; pharmacological and chemical properties similar to those of amphetamines. The mechanism of action of diethylpropion in reducing appetite appears to be secondary to CNS effects, specifically stimulation of the hypothalamus to release catecholamines into the central nervous system; anorexiant effects are mediated via norepinephrine and dopamine metabolism. An increase in physical activity and metabolic effects (inhibition of lipogenesis and enhancement of lipolysis) may also contribute to weight loss.	Tablet: 25 mg 3 times/day before meals or food Tablet, controlled release: 75 mg at midmorning

Medications for the Treatment of Obesity *(continued)*

Generic (Trade) Name	Therapeutic Category / Mechanism of Action	Usual Adult Dosage
Mazindol (Mazanor®, Sanorex®)	Anorexiant; an isoindole with pharmacologic activity similar to amphetamine; produces CNS stimulation in humans and animals and appears to work primarily in the limbic system	Initial dose: 1 mg once daily and adjust to patient response; usual dose: 1 mg 3 times/day, 1 hour before meals, or 2 mg once daily, 1 hour before lunch; take with meals to avoid GI discomfort
Methamphetamine (Desoxyn®)	A sympathomimetic amine related to ephedrine and amphetamine with CNS stimulant activity	5 mg, 30 minutes before each meal; long-acting formulation: 10-15 mg in morning; treatment duration should not exceed a few weeks
Phentermine (Adipex-P®, Fastin®, Ionamin®, Zantryl®)	Anorexiant; structurally similar to dextroamphetamine and is comparable to dextroamphetamine as an appetite suppressant, but is generally associated with a lower incidence and severity of CNS side effects. Stimulates the hypothalamus to result in decreased appetite; anorexiant effects are most likely mediated via norepinephrine and dopamine metabolism. However, other CNS effects or metabolic effects may be involved.	8 mg 3 times/day 30 minutes before meals or food or 15-37.5 mg/day before breakfast or 10-14 hours before retiring
Sibutramine (Meridia™)	Anorexiant; blocks the neuronal uptake of norepinephrine and, to a lesser extent, serotonin and dopamine	Initial: 10 mg once daily; after 4 weeks may titrate up to 15 mg once daily as needed and tolerated

OSTEOPOROSIS MANAGEMENT

PREVALENCE

Osteoporosis effects 25 million Americans of which 80% are women; 27% of American women >80 years of age have osteopenia and 70% of American women >80 years of age have osteoporosis.

CONSEQUENCES

1.3 million bone fractures annually (low impact/nontraumatic) and pain, pulmonary insufficiency, decreased quality of life, and economic costs; >250,000 hip fractures per year with a 20% mortality rate.

RISK FACTORS

Advanced age, female, chronic renal disease, hyperparathyroidism, Cushing's disease, hypogonadism/anorexia, hyperprolactinemia, cancer, large and prolonged dose heparin or glucocorticoids, anticonvulsants, hyperthyroidism (current or history, or excessive thyroid supplements), sedentary, excessive exercise, early menopause, oophorectomy without hormone replacement, excessive aluminum-containing antacid, smoking, methotrexate.

DIAGNOSIS/MONITORING

DXA bone density, history of fracture (low impact or nontraumatic), compressed vertebrae, decreased height, hump-back appearance. Osteomark™ urine assay measures bone breakdown fragments and may help assess therapy response earlier than DXA but diagnostic value is uncertain as Osteomark™ doesn't reveal extent of bone loss. Bone markers may be tested to evaluate effectiveness of antiresorptive urine therapy.

PREVENTION

1. Adequate dietary calcium (eg, dairy products)
2. Vitamin D (eg, fortified dairy products, cod, fatty fish)
3. Weight-bearing exercise (eg, walking) as tolerated
4. Calcium supplement of 1000-1500 mg elemental calcium daily (divided in 500 mg increments); women >65 years on estrogen replacement therapy supplement 1000 mg elemental calcium; women >65 not receiving estrogens and men >55 years supplement 1500 mg elemental calcium. To minimize constipation add fiber and start with 500 mg/day for several months, then increase to 500 mg twice daily taken at different times than fiber. Chewable and liquid products are available. Calcium carbonate is given with food to enhance bioavailability. Calcium citrate may be given without regards to meals.
   - Contraindications: Hypercalcemia, ventricular fibrillation
   - Side effects: Constipation, anorexia
   - Drug interactions: Fiber, tetracycline, iron supplement, minerals
5. Vitamin D Supplement: 400-800 units daily (often satisfied by 1-2 multivitamins or fortified milk) in addition to calcium or a combined calcium and vitamin D supplement and/or >15 minutes direct sunlight/day. Some elderly, especially with significant renal or liver disease can't metabolize (activate) vitamin D and require calcitriol 0.25 mcg orally twice daily or adjusted per serum calcium level, the active form of vitamin D; can check 1,25 OH vitamin D level to confirm need for calcitriol.
   - Contraindications: Hypercalcemia (weakness, headache, drowsiness, nausea, diarrhea), hypercalciuria and renal stones
   - Side effects (uncommon): Hypercalcemia (see above)
   - Monitor 24-hour urine and serum calcium if using >1000 units/day
6. Estrogen: Especially useful if bone density <80% of average plus symptoms of estrogen deficiency or cardiac disease. Bone density increases over 1-2 years then plateaus. This is considered 1st line therapy unless contraindicated due to medicinal history (see below) or risk:benefit assessment which leads to decision to avoid HRT (hormone replacement therapy). **Note:** Estrogens should not be used to prevent coronary heart disease.

- Contraindications: Pregnancy, breast or estrogen-dependent cancer, undiagnosed abnormal genital bleeding, active thrombophlebitis, or history of thromboembolism during previous estrogen or oral contraceptive therapy or pregnancy. Pretreatment mammogram, gynecological exam are advised along with routine breast exam because of an increased risk of breast cancer with long-term use.
- Dose: Conjugated estrogen of 0.625 mg/day or its equivalent (continuous therapy preferred).
- Side effects: Vaginal spotting/bleeding, nausea, vomiting, breast tenderness/ enlargement, amenorrheic with extended use.
  Initiate therapy slowly (side effects are more common and severe in women without estrogen for many years). Administer with medroxyprogesterone acetate (MPA) 2.5-5 mg daily, or another oral progesterone, in women with uterus (unopposed estrogen can cause endometrial cancer). MPA can increase vaginal bleeding, increase weight, edema, mood changes.
- Drug Interactions: May increase corticosteroid effect, monitor for need to decrease corticosteroid dose.

7. Selective estrogen receptor modulators: Selective-estrogen receptor modulators (SERMs) are nonsteroidal modulators of estrogen-receptor mediated reactions. The key difference between these agents and estrogen replacement therapies is the potential to exert tissue specific effects. Due to their chemical differences, these agents retain some of estrogen's beneficial effects on bone metabolism and lipid levels, but differ in their actions on breast and endometrial tissues, potentially limiting adverse effects related to nonspecific hormone stimulation. Among the SERMs, tamoxifen retains stimulatory effects in endometrial tissue, while raloxifene does not stimulate endometrial or breast tissue, limiting the potential for endometrial or breast cancer related to this agent. Raloxifene is the only SERM which has been approved by the FDA for osteoporosis prevention.

   It should be noted that the effects on bone observed with SERMs appear to be less than that observed with estrogen replacement. In one study, the effect of raloxifene on hip bone mineral density was approximately half of that observed with conjugated estrogens. In addition, the effects on lipid profiles are less than with estrogen replacement. Finally, SERMs do not block the vasomotor effects observed with menopause, which may limit compliance with therapy. As with estrogen replacement, reloxifene has been associated with an increased risk of thromboembolism and is contraindicated in patients with a history of thromboembolic disease.

8. Estradiol, as well as various combination therapies, including ethinyl estradiol with norethindrone (Femhrt®) and ethinyl with norgestimate (Ortho-Prefest™), have been approved for the prevention of osteoporosis.

TREATMENT

1. Calcium, vitamin D, exercise, and estrogen: As above
2. Bisphosphonates:

   Consider if patient is intolerant of, or refuses estrogen or it is contraindicated, especially if severe osteoporosis (ie, ≥2.5 standard deviations below average young adult bone density, T-score, or history of low impact or nontraumatic fracture). Increasing bone density of hip and spine observed for at least 3 years (ie, no plateau as seen with estrogen).

   Contraindications: Hypocalcemia, not advised if existing gastrointestinal disorders (eg, esophageal disorders such as reflux, sensitive stomach).

   - Alendronate (Fosamax®): Dose: 10 mg once daily or 70 mg/week (treatment dose for osteoporosis; not recommended if creatinine clearance <35 mL/ minute). Osteopenia: 5 mg per day or 35 mg/week for prevention.
   - Risedronate (Actonel®: Dose: 5 mg daily or 35 mg/week for treatment or prevention

   Take before breakfast on an empty stomach with 6-8 ounces tap water (not mineral water, coffee, or juice) and remain upright or raise head of bed for bedridden patients at least 30 degree angle for at least 30 minutes (otherwise may cause ulcerative esophagitis) before eating or drinking.

   Therapy with calcium and vitamin D is advised, but must be given at a different time of day than alendronate.

   - Side effects (well tolerated): Difficulty swallowing, heartburn, abdominal discomfort, nausea (GI side effects increase with aspirin products), arthralgia/ myalgia, constipation, diarrhea, headache, esophagitis.
   - Drug interactions: None known to date.

OSTEOPOROSIS MANAGEMENT *(Continued)*

3. Etidronate: Not FDA approved for postmenopausal osteoporosis and can decrease the quality of bone formation, therefore, change to alendronate.
4. Calcitonin (nasal; Miacalcin®): Indicated if estrogen refused, intolerant, or contraindicated. Potential analgesic effect.
   - Contraindications: Hypersensitivity to salmon protein or gelatin diluent; 1 spray (200 units) into 1 nostril daily (alternate right and left nostril daily); 5 days on and 2 days off is also effective; alternate day administration not effective. If used only for pain, can decrease dose once pain is controlled.
   - Side effects (few): Nasal dryness and irritation (periodically inspect); adequate dietary or supplemental calcium + vitamin D is essential.

   Subcutaneous route (100 units daily): Many side effects (eg, nausea, flushing, anorexia) and the discomfort/inconvenience of injection.
5. Fall prevention: Minimize psychoactive and cardiovascular drugs (monitor BP for orthostasis), give diuretics early in the day, environmental safety check.

	% Elemental Calcium	Elemental Calcium
Calcium gluconate (various)	9	500 mg = 45 mg
Calcium glubionate (Neo-Calglucon®)	6.5	1.8 g = 115 g/5 mL
Calcium lactate (various)	13	325 mg = 42.25 mg
Calcium citrate (Citrical®)	21	950 mg = 200 mg
Effervescent tabs (Citrical Liquitab®)		2376 mg = 500 mg
Calcium acetate		
Phos-Ex 250®	25	1000 mg = 250 mg
Phos-Lo®		667 mg = 169 mg
Tricalcium phosphate (Posture®)	39	1565.2 mg = 600 mg
Calcium carbonate		
Tums®	40	1.2 g = 500 mg
Oscal-500® oral suspension		1.2 g/5 mL = 500 mg
Caltrate 600®		1.5 g = 600 mg

References

Ashworth L, "Focus on Alendronate. A Nonhormonal Option for the Treatment of Osteoporosis in Postmenopausal Women," *Formulary*, 1996, 31:23-30.

Johnson SR, "Should Older Women Use Estrogen Replacement," *J Am Geriatr Soc*, 1996, 44:89-90.

Liberman UA, Weiss SR, and Brool J, "Effect of Oral Alendronate on Bone-Mineral Density and the Incidence of Fracture in Postmenopausal Osteoporosis," *N Engl J Med*, 1995, 333:1437-43.

"New Drugs for Osteoporosis," *Med Lett Drugs Ther*, 1996, 38:1-3.

NIH Consensus Development Panel on Optimal Calcium Intake, *JAMA*, 1994, 272:1942-8.

PHARMACOTHERAPY OF URINARY INCONTINENCE

Incontinence Type	Drug Class	Drug Therapy	Adverse Effects and Precautions	Comments
Urge incontinence	Anticholinergic agents	Oxybutynin (2.5-5 mg bid-qid or extended release 5-20 mg qd), propantheline (7.5-30 mg at least tid), dicyclomine (10-20 mg tid)	Dry mouth, visual disturbances, constipation, dry skin, confusion	Anticholinergics are the first-line drug therapy (oxybutynin is preferred); propantheline is a second-line therapy
		Tolterodine (1-2 mg bid; extended release capsule: 2-4 mg once daily)	Dry mouth, visual disturbances, constipation, dry skin, confusion	**Note:** Tolterodine was not included in practice guideline; no comment may be made concerning placement in therapy
	Tricyclic antidepressants (TCAs)	Imipramine, desipramine, nortriptyline (25-100 mg/day)	Anticholinergic effects (as above), orthostatic hypotension, and cardiac dysrhythmia	TCAs are generally reserved for patients with an additional indication (eg, depression, neuralgia) at an initial dose of 10-25 mg 1-3 times/day
Stress incontinence	Alpha-adrenergic agonists	Pseudoephedrine (15-60 mg tid)	Anxiety, insomnia, agitation, respiratory difficulty, sweating, cardiac dysrhythmia, hypertension, tremor; should not be used in obstructive syndromes and/or hypertension	PPA (preferred) or pseudoephedrine are first-line therapy for women with no contraindication (notably hypertension)
Stress or combined urge/stress incontinence	Estrogen replacement agents	Conjugated estrogens (0.3-0.625 mg/day orally or 1 g vaginal cream at bedtime)	Should not be used if suspected or confirmed breast or endometrial cancer, active or past thromboembolism with past oral contraceptive, estrogen, or pregnancy; headache, spotting, edema, breast tenderness, possible depression	Estrogen (oral or vaginal) is an adjunctive therapy for postmenopausal women as it augments alpha-agonists such as PPA or pseudoephedrine
			Give progesterone with estrogen if uterus is present; pretreatment/periodic mammogram, gynecologic, breast exam advised	Progestin (eg, medroxyprogesterone 2.5-10 mg/day) continuously or intermittently; combined oral or vaginal estrogen and PPA in postmenopausal women if single drug is inadequate; imipramine is an alternative therapy when first-line therapy is inadequate
	Imipramine (10-25 mg tid)		May worsen cardiac conduction abnormalities, postural hypotension, anticholinergic effects	
Overflow	Alpha-adrenergic antagonists	Terazosin (1 mg at bedtime with first dose in supine position and increase by 1 mg every 4 days to 5 mg/day)	Postural hypotension, dizziness, vertigo, heart palpitations, edema, headache, anticholinergic effects	Possible benefit in men with obstructive symptoms of benign prostatic hyperplasia; monitor postural vital signs with first dose/each dose increase; may worsen female stress incontinence
		Doxazosin (1 mg at bedtime with first dose in supine position and increase by 1 mg every 7-14 days to 5 mg/day)	Same as terazosin (may be smaller incidence of hypotension)	Same as terazosin

"Urinary Incontinence," *Clinical Practice Guideline* , 1996, American Medical Directors Association, reprinted with permission. For more information call 1-800-876-2632.

SEIZURE TREATMENT

Seizure Type	Age	Commonly Used	Alternatives
Primary generalized tonic-clonic	1 mo - 6 y	Carbamazepine, phenytoin, phenobarbital	Valproate
	6-11 y	Carbamazepine	Valproate, phenytoin, phenobarbital, lamotrigine, primidone
Primary generalized tonic-clonic with absence or with myoclonic	1 mo - 18 y	Valproate	Phenytoin, phenobarbital, carbamazepine, primidone
Partial seizures (with or without secondary generalization)	1-12 mo	Phenobarbital	Carbamazepine, phenytoin
	1-6 y	Carbamazepine	Phenytoin, phenobarbital, valproate, lamotrigine, gabapentin, oxcarbazepine (>4 y), primidone
	>6 y	Carbamazepine	Lamotrigine, levetiracetam, oxcarbazepine, phenytoin, phenobarbital, tiagabine, topiramate, valproate, primidone, zonisamide (>16 y)
Absence seizures	<10 y	Ethosuximide, valproate	Clonazepam, acetazolamide, lamotrigine
	>10 y	Valproate	Ethosuximide, acetazolamide, clonazepam
Juvenile myoclonic		Valproate	Phenobarbital, primidone, clonazepam; consider: carbamazepine, phenytoin, acetazolamide
Progressive myoclonic		Valproate	Valproate plus clonazepam, phenobarbital
Lennox-Gastaut and related syndromes		Valproate	lamotrigine, phenobarbital, clonazepam, ethosuximide; consider: steroids, ketogenic diet
Infantile spasms		ACTH, steroids	Valproate; consider: clonazepam, vigabatrin, pyridoxine
Neonatal seizures		Phenobarbital	Phenytoin; consider: clonazepam, primidone, valproate, pyridoxine

TREATMENT OF SEXUALLY-TRANSMITTED DISEASES

Type or Stage	Drug of Choice	Alternatives
CHLAMYDIAL INFECTION AND RELATED CLINICAL SYNDROMES[1]		
Urethritis, cervicitis, conjunctivitis, or proctitis (except lymphogranuloma venereum)		
	Azithromycin 1 g oral once **or** Doxycycline[2,3] 100 mg oral bid x 7 d	Ofloxacin[3] 300 mg oral bid x 7 d **or** Erythromycin[4] 500 mg oral qid x 7 d **or** Erythromycin ethylsuccinate 800 mg oral qid x 7 d **or** Levofloxacin 500 mg oral qd x 7 d
Recurrent/persistent		
	Metronidazole 2 g oral **plus** Erythromycin 500 mg oral qid x 7 d **or** Erythromycin ethylsuccinate 800 mg oral qid x 7 d	
Infection in pregnancy		
	Amoxicillin 500 mg oral tid x 7 d **or** Erythromycin[4] 500 mg oral qid x 7 d	Azithromycin[5] 1 g oral once **or** Erythromycin base 250 mg oral qid x 14 d **or** Erythromycin ethylsuccinate 800 mg oral qid x 7 d **or** Erythromycin ethylsuccinate 400 mg oral qid x 14 d
Neonatal		
Ophthalmia	Erythromycin (base or ethylsuccinate) 12.5 mg/kg oral qid x 10-14 d	
Pneumonia	Erythromycin (base or ethylsuccinate) 12.5 mg/kg oral or I.V. qid x 14 d	
Lymphogranuloma venereum		
	Doxycycline[2,3] 100 mg oral bid x 21 d	Erythromycin[4] 500 mg oral qid x 21 d
GONORRHEA[6]		
Urethral, cervical, rectal, or pharyngeal		
	Cefixime 400 mg oral once **or** Ceftriaxone 125 mg I.M. once **or** Ciprofloxacin[3] 500 mg oral once **or** Ofloxacin[3] 400 mg oral once **plus** (if chlamydial infection is not ruled out) Azithromycin 1 g oral once **or** Doxycycline 100 mg oral bid x 7 d	Spectinomycin 2 g I.M. once[7] **or** Lomefloxacin 400 mg oral once **or** Norfloxacin 800 mg oral once **or** Gatifloxacin 400 mg oral once

TREATMENT OF SEXUALLY-TRANSMITTED DISEASES *(Continued)*

Type or Stage	Drug of Choice	Alternatives
Disseminated gonococcal infection		
	Ceftriaxone 1 g I.M. or I.V. q24h	Cefotaxime 1 g I.V. q8h **or** Ceftizoxime 1 g I.V. q8h **or** **For persons allergic to β-lactam drugs:** Ciprofloxacin 500 mg I.V. q12h **or** Levofloxacin 250 mg I.V. once daily **or** Ofloxacin 400 mg I.V. q12h **or** Spectinomycin 2 g I.M. q12h All regimens should be continued for 24-48 hours after improvement begins, at which time therapy may be switched to one of the following regimens to complete a full week of antimicrobial therapy: Cefixime 400 mg oral bid **or** Ciprofloxacin 500 mg oral bid **or** Levofloxacin 500 mg oral once daily **or** Ofloxacin 400 mg oral bid
Gonococcal meningitis and endocarditis		
	Ceftriaxone 1-2 g I.V. q12h	
EPIDIDYMITIS		
Most likely caused by enteric organisms, or in patients allergic to cephalosporins and/or tetracyclines		
	Ofloxacin 300 mg bid x 10 d **or** Levofloxacin 500 mg oral once daily x 10 d	
Most likely caused by gonorrhea or chlamydial		
	Ceftriaxone 250 mg I.M. once **followed by** Doxycycline[2] 100 mg oral bid x 10 d	
PELVIC INFLAMMATORY DISEASE		
– Inpatients	**Parenteral Regimen A** Cefotetan 2 g I.V. q12h **or** Cefoxitin 2 g I.V. q6h **plus** Doxycycline 100 mg oral or I.V. q12h (see Note) **Parenteral Regimen B** Clindamycin 900 mg I.V. q8h **plus** Gentamicin loading dose I.V. or I.M. (2 mg/kg of body weight) followed by maintenance dose (1.5 mg/kg) q8h. Single daily dosing may be substituted. **Note:** Because of pain associated with infusion, doxycycline should be administered orally when possible, even when the patient is hospitalized. Both oral and I.V. administration of doxycycline provide similar bioavailability. Parenteral therapy may be discontinued 24 hours after a patient improves clinically, and oral therapy with doxycycline (100 mg twice daily) should continue to complete 14 days of therapy. When tubo-ovarian abscess is present, many healthcare providers use clindamycin or metronidazole with doxycycline for continued therapy rather than doxycycline alone, because it provides more effective anaerobic coverage.	Ofloxacin 400 mg I.V. q12h **or** Levofloxacin 500 mg I.V. once daily **with or without** Metronidazole 500 mg I.V. q8h **or** Ampicillin/sulbactam 3 g I.V. q6h **plus** Doxycycline 100 mg oral or I.V. q12h

Type or Stage	Drug of Choice	Alternatives
– Outpatients	**Regimen A** Ofloxacin 400 mg oral bid x 14 d **or** Levofloxacin 500 mg oral once daily x 14 d **with or without** Metronidazole 500 mg oral bid x 14 d **Regimen B** Ceftriaxone 250 mg I.M. once **or** Cefoxitin 2 g I.M. once and Probenecid 1 g oral once administered concurrently **or** Other parenteral 3rd generation cephalosporin (eg, ceftizoxime or cefotaxime) **plus** Doxycycline 100 mg oral bid x 14 d **with or without** Metronidazole 500 mg oral bid x 14 d If the healthcare provider prescribes outpatient oral or parenteral therapy, a follow-up examination should be performed within 72 hours using the criteria for clinical improvement described previously. If the patient has not improved, hospitalization for parenteral therapy and further evaluation are recommended.	
VAGINAL INFECTION		
Trichomoniasis		
	Metronidazole 2 g oral once	Metronidazole 500 mg oral bid x 7 d
Bacterial vaginosis		
	Metronidazole 500 mg oral bid x 7 d **or** Metronidazole gel 0.75% 5 g intravaginally once or twice daily x 5 d **or** Clindamycin 2% cream 5 g intravaginally qhs x 3-7 d	Clindamycin 100 g intravaginally at bedtime x 3 d **or** Clindamycin 300 mg oral bid x 7 d **or** Metronidazole 2 g oral once[8]
Vulvovaginal candidiasis		
	Intravaginal butoconazole, clotrimazole, miconazole, terconazole, or tioconazole[9] **or** Fluconazole 150 mg oral once	Nystatin 100,000 unit vaginal tablet once daily x 14 d
SYPHILIS		
Early (primary, secondary, or latent <1 y)		
	Penicillin G benzathine 2.4 million units I.M. once[10]	Doxycycline[3] 100 mg oral bid x 14 d **or** Tetracycline 500 mg oral qid x 24 d
Late (>1 year's duration, cardiovascular, gumma, late-latent)		
	Penicillin G benzathine 2.4 million units I.M. weekly x 3 wk	Doxycycline[3] 100 mg oral bid x 4 wk
Neurosyphilis[11]		
	Penicillin G 3-4 million units I.V. q4h x 10-14 d	Penicillin G procaine 2.4 million units I.M. daily, **plus** Probenecid 500 mg qid oral, both x 10-14 d
Congenital		
	Penicillin G 50,000 units/kg I.V. q8-12h (q12h during first 7 d of life, then q8h for total of 10 d) **or** Penicillin G procaine 50,000 units/kg I.M. daily for 10 d	

TREATMENT OF SEXUALLY-TRANSMITTED DISEASES *(Continued)*

Type or Stage	Drug of Choice	Alternatives
CHANCROID[12]		
	Azithromycin 1 g oral once **or** Ceftriaxone 250 mg I.M. once **or** Ciprofloxacin[3] 500 mg oral bid x 3 d **or** Erythromycin[4] 500 mg oral qid x 7 d	
GENITAL HERPES		
First episode		
	Acyclovir 400 mg oral tid x 7-10 d[13] **or** Famciclovir 250 mg oral tid x 7-10 d **or** Valacyclovir 1 g oral bid x 7-10 d	Acyclovir 200 mg oral 5 times/d x 7-10 d[13]
Recurrent[14]		
	Acyclovir 400 mg oral tid x 5 d **or** Famciclovir 125 mg oral bid x 5 d **or** Valacyclovir 500 mg oral bid x 5 d	Acyclovir 200 mg orally 5 times/day for 5 d **or** Acyclovir 800 mg oral bid x 5 d
Severe (hospitalized patients)		
	Acyclovir 5-10 mg/kg I.V. q8h x 5-7 d	
Suppression of recurrence[15]		
	Valacyclovir 500 mg - 1 g once daily[16] **or** Acyclovir 400 mg oral bid **or** Famciclovir 250 mg oral bid	
GRANULOMA INGUINALE		
	TMP-SMZ 1 double-strength tablet oral bid for a minimum of 3 wk **or** Doxycycline 100 oral bid for a minimum of 3 wk	Ciprofloxacin 750 mg oral bid for a minimum of 3 wk **or** Erythromycin base 500 mg oral qid for a minimum of 3 wk **or** Azithromycin 1 g oral once per week for minimum of 3 weeks

[1]Related clinical syndromes include nonchlamydial nongonococcal urethritis and cervicitis.
[2]Or tetracycline 500 mg oral qid or minocycline 100 mg oral bid.
[3]Contraindicated in pregnancy.
[4]Erythromycin estolate is contraindicated in pregnancy.
[5]Safety in pregnancy not established.
[6]All patients should also receive a course of treatment effective for *Chlamydia.*
[7]Recommended only for use during pregnancy in patients allergic to beta-lactams. Not effective for pharyngeal infection.
[8]Higher relapse rate with single dose, but useful for patients who may not comply with multiple-dose therapy.
[9]For preparations and dosage of topical products, see *Medical Letter*, 36:81,1994; single-dose therapy is not recommended.
[10]Some experts recommend repeating this regimen after 7 days, especially in patients with HIV infection.
[11]Patients allergic to penicillin should be desensitized.
[12]All regimens, especially single-dose ceftriaxone, are less effective in HIV-infected patients.
[13]For first-episode proctitis, use acyclovir 800 mg oral tid or 400 mg oral 5 times/day.
[14]Antiviral therapy is variably effective for treatment of recurrences; only effective if started early.
[15]Preventive treatment should be discontinued for 1-2 months once a year to reassess the frequency of recurrence.
[16]Use 500 mg qd in patients with <10 recurrences per year and 500 mg bid or 1 g daily in patients with ≥ 10 recurrences per year.

Adapted from "Sexually Transmitted Diseases Treatment Guidelines 2002," *MMWR Morb Mortal Wkly Rep*, 2002, 51(RR-6).

TUBERCULOSIS

TESTING

Tuberculin Skin Test Recommendations[1]

Children for whom immediate skin testing is indicated:

- Contacts of persons with confirmed or suspected infectious tuberculosis (contact investigation); this includes children identified as contacts of family members or associates in jail or prison in the last 5 years
- Children with radiographic or clinical findings suggesting tuberculosis
- Children immigrating from endemic countries (eg, Asia, Middle East, Africa, Latin America)
- Children with travel histories to endemic countries and/or significant contact with indigenous persons from such countries

Children who should be tested annually for tuberculosis[2]:

- Children infected with HIV or living in household with HIV-infected persons
- Incarcerated adolescents

Children who should be tested every 2-3 years[2]:

- Children exposed to the following individuals: HIV-infected, homeless, residents of nursing homes, institutionalized adolescents or adults, users of illicit drugs, incarcerated adolescents or adults, and migrant farm workers. Foster children with exposure to adults in the preceding high-risk groups are included.

Children who should be considered for tuberculin skin testing at ages 4-6 and 11-16 years:

- Children whose parents immigrated (with unknown tuberculin skin test status) from regions of the world with high prevalence of tuberculosis; continued potential exposure by travel to the endemic areas and/or household contact with persons from the endemic areas (with unknown tuberculin skin test status) should be an indication for repeat tuberculin skin testing
- Children without specific risk factors who reside in high-prevalence areas; in general, a high-risk neighborhood or community does not mean an entire city is at high risk; rates in any area of the city may vary by neighborhood, or even from block to block; physicians should be aware of these patterns in determining the likelihood of exposure; public health officials or local tuberculosis experts should help clinicians identify areas that have appreciable tuberculosis rates

Children at increased risk of progression of infection to disease: Those with other medical risk factors, including diabetes mellitus, chronic renal failure, malnutrition, and congenital or acquired immunodeficiencies deserve special consideration. Without recent exposure, these persons are not at increased risk of acquiring tuberculosis infection. Underlying immune deficiencies associated with these conditions theoretically would enhance the possibility for progression to severe disease. Initial histories of potential exposure to tuberculosis should be included on all of these patients. If these histories or local epidemiologic factors suggest a possibility of exposure, immediate and periodic tuberculin skin testing should be considered. An initial Mantoux tuberculin skin test should be performed before initiation of immunosuppressive therapy in any child with an underlying condition that necessitates immunosuppressive therapy.

---

[1]BCG immunization is not a contraindication to tuberculin skin testing.

[2]Initial tuberculin skin testing is at the time of diagnosis or circumstance, beginning as early as at age 3 months.

TUBERCULOSIS *(Continued)*

Changes From Prior Recommendations on Tuberculin Testing and Treatment of Latent Tuberculosis Infection (LTBI)

Tuberculin Testing

- Emphasis on targeted tuberculin testing among persons at high risk for recent LTBI or with clinical conditions that increase the risk for tuberculosis (TB), regardless of age; testing is discouraged among persons at lower risk.
- For patients with organ transplant and other immunosuppressed patients (eg, persons receiving the equivalent of ≥15 mg/day prednisone for 1 month or more), 5 mm of induration rather than 10 mm of induration as a cut-off level for tuberculin positivity.
- A tuberculin skin test conversion is defined as an increase of ≥10 mm of induration within a 2-year period, regardless of age.

Treatment of Latent Tuberculosis Infection

- For HIV-negative persons, isoniazid given for 9 months is preferred over 6-month regimens.
- For HIV-positive persons and those with fibrotic lesions on chest x-ray consistent with previous TB, isoniazid should be given for 9 months instead of 12 months.
- For HIV-negative and HIV-positive persons, rifampin and pyrazinamide should be given for 2 months.
- For HIV-negative and HIV-positive persons, rifampin should be given for 4 months.

Clinical and Laboratory Monitoring

- Routine baseline and follow-up laboratory monitoring can be eliminated in most persons with LTBI, except for those with HIV infection, pregnant women (or those in the immediate postpartum period), and persons with chronic liver disease or those who use alcohol regularly.
- Emphasis on clinical monitoring for signs and symptoms of possible adverse effects, with prompt evaluation and changes in treatment, as indicated.

Modified from *MMWR Morb Mortal Wkly Rep*, 2000, 49(RR-6).

Criteria for Tuberculin Positivity, by Risk Group

Reaction ≥5 mm of Induration	Reaction ≥10 mm of Induration	Reaction ≥15 mm of Induration
HIV-positive persons	Recent immigrants (ie, within the last 5 years) from high prevalence countries	Persons with no risk factors for TB
Recent contacts of tuberculosis (TB) case patients	Injection drug users	
Fibrotic changes on chest radiograph consistent with prior TB	Residents and employees[1] of the following high risk congregate settings: prisons and jails, nursing homes and other long-term facilities for the elderly, hospitals and other healthcare facilities, residential facilities for patients with AIDS, and homeless shelters	
Patients with organ transplant and other immunosuppressed patients (receiving the equivalent of ≥15 mg/day of prednisone for 1 month of more)[2]	Mycobacteriology laboratory personnel	
	Persons with the following clinical conditions that place them at high risk: silicosis, diabetes mellitus, chronic renal failure, some hematologic disorders (eg, leukemias and lymphomas), other specific malignancies (eg, carcinoma of the head or neck and lung), weight loss of ≥10% of ideal body weight, gastrectomy, and jejunoileal bypass	
	Children <4 years of age or infants, children, and adolescents exposed to adults at high-risk	

[1]For persons who are otherwise at low risk and are tested at the start of employment, a reaction of ≥15 mm induration is considered positive.

[2]Risk of TB in patients treated with corticosteroids increases with higher dose and longer duration.

Modified from *MMWR Morb Mortal Wkly Rep*, 2000, 49(RR-6).

Recommendations, Rankings, and Performance Indicators for Treatment of Patients With Tuberculosis (TB)

Recommendation	Ranking[1] (Evidence)[2]	Performance Indicator
Obtain bacteriologic confirmation and susceptibility testing for patients with TB or suspected of having TB	A (II)	90% of adults with or suspected of having TB have 3 cultures for mycobacteria obtained before initiation of antituberculosis therapy (50% of children 0-12 y)
Place persons with suspected or confirmed smear-positive pulmonary or laryngeal TB in respiratory isolation until noninfectious	A (II)	90% of persons with sputum smear-positive TB remain in respiratory isolation until smear converts to negative
Begin treatment of patients with confirmed or suspected TB disease with one of the following drug combinations, depending on local resistance patterns: INH + RIF + PZA **or** INH + RIF + PZA + EMB **or** INH + RIF + PZA + SM	A (III)	90% of all patients with TB are started on INH + RIF + PZA + EMB or SM in geographic areas where >4% of TB isolates are resistant to INH
Report each case of TB promptly to the local public health department	A (III)	100% of persons with active TB are reported to the local public health department within 1 week of diagnosis
Perform HIV testing for all patients with TB	A (III)	80% of all patients with TB have HIV status determined within 2 months of a diagnosis of TB
Treat patients with TB caused by a susceptible organism for 6 months, using an ATS/CDC-approved regimen	A (I)	90% of all patients with TB complete 6 months of therapy with 12 months of beginning treatment
Re-evaluate patients with TB who are smear positive at 3 months for possible nonadherence or infection with drug-resistant bacilli	A (III)	90% of all patients with TB who are smear positive at 3 months have sputum culture/susceptibility testing performed within 1 month of the 3-month visit
Add ≥2 new antituberculosis agents when TB treatment failure is suspected	A (II)	100% of patients with TB with suspected treatment failure are prescribed ≥2 new antituberculosis agents
Perform tuberculin skin testing on all patients with a history of ≥1 of the following: HIV infection, I.V. drug use, homelessness, incarceration, or contact with a person with pulmonary TB	A (II)	80% of persons in the indicated population groups receive tuberculin skin test and return for reading
Administer treatment for latent TB infection to all persons with latent TB infection, unless it can be documented that they received such treatment previously	A (I)	75% of patients with positive tuberculin skin tests who are candidates for treatment for latent TB infection complete a course of therapy within 12 months of initiation

Adapted from the Infectious Diseases Society of America, *Clinical Infectious Diseases,* 2000, 31:633-9.

Note: ATS/CDC = American Thoracic Society and Centers for Disease Control and Prevention; EMB = ethambutol; INH = isoniazid; PZA = pyrazinamide; RIF = rifampin; SM = streptomycin.

[1]Strength of recommendation: A = preferred; B = acceptable alternative; C = offer when A and B cannot be given.

[2]Quality of evidence: I = randomized clinical trial data; II = data from clinical trials that are not randomized or were conducted in other populations; III = expert opinion.

TUBERCULOSIS *(Continued)*

PROPHYLAXIS

Specific Circumstances/ Organism	Comments	Regimen
Category I. Exposure (Household members and other close contacts of potentially infectious cases) (Exposee tuberculin test negative)[1]		
Neonate	Rx essential	INH (10 mg/kg/d) for 3 months, then repeat tuberculin test (TBnT). If mother's smear negative and infant's TBnT negative and chest x-ray (CXR) are normal, stop INH. In the United Kingdom, BCG is then given (*Lancet*, 1990, 2:1479), unless mother is HIV-positive. If infant's repeat TBnT is positive and/or CXR abnormal (hilar adenopathy and/or infiltrate), administer INH + RIF (10-20 mg/kg/d) (or streptomycin) for a total of 6 months. If mother is being treated, separation from mother is not indicated.
Children <5 y	Rx indicated	As for neonate first 3 months. If repeat TBnT is negative, stop. If repeat TBnT is positive, continue INH for a total of 9 months. If INH is not given initially, repeat TBnT at 3 months; if positive, treat with INH for 9 months (see Category II below).
Older children and adults	No Rx	Repeat TBnT at 3 months, if positive, treat with INH for 6 months (see Category II below)
Category II. Infection Without Disease (Positive tuberculin test)[1]		
Regardless of age (see INH Preventive Therapy)	Rx indicated	INH (5 mg/kg/d, maximum: 300 mg/d for adults, 10 mg/kg/d not to exceed 300 mg/d for children). Results with 6 months of treatment are nearly as effective as 12 months (65% vs 75% reduction in disease). *Am Thoracic Society* (6 months), *Am Acad Pediatrics*, 1991 (9 months). If CXR is abnormal, treat for 12 months. In HIV-positive patient, treatment for a minimum of 12 months, some suggest longer. Monitor transaminases monthly (*MMWR Morb Mortal Wkly Rep* 1989, 38:247).
Age <35 y	Rx indicated	Reanalysis of earlier studies favors INH prophylaxis for 6 months (if INH-related hepatitis case fatality rate is <1% and TB case fatality is ≥6.7%, which appears to be the case, monitor transaminases monthly (*Arch Int Med*, 1990, 150:2517).
INH-resistant organisms likely	Rx indicated	Data on efficacy of alternative regimens is currently lacking. Regimens include ETB + RIF daily for 6 months. PZA + RIF daily for 2 months, then INH + RIF daily until sensitivities from index case (if available) known, then if INH-CR, discontinue INH and continue RIF for 9 months, otherwise INH + RIF for 9 months (this latter is *Am Acad Pediatrics*, 1991 recommendation).
INH + RIF resistant organisms likely	Rx indicated	Efficacy of alternative regimens is unknown; PZA (25-30 mg/kg/d P.O.) + ETB (15-25 mg/kg/d P.O.) (at 25 mg/kg ETB, monitoring for retrobulbar neuritis required), for 6 months unless HIV-positive, then 12 months; PZA + ciprofloxacin (750 mg P.O. bid) or ofloxacin (400 mg P.O. bid) x 6-12 months *(MMWR Morb Mortal Wkly Rep*, 1992, 41(RR11):68).

INH = isoniazid; RIF = rifampin; KM = kanamycin; ETB = ethambutol.

SM = streptomycin; CXR = chest x-ray; Rx = treatment.

See also guidelines for interpreting PPD in "Skin Testing for Delayed Hypersensitivity."

[1]Tuberculin test (TBnT). The standard is the Mantoux test, 5 TU PPD in 0.1 mL diluent stabilized with Tween 80. Read at 48-72 hours measuring maximum diameter of induration. A reaction ≥5 mm is defined as positive in the following: positive HIV or risk factors, recent close case contacts, CXR consistent with healed TBc. ≥10 mm is positive in foreign-born in countries of high prevalence, injection drug users, low income populations, nursing home residents, patients with medical conditions which increase risk (see above, preventive treatment). ≥15 mm is positive in all others (*Am Rev Resp Dis*, 1990, 142:725). Two-stage TBnT: Use in individuals to be tested regularly (ie, healthcare workers). TBn reactivity may decrease over time but be boosted by skin testing. If unrecognized, individual may be incorrectly diagnosed as recent converter. If first TBnT is reactive but <10 mm, repeat 5 TU in 1 week, if then ≥10 mm = positive, not recent conversion (*Am Rev Resp Dis*, 1979, 119:587).

TREATMENT

Recommended Treatment Regimens for Drug-Susceptible Tuberculosis in Infants, Children, and Adolescents

Infection or Disease Category	Regimen	Remarks
Latent tuberculosis infection (positive skin test, no disease):		If daily therapy is not possible, therapy twice a week directly observed therapy may be used for 9 months. HIV-infected children should be treated for 9-12 months.
• Isoniazid-susceptible	9 months of isoniazid once daily	
• Isoniazid-resistant	6 months of rifampin once daily	
• Isoniazid-rifampin-resistant[1]	Consult a tuberculosis specialist	
Pulmonary	**6-Month Regimens** 2 months of isoniazid, rifampin, and pyrazinamide once daily, followed by 4 months of isoniazid and rifampin daily	If possible drug resistance is a concern (see text), another drug (ethambutol or streptomycin) is added to the initial 3-drug therapy until drug susceptibilities are determined.
	OR	
	2 months of isoniazid, rifampin, and pyrazinamide daily, followed by 4 months of isoniazid and rifampin twice a week	Drugs can be given 2 or 3 times per week under direct observation in the initial phase if nonadherence is likely.
	9-Month Alternative Regimens (for hilar adenopathy only) 9 months of isoniazid and rifampin once daily **OR** 1 month of isoniazid and rifampin once daily, followed by 8 months of isoniazid and rifampin twice a week	Regimens consisting of 6 months of isoniazid and rifampin once daily, and 1 month of isoniazid and rifampin once daily, followed by 5 months of isoniazid and rifampin directly observed therapy twice a week, have been successful in areas where drug resistance is rare.
Extrapulmonary meningitis, disseminated (miliary), bone/joint disease	2 months of isoniazid, rifampin, pyrazinamide, and streptomycin once daily, followed by 7-10 months of isoniazid and rifampin once daily (9-12 months total)	Streptomycin is given with initial therapy until drug susceptibility is known.
	OR	
	2 months of isoniazid, rifampin, pyrazinamide, and streptomycin once daily, followed by 7-10 months of isoniazid and rifampin twice a week (9-12 months total)	For patients who may have acquired tuberculosis in geographic areas where resistance to streptomycin is common, capreomycin (15-30 mg/kg/d) or kanamycin (15-30 mg/kg/d) may be used instead of streptomycin.
Other (eg, cervical lymphadenopathy)	Same as for pulmonary disease	See Pulmonary.

[1]Duration of therapy is longer in HIV-infected persons and additional drugs may be indicated.

Adapted from "Report of the Committee on Infectious Diseases," *2000 Red Book®*, 25th ed.

TUBERCULOSIS *(Continued)*

Commonly Used Drugs for the Treatment of Tuberculosis in Infants, Children, and Adolescents

Drugs	Dosage Forms	Daily Dose (mg/kg/d)	Twice a Week Dose (mg/kg per dose)	Maximum Dose	Adverse Reactions
Ethambutol	Tablets 100 mg 400 mg	15-25	50	2.5 g	Optic neuritis (usually reversible), decreased visual acuity, decreased red-green color discrimination, gastrointestinal disturbances, hypersensitivity
Isoniazid[1]	Scored tablets 100 mg 300 mg Syrup 10 mg/mL	10-15[2]	20-30	Daily, 300 mg Twice a week, 900 mg	Mild hepatic enzyme elevation, hepatitis,[2] peripheral neuritis, hypersensitivity
Pyrazinamide[1]	Scored tablets 500 mg	20-40	50	2 g	Hepatotoxicity, hyperuricemia
Rifampin[1]	Capsules 150 mg 300 mg Syrup formulated in syrup from capsules	10-20	10-20	600 mg	Orange discoloration of secretions/urine, staining contact lenses, vomiting, hepatitis, flu-like reaction, and thrombocytopenia; may render birth-control pills ineffective
Streptomycin (I.M. administration)	Vials 1 g 4 g	20-40	20-40	1 g	Auditory and vestibular toxicity, nephrotoxicity, rash

[1]Rifamate® is a capsule containing 150 mg of isoniazid and 300 mg of rifampin. Two capsules provide the usual adult (>50 kg body weight) daily doses of each drug. Rifater® is a capsule containing 50 mg of isoniazid, 120 mg of rifampin, and 300 mg of pyrazinamide.

[2]When isoniazid in a dosage exceeding 10 mg/kg/day is used in combination with rifampin, the incidence of hepatotoxicity may be increased.

Adapted from "Report of the Committee on Infectious Diseases," *2000 Red Book®*, 25th ed.

Rifampin is a bactericidal agent. It is metabolized by the liver and affects the pharmacokinetics of many other drugs, affecting their serum concentrations. Mycobacterium tuberculosis, initially resistant to rifampin, remains relatively uncommon in most areas of the United States. Rifampin is excreted in bile and urine and can cause orange urine, sweat and tears. It can also cause discoloration of soft contact lenses and render oral contraceptives ineffective. Hepatotoxicity occurs rarely. Blood dyscrasia accompanied by influenza-like symptoms can occur if doses are taken sporadically.

Less Commonly Used Drugs for Treatment of Drug-Resistant Tuberculosis in Infants, Children, and Adolescents[1]

Drugs	Dosage Forms	Daily Dose (mg/kg/d)	Maximum Dose	Adverse Reactions
Capreomycin	Vials 1 g	15-30 I.M.	1 g	Ototoxicity, nephrotoxicity
Ciprofloxacin[2]	Tablets 250 mg 500 mg 750 mg	Adults 500-1500 mg total per day (twice daily)	1.5 g	Theoretical effect on growing cartilage, gastrointestinal tract disturbances, rash, headache
Cycloserine	Capsules 250 mg	10-20	1 g	Psychosis, personality changes, seizures, rash
Ethionamide	Tablets 250 mg	15-20 given in 2-3 divided doses	1 g	Gastrointestinal tract disturbances, hepatotoxicity, hypersensitive reactions
Kanamycin	Vials 75 mg/2 mL 500 mg/2 mL 1 g/3 mL	15-30 I.M.	1 g	Auditory and vestibular toxic effects, nephrotoxicity
Levofloxacin[2]	Tablets 250 mg 500 mg Vials 25 mg/mL	Adults 500-1000 mg once daily	1 g	Theoretical effect on growing cartilage, gastrointestinal tract disturbances, rash, headache
Ofloxacin[2]	Tablets 200 mg 300 mg 400 mg	Adults 400-800 mg total per day (twice daily)	0.8 g	Theoretical effect on growing cartilage, gastrointestinal tract disturbances, rash, headache
Para-amino salicylic acid (PAS)	Tablets 500 mg	200-300 (3-4 times/day)	10 g	Gastrointestinal tract disturbances, hypersensitivity, hepatotoxicity

[1]These drugs should be used in consultation with a specialist in tuberculosis.

[2]Fluoroquinolones are not currently approved for use in persons <18 years; their use in younger patients necessitates assessment of the potential risks and benefits.

Adapted from "Report of the Committee on Infectious Diseases," *2000 Red Book*®, 25th ed.

TUBERCULOSIS *(Continued)*

TB Drugs in Special Situations

Drug	Pregnancy	CNS TB Disease	Renal Insufficiency
Isoniazid	Safe	Good penetration	Normal clearance
Rifampin	Safe	Fair penetration Penetrates inflamed meninges (10% to 20%)	Normal clearance
Pyrazinamide	Avoid	Good penetration	Clearance reduced Decrease dose or prolong interval
Ethambutol	Safe	Penetrates inflamed meninges only (4% to 64%)	Clearance reduced Decrease dose or prolong interval
Streptomycin	Avoid	Penetrates inflamed meninges only	Clearance reduced Decrease dose or prolong interval
Capreomycin	Avoid	Penetrates inflamed meninges only	Clearance reduced Decrease dose or prolong interval
Kanamycin	Avoid	Penetrates inflamed meninges only	Clearance reduced Decrease dose or prolong interval
Ethionamide	Do not use	Good penetration	Normal clearance
Para-aminosalicylic acid	Safe	Penetrates inflamed meninges only (10% to 50%)	Incomplete data on clearance
Cycloserine	Avoid	Good penetration	Clearance reduced Decrease dose or prolong interval
Ciprofloxacin	Do not use	Fair penetration (5% to 10%) Penetrates inflamed meninges (50% to 90%)	Clearance reduced Decrease dose or prolong interval
Ofloxacin	Do not use	Fair penetration (5% to 10%) Penetrates inflamed meninges (50% to 90%)	Clearance reduced Decrease dose or prolong interval
Amikacin	Avoid	Penetrates inflamed meninges only	Clearance reduced Decrease dose or prolong interval
Clofazimine	Avoid	Penetration unknown	Clearance probably normal

Safe = the drug has not been demonstrated to have teratogenic effects.

Avoid = data on the drug's safety are limited, or the drug is associated with mild malformations (as in the aminoglycosides).

Do not use = studies show an association between the drug and premature labor, congenital malformations, or teratogenicity.

Recommendations for Coadministering Different Antiretroviral Drugs With the Antimycobacterial Drugs Rifabutin and Rifampin

Antiretroviral	Use in Combination with Rifabutin	Use in Combination with Rifampin	Comments
Saquinavir[1]			
Hard-gel capsules (HGC)	Possibly[2], if antiretroviral regimen also includes ritonavir	Possibly, if antiretroviral regimen also includes ritonavir	Coadministration of saquinavir SGC with usual-dose rifabutin (300 mg/day or 2-3 times/week) is a possibility. However, the pharmacokinetic data and clinical experience for this combination are limited.
Soft-gel capsules (SGC)	Probably[3]	Possibly, if antiretroviral regimen also includes ritonavir	The combination of saquinavir SGC or saquinavir HGC and ritonavir, coadministered with 1) usual-dose rifampin (600 mg/day or 2-3 times/week), or 2) reduced-dose rifabutin (150 mg 2-3 times/week) is a possibility. However, the pharmacokinetic data and clinical experience for these combinations are limited. Coadministration of saquinavir or saquinavir SGC with rifampin is not recommended because rifampin markedly decreases concentrations of saquinavir.
Ritonavir	Probably	Probably	If the combination of ritonavir and rifabutin is used, then a substantially reduced-dose rifabutin regimen (150 mg 2-3 times/week) is recommended. Coadministration of ritonavir with usual-dose rifampin (600 mg/day or 2-3 times/week) is a possibility, though pharmacokinetic data and clinical experience are limited.
Indinavir	Yes	No	There is limited, but favorable, clinical experience with coadministration of indinavir[4] with a reduced daily dose of rifabutin (150 mg) or with the usual dose of rifabutin (300 mg 2-3 times/week). Coadministration of indinavir with rifampin is not recommended because rifampin markedly decreases concentrations of indinavir.
Nelfinavir	Yes	No	There is limited, but favorable, clinical experience with coadministration of nelfinavir[5] with a reduced daily dose of rifabutin (150 mg) or with the usual dose of rifabutin (300 mg 2-3 times/week). Coadministration of nelfinavir with rifampin is not recommended because rifampin markedly decreases concentrations of nelfinavir.
Amprenavir	Yes	No	Coadministration of amprenavir with a reduced daily dose of rifabutin (150 mg) or with the usual dose of rifabutin (300 mg 2-3 times/week) is a possibility, but there is no published clinical experience. Coadministration of amprenavir with rifampin is not recommended because rifampin markedly decreases concentrations of amprenavir.

TUBERCULOSIS *(Continued)*

Recommendations for Coadministering Different Antiretroviral Drugs With the Antimycobacterial Drugs Rifabutin and Rifampin *(continued)*

Antiretroviral	Use in Combination with Rifabutin	Use in Combination with Rifampin	Comments
Nevirapine	Yes	Possibly	Coadministration of nevirapine with usual-dose rifabutin (300 mg/day or 2-3 times/week) is a possibility based on pharmacokinetic study data. However, there is no published clinical experience for this combination. Data are insufficient to assess whether dose adjustments are necessary when rifampin is coadministered with nevirapine. Therefore, rifampin and nevirapine should be used only in combination if clearly indicated and with careful monitoring.
Delavirdine	No	No	Contraindicated because of the marked decrease in concentrations of delavirdine when administered with either rifabutin or rifampin.
Efavirenz	Probably	Probably	Coadministration of efavirenz with increased-dose rifabutin (450 mg/day or 600 mg/day, or 600 mg 2-3 times/week) is a possibility, though there is no published clinical experience. Coadministration of efavirenz[6] with usual-dose rifampin (600 mg/day or 2-3 times/week) is a possibility, though there is no published clinical experience.

[1]Usual recommended doses are 400 mg twice daily for each of these protease inhibitors and 400 mg of ritonavir.

[2]Despite limited data and clinical experience, the use of this combination is potentially successful.

[3]Based on available data and clinical experience, the successful use of this combination is likely.

[4] Usual recommended dose is 800 mg every 8 hours; some experts recommend increasing the indinavir dose to 1000 mg every 8 hours if indinavir is used in combination with rifabutin.

[5]Usual recommended dose is 750 mg 3 times/day or 1250 mg twice daily; some experts recommend increasing the nelfinavir dose to 1000 mg if the 3-times/day dosing is used and nelfinavir is used in combination with rifabutin.

[6]Usual recommended dose is 600 mg/day; some experts recommend increasing the efavirenz dose to 800 mg/day if efavirenz is used in combination with rifampin.

Updated March 2000 from www.hivatis.org -"Updated Guidelines for the Use of Rifabutin or Rifampin for the Treatment and Prevention of Tuberculosis Among HIV-Infected Patients Taking Protease Inhibitors or Non-nucleoside Reverse Transcriptase Inhibitors," *MMWR*, March 10, 2000, 49(09):185-9.

Recommended Drug Regimens for Treatment of Latent Tuberculosis (TB) Infection in Adults

Drug	Interval and Duration	Comments	Rating[1] (Evidence)[2] HIV⁻	HIV⁺
Isoniazid	Daily for 9 months[3,4]	In HIV-infected patients, isoniazid may be administered concurrently with nucleoside reverse transcriptase inhibitors (NRTIs), protease inhibitors, or non-nucleoside reverse transcriptase inhibitors (NNRTIs)	A (II)	A (II)
	Twice weekly for 9 months[3,4]	Directly observed therapy (DOT) must be used with twice-weekly dosing	B (II)	B (II)
Isoniazid	Daily for 6 months[4]	Not indicated for HIV-infected persons, those with fibrotic lesions on chest radiographs, or children	B (I)	C (I)
	Twice weekly for 6 months[4]	DOT must be used with twice-weekly dosing	B (II)	C (I)
Rifampin plus pyrazinamide	Daily for 2 months	May also be offered to persons who are contacts of pyrazinamide patients with isoniazid-resistant, rifampin-susceptible TB	B (II)	A (II)
		In HIV-infected persons, protease inhibitors or NNRTIs should generally not be administered concurrently with rifampin; rifabutin can be used as an alternative for patients treated with indinavir, nelfinavir, amprenavir, ritonavir, or efavirenz, and possibly with nevirapine or soft-gel saquinavir[5]		
	Twice weekly for 2-3 months	DOT must be used with twice-weekly dosing	C (II)	C (I)
Rifampin	Daily for 4 months	For persons who cannot tolerate pyrazinamide	B (II)	B (III)
		For persons who are contacts of patients with isoniazid-resistant rifampin-susceptible TB who cannot tolerate pyrazinamide		

[1]Strength of recommendation: A = preferred; B = acceptable alternative; C = offer when A and B cannot be given.

[2]Quality of evidence: I = randomized clinical trial data; II = data from clinical trials that are not randomized or were conducted in other populations; III = expert opinion.

[3]Recommended regimen for children <18 years of age.

[4]Recommended regimens for pregnant women. Some experts would use rifampin and pyrazinamide for 2 months as an alternative regimen for HIV-infected pregnant women, although pyrazinamide should be avoided during the first trimester.

[5]Rifabutin should not be used with hard-gel saquinavir or delavirdine. When used with other protease inhibitors or NNRTIs, dose adjustment of rifabutin may be required.

Modified from *MMWR Morb Mortal Wkly Rep*, 2000, 49(RR-6).

NOTES

NOTES

NOTES

Other titles offered by

LEXI-COMP, INC

DRUG INFORMATION HANDBOOK (International edition available)

by Charles Lacy, RPh, PharmD, FCSHP; Lora L. Armstrong, RPh, PharmD, BCPS; Morton P. Goldman, PharmD, BCPS; and Leonard L. Lance, RPh, BSPharm

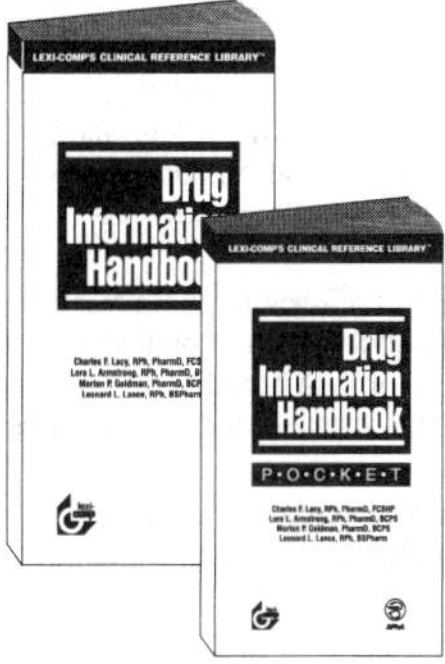

Specifically compiled and designed for the healthcare professional requiring quick access to concisely-stated comprehensive data concerning clinical use of medications.

The Drug Information Handbook is an ideal portable drug information resource, providing the reader with up to 34 key points of data concerning clinical use and dosing of the medication. Material provided in the Appendix section is recognized by many users to be, by itself, well worth the purchase of the handbook.

All medications found in the *Drug Information Handbook,* are included in the abridged *Pocket* edition (select fields were extracted to maintain portability).

PEDIATRIC DOSAGE HANDBOOK (International edition available)

by Carol K. Taketomo, PharmD; Jane Hurlburt Hodding, PharmD; and Donna M. Kraus, PharmD

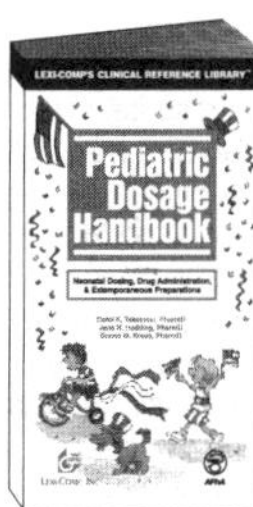

Special considerations must frequently be taken into account when dosing medications for the pediatric patient. This highly regarded quick reference handbook is a compilation of recommended pediatric doses based on current literature, as well as the practical experience of the authors and their many colleagues who work every day in the pediatric clinical setting.

Includes neonatal dosing, drug administration, and (in select monographs) extemporaneous preparations for medications used in pediatric medicine.

GERIATRIC DOSAGE HANDBOOK

by Todd P. Semla, PharmD, BCPS, FCCP; Judith L. Beizer, PharmD, FASCP; and Martin D. Higbee, PharmD, CGP

2000 "Book of the Year" — *American Journal of Nursing*

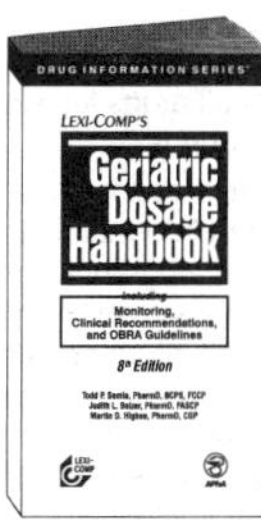

Many physiologic changes occur with aging, some of which affect the pharmacokinetics or pharmacodynamics of medications. Strong consideration should also be given to the effect of decreased renal or hepatic functions in the elderly, as well as the probability of the geriatric patient being on multiple drug regimens.

Healthcare professionals working with nursing homes and assisted living facilities will find the drug information contained in this handbook to be an invaluable source of helpful information.

An International Brand Name Index with names from 58 different countries is also included.

Other titles offered by

LEXI-COMP, INC

DRUG INFORMATION HANDBOOK FOR THE ALLIED HEALTH PROFESSIONAL

by Leonard L. Lance, RPh, BSPharm; Charles Lacy, RPh, PharmD, FCSHP; Lora L. Armstrong, RPh, PharmD, BCPS; and Morton P. Goldman, PharmD, BCPS

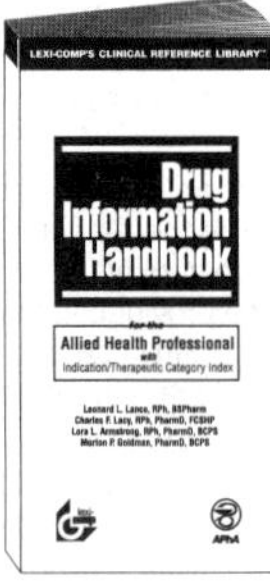

Working with clinical pharmacists, hospital pharmacy and therapeutics committees, and hospital drug information centers, the authors have assisted hundreds of hospitals in developing institution-specific formulary reference documentation.

The most current basic drug and medication data from those clinical settings have been reviewed, coalesced, and cross-referenced to create this unique handbook. The handbook offers quick access to abbreviated monographs for generic drugs.

This is a great tool for physician assistants, medical records personnel, medical transcriptionists and secretaries, pharmacy technicians, and other allied health professionals.

NATURAL THERAPEUTICS POCKET GUIDE

by Daniel L. Krinsky, RPh, MS; James B. LaValle, RPh, DHM, NMD, CCN; Ernest B. Hawkins, RPh, MS; Ross Pelton, RPh, PhD, CCN; Nancy Ashbrook Willis, BA, JD

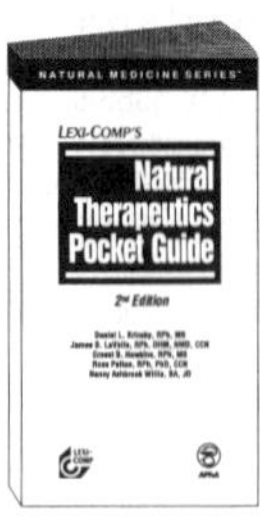

Provides condition-specific information on common uses of natural therapies. Each condition discussed includes the following: review of condition, decision tree, list of commonly recommended herbals, nutritional supplements, homeopathic remedies, lifestyle modifications, and special considerations.

Provides herbal/nutritional/nutraceutical monographs with over 10 fields including references, reported uses, dosage, pharmacology, toxicity, warnings & interactions, and cautions & contraindications.

The Appendix includes: drug-nutrient depletion, herb-drug interactions, drug-nutrient interaction, herbal medicine use in pediatrics, unsafe herbs, and reference of top herbals.

DRUG-INDUCED NUTRIENT DEPLETION HANDBOOK

by Ross Pelton, RPh, PhD, CCN; James B. LaValle, RPh, DHM, NMD, CCN; Ernest B. Hawkins, RPh, MS; Daniel L. Krinsky, RPh, MS

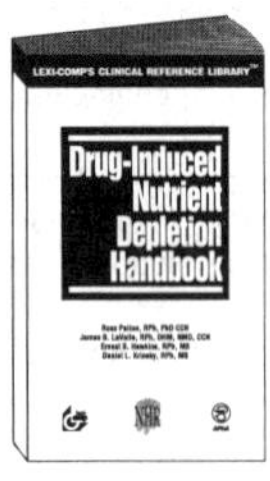

A complete and up-to-date listing of all drugs known to deplete the body of nutritional compounds.

This book is alphabetically organized and provides extensive cross-referencing to related information in the various sections of the book. Drug monographs identify the nutrients depleted and provide cross-references to the nutrient monographs for more detailed information on Effects of Depletion, Biological Function & Effect, Side Effects & Toxicity, RDA, Dosage Range, and Dietary Sources. This book also contains a Studies & Abstracts section, a valuable Appendix, and Alphabetical & Pharmacological Indexes.

To order call toll free anywhere in the U.S.: 1-800-837-LEXI (5394)
Outside of the U.S. call: 330-650-6506 or online at www.lexi.com

Other titles offered by

LEXI-COMP, INC

DRUG INFORMATION HANDBOOK FOR NURSING

by Beatrice B. Turkoski, RN, PhD; Brenda R. Lance, RN, MSN; and Mark F. Bonfiglio, PharmD

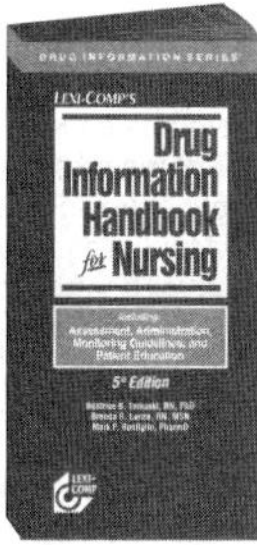

Registered Professional Nurses and upper-division nursing students involved with drug therapy will find this handbook provides quick access to drug data in a concise easy-to-use format.

Over 4000 U.S., Canadian, and Mexican medications are covered with up to 43 key points of information in each monograph. The handbook contains basic pharmacology concepts and nursing issues such as patient factors that influence drug therapy (ie, pregnancy, age, weight, etc) and general nursing issues (ie, assessment, administration, monitoring, and patient education). The Appendix contains over 230 pages of valuable information.

ANESTHESIOLOGY & CRITICAL CARE DRUG HANDBOOK

by Andrew J. Donnelly, PharmD; Francesca E. Cunningham, PharmD; and Verna L. Baughman, MD

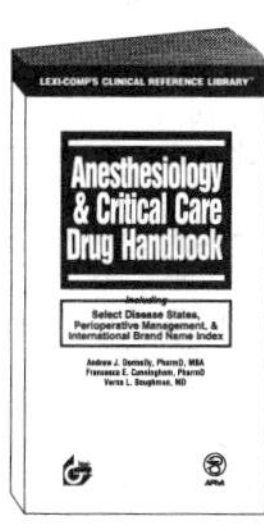

Contains the most commonly used drugs in the perioperative and critical care setting. This handbook also contains the following Special Issues and Topics: Allergic Reaction, Anesthesia for Cardiac Patients in Noncardiac Surgery, Anesthesia for Obstetric Patients in Nonobstetric Surgery, Anesthesia for Patients With Liver Disease, Chronic Pain Management, Chronic Renal Failure, Conscious Sedation, Perioperative Management of Patients on Antiseizure Medication, and Substance Abuse and Anesthesia.

The Appendix includes Abbreviations & Measurements, Anesthesiology Information, Assessment of Liver & Renal Function, Comparative Drug Charts, Infectious Disease-Prophylaxis & Treatment, Laboratory Values, Therapy Recommendations, Toxicology information, *and much more.*

International Brand Name Index with names from over 58 different countries is also included.

DRUG INFORMATION HANDBOOK FOR ONCOLOGY

by Dominic A. Solimando, Jr, MA; Linda R. Bressler, PharmD, BCOP; Polly E. Kintzel, PharmD, BCPS, BCOP; and Mark C. Geraci, PharmD, BCOP

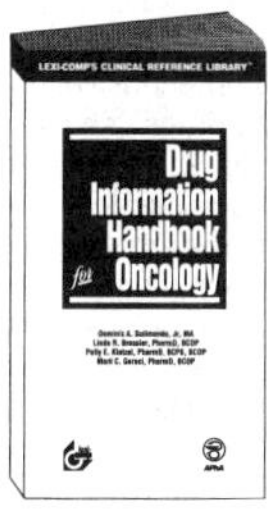

Presented in a concise and uniform format, this book contains the most comprehensive collection of oncology-related drug information available. Organized like a dictionary for ease of use, drugs can be found by looking up the *brand or generic name*!

This book contains individual monographs for both Antineoplastic Agents and Ancillary Medications.

The fields of information per monograph include: Use, U.S. Investigational, Bone Marrow/Blood Cell Transplantation, Vesicant, Emetic Potential. A Special Topics Section, Appendix, and Therapeutic Category & Key Word Index are valuable features to this book, as well.

To order call toll free anywhere in the U.S.: 1-800-837-LEXI (5394)

Outside of the U.S. call: 330-650-6506 or online at www.lexi.com

Other titles offered by

LEXI-COMP, INC

INFECTIOUS DISEASES HANDBOOK

by Carlos M. Isada, MD; Bernard L. Kasten Jr., MD; Morton P. Goldman, PharmD; Larry D. Gray, PhD; and Judith A. Aberg, MD

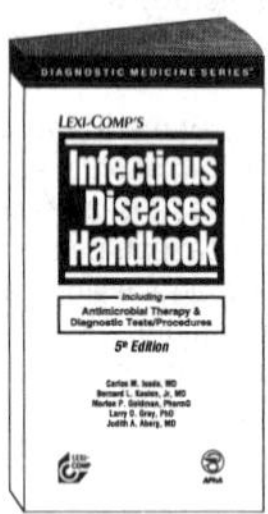

A four-in-one quick reference concerned with the identification and treatment of infectious diseases. Each of the four sections of the book contain related information and cross-referencing to one or more of the other three sections. The Disease Syndrome section provides the clinical presentation, differential diagnosis, diagnostic tests, and drug therapy recommended for treatment of more common infectious diseases. The Organism section presents the microbiology, epidemiology, diagnosis, and treatment of each organism. The Laboratory Diagnosis section describes performance of specific tests and procedures. The Antimicrobial Therapy section presents important facts and considerations regarding each drug recommended for specific diseases of organisms. Also contains an International Brand Name Index with names from 58 different countries.

DIAGNOSTIC PROCEDURE HANDBOOK by Frank Michota, MD

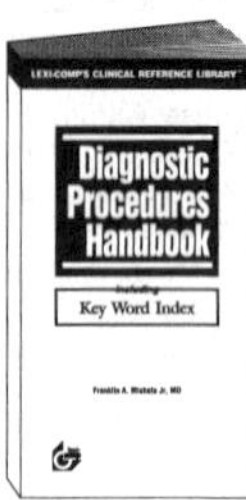

A comprehensive, yet concise, quick reference source for physicians, nurses, students, medical records personnel, or anyone needing quick access to diagnostic procedure information. This handbook is an excellent source of information in the following areas: allergy, rheumatology, and infectious disease; cardiology; computed tomography; diagnostic radiology; gastroenterology; invasive radiology; magnetic resonance imaging; nephrology, urology, and hematology; neurology; nuclear medicine; pulmonary function; pulmonary medicine and critical care; ultrasound; and women's health.

POISONING & TOXICOLOGY HANDBOOK

by Jerrold B. Leikin, MD and Frank P. Paloucek, PharmD

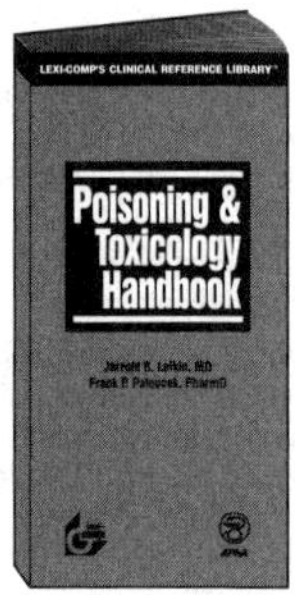

It's back by popular demand! The small size of our Poisoning & Toxicology Handbook is once again available. Better than ever, this comprehensive, portable reference contains 80 antidotes and drugs used in toxicology with 694 medicinal agents, 287 nonmedicinal agents, 291 biological agents, 57 herbal agents, and more than 200 laboratory tests. Monographs are extensively referenced and contain valuable information on overdose symptomatology and treatment considerations, as well as, admission criteria and impairment potential of select agents. Designed for quick reference with monographs arranged alphabetically, plus a cross-referencing index. The authors have expanded current information on drugs of abuse and use of antidotes, while providing concise tables, graphics, and other pertinent toxicology text.

To order call toll free anywhere in the U.S.: 1-800-837-LEXI (5394)
Outside of the U.S. call: 330-650-6506 or online at www.lexi.com

Other titles offered by
LEXI-COMP, INC

CLINICIAN'S GUIDE TO LABORATORY MEDICINE—A Practical Approach by Samir P. Desai, MD and Sana Isa-Pratt, MD

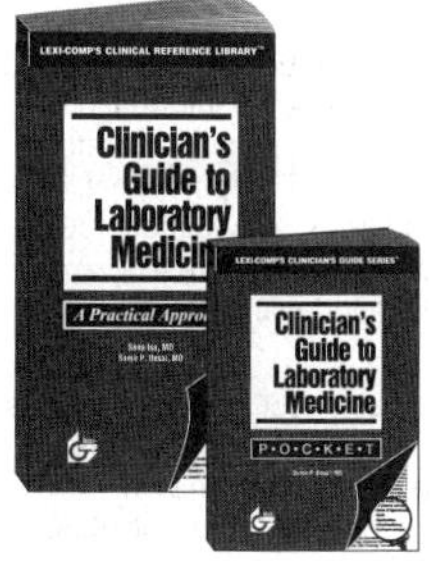

When faced with the patient presenting with abnormal laboratory tests, the clinician can now turn to the *Clinician's Guide to Laboratory Medicine: A Practical Approach.* This source is unique in its ability to lead the clinician from laboratory test abnormality to clinical diagnosis. Written for the busy clinician, this concise handbook will provide rapid answers to the questions that busy clinicians face in the care of their patients. No longer does the clinician have to struggle in an effort to find this information - *it's all here.*
Included is a **FREE** copy of *Clinician's Guide to Laboratory Medicine - Pocket.* Great to carry in your pocket! Perfect for use *"in the trenches".*

CLINICIAN'S GUIDE TO INTERNAL MEDICINE—A Practical Approach by Samir P. Desai, MD

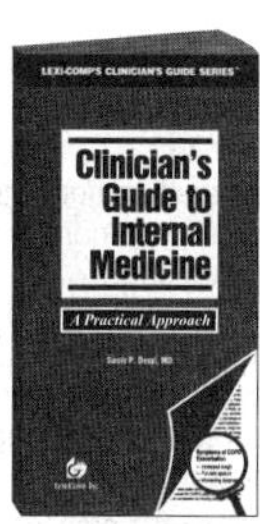

Provides quick access to essential information covering diagnosis, treatment, and management of commonly encountered patient problems in Internal Medicine.

- Up-to-date information in an easy-to-read format
- Clinically relevant information that is easily accessible
- Practical approaches that are not readily available in standard textbooks
- Algorithms to help you establish the diagnosis and select the appropriate therapy
- Numerous tables and boxes that summarize diagnostic and therapeutic strategies
- Ideal reference for use at the point-of-care

This is a reference companion that will provide you with the tools necessary to tackle even the most challenging problems in Internal Medicine.

CLINICIAN'S GUIDE TO DIAGNOSIS—A Practical Approach
by Samir Desai, MD

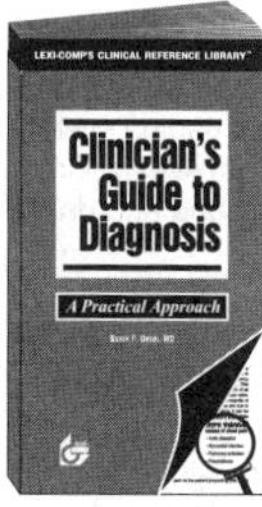

Symptoms are what prompt patients to seek medical care. In the evaluation of a patient's symptom, it is not unusual for healthcare professionals to ask "What do I do next?" This is precisely the question for which the *Clinician's Guide to Diagnosis: A Practical Approach* provides the answer. It will lead you from symptom to diagnosis through a series of steps designed to mimic the logical thought processes of seasoned clinicians. For the young clinician, this is an ideal book to help bridge the gap between the classroom and actual patient care. For the experienced clinician, this concise handbook offers rapid answers to the questions that are commonly encountered on a day-to-day basis. Let this guide become your companion, providing you with the tools necessary to tackle even the most challenging symptoms.

To order call toll free anywhere in the U.S.: 1-800-837-LEXI (5394)
Outside of the U.S. call: 330-650-6506 or online at www.lexi.com

Other titles offered by

LEXI-COMP, INC

***LABORATORY TEST HANDBOOK** & **CONCISE** version*

by David S. Jacobs MD, FACP; Wayne R. DeMott, MD, FACP; and Dwight K. Oxley, MD, FACP

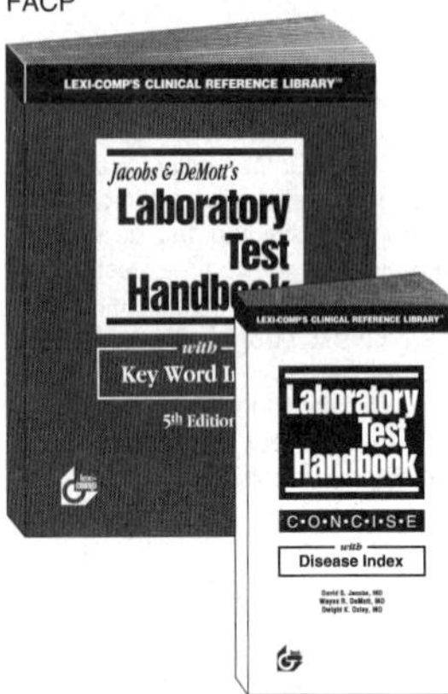

Contains over 900 clinical laboratory tests and is an excellent source of laboratory information for physicians of all specialties, nurses, laboratory professionals, students, medical personnel, or anyone who needs quick access to most routine and many of the more specialized testing procedures available in today's clinical laboratory.

Each monograph contains test name, synonyms, patient care, specimen requirements, reference ranges, and interpretive information with footnotes, references, and selected websites.

The *Laboratory Test Handbook Concise* is a portable, abridged (800 tests) version and is an ideal, quick reference for anyone requiring information concerning patient preparation, specimen collection and handling, and test result interpretation.

POISONING & TOXICOLOGY COMPENDIUM

by Jerrold B. Leikin, MD and Frank P. Paloucek, PharmD

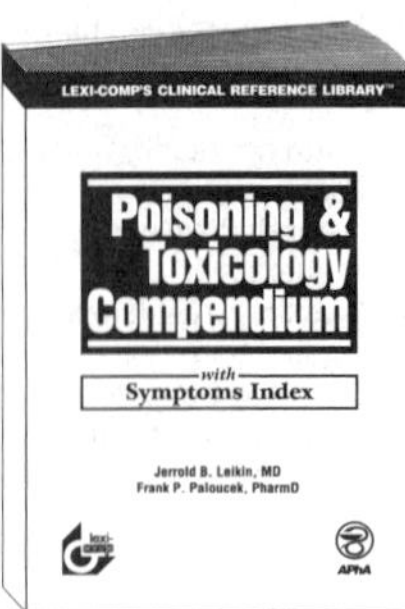

A six-in-one reference wherein each major entry contains information relative to one or more of the other sections. This compendium offers comprehensive, concisely-stated monographs covering 645 medicinal agents, 256 nonmedicinal agents, 273 biological agents, 49 herbal agents, 254 laboratory tests, 79 antidotes, and 222 pages of exceptionally useful appendix material.

A truly unique reference that presents signs and symptoms of acute overdose along with considerations for overdose treatment. Ideal reference for emergency situations.

DENTAL OFFICE MEDICAL EMERGENCIES

by Timothy F. Meiller, DDS, PhD; Richard L. Wynn, BSPharm, PhD; Ann Marie McMullin, MD; Cynthia Biron, RDH, EMT, MA; and Harold L. Crossley, DDS, PhD

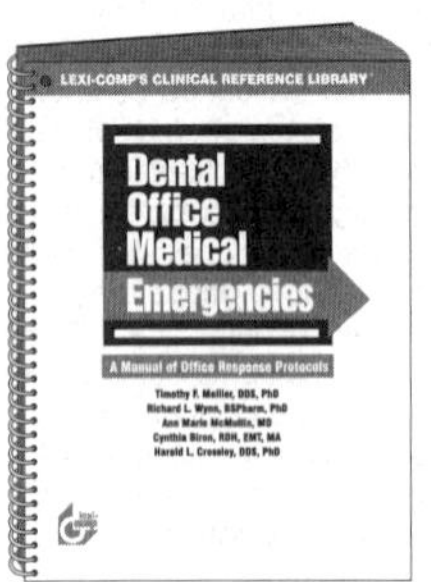

Designed specifically for general dentists during times of emergency. A tabbed paging system allows for quick access to specific crisis events. Created with urgency in mind, it is spiral bound and drilled with a hole for hanging purposes.

- Basic Action Plan for Stabilization
- Allergic / Drug Reactions
- Loss of Consciousness / Respiratory Distress / Chest Pain
- Altered Sensation / Changes in Affect
- Management of Acute Bleeding
- Office Preparedness / Procedures and Protocols
- Automated External Defibrillator (AED)
- Oxygen Delivery

To order call toll free anywhere in the U.S.: 1-800-837-LEXI (5394)

Outside of the U.S. call: 330-650-6506 or online at www.lexi.com